1995–96 AHA Guide Code Chart

Hospital, Address, Telephone, Administrator, Approval, Facility, and Physician Codes, Health Care System	Classification Codes		Utilization Data					Expense (thousands) of dollars		
★ American Hospital Association (AHA) membership ☐ Joint Commission on Accreditation of Healthcare Organizations (JCAHO) accreditation + American Osteopathic Hospital Association (AOHA) membership ○ American Osteopathic Association (AOA) accreditation △ Commission on Accreditation of Rehabilitation Facilities (CARF) accreditation Control codes 61, 63, 64, 71, 72 and 73 indicate hospitals listed by AOHA, but not registered by AHA. For definition of numerical codes, see page A6	Control	Service	Beds	Admissions	Census	Outpatient Visits	Births	Total	Payroll	Personnel
★ ANYTOWN—Universal County COMMUNITY HOSPITAL, First Street and Main Avenue Zip 62835; tel 204/391–2345; Jane Doe, Administrator **A**1 2 3 4 6 9 10 **F**1 2 3 4 5 6 8 9 10 23 24 34; **P**1 2 3 4; **S**1234 Acme HCS	23	10	346	10778	248	75953	1693	20695	9973	796

       ⎣__1__⎦ ⎣__2__⎦ ⎣__3__⎦

1 Approval Codes

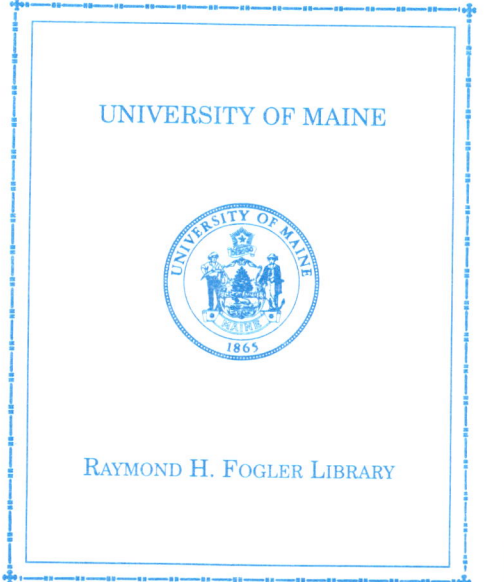

6 Hospital–controlled professional nursing school, reported by National League for Nursing (January 1995).
7 Accreditation by Commission on Accreditation of Rehabilitation Facilities (January 1995).
8 Member of Council of Teaching Hospitals of the Association of American Medical Colleges (January 1995).
9 Hospital contracting or participating in Blue Cross Plan, reported by Blue Cross Association (January 1995).
10 Certified for participation in the Health Insurance for the Aged (Medicare) Program by the U.S. Department of Health and Human Services (January 1995).
11 Accreditation by American Osteopathic Association (January 1995).
12 Internship approved by American Osteopathic Association (January 1995).
13 Residency approved by American Osteopathic Association (January 1995).

Nonreporting indicates that the 1994 Annual Survey questionnaire for the hospital had not been received by April 30, 1995, the cutoff date for statistical processing.

Newly Registered indicates that the hospital was registered after the mailing of the 1994 Annual Survey.

5 Arthritis treatment center
6 Assisted living
7 Birthing room–LDR room–LDRP room
8 Breast cancer screening/mammograms
9 Burn care unit
10 Cardiac catheterization laboratory
11 Cardiac intensive care unit
12 Case management
13 Children wellness program
14 Community health reporting
15 Community health status assessment
16 Community health status based service planning
17 Community outreach
18 Crisis prevention
19 CT scanner
20 Dental services
21 Diagnostic radioisotope facility
22 Emergency department
23 Extracorporeal shock wave lithotripter (ESWL)
24 Fitness center
25 Freestanding outpatient care center
26 Geriatric services
27 Health facility transportation (to/from)
28 Health fair
29 Health information center
30 Health screenings
31 HIV–AIDS services
32 Home health services
33 Hospice
34 Hospital–based outpatient care center–services
35 Magnetic resonance imaging (MRI)
36 Meals on wheels
37 Medical surgical intensive care unit
38 Neonatal intensive care unit
39 Nutrition programs
40 Obstetrics unit
41 Occupational health services
42 Oncology services
43 Open heart surgery
44 Outpatient surgery
45 Patient education center
46 Patient representative services
47 Pediatric intensive care unit
48 Physical rehabilitation inpatient unit
49 Physical rehabilitation outpatient services
50 Positron emission tomography scanner (PET)
51 Primary care department
52 Psychiatric acute inpatient unit
53 Psychiatric child adolescent services
54 Psychiatric consultation–liaison services
55 Psychiatric education services
56 Psychiatric emergency services
57 Psychiatric geriatric services
58 Psychiatric outpatient services
59 Psychiatric partial hospitalization program
60 Radiation therapy
61 Reproductive health services
62 Retirement housing
63 Single photon emission computerized tomography (SPECT)
64 Skilled nursing or other long–term care unit
65 Social work services
66 Sports medicine
67 Support groups
68 Teen outreach services
69 Transplant services
70 Trauma center (certified)
71 Ultrasound
72 Urgent care center
73 Volunteer services department
74 Women's health center/services

3 Physician Codes

Actually available within, and reported by the institution; for definitions, see page A11.

(Alphabetical/Numerical Order)

1 Closed physician–hospital organization (PHO)
2 Equity model
3 Foundation
4 Group practice without walls
5 Independent practice association (IPA)
6 Integrated salary model
7 Management service organization (MSO)
8 Open physician–hospital organization (PHO)

Hospital, Address, Telephone, Administrator, Approval, Facility, and Physician Codes, Health Care System	Classification Codes		Utilization Data					Expense (thousands) of dollars		Personnel
	Control	Service	Beds	Admissions	Census	Outpatient Visits	Births	Total	Payroll	

★ American Hospital Association (AHA) membership
☐ Joint Commission on Accreditation of Healthcare Organizations (JCAHO) accreditation
+ American Osteopathic Hospital Association (AOHA) membership
○ American Osteopathic Association (AOA) accreditation
△ Commission on Accreditation of Rehabilitation Facilities (CARF) accreditation
Control codes 61, 63, 64, 71, 72 and 73 indicate hospitals listed by AOHA, but not registered by AHA. For definition of numerical codes, see page A6

ANYTOWN—Universal County
★ COMMUNITY HOSPITAL, First Street and Main Avenue Zip 62835; tel 204/391-2345; Jane Doe, Administrator **A**1 2 3 4 6 9 10 **F**1 2 3 4 5 6 8 9 10 23 24 34; **P**1 2 3 4; **S**1234 Acme HCS 23 10 346 10778 248 75953 1693 20695 9973 796

4 Health Care System Code and Name

A code number has been assigned to each health care system headquarters. The inclusion of one of these codes (1) indicates that the hospital belongs to a health care system and (2) identifies the specific system to which the hospital belongs.

5 Classification Codes

Control

Government, nonfederal
12 State
13 County
14 City
15 City–county
16 Hospital district or authority

Nongovernment not–for–profit
21 Church operated
23 Other

Investor–owned (for–profit)
31 Individual
32 Partnership
33 Corporation

Government, federal
41 Air Force
42 Army
43 Navy
44 Public Health Service other than 47

45 Veterans Administration
46 Federal other than 41–45, 47–48
47 Public Health Service Indian Service
48 Department of Justice

Osteopathic
61 Church operated
63 Other not–for–profit
64 Other
71 Individual for–profit
72 Partnership for–profit
73 Corporation for–profit

Service
10 General medical and surgical
11 Hospital unit of an institution (prison hospital, college infirmary, etc.)
12 Hospital unit within an institution for the mentally retarded
22 Psychiatric
33 Tuberculosis and other respiratory diseases

44 Obstetrics and gynecology
45 Eye, ear, nose, and throat
46 Rehabilitation
47 Orthopedic
48 Chronic disease
49 Other specialty
50 Children's general
51 Children's hospital unit of an institution
52 Children's psychiatric
53 Children's tuberculosis and other respiratory diseases
55 Children's eye, ear, nose, and throat
56 Children's rehabilitation
57 Children's orthopedic
58 Children's chronic disease
59 Children's other specialty
62 Institution for mental retardation
82 Alcoholism and other chemical dependency

* Control codes 61, 63, 64, 71, 72 and 73 indicate hospitals listed by the AOHA but not registered by AHA.
When a hospital restricts its service to a specialty not defined by a specific code, it is coded 49 (59 if a children's hospital) and the specialty is indicated in parentheses following the name of the hospital.

6 Headings

Definitions are based on the American Hospital Association's Hospital Administration Terminology. Where a 12–month period is specified, hospitals were requested to report on the Annual Survey of Hospitals for the 12 months ending September 30, 1994. Hospitals reporting for less than a 12–month period are so designated.

Utilization Data:

Beds–Number of beds regularly maintained (set up and staffed for use) for inpatients as of the close of the reporting period.

Admissions–Number of patients accepted for inpatient service during a 12–month period; does not include newborn.

Census–Average number of inpatients receiving care each day during the 12–month reporting period; does not include newborn.

Outpatient Visits–An outpatient visit is a visit by a patient who is not lodged in the hospital while receiving medical, dental, or other services. Each appearance of an outpatient in each unit constitutes one visit regardless of the number of diagnostic and/or therapeutic treatments that a patient receives.

Births–Number of infants born in the hospital and accepted for service in a newborn infant bassinet during a 12–month period; excludes stillbirths.

Expense: Expense for a 12–month period; both total expense and payroll components are shown. Payroll expenses include all salaries and wages except those paid to medical and dental interns and residents, and other trainees (e.g., medical technology trainees, x–ray therapy trainees, administrative residents, etc.).

Personnel: Includes persons on payroll on September 30, 1994; includes full–time equivalents of part–time personnel, but excludes medical and dental interns and residents and other trainees. Full-time equivalents were calculated on the basis that two part–time persons equal one full–time person.

AHA Guide Evaluation Questionnaire

In order to present you with the most valuable information, please take some time to fill out this questionnaire.

Name and Title: _____

Organization Name: _____

Address: _____

City/State/Zip: _____

Phone Number: (_____) - _____

I. Please rank the following items.

Section A   Hospitals

	Use Almost Always	Sometimes Use	Never Use
1. State Population Information	( )	( )	( )
2. Beds	( )	( )	( )
3. Facilities and Services	( )	( )	( )
4. Approval Codes	( )	( )	( )
5. Physician Codes	( )	( )	( )
6. Births	( )	( )	( )
7. Expenses	( )	( )	( )
8. Payroll	( )	( )	( )
9. FTE	( )	( )	( )

Section B   Integrated Health Delivery Networks, Health Care Systems and Alliances

1. Integrated Health Delivery Networks	( )	( )	( )
2. Health Care Systems	( )	( )	( )
3. Alliances	( )	( )	( )

Section C   Health Organizations, Agencies and Providers

1. National Organizations	( )	( )	( )
2. Healthfinder	( )	( )	( )
3. International Organizations	( )	( )	( )
4. U.S. Government Agencies	( )	( )	( )
5. Blue Cross-Blue Shield Plans	( )	( )	( )
6. Health Systems Agencies	( )	( )	( )
7. Hospital Associations	( )	( )	( )

	Use Almost Always	Sometimes Use	Never Use
8. Hospital Licensure Agencies	( )	( )	( )
9. Medical and Nursing Licensure Agencies	( )	( )	( )
10. Peer Review Organizations	( )	( )	( )
11. State Health Planning and Development Agencies	( )	( )	( )
12. State and Provincial Government Agencies	( )	( )	( )
13. Health Maintenance Organizations	( )	( )	( )
14. State Government Agencies for Health Maintenance Organizations	( )	( )	( )
15. Freestanding Ambulatory Surgery Centers	( )	( )	( )
16. State Government Agencies for Freestanding Ambulatory Surgery Centers	( )	( )	( )
17. Freestanding Hospices	( )	( )	( )
18. State Government Agencies for Freestanding Hospices	( )	( )	( )
19. Accredited Freestanding Long-Term Care Facilities	( )	( )	( )
20. Accredited Freestanding Psychiatric Facilities	( )	( )	( )
21. Accredited Freestanding Substance Abuse Programs	( )	( )	( )

II. Please complete the following regarding use issues.

1. Are you a first time purchaser of the AHA Guide? __YES (Please go to question 4)   __NO (Please go to question 2)
2. How often have you purchased the AHA Guide?_____
3. What do you find most valuable about this book? _____
_____
_____
4. What additional information would make this publication more useful to you and your organization? _____
_____
_____
5. What information in this publication is not useful to you and your organization?_____
_____
_____

III. Additional comments

Additional comments:_____
_____
_____
_____
_____

Thank you for taking the time to complete our questionnaire. Your input will help us to improve this publication in the future.

American Hospital Association Guide to the Health Care Field

1995–96 Edition

American Hospital Association
One North Franklin
Chicago, IL 60606–3401

AHA Institutional Members $75
Nonmembers $195
AHA catalog NUMBER C–010095
Telephone ORDERS 1–800–AHA–2626

ISSN 0094–8969
ISBN 0–87258–681–2

Copyright 1995 by the
American Hospital Association
One North Franklin
Chicago, IL 60606–3401

All rights reserved
Printed in the U.S.A.

Contents

Section

		v	Acknowledgements and Advisements
		vi	Introduction
A	Hospitals	A1	Contents of Section A
		2	AHA Offices, Officers, and Historical Data
		4	Registration Requirements for Hospitals
		6	Explanation of Hospital Listings
		8	Annual Survey
		13	Hospitals in the United States, by State
		443	Hospitals in Areas Associated with the United States, by Area
		447	U.S. Government Hospitals Outside the United States, by Area
		448	All U.S. Hospitals, Alphabetically
		483	AHA Membership Categories
		484	Institutional Members
		489	Associate Members
B	Health Care Systems, Integrated Health Delivery Networks and Alliances	B1	Contents of Section B
		2	Introduction
		3	Integrated Health Delivery Networks
		8	Statistics for Multihospital Health Care Systems and Their Hospitals
		9	Health Care Systems and Their Hospitals
		84	Headquarters of Health Care Systems, Alphabetically
		85	Headquarters of Health Care Systems, by System Code
		92	Headquarters of Health Care Systems, Geographically
		100	Alliances

© 1995 AHA Guide

Section

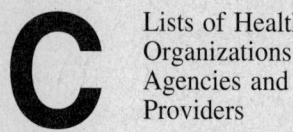 Lists of Health Organizations, Agencies and Providers

C1	Contents of Section C
2	Description of Lists
3	National Organizations
13	Healthfinder List
25	International Organizations
27	U.S. Government Agencies
28	Blue Cross–Blue Shield Plans
30	Health Systems Agencies
31	Hospital Associations
34	Hospital Licensure Agencies
36	Medical and Nursing Licensure Agencies
39	Peer Review Organizations
41	State Health Planning and Development Agencies
43	State and Provincial Government Agencies
60	Health Maintenance Organizations
73	State Government Agencies for Health Maintenance Organizations
75	Freestanding Ambulatory Surgery Centers
99	State Government Agencies for Freestanding Ambulatory Surgery Centers
101	Freestanding Hospices
120	State Government Agencies for Freestanding Hospices
122	Accredited Freestanding Long–Term Care Facilities†
128	Accredited Freestanding Psychiatric Facilities†
140	Accredited Freestanding Substance Abuse Programs†

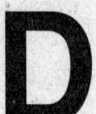 Indexes

D1	Index
2	Abbreviations Used in the AHA Guide

† List supplied by the Joint Commission on Accreditation of Healthcare Organizations

Acknowledgements and Advisements

Acknowledgements

The American Hospital Association Guide to the Health Care Field is published annually by the American Hospital Association, Richard J. Davidson, President. Contributions made by the AHA Communications Group, Computer Application Services, Constituency Sections, Health Statistics Group, Member Relations, Printing Services Group, Resource Center, Special Membership Services and Tools for Change.

The American Hospital Association acknowledges the cooperation given by many professional groups and government agencies in the health care field, particularly the following: American College of Surgeons; American Medical Association; American Osteopathic Hospital Association; Blue Cross–Blue Shield Association; Council of Teaching Hospitals of the Association of American Medical Colleges; Joint Commission on Accreditation of Healthcare Organizations; National League for Nursing; Commission on Accreditation of Rehabilitation Facilities; American Osteopathic Association; Health Care Financing Administration; and various offices within the U.S. Department of Health and Human Services.

Advisements

The data published here should be used with the following advisements: The data are based on replies to an annual survey that seeks a variety of information, not all of which is published in this book. The information gathered by the survey includes specific services, but not all of each hospital's services. Therefore, the data do not reflect an exhaustive list of all services offered by all hospitals. For information on the availability of additional data, please contact the American Hospital Association's Health Statistics Group, 312/422–3990.

The American Hospital Association does not assume responsibility for the accuracy of information voluntarily reported by the individual institutions surveyed. The purpose of this publication is to provide basic data reflecting the delivery of health care in the United States and associated areas, and is not to serve as an official and all inclusive list of services offered by individual hospitals.

Introduction

Each of the three major sections of the AHA Guide begins with its own table of contents and pertinent definitions or explanatory information. Sections B, C and indices have black bleed bar tabs for easy identification. The three major sections are:
- Hospitals
- Integrated Health Delivery Networks, Health Care Systems and Alliances
- Health Organizations, Agencies and Providers

Hospitals
This section lists:
- AHA–registered and osteopathic hospitals in the U.S. and associated areas, by state within city.
- U.S. government hospitals outside the United States.
- Alphabetical index of all U.S. hospitals.
- AHA Associate members.

AHA member hospitals are identified by a star (★). Hospitals accredited under one of the programs of the Joint Commission on Accreditation of Healthcare Organizations are identified by a hollow box (□). Preceding the list of hospitals is a statement of the formal requirements for registration by the AHA.

The lists provide a variety of information about each hospital, including the administrator's name; various approvals; selected facilities and services; relationship to a health care system; classification by control, service; physician arrangement relationships and other selected statistical data from the 1994 AHA Annual Survey.

Also new in this edition of the *AHA Guide* is the inclusion of state population data from the U.S. Bureau of the Census, *Statistical Abstract of the United States: 1994* (114th edition.) Washington, DC, 1994. They include the following:
- Total resident population (in thousands)
- Percent of resident population in metro areas
- Birth rate per 1,000 population
- Percent of population 65 years and over
- Percent of persons without health insurance

Some of this information is coded. These include approval, facility, health care system and classification codes.

Approval codes refer to approvals held by a hospital; they represent information supplied by various national approving and reporting bodies. For example, code A–1 indicates accreditation under one of the programs of the Joint Commission on Accreditation of Healthcare Organizations – formal evidence that a hospital meets established standards for quality of patient care.

Physician codes refer to the different types of physician arrangements the hospital participates in.

Health care system codes and system name reference specific health care system headquarters. The presence of the system code and system name indicate the hospital belongs to a health care system and identifies the system to which the hospital belongs. Absence of a system code and system name indicate that the hospital does not belong to a health care system.

Classification codes indicate the type of organization that controls or operates the hospital and type of service. Code numbers in the 10s denote nonfederal (states and local) government hospitals; in the 20s, nongovernment not–for–profit hospitals; in the 40s, federal government hospitals; and in the 60s and 70s, nonregistered osteopathic hospitals.

Among **service codes,** the most common code is 10, indicating a general hospital. Other numbers designate various special services. For example, code 22 indicates psychiatric hospitals and codes in the 50s indicate different types of children's hospitals.

Facility codes refer to facilities and services available within the hospital.

(For easy reference, there is a alphabetical/numerical list for all of the codes on page A6).

Names of osteopathic hospitals, supplied by the American Osteopathic Hospital Association are interfiled in the list of hospitals. Codes and symbols identifying these institutions are explained on page A6 and in the headnote at the top of each page of the list of hospitals. Also included in this section is an **index of all U.S. hospitals** in alphabetical order by hospital name, followed by the city and state and the page reference to the hospital's listing in Section A. This section is designated by black tabs along the side of the pages.

This section also lists **other AHA institution members** not listed elsewhere in the AHA Guide and **AHA associate members.** The list of AHA institutional members include Canadian hospitals, associated university programs in health administration, hospital schools of nursing, nonhospital preacute and postacute care facilities, and provisional members. The list of associate members includes ambulatory centers and home care agencies, Blue Cross plans, health maintenance organizations/health care corporations, health system agencies, other inpatient care institutions, shared services organizations and other associate members.

Integrated Health Delivery Networks, Health Care Systems and Alliances

Integrated Health Delivery Networks
New in this edition of the *AHA Guide* is a listing of the names and addresses of Integrated Health Delivery Networks by state, alphabetically by name. An update card is also provided in this section for additions, corrections or updates to the listings. We encourage you to use this card if you have any corrections or updates to this listing. Please see page B2 for more information.

Health Care Systems
This is an alphabetical list of health care systems and their hospitals. Data on bed size for each hospital in the system is provided along with an indication of whether the hospital is owned, leased, sponsored or contract–managed.

Following are three indices for health care system headquarters: by system code number; alphabetically by system name; and geographically by state. These indices are useful for cross–referencing the system codes and system names included in the Hospitals Section.

Alliances
Alliances provide information on multistate alliances and their members. Alliances are listed alphabetically by name. Members are listed alphabetically by state, city and then by name.

Health Organizations, Agencies and Providers
There are four major categories in this section.

First is an alphabetical listing of national, international, and regional organizations. Many voluntary organizations that are interested in, or of interest to the health care field are included. New in this edition of the *AHA Guide* is the inclusion of the Health Finder listing.

The second lists United States government agencies.

The third presents a list of state and local organizations and government agencies. The list for states and provinces include Blue Cross and Blue Shield plans, health systems agencies, hospital associations and councils, hospital licensure agencies, medical and nursing licensure agencies, peer review organizations, state health planning and development agencies, and state and provincial government agencies.

The fourth consists of lists of various health care providers including JCAHO accredited freestanding long–term care facilities, JCAHO accredited freestanding substance abuse programs, and JCAHO accredited freestanding psychiatric facilities, freestanding hospices, freestanding ambulatory surgery centers and health maintenance organizations (HMOs).

Index
This index helps the reader locate specific information quickly. It lists alphabetically the

subjects covered in the various sections and where they can be found.

Abbreviations
This is an alphabetical list of all abbreviations used in the *AHA Guide*. In some cases an abbreviation may stand for more than one word or term. In such cases, the meaning will be determined by the context.

We hope you find the *AHA Guide* a valuable resource. If you have any questions or comments, please call the Health Statistics Group at 312/422–3990.

A   Hospitals

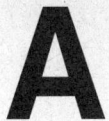

- A2   AHA Offices, Officers, and Historical Data
- 4   Registration Requirements for Hospitals
- 6   Explanation of Hospital Listings
- 8   Annual Survey
- 13   Hospitals in the United States, by State*
- 447   Hospitals in Areas Associated with the United States, by Area
- 451   U.S. Government Hospitals Outside the United States, by Area
- 452   All U.S. Hospitals, Alphabetically
- 486   AHA Membership Categories

- 487   Institutional Members
- 487   *Types I and II Hospitals*
- 487   *Type III Health Care Systems*
- 488   *Type IV Members*
- 488   *Associated University Programs in Health Administration*
- 489   *Hospital Schools of Nursing*
- 490   *Nonhospital Preacute and Postacute Care Facilities*
- 491   *Provisional*

- 492   Associate Members
- 492   *Ambulatory Centers and Home Care Agencies*
- 492   *Blue Cross Plans*
- 493   *Health Maintenance Organizations/Health Care Corporations*
- 493   *Health System Agencies*
- 493   *Other Inpatient Care Institutions*
- 493   *Shared Services Organizations*
- 494   *Other Associate Members*

*AHA–registered hospitals in the United States and associated areas are approved for registration by the Executive Committee of the Board of Trustees of the American Hospital Association. This list of registered hospitals is complete as of June 1, 1995. The list of osteopathic hospitals, integrated in this section, is supplied by the American Osteopathic Hospital Association.

AHA Offices, Officers, and Historical Data

Chicago: One North Franklin, Chicago, IL 60606-3401; tel. 312/422-3000

Washington: 325 Seventh Street, N.W., Suite 700, Washington, DC 20004; tel. 202/638-1100

Speaker of the House of Delegates: Carolyn C. Roberts, Copley Hospital, Washington Highway, Morrisville, VT 05661

Chairman of the Board of Trustees: Gail L. Warden, Henry Ford Health System, 1 Ford Place, Detroit, MI 48202-3450

Chairman-Elect of the Board of Trustees: Gordon M. Sprenger, Allina Health System, Gateway Building, 10th Floor, 5601 Smetana Drive, Minnetonka, MN 55343

President: Richard J. Davidson, 325 Seventh Street, N.W., Suite 700, Washington, DC 20004; tel. 202/638-1100

Vice President and Secretary: Michael P. Guerin, One North Franklin, Chicago, IL 60606-3401

Vice President, Finance and Assistant Treasurer: Sidney Jacob, One North Franklin, Chicago, IL 60606-3401

Past Presidents/Chairmen†

Year	Name	Year	Name	Year	Name
1899	★James S. Knowles	1931	★Lewis A. Sexton, M.D.	1963	T. Stewart Hamilton, M.D.
1900	★James S. Knowles	1932	★Paul H. Fesler	1964	Stanley A. Ferguson
1901	★Charles S. Howell	1933	★George F. Stephens, M.D.	1965	Clarence E. Wonnacott
1902	★J. T. Duryea	1934	★Nathaniel W. Faxon, M.D.	1966	Philip D. Bonnet, M.D.
1903	★John Fehrenbatch	1935	★Robert Jolly	1967	George E. Cartmill
1904	★Daniel D. Test	1936	★Robin C. Buerki, M.D.	1968	★David B. Wilson, M.D.
1905	★George H. M. Rowe, M.D.	1937	★Claude W. Munger, M.D.	1969	George William Graham, M.D.
1906	★George P. Ludlam	1938	★Robert E. Neff	1970	★Mark Berke
1907	★Renwick R. Ross, M.D.	1939	★G. Harvey Agnew, M.D.	1971	Jack A. L. Hahn
1908	★Sigismund S. Goldwater, M.D.	1940	★Fred G. Carter, M.D.	1972	Stephen M. Morris
1909	★John M. Peters, M.D.	1941	★B. W. Black, M.D.	1973	★John W. Kauffman
1910	★H. B. Howard, M.D.	1942	★Basil C. MacLean, M.D.	1974	Horace M. Cardwell
1911	★W. L. Babcock, M.D.	1943	★James A. Hamilton	1975	Wade Mountz
1912	★Henry M. Hurd, M.D.	1944	★Frank J. Walter	1976	H. Robert Cathcart
1913	★F. A. Washburn, M.D.	1945	★Donald C. Smelzer, M.D.	1977	John M. Stagl
1914	★Thomas Howell, M.D.	1946	★Peter D. Ward, M.D.	1978	★Samuel J. Tibbitts
1915	★William O. Mann, M.D.	1947	★John H. Hayes	1979	W. Daniel Barker
1916	★Winford H. Smith, M.D.	1948	★Graham L. Davis	1980	Sister Irene Kraus
1917	★Robert J. Wilson, M.D.	1949	★Joseph G. Norby	1981	Bernard J. Lachner
1918	★A. B. Ancker, M.D.	1950	★John H. Hatfield	1982	Stanley R. Nelson
1919	★A. R. Warner, M.D.	1951	★Charles F. Wilinsky, M.D.	1983	Elbert E. Gilbertson
1920	★Joseph B. Howland, M.D.	1952	★Anthony J. J. Rourke, M.D.	1984	Thomas R. Matherlee
1921	★Louis B. Baldwin, M.D.	1953	★Edwin L. Crosby, M.D.	1985	Jack A. Skarupa
1922	★George O'Hanlon, M.D.	1954	★Ritz E. Heerman	1986	Scott S. Parker
1923	★Asa S. Bacon	1955	★Frank R. Bradley	1987	Donald C. Wegmiller
1924	★Malcolm T. MacEachern, M.D.	1956	★Ray E. Brown	1988	Eugene W. Arnett
1925	★E. S. Gilmore	1957	★Albert W. Snoke, M.D.	1989	Edward J. Connors
1926	★Arthur C. Bachmeyer, M.D.	1958	★Tol Terrell	1990	David A. Reed
1927	★R. G. Brodrick, M.D.	1959	★Ray Amberg	1991	C. Thomas Smith
1928	★Joseph C. Doane, M.D.	1960	Russell A. Nelson, M.D.	1992	D. Kirk Oglesby, Jr.
1929	★Louis H. Burlingham, M.D.	1961	★Frank S. Groner	1993	Larry L. Mathis
1930	★Christopher G. Parnall, M.D.	1962	★Jack Masur, M.D.	1994	Carolyn C. Roberts

Chief Executive Officers

Years	Name	Years	Name	Years	Name
1917-18	★William H. Walsh, M.D.	1943-54	George Bugbee	1986-91	Carol M. McCarthy, Ph.D., J.D.
1919-24	★Andrew Robert Warner, M.D.	1954-72	★Edwin L. Crosby, M.D.	1991	Jack W. Owen (acting)
1925-27	★William H. Walsh, M.D.	1972	Madison B. Brown, M.D. (acting)	1991	Richard J. Davidson
1928-42	★Bert W. Caldwell, M.D.	1972-86	J. Alexander McMahon		

Distinguished Service Award

Year	Name	Year	Name	Year	Name
1934	★Matthew O. Foley	1958	★John N. Hatfield	1978	★Richard J. Stull
1939	★Malcolm T. MacEachern, M.D.	1959	★Edwin L. Crosby, M.D.	1979	Horace M. Cardwell
1940	★Sigismund S. Goldwater, M.D.	1960	★Oliver G. Pratt	1980	Donald W. Cordes
1941	★Frederic A. Washburn, M.D.	1961	★E. M. Bluestone, M.D.	1981	★Sister Mary Brigh Cassidy
1942	★Winford H. Smith, M.D.	1962	Mother Loretto Bernard, S.C., R.N.	1982	R. Zach Thomas, Jr.
1943	★Arthur C. Bachmeyer, M.D.	1963	★Ray E. Brown	1983	H. Robert Cathcart
1944	★Rt. Rev. Msgr. Maurice F. Griffin, LL.D.	1964	Russell A. Nelson, M.D.	1984	Matthew F. McNulty, Jr., Sc.D.
1945	★Asa S. Bacon	1965	★Albert W. Snoke, M.D.	1985	J. Alexander McMahon
1946	★George F. Stephens, M.D.	1966	★Frank S. Groner	1986	Sister Irene Kraus
1947	★Robin C. Buerki, M.D.	1967	★Rev. John J. Flanagan, S.J.	1987	W. Daniel Barker
1948	★James A. Hamilton	1968	Stanley W. Martin	1988	Elbert E. Gilbertson
1949	★Claude W. Munger, M.D.	1969	T. Stewart Hamilton, M.D.	1989	Donald G. Shropshire
1950	★Nathaniel W. Faxon, M.D.	1970	★Charles Patteson Cladwell, Jr.	1990	John W. Colloton
1951	★Bert W. Caldwell, M.D.	1971	★Mark Berke	1991	Carol M. McCarthy, Ph.D., J.D.
1952	★Fred G. Carter, M.D.	1972	Stanley A. Ferguson	1992	David H. Hitt
1953	★Basil C. MacLean, M.D.	1973	Jack A. L. Hahn	1993	Edward J. Connors
1954	George Bugbee	1974	George William Graham, M.D.		Jack W. Owen
1955	★Joseph G. Norby	1975	George E. Cartmill	1994	George Adams
1956	★Charles F. Wilinsky, M.D.	1976	D. O. McClusky, Jr.	1995	Scott S. Parker
1957	★John H. Hayes	1977	Boone Powell		

★Deceased

†On June 3, 1972, the House of Delegates changed the title of the chief elected officer to chairman of the Board of Trustees, and the title of president was conferred on the chief executive officer of the Association.

AHA Offices, Officers, and Historical Data

Award of Honor
1966 ★Senator Lister Hill	1990 Joyce C. Clifford, R.N.	William A. Spencer, M.D.
1967 ★Emory W. Morris, D.D.S.	1991 ★Haynes Rice	1994 Robert A. Derzon
1971 Special Committee on Provision of Health Services (staff also)	1992 Donald W. Dunn Ira M. Lane, Jr.	1995 Russell G. Mawby, Ph.D. John K. Springer
1982 Walter J. McNemey	1993 Elliott C. Roberts, Sr.	
1989 Ruth M. Rothstein		

Justin Ford Kimball Award
1958 ★E. A. van Steenwyk	1970 ★Edwin L. Crosby, M.D.	1982 Robert E. Rinehimer
1959 George A. Newbury	1971 ★H. Charles Abbott	1983 John B. Morgan, Jr.
1960 ★C. Rufus Rorem, Ph.D.	1972 ★John R. Mannix	1984 Joseph F. Duplinsky
1961 ★James E. Stuart	1973 Herman M. Somers	1985 David W. Stewart
1962 Frank Van Dyk	1974 William H. Ford, Ph.D.	1988 ★Ernest W. Saward, M.D.
1963 ★William S. McNary	1975 Earl H. Kammer	1990 James A. Vohs
1964 ★Frank S. Groner	1976 J. Ed McConnell	1993 John C. Lewin, M.D.
1965 ★J. Douglas Colman	1978 Edwin R. Werner	1994 Donald A. Brennan
1967 Walter J. McNemey	1979 ★Robert M. Cunningham, Jr.	1995 E. George Middleton, Jr.
1968 John W. Paynter	1981 ★Maurice J. Norby	Glenn R. Mitchell

Trustees Award
1959 ★Joseph V. Friel ★John H. Hayes	1974 ★James E. Hague Sister Marybelle	1986 Rex N. Olsen
1960 Duncan D. Sutphen, Jr.	1975 Helen T. Yast	1987 Michael Lesparre
1963 Eleanor C. Lambertsen, R.N., Ed.D.	1976 Boynton P. Livingston James Ludlam ★Helen McGuire	1988 Barbara A. Donaho, R.N.
1964 ★John R. Mannix		1989 Walter H. MacDonald Donald R. Newkirk
1965 ★Albert G. Hahn ★Maurice J. Norby	1979 ★Newton J. Jacobson Edward W. Weimer	1990 William T. Robinson
1966 Madison B. Brown, M.D. Kenneth Williamson	1980 ★Robert B. Hunter, M.D. ★Samuel J. Tibbitts	1992 Jack C. Bills Anne Hall Davis
1967 Alanson W. Wilcox	1981 Vernon A. Knutson John E. Sullivan	1993 Theodore C. Eickhoff, M.D. Stephen W. Gamble Yoshi Honkawa
1968 ★E. Dwight Barnett, M.D.		
1969 ★Vane M. Hoge, M.D. Joseph H. McNinch, M.D.	1982 John Bigelow Robert W. O'Leary Jack W. Owen	1994 Roger M. Busfield, Jr., Ph.D.
1972 David F. Drake, Ph.D. Paul W. Earle Michael Lesparre Andrew Pattullo	1984 Howard J. Berman O. Ray Hurst James R. Neely	1995 Stephen E. Dorn William L. Yates
1973 Tilden Cummings Edmond J. Lanigan	1985 ★James E. Ferguson Cleveland Rodgers	

Citation for Meritorious Service•
1968 ★F. R. Knautz Sister Conrad Mary, R.N.	Gordon McLachlan	1983 ★David M. Kinzer
1971 Hospital Council of Southern California	1977 Theodore Cooper, M.D.	1984 Donald L. Custis, M.D.
1972 College of Misericordia, Dallas, PA	1979 Norman D. Burkett John L. Quigley ★William M. Whelan	1985 John A. D. Cooper, M.D. Imperial Council of the Ancient Arabic Order of the Nobles of the Mystic Shrine for North America
1973 Madison B. Brown, M.D. ★Samuel J. Tibbitts		
1975 ★Kenneth B. Babcock, M.D. Sister Mary Maurita Sengelaube	1980 ★Sister Grace Marie Hiltz Leo J. Gehrig, M.D.	1986 Howard F. Cook
1976 Chaiker Abbis ★Susan Jenkins	1981 Richard Davi Pearl S. Fryar	1987 David H. Hitt ★Lucile Packard
	1982 Jorge Brull Nater	

Conventions
1	1899	Cleveland, September 12–13	34	1932	Detroit, September 12–16	67	1965	San Francisco, August 30–September 2
2	1900	Pittsburgh, August 21–23	35	1933	Milwaukee, September 11–15	68	1966	Chicago, August 29–September 1
3	1901	New York, September 10–12	36	1934	Philadelphia, September 24–28	69	1967	Chicago, August 21–24
4	1902	Philadelphia, October 14–16	37	1935	St. Louis, September 30–October 4	70	1968	Atlantic City, September 16–19
5	1903	Cincinnati, October 20–22	38	1936	Cleveland, September 28–October 2	71	1969	Chicago, August 18–21
6	1904	Atlantic City, September 21–23	39	1937	Atlantic City, September 13–17	72	1970	Houston, September 14–17
7	1905	Boston, September 26–29	40	1938	Dallas, September 26–30	73	1971	Chicago, August 23–26
8	1906	Buffalo, September 18–21	41	1939	Toronto, September 25–29		1972	Chicago, August 7–10 American
9	1907	Chicago, September 17–20	42	1940	Boston, September 16–20		1973	Chicago, August 20–23 Health
10	1908	Toronto, September 29–October 2	43	1941	Atlantic City, September 15–19		1974	Chicago, August 12–15 Congress
11	1909	Washington, September 21–24	44	1942	St. Louis, October 12–16	74	1975	Chicago, August 18–21
12	1910	St. Louis, September 20–23	45	1943	Buffalo, September 13–17	75	1976	Dallas, September 20–23
13	1911	New York, September 19–22	46	1944	Cleveland, October 2–6	76	1977	Atlanta, August 29–September 1
14	1912	Detroit, September 24–27	47	1945	Chicago, November 6–7 (House only)	77	1978	Anaheim, September 11–14
15	1913	Boston, August 26–29	48	1946	Philadelphia, September 30–October 3	78	1979	Chicago, August 27–30
16	1914	St. Paul, August 25–28	49	1947	St. Louis, September 22–25	79	1980	Montreal, July 28–31
17	1915	San Francisco, June 22–25	50	1948	Atlantic City, September 20–23	80	1981	Philadelphia, August 31–September 3
18	1916	Philadelphia, September 26–30	51	1949	Cleveland, September 26–29	81	1982	Atlanta, August 30–September 1
19	1917	Cleveland, September 10–15	52	1950	Atlantic City, September 18–21	82	1983	Houston, August 1–3
20	1918	Atlantic City, September 24–28	53	1951	St. Louis, September 17–20	83	1984	Denver, August 13–15
21	1919	Cincinnati, September 8–12	54	1952	Philadelphia, September 15–18	84	1985	Chicago, July 29–31
22	1920	Montreal, October 4–8	55	1953	San Francisco, August 31–September 3	85	1986	Toronto, August 4–6
23	1921	West Baden, IN, September 12–16	56	1954	Chicago, September 13–16	86	1987	Atlanta, July 27–29
24	1922	Atlantic City, September 25–28	57	1955	Atlantic City, September 19–22	87	1988	New Orleans, August 8–10
25	1923	Milwaukee, October 27–November 3	58	1956	Chicago, September 17–20	88	1989	Chicago, July 31–August 2
26	1924	Buffalo, October 6–10	59	1957	Atlantic City, September 30–October 2	89	1990	Washington, July 30–August 1
27	1925	Louisville, October 19–23	60	1958	Chicago, August 18–21	90	1991	Anaheim, July 29–31
28	1926	Atlantic City, September 22–October 1	61	1959	New York, August 24–27	91	1992	Denver, July 27–29
29	1927	Minneapolis, October 10–14	62	1960	San Francisco, August 29–September 1	92	1993	Orlando, August 9–11
30	1928	San Francisco, August 6–10	63	1961	Atlantic City, September 25–28	93	1994	Dallas, August 8–10
31	1929	Atlantic City, June 17–21	64	1962	Chicago, September 17–20	94	1995	San Francisco, August 21–23
32	1930	New Orleans, October 20–24	65	1963	New York, August 26–29	95	1996	Philadelphia, August 5–7
33	1931	Toronto, September 28–October 2	66	1964	Chicago, August 24–27			

★Deceased
•This citation is no longer awarded

© 1995 AHA Guide

Registration Requirements for Hospitals

This directory includes hospitals registered by the American Hospital Association and osteopathic hospitals listed by the American Osteopathic Association. Identification codes for both types of hospitals are explained fully on pages A6–8. For the reader's convenience, the codes for osteopathic hospitals are also summarized in the notes at the top of each page of this section. Beginning in November 1970, osteopathic hospitals became eligible to apply for registration with the American Hospital Association. Registered osteopathic hospitals carry the same codes as all other hospitals registered by the American Hospital Association.

The following requirements were approved by the Executive Committee of the Board of Trustees, May 13, 1986.

AHA–Registered Hospitals

Any institution that can be classified as a hospital according to the requirements may be registered if it so desires. Membership in the American Hospital Association is not a prerequisite.

The American Hospital Association may, at the sole discretion of the Executive Committee of the Board of Trustees, grant, deny, or withdraw the registration of an institution.

An Institution may be registered by the American Hospital Association as a hospital if it is accredited as a hospital by the Joint Commission on Accreditation of Healthcare Organizations or is certified as a provider of acute services under Title 18 of the Social Security Act and has provided the Association with documents verifying the accreditation or certification.

In lieu of the preceding accreditation or certification, an institution licensed as a hospital by the appropriate state agency may be registered by AHA as a hospital by meeting the following alternative requirements:

Function: The primary function of the institution is to provide patient services, diagnostic and therapeutic, for particular or general medical conditions.

1. The institution shall maintain at lease six inpatient beds, which shall be continuously available for the care of patients who are nonrelated and who stay on the average in excess of 24 hours per admission.

2. The institution shall be constructed, equipped, and maintained to ensure the health and safety of patients and to provide uncrowded, sanitary facilities for the treatment of patients.

3. There shall be an identifiable governing authority legally and morally responsible for the conduct of the hospital.

4. There shall be a chief executive to whom the governing authority delegates the continuous responsibility for the operation of the hospital in accordance with established policy.

5. There shall be an organized medical staff of fully licensed physicians* that may include other licensed individuals permitted by law and by the hospital to provide patient care services independently in the hospital. The medical staff shall be accountable to the governing authority for maintaining proper standards of medical care, and it shall be governed by bylaws adopted by said staff and approved by the governing authority.

6. Each patient shall be admitted on the authority of a member of the medical staff who has been granted the privilege to admit patients to inpatient services in accordance with state law and criteria for standards of medical care established by the individual medical staff. Each patient's general medical condition is the responsibility of a qualified physician member of the medical staff. When nonphysician members of the medical staff are granted privileges to admit patients, provision is made for prompt medical evaluation of these patients by a qualified physician. Any graduate of a foreign medical school who is permitted to assume responsibilities for patient care shall possess a valid license to practice medicine, or shall be certified by the Educational Commission for Foreign Medical Graduates, or shall have qualified for and have successfully completed an academic year of supervised clinical training under the direction of a medical school approved by the Liaison Committee on Medical Education.

7. Registered nurse supervision and other nursing services are continuous.

8. A current and complete‡ medical record shall be maintained by the institution for each patient and shall be available for reference.

9. Pharmacy service shall be maintained in the institution and shall be supervised by a registered pharmacist.

10. The institution shall provide patients with food service that meets their nutritional and therapeutic requirements; special diets shall also be available.

*Physician–Term used to describe an individual with an M.D. or D.O. degree who is fully licensed to practice medicine in all its phases.

‡The completed records in general shall contain at least the following: the patient's identifying data and consent forms, medical history, record of physical examination, physicians' progress notes, operative notes, nurses' notes, routine x–ray and laboratory reports, doctors' orders, and final diagnosis.

Registration Requirements for Hospitals

Types of Hospitals

In addition to meeting these 10 general registration requirements, hospitals are registered as one of four types of hospitals: general, special, rehabilitation and chronic disease, or psychiatric. The following definitions of function by type of hospital and special requirements for registration are employed:

General

The primary function of the institution is to provide patient services, diagnostic and therapeutic, for a variety of medical conditions. A general hospital also shall provide:
- diagnostic x–ray services with facilities and staff for a variety of procedures
- clinical laboratory service with facilities and staff for a variety of procedures and with anatomical pathology services regularly and conveniently available
- operating room service with facilities and staff.

Special

The primary function of the institution is to provide diagnostic and treatment services for patients who have specified medical conditions, both surgical and nonsurgical. A special hospital also shall provide:
- such diagnostic and treatment services as may be determined by the Executive Committee of the Board of Trustees of the American Hospital Association to be appropriate for the specified medical conditions for which medical services are provided shall be maintained in the institution with suitable facilities and staff. If such conditions do not normally require diagnostic x–ray service, laboratory service, or operating room service, and if any such services are therefore not maintained in the institution, there shall be written arrangements to make them available to patients requiring them.
- clinical laboratory services capable of providing tissue diagnosis when offering pregnancy termination services.

Rehabilitation and Chronic Disease

The primary function of the institution is to provide diagnostic and treatment services to handicapped or disabled individuals requiring restorative and adjustive services. A rehabilitation and chronic disease hospital also shall provide:
- arrangements for diagnostic x–ray services, as required, on a regular and conveniently available basis
- arrangements for clinical laboratory service, as required on a regular and conveniently available basis
- arrangements for operating room service, as required, on a regular and conveniently available basis
- a physical therapy service with suitable facilities and staff in the institution
- an occupational therapy service with suitable facilities and staff in the institution
- arrangements for psychological and social work services on a regular and conveniently available basis
- arrangements for educational and vocational services on a regular and conveniently available basis
- written arrangements with a general hospital for the transfer of patients who require medical, obstetrical, or surgical services not available in the institution.

Psychiatric

The primary function of the institution is to provide diagnostic and treatment services for patients who have psychiatric–related illnesses. A psychiatric hospital also shall provide:
- arrangements for clinical laboratory service, as required, on a regular and conveniently available basis
- arrangements for diagnostic x–ray services, as required on a regular and conveniently available basis
- psychiatric, psychological, and social work service with facilities and staff in the institution
- arrangements for electroencephalo–graph services, as required, on a regular and conveniently available basis
- written arrangements with a general hospital for the transfer of patients who require medical, obstetrical, or surgical services not available in the institution.

The American Hospital Association may, at the sole discretion of the Executive Committee of the Board of Trustees, grant, deny, or withdraw the registration of an institution.

AOHA–Listed Hospitals

The list of osteopathic hospitals includes both members and nonmembers of the American Osteopathic Hospital Association.

---

*Physician–Term used to describe an individual with an M.D. or D.O. degree who is fully licensed to practice medicine in all its phases.

‡The completed records in general shall contain at least the following: the patient's identifying data and consent forms, medical history, record of physical examination, physicians' progress notes, operative notes, nurses' notes, routine x–ray and laboratory reports, doctors' orders, and final diagnosis.

Explanation of Hospital Listings

Hospital, Address, Telephone, Administrator, Approval, Facility, and Physician Codes, Health Care System	Classi-fication Codes		Utilization Data					Expense (thousands) of dollars		
	Control	Service	Beds	Admissions	Census	Outpatient Visits	Births	Total	Payroll	Personnel
★ American Hospital Association (AHA) membership □ Joint Commission on Accreditation of Healthcare Organizations (JCAHO) accreditation + American Osteopathic Hospital Association (AOHA) membership ○ American Osteopathic Association (AOA) accreditation △ Commission on Accreditation of Rehabilitation Facilities (CARF) accreditation Control codes 61, 63, 64, 71, 72 and 73 indicate hospitals listed by AOHA, but not registered by AHA. For definition of numerical codes, see page A6										
ANYTOWN—Universal County ★ COMMUNITY HOSPITAL, First Street and Main Avenue Zip 62835; tel 204/391–2345; Jane Doe, Administrator **A**1 2 3 4 6 9 10 **F**1 2 3 4 5 6 8 9 10 23 24 34; **P**1 2 3 4; **S**1234 Acme HCS	23	10	346	10778	248	75953	1693	20695	9973	796

(groupings labeled: **1** = Approval codes **A**..., **2** = Facility codes **F**..., **3** = Physician codes **P**...)

1 Approval Codes

Reported by the approving bodies specified, as of the dates noted.

1. Accreditation under the hospital program of the Joint Commission on Accreditation of Healthcare Organizations (January 1995).
2. Cancer program approved by American College of Surgeons (January 1995).
3. Approval to participate in residency training, by the Accreditation Council for Graduate Medical Education (January 1995). As of June 30, 1975, internship (formerly code 4) was included under residency, code 3.
5. Medical school affiliation reported to the American Medical Association (January 1995).
6. Hospital-controlled professional nursing school, reported by National League for Nursing (January 1995).
7. Accreditation by Commission on Accreditation of Rehabilitation Facilities (January 1995).
8. Member of Council of Teaching Hospitals of the Association of American Medical Colleges (January 1995).
9. Hospital contracting or participating in Blue Cross Plan, reported by Blue Cross Association (January 1995).
10. Certified for participation in the Health Insurance for the Aged (Medicare) Program by the U.S. Department of Health and Human Services (January 1995).
11. Accreditation by American Osteopathic Association (January 1995).
12. Internship approved by American Osteopathic Association (January 1995).
13. Residency approved by American Osteopathic Association (January 1995).

Nonreporting indicates that the 1994 Annual Survey questionnaire for the hospital had not been received by April 30, 1995, the cutoff date for statistical processing.

Newly Registered indicates that the hospital was registered after the mailing of the 1994 Annual Survey.

2 Facility Codes

Actually available within, and reported by the institution; for definitions, see page A8.

(Alphabetical/Numerical Order)

1. Adult day care program
2. Alcoholism–drug abuse or dependency inpatient unit
3. Alcoholism–drug abuse or dependency outpatient services
4. Angioplasty
5. Arthritis treatment center
6. Assisted living
7. Birthing room–LDR room–LDRP room
8. Breast cancer screening/mammograms
9. Burn care unit
10. Cardiac catheterization laboratory
11. Cardiac intensive care unit
12. Case management
13. Children wellness program
14. Community health reporting
15. Community health status assessment
16. Community health status based service planning
17. Community outreach
18. Crisis prevention
19. CT scanner
20. Dental services
21. Diagnostic radioisotope facility
22. Emergency department
23. Extracorporeal shock wave lithotripter (ESWL)
24. Fitness center
25. Freestanding outpatient care center
26. Geriatric services
27. Health facility transportation (to/from)
28. Health fair
29. Health information center
30. Health screenings
31. HIV–AIDS services
32. Home health services
33. Hospice
34. Hospital-based outpatient care center–services
35. Magnetic resonance imaging (MRI)
36. Meals on wheels
37. Medical surgical intensive care unit
38. Neonatal intensive care unit
39. Nutrition programs
40. Obstetrics unit
41. Occupational health services
42. Oncology services
43. Open heart surgery
44. Outpatient surgery
45. Patient education center
46. Patient representative services
47. Pediatric intensive care unit
48. Physical rehabilitation inpatient unit
49. Physical rehabilitation outpatient services
50. Positron emission tomography scanner (PET)
51. Primary care department
52. Psychiatric acute inpatient unit
53. Psychiatric child adolescent services
54. Psychiatric consultation–liaison services
55. Psychiatric education services
56. Psychiatric emergency services
57. Psychiatric geriatric services
58. Psychiatric outpatient services
59. Psychiatric partial hospitalization program
60. Radiation therapy
61. Reproductive health services
62. Retirement housing
63. Single photon emission computerized tomography (SPECT)
64. Skilled nursing or other long-term care unit
65. Social work services
66. Sports medicine
67. Support groups
68. Teen outreach services
69. Transplant services
70. Trauma center (certified)
71. Ultrasound
72. Urgent care center
73. Volunteer services department
74. Women's health center/services

3 Physician Codes

Actually available within, and reported by the institution; for definitions, see page A11.

(Alphabetical/Numerical Order)

1. Closed physician–hospital organization (PHO)
2. Equity model
3. Foundation
4. Group practice without walls
5. Independent practice association (IPA)
6. Integrated salary model
7. Management service organization (MSO)
8. Open physician–hospital organization (PHO)

Explanation of Hospital Listings

Hospital, Address, Telephone, Administrator, Approval, Facility, and Physician Codes, Health Care System	Classi-fication Codes		Utilization Data					Expense (thousands) of dollars		
	Control	Service	Beds	Admissions	Census	Outpatient Visits	Births	Total	Payroll	Personnel

★ American Hospital Association (AHA) membership
☐ Joint Commission on Accreditation of Healthcare Organizations (JCAHO) accreditation
+ American Osteopathic Hospital Association (AOHA) membership
○ American Osteopathic Association (AOA) accreditation
△ Commission on Accreditation of Rehabilitation Facilities (CARF) accreditation
Control codes 61, 63, 64, 71, 72 and 73 indicate hospitals listed by AOHA, but not registered by AHA. For definition of numerical codes, see page A6

ANYTOWN—Universal County
★ COMMUNITY HOSPITAL, First Street and Main Avenue Zip 62835; tel 204/391–2345; Jane Doe, Administrator **A**1 2 3 4 6 9 10 **F**1 2 3 4 5 6 8 9 10 23 24 34; **P**1 2 3 4; **S**1234 Acme HCS   23   10   346   10778   248   75953   1693   20695   9973   796

(4 = Control/Service codes area; 5 = Classification Codes area; 6 = Utilization and Expense data area)

4 Health Care System Code and Name

A code number has been assigned to each health care system headquarters. The inclusion *of one of these codes (1) indicates that the hospital belongs to a health care system and* *(2) identifies the specific system to which the hospital belongs.*

5 Classification Codes

Control

Government, nonfederal
12 State
13 County
14 City
15 City–county
16 Hospital district or authority

Nongovernment not–for–profit
21 Church operated
23 Other

Investor–owned (for–profit)
31 Individual
32 Partnership
33 Corporation

Government, federal
41 Air Force
42 Army
43 Navy
44 Public Health Service other than 47
45 Veterans Administration
46 Federal other than 41–45, 47–48
47 Public Health Service Indian Service
48 Department of Justice

Osteopathic
61 Church operated
63 Other not–for–profit
64 Other
71 Individual for–profit
72 Partnership for–profit
73 Corporation for–profit

Service
10 General medical and surgical
11 Hospital unit of an institution (prison hospital, college infirmary, etc.)
12 Hospital unit within an institution for the mentally retarded
22 Psychiatric
33 Tuberculosis and other respiratory diseases
44 Obstetrics and gynecology
45 Eye, ear, nose, and throat
46 Rehabilitation
47 Orthopedic
48 Chronic disease
49 Other specialty
50 Children's general
51 Children's hospital unit of an institution
52 Children's psychiatric
53 Children's tuberculosis and other respiratory diseases
55 Children's eye, ear, nose, and throat
56 Children's rehabilitation
57 Children's orthopedic
58 Children's chronic disease
59 Children's other specialty
62 Institution for mental retardation
82 Alcoholism and other chemical dependency

* Control codes 61, 63, 64, 71, 72 and 73 indicate hospitals listed by the AOHA but not registered by AHA.
When a hospital restricts its service to a specialty not defined by a specific code, it is coded 49 (59 if a children's hospital) and the specialty is indicated in parentheses following the name of the hospital.

6 Headings

Definitions are based on the American Hospital Association's Hospital Administration Terminology. Where a 12–month period is specified, hospitals were requested to report on the Annual Survey of Hospitals for the 12 months ending September 30, 1994. Hospitals reporting for less than a 12–month period are so designated.

Utilization Data:

Beds–Number of beds regularly maintained (set up and staffed for use) for inpatients as of the close of the reporting period.

Admissions–Number of patients accepted for inpatient service during a 12–month period; does not include newborn.

Census–Average number of inpatients receiving care each day during the 12–month reporting period; does not include newborn.

Outpatient Visits–An outpatient visit is a visit by a patient who is not lodged in the hospital while receiving medical, dental, or other services. Each appearance of an outpatient in each unit constitutes one visit regardless of the number of diagnostic and/or therapeutic treatments that a patient receives.

Births–Number of infants born in the hospital and accepted for service in a newborn infant bassinet during a 12–month period; excludes stillbirths.

Expense: Expense for a 12–month period; both total expense and payroll components are shown. Payroll expenses include all salaries and wages except those paid to medical and dental interns and residents, and other trainees (e.g., medical technology trainees, x–ray therapy trainees, administrative residents, etc.).

Personnel: Includes persons on payroll on September 30, 1994; includes full–time equivalents of part–time personnel, but excludes medical and dental interns and residents and other trainees. Full–time equivalents were calculated on the basis that two part–time persons equal one full–time person.

© 1995 AHA Guide

Annual Survey

Each year, an annual survey of hospitals is conducted by the Health Statistics Group of the American Hospital Association (AHA).

Until the 1981 edition, this publication included a copy of both the Annual Survey and instructions and definitions that accompanied the survey instrument. However, because of their size, the questionnaire and associated definitions are no longer reproduced. The definitions of facility codes are presented instead.

The American Hospital Association Guide to the Health Care Field does not include all data collected from the 1994 Annual Survey. Requests for purchasing other Annual Survey data should be directed to the Health Statistics Group, American Hospital Association, One North Franklin, Chicago, IL 60606–3401, 312/422–3990.

Definitions of Facility Codes

1. **Adult day care program** Program providing supervision, medical and psychological care, and social activities for older adults who live at home or in another family setting, but cannot be alone or prefer to be with others during the day. May include intake assessment, health monitoring, occupational therapy, personal care, noon meal, and transportation services.

2. **Alcoholism–drug abuse or dependency inpatient services** Provides, diagnosis and therapeutic services to patients with alcoholism or other drug dependencies. Includes care for inpatient/residential treatment for patients whose course of treatment involves more intensive care than provided in an outpatient setting or where patient requires supervised withdrawal.

3. **Alcoholism–drug abuse or dependency outpatient services** Organized hospital services that provide medical care and/or rehabilitative treatment services to outpatients for whom the primary diagnosis is alcoholism or other chemical dependency.

4. **Angioplasty** The reconstruction of restructuring of a blood vessel by operative means or by nonsurgical techniques such as balloon dilation or laser.

5. **Arthritis treatment center** Specifically equipped and staffed center for the diagnosis and treatment of arthritis and other joint disorders.

6. **Assisted living** A special combination of housing, supportive services, personalized assistance and health care designed to respond to the individual needs of those who need help in activities of daily living and instrumental activities of daily living. Supportive services are available, 24 hours a day, to meet scheduled and unscheduled needs, in a way that promotes maximum independence and dignity for each resident and encourages the involvement of a resident's family, neighbor and friends.

7. **Birthing room–LDR room–LDRP room** A single room–type of maternity care with a more homelike setting for families than the traditional three–room unit (labor/delivery/recovery) with a separate postpartum area. A birthing room combines labor and delivery in one room. An LDR room accommodates three stages in the birthing process—labor, delivery, and recovery. An LDRP room accommodates all four stages of the birth process—labor, delivery, recovery and postpartum.

8. **Breast cancer screening/mammograms** Mammography screening The use of breast x–ray to detect unsuspected breast cancer in asymptomatic women. Diagnostic mammography The x–ray imaging of breast tissue in symptomatic women who are considered to have a substantial likelihood of having breast cancer already.

9. **Burn care unit** Provides care to severely burned patients. Severely burned patients are those with any of the following: 1. Second–degree burns of more than 25% total body surface area for adults or 20% total body surface area for children; 2. Third–degree burns of more than 10% total body surface area; 3. Any severe burns of the hands, face, eyes, ears or feet or; 4. All inhalation injuries, electrical burns, complicated burn injuries involving fractures and other major traumas, and all other poor risk factors.

10. **Cardiac catheterization laboratory** Facilities offering special diagnostic procedures for cardiac patients. Available procedures must include, but need not be limited to, introduction of a catheter into the interior of the heart by way of a vein or artery or by direct needle puncture. Procedures must be performed in a laboratory or a special procedure room.

11. **Cardiac intensive care unit** Provides patient care of a more specialized nature than the usual medical and surgical care, on the basis of physicians' orders and approved nursing care plans. The unit is staffed with specially trained nursing personnel and contains monitoring and specialized support or treatment equipment for patients who, because of heart seizure, open–heart surgery, or other life–threatening conditions, require intensified, comprehensive observation and care. May include myocardial infarction, pulmonary care, and heart transplant units.

12. **Case management** A system of assessment, treatment planning, referral and follow–up that ensures the provision of comprehensive and continuous services and the coordination of payment and reimbursement for care.

13. **Children wellness program** A program that encourages improved health status and a healthful lifestyle of children through health education, exercise, nutrition and health promotion.

14. **Community health reporting** Does your hospital either by itself or in conjunction with others disseminate reports to the community on the quality and costs of health care services?

15. **Community health status assessment** Does your hospital work with other providers, public agencies, or community representatives to conduct a health status assessment of the community?

16. **Community health status based service planning** Does your hospital use health status indicators (such as rates of health problems or surveys of self–reported health) for defined populations to design new services or modify existing services?

17. **Community outreach** A program that systematically interacts with the community to identify those in need of services, alerting persons and their families to the availability of services, locating needed services, and enabling persons to enter the service delivery system.

18. **Crisis prevention** Services provided in order to promote physical and mental well being and the early identification of disease and ill health prior to the onset and recognition of symptoms so as to permit early treatment.

19. **CT scanner** Computed tomographic scanner for head or whole body scans.

20. **Dental services** An organized dental service, not necessarily involving special facilities, that provides dental or oral services to inpatients or outpatients.

21. **Diagnostic radioisotope facility** The use of radioactive isotopes (Radiopharmaceutical) as tracers or indicators to detect an abnormal condition or disease.

22. **Emergency department** Hospital facilities for the provision of unscheduled outpatient services to patients whose conditions require immediate care. Must be staffed 24 hours a day.

23. **Extracorporeal shock wave lithotripter (ESWL)** A medical device used for treating stones in the kidney or ureter. The device disintegrates kidney stones noninvasively through the transmission of acoustic shock waves directed at the stones.

24. **Fitness center** Provides exercise, testing, or evaluation programs and fitness activities to the community and hospital employees.

25. **Freestanding outpatient care center** A facility owned and operated by the hospital, but physically separate from the hospital, that provides various medical treatments on an outpatient basis only. May be any of the following three types of center, depending on the level of care it is equipped to provide; freestanding emergency center, freestanding urgent care center, or primary care center. In addition to treating minor illnesses or injuries, the center will stabilize seriously ill or injured patients before transporting them to a hospital. Laboratory and radiology services are usually available.

26. **Geriatric services** The branch of medicine dealing with the physiology of aging and the diagnosis and treatment of disease affecting the aged. Services could include: Adult day care program; Alzheimer's diagnostic–assessment services; Comprehensive geriatric assessment; Emergency response system; Geriatric acute care unit; and/or Geriatric clinics.

27. **Health facility transportation (to/from)** A long–term care support service designed to assist the mobility of the elderly. Some programs offer improved financial access by offering reduced rates and barrier–free buses or vans with ramps and lifts to assist the elderly or handicapped; others offer subsidies for public transport systems or operate mini–bus services exclusively for use by senior citizens.

28. **Health fair** Community health education events that focus on the prevention of disease and promotion of health through such activities as audiovisual exhibits and free diagnostic services.

29. **Health information center** Education which is directed at increasing the information of individuals and populations. It is intended to increase the ability to make informed personal, family and community health decision by providing consumers with informed choices about health matters with the objective of improving health status.

30. **Health screenings** A preliminary procedure, such as a test or examination to detect the most characteristic sign or signs of a disorder that may require further investigation.

31. **HIV–AIDS services** Services may include one or more of the following: HIV–AIDS unit (special unit or team designated and equipped specifically for diagnosis, treatment, continuing care planning, and counseling services for HIV–AIDS patients and their families.), General inpatient care for HIV–AIDS (inpatient diagnosis and treatment for human immunodeficiency virus and acquired immunodeficiency syndrome patients, but dedicated unit is not available.) Specialized outpatient program for HIV–AIDS (special outpatient program providing diagnostic, treatment, continuing care planning, and counseling for HIV–AIDS patients and their families.)

32. **Home health services** Service providing nursing, therapy, and health–related homemaker or social services in the patient's home.

33. **Hospice** A program providing palliative care, chiefly medical relief of pain and supportive services, addressing the emotional, social, financial, and legal needs of terminally ill patients and their families. Care can be provided in a variety of settings, both inpatient and at home.

34. **Hospital–based outpatient care center–services** Organized hospital health care services offered by appointment on an ambulatory basis. Services may include outpatient surgery, examination, diagnosis, and treatment of a variety of medical conditions on a nonemergency basis, and laboratory and other diagnostic testing as ordered by staff or outside physician referral.

35. **Magnetic resonance imaging (MRI)** The use of a uniform magnetic field and radio frequencies to study tissue and structure of the body. This procedure enables the visualization of biochemical activity of the cell in vivo without the use of ionizing radiation, radioisotopic substances, or high–frequency sound.

36. **Meals on wheels** A hospital sponsored program which delivers meals to people, usually the elderly, who are unable to prepare their own meals. Low cost, nutritional meals are delivered to individuals' homes on a regular basis.

37. **Medical surgical intensive care unit** Provides patient care of a more intensive nature than the usual medical and surgical care, on the basis of physicians' orders and approved nursing care plans. These units are staffed with specially trained nursing personnel and contain monitoring and specialized support equipment of patients who, because of shock, trauma, or other life–threatening conditions, require intensified, comprehensive observation and care. Includes mixed intensive care units.

38. **Neonatal intensive care unit** A unit that must be separate from the newborn nursery providing intensive care to all sick infants including those with the very lowest birth weights (less that 1500 grams). NICU has potential for providing mechanical ventilation, neonatal surgery, and special care for the sickest infants born in the hospital or transferred from another institution. A full–time neonatologist serves as director of the NICU.

39. **Nutrition programs** Those services within a health care facility which are designed to provide inexpensive, nutritionally sound meals to patients.

40. **Obstetrics unit** Levels should be designated: (1) unit provides services for uncomplicated maternity and newborn cases; (2) unit provides services for uncomplicated cases, the majority of complicated problems, and special neonatal services; and (3) unit provides services for all serious illnesses and abnormalities and is supervised by a full–time maternal/fetal specialist.

41. **Occupational health services** Includes services designed to protect the safety of employees from hazards in the work environment.

42. **Oncology services** An organized program for the treatment of cancer by the use of drugs or chemicals.

43. **Open heart surgery** Heart surgery where the chest has been opened and the blood recirculated and oxygenated with the proper equipment and the necessary staff to perform the surgery.

44. **Outpatient surgery** Scheduled surgical services provided to patients who do not remain in the hospital overnight. The surgery may be performed in operating suites also used for inpatient surgery, specially designated surgical suites for outpatient surgery, or procedure rooms within an outpatient care facility.

45. **Patient education center** Written goals and objectives for the patient and/or family related to therapeutic regimens, medical procedures, and self care.

46. **Patient representative services** Organized hospital services providing personnel through whom patients and staff can seek solutions to institutional problems affecting the delivery of high-quality care and services.

47. **Pediatric intensive care unit** Provides care to pediatric patients that is of a more intensive nature than that usually provided to pediatric patients. The unit is staffed with specially trained personnel and contains monitoring and specialized support equipment for treatment of patients who, because of shock, trauma, or other life-threatening conditions, require intensified, comprehensive observation and care.

48. **Physical rehabilitation inpatient unit** Provides care encompassing a comprehensive array of restoration services for the disabled and all support services necessary to help patients attain their maximum functional capacity.

49. **Physical rehabilitation outpatient services** Outpatient program providing medical, health-related, therapy, social, and/or vocational services to help disabled persons attain or retain their maximum functional capacity.

50. **Positron emission tomography scanner (PET)** is a nuclear medicine imaging technology which uses radioactive (positron emitting) isotopes created in a cyclotron or generator and computers to produce composite pictures of the brain and heart at work. PET scanning produces sectional images depicting metabolic activity or blood flow rather than anatomy.

51. **Primary care department** A unit of clinic within the hospital that provides primary care services (e.g. general pediatric care, general internal medicine, family practice and gynecology) through hospital-salaried medical and or nursing staff, focusing on evaluating and diagnosing medical problems and providing medical treatment on an outpatient basis.

52. **Psychiatric acute inpatient unit** Provides acute or long-term care to emotionally disturbed patients, including patients admitted for diagnosis and those admitted for treatment of psychiatric problems, on the basis of physicians' orders and approved nursing care plans. Long-term care may include intensive supervision to the chronically mentally ill, mentally disordered, or other mentally incompetent persons.

53. **Psychiatric child adolescent services** Provides care to emotionally disturbed children and adolescents, including those admitted for diagnosis and those admitted for treatment.

54. **Psychiatric consultation-liaison services** Provides organized psychiatric consultation/liaison services to nonpsychiatric hospital staff and/or department on psychological aspects of medical care that may be generic or specific to individual patients.

55. **Psychiatric education services** Provides psychiatric educational services to community agencies and workers such as schools, police, courts, public health nurses, welfare agencies, clergy and so forth. The purpose is to expand the mental health knowledge and competence of personnel not working in the mental health field and to promote good mental health through improved understanding, attitudes, and behavioral patterns.

56. **Psychiatric emergency services** Services or facilities available on a 24-hour basis to provide immediate unscheduled outpatient care, diagnosis, evaluation, crisis intervention, and assistance to persons suffering acute emotional or mental distress.

57. **Psychiatric geriatric services** Provides care to emotionally disturbed elderly patients, including those admitted for diagnosis and those admitted for treatment.

58. **Psychiatric outpatient services** Provides medical care, including diagnosis and treatment of psychiatric outpatients.

59. **Psychiatric partial hospitalization program** Organized hospital services of intensive day/evening outpatient services of three hours or more duration, distinguished from other outpatient visits of one hour.

60. **Radiation therapy** The branch of medicine concerned with radioactive substances and using various techniques of visualization, with the diagnosis and treatment of disease using any of the various sources of radiant energy. Services could include: megavoltage radiation therapy; radioactive implants; stereotactic radiosurgery; therapeutic radioisotope facility; X-ray radiation therapy.

61. **Reproductive health services** Services that include any or all of the following:

    Fertility counseling A service that counsels and educates on infertility problems and includes laboratory and surgical workup and management for individuals having problems conceiving children.

    In vitro fertilization Program providing for the induction of fertilization of a surgically removed ovum by donated sperm in a culture medium followed by a short incubation period. The embryo is then reimplanted in the womb.

62. **Retirement housing** A facility which provides social activities to senior citizens, usually retired persons, who do not require health care but some short-term skilled nursing care may be provided. A retirement center may furnish housing and may also have acute hospital and long-term care facilities, or it may arrange for acute and long term care through affiliated institutions.

63. **Single photon emission computerized tomography (SPECT)** is a nuclear medicine imaging technology that combines existing technology of gamma camera imaging with computed tomographic imaging technology to provide a more precise and clear image.

64. **Skilled nursing or other long-term care unit** Provides non-acute medical and skilled nursing care services, therapy, and social services under the supervision of a licensed registered nurse on a 24-hour basis.

65. **Social work services** Services may include one or more of the following: Organized social work services (services that are properly directed and sufficiently staffed by qualified individuals who provide assistance and counseling to patients and their families in dealing with social, emotional, and environmental problems associated with illness or disability, often in the context of financial or discharge planning coordination.), Outpatient social work services (social work services provided in ambulatory care areas.) Emergency department social work services (social work services provided to emergency department patients by social workers dedicated to the emergency department or on call.)

66. **Sports medicine** Provision of diagnostic screening and assessment and clinical and rehabilitation services for the prevention and treatment of sports-related injuries.

67. **Support groups** A hospital sponsored program which allows a group of individuals with the same or similar problems who meet periodically to share experiences, problems, and solutions, in order to support each other.

68. **Teen outreach services** A program focusing on the teenager which encourages an improved health status and a healthful lifestyle including physical, emotional, mental, social, spiritual and economic through health education, exercise, nutrition and health promotion.

69. **Transplant services** The branch of medicine that transfers an organ or tissue from one person to another or from one body part to another to replace a diseased structure or to restore function or to change appearance. Services could includes: Bone marrow transplant program; kidney transplant; organ transplant (other than kidney); tissue transplant.

70. **Trauma center (certified)** A facility certified to provide emergency and specialized intensive care to critically ill and injured patients.

71. **Ultrasound** The use of acoustic waves above the range of 20,000 cycles per second to visualize internal body structures.

72. **Urgent care center** A facility that provides care and treatment for problems that are not life-threatening but require attention over the short term. These units function like emergency rooms but are separate from hospitals with which they may have backup affiliation arrangements.

73. **Volunteer services department** An organized hospital department responsible for coordinating the services of volunteers working within the institution.

74. **Women's health center/services** An area set aside for coordinated education and treatment services specifically for and promoted by women as provided by this special unit. Services may or may not include obstetrics but include a range of services other than OB.

Definitions of Physician Codes

1. **Closed physician-hospital organization (PHO)** A PHO that restricts physician membership to those practitioners who meet criteria for cost effectiveness and/or high quality.

2. **Equity model** Allows established practitioners to become shareholders in a professional corporation in exchange for tangible and intangible assets of their existing practices.

3. **Foundation** A corporation, organized either as a hospital affiliate or subsidiary, which purchases both the tangible and intangible assets of one or more medical group practices. Physicians remain in a separate corporate entity but sign a professional services agreement with the foundation.

4. **Group practice without walls** Hospital sponsors the formation of, or provides capital to physicians to establish, a "quasi" group to share administrative expenses while remaining independent practitioners.

5. **Independent practice association (IPA)** An IPA is a legal entity that hold managed care contracts. The IPA then contracts with physicians, usually in solo practice, to provide care either on a fee-for-services or capitated basis. The purpose of an IPA is to assist solo physicians in obtaining managed care contracts.

6. **Integrated salary model** Physicians are salaried by the hospital or another entity of a health system to provide medical services for primary care and specialty care.

7. **Management services organization (MSO)** A corporation, owned by the hospital or a physician/hospital joint venture, that provides management services to one or more medical group practices. The MSO purchases the tangible assets of the practices and leases them back as part of a full-service management agreement, under which the MSO employs all non-physician staff and provides all supplies/administrative systems for a fee.

8. **Open physician-hospital organization (PHO)** A joint venture between the hospital and all members of the medical staff who wish to participate. The PHO can act as a unified agent in managed care contracting, own a managed care plan, own and operate ambulatory care centers or ancillary services projects, or provide administrative services to physician members.

Hospitals in the United States, by State

ALABAMA

Resident population 4,187 (in thousands)
Resident population in metro areas 67.4%
Birth rate per 1,000 population 15.4
65 years and over 13.0%
Percent of persons without health insurance 17.3%

★ American Hospital Association (AHA) membership
☐ Joint Commission on Accreditation of Healthcare Organizations (JCAHO) accreditation
+ American Osteopathic Hospital Association (AOHA) membership
○ American Osteopathic Association (AOA) accreditation
△ Commission on Accreditation of Rehabilitation Facilities (CARF) accreditation
Control codes 61, 63, 64, 71, 72 and 73 indicate hospitals listed by AOHA, but not registered by AHA. For definition of numerical codes, see page A6

Hospital, Address, Telephone, Administrator, Approval, Facility, and Physician Codes, Health Care System	Classification Codes		Utilization Data					Expense (thousands) of dollars		
	Control	Service	Beds	Admissions	Census	Outpatient Visits	Births	Total	Payroll	Personnel
ALABASTER—Shelby County ★ SHELBY MEDICAL CENTER, 1000 First Street North, Zip 35007–0488, Mailing Address: Box 488, Zip 35007–0488; tel. 205/620–8100; Charles C. Colvert, President (Nonreporting) **A**1 9 10 **S**0345 Baptist Health System	13	10	228	—	—	—	—	—	—	—
ALEXANDER CITY—Tallapoosa County ★ RUSSELL HOSPITAL, U.S. 280 By–Pass, Zip 35010, Mailing Address: P.O. Box 939, Zip 35010–0939; tel. 205/329–7100; Frank W. Harris, President and Chief Executive Officer **A**1 9 10 **F**8 14 15 16 19 22 30 32 33 34 35 36 37 40 42 44 45 46 49 65 71 73 74 **P**7	23	10	75	3371	35	50990	369	19385	8864	365
ANDALUSIA—Covington County ★ ANDALUSIA HOSPITAL, South Three Notch Street, Zip 36420–0760, Mailing Address: Box 760, Zip 36420; tel. 205/222–8466; Joel O. Montgomery, Interim Chief Executive Officer **A**1 9 10 **F**7 8 14 15 16 19 21 22 24 30 31 32 34 35 36 37 40 44 54 65 71 73 **S**0048 Columbia/HCA Healthcare Corporation	33	10	101	2830	30	25429	433	13756	5638	249
ANNISTON—Calhoun County ★ NORTHEAST ALABAMA REGIONAL MEDICAL CENTER, 400 East Tenth Street, Zip 36209, Mailing Address: Box 2208, Zip 36202; tel. 205/235–5121; Allen P. Fletcher, President **A**1 2 9 10 **F**7 8 10 14 15 16 19 21 22 30 31 32 33 34 35 37 40 41 42 44 46 49 52 54 55 56 57 60 65 66 70 71 73	16	10	284	12776	177	96639	1450	67408	30078	1136
☐ STRINGFELLOW MEMORIAL HOSPITAL, 301 East 18th Street, Zip 36201; tel. 205/235–8900; Michael E. Cassidy, Administrator and Chief Executive Officer **A**1 9 10 **F**1 2 6 8 10 12 15 19 20 21 22 28 30 32 33 35 36 37 39 40 41 42 44 45 46 48 49 52 60 61 63 64 65 67 71 73 **P**3 **S**1775 Health Management Associates	23	10	45	1629	24	22747	0	—	—	285
ASHLAND—Clay County ☐ CLAY COUNTY HOSPITAL AND NURSING HOME, 544 East First Avenue, Zip 36251, Mailing Address: Box 10, Zip 36251–0277; tel. 205/354–2131; Linda Barnes, Administrator (Nonreporting) **A**1 9 10	13	10	106	—	—	—	—	—	—	—
ATHENS—Limestone County ★ ATHENS–LIMESTONE HOSPITAL, 700 West Market Street, Zip 35611, Mailing Address: Box 999, Zip 35611; tel. 205/233–9292; Philip E. Dotson, Chief Executive Officer **A**1 9 10 **F**7 8 12 15 16 19 21 22 26 27 28 30 32 37 39 40 44 45 49 65 71 73 74 **P**6	16	10	101	4350	52	39307	389	27407	11783	423
ATMORE—Escambia County ☐ ATMORE COMMUNITY HOSPITAL, 401 Medical Park Drive, Zip 36502; tel. 205/368–2500; Lavon Henley, Administrator (Nonreporting) **A**1 9 10 **S**1255 Escambia County Health Care Authority	13	10	51	—	—	—	—	—	—	—
BAY MINETTE—Baldwin County ★ NORTH BALDWIN HOSPITAL, 1815 Hand Avenue, Zip 36507, Mailing Address: P.O. Box 1409, Zip 36507; tel. 205/937–5521; Gary W. Farrow, Administrator (Nonreporting) **A**1 9 10	13	10	55	—	—	—	—	—	—	—
BESSEMER—Jefferson County ★ BESSEMER CARRAWAY MEDICAL CENTER, U.S. Highway 11 South, Zip 35023, Mailing Address: Box 847, Zip 35021–0847; tel. 205/481–7000; Dan M. Eagar Jr., Administrator **A**1 2 9 10 **F**2 7 8 10 11 12 14 17 19 21 27 28 33 37 39 41 42 44 48 49 52 54 55 56 57 65 67 70 71 73 74 **P**4	23	10	210	6051	107	63032	271	40819	17892	677
BIRMINGHAM—Jefferson County ★ BIRMINGHAM BAPTIST MEDICAL CENTER–MONTCLAIR CAMPUS, 800 Montclair Road, Zip 35213; tel. 205/592–1000; Dana S. Hensley, President (Nonreporting) **A**1 2 3 5 8 9 10 **S**0345 Baptist Health System	21	10	596	—	—	—	—	—	—	—
★ BIRMINGHAM BAPTIST MEDICAL CENTER–PRINCETON, (Formerly Princeton Baptist Medical Center) 701 Princeton Avenue S.W., Zip 35211–1305; tel. 205/783–3000; Dana S. Hensley, President and Chief Executive Officer (Nonreporting) **A**1 2 3 5 8 9 10 **S**0345 Baptist Health System	23	10	356	—	—	—	—	—	—	—
BRADFORD PARKSIDE AT BIRMINGHAM, (Formerly Bradford at Birmingham–Adults) 1221 Alton Drive, Zip 35210; tel. 205/833–4000; W. Clay Simmons, Executive Director (Nonreporting) **A**9 **S**2455 Bradford Parkside	33	82	90	—	—	—	—	—	—	—
★ BROOKWOOD MEDICAL CENTER, 2010 Brookwood Medical Center Drive, Zip 35209; tel. 205/877–1000; Gregory H. Burfitt, Chief Executive Officer (Nonreporting) **A**1 2 9 10 **S**0063 TENET Healthcare Corporation	33	10	515	—	—	—	—	—	—	—
★ △ CARRAWAY METHODIST MEDICAL CENTER, 1600 Carraway Boulevard, Zip 35234–1990; tel. 205/226–6000; Warren E. Callaway FACHE, Administrator **A**1 2 3 5 7 8 9 10 **F**2 4 7 8 10 11 12 14 15 16 17 19 20 21 22 23 26 28 30 31 32 33 34 35 37 39 40 41 42 43 44 45 46 48 49 51 52 53 54 55 56 57 58 59 60 65 67 70 71 73 **P**6 8	23	10	390	13590	237	202769	511	121946	48969	1709

© 1995 AHA Guide

Hospitals, U.S. / ALABAMA

Hospital, Address, Telephone, Administrator, Approval, Facility, and Physician Codes, Health Care System	Classification Codes		Utilization Data					Expense (thousands) of dollars		
★ American Hospital Association (AHA) membership □ Joint Commission on Accreditation of Healthcare Organizations (JCAHO) accreditation + American Osteopathic Hospital Association (AOHA) membership ○ American Osteopathic Association (AOA) accreditation △ Commission on Accreditation of Rehabilitation Facilities (CARF) accreditation Control codes 61, 63, 64, 71, 72 and 73 indicate hospitals listed by AOHA, but not registered by AHA. For definition of numerical codes, see page A6	Control	Service	Beds	Admissions	Census	Outpatient Visits	Births	Total	Payroll	Personnel
★ CHILDREN'S HOSPITAL OF ALABAMA, 1600 Seventh Avenue South, Zip 35233–1785; tel. 205/939–9100; Jim Dearth M.D., Chief Executive Officer **A**1 3 5 9 10 **F**9 12 13 14 15 16 17 19 20 21 22 25 29 31 34 35 38 41 42 44 45 46 47 49 52 53 54 56 58 65 66 67 70 71 72 73 **P**5 7 8	23	50	218	10073	155	185003	0	113900	54773	1727
□ COOPER GREEN HOSPITAL, 1515 Sixth Avenue South, Zip 35233; tel. 205/930–3600; Max Michael M.D., Chief Executive Officer and Medical Director **A**1 3 5 9 10 **F**4 7 8 10 12 14 15 16 19 21 22 23 28 31 33 34 35 37 40 41 42 43 44 49 52 53 54 56 58 60 61 65 71 73 74 **P**8	13	10	168	7355	108	122399	1915	59122	22740	679
★ EYE FOUNDATION HOSPITAL, 1720 University Boulevard, Zip 35233–1816; tel. 205/325–8100; Gordon L. Smith, Executive Director **A**1 3 5 9 10 **F**15 16 17 19 21 22 30 34 35 41 44 65 71 73	23	45	91	1339	5	17298	0	12608	4618	173
★ HEALTHSOUTH MEDICAL CENTER, 1201 11th Avenue South, Zip 35205; tel. 205/930–7000; Frank R. Gannon, Administrator (Nonreporting) **A**1 9 10 **S**0023 Healthsouth Corporation	23	10	177	—	—	—	—	—	—	—
□ HILL CREST BEHAVIORAL HEALTH SERVICES, 6869 Fifth Avenue South, Zip 35212; tel. 205/833–9000; Guy A. Barg, Chief Executive Officer **A**1 9 10 **F**2 3 52 53 54 55 56 57 58 59 65 **P**4 5 **S**0405 Ramsay Health Care, Inc.	32	22	130	964	38	0	0	—	—	182
★ △ LAKESHORE HOSPITAL, 3800 Ridgeway Drive, Zip 35209; tel. 205/868–2000; Thomas P. Kent Jr., Administrator and Chief Executive Officer **A**1 7 9 10 **F**12 14 15 16 30 41 48 49 65 67 73 **P**5	23	46	100	1659	79	—	0	—	—	325
★ LLOYD NOLAND HOSPITAL AND AMBULATORY CENTER, (Formerly Listed Under Fairfield) 701 Lloyd Noland Parkway, Fairfield, Zip 35064–2699; tel. 205/783–5121; Gary M. Glasscock, Administrator (Nonreporting) **A**1 2 3 5 9 10	23	10	222	—	—	—	—	—	—	—
★ △ MEDICAL CENTER EAST, 50 Medical Park East Drive, Zip 35235–9987; tel. 205/838–3000; Robert C. Chapman FACHE, President and Chief Executive Officer **A**1 2 3 5 7 9 10 **F**1 4 6 7 8 10 11 12 14 15 16 17 19 21 22 25 27 28 29 30 31 32 33 34 35 37 38 39 40 41 42 43 44 45 46 48 49 51 56 60 62 64 65 67 69 70 71 73 74 **P**5 7	23	10	271	11807	184	96032	817	77138	33176	909
PRINCETON BAPTIST MEDICAL CENTER See Birmingham Baptist Medical Center–Princeton										
★ ST. VINCENT'S HOSPITAL, 810 St. Vincent's Drive, Zip 35205, Mailing Address: P.O. Box 12407, Zip 35202–2407; tel. 205/939–7000; Vincent Caponi, President **A**1 2 3 5 9 10 **F**4 5 7 8 10 11 15 16 17 18 19 21 22 24 25 26 27 28 29 30 31 32 33 34 35 36 37 38 39 40 41 42 43 44 45 46 49 52 54 55 56 57 60 63 65 67 71 73 **P**5 **S**1855 Daughters of Charity National Health System	23	10	338	14094	215	80998	2184	110105	49993	1652
★ UNIVERSITY OF ALABAMA HOSPITAL, 619 South 19th Street, Zip 35233–6505; tel. 205/975–7545; Kevin E. Lofton, Executive Director and Chief Executive Officer **A**1 2 3 5 8 9 10 12 **F**2 3 4 5 7 8 9 10 11 12 14 16 17 19 20 21 22 23 24 26 27 29 31 32 33 34 35 37 38 39 40 41 42 43 44 45 46 48 49 51 52 53 54 55 56 57 58 59 60 61 65 69 70 71 73 74 **P**2 3 7 **S**9105 University of Alabama Hospitals	12	10	783	34577	633	84606	3374	391079	156498	5167
★ VETERANS AFFAIRS MEDICAL CENTER, 700 South 19th Street, Zip 35233–1996; tel. 205/933–8101; William A. Mountcastle, Director **A**1 2 3 5 8 9 **F**3 4 5 8 10 11 19 20 21 24 25 27 28 29 30 31 32 34 35 37 39 41 42 43 44 45 46 49 51 54 56 58 60 67 69 71 73 74 **S**9295 Department of Veterans Affairs	45	10	257	7256	182	166437	0	107003	57716	1381
BOAZ—Marshall County										
★ BOAZ–ALBERTVILLE MEDICAL CENTER, U.S. Highway 431 North, Zip 35957–0999, Mailing Address: Drawer Z, Zip 35957–0999; tel. 205/593–8310; Marlin Hanson, Administrator **A**1 9 10 **F**7 8 15 16 17 19 21 22 28 29 30 33 34 37 40 42 44 54 63 65 66 71 73 74 **S**1975 Marshall County Health Care Authority	13	10	102	4446	69	104981	182	27664	13138	516
BREWTON—Escambia County										
★ D. W. MCMILLAN MEMORIAL HOSPITAL, 1301 Belleville Avenue, Zip 36426, Mailing Address: Box 908, Zip 36427; tel. 334/867–8061; Phillip L. Parker, Administrator **A**1 9 10 **F**7 8 14 19 22 34 35 37 40 42 44 46 49 65 73 **P**4 **S**1255 Escambia County Health Care Authority	13	10	83	2750	30	30061	301	11321	6728	267
BRIDGEPORT—Jackson County										
□ NORTH JACKSON HOSPITAL, Mailing Address: 47005 U.S. Highway 72, Zip 35740–9732; tel. 205/437–2101; Rodney C. Watford, Administrator (Nonreporting) **A**1 9 10	16	10	109	—	—	—	—	—	—	—
CAMDEN—Wilcox County										
J. PAUL JONES HOSPITAL, 317 McWilliams Avenue, Zip 36726; tel. 205/682–4131; Arden Chesnut, Administrator (Nonreporting) **A**9 10	15	10	30	—	—	—	—	—	—	—
CARROLLTON—Pickens County										
□ PICKENS COUNTY MEDICAL CENTER, Route 2, Zip 35447, Mailing Address: P.O. Box 478, Zip 35447–0478; tel. 205/367–8111; William H. Lang Jr., Administrator (Nonreporting) **A**1 9 10	13	10	45	—	—	—	—	—	—	—
CENTRE—Cherokee County										
★ CHEROKEE BAPTIST MEDICAL CENTER, 400 Northwood Drive, Zip 35960–1023; tel. 205/927–5531; Barry S. Cochran, President **A**1 9 10 **F**8 11 14 16 17 19 21 22 28 29 30 32 34 44 45 51 71 73 **S**0345 Baptist Health System	23	10	45	1570	19	33744	0	11063	3598	162
CENTREVILLE—Bibb County										
BIBB MEDICAL CENTER, 164 Pierson Avenue, Zip 35042; tel. 205/926–4881; Terry J. Smith, Administrator (Total facility includes 103 beds in nursing home–type unit) **A**9 10 **F**15 16 19 22 32 62 64 71	13	10	128	964	110	18953	0	7399	3503	193

Hospitals, U.S. / ALABAMA

Hospital, Address, Telephone, Administrator, Approval, Facility, and Physician Codes, Health Care System	Classification Codes		Utilization Data					Expense (thousands) of dollars		
★ American Hospital Association (AHA) membership ☐ Joint Commission on Accreditation of Healthcare Organizations (JCAHO) accreditation + American Osteopathic Hospital Association (AOHA) membership ○ American Osteopathic Association (AOA) accreditation △ Commission on Accreditation of Rehabilitation Facilities (CARF) accreditation Control codes 61, 63, 64, 71, 72 and 73 indicate hospitals listed by AOHA, but not registered by AHA. For definition of numerical codes, see page A6	Control	Service	Beds	Admissions	Census	Outpatient Visits	Births	Total	Payroll	Personnel
CHATOM—Washington County										
WASHINGTON COUNTY INFIRMARY AND NURSING HOME, St. Stephens Avenue, Zip 36518, Mailing Address: Box 597, Zip 36518–0597; tel. 334/847–2223; Howard C. Holcomb, Administrator (Nonreporting) A9 10 S2025 Infirmary Health System, Inc.	13	10	103	—	—	—	—	—	—	—
CLANTON—Chilton County										
☐ VAUGHAN CHILTON MEDICAL CENTER, 1010 Lay Dam Road, Zip 35045; tel. 205/755–2500; Jeffrey Potts, Administrator A1 9 10 F8 12 14 15 17 19 22 25 28 32 34 36 46 51 64 65 71 73 S2795 Healthcorp of Tennessee, Inc.	23	10	25	948	10	29162	0	5464	3027	181
CULLMAN—Cullman County										
CULLMAN MEDICAL CENTER See Cullman Regional Medical Center										
✴ CULLMAN REGIONAL MEDICAL CENTER, (Formerly Cullman Medical Center) 1912 Alabama Highway 157, Zip 35055, Mailing Address: P.O. Box 1108, Zip 35056–1108; tel. 205/737–2000; Jesse O. Weatherly, President A1 9 10 F7 8 10 12 14 15 16 17 19 21 22 24 28 30 32 33 34 35 37 40 41 42 44 46 49 51 60 62 65 66 67 71 72 73 74 P3 S0345 Baptist Health System	23	10	99	5724	64	108213	574	28327	12310	—
☐ WOODLAND COMMUNITY HOSPITAL, 1910 Cherokee Avenue S.W., Zip 35055; tel. 205/739–3500; Lowell Benton, Executive Director (Nonreporting) A1 9 10 S5895 Hallmark Healthcare Corporation	33	10	100	—	—	—	—	—	—	—
DADEVILLE—Tallapoosa County										
★ LAKESHORE COMMUNITY HOSPITAL, 201 Mariarden Road, Zip 36853, Mailing Address: P.O. Box 248, Zip 36853; tel. 205/825–7821; Mavis B. Halko, Administrator A9 10 F15 19 22 32 33 65 71 73 S2795 Healthcorp of Tennessee, Inc.	23	10	27	1287	12	9563	0	3930	2023	86
DAPHNE—Baldwin County										
✴ MERCY MEDICAL, 101 Villa Drive, Zip 36526, Mailing Address: P.O. Box 1090, Zip 36526; tel. 334/626–2694; Sister Mary Eileen Wilhelm, President and Chief Executive Officer (Total facility includes 132 beds in nursing home–type unit) A1 10 F1 6 12 15 16 17 20 22 26 31 32 33 34 36 39 42 49 62 64 65 67 73 S3595 Eastern Mercy Health System	21	46	157	1272	128	4237	0	21546	11110	621
DECATUR—Morgan County										
CHARTER RETREAT HOSPITAL See Decatur General Hospital–West										
✴ DECATUR GENERAL HOSPITAL, 1201 Seventh Street S.E., Zip 35601, Mailing Address: Box 2239, Zip 35609–2239; tel. 205/552–0055; Robert L. Smith, President and Chief Executive Officer A1 9 10 F4 7 8 10 11 15 16 19 21 22 28 29 30 32 34 35 37 40 42 44 45 46 52 53 54 55 56 57 58 59 60 63 65 71 73	16	10	260	7977	127	103470	1833	61020	25212	917
☐ DECATUR GENERAL HOSPITAL–WEST, (Formerly Charter Retreat Hospital) 2205 Beltline Road S.W., Zip 35602, Mailing Address: P.O. Box 2240, Zip 35609–2240; tel. 205/350–1450; Dennis Griffith, Vice President (Nonreporting) A1 9 10	33	22	64	—	—	—	—	—	—	—
☐ PARKWAY MEDICAL CENTER HOSPITAL, 1874 Beltline Road S.W., Zip 35601, Mailing Address: P.O. Box 2211, Zip 35609; tel. 205/350–2211; Philip J. Mazzuca, Managing Director (Nonreporting) A1 9 10 S5895 Hallmark Healthcare Corporation	33	10	94	—	—	—	—	—	—	—
DEMOPOLIS—Marengo County										
✴ BRYAN W. WHITFIELD MEMORIAL HOSPITAL, Highway 80, Zip 36732, Mailing Address: Box 890, Zip 36732; tel. 334/289–4000; Charles E. Nabors, Chief Executive Officer and Administrator A1 9 10 F1 8 14 15 16 17 19 21 22 24 30 32 37 40 44 63 71 73 P5	14	10	99	4138	51	16570	543	14712	6602	304
DOTHAN—Houston County										
☐ CHARTER WOODS BEHAVIORAL HEALTH SYSTEM, (Formerly Charter Woods Hospital) 700 Cottonwood Road, Zip 36301, Mailing Address: P.O. Box 6138, Zip 36302; tel. 334/794–4357; Charles Whitson, Chief Executive Officer A1 9 F2 3 14 19 35 52 53 54 55 57 58 59 63 65 67 71 S0695 Charter Medical Corporation	33	22	75	1029	24	1550	0	—	—	78
☐ FLOWERS HOSPITAL, 3228 West Main Street, Zip 36301, Mailing Address: Box 6907, Zip 36302–6907; tel. 334/793–5000; Keith Granger, Administrator (Nonreporting) A1 9 10	33	10	215	—	—	—	—	—	—	—
☐ SOUTHEAST ALABAMA MEDICAL CENTER, 1108 Ross Clark Circle, Zip 36301, Mailing Address: P.O. Drawer 6987, Zip 36302; tel. 334/793–8111; James R. Blackmon, Chief Executive Officer A1 2 9 10 F4 7 8 10 11 12 14 19 21 22 23 26 28 29 30 31 32 34 35 37 39 40 41 42 43 44 45 46 49 51 52 54 55 56 57 60 63 65 66 69 70 71 73	16	10	400	16951	261	121227	1232	121124	49531	1965
ELBA—Coffee County										
☐ ELBA GENERAL HOSPITAL, 987 Drayton Street, Zip 36323; tel. 205/897–2257; Ellen Briley, Administrator (Nonreporting) A9 10	16	10	116	—	—	—	—	—	—	—
ENTERPRISE—Coffee County										
✴ MEDICAL CENTER ENTERPRISE, 400 North Edwards Street, Zip 36330–9981; tel. 334/347–0584; John L. Robertson, Chief Executive Officer A1 9 10 F7 8 15 16 17 19 21 22 35 37 44 46 49 65 71 73 P5 S0002 Quorum Health Group/Quorum Health Resources	33	10	113	3947	44	32915	920	—	—	295
EUFAULA—Barbour County										
☐ LAKEVIEW COMMUNITY HOSPITAL, 820 West Washington Street, Zip 36027; tel. 205/687–5761; Carl D. Brown, Associate Administrator (Nonreporting) A1 9 10 S2795 Healthcorp of Tennessee, Inc.	33	10	74	—	—	—	—	—	—	—

© 1995 AHA Guide

Hospitals, U.S. / ALABAMA

Hospital, Address, Telephone, Administrator, Approval, Facility, and Physician Codes, Health Care System	Classification Codes		Utilization Data					Expense (thousands) of dollars		
	Control	Service	Beds	Admissions	Census	Outpatient Visits	Births	Total	Payroll	Personnel

★ American Hospital Association (AHA) membership
□ Joint Commission on Accreditation of Healthcare Organizations (JCAHO) accreditation
+ American Osteopathic Hospital Association (AOHA) membership
○ American Osteopathic Association (AOA) accreditation
△ Commission on Accreditation of Rehabilitation Facilities (CARF) accreditation
Control codes 61, 63, 64, 71, 72 and 73 indicate hospitals listed by AOHA, but not registered by AHA. For definition of numerical codes, see page A6

EUTAW—Greene County

Hospital	Control	Service	Beds	Admissions	Census	Outpatient Visits	Births	Total	Payroll	Personnel
GREENE COUNTY HOSPITAL, 509 Wilson Avenue, Zip 35462; tel. 205/372-3388; Robert J. Coker Jr., Administrator (Nonreporting) **A**9 10	13	10	44	—	—	—	—	—	—	—

FAIRFIELD—Jefferson County

LLOYD NOLAND HOSPITAL AND AMBULATORY CENTER See Birmingham

FAIRHOPE—Baldwin County

Hospital	Control	Service	Beds	Admissions	Census	Outpatient Visits	Births	Total	Payroll	Personnel
★ THOMAS HOSPITAL, 750 Morphy Avenue, Zip 36532-1812, Mailing Address: Drawer 929, Zip 36533-0929; tel. 205/928-2375; Owen Bailey, Administrator **A**1 9 10 **F**3 7 8 17 19 22 28 31 34 35 37 40 41 44 46 52 54 55 56 58 65 71 **P**1	16	10	105	4513	53	35079	474	23608	10098	410

FAYETTE—Fayette County

Hospital	Control	Service	Beds	Admissions	Census	Outpatient Visits	Births	Total	Payroll	Personnel
★ FAYETTE COUNTY HOSPITAL AND NURSING HOME, 1653 Temple Avenue North, Zip 35555, Mailing Address: P.O. Drawer 878, Zip 35555; tel. 205/932-5966; Harold Reed, Administrator (Total facility includes 122 beds in nursing home-type unit) **A**1 9 10 **F**8 19 21 22 28 30 32 33 34 35 37 41 42 44 49 63 65 67 71 73 **S**1825 DCH Healthcare Authority	16	10	166	1537	124	23551	0	12408	7686	252

FLORALA—Covington County

Hospital	Control	Service	Beds	Admissions	Census	Outpatient Visits	Births	Total	Payroll	Personnel
FLORALA MEMORIAL HOSPITAL, 515 East Fifth, Zip 36442-0206, Mailing Address: Box 206, Zip 36442-0206; tel. 205/858-3287; James N. York, Administrator (Nonreporting) **A**9 10 **S**1765 United Hospital Corporation	33	10	23	—	—	—	—	—	—	—

FLORENCE—Lauderdale County

Hospital	Control	Service	Beds	Admissions	Census	Outpatient Visits	Births	Total	Payroll	Personnel
★ ELIZA COFFEE MEMORIAL HOSPITAL, (Includes Mitchell-Hollingsworth Annex) 205 Marengo Street, Zip 35630, Mailing Address: Box 818, Zip 35631; tel. 205/767-9191; Richard H. Peck, Administrator (Total facility includes 214 beds in nursing home-type unit) **A**1 9 10 **F**4 7 8 10 11 19 21 22 26 31 34 35 37 40 42 43 44 45 46 49 52 53 54 55 56 57 59 64 65 67 71 73	16	10	510	10980	377	38102	1289	61685	29314	1211
★ FLORENCE HOSPITAL, 2111 Cloyd Boulevard, Zip 35630, Mailing Address: Box 2010, Zip 35631; tel. 205/766-5091; Glen M. Jones, Chief Executive Officer (Nonreporting) **A**1 9 10 **S**0048 Columbia/HCA Healthcare Corporation	33	10	155	—	—	—	—	—	—	—

FOLEY—Baldwin County

Hospital	Control	Service	Beds	Admissions	Census	Outpatient Visits	Births	Total	Payroll	Personnel
★ SOUTH BALDWIN HOSPITAL, 1613 North McKenzie Street, Zip 36535-2299; tel. 334/952-3400; Robert F. Jernigan Jr., Administrator **A**1 9 10 **F**7 8 14 17 19 22 32 34 35 37 39 40 42 44 45 49 65 67 71 73	13	10	76	3497	42	24050	359	15670	7756	314

FORT MCCLELLAN—Anniston County

Hospital	Control	Service	Beds	Admissions	Census	Outpatient Visits	Births	Total	Payroll	Personnel
★ NOBLE ARMY COMMUNITY HOSPITAL, Zip 36205-5083; tel. 205/848-2232; Lieutenant Colonel Ed Wacy, Deputy Commander Administration **A**1 **F**1 2 3 4 5 6 7 8 9 10 11 12 13 14 15 16 17 18 19 20 21 22 23 24 25 26 27 28 29 30 31 32 33 34 35 36 37 38 39 40 41 42 43 44 45 46 47 48 49 50 51 52 53 54 55 57 58 59 60 61 62 63 64 65 66 67 68 69 70 71 72 73 74 **P**1 2 3 4 5 6 7 8 **S**9395 Department of the Army	42	10	48	2210	13	172201	0	18825	6038	209

FORT PAYNE—De Kalb County

Hospital	Control	Service	Beds	Admissions	Census	Outpatient Visits	Births	Total	Payroll	Personnel
★ DEKALB BAPTIST MEDICAL CENTER, 200 Medical Center Drive, Zip 35967, Mailing Address: P.O. Box 778, Zip 35967-0778; tel. 205/845-3150; Barry S. Cochran, President **A**1 9 10 **F**2 8 12 14 15 16 17 19 21 22 24 26 30 31 32 33 35 37 40 41 44 46 62 65 66 68 70 71 73 74 **P**3 5 7 **S**0345 Baptist Health System	21	10	103	3735	48	54266	542	24374	9337	348

FORT RUCKER—Coffee County

Hospital	Control	Service	Beds	Admissions	Census	Outpatient Visits	Births	Total	Payroll	Personnel
★ LYSTER U.S. ARMY COMMUNITY HOSPITAL, U.S. Army Aeromedical Center, Zip 36362-5333; tel. 334/255-7360; Colonel Glenn W. Mitchell M.D., Commander **A**1 **F**1 2 3 4 5 6 7 8 9 10 11 12 13 14 15 16 17 18 19 20 21 22 23 24 25 26 27 28 29 30 31 32 33 34 35 36 37 38 39 40 41 42 43 44 45 46 47 48 49 50 51 52 53 54 55 56 57 58 59 60 61 62 63 64 65 66 67 68 69 70 71 72 73 74 **P**1 2 3 4 5 6 7 8 **S**9395 Department of the Army	42	10	58	4808	14	237524	0	31568	19231	493

GADSDEN—Etowah County

Hospital	Control	Service	Beds	Admissions	Census	Outpatient Visits	Births	Total	Payroll	Personnel
★ GADSDEN REGIONAL MEDICAL CENTER, 1007 Goodyear Avenue, Zip 35999; tel. 205/494-4648; Michael R. Blackburn, Chief Executive Officer **A**1 2 9 10 **F**4 7 8 10 11 12 16 17 19 21 22 23 28 30 32 33 34 35 37 39 40 41 42 43 44 45 46 49 52 56 60 63 65 67 71 73 74 **S**0002 Quorum Health Group/Quorum Health Resources	33	10	287	12234	193	139127	1385	78535	31278	1154
□ MOUNTAIN VIEW HOSPITAL, 3001 Scenic Highway, Zip 35901-9956, Mailing Address: P.O. Box 8406, Zip 35902-8406; tel. 205/546-9265; Jon Orr, Administrator (Nonreporting) **A**1 9 10	33	22	68	—	—	—	—	—	—	—
□ RIVERVIEW REGIONAL MEDICAL CENTER, 600 South Third Street, Zip 35901, Mailing Address: P.O. Box 268, Zip 35999-0268; tel. 205/543-5200; Jon P. Vollmer, Executive Director **A**1 9 10 **F**4 7 8 10 11 12 17 19 21 22 26 28 29 30 32 34 35 36 37 39 40 41 42 43 44 45 46 49 60 63 65 66 70 71 73 74 **S**1775 Health Management Associates	33	10	281	6416	117	44037	260	—	—	539

GENEVA—Geneva County

Hospital	Control	Service	Beds	Admissions	Census	Outpatient Visits	Births	Total	Payroll	Personnel
★ WIREGRASS HOSPITAL, 1200 West Maple Avenue, Zip 36340; tel. 334/684-3655; H. Randolph Smith, Administrator (Total facility includes 86 beds in nursing home-type unit) **A**1 9 10 **F**8 19 22 28 34 37 44 49 65 71 **S**0002 Quorum Health Group/Quorum Health Resources	13	10	151	2398	112	—	0	11279	5116	250

GEORGIANA—Butler County

Hospital	Control	Service	Beds	Admissions	Census	Outpatient Visits	Births	Total	Payroll	Personnel
GEORGIANA DOCTORS HOSPITAL, Jones and Miranda Streets, Zip 36033, Mailing Address: Box 548, Zip 36033; tel. 205/376-2205; Harry Cole, Administrator (Nonreporting) **A**9 10	33	10	22	—	—	—	—	—	—	—

Hospitals, U.S. / ALABAMA

Hospital, Address, Telephone, Administrator, Approval, Facility, and Physician Codes, Health Care System	Classification Codes		Utilization Data					Expense (thousands) of dollars		
	Control	Service	Beds	Admissions	Census	Outpatient Visits	Births	Total	Payroll	Personnel

★ American Hospital Association (AHA) membership
☐ Joint Commission on Accreditation of Healthcare Organizations (JCAHO) accreditation
+ American Osteopathic Hospital Association (AOHA) membership
○ American Osteopathic Association (AOA) accreditation
△ Commission on Accreditation of Rehabilitation Facilities (CARF) accreditation
Control codes 61, 63, 64, 71, 72 and 73 indicate hospitals listed by AOHA, but not registered by AHA. For definition of numerical codes, see page A6

Hospital	Control	Service	Beds	Admissions	Census	Outpatient Visits	Births	Total	Payroll	Personnel
GRAYSVILLE—Jefferson County LONGVIEW GENERAL HOSPITAL, 1100 Bankhead Highway S.W., Zip 35073; tel. 205/674-9422; David G. Stoves, Administrator (Nonreporting) **A**9 10	33	10	50	—	—	—	—	—	—	—
GREENSBORO—Hale County HALE COUNTY HOSPITAL, First and Greene Streets, Zip 36744; tel. 334/624-3024; James F. Stegall, Administrator (Nonreporting) **A**9 10	13	10	32	—	—	—	—	—	—	—
GREENVILLE—Butler County L. V. STABLER MEMORIAL HOSPITAL, Highway 10 West, Zip 36037-0915, Mailing Address: Box 1000, Zip 36037-0915; tel. 334/382-2671; Steve Southerland, Executive Director (Nonreporting) **A**9 10 **S**5895 Hallmark Healthcare Corporation	33	10	67	—	—	—	—	—	—	—
GROVE HILL—Clarke County ★ GROVE HILL MEMORIAL HOSPITAL, Jackson Highway, Zip 36451, Mailing Address: P.O. Box 935, Zip 36451; tel. 205/275-3191; Darrell M. Butler, Administrator **A**1 9 10 **F**7 8 19 22 32 34 39 40 41 44 48 49 71 73 **S**2025 Infirmary Health System, Inc.	14	10	32	1013	11	13819	187	3660	1383	96
GUNTERSVILLE—Marshall County ★ GUNTERSVILLE-ARAB MEDICAL CENTER, 8000 Alabama Highway 69, Zip 35976; tel. 205/753-8000; Gary R. Gore, Administrator **A**1 9 10 **F**7 8 12 14 15 16 19 21 22 24 28 29 30 31 32 34 37 40 41 44 46 49 54 63 65 70 71 73 74 **S**1975 Marshall County Health Care Authority	16	10	90	4214	52	44061	651	22536	7854	357
HALEYVILLE—Winston County ★ BURDICK-WEST MEMORIAL HOSPITAL, Highway 195 East, Zip 35565, Mailing Address: Box 780, Zip 35565-0780; tel. 205/486-5213; Tillman L. Hill, Administrator **A**1 9 10 **F**19 21 22 32 33 35 37 44 45 49 65 71	13	10	47	2156	31	23527	0	9042	3915	155
HAMILTON—Marion County ★ MARION BAPTIST MEDICAL CENTER, 1315 Military Street South, Zip 35570; tel. 205/921-7861; (Nonreporting) **A**1 9 10 **S**0345 Baptist Health System	16	10	126	—	—	—	—	—	—	—
HARTSELLE—Morgan County ☐ HARTSELLE MEDICAL CENTER, 201 Pine Street N.W., Zip 35640, Mailing Address: P.O. Box 969, Zip 35640; tel. 205/773-6511; David E. Loving, Managing Director (Nonreporting) **A**1 9 10 **S**5895 Hallmark Healthcare Corporation	33	10	119	—	—	—	—	—	—	—
HUNTSVILLE—Madison County ★ CRESTWOOD HOSPITAL, One Hospital Drive, Zip 35801-3403; tel. 205/882-3100; Thomas M. Weiss, Chief Executive Officer (Nonreporting) **A**1 9 10 **S**0048 Columbia/HCA Healthcare Corporation	33	10	120	—	—	—	—	—	—	—
FOX ARMY COMMUNITY HOSPITAL See Redstone Arsenal										
★ HUNTSVILLE HOSPITAL, 101 Sivley Road, Zip 35801-9990; tel. 205/517-8123; Ronald S. Owen, Chief Executive Officer **A**1 2 3 5 9 10 **F**4 7 8 10 11 12 14 15 16 19 21 22 23 24 25 27 28 32 34 35 37 38 39 40 41 42 43 44 45 46 47 49 52 54 55 56 57 58 59 60 65 67 70 71 73 74	16	10	558	26414	363	133042	3663	178868	72506	2581
☐ HUNTSVILLE HOSPITAL EAST, (Formerly Medical Center Hospital) 911 Big Cove Road S.E., Zip 35801-3784; tel. 205/532-5600; L. Joe Austin, Administrator (Data for 190 days) **A**1 9 10 **F**4 7 8 10 12 14 15 16 19 21 22 23 24 25 27 32 34 35 37 39 40 41 42 43 44 45 46 49 54 55 56 57 58 59 60 65 67 70 71 73 74	16	10	197	9293	79	20859	437	22158	9740	670
MEDICAL CENTER HOSPITAL See Huntsville Hospital East										
NORTH ALABAMA REHABILITATION HOSPITAL, 107 Governors Drive, Zip 35801; tel. 205/535-2300; Rod Moss, Chief Executive Officer (Nonreporting) **A**10	33	46	50	—	—	—	—	—	—	—
JACKSON—Clarke County RIVERSIDE MEDICAL CENTER, 220 Hospital Drive, Zip 36545, Mailing Address: Box 428, Zip 36545; tel. 205/246-9021; Tony Jeselnik, Interim Administrator (Nonreporting) **A**10	33	10	35	—	—	—	—	—	—	—
JACKSONVILLE—Calhoun County ★ JACKSONVILLE HOSPITAL, 1701 Pelham Road South, Zip 36265, Mailing Address: P.O. Box 999, Zip 36265; tel. 205/435-4970; Richard L. McConahy, Administrator **A**9 10 **F**7 8 19 22 31 34 35 36 37 40 44 49 61 71 73 **P**1 **S**0002 Quorum Health Group/Quorum Health Resources	16	10	56	2099	22	25940	312	13335	5101	175
JASPER—Walker County ★ WALKER BAPTIST MEDICAL CENTER, 3400 Highway 78 East, Zip 35501, Mailing Address: Box 3547, Zip 35502-3547; tel. 205/387-4000; Jeff Brewer, President **A**1 9 10 **F**2 3 4 6 7 8 10 12 15 16 17 19 21 22 24 25 32 33 34 35 37 38 40 42 43 44 46 47 48 49 52 64 65 71 73 74 **P**7 **S**0345 Baptist Health System	21	10	267	8704	124	50366	693	39571	15699	693
LUVERNE—Crenshaw County ★ CRENSHAW BAPTIST HOSPITAL, 1625 South Forrest Avenue, Zip 36049, Mailing Address: Box 432, Zip 36049; tel. 205/335-3374; Wayne Sasser, Administrator (Nonreporting) **A**1 9 10	13	10	65	—	—	—	—	—	—	—
MADISON—Madison County BRADFORD PARKSIDE AT MADISON, 1600 Browns Ferry Road, Zip 35758, Mailing Address: P.O. Box 176, Zip 35758-0176; tel. 205/461-7272; Bob Hinds, Executive Director **A**9 **F**2 25 **P**6 **S**2455 Bradford Parkside	33	82	84	1258	42	1200	0	—	—	87
MARION—Perry County VAUGHAN PERRY HOSPITAL, (Formerly Perry County Hospital) East Lafayette Street, Zip 36756-0149, Mailing Address: P.O. Box 149, Zip 36756-0149; tel. 205/683-9696; Donald J. Jones, Administrator (Nonreporting) **A**9 10	13	10	66	—	—	—	—	—	—	—

Hospitals, U.S. / ALABAMA

Hospital, Address, Telephone, Administrator, Approval, Facility, and Physician Codes, Health Care System ★ American Hospital Association (AHA) membership □ Joint Commission on Accreditation of Healthcare Organizations (JCAHO) accreditation + American Osteopathic Hospital Association (AOHA) membership ○ American Osteopathic Association (AOA) accreditation △ Commission on Accreditation of Rehabilitation Facilities (CARF) accreditation Control codes 61, 63, 64, 71, 72 and 73 indicate hospitals listed by AOHA, but not registered by AHA. For definition of numerical codes, see page A6	Classification Codes		Utilization Data					Expense (thousands) of dollars		Personnel
	Control	Service	Beds	Admissions	Census	Outpatient Visits	Births	Total	Payroll	
MOBILE—Mobile County										
□ CHARTER HOSPITAL OF MOBILE, 5800 Southland Drive, Zip 36693, Mailing Address: P.O. Box 991800, Zip 36691; tel. 205/661–3001; Keith Cox, Chief Executive Officer **A**1 9 10 **F**3 52 53 54 55 56 57 58 59 **P**5 **S**0695 Charter Medical Corporation	33	22	84	1227	41	—	0	—	—	97
★ MOBILE INFIRMARY MEDICAL CENTER, (Includes Rotary Rehabilitation Hospital, Mobile, Alabama) 5 Mobile Infirmary Circle, Zip 36607, Mailing Address: P.O. Box 2144, Zip 36652–2144; tel. 334/431–2408; E. Chandler Bramlett Jr., President and Chief Executive Officer (Nonreporting) **A**1 2 5 9 10 **S**2025 Infirmary Health System, Inc.	72	10	633	—	—	—	—	—	—	—
★ PROVIDENCE HOSPITAL, 6801 Airport Boulevard, Zip 36608, Mailing Address: P.O. Box 850429, Zip 36685; tel. 334/633–1000; John R. Roeder, President and Chief Executive Officer **A**1 2 9 10 **F**4 7 8 10 11 16 17 19 21 22 23 24 25 30 31 32 33 34 35 37 40 42 43 44 46 49 60 65 67 71 73 **P**5 6 7 **S**1855 Daughters of Charity National Health System	21	10	349	15307	242	129261	1028	100674	40638	1444
ROTARY REHABILITATION HOSPITAL See Mobile Infirmary Medical Center										
□ SPRINGHILL MEMORIAL HOSPITAL, 3719 Dauphin Street, Zip 36608–1798, Mailing Address: Box 8246, Zip 36608; tel. 205/344–9630; Bill A. Mason, President and Chief Executive Officer **A**1 9 10 **F**8 19 21 24 31 34 35 40 44 45 46 60 65 70 71 74	31	10	208	9804	135	53599	1379	—	—	812
★ UNIVERSITY OF SOUTH ALABAMA DOCTORS HOSPITAL, 1700 Center Street, Zip 36604–3391; tel. 205/415–1000; Thomas J. Gibson, Administrator **A**1 3 5 9 10 13 **F**4 7 8 9 10 11 19 21 22 31 34 35 37 38 40 41 42 43 44 46 47 48 49 52 57 60 61 65 70 71 73 **P**3 **S**0057 University of South Alabama Hospitals	12	10	124	3126	43	31425	0	20303	10480	572
★ UNIVERSITY OF SOUTH ALABAMA KNOLLWOOD PARK HOSPITAL, 5600 Girby Road, Zip 36693–3398; tel. 205/660–5120; Stanley K. Hammack, Administrator **A**1 3 5 9 10 13 **F**8 16 17 19 21 22 24 31 35 37 41 44 49 53 63 65 71 73 **S**0057 University of South Alabama Hospitals	12	10	201	3029	89	40508	0	32792	13552	498
★ UNIVERSITY OF SOUTH ALABAMA MEDICAL CENTER, 2451 Fillingim Street, Zip 36617; tel. 205/471–7000; Stephen H. Simmons, Senior Administrator **A**1 2 3 5 8 9 10 **F**4 7 9 10 11 16 19 21 22 31 35 37 38 40 42 44 46 60 63 65 69 70 71 73 74 **S**0057 University of South Alabama Hospitals	12	10	316	12472	261	74639	4247	103809	54168	1791
MONROEVILLE—Monroe County										
□ MONROE COUNTY HOSPITAL, 1901 South Alabama Avenue, Zip 36460, Mailing Address: P.O. Box 886, Zip 36461–0886; tel. 334/575–3111; Floyd N. Price, Administrator **A**1 9 10 **F**7 8 12 14 15 16 19 22 32 34 37 40 44 45 46 49 65 71 73	15	10	59	2859	30	28749	287	10758	4494	180
MONTGOMERY—Montgomery County										
★ BAPTIST MEDICAL CENTER, 2105 East South Boulevard, Zip 36116–2498, Mailing Address: Box 11010, Zip 36111–1101; tel. 334/288–2100; Michael D. DeBoer, President and Chief Executive Officer **A**1 3 5 9 10 **F**2 3 4 7 8 10 11 12 13 15 16 17 19 21 22 23 24 25 26 28 29 30 32 33 34 35 37 38 39 40 41 42 43 44 45 46 49 51 52 54 55 56 57 58 61 62 65 67 71 72 73 74 **P**3 7	21	10	288	14378	209	64156	2154	86648	35199	1398
★ EAST MONTGOMERY MEDICAL CENTER, 400 Taylor Road, Zip 36117, Mailing Address: P.O. Box 241267, Zip 36124–1267; tel. 334/277–8330; John W. Melton, Chief Executive Officer (Nonreporting) **A**1 9 10 **S**0048 Columbia/HCA Healthcare Corporation	33	10	150	—	—	—	—	—	—	—
□ △ HEALTHSOUTH REHABILITATION HOSPITAL OF MONTGOMERY, 4465 Narrow Lane Road, Zip 36116; tel. 334/284–7700; Arnold F. McRae, Administrator and Chief Executive Officer **A**1 7 10 **F**5 12 14 15 16 19 21 22 24 25 26 27 28 29 30 34 35 39 41 45 48 49 50 63 65 66 67 71 73 **S**0023 Healthsouth Corporation	33	46	80	1155	75	6804	0	15180	8031	250
★ JACKSON HOSPITAL AND CLINIC, 1235 Forest Avenue, Zip 36106–1125; tel. 205/293–8000; Donald M. Ball, President **A**1 2 9 10 **F**7 10 11 15 22 23 30 33 34 35 37 39 40 42 44 46 49 52 54 56 60 65 66 71 73 **P**6	23	10	268	11534	167	71918	760	55445	30597	1209
★ MAXWELL HOSPITAL, 330 Kirkpatrick Avenue East, Zip 36112–6219; tel. 205/953–7801; James J. Gallman, Administrator (Nonreporting) **A**1 **S**9495 Department of the Air Force	41	10	40	—	—	—	—	—	—	—
★ MONTGOMERY REGIONAL MEDICAL CENTER, 301 South Ripley Street, Zip 36104–4495; tel. 205/269–8000; Larry Montgomery, Interim Chief Executive Officer **A**1 3 5 9 10 **F**2 4 7 8 10 11 12 17 19 21 22 26 28 29 30 34 35 37 40 42 43 44 45 46 49 50 52 54 63 65 71 73 **P**5 8 **S**0048 Columbia/HCA Healthcare Corporation	33	10	250	7986	119	97317	1267	—	—	797
★ VETERANS AFFAIRS MEDICAL CENTER, 215 Perry Hill Road, Zip 36109–3798; tel. 334/272–4670; John R. Rowan, Director **A**1 9 **F**19 20 22 33 34 37 44 46 49 51 65 71 73 74 **S**9295 Department of Veterans Affairs	45	10	162	3553	127	45310	0	42569	18909	547
MOULTON—Lawrence County										
□ LAWRENCE BAPTIST MEDICAL CENTER, (Formerly Lawrence County Hospital) 202 Hospital Street, Zip 35650–0039, Mailing Address: P.O. Box 39, Zip 35650–0039; tel. 205/974–2200; Ronald L. Sparkman, Administrator **A**1 9 10 **F**8 13 14 15 16 17 19 22 25 28 30 31 32 33 34 39 44 45 46 49 65 71 73 **P**5 **S**0345 Baptist Health System	13	10	30	2521	31	23575	0	9515	3980	—
MOUNT VERNON—Mobile County										
□ SEARCY HOSPITAL, Mailing Address: P.O. Box 1001, Zip 36560–1001; tel. 334/829–9411; John T. Bartlett, Director (Nonreporting) **A**1 3 10	12	22	610	—	—	—	—	—	—	—

Hospitals, U.S. / ALABAMA

Hospital, Address, Telephone, Administrator, Approval, Facility, and Physician Codes, Health Care System	Classification Codes		Utilization Data					Expense (thousands) of dollars		
★ American Hospital Association (AHA) membership ☐ Joint Commission on Accreditation of Healthcare Organizations (JCAHO) accreditation + American Osteopathic Hospital Association (AOHA) membership ○ American Osteopathic Association (AOA) accreditation △ Commission on Accreditation of Rehabilitation Facilities (CARF) accreditation Control codes 61, 63, 64, 71, 72 and 73 indicate hospitals listed by AOHA, but not registered by AHA. For definition of numerical codes, see page A6	Control	Service	Beds	Admissions	Census	Outpatient Visits	Births	Total	Payroll	Personnel
MUSCLE SHOALS—Colbert County ※ MEDICAL CENTER SHOALS, 201 Avalon Avenue, Zip 35661, Mailing Address: P.O. Box 3359, Zip 35662; tel. 205/386–1600; Connie Hawthorne, Chief Executive Officer (Nonreporting) **A**1 9 10 **S**0048 Columbia/HCA Healthcare Corporation	33	10	128	—	—	—	—	—	—	—
NORTHPORT—Tuscaloosa County ※ NORTHPORT HOSPITAL–DCH, 2700 Hospital Drive, Zip 35476; tel. 205/333–4500; Wendell Briggs, Administrator **A**1 9 10 **F**2 4 7 8 10 11 12 14 15 17 18 19 21 22 23 24 25 26 28 29 30 31 32 34 35 37 38 40 41 42 43 44 45 46 47 48 49 52 54 55 56 57 60 65 66 67 70 71 73 74 **P**3 **S**1825 DCH Healthcare Authority	23	10	133	4906	78	62952	585	34931	14775	467
ONEONTA—Blount County BLOUNT MEMORIAL HOSPITAL, 1000 Lincoln Avenue, Zip 35121, Mailing Address: P.O. Box 220, Zip 35121; tel. 205/625–3511; George McGowan, Chief Executive Officer **A**9 10 **F**8 13 14 15 16 19 21 22 28 29 30 32 34 37 39 42 44 46 49 65 71 73	13	10	57	2090	27	30253	0	10257	4357	191
OPELIKA—Lee County EAST ALABAMA MEDICAL CENTER, 2000 Pepperell Parkway, Zip 36802–3201; tel. 205/749–3411; Terry W. Andrus, President (Total facility includes 24 beds in nursing home–type unit) **A**1 2 9 10 **F**2 4 7 8 10 11 12 14 19 21 22 26 31 32 33 34 35 37 39 40 42 43 44 45 49 52 53 56 60 64 65 70 71 73 **P**8	16	10	302	12994	216	141801	1417	85396	36444	1374
OPP—Covington County ★ MIZELL MEMORIAL HOSPITAL, 702 Main Street, Zip 36467–1626, Mailing Address: P.O. Box 429, Zip 36467–0429; tel. 205/493–3541; Allen Foster, Interim Administrator **A**9 10 **F**7 8 11 15 16 19 21 22 28 31 32 34 35 40 41 44 49 65 71 **S**0185 Baptist Health Care Corporation	23	10	57	1864	22	14575	91	7191	3041	157
OZARK—Dale County ☐ DALE MEDICAL CENTER, 100 Hospital Avenue, Zip 36360; tel. 205/774–2601; James L. Armour, Administrator **A**1 9 10 **F**7 8 19 21 22 28 30 32 34 37 40 44 45 46 49 65 71	16	10	85	3041	38	26832	324	14682	6160	292
PELHAM—Shelby County BRADFORD–PARKSIDE ADOLESCENT AT OAK MOUNTAIN, 2280 Highway 35, Zip 35124; tel. 205/664–3460; Joseph Roche, Acting Executive Director **A**9 **F**2 3 **P**6 **S**2455 Bradford Parkside	33	82	84	759	54	700	0	—	—	102
PELL CITY—St. Clair County ★ ST. CLAIR REGIONAL HOSPITAL, 2805 Hospital Drive, Zip 35125; tel. 205/338–3301; Martin Nowak, Administrator **A**9 10 **F**8 12 19 22 28 31 32 37 40 44 63 65 71 73 **P**5 8 **S**9105 University of Alabama Hospitals	13	10	72	1804	25	30174	294	9013	4428	187
PHENIX CITY—Russell County ※ PHENIX REGIONAL HOSPITAL, (Formerly Phenix Medical Park Hospital) 1707 21st Avenue, Zip 36867, Mailing Address: Box 190, Zip 36868–0190; tel. 334/291–8502; Lance B. Duke FACHE, President and Chief Executive Officer (Nonreporting) **A**1 9 10	14	10	175	—	—	—	—	—	—	—
PRATTVILLE—Autauga County ☐ AUTAUGA MEDICAL CENTER, 124 South Memorial Drive, Zip 36067; tel. 334/365–0651; William C. Bentley, Administrator **A**1 9 10 **F**8 19 22 37 44 65 71 73 **S**0985 Amerihealth, Inc.	33	10	50	1635	21	32792	0	12929	4053	159
RED BAY—Franklin County RED BAY HOSPITAL, 211 Hospital Road, Zip 35582, Mailing Address: Box 490, Zip 35582; tel. 205/356–9532; Ralph J. Wilson, Administrator **A**9 10 **F**14 19 32 44 71	13	10	31	993	10	9792	0	2745	1444	73
REDSTONE ARSENAL—Madison County ※ FOX ARMY COMMUNITY HOSPITAL, Zip 35809–7000; tel. 205/876–4147; Lieutenant Colonel Cary J. Payne, Deputy Commander Administration; Major Alan C. Shero MSC, USA, Director Logistics Division **A**1 **F**3 8 12 19 20 21 22 27 28 31 34 35 37 40 41 44 46 48 49 51 58 61 63 65 71 72 73 74 **S**9395 Department of the Army	42	10	41	1556	11	150300	0	33614	—	358
ROANOKE—Randolph County ★ RANDOLPH COUNTY HOSPITAL, 1000 Wadley Highway, Zip 36274, Mailing Address: Box 669, Zip 36274; tel. 205/863–4111; Sandy D. McGill, Interim Administrator (Nonreporting) **A**9 10	13	10	66	—	—	—	—	—	—	—
RUSSELLVILLE—Franklin County ※ NORTHWEST MEDICAL CENTER, Highway 43 By-Pass, Zip 35653, Mailing Address: P.O. Box 1089, Zip 35653; tel. 205/332–1611; Christine R. Stewart, Chief Executive Officer (Nonreporting) **A**1 9 10 **S**0048 Columbia/HCA Healthcare Corporation	33	10	100	—	—	—	—	—	—	—
SCOTTSBORO—Jackson County ☐ JACKSON COUNTY HOSPITAL, Woods Cove Road, Zip 35768, Mailing Address: Box 1050, Zip 35768; tel. 205/259–4444; James K. Mason, Chief Executive Officer (Total facility includes 50 beds in nursing home–type unit) **A**1 9 10 **F**7 11 14 15 16 19 22 32 40 44 65 71 73	13	10	140	4166	98	61249	423	19310	9805	376
SELMA—Dallas County ※ FOUR RIVERS MEDICAL CENTER, 1015 Medical Center Parkway, Zip 36701; tel. 334/872–8461; J. Glenn Brown Jr., Chief Executive Officer **A**1 2 3 5 9 10 **F**7 8 10 12 15 16 17 19 21 22 28 30 34 37 44 49 52 60 65 67 71 73 **P**8 **S**0048 Columbia/HCA Healthcare Corporation	33	10	214	4963	83	47410	0	24014	10398	416
※ VAUGHAN REGIONAL MEDICAL CENTER, 1050 West Dallas Avenue, Zip 36701, Mailing Address: Box 328, Zip 36702–0328; tel. 334/418–6000; Robert E. Morrow, President **A**1 3 5 9 10 **F**7 8 11 12 15 16 17 19 21 22 24 27 32 35 37 40 44 45 46 49 63 65 67 71 73	23	10	125	5814	70	35651	1343	21890	11103	522

© 1995 AHA Guide

Hospitals, U.S. / ALABAMA

Hospital, Address, Telephone, Administrator, Approval, Facility, and Physician Codes, Health Care System	Classification Codes		Utilization Data					Expense (thousands) of dollars		
★ American Hospital Association (AHA) membership □ Joint Commission on Accreditation of Healthcare Organizations (JCAHO) accreditation + American Osteopathic Hospital Association (AOHA) membership ○ American Osteopathic Association (AOA) accreditation △ Commission on Accreditation of Rehabilitation Facilities (CARF) accreditation Control codes 61, 63, 64, 71, 72 and 73 indicate hospitals listed by AOHA, but not registered by AHA. For definition of numerical codes, see page A6	Control	Service	Beds	Admissions	Census	Outpatient Visits	Births	Total	Payroll	Personnel
SHEFFIELD—Colbert County										
★ HELEN KELLER HOSPITAL, 1300 South Montgomery Avenue, Zip 35660, Mailing Address: Box 610, Zip 35660; tel. 205/386-4556; Ralph Clark Jr., President **A**1 9 10 **F**2 3 7 8 10 11 19 22 27 28 35 37 40 44 46 48 52 71 73 74	16	10	152	5009	79	52666	630	35126	12832	509
SYLACAUGA—Talladega County										
★ COOSA VALLEY BAPTIST MEDICAL CENTER, (Formerly Coosa Valley Medical Center) 315 West Hickory Street, Zip 35150-2996; tel. 205/249-5000; Steven M. Johnson, Administrator (Nonreporting) **A**1 6 9 10 **S**0345 Baptist Health System	16	10	178	—	—	—	—	—	—	—
TALLADEGA—Talladega County										
★ CITIZENS BAPTIST MEDICAL CENTER, 604 Stone Avenue, Zip 35160, Mailing Address: P.O. Box 978, Zip 35160; tel. 205/362-8111; Jack B. Hethcox, President **A**1 9 10 **F**2 3 7 8 12 15 17 19 20 21 22 29 30 31 32 34 37 39 40 41 42 44 45 49 51 65 67 71 73 74 **P**3 5 **S**0345 Baptist Health System	23	10	97	3879	46	27607	483	16185	6800	343
TALLASSEE—Elmore County										
□ COMMUNITY HOSPITAL, Friendship Road, Zip 36078, Mailing Address: Box 707, Zip 36078-0707; tel. 205/283-6541; K. Byron Lowery, Administrator **A**1 9 10 **F**16 19 22 28 30 32 35 37 44 46 49 65 71 73	23	10	69	2149	31	26516	0	9724	4584	181
THOMASVILLE—Clarke County										
□ THOMASVILLE HOSPITAL, Highway 43 North, Zip 36784, Mailing Address: Drawer 429, Zip 36784; tel. 334/636-4431; Benny Ray Stephens, Administrator (Nonreporting) **A**1 9 10	33	10	37	—	—	—	—	—	—	—
TROY—Pike County										
★ EDGE REGIONAL MEDICAL CENTER, 1330 Highway 231 South, Zip 36081-1224; tel. 205/670-5000; Calvin Green, Administrator and Chief Executive Officer (Nonreporting) **A**1 9 10	14	10	87	—	—	—	—	—	—	—
TUSCALOOSA—Tuscaloosa County										
□ BRYCE HOSPITAL, 200 University Boulevard, Zip 35401; tel. 205/759-0799; James F. Reddoch Jr., Director (Total facility includes 414 beds in nursing home-type unit) **A**1 10 **F**8 15 16 19 20 21 31 35 37 41 44 49 52 53 54 55 56 57 58 59 64 65 67 71 73	12	22	1065	789	1065	0	0	64327	35633	1889
★ DCH REGIONAL MEDICAL CENTER, 809 University Boulevard East, Zip 35401-9961; tel. 205/759-7111; J. H. Ford Jr., Chief Executive Officer **A**1 2 3 5 9 10 **F**2 4 7 8 10 11 12 14 17 18 19 21 22 23 24 25 28 30 31 32 33 34 35 37 38 40 41 42 43 44 45 46 47 48 49 52 54 55 56 57 60 65 66 67 70 71 73 74 **P**3 **S**1825 DCH Healthcare Authority	23	10	523	21560	402	163357	2166	148060	71882	2435
★ DCH REHABILITATION PAVILION, 1101 Sixth Avenue East, Zip 35401-3297; tel. 205/759-7375; Ann Loggins, Vice President Rehabilitation Services **A**1 9 10 **F**2 3 4 7 8 10 11 12 14 16 17 18 19 21 22 23 24 25 28 30 31 32 33 34 35 37 38 40 41 42 43 44 45 46 47 48 49 52 54 55 56 57 58 60 65 66 67 70 71 73 74 **P**3 **S**1825 DCH Healthcare Authority	23	10	65	643	55	2733	0	10336	5572	203
★ VETERANS AFFAIRS MEDICAL CENTER, 3701 Loop Road, Zip 35404-9983; tel. 205/554-2000; Robert P. Blair, Director (Total facility includes 181 beds in nursing home-type unit) **A**1 9 **F**1 2 3 4 8 10 17 18 19 20 21 22 26 29 30 31 33 35 37 39 41 42 44 45 46 48 49 51 52 54 55 56 57 58 59 60 64 65 67 71 73 74 **P**6 **S**9295 Department of Veterans Affairs	45	22	649	3630	596	65525	0	65489	40923	860
TUSKEGEE—Macon County										
★ VETERANS AFFAIRS MEDICAL CENTER, 2400 Hospital Road, Zip 36083-5001; tel. 334/727-0550; Jim Clay, Director (Total facility includes 152 beds in nursing home-type unit) **A**1 2 3 5 9 13 **F**2 3 11 12 17 19 20 21 22 25 26 27 31 32 34 35 37 41 42 44 45 46 48 49 50 52 54 55 56 57 58 63 64 65 67 71 73 74 **S**9295 Department of Veterans Affairs	45	10	769	5339	656	85639	0	72456	45347	1324
UNION SPRINGS—Bullock County										
BULLOCK COUNTY HOSPITAL, 102 West Conecuh Avenue, Zip 36089; tel. 205/738-2140; Roger Long, Administrator (Nonreporting) **A**9 10	13	10	62	—	—	—	—	—	—	—
VALLEY—Chambers County										
□ GEORGE H. LANIER MEMORIAL HOSPITAL AND NURSING HOME, 4800 48th Street, Zip 36854-3666; tel. 205/756-3111; Robert J. Humphrey, Administrator (Total facility includes 75 beds in nursing home-type unit) **A**1 9 10 **F**2 3 4 7 8 14 16 19 20 21 22 23 26 28 29 30 31 32 33 34 35 37 39 40 42 44 45 46 56 64 65 67 71 73	23	10	182	3842	127	28905	391	16519	8525	408
VERNON—Lamar County										
LAMAR COMMUNITY HOSPITAL, 110 Hospital Drive, Zip 35592; tel. 205/695-7111; Paul E. Majors Jr., Administrator (Nonreporting) **A**9 10	33	10	33	—	—	—	—	—	—	—
WEDOWEE—Randolph County										
WEDOWEE HOSPITAL, 301 North Main Street, Zip 36278, Mailing Address: Box 307, Zip 36278; tel. 205/357-2111; Kerlene Mitchell, Administrator (Nonreporting) **A**9 10	23	10	34	—	—	—	—	—	—	—
WETUMPKA—Elmore County										
★ ELMORE COMMUNITY HOSPITAL, 500 Hospital Drive, Zip 36092, Mailing Address: P.O. Box 120, Zip 36092-0120; tel. 334/567-4311; Thomas J. Enright, Administrator **A**9 10 **F**2 3 12 14 15 16 19 21 22 25 28 29 30 32 34 37 44 49 65 66 67 71 72 **P**1 3 5 7	13	10	69	1815	28	17499	0	6508	3043	150
WINFIELD—Marion County										
★ CARRAWAY NORTHWEST MEDICAL CENTER, Highway 78 West, Zip 35594, Mailing Address: Box 130, Zip 35594-0130; tel. 205/487-4234; Robert E. Henger, Administrator **A**1 9 10 **F**7 8 12 15 17 19 21 22 28 30 32 33 34 37 40 42 44 49 65 71	21	10	63	1929	26	24612	410	9639	3951	182

ALASKA

Resident population 599 (in thousands)
Resident population in metro areas 41.8%
Birth rate per 1,000 population 20.5
65 years and over 4.4%
Percent of persons without health insurance 14.9%

★ American Hospital Association (AHA) membership
☐ Joint Commission on Accreditation of Healthcare Organizations (JCAHO) accreditation
+ American Osteopathic Hospital Association (AOHA) membership
○ American Osteopathic Association (AOA) accreditation
△ Commission on Accreditation of Rehabilitation Facilities (CARF) accreditation
Control codes 61, 63, 64, 71, 72 and 73 indicate hospitals listed by AOHA, but not registered by AHA. For definition of numerical codes, see page A6

Hospital, Address, Telephone, Administrator, Approval, Facility, and Physician Codes, Health Care System	Classification Codes		Utilization Data					Expense (thousands) of dollars		
	Control	Service	Beds	Admissions	Census	Outpatient Visits	Births	Total	Payroll	Personnel
ANCHORAGE—2nd Judicial Division										
☐ ALASKA PSYCHIATRIC HOSPITAL, 2900 Providence Drive, Zip 99508–4677; tel. 907/269–7100; Daniel J. Meddleton, Administator (Nonreporting) **A**1 9 10	12	22	114	—	—	—	—	—	—	—
★ ALASKA REGIONAL HOSPITAL, 2801 Debarr Road, Zip 99508, Mailing Address: P.O. Box 143889, Zip 99514–3189; tel. 907/276–1131; Sharon A. Anderson, Chief Executive Officer (Nonreporting) **A**1 9 10 **S**0048 Columbia/HCA Healthcare Corporation	33	10	238	—	—	—	—	—	—	—
☐ CHARTER NORTH HOSPITAL, 2530 Debarr Road, Zip 99508; tel. 907/258–7575; Kathleen Cronen, Administrator (Nonreporting) **A**1 9 10 **S**0695 Charter Medical Corporation	33	22	80	—	—	—	—	—	—	—
☐ NORTH STAR HOSPITAL AND COUNSELING CENTER, 1650 South Bragaw, Zip 99508–3467; tel. 907/277–1522; Bob Marshall, Administrator (Nonreporting) **A**1 10 **S**0044 Sterling Healthcare Corporation	33	52	34	—	—	—	—	—	—	—
★ PROVIDENCE ALASKA MEDICAL CENTER, 3200 Providence Drive, Zip 99508, Mailing Address: P.O. Box 196604, Zip 99519–6604; tel. 907/562–2211; Douglas A. Bruce, Chief Executive **A**1 9 10 **F**2 3 4 7 8 9 10 11 14 15 16 17 19 20 21 22 23 28 32 34 35 37 38 39 40 42 43 44 45 46 47 48 49 50 52 53 54 56 58 59 60 63 65 67 71 73 **S**5275 Sisters of Providence Health System	21	10	341	12763	198	254796	2551	157312	74322	1541
★ U.S. PUBLIC HEALTH SERVICE ALASKA NATIVE MEDICAL CENTER, 255 Gambell Street, Zip 99501, Mailing Address: P.O. Box 107741, Zip 99510; tel. 907/279–6661; Frank H. Williams, Executive Officer **A**1 10 **F**4 5 7 8 9 10 12 13 15 16 19 20 21 22 23 26 27 28 29 30 31 34 35 37 38 39 40 42 43 44 45 46 48 50 51 52 53 54 56 57 58 60 65 69 71 72 73 **S**9195 U.S. Public Health Service Indian Health Service	47	10	146	4980	94	169064	883	65533	30058	820
BARROW—4th Judicial District County										
★ U.S. PUBLIC HEALTH SERVICE ALASKA NATIVE HOSPITAL, Zip 99723; tel. 907/852–4611; (Nonreporting) **A**1 10 **S**9195 U.S. Public Health Service Indian Health Service	47	10	15	—	—	—	—	—	—	—
BETHEL—1st Judicial Division										
★ YUKON–KUSKOKWIM DELTA REGIONAL HOSPITAL, P.O. Box 528, Zip 99559–3000; tel. 907/543–2220; Edwin L. Hansen, Administrator (Nonreporting) **A**1 10 **S**9195 U.S. Public Health Service Indian Health Service	47	10	50	—	—	—	—	—	—	—
CORDOVA—2nd Judicial Division										
★ CORDOVA COMMUNITY HOSPITAL, 602 Chase Avenue, Zip 99574, Mailing Address: Box 160, Zip 99574; tel. 907/424–8000; Greg Porter, Administrator (Nonreporting) **A**9 10	14	10	23	—	—	—	—	—	—	—
DILLINGHAM—1st Judicial Division										
★ KANAKANAK HOSPITAL, Mailing Address: P.O. Box 130, Zip 99576; tel. 907/842–5201; Darrel C. Richardson, Administrator (Nonreporting) **A**1 9 10 **S**9195 U.S. Public Health Service Indian Health Service	47	10	16	—	—	—	—	—	—	—
ELMENDORF AIR FORCE BASE—2nd Judicial Division										
★ U.S. AIR FORCE REGIONAL HOSPITAL, 24800 Hospital Drive, Zip 99506–3700; tel. 907/552–4033; Colonel Larry J. Sutterer MSC, Administrator **A**1 5 **F**2 7 8 12 14 15 16 18 19 20 21 22 28 29 30 31 34 35 37 38 39 40 41 44 46 51 52 53 54 56 58 59 61 65 67 71 **S**9495 Department of the Air Force	41	10	75	4795	44	263398	892	—	—	904
FAIRBANKS—1st Judicial Division										
★ BASSETT ARMY COMMUNITY HOSPITAL, Fort Wainwright, Zip 99703–7300; tel. 907/353–5108; Colonel Charles C. Franz, Deputy Commander for Administration **A**1 **F**3 7 8 12 14 15 16 19 20 22 25 31 34 39 40 41 44 46 51 54 55 56 58 59 61 65 71 73 **S**9395 Department of the Army	42	10	43	2776	17	143990	702	—	—	521
★ FAIRBANKS MEMORIAL HOSPITAL, 1650 Cowles Street, Zip 99701; tel. 907/452–8181; James Gingerich, Administrator (Total facility includes 90 beds in nursing home–type unit) **A**1 2 9 10 **F**1 3 4 7 8 9 12 14 15 16 17 19 21 22 26 27 28 30 31 32 34 35 36 37 38 39 40 41 44 45 46 49 52 53 54 55 56 57 58 59 60 63 64 65 71 73 74 **S**2235 Lutheran Health Systems	23	10	206	5621	137	169151	1019	62120	29236	768
HOMER—3rd Judicial Division										
★ SOUTH PENINSULA HOSPITAL, 4300 Bartlett Street, Zip 99603; tel. 907/235–8101; Ronald A. Pavellas, Administrator (Total facility includes 18 beds in nursing home–type unit) **A**9 10 **F**7 11 12 15 21 22 28 31 32 37 40 44 49 64 65 71	23	10	38	890	25	15859	145	11141	5257	396
JUNEAU—3rd Judicial Division										
★ BARTLETT MEMORIAL HOSPITAL, 3260 Hospital Drive, Zip 99801; tel. 907/586–8438; Robert F. Valliant, Administrator (Nonreporting) **A**1 9 10 **S**0002 Quorum Health Group/Quorum Health Resources	15	10	64	—	—	—	—	—	—	—
KETCHIKAN—3rd Judicial Division										
★ KETCHIKAN GENERAL HOSPITAL, 3100 Tongass Avenue, Zip 99901–5746; tel. 907/225–5171; Edward F. Mahn, Chief Executive Officer (Total facility includes 26 beds in nursing home–type unit) **A**1 9 10 **F**3 7 8 14 15 16 19 21 22 28 33 34 37 39 40 41 44 49 56 64 65 71 73 **S**5415 PeaceHealth	23	10	60	1655	35	46551	312	20844	10944	260

© 1995 AHA Guide

Hospitals, U.S. / ALASKA

Hospital, Address, Telephone, Administrator, Approval, Facility, and Physician Codes, Health Care System	Classification Codes		Utilization Data					Expense (thousands of dollars)		
★ American Hospital Association (AHA) membership ☐ Joint Commission on Accreditation of Healthcare Organizations (JCAHO) accreditation + American Osteopathic Hospital Association (AOHA) membership ○ American Osteopathic Association (AOA) accreditation △ Commission on Accreditation of Rehabilitation Facilities (CARF) accreditation Control codes 61, 63, 64, 71, 72 and 73 indicate hospitals listed by AOHA, but not registered by AHA. For definition of numerical codes, see page A6	Control	Service	Beds	Admissions	Census	Outpatient Visits	Births	Total	Payroll	Personnel
KODIAK—2nd Judicial Division										
★ KODIAK ISLAND HOSPITAL AND CARE CENTER, 1915 East Rezanof Drive, Zip 99615; tel. 907/486–3281; Edmon W. Myers, Administrator (Nonreporting) **A**9 10 **S**2235 Lutheran Health Systems	13	10	44	—	—	—	—	—	—	—
KOTZEBUE—2nd Judicial Division										
✠ MANIILAQ HEALTH CENTER, Zip 99752–0043; tel. 907/442–3321; Jan Harris, Administrator (Nonreporting) **A**1 10 **S**9195 U.S. Public Health Service Indian Health Service	47	10	25	—	—	—	—	—	—	—
NOME—4th Judicial Division										
✠ NORTON SOUND REGIONAL HOSPITAL, Bering Street, Zip 99762, Mailing Address: Box 966, Zip 99762; tel. 907/443–3311; Gail Atchnson, Administrator (Nonreporting) **A**1 9 10 **S**9195 U.S. Public Health Service Indian Health Service	23	10	34	—	—	—	—	—	—	—
PALMER—2nd Judicial Division										
★ VALLEY HOSPITAL, 515 East Dahlia Street, Zip 99645, Mailing Address: P.O. Box 1687, Zip 99645; tel. 907/352–2860; James G. Walsh, Executive Director (Nonreporting) **A**9 10	23	10	36	—	—	—	—	—	—	—
PETERSBURG—3rd Judicial Division										
PETERSBURG MEDICAL CENTER, 103 Fram Street, Zip 99833, Mailing Address: Box 589, Zip 99833–0589; tel. 907/772–4291; Gary W. Grandy, Administrator (Total facility includes 14 beds in nursing home–type unit) **A**9 10 **F**7 8 14 15 21 22 32 34 37 40 44 52 56 71	14	10	25	138	13	9868	17	3426	1669	50
SEWARD—2nd Judicial Division										
★ SEWARD GENERAL HOSPITAL, 417 First Avenue, Zip 99664, Mailing Address: P.O. Box 365, Zip 99664–0365; tel. 907/224–5205; Richard W. Jones, Administrator and Chief Executive Officer (Nonreporting) **A**9 10	14	10	20	—	—	—	—	—	—	—
SITKA—3rd Judicial Division										
✠ SEARHC MOUNTAIN EDGECUMBE HOSPITAL, 222 Tongass Drive, Zip 99835–9416; tel. 907/966–2411; Arthur C. Willman, Vice President Operations **A**1 5 10 **F**2 7 8 15 16 20 22 24 27 28 34 40 44 52 53 54 56 57 58 65 67 71 74 **S**9195 U.S. Public Health Service Indian Health Service	47	10	72	1843	35	28186	112	—	—	266
✠ SITKA COMMUNITY HOSPITAL, 209 Moller Avenue, Zip 99835–7145; tel. 907/747–3241; J. Kay Hawks, Chief Executive Officer (Nonreporting) **A**1 9 10	15	10	24	—	—	—	—	—	—	—
SOLDOTNA—3rd Judicial Division										
★ CENTRAL PENINSULA GENERAL HOSPITAL, 250 Hospital Place, Zip 99669; tel. 907/262–4404; Randy Wirick, Administrator (Nonreporting) **A**10 **S**2235 Lutheran Health Systems	23	10	62	—	—	—	—	—	—	—
VALDEZ—3rd Judicial Division										
VALDEZ COMMUNITY HOSPITAL, 911 Meals Avenue, Zip 99686–0550, Mailing Address: Box 550, Zip 99686–0550; tel. 907/835–2249; Daniel R. Mohler, Administrator (Nonreporting) **A**9 10 **S**2235 Lutheran Health Systems	15	10	15	—	—	—	—	—	—	—
WRANGELL—3rd Judicial Division										
★ WRANGELL GENERAL HOSPITAL AND LONG TERM CARE FACILITY, First Avenue and Bennett Street, Zip 99929, Mailing Address: P.O. Box 1081, Zip 99929; tel. 907/874–3356; (Total facility includes 14 beds in nursing home–type unit) **A**9 10 **F**1 3 7 8 11 22 26 27 28 29 34 39 40 44 45 49 64 71	14	10	22	228	13	7303	24	2988	1379	44

Hospitals, U.S. / ARIZONA

ARIZONA

Resident population 3,936 (in thousands)
Resident population in metro areas 84.7%
Birth rate per 1,000 population 18.2
65 years and over 13.4%
Percent of persons without health insurance 15.8%

- ★ American Hospital Association (AHA) membership
- □ Joint Commission on Accreditation of Healthcare Organizations (JCAHO) accreditation
- + American Osteopathic Hospital Association (AOHA) membership
- ○ American Osteopathic Association (AOA) accreditation
- △ Commission on Accreditation of Rehabilitation Facilities (CARF) accreditation

Control codes 61, 63, 64, 71, 72 and 73 indicate hospitals listed by AOHA, but not registered by AHA. For definition of numerical codes, see page A6

Hospital, Address, Telephone, Administrator, Approval, Facility, and Physician Codes, Health Care System	Classification Codes		Utilization Data					Expense (thousands) of dollars		Personnel
	Control	Service	Beds	Admissions	Census	Outpatient Visits	Births	Total	Payroll	
BENSON—Cochise County □ BENSON HOSPITAL, 450 South Ocotillo Street, Zip 85602, Mailing Address: P.O. Box 2290, Zip 85602-2290; tel. 602/586-2261; Ronald A. McKinnon, Administrator **A**1 9 10 **F**8 14 15 16 22 32 34 40 44 64 71	23	10	22	321	7	53249	0	2816	1458	67
BISBEE—Cochise County □ COPPER QUEEN COMMUNITY HOSPITAL, 101 Cole Avenue, Zip 85603-1399; tel. 520/432-5383; Jim Tavary, Chief Executive Officer (Total facility includes 21 beds in nursing home–type unit) **A**1 9 10 **F**7 8 14 15 16 17 20 22 28 32 33 34 40 41 44 49 51 56 64 65 66 67 71 73 **P**5	23	10	49	540	27	11636	50	4829	2419	117
BULLHEAD CITY—Mohave County ★ BULLHEAD COMMUNITY HOSPITAL, 2735 Silver Creek Road, Zip 86442; tel. 602/763-2273; Ronald W. Tenbarge, Executive Vice President and Chief Executive Officer **A**1 9 10 **F**3 7 8 12 19 22 28 29 30 32 34 35 37 40 41 44 49 64 65 71 73 **P**5 **S**8810 Baptist Hospitals and Health Systems, Inc.	23	10	62	2591	27	36340	76	21960	7504	289
★ MOHAVE VALLEY HOSPITAL AND MEDICAL CENTER, 1225 East Hancock Road, Zip 86442; tel. 520/758-3931; Gordon L. Ritter, President and Medical Director (Newly Registered) **A**10	33	10	12	—	—	—	—	—	—	—
CASA GRANDE—Pinal County ★ CASA GRANDE REGIONAL MEDICAL CENTER, 1800 East Florence Boulevard, Zip 85222; tel. 602/426-6300; Robert F. Theilmann, Chief Executive Officer (Total facility includes 128 beds in nursing home–type unit) **A**1 9 10 **F**7 8 12 14 15 16 19 22 23 24 27 28 29 30 32 33 34 35 37 39 40 41 44 45 49 64 65 67 70 71 73 74	23	10	228	4711	167	47879	739	34593	14238	534
CHANDLER—Maricopa County ★ CHANDLER REGIONAL HOSPITAL, 475 South Dobson Road, Zip 85224-4230; tel. 602/963-4561; Kaylor E. Shemberger, President and Chief Executive Officer **A**1 9 10 **F**7 8 12 14 15 16 17 19 21 22 25 28 30 31 32 34 35 36 37 40 41 42 44 45 46 49 61 65 69 70 71 72 73 **P**1 3 5	23	10	120	9121	81	76774	2424	54018	20196	840
□ CHARTER BEHAVIORAL HEALTH SYSTEM, 2190 North Grace Boulevard, Zip 85224; tel. 602/899-8989; Kim Hall, Administrator **A**1 9 10 **F**2 3 12 14 52 53 54 55 56 57 58 59 65 **S**0695 Charter Medical Corporation	33	22	80	1051	44	4267	0	—	—	110
CHINLE—Apache County ★ CHINLE COMPREHENSIVE HEALTH CARE FACILITY, Highway 191, Zip 86503, Mailing Address: P.O. Drawer PH, Zip 86503; tel. 602/674-5281; Ronald Tso, Chief Executive Officer **A**1 9 10 **F**3 7 8 14 15 16 20 22 25 27 31 34 37 39 40 44 46 49 58 65 67 68 71 **P**6 **S**9195 U.S. Public Health Service Indian Health Service	47	10	60	2965	34	136428	723	—	—	465
CLAYPOOL—Gila County ★ COBRE VALLEY COMMUNITY HOSPIAL, One Hospital Drive, Zip 85532, Mailing Address: P.O. Box 3261, Zip 85532-3261; tel. 602/425-3261; John L. Hoopes, Chief Executive Officer and Administrator **A**1 9 10 **F**7 8 11 16 19 22 28 35 37 40 44 65 67 71 73 74 **P**3 **S**0585 Brim, Inc.	23	10	42	2087	21	30937	399	12132	4428	212
COTTONWOOD—Yavapai County ★ MARCUS J. LAWRENCE MEDICAL CENTER, 202 South Willard Street, Zip 86326; tel. 602/634-2251; Reid M. Wood, President and Chief Executive Officer **A**1 9 10 **F**4 7 8 12 14 15 19 21 22 28 30 31 32 33 34 35 37 40 41 42 44 45 49 54 63 65 70 71 73	23	10	75	3464	37	45432	468	23972	9578	344
DAVIS-MONTHAN AIR FORCE BASE—Maricopa County ★ U.S. AIR FORCE HOSPITAL, 4175 South Alamo Avenue, Zip 85707-4405; tel. 520/750-2930; Colonel Richard C. Storey Jr. USAF, MSC, Commander **A**1 9 **F**3 7 8 12 14 16 17 19 20 22 28 29 30 34 37 39 40 41 44 46 51 53 54 55 56 57 58 61 65 67 68 71 73 74 **S**9495 Department of the Air Force	41	10	30	2016	13	231704	198	18603	—	549
DOUGLAS—Cochise County □ SOUTHEAST ARIZONA MEDICAL CENTER, Rural Route 1, Box 30, Zip 85607; tel. 520/364-7931; Robert C. Benjamin, Executive Director (Total facility includes 43 beds in nursing home–type unit) **A**1 9 10 **F**1 14 17 19 22 24 26 27 30 32 37 40 41 42 44 46 49 64 65 71	23	10	75	1539	41	41885	428	9730	4476	182
FLAGSTAFF—Coconino County ★ ASPEN HILL HOSPITAL, 305 West Forest Avenue, Zip 86001-1464; tel. 602/773-1060; Linda Cowan, Administrator (Nonreporting) **A**1 9 10	33	22	26	—	—	—	—	—	—	—
★ △ FLAGSTAFF MEDICAL CENTER, 1200 North Beaver Street, Zip 86001; tel. 602/779-3366; Joseph M. Kortum, President and Chief Executive Officer (Total facility includes 18 beds in nursing home–type unit) **A**1 7 9 10 **F**7 12 15 16 19 21 22 25 28 29 31 32 33 34 35 37 40 41 42 44 45 46 48 49 51 60 63 64 65 67 71 72 73 **P**3	23	10	128	7498	91	—	1275	56956	—	816
FLORENCE—Pinal County □ CENTRAL ARIZONA MEDICAL CENTER, Adamsville Road, Zip 85232, Mailing Address: Box 2080, Zip 85232; tel. 520/868-2003; Darrold Bertsch, Administrator (Total facility includes 27 beds in nursing home–type unit) **A**1 9 10 **F**14 16 19 22 24 26 28 30 34 40 44 52 54 56 57 58 64 71	23	10	77	1450	20	—	74	9773	4146	90

© 1995 AHA Guide

Hospitals, U.S. / ARIZONA

Hospital, Address, Telephone, Administrator, Approval, Facility, and Physician Codes, Health Care System	Classi-fication Codes		Utilization Data					Expense (thousands) of dollars		
★ American Hospital Association (AHA) membership ☐ Joint Commission on Accreditation of Healthcare Organizations (JCAHO) accreditation + American Osteopathic Hospital Association (AOHA) membership ○ American Osteopathic Association (AOA) accreditation △ Commission on Accreditation of Rehabilitation Facilities (CARF) accreditation Control codes 61, 63, 64, 71, 72 and 73 indicate hospitals listed by AOHA, but not registered by AHA. For definition of numerical codes, see page A6	Control	Service	Beds	Admissions	Census	Outpatient Visits	Births	Total	Payroll	Personnel
FORT DEFIANCE—Apache County										
★ U.S. PUBLIC HEALTH SERVICE FORT DEFIANCE INDIAN HEALTH SERVICE HOSPITAL, Mailing Address: P.O. Box 649, Zip 86504; tel. 602/729-3223; Franklin Freeland Ph.D., Ed.D., Chief Executive Officer (Nonreporting) **A**1 9 10 **S**9195 U.S. Public Health Service Indian Health Service	47	10	49	—		—		—	—	—
FORT HUACHUCA—Cochise County										
★ RAYMOND W. BLISS ARMY COMMUNITY HOSPITAL, Zip 85613-7040; tel. 602/533-2026; Lieutenant Colonel Al Santos, Deputy Commander, Administration **A**1 9 **F**3 8 12 13 15 16 17 18 20 22 30 31 32 34 39 41 44 45 46 51 54 58 65 71 73 **S**9395 Department of the Army	42	10	30	1724	10	173847	0	—	—	608
GANADO—Apache County										
☐ SAGE MEMORIAL HOSPITAL, Highway 264, Zip 86505, Mailing Address: P.O. Box 457, Zip 86505; tel. 602/755-3411; Jeffrey J. Hamblen, Chief Executive Officer **A**1 9 10 **F**9 11 20 22 24 25 34 37 38 40 46 47 48 51 52 65 71	23	10	45	803	8	58929	72	10394	5229	243
GLENDALE—Maricopa County										
★ ARROWHEAD COMMUNITY HOSPITAL AND MEDICAL CENTER, 18701 North 67th Avenue, Zip 85308-5722; tel. 602/561-1000; Richard S. Alley, Administrator **A**1 9 10 **F**2 3 4 7 8 9 10 11 12 19 21 22 23 28 29 30 33 35 37 38 40 42 43 44 47 48 49 50 51 52 53 54 55 56 57 58 59 60 62 64 65 66 67 69 70 71 72 73 74 **P**5 8 **S**8810 Baptist Hospitals and Health Systems, Inc.	23	10	80	3652	33	35564	1043	26049	8740	279
☐ CHARTER BEHAVIORAL HEALTH SYSTEM, (Formerly Charter Hospital of Glendale) 6015 West Peoria Avenue, Zip 85302; tel. 602/878-7878; Kimbrough Hall, Chief Executive Officer **A**1 9 10 **F**2 3 12 14 52 53 54 55 56 57 58 59 **S**0695 Charter Medical Corporation	33	22	90	1604	61	11938	0	—	—	160
CHARTER HOSPITAL OF GLENDALE See Charter Behavioral Health System										
☐ △ NOVACARE VALLEY OF THE SUN REHABILITATION HOSPITAL, 13460 North 67th Avenue, Zip 85304; tel. 602/878-8800; Michael S. Wallace, Chief Executive Officer **A**1 7 10 **F**5 12 14 15 16 17 20 25 28 30 34 48 49 67 73 **P**8	12	46	42	603	33	5820	0	9697	3795	93
SAMARITAN BEHAVIORAL HEALTH CENTER See Thunderbird Samaritan Medical Center										
★ THUNDERBIRD SAMARITAN MEDICAL CENTER, (Includes Samaritan Behavioral Health Center–Thunderbird Samaritan Campus, Glendale, Arizona) 5555 West Thunderbird Road, Zip 85306; tel. 602/588-5555; Robert H. Curry Sr., Senior Vice President and Chief Executive Officer (Nonreporting) **A**1 9 10 **F**1 3 4 6 7 8 9 10 12 13 14 15 16 17 18 19 20 21 22 23 25 26 28 30 31 32 33 34 35 36 39 40 41 42 43 44 45 46 49 50 51 52 55 56 57 58 59 60 61 62 63 65 66 67 68 69 71 72 73 74 **P**1 5 7 **S**2535 Samaritan Health System	23	10	290	10944	119	71906	2677	77095	33425	972
★ U.S. AIR FORCE HOSPITAL LUKE, Luke Air Force Base, Zip 85309-1525; tel. 602/856-7501; Colonel Robert P. Edwards, Administrator (Nonreporting) **A**1 9 **S**9495 Department of the Air Force	41	10	40	—		—		—	—	—
KEAMS CANYON—Navajo County										
★ U.S. PUBLIC HEALTH SERVICES INDIAN HOSPITAL, Mailing Address: P.O. Box 98, Zip 86034; tel. 602/738-2211; Taylor Satala, Service Unit Director (Nonreporting) **A**1 9 10 **S**9195 U.S. Public Health Service Indian Health Service	47	10	26	—		—		—	—	—
KINGMAN—Mohave County										
★ KINGMAN REGIONAL MEDICAL CENTER, 3269 Stockton Hill Road, Zip 86401; tel. 520/757-2101; Brian Turney, Chief Executive Officer (Total facility includes 14 beds in nursing home–type unit) **A**1 9 10 **F**7 8 10 19 21 32 33 34 35 37 39 40 41 42 44 45 46 49 63 64 65 67 71 73	23	10	124	4845	58	49608	1053	27132	10782	527
LAKE HAVASU CITY—Mohave County										
★ HAVASU SAMARITAN REGIONAL HOSPITAL, 101 Civic Center Lane, Zip 86403; tel. 602/855-8185; Dennis G. Zielinski, Vice President and Chief Executive Officer (Total facility includes 19 beds in nursing home–type unit) **A**1 9 10 **F**7 8 14 15 16 17 19 21 22 23 26 27 31 32 34 35 37 40 41 42 44 45 46 49 58 61 63 64 65 71 73 **P**3 5 7 **S**2535 Samaritan Health System	23	10	118	3782	49	31677	624	30618	11847	407
MESA—Maricopa County										
★ DESERT SAMARITAN MEDICAL CENTER, 1400 South Dobson Road, Zip 85202-9879; tel. 602/835-3000; Steven L. Seiler, Senior Vice President and Chief Executive Officer **A**1 2 9 10 **F**1 3 4 5 7 8 10 14 15 16 19 21 22 29 31 32 34 35 39 40 41 42 43 44 49 50 52 53 54 55 58 59 61 63 65 69 70 71 73 **P**3 5 7 **S**2535 Samaritan Health System	23	10	324	19151	188	83665	5622	125247	50829	1383
☐ DESERT VISTA HOSPITAL, 570 West Brown Road, Zip 85201; tel. 602/962-3900; Allen S. Nohre, Chief Executive Officer (Nonreporting) **A**1 9 10 **S**0405 Ramsay Health Care, Inc.	33	22	98	—		—		—	—	—
☐ ○ MESA GENERAL HOSPITAL MEDICAL CENTER, 515 North Mesa Drive, Zip 85201; tel. 602/969-9111; Jeffrey A. Ashin, Chief Executive Officer (Total facility includes 13 beds in nursing home–type unit) **A**1 9 10 11 12 13 **F**4 7 8 10 12 14 16 17 19 21 22 25 28 30 32 33 34 35 37 39 40 42 43 44 63 64 65 71 73 74 **P**4 5 7 **S**6525 Ornda Healthcorp	33	10	138	6103	64	48923	0	37453	13921	451
★ △ MESA LUTHERAN HOSPITAL, 525 West Brown Road, Zip 85201-3299; tel. 602/834-1211; Robert A. Rundio, Executive Director (Total facility includes 60 beds in nursing home–type unit) **A**1 2 5 7 9 10 **F**4 7 8 10 12 14 16 17 18 19 20 21 22 23 26 27 28 29 30 32 33 35 36 37 39 40 41 42 43 44 45 46 47 48 49 52 57 59 60 64 65 67 70 71 73 74 **P**5 7 8 **S**2235 Lutheran Health Systems	23	10	278	8893	110	46823	2045	75821	33190	944

Hospitals, U.S. / ARIZONA

Hospital, Address, Telephone, Administrator, Approval, Facility, and Physician Codes, Health Care System	Classification Codes		Utilization Data					Expense (thousands) of dollars		Personnel
	Control	Service	Beds	Admissions	Census	Outpatient Visits	Births	Total	Payroll	

Key:
- ★ American Hospital Association (AHA) membership
- ☐ Joint Commission on Accreditation of Healthcare Organizations (JCAHO) accreditation
- + American Osteopathic Hospital Association (AOHA) membership
- ○ American Osteopathic Association (AOA) accreditation
- △ Commission on Accreditation of Rehabilitation Facilities (CARF) accreditation

Control codes 61, 63, 64, 71, 72 and 73 indicate hospitals listed by AOHA, but not registered by AHA. For definition of numerical codes, see page A6.

Hospital	Control	Service	Beds	Admissions	Census	Outpatient Visits	Births	Total	Payroll	Personnel
★ SAMARITAN BEHAVIORAL HEALTH CENTER – DESERT SAMARITAN CAMPUS, 2225 West Southern Avenue, Zip 85202; tel. 602/464–4000; Steven L. Seiler, Senior Vice President and Chief Executive Officer (Nonreporting) A9 10 S2535 Samaritan Health System	23	22	26	—	—	—	—	—	—	—
★ VALLEY LUTHERAN HOSPITAL, 6644 Baywood Avenue, Zip 85206; tel. 602/981–4100; Robert A. Rundio, Executive Director A1 9 10 F4 7 8 10 12 16 17 18 19 20 21 22 23 26 27 28 29 30 32 33 34 35 36 37 39 40 41 42 43 44 45 48 49 52 57 59 60 64 65 67 70 71 73 74 P1 5 7 8 S2235 Lutheran Health Systems	23	10	172	7387	107	50141	0	52530	21025	778
NOGALES—Santa Cruz County										
★ CARONDOLET HOLY CROSS HOSPITAL, 1171 Target Range Road, Zip 85621; tel. 520/287–2771; C. Ray Honaker, Administrator (Total facility includes 49 beds in nursing home–type unit) A1 9 10 F8 14 15 16 19 22 30 33 35 37 40 44 46 49 64 65 71 73 74 S5945 Carondelet Health System	21	10	80	1827	61	18263	750	10974	5093	187
PAGE—Coconino County										
★ PAGE HOSPITAL, North Navajo Drive and Vista Avenue, Zip 86040, Mailing Address: P.O. Box 1447, Zip 86040; tel. 602/645–2424; Kevin P. Poorten, Chief Executive Officer A1 9 10 F7 8 14 15 16 19 22 31 34 40 44 45 46 49 61 71 73 P3 5 7 S2535 Samaritan Health System	23	10	25	530	4	7487	186	5037	2353	72
PARKER—La Paz County										
★ ○ PARKER COMMUNITY HOSPITAL, 1200 Mohave Road, Zip 85344, Mailing Address: Box 1149, Zip 85344; tel. 520/669–9201; William G. Coe, Chief Executive Officer A9 10 11 F8 14 15 19 21 22 25 29 31 34 37 44 45 46 49 65 67 70 71 73	23	10	39	1103	12	16049	0	8953	3193	140
★ U.S. PUBLIC HEALTH SERVICE INDIAN HOSPITAL, Mailing Address: Route 1, Box 12, Zip 85344; tel. 602/669–2137; (Nonreporting) A1 9 10 S9195 U.S. Public Health Service Indian Health Service	47	10	20	—	—	—	—	—	—	—
PAYSON—Gila County										
★ PAYSON REGIONAL MEDICAL CENTER, 807 South Ponderosa Street, Zip 85541; tel. 602/474–3222; Donald J. Logue, President and Chief Executive Officer A1 9 10 F7 8 17 19 22 26 28 32 34 35 40 44 65 66 71 73 P3 5	23	10	38	1686	17	19349	123	11580	5156	197
PHOENIX—Maricopa County										
☐ ARIZONA STATE HOSPITAL, 2500 East Van Buren Street, Zip 85008; tel. 602/244–1331; John R. Migliaro Ph.D., Chief Executive Officer A1 9 10 F1 2 3 4 5 6 7 8 9 10 11 12 13 14 15 16 17 18 19 20 21 22 23 24 26 27 28 29 30 31 32 33 34 35 37 38 39 40 41 42 43 44 45 46 47 48 49 50 51 52 53 54 56 57 58 59 60 61 62 63 64 65 66 67 68 69 70 71 73 74	12	22	489	764	456	0	0	39715	20712	745
★ CARL T. HAYDEN VETERANS AFFAIRS MEDICAL CENTER, 650 East Indian School Road, Zip 85012–1894; tel. 602/277–5551; John R. Fears, Director (Total facility includes 120 beds in nursing home–type unit) A1 2 3 5 9 F1 2 3 4 8 10 12 14 16 19 20 21 22 24 25 26 27 30 31 32 34 37 39 41 42 44 45 46 48 49 51 52 54 55 58 59 63 64 65 67 71 73 74 S9295 Department of Veterans Affairs	45	10	530	10262	402	233417	0	103200	75200	1642
COLUMBIA DOCTORS HOSPITAL See Paradise Valley Hospital										
☐ ○ COMMUNITY HOSPITAL MEDICAL CENTER, 6501 North 19th Avenue, Zip 85015; tel. 602/249–3434; Michael Miglis, Chief Executive Officer A1 9 10 11 12 F7 14 15 19 21 22 31 34 35 37 40 42 44 49 65 72 73 P5 7 8 S6525 Ornda Healthcorp	33	10	59	2235	28	17463	609	15644	7175	176
★ △ GOOD SAMARITAN REGIONAL MEDICAL CENTER, 1111 East McDowell Road, Zip 85006, Mailing Address: Box 2989, Zip 85062; tel. 602/239–2000; Steven L. Seiler, Senior Vice President and Chief Executive Officer (Total facility includes 20 beds in nursing home–type unit) A1 2 3 5 7 8 9 10 F1 3 4 5 7 8 10 11 14 15 16 19 21 22 23 26 29 31 32 34 35 37 39 40 41 42 43 44 48 49 50 52 53 54 55 57 58 59 60 61 63 64 65 67 70 71 73 74 P3 5 7 S2535 Samaritan Health System	23	10	576	27763	372	181217	7294	250828	105050	3474
★ HEALTHWEST REGIONAL MEDICAL CENTER, 1947 East Thomas Road, Zip 85016; tel. 602/241–7600; John D. Hicks, Chief Executive Officer (Total facility includes 13 beds in nursing home–type unit) A1 9 10 F4 7 8 10 11 12 16 19 20 21 22 23 34 35 37 40 41 42 43 44 48 49 54 63 64 65 69 71 73 S0048 Columbia/HCA Healthcare Corporation	33	10	302	8201	138	24283	0	69600	26648	668
★ △ JOHN C. LINCOLN HOSPITAL AND HEALTH CENTER, 250 East Dunlap Avenue, Zip 85020–2446; tel. 602/943–2381; Dan C. Coleman, President and Chief Executive Officer A1 7 9 10 F1 4 7 8 10 11 12 15 19 21 22 24 28 32 33 34 35 37 40 42 43 44 45 48 49 54 62 63 64 65 66 67 70 71 73 74 P1 5 7 8	23	10	240	9887	119	56548	858	85903	37881	1065
★ MARICOPA MEDICAL CENTER, 2601 East Roosevelt Street, Zip 85008, Mailing Address: P.O. Box 5099, Zip 85010; tel. 602/267–5011; Anthony Rodgers, Director A1 2 3 5 8 9 10 F1 3 4 7 8 9 11 12 13 15 17 18 19 20 25 26 27 28 29 30 31 32 33 34 35 37 38 39 40 42 43 44 45 46 47 49 51 52 53 54 55 56 57 58 59 60 61 63 65 69 70 71 72 73 74 P3	13	10	474	22449	313	436197	3838	212438	95259	2801
★ MARYVALE SAMARITAN MEDICAL CENTER, 5102 West Campbell Avenue, Zip 85031; tel. 602/848–5101; Robert H. Curry Sr., Senior Vice President and Chief Executive Officer A1 2 9 10 F1 4 7 8 10 14 15 16 19 21 22 31 32 34 35 38 40 42 44 45 49 50 60 63 65 69 70 71 P3 5 7 S2535 Samaritan Health System	23	10	213	8399	77	56842	2142	53765	24691	685
★ PARADISE VALLEY HOSPITAL, (Formerly Columbia Doctors Hospital) 3929 East Bell Road, Zip 85032; tel. 602/867–1881; Gary Grover, Chief Executive Officer (Nonreporting) A1 2 9 10 S0048 Columbia/HCA Healthcare Corporation	33	10	140	—	—	—	—	—	—	—
★ PHOENIX BAPTIST HOSPITAL AND MEDICAL CENTER, 6025 North 20th Avenue, Zip 85015; tel. 602/249–0212; Michael Purvis, Chief Executive Officer A1 2 3 5 9 F1 2 3 4 7 8 10 11 12 14 15 17 18 19 20 21 22 23 25 26 27 28 29 30 32 34 35 37 38 39 40 42 43 44 45 47 48 49 50 51 52 53 54 55 56 57 58 59 60 61 62 63 64 65 66 67 69 70 71 73 74 P5 6 8 S8810 Baptist Hospitals and Health Systems, Inc.	23	10	222	9692	122	104967	1468	76173	31328	955

© 1995 AHA Guide

Hospitals, U.S. / ARIZONA

- ★ American Hospital Association (AHA) membership
- ☐ Joint Commission on Accreditation of Healthcare Organizations (JCAHO) accreditation
- + American Osteopathic Hospital Association (AOHA) membership
- ○ American Osteopathic Association (AOA) accreditation
- △ Commission on Accreditation of Rehabilitation Facilities (CARF) accreditation

Control codes 61, 63, 64, 71, 72 and 73 indicate hospitals listed by AOHA, but not registered by AHA. For definition of numerical codes, see page A6.

Hospital, Address, Telephone, Administrator, Approval, Facility, and Physician Codes, Health Care System	Classification Codes		Utilization Data					Expense (thousands) of dollars		Personnel
	Control	Service	Beds	Admissions	Census	Outpatient Visits	Births	Total	Payroll	
★ PHOENIX CHILDREN'S HOSPITAL, 1111 East McDowell Road, Zip 85006, Mailing Address: 1300 North 12th St, Ste 404, Zip 85006; tel. 602/239–5920; Leland G. Clabots, President and Chief Executive Officer **A**1 3 9 13 **F**10 14 17 19 20 21 22 25 27 28 29 30 31 32 34 35 39 41 42 43 44 45 46 47 49 50 52 53 54 55 56 58 60 65 67 70 71 73	23	50	113	8353	146	30542	0	79173	30923	561
★ ○ PHOENIX GENERAL HOSPITAL AND MEDICAL CENTER, 19829 North 27th Avenue, Zip 85027–4002; tel. 602/879–6100; Robert Duncan, Chief Executive Officer (Total facility includes 23 beds in nursing home–type unit) **A**9 10 11 12 13 **F**4 7 8 10 11 12 13 15 17 19 20 21 22 28 29 30 31 34 35 37 39 40 41 42 43 44 45 46 48 49 54 57 58 60 64 65 71 73 **P**3 **S**0002 Quorum Health Group/Quorum Health Resources	23	10	97	2550	33	17891	388	28578	9884	284
PHOENIX MEMORIAL HOSPITAL See PMH Health Services Network										
★ PMH HEALTH SERVICES NETWORK, (Formerly Phoenix Memorial Hospital) 1201 South Seventh Avenue, Zip 85007–3995; tel. 602/258–5111; Jeffrey Norman, Chief Executive Officer **A**1 2 9 10 **F**1 2 3 4 5 6 7 8 9 10 11 12 13 14 15 16 17 18 19 20 21 22 23 25 26 27 28 29 30 31 32 33 34 35 36 37 38 39 40 41 42 43 44 45 46 47 48 49 51 52 53 54 55 56 57 58 59 60 61 62 63 64 65 66 67 68 70 71 72 73 74 **P**1 4 5 6 7 8 **S**0034 PMH Health Resources, Inc.	23	10	183	10035	100	158877	1316	101677	27145	704
★ SAMARITAN–WENDY PAINE O'BRIEN TREATMENT CENTER, 5055 North 34th Street, Zip 85018; tel. 602/955–6200; Mike Todd, Chief Executive Officer **A**9 10 **F**3 14 52 54 55 58 59 **P**3 5 7 **S**2535 Samaritan Health System	23	22	23	129	14	1057	0	1692	984	28
★ △ ST. JOSEPH'S HOSPITAL AND MEDICAL CENTER, 350 West Thomas Road, Zip 85013, Mailing Address: Box 2071, Zip 85001–2071; tel. 602/285–3000; Mary G. Yarbrough, Chief Executive Officer **A**1 2 3 5 7 8 9 10 **F**1 3 4 7 8 10 11 12 13 14 15 17 18 19 20 21 22 23 24 25 26 27 28 29 30 31 32 33 34 35 37 38 39 40 41 42 43 44 45 46 47 48 49 50 51 52 53 54 55 56 58 59 60 61 64 65 66 67 68 69 70 71 73 74 **P**1 4 6 8 **S**5205 Catholic Healthcare West	21	10	493	24622	369	345512	4958	275401	118753	3102
★ ST. LUKE'S BEHAVIORAL HEALTH CENTER, 1800 East Van Buren, Zip 85006–3742; tel. 602/251–8484; Edward H. Lamb, Chief Executive Officer **A**1 9 10 **F**1 2 3 7 8 10 11 12 14 15 16 17 18 19 22 25 26 28 29 30 32 33 34 35 37 38 40 41 42 43 44 45 46 47 49 52 53 54 55 56 57 58 59 60 64 65 73 74 **S**6525 Ornda Healthcorp	23	22	86	2452	60	13452	0	12655	4975	154
★ ST. LUKE'S MEDICAL CENTER, 1800 East Van Buren Street, Zip 85006–3742; tel. 602/251–8100; Mary Starmann–Harrison FACHE, President (Nonreporting) **A**1 9 10 **S**6525 Ornda Healthcorp	23	10	296	—	—	—	—	—	—	—
★ U.S. PUBLIC HEALTH SERVICE PHOENIX INDIAN MEDICAL CENTER, 4212 North 16th Street, Zip 85016–5389; tel. 602/263–1200; Anna Albert, Chief Executive Officer **A**1 3 5 10 **F**1 3 4 5 6 7 8 10 12 15 16 17 18 19 20 21 22 23 25 26 27 28 29 30 31 32 33 34 35 37 39 40 41 42 43 44 45 46 49 50 51 52 53 54 55 56 58 60 61 65 68 69 70 71 72 73 74 **P**6 **S**9195 U.S. Public Health Service Indian Health Service	44	10	147	5640	82	139534	533	39425	27385	721
☐ VENCOR HOSPITAL – PHOENIX, 40 East Indianola, Zip 85012; tel. 602/280–7000; John L. Harrington Jr. FACHE, Administrator (Nonreporting) **A**1 10 **S**0026 Vencor, Incorporated	23	10	104	—	—	—	—	—	—	—
WESTBRIDGE TREATMENT CENTER, 1830 East Roosevelt, Zip 85006; tel. 602/254–0884; Jeffrey M. Kaplan, Chief Executive Officer (Nonreporting) **A**9 10 **S**0665 Century Healthcare Corporation	33	52	83	—	—	—	—	—	—	—
WESTBRIDGE TREATMENT CENTER – NORTH CAMPUS, 720 East Montebello, Zip 85014–2599; tel. 602/277–KIDS; Jeffrey M. Kaplan, Chief Executive Officer (Nonreporting) **S**0665 Century Healthcare Corporation	33	52	45	—	—	—	—	—	—	—
PRESCOTT—Yavapai County										
★ VETERANS AFFAIRS MEDICAL CENTER, 500 Highway 89 North, Zip 86313; tel. 520/445–4860; Patricia A. McKlem, Director (Nonreporting) **A**1 9 **S**9295 Department of Veterans Affairs	45	10	369	—	—	—	—	—	—	—
☐ YAVAPAI REGIONAL MEDICAL CENTER, 1003 Willow Creek Road, Zip 86301; tel. 602/445–2700; Timothy Barnett, Chief Executive Officer **A**1 9 10 **F**7 8 11 15 17 19 21 22 24 32 33 34 35 40 41 42 44 46 49 56 63 65 67 70 71 73 **P**1	23	10	87	5088	53	47211	625	32626	14191	612
SACATON—Maricopa County										
★ HUHUKAM MEMORIAL HOSPITAL, Seed Farm Road, Zip 85247–0038, Mailing Address: P.O. Box 38, Zip 85247; tel. 602/562–3321; Viola Johnson, Service Unit Director (Nonreporting) **A**1 9 10 **S**9195 U.S. Public Health Service Indian Health Service	47	10	20	—	—	—	—	—	—	—
SAFFORD—Graham County										
★ MOUNT GRAHAM COMMUNITY HOSPITAL, 1600 20th Avenue, Zip 85546; tel. 520/348–4000; Karl E. Johnson, Chief Executive Officer **A**1 9 10 **F**7 19 21 22 31 32 33 34 40 44 **P**3 5 8	16	10	36	2189	14	30688	475	8009	3738	169
SCOTTSDALE—Maricopa County										
☐ △ NOVACARE MERIDIAN POINT REHABILITATION HOSPITAL, 11250 North 92nd Street, Zip 85260–6148; tel. 602/860–0671; Michael J. Soisson, Administrator **A**1 7 9 10 **F**5 6 12 15 16 29 34 41 45 46 48 49 65 66 67	33	46	43	417	25	7409	0	8859	3259	78
★ SAMARITAN BEHAVIORAL HEALTH CENTER – SCOTTSDALE, 7575 East Earll Drive, Zip 85251–6998; tel. 602/941–7500; Robert F. Meyer M.D., Vice President, Chief Executive Officer and Medical Director **A**1 9 **F**1 3 12 14 15 16 52 53 55 56 57 58 59 **P**1 4 5 7 **S**2535 Samaritan Health System	23	22	60	1501	30	0	0	7121	3409	123
★ △ SCOTTSDALE MEMORIAL HOSPITAL, 7400 East Osborn Road, Zip 85251; tel. 602/481–4000; David R. Carpenter, Senior Vice President and Administrator (Total facility includes 60 beds in nursing home–type unit) **A**1 2 3 5 7 9 10 **F**1 4 7 8 9 10 11 12 13 14 15 16 19 21 22 24 25 26 27 28 31 32 33 35 36 37 38 39 40 41 42 43 44 45 46 47 48 49 54 55 56 60 61 63 64 65 67 70 71 73 **P**1 7 **S**0037 Scottsdale Memorial Health Systems, Inc.	23	10	318	12623	204	63850	1127	101458	39445	1330

Hospitals, U.S. / ARIZONA

Hospital, Address, Telephone, Administrator, Approval, Facility, and Physician Codes, Health Care System	Classification Codes		Utilization Data					Expense (thousands) of dollars		
★ American Hospital Association (AHA) membership ☐ Joint Commission on Accreditation of Healthcare Organizations (JCAHO) accreditation + American Osteopathic Hospital Association (AOHA) membership ○ American Osteopathic Association (AOA) accreditation △ Commission on Accreditation of Rehabilitation Facilities (CARF) accreditation Control codes 61, 63, 64, 71, 72 and 73 indicate hospitals listed by AOHA, but not registered by AHA. For definition of numerical codes, see page A6	Control	Service	Beds	Admissions	Census	Outpatient Visits	Births	Total	Payroll	Personnel
☐ SCOTTSDALE MEMORIAL HOSPITAL–NORTH, 10450 North 92nd Street, Zip 85258–4514, Mailing Address: P.O. Box 4500, Zip 85261–9930; tel. 602/860–3000; Thomas J. Sadvary, Senior Vice President and Administrator **A**1 3 5 9 10 **F**1 2 3 4 5 6 7 8 9 10 11 12 13 14 15 16 17 18 19 20 21 22 23 24 25 26 27 28 29 30 31 32 33 34 35 36 37 38 39 40 41 42 43 44 45 46 47 48 49 52 56 60 61 63 64 65 67 68 69 70 71 72 73 74 **P**1 6 7 8 **S**0037 Scottsdale Memorial Health Systems, Inc.	23	10	242	11926	152	40317	1662	95192	33682	1115
SELLS—Pima County										
★ U.S. PUBLIC HEALTH SERVICE INDIAN HOSPITAL, Mailing Address: P.O. Box 548, Zip 85634; tel. 602/383–7251; Darrell Rumley, Director **A**1 9 10 **F**2 3 8 9 11 15 16 20 22 24 25 34 37 38 40 44 47 51 52 65 **S**9195 U.S. Public Health Service Indian Health Service	47	10	36	650	12	45000	8	—	—	195
SHOW LOW—Navajo County										
★ NAVAPACHE REGIONAL MEDICAL CENTER, 2200 Show Low Lake Road, Zip 85901; tel. 602/537–4375; Leigh Cox, Chief Executive Officer **A**1 9 10 **F**7 8 11 15 17 19 22 24 30 32 34 40 44 45 49 63 65 67 71 73 **P**3 **S**0585 Brim, Inc.	23	10	44	2863	25	25937	647	14909	6604	224
SIERRA VISTA—Cochise County										
☐ SIERRA VISTA COMMUNITY HOSPITAL, 300 El Camino Real, Zip 85635; tel. 602/458–4641; Dale A. Decker, Chief Executive Officer (Nonreporting) **A**1 9 10	23	10	87	—	—	—	—	—	—	—
SPRINGERVILLE—Apache County										
★ WHITE MOUNTAIN COMMUNITIES HOSPITAL, (Formerly Samaritan Medical Center–White Mountain) 118 South Mountain Avenue, Zip 85938, Mailing Address: Box 880, Zip 85938–0471; tel. 602/333–4368; (Nonreporting) **A**1 9 10	23	10	25	—	—	—	—	—	—	—
SUN CITY—Maricopa County										
★ WALTER O. BOSWELL MEMORIAL HOSPITAL, 10401 West Thunderbird Boulevard, Zip 85351, Mailing Address: Box 1690, Zip 85372; tel. 602/977–7211; George Perez, Executive Vice President and Chief Executive Officer (Total facility includes 20 beds in nursing home–type unit) **A**1 2 9 10 **F**3 4 6 8 10 11 12 15 16 17 19 21 22 24 26 27 32 33 35 36 37 41 42 43 44 48 49 51 54 55 56 57 58 60 63 64 65 67 71 73 **P**1 **S**0030 Sun Health Corporation	23	10	317	11573	197	18671	0	73880	30890	932
SUN CITY WEST—Maricopa County										
★ DEL E. WEBB MEMORIAL HOSPITAL, 14502 West Meeker Boulevard, Zip 85375, Mailing Address: P.O. Box 5169, Zip 85375; tel. 602/214–4000; Thomas C. Dickson, Chief Operating Officer and Executive Vice President (Total facility includes 40 beds in nursing home–type unit) **A**1 9 10 **F**1 3 4 8 10 11 12 15 17 19 21 22 26 27 28 29 30 31 32 33 34 35 36 39 41 42 43 44 45 46 48 49 52 54 55 56 57 58 59 60 63 64 65 67 70 71 73 **P**1 5 **S**0030 Sun Health Corporation	23	10	241	3823	88	29544	0	31033	12981	324
TEMPE—Maricopa County										
★ TEMPE ST. LUKE'S HOSPITAL, 1500 South Mill Avenue, Zip 85281–6699; tel. 602/968–9411; Brian S. Bentley, President **A**1 9 10 12 13 **F**2 3 4 7 8 10 11 16 17 18 19 21 22 25 27 30 31 32 33 34 36 37 39 40 41 42 43 44 45 46 48 49 51 52 53 54 55 56 58 59 61 63 64 65 66 71 73 74 **P**1 5 6 7 **S**6525 Ornda Healthcorp	33	10	102	3716	40	27261	523	25895	8998	197
TUBA CITY—Coconino County										
★ TUBA CITY INDIAN MEDICAL CENTER, Main Street, Zip 86045–6211, Mailing Address: P.O. Box 600, Zip 86045–6211; tel. 602/283–7201; Rosalyn Curtis, Chief Executive Officer (Nonreporting) **A**1 9 10 **S**9195 U.S. Public Health Service Indian Health Service	47	10	85	—	—	—	—	—	—	—
TUCSON—Pima County										
★ △ CARONDELET ST. JOSEPH'S HOSPITAL, 350 North Wilmot Road, Zip 85711; tel. 520/296–3211; Thomas C. Gagen, Chief Operating Officer **A**1 7 9 10 **F**4 8 10 11 12 14 15 16 19 21 22 29 30 32 33 35 37 40 41 42 43 44 46 48 49 52 54 55 56 57 58 59 63 65 67 71 73 74 **P**1 2 6 7 **S**5945 Carondelet Health System	21	10	223	11478	134	77874	1985	75493	31723	906
★ △ CARONDELET ST. MARY'S HOSPITAL, 1601 West St. Mary's Road, Zip 85745–2682; tel. 602/622–5833; Sister St. Joan Willert, President and Chief Executive Officer **A**1 5 7 9 10 **F**4 8 9 10 11 12 14 15 16 19 21 22 29 30 32 33 34 35 37 41 42 43 44 46 48 49 52 54 55 56 57 58 59 63 65 67 71 73 74 **P**1 2 6 7 **S**5945 Carondelet Health System	21	10	332	15936	225	64605	0	103284	44947	1317
☐ CHARTER BEHAVIORAL HEALTH SYSTEM–TUCSON, (Formerly Tucson Psychiatric Institute) 7220 East Rosewood Street, Zip 85710; tel. 520/745–5100; Mary Jean Geroulo, Chief Executive Officer (Nonreporting) **A**1 9 10 **S**0695 Charter Medical Corporation	33	22	54	—	—	—	—	—	—	—
☐ DESERT HILLS CENTER FOR YOUTH AND FAMILIES, 2797 North Introspect Drive, Zip 85745; tel. 602/622–5437; Fletcher McCasker, Chief Executive Officer (Nonreporting) **A**1 3 9	33	52	108	—	—	—	—	—	—	—
★ EL DORADO HOSPITAL AND MEDICAL CENTER, 1400 North Wilmot, Zip 85712, Mailing Address: Box 13070, Zip 85732; tel. 520/886–6361; Rhonda Dean, Chief Executive Officer (Total facility includes 31 beds in nursing home–type unit) **A**1 9 10 **F**4 8 10 11 12 14 15 16 19 22 26 32 34 35 37 41 43 44 48 49 52 57 64 65 71 73 **P**1 7 **S**0048 Columbia/HCA Healthcare Corporation	33	10	166	4727	77	22847	0	36583	13013	505
☐ KINO COMMUNITY HOSPITAL, 2800 East Ajo Way, Zip 85713; tel. 602/573–2815; (Total facility includes 20 beds in nursing home–type unit) **A**1 3 5 9 10 **F**7 8 13 14 15 16 19 20 22 28 31 34 37 39 40 41 42 44 46 49 51 52 53 54 55 57 58 61 64 65 67 71 72 73 74	13	10	135	4658	71	119034	751	47401	20305	797

Hospitals, U.S. / ARIZONA

Hospital, Address, Telephone, Administrator, Approval, Facility, and Physician Codes, Health Care System	Classification Codes		Utilization Data					Expense (thousands) of dollars		
★ American Hospital Association (AHA) membership □ Joint Commission on Accreditation of Healthcare Organizations (JCAHO) accreditation + American Osteopathic Hospital Association (AOHA) membership ○ American Osteopathic Association (AOA) accreditation △ Commission on Accreditation of Rehabilitation Facilities (CARF) accreditation Control codes 61, 63, 64, 71, 72 and 73 indicate hospitals listed by AOHA, but not registered by AHA. For definition of numerical codes, see page A6	Control	Service	Beds	Admissions	Census	Outpatient Visits	Births	Total	Payroll	Personnel
★ NORTHWEST HOSPITAL, 6200 North La Cholla Boulevard, Zip 85741; tel. 602/742–9000; Mark T. Brenzel, Chief Executive Officer (Total facility includes 16 beds in nursing home–type unit) **A**1 9 10 **F**4 7 8 10 12 15 16 17 19 21 22 26 27 28 30 32 34 35 37 40 41 42 43 44 49 60 64 65 67 71 72 73 **P**1 5 7 **S**0048 Columbia/HCA Healthcare Corporation	33	10	144	6821	83	54424	295	46852	17806	621
SIERRA TUCSON, 16500 North Lago Del Oro Parkway, Zip 85737; tel. 602/624–4000; John H. Schmitz, President **A**9 **F**2 12 14 16 17 20 22 24 27 39 45 46 52 65 67 **P**6	33	22	102	720	44	0	0	9428	4532	168
□ ○ TUCSON GENERAL HOSPITAL, 3838 North Campbell Avenue, Zip 85719–1497, Mailing Address: P.O. Box 40360, Zip 85717–0360; tel. 520/318–6302; William C. Behnke Jr., Chief Executive Officer (Nonreporting) **A**1 9 10 11 12 13 **S**6525 Ornda Healthcorp	33	10	94	—	—	—	—	—	—	—
★ TUCSON MEDICAL CENTER, (Includes Palo Verde Hospital, 2695 North Craycroft, Tucson, Arizona, Zip 85712, Mailing Address: P.O. Box 40030, Zip 85717–0030; tel. 602/322–4390) 5301 East Grant Road, Zip 85712–2874, Mailing Address: Box 42195, Zip 85733–2195; tel. 602/327–5461; Rodrigo A. Pascualy, Administrator (Total facility includes 50 beds in nursing home–type unit) **A**1 2 3 5 9 10 **F**4 5 7 8 10 11 12 14 15 16 17 19 21 22 23 24 29 30 31 32 33 34 35 36 37 38 39 40 41 42 43 44 45 46 47 49 60 63 65 67 68 70 71 72 73 74 **P**3 TUCSON PSYCHIATRIC INSTITUTE See Charter Behavioral Health System–Tucson	23	10	511	25533	302	110481	4546	174996	78641	2551
★ UNIVERSITY MEDICAL CENTER, 1501 North Campbell Avenue, Zip 85724; tel. 602/694–0111; Gregory A. Pivirotto, President and Chief Executive Officer **A**1 2 3 5 8 9 10 **F**4 7 8 10 11 15 16 19 21 22 23 26 28 30 31 32 34 35 37 38 39 40 41 42 43 44 46 49 52 55 56 57 58 60 61 65 69 70 71 73 **P**5	23	10	297	15456	220	327333	3432	156332	69787	2285
★ VETERANS AFFAIRS MEDICAL CENTER, 3601 South 6th Avenue, Zip 85723; tel. 520/792–1450; Jonathan H. Gardner, Director (Nonreporting) **A**1 3 5 8 9 **S**9295 Department of Veterans Affairs	45	10	286	—	—	—	—	—	—	—
WHITERIVER—Navajo County										
★ U.S. PUBLIC HEALTH SERVICE INDIAN HOSPITAL, State Route 73, Box 860, Zip 85941–0860; tel. 520/338–4911; Carla Alchesay–Nachu, Service Unit Director **A**1 9 **F**2 3 4 5 6 7 8 9 10 11 12 13 14 15 16 17 18 19 20 21 22 23 24 25 26 27 28 29 30 31 32 33 34 35 37 38 39 40 41 42 43 44 45 46 47 48 49 50 51 52 53 54 55 56 57 58 59 60 61 63 65 66 67 68 69 70 71 72 73 74 **P**6 **S**9195 U.S. Public Health Service Indian Health Service	44	10	45	1955	21	83684	162	16573	9170	278
WICKENBURG—Maricopa County										
★ WICKENBURG COMMUNITY HOSPITAL, 520 Rose Lane, Zip 85390, Mailing Address: 520 Roase Lane, Zip 85390; tel. 520/684–5421; Carol Schmoyer, Administrator (Total facility includes 57 beds in nursing home–type unit) **A**1 9 10 **F**8 9 14 15 17 19 22 28 29 31 34 37 44 49 64 65 71 73	23	10	80	624	58	6574	7	5394	2713	119
WILLCOX—Graham County										
NORTHERN COCHISE COMMUNITY HOSPITAL, 901 West Rex Allen Drive, Zip 85643, Mailing Address: P.O. Drawer D, Zip 85643; tel. 520/384–3541; Chris Cronberg, Interim Chief Executive Officer (Total facility includes 24 beds in nursing home–type unit) **A**9 10 **F**7 8 12 15 16 19 22 26 28 33 34 39 40 44 46 49 64 65 71 73 **S**0585 Brim, Inc.	16	10	48	660	32	11091	54	2748	1802	95
WINSLOW—Navajo County										
★ WINSLOW MEMORIAL HOSPITAL, 1501 Williamson Avenue, Zip 86047; tel. 602/289–4691; Michael King, Administrator **A**9 10 **F**7 8 14 16 19 20 22 30 32 33 34 40 44 64 71	23	10	34	1208	12	13325	253	6839	2863	118
YUMA—Yuma County										
U.S. PUBLIC HEALTH SERVICE INDIAN HOSPITAL See Winterhaven, California										
★ YUMA REGIONAL MEDICAL CENTER, 2400 Avenue A, Zip 85364–7170; tel. 602/344–2000; Robert T. Olsen, Chief Executive Officer **A**1 9 10 **F**7 8 16 19 20 21 22 23 24 26 28 31 34 35 37 38 39 40 42 44 49 56 60 65 67 70 71 73 **P**8	23	10	226	11349	131	80821	2986	55735	28414	787

Hospitals, U.S. / ARKANSAS

ARKANSAS

Resident population 2,424 (in thousands)
Resident population in metro areas 44.7%
Birth rate per 1,000 population 15.0
65 years and over 15.0%
Percent of persons without health insurance 17.6%

Hospital, Address, Telephone, Administrator, Approval, Facility, and Physician Codes, Health Care System	Classification Codes		Utilization Data					Expense (thousands) of dollars		Personnel
★ American Hospital Association (AHA) membership ☐ Joint Commission on Accreditation of Healthcare Organizations (JCAHO) accreditation + American Osteopathic Hospital Association (AOHA) membership ○ American Osteopathic Association (AOA) accreditation △ Commission on Accreditation of Rehabilitation Facilities (CARF) accreditation Control codes 61, 63, 64, 71, 72 and 73 indicate hospitals listed by AOHA, but not registered by AHA. For definition of numerical codes, see page A6	Control	Service	Beds	Admissions	Census	Outpatient Visits	Births	Total	Payroll	
ARKADELPHIA—Clark County ★ BAPTIST MEDICAL CENTER ARKADELPHIA, 3050 Twin Rivers Drive, Zip 71923; tel. 501/245–1100; Dan Gathright, Senior Vice President and Administrator **A**1 9 10 **F**7 8 12 15 16 19 21 22 27 30 31 32 33 35 37 40 41 44 49 65 71 73 **P**1 3 4 5 6 7 **S**0355 Baptist Medical System	23	10	57	1741	18	18679	296	10050	3784	197
ASHDOWN—Little River County ★ LITTLE RIVER MEMORIAL HOSPITAL, Fifth and Locke Streets, Zip 71822–0577, Mailing Address: Box 577, Zip 71822; tel. 501/898–5011; Judy Adams, Administrator **A**9 10 **F**8 15 16 19 22 32 33 44 71 **P**5	13	10	42	968	13	8455	0	—	—	103
BATESVILLE—Independence County ★ WHITE RIVER MEDICAL CENTER, 1710 Harrison Street, Zip 72501, Mailing Address: P.O. Box 2197, Zip 72503–2197; tel. 501/793–1200; Gary Bebow, Administrator and Chief Executive Officer **A**1 9 10 **F**7 8 10 11 12 14 15 16 19 21 22 25 28 30 31 32 33 34 35 37 40 41 42 44 46 49 52 57 63 64 65 71 73 **P**1 2	23	10	146	5869	90	58594	227	30927	12089	525
BENTON—Saline County ☐ RIVENDELL PSYCHIATRIC CENTER, 100 Rivendell Drive, Zip 72015; tel. 501/794–1255; Laura Davis, Director Clinical Operations (Nonreporting) **A**1 9 10	33	52	64	—	—	—	—	—	—	—
★ SALINE MEMORIAL HOSPITAL, 1 Medical Park Drive, Zip 72015; tel. 501/776–6000; Terry G. Whittington, Chief Executive Officer (Total facility includes 10 beds in nursing home–type unit) **A**1 9 10 **F**7 8 12 19 22 32 34 35 37 40 44 52 57 64 65 71 73 **S**0002 Quorum Health Group/Quorum Health Resources	13	10	141	3993	69	27684	229	24409	9459	447
BENTONVILLE—Benton County ★ BATES MEDICAL CENTER, 602 North Walton Boulevard, Zip 72712; tel. 501/273–2481; Thomas P. O'Neal, President **A**1 9 10 **F**8 10 11 12 14 15 16 17 19 21 22 23 24 26 28 29 30 32 33 35 37 39 41 42 44 45 49 52 57 59 63 65 67 71 72 73 74 **P**5 **S**0002 Quorum Health Group/Quorum Health Resources	23	10	40	2017	25	22463	0	12621	5001	222
BERRYVILLE—Carroll County ★ CARROLL REGIONAL MEDICAL CENTER, 214 Carter Street, Zip 72616, Mailing Address: P.O. Box 387, Zip 72616; tel. 501/423–3355; J. Rudy Darling, President and Chief Executive Officer **A**9 10 **F**7 8 15 17 19 22 30 32 33 35 37 40 41 42 44 65 67 70 71 73	23	10	46	1833	17	13495	254	8406	4098	177
BLYTHEVILLE—Mississippi County ★ BAPTIST MEMORIAL HOSPITAL–BLYTHEVILLE, 1520 North Division Street, Zip 72315, Mailing Address: P.O. Box 108, Zip 72316–0108; tel. 501/762–3300; Randy King, Administrator (Total facility includes 70 beds in nursing home–type unit) **A**1 9 10 **F**8 11 12 13 14 15 16 17 19 21 22 28 29 30 31 32 35 37 39 40 41 44 45 46 49 52 65 67 71 73 **P**3 7 **S**1625 Baptist Memorial Health Care System, Inc.	21	10	198	3060	103	24646	622	13922	6064	219
BOONEVILLE—Logan County ★ BOONEVILLE COMMUNITY HOSPITAL, 880 West Main, Zip 72927, Mailing Address: P.O. Box 290, Zip 72927; tel. 501/675–2800; Robert R. Bash, Administrator **A**9 10 **F**8 19 22 30 32 34 44 48 49 71 73 **P**1 3	23	10	26	688	12	18179	0	2506	1408	74
CALICO ROCK—Izard County MEDICAL CENTER OF CALICO ROCK, 103 Grasse Street, Zip 72519; tel. 501/297–3726; Terry Amstutz, Chief Executive Officer **A**9 10 **F**7 8 11 12 19 22 25 27 28 32 33 34 37 39 40 44 49 65 71 73	23	10	26	817	11	1779	52	—	—	78
CAMDEN—Ouachita County ★ OUACHITA MEDICAL CENTER, 638 California Street, Zip 71701, Mailing Address: Box 797, Zip 71701; tel. 501/836–1000; C. C. McAllister, Administrator and Chief Executive Officer **A**1 9 10 **F**1 2 3 7 8 15 16 17 19 21 22 23 26 27 28 30 32 33 34 37 40 44 45 46 49 52 57 63 65 71 73 **P**5	15	10	118	3208	47	21414	368	15213	7272	411
CHEROKEE VILLAGE—Sharp County ★ BAPTIST MEMORIAL HOSPITAL–EASTERN OZARKS, 122 South Allegheny Drive, Zip 72542; tel. 501/257–4101; Jerry L. Lee, Administrator **A**1 10 **F**8 19 22 28 32 44 65 67 71 73 **P**1 3 7 **S**1625 Baptist Memorial Health Care System, Inc.	21	10	40	1029	15	14515	0	4803	1500	109
CLARKSVILLE—Johnson County ★ JOHNSON COUNTY REGIONAL HOSPITAL, 1100 East Poplar Street, Zip 72830, Mailing Address: P.O. Box 738, Zip 72830–0738; tel. 501/754–5454; Kenneth R. Wood, Administrator (Nonreporting) **A**9 10	13	10	68	—	—	—	—	—	—	—
CLINTON—Van Buren County VAN BUREN COUNTY MEMORIAL HOSPITAL, Highway 65 South, Zip 72031, Mailing Address: Box 206, Zip 72031; tel. 501/745–2401; Alan Finley, Administrator (Nonreporting) **A**9 10 **S**1765 United Hospital Corporation	13	10	152	—	—	—	—	—	—	—
CONWAY—Faulkner County ★ CONWAY REGIONAL MEDICAL CENTER, 2302 College Avenue, Zip 72032–6297; tel. 501/329–3831; James A. Summersett III FACHE, President and Chief Executive Officer **A**1 9 10 **F**7 8 10 11 15 19 20 21 22 23 24 28 32 33 34 35 37 40 41 44 46 49 52 57 65 66 67 71 **P**8	23	10	116	5055	62	43952	903	30688	11298	509

© 1995 AHA Guide

Hospitals, U.S. / ARKANSAS

Hospital, Address, Telephone, Administrator, Approval, Facility, and Physician Codes, Health Care System

- ★ American Hospital Association (AHA) membership
- ☐ Joint Commission on Accreditation of Healthcare Organizations (JCAHO) accreditation
- + American Osteopathic Hospital Association (AOHA) membership
- ○ American Osteopathic Association (AOA) accreditation
- △ Commission on Accreditation of Rehabilitation Facilities (CARF) accreditation

Control codes 61, 63, 64, 71, 72 and 73 indicate hospitals listed by AOHA, but not registered by AHA. For definition of numerical codes, see page A6

Hospital	Classification Codes		Utilization Data					Expense (thousands) of dollars		Personnel
	Control	Service	Beds	Admissions	Census	Outpatient Visits	Births	Total	Payroll	
CROSSETT—Ashley County										
★ ASHLEY MEMORIAL HOSPITAL, 400 Main Street, Zip 71635, Mailing Address: Box 400, Zip 71635; tel. 501/364–4111; Willis Bultje, Administrator **A**9 10 **F**11 19 21 22 24 30 32 35 37 40 41 44 49 52 57 58 62 65 71 73	23	10	44	1470	18	15265	74	8761	3553	130
DANVILLE—Yell County										
★ CHAMBERS MEMORIAL HOSPITAL, Highway 10 at Detroit, Zip 72833, Mailing Address: P.O. Box 639, Zip 72833–0639; tel. 501/495–2241; Scott Peek, Administrator **A**9 10 **F**19 22 32 40 44 49 64 65 71	13	10	41	1128	10	12341	101	4714	1836	101
DARDANELLE—Yell County										
DARDANELLE HOSPITAL, 200 North Third Street, Zip 72834, Mailing Address: Box 578, Zip 72834; tel. 501/229–4677; Donald T. Cline, Administrator **A**9 10 **F**11 14 22 44 49 64 71	13	10	44	963	11	4156	0	3026	1185	72
DE QUEEN—Sevier County										
★ DE QUEEN REGIONAL MEDICAL CENTER, Collins Raye Drive, Zip 71832–2198; tel. 501/584–4111; Steve Nichols, Chief Executive Officer **A**9 10 **F**7 8 12 16 19 20 21 23 28 29 30 32 33 34 35 37 39 40 44 48 49 65 69 71 73 **P**7 8 **S**0048 Columbia/HCA Healthcare Corporation	33	10	75	2075	28	—	147	9656	4061	218
DE WITT—Arkansas County										
DEWITT CITY HOSPITAL, Highway 1 and Madison Street, Zip 72042, Mailing Address: Box 32, Zip 72042; tel. 501/946–3571; Darren Caldwell, Administrator (Total facility includes 54 beds in nursing home–type unit) **A**9 10 **F**22 32 64 71	14	10	88	783	62	8619	0	4024	1799	89
DUMAS—Lincoln County										
★ DELTA MEMORIAL HOSPITAL, 300 East Pickens Street, Zip 71639, Mailing Address: Box 128, Zip 71639–0126; tel. 501/382–4303; Rodney McPherson, Administrator (Nonreporting) **A**9 10 **S**0002 Quorum Health Group/Quorum Health Resources	23	10	35	—	—	—	—	—	—	—
EL DORADO—Union County										
★ MEDICAL CENTER OF SOUTH ARKANSAS, (Includes Union Medical Center, 700 West Grove Street, El Dorado, Arkansas, Zip 71730; tel. 501/864–3200; Warner Brown Hospital, 460 West Oak Street, El Dorado, Arkansas, Zip 71730; tel. 501/863–2000) 700 West Grove Street, Zip 71730, Mailing Address: P.O. Box 1998, Zip 71731–1998; tel. 501/864–3200; Luther J. Lewis, President and Administrator **A**1 3 5 9 10 **F**3 7 8 10 12 14 15 16 17 19 21 22 23 26 28 29 30 31 32 33 34 35 37 38 39 40 41 42 44 45 46 48 49 52 54 55 56 57 58 59 60 63 64 65 66 67 68 71 73 74 **P**3 8	23	10	213	7468	127	33734	908	39784	16601	736
UNION MEDICAL CENTER See Medical Center of South Arkansas										
WARNER BROWN HOSPITAL See Medical Center of South Arkansas										
EUREKA SPRINGS—Carroll County										
★ EUREKA SPRINGS HOSPITAL, 24 Norris Street, Zip 72632; tel. 501/253–7400; Joe Hammond, Administrator **A**9 10 **F**8 17 22 28 30 31 32 33 34 44 46 49 51 65 71 73	23	10	18	560	7	4601	0	3413	1919	108
FAYETTEVILLE—Washington County										
☐ CHARTER VISTA HOSPITAL, 4253 Crossover Road, Zip 72702; tel. 501/521–5731; Lucinda DeBruce, Administrator **A**1 9 10 **F**3 14 18 25 52 53 54 55 56 58 59 65 67 **S**0695 Charter Medical Corporation	33	22	65	820	48	0	0	—	—	104
FAYETTEVILLE CITY HOSPITAL, 221 South School Street, Zip 72701; tel. 501/442–5100; Michael A. McLean R.N., Administrator (Nonreporting) **A**9 10	23	10	144	—	—	—	—	—	—	—
△ NORTHWEST ARKANSAS REHABILITATION HOSPITAL, 153 Monte Painter Drive, Zip 72703; tel. 501/444–2200; Dennis R. Shelby, Administrator (Nonreporting) **A**7 9 10 **S**1715 Continental Medical Systems, Inc.	32	46	60	—	—	—	—	—	—	—
★ VETERANS AFFAIRS MEDICAL CENTER, 1100 North College Avenue, Zip 72703–6995; tel. 501/443–4301; Richard F. Robinson, Director **A**1 9 **F**3 19 20 22 25 26 27 29 30 31 33 34 35 37 41 42 44 45 46 49 51 52 58 60 65 71 73 74 **S**9295 Department of Veterans Affairs	45	10	152	3649	78	76726	0	32366	18048	523
★ WASHINGTON REGIONAL MEDICAL CENTER, 1125 North College Avenue, Zip 72703; tel. 501/442–1000; Patrick D. Flynn, President and Chief Executive Officer (Nonreporting) **A**1 2 3 5 9 10	23	10	223	—	—	—	—	—	—	—
FORDYCE—Dallas County										
DALLAS COUNTY HOSPITAL, 201 Clifton Street, Zip 71742; tel. 501/352–3155; Greg R. McNeil, Administrator (Nonreporting) **A**9 10 **S**2795 Healthcorp of Tennessee, Inc.	33	10	83	—	—	—	—	—	—	—
FORREST CITY—St. Francis County										
★ BAPTIST MEMORIAL HOSPITAL–FORREST CITY, 1601 Newcastle Road, Zip 72335, Mailing Address: P.O. Box 667, Zip 72335; tel. 501/633–2020; George S. Fray, Administrator (Nonreporting) **A**1 9 10 **S**1625 Baptist Memorial Health Care System, Inc.	21	10	76	—	—	—	—	—	—	—
FORT SMITH—Sebastian County										
HARBOR VIEW MERCY HOSPITAL, 10301 Mayo Road, Zip 72903, Mailing Address: P.O. Box 17000, Zip 72917–7000; tel. 501/484–5550; Ron Summerhill, Administrator; Sister Judith Marie Keith, President and Chief Executive Officer **A**9 10 **F**2 3 15 16 19 22 26 32 34 35 52 53 54 55 56 57 58 59 65 67 71 73 **S**5185 Sisters of Mercy Health System–St. Louis	21	22	80	986	47	9111	0	5401	3014	115
★ △ HEALTHSOUTH REHABILITATION HOSPITAL OF FORT SMITH, 1401 South J Street, Zip 72901; tel. 501/785–3300; Stan Johnson, Administrator and Chief Executive Officer **A**1 7 9 10 **F**12 14 15 16 28 29 30 32 41 45 46 48 49 65 66 **S**0023 Healthsouth Corporation	33	46	80	1050	69	19674	0	16320	6794	221

Hospitals, U.S. / ARKANSAS

Hospital, Address, Telephone, Administrator, Approval, Facility, and Physician Codes, Health Care System	Classification Codes		Utilization Data					Expense (thousands) of dollars		
	Control	Service	Beds	Admissions	Census	Outpatient Visits	Births	Total	Payroll	Personnel

★ American Hospital Association (AHA) membership
☐ Joint Commission on Accreditation of Healthcare Organizations (JCAHO) accreditation
+ American Osteopathic Hospital Association (AOHA) membership
○ American Osteopathic Association (AOA) accreditation
△ Commission on Accreditation of Rehabilitation Facilities (CARF) accreditation
Control codes 61, 63, 64, 71, 72 and 73 indicate hospitals listed by AOHA, but not registered by AHA. For definition of numerical codes, see page A6

Hospital	Control	Service	Beds	Admissions	Census	Outpatient Visits	Births	Total	Payroll	Personnel
★ SPARKS REGIONAL MEDICAL CENTER, 1311 South I Street, Zip 72901–4995, Mailing Address: P.O. Box 17006, Zip 72917–7006; tel. 501/441–4000; Charles R. Shuffield, President (Nonreporting) A1 2 3 5 9 10	23	10	442	—	—	—	—	—	—	—
★ ST. EDWARD MERCY MEDICAL CENTER, 7301 Rogers Avenue, Zip 72903, Mailing Address: P.O. Box 17000, Zip 72917–7000; tel. 501/484–6000; Sister Judith Marie Keith, President and Chief Executive Officer A1 2 9 10 F1 3 4 7 8 10 14 15 16 19 20 21 22 24 25 26 29 31 32 33 34 35 37 40 41 42 44 49 52 53 54 55 56 57 58 59 60 63 64 65 67 69 71 72 73 P8 S5185 Sisters of Mercy Health System–St. Louis	21	10	260	12880	227	75839	1425	75785	31298	1165
GRAVETTE—Benton County										
GRAVETTE MEDICAL CENTER HOSPITAL, 1101 Jackson Street S.W., Zip 72736–0470, Mailing Address: P.O. Box 470, Zip 72736–0470; tel. 501/787–5291; John F. Phillips, Administrator A9 10 F8 11 14 19 21 22 28 34 40 44 46 71	23	10	58	2281	24	—	356	5971	3202	161
HARRISON—Boone County										
★ NORTH ARKANSAS MEDICAL CENTER, 620 North Willow Street, Zip 72601; tel. 501/365–2000; Brian L. Clemens, Chief Executive Officer (Total facility includes 14 beds in nursing home–type unit) A9 10 F7 8 10 11 12 14 15 17 19 21 22 23 28 30 32 33 35 37 39 40 41 42 44 45 46 47 49 50 60 63 64 65 71 73 74	13	10	174	3991	52	139329	461	23544	10340	553
HEBER SPRINGS—Cleburne County										
☐ CLEBURNE MEMORIAL HOSPITAL, Highway 110 West, Zip 72543–1087, Mailing Address: P.O. Box 1087, Zip 72543–1087; tel. 501/362–3121; Harrell E. Clendenin, President and Chief Executive Officer (Nonreporting) A1 9 10	23	10	25	—	—	—	—	—	—	—
HELENA—Phillips County										
★ HELENA REGIONAL MEDICAL CENTER, 1801 Martin Luther King Jr., Zip 72342, Mailing Address: Box 788, Zip 72342–0788; tel. 501/338–5800; Steve Reeder, Chief Executive Officer (Nonreporting) A1 9 10 S0002 Quorum Health Group/Quorum Health Resources	23	10	100	—	—	—	—	—	—	—
HOPE—Hempstead County										
★ MEDICAL PARK HOSPITAL, 2001 South Main Street, Zip 71801; tel. 501/777–2323; Allen Golson, Executive Director (Nonreporting) A1 9 10 S0048 Columbia/HCA Healthcare Corporation	33	10	91	—	—	—	—	—	—	—
HOT SPRINGS—Garland County										
AMI NATIONAL PARK MEDICAL CENTER See National Park Medical Center										
★ NATIONAL PARK MEDICAL CENTER, (Formerly AMI National Park Medical Center) 1910 Malvern Avenue, Zip 71901; tel. 501/321–1000; Jerry D. Mabry, Executive Director A1 9 10 F7 8 10 12 16 19 21 22 23 28 29 32 33 34 35 37 40 42 44 48 52 55 56 57 63 64 65 71 73 74 P1 2 4 5 7 8 S0063 TENET Healthcare Corporation	33	10	166	5239	93	34605	566	30613	11333	614
★ ST. JOSEPH'S REGIONAL HEALTH CENTER, 300 Werner Street, Zip 71913; tel. 501/622–1000; Randall J. Fale, President and Chief Executive Officer (Total facility includes 40 beds in nursing home–type unit) A1 2 9 10 F4 7 8 10 12 15 16 17 19 22 26 27 28 29 30 32 34 36 39 40 41 42 43 44 45 46 48 49 60 64 65 66 67 71 73 74 P7 S5185 Sisters of Mercy Health System–St. Louis	21	10	276	11853	203	141501	670	82718	33414	1296
HOT SPRINGS NATIONAL PARK—Garland County										
★ LEVI HOSPITAL, 300 Prospect Avenue, Hot Springs Natl Pk, Zip 71901, Mailing Address: P.O. Box 850, Zip 71902; tel. 501/624–1281; Patrick McCabe Jr., Executive Director (Nonreporting) A1 9 10	23	46	86	—	—	—	—	—	—	—
JACKSONVILLE—Pulaski County										
★ △ REBSAMEN REGIONAL MEDICAL CENTER, 1400 West Braden Street, Zip 72076, Mailing Address: Box 159, Zip 72078–0159; tel. 501/985–7000; Thomas R. Siemers, Administrator (Nonreporting) A1 7 9 10 S0002 Quorum Health Group/Quorum Health Resources	14	10	113	—	—	—	—	—	—	—
★ U.S. AIR FORCE HOSPITAL LITTLE ROCK, Little Rock Air Force Base, Zip 72099–5057; tel. 501/988–7411; Colonel Norman L. Sims MSC, USAF, Commander A1 9 F14 15 16 34 44 51 71 S9495 Department of the Air Force	41	10	20	1131	9	167448	0	—	—	378
JONESBORO—Craighead County										
☐ GREENLEAF CENTER, 2712 East Johnson, Zip 72401; tel. 501/932–2800; John S. Hart, Administrator (Nonreporting) A1 10 S1155 Greenleaf Health Systems, Inc.	33	22	48	—	—	—	—	—	—	—
★ METHODIST HOSPITAL OF JONESBORO, 3024 Stadium Boulevard, Zip 72401; tel. 501/972–7000; Philip H. Walkley Jr., Administrator A1 9 10 F7 8 10 11 12 17 19 20 21 22 26 28 29 30 32 35 38 39 40 44 45 46 49 54 65 67 69 71 73 74 P8 S9345 Methodist Health Systems, Inc.	21	10	104	4562	52	26175	1143	18841	6563	339
★ △ NORTHEAST ARKANSAS REHABILITATION HOSPITAL, 1201 Fleming Avenue, Zip 72401, Mailing Address: P.O. Box 1680, Zip 72403–1680; tel. 501/932–0440; Wayne A. Sensor, Chief Executive Officer A1 7 9 10 F12 15 16 17 19 25 28 30 34 48 49 65 66 67 69 71 P8	33	46	54	889	52	8844	0	10280	4575	174
★ ST. BERNARDS REGIONAL MEDICAL CENTER, 224 East Matthews Street, Zip 72401, Mailing Address: P.O. Box 9320, Zip 72403–9320; tel. 501/972–4100; Ben E. Owens, President (Total facility includes 18 beds in nursing home–type unit) A1 2 3 5 9 10 F4 7 8 10 11 12 13 14 15 16 17 19 21 22 23 24 27 29 30 31 32 33 34 35 37 40 41 42 43 44 45 49 51 60 64 65 66 67 69 71 73 74 P8	21	10	291	14658	226	61684	1114	—	—	1257

© 1995 AHA Guide

Hospitals, U.S. / ARKANSAS

Hospital, Address, Telephone, Administrator, Approval, Facility, and Physician Codes, Health Care System	Classification Codes		Utilization Data					Expense (thousands) of dollars		Personnel
	Control	Service	Beds	Admissions	Census	Outpatient Visits	Births	Total	Payroll	

★ American Hospital Association (AHA) membership
□ Joint Commission on Accreditation of Healthcare Organizations (JCAHO) accreditation
+ American Osteopathic Hospital Association (AOHA) membership
○ American Osteopathic Association (AOA) accreditation
△ Commission on Accreditation of Rehabilitation Facilities (CARF) accreditation
Control codes 61, 63, 64, 71, 72 and 73 indicate hospitals listed by AOHA, but not registered by AHA. For definition of numerical codes, see page A6

Hospital	Control	Service	Beds	Admissions	Census	Outpatient Visits	Births	Total	Payroll	Personnel
LAKE VILLAGE—Chicot County										
★ CHICOT MEMORIAL HOSPITAL, Highway 65 and 82, Zip 71653-0000, Mailing Address: Box 512, Zip 71653-0441; tel. 501/265-5351; Robert R. Reddish, Administrator A9 10 F7 8 11 14 19 22 28 32 33 34 37 40 44 45 53 56 57 65 67 71 73 P3 S0002 Quorum Health Group/Quorum Health Resources	13	10	54	2382	29	14269	203	7961	3891	170
LITTLE ROCK—Pulaski County										
★ △ ARKANSAS CHILDREN'S HOSPITAL, 800 Marshall Street, Zip 72202-3591; tel. 501/320-1100; Jonathan R. Bates M.D., Chief Executive Officer A1 3 5 7 8 9 10 F4 9 10 11 12 14 19 20 22 24 25 27 28 30 31 34 35 38 39 42 43 44 46 47 48 49 51 52 53 54 56 58 59 63 65 67 69 71 73 P8	23	50	268	9342	200	253300	0	150581	70602	2376
★ ARKANSAS STATE HOSPITAL, 4313 West Markham Street, Zip 72205-4096; tel. 501/686-9000; Bob Davis, Administrator (Nonreporting) A1 3 5 9 10	12	22	192	—	—	—	—	—	—	—
★ BAPTIST MEDICAL CENTER, 9601 Interstate 630, Exit 7, Zip 72205-7299; tel. 501/227-2000; Steven B. Lampkin, Senior Vice President and Administrator A1 3 5 6 9 10 F2 3 4 7 8 10 11 12 13 15 16 17 18 19 20 21 22 23 24 25 26 27 28 29 30 31 32 33 34 35 37 38 39 40 41 42 43 44 45 46 48 52 53 54 55 56 57 60 61 63 64 65 66 67 68 69 70 71 72 73 74 P1 5 7 S0355 Baptist Medical System	23	10	641	26225	461	175591	2207	205176	77759	2643
★ △ BAPTIST REHABILITATION INSTITUTE OF ARKANSAS, 9601 Interstate 630, Exit 7, Zip 72205-7249; tel. 501/223-7000; Doug Weeks, Vice President and Administrator A1 3 5 7 9 10 F2 3 4 5 7 8 9 10 11 12 14 15 16 17 19 21 22 23 24 27 28 29 30 31 32 33 34 35 37 38 39 40 41 42 43 44 45 46 47 48 49 51 52 53 54 55 56 57 58 59 60 62 63 64 65 66 67 68 69 70 71 72 73 74 P7 S0355 Baptist Medical System	23	46	120	1286	67	65500	0	14956	7210	221
★ COLUMBIA DOCTORS HOSPITAL, (Formerly Doctors Hospital) 6101 West Capitol, Zip 72205-5331; tel. 501/661-4000; W. Perry Kinder, President and Chief Executive Officer A1 9 10 F4 7 8 10 11 12 14 15 16 19 21 22 29 30 35 37 38 40 41 42 43 44 45 46 48 49 52 59 63 64 65 67 71 73 74 P4 5 S0048 Columbia/HCA Healthcare Corporation	33	10	189	7286	103	24668	2041	—	—	584
□ CPC PINNACLE POINTE HOSPITAL, 11501 Financial Center Parkway, Zip 72211-3715; tel. 501/223-3322; Pat Perry, Chief Executive Officer A1 10 F2 3 12 16 17 27 29 41 52 53 54 55 56 57 58 59 65 67 S0785 Community Psychiatric Centers	33	22	102	803	62	2916	0	—	—	83
DOCTORS HOSPITAL See Columbia Doctors Hospital										
□ SOUTHWEST HOSPITAL, 11401 Interstate 30, Zip 72209; tel. 501/455-7100; Timothy E. Hill, President and Chief Executive Officer A1 9 10 F8 10 11 15 16 19 21 22 26 27 30 35 40 41 44 46 49 51 52 57 64 65 71 73 74 P6	23	10	125	2684	46	23018	239	17546	7798	294
★ ST. VINCENT INFIRMARY MEDICAL CENTER, Two St. Vincent Circle, Zip 72205-5499; tel. 501/660-3000; Thomas L. Feurig, President and Chief Executive Officer (Total facility includes 52 beds in nursing home-type unit) A1 2 3 5 9 10 F2 3 4 7 8 10 11 12 13 14 15 16 17 19 20 21 22 23 25 27 28 29 30 31 32 33 34 35 37 38 40 42 43 44 45 46 47 48 49 52 54 55 56 57 58 59 63 64 65 66 67 70 71 73 74 P2 4 7 8 S3045 Sisters of Charity of Nazareth Health System	21	10	566	20119	404	135732	726	178355	75943	2510
★ UNIVERSITY HOSPITAL OF ARKANSAS, 4301 West Markham Street, Zip 72205; tel. 501/686-7000; Richard Pierson, Vice Chancellor Clinical Program (Nonreporting) A1 2 3 5 8 9 10	12	10	325	—	—	—	—	—	—	—
★ VETERANS AFFAIRS MEDICAL CENTER, (Includes Little Rock Division) 4300 West Seventh Street, Zip 72205-5484; tel. 501/661-1202; Robert D. Shimp, Associate Director (Total facility includes 196 beds in nursing home-type unit) A1 2 3 5 8 9 F1 2 3 4 5 6 8 10 11 12 17 19 20 21 22 24 26 28 30 31 32 33 34 35 37 39 41 42 43 44 45 46 48 49 51 52 54 55 56 57 58 59 60 63 64 65 67 71 73 74 P6 S9295 Department of Veterans Affairs	45	10	958	16421	803	288128	0	209212	107568	2048
LITTLE ROCK AIR FORCE BASE—Pulaski County										
U.S. AIR FORCE HOSPITAL See Little Rock										
MAGNOLIA—Columbia County										
★ MAGNOLIA HOSPITAL, 101 Hospital Drive, Zip 71753-2416, Mailing Address: Box 629, Zip 71753-0629; tel. 501/235-3000; William D. Hedden, Administrator A1 9 10 F19 22 32 34 37 39 40 44 45 65 71 73	14	10	65	2245	31	15562	196	8876	5462	221
MALVERN—Hot Spring County										
★ HOT SPRING COUNTY MEMORIAL HOSPITAL, 1001 Schneider Drive, Zip 72104; tel. 501/337-4911; Jeff Curtis, Administrator A9 10 F7 8 11 19 21 22 28 32 37 40 44 51 52 54 56 57 71 73 P8	15	10	77	2867	46	53179	97	12311	6148	338
MAUMELLE—Pulaski County										
□ CHARTER HOSPITAL OF LITTLE ROCK, 1601 Murphy Drive, Zip 72113; tel. 501/851-8700; Joseph Fischer, Administrator (Nonreporting) A1 10 S0695 Charter Medical Corporation	33	22	60	—	—	—	—	—	—	—
MCGEHEE—Desha County										
★ MCGEHEE-DESHA COUNTY HOSPITAL, 900 South Third, Zip 71654-0351, Mailing Address: Box 351, Zip 71654-0351; tel. 501/222-5600; William A. Conway, Administrator (Nonreporting) A1 9 10	13	10	34	—	—	—	—	—	—	—
MENA—Polk County										
□ MENA MEDICAL CENTER, 311 North Morrow Street, Zip 71953; tel. 501/394-6100; Albert Pilkington III, Administrator and Chief Executive Officer A1 9 10 F7 14 19 22 32 34 37 44 49 71	14	10	36	1524	15	37234	221	6436	2875	149

Hospitals, U.S. / ARKANSAS

Hospital, Address, Telephone, Administrator, Approval, Facility, and Physician Codes, Health Care System	Classification Codes		Utilization Data					Expense (thousands) of dollars		Personnel
	Control	Service	Beds	Admissions	Census	Outpatient Visits	Births	Total	Payroll	

★ American Hospital Association (AHA) membership
☐ Joint Commission on Accreditation of Healthcare Organizations (JCAHO) accreditation
+ American Osteopathic Hospital Association (AOHA) membership
○ American Osteopathic Association (AOA) accreditation
△ Commission on Accreditation of Rehabilitation Facilities (CARF) accreditation
Control codes 61, 63, 64, 71, 72 and 73 indicate hospitals listed by AOHA, but not registered by AHA. For definition of numerical codes, see page A6

Hospital	Control	Service	Beds	Admissions	Census	Outpatient Visits	Births	Total	Payroll	Personnel
MONTICELLO—Drew County ★ DREW MEMORIAL HOSPITAL, 778 Scogin Drive, Zip 71655–5728; tel. 501/367–2411; Jerry W. Bradshaw, Chief Executive Officer (Nonreporting) A9 10 S0002 Quorum Health Group/Quorum Health Resources	13	10	50	—	—	—	—	—	—	—
MORRILTON—Conway County ★ CONWAY COUNTY HOSPITAL, 4 Hospital Drive, Zip 72110–4510; tel. 501/354–3512; Johnson L. Smith, Chief Executive Officer and Administrator A9 10 F7 11 16 19 22 32 34 37 44 49 65 71 73	21	10	52	1738	24	16928	97	8325	3917	205
MOUNTAIN HOME—Baxter County ▣ BAXTER COUNTY REGIONAL HOSPITAL, 624 Hospital Drive, Zip 72653; tel. 501/424–1000; H. William Anderson, Administrator (Total facility includes 25 beds in nursing home–type unit) A1 2 9 10 F7 8 10 12 14 19 21 22 23 28 32 33 34 35 37 40 41 42 44 45 49 60 64 65 66 67 71 73 74 P1	23	10	197	8804	124	52769	568	44666	19743	878
MOUNTAIN VIEW—Stone County STONE COUNTY MEDICAL CENTER, Highway 14 East, Zip 72560–0510, Mailing Address: P.O. Box 510, Zip 72560; tel. 501/269–4361; Stanley Townsend, Administrator A9 10 F8 19 21 22 32 33 44 65 71 P5	33	10	48	912	17	12116	34	4098	1798	78
MURFREESBORO—Pike County PIKE COUNTY MEMORIAL HOSPITAL, 315 East 13th Street, Zip 71958; tel. 501/285–3182; Dolly Wylie, Administrator A9 10 F11 19 22 34 64 71	13	10	32	541	7	4554	0	1530	852	46
NASHVILLE—Howard County ★ HOWARD MEMORIAL HOSPITAL, 800 West Leslie Street, Zip 71852–0381, Mailing Address: Box 381, Zip 71852 0381; tel. 501/845–4400; Lynn Crowell, Chief Executive Officer A9 10 F8 15 16 19 21 22 28 29 30 32 33 37 39 44 46 49 69 71 73 P3 S0002 Quorum Health Group/Quorum Health Resources	23	10	50	1052	15	25008	0	7203	2839	143
NEWPORT—Jackson County ☐ HARRIS HOSPITAL, 1205 McLain Street, Zip 72112; tel. 501/523–8911; Ronald T. Seal, Executive Director A1 9 10 F8 11 12 14 15 16 17 19 20 21 22 26 32 35 39 44 46 52 57 61 65 71 73 74 S5895 Hallmark Healthcare Corporation	33	10	88	2906	40	14871	450	13154	4894	187
★ NEWPORT HOSPITAL AND CLINIC, 2000 McLain Street, Zip 72112; tel. 501/523–6721; Eugene Zuber, Administrator A9 10 F8 10 11 17 19 21 22 28 30 31 32 34 40 42 44 71 73	33	10	86	2462	33	14230	169	8432	3636	167
NORTH LITTLE ROCK—Pulaski County ▣ BAPTIST MEMORIAL MEDICAL CENTER, One Pershing Circle, Zip 72114–1899; tel. 501/771–3000; Harrison M. Dean, Senior Vice President & Administrator A1 9 10 F4 7 8 10 11 12 13 14 16 17 19 21 22 23 24 28 29 30 31 32 33 34 35 37 39 40 41 42 43 44 45 46 49 51 52 55 56 58 60 62 64 65 66 67 69 71 72 73 74 P1 5 7 S0355 Baptist Medical System	23	10	200	7979	108	63590	586	50935	19152	452
☐ BRIDGEWAY, 21 Bridgeway Road, Zip 72113; tel. 501/771–1500; Barry Pipkin, Director (Nonreporting) A1 9 10 S9555 Universal Health Services, Inc.	33	22	70	—	—	—	—	—	—	—
VETERANS AFFAIRS HOSPITAL See Veterans Affairs Medical Center, Little Rock										
OSCEOLA—Mississippi County ▣ BAPTIST MEMORIAL HOSPITAL–OSCEOLA, 611 West Lee Avenue, Zip 72370, Mailing Address: Box 607, Zip 72370–0607; tel. 501/563–7000; Al Sypniewski, Administrator (Nonreporting) A1 9 10 S1625 Baptist Memorial Health Care System, Inc.	21	10	72	—	—	—	—	—	—	—
OZARK—Franklin County ★ MERCY HOSPITAL–TURNER MEMORIAL, 801 West River, Zip 72949; tel. 501/667–4138; Sister Mary Werner Keith, Administrator A9 10 F2 3 4 7 8 10 11 14 15 16 19 21 22 25 27 28 31 32 33 34 35 37 38 39 40 41 42 43 44 47 52 53 54 55 56 57 58 59 60 62 64 65 71 73 P1 S5185 Sisters of Mercy Health System–St. Louis	23	10	39	553	8	6819	0	2333	1089	51
PARAGOULD—Greene County ▣ ARKANSAS METHODIST HOSPITAL, 900 West Kingshighway, Zip 72450, Mailing Address: Box 339, Zip 72450; tel. 501/239–7000; Ronald K. Rooney, President A1 9 10 F7 8 10 12 14 16 19 22 28 30 32 33 34 35 37 39 40 44 45 46 49 65 71 73	23	10	129	3867	53	—	386	16945	6864	0
PARIS—Logan County ★ NORTH LOGAN MERCY HOSPITAL, 500 East Academy, Zip 72855–4099; tel. 501/963–6101; Jim L. Maddox, Chief Administrative Officer A9 10 F2 3 4 7 8 9 10 11 14 15 16 19 20 21 22 25 28 30 31 32 33 34 35 37 38 39 40 41 42 43 44 47 50 52 53 54 55 56 57 58 59 60 64 65 69 71 73 P1 S5185 Sisters of Mercy Health System–St. Louis	21	10	16	472	6	8358	0	2283	916	43
PIGGOTT—Clay County ★ PIGGOTT COMMUNITY HOSPITAL, 1206 Highway 62 West, Zip 72454; tel. 501/598–3881; Betty J. Reams, Executive Director A9 10 F19 22 27 32 44 49 65 67 71	14	10	35	1037	16	5300	0	4689	2314	107
PINE BLUFF—Jefferson County ▣ JEFFERSON REGIONAL MEDICAL CENTER, 1515 West 42nd Avenue, Zip 71603–7089; tel. 501/541–7100; Robert P. Atkinson, President and Chief Executive Officer (Total facility includes 109 beds in nursing home–type unit) A1 2 3 5 6 9 10 F2 3 4 6 7 8 10 11 12 13 14 15 16 17 18 19 21 22 23 24 25 26 27 28 29 30 31 32 33 34 35 37 38 39 40 41 42 43 44 45 46 48 49 51 52 53 54 55 56 57 58 59 60 61 63 64 65 66 67 68 70 71 72 73 74 P7	23	10	481	12655	310	80096	1624	85972	35875	1459

© 1995 AHA Guide

Hospitals, U.S. / ARKANSAS

Hospital, Address, Telephone, Administrator, Approval, Facility, and Physician Codes, Health Care System	Classification Codes		Utilization Data					Expense (thousands) of dollars		
★ American Hospital Association (AHA) membership □ Joint Commission on Accreditation of Healthcare Organizations (JCAHO) accreditation + American Osteopathic Hospital Association (AOHA) membership ○ American Osteopathic Association (AOA) accreditation △ Commission on Accreditation of Rehabilitation Facilities (CARF) accreditation Control codes 61, 63, 64, 71, 72 and 73 indicate hospitals listed by AOHA, but not registered by AHA. For definition of numerical codes, see page A6	Control	Service	Beds	Admissions	Census	Outpatient Visits	Births	Total	Payroll	Personnel
POCAHONTAS—Randolph County □ RANDOLPH COUNTY MEDICAL CENTER, 2801 Medical Center Drive, Zip 72455; tel. 501/892–4511; Michael J. McBride, Executive Director **A**1 9 10 **F**19 21 22 28 32 34 37 44 49 52 57 65 71 **S**5895 Hallmark Healthcare Corporation	33	10	50	1004	16	13132	0	7403	2281	114
PRESCOTT—Nevada County NEVADA COUNTY HOSPITAL, 1467 West First North, Zip 71857, Mailing Address: Box 707, Zip 71857; tel. 501/887–2681; Karen Ward, Administrator **A**9 10 **F**2 22 32 44 49 71	13	10	49	920	12	3601	0	3149	1518	108
ROGERS—Benton County ★ ST. MARY–ROGERS MEMORIAL HOSPITAL, 1200 West Walnut Street, Zip 72756–3599; tel. 501/636–0200; Sister Sharon Therese Zayac, President **A**1 2 9 10 **F**1 7 8 10 11 12 14 15 16 17 19 21 22 24 28 30 32 33 34 35 36 38 39 40 42 44 49 63 64 65 67 71 73 **P**5 **S**1295 Dominican Sisters of Springfield	21	10	92	5973	68	40663	1065	31952	16294	605
RUSSELLVILLE—Pope County ★ △ ST. MARY'S REGIONAL MEDICAL CENTER, (Formerly AMI St. Mary's Regional Medical Center) 1808 West Main Street, Zip 72801; tel. 501/968–2841; William L. Bradley, Executive Director **A**1 7 10 **F**7 8 10 11 12 14 16 17 19 20 21 22 23 25 30 32 33 34 35 37 39 40 41 42 44 46 48 49 54 56 60 63 65 66 71 73 74 **P**6 7 **S**0063 TENET Healthcare Corporation	33	10	155	5221	81	29727	954	29353	8236	396
SALEM—Fulton County FULTON COUNTY HOSPITAL, Highway 9, Zip 72576, Mailing Address: P.O. Box 517, Zip 72576; tel. 501/895–2691; Franklin E. Wise, Administrator **A**9 10 **F**8 19 22 32 40 44 64 71	13	10	30	862	10	15388	86	3032	1523	89
SEARCY—White County ★ CENTRAL ARKANSAS HOSPITAL, 1200 South Main, Zip 72143; tel. 501/278–3131; David C. Laffoon, Executive Director **A**1 2 9 10 **F**7 10 11 12 14 15 16 19 22 32 35 37 38 40 42 44 48 60 65 71 74 **P**6 7 8 **S**0063 TENET Healthcare Corporation	33	10	149	5291	72	53226	474	20050	8922	352
★ WHITE COUNTY MEMORIAL HOSPITAL, 3214 East Race, Zip 72143–4847; tel. 501/268–6121; Raymond W. Montgomery II, Administrator and Chief Executive Officer **A**1 2 9 10 **F**7 10 11 12 15 19 21 22 28 30 31 32 33 35 37 40 42 44 45 46 49 65 66 71	13	10	95	5020	58	28136	651	18955	8675	433
SHERWOOD—Pulaski County □ △ CENTRAL ARKANSAS REHABILITATION HOSPITAL, 2201 Wildwood Avenue, Zip 72116, Mailing Address: P.O. Box 6930, North Little Rock Zip 72116–6930; tel. 501/834–1800; Douglas W. Parker, Chief Executive Officer **A**1 7 9 10 **F**12 15 48 49 66 73 **P**5 **S**1715 Continental Medical Systems, Inc.	32	46	60	740	46	8000	0	11144	4467	148
SILOAM SPRINGS—Benton County ★ MEMORIAL HOSPITAL, 205 East Jefferson Street, Zip 72761; tel. 501/524–4141; Donald E. Patterson, Administrator **A**1 9 10 **F**7 8 11 19 21 22 30 32 34 37 40 44 46 64 65 67 71 73 **S**0002 Quorum Health Group/Quorum Health Resources	14	10	73	1971	29	15559	116	9934	4228	218
SPRINGDALE—Washington County ★ NORTHWEST MEDICAL CENTER, 607 Maple Street, Zip 72764, Mailing Address: P.O. Box 47, Zip 72765; tel. 501/751–5711; Hugh D. Means, Chief Executive Officer (Total facility includes 18 beds in nursing home–type unit) **A**1 2 9 10 **F**4 7 8 10 11 12 15 16 17 19 20 21 22 26 28 29 30 32 33 34 35 37 38 39 40 42 43 44 45 48 49 52 53 56 58 59 60 61 63 64 65 67 71 73 74 **P**3 5	23	10	204	7409	112	50519	448	55781	23474	1084
STUTTGART—Arkansas County ★ STUTTGART MEMORIAL HOSPITAL, North Buerkle Road, Zip 72160, Mailing Address: Box 1905, Zip 72160; tel. 501/673–3511; Jim E. Bushmaier, Administrator and Chief Executive Officer (Nonreporting) **A**1 9 10	23	10	89	—	—	—	—	—	—	—
VAN BUREN—Crawford County □ CRAWFORD MEMORIAL HOSPITAL, East Main & South 20th Streets, Zip 72956, Mailing Address: Box 409, Zip 72956; tel. 501/474–3401; J. Phillip Young, Administrator (Nonreporting) **A**1 9 10 **S**1775 Health Management Associates	33	10	103	—	—	—	—	—	—	—
WALDRON—Scott County ★ MERCY HOSPITAL OF SCOTT COUNTY, (Formerly Mercy Hospital) Highways 71 and 80, Zip 72958–9984, Mailing Address: Box 2230, Zip 72958–2230; tel. 501/637–4135; Sister Mary Alvera Simon, Administrator (Total facility includes 105 beds in nursing home–type unit) **A**9 10 **F**8 14 15 19 22 29 30 32 34 44 64 65 71 73 **P**3 **S**5185 Sisters of Mercy Health System–St. Louis	21	10	129	492	109	9754	0	2678	1074	49
WALNUT RIDGE—Lawrence County □ LAWRENCE MEMORIAL HOSPITAL, (Includes Lawrence Hall Nursing Home) 1309 West Main, Zip 72476–0839, Mailing Address: Box 839, Zip 72476; tel. 501/886–1200; Larry Morse, Administration (Nonreporting) **A**1 9 10	13	10	194	—	—	—	—	—	—	—
WARREN—Bradley County ★ BRADLEY COUNTY MEMORIAL HOSPITAL, 404 South Bradley Street, Zip 71671; tel. 501/226–3731; Harry H. Stevens, Administrator **A**1 9 10 **F**7 8 11 12 15 16 17 19 20 21 22 32 33 34 44 46 49 61 65 67 71 73	13	10	49	1762	20	13920	157	6777	3248	185
WEST MEMPHIS—Crittenden County □ CRITTENDEN MEMORIAL HOSPITAL, 200 Tyler Street, Zip 72301, Mailing Address: Box 2248, Zip 72303–2248; tel. 501/735–1500; Ross Hooper, Chief Executive Officer **A**1 9 10 **F**14 15 17 19 21 22 24 25 27 28 30 32 33 34 35 37 44 46 48 49 56 65 69 71 73	23	10	113	3625	60	30742	0	24869	12031	471

Hospitals, U.S. / ARKANSAS

Hospital, Address, Telephone, Administrator, Approval, Facility, and Physician Codes, Health Care System	Classi-fication Codes		Utilization Data					Expense (thousands) of dollars		
★ American Hospital Association (AHA) membership ☐ Joint Commission on Accreditation of Healthcare Organizations (JCAHO) accreditation + American Osteopathic Hospital Association (AOHA) membership ○ American Osteopathic Association (AOA) accreditation △ Commission on Accreditation of Rehabilitation Facilities (CARF) accreditation Control codes 61, 63, 64, 71, 72 and 73 indicate hospitals listed by AOHA, but not registered by AHA. For definition of numerical codes, see page A6	Control	Service	Beds	Admissions	Census	Outpatient Visits	Births	Total	Payroll	Personnel
WYNNE—Cross County ★ CROSS COUNTY HOSPITAL, 310 South Falls Boulevard, Zip 72396, Mailing Address: P.O. Drawer H, Zip 72396; tel. 501/238–3300; Harry M. Baker, Chief Executive Officer **A**9 10 **F**11 15 19 22 32 40 44 65 71	13	10	53	1737	23	12601	159	6354	2925	148

Hospitals, U.S. / CALIFORNIA

CALIFORNIA

Resident population 31,211 (in thousands)
Resident population in metro areas 96.7%
Birth rate per 1,000 population 20.1
65 years and over 10.6%
Percent of persons without health insurance 19.0%

Hospital, Address, Telephone, Administrator, Approval, Facility, and Physician Codes, Health Care System	Classification Codes		Utilization Data					Expense (thousands) of dollars		
	Control	Service	Beds	Admissions	Census	Outpatient Visits	Births	Total	Payroll	Personnel

★ American Hospital Association (AHA) membership
☐ Joint Commission on Accreditation of Healthcare Organizations (JCAHO) accreditation
+ American Osteopathic Hospital Association (AOHA) membership
○ American Osteopathic Association (AOA) accreditation
△ Commission on Accreditation of Rehabilitation Facilities (CARF) accreditation
Control codes 61, 63, 64, 71, 72 and 73 indicate hospitals listed by AOHA, but not registered by AHA. For definition of numerical codes, see page A6

ALAMEDA—Alameda County

★ ALAMEDA HOSPITAL, 2070 Clinton Avenue, Zip 94501; tel. 510/522–3700; William J. Dal Cielo, Chief Executive Officer (Total facility includes 23 beds in nursing home–type unit) **A**1 9 10 **F**7 8 11 16 19 21 22 26 28 29 31 32 33 34 35 37 39 40 41 42 44 45 48 49 52 57 63 64 71 73 **P**1 4 5 6 7	23	10	98	3293	58	33187	406	33106	18264	385

ALHAMBRA—Los Angeles County

☐ ALHAMBRA HOSPITAL, 100 South Raymond Avenue, Zip 91801, Mailing Address: Box 510, Zip 91802–0510; tel. 818/570–1606; Timothy McGlew, Acting Chief Executive Officer (Nonreporting) **A**1 2 9 10	32	10	59	—	—	—	—	—	—	—

ALTURAS—Modoc County

★ MODOC MEDICAL CENTER, 228 McDowell Street, Zip 96101; tel. 916/233–5131; Donna M. Donald, Chief Executive Officer (Total facility includes 71 beds in nursing home–type unit) **A**9 10 **F**7 8 13 15 17 22 28 30 32 34 44 49 64 65 71	13	10	87	379	64	20085	64	6135	2567	130

ANAHEIM—Orange County

☐ ANAHEIM GENERAL HOSPITAL, 3350 West Ball Road, Zip 92804–9998; tel. 714/827–6700; Peter A. Szekrenyi Ph.D., Executive Director **A**1 9 10 **F**4 8 11 12 15 19 22 26 27 31 32 34 35 37 39 40 41 42 44 49 51 65 71 74 **P**5 **S**0435 Pacific Health Corporation	32	10	99	3398	45	—	592	16358	9761	291
★ ANAHEIM MEMORIAL HOSPITAL, 1111 West La Palma Avenue, Zip 92801, Mailing Address: Box 3005, Zip 92803; tel. 714/774–1450; Chris D. Van Gorder, President and Chief Executive Officer **A**1 2 9 10 **F**4 7 8 10 11 12 17 18 19 21 22 27 28 29 30 32 33 34 35 37 38 39 40 41 42 43 44 45 46 49 64 65 66 67 71 73 **P**5 7	23	10	173	6367	97	40175	0	62394	26231	785
★ KAISER FOUNDATION HOSPITAL, 441 North Lakeview Avenue, Zip 92807; tel. 714/978–4100; Gerald A. McCall, Administrator **A**1 2 3 9 10 **F**2 3 4 7 8 9 10 11 12 13 14 15 16 17 18 19 21 22 23 28 29 30 31 32 33 35 37 38 39 40 41 42 43 44 45 46 47 48 49 51 52 53 54 55 57 58 59 60 61 63 64 65 67 68 69 71 72 73 **P**4 **S**2105 Kaiser Foundation Hospitals	23	10	158	8549	89	51014	2529	—	—	840
★ MARTIN LUTHER HOSPITAL– ANEHEIM, 1830 West Romneya Drive, Zip 92801–1854, Mailing Address: Box 3304, Zip 92803–3304; tel. 714/491–5200; John R. Cochran III, President and Chief Executive Officer (Total facility includes 22 beds in nursing home–type unit) **A**1 2 9 10 **F**1 3 4 7 8 9 10 11 12 13 15 16 17 18 19 20 21 23 27 28 29 30 32 33 35 37 38 39 40 41 42 43 44 45 46 48 49 51 53 54 55 56 57 58 59 60 61 64 65 66 67 68 69 70 71 72 73 74 **P**3 5 7 **S**2315 UniHealth	23	10	200	6947	81	53534	2311	50509	22580	571
★ WEST ANAHEIM MEDICAL CENTER, 3033 West Orange Avenue, Zip 92804–3184; tel. 714/827–3000; David Culberson, Chief Executive Officer (Total facility includes 22 beds in nursing home–type unit) **A**1 2 9 10 **F**5 7 8 10 11 12 15 16 19 22 27 28 30 32 33 34 35 37 40 41 42 43 44 45 49 61 64 65 67 70 71 73 **P**5 **S**0048 Columbia/HCA Healthcare Corporation	33	10	243	7647	85	26660	1398	—	—	519
★ WESTERN MEDICAL CENTER HOSPITAL ANAHEIM, 1025 South Anaheim Boulevard, Zip 92805; tel. 714/533–6220; Daniel L. Frank, Chief Executive Officer **A**1 9 10 **F**4 7 10 12 14 15 16 19 21 22 28 32 35 37 40 41 43 44 46 48 49 52 53 54 55 56 58 59 65 71 73 **P**4 7 **S**2085 United Western Medical Centers	23	10	171	4842	85	55830	1378	50387	15479	525

ANTIOCH—Contra Costa County

☐ DELTA MEMORIAL HOSPITAL, 3901 Lone Tree Way, Zip 94509; tel. 510/779–7200; Linda Horn, Administrator **A**1 9 10 **F**1 2 3 4 7 8 10 11 12 13 14 15 16 17 18 19 20 21 22 23 24 25 26 27 28 29 30 31 32 33 34 35 36 37 38 39 40 41 42 43 44 45 46 47 48 49 51 52 60 61 64 65 66 67 69 70 71 72 73 74 **P**2 3 4 5 6 7 8 **S**8795 Sutter Health	23	10	111	4848	52	23821	1110	39543	16558	325

APPLE VALLEY—San Bernardino County

★ ST. MARY DESERT VALLEY HOSPITAL, 18300 Highway 18, Zip 92307–0725, Mailing Address: Box 7025, Zip 92307–0725; tel. 619/242–2311; Thomas G. Neff, President **A**1 2 9 10 **F**7 8 10 12 15 16 17 19 21 22 26 28 29 30 31 32 33 34 35 37 40 42 44 45 49 60 63 65 67 71 73 **P**3 5 **S**5425 St. Joseph Health System	21	10	109	8732	85	50942	1923	42798	15433	435

ARCADIA—Los Angeles County

★ METHODIST HOSPITAL OF SOUTHERN CALIFORNIA, 300 West Huntington Drive, Zip 91007, Mailing Address: P.O. Box 60016, Zip 91066–6016; tel. 818/445–4441; Dennis M. Lee, President (Total facility includes 26 beds in nursing home–type unit) **A**1 2 9 10 **F**4 7 8 10 11 12 17 19 21 22 28 30 32 33 34 36 37 38 39 40 41 42 43 44 48 49 52 54 55 56 57 58 59 60 64 65 66 67 70 71 73 **P**1 3 5 7	23	10	304	10639	157	62403	896	77522	35902	882

ARCATA—Humboldt County

☐ MAD RIVER COMMUNITY HOSPITAL, 3800 Janes Road, Zip 95521, Mailing Address: P.O. Box 1115, Zip 95521–1115; tel. 707/822–3621; Michael Young, Administrator (Nonreporting) **A**1 9 10	33	10	78	—	—	—	—	—	—	—

ARROYO GRANDE—San Luis Obispo County

☐ ARROYO GRANDE COMMUNITY HOSPITAL, 345 South Halcyon Road, Zip 93420; tel. 805/489–4261; Richard N. Woolslayer, Chief Executive Officer **A**1 9 10 **F**4 8 15 19 21 22 26 28 31 33 34 35 37 42 44 49 65 66 71	23	10	34	2404	28	43828	0	17187	5900	212

Hospitals, U.S. / CALIFORNIA

Hospital, Address, Telephone, Administrator, Approval, Facility, and Physician Codes, Health Care System	Classification Codes		Utilization Data					Expense (thousands) of dollars		
★ American Hospital Association (AHA) membership ☐ Joint Commission on Accreditation of Healthcare Organizations (JCAHO) accreditation + American Osteopathic Hospital Association (AOHA) membership ○ American Osteopathic Association (AOA) accreditation △ Commission on Accreditation of Rehabilitation Facilities (CARF) accreditation Control codes 61, 63, 64, 71, 72 and 73 indicate hospitals listed by AOHA, but not registered by AHA. For definition of numerical codes, see page A6	Control	Service	Beds	Admissions	Census	Outpatient Visits	Births	Total	Payroll	Personnel
ARTESIA—Los Angeles County ☐ PIONEER HOSPITAL, 17831 South Pioneer Boulevard, Zip 90701; tel. 310/865–6291; Sharon L. Jose R.N., MS, Administrator **A**1 9 10 **F**2 4 7 8 10 14 15 16 17 18 19 20 22 26 29 30 31 32 35 37 38 39 40 41 42 43 44 45 47 48 49 52 53 54 56 57 60 64 65 71 72 73 74 **P**5 7	32	10	99	5207	47	17893	1859	—	—	294
ATASCADERO—San Luis Obispo County ☐ ATASCADERO STATE HOSPITAL, 10333 El Camino Real, Zip 93422–7001, Mailing Address: P.O. Box 7001, Zip 93423–7001; tel. 805/461–2000; Jon Demorales, Executive Director **A**1 5 **F**4 10 11 16 19 20 21 22 27 31 35 37 41 44 46 52 54 55 56 57 60 65 71 73	12	22	946	1091	892	0	0	87294	54275	1526
ATWATER—Merced County BLOSS MEMORIAL HOSPITAL DISTRICT, 1691 Third Street, Zip 95301; tel. 209/358–8201; David Young, Administrator and Chief Executive Officer **A**9 10 **F**8 22 34 39 65 71 73	16	10	6	310	4	32052	0	4487	1938	94
AUBURN—Placer County ★ AUBURN FAITH COMMUNITY HOSPITAL, 11815 Education Street, Zip 95604, Mailing Address: Box 8992, Zip 95604–8992; tel. 916/888–4518; Joel E. Grey, Administrator **A**1 9 10 **F**7 8 11 12 15 16 19 21 22 23 27 28 32 34 35 37 39 40 41 42 44 46 48 49 50 63 65 71 73 **S**8795 Sutter Health	23	10	106	5051	61	35185	694	42455	18795	463
AVALON—Los Angeles County AVALON MUNICIPAL HOSPITAL AND CLINIC, 100 Falls Canyon Road, Zip 90704, Mailing Address: Box 1563, Zip 90704–1563; tel. 310/510–0700; Karla Parsons R.N., Chief Executive Officer (Nonreporting) **A**9 10	23	10	12	—						
BAKERSFIELD—Kern County ★ BAKERSFIELD MEMORIAL HOSPITAL, 420 34th Street, Zip 93301, Mailing Address: Box 1888, Zip 93303–1888; tel. 805/327–1792; C. Larry Carr, President **A**1 2 9 10 **F**1 2 3 4 7 8 10 11 12 15 18 19 21 22 23 31 32 35 37 38 40 41 42 43 44 49 52 53 54 55 57 58 59 65 67 71 72 **P**5	23	10	233	10223	156	55826	2587	91432	32607	1098
GOOD SAMARITAN HOSPITAL, 901 Olive Drive, Zip 93308–4137; tel. 805/399–4461; Michael H. Keisling, Chief Executive Officer (Nonreporting) **A**10	32	10	64							
☐ KERN MEDICAL CENTER, 1830 Flower Street, Zip 93305–4197; tel. 805/326–2000; Gerald A. Starr, Chief Executive Officer **A**1 2 3 5 8 9 10 **F**4 7 8 10 15 16 17 19 21 28 31 32 33 35 37 38 40 41 42 43 44 45 51 52 53 54 55 56 57 58 59 60 61 63 64 65 69 70 71 73 74 **P**4 6	13	10	236	13379	151	183481	3845	108892	52192	1575
☐ MEMORIAL CENTER, 5201 White Lane, Zip 93309; tel. 805/398–1800; Martin Bragg Ph.D., Chief Executive Officer (Nonreporting) **A**1 9 10	23	22	60	—	—	—	—	—	—	—
★ MERCY HOSPITAL, 2215 Truxtun Avenue, Zip 93301, Mailing Address: Box 119, Zip 93302; tel. 805/632–5000; Bernard J. Herman, President (Total facility includes 50 beds in nursing home–type unit) **A**1 2 9 10 **F**7 8 10 15 16 17 19 22 23 30 31 32 34 35 37 38 39 40 42 44 45 46 49 60 64 65 71 72 73 74 **P**3 5 7 **S**5205 Catholic Healthcare West	21	10	261	9909	181	101533	1954	93784	37979	1113
★ SAN JOAQUIN COMMUNITY HOSPITAL, 2615 Eye Street, Zip 93301, Mailing Address: Box 2615, Zip 93303–2615; tel. 805/395–3000; Fred Manchur, President (Nonreporting) **A**1 2 9 10 **S**0235 Adventist Health System/West	23	10	178							
BANNING—Riverside County ★ SAN GORGONIO MEMORIAL HOSPITAL, 600 North Highland Springs Avenue, Zip 92220; tel. 909/845–1121; Kay Lang, Chief Executive Officer **A**1 9 10 **F**8 14 15 16 19 21 22 28 31 32 33 34 37 40 44 49 59 63 65 68 71 73	23	10	68	2823	31	28199	415	15095	7135	222
BARSTOW—San Bernardino County ☐ BARSTOW COMMUNITY HOSPITAL, 555 South Seventh Avenue, Zip 92311; tel. 619/256–1761; John V. Villanueva, Executive Director (Nonreporting) **A**1 2 9 10 **S**0875 Community Health Systems, Inc.	33	10	48							
BEALE AIR FORCE BASE—Riverside County ★ U.S. AIR FORCE HOSPITAL, 15301 Warren Shingle Road, Zip 95903–1907; tel. 916/634–4838; Major Ty J. Obenoskey MSC, USAF, Administrator **F**3 14 15 16 20 27 28 29 30 39 41 44 46 49 51 58 65 71 **S**9495 Department of the Air Force	41	10	9	702	4	78971	102	—	—	261
BELLFLOWER—Los Angeles County ☐ BELLFLOWER MEDICAL CENTER, 9542 East Artesia Boulevard, Zip 90706; tel. 310/925–8355; Stanley Otake, Administrator and Chief Executive Officer **A**1 9 10 **F**8 19 21 22 27 35 37 39 40 44 49 52 58 65 71 73 **P**5 **S**0435 Pacific Health Corporation	33	10	145	4301	59	16509	963	29950	7808	—
☐ BELLWOOD GENERAL HOSPITAL, 10250 East Artesia Boulevard, Zip 90706; tel. 310/866–9028; Roger W. Wessels, Chief Executive Officer and Administrator **A**1 2 9 10 **F**1 2 3 4 7 8 11 12 17 19 21 22 27 28 30 34 35 37 40 42 43 44 46 49 51 52 53 54 55 58 59 67 70 71 72 73 **P**2 5 7 **S**5765 Paracelsus Healthcare Corporation	33	10	85	3288	46	13157	878	28858	9387	199
★ KAISER FOUNDATION HOSPITAL, (Includes Kaiser Foundation Hospital, Norwalk, California) 9400 East Rosecrans Avenue, Zip 90706–2246; tel. 310/461–3000; Timothy A. Reed, Administrator **A**1 2 9 10 **F**2 3 4 7 8 9 10 12 15 16 18 19 21 22 25 28 29 30 31 32 33 35 36 37 38 39 40 41 42 43 44 45 46 47 48 49 51 52 53 54 55 56 57 58 59 60 61 63 64 65 67 69 71 72 73 74 **P**6 **S**2105 Kaiser Foundation Hospitals	23	10	210	15735	148	—	4801	—	—	1573

© 1995 AHA Guide

Hospitals, U.S. / CALIFORNIA

Hospital, Address, Telephone, Administrator, Approval, Facility, and Physician Codes, Health Care System	Classification Codes		Utilization Data					Expense (thousands) of dollars		
★ American Hospital Association (AHA) membership □ Joint Commission on Accreditation of Healthcare Organizations (JCAHO) accreditation + American Osteopathic Hospital Association (AOHA) membership ○ American Osteopathic Association (AOA) accreditation △ Commission on Accreditation of Rehabilitation Facilities (CARF) accreditation Control codes 61, 63, 64, 71, 72 and 73 indicate hospitals listed by AOHA, but not registered by AHA. For definition of numerical codes, see page A6	Control	Service	Beds	Admissions	Census	Outpatient Visits	Births	Total	Payroll	Personnel
BELMONT—San Mateo County □ CPC BELMONT HILLS HOSPITAL, 1301 Ralston Avenue, Zip 94002; tel. 415/593–2143; Bill Bay, Administrator (Nonreporting) **A**1 9 10 **S**0785 Community Psychiatric Centers	33	22	53	—	—	—	—	—	—	—
BERKELEY—Alameda County ★ ALTA BATES MEDICAL CENTER–ASHBY CAMPUS, (Includes Alta Bates Medical Center–Herrick Campus, 2001 Dwight Way, Berkeley, California, Zip 94704; tel. 415/845–0130) 2450 Ashby Avenue, Zip 94705; tel. 510/204–4444; Albert Lawrence Greene, President and Chief Executive Officer (Total facility includes 63 beds in nursing home–type unit) **A**1 2 9 10 **F**4 7 8 9 10 11 12 16 17 19 21 22 23 26 27 28 29 30 31 32 33 34 35 37 38 39 40 41 42 43 44 48 49 52 53 54 55 57 59 60 61 63 64 65 66 67 69 71 73 74 **P**3 5 7	23	10	499	19462	367	110270	4057	227395	99547	1907
BIG BEAR LAKE—San Bernardino County ★ BEAR VALLEY COMMUNITY HOSPITAL, 41870 Garstin Road, Zip 92315, Mailing Address: P.O. Box 1649, Zip 92315–1649; tel. 909/866–6501; Robert M. Baden, Chief Executive Officer (Total facility includes 15 beds in nursing home–type unit) **A**1 9 10 **F**15 19 22 34 36 44 49 64 65 67 71 73 **S**0585 Brim, Inc.	16	10	30	387	17	14395	0	5177	2443	83
BISHOP—Inyo County ★ NORTHERN INYO HOSPITAL, 150 Pioneer Lane, Zip 93514–2599; tel. 619/873–5811; Herman J. Spencer, Administrator **A**1 9 10 **F**7 19 22 33 34 37 40 44 49 65 71	16	10	32	1656	12	13656	333	14783	6744	209
BLYTHE—Riverside County ★ PALO VERDE HOSPITAL, 250 North First Street, Zip 92225, Mailing Address: P.O. Drawer Z, Zip 92226; tel. 619/922–4115; Vern Reed, Chief Executive Officer **A**9 10 **F**7 8 19 22 32 34 37 40 44 71 73 **S**0585 Brim, Inc.	33	10	55	1588	13	18802	354	9201	3179	146
BRAWLEY—Imperial County ★ PIONEERS MEMORIAL HOSPITAL, 207 West Legion Road, Zip 92227–9699; tel. 619/351–3333; William W. Daniel, Administrator and Chief Executive Officer **A**1 9 10 **F**7 8 14 15 16 19 20 22 28 30 33 34 35 37 38 40 44 49 56 60 65 67 71 73 **P**4 5 7 **S**0585 Brim, Inc.	16	10	80	4241	43	38833	1390	27427	12514	405
BREA—Orange County □ BREA COMMUNITY HOSPITAL, 380 West Central Avenue, Zip 92621; tel. 714/529–0211; Joseph S. Noviello, President (Nonreporting) **A**1 2 5 9 10	32	10	147	—	—	—	—	—	—	—
BUENA PARK—Orange County □ BUENA PARK MEDICAL CENTER, 5742 Beach Boulevard, Zip 90621; tel. 714/521–4770; (Nonreporting) **A**1 9 10 **S**0435 Pacific Health Corporation	33	10	58	—	—	—	—	—	—	—
□ ORANGE COUNTY COMMUNITY HOSPITAL OF BUENA PARK, 6850 Lincoln Avenue, Zip 90620–5703; tel. 714/827–1161; Joseph Sharp, Acting Administrator (Nonreporting) **A**1 9 10 **S**5765 Paracelsus Healthcare Corporation	33	10	159	—	—	—	—	—	—	—
BURBANK—Los Angeles County ★ SAINT JOSEPH MEDICAL CENTER, 501 South Buena Vista Street, Zip 91505–4866; tel. 818/843–5111; Michael J. Madden, Administrator and Chief Executive Officer (Total facility includes 121 beds in nursing home–type unit) **A**1 2 9 10 **F**4 7 8 10 11 12 13 14 15 16 17 19 20 21 22 23 24 26 28 29 30 31 32 33 34 35 37 38 39 40 41 42 43 44 45 46 48 60 64 65 67 68 71 73 **P**5 **S**5275 Sisters of Providence Health System	21	10	423	18372	303	272842	2806	164354	65494	1659
□ THOMPSON MEMORIAL MEDICAL CENTER, 466 East Olive Avenue, Zip 91501, Mailing Address: P.O. Box 4501, Zip 91503; tel. 818/953–6500 **A**1 9 10 **F**11 19 22 31 35 41 44 59 65 71 73	32	10	105	1957	26	8510	0	14912	5164	165
BURLINGAME—San Mateo County ★ △ MILLS–PENINSULA HOSPITALS, (Includes Mills Hospital, 100 South San Mateo Drive, San Mateo, California, Zip 94401; tel. 415/696–4400; Peninsula Hospital, 1783 El Camino Real, Burlingame, California, Zip 94010–3205; tel. 415/696–5400) 1783 El Camino Real, Zip 94010–3205; tel. 415/696–5400; Charles H. Mason Jr., President and Chief Executive Officer (Total facility includes 111 beds in nursing home–type unit) **A**1 2 7 9 10 **F**1 2 3 4 5 7 8 10 11 15 16 18 19 21 22 23 24 26 28 29 30 32 34 35 37 39 40 41 42 43 44 45 46 48 49 52 54 55 56 57 58 59 60 63 64 65 67 71 74 **P**5 7	23	10	438	16318	280	286036	2508	174572	90160	1701
CALEXICO—Imperial County CALEXICO HOSPITAL, 450 Birch Street, Zip 92231; tel. 619/357–1191; Darrell J. Carter, Administrator (Nonreporting) **A**9 10	16	10	34	—	—	—	—	—	—	—
CAMARILLO—Ventura County □ CAMARILLO STATE HOSPITAL AND DEVELOPMENT CENTER, 1878 South Lewis Road, Zip 93012, Mailing Address: P.O. Box 6022, Zip 93011–6022; tel. 805/484–3661; David Freehauf, Executive Director (Nonreporting) **A**1 9 10	12	22	1114	—	—	—	—	—	—	—
★ ST. JOHN'S PLEASANT VALLEY HOSPITAL, 2309 Antonio Avenue, Zip 93010–1459; tel. 805/389–5800; Charles Padilla, Vice President and Administrator (Total facility includes 99 beds in nursing home–type unit) **A**1 9 10 **F**7 8 11 15 16 17 19 21 22 28 29 30 32 34 35 37 40 44 45 46 49 63 64 65 67 71 73 **P**3 5 7 **S**5205 Catholic Healthcare West	23	10	158	3705	201	35988	734	31706	13187	325
CAMP PENDLETON—San Diego County ★ NAVAL HOSPITAL, Mailing Address: Box 555191, Zip 92055–5191; tel. 619/725–1288; Captain James Staiger, Commanding Officer **A**1 3 5 **F**2 3 4 7 8 10 11 12 13 17 18 19 20 21 22 23 25 26 27 28 29 30 31 32 34 35 37 38 39 40 41 42 43 44 46 47 48 49 50 51 52 53 54 56 57 58 59 60 61 63 64 65 66 69 71 72 73 **P**1 **S**9655 Department of Navy	43	10	127	9076	93	550872	1139	50521	11796	1520

Hospitals, U.S. / CALIFORNIA

Hospital, Address, Telephone, Administrator, Approval, Facility, and Physician Codes, Health Care System	Classification Codes		Utilization Data					Expense (thousands) of dollars		
	Control	Service	Beds	Admissions	Census	Outpatient Visits	Births	Total	Payroll	Personnel

★ American Hospital Association (AHA) membership
☐ Joint Commission on Accreditation of Healthcare Organizations (JCAHO) accreditation
+ American Osteopathic Hospital Association (AOHA) membership
○ American Osteopathic Association (AOA) accreditation
△ Commission on Accreditation of Rehabilitation Facilities (CARF) accreditation
Control codes 61, 63, 64, 71, 72 and 73 indicate hospitals listed by AOHA, but not registered by AHA. For definition of numerical codes, see page A6

CAMPBELL—Santa Clara County

☐ CHEMICAL DEPENDENCY INSTITUTE OF NORTHERN CALIFORNIA, 3333 South Bascom Avenue, Zip 95008; tel. 408/559–2000; Roy R. Shelden, Administrator and Chief Executive Officer (Nonreporting)	33	82	40	—	—	—	—	—	—	—

CANOGA PARK–Los Angeles County, See Los Angeles

CARMICHAEL—Sacramento County

MERCY AMERICAN RIVER HOSPITAL See Mercy Healthcare Sacramento

★ MERCY HEALTHCARE SACRAMENTO, (Includes Mercy American River Hospital, 4747 Engle Road, Carmichael, California, Zip 95608; tel. 916/484–2222; Mercy San Juan Hospital, Carmichael, California) 6501 Coyle Avenue, Zip 95608, Mailing Address: P.O. Box 479, Zip 95608; tel. 916/537–5000; Sister Bridget McCarthy, President **A**1 5 9 10 **F**4 7 10 11 12 16 19 22 23 28 30 31 32 33 34 35 37 38 39 40 41 42 43 44 49 50 64 65 71 72 73 74 **P**3 5 **S**5205 Catholic Healthcare West	21	10	354	18132	248	109698	2859	139197	68391	1641

MERCY SAN JUAN HOSPITAL See Mercy Healthcare Sacramento

CASTRO VALLEY—Alameda County

☐ EDEN HOSPITAL MEDICAL CENTER, 20103 Lake Chabot Road, Zip 94546; tel. 510/537–1234; Edward Schreck, President and Chief Executive Officer (Nonreporting) **A**1 2 9 10	16	10	259	—	—	—	—	—	—	—

CATHEDRAL CITY—Riverside County

☐ CANYON SPRINGS HOSPITAL, 69–696 Ramon Road, Zip 92234; tel. 619/321–2000; Michael A. Dougherty Ph.D., Chief Executive Officer (Nonreporting) **A**1 10 **S**0695 Charter Medical Corporation	33	22	80	—	—	—	—	—	—	—

CEDARVILLE—Modoc County

SURPRISE VALLEY COMMUNITY HOSPITAL, Main and Washington Streets, Zip 96104, Mailing Address: P.O. Box 246, Zip 96104–0246; tel. 916/279–6111; Joyce Gysin, Administrator (Total facility includes 14 beds in nursing home–type unit) **A**10 **F**14 15 22 26 28 30 32 34 36 39 64 71 73	16	10	18	77	17	7023	9	2021	—	54

CERES—Stanislaus County

MEMORIAL HOSPITAL–CERES See Memorial Hospital Association, Modesto

CERRITOS—Los Angeles County

☐ COLLEGE HOSPITAL, 10802 College Place, Zip 90703–1579; tel. 310/924–9581; Stephen Witt, Aministrator and Chief Operating Officer **A**1 2 9 10 **F**15 16 26 52 53 55 56 57 59 65 **P**5	31	22	106	2894	58	21078	0	14298	6549	188

CHESTER—Plumas County

SENECA DISTRICT HOSPITAL, 130 Brentwood Drive, Zip 96020, Mailing Address: Box 737, Zip 96020; tel. 916/258–2151; Bernard G. Hietpas, Administrator (Total facility includes 16 beds in nursing home–type unit) **A**9 10 **F**7 8 22 28 31 33 34 40 44 64 65 71 73	16	10	26	463	19	10796	65	5362	2658	86

CHICO—Butte County

☐ △ CHICO COMMUNITY HOSPITAL, 560 Cohasset Road, Zip 95926; tel. 916/896–5000; Fredrick W. Hodges, Chief Executive Officer (Nonreporting) **A**1 7 9 10 **S**5765 Paracelsus Healthcare Corporation	33	10	129	—	—	—	—	—	—	—
★ N. T. ENLOE MEMORIAL HOSPITAL, West Fifth Avenue and Esplanade, Zip 95926–3386; tel. 916/891–7300; James P. Sweeney, Executive Director **A**1 2 9 10 **F**4 7 8 10 11 14 15 17 19 21 22 25 28 30 31 32 33 34 35 36 37 38 39 40 41 42 43 44 45 51 65 67 70 71 72 73	23	10	208	10433	146	109892	1677	98803	48357	1392

CHINO—San Bernardino County

☐ CANYON RIDGE HOSPITAL, 5353 G Street, Zip 91710; tel. 909/590–3700; Diana L. Goulet, Administrator **A**1 10 **F**1 3 16 27 52 53 54 55 56 57 58 59 62 67 68	33	22	59	2066	37	4683	0	6203	3514	91
★ CHINO VALLEY MEDICAL CENTER, 5451 Walnut Avenue, Zip 91710; tel. 909/464–8600; Kenneth Westbrook, Chief Executive Officer (Total facility includes 14 beds in nursing home–type unit) **A**1 9 10 **F**1 3 4 5 6 7 8 10 12 13 15 17 18 19 20 21 22 23 24 25 26 27 28 29 30 31 32 33 34 35 36 37 39 40 41 42 43 44 45 46 49 50 51 53 54 55 56 57 58 59 60 62 63 64 65 66 67 68 69 70 71 72 73 74 **S**0048 Columbia/HCA Healthcare Corporation	33	10	126	4159	47	54379	625	32462	12304	394
HOSPITAL OF THE CALIFORNIA INSTITUTION FOR MEN, 14901 Central Avenue, Zip 91710, Mailing Address: Box 128, Zip 91710; tel. 909/597–1821; M. Sundareson M.D., Chief Medical Officer **F**1 2 3 4 5 6 9 10 11 12 18 19 20 21 22 23 24 25 26 27 28 29 30 31 32 33 34 35 37 39 42 43 44 45 46 48 49 50 51 54 55 56 57 58 59 60 63 64 65 66 69 70 71 72 **P**6	12	11	80	1171	57	90133	0	—	—	258

CHOWCHILLA—Madera County

CHOWCHILLA DISTRICT MEMORIAL HOSPITAL, 1104 Ventura Avenue, Zip 93610, Mailing Address: Box 1027, Zip 93610; tel. 209/665–3781; Julia Kiil, Administrator (Nonreporting) **A**9 10	16	10	23	—	—	—	—	—	—	—

CHULA VISTA—San Diego County

☐ BAYVIEW HOSPITAL, (Formerly Southwood Treatment Centers) 330 Moss Street, Zip 91911–2005; tel. 619/426–6310; James Plummer, Chief Executive Officer (Nonreporting) **A**1 9 10	33	22	108	—	—	—	—	—	—	—
★ SCRIPPS MEMORIAL HOSPITAL–CHULA VISTA, 435 H Street, Zip 91912–1537, Mailing Address: Box 1537, Zip 91910–1537; tel. 619/691–7000; Thomas A. Gammiere, Vice President, Administration **A**1 9 10 **F**1 2 3 4 6 7 8 10 11 12 14 15 16 17 19 21 22 23 24 25 26 27 28 29 31 33 34 35 36 37 38 39 40 41 42 43 44 45 46 47 48 49 50 52 53 54 55 56 57 58 59 60 63 64 65 66 67 68 69 70 71 72 73 74 **P**3 4 5 7 **S**1505 Scripps Hospitals	23	10	159	8798	108	51305	2605	49502	22126	706

© 1995 AHA Guide

Hospitals, U.S. / CALIFORNIA

Hospital, Address, Telephone, Administrator, Approval, Facility, and Physician Codes, Health Care System	Classification Codes		Utilization Data					Expense (thousands) of dollars		Personnel
★ American Hospital Association (AHA) membership ☐ Joint Commission on Accreditation of Healthcare Organizations (JCAHO) accreditation + American Osteopathic Hospital Association (AOHA) membership ○ American Osteopathic Association (AOA) accreditation △ Commission on Accreditation of Rehabilitation Facilities (CARF) accreditation Control codes 61, 63, 64, 71, 72 and 73 indicate hospitals listed by AOHA, but not registered by AHA. For definition of numerical codes, see page A6	Control	Service	Beds	Admissions	Census	Outpatient Visits	Births	Total	Payroll	
★ SHARP CHULA VISTA MEDICAL CENTER, 751 Medical Center Court, Zip 91911, Mailing Address: Box 1297, Zip 91912; tel. 619/482–5800; Thomas F. Spindler, Chief Executive Officer (Total facility includes 133 beds in nursing home–type unit) **A**1 2 9 10 **F**1 3 4 5 6 7 8 10 11 12 14 15 16 17 19 21 22 23 24 25 26 27 29 30 31 32 34 37 38 39 40 41 42 43 44 45 46 48 49 51 52 54 55 56 57 58 59 60 61 63 64 65 66 67 69 70 71 72 73 74 **P**1 5 **S**2065 Sharp Healthcare	23	10	306	8578	230	23881	1973	64413	25985	745
SOUTHWOOD TREATMENT CENTERS See Bayview Hospital										
VISTA HILL HOSPITAL, 730 Medical Center Court, Zip 91911–6618; tel. 619/421–6900; Shawn Miyake, Administrator (Nonreporting) **A**9 **S**8895 Vista Hill Foundation	23	22	77	—	—	—	—	—	—	—
CLEARLAKE—Lake County										
☐ REDBUD COMMUNITY HOSPITAL, 18th Avenue and Highway 53, Zip 95422, Mailing Address: Box 6720, Zip 95422; tel. 707/994–6486; David Coffler, Chief Executive Officer **A**1 9 10 **F**7 8 15 16 19 21 22 28 32 33 34 35 37 39 40 41 43 44 45 53 54 56 58 59 63 65 71 73	16	10	36	1460	14	32594	227	16837	3443	188
CLOVIS—Fresno County										
☐ CLOVIS COMMUNITY HOSPITAL, 2755 Herndon Avenue, Zip 93611; tel. 209/323–4060; Paul F. Dyer, Administrator **A**1 9 10 **F**1 2 3 4 7 8 10 11 14 15 16 17 19 21 22 23 25 26 28 29 30 31 32 33 34 35 37 38 39 40 41 42 43 44 45 46 49 50 52 53 54 55 56 57 58 59 60 61 63 65 69 71 73 74 **P**2 5 7 8 **S**1085 Community Hospitals of Central California	23	10	143	5043	73	31400	2643	37581	14254	342
COALINGA—Fresno County										
COALINGA REGIONAL MEDICAL CENTER, 1191 Phelps Avenue, Zip 93210; tel. 209/935–6562; James J. Dickson, Administrator and Chief Executive Officer (Total facility includes 54 beds in nursing home–type unit) **A**9 10 **F**7 8 19 35 40 44 49 64 66 71 72	16	10	78	1070	43	24180	30	12722	6101	180
COLUSA—Colusa County										
☐ COLUSA COMMUNITY HOSPITAL, 199 East Webster Street, Zip 95932, Mailing Address: P.O. Box 331, Zip 95932–0331; tel. 916/458–5821; Edward C. Bland, Chief Executive Officer **A**1 9 10 **F**7 8 12 14 15 17 19 22 28 29 30 31 32 34 37 40 41 44 49 67 71 72 73	23	10	36	1147	14	17114	249	9348	3697	126
CONCORD—Contra Costa County										
★ MOUNT DIABLO MEDICAL CENTER, 2540 East Street, Zip 94520, Mailing Address: P.O. Box 4110, Zip 94524–4110; tel. 510/682–8200; Michael L. Wall, President and Chief Executive Officer **A**1 2 9 10 **F**1 3 4 5 7 8 10 11 12 14 15 18 19 20 21 22 23 24 25 27 28 29 30 31 32 34 35 37 38 40 41 42 43 44 45 46 49 51 54 56 57 58 59 60 61 63 65 66 67 71 73 **P**5	16	10	273	7943	104	244506	657	—	—	1005
CORCORAN—Kings County										
CORCORAN DISTRICT HOSPITAL, 1310 Hanna Avenue, Zip 93212, Mailing Address: Box 758, Zip 93212; tel. 209/992–5051; Rod Vieira, Acting Administrator (Nonreporting) **A**9 10	16	10	32	—	—	—	—	—	—	—
CORONA—Riverside County										
☐ CHARTER BEHAVIORAL HEALTH SYSTEM OF THE INLAND EMPIRE, 2055 Kellogg Avenue, Zip 91719; tel. 909/735–2910; Diana C. Hanyak, Chief Executive Officer (Nonreporting) **A**1 9 10 **S**0695 Charter Medical Corporation	33	22	158	—	—	—	—	—	—	—
☐ △ CORONA REGIONAL MEDICAL CENTER, (Includes Corona Regional Medical Center–Rehabilitation, 730 Magnolia Avenue, Corona, California, Zip 91719; tel. 909/736–7200) 800 South Main Street, Zip 91720; tel. 909/736–6240; Marlene Woodworth, Chief Executive Officer **A**1 2 7 9 10 **F**4 7 8 9 10 11 12 14 15 16 19 22 23 27 28 30 32 33 34 35 37 38 40 41 42 43 44 46 47 48 49 52 57 59 60 65 67 69 71 73 74 **P**5	23	10	225	7914	98	53193	1751	54698	20279	658
CORONA REGIONAL MEDICAL CENTER–REHABILITATION See Corona Regional Medical Center										
CORONADO—San Diego County										
★ CORONADO HOSPITAL, 250 Prospect Place, Zip 92118; tel. 619/435–6251; Lowell B. Hanks, Administrator and Chief Executive Officer (Nonreporting) **A**1 9 10	23	10	195	—	—	—	—	—	—	—
COSTA MESA—Orange County										
☐ COLLEGE HOSPITAL COSTA MESA, 301 Victoria Street, Zip 92627; tel. 714/642–2734; Kenneth W. Lukhard, Chief Executive Officer (Nonreporting) **A**1 9 10	33	22	125	—	—	—	—	—	—	—
COVINA—Los Angeles County										
★ CHARTER BEHAVIORAL HEALTH SYSTEM OF SOUTHERN CALIFORNIA–CHARTER OAK, (Formerly Charter Oak Hospital) 1161 East Covina Boulevard, Zip 91724–1161; tel. 818/966–1632; Todd A. Smith, Chief Executive Officer (Nonreporting) **A**1 9 10 **S**0695 Charter Medical Corporation	33	22	95	—	—	—	—	—	—	—
☐ INTER–COMMUNITY MEDICAL CENTER, 210 West San Bernardino Road, Zip 91723–1901; tel. 818/331–7331; Peter E. Makowski, President and Chief Executive Officer **A**1 2 9 10 **F**4 7 8 10 11 12 14 15 16 17 19 21 22 28 30 32 33 34 35 36 37 38 39 40 41 42 43 44 45 46 49 52 60 63 64 65 67 71 73 **P**1 5 7	23	10	268	7509	113	49469	557	63297	23525	746
CRESCENT CITY—Del Norte County										
☐ SUTTER COAST HOSPITAL, 800 East Washington Boulevard, Zip 95531; tel. 707/464–8511; John E. Menaugh, Administrator **A**1 9 10 **F**7 8 13 17 19 22 28 30 31 32 33 34 35 37 40 41 44 45 49 65 70 71 73 74 **P**5 **S**8795 Sutter Health	23	10	47	2518	31	75540	335	—	—	292

Hospitals, U.S. / CALIFORNIA

Hospital, Address, Telephone, Administrator, Approval, Facility, and Physician Codes, Health Care System	Classification Codes		Utilization Data					Expense (thousands) of dollars		
	Control	Service	Beds	Admissions	Census	Outpatient Visits	Births	Total	Payroll	Personnel

★ American Hospital Association (AHA) membership
☐ Joint Commission on Accreditation of Healthcare Organizations (JCAHO) accreditation
+ American Osteopathic Hospital Association (AOHA) membership
○ American Osteopathic Association (AOA) accreditation
△ Commission on Accreditation of Rehabilitation Facilities (CARF) accreditation
Control codes 61, 63, 64, 71, 72 and 73 indicate hospitals listed by AOHA, but not registered by AHA. For definition of numerical codes, see page A6

CULVER CITY—Los Angeles County
☐ BROTMAN MEDICAL CENTER, 3828 Delmas Terrace, Zip 90231-2459, Mailing Address: Box 2459, Zip 90231-2459; tel. 310/836-7000; Daniel P. McLean, Chief Executive Officer (Total facility includes 21 beds in nursing home-type unit) **A**1 9 10 **F**2 3 4 7 8 10 11 12 14 15 16 17 18 19 20 21 22 23 26 27 28 29 30 31 32 34 35 37 39 40 41 42 43 44 45 46 49 52 54 55 56 57 60 63 64 65 67 71 73 74 **P**2 5 **S**6525 Ornda Healthcorp — 33 10 240 9436 206 102242 654 80146 38004 950

☐ WASHINGTON MEDICAL CENTER, 12101 West Washington Boulevard, Zip 90231, Mailing Address: Box 2787, Zip 90231; tel. 310/391-0601; Peter Friedman, Administrator (Nonreporting) **A**1 9 10 — 33 10 99

DALY CITY—San Mateo County
★ SETON MEDICAL CENTER, 1900 Sullivan Avenue, Zip 94015-2229; tel. 415/992-4000; Deborah E. Stebbins FACHE, Acting President and Chief Executive Officer (Total facility includes 66 beds in nursing home-type unit) **A**1 2 3 5 9 10 **F**4 7 8 10 11 12 14 16 17 18 19 21 22 25 26 27 28 29 30 31 32 33 34 35 37 38 39 40 41 42 43 44 45 46 49 51 52 54 55 56 57 58 59 60 63 64 65 67 71 73 74 **P**5 7 **S**1855 Daughters of Charity National Health System — 21 10 275 10768 204 230005 1082 120688 51819 881

DANA POINT—Orange County
☐ CAPISTRANO BY THE SEA HOSPITAL, 34000 Capistrano by the Sea Drive, Zip 92629-2104, Mailing Address: Box 398, Zip 92629-2104; tel. 714/496-5702; Harold E. Day, Administrator and Chief Executive Officer (Nonreporting) **A**1 9 10 — 33 22 82

DAVIS—Yolo County
☐ SUTTER DAVIS HOSPITAL, 2000 Sutter Place, Zip 95616, Mailing Address: P.O. Box 1617, Zip 95617; tel. 916/756-6440; Lawrence A. Maas, Administrator **A**1 9 10 **F**15 16 19 22 32 35 37 42 44 71 72 **P**3 **S**8795 Sutter Health — 23 10 48 1764 19 19026 0 13771 7470 197

DEER PARK—Napa County
☐ ST. HELENA HOSPITAL, 650 Sanitarium Road, Zip 94576, Mailing Address: P.O. Box 250, Zip 94576; tel. 707/963-3611; Lenard Heffner M.D., President and Chief Executive Officer (Nonreporting) **A**1 9 10 **S**0235 Adventist Health System/West — 21 10 168

DELANO—Kern County
☐ DELANO REGIONAL MEDICAL CENTER, 1401 Garces Highway, Zip 93215, Mailing Address: Box 460, Zip 93216; tel. 805/725-4800; Sean O'Neal, Executive Director (Total facility includes 28 beds in nursing home-type unit) **A**1 9 10 **F**7 8 10 12 14 15 16 17 19 20 21 22 27 28 30 31 32 34 37 39 40 44 45 46 49 59 64 65 71 73 **P**5 — 23 10 128 4122 77 27824 1236 25757 9455 415

DINUBA—Tulare County
★ ALTA DISTRICT HOSPITAL, 500 Adelaide Way, Zip 93618-1698; tel. 209/591-4171; Robert M. Montion, Administrator (Total facility includes 18 beds in nursing home-type unit) **A**9 10 **F**15 19 20 22 32 34 35 36 44 64 65 71 73 — 16 10 50 1402 23 34613 0 8168 3075 128

DOS PALOS—Merced County
DOS PALOS MEMORIAL HOSPITAL, 2118 Marguerite Street, Zip 93620; tel. 209/392-6106; Howard Sager, Administrator (Nonreporting) **A**9 10 — 23 10 15 — — — — — — —

DOWNEY—Los Angeles County
★ △ DOWNEY COMMUNITY HOSPITAL FOUNDATION, (Includes Downey Community Hospital, 11500 Brookshire Avenue, Downey, California, Zip 90241-4990, Mailing Address: P.O. Box 7010, Zip 90241-7010; tel. 310/904-5000; Rio Hondo Memorial Hospital, 8300 East Telegraph Road, Downey, California, Zip 90240, Mailing Address: P.O. Box 7020, Zip 90241-7020; tel. 310/806-1821) 11500 Brookshire Avenue, Zip 90241-4990; tel. 310/904-5000; Allen R. Korneff, President and Chief Executive Officer (Total facility includes 20 beds in nursing home-type unit) **A**1 2 7 9 10 **F**4 7 8 10 11 19 21 22 23 24 26 27 28 30 35 36 37 38 40 42 43 44 48 49 60 63 64 65 67 71 73 **P**3 7 — 23 10 227 11904 141 99860 1829 105096 45560 1298

★ △ LAC-RANCHO LOS AMIGOS MEDICAL CENTER, 7601 East Imperial Highway, Zip 90242; tel. 310/940-7022; Consuelo C. Diaz, Chief Executive Officer (Total facility includes 20 beds in nursing home-type unit) **A**1 3 5 7 9 10 **F**1 2 3 4 5 7 8 9 10 11 12 13 14 15 17 18 19 20 21 22 23 25 26 27 28 29 30 31 32 34 35 37 38 39 40 41 42 43 44 45 46 47 48 49 51 52 53 54 55 56 57 58 59 60 61 63 64 65 66 68 69 70 71 72 73 74 **P**3 5 6 **S**5755 Los Angeles County–Department of Health Services — 13 46 369 4550 365 93157 0 259569 86003 2404

DUARTE—Los Angeles County
★ CITY OF HOPE NATIONAL MEDICAL CENTER, (Cancer, Genetic, Respiratory, Blood Dyscrasia and Metabolic Diseases) 1500 East Duarte Road, Zip 91010-3000; tel. 818/359-8111; Sanford M. Shapero, President and Chief Executive Officer **A**1 2 3 5 9 10 **F**8 10 15 16 19 20 21 29 31 32 34 35 37 41 42 44 46 49 60 65 67 71 73 **P**5 7 — 23 49 147 3858 104 93136 0 152513 67244 1642

☐ SANTA TERESITA HOSPITAL, 819 Buena Vista Street, Zip 91010-1703; tel. 818/359-3243; Michael J. Costello Jr., Chief Executive Officer (Nonreporting) **A**1 2 9 10 — 21 10 283

EDWARDS AIR FORCE BASE—Mendocino County
★ U.S. AIR FORCE HOSPITAL, Mailing Address: Building 5500, Zip 93524-1730; tel. 805/277-2010; Colonel Paul H. Lilly Jr. USAF, MC, Commander (Nonreporting) **S**9495 Department of the Air Force — 41 10 28

EL CAJON—San Diego County
KAISER FOUNDATION HOSPITAL See Kaiser Foundation Hospital, San Diego
★ SCRIPPS HOSPITAL–EAST COUNTY, 1688 East Main Street, Zip 92021; tel. 619/440-1122; Robin B. Brown, Vice President and Administrator (Total facility includes 41 beds in nursing home-type unit) **A**1 9 10 **F**4 8 10 11 12 17 19 22 27 28 32 34 35 37 40 41 42 43 44 48 49 52 57 59 64 65 69 70 71 73 74 **P**5 7 **S**1505 Scripps Hospitals — 23 10 158 3897 67 36684 0 — — 378

Hospitals, U.S. / CALIFORNIA

Hospital, Address, Telephone, Administrator, Approval, Facility, and Physician Codes, Health Care System	Classification Codes		Utilization Data					Expense (thousands) of dollars		
	Control	Service	Beds	Admissions	Census	Outpatient Visits	Births	Total	Payroll	Personnel

★ American Hospital Association (AHA) membership
☐ Joint Commission on Accreditation of Healthcare Organizations (JCAHO) accreditation
+ American Osteopathic Hospital Association (AOHA) membership
○ American Osteopathic Association (AOA) accreditation
△ Commission on Accreditation of Rehabilitation Facilities (CARF) accreditation
Control codes 61, 63, 64, 71, 72 and 73 indicate hospitals listed by AOHA, but not registered by AHA. For definition of numerical codes, see page A6

EL CENTRO—Imperial County
★ EL CENTRO REGIONAL MEDICAL CENTER, 1415 Ross Avenue, Zip 92243; tel. 619/339–7100; Ted Fox, Administrator **A**1 9 10 **F**8 19 22 23 28 34 35 37 38 40 44 45 46 56 60 63 65 71 73 **P**4 5 — 14 10 107 5674 59 56107 1332 32031 14108 495

ELDRIDGE—Sonoma County
SONOMA DEVELOPMENTAL CENTER, 15000 Arnold Drive, Zip 95431; tel. 707/938–6000; Timothy L. Meeker, Executive Director (Nonreporting) **A**10 — 12 62 1423 — — — — — — —

ENCINITAS—San Diego County
☐ CPC SAN LUIS REY HOSPITAL, 335 Saxony Road, Zip 92024–2723; tel. 619/753–1245; William T. Sparrow, Administrator (Nonreporting) **A**1 9 10 **S**0785 Community Psychiatric Centers — 33 22 123 — — — — — — —

★ △ SCRIPPS MEMORIAL HOSPITAL–ENCINITAS, 354 Santa Fe Drive, Zip 92023; Mailing Address: P.O. Box 817, Zip 92023; tel. 619/753–6501; Steven J. Goe, Vice President and Administrator **A**1 2 7 9 10 **F**2 3 4 7 8 10 11 12 14 15 16 17 19 20 21 22 23 24 27 28 29 30 32 35 36 37 38 40 41 42 43 44 45 46 48 49 52 53 56 60 61 63 64 65 66 67 69 70 71 73 74 **P**3 5 7 **S**1505 Scripps Hospitals — 23 10 145 5405 74 39133 558 49034 15696 463

ENCINO–Los Angeles County, See Los Angeles

ESCONDIDO—San Diego County
★ PALOMAR MEDICAL CENTER, 555 East Valley Parkway, Zip 92025–3084; tel. 619/739–3000; Victoria M. Penland, Administrator and Chief Operating Officer (Total facility includes 96 beds in nursing home–type unit) **A**1 2 9 10 **F**3 4 7 8 10 17 19 21 22 23 24 25 26 27 28 29 30 31 32 33 34 35 37 38 40 41 42 43 44 45 46 49 51 52 54 56 57 58 60 61 63 64 65 66 70 71 73 **P**6 7 **S**7555 Palomar Pomerado Health System — 16 10 395 15067 261 102317 3207 129553 47978 1309

EUREKA—Humboldt County
★ △ GENERAL HOSPITAL, 2200 Harrison Avenue, Zip 95501; tel. 707/445–5111; Gary A. McCormack, Chief Executive Officer **A**1 7 9 10 **F**7 8 12 19 20 21 22 23 25 28 31 32 33 34 35 37 38 40 41 44 48 49 51 56 61 63 65 71 72 73 **S**0585 Brim, Inc. — 33 10 83 2323 29 33338 620 27843 12151 398

★ ST. JOSEPH HOSPITAL, 2700 Dolbeer Street, Zip 95501; tel. 707/445–8121; Paul J. Chodkowski, President and Chief Executive Officer **A**1 2 9 10 **F**2 3 8 9 10 11 12 14 15 16 17 19 21 22 27 28 29 30 31 32 33 34 35 37 40 41 42 44 45 46 49 60 65 67 71 73 74 **P**3 5 7 8 **S**5425 St. Joseph Health System — 21 10 65 3313 44 130847 0 33622 11305 344

EXETER—Tulare County
☐ MEMORIAL HOSPITAL AT EXETER, 215 Crespi Avenue, Zip 93221–1399; tel. 209/592–2151; Sally Brewer, Administrator (Total facility includes 66 beds in nursing home–type unit) **A**1 9 10 **F**8 13 15 16 19 20 21 22 28 34 41 44 64 65 67 71 72 **P**5 6 — 23 10 80 259 58 9605 0 7596 3327 142

FAIRFIELD—Solano County
★ NORTHBAY MEDICAL CENTER, 1200 B. Gale Wilson Boulevard, Zip 94533–3587; tel. 707/429–3600; Deborah Sugiyama, Administrator (Total facility includes 11 beds in nursing home–type unit) **A**1 9 10 **F**7 8 10 11 12 15 19 21 22 28 32 33 35 36 37 38 39 40 41 42 44 49 60 64 65 66 67 71 72 73 **P**3 5 **S**2075 NorthBay Healthcare System — 23 10 89 5012 51 66702 1585 49397 19203 339

FALL RIVER MILLS—Shasta County
MAYERS MEMORIAL HOSPITAL DISTRICT, Highway 299 East, Zip 96028, Mailing Address: Box 459, Zip 96028; tel. 916/336–5511; Everett L. Beck, Administrator (Nonreporting) **A**10 — 16 10 72 — — — — — — —

FALLBROOK—San Diego County
★ FALLBROOK HOSPITAL DISTRICT, 624 East Elder Street, Zip 92028; tel. 619/728–1191; Donald N. Larkin, Chief Executive Officer (Total facility includes 99 beds in nursing home–type unit) **A**1 9 10 **F**7 8 11 14 15 17 19 21 22 25 27 28 29 30 31 32 33 34 35 37 39 40 41 42 44 45 49 51 54 63 64 65 66 67 71 73 74 **P**4 5 7 8 — 16 10 149 2557 45 41216 649 22000 12450 364

FOLSOM—Sacramento County
★ MERCY HOSPITAL OF FOLSOM, 1650 Creekside Drive, Zip 95630–3405; tel. 916/983–7400; Donald C. Hudson, Vice President and Chief Operating Officer (Nonreporting) **A**1 9 10 **S**5205 Catholic Healthcare West — 21 10 89 — — — — — — —

☐ VENCOR HOSPITAL–SACRAMENTO, 223 Fargo Way, Zip 95630; tel. 916/351–9151; Kenneth H. Smith, Administrator (Nonreporting) **A**1 10 **S**0026 Vencor, Incorporated — 33 10 32 — — — — — — —

FONTANA—San Bernardino County
☐ CPC RANCHO LINDO HOSPITAL, 7625 East Avenue, Zip 92336; tel. 714/899–3233; Bruce Waldo, Chief Executive Officer (Nonreporting) **A**1 9 10 **S**0785 Community Psychiatric Centers — 33 22 74 — — — — — — —

★ KAISER FOUNDATION HOSPITAL, 9961 Sierra Avenue, Zip 92335–6794; tel. 909/427–5000; Patricia Siegel, Administrator **A**1 2 3 5 9 10 **F**2 3 4 7 9 10 11 14 15 16 19 21 22 23 25 29 30 31 32 33 35 37 38 40 41 42 43 45 46 48 52 53 54 55 56 57 58 59 60 61 63 64 65 66 67 68 69 71 72 73 **S**2105 Kaiser Foundation Hospitals — 23 10 233 19476 209 56255 3518 — — 2183

FORT BRAGG—Mendocino County
★ MENDOCINO COAST DISTRICT HOSPITAL, 700 River Drive, Zip 95437; tel. 707/961–1234; Elizabeth MacGard, Chief Executive Officer **A**1 9 10 **F**7 8 11 12 16 17 19 21 22 26 28 29 30 31 32 33 34 35 36 37 39 40 41 42 44 45 46 49 60 63 64 65 67 68 71 73 **P**3 — 16 10 54 1956 25 — 241 18813 8557 231

Hospitals, U.S. / CALIFORNIA

Hospital, Address, Telephone, Administrator, Approval, Facility, and Physician Codes, Health Care System	Classification Codes		Utilization Data					Expense (thousands) of dollars		
★ American Hospital Association (AHA) membership ☐ Joint Commission on Accreditation of Healthcare Organizations (JCAHO) accreditation + American Osteopathic Hospital Association (AOHA) membership ○ American Osteopathic Association (AOA) accreditation △ Commission on Accreditation of Rehabilitation Facilities (CARF) accreditation Control codes 61, 63, 64, 71, 72 and 73 indicate hospitals listed by AOHA, but not registered by AHA. For definition of numerical codes, see page A6	Control	Service	Beds	Admissions	Census	Outpatient Visits	Births	Total	Payroll	Personnel
FORT IRWIN—San Bernardino County										
★ WEED ARMY COMMUNITY HOSPITAL, Zip 92310–5065; tel. 619/380–3108; Colonel Alan Mease, Commander (Nonreporting) A1 S9395 Department of the Army	42	10	27	—	—	—	—	—	—	—
FORTUNA—Humboldt County										
★ REDWOOD MEMORIAL HOSPITAL, 3300 Renner Drive, Zip 95540; tel. 707/725–3361; Paul J. Chodkowski, President and Chief Executive Officer A1 2 9 10 F7 8 15 16 19 21 22 29 32 33 37 40 44 45 46 47 71 S5425 St. Joseph Health System	21	10	35	2085	22	32172	480	12830	5069	167
FOUNTAIN VALLEY—Orange County										
★ FHP HOSPITAL – FOUNTAIN VALLEY, 9920 Talbert Avenue, Zip 92728; tel. 714/962–4677; Marcia Manker, Administrator A1 3 10 F2 3 4 7 8 10 11 12 13 15 16 19 20 21 22 25 26 27 28 29 30 32 33 34 35 37 38 39 40 41 42 43 44 45 46 48 49 50 51 52 53 54 55 56 57 58 59 60 64 65 67 69 70 71 72 73 74 P1 2 4 5 6 7 8	33	10	230	8100	83	45217	1204	—	—	577
☐ FOUNTAIN VALLEY REGIONAL HOSPITAL AND MEDICAL CENTER, 17100 Euclid, Zip 92708; tel. 714/966–7200; Richard Butler, Administrator (Nonreporting) A1 2 9 10 S6525 Ornda Healthcorp	33	10	359	—	—	—	—	—	—	—
FREMONT—Alameda County										
☐ CPC FREMONT HOSPITAL, 39001 Sundale Drive, Zip 94538; tel. 510/796–1100; Alan M. Gitlin, Chief Executive Officer A1 10 F1 3 12 17 20 22 52 53 54 55 56 57 58 59 65 S0785 Community Psychiatric Centers	33	22	78	1650	46	5694	0	—	—	102
★ WASHINGTON HOSPITAL, 2000 Mowry Avenue, Zip 94538–1716; tel. 510/797–1111; Nancy D. Farber, Chief Executive Officer A1 2 9 10 F4 7 8 10 11 12 13 14 15 16 17 18 19 21 22 28 29 30 32 33 34 35 37 39 40 41 42 43 44 46 49 52 54 56 57 59 60 63 65 67 71 72 73 P5 7	16	10	202	11763	135	125379	2230	106433	50865	741
FRENCH CAMP—Santa Clara County										
△ SAN JOAQUIN GENERAL HOSPITAL, 500 West Hospital Road, Zip 95231, Mailing Address: P.O. Box 1020, Stockton Zip 95201; tel. 209/468–6600; Michael N. Smith, Director Healthcare Services A3 5 7 9 10 12 F3 4 7 8 10 11 12 15 16 17 18 19 20 21 22 25 26 27 28 31 32 33 34 35 37 38 39 40 42 43 44 46 48 49 51 53 54 55 56 57 58 60 63 65 67 68 69 71 72 73 P6	13	10	194	8068	136	183263	2128	83784	36068	1360
FRESNO—Fresno County										
☐ CEDAR VISTA HOSPITAL PSYCHIATRIC SERVICES, 7171 North Cedar Avenue, Zip 93720; tel. 209/449–8000; Lynn M. Horton, Administrator (Nonreporting) A1 9 10	33	22	60	—	—	—	—	—	—	—
★ △ FRESNO COMMUNITY HOSPITAL AND MEDICAL CENTER, Fresno and R Streets, Zip 93721, Mailing Address: Box 1232, Zip 93715; tel. 209/442–6000; Bruce M. Perry, Chief Executive Officer A1 2 7 9 10 F1 2 3 4 7 8 10 11 14 15 16 17 19 21 22 23 25 26 28 29 30 31 32 33 34 35 37 38 39 40 41 42 43 44 45 46 48 49 50 52 53 54 55 56 57 58 59 60 61 63 65 69 71 73 74 P2 5 7 8 S1085 Community Hospitals of Central California	23	10	359	19021	227	199763	5126	148707	65650	1794
☐ KAISER FOUNDATION HOSPITAL, 7300 North Fresno Street, Zip 93720; tel. 209/448–4000; Edward S. Glavis, Vice President and Area Administrator (Newly Registered) A1 10 S2105 Kaiser Foundation Hospitals	23	10	41	—	—	—	—	—	—	—
★ SIERRA COMMUNITY HOSPITAL, 2025 East Dakota Avenue, Zip 93726–4896; tel. 209/221–5600; Bruce M. Perry, Chief Executive Officer A1 9 10 F1 2 3 4 7 8 10 11 14 15 16 17 19 21 22 23 25 26 28 29 30 31 32 33 34 35 37 38 39 40 41 42 43 44 45 46 49 50 52 53 54 55 56 57 58 59 60 61 63 65 69 71 73 74 P2 5 7 8 S1085 Community Hospitals of Central California	23	10	77	2049	21	31037	0	22562	8635	230
★ ST. AGNES MEDICAL CENTER, 1303 East Herndon Avenue, Zip 93720–3397; tel. 209/449–3000; Sister Ruth Marie Nickerson, President A1 2 9 10 F1 4 7 8 10 11 15 16 19 22 28 30 31 32 33 34 35 37 38 39 40 41 42 43 44 49 53 54 55 56 57 58 59 60 62 65 66 67 68 70 71 72 73 74 P1 5 7 S5585 Holy Cross Health System Corporation	21	10	326	19215	221	259180	3370	177637	67525	1863
☐ △ VALLEY CHILDREN'S HOSPITAL, 3151 North Millbrook, Zip 93703–1497; tel. 209/225–3000; Rex Riley, Acting Administrator A1 3 5 7 9 10 F10 13 15 16 17 19 21 22 25 28 30 34 35 38 41 42 43 44 46 47 48 49 51 58 60 65 67 71 72 73	23	50	184	8064	140	135206	0	102371	50301	1572
☐ VALLEY MEDICAL CENTER OF FRESNO, 445 South Cedar Avenue, Zip 93702–2907; tel. 209/453–4000 A1 2 3 5 8 9 10 F4 8 9 10 15 16 19 20 21 22 23 28 29 31 32 34 35 37 38 40 41 42 43 44 45 46 47 49 51 52 54 55 56 58 60 61 63 64 65 68 70 71 73 P6	13	10	257	11612	183	171172	3191	127204	63195	1849
★ VETERANS AFFAIRS MEDICAL CENTER, 2615 East Clinton Avenue, Zip 93703; tel. 209/225–6100; James C. DeNiro, Director (Total facility includes 60 beds in nursing home–type unit) A1 2 3 5 F2 3 6 10 15 16 19 20 21 22 26 27 28 30 31 32 33 34 35 37 39 41 42 45 46 47 51 52 54 56 57 58 60 65 71 73 74 S9295 Department of Veterans Affairs	45	10	219	4687	164	132960	0	62083	—	861
FULLERTON—Orange County										
★ △ ST. JUDE MEDICAL CENTER, 101 East Valencia Mesa Drive, Zip 92635; tel. 714/992–3000; Patty Maysent, President and Chief Executive Officer A1 2 7 9 10 F1 3 4 7 8 10 11 12 13 15 16 17 18 19 21 22 23 26 27 28 29 30 31 32 33 34 35 37 38 40 41 42 43 44 45 46 48 49 51 52 54 55 56 57 58 59 60 63 65 67 68 71 72 73 74 P3 5 7 S5425 St. Joseph Health System	21	10	317	12768	194	141132	2294	112243	43157	1254

Hospitals, U.S. / CALIFORNIA

Hospital, Address, Telephone, Administrator, Approval, Facility, and Physician Codes, Health Care System	Classification Codes		Utilization Data					Expense (thousands of dollars)		
	Control	Service	Beds	Admissions	Census	Outpatient Visits	Births	Total	Payroll	Personnel

★ American Hospital Association (AHA) membership
☐ Joint Commission on Accreditation of Healthcare Organizations (JCAHO) accreditation
+ American Osteopathic Hospital Association (AOHA) membership
○ American Osteopathic Association (AOA) accreditation
△ Commission on Accreditation of Rehabilitation Facilities (CARF) accreditation
Control codes 61, 63, 64, 71, 72 and 73 indicate hospitals listed by AOHA, but not registered by AHA. For definition of numerical codes, see page A6

Hospital	Control	Service	Beds	Admissions	Census	Outpatient Visits	Births	Total	Payroll	Personnel
GARBERVILLE—Humboldt County SOUTHERN HUMBOLDT COMMUNITY HOSPITAL DISTRICT, 733 Cedar Street, Zip 95542–3292; tel. 707/923–3921; Dian Pecora, Administrator (Total facility includes 8 beds in nursing home-type unit) **A**9 10 **F**2 4 7 8 9 10 11 12 16 17 19 20 22 28 29 30 31 32 33 35 36 38 40 41 42 43 44 47 48 51 52 60 65 67 71 **P**3 5	16	10	18	445	10	6581	59	2834	1468	67
GARDEN GROVE—Orange County ★ GARDEN GROVE HOSPITAL AND MEDICAL CENTER, (Formerly AMI Garden Grove Hospital and Medical Center) 12601 Garden Grove Boulevard, Zip 92643–1959; tel. 714/741–2700; Timothy Smith, Executive Director (Total facility includes 12 beds in nursing home–type unit) **A**1 9 10 **F**7 12 16 19 21 22 23 26 28 30 31 32 33 34 35 37 38 39 40 41 42 44 49 63 64 65 71 73 **P**5 7 **S**0063 TENET Healthcare Corporation	33	10	167	8714	81	34286	3381	38629	17234	549
GARDENA—Los Angeles County ☐ COMMUNITY HOSPITAL OF GARDENA, 1246 West 155th Street, Zip 90247–4062; tel. 310/323–5330; Raymond N. Smith, Chief Executive Officer (Nonreporting) **A**1 9 10	33	10	55	—	—	—	—	—	—	—
☐ MEMORIAL HOSPITAL OF GARDENA, 1145 West Redondo Beach Boulevard, Zip 90247; tel. 310/532–4200; Ursula Durity, Administrator and Chief Executive Officer (Nonreporting) **A**1 9 10	33	10	107	—	—	—	—	—	—	—
GILROY—Santa Clara County ★ SOUTH VALLEY HOSPITAL, 9400 No Name Uno, Zip 95020–2368; tel. 408/848–2000; James M. Davis, Vice President and Administrator (Total facility includes 21 beds in nursing home–type unit) **A**1 10 **F**3 6 7 8 10 11 12 13 15 17 18 19 21 22 23 25 26 27 28 29 30 31 32 33 34 35 36 37 38 39 40 41 42 43 44 45 46 47 48 49 51 53 54 55 56 57 58 59 60 61 63 64 65 66 67 68 70 71 73 74 **P**3 **S**0965 Good Samaritan Health System	23	10	93	3084	41	33401	664	26662	9937	179
GLENDALE—Los Angeles County ☐ △ GLENDALE ADVENTIST MEDICAL CENTER, 1509 Wilson Terrace, Zip 91206–4007; tel. 818/409–8000; Robert G. Carmen, President (Nonreporting) **A**1 2 3 5 7 9 10 **S**0235 Adventist Health System/West	21	10	463	—	—	—	—	—	—	—
★ △ GLENDALE MEMORIAL HOSPITAL AND HEALTH CENTER, 1420 South Central Avenue, Zip 91204; tel. 818/502–1900; Roger E. Seaver, President and Chief Executive Officer **A**1 2 7 9 10 **F**3 4 7 8 10 11 12 16 17 18 19 21 22 24 27 28 29 30 32 34 36 37 39 40 41 42 43 44 45 48 49 52 54 56 59 60 63 64 65 67 71 73 **P**3 4 5 7 **S**2315 UniHealth	23	10	273	10124	166	44685	901	77308	36671	1008
☐ VERDUGO HILLS HOSPITAL, 1812 Verdugo Boulevard, Zip 91208, Mailing Address: P.O. Box 1431, Zip 91209–1431; tel. 818/790–7100; Bernard Glossy, President and Chief Executive Officer **A**1 2 9 10 **F**7 8 11 12 13 16 19 20 21 22 24 26 28 29 32 34 35 37 40 42 44 45 49 64 65 67 71 73 **P**5	23	10	148	5103	64	33457	1135	39791	15795	410
GLENDORA—Los Angeles County ★ FOOTHILL PRESBYTERIAN HOSPITAL–MORRIS L. JOHNSTON MEMORIAL, 250 South Grand Avenue, Zip 91741; tel. 818/963–8411; Bryan R. Rogers, President and Chief Executive Officer **A**1 2 9 10 **F**4 7 8 10 11 14 15 16 19 22 28 29 30 32 34 36 37 40 42 44 46 49 63 65 66 67 71 73 74 **P**3 5	23	10	107	4601	44	52167	1233	31447	12931	411
☐ HUNTINGTON EAST VALLEY HOSPITAL, 150 West Alosta Avenue, Zip 91740–4398; tel. 818/335–0231; James W. Maki, Interim Chief Executive Officer (Nonreporting) **A**1 9 10	32	10	138	—	—	—	—	—	—	—
GRANADA HILLS–Los Angeles County, See Los Angeles										
GRASS VALLEY—Nevada County ★ SIERRA NEVADA MEMORIAL HOSPITAL, 155 Glasson Way, Zip 95945–5792, Mailing Address: Box 1029, Zip 95945–5792; tel. 916/274–6000; C. Thomas Collier, Chief Executive Officer **A**1 9 10 **F**7 12 14 15 16 19 22 31 32 33 34 35 36 37 39 40 44 45 49 71	23	10	110	4916	55	89565	480	39417	14350	450
GREENBRAE—Marin County ★ MARIN GENERAL HOSPITAL, 250 Bon Air Road, Zip 94904, Mailing Address: Box 8010, San Rafael Zip 94912–8010; tel. 415/925–7000; Henry J. Buhrmann, President and Chief Executive Officer **A**1 2 9 10 **F**4 7 8 10 11 12 14 16 19 21 22 23 24 31 32 34 35 37 38 40 41 42 43 44 45 49 52 53 54 55 56 57 58 59 60 65 71 73 74 **P**1 7	23	10	91	9651	106	101506	1600	103388	42205	887
GREENVILLE—Plumas County INDIAN VALLEY HOSPITAL DISTRICT, 174 Hot Springs Road, Zip 95947; tel. 916/284–7191; Kent Aland, Administrator and Chief Executive Officer (Nonreporting) **A**9 10	16	10	26	—	—	—	—	—	—	—
GRIDLEY—Butte County BIGGS–GRIDLEY MEMORIAL HOSPITAL, 240 Spruce Street, Zip 95948, Mailing Address: Box 97, Zip 95948; tel. 916/846–5671; Charles R. Norton, Administrator (Nonreporting) **A**9 10	23	10	55	—	—	—	—	—	—	—
HANFORD—Kings County ☐ CENTRAL VALLEY GENERAL HOSPITAL, 1025 North Douty Street, Zip 93230, Mailing Address: Box 480, Zip 93232; tel. 209/583–2100; Gary K. Wiggins, Chief Executive Officer (Nonreporting) **A**1 9 10	21	10	66	—	—	—	—	—	—	—
★ HANFORD COMMUNITY MEDICAL CENTER, 450 Greenfield Avenue, Zip 93230–0240; Mailing Address: Box 240, Zip 93232–0240; tel. 209/582–9000; Stan B. Berry FACHE, Chief Executive Officer **A**1 9 10 **F**7 8 10 12 14 15 16 19 22 23 25 28 30 32 33 34 35 37 39 40 41 44 45 46 51 60 65 70 71 72 73 **P**3 **S**0235 Adventist Health System/West	21	10	54	4448	43	128325	1152	40994	15320	455

A44 Hospitals © 1995 AHA Guide

Hospitals, U.S. / CALIFORNIA

Hospital, Address, Telephone, Administrator, Approval, Facility, and Physician Codes, Health Care System	Classification Codes		Utilization Data					Expense (thousands) of dollars		
★ American Hospital Association (AHA) membership ☐ Joint Commission on Accreditation of Healthcare Organizations (JCAHO) accreditation + American Osteopathic Hospital Association (AOHA) membership ○ American Osteopathic Association (AOA) accreditation △ Commission on Accreditation of Rehabilitation Facilities (CARF) accreditation Control codes 61, 63, 64, 71, 72 and 73 indicate hospitals listed by AOHA, but not registered by AHA. For definition of numerical codes, see page A6	Control	Service	Beds	Admissions	Census	Outpatient Visits	Births	Total	Payroll	Personnel

HARBOR CITY–Los Angeles County, See Los Angeles

HAWAIIAN GARDENS—Los Angeles County

☐ CHARTER COMMUNITY HOSPITAL, 21530 South Pioneer Boulevard, Zip 90716; tel. 310/860–0401; Warren J. Kirk, Administrator **A**1 9 10 **F**3 4 7 8 10 12 13 15 18 19 20 21 22 25 26 27 28 29 30 31 32 33 34 35 36 37 39 41 42 43 44 45 46 49 50 51 53 54 55 56 57 58 59 60 61 62 63 65 66 67 68 69 70 71 72 73 74 **P**6 | 33 | 10 | 125 | 6718 | 91 | 17539 | 1 | 34367 | 15137 | 445

HAWTHORNE—Los Angeles County

☐ HAWTHORNE HOSPITAL, 13300 South Hawthorne Boulevard, Zip 90250; tel. 310/679–3321; Marvin Herschberg, Administrator (Nonreporting) **A**1 10 **S**0435 Pacific Health Corporation | 33 | 10 | 73 | — | — | — | — | — | — | —

★ ROBERT F. KENNEDY MEDICAL CENTER, 4500 West 116th Street, Zip 90250; tel. 310/973–1711; Patricia E. Cunningham R.N., President and Chief Executive Officer (Total facility includes 34 beds in nursing home–type unit) **A**1 9 10 **F**8 11 12 15 16 17 19 20 21 22 27 28 29 30 31 34 35 37 39 41 42 44 45 46 49 52 54 55 56 57 59 60 63 64 65 67 69 71 73 **P**5 | 23 | 10 | 196 | 5126 | 122 | 38550 | 0 | 43521 | 21324 | 565

HAYWARD—Alameda County

★ KAISER FOUNDATION HOSPITAL, 27400 Hesperian Boulevard, Zip 94545–4297; tel. 510/784–4313 **A**1 10 **F**3 8 10 11 12 14 15 16 17 19 21 22 23 29 31 32 33 37 38 39 40 42 43 44 45 46 49 51 53 54 55 56 57 58 59 60 65 67 71 72 73 **P**3 **S**2105 Kaiser Foundation Hospitals | 23 | 10 | 224 | 13729 | 147 | 761013 | 3052 | — | — | 1809

☐ ST. ROSE HOSPITAL, 27200 Calaroga Avenue, Zip 94545–4383; tel. 510/264–4000; Michael P. Mahoney, President and Chief Executive Officer (Nonreporting) **A**1 2 9 10 **S**5435 CSJ Health System of Wichita | 21 | 10 | 175 | — | — | — | — | — | — | —

HEALDSBURG—Sonoma County

★ HEALDSBURG GENERAL HOSPITAL, 1375 University Street, Zip 95448; tel. 707/431–6500; Brad Mitchell, Executive Director (Nonreporting) **A**1 9 10 **S**0048 Columbia/HCA Healthcare Corporation | 33 | 10 | 49 | — | — | — | — | — | — | —

HEMET—Riverside County

☐ HEMET VALLEY MEDICAL CENTER, 1117 East Devonshire Avenue, Zip 92543; tel. 909/652–2811; Edward C. Burke, Administrator **A**1 9 10 **F**3 8 10 11 12 15 16 19 21 22 23 26 27 28 29 33 34 35 37 40 41 42 44 45 46 49 52 57 58 59 60 65 71 73 **P**4 5 **S**0043 Valley Health System | 16 | 10 | 295 | 12674 | 165 | 107938 | 1237 | 70673 | 26528 | 742

HOLLISTER—San Benito County

HAZEL HAWKINS CONVALESCENT HOSPITAL–SOUTHSIDE See San Benito Hospital District

HAZEL HAWKINS MEMORIAL HOSPITAL See San Benito Hospital District

☐ SAN BENITO HOSPITAL DISTRICT, (Includes Hazel Hawkins Convalescent Hospital–Southside, 3110 Southside Road, Hollister, California, Zip 95023; tel. 408/637–5711; Hazel Hawkins Memorial Hospital, 911 Sunset Drive, Hollister, California, Zip 95023; tel. 408/637–5711) 911 Sunset Drive, Zip 95023–5695; tel. 408/637–5711; Louis D. Kraml, Administrator (Nonreporting) **A**1 **S**0585 Brim, Inc. | 16 | 10 | 86 | — | — | — | — | — | — | —

HOLLYWOOD–Los Angeles County, See Los Angeles

HUNTINGTON BEACH—Orange County

★ HUNTINGTON BEACH HOSPITAL AND MEDICAL CENTER, (Formerly Huntington Beach Medical Center) 17772 Beach Boulevard, Zip 92647–9932; tel. 714/842–1473; Carol B. Freeman, Chief Executive Officer **A**1 9 10 **F**4 7 8 11 15 16 17 18 19 21 22 23 27 28 35 37 39 40 41 42 44 49 52 59 65 71 73 **P**5 **S**0048 Columbia/HCA Healthcare Corporation | 33 | 10 | 135 | 3145 | 40 | — | 327 | 26100 | 12449 | 349

☐ PACIFICA HOSPITAL, (Formerly Pacifica Community Hospital) 18800 Delaware Street, Zip 92648; tel. 714/842–0611; Barbara J. Foster, Chief Operating Officer (Nonreporting) **A**1 9 10 | 33 | 10 | 103 | — | — | — | — | — | — | —

HUNTINGTON PARK—Los Angeles County

☐ COMMUNITY AND MISSION HOSPITALS OF HUNTINGTON, (Includes Community Hospital of Huntington Park, 2623 East Slauson Avenue, Huntington Park, California, Zip 90255; tel. 213/583–1931; Mission Hospital, 3111 East Florence Avenue, Huntington Park, California, Zip 90255; tel. 213/582–8261) 2623 East Slauson Avenue, Zip 90255; tel. 213/583–1931; Jeffrey K. Stadnik, Administrator (Nonreporting) **A**1 9 10 **S**6525 Ornda Healthcorp | 33 | 10 | 226 | — | — | — | — | — | — | —

COMMUNITY HOSPITAL OF HUNTINGTON PARK See Community and Mission Hospitals of Huntington

MISSION HOSPITAL See Community and Mission Hospital of Huntington

INDIO—Riverside County

☐ JOHN F. KENNEDY MEMORIAL HOSPITAL, 47–111 Monroe Street, Zip 92201, Mailing Address: P.O. Drawer LLLL, Zip 92202–2558; tel. 619/347–6191; Barry A. Wolfman, Chief Executive Officer (Nonreporting) **A**1 9 10 | 33 | 10 | 130 | — | — | — | — | — | — | —

INGLEWOOD—Los Angeles County

★ △ CENTINELA HOSPITAL MEDICAL CENTER, 555 East Hardy Street, Zip 90301–4073, Mailing Address: Box 720, Zip 90307–0720; tel. 310/673–4660; Russell S. Stromberg, President (Total facility includes 24 beds in nursing home–type unit) **A**1 2 3 7 9 10 **F**4 5 8 10 12 14 15 16 17 19 21 22 23 24 25 27 28 29 30 31 32 34 35 37 38 40 41 42 43 44 45 46 48 49 51 60 61 63 64 65 66 71 72 73 74 **P**5 7 | 23 | 10 | 375 | 13457 | 203 | 136899 | 2879 | 122348 | 56500 | 1435

Hospitals, U.S. / CALIFORNIA

Hospital, Address, Telephone, Administrator, Approval, Facility, and Physician Codes, Health Care System	Classification Codes		Utilization Data					Expense (thousands) of dollars		
★ American Hospital Association (AHA) membership ☐ Joint Commission on Accreditation of Healthcare Organizations (JCAHO) accreditation + American Osteopathic Hospital Association (AOHA) membership ○ American Osteopathic Association (AOA) accreditation △ Commission on Accreditation of Rehabilitation Facilities (CARF) accreditation Control codes 61, 63, 64, 71, 72 and 73 indicate hospitals listed by AOHA, but not registered by AHA. For definition of numerical codes, see page A6.	Control	Service	Beds	Admissions	Census	Outpatient Visits	Births	Total	Payroll	Personnel
★ △ DANIEL FREEMAN MEMORIAL HOSPITAL, 333 North Prairie Avenue, Zip 90301–4514; tel. 310/674–7050; Peter F. Bastone, Chief Executive Officer (Nonreporting) **A**1 5 7 9 10 **S**5945 Carondelet Health System	21	10	181	—	—	—	—	—	—	—
IRVINE—Orange County										
★ IRVINE MEDICAL CENTER, 16200 Sand Canyon Avenue, Zip 92718–3701; tel. 714/753–2000; Robert C. Shaw, Executive Director (Nonreporting) **A**1 10 **S**0063 TENET Healthcare Corporation	33	10	176	—	—	—	—	—	—	—
JACKSON—Amador County										
☐ SUTTER AMADOR HOSPITAL, 810 Court Street, Zip 95642–2379; tel. 209/223–7500; Scott Stenberg, Administrator (Total facility includes 44 beds in nursing home–type unit) **A**1 9 10 **F**7 8 15 19 21 22 26 29 30 31 34 35 37 40 42 44 63 64 65 71 73 **P**3 5 **S**8795 Sutter Health	23	10	85	2359	59	29254	201	17801	7903	210
JOSHUA TREE—San Bernardino County										
★ HI-DESERT MEDICAL CENTER, 6601 White Feather Road, Zip 92252–6601; tel. 619/366–3711; James R. Larson, President and Chief Executive Officer (Total facility includes 73 beds in nursing home–type unit) **A**1 9 10 **F**8 12 17 19 20 21 22 25 26 28 30 32 33 34 35 37 39 41 44 45 46 49 64 65 67 71 73	16	10	109	2926	109	43294	0	27630	9755	335
KENTFIELD—Marin County										
★ △ KENTFIELD REHABILITATION HOSPITAL, 1125 Sir Francis Drake Boulevard, Zip 94904, Mailing Address: P.O. Box 338, Zip 94914–0338; tel. 415/456–9680; William O. Mitchell Jr., Administrator (Nonreporting) **A**1 7 9 10 **S**1715 Continental Medical Systems, Inc.	33	46	60	—	—	—	—	—	—	—
☐ ROSS HOSPITAL, 1111 Sir Francis Drake Boulevard, Zip 94904; tel. 415/258–6900; Judy G. House, Administrator **A**1 10 **F**2 3 15 19 21 35 50 52 53 57 59 63	33	22	57	952	25	9178	0	6608	3981	54
KING CITY—Monterey County										
GEORGE L. MEE MEMORIAL HOSPITAL, 300 Canal Street, Zip 93930–3410; tel. 408/385–6000; Linda B. Stireman, Chief Executive Officer (Nonreporting) **A**9 10	23	10	42	—	—	—	—	—	—	—
KINGSBURG—Fresno County										
☐ KINGSBURG DISTRICT HOSPITAL, 1200 Smith Street, Zip 93631; tel. 209/897–5841; Larry E. Kast, Administrator (Total facility includes 20 beds in nursing home–type unit) **A**1 9 10 **F**14 15 16 34 44 64 71 72 73	16	10	35	134	19	14768	0	3451	1630	58
LA HABRA—Orange County										
★ FRIENDLY HILLS REGIONAL MEDICAL CENTER, 1251 West Lambert Road, Zip 90631; tel. 310/694–3838; Robert E. Hanna, Executive Director and Senior Vice President **A**1 9 10 **F**3 4 7 8 10 12 13 15 16 17 19 21 22 23 27 29 30 32 33 34 35 36 37 38 39 40 41 42 43 44 45 46 49 51 53 54 55 56 57 58 59 60 61 64 65 67 69 71 72 73 74 **P**3 5 6	23	10	226	7112	78	23421	1742	94509	27695	692
LA JOLLA—San Diego County										
★ GREEN HOSPITAL OF SCRIPPS CLINIC, 10666 North Torrey Pines Road, Zip 92037–1093; tel. 619/455–9100; Glenn W. Chong, Senior Vice President and Director **A**1 2 5 8 9 10 **F**2 3 4 7 8 10 12 16 17 19 20 21 22 23 24 25 26 27 28 29 30 31 32 34 35 37 38 39 40 41 42 43 44 45 48 49 52 53 54 55 56 57 58 59 60 61 63 64 65 66 67 69 70 71 72 73 74 **P**3 5 7 **S**1505 Scripps Hospitals	23	10	165	7769	93	118786	0	94295	31343	829
★ △ SCRIPPS MEMORIAL HOSPITAL – LA JOLLA, 9888 Genesee Avenue, Zip 92037–1276, Mailing Address: Box 28, Zip 92038–0028; tel. 619/457–4123; (Nonreporting) **A**1 2 7 9 10 **S**1505 Scripps Hospitals	23	10	433	—	—	—	—	—	—	—
LA MESA—San Diego County										
★ △ GROSSMONT HOSPITAL, 5555 Grossmont Center Drive, Zip 91942, Mailing Address: Box 158, Zip 91944–0158; tel. 619/465–0711; Thomas F. Spindler, Interim Chief Executive Officer **A**1 2 3 7 9 10 **F**4 7 8 10 12 16 17 19 20 21 22 23 25 26 27 31 32 33 34 35 36 37 38 39 40 41 42 43 44 46 48 49 51 52 54 55 56 57 58 59 60 61 64 65 66 67 68 69 70 71 72 73 74 **P**5 7 **S**2065 Sharp Healthcare	23	10	377	18036	233	184944	3136	143163	63893	1738
LA PALMA—Orange County										
★ △ LA PALMA INTERCOMMUNITY HOSPITAL, 7901 Walker Street, Zip 90623–5850, Mailing Address: P.O. Box 5850, Buena Park Zip 90622; tel. 714/670–7400; Stephen Dixon, President and Chief Executive Officer **A**1 2 7 9 10 **F**1 3 4 7 8 10 12 14 15 16 17 19 21 22 27 28 31 32 33 34 35 36 37 39 40 41 42 43 44 46 48 49 52 57 58 59 60 63 65 67 71 72 73 74 **P**3 5 7 **S**2315 UniHealth	23	10	139	4059	61	48133	860	35441	15034	406
LAGUNA BEACH—Orange County										
☐ LAGUNA HILLS HOSPITAL AND MENTAL HEALTH CENTER, 24552 Pacific Park Drive, Zip 92656; tel. 714/831–1800; Gilbert Carmona, Regional Chief Executive Officer (Nonreporting) **A**1 9 10 **S**0785 Community Psychiatric Centers	33	22	78	—	—	—	—	—	—	—
LAGUNA HILLS—Orange County										
☐ △ SADDLEBACK MEMORIAL MEDICAL CENTER, 24451 Health Center Drive, Zip 92653; tel. 714/837–4500; Nolan Draney, Executive Vice President (Nonreporting) **A**1 2 7 9 10	23	10	221	—	—	—	—	—	—	—
LAKE ARROWHEAD—San Bernardino County										
☐ MOUNTAINS COMMUNITY HOSPITAL, 29101 Hospital Road, Zip 92352, Mailing Address: Box 70, Zip 92352; tel. 909/336–3651; John J. McCormick, Chief Executive Officer (Total facility includes 18 beds in nursing home–type unit) **A**1 9 10 **F**7 8 14 19 22 32 36 41 44 49 64 65 71 **P**3	16	10	36	653	21	15672	138	8884	3920	123
LAKE ISABELLA—Kern County										
KERN VALLEY HOSPITAL DISTRICT, 6412 Laurel Avenue, Zip 93240, Mailing Address: P.O. Box 1628, Zip 93240; tel. 619/379–2681; L. Ned Miller, Chief Executive Officer (Total facility includes 74 beds in nursing home–type unit) **A**9 10 **F**14 15 16 17 19 22 28 30 32 34 37 44 46 64 67 71 73	16	10	101	1275	77	15924	5	12137	4539	131

Hospitals, U.S. / CALIFORNIA

Hospital, Address, Telephone, Administrator, Approval, Facility, and Physician Codes, Health Care System ★ American Hospital Association (AHA) membership ☐ Joint Commission on Accreditation of Healthcare Organizations (JCAHO) accreditation + American Osteopathic Hospital Association (AOHA) membership ○ American Osteopathic Association (AOA) accreditation △ Commission on Accreditation of Rehabilitation Facilities (CARF) accreditation Control codes 61, 63, 64, 71, 72 and 73 indicate hospitals listed by AOHA, but not registered by AHA. For definition of numerical codes, see page A6	Classification Codes		Utilization Data					Expense (thousands) of dollars		
	Control	Service	Beds	Admissions	Census	Outpatient Visits	Births	Total	Payroll	Personnel
LAKEPORT—Lake County ★ SUTTER LAKESIDE HOSPITAL, 5176 Hill Road East, Zip 95453-6112; tel. 707/262-5001; Paul J. Hensler, Administrator (Nonreporting) A1 10 S8795 Sutter Health	23	10	50	—	—	—	—	—	—	—
LAKEWOOD—Los Angeles County DOCTORS HOSPITAL OF LAKEWOOD See Lakewood Regional Medical Center ☐ LAKEWOOD REGIONAL MEDICAL CENTER, (Includes Doctors Hospital of Lakewood, 3700 East South Street, Lakewood, California, Zip 90712; tel. 213/531-2550; Michael Kerr, Chief Executive Officer; New Beginnings Doctors Hospital of Lakewood-Clark, 5300 Clark Avenue, Lakewood, California, Zip 90712; tel. 213/866-9711) 3700 East South Street, Zip 90712; tel. 310/531-2550; Gustavo A. Valdespino, Chief Executive Officer A1 2 9 10 F1 3 4 6 7 8 10 11 12 14 15 16 17 18 19 21 22 28 29 30 33 34 35 37 39 40 41 42 43 44 45 46 49 50 51 63 65 66 71 73 74 P5 S0063 TENET Healthcare Corporation NEW BEGINNINGS DOCTORS HOSPITAL OF LAKEWOOD-CLARK See Lakewood Regional Medical Center	33	10	175	6453	89	41774	846	46568	18157	514
LANCASTER—Los Angeles County ★ ANTELOPE VALLEY HOSPITAL MEDICAL CENTER, 1600 West Avenue J, Zip 93534-2894; tel. 805/949-5000; Robert J. Harenski, Chief Executive Officer (Nonreporting) A1 9 10	16	10	281	—	—	—	—	—	—	—
★ LAC-HIGH DESERT HOSPITAL, 44900 North 60th Street West, Zip 93536; tel. 805/945-8461; A. Roy Fleischman, Administrator (Total facility includes 70 beds in nursing home-type unit) A1 9 10 F7 8 12 17 19 20 21 23 25 30 31 32 34 35 37 38 40 41 42 44 45 46 48 49 51 64 65 71 73 74 P6 S5755 Los Angeles County-Department of Health Services	13	10	114	1906	99	74331	0	55126	23808	694
☐ LANCASTER COMMUNITY HOSPITAL, 43830 North Tenth Street West, Zip 93534; tel. 805/948-4781; Steve Schmidt, Chief Executive Officer (Nonreporting) A1 9 10 S5765 Paracelsus Healthcare Corporation	33	10	132	—	—	—	—	—	—	—
LEMOORE—Kings County ★ NAVAL HOSPITAL, 930 Franklin Avenue, Zip 93246-5000; tel. 209/998-4201; Lieutenant Commander Sharon R. Thomas MSC, Administrator A1 F7 8 12 17 19 20 21 27 28 30 32 34 40 41 44 46 49 51 54 56 58 65 71 73 S9655 Department of Navy	43	10	29	1279	8	103467	320	—	—	344
LINDSAY—Tulare County ★ LINDSAY HOSPITAL MEDICAL CENTER, 740 North Sequoia Avenue, Zip 93247, Mailing Address: Box 40, Zip 93247; tel. 209/562-4955; Frank F. Jordan, President and Chief Executive Officer (Total facility includes 53 beds in nursing home-type unit) A1 9 10 F7 15 16 19 21 22 26 30 35 37 39 40 41 44 64 65 71 73 74 S2315 UniHealth	23	10	106	2236	71	46403	777	13421	6150	213
LIVERMORE—Alameda County ☐ VALLEY MEMORIAL HOSPITAL, 1111 East Stanley Boulevard, Zip 94550; tel. 510/447-7000; Robert H. Fish, President and Chief Executive Officer (Nonreporting) A1 2 9 10	23	10	110	—	—	—	—	—	—	—
★ VETERANS AFFAIRS MEDICAL CENTER, 4951 Arroyo Road, Zip 94550; tel. 510/447-2560; Clarence H. Nixon, Director (Nonreporting) A1 3 5 S9295 Department of Veterans Affairs	45	10	165	—	—	—	—	—	—	—
LODI—San Joaquin County ★ △ LODI MEMORIAL HOSPITAL, (Includes Lodi Memorial Hospital West, 800 South Lower Sacramento Road, Zip 95242; tel. 209/333-0211) 975 South Fairmont Avenue, Zip 95240-5179, Mailing Address: P.O. Box 3004, Zip 95241-1908; tel. 209/334-3411; Joseph P. Harrington, Administrator and Chief Executive Officer (Total facility includes 41 beds in nursing home-type unit) A1 7 9 10 F1 7 8 10 12 14 16 19 22 23 24 26 27 28 32 33 34 35 36 37 39 40 42 44 45 46 48 49 64 65 67 71 72 P5	23	10	154	5763	86	86394	1130	43961	22091	597
LOMA LINDA—San Bernardino County ★ JERRY L. PETTIS MEMORIAL VETERANS HOSPITAL, 11201 Benton Street, Zip 92357; tel. 909/825-7084; Dean R. Stordahl, Director (Total facility includes 108 beds in nursing home-type unit) A1 3 5 8 F2 3 4 5 8 10 11 12 14 18 19 20 21 22 26 27 28 30 31 32 34 35 37 39 41 42 43 44 45 46 48 49 51 52 54 56 57 58 60 64 65 67 69 71 72 73 74 S9295 Department of Veterans Affairs	45	10	393	7679	288	198300	0	103471	69454	1313
★ △ LOMA LINDA UNIVERSITY COMMUNITY MEDICAL CENTER, (Includes Loma Linda Community Hospital, 25333 Barton Road, Zip 92354; tel. 909/796-0167) 11234 Anderson Street, Zip 92354-2870, Mailing Address: P.O. Box 2000, Zip 92354-0200; tel. 909/824-0800; J. David Moorhead M.D., President and Chief Executive Officer A1 2 3 5 7 8 9 10 F1 2 3 4 5 6 7 8 9 10 11 12 13 15 16 17 18 19 20 21 22 23 24 25 26 27 28 29 30 31 32 33 34 35 36 37 38 39 41 42 43 44 45 46 47 48 49 50 51 52 53 54 55 56 57 58 59 60 61 63 65 66 67 68 69 70 71 72 73 74 P3 4 5 7 S2175 Adventist Health System-Loma Linda	21	10	850	31374	518	212585	2539	419697	142671	5409
LOMPOC—Santa Barbara County ☐ LOMPOC DISTRICT HOSPITAL, 508 East Hickory Street, Zip 93436, Mailing Address: Box 1058, Zip 93438; tel. 805/737-3300; Scott Rhine, Administrator and Chief Executive Officer (Nonreporting) A1 9 10	16	10	170	—	—	—	—	—	—	—
LONE PINE—Inyo County SOUTHERN INYO HOSPITAL, 501 East Locust Street, Zip 93545, Mailing Address: Box 1009, Zip 93545; tel. 619/876-5501; Walter Beck, Administrator (Nonreporting) A9 10	16	10	37	—	—	—	—	—	—	—

Hospitals, U.S. / CALIFORNIA

Hospital, Address, Telephone, Administrator, Approval, Facility, and Physician Codes, Health Care System	Classification Codes		Utilization Data					Expense (thousands) of dollars		Personnel
★ American Hospital Association (AHA) membership ☐ Joint Commission on Accreditation of Healthcare Organizations (JCAHO) accreditation + American Osteopathic Hospital Association (AOHA) membership ○ American Osteopathic Association (AOA) accreditation △ Commission on Accreditation of Rehabilitation Facilities (CARF) accreditation Control codes 61, 63, 64, 71, 72 and 73 indicate hospitals listed by AOHA, but not registered by AHA. For definition of numerical codes, see page A6	Control	Service	Beds	Admissions	Census	Outpatient Visits	Births	Total	Payroll	

LONG BEACH—Los Angeles County

☐ CHARTER BEHAVIORAL HEALTH SYSTEM OF SOUTHERN CALIFORNIA–LONG BEACH, (Formerly Charter Hospital of Long Beach) 6060 Paramount Boulevard, Zip 90805; tel. 310/220–1000; (Nonreporting) A1 9 10 S0695 Charter Medical Corporation	33	22	50	—	—	—	—	—	—	—
☐ CHARTER BEHAVIORAL HEALTH SYSTEM OF SOUTHERN CALIFORNIA–LOS ALTOS, (Formerly Los Altos Hospital and Mental Health Center) 3340 Los Coyotes Diagonal, Zip 90808–3999; tel. 310/421–9311; Larry Steudle, Chief Executive Officer (Nonreporting) A1 9 10 S0695 Charter Medical Corporation	33	22	46	—	—	—	—	—	—	—
CHARTER HOSPITAL OF LONG BEACH See Charter Behavioral Health System of Southern California–Long Beach										
★ LONG BEACH COMMUNITY HOSPITAL AND MEDICAL CENTER, 1720 Termino Avenue, Zip 90804; tel. 310/498–1000; Janet Parodi, President and Chief Executive Officer A1 2 9 10 F1 4 7 8 10 11 12 14 15 16 17 19 21 22 23 26 27 28 30 31 32 33 34 35 37 38 39 40 41 42 43 44 45 46 47 49 51 52 54 55 56 57 58 59 60 63 64 65 67 71 73 74 P1 2 3 4 5 7 S2315 UniHealth	23	10	302	16745	148	66671	3205	84327	35091	975
☐ LONG BEACH DOCTORS HOSPITAL, 1725 Pacific Avenue, Zip 90813–1798; tel. 310/599–3551; Lenore M. Cullman R.N., Administrator and Chief Executive Officer (Nonreporting) A1 9 10	33	10	43	—	—	—	—	—	—	—
☐ △ LONG BEACH MEMORIAL MEDICAL CENTER, 2801 Atlantic Avenue, Zip 90806, Mailing Address: Box 1428, Zip 90801–1428; tel. 310/933–2000; Thomas J. Collins, President and Chief Executive Officer (Nonreporting) A1 2 3 5 7 8 9 10	23	10	729	—	—	—	—	—	—	—
LOS ALTOS HOSPITAL AND MENTAL HEALTH CENTER See Charter Behavioral Health System of Southern California–Los Altos										
☐ ○ PACIFIC HOSPITAL OF LONG BEACH, 2776 Pacific Avenue, Zip 90806–2699, Mailing Address: P.O. Box 1268, Zip 90801; tel. 310/595–1911; Gerald S. Goldberg, Administrator and Chief Executive Officer (Total facility includes 27 beds in nursing home–type unit) A1 9 10 11 12 13 F8 12 13 15 16 17 19 20 22 26 27 28 31 32 33 34 35 37 40 41 44 49 52 56 57 59 64 65 69 71 73 P3 5	23	10	179	3449	68	42892	777	26889	12719	387
REDGATE MEMORIAL HOSPITAL, 1775 Chestnut Avenue, Zip 90813; tel. 310/599–8444; Robert Worrell, Administrator (Nonreporting)	23	82	63	—	—	—	—	—	—	—
★ ST. MARY MEDICAL CENTER, 1050 Linden Avenue, Zip 90801, Mailing Address: P.O. Box 887, Zip 90801; tel. 310/491–9000; David Tillman M.D., President (Total facility includes 80 beds in nursing home–type unit) A1 2 3 5 9 10 F1 2 3 4 6 7 8 10 12 15 16 17 19 21 22 24 25 26 30 31 32 33 34 35 37 38 40 41 42 43 44 46 47 48 49 50 51 52 57 58 59 60 63 64 65 69 70 71 72 73 P5 7 S0605 Sisters of Charity of the Incarnate Word Healthcare System	21	10	484	12457	268	173311	2817	135440	56928	1693
★ VETERANS AFFAIRS MEDICAL CENTER, 5901 East Seventh Street, Zip 90822–5201; tel. 310/494–5400; Jerry B. Boyd, Director (Nonreporting) A1 2 3 5 8 S9295 Department of Veterans Affairs	45	10	1131	—	—	—	—	—	—	—
☐ WOODRUFF COMMUNITY HOSPITAL, 3800 Woodruff Avenue, Zip 90808; tel. 310/421–8241; Robert Glass, Administrator A1 9 10 F11 16 19 22 35 37 44 49 65 71 73 74 P5 7 S6525 Ornda Healthcorp	33	10	96	1478	42	5369	0	16874	6341	192

LOS ALAMITOS—Orange County

☐ LOS ALAMITOS MEDICAL CENTER, 3751 Katella Avenue, Zip 90720; tel. 310/598–1311; Gustavo A. Valdespino, Executive Director (Nonreporting) A1 2 9 10 S0063 TENET Healthcare Corporation	33	10	173	—	—	—	—	—	—	—

LOS ANGELES—Los Angeles County
(Mailing Addresses – Canoga Park, Encino, Granada Hills, Harbor City, Hollywood, Mission Hills, North Hollywood, Northridge, Panorama City, San Pedro, Sepulveda, Sherman Oaks, Sun Valley, Sylmar, Tarzana, Van Nuys, West Hills, West Los Angeles, Woodland Hills)

★ BARLOW RESPIRATORY HOSPITAL, 2000 Stadium Way, Zip 90026–2696; tel. 213/250–4200; Margaret W. Crane, Chief Executive Officer A1 3 5 9 10 F15 16 19 20 21 34 37 41 49 65 67 71	23	33	49	312	38	700	0	19940	8274	188
★ BAY HARBOR HOSPITAL, 1437 West Lomita Boulevard, Harbor City, Zip 90710–2097; tel. 310/325–1221; Jack W. Weiblen FACHE, Chief Executive Officer (Total facility includes 212 beds in nursing home–type unit) A1 2 9 10 F2 4 8 9 10 11 12 17 19 22 28 32 34 35 37 38 40 42 43 44 45 47 49 51 52 60 64 71 73 P3	23	10	362	6342	222	36085	704	49768	23381	871
★ CALIFORNIA HOSPITAL MEDICAL CENTER, 1401 South Grand Avenue, Zip 90015; tel. 213/748–2411; James T. Yoshioka, President and Chief Executive Officer (Total facility includes 19 beds in nursing home–type unit) A1 2 3 5 9 10 F7 8 10 11 12 17 19 21 22 27 28 30 32 34 37 38 40 41 42 44 47 48 49 51 52 54 58 60 61 64 65 67 68 71 72 73 74 P3 4 5 6 7 S2315 UniHealth	23	10	279	13518	164	81359	4748	97561	42309	1139
★ CEDARS–SINAI MEDICAL CENTER, 8700 Beverly Boulevard, Zip 90048–0750, Mailing Address: Box 48750, Zip 90048–0750; tel. 310/855–5000; Thomas M. Priselac, President and Chief Executive Officer A1 2 3 5 8 9 10 F2 3 4 5 7 8 10 11 12 13 14 15 16 17 18 19 20 21 22 23 26 27 28 29 30 31 32 33 34 35 36 37 39 40 41 42 43 44 45 46 47 48 49 51 52 53 54 55 56 57 58 60 61 63 64 65 67 68 69 70 71 73 74 P3 5 8	23	10	815	39154	625	—	6870	558420	—	5671
☐ CENTURY CITY HOSPITAL, 2070 Century Park East, Zip 90067; tel. 310/553–6211; Kenneth Berg, Chief Executive Officer A1 5 9 10 F1 7 8 12 15 16 17 19 21 22 25 26 27 28 30 31 32 34 35 37 39 42 44 45 46 49 52 54 55 57 59 60 61 65 66 67 71 73 74 P5 7 S0063 TENET Healthcare Corporation	33	10	135	4452	77	19196	0	61304	22406	584

Hospitals, U.S. / CALIFORNIA

Hospital, Address, Telephone, Administrator, Approval, Facility, and Physician Codes, Health Care System	Classification Codes		Utilization Data					Expense (thousands) of dollars		
★ American Hospital Association (AHA) membership □ Joint Commission on Accreditation of Healthcare Organizations (JCAHO) accreditation + American Osteopathic Hospital Association (AOHA) membership ○ American Osteopathic Association (AOA) accreditation △ Commission on Accreditation of Rehabilitation Facilities (CARF) accreditation Control codes 61, 63, 64, 71, 72 and 73 indicate hospitals listed by AOHA, but not registered by AHA. For definition of numerical codes, see page A6	Control	Service	Beds	Admissions	Census	Outpatient Visits	Births	Total	Payroll	Personnel
★ CHILDRENS HOSPITAL OF LOS ANGELES, 4650 Sunset Boulevard, Zip 90027–6089; Mailing Address: Box 54700, Zip 90054–0700; tel. 213/660–2450; Walter W. Noce Jr., President **A**1 2 3 5 9 10 **F**4 5 10 12 15 16 17 19 20 21 22 31 32 34 35 38 42 43 44 46 47 48 49 51 53 60 65 67 68 69 70 71 72 73 **P**5	23	50	330	11527	218	186194	0	217727	100585	2490
★ DOHENY EYE INSTITUTE, (Ophthalmology) 1450 San Pablo Street, Zip 90033–1059; tel. 213/342–6500; Lise Luttgens–Santulli, Chief Operating Officer and Administrator **A**1 9 10 **F**14 15 16 17 19 34 35 44 50 65 71 **P**4 5	23	49	25	357	2	—	0	5068	1734	57
□ EAST LOS ANGELES DOCTORS HOSPITAL, 4060 Whittier Boulevard, Zip 90023; tel. 213/268–5514; Sandy Hazel, Chief Executive Officer (Total facility includes 25 beds in nursing home–type unit) **A**1 9 10 **F**7 8 19 20 22 27 28 32 34 35 37 40 41 44 46 49 64 65 67 71 73 **P**5 8	33	10	127	2740	58	16906	851	23863	10558	324
□ EDGEMONT HOSPITAL, 4841 Hollywood Boulevard, Zip 90027; tel. 213/913–9000; Jack Freinhar, Administrator (Nonreporting) **A**1 9 10	33	22	61	—	—	—	—	—	—	—
★ ENCINO–TARZANA REGIONAL MEDICAL CENTER, (Includes Encino–Tarzana Regional Medical Center, 16237 Ventura Boulevard, Los Angeles, California, Zip 91436–2201; tel. 818/995–5000) 18321 Clark Street, Encino, Zip 91356; tel. 818/881–0800; William H. Comte, Chief Executive Officer (Nonreporting) **A**1 2 3 5 9 10 **S**0063 TENET Healthcare Corporation	33	10	391	—	—	—	—	—	—	—
□ GATEWAYS HOSPITAL AND MENTAL HEALTH CENTER, 1891 Effie Street, Zip 90026–1711; tel. 213/644–2000; Saul Goldfarb, Chief Executive Officer **A**1 9 10 **F**52 53 57 58 59	23	22	55	449	25	0	0	6796	3850	115
★ GRANADA HILLS COMMUNITY HOSPITAL, 10445 Balboa Boulevard, Granada Hills, Zip 91394–9400; tel. 818/360–1021; Richard A. Gold, President and Chief Executive Officer **A**1 9 10 **F**4 8 10 11 12 15 16 19 21 22 24 26 34 35 37 40 41 43 44 64 65 71 73 74 **P**5 7 8	23	10	129	4979	67	22971	1455	36101	15163	440
□ HOLLYWOOD COMMUNITY HOSPITAL OF HOLLYWOOD, 6245 De Longpre Avenue, Hollywood, Zip 90028; tel. 213/462–2271; Maxine Cooper, Chief Executive Officer **A**1 9 10 **F**1 4 10 11 15 16 17 18 19 20 21 22 26 31 32 33 34 35 37 39 42 43 44 51 52 56 57 58 59 60 65 67 68 71 **S**5765 Paracelsus Healthcare Corporation	33	10	99	1423	23	6266	0	24054	8014	187
HOLLYWOOD COMMUNITY HOSPITAL OF VAN NUYS, 14433 Emelita Street, Van Nuys, Zip 91401, Mailing Address: P.O. Box 2698, Zip 91401; tel. 818/787–1511; Elizabeth Scarcelli, Administrator **A**9 **F**15 16 52 54 55 57 59 65 **S**5765 Paracelsus Healthcare Corporation	33	22	61	548	22	10190	0	8796	2540	65
★ △ HOLY CROSS MEDICAL CENTER, 15031 Rinaldi Street, Mission Hills, Zip 91345–1285; tel. 818/365–8051; Carl W. Fitch Sr., President and Chief Executive Officer **A**1 2 7 10 **F**7 8 10 14 15 16 17 19 21 22 28 30 31 32 34 35 37 38 40 41 42 43 44 45 49 60 63 64 65 70 71 72 73 **P**7 **S**5585 Holy Cross Health System Corporation	21	10	257	9707	152	82430	1418	79037	29633	839
□ △ HOSPITAL OF THE GOOD SAMARITAN, 616 South Witmer Street, Zip 90017–2395; tel. 213/977–2121; Mirion P. Bowers, President and Chief Executive Officer (Nonreporting) **A**1 2 5 7 8 9 10	23	10	377	—	—	—	—	—	—	—
★ KAISER FOUNDATION HOSPITAL, (Includes Kaiser Foundation Mental Health Center, 765 West College Street, Los Angeles, California, Zip 90012; tel. 213/580–7200) 4867 Sunset Boulevard, Zip 90027; tel. 213/667–4011; Joseph William Hummel, Administrator **A**1 2 3 5 9 10 **F**3 4 8 10 11 14 15 16 19 21 22 26 28 31 32 33 35 37 38 40 41 42 43 44 45 47 49 52 53 54 55 56 58 59 60 61 63 65 69 71 73 **S**2105 Kaiser Foundation Hospitals	23	10	496	21310	255	—	2890	—	—	1759
★ KAISER FOUNDATION HOSPITAL, 25825 South Vermont Avenue, Harbor City, Zip 90710; tel. 310/517–2770; Mary Ann Barnes, Administrator **A**1 2 9 10 **F**2 3 4 7 8 10 11 12 14 15 16 19 21 22 23 25 26 28 30 31 32 33 34 35 37 39 40 41 42 43 44 45 46 49 51 53 54 55 56 57 58 60 61 63 65 69 71 72 73 **S**2105 Kaiser Foundation Hospitals	23	10	223	10246	105	68666	1900	—	—	748
★ KAISER FOUNDATION HOSPITAL, 13652 Cantara Street, Panorama City, Zip 91402; tel. 818/375–2000; Dev Mahadevan, Administrator **A**1 2 5 9 10 **F**3 4 7 8 11 12 13 14 15 16 17 18 19 21 22 26 27 28 29 30 31 32 33 34 35 37 38 40 41 42 43 44 45 46 49 50 51 53 54 55 56 57 58 59 61 63 65 66 67 68 69 71 72 **P**4 **S**2105 Kaiser Foundation Hospitals	23	10	269	9854	101	20832	1899	—	—	—
★ KAISER FOUNDATION HOSPITAL, 5601 DeSoto Avenue, Woodland Hills, Zip 91365–4084; tel. 818/719–2000; James L. Breeden, Administrator **A**1 3 5 10 **F**2 3 4 7 8 10 11 12 13 14 15 16 17 19 21 22 23 25 26 27 28 29 30 31 32 33 35 37 38 39 40 41 42 44 45 48 49 50 51 52 53 54 55 56 58 61 63 64 65 66 67 68 69 71 72 73 74 **S**2105 Kaiser Foundation Hospitals	23	10	134	8791	89	34076	1867	—	—	718
★ KAISER FOUNDATION HOSPITAL–WEST LOS ANGELES, 6041 Cadillac Avenue, Zip 90034; tel. 213/857–2201; Ivette Estrada, Administrator **A**1 2 3 5 9 10 **F**1 2 3 4 5 6 7 8 9 10 11 12 13 14 15 16 17 18 19 20 21 22 23 24 25 26 27 29 30 31 32 33 34 35 36 37 38 39 40 41 42 43 44 45 46 47 48 49 50 51 52 53 54 55 56 57 58 59 60 61 62 63 64 65 66 67 68 69 70 71 72 73 74 **P**3 **S**2105 Kaiser Foundation Hospitals	23	10	191	10618	99	63950	1749	—	—	1031
★ LAC UNIVERSITY OF SOUTHERN CALIFORNIA MEDICAL CENTER, (Includes General Hospital, 1200 North State Street, Los Angeles, California, Zip 90033; Women's and Children's Hospital, 1240 North Mission Road, Los Angeles, California, Zip 90033) 1200 North State Street, Zip 90033–1084; tel. 213/226–2622 **A**1 2 3 5 6 8 9 10 **F**3 4 5 7 8 9 10 11 12 13 14 15 16 17 18 19 20 21 22 23 25 28 30 31 32 34 35 37 38 40 41 43 44 45 46 47 48 49 51 52 53 54 55 56 57 58 59 61 63 64 65 66 69 70 71 73 74 **P**6 **S**5755 Los Angeles County–Department of Health Services	13	10	1236	60789	993	860655	10868	1231235	338226	8295

Hospitals, U.S. / CALIFORNIA

Hospital, Address, Telephone, Administrator, Approval, Facility, and Physician Codes, Health Care System

★ American Hospital Association (AHA) membership
☐ Joint Commission on Accreditation of Healthcare Organizations (JCAHO) accreditation
+ American Osteopathic Hospital Association (AOHA) membership
○ American Osteopathic Association (AOA) accreditation
△ Commission on Accreditation of Rehabilitation Facilities (CARF) accreditation
Control codes 61, 63, 64, 71, 72 and 73 indicate hospitals listed by AOHA, but not registered by AHA. For definition of numerical codes, see page A6

Hospital	Classification Codes		Utilization Data					Expense (thousands) of dollars		
	Control	Service	Beds	Admissions	Census	Outpatient Visits	Births	Total	Payroll	Personnel
★ LAC–KING–DREW MEDICAL CENTER, 12021 South Wilmington Avenue, Zip 90059; tel. 310/668–5201; Jaron Gammons, Administrator **A**1 2 3 5 8 9 10 **F**3 4 5 6 7 8 10 11 12 13 14 15 16 17 18 19 20 21 22 24 25 26 27 28 29 30 31 32 33 34 35 37 38 39 40 41 42 43 44 45 46 47 48 49 51 52 53 54 55 56 57 58 59 60 61 63 65 67 70 71 72 73 74 **P**1 3 **S**5755 Los Angeles County–Department of Health Services	13	10	444	20341	299	216109	5532	420984	132864	3538
LINCOLN HOSPITAL MEDICAL CENTER, 443 South Soto Street, Zip 90033; tel. 213/261–1181; Tim Kollars, Chief Executive Officer (Nonreporting) **A**9	33	10	61	—	—	—	—	—	—	—
☐ LOS ANGELES COMMUNITY HOSPITAL, 4081 East Olympic Boulevard, Zip 90023; tel. 213/267–0477; Sandra J. Anaya R.N., Administrator (Nonreporting) **A**1 9 10 **S**5765 Paracelsus Healthcare Corporation	33	10	136	—	—	—	—	—	—	—
LOS ANGELES COUNTY CENTRAL JAIL HOSPITAL, 441 Bauchet Street, Zip 90012; tel. 213/974–5045; Tom Flaherty, Assistant Administrator (Nonreporting)	13	11	190	—	—	—	—	—	—	—
☐ LOS ANGELES METROPOLITAN MEDICAL CENTER, 2231 South Western Avenue, Zip 90018–1399; tel. 213/737–7372; Marvin Herschberg, Chief Executive Officer (Nonreporting) **A**1 9 10 **S**0435 Pacific Health Corporation	32	10	100	—	—	—	—	—	—	—
★ MEDICAL CENTER OF NORTH HOLLYWOOD, 12629 Riverside Drive, North Hollywood, Zip 91607–3495; tel. 818/980–9200; Dale Surowitz, Chief Executive Officer (Nonreporting) **A**1 9 10 **S**0063 TENET Healthcare Corporation	33	10	163	—	—	—	—	—	—	—
☐ MIDWAY HOSPITAL MEDICAL CENTER, 5925 San Vicente Boulevard, Zip 90019, Mailing Address: Box 35909, Zip 90035; tel. 213/938–3161; John V. Fenton, Chief Executive Officer **A**1 9 10 **F**1 2 3 4 5 6 7 8 9 10 11 12 13 15 16 17 18 19 20 21 22 23 24 25 26 27 28 29 30 31 32 33 34 35 36 37 38 39 40 41 42 43 44 46 47 48 49 50 51 52 53 54 55 56 57 58 59 60 61 63 64 65 66 67 68 69 70 71 72 73 74 **P**1 2 3 4 5 6 7 8 **S**6525 Ornda Healthcorp	33	10	225	5311	86	31148	0	68457	24333	589
MISSION COMMUNITY HOSPITAL–PANORAMA CITY CAMPUS See Mission Community Hospital–San Fernando Campus, San Fernando										
★ MOTION PICTURE AND TELEVISION FUND HOSPITAL AND RESIDENTIAL SERVICES, 23388 Mulholland Drive, Woodland Hills, Zip 91364–2792; tel. 818/876–1888; William F. Haug FACHE, Chief Executive Officer (Total facility includes 165 beds in nursing home–type unit) **A**1 9 10 **F**4 6 7 8 10 11 12 13 15 16 17 18 19 21 22 23 25 26 28 29 30 31 32 34 35 37 38 39 40 41 42 43 44 45 46 47 48 49 51 58 60 61 62 64 65 66 71 73 74 **P**4 5 6	23	10	218	971	170	37778	0	44995	18438	552
★ △ NORTHRIDGE HOSPITAL MEDICAL CENTER, 18300 Roscoe Boulevard, Northridge, Zip 91328; tel. 818/885–8500; Jeffery E. Flocken, President and Chief Executive Officer (Total facility includes 31 beds in nursing home–type unit) **A**1 2 3 5 7 9 10 **F**1 3 4 7 8 10 12 15 17 18 19 21 22 24 26 27 28 30 31 32 34 35 37 38 39 40 41 42 43 44 45 46 47 48 49 52 53 54 55 56 57 58 59 60 61 63 64 65 67 68 70 71 73 74 **P**3 5 **S**2315 UniHealth	23	10	385	14634	261	157267	2695	145907	61671	1567
★ OLIVE VIEW MEDICAL CENTER, 14445 Olive View Drive, Sylmar, Zip 91342–1495; tel. 818/364–1555; Melinda Anderson, Acting Administrator **A**1 3 5 9 10 **F**4 7 8 9 10 11 12 13 17 18 19 20 21 22 23 25 26 27 28 29 30 31 32 33 34 35 37 38 39 40 41 42 43 44 45 46 47 48 49 51 52 53 54 55 56 57 58 59 60 61 63 64 65 68 69 70 71 72 73 74 **P**3 6 8 **S**5755 Los Angeles County–Department of Health Services	13	10	253	16131	246	199512	6036	366173	92470	2436
☐ ORTHOPAEDIC HOSPITAL, 2400 South Flower Street, Zip 90007, Mailing Address: Box 60132, Terminal Annex, Zip 90060; tel. 213/742–1000; James V. Luck Jr. M.D., Chief Executive Officer (Nonreporting) **A**1 2 3 5 9 10	23	47	152	—	—	—	—	—	—	—
★ PACIFIC ALLIANCE MEDICAL CENTER, 531 West College Street, Zip 90012; tel. 213/624–8411; John R. Edwards, Administrator and Chief Executive Officer (Nonreporting) **A**1 10	32	10	89	—	—	—	—	—	—	—
☐ PACIFICA HOSPITAL OF THE VALLEY, 9449 San Fernando Road, Sun Valley, Zip 91352; tel. 818/767–3310; Ermanno Mariani, Executive Director (Nonreporting) **A**1 9 10	33	10	110	—	—	—	—	—	—	—
☐ PINE GROVE HOSPITAL AND MENTAL HEALTH CENTER, 7011 Shoup Avenue, Canoga Park, Zip 91307; tel. 818/348–0500; David Lisonbee, Chief Executive Officer (Nonreporting) **A**1 9 10	33	22	82	—	—	—	—	—	—	—
☐ QUEEN OF ANGELS–HOLLYWOOD PRESBYTERIAN MEDICAL CENTER, 1300 North Vermont Avenue, Zip 90027–0069; tel. 213/413–3000; Sylvester Graff, President and Chief Executive Officer (Total facility includes 89 beds in nursing home–type unit) **A**1 10 **F**7 8 11 15 16 19 21 22 27 31 32 34 35 37 38 40 41 42 44 45 46 48 49 51 60 64 65 71 72 73 74 **P**5 7	23	10	411	16792	300	82850	6178	112424	45468	1335
★ SAN PEDRO PENINSULA HOSPITAL, 1300 West Seventh Street, San Pedro, Zip 90732; tel. 310/832–3311; John M. Wilson, President and Chief Executive Officer (Total facility includes 128 beds in nursing home–type unit) **A**1 2 9 10 **F**2 3 7 8 10 11 12 19 21 22 23 25 26 27 31 32 33 34 35 37 38 40 41 42 43 44 48 49 52 54 57 60 64 65 71 73 **P**5	23	10	359	5549	195	94953	507	57321	28144	781
★ SANTA MARTA HOSPITAL, 319 North Humphreys Avenue, Zip 90022; tel. 213/266–6500; Wilfred G. Mallari, President and Chief Executive Officer (Nonreporting) **A**1 10 **S**5945 Carondelet Health System	21	10	110	—	—	—	—	—	—	—
☐ SHERMAN OAKS HOSPITAL AND HEALTH CENTER, 4929 Van Nuys Boulevard, Van Nuys, Zip 91403; tel. 818/981–7111; (Nonreporting) **A**1 9 10	23	10	105	—	—	—	—	—	—	—
★ SHRINERS HOSPITALS FOR CRIPPLED CHILDREN, LOS ANGELES UNIT, 3160 Geneva Street, Zip 90020–1199; tel. 213/388–3151; Paul D. Hargis, Administrator **A**1 3 5 **F**15 17 19 21 22 34 35 41 47 48 51 56 65 69 70 71 73 **P**6 **S**4125 Shriners Hospitals for Crippled Children	23	57	50	1620	34	13829	0	—	—	224

Hospitals, U.S. / CALIFORNIA

Hospital, Address, Telephone, Administrator, Approval, Facility, and Physician Codes, Health Care System	Classification Codes		Utilization Data					Expense (thousands) of dollars		
★ American Hospital Association (AHA) membership ☐ Joint Commission on Accreditation of Healthcare Organizations (JCAHO) accreditation + American Osteopathic Hospital Association (AOHA) membership ○ American Osteopathic Association (AOA) accreditation △ Commission on Accreditation of Rehabilitation Facilities (CARF) accreditation Control codes 61, 63, 64, 71, 72 and 73 indicate hospitals listed by AOHA, but not registered by AHA. For definition of numerical codes, see page A6	Control	Service	Beds	Admissions	Census	Outpatient Visits	Births	Total	Payroll	Personnel
★ ST. VINCENT MEDICAL CENTER, 2131 West Third Street, Zip 90057–0992, Mailing Address: P.O. Box 57992, Zip 90057; tel. 213/484–7111; Vincent F. Guinan, President (Total facility includes 24 beds in nursing home–type unit) **A**1 2 3 5 9 10 **F**4 8 10 11 12 15 16 17 19 21 25 26 27 30 31 32 33 34 35 36 37 39 41 42 43 44 45 46 49 60 63 64 65 66 67 68 69 71 72 73 **P**5 7 8 **S**1855 Daughters of Charity National Health System	21	10	313	10159	189	30113	0	107625	44228	1115
☐ TEMPLE COMMUNITY HOSPITAL, 235 North Hoover Street, Zip 90004; tel. 213/382–7252; Herbert G. Needman, Administrator and Chief Executive Officer (Total facility includes 11 beds in nursing home–type unit) **A**1 9 10 **F**8 11 19 20 21 31 35 37 44 45 60 64 65 73 **P**5	33	10	130	3055	67	8000	0	25783	8569	279
★ UNIVERSITY OF CALIFORNIA LOS ANGELES MEDICAL CENTER, 10833 Le Conte Avenue, Zip 90024–1730; tel. 310/825–5041; Raymond G. Schultze M.D., Director **A**1 2 3 5 8 9 10 **F**4 7 8 10 11 15 16 17 18 19 20 22 23 24 26 28 30 31 32 34 35 37 38 39 40 41 42 43 44 46 47 49 50 51 54 60 63 65 66 69 70 71 73 74 **P**1 **S**6405 University of California–Systemwide Administration	23	10	610	22532	377	355816	1752	429289	184111	4372
★ UNIVERSITY OF CALIFORNIA LOS ANGELES NEUROPSYCHIATRIC HOSPITAL, 760 Westwood Plaza, Zip 90024–1759; tel. 310/825–9548; Don A. Rockwell M.D., Director (Nonreporting) **A**1 3 5 9 10 **S**6405 University of California–Systemwide Administration	23	49	117	—	—	—	—	—	—	—
★ UNIVERSITY OF SOUTHERN CALIFORNIA–KENNETH NORRIS JR. CANCER HOSPITAL, 1441 Eastlake Avenue, Zip 90033–0804, Mailing Address: P.O. Box 33804, Zip 90033; tel. 213/764–3000; G. Peter Shostak, Administrator **A**1 2 3 5 9 10 **F**8 15 16 17 19 21 23 29 30 31 32 34 35 37 42 44 45 50 54 60 63 65 67 69 71 73 74	23	49	60	2127	33	39455	0	45453	15496	357
★ △ VALLEY HOSPITAL MEDICAL CENTER, 14500 Sherman Circle, Van Nuys, Zip 91405; tel. 818/997–0101; Richard D. Lyons, President and Chief Executive Officer (Total facility includes 38 beds in nursing home–type unit) **A**1 7 9 10 **F**1 3 4 6 7 8 10 12 13 15 17 18 19 21 22 23 24 25 26 27 28 29 30 31 32 34 35 37 39 41 42 43 44 45 46 48 49 51 52 53 54 55 56 57 58 59 60 61 62 63 64 65 67 70 71 73 74 **P**1 3 4 5 7 8 **S**2315 UniHealth	23	10	163	4716	79	46184	0	40135	17661	437
★ VALLEY PRESBYTERIAN HOSPITAL, 15107 Vanowen Street, Van Nuys, Zip 91405; tel. 818/782–6600; Robert C. Bills, President and Vice Chairman (Nonreporting) **A**1 2 9 10	23	10	313	—	—	—	—	—	—	—
☐ VAN NUYS HOSPITAL, 15220 Vanowen Street, Van Nuys, Zip 91405; tel. 818/787–0123; Brent Lamb, Administrator **A**1 10 **F**52 53 58 **P**5	33	22	41	988	32	0	0	—	—	86
★ VETERANS AFFAIRS MEDICAL CENTER–WEST LOS ANGELES, 11301 Wilshire Boulevard, Zip 90073–0275; tel. 310/824–3132; Kenneth Clark, Director (Total facility includes 240 beds in nursing home–type unit) **A**1 3 5 8 **F**1 2 3 4 5 6 8 10 11 12 14 15 16 17 18 19 20 21 22 24 25 26 27 28 29 30 31 32 33 34 35 36 37 39 41 42 43 44 45 46 48 49 50 51 52 54 55 56 57 58 59 60 61 63 64 65 67 69 71 72 73 74 **S**9295 Department of Veterans Affairs	45	10	1588	15759	1224	408834	0	308643	145065	4419
★ WEST HILLS REGIONAL MEDICAL CENTER, 7300 Medical Center Drive, West Hills, Zip 91307, Mailing Address: P.O. Box 7937, Zip 91309–7937; tel. 818/712–4110; Dan Brothman, Chief Executive Officer **A**1 10 **F**1 2 3 4 7 8 9 10 11 12 13 14 19 21 22 24 25 26 27 28 29 30 32 33 34 35 37 38 39 40 41 42 43 44 45 47 48 49 51 52 60 61 64 65 69 71 72 73 74 **P**5 **S**0048 Columbia/HCA Healthcare Corporation	33	10	236	7076	86	28490	1435	51164	24186	651
★ WESTSIDE HOSPITAL, 910 South Fairfax Avenue, Zip 90036; tel. 213/938–3431; Jerry Gillman, President and Chief Executive Officer (Nonreporting) **A**1 9 10 **S**0048 Columbia/HCA Healthcare Corporation	33	10	66	—	—	—	—	—	—	—
☐ △ WHITE MEMORIAL MEDICAL CENTER, 1720 Brooklyn Avenue, Zip 90033–2481; tel. 213/268–5000; (Total facility includes 41 beds in nursing home–type unit) **A**1 3 5 7 9 10 **F**7 8 10 11 12 14 15 16 17 19 22 24 28 30 32 34 35 37 38 40 41 42 43 44 46 47 48 49 52 54 57 58 59 60 64 65 70 71 73 74 **P**3 **S**0235 Adventist Health System/West	21	10	354	15487	241	132719	4724	115369	49267	1345
LOS BANOS—Merced County										
☐ LOS BANOS COMMUNITY HOSPITAL, 520 West I Street, Zip 93635; tel. 209/826–0591; Darline Kiley R.N., Co-Administrator (Nonreporting) **A**1 9 10	23	10	48	—	—	—	—	—	—	—
LOS GATOS—Santa Clara County										
☐ △ COMMUNITY HOSPITAL AND REHABILITATION CENTER OF LOS GATOS–SARATOGA, 815 Pollard Road, Zip 95030; tel. 408/378–6131; Truman L. Gates, Chief Executive Officer (Nonreporting) **A**1 7 9 10 **S**0063 TENET Healthcare Corporation	33	10	209	—	—	—	—	—	—	—
GOOD SAMARITAN HOSPITAL–MISSION OAKS, 15891 Los Gatos–Almaden Road, Zip 95032; tel. 408/356–4111; Michael B. Guthrie M.D., President and Chief Executive Officer (Nonreporting) **A**2 9 **S**0965 Good Samaritan Health System	23	10	551	—	—	—	—	—	—	—
LOYALTON—Sierra County										
SIERRA VALLEY DISTRICT HOSPITAL, 700 Third Street, Zip 96118, Mailing Address: Box 178, Zip 96118; tel. 916/993–1225; Billie Weatherson, Administrator (Total facility includes 34 beds in nursing home–type unit) **A**9 10 **F**3 8 13 14 15 17 18 22 28 30 32 33 34 36 39 46 49 54 56 58 64 65 66 **P**6	16	10	40	72	33	3818	2	3154	1455	62
LYNWOOD—Los Angeles County										
★ ST. FRANCIS MEDICAL CENTER, 3630 East Imperial Highway, Zip 90262; tel. 310/603–6000; Sister Elizabeth Joseph Keaveney, President and Chief Executive Officer (Total facility includes 30 beds in nursing home–type unit) **A**1 9 10 **F**4 7 8 10 12 15 16 17 19 20 21 22 25 27 28 30 31 32 34 35 37 38 40 41 42 43 44 45 46 49 51 52 56 58 59 60 63 64 65 67 71 72 73 **P**4 5 6 **S**1855 Daughters of Charity National Health System	21	10	356	17372	249	174018	5745	110583	55168	1539

Hospitals, U.S. / CALIFORNIA

Hospital, Address, Telephone, Administrator, Approval, Facility, and Physician Codes, Health Care System	Classification Codes		Utilization Data					Expense (thousands) of dollars		
★ American Hospital Association (AHA) membership ☐ Joint Commission on Accreditation of Healthcare Organizations (JCAHO) accreditation + American Osteopathic Hospital Association (AOHA) membership ○ American Osteopathic Association (AOA) accreditation △ Commission on Accreditation of Rehabilitation Facilities (CARF) accreditation Control codes 61, 63, 64, 71, 72 and 73 indicate hospitals listed by AOHA, but not registered by AHA. For definition of numerical codes, see page A6	Control	Service	Beds	Admissions	Census	Outpatient Visits	Births	Total	Payroll	Personnel
MADERA—Madera County ☐ MADERA COMMUNITY HOSPITAL, 1250 East Almond Avenue, Zip 93637–5696, Mailing Address: Box 1328, Zip 93639–1328; tel. 209/675–5501; Robert C. Kelley, Chief Executive Officer **A**1 9 10 **F**7 8 11 15 16 19 21 22 25 30 32 37 40 41 44 46 47 49 65 71 73	23	10	100	4130	47	61018	1100	25332	11446	419
MAMMOTH LAKES—Mono County ☐ MAMMOTH HOSPITAL, 85 Sierra Park Road, Zip 93546, Mailing Address: P.O. Box 660, Zip 93546; tel. 619/934–3311; Gary Myers, Administrator (Nonreporting) **A**1 9 10	23	10	15	—	—	—	—	—	—	—
MANTECA—San Joaquin County ☐ DOCTORS HOSPITAL OF MANTECA, 1205 East North Street, Zip 95336, Mailing Address: Box 191, Zip 95336; tel. 209/823–3111; Richard H. Robinson, Administrator **A**1 9 10 **F**2 3 4 7 8 9 10 11 12 15 16 19 21 22 24 25 26 27 28 29 30 32 33 34 35 36 37 38 40 41 42 43 44 45 46 47 48 49 51 52 54 55 56 58 59 60 61 64 65 66 67 70 71 72 73 74 **P**1 5 7 8 **S**0063 TENET Healthcare Corporation	33	10	73	2839	31	38747	523	23417	9800	275
MARCH AIR FORCE BASE—Riverside Valley County ★ U.S. AIR FORCE REGIONAL HOSPITAL, 1500 Hospital Way, Suite 1019, Zip 92518–2032; tel. 909/655–4461; Lieutenant Colonel George W. Sherman MSC, USAF, Administrator (Nonreporting) **S**9495 Department of the Air Force	41	10	70	—	—	—	—	—	—	—
MARINA DEL REY—Los Angeles County ★ DANIEL FREEMAN MARINA HOSPITAL, 4650 Lincoln Boulevard, Zip 90292–6360; tel. 310/823–8911; Joseph W. Dunn Ph.D., Administrator **A**1 9 10 **F**2 3 4 8 10 12 15 16 17 18 19 21 22 23 24 26 27 28 30 31 32 34 35 36 37 39 41 42 43 44 45 46 49 52 54 55 56 57 58 59 60 64 65 66 67 68 71 72 73 **P**5 7 **S**5945 Carondelet Health System	21	10	179	4126	93	20842	0	37057	18597	289
MARIPOSA—Mariposa County JOHN C. FREMONT HEALTHCARE DISTRICT, 5189 Hospital Road, Zip 95338, Mailing Address: Box 216, Zip 95338; tel. 209/966–3631; Mary Mennig, Administrator (Nonreporting) **A**5 9 10	16	10	30	—	—	—	—	—	—	—
MARTINEZ—Contra Costa County ★ KAISER FOUNDATION HOSPITAL, 200 Muir Road, Zip 94553–4696; tel. 510/372–1000; Joyce M. Berger, Administrator (Nonreporting) **A**1 10 **S**2105 Kaiser Foundation Hospitals	23	10	134	—	—	—	—	—	—	—
☐ MERRITHEW MEMORIAL HOSPITAL, 2500 Alhambra Avenue, Zip 94553; tel. 510/370–5000; Frank J. Puglisi Jr., Executive Director (Nonreporting) **A**1 2 3 5 10	13	10	137	—	—	—	—	—	—	—
MARYSVILLE—Yuba County RIDEOUT MEMORIAL HOSPITAL, 726 Fourth Street, Zip 95901–2128, Mailing Address: Box 2128, Zip 95901–2128; tel. 916/749–4300; Thomas P. Hayes, Chief Executive Officer (Total facility includes 11 beds in nursing home–type unit) **A**9 10 **F**10 15 16 19 22 32 33 34 35 37 41 42 44 45 49 64 65 71 73 **P**5 **S**2115 Fremont–Rideout Health Group	23	10	128	4383	78	97361	0	39270	15753	431
MATHER AIR FORCE BASE—San Diego County ★ U.S. AIR FORCE HOSPITAL, 10535 Hospital Way, Zip 95655–1200; tel. 916/643–7166; Richard Davis, Foreman Biomedical Equipment Maintenance (Newly Registered) **A**1	41	10	40	—	—	—	—	—	—	—
MERCED—Merced County ☐ MERCED COMMUNITY MEDICAL CENTER, 301 East 13th Street, Zip 95340–6211, Mailing Address: Box 231, Zip 95341–0231; tel. 209/385–7000; William L. Gilbert, Chief Executive Officer **A**1 3 5 9 10 **F**2 8 9 10 11 12 13 14 15 16 17 19 21 22 28 29 30 32 33 34 35 37 38 40 44 45 46 47 48 49 51 52 56 60 64 65 67 71 73 **P**8	13	10	154	7170	77	83673	2230	51312	22980	697
★ MERCY HOSPITAL AND HEALTH SERVICES, 2740 M Street, Zip 95340–2880; tel. 209/384–6444; Kelly C. Morgan, President and Chief Executive Officer **A**1 9 10 **F**7 8 11 14 15 16 17 19 22 23 25 26 32 34 35 40 42 44 49 65 71 73 **S**5175 Catholic Health Corporation	21	10	101	5224	64	38835	1059	30483	13797	446
MISSION HILLS–Los Angeles County, See Los Angeles										
MISSION VIEJO—Orange County ☐ CHARTER HOSPITAL OF MISSION VIEJO, 23228 Madero, Zip 92691; tel. 714/830–4800; Jeffrey A. Thrash, Administrator (Nonreporting) **A**1 10 **S**0695 Charter Medical Corporation	33	22	80	—	—	—	—	—	—	—
★ MISSION HOSPITAL REGIONAL MEDICAL CENTER, 27700 Medical Center Road, Zip 92691; tel. 714/364–1400; Reynold R. Welch, President **A**1 2 9 10 **F**4 7 8 10 11 12 13 14 15 16 17 19 21 22 23 24 25 26 29 30 32 34 35 37 38 39 40 41 42 43 44 45 46 47 48 49 63 65 66 70 71 73 **P**1 3 5 7 **S**5425 St. Joseph Health System	21	10	202	11124	122	100549	2906	104501	38242	1056
MODESTO—Stanislaus County ☐ △ DOCTORS MEDICAL CENTER, 1441 Florida Avenue, Zip 95350–4418, Mailing Address: P.O. Box 4138, Zip 95352–4138; tel. 209/578–1211; Chris DiCicco, Chief Executive Officer (Nonreporting) **A**1 7 9 10 **S**0063 TENET Healthcare Corporation	33	10	364	—	—	—	—	—	—	—
☐ MEMORIAL HOSPITALS ASSOCIATION, (Includes Memorial Hospital, Ceres, California; Memorial Medical Center, Modesto, California) 1800 Coffee Road, Zip 95355, Mailing Address: P.O. Box 942, Zip 95353; tel. 209/526–4500; David P. Benn, President and Chief Executive Officer (Nonreporting) **A**1 2 9 10	23	10	373	—	—	—	—	—	—	—

Hospitals, U.S. / CALIFORNIA

Hospital, Address, Telephone, Administrator, Approval, Facility, and Physician Codes, Health Care System	Classification Codes		Utilization Data					Expense (thousands) of dollars		
★ American Hospital Association (AHA) membership □ Joint Commission on Accreditation of Healthcare Organizations (JCAHO) accreditation + American Osteopathic Hospital Association (AOHA) membership ○ American Osteopathic Association (AOA) accreditation △ Commission on Accreditation of Rehabilitation Facilities (CARF) accreditation Control codes 61, 63, 64, 71, 72 and 73 indicate hospitals listed by AOHA, but not registered by AHA. For definition of numerical codes, see page A6	Control	Service	Beds	Admissions	Census	Outpatient Visits	Births	Total	Payroll	Personnel
STANISLAUS BEHAVIORAL HEALTH CENTER, 1501 Claus Road, Zip 95355; tel. 209/524–4888; (Nonreporting) A10	13	22	70	—	—	—	—	—	—	—
□ STANISLAUS MEDICAL CENTER, 830 Scenic Drive, Zip 95350, Mailing Address: Box 3271, Zip 95353; tel. 209/558–7000; Beverly M. Finley, Chief Executive Officer (Nonreporting) A1 3 5 9 10	13	10	84	—	—	—	—	—	—	—
MONROVIA—Los Angeles County □ MONROVIA COMMUNITY HOSPITAL, 323 South Heliotrope Avenue, Zip 91016, Mailing Address: Box 707, Zip 91017-0707; tel. 818/359–8341; Steve Courtier, Administrator A1 9 10 F14 16 19 21 22 32 34 35 36 37 44 49 65 71 S5765 Paracelsus Healthcare Corporation	32	10	49	1872	24	4374	0	14022	4290	124
MONTCLAIR—San Bernardino County □ DOCTORS' HOSPITAL OF MONTCLAIR, 5000 San Bernardino Street, Zip 91763; tel. 714/625–5411; Charles L. Baker, Administrator and Chief Executive Officer (Nonreporting) A1 9 10 12 13	33	10	102	—	—	—	—	—	—	—
MONTEBELLO—Los Angeles County ★ BEVERLY HOSPITAL, 309 West Beverly Boulevard, Zip 90640; tel. 213/726–1222; James G. Ovieda, Administrator A1 2 9 10 F4 7 8 10 11 19 21 22 27 28 30 35 37 40 43 44 45 49 60 63 65 67 71 73 P4 5 7 8	23	10	212	9410	117	48396	2511	64213	28963	846
MONTEREY—Monterey County ★ COMMUNITY HOSPITAL OF THE MONTEREY PENINSULA, 23625 Holman Highway, Zip 93940, Mailing Address: Box H, Zip 93942–1085; tel. 408/624–5311; Jay Hudson, President and Chief Executive Officer A1 9 10 F1 3 7 8 14 15 16 19 21 22 31 34 35 37 40 41 42 44 52 53 54 56 57 58 59 60 63 71 73	23	10	174	10717	135	167641	1885	113855	48318	980
MONTEREY PARK—Los Angeles County □ △ GARFIELD MEDICAL CENTER, 525 North Garfield Avenue, Zip 91754; tel. 818/573–2222; Arnold R. Schaffer, Chief Executive Officer A1 2 7 9 10 F1 2 3 4 7 8 10 11 12 14 15 16 17 19 21 22 23 25 27 28 30 31 32 33 34 35 37 38 39 40 41 42 43 44 45 46 48 49 52 53 54 55 56 58 59 60 61 64 65 66 68 69 71 73 74 P5 S0063 TENET Healthcare Corporation	33	10	223	11036	210	38852	3953	—	—	753
□ MONTEREY PARK HOSPITAL, 900 South Atlantic Boulevard, Zip 91754; tel. 818/570–9000; Dan F. Ausman, Chief Executive Officer (Nonreporting) A1 2 10 S6525 Ornda Healthcorp	33	10	95	—	—	—	—	—	—	—
MORENO VALLEY—Riverside County □ MORENO VALLEY COMMUNITY HOSPITAL, 27300 Iris Avenue, Zip 92555; tel. 909/243–0811; Thomas McClintock, Administrator A1 10 F3 8 11 12 15 16 19 21 22 26 28 29 34 35 37 40 41 44 45 46 65 73 P4 5 S0043 Valley Health System	16	10	66	3409	31	37210	1003	22524	7028	150
MORGAN HILL—Santa Clara County ★ SAINT LOUISE HOSPITAL, 18500 Saint Louise Drive, Zip 95037; tel. 408/779–1500; William C. Finlayson, President and Chief Executive Officer (Total facility includes 19 beds in nursing home–type unit) A1 10 F1 2 3 4 7 8 9 10 11 15 16 17 18 19 20 21 22 23 24 27 28 29 30 31 32 33 34 35 36 37 38 39 40 41 42 43 44 45 46 47 49 53 54 55 56 57 58 59 60 63 64 65 67 68 69 71 73 74 P1 3 4 5 7 8 S1855 Daughters of Charity National Health System	21	10	32	2075	31	24430	497	18964	6445	152
MOSS BEACH—San Mateo County ★ SETON MEDICAL CENTER COASTSIDE, 600 Marine Boulevard, Zip 94038; tel. 415/728–5521; Deborah E. Stebbins FACHE, Acting President and Chief Executive Officer (Total facility includes 116 beds in nursing home–type unit) A1 9 10 F8 12 14 16 17 22 26 27 28 30 31 34 39 45 46 49 51 64 65 67 73 P5 7 S1855 Daughters of Charity National Health System	21	10	123	181	113	7465	0	7625	4019	99
MOUNT SHASTA—Siskiyou County ★ MERCY MEDICAL CENTER MOUNT SHASTA, 914 Pine Street, Zip 96067, Mailing Address: P.O. Box 239, Zip 96067–0239; tel. 916/926–6111; James R. Hoss, President (Total facility includes 47 beds in nursing home–type unit) A1 9 10 F7 8 15 17 19 22 24 25 26 28 31 32 33 34 35 37 39 40 41 42 44 56 64 65 66 70 71 73 P4 5 S5205 Catholic Healthcare West	21	10	80	1655	59	30415	139	16759	6987	252
MOUNTAIN VIEW—Santa Clara County ★ CAMINO HEALTHCARE, (Formerly El Camino Hospital) 2500 Grant Road, Zip 94040, Mailing Address: P.O. Box 7025, Zip 94039; tel. 415/940–7000; Richard R. Pettingill, President and Chief Executive Officer (Nonreporting) A1 9 10	16	10	290	—	—	—	—	—	—	—
MURRIETA—Riverside County ★ SHARP HEALTHCARE MURRIETA, 25500 Medical Center Drive, Zip 92562–5966; tel. 909/696–6000; Robert M. Edwards, Senior Vice President and Chief Executive Officer (Total facility includes 42 beds in nursing home–type unit) A10 F1 3 4 7 8 10 11 12 14 15 16 17 19 21 22 23 24 25 26 27 29 30 31 32 34 35 37 38 39 40 41 42 43 44 45 46 48 49 51 52 54 55 56 57 58 59 60 61 64 65 66 67 69 70 71 72 73 74 P5 8 S2065 Sharp Healthcare	23	10	91	4210	73	26710	1503	27185	12179	369
NAPA—Napa County □ NAPA STATE HOSPITAL, 2100 Napa–Vallejo Highway, Zip 94558; tel. 707/253–5454; Sidney F. Herndon, Executive Director (Nonreporting) A1 3 10	12	22	1075	—	—	—	—	—	—	—
★ QUEEN OF THE VALLEY HOSPITAL, 1000 Trancas Street, Zip 94558, Mailing Address: Box 2340, Zip 94558; tel. 707/252–4411; Joseph A. Stewart, President and Chief Executive Officer (Total facility includes 24 beds in nursing home–type unit) A1 2 9 10 F4 7 8 10 12 15 16 17 19 20 21 22 23 24 26 27 28 29 30 31 32 33 34 35 37 38 40 41 42 43 44 46 48 60 64 65 67 70 71 72 73 74 P3 5 S5425 St. Joseph Health System	21	10	176	7318	93	251381	477	75781	27372	776

© 1995 AHA Guide

Hospitals, U.S. / CALIFORNIA

Hospital, Address, Telephone, Administrator, Approval, Facility, and Physician Codes, Health Care System ★ American Hospital Association (AHA) membership □ Joint Commission on Accreditation of Healthcare Organizations (JCAHO) accreditation + American Osteopathic Hospital Association (AOHA) membership ○ American Osteopathic Association (AOA) accreditation △ Commission on Accreditation of Rehabilitation Facilities (CARF) accreditation Control codes 61, 63, 64, 71, 72 and 73 indicate hospitals listed by AOHA, but not registered by AHA. For definition of numerical codes, see page A6	Classification Codes		Utilization Data					Expense (thousands) of dollars		
	Control	Service	Beds	Admissions	Census	Outpatient Visits	Births	Total	Payroll	Personnel
NATIONAL CITY—San Diego County										
□ △ PARADISE VALLEY HOSPITAL, 2400 East Fourth Street, Zip 91950; tel. 619/470–4321; Fred M. Harder, President (Nonreporting) **A**1 7 9 10 **S**0235 Adventist Health System/West	21	10	130	—	—	—	—	—	—	—
NEEDLES—San Bernardino County										
★ NEEDLES–DESERT COMMUNITIES HOSPITAL, 1401 Bailey Avenue, Zip 92363; tel. 619/326–4531; Patricia Rahnema, Administrator **A**1 9 10 **F**7 8 12 14 15 16 19 21 22 28 34 36 37 40 44 49 65 71 **P**5	14	10	39	1314	12	5811	119	10121	4545	147
NEWHALL—Los Angeles County										
NEWHALL COMMUNITY HOSPITAL, 22607 6th Street, Zip 91322–1328, Mailing Address: Box 221328, Zip 91321–1328; tel. 805/259–4555; Bienvenido Tan M.D., Administrator (Nonreporting) **A**9 10	12	10	13	—	—	—	—	—	—	—
NEWPORT BEACH—Orange County										
★ HOAG MEMORIAL HOSPITAL PRESBYTERIAN, 301 Newport Boulevard, Zip 92663–4120, Mailing Address: Box 6100, Zip 92658–6100; tel. 714/645–8600; Michael D. Stephens, President and Chief Executive Officer **A**1 2 9 10 **F**1 2 3 4 7 8 10 11 12 14 15 17 19 21 22 23 25 26 28 30 32 33 34 35 36 37 38 39 40 41 42 43 44 45 46 48 49 54 60 61 63 65 67 71 72 73 74 **P**5 7	23	10	355	19573	236	180718	3752	216548	80054	2674
NORTH HOLLYWOOD–Los Angeles County, See Los Angeles										
NORTHRIDGE–Los Angeles County, See Los Angeles										
NORWALK–Los Angeles County										
□ COAST PLAZA DOCTORS HOSPITAL, 13100 Studebaker Road, Zip 90650; tel. 310/868–3751; (Nonreporting) **A**1 9 10 12	32	10	108	—	—	—	—	—	—	—
KAISER FOUNDATION HOSPITAL, NORWALK See Kaiser Foundation Hospital, Bellflower										
□ LOS ANGELES COMMUNITY HOSPITAL OF NORWALK, (Formerly Norwalk Community Hospital) 13222 Bloomfield Avenue, Zip 90650; tel. 310/863–4763; Sandra J. Anaya R.N., Administrator (Nonreporting) **A**1 9 **S**5765 Paracelsus Healthcare Corporation	33	10	50	—	—	—	—	—	—	—
□ METROPOLITAN STATE HOSPITAL, 11400 Norwalk Boulevard, Zip 90650; tel. 310/863–7011; William G. Silva, Administrator **A**1 10 **F**20 24 30 39 41 45 46 52 55 59 65 67 73	12	22	834	1663	646	0	0	—	—	1378
NORWALK COMMUNITY HOSPITAL See Los Angeles Community Hospital of Norwalk										
NOVATO—Marin County										
★ NOVATO COMMUNITY HOSPITAL, 1625 Hill Road, Zip 94947, Mailing Address: P.O. Box 1108, Zip 94948; tel. 415/897–3111; Lowell W. Smith, Administrator **A**1 9 10 **F**7 8 12 15 16 19 21 22 27 28 29 30 31 32 33 34 35 37 38 40 42 44 47 48 65 71 73 **P**1 3 4 5 7 **S**8795 Sutter Health	23	10	52	2020	23	29583	278	19515	9049	183
OAKDALE—Stanislaus County										
□ OAK VALLEY DISTRICT HOSPITAL, 350 South Oak Street, Zip 95361; tel. 209/847–3011; Gary D. Rapaport, Administrator and Chief Executive Officer (Total facility includes 99 beds in nursing home–type unit) **A**1 9 10 **F**7 8 11 15 16 17 19 22 25 30 34 35 37 39 40 41 44 46 49 64 65 67 71 73 74 **P**5	16	10	138	1985	112	45459	326	18686	7404	270
OAKLAND—Alameda County										
□ CHILDREN'S HOSPITAL – OAKLAND, 747 52nd Street, Zip 94609; tel. 510/428–3000; Antonie H. Paap, President and Chief Executive Officer **A**1 3 5 9 10 **F**4 10 12 13 14 15 16 17 19 20 21 22 25 28 29 30 31 32 33 34 35 38 39 42 43 44 45 47 48 49 51 53 54 55 56 58 60 65 66 67 68 70 71 72 73 **P**5 8	23	50	193	9017	153	150892	0	145791	70980	1458
HIGHLAND GENERAL HOSPITAL, 1411 East 31st Street, Zip 94602; tel. 510/437–4397; Ophelia Long R.N., Administrator **A**3 5 **F**1 3 4 5 7 8 10 12 13 14 15 16 17 18 19 21 22 23 25 26 27 28 29 30 31 34 35 37 38 39 40 41 42 44 45 46 48 49 50 51 52 53 54 55 56 57 58 59 60 63 64 65 67 68 70 71 72 73 74 **P**6 **S**0225 Alameda County Health Care Services Agency	13	10	247	14778	213	187800	2011	158744	98692	1737
★ KAISER FOUNDATION HOSPITAL, 280 West MacArthur Boulevard, Zip 94611; tel. 510/596–1000; Donald Oxley, Vice President and Area Manager **A**1 3 5 10 **F**4 7 8 10 14 16 17 19 21 22 24 26 27 28 29 30 31 32 33 34 35 37 38 39 40 41 42 43 44 45 46 47 49 51 53 54 55 56 57 58 59 60 61 65 66 67 68 69 71 72 73 74 **P**1 **S**2105 Kaiser Foundation Hospitals	23	10	220	15991	165	565416	2434	—	—	1064
★ NAVAL HOSPITAL, Zip 94627; tel. 510/633–5019; Captain R. E. McKee MSC, USN, Director Administration (Nonreporting) **A**1 2 3 5 **S**9655 Department of Navy	43	10	260	—	—	—	—	—	—	—
PROVIDENCE HOSPITAL See Summit Medical Center										
SAMUEL MERRITT HOSPITAL See Summit Medical Center										
□ SUMMIT MEDICAL CENTER, (Includes Providence Hospital, 3100 Summit Street, Oakland, California, Zip 94609–3410, Mailing Address: Box 23020, Zip 94623–2302; tel. 510/835–4500; Samuel Merritt Hospital, Hawthorne Avenue & Webster Street, Oakland, California, Zip 94609; tel. 415/655–4000) Hawthorne Avenue & Webster Street, Zip 94609; tel. 510/655–4000; Irwin C. Hansen, President and Chief Executive Officer (Total facility includes 48 beds in nursing home–type unit) **A**1 2 9 10 **F**1 2 3 4 7 8 10 11 12 15 16 17 19 21 22 23 26 27 28 29 30 31 32 33 34 35 37 38 40 42 43 44 46 49 60 64 65 67 71 73 74 **P**5 7	23	10	420	18179	220	137901	2934	186221	86707	2052
OCEANSIDE—San Diego County										
★ TRI-CITY MEDICAL CENTER, 4002 Vista Way, Zip 92056–4593; tel. 619/724–8411; John P. Lauri, President and Chief Executive Officer **A**1 2 9 10 **F**1 4 7 8 10 11 12 14 15 16 17 19 20 22 23 27 28 30 32 33 34 35 37 38 40 41 42 43 44 45 46 48 49 52 53 54 55 56 57 58 59 60 65 71 72 73 74 **P**3 5 8	16	10	371	17978	205	170677	4453	110445	53346	1517

Hospitals, U.S. / CALIFORNIA

Hospital, Address, Telephone, Administrator, Approval, Facility, and Physician Codes, Health Care System	Classification Codes		Utilization Data					Expense (thousands) of dollars		
★ American Hospital Association (AHA) membership ☐ Joint Commission on Accreditation of Healthcare Organizations (JCAHO) accreditation + American Osteopathic Hospital Association (AOHA) membership ○ American Osteopathic Association (AOA) accreditation △ Commission on Accreditation of Rehabilitation Facilities (CARF) accreditation Control codes 61, 63, 64, 71, 72 and 73 indicate hospitals listed by AOHA, but not registered by AHA. For definition of numerical codes, see page A6	Control	Service	Beds	Admissions	Census	Outpatient Visits	Births	Total	Payroll	Personnel
OJAI—Ventura County										
★ OJAI VALLEY COMMUNITY HOSPITAL, 1306 Maricopa Highway, Zip 93023–3180; tel. 805/646–1401; James Van Duzer, Chief Executive Officer (Nonreporting) **A**1 9 10 **S**0585 Brim, Inc.	33	10	116	—	—	—	—	—	—	—
ONTARIO—San Bernardino County										
ONTARIO COMMUNITY HOSPITAL, 550 North Monterey, Zip 91764; tel. 714/984–2201; Charles L. Baker, Administrator and Chief Executive Officer (Nonreporting) **A**9 10 12 13	33	10	100	—	—	—	—	—	—	—
ORANGE—Orange County										
☐ CHAPMAN GENERAL HOSPITAL, 2601 East Chapman Avenue, Zip 92669; tel. 714/633–0011; Howard H. Levine, Executive Director **A**1 9 10 **F**4 5 7 8 10 11 12 14 15 16 17 19 21 22 25 26 27 28 29 30 31 32 33 34 35 37 38 39 40 41 42 43 44 45 46 47 48 49 51 52 54 57 60 61 63 64 65 66 67 71 73 74 **P**3 4 5 7 8 **S**6525 Ornda Healthcorp	33	10	104	2462	32	17373	647	—	—	209
★ CHILDREN'S HOSPITAL OF ORANGE COUNTY, 455 South Main Street, Zip 92668–3874; tel. 714/997–3000; Thomas Penn Jones, President and Chief Executive Officer (Nonreporting) **A**1 2 3 5 9 10	23	50	192	—	—	—	—	—	—	—
★ ST. JOSEPH HOSPITAL, 1100 West Stewart Drive, Zip 92668, Mailing Address: P.O. Box 5600, Zip 92613–5600; tel. 714/633–9111; Larry K. Ainsworth, Chief Executive Officer **A**1 2 3 5 9 10 **F**1 2 3 4 6 7 8 9 10 11 12 13 15 16 17 18 19 21 22 23 24 25 26 27 28 30 31 32 34 35 36 37 38 39 40 41 42 43 44 45 46 47 48 49 52 54 55 56 57 58 59 60 63 64 65 67 69 71 72 73 74 **P**3 5 7 **S**5425 St. Joseph Health System	21	10	411	17172	223	160887	4862	160240	66531	1844
★ UNIVERSITY OF CALIFORNIA, IRVINE MEDICAL CENTER, 101 The City Drive, Zip 92668–3298; tel. 714/456–5678; Mary A. Piccione, Executive Director **A**1 2 3 5 8 9 10 **F**4 5 7 8 9 10 11 12 13 14 15 16 17 18 19 21 22 23 25 26 28 29 30 31 32 33 34 35 37 38 39 40 41 42 43 44 45 46 47 48 49 51 52 53 54 55 56 57 58 59 60 61 65 66 67 68 69 70 71 72 73 74 **P**5 **S**6405 University of California–Systemwide Administration	23	10	383	14875	273	170284	2592	196429	86445	2075
OROVILLE—Butte County										
☐ OROVILLE HOSPITAL, 2767 Olive Highway, Zip 95966–6185; tel. 916/533–8500; Robert J. Wentz, Administrator and Chief Executive Officer (Total facility includes 20 beds in nursing home–type unit) **A**1 9 10 **F**7 8 15 16 19 20 21 22 24 25 26 28 30 31 32 34 35 37 39 40 41 44 46 49 51 61 63 64 65 67 69 70 71 72 73 74 **P**7	23	10	120	4595	56	163978	735	43557	20757	579
OXNARD—Ventura County										
★ △ ST. JOHN'S REGIONAL MEDICAL CENTER, 1600 North Rose Avenue, Zip 93030; tel. 805/988–2500; Daniel R. Herlinger, President and Chief Executive Officer **A**1 7 9 10 **F**4 7 8 10 11 15 16 17 19 21 22 23 28 29 30 32 34 35 37 38 40 41 43 44 45 46 48 49 60 63 65 67 71 73 **P**3 5 7 **S**5205 Catholic Healthcare West	23	10	240	10876	162	84165	2147	93929	31840	1112
PALM SPRINGS—Riverside County										
★ △ DESERT HOSPITAL, 1150 North Indian Canyon Drive, Zip 92262, Mailing Address: Box 2739, Zip 92263; tel. 619/323–6511; David A. Seeley, President (Nonreporting) **A**1 2 7 9 10	23	10	348	—	—	—	—	—	—	—
PALMDALE—Los Angeles County										
☐ DESERT PALMS COMMUNITY HOSPITAL, (Formerly Palmdale Hospital Medical Center) 1212 East Avenue South, Zip 93550; tel. 805/273–2211; Elizabeth Scarcelli, Interim Administrator **A**1 9 10 **F**8 15 18 19 22 37 40 44 52 53 54 55 56 57 58 59 71 73 **S**5765 Paracelsus Healthcare Corporation	33	10	123	2551	42	35502	190	16146	8055	214
PALO ALTO—Santa Clara County										
★ LUCILE SALTER PACKARD CHILDREN'S HOSPITAL AT STANFORD, 725 Welch Road, Zip 94304; tel. 415/497–8000; Lorraine Zippiroli, President **A**1 3 5 9 10 **F**4 5 10 12 13 14 15 16 17 19 21 22 23 27 29 30 31 32 34 35 38 42 43 44 45 46 47 50 51 53 54 55 56 58 59 60 65 67 69 70 71 73	23	50	156	5100	112	56994	0	113825	47930	1074
★ VETERANS AFFAIRS MEDICAL CENTER, 3801 Miranda Avenue, Zip 94304–1207; tel. 415/493–5000; James A. Goff FACHE, Director (Total facility includes 270 beds in nursing home–type unit) **A**1 2 3 5 8 **F**1 2 3 4 5 8 10 11 19 20 21 22 23 25 26 27 30 31 32 33 35 37 42 43 44 45 46 48 49 50 51 52 54 55 56 57 58 59 60 64 65 67 69 71 73 74 **P**6 **S**9295 Department of Veterans Affairs	45	10	1062	11791	762	322214	0	—	—	3269
PANORAMA CITY–Los Angeles County, See Los Angeles										
PARADISE—Butte County										
☐ FEATHER RIVER HOSPITAL, 5974 Pentz Road, Zip 95969–5593; tel. 916/877–9361; George Pifer, President (Nonreporting) **A**1 9 10 **S**0235 Adventist Health System/West	21	10	121	—	—	—	—	—	—	—
PARAMOUNT—Los Angeles County										
★ SUBURBAN MEDICAL CENTER, 16453 South Colorado Avenue, Zip 90723; tel. 310/531–3110; Marc A. Furstman, Chief Executive Officer (Nonreporting) **A**1 9 **S**6525 Ornda Healthcorp	33	10	140	—	—	—	—	—	—	—
PASADENA—Los Angeles County										
★ HUNTINGTON MEMORIAL HOSPITAL, 100 West California Boulevard, Zip 91105, Mailing Address: P.O. Box 7013, Zip 91109–7013; tel. 818/397–5555; Stephen A. Ralph, President (Total facility includes 75 beds in nursing home–type unit) **A**1 2 3 5 8 9 10 **F**4 7 8 10 11 12 15 16 17 19 21 22 23 26 28 30 31 32 34 35 37 38 40 41 42 44 47 48 49 51 52 54 55 56 57 58 59 60 61 64 65 70 71 73 **P**1 3 4 5 7 8	23	10	554	22505	389	203780	4702	209744	92061	2399

© 1995 AHA Guide

Hospitals, U.S. / CALIFORNIA

Hospital, Address, Telephone, Administrator, Approval, Facility, and Physician Codes, Health Care System	Classification Codes		Utilization Data					Expense (thousands) of dollars		
★ American Hospital Association (AHA) membership ☐ Joint Commission on Accreditation of Healthcare Organizations (JCAHO) accreditation + American Osteopathic Hospital Association (AOHA) membership ○ American Osteopathic Association (AOA) accreditation △ Commission on Accreditation of Rehabilitation Facilities (CARF) accreditation Control codes 61, 63, 64, 71, 72 and 73 indicate hospitals listed by AOHA, but not registered by AHA. For definition of numerical codes, see page A6	Control	Service	Beds	Admissions	Census	Outpatient Visits	Births	Total	Payroll	Personnel
IMPACT DRUG AND ALCOHOL TREATMENT CENTER, 1680 North Fair Oaks Avenue, Zip 91103; tel. 818/681-2575; James M. Stillwell, Director (Nonreporting)	23	82	130	—	—	—	—	—	—	—
★ LAS ENCINAS HOSPITAL, 2900 East Del Mar Boulevard, Zip 91107-4375; tel. 818/795-9901; Roland Metivier, Chief Executive Officer (Nonreporting) **A**1 9 10 **S**0048 Columbia/HCA Healthcare Corporation	33	22	147	—	—	—	—	—	—	—
☐ ST. LUKE MEDICAL CENTER, 2632 East Washington Boulevard, Zip 91107-1494, Mailing Address: Bin 7021, Zip 91109; tel. 818/797-1141; Robert S. Freymuller, Chief Executive Officer (Total facility includes 18 beds in nursing home–type unit) **A**1 2 9 10 **F**3 7 11 16 19 22 27 31 32 35 37 39 40 41 44 45 46 49 64 65 67 71 73 **P**5 7 **S**6525 Ornda Healthcorp	33	10	120	5165	75	37966	661	35343	14469	411
PATTERSON—Stanislaus County										
DEL PUERTO HOSPITAL, South Ninth Street, Zip 95363-0187, Mailing Address: Box 187, Zip 95363-0187; tel. 209/892-8781; Thomas Avery, Administrator (Total facility includes 23 beds in nursing home–type unit) **A**9 10 **F**8 12 14 15 16 22 26 30 34 41 44 48 49 64 65 71 73	16	10	30	187	23	7923	0	4250	—	78
PATTON—San Bernardino County										
☐ PATTON STATE HOSPITAL, 3102 East Highland Avenue, Zip 92369; tel. 909/425-7000; William L. Summers, Executive Director **A**1 **F**3 4 5 7 8 10 12 18 19 20 21 22 28 29 30 31 35 39 41 42 43 44 45 46 49 50 52 53 54 57 60 61 63 65 69 70 71 72 73 **P**6	12	22	1018	806	1018	0	0	—	—	1478
PETALUMA—Sonoma County										
☐ PETALUMA VALLEY HOSPITAL, 400 North McDowell Boulevard, Zip 94954-2339; tel. 707/778-1111; Neil Martin, Administrator (Total facility includes 14 beds in nursing home–type unit) **A**1 2 9 10 **F**7 11 12 13 17 19 22 28 29 30 32 33 34 35 37 39 40 41 42 44 45 46 49 67 71 73 **P**3 5 8	16	10	82	3649	44	53900	547	30597	12358	440
PINOLE—Contra Costa County										
☐ DOCTORS HOSPITAL OF PINOLE, 2151 Appian Way, Zip 94564; tel. 510/724-5000; Gary Sloan, Chief Executive Officer (Total facility includes 24 beds in nursing home–type unit) **A**1 9 10 **F**2 3 4 7 8 10 11 12 15 17 19 21 22 26 28 29 30 31 32 33 34 35 37 42 43 44 46 49 53 57 58 60 63 64 65 67 69 71 73 74 **P**5 **S**0063 TENET Healthcare Corporation	33	10	137	3868	76	27775	2	42590	19580	408
PITTSBURG—Contra Costa County										
LOS MEDANOS COMMUNITY HOSPITAL, 2311 Loveridge Road, Zip 94565; tel. 510/432-2200; James K. Osborn, Interim Chief Executive Officer (Nonreporting) **A**9	16	10	188	—	—	—	—	—	—	—
PLACENTIA—Orange County										
☐ PLACENTIA–LINDA COMMUNITY HOSPITAL, 1301 Rose Drive, Zip 92670; tel. 714/993-2000; Michael A. Kelly, Chief Executive Officer (Nonreporting) **A**1 9 10 **S**0063 TENET Healthcare Corporation	33	10	114	—	—	—	—	—	—	—
PLACERVILLE—El Dorado County										
★ MARSHALL HOSPITAL, Marshall Way, Zip 95667-3439; tel. 916/622-1441; Frank Nachtman, Administrator **A**1 9 10 **F**7 8 15 16 17 19 21 22 28 30 32 33 34 35 37 39 40 41 42 44 45 46 60 63 64 65 71 73 **P**3 5	23	10	107	5041	62	107283	705	47380	18649	576
POMONA—Los Angeles County										
★ △ CASA COLINA HOSPITAL FOR REHABILITATIVE MEDICINE, 255 East Bonita Avenue, Zip 91767-9966, Mailing Address: P.O. Box 6001, Zip 91769-6001; tel. 909/593-7521; Judy Cummings, Administrator and Vice President Hospital Services **A**1 7 9 10 **F**1 12 14 17 24 25 26 32 34 41 45 48 49 65 67 73	23	46	64	425	29	13819	0	10561	7364	201
LANTERMAN DEVELOPMENTAL CENTER, 3530 Pomona Boulevard, Zip 91768, Mailing Address: P.O. Box 100, Zip 91769; tel. 714/595-1221; David Bourne, Executive Director **A**10 **F**1 12 20 22 24 27 28 30 39 41 45 46 54 64 65 73 **P**6	12	62	980	400	14	0	0	75000	50572	1443
★ POMONA VALLEY HOSPITAL MEDICAL CENTER, 1798 North Garey Avenue, Zip 91767-2918; tel. 909/865-9885; Richard E. Yochum, President and Chief Executive Officer (Total facility includes 38 beds in nursing home–type unit) **A**1 2 9 10 **F**4 7 8 10 11 12 15 16 17 19 20 21 22 23 24 25 28 29 30 31 34 35 36 37 38 39 40 41 42 43 44 45 46 60 64 65 66 67 68 71 72 73 74 **P**5	23	10	449	20589	255	269530	6270	164512	72978	1895
PORT HUENEME—Ventura County										
☐ ANACAPA HOSPITAL, 307 East Clara Street, Zip 93041; tel. 805/488-3661; Dennis N. Fliegelman, Administrator (Nonreporting) **A**1 9 10 **S**0235 Adventist Health System/West	21	22	24	—	—	—	—	—	—	—
PORTERVILLE—Tulare County										
PORTERVILLE DEVELOPMENTAL CENTER, 26501 Avenue 140, Zip 93257-9430, Mailing Address: Box 2000, Zip 93258-2000; tel. 209/782-2222; Ruth Maples, Executive Director (Nonreporting) **A**10	12	62	1177	—	—	—	—	—	—	—
SIERRA VIEW DISTRICT HOSPITAL, 465 West Putnam Avenue, Zip 93257-3320; tel. 209/784-1110; David S. Wanger, Administrator **A**10 **F**7 8 11 12 15 16 17 19 21 22 25 28 29 30 32 34 35 37 38 40 42 44 45 46 47 51 60 64 65 71 **P**5 8	16	10	93	5456	61	39499	1075	32652	12052	448
PORTOLA—Plumas County										
EASTERN PLUMAS DISTRICT HOSPITAL, 500 First Avenue, Zip 96122; tel. 916/832-4277; Charles Gunther, Chief Executive Officer (Nonreporting) **A**9 10 **S**0585 Brim, Inc.	16	10	24	—	—	—	—	—	—	—
POWAY—San Diego County										
★ POMERADO HOSPITAL, 15615 Pomerado Road, Zip 92064; tel. 619/485-4600; Mark R. Middlebrook, Administrator and Chief Operating Officer (Total facility includes 149 beds in nursing home–type unit) **A**1 2 9 10 **F**3 4 7 8 11 12 14 15 16 17 19 21 22 27 29 30 31 32 33 34 35 37 38 40 41 42 44 45 46 49 59 61 63 64 65 71 73 74 **P**3 5 **S**7555 Palomar Pomerado Health System	16	10	279	5443	187	48359	1470	42102	13487	389

Hospitals, U.S. / CALIFORNIA

Hospital, Address, Telephone, Administrator, Approval, Facility, and Physician Codes, Health Care System	Classi-fication Codes		Utilization Data					Expense (thousands) of dollars		
★ American Hospital Association (AHA) membership □ Joint Commission on Accreditation of Healthcare Organizations (JCAHO) accreditation + American Osteopathic Hospital Association (AOHA) membership ○ American Osteopathic Association (AOA) accreditation △ Commission on Accreditation of Rehabilitation Facilities (CARF) accreditation Control codes 61, 63, 64, 71, 72 and 73 indicate hospitals listed by AOHA, but not registered by AHA. For definition of numerical codes, see page A6	Control	Service	Beds	Admissions	Census	Outpatient Visits	Births	Total	Payroll	Personnel
QUINCY—Plumas County										
□ PLUMAS DISTRICT HOSPITAL, 1065 Bucks Lake Road, Zip 95971–9599; tel. 916/283–2121; R. Michael Barry, Administrator (Nonreporting) A1 9 10 S8795 Sutter Health	16	10	32	—						
RANCHO MIRAGE—Riverside County										
□ EISENHOWER MEMORIAL HOSPITAL AT EISENHOWER MEDICAL CENTER, 39000 Bob Hope Drive, Zip 92270; tel. 619/340–3911; Nancy Wilson, Executive Vice President and Administrator A1 2 5 9 10 F1 3 4 5 7 8 10 11 12 15 19 21 22 24 25 29 32 33 34 35 37 38 39 40 41 42 43 44 49 60 65 66 67 71 72 73 74 P5	23	10	261	10506	161	115630	308	133046	43356	1226
RED BLUFF—Tehama County										
★ ST. ELIZABETH COMMUNITY HOSPITAL, 2550 Sister Mary Columba Drive, Zip 96080–4397; tel. 916/529–8005; Thomas F. Grimes III, Executive Vice President and Chief Operating Officer A1 9 10 F7 8 12 13 15 19 21 22 23 24 25 27 28 32 33 34 35 37 40 41 44 47 48 49 56 65 67 68 70 71 73 74	21	10	71	3087	31	38574	670	25250	10884	372
REDDING—Shasta County										
★ MERCY MEDICAL CENTER, 2175 Rosaline Avenue, Zip 96001, Mailing Address: Box 496009, Zip 96049–6009; tel. 916/225–6000; George A. Govier, President A1 2 3 5 9 10 F4 7 8 10 11 15 16 19 21 22 23 24 25 27 29 30 31 32 33 34 35 36 37 38 39 40 41 42 43 44 49 60 63 64 65 67 70 71 73 74 P3 5 S5205 Catholic Healthcare West	21	10	220	9456	124	93451	1826	99047	39386	1141
□ REDDING MEDICAL CENTER, 1100 Butte Street, Zip 96001–0853, Mailing Address: Box 496072, Zip 96049–6072; tel. 916/244–5454; Stephen Corbeil, Chief Executive Officer A1 9 10 F2 3 4 5 7 8 9 10 11 12 14 15 16 17 18 19 20 21 22 23 24 27 28 29 30 32 33 34 35 36 37 38 39 40 42 43 44 45 47 48 49 52 53 54 57 58 59 60 61 63 64 65 67 68 69 70 71 72 73 74 P4 5 6	33	10	164	6901	107	41852	0	73229	28258	808
REDLANDS—San Bernardino County										
□ LOMA LINDA UNIVERSITY BEHAVIORAL MEDICINE CENTER, 1710 Barton Road, Zip 92373; tel. 714/793–9333; Edward H. Weiss, Administrator (Nonreporting) A1 S2175 Adventist Health System—Loma Linda	21	22	89	—	—	—	—	—	—	—
□ REDLANDS COMMUNITY HOSPITAL, 350 Terracina Boulevard, Zip 92373, Mailing Address: Box 3391, Zip 92373–0742; tel. 909/335–5500; James R. Holmes, President (Nonreporting) A1 2 9 10	23	10	194	—	—	—	—	—	—	—
REDONDO BEACH—Los Angeles County										
★ SOUTH BAY MEDICAL CENTER, (Formerly AMI South Bay Hospital) 514 North Prospect Avenue, Zip 90277; tel. 310/376–9474; Jerald R. Happel, Administrator (Total facility includes 30 beds in nursing home–type unit) A1 9 10 F7 8 11 15 16 19 21 22 24 28 34 36 37 38 39 40 44 46 48 49 52 61 63 64 65 71 73 P4 5 7 S0063 TENET Healthcare Corporation	33	10	201	4341	67	15710	900	40259	10699	250
REDWOOD CITY—San Mateo County										
★ KAISER FOUNDATION HOSPITAL, 1150 Veterans Boulevard, Zip 94063–2087; tel. 415/299–2000; Carol Kiecker, Administrator A1 3 5 10 F2 3 4 7 8 10 11 12 13 17 18 22 25 26 28 29 30 31 32 33 37 38 39 40 41 42 43 44 45 46 47 48 49 52 53 54 55 56 61 65 73 P3 S2105 Kaiser Foundation Hospitals	23	10	147	7747	90	496728	1849	—	—	1116
★ SEQUOIA HOSPITAL DISTRICT, 170 Alameda De Las Pulgas, Zip 94062–2799; tel. 415/367–5561; Arthur J. Faro, Chief Executive Officer (Total facility includes 44 beds in nursing home–type unit) A1 2 9 10 F2 3 4 7 8 10 11 12 15 16 17 18 19 21 22 28 30 31 32 34 35 37 38 40 41 42 43 44 48 49 52 56 59 60 64 65 66 67 71 73 P5 6	16	10	229	10827	164	84463	1164	132505	52146	1129
REEDLEY—Fresno County										
★ SIERRA–KINGS DISTRICT HOSPITAL, 372 West Cypress Avenue, Zip 93654; tel. 209/638–8155; Daniel DeSantis, Administrator A1 9 10 F7 8 19 22 24 32 34 40 44 49 65 71 73	16	10	36	1585	11	35427	890	9286	3745	132
RICHMOND—Contra Costa County										
□ EAST BAY HOSPITAL, 820 23rd Street, Zip 94804–1397; tel. 510/234–2525; Lois K. Patsey, Administrator A1 10 F41 44 52 55 59 65 73	33	22	87	1939	70	2995	0	11235	3779	129
★ KAISER FOUNDATION HOSPITAL, 1330 Cutting Boulevard, Zip 94804–2555; tel. 510/596–6000; Donald Oxley, Administrator (Nonreporting) A1 10 S2105 Kaiser Foundation Hospitals	23	10	43	—	—	—	—	—	—	—
RIDGECREST—Kern County										
★ RIDGECREST COMMUNITY HOSPITAL, 1081 North China Lake Boulevard, Zip 93555; tel. 619/446–3551; David A. Mechtenberg, Administrator A1 9 10 F7 11 15 19 22 28 32 34 35 36 37 40 41 44 45 46 49 65 71 73	23	10	80	2140	22	37601	530	18690	8025	250
RIVERSIDE—Riverside County										
★ KAISER FOUNDATION HOSPITAL–RIVERSIDE, 10800 Magnolia Avenue, Zip 92505–3000; tel. 909/353–4600; Robert S. Lund, Administrator A1 3 10 F3 4 7 8 10 21 22 31 32 33 35 37 40 41 42 43 45 46 53 54 55 56 58 63 65 69 71 72 73 74 S2105 Kaiser Foundation Hospitals	23	10	215	8064	76	25306	2417	—	—	766
□ PARKVIEW COMMUNITY HOSPITAL MEDICAL CENTER, 3865 Jackson Street, Zip 92503; tel. 909/688–2211; Kenneth L. Willes, President A1 2 9 10 F7 8 10 11 12 14 15 16 19 21 22 28 30 35 37 38 40 41 42 43 44 46 49 65 71 73 P7	23	10	193	12416	117	68036	4664	79522	27845	746
□ RIVERSIDE COMMUNITY HOSPITAL, 4445 Magnolia Avenue, Zip 92501–1669, Mailing Address: Box 1669, Zip 92502–1669; tel. 909/788–3000; Nancy J. Bitting, President and Chief Executive Officer A1 9 10 F4 7 8 10 12 15 16 19 21 22 23 27 28 29 30 31 32 34 35 36 37 38 39 40 41 42 43 44 45 46 49 65 70 71 72 73 74 P4 5	23	10	245	9734	125	71372	1516	79333	29942	741

© 1995 AHA Guide

Hospitals, U.S. / CALIFORNIA

★ American Hospital Association (AHA) membership
□ Joint Commission on Accreditation of Healthcare Organizations (JCAHO) accreditation
+ American Osteopathic Hospital Association (AOHA) membership
○ American Osteopathic Association (AOA) accreditation
△ Commission on Accreditation of Rehabilitation Facilities (CARF) accreditation
Control codes 61, 63, 64, 71, 72 and 73 indicate hospitals listed by AOHA; but not registered by AHA. For definition of numerical codes, see page A6

Hospital, Address, Telephone, Administrator, Approval, Facility, and Physician Codes, Health Care System	Classification Codes		Utilization Data					Expense (thousands) of dollars		
	Control	Service	Beds	Admissions	Census	Outpatient Visits	Births	Total	Payroll	Personnel
□ RIVERSIDE GENERAL HOSPITAL–UNIVERSITY MEDICAL CENTER, 9851 Magnolia Avenue, Zip 92503; tel. 909/358-5030; Kenneth B. Cohen, Director (Nonreporting) A1 3 5 9 10	13	10	263	—	—	—	—	—	—	—
ROSEMEAD—Los Angeles County										
□ CPC ALHAMBRA HOSPITAL, 4619 North Rosemead Boulevard, Zip 91770–1498, Mailing Address: P.O. Box 369, Zip 91770; tel. 818/286-1191; Peggy Minnick, Administrator (Nonreporting) A1 9 10 S0785 Community Psychiatric Centers	33	22	98	—	—	—	—	—	—	—
□ INGLESIDE HOSPITAL, 7500 East Hellman Avenue, Zip 91770; tel. 818/288-1160; Clark D. Todd Jr., Chief Executive Officer A1 9 10 F1 3 12 14 15 16 41 52 53 54 55 56 58 59 65	33	22	126	1217	33	19612	0	—	—	128
ROSEVILLE—Placer County										
★ ROSEVILLE HOSPITAL, 333 Sunrise Avenue, Zip 95661–3477; tel. 916/781-1000; W. Jefferson Comer, Administrator A1 2 9 10 F4 7 8 10 11 12 15 16 17 19 20 21 22 23 26 29 30 31 32 33 34 35 37 39 40 41 42 43 44 45 46 49 60 63 65 66 67 71 73 P3 5 7 S8795 Sutter Health	23	10	201	9303	115	143441	1546	77484	35845	709
SACRAMENTO—Sacramento County										
★ CPC HERITAGE OAKS HOSPITAL, 4250 Auburn Boulevard, Zip 95841; tel. 916/489-3336; Ingrid L. Whipple, Chief Executive Officer A1 9 10 F52 53 57 58 59 S0785 Community Psychiatric Centers	33	22	76	1508	49	10366	0	—	—	110
□ CPC SIERRA VISTA HOSPITAL, 8001 Bruceville Road, Zip 95823; tel. 916/423-2000; Kenneth A. Meibert, Chief Executive Officer (Nonreporting) A1 9 10 S0785 Community Psychiatric Centers	33	22	72	—	—	—	—	—	—	—
★ KAISER FOUNDATION HOSPITAL, 2025 Morse Avenue, Zip 95825–2115; tel. 916/973-5000; Sarah Krevans, Area Manager (Nonreporting) A1 3 5 10 S2105 Kaiser Foundation Hospitals	23	10	304	—	—	—	—	—	—	—
★ KAISER FOUNDATION HOSPITAL, 6600 Bruceville Road, Zip 95823; tel. 916/688-2430; Sarah Krevans, Area Manager A1 3 10 F4 7 8 9 10 11 12 14 19 21 22 23 24 29 30 31 32 33 34 35 37 40 41 43 44 47 49 52 53 54 56 58 59 60 63 64 65 70 71 72 73 P3 S2105 Kaiser Foundation Hospitals	23	10	221	9477	89	30796	1916	—	—	1057
★ MERCY GENERAL HOSPITAL, 4001 J Street, Zip 95819; tel. 916/453-4950; Thomas A. Petersen, Vice President and Chief Operating Officer (Total facility includes 117 beds in nursing home–type unit) A1 2 9 10 F4 7 8 10 11 12 14 15 16 19 21 22 23 24 26 28 29 30 31 32 33 34 35 37 39 40 41 42 43 44 46 48 49 60 62 64 65 69 71 73 74 P3 5 S5205 Catholic Healthcare West	21	10	404	16674	248	107329	3715	144142	57831	1183
★ METHODIST HOSPITAL, 7500 Hospital Drive, Zip 95823–5477; tel. 916/423-3000; Stanley C. Oppegard, Vice President and Chief Operating Officer (Total facility includes 140 beds in nursing home–type unit) A1 9 10 F4 5 7 8 10 11 12 14 15 16 17 19 20 21 22 23 24 25 26 27 28 29 30 31 32 33 34 35 37 38 39 40 41 42 43 44 45 46 49 50 51 53 54 55 56 57 58 59 60 63 64 65 66 67 69 70 71 72 73 74 P3 5 S5205 Catholic Healthcare West	23	10	309	6195	203	48882	759	53688	22880	657
SUTTER CENTER FOR PSYCHIATRY, 7700 Folsom Boulevard, Zip 95826–2608; tel. 916/386-3000; Diane Gail Stewart, Administrator A10 F1 3 4 6 7 8 10 11 12 13 17 18 19 20 21 22 23 24 25 26 27 28 29 30 31 32 33 34 35 37 38 39 40 41 42 43 44 45 46 47 48 49 50 51 52 53 54 55 56 57 58 59 60 61 62 63 64 65 66 67 68 69 70 71 72 73 74 P1 3 4 5 6 7 S8795 Sutter Health	23	22	69	2017	45	21338	0	11024	5744	121
★ SUTTER GENERAL HOSPITAL, 2801 L Street, Zip 95816; tel. 916/454-2222; Patrick E. Fry, Administrator (Total facility includes 230 beds in nursing home–type unit) A1 3 5 9 10 F1 2 3 4 7 8 10 11 12 14 15 16 17 19 20 21 22 23 25 26 28 29 30 31 32 33 34 35 37 38 40 41 42 43 44 45 46 47 50 52 53 54 55 56 57 58 59 60 61 62 63 64 65 67 68 69 70 71 72 73 74 P3 4 5 6 7 S8795 Sutter Health	23	10	438	10766	270	73151	0	106190	40110	1443
★ SUTTER MEMORIAL HOSPITAL, 5151 F Street, Zip 95819–3295; tel. 916/454-3333; Patrick E. Fry, Chief Operating Officer A1 2 9 10 F1 2 3 4 7 8 10 11 12 14 15 16 17 19 20 21 22 23 25 26 28 29 30 31 32 33 34 35 37 38 40 42 43 44 46 47 50 52 53 54 55 56 57 58 59 60 61 62 63 64 65 67 68 69 70 71 72 73 74 P3 4 5 6 7 S8795 Sutter Health	23	10	346	17472	254	58632	6060	153989	65157	1847
★ UNIVERSITY OF CALIFORNIA, DAVIS MEDICAL CENTER, 2315 Stockton Boulevard, Zip 95817–2282; tel. 916/734-3096; Frank J. Loge, Director A1 2 3 5 8 9 10 F4 7 8 9 10 11 14 15 16 17 19 22 23 25 26 28 29 31 32 33 34 35 37 38 40 41 42 43 44 45 46 47 48 49 51 54 56 58 60 61 65 66 67 69 70 71 72 73 74 P6 S6405 University of California–Systemwide Administration	12	10	474	21082	364	300757	1107	365433	181120	4983
SALINAS—Monterey County										
★ NATIVIDAD MEDICAL CENTER, 1330 Natividad Road, Zip 93906, Mailing Address: Box 81611, Zip 93912-1611; tel. 408/755-4111; Howard H. Classen, Chief Executive Officer (Total facility includes 52 beds in nursing home–type unit) A1 3 5 10 F3 4 7 8 12 13 15 16 17 18 19 20 22 26 29 30 31 32 33 34 35 36 37 38 39 40 41 42 43 44 49 51 52 56 64 65 66 71 73 74 P5	13	10	211	5719	101	126380	1843	58235	24451	499
★ SALINAS VALLEY MEMORIAL HOSPITAL, 450 East Romie Lane, Zip 93901–4098; tel. 408/757-4333; Samuel W. Downing, Chief Executive Officer (Nonreporting) A1 2 9 10	16	10	232	—	—	—	—	—	—	—
SAN ANDREAS—Calaveras County										
□ MARK TWAIN ST. JOSEPH'S HOSPITAL, 768 Mountain Ranch Road, Zip 95249–9710; tel. 209/754-3521; Kathy Yarbrough, Administrator (Nonreporting) A1 9 10	23	10	33	—	—	—	—	—	—	—

Hospitals, U.S. / CALIFORNIA

Hospital, Address, Telephone, Administrator, Approval, Facility, and Physician Codes, Health Care System	Classification Codes		Utilization Data					Expense (thousands) of dollars		
★ American Hospital Association (AHA) membership □ Joint Commission on Accreditation of Healthcare Organizations (JCAHO) accreditation + American Osteopathic Hospital Association (AOHA) membership ○ American Osteopathic Association (AOA) accreditation △ Commission on Accreditation of Rehabilitation Facilities (CARF) accreditation Control codes 61, 63, 64, 71, 72 and 73 indicate hospitals listed by AOHA, but not registered by AHA. For definition of numerical codes, see page A6	Control	Service	Beds	Admissions	Census	Outpatient Visits	Births	Total	Payroll	Personnel
SAN BERNARDINO—San Bernardino County										
□ COMMMUNITY HOSPITAL OF SAN BERNARDINO, (Formerly San Bernardino Community Hospital) 1805 Medical Center Drive, Zip 92411; tel. 909/887–6333; Bruce G. Satzger, Administrator and Chief Executive Officer (Total facility includes 99 beds in nursing home–type unit) **A**1 9 10 **F**1 7 8 10 11 12 15 16 19 21 22 27 28 29 31 32 34 35 36 37 38 39 40 41 42 44 45 46 48 49 52 53 54 56 57 58 61 64 65 67 71 73 74 **P**5 7	23	10	390	9626	237	100767	2702	67606	26946	1059
SAN BERNARDINO COMMUNITY HOSPITAL See Commmunity Hospital of San Bernardino										
★ SAN BERNARDINO COUNTY MEDICAL CENTER, 780 East Gilbert Street, Zip 92415–0935; tel. 909/387–8111; Charles R. Jervis, Administrator **A**1 2 3 5 9 10 12 **F**3 4 7 9 10 12 14 19 20 21 22 26 28 31 32 34 35 37 38 40 41 42 44 45 51 52 53 55 56 57 58 59 60 61 63 65 69 70 71 72 73 **P**5	13	10	293	14848	203	196076	2087	133751	64599	1786
★ ST. BERNARDINE MEDICAL CENTER, 2101 North Waterman Avenue, Zip 92404; tel. 909/883–8711; Gregory A. Adams, Administrator and Chief Executive Officer (Total facility includes 29 beds in nursing home–type unit) **A**1 2 9 10 **F**4 7 8 10 11 19 21 22 23 24 25 28 29 30 31 32 33 34 35 37 38 39 40 41 42 43 44 45 46 48 49 50 51 52 60 63 64 65 67 68 69 71 73 **P**2 5 7 **S**0605 Sisters of Charity of the Incarnate Word Healthcare System	23	10	447	14890	207	262451	2961	—	—	1285
SAN CLEMENTE—Orange County										
★ SAMARITAN MEDICAL CENTER SAN CLEMENTE, 654 Camino De Los Mares, Zip 92673; tel. 714/496–1122; Tony Struthers, Chief Executive Officer **A**1 9 10 **F**7 8 12 13 15 17 19 21 23 27 28 29 30 32 34 35 36 37 39 40 41 42 44 45 46 49 59 65 67 71 73 **P**5 **S**2535 Samaritan Health System	23	10	86	2416	21	15107	571	22455	9291	279
SAN DIEGO—San Diego County										
□ ALVARADO HOSPITAL MEDICAL CENTER, 6655 Alvarado Road, Zip 92120–5298; tel. 619/229–3100; Barry G. Weinbaum, Executive Director **A**1 9 10 **F**4 7 8 10 11 12 14 16 17 19 21 22 25 26 27 28 29 30 31 32 34 35 37 38 40 41 42 43 44 45 48 49 53 54 55 56 57 58 59 60 61 63 64 65 66 67 71 73 74 **P**1 2 3 4 5 6 7 8 **S**0063 TENET Healthcare Corporation	33	10	231	9079	115	54223	1255	—	—	900
□ CHILDREN'S HOSPITAL AND HEALTH CENTER, 3020 Children's Way, Zip 92123–4282; tel. 619/576–1700; Blair L. Sadler, President (Total facility includes 59 beds in nursing home–type unit) **A**1 2 3 5 9 10 **F**5 10 15 16 17 19 21 22 25 28 31 32 33 34 35 38 39 41 42 43 44 46 47 48 49 53 54 58 64 65 67 69 70 71 72 73 **P**5	23	50	271	9968	187	189896	0	135811	58490	1715
□ HARBOR VIEW MEDICAL CENTER, 120 Elm Street, Zip 92101; tel. 619/235–3102; Roger W. Kielman, Administrator **A**1 9 10 **F**4 5 7 8 9 10 11 12 13 15 16 17 19 20 21 22 23 25 26 27 28 29 30 31 32 34 35 37 38 39 40 41 42 43 44 46 47 49 50 51 52 53 54 55 56 57 58 59 60 63 65 66 67 68 69 70 71 72 73 74 **P**5 7 **S**6525 Ornda Healthcorp	32	10	130	3328	75	39633	0	29774	13213	294
★ KAISER FOUNDATION HOSPITAL, (Includes Kaiser Foundation Hospital, 203 Travelodge Drive, El Cajon, California, Zip 92020; tel. 619/528–5000) 4647 Zion Avenue, Zip 92120; tel. 619/528–5000; Kenneth F. Colling, Administrator **A**1 2 3 5 9 10 **F**4 7 8 12 14 15 16 19 21 22 23 28 29 31 32 33 35 41 43 44 45 46 49 51 65 71 73 **S**2105 Kaiser Foundation Hospitals	23	10	326	21630	213	—	4703	—	—	—
★ MERCY HOSPITAL AND MEDICAL CENTER, 4077 Fifth Avenue, Zip 92103–2180; tel. 619/294–8111; Ralph George M.D., President and Chief Executive Officer (Nonreporting) **A**1 2 3 5 9 10 **S**5205 Catholic Healthcare West	21	10	417	—	—	—	—	—	—	—
□ MESA VISTA HOSPITAL, 7850 Vista Hill Avenue, Zip 92123–2790; tel. 619/694–8300; Donald K. Allen, Administrator and Chief Executive Officer (Nonreporting) **A**1 9 10 **S**8895 Vista Hill Foundation	23	22	150	—	—	—	—	—	—	—
★ MISSION BAY MEMORIAL HOSPITAL, 3030 Bunker Hill Street, Zip 92109–5780; tel. 619/274–7721; Britt Berrett, Chief Executive Officer (Total facility includes 26 beds in nursing home–type unit) **A**1 9 10 **F**8 10 11 12 14 16 17 19 26 27 28 30 32 35 37 44 46 52 57 59 63 64 65 71 73 **P**5 7 **S**0048 Columbia/HCA Healthcare Corporation	33	10	128	2678	39	71645	0	37327	12322	333
★ NAVAL MEDICAL CENTER, Zip 92134–5000; tel. 619/532–6400; Rear Admiral R. A. Nelson MC, USN, Commander (Nonreporting) **A**1 2 3 5 **S**9655 Department of Navy	43	10	422	—	—	—	—	—	—	—
SAN DIEGO COUNTY LOMA PORTAL MENTAL HEALTH FACILITY, 3485 Kenyon Street, Zip 92110, Mailing Address: Box 85524, Zip 92138; tel. 619/692–5501; Eric Eliason, Administrator and Chief Executive Officer (Nonreporting) **A**10	13	52	32	—	—	—	—	—	—	—
□ SAN DIEGO COUNTY PSYCHIATRIC HOSPITAL, 3851 Rosecrans Street, Zip 92110, Mailing Address: P.O. Box 85524, Zip 92138–5524; tel. 619/692–8211; Karen C. Hogan, Administrator and Chief Executive Officer **A**1 9 10 **F**14 15 16 22 52 59	13	22	109	980	105	—	0	—	—	182
★ SAN DIEGO HOSPICE, (Acute Hospice Care) 4311 Third Avenue, Zip 92103; tel. 619/688–1600; Virginia S. Mackey, President (Nonreporting) **A**10	23	49	24	—	—	—	—	—	—	—
★ SHARP CABRILLO HOSPITAL, 3475 Kenyon Street, Zip 92110–5067; tel. 619/221–3400; James M. Schibanoff M.D., Chief Executive Officer (Total facility includes 79 beds in nursing home–type unit) **A**1 2 9 10 **F**1 3 4 7 8 10 11 12 14 15 16 17 19 21 22 23 24 25 26 27 29 30 31 32 34 35 37 38 39 40 41 42 43 44 45 46 48 49 51 52 53 54 55 56 57 58 59 60 61 64 65 66 67 69 71 72 73 74 **P**5 8 **S**2065 Sharp Healthcare	23	10	227	4899	113	25604	0	44879	19367	488
★ △ SHARP MEMORIAL HOSPITAL, 7901 Frost Street, Zip 92123–2788; tel. 619/541–3400; James M. Schibanoff M.D., Chief Executive Officer **A**1 2 3 7 9 **F**1 3 4 7 8 10 11 12 14 15 16 17 19 21 22 23 24 25 26 27 29 30 31 32 34 35 37 38 39 40 41 42 44 45 46 49 51 52 54 55 56 57 58 59 60 61 63 64 65 66 67 69 70 71 72 73 74 **P**1 5 **S**2065 Sharp Healthcare	23	10	488	22981	293	63626	8570	205905	87270	2236

© 1995 AHA Guide

Hospitals, U.S. / CALIFORNIA

Hospital, Address, Telephone, Administrator, Approval, Facility, and Physician Codes, Health Care System

- ★ American Hospital Association (AHA) membership
- ☐ Joint Commission on Accreditation of Healthcare Organizations (JCAHO) accreditation
- \+ American Osteopathic Hospital Association (AOHA) membership
- ○ American Osteopathic Association (AOA) accreditation
- △ Commission on Accreditation of Rehabilitation Facilities (CARF) accreditation

Control codes 61, 63, 64, 71, 72 and 73 indicate hospitals listed by AOHA, but not registered by AHA. For definition of numerical codes, see page A6.

	Classification Codes		Utilization Data					Expense (thousands) of dollars		
Hospital	Control	Service	Beds	Admissions	Census	Outpatient Visits	Births	Total	Payroll	Personnel
★ UNIVERSITY OF CALIFORNIA SAN DIEGO MEDICAL CENTER, 200 West Arbor Drive, Zip 92103–8970; tel. 619/543–6222; Michael R. Stringer, Director (Nonreporting) A1 2 3 5 8 9 10 S6405 University of California–Systemwide Administration	12	10	412	—	—	—	—	—	—	—
☐ VENCOR HOSPITAL–SAN DIEGO, 1940 El Cajon Boulevard, Zip 92104; tel. 619/543–4500; (Nonreporting) A1 9 10 S0026 Vencor, Incorporated	23	10	133	—	—	—	—	—	—	—
★ VETERANS AFFAIRS MEDICAL CENTER, 3350 LaJolla Village Drive, Zip 92161; tel. 619/552–8585; Leonard C. Rogers, Director (Total facility includes 44 beds in nursing home–type unit) A1 3 5 8 F1 2 3 4 5 6 8 9 10 11 12 14 15 16 17 18 19 20 21 22 24 25 26 27 28 29 30 31 32 33 34 35 37 39 42 43 44 45 46 48 49 51 52 54 55 56 57 58 59 64 65 67 71 72 73 74 P6 S9295 Department of Veterans Affairs	45	10	336	8308	256	261498	0	137309	69555	1919
☐ VILLAVIEW COMMUNITY HOSPITAL, 5550 University Avenue, Zip 92105, Mailing Address: P.O. Box 5587, Zip 92105; tel. 619/582–3516; Ted N. Pendleton, President (Nonreporting) A1 10	23	10	100	—	—	—	—	—	—	—

SAN DIMAS—Los Angeles County

Hospital	Control	Service	Beds	Admissions	Census	Outpatient Visits	Births	Total	Payroll	Personnel
★ SAN DIMAS COMMUNITY HOSPITAL, (Formerly AMI San Dimas Community Hospital) 1350 West Covina Boulevard, Zip 91773–0308; tel. 909/599–6811; Larry Peterson, Chief Executive Officer A1 2 9 10 F8 11 12 19 21 22 27 28 30 34 35 39 41 44 49 50 60 65 71 72 73 P5 S0063 TENET Healthcare Corporation	33	10	99	2720	26	22789	573	18394	7858	284

SAN FERNANDO—Los Angeles County

Hospital	Control	Service	Beds	Admissions	Census	Outpatient Visits	Births	Total	Payroll	Personnel
★ MISSION COMMUNITY HOSPITAL–SAN FERNANDO CAMPUS, (Formerly San Fernando Community Hospital) (Includes Mission Community Hospital–Panorama City Campus, 14850 Roscoe Boulevard, Panorama City, California, Zip 91402–4618; tel. 818/787–2222) 700 Chatsworth Drive, Zip 91340–4299; tel. 818/361–7331; Cathy Fickes, Chief Executive Officer A1 9 10 F8 10 11 12 18 19 20 21 22 26 27 30 37 40 44 49 52 54 55 56 59 65 71 73 P3 5 7	23	10	152	3339	65	10600	0	35557	—	209

SAN FERNANDO COMMUNITY HOSPITAL See Mission Community Hospital–San Fernando Campus

SAN FRANCISCO—San Francisco County

Hospital	Control	Service	Beds	Admissions	Census	Outpatient Visits	Births	Total	Payroll	Personnel
★ CALIFORNIA PACIFIC MEDICAL CENTER, Clay at Buchanan Street, Zip 94115, Mailing Address: P.O. Box 7999, Zip 94120; tel. 415/563–4321; Martin Brotman M.D., President (Total facility includes 91 beds in nursing home–type unit) A1 2 3 5 8 10 F1 2 4 7 8 10 11 12 13 14 15 16 17 19 20 21 22 23 26 27 29 30 31 32 33 34 35 36 37 38 39 40 41 42 43 44 45 46 47 48 49 51 52 53 54 55 56 57 58 59 60 63 64 65 66 67 68 69 71 73 74 P2 5 7	23	10	508	22807	368	442510	3912	348855	147663	3847
★ CHINESE HOSPITAL, 845 Jackson Street, Zip 94133–4899; tel. 415/982–2400; Thomas M. Harlan, Chief Executive Officer A1 9 10 F4 7 8 10 12 15 17 19 21 22 23 28 29 31 32 33 34 35 37 39 40 41 42 43 44 45 49 50 53 54 58 60 61 63 65 67 69 71 72 73 P5	23	10	59	2111	31	32076	336	19251	8120	204
★ DAVIES MEDICAL CENTER, Castro and Duboce Streets, Zip 94114; tel. 415/565–6003; Greg Monardo, President (Total facility includes 35 beds in nursing home–type unit) A1 3 5 9 10 F8 11 12 14 15 16 17 19 21 22 31 33 34 35 39 41 42 44 46 48 49 52 54 55 57 60 64 65 66 67 71 72 73 74 P5	23	10	153	2606	88	100890	0	55642	27799	660
★ KAISER FOUNDATION HOSPITAL, 2425 Geary Boulevard, Zip 94115; tel. 415/202–2000; Frank D. Alvarez, Administrator A1 3 5 10 F3 4 7 8 10 11 12 14 15 16 17 19 20 21 22 23 24 25 28 29 31 32 33 34 35 37 38 39 40 41 42 43 44 45 46 47 49 51 52 53 54 55 56 58 59 60 61 63 65 66 67 69 70 71 72 73 P1 S2105 Kaiser Foundation Hospitals	23	10	149	17033	95	822256	2574	—	—	3139
★ LAGUNA HONDA HOSPITAL AND REHABILITATION CENTER, 375 Laguna Honda Boulevard, Zip 94116–1499; tel. 415/664–1580; Anthony G. Wagner, Executive Administrator (Total facility includes 1145 beds in nursing home–type unit) A9 10 F1 2 3 4 8 9 10 11 16 18 19 20 22 26 27 28 31 32 33 34 35 37 38 39 40 41 42 43 44 45 47 48 49 51 52 53 54 56 57 58 60 61 64 65 67 71 72 73 P6	15	48	1193	1321	1121	0	0	101746	71081	1619
★ MOUNT ZION MEDICAL CENTER OF UNIVERSITY OF CALIFORNIA–SAN FRANCISCO, 1600 Divisadero Street, Zip 94115, Mailing Address: Box 7921, Zip 94120; tel. 415/567–6600; Martin H. Diamond, Director (Nonreporting) A1 2 3 5 9 10 S6405 University of California–Systemwide Administration	12	10	290	—	—	—	—	—	—	—
☐ PACIFIC COAST HOSPITAL, (Podiatry) 1210 Scott Street, Zip 94115–4000; tel. 415/563–3444; Deborah J. Black M.P.A., R.N., Administrator (Nonreporting) A1 9 10	23	49	28	—	—	—	—	—	—	—
★ SAINT FRANCIS MEMORIAL HOSPITAL, 900 Hyde Street, Zip 94109, Mailing Address: Box 7726, Zip 94120–7726; tel. 415/353–6000; John G. Williams, President (Total facility includes 34 beds in nursing home–type unit) A1 2 3 9 10 F4 8 9 10 11 12 14 17 19 21 22 27 28 30 31 32 34 35 37 39 41 42 44 45 46 48 49 52 54 55 56 57 60 64 65 66 67 71 73 P4 5 7 S5205 Catholic Healthcare West	23	10	221	6267	118	167811	0	67347	26573	740
☐ SAN FRANCISCO GENERAL HOSPITAL MEDICAL CENTER, 1001 Potrero Avenue, Zip 94110; tel. 415/206–8000; Richard Cordova, Executive Director A1 2 3 5 9 10 F3 4 7 8 10 11 15 16 17 18 19 20 22 25 28 29 30 31 32 33 34 35 36 37 38 39 40 41 42 43 46 47 49 51 52 53 54 56 57 58 59 60 61 63 65 66 67 69 70 71 72 73 74 P1 6	15	10	340	17270	273	321705	1696	250579	101566	3918
★ SHRINERS HOSPITALS FOR CRIPPLED CHILDREN, SAN FRANCISCO UNIT, 1701 19th Avenue, Zip 94122–4599; tel. 415/759–4000; Margaret Bryan–Williams, Administrator A1 3 5 F9 12 19 21 28 34 35 39 41 45 46 48 49 65 67 71 73 P6 S4125 Shriners Hospitals for Crippled Children	23	56	48	765	23	9565	0	—	—	165

Hospitals, U.S. / CALIFORNIA

Hospital, Address, Telephone, Administrator, Approval, Facility, and Physician Codes, Health Care System	Classi-fication Codes		Utilization Data					Expense (thousands) of dollars		
★ American Hospital Association (AHA) membership ☐ Joint Commission on Accreditation of Healthcare Organizations (JCAHO) accreditation + American Osteopathic Hospital Association (AOHA) membership ○ American Osteopathic Association (AOA) accreditation △ Commission on Accreditation of Rehabilitation Facilities (CARF) accreditation Control codes 61, 63, 64, 71, 72 and 73 indicate hospitals listed by AOHA, but not registered by AHA. For definition of numerical codes, see page A6	Control	Service	Beds	Admissions	Census	Outpatient Visits	Births	Total	Payroll	Personnel
★ ST. MARY'S MEDICAL CENTER, 450 Stanyan Street, Zip 94117–1079; tel. 415/668–1000; Mary Ann Thode, President and Chief Executive Officer **A**1 2 3 5 8 9 10 **F**1 2 3 4 8 9 10 12 15 16 17 19 21 22 26 27 30 31 32 34 35 37 42 43 44 46 48 49 52 53 54 56 57 58 59 60 64 65 66 67 71 73 74 **P**3 4 5 7 **S**5205 Catholic Healthcare West	21	10	309	9205	213	127420	0	127442	59287	1222
☐ ST. LUKE'S HOSPITAL, 3555 Army Street, Zip 94110; tel. 415/647–8600; Jack Fries, President (Nonreporting) **A**1 9 10	23	10	239	—	—	—	—	—	—	—
★ UNIVERSITY OF CALIFORNIA SAN FRANCISCO MEDICAL CENTER, (Includes Langley Porter Psychiatric Hospital, 401 Parnassus Avenue, San Francisco, California, Zip 94143–0984, Mailing Address: Box F–0984, Zip 94143–0984; tel. 415/476–7347) 500 Parnassus, Zip 94143–0296; tel. 415/476–1000; William B. Kerr, Director **A**1 2 3 5 8 9 10 **F**1 3 4 5 7 8 10 11 12 13 14 17 18 19 20 21 22 23 24 25 26 27 30 31 32 34 35 37 38 39 40 41 42 43 44 45 46 47 48 49 50 51 53 54 55 56 57 58 59 60 61 63 64 65 66 67 68 69 70 71 72 73 74 **P**1 4 5 6 **S**6405 University of California–Systemwide Administration	23	10	706	25477	468	387917	1680	454473	206716	3479
★ VETERANS AFFAIRS MEDICAL CENTER, 4150 Clement Street, Zip 94121–1598; tel. 415/750–2041; Lawrence C. Stewart, Director (Total facility includes 120 beds in nursing home–type unit) **A**1 3 5 8 **F**1 2 3 4 8 10 11 16 19 20 21 22 26 27 28 31 32 33 34 35 37 39 41 42 43 44 45 46 48 49 51 52 54 56 58 60 63 64 65 67 71 73 74 **P**6 **S**9295 Department of Veterans Affairs	45	10	372	7703	268	378863	0	151299	98525	1732
SAN GABRIEL—Los Angeles County										
★ SAN GABRIEL VALLEY MEDICAL CENTER, 218 South Santa Anita Street, Zip 91776, Mailing Address: P.O. Box 1507, Zip 91778–1507; tel. 818/289–5454; Makoto Nakayama, President (Total facility includes 41 beds in nursing home–type unit) **A**1 9 10 **F**7 8 10 11 12 15 17 19 21 22 23 27 30 32 34 35 37 38 39 40 41 42 44 45 46 49 52 57 59 60 63 64 65 67 71 73 **P**5 7 **S**2315 UniHealth	23	10	266	7192	140	62430	596	61726	25000	737
SAN JOSE—Santa Clara County										
☐ ALEXIAN BROTHERS HOSPITAL, 225 North Jackson Avenue, Zip 95116–1691; tel. 408/259–5000; Steven R. Barron, Chief Executive Officer **A**1 9 10 **F**7 8 10 12 15 16 17 19 21 22 26 28 31 32 34 35 37 38 40 41 42 44 45 46 49 65 71 73 **P**5 7 **S**0065 Alexian Brothers Health System, Inc.	21	10	188	10951	119	76402	2797	76296	37104	871
★ GOOD SAMARITAN HOSPITAL OF SANTA CLARA VALLEY, 2425 Samaritan Drive, Zip 95124; tel. 408/559–2011; Joan White, Vice President and Administrator **A**1 9 10 **F**1 2 3 4 6 7 8 10 11 12 13 15 18 19 22 23 24 25 26 27 28 29 30 31 32 33 34 35 36 37 38 39 40 41 42 43 44 45 46 49 51 52 53 54 55 56 57 58 59 60 61 65 66 67 68 70 71 73 74 **P**3 **S**0965 Good Samaritan Health System	23	10	348	17176	208	89903	4100	164407	67923	1195
★ O'CONNOR HOSPITAL, 2105 Forest Avenue, Zip 95128–1471; tel. 408/947–2500; William C. Finlayson, President and Chief Executive Officer (Total facility includes 15 beds in nursing home–type unit) **A**1 2 9 10 **F**2 3 4 7 8 9 10 11 12 15 16 17 18 19 20 21 22 23 24 25 26 27 28 29 30 31 32 33 34 35 37 38 39 40 41 42 43 44 45 46 47 48 49 50 52 53 54 56 57 58 59 60 63 64 65 66 67 68 69 70 71 73 74 **P**2 3 5 6 7 **S**1855 Daughters of Charity National Health System	21	10	138	11430	135	157545	2775	101078	44672	940
★ SAN JOSE MEDICAL CENTER, 675 East Santa Clara Street, Zip 95112; tel. 408/998–3212; (Total facility includes 26 beds in nursing home–type unit) **A**1 2 3 5 9 10 **F**3 4 7 8 10 11 12 15 19 21 22 23 26 31 32 33 34 35 37 38 39 40 41 42 43 44 47 48 49 51 52 53 57 60 64 65 70 71 72 73 74 **P**3 **S**0965 Good Samaritan Health System	23	10	327	7960	145	75131	1877	111406	37120	860
★ △ SANTA CLARA VALLEY MEDICAL CENTER, 751 South Bascom Avenue, Zip 95128; tel. 408/299–5100; Robert Sillen, Executive Director (Nonreporting) **A**1 2 3 5 7 10	13	10	388	—	—	—	—	—	—	—
★ SANTA TERESA COMMUNITY HOSPITAL, 250 Hospital Parkway, Zip 95119; tel. 408/972–7000; Nancy Madsen R.N., Patient Care Services Leader **A**1 9 10 **F**2 3 4 6 7 8 9 10 11 12 13 14 16 17 18 19 20 21 22 23 24 25 26 28 29 30 31 32 33 34 35 37 38 39 40 41 42 43 44 45 46 47 48 49 50 51 52 53 54 56 57 58 59 60 61 63 64 65 66 67 68 69 70 71 72 73 74 **S**2105 Kaiser Foundation Hospitals	23	10	208	9275	116	—	2565	—	—	608
SAN LEANDRO—Alameda County										
FAIRMONT HOSPITAL, (SNF with Rehabilitation and Medical Acute) 15400 Foothill Boulevard, Zip 94578–1091; tel. 510/667–7800; Mike Smart, Administrator (Total facility includes 119 beds in nursing home–type unit) **A**9 **F**1 3 4 5 7 8 10 12 13 14 15 16 17 18 19 20 21 22 23 25 26 27 28 29 30 31 33 34 35 37 38 39 40 41 42 44 45 46 48 49 50 51 52 53 54 55 56 57 58 59 60 61 63 64 65 67 68 70 71 72 73 74 **P**6 **S**0225 Alameda County Health Care Services Agency	13	49	193	1478	192	54261	0	47606	26843	560
★ SAN LEANDRO HOSPITAL, 13855 East 14th Street, Zip 94578–0398; tel. 510/667–4510; Steve Monaghan, President and Chief Executive Officer (Nonreporting) **A**1 9 10 **S**0048 Columbia/HCA Healthcare Corporation	33	10	136	—	—	—	—	—	—	—
☐ VENCOR HOSPITAL–SAN LEANDRO, 2800 Benedict Drive, Zip 94577; tel. 510/357–8300; Jan E. Nielsen, Administrator **A**1 9 10 **F**14 15 19 22 35 37 45 65 67 71 **S**0026 Vencor, Incorporated	33	10	62	300	36	0	0	12160	6247	150
SAN LUIS OBISPO—San Luis Obispo County										
AMI SIERRA VISTA REGIONAL MEDICAL CENTER See Tenet Sierra Vista Regional Medical Center										
CALIFORNIA MENS COLONY HOSPITAL, Johnson Avenue, Zip 93409–8101, Mailing Address: P.O. Box 8101, Zip 93409–8101; tel. 805/547–7913; Galen Kirn, Administrator **F**10 19 20 21 22 31 34 35 42 43 44 50 54 55 56 58 60 65 67 71 72	12	10	39	561	30	41223	0	—	—	200

© 1995 AHA Guide

Hospitals, U.S. / CALIFORNIA

Hospital, Address, Telephone, Administrator, Approval, Facility, and Physician Codes, Health Care System	Classification Codes		Utilization Data					Expense (thousands) of dollars		
★ American Hospital Association (AHA) membership ☐ Joint Commission on Accreditation of Healthcare Organizations (JCAHO) accreditation + American Osteopathic Hospital Association (AOHA) membership ○ American Osteopathic Association (AOA) accreditation △ Commission on Accreditation of Rehabilitation Facilities (CARF) accreditation Control codes 61, 63, 64, 71, 72 and 73 indicate hospitals listed by AOHA, but not registered by AHA. For definition of numerical codes, see page A6	Control	Service	Beds	Admissions	Census	Outpatient Visits	Births	Total	Payroll	Personnel
☐ FRENCH HOSPITAL MEDICAL CENTER, 1911 Johnson Avenue, Zip 93401; tel. 805/543-5353; (Nonreporting) **A**1 9 **S**6525 Ornda Healthcorp	33	10	124	—	—	—	—	—	—	—
☐ SAN LUIS OBISPO GENERAL HOSPITAL, 2180 Johnson Avenue, Zip 93401, Mailing Address: Box 8113, Zip 93403-8113; tel. 805/781-4800; Marc Goldberg, Chief Executive Officer **A**1 9 10 **F**3 7 12 13 14 15 16 18 19 20 22 26 28 29 30 31 32 33 34 35 36 37 39 40 41 42 43 44 45 46 49 51 52 53 54 55 56 57 58 60 61 65 67 71 72 73	13	10	60	3028	30	58531	863	22966	10468	333
★ △ TENET SIERRA VISTA REGIONAL MEDICAL CENTER, (Formerly AMI Sierra Vista Regional Medical Center) 1010 Murray Street, Zip 93405, Mailing Address: Box 1367, Zip 93406-1367; tel. 805/546-7600; Philip R. Wolfe, Executive Director **A**1 7 9 10 **F**7 8 11 12 15 16 19 21 22 25 30 34 35 37 38 40 41 42 44 46 48 49 60 65 67 71 73 **P**7 **S**0063 TENET Healthcare Corporation	33	10	178	5945	80	31269	1080	33486	14196	401

SAN MATEO—San Mateo County

☐ SAN MATEO COUNTY GENERAL HOSPITAL, 222 West 39th Avenue, Zip 94403-4398; tel. 415/573-2222; Timothy B. McMurdo, Chief Executive Officer (Total facility includes 124 beds in nursing home-type unit) **A**1 3 9 10 **F**8 12 15 16 19 20 21 22 27 28 29 30 31 34 35 36 37 39 42 44 45 46 49 51 52 54 56 57 58 60 63 64 65 71 73	13	10	238	3900	191	133049	0	74356	31152	663

SAN PABLO—Contra Costa County

☐ BROOKSIDE HOSPITAL, 2000 Vale Road, Zip 94806; tel. 510/235-7006; Michael P. Lawson, President and Chief Executive Officer (Total facility includes 114 beds in nursing home-type unit) **A**1 2 9 10 **F**4 7 8 9 10 11 12 14 15 16 17 19 21 22 25 27 28 29 30 32 34 35 37 38 40 42 43 44 45 46 49 51 60 64 65 67 71 72 73 74 **P**4 5	16	10	286	7160	175	112321	1161	74053	40207	676

SAN PEDRO–Los Angeles County, See Los Angeles

SAN RAFAEL—Marin County

★ KAISER FOUNDATION HOSPITAL, 99 Montecillo Road, Zip 94903-3397; tel. 415/499-2227; Pete Delgado, Vice President and Area Manager **A**1 10 **F**4 8 9 10 11 14 19 21 23 29 31 32 33 34 35 37 38 39 40 41 43 44 45 46 47 48 49 52 53 54 63 64 65 69 71 73 **S**2105 Kaiser Foundation Hospitals	23	10	119	4338	51	282745	0	—	—	312

SAN RAMON—Contra Costa County

☐ SAN RAMON REGIONAL MEDICAL CENTER, 6001 Norris Canyon Road, Zip 94583; tel. 510/275-9200; Philip A. Cohen, Chief Executive Officer **A**1 10 **F**2 3 7 8 10 11 12 14 15 16 19 22 30 34 35 37 38 40 41 42 44 45 46 61 63 70 71 73 74	33	10	123	3526	43	34694	823	—	—	335

SANGER—Fresno County

★ SANGER GENERAL HOSPITAL, 2558 Jensen Avenue, Zip 93657-2296; tel. 209/875-6571; Jessie E. Hudgins, Chief Executive Officer **A**1 9 10 **F**7 8 19 30 34 35 40 44 65 71	32	10	25	1454	14	18688	886	4982	2406	102

SANTA ANA—Orange County

☐ COASTAL COMMUNITIES HOSPITAL, 2701 South Bristol Street, Zip 92704-9911, Mailing Address: P.O. Box 5240, Zip 92704-0240; tel. 714/754-5454; (Total facility includes 46 beds in nursing home-type unit) **A**1 9 10 **F**8 12 15 16 19 20 21 22 34 37 39 40 41 44 46 51 52 57 60 63 64 65 71 73 74 **P**2 4 5 7 **S**6525 Ornda Healthcorp	32	10	165	5016	67	—	2259	—	—	391
☐ CPC SANTA ANA HOSPITAL, 2212 East Fourth Street, Zip 92705-3873; tel. 714/543-8481; Gilbert Carmona, Regional Chief Executive Officer (Nonreporting) **A**1 9 10 **S**0785 Community Psychiatric Centers	33	22	100	—	—	—	—	—	—	—
☐ DOCTORS HOSPITAL OF SANTA ANA, 1901 North College Avenue, Zip 92706; tel. 714/547-2565; R. Michael Hartman, Chief Executive Officer (Nonreporting) **A**1 9 **S**6525 Ornda Healthcorp	33	10	54	—	—	—	—	—	—	—
SANTA ANA HOSPITAL MEDICAL CENTER, 1901 North Fairview Street, Zip 92706; tel. 714/554-1653; R. Michael Hartman, Chief Executive Officer (Nonreporting) **A**9 10 **S**6525 Ornda Healthcorp	33	10	99	—	—	—	—	—	—	—
☐ WESTERN MEDICAL CENTER–SANTA ANA, 1001 North Tustin Avenue, Zip 92705-3502; tel. 714/835-3555; Daniel L. Frank, Chief Executive Officer **A**1 2 3 5 9 10 **F**2 3 4 7 8 10 11 12 14 15 17 19 20 21 22 23 27 28 30 32 34 35 37 38 39 40 41 42 43 44 46 47 48 49 52 53 54 56 57 60 64 65 67 69 70 71 73 **P**5 **S**2085 United Western Medical Centers	23	10	288	12305	132	62501	4159	44633	—	1061

SANTA BARBARA—Santa Barbara County

ALAMAR HOSPITAL, 45 East Alamar, Zip 93105-3495; tel. 805/687-2411; Pamela J. Pratt, Administrator and Chief Executive Officer (Nonreporting) **A**9 **S**0575 Schick Laboratories, Inc.	33	22	30	—	—	—	—	—	—	—
☐ GOLETA VALLEY COMMUNITY HOSPITAL, 351 South Patterson Avenue, Zip 93111, Mailing Address: Box 6306, Zip 93160; tel. 805/967-3411; David C. Bigelow, President (Nonreporting) **A**1 9 10	23	10	70	—	—	—	—	—	—	—
★ △ REHABILITATION INSTITUTE AT SANTA BARBARA, 427 Camino Del Remedio, Zip 93110; tel. 805/683-3788; Rusty Pollock, President and Chief Executive Officer (Nonreporting) **A**1 7 9 10	23	46	40	—	—	—	—	—	—	—
★ SANTA BARBARA COTTAGE HOSPITAL, (Includes Santa Barbara Cottage Care Center, Santa Barbara, California) Pueblo at Bath Streets, Zip 93105, Mailing Address: Box 689, Zip 93102; tel. 805/682-7111; James L. Ash, President (Nonreporting) **A**1 2 3 5 9 10	23	10	332	—	—	—	—	—	—	—
☐ ST. FRANCIS MEDICAL CENTER OF SANTA BARBARA, 601 East Micheltorena Street, Zip 93103; tel. 805/962-7661; Ron Biscaro, President (Nonreporting) **A**1 9 10	21	10	98	—	—	—	—	—	—	—

Hospitals, U.S. / CALIFORNIA

Hospital, Address, Telephone, Administrator, Approval, Facility, and Physician Codes, Health Care System	Classification Codes		Utilization Data					Expense (thousands) of dollars		
	Control	Service	Beds	Admissions	Census	Outpatient Visits	Births	Total	Payroll	Personnel

★ American Hospital Association (AHA) membership
☐ Joint Commission on Accreditation of Healthcare Organizations (JCAHO) accreditation
+ American Osteopathic Hospital Association (AOHA) membership
○ American Osteopathic Association (AOA) accreditation
△ Commission on Accreditation of Rehabilitation Facilities (CARF) accreditation
Control codes 61, 63, 64, 71, 72 and 73 indicate hospitals listed by AOHA, but not registered by AHA. For definition of numerical codes, see page A6

SANTA CLARA—Santa Clara County

★ KAISER FOUNDATION HOSPITAL, 900 Kiely Boulevard, Zip 95051-5386; tel. 408/236-6400; Carol Kiecker, Vice President and Area Manager **A**1 3 5 10 **F**2 3 4 8 9 11 12 15 19 22 25 26 29 30 31 32 33 34 35 37 38 39 40 41 42 43 44 45 46 47 48 49 51 52 53 54 55 56 57 58 60 61 64 65 66 67 68 69 71 72 73 74 **P**6 **S**2105 Kaiser Foundation Hospitals	23	10	287	17193	165	—	3146	—	—	1041

SANTA CRUZ—Santa Cruz County

★ DOMINICAN SANTA CRUZ HOSPITAL, 1555 Soquel Drive, Zip 95065-1794; tel. 408/462-7700; Sister Julie Hyer, President and Chief Executive Officer **A**1 9 10 **F**3 4 6 7 8 10 11 12 13 14 15 16 17 19 22 24 25 30 32 34 35 37 40 41 42 43 44 45 46 48 49 52 54 56 60 62 64 65 66 67 71 72 73 **P**3 5 7 8 **S**5205 Catholic Healthcare West	21	10	284	12238	194	104651	1756	97956	40988	858

SANTA MARIA—Santa Barbara County

★ MARIAN MEDICAL CENTER, 1400 East Church Street, Zip 93454, Mailing Address: Box 1238, Zip 93456; tel. 805/922-5811; Charles J. Cova, Executive Vice President (Total facility includes 95 beds in nursing home-type unit) **A**1 9 10 **F**4 7 8 10 11 12 14 15 16 17 18 19 20 21 22 23 26 28 29 30 31 32 33 34 35 39 40 41 42 43 44 45 46 49 54 56 60 64 65 67 70 71 73 74 **P**7	21	10	225	6903	147	78439	1874	51211	21733	638
☐ VALLEY COMMUNITY HOSPITAL, 505 East Plaza Drive, Zip 93454-9943; tel. 805/925-0935; William C. Rasmussen, Chief Executive Officer (Nonreporting) **A**1 9 10 **S**6525 Ornda Healthcorp	33	10	70	—	—	—	—	—	—	—

SANTA MONICA—Los Angeles County

★ SAINT JOHN'S HOSPITAL AND HEALTH CENTER, 1328 22nd Street, Zip 90404; tel. 310/829-5511; Sister Marie Madeleine Shonka, President (Data for 234 days) **A**1 2 9 10 **F**2 3 4 7 8 10 11 15 19 21 22 28 29 30 32 33 34 35 36 37 38 39 40 41 42 43 44 45 49 52 54 55 56 57 58 59 60 64 65 66 71 73 74 **P**5 7 **S**5095 Sisters of Charity of Leavenworth Health Services Corporation	21	10	353	8579	221	137051	941	98144	50081	1093
★ SANTA MONICA HOSPITAL MEDICAL CENTER, 1250 16th Street, Zip 90404-1200; tel. 310/319-4000; William D. Parente, President and Chief Executive Officer **A**1 2 3 5 9 10 **F**4 7 10 12 15 17 18 19 20 21 22 24 28 30 31 32 33 34 35 37 38 40 41 42 43 44 49 60 61 64 65 71 73 **P**3 4 5 7 **S**2315 UniHealth	23	10	178	10500	122	60047	2937	97474	37944	870

SANTA PAULA—Ventura County

☐ SANTA PAULA MEMORIAL HOSPITAL, 825 North Tenth Street, Zip 93060-0270, Mailing Address: P.O. Box 270, Zip 93060; tel. 805/525-7171; Rulon J. Barlow, President and Chief Executive Officer (Nonreporting) **A**1 9 10	23	10	60	—	—	—	—	—	—	—

SANTA ROSA—Sonoma County

☐ COMMUNITY HOSPITAL, 3325 Chanate Road, Zip 95404; tel. 707/576-4000; Jimmy M. Knight, Chief Executive Officer (Nonreporting) **A**1 3 5 9 10	13	10	98	—	—	—	—	—	—	—
★ KAISER FOUNDATION HOSPITAL, 401 Bicentennial Way, Zip 95403; tel. 707/571-4000; Pete Delgado, Vice President and Area Manager **A**1 10 **F**3 4 7 8 10 12 13 19 22 24 25 29 30 31 32 33 34 35 37 39 40 41 42 43 44 46 49 51 53 54 55 56 58 59 60 61 65 67 68 69 71 72 73 **P**6 **S**2105 Kaiser Foundation Hospitals	23	10	110	5958	57	468511	1496	—	—	1360
☐ △ NORTH COAST REHABILITATION CENTER, 151 Sotoyome Street, Zip 95405; tel. 707/542-2771; Pamela J. McFadden, President and Chief Executive Officer **A**1 7 9 10 **F**5 12 15 16 19 21 22 24 25 26 31 32 34 35 39 41 42 48 49 52 57 59 60 65 71 73	33	46	119	1178	50	20650	0	13268	6998	—
★ SANTA ROSA MEMORIAL HOSPITAL, 1165 Montgomery Drive, Zip 95405, Mailing Address: Box 522, Zip 95402; tel. 707/546-3210; James P. Houser, Regional President **A**1 2 9 10 **F**4 7 8 10 11 12 15 16 17 19 20 22 23 25 28 32 34 35 37 38 40 42 43 44 49 63 67 69 71 72 73 **P**5 **S**5425 St. Joseph Health System	23	10	225	11883	163	55193	1352	89201	39723	737
☐ WARRACK MEDICAL CENTER HOSPITAL, 2449 Summerfield Road, Zip 95405; tel. 707/542-9030; Dale E. Iversen, Administrator (Nonreporting) **A**1 9 10	33	10	79	—	—	—	—	—	—	—

SEBASTOPOL—Sonoma County

★ PALM DRIVE HOSPITAL, 501 Petaluma Avenue, Zip 95472; tel. 707/823-8511; Brian E. Dunn, Chief Executive Officer (Nonreporting) **A**1 9 10 **S**0048 Columbia/HCA Healthcare Corporation	33	10	48	—	—	—	—	—	—	—

SELMA—Fresno County

☐ SELMA DISTRICT HOSPITAL, 1141 Rose Avenue, Zip 93662-3293; tel. 209/891-1000; Jerry Sullivan, Chief Executive Officer (Total facility includes 14 beds in nursing home-type unit) **A**1 9 10 **F**7 8 14 16 19 21 22 35 40 44 64 65 71 **P**3	16	10	57	2201	29	43077	718	11948	4653	198

SEPULVEDA—Los Angeles County, See Los Angeles

SHERMAN OAKS—Los Angeles County, See Los Angeles

SIMI VALLEY—Ventura County

☐ SIMI VALLEY HOSPITAL AND HEALTH CARE SERVICES, (Includes Simi Valley Hospital and Health Care Services-South Campus, 1850 Heywood Street, Simi Valley, California, Zip 93065; tel. 805/582-5050) 2975 North Sycamore Drive, Zip 93065-1277; tel. 805/527-2462; Alan J. Rice, President and Chief Executive Officer (Nonreporting) **A**1 9 10 **S**0235 Adventist Health System/West	21	10	209	—	—	—	—	—	—	—

SOLVANG—Santa Barbara County

☐ SANTA YNEZ VALLEY HOSPITAL, 700 Alamo Pintado Road, Zip 93463; tel. 805/688-6431; Harris R. Sherline, Chief Executive Officer **A**1 9 10 **F**8 17 19 22 28 34 41 44 49 64 71 73	23	10	20	436	4	12972	0	5703	2210	65

© 1995 AHA Guide

Hospitals, U.S. / CALIFORNIA

Hospital, Address, Telephone, Administrator, Approval, Facility, and Physician Codes, Health Care System	Classification Codes		Utilization Data					Expense (thousands) of dollars		
★ American Hospital Association (AHA) membership □ Joint Commission on Accreditation of Healthcare Organizations (JCAHO) accreditation + American Osteopathic Hospital Association (AOHA) membership ○ American Osteopathic Association (AOA) accreditation △ Commission on Accreditation of Rehabilitation Facilities (CARF) accreditation Control codes 61, 63, 64, 71, 72 and 73 indicate hospitals listed by AOHA, but not registered by AHA. For definition of numerical codes, see page A6	Control	Service	Beds	Admissions	Census	Outpatient Visits	Births	Total	Payroll	Personnel
SONOMA—Sonoma County										
□ SONOMA VALLEY HOSPITAL, 347 Andrieux Street, Zip 95476–6811, Mailing Address: Box 600, Zip 95476–0600; tel. 707/935–5000; Dennis R. Burns, Administrator and Chief Executive Officer (Nonreporting) **A**1 9 10	16	10	86	—	—	—	—	—	—	—
SONORA—Tuolumne County										
□ SONORA COMMUNITY HOSPITAL, 1 South Forest Road, Zip 95370; tel. 209/532–3161; Lary Davis, President (Total facility includes 62 beds in nursing home–type unit) **A**1 9 10 **F**7 8 11 15 17 19 22 25 26 28 29 30 34 35 37 39 40 41 44 45 46 49 51 64 65 66 67 71 72 73 **S**0235 Adventist Health System/West	21	10	112	3331	88	76532	580	32152	14071	376
□ TUOLUMNE GENERAL HOSPITAL, 101 Hospital Road, Zip 95370; tel. 209/533–7100; Clifton T. White, Interim Administrator (Nonreporting) **A**1 9 10	13	10	77	—	—	—	—	—	—	—
SOUTH EL MONTE—Los Angeles County										
□ GREATER EL MONTE COMMUNITY HOSPITAL, 1701 South Santa Anita Avenue, Zip 91733–9918; tel. 818/579–7777; Sandra M. Chester, Chief Executive Officer **A**1 9 10 **F**4 7 8 10 11 12 13 15 16 17 19 21 22 23 27 28 30 31 32 34 35 37 40 42 44 45 46 49 52 54 55 58 59 60 63 64 65 66 67 68 71 72 73 74 **P**1 5 7 **S**6525 Ornda Healthcorp	33	10	115	4948	47	21938	1932	22427	10272	246
SOUTH LAGUNA—Orange County										
★ SOUTH COAST MEDICAL CENTER, 31872 Coast Highway, Zip 92677; tel. 714/499–1311; T. Michael Murray, President (Total facility includes 29 beds in nursing home–type unit) **A**1 9 10 **F**2 3 7 8 12 17 18 19 21 22 25 26 27 28 29 30 31 34 35 36 37 38 39 40 41 42 44 49 52 56 57 58 59 60 64 65 67 71 73 74 **P**2 4 5 7 8	23	10	210	4521	56	25264	700	37590	16495	480
SOUTH LAKE TAHOE—El Dorado County										
□ BARTON MEMORIAL HOSPITAL, Fourth and South Streets, Zip 96158, Mailing Address: Box 9578, Zip 96158; tel. 916/541–3420; William G. Gordon, Chief Executive Officer (Nonreporting) **A**1 9 10	23	10	81	—	—	—	—	—	—	—
SOUTH SAN FRANCISCO—San Mateo County										
★ KAISER FOUNDATION HOSPITAL, 1200 El Camino Real, Zip 94080–3299; tel. 415/742–2547; Frank D. Alvarez, Administrator **A**1 10 **F**14 15 16 19 22 29 30 32 33 34 35 37 42 44 45 46 51 60 65 67 71 72 73 **P**1 **S**2105 Kaiser Foundation Hospitals	23	10	127	3150	42	47062	2	—	—	276
STANFORD—Santa Clara County										
★ △ STANFORD UNIVERSITY HOSPITAL, 300 Pasteur Drive, Zip 94305–5584; tel. 415/723–4000; Peter Van Etter, President and Chief Executive Officer (Total facility includes 22 beds in nursing home–type unit) **A**1 3 5 7 8 9 10 **F**4 7 8 10 11 12 15 16 17 19 21 22 26 27 28 29 30 31 32 34 35 37 38 40 42 43 44 45 46 47 48 49 52 54 55 56 57 58 59 60 61 63 64 65 66 67 69 70 71 72 73 **P**3 5 6	23	10	469	23232	344	—	4226	403851	162139	4512
STOCKTON—San Joaquin County										
★ DAMERON HOSPITAL, 525 West Acacia Street, Zip 95203; tel. 209/944–5550; Luis Arismendi M.D., Administrator **A**1 9 10 **F**4 7 8 9 10 11 15 19 21 22 23 28 32 34 35 37 38 39 40 41 42 43 44 46 49 63 65 67 69 71 73 **P**5	23	10	211	10297	122	109068	2634	69973	30654	803
□ ST. JOSEPH'S BEHAVIORAL HEALTH CENTER, 2510 North California Street, Zip 95204–5568; tel. 209/948–2100; John Walton, Administrator **A**1 9 10 **F**2 3 15 19 26 29 35 52 54 55 56 57 58 59	23	22	35	934	23	2234	0	4763	2716	—
★ ST. JOSEPH'S MEDICAL CENTER, 1800 North California Street, Zip 95204–6088, Mailing Address: P.O. Box 213008, Zip 95213–9008; tel. 209/943–2000; Edward G. Schroeder, President (Total facility includes 27 beds in nursing home–type unit) **A**1 2 9 10 **F**2 3 4 6 7 8 10 11 12 13 14 15 16 17 18 19 20 21 22 23 24 25 26 27 28 29 30 31 32 33 34 35 37 38 39 40 41 42 43 44 45 46 49 52 54 55 56 57 58 59 60 62 64 65 66 67 71 72 73 74 **P**5 7 **S**1195 Dominican Sisters Congregation of the Most Holy Name	21	10	319	15374	201	275137	2025	128285	60132	1412
SUN CITY—Riverside County										
MENIFEE VALLEY MEDICAL CENTER, 28400 McCall Boulevard, Zip 92585–9537; tel. 909/679–8888; Susan Ballard, Administrator **A**10 **F**3 8 11 12 15 16 19 21 22 26 28 29 34 37 41 44 49 65 73 **P**4 5 **S**0043 Valley Health System	16	10	84	4145	53	33748	0	25422	9124	259
SUN VALLEY—Los Angeles County, See Los Angeles										
SUSANVILLE—Lassen County										
□ LASSEN COMMUNITY HOSPITAL, 560 Hospital Lane, Zip 96130–4809; tel. 916/257–5325; David S. Anderson FACHE, Chief Executive Officer (Total facility includes 31 beds in nursing home–type unit) **A**1 9 10 **F**7 8 15 16 19 22 34 35 40 44 64 65 71 73	21	10	59	1118	29	39708	251	8647	3854	127
SYLMAR—Los Angeles County, See Los Angeles										
TAFT—Kern County										
WEST SIDE DISTRICT HOSPITAL, 110 East North Street, Zip 93268; tel. 805/763–4211; Margo Arnold, Administrator (Nonreporting) **A**9 10	16	10	72	—	—	—	—	—	—	—
TARZANA—Los Angeles County, See Los Angeles										
TEHACHAPI—Kern County										
TEHACHAPI HOSPITAL, 115 West E Street, Zip 93561, Mailing Address: Box 648, Zip 93581; tel. 805/822–3241; David P. Jacobsen, Chief Executive Officer **A**9 10 **F**8 15 16 22 28 34 44 65 71 73	16	10	21	241	13	12123	0	5026	2033	53
TEMPLETON—San Luis Obispo County										
□ TWIN CITIES COMMUNITY HOSPITAL, 1100 Las Tablas Road, Zip 93465; tel. 805/434–3500; Harold E. Chilton, Chief Executive Officer **A**1 9 10 **F**7 10 14 15 19 21 22 28 32 37 40 42 44 65 71 73 **P**5 **S**0063 TENET Healthcare Corporation	33	10	84	4090	50	76204	387	—	—	376

Hospitals, U.S. / CALIFORNIA

Hospital, Address, Telephone, Administrator, Approval, Facility, and Physician Codes, Health Care System	Classification Codes		Utilization Data					Expense (thousands) of dollars		
★ American Hospital Association (AHA) membership ☐ Joint Commission on Accreditation of Healthcare Organizations (JCAHO) accreditation + American Osteopathic Hospital Association (AOHA) membership ○ American Osteopathic Association (AOA) accreditation △ Commission on Accreditation of Rehabilitation Facilities (CARF) accreditation Control codes 61, 63, 64, 71, 72 and 73 indicate hospitals listed by AOHA, but not registered by AHA. For definition of numerical codes, see page A6	Control	Service	Beds	Admissions	Census	Outpatient Visits	Births	Total	Payroll	Personnel
THOUSAND OAKS—Los Angeles County										
★ CHARTER BEHAVIORAL HEALTH SYSTEM OF SOUTHERN CALIFORNIA–THOUSAND OAKS, 150 Via Merida, Zip 91361; tel. 805/495–3292; Michelle Egerer, Chief Executive Officer **A**1 10 **F**1 2 3 12 15 16 17 18 26 34 52 53 54 55 56 57 58 59 65 67 68 **P**5 **S**0695 Charter Medical Corporation	33	22	35	1190	26	6275	0	7190	3652	81
★ LOS ROBLES REGIONAL MEDICAL CENTER, 215 West Janss Road, Zip 91360–1899; tel. 805/497–2727; Ronald C. Phelps, Chief Executive Officer (Nonreporting) **A**1 2 9 10 **S**0048 Columbia/HCA Healthcare Corporation	33	10	187	—	—	—	—	—	—	—
TORRANCE—Los Angeles County										
☐ DEL AMO HOSPITAL, 23700 Camino Del Sol, Zip 90505; tel. 310/530–1151; Michael Hunn, Administrator and Chief Executive Officer (Nonreporting) **A**1 9 10 **S**9555 Universal Health Services, Inc.	33	22	166	—	—	—	—	—	—	—
★ LAC–HARBOR–UNIVERSITY OF CALIFORNIA AT LOS ANGELES MEDICAL CENTER, 1000 West Carson Street, Zip 90509; tel. 310/222–2101; Tecla A. Mickoseff, Administrator **A**1 2 3 5 9 10 **F**4 8 10 11 16 19 21 22 23 29 31 32 34 35 37 38 39 40 41 42 43 44 45 47 52 54 56 58 60 61 63 65 66 69 70 71 72 73 74 **P**6 **S**5755 Los Angeles County–Department of Health Services	13	10	493	24288	380	316561	4062	470667	145910	3455
★ LITTLE COMPANY OF MARY HEALTH SERVICES, 4101 Torrance Boulevard, Zip 90503–4698; tel. 310/540–7676; Mark Costa, President (Nonreporting) **A**1 2 9 10 **S**2295 Little Company of Mary Sisters Healthcare System	23	10	345	—	—	—	—	—	—	—
★ TORRANCE MEMORIAL MEDICAL CENTER, 3330 Lomita Boulevard, Zip 90505–5073; tel. 310/325–9110; George W. Graham, President **A**1 2 9 10 **F**3 4 7 8 9 10 14 15 16 17 19 21 22 23 25 26 27 28 29 30 31 34 35 37 38 40 41 42 43 44 45 46 49 51 52 54 55 56 57 58 59 60 65 71 72 73 74 **P**5	23	10	320	16938	194	82124	4168	112391	47483	1415
TRACY—San Joaquin County										
★ TRACY COMMUNITY MEMORIAL HOSPITAL, 1420 North Tracy Boulevard, Zip 95376–3497; tel. 209/835–1500; Terry G. Mack, Vice President and Administrator (Total facility includes 11 beds in nursing home–type unit) **A**1 9 10 **F**6 7 8 13 14 15 16 17 19 21 22 26 28 30 31 32 33 34 35 37 40 41 42 44 45 49 50 63 64 65 71 72 73 **P**3 **S**8795 Sutter Health	23	10	79	2700	29	67616	491	23511	9697	301
TRAVIS AIR FORCE BASE—Solano County										
★ DAVID GRANT MEDICAL CENTER, 101 Bodin Circle, Zip 94535–1800; tel. 707/423–7300; Colonel P. E. Jacobson Jr. USAF, MSC, Administrator **A**1 2 3 5 **F**2 3 7 8 10 11 12 14 15 16 17 18 19 20 21 22 28 29 30 34 35 37 38 39 40 41 42 44 45 46 49 51 52 53 54 55 56 57 58 59 60 63 65 71 73 **S**9495 Department of the Air Force	41	10	195	11330	146	405372	993	—	—	1825
TRUCKEE—Nevada County										
☐ TAHOE FOREST HOSPITAL DISTRICT, 10121 Pine Avenue, Zip 96161, Mailing Address: Box 759, Zip 96160; tel. 916/582–3481; Lawrence C. Long, Chief Executive Officer (Total facility includes 30 beds in nursing home–type unit) **A**1 10 **F**3 7 8 12 15 16 17 19 22 23 28 29 30 32 33 34 35 36 37 39 40 41 42 44 46 49 64 65 66 67 71 73 **P**5 7 8	16	10	72	1951	47	59631	415	29009	9912	319
TULARE—Tulare County										
★ TULARE DISTRICT HOSPITAL, 869 Cherry Street, Zip 93274–2287; tel. 209/688–0821; Jerry W. Boyter, Administrator **A**1 9 10 **F**7 8 12 19 21 22 23 35 37 40 42 44 46 49 65 71 73 74 **P**5 8	16	10	77	3682	40	47539	923	28233	14488	480
TURLOCK—Stanislaus County										
★ EMANUEL MEDICAL CENTER, 825 Delbon Avenue, Zip 95382, Mailing Address: Box 2120, Zip 95381–2120; tel. 209/667–4200; Robert A. Moen, President and Chief Executive Officer (Total facility includes 145 beds in nursing home–type unit) **A**1 9 10 **F**3 6 7 8 12 15 18 19 22 23 25 27 28 29 30 32 33 34 35 36 37 38 39 40 41 42 44 45 46 49 60 64 65 67 71 72 73 74	21	10	333	8040	263	84094	1711	50206	20587	768
TUSTIN—Orange County										
☐ TUSTIN HOSPITAL, 14662 Newport Avenue, Zip 92680; tel. 714/838–9600; Wayne M. Lingenfelter, Chief Executive Officer (Nonreporting) **A**1 9 10	33	10	117	—	—	—	—	—	—	—
☐ △ TUSTIN REHABILITATION HOSPITAL, 14851 Yorba Street, Zip 92680; tel. 714/832–9200; Patricia Keller, Chief Executive Officer (Nonreporting) **A**1 7 10	33	46	117	—	—	—	—	—	—	—
TWENTYNINE PALMS—San Bernardino County										
★ NAVAL HOSPITAL, Mailing Address: Box 788250, MCAGCC, Zip 92278–8250; tel. 619/830–2188; Captain C. S. Chitwood MSC, USN, Commanding Officer **F**7 8 13 14 15 16 19 22 28 30 34 39 40 41 44 45 46 49 51 53 56 58 65 71 **S**9655 Department of Navy	43	10	29	2633	17	157000	580	—	—	465
UKIAH—Mendocino County										
★ UKIAH VALLEY MEDICAL CENTER, (Includes Ukiah Valley Medical Center–Dora Street, Ukiah, California, Mailing Address: 275 Hospital Drive, Zip 95482; Ukiah Valley Medical Center–Hospital Drive, Ukiah, California) 275 Hospital Drive, Zip 95482; tel. 707/462–3111; ValGene Devitt, President and Chief Executive Officer **A**1 9 10 **F**3 7 8 10 11 12 14 15 16 19 20 21 22 23 28 29 30 31 34 35 36 37 38 39 40 41 42 44 45 46 49 58 60 61 63 64 65 67 71 73 74 **P**1 3 4 5 7 **S**0235 Adventist Health System/West	21	10	116	3956	43	64372	815	32541	13675	435
UPLAND—San Bernardino County										
★ SAN ANTONIO COMMUNITY HOSPITAL, 999 San Bernardino Road, Zip 91786–4920, Mailing Address: Box 5001, Zip 91785–0016; tel. 714/985–2811; George A. Kuykendall, President **A**1 2 9 10 **F**2 3 4 7 8 10 11 12 14 15 19 21 22 25 32 34 35 37 38 40 41 43 44 46 49 52 58 59 60 61 63 65 67 71 72 73 **P**5 7	23	10	190	15683	173	140823	3909	123076	52225	1763

© 1995 AHA Guide

Hospitals, U.S. / CALIFORNIA

Hospital, Address, Telephone, Administrator, Approval, Facility, and Physician Codes, Health Care System	Classification Codes		Utilization Data					Expense (thousands) of dollars		
★ American Hospital Association (AHA) membership ☐ Joint Commission on Accreditation of Healthcare Organizations (JCAHO) accreditation + American Osteopathic Hospital Association (AOHA) membership ○ American Osteopathic Association (AOA) accreditation △ Commission on Accreditation of Rehabilitation Facilities (CARF) accreditation Control codes 61, 63, 64, 71, 72 and 73 indicate hospitals listed by AOHA, but not registered by AHA. For definition of numerical codes, see page A6	Control	Service	Beds	Admissions	Census	Outpatient Visits	Births	Total	Payroll	Personnel
VACAVILLE—Solano County										
CALIFORNIA MEDICAL FACILITY, 1600 California Drive, Zip 95687–2000; tel. 707/448–6841; Velma Alcorn, Administrator **F**1 4 10 11 19 20 21 22 31 33 34 35 41 42 43 44 49 52 54 56 58 60 65 69 70 71	12	11	215	1590	188	430649	0	—	—	446
★ VACAVALLEY HOSPITAL, 1000 Nut Tree Road, Zip 95687; tel. 707/446–5716; Deborah Sugiyama, Administrator **A**9 10 **F**7 8 10 11 12 15 19 21 22 23 28 32 33 35 36 37 39 40 41 42 44 49 60 64 65 66 67 71 72 73 **P**3 5 **S**2075 NorthBay Healthcare System	23	10	35	1681	17	25397	0	22053	7430	115
VALENCIA—Los Angeles County										
★ HENRY MAYO NEWHALL MEMORIAL HOSPITAL, 23845 McBean Parkway, Zip 91355; tel. 805/253–8000; Duffy Watson, President and Chief Executive Officer (Total facility includes 62 beds in nursing home–type unit) **A**1 2 9 10 **F**1 7 8 11 12 14 15 16 17 18 19 20 21 22 25 26 27 28 29 30 31 32 33 34 35 37 39 40 41 42 44 45 46 48 49 52 56 57 58 59 60 63 64 65 67 70 71 73 74	23	10	227	8119	140	53509	1503	65320	21786	506
VALLEJO—Solano County										
☐ FIRST HOSPITAL VALLEJO, 525 Oregon Street, Zip 94590; tel. 707/648–2200; Bill F. Dye, Chief Executive Officer and Administrator **A**1 10 **F**3 15 18 19 21 22 35 52 53 54 55 56 57 59 65 67 71 **P**7 **S**2635 First Hospital Corporation	33	22	61	1382	37	1985	0	6959	4028	89
★ KAISER FOUNDATION HOSPITAL AND REHABILITATION CENTER, 975 Sereno Drive, Zip 94589; tel. 707/648–6230; Joyce M. Berger, Area Manager (Nonreporting) **A**1 10 **S**2105 Kaiser Foundation Hospitals	23	10	231	—						
★ SUTTER SOLANO MEDICAL CENTER, 300 Hospital Drive, Zip 94589–2517, Mailing Address: P.O. Box 3189, Zip 94589; tel. 707/554–4444; Patrick R. Brady, Administrator **A**1 9 10 **F**7 8 10 12 14 15 16 19 21 22 30 32 34 35 36 37 40 41 42 44 49 63 65 71 73 74 **P**3 **S**8795 Sutter Health	23	10	108	3962	40	68426	843	37586	15933	331
VAN NUYS–Los Angeles County, See Los Angeles										
VANDENBERG AIR FORCE BASE—Hillsborough County										
★ U.S. AIR FORCE HOSPITAL, 338 South Dakota, Zip 93437–6307; tel. 805/734–8232; Colonel Claude H. Chan MSC, Commander **A**1 **F**3 7 8 15 20 21 22 27 34 39 40 44 49 51 53 56 57 58 61 65 71 73 **P**6 **S**9495 Department of the Air Force	41	10	32	1860	14	159403	231	—	—	331
VENTURA—Ventura County										
★ COMMUNITY MEMORIAL HOSPITAL OF SAN BUENAVENTURA, Loma Vista Road at Brent, Zip 93003–2854; tel. 805/652–5011; Michael D. Bakst Ph.D., Executive Director **A**1 9 10 **F**4 7 8 10 11 14 15 16 17 19 21 22 24 25 29 30 34 35 37 40 43 44 63 64 65 67 71 **P**5 7	23	10	230	9646	127	66358	2032	63493	28352	860
☐ CPC VISTA DEL MAR HOSPITAL, 801 Seneca Street, Zip 93001; tel. 805/653–6434; Jerry Conway, Chief Executive Officer (Nonreporting) **A**1 9 10 **S**0785 Community Psychiatric Centers	33	22	87	—	—	—	—	—	—	—
☐ VENTURA COUNTY MEDICAL CENTER, 3291 Loma Vista Road, Zip 93003; tel. 805/652–6058; Pierre Durand, Administrator (Nonreporting) **A**1 3 9 10	13	10	110							
VICTORVILLE—San Bernardino County										
☐ VICTOR VALLEY COMMUNITY HOSPITAL, 15248 11th Street, Zip 92392; tel. 619/245–8691; Ralph L. Parks, Administrator and Chief Executive Officer (Nonreporting) **A**1 2 9 10	23	10	119							
VISALIA—Tulare County										
★ KAWEAH DELTA HEALTHCARE DISTRICT, 400 West Mineral King Avenue, Zip 93291; tel. 209/625–2211; Thomas M. Johnson, Chief Executive Officer (Total facility includes 12 beds in nursing home–type unit) **A**1 2 9 10 **F**7 8 10 15 16 17 18 19 21 22 23 24 28 29 30 32 33 34 35 37 38 40 41 42 44 45 48 49 60 64 65 67 71 73 **P**5 7	16	10	212	12319	175	233083	3180	96490	44815	1486
★ VISALIA COMMUNITY HOSPITAL, 1633 South Court Street, Zip 93277, Mailing Address: Box 911, Zip 93277; tel. 209/733–1333; Lindsay K. Mann, Administrator **A**1 9 10 **F**7 12 14 15 16 19 22 32 34 35 37 40 41 44 65 71 73 **P**1	16	10	52	2230	21	25119	573	15499	7020	191
WALNUT CREEK—Contra Costa County										
☐ CPC WALNUT CREEK HOSPITAL, 175 La Casa Via, Zip 94598; tel. 510/933–7990; Lee L. Haber, Chief Executive Officer (Nonreporting) **A**1 9 10 **S**0785 Community Psychiatric Centers	33	22	108	—	—	—	—	—	—	—
☐ △ JOHN MUIR MEDICAL CENTER, 1601 Ygnacio Valley Road, Zip 94598–3194; tel. 510/939–3000; J. Kendall Anderson, President and Chief Executive Officer (Total facility includes 29 beds in nursing home–type unit) **A**1 2 7 9 10 **F**4 7 8 10 11 12 15 17 19 21 22 23 26 28 29 32 33 34 35 37 38 40 42 43 44 48 49 60 64 65 67 69 70 71 73 74 **P**5 7	23	10	256	12881	176	68748	1999	147840	63586	1331
★ KAISER FOUNDATION HOSPITAL, 1425 South Main Street, Zip 94596; tel. 510/295–4000 **A**1 5 10 **F**3 4 7 11 14 15 16 19 21 22 23 31 32 33 34 35 37 38 40 41 42 43 44 45 46 49 53 54 57 58 59 60 63 64 65 69 71 73 **S**2105 Kaiser Foundation Hospitals	23	10	134	11851	121	58915	3518	—	—	1327
WATSONVILLE—Santa Cruz County										
☐ WATSONVILLE COMMUNITY HOSPITAL, 298 Green Valley Road, Zip 95076; tel. 408/724–4741; John P. Friel, President and Chief Executive Officer (Total facility includes 13 beds in nursing home–type unit) **A**1 9 10 **F**2 3 7 8 10 11 15 16 17 19 21 22 23 25 26 28 30 31 32 34 35 37 39 40 41 42 44 46 64 65 66 67 68 71 72 73 **P**5	23	10	125	5547	72	58242	1840	47670	24026	600

Hospitals, U.S. / CALIFORNIA

Hospital, Address, Telephone, Administrator, Approval, Facility, and Physician Codes, Health Care System	Classification Codes		Utilization Data					Expense (thousands) of dollars		
	Control	Service	Beds	Admissions	Census	Outpatient Visits	Births	Total	Payroll	Personnel

★ American Hospital Association (AHA) membership
☐ Joint Commission on Accreditation of Healthcare Organizations (JCAHO) accreditation
+ American Osteopathic Hospital Association (AOHA) membership
○ American Osteopathic Association (AOA) accreditation
△ Commission on Accreditation of Rehabilitation Facilities (CARF) accreditation
Control codes 61, 63, 64, 71, 72 and 73 indicate hospitals listed by AOHA, but not registered by AHA. For definition of numerical codes, see page A6

WEAVERVILLE—Trinity County

Hospital	Control	Service	Beds	Admissions	Census	Outpatient Visits	Births	Total	Payroll	Personnel
TRINITY HOSPITAL, 410 North Taylor Street, Zip 96093, Mailing Address: P.O. Box 1229, Zip 96093–1229; tel. 916/623–5541; Patricia Menning, Administrator (Nonreporting) **A**9 10	13	10	65	—	—	—	—	—	—	—

WEST COVINA—Los Angeles County

Hospital	Control	Service	Beds	Admissions	Census	Outpatient Visits	Births	Total	Payroll	Personnel
☐ COVINA VALLEY COMMUNITY HOSPITAL, 845 North Lark Ellen Avenue, Zip 91791; tel. 818/339–5451; John Hogue, Administrator **A**1 9 10 **F**1 15 16 19 22 34 35 37 41 44 46 49 59 65 71 **P**5	32	10	76	1249	13	5578	0	6784	2636	96
☐ DOCTORS HOSPITAL OF WEST COVINA, 725 South Orange Avenue, Zip 91790–2614; tel. 818/338–8481; Gerald H. Wallman, Administrator (Nonreporting) **A**1 9 10	33	10	47	—	—	—	—	—	—	—
☐ QUEEN OF THE VALLEY HOSPITAL, 1115 South Sunset Avenue, Zip 91790, Mailing Address: Box 1980, Zip 91793; tel. 818/962–4011; Peter E. Makowski, President and Chief Executive Officer (Total facility includes 23 beds in nursing home–type unit) **A**1 2 9 10 **F**4 8 10 11 12 13 15 16 17 19 21 22 23 28 29 30 31 32 33 34 35 36 37 38 39 40 41 42 43 44 46 48 49 64 65 67 68 71 72 73 74	23	10	263	17271	210	—	5195	90491	42926	1106

WEST HILLS–Los Angeles County, See Los Angeles

WEST LOS ANGELES–Los Angeles County, See Los Angeles

WESTLAKE VILLAGE—Los Angeles County

Hospital	Control	Service	Beds	Admissions	Census	Outpatient Visits	Births	Total	Payroll	Personnel
☐ WESTLAKE MEDICAL CENTER, 4415 South Lakeview Canyon Road, Zip 91361; tel. 818/706–8000; K. D. Justyn, Managing Director **A**1 9 10 **F**7 8 11 12 19 21 22 28 29 30 34 35 36 37 39 40 41 42 44 45 46 49 50 60 63 65 67 69 70 71 73 74 **S**9555 Universal Health Services, Inc.	33	10	60	2807	29	24443	793	30026	14138	276

WHITTIER—Los Angeles County

Hospital	Control	Service	Beds	Admissions	Census	Outpatient Visits	Births	Total	Payroll	Personnel
★ PRESBYTERIAN INTERCOMMUNITY HOSPITAL, 12401 Washington Boulevard, Zip 90602–1099; tel. 310/698–0811; Daniel F. Adams, President and Chief Executive Officer **A**1 2 3 5 9 10 **F**2 3 4 8 10 11 12 15 17 19 20 21 22 25 27 28 30 31 32 33 34 36 37 38 39 40 41 42 43 44 45 46 48 49 51 52 56 59 60 63 65 67 71 73 74 **P**3 5	23	10	302	10583	139	163433	3331	97490	41672	1013
☐ WHITTIER HOSPITAL MEDICAL CENTER, 15151 Janine Drive, Zip 90605; tel. 310/945–3561; Michael H. Sussman, Chief Executive Officer (Total facility includes 39 beds in nursing home–type unit) **A**1 9 10 **F**7 8 11 14 16 17 19 21 22 26 27 28 30 32 34 35 37 39 40 41 44 46 49 61 64 65 71 73 74 **P**5 **S**6525 Ornda Healthcorp	33	10	159	5523	55	32794	1987	36504	12885	437

WILDOMAR—Riverside County

Hospital	Control	Service	Beds	Admissions	Census	Outpatient Visits	Births	Total	Payroll	Personnel
★ INLAND VALLEY REGIONAL MEDICAL CENTER, 36485 Inland Valley Drive, Zip 92595; tel. 909/677–1111; B. Ann Kuss, Chief Executive Officer and Managing Director (Nonreporting) **A**1 10 **S**9555 Universal Health Services, Inc.	33	10	80	—	—	—	—	—	—	—

WILLITS—Mendocino County

Hospital	Control	Service	Beds	Admissions	Census	Outpatient Visits	Births	Total	Payroll	Personnel
☐ FRANK R. HOWARD MEMORIAL HOSPITAL, Madrone and Manzanita Streets, Zip 95490, Mailing Address: Box 1430, Zip 95490; tel. 707/459–6801; Robert J. Walker, President (Nonreporting) **A**1 9 10 **S**0235 Adventist Health System/West	21	10	28	—	—	—	—	—	—	—

WILLOWS—Glenn County

Hospital	Control	Service	Beds	Admissions	Census	Outpatient Visits	Births	Total	Payroll	Personnel
GLENN GENERAL HOSPITAL, 1133 West Sycamore Street, Zip 95988; tel. 916/934–6461; Chase W. Mearian, Administrator **A**9 10 **F**8 17 22 34 44 49 65 71 **P**6	13	10	27	281	2	38194	0	5517	2049	87

WINTERHAVEN—Imperial County

Hospital	Control	Service	Beds	Admissions	Census	Outpatient Visits	Births	Total	Payroll	Personnel
★ U.S. PUBLIC HEALTH SERVICE INDIAN HOSPITAL, Mailing Address: P.O. Box 1368, Yuma, AZ Zip 85366–8368; tel. 619/572–0217; Kenneth W. Hernasy M.P.H., Service Unit Director (Nonreporting) **A**1 9 10 **S**9195 U.S. Public Health Service Indian Health Service	47	10	17	—	—	—	—	—	—	—

WOODLAND—Yolo County

Hospital	Control	Service	Beds	Admissions	Census	Outpatient Visits	Births	Total	Payroll	Personnel
★ WOODLAND MEMORIAL HOSPITAL, 1325 Cottonwood Street, Zip 95695–5199; tel. 916/662–3961; Jack Hudock, Administrator **A**1 9 10 **F**5 7 8 10 13 14 16 19 20 21 22 23 25 28 30 31 32 34 35 37 40 41 42 44 45 46 49 52 53 54 56 57 58 65 66 67 71 72 73 74 **P**7 8	23	10	103	5857	52	365289	1677	73309	—	665

WOODLAND HILLS–Los Angeles County, See Los Angeles

YOUNTVILLE—Napa County

Hospital	Control	Service	Beds	Admissions	Census	Outpatient Visits	Births	Total	Payroll	Personnel
★ VETERANS HOME OF CALIFORNIA, Mailing Address: P.O. Box 1200, Zip 94599–1297; tel. 707/944–4600; James D. Helzer, Administrator (Nonreporting)	12	10	540	—	—	—	—	—	—	—

YREKA—Siskiyou County

Hospital	Control	Service	Beds	Admissions	Census	Outpatient Visits	Births	Total	Payroll	Personnel
☐ SISKIYOU GENERAL HOSPITAL, 818 South Main Street, Zip 96097; tel. 916/842–4121; Kenneth E. Monfore Jr., Administrator (Nonreporting) **A**1 10	23	10	48	—	—	—	—	—	—	—

YUBA CITY—Sutter County

Hospital	Control	Service	Beds	Admissions	Census	Outpatient Visits	Births	Total	Payroll	Personnel
☐ FREMONT MEDICAL CENTER, 970 Plumas Street, Zip 95991; tel. 916/751–4000; Thomas P. Hayes, Chief Executive Officer **A**1 10 **F**7 10 15 16 19 22 34 35 37 40 41 44 45 49 65 71 73 **P**5 **S**2115 Fremont–Rideout Health Group	23	10	132	6963	71	46880	2125	36377	14573	388

© 1995 AHA Guide

Hospitals, U.S. / COLORADO

COLORADO

Resident population 3,566 (in thousands)
Resident population in metro areas 81.8%
Birth rate per 1,000 population 15.9
65 years and over 10.0%
Percent of persons without health insurance 12.4%

Hospital, Address, Telephone, Administrator, Approval, Facility, and Physician Codes, Health Care System

★ American Hospital Association (AHA) membership
□ Joint Commission on Accreditation of Healthcare Organizations (JCAHO) accreditation
+ American Osteopathic Hospital Association (AOHA) membership
○ American Osteopathic Association (AOA) accreditation
△ Commission on Accreditation of Rehabilitation Facilities (CARF) accreditation
Control codes 61, 63, 64, 71, 72 and 73 indicate hospitals listed by AOHA, but not registered by AHA. For definition of numerical codes, see page A6

Hospital	Control	Service	Beds	Admissions	Census	Outpatient Visits	Births	Total	Payroll	Personnel
ALAMOSA—Alamosa County										
★ SAN LUIS VALLEY REGIONAL MEDICAL CENTER, 106 Blanca Avenue, Zip 81101–2393; tel. 719/589–2511; Paul Herman, Administrator **A**1 9 10 **F**6 7 8 12 14 15 16 19 20 21 22 23 27 31 33 34 35 37 40 42 44 46 49 65 67 68 69 71 72 73 **P**3	21	10	85	3256	27	27187	569	12198	5397	231
ASPEN—Pitkin County										
★ ASPEN VALLEY HOSPITAL DISTRICT, 0401 Castle Creek Road, Zip 81611; tel. 303/925–1120; Michael Kerr, Administrator **A**1 9 10 **F**6 7 8 12 13 14 17 19 20 21 22 28 32 33 34 35 36 37 39 40 41 42 44 45 46 49 51 56 66 71 73 **P**3 8	16	10	27	1392	11	28382	224	15298	6320	212
AURORA—Adams County										
★ AURORA PRESBYTERIAN HOSPITAL, 700 Potomac Street, Zip 80011–6792; tel. 303/363–7200; H. Phil Herre, Administrator (Nonreporting) **A**2 9 10 **S**0935 HealthONE Healthcare System	23	10	138	—	—	—	—	—	—	—
★ AURORA REGIONAL MEDICAL CENTER, 1501 South Potomac, Zip 80012; tel. 303/695–2600; William K. Atkinson, Chief Executive Officer (Nonreporting) **A**1 9 10 **S**0048 Columbia/HCA Healthcare Corporation	33	10	180	—	—	—	—	—	—	—
★ FITZSIMONS ARMY MEDICAL CENTER, Zip 80045–5000; tel. 303/361–8313; Colonel Van R. Booth, Chief of Staff **A**1 2 3 5 **F**3 4 5 7 8 9 10 11 12 13 16 19 20 21 22 25 29 30 31 32 34 35 37 38 39 40 41 42 43 44 45 46 48 49 51 52 53 54 56 58 60 63 65 66 67 71 73 **S**9395 Department of the Army	42	10	237	9428	143	531594	542	—	—	2600
□ △ ROCKY MOUNTAIN REHABILITATION INSTITUTE, 900 Potomac Street, Zip 80011–6716; tel. 303/367–1166; Russell W. York, President and Chief Executive Officer (Nonreporting) **A**1 7 10 **S**0935 HealthONE Healthcare System	33	46	76	—	—	—	—	—	—	—
BOULDER—Boulder County										
★ △ BOULDER COMMUNITY HOSPITAL, 1100 Balsam, Zip 80304–3496, Mailing Address: P.O. Box 9019, Zip 80301–9019; tel. 303/440–2273; David P. Gehant, President **A**1 2 7 9 10 **F**2 3 4 5 7 8 10 11 12 13 14 15 19 21 22 24 25 26 29 30 31 32 33 34 35 37 40 41 42 43 44 45 46 48 49 52 53 54 55 56 57 58 59 60 63 65 66 67 68 70 71 72 73 74 **P**4 7 8	23	10	206	8679	107	125954	1676	82432	37062	1203
BRIGHTON—Adams County										
★ PLATTE VALLEY MEDICAL CENTER, 1850 Egbert Street, Zip 80601, Mailing Address: P.O. Box 98, Zip 80601; tel. 303/659–1531; John Sackett, President **A**1 9 10 **F**7 8 11 13 15 16 17 19 21 22 24 27 28 30 32 33 34 35 36 37 39 40 41 42 44 49 51 65 66 67 71 73 **P**3 4 5	21	10	49	1595	11	21657	661	14138	6484	202
BRUSH—Morgan County										
★ EAST MORGAN COUNTY HOSPITAL, 2400 West Edison, Zip 80723; tel. 303/842–5151; Anne Platt, Administrator (Nonreporting) **A**1 9 10 **S**2235 Lutheran Health Systems	23	10	29	—	—	—	—	—	—	—
BURLINGTON—Kit Carson County										
★ KIT CARSON COUNTY MEMORIAL HOSPITAL, 286 16th Street, Zip 80807–1697; tel. 719/346–5311; DeAnn K. Cure, Chief Executive Officer **A**9 10 **F**7 8 10 14 15 16 19 21 22 32 34 35 39 40 44 49 67 71	13	10	24	474	4	9528	84	3200	1553	85
CANON CITY—Fremont County										
★ ST. THOMAS MORE HOSPITAL AND PROGRESSIVE CARE CENTER, 1338 Phay Avenue, Zip 81212–2221; tel. 719/269–2021; William A. Burns, Chief Executive Officer (Total facility includes 163 beds in nursing home–type unit) **A**1 9 10 **F**2 7 14 15 16 19 21 22 24 32 37 40 44 46 49 64 65 71 73 **S**5115 Sisters of Charity Health Care Systems, Inc.	21	10	218	3040	186	73699	330	21523	10570	355
CHEYENNE WELLS—Cheyenne County										
★ KEEFE MEMORIAL HOSPITAL, 602 North Sixth Street West, Zip 80810, Mailing Address: P.O. Box 578, Zip 80810; tel. 719/767–5661; Linda Roth, Administrator **A**1 9 10 **F**8 13 16 19 22 26 28 29 30 32 35 39 42 44 45 46 49 51 65 66 67 71 73 74	13	10	16	226	3	9207	0	2422	978	60
COLORADO SPRINGS—El Paso County										
□ CEDAR SPRINGS PSYCHIATRIC HOSPITAL, 2135 Southgate Road, Zip 80906, Mailing Address: Box 640, Zip 80901; tel. 719/633–4114; (Nonreporting) **A**1 10 **S**0395 Healthcare International, Inc.	33	22	100	—	—	—	—	—	—	—
★ MEMORIAL HOSPITAL, 1400 East Boulder Street, Zip 80909–5599, Mailing Address: Box 1326, Zip 80901; tel. 719/475–5000; J. Robert Peters, Executive Director **A**1 2 9 10 **F**4 7 8 10 11 14 15 16 17 19 21 22 25 26 28 29 30 31 32 34 35 37 38 39 40 41 42 43 44 45 46 47 49 51 54 60 63 65 67 70 71 72 73 74 **P**5 7	14	10	340	15000	186	167316	2641	150778	69148	2337
PENROSE HOSPITALS See Penrose–St. Francis Healthcare System										
★ PENROSE–ST. FRANCIS HEALTHCARE SYSTEM, (Includes Penrose Hospital, 2215 North Cascade Avenue, Colorado Springs, Colorado, Zip 80907, Mailing Address: P.O. Box 7021, Zip 80933–7021; tel. 719/776–5000; Penrose Community Hospital, 3205 North Academy, Colorado Springs, Colorado, Zip 80907, Mailing Address: P.O. Box 7021, Zip 80933–7021; tel. 719/776–3000; St. Francis Health Center, 825 East Pikes Peak Avenue, Colorado Springs, Colorado, Zip 80903, Mailing Address: P.O. Box 7021, Zip 80933–7021; tel. 719/776–8800) Leonard A. Farr, President and Chief Executive Officer (Total facility includes 64 beds in nursing home–type unit) **A**1 2 3 5 9 10 **F**1 2 3 4 7 8 9 10 11 12 13 14 15 16 17 18 19 20 21 22 23 24 25 26 27 28 29 30 31 32 34 35 36 37 38 39 40 41 42 43 46 47 48 49 51 52 53 54 55 56 57 58 59 60 61 63 64 65 66 69 70 71 72 73 74 **P**1 3 7 **S**5115 Sisters of Charity Health Care Systems, Inc.	21	10	522	19743	352	175671	2816	169535	73252	2534

Hospitals, U.S. / COLORADO

Hospital, Address, Telephone, Administrator, Approval, Facility, and Physician Codes, Health Care System	Classification Codes		Utilization Data					Expense (thousands) of dollars		
	Control	Service	Beds	Admissions	Census	Outpatient Visits	Births	Total	Payroll	Personnel

★ American Hospital Association (AHA) membership
☐ Joint Commission on Accreditation of Healthcare Organizations (JCAHO) accreditation
+ American Osteopathic Hospital Association (AOHA) membership
○ American Osteopathic Association (AOA) accreditation
△ Commission on Accreditation of Rehabilitation Facilities (CARF) accreditation
Control codes 61, 63, 64, 71, 72 and 73 indicate hospitals listed by AOHA, but not registered by AHA. For definition of numerical codes, see page A6

CORTEZ—Montezuma County

★ MONTEZUMA COUNTY HOSPITAL DISTRICT, 1311 North Mildred Road, Zip 81321; tel. 303/565–6666; Stephen R. Selzer, Administrator (Total facility includes 76 beds in nursing home–type unit) **A**1 9 10 **F**7 8 12 14 15 16 17 19 20 22 30 31 33 35 36 37 39 40 41 44 45 46 49 60 64 65 67 71 73 **P**3 8 **S**0002 Quorum Health Group/Quorum Health Resources — 16 10 123 2685 169 20318 250 17058 7265 223

CRAIG—Moffat County

★ MEMORIAL HOSPITAL, 785 Russell Street, Zip 81625–9906; tel. 303/824–9411; M. Randell Phelps, Administrator (Nonreporting) **A**1 9 10 **S**0002 Quorum Health Group/Quorum Health Resources — 13 10 27 — — — — — — —

DELTA—Delta County

★ DELTA COUNTY MEMORIAL HOSPITAL, 100 Stafford Lane, Zip 81416–5003, Mailing Address: P.O. Box 10100, Zip 81416–5003; tel. 303/874–7681; Kevin McMullan, Administrator **A**1 9 10 **F**8 14 19 21 22 28 32 37 40 41 42 44 49 65 71 73 **P**5 **S**3505 Presbyterian Healthcare Services — 16 10 44 2127 23 26686 281 12952 6102 269

DENVER—Denver and Adams County

BEHAVIORAL HEALTH SERVICES See HealthONE–Behavioral Health Services, Bethesda Campus

★ CHILDREN'S HOSPITAL, 1056 East 19th Avenue, Zip 80218–1088; tel. 303/861–8888; Lua R. Blankenship Jr., President and Chief Executive Officer **A**1 3 5 9 10 **F**4 5 9 10 12 13 14 15 16 17 18 19 20 21 25 29 31 32 34 35 38 39 41 42 43 44 46 47 48 49 51 52 53 54 55 56 58 59 60 65 67 68 69 71 72 73 **P**4 — 23 50 209 7706 147 267158 1385 140148 67621 1800

☐ COLORADO MENTAL HEALTH INSTITUTE AT FORT LOGAN, 3520 West Oxford Avenue, Zip 80236; tel. 303/761–0220; Allan Brock Willett M.D., Director **A**1 9 10 **F**1 2 3 4 5 6 7 8 9 10 11 12 13 14 15 16 17 18 19 20 21 22 23 24 25 26 27 28 29 30 31 32 33 34 35 36 37 38 39 40 41 42 43 44 45 46 47 48 49 50 51 52 53 54 55 56 57 58 59 60 61 62 63 64 65 66 67 68 69 70 71 72 73 74 **P**4 6 — 12 22 347 589 309 2250 0 25753 18392 504

☐ DENVER HEALTH AND HOSPITALS, 777 Bannock Street, Zip 80204–4507; tel. 303/893–6000; Tom Moe, Manager **A**1 3 5 9 10 **F**2 3 4 7 8 10 11 14 15 16 17 19 20 21 22 25 26 27 31 32 34 35 37 38 39 40 41 42 43 44 45 46 47 48 49 51 52 53 54 55 56 57 58 59 60 61 63 65 69 70 71 72 73 74 — 15 10 313 15596 215 394422 2617 — — 2476

★ HEALTHONE–BEHAVIORAL HEALTH SERVICES, BETHESDA CAMPUS, (Formerly Behavioral Health Services) 4400 East Iliff Avenue, Zip 80222; tel. 303/758–1514; William Kent Ph.D., Vice President Behavioral Health (Nonreporting) **A**1 9 **S**0935 HealthONE Healthcare System — 23 22 82 — — — — — — —

★ NATIONAL JEWISH CENTER FOR IMMUNOLOGY AND RESPIRATORY MEDICINE, 1400 Jackson Street, Zip 80206–2762; tel. 303/398–1031; Lynn M. Taussig, President **A**1 3 5 9 10 **F**12 14 16 17 19 21 22 27 34 39 41 44 46 49 53 54 55 58 63 65 72 73 **P**6 — 23 49 98 1049 37 23024 0 78155 49788 1083

★ PORTER CARE HOSPITAL, (Formerly Porter Memorial Hospital) 2525 South Downing Street, Zip 80210–5876; tel. 303/778–1955; Richard C. Hale, Administrator (Total facility includes 30 beds in nursing home–type unit) **A**1 2 3 5 9 10 **F**3 4 7 8 10 11 12 15 16 17 19 21 22 24 29 30 31 32 33 34 35 37 39 40 41 42 43 44 45 46 47 48 49 52 54 55 56 57 58 59 60 61 63 64 65 66 67 69 71 73 74 **P**1 3 5 7 — 21 10 339 11540 183 93176 1012 120823 43315 1599

★ PRESBYTERIAN–ST. LUKE'S MEDICAL CENTER, (Includes Presbyterian–Denver Hospital, 1719 East 19th Avenue, Denver, Colorado, Zip 80218–1124; tel. 303/839–6100) 1719 East 19th Avenue, Zip 80218; tel. 303/839–6000; H. Phil Herre, Chief Operating Officer (Nonreporting) **A**1 2 3 5 9 10 12 13 **S**0935 HealthONE Healthcare System — 23 10 558 — — — — — — —

★ PROVENANT ST. ANTHONY HOSPITAL CENTRAL, 4231 West 16th Avenue, Zip 80204–4098; tel. 303/629–3511; Michael H. Erne, Chief Executive Officer and Executive Vice President (Nonreporting) **A**2 3 5 10 **S**5115 Sisters of Charity Health Care Systems, Inc. — 21 10 364 — — — — — — —

★ ROSE MEDICAL CENTER, 4567 East Ninth Avenue, Zip 80220; tel. 303/320–2121; Philip A. Kalin, Executive Vice President **A**1 2 3 5 9 10 **F**4 5 7 8 10 12 13 14 15 16 17 19 21 22 25 26 29 30 31 32 34 35 37 40 41 42 43 44 45 46 48 49 51 53 54 55 56 57 58 59 60 61 64 65 66 67 68 71 72 73 74 **P**4 7 **S**0048 Columbia/HCA Healthcare Corporation — 23 10 285 8799 124 107076 3367 111794 45286 1609

★ SAINT JOSEPH HOSPITAL, 1835 Franklin Street, Zip 80218; tel. 303/837–7111; Sister Marianna Bauder, President and Chief Executive Officer **A**1 2 3 9 10 **F**3 4 7 8 10 11 14 15 16 17 19 20 21 22 23 26 29 30 31 34 35 37 38 39 40 41 42 43 44 45 46 49 51 52 54 55 56 57 58 59 60 63 64 65 66 67 68 71 72 73 74 **P**1 6 **S**5095 Sisters of Charity of Leavenworth Health Services Corporation — 21 10 437 25234 321 226294 5016 161101 80719 1891

★ △ SPALDING REHABILITATION HOSPITAL, 4500 East Iliff Avenue, Zip 80222–6021, Mailing Address: 900 Potomac Street, Aurora Zip 80011; tel. 303/363–5189; Russell W. York, President and Chief Executive Officer (Total facility includes 32 beds in nursing home–type unit) **A**1 7 9 10 **F**1 2 3 4 5 7 8 10 11 12 14 16 17 18 19 21 22 24 25 26 27 28 29 30 31 32 33 34 35 37 38 39 40 41 42 43 44 45 46 47 48 49 50 51 52 53 54 55 56 57 58 59 60 61 62 64 65 66 67 68 69 70 71 72 73 74 **P**1 2 4 5 6 7 8 — 23 46 146 2849 82 — 0 25336 9748 202

★ UNIVERSITY HOSPITAL, 4200 East Ninth Avenue, Zip 80262; tel. 303/399–1211; Dennis C. Brimhall, President **A**1 2 5 8 9 10 **F**3 4 5 7 8 9 10 12 14 15 16 17 18 19 20 21 22 24 25 28 29 31 35 38 39 40 41 42 43 44 45 46 48 49 51 53 54 55 56 57 58 59 60 61 63 65 66 67 69 70 71 73 74 **P**4 — 16 10 316 14166 214 244985 1920 186077 66957 1981

© 1995 AHA Guide

Hospitals, U.S. / COLORADO

Hospital, Address, Telephone, Administrator, Approval, Facility, and Physician Codes, Health Care System

- ★ American Hospital Association (AHA) membership
- □ Joint Commission on Accreditation of Healthcare Organizations (JCAHO) accreditation
- + American Osteopathic Hospital Association (AOHA) membership
- ○ American Osteopathic Association (AOA) accreditation
- △ Commission on Accreditation of Rehabilitation Facilities (CARF) accreditation

Control codes 61, 63, 64, 71, 72 and 73 indicate hospitals listed by AOHA, but not registered by AHA. For definition of numerical codes, see page A6.

Hospital	Classification Codes		Utilization Data					Expense (thousands) of dollars		Personnel
	Control	Service	Beds	Admissions	Census	Outpatient Visits	Births	Total	Payroll	
★ VETERANS AFFAIRS MEDICAL CENTER, 1055 Clermont Street, Zip 80220-3877; tel. 303/393-2800; Thomas A. Trujillo, Director (Total facility includes 60 beds in nursing home-type unit) **A**1 2 3 5 **F**2 3 4 8 10 11 14 15 16 19 20 23 26 31 32 33 34 35 37 41 42 43 44 45 46 48 49 50 52 56 58 60 64 65 69 71 73 **P**6 **S**9295 Department of Veterans Affairs	45	10	336	7675	199	186429	0	114249	58019	1806
DURANGO—La Plata County										
DURANGO CENTER FOR BEHAVIORAL HEALTH See Mercy Behavioral Health										
MERCY BEHAVIORAL HEALTH, (Formerly Durango Center for Behavioral Health) 3801 North Main Avenue, Zip 81301; tel. 970/382-2440; Jerry Brown, Manager (Nonreporting) **A**9	16	22	20	—	—	—	—	—	—	—
★ MERCY MEDICAL CENTER, 375 East Park Avenue, Zip 81301; tel. 303/247-4311; G. Dale Jessup, President and Chief Executive Officer (Total facility includes 11 beds in nursing home-type unit) **A**1 9 10 **F**3 4 7 8 10 12 14 19 21 22 23 28 30 31 32 33 34 35 36 37 38 39 40 41 42 44 46 49 51 52 53 56 58 64 66 67 70 71 73 74 **P**8 **S**5175 Catholic Health Corporation	21	10	105	4901	67	107790	669	35570	17431	543
EADS—Kiowa County										
★ WEISBROD MEMORIAL HOSPITAL, 1208 Luther Street, Zip 81036, Mailing Address: P.O. Box 817, Zip 81036-0817; tel. 719/438-5401; Gerald L. Tipsword, Administrator (Total facility includes 34 beds in nursing home-type unit) **A**9 10 **F**1 14 15 22 27 28 30 32 34 36 44 46 54 65 73 **P**2	16	10	42	92	25	3702	0	—	—	48
ENGLEWOOD—Arapahoe County										
★ △ CRAIG HOSPITAL, 3425 South Clarkson, Zip 80110; tel. 303/789-8000; Dennis O'Malley, President **A**1 7 9 10 **F**12 14 16 17 19 20 21 22 23 24 34 39 41 44 45 46 48 49 50 60 63 65 67 70 71 73	23	46	70	482	62	5622	0	27673	12261	383
★ SWEDISH MEDICAL CENTER, 501 East Hampden Avenue, Zip 80110-0101, Mailing Address: P.O. Box 2901, Zip 80150-0101; tel. 303/788-5000; Margaret D. Sabin, Vice President and Administrator (Nonreporting) **A**1 2 3 5 9 10 **S**0935 HealthONE Healthcare System	23	10	310	—	—	—	—	—	—	—
ESTES PARK—Larimer County										
★ ESTES PARK MEDICAL CENTER, 555 Prospect, Zip 80517, Mailing Address: P.O. Box 2740, Zip 80517-2740; tel. 303/586-2317; Andrew Wills, Chief Executive Officer (Total facility includes 60 beds in nursing home-type unit) **A**9 10 **F**2 7 8 12 14 15 22 26 28 29 30 32 33 34 40 41 42 44 49 62 64 65 71 **P**7	16	10	77	341	51	29069	62	5065	2083	98
FORT CARSON—El Paso County										
★ EVANS U.S. ARMY COMMUNITY HOSPITAL, Zip 80913-5101; tel. 719/526-7200; Colonel Homer J. Wright MC, Commander **A**1 2 **F**3 7 8 12 14 15 16 17 19 20 21 22 24 25 28 29 30 31 32 34 37 39 40 41 42 44 46 48 49 51 52 53 54 56 57 58 59 61 65 67 71 73 74 **P**5 6 **S**9395 Department of the Army	42	10	139	8342	68	554599	1666	52662	20770	1197
FORT COLLINS—Larimer County										
□ MOUNTAIN CREST HOSPITAL, 4601 Corbett Drive, Zip 80525; tel. 303/225-9191; Frank Baumann, Administrator (Nonreporting) **A**1 10	33	22	60	—	—	—	—	—	—	—
★ POUDRE VALLEY HOSPITAL, 1024 Lemay Avenue, Zip 80524-3998; tel. 303/495-7000; Karna Kruckenberg Schofer R.N., Ph.D., Chief Executive Officer **A**1 2 3 9 10 **F**1 4 7 8 10 15 19 21 22 24 26 27 28 29 30 32 34 35 36 37 39 40 41 42 43 44 45 46 47 48 49 51 52 53 54 55 56 57 58 59 60 61 65 67 70 71 72 73 74 **P**5 8	16	10	224	11929	133	280795	2100	105592	46515	1204
FORT LYON—Bent County										
★ VETERANS AFFAIRS MEDICAL CENTER, Zip 81038; tel. 719/456-1260; W. David Smith, Director (Total facility includes 155 beds in nursing home-type unit) **F**15 16 20 22 26 29 30 33 41 45 46 49 51 52 54 58 64 65 71 73 74 **P**6 **S**9295 Department of Veterans Affairs	45	22	289	759	268	37583	0	34771	19223	498
FORT MORGAN—Morgan County										
★ COLORADO PLAINS MEDICAL CENTER, 1000 Lincoln Street, Zip 80701; tel. 303/867-3391; Keith Mesmer, Administrator and Chief Executive Officer **A**1 9 10 **F**4 7 8 10 14 15 16 17 19 21 22 28 29 30 32 33 34 35 37 40 41 42 44 45 46 49 65 67 70 71 73 **P**1 **S**0585 Brim, Inc.	33	10	40	2197	22	67103	368	13293	5324	221
FRUITA—Mesa County										
FAMILY HEALTH WEST, 228 North Cherry Street, Zip 81521, Mailing Address: Box 130, Zip 81521-0130; tel. 303/858-9871; Dennis E. Ficklin, Executive Director (Total facility includes 352 beds in nursing home-type unit) **A**9 10 **F**15 16 22 49 62 64 65 73 **P**3	23	10	358	278	336	6723	0	5702	3561	157
GLENWOOD SPRINGS—Garfield County										
★ VALLEY VIEW HOSPITAL, 1906 Blake Avenue, Zip 81601, Mailing Address: Box 1970, Zip 81602; tel. 303/945-6535; Norman L. McBride, Chief Executive Officer **A**1 9 10 **F**2 7 8 15 16 19 21 22 32 34 35 36 37 39 40 41 42 44 46 49 63 65 66 70 71 73 **P**5 **S**0002 Quorum Health Group/Quorum Health Resources	23	10	59	2898	32	—	504	23444	10876	364
GRAND JUNCTION—Mesa County										
□ + ○ COMMUNITY HOSPITAL, 2021 North 12th Street, Zip 81501; tel. 303/242-0920; Roger C. Zumwalt, Executive Director **A**1 9 10 11 **F**1 3 4 6 7 8 10 11 12 14 15 16 17 19 21 22 25 26 28 29 30 31 32 33 34 35 36 39 40 41 42 43 44 45 46 49 54 55 56 57 59 60 61 62 63 65 66 67 68 71 73 74 **P**8	23	10	51	1696	18	99860	298	15343	6464	258
□ HILLTOP REHABILITATION CENTER, 1100 Patterson Road, Zip 81506; tel. 303/244-6007; Dennis Stahl, Administrator (Total facility includes 22 beds in nursing home-type unit) **A**1 9 10 **F**14 15 16 27 28 32 39 41 45 46 48 49 64 65 66 67 73 **P**5	23	46	50	749	28	17722	0	9758	5406	213

Hospitals, U.S. / COLORADO

Hospital, Address, Telephone, Administrator, Approval, Facility, and Physician Codes, Health Care System	Classi-fication Codes		Utilization Data					Expense (thousands) of dollars		
★ American Hospital Association (AHA) membership □ Joint Commission on Accreditation of Healthcare Organizations (JCAHO) accreditation + American Osteopathic Hospital Association (AOHA) membership ○ American Osteopathic Association (AOA) accreditation △ Commission on Accreditation of Rehabilitation Facilities (CARF) accreditation Control codes 61, 63, 64, 71, 72 and 73 indicate hospitals listed by AOHA, but not registered by AHA. For definition of numerical codes, see page A6	Control	Service	Beds	Admissions	Census	Outpatient Visits	Births	Total	Payroll	Personnel
⚹ ST. MARY'S HOSPITAL AND MEDICAL CENTER, 2635 North 7th Street, Zip 81501-1628, Mailing Address: P.O. Box 3433, Zip 81502; tel. 303/244-2273; Sister Lynn Casey, President **A**1 2 3 5 9 10 **F**3 4 7 8 10 11 12 13 14 15 16 17 18 19 21 22 24 26 27 28 30 31 32 33 34 35 36 37 38 39 40 41 42 43 44 45 46 49 52 53 54 55 56 57 58 59 60 61 63 65 66 67 68 70 71 72 73 74 **P**3 5 **S**5095 Sisters of Charity of Leavenworth Health Services Corporation	21	10	200	10471	136	211122	1236	83006	36600	1176
⚹ VETERANS AFFAIRS MEDICAL CENTER, 2121 North Avenue, Zip 81501-6499; tel. 970/242-0731; Robert R. Rhyne D.D.S., Director (Total facility includes 36 beds in nursing home-type unit) **A**1 **F**2 3 8 14 15 16 17 19 20 21 22 26 27 29 30 31 33 34 35 37 39 41 42 44 46 49 51 52 54 56 57 58 60 64 65 67 71 73 74 **S**9295 Department of Veterans Affairs	45	10	126	2428	87	45280	0	24066	12534	330
GREELEY—Weld County										
⚹ NORTH COLORADO MEDICAL CENTER, 1801 16th Street, Zip 80631-5199; tel. 970/352-4121; Karl Benjamin Gills, Administrator **A**1 2 3 9 10 **F**3 4 7 8 9 10 12 14 15 16 17 19 21 22 23 25 26 27 29 30 31 32 33 34 35 37 39 40 41 42 43 44 45 46 48 49 51 52 53 54 55 56 57 58 59 60 63 64 65 66 67 70 71 73 74 **P**5 7 8 **S**2235 Lutheran Health Systems	23	10	326	12590	168	206930	1739	109876	51080	1516
GUNNISON—Gunnison County										
GUNNISON VALLEY HOSPITAL, 214 East Denver Avenue, Zip 81230; tel. 970/641-1456; Robert S. Austin, President **A**9 10 **F**7 8 11 15 17 19 22 28 29 32 34 35 37 40 44 47 49 65 71 73	13	10	24	566	5	15642	109	4998	2066	80
HAXTUN—Phillips County										
★ HAXTUN HOSPITAL DISTRICT, 235 West Fletcher Street, Zip 80731-0308, Mailing Address: Box 308, Zip 80731-0308; tel. 303/774-6123; James R. Beeler, Administrator (Nonreporting) **A**9 10	16	10	48	—	—	—	—	—	—	—
HOLYOKE—Phillips County										
★ MELISSA MEMORIAL HOSPITAL, 505 South Baxter Avenue, Zip 80734-1496; tel. 303/854-2241; Acel K. Thacker, Administrator **A**9 10 **F**7 8 14 15 17 19 20 22 24 27 28 32 34 40 44 45 49 65 71 73 **P**6	16	10	18	266	3	7250	30	2655	1197	63
HUGO—Lincoln County										
★ LINCOLN COMMUNITY HOSPITAL AND NURSING HOME, 111 Sixth Street, Zip 80821, Mailing Address: Box 248, Zip 80821; tel. 719/743-2421; Mary L. Thompson, Administartor (Total facility includes 35 beds in nursing home-type unit) **A**9 10 **F**7 19 35 40 44 49 64 65 71	13	10	56	318	31	6728	49	1847	718	82
JULESBURG—Sedgwick County										
SEDGWICK COUNTY MEMORIAL HOSPITAL, 900 Cedar Street, Zip 80737; tel. 970/474-3323; Aloha Kier, Administrator (Total facility includes 32 beds in nursing home-type unit) **A**9 10 **F**7 8 16 19 22 24 31 32 34 35 44 64 71	13	10	58	180	33	5267	18	—	—	28
KREMMLING—Grand County										
KREMMLING MEMORIAL HOSPITAL, Fourth and Grand Avenue, Zip 80459, Mailing Address: Box 399, Zip 80459-0399; tel. 303/724-3442; Lorraine Caposole, Chief Executive Officer (Total facility includes 8 beds in nursing home-type unit) **A**9 10 **F**6 14 15 16 21 24 26 28 32 34 44 64 65 67 70 71 73 **P**6	16	10	19	230	10	14554	0	—	—	47
LA JARA—Conejos County										
□ CONEJOS COUNTY HOSPITAL, Mailing Address: Box 639, Zip 81140-0639; tel. 719/274-5121; Monica Morris, Administrator (Total facility includes 34 beds in nursing home-type unit) **A**1 9 10 **F**6 7 13 22 28 30 33 34 40 41 44 49 51 64 65 71 73	16	10	49	742	36	3605	31	2336	1865	90
LA JUNTA—Otero County										
⚹ ARKANSAS VALLEY REGIONAL MEDICAL CENTER, 1100 Carson Avenue, Zip 81050; tel. 719/384-5412; Dale D. Stoll, Chief Executive Officer (Total facility includes 143 beds in nursing home-type unit) **A**1 9 10 **F**7 8 10 12 19 22 31 32 34 35 37 40 42 44 46 49 64 65 71 **P**4 5 8	21	10	206	2863	165	45206	324	20674	8923	342
LAMAR—Prowers County										
⚹ PROWERS MEDICAL CENTER, 401 Kendall Drive, Zip 81052-3993; tel. 719/336-4343; Earl J. Steinhoff, Chief Executive Officer **A**1 9 10 **F**1 2 3 4 7 8 9 10 11 15 17 19 20 21 22 23 25 26 27 28 29 30 32 33 34 35 36 37 38 39 40 41 42 43 44 45 46 47 48 49 50 51 53 54 55 56 57 58 59 60 61 63 64 65 69 70 71 73 74 **S**0002 Quorum Health Group/Quorum Health Resources	16	10	40	1215	13	21530	175	7415	2768	128
LEADVILLE—Lake County										
★ ST. VINCENT GENERAL HOSPITAL, 822 West Fourth Street, Zip 80461-3897; tel. 719/486-0230; Glade R. Hamilton, Administrator **A**9 10 **F**7 8 12 13 17 18 19 21 22 25 40 44 46 56 61 64 65 71 74	16	10	31	814	21	8045	124	4767	2188	101
LITTLETON—Arapahoe County										
⚹ COLUMBINE PSYCHIATRIC CENTER, 8565 South Poplar Way, Zip 80126; tel. 303/470-9500; Jonathan Bartlett, Chief Financial Officer and Interim Chief Executive Officer (Nonreporting) **A**1 9 10 **S**0048 Columbia/HCA Healthcare Corporation	33	22	70	—	—	—	—	—	—	—
LITTLETON HOSPITAL-PORTER See Porter Care Hospital-Littleton										
⚹ PORTER CARE HOSPITAL-LITTLETON, (Formerly Littleton Hospital-Porter) 7700 South Broadway, Zip 80122; tel. 303/730-8900; Richard C. Hale, Administrator **A**1 9 **F**2 3 4 7 8 10 11 12 16 17 18 19 22 23 33 34 35 37 38 39 40 41 42 43 44 45 46 48 49 52 53 54 55 56 57 58 59 60 61 64 65 67 68 69 71 73 74 **P**1 2 7	21	10	105	5212	48	50080	1549	38420	13281	415

© 1995 AHA Guide

Hospitals, U.S. / COLORADO

Hospital, Address, Telephone, Administrator, Approval, Facility, and Physician Codes, Health Care System

- ★ American Hospital Association (AHA) membership
- ☐ Joint Commission on Accreditation of Healthcare Organizations (JCAHO) accreditation
- + American Osteopathic Hospital Association (AOHA) membership
- ○ American Osteopathic Association (AOA) accreditation
- △ Commission on Accreditation of Rehabilitation Facilities (CARF) accreditation

Control codes 61, 63, 64, 71, 72 and 73 indicate hospitals listed by AOHA, but not registered by AHA. For definition of numerical codes, see page A6.

Hospital	Control	Service	Beds	Admissions	Census	Outpatient Visits	Births	Total	Payroll	Personnel
LONGMONT—Boulder County										
★ LONGMONT UNITED HOSPITAL, 1950 West Mountain View Avenue, Zip 80501–3162, Mailing Address: Box 1659, Zip 80502–1659; tel. 303/651–5111; Kenneth R. Huey, President and Chief Executive Officer **A**1 2 9 10 **F**1 3 7 8 12 14 19 20 21 22 26 32 33 35 37 39 40 44 45 46 48 49 52 53 54 55 56 57 58 59 60 65 66 70 71 73 **P**8	23	10	110	4704	55	117301	709	41334	17702	726
LOUISVILLE—Boulder County										
★ AVISTA HOSPITAL, 100 Health Park Drive, Zip 80027–9583; tel. 303/673–1000 **A**1 3 9 10 **F**7 8 10 12 13 14 15 17 19 21 22 28 29 30 32 33 34 35 37 39 40 41 42 44 45 46 49 61 65 66 71 73 **P**3 5	21	10	58	3198	25	37499	1109	25175	9006	332
☐ CHARTER BEHAVIORAL HEALTH SYSTEM AT CENTENNIAL PEAKS, (Formerly Centennial Peaks Hospital) 2255 South 88th Street, Zip 80027; tel. 303/673–9990; Sharon Worsham, Administrator (Nonreporting) **A**1 9 10 **S**0695 Charter Medical Corporation	33	22	72	—	—	—	—	—	—	—
LOVELAND—Larimer County										
★ MCKEE MEDICAL CENTER, 2000 Boise Avenue, Zip 80538–4281; tel. 303/635–4000; Charles F. Harms, Administrator **A**1 9 10 **F**7 8 12 14 15 16 17 18 19 22 23 28 30 31 32 33 34 35 37 39 40 41 44 45 46 48 49 56 65 70 71 73 **P**1 **S**2235 Lutheran Health Systems	23	10	106	4979	61	47869	638	38574	16524	652
MEEKER—Rio Blanco County										
★ PIONEERS HOSPITAL OF RIO BLANCO COUNTY, (Includes Walbridge Memorial Convalescent Wing) 345 Cleveland Street, Zip 81641–0000; tel. 303/878–5047; Jim Murphy, Administrator (Total facility includes 25 beds in nursing home–type unit) **A**9 10 **F**1 7 8 14 15 20 22 25 26 27 28 32 34 36 39 44 49 64 65 71 73 74 **P**1 **S**0002 Quorum Health Group/Quorum Health Resources	13	10	42	285	30	6900	2	4186	1857	90
MONTROSE—Montrose County										
★ MONTROSE MEMORIAL HOSPITAL, 800 South Third Street, Zip 81401–4291; tel. 303/249–2211; Tyler Erickson, Administrator **A**1 9 10 **F**2 3 7 8 11 15 17 19 20 21 22 23 24 26 28 29 30 34 35 37 39 40 41 42 44 45 46 48 49 52 53 54 55 56 57 58 63 65 66 67 71 73 74 **P**5 8 **S**0002 Quorum Health Group/Quorum Health Resources	13	10	68	3312	36	43798	373	21785	9775	327
PUEBLO—Pueblo County										
☐ COLORADO MENTAL HEALTH INSTITUTE AT PUEBLO, 1600 West 24th Street, Zip 81003–1499; tel. 719/546–4000; Harold Carmel M.D., Superintendent **A**1 9 10 **F**3 24 26 41 44 45 46 52 53 54 55 56 57 58 65 73	12	22	605	2156	616	—	0	59051	43146	1228
★ PARKVIEW EPISCOPAL MEDICAL CENTER, 400 West 16th Street, Zip 81003; tel. 719/584–4000; C. W. Smith, President and Chief Operating Officer **A**1 9 10 **F**1 2 3 4 7 8 10 12 14 15 16 17 18 19 22 23 26 31 32 35 37 40 41 42 43 44 45 46 48 49 52 53 54 55 56 57 58 59 64 65 66 70 71 73 **P**3 7 **S**0002 Quorum Health Group/Quorum Health Resources	23	10	249	7765	117	55530	840	52477	23565	894
★ ST. MARY–CORWIN REGIONAL MEDICAL CENTER, 1008 Minnequa Avenue, Zip 81004–3798; tel. 719/560–4000; William G. Turman M.D., President and Chief Executive Officer (Nonreporting) **A**1 2 3 9 10 **S**5115 Sisters of Charity Health Care Systems, Inc.	21	10	307	—	—	—	—	—	—	—
RANGELY—Rio Blanco County										
★ RANGELY DISTRICT HOSPITAL, 511 South White Avenue, Zip 81648–2104; tel. 970/675–5011; Julie Standen, Chief Executive Officer **A**9 10 **F**8 15 22 28 30 34 44 46 49 51 71 **P**6	16	10	22	90	12	6987	0	2726	1215	45
RIFLE—Garfield County										
★ CLAGETT MEMORIAL HOSPITAL, 701 East Fifth Street, Zip 81650–2970, Mailing Address: P.O. Box 912, Zip 81650–0912; tel. 303/625–1510; Edwin A. Gast, Administrator (Total facility includes 57 beds in nursing home–type unit) **A**9 10 **F**7 8 16 17 22 26 28 29 30 32 33 34 36 39 40 44 49 51 64 65 71 73 **P**6 8 **S**0002 Quorum Health Group/Quorum Health Resources	16	10	75	347	57	10812	14	5770	2816	114
SALIDA—Chaffee County										
★ HEART OF THE ROCKIES REGIONAL MEDICAL CENTER, 448 East First Street, Zip 81201–0429, Mailing Address: P.O. Box 429, Zip 81201–0429; tel. 719/539–6661; Howard D. Turner, Administrator and Chief Executive Officer **A**9 10 **F**7 8 19 22 28 32 33 36 37 40 42 44 46 49 65 71 73 **P**3 8 **S**0002 Quorum Health Group/Quorum Health Resources	16	10	35	1213	12	22925	119	8344	3458	156
SPRINGFIELD—Baca County										
★ SOUTHEAST COLORADO HOSPITAL AND LONG TERM CARE, 373 East Tenth Avenue, Zip 81073; tel. 719/523–4501; Annie L. Dukes B.S.N., M.B.A., J.D., Chief Executive Officer (Total facility includes 40 beds in nursing home–type unit) **A**9 10 **F**8 14 15 16 22 26 27 28 31 32 33 44 45 49 65 67 73 74	16	10	65	326	43	11291	0	3877	2046	115
STEAMBOAT SPRINGS—Routt County										
★ ROUTT MEMORIAL HOSPITAL, 80 Park Avenue, Zip 80487–5010; tel. 303/879–1322; Robert L. Brandt, Chief Executive Officer (Total facility includes 50 beds in nursing home–type unit) **A**1 9 10 **F**3 7 8 14 15 19 21 22 26 28 34 35 37 40 44 49 53 54 55 56 57 58 59 63 64 65 66 70 71 74 **P**8	23	10	72	1026	52	34016	177	12462	6067	202
STERLING—Logan County										
★ STERLING REGIONAL MEDCENTER, 615 Fairhurst, Zip 80751–0500, Mailing Address: Box 3500, Zip 80751; tel. 303/522–0122; James O. Pernau, Administrator **A**1 9 10 **F**7 8 14 19 21 22 30 32 34 35 36 37 40 44 45 46 49 51 65 71 73 **P**3 **S**2235 Lutheran Health Systems	23	10	36	1728	20	81016	267	18806	7386	294

Hospitals, U.S. / COLORADO

Hospital, Address, Telephone, Administrator, Approval, Facility, and Physician Codes, Health Care System	Classification Codes		Utilization Data					Expense (thousands) of dollars		Personnel
★ American Hospital Association (AHA) membership □ Joint Commission on Accreditation of Healthcare Organizations (JCAHO) accreditation + American Osteopathic Hospital Association (AOHA) membership ○ American Osteopathic Association (AOA) accreditation △ Commission on Accreditation of Rehabilitation Facilities (CARF) accreditation Control codes 61, 63, 64, 71, 72 and 73 indicate hospitals listed by AOHA, but not registered by AHA. For definition of numerical codes, see page A6	Control	Service	Beds	Admissions	Census	Outpatient Visits	Births	Total	Payroll	
THORNTON—Adams County □ △ MEDIPLEX REHABILITATION–DENVER, 8451 Pearl Street, Zip 80229; tel. 303/288–3000; Jude Torchia, Administrator and Chief Executive Officer (Nonreporting) **A**1 5 7 10	33	46	70	—	—	—	—	—	—	—
★ NORTH SUBURBAN MEDICAL CENTER, 9191 Grant Street, Zip 80229; tel. 303/451–7800; Jay S. Weinstein, Chief Executive Officer (Nonreporting) **A**1 9 10 **S**0048 Columbia/HCA Healthcare Corporation	33	10	160	—	—	—	—	—	—	—
TRINIDAD—Las Animas County ★ MOUNT SAN RAFAEL HOSPITAL, 410 Benedicta Avenue, Zip 81082–2093; tel. 719/846–9213; James P. D'Agostino, Chief Executive Officer **A**1 9 10 **F**8 14 19 21 22 32 35 40 44 46 49 71 **S**0002 Quorum Health Group/Quorum Health Resources	23	10	31	1266	16	35685	153	6755	2819	128
USAF ACADEMY—Sedgwick County ★ U.S. AIR FORCE ACADEMY HOSPITAL, 4102 Pinion Drive, Zip 80840–4000; tel. 719/472–5101; Colonel Charles K. Maffet MC, Commander **A**1 **F**7 8 12 14 15 16 19 20 22 24 27 28 29 30 34 35 37 39 40 41 44 45 46 48 49 51 53 54 55 56 57 58 59 61 65 66 67 70 71 73 **S**9495 Department of the Air Force	41	10	82	5686	38	284954	611	—	—	703
VAIL—Eagle County ★ VAIL VALLEY MEDICAL CENTER, 181 West Meadow Drive, Zip 81657; tel. 303/476–2451; Ray McMahan, Chief Executive Officer **A**1 3 9 10 **F**4 7 8 12 14 15 16 19 21 22 28 31 32 33 35 37 39 40 41 44 48 51 65 66 67 68 71 73 74 **P**5	23	10	49	2077	16	34918	356	23472	9757	291
WALSENBURG—Huerfano County ★ HUERFANO MEDICAL CENTER, 23500 U.S. Highway 160, Zip 81089; tel. 719/738–5100; Michael J. Lockwood, President and Chief Executive Officer **A**9 10 **F**3 5 8 15 16 17 19 20 22 26 27 28 29 30 31 32 33 34 35 39 41 44 45 46 49 65 66 71 73 74	16	10	24	752	13	20852	0	5342	1580	149
WESTMINSTER—Jefferson County ★ CLEO WALLACE CENTER HOSPITAL, 8405 West 100th Avenue, Zip 80021; tel. 303/466–7391; James M. Cole, President and Chief Executive Officer **A**1 5 9 10 **F**12 16 20 22 39 45 46 52 53 55 56 58 59 65 67 **P**8	23	52	146	1065	40	—	0	—	—	241
★ PROVENANT ST. ANTHONY HOSPITAL NORTH, (Formerly St. Anthony Hospital North) 2551 West 84th Avenue, Zip 80030; tel. 303/426–2151; Michael H. Erne, Chief Executive Officer and Executive Vice President (Nonreporting) **A**10 **S**5115 Sisters of Charity Health Care Systems, Inc.	21	10	130	—	—	—	—	—	—	—
ST. ANTHONY HOSPITAL NORTH See Provenant St. Anthony Hospital North										
WHEAT RIDGE—Jefferson County ★ LUTHERAN MEDICAL CENTER, 8300 West 38th Avenue, Zip 80033–6005; tel. 303/425–4500; Kay R. Phillips, President and Chief Executive Officer (Total facility includes 18 beds in nursing home–type unit) **A**1 2 9 10 **F**2 3 4 6 7 8 10 11 12 13 14 15 17 19 21 22 25 26 28 29 30 32 33 34 35 37 38 40 41 42 43 44 45 46 48 49 52 53 54 55 56 57 58 59 60 61 62 64 65 67 70 71 73 74 **P**4 5 6 7 8	23	10	339	14092	149	139630	1932	127288	65043	1829
WEST PINES AT LUTHERAN MEDICAL CENTER, 3400 Lutheran Parkway, Zip 80033; tel. 303/239–4000; Edward A. Ross, Administrator (Nonreporting) **A**9 10	23	22	64	—	—	—	—	—	—	—
WRAY—Yuma County ★ WRAY COMMUNITY DISTRICT HOSPITAL, 340 Birch Street, Zip 80758, Mailing Address: Box 65, Zip 80758–0065; tel. 303/332–4811; Daniel Dennis, Administrator (Nonreporting) **A**3 9 10	16	10	25	—	—	—	—	—	—	—
YUMA—Yuma County ★ YUMA DISTRICT HOSPITAL, 910 South Main Street, Zip 80759–3098, Mailing Address: P.O. Box 306, Zip 80759–0306; tel. 303/848–5405; S. A. Thomas, Administrator **A**9 10 **F**7 8 14 15 19 22 28 31 32 35 39 40 44 49 71 73	16	10	14	185	2	9822	25	1776	923	56

© 1995 AHA Guide

Hospitals, U.S. / CONNECTICUT

CONNECTICUT

Resident population 3,277 (in thousands)
Resident population in metro areas 95.7%
Birth rate per 1,000 population 14.8
65 years and over 14.1%
Percent of persons without health insurance 7.5%

Hospital, Address, Telephone, Administrator, Approval, Facility, and Physician Codes, Health Care System	Classification Codes		Utilization Data					Expense (thousands) of dollars		
	Control	Service	Beds	Admissions	Census	Outpatient Visits	Births	Total	Payroll	Personnel

★ American Hospital Association (AHA) membership
☐ Joint Commission on Accreditation of Healthcare Organizations (JCAHO) accreditation
+ American Osteopathic Hospital Association (AOHA) membership
○ American Osteopathic Association (AOA) accreditation
△ Commission on Accreditation of Rehabilitation Facilities (CARF) accreditation
Control codes 61, 63, 64, 71, 72 and 73 indicate hospitals listed by AOHA, but not registered by AHA. For definition of numerical codes, see page A6

BETHLEHEM—Litchfield County

★ WELLSPRING FOUNDATION, 21 Arch Bridge Road, Zip 06751–1612, Mailing Address: P.O. Box 370, Zip 06751–0370; tel. 203/266–7235; Herbert L. Hall, Chief Executive Officer **F**8 9 10 19 21 22 27 29 30 31 35 37 39 40 44 45 47 52 53 54 55 58 59 60 65 67 70 71 **P**6	23	22	34	62	24	—	0	3041	2235	58

BRIDGEPORT—Fairfield County

★ BRIDGEPORT HOSPITAL, 267 Grant Street, Zip 06610–2875, Mailing Address: P.O. Box 5000, Zip 06610; tel. 203/384–3000; Robert J. Trefry, President and Chief Executive Officer **A**1 2 3 5 6 8 9 10 **F**4 7 8 9 10 11 12 13 17 19 21 22 25 27 28 29 30 31 32 33 34 35 36 37 38 39 40 41 42 43 44 45 46 47 48 49 51 52 53 54 55 56 57 58 59 60 61 65 66 67 68 69 71 72 73 74 **P**8	23	10	441	17787	336	138267	2748	176202	88208	2099
GREATER BRIDGEPORT COMMUNITY MENTAL HEALTH CENTER, 1635 Central Avenue, Zip 06610–0902, Mailing Address: Box 5117, Zip 06610; tel. 203/579–6646; James M. Lehane III, Director **A**10 **F**6 12 15 16 17 18 30 39 45 52 54 55 56 57 58 59 65 67 73 **S**0014 Connecticut State Department of Mental Health	12	22	22	366	17	75281	0	—	—	324
★ ST. VINCENT'S MEDICAL CENTER, 2800 Main Street, Zip 06606–4201; tel. 203/576–6000; William J. Riordan, President and Chief Executive Officer **A**1 2 3 5 8 9 10 **F**1 2 4 7 8 10 11 14 15 17 19 21 25 26 28 29 30 31 32 34 35 37 39 40 41 42 43 44 46 49 51 52 54 56 58 59 60 65 67 68 70 71 72 73 **P**5 7 8 **S**1855 Daughters of Charity National Health System	21	10	289	16138	308	92636	1896	134265	67525	1524

BRISTOL—Hartford County

★ BRISTOL HOSPITAL, P.O. Box 529, Brewster Road, Zip 06011–0529; tel. 203/585–3000; Thomas D. Kennedy III, President and Chief Executive Officer **A**1 2 5 9 10 **F**3 7 8 12 13 17 18 19 21 22 30 32 33 34 35 37 39 40 41 42 44 46 49 51 52 54 58 63 65 71 73 74	23	10	190	7915	120	162435	984	69278	36565	1157

DANBURY—Fairfield County

★ DANBURY HOSPITAL, 24 Hospital Avenue, Zip 06810–6099; tel. 203/797–7000; Frank J. Kelly, President and Chief Executive Officer **A**1 2 3 5 8 9 10 **F**3 4 5 7 8 10 11 12 13 14 15 16 17 18 19 20 21 22 24 26 28 29 30 31 32 33 34 35 37 38 39 40 41 42 44 45 46 48 49 51 52 53 54 56 58 59 60 61 63 65 67 68 70 71 73 74 **P**1	23	10	357	16662	302	215074	2319	171268	82902	1984

DERBY—New Haven County

★ GRIFFIN HOSPITAL, 130 Division Street, Zip 06418; tel. 203/735–7421; John Bustelos Jr., President **A**1 2 3 5 9 10 **F**3 7 8 12 14 15 16 19 20 21 22 28 29 30 35 37 41 42 44 45 46 49 51 52 56 58 59 61 65 71 72 73 74 **P**5	23	10	160	5806	107	94567	782	59132	28511	718

FARMINGTON—Hartford County

★ UNIVERSITY OF CONNECTICUT HEALTH CENTER, JOHN DEMPSEY HOSPITAL, 263 Farmington Avenue, Zip 06030–3802; tel. 203/679–2000; Andria Martin MS, Director **A**1 2 3 5 8 9 10 **F**2 4 5 8 10 12 13 14 19 20 22 23 26 28 30 31 34 35 36 37 38 39 40 41 42 43 44 45 46 47 49 51 52 54 55 56 58 59 60 61 65 66 67 69 71 73 **P**5 7	12	10	232	6479	120	424170	330	110600	45830	1055

GREENWICH—Fairfield County

★ GREENWICH HOSPITAL, 5 Perryridge Road, Zip 06830–4697; tel. 203/863–3901; Frank A. Corvino, President **A**1 2 3 5 9 10 **F**2 3 4 7 8 10 11 12 13 15 16 17 18 19 20 21 22 24 25 26 28 29 30 31 32 33 34 35 37 38 39 40 41 42 44 46 47 49 51 53 54 56 58 60 61 63 65 67 68 71 73 **P**5	23	10	247	7109	121	180066	1301	94159	49971	1293

GROTON—New London County

★ NAVAL HOSPITAL, Zip 06349–5600; tel. 203/449–3261; Lieutenant, Junior Grade T. L. Sauvigne' MSC, U.S.N.R., Administrator **A**1 5 9 **F**8 12 14 15 16 18 19 20 22 24 28 29 30 35 36 37 39 41 44 45 46 49 65 67 71 72 73 **S**9655 Department of Navy	43	10	25	1826	12	216427	0	14638	3884	528

HARTFORD—Hartford County

★ HARTFORD HOSPITAL, 80 Seymour Street, Zip 06102–5037, Mailing Address: P.O. Box 5037, Zip 06102–5037; tel. 203/545–5555; John J. Meehan Jr., President and Chief Executive Officer (Total facility includes 104 beds in nursing home–type unit) **A**1 3 5 8 9 10 **F**1 3 4 7 8 10 11 14 16 19 20 21 22 26 30 31 33 34 35 36 37 38 40 41 42 43 44 45 46 47 48 49 50 51 52 53 54 55 56 57 58 59 60 61 64 65 66 69 70 71 73 74 **P**4 5 8	23	10	934	34513	667	229846	5203	413742	194992	3984
★ INSTITUTE OF LIVING, 400 Washington Street, Zip 06106–3392; tel. 203/241–8015; William A. Himmelsbach Jr., President and Chief Executive Officer (Nonreporting) **A**1 3 5 9 10	23	22	120	—	—	—	—	—	—	—
★ MOUNT SINAI HOSPITAL, 500 Blue Hills Avenue, Zip 06112–1596; tel. 203/286–4600; David D'Eramo Ph.D., President and Chief Executive Officer **A**1 2 3 5 9 10 **F**2 3 4 7 8 10 12 13 14 15 16 17 19 20 21 22 24 25 26 28 29 30 31 32 33 34 35 37 38 40 41 42 43 44 45 46 48 49 50 51 52 53 54 55 56 57 58 59 60 61 63 65 66 67 68 70 71 72 73 74 **P**8	23	10	218	7203	131	171537	1012	83631	42950	909

Hospitals, U.S. / CONNECTICUT

Hospital, Address, Telephone, Administrator, Approval, Facility, and Physician Codes, Health Care System	Control	Service	Beds	Admissions	Census	Outpatient Visits	Births	Total	Payroll	Personnel
★ SAINT FRANCIS HOSPITAL AND MEDICAL CENTER, 114 Woodland Street, Zip 06105–1299; tel. 203/548–4000; David D'Eramo Ph.D., President and Chief Executive Officer **A**1 2 3 5 6 8 9 10 **F**2 3 4 7 8 10 12 13 14 15 16 17 19 20 21 22 24 25 26 28 29 30 31 32 33 34 35 37 38 40 41 42 43 44 45 46 48 49 51 52 53 54 55 56 57 58 59 60 61 63 65 66 67 68 70 71 72 73 74 **P**8	21	10	456	19856	353	219641	2630	217495	104301	2489
MANCHESTER—Hartford County										
★ MANCHESTER MEMORIAL HOSPITAL, 71 Haynes Street, Zip 06040–4188; tel. 203/646–1222; Michael R. Gallacher, President **A**1 5 9 10 **F**7 8 12 14 15 16 17 18 19 20 21 22 26 28 30 31 32 33 34 35 36 37 39 40 41 42 44 45 46 49 52 53 54 55 56 57 58 59 61 63 65 67 68 71 72 73 74 **P**4 5 8	23	10	201	8779	133	122197	1136	88965	45040	978
MANSFIELD CENTER—Tolland County										
□ NATCHAUG HOSPITAL, 189 Storrs Road, Zip 06250–1638; tel. 203/456–1311; Stephen W. Larcen Ph.D., Chief Executive Officer **A**1 9 10 **F**3 52 53 54 55 56 57 58 59	23	22	56	1131	42	28606	0	12390	6463	192
MERIDEN—New Haven County										
HENRY D. ALTOBELLO CHILDREN AND YOUTH CENTER, Undercliff Road, Zip 06450; tel. 203/238–6351; Margery S. Stahl, Superintendent (Nonreporting) **A**9	12	52	34	—	—	—	—	—	—	—
★ VETERANS MEMORIAL MEDICAL CENTER, (Includes East Campus, 883 Paddock Avenue, Meriden, Connecticut, Zip 06450–7094; tel. 203/238–8200) One King Place, Zip 06450–1009, Mailing Address: P.O. Box 1009, Zip 06450–1009; tel. 203/238–8200; Theodore H. Horwitz, President **A**1 2 9 10 **F**3 11 15 16 19 21 22 24 26 28 30 33 34 35 37 39 40 41 42 44 46 52 53 54 55 56 57 58 59 60 65 71 72 73 74 **P**5 8	23	10	154	8354	127	115741	1247	94604	49873	1467
MIDDLETOWN—Middlesex County										
□ CONNECTICUT VALLEY HOSPITAL, Eastern Drive, Zip 06457–7023, Mailing Address: P.O. Box 351, Zip 06457–7024; tel. 203/344–2666; Judith Normandin, Chief Executive Officer (Nonreporting) **A**1 3 5 9 10 **S**0014 Connecticut State Department of Mental Health	12	22	318	—	—	—	—	—	—	—
★ MIDDLESEX HOSPITAL, 28 Crescent Street, Zip 06457–3650; tel. 203/344–6000; Robert Gerard Kiely, President and Chief Executive Officer **A**1 2 3 5 9 10 **F**3 7 8 12 13 14 15 17 18 19 20 21 22 25 26 27 28 29 30 31 32 33 34 35 37 39 40 41 42 44 45 49 51 52 53 54 55 56 57 58 59 60 61 63 65 66 67 68 71 72 73 **P**5	23	10	195	9576	140	224074	1296	110668	58986	1229
RIVERVIEW HOSPITAL FOR CHILDREN, River Road, Zip 06457, Mailing Address: Box 621, Zip 06457; tel. 203/344–2700; Richard J. Wiseman Ph.D., Superintendent (Nonreporting) **A**3 9	12	52	55	—	—	—	—	—	—	—
□ WHITING FORENSIC INSTITUTE, O'Brien Drive, Zip 06457, Mailing Address: Box 70, Zip 06457–3942; tel. 203/344–2541; Michael A. Norko M.D., Director **A**1 **F**2 8 10 11 14 15 16 17 19 20 21 22 28 29 30 31 35 37 39 45 48 52 54 55 56 57 58 59 65 67 70 71 **P**6 **S**0014 Connecticut State Department of Mental Health	12	22	100	53	82	0	0	—	—	249
MILFORD—New Haven County										
★ MILFORD HOSPITAL, 2047 Bridgeport Avenue, Zip 06460–4606; tel. 203/876–4000; Paul E. Moss, President **A**1 2 9 10 **F**7 14 19 21 22 28 30 32 34 35 37 40 42 44 46 63 65 67 71 73 **P**5	23	10	96	4241	66	45023	672	37398	19436	419
NEW BRITAIN—Hartford County										
★ △ HOSPITAL FOR SPECIAL CARE, (Chronic Disease and Rehabilitation) 2150 Corbin Avenue, Zip 06053–2263; tel. 203/827–4761; Katherine C. III M.D., President and Chief Executive Officer **A**1 7 9 10 **F**12 15 17 20 24 25 26 34 39 41 48 49 54 65 66 67 73 **P**6	23	49	171	376	162	11921	0	44040	26121	681
★ NEW BRITAIN GENERAL HOSPITAL, 100 Grand Street, Zip 06052–2000, Mailing Address: P.O. Box 100, Zip 06050–0100; tel. 203/224–5011; Laurence A. Tanner, President and Chief Executive Officer **A**1 2 3 5 8 9 10 **F**1 2 3 4 7 8 10 11 12 14 15 16 17 18 19 21 22 23 24 25 26 30 31 32 33 34 35 37 38 39 40 41 42 43 44 46 48 49 51 52 53 54 55 56 57 58 59 60 61 63 65 66 67 70 71 73 74 **P**5 8	23	10	294	13435	212	237145	2101	124613	71239	1818
NEW CANAAN—Fairfield County										
★ SILVER HILL HOSPITAL, 208 Valley Road, Zip 06840–3899; tel. 203/966–3561; Michael Sheehy M.D., President and Medical Director **A**1 9 **F**2 3 14 34 52 53 55 58 59	23	22	76	924	49	6840	0	16295	8363	221
NEW HAVEN—New Haven County										
□ CONNECTICUT MENTAL HEALTH CENTER, 34 Park Street, Zip 06519, Mailing Address: Box 1842, Zip 06508–1842; tel. 203/789–7290; Ezra Griffith M.D., Director **A**1 3 5 9 10 **F**2 3 12 17 18 19 20 21 22 35 39 46 52 53 55 56 58 59 65 67 71 **S**0014 Connecticut State Department of Mental Health	12	22	54	739	47	66431	0	—	—	480
★ HOSPITAL OF SAINT RAPHAEL, 1450 Chapel Street, Zip 06511–4444; tel. 203/789–3000; James J. Cullen, President **A**1 2 3 5 8 9 10 **F**1 3 4 7 8 10 11 12 13 15 16 17 18 19 21 22 26 27 28 29 30 31 32 34 35 37 39 40 41 42 43 44 45 46 48 49 52 53 55 56 58 59 61 63 65 67 68 70 71 73 74 **P**1 9	21	10	491	20197	433	113104	1424	271242	119139	2855
□ YALE PSYCHIATRIC INSTITUTE, 184 Liberty Street, Zip 06519, Mailing Address: Box 208038, Zip 06520–8038; tel. 203/785–7200; Thomas H. McGlashan M.D., Director (Nonreporting) **A**1 3 5 9 10	23	22	66	—	—	—	—	—	—	—
★ YALE–NEW HAVEN HOSPITAL, 20 York Street, Zip 06504–1001; tel. 203/785–4242; Joseph A. Zaccagnino, President and Chief Executive Officer **A**1 2 3 5 8 9 10 **F**4 7 8 10 11 12 14 15 16 17 19 20 21 22 23 26 27 28 30 31 32 34 35 37 38 40 41 42 43 44 46 47 48 49 50 51 52 53 54 55 56 57 58 59 60 61 63 65 66 67 68 69 70 71 73 74 **P**5 7 8	23	10	725	32672	626	330209	5505	407643	194988	4591

Hospitals, U.S. / CONNECTICUT

Hospital, Address, Telephone, Administrator, Approval, Facility, and Physician Codes, Health Care System	Classification Codes		Utilization Data					Expense (thousands) of dollars		
★ American Hospital Association (AHA) membership ☐ Joint Commission on Accreditation of Healthcare Organizations (JCAHO) accreditation + American Osteopathic Hospital Association (AOHA) membership ○ American Osteopathic Association (AOA) accreditation △ Commission on Accreditation of Rehabilitation Facilities (CARF) accreditation Control codes 61, 63, 64, 71, 72 and 73 indicate hospitals listed by AOHA, but not registered by AHA. For definition of numerical codes, see page A6	Control	Service	Beds	Admissions	Census	Outpatient Visits	Births	Total	Payroll	Personnel
NEW LONDON—New London County										
★ LAWRENCE AND MEMORIAL HOSPITAL, 365 Montauk Avenue, Zip 06320–4769; tel. 203/442–0711; William T. Christopher, President and Chief Executive Officer **A**1 9 10 **F**3 7 8 10 11 12 19 22 23 25 31 32 34 35 37 38 39 40 41 42 44 45 46 48 49 52 53 54 55 56 58 59 65 71 73 **P**4 8	23	10	258	11624	193	92234	1996	112156	60289	1229
NEW MILFORD—Litchfield County										
★ NEW MILFORD HOSPITAL, 21 Elm Street, Zip 06776–2993; tel. 203/355–2611; Richard E. Pugh, President and Chief Executive Officer **A**1 9 10 **F**8 12 14 19 20 21 22 24 28 30 31 34 35 37 39 40 41 42 44 46 49 56 58 63 65 67 71 73 **P**8	23	10	85	2941	42	50220	449	33699	15857	333
NEWINGTON—Hartford County										
☐ CEDARCREST REGIONAL HOSPITAL, 525 Russell Road, Zip 06111–1595; tel. 203/666–4613; David E. K. Hunter Ph.D., Superintendent **A**1 9 10 **F**1 2 3 4 5 6 8 9 10 11 12 14 16 17 18 19 20 21 22 23 24 25 26 27 28 29 30 31 32 33 34 35 36 37 38 39 40 41 42 43 44 45 46 48 49 50 51 52 53 54 55 56 57 58 59 60 61 62 63 64 65 66 67 69 70 71 72 73 74 **P**1 **S**0014 Connecticut State Department of Mental Health	12	22	73	884	65	—	0	15998	10398	228
★ NEWINGTON CHILDREN'S HOSPITAL, 181 East Cedar Street, Zip 06111–1540; tel. 203/667–5580; Scott Winans Goodspeed, President and Chief Executive Officer (Nonreporting) **A**1 3 5 9 10	23	50	76	—	—	—	—	—	—	—
★ VETERANS AFFAIRS MEDICAL CENTER, 555 Willard Avenue, Zip 06111–2600; tel. 203/666–6951; Vincent Ng, Director **A**1 3 5 8 9 **F**1 2 3 4 8 10 15 16 17 19 20 21 22 26 27 28 30 31 32 33 34 35 39 42 43 44 46 49 50 51 52 54 56 57 58 59 60 63 65 67 69 71 73 74 **S**9295 Department of Veterans Affairs	45	10	101	2600	95	80425	0	47178	27002	444
NEWTOWN—Fairfield County										
☐ FAIRFIELD HILLS HOSPITAL, Mile Hill Road, Zip 06470–5525, Mailing Address: Box 5525, Zip 06470–5525; tel. 203/426–2531; Andrew J. Phillips Ed.D., Superintendent **A**1 9 10 **F**2 4 6 8 9 11 12 15 16 17 18 19 20 21 22 26 27 28 29 31 32 33 34 35 36 37 39 40 41 42 43 44 45 46 50 52 54 55 56 57 58 59 60 61 63 65 67 69 71 73 **P**6 **S**0014 Connecticut State Department of Mental Health	12	22	212	341	252	0	0	32148	27301	592
HOUSATONIC ADOLESCENT HOSPITAL, Mile Hill Road, Zip 06470, Mailing Address: Box 5525, Zip 06470; tel. 203/270–2700; Brenda McGavran, Superintendent (Nonreporting) **A**9	12	52	35	—	—	—	—	—	—	—
NORWALK—Fairfield County										
★ △ NORWALK HOSPITAL, Maple Street, Zip 06856–5050; tel. 203/852–2000; David W. Osborne, President and Chief Executive Officer **A**1 2 3 5 7 9 10 **F**2 3 7 8 10 11 12 13 16 17 18 19 20 21 22 25 26 28 29 30 31 32 33 34 35 37 38 39 40 41 42 44 45 48 49 51 52 53 54 55 56 57 58 59 60 61 65 67 68 70 71 73 74 **P**5 8	23	10	311	13224	241	121460	1850	160539	85479	1821
NORWICH—New London County										
★ NORWICH HOSPITAL, Route 12, Zip 06360, Mailing Address: Box 508, Zip 06360–0508; tel. 203/823–5200; Garrell S. Mullaney, Superintendent (Nonreporting) **A**1 3 9 10 **S**0014 Connecticut State Department of Mental Health	12	22	314	—	—	—	—	—	—	—
★ UNCAS ON THAMES HOSPITAL, 401 West Thames Street, Zip 06360–0711; tel. 203/823–4617; Marta M. Smith, Director (Nonreporting) **A**1 3 5 9 10	12	48	29	—	—	—	—	—	—	—
★ WILLIAM W. BACKUS HOSPITAL, 326 Washington Street, Zip 06360–2742; tel. 203/889–8331; Thomas P. Pipicelli, President **A**1 3 9 10 **F**7 8 10 12 14 16 19 21 22 28 29 30 31 32 34 35 37 38 39 40 41 42 44 45 49 52 54 56 58 59 60 65 67 71 73	23	10	183	9419	136	126617	1317	77858	39933	1007
PORTLAND—Middlesex County										
☐ ELMCREST PSYCHIATRIC INSTITUTE, 25 Marlborough Street, Zip 06480; tel. 203/342–0480; Ralph Sperry, Chief Executive Officer (Nonreporting) **A**1 9 10 **S**0695 Charter Medical Corporation	32	22	105	—	—	—	—	—	—	—
PUTNAM—Windham County										
★ DAY KIMBALL HOSPITAL, 320 Pomfret Street, Zip 06260, Mailing Address: P.O. Box 6001, Zip 06260–9417; tel. 203/928–6541; Charles F. Schneider, President **A**1 9 10 **F**3 7 8 12 13 15 16 17 18 19 21 22 25 26 27 28 29 30 32 33 34 35 37 39 40 41 42 44 45 46 49 52 54 55 56 57 58 59 61 63 65 66 67 68 71 72 73 74 **P**8	23	10	124	4522	63	222411	600	43784	22995	498
ROCKY HILL—Hartford County										
☐ VETERANS HOME AND HOSPITAL, 287 West Street, Zip 06067; tel. 203/529–2571; Sharon R. Wood, Administrator (Nonreporting) **A**1 10	12	48	266	—	—	—	—	—	—	—
SHARON—Litchfield County										
★ SHARON HOSPITAL, 50 Hospital Hill Road, Zip 06069–0789, Mailing Address: P.O. Box 789, Zip 06069–0789; tel. 203/364–4141 **A**1 2 9 10 **F**7 8 14 15 17 19 21 22 29 30 33 34 35 37 39 40 42 44 46 49 63 65 67 71 73 **P**1 5	23	10	78	3344	46	35661	403	28524	13496	336
SOMERS—Tolland County										
CONNECTICUT DEPARTMENT OF CORRECTION'S HOSPITAL, Mailing Address: Box 100, Zip 06071; tel. 203/749–8391; Edward A. Blanchette M.D., Director (Nonreporting)	12	11	29	—	—	—	—	—	—	—
SOUTHINGTON—Hartford County										
★ BRADLEY MEMORIAL HOSPITAL AND HEALTH CENTER, 81 Meriden Avenue, Zip 06489–3297; tel. 203/276–5000; Clarence J. Silvia, President **A**1 9 10 **F**8 12 14 15 17 18 19 22 26 28 29 30 33 34 35 37 39 41 42 44 45 49 55 56 63 65 67 71 73 74 **P**8	23	10	74	2490	44	33141	0	25558	12098	317

Hospitals, U.S. / CONNECTICUT

Hospital, Address, Telephone, Administrator, Approval, Facility, and Physician Codes, Health Care System	Classification Codes		Utilization Data					Expense (thousands) of dollars		
★ American Hospital Association (AHA) membership ☐ Joint Commission on Accreditation of Healthcare Organizations (JCAHO) accreditation + American Osteopathic Hospital Association (AOHA) membership ○ American Osteopathic Association (AOA) accreditation △ Commission on Accreditation of Rehabilitation Facilities (CARF) accreditation Control codes 61, 63, 64, 71, 72 and 73 indicate hospitals listed by AOHA, but not registered by AHA. For definition of numerical codes, see page A6	Control	Service	Beds	Admissions	Census	Outpatient Visits	Births	Total	Payroll	Personnel
STAFFORD SPRINGS—Tolland County ☐ JOHNSON MEMORIAL HOSPITAL, 201 Chestnut Hill Road, Zip 06076-0860, Mailing Address: P.O. Box 860, Zip 06076-0860; tel. 203/684-4251; Alfred A. Lerz, President and Chief Executive Officer **A**1 9 10 **F**3 7 8 12 13 15 16 17 19 21 22 28 29 30 31 32 33 34 35 37 40 41 42 44 45 49 52 54 55 56 57 58 59 65 67 71 73 74 **P**5	23	10	89	3616	61	38540	104	32583	16951	403
STAMFORD—Fairfield County ★ ST. JOSEPH MEDICAL CENTER, 128 Strawberry Hill Avenue, Zip 06904-1222, Mailing Address: P.O. Box 1222, Zip 06904-1222; tel. 203/353-2000; William J. Riordan, President and Chief Executive Officer (Nonreporting) **A**1 3 9 10	21	10	180	—	—	—	—	—	—	—
★ STAMFORD HOSPITAL, Shelburne Road and West Broad Street, Zip 06902, Mailing Address: P.O. Box 9317, Zip 06904-9317; tel. 203/325-7000; Philip D. Cusano, President and Chief Executive Officer **A**1 2 3 5 8 9 10 **F**3 7 8 10 12 15 16 19 20 21 22 26 28 29 30 31 32 33 34 35 37 38 39 40 41 42 44 45 46 49 51 52 53 54 55 56 57 58 59 60 61 63 65 67 69 70 71 73 74 **P**7 8	23	10	266	10872	192	114118	1970	112223	56167	1139
TORRINGTON—Litchfield County ★ CHARLOTTE HUNGERFORD HOSPITAL, 540 Litchfield Street, Zip 06790, Mailing Address: Box 988, Zip 06790-0988; tel. 203/496-6666; David R. Newton, President and Executive Director **A**1 2 9 10 **F**7 8 11 12 14 15 16 17 18 19 20 21 22 25 28 30 31 32 33 34 35 37 40 41 42 44 49 53 54 56 58 59 60 64 65 66 71 72 73 **P**1	23	10	133	5736	99	149318	617	53874	28592	742
VERNON ROCKVILLE—Hartford County ★ ROCKVILLE GENERAL HOSPITAL, 31 Union Street, Zip 06066; tel. 203/872-0501; Barry G. Beeman, President and Chief Executive Officer (Nonreporting) **A**1 9 10	23	10	95	—	—	—	—	—	—	—
WALLINGFORD—New Haven County ★ △ GAYLORD HOSPITAL, Gaylord Farm Road, Zip 06492, Mailing Address: P.O. Box 400, Zip 06492-0400; tel. 203/284-2801; Paul H. Johnson, President and Chief Executive Officer **A**1 5 7 9 10 **F**2 3 41 48 49 66 **P**6	23	46	121	1334	93	58433	0	34860	20010	438
★ MASONIC HOME AND HOSPITAL, (Chronic Disease Hospital with Skilled Nursing Facility) 22 Masonic Avenue, Zip 06492-3048, Mailing Address: P.O. Box 70, Zip 06492-7002; tel. 203/284-3900; Barry M. Spero, President (Total facility includes 468 beds in nursing home-type unit) **A**1 9 10 **F**6 8 12 16 17 20 22 26 27 28 29 30 32 34 36 39 41 44 45 46 49 51 52 54 55 57 58 62 64 65 67 71 73 **P**6	23	49	493	1220	480	0	0	31532	18555	663
WATERBURY—New Haven County ★ ST. MARY'S HOSPITAL, 56 Franklin Street, Zip 06706-1200; tel. 203/574-6000; Sister Marguerite Waite, President and Chief Executive Officer **A**1 2 3 5 6 8 9 10 **F**3 5 7 8 10 11 12 13 15 16 17 18 19 20 21 22 25 26 28 29 30 31 33 34 35 36 37 39 40 41 42 44 45 46 49 51 52 54 55 56 58 59 60 63 65 67 71 72 73 **P**5 8	21	10	272	11694	192	156823	1467	122873	64394	1528
★ WATERBURY HOSPITAL, 64 Robbins Street, Zip 06721, Mailing Address: P.O. Box 1589, Zip 06721-1589; tel. 203/573-6000; John H. Tobin, President **A**1 2 3 5 9 10 **F**5 7 8 10 11 12 15 16 17 18 19 20 21 22 24 28 29 30 31 33 34 35 37 40 41 42 44 48 49 51 52 53 54 55 56 57 58 59 60 61 65 67 69 71 72 73 74 **P**8	23	10	262	12615	202	700949	1543	124253	63012	1401
WEST HARTFORD—Hartford County ★ HEBREW HOME AND HOSPITAL, (Long-term Care, Chronic Disease, Geriatric Skilled Nursing Facility) 1 Abrahms Boulevard, Zip 06117-1525; tel. 203/523-3800; Irving Kronenberg, President and Executive Director (Total facility includes 293 beds in nursing home-type unit) **A**5 9 10 **F**1 5 12 17 19 20 21 26 27 29 30 32 33 34 35 36 39 42 45 46 49 54 55 56 57 58 64 65 67 69 71 73 **P**3	23	49	334	628	331	0	0	26858	15823	393
WEST HAVEN—New Haven County ★ VETERANS AFFAIRS MEDICAL CENTER, 950 Campbell Avenue, Zip 06516-2700; tel. 203/932-5711; Vincent Ng, Director (Total facility includes 90 beds in nursing home-type unit) **A**1 3 5 8 9 **F**2 3 4 6 8 10 11 15 17 19 20 21 22 23 26 27 30 31 32 33 34 35 37 41 42 43 44 45 46 49 50 51 52 54 55 56 57 58 59 60 61 63 64 65 67 69 70 71 73 74 **P**5 **S**9295 Department of Veterans Affairs	45	10	550	7036	449	178867	0	128027	70443	1746
WESTPORT—Fairfield County ★ HALL-BROOKE HOSPITAL, A DIVISION OF HALL-BROOKE FOUNDATION, 47 Long Lots Road, Zip 06880-3800; tel. 203/227-1251; Rosalie Aberman, Executive Director **A**1 9 10 **F**1 2 3 14 15 16 26 52 53 54 57 58 59 65 73 **P**1	23	22	52	541	27	17731	0	8062	4796	132
WILLIMANTIC—Windham County ☐ WINDHAM COMMUNITY MEMORIAL HOSPITAL, 112 Mansfield Avenue, Zip 06226-2082; tel. 203/456-9116; Duane A. Carlberg, President **A**1 9 10 **F**7 8 12 17 19 20 21 22 25 28 31 34 35 37 40 41 44 45 49 54 61 63 65 68 70 71 73	23	10	82	4128	59	82526	433	41887	19252	500
WINSTED—Litchfield County ☐ WINSTED MEMORIAL HOSPITAL, 115 Spencer Street, Zip 06098-1191, Mailing Address: P.O. Box 749, Zip 06098-0749; tel. 203/738-6616; James E. Sok, President **A**1 9 10 **F**8 11 13 14 15 17 19 21 22 29 30 34 35 37 44 56 65 71 73 **P**5	23	10	30	1421	22	38577	1	15866	6093	195

DELAWARE

Resident population 700 (in thousands)
Resident population in metro areas 82.7%
Birth rate per 1,000 population 16.5
65 years and over 12.4%
Percent of persons without health insurance 12.7%

Hospital, Address, Telephone, Administrator, Approval, Facility, and Physician Codes, Health Care System	Classification Codes		Utilization Data					Expense (thousands) of dollars		Personnel
★ American Hospital Association (AHA) membership ☐ Joint Commission on Accreditation of Healthcare Organizations (JCAHO) accreditation + American Osteopathic Hospital Association (AOHA) membership ○ American Osteopathic Association (AOA) accreditation △ Commission on Accreditation of Rehabilitation Facilities (CARF) accreditation Control codes 61, 63, 64, 71, 72 and 73 indicate hospitals listed by AOHA, but not registered by AHA. For definition of numerical codes, see page A6	Control	Service	Beds	Admissions	Census	Outpatient Visits	Births	Total	Payroll	
DOVER—Kent County										
★ KENT GENERAL HOSPITAL, 640 South State Street, Zip 19901–3597; tel. 302/674–4700; Dennis E. Klima, President **A**1 2 9 10 **F**1 2 7 8 11 15 16 17 19 21 22 23 24 25 28 29 30 31 32 34 35 37 38 39 40 41 42 44 45 46 49 51 52 53 54 55 56 57 59 60 61 63 65 66 67 70 71 72 73 74	23	10	203	9271	143	153668	1289	71128	30879	1060
DOVER AIR FORCE BASE—San Francisco County										
★ U.S. AIR FORCE HOSPITAL DOVER, 307 Dover Street, Zip 19902–7307; tel. 302/677–2525; Lieutenant Colonel Larry W. Thornhill MSC, Administrator **F**7 8 20 22 27 28 34 39 40 44 46 49 51 55 56 58 67 71 73 74 **S**9495 Department of the Air Force	41	10	31	1676	11	153392	392	—	—	427
LEWES—Sussex County										
★ BEEBE MEDICAL CENTER, 424 Savannah Road, Zip 19958–0226; tel. 302/645–3300; Jeffrey M. Fried FACHE, President and Chief Executive Officer **A**1 2 6 9 10 **F**1 3 4 7 8 11 12 17 19 21 22 23 25 30 31 32 33 34 35 37 39 40 41 42 44 49 51 52 53 54 55 56 57 58 59 63 67 71 72 73 74	23	10	124	6252	90	54621	646	51081	21990	770
MILFORD—Sussex County										
★ MILFORD MEMORIAL HOSPITAL, Clarke Avenue, Zip 19963, Mailing Address: P.O. Box 199, Zip 19963–0199; tel. 302/424–5738; L. Glenn Davis, Administrator **A**1 2 9 10 **F**7 8 15 17 19 21 22 24 25 28 29 30 32 33 34 35 37 39 40 41 42 44 45 46 48 49 63 65 66 67 71 73 74 **P**4 6	23	10	109	5380	97	120121	387	40253	17886	691
NEW CASTLE—New Castle County										
☐ DELAWARE STATE HOSPITAL, DuPont Highway, Zip 19720–1199; tel. 302/577–4381; Jiro R. Shimono, Director (Total facility includes 59 beds in nursing home–type unit) **A**1 3 9 10 **F**12 19 20 21 22 26 29 35 39 41 45 46 49 50 52 56 57 63 65 67 71 73 **P**6	12	22	336	1471	323	0	0	27701	15934	691
☐ MEADOW WOOD HOSPITAL, 575 South DuPont Highway, Zip 19720; tel. 302/328–3330; Arris S. Veronie, Administrator and Chief Executive Officer **A**1 10 **F**52 53 54 56 57 58 59 65 **S**0455 Hospital Group of America	33	52	50	951	38	4393	0	8905	4265	121
NEWARK—New Castle County										
★ ROCKFORD CENTER, 100 Rockford Drive, Zip 19713; tel. 302/996–5480; Walter J. Yokobosky Jr., Chief Executive Officer (Nonreporting) **A**1 9 10 **S**0048 Columbia/HCA Healthcare Corporation	33	22	74	—	—	—	—	—	—	—
SEAFORD—Sussex County										
★ NANTICOKE MEMORIAL HOSPITAL, 801 Middleford Road, Zip 19973–3698; tel. 302/629–6611; Edward H. Hancock, President (Total facility includes 82 beds in nursing home–type unit) **A**1 9 10 **F**2 3 4 7 8 10 12 14 15 16 17 19 22 24 27 28 30 32 35 37 39 40 41 42 44 45 46 49 52 56 58 59 64 65 66 67 71 73 74 **P**1 5 6 7	23	10	208	5798	164	56945	675	43920	18813	586
WILMINGTON—New Castle County										
★ △ ALFRED I. DUPONT INSTITUTE, 1600 Rockland Road, Zip 19803–3616, Mailing Address: Box 269, Zip 19899–0269; tel. 302/651–4000; Thomas P. Ferry, Administrator **A**1 3 5 7 9 10 **F**12 13 14 15 16 19 20 21 22 24 25 34 35 38 39 42 44 47 48 49 51 53 54 58 65 66 69 71 73 **P**3	23	50	128	4400	76	161885	0	86100	44126	1101
CHRISTIANA HOSPITAL See Medical Center of Delaware										
EUGENE DUPONT MEMORIAL HOSPITAL See Medical Center of Delaware										
★ △ MEDICAL CENTER OF DELAWARE, (Includes Christiana Hospital, Wilmington, Delaware; Eugene DuPont Memorial Hospital, Wilmington, Delaware; Wilmington Hospital, Wilmington, Delaware) 501 West 14th Street, Zip 19801, Mailing Address: P.O. Box 1668, Zip 19899–1668; tel. 302/733–1000; Allen L. Johnson, President and Chief Executive Officer **A**1 2 3 5 7 8 9 10 **F**4 7 8 10 11 16 17 19 20 21 22 23 25 29 31 32 34 35 37 38 39 40 41 42 43 44 45 46 47 48 49 51 52 53 54 56 58 59 60 61 63 65 67 70 71 73 74 **P**8	23	10	609	34618	613	376980	6081	398335	191358	4661
★ + ○ RIVERSIDE HOSPITAL, 700 Lea Boulevard, Zip 19802, Mailing Address: Box 845, Zip 19899; tel. 302/764–6120; Norval R. Copeland, President (Total facility includes 99 beds in nursing home–type unit) **A**9 10 11 12 13 **F**1 3 8 14 19 21 22 24 26 28 30 32 33 34 35 37 39 41 42 44 45 46 49 53 54 55 56 57 58 59 60 64 65 66 70 71 73 74	23	10	145	2059	113	36683	0	30631	14052	362
★ ST. FRANCIS HOSPITAL, Seventh and Clayton Streets, Zip 19805–0500, Mailing Address: P.O. Box 2500, Zip 19805–0500; tel. 302/575–8301; Paul C. King Jr., President **A**1 2 3 5 9 10 **F**5 7 8 10 12 14 15 16 17 19 20 21 22 25 26 29 30 31 32 33 34 35 36 37 39 40 41 42 44 48 49 51 52 54 55 57 63 64 65 67 71 72 73 74 **S**5325 Franciscan Health System	21	10	283	11702	213	262351	1352	103008	48169	1293
★ VETERANS AFFAIRS MEDICAL CENTER, 1601 Kirkwood Highway, Zip 19805–4989; tel. 302/633–5201; Dexter D. Dix, Director (Total facility includes 60 beds in nursing home–type unit) **A**1 3 5 8 9 **F**2 8 14 16 19 21 22 26 27 30 31 34 37 41 42 44 46 48 49 51 52 58 60 63 64 65 71 73 74 **S**9295 Department of Veterans Affairs	45	10	210	3096	171	80038	0	51211	27790	675
WILMINGTON HOSPITAL See Medical Center of Delaware										

DISTRICT OF COLUMBIA

Resident population 578 (in thousands)
Resident population in metro areas 100.0%
Birth rate per 1,000 population 19.7
65 years and over 13.3%
Percent of persons without health insurance 22.0%

Hospital, Address, Telephone, Administrator, Approval, Facility, and Physician Codes, Health Care System	Classification Codes		Utilization Data					Expense (thousands) of dollars		
	Control	Service	Beds	Admissions	Census	Outpatient Visits	Births	Total	Payroll	Personnel

- ★ American Hospital Association (AHA) membership
- ☐ Joint Commission on Accreditation of Healthcare Organizations (JCAHO) accreditation
- + American Osteopathic Hospital Association (AOHA) membership
- ○ American Osteopathic Association (AOA) accreditation
- △ Commission on Accreditation of Rehabilitation Facilities (CARF) accreditation

Control codes 61, 63, 64, 71, 72 and 73 indicate hospitals listed by AOHA, but not registered by AHA. For definition of numerical codes, see page A6.

WASHINGTON—Baltimore City County

MALCOLM GROW MEDICAL CENTER See Andrews Air Force Base, MD

Hospital	Control	Service	Beds	Admissions	Census	Outpatient Visits	Births	Total	Payroll	Personnel
★ CHILDREN'S NATIONAL MEDICAL CENTER, 111 Michigan Avenue N.W., Zip 20010-2970; tel. 202/884-5000; Edwin K. Zechman Jr., President and Chief Executive Officer **A**1 3 5 8 9 10 **F**4 5 9 10 12 14 15 17 19 20 21 22 25 27 30 31 32 33 34 35 38 39 41 42 43 44 46 47 49 51 52 53 54 55 56 58 59 63 65 66 67 68 69 70 71 73 **P**6	23	50	185	10412	173	167327	0	162124	74159	1833
★ COLUMBIA HOSPITAL FOR WOMEN MEDICAL CENTER, 2425 L. Street N.W., Zip 20037-1433; tel. 202/293-6500; Charles R. Loar, Acting President and Chief Executive Officer **A**1 9 10 **F**7 8 14 15 16 17 21 28 30 34 38 39 40 44 46 51 60 61 65 67 68 71 73 74	23	44	100	12469	72	44257	4899	66430	29837	746
★ DISTRICT OF COLUMBIA GENERAL HOSPITAL, 19th Street and Massachusetts Avenue S.E., Zip 20003; tel. 202/675-5000; John A. Fairman, Executive Director **A**1 3 5 9 10 **F**7 8 10 11 13 14 15 16 17 19 20 21 22 27 29 30 31 34 37 38 40 41 42 44 46 49 54 56 60 61 65 70 71 73 **P**6	14	10	338	13664	285	194221	1593	150779	86671	2341
★ GEORGE WASHINGTON UNIVERSITY HOSPITAL, 901 23rd Street N.W., Zip 20037; tel. 202/994-1000; Thomas W. Chapman, Chief Executive Officer **A**1 2 3 5 8 9 10 **F**4 7 10 11 14 15 16 17 19 21 22 25 26 31 32 34 35 37 38 40 41 42 44 45 46 48 49 52 53 54 55 56 57 58 59 60 61 63 65 66 69 70 71 73 74 **P**4	23	10	353	16495	286	118036	1334	197328	82609	2271
★ GEORGETOWN UNIVERSITY HOSPITAL, 3800 Reservoir Road N.W., Zip 20007-2197; tel. 202/784-3000; Dan J. Oldani, Administrator **A**1 2 3 5 8 9 10 **F**4 7 8 10 11 12 13 17 19 20 21 22 23 31 34 35 37 38 39 40 42 43 44 47 49 51 52 53 54 55 56 57 58 59 60 61 65 66 67 69 70 71 73 74	21	10	409	17784	353	176734	1355	230246	104189	2825
★ GREATER SOUTHEAST COMMUNITY HOSPITAL, 1310 Southern Avenue S.E., Zip 20032-4699; tel. 202/574-6000; David E. Brown, President (Total facility includes 24 beds in nursing home–type unit) **A**1 2 3 5 9 10 **F**1 7 8 10 11 12 14 15 16 17 19 21 22 25 26 27 28 30 32 34 36 37 38 39 40 41 42 44 45 46 48 49 51 52 53 54 55 57 59 60 62 64 65 68 71 72 73 74 **P**8	23	10	418	14059	283	67850	1551	116592	54360	1467
☐ HADLEY MEMORIAL HOSPITAL, 4601 Martin Luther King Jr. Avenue S.W., Zip 20032; tel. 202/574-5700; (Total facility includes 31 beds in nursing home–type unit) **A**1 9 10 **F**8 15 19 21 22 25 28 37 44 64 65 **P**4 5 7	33	10	103	2378	58	—	0	—	—	473
★ HOSPITAL FOR SICK CHILDREN, 1731 Bunker Hill Road N.E., Zip 20017; tel. 202/635-6125; Vernell P. DeWitty, Acting Chief Executive Officer **A**1 5 9 **F**12 14 17 20 28 31 41 42 45 46 54 65 67 68 73 **P**6	23	56	130	205	106	0	0	—	—	394
★ HOWARD UNIVERSITY HOSPITAL, 2041 Georgia Avenue N.W., Zip 20060; tel. 202/865-6100; Marie Cameron, Interim Executive Director (Nonreporting) **A**1 2 3 5 8 9 10	23	10	437	—	—	—	—	—	—	—
★ △ NATIONAL REHABILITATION HOSPITAL, 102 Irving Street N.W., Zip 20010-2949; tel. 202/877-1000; Edward A. Eckenhoff, President and Chief Executive Officer **A**1 3 5 7 9 10 **F**2 3 4 5 8 9 10 11 12 13 14 16 17 19 20 21 22 25 26 27 28 29 30 31 32 33 34 35 37 38 39 40 41 42 43 44 45 46 47 48 49 50 52 53 54 55 56 57 58 59 60 61 64 65 66 67 69 70 71 72 73 74 **P**6 8 **S**6615 Medlantic Healthcare Group	23	46	160	1559	118	55022	0	55076	27635	829
★ PROVIDENCE HOSPITAL, 1150 Varnum Street N.E., Zip 20017-2180; tel. 202/269-7000; Sister Carol Keehan, President **A**1 3 5 9 10 **F**2 3 7 8 10 11 14 15 16 17 18 19 22 24 25 26 27 28 29 30 33 34 35 36 37 38 39 40 41 42 44 45 49 51 52 54 55 56 57 58 59 61 65 67 71 72 73 74 **S**1855 Daughters of Charity National Health System	21	10	333	12301	246	74585	1721	105330	53010	1563
☐ PSYCHIATRIC INSTITUTE OF WASHINGTON, 4228 Wisconsin Avenue N.W., Zip 20016; tel. 202/965-8550; Nancy R. Cassidy, Acting Administrator (Nonreporting) **A**1 5 9 10	33	22	99	—	—	—	—	—	—	—
★ SIBLEY MEMORIAL HOSPITAL, 5255 Loughboro Road N.W., Zip 20016; tel. 202/537-4000; Robert L. Sloan, Chief Executive Officer (Total facility includes 18 beds in nursing home–type unit) **A**1 3 5 9 10 **F**7 8 10 12 16 17 19 21 22 23 26 28 30 31 32 34 35 37 39 40 41 42 44 45 46 49 52 53 55 56 57 60 61 64 65 66 67 69 71 73	23	10	362	12448	195	61635	896	89115	44230	1116
★ ST. ELIZABETHS HOSPITAL, 2700 Martin Luther King Jr. Avenue S.E., Zip 20032; tel. 202/373-7166; Guido R. Zanni Ph.D., Acting Commissioner **A**3 5 10 **F**1 2 14 15 16 17 18 19 20 34 35 37 44 52 53 54 55 56 57 58 59 65 73	14	22	1024	2781	1057	285878	0	205317	108564	3516
★ VETERANS AFFAIRS MEDICAL CENTER, 50 Irving Street N.W., Zip 20422; tel. 202/745-8000; Sanford M. Garfunkel, Director (Total facility includes 120 beds in nursing home–type unit) **A**1 2 3 5 8 9 **F**1 2 3 4 8 10 14 15 16 17 19 20 21 22 23 26 27 28 29 30 32 35 37 39 41 42 43 44 45 46 49 52 54 55 56 57 58 59 60 64 65 67 71 73 74 **S**9295 Department of Veterans Affairs	45	10	699	9184	520	241504	0	—	—	1994
★ WALTER REED ARMY MEDICAL CENTER, Zip 20307-5001; tel. 202/782-1104; Major General Ronald R. Blanck MS, Commander **A**1 2 3 5 **F**3 4 5 7 8 10 11 12 13 14 15 17 18 19 20 21 22 23 24 25 28 29 30 31 34 35 37 38 39 40 41 42 43 44 45 46 47 49 51 52 53 54 55 56 57 58 59 60 61 65 66 67 69 71 73 **S**9395 Department of the Army	42	10	738	24848	536	539295	706	—	—	5643

Hospitals, U.S. / DISTRICT OF COLUMBIA

Hospital, Address, Telephone, Administrator, Approval, Facility, and Physician Codes, Health Care System	Classification Codes		Utilization Data					Expense (thousands) of dollars		
	Control	Service	Beds	Admissions	Census	Outpatient Visits	Births	Total	Payroll	Personnel

★ American Hospital Association (AHA) membership
☐ Joint Commission on Accreditation of Healthcare Organizations (JCAHO) accreditation
+ American Osteopathic Hospital Association (AOHA) membership
○ American Osteopathic Association (AOA) accreditation
△ Commission on Accreditation of Rehabilitation Facilities (CARF) accreditation
Control codes 61, 63, 64, 71, 72 and 73 indicate hospitals listed by AOHA, but not registered by AHA. For definition of numerical codes, see page A6

Hospital	Control	Service	Beds	Admissions	Census	Outpatient Visits	Births	Total	Payroll	Personnel
★ WASHINGTON HOSPITAL CENTER, 110 Irving Street N.W., Zip 20010–2975; tel. 202/877–7000; Kenneth A. Samet, President **A**1 2 3 5 8 9 10 **F**2 4 8 9 10 11 12 15 16 17 19 21 22 26 27 28 30 31 32 34 35 37 38 39 40 41 42 43 44 45 46 48 49 51 52 60 61 63 65 66 67 69 70 71 73 74 **P**3 8 **S**6615 Medlantic Healthcare Group	23	10	874	31318	618	105180	2812	408424	205840	4157

Hospitals, U.S. / FLORIDA

FLORIDA

Resident population 13,679 (in thousands)
Resident population in metro areas 93.0%
Birth rate per 1,000 population 14.6
65 years and over 18.6%
Percent of persons without health insurance 18.7%

Hospital, Address, Telephone, Administrator, Approval, Facility, and Physician Codes, Health Care System	Classification Codes		Utilization Data					Expense (thousands) of dollars		
★ American Hospital Association (AHA) membership ☐ Joint Commission on Accreditation of Healthcare Organizations (JCAHO) accreditation + American Osteopathic Hospital Association (AOHA) membership ○ American Osteopathic Association (AOA) accreditation △ Commission on Accreditation of Rehabilitation Facilities (CARF) accreditation Control codes 61, 63, 64, 71, 72 and 73 indicate hospitals listed by AOHA, but not registered by AHA. For definition of numerical codes, see page A6	Control	Service	Beds	Admissions	Census	Outpatient Visits	Births	Total	Payroll	Personnel
ALTAMONTE SPRINGS—Seminole County FLORIDA HOSPITAL–ALTAMONTE See Florida Hospital Medical Center, Orlando										
APALACHICOLA—Franklin County EMERALD COAST HOSPITAL, Washington Square, Zip 32320, Mailing Address: P.O. Box 610, Zip 32329; tel. 904/653-8853; Kenneth E. Dykes Sr., Administrator (Nonreporting) **A**9 10	33	10	29	—	—	—	—	—	—	—
APOPKA—Orange County FLORIDA HOSPITAL–APOPKA See Florida Hospital Medical Center, Orlando										
ARCADIA—De Soto County ★ DESOTO MEMORIAL HOSPITAL, 900 North Robert Avenue, Zip 33821-2180, Mailing Address: P.O. Box 2180, Zip 33821-2180; tel. 813/494-3535; Gary M. Moore, Administrator; Cindy Peck, Vice President Nursing and Clinical Services **A**1 9 10 **F**7 8 12 15 16 17 19 22 28 30 32 34 35 37 39 40 44 46 49 51 65 71 73 **S**0002 Quorum Health Group/Quorum Health Resources	23	10	82	2702	29	32911	478	14821	6393	232
☐ G. PIERCE WOOD MEMORIAL HOSPITAL, 5847 Southeast Highway 31, Zip 33821-9627; tel. 813/494-3323; Richard J. Bradley, Administrator (Nonreporting) **A**1 10	12	22	500	—	—	—	—	—	—	—
ATLANTIS—Palm Beach County ★ JFK MEDICAL CENTER, 5301 South Congress Avenue, Zip 33462; tel. 407/965-7300; Richard C. Cascio, President and Chief Executive Officer **A**1 2 10 **F**2 4 8 10 11 12 14 15 16 17 19 21 22 25 28 30 32 34 35 37 39 41 42 43 44 46 49 52 60 65 67 71 72 73 **P**3 4 5 7	23	10	369	12235	188	115537	0	110217	39559	1148
AVON PARK—Highlands County FLORIDA CENTER FOR ADDICTIONS AND DUAL DISORDERS, 100 West College Drive, Zip 33825; tel. 813/453-3151; Arthur J. Cox Sr., Director (Nonreporting) **A**9	23	82	50	—	—	—	—	—	—	—
★ FLORIDA HOSPITAL–WALKER, 2501 U.S. Highway 27 North, Zip 33825-1200, Mailing Address: P.O. Box 1200, Zip 33825-1200; tel. 813/453-7511; Samuel Leonor, President **A**1 9 10 **F**11 12 15 19 21 22 24 28 30 35 37 40 41 44 49 52 54 55 56 57 60 63 67 71 73 **P**5 7 **S**4165 Adventist Health System–Sunbelt Health Care Corporation	21	10	151	7188	99	71607	922	50510	19028	774
BARTOW—Polk County ★ BARTOW MEMORIAL HOSPITAL, 1239 East Main Street, Zip 33830-5005, Mailing Address: Box 1050, Zip 33830-1050; tel. 813/533-8111; David M. Klein, Administrator **A**1 9 10 **F**1 2 3 4 7 8 10 11 12 14 15 16 17 19 21 22 23 24 26 27 28 29 30 31 32 33 34 35 37 38 39 41 42 43 44 45 46 47 48 49 50 51 52 53 54 55 56 58 60 61 63 64 65 66 69 70 71 72 73 **P**3 **S**0002 Quorum Health Group/Quorum Health Resources	23	10	56	2105	26	19754	198	13865	5829	190
★ POLK GENERAL HOSPITAL, (Includes Rohr Nursing Home) 2010 East Georgia Street, Zip 33830-0816; tel. 813/533-1111; Walter P. Donalson III, Chief Executive Officer (Nonreporting) **A**1 9 10	13	10	191	—	—	—	—	—	—	—
BAY PINES—Pinellas County ★ VETERANS AFFAIRS MEDICAL CENTER, 10000 Bay Pines Boulevard, Zip 33504; tel. 813/398-6661; Thomas H. Weaver, Director (Total facility includes 440 beds in nursing home–type unit) **A**1 3 5 **F**2 3 6 8 11 12 15 16 17 19 20 21 22 24 25 26 27 28 29 30 31 32 33 34 35 37 39 41 42 44 45 46 48 49 51 52 54 55 56 57 58 61 63 64 65 67 71 73 74 **P**1 **S**9295 Department of Veterans Affairs	45	10	1021	11770	777	204000	0	152618	79420	2174
BELLE GLADE—Palm Beach County ★ GLADES GENERAL HOSPITAL, 1201 South Main Street, Zip 33430-8002, Mailing Address: Box 8002, Zip 33430-8002; tel. 407/996-6571; Neil Whipkey, Administrator **A**1 9 10 **F**7 8 9 11 14 15 16 19 21 22 30 31 33 35 37 38 40 43 44 45 48 49 61 65 70 71 **S**0002 Quorum Health Group/Quorum Health Resources	16	10	73	2725	33	26578	483	20460	7777	269
BLOUNTSTOWN—Calhoun County CALHOUN–LIBERTY HOSPITAL, 424 Burns Avenue, Zip 32424-0250, Mailing Address: P.O. Box 250, Zip 32424-0250; tel. 904/674-5411; Margaret Brock, President and Chief Executive Officer (Nonreporting) **A**9 10	23	10	36	—	—	—	—	—	—	—
BOCA RATON—Palm Beach County ★ BOCA RATON COMMUNITY HOSPITAL, 800 Meadows Road, Zip 33486-2368; tel. 407/395-7100; Nat West, President **A**1 2 9 10 **F**7 8 10 11 12 14 15 16 17 19 20 21 22 23 24 27 28 29 30 31 32 33 34 35 37 40 41 42 44 45 46 49 56 60 61 63 65 67 71 73 74 **P**1	23	10	342	14204	226	—	645	129162	54581	1624
☐ WEST BOCA MEDICAL CENTER, 21644 State Road 7, Zip 33428-1899; tel. 407/488-8000; Richard S. Freeman, Chief Executive Officer **A**1 9 10 **F**4 7 8 12 19 21 22 23 30 32 34 35 37 38 39 40 42 44 47 49 65 71 73 74 **P**5 **S**0063 TENET Healthcare Corporation	33	10	185	7855	93	45903	1825	56725	20188	581
BONIFAY—Holmes County ☐ DOCTORS MEMORIAL HOSPITAL, 401 East Byrd Avenue, Zip 32425, Mailing Address: Box 188, Zip 32425; tel. 904/547-1120; Robert E. Winkler, Administrator (Nonreporting) **A**1 9 10 **S**5895 Hallmark Healthcare Corporation	33	10	34	—	—	—	—	—	—	—

© 1995 AHA Guide

Hospitals, U.S. / FLORIDA

Hospital, Address, Telephone, Administrator, Approval, Facility, and Physician Codes, Health Care System	Classification Codes		Utilization Data					Expense (thousands) of dollars		
	Control	Service	Beds	Admissions	Census	Outpatient Visits	Births	Total	Payroll	Personnel

★ American Hospital Association (AHA) membership
☐ Joint Commission on Accreditation of Healthcare Organizations (JCAHO) accreditation
+ American Osteopathic Hospital Association (AOHA) membership
○ American Osteopathic Association (AOA) accreditation
△ Commission on Accreditation of Rehabilitation Facilities (CARF) accreditation
Control codes 61, 63, 64, 71, 72 and 73 indicate hospitals listed by AOHA, but not registered by AHA. For definition of numerical codes, see page A6

BOYNTON BEACH—Palm Beach County

★ BETHESDA MEMORIAL HOSPITAL, 2815 South Seacrest Boulevard, Zip 33435; tel. 407/737-7733; Robert B. Hill, President **A**1 2 9 10 **F**7 8 10 11 17 19 22 23 24 26 27 28 30 32 33 34 35 37 38 39 40 41 42 44 49 52 54 55 57 58 59 60 63 65 66 67 71 73 74 **P**6 7	23	10	362	11868	166	74897	2399	94035	40995	1413

BRADENTON—Manatee County

★ △ L. W. BLAKE HOSPITAL, 2020 59th Street West, Zip 34209, Mailing Address: P.O. Box 25004, Zip 34206-5004; tel. 813/792-6611; Lindell W. Orr, Chief Executive Officer **A**1 2 7 9 10 **F**4 7 8 10 11 12 13 14 15 16 17 19 21 22 24 28 30 32 34 37 39 40 41 42 43 44 45 49 60 65 67 71 73 74 **S**0048 Columbia/HCA Healthcare Corporation	33	10	292	10672	182	56586	472	73992	32412	952
★ MANATEE MEMORIAL HOSPITAL, 206 Second Street East, Zip 34208; tel. 813/746-5111; Karl R. Tague, President and Chief Executive Officer **A**1 2 9 10 **F**2 4 7 8 10 11 12 14 15 16 17 19 21 22 24 25 26 28 29 30 31 32 33 34 35 37 38 39 40 41 42 43 44 46 49 52 53 55 56 57 59 60 63 65 66 67 71 72 73 74 **P**8 **S**8810 Baptist Hospitals and Health Systems, Inc.	23	10	512	13577	215	65455	1887	97919	35466	1227

BRANDON—Hillsborough County

★ BRANDON HOSPITAL, 119 Oakfield Drive, Zip 33511-5799; tel. 813/681-5551; H. Rex Etheredge, Chief Executive Officer (Nonreporting) **A**1 9 10 **S**0048 Columbia/HCA Healthcare Corporation	33	10	250	—	—	—	—	—	—	—

BROOKSVILLE—Hernando County

★ BROOKSVILLE REGIONAL HOSPITAL, 55 Ponce De Leon Boulevard, Zip 34601-0037, Mailing Address: Box 37, Zip 34605-0037; tel. 904/796-5111; Hal W. Leftwich FACHE, Administrator **A**1 9 10 **F**8 10 15 16 17 19 21 22 25 29 34 35 37 44 45 49 51 60 63 65 71 72 73 **P**3 6 **S**0002 Quorum Health Group/Quorum Health Resources	23	10	91	3231	50	22456	1	20774	6538	247

BUNNELL—Flagler County

★ MEMORIAL HOSPITAL–FLAGLER, Moody Boulevard, Zip 32110, Mailing Address: HCR1, Box 2, Zip 32110; tel. 904/437-2211; Clark P. Christianson, Senior Vice President and Administrator (Nonreporting) **A**10 **S**2615 Memorial Health Systems	23	10	81	—	—	—	—	—	—	—

CAPE CORAL—Lee County

☐ CAPE CORAL HOSPITAL, 636 Del Prado Boulevard, Zip 33990, Mailing Address: P.O. Box 150010, Zip 33915; tel. 813/574-2323; Jeff Myers, Acting Chief Executive Officer (Nonreporting) **A**1 2 9 10	23	10	201	—	—	—	—	—	—	—

CHATTAHOOCHEE—Gadsden County

FLORIDA STATE HOSPITAL, 612 Morgan Avenue, Zip 32324-1000, Mailing Address: P.O. Box 1000, Zip 32324-1000; tel. 904/663-7536; Robert B. Williams, Administrator (Total facility includes 109 beds in nursing home–type unit) **A**10 **F**4 8 10 11 12 19 20 21 22 23 26 28 29 30 31 35 37 39 40 41 42 43 50 52 54 56 57 60 63 64 65 67 70 71 73 74 **P**2	12	22	1087	842	954	0	0	96541	53668	2568

CHIPLEY—Washington County

★ NORTHWEST FLORIDA COMMUNITY HOSPITAL, 1360 Brickyard Road, Zip 32428-5010, Mailing Address: Drawer K, Zip 32428; tel. 904/638-1610; Stephen D. Mason, Administrator **A**1 9 10 **F**11 15 19 21 22 27 28 30 32 33 34 35 44 54 65 71 73	13	10	45	1466	24	52502	0	9390	3852	184

CLEARWATER—Pinellas County

★ CLEARWATER COMMUNITY HOSPITAL, 1521 East Druid Road, Zip 34616-6193; tel. 813/447-4571; Richard H. Katzeff, Executive Director (Total facility includes 20 beds in nursing home–type unit) **A**1 9 10 **F**4 8 10 12 14 16 17 19 21 22 26 28 29 30 32 34 35 37 41 42 43 44 51 64 65 69 71 72 73 **P**6 8 **S**0048 Columbia/HCA Healthcare Corporation	32	10	133	4883	79	17957	0	—	—	563
☐ HORIZON HOSPITAL, 11300 U.S. 19 North, Zip 34624; tel. 813/541-2646; John R. Picciano, President and Chief Executive Officer (Nonreporting) **A**1 9 10	33	22	167	—	—	—	—	—	—	—
☐ MORTON PLANT HOSPITAL, 323 Jeffords Street, Zip 34616-3892, Mailing Address: Box 210, Zip 34617-0210; tel. 813/462-7000; Frank V. Murphy III, President and Chief Executive Officer (Total facility includes 126 beds in nursing home–type unit) **A**1 2 9 10 **F**1 4 5 6 7 8 10 11 13 15 16 17 19 21 22 24 25 26 27 28 29 30 32 34 35 37 38 40 41 42 43 44 48 49 51 52 53 54 55 57 58 59 60 62 65 66 67 71 73 74 **P**1 4 6 7 8	23	10	742	23008	448	—	2477	163727	66693	2221

CLERMONT—Lake County

★ SOUTH LAKE MEMORIAL HOSPITAL, 847 Eighth Street, Zip 34711; tel. 904/394-4071; P. Shannon Elswick, Administrator and Chief Executive Officer **A**1 9 10 **F**8 12 14 15 16 19 21 22 28 29 30 32 34 35 37 41 44 45 49 65 66 71 73 **S**0002 Quorum Health Group/Quorum Health Resources	16	10	68	1959	27	19188	0	13283	5460	178

CLEWISTON—Hendry County

★ HENDRY GENERAL HOSPITAL, 500 West Sugarland Highway, Zip 33440; tel. 813/983-9121; J. Rudy Reinhardt, Administrator **A**1 9 10 **F**8 14 15 17 19 20 21 22 26 28 29 30 31 33 34 35 37 39 41 42 44 45 49 51 56 65 67 71 73 **S**0002 Quorum Health Group/Quorum Health Resources	16	10	48	1174	15	16594	0	8339	3579	129

COCOA BEACH—Brevard County

★ CAPE CANAVERAL HOSPITAL, 701 West Cocoa Beach Causeway, Zip 32931, Mailing Address: P.O. Box 320069, Zip 32932-0069; tel. 407/799-7111; Larry F. Garrison, President **A**1 9 10 **F**7 8 10 16 17 19 21 22 23 24 25 27 28 29 30 31 32 33 35 37 40 41 42 44 45 49 60 65 67 71 72 73 74	23	10	128	6228	81	61403	991	49200	20440	741

Hospitals, U.S. / FLORIDA

Hospital, Address, Telephone, Administrator, Approval, Facility, and Physician Codes, Health Care System	Classification Codes		Utilization Data					Expense (thousands) of dollars		
	Control	Service	Beds	Admissions	Census	Outpatient Visits	Births	Total	Payroll	Personnel

* ★ American Hospital Association (AHA) membership
* ☐ Joint Commission on Accreditation of Healthcare Organizations (JCAHO) accreditation
* + American Osteopathic Hospital Association (AOHA) membership
* ○ American Osteopathic Association (AOA) accreditation
* △ Commission on Accreditation of Rehabilitation Facilities (CARF) accreditation
* Control codes 61, 63, 64, 71, 72 and 73 indicate hospitals listed by AOHA, but not registered by AHA. For definition of numerical codes, see page A6

CORAL GABLES—Dade County

☐ CORAL GABLES HOSPITAL, 3100 Douglas Road, Zip 33134–6990; tel. 305/445–8461; Nick Bianco, Chief Executive Officer (Nonreporting) **A**1 9 10 **S**6525 Ornda Healthcorp	33	10	205	—	—	—	—	—	—	—
★ HEALTHSOUTH DOCTORS' HOSPITAL, 5000 University Drive, Zip 33146–2094; tel. 305/666–2111; E. Tim Cook, Chief Executive Officer (Nonreporting) **A**1 3 9 10 **S**0023 Healthsouth Corporation	33	10	157	—	—	—	—	—	—	—
VENCOR HOSPITAL–CORAL GABLES, 5190 Southwest Eighth Street, Zip 33134; tel. 305/445–1364; Theodore Welding, Chief Executive Officer (Nonreporting) **A**1 9 10 **S**0026 Vencor, Incorporated	33	10	53	—	—	—	—	—	—	—

CORAL SPRINGS—Broward County

★ CORAL SPRINGS MEDICAL CENTER, 3000 Coral Hills Drive, Zip 33065; tel. 305/344–3000; Jason H. Moore, Administrator **A**1 10 **F**4 5 7 8 10 11 12 14 15 16 17 19 21 22 23 24 25 27 28 29 30 31 32 33 34 35 37 38 39 40 41 42 43 44 45 46 47 48 49 50 51 52 54 56 57 60 63 64 65 66 67 70 71 72 73 74 **P**6 8 **S**3115 North Broward Hospital District	16	10	167	8488	106	79145	2291	64125	25428	718

CRESTVIEW—Okaloosa County

★ NORTH OKALOOSA MEDICAL CENTER, 151 Redstone Avenue S.E., Zip 32539–7304; tel. 904/689–8100; Rodney R. Smith, Chief Executive Officer **A**1 9 10 **F**7 8 12 14 15 16 19 22 28 29 30 32 33 34 35 37 40 41 44 45 46 49 51 65 71 73 74 **P**7 8 **S**0048 Columbia/HCA Healthcare Corporation	33	10	110	3082	45	45498	346	19984	7459	379

CRYSTAL RIVER—Citrus County

☐ + SEVEN RIVERS COMMUNITY HOSPITAL, 6201 North Suncoast Boulevard, Zip 34428; tel. 904/795–6560; Frank T. Beirne, Chief Executive Officer **A**1 9 10 **F**7 8 10 11 12 17 19 21 22 23 24 28 29 30 35 37 39 40 41 42 44 45 48 49 52 54 55 56 57 63 65 67 71 73 74 **S**0063 TENET Healthcare Corporation	33	10	128	5342	83	33878	210	34453	12261	406

DADE CITY—Pasco County

★ DADE CITY HOSPITAL, 1550 Fort King Road, Zip 33525–5294; tel. 904/521–1100; Robert Meade, Chief Executive Officer (Nonreporting) **A**1 10 **S**0048 Columbia/HCA Healthcare Corporation	33	10	120	—	—	—	—	—	—	—

DAYTONA BEACH—Volusia County

★ DAYTONA MEDICAL CENTER, 400 North Clyde Morris Boulevard, Zip 32114, Mailing Address: Box 9000, Zip 32120; tel. 904/239–5000; (Nonreporting) **A**1 10 **S**0048 Columbia/HCA Healthcare Corporation	33	10	214	—	—	—	—	—	—	—
HALIFAX BEHAVIORAL CENTER See Halifax Medical Center										
★ HALIFAX MEDICAL CENTER, (Includes Halifax Behavioral Center, 841 Jimmy Ann Drive, Daytona Beach, Florida, Zip 32117–4599; tel. 904/274–5333) 303 North Clyde Morris Boulevard, Zip 32114; tel. 904/254–4065; Ron R. Rees, Administrator **A**1 2 3 5 9 10 **F**7 8 10 12 14 15 16 17 19 21 22 23 24 25 27 28 29 30 31 32 33 34 35 37 38 39 40 41 42 44 45 46 49 51 52 53 54 56 57 58 59 60 61 63 65 66 67 68 70 71 72 73 74 **P**6 7 8	16	10	450	19539	284	235992	2712	162771	59196	2188

DE FUNIAK SPRINGS—Walton County

WALTON REGIONAL HOSPITAL, 336 College Avenue, Zip 32433; tel. 904/892–5171; James C. Thomas, Administrator **A**9 10 **F**8 19 22 32 34 37 39 44 46 65 71 73 **P**6	33	10	50	1015	14	16386	0	7126	2524	137

DE LAND—Volusia County

★ MEMORIAL HOSPITAL–WEST VOLUSIA, 701 West Plymouth Avenue, Zip 32720, Mailing Address: Box 509, Zip 32721–0509; tel. 904/734–3320; Mark B. Van Fleet, Chief Executive Officer **A**1 9 10 **F**3 4 7 8 10 12 14 15 16 19 21 22 23 27 28 30 32 33 35 37 40 42 44 48 49 56 57 65 71 73 **P**7 **S**2615 Memorial Health Systems	23	10	138	7782	101	67987	1009	52192	26316	—

DELRAY—Palm Beach County

☐ △ PINECREST REHABILITATION HOSPITAL, 5360 Linton Boulevard, Zip 33484; tel. 407/495–0400; Paul D. Echelard, Administrator (Nonreporting) **A**1 7 9 10	33	46	90	—	—	—	—	—	—	—

DELRAY BEACH—Palm Beach County

☐ DELRAY COMMUNITY HOSPITAL, 5352 Linton Boulevard, Zip 33484; tel. 407/498–4440 **A**1 9 10 **F**3 4 7 8 10 11 12 17 18 19 21 26 27 28 29 30 31 32 35 37 39 41 42 43 44 45 46 49 50 51 53 54 55 56 57 58 59 61 63 65 66 67 71 73 74 **S**0063 TENET Healthcare Corporation	33	10	211	9602	163	56930	0	83831	29910	950
☐ FAIR OAKS HOSPITAL AT BOCA DELRAY, 5440 Linton Boulevard, Zip 33484; tel. 407/495–1000; Michael B. Gittelman, Chief Executive Officer (Nonreporting) **A**1 9 10	33	22	102	—	—	—	—	—	—	—

DUNEDIN—Pinellas County

☐ MEASE HOSPITAL DUNEDIN, 601 Main Street, Zip 34698, Mailing Address: P.O. Box 760, Zip 34697–0760; tel. 813/733–1111; Philip K. Beauchamp FACHE, President and Chief Executive Officer (Total facility includes 20 beds in nursing home-type unit) **A**1 2 9 10 **F**7 8 10 12 15 17 19 21 22 28 29 30 31 32 34 35 37 38 39 40 41 42 44 45 46 49 52 53 54 55 56 57 60 63 64 65 67 71 73 74 **P**8 **S**1335 Mease Health Care	23	10	258	8322	118	—	1749	54811	22879	696

EGLIN AIR FORCE BASE—Okaloosa County

★ U.S. AIR FORCE REGIONAL HOSPITAL, 307 Boatner Road, Suite 114, Zip 32542–1282; tel. 904/882–7221; Colonel Joseph E. Melchiorre Jr. MSC, Administrator **A**1 3 **F**2 3 8 12 19 20 21 22 27 28 29 30 34 37 39 40 41 42 46 49 50 51 52 54 58 61 63 64 65 71 73 **S**9495 Department of the Air Force	41	10	105	6243	63	412373	1088	—	—	1061

© 1995 AHA Guide

Hospitals, U.S. / FLORIDA

Hospital, Address, Telephone, Administrator, Approval, Facility, and Physician Codes, Health Care System	Classification Codes		Utilization Data					Expense (thousands) of dollars		
★ American Hospital Association (AHA) membership □ Joint Commission on Accreditation of Healthcare Organizations (JCAHO) accreditation + American Osteopathic Hospital Association (AOHA) membership ○ American Osteopathic Association (AOA) accreditation △ Commission on Accreditation of Rehabilitation Facilities (CARF) accreditation Control codes 61, 63, 64, 71, 72 and 73 indicate hospitals listed by AOHA, but not registered by AHA. For definition of numerical codes, see page A6	Control	Service	Beds	Admissions	Census	Outpatient Visits	Births	Total	Payroll	Personnel
ENGLEWOOD—Sarasota County										
★ ENGLEWOOD COMMUNITY HOSPITAL, 700 Medical Boulevard, Zip 34223; tel. 813/475-6571; Terry L. Moore, Chief Executive Officer (Nonreporting) **A**1 9 10 **S**0048 Columbia/HCA Healthcare Corporation	33	10	100	—	—	—	—	—	—	—
EUSTIS—Lake County										
□ FLORIDA HOSPITAL-WATERMAN, 201 North Eustis, Zip 32726, Mailing Address: P.O. Box B, Zip 32727-0377; tel. 904/589-3333; Royce C. Thompson, President (Total facility includes 29 beds in nursing home-type unit) **A**1 9 10 **F**7 8 10 12 15 17 19 21 22 23 24 25 27 28 30 31 32 33 34 35 37 39 40 42 44 46 49 63 64 65 66 67 68 71 73 74 **P**1 6 7 **S**4165 Adventist Health System-Sunbelt Health Care Corporation	21	10	182	7427	119	120567	658	61008	29662	980
FERNANDINA BEACH—Nassau County										
★ BAPTIST MEDICAL CENTER-NASSAU, (Formerly Nassau General Hospital) 1250 South 18th Street, Zip 32034; tel. 904/261-3627; Jim L. Mayo, Administrator (Nonreporting) **A**1 9 10	16	10	54	—	—	—	—	—	—	—
FORT LAUDERDALE—Broward County										
★ BROWARD GENERAL MEDICAL CENTER, 1600 South Andrews Avenue, Zip 33316-2510; tel. 305/355-5610; Ruth A. Eldridge R.N., Interim Vice President, Hospital Administration **A**1 2 9 10 **F**4 7 8 10 11 12 15 16 17 19 21 22 23 24 25 27 28 29 30 31 33 34 35 37 38 39 40 41 42 43 44 45 46 47 48 49 50 51 52 54 56 57 60 63 65 66 70 71 72 73 74 **P**1 6 **S**3115 North Broward Hospital District	16	10	577	19588	402	186305	3532	175913	74441	2039
□ CLEVELAND CLINIC HOSPITAL, 2835 North Ocean Boulevard, Zip 33308; tel. 305/568-1000; Kenneth H. Kozloff FACHE, Chief Administrative Officer **A**1 3 9 10 **F**8 10 12 14 15 16 17 19 21 22 24 26 27 29 30 31 32 33 34 35 37 39 41 43 44 45 46 49 51 60 65 66 67 71 73 74 **P**3 5	23	10	120	4209	73	25031	0	44115	14542	427
□ CORAL RIDGE PSYCHIATRIC HOSPITAL, 4545 North Federal Highway, Zip 33308; tel. 305/771-2711; Michael J. Held, Administrator **A**1 9 10 **F**2 15 52 53 54 55 57 58 59 65 67 68	31	22	86	995	40	0	0	—	—	115
□ CPC FORT LAUDERDALE HOSPITAL, 1601 East Las Olas Boulevard, Zip 33301-2393; tel. 305/463-4321; Eric Trafals, Chief Executive Officer **A**1 9 10 **F**1 3 12 14 15 16 17 18 30 34 52 53 54 55 56 57 58 59 **S**0785 Community Psychiatric Centers	33	22	100	1198	35	2603	0	4426	2508	137
□ FLORIDA MEDICAL CENTER HOSPITAL, 5000 West Oakland Park Boulevard, Zip 33313-1585; tel. 305/735-6000; Denny De Narvaez, Chief Executive Officer **A**1 10 **F**4 10 11 12 14 19 21 22 26 27 32 33 35 37 41 42 43 44 46 48 49 52 53 55 56 57 60 61 63 65 66 71 73 **S**6525 Ornda Healthcorp	32	10	459	11621	235	70280	0	105789	39102	1140
HEALTHSOUTH SUNRISE REHABILITATION HOSPITAL, 4399 Nob Hill Road, Zip 33351-5899; tel. 305/749-0300; Barbara D. Hayes, Administrator (Nonreporting) **A**10 **S**0023 Healthsouth Corporation	33	46	108	—	—	—	—	—	—	—
□ △ HOLY CROSS HOSPITAL, 4725 North Federal Highway, Zip 33308, Mailing Address: Box 23460, Zip 33307; tel. 305/771-8000; Ray Budrys, President and Chief Executive Officer (Nonreporting) **A**1 7 9 10 **S**3595 Eastern Mercy Health System	21	10	437	—	—	—	—	—	—	—
★ IMPERIAL POINT MEDICAL CENTER, 6401 North Federal Highway, Zip 33308-1495; tel. 305/776-8500; A. Gary Muller, Administrator **A**1 9 10 **F**4 5 7 8 10 12 14 15 16 17 19 22 23 24 26 28 30 31 32 33 34 35 37 39 41 42 43 44 49 51 52 56 57 58 60 66 70 71 74 **P**6 **S**3115 North Broward Hospital District	16	10	154	5677	117	30041	0	47391	21193	554
★ NORTH RIDGE MEDICAL CENTER, 5757 North Dixie Highway, Zip 33334; tel. 305/776-6000; Don S. Steigman, Executive Director (Nonreporting) **A**1 9 10 **S**0063 TENET Healthcare Corporation	33	10	280	—	—	—	—	—	—	—
□ VENCOR HOSPITAL-FORT LAUDERDALE, 1516 East Las Olas Boulevard, Zip 33301-2399; tel. 305/764-8900; Lewis A. Ransdell, Administrator (Nonreporting) **A**1 10 **S**0026 Vencor, Incorporated	33	10	64	—	—	—	—	—	—	—
FORT MYERS—Lee County										
□ CHARTER GLADE BEHAVIORAL HEALTH SYSTEM, (Formerly Charter Glade Hospital) 3550 Colonial Boulevard, Zip 33912, Mailing Address: P.O. Box 06120, Zip 33906; tel. 813/939-0403; Martin Schappell, Administrator (Nonreporting) **A**1 9 10 **S**0695 Charter Medical Corporation	33	22	104	—	—	—	—	—	—	—
★ ○ GULF COAST HOSPITAL, 13681 Doctors Way, Zip 33912; tel. 813/768-5000; Denny W. Powell, Chief Executive Officer **A**1 11 **F**1 2 3 4 7 8 10 11 12 15 16 19 21 22 23 24 26 27 28 29 30 31 32 33 34 35 37 40 41 42 43 44 45 46 47 48 49 51 61 65 69 71 73 74 **P**2 7 8 **S**0048 Columbia/HCA Healthcare Corporation	33	10	120	3195	35	21400	617	30346	10912	271
★ △ LEE MEMORIAL HOSPITAL, 2776 Cleveland Avenue, Zip 33901, Mailing Address: P.O. Box 2218, Zip 33902; tel. 813/332-1111; James R. Nathan, President (Total facility includes 88 beds in nursing home-type unit) **A**1 2 7 9 10 **F**4 7 8 10 11 12 14 15 17 19 21 22 24 26 29 30 31 32 34 35 37 38 39 40 41 42 43 44 45 48 49 60 61 63 64 65 66 67 69 70 71 73 **P**6 8	16	10	621	25016	348	128345	2919	174768	73351	2880
★ SOUTHWEST FLORIDA REGIONAL MEDICAL CENTER, 2727 Winkler Avenue, Zip 33901-9396; tel. 813/939-1147; Nick Carbone, Chief Executive Officer (Nonreporting) **A**1 2 10 **S**0048 Columbia/HCA Healthcare Corporation	33	10	400	—	—	—	—	—	—	—
FORT PIERCE—St. Lucie County										
HARBOUR SHORES OF LAWNWOOD See Lawnwood Regional Medical Center										
★ LAWNWOOD REGIONAL MEDICAL CENTER, (Includes Harbour Shores of Lawnwood, 1860 North Lawnwood Circle, Fort Pierce, Florida, Zip 34950, Mailing Address: P.O. Box 1540, Zip 34954-1540; tel. 407/466-1500; Joel Engles, Administrator 1700 South 23rd Street, Zip 34950-0188; tel. 407/461-4000; Jon C. Trezona, Chief Executive Officer (Total facility includes 33 beds in nursing home-type unit) **A**1 9 **F**2 3 4 8 10 11 12 14 15 16 19 22 23 24 28 31 32 34 35 37 40 42 44 45 46 52 53 55 58 59 60 64 65 66 71 73 74 **S**0048 Columbia/HCA Healthcare Corporation	33	10	320	10660	196	70730	1488	72872	33988	—

Hospitals, U.S. / FLORIDA

Hospital, Address, Telephone, Administrator, Approval, Facility, and Physician Codes, Health Care System	Classification Codes		Utilization Data					Expense (thousands) of dollars		
★ American Hospital Association (AHA) membership ☐ Joint Commission on Accreditation of Healthcare Organizations (JCAHO) accreditation + American Osteopathic Hospital Association (AOHA) membership ○ American Osteopathic Association (AOA) accreditation △ Commission on Accreditation of Rehabilitation Facilities (CARF) accreditation Control codes 61, 63, 64, 71, 72 and 73 indicate hospitals listed by AOHA, but not registered by AHA. For definition of numerical codes, see page A6	Control	Service	Beds	Admissions	Census	Outpatient Visits	Births	Total	Payroll	Personnel
FORT WALTON BEACH—Okaloosa County										
★ FORT WALTON BEACH MEDICAL CENTER, 1000 Mar–Walt Drive, Zip 32547–6708; tel. 904/862–1111; David A. McClellan, Chief Executive Officer **A**1 9 10 **F**4 7 8 10 12 14 15 16 17 19 21 22 23 31 32 34 37 40 41 42 44 45 49 52 55 56 57 59 63 66 71 73 74 **S**0048 Columbia/HCA Healthcare Corporation	33	10	247	7658	123	62918	971	—	—	668
HARBOR OAKS HOSPITAL, 1015 Mar–Walt Drive, Zip 32547; tel. 904/863–4160; James M. Hunt, Chief Executive Officer and Administrator (Nonreporting) **A**10	33	52	79	—	—	—	—	—	—	—
GAINESVILLE—Alachua County										
★ ALACHUA GENERAL HOSPITAL, (Includes Vista Pavilion, 8900 N.E. 39th Avenue, Gainesville, Florida, Zip 32606, Mailing Address: P.O. Box 24059, Zip 32602; tel. 904/338–0097) 801 S.W. Second Avenue, Zip 32601; tel. 904/372–4321; Les C. Rankin, Chief Executive Officer **A**1 2 3 5 9 10 **F**1 2 3 4 7 8 10 11 14 15 16 19 21 22 23 24 28 29 30 31 32 33 34 35 36 37 38 39 40 41 42 43 44 45 46 48 49 52 53 54 55 56 57 58 59 60 63 65 67 71 72 **S**7895 AvMed–Santa Fe	23	10	350	10143	174	423002	676	78410	31242	1228
★ NORTH FLORIDA REGIONAL MEDICAL CENTER, 6500 Newberry Road, Zip 32605–4392, Mailing Address: P.O. Box 147006, Zip 32614–7006; tel. 904/333–4000; Patrick J. Gray, Chief Executive Officer **A**1 9 10 **F**3 4 5 7 8 10 11 12 14 16 17 19 21 22 23 24 25 28 30 32 34 35 37 39 40 41 42 43 44 46 49 58 60 65 66 67 71 72 73 74 **P**6 8 **S**0048 Columbia/HCA Healthcare Corporation	33	10	267	13476	187	75901	1535	76952	30149	1124
★ SHANDS HOSPITAL AT THE UNIVERSITY OF FLORIDA, 1600 Southwest Archer Road, Zip 32610–0366; tel. 904/395–0111; Paul E. Metts, Executive Vice President (Nonreporting) **A**1 2 3 5 8 9 10	23	10	546	—	—	—	—	—	—	—
★ △ UPREACH REHABILITATION HOSPITAL, (Formerly Upreach Pavilion) 8900 Northwest 39th Avenue, Zip 32606–5625; tel. 904/338–0091; Barry G. Wagner, Chief Executive Officer (Nonreporting) **A**1 7 10 **S**7895 AvMed–Santa Fe	23	46	40	—	—	—	—	—	—	—
★ VETERANS AFFAIRS MEDICAL CENTER, 1601 Southwest Archer Road, Zip 32608–1197; tel. 904/376–1611; Malcom Randall, Director (Total facility includes 120 beds in nursing home–type unit) **A**1 3 5 8 **F**1 2 3 4 10 16 17 18 19 20 21 23 25 26 27 28 29 30 31 32 33 34 35 37 39 41 42 43 44 46 49 51 52 54 55 56 57 58 59 60 63 65 67 71 73 74 **P**1 **S**9295 Department of Veterans Affairs	45	10	469	9426	384	—	0	122203	61179	2101
VISTA PAVILION See Alachua General Hospital										
GRACEVILLE—Jackson County										
CAMPBELLTON GRACEVILLE HOSPITAL, 5429 College Drive, Zip 32440; tel. 904/263–4431; H. D. Cannington, Administrator **A**9 10 **F**8 15 19 21 22 28 30 32 33 34 46 51 64 65 71	16	10	22	727	8	5044	0	3646	1722	90
GULF BREEZE—Santa Rosa County										
☐ GULF BREEZE HOSPITAL, 1110 Gulf Breeze Parkway, Zip 32561–1110, Mailing Address: P.O. Box 159, Zip 32562–0159; tel. 904/934–2000; Richard C. Fulford, Administrator **A**1 9 10 **F**2 3 4 7 8 9 10 11 12 13 14 15 16 19 21 22 23 26 27 28 31 32 33 35 37 38 39 40 41 42 43 44 45 46 47 48 49 51 52 53 54 55 56 57 58 59 60 61 62 63 64 65 66 67 70 71 72 73 74 **P**4 5 7 **S**0185 Baptist Health Care Corporation	23	10	43	1899	26	23879	0	14055	4825	165
THE FRIARY OF BAPTIST HEALTH CENTER, 4400 Hickory Shores Boulevard, Zip 32561; tel. 904/932–9375; Leo J. Donnelly, Executive Director **A**9 **F**2	23	82	28	260	7	2044	0	—	—	32
HAINES CITY—Polk County										
☐ HEART OF FLORIDA HOSPITAL, Tenth Street and Wood Avenue, Zip 33844, Mailing Address: Box 67, Zip 33844; tel. 813/422–4971; Robert Mahaffey, Administrator **A**1 9 10 **F**8 14 16 19 21 22 26 30 34 35 37 44 45 46 49 65 66 71 73 **P**5	33	10	51	1833	22	16698	0	9681	4068	153
HIALEAH—Dade County										
AMI PALMETTO GENERAL HOSPITAL See Palmetto General Hospital										
★ HIALEAH HOSPITAL, 651 East 25th Street, Zip 33013–3878; tel. 305/693–6100; Clifford J. Bauer, Chief Executive Officer (Nonreporting) **A**1 9 10 **S**0002 Quorum Health Group/Quorum Health Resources	23	10	411	—	—	—	—	—	—	—
☐ PALM SPRINGS GENERAL HOSPITAL, 1475 West 49th Street, Zip 33012, Mailing Address: Box 2804, Zip 33012; tel. 305/558–2500; Carlos Milanes, Executive Vice President and Administrator **A**1 9 10 **F**8 16 19 21 22 26 34 35 37 39 44 46 49 65 71 73 **P**5	33	10	180	7240	114	20302	0	—	—	550
★ PALMETTO GENERAL HOSPITAL, (Formerly AMI Palmetto General Hospital) 2001 West 68th Street, Zip 33016; tel. 305/823–5000; (Nonreporting) **A**1 9 10 12 **S**0063 TENET Healthcare Corporation	33	10	360	—	—	—	—	—	—	—
☐ SOUTHERN WINDS HOSPITAL, 4225 West 20th Street, Zip 33012; tel. 305/558–9700; Michael J. Gerber, Chief Executive Officer (Nonreporting) **A**1 10	33	22	60	—	—	—	—	—	—	—
HOLLYWOOD—Broward County										
☐ HOLLYWOOD MEDICAL CENTER, 3600 Washington Street, Zip 33021; tel. 305/966–4500; Holly L. Lerner, Chief Executive Officer (Nonreporting) **A**1 9 10 **S**0063 TENET Healthcare Corporation	33	10	334	—	—	—	—	—	—	—
☐ HOLLYWOOD PAVILION, 1201 North 37th Avenue, Zip 33021; tel. 305/962–1355; Karen Kallen, Administrator (Nonreporting) **A**1 10	33	22	46	—	—	—	—	—	—	—
★ △ MEMORIAL HOSPITAL, 3501 Johnson Street, Zip 33021–5421; tel. 305/987–2000; Frank V. Sacco, Chief Executive Officer (Total facility includes 85 beds in nursing home–type unit) **A**1 2 3 7 9 10 **F**1 2 3 4 7 9 10 11 12 13 15 16 17 19 21 22 23 24 25 26 27 28 29 30 31 32 33 34 35 37 38 39 40 41 42 43 44 45 46 47 48 49 51 52 53 54 55 56 57 58 59 60 61 63 64 65 67 66 68 69 70 71 72 73 74 **P**1 7	16	10	739	25132	530	218603	3209	264318	113135	3316

© 1995 AHA Guide

Hospitals, U.S. / FLORIDA

Hospital, Address, Telephone, Administrator, Approval, Facility, and Physician Codes, Health Care System

★ American Hospital Association (AHA) membership
□ Joint Commission on Accreditation of Healthcare Organizations (JCAHO) accreditation
+ American Osteopathic Hospital Association (AOHA) membership
○ American Osteopathic Association (AOA) accreditation
△ Commission on Accreditation of Rehabilitation Facilities (CARF) accreditation
Control codes 61, 63, 64, 71, 72 and 73 indicate hospitals listed by AOHA, but not registered by AHA. For definition of numerical codes, see page A6

Hospital	Classification Codes		Utilization Data					Expense (thousands of dollars)		
	Control	Service	Beds	Admissions	Census	Outpatient Visits	Births	Total	Payroll	Personnel
HOMESTEAD—Dade County										
★ SMH HOMESTEAD HOSPITAL, 160 Northwest 13th Street, Zip 33030–4299; tel. 305/248–3232; Bo Boulenger, Administrator A1 9 10 F2 3 7 8 10 11 12 13 14 15 16 17 19 21 22 25 26 27 28 29 30 31 32 35 37 38 39 40 41 42 43 44 45 46 47 48 49 50 51 52 60 61 64 65 67 68 71 72 73 74 P1 5 7	23	10	103	5145	71	43834	1246	28313	12224	431
HUDSON—Pasco County										
★ COLUMBIA REGIONAL MEDICAL CENTER AT BAYONET POINT, (Formerly Bayonet Point–Medical Center) 14000 Fivay Road, Zip 34667–7199; tel. 813/863–2411; J. Daniel Miller, President and Chief Executive Officer (Nonreporting) A1 9 10 S0048 Columbia/HCA Healthcare Corporation	33	10	256	—	—	—	—	—	—	—
INVERNESS—Citrus County										
★ CITRUS MEMORIAL HOSPITAL, 502 Highland Boulevard, Zip 34452–4754; tel. 904/726–1551; Charles A. Blasband, Chief Executive Officer A1 9 10 F7 8 10 14 15 19 21 22 25 28 30 32 34 37 39 40 44 49 51 65 67 71 73 P6 7	23	10	171	8100	114	108298	613	53096	18284	742
JACKSONVILLE—Duval County										
★ BAPTIST MEDICAL CENTER, 800 Prudential Drive, Zip 32207–8203; tel. 904/393–2000; William C. Mason, President and Chief Executive Officer A1 3 5 9 10 F2 4 7 8 10 11 13 17 18 19 20 21 22 23 24 25 26 28 29 30 31 32 34 35 37 38 39 40 41 42 43 44 45 46 47 49 52 53 55 56 57 58 60 61 65 66 67 69 71 73 74 P5 6	23	10	501	20256	319	232912	3501	189821	72300	2561
□ CHARTER HOSPITAL OF JACKSONVILLE, 3947 Salisbury Road, Zip 32216; tel. 904/296–2447; Douglas Joiner, Chief Executive Officer (Nonreporting) A1 10 S0695 Charter Medical Corporation	33	22	64	—	—	—	—	—	—	—
□ CPC ST. JOHNS RIVER HOSPITAL, 6300 Beach Boulevard, Zip 32216; tel. 904/724–9202; Doug Gifford, Administrator (Nonreporting) A1 9 10 S0785 Community Psychiatric Centers	33	22	99	—	—	—	—	—	—	—
★ MEMORIAL HOSPITAL JACKSONVILLE, 3625 University Boulevard S, Zip 32216, Mailing Address: Box 16325, Zip 32216; tel. 904/399–6111; Winston Rushing, President A1 9 10 F4 7 8 10 11 12 14 16 17 19 21 22 23 24 25 28 30 33 34 35 37 38 40 41 42 43 44 46 48 49 50 51 54 60 61 65 67 70 71 73 74 P3 8 S0048 Columbia/HCA Healthcare Corporation	23	10	311	16849	252	106654	2943	146536	54700	1664
MEMORIAL REGIONAL REHABILITATION CENTER See Memorial Rehabilitation Hospital										
★ △ MEMORIAL REHABILITATION HOSPITAL, (Formerly Memorial Regional Rehabilitation Center) 3599 University Boulevard South, Zip 32216–4211, Mailing Address: P.O. Box 16406, Zip 32245–6406; tel. 904/399–6819; Stephen K. Wilson, Administrator A1 2 7 10 F15 16 48 49	23	46	95	1148	77	0	0	22021	8423	319
★ METHODIST MEDICAL CENTER, 580 West Eighth Street, Zip 32209–6553; tel. 904/798–8000; Marcus E. Drewa, President A1 9 F2 3 8 10 11 14 15 16 19 21 22 25 28 30 31 32 33 34 35 37 40 41 44 45 49 65 67 69 71 73 P6 S2715 Methodist Health System	23	10	269	6578	116	30958	0	66612	21047	824
METHODIST PATHWAY CENTER, 580 West Eighth Street, Zip 32209–6553; tel. 904/798–8250; Marcus E. Drewa, President A10 F2 3 14 15 16 41 65 67 73 S2715 Methodist Health System	23	82	25	157	3	—	0	—	—	13
★ NAVAL HOSPITAL, 2080 Child Street, Zip 32214–5000; tel. 904/777–7300; Captain D. Vertrees Hollingsworth MSC, USN, Commanding Officer (Nonreporting) A1 3 5 S9655 Department of Navy	43	10	117	—	—	—	—	—	—	—
★ RIVERSIDE HOSPITAL, 2033 Riverside Avenue, Zip 32204; tel. 904/387–7000; Charles S. Kinney, Executive Vice President A1 9 10 F4 7 8 10 11 15 17 19 21 22 23 25 29 30 31 32 33 35 37 38 40 43 44 47 49 52 60 64 65 66 67 71 73 74 S1855 Daughters of Charity National Health System	23	10	108	3718	72	20994	0	28982	11204	364
★ SPECIALTY HOSPITAL JACKSONVILLE, (Long–term Acute Care) 4901 Richard Street, Zip 32207; tel. 904/737–3120; W. Raymond C. Ford, Administrator A1 9 10 F4 7 8 10 11 12 14 15 16 18 19 21 22 24 28 29 30 32 33 34 35 37 39 40 41 42 43 44 45 46 48 49 50 61 65 67 70 71 73 74 P3 7 8	33	49	25	337	19	0	0	11623	2165	68
★ ST. LUKE'S HOSPITAL, 4201 Belfort Road, Zip 32216; tel. 904/296–3700; J. Larry Read, President A1 3 5 8 9 10 F4 8 10 11 12 17 19 20 21 22 23 25 28 30 34 35 37 41 42 43 44 48 49 51 60 61 63 65 66 67 69 71 73 P3 6 S1875 Mayo Foundation	23	10	226	7141	129	45938	0	96267	33042	1249
★ ST. VINCENT'S MEDICAL CENTER, 1800 Barrs Street, Zip 32204, Mailing Address: P.O. Box 2982, Zip 32203–2982; tel. 904/387–7300; Everett M. Devaney, President (Total facility includes 34 beds in nursing home–type unit) A1 2 3 5 9 10 F4 7 8 10 11 14 15 16 17 19 20 21 22 23 28 29 30 31 32 33 34 35 37 39 40 41 42 43 44 45 48 49 52 54 56 57 59 60 64 65 67 71 72 73 P1 2 4 5 7 8 S1855 Daughters of Charity National Health System	21	10	528	18515	287	208501	2186	161356	64805	2298
★ UNIVERSITY MEDICAL CENTER, 655 West Eighth Street, Zip 32209; tel. 904/549–5000; John F. Gregg, President and Chief Executive Officer A1 2 3 5 8 9 10 F4 7 8 10 11 12 15 17 18 19 20 21 22 26 27 28 30 31 34 35 37 38 40 41 42 43 44 45 46 47 49 51 52 53 54 55 56 57 58 59 60 61 63 65 67 68 69 70 71 72 73 74 P7	23	10	500	17551	315	196321	3042	190369	68830	2366
JACKSONVILLE BEACH—Duval County										
★ BAPTIST MEDICAL CENTER–BEACHES, 1350 13th Avenue South, Zip 32250–3205; tel. 904/247–2900; Jerry L. Miller, Administrator A1 9 10 F8 11 12 19 21 22 28 30 32 33 35 37 41 42 44 45 49 54 56 63 69 71 73	23	10	76	2695	42	40622	0	23092	8640	397

Hospitals, U.S. / FLORIDA

Hospital, Address, Telephone, Administrator, Approval, Facility, and Physician Codes, Health Care System	Classification Codes		Utilization Data					Expense (thousands) of dollars		
★ American Hospital Association (AHA) membership □ Joint Commission on Accreditation of Healthcare Organizations (JCAHO) accreditation + American Osteopathic Hospital Association (AOHA) membership ○ American Osteopathic Association (AOA) accreditation △ Commission on Accreditation of Rehabilitation Facilities (CARF) accreditation Control codes 61, 63, 64, 71, 72 and 73 indicate hospitals listed by AOHA, but not registered by AHA. For definition of numerical codes, see page A6	Control	Service	Beds	Admissions	Census	Outpatient Visits	Births	Total	Payroll	Personnel
JASPER—Hamilton County HAMILTON MEMORIAL HOSPITAL, (Formerly Hamilton County Memorial Hospital) 506 Northwest Fourth Street, Zip 32052–1300, Mailing Address: Box 1300, Zip 32052–1300; tel. 904/792–2101; Amelia Tuten R.N., Administrator **A**9 10 **F**19 22 32 44 71 **S**0048 Columbia/HCA Healthcare Corporation	13	10	42	541	6	7048	0	4479	2310	103
JAY—Santa Rosa County JAY HOSPITAL, 221 South Alabama Street, Zip 32565; tel. 904/675–4532; William Allen Foster, Administrator (Nonreporting) **A**9 10 **S**0185 Baptist Health Care Corporation	23	10	36	—	—	—	—	—	—	—
JUPITER—Palm Beach County ★ JUPITER MEDICAL CENTER, 1210 South Old Dixie Highway, Zip 33458; tel. 407/747–2234; Donald A. Mayer, Chief Executive Officer (Total facility includes 120 beds in nursing home–type unit) **A**1 2 9 10 **F**8 19 21 22 31 34 35 37 44 65 71 73 **S**0002 Quorum Health Group/Quorum Health Resources	23	10	276	5954	204	34285	0	59939	24996	694
KEY WEST—Monroe County DE POO HOSPITAL See Lower Florida Keys Health System FLORIDA KEYS MEMORIAL HOSPITAL See Lower Florida Keys Health System ★ LOWER FLORIDA KEYS HEALTH SYSTEM, (Includes De Poo Hospital, 1200 Kennedy Drive, Key West, Florida, Zip 33041; tel. 305/294–4692; Florida Keys Memorial Hospital, 5900 College Road, Key West, Florida, Zip 33040; tel. 305/294–5531) 5900 College Road, Zip 33040, Mailing Address: P.O. Box 1119, Zip 33041; tel. 305/294–5531; James K. Simon FACHE, President and Chief Executive Officer **A**1 9 10 **F**1 2 3 6 7 8 11 13 14 15 16 17 18 19 20 21 22 26 27 28 29 30 31 32 33 35 36 39 40 41 42 44 45 46 49 51 52 53 55 56 57 58 59 61 63 64 65 66 67 68 69 71 73	23	10	169	4695	76	38411	690	31892	15790	425
KISSIMMEE—Osceola County □ CHARTER HOSPITAL ORLANDO SOUTH, 206 Park Place Drive, Zip 34741; tel. 407/846–0444; Michael L. Harrington, Group Chief Executive Officer (Nonreporting) **A**1 10 **S**0695 Charter Medical Corporation	33	22	60	—	—	—	—	—	—	—
FLORIDA HOSPITAL KISSIMMEE, 200 Hilda Street, Zip 34741–2301; tel. 407/933–6600; Eugene K. Wedel, Administrator (Nonreporting) **A**9 **S**4165 Adventist Health System–Sunbelt Health Care Corporation	33	10	120	—	—	—	—	—	—	—
★ OSCEOLA REGIONAL HOSPITAL, 700 West Oak Street, Zip 34741, Mailing Address: P.O. Box 422589, Zip 34742–2589; tel. 407/846–2266; Mark Aanonson, Chief Executive Officer (Nonreporting) **A**1 10 **S**0048 Columbia/HCA Healthcare Corporation	33	10	169	—	—	—	—	—	—	—
LAKE BUTLER—Union County NORTH FLORIDA RECEPTION CENTER HOSPITAL, Mailing Address: P.O. Box 628, Zip 32054; tel. 904/496–2222; Mikeal Eberhard, Administrator (Nonreporting)	12	11	153	—	—	—	—	—	—	—
LAKE CITY—Columbia County ★ LAKE CITY MEDICAL CENTER, 1701 West Duval Street, Zip 32055; tel. 904/752–2922; David P. Steitz, Chief Executive Officer (Total facility includes 5 beds in nursing home–type unit) **A**1 9 10 **F**8 15 16 19 22 23 27 31 32 33 34 35 37 41 44 45 49 52 54 55 63 64 65 71 73 **P**7 8 **S**0048 Columbia/HCA Healthcare Corporation	33	10	75	2732	45	30909	0	21187	8999	361
★ LAKE SHORE HOSPITAL, 560 East Franklin Street, Zip 32055, Mailing Address: Box 1989, Zip 32056–1989; tel. 904/755–3200; Linda A. McKnew R.N., Chief Operating Officer **A**1 9 10 **F**7 15 16 17 19 21 22 28 29 30 32 33 34 35 37 40 42 44 45 49 65 71 **P**5 **S**7895 AvMed–Santa Fe	23	10	60	2914	29	21405	305	19552	8024	249
★ VETERANS AFFAIRS MEDICAL CENTER, 801 South Marion Street, Zip 32025–5898; tel. 904/755–3016; Alline L. Norman, Director (Total facility includes 115 beds in nursing home–type unit) **A**1 3 5 **F**3 4 6 8 10 11 12 17 19 20 21 22 24 25 26 27 28 30 31 32 33 34 35 37 39 41 42 43 44 46 49 50 51 52 54 56 57 58 60 61 63 65 69 70 71 73 **P**5 **S**9295 Department of Veterans Affairs	45	10	387	5912	335	59544	0	57723	31806	728
LAKE WALES—Polk County ★ LAKE WALES MEDICAL CENTERS, 410 South 11th Street, Zip 33853, Mailing Address: P.O. Box 3460, Zip 33859–3460; tel. 813/676–1433; Joe M. Connell, Chief Executive Officer (Total facility includes 177 beds in nursing home–type unit) **A**1 9 10 **F**7 17 19 22 32 33 36 37 40 44 45 46 49 64 65 67 71 73 **P**6	23	10	260	2302	148	39835	127	18607	9641	401
LAKE WORTH—Palm Beach County ★ PALM BEACH REGIONAL HOSPITAL, 2829 Tenth Avenue North, Zip 33461; tel. 407/967–7800; Wayne Campbell, Chief Executive Officer **A**1 9 10 **F**7 8 10 12 14 15 19 22 23 28 30 35 37 40 41 44 46 49 51 64 65 71 73 **P**8 **S**0048 Columbia/HCA Healthcare Corporation	33	10	200	4617	68	46442	36	37169	13621	477
LAKELAND—Polk County ★ LAKELAND REGIONAL MEDICAL CENTER, 1324 Lakeland Hills Boulevard, Zip 33805–4543, Mailing Address: P.O. Box 95448, Zip 33804–5448; tel. 813/687–1100; Jack T. Stephens Jr., President and Chief Executive Officer **A**1 2 9 10 **F**3 4 7 10 11 12 13 14 15 16 17 18 19 21 22 23 26 29 30 31 34 37 39 40 42 43 44 45 46 49 51 52 53 54 55 56 57 58 59 60 65 66 67 71 72 73 74	23	10	633	23364	404	120786	2119	191440	86096	2473
□ PALMVIEW HOSPITAL, 2510 North Florida Avenue, Zip 33805; tel. 813/682–6105; Michael Terry, Administrator and Chief Executive Officer (Nonreporting) **A**1 10 **S**1775 Health Management Associates	33	22	66	—	—	—	—	—	—	—

© 1995 AHA Guide

Hospitals, U.S. / FLORIDA

Hospital, Address, Telephone, Administrator, Approval, Facility, and Physician Codes, Health Care System	Classification Codes		Utilization Data					Expense (thousands) of dollars		
★ American Hospital Association (AHA) membership □ Joint Commission on Accreditation of Healthcare Organizations (JCAHO) accreditation + American Osteopathic Hospital Association (AOHA) membership ○ American Osteopathic Association (AOA) accreditation △ Commission on Accreditation of Rehabilitation Facilities (CARF) accreditation Control codes 61, 63, 64, 71, 72 and 73 indicate hospitals listed by AOHA, but not registered by AHA. For definition of numerical codes, see page A6	Control	Service	Beds	Admissions	Census	Outpatient Visits	Births	Total	Payroll	Personnel
LANTANA—Palm Beach County										
A. G. HOLLEY STATE HOSPITAL, 1199 West Lantana Road, Zip 33462, Mailing Address: Box 3084, Zip 33465–3084; tel. 407/582–5666; Jorge A. Manas M.D., Executive Director **A**10 **F**2 14 15 20 27 31 45 54 65 **P**6	12	33	50	100	46	0	0	—	—	173
LARGO—Pinellas County										
□ CHARTER BEHAVIORAL HEALTH SYSTEM AT MEDFIELD, (Formerly Medfield Hospital) 12891 Seminole Boulevard, Zip 34648–2300; tel. 813/587–6000; Laura M. Schuck, Chief Executive Officer (Nonreporting) **A**1 9 10 **S**0695 Charter Medical Corporation	33	22	64	—	—	—	—	—	—	—
□ △ HEALTHSOUTH REHABILITATION HOSPITAL, 901 North Clearwater–Largo Rd, Zip 34640–1955; tel. 813/586–2999; Vincent O. Nico, Administrator (Nonreporting) **A**1 7 10 **S**0023 Healthsouth Corporation	33	46	40	—	—	—	—	—	—	—
★ LARGO MEDICAL CENTER, (Formerly Medical Center Hospital–Largo) 201 14th Street S.W., Zip 34640, Mailing Address: P.O. Box 2905, Zip 34649–2905; tel. 813/586–1411; Jon C. Trezona, Administrator **A**1 2 9 10 **F**4 8 10 11 12 14 15 16 17 19 21 22 24 28 30 32 34 35 37 41 42 43 44 45 49 51 55 63 65 67 71 **S**0048 Columbia/HCA Healthcare Corporation	33	10	256	9206	165	41124	0	56446	19928	676
MEDFIELD HOSPITAL See Charter Behavioral Health System at Medfield										
MEDICAL CENTER HOSPITAL–LARGO See Largo Medical Center										
+ ○ SUN COAST HOSPITAL, 2025 Indian Rocks Road, Zip 34644, Mailing Address: Box 2025, Zip 34649–2025; tel. 813/581–9474; Jeffrey A. Collins, Chief Executive Officer (Total facility includes 14 beds in nursing home–type unit) **A**2 9 10 11 12 13 **F**2 3 5 7 8 15 17 19 20 22 23 27 30 31 32 35 37 40 41 42 44 48 49 51 52 59 64 65 67 71 73 74	23	10	241	7454	138	73682	410	53259	23896	961
LECANTO—Citrus County										
□ HERITAGE BEVERLY HILLS HOSPITAL, 2804 West Marc Knighton Court, Zip 34461; tel. 904/746–9000; Charles Visalli, Administrator (Nonreporting) **A**1 10	33	22	88	—	—	—	—	—	—	—
LEESBURG—Lake County										
★ △ LEESBURG REGIONAL MEDICAL CENTER, 600 East Dixie Avenue, Zip 34748; tel. 904/323–5000; James R. Giffin, President and Chief Executive Officer (Total facility includes 120 beds in nursing home–type unit) **A**1 7 9 10 **F**7 8 10 12 14 15 19 21 22 23 24 25 26 28 30 32 33 35 37 40 41 42 44 46 48 49 60 63 64 65 71 72 73 **S**0002 Quorum Health Group/Quorum Health Resources	23	10	414	9737	257	58806	1147	67069	26906	992
LEHIGH ACRES—Lee County										
★ EAST POINTE HOSPITAL, 1500 Lee Boulevard, Zip 33936; tel. 813/369–2101; Valerie A. Jackson, Chief Executive Officer (Total facility includes 13 beds in nursing home–type unit) **A**1 9 10 **F**4 7 8 10 11 12 14 15 16 17 19 21 22 27 28 30 31 32 33 34 35 36 37 38 39 40 41 42 43 44 45 46 47 49 59 60 61 63 64 65 66 67 69 70 71 72 73 74 **P**8 **S**0048 Columbia/HCA Healthcare Corporation	33	10	75	2464	37	22756	235	15462	6432	—
LIVE OAK—Suwannee County										
★ SUWANNEE HOSPITAL, 1100 Southwest 11th Avenue, Zip 32060, Mailing Address: P.O. Drawer X, Zip 32060; tel. 904/362–1413; Rhonda Sherrod, Administrator (Nonreporting) **A**1 9 10 **S**7895 AvMed-Santa Fe	23	10	16	—	—	—	—	—	—	—
LONGWOOD—Seminole County										
★ SOUTH SEMINOLE HOSPITAL, 555 West State Road 434, Zip 32750; tel. 407/767–1200; Steve Grimm, Executive Director and Chief Executive Officer **A**1 **F**2 3 4 7 8 9 10 11 13 17 19 21 22 23 24 26 27 31 32 33 34 35 37 38 40 42 43 44 47 48 52 53 54 55 56 58 60 63 64 65 70 71 73 74 **P**5 **S**0048 Columbia/HCA Healthcare Corporation	32	10	206	5490	81	65887	805	38401	13430	452
LOXAHATCHEE—Palm Beach County										
★ PALMS WEST HOSPITAL, 13001 Southern Boulevard, Zip 33470–1150; tel. 305/798–3300; Paul M. Pugh, Chief Executive Officer **A**1 10 **F**7 8 10 12 14 15 16 17 19 21 22 23 26 27 28 29 30 31 32 34 35 37 39 40 41 42 44 45 46 49 56 64 65 66 67 71 73 74 **P**7 **S**0048 Columbia/HCA Healthcare Corporation	33	10	117	4117	45	19340	669	25931	10122	350
LUTZ—Hillsborough County										
□ CHARTER HOSPITAL OF PASCO, 21808 State Road 54, Zip 33549; tel. 813/948–2441; Miriam K. Williams, Administrator **A**1 10 **F**15 34 52 54 55 56 57 58 59 **S**0695 Charter Medical Corporation	33	22	72	1448	44	6723	0	—	—	97
MACCLENNY—Baker County										
ED FRASER MEMORIAL HOSPITAL, 159 North Third Street, Zip 32063–0484; tel. 904/259–3151; Dennis R. Markos, Chief Executive Officer (Nonreporting) **A**9 10	23	10	68	—	—	—	—	—	—	—
MACDILL AIR FORCE BASE—Hillsborough County										
★ U.S. AIR FORCE HOSPITAL, 8415 Bayshore Boulevard, Zip 33621–1607; tel. 813/828–3258; Colonel Roger H. Bower USAF, MC, Commander **F**7 8 19 20 22 24 27 28 29 30 31 34 35 37 39 40 41 44 46 49 51 59 65 67 71 73 **S**9495 Department of the Air Force	41	10	50	5398	31	332758	426	—	—	784
MADISON—Madison County										
MADISON COUNTY MEMORIAL HOSPITAL, 201 East Marion Street, Zip 32340; tel. 904/973–2271; Roberta Agner R.N., Interim Administrator (Nonreporting) **A**9 10	23	10	23	—	—	—	—	—	—	—
MARATHON—Monroe County										
□ FISHERMEN'S HOSPITAL, 3301 Overseas Highway, Zip 33050–0068; tel. 305/743–5533; Kevin Van Hoose, Administrator (Nonreporting) **A**1 9 10 **S**1775 Health Management Associates	33	10	58	—	—	—	—	—	—	—

Hospitals, U.S. / FLORIDA

Hospital, Address, Telephone, Administrator, Approval, Facility, and Physician Codes, Health Care System	Classification Codes		Utilization Data					Expense (thousands) of dollars		
★ American Hospital Association (AHA) membership □ Joint Commission on Accreditation of Healthcare Organizations (JCAHO) accreditation + American Osteopathic Hospital Association (AOHA) membership ○ American Osteopathic Association (AOA) accreditation △ Commission on Accreditation of Rehabilitation Facilities (CARF) accreditation Control codes 61, 63, 64, 71, 72 and 73 indicate hospitals listed by AOHA, but not registered by AHA. For definition of numerical codes, see page A6	Control	Service	Beds	Admissions	Census	Outpatient Visits	Births	Total	Payroll	Personnel

MARGATE—Broward County

★ NORTHWEST MEDICAL CENTER, (Formerly Northwest Regional Hospital) 2801 North State Road 7, Zip 33063, Mailing Address: P.O. Box 639002, Zip 33063–9002; tel. 305/978–4000; Kenneth H. Feiler, Chief Executive Officer **A**1 9 10 **F**1 2 3 4 5 6 7 8 9 10 11 12 13 15 17 18 19 20 21 22 23 24 25 26 27 28 29 30 31 32 33 34 35 36 37 38 39 40 41 42 43 44 45 46 47 48 49 50 51 52 53 54 55 56 57 58 59 60 61 62 63 64 65 66 67 68 69 70 71 72 73 74 **P**1 2 3 4 5 6 7 8 **S**0048 Columbia/HCA Healthcare Corporation	33	10	150	4742	71	24024	432	39716	15688	413

MARIANNA—Jackson County

★ JACKSON HOSPITAL, 4250 Hospital Drive, Zip 32446, Mailing Address: P.O. Box 1608, Zip 32447–1608; tel. 904/526–2200; Chuck Ellis, Administrator **A**1 9 10 **F**7 8 15 17 19 21 22 23 24 28 30 31 34 35 37 40 44 45 46 49 65 66 71 73 **P**3 **S**0002 Quorum Health Group/Quorum Health Resources	16	10	107	3490	49	37869	619	19761	7476	268

MELBOURNE—Brevard County

□ CIRCLES OF CARE, 400 East Sheridan Road, Zip 32901–3184; tel. 407/722–5200; James B. Whitaker, President **A**1 10 **F**1 2 3 12 14 15 16 17 18 25 27 41 52 53 54 55 56 57 58 59 65 67 68	23	22	72	3890	49	—	0	15354	9104	432
★ DEVEREUX HOSPITAL AND CHILDREN'S CENTER OF FLORIDA, 8000 Devereux Drive, Zip 32940–7907; tel. 407/242–9100; James E. Colvin, Administrator (Nonreporting) **S**0845 Devereux Foundation	23	52	100	—	—	—	—	—	—	—
□ △ HEALTHSOUTH SEA PINES REHABILITATION HOSPITAL, 101 East Florida Avenue, Zip 32901–9966; tel. 407/984–4600; Robert M. Smart, Administrator and Chief Executive Officer **A**1 7 10 **F**5 12 14 15 16 17 21 25 27 34 41 42 45 48 49 54 58 66 67 73 **S**0023 Healthsouth Corporation	32	46	80	1319	77	17484	0	18757	8131	238
★ HOLMES REGIONAL MEDICAL CENTER, 1350 South Hickory Street, Zip 32901; tel. 407/727–7000; Michael D. Means, President and Chief Executive Officer **A**1 2 9 10 **F**4 7 8 10 11 12 13 14 15 16 17 19 20 21 22 23 24 27 28 29 30 31 32 33 34 35 37 38 39 40 41 42 43 44 45 46 49 51 53 54 55 56 57 58 59 60 61 63 64 65 67 68 71 72 73 74	23	10	491	22826	340	211379	2320	172004	73801	2722

MIAMI—Dade County

★ AVENTURA HOSPITAL AND MEDICAL CENTER, 20900 Biscayne Boulevard, Zip 33180–1407; tel. 305/932–0250; Davide M. Carbone, Chief Executive Officer **A**10 **F**2 3 7 8 10 11 12 13 14 15 16 17 18 19 21 22 23 24 25 26 27 28 29 30 31 32 33 34 35 37 38 39 40 41 42 43 44 45 46 47 48 49 51 52 53 54 55 56 57 58 59 60 61 63 64 65 66 67 68 69 70 72 73 74 **S**0048 Columbia/HCA Healthcare Corporation	33	10	458	8517	136	44096	0	51157	21110	770
★ △ BAPTIST HOSPITAL OF MIAMI, 8900 North Kendall Drive, Zip 33176–2197; tel. 305/596–6503; Brian E. Keeley, President and Chief Executive Officer **A**1 2 3 7 9 10 **F**2 3 4 5 7 8 10 12 14 15 16 17 19 21 22 24 25 26 27 28 29 30 31 32 34 35 37 38 40 41 42 43 44 45 46 47 48 49 50 60 61 63 65 66 67 69 71 72 73 74 **P**1 6 7	23	10	429	21987	310	100270	3812	197201	82979	2560
★ BASCOM PALMER EYE INSTITUTE–ANNE BATES LEACH EYE HOSPITAL, 900 Northwest 17th Street, Zip 33136–1199, Mailing Address: Box 016880, Zip 33101–6880; tel. 305/326–6000; David Bixler, Administrator **A**1 3 5 9 10 **F**22 27 31 34 39 41 44 45 46 60 65 69 71 73 **P**6 **S**0002 Quorum Health Group/Quorum Health Resources	23	45	34	1406	7	117853	0	26140	11512	407
★ CEDARS MEDICAL CENTER, (Includes Victoria Pavilion, 955 Northwest Third Street, Miami, Florida, Zip 33128, Mailing Address: Box 016216, Flagler Station, Zip 33101; tel. 305/545–8050) 1400 Northwest 12th Avenue, Zip 33136–1003; tel. 305/325–5511; Ralph A. Aleman, Chief Executive Officer (Nonreporting) **A**1 2 3 5 10 **S**0048 Columbia/HCA Healthcare Corporation	23	10	885	—	—	—	—	—	—	—
□ CHARTER HOSPITAL OF MIAMI, 11100 Northwest 27th Street, Zip 33172; tel. 305/591–3230; Amanda Hopkins-Alexiadis, Chief Executive Officer **A**1 10 **F**1 2 3 15 16 18 52 53 55 56 57 58 59 65 **P**8 **S**0695 Charter Medical Corporation	33	22	88	1266	47	5878	0	7622	3945	89
★ DEERING HOSPITAL, 9333 Southwest 152nd Street, Zip 33157; tel. 305/251–2500; Anthony Degina, Chief Executive Officer **A**1 9 10 **F**7 8 10 11 12 14 15 16 19 21 22 23 27 28 31 33 34 35 37 39 40 42 44 45 46 49 52 53 55 56 57 58 59 60 65 67 71 73 74 **S**0048 Columbia/HCA Healthcare Corporation	32	10	233	4887	99	27545	170	—	—	616
□ GOLDEN GLADES REGIONAL MEDICAL CENTER, 17300 Northwest Seventh Avenue, Zip 33169; tel. 305/652–4200; Martha Garcia, Acting Chief Executive Officer (Nonreporting) **A**1 10 **S**6525 Ornda Healthcorp	33	10	128	—	—	—	—	—	—	—
★ GRANT CENTER OF DEERING HOSPITAL, 20601 Southwest 157th Avenue, Zip 33187, Mailing Address: Box 1159, Zip 33187–1159; tel. 305/251–0710; Anthony Degina, Chief Executive Officer (Nonreporting) **A**1 9 10 **S**0048 Columbia/HCA Healthcare Corporation	33	22	140	—	—	—	—	—	—	—
□ HARBOR VIEW, 1861 Northwest South River Drive, Zip 33125; tel. 305/642–3555; Nelson Rodney, Administrator (Nonreporting) **A**1 9 10	33	22	94	—	—	—	—	—	—	—
HIGHLAND PARK HOSPITAL See Jackson Memorial Hospital										
★ △ JACKSON MEMORIAL HOSPITAL, (Includes Highland Park Hospital, 1660 Northwest Seventh Court, Miami, Florida, Zip 33136; tel. 305/324–8111; Stuart Podolnick, Administrator) 1611 Northwest 12th Avenue, Zip 33136–1094; tel. 305/585–6754; Ira C. Clark, President **A**1 2 3 6 7 8 9 10 **F**1 2 3 4 5 7 8 9 10 11 12 14 15 16 17 18 19 20 21 22 23 24 25 26 27 28 29 30 31 32 33 34 35 37 38 39 40 41 42 43 44 45 46 47 48 49 51 52 53 54 55 56 57 58 59 60 61 65 66 69 70 71 72 73 74	13	10	1446	50827	1043	433698	7675	642253	282427	8674

© 1995 AHA Guide

Hospitals, U.S. / FLORIDA

Hospital, Address, Telephone, Administrator, Approval, Facility, and Physician Codes, Health Care System

★ American Hospital Association (AHA) membership
□ Joint Commission on Accreditation of Healthcare Organizations (JCAHO) accreditation
+ American Osteopathic Hospital Association (AOHA) membership
○ American Osteopathic Association (AOA) accreditation
△ Commission on Accreditation of Rehabilitation Facilities (CARF) accreditation

Control codes 61, 63, 64, 71, 72 and 73 indicate hospitals listed by AOHA, but not registered by AHA. For definition of numerical codes, see page A6

Hospital	Classification Codes		Utilization Data					Expense (thousands) of dollars		Personnel
	Control	Service	Beds	Admissions	Census	Outpatient Visits	Births	Total	Payroll	
★ KENDALL REGIONAL MEDICAL CENTER, 11750 Bird Road, Zip 33175–3530; tel. 305/223–3000; Victor Maya, Chief Executive Officer **A**1 10 **F**4 8 10 11 12 14 16 19 21 22 27 28 32 33 34 35 37 41 42 43 44 46 49 65 71 73 **S**0048 Columbia/HCA Healthcare Corporation	32	10	230	7884	139	35409	0	—	—	763
★ △ MERCY HOSPITAL, 3663 South Miami Avenue, Zip 33133–4237; tel. 305/854–4400; Edward J. Rosasco Jr., President **A**1 2 7 9 10 **F**3 4 5 7 8 10 11 12 14 15 16 17 18 19 21 22 23 25 26 27 28 29 30 31 32 33 34 35 37 38 39 40 41 42 43 44 46 48 49 50 52 54 55 57 58 59 60 61 63 64 65 66 67 68 69 71 72 73 74 **P**4 5 8	21	10	365	14983	271	115032	1934	140614	57136	1766
★ MIAMI CHILDREN'S HOSPITAL, 3100 Southwest 62nd Avenue, Zip 33155–3009; tel. 305/666–6511; William A. McDonald, President and Chief Executive Officer **A**1 3 5 10 **F**2 3 4 5 6 7 8 10 12 13 14 17 18 19 20 21 22 23 24 25 26 27 28 31 32 33 34 35 37 38 40 41 42 43 44 45 46 47 48 49 51 52 53 54 55 56 57 58 59 60 61 65 67 68 69 70 71 72 73 74 **P**1 7	23	50	225	9263	171	136561	0	148464	67332	2054
★ MIAMI HEART INSTITUTE, (Includes Miami Heart Institute – South, 250 63rd Street, Miami, Florida, Zip 33141; tel. 305/672–1111) 4701 Meridian Avenue, Zip 33140–2910; tel. 305/672–1111; Stephen Bernstein, Chief Executive Officer (Nonreporting) **A**1 9 10 **S**0048 Columbia/HCA Healthcare Corporation	33	10	531	—	—	—	—	—	—	—
MIAMI HEART INSTITUTE – SOUTH See Miami Heart Institute										
★ MIAMI JEWISH HOME AND HOSPITAL FOR AGED, (Gerontology) 5200 Northeast Second Avenue, Zip 33137–2706; tel. 305/751–8626; Terry Goodman, Executive Director (Total facility includes 462 beds in nursing home–type unit) **A**1 3 9 10 **F**1 6 12 15 16 17 20 25 26 27 32 33 39 45 46 49 53 54 55 56 57 58 64 65 67 73	23	49	494	547	381	7200	0	28686	15202	908
★ NORTH SHORE MEDICAL CENTER, 1100 Northwest 95th Street, Zip 33150–2098; tel. 305/835–6000; Don E. Friedewald, President **A**1 2 9 10 **F**1 3 5 6 7 8 9 10 11 12 13 14 15 16 17 18 19 22 23 24 25 26 27 28 29 30 31 32 33 34 35 37 38 39 40 41 42 43 44 45 46 47 48 49 50 51 52 53 54 55 56 57 58 59 60 61 62 63 64 65 66 67 68 69 70 71 72 73 74 **P**1 7	23	10	286	10950	157	79677	2380	80255	35624	1179
★ PAN AMERICAN HOSPITAL, 5959 Northwest Seventh Street, Zip 33126–3198; tel. 305/264–1000; Carolina Calderin, Chief Executive Officer **A**1 9 10 **F**3 4 7 8 10 11 12 14 15 16 17 19 20 22 27 28 30 32 33 34 35 37 41 42 43 44 45 46 49 54 59 60 61 63 65 71 73 74 **P**1 4 5 7	23	10	146	5655	111	20146	0	41348	19239	724
★ △ SOUTH MIAMI HOSPITAL, 6200 Southwest 73rd Street, Zip 33143–9990; tel. 305/661–4611; John Geanes, President and Chief Executive Officer **A**1 2 7 9 10 **F**2 3 4 7 8 10 11 14 17 19 21 22 26 27 28 29 30 31 32 33 34 37 38 40 41 42 43 44 45 46 48 49 60 62 63 64 66 71 72 73 74 **P**8	23	10	411	14205	193	114368	3698	119533	52290	1330
★ UNIVERSITY OF MIAMI HOSPITAL AND CLINICS, 1475 Northwest 12th Avenue, Zip 33136–1002; tel. 305/548–4382; David L. Stansberry, Administrator **A**1 3 5 9 10 **F**8 12 14 15 16 17 19 20 21 22 27 28 30 31 34 35 42 45 46 51 54 58 60 63 65 67 71 73 **P**1 **S**0002 Quorum Health Group/Quorum Health Resources	23	10	40	1109	21	116201	0	47226	12283	451
★ VETERANS AFFAIRS MEDICAL CENTER, 1201 Northwest 16th Street, Zip 33125–1624; tel. 305/324–4455; Thomas C. Doherty, Medical Director (Total facility includes 240 beds in nursing home–type unit) **A**1 3 5 8 **F**1 2 3 4 8 10 11 15 16 17 18 19 20 21 22 25 26 28 29 30 31 32 33 34 37 39 41 42 43 44 45 46 48 49 51 52 54 55 56 57 58 59 60 63 64 65 67 69 71 73 74 **S**9295 Department of Veterans Affairs	45	10	870	11721	658	396341	0	185925	98942	2584
VICTORIA PAVILION See Cedars Medical Center										
+ ○ WESTCHESTER GENERAL HOSPITAL, 2500 Southwest 75th Avenue, Zip 33155–9947; tel. 305/264–5252; Gilda Baldwin, Chief Administrative Officer (Nonreporting) **A**9 10 11 12 13	33	10	110	—	—	—	—	—	—	—
MIAMI BEACH—Dade County										
□ △ MOUNT SINAI MEDICAL CENTER, 4300 Alton Road, Zip 33140–2800; tel. 305/674–2121; Fred D. Hirt, President (Nonreporting) **A**1 2 3 5 7 8 9 10	23	10	585	—	—	—	—	—	—	—
★ SOUTH SHORE HOSPITAL AND MEDICAL CENTER, 630 Alton Road, Zip 33139; tel. 305/672–2100; William Zubkoff Ph.D., Chief Executive Officer **A**1 3 9 10 **F**14 15 16 17 19 21 22 26 27 29 31 32 33 34 37 41 44 45 46 49 52 57 59 65 71 72 73 **P**5	23	10	178	4066	137	12310	0	29484	13267	668
MILTON—Santa Rosa County										
★ SANTA ROSA MEDICAL CENTER, 1450 Berryhill Road, Zip 32570, Mailing Address: P.O. Box 648, Zip 32572; tel. 904/626–7762; Barbara H. Thames, Chief Executive Officer (Total facility includes 10 beds in nursing home–type unit) **A**1 9 10 **F**4 7 8 14 15 16 19 21 22 26 28 29 30 33 34 35 37 39 40 41 42 44 45 46 49 64 65 66 67 68 71 73 74 **P**7 8 **S**0048 Columbia/HCA Healthcare Corporation	33	10	129	3425	45	39618	519	21816	7456	325
NAPLES—Collier County										
★ NAPLES COMMUNITY HOSPITAL, 350 Seventh Street North, Zip 33940–5791, Mailing Address: P.O. Box 413029, Zip 33941–3029; tel. 813/436–5000; William G. Crone, President **A**1 2 7 9 10 **F**7 8 10 11 12 13 17 19 21 22 23 24 25 26 28 29 30 31 32 34 35 37 39 40 41 42 44 45 46 48 49 52 54 56 57 60 63 65 66 67 68 71 72 73 74	23	10	434	20030	301	178543	2340	153100	68797	2126
WILLOUGH AT NAPLES, 9001 Tamiami Trail East, Zip 33962–3316; tel. 813/775–4500; James G. Brown, Executive Director (Nonreporting) **A**10	33	22	64	—	—	—	—	—	—	—
NEW PORT RICHEY—Pasco County										
★ NEW PORT RICHEY HOSPITAL, 5637 Marine Parkway, Zip 34652, Mailing Address: Box 996, Zip 34656–0996; tel. 813/848–1733; Andrew Oravec Jr., Administrator (Nonreporting) **A**1 10 **S**0048 Columbia/HCA Healthcare Corporation	33	10	414	—	—	—	—	—	—	—

Hospitals, U.S. / FLORIDA

Hospital, Address, Telephone, Administrator, Approval, Facility, and Physician Codes, Health Care System	Classification Codes		Utilization Data					Expense (thousands) of dollars		
★ American Hospital Association (AHA) membership ☐ Joint Commission on Accreditation of Healthcare Organizations (JCAHO) accreditation + American Osteopathic Hospital Association (AOHA) membership ○ American Osteopathic Association (AOA) accreditation △ Commission on Accreditation of Rehabilitation Facilities (CARF) accreditation Control codes 61, 63, 64, 71, 72 and 73 indicate hospitals listed by AOHA, but not registered by AHA. For definition of numerical codes, see page A6	Control	Service	Beds	Admissions	Census	Outpatient Visits	Births	Total	Payroll	Personnel
☐ NORTH BAY MEDICAL CENTER, 6600 Madison Street, Zip 34652; tel. 813/842-8468; Michael G. Layfield, Administrator (Nonreporting) **A**1 10 **S**6525 Ornda Healthcorp	33	10	122	—	—	—	—	—	—	—
NEW SMYRNA BEACH—Volusia County										
★ BERT FISH MEDICAL CENTER, 401 Palmetto, Zip 32168; tel. 904/427-3401; James R. Foster, Administrator **A**1 9 10 **F**8 14 15 16 19 21 22 26 28 29 30 32 33 34 35 37 42 44 49 51 65 67 71 **P**7 **S**0002 Quorum Health Group/Quorum Health Resources	16	10	82	2890	43	111583	0	26388	10504	399
NICEVILLE—Okaloosa County										
★ TWIN CITIES HOSPITAL, 2190 Highway 85 North, Zip 32578; tel. 904/678-4131; David Whalen, Chief Executive Officer **A**1 10 **F**8 12 14 15 16 19 21 22 37 44 45 49 51 63 71 **S**0048 Columbia/HCA Healthcare Corporation	33	10	75	2016	30	22272	0	14404	5578	230
NORTH MIAMI—Dade County										
★ △ VILLA MARIA NURSING AND REHABILITATION CENTER, (Formerly Bon Secours Hospital) 1050 Northeast 125th Street, Zip 33161; tel. 305/891-8850; Sherry L. Brunner, Chief Executive Officer (Nonreporting) **A**1 7 9 10	21	46	272	—	—	—	—	—	—	—
NORTH MIAMI BEACH—Dade County										
☐ △ PARKWAY REGIONAL MEDICAL CENTER, 160 Northwest 170th Street, Zip 33169; tel. 305/654-5050; David S. Catlin, Chief Executive Officer (Nonreporting) **A**1 7 9 **S**6525 Ornda Healthcorp	32	10	299	—	—	—	—	—	—	—
OCALA—Marion County										
☐ CHARTER SPRINGS HOSPITAL, 3130 Southwest 27th Avenue, Zip 34474, Mailing Address: P.O. Box 3338, Zip 34478; tel. 904/237-7293; James Duff, Administrator **A**1 9 10 **F**1 2 3 6 12 13 17 18 26 29 30 49 52 53 54 55 56 57 58 59 65 67 68 **S**0695 Charter Medical Corporation	33	22	92	1136	39	—	0	—	—	111
★ MARION COMMUNITY HOSPITAL, 1431 Southwest First Avenue, Zip 34474, Mailing Address: Box 2200, Zip 34478-2200; tel. 904/732-2700; Terry Upton, Chief Executive Officer **A**1 2 9 10 **F**4 7 8 10 11 12 14 19 21 22 37 39 40 41 42 43 44 45 49 60 63 65 66 71 72 73 **P**8 **S**0048 Columbia/HCA Healthcare Corporation	33	10	230	8389	143	55055	188	70204	23421	863
★ MUNROE REGIONAL MEDICAL CENTER, 131 Southwest 15th Street, Zip 34474, Mailing Address: Box 6000, Zip 34478; tel. 904/351-7200; Dyer T. Michell, President **A**1 2 9 10 **F**4 7 8 10 11 14 15 16 19 21 22 23 24 26 28 29 30 31 32 33 34 35 37 39 40 41 43 44 46 49 51 65 66 71 72 73 74 **P**8	23	10	296	14037	208	79394	1980	102866	39559	1241
OCOEE—Orange County										
★ HEALTH CENTRAL, 10000 West Colonial Drive, Zip 34761, Mailing Address: P.O. Box 614007, Orlando Zip 32861-4007; tel. 407/296-1000; Richard M. Irwin Jr., President and Chief Executive Officer (Total facility includes 228 beds in nursing home-type unit) **A**1 9 10 **F**1 4 7 8 10 11 15 17 19 21 22 27 28 30 31 32 33 34 35 39 40 41 42 43 44 45 46 49 60 65 66 69 70 71 72 73 74	16	10	141	4149	42	31538	508	30473	10346	325
OKEECHOBEE—Okeechobee County										
★ RAULERSON HOSPITAL, 1796 Highway 441 North, Zip 34972, Mailing Address: Box 1307, Zip 34973-1307; tel. 813/763-2151; Frank Irby, Chief Executive Officer **A**1 9 10 **F**8 10 12 15 16 19 21 22 23 28 32 33 34 35 37 42 44 49 60 71 73 **S**0048 Columbia/HCA Healthcare Corporation	33	10	101	3517	55	38634	0	20769	9070	303
ORANGE PARK—Clay County										
★ ORANGE PARK MEDICAL CENTER, 2001 Kingsley Avenue, Zip 32073-5156; tel. 904/276-8500; Robert M. Krieger, Chief Executive Officer (Nonreporting) **A**1 9 10 **S**0048 Columbia/HCA Healthcare Corporation	33	10	224	—	—	—	—	—	—	—
ORLANDO—Orange County										
★ △ COLUMBIA PARK MEDICAL CENTER, (Formerly Lucerne Medical Center) 818 South Main Lane, Zip 32801-9964; tel. 407/649-6111; Roy C. Vinson, Chief Executive Officer (Nonreporting) **A**1 7 10 **S**0048 Columbia/HCA Healthcare Corporation	33	10	267	—	—	—	—	—	—	—
FLORIDA HOSPITAL EAST ORLANDO See Florida Hospital Medical Center										
★ ○ △ FLORIDA HOSPITAL MEDICAL CENTER, (Includes Florida Hospital East Orlando, 7727 Lake Underhill Drive, Orlando, Florida, Zip 32822; tel. 407/277-8110; Florida Hospital–Altamonte, 601 East Altamonte Drive, Altamonte Springs, Florida, Zip 32701; tel. 407/830-4321; Florida Hospital–Apopka, 201 North Park Avenue, Apopka, Florida, Zip 32703; tel. 305/889-2566) 601 East Rollins Street, Zip 32803-1489; tel. 407/896-6611; Thomas L. Werner, President **A**1 2 3 5 7 9 10 11 12 13 **F**2 4 7 8 10 11 12 14 15 16 17 19 21 22 23 26 29 30 31 32 34 35 37 38 39 40 41 42 43 44 45 46 47 48 49 50 51 52 53 54 55 56 57 60 63 64 65 67 69 71 73 74 **P**1 4 7 8 **S**4165 Adventist Health System–Sunbelt Health Care Corporation	21	10	1394	52408	829	346706	6663	522838	219701	7256
HOLIDAY HOSPITAL See Orlando Regional Medical Center										
☐ LAUREL OAKS HOSPITAL, 6601 Central Florida Parkway, Zip 32821; tel. 407/345-5000; Steve McCabe, Chief Executive Officer **A**1 9 **F**2 3 12 13 14 15 16 17 18 52 53 54 55 56 58 59 **S**0069 Behavioral Healthcare Corporation	33	22	80	368	38	193	0	6026	2750	124
LUCERNE MEDICAL CENTER See Columbia Park Medical Center										
★ NAVAL HOSPITAL, Zip 32813-8221; tel. 407/643-2477; (Nonreporting) **A**5 **S**9655 Department of Navy	43	10	143	—	—	—	—	—	—	—
ORANGE MEMORIAL HOSPITAL See Orlando Regional Medical Center										
★ ORLANDO REGIONAL MEDICAL CENTER, (Includes Holiday Hospital, Orlando, Florida; Orange Memorial Hospital, Orlando, Florida) 1414 Kuhl Avenue, Zip 32806-2093; tel. 407/841-5111; J. Gary Strack, President and Chief Executive Officer **A**1 2 3 5 8 9 10 **F**2 3 4 7 8 9 10 11 12 13 15 16 17 18 19 20 21 22 23 24 25 26 27 28 29 30 31 32 33 34 35 37 38 39 40 41 42 43 44 45 46 47 48 49 51 52 53 54 55 56 57 58 59 60 61 63 65 66 67 70 71 72 73 74 **P**2 5 7 **S**3355 Orlando Regional Healthcare System	23	10	790	36620	532	341905	6466	328689	152115	5406

Hospitals, U.S. / FLORIDA

Hospital, Address, Telephone, Administrator, Approval, Facility, and Physician Codes, Health Care System	Classification Codes		Utilization Data					Expense (thousands) of dollars		
AHA membership symbols legend	Control	Service	Beds	Admissions	Census	Outpatient Visits	Births	Total	Payroll	Personnel
☐ PRINCETON HOSPITAL, 1800 Mercy Drive, Zip 32808–5694; tel. 407/295–5151; Teresa B. Soderlund, President and Chief Executive Officer **A**1 10 **F**7 8 10 11 12 15 19 21 22 23 26 28 30 31 33 34 35 37 39 40 42 44 49 52 54 55 56 57 59 61 65 67 71 73 74 **P**8	23	10	150	3918	61	28529	587	34983	10190	401
ORMOND BEACH—Volusia County										
✦ MEMORIAL HOSPITAL–ORMOND BEACH, 875 Sterthaus Avenue, Zip 32174–5197; tel. 904/676–6000; Clark P. Christianson, Senior Vice President and Administrator (Nonreporting) **A**1 9 10 **S**2615 Memorial Health Systems	23	10	205	—	—	—	—	—	—	—
☐ ○ PENINSULA MEDICAL CENTER, 264 South Atlantic Avenue, Zip 32176–8192; tel. 904/672–4161; Peter A. Marmerstein, Chief Executive Officer **A**1 10 11 12 13 **F**8 11 12 14 16 17 19 21 22 26 28 29 30 32 34 35 37 39 44 45 46 48 49 63 64 65 71 73 **S**5765 Paracelsus Healthcare Corporation	33	10	119	3007	63	21622	0	—	—	329
PAHOKEE—Palm Beach County										
☐ EVERGLADES REGIONAL MEDICAL CENTER, 200 South Barfield Highway, Zip 33476–1897; tel. 407/924–5200; Donald A. Anderson, President and Chief Executive Officer (Nonreporting) **A**1 9 10 **S**0585 Brim, Inc.	23	10	63	—	—	—	—	—	—	—
PALATKA—Putnam County										
✦ PUTNAM COMMUNITY HOSPITAL, Highway 20 West, Zip 32177, Mailing Address: P.O. Box 778, Zip 32178–0778; tel. 904/328–5711; Rick Palombo, Chief Executive Officer **A**1 9 10 **F**7 8 10 12 14 15 16 19 21 22 25 28 29 30 32 35 37 41 42 44 45 46 49 52 54 55 56 57 59 60 63 64 65 70 71 73 **P**8 **S**0048 Columbia/HCA Healthcare Corporation	33	10	161	6052	89	0	491	—	—	525
PALM BAY—Brevard County										
☐ CPC PALM BAY HOSPITAL, 4400 Dixie Highway N.E., Zip 32905–4396; tel. 407/729–0500; Harold G. Marohn, Administrator (Nonreporting) **A**1 9 **S**0785 Community Psychiatric Centers	33	22	60	—	—	—	—	—	—	—
PALM BEACH GARDENS—Palm Beach County										
✦ PALM BEACH GARDENS MEDICAL CENTER, (Formerly AMI Palm Beach Gardens Medical Center) 3360 Burns Road, Zip 33410–4304; tel. 407/622–1411; Thomas G. Hennessy, Chief Executive Officer **A**1 9 10 **F**4 7 10 12 14 19 21 22 23 28 31 34 35 36 37 38 39 40 41 43 44 45 46 49 63 65 67 71 73 74 **P**8 **S**0063 TENET Healthcare Corporation	33	10	189	7794	128	35527	663	73030	24456	745
PANAMA CITY—Bay County										
✦ BAY MEDICAL CENTER, 615 North Bonita Avenue, Zip 32401–2515, Mailing Address: P.O. Box 2515, Zip 32402; tel. 904/769–1511; Ronald V. Wolff, President and Chief Executive Officer **A**1 9 10 **F**4 7 8 10 17 19 21 22 25 27 31 32 33 34 35 37 40 41 42 43 44 46 48 49 52 60 63 64 65 71 73	13	10	353	11692	216	94369	707	95185	38416	1428
✦ GULF COAST HOSPITAL, 449 West 23rd Street, Zip 32405, Mailing Address: P.O. Box 15309, Zip 32406–5309; tel. 904/769–8341; Donald E. Butts, Chief Executive Officer **A**1 9 10 **F**7 8 10 11 12 17 19 21 22 23 24 28 29 35 37 39 40 42 44 46 49 63 65 71 73 74 **S**0048 Columbia/HCA Healthcare Corporation	33	10	176	6735	91	70511	1282	—	—	627
✦ U.S. AIR FORCE HOSPITAL, Tyndall Air Force Base, Zip 32403–5300; tel. 904/283–7515; Colonel Forrest Giles MSC, USAF, Commander **A**1 **F**7 8 12 17 18 19 20 24 25 28 29 30 34 39 41 44 45 46 49 51 52 54 55 56 58 60 65 71 72 73 74 **P**6 **S**9495 Department of the Air Force	41	10	25	1982	17	161758	414	—	—	465
PATRICK AIR FORCE BASE—Citrus County										
★ U.S. AIR FORCE HOSPITAL, 1381 South Patrick Drive, Zip 32925–3606; tel. 407/494–8102; Colonel William Trent MSC, Commanding Officer **F**8 13 15 17 20 22 28 29 30 31 39 41 44 51 56 58 65 71 **S**9495 Department of the Air Force	41	10	15	1263	8	136151	0	13269	3060	87
PEMBROKE PINES—Broward County										
✦ MEMORIAL HOSPITAL PEMBROKE, (Formerly Pembroke Pines Hospital) 2301 University Drive, Zip 33024; tel. 305/962–9650; J. E. Piriz, Administrator **A**1 9 10 12 **F**1 2 3 4 5 6 7 8 10 12 13 14 15 16 17 18 19 20 21 22 23 24 25 26 27 28 29 30 31 32 33 34 35 37 38 39 40 41 42 43 44 45 46 47 48 49 50 52 53 54 55 56 57 58 59 60 61 63 64 65 66 67 68 69 70 71 72 73 74 **P**7 **S**0048 Columbia/HCA Healthcare Corporation	33	10	301	4265	61	17230	0	29914	12695	465
★ MEMORIAL HOSPITAL WEST, 703 North Flamingo Road, Zip 33028; tel. 305/436–5000; Zeff Ross, Administrator **A**10 **F**1 2 3 4 7 8 9 10 11 12 13 14 15 16 17 18 19 20 21 22 23 24 25 26 27 28 29 30 31 32 33 34 35 36 37 38 39 40 41 42 43 44 47 48 49 50 51 52 53 54 55 56 57 58 59 60 61 63 64 65 66 67 68 69 70 71 72 73 74 **P**1 3 7	16	10	100	6475	71	75854	2050	42758	18106	456
PEMBROKE PINES HOSPITAL See Memorial Hospital Pembroke										
SOUTH FLORIDA STATE HOSPITAL, 1000 Southwest 84th Avenue, Zip 33025; tel. 305/967–7000; Anne M. Brennan, Administrator (Nonreporting) **A**10	12	22	355	—	—	—	—	—	—	—
PENSACOLA—Escambia County										
✦ BAPTIST HOSPITAL, 1000 West Moreno, Zip 32501–2393, Mailing Address: P.O. Box 17500, Zip 32522–7500; tel. 904/434–4011; Alfred G. Stubblefield, Senior Vice President and Administrator (Total facility includes 62 beds in nursing home–type unit) **A**1 2 9 10 **F**2 3 4 7 8 10 12 14 15 16 17 18 19 22 23 25 26 27 28 29 30 31 32 34 35 37 40 41 42 44 45 46 49 51 52 53 54 55 57 58 59 60 61 62 63 64 65 67 68 71 72 73 74 **P**4 5 7 **S**0185 Baptist Health Care Corporation	23	10	546	13796	275	115518	1372	106602	38801	1567
✦ NAVAL HOSPITAL, 6000 West Highway 98, Zip 32512–0003; tel. 904/452–6611; Commander H. M. Chinnery, Director, Administration (Nonreporting) **A**1 3 5 **S**9655 Department of Navy	43	10	104	—	—	—	—	—	—	—
REHABILITATION INSTITUTE OF WEST FLORIDA See West Florida Regional Medical Center										

Hospitals, U.S. / FLORIDA

Hospital, Address, Telephone, Administrator, Approval, Facility, and Physician Codes, Health Care System	Classification Codes		Utilization Data					Expense (thousands) of dollars		
★ American Hospital Association (AHA) membership □ Joint Commission on Accreditation of Healthcare Organizations (JCAHO) accreditation + American Osteopathic Hospital Association (AOHA) membership ○ American Osteopathic Association (AOA) accreditation △ Commission on Accreditation of Rehabilitation Facilities (CARF) accreditation Control codes 61, 63, 64, 71, 72 and 73 indicate hospitals listed by AOHA, but not registered by AHA. For definition of numerical codes, see page A6	Control	Service	Beds	Admissions	Census	Outpatient Visits	Births	Total	Payroll	Personnel
★ SACRED HEART HOSPITAL OF PENSACOLA, 5151 North Ninth Avenue, Zip 32504, Mailing Address: P.O. Box 2700, Zip 32513–2700; tel. 904/474–7000; Sister Irene Kraus, President and Chief Executive Officer (Total facility includes 89 beds in nursing home–type unit) **A**1 2 3 5 9 10 **F**4 7 8 10 11 12 13 15 16 17 19 21 22 23 24 25 27 28 30 32 34 35 37 38 40 42 43 44 45 46 47 49 51 53 60 63 65 67 71 72 73 74 **P**7 **S**1855 Daughters of Charity National Health System	21	10	391	18762	282	299850	2321	131630	59694	1983
WEST FLORIDA HOSPITAL See West Florida Regional Medical Center										
★ △ WEST FLORIDA REGIONAL MEDICAL CENTER, (Includes Rehabilitation Institute of West Florida, 8383 North Davis Highway, Florida, Zip 32514, Mailing Address: P.O. Box 18900, Zip 32523; tel. 904/494–6000; The Pavilion; tel. 904/494–5000; West Florida Hospital; tel. 904/478–4460; John Kausch, Administrator) 8383 North Davis Highway, Zip 32514, Mailing Address: P.O. Box 18900, Zip 32523–8900; tel. 904/494–4000; John Kausch, Chief Executive Officer (Total facility includes 19 beds in nursing home–type unit) **A**1 2 7 9 10 **F**2 3 4 7 8 10 11 12 14 16 17 19 21 23 24 26 27 28 29 30 32 35 36 37 39 40 41 42 43 44 45 48 49 52 53 54 56 57 58 59 60 63 64 65 66 67 70 71 73 74 **S**0048 Columbia/HCA Healthcare Corporation	33	10	547	12760	265	130791	833	100052	40862	1513
PERRY—Taylor County										
DOCTOR'S MEMORIAL HOSPITAL, 407 East Ash Street, Zip 32347, Mailing Address: P.O. Box 1847, Zip 32347–1847; tel. 904/584–0800; Thomas O. Logue Jr. Ph.D., Administrator and Chief Executive Officer (Nonreporting) **A**9 10	23	10	44							
PINELLAS PARK—Hillsborough County										
○ PINELLAS COMMUNITY HOSPITAL, (Formerly Metropolitan General Hospital) 7950 66th Street North, Zip 34665–2105, Mailing Address: Box 30, Zip 34665–0030; tel. 813/546–9871; Emil Miller, Administrator and Chief Executive Officer **A**9 10 11 12 13 **F**2 3 4 7 8 10 12 16 19 21 22 27 30 31 32 33 34 35 37 42 44 46 49 57 58 59 61 65 69 71 73 74 **P**8	33	10	98	2536	43	15708	0	18986	7010	261
PLANT CITY—Hillsborough County										
★ SOUTH FLORIDA BAPTIST HOSPITAL, 301 North Alexander Street, Zip 33566–9058, Mailing Address: Drawer H, Zip 33564–9058; tel. 813/757–1200; William H. Anderson, Administrator and Chief Executive Officer (Total facility includes 15 beds in nursing home–type unit) **A**1 9 10 **F**4 7 8 10 11 14 15 16 17 19 21 22 23 25 28 30 31 32 35 37 38 40 41 42 43 44 47 49 50 52 53 56 58 60 63 64 65 70 71 72 74 **P**8	23	10	100	4098	55	—	443	—	—	480
PLANTATION—Broward County										
★ PLANTATION GENERAL HOSPITAL, 401 Northwest 42nd Avenue, Zip 33317–2882; tel. 305/587–5010 **A**1 9 10 **F**4 7 8 10 11 12 14 15 16 17 19 21 22 23 28 29 30 34 35 37 38 39 40 41 44 45 46 47 48 49 61 65 67 71 73 74 **P**1 7 **S**0048 Columbia/HCA Healthcare Corporation	33	10	264	9234	124	52251	2886	71095	22715	573
□ ○ UNIVERSAL MEDICAL CENTER, 6701 West Sunrise Boulevard, Zip 33313; tel. 305/581–7800; Gregory E. Boyer, Administrator **A**1 10 11 12 **F**4 8 11 12 15 16 18 19 22 23 27 28 29 30 33 34 35 37 41 42 43 44 45 46 49 50 56 60 65 66 67 71 73 **S**9555 Universal Health Services, Inc.	33	10	80	3185	43	20479	0	22645	11264	320
★ WESTSIDE REGIONAL MEDICAL CENTER, 8201 West Broward Boulevard, Zip 33324–9937; tel. 305/473–6600; David E. Bussone, Chief Executive Officer **A**1 10 **F**2 3 4 5 7 8 10 11 12 13 15 16 17 19 20 21 22 23 25 26 27 28 31 32 33 34 35 37 38 39 40 41 42 43 44 45 47 48 49 51 52 53 54 55 56 57 58 59 60 61 64 65 66 67 68 71 72 73 74 **P**4 5 8 **S**0048 Columbia/HCA Healthcare Corporation	33	10	204	9659	111	57982	1422	54013	20185	624
POMPANO BEACH—Broward County										
★ △ NORTH BROWARD MEDICAL CENTER, 201 Sample Road, Zip 33064–3502; tel. 305/941–8300; James R. Chromik, Administrator **A**1 7 9 10 **F**3 4 7 8 10 11 12 13 15 16 17 18 19 21 22 23 24 26 27 28 29 30 31 32 33 34 35 37 39 41 42 43 44 45 46 48 49 50 51 53 54 55 56 57 58 59 60 61 63 65 66 67 68 70 71 72 73 **P**3 **S**3115 North Broward Hospital District	16	10	316	9799	195	—	0	98349	45426	962
★ POMPANO BEACH MEDICAL CENTER, 600 Southwest Third Street, Zip 33060–6979; tel. 305/782–2000; Heather J. Rohan, Chief Executive Officer **A**1 10 **F**8 10 11 12 14 15 16 17 19 21 22 23 27 28 29 30 31 32 33 34 35 37 39 41 42 44 45 46 49 61 63 65 67 71 72 73 74 **P**2 **S**0048 Columbia/HCA Healthcare Corporation	33	10	273	5844	82	32836	0	35949	15656	504
PORT CHARLOTTE—Charlotte County										
★ BON SECOURS–ST. JOSEPH HOSPITAL, 2500 Harbor Boulevard, Zip 33952–5396; tel. 813/625–4122; Kevin T. Potter, Chief Executive Officer (Total facility includes 104 beds in nursing home–type unit) **A**1 10 **F**4 7 8 10 15 17 18 19 21 22 24 26 27 28 29 30 31 32 34 35 37 39 40 41 42 44 45 46 49 56 61 63 64 65 67 71 73 74 **P**8 **S**5085 Bon Secours Health System, Inc.	21	10	216	8013	211	47004	1006	51838	17666	578
★ △ FAWCETT MEMORIAL HOSPITAL, 21298 Olean Boulevard, Zip 33952–6765; tel. 813/629–1181; Ward Boston, Chief Executive Officer (Total facility includes 8 beds in nursing home–type unit) **A**1 7 10 **F**5 8 10 12 15 16 19 21 22 23 25 26 27 28 29 30 32 34 35 37 39 42 44 45 46 48 49 59 60 64 65 66 71 73 **P**8 **S**0048 Columbia/HCA Healthcare Corporation	33	10	249	6321	111	42149	0	63807	24157	925
PORT SAINT JOE—Gulf County										
GULF PINES HOSPITAL, 102 20th Street, Zip 32456, Mailing Address: P.O. Box 40, Zip 32456; tel. 904/227–1121; Brian Upton, Chief Executive Officer (Nonreporting) **A**9 10	33	10	45	—	—	—	—	—	—	—

Hospitals, U.S. / FLORIDA

Hospital, Address, Telephone, Administrator, Approval, Facility, and Physician Codes, Health Care System

- ★ American Hospital Association (AHA) membership
- ☐ Joint Commission on Accreditation of Healthcare Organizations (JCAHO) accreditation
- + American Osteopathic Hospital Association (AOHA) membership
- ⊙ American Osteopathic Association (AOA) accreditation
- △ Commission on Accreditation of Rehabilitation Facilities (CARF) accreditation

Control codes 61, 63, 64, 71, 72 and 73 indicate hospitals listed by AOHA, but not registered by AHA. For definition of numerical codes, see page A6.

Classification Codes		Utilization Data					Expense (thousands) of dollars		
Control	Service	Beds	Admissions	Census	Outpatient Visits	Births	Total	Payroll	Personnel

PORT SAINT LUCIE—St. Lucie County

★ MEDICAL CENTER OF PORT ST. LUCIE, 1800 Southeast Tiffany Avenue, Zip 34952–7580; tel. 407/335–4000; Michael P. Joyce, Chief Executive Officer (Nonreporting) **A**1 9 10 **S**0048 Columbia/HCA Healthcare Corporation — 33, 10, 150, —, —, —, —, —, —, —

☐ SAVANNAS HOSPITAL, 2550 Southeast Walton Road, Zip 34952; tel. 407/335–0400; Patricia W. Brown, Executive Director (Nonreporting) **A**1 10 — 33, 22, 70, —, —, —, —, —, —, —

PUNTA GORDA—Charlotte County

★ CHARLOTTE REGIONAL MEDICAL CENTER, (Formerly Medical Center Hospital) 809 East Marion Avenue, Zip 33950–3898; tel. 813/637–3128; William Heburn, Executive Director (Nonreporting) **A**1 9 10 — 21, 10, 148, —, —, —, —, —, —, —

QUINCY—Gadsden County

GADSDEN MEMORIAL HOSPITAL, 418 North Ninth Street, Zip 32353, Mailing Address: P.O. Box 819, Zip 32353; tel. 904/875–1100; Jon Hufstedler, Administrator (Nonreporting) **A**9 10 — 23, 10, 51, —, —, —, —, —, —, —

ROCKLEDGE—Brevard County

☐ WUESTHOFF HOSPITAL, 110 Longwood Avenue, Zip 32955, Mailing Address: P.O. Box 565002, Mail Stop 1, Zip 32956–5002; tel. 407/636–2211; Robert O. Carman, President **A**1 2 9 10 **F**1 3 4 7 8 10 11 12 14 15 19 21 22 23 24 26 28 29 30 32 33 34 35 37 39 40 41 42 43 44 45 46 49 52 53 54 55 57 58 63 65 66 67 71 73 74 — 23, 10, 241, 10214, 158, 105123, 931, 87090, 41060, 1320

SAFETY HARBOR—Pinellas County

MEASE COUNTRYSIDE HOSPITAL, 3231 McMullen–Booth Road, Zip 34695–1098, Mailing Address: P.O. 1098, Zip 34695–1098; tel. 813/725–6222; James A. Pfeiffer, Chief Administrative Officer **A**10 **F**8 10 12 15 17 19 21 22 26 28 29 30 31 32 34 35 37 39 41 42 44 45 46 49 63 65 66 67 71 73 **P**8 **S**1335 Mease Health Care — 23, 10, 100, 5615, 81, —, 0, 34276, 13318, 379

SAINT AUGUSTINE—St. Johns County

★ FLAGLER HOSPITAL, (Includes Flagler Hospital–West, 1955 U.S. 1 South, Saint Augustine, Florida, Zip 32086; tel. 904/826–4700) 400 Health Park Boulevard, Zip 32086; tel. 904/825–4400; James D. Conzemius, President **A**1 10 **F**7 10 19 21 22 28 30 32 34 35 37 40 44 49 63 65 71 73 **P**3 — 23, 10, 230, 6928, 113, 79508, 1216, 50587, 20956, 637

☐ ST. AUGUSTINE PSYCHIATRIC CENTER, 200 River Haven Way, Zip 32086; tel. 904/824–9800; Greg Steele, Administrator (Nonreporting) **A**1 10 **S**2635 First Hospital Corporation — 33, 22, 50, —, —, —, —, —, —, —

SAINT CLOUD—Lowndes County

★ ST. CLOUD HOSPITAL, A DIVISION OF ORLANDO REGIONAL HEALTHCARE SYSTEM, 2906 17th Street, Zip 34769–6099; tel. 407/892–2135; Jim Norris, Executive Director **A**1 9 10 **F**4 7 8 9 10 11 12 13 14 15 16 17 18 19 20 21 22 23 24 25 26 27 28 29 30 31 32 33 34 35 37 38 39 40 41 42 43 44 45 46 47 48 49 51 52 53 54 55 56 57 58 59 60 61 63 65 66 67 70 71 72 73 74 **S**3355 Orlando Regional Healthcare System — 23, 10, 68, 3043, 41, 31485, 0, 17171, 8206, —

SAINT PETERSBURG—Pinellas County

★ ALL CHILDREN'S HOSPITAL, 801 Sixth Street South, Saint Petersburg, Zip 33701–4899; tel. 813/898–7451; J. Dennis Sexton, President **A**1 3 5 8 9 10 **F**4 10 12 13 14 15 16 17 19 20 22 24 25 27 28 30 31 34 35 37 38 39 41 42 43 44 45 49 51 65 67 69 71 73 — 23, 50, 168, 6321, 130, 51196, 0, 107463, 48226, 1463

★ △ BAYFRONT MEDICAL CENTER, 701 Sixth Street South, Saint Petersburg, Zip 33701–4891; tel. 813/823–1234; Sue G. Brody, President (Nonreporting) **A**1 2 5 7 9 10 — 23, 10, 409, —, —, —, —, —, —, —

★ EDWARD WHITE HOSPITAL, 2323 Ninth Avenue North, Saint Petersburg, Zip 33713, Mailing Address: P.O. Box 12018, Zip 33733–2018; tel. 813/323–1111; Lindell W. Orr, Chief Executive Officer **A**1 9 10 **F**4 5 8 10 12 14 19 22 24 28 30 32 34 35 37 41 42 44 49 64 65 66 71 72 **P**7 8 **S**0048 Columbia/HCA Healthcare Corporation — 33, 10, 167, 3881, 70, 56219, 0, 31167, 11847, 380

GULF COAST HOSPITAL AND ORTHOPEDIC INSTITUTE See Physicians Community Hospital

★ NORTHSIDE HOSPITAL, 6000 49th Street North, Saint Petersburg, Zip 33709; tel. 813/521–4411; Bradley K. Grover Sr., Chief Executive Officer **A**1 10 **F**10 11 12 16 17 19 20 22 23 26 28 29 30 31 32 35 37 39 41 42 44 49 65 71 73 **P**5 7 **S**0048 Columbia/HCA Healthcare Corporation — 33, 10, 301, 5575, 111, 0, 0, —, —, 574

☐ PALMS OF PASADENA HOSPITAL, 1501 Pasadena Avenue South, Saint Petersburg, Zip 33707; tel. 813/381–1000; Daniel J. Bonk, Interim Chief Executive Officer **A**1 9 10 **F**4 8 10 11 12 15 17 19 20 21 22 23 26 27 28 29 30 32 34 35 37 39 41 42 44 45 46 49 51 60 63 65 66 67 71 73 **P**5 7 **S**0063 TENET Healthcare Corporation — 33, 10, 276, 7601, 142, 109241, 0, 62463, 24394, 789

☐ PHYSICIANS COMMUNITY HOSPITAL, (Formerly Gulf Coast Hospital and Orthopedic Institute) 3030 6th Street South, Saint Petersburg, Zip 33705; tel. 813/823–1122 **A**1 **F**8 10 14 15 16 17 19 22 25 27 28 30 32 33 35 36 37 39 41 43 44 46 58 59 65 67 71 73 **P**5 — 12, 10, 30, 848, 15, 7965, 0, 8766, 4078, 85

★ ST. ANTHONY'S HOSPITAL, 1200 Seventh Avenue North, Saint Petersburg, Zip 33705, Mailing Address: P.O. Box 12588, Zip 33733; tel. 813/825–1100; Revonda L. Shumaker R.N., President (Total facility includes 30 beds in nursing home–type unit) **A**1 2 9 10 **F**2 7 8 10 11 12 16 17 18 19 20 21 22 24 25 28 29 30 31 32 33 34 35 37 38 39 40 41 42 43 44 45 46 48 49 52 54 55 56 57 58 60 63 64 65 66 67 70 71 72 73 74 **P**1 5 7 **S**1385 Allegany Health System — 21, 10, 279, 9810, 178, 242486, 401, 93975, 35433, 1200

Hospitals, U.S. / FLORIDA

Hospital, Address, Telephone, Administrator, Approval, Facility, and Physician Codes, Health Care System

★ American Hospital Association (AHA) membership
☐ Joint Commission on Accreditation of Healthcare Organizations (JCAHO) accreditation
+ American Osteopathic Hospital Association (AOHA) membership
○ American Osteopathic Association (AOA) accreditation
△ Commission on Accreditation of Rehabilitation Facilities (CARF) accreditation
Control codes 61, 63, 64, 71, 72 and 73 indicate hospitals listed by AOHA, but not registered by AHA. For definition of numerical codes, see page A6

Hospital	Control	Service	Beds	Admissions	Census	Outpatient Visits	Births	Total	Payroll	Personnel
✠ ST. PETERSBURG GENERAL HOSPITAL, 6500 38th Avenue North, Saint Petersburg, Zip 33710; tel. 813/384-1414; Thomas L. Herron, Chief Executive Officer (Nonreporting) A1 9 10 S0048 Columbia/HCA Healthcare Corporation	33	10	219	—	—	—	—	—	—	—
SANFORD—Seminole County										
✠ CENTRAL FLORIDA REGIONAL HOSPITAL, 1401 West Seminole Boulevard, Zip 32771-6764; tel. 407/321-4500; Doug Sills, President and Chief Executive Officer (Nonreporting) A1 9 10 S0048 Columbia/HCA Healthcare Corporation	33	10	226	—	—	—	—	—	—	—
SARASOTA—Sarasota County										
✠ DOCTORS HOSPITAL OF SARASOTA, 5731 Bee Ridge Road, Zip 34233; tel. 813/342-1100; William C. Lievense, Chief Executive Officer (Nonreporting) A1 9 10 S0048 Columbia/HCA Healthcare Corporation	32	10	168	—	—	—	—	—	—	—
☐ △ HEALTHSOUTH REHABILITATION INSTITUTE OF SARASOTA, 3251 Proctor Road, Zip 34231-8538; tel. 813/921-8600; Jeff Garber, Administrator and Chief Executive Officer (Nonreporting) A1 7 10 S0023 Healthsouth Corporation	33	46	60	—	—	—	—	—	—	—
✠ △ SARASOTA MEMORIAL HOSPITAL, 1700 South Tamiami Trail, Zip 34239-3555; tel. 813/917-1300; Michael H. Covert FACHE, President and Chief Executive Officer (Nonreporting) A1 2 5 7 9 10	16	10	807	—	—	—	—	—	—	—
SEBASTIAN—Indian River County										
☐ SEBASTIAN RIVER MEDICAL CENTER, 13695 North U.S. Hwy 1, Zip 32958, Mailing Address: Box 780838, Zip 32978; tel. 407/589-3186; David McCormack, Executive Director A1 9 10 F2 7 8 12 14 15 16 17 19 21 22 25 27 28 30 34 37 39 40 41 42 44 49 60 65 71 72 73 74 P7 8 S1775 Health Management Associates	33	10	133	2682	48	24740	32	19440	8092	288
SEBRING—Highlands County										
☐ HIGHLANDS REGIONAL MEDICAL CENTER, 3600 South Highlands Avenue, Zip 33870-5495, Mailing Address: Drawer 2066, Zip 33871-2066; tel. 813/385-6101; C. Scott Campbell, Executive Director (Nonreporting) A1 9 10 S1775 Health Management Associates	33	10	126	—	—	—	—	—	—	—
SEMINOLE—Pasco County										
☐ ○ UNIVERSITY GENERAL HOSPITAL, 10200 Seminole Boulevard, Zip 34642-0005, Mailing Address: P.O. Box 4005, Zip 34642-0005; tel. 813/397-5511; Emil Miller, Chief Executive Officer (Nonreporting) A1 9 10 11 12 13 S0875 Community Health Systems, Inc.	33	10	140	—	—	—	—	—	—	—
☐ WOMEN'S HOSPITAL AND MEDICAL CENTER, 9675 Seminole Boulevard, Zip 34642-2526, Mailing Address: P.O. Box 4001, Zip 34642; tel. 813/393-4646; Emil Miller, Chief Executive Officer (Nonreporting) A1 10 S0875 Community Health Systems, Inc.	33	10	99	—	—	—	—	—	—	—
SOUTH MIAMI—Dade County										
☐ HEALTHSOUTH LARKIN HOSPITAL, 7031 S.W. 62nd Avenue, Zip 33143; tel. 305/284-7700; Mel D. Deutsch, Administrator (Nonreporting) A1 9 10 S0023 Healthsouth Corporation	33	10	112	—	—	—	—	—	—	—
SPRING HILL—Hernando County										
✠ OAK HILL HOSPITAL, 11375 Cortez Boulevard, Zip 34613, Mailing Address: P.O. Box 5300, Zip 34606; tel. 904/596-6632; Robert K. Peterson, Administrator (Nonreporting) A1 9 10 S0048 Columbia/HCA Healthcare Corporation	33	10	150	—	—	—	—	—	—	—
★ SPRING HILL REGIONAL HOSPITAL, 10461 Quality Drive, Zip 34609; tel. 904/688-3053; Michael J. Stenger, Administrator and Chief Executive Officer A10 F7 8 10 12 15 16 17 19 21 22 25 28 29 30 31 34 35 36 37 39 40 44 45 49 63 65 66 67 71 72 73 S0002 Quorum Health Group/Quorum Health Resources	23	10	75	2867	34	25156	451	18772	6000	240
STARKE—Bradford County										
✠ BRADFORD HOSPITAL, 922 East Call Street, Zip 32091, Mailing Address: P.O. Box 1210, Zip 32091-1210; tel. 904/964-6000; Jeannie Baker, Chief Operating Officer A1 9 10 F8 19 22 26 28 30 32 33 44 48 49 51 71 S7895 AvMed–Santa Fe	23	10	23	932	12	0	0	6990	2124	136
STUART—Martin County										
✠ MARTIN MEMORIAL MEDICAL CENTER, 300 S.E. Hospital Drive, Zip 34994, Mailing Address: P.O. Box 9010, Zip 34995-9010; tel. 407/287-5200; Richmond M. Harman, President and Chief Executive Officer A1 2 9 10 F5 7 8 10 12 14 15 16 17 19 21 22 23 24 25 26 27 28 29 30 31 32 33 34 35 36 37 39 40 41 42 44 45 46 49 51 54 60 63 65 66 67 71 72 73 74 P1 3	23	10	254	13143	168	114304	1432	104882	45797	1672
SUN CITY CENTER—Hillsborough County										
✠ SOUTH BAY HOSPITAL, 4016 State Road 674, Zip 33573-5298; tel. 813/634-3301; Tracy A. Chelf, Chief Executive Officer (Total facility includes 16 beds in nursing home-type unit) A1 9 10 F8 12 14 15 16 17 19 20 21 22 24 25 26 28 30 31 32 34 35 36 37 39 41 42 44 45 46 49 64 65 67 70 71 73 P6 7 8 S0048 Columbia/HCA Healthcare Corporation	33	10	112	3616	66	49124	0	22919	9462	355
TALLAHASSEE—Leon County										
☐ △ HEALTHSOUTH REHABILITATION HOSPITAL OF TALLAHASSEE, (Formerly Healthsouth Capital Rehabilitation Hospital) 1675 Riggins Road, Zip 32308-5315; tel. 904/656-4800; Mike Marshall, Chief Executive Officer (Nonreporting) A1 7 10 S0023 Healthsouth Corporation	33	46	70	—	—	—	—	—	—	—
✠ TALLAHASSEE COMMUNITY HOSPITAL, 2626 Capital Medical Boulevard, Zip 32308; tel. 904/656-5000; Gary L. Brewer, Chief Executive Officer A1 9 10 F3 4 7 8 10 11 12 14 15 16 19 21 22 24 25 27 28 30 31 35 37 40 41 42 43 44 49 51 65 71 73 P6 S0048 Columbia/HCA Healthcare Corporation	33	10	180	6978	98	—	1045	38979	16379	621

© 1995 AHA Guide

Hospitals, U.S. / FLORIDA

Hospital, Address, Telephone, Administrator, Approval, Facility, and Physician Codes, Health Care System	Classification Codes		Utilization Data					Expense (thousands) of dollars		Personnel
	Control	Service	Beds	Admissions	Census	Outpatient Visits	Births	Total	Payroll	

★ American Hospital Association (AHA) membership
□ Joint Commission on Accreditation of Healthcare Organizations (JCAHO) accreditation
+ American Osteopathic Hospital Association (AOHA) membership
○ American Osteopathic Association (AOA) accreditation
△ Commission on Accreditation of Rehabilitation Facilities (CARF) accreditation
Control codes 61, 63, 64, 71, 72 and 73 indicate hospitals listed by AOHA, but not registered by AHA. For definition of numerical codes, see page A6

Hospital	Control	Service	Beds	Admissions	Census	Outpatient Visits	Births	Total	Payroll	Personnel
★ TALLAHASSEE MEMORIAL REGIONAL MEDICAL CENTER, Miccosukee Road & Magnolia Drive, Zip 32308–5093; tel. 904/681–1155; Duncan Moore, President (Total facility includes 110 beds in nursing home–type unit) **A**1 2 3 9 10 **F**4 7 8 10 11 14 15 16 17 19 21 22 23 24 26 27 28 30 31 32 34 35 37 38 39 40 41 42 43 44 45 46 47 49 51 52 53 54 55 56 57 58 59 60 63 64 65 66 67 69 71 73 74	23	10	611	23477	477	169158	3350	171352	79744	2670

TAMARAC—Broward County

Hospital	Control	Service	Beds	Admissions	Census	Outpatient Visits	Births	Total	Payroll	Personnel
★ UNIVERSITY HOSPITAL, (Includes University Pavilion, 7425 North University Drive, Tamarac, Florida, Zip 33328; tel. 305/722–9933) 7201 North University Drive, Zip 33321; tel. 305/721–2200; Robert L. Newman, Chief Executive Officer **A**1 10 **F**1 2 3 4 5 7 8 10 11 12 14 15 16 19 21 22 23 26 27 28 30 32 33 35 37 38 40 41 42 43 44 46 47 48 49 52 53 54 55 56 57 58 59 60 61 65 66 67 71 73 74 **P**8 **S**0048 Columbia/HCA Healthcare Corporation	33	10	211	5665	101	41923	0	40989	17088	605

TAMPA—Hillsborough County

AMI MEMORIAL HOSPITAL OF TAMPA See Memorial Hospital of Tampa
AMI TOWN AND COUNTRY HOSPITAL See Town and Country Hospital

Hospital	Control	Service	Beds	Admissions	Census	Outpatient Visits	Births	Total	Payroll	Personnel
□ CHARTER HOSPITAL OF TAMPA BAY, 4004 North Riverside Drive, Zip 33603; tel. 813/238–8671; Terry Fields, Administrator **A**1 9 10 **F**3 12 15 52 53 54 55 56 57 58 59 65 67 **S**0695 Charter Medical Corporation	33	22	146	3016	91	11873	0	—	—	112
★ H. LEE MOFFITT CANCER CENTER, 12902 Magnolia Drive, Zip 33612–9497; tel. 813/972–4673; John C. Ruckdeschel M.D., Director and Chief Executive Officer **A**1 2 3 5 10 **F**8 16 19 20 21 26 30 31 33 34 37 39 42 44 45 46 49 54 55 58 60 65 67 69 71 73 74	23	49	120	4057	95	70418	0	103436	39585	1470
★ JAMES A. HALEY VETERANS HOSPITAL, 13000 Bruce B. Downs Boulevard, Zip 33612–4798; tel. 813/972–2000; Richard A. Silver, Director (Total facility includes 240 beds in nursing home–type unit) **A**1 3 5 8 **F**2 3 4 8 10 11 12 19 20 21 23 24 25 26 27 28 29 30 31 32 33 34 35 37 39 41 42 43 44 45 46 48 49 51 52 54 55 56 57 58 59 60 63 65 67 71 72 73 74 **S**9295 Department of Veterans Affairs	45	10	778	12169	607	371242	0	—	—	2373
★ MEMORIAL HOSPITAL OF TAMPA, (Formerly AMI Memorial Hospital of Tampa) 2901 Swann Avenue, Zip 33609–4057; tel. 813/873–6400; Keith Henthorne, President **A**1 9 10 **F**3 4 7 8 10 12 16 19 21 22 31 32 34 35 37 41 42 44 52 56 58 59 63 65 71 73 74 **P**8 **S**0063 TENET Healthcare Corporation	32	10	174	4744	94	24465	0	30724	12193	489
★ SHRINERS HOSPITALS FOR CRIPPLED CHILDREN, TAMPA UNIT, 12502 North Pine Drive, Zip 33612–9499; tel. 813/972–2250; John Holtz, Administrator **A**1 3 5 **F**14 15 19 27 34 35 44 49 65 71 73 **S**4125 Shriners Hospitals for Crippled Children	23	57	60	1245	34	12215	0	—	—	255
★ ST. JOSEPH'S HOSPITALS, (Includes St. Joseph's Children's Hospital, 3001 West Martin Luther King Jr. Boulevard, Tampa, Florida, Zip 33607–6387; tel. 813/870–4662; Michael D. Aubin, Administrator; St. Joseph's Women's Hospital – Tampa, 3030 West Dr. Martin Luther King Jr. Boulevard, Tampa, Florida, Zip 33607–6394; tel. 813/879–4730; Michael D. Aubin, Administrator) 3001 West Martin Luther King Jr. Boulevard, Zip 33607–6387, Mailing Address: P.O. Box 4227, Zip 33677–4227; tel. 813/870–4000; Charles Francis Scott, President **A**1 2 5 9 10 **F**4 6 7 8 10 11 16 17 19 21 22 24 26 29 31 32 35 37 38 40 41 42 43 44 46 47 49 52 54 55 56 57 58 59 60 63 65 67 70 71 73 74 **P**7 8 **S**1385 Allegany Health System	21	10	883	32046	550	0	5903	264019	106750	3275
★ △ TAMPA GENERAL HEALTHCARE, (Includes TGH–University Psychiatry Center, 3515 East Fletcher Avenue, Tampa, Florida, Zip 33613–4788; tel. 813/972–3000; Davis Islands, Zip 33606, Mailing Address: P.O. Box 1289, Zip 33601; tel. 813/251–7000; Frederick B. Karl, President and Chief Executive Officer (Total facility includes 24 beds in nursing home–type unit) **A**1 2 3 5 7 8 9 10 **F**3 4 5 7 8 9 10 11 12 13 14 15 16 17 18 19 21 22 23 24 25 26 28 29 30 31 32 34 35 37 38 40 41 42 43 44 45 46 47 48 49 51 52 53 54 55 56 57 58 59 60 61 64 65 66 67 68 69 70 71 72 73 74 **P**4	16	10	686	21597	477	215637	3226	284939	106529	3097
TGH–UNIVERSITY PSYCHIATRY CENTER See Tampa General Healthcare										
★ TOWN AND COUNTRY HOSPITAL, (Formerly AMI Town and Country Hospital) 6001 Webb Road, Zip 33615–3291; tel. 813/885–6666; Keith Henthorne, Executive Director (Nonreporting) **A**1 9 10 **S**0063 TENET Healthcare Corporation	33	10	148							
□ UNIVERSITY COMMUNITY HOSPITAL, 3100 East Fletcher Avenue, Zip 33613–4688; tel. 813/971–6000; Norman V. Stein, President (Total facility includes 20 beds in nursing home–type unit) **A**1 2 9 10 **F**4 7 8 10 11 12 14 17 19 20 21 22 24 26 27 28 29 30 31 32 34 35 37 38 39 40 41 42 43 44 45 46 47 48 49 60 61 63 64 65 67 71 72 73 74	23	10	424	15547	242	—	2100	122066	56998	1574
□ ○ UNIVERSITY COMMUNITY HOSPITAL – CARROLLWOOD, 7171 North Dale Mabry Highway, Zip 33614–2699; tel. 813/932–2222; Steven R. Baratta, Administrator and Senior Vice President (Nonreporting) **A**1 10 11 12 13	33	10	120	—	—	—	—	—	—	—
□ VENCOR HOSPITAL – TAMPA, 4555 South Manhattan Avenue, Zip 33611; tel. 813/839–6341; Frank J. Battafarano, Administrator (Nonreporting) **A**1 3 10 **S**0026 Vencor, Incorporated	33	48	73	—	—	—	—	—	—	—

TARPON SPRINGS—Pinellas County

Hospital	Control	Service	Beds	Admissions	Census	Outpatient Visits	Births	Total	Payroll	Personnel
★ HELEN ELLIS MEMORIAL HOSPITAL, 1395 South Pinellas Avenue, Zip 34689–3721, Mailing Address: P.O. Box 1487, Zip 34688–1487; tel. 813/942–5000; Joseph N. Kiefer, Administrator **A**1 9 10 **F**7 8 10 11 16 17 19 21 22 25 26 28 30 31 34 35 37 39 40 41 42 44 45 46 49 60 63 65 67 71 73 74	23	10	150	6132	109	37760	112	41242	15763	559

Hospitals, U.S. / FLORIDA

Hospital, Address, Telephone, Administrator, Approval, Facility, and Physician Codes, Health Care System	Classi-fication Codes		Utilization Data					Expense (thousands) of dollars		
★ American Hospital Association (AHA) membership ☐ Joint Commission on Accreditation of Healthcare Organizations (JCAHO) accreditation + American Osteopathic Hospital Association (AOHA) membership ○ American Osteopathic Association (AOA) accreditation △ Commission on Accreditation of Rehabilitation Facilities (CARF) accreditation Control codes 61, 63, 64, 71, 72 and 73 indicate hospitals listed by AOHA, but not registered by AHA. For definition of numerical codes, see page A6	Control	Service	Beds	Admissions	Census	Outpatient Visits	Births	Total	Payroll	Personnel
★ THE MANORS, 1527 Riverside Drive, Zip 34689–2023; tel. 813/937–4211; F. Dee Goldberg, President and Chief Executive Officer (Total facility includes 16 beds in nursing home–type unit) **A**1 9 10 **F**2 15 16 27 52 53 54 55 56 57 58 59 65	32	22	130	1419	89	16957	0	13564	6378	255
TAVERNIER—Monroe County										
★ MARINERS HOSPITAL, 50 High Point Road, Zip 33070; tel. 305/852–4418; Robert H. Luse, President **A**1 9 10 **F**15 16 19 22 35 37 44 63 65 71	23	10	42	1048	13	16759	0	10380	3832	131
TEQUESTA—Martin County										
☐ SANDYPINES, 11301 Southeast Tequesta Terrace, Zip 33469; tel. 407/744–0211; David L. Beardsley, Administrator **A**1 10 **F**1 12 14 15 16 17 18 46 52 53 54 55 56 57 58 59 65 67 **P**8	33	22	60	346	14		0	5007	1975	73
TITUSVILLE—Brevard County										
☐ PARRISH MEDICAL CENTER, 951 North Washington Avenue, Zip 32796–2194; tel. 407/268–6100; Rod L. Baker, President and Chief Executive Officer **A**1 2 9 10 **F**4 7 8 10 14 15 16 19 21 22 23 24 25 28 29 30 31 33 34 35 37 40 42 44 45 46 49 56 60 65 69 71 73	16	10	176	8130	116	66745	662	48454	20771	674
VENICE—Sarasota County										
★ VENICE HOSPITAL, 540 the Rialto, Zip 34285; tel. 813/485–7711; Jack A. Norman, President and Chief Executive Officer (Total facility includes 120 beds in nursing home–type unit) **A**1 2 9 10 **F**3 8 10 11 12 15 16 17 19 20 21 22 25 26 27 28 29 30 32 34 35 37 39 42 44 46 49 52 60 64 65 71 72 73 **P**8	23	10	387	9601	280	51773	0	79274	33931	995
VERO BEACH—Indian River County										
☐ △ HEALTHSOUTH TREASURE COAST REHABILITATION HOSPITAL, 1600 37th Street, Zip 32960–6549; tel. 407/778–2100; Mark J. Tarr, Administrator and Chief Executive Officer (Nonreporting) **A**1 7 10 **S**0023 Healthsouth Corporation	33	46	70	—	—	—	—	—	—	—
★ INDIAN RIVER MEMORIAL HOSPITAL, 1000 36th Street, Zip 32960–6592; tel. 407/567–4311; Michael J. O'Grady Jr., President and Chief Executive Officer **A**1 2 9 10 **F**2 3 7 8 10 11 12 14 15 16 17 19 21 22 23 26 27 28 29 30 31 32 33 35 37 39 40 41 42 44 45 46 49 51 52 53 54 55 56 57 58 59 60 65 66 67 71 73 74	23	10	347	10656	213	51908	958	88481	36796	1010
WEST PALM BEACH—Palm Beach County										
45TH STREET MENTAL HEALTH CENTER, 1041 45th Street, Zip 33407; tel. 407/844–9741; Terry H. Allen, Executive Director (Nonreporting) **A**10	23	22	44	—	—	—	—	—	—	—
★ ○ COLUMBIA HOSPITAL, (Formerly Palm Beaches Medical Center) 2201 45th Street, Zip 33407–2069; tel. 407/842–6141; Michael M. Fencel, Chief Executive Officer **A**1 10 11 12 **F**3 7 8 10 12 14 16 17 18 19 21 22 23 26 28 30 31 32 34 35 37 39 40 41 42 44 45 49 52 53 55 56 57 58 59 63 64 65 71 73 **S**0048 Columbia/HCA Healthcare Corporation	33	10	250	5196	93	26326	0	32041	14954	604
★ GOOD SAMARITAN MEDICAL CENTER, Flagler Drive at Palm Beach Lakes Boulevard, Zip 33401; tel. 407/655–5511; Michael French, President and Chief Executive Officer **A**1 2 9 10 **F**7 8 10 11 15 16 19 21 22 23 24 25 28 29 30 32 34 35 37 38 39 40 41 42 44 45 47 48 49 51 52 60 63 65 67 70 71 73 **P**6 8	23	10	276	10889	172	94211	1657	90892	33241	1109
HOSPICE OF PALM BEACH COUNTY, 5300 East Avenue, Zip 33407–2352; tel. 407/848–5200; Deborah S. Dailey, President and Chief Executive Officer **F**14 15 16 32 33 **P**5	23	49	24	1959	24	0	0	9622	—	134
PALM BEACHES MEDICAL CENTER See Columbia Hospital										
★ △ ST. MARY'S HOSPITAL, 901 45th Street, Zip 33407–2495, Mailing Address: P.O. Box 24620, Zip 33416–4620; tel. 407/844–6300; Michael French, President and Chief Executive **A**1 2 7 9 10 **F**3 7 8 10 11 14 17 19 22 23 28 30 31 32 33 34 35 37 38 40 41 42 43 44 47 48 49 52 54 55 56 57 58 59 60 65 67 70 71 72 73 74 **P**8 **S**1385 Allegany Health System	23	10	430	18804	294	0	4794	155929	64050	1929
☐ ○ WELLINGTON REGIONAL MEDICAL CENTER, 10101 Forest Hill Boulevard, Zip 33414; tel. 407/798–8500; Michael Marquez, Chief Executive Officer **A**1 10 11 12 13 **F**2 3 7 8 12 15 16 17 18 19 21 22 23 27 28 29 30 31 32 33 34 35 37 39 40 41 42 44 46 49 60 61 65 67 69 71 73 **S**9555 Universal Health Services, Inc.	33	10	87	2913	39	33896	291	31509	12124	285
WILLISTON—Levy County										
★ NATURE COAST REGIONAL HOSPITAL, 125 Southwest Seventh Street, Zip 32696, Mailing Address: P.O. Drawer 550, Zip 32696; tel. 904/528–2801; John H. Byrd Jr. CPA, Administrator **A**1 9 10 **F**8 12 14 15 16 19 20 22 27 28 30 32 33 34 36 37 39 41 44 46 49 53 54 57 65 67 71 73	23	10	30	958	14	22096	0	—	—	110
WINTER GARDEN—Orange County										
HEALTH CENTRAL See Ocoee										
WINTER HAVEN—Polk County										
★ WINTER HAVEN HOSPITAL, 200 Avenue F N.E., Zip 33881; tel. 813/297–1899; Lance W. Anastasio, President (Nonreporting) **A**1 9 10	23	10	438	—	—	—	—	—	—	—
WINTER PARK—Orange County										
★ WINTER PARK MEMORIAL HOSPITAL, (Includes Winter Park Psychiatric Care Center, 1600 Dodd Road, Winter Park, Florida, Zip 32792; tel. 407/677–6842) 200 North Lakemont Avenue, Zip 32792–3273; tel. 407/646–7000; Pete Lawson, Chief Executive Officer (Nonreporting) **A**1 9 10 **S**0048 Columbia/HCA Healthcare Corporation	23	10	339	—	—	—	—	—	—	—
WINTER PARK PSYCHIATRIC CARE CENTER See Winter Park Memorial Hospital										
ZEPHYRHILLS—Pasco County										
★ EAST PASCO MEDICAL CENTER, 7050 Gall Boulevard, Zip 33541–1399; tel. 813/788–0411; Bob A. Dodd, President (Total facility includes 11 beds in nursing home–type unit) **A**1 9 10 **F**7 8 10 14 15 16 17 19 22 24 26 28 30 32 34 35 37 40 41 44 46 49 54 56 60 63 64 65 67 71 73 74 **S**4165 Adventist Health System–Sunbelt Health Care Corporation	21	10	96	5564	75	—	481	50930	21031	798

© 1995 AHA Guide

Hospitals, U.S. / GEORGIA

GEORGIA

Resident population 6,917 (in thousands)
Resident population in metro areas 67.7%
Birth rate per 1,000 population 16.7
65 years and over 10.1%
Percent of persons without health insurance 16.1%

Hospital, Address, Telephone, Administrator, Approval, Facility, and Physician Codes, Health Care System	Classification Codes		Utilization Data					Expense (thousands) of dollars		
★ American Hospital Association (AHA) membership ☐ Joint Commission on Accreditation of Healthcare Organizations (JCAHO) accreditation + American Osteopathic Hospital Association (AOHA) membership ○ American Osteopathic Association (AOA) accreditation △ Commission on Accreditation of Rehabilitation Facilities (CARF) accreditation Control codes 61, 63, 64, 71, 72 and 73 indicate hospitals listed by AOHA, but not registered by AHA. For definition of numerical codes, see page A6	Control	Service	Beds	Admissions	Census	Outpatient Visits	Births	Total	Payroll	Personnel
ADEL—Cook County MEMORIAL HOSPITAL OF ADEL, 706 North Parrish Avenue, Zip 31620–0677, Mailing Address: Box 677, Zip 31620–0677; tel. 912/896–2251; James E. Cunningham, Administrator (Total facility includes 95 beds in nursing home–type unit) **A**9 10 **F**7 14 15 16 17 19 22 32 34 37 40 44 46 49 71 73 **S**2335 Memorial Health Services	33	10	161	2787	123	18343	325	11198	4672	272
ALBANY—Dougherty County ★ PALMYRA MEDICAL CENTERS, 2000 Palmyra Road, Zip 31701, Mailing Address: Box 1908, Zip 31702–1908; tel. 912/434–2000; Douglas M. Parker, Chief Executive Officer **A**1 9 10 **F**8 11 12 15 16 19 21 22 23 28 29 30 34 35 37 39 41 42 44 45 48 49 65 66 67 70 71 73 **S**0048 Columbia/HCA Healthcare Corporation	33	10	145	4627	100	44684	0	43643	14811	545
★ PHOEBE PUTNEY MEMORIAL HOSPITAL, 417 Third Avenue, Zip 31701–1943, Mailing Address: P.O. Box 1828, Zip 31703–6801; tel. 912/883–1800; Joel Wernick, President and Chief Executive Officer **A**1 3 5 9 10 **F**1 2 3 4 7 8 10 11 12 15 16 17 18 19 21 22 23 26 29 30 33 35 37 38 40 42 43 44 46 49 52 58 59 60 65 71 73 74 **P**3	23	10	418	17315	288	152582	2674	—	—	2097
ALMA—Bacon County BACON COUNTY HOSPITAL, 302 South Wayne Street, Zip 31510, Mailing Address: P.O. Drawer 1987, Zip 31510; tel. 912/632–8961; Jeff Kinlaw, Administrator (Total facility includes 88 beds in nursing home–type unit) **A**9 10 **F**7 8 14 15 16 17 19 22 26 30 31 35 37 40 41 44 45 46 49 57 61 64 65 71 73 74 **P**8	16	10	131	1614	107	14008	76	6918	2743	222
AMERICUS—Sumter County ★ SUMTER REGIONAL HOSPITAL, 100 Wheatley Drive, Zip 31709; tel. 912/924–6011; Jerry W. Adams, Administrator **A**1 9 10 **F**7 8 11 15 16 17 19 21 22 23 27 28 29 30 31 33 34 35 37 39 40 42 44 45 46 48 49 51 52 56 57 65 67 71 73 **P**8	16	10	152	5465	75	39342	914	26923	11167	475
ARLINGTON—Calhoun County CALHOUN MEMORIAL HOSPITAL, 209 Academy & Carswell Streets, Zip 31713, Mailing Address: Drawer R, Zip 31713; tel. 912/725–4272; Newana Williams, Administrator (Nonreporting) **A**9 10	16	10	24	—	—	—	—	—	—	—
ATHENS—Clarke County ★ ATHENS REGIONAL MEDICAL CENTER, 1199 Prince Avenue, Zip 30606–2793; tel. 706/549–9977; John A. Drew, President and Chief Executive Officer **A**1 9 10 **F**2 3 4 7 8 10 11 15 16 17 18 19 21 22 23 25 28 30 31 32 33 35 37 38 40 41 42 43 44 46 49 52 53 54 55 56 57 61 65 66 67 71 73	16	10	305	15671	234	85795	1493	108642	47010	1507
☐ CHARTER WINDS HOSPITAL, 240 Mitchell Bridge Road, Zip 30606, Mailing Address: P.O. Box 6297, Zip 30604; tel. 706/546–7277; Mark Snow, Chief Executive Officer **A**1 9 10 **F**1 2 3 14 16 19 22 25 26 35 44 48 50 52 53 54 55 56 57 58 59 65 67 **P**8 **S**0695 Charter Medical Corporation	33	22	80	898	28	1159	0	8003	2736	89
★ ST. MARY'S HEALTH CARE SYSTEM, 1230 Baxter Street, Zip 30606–3791; tel. 706/548–7581; Edward J. Fechtel Jr., Administrator (Total facility includes 120 beds in nursing home–type unit) **A**1 9 10 **F**7 11 14 15 16 19 21 22 24 26 27 29 31 32 33 34 35 37 39 40 41 42 44 45 46 48 49 60 63 64 65 66 67 71 73	23	10	301	7545	220	66195	912	69504	33868	1039
ATLANTA—Fulton and De Kalb Counties ★ ANCHOR HOSPITAL, 5454 Yorktowne Drive, Zip 30349–5305; tel. 404/991–6044; Benjamin H. Underwood CHE, FAAMA, President and Chief Executive Officer **A**10 **F**2 3 14 15 16 17 20 21 24 27 34 45 46 49 52 53 54 55 56 57 58 59 65 67 **P**6	33	82	84	1496	38	4914	0	8091	3526	137
CHARTER BROOK HOSPITAL See Charter Peachford Hospital										
CHARTER PEACHFORD HOSPITAL, (Includes Charter Brook Hospital, Atlanta, Georgia) 2151 Peachford Road, Zip 30338; tel. 404/455–3200; James F. Button, Administrator (Nonreporting) **A**10 **S**0695 Charter Medical Corporation	33	22	294	—	—	—	—	—	—	—
☐ CPC PARKWOOD HOSPITAL, 1999 Cliff Valley Way N.E., Zip 30329–2448; tel. 404/633–8431; J. Shawn O'Connor, Administrator and Chief Executive Officer **A**1 5 9 10 **F**2 3 12 16 17 18 19 21 22 25 26 27 30 32 34 35 45 46 50 52 53 54 55 56 57 58 59 63 65 67 68 71 73 **P**8 **S**0785 Community Psychiatric Centers	33	22	145	1205	31	6805	0	8360	3860	66
★ CRAWFORD LONG HOSPITAL OF EMORY UNIVERSITY, 550 Peachtree Street N.E., Zip 30365–2225; tel. 404/686–2445; John Dunklin Henry Sr., Chief Executive Officer **A**1 2 3 5 8 9 10 **F**4 7 8 10 11 12 14 17 19 21 22 23 25 30 31 32 33 34 35 37 38 40 42 43 44 49 50 51 54 60 61 63 65 67 71 74 **P**3	21	10	416	18657	329	78200	2470	173864	65953	2050
★ DUNWOODY MEDICAL CENTER, 4575 North Shallowford Road, Zip 30338; tel. 404/454–2000; Thomas D. Gilbert, President and Chief Executive Officer **A**1 9 10 **F**7 8 10 12 14 15 16 17 18 19 21 22 25 28 29 30 32 34 35 37 38 39 40 41 44 45 46 49 53 54 55 56 57 58 59 61 63 65 66 67 70 71 72 73 74 **P**1 2 4 8 **S**0048 Columbia/HCA Healthcare Corporation	33	10	168	5477	58	21427	1242	—	—	539
★ EGLESTON CHILDREN'S HOSPITAL AT EMORY UNIVERSITY, 1405 Clifton Road N.E., Zip 30322–1101; tel. 404/325–6000; Alan J. Gayer, President **A**1 3 5 8 9 10 **F**4 10 11 13 15 16 17 19 20 21 22 23 24 25 27 28 29 30 31 32 34 35 38 39 42 43 44 45 46 47 48 49 51 63 65 68 69 70 71 72 73 **P**1	23	50	196	8512	149	144092	0	139845	66914	1532
★ △ EMORY UNIVERSITY HOSPITAL, 1364 Clifton Road N.E., Zip 30322–1102; tel. 404/727–7021; John Dunklin Henry Sr., Chief Executive Officer **A**1 2 3 5 7 8 9 10 **F**2 3 4 7 8 10 11 12 14 16 17 19 21 22 23 25 26 28 29 30 31 33 34 35 37 38 39 41 42 43 44 45 46 49 50 51 52 55 56 57 58 59 60 61 63 65 67 69 71 72 73 74 **P**1 3	23	10	523	18748	392	79054	0	272646	98543	2557

Hospitals, U.S. / GEORGIA

Hospital, Address, Telephone, Administrator, Approval, Facility, and Physician Codes, Health Care System	Classification Codes		Utilization Data					Expense (thousands) of dollars		
★ American Hospital Association (AHA) membership □ Joint Commission on Accreditation of Healthcare Organizations (JCAHO) accreditation + American Osteopathic Hospital Association (AOHA) membership ○ American Osteopathic Association (AOA) accreditation △ Commission on Accreditation of Rehabilitation Facilities (CARF) accreditation Control codes 61, 63, 64, 71, 72 and 73 indicate hospitals listed by AOHA, but not registered by AHA. For definition of numerical codes, see page A6	Control	Service	Beds	Admissions	Census	Outpatient Visits	Births	Total	Payroll	Personnel
★ △ GEORGIA BAPTIST MEDICAL CENTER, 300 Boulevard N.E., Zip 30312; tel. 404/265–4000; David Harrell, Chief Executive Officer (Total facility includes 219 beds in nursing home–type unit) **A**1 2 3 5 7 8 9 10 **F**1 4 7 8 10 11 12 14 15 16 17 19 21 22 23 24 25 26 27 28 31 32 33 34 35 37 38 40 41 42 43 44 46 48 49 51 52 54 58 59 60 61 65 67 71 72 73 74 **P**7 8	21	10	592	14818	443	115963	2744	178877	75750	2130
□ GEORGIA MENTAL HEALTH INSTITUTE, 1256 Briarcliff Road N.E., Zip 30306; tel. 404/894–5911; B. C. Robbins, Superintendent (Nonreporting) **A**1 3 10	12	22	246	—	—	—	—	—	—	—
★ GRADY MEMORIAL HOSPITAL, 80 Butler Street S.E., Zip 30335–3801, Mailing Address: P.O. Box 26189, Zip 30335–3801; tel. 404/616–4307; Edward J. Renford, President and Chief Executive Officer (Total facility includes 354 beds in nursing home–type unit) **A**1 2 3 5 8 9 10 **F**3 4 5 7 8 9 10 11 12 13 14 15 16 17 18 19 20 21 22 25 27 28 31 33 34 35 37 38 40 41 42 43 44 45 46 47 49 51 52 53 54 56 57 58 59 60 61 63 64 65 67 68 69 70 71 72 73 74	16	10	1273	33216	962	756966	4903	401958	173492	5509
★ HILLSIDE HOSPITAL, 690 Courtney Drive N.E., Zip 30306–0206, Mailing Address: P.O. Box 8206, Zip 31106–0206; tel. 404/875–4551; Thomas Corbett, Executive Director **F**14 15 16 52 53 55 56 58 59 65 67	23	52	61	21	61	0	0	6158	3270	129
JOSEPH B. WHITEHEAD MEMORIAL INFIRMARY, GEORGIA INSTITUTE OF TECHNOLOGY, 275 Fifth Street N.W., Zip 30318; tel. 404/894–2584; J. Nicholas Gordon M.D., Director (Nonreporting)	12	11	70	—	—	—	—	—	—	—
★ METROPOLITAN HOSPITAL, (Specialty Surgery, Plastic Surgery, Orthopedics, Urology, Eye, Ear, Nose, Throat, Dental, Hand Surgery and Women's Center) 3223 Howell Mill Road N.W., Zip 30327; tel. 404/351–0500; R. Stan Lentz, Chief Executive Officer **A**1 9 10 **F**8 21 30 34 44 45 46 49 60 63 65 66 69 71 **P**4 **S**0048 Columbia/HCA Healthcare Corporation	33	49	64	857	3	4590	0	—	—	94
★ + ○ NORTHLAKE REGIONAL MEDICAL CENTER, 1455 Montreal Road, Zip 30084, Mailing Address: P.O. Box 450000, Zip 31145; tel. 404/270–3000; Michael K. Kerner, Chief Executive Officer **A**1 2 9 10 11 12 13 **F**7 8 11 19 22 30 31 34 35 37 38 39 40 41 42 44 48 49 65 66 71 73 74 **S**0048 Columbia/HCA Healthcare Corporation	33	10	120	3273	45	27124	467	—	—	403
★ NORTHSIDE HOSPITAL, 1000 Johnson Ferry Road N.E., Zip 30342–1611; tel. 404/851–8700; Sidney Kirschner, President and Chief Executive Officer **A**1 2 9 10 **F**2 3 7 8 10 11 12 14 15 16 17 18 19 21 22 23 24 25 28 29 30 31 32 33 34 35 38 39 40 41 42 44 45 46 49 51 52 54 55 56 58 59 60 61 63 65 67 69 71 72 73 74 **P**7	23	44	352	24671	231	109385	9196	205672	82523	2258
★ PIEDMONT HOSPITAL, 1968 Peachtree Road N.W., Zip 30309–1231; tel. 404/605–5000; Richard B. Hubbard III, President and Chief Executive Officer (Total facility includes 37 beds in nursing home–type unit) **A**1 2 3 5 9 10 **F**4 5 7 8 10 11 14 17 19 21 22 24 25 26 27 28 29 30 31 33 34 35 37 38 39 40 41 42 43 44 45 48 49 60 61 64 65 66 67 69 70 71 72 73 74 **P**1 3 6	23	10	444	21859	316	141091	3194	—	—	2282
□ PSYCHIATRIC INSTITUTE OF ATLANTA, 811 Juniper Street N.E., Zip 30308; tel. 404/881–5800; Dennis Workman M.D., Medical Director (Nonreporting) **A**1 10 **S**0695 Charter Medical Corporation	33	22	40	—	—	—	—	—	—	—
★ SAINT JOSEPH'S HOSPITAL OF ATLANTA, 5665 Peachtree Dunwoody Road N.E., Zip 30342–1764; tel. 404/851–7001; Kathryn J. McDonagh, President **A**1 2 9 10 **F**4 8 10 11 13 15 16 17 18 19 20 21 22 26 27 28 29 30 31 34 35 36 37 39 41 42 43 44 45 46 49 50 51 54 60 63 65 67 69 71 73 **S**3595 Eastern Mercy Health System	23	10	346	17675	255	102434	0	177123	68707	1881
★ △ SCOTTISH RITE CHILDREN'S MEDICAL CENTER, 1001 Johnson Ferry Road N.E., Zip 30342; tel. 404/256–5252; James E. Tally Ph.D., President and Chief Executive Officer **A**1 3 5 7 9 **F**12 13 15 16 17 19 20 21 22 25 27 29 34 35 39 41 42 44 45 46 47 48 49 51 60 65 66 67 68 70 71 73	23	50	165	7977	114	104537	0	93747	46572	1380
★ SHEPHERD CENTER, 2020 Peachtree Road N.W., Zip 30309–1402; tel. 404/352–2020; Gary R. Ulicny Ph.D., President and Chief Executive Officer **A**1 5 10 **F**12 14 15 17 19 20 22 27 34 35 37 39 45 46 48 49 53 54 58 61 65 67 70 71 73 **P**6	23	46	100	625	76	7704	0	36830	18915	481
□ SOUTHWEST HOSPITAL AND MEDICAL CENTER, 501 Fairburn Road S.W., Zip 30331–1437; tel. 404/699–1111; Michael R. Burroughs, President and Chief Executive Officer **A**1 3 5 9 10 **F**7 8 15 16 19 21 22 28 29 30 34 37 40 44 46 49 51 65 71 73 **P**6	23	10	80	2428	33	30125	425	20325	9996	301
□ VENCOR HOSPITAL–ATLANTA, (Long–term Acute Care) 705 Juniper Street N.E., Zip 30365; tel. 404/873–2871; Skip Wright, Administrator **A**1 9 10 **F**12 14 19 21 22 27 35 65 71 **S**0026 Vencor, Incorporated	33	49	66	248	53	0	0	36503	5789	262
★ WESLEY WOODS GERIATRIC HOSPITAL, 1821 Clifton Road N.E., Zip 30329–5102; tel. 404/728–6200; William L. Minnix, Chief Executive Officer **A**1 3 5 9 10 **F**3 4 8 10 11 12 17 19 20 21 22 26 27 29 30 33 34 35 37 39 41 42 43 44 45 46 48 49 50 51 52 54 55 56 57 58 59 60 62 63 64 65 67 69 71 73	23	22	93	1553	63	23391	0	22277	8485	305
★ WEST PACES MEDICAL CENTER, 3200 Howell Mill Road N.W., Zip 30327–4101; tel. 404/351–0351; Stuart Voelpel, President and Chief Executive Officer **A**1 2 3 9 10 **F**2 3 7 8 10 11 14 15 18 19 21 22 23 25 26 28 29 30 31 34 35 37 38 39 40 42 44 46 49 52 53 54 56 58 59 65 66 67 68 71 72 73 74 **S**0048 Columbia/HCA Healthcare Corporation	33	10	294	8669	111	36888	1876	72884	26141	707

AUGUSTA—Richmond County

★ AUGUSTA REGIONAL MEDICAL CENTER, 3651 Wheeler Road, Zip 30909–1499; tel. 706/863–3232; Jesse G. Smith, Chief Executive Officer **A**1 9 10 **F**2 3 7 8 9 10 11 12 13 15 16 17 18 19 20 23 29 30 31 34 35 37 40 41 42 44 45 46 49 51 52 53 54 57 60 65 67 69 71 72 73 74 **P**1 6 7 **S**0048 Columbia/HCA Healthcare Corporation	33	10	252	9095	135	65237	1080	74729	29486	1010

© 1995 AHA Guide

Hospitals, U.S. / GEORGIA

Hospital, Address, Telephone, Administrator, Approval, Facility, and Physician Codes, Health Care System	Classification Codes		Utilization Data					Expense (thousands) of dollars		
★ American Hospital Association (AHA) membership □ Joint Commission on Accreditation of Healthcare Organizations (JCAHO) accreditation + American Osteopathic Hospital Association (AOHA) membership ○ American Osteopathic Association (AOA) accreditation △ Commission on Accreditation of Rehabilitation Facilities (CARF) accreditation Control codes 61, 63, 64, 71, 72 and 73 indicate hospitals listed by AOHA, but not registered by AHA. For definition of numerical codes, see page A6	Control	Service	Beds	Admissions	Census	Outpatient Visits	Births	Total	Payroll	Personnel
□ GEORGIA REGIONAL HOSPITAL AT AUGUSTA, 3405 Old Savannah Road, Zip 30906; tel. 706/790–2600; Ronald C. Hogan, Superintendent **A**1 3 10 **F**1 2 3 4 5 6 7 8 9 10 11 12 13 14 17 18 19 20 21 22 23 24 25 26 27 28 29 30 31 32 33 34 35 36 37 38 39 40 41 42 43 44 45 46 47 48 49 50 51 52 53 54 55 56 57 58 59 60 61 62 63 64 65 66 67 68 69 70 71 72 73 74 **P**3 6	12	22	262	3646	243	0	0	24868	14838	543
★ MEDICAL COLLEGE OF GEORGIA HOSPITAL AND CLINICS, 1120 15th Street, Zip 30912–5000; tel. 706/721–0211; Patricia Findling–Sodomka, Executive Director **A**1 2 3 5 8 9 10 **F**4 7 8 9 10 11 15 16 17 19 20 21 22 23 26 27 28 31 34 35 37 38 39 40 41 42 43 44 46 47 49 52 53 54 55 56 57 58 60 61 63 65 66 67 69 70 71 73 74 **P**6	12	10	488	17089	329	373772	1187	209991	—	3185
★ ST. JOSEPH HOSPITAL, 2260 Wrightsboro Road, Zip 30904–4726; tel. 706/481–7000; J. William Paugh, President and Chief Executive Officer **A**1 9 10 **F**7 8 10 12 14 15 16 17 19 22 23 25 28 29 30 33 34 35 37 38 39 40 42 44 45 49 51 62 65 67 71 73 74 **P**8 **S**5945 Carondelet Health System	21	10	148	6049	94	420953	1231	65365	30372	954
★ UNIVERSITY HOSPITAL, 1350 Walton Way, Zip 30901–2629; tel. 706/722–9011; Donald C. Bray, President and Chief Executive Officer (Data for 364 days) **A**1 2 3 5 9 10 **F**1 2 3 4 5 6 7 8 9 10 11 12 14 15 16 17 18 19 20 21 22 23 24 25 26 28 29 30 31 32 34 35 37 38 39 40 41 42 43 44 45 46 47 48 49 51 52 54 55 56 57 58 59 60 61 62 63 64 65 66 67 68 71 72 73 74 **P**2 6 8	23	10	613	21678	396	206660	2737	204245	89207	3335
★ VETERANS AFFAIRS MEDICAL CENTER, 1 Freedom Way, Zip 30904–6285; tel. 706/733–0188; Thomas L. Ayres, Director (Nonreporting) **A**1 2 3 5 8 9 **S**9295 Department of Veterans Affairs	45	10	732	—						
★ △ WALTON REHABILITATION HOSPITAL, 1355 Independence Drive, Zip 30901–1037; tel. 706/823–8505; Dennis B. Skelley, President and Chief Executive Officer **A**1 7 9 10 **F**14 15 16 19 27 28 30 34 35 41 45 48 49 65 66 67 68 73 **P**4 5 6 7 8 **S**5945 Carondelet Health System	23	46	58	830	47	68786	0	15856	7851	229
AUSTELL—Cobb County										
★ COBB HOSPITAL AND MEDICAL CENTER, 3950 Austell Road, Zip 30001–1121; tel. 404/732–4000; Paul F. Johnson, President **A**1 2 7 9 10 **F**3 6 7 8 10 11 12 14 15 17 18 19 20 21 22 24 25 26 28 29 30 31 32 33 34 35 37 38 39 40 41 42 44 45 46 48 49 50 51 52 53 54 55 56 57 58 59 61 62 65 66 67 70 71 72 73 74 **P**1 3 7 **S**0995 Promina Northwest Health System	23	10	303	14326	201	126539	2516	87157	36585	1239
BAINBRIDGE—Decatur County										
★ MEMORIAL HOSPITAL AND MANOR, 1500 East Shotwell Street, Zip 31717; tel. 912/246–3500; Raymond W. Wright, Director (Nonreporting) **A**1 9 10	16	10	187	—	—	—	—	—	—	—
BAXLEY—Appling County										
APPLING GENERAL HOSPITAL, 301 East Tollison Street, Zip 31513; tel. 912/367–9841; Luther E. Reeves, Chief Executive Officer (Total facility includes 101 beds in nursing home–type unit) **A**9 10 **F**7 8 17 19 22 27 28 30 35 40 44 64 71	16	10	141	1428	116	17850	68	8047	4331	215
BLAIRSVILLE—Union County										
★ UNION GENERAL HOSPITAL, 214 Hospital Drive, Zip 30512; tel. 706/745–2111; Rebecca T. Dyer, Administrator (Total facility includes 105 beds in nursing home–type unit) **A**9 10 **F**8 11 15 16 19 21 22 28 30 31 34 37 40 44 56 59 63 64 65 71 73	16	10	150	1849	118	—	203	9786	—	225
BLAKELY—Early County										
★ EARLY MEMORIAL HOSPITAL, 630 Columbia Street, Zip 31723; tel. 912/723–4241; Jackie Frith, Acting Administrator (Total facility includes 127 beds in nursing home–type unit) **A**1 9 10 **F**7 8 14 15 16 19 22 26 28 30 34 40 44 45 64 71 **P**4	16	10	176	747	133	11930	100	7549	3377	123
BLUE RIDGE—Fannin County										
□ FANNIN REGIONAL HOSPITAL, Highway 5 North, Zip 30513, Mailing Address: Box 1549, Zip 30513; tel. 706/632–3711; Marvin Stern, Administrator (Nonreporting) **A**1 9 10 **S**0875 Community Health Systems, Inc.	33	10	51	—	—	—	—	—	—	—
BOWDON—Carroll County										
BOWDON AREA HOSPITAL, 501 Mitchell Avenue, Zip 30108; tel. 404/258–7207; Yvonne Willis, Administrator **A**9 10 **F**8 15 19 22 23 28 33 34 35 39 44 48 49 65 71	33	10	41	854	14	4143	0	3937	1217	51
BREMEN—Haralson County										
★ HIGGINS GENERAL HOSPITAL, 200 Allen Memorial Drive, Zip 30110, Mailing Address: Box 655, Zip 30110; tel. 404/537–5851; Robbie Smith, Administrator **A**9 10 **F**8 10 19 22 28 37 44 65	15	10	59	1335	20	13478	0	7578	3118	136
BRUNSWICK—Glynn County										
★ SOUTHEAST GEORGIA REGIONAL MEDICAL CENTER, 3100 Kemble Avenue, Zip 31520, Mailing Address: Box 1518, Zip 31521; tel. 912/264–7000; Ted R. Whitten, Acting Chief Executive Officer **A**1 9 10 **F**7 8 10 11 15 19 21 22 23 28 29 30 31 33 34 35 37 40 41 42 44 45 46 49 52 56 58 59 60 65 67 71 73 **P**3 **S**0002 Quorum Health Group/Quorum Health Resources	16	10	337	11956	209	86819	1229	86044	35258	1257
CAIRO—Grady County										
□ GRADY GENERAL HOSPITAL, 1155 Fifth Street S.E., Zip 31728, Mailing Address: P.O. Box 360, Zip 31728; tel. 912/377–1150; W. Douglas Arnold, Administrator **A**1 9 10 **F**7 8 17 19 22 28 37 40 44 49 71	23	10	45	1472	23	16812	230	7393	3462	147
CALHOUN—Gordon County										
★ GORDON HOSPITAL, 1035 Red Bud Road, Zip 30701, Mailing Address: P.O. Box 12938, Zip 30703–7013; tel. 706/629–2895; Dennis Kiley, President **A**1 9 10 **F**8 10 12 17 19 21 22 23 26 28 30 34 35 37 40 44 45 49 63 65 67 71 72 73 **S**4165 Adventist Health System–Sunbelt Health Care Corporation	21	10	50	2880	29	56558	305	19066	7605	301

Hospitals, U.S. / GEORGIA

Hospital, Address, Telephone, Administrator, Approval, Facility, and Physician Codes, Health Care System ★ American Hospital Association (AHA) membership ☐ Joint Commission on Accreditation of Healthcare Organizations (JCAHO) accreditation + American Osteopathic Hospital Association (AOHA) membership ○ American Osteopathic Association (AOA) accreditation △ Commission on Accreditation of Rehabilitation Facilities (CARF) accreditation Control codes 61, 63, 64, 71, 72 and 73 indicate hospitals listed by AOHA, but not registered by AHA. For definition of numerical codes, see page A6	Classification Codes		Utilization Data					Expense (thousands) of dollars		
	Control	Service	Beds	Admissions	Census	Outpatient Visits	Births	Total	Payroll	Personnel
CAMILLA—Mitchell County ☐ MITCHELL COUNTY HOSPITAL, 90 Stevens Street, Zip 31730, Mailing Address: P.O. Box 639, Zip 31730; tel. 912/336-5284; Gerald Trevisol, Administrator (Total facility includes 156 beds in nursing home–type unit) **A**1 9 10 **F**7 8 15 19 22 33 34 44 64 65 71	23	10	182	748	166	18727	153	8834	4245	205
CANTON—Cherokee County ★ PROMINA R. T. JONES HOSPITAL, (Formerly R. T. Jones Regional Hospital) 201 Hospital Road, Zip 30114, Mailing Address: P.O. Box 906, Zip 30114; tel. 404/720-5100; Duane Thompson, Chief Executive Officer **A**1 9 10 **F**3 6 7 8 10 11 12 14 15 17 18 19 20 21 22 24 25 26 28 29 30 31 32 33 34 35 37 38 39 40 41 42 44 45 46 48 49 50 51 52 53 54 55 56 57 58 59 60 61 62 65 66 67 70 71 72 73 74 **P**1 3 7 **S**0995 Promina Northwest Health System	16	10	84	2486	32	29083	123	18571	7805	241
CARROLLTON—Carroll County ★ TANNER MEDICAL CENTER, 705 Dixie Street, Zip 30117-3818; tel. 404/836-9666; Loy M. Howard, Chief Executive Officer **A**1 9 10 **F**7 8 10 15 17 19 20 21 22 23 28 30 34 35 37 40 41 42 44 46 48 52 59 60 63 65 67 71 73 74 **P**8 **S**0002 Quorum Health Group/Quorum Health Resources	23	10	183	7383	103	46508	1086	41600	18428	689
CARTERSVILLE—Bartow County ★ CARTERSVILLE MEDICAL CENTER, 960 Joe Frank Harris Parkway, Zip 30120, Mailing Address: Box 1008, Zip 30120; tel. 404/382-1530; Keith Sandlin, Chief Executive Officer (Nonreporting) **A**1 9 10 **S**0048 Columbia/HCA Healthcare Corporation	33	10	80	—	—	—	—	—	—	—
CEDARTOWN—Polk County ★ POLK GENERAL HOSPITAL, 424 North Main Street, Zip 30125; tel. 404/748-2500; Elder B. Perdue, Administrator **A**1 9 10 **F**8 15 19 22 32 44 45 65 71 73 **P**5	16	10	35	907	10	29818	0	5746	2354	122
CHATSWORTH—Murray County ★ MURRAY MEDICAL CENTER, 707 Old Ellijay Road, Zip 30705, Mailing Address: P.O. Box 1406, Zip 30705; tel. 706/695-4564; Richard Cook, Administrator (Nonreporting) **A**9 10 **S**0048 Columbia/HCA Healthcare Corporation	16	10	42	—	—	—	—	—	—	—
CLAXTON—Evans County ☐ EVANS MEMORIAL HOSPITAL, 200 North River Street, Zip 30417, Mailing Address: Box 518, Zip 30417; tel. 912/739-2611; Eston Price Jr., Administrator (Nonreporting) **A**1 9 10	16	10	32	—	—	—	—	—	—	—
CLAYTON—Rabun County ★ RABUN COUNTY MEMORIAL HOSPITAL, South Main Street, Zip 30525, Mailing Address: Box 705, Zip 30525-0705; tel. 706/782-4233; Richard B. Wallace, Chief Executive Officer **A**9 10 **F**15 19 22 31 32 33 34 44 49 54 65 71	16	10	26	932	12	13404	0	2657	1033	53
★ RIDGECREST HOSPITAL, 393 Ridgecrest Circle, Zip 30525; tel. 706/782-4297; Gerald E. Knepp, Chief Executive Officer **A**1 9 10 **F**3 15 19 22 28 30 32 44 54 56 63 65 71 **P**6 **S**0002 Quorum Health Group/Quorum Health Resources	23	10	45	1902	20	12398	0	—	—	125
★ WOODRIDGE HOSPITAL, 394 Ridgecrest Circle, Zip 30525; tel. 706/782-3100; Gerald E. Knepp, Chief Executive Officer **A**1 9 10 **F**2 3 15 16 18 26 29 52 53 54 55 56 57 58 59 **S**0002 Quorum Health Group/Quorum Health Resources	23	82	42	793	25	1363	0	6658	2146	93
COCHRAN—Bleckley County BLECKLEY MEMORIAL HOSPITAL, 408 Peacock Street, Zip 31014-1559, Mailing Address: Box 536, Zip 31014-0536; tel. 912/934-6211; Henry T. Gibbs, Administrator **A**9 10 **F**3 15 19 20 22 27 28 30 39 41 44 46 49 65 67 71 73 **P**5 **S**2335 Memorial Health Services	16	10	45	871	9	4445	1	3821	1483	90
COLQUITT—Miller County MILLER COUNTY HOSPITAL, 209 North Cuthbert Street, Zip 31737; tel. 912/758-3385; Colleen B. Houston, Administrator (Total facility includes 97 beds in nursing home–type unit) **A**9 10 **F**15 16 19 22 34 40 44 64 71	16	10	135	466	101	4960	56	4055	2179	64
COLUMBUS—Muscogee County ★ BRADLEY CENTER, 2000 16th Avenue, Zip 31906-0308; tel. 706/649-6450 **A**1 9 10 **F**3 16 52 53 54 55 59	21	22	54	641	22	0	0	9393	3220	110
★ DOCTORS HOSPITAL, 616 19th Street, Zip 31901-1528, Mailing Address: P.O. Box 2188, Zip 31902-2188; tel. 706/571-4262; Kent Vaughn, Chief Executive Officer **A**1 9 10 **F**3 8 10 12 19 21 22 23 26 28 29 30 33 34 35 37 39 41 42 44 45 46 49 51 52 55 56 57 58 59 60 61 63 65 67 71 73 74 **P**8 **S**0048 Columbia/HCA Healthcare Corporation	33	10	248	4685	85	31547	0	42075	11810	423
★ HUGHSTON SPORTS MEDICINE HOSPITAL, 100 Frist Court, Zip 31908-7188, Mailing Address: P.O. Box 7188, Zip 31908-7188; tel. 706/576-2100; Charles Keaton, Chief Executive Officer **A**1 3 5 9 10 **F**15 16 19 21 22 35 37 41 44 46 48 49 65 66 **S**0048 Columbia/HCA Healthcare Corporation	33	47	100	3141	40	6124	0	15856	6557	297
★ ST. FRANCIS HOSPITAL, Manchester Expressway & Woodruff Road, Zip 31904-6878, Mailing Address: Box 7000, Zip 31908-7000; tel. 706/596-4000; Michael E. Garrigan, President **A**1 9 10 **F**2 3 4 10 11 16 19 21 22 28 30 31 34 35 37 39 43 44 46 49 65 67 71 **S**5455 SSM Health Care System	21	10	201	7399	134	58405	0	58639	25899	1108
★ THE MEDICAL CENTER, 710 Center Street, Zip 31901, Mailing Address: Box 951, Zip 31994-2299; tel. 706/571-1000; Lance B. Duke FACHE, President and Chief Executive Officer (Total facility includes 150 beds in nursing home–type unit) **A**1 2 3 5 9 10 **F**2 3 6 7 8 10 12 15 16 17 18 19 21 22 26 27 28 29 30 31 32 34 35 37 38 40 41 42 44 45 46 47 48 49 51 52 54 55 56 60 63 64 65 67 68 70 71 72 73 74 **P**8	23	10	606	15106	388	122611	3375	95952	40080	1269

© 1995 AHA Guide

Hospitals, U.S. / GEORGIA

Hospital, Address, Telephone, Administrator, Approval, Facility, and Physician Codes, Health Care System	Classification Codes		Utilization Data					Expense (thousands) of dollars		
★ American Hospital Association (AHA) membership ☐ Joint Commission on Accreditation of Healthcare Organizations (JCAHO) accreditation + American Osteopathic Hospital Association (AOHA) membership ○ American Osteopathic Association (AOA) accreditation △ Commission on Accreditation of Rehabilitation Facilities (CARF) accreditation Control codes 61, 63, 64, 71, 72 and 73 indicate hospitals listed by AOHA, but not registered by AHA. For definition of numerical codes, see page A6	Control	Service	Beds	Admissions	Census	Outpatient Visits	Births	Total	Payroll	Personnel
COMMERCE—Jackson County										
★ B.J.C. MEDICAL CENTER, 70 Medical Center Drive, Zip 30529–9989; tel. 706/335–1000; J. David Lawrence Jr., Chief Executive Officer (Total facility includes 167 beds in nursing home–type unit) **A**9 10 **F**7 8 19 21 22 26 37 40 44 46 48 49 64 65 71 73	16	10	257	2045	186	16754	119	13659	6350	207
CONYERS—Rockdale County										
☒ ROCKDALE HOSPITAL, 1412 Milstead Avenue N.E., Zip 30207–9990; tel. 404/918–3101; Archer R. Rose, President and Chief Executive Officer **A**1 2 9 10 **F**7 8 11 12 14 15 19 21 22 31 34 35 37 40 41 42 44 49 61 65 71 73 74	23	10	107	5697	64	75167	1253	41344	16106	562
CORDELE—Crisp County										
☐ CRISP REGIONAL HOSPITAL, 902 North Seventh Street, Zip 31015–5007; tel. 912/276–3100; Wayne T. Martin, Administrator (Nonreporting) **A**1 9 10	16	10	65	—	—	—	—	—	—	—
COVINGTON—Newton County										
☒ NEWTON GENERAL HOSPITAL, 5126 Hospital Drive, Zip 30209; tel. 404/786–7053; James F. Weadick, Administrator and Chief Executive Officer **A**1 9 10 **F**7 8 15 17 19 22 23 28 29 30 33 34 35 37 40 41 44 45 56 63 65 67 69 71 73	16	10	90	3128	33	55601	394	22157	9865	468
CUMMING—Forsyth County										
☐ BAPTIST NORTH HOSPITAL, 133 Samaritan Drive, Zip 30130, Mailing Address: Box 768, Zip 30130; tel. 404/887–2355; John M. Herron, Administrator **A**1 9 10 **F**1 4 7 8 10 11 12 14 15 16 17 19 21 22 23 24 26 28 29 30 31 32 33 34 35 37 38 40 41 42 43 44 46 48 49 51 52 54 58 59 60 61 65 71 73 74 **P**7 8	21	10	28	1200	15	20078	0	10243	3967	138
CUTHBERT—Randolph County										
★ PATTERSON HOSPITAL, 109 Randolph Street, Zip 31740–1338; tel. 912/732–2181; Earnest E. Benton, Chief Executive Officer (Total facility includes 80 beds in nursing home–type unit) **A**9 10 **F**19 22 34 40 44 46 64 71	16	10	120	955	52	12336	88	5623	3348	166
DAHLONEGA—Lumpkin County										
☒ SAINT JOSEPH'S HOSPITAL OF DAHLONEGA, 1111 Mountain Drive, Zip 30533; tel. 706/864–6136; Richard B. Maxwell III, President **A**1 9 10 **F**7 8 14 15 16 17 19 21 22 28 30 37 44 65 71	21	10	52	1376	14	21912	202	12399	5488	195
DALLAS—Paulding County										
☒ PROMINA PAULDING MEMORIAL MEDICAL CENTER, (Formerly Paulding Memorial Medical Center) 600 West Memorial Drive, Zip 30132–1335; tel. 404/445–4411; James Roy Orr Jr., Administrator (Total facility includes 136 beds in nursing home–type unit) **A**1 9 10 **F**3 6 7 8 10 11 12 14 15 17 18 19 20 21 22 24 25 26 28 29 30 31 32 33 34 35 37 38 39 40 41 42 44 45 46 48 49 50 51 52 53 54 55 56 57 58 59 60 61 62 64 65 66 67 70 71 72 73 74 **P**1 3 7 **S**0995 Promina Northwest Health System	16	10	175	1232	149	23958	0	12918	6067	251
DALTON—Whitfield County										
☒ HAMILTON MEDICAL CENTER, 1200 Memorial Drive, Zip 30720, Mailing Address: P.O. Box 1168, Zip 30722–1168; tel. 706/272–6000; Ned B. Wilford, President and Chief Executive Officer **A**1 2 9 10 **F**2 3 6 7 8 10 11 15 17 19 21 22 23 24 27 28 30 31 32 33 34 35 37 38 39 40 41 42 44 46 49 52 53 54 55 56 57 58 60 62 65 67 70 71 72 73 **P**8	23	10	282	11353	147	176920	2057	79094	36954	1162
DECATUR—De Kalb County										
☒ DECATUR HOSPITAL, 450 North Candler Street, Zip 30030, Mailing Address: Box 40, Zip 30031; tel. 404/377–0221; Carol Nickola R.N., Chief Executive Officer (Nonreporting) **A**1 9 10	23	10	83	—	—	—	—	—	—	—
☒ △ DEKALB MEDICAL CENTER, 2701 North Decatur Road, Zip 30033; tel. 404/501–1000; Charles B. Eberhart, Chief Executive Officer (Total facility includes 48 beds in nursing home–type unit) **A**1 2 7 9 10 **F**2 3 5 7 8 10 11 12 15 16 17 18 19 20 21 22 23 24 25 26 27 28 29 30 31 32 33 34 35 37 38 39 40 41 42 44 45 46 48 49 51 52 54 55 56 57 58 59 60 61 63 64 65 66 67 68 69 70 71 72 73 74 **P**1 6 7	23	10	427	19356	274	158961	4064	156235	67204	2028
☐ GEORGIA REGIONAL HOSPITAL AT ATLANTA, 3073 Panthersville Road, Zip 30034–3828; tel. 404/243–2100; Richard A. Fields M.D., Superintendent (Total facility includes 67 beds in nursing home–type unit) **A**1 3 5 10 **F**1 2 3 4 5 6 7 8 9 10 11 12 13 15 16 17 18 19 20 21 22 23 24 25 26 27 28 29 30 31 32 33 34 35 36 37 38 39 40 41 42 43 44 45 46 47 48 49 50 51 52 53 54 55 56 57 58 59 60 63 64 65 67 68 69 70 71 72 73 74 **P**6	12	22	353	6307	302	0	0	28332	17550	586
☒ VETERANS AFFAIRS MEDICAL CENTER, 1670 Clairmont Road, Zip 30033–4098; tel. 404/728–7600; Larry R. Deal, Medical Director (Total facility includes 120 beds in nursing home–type unit) **A**1 3 5 8 9 **F**2 3 4 5 8 10 11 12 19 20 21 22 23 26 27 30 31 32 33 34 35 37 39 41 42 43 44 45 46 48 49 50 51 52 54 55 56 57 58 59 60 63 64 65 67 70 71 73 74 **S**9295 Department of Veterans Affairs	45	10	486	8512	360	180544	0	133519	78884	1701
DEMOREST—Habersham County										
☒ HABERSHAM COUNTY MEDICAL CENTER, Highway 441, Zip 30535, Mailing Address: Box 37, Zip 30535; tel. 706/754–2161; C. Richard Dwozan, President (Nonreporting) **A**1 9 10 **S**0002 Quorum Health Group/Quorum Health Resources	16	10	137	—	—	—	—	—	—	—
DONALSONVILLE—Seminole County										
☒ DONALSONVILLE HOSPITAL, Hospital Circle, Zip 31745, Mailing Address: Box 677, Zip 31745; tel. 912/524–5217; Charles H. Orrick, Administrator (Total facility includes 62 beds in nursing home–type unit) **A**9 10 **F**4 8 10 14 19 22 31 33 34 42 43 44 64 71 **P**5	23	10	127	1823	79	6367	0	8115	3254	133

Hospitals, U.S. / GEORGIA

Hospital, Address, Telephone, Administrator, Approval, Facility, and Physician Codes, Health Care System	Classification Codes		Utilization Data					Expense (thousands) of dollars		Personnel
	Control	Service	Beds	Admissions	Census	Outpatient Visits	Births	Total	Payroll	

★ American Hospital Association (AHA) membership
☐ Joint Commission on Accreditation of Healthcare Organizations (JCAHO) accreditation
+ American Osteopathic Hospital Association (AOHA) membership
○ American Osteopathic Association (AOA) accreditation
△ Commission on Accreditation of Rehabilitation Facilities (CARF) accreditation
Control codes 61, 63, 64, 71, 72 and 73 indicate hospitals listed by AOHA, but not registered by AHA. For definition of numerical codes, see page A6

Hospital	Control	Service	Beds	Admissions	Census	Outpatient Visits	Births	Total	Payroll	Personnel
DOUGLAS—Coffee County										
★ COFFEE REGIONAL MEDICAL CENTER, 1101 Ocilla Road, Zip 31533–1248, Mailing Address: P.O. Box 1248, Zip 31533; tel. 912/384–1900; George L. Heck III, President and Chief Executive Officer **A**1 9 10 **F**8 11 14 15 16 17 19 20 21 22 23 26 27 28 30 34 35 37 38 40 41 44 45 46 48 49 63 65 67 71 73	16	10	145	6728	68	71079	845	29438	13210	495
DOUGLASVILLE—Douglas County										
DOUGLAS GENERAL HOSPITAL See Promina Douglas Hospital										
INNER HARBOUR HOSPITALS, 4685 Dorsett Shoals Road, Zip 30135; tel. 404/942–2391; Steve Izenour, Chief Executive Officer **A**9 **F**12 20 22 46 52 53 54 55 59 65 70 73 **P**6	23	52	129	388	125	1008	0	11447	6498	286
★ PROMINA DOUGLAS HOSPITAL, (Formerly Douglas General Hospital) 8954 Hospital Drive, Zip 30134–2282; tel. 404/949–1500; T. Mark Haney, President and Chief Executive Officer **A**1 9 10 **F**3 6 7 8 10 11 12 14 15 17 18 19 20 21 22 24 25 26 28 29 30 31 32 33 34 35 37 38 39 40 41 42 44 45 46 48 49 50 51 52 53 54 55 56 57 58 59 60 61 62 65 66 67 70 71 72 73 74 **P**1 3 7 **S**0995 Promina Northwest Health System	23	10	98	3787	41	36822	202	20077	8777	291
DUBLIN—Laurens County										
★ FAIRVIEW PARK HOSPITAL, 200 Industrial Boulevard, Zip 31021, Mailing Address: Box 1408, Zip 31040; tel. 912/275–2000; Steve C. Hoelscher, Chief Executive Officer **A**1 2 9 10 **F**11 14 15 16 19 21 22 23 24 35 37 40 44 45 48 49 50 63 65 66 71 **S**0048 Columbia/HCA Healthcare Corporation	33	10	190	8630	113	52109	989	—	—	554
★ VETERANS AFFAIRS MEDICAL CENTER, 1826 Veterans Boulevard, Zip 31021; tel. 912/272–1210; William O. Edgar, Director (Nonreporting) **A**1 3 9 **S**9295 Department of Veterans Affairs	45	10	722	—	—	—	—	—	—	—
DULUTH—Gwinnett County										
JOAN CLANCY MEMORIAL HOSPITAL See Promina Gwinnett Hospital System, Lawrenceville										
EAST POINT—Fulton County										
★ SOUTH FULTON MEDICAL CENTER, 1170 Cleveland Avenue, Zip 30344; tel. 404/305–3500; H. Neil Copelan, President and Chief Executive Officer (Total facility includes 36 beds in nursing home–type unit) **A**1 2 9 10 **F**7 8 10 11 12 17 19 21 22 24 28 29 30 35 37 39 40 41 42 44 46 48 49 60 63 65 68 71 73 74	23	10	369	11355	173	73767	1813	85957	37801	1283
EASTMAN—Dodge County										
☐ DODGE COUNTY HOSPITAL, 715 Griffin Street, Zip 31023, Mailing Address: Box 4309, Zip 31023; tel. 912/374–4000; Hal W. Sanders, Administrator **A**1 9 10 **F**8 17 19 21 22 34 35 36 37 40 44 52 57 67 71 73	16	10	84	2795	46	21328	196	11970	5153	223
EATONTON—Putnam County										
PUTNAM GENERAL HOSPITAL, Greensboro Highway, Zip 31024–4330, Mailing Address: Box 4330, Zip 31024–4330; tel. 706/485–2711; Darrell M. Oglesby, Administrator **A**9 10 **F**15 19 22 37 39 44 45 46 49 65 71 73 **P**5	16	10	50	992	10	9814	0	6451	2526	113
ELBERTON—Elbert County										
★ ELBERT MEMORIAL HOSPITAL, 4 Medical Drive, Zip 30635–1897; tel. 706/283–3151; Tim Merritt, Administrator (Nonreporting) **A**1 9 10 **S**0002 Quorum Health Group/Quorum Health Resources	16	10	53	—	—	—	—	—	—	—
ELLIJAY—Gilmer County										
☐ NORTH GEORGIA MEDICAL CENTER AND GILMER NURSING HOME, Jasper Road, Zip 30540–0346, Mailing Address: Box 346, Zip 30540–0346; tel. 706/276–4741; Mickey M. Rabuka, Administrator (Total facility includes 84 beds in nursing home–type unit) **A**1 9 10 **F**8 19 21 22 27 28 35 37 44 63 64 71	33	10	134	2252	109	15987	0	10845	3761	178
FITZGERALD—Ben Hill County										
★ DORMINY MEDICAL CENTER, Perry House Road, Zip 31750, Mailing Address: Drawer 1447, Zip 31750–1447; tel. 912/424–7100; Steve Barber, Administrator **A**1 9 10 **F**8 14 19 21 22 34 35 37 39 40 44 49 63 65 71 73	16	10	60	2211	29	20351	216	9369	4797	253
FOLKSTON—Charlton County										
CHARLTON MEMORIAL HOSPITAL, 1203 Third Street, Zip 31537, Mailing Address: Box 188, Zip 31537; tel. 912/496–2531; James L. Leis Jr., Administrator and Chief Executive Officer **A**9 10 **F**8 11 14 15 19 21 22 29 34 37 44 45 71 **P**6 **S**0985 Amerihealth, Inc.	16	10	50	547	6	3780	0	3132	1488	68
FORSYTH—Monroe County										
☐ MONROE COUNTY HOSPITAL, 88 Martin Luther King Jr. Drive, Zip 31029, Mailing Address: Box 1068, Zip 31029–1068; tel. 912/994–2521; Gale V. Tanner, Administrator **A**1 9 10 **F**8 19 22 31 34 35 42 44 65 71	16	10	40	968	13	18929	0	5946	—	115
FORT BENNING—Muscogee County										
★ MARTIN ARMY COMMUNITY HOSPITAL, Zip 31905–6100; tel. 706/544–2041; Colonel Ira F. Walton III MSC, USA, Deputy Commander for Administration **A**1 2 3 5 **F**3 8 11 12 15 16 19 21 22 23 25 26 28 29 30 31 34 37 39 40 41 44 45 46 49 51 52 53 54 55 56 57 58 61 63 65 66 71 73 **S**9395 Department of the Army	42	10	152	8241	83	634444	1128	93542	39800	1567
FORT GORDON—Richmond County										
★ DWIGHT DAVID EISENHOWER ARMY MEDICAL CENTER, Zip 30905–5650; tel. 706/787–8192; Colonel John E. Vigna, Chief of Staff (Nonreporting) **A**1 2 3 5 **S**9395 Department of the Army	42	10	396	—	—	—	—	—	—	—
FORT OGLETHORPE—Catoosa County										
GREENLEAF CENTER, 500 Greenleaf Circle, Zip 30742; tel. 706/861–4357; Richard A. Waxler, Administrator (Nonreporting) **A**9 10 **S**1155 Greenleaf Health Systems, Inc.	33	22	90	—	—	—	—	—	—	—

© 1995 AHA Guide

Hospitals, U.S. / GEORGIA

Hospital, Address, Telephone, Administrator, Approval, Facility, and Physician Codes, Health Care System

★ American Hospital Association (AHA) membership
□ Joint Commission on Accreditation of Healthcare Organizations (JCAHO) accreditation
+ American Osteopathic Hospital Association (AOHA) membership
○ American Osteopathic Association (AOA) accreditation
△ Commission on Accreditation of Rehabilitation Facilities (CARF) accreditation
Control codes 61, 63, 64, 71, 72 and 73 indicate hospitals listed by AOHA, but not registered by AHA. For definition of numerical codes, see page A6

Hospital	Control	Service	Beds	Admissions	Census	Outpatient Visits	Births	Total	Payroll	Personnel
★ HUTCHESON MEDICAL CENTER, 100 Gross Crescent Circle, Zip 30742; tel. 706/858-2000; John W. Taylor, Administrator and Chief Executive Officer (Total facility includes 109 beds in nursing home-type unit) A1 9 10 F1 2 3 7 8 10 11 12 14 15 16 19 21 22 28 30 31 32 33 35 37 38 40 42 44 49 52 53 54 55 56 57 58 59 64 65 66 70 71 73 74 P3	16	10	297	8550	220	56910	1188	69152	30260	1053
FORT STEWART—Bryan County										
★ WINN ARMY COMMUNITY HOSPITAL, Zip 31314-5300; tel. 912/767-6001 A1 5 F3 8 12 13 14 17 18 19 20 22 28 30 31 34 37 39 40 41 44 46 51 52 53 54 56 58 65 67 69 S9395 Department of the Army	42	10	100	6421	49	401091	1335	—	—	1103
FORT VALLEY—Peach County										
□ PEACH COUNTY HOSPITAL, 601 North Camellia Boulevard, Zip 31030-4599; tel. 912/825-8691; Charles E. Hill, Administrator (Nonreporting) A1 9 10	16	10	61	—	—	—	—	—	—	—
GAINESVILLE—Hall County										
★ LANIER PARK REGIONAL HOSPITAL, 675 White Sulphur Road, Zip 30505, Mailing Address: P.O. Box 1354, Zip 30503; tel. 404/503-3000; Jerry Fulks, Chief Executive Officer A1 9 10 F8 10 12 16 19 21 22 23 28 30 34 35 37 41 42 44 48 49 63 65 66 71 73 74 P8 S0048 Columbia/HCA Healthcare Corporation	33	10	124	3657	57	50671	0	32138	10650	393
★ NORTHEAST GEORGIA MEDICAL CENTER, 743 Spring Street N.E., Zip 30501-3899; tel. 404/535-3553; John A. Ferguson Jr. FACHE, President (Total facility includes 15 beds in nursing home-type unit) A1 2 9 10 F2 5 7 8 10 11 12 13 14 15 16 17 18 19 20 21 22 24 25 26 27 28 29 30 31 32 33 34 35 37 38 39 40 41 42 44 45 46 48 49 51 52 55 56 57 58 59 60 62 64 65 66 67 69 71 72 73 74 P6 7 8	23	10	338	13997	232	107386	2337	107581	43344	1443
GLENWOOD—Wheeler County										
WHEELER COUNTY HOSPITAL, Third Street, Zip 30428, Mailing Address: P.O. Box 398, Zip 30428; tel. 912/523-5113; Charles M. Mayo, Administrator (Nonreporting) A9 10	33	10	30	—	—	—	—	—	—	—
GRACEWOOD—Richmond County										
GRACEWOOD STATE SCHOOL AND HOSPITAL, Zip 30812; tel. 706/790-2030; Joanne P. Miklas Ph.D., Superintendent (Nonreporting) A10	12	12	71	—	—	—	—	—	—	—
GREENSBORO—Greene County										
MINNIE G. BOSWELL MEMORIAL HOSPITAL, Siloam Road, Zip 30642, Mailing Address: P.O. Box 329, Zip 30642; tel. 706/453-7331; Larry W. Anderson, Administrator (Nonreporting) A9 10	16	10	58	—	—	—	—	—	—	—
GRIFFIN—Spalding County										
★ SPALDING REGIONAL HOSPITAL, (Formerly AMI Spalding Regional Hospital) South Eighth Street, Zip 30223, Mailing Address: P.O. Drawer V, Zip 30224-1168; tel. 404/228-2721; Phil Shaw, Executive Director (Nonreporting) A1 9 10 S0063 TENET Healthcare Corporation	33	10	162	—	—	—	—	—	—	—
HAHIRA—Lowndes County										
SMITH HOSPITAL, 117 East Main Street, Zip 31632; tel. 912/794-2502; Amanda M. Hall, Administrator A9 10 F2 8 15 16 17 19 20 27 29 35 44 49 51 65 71 73 S2335 Memorial Health Services	33	10	71	3711	52	9818	64	6426	2780	196
HARTWELL—Hart County										
★ HART COUNTY HOSPITAL, Gibson and Cade Streets, Zip 30643-0280, Mailing Address: P.O. Box 280, Zip 30643-0280; tel. 706/376-3921; Max R. Milford, Administrator A1 9 10 F8 14 15 16 17 19 21 22 23 34 37 44 46 49 51 65 67 71 73	16	10	53	1115	14	19814	0	7292	2962	120
HAWKINSVILLE—Pulaski County										
★ TAYLOR REGIONAL HOSPITAL, Macon Highway, Zip 31036; tel. 912/783-0200; Dan S. Maddock, President (Nonreporting) A1 9 10	23	10	56	—	—	—	—	—	—	—
HAZLEHURST—Jeff Davis County										
JEFF DAVIS HOSPITAL, 1215 South Tallahassee Street, Zip 31539, Mailing Address: Box 1200, Zip 31539; tel. 912/375-7781; Oreta Williams, Administrator A9 10 F7 8 14 19 21 22 28 30 34 35 37 40 44 51 63 71 73	16	10	50	1013	11	10443	93	5240	2947	112
HIAWASSEE—Towns County										
CHATUGE REGIONAL HOSPITAL AND NURSING HOME, (Formerly Hospital Authority of Towns County) 110 Main Street, Zip 30546, Mailing Address: Box 509, Zip 30546-0509; tel. 706/896-2222; Robert R. Gora, President and Chief Executive Officer (Total facility includes 76 beds in nursing home-type unit) A9 F8 16 19 21 22 28 30 32 33 34 37 41 44 46 49 51 63 64 65 71 73	33	10	116	882	84	5612	0	3287	1722	158
HINESVILLE—Liberty County										
LIBERTY REGIONAL MEDICAL CENTER, (Formerly Liberty Memorial Hospital) 112 East Oglethorpe Boulevard, Zip 31313, Mailing Address: Box 919, Zip 31313; tel. 912/369-9400; H. Scott Kroell Jr., Chief Executive Officer A9 10 F7 8 15 16 19 22 27 28 30 34 35 39 40 44 45 46 49 65 66 71 73	16	10	41	1464	14	21761	13	6216	2245	154
HOMERVILLE—Clinch County										
★ CLINCH MEMORIAL HOSPITAL, 524 Carswell Street, Zip 31634, Mailing Address: P.O. Box 516, Zip 31634; tel. 912/487-5211; Patricia W. Busbin, Administrator A9 10 F8 15 16 19 20 22 34 44 46 49 65 71 73 P6	16	10	36	898	12	8278	2	3890	1844	112
JACKSON—Butts County										
SYLVAN GROVE HOSPITAL, 1050 McDonough Road, Zip 30233; tel. 404/775-7861; Jack S. Frayer, Administrator (Nonreporting) A9 10 S1585 Healthcare Management Group, Inc.	16	10	28	—	—	—	—	—	—	—

Hospitals, U.S. / GEORGIA

Hospital, Address, Telephone, Administrator, Approval, Facility, and Physician Codes, Health Care System	Classification Codes		Utilization Data					Expense (thousands) of dollars		
★ American Hospital Association (AHA) membership ☐ Joint Commission on Accreditation of Healthcare Organizations (JCAHO) accreditation + American Osteopathic Hospital Association (AOHA) membership ○ American Osteopathic Association (AOA) accreditation △ Commission on Accreditation of Rehabilitation Facilities (CARF) accreditation Control codes 61, 63, 64, 71, 72 and 73 indicate hospitals listed by AOHA, but not registered by AHA. For definition of numerical codes, see page A6	Control	Service	Beds	Admissions	Census	Outpatient Visits	Births	Total	Payroll	Personnel
JESUP—Wayne County ★ WAYNE MEMORIAL HOSPITAL, 865 South First Street, Zip 31545, Mailing Address: Box 408, Zip 31545; tel. 912/427–6811; Charles R. Morgan, Administrator **A**1 2 9 10 **F**7 15 19 21 22 34 35 37 40 44 71 **S**0002 Quorum Health Group/Quorum Health Resources	16	10	138	4520	64	36368	409	19742	9457	395
KENNESAW—Cobb County DEVEREUX CENTER–GEORGIA, 1291 Stanley Road, Zip 30144–4359; tel. 404/427–0147; Ralph L. Comerford, Director **F**14 15 16 22 52 53 55 65 **P**6 **S**0845 Devereux Foundation	23	52	115	73	108	0	0	12026	6402	267
LA GRANGE—Troup County ★ WEST GEORGIA MEDICAL CENTER, 1514 Vernon Road, Zip 30240–4199; tel. 706/882–1411; Charles L. Foster Jr. FACHE, President and Chief Executive Officer (Total facility includes 150 beds in nursing home–type unit) **A**1 2 9 10 **F**2 3 7 8 10 11 12 14 16 19 21 22 23 28 30 31 32 33 34 40 42 44 51 52 54 55 56 57 58 59 60 61 64 65 67 71 72 73 74 **P**5 6 7 8	15	10	363	9244	270	—	1077	59481	28480	1128
LAKELAND—Lanier County ★ LOUIS SMITH MEMORIAL HOSPITAL, 852 West Thigpen Avenue, Zip 31635–1099; tel. 912/482–3110; Neil W. Ginty, Interim Administrator (Total facility includes 62 beds in nursing home–type unit) **A**1 9 10 **F**7 15 16 22 34 40 44 46 49 64 65 71	23	10	102	841	72	8266	34	4982	2393	142
LAWRENCEVILLE—Gwinnett County ★ PROMINA GWINNETT HOSPITAL SYSTEM, (Formerly Gwinnett Hospital System) (Includes Gwinnett Medical Center, Lawrenceville, Georgia; Joan Glancy Memorial Hospital, McClure Bridge Road, Duluth, Georgia, Zip 30136; tel. 770/497–4800; Lea Capone, Administrator; Summitridge, 250 Scenic Highway, Lawrenceville, Georgia, Zip 30245; tel. 770/822–2200; David Lowry, Administrator) 1000 Medical Center Boulevard, Zip 30245, Mailing Address: Box 348, Zip 30246–0348; tel. 770/995–4321; Franklin M. Rinker, President and Chief Executive Officer (Nonreporting) **A**1 2 9 10	16	10	406	—	—	—	—	—	—	—
LITHIA SPRINGS—Douglas County ★ PARKWAY MEDICAL CENTER, 1000 Thornton Road, Zip 30057, Mailing Address: P.O. Box 570, Zip 30057; tel. 404/732–7777; Deborah S. Guthrie, Chief Operating Officer **A**1 2 9 10 **F**2 3 7 8 10 12 14 15 16 17 18 19 21 22 23 24 26 28 30 34 35 37 38 40 41 42 44 46 48 49 51 52 53 54 55 56 57 58 59 60 61 65 66 67 68 71 73 74 **P**5 **S**0048 Columbia/HCA Healthcare Corporation	33	10	233	4987	72	38600	942	33327	13748	482
LOUISVILLE—Jefferson County ☐ JEFFERSON HOSPITAL, 1067 Peachtree Street, Zip 30434; tel. 912/625–7000; Rita Culvern, Administrator **A**1 9 10 **F**14 15 16 19 22 24 30 34 44 71 73	16	10	37	798	9	15415	5	4046	1621	78
MACON—Bibb County CHARTER LAKE HOSPITAL, 3500 Riverside Drive, Zip 31210; tel. 912/474–6200; Blair R. Johanson, Administrator (Nonreporting) **A**9 10 **S**0695 Charter Medical Corporation	33	22	118	—	—	—	—	—	—	—
★ COLISEUM MEDICAL CENTERS, 350 Hospital Drive, Zip 31213; tel. 912/745–9461; Michael S. Boggs, Chief Executive Officer **A**1 9 10 **F**3 7 8 10 12 13 16 19 21 22 23 25 28 29 30 34 35 37 38 40 41 42 44 45 46 48 49 51 52 53 54 55 58 59 60 61 65 71 72 73 74 **P**1 7 **S**0048 Columbia/HCA Healthcare Corporation	33	10	188	7794	112	126537	1295	—	—	903
★ COLISEUM PSYCHIATRIC HOSPITAL, 340 Hospital Drive, Zip 31201–8002; tel. 912/741–1355; James G. Helgeson, Chief Executive Officer **A**1 9 10 **F**2 3 7 8 10 11 12 13 15 16 17 18 19 22 23 25 27 28 29 30 34 35 37 38 39 40 41 42 44 45 46 49 51 52 53 54 55 56 57 58 59 60 65 67 68 71 72 73 74 **P**1 6 7 **S**0048 Columbia/HCA Healthcare Corporation	33	22	92	1213	43	7411	0	9292	3662	122
★ MACON NORTHSIDE HOSPITAL, 400 Charter Boulevard, Zip 31210, Mailing Address: P.O. Box 4627, Zip 31208; tel. 912/757–8200; Richard Gaston, Administrator **A**1 9 10 **F**2 3 7 8 10 12 19 21 22 23 25 28 29 30 33 34 35 37 38 39 40 41 44 45 46 49 51 52 53 54 55 56 58 59 60 63 65 71 72 73 74	33	10	103	2651	39	31352	0	—	—	391
★ MEDICAL CENTER OF CENTRAL GEORGIA, 777 Hemlock Street, Zip 31201, Mailing Address: Box 6000, Zip 31208; tel. 912/633–1000; Damon D. King FACHE, President **A**1 2 3 5 8 9 10 **F**2 3 4 7 8 10 11 12 16 17 19 21 22 24 25 26 28 30 31 33 34 35 37 38 39 40 41 42 43 44 46 47 48 49 51 52 53 54 55 56 57 58 59 60 61 65 67 71 72 73 74 **P**1 7	16	10	518	21535	340	277923	3154	213970	94675	3367
★ MIDDLE GEORGIA HOSPITAL, 888 Pine Street, Zip 31201, Mailing Address: Box 6278, Zip 31208–6278; tel. 912/751–1111; William W. Fox III, Chief Executive Officer (Nonreporting) **A**1 9 10	33	10	119	—	—	—	—	—	—	—
MADISON—Morgan County MORGAN MEMORIAL HOSPITAL, Canterbury Park, Zip 30650, Mailing Address: Box 860, Zip 30650; tel. 706/342–1667; Shirley C. Harridge, Administrator **A**9 10 **F**14 15 22 34 44 71 **P**5 **S**1585 Healthcare Management Group, Inc.	33	10	26	270	3	8120	0	2287	903	42
MARIETTA—Cobb County ★ KENNESTONE HOSPITAL, 677 Church Street, Zip 30060; tel. 404/793–5000; Edward J. Bonn, President **A**1 9 10 **F**3 6 7 8 10 11 12 14 15 17 18 19 20 21 22 24 25 28 29 30 31 32 35 36 37 38 40 41 42 44 45 46 47 48 49 50 51 52 53 54 55 56 57 58 59 60 61 62 65 66 67 70 71 72 73 74 **P**1 3 7 **S**0995 Promina Northwest Health System KENNESTONE HOSPITAL AT WINDY HILL See Promina Windy Hill Hospital	23	10	505	22416	307	190367	4010	153080	66568	2307

Hospitals, U.S. / GEORGIA

Hospital, Address, Telephone, Administrator, Approval, Facility, and Physician Codes, Health Care System	Classification Codes		Utilization Data					Expense (thousands) of dollars		Personnel
★ American Hospital Association (AHA) membership □ Joint Commission on Accreditation of Healthcare Organizations (JCAHO) accreditation + American Osteopathic Hospital Association (AOHA) membership ○ American Osteopathic Association (AOA) accreditation △ Commission on Accreditation of Rehabilitation Facilities (CARF) accreditation Control codes 61, 63, 64, 71, 72 and 73 indicate hospitals listed by AOHA, but not registered by AHA. For definition of numerical codes, see page A6	Control	Service	Beds	Admissions	Census	Outpatient Visits	Births	Total	Payroll	
★ △ PROMINA WINDY HILL HOSPITAL, (Formerly Kennestone Hospital at Windy Hill) 2540 Windy Hill Road, Zip 30067; tel. 404/644–1000; John H. Richards, Administrator **A**1 2 7 9 10 **F**3 6 7 8 10 11 12 14 15 17 18 19 20 21 22 24 25 26 28 30 31 32 33 34 35 37 38 39 40 41 42 44 45 46 48 49 50 51 52 53 54 55 56 57 58 59 60 61 62 65 66 67 70 71 72 73 74 **P**1 3 7 **S**0995 Promina Northwest Health System	23	10	100	3138	39	47106	0	29787	11721	365
MCRAE—Laurens County										
TELFAIR COUNTY HOSPITAL, U.S. 341 South, Zip 31055, Mailing Address: P.O. Box 150, Zip 31055; tel. 912/868–5621; Gail B. Norris, Administrator **A**9 10 **F**15 16 19 22 28 37 44 46 65 71 **S**2335 Memorial Health Services	33	10	52	996	12	5145	0	4443	1553	85
METTER—Candler County										
★ CANDLER COUNTY HOSPITAL, Cedar Road, Zip 30439, Mailing Address: Box 597, Zip 30439–0597; tel. 912/685–5741; Charles Balkcom, President **A**9 10 **F**8 12 14 15 17 19 22 27 28 30 31 33 34 44 46 49 71 **P**5	16	10	47	1719	29	14477	0	7165	3351	153
MILLEDGEVILLE—Baldwin County										
□ CENTRAL STATE HOSPITAL, (Mental Health, Mental Retardation, and Substance Abuse) Zip 31062–9989; tel. 912/453–4128; Britton B. Dennis Sr., Superintendent (Total facility includes 1301 beds in nursing home–type unit) **A**1 10 **F**3 8 10 12 15 16 19 20 21 22 26 28 31 34 35 37 41 42 44 45 46 50 52 53 54 55 56 57 58 64 65 67 71 73 **P**6	12	49	1983	3405	1833	46182	0	135571	82231	3604
★ OCONEE REGIONAL MEDICAL CENTER, 821 North Cobb Street, Zip 31061, Mailing Address: Box 690, Zip 31061; tel. 912/454–3500; Brian L. Riddle, Chief Executive Officer **A**1 9 10 **F**4 7 8 14 15 16 17 19 21 22 23 24 28 30 31 33 34 35 36 37 40 44 45 46 49 60 65 70 71 73 **S**0002 Quorum Health Group/Quorum Health Resources	16	10	145	4670	57	51927	671	33603	14060	547
MILLEN—Jenkins County										
★ JENKINS COUNTY HOSPITAL, 515 East Winthrope Avenue, Zip 30442; tel. 912/982–4221; Watson W. Rocker, President and Chief Executive Officer **A**9 10 **F**7 8 17 18 20 22 28 29 30 31 34 39 40 44 45 46 51 56 64 71	16	10	40	1132	10	10275	33	2956	1488	79
MONROE—Walton County										
★ WALTON MEDICAL CENTER, 330 Alcova Street, Zip 30655, Mailing Address: Box 1346, Zip 30655; tel. 404/267–8461; Edgar L. Belcher, Administrator (Total facility includes 58 beds in nursing home–type unit) **A**1 9 10 **F**7 8 16 19 20 21 22 23 24 35 37 40 44 46 64 65 71 73 74 **S**0002 Quorum Health Group/Quorum Health Resources	16	10	115	2349	83	34174	149	18088	7927	267
MONTEZUMA—Macon County										
★ FLINT RIVER COMMUNITY HOSPITAL, 509 Sumter Street, Zip 31063–0770, Mailing Address: P.O. Box 770, Zip 31063–0770; tel. 912/472–3100; Michael Clark, Administrator **A**9 10 **F**8 19 21 22 31 34 35 44 70 71 **S**5765 Paracelsus Healthcare Corporation	33	10	50	1111	12	15164	0	6358	2264	83
MONTICELLO—Jasper County										
JASPER MEMORIAL HOSPITAL, 898 College Street, Zip 31064; tel. 706/468–6411; Donna Holman, Administrator (Total facility includes 44 beds in nursing home–type unit) **A**9 10 **F**14 15 16 17 19 22 27 29 30 31 32 34 35 37 41 49 64 65 71 73 **P**5	16	10	72	239	51	4678	0	—	—	72
MOODY AIR FORCE BASE—Lowndes County										
★ U.S. AIR FORCE HOSPITAL MOODY, 3278 Mitchell Boulevard, Zip 31699–1500; tel. 912/333–3772; Colonel P. R. Martin MC, USAF, Commander (Nonreporting) **A**1 **S**9495 Department of the Air Force	41	10	30							
MOULTRIE—Colquitt County										
★ COLQUITT REGIONAL MEDICAL CENTER, 3131 South Main Street, Zip 31768–6701, Mailing Address: Box 40, Zip 31776–0040; tel. 912/985–3420; James R. Lowry FACHE, Chief Executive Officer **A**1 9 10 **F**7 8 10 11 14 15 16 17 19 20 21 22 23 26 27 28 29 30 31 32 34 35 37 39 40 42 44 45 46 49 51 58 61 63 65 67 71 73 74 **P**3	16	10	155	4181	52	65614	511	25610	11188	430
TURNING POINT HOSPITAL, 319 By–Pass, Zip 31776, Mailing Address: P.O. Box 1177, Zip 31768; tel. 912/985–4815; Larry J. Burge, Managing Director (Nonreporting) **A**9 10 **S**9555 Universal Health Services, Inc.	33	82	59	—	—	—	—	—	—	—
NASHVILLE—Berrien County										
□ BERRIEN COUNTY HOSPITAL, 1221 East McPherson Street, Zip 31639, Mailing Address: P.O. Box 665, Zip 31639; tel. 912/686–7471; James P. Seward Jr., Executive Director (Total facility includes 108 beds in nursing home–type unit) **A**1 9 10 **F**8 12 15 19 21 22 32 34 35 44 46 53 57 59 64 65 71 **S**5895 Hallmark Healthcare Corporation	33	10	167	1223	121	11056	0	8253	4469	210
NEWNAN—Coweta County										
★ NEWNAN HOSPITAL, 80 Jackson Street, Zip 30263–1941, Mailing Address: Box 997, Zip 30264–0997; tel. 404/253–2330; Glenn M. Flake, Administrator (Total facility includes 143 beds in nursing home–type unit) **A**1 9 10 **F**8 10 11 12 19 20 21 22 23 24 30 31 35 37 44 45 46 49 64 65 66 71 73	23	10	253	4317	215	45240	0	32498	11478	411
★ PEACHTREE REGIONAL HOSPITAL, 60 Hospital Road, Zip 30263, Mailing Address: Box 2228, Zip 30264; tel. 404/253–1912; Linda Jubinsky, Chief Executive Officer (Nonreporting) **A**1 9 10 **S**0048 Columbia/HCA Healthcare Corporation	33	10	144	—	—	—	—	—	—	—
OCILLA—Irwin County										
★ IRWIN COUNTY HOSPITAL, 710 North Irwin Avenue, Zip 31774; tel. 912/468–7411; H. Richard Murphy, Administrator (Nonreporting) **A**9 10 **S**2335 Memorial Health Services	16	10	64							

Hospitals, U.S. / GEORGIA

Hospital, Address, Telephone, Administrator, Approval, Facility, and Physician Codes, Health Care System	Classification Codes		Utilization Data					Expense (thousands) of dollars		
★ American Hospital Association (AHA) membership ☐ Joint Commission on Accreditation of Healthcare Organizations (JCAHO) accreditation + American Osteopathic Hospital Association (AOHA) membership ○ American Osteopathic Association (AOA) accreditation △ Commission on Accreditation of Rehabilitation Facilities (CARF) accreditation Control codes 61, 63, 64, 71, 72 and 73 indicate hospitals listed by AOHA, but not registered by AHA. For definition of numerical codes, see page A6	Control	Service	Beds	Admissions	Census	Outpatient Visits	Births	Total	Payroll	Personnel
PERRY—Houston County ★ PERRY HOSPITAL, 1120 Morningside Drive, Zip 31069, Mailing Address: Drawer 1004, Zip 31069–1004; tel. 912/987–3600; Nadine L. Weems, Administrator **A**1 9 10 **F**2 3 7 8 10 12 13 14 15 16 17 18 19 20 22 26 27 28 29 30 31 32 33 34 35 36 37 39 40 44 45 46 49 51 52 54 56 65 66 67 68 71 72 73 **P**8	16	10	45	1962	22	30431	362	12420	5692	164
QUITMAN—Brooks County ☐ BROOKS COUNTY HOSPITAL, 903 North Court Street, Zip 31643, Mailing Address: P.O. Box 5000, Zip 31643; tel. 912/263–4171; Kim Bird, Administrator **A**1 9 10 **F**12 19 22 27 28 29 30 32 33 71	23	10	35	693	13	12385	0	2442	1450	52
REIDSVILLE—Tattnall County TATTNALL MEMORIAL HOSPITAL, Highway 121 South, Zip 30453, Mailing Address: Route 1, Box 261, Zip 30453; tel. 912/557–4731; Ken Ford, Administrator **A**9 10 **F**7 15 16 22 40 44 71	16	10	40	701	8	12827	51	3427	1539	72
RICHLAND—Stewart County STEWART–WEBSTER HOSPITAL, 300 Alston Street, Zip 31825, Mailing Address: Box 190, Zip 31825; tel. 912/887–3366; Edwin Bennett, Administrator **A**9 10 **F**19 22 44 65 71	33	10	32	659	11	7721	0	2714	914	49
RIVERDALE—Clayton County ★ SOUTHERN REGIONAL MEDICAL CENTER, 11 Upper Riverdale Road S.W., Zip 30274–2600; tel. 404/991–8000; Donald B. Logan, President and Chief Executive Officer **A**1 2 9 10 **F**2 7 8 10 11 12 14 15 16 17 18 19 21 22 23 25 26 28 29 30 31 32 33 34 35 37 38 39 40 41 42 44 45 46 49 52 53 54 55 56 57 58 59 60 61 62 65 67 71 73 74 **P**6	23	10	323	14289	215	111502	1742	108811	47284	1507
ROBINS AIR FORCE BASE—Houston County ★ U.S. AIR FORCE HOSPITAL ROBINS, Zip 31098–2227; tel. 912/926–9381; Lieutenant Colonel Don C. Brown MSC, USAF, Administrator (Nonreporting) **A**1 **S**9495 Department of the Air Force	41	10	32	—	—	—	—	—	—	—
ROME—Floyd County ★ △ FLOYD MEDICAL CENTER, 304 Turner McCall Boulevard, Zip 30165, Mailing Address: Box 233, Zip 30162–0233; tel. 706/802–2000; Bill G. Waters, President and Chief Executive Officer **A**1 2 3 7 9 10 **F**7 8 10 11 12 14 16 18 19 22 23 28 29 30 32 33 34 35 37 39 40 41 42 44 46 48 49 51 52 54 55 56 57 58 59 60 65 66 67 70 71 72 73 74 **P**1 6	16	10	304	12143	163	138733	2015	88280	34081	1503
☐ NORTHWEST GEORGIA REGIONAL HOSPITAL, 1305 Redmond Circle, Zip 30161; tel. 706/295–6246; Robert L. Pulliam, Superintendent (Nonreporting) **A**1 10	12	22	343	—	—	—	—	—	—	—
★ REDMOND REGIONAL MEDICAL CENTER, 501 Redmond Road, Zip 30165–7001, Mailing Address: Box 107001, Zip 30164–7001; tel. 706/291–0291; James R. Thomas, Chief Executive Officer **A**1 2 9 10 **F**8 10 11 12 15 16 19 21 22 23 25 28 35 37 42 43 44 45 63 65 67 70 71 **S**0048 Columbia/HCA Healthcare Corporation	33	10	201	8649	123	83448	0	53003	20753	836
ROSWELL—Fulton County ★ NORTH FULTON REGIONAL HOSPITAL, 3000 Hospital Boulevard, Zip 30076–9930; tel. 404/751–2500; Frederick R. Bailey, Chief Executive Officer (Nonreporting) **A**1 9 10 **S**0063 TENET Healthcare Corporation	33	10	168	—	—	—	—	—	—	—
ROYSTON—Franklin County ★ COBB MEMORIAL HOSPITAL, (Includes Brown Memorial Convalescent Center, Cobb Health Care Center) 577 Franklin Springs Street, Zip 30662, Mailing Address: Box 589, Zip 30662–0589; tel. 706/245–5034; H. Thomas Brown, Administrator (Total facility includes 260 beds in nursing home–type unit) **A**1 9 10 **F**6 7 12 13 14 15 16 17 19 21 22 28 32 36 37 39 40 41 44 46 62 64 65 71 73	23	10	331	2671	296	30387	202	17484	8552	458
SAINT MARYS—De Kalb County ★ CAMDEN MEDICAL CENTER, 2000 Dan Proctor Drive, Saint Marys, Zip 31558–0805, Mailing Address: Box 805, Zip 31558–0805; tel. 912/576–4200 **A**9 10 **F**2 3 4 7 8 10 11 15 16 19 28 31 33 34 35 38 39 40 41 42 44 46 47 48 49 51 52 53 54 55 56 58 59 60 65 71 73 **P**5 8 **S**0002 Quorum Health Group/Quorum Health Resources	23	10	40	2018	17	15220	371	13948	3724	181
SAINT SIMONS ISLAND—Benton County ☐ CHARTER BY–THE–SEA HOSPITAL, 2927 Demere Road, Saint Simons Island, Zip 31522–1620; tel. 912/638–1999; Olivia A. Erbele, Chief Executive Officer (Nonreporting) **A**1 9 10 **S**0695 Charter Medical Corporation	33	22	101	—	—	—	—	—	—	—
SANDERSVILLE—Washington County ★ MEMORIAL HOSPITAL OF WASHINGTON COUNTY, 610 Sparta Highway, Zip 31082, Mailing Address: Box 636, Zip 31082; tel. 912/552–3901; Shirley R. Roberts, Administrator (Total facility includes 60 beds in nursing home–type unit) **A**1 9 10 **F**3 8 15 16 17 19 21 22 24 26 28 30 35 37 39 42 44 45 46 49 54 55 57 58 64 65 71 73	16	10	116	2075	91	—	9	13348	5791	199
SAVANNAH—Chatham County ★ △ CANDLER HOSPITAL, 5353 Reynolds Street, Zip 31405, Mailing Address: Box 9787, Zip 31412–9787; tel. 912/692–6000; Kenneth W. Wood, President and Chief Executive Officer **A**1 7 9 10 **F**1 2 3 4 7 8 10 11 14 15 16 17 19 20 21 22 24 26 28 30 31 32 33 34 35 37 39 40 42 44 45 46 48 49 60 61 63 65 66 67 69 71 73 74 **P**5 7	23	10	335	13378	223	—	2044	111310	44922	1607
☐ CHARTER SAVANNAH BEHAVIORAL HEALTH SYSTEM, (Formerly Charter Hospital of Savannah) 1150 Cornell Avenue, Zip 31406, Mailing Address: P.O. Box 13817, Zip 31416; tel. 912/354–3911; Ron Fincher, Chief Executive Officer (Nonreporting) **A**1 9 10 **S**0695 Charter Medical Corporation	33	22	112	—	—	—	—	—	—	—

Hospitals, U.S. / GEORGIA

Hospital, Address, Telephone, Administrator, Approval, Facility, and Physician Codes, Health Care System	Classification Codes		Utilization Data					Expense (thousands) of dollars		
★ American Hospital Association (AHA) membership □ Joint Commission on Accreditation of Healthcare Organizations (JCAHO) accreditation + American Osteopathic Hospital Association (AOHA) membership ○ American Osteopathic Association (AOA) accreditation △ Commission on Accreditation of Rehabilitation Facilities (CARF) accreditation Control codes 61, 63, 64, 71, 72 and 73 indicate hospitals listed by AOHA, but not registered by AHA. For definition of numerical codes, see page A6	Control	Service	Beds	Admissions	Census	Outpatient Visits	Births	Total	Payroll	Personnel
□ GEORGIA REGIONAL HOSPITAL AT SAVANNAH, Eisenhower Drive at Varnedoe, Zip 31406, Mailing Address: Box 13607, Zip 31416-0607; tel. 912/356-2011; Walter M. Lawson III, Superintendent **A**1 5 10 **F**14 15 16 20 52 53 56 57 65 73 **P**6	12	22	226	2126	203	0	0	18028	11140	504
✠ MEMORIAL MEDICAL CENTER, 4700 Waters Avenue, Zip 31404, Mailing Address: Box 23089, Zip 31403-3089; tel. 912/350-8000; Kathy H. Jones, Interim President and Chief Executive Officer (Nonreporting) **A**1 2 3 5 8 9 10	16	10	529	—	—	—	—	—	—	—
✠ ST. JOSEPH'S HOSPITAL, 11705 Mercy Boulevard, Zip 31419-1791; tel. 912/927-5404; Paul H. Hinchey, President and Chief Executive Officer **A**1 2 9 10 **F**4 7 8 10 11 12 14 15 16 17 19 20 21 22 24 25 27 28 29 30 31 32 33 34 35 37 39 40 41 42 43 44 45 46 48 49 51 54 55 56 57 60 61 65 66 67 71 72 73 **P**1 3 5 7 **S**6015 Sisters of Mercy of the Americas–Regional Community of Baltimore	21	10	305	8747	150	48061	501	71558	32036	1041
SMYRNA—Cobb County										
BRAWNER NORTH, 3180 Atlanta Street S.E., Zip 30080; tel. 404/436-0081; John J. Cascone, Chief Executive Officer (Nonreporting) **A**3 9 10 **S**0054 Healthtrust, Inc	33	22	108	—	—	—	—	—	—	—
✠ RIDGEVIEW INSTITUTE, 3995 South Cobb Drive, Zip 30080; tel. 404/434-4567; John E. Gronewald, Executive Vice President Operations **A**1 3 5 9 10 **F**2 3 12 15 19 52 53 54 55 56 57 58 59 65 74	23	22	144	2271	69	20979	0	20964	7712	251
✠ SMYRNA HOSPITAL, 3949 South Cobb Drive, Zip 30080; tel. 404/434-0710; (Total facility includes 12 beds in nursing home–type unit) **A**1 9 10 **F**10 14 19 20 21 22 23 25 29 30 31 34 35 37 39 41 44 45 46 63 64 65 71 72 73 **S**4165 Adventist Health System–Sunbelt Health Care Corporation	21	10	100	1789	29	30956	0	19279	7116	234
SNELLVILLE—Gwinnett County										
✠ EASTSIDE MEDICAL CENTER, 1700 Medical Way, Zip 30278, Mailing Address: P.O. Box 587, Zip 30278; tel. 404/736-2498; Michael K. Kerner, Chief Executive Officer (Nonreporting) **A**1 9 10 **S**0048 Columbia/HCA Healthcare Corporation	33	10	114	—	—	—	—	—	—	—
SPARTA—Hancock County										
★ HANCOCK MEMORIAL HOSPITAL, 453 Boland Street, Zip 31087, Mailing Address: P.O. Box 490, Zip 31087; tel. 706/444-7006; Daniel D. Holtz FACHE, Administrator and Chief Executive Officer **A**9 10 **F**14 19 21 22 27 34 35 37 44 49 65 71 **S**0002 Quorum Health Group/Quorum Health Resources	23	10	30	1582	16	5979	0	5149	2186	116
SPRINGFIELD—Effingham County										
✠ EFFINGHAM HOSPITAL, 459 Highway 119 South, Zip 31329, Mailing Address: Box 386, Zip 31329-0386; tel. 912/754-6451; Norma J. Morgan, Administrator (Total facility includes 103 beds in nursing home–type unit) **A**1 9 10 **F**15 16 19 22 24 28 32 33 35 41 44 49 64 65 71 73	16	10	144	813	113	76882	0	6843	4804	133
STATESBORO—Bulloch County										
✠ BULLOCH MEMORIAL HOSPITAL, 500 East Grady Street, Zip 30459, Mailing Address: P.O. Box 1048, Zip 30459-1048; tel. 912/764-6671; Ramsey Jennings, Administrator **A**1 2 9 10 **F**7 8 14 16 19 20 21 22 23 26 28 29 30 33 34 35 37 39 40 44 45 49 63 65 70 71 73	16	10	119	5396	74	42202	1167	30097	12448	463
✠ WILLINGWAY HOSPITAL, 311 Jones Mill Road, Zip 30458; tel. 912/764-6236; Rodney Battles, Administrator **A**1 9 **F**2 3 22	33	82	40	406	30	0	0	4882	2745	100
STOCKBRIDGE—Henry County										
✠ HENRY GENERAL HOSPITAL, 1133 Eagle's Landing Parkway, Zip 30281-5099; tel. 404/389-2200; Joseph G. Brum, President and Chief Executive Officer **A**1 9 10 **F**7 8 10 11 14 15 19 21 22 28 30 34 35 37 40 42 44 60 63 65 67 70 71 73 74	16	10	124	6902	89	47285	1257	58547	21599	660
SUMMERVILLE—Chattooga County										
CHATTOOGA COUNTY HOSPITAL, 1010 Highland Avenue, Zip 30747, Mailing Address: Box 449, Zip 30747-0449; tel. 706/857-4761; David C. Hortman, Executive Director (Nonreporting) **A**9 10	16	10	172	—	—	—	—	—	—	—
SWAINSBORO—Emanuel County										
✠ EMANUEL COUNTY HOSPITAL, 117 Kite Road, Zip 30401, Mailing Address: P.O. Box 879, Zip 30401; tel. 912/237-9911; James Jarrett, Administrator (Nonreporting) **A**1 9 10 **S**0002 Quorum Health Group/Quorum Health Resources	16	10	119	—	—	—	—	—	—	—
SYLVANIA—Screven County										
★ SCREVEN COUNTY HOSPITAL, 215 Mims Road, Zip 30467; tel. 912/564-7426; Samuel A. Strickland, Administrator (Nonreporting) **A**9 10	16	10	40	—	—	—	—	—	—	—
SYLVESTER—Worth County										
✠ WORTH COUNTY HOSPITAL, 807 South Isabella Street, Zip 31791-0545, Mailing Address: Box 545, Zip 31791-0545; tel. 912/776-6961; Loron H. Coxwell, Administrator **A**1 9 10 **F**15 16 17 19 22 40 44 46 71 73 **S**2335 Memorial Health Services	33	10	50	1376	15	13005	69	4458	1846	99
THOMASTON—Upson County										
✠ UPSON REGIONAL MEDICAL CENTER, 801 West Gordon Street, Zip 30286-2831, Mailing Address: Box 1059, Zip 30286; tel. 706/647-8111; Samuel S. Gregory, Administrator **A**1 9 10 **F**14 15 16 17 19 21 22 23 35 37 40 44 49 65 71 73 **S**0002 Quorum Health Group/Quorum Health Resources	23	10	119	4859	50	46707	797	28339	12138	478
THOMASVILLE—Thomas County										
✠ JOHN D. ARCHBOLD MEMORIAL HOSPITAL, Gordon Avenue and Mimosa Drive, Zip 31799-1018, Mailing Address: P.O. Box 1018, Zip 31799; tel. 912/228-2000; Ken B. Beverly, President and Chief Executive Officer **A**1 2 9 10 **F**3 4 7 8 10 11 12 14 15 16 17 18 19 20 21 22 23 25 26 27 28 29 30 31 32 33 34 35 37 39 40 41 42 44 45 46 48 49 50 51 52 53 54 55 56 57 58 59 60 61 63 65 66 67 69 70 71 72 73 **P**8	23	10	264	9311	165	112708	857	71249	29799	1355

Hospitals, U.S. / GEORGIA

Hospital, Address, Telephone, Administrator, Approval, Facility, and Physician Codes, Health Care System	Classification Codes		Utilization Data					Expense (thousands) of dollars		
★ American Hospital Association (AHA) membership ☐ Joint Commission on Accreditation of Healthcare Organizations (JCAHO) accreditation + American Osteopathic Hospital Association (AOHA) membership ○ American Osteopathic Association (AOA) accreditation △ Commission on Accreditation of Rehabilitation Facilities (CARF) accreditation Control codes 61, 63, 64, 71, 72 and 73 indicate hospitals listed by AOHA, but not registered by AHA. For definition of numerical codes, see page A6	Control	Service	Beds	Admissions	Census	Outpatient Visits	Births	Total	Payroll	Personnel
THOMSON—McDuffie County										
★ MCDUFFIE COUNTY HOSPITAL, 521 Hill Street S.W., Zip 30824; tel. 706/595-1411; Douglas C. Keir, Chief Executive Officer **A**9 10 **F**8 14 15 16 17 19 22 24 28 35 37 39 44 46 49 51 65 71 73 **P**6 **S**0002 Quorum Health Group/Quorum Health Resources	16	10	47	2066	26	18869	0	10370	4687	226
TIFTON—Tift County										
★ TIFT GENERAL HOSPITAL, 901 East 18th Street, Zip 31794, Mailing Address: Drawer 747, Zip 31793; tel. 912/382-7120; William T. Richardson, Administrator **A**1 9 10 **F**7 8 10 12 14 15 16 17 19 21 22 23 28 33 35 36 37 41 44 45 46 48 49 54 61 65 71 73 74 **P**8	16	10	181	7658	100	64511	1045	48042	15936	735
TOCCOA—Stephens County										
★ STEPHENS COUNTY HOSPITAL, Falls Road, Zip 30577, Mailing Address: Box 947, Zip 30577-0947; tel. 706/886-6841; Edward C. Gambrell Jr., Administrator (Total facility includes 82 beds in nursing home–type unit) **A**1 9 10 **F**6 7 8 14 16 17 19 21 22 23 28 30 35 37 40 41 44 45 49 62 63 65 67 69 70 71 73	16	10	178	3366	107	28878	325	21688	10162	357
VALDOSTA—Lowndes County										
☐ GREENLEAF CENTER, 2209 Pineview Drive, Zip 31602; tel. 912/247-4357; Michael Lane, Administrator and Chief Executive Officer (Nonreporting) **A**1 9 10 **S**1155 Greenleaf Health Systems, Inc.	33	22	70	—	—	—	—	—	—	—
★ SOUTH GEORGIA MEDICAL CENTER, 2501 North Patterson Street, Zip 31602, Mailing Address: Box 1727, Zip 31603-1727; tel. 912/333-1000; John S. Bowling, President and Chief Executive Officer **A**1 2 9 10 **F**6 7 8 10 12 14 15 16 17 19 20 21 22 23 25 28 30 33 34 35 37 38 39 40 41 42 44 46 48 49 51 52 53 54 56 60 62 63 65 66 67 70 71 72 73 74 **P**8	16	10	288	11955	186	110442	1763	85021	30846	1349
VIDALIA—Toombs County										
★ MEADOWS REGIONAL MEDICAL CENTER, (Formerly Dr. John M. Meadows Memorial Hospital) 1703 Meadows Lane, Zip 30474, Mailing Address: P.O. Box 1048, Zip 30474; tel. 912/537-8921; Ronald E. Williams, Interim Administrator (Total facility includes 35 beds in nursing home–type unit) **A**9 **F**7 8 10 11 14 15 16 17 19 21 22 23 25 28 30 31 34 35 37 39 40 41 44 45 46 49 64 65 67 71 72 73	16	10	122	4335	93	34843	518	24342	9799	342
VIENNA—Dooly County										
☐ DOOLY MEDICAL CENTER, 1300 Union Street, Zip 31092, Mailing Address: Box 278, Zip 31092; tel. 912/268-4141; Kevin Paul, Administrator (Nonreporting) **A**1 9 10	16	10	38	—	—	—	—	—	—	—
VILLA RICA—Carroll County										
★ TANNER MEDICAL CENTER–VILLA RICA, 601 Dallas Road, Zip 30180, Mailing Address: Box 638, Zip 30180; tel. 404/459-7100; J. M. McCollum, Administrator **A**1 9 10 **F**7 8 10 11 15 16 17 19 22 23 35 37 38 40 42 44 46 48 60 65 71 73 74 **S**0002 Quorum Health Group/Quorum Health Resources	16	10	53	1505	15	15155	217	7633	3448	112
WARM SPRINGS—Meriwether County										
MERIWETHER MEMORIAL HOSPITAL, Mailing Address: P.O. Box 8, Zip 31830; tel. 706/655-3331; William E. Daniel, Administrator (Total facility includes 58 beds in nursing home–type unit) **A**9 10 **F**14 15 16 19 22 31 33 34 40 44 49 56 65 71	13	10	96	603	58	7427	50	—	—	49
☐ △ ROOSEVELT WARM SPRINGS INSTITUTE FOR REHABILITATION, Mailing Address: P.O. Box 1000, Zip 31830-0268; tel. 706/655-5001; Frank C. Ruzycki, Executive Director; Paul E. Peach, Medical Director (Nonreporting) **A**1 7 9 10	12	46	78	—	—	—	—	—	—	—
WARNER ROBINS—Houston County										
★ HOUSTON MEDICAL CENTER, 1601 Watson Boulevard, Zip 31093-3431, Mailing Address: Box 2886, Zip 31099-2886; tel. 912/922-4281; Arthur P. Christie, Administrator **A**1 9 10 **F**7 8 10 14 15 16 19 20 21 22 25 28 30 33 34 35 36 37 38 39 40 44 45 46 49 52 54 55 56 57 58 59 65 66 67 71 72 73	16	10	186	9669	112	71919	904	50862	22295	806
WASHINGTON—Wilkes County										
WILLS MEMORIAL HOSPITAL, 120 Gordon Street, Zip 30673, Mailing Address: Box 370, Zip 30673-0370; tel. 706/678-2151; Marshall L. Nero, Administrator (Nonreporting) **A**9 10	16	10	51	—	—	—	—	—	—	—
WAYCROSS—Ware County										
★ SATILLA REGIONAL MEDICAL CENTER, 410 Darling Avenue, Zip 31501, Mailing Address: P.O. Box 139, Zip 31502-0139; tel. 912/283-3030; Eugene Johnson, President and Chief Executive Officer (Nonreporting) **A**1 9 10	23	10	125	—	—	—	—	—	—	—
WAYNESBORO—Burke County										
☐ BURKE COUNTY HOSPITAL, 351 Liberty Street, Zip 30830; tel. 706/554-4435; Gloria Cochran, Administrator **A**1 9 10 **F**7 8 15 16 19 22 28 37 40 41 44 46 49 65 71 73 **S**2335 Memorial Health Services	13	10	40	1426	17	11792	180	6312	2330	118
WILDWOOD—Dade County										
WILDWOOD LIFESTYLE CENTER AND HOSPITAL, Lifestyle Lane, Zip 30757; tel. 706/820-1493; Dean D. Sigsworth, Administrator (Nonreporting)	23	10	13	—	—	—	—	—	—	—
WINDER—Barrow County										
★ BARROW MEDICAL CENTER, 316 North Broad Street, Zip 30680, Mailing Address: Box 768, Zip 30680; tel. 404/867-3400; Jeffrey T. Whitehorn, Chief Executive Officer (Nonreporting) **A**1 9 10 **S**0048 Columbia/HCA Healthcare Corporation	33	10	60	—	—	—	—	—	—	—

Hospitals, U.S. / HAWAII

HAWAII

Resident population 1,172 (in thousands)
Resident population in metro areas 74.7%
Birth rate per 1,000 population 17.6
65 years and over 11.7%
Percent of persons without health insurance 6.8%

- ★ American Hospital Association (AHA) membership
- ☐ Joint Commission on Accreditation of Healthcare Organizations (JCAHO) accreditation
- + American Osteopathic Hospital Association (AOHA) membership
- ○ American Osteopathic Association (AOA) accreditation
- △ Commission on Accreditation of Rehabilitation Facilities (CARF) accreditation

Control codes 61, 63, 64, 71, 72 and 73 indicate hospitals listed by AOHA, but not registered by AHA. For definition of numerical codes, see page A6

Hospital, Address, Telephone, Administrator, Approval, Facility, and Physician Codes, Health Care System	Classification Codes		Utilization Data					Expense (thousands) of dollars		
	Control	Service	Beds	Admissions	Census	Outpatient Visits	Births	Total	Payroll	Personnel
HANA—Maui County										
HANA MEDICAL CENTER See Maui Memorial Hospital, Wailuku										
HILO—Hawaii County										
★ HILO MEDICAL CENTER, 1190 Waianuenue Avenue, Zip 96720–2095; tel. 808/969–4111; John H. Westerman, Administrator (Total facility includes 108 beds in nursing home–type unit) A1 9 10 F7 8 11 14 15 16 19 20 21 22 25 26 29 31 32 33 35 40 41 44 45 49 52 54 55 56 57 59 60 64 65 71 73 S3555 State of Hawaii, Department of Health	12	10	274	9038	237	—	1324	58421	24173	751
HONOKAA—Hawaii County										
★ HONOKAA HOSPITAL, Mailing Address: P.O. Box 237, Zip 96727–0237; tel. 808/775–7211; Ivan S. Yamamoto, Administrator A9 10 F21 32 33 40 44 64 S3555 State of Hawaii, Department of Health	12	10	30	254	19	2197	2	4629	1881	53
HONOLULU—Honolulu County										
★ KAISER FOUNDATION HOSPITAL, 3288 Moanalua Road, Zip 96819; tel. 808/834–5333; Bruce Behnke, Administrator (Total facility includes 55 beds in nursing home–type unit) A1 2 3 5 10 F3 4 8 10 12 13 14 16 17 19 21 22 23 26 27 30 31 32 33 34 35 37 38 39 40 41 42 43 44 45 46 49 51 53 54 55 57 58 59 60 64 65 67 68 69 70 71 72 73 74 P4 S2105 Kaiser Foundation Hospitals	23	10	194	10336	164	1100553	2179	—	—	—
★ KAPIOLANI MEDICAL CENTER FOR WOMEN AND CHILDREN, 1319 Punahou Street, Zip 96826–1032; tel. 808/973–8511; Frances A. Hallonquist, Chief Executive Officer A1 3 5 10 F7 8 10 12 13 14 15 16 17 18 19 21 22 25 27 28 29 30 31 32 34 36 37 38 39 40 41 42 43 44 45 46 47 49 51 53 54 55 56 58 59 60 61 65 66 67 68 69 70 71 72 73 74 P6	23	44	276	13103	164	103698	5790	130682	55593	1471
★ KUAKINI MEDICAL CENTER, 347 North Kuakini Street, Zip 96817–2381; tel. 808/536–2236; Gary K. Kajiwara, President and Chief Executive Officer A1 2 3 5 9 10 F1 4 8 10 11 12 14 15 16 19 21 22 23 26 28 29 30 32 33 34 35 37 39 41 42 43 44 45 46 49 60 63 64 65 71 73	23	10	190	5786	155	37663	0	90980	45961	1386
★ LEAHI HOSPITAL, 3675 Kilauea Avenue, Zip 96816; tel. 808/733–8000; Fred D. Horwitz, Administrator (Total facility includes 179 beds in nursing home–type unit) A3 5 9 10 F1 16 19 20 21 34 35 41 50 57 63 64 65 71 P6 S3555 State of Hawaii, Department of Health	12	33	192	70	174	119	0	15432	7304	307
★ QUEEN'S MEDICAL CENTER, 1301 Punchbowl Street, Zip 96813; tel. 808/538–9011; Arthur A. Ushijima, President and Chief Executive Officer (Total facility includes 30 beds in nursing home–type unit) A1 2 3 5 8 9 10 F3 4 6 7 8 10 11 14 15 16 17 18 19 20 21 22 23 25 26 28 29 30 31 34 35 36 37 39 40 41 42 43 44 46 49 51 52 53 54 55 56 57 58 59 60 61 63 65 67 69 70 71 73 74 P5 S0040 Queen's Health Systems	23	10	541	19926	447	186264	2454	272417	122301	3062
★ △ REHABILITATION HOSPITAL OF THE PACIFIC, 226 North Kuakini Street, Zip 96817–9881; tel. 808/531–3511; Lester M. Fujitake, President and Chief Executive Officer A1 7 9 10 F6 12 14 15 16 19 21 25 27 32 34 35 36 39 41 46 48 49 54 57 58 65 66 67 71 73 P6	23	46	87	1241	75	44328	0	26371	17202	403
★ SHRINERS HOSPITALS FOR CRIPPLED CHILDREN, HONOLULU UNIT, 1310 Punahou Street, Zip 96826; tel. 808/941–4466; James B. Brasel, Administrator A1 3 5 F34 41 49 65 73 S4125 Shriners Hospitals for Crippled Children	23	57	40	421	25	4436	0	—	—	120
★ ST. FRANCIS MEDICAL CENTER, 2230 Liliha Street, Zip 96817–9979, Mailing Address: P.O. Box 30100, Zip 96820–0100; tel. 808/547–6011; Sister Beatrice Tom, President and Chief Executive Officer (Total facility includes 38 beds in nursing home–type unit) A1 2 3 5 9 10 F2 3 4 7 8 10 15 16 17 19 20 21 22 28 30 32 33 35 37 39 40 41 42 43 44 45 46 49 54 60 64 65 67 69 70 71 73 P3 S5955 Sisters of the 3rd Franciscan Order	21	10	217	5022	194	290064	0	114580	53742	1461
☐ STRAUB CLINIC AND HOSPITAL, 888 South King Street, Zip 96813; tel. 808/522–4000; Blake E. Waterhouse M.D., President and Chief Executive Officer (Nonreporting) A1 2 3 5 10	33	10	143	—	—	—	—	—	—	—
★ TRIPLER ARMY MEDICAL CENTER, Zip 96859–5000; tel. 808/433–5716; Brigadier General James E. Hastings, Commanding General A1 2 3 5 F2 3 4 7 8 10 11 12 13 17 18 19 20 21 22 24 25 28 30 31 32 34 35 37 38 39 40 41 42 43 44 45 46 49 51 52 53 54 55 56 58 59 60 61 65 66 67 70 71 73 S9395 Department of the Army	42	10	358	18736	300	868490	2963	—	—	3247
KAHUKU—Honolulu County										
★ KAHUKU HOSPITAL, Mailing Address: P.O. Box 219, Zip 96731; tel. 808/293–9221; Mark Fukuhara, Chief Executive Officer A1 9 10 F7 8 16 22 32 34 36 40 44 64 71 P6	23	10	25	558	8	7048	184	5231	2224	57
KAILUA—Honolulu County										
★ CASTLE MEDICAL CENTER, 640 Ulukahiki Street, Zip 96734–4498; tel. 808/263–5500; Kenneth A. Finch, President and Administrator A1 9 10 F2 3 7 8 14 15 16 17 19 21 22 28 29 30 32 35 37 40 41 42 44 46 49 52 53 56 58 59 64 65 71 73 74 P5 S0235 Adventist Health System/West	21	10	160	6489	112	73918	616	54349	26048	564

Hospitals, U.S. / HAWAII

Hospital, Address, Telephone, Administrator, Approval, Facility, and Physician Codes, Health Care System

★ American Hospital Association (AHA) membership
☐ Joint Commission on Accreditation of Healthcare Organizations (JCAHO) accreditation
+ American Osteopathic Hospital Association (AOHA) membership
○ American Osteopathic Association (AOA) accreditation
△ Commission on Accreditation of Rehabilitation Facilities (CARF) accreditation
Control codes 61, 63, 64, 71, 72 and 73 indicate hospitals listed by AOHA, but not registered by AHA. For definition of numerical codes, see page A6

Hospital	Classification Codes		Utilization Data					Expense (thousands) of dollars		Personnel
	Control	Service	Beds	Admissions	Census	Outpatient Visits	Births	Total	Payroll	
KANEOHE—Honolulu County HAWAII STATE HOSPITAL, 45–710 Keaahala Road, Zip 96744–3597; tel. 808/247–2191; Marvin O. St. Clair, Administrator **A**3 5 **F**1 3 6 11 15 16 17 18 20 22 26 27 31 37 46 52 54 55 57 58 65 67 73	12	22	187	273	196	0	0	—	—	494
KAPAA—Kauai County ★ SAMUEL MAHELONA MEMORIAL HOSPITAL, (Acute Care, Psychiatric, Nursing Hospice) 4800 Kawaihau Road, Zip 96746–1998; tel. 808/822–4961; Neva M. Olson, Administrator (Nonreporting) **A**9 10 **S**3555 State of Hawaii, Department of Health	12	49	82	—	—	—	—	—	—	—
KAUNAKAKAI—Maui County ★ MOLOKAI GENERAL HOSPITAL, Mailing Address: P.O. Box 408, Zip 96748–0408; tel. 808/553–5331; W. C. McElhannon, President and Chief Executive Officer (Total facility includes 22 beds in nursing home–type unit) (Data for 364 days) **A**1 9 10 **F**4 7 8 9 10 11 14 15 16 17 19 20 21 22 23 25 28 29 31 32 33 34 35 36 37 40 42 43 44 45 48 49 51 52 54 55 56 58 59 60 61 64 65 70 71 72 73 74 **P**1 4 **S**0040 Queen's Health Systems	23	10	30	204	18	9487	54	5280	2247	67
KEALAKEKUA—Hawaii County ★ KONA COMMUNITY HOSPITAL, Mailing Address: P.O. Box 69, Zip 96750–0069; tel. 808/322–4429; David W. Patton, President (Total facility includes 22 beds in nursing home–type unit) **A**1 9 10 **F**7 15 19 22 34 37 40 41 44 59 64 65 71 73 **S**3555 State of Hawaii, Department of Health	12	10	71	3280	59	30556	605	24149	10713	315
KOHALA—Hawaii County ★ KOHALA HOSPITAL, Mailing Address: P.O. Box 10, Kapaau Zip 96755–0010; tel. 808/889–6211; Manuel Anduha, Administrator **A**9 10 **F**1 2 3 4 5 6 7 8 9 10 11 12 13 15 16 17 18 19 20 21 22 23 24 25 26 27 28 29 30 31 32 33 34 35 36 37 38 39 40 41 42 43 44 45 46 47 48 49 50 51 52 53 54 55 56 57 58 59 60 61 62 63 64 65 66 67 68 69 70 71 72 73 74 **P**1 2 3 4 5 6 7 8 **S**3555 State of Hawaii, Department of Health	12	10	26	56	23	1934	0	—	—	43
KULA—Maui County ★ KULA HOSPITAL, (Long–term Skilled Nursing Facility, Intermediate Care Facility and Mental Retardation) 204 Kula Highway, Zip 96790–9499; tel. 808/878–1221; Shirley K. Takahashi R.N., Administrator (Total facility includes 103 beds in nursing home–type unit) **A**9 10 **F**15 65 **S**3555 State of Hawaii, Department of Health	12	49	105	31	97	709	0	10611	5081	179
LANAI CITY—Maui County ★ LANAI COMMUNITY HOSPITAL, 628 Seventh Street, Zip 96763–0797, Mailing Address: P.O. Box 797, Zip 96763–0797; tel. 808/565–6411; Herbert K. Yim, Administrator **A**9 10 **F**7 14 15 16 22 **S**3555 State of Hawaii, Department of Health	12	10	14	38	8	2787	2	2052	1001	29
LIHUE—Kauai County ★ WILCOX MEMORIAL HOSPITAL, 3420 Kuhio Highway, Zip 96766; tel. 808/245–1100; Kenneth T. Ono, President and Chief Executive Officer (Total facility includes 110 beds in nursing home–type unit) **A**1 2 9 10 **F**1 7 8 10 15 16 19 20 21 22 25 26 27 28 29 30 31 32 33 34 37 39 40 41 42 44 45 49 51 61 63 64 65 68 71 73 **P**5 6	23	10	177	3958	166	—	827	40837	18742	526
PAHALA—Hawaii County ★ KAU HOSPITAL, Mailing Address: P.O. Box 40, Zip 96777; tel. 808/928–8331; Dawn S. Pung, Administrator **A**9 10 **F**1 16 22 **S**3555 State of Hawaii, Department of Health	12	10	15	38	13	5523	0	2354	1086	33
WAHIAWA—Honolulu County ★ WAHIAWA GENERAL HOSPITAL, 128 Lehua Street, Zip 96786, Mailing Address: P.O. Box 580, Zip 96786–0580; tel. 808/621–8411; David L. Hill, President and Chief Executive Officer (Nonreporting) **A**1 3 5 10	23	10	162	—	—	—	—	—	—	—
WAILUKU—Maui County ★ MAUI MEMORIAL HOSPITAL, (Includes Hana Medical Center, Hana) 221 Mahalani Street, Zip 96793–2581; tel. 808/244–9056; Marian Hanlon M.D., Acting Administrator (Nonreporting) **A**1 2 9 10 **S**3555 State of Hawaii, Department of Health	12	10	145	—	—	—	—	—	—	—
WAIMEA—Kauai County ★ KAUAI VETERANS MEMORIAL HOSPITAL, Waimea Canyon Road, Zip 96796, Mailing Address: Box 337, Zip 96796–0337; tel. 808/338–9431; Orianna A. Skomoroch, Administrator (Total facility includes 20 beds in nursing home–type unit) **A**1 9 10 **F**7 8 11 12 14 15 16 22 28 39 40 44 46 65 71 **S**3555 State of Hawaii, Department of Health	12	10	49	725	27	8130	69	10253	4635	127

© 1995 AHA Guide

Hospitals, U.S. / IDAHO

IDAHO

Resident population 1,099 (in thousands)
Resident population in metro areas 30.0%
Birth rate per 1,000 population 16.2
65 years and over 11.8%
Percent of persons without health insurance 16.4%

Hospital, Address, Telephone, Administrator, Approval, Facility, and Physician Codes, Health Care System	Classification Codes		Utilization Data					Expense (thousands) of dollars		
★ American Hospital Association (AHA) membership □ Joint Commission on Accreditation of Healthcare Organizations (JCAHO) accreditation + American Osteopathic Hospital Association (AOHA) membership ○ American Osteopathic Association (AOA) accreditation △ Commission on Accreditation of Rehabilitation Facilities (CARF) accreditation Control codes 61, 63, 64, 71, 72 and 73 indicate hospitals listed by AOHA, but not registered by AHA. For definition of numerical codes, see page A6	Control	Service	Beds	Admissions	Census	Outpatient Visits	Births	Total	Payroll	Personnel
AMERICAN FALLS—Power County										
★ HARMS MEMORIAL HOSPITAL DISTRICT, 510 Roosevelt, Zip 83211–0420, Mailing Address: P.O. Box 420, Zip 83211–0420; tel. 208/226–2327; Dale E. Polla, Administrator (Total facility includes 31 beds in nursing home–type unit) **A**9 10 **F**7 8 14 15 22 26 34 37 40 41 46 49 64 65 73 **P**5	16	10	40	238	25	13769	42	1539	1081	100
ARCO—Butte County										
★ LOST RIVERS DISTRICT HOSPITAL, 551 Highland Drive, Zip 83213, Mailing Address: P.O. Box 145, Zip 83213; tel. 208/527–8206; Thomas Packer, Administrator (Nonreporting) **A**9 10	16	10	41	—	—	—	—	—	—	—
BLACKFOOT—Bingham County										
✠ BINGHAM MEMORIAL HOSPITAL, 98 Poplar Street, Zip 83221–1799; tel. 208/785–4100; Robert M. Peterson, Administrator (Total facility includes 66 beds in nursing home–type unit) **A**1 9 10 **F**7 8 15 16 17 19 21 22 26 28 29 30 35 37 39 40 41 44 45 46 49 63 64 65 67 68 73 **P**8 **S**0002 Quorum Health Group/Quorum Health Resources	13	10	120	1456	73	40876	316	11031	4252	145
STATE HOSPITAL SOUTH, 700 East Alice Street, Zip 83221–0400, Mailing Address: Box 400, Zip 83221–0400; tel. 208/785–1200; Stephen C. Weeg, Administrative Director (Total facility includes 30 beds in nursing home–type unit) **F**52 53 54 55 56 57 64 **P**6	12	22	136	164	55	0	0	11570	7396	240
BOISE—Ada County										
□ CPC INTERMOUNTAIN HOSPITAL OF BOISE, 303 North Allumbaugh Street, Zip 83704–9266; tel. 208/377–8400; Vernon G. Garrett, Administrator (Nonreporting) **A**1 9 10 **S**0785 Community Psychiatric Centers	33	22	75	—	—	—	—	—	—	—
★ △ IDAHO ELKS REHABILITATION HOSPITAL, 204 Fort Place, Zip 83702–4597, Mailing Address: Box 1100, Zip 83701–1100; tel. 208/343–2583; Joseph P. Caroselli, Administrator (Total facility includes 10 beds in nursing home–type unit) **A**7 9 10 **F**12 15 16 17 24 48 49 53 64 65 66 67 73	23	46	60	1162	38	31980	0	10956	6378	216
✠ △ SAINT ALPHONSUS REGIONAL MEDICAL CENTER, 1055 North Curtis Road, Zip 83706–1370; tel. 208/378–2121; Chris J. Anton, President **A**1 2 3 5 7 9 10 **F**3 4 8 10 12 14 15 16 17 18 19 21 22 26 27 29 30 32 34 35 37 39 42 44 45 46 48 49 52 54 55 56 57 60 65 67 69 70 71 73 **S**5585 Holy Cross Health System Corporation	23	10	248	12947	162	154670	0	101575	40232	1514
✠ ST. LUKE'S REGIONAL MEDICAL CENTER, 190 East Bannock Street, Zip 83712–6297; tel. 208/386–2222; Edwin E. Dahlberg, President **A**1 2 3 5 9 10 **F**4 7 8 10 11 13 14 15 16 17 19 20 21 22 23 24 25 26 28 29 30 31 32 33 35 37 38 39 40 41 42 43 44 45 46 47 49 50 54 56 60 63 65 67 69 71 73 74 **P**6	23	10	267	15090	166	193999	3950	119305	50868	1638
✠ VETERANS AFFAIRS MEDICAL CENTER, 500 West Fort Street, Zip 83702–4598; tel. 208/336–5100; Wayne C. Tippets, Director (Nonreporting) **A**1 3 5 9 **S**9295 Department of Veterans Affairs	45	10	181	—	—	—	—	—	—	—
BONNERS FERRY—Boundary County										
★ COMMUNITY HOSPITAL, (Includes Boundary County Nursing Home) 6640 Kaniksu Street, Zip 83805, Mailing Address: HCR 61, Box 61A, Zip 83805; tel. 208/267–3141; William T. McClintock FACHE, Chief Executive Officer (Total facility includes 52 beds in nursing home–type unit) **A**9 10 **F**1 3 8 12 15 16 17 20 22 26 27 28 30 32 33 34 37 39 44 49 64 65 67 73 **P**8	13	10	62	460	46	18729	0	3900	2264	129
BURLEY—Cassia County										
✠ CASSIA REGIONAL MEDICAL CENTER, (Formerly Cassia Memorial Hospital and Medical Center) 1501 Hiland Avenue, Zip 83318, Mailing Address: Box 489, Zip 83318; tel. 208/678–4444; Richard Packer, Administrator (Nonreporting) **A**1 2 9 10 **S**1815 Intermountain Health Care, Inc.	23	10	83	—	—	—	—	—	—	—
CALDWELL—Canyon County										
✠ WEST VALLEY MEDICAL CENTER, 1717 Arlington, Zip 83605–4864; tel. 208/459–4641; Mark Adams, Chief Executive Officer (Total facility includes 16 beds in nursing home–type unit) **A**1 9 10 **F**7 8 10 11 15 16 17 18 19 20 21 22 23 25 26 28 30 32 33 34 35 36 37 39 40 41 42 44 45 46 49 52 53 55 56 57 58 63 64 65 66 67 71 73 74 **S**0048 Columbia/HCA Healthcare Corporation	33	10	118	3283	35	54602	512	22593	8687	319
CASCADE—Valley County										
★ VALLEY COUNTY HOSPITAL, 402 Old State Highway, Zip 83611, Mailing Address: P.O. Box 151, Zip 83611; tel. 208/382–4242; Richard Holm, Administrator (Nonreporting) **A**9 10 **S**5585 Holy Cross Health System Corporation	13	10	10	—	—	—	—	—	—	—
COEUR D'ALENE—Kootenai County										
COEUR D'ALENE GENERAL HOSPITAL See Kootenai Medical Center										
✠ KOOTENAI MEDICAL CENTER, (Includes Coeur D'Alene General Hospital, 725 Hazel Avenue, Coeur D'Alene, Idaho, Zip 83814; tel. 208/664–9141; John L. Brophy, Administrator; Lake City General Hospital, 412 Lakeside Avenue, Coeur D'Alene, Idaho, Zip 83814; tel. 208/664–8161; James C. Evenden, Administrator) 2003 Lincoln Way, Zip 83814; tel. 208/666–2000; Joe Morris, Chief Executive Officer (Total facility includes 25 beds in nursing home–type unit) **A**1 2 9 10 **F**2 7 8 10 11 15 16 17 18 19 21 22 26 30 34 35 37 39 40 41 42 44 45 46 48 49 52 53 54 55 56 58 59 60 64 65 67 70 71 72 73 **P**1	16	10	212	9459	98	71288	1181	48995	22250	753
LAKE CITY GENERAL HOSPITAL See Kootenai Medical Center										

Hospitals, U.S. / IDAHO

Hospital, Address, Telephone, Administrator, Approval, Facility, and Physician Codes, Health Care System	Classification Codes		Utilization Data					Expense (thousands) of dollars		Personnel
★ American Hospital Association (AHA) membership ☐ Joint Commission on Accreditation of Healthcare Organizations (JCAHO) accreditation + American Osteopathic Hospital Association (AOHA) membership ○ American Osteopathic Association (AOA) accreditation △ Commission on Accreditation of Rehabilitation Facilities (CARF) accreditation Control codes 61, 63, 64, 71, 72 and 73 indicate hospitals listed by AOHA, but not registered by AHA. For definition of numerical codes, see page A6	Control	Service	Beds	Admissions	Census	Outpatient Visits	Births	Total	Payroll	
☐ PINE CREST HOSPITAL AND COUNSELING CENTER, 2301 North Ironwood Place, Zip 83814; tel. 208/666–1441; Ron Mays, Administrator **A**1 10 **F**2 3 12 16 17 18 30 52 53 54 55 56 58 59 65 **S**0044 Sterling Healthcare Corporation	33	22	48	669	29	0	0	5202	2343	83
COTTONWOOD—Idaho County										
★ ST. MARY'S HOSPITAL, Lewiston and North Streets, Zip 83522, Mailing Address: P.O. Box 137, Zip 83522–0137; tel. 208/962–3251; Casey Uhling, Administrator (Nonreporting) **A**9 10 **S**0515 Benedictine Health System	21	10	28	—	—	—	—	—	—	—
COUNCIL—Adams County										
COUNCIL COMMUNITY HOSPITAL AND NURSING HOME, 205 North Berkley Street, Zip 83612; tel. 208/253–4242; Joseph B. Rudd, Administrator (Nonreporting) **A**9 10	16	10	26	—	—	—	—	—	—	—
DRIGGS—Teton County										
★ TETON VALLEY HOSPITAL, 283 North First East, Zip 83422–0728, Mailing Address: P.O. Box 728, Zip 83422–0728; tel. 208/354–2383; Susan Kunz, Administrator **A**9 10 **F**7 8 13 14 15 16 17 18 20 22 26 28 29 30 31 32 33 34 37 39 40 41 44 45 46 49 51 62 65 71 72 73 **P**3	13	10	13	335	3	3515	30	2341	964	55
EMMETT—Gem County										
WALTER KNOX MEMORIAL HOSPITAL, 1202 East Locust Street, Zip 83617; tel. 208/365–3561; Max Long, Chief Executive Officer **A**9 10 **F**7 19 22 28 32 34 40 44 71 **P**6	13	10	22	459	3	12250	25	2932	1676	76
GOODING—Gooding County										
GOODING COUNTY MEMORIAL HOSPITAL, 1120 Montana Street, Zip 83330; tel. 208/934–4433; Kenneth W. Archer, Administrator (Nonreporting) **A**9 10	16	10	27	—	—	—	—	—	—	—
WALKER CENTER, 1120A Montana Street, Zip 83330–1858; tel. 208/934–8461; Vayle Mauldin, Treatment Coordinator **A**9 10 **F**2 3 15 16 20 22 52	23	82	20	198	8	959	0	—	—	23
GRANGEVILLE—Idaho County										
SYRINGA GENERAL HOSPITAL, 607 West Main Street, Zip 83530–1396; tel. 208/983–1700; Jess Hawley, Administrator (Nonreporting) **A**9 10	16	10	16	—	—	—	—	—	—	—
HAILEY—Blaine County										
BLAINE COUNTY MEDICAL CENTER See Wood River Medical Center, Sun Valley										
IDAHO FALLS—Bonneville County										
★ EASTERN IDAHO REGIONAL MEDICAL CENTER, 3100 Channing Way, Zip 83404, Mailing Address: P.O. Box 2077, Zip 83403–2077; tel. 208/529–6111; Ronald G. Butler, Chief Executive Officer **A**1 9 10 **F**2 3 4 7 8 10 12 14 15 16 17 18 19 20 21 24 25 28 29 30 31 32 33 34 35 37 38 39 40 41 42 43 44 45 48 49 51 52 53 54 55 56 58 61 63 64 65 66 67 70 71 72 73 74 **S**0048 Columbia/HCA Healthcare Corporation	33	10	286	9981	140	131796	1726	65279	26062	891
JEROME—Jerome County										
★ ST. BENEDICTS FAMILY MEDICAL CENTER, 709 North Lincoln Avenue, Zip 83338, Mailing Address: Box 586, Zip 83338–0586; tel. 208/324–4301; David Farnes, Administrator (Nonreporting) **A**9 10 **S**5585 Holy Cross Health System Corporation	21	10	80	—	—	—	—	—	—	—
KELLOGG—Shoshone County										
★ SHOSHONE MEDICAL CENTER, Jacobs Gulch, Zip 83837–2096; tel. 208/784–1221; Robert A. Morasko, Chief Executive Officer (Total facility includes 20 beds in nursing home–type unit) **A**1 9 10 **F**15 16 19 22 24 27 32 37 44 49 64 67 71 73 **P**3 5 8	16	10	46	1046	26	16255	89	6211	2388	107
LEWISTON—Nez Perce County										
★ ST. JOSEPH REGIONAL MEDICAL CENTER, 415 Sixth Street, Zip 83501–0816; tel. 208/743–2511; Howard A. Hayes, President and Chief Executive Officer **A**1 2 9 10 **F**7 8 13 14 15 16 17 18 19 20 21 22 26 27 28 29 30 31 32 33 34 35 36 37 38 39 40 41 42 44 45 46 47 49 52 54 55 56 57 58 59 60 63 65 66 67 69 70 71 72 73 74 **S**5945 Carondelet Health System	21	10	141	6366	81	96464	778	44728	19257	599
MALAD CITY—Oneida County										
ONEIDA COUNTY HOSPITAL, 150 North 200 West, Zip 83252–0126, Mailing Address: Box 126, Zip 83252–0126; tel. 208/766–2231; Robert O. Kent, Administrator and Chief Executive Officer (Nonreporting) **A**9 10	13	10	52	—	—	—	—	—	—	—
MCCALL—Ada County										
★ MCCALL MEMORIAL HOSPITAL, 1000 State Street, Zip 83638, Mailing Address: P.O. Box 906, Zip 83638; tel. 208/634–2221; Karen J. Kellie, President **A**9 10 **F**8 14 19 22 28 32 33 37 39 40 44 45 49 71 73 **P**3 **S**5585 Holy Cross Health System Corporation	16	10	17	656	5	14482	117	4490	1756	74
MONTPELIER—Bear Lake County										
★ BEAR LAKE MEMORIAL HOSPITAL, 164 South Fifth Street, Zip 83254; tel. 208/847–1630; Rod Jacobson, Administrator (Total facility includes 37 beds in nursing home–type unit) **A**9 10 **F**11 14 15 16 19 22 27 28 30 32 35 44 46 49 64 65 71 73	13	10	58	383	39	11094	82	3664	1943	112
MOSCOW—Latah County										
★ GRITMAN MEDICAL CENTER, 700 South Washington Street, Zip 83843; tel. 208/882–4511; Robert A. Colvin, President and Chief Executive Officer **A**1 9 10 **F**7 8 11 13 14 15 16 17 19 21 22 23 28 30 32 33 34 35 37 39 40 41 44 49 52 56 63 64 65 71 73 74 **P**3 8 **S**0002 Quorum Health Group/Quorum Health Resources	23	10	45	1783	17	30287	396	13040	5673	238
MOUNTAIN HOME—Elmore County										
★ ELMORE MEDICAL CENTER, 895 North Sixth East Street, Zip 83647, Mailing Address: P.O. Box 1270, Zip 83647–0348; tel. 208/587–8401; Jan G. Cox, Administrator (Total facility includes 55 beds in nursing home–type unit) **A**9 10 **F**7 8 14 19 22 28 44 49 64 71 **S**5585 Holy Cross Health System Corporation	16	10	75	1211	61	15334	91	6669	3624	87

© 1995 AHA Guide

Hospitals, U.S. / IDAHO

Hospital, Address, Telephone, Administrator, Approval, Facility, and Physician Codes, Health Care System	Classification Codes		Utilization Data					Expense (thousands) of dollars		
★ American Hospital Association (AHA) membership □ Joint Commission on Accreditation of Healthcare Organizations (JCAHO) accreditation + American Osteopathic Hospital Association (AOHA) membership ○ American Osteopathic Association (AOA) accreditation △ Commission on Accreditation of Rehabilitation Facilities (CARF) accreditation Control codes 61, 63, 64, 71, 72 and 73 indicate hospitals listed by AOHA, but not registered by AHA. For definition of numerical codes, see page A6	Control	Service	Beds	Admissions	Census	Outpatient Visits	Births	Total	Payroll	Personnel
MOUNTAIN HOME AIR FORCE BASE—Elmore County										
✠ U.S. AIR FORCE HOSPITAL MOUNTAIN HOME, Zip 83648–5300; tel. 208/828–7600; Lieutenant Colonel Roy U. Tweedle, Administrator **A**1 **F**7 8 14 15 16 20 22 29 30 34 40 44 46 51 58 65 71 73 **S**9495 Department of the Air Force	41	10	20	2189	11	111405	321	—	—	339
NAMPA—Canyon County										
✠ MERCY MEDICAL CENTER, 1512 12th Avenue Road, Zip 83686–6008; tel. 208/467–1171; Robert A. Fale, President and Chief Executive Officer **A**1 2 9 10 **F**2 3 4 7 8 10 14 15 16 19 22 27 32 33 35 36 37 40 41 44 49 65 66 71 73 **S**5175 Catholic Health Corporation	21	10	152	6038	66	154515	1201	31285	14510	497
OROFINO—Clearwater County										
★ CLEARWATER VALLEY HOSPITAL, 301 Cedar, Zip 83544–9029; tel. 208/476–4555; Warner H. Bartleson, Administrator (Nonreporting) **A**9 10 **S**0585 Brim, Inc.	13	10	26	—	—	—	—	—	—	—
STATE HOSPITAL NORTH, 300 Hospital Drive, Zip 83544; tel. 208/476–4511; Marvin Lambrecht, Administrative Director **F**14 15 16 52 65	12	22	30	188	26	0	0	2998	1221	50
POCATELLO—Bannock County										
✠ BANNOCK REGIONAL MEDICAL CENTER, 651 Memorial Drive, Zip 83201; tel. 208/239–1000; Fred R. Eaton, Administrator (Total facility includes 120 beds in nursing home–type unit) **A**1 2 3 9 10 **F**7 8 12 13 15 16 17 19 22 23 25 26 28 29 30 31 32 34 35 37 38 39 40 41 42 44 45 46 47 49 60 64 65 66 67 69 70 71 72 73 74 **P**3 5	13	10	267	5096	149	103921	1436	36459	14714	584
✠ △ POCATELLO REGIONAL MEDICAL CENTER, 777 Hospital Way, Zip 83201; tel. 208/234–0777; Earl L. Christison, Administrator (Total facility includes 9 beds in nursing home–type unit) **A**1 3 7 9 10 **F**8 10 11 12 15 16 17 19 22 28 32 35 44 46 48 49 63 64 65 71 73 **S**1815 Intermountain Health Care, Inc.	23	10	110	2394	32	94895	0	28753	11257	404
PRESTON—Franklin County										
FRANKLIN COUNTY MEDICAL CENTER, 44 North First East Street, Zip 83263; tel. 208/852–0137; Michael G. Andrus, Administrator and Chief Executive Officer (Nonreporting) **A**9 10	13	10	65	—	—	—	—	—	—	—
REXBURG—Madison County										
★ MADISON MEMORIAL HOSPITAL, 400 East Main, Zip 83440, Mailing Address: Box 310, Zip 83440–0310; tel. 208/356–3691; Keith M. Steiner, Chief Executive Officer **A**9 10 **F**7 8 14 16 19 21 22 28 29 31 32 37 39 40 44 45 55 58 60 65 71 73	13	10	52	2947	21	25552	895	11051	4676	193
RUPERT—Minidoka County										
MINIDOKA MEMORIAL HOSPITAL AND EXTENDED CARE FACILITY, 1224 Eighth Street, Zip 83350; tel. 208/436–0481; Randall G. Holom, Administrator (Total facility includes 78 beds in nursing home–type unit) **A**10 **F**8 15 16 19 21 22 26 28 30 31 32 34 35 37 40 41 44 46 51 63 65 71 73	13	10	103	1182	78	30586	175	10085	4509	139
SAINT MARIES—Benewah County										
★ BENEWAH COMMUNITY HOSPITAL, 229 South Seventh Street, Zip 83861; tel. 208/245–5551; J. Michael Boyd, Administrator **A**9 10 **F**7 8 14 15 16 18 19 22 25 28 33 37 39 40 41 44 49 51 65 67 71 73 **P**8	13	10	23	795	7	11761	71	5738	2370	105
SALMON—Lemhi County										
★ STEELE MEMORIAL HOSPITAL, Main and Daisy Streets, Zip 83467, Mailing Address: Box 700, Zip 83467; tel. 208/756–4291; Kay H. Springer, Administrator **A**9 10 **F**7 8 22 34 37 40 44 56 71	13	10	28	688	7	10334	85	2595	1503	57
SANDPOINT—Bonner County										
✠ BONNER GENERAL HOSPITAL, 520 North Third Avenue, Zip 83864–0877, Mailing Address: Box 1448, Zip 83864–0877; tel. 208/263–1441; Gene Tomt, Chief Executive Officer **A**1 9 10 **F**7 8 11 17 19 22 28 30 31 32 33 34 40 41 44 46 49 56 59 65 67 71 73 **P**3 8	23	10	54	2267	15	20239	401	9757	4837	163
SODA SPRINGS—Caribou County										
★ CARIBOU MEMORIAL HOSPITAL AND NURSING HOME, 300 South Third West Street, Zip 83276; tel. 208/547–3341; Arthur J. Phillips, Administrator (Nonreporting) **A**9 10	13	10	66	—	—	—	—	—	—	—
SUN VALLEY—Blaine County										
MORITZ COMMUNITY HOSPITAL See Wood River Medical Center										
★ WOOD RIVER MEDICAL CENTER, (Includes Blaine County Medical Center, 706 South Main Street, Hailey, Idaho, Zip 83333, Mailing Address: Box 927, Zip 83333; tel. 208/788–2222; Moritz Community Hospital, Sun Valley, Idaho, Mailing Address: P.O. Box 86, Zip 83353; tel. 208/622–3333) Sun Valley Road, Zip 83353, Mailing Address: P.O. Box 86, Zip 83353; tel. 208/622–3333; Alan Stevenson, Administrator (Total facility includes 25 beds in nursing home–type unit) **A**9 **F**7 8 14 15 19 21 22 24 33 34 35 41 44 48 49 64 65 66 71 73 74	15	10	67	1942	40	18687	227	14010	6350	199
TWIN FALLS—Twin Falls County										
✠ MAGIC VALLEY REGIONAL MEDICAL CENTER, 650 Addison Avenue West, Zip 83301, Mailing Address: Box 409, Zip 83303–0409; tel. 208/737–2000; John Bingham, Administrator (Total facility includes 20 beds in nursing home–type unit) **A**1 2 9 10 **F**7 8 15 16 19 21 22 26 30 32 33 35 37 38 40 41 42 44 46 47 49 60 64 65 70 71 72 73 **P**1 5 **S**0002 Quorum Health Group/Quorum Health Resources	13	10	147	4878	53	69786	1099	38723	15832	421
TWIN FALLS CLINIC HOSPITAL, 666 Shoshone Street East, Zip 83301, Mailing Address: Box 1233, Zip 83301; tel. 208/733–3700; Marley D. Jackman, Administrator (Nonreporting) **A**9 10	33	10	40	—	—	—	—	—	—	—

Hospital, Address, Telephone, Administrator, Approval, Facility, and Physician Codes, Health Care System	Classi- fication Codes		Utilization Data					Expense (thousands) of dollars		
★ American Hospital Association (AHA) membership □ Joint Commission on Accreditation of Healthcare Organizations (JCAHO) accreditation + American Osteopathic Hospital Association (AOHA) membership ○ American Osteopathic Association (AOA) accreditation △ Commission on Accreditation of Rehabilitation Facilities (CARF) accreditation Control codes 61, 63, 64, 71, 72 and 73 indicate hospitals listed by AOHA, but not registered by AHA. For definition of numerical codes, see page A6	Control	Service	Beds	Admissions	Census	Outpatient Visits	Births	Total	Payroll	Personnel
WEISER—Washington County ★ MEMORIAL HOSPITAL, 645 East Fifth Street, Zip 83672, Mailing Address: Box 550, Zip 83672; tel. 208/549-0370; Phillip Lowe, Administrator **A**9 10 **F**7 8 16 22 32 44 71	16	10	18	624	4	11434	92	2589	1422	56

Hospitals, U.S. / ILLINOIS

ILLINOIS

Resident population 11,697 (in thousands)
Resident population in metro areas 84.0%
Birth rate per 1,000 population 16.8
65 years and over 12.6%
Percent of persons without health insurance 11.8%

Hospital, Address, Telephone, Administrator, Approval, Facility, and Physician Codes, Health Care System	Classification Codes		Utilization Data					Expense (thousands) of dollars		
	Control	Service	Beds	Admissions	Census	Outpatient Visits	Births	Total	Payroll	Personnel

★ American Hospital Association (AHA) membership
□ Joint Commission on Accreditation of Healthcare Organizations (JCAHO) accreditation
+ American Osteopathic Hospital Association (AOHA) membership
○ American Osteopathic Association (AOA) accreditation
△ Commission on Accreditation of Rehabilitation Facilities (CARF) accreditation
Control codes 61, 63, 64, 71, 72 and 73 indicate hospitals listed by AOHA, but not registered by AHA. For definition of numerical codes, see page A6

ALEDO—Mercer County

★ MERCER COUNTY HOSPITAL, 409 Northwest Ninth Avenue, Zip 61231; tel. 309/582–5301; Bruce D. Peterson, Administrator (Total facility includes 18 beds in nursing home–type unit) **A**9 10 **F**8 15 16 19 22 30 31 32 36 37 40 41 44 48 51 58 64 65 69 71 73 **P**3 | 13 | 10 | 45 | 786 | 20 | 33491 | 51 | 6748 | 3123 | 168

ALTON—Madison County

★ ALTON MEMORIAL HOSPITAL, One Memorial Drive, Zip 62002–6722; tel. 618/463–7311; Ronald B. McMullen, President (Total facility includes 64 beds in nursing home–type unit) **A**1 2 9 10 **F**7 8 10 14 19 21 22 28 30 31 32 33 34 35 36 37 40 42 44 60 63 64 65 67 70 71 73 **P**3 4 5 7 8 **S**0051 BJC Health System | 23 | 10 | 232 | 5981 | 144 | 83668 | 635 | 50997 | 23621 | 756

□ ALTON MENTAL HEALTH CENTER, 4500 College Avenue, Zip 62002–5099; tel. 618/465–5593; Karl Kruckeberg, Director **A**1 10 **F**14 15 52 | 12 | 22 | 203 | 761 | 248 | 0 | 0 | — | — | 404

★ SAINT ANTHONY'S HEALTH CENTER, (Includes Saint Clare's Hospital, 915 East Fifth Street, Alton, Illinois, Zip 62002–6434; tel. 618/463–5151) Saint Anthony's Way, Zip 62002, Mailing Address: P.O. Box 340, Zip 62002–0340; tel. 618/465–2571; William E. Kessler, President (Total facility includes 30 beds in nursing home–type unit) **A**1 2 9 10 **F**1 2 3 4 7 8 9 10 11 12 13 14 15 16 17 18 19 20 21 22 23 24 26 27 28 29 30 31 32 33 34 35 36 37 38 39 40 41 42 43 44 45 47 48 49 52 53 54 55 56 57 58 59 60 61 63 64 65 66 67 68 69 71 72 73 74 **P**2 3 5 7 8 | 23 | 10 | 210 | 6778 | 127 | 114474 | 764 | 55284 | 23414 | 741

SAINT CLARE'S HOSPITAL See Saint Anthony's Health Center

ANNA—Union County

□ CHOATE MENTAL HEALTH AND DEVELOPMENTAL CENTER, 1000 North Main Street, Zip 62906–1699; tel. 618/833–5161; Shawn E. Jeffers, Facility Director **A**1 5 **F**14 15 19 21 22 31 35 50 52 53 54 55 56 57 58 63 65 71 73 | 12 | 22 | 385 | 705 | 403 | 0 | 0 | 23630 | 18797 | 580

★ UNION COUNTY HOSPITAL DISTRICT, 517 North Main Street, Zip 62906–1696; tel. 618/833–4511; Carol L. Goodman, Administrator (Total facility includes 60 beds in nursing home–type unit) **A**1 9 10 **F**15 17 19 21 22 28 33 34 44 45 46 49 51 64 65 71 | 16 | 10 | 100 | 1358 | 69 | 26157 | 0 | 8148 | 4215 | 222

ARLINGTON HEIGHTS—Cook County

★ NORTHWEST COMMUNITY HOSPITAL, 800 West Central Road, Zip 60005–2392; tel. 708/259–1000; Bruce K. Crowther, President and Chief Executive Officer **A**1 2 9 10 **F**1 4 7 8 10 11 12 15 17 19 21 22 23 24 26 28 29 30 32 33 34 35 37 39 40 41 42 43 44 45 46 49 52 53 54 55 56 57 58 59 60 63 65 66 67 70 71 72 73 74 **P**1 | 23 | 10 | 401 | 19719 | 269 | 418887 | 2899 | 158740 | 73472 | 1934

AURORA—Du Page County

★ △ COPLEY MEMORIAL HOSPITAL, 502 South Lincoln Avenue, Zip 60505–4690; tel. 708/844–1030; D. Chet McKee, President **A**1 2 5 7 9 10 **F**2 3 4 7 8 10 12 14 16 17 19 21 22 24 26 27 28 29 30 31 32 33 34 35 37 39 40 41 42 43 44 45 46 48 49 50 52 53 54 55 56 57 58 59 60 63 64 65 66 69 71 73 74 **P**3 5 6 **S**3855 Rush–Presbyterian–St. Luke's Medical Center | 23 | 10 | 152 | 5741 | 85 | 59966 | 833 | 50165 | 23273 | 615

★ MERCY CENTER FOR HEALTH CARE SERVICES, 1325 North Highland Avenue, Zip 60506; tel. 708/801–2601; Sister Dorothy Burns, President **A**1 2 5 9 10 **F**2 3 4 7 8 10 15 16 19 22 26 28 30 31 32 34 35 36 37 40 41 42 43 44 45 46 49 52 53 56 57 58 59 65 70 71 73 **S**5215 Mercy–Chicago Region Healthcare System | 21 | 10 | 262 | 9130 | 129 | 87064 | 1771 | 64360 | 30548 | 813

BARRINGTON—Lake County

★ GOOD SHEPHERD HOSPITAL, (Formerly EHS Good Shepherd Hospital) 450 West Highway 22, Zip 60010–1999; tel. 708/381–9600; Russell E. Feurer, Chief Executive **A**1 2 9 10 **F**15 16 19 21 27 35 37 40 44 46 49 52 53 54 58 59 63 65 66 67 71 73 74 **P**3 4 5 7 8 **S**0064 Advocate Health Care | 21 | 10 | 154 | 7655 | 80 | 75453 | 2153 | 65200 | 26040 | 735

BELLEVILLE—St. Clair County

★ MEMORIAL HOSPITAL, 4500 Memorial Drive, Zip 62223–5399; tel. 618/233–7750; Harry R. Maier, President (Total facility includes 108 beds in nursing home–type unit) **A**1 2 3 5 9 10 **F**3 4 7 8 10 16 19 21 22 23 24 28 30 32 33 34 37 40 41 42 43 44 45 46 49 52 56 58 60 64 65 66 67 71 73 | 23 | 10 | 449 | 14531 | 299 | 150374 | 1371 | 104108 | 45419 | 1655

★ △ ST. ELIZABETH'S HOSPITAL, 211 South Third Street, Zip 62222–0694; tel. 618/234–2120; Gerald M. Harman, Chief Executive Officer and Executive Vice President **A**1 2 3 5 7 9 10 **F**1 2 3 4 5 6 7 8 9 10 11 12 13 14 15 17 18 19 20 21 22 23 24 25 26 28 29 30 31 32 33 34 35 36 37 39 40 41 42 43 44 45 46 47 48 49 52 54 56 57 58 59 60 64 65 66 67 68 70 71 73 **P**8 **S**5355 Hospital Sisters Health System | 21 | 10 | 379 | 12929 | 242 | 127999 | 776 | 93785 | 39405 | 1405

BELVIDERE—Boone County

□ HIGHLAND HOSPITAL, 1625 South State Street, Zip 61008; tel. 815/547–5441; Gregory A. Olson, Administrator and Chief Executive Officer (Nonreporting) **A**1 9 10 | 23 | 10 | 69 | — | — | — | — | — | — | —

★ SAINT JOSEPH HOSPITAL, 1005 Julien Street, Zip 61008–9932; tel. 815/544–3411; Kevin D. Schoplein, Administrator (Total facility includes 15 beds in nursing home–type unit) **A**1 9 10 **F**19 22 36 44 64 71 72 73 **P**6 **S**5335 OSF Healthcare System | 21 | 10 | 48 | 1531 | 28 | 18459 | 0 | 10020 | 4336 | 173

Hospitals, U.S. / ILLINOIS

Hospital, Address, Telephone, Administrator, Approval, Facility, and Physician Codes, Health Care System	Classification Codes		Utilization Data					Expense (thousands) of dollars		
	Control	Service	Beds	Admissions	Census	Outpatient Visits	Births	Total	Payroll	Personnel

★ American Hospital Association (AHA) membership
□ Joint Commission on Accreditation of Healthcare Organizations (JCAHO) accreditation
+ American Osteopathic Hospital Association (AOHA) membership
○ American Osteopathic Association (AOA) accreditation
△ Commission on Accreditation of Rehabilitation Facilities (CARF) accreditation
Control codes 61, 63, 64, 71, 72 and 73 indicate hospitals listed by AOHA, but not registered by AHA. For definition of numerical codes, see page A6

BENTON—Franklin County

★ FRANKLIN HOSPITAL AND SKILLED NURSING CARE UNIT, 201 Bailey Lane, Zip 62812; tel. 618/439–3161; Ron Slaviero, Administrator (Total facility includes 83 beds in nursing home–type unit) **A**1 9 10 **F**8 14 15 16 19 21 22 26 30 32 33 34 36 37 39 41 44 45 49 51 64 65 71 **P**3 — 16 10 158 1393 98 29790 0 10515 4181 240

BERWYN—Cook County

★ MACNEAL HOSPITAL, 3249 South Oak Park Avenue, Zip 60402; tel. 708/795–9100; Luke McGuinness, President **A**1 2 3 5 8 9 10 **F**2 3 4 7 8 10 11 12 14 15 16 17 18 19 20 21 22 23 25 26 27 28 29 30 31 32 33 34 35 36 37 39 40 41 42 43 44 49 51 52 53 54 55 56 57 58 59 60 61 63 65 66 67 68 70 71 73 74 **P**5 6 — 23 10 427 16590 207 83062 2200 115236 53671 1898

BLOOMINGTON—McLean County

BROMENN HEALTHCARE See Normal
BROMENN LIFECARE CENTER See Bromenn Healthcare, Normal

★ ST. JOSEPH MEDICAL CENTER, 2200 East Washington Street, Zip 61701–4364, Mailing Address: Box 1287, Zip 61702–1287; tel. 309/662–3311; Kenneth J. Natzke, Administrator (Total facility includes 13 beds in nursing home–type unit) **A**1 2 9 10 **F**4 7 8 10 12 14 15 16 19 21 22 23 25 28 29 30 31 32 33 34 35 37 39 40 41 42 43 44 46 49 60 63 64 65 67 70 71 72 73 74 **P**6 **S**5335 OSF Healthcare System — 21 10 164 5254 67 54849 726 54348 22819 699

BLUE ISLAND—Cook County

★ ST. FRANCIS HOSPITAL AND HEALTH CENTER, 12935 South Gregory Street, Zip 60406–2470; tel. 708/597–2000; Jay E. Kreuzer, President **A**1 2 9 10 **F**4 5 7 8 10 12 14 17 18 19 21 22 24 25 28 29 30 31 32 33 34 35 36 37 39 40 41 42 43 44 45 46 49 54 60 63 65 67 71 72 73 74 **P**6 8 **S**5455 SSM Health Care System — 21 10 306 12832 204 73806 1302 107651 50166 1609

BREESE—Clinton County

★ ST. JOSEPH'S HOSPITAL, 9515 Holy Cross Lane, Zip 62230–0099, Mailing Address: P.O. Box 99, Zip 62230–0099; tel. 618/526–4511; Jacolyn M. Schlautman, Executive Vice President and Administrator **A**1 9 10 **F**7 8 14 15 16 19 21 22 28 30 32 33 34 35 37 40 44 49 63 65 67 71 73 **S**5355 Hospital Sisters Health System — 21 10 85 2595 32 38028 571 13388 6193 230

CANTON—Fulton County

★ GRAHAM HOSPITAL, 210 West Walnut Street, Zip 61520; tel. 309/647–5240; D. Ray Slaubaugh, President (Total facility includes 54 beds in nursing home–type unit) **A**1 6 9 10 **F**7 8 12 14 15 16 17 19 21 22 28 30 32 33 35 37 40 42 44 46 64 65 67 71 73 — 23 10 131 3210 86 36203 281 25529 11729 479

CARBONDALE—Jackson County

★ MEMORIAL HOSPITAL OF CARBONDALE, 405 West Jackson Street, Zip 62902, Mailing Address: P.O. Box 10000, Zip 62902–9000; tel. 618/549–0721; George Maroney, Administrator **A**1 2 3 5 9 10 **F**7 10 15 16 17 19 21 22 23 32 33 35 37 38 40 42 44 45 49 60 63 65 70 71 73 **S**4175 Southern Illinois Hospital Services — 23 10 137 6585 70 96548 1832 42768 18930 608

CARLINVILLE—Macoupin County

★ CARLINVILLE AREA HOSPITAL, 1001 East Morgan Street, Zip 62626–1499; tel. 217/854–3141; Robert W. Porteus, President and Chief Executive Officer (Nonreporting) **A**1 9 10 — 23 10 31 — — — — — — —

CARMI—White County

★ WHITE COUNTY HOSPITAL, 400 Plum Street, Zip 62821–1799; tel. 618/382–4171; Craig A. Jesiolowski, Chief Executive Officer (Total facility includes 98 beds in nursing home–type unit) **A**1 9 10 **F**8 12 19 21 22 28 30 33 37 44 64 71 **S**0002 Quorum Health Group/Quorum Health Resources — 16 10 130 812 102 31344 0 6775 3143 93

CARROLLTON—Greene County

★ THOMAS H. BOYD MEMORIAL HOSPITAL, (Includes Reisch Memorial Nursing Home) 800 School Street, Zip 62016–1498; tel. 217/942–6946; Deborah Campbell, Administrator (Total facility includes 40 beds in nursing home–type unit) **A**9 10 **F**8 15 22 28 30 33 44 64 — 23 10 69 425 41 16081 0 3190 1589 80

CARTHAGE—Hancock County

★ MEMORIAL HOSPITAL, South Adams Street, Zip 62321, Mailing Address: P.O. Box 160, Zip 62321; tel. 217/357–3131; Joseph Murrell, Chief Executive Officer **A**1 9 10 **F**1 3 7 8 10 12 19 21 22 28 29 32 33 34 35 40 41 42 44 45 49 65 67 71 73 **S**0002 Quorum Health Group/Quorum Health Resources — 23 10 67 1328 13 12594 82 7768 3328 150

CENTRALIA—Marion County

★ ST. MARY'S HOSPITAL, 400 North Pleasant Avenue, Zip 62801–3091; tel. 618/532–6731; James W. McDowell, President and Chief Executive Officer **A**1 2 9 10 **F**1 2 3 7 8 12 17 19 20 21 22 26 27 30 31 33 34 35 37 39 40 41 42 44 46 49 52 53 54 55 56 57 58 59 60 63 65 67 69 71 73 — 21 10 276 8689 169 96561 605 51965 21570 874

CENTREVILLE—St. Clair County

★ TOUCHETTE REGIONAL HOSPITAL, 5900 Bond Avenue, Zip 62207; tel. 618/332–3060; Mark S. Brodeur, President and Chief Executive Officer **A**1 10 — 23 10 105 2950 32 35288 1192 19988 8999 313

CHAMPAIGN—Champaign County

BURNHAM HOSPITAL See Medical Center, Urbana

□ THE PAVILION, (Formerly Carle Pavilion) 809 West Church Street, Zip 61820; tel. 217/373–1700; Nina Wanchic Eisner, Chief Executive Officer **A**1 9 10 **F**2 3 12 14 15 16 17 22 52 53 54 55 56 57 58 59 **P**4 **S**2575 Carle Foundation — 23 22 38 810 22 3120 0 6372 2350 82

© 1995 AHA Guide

Hospitals, U.S. / ILLINOIS

Hospital, Address, Telephone, Administrator, Approval, Facility, and Physician Codes, Health Care System	Classi-fication Codes		Utilization Data					Expense (thousands) of dollars		
	Control	Service	Beds	Admissions	Census	Outpatient Visits	Births	Total	Payroll	Personnel

★ American Hospital Association (AHA) membership
☐ Joint Commission on Accreditation of Healthcare Organizations (JCAHO) accreditation
+ American Osteopathic Hospital Association (AOHA) membership
○ American Osteopathic Association (AOA) accreditation
△ Commission on Accreditation of Rehabilitation Facilities (CARF) accreditation
Control codes 61, 63, 64, 71, 72 and 73 indicate hospitals listed by AOHA, but not registered by AHA. For definition of numerical codes, see page A6

CHESTER—Randolph County

Hospital	Control	Service	Beds	Admissions	Census	Outpatient Visits	Births	Total	Payroll	Personnel
☐ CHESTER MENTAL HEALTH CENTER, Chester Road, Zip 62233–0031, Mailing Address: Box 31, Zip 62233–0031; tel. 618/826–4571; Stephen L. Hardy Ph.D., Facility Director (Nonreporting) **A**1	12	22	314	—	—	—	—	—	—	—
★ MEMORIAL HOSPITAL, 1900 State Street, Zip 62233–0609, Mailing Address: Box 609, Zip 62233; tel. 618/826–4581; Eric Freeburg, Administrator **A**1 9 10 **F**2 3 8 11 14 15 19 21 22 23 28 30 32 33 35 36 39 40 42 44 46 49 54 58 64 65 67 71 73	16	10	55	1262	17	39827	75	8893	3995	182

CHICAGO—Cook County

Hospital	Control	Service	Beds	Admissions	Census	Outpatient Visits	Births	Total	Payroll	Personnel
BELMONT COMMUNITY HOSPITAL See THC–Chicago										
BERNARD MITCHELL HOSPITAL See University of Chicago Hospitals										
★ BETHANY HOSPITAL, (Formerly EHS Bethany Hospital) 3435 West Van Buren, Zip 60624; tel. 312/265–7700; Johnny C. Brown, President **A**1 9 10 **F**2 3 7 8 12 13 17 18 19 20 21 22 25 26 27 28 30 34 37 39 40 41 42 44 49 51 52 54 60 61 65 71 73 **P**6 8 **S**0064 Advocate Health Care	23	10	138	6104	77	44982	1117	44777	19556	490
☐ CHARTER BARCLAY HOSPITAL, 4700 North Clarendon Avenue, Zip 60640; tel. 312/728–7100; John F. Buckley, Administrator (Nonreporting) **A**1 9 10 **S**0695 Charter Medical Corporation	33	22	123	—	—	—	—	—	—	—
★ CHICAGO LAKESHORE HOSPITAL, (Formerly HCA Chicago Lakeshore Hospital) 4840 North Marine Drive, Zip 60640; tel. 312/878–9700; Marcia S. Shapiro, Chief Executive Officer **A**1 3 9 10 **F**2 3 14 15 17 18 21 34 35 52 53 54 55 56 57 58 59 67 **S**0048 Columbia/HCA Healthcare Corporation	33	22	102	1486	66	3393	0	9848	5155	131
CHICAGO LYING–IN HOSPITAL See University of Chicago Hospitals										
+ ○ CHICAGO OSTEOPATHIC HOSPITAL AND MEDICAL CENTERS, 5200 South Ellis Avenue, Zip 60615–4399; tel. 312/947–3000; (Nonreporting) **A**9 10 11 12 13	23	10	262	—	—	—	—	—	—	—
CHICAGO–READ MENTAL HEALTH CENTER, 4200 North Oak Park Avenue, Zip 60634; tel. 312/794–4000; Thomas Simpatico M.D., Medical and Facility Director **A**10 **F**2 4 5 7 8 9 10 11 15 16 18 19 20 21 22 23 31 32 35 37 40 41 42 43 44 45 46 48 49 50 51 52 54 55 56 57 58 60 61 63 64 65 66 67 70 71 73 74	12	22	328	2867	318	0	0	38501	30374	609
★ CHILDREN'S MEMORIAL HOSPITAL, 2300 Children's Plaza, Zip 60614; tel. 312/880–4000; Jan R. Jennings, President and Chief Executive Officer **A**1 2 3 5 8 9 10 **F**4 5 10 13 15 16 17 19 20 21 22 23 29 30 31 32 34 35 38 39 42 43 44 45 46 47 49 51 52 53 54 55 56 58 59 60 63 65 67 69 70 71 73	23	50	243	10566	180	200554	0	191841	87052	2385
★ COLUMBUS HOSPITAL, 2520 North Lakeview Avenue, Zip 60614; tel. 312/883–7300; Lee Domanico, Chief Executive Officer **A**1 2 3 5 9 10 **F**2 3 4 7 8 10 13 19 21 22 26 30 31 34 35 37 38 40 41 42 43 44 46 48 49 60 65 67 71 73 74 **P**8 **S**8805 Columbus–Cabrini Medical Center	21	10	290	10554	174	81251	1456	107386	39864	1203
★ COOK COUNTY HOSPITAL, 1835 West Harrison Street, Zip 60612; tel. 312/633–6000; Ruth M. Rothstein, Director **A**1 2 3 5 8 9 10 **F**3 4 5 7 8 9 10 11 12 13 14 15 16 17 18 19 20 21 22 23 25 26 27 28 29 30 31 33 34 35 37 38 39 40 41 42 43 44 45 46 47 48 49 51 52 53 54 55 56 57 58 60 61 62 64 65 67 68 69 70 71 73 74 **P**6 **S**0016 Cook County Bureau of Health Services	13	10	842	33044	552	686382	2883	463194	269934	5868
☐ DOCTORS HOSPITAL OF HYDE PARK, 5800 South Stony Island Avenue, Zip 60637–2099; tel. 312/643–9200; Stephen M. Weinstein, President and Chief Executive Officer (Nonreporting) **A**1 9 10	32	10	177	—	—	—	—	—	—	—
★ EDGEWATER MEDICAL CENTER, 5700 North Ashland Avenue, Zip 60660–4086; tel. 312/878–6000; Peter G. Rogan, Chief Executive Officer **A**1 2 3 9 10 **F**4 8 10 14 15 16 19 21 22 26 29 30 31 33 34 37 41 42 43 44 46 49 54 56 60 65 71 **P**5	23	10	201	6855	147	29848	0	54137	20361	660
EHS BETHANY HOSPITAL See Bethany Hospital										
EHS TRINITY HOSPITAL See Trinity Hospital										
★ △ GRANT HOSPITAL, 550 West Webster Avenue, Zip 60614–9980; tel. 312/883–2000; Timothy J. Crowley, Chief Executive Officer (Total facility includes 33 beds in nursing home–type unit) (Data for 337 days) **A**1 3 5 7 9 10 **F**2 3 4 7 8 10 11 13 14 15 16 17 18 19 20 21 22 23 27 28 29 30 31 32 34 35 37 38 40 41 42 43 44 48 49 51 52 53 54 55 56 57 58 59 60 61 64 65 66 67 68 70 71 73 74 **P**5 **S**0048 Columbia/HCA Healthcare Corporation	33	10	232	8451	165	75097	566	58897	28621	890
☐ HARTGROVE HOSPITAL, 520 North Ridgeway Avenue, Zip 60624; tel. 312/722–3113; Karen E. Johnson, Administrator (Nonreporting) **A**1 9 10 **S**0455 Hospital Group of America	33	22	109	—	—	—	—	—	—	—
HCA CHICAGO LAKESHORE HOSPITAL See Chicago Lakeshore Hospital										
★ △ HOLY CROSS HOSPITAL, 2701 West 68th Street, Zip 60629–1882; tel. 312/471–8000; Mark C. Clement, President and Chief Executive Officer (Total facility includes 37 beds in nursing home–type unit) **A**1 2 7 9 **F**8 10 11 12 15 16 17 19 21 22 32 33 34 35 37 40 42 44 45 48 64 65 71 73 **P**3 5	23	10	263	11253	209	98003	691	80541	42709	1292
★ ILLINOIS MASONIC MEDICAL CENTER, 836 West Wellington Avenue, Zip 60657–5193; tel. 312/975–1600; Bruce C. Campbell, President (Total facility includes 255 beds in nursing home–type unit) **A**1 2 3 5 8 9 10 **F**3 4 7 8 10 11 12 13 14 15 16 17 18 19 20 21 22 25 26 27 28 29 30 31 32 33 34 35 37 38 39 40 41 42 43 44 45 46 47 49 51 52 53 54 55 56 57 58 59 60 61 63 64 65 67 69 70 71 73 74 **P**5 6	23	10	620	18107	523	330220	3621	234150	119020	2763
ILLINOIS STATE PSYCHIATRIC INSTITUTE, 1153 North Laverne Street, Zip 60612–4310; tel. 312/854–6300; James T. Barter M.D., Director (Nonreporting) **A**5	12	22	182	—	—	—	—	—	—	—

Hospitals, U.S. / ILLINOIS

Hospital, Address, Telephone, Administrator, Approval, Facility, and Physician Codes, Health Care System	Classification Codes		Utilization Data					Expense (thousands) of dollars		
	Control	Service	Beds	Admissions	Census	Outpatient Visits	Births	Total	Payroll	Personnel

★ American Hospital Association (AHA) membership
☐ Joint Commission on Accreditation of Healthcare Organizations (JCAHO) accreditation
+ American Osteopathic Hospital Association (AOHA) membership
○ American Osteopathic Association (AOA) accreditation
△ Commission on Accreditation of Rehabilitation Facilities (CARF) accreditation
Control codes 61, 63, 64, 71, 72 and 73 indicate hospitals listed by AOHA, but not registered by AHA. For definition of numerical codes, see page A6

Hospital	Control	Service	Beds	Admissions	Census	Outpatient Visits	Births	Total	Payroll	Personnel
☐ JACKSON PARK HOSPITAL, 7531 Stony Island Avenue, Zip 60649–3993; tel. 312/947–7500; Peter E. Friedell M.D., President (Nonreporting) **A**1 2 3 9	23	10	225	—	—	—	—	—	—	—
JOHNSTON R. BOWMAN HEALTH CENTER See Rush–Presbyterian–St. Luke's Medical Center										
★ LARABIDA CHILDREN'S HOSPITAL AND RESEARCH CENTER, (Pediatric Chronic Disease) East 65th St at Lake Michigan, Zip 60649–1395; tel. 312/363–6700; Arthur F. Kohrman M.D., President **A**1 9 10 **F**14 22 34 45 49 65 73	23	59	62	1294	44	19130	0	25374	12439	412
LINCOLN WEST HOSPITAL See Vencor Hospital–Chicago North										
☐ LORETTO HOSPITAL, 645 South Central Avenue, Zip 60644–5088; tel. 312/626–4300; Dallas Keith Larson, President and Chief Executive Officer **A**1 9 10 **F**1 2 3 8 9 11 12 15 19 21 22 27 28 30 31 32 33 34 37 38 40 41 44 46 47 48 49 51 52 54 56 58 64 65 67 71 **P**5 **S**0905 Summit Medical Management, Inc.	23	10	222	5858	158	43665	0	32807	15157	538
★ LOUIS A. WEISS MEMORIAL HOSPITAL, 4646 North Marine Drive, Zip 60640–1501; tel. 312/878–8700; Dean M. Harrison, President and Chief Executive Officer **A**1 2 3 5 9 10 **F**2 3 4 7 8 10 11 12 14 15 16 17 19 21 22 26 27 28 30 31 35 37 39 40 41 42 43 44 46 49 51 60 65 66 69 71 73 74 **P**5 6 7	23	10	222	6954	126	117220	404	76951	38310	925
★ MERCY HOSPITAL AND MEDICAL CENTER, Stevenson Expwy at King Drive, Zip 60616–2477; tel. 312/567–2100; Winkle Lee, Chief Executive Officer (Total facility includes 28 beds in nursing home–type unit) **A**1 2 3 5 8 9 10 **F**2 3 4 5 7 8 10 11 12 13 14 15 17 18 19 21 22 24 25 27 28 29 30 31 33 34 35 37 38 39 40 41 42 43 44 45 46 48 49 52 53 54 55 56 57 58 59 60 64 65 66 67 68 69 71 73 **P**8 **S**5215 Mercy–Chicago Region Healthcare System	21	10	487	16282	265	263980	2641	148270	74759	2008
☐ METHODIST HOSPITAL OF CHICAGO, 5025 North Paulina Street, Zip 60640–2797; tel. 312/271–9040; Steven H. Friedman Ph.D., Executive Vice President (Nonreporting) **A**1 2 9 10	23	10	189	—	—	—	—	—	—	—
★ △ MICHAEL REESE HOSPITAL AND MEDICAL CENTER, 2929 South Ellis Avenue, Zip 60616; tel. 312/791–2000; Nancy S. Carlstedt, Chief Executive Officer **A**1 2 3 5 7 8 9 10 **F**4 7 8 10 11 12 13 16 17 19 20 21 22 23 25 27 28 31 32 33 34 35 37 38 40 41 42 43 44 46 47 48 49 51 52 54 56 57 58 59 60 61 63 65 67 69 71 73 74 **P**5 **S**0048 Columbia/HCA Healthcare Corporation	33	10	565	18339	305	—	2729	190620	79519	2417
★ MOUNT SINAI HOSPITAL MEDICAL CENTER OF CHICAGO, California Avenue and 15th Street, Zip 60608–1610; tel. 312/542–2000; Benn Greenspan, President and Chief Executive Officer **A**1 2 3 8 9 10 **F**2 3 4 7 8 10 11 12 14 15 16 17 19 20 21 22 23 25 26 27 28 30 31 32 34 35 37 38 39 40 41 42 43 44 45 46 48 49 51 52 53 54 55 56 57 58 59 60 61 64 65 66 67 68 69 70 71 72 73 74 **P**6	23	10	356	14841	270	786064	3339	130213	66463	2360
NORMAN AND IDA STONE INSTITUTE OF PSYCHIATRY See Northwestern Memorial Hospital										
★ NORTHWESTERN MEMORIAL HOSPITAL, (Includes Norman and Ida Stone Institute of Psychiatry, 320 East Huron Street, Chicago, Illinois, Zip 60611; Olson Pavilion, 707 North Fairbanks Court, Chicago, Illinois, Zip 60611; Passavant Pavilion, 303 East Superior Street, Chicago, Illinois, Zip 60611; tel. 312/908–2000; Prentice Women's Hospital, 333 East Superior Street, Chicago, Illinois, Zip 60611; tel. 312/908–2000; Wesley Pavilion, 250 East Superior Street, Chicago, Illinois, Zip 60611; tel. 312/908–2000) Superior Street and Fairbanks Court, Chicago, Illinois, Zip 60611–2950; tel. 312/908–2000; Gary A. Mecklenburg, President and Chief Executive Officer **A**1 2 3 5 8 9 10 **F**3 4 5 7 8 10 12 13 14 15 16 17 18 19 20 21 22 23 24 26 27 28 29 30 31 32 33 34 35 37 38 39 40 41 42 43 44 45 46 47 49 51 52 53 54 55 56 57 58 59 60 61 63 65 67 69 70 71 73 74 **P**4 5 7 8	23	10	708	31704	436	189710	5064	347157	159659	3995
★ NORWEGIAN–AMERICAN HOSPITAL, 1044 North Francisco Avenue, Zip 60622; tel. 312/292–8200; Clarence A. Nagelvoort, President and Chief Executive Officer **A**1 9 10 **F**7 8 12 13 15 17 19 20 22 25 30 34 35 37 38 40 41 44 46 49 51 65 71 73 **P**1 6	23	10	230	9794	97	83345	3546	51284	24524	732
★ OUR LADY OF THE RESURRECTION MEDICAL CENTER, 5645 West Addison Street, Zip 60634–4455; tel. 312/282–7000; John Sullivan, Chief Executive Officer (Total facility includes 46 beds in nursing home–type unit) **A**1 9 10 **F**2 3 4 6 7 8 9 10 11 12 15 16 17 19 20 21 22 24 25 27 28 29 30 32 33 34 35 37 38 39 40 41 42 43 44 45 46 48 49 51 60 62 63 64 65 67 71 72 73 74 **P**5 6	21	10	273	9571	209	89905	0	64133	28825	1007
PASSAVANT PAVILION See Northwestern Memorial Hospital										
PRENTICE WOMEN'S HOSPITAL See Northwestern Memorial Hospital										
★ PROVIDENT HOSPITAL OF COOK COUNTY, 500 East 51st Street, Zip 60615; tel. 312/572–1200; Shirley Bomar-Cole, Acting Chief Operating Officer **A**1 10 **F**2 3 4 5 7 8 9 10 11 12 13 14 15 16 17 18 19 20 21 22 23 25 26 28 29 30 31 34 35 37 38 39 40 41 42 43 44 45 46 47 48 49 51 52 53 64 65 66 67 68 69 70 71 72 73 74 **P**6 **S**0016 Cook County Bureau of Health Services	13	10	96	4353	58	58945	651	69671	29692	775
★ △ RAVENSWOOD HOSPITAL MEDICAL CENTER, 4550 North Winchester Avenue, Zip 60640–5205; tel. 312/878–4300; John E. Blair, President (Total facility includes 38 beds in nursing home–type unit) **A**1 2 3 5 6 7 9 10 **F**3 4 5 7 8 10 11 12 13 16 17 18 19 21 22 25 27 29 30 31 32 33 34 35 37 39 40 41 42 43 44 46 48 52 53 54 55 56 57 58 59 60 61 63 64 65 67 71 73 74 **P**1 3 6 **S**0064 Advocate Health Care	23	10	321	11943	223	133705	2294	97791	50074	1556
★ △ REHABILITATION INSTITUTE OF CHICAGO, 345 East Superior Street, Zip 60611–4496; tel. 312/908–6017; Henry B. Betts M.D., President and Chief Executive Officer **A**1 3 5 7 9 10 **F**5 16 17 19 20 21 22 25 26 29 34 35 42 44 45 46 48 49 53 54 56 60 61 65 66 67 71 73 74 **P**6	23	46	176	2278	139	66000	0	61134	34500	966

© 1995 AHA Guide

Hospitals, U.S. / ILLINOIS

Hospital, Address, Telephone, Administrator, Approval, Facility, and Physician Codes, Health Care System	Classification Codes		Utilization Data					Expense (thousands of dollars)		Personnel
★ American Hospital Association (AHA) membership ☐ Joint Commission on Accreditation of Healthcare Organizations (JCAHO) accreditation + American Osteopathic Hospital Association (AOHA) membership ○ American Osteopathic Association (AOA) accreditation △ Commission on Accreditation of Rehabilitation Facilities (CARF) accreditation Control codes 61, 63, 64, 71, 72 and 73 indicate hospitals listed by AOHA, but not registered by AHA. For definition of numerical codes, see page A6	Control	Service	Beds	Admissions	Census	Outpatient Visits	Births	Total	Payroll	
★ RESURRECTION MEDICAL CENTER, 7435 West Talcott Avenue, Zip 60631–3746; tel. 312/774–8000; Sister Donna Marie, Executive Vice President and Chief Executive Officer (Total facility includes 275 beds in nursing home–type unit) **A**1 2 3 5 9 10 **F**3 4 7 8 10 15 16 17 19 21 22 24 29 31 32 34 35 37 38 40 41 42 43 44 45 48 49 53 54 55 56 57 58 59 60 64 65 66 67 71 74 **P**1 5 6 7	21	10	623	16760	574	—	1233	146725	57230	2431
★ ROSELAND COMMUNITY HOSPITAL, 45 West 111th Street, Zip 60628; tel. 312/995–3000; Denise R. Williams, President **A**1 9 10 **F**14 15 16 19 22 25 34 35 37 38 39 40 44 46 65 71 73 **P**1	23	10	128	4947	81	51998	1087	29181	14081	495
★ △ RUSH–PRESBYTERIAN–ST. LUKE'S MEDICAL CENTER, (Includes Johnston R. Bowman Health Center, 700 South Paulina, Chicago, Illinois, Zip 60612; tel. 312/942–7000; James T. Frankenbach, President) 1653 West Congress Parkway, Zip 60612–3833; tel. 312/942–5000; Leo M. Henikoff M.D., President and Chief Executive Officer (Total facility includes 44 beds in nursing home–type unit) **A**1 2 3 5 7 8 9 10 **F**1 2 3 4 5 6 7 8 10 11 14 17 19 20 21 22 23 26 28 30 31 32 34 35 37 38 40 41 42 43 44 46 47 48 49 50 51 52 53 54 55 56 57 58 59 60 61 63 64 65 66 67 69 71 73 74 **P**5 6 **S**3855 Rush-Presbyterian–St. Luke's Medical Center	23	10	829	29301	658	270453	2416	408432	195404	7077
☐ SACRED HEART HOSPITAL, 3240 West Franklin Boulevard, Zip 60624–1599; tel. 312/722–3020; Edward Novak, President and Chief Executive Officer (Nonreporting) **A**1 9 10	33	10	96							
★ SAINT ANTHONY HOSPITAL, 2875 West 19th Street, Zip 60623; tel. 312/521–1710; F. Scott Winslow, Regional Chief Operating Officer (Total facility includes 12 beds in nursing home–type unit) **A**1 9 10 **F**3 4 7 8 10 13 19 21 22 26 28 30 32 34 35 37 40 41 42 43 44 46 49 51 52 54 55 56 58 59 60 64 65 67 71 74 **P**8 **S**8805 Columbus–Cabrini Medical Center	21	10	159	5707	92	39145	1548	32618	15322	460
SAINT CABRINI HOSPITAL, 811 South Lytle Street, Zip 60607; tel. 312/883–4300; F. Scott Winslow, Chief Operating Officer **A**3 9 10 **F**3 4 7 8 10 13 19 21 22 26 28 30 31 34 35 37 40 41 42 43 44 49 60 65 67 71 73 74 **P**8 **S**8805 Columbus–Cabrini Medical Center	21	10	190	6078	85	27522	1590	35824	13420	413
★ SAINT MARY OF NAZARETH HOSPITAL CENTER, 2233 West Division Street, Zip 60622–3086; tel. 312/770–2000; Sister Stella Louise, President and Chief Executive Officer **A**1 2 3 9 10 **F**1 4 8 10 11 12 14 15 16 17 19 20 21 23 25 28 30 31 32 33 34 35 37 39 40 41 42 43 44 45 46 49 51 52 53 54 55 56 57 58 59 60 65 67 71 73 74 **P**5 8 **S**5575 Sisters of the Holy Family of Nazareth–Sacred Heart Province	21	10	305	12419	234	159835	1994	99754	48382	1292
★ △ SCHWAB REHABILITATION HOSPITAL AND CARE NETWORK, 1401 South California Boulevard, Zip 60608–1612; tel. 312/522–2010; Kathleen C. Yosko, President and Chief Executive Officer **A**1 3 7 8 9 10 **F**2 3 4 7 8 10 11 12 17 19 20 21 27 31 32 34 35 37 38 39 40 41 42 43 44 46 47 48 49 51 52 53 54 55 56 59 60 61 64 65 67 68 70 71 73	23	46	85	1051	73	38404	0	20889	12234	301
★ SHRINERS HOSPITALS FOR CRIPPLED CHILDREN, CHICAGO UNIT, 2211 North Oak Park Avenue, Zip 60635–3392; tel. 312/622–5400; A. James Spang, Administrator **A**1 3 5 **F**5 12 15 16 17 19 20 21 27 34 35 39 41 44 45 47 48 49 53 54 56 65 67 71 73 **P**6 **S**4125 Shriners Hospitals for Crippled Children	23	57	60	1491	25	14633	0	—		264
★ SOUTH SHORE HOSPITAL, 8012 South Crandon Avenue, Zip 60617–1199; tel. 312/768–0810; John D. Harper, Administrator (Nonreporting) **A**1 9 10	23	10	124							
☐ ST. BERNARD HOSPITAL, 64th & Dan Ryan Expressway, Zip 60621; tel. 312/962–3900; Sister Elizabeth Van Straten, President and Chief Executive Officer (Nonreporting) **A**1 9 10	21	10	194							
★ ST. ELIZABETH'S HOSPITAL, 1431 North Claremont Avenue, Zip 60622; tel. 312/633–5930; Joann Birdzell, President (Total facility includes 27 beds in nursing home–type unit) **A**1 2 3 9 10 **F**2 3 8 10 14 15 16 17 19 20 21 22 23 25 28 30 31 32 33 34 35 36 37 41 42 44 45 46 48 49 52 58 59 64 65 71 **P**3 5 7 8 **S**0135 Ancilla Systems Inc.	21	10	240	9186	186	91876	0	59655	27240	894
★ ST. JOSEPH HEALTH CENTERS AND HOSPITAL, (Formerly St. Joseph Hospital and Health Care Center) 2900 North Lake Shore Drive, Zip 60657–6274; tel. 312/665–3000; Sister Theresa Peck, President and Chief Executive Officer (Total facility includes 68 beds in nursing home–type unit) **A**1 2 3 5 9 10 **F**4 5 7 8 10 12 13 14 15 16 17 19 20 21 22 25 26 27 28 29 30 31 32 33 34 35 37 40 41 42 43 44 45 46 48 49 51 52 54 56 57 60 61 62 64 65 66 67 71 73 74 **P**5 **S**1855 Daughters of Charity National Health System	21	10	493	11272	231	104342	1460	109016	55015	1626
★ SWEDISH COVENANT HOSPITAL, 5145 North California Avenue, Zip 60625–3688; tel. 312/878–8200; Edward A. Cucci, President **A**1 2 3 5 9 10 **F**4 7 8 10 12 13 14 15 16 17 19 20 21 22 23 24 26 27 28 29 30 32 33 35 37 40 41 42 43 44 45 46 48 49 51 52 55 56 57 58 60 62 63 64 65 66 67 69 70 71 72 73 74 **P**5	21	10	292	10112	216	144307	1019	83105	40313	1279
☐ THC–CHICAGO, (Formerly Belmont Community Hospital) 4058 West Melrose Street, Zip 60641; tel. 312/736–7000; Darryl L. Duncan, Chief Executive Officer (Data for 343 days) **A**1 9 10 **F**12 14 16 19 20 22 26 27 31 33 34 35 37 39 41 44 54 65 71	33	10	55	174	19	0	0	8554	2813	158
★ THOREK HOSPITAL AND MEDICAL CENTER, 850 West Irving Park Road, Zip 60613; tel. 312/525–6780; Frank A. Solare, President and Chief Executive Officer **A**1 3 9 10 **F**8 14 15 17 19 21 22 27 28 30 31 33 36 37 41 42 44 46 49 51 60 65 67 71 73 **P**5 6	23	10	158	4858	78	89819	0	37571	15141	479
★ TRINITY HOSPITAL, (Formerly EHS Trinity Hospital) 2320 East 93rd Street, Zip 60617; tel. 312/978–2000; John N. Schwartz, Chief Executive Officer **A**1 9 10 **F**2 3 7 8 10 12 15 17 19 20 21 22 27 28 29 30 32 33 34 35 37 39 40 41 42 44 45 46 49 51 54 58 62 65 67 71 73 74 **P**1 2 6 7 **S**0064 Advocate Health Care	21	10	228	9948	132	70134	1915	71987	29917	994

Hospitals, U.S. / ILLINOIS

Hospital, Address, Telephone, Administrator, Approval, Facility, and Physician Codes, Health Care System	Classification Codes		Utilization Data					Expense (thousands) of dollars		
★ American Hospital Association (AHA) membership □ Joint Commission on Accreditation of Healthcare Organizations (JCAHO) accreditation + American Osteopathic Hospital Association (AOHA) membership ○ American Osteopathic Association (AOA) accreditation △ Commission on Accreditation of Rehabilitation Facilities (CARF) accreditation Control codes 61, 63, 64, 71, 72 and 73 indicate hospitals listed by AOHA, but not registered by AHA. For definition of numerical codes, see page A6	Control	Service	Beds	Admissions	Census	Outpatient Visits	Births	Total	Payroll	Personnel
□ UNIVERSITY HOSPITAL, 1116 North Kedzie Avenue, Zip 60651; tel. 312/276–5200; Anthony M. DeJoseph Psy.D., Administrator and Chief Executive Officer (Nonreporting) **A**1 9 10	33	22	110	—	—	—	—	—	—	—
★ UNIVERSITY OF CHICAGO HOSPITALS, (Includes Bernard Mitchell Hospital, Chicago, Illinois; Chicago Lying–In Hospital, Chicago, Illinois; Wyler Children's Hospital, Chicago, Illinois; tel. 312/702–6168) 5841 South Maryland, Zip 60637–1470; tel. 312/702–1000; Ralph W. Muller, President and Chief Executive Officer **A**1 2 3 5 8 9 10 **F**4 5 7 8 9 10 11 12 13 14 17 19 20 21 22 23 24 26 27 28 30 32 34 35 37 38 39 40 41 42 43 44 45 46 47 49 50 51 52 53 54 55 56 57 58 59 60 61 63 65 67 69 70 71 73 74 **P**5	23	10	572	24242	457	406081	3109	386981	166191	4675
★ △ UNIVERSITY OF ILLINOIS AT CHICAGO MEDICAL CENTER, 1740 West Taylor Street, Zip 60612–4348; tel. 312/996–3900; Sidney E. Mitchell, Director **A**1 2 3 5 7 8 9 10 **F**3 4 5 7 8 10 11 12 13 14 15 16 17 19 20 21 22 23 25 26 27 28 29 30 31 34 35 37 38 40 41 42 43 44 45 46 47 48 49 51 52 53 54 55 56 57 58 59 60 61 65 67 68 69 70 71 73 74 **P**4 6	12	10	429	17460	313	382899	3335	273019	123606	2910
□ VENCOR HOSPITAL–CHICAGO NORTH, (Formerly Lincoln West Hospital) 2544 West Montrose Avenue, Zip 60618; tel. 312/267–2200; Jack Nathan Shapiro, Administrator **A**1 10 **F**8 15 16 19 21 22 30 34 35 37 41 44 52 54 55 57 63 65 71 73 **P**5 **S**0026 Vencor, Incorporated	33	10	94	2366	62	11784	0	—	—	263
★ VETERANS AFFAIRS LAKESIDE MEDICAL CENTER, 333 East Huron Street, Zip 60611–3004; tel. 312/640–2100; Joseph L. Moore, Director **A**1 3 5 8 **F**2 3 4 5 6 8 10 11 12 14 15 16 17 18 19 20 21 22 23 25 26 27 28 29 30 31 32 33 34 35 37 39 41 42 43 44 45 46 48 49 51 52 54 55 56 57 58 59 60 65 67 69 71 73 74 **S**9295 Department of Veterans Affairs	45	10	252	6500	191	192180	0	94405	—	1159
★ VETERANS AFFAIRS WEST SIDE MEDICAL CENTER, 820 South Damen Avenue, Zip 60612, Mailing Address: Box 8195, Zip 60680; tel. 312/666–6500; John J. DeNardo, Director **A**1 2 3 5 8 **F**1 2 3 4 6 8 10 11 12 14 15 16 17 18 19 20 21 23 24 26 27 28 29 30 31 32 33 34 35 37 39 41 42 43 44 45 46 48 49 50 51 52 54 55 56 57 58 59 60 61 63 64 65 67 69 71 73 74 **S**9295 Department of Veterans Affairs	45	10	337	7892	265	265084	0	119431	78615	1578
WESLEY PAVILION See Northwestern Memorial Hospital										
WYLER CHILDREN'S HOSPITAL See University of Chicago Hospitals										
CHICAGO HEIGHTS—Cook County										
★ ST. JAMES HOSPITAL AND HEALTH CENTERS, 1423 Chicago Road, Zip 60411–9934; tel. 708/756–1000; Peter J. Murphy, President and Chief Executive Officer (Total facility includes 101 beds in nursing home–type unit) **A**1 2 9 10 **F**7 8 10 11 15 19 21 22 25 26 27 28 29 30 32 33 34 35 36 37 39 40 41 42 44 45 46 49 60 64 65 67 71 73 74 **P**5 6 8 **S**5345 Sisters of St. Francis Health Services, Inc.	21	10	348	11962	239	63229	1405	87823	37349	1167
CLIFTON—Iroquois County										
★ CENTRAL COMMUNITY HOSPITAL, 335 East Fifth Avenue, Zip 60927, Mailing Address: Box 68, Zip 60927; tel. 815/694–2392; John F. Kuhn, Chief Executive Officer **A**1 9 10 **F**19 21 22 25 26 28 30 33 34 36 41 44 45 65 71 **S**4025 Servantcor	23	10	33	504	5	7157	0	2660	963	53
CLINTON—Dewitt County										
★ DR. JOHN WARNER HOSPITAL, 422 West White Street, Zip 61727–2199; tel. 217/935–9571; Brian K. Klitzing, Chief Executive Officer and Chief Financial Officer (Total facility includes 9 beds in nursing home–type unit) **A**9 10 **F**8 11 15 19 20 22 32 34 42 44 45 54 64 65 66 71	14	10	37	1090	15	19926	0	7504	3409	152
DANVILLE—Vermilion County										
★ UNITED SAMARITANS MEDICAL CENTER, (Includes United Samaritans Medical Center, 812 North Logan Avenue, Danville, Illinois, Zip 61832; tel. 217/443–5000; United Samaritans Medical Center, 600 Sager Avenue, Danville, Illinois, Zip 61832; tel. 217/442–6300) Dennis J. Doran, President **A**1 2 9 **F**2 3 7 8 12 15 16 19 23 32 35 37 40 41 42 44 49 52 53 57 58 60 64 65 70 71 73 **P**3 **S**1415 Franciscan Sisters Health Care Corporation	21	10	332	5603	99	—	1186	77334	31858	1353
★ VETERANS AFFAIRS MEDICAL CENTER, 1900 East Main Street, Zip 61832; tel. 217/442–8000; James S. Jones, Director (Total facility includes 180 beds in nursing home–type unit) **A**1 3 5 **F**1 2 3 14 15 16 19 20 21 22 26 27 28 29 30 31 32 34 37 39 41 44 45 46 48 49 51 52 54 55 57 58 64 65 67 71 73 **P**6 **S**9295 Department of Veterans Affairs	45	10	776	5817	457	122191	0	84157	47006	1342
DE KALB—De Kalb County										
★ KISHWAUKEE COMMUNITY HOSPITAL, 626 Bethany Road, Zip 60115, Mailing Address: Box 707, Zip 60115; tel. 815/756–1521; Robert S. Thebeau, President (Nonreporting) **A**1 2 9 10	23	10	111	—	—	—	—	—	—	—
DECATUR—Macon County										
□ ADOLF MEYER MENTAL HEALTH CENTER, 2310 East Mound Road, Zip 62526–9359; tel. 217/875–8710; Christopher T. Power Ph.D., Director **A**1 **F**14 15 16 19 35 52 53 54 56 57 65	12	22	114	387	123	0	0	8238	5719	175
★ DECATUR MEMORIAL HOSPITAL, 2300 North Edward Street, Zip 62526; tel. 217/876–2116; Kenneth L. Smithmier, Chief Executive Officer (Total facility includes 59 beds in nursing home–type unit) **A**1 2 3 5 9 10 **F**7 8 10 14 15 16 17 19 21 22 26 27 28 29 30 31 32 33 37 39 40 41 42 44 47 49 51 52 54 55 56 57 60 61 63 64 65 67 71 72 73 74 **P**3 6	23	10	305	10261	169	160000	1040	81076	33925	1283

© 1995 AHA Guide

Hospitals, U.S. / ILLINOIS

Hospital, Address, Telephone, Administrator, Approval, Facility, and Physician Codes, Health Care System

- ★ American Hospital Association (AHA) membership
- □ Joint Commission on Accreditation of Healthcare Organizations (JCAHO) accreditation
- + American Osteopathic Hospital Association (AOHA) membership
- ○ American Osteopathic Association (AOA) accreditation
- △ Commission on Accreditation of Rehabilitation Facilities (CARF) accreditation

Control codes 61, 63, 64, 71, 72 and 73 indicate hospitals listed by AOHA, but not registered by AHA. For definition of numerical codes, see page A6

	Classification Codes		Utilization Data					Expense (thousands) of dollars		
	Control	Service	Beds	Admissions	Census	Outpatient Visits	Births	Total	Payroll	Personnel

★ ST. MARY'S HOSPITAL, 1800 East Lake Shore Drive, Zip 62521–3883; tel. 217/464–2966; Rex D. Conger, Acting Administrator (Total facility includes 40 beds in nursing home–type unit) **A**1 2 3 5 9 10 **F**1 3 7 8 12 13 14 15 16 17 19 21 22 23 27 28 29 30 33 34 35 36 37 40 41 42 44 45 46 47 49 51 52 53 55 58 59 60 63 64 65 67 68 71 72 73 **S**5355 Hospital Sisters Health System
— 21 | 10 | 290 | 8643 | 179 | 152018 | 912 | 68064 | 31399 | 1010

DES PLAINES—Cook County

★ FOREST HOSPITAL, 555 Wilson Lane, Zip 60016–4794; tel. 708/635–4100; Dennis Regnier, Administrator **A**1 9 10 **F**1 2 3 14 15 16 17 18 26 52 53 54 55 56 57 58 59 65 74 **P**3 7 8
— 31 | 22 | 80 | 2177 | 80 | 9087 | 0 | — | — | 272

★ HOLY FAMILY MEDICAL CENTER, (Formerly Holy Family Hospital) 100 North River Road, Zip 60016; tel. 708/297–1800; Sister Patricia Ann Koschalke, President and Chief Executive Officer **A**1 2 5 9 10 **F**2 3 4 5 6 7 8 10 12 13 14 15 16 17 18 19 20 21 22 25 26 27 28 29 30 31 32 33 34 35 36 37 39 40 41 42 43 44 45 46 49 50 53 54 55 56 57 58 59 60 61 62 63 65 66 67 68 69 70 71 72 73 74 **P**5 8 **S**5575 Sisters of the Holy Family of Nazareth–Sacred Heart Province
— 23 | 10 | 183 | 7058 | 95 | 51423 | 553 | 62859 | 24681 | 815

DIXON—Lee County

★ KATHERINE SHAW BETHEA HOSPITAL, 403 East First Street, Zip 61021; tel. 815/288–5531; Darryl L. Vandervort, Chief Executive Officer (Total facility includes 15 beds in nursing home–type unit) **A**1 2 9 10 **F**7 8 11 12 14 15 19 21 22 24 26 28 30 32 35 36 37 40 41 42 44 45 46 49 51 52 53 54 55 56 57 58 59 60 63 64 65 67 71 73 **P**4 6
— 23 | 10 | 122 | 3505 | 52 | 50107 | 267 | 27230 | 11208 | 400

DOWNERS GROVE—Du Page County

★ GOOD SAMARITAN HOSPITAL, (Formerly EHS Good Samaritan Hospital) 3815 Highland Avenue, Zip 60515; tel. 708/275–5900; David M. McConkey, President (Total facility includes 20 beds in nursing home–type unit) **A**1 2 9 10 **F**1 4 7 8 10 11 12 15 16 17 18 19 21 22 23 24 25 26 27 28 29 30 31 32 33 34 35 37 38 39 40 41 44 45 49 51 52 53 54 55 56 57 58 59 61 62 63 64 65 66 67 70 71 72 73 **P**1 5 6 7 **S**0064 Advocate Health Care
— 21 | 10 | 307 | 13500 | 184 | 125260 | 2657 | 133303 | 49767 | 1428

DU QUOIN—Perry County

★ MARSHALL BROWNING HOSPITAL, 900 North Washington Street, Zip 62832, Mailing Address: Box 192, Zip 62832–0192; tel. 618/542–2146; William J. Huff, Interim Chief Executive Officer **A**1 9 10 **F**8 14 16 19 22 25 34 36 40 44 49 65 71 73
— 23 | 10 | 33 | 1074 | 11 | 47039 | 134 | 7253 | 3281 | 143

EAST SAINT LOUIS—St. Clair County

★ ST. MARY'S HOSPITAL, 129 North Eighth Street, Zip 62201–2999; tel. 618/274–1900; Richard J. Mark, President and Chief Executive Officer **A**1 9 10 **F**2 3 8 15 16 17 18 19 20 21 22 25 26 28 30 31 32 34 36 37 39 44 45 46 49 51 52 53 54 55 56 65 66 67 70 71 72 73 74 **S**0135 Ancilla Systems Inc.
— 21 | 10 | 135 | 4113 | 77 | 52229 | 0 | 28483 | 13522 | 506

EFFINGHAM—Effingham County

★ ST. ANTHONY'S MEMORIAL HOSPITAL, 503 North Maple Street, Zip 62401–2099; tel. 217/342–2121; Anthony D. Pfitzer, Executive Vice President and Chief Executive Officer **A**1 2 9 10 **F**7 8 14 15 16 19 21 22 23 34 35 36 37 39 40 42 44 49 60 63 65 71 73 **S**5355 Hospital Sisters Health System
— 21 | 10 | 146 | 5752 | 77 | 137000 | 730 | 33209 | 13816 | 470

ELDORADO—Saline County

FERRELL HOSPITAL, 1201 Pine Street, Zip 62930; tel. 618/273–3361; Todd R. Kranpitz, Administrator (Nonreporting) **A**9 10
— 33 | 10 | 51 | — | | | | | |

ELGIN—Kane County

□ ELGIN MENTAL HEALTH CENTER, 750 South State Street, Zip 60123–7692; tel. 708/742–1040; Angelo J. Campagna, Director **A**1 **F**3 4 8 9 10 11 12 14 15 16 17 18 19 20 21 22 28 29 30 31 35 37 39 41 42 45 46 48 51 52 53 54 55 56 57 58 59 60 65 67 68 69 70 71 73 **P**6
— 12 | 22 | 708 | 1539 | 665 | 0 | 0 | 49496 | 39491 | 1174

★ SAINT JOSEPH HOSPITAL, 77 North Airlite Street, Zip 60123–4912; tel. 708/695–3200; Larry Narum, President **A**1 2 9 10 **F**3 7 8 10 12 15 16 17 18 19 21 22 25 26 27 29 30 31 32 33 34 35 36 37 39 40 41 42 44 45 49 52 53 54 55 56 57 58 59 60 65 67 70 71 72 73 **P**3 5 8 **S**1415 Franciscan Sisters Health Care Corporation
— 21 | 10 | 97 | 6653 | 103 | 213788 | 665 | 59394 | 26823 | 759

★ SHERMAN HOSPITAL, 934 Center Street, Zip 60120–2198; tel. 708/742–9800; John A. Graham, President **A**1 2 9 10 **F**2 3 4 7 8 10 11 12 13 15 16 17 19 21 22 25 27 28 29 30 31 32 33 34 35 36 37 39 40 41 42 43 44 49 56 63 64 65 67 71 72 73 74 **P**5
— 23 | 10 | 331 | 13298 | 166 | 143736 | 3207 | 112234 | 42186 | 1246

ELK GROVE VILLAGE—Cook County

★ △ ALEXIAN BROTHERS MEDICAL CENTER, 800 Biesterfield Road, Zip 60007–3397; tel. 708/437–5500; Brother Philip Kennedy, President and Chief Executive Officer **A**1 2 5 7 9 10 **F**2 3 4 6 7 8 10 11 12 13 15 16 17 18 19 20 21 22 26 27 28 29 30 31 32 33 34 35 36 37 39 40 41 42 43 44 46 48 49 51 52 53 54 55 56 57 58 59 60 61 64 65 67 68 70 71 72 73 74 **P**5 6 7 8 **S**0065 Alexian Brothers Health System, Inc.
— 21 | 10 | 378 | 15468 | 229 | 148674 | 2557 | 131214 | 55229 | 1731

ELMHURST—Du Page County

★ ELMHURST MEMORIAL HOSPITAL, 200 Berteau Avenue, Zip 60126–2989; tel. 708/833–1400; Leo F. Fronza Jr., President and Chief Executive Officer **A**1 2 9 10 **F**3 4 7 8 10 11 15 19 21 22 23 24 26 29 30 31 32 33 34 35 36 37 38 39 40 41 42 43 44 45 46 49 52 54 55 56 57 58 59 60 61 63 65 67 69 70 71 73 74 **P**5
— 23 | 10 | 308 | 13586 | 226 | 130512 | 1875 | 144956 | 68439 | 2120

EUREKA—Woodford County

EUREKA COMMUNITY HOSPITAL See Bromenn Healthcare, Normal

Hospitals, U.S. / ILLINOIS

Hospital, Address, Telephone, Administrator, Approval, Facility, and Physician Codes, Health Care System	Classification Codes		Utilization Data					Expense (thousands) of dollars		
	Control	Service	Beds	Admissions	Census	Outpatient Visits	Births	Total	Payroll	Personnel

★ American Hospital Association (AHA) membership
☐ Joint Commission on Accreditation of Healthcare Organizations (JCAHO) accreditation
+ American Osteopathic Hospital Association (AOHA) membership
○ American Osteopathic Association (AOA) accreditation
△ Commission on Accreditation of Rehabilitation Facilities (CARF) accreditation
Control codes 61, 63, 64, 71, 72 and 73 indicate hospitals listed by AOHA, but not registered by AHA. For definition of numerical codes, see page A6

EVANSTON—Cook County

★ △ EVANSTON HOSPITAL, (Includes Glenbrook Hospital, 2100 Pfingsten Road, Glenview, Illinois, Zip 60025; tel. 708/657–5800) 2650 Ridge Avenue, Zip 60201; tel. 708/570–2000; Mark R. Neaman, President and Chief Executive Officer **A**1 2 3 5 7 8 9 10 **F**1 2 3 4 5 7 8 9 10 11 12 14 15 16 17 18 19 20 21 22 23 24 25 26 28 29 30 31 32 33 34 35 36 37 38 39 40 41 42 43 44 45 46 48 49 51 52 53 54 55 56 57 58 59 60 61 63 65 66 67 68 69 70 71 73 74 **P**1 3 5 6 7	23	10	457	26116	383	715960	3829	230263	100128	3090
NORTHWESTERN UNIVERSITY STUDENT HEALTH SERVICE HOSPITAL, 633 Emerson Street, Zip 60208–4000; tel. 708/491–8100; Mark Gardner M.D., Medical Director (Nonreporting) **A**9	23	11	16	—	—	—	—	—	—	—
★ ST. FRANCIS HOSPITAL, 355 Ridge Avenue, Zip 60202–3399; tel. 708/316–4000; James C. Gizzi, President and Chief Executive Officer (Total facility includes 159 beds in nursing home–type unit) **A**1 2 3 5 6 9 **F**3 4 7 8 10 11 12 14 15 16 18 19 21 25 26 27 28 30 32 33 34 35 36 37 38 40 41 42 43 44 49 51 52 53 54 55 56 57 58 59 60 63 64 66 67 70 71 72 73 74 **P**1 5 7 **S**5345 Sisters of St. Francis Health Services, Inc.	21	10	555	13916	219	242735	1333	—	—	1275

EVERGREEN PARK—Cook County

★ LITTLE COMPANY OF MARY HOSPITAL AND HEALTH CARE CENTERS, 2800 West 95th Street, Zip 60642–2795; tel. 708/422–6200; Sister Kathleen McIntyre, President **A**1 2 9 10 **F**1 2 3 5 7 8 10 11 12 14 15 16 17 19 21 22 25 26 28 30 31 32 33 34 35 37 38 40 41 42 44 45 46 47 49 52 53 54 55 56 57 58 59 60 63 65 67 71 72 73 74 **P**1 3 7 **S**2295 Little Company of Mary Sisters Healthcare System	21	10	367	21099	253	203338	2264	121008	57955	2046

FAIRBURY—Livingston County

★ FAIRBURY HOSPITAL, (Includes Helen Lewis Smith Pavilion) 519 South Fifth Street, Zip 61739; tel. 815/692–2346; (Total facility includes 49 beds in nursing home–type unit) **A**9 **F**8 19 21 33 36 42 44 49 58 65 70 71 73	23	10	94	458	57	9616	0	5463	2222	—

FAIRFIELD—Wayne County

★ FAIRFIELD MEMORIAL HOSPITAL, 303 Northwest 11th Street, Zip 62837; tel. 618/842–2611; Albert Ban Jr., Chief Executive Officer (Total facility includes 104 beds in nursing home–type unit) **A**1 9 **F**7 8 15 16 19 22 26 27 28 32 33 34 35 37 40 42 44 49 64 65 71 **P**3 **S**2285 Alliant Health System	23	10	185	1618	116	16804	264	9016	4049	242

FLORA—Clay County

★ CLAY COUNTY HOSPITAL, 700 North Mill Street, Zip 62839, Mailing Address: P.O. Box 280, Zip 62839; tel. 618/662–2131; John E. Monnahan, Administrator **A**1 9 10 **F**7 8 15 19 22 28 30 33 36 40 44 46 49 71 **S**0051 BJC Health System	13	10	40	1132	14	21330	78	5481	2291	126

FOREST PARK—Cook County

★ RIVEREDGE HOSPITAL, 8311 West Roosevelt Road, Zip 60130–2500; tel. 708/771–7000; Joyce W. Washington, President and Chief Executive Officer **A**1 5 9 10 **F**2 13 15 16 17 18 19 35 52 53 55 56 57 59 65 67 71 **S**0048 Columbia/HCA Healthcare Corporation	33	22	164	1892	85	7170	0	17317	7957	219

FREEPORT—Stephenson County

★ FREEPORT MEMORIAL HOSPITAL, 1045 West Stephenson Street, Zip 61032; tel. 815/235–4131; Dennis L. Hamilton, President (Total facility includes 33 beds in nursing home–type unit) **A**1 2 9 10 **F**7 8 10 13 14 15 16 17 19 21 22 23 24 27 28 29 30 32 33 35 36 37 39 40 41 42 44 48 49 60 64 65 66 67 71 73 74 **P**3	23	10	165	6117	93	79011	713	35694	14726	583

GALENA—Jo Daviess County

★ GALENA-STAUSS HOSPITAL, 215 Summit Street, Zip 61036–1697; tel. 815/777–1340; Roger D. Hervey, Administrator (Total facility includes 60 beds in nursing home–type unit) **A**1 9 10 **F**1 15 19 22 28 30 44 49 64 65 71	16	10	85	424	69	16589	0	3901	1752	95

GALESBURG—Knox County

★ GALESBURG COTTAGE HOSPITAL, 695 North Kellogg Street, Zip 61401; tel. 309/343–8131; Steven J. West, President and Chief Executive Officer **A**1 9 10 **F**2 3 7 8 11 15 19 21 22 30 32 33 35 36 37 40 41 42 44 49 52 54 55 56 58 63 64 65 70 71 73 **P**6	23	10	193	5557	83	44124	352	34626	13583	513
★ ST. MARY MEDICAL CENTER, 3333 North Seminary Street, Zip 61401–1299; tel. 309/344–3161; Richard S. Kowalski, Chief Executive Officer (Total facility includes 14 beds in nursing home–type unit) **A**1 2 9 10 **F**4 7 8 10 11 15 16 17 19 21 22 23 30 32 35 37 40 41 42 44 49 64 65 66 70 71 73 74 **P**6 **S**5335 OSF Healthcare System	21	10	156	4733	60	47028	482	31419	12486	446

GENESEO—Henry County

★ HAMMOND–HENRY HOSPITAL, 210 West Elk Street, Zip 61254–1099; tel. 309/944–6431; William Price, Interim Administrator (Total facility includes 60 beds in nursing home–type unit) **A**1 9 10 **F**7 11 14 16 19 22 32 34 40 44 64 65 71 73 **S**0585 Brim, Inc.	16	10	105	1034	96	37685	121	11364	5622	205

GENEVA—Kane County

★ DELNOR–COMMUNITY HOSPITAL, 300 Randall Road, Zip 60134–4200; tel. 708/208–3000; Craig A. Livermore, President and Chief Executive Officer **A**1 2 9 10 **F**7 8 10 12 13 14 15 16 17 19 21 22 24 28 29 30 34 35 37 39 40 41 42 44 45 46 49 53 65 66 67 70 71 73 74	23	10	118	6371	73	67288	1238	55082	23060	673

GIBSON CITY—Ford County

★ GIBSON COMMUNITY HOSPITAL, (Includes Gibson Community Hospital Annex) 1120 North Melvin Street, Zip 60936, Mailing Address: P.O. Box 429, Zip 60936–0429; tel. 217/784–4251; Terry Thompson, Administrator (Total facility includes 42 beds in nursing home–type unit) **A**1 9 10 **F**7 8 16 19 20 21 22 26 28 30 32 33 34 37 39 40 41 44 64 65 67 71 **S**0002 Quorum Health Group/Quorum Health Resources	23	10	82	1071	52	18656	99	7839	3253	170

© 1995 AHA Guide

Hospitals, U.S. / ILLINOIS

Hospital, Address, Telephone, Administrator, Approval, Facility, and Physician Codes, Health Care System	Classification Codes		Utilization Data					Expense (thousands) of dollars		
★ American Hospital Association (AHA) membership □ Joint Commission on Accreditation of Healthcare Organizations (JCAHO) accreditation + American Osteopathic Hospital Association (AOHA) membership ○ American Osteopathic Association (AOA) accreditation △ Commission on Accreditation of Rehabilitation Facilities (CARF) accreditation Control codes 61, 63, 64, 71, 72 and 73 indicate hospitals listed by AOHA, but not registered by AHA. For definition of numerical codes, see page A6	Control	Service	Beds	Admissions	Census	Outpatient Visits	Births	Total	Payroll	Personnel
GLENDALE HEIGHTS—Du Page County										
★ GLENOAKS HOSPITAL AND MEDICAL CENTER, 701 Winthrop Avenue, Zip 60139; tel. 708/858–9700; Gary G. Irish, President **A**1 9 10 **F**7 8 11 12 13 14 15 16 17 18 19 21 22 27 28 29 30 31 34 35 37 38 39 40 41 44 48 49 52 53 54 55 56 58 59 65 70 71 73 74 **P**3 5 7 8	21	10	115	3599	52	28133	785	36238	13530	489
GLENVIEW—Cook County GLENBROOK HOSPITAL See Evanston Hospital, Evanston										
GRANITE CITY—Madison County										
★ ST. ELIZABETH MEDICAL CENTER, 2100 Madison Avenue, Zip 62040; tel. 618/798–3000; Ted Eilerman, President **A**1 2 3 5 9 10 **F**2 3 7 8 10 12 13 14 15 16 17 18 19 21 22 24 27 28 29 30 32 33 34 35 36 37 39 40 41 42 44 45 46 49 51 52 53 54 55 56 57 58 59 63 64 65 66 67 68 71 73 74 **P**4 6 8	21	10	276	7768	175	150217	465	66875	28974	1103
GREAT LAKES—Lake County										
★ NAVAL HOSPITAL, Zip 60088–5230; tel. 708/688–4560 **A**1 2 **F**2 3 4 7 8 10 12 13 14 15 16 17 18 19 20 22 23 24 25 28 29 30 31 32 33 34 35 36 37 39 41 42 43 44 45 46 49 51 52 53 54 56 58 65 67 71 73 74 **P**5 **S**9655 Department of Navy	43	10	136	3556	51	212278	0	95483	42204	1424
GREENVILLE—Bond County										
★ EDWARD A. UTLAUT MEMORIAL HOSPITAL, (Includes Fair Oaks) 200 Health Care Drive, Zip 62246; tel. 618/664–1230; Charles Bouis, President and Chief Executive Officer (Total facility includes 139 beds in nursing home–type unit) **A**1 9 10 **F**7 8 19 22 28 34 35 40 42 44 45 49 64 65 66 71 73	23	10	189	1568	142	37346	79	10095	4600	164
HARRISBURG—Saline County										
★ HARRISBURG MEDICAL CENTER, 17 Country Club Court, Zip 62946–0017, Mailing Address: P.O. Box 428, Zip 62946–0428; tel. 618/253–7671; John T. Graves, Chief Executive Officer **A**1 10 **F**14 15 16 19 21 22 32 37 39 41 44 48 49 52 56 63 65 71 73 **P**7 **S**0002 Quorum Health Group/Quorum Health Resources	23	10	78	2910	43	38682	0	14250	6037	311
HARVARD—McHenry County										
★ HARVARD COMMUNITY MEMORIAL HOSPITAL, Grant and McKinley Streets, Zip 60033–1898; tel. 815/943–5431; Bruce B. Berg, Administrator (Total facility includes 45 beds in nursing home–type unit) **A**1 9 10 **F**1 2 3 4 5 6 7 8 9 10 11 12 13 15 17 18 19 20 21 22 23 24 25 26 27 28 29 30 31 32 33 34 35 36 37 38 39 40 41 42 43 44 45 46 47 48 49 50 51 52 53 54 55 56 57 58 59 60 61 62 63 64 65 66 67 68 69 70 71 72 73 74	16	10	78	930	44	4184	141	5278	2616	119
HARVEY—Cook County										
★ △ INGALLS MEMORIAL HOSPITAL, One Ingalls Drive, Zip 60426–3591; tel. 708/333–2300; Robert L. Harris, President and Chief Executive Officer **A**1 2 7 9 10 **F**2 3 4 7 8 10 11 14 15 16 17 18 19 20 21 22 24 25 26 27 28 29 30 31 32 33 34 35 37 38 39 40 41 42 43 44 45 46 48 49 51 52 54 55 56 57 58 59 60 61 65 66 67 71 72 73 74 **P**1 3 4 7	23	10	429	19014	293	211264	2671	157439	71358	1916
HAVANA—Mason County										
★ MASON DISTRICT HOSPITAL, 520 East Franklin Street, Zip 62644–0530, Mailing Address: Box 530, Zip 62644–0530; tel. 309/543–4431; Norman K. Reynolds, Administrator **A**1 9 10 **F**8 11 14 19 21 22 28 30 32 35 36 37 44 49 65 71 **P**3	16	10	32	790	12	24761	0	6952	3134	156
HAZEL CREST—Cook County										
★ SOUTH SUBURBAN HOSPITAL, 17800 South Kedzie Avenue, Zip 60429; tel. 708/799–8000; Robert Rutkowski, President and Chief Executive Officer (Total facility includes 31 beds in nursing home–type unit) **A**1 2 9 10 **F**7 8 10 12 14 17 19 21 22 25 28 30 32 33 34 35 37 40 41 42 44 46 49 63 64 65 66 67 71 73 **P**1 7 **S**0064 Advocate Health Care	23	10	240	10323	154	84657	1063	86160	38521	850
HERRIN—Williamson County										
★ HERRIN HOSPITAL, 201 South 14th Street, Zip 62948; tel. 618/942–2171; Virgil Hannig, Administrator (Total facility includes 13 beds in nursing home–type unit) **A**1 9 10 **F**7 8 15 19 21 22 28 31 32 33 34 37 40 44 45 46 49 64 65 67 71 73 74 **P**8 **S**4175 Southern Illinois Hospital Services	23	10	78	3721	56	50784	275	21800	10208	—
HIGHLAND—Madison County										
★ ST. JOSEPH'S HOSPITAL, 1515 Main Street, Zip 62249–1656; tel. 618/654–7421; Anthony G. Mastrangelo, Executive Vice President and Chief Executive Officer (Total facility includes 30 beds in nursing home–type unit) **A**1 9 10 **F**8 13 15 17 19 21 22 27 28 29 30 31 32 33 34 35 36 37 42 44 51 64 65 66 67 71 73 **S**5355 Hospital Sisters Health System	21	10	76	1358	45	35685	0	11482	4817	167
HIGHLAND PARK—Lake County										
★ HIGHLAND PARK HOSPITAL, 718 Glenview Avenue, Zip 60035–2497; tel. 708/432–8000; Ronald G. Spaeth, President (Total facility includes 28 beds in nursing home–type unit) **A**1 2 9 10 **F**1 3 7 8 10 11 12 14 15 16 17 19 20 21 22 23 26 28 29 30 32 33 34 35 36 37 39 40 41 42 43 44 45 46 48 49 52 53 54 55 56 57 58 59 60 61 63 64 65 67 69 70 71 73 74 **P**1 5 7	23	10	225	8974	133	168476	1898	74881	33135	975
HILLSBORO—Montgomery County										
□ HILLSBORO AREA HOSPITAL, 1200 East Tremont Street, Zip 62049; tel. 217/532–6111; Rex H. Brown, President (Total facility includes 40 beds in nursing home–type unit) **A**1 9 10 **F**7 8 12 14 19 20 21 22 26 28 30 32 33 34 35 37 39 40 42 44 45 49 64 65 66 67 71 73 **S**0585 Brim, Inc.	23	10	100	2024	41	15287	111	8816	3784	194
HINES—Cook County										
□ JOHN J. MADDEN MENTAL HEALTH CENTER, 1200 South First Avenue, Zip 60141; tel. 708/338–7202; Ugo Formigoni, Director **A**1 5 10 **F**14 15 16 52 56	12	22	240	1776	179	0	0	—	—	432

Hospitals, U.S. / ILLINOIS

Hospital, Address, Telephone, Administrator, Approval, Facility, and Physician Codes, Health Care System	Classification Codes		Utilization Data					Expense (thousands) of dollars		Personnel
★ American Hospital Association (AHA) membership □ Joint Commission on Accreditation of Healthcare Organizations (JCAHO) accreditation + American Osteopathic Hospital Association (AOHA) membership ○ American Osteopathic Association (AOA) accreditation △ Commission on Accreditation of Rehabilitation Facilities (CARF) accreditation Control codes 61, 63, 64, 71, 72 and 73 indicate hospitals listed by AOHA, but not registered by AHA. For definition of numerical codes, see page A6	Control	Service	Beds	Admissions	Census	Outpatient Visits	Births	Total	Payroll	
★ VETERANS AFFAIRS EDWARD HINES, JR. HOSPITAL, Fifth Avenue & Roosevelt Road, Zip 60141–5000, Mailing Address: P.O. Box 5000, Zip 60141–5000; tel. 708/343–7200; Joan E. Cummings M.D., Director (Total facility includes 240 beds in nursing home–type unit) **A**1 3 5 8 9 **F**1 2 3 4 5 8 10 11 12 15 16 18 19 20 22 23 24 26 30 31 32 33 34 35 37 39 41 42 43 44 45 46 48 49 52 54 55 56 57 58 60 63 64 65 67 69 71 73 74 **S**9295 Department of Veterans Affairs	45	10	1022	12721	801	279908	0	228804	132909	3060
HINSDALE—Du Page County										
★ △ HINSDALE HOSPITAL, 120 North Oak Street, Zip 60521; tel. 708/856–9000; Ronald Sackett, President **A**1 2 3 5 7 9 10 **F**2 3 4 7 8 10 11 12 13 14 19 21 22 24 25 28 29 30 32 33 34 35 37 40 41 42 43 44 45 46 48 49 51 52 53 54 55 56 57 58 59 60 61 65 67 68 69 70 71 72 73 **P**3 5	21	10	417	14248	197	183593	3005	157843	66090	1839
□ SUBURBAN HOSPITAL, 55th Street & County Line Road, Zip 60521–8900; tel. 708/323–5800; Jeffrey Steadman, Chief Executive Officer **A**1 9 10 **F**12 14 17 19 21 22 25 26 27 28 29 30 31 32 33 35 37 41 42 44 45 46 48 49 51 54 63 64 65 67 71 72 73 **P**5	16	10	81	2078	51	6072	0	24503	9646	233
HOFFMAN ESTATES—Cook County										
★ HOFFMAN ESTATES MEDICAL CENTER, 1555 North Barrington Road, Zip 60194; tel. 708/843–2000; Edward Goldberg, Chief Executive Officer (Total facility includes 21 beds in nursing home–type unit) **A**1 2 9 10 **F**4 7 8 10 11 12 14 15 16 19 21 22 27 30 33 34 35 37 40 42 44 45 46 49 64 65 67 68 70 71 73 74 **P**5 **S**0048 Columbia/HCA Healthcare Corporation	33	10	193	8954	103	50391	2249	62865	26947	779
★ WOODLAND HOSPITAL, 1650 Moon Lake Boulevard, Zip 60194–5000; tel. 708/882–1600; Patrick Waugh, Chief Executive Officer **A**1 9 10 **F**2 3 16 27 52 53 57 58 59 65 67 **P**7 **S**0048 Columbia/HCA Healthcare Corporation	33	22	100	1358	49	4985	0	9688	4234	141
HOOPESTON—Vermilion County										
★ HOOPESTON COMMUNITY MEMORIAL HOSPITAL, 701 East Orange Street, Zip 60942; tel. 217/283–5531; Rod Burkett, Administrator (Nonreporting) **A**1 9 10	23	10	76	—	—	—	—	—	—	—
HOPEDALE—Tazewell County										
HOPEDALE MEDICAL COMPLEX, (Formerly Hopedale Hospital) 107 Tremont Street, Zip 61747; tel. 309/449–3321; L. J. Rossi M.D., Chief Executive Officer (Nonreporting) **A**9 10	23	10	119	—	—	—	—	—	—	—
JACKSONVILLE—Morgan County										
★ PASSAVANT AREA HOSPITAL, 1600 West Walnut Street, Zip 62650; tel. 217/245–9541; Chester A. Wynn, President and Chief Executive Officer **A**1 2 9 10 **F**3 4 7 8 16 17 19 21 22 24 28 29 30 31 32 35 36 37 39 40 42 44 45 46 49 63 65 66 67 70 71 73 **P**1	23	10	146	4696	73	70257	405	33793	15328	603
JERSEYVILLE—Jersey County										
□ JERSEY COMMUNITY HOSPITAL, 400 Maple Summit Road, Zip 62052, Mailing Address: P.O. Box 426, Zip 62052; tel. 618/498–6402; Lawrence P. Bear, Chief Executive Officer **A**1 9 10 **F**7 8 11 14 15 16 19 20 22 28 30 31 33 35 36 37 39 40 42 44 46 49 61 65 66 67 71 73	16	10	67	1539	16	24959	288	10010	4657	187
JOLIET—Will County										
★ △ SAINT JOSEPH MEDICAL CENTER, 333 North Madison Street, Zip 60435–6595; tel. 815/725–7133; David W. Benfer, President and Chief Executive Officer **A**1 2 5 7 9 10 **F**3 4 7 8 10 11 14 15 16 17 18 19 20 21 22 25 26 27 28 29 30 31 32 33 34 35 37 38 40 41 42 43 44 45 48 49 52 53 54 55 56 57 58 59 60 63 65 66 67 70 71 73 74 **P**8 **S**1415 Franciscan Sisters Health Care Corporation	21	10	500	16629	265	313019	1509	131541	56287	1487
★ SILVER CROSS HOSPITAL, 1200 Maple Road, Zip 60432; tel. 815/740–1100; Paul Pawlak, President **A**1 2 9 10 **F**1 3 4 5 6 7 8 9 10 12 13 15 16 17 18 19 20 21 22 23 24 25 26 27 28 29 30 31 32 33 34 35 36 37 38 39 40 41 42 43 44 45 46 47 48 49 50 52 53 54 55 56 57 58 59 60 61 62 63 64 65 66 67 68 69 70 71 **P**3 6 7 8	23	10	231	10948	152	131173	1433	80702	33856	853
KANKAKEE—Kankakee County										
★ △ RIVERSIDE MEDICAL CENTER, 350 North Wall Street, Zip 60901–0749; tel. 815/933–1671; Dennis C. Millirons, President and Chief Executive Officer (Total facility includes 14 beds in nursing home–type unit) **A**1 2 7 9 10 **F**2 3 6 7 8 10 11 12 13 15 17 19 20 21 22 23 26 27 28 29 30 31 32 33 34 35 36 37 39 40 41 42 44 45 46 49 52 53 54 55 56 57 58 59 60 61 62 63 64 65 66 67 68 69 70 71 73 74 **P**6 8	23	10	295	8933	173	120656	1164	66833	29247	1185
★ ST. MARY'S HOSPITAL OF KANKAKEE, 500 West Court Street, Zip 60901; tel. 815/937–2400; Allan C. Sonduck, President and Chief Executive Officer (Total facility includes 13 beds in nursing home–type unit) **A**1 2 9 10 **F**1 4 5 7 8 10 12 15 16 17 19 21 22 23 24 26 27 28 29 30 31 32 33 34 35 37 39 40 41 42 43 44 45 46 49 50 51 52 53 54 55 56 57 58 59 60 61 63 64 65 66 69 70 71 73 74 **P**8 **S**4025 Servantcor	21	10	214	6977	123	123283	613	54807	19785	818
KEWANEE—Henry County										
★ KEWANEE HOSPITAL, 719 Elliott Street, Zip 61443–2711, Mailing Address: P.O. Box 747, Zip 61443–0747; tel. 309/853–3361; Charles Duffy, President (Total facility includes 14 beds in nursing home–type unit) **A**1 9 10 **F**7 8 11 15 19 22 30 32 33 36 37 40 42 44 49 64 65 67 71 73 **P**6 **S**0002 Quorum Health Group/Quorum Health Resources	23	10	55	2453	34	52202	223	18720	8083	338
LA GRANGE—Cook County										
★ LA GRANGE MEMORIAL HOSPITAL, 5101 South Willow Springs Road, Zip 60525–2680; tel. 708/352–1200; Thomas Alfred Beckett, President and Chief Executive Officer (Total facility includes 43 beds in nursing home–type unit) **A**1 2 3 5 9 10 **F**4 7 8 10 11 14 15 16 17 19 21 22 26 27 28 29 30 31 32 33 34 35 37 39 40 41 42 43 44 45 46 49 60 63 64 65 66 67 70 71 73 74 **P**5 6 7 8	23	10	227	9531	153	117795	948	99646	40600	1023

© 1995 AHA Guide

Hospitals, U.S. / ILLINOIS

Hospital, Address, Telephone, Administrator, Approval, Facility, and Physician Codes, Health Care System	Classi-fication Codes		Utilization Data					Expense (thousands) of dollars		
★ American Hospital Association (AHA) membership □ Joint Commission on Accreditation of Healthcare Organizations (JCAHO) accreditation + American Osteopathic Hospital Association (AOHA) membership ○ American Osteopathic Association (AOA) accreditation △ Commission on Accreditation of Rehabilitation Facilities (CARF) accreditation Control codes 61, 63, 64, 71, 72 and 73 indicate hospitals listed by AOHA, but not registered by AHA. For definition of numerical codes, see page A6	Control	Service	Beds	Admissions	Census	Outpatient Visits	Births	Total	Payroll	Personnel
LAKE FOREST—Lake County ★ △ LAKE FOREST HOSPITAL, 660 North Westmoreland Road, Zip 60045–1696; tel. 708/234–5600; William G. Ries, President (Total facility includes 88 beds in nursing home–type unit) **A**1 2 7 9 10 **F**1 5 7 8 12 14 15 17 19 21 22 24 26 28 30 31 32 33 34 35 36 37 39 40 41 42 44 45 46 49 51 54 60 61 63 64 65 66 67 70 71 73 **P**1	23	10	261	6541	158	158023	1547	77753	35290	939
LAWRENCEVILLE—Lawrence County ★ LAWRENCE COUNTY MEMORIAL HOSPITAL, West State Street, Zip 62439; tel. 618/943–1000; Gerald E. Waldroup, Administrator **A**1 9 10 **F**7 8 11 14 15 16 17 19 22 28 29 33 34 35 37 39 40 44 49 52 53 54 55 56 57 59 63 65 67 71 73 **P**5	13	10	59	1484	24	24234	64	6427	2992	139
LIBERTYVILLE—Lake County ★ CONDELL MEDICAL CENTER, 900 Garfield, Zip 60048–3199; tel. 708/362–2900; Eugene Pritchard, President **A**1 2 9 10 **F**1 3 7 8 16 19 21 22 24 25 32 33 34 35 37 40 42 44 46 49 52 57 58 59 60 63 65 66 67 70 71 72 73 **P**1 5	23	10	175	7578	89	167283	1504	62888	26968	1029
LINCOLN—Logan County ★ ABRAHAM LINCOLN MEMORIAL HOSPITAL, 315 Eighth Street, Zip 62656–2698, Mailing Address: P.O. Box 569, Zip 62656–2698; tel. 217/732–2161; D. David Sniff, President and Chief Executive Officer **A**1 9 **F**1 3 8 14 15 16 19 20 21 22 25 28 31 33 35 37 39 40 42 44 46 49 56 58 65 67 71 73	23	10	66	2920	24	35234	290	15536	6658	293
LINCOLN DEVELOPMENTAL CENTER, 861 South State Street, Zip 62656–2599; tel. 217/735–2361; Martin Downs, Facility Director (Nonreporting)	12	62	508	—	—	—	—	—	—	—
LITCHFIELD—Montgomery County ★ ST. FRANCIS HOSPITAL, 1215 East Union Avenue, Zip 62056–1215, Mailing Address: P.O. Box 1215, Zip 62056–1215; tel. 217/324–2191; Michael Sipkoski, Executive Vice President (Total facility includes 35 beds in nursing home–type unit) **A**1 9 10 **F**7 8 11 14 15 16 19 22 30 32 33 35 37 39 40 41 44 45 63 64 65 67 71 73 **S**5355 Hospital Sisters Health System	21	10	101	3465	50	52611	404	17767	7593	322
MACOMB—McDonough County ★ MCDONOUGH DISTRICT HOSPITAL, 525 East Grant Street, Zip 61455; tel. 309/833–4101; Stephen R. Hopper, President and Chief Executive Officer (Total facility includes 16 beds in nursing home–type unit) **A**1 2 9 10 **F**1 3 7 8 14 15 19 21 22 24 26 28 29 30 32 33 35 37 39 40 41 42 44 46 53 56 57 58 64 65 67 71 73 74 **P**8	16	10	144	4443	69	37490	341	28969	13387	462
MARION—Williamson County ★ MARION MEMORIAL HOSPITAL, 917 West Main Street, Zip 62959; tel. 618/997–5341; Richard V. Livengood FACHE, President and Chief Executive Officer **A**1 9 10 **F**8 12 15 16 17 19 21 22 26 27 28 29 30 31 33 34 36 37 38 39 40 41 42 44 45 46 47 49 51 54 55 56 63 65 66 67 68 71 73 **P**6	14	10	84	2678	40	47984	183	19593	8492	344
★ VETERANS AFFAIRS MEDICAL CENTER, 2401 West Main Street, Zip 62959–1194; tel. 618/997–5311; Linda K. Kurz, Director (Total facility includes 60 beds in nursing home–type unit) **A**1 5 **F**3 8 16 19 20 21 22 25 26 27 31 32 33 34 35 37 41 42 44 46 49 51 54 58 64 65 67 71 73 74 **S**9295 Department of Veterans Affairs	45	10	163	4820	158	93357	0	38046	20606	513
MARYVILLE—Madison County ★ ANDERSON HOSPITAL, Route 162, Zip 62062; tel. 618/288–5711; R. Coert Shepard, President **A**1 9 10 **F**4 7 8 10 14 16 17 19 21 22 26 28 30 32 33 34 35 37 40 44 45 46 50 56 65 67 71 73	23	10	130	4203	54	53014	621	25707	11879	375
MATTOON—Coles County ★ SARAH BUSH LINCOLN HEALTH SYSTEM, 1000 Health Center Drive, Zip 61938–0372, Mailing Address: P.O. Box 372, Zip 61938; tel. 217/258–2525; Eugene A. Leblond FACHE, President and Chief Executive Officer (Total facility includes 23 beds in nursing home–type unit) **A**1 2 9 10 **F**7 11 12 19 20 21 22 23 24 26 28 30 31 34 35 37 39 40 41 42 44 45 46 49 52 53 54 55 56 57 59 60 63 64 65 66 67 70 71 73 74 **P**4 5 6 7	23	10	174	7429	96	149140	864	51831	22966	769
MAYWOOD—Cook County ★ LOYOLA UNIVERSITY MEDICAL CENTER, (Formerly Foster F. G. Mcgaw Hospital, Loyola University of Chicago) 2160 South First Avenue, Zip 60153–5585; tel. 708/216–9000; Anthony L. Barbato M.D., Executive Vice President and Chief Executive Officer **A**1 2 3 5 8 9 **F**3 4 7 8 9 10 11 12 13 15 17 19 20 21 22 23 26 28 30 31 32 33 34 35 37 38 39 40 41 42 43 44 45 46 47 48 49 51 52 53 54 55 56 57 58 60 61 63 65 66 67 69 70 71 73 74 **P**1 3 5 7	23	10	536	19494	366	282299	1631	371950	132015	3855
MCHENRY—Cook County ★ △ NORTHERN ILLINOIS MEDICAL CENTER, 4201 Medical Center Drive, Zip 60050–9506; tel. 815/344–5000; Paul E. Laudick, President and Chief Executive Officer **A**1 2 7 9 10 **F**7 8 10 12 14 15 16 17 19 20 22 23 25 26 27 28 29 30 32 33 34 35 36 37 39 40 41 44 45 48 49 52 54 55 56 57 58 60 64 65 67 70 71 73 74	23	10	154	7059	105	131269	850	63275	22866	642
MCLEANSBORO—Du Page County ★ HAMILTON MEMORIAL HOSPITAL DISTRICT, 611 South Marshall Avenue, Zip 62859; tel. 618/643–2361; James M. Hayes, Chief Executive Officer (Total facility includes 60 beds in nursing home–type unit) **A**1 9 10 **F**15 16 19 21 22 28 32 34 35 44 45 46 49 65 71	16	10	91	1299	75	13851	0	7430	3942	72
MELROSE PARK—Cook County ★ GOTTLIEB MEMORIAL HOSPITAL, 701 West North Avenue, Zip 60160–1692; tel. 708/681–3200; John Morgan, President (Total facility includes 34 beds in nursing home–type unit) **A**1 9 10 **F**4 5 7 8 10 11 12 15 17 18 19 21 22 26 27 28 29 30 31 32 33 34 35 37 39 40 41 42 43 44 45 46 55 65 66 67 70 71 73 74 **P**5	23	10	208	9102	130	92155	917	71603	34614	1032

Hospitals, U.S. / ILLINOIS

Hospital, Address, Telephone, Administrator, Approval, Facility, and Physician Codes, Health Care System	Classification Codes		Utilization Data					Expense (thousands) of dollars		
★ American Hospital Association (AHA) membership □ Joint Commission on Accreditation of Healthcare Organizations (JCAHO) accreditation + American Osteopathic Hospital Association (AOHA) membership ○ American Osteopathic Association (AOA) accreditation △ Commission on Accreditation of Rehabilitation Facilities (CARF) accreditation Control codes 61, 63, 64, 71, 72 and 73 indicate hospitals listed by AOHA, but not registered by AHA. For definition of numerical codes, see page A6	Control	Service	Beds	Admissions	Census	Outpatient Visits	Births	Total	Payroll	Personnel
★ △ WESTLAKE COMMUNITY HOSPITAL, 1225 Lake Street, Zip 60160; tel. 708/681–3000; David R. Hey, Chief Operating Officer (Total facility includes 17 beds in nursing home–type unit) **A**1 3 7 9 10 **F**2 3 4 5 7 8 10 11 15 16 17 18 19 21 22 24 26 27 28 30 32 33 34 35 36 37 38 39 40 41 42 43 44 45 46 48 49 52 54 55 56 57 58 60 63 64 65 66 67 71 73 **P**2 5 7	23	10	250	8309	166	—	996	71947	33090	972
MENDOTA—La Salle County										
★ MENDOTA COMMUNITY HOSPITAL, 1315 Memorial Drive, Zip 61342; tel. 815/539–7461; Gareth D. Weeks, President **A**1 9 10 **F**3 7 8 19 21 22 30 34 36 37 39 40 41 42 44 46 65 67 71 73	23	10	68	1799	19	45358	116	9939	5023	159
METROPOLIS—Massac County										
★ MASSAC MEMORIAL HOSPITAL, 28 Chick Street, Zip 62960–2481, Mailing Address: P.O. Box 850, Zip 62960–0850; tel. 618/524–2176; Jim Marshall, Interim Chief Executive Officer **A**1 9 10 **F**19 21 22 33 44 65 71 **S**2285 Alliant Health System	16	10	31	1489	18	20030	0	7456	3366	161
MOLINE—Rock Island County										
TRINITY MEDICAL CENTER–EAST CAMPUS See Trinity Medical Center–West Campus, Rock Island										
MONMOUTH—Warren County										
COMMUNITY MEMORIAL HOSPITAL, 1000 West Harlem Avenue, Zip 61462–1099; tel. 309/734–3141; Mary K. Robbins, Co-Administrator (Nonreporting) **A**9 10 **S**8875 Methodist Health Services Corporation	14	10	69	—	—	—	—	—	—	—
MONTICELLO—Piatt County										
★ JOHN AND MARY KIRBY HOSPITAL, 1111 North State Street, Zip 61856; tel. 217/762–2115; Thomas D. Dixon, Administrator **A**1 9 10 **F**8 14 15 16 19 22 28 29 30 32 33 34 35 42 44 49 53 54 55 56 57 58 59 60 64 65 71 73 **P**6	23	10	18	508	7	29818	0	3879	1547	80
MORRIS—Grundy County										
★ MORRIS HOSPITAL, 150 West High Street, Zip 60450; tel. 815/942–2932; Clifford L. Corbett, President and Chief Executive Officer **A**1 2 9 10 **F**3 7 8 11 15 16 17 18 19 20 21 22 26 28 29 30 32 33 34 36 37 39 40 41 42 44 46 49 50 53 54 55 56 57 58 65 66 67 70 71 73	23	10	82	3393	39	70062	191	29045	13304	370
MORRISON—Whiteside County										
★ MORRISON COMMUNITY HOSPITAL, 303 North Jackson Street, Zip 61270–3042; tel. 815/772–4003; Mark F. Fedyk, Chief Executive Officer (Nonreporting) **A**9 10 **S**5165 Mercy Health Services	16	10	114	—	—	—	—	—	—	—
MOUNT CARMEL—Wabash County										
★ WABASH GENERAL HOSPITAL DISTRICT, 1418 College Drive, Zip 62863; tel. 618/262–8621; J. Jay Purvis, Interim Chief Executive Officer **A**1 9 10 **F**8 12 15 19 22 28 30 32 33 35 37 42 44 46 49 65 71 73 **S**2285 Alliant Health System	16	10	56	1394	17	18638	0	7003	2751	143
MOUNT VERNON—Jefferson County										
CROSSROADS COMMUNITY HOSPITAL, 8 Doctors Park, Zip 62864; tel. 618/244–5500; Chris Wearmouth, Managing Director (Nonreporting) **A**10 **S**5895 Hallmark Healthcare Corporation	33	10	49	—	—	—	—	—	—	—
★ GOOD SAMARITAN REGIONAL HEALTH CENTER, 605 North 12th Street, Zip 62864; tel. 618/242–4600; Leo F. Childers Jr. FACHE, President **A**1 2 9 10 **F**4 7 8 10 11 14 15 16 19 20 21 22 23 24 26 28 29 30 32 33 34 35 37 39 40 42 44 45 48 49 60 63 65 67 71 73 **P**2 3 5 6 7 8 **S**5455 SSM Health Care System	21	10	141	4925	74	42480	586	44142	18558	691
MURPHYSBORO—Jackson County										
★ ST. JOSEPH MEMORIAL HOSPITAL, 800 North Second Street, Zip 62966, Mailing Address: P.O. Box 580, Zip 62966–0580; tel. 618/684–3156; Virgil Hannig, President **A**1 9 10 **F**7 8 19 22 31 34 40 44 45 65 67 71 73 **S**4175 Southern Illinois Hospital Services	21	10	59	2023	24	21059	328	10753	4968	222
NAPERVILLE—Du Page County										
★ EDWARD HOSPITAL, 801 South Washington Street, Zip 60566–7060; tel. 708/355–0450; Pamela Meyer Davis, President and Chief Executive Officer **A**1 2 9 10 **F**3 4 7 8 10 12 13 14 15 16 17 18 19 20 22 24 25 28 29 30 32 34 35 37 39 40 41 42 43 44 45 46 49 51 53 54 55 56 57 58 59 61 65 67 70 71 73 74 **P**8	23	10	159	8915	101	107769	1885	94332	33594	949
NASHVILLE—Washington County										
★ WASHINGTON COUNTY HOSPITAL, 705 South Grand Street, Zip 62263–1532; tel. 618/327–8236; Michael P. Ellermann, Administrator and Chief Executive Officer (Total facility includes 20 beds in nursing home–type unit) **A**1 9 10 **F**3 4 5 7 8 9 10 11 12 13 17 18 19 20 21 22 25 27 28 29 30 31 32 33 34 35 37 38 39 40 41 42 43 44 45 47 48 51 52 53 54 55 56 57 58 59 60 61 63 64 65 66 67 69 70 71 72 73 74 **P**1 6 7 **S**5455 SSM Health Care System	16	10	56	819	25	18335	61	5111	2150	95
NORMAL—McLean County										
★ BROMENN HEALTHCARE, (Formerly Listed Under Bloomington) (Includes Bromenn Lifecare Center, 807 North Main Street, Bloomington, Illinois, Zip 61702, Mailing Address: P.O. Box 2850, Zip 61702–2850; tel. 309/454–1400; Bromenn Regional Medical Center, Virginia and Franklin Streets, Normal, Illinois, Zip 61761, Mailing Address: P.O. Box 2850, Bloomington, Zip 61702–2850; tel. 309/454–1400; Eureka Community Hospital, 101 South Major Street, Eureka, Illinois, Zip 61530, Mailing Address: P.O. Box 203, Zip 61530; tel. 309/467–2361; Michael Milbrath, Administrator) Virginia and Franklin Streets, Zip 61761, Mailing Address: P.O. Box 2850, Bloomington Zip 61702–2850; tel. 309/454–0700; Dale S. Strassheim, President (Total facility includes 108 beds in nursing home–type unit) **A**1 2 9 10 **F**1 2 3 7 8 10 12 13 15 16 17 18 19 21 22 23 24 25 26 27 28 29 30 31 32 33 34 35 36 37 38 39 40 41 42 44 46 48 49 51 52 53 54 55 56 57 58 59 61 63 64 65 67 68 70 71 73 **P**6 7 8 BROMENN REGIONAL MEDICAL CENTER See Bromenn Healthcare	21	10	416	9245	260	84519	1306	90290	40940	1203

© 1995 AHA Guide

Hospitals, U.S. / ILLINOIS

Hospital, Address, Telephone, Administrator, Approval, Facility, and Physician Codes, Health Care System	Classification Codes		Utilization Data					Expense (thousands) of dollars		
★ American Hospital Association (AHA) membership □ Joint Commission on Accreditation of Healthcare Organizations (JCAHO) accreditation + American Osteopathic Hospital Association (AOHA) membership ○ American Osteopathic Association (AOA) accreditation △ Commission on Accreditation of Rehabilitation Facilities (CARF) accreditation Control codes 61, 63, 64, 71, 72 and 73 indicate hospitals listed by AOHA, but not registered by AHA. For definition of numerical codes, see page A6	Control	Service	Beds	Admissions	Census	Outpatient Visits	Births	Total	Payroll	Personnel
NORTH CHICAGO—Lake County										
★ VETERANS AFFAIRS MEDICAL CENTER, 3001 Green Bay Road, Zip 60064; tel. 708/578–3700; Alfred S. Pate, Director (Total facility includes 373 beds in nursing home–type unit) **A**1 3 5 9 **F**1 2 3 4 5 6 8 10 12 17 18 19 20 21 22 24 25 26 27 28 29 30 31 32 33 34 35 37 39 41 43 44 45 46 48 49 50 51 52 54 55 56 57 58 59 60 63 65 67 69 71 72 73 74 **P**6 **S**9295 Department of Veterans Affairs	45	22	947	4374	799	158402	0	—	—	1671
OAK FOREST—Cook County										
★ △ OAK FOREST HOSPITAL OF COOK COUNTY, 15900 South Cicero Avenue, Zip 60452; tel. 708/687–7200; Patricia Rush M.D., Director **A**1 3 5 7 9 10 **F**3 8 10 13 14 15 16 19 20 21 22 25 26 27 29 30 31 33 34 36 37 39 41 42 43 44 45 46 48 49 51 54 57 58 63 64 65 67 71 73 **P**6 **S**0016 Cook County Bureau of Health Services	13	48	838	3009	745	47940	0	106075	66205	1821
OAK LAWN—Cook County										
★ △ CHRIST HOSPITAL AND MEDICAL CENTER, (Formerly EHS Christ Hospital and Medical Center) 4440 West 95th Street, Zip 60453–2699; tel. 708/425–8000; Carol Schneider, Chief Executive (Nonreporting) **A**1 2 3 5 7 9 10 **S**0064 Advocate Health Care	21	10	827	—	—	—	—	—	—	—
OAK PARK—Cook County										
★ △ OAK PARK HOSPITAL, 520 South Maple Avenue, Zip 60304–1097; tel. 708/383–9300; Leonard J. Muller, President (Total facility includes 47 beds in nursing home–type unit) **A**1 2 5 7 9 10 **F**2 3 4 5 7 8 10 15 16 17 18 19 20 22 24 25 26 27 28 30 31 32 33 34 35 36 37 38 39 40 41 42 43 44 45 46 48 49 50 52 54 55 56 57 58 60 63 64 65 66 67 69 71 73 **P**2 5 7 **S**6745 Wheaton Franciscan Services, Inc.	21	10	186	5114	125	—	0	46251	20241	605
★ WEST SUBURBAN HOSPITAL MEDICAL CENTER, Erie at Austin, Zip 60302–2599; tel. 708/383–6200; Douglas F. Dean Jr., President (Total facility includes 20 beds in nursing home–type unit) **A**1 2 3 5 9 10 **F**4 5 7 8 10 11 12 13 14 16 17 19 20 21 22 25 26 28 29 30 32 33 34 35 37 38 39 40 41 42 43 44 45 46 49 51 54 56 60 61 63 64 65 66 67 71 73 **P**6 7 8	23	10	255	11264	154	180086	1980	101457	53595	1509
OLNEY—Richland County										
★ RICHLAND MEMORIAL HOSPITAL, 800 East Locust Street, Zip 62450–2598; tel. 618/395–2131; Harvey H. Pettry, Administrator (Total facility includes 28 beds in nursing home–type unit) **A**1 2 9 10 **F**7 8 14 15 16 19 20 21 22 27 28 29 30 32 33 34 35 36 37 39 40 41 42 44 45 49 50 52 54 56 59 64 65 66 67 71 73 **P**3	13	10	134	3213	58	47743	396	18677	7956	368
OLYMPIA FIELDS—Cook County										
○ OLYMPIA FIELDS HOSPITAL AND MEDICAL CENTER, 20201 Crawford Avenue, Zip 60461–1080; tel. 708/747–4000 **A**9 11 **F**4 5 7 8 10 11 12 13 14 16 17 19 21 22 23 25 26 28 29 30 32 34 35 37 39 40 41 42 43 44 45 46 48 49 51 52 53 54 55 56 57 58 59 60 61 65 66 67 70 71 72 73 74 **P**5	23	10	174	7230	101	135443	722	85828	32923	820
OTTAWA—La Salle County										
★ + COMMUNITY HOSPITAL OF OTTAWA, 1100 East Norris Drive, Zip 61350; tel. 815/433–3100; Robert Schmelter, President **A**1 9 10 **F**1 2 4 6 7 8 10 11 15 19 20 21 22 23 26 27 28 29 30 32 33 36 39 40 42 44 45 49 52 53 54 56 57 58 65 67 69 70 71 73 **P**3	23	10	124	3693	58	63872	416	23678	11030	417
PALOS HEIGHTS—Cook County										
★ PALOS COMMUNITY HOSPITAL, 12251 South 80th Avenue, Zip 60463–0930; tel. 708/923–4000; Sister Margaret Wright, President **A**1 2 9 10 **F**2 3 5 7 8 10 11 16 19 21 22 25 31 32 34 35 36 37 39 40 41 42 44 45 49 52 53 54 56 57 58 63 65 66 67 71 72 73	23	10	337	16279	221	158682	2329	137487	68869	1657
PANA—Christian County										
★ PANA COMMUNITY HOSPITAL, South Locust Street, Zip 62557–0169; tel. 217/562–2131; David Faulkner, Administrator and Chief Executive Officer **A**1 9 10 **F**8 12 14 15 16 19 21 22 29 31 32 33 34 36 37 42 44 45 46 49 51 54 65 71 **P**3 **S**0002 Quorum Health Group/Quorum Health Resources	23	10	44	910	10	16599	0	6095	2590	126
PARIS—Edgar County										
★ PARIS COMMUNITY HOSPITAL, 721 East Court Street, Zip 61944–2420; tel. 217/465–4141; John M. Dillon, Chief Executive Officer **A**1 9 10 **F**8 17 19 22 30 34 36 37 39 42 44 49 65 67 71 73 **P**6 **S**2285 Alliant Health System	23	10	49	1024	18	10144	0	8367	3306	131
PARK RIDGE—Cook County										
★ △ LUTHERAN GENERAL HOSPITAL, 1775 Dempster Street, Zip 60068–1174; tel. 708/696–8446; Kenneth J. Rojek, Chief Executive (Total facility includes 188 beds in nursing home–type unit) **A**1 2 3 5 7 8 9 10 **F**1 2 3 4 5 6 7 8 10 11 12 15 16 19 22 24 26 31 32 33 34 36 37 38 39 40 41 42 43 44 46 47 48 49 52 53 54 55 57 58 59 60 61 62 64 65 66 67 69 70 71 73 **P**1 4 5 6 8 **S**0064 Advocate Health Care	21	10	800	25004	433	198446	4811	308947	120059	3872
PEKIN—Tazewell County										
★ PEKIN HOSPITAL, 600 South 13th Street, Zip 61554–5098; tel. 309/353–0791; David A. Schertz, Chief Executive Officer (Total facility includes 10 beds in nursing home–type unit) **A**1 9 10 **F**2 3 4 7 8 10 12 14 15 16 17 18 19 20 21 22 23 24 26 28 29 30 31 32 34 35 37 39 40 41 42 43 44 45 46 49 51 52 53 54 55 56 57 58 59 60 61 63 64 65 66 67 68 69 70 71 73 74 **P**5 8	23	10	144	4379	58	61398	522	33962	14486	561
PEORIA—Peoria County										
□ GEORGE A. ZELLER MENTAL HEALTH CENTER, 5407 North University Street, Zip 61614–4785; tel. 309/693–5228; Robert W. Vyverberg Ed.D., Director **A**1 10 **F**8 11 15 19 20 21 35 37 44 48 52 53 65 **P**6	12	22	154	482	135	59	0	13679	11056	312

Hospitals, U.S. / ILLINOIS

Hospital, Address, Telephone, Administrator, Approval, Facility, and Physician Codes, Health Care System	Classification Codes		Utilization Data					Expense (thousands) of dollars		
★ American Hospital Association (AHA) membership □ Joint Commission on Accreditation of Healthcare Organizations (JCAHO) accreditation + American Osteopathic Hospital Association (AOHA) membership ○ American Osteopathic Association (AOA) accreditation △ Commission on Accreditation of Rehabilitation Facilities (CARF) accreditation Control codes 61, 63, 64, 71, 72 and 73 indicate hospitals listed by AOHA, but not registered by AHA. For definition of numerical codes, see page A6	Control	Service	Beds	Admissions	Census	Outpatient Visits	Births	Total	Payroll	Personnel
★ △ METHODIST MEDICAL CENTER OF ILLINOIS, 221 Northeast Glen Oak Avenue, Zip 61636; tel. 309/672-5522; James K. Knoble, President **A**1 2 3 5 6 7 9 **F**1 3 4 7 8 10 12 14 16 19 21 22 23 24 26 28 30 31 32 33 34 35 37 39 40 41 42 43 44 45 46 48 49 50 51 52 53 54 55 57 59 60 62 63 64 65 67 68 69 70 71 73 74 **P**1 7 **S**8875 Methodist Health Services Corporation	23	10	346	12005	234	193800	1777	148394	63850	2356
★ PROCTOR HOSPITAL, 5409 North Knoxville Avenue, Zip 61614-5094; tel. 309/691-1000; Norman H. LaConte, President and Chief Executive Officer (Total facility includes 30 beds in nursing home-type unit) **A**1 9 10 **F**2 3 4 7 8 10 12 14 16 19 21 22 24 28 29 30 34 35 36 37 39 40 41 42 43 44 46 49 61 63 64 65 70 71 73 **P**3	23	10	185	5528	104	142416	619	52959	19769	786
★ △ SAINT FRANCIS MEDICAL CENTER, 530 Northeast Glen Oak Avenue, Zip 61637; tel. 309/655-2000; Sister M. Canisia, Administrator **A**1 2 3 5 7 9 10 **F**1 2 3 4 5 6 7 8 9 10 11 12 13 14 15 16 17 18 19 20 21 22 23 24 25 26 27 28 29 30 31 32 33 34 35 36 37 38 39 40 41 42 43 44 45 46 47 48 49 50 51 52 53 54 55 56 57 58 59 60 61 62 63 64 65 66 67 68 69 70 71 72 73 74 **P**1 4 5 **S**5335 OSF Healthcare System	21	10	560	20276	373	373466	2339	240605	96274	3655

PERU—La Salle County

★ ILLINOIS VALLEY COMMUNITY HOSPITAL, 925 West Street, Zip 61354-2799; tel. 815/223-3300; Ralph B. Berkley, Administrator **A**1 9 10 **F**1 7 8 10 15 16 19 21 22 23 26 28 29 30 31 32 33 35 36 37 39 40 41 42 44 45 46 49 52 53 54 56 57 64 65 66 67 71 73 74 **P**8	23	10	104	3593	57	64015	362	25278	10904	434

PINCKNEYVILLE—Perry County

★ PINCKNEYVILLE COMMUNITY HOSPITAL, 101 North Walnut Street, Zip 62274; tel. 618/357-2187; John Bennett, Administrator (Nonreporting) **A**1 9 10	16	10	92	—	—	—	—	—	—	—

PITTSFIELD—Pike County

★ ILLINI COMMUNITY HOSPITAL, 640 West Washington Street, Zip 62363; tel. 217/285-2113; Kathleen E. Millgard, President and Chief Executive Officer **A**1 9 10 **F**8 11 19 22 24 32 33 36 37 40 44 46 49 65 71 73 **S**0002 Quorum Health Group/Quorum Health Resources	23	10	48	1361	17	29642	51	7592	3041	141

PONTIAC—Livingston County

★ SAINT JAMES HOSPITAL, 610 East Water Street, Zip 61764; tel. 815/842-2828; David Ochs, Administrator (Total facility includes 16 beds in nursing home-type unit) **A**1 9 10 **F**7 8 10 12 13 14 15 16 17 19 21 22 26 28 29 30 32 33 34 35 36 37 39 40 41 42 44 49 56 63 64 65 66 67 70 71 72 73 74 **P**5 6 7 **S**5335 OSF Healthcare System	21	10	84	3035	36	67339	353	21949	9179	327

PRINCETON—Bureau County

★ PERRY MEMORIAL HOSPITAL, 530 Park Avenue East, Zip 61356-2598; tel. 815/875-2811; William H. Spitler III, President (Total facility includes 15 beds in nursing home-type unit) **A**1 9 10 **F**7 8 17 19 21 22 30 32 33 35 36 37 39 40 41 42 44 49 53 54 56 58 64 65 67 71 **P**3	14	10	98	2720	40	36510	145	15641	6803	225

QUINCY—Adams County

★ BLESSING HOSPITAL, (Includes Blessing Hospital, Broadway & 14th Street, Quincy, Illinois, Zip 62301, Mailing Address: P.O. Box 7005, Zip 62305-7005; tel. 217/223-1200) Broadway At 11th Street, Zip 62301, Mailing Address: P.O. Box 7005, Zip 62305-7005; tel. 217/223-5811; Lawrence L. Swearingen, President (Total facility includes 44 beds in nursing home-type unit) **A**1 2 3 5 9 10 **F**1 2 5 7 8 10 12 14 15 16 19 21 22 23 24 26 27 28 29 30 31 32 33 35 36 37 39 40 41 42 44 45 46 48 49 52 53 56 60 63 64 65 66 67 70 71 72 73 74 **P**1 8	23	10	330	13153	67	201899	1318	73730	34077	1398

RED BUD—Randolph County

★ ST. CLEMENT HOSPITAL, 1 St. Clement Boulevard, Zip 62278-1194; tel. 618/282-3831; Michael Thomas McManus, President (Total facility includes 40 beds in nursing home-type unit) **A**1 9 10 **F**7 8 14 15 16 19 20 21 22 25 28 30 32 33 34 35 37 39 40 42 44 64 65 67 71 **S**0205 ASC Health System	21	10	105	1836	55	47955	138	11669	5548	238

ROBINSON—Crawford County

★ CRAWFORD MEMORIAL HOSPITAL, 1000 North Allen Street, Zip 62454, Mailing Address: P.O. Box 151, Zip 62454; tel. 618/544-3131; Roger D. Feldt, Chief Executive Officer (Total facility includes 46 beds in nursing home-type unit) **A**1 9 10 **F**7 8 13 14 15 16 18 19 22 27 28 30 32 33 35 36 37 39 40 41 42 44 46 49 64 65 67 71 **S**0002 Quorum Health Group/Quorum Health Resources	16	10	107	2009	61	26150	256	10851	4152	214

ROCHELLE—Ogle County

★ ROCHELLE COMMUNITY HOSPITAL, 900 North Second Street, Zip 61068-0330; tel. 815/562-2181; Roland R. Carlson, President and Chief Executive Officer **A**1 9 10 **F**7 8 12 15 16 19 21 22 24 30 31 32 34 37 40 44 49 51 64 65 67 71 72 **P**5 8	23	10	42	1268	15	68490	132	8648	3743	150

ROCK ISLAND—Rock Island County

★ △ TRINITY MEDICAL CENTER—WEST CAMPUS, (Includes Trinity Medical Center—East Campus, 501 Tenth Avenue, Moline, Illinois, Zip 61265; tel. 309/757-3131) 2701 17th Street, Zip 61201; tel. 309/757-3822; Eric Crowell, President and Chief Executive Officer (Total facility includes 29 beds in nursing home-type unit) **A**1 2 6 7 9 10 **F**2 3 4 7 8 9 10 11 12 14 15 16 17 19 21 22 23 24 25 26 27 28 29 30 31 32 33 34 35 37 38 39 40 41 42 44 45 46 48 49 52 53 54 55 56 57 58 59 60 61 63 64 65 66 67 70 71 73 74 **P**8	23	10	415	16025	267	188352	1846	120580	51622	1583

ROCKFORD—Winnebago County

□ H. DOUGLAS SINGER MENTAL HEALTH AND DEVELOPMENTAL CENTER, 4402 North Main Street, Zip 61103-1278; tel. 815/987-7096; Richard F. Kunnert, Director **A**1 10 **F**4 7 8 9 10 11 15 19 20 21 22 31 35 37 38 40 41 42 43 45 46 47 48 49 50 52 53 55 56 57 60 63 65 71 73	12	22	190	863	163	0	0	12778	9641	258

© 1995 AHA Guide

Hospitals, U.S. / ILLINOIS

Hospital, Address, Telephone, Administrator, Approval, Facility, and Physician Codes, Health Care System

- ★ American Hospital Association (AHA) membership
- □ Joint Commission on Accreditation of Healthcare Organizations (JCAHO) accreditation
- + American Osteopathic Hospital Association (AOHA) membership
- ○ American Osteopathic Association (AOA) accreditation
- △ Commission on Accreditation of Rehabilitation Facilities (CARF) accreditation

Control codes 61, 63, 64, 71, 72 and 73 indicate hospitals listed by AOHA, but not registered by AHA. For definition of numerical codes, see page A6.

Hospital	Control	Service	Beds	Admissions	Census	Outpatient Visits	Births	Total	Payroll	Personnel
★ △ ROCKFORD MEMORIAL HOSPITAL, 2400 North Rockton Avenue, Zip 61103–3692; tel. 815/968–6861; Thomas David DeFauw, President **A**1 2 5 7 9 **F**2 3 4 7 8 11 14 15 16 17 19 21 22 26 28 29 30 31 32 33 36 37 38 39 40 41 42 43 44 45 46 47 48 49 51 52 53 54 55 56 57 58 59 60 61 65 66 67 70 71 72 73 74 **P**3	23	10	451	14190	285	—	1884	156962	68604	1932
★ SAINT ANTHONY MEDICAL CENTER, 5666 East State Street, Zip 61108–2472; tel. 815/226–2000; Jerry A. Nash, Administrator **A**1 2 3 5 9 10 **F**4 7 8 9 10 11 12 14 15 16 17 19 21 22 23 24 26 27 28 29 30 31 32 33 34 35 36 37 39 40 41 42 43 45 46 49 51 56 60 63 64 65 66 67 69 70 71 72 73 **P**6 7 **S**5335 OSF Healthcare System	21	10	210	8464	128	110887	901	88015	36108	1174
★ SWEDISHAMERICAN HOSPITAL, 1400 Charles Street, Zip 61104–2298; tel. 815/968–4400; Robert B. Klint M.D., President **A**1 2 3 5 9 10 **F**3 4 5 7 8 10 11 12 13 14 15 16 17 18 19 20 21 22 24 26 30 31 32 33 34 35 37 39 40 41 42 43 44 45 46 47 49 52 53 54 55 56 57 58 59 60 63 64 65 66 67 68 70 71 72 73 74 **P**3 7 8	23	10	298	12099	182	112857	1798	105659	45413	1596
ROSICLARE—Hardin County										
★ HARDIN COUNTY GENERAL HOSPITAL, Ferrell Road, Zip 62982; tel. 618/285–6634; Roby D. Williams, Administrator (Nonreporting) **A**1 9 10	23	10	48	—	—	—	—	—	—	—
RUSHVILLE—Schuyler County										
★ SARAH D. CULBERTSON MEMORIAL HOSPITAL, 238 South Congress Street, Zip 62681, Mailing Address: P.O. Box 440, Zip 62681; tel. 217/322–4321; Michael C. O'Brien, Administrator (Total facility includes 25 beds in nursing home–type unit) **A**9 10 **F**7 8 17 19 22 28 30 33 34 36 39 40 42 44 49 64 67 71 73 **P**6	16	10	53	865	34	17064	141	4938	1880	111
SALEM—Marion County										
★ PUBLIC HOSPITAL OF THE TOWN OF SALEM, One Bryan Memorial Park, Zip 62881–6250, Mailing Address: P.O. Box 1250, Zip 62881–1250; tel. 618/548–3194; Clarence E. Lay, Chief Executive Officer **A**1 9 10 **F**8 14 15 16 17 19 22 25 28 30 32 36 37 44 49 71 73	14	10	52	1755	23	30147	0	9270	3828	186
SANDWICH—De Kalb County										
★ SANDWICH COMMUNITY HOSPITAL, 11 East Pleasant Avenue, Zip 60548–0901; tel. 815/786–8484; Loren D. Slade, Administrator **A**9 10 **F**7 8 19 21 22 28 30 34 35 37 39 40 41 44 45 49 65 71 73 **S**0002 Quorum Health Group/Quorum Health Resources	23	10	50	1301	14	42174	67	9213	3766	118
SCOTT AIR FORCE BASE—St. Clair County										
★ SCOTT MEDICAL CENTER, (Formerly U.S. Air Force Medical Center) Zip 62225–5252; tel. 618/256–7012; Colonel Talbot N. Vivian MSC, USAF, Administrator **A**1 2 3 5 **F**2 3 4 7 8 9 10 11 12 13 15 16 18 19 20 21 24 28 29 30 35 37 38 39 40 41 42 43 44 46 48 49 50 51 52 53 55 58 60 61 64 65 66 68 70 71 73 74 **S**9495 Department of the Air Force	41	10	85	5972	54	338490	671	—	—	1308
SHELBYVILLE—Shelby County										
★ SHELBY MEMORIAL HOSPITAL, 200 South Cedar Street, Zip 62565–1899; tel. 217/774–3961; Roger L. Holloway, President and Chief Executive Officer (Total facility includes 15 beds in nursing home–type unit) **A**1 9 10 **F**8 11 15 16 19 21 22 31 33 34 35 37 41 42 44 49 64 65 66 71	23	10	64	2057	38	28637	0	9124	3905	196
SILVIS—Rock Island County										
★ ILLINI HOSPITAL, 801 Hospital Road, Zip 61282; tel. 309/792–9363; Gary E. Larson, Chief Executive Officer **A**1 9 10 **F**6 7 8 19 21 22 24 25 26 28 29 30 32 35 37 40 41 44 45 62 63 65 71 72 73 **P**6 7 8	23	10	133	4372	54	89370	656	30618	13000	477
SKOKIE—Cook County										
□ CPC OLD ORCHARD HOSPITAL, 9700 North Kenton Avenue, Zip 60076–1218; tel. 708/679–0760; Sheila Mishler, Chief Executive Officer (Nonreporting) **A**1 9 10 **S**0785 Community Psychiatric Centers	33	22	133	—	—	—	—	—	—	—
★ RUSH NORTH SHORE MEDICAL CENTER, 9600 Gross Point Road, Zip 60076–1257; tel. 708/677–9600; John S. Frigo, President (Data for 242 days) **A**1 2 3 5 9 10 **F**4 5 7 8 10 14 19 21 22 26 34 35 36 40 42 43 44 46 49 52 54 55 56 57 58 59 60 63 65 70 71 73 74 **P**8 **S**3855 Rush–Presbyterian–St. Luke's Medical Center	23	10	245	6927	192	232541	506	63571	28889	1060
SPARTA—Randolph County										
★ SPARTA COMMUNITY HOSPITAL, 818 East Broadway Street, Zip 62286–0000; tel. 618/443–2177; Donald G. Brown, Administrator **A**9 10 **F**1 7 8 12 14 15 16 17 19 22 25 28 30 33 34 40 41 42 44 46 49 51 65 67 71 73 74 **P**6	16	10	43	1002	11	27029	176	7073	2886	145
SPRING VALLEY—Bureau County										
★ ST. MARGARET'S HOSPITAL, 600 East First Street, Zip 61362–2034; tel. 815/664–5311; Tim Muntz, President (Total facility includes 33 beds in nursing home–type unit) **A**1 2 9 10 **F**1 7 8 10 14 15 16 19 21 22 23 24 27 30 32 33 35 37 39 40 41 42 44 48 49 60 62 64 65 66 67 71 73 74 **P**6 **S**5805 Sisters of Mary of the Presentation Health Corporation	21	10	127	3254	59	70497	392	21400	8500	249
SPRINGFIELD—Sangamon County										
□ ANDREW MCFARLAND MENTAL HEALTH CENTER, 901 Southwind Road, Zip 62703; tel. 217/786–6994; Nieves Tan–Lachica M.D., Superintendent (Nonreporting) **A**1	12	22	146	—	—	—	—	—	—	—
□ DOCTORS HOSPITAL, 5230 South Sixth Street, Zip 62703, Mailing Address: P.O. Box 19254, Zip 62794–9254; tel. 217/529–7151; Jim Bohl, President and Chief Executive Officer (Nonreporting) **A**1 9 10	33	10	150	—	—	—	—	—	—	—
★ △ MEMORIAL MEDICAL CENTER, 800 North Rutledge Street, Zip 62781–0001; tel. 217/788–3000; Robert T. Clarke, President and Chief Executive Officer **A**1 2 3 5 7 8 9 10 **F**3 4 7 8 9 10 11 15 16 19 21 22 25 26 29 31 32 33 34 35 37 40 41 42 43 44 45 46 48 49 50 52 53 54 55 56 57 58 59 60 61 63 65 66 69 70 71 73 74 **P**6 7	23	10	520	17550	333	244786	1559	182946	83361	2514

Hospitals, U.S. / ILLINOIS

Hospital, Address, Telephone, Administrator, Approval, Facility, and Physician Codes, Health Care System	Classification Codes		Utilization Data					Expense (thousands) of dollars		
	Control	Service	Beds	Admissions	Census	Outpatient Visits	Births	Total	Payroll	Personnel

★ American Hospital Association (AHA) membership
☐ Joint Commission on Accreditation of Healthcare Organizations (JCAHO) accreditation
+ American Osteopathic Hospital Association (AOHA) membership
○ American Osteopathic Association (AOA) accreditation
△ Commission on Accreditation of Rehabilitation Facilities (CARF) accreditation
Control codes 61, 63, 64, 71, 72 and 73 indicate hospitals listed by AOHA, but not registered by AHA. For definition of numerical codes, see page A6

Hospital	Control	Service	Beds	Admissions	Census	Outpatient Visits	Births	Total	Payroll	Personnel
★ ST. JOHN'S HOSPITAL, 800 East Carpenter Street, Zip 62769; tel. 217/544–6464; Allison C. Laabs, Executive Vice President (Total facility includes 51 beds in nursing home–type unit) **A**1 2 3 5 8 9 10 **F**1 3 4 8 10 19 21 22 26 28 30 32 33 34 35 36 37 38 40 42 43 44 46 47 49 52 57 58 59 60 64 65 67 70 71 73 **S**5355 Hospital Sisters Health System	21	10	633	24078	468	200579	2327	214039	94133	3414
STAUNTON—Macoupin County										
★ COMMUNITY MEMORIAL HOSPITAL, 400 Caldwell Street, Zip 62088–1499; tel. 618/635–2200; Patrick B. Heise, Chief Executive Officer **A**1 9 10 **F**8 19 32 34 44 65 71 73 **P**3 **S**0002 Quorum Health Group/Quorum Health Resources	23	10	57	914	11	16129	0	5994	2468	116
STERLING—Whiteside County										
★ CGH MEDICAL CENTER, 100 East LeFevre Road, Zip 61081–1279; tel. 815/625–0400; Darryl Wahler, President (Total facility includes 10 beds in nursing home–type unit) **A**1 2 9 10 **F**7 8 14 16 17 19 21 22 23 28 29 30 31 32 33 35 37 39 40 41 42 44 46 49 60 63 64 65 66 70 71 73 **P**5	14	10	143	6232	74	64171	780	38509	17548	716
STREAMWOOD—Cook County										
☐ CPC STREAMWOOD HOSPITAL, 1400 East Irving Park Road, Zip 60107; tel. 708/837–9000; Suzanne Barry, Administrator **A**1 9 10 **F**3 15 28 29 52 53 54 55 56 58 67 **S**0785 Community Psychiatric Centers	33	22	100	515	51	0	0	9286	4605	142
STREATOR—La Salle County										
★ ST. MARY'S HOSPITAL, 111 East Spring Street, Zip 61364; tel. 815/673–2311; Jimmie D. Lansford, Executive Vice President (Total facility includes 30 beds in nursing home–type unit) **A**1 9 10 **F**1 3 7 8 14 15 16 17 19 21 22 24 27 28 30 32 33 34 35 37 40 41 42 44 49 60 63 64 65 67 71 73 **S**5355 Hospital Sisters Health System	21	10	170	4298	83	35667	342	26229	13506	430
SYCAMORE—De Kalb County										
☐ VENCOR HOSPITAL–SYCAMORE, 225 Edward Street, Zip 60178; tel. 815/895–2144; Donald Van Voorhis, Administrator (Nonreporting) **A**1 9 10 **S**0026 Vencor, Incorporated	14	10	50	—	—	—	—	—	—	—
TAYLORVILLE—Christian County										
★ ST. VINCENT MEMORIAL HOSPITAL, 201 East Pleasant Street, Zip 62568–1597; tel. 217/824–3331; Dan Colby, President and Chief Executive Officer (Nonreporting) **A**1 9 10 **S**0205 ASC Health System	21	10	152	—	—	—	—	—	—	—
TINLEY PARK—Cook County										
☐ TINLEY PARK MENTAL HEALTH CENTER, 7400 West 183rd Street, Zip 60477–3695; tel. 708/614–4000; Delores Newman MS, Director **A**1 10 **F**1 2 3 14 15 16 20 22 44 52 55 56 57 58 59 65 70 73	12	22	355	2816	258	1245	0	—	—	497
URBANA—Champaign County										
★ △ CARLE FOUNDATION HOSPITAL, 611 West Park Street, Zip 61801–2595; tel. 217/383–3311; Michael H. Fritz, President (Total facility includes 240 beds in nursing home–type unit) **A**1 2 3 5 7 9 10 **F**2 4 7 8 10 14 15 16 19 22 23 26 28 29 30 31 32 33 34 35 37 38 39 40 41 42 43 44 45 46 48 49 62 63 64 65 67 70 71 72 73 **P**5 **S**2575 Carle Foundation	23	10	540	12361	334	44129	1553	98440	40099	1260
★ △ COVENANT MEDICAL CENTER, (Includes Burnham Hospital, 407 South Fourth Street, Champaign, Illinois, Zip 61820; tel. 217/337–2500; Mercy Hospital, Urbana, Illinois) 1400 West Park Street, Zip 61801; tel. 217/337–2000; Joseph W. Beard, President **A**1 2 3 5 7 9 10 **F**4 7 10 12 16 17 19 21 22 23 24 26 30 32 33 34 35 37 38 39 40 41 42 43 44 48 49 52 54 55 56 58 59 60 63 65 67 71 73 **P**3 4 **S**4025 Servantcor	21	10	268	11591	174	113217	1594	86246	34739	1463
MERCY HOSPITAL See Covenant Medical Center										
VANDALIA—Fayette County										
★ FAYETTE COUNTY HOSPITAL, Seventh and Taylor Streets, Zip 62471–1296; tel. 618/283–1231; Jerome J. Bozek, Administrator (Total facility includes 92 beds in nursing home–type unit) **A**1 9 10 **F**8 14 15 16 19 20 21 22 28 33 36 41 42 44 45 46 49 50 56 64 65 71 73 **P**1 5 6 7 8 **S**0051 BJC Health System	16	10	133	1631	94	23944	0	10405	4466	208
WATSEKA—Iroquois County										
★ IROQUOIS MEMORIAL HOSPITAL AND RESIDENT HOME, 200 Fairman Avenue, Zip 60970–1644; tel. 815/432–5841; Melvin H. Fahs, President (Total facility includes 46 beds in nursing home–type unit) **A**1 9 10 **F**7 8 14 15 16 19 20 21 22 26 30 32 34 36 37 38 40 41 42 44 45 49 58 64 65 67 71 73	23	10	112	2117	73	26394	185	15282	6842	224
WAUKEGAN—Lake County										
★ SAINT THERESE MEDICAL CENTER, 2615 Washington Street, Zip 60085–4988; tel. 708/249–3900; Timothy P. Selz, President (Total facility includes 25 beds in nursing home–type unit) **A**1 2 9 10 **F**3 4 7 8 10 11 12 13 14 15 16 17 18 19 20 21 22 23 24 25 26 27 28 29 30 31 32 33 34 39 40 41 42 44 45 46 48 49 51 52 53 54 55 56 58 59 63 64 65 66 67 68 70 71 72 73 74 **P**5 7 8 **S**1415 Franciscan Sisters Health Care Corporation	21	10	254	9072	139	222530	1271	69588	30244	822
★ VICTORY MEMORIAL HOSPITAL, 1324 North Sheridan Road, Zip 60085–2181; tel. 708/360–3000; Timothy Harrington, President **A**1 2 9 10 **F**1 2 3 4 7 8 10 12 14 15 16 19 21 22 24 25 26 28 30 32 33 34 35 36 37 39 40 41 42 43 44 45 46 52 54 55 56 57 58 59 60 64 65 67 71 73 **P**5 7 8	23	10	277	9316	129	90677	1496	67681	29693	927
WEST FRANKFORT—Franklin County										
★ WEST FRANKFORT UNITED MINE WORKERS OF AMERICA UNION HOSPITAL, 507 West St Louis Street, Zip 62896–1999; tel. 618/932–2155; John D. Groves, Chief Executive Officer **A**9 10 **F**19 32 44 70 71 73 **S**2285 Alliant Health System	23	10	34	885	12	—	0	5109	2084	118

© 1995 AHA Guide

Hospitals, U.S. / ILLINOIS

Hospital, Address, Telephone, Administrator, Approval, Facility, and Physician Codes, Health Care System	Classification Codes		Utilization Data					Expense (thousands) of dollars		
★ American Hospital Association (AHA) membership □ Joint Commission on Accreditation of Healthcare Organizations (JCAHO) accreditation + American Osteopathic Hospital Association (AOHA) membership ○ American Osteopathic Association (AOA) accreditation △ Commission on Accreditation of Rehabilitation Facilities (CARF) accreditation Control codes 61, 63, 64, 71, 72 and 73 indicate hospitals listed by AOHA, but not registered by AHA. For definition of numerical codes, see page A6	Control	Service	Beds	Admissions	Census	Outpatient Visits	Births	Total	Payroll	Personnel
WHEATON—Du Page County										
★ △ MARIANJOY REHABILITATION HOSPITAL AND CLINICS, 26 West 171 Roosevelt Road, Zip 60187, Mailing Address: P.O. Box 795, Zip 60189-0795; tel. 708/462-4000; Bruce A. Schurman, President **A**1 3 5 7 9 10 **F**5 17 19 20 21 22 24 25 27 29 32 34 35 41 45 46 48 49 50 54 62 63 65 66 67 71 73 **P**1 **S**6745 Wheaton Franciscan Services, Inc.	21	46	107	1599	99	18370	0	39718	19348	606
WINFIELD—Du Page County										
ALCOHOLISM TREATMENT CENTER, 27 West 350 High Lake Road, Zip 60190; tel. 708/653-4000; David Fox, President (Nonreporting)	23	82	52	—	—	—	—	—	—	—
★ CENTRAL DUPAGE HOSPITAL, 25 North Winfield Road, Zip 60190; tel. 708/682-1600; George G. Holzhauer, President **A**1 2 9 10 **F**1 2 3 4 6 7 8 10 11 12 15 16 17 19 20 21 22 23 25 26 28 30 31 32 33 34 35 36 37 38 39 40 41 42 43 44 45 46 52 54 55 57 58 59 60 62 64 65 67 70 71 72 73 **P**6	23	10	317	14133	163	140786	3229	134717	53889	1384
WOOD RIVER—Madison County										
★ WOOD RIVER TOWNSHIP HOSPITAL, 101 East Edwardsville Road, Zip 62095-1332; tel. 618/254-3821; Jerry L. Bolandis, President **A**1 9 10 **F**3 7 8 10 12 13 14 15 16 17 18 19 21 22 26 27 28 29 30 31 32 33 34 35 36 37 38 39 40 41 44 45 46 47 48 49 51 52 54 55 56 57 60 64 65 66 67 68 71 73 74	16	10	131	1756	45	18913	245	17003	7404	301
WOODSTOCK—Mchenry County										
★ MEMORIAL MEDICAL CENTER, (Formerly Memorial Hospital) Highway 14 and Doty Road, Zip 60098-3797, Mailing Address: P.O. Box 1990, Zip 60098; tel. 815/338-2500; Jim D. Redding, Chief Executive Officer **A**1 2 9 10 **F**2 3 7 8 12 14 15 16 17 18 19 21 22 23 26 30 32 33 34 35 36 37 39 40 41 44 46 49 52 53 54 55 56 57 58 59 60 63 64 65 66 67 68 71 73 74	23	10	146	4000	63	44195	536	34168	15294	501
ZION—Lake County										
□ MIDWESTERN REGIONAL MEDICAL CENTER, 2501 Emmaus Avenue, Zip 60099-2587; tel. 708/872-4561; Donald L. Maloney II, President and Chief Executive Officer **A**1 2 9 10 **F**8 17 19 20 21 22 25 27 28 29 30 31 32 34 35 36 37 39 41 42 44 45 46 49 54 60 63 65 69 71 73	33	10	70	2152	36	18144	0	46291	11075	277

INDIANA

Resident population 5,713 (in thousands)
Resident population in metro areas 71.6%
Birth rate per 1,000 population 15.3
65 years and over 12.7%
Percent of persons without health insurance 11.5%

Hospital, Address, Telephone, Administrator, Approval, Facility, and Physician Codes, Health Care System

★ American Hospital Association (AHA) membership
□ Joint Commission on Accreditation of Healthcare Organizations (JCAHO) accreditation
+ American Osteopathic Hospital Association (AOHA) membership
○ American Osteopathic Association (AOA) accreditation
△ Commission on Accreditation of Rehabilitation Facilities (CARF) accreditation
Control codes 61, 63, 64, 71, 72 and 73 indicate hospitals listed by AOHA, but not registered by AHA. For definition of numerical codes, see page A6

Hospital	Control	Service	Beds	Admissions	Census	Outpatient Visits	Births	Total	Payroll	Personnel
ANDERSON—Madison County										
★ COMMUNITY HOSPITAL OF ANDERSON AND MADISON COUNTY, (Includes Crestview Center, 2211 Hillcrest Drive, Anderson, Indiana, Zip 46012) 1515 North Madison Avenue, Zip 46011–3453; tel. 317/642–8011; (Total facility includes 30 beds in nursing home–type unit) **A**1 9 10 **F**2 3 7 8 10 12 13 14 15 16 17 18 19 21 22 23 24 25 26 27 28 29 30 31 34 35 37 39 40 41 42 44 45 46 49 52 53 56 58 59 64 65 67 68 71 73 74 **P**6 8	23	10	207	7461	114	104614	1013	54030	22984	723
CRESTVIEW CENTER See Community Hospital of Anderson and Madison County										
★ SAINT JOHN'S HEALTH SYSTEM, 2015 Jackson Street, Zip 46016–4339; tel. 317/649–2511; James H. Stephens, President and Chief Executive Officer (Total facility includes 29 beds in nursing home–type unit) **A**1 2 9 10 **F**1 2 3 7 8 12 14 15 16 17 19 20 21 22 23 26 27 28 29 30 31 32 33 34 35 37 39 40 41 42 44 45 48 49 52 53 54 55 56 57 58 59 60 63 64 65 66 67 71 73 74 **P**8 **S**5585 Holy Cross Health System Corporation	21	10	371	8507	154	188495	529	75589	29876	1105
ANGOLA—Steuben County										
★ CAMERON MEMORIAL COMMUNITY HOSPITAL, (Includes Elmhurst Hospital, 909 West Maumee Street, Angola, Indiana, Zip 46703; tel. 219/665–3151; Ronald Showalter, Administrator) 416 East Maumee Street, Zip 46703; tel. 219/665–2141; Dennis L. Knapp, President **A**9 10 **F**2 3 7 8 14 19 21 22 29 30 32 33 34 35 36 37 39 40 41 44 46 49 65 67 71 73	23	10	61	1563	14	58674	313	12587	6193	242
ELMHURST HOSPITAL See Cameron Memorial Community Hospital										
AUBURN—De Kalb County										
★ DEKALB MEMORIAL HOSPITAL, 1316 East Seventh Street, Zip 46706–0542, Mailing Address: P.O. Box 542, Zip 46706; tel. 219/925–4600; Jack M. Corey, President **A**1 9 10 **F**7 8 11 14 15 16 17 19 21 22 29 30 32 34 36 37 39 40 41 42 44 45 46 49 65 67 71 72 73 **P**6 7	23	10	47	2297	23	80384	447	17350	8042	306
BATESVILLE—Franklin County										
★ MARGARET MARY COMMUNITY HOSPITAL, 321 Mitchell Avenue, Zip 47006–8953, Mailing Address: P.O. Box 226, Zip 47006–0226; tel. 812/934–6624; James L. Amos, President (Total facility includes 35 beds in nursing home–type unit) **A**1 9 10 **F**7 8 19 20 21 22 26 28 30 32 34 35 36 37 39 40 41 42 44 49 63 64 65 66 67 71 73	23	10	94	1980	45	81154	416	15103	7031	268
BEDFORD—Lawrence County										
★ BEDFORD REGIONAL MEDICAL CENTER, (Formerly Bedford Medical Center) 2900 West 16th Street, Zip 47421; tel. 812/275–1200; Richard D. Hawkins M.D., President and Chief Executive Officer **A**1 9 10 **F**3 7 8 10 14 15 16 17 19 21 22 28 30 31 32 33 34 35 37 40 42 44 46 49 51 63 65 66 71 73 **P**6	23	10	60	2800	27	88521	437	20895	9032	502
★ DUNN MEMORIAL HOSPITAL, 1600 23rd Street, Zip 47421–4704; tel. 812/275–3331; Richard Hahn, Executive Director **A**1 9 10 **F**1 7 8 10 11 13 17 19 20 21 22 27 28 29 30 31 32 33 34 37 39 40 42 44 45 46 49 51 65 71 73 74 **P**3	13	10	106	2747	33	38703	267	20274	9684	420
BEECH GROVE—Marion County										
★ ST. FRANCIS HOSPITAL AND HEALTH CENTERS, 1600 Albany Street, Zip 46107–1593; tel. 317/787–3311; Kevin D. Leahy, President and Chief Executive Officer (Nonreporting) **A**1 2 3 5 9 10 **S**5345 Sisters of St. Francis Health Services, Inc.	21	10	428	—	—	—	—	—	—	—
BLOOMINGTON—Monroe County										
★ BLOOMINGTON HOSPITAL, 601 West Second Street, Zip 47403–2317, Mailing Address: Box 1149, Zip 47402–1149; tel. 812/336–6821; Roland E. Kohr, President **A**1 9 10 **F**1 2 3 4 7 8 10 11 12 15 17 19 21 22 23 25 26 27 28 30 31 33 34 35 36 37 39 40 41 42 43 44 45 46 48 49 52 54 56 57 58 59 60 63 65 66 67 71 73 **P**7 8	23	10	245	13741	170	279742	1695	99406	45957	1572
BLUFFTON—Wells County										
★ CAYLOR–NICKEL MEDICAL CENTER, One Caylor–Nickel Square, Zip 46714; tel. 219/824–3500; William F. Brockmann, President and Chief Executive Officer (Total facility includes 19 beds in nursing home–type unit) **A**1 2 9 10 **F**3 5 7 8 10 11 12 14 15 16 17 19 20 21 22 24 25 26 30 32 34 35 37 39 40 41 42 44 45 46 49 51 52 53 54 56 57 58 60 64 65 67 71 73 **P**1	23	10	99	2961	36	58585	291	26344	10751	520
★ WELLS COMMUNITY HOSPITAL, 1100 South Main Street, Zip 46714; tel. 219/824–3210; Martin P. Braaksma, Executive Director (Nonreporting) **A**1 9 10	15	10	45	—	—	—	—	—	—	—
BOONVILLE—Warrick County										
★ WARRICK HOSPITAL, 1116 Millis Avenue, Zip 47601–0629, Mailing Address: Box 629, Zip 47601–0629; tel. 812/897–4800; John D. O'Neil, Chief Operating Officer **A**1 9 10 **F**8 15 17 19 20 22 28 31 32 37 41 44 49 64 65 71 73 **S**1855 Daughters of Charity National Health System	23	10	36	1388	15	10349	0	8961	4550	252
BRAZIL—Clay County										
★ CLAY COUNTY HOSPITAL, 1206 East National Avenue, Zip 47834–2797; tel. 812/448–2675; Jay P. Jolly, Chief Executive Officer **A**1 9 10 **F**7 8 17 19 21 22 28 31 34 35 37 40 41 42 44 45 46 49 61 65 71 73 74 **S**2285 Alliant Health System	13	10	53	1015	14	21096	116	8002	3421	156

© 1995 AHA Guide

Hospitals, U.S. / INDIANA

Hospital, Address, Telephone, Administrator, Approval, Facility, and Physician Codes, Health Care System	Classification Codes		Utilization Data					Expense (thousands) of dollars		Personnel
★ American Hospital Association (AHA) membership ☐ Joint Commission on Accreditation of Healthcare Organizations (JCAHO) accreditation + American Osteopathic Hospital Association (AOHA) membership ○ American Osteopathic Association (AOA) accreditation △ Commission on Accreditation of Rehabilitation Facilities (CARF) accreditation Control codes 61, 63, 64, 71, 72 and 73 indicate hospitals listed by AOHA, but not registered by AHA. For definition of numerical codes, see page A6	Control	Service	Beds	Admissions	Census	Outpatient Visits	Births	Total	Payroll	
BREMEN—Marshall County ★ COMMUNITY HOSPITAL OF BREMEN, 411 South Whitlock Street, Zip 46506–1699; tel. 219/546–2211; Scott R. Graybill, Administrator and Chief Executive Officer (Nonreporting) **A**9 10 **S**0135 Ancilla Systems Inc.	23	10	28	—	—	—	—	—	—	—
CARMEL—Hamilton County ST. VINCENT CARMEL HOSPITAL See St. Vincent Hospital and Health Care Center, Indianapolis										
CHARLESTOWN—Clark County ☐ MEDICAL CENTER OF SOUTHERN INDIANA, 2200 Market Street, Zip 47111–0069, Mailing Address: P.O. Box 69, Zip 47111–0069; tel. 812/256–3301; Kevin J. Miller, Chief Executive Officer (Total facility includes 24 beds in nursing home–type unit) **A**1 10 **F**4 6 7 8 9 10 12 13 14 15 19 20 21 22 23 25 26 28 29 30 31 32 35 37 38 39 40 41 42 43 44 45 46 47 48 49 50 51 52 57 58 59 60 61 63 64 65 66 67 69 70 71 72 73 74 **P**4	23	10	70	1471	31	13524	0	6199	13575	240
CLINTON—Vermillion County ☐ VERMILLION COUNTY HOSPITAL, 801 South Main Street, Zip 47842–0349; tel. 317/832–2451; John F. Ling Jr., President and Chief Executive Officer (Nonreporting) **A**1 9 10	13	10	56	—	—	—	—	—	—	—
COLUMBIA CITY—Whitley County ☐ WHITLEY COUNTY MEMORIAL HOSPITAL, 353 North Oak Street, Zip 46725; tel. 219/244–6191; John M. Hatcher, President (Total facility includes 82 beds in nursing home–type unit) **A**1 9 10 **F**7 8 11 15 16 19 21 22 24 28 30 32 33 35 36 39 40 41 44 46 48 49 64 71 **P**3 6	13	10	129	1788	82	34437	338	18893	7947	296
COLUMBUS—Bartholomew County ★ △ COLUMBUS REGIONAL HOSPITAL, 2400 East 17th Street, Zip 47201–5360; tel. 812/379–4441; John C. McGinty Jr., President and Chief Executive Officer **A**1 2 7 9 10 **F**3 5 7 8 10 12 14 15 16 17 19 20 21 22 23 28 29 30 31 32 33 34 35 36 37 38 39 40 41 42 44 46 48 49 51 52 53 54 55 56 57 58 59 60 63 65 66 67 71 73 74 **P**3 5 6 7	13	10	237	10144	131	109905	1241	86014	37139	1364
☐ KOALA HOSPITAL AND COUNSELING CENTER, 2223 Poshard Drive, Zip 47203; tel. 812/376–1711; Thomas N. Theroult, Administrator (Nonreporting) **A**1 9 10 **S**0044 Sterling Healthcare Corporation	33	22	60	—	—	—	—	—	—	—
CONNERSVILLE—Fayette County ★ FAYETTE MEMORIAL HOSPITAL, 1941 Virginia Avenue, Zip 47331–9990; tel. 317/825–5131; Craig C. Kinyon, Chief Financial Officer and Acting Chief Executive Officer (Nonreporting) **A**1 9 10	23	10	81	—	—	—	—	—	—	—
CORYDON—Harrison County ★ HARRISON COUNTY HOSPITAL, 245 Atwood Street, Zip 47112–0245; tel. 812/738–4251; Steven L. Taylor, Chief Executive Officer **A**1 9 10 **F**7 8 14 15 16 17 19 21 22 28 30 32 33 34 35 37 39 40 41 42 44 46 49 51 63 65 66 71 **P**6 7 **S**2285 Alliant Health System	13	10	50	1360	15	28952	185	10816	4523	223
CRAWFORDSVILLE—Montgomery County ★ CULVER UNION HOSPITAL, (Formerly AMI Culver Union Hospital) 1710 Lafayette Road, Zip 47933; tel. 317/362–2800; Michael Collins, Executive Director (Total facility includes 17 beds in nursing home–type unit) **A**1 10 **F**7 8 10 12 19 21 22 28 30 31 32 35 36 37 40 42 44 45 46 49 58 64 65 66 67 71 73 **P**1 2 4 5 6 7 8 **S**0063 TENET Healthcare Corporation	33	10	101	3615	48	34023	359	22374	6595	294
CROWN POINT—Lake County ★ ST. ANTHONY MEDICAL CENTER, 1201 South Main Street, Zip 46307–8483; tel. 219/757–6106; Stephen O. Leurck, President **A**1 2 10 **F**4 7 8 10 11 12 15 16 17 19 21 22 24 25 26 28 29 30 31 32 33 35 36 39 40 41 42 43 44 45 48 49 52 54 55 56 57 60 63 64 65 67 71 72 73 **P**3 4 6 7	21	10	275	8122	135	83624	821	80808	35406	853
DANVILLE—Hendricks County ★ HENDRICKS COMMUNITY HOSPITAL, 1000 East Main Street, Zip 46122–0409, Mailing Address: P.O. Box 409, Zip 46122–0409; tel. 317/745–4451; Dennis W. Dawes, President **A**1 9 10 **F**2 7 8 12 14 19 20 21 22 28 29 30 31 32 34 35 36 37 39 40 41 42 44 45 51 52 54 55 56 57 65 66 67 71 72 73 74 **P**6 8	13	10	127	5204	63	127235	637	34870	16417	478
DECATUR—Adams County ★ ADAMS COUNTY MEMORIAL HOSPITAL, 805 High Street, Zip 46733, Mailing Address: P.O. Box 151, Zip 46733; tel. 219/724–2145; Marvin L. Baird, Executive Director (Total facility includes 14 beds in nursing home–type unit) **A**9 10 **F**7 8 11 12 14 15 16 19 21 22 32 34 35 40 42 44 49 52 64 71	13	10	87	2334	39	49409	283	14725	6387	209
DYER—Lake County SAINT MARGARET MERCY HEALTHCARE CENTERS–SOUTH CAMPUS See Saint Margaret Mercy Healthcare Centers, Hammond										
EAST CHICAGO—Lake County ★ ST. CATHERINE HOSPITAL, 4321 Fir Street, Zip 46312; tel. 219/392–7000; Joseph M. Mark, President and Chief Executive Officer **A**1 9 10 **F**4 7 8 10 12 15 16 17 19 21 22 23 24 28 29 32 33 34 35 37 39 40 41 42 43 44 45 46 49 52 56 60 63 65 71 73 **P**2 3 6 7 8 **S**0135 Ancilla Systems Inc.	21	10	158	7577	149	45512	475	67458	25622	730
ELKHART—Elkhart County ★ ELKHART GENERAL HOSPITAL, 600 East Boulevard, Zip 46514, Mailing Address: Box 1329, Zip 46515; tel. 219/294–2621; Gregory W. Lintjer, President (Total facility includes 42 beds in nursing home–type unit) **A**1 9 10 **F**3 7 8 10 12 17 19 21 22 23 28 30 31 32 33 34 35 36 37 38 39 40 41 44 48 49 52 53 54 55 56 58 59 64 65 71 73 **P**5	23	10	312	11696	199	77239	1774	80371	33770	1343

Hospitals, U.S. / INDIANA

Hospital, Address, Telephone, Administrator, Approval, Facility, and Physician Codes, Health Care System	Classification Codes		Utilization Data					Expense (thousands) of dollars		
★ American Hospital Association (AHA) membership □ Joint Commission on Accreditation of Healthcare Organizations (JCAHO) accreditation + American Osteopathic Hospital Association (AOHA) membership ○ American Osteopathic Association (AOA) accreditation △ Commission on Accreditation of Rehabilitation Facilities (CARF) accreditation Control codes 61, 63, 64, 71, 72 and 73 indicate hospitals listed by AOHA, but not registered by AHA. For definition of numerical codes, see page A6	Control	Service	Beds	Admissions	Census	Outpatient Visits	Births	Total	Payroll	Personnel
ELWOOD—Madison County										
★ ST. VINCENT MERCY HOSPITAL, (Formerly Mercy Hospital) 1331 South A Street, Zip 46036–1942; tel. 317/552–3336; James E. Baer, Administrator **A**1 9 10 **F**7 8 11 15 17 19 20 21 22 31 34 35 37 40 41 42 44 49 51 61 65 71 73 **P**1 3 8	21	10	30	1712	23	25199	114	10488	4466	200
EVANSVILLE—Vanderburgh County										
★ △ DEACONESS HOSPITAL, 600 Mary Street, Zip 47747–0001; tel. 812/426–3000; Thomas H. Kramer, President **A**1 2 3 5 7 9 10 **F**3 4 7 8 10 11 14 17 19 21 22 23 24 26 27 28 29 30 31 32 33 34 35 36 37 39 40 41 42 43 44 46 47 48 49 51 52 54 56 60 61 62 63 65 67 70 71 73 74	23	10	380	16993	258	174594	1167	127567	58273	1875
□ EVANSVILLE STATE HOSPITAL, 3400 Lincoln Avenue, Zip 47714–0146; tel. 812/473–2222; Ralph Nichols, Superintendent (Nonreporting) **A**1 9	12	22	418	—	—	—	—	—	—	—
★ ST. MARY'S MEDICAL CENTER OF EVANSVILLE, 3700 Washington Avenue, Zip 47750; tel. 812/479–4000; Richard C. Breon, President and Chief Executive Officer (Total facility includes 128 beds in nursing home–type unit) **A**1 2 3 5 9 10 **F**3 4 7 8 10 11 12 14 15 16 17 19 21 22 23 24 25 28 30 32 34 35 37 38 41 42 43 44 47 49 52 54 55 56 57 58 59 60 61 64 65 66 67 71 72 73 74 **P**7 **S**1855 Daughters of Charity National Health System	21	10	575	13393	352	221151	2277	124310	53685	2007
★ △ TRI-STATE REGIONAL REHABILITATION HOSPITAL, 4100 Covert Avenue, Zip 47714, Mailing Address: P.O. Box 5349, Zip 47716–5349; tel. 812/476–9983; Gerald F. Vozel, Chief Executive Officer **A**1 7 9 10 **F**12 15 16 19 27 32 34 35 48 49 65 67 71 73	33	46	80	725	54	3729	0	15553	7580	184
★ △ WELBORN MEMORIAL BAPTIST HOSPITAL, 401 Southeast Sixth Street, Zip 47713–1299; tel. 812/426–8000; Marjorie Z. Soyugenc, President **A**1 2 7 9 10 **F**2 3 4 7 8 10 11 12 14 15 19 21 22 23 24 26 28 29 30 31 32 33 35 36 37 38 39 40 41 42 43 44 45 46 47 48 49 52 53 54 55 56 58 59 60 61 63 65 67 69 71 73 **P**1 3 6	23	10	350	9992	183	40490	896	77255	39654	1228
FORT WAYNE—Allen County										
□ CHARTER BEACON, 1720 Beacon Street, Zip 46805; tel. 219/423–3651; Wendy Swisher, Chief Executive Officer (Nonreporting) **A**1 9 10 **S**0695 Charter Medical Corporation	33	22	97	—	—	—	—	—	—	—
★ LUTHERAN HOSPITAL OF INDIANA, 7950 West Jefferson Boulevard, Zip 46804–1677; tel. 219/435–7001; Frederick H. Kerr, President and Chief Executive Officer **A**1 3 5 9 10 **F**2 3 4 7 8 10 11 14 15 16 18 19 20 21 22 23 24 26 27 28 29 30 31 32 33 34 35 36 37 38 39 40 41 42 43 44 47 48 49 54 55 56 57 58 59 60 61 63 64 65 66 69 71 72 73 74 **P**1 5 7	21	10	330	13217	190	134674	1703	130107	49302	1598
★ △ PARKVIEW MEMORIAL HOSPITAL, 2200 Randallia Drive, Zip 46805; tel. 219/484–6636; David S. Ridderheim, President and Chief Executive Officer **A**1 3 5 7 9 10 **F**3 4 6 7 8 10 11 12 14 15 16 17 18 19 21 22 24 25 27 28 30 32 34 35 37 41 42 43 44 45 46 47 48 49 51 52 53 54 55 56 57 58 59 60 64 65 67 68 71 72 73 74 **P**5 6 7 8	23	10	580	21790	354	100892	3869	180417	83742	2477
★ △ ST. JOSEPH MEDICAL CENTER OF FORT WAYNE, 700 Broadway, Zip 46802; tel. 219/425–3000; John T. Farrell Sr., President and Chief Executive Officer **A**1 3 5 7 9 10 **F**4 7 8 9 10 11 12 13 14 15 16 17 19 20 21 22 23 24 25 26 27 28 29 30 31 32 33 34 35 37 39 40 41 42 43 44 45 46 48 49 51 56 57 58 61 63 65 67 68 70 71 72 73 74 **P**6 8 **S**0135 Ancilla Systems Inc.	21	10	262	8325	144	115246	751	77361	30544	970
★ VETERANS AFFAIRS MEDICAL CENTER, 2121 Lake Avenue, Zip 46805–5347; tel. 219/426–5431; Jonathan D. Hawk, Director (Total facility includes 53 beds in nursing home–type unit) **A**1 **F**3 8 15 19 20 22 26 31 32 33 34 35 37 39 42 44 46 49 51 54 58 60 64 65 71 73 **S**9295 Department of Veterans Affairs	45	10	151	3118	117	37560	0	31186	14098	344
FRANKFORT—Clinton County										
★ CLINTON COUNTY HOSPITAL, 1300 South Jackson Street, Zip 46041–3394, Mailing Address: P.O. Box 669, Zip 46041–0669; tel. 317/659–4731; Brian R. Zeh, Executive Director **A**1 9 10 **F**7 8 14 19 20 21 22 24 26 27 28 29 30 31 32 34 35 37 39 40 41 42 44 45 46 49 54 63 65 66 71 73 74 **P**1 6	13	10	53	1702	11	34958	300	12813	5381	214
FRANKLIN—Johnson County										
★ JOHNSON MEMORIAL HOSPITAL, 1125 West Jefferson Street, Zip 46131–2140, Mailing Address: P.O. Box 549, Zip 46131–0549; tel. 317/736–3300; Gregg A. Bechtold, President and Chief Executive Officer (Total facility includes 69 beds in nursing home–type unit) **A**1 9 10 **F**1 7 8 14 15 16 19 21 22 28 29 30 34 35 37 40 41 42 44 46 49 64 65 67 71 73 **P**8	13	10	142	3750	95	49144	529	27107	11872	448
GARY—Lake County										
★ △ METHODIST HOSPITALS, (Includes Broadway Methodist Hospital, 8701 Broadway, Merrillville, Indiana, Zip 46410; tel. 219/738–5500; Northlake Campus, 600 Grant Street, Gary, Indiana, Zip 46402; tel. 219/886–4000) John H. Betjemann, President **A**1 2 3 5 7 9 10 **F**1 2 3 4 5 7 8 10 11 15 19 21 22 23 26 28 29 30 32 33 34 35 37 38 39 40 41 42 43 44 48 49 52 53 54 56 57 58 60 61 63 65 67 71 72 73 74 **P**5 7	23	10	617	21214	424	220262	2441	189165	82284	2396
NORTHLAKE CAMPUS See Methodist Hospitals										
NORTHWEST FAMILY HOSPITAL, 501 Family Plaza, Zip 46402; tel. 219/882–9411; Willie C. White III, President and Chief Executive Officer (Nonreporting) **A**9 10 **S**0905 Summit Medical Management, Inc.	21	10	140	—	—	—	—	—	—	—
GOSHEN—Elkhart County										
★ GOSHEN GENERAL HOSPITAL, 200 High Park Avenue, Zip 46526, Mailing Address: P.O. Box 139, Zip 46527; tel. 219/533–2141; James O. Dague, President **A**1 10 **F**7 8 14 15 16 19 20 21 22 23 25 29 32 33 34 35 37 40 41 42 44 46 49 65 71 73 **P**8	23	10	90	4926	51	50202	1223	33737	17335	599

© 1995 AHA Guide

Hospitals, U.S. / INDIANA

Hospital, Address, Telephone, Administrator, Approval, Facility, and Physician Codes, Health Care System	Classification Codes		Utilization Data					Expense (thousands) of dollars		Personnel
	Control	Service	Beds	Admissions	Census	Outpatient Visits	Births	Total	Payroll	

★ American Hospital Association (AHA) membership
☐ Joint Commission on Accreditation of Healthcare Organizations (JCAHO) accreditation
+ American Osteopathic Hospital Association (AOHA) membership
○ American Osteopathic Association (AOA) accreditation
△ Commission on Accreditation of Rehabilitation Facilities (CARF) accreditation
Control codes 61, 63, 64, 71, 72 and 73 indicate hospitals listed by AOHA, but not registered by AHA. For definition of numerical codes, see page A6

Hospital	Control	Service	Beds	Admissions	Census	Outpatient Visits	Births	Total	Payroll	Personnel
★ OAKLAWN PSYCHIATRIC CENTER, INC., 330 Lakeview Drive, Zip 46526-9365, Mailing Address: P.O. Box 809, Zip 46527-0809; tel. 219/533-1234; Harold C. Loewen, President **A**1 10 **F**3 12 15 16 17 26 27 34 52 53 54 56 57 58 59 65 73 **P**1 6	21	22	48	1239	34	0	0	9622	4637	305
GREENCASTLE—Putnam County										
☐ PUTNAM COUNTY HOSPITAL, 1542 Bloomington Street, Zip 46135; tel. 317/653-5121; John D. Fajt, Executive Director **A**1 2 9 10 **F**7 8 14 17 19 20 21 22 26 30 35 37 39 40 41 42 44 49 56 65 67 71	13	10	85	2054	28	46052	284	11808	5559	231
GREENFIELD—Hancock County										
★ HANCOCK MEMORIAL HOSPITAL, 801 North State Street, Zip 46140-2537, Mailing Address: Box 827, Zip 46140; tel. 317/462-5544; Robert C. Keen Ph.D., President and Chief Executive Officer **A**1 9 10 **F**7 8 10 11 14 15 16 17 19 20 21 22 28 30 32 33 34 35 36 37 39 40 41 42 44 46 48 49 51 65 66 67 70 71 73 74 **P**2 3	13	10	87	3424	42	119994	496	32489	13550	420
GREENSBURG—Decatur County										
★ DECATUR COUNTY MEMORIAL HOSPITAL, 720 North Lincoln Street, Zip 47240-1398; tel. 812/663-4331; Dalton L. Smart, Chief Executive Director **A**1 9 10 **F**7 8 16 19 20 21 22 27 28 32 33 34 35 36 37 40 41 42 45 46 48 49 63 65 67 71 73 **P**3 **S**2285 Alliant Health System	13	10	71	1685	34	48727	317	11581	5264	278
GREENWOOD—Johnson County										
☐ CPC VALLE VISTA HOSPITAL, 898 East Main Street, Zip 46143; tel. 317/887-1348 **A**1 9 10 **F**1 2 3 12 14 15 16 17 25 27 31 34 52 53 54 56 57 58 59 65 67 68 **P**7 **S**0785 Community Psychiatric Centers	33	22	96	635	68	2798	0	—	—	154
HAMMOND—Lake County										
★ SAINT MARGARET MERCY HEALTHCARE CENTERS, (Includes Saint Margaret Mercy Healthcare Centers–North Campus, Hammond, Indiana; Saint Margaret Mercy Healthcare Centers–South Campus, 24 Joliet Street, Dyer, Indiana, Zip 46311-1799; tel. 219/865-2141) 5454 Hohman Avenue, Zip 46320; tel. 219/933-2074; Gene Diamond, President and Chief Executive Officer (Total facility includes 20 beds in nursing home–type unit) **A**1 2 3 9 10 **F**2 3 4 7 8 10 11 12 13 14 15 16 17 19 20 21 22 27 28 29 30 32 34 35 36 37 38 39 40 42 43 44 45 46 48 49 51 52 53 54 55 56 57 58 59 60 64 65 67 71 73 74 **P**8 **S**5345 Sisters of St. Francis Health Services, Inc.	21	10	592	21269	365	579300	1677	162513	70280	2263
HARTFORD CITY—Blackford County										
★ BLACKFORD COUNTY HOSPITAL, 503 East Van Cleve Street, Zip 47348; tel. 317/348-0300; Mark A. Edwards, Chief Executive Officer **A**1 10 **F**3 8 12 14 16 19 20 21 22 28 32 34 37 40 41 44 49 65 71 **P**3 6 **S**2285 Alliant Health System	13	10	36	1240	14	17414	88	6052	2683	119
HOBART—Lake County										
☐ CHARTER BEHAVIORAL HEALTH SYSTEM OF NORTHWEST INDIANA, (Formerly Charter Hospital of Northwest Indiana) 101 West 61st Avenue & State Road 51, Zip 46342; tel. 219/947-4464; Barry W. Woodward, Chief Executive Officer (Nonreporting) **A**1 10 **S**0695 Charter Medical Corporation	33	22	60	—	—	—	—	—	—	—
★ ST. MARY MEDICAL CENTER, 1500 South Lake Park Avenue, Zip 46342; tel. 219/947-6000; Joseph M. Mark, President and Chief Executive Officer (Nonreporting) **A**1 10 **S**0135 Ancilla Systems Inc.	21	10	179	—	—	—	—	—	—	—
HUNTINGBURG—Dubois County										
☐ ST. JOSEPH'S HOSPITAL, 1900 Medical Arts Drive, Zip 47542-9521, Mailing Address: P.O. Box 148, Zip 47542-0148; tel. 812/683-2121; Dale R. Mulder, President and Chief Executive Officer (Nonreporting) **A**1 10	23	10	76	—	—	—	—	—	—	—
HUNTINGTON—Huntington County										
★ HUNTINGTON MEMORIAL HOSPITAL, 1215 Etna Avenue, Zip 46750-3696; tel. 219/356-3000; L. Kent McCoy, President (Nonreporting) **A**1 9 10	23	10	68	—	—	—	—	—	—	—
INDIANAPOLIS—Marion County										
★ CHARTER INDIANAPOLIS BEHAVIORAL HEALTH SYSTEM, (Formerly Charter Hospital of Indianapolis) 5602 Caito Drive, Zip 46226; tel. 317/545-2111; Daniel J. Body, Chief Executive Officer **A**1 9 10 **F**2 3 14 15 16 52 53 54 55 56 58 59 65 **S**0695 Charter Medical Corporation	33	22	60	1159	30	0	0	—	—	—
☐ △ COMMUNITY HOSPITALS OF INDIANAPOLIS, (Includes Community Hospital South, 1402 East County Line Road South, Indianapolis, Indiana, Zip 46227; tel. 317/887-7000) 1500 North Ritter Avenue, Zip 46219-3095; tel. 317/355-1411; William E. Corley, President (Nonreporting) **A**1 2 3 5 7 9 10	23	10	822	—	—	—	—	—	—	—
★ FAIRBANKS HOSPITAL, 8102 Clearvista Parkway, Zip 46256-4698; tel. 317/849-8222; Timothy L. Boruff, Administrator (Nonreporting) **A**9 10	23	82	86	—	—	—	—	—	—	—
★ HAWLEY U.S. ARMY COMMUNITY HOSPITAL, Fort Benjamin Harrison, Zip 46216-7000; tel. 317/549-5153; Charles H. Lewis, Deputy Commander Administration (Nonreporting) **S**9395 Department of the Army	42	10	20	—	—	—	—	—	—	—
★ INDIANA UNIVERSITY MEDICAL CENTER, (Includes Riley University Hospital and Outpatient Center, Indianapolis, Indiana; University Hospital and Outpatient Center, Indianapolis, Indiana) 550 North University Boulevard, Zip 46202-5262; tel. 317/274-5000; David J. Handel, Director **A**1 3 5 8 9 10 **F**4 5 7 8 9 10 11 12 13 14 15 16 17 19 20 21 22 23 30 31 32 34 35 37 38 39 40 41 42 43 44 46 47 49 50 51 52 53 54 55 56 57 58 60 61 63 65 69 70 71 73 74	12	10	611	20838	436	339419	1215	315301	128889	4177
☐ LARUE D. CARTER MEMORIAL HOSPITAL, 1315 West Tenth Street, Zip 46202; tel. 317/634-8401; Diana Haugh MS, Superintendent **A**1 3 5 9 10 **F**14 29 30 34 41 45 46 52 53 55 57 58 65 67 73 **P**1	12	22	146	232	97	3906	0	14854	7075	371

Hospitals, U.S. / INDIANA

Hospital, Address, Telephone, Administrator, Approval, Facility, and Physician Codes, Health Care System	Classification Codes		Utilization Data					Expense (thousands) of dollars		Personnel
★ American Hospital Association (AHA) membership ☐ Joint Commission on Accreditation of Healthcare Organizations (JCAHO) accreditation + American Osteopathic Hospital Association (AOHA) membership ○ American Osteopathic Association (AOA) accreditation △ Commission on Accreditation of Rehabilitation Facilities (CARF) accreditation Control codes 61, 63, 64, 71, 72 and 73 indicate hospitals listed by AOHA, but not registered by AHA. For definition of numerical codes, see page A6	Control	Service	Beds	Admissions	Census	Outpatient Visits	Births	Total	Payroll	
★ METHODIST HOSPITAL OF INDIANA, 1701 North Senate Boulevard, Zip 46202, Mailing Address: P.O. Box 1367, Zip 46206–1367; tel. 317/929–2000; William J. Loveday, President and Chief Executive Officer **A**1 2 3 5 8 9 10 **F**2 3 4 5 7 8 10 11 12 13 14 15 16 17 18 19 21 22 23 24 25 26 27 28 29 30 31 32 33 34 35 36 37 38 39 40 41 42 43 44 45 46 47 49 51 52 53 54 55 56 57 58 59 60 61 63 64 65 66 67 68 69 70 71 72 73 74 **P**5 6 7 8	23	10	923	41335	667	365593	3932	407460	188973	4984
★ △ REHABILITATION HOSPITAL OF INDIANA, 4141 Shore Drive, Zip 46254–2607; tel. 317/329–2000; Kim D. Eicher, Administrator and Chief Executive Officer (Nonreporting) **A**1 7	23	46	80	—		—		—	—	—
★ RICHARD L. ROUDEBUSH VETERANS AFFAIRS MEDICAL CENTER, 1481 West Tenth Street, Zip 46202; tel. 317/635–7401; (Total facility includes 58 beds in nursing home–type unit) **A**1 3 5 8 9 **F**1 2 3 4 5 6 8 10 11 12 14 15 16 17 19 20 21 22 23 24 26 27 28 29 30 31 32 33 34 35 37 39 41 42 43 44 45 46 48 49 50 51 52 54 55 56 57 58 59 60 61 63 64 65 67 69 71 72 73 74 **S**9295 Department of Veterans Affairs	45	10	354	7752	228	183679	0	137332	80124	2267
RILEY UNIVERSITY HOSPITAL AND OUTPATIENT CENTER See Indiana University Medical Center										
★ ST. VINCENT HOSPITAL AND HEALTH CARE CENTER, (Includes St. Vincent Carmel Hospital, 13500 North Meridian Street, Carmel, Indiana, Zip 46032; tel. 317/582–7000; St. Vincent Stress Center, 8401 Harcourt Road, Indianapolis, Indiana, Zip 46260, Mailing Address: P.O. Box 80160, Zip 46280; tel. 317/338–4600; Anita J. Harden, Administrator) 2001 West 86th Street, Zip 46260, Mailing Address: Box 40970, Zip 46240–0970; tel. 317/338–2345; Douglas D. French, President and Chief Executive Officer **A**1 2 3 5 9 10 **F**2 3 4 6 7 8 10 11 13 14 15 16 17 18 19 20 21 22 23 24 25 26 27 28 29 30 31 32 33 34 35 37 38 39 40 41 42 43 44 45 46 48 49 51 52 53 54 55 56 57 58 59 60 63 65 66 67 69 70 71 72 73 74 **P**5 6 8 **S**1855 Daughters of Charity National Health System	21	10	836	32226	548	485917	3945	368566	161754	4717
ST. VINCENT STRESS CENTER See St. Vincent Hospital and Health Care Center										
UNIVERSITY HOSPITAL AND OUTPATIENT CENTER See Indiana University Medical Center										
+ ○ WESTVIEW HOSPITAL, 3630 Guion Road, Zip 46222–1699; tel. 317/924–6661; David C. Dyar, President and Administrator (Nonreporting) **A**9 10 11 12	23	10	67	—		—		—	—	—
★ WILLIAM N. WISHARD MEMORIAL HOSPITAL, 1001 West 10th Street, Zip 46202–2879; tel. 317/630–7356; John F. Williams Jr. M.D., Director **A**1 3 5 8 9 10 **F**3 4 5 7 8 9 10 14 15 16 17 18 19 20 21 23 25 26 28 30 31 34 35 36 37 38 39 40 41 42 43 44 46 49 50 51 52 53 54 55 56 57 58 59 60 61 63 65 67 68 69 70 71 72 73 **P**6	15	10	328	14356	228	597675	2466	182986	76194	2833
☐ △ WINONA MEMORIAL HOSPITAL, 3232 North Meridian Street, Zip 46208–4693; tel. 317/924–3392; Keith R. King, Chief Executive Officer (Total facility includes 28 beds in nursing home–type unit) **A**1 7 10 **F**2 3 4 8 10 14 15 16 19 21 22 26 28 30 31 32 33 34 35 36 37 39 41 42 44 45 46 48 49 52 55 56 57 58 59 64 65 67 70 71 72 73 **P**1 5 6 7 **S**6525 Ornda Healthcorp	32	10	170	3252	86	43245	0	—	—	432
★ WOMEN'S HOSPITAL–INDIANAPOLIS, 8111 Township Line Road, Zip 46260–8043; tel. 317/875–5994; Steven B. Reed, President and Chief Executive Officer **A**1 9 10 **F**7 8 19 38 40 41 44 45 52 57 61 65 71 73 74 **S**0048 Columbia/HCA Healthcare Corporation	33	10	132	4249	43	18853	2559	22665	10634	389
JASPER—Dubois County										
★ MEMORIAL HOSPITAL AND HEALTH CARE CENTER, 800 West Ninth Street, Zip 47546–2516; tel. 812/482–2345; Sister M. Adrian Davis Ph.D., President and Chief Executive Officer (Total facility includes 24 beds in nursing home–type unit) **A**1 9 10 **F**7 8 10 11 14 15 16 18 19 21 22 26 28 29 30 32 33 34 35 37 39 40 41 42 44 45 49 51 52 53 54 55 56 57 60 63 64 65 66 67 71 73 **P**3 **S**2295 Little Company of Mary Sisters Healthcare System	21	10	122	4320	76	87696	491	31691	16420	514
JEFFERSONVILLE—Clark County										
★ △ CLARK MEMORIAL HOSPITAL, 1220 Missouri Avenue, Zip 47130–3743, Mailing Address: Box 69, Zip 47131–0069; tel. 812/282–6631; Merle E. Stepp, President (Total facility includes 52 beds in nursing home–type unit) **A**1 7 9 10 **F**7 8 10 17 19 21 22 28 29 30 31 32 33 34 35 37 40 41 42 44 45 46 48 49 52 53 54 55 56 57 59 60 63 64 65 71 73 **P**4 **S**0052 Jewish Hospital Healthcare Services	13	10	280	9297	202	85648	918	64814	30969	1088
KENDALLVILLE—Noble County										
★ MCCRAY MEMORIAL HOSPITAL, 951 East Hospital Drive, Zip 46755, Mailing Address: P.O. Box 249, Zip 46755; tel. 219/347–1100; John Berhow, Administrator **A**1 9 10 **F**7 14 15 17 19 20 21 22 24 25 26 27 28 30 32 33 35 37 39 40 41 42 44 46 49 52 56 57 63 65 67 71 72 73 **P**7	15	10	51	1881	25	359957	277	29653	16165	708
KNOX—Starke County										
★ STARKE MEMORIAL HOSPITAL, 102 East Culver Road, Zip 46534–2299; tel. 219/772–6231; Leonard W. Daugherty, Executive Director **A**1 10 **F**3 7 8 13 15 16 19 22 26 31 32 33 34 35 37 39 40 41 42 45 46 49 54 55 65 67 71 73 **P**3 **S**0002 Quorum Health Group/Quorum Health Resources	13	10	35	1437	12	32525	190	11470	5279	229
KOKOMO—Howard County										
★ HOWARD COMMUNITY HOSPITAL, 3500 South La Fountain Street, Zip 46904–9011; tel. 317/453–0702; James C. Bigogno, President (Total facility includes 27 beds in nursing home–type unit) **A**1 9 10 **F**7 8 10 14 15 16 19 21 22 23 26 29 30 32 34 35 37 39 40 42 44 45 49 51 52 53 54 55 56 57 58 59 60 64 65 67 68 71 73 74 **P**8	13	10	132	4673	72	223532	347	39865	18626	686

© 1995 AHA Guide

Hospitals, U.S. / INDIANA

Hospital, Address, Telephone, Administrator, Approval, Facility, and Physician Codes, Health Care System	Classification Codes		Utilization Data					Expense (thousands) of dollars		
★ American Hospital Association (AHA) membership □ Joint Commission on Accreditation of Healthcare Organizations (JCAHO) accreditation + American Osteopathic Hospital Association (AOHA) membership ○ American Osteopathic Association (AOA) accreditation △ Commission on Accreditation of Rehabilitation Facilities (CARF) accreditation Control codes 61, 63, 64, 71, 72 and 73 indicate hospitals listed by AOHA, but not registered by AHA. For definition of numerical codes, see page A6	Control	Service	Beds	Admissions	Census	Outpatient Visits	Births	Total	Payroll	Personnel
□ KOKOMO REHABILITATION HOSPITAL, 829 North Dixon Road, Zip 46901; tel. 317/452–6700; Jackie Hoelter, Interim Chief Executive Officer (Nonreporting) A1 10	33	46	60	—	—	—	—	—	—	—
★ SAINT JOSEPH HOSPITAL AND HEALTH CENTER, 1907 West Sycamore Street, Zip 46901–9010; tel. 317/452–5611; Sister M. Martin McEntee, President and Chief Executive Officer A1 9 10 F2 3 7 8 10 12 14 15 16 17 19 20 21 22 23 25 26 28 30 31 32 34 35 36 37 39 40 42 44 46 48 49 51 52 53 54 55 56 58 59 60 64 65 66 67 71 72 73 74 S1855 Daughters of Charity National Health System	21	10	160	6888	107	993071	1061	51161	23878	893
LA PORTE—La Porte County										
★ LA PORTE HOSPITAL, State and Madison Streets, Zip 46350–0250, Mailing Address: P.O. Box 250, Zip 46352–0250; tel. 219/326–1234; Leigh E. Morris, President (Total facility includes 55 beds in nursing home–type unit) A1 2 9 10 F3 7 8 10 14 15 16 17 19 20 21 22 23 26 27 28 29 30 31 32 33 34 35 36 37 39 40 41 42 44 45 46 48 49 52 53 54 55 56 57 58 59 61 64 65 66 67 71 73 P5	23	10	227	6397	135	53620	651	44531	20986	757
LAFAYETTE—Tippecanoe County										
□ CHARTER BEHAVIORAL HEALTH SYSTEMS, (Formerly Charter Hospital of Lafayette) 3700 Rome Drive, Zip 47905, Mailing Address: P.O. Box 5969, Zip 47903; tel. 317/448–6999; Stewart Graham, Administrator A1 10 F2 12 14 15 16 17 18 34 52 53 54 55 56 58 59 65 S0695 Charter Medical Corporation	33	22	64	933	28	0	0	—	—	67
★ LAFAYETTE HOME HOSPITAL, 2400 South Street, Zip 47904; tel. 317/447–6811; John R. Walling, President and Chief Executive Officer (Total facility includes 21 beds in nursing home–type unit) A1 9 10 F6 7 8 10 12 15 16 19 20 21 22 23 24 26 28 29 30 31 32 34 35 36 37 38 39 40 41 42 44 45 46 48 49 52 54 56 57 58 61 62 63 64 65 66 67 71 73 74	23	10	276	9667	148	81418	2116	71386	31695	1178
★ ST. ELIZABETH HOSPITAL MEDICAL CENTER, 1501 Hartford Street, Zip 47904–2126, Mailing Address: Box 7501, Zip 47903–7501; tel. 317/423–6011; Douglas W. Eberle, President and Chief Executive Officer (Total facility includes 24 beds in nursing home–type unit) A1 2 6 9 10 F4 7 8 10 11 14 15 16 17 19 21 22 25 26 31 32 33 34 35 37 39 40 41 42 44 45 49 56 57 60 63 64 65 66 67 71 73 74 S5345 Sisters of St. Francis Health Services, Inc.	21	10	212	6147	95	81672	429	73639	32747	1041
LAGRANGE—Vermillion County										
□ VENCOR HOSPITAL–LAGRANGE, 0300N 00EW Townline Road, Zip 46761; tel. 219/463–2143; Joseph A. Stuber, Administrator A1 9 10 F7 12 14 15 16 19 22 34 35 40 42 44 48 49 65 71 73 S0026 Vencor, Incorporated	33	10	62	1668	19	20763	432	—	—	140
LAWRENCEBURG—Dearborn County										
★ DEARBORN COUNTY HOSPITAL, 600 Wilson Creek Road, Zip 47025–1199; tel. 812/537–1010; Peter V. Resnick, Executive Director A1 9 10 F7 8 12 13 15 16 19 20 21 22 23 28 30 32 33 35 37 40 42 44 49 60 63 65 66 67 71 73 P3	13	10	76	2919	36	83423	298	22440	9785	335
LEBANON—Boone County										
□ WITHAM MEMORIAL HOSPITAL, 1124 North Lebanon Street, Zip 46052–1776, Mailing Address: P.O. Box 1200, Zip 46052–3005; tel. 317/482–2700; John B. Riekena, President and Chief Executive Officer (Nonreporting) A1 9 10	13	10	60	—	—	—	—	—	—	—
LINTON—Greene County										
★ GREENE COUNTY GENERAL HOSPITAL, Rural Route 1, Box 555, Zip 47441–9457; tel. 812/847–2281; Jonas S. Uland, Executive Director A1 9 10 F8 11 14 15 16 17 19 21 22 26 28 32 34 37 40 42 44 45 49 56 57 65 71 73 P3	13	10	76	1695	22	—	95	10084	3832	207
LOGANSPORT—Cass County										
□ LOGANSPORT STATE HOSPITAL, Rural Route 2, Box 38, Zip 46947–9699; tel. 219/722–4141; Jeffrey H. Smith Ph.D., Superintendent A1 9 F14 19 20 22 23 26 30 31 35 39 45 46 52 54 55 56 57 64 65 70 71 73	12	22	490	387	451	0	0	31013	19190	738
★ MEMORIAL HOSPITAL, 1101 Michigan Avenue, Zip 46947–1596, Mailing Address: P.O. Box 7013, Zip 46947–7013; tel. 219/753–7541; George W. Poor, President A1 9 10 F3 7 8 14 15 16 19 21 22 30 32 33 35 36 37 39 40 42 44 46 49 52 53 56 57 58 59 63 65 67 71 73 P3	13	10	104	3532	43	44226	554	25484	11503	435
MADISON—Jefferson County										
★ KING'S DAUGHTERS' HOSPITAL, One King's Daughters' Drive, Zip 47250, Mailing Address: Box 447, Zip 47250; tel. 812/265–5211; Roger J. Allman, Chief Executive Officer (Total facility includes 15 beds in nursing home–type unit) A1 9 10 F7 8 10 11 14 16 17 19 21 22 23 25 27 28 30 32 33 34 35 39 40 41 42 44 49 60 64 65 66 67 71 73	23	10	119	5131	90	40143	451	32975	15003	532
□ MADISON STATE HOSPITAL, 711 Green Road, Zip 47250; tel. 812/265–2611; Jerry Thaden, Superintendent A1 9 10 F2 15 20 52 53 57 65 73 P6	12	22	370	249	342	0	0	32379	12164	545
MARION—Grant County										
★ MARION GENERAL HOSPITAL, 441 North Wabash Avenue, Zip 46952–2690; tel. 317/662–1441; Albert C. Knauss, President and Chief Executive Officer (Total facility includes 21 beds in nursing home–type unit) A1 9 10 F7 8 10 11 15 16 19 21 22 28 30 32 33 34 35 37 39 40 41 42 44 46 49 64 65 66 67 71 73 74 P6	23	10	212	8635	108	177072	752	57537	27120	945
★ VETERANS AFFAIRS MEDICAL CENTER, East 38th Street, Zip 46953–4589; tel. 317/674–3321; Jon E. Crisman, Director (Nonreporting) A1 9 S9295 Department of Veterans Affairs	45	22	580	—	—	—	—	—	—	—
MARTINSVILLE—Morgan County										
★ MORGAN COUNTY MEMORIAL HOSPITAL, 2209 John R Wooden Drive, Zip 46151, Mailing Address: P.O. Box 1717, Zip 46151; tel. 317/342–8441; S. Dean Melton, Administrator A9 10 F7 8 10 15 16 19 21 22 28 29 30 32 34 35 36 37 39 40 41 42 44 45 49 51 65 71 73 P6 8	13	10	86	2054	31	77118	184	17583	7711	284

Hospitals, U.S. / INDIANA

Hospital, Address, Telephone, Administrator, Approval, Facility, and Physician Codes, Health Care System	Classification Codes		Utilization Data					Expense (thousands) of dollars		
★ American Hospital Association (AHA) membership ☐ Joint Commission on Accreditation of Healthcare Organizations (JCAHO) accreditation + American Osteopathic Hospital Association (AOHA) membership ○ American Osteopathic Association (AOA) accreditation △ Commission on Accreditation of Rehabilitation Facilities (CARF) accreditation Control codes 61, 63, 64, 71, 72 and 73 indicate hospitals listed by AOHA, but not registered by AHA. For definition of numerical codes, see page A6	Control	Service	Beds	Admissions	Census	Outpatient Visits	Births	Total	Payroll	Personnel
MERRILLVILLE—Lake County BROADWAY METHODIST HOSPITAL See Methodist Hospitals, Gary										
MICHIGAN CITY—La Porte County ☐ CHARTER BEHAVIORAL HEALTH SYSTEM OF MICHIGAN CITY, (Formerly Kingwood Hospital) 3714 South Franklin Street, Zip 46360; tel. 219/872–0531; Michael J. Brown, Administrator (Nonreporting) **A**1 10 **S**0695 Charter Medical Corporation KINGWOOD HOSPITAL See Charter Behavioral Health System of Michigan City	33	22	89	—	—	—	—	—	—	—
★ MEMORIAL HOSPITAL OF MICHIGAN CITY, 515 Pine Street, Zip 46360–3370; tel. 219/879–0202; Norman D. Steider, President **A**1 10 **F**2 3 4 7 8 12 15 16 17 18 19 20 21 22 24 28 29 30 31 33 34 35 36 37 39 40 41 42 44 45 46 48 49 60 63 65 66 67 68 71 73	23	10	102	1981	31	14616	233	19826	6983	231
★ △ SAINT ANTHONY HOSPITAL AND HEALTH CENTERS, 301 West Homer Street, Zip 46360–4358; tel. 219/879–8511; Edel Dunne–O'Toole, President and Chief Executive Officer **A**1 7 9 10 **F**7 8 10 12 13 14 15 16 17 19 21 22 23 25 26 28 29 30 32 33 34 35 36 37 39 40 41 42 44 45 46 48 49 51 60 63 64 65 67 68 71 73 74 **P**7 8 **S**5345 Sisters of St. Francis Health Services, Inc.	21	10	141	5659	86	83244	487	44596	17796	646
MISHAWAKA—St. Joseph County ★ ST. JOSEPH HOSPITAL, 215 West Fourth Street, Zip 46544; tel. 219/259–2431; Douglas L. Elwell, President and Chief Executive Officer **A**1 9 10 **F**3 4 7 8 10 12 13 14 15 16 17 18 19 21 22 23 25 26 28 29 30 32 33 34 35 37 39 40 41 42 44 45 46 49 51 52 53 54 55 56 57 58 59 61 63 64 65 66 67 68 71 73 **P**1 2 3 5 6 7 **S**0135 Ancilla Systems Inc.	21	10	117	4248	65	49371	714	38149	15851	375
MONTICELLO—White County ★ WHITE COUNTY MEMORIAL HOSPITAL, 1101 O'Connor Boulevard, Zip 47960; tel. 219/583–7111; John M. Avers, Chief Executive Officer **A**1 9 10 **F**8 11 14 15 16 17 19 21 22 26 28 29 30 31 34 35 37 39 40 42 44 45 46 51 65 67 71 73 **P**6	15	10	59	1584	18	39371	131	9662	4121	170
MOORESVILLE—Morgan County ☐ KENDRICK MEMORIAL HOSPITAL, 1201 Hadley Road N.W., Zip 46158–1789; tel. 317/831–1160; Charles D. Swisher, Director (Nonreporting) **A**1 9 10	23	10	60	—	—	—	—	—	—	—
MUNCIE—Delaware County ★ △ BALL MEMORIAL HOSPITAL, 2401 University Avenue, Zip 47303–3499; tel. 317/747–3111; Robert T. Brodhead, President and Chief Executive Officer (Total facility includes 30 beds in nursing home–type unit) **A**1 3 5 7 9 10 **F**2 4 7 8 10 11 14 15 16 17 19 20 21 22 23 24 28 30 31 32 33 34 35 36 37 38 39 40 42 43 44 45 46 48 49 52 54 55 56 57 60 63 64 65 71 73 **P**6	23	10	438	17498	286	157861	1821	126888	57307	2072
MUNSTER—Lake County ☐ COMMUNITY HOSPITAL, 901 MacArthur Boulevard, Zip 46321–2959; tel. 219/836–1600; Edward P. Robinson, Administrator (Nonreporting) **A**1 2 9 10	23	10	292	—	—	—	—	—	—	—
NEW ALBANY—Floyd County ★ FLOYD MEMORIAL HOSPITAL AND HEALTHCARE SERVICES, 1850 State Street, Zip 47150; tel. 812/949–5500; Bryant R. Hanson, President **A**1 2 9 10 **F**7 8 10 11 12 14 15 19 21 22 23 32 35 37 39 40 41 42 44 46 49 60 64 65 67 70 71 72 73 74 **P**1	13	10	213	8745	132	96038	835	60233	28789	884
NEW CASTLE—Henry County ★ HENRY COUNTY MEMORIAL HOSPITAL, 1000 North 16th Street, Zip 47362–4319, Mailing Address: Box 490, Zip 47362–0490; tel. 317/521–0890; Jack Basler, President **A**1 9 10 **F**7 8 15 16 17 19 21 22 31 34 35 37 40 42 44 46 65 71 73 **P**8	13	10	107	3306	40	47963	346	25028	10999	549
NOBLESVILLE—Hamilton County ★ RIVERVIEW HOSPITAL, 395 Westfield Road, Zip 46060–1425, Mailing Address: P.O. Box 220, Zip 46060–0220; tel. 317/773–0760; Seward Horner, President **A**1 9 10 **F**4 7 8 10 12 17 19 22 27 28 30 32 34 35 36 37 40 42 44 46 48 49 56 60 61 63 65 66 67 71 73 74 **P**6 7 8	13	10	111	4361	54	114000	684	42867	19374	667
NORTH VERNON—Jennings County ★ JENNINGS COMMUNITY HOSPITAL, 301 Henry Street, Zip 47265; tel. 812/346–6200; Todd L. Stallings, Chief Executive Officer (Nonreporting) **A**10 **S**2285 Alliant Health System	23	10	48	—	—	—	—	—	—	—
OAKLAND CITY—Gibson County ★ + WIRTH OSTEOPATHIC HOSPITAL, Highway 64 West, Zip 47660–9379, Mailing Address: Rural Route 3, Box 14A, Zip 47660–9379; tel. 812/749–6111; James A. Schindler, Administrator **A**10 **F**15 20 22 40 44 71 **S**0585 Brim, Inc.	23	10	11	541	7	13615	18	2921	1371	77
PAOLI—Orange County ★ ORANGE COUNTY HOSPITAL, 642 West Hospital Road, Zip 47454; tel. 812/723–2811; James W. Pope, Chief Executive Officer **A**9 10 **F**7 8 11 16 17 19 22 28 29 30 32 34 37 40 41 44 49 67 71 73	13	10	37	1092	11	26020	146	6871	3499	149
PERU—Miami County ★ DUKES MEMORIAL HOSPITAL, Grant and Boulevard, Zip 46970–1698; tel. 317/473–6621; R. Joe Johnston, President and Chief Executive Officer (Total facility includes 35 beds in nursing home–type unit) **A**1 9 10 **F**7 8 11 14 15 16 17 19 21 22 24 26 28 30 31 32 33 34 35 36 39 40 41 42 44 45 46 49 63 64 65 67 68 71 73 **P**6	15	10	105	1949	51	34933	354	15430	6862	280
PLYMOUTH—Marshall County ☐ KOALA HOSPITAL AND COUNSELING CENTER, 1800 North Oak Road, Zip 46563; tel. 219/936–3784; Wayne T. Miller, Administrator (Nonreporting) **A**1 10 **S**0044 Sterling Healthcare Corporation	33	22	80	—	—	—	—	—	—	—

Hospitals, U.S. / INDIANA

Hospital, Address, Telephone, Administrator, Approval, Facility, and Physician Codes, Health Care System	Classification Codes		Utilization Data					Expense (thousands) of dollars		
★ American Hospital Association (AHA) membership □ Joint Commission on Accreditation of Healthcare Organizations (JCAHO) accreditation + American Osteopathic Hospital Association (AOHA) membership ○ American Osteopathic Association (AOA) accreditation △ Commission on Accreditation of Rehabilitation Facilities (CARF) accreditation Control codes 61, 63, 64, 71, 72 and 73 indicate hospitals listed by AOHA, but not registered by AHA. For definition of numerical codes, see page A6	Control	Service	Beds	Admissions	Census	Outpatient Visits	Births	Total	Payroll	Personnel
★ ST. JOSEPH'S HOSPITAL OF MARSHALL COUNTY, 1915 Lake Avenue, Zip 46563–9905, Mailing Address: P.O. Box 670, Zip 46563–9905; tel. 219/936–3181; Brian E. Dietz, President **A**1 10 **F**1 4 6 7 8 10 12 14 15 16 19 21 22 23 24 26 27 28 31 33 35 36 37 40 41 42 43 44 47 48 49 60 64 65 70 71 73 74 **P**7 8 **S**5585 Holy Cross Health System Corporation	21	10	58	1694	17	27379	232	13705	4534	185
PORTLAND—Jay County ★ JAY COUNTY HOSPITAL, 500 West Votaw Street, Zip 47371–1322; tel. 219/726–7131; Thomas J. Valerius, Chief Executive Officer **A**1 10 **F**7 8 11 15 17 19 21 22 28 30 32 34 35 37 39 40 44 46 48 49 65 67 71 73 74 **P**8 **S**2285 Alliant Health System	13	10	55	1733	18	24940	183	9036	3428	142
PRINCETON—Gibson County ★ GIBSON GENERAL HOSPITAL, 1808 Sherman Drive, Zip 47670–1000; tel. 812/385–3401; Michael J. Budnick, Administrator and Chief Executive Officer (Total facility includes 45 beds in nursing home–type unit) **A**1 9 10 **F**3 7 8 14 17 19 21 22 26 28 29 30 31 34 37 40 42 45 48 49 52 53 54 55 56 57 58 59 60 64 65 67 71 73 **P**3 **S**2285 Alliant Health System	23	10	109	1812	62	25200	181	10779	4773	213
RENSSELAER—Jasper County ★ JASPER COUNTY HOSPITAL, 1104 East Grace Street, Zip 47978–3296; tel. 219/866–5141; Timothy M. Schreeg, President and Chief Executive Officer (Total facility includes 21 beds in nursing home–type unit) **A**9 10 **F**7 8 14 17 19 20 21 22 23 26 27 28 29 30 31 32 33 34 35 36 37 39 40 41 42 44 45 46 49 53 54 55 56 57 58 59 65 66 67 71 73 **P**6	13	10	69	1871	44	41519	168	12554	6195	264
RICHMOND—Wayne County ★ REID HOSPITAL AND HEALTH CARE SERVICES, 1401 Chester Boulevard, Zip 47374; tel. 317/983–3000; Barry S. MacDowell, President **A**1 2 9 10 **F**2 3 4 8 10 11 14 19 21 22 23 32 33 35 36 37 40 41 42 44 46 49 50 52 53 58 65 67 71 73	23	10	257	10593	144	111722	932	68627	30465	987
□ RICHMOND STATE HOSPITAL, 498 Northwest 18th Street, Zip 47374–2898; tel. 317/966–0511; Gene Darby, Superintendent (Nonreporting) **A**1 10	12	22	410	—	—	—	—	—	—	—
ROCHESTER—Fulton County ★ WOODLAWN HOSPITAL, 1400 East Ninth Street, Zip 46975–8937; tel. 219/223–3141; Michael L. Gordon, President (Nonreporting) **A**9 10	13	10	49	—	—	—	—	—	—	—
RUSHVILLE—Rush County ★ RUSH MEMORIAL HOSPITAL, 1300 North Main Street, Zip 46173–1198; tel. 317/932–4111; H. William Hartley, Chief Executive Officer **A**9 10 **F**8 19 22 30 32 34 35 37 39 42 44 49 51 71 **S**2285 Alliant Health System	13	10	52	813	23	42452	0	7434	3424	156
SALEM—Washington County ★ WASHINGTON COUNTY MEMORIAL HOSPITAL, 911 North Shelby Street, Zip 47167; tel. 812/883–5881; Rodney M. Coats, Executive Director (Nonreporting) **A**1 9 10 **S**0052 Jewish Hospital Healthcare Services	13	10	70	—	—	—	—	—	—	—
SCOTTSBURG—Scott County ★ SCOTT MEMORIAL HOSPITAL, 1415 North Gardner Street, Zip 47170–0456, Mailing Address: Box 456, Zip 47170–0456; tel. 812/752–8500; Clifford D. Nay, Administrator **A**1 9 10 **F**7 8 16 17 19 21 22 28 30 32 33 34 37 40 42 44 65 67 71 **S**0052 Jewish Hospital Healthcare Services	13	10	40	1081	12	14043	67	8239	—	129
SEYMOUR—Jackson County ★ MEMORIAL HOSPITAL, 411 West Tipton Street, Zip 47274–5000, Mailing Address: P.O. Box 2349, Zip 47274–0490; tel. 812/522–2349; George H. James Jr., Administrator and Chief Executive Officer **A**1 2 9 10 **F**7 8 14 15 16 19 21 22 23 28 30 32 33 34 35 36 37 40 42 44 45 46 49 63 65 67 71 73	13	10	107	4376	52	105016	676	29274	12342	474
SHELBYVILLE—Shelby County ★ MAJOR HOSPITAL, 150 West Washington Street, Zip 46176–1236, Mailing Address: Box 10, Zip 46176–0010; tel. 317/392–3211; Anthony B. Lennen, President and Chief Executive Officer **A**1 9 10 **F**7 12 14 17 19 21 22 28 29 34 36 37 39 40 41 42 44 45 49 63 66 71 73	15	10	59	2385	30	37371	251	16980	7401	256
SOUTH BEND—St. Joseph County ★ HEALTHWIN HOSPITAL, 20531 Darden Road, Zip 46637, Mailing Address: P.O. Box 4136, Zip 46634–4136; tel. 219/272–0100; Michael Roman, Chief Executive Officer (Total facility includes 131 beds in nursing home–type unit) **A**9 10 **F**12 20 26 34 48 49 64 65 67 73	23	48	163	149	134	3263	0	—	—	257
★ △ MEMORIAL HOSPITAL OF SOUTH BEND, 615 North Michigan Street, Zip 46601–9986; tel. 219/234–9041; Philip A. Newbold, President and Chief Executive Officer **A**1 2 3 5 7 9 10 **F**2 3 4 7 8 10 11 13 14 15 16 17 18 19 20 21 22 23 24 26 27 28 29 30 31 34 35 37 38 39 40 41 42 43 44 46 47 48 49 50 52 53 54 55 56 57 58 59 60 61 63 65 66 67 70 71 72 73 74 **P**1 6	23	10	351	13487	217	90268	2291	138920	55831	1699
+ ○ MICHIANA COMMUNITY HOSPITAL, 2515 East Jefferson Boulevard, Zip 46615–2691; tel. 219/288–8311; Stephen Crain, President **A**9 10 11 12 13 **F**7 8 10 11 14 15 16 19 22 25 28 29 30 31 34 35 37 40 41 42 44 45 46 48 52 54 56 58 59 63 64 65 71 73 **P**1 3 6 7 **S**0135 Ancilla Systems Inc.	23	10	90	2956	39	56517	652	24129	10933	330
★ △ ST. JOSEPH'S MEDICAL CENTER, 801 East LaSalle, Zip 46617, Mailing Address: Box 1935, Zip 46634; tel. 219/237–7111; Dennis W. Heck, Chief Executive Officer **A**1 2 3 5 7 9 10 **F**1 4 6 7 8 10 11 12 13 14 15 16 17 19 21 22 23 24 26 28 29 30 32 33 34 35 36 37 39 40 41 42 43 44 45 47 48 49 51 60 61 62 65 66 67 68 71 72 73 74 **P**5 7 8 **S**5585 Holy Cross Health System Corporation	21	10	297	11791	191	116231	1017	129521	43033	1393

Hospitals, U.S. / INDIANA

Hospital, Address, Telephone, Administrator, Approval, Facility, and Physician Codes, Health Care System	Classification Codes		Utilization Data					Expense (thousands) of dollars		
* American Hospital Association (AHA) membership □ Joint Commission on Accreditation of Healthcare Organizations (JCAHO) accreditation + American Osteopathic Hospital Association (AOHA) membership ○ American Osteopathic Association (AOA) accreditation △ Commission on Accreditation of Rehabilitation Facilities (CARF) accreditation Control codes 61, 63, 64, 71, 72 and 73 indicate hospitals listed by AOHA, but not registered by AHA. For definition of numerical codes, see page A6	Control	Service	Beds	Admissions	Census	Outpatient Visits	Births	Total	Payroll	Personnel
SULLIVAN—Sullivan County ★ MARY SHERMAN HOSPITAL, 320 North Section Street, Zip 47882, Mailing Address: P.O. Box 10, Zip 47882-0010; tel. 812/268-4311; Thomas J. Hudgins, Administrator **A**1 9 10 **F**8 12 13 14 15 16 17 18 19 20 21 22 26 28 29 30 31 37 39 40 41 42 44 45 46 49 53 54 55 56 57 58 65 66 67 68 71 73 74 **S**0002 Quorum Health Group/Quorum Health Resources	13	10	53	1700	21	31888	103	8531	3440	159
TELL CITY—Perry County ★ PERRY COUNTY MEMORIAL HOSPITAL, 1 Hospital Road, Zip 47586-0362; tel. 812/547-7011; Bradford W. Dykes, Administrator **A**1 9 10 **F**2 8 14 15 16 17 19 22 25 26 28 29 30 32 33 34 35 37 39 40 42 44 45 46 49 54 56 58 61 65 67 71 73 **S**2285 Alliant Health System	13	10	38	1113	13	46275	91	8493	3764	170
TERRE HAUTE—Vigo County HAMILTON CENTER, 620 Eighth Avenue, Zip 47804-0323; tel. 812/231-8323; Galen Goode, Administrator **A**9 10 **F**2 3 12 13 14 15 16 17 18 52 53 54 55 56 57 58 59 65	23	22	45	491	15	0	0	—	—	435
★ TERRE HAUTE REGIONAL HOSPITAL, 3901 South Seventh Street, Zip 47802-4299; tel. 812/232-0021; Jerry Dooley, Chief Executive Officer (Total facility includes 25 beds in nursing home–type unit) **A**1 10 **F**2 3 4 7 8 10 11 12 14 16 19 21 22 24 26 28 29 30 31 32 34 35 36 37 38 39 40 41 42 43 44 45 48 49 50 51 52 54 55 56 57 58 60 61 63 64 66 67 71 72 73 74 **P**8 **S**0048 Columbia/HCA Healthcare Corporation	33	10	236	6449	110	59888	799	42212	15359	661
★ △ UNION HOSPITAL, 1606 North Seventh Street, Zip 47804-2780; tel. 812/238-7000; Frank Shelton, President **A**1 2 3 5 7 9 10 **F**4 7 8 10 11 14 15 16 17 19 20 21 22 23 24 25 28 29 30 31 32 33 34 35 37 38 39 40 41 42 43 44 45 46 48 49 51 53 56 58 59 60 61 64 65 66 67 71 72 73 **P**5 6	23	10	298	12418	217	227285	1698	111726	49477	1709
TIPTON—Tipton County ★ TIPTON COUNTY MEMORIAL HOSPITAL, 1000 South Main Street, Zip 46072-9799; tel. 317/675-8500; Alfonso W. Gatmaitan, Chief Executive Officer (Total facility includes 39 beds in nursing home–type unit) **A**1 9 10 **F**7 8 12 19 21 22 26 28 30 32 35 36 37 39 40 41 42 44 46 49 50 63 64 65 66 71 73 74 **P**3 8	13	10	89	3175	53	33696	154	14702	7082	282
VALPARAISO—Porter County ★ PORTER MEMORIAL HOSPITAL, 814 La Porte Avenue, Zip 46383-5898; tel. 219/465-4600; Wiley N. Carr, President and Chief Executive Officer **A**1 9 10 **F**4 7 8 10 14 16 18 19 20 21 22 23 28 34 35 37 38 40 41 42 43 44 45 49 53 58 60 63 65 70 71 72 73 **P**8	13	10	360	12226	199	266064	1184	96225	41799	1416
VINCENNES—Knox County ★ GOOD SAMARITAN HOSPITAL, 520 South Seventh Street, Zip 47591-1098; tel. 812/882-5220; A. John Hidde, President and Chief Executive Officer (Total facility includes 26 beds in nursing home–type unit) **A**1 2 9 10 **F**3 4 7 8 10 11 13 15 19 20 21 22 23 24 28 29 30 33 34 35 37 39 40 41 42 43 44 45 52 53 54 55 56 57 58 59 60 63 64 65 67 69 71 73	13	10	254	8932	140	111333	459	69676	31949	1291
WABASH—Wabash County ★ WABASH COUNTY HOSPITAL, 710 North East Street, Zip 46992, Mailing Address: Box 548, Zip 46992-0548; tel. 219/563-3131; Jerome H. Horn CPA, Executive Director (Nonreporting) **A**1 2 9 10	13	10	94	—	—	—	—	—	—	—
WARSAW—Kosciusko County ★ KOSCIUSKO COMMUNITY HOSPITAL, 2101 East Dubois Drive, Zip 46580; tel. 219/267-3200; Wayne Hendrix, President (Total facility includes 64 beds in nursing home–type unit) **A**1 9 10 **F**2 3 7 8 12 13 14 15 16 19 22 26 32 33 35 37 40 41 42 44 45 46 49 52 64 65 66 67 71 73 **P**6 8	23	10	161	3570	113	34144	654	27879	11524	402
WASHINGTON—Daviess County ★ DAVIESS COUNTY HOSPITAL, 1314 Grand Avenue, Zip 47501-2198, Mailing Address: P.O. Box 760, Zip 47501-0760; tel. 812/254-2760; Marc Chircop, Chief Executive Officer (Total facility includes 29 beds in nursing home–type unit) **A**1 9 10 **F**7 8 11 12 15 16 17 19 21 22 32 34 35 36 37 39 40 41 42 44 45 49 53 55 56 57 58 63 64 65 66 67 71 73 **P**3 7 **S**0002 Quorum Health Group/Quorum Health Resources	13	10	85	2716	51	34851	398	16092	7240	320
WEST LAFAYETTE—Tippecanoe County ★ WABASH VALLEY HOSPITAL, 2900 North River Road, Zip 47906-3766; tel. 317/463-2555; R. Craig Lysinger, Administrator (Nonreporting) **A**9 10	23	22	70	—	—	—	—	—	—	—
WILLIAMSPORT—Warren County ★ COMMUNITY HOSPITAL, 412 North Monroe Street, Zip 47993-0215; tel. 317/762-2496; Jane Craigin, Chief Executive Officer (Nonreporting) **A**9 10 **S**2285 Alliant Health System	23	10	35	—	—	—	—	—	—	—
WINAMAC—Pulaski County ★ PULASKI MEMORIAL HOSPITAL, 616 East 13th Street, Zip 46996-1117; tel. 219/946-6131; Richard H. Mynark, Administrator **A**1 9 10 **F**7 8 14 15 17 19 20 22 26 29 30 32 35 37 39 40 41 42 44 45 49 58 65 67 71 73	15	10	52	1138	14	14320	164	9122	4173	187
WINCHESTER—Randolph County ★ RANDOLPH COUNTY HOSPITAL, 325 South Oak Street, Zip 47394, Mailing Address: P.O. Box 407, Zip 47394; tel. 317/584-9001; James M. Full, Chief Executive Officer **A**9 10 **F**7 8 13 15 16 17 19 22 28 30 32 34 37 40 41 42 44 46 49 65 66 71 73 **P**3 **S**2285 Alliant Health System	13	10	27	926	10	19928	85	7014	2516	118

© 1995 AHA Guide

Hospitals, U.S. / IOWA

IOWA

Resident population 2,814 (in thousands)
Resident population in metro areas 43.8%
Birth rate per 1,000 population 13.9
65 years and over 15.5%
Percent of persons without health insurance 9.0%

Hospital, Address, Telephone, Administrator, Approval, Facility, and Physician Codes, Health Care System	Classification Codes		Utilization Data					Expense (thousands) of dollars		
	Control	Service	Beds	Admissions	Census	Outpatient Visits	Births	Total	Payroll	Personnel

★ American Hospital Association (AHA) membership
☐ Joint Commission on Accreditation of Healthcare Organizations (JCAHO) accreditation
+ American Osteopathic Hospital Association (AOHA) membership
○ American Osteopathic Association (AOA) accreditation
△ Commission on Accreditation of Rehabilitation Facilities (CARF) accreditation
Control codes 61, 63, 64, 71, 72 and 73 indicate hospitals listed by AOHA, but not registered by AHA. For definition of numerical codes, see page A6

Hospital	Control	Service	Beds	Admissions	Census	Outpatient Visits	Births	Total	Payroll	Personnel
ALBIA—Monroe County MONROE COUNTY HOSPITAL, RFD 3, Zip 52531; tel. 515/932–2134; Gregory A. Paris, Administrator **A**9 10 **F**15 16 19 22 28 30 32 33 34 35 36 44 49 67 71 **P**3 5	13	10	46	388	21	28056	0	4368	2064	97
ALGONA—Kossuth County ★ KOSSUTH COUNTY HOSPITAL, 1515 South Phillips Street, Zip 50511; tel. 515/295–2451; James G. Fitzpatrick, Administrator **A**9 10 **F**8 12 14 15 16 17 19 22 26 28 30 31 32 33 34 35 36 37 39 40 41 42 44 45 48 49 58 64 65 66 67 71 73 **P**6 **S**5165 Mercy Health Services	13	10	29	706	10	13409	84	4840	1924	76
AMES—Story County ✠ MARY GREELEY MEDICAL CENTER, 111 Duff Avenue, Zip 50010; tel. 515/239–2011; Kimberly A. Russel, President and Chief Executive Officer (Total facility includes 20 beds in nursing home–type unit) **A**1 2 9 10 **F**7 8 10 14 17 18 19 21 22 26 28 30 31 32 33 34 35 36 37 38 39 40 41 42 44 45 48 49 52 53 54 55 56 57 58 59 60 61 63 64 65 66 67 71 73	14	10	216	8649	131	32616	993	54573	25308	908
ANAMOSA—Jones County ✠ ANAMOSA COMMUNITY HOSPITAL, 104 Broadway Place, Zip 52205; tel. 319/462–6131; Julie May, Administrator **A**1 9 10 **F**1 7 14 15 16 17 19 22 28 30 32 33 34 40 44 49 65 73 **P**5 **S**0061 Iowa Health System	23	10	24	519	8	13241	40	2933	1154	79
ATLANTIC—Cass County ✠ CASS COUNTY MEMORIAL HOSPITAL, 1501 East Tenth Street, Zip 50022–1997; tel. 712/243–3250; Patricia Markham, Administrator (Total facility includes 10 beds in nursing home–type unit) **A**1 9 10 **F**1 7 21 22 28 32 33 34 35 36 37 40 41 42 44 52 53 56 57 58 59 64 65 71 **P**8	13	10	71	1564	27	28807	215	10672	5368	227
AUDUBON—Audubon County AUDUBON COUNTY MEMORIAL HOSPITAL, 515 Pacific Street, Zip 50025–1099; tel. 712/563–2611; Rebecca L. Cooper, Administrator **A**9 10 **F**8 14 15 19 21 22 28 30 33 34 35 40 42 44 49 63 71 **P**3	13	10	29	543	6	13452	38	3010	1323	56
BELMOND—Wright County ★ BELMOND COMMUNITY HOSPITAL, 403 First Street S.E., Zip 50421–0326, Mailing Address: P.O. Box 326, Zip 50421; tel. 515/444–3223; Douglas E. Morse, Interim Administrator **A**9 10 **F**3 8 14 16 17 19 22 28 30 31 32 36 39 44 48 49 53 54 55 58 71 73 **P**1 2 3 4 5 6 7 8 **S**5165 Mercy Health Services	14	10	22	325	5	6072	0	2163	1038	48
BLOOMFIELD—Davis County DAVIS COUNTY HOSPITAL, 507 North Madison Street, Zip 52537–1299; tel. 515/664–2145; Wallace Simmons, Administrator (Total facility includes 32 beds in nursing home–type unit) **A**9 10 **F**3 7 8 13 15 16 19 20 22 24 28 30 31 32 33 34 35 36 37 39 40 42 44 45 49 53 54 55 56 58 65 71 73	13	10	80	1123	46	10896	72	7064	3225	167
BOONE—Boone County ✠ BOONE COUNTY HOSPITAL, 1015 Union Street, Zip 50036–4898; tel. 515/432–3140; Joseph S. Smith, Chief Executive Officer **A**1 9 10 **F**7 8 11 14 19 22 24 28 30 32 34 35 36 39 40 44 46 49 71 73 **P**3 **S**0002 Quorum Health Group/Quorum Health Resources	13	10	57	1529	26	9684	135	12664	5330	210
BRITT—Hancock County ★ HANCOCK COUNTY MEMORIAL HOSPITAL, 531 Second Street N.W., Zip 50423, Mailing Address: Box 68, Zip 50423–0068; tel. 515/843–3801; Lawrence N. Crail, Administrator **A**9 10 **F**1 7 8 14 15 17 20 22 27 30 33 34 36 40 41 44 46 65 67 71 **P**6 **S**5165 Mercy Health Services	13	10	30	553	8	12314	27	3164	1508	58
BURLINGTON—Des Moines County ✠ BURLINGTON MEDICAL CENTER, (Includes Burlington Medical Center–Klein Unit, 2910 Madison Road, Burlington, Iowa, Zip 52601; tel. 319/752–5461; Richard Miller, Administrator) 602 North Third Street, Zip 52601–5088; tel. 319/753–3011; Glen L. Heagle, President and Chief Executive Officer (Total facility includes 159 beds in nursing home–type unit) **A**1 9 10 **F**2 3 4 8 10 12 13 14 15 16 17 18 19 21 22 23 24 28 29 30 31 32 33 35 36 37 39 40 41 42 44 45 46 48 49 52 53 54 55 56 57 58 60 63 64 65 66 67 71 73	23	10	388	7089	248	86130	731	50719	22175	671
CARROLL—Carroll County ✠ ST. ANTHONY REGIONAL HOSPITAL, South Clark Street, Zip 51401; tel. 712/792–8231; Gary P. Riedmann, President and Chief Executive Officer (Total facility includes 79 beds in nursing home–type unit) **A**1 9 10 **F**7 8 12 14 15 16 17 19 20 21 22 26 28 29 30 31 32 33 34 37 39 40 41 42 44 45 46 49 51 52 53 54 55 56 57 58 59 60 62 64 65 66 67 68 71 73 **P**5	21	10	142	2242	108	35026	234	13824	6330	236
CEDAR FALLS—Black Hawk County ✠ SARTORI MEMORIAL HOSPITAL, 515 College Street, Zip 50613–2599; tel. 319/266–3584; Verna M. Klinkenborg, President (Total facility includes 18 beds in nursing home–type unit) **A** 9 10 **F**8 12 15 17 19 20 22 24 30 32 33 34 36 37 39 41 44 49 51 64 65 66 67 71 73	14	10	101	1743	24	71595	0	17383	7577	241

Hospitals, U.S. / IOWA

Hospital, Address, Telephone, Administrator, Approval, Facility, and Physician Codes, Health Care System	Classification Codes		Utilization Data					Expense (thousands) of dollars		Personnel
	Control	Service	Beds	Admissions	Census	Outpatient Visits	Births	Total	Payroll	

★ American Hospital Association (AHA) membership
☐ Joint Commission on Accreditation of Healthcare Organizations (JCAHO) accreditation
+ American Osteopathic Hospital Association (AOHA) membership
○ American Osteopathic Association (AOA) accreditation
△ Commission on Accreditation of Rehabilitation Facilities (CARF) accreditation
Control codes 61, 63, 64, 71, 72 and 73 indicate hospitals listed by AOHA, but not registered by AHA. For definition of numerical codes, see page A6

CEDAR RAPIDS—Linn County

★ MERCY MEDICAL CENTER, 701 Tenth Street S.E., Zip 52403; tel. 319/398–6011; A. James Tinker, President and Chief Executive Officer (Total facility includes 91 beds in nursing home–type unit) **A**1 2 3 9 10 **F**2 3 4 7 8 10 12 13 14 15 16 17 18 19 21 22 24 26 27 28 29 30 31 32 33 34 35 37 39 40 41 42 43 44 45 46 47 49 51 52 53 54 55 56 57 58 59 60 63 64 65 67 68 71 73 74	21	10	444	8431	233	96545	984	76659	34080	1198
★ △ ST. LUKE'S HOSPITAL, (Formerly St. Luke's Methodist Hospital) 1026 A Avenue N.E., Zip 52402–3026, Mailing Address: P.O. Box 3026, Zip 52406–3026; tel. 319/369–7211; Samuel T. Wallace, President (Total facility includes 28 beds in nursing home–type unit) **A**1 3 7 9 10 **F**3 4 7 8 10 11 12 14 15 16 17 19 20 21 22 23 24 25 26 27 28 29 30 31 32 33 34 35 36 37 38 39 40 41 42 43 44 45 46 47 48 49 51 52 53 54 55 56 57 58 59 60 61 64 65 66 67 68 70 71 72 73 74 **P**3 7 8 **S**0061 Iowa Health System	23	10	428	14807	251	194742	2240	113720	51058	1764

CENTERVILLE—Appanoose County

★ ST. JOSEPH'S MERCY HOSPITAL, 1 St. Joseph's Drive, Zip 52544; tel. 515/437–4111; William C. Assell, President and Chief Executive Officer (Total facility includes 24 beds in nursing home–type unit) **A**1 9 10 **F**7 8 14 15 16 19 21 22 26 28 29 30 32 33 34 35 36 37 39 40 42 44 45 51 65 67 71 73 **S**5175 Catholic Health Corporation	21	10	58	1214	49	30941	106	7398	3574	162

CHARITON—Lucas County

★ LUCAS COUNTY HEALTH CENTER, 1200 North Seventh Street, Zip 50049; tel. 515/774–3000; Billy J. Bruce Jr., Chief Executive Officer **A**9 10 **F**1 2 3 6 7 8 15 16 19 21 22 26 27 28 30 32 33 34 35 41 44 48 49 51 53 54 55 56 57 58 59 61 62 64 65 66 67 70 71 72 73 **P**7	13	10	56	591	7	11899	61	5699	2442	137

CHARLES CITY—Floyd County

★ FLOYD COUNTY MEMORIAL HOSPITAL, 700 Eleventh Street, Zip 50616–3499; tel. 515/228–6830; Bill D. Faust, Administrator **A**9 10 **F**7 8 11 14 15 16 19 22 28 29 30 32 33 34 36 37 39 40 41 42 44 51 53 57 58 65 66 67 71	13	10	38	1199	15	30968	89	7870	3327	151

CHEROKEE—Cherokee County

☐ MENTAL HEALTH INSTITUTE, 1200 West Cedar Street, Zip 51012; tel. 712/225–2594; Tom Deiker Ph.D., Superintendent **A**1 10 13 **F**12 14 34 45 52 53 54 55 56 58 59 65 **P**6	12	22	174	1017	117	1734	0	14491	10193	319
★ SIOUX VALLEY MEMORIAL HOSPITAL, 300 Sioux Valley Drive, Zip 51012; tel. 712/225–5101; Douglas Krauth, Chief Executive Officer **A**9 10 **F**3 7 8 11 12 14 15 17 19 20 22 24 26 28 29 30 31 32 33 34 36 39 40 41 42 44 45 46 49 51 64 65 66 67 71 73 **P**4 6	23	10	67	1033	14	19937	123	7145	3651	170

CLARINDA—Page County

★ CLARINDA MUNICIPAL HOSPITAL, 17th And Wells Streets, Zip 51632, Mailing Address: P.O. Box 217, Zip 51632–0217; tel. 712/542–2176 **A**9 10 **F**8 14 15 16 17 19 21 22 26 28 30 31 34 36 39 40 42 44 46 49 58 65 67 71 73	14	10	26	590	11	27302	64	3698	1736	96
MENTAL HEALTH INSTITUTE, Mailing Address: Box 338, Zip 51632–0338; tel. 712/542–2161; Mark Lund, Superintendent (Total facility includes 63 beds in nursing home–type unit) **F**2 3 4 10 11 14 15 16 19 20 21 25 26 31 35 37 40 41 42 43 44 48 50 52 54 55 56 57 58 60 63 65 71 73	12	22	83	193	68	0	0	6118	—	175

CLARION—Wright County

★ COMMUNITY MEMORIAL HOSPITAL, 1316 South Main Street, Zip 50525–0429; tel. 515/532–2811; Richard W. Rhiner, Interim Administrator **A**9 10 **F**7 8 14 17 19 20 22 30 32 33 34 35 36 39 40 41 42 44 49 62 64 65 67 71 73 **P**7 8 **S**0061 Iowa Health System	14	10	33	655	17	17918	98	3553	1626	84

CLINTON—Clinton County

★ SAMARITAN HEALTH SYSTEM, (Includes Samaritan Hospital North, 1410 North Fourth Street, Clinton, Iowa, Zip 52732; Samaritan Intermediate Care, 600 14th Avenue North, Clinton, Iowa, Zip 52732; tel. 319/243–3200) 1410 North Fourth Street, Zip 52732, Mailing Address: P.O. Box 2960, Zip 52733–2960; tel. 319/244–5555; Thomas J. Hesselmann, President (Total facility includes 23 beds in nursing home–type unit) **A**1 9 10 **F**3 7 8 10 11 15 16 17 19 21 22 23 26 28 30 32 33 34 35 36 39 40 41 42 44 45 46 49 52 53 54 55 56 57 60 64 65 67 71 73 **P**1 **S**5165 Mercy Health Services	21	10	194	5531	97	36673	444	33450	14681	619

CORNING—Adams County

★ MERCY HOSPITAL, Rosary Drive, Zip 50841, Mailing Address: Box 368, Zip 50841; tel. 515/322–3121; James C. Ruppert, President **A**1 9 10 **F**8 12 14 15 16 19 22 28 29 30 32 33 35 36 39 40 41 42 44 49 58 65 71 73 **P**6 **S**5175 Catholic Health Corporation	21	10	22	551	8	24420	80	4101	1729	105

CORYDON—Wayne County

★ WAYNE COUNTY HOSPITAL, 417 South East Street, Zip 50060; tel. 515/872–2260; Bill D. Wilson, Administrator **A**9 10 **F**1 2 3 4 5 6 7 8 9 10 11 12 13 14 15 16 17 18 19 20 21 22 23 24 25 26 27 28 29 30 31 32 33 34 35 36 37 38 39 40 41 42 43 44 45 46 47 48 49 50 51 52 53 54 55 56 57 58 59 60 61 62 63 64 65 66 67 68 69 70 71 72 73 74 **P**8	13	10	28	855	13	9986	81	3531	1645	90

COUNCIL BLUFFS—Pottawattamie County

★ JENNIE EDMUNDSON MEMORIAL HOSPITAL, 933 East Pierce Street, Zip 51503–4652, Mailing Address: P.O. Box 2C, Zip 51502–3002; tel. 712/328–6000; David M. Holcomb, President and Chief Executive Officer (Total facility includes 25 beds in nursing home–type unit) **A**1 6 9 10 **F**1 3 7 8 10 12 17 19 21 22 23 30 31 32 33 34 35 36 37 39 40 41 42 44 46 49 52 53 54 55 56 57 58 59 60 63 64 65 66 67 71 73 **P**3 8	23	10	220	5325	100	61675	615	42983	19843	661

© 1995 AHA Guide

Hospitals, U.S. / IOWA

Hospital, Address, Telephone, Administrator, Approval, Facility, and Physician Codes, Health Care System	Classification Codes		Utilization Data					Expense (thousands) of dollars		
★ American Hospital Association (AHA) membership ☐ Joint Commission on Accreditation of Healthcare Organizations (JCAHO) accreditation + American Osteopathic Hospital Association (AOHA) membership ○ American Osteopathic Association (AOA) accreditation △ Commission on Accreditation of Rehabilitation Facilities (CARF) accreditation Control codes 61, 63, 64, 71, 72 and 73 indicate hospitals listed by AOHA, but not registered by AHA. For definition of numerical codes, see page A6	Control	Service	Beds	Admissions	Census	Outpatient Visits	Births	Total	Payroll	Personnel
★ MERCY HOSPITAL, 800 Mercy Drive, Zip 51503, Mailing Address: Box 1C, Zip 51502; tel. 712/328-5000; Richard A. Hachten II, President (Total facility includes 24 beds in nursing home–type unit) A1 9 10 F1 2 3 4 6 7 8 10 11 12 14 15 16 17 18 19 20 21 22 23 24 25 26 27 28 29 30 31 32 33 34 35 36 37 38 39 40 41 42 43 44 45 46 48 49 51 52 53 54 55 56 57 58 59 60 61 62 63 64 65 66 67 68 70 71 72 73 74 P6 8 S5175 Catholic Health Corporation	21	10	210	5689	94	42892	477	42878	18312	726
CRESCO—Howard County										
★ HOWARD COUNTY HOSPITAL, 235 Eighth Avenue West, Zip 52136-1098; tel. 319/547-2101; Elizabeth Doty, Administrator A1 9 10 F7 8 15 16 19 21 22 30 34 40 44 49 71 73 P6 S5165 Mercy Health Services	13	10	42	490	5	16257	109	4012	1838	88
CRESTON—Union County										
★ GREATER COMMUNITY HOSPITAL, 1700 West Townline, Zip 50801-1099; tel. 515/782-7091; Marlys Scherlin, Administrator A1 9 10 F7 8 12 15 19 20 22 27 28 29 30 31 33 34 35 36 37 39 40 41 42 44 49 50 54 56 58 59 60 63 65 67 69 71 73	13	10	53	1365	17	26321	183	9140	4288	192
DAVENPORT—Scott County										
☐ ○ DAVENPORT MEDICAL CENTER, 1111 West Kimberly Road, Zip 52806; tel. 319/391-2020; Richard A. Seidler, Chief Executive Officer (Data for 352 days) A1 9 10 11 12 13 F7 8 12 14 15 16 19 20 22 26 32 34 35 37 40 41 42 44 45 46 49 61 65 67 71 72 73 74 P5 S6525 Ornda Healthcorp	33	10	150	1902	24	29130	263	—	—	225
★ △ GENESIS MEDICAL CENTER, (Includes Genesis Medical Center–East Campus (Formerly St. Luke's Hospital), 1227 East Rusholme Street, Davenport, Iowa, Zip 52803; tel. 319/326-6512; Genesis Medical Center–West Campus (Formerly Mercy Hospital), 1401 West Central Park, Davenport, Iowa, Zip 52804-1769; tel. 319/383-1000) 1227 East Rusholme Street, Zip 52803; tel. 319/326-6512; Leo A. Bressanelli, President and Chief Executive Officer (Total facility includes 41 beds in nursing home–type unit) A1 2 5 7 9 10 F2 3 4 7 8 10 11 12 15 19 21 22 23 27 28 29 30 31 32 33 34 35 37 38 40 41 42 43 44 46 47 48 49 51 52 53 54 56 58 60 64 65 67 71 72 73 74 P5	23	10	502	20305	337	190938	2177	147938	58420	2055
GENESIS MEDICAL CENTER–EAST CAMPUS See Genesis Medical Center										
GENESIS MEDICAL CENTER–WEST CAMPUS See Genesis Medical Center										
MERCY HOSPITAL See Genesis Medical Center										
DEWITT—Clinton County										
★ DEWITT COMMUNITY HOSPITAL, 1118 11th Street, De Witt, Zip 52742; tel. 319/659-3241; C. J. Christensen, Chief Executive Officer (Total facility includes 77 beds in nursing home–type unit) A1 9 10 F7 8 9 13 14 15 16 19 22 26 28 30 33 34 36 44 51 65 71 72 73	23	10	101	371	83	12046	1	4262	1940	155
DECORAH—Winneshiek County										
★ WINNESHIEK COUNTY MEMORIAL HOSPITAL, 901 Montgomery Street, Zip 52101; tel. 319/382-2911; Paul J. Anderson, Administrator A1 9 10 F7 8 11 12 15 17 19 21 22 28 30 31 32 33 37 39 40 42 44 45 49 63 65 66 71 73	13	10	83	1267	15	26652	204	7595	3924	161
DENISON—Crawford County										
☐ CRAWFORD COUNTY MEMORIAL HOSPITAL, 2020 First Avenue South, Zip 51442; tel. 712/263-5021; Kenneth A. Ewen II, Administrator A1 9 10 F3 7 8 14 15 16 17 18 19 20 21 22 24 26 27 28 30 31 32 33 34 35 40 41 42 44 45 46 49 51 53 54 55 56 57 58 59 61 62 65 66 67 68 71 72 73 74	13	10	72	930	13	17442	139	5517	2538	109
DES MOINES—Polk County										
★ BROADLAWNS MEDICAL CENTER, 1801 Hickman Road, Zip 50314-1597; tel. 515/282-2200; Willis F. Fry, Executive Director A1 3 5 9 10 F1 2 3 7 8 12 14 15 16 17 18 19 20 21 22 27 28 31 33 34 35 37 38 39 40 41 43 44 46 49 51 52 53 54 56 58 59 65 67 71 72 73 P6	13	10	200	5028	81	205759	504	51455	24840	830
★ + ○ DES MOINES GENERAL HOSPITAL, 603 East 12th Street, Zip 50309-5515; tel. 515/263-4200; Roy W. Wright, Chief Executive Officer (Total facility includes 15 beds in nursing home–type unit) A9 10 11 12 13 F2 3 4 7 8 10 14 15 16 17 19 22 24 26 28 29 31 32 34 35 37 40 42 43 44 45 46 49 64 65 71 73 P8 S0002 Quorum Health Group/Quorum Health Resources	23	10	113	4487	91	31269	368	38671	15643	678
★ IOWA LUTHERAN HOSPITAL, 700 East University Avenue, Zip 50316-2392; tel. 515/263-5612; James H. Skogsbergh, President A1 3 5 9 10 F1 2 3 4 7 8 9 10 11 12 14 15 16 17 18 19 21 22 23 24 26 27 28 29 30 31 32 33 34 35 37 38 39 40 41 42 43 44 45 46 47 49 51 52 53 54 55 56 57 58 59 60 61 63 64 65 66 67 68 69 70 71 72 73 P1 2 3 6 S0061 Iowa Health System	23	10	275	9189	94	183701	1515	77463	36808	1431
★ △ IOWA METHODIST MEDICAL CENTER, (Includes Powell Convalescent Center, Des Moines, Iowa; Raymond Blank Memorial Hospital for Children, Des Moines, Iowa; Younker Memorial Rehabilitation Center, 1200 Pleasant Road, Des Moines, Iowa) 1200 Pleasant Street, Zip 50309-9976; tel. 515/241-6212; James H. Skogsbergh, President A1 2 3 5 6 7 9 10 F1 2 3 4 7 8 9 10 11 12 14 15 16 17 18 19 21 22 23 24 26 27 28 29 30 31 32 33 34 35 37 38 39 40 41 42 43 44 45 46 47 48 49 51 52 53 54 57 58 59 60 61 63 64 65 66 67 68 69 70 71 72 73 P1 2 3 6 S0061 Iowa Health System	23	10	573	19932	368	190551	2088	201545	87851	3154
MERCY FRANKLIN CENTER See Mercy Hospital Medical Center										
★ MERCY HOSPITAL MEDICAL CENTER, (Includes Mercy Franklin Center, 1818 48th Street, Des Moines, Iowa, Zip 50310; tel. 515/271-6000) 400 University Avenue, Zip 50314; tel. 515/247-4278; Thomas A. Reitinger, President and Chief Executive Officer (Total facility includes 35 beds in nursing home–type unit) A1 2 3 6 9 10 F1 3 4 5 6 7 8 10 11 12 14 15 16 17 18 19 20 21 22 23 24 25 26 28 30 31 32 33 34 35 37 38 39 40 41 42 43 44 47 49 51 52 53 54 55 56 57 58 59 60 62 64 65 66 67 69 71 72 73 P1 S5175 Catholic Health Corporation	21	10	638	24395	370	—	2401	219135	82569	3273

Hospitals, U.S. / IOWA

Hospital, Address, Telephone, Administrator, Approval, Facility, and Physician Codes, Health Care System	Classification Codes		Utilization Data					Expense (thousands) of dollars		
★ American Hospital Association (AHA) membership ☐ Joint Commission on Accreditation of Healthcare Organizations (JCAHO) accreditation + American Osteopathic Hospital Association (AOHA) membership ○ American Osteopathic Association (AOA) accreditation △ Commission on Accreditation of Rehabilitation Facilities (CARF) accreditation Control codes 61, 63, 64, 71, 72 and 73 indicate hospitals listed by AOHA, but not registered by AHA. For definition of numerical codes, see page A6	Control	Service	Beds	Admissions	Census	Outpatient Visits	Births	Total	Payroll	Personnel
★ VETERANS AFFAIRS MEDICAL CENTER, 3600 30th Street, Zip 50310–5774; tel. 515/255–2173; Ellen DeGeorge–Smith, Director **A**1 2 3 5 **F**2 3 4 8 10 11 18 19 20 21 22 23 26 27 29 30 31 32 33 34 35 37 39 41 42 43 44 46 48 49 51 52 54 55 56 57 58 59 60 63 64 65 67 69 70 71 73 74 **S**9295 Department of Veterans Affairs	45	10	129	3933	98	79573	0	48603	28159	801
DUBUQUE—Dubuque County ★ FINLEY HOSPITAL, 350 North Grandview Avenue, Zip 52001–6392; tel. 319/582–1881; Kevin L. Rogols, President and Chief Executive Officer (Total facility includes 17 beds in nursing home–type unit) **A**1 2 9 10 **F**7 8 12 14 15 16 17 19 21 22 23 24 26 27 28 29 30 31 32 33 34 35 36 37 39 40 41 42 44 45 46 49 60 61 63 64 65 66 67 70 71 72 73 74 **P**1 5	23	10	141	4618	63	40680	578	38668	15855	614
★ △ MERCY HEALTH CENTER, (Includes Mercy Health Center–St. Mary's Unit, 1111 Third Street S.W., Dyersville, Iowa, Zip 52040; tel. 319/875–7101) 250 Mercy Drive, Zip 52001–7360; tel. 319/589–8000; Sister Helen Huewe, President (Total facility includes 63 beds in nursing home–type unit) **A**1 7 9 10 **F**2 3 4 7 8 10 12 13 15 16 17 19 20 21 22 23 26 27 28 29 30 31 32 34 35 37 38 39 40 41 42 43 44 45 48 49 52 53 54 55 56 57 58 59 60 63 64 65 66 67 68 69 70 71 72 73 74 **S**5165 Mercy Health Services	21	10	363	10549	209	50671	1062	71135	30715	1161
DYERSVILLE—Dubuque County MERCY HEALTH CENTER–ST. MARY'S UNIT See Mercy Health Center										
ELDORA—Hardin County ★ ELDORA REGIONAL MEDICAL CENTER, 2413 Edgington Avenue, Zip 50627–1541; tel. 515/858–5416; Jeffrey C. Brittain, Administrator **A**9 10 **F**8 15 16 19 22 28 30 33 34 44 46 49 60 70 71 73 **P**6 **S**5165 Mercy Health Services	14	10	18	339	4	9196	3	2171	938	50
ELKADER—Clayton County CENTRAL COMMUNITY HOSPITAL, 901 Davidson Street N.W., Zip 52043–9799, Mailing Address: Rural Route 1, Box 269A, Zip 52043–9799; tel. 319/245–2250; Lisa Manson, Co–Administrator **A**9 10 **F**7 8 15 16 19 22 24 26 28 29 30 33 34 40 44 45 49 64 67 71 73 74 **P**3 **S**2235 Lutheran Health Systems	23	10	29	348	6	7148	35	2293	856	56
EMMETSBURG—Palo Alto County PALO ALTO COUNTY HOSPITAL, 3201 West First Street, Zip 50536; tel. 712/852–2434; Darrell E. Vondrak, Administrator (Total facility includes 22 beds in nursing home–type unit) **A**9 10 **F**7 8 14 15 16 17 19 22 26 27 28 30 31 32 33 34 35 36 37 39 40 41 44 45 46 49 66 67 71	13	10	54	786	32	14866	100	4445	2266	107
ESTHERVILLE—Emmet County ★ HOLY FAMILY HOSPITAL, 826 North Eighth Street, Zip 51334–1598; tel. 712/362–2631; Thomas Nordwick, President and Chief Executive Officer **A**1 9 10 **F**1 2 3 6 7 8 13 15 17 19 22 26 27 28 30 31 32 33 34 35 36 37 39 40 41 44 49 65 67 71 **S**5305 Sisters of the Sorrowful Mother United States Health System	21	10	58	1134	21	25821	105	7936	3657	160
FAIRFIELD—Jefferson County ★ JEFFERSON COUNTY HOSPITAL, 400 Highland Avenue, Zip 52556, Mailing Address: Box 588, Zip 52556; tel. 515/472–4111; Walter W. Brownlee, President (Total facility includes 16 beds in nursing home–type unit) **A**9 10 **F**7 11 19 22 30 34 37 39 40 41 44 49 52 53 54 56 58 64 65 71	13	10	83	1681	46	23321	27	9197	4487	163
FORT DODGE—Webster County ★ TRINITY REGIONAL HOSPITAL, 802 Kenyon Road, Zip 50501; tel. 515/573–3101; Tom Tibbitts, President (Total facility includes 12 beds in nursing home–type unit) **A**1 9 10 **F**2 3 7 8 12 14 15 16 17 19 20 21 22 23 24 27 28 29 30 31 32 33 34 35 37 39 40 41 44 46 49 52 53 54 55 56 57 58 59 61 64 65 66 67 71 73 **P**7	23	10	182	5001	91	63742	616	40918	19136	727
FORT MADISON—Lee County ★ FORT MADISON COMMUNITY HOSPITAL, 5445 Avenue O, Zip 52627–0174, Mailing Address: P.O. Box 174, Zip 52627–0174; tel. 319/372–6530; C. James Platt, Administrator **A**1 9 10 **F**7 8 14 15 16 19 22 24 27 30 34 35 37 40 41 42 44 45 46 48 49 60 63 64 65 71 73 74 **S**0002 Quorum Health Group/Quorum Health Resources	23	10	50	1923	25	28871	145	12599	4925	175
GLENWOOD—Mills County GLENWOOD STATE HOSPITAL SCHOOL, Zip 51534; tel. 712/527–4811; William E. Campbell Ph.D., Superintendent **F**1 2 3 4 5 6 11 20 24 36 37 41 48 52 53 54 57 65 73	12	62	575	25	445	0	0	36910	25112	898
GREENFIELD—Adair County ADAIR COUNTY MEMORIAL HOSPITAL, 609 Southeast Kent Street, Zip 50849, Mailing Address: Rural Route 2, Box 100, Zip 50849; tel. 515/743–2123; Joseph Rivera, Administrator **A**9 10 **F**8 15 16 19 22 27 30 35 36 40 44 49 71 **P**5	13	10	31	512	7	7230	43	2274	1070	49
GRINNELL—Poweshiek County ★ GRINNELL REGIONAL MEDICAL CENTER, 210 Fourth Avenue, Zip 50112–1833; tel. 515/236–7511; Todd C. Linden, President and Chief Executive Officer **A**1 9 10 **F**7 8 12 13 14 15 16 19 22 28 29 30 31 32 33 34 35 37 39 40 41 42 44 45 46 49 63 65 67 71 73 **P**7	23	10	46	2371	26	31459	232	15219	6879	250
GRUNDY CENTER—Grundy County GRUNDY COUNTY MEMORIAL HOSPITAL, East J Avenue, Zip 50638; tel. 319/824–5421; (Total facility includes 55 beds in nursing home–type unit) **A**9 10 **F**7 8 12 14 15 16 17 19 22 30 64 65 71 72 **P**3	13	10	88	428	61	33730	26	3251	1697	100
GUTHRIE CENTER—Guthrie County ★ GUTHRIE COUNTY HOSPITAL, 710 North 12th Street, Zip 50115; tel. 515/747–2201; Dwight P. Daniels, Administrator **A**9 10 **F**7 8 14 15 16 17 19 20 22 30 33 34 35 37 40 41 42 44 49 53 54 56 57 58 65 71 73	13	10	26	617	6	7938	18	2611	1115	39

© 1995 AHA Guide

Hospitals, U.S. / IOWA

Hospital, Address, Telephone, Administrator, Approval, Facility, and Physician Codes, Health Care System	Classification Codes		Utilization Data					Expense (thousands) of dollars		Personnel
★ American Hospital Association (AHA) membership □ Joint Commission on Accreditation of Healthcare Organizations (JCAHO) accreditation + American Osteopathic Hospital Association (AOHA) membership ○ American Osteopathic Association (AOA) accreditation △ Commission on Accreditation of Rehabilitation Facilities (CARF) accreditation Control codes 61, 63, 64, 71, 72 and 73 indicate hospitals listed by AOHA, but not registered by AHA. For definition of numerical codes, see page A6	Control	Service	Beds	Admissions	Census	Outpatient Visits	Births	Total	Payroll	
GUTTENBERG—Clayton County										
★ GUTTENBERG MUNICIPAL HOSPITAL, Second and Main Street, Zip 52052-0550, Mailing Address: Box 550, Zip 52052-0550; tel. 319/252-1121; Timothy J. Wick, Chief Executive Officer **A**9 10 **F**7 8 11 19 21 22 26 28 30 32 33 36 39 40 42 44 66 71 **S**0585 Brim, Inc.	14	10	29	585	7	11680	50	3098	1307	61
HAMBURG—Fremont County										
GRAPE COMMUNITY HOSPITAL, (Formerly Grape Community Hospital–Southwest Medical Center) Highway 275 North, Zip 51640, Mailing Address: P.O. Box 246, Zip 51640-0246; tel. 712/382-1515; David E. Schultz, Administrator **A**9 10 **F**7 8 15 19 21 22 30 32 34 35 36 37 39 40 41 42 44 45 49 50 63 65 71 73	23	10	49	648	23	8725	56	—	—	90
HAMPTON—Franklin County										
★ FRANKLIN GENERAL HOSPITAL, 1720 Central Avenue East, Zip 50441-0417, Mailing Address: P.O. Box 417, Zip 50441-0417; tel. 515/456-4721; Scott Curtis, Interim Chief Executive Officer (Total facility includes 52 beds in nursing home–type unit) **A**9 10 **F**8 14 15 16 18 19 20 22 26 28 30 31 32 33 34 37 39 41 42 44 45 49 65 71 73 **P**6 **S**5165 Mercy Health Services	13	10	92	506	61	18822	0	5143	2474	103
HARLAN—Shelby County										
□ MYRTUE MEMORIAL HOSPITAL, 1213 Garfield Avenue, Zip 51537; tel. 712/755-5161; Stephen L. Goeser, Administrator **A**1 9 10 **F**7 8 13 14 15 16 18 19 22 24 28 32 33 34 35 36 37 40 41 42 44 49 51 53 54 56 58 63 67 68 71 73 **P**3 8	13	10	52	1092	16	20853	89	7622	3112	132
HAWARDEN—Sioux County										
HAWARDEN COMMUNITY HOSPITAL, 1111 11th Street, Zip 51023; tel. 712/552-1121; Omar L. Voran, Administrator **A**10 **F**8 14 19 21 22 30 32 33 34 39 40 42 44 46 54 58 64 71 **S**5165 Mercy Health Services	14	10	19	192	6	10361	7	1477	641	35
HUMBOLDT—Humboldt County										
HUMBOLDT COUNTY MEMORIAL HOSPITAL, 1000 North 15th Street, Zip 50548; tel. 515/332-4200; Kari L. Engholm, Administrator **A**10 **F**7 8 17 19 21 22 28 29 30 33 34 35 36 39 40 41 44 49 65 71 **P**3	13	10	49	568	30	15031	58	4195	2060	102
IDA GROVE—Ida County										
★ HORN MEMORIAL HOSPITAL, 700 East Second Street, Zip 51445; tel. 712/364-3311; John Blanco, Administrator **A**9 10 **F**8 14 19 22 32 34 36 40 42 44 51 65 71 73	23	10	36	685	10	18688	100	3337	1978	71
INDEPENDENCE—Buchanan County										
□ MENTAL HEALTH INSTITUTE, First Street East, Zip 50644, Mailing Address: Box 111, Zip 50644; tel. 319/334-2583; B. J. Dave M.D., Superintendent **A**1 10 **F**14 15 16 20 22 27 45 46 51 52 53 54 55 56 65 67 73 **P**6	12	22	213	1112	172	15	0	17675	13206	397
★ PEOPLE'S MEMORIAL HOSPITAL, 1600 First Street East, Zip 50644-3155; tel. 319/334-6071; Robert J. Richard, Administrator (Total facility includes 59 beds in nursing home–type unit) **A**9 10 **F**7 8 14 15 16 19 28 31 32 33 36 40 44 49 65 71	13	10	109	662	64	22559	42	5269	2492	119
IOWA CITY—Johnson County										
✦ MERCY HOSPITAL, 500 East Market Street, Zip 52245; tel. 319/339-0300; (Total facility includes 12 beds in nursing home–type unit) **A**1 2 3 5 9 10 **F**4 7 8 10 12 13 14 15 16 17 18 19 20 21 22 23 26 28 29 30 31 32 34 35 37 38 39 40 41 42 43 44 45 46 47 48 49 52 54 55 56 57 60 64 65 67 71 73 **P**3 6 8 **S**5215 Mercy–Chicago Region Healthcare System	21	10	240	8404	135	157599	1198	58568	26963	829
UNIVERSITY HOSPITAL SCHOOL See University of Iowa Hospitals and Clinics										
✦ UNIVERSITY OF IOWA HOSPITALS AND CLINICS, (Includes Chemical Dependency Center, Oakdale, Iowa, Zip 52319; tel. 319/335-4165; State Psychiatric Hospital, 200 Hawkins Drive, Iowa City, Iowa, Zip 52242; tel. 319/356-4658; Robert R. Robinson M.D., Professor and Head; University Hospital School, 200 Hawkins Drive, Iowa City, Iowa, Zip 52242; tel. 319/353-6456) 200 Hawkins Drive, Zip 52242-1009; tel. 319/356-1616; R. Edward Howell, Director and Chief Executive Officer **A**1 2 3 5 8 9 10 **F**2 3 4 5 7 8 9 10 11 12 13 14 15 16 17 18 19 20 21 22 23 25 26 27 28 29 30 31 32 33 34 35 37 38 39 40 41 42 43 44 46 47 48 49 50 51 52 53 54 55 56 57 58 59 60 61 63 65 66 67 69 70 71 73 74	12	10	858	33649	649	483306	1498	382119	169459	5118
✦ VETERANS AFFAIRS MEDICAL CENTER, Highway 6 West, Zip 52246-2208; tel. 319/338-0581; Gary L. Wilkinson, Director **A**1 3 5 8 **F**1 3 4 8 10 19 20 21 22 26 27 28 30 31 32 33 34 35 37 39 41 42 45 46 49 51 52 54 55 56 58 60 63 65 67 69 71 73 74 **S**9295 Department of Veterans Affairs	45	10	198	6398	147	108731	0	80254	40689	957
IOWA FALLS—Hardin County										
✦ ELLSWORTH MUNICIPAL HOSPITAL, 110 Rocksylvania Avenue, Zip 50126-2431; tel. 515/648-4631; William L. Sword, Administrator and Chief Executive Officer **A**1 2 9 10 **F**1 3 7 8 11 14 15 16 19 22 24 28 29 30 34 37 39 40 41 42 44 45 46 49 51 52 53 54 55 56 58 65 67 71 73 **P**6	14	10	42	1114	15	13461	130	5645	2962	129
JEFFERSON—Greene County										
✦ GREENE COUNTY MEDICAL CENTER, 1000 West Lincolnway, Zip 50129-1697; tel. 515/386-2114; Karen L. Bossard R.N., Interim Administrator (Total facility includes 62 beds in nursing home–type unit) **A**1 9 10 **F**1 7 8 11 12 13 14 15 16 17 18 19 21 22 26 28 29 30 31 32 33 34 35 39 40 41 44 45 49 62 65 66 67 68 71 73 **P**5	13	10	115	709	85	22987	97	7441	3875	182
KEOKUK—Lee County										
✦ KEOKUK AREA HOSPITAL, 1600 Morgan Street, Zip 52632; tel. 319/524-7150; Allan Zastrow, Chief Executive Officer (Total facility includes 20 beds in nursing home–type unit) **A**1 9 10 **F**3 7 8 11 14 15 16 17 19 21 22 23 28 29 30 32 33 34 35 40 44 45 46 49 52 53 54 55 56 61 64 65 66 67 71 73	23	10	113	4276	70	18536	291	19644	9056	385

Hospitals, U.S. / IOWA

Hospital, Address, Telephone, Administrator, Approval, Facility, and Physician Codes, Health Care System	Classification Codes		Utilization Data					Expense (thousands) of dollars		
★ American Hospital Association (AHA) membership ☐ Joint Commission on Accreditation of Healthcare Organizations (JCAHO) accreditation + American Osteopathic Hospital Association (AOHA) membership ○ American Osteopathic Association (AOA) accreditation △ Commission on Accreditation of Rehabilitation Facilities (CARF) accreditation Control codes 61, 63, 64, 71, 72 and 73 indicate hospitals listed by AOHA, but not registered by AHA. For definition of numerical codes, see page A6	Control	Service	Beds	Admissions	Census	Outpatient Visits	Births	Total	Payroll	Personnel
KEOSAUQUA—Van Buren County ★ VAN BUREN COUNTY HOSPITAL, Highway 1 North, Zip 52565, Mailing Address: Box 70, Zip 52565; tel. 319/293–3171; Lisa Wagner Schnedler, Administrator **A**9 10 **F**1 7 8 14 15 16 17 19 22 28 34 40 41 42 44 45 46 49 54 58 60 61 65 71 73 74 **S**5805 Sisters of Mary of the Presentation Health Corporation	13	10	40	670	19	8184	55	3678	1657	100
KNOXVILLE—Marion County ☐ KNOXVILLE AREA COMMUNITY HOSPITAL, 1002 South Lincoln Street, Zip 50138–3121; tel. 515/842–2151; Terry R. Lambert, Administrator (Total facility includes 14 beds in nursing home–type unit) **A**1 9 10 **F**7 8 11 15 16 19 21 22 28 30 33 34 35 37 40 41 44 45 49 56 63 65 66 67 71 73 **P**8 **S**0002 Quorum Health Group/Quorum Health Resources	23	10	59	1489	31	13790	113	7720	2857	141
☐ VETERANS AFFAIRS MEDICAL CENTER, 1515 West Pleasant, Zip 50138–3399; tel. 515/842–3101; Donald D. Ziska, Director (Total facility includes 260 beds in nursing home–type unit) **A**1 **F**1 2 3 15 20 22 26 30 31 32 34 35 41 46 48 49 52 54 55 56 57 58 64 65 71 73 **S**9295 Department of Veterans Affairs	45	22	637	2585	537	55620	0	50278	30230	897
LAKE CITY—Calhoun County ★ STEWART MEMORIAL COMMUNITY HOSPITAL, 1301 West Main, Zip 51449–1585; tel. 712/464–3171; Edward R. Maahs, Chief Executive Officer **A**10 **F**7 8 14 19 22 29 30 32 33 34 35 36 37 40 41 42 44 45 49 56 71 **P**6	23	10	49	1858	22	36702	153	7915	3709	166
LE MARS—Plymouth County FLOYD VALLEY HOSPITAL, Highway 3 East, Zip 51031, Mailing Address: P.O. Box 10, Zip 51031; tel. 712/546–7871; G. Frank Labonte, Chief Executive Officer **A**10 **F**3 7 8 11 13 15 16 17 18 19 22 24 28 29 30 32 33 34 35 36 39 40 41 42 44 45 46 49 56 65 66 67 71 73 **P**5 **S**5845 St. Luke's Health System, Inc.	14	10	44	1015	17	29915	136	6330	2844	108
LEON—Decatur County ☐ DECATUR COUNTY HOSPITAL, 1405 Northwest Church Street, Zip 50144–1299; tel. 515/446–4871; Neil Davenport, Administrator **A**1 9 10 **F**8 14 15 16 19 21 22 28 34 39 40 41 42 44 45 46 49 53 54 55 56 57 58 59 65 71 73	13	10	49	708	11	10555	90	3948	1806	96
MANCHESTER—Delaware County DELAWARE COUNTY MEMORIAL HOSPITAL, 709 West Main Street, Zip 52057–0359; tel. 319/927–3232; Lon D. Butikofer R.N., Ph.D., Administrator and Chief Executive Officer (Total facility includes 15 beds in nursing home–type unit) **A**9 10 **F**7 8 12 15 17 18 19 20 22 24 28 30 31 32 33 34 37 39 40 44 45 46 49 53 54 55 56 57 65 66 67 71 **P**5	13	10	56	1022	60	45522	200	9671	5152	173
MANNING—Carroll County MANNING GENERAL HOSPITAL, 410 Main Street, Zip 51455; tel. 712/653–2072; Jeffrey A. Livingston, Administrator (Total facility includes 12 beds in nursing home–type unit) **A**10 **F**1 2 3 7 8 18 19 21 22 26 29 30 31 34 35 40 41 44 45 46 51 54 56 58 65 67 71 73 **P**3	23	10	41	533	17	5525	26	2685	1261	82
MAQUOKETA—Jackson County ☐ JACKSON COUNTY PUBLIC HOSPITAL, 700 West Grove Street, Zip 52060–0910; tel. 319/652–2474; Harold S. Geller, Administrator (Total facility includes 18 beds in nursing home–type unit) **A**1 9 10 **F**3 7 8 19 21 22 30 32 34 36 37 39 40 44 45 64 65 71 73	13	10	61	1498	29	28660	178	8402	4220	186
MARENGO—Iowa County MARENGO MEMORIAL HOSPITAL, 300 West May Street, Zip 52301, Mailing Address: Box 228, Zip 52301; tel. 319/642–5543; James H. Ragland, Administrator **A**9 10 **F**16 19 22 27 28 30 33 36 39 44 49 65 71 73 **P**6	14	10	44	198	33	9476	0	2962	1333	78
MARSHALLTOWN—Marshall County ☐ MARSHALLTOWN MEDICAL AND SURGICAL CENTER, 3 South Fourth Avenue, Zip 50158; tel. 515/754–5151; Robert Cooper, Chief Executive Officer (Total facility includes 26 beds in nursing home–type unit) **A**1 9 10 **F**7 8 13 14 15 16 17 19 20 21 22 24 25 26 27 28 29 30 31 32 33 34 35 36 37 39 40 41 42 44 46 49 56 63 64 65 66 67 71 73	23	10	140	4292	64	135626	978	30101	15258	501
MASON CITY—Cerro Gordo County ☐ NORTH IOWA MERCY HEALTH CENTER, 84 Beaumont Drive, Zip 50401–2999; tel. 515/424–7211; David H. Vellinga, President and Chief Executive Officer (Total facility includes 30 beds in nursing home–type unit) **A**1 2 3 **F**1 3 4 7 8 10 12 13 15 16 17 18 19 20 21 22 23 24 26 27 28 29 30 31 32 33 34 35 36 37 38 39 40 41 42 43 44 45 46 49 51 52 53 54 55 56 57 58 59 60 62 64 65 66 67 68 70 71 73 74 **P**6 **S**5165 Mercy Health Services	21	10	285	11304	180	331064	1272	102745	41601	1563
MISSOURI VALLEY—Harrison County ☐ COMMUNITY MEMORIAL HOSPITAL, 631 North Eighth Street, Zip 51555–1199; tel. 712/642–2784; James A. Seymour, President and Chief Executive Officer **A**1 10 **F**8 15 16 19 22 28 29 30 32 34 35 39 41 42 44 45 49 53 55 56 58 65 67 71 **P**1 3	23	10	35	731	9	16139	0	4808	2264	80
MOUNT AYR—Ringgold County RINGGOLD COUNTY HOSPITAL, 211 Shellway Drive, Zip 50854; tel. 515/464–3226; Gordon W. Winkler, Administrator **A**9 10 **F**2 3 7 8 19 22 27 30 33 40 41 42 44 71 **P**6	13	10	36	318	8	10670	0	3002	1371	73
MOUNT PLEASANT—Henry County ★ HENRY COUNTY HEALTH CENTER, Saunders Park, Zip 52641–2299; tel. 319/385–3141; Robert Miller, Chief Executive Officer (Total facility includes 31 beds in nursing home–type unit) **A**9 10 **F**7 8 11 12 13 14 15 16 17 18 19 20 21 22 23 26 27 28 29 30 32 34 37 39 40 41 42 44 45 49 54 56 64 65 66 67 71 73 74 **P**3 5	13	10	61	1552	50	29910	193	10633	4889	201

© 1995 AHA Guide

Hospitals, U.S. / IOWA

Hospital, Address, Telephone, Administrator, Approval, Facility, and Physician Codes, Health Care System	Classification Codes		Utilization Data					Expense (thousands) of dollars		
★ American Hospital Association (AHA) membership ☐ Joint Commission on Accreditation of Healthcare Organizations (JCAHO) accreditation + American Osteopathic Hospital Association (AOHA) membership ○ American Osteopathic Association (AOA) accreditation △ Commission on Accreditation of Rehabilitation Facilities (CARF) accreditation Control codes 61, 63, 64, 71, 72 and 73 indicate hospitals listed by AOHA, but not registered by AHA. For definition of numerical codes, see page A6	Control	Service	Beds	Admissions	Census	Outpatient Visits	Births	Total	Payroll	Personnel
MENTAL HEALTH INSTITUTE, 1200 East Washington Street, Zip 52641; tel. 319/385-7231; David J. Scurr, Superintendent **A**10 **F**2 20 45 52 65 73	12	82	88	1058	73	0	0	4749	3128	77
MUSCATINE—Muscatine County										
☐ MUSCATINE GENERAL HOSPITAL, 1518 Mulberry Avenue, Zip 52761-3499; tel. 319/264-9100; Jonathan R. Goble, Chief Executive Officer (Total facility includes 8 beds in nursing home–type unit) **A**1 9 10 **F**3 7 8 14 17 19 21 22 26 30 33 35 36 37 39 40 41 44 49 64 65 67 71	13	10	66	2799	35	21756	485	18985	8505	321
NEVADA—Story County										
★ STORY COUNTY HOSPITAL AND LONG TERM CARE FACILITY, 630 Sixth Street, Zip 50201; tel. 515/382-2111; Todd Willert, Administrator (Total facility includes 80 beds in nursing home–type unit) **A**9 10 **F**8 15 19 20 22 24 26 27 28 30 32 33 34 36 37 39 41 42 44 48 49 51 64 65 66 71 73	13	10	122	298	85	11302	0	4909	2194	159
NEW HAMPTON—Chickasaw County										
★ SAINT JOSEPH COMMUNITY HOSPITAL, 308 North Maple Avenue, Zip 50659; tel. 515/394-4121; Thomas Thompson, President (Total facility includes 35 beds in nursing home–type unit) **A**1 9 10 **F**1 7 8 12 13 15 16 17 18 19 22 26 28 29 30 31 32 33 34 39 40 41 44 45 49 63 65 66 67 71 74 **P**6 7 8 **S**5165 Mercy Health Services	21	10	55	926	43	16550	121	5821	2724	118
NEWTON—Jasper County										
★ SKIFF MEDICAL CENTER, 204 North Fourth Avenue East, Zip 50208; tel. 515/792-1273; Ronald R. Ross, Chief Executive Officer **A**1 9 10 **F**13 15 16 19 22 32 33 34 35 37 40 44 52 53 54 56 57 59 63 71	14	10	68	1916	31	44192	154	14208	7155	280
OAKDALE—Johnson County										
CHEMICAL DEPENDENCY CENTER See University of Iowa Hospitals and Clinics, Iowa City										
IOWA MEDICAL AND CLASSIFICATION CENTER, Zip 52319; tel. 319/626-2391; R. E. Rogerson, Warden **A**9 **F**1 2 3 4 5 6 7 8 9 10 11 12 13 17 18 19 20 21 22 23 24 25 26 28 29 30 31 32 33 34 35 37 38 39 40 41 42 43 44 45 47 48 49 50 51 52 53 54 55 56 57 58 60 61 63 64 65 66 67 68 69 70 71 72 73 74	12	22	46	201	39	0	0	2441	1673	—
OELWEIN—Fayette County										
★ MERCY HOSPITAL OF FRANCISCAN SISTERS, 201 Eighth Avenue S.E., Zip 50662; tel. 319/283-2314; Judith Blake, President and Chief Executive Officer (Total facility includes 39 beds in nursing home–type unit) **A**1 9 10 **F**3 7 8 14 15 17 19 22 26 27 28 30 32 33 34 36 37 40 41 44 49 63 64 65 68 71 **P**6 **S**6745 Wheaton Franciscan Services, Inc.	21	10	64	1039	50	43066	73	6447	2882	119
ONAWA—Monona County										
★ BURGESS MEMORIAL HOSPITAL, 1600 Diamond Street, Zip 51040-1548; tel. 712/423-2311; Karmon T. Bjella, President **A**1 9 10 **F**3 7 8 13 14 15 17 19 21 22 24 26 28 30 32 34 37 40 42 44 45 46 49 51 53 54 57 58 64 65 67 71 73 74	23	10	38	1356	17	16626	87	7700	3553	146
ORANGE CITY—Sioux County										
ORANGE CITY MUNICIPAL HOSPITAL, 400 Central Avenue N.W., Zip 51041-1398; tel. 712/737-4984; Martin W. Guthmiller, Administrator (Total facility includes 33 beds in nursing home–type unit) **A**10 **F**7 8 13 14 15 16 17 18 19 20 21 22 28 29 30 33 34 35 36 37 39 40 41 42 44 45 46 58 65 66 67 71 73 74 **P**8 **S**5845 St. Luke's Health System, Inc.	14	10	63	1046	47	23698	152	6701	2273	117
OSAGE—Mitchell County										
★ MITCHELL COUNTY REGIONAL HEALTH CENTER, (Formerly Mitchell County Memorial Hospital) 616 North Eighth Street, Zip 50461-1498; tel. 515/732-3781; Richard C. Hamilton, Chief Executive Officer **A**9 10 **F**7 8 15 16 19 22 32 33 36 37 39 40 41 42 44 49 51 65 71 73 **P**1 **S**5165 Mercy Health Services	13	10	40	781	9	7083	54	4099	1803	56
OSCEOLA—Clarke County										
★ CLARKE COUNTY HOSPITAL, 800 South Fillmore Street, Zip 50213-0427, Mailing Address: P.O. Box 427, Zip 50213-0427; tel. 515/342-2184; Kris Baumgart, Administrator **A**9 10 **F**8 14 15 16 19 21 22 24 30 33 36 37 42 44 49 71 **S**0061 Iowa Health System	13	10	48	576	37	11991	0	3660	1592	94
OSKALOOSA—Mahaska County										
★ MAHASKA COUNTY HOSPITAL, 1229 C Avenue East, Zip 52577; tel. 515/673-3431; David E. Rutter, Administrator **A**1 9 10 **F**1 3 4 7 8 10 11 12 13 14 15 16 17 18 19 20 21 22 23 24 25 26 27 28 29 30 31 32 33 34 35 36 39 40 41 42 43 44 45 46 49 50 51 53 54 55 56 57 58 59 60 61 63 65 66 67 68 69 70 71 72 74 **P**1 **S**0061 Iowa Health System	13	10	53	1582	16	58381	204	8413	3863	173
OTTUMWA—Wapello County										
★ OTTUMWA REGIONAL HEALTH CENTER, (Includes St. Joseph Health and Rehabilitation Center, 312 East Alta Vista Avenue, Ottumwa, Iowa, Zip 52501; tel. 515/684-4651) 1001 Pennsylvania Avenue, Zip 52501-2186; tel. 515/682-7511; Clarence Cory, President (Total facility includes 14 beds in nursing home–type unit) **A**1 2 9 10 **F**1 2 3 7 8 14 15 19 21 22 23 28 29 30 32 33 34 35 36 37 40 41 42 44 46 49 52 56 58 59 60 63 64 65 67 71 73 **P**8	23	10	94	6190	108	47604	775	39921	17646	706
PELLA—Marion County										
★ PELLA COMMUNITY HOSPITAL, 404 Jefferson Street, Zip 50219; tel. 515/628-3150; Robert D. Kroese, Chief Executive Officer (Total facility includes 109 beds in nursing home–type unit) **A**9 10 **F**1 8 14 15 16 17 19 22 29 30 32 33 34 35 37 39 40 41 42 44 49 61 65 67 69 71 73 **P**1	23	10	156	1284	139	93078	237	11103	5243	243

Hospitals, U.S. / IOWA

Hospital, Address, Telephone, Administrator, Approval, Facility, and Physician Codes, Health Care System	Classi-fication Codes		Utilization Data					Expense (thousands) of dollars		Personnel
	Control	Service	Beds	Admissions	Census	Outpatient Visits	Births	Total	Payroll	

★ American Hospital Association (AHA) membership
☐ Joint Commission on Accreditation of Healthcare Organizations (JCAHO) accreditation
+ American Osteopathic Hospital Association (AOHA) membership
○ American Osteopathic Association (AOA) accreditation
△ Commission on Accreditation of Rehabilitation Facilities (CARF) accreditation
Control codes 61, 63, 64, 71, 72 and 73 indicate hospitals listed by AOHA, but not registered by AHA. For definition of numerical codes, see page A6

Hospital	Control	Service	Beds	Admissions	Census	Outpatient Visits	Births	Total	Payroll	Personnel
PERRY—Dallas County ★ DALLAS COUNTY HOSPITAL, 610 10th Street, Zip 50220, Mailing Address: P.O. Box 608, Zip 50220; tel. 515/465–3547; Vernette Riley, Administrator **A**9 10 **F**1 7 8 19 22 40 42 44 65 67 71 73 **S**0061 Iowa Health System	13	10	30	678	9	21153	48	5178	2152	114
POCAHONTAS—Pocahontas County ★ POCAHONTAS COMMUNITY HOSPITAL, 606 Northwest Seventh, Zip 50574; tel. 712/335–3501; Carolyn K. Hess, Administrator **A**10 **F**8 11 12 16 17 19 22 28 30 32 33 34 37 41 44 49 64 65 67 71 **P**6	14	10	20	397	5	18645	8	2427	1208	63
PRIMGHAR—Obrien County ★ BAUM HARMON MEMORIAL HOSPITAL, 255 North Welch Avenue, Zip 51245; tel. 712/757–3905; Dan Ellis, Administrator **A**10 **F**8 12 16 19 22 24 28 30 32 33 34 35 36 37 40 41 42 44 49 65 66 67 71 **P**8 **S**5165 Mercy Health Services	14	10	19	300	4	7793	41	2010	774	42
RED OAK—Montgomery County ★ MONTGOMERY COUNTY MEMORIAL HOSPITAL, 2301 Eastern Avenue, Zip 51566; tel. 712/623–7000; Allen E. Pohren, Administrator **A**9 10 **F**7 14 16 19 22 23 32 33 34 35 36 37 39 40 41 42 44 49 58 63 65 71 73	13	10	40	1757	26	25443	103	10302	4603	188
ROCK RAPIDS—Lyon County ★ MERRILL PIONEER COMMUNITY HOSPITAL, 801 South Greene Street, Zip 51246–1998; tel. 712/472–2591; Gordon Smith, Administrator **A**10 **F**7 8 19 22 28 33 40 42 44 49 71 **P**6 7	23	10	30	277	3	8435	45	2097	956	56
ROCK VALLEY—Sioux County ★ HEGG MEMORIAL HEALTH CENTER, 1202 21st Avenue, Zip 51247–1497; tel. 712/476–5305; Terry Dejong, Administrator (Total facility includes 95 beds in nursing home–type unit) **A**10 **F**6 7 8 12 14 15 16 17 19 20 22 24 28 30 32 33 34 37 39 40 41 44 49 51 62 64 65 71 73 **P**8	23	10	123	348	93	8901	47	3662	2149	49
SAC CITY—Sac County ★ LORING HOSPITAL, Highland Avenue, Zip 50583–0217; tel. 712/662–7105; Greg Miner, Administrator (Total facility includes 21 beds in nursing home–type unit) **A**9 10 **F**3 4 5 7 8 10 11 13 14 15 16 17 19 22 23 26 28 29 30 31 32 33 34 35 39 40 42 43 44 45 46 49 51 53 54 55 56 57 58 59 60 64 65 66 67 69 71 73 **S**0061 Iowa Health System	23	10	54	689	29	7897	30	2950	1590	76
SHELDON—Obrien County ★ NORTHWEST IOWA HEALTH CENTER, 118 North Seventh Avenue, Zip 51201; tel. 712/324–5041; Charles R. Miller, Chief Executive Officer (Total facility includes 70 beds in nursing home–type unit) **A**9 10 **F**3 8 16 17 18 19 20 22 26 28 30 32 33 34 35 36 39 40 41 42 44 45 46 49 53 54 55 56 57 58 65 66 67 71 73 **P**6	23	10	95	1011	78	21719	110	6303	2841	150
SHENANDOAH—Page County ★ SHENANDOAH MEMORIAL HOSPITAL, 300 Pershing Avenue, Zip 51601; tel. 712/246–1230; Charles L. Millburg CHE, Chief Executive Officer (Total facility includes 62 beds in nursing home–type unit) **A**9 10 **F**7 8 17 19 21 22 24 28 34 35 36 37 41 42 44 45 46 49 58 60 65 71 73	23	10	106	1029	73	16747	99	5665	2455	163
SIBLEY—Osceola County ★ OSCEOLA COMMUNITY HOSPITAL, Ninth Avenue North, Zip 51249–0258, Mailing Address: P.O. Box 258, Zip 51249–0258; tel. 712/754–2574; Janet Dykstra, Chief Executive Officer **A**10 **F**2 7 8 13 14 15 16 17 19 21 22 26 28 29 30 31 32 33 34 35 37 39 40 42 44 45 48 58 64 65 66 67 71	23	10	32	482	7	10242	72	2920	1430	68
SIGOURNEY—Keokuk County KEOKUK COUNTY HEALTH CENTER, 1312 South Stuart Street, Zip 52591–0286, Mailing Address: P.O. Box 286, Zip 52591–0286; tel. 515/622–2720; Douglas A. Sheetz, Chief Executive Officer **A**9 10 **F**15 16 19 22 30 44 71	13	10	33	137	15	5081	0	1619	839	42
SIOUX CENTER—Sioux County ★ SIOUX CENTER COMMUNITY HOSPITAL, 605 South Main Avenue, Zip 51250; tel. 712/722–1271; Timothy F. Weyers, Administrator (Total facility includes 69 beds in nursing home–type unit) **A**10 **F**7 8 11 15 19 21 22 28 30 32 33 34 35 39 40 41 44 49 64 65 66 71	23	10	90	517	83	22284	200	4851	2424	159
SIOUX CITY—Woodbury County ★ △ MARIAN HEALTH CENTER, (Includes Marian Behavioral Health Center, 4301 Sergeant Road, Sioux City, Iowa, Zip 51106; tel. 712/279–2446; St. Vincent Hospital, 624 Jones Street, Sioux City, Iowa, Zip 51105, Mailing Address: Box 3168, Zip 51102; tel. 712/279–2010) 801 Fifth Street, Zip 51101, Mailing Address: Box 3168, Zip 51102; tel. 712/279–2010; Douglas V. Johnson, President **A**1 2 3 5 7 9 10 **F**1 2 3 4 7 8 10 11 12 13 15 16 17 19 21 22 23 25 26 27 28 29 31 33 34 35 36 37 39 40 41 42 43 44 45 46 48 49 51 52 53 54 55 56 57 58 59 60 65 67 70 71 72 73 **P**4 5 8 **S**5165 Mercy Health Services	21	10	328	10539	188	226412	775	110933	43221	1444
★ ST. LUKE'S REGIONAL MEDICAL CENTER, 2720 Stone Park Boulevard, Zip 51104–2000; tel. 712/279–3500; David O. Biorn FACHE, President and Chief Executive Officer (Total facility includes 25 beds in nursing home–type unit) **A**1 2 3 5 6 10 **F**1 2 3 6 7 8 9 10 11 12 17 19 20 21 22 23 24 26 27 29 30 32 33 34 35 36 37 38 39 40 41 44 47 49 52 54 56 59 60 62 63 64 65 67 71 73 **P**1 **S**5845 St. Luke's Health System, Inc.	23	10	242	10611	145	87925	1677	73412	29155	1199
SPENCER—Clay County ★ SPENCER MUNICIPAL HOSPITAL, 1200 First Avenue East, Zip 51301–4330; tel. 712/264–6198; James L. Striepe, Administrator (Total facility includes 21 beds in nursing home–type unit) **A**10 **F**3 7 8 11 12 15 16 17 19 20 21 27 35 40 44 46 49 52 54 56 57 61 63 64 65 66 67 71 73	14	10	95	2812	42	22661	234	17167	7997	323

© 1995 AHA Guide

Hospitals, U.S. / IOWA

Hospital, Address, Telephone, Administrator, Approval, Facility, and Physician Codes, Health Care System	Classification Codes		Utilization Data					Expense (thousands) of dollars		
★ American Hospital Association (AHA) membership □ Joint Commission on Accreditation of Healthcare Organizations (JCAHO) accreditation + American Osteopathic Hospital Association (AOHA) membership ○ American Osteopathic Association (AOA) accreditation △ Commission on Accreditation of Rehabilitation Facilities (CARF) accreditation Control codes 61, 63, 64, 71, 72 and 73 indicate hospitals listed by AOHA, but not registered by AHA. For definition of numerical codes, see page A6	Control	Service	Beds	Admissions	Census	Outpatient Visits	Births	Total	Payroll	Personnel
SPIRIT LAKE—Dickinson County										
□ DICKINSON COUNTY MEMORIAL HOSPITAL, Highway 71 South, Zip 51360, Mailing Address: Box AB, Zip 51360; tel. 712/336–1230; Richard C. Kielman, President and Chief Executive Officer **A**1 10 **F**8 14 15 16 22 27 30 31 37 40 42 44 46 48 64 65 67 71 73 **P**5	13	10	49	1593	18	20099	136	7988	3567	145
STORM LAKE—Buena Vista County										
★ BUENA VISTA COUNTY HOSPITAL, 1525 West Fifth Street, Zip 50588–0309; tel. 712/732–4030; James O. Nelson, Administrator **A**1 10 **F**1 3 11 12 14 15 16 19 22 24 28 30 32 33 34 35 36 37 40 42 44 49 65 67 71 **P**3	13	10	31	1585	18	22364	316	9325	4613	274
STORY CITY—Story County										
★ STORY CITY MEMORIAL HOSPITAL, 812 Elm Street, Zip 50248–1310; tel. 515/733–5121; James Mullen, Administrator **A**9 10 **F**7 15 19 21 22 32 34 36 40 44 49 51 65 71	14	10	36	232	14	6000	24	1862	900	55
SUMNER—Bremer County										
COMMUNITY MEMORIAL HOSPITAL, 909 West First Street, Zip 50674, Mailing Address: Box 148, Zip 50674–0148; tel. 319/578–3275; Scott Knode, Associate Administrator, General Services **A**9 10 **F**7 8 19 21 22 26 32 33 34 36 39 40 41 42 44 54 65 69 71	23	10	29	434	5	11556	29	2698	1215	52
VINTON—Benton County										
★ VIRGINIA GAY HOSPITAL, 502 North Ninth Avenue, Zip 52349; tel. 319/472–2348; Michael J. Riege, Administrator (Total facility includes 58 beds in nursing home–type unit) **A**9 10 **F**8 10 14 15 16 17 19 22 26 27 28 29 30 31 32 33 34 35 39 41 42 44 45 49 51 53 54 55 56 57 58 59 60 65 71 73 **P**3 **S**0061 Iowa Health System	23	10	87	324	63	12065	0	4573	1520	74
WASHINGTON—Washington County										
★ WASHINGTON COUNTY HOSPITAL, 400 East Polk Street, Zip 52353, Mailing Address: P.O. Box 909, Zip 52353; tel. 319/653–5481; E. Patrick Smith III, Administrator (Total facility includes 43 beds in nursing home–type unit) **A**9 10 **F**7 8 11 12 15 19 22 28 30 34 36 40 44 45 49 65 71 73 **S**0002 Quorum Health Group/Quorum Health Resources	13	10	83	1354	59	29279	148	7973	3794	147
WATERLOO—Black Hawk County										
★ ALLEN MEMORIAL HOSPITAL, 1825 Logan Avenue, Zip 50703; tel. 319/235–3941; Larry W. Pugh, President and Chief Executive Officer (Total facility includes 20 beds in nursing home–type unit) **A**1 3 5 6 9 10 **F**3 4 7 8 10 14 15 16 17 19 21 22 23 24 25 26 28 30 31 32 33 34 35 37 40 41 42 43 44 45 46 49 51 52 53 54 55 56 57 58 59 60 64 65 67 68 71 73 74 **P**4	23	10	194	8405	134	186076	826	60705	26968	938
★ △ COVENANT MEDICAL CENTER, (Includes Kimball–Ridge Center, 2101 Kimball Avenue, Waterloo, Iowa, Zip 50702) 3421 West Ninth Street, Zip 50702–5499; tel. 319/236–4111; Raymond F. Burfeind, President (Total facility includes 44 beds in nursing home–type unit) **A**1 3 5 7 9 10 **F**2 3 4 6 7 8 12 15 16 17 18 19 20 21 22 23 24 26 27 28 29 30 31 32 33 34 35 37 38 39 40 41 42 44 45 48 49 51 52 53 54 55 56 57 58 59 60 62 63 64 65 66 67 70 71 73 74 **P**6 7 8 **S**6745 Wheaton Franciscan Services, Inc.	21	10	346	11033	174	239811	1517	82750	37504	1369
WAUKON—Allamakee County										
□ VETERANS MEMORIAL HOSPITAL, 40 First Street S.E., Zip 52172–2099; tel. 319/568–3411; Daniel J. Woods, Administrator **A**1 9 10 **F**7 8 14 15 16 17 19 22 24 26 28 29 30 33 40 44 49 66 67 68 71 72	14	10	25	709	8	14523	49	3213	1590	87
WAVERLY—Bremer County										
★ WAVERLY MUNICIPAL HOSPITAL, 312 Ninth Street S.W., Zip 50677; tel. 319/352–4120; Arnold Flessner, Administrator **A**1 9 10 **F**7 8 14 15 22 24 32 33 34 41 44 49 65 71	14	10	38	1094	13	14819	115	5998	2738	114
WEBSTER CITY—Hamilton County										
□ HAMILTON COUNTY PUBLIC HOSPITAL, 800 Ohio Street, Zip 50595; tel. 515/832–9400; Roger W. Lenz, Administrator **A**1 9 10 **F**7 8 19 22 28 35 36 39 40 44 49 65 71 73	13	10	40	2106	23	15502	152	9642	4926	192
WEST UNION—Fayette County										
★ PALMER LUTHERAN HEALTH CENTER, 112 Jefferson Street, Zip 52175–1064; tel. 319/422–3811; Jeanine Matt, President **A**1 9 10 **F**3 7 8 10 12 15 17 18 19 20 21 22 24 28 30 32 33 34 35 39 40 42 44 46 49 53 54 56 57 59 60 61 62 63 65 66 67 68 71 73 74 **P**3	23	10	30	1034	11	49464	139	6245	2674	128
WINTERSET—Madison County										
MADISON COUNTY MEMORIAL HOSPITAL, 300 Hutchings Street, Zip 50273–2199; tel. 515/462–2373; Robert Young, Administrator **A**9 10 **F**3 8 12 17 19 22 26 30 31 32 34 35 37 39 41 42 44 45 48 49 51 65 66 67 68 71 73 **P**6	13	10	31	628	12	31119	0	4290	1587	76
WOODWARD—Dallas County										
WOODWARD STATE HOSPITAL–SCHOOL, Zip 50276–9999; tel. 515/438–2600; Michael J. Davis Ph.D., Superintendent **F**4 5 8 9 10 11 19 20 21 22 23 27 31 35 37 39 41 42 43 44 47 50 52 53 54 55 56 57 58 60 63 65 70 71 73	12	62	306	24	327	0	0	31444	22010	759

Hospitals, U.S. / KANSAS

KANSAS

Resident population 2,531 (in thousands)
Resident population in metro areas 54.6%
Birth rate per 1,000 population 15.2
65 years and over 13.9%
Percent of persons without health insurance 11.0%

★ American Hospital Association (AHA) membership
☐ Joint Commission on Accreditation of Healthcare Organizations (JCAHO) accreditation
+ American Osteopathic Hospital Association (AOHA) membership
○ American Osteopathic Association (AOA) accreditation
△ Commission on Accreditation of Rehabilitation Facilities (CARF) accreditation
Control codes 61, 63, 64, 71, 72 and 73 indicate hospitals listed by AOHA, but not registered by AHA. For definition of numerical codes, see page A6

Hospital, Address, Telephone, Administrator, Approval, Facility, and Physician Codes, Health Care System	Classification Codes		Utilization Data					Expense (thousands) of dollars		
	Control	Service	Beds	Admissions	Census	Outpatient Visits	Births	Total	Payroll	Personnel
ABILENE—Dickinson County ✦ MEMORIAL HOSPITAL, 511 Northeast Tenth Street, Zip 67410, Mailing Address: P.O. Box 219, Zip 67410-0219; tel. 913/263-2100; Leon J. Boor, Chief Executive Officer **A**1 9 10 **F**7 8 15 19 22 30 32 33 34 36 39 40 42 44 49 64 65 71 73	16	10	30	842	11	10853	65	5214	2502	107
ANTHONY—Harper County HOSPITAL DISTRICT NUMBER SIX OF HARPER COUNTY, 1101 East Spring Street, Zip 67003; tel. 316/842-5111; Cindy McCray, Administrator (Total facility includes 15 beds in nursing home-type unit) **A**9 10 **F**8 22 30 33 34 42 44 51 61 64 65 71 **P**6	16	10	37	392	17	—	0	3562	1667	72
ARKANSAS CITY—Cowley County ✦ ARKANSAS CITY MEMORIAL HOSPITAL, 216 West Birch Avenue, Zip 67005, Mailing Address: P.O. Box 1107, Zip 67005; tel. 316/442-2500; Webster Russell, Chief Executive Officer (Total facility includes 10 beds in nursing home-type unit) **A**1 9 10 **F**7 8 11 14 15 16 17 19 22 29 32 34 35 36 37 39 40 42 44 46 48 64 71 73	14	10	70	1474	21	62754	184	7824	3655	171
ASHLAND—Clark County ★ ASHLAND DISTRICT HOSPITAL, 709 Oak Street, Zip 67831, Mailing Address: P.O. Box 188, Zip 67831; tel. 316/635-2241; Leanne Pike, Administrator (Total facility includes 36 beds in nursing home-type unit) **A**9 10 **F**1 8 20 22 27 33 34 41 44 46 49 54 56 58 65 71 **S**1535 Great Plains Health Alliance, Inc.	16	10	52	89	34	3622	0	1626	838	48
ATCHISON—Atchison County ✦ ATCHISON HOSPITAL, 1301 North Second Street, Zip 66002; tel. 913/367-2131; Edward M. Hackman Ph.D., President and Chief Executive Officer (Total facility includes 59 beds in nursing home-type unit) **A**1 9 10 **F**7 8 15 16 17 19 21 22 23 27 28 30 32 33 34 35 37 40 44 46 48 49 51 54 64 65 66 67 71 73 **P**4 7	23	10	131	2468	60	40032	201	13783	6716	269
ATWOOD—Rawlins County RAWLINS COUNTY HOSPITAL, 707 Grant Street, Zip 67730-4700, Mailing Address: Box 47, Zip 67730-4700; tel. 913/626-3211; Donald J. Kessen, Administrator **A**9 10 **F**3 7 8 14 15 16 17 19 20 22 26 30 31 32 34 35 44 49 65 71	13	10	24	162	2	6571	6	1477	732	38
AUGUSTA—Butler County AUGUSTA MEDICAL COMPLEX, 2101 Dearborn Street, Zip 67010-0430, Mailing Address: Box 430, Zip 67010-0430; tel. 316/775-5421; Larry D. Wilkerson, Chief Executive Officer (Total facility includes 107 beds in nursing home-type unit) **A**9 10 **F**2 3 8 14 19 21 22 27 28 30 32 33 34 41 42 44 49 64 65 67 71	23	10	147	415	98	—	0	5913	2839	166
BELLEVILLE—Republic County ✦ REPUBLIC COUNTY HOSPITAL, 2420 G Street, Zip 66935; tel. 913/527-2255; Charles A. Westin FACHE, Administrator (Total facility includes 38 beds in nursing home-type unit) **A**1 9 10 **F**1 7 17 19 20 22 26 34 42 44 45 49 65 71 **S**1535 Great Plains Health Alliance, Inc.	23	10	86	1093	53	5303	84	5441	2473	129
BELOIT—Mitchell County ✦ MITCHELL COUNTY COMMUNITY HOSPITAL, 400 West Eighth, Zip 67420, Mailing Address: P.O. Box 399, Zip 67420; tel. 913/738-2266; Jeffrey S. Tarrant, Administrator (Total facility includes 40 beds in nursing home-type unit) **A**1 9 10 **F**7 8 17 19 20 22 24 26 32 33 34 35 36 41 44 45 49 65 71 **S**1535 Great Plains Health Alliance, Inc.	23	10	89	1512	61	13240	88	7359	3647	144
BURLINGTON—Coffey County COFFEY COUNTY HOSPITAL, 801 North Fourth Street, Zip 66839, Mailing Address: Box 189, Zip 66839-0189; tel. 316/364-2121; Dennis L. George, Administrator **A**9 10 **F**7 8 11 15 19 22 25 28 32 34 37 40 41 44 62 64 71 73 **P**6	13	10	20	543	6	7123	32	6642	3451	116
CALDWELL—Sumner County ★ SUMNER COUNTY HOSPITAL DISTRICT ONE, 601 South Osage Street, Zip 67022; tel. 316/845-6492; Jeffrey R. Lebeda, Administrator **A**9 10 **F**8 22 33 34 44 71	16	10	27	225	3	4336	0	1530	795	34
CEDAR VALE—Chautauqua County CEDAR VALE REGIONAL HOSPITAL, 501 Cedar Street, Zip 67024, Mailing Address: Box 398, Zip 67024; tel. 316/758-2266; Judy Curry, Administrator (Nonreporting) **A**9 10	23	10	35	—	—	—	—	—	—	—
CHANUTE—Neosho County ✦ NEOSHO MEMORIAL REGIONAL MEDICAL CENTER, 629 South Plummer, Zip 66720; tel. 316/431-4000; Murray L. Brown, Administrator **A**1 9 10 **F**7 8 15 19 20 21 22 23 27 28 32 33 34 35 37 40 44 49 65 67 71 **S**0002 Quorum Health Group/Quorum Health Resources	13	10	60	2578	35	13188	283	11256	5070	213
CLAY CENTER—Clay County ★ CLAY COUNTY HOSPITAL, 617 Liberty Street, Zip 67432; tel. 913/632-2144; John F. Wiebe, Chief Executive Officer **A**9 10 **F**8 15 19 22 28 33 34 39 44 45 49 65 67 71	13	10	35	834	10	16707	70	4932	2083	101
COFFEYVILLE—Montgomery County ✦ COFFEYVILLE REGIONAL MEDICAL CENTER, 1400 West Fourth, Zip 67337-3306; tel. 316/251-1200; Jerry Marquette Jr., Administrator (Total facility includes 33 beds in nursing home-type unit) **A**1 2 9 10 **F**3 8 14 15 16 19 21 22 27 28 30 31 32 33 34 35 37 40 42 44 49 52 53 57 58 60 64 65 71 73 74 **P**8 **S**0002 Quorum Health Group/Quorum Health Resources	14	10	123	3343	69	16329	235	17194	8230	343

© 1995 AHA Guide

Hospitals, U.S. / KANSAS

Hospital, Address, Telephone, Administrator, Approval, Facility, and Physician Codes, Health Care System ★ American Hospital Association (AHA) membership □ Joint Commission on Accreditation of Healthcare Organizations (JCAHO) accreditation + American Osteopathic Hospital Association (AOHA) membership ○ American Osteopathic Association (AOA) accreditation △ Commission on Accreditation of Rehabilitation Facilities (CARF) accreditation Control codes 61, 63, 64, 71, 72 and 73 indicate hospitals listed by AOHA, but not registered by AHA. For definition of numerical codes, see page A6	Classification Codes		Utilization Data					Expense (thousands) of dollars		
	Control	Service	Beds	Admissions	Census	Outpatient Visits	Births	Total	Payroll	Personnel
COLBY—Thomas County										
□ CITIZENS MEDICAL CENTER, 100 East College Drive, Zip 67701–3912; tel. 913/462–7511; Kevan Trenkle, Interim Chief Executive Officer **A**1 9 10 **F**7 8 11 19 21 22 29 32 33 34 36 37 40 42 44 45 46 49 51 64 65 67 71 73 **P**6	23	10	40	815	10	8090	124	6039	2522	114
COLDWATER—Comanche County										
COMANCHE COUNTY HOSPITAL, Second and Frisco Streets, Zip 67029, Mailing Address: HC 65, Box 8A, Zip 67029; tel. 316/582–2144; Nancy Zimmerman, Administrator **A**9 10 **F**8 20 22 24 28 29 30 31 40 41 42 44 49 56 64 70 71	13	10	14	236	3	2744	17	1218	526	30
COLUMBUS—Cherokee County										
★ MAUDE NORTON MEMORIAL CITY HOSPITAL, 220 North Pennsylvania Street, Zip 66725–1197; tel. 316/429–2545; Jim Robertson Jr. CHE, Administrator **A**9 10 **F**8 17 19 22 28 29 30 31 32 34 36 41 44 45 46 49 65 69 71 73	14	10	39	273	4	7463	0	2349	1160	49
CONCORDIA—Cloud County										
★ ST. JOSEPH HOSPITAL, 1100 Highland Drive, Zip 66901–3997; tel. 913/243–8500; Daniel R. Bartz, Acting Administrator **A**1 9 10 **F**8 15 16 17 19 20 21 22 26 27 28 30 31 33 34 36 37 39 41 44 45 46 49 50 51 53 54 55 56 57 58 59 64 65 67 70 71 73 **S**5435 CSJ Health System of Wichita	21	10	57	1595	30	27483	0	8119	3966	150
COUNCIL GROVE—Morris County										
MORRIS COUNTY HOSPITAL, 600 North Washington Street, Zip 66846, Mailing Address: P.O. Box 275, Zip 66846; tel. 316/767–6811; Gary L. Tiller, Administrator **A**9 10 **F**1 7 8 11 13 15 16 17 22 26 28 30 31 32 33 34 39 40 42 44 48 49 67 71 73	13	10	29	660	7	9938	91	3286	1523	78
DIGHTON—Lane County										
★ LANE COUNTY HOSPITAL, 243 South Second, Zip 67839, Mailing Address: Box 969, Zip 67839; tel. 316/397–5321; Donna McGowan R.N., Administrator (Total facility includes 21 beds in nursing home-type unit) **A**9 10 **F**1 8 15 19 22 26 28 34 35 41 49 65 71 **S**1535 Great Plains Health Alliance, Inc.	13	10	31	196	20	3231	0	1533	745	45
DODGE CITY—Ford County										
★ WESTERN PLAINS REGIONAL HOSPITAL, 3001 Avenue A, Zip 67801, Mailing Address: Box 1478, Zip 67801; tel. 316/225–8401; Greg J. Simmons, Interim President and Chief Executive Officer **A**1 9 10 **F**8 12 14 15 16 17 19 20 22 23 25 28 30 32 34 35 37 39 40 42 44 45 46 48 51 65 67 71 73 74 **S**0048 Columbia/HCA Healthcare Corporation	33	10	84	3245	37	15560	689	16323	6583	248
EL DORADO—Butler County										
★ SUSAN B. ALLEN MEMORIAL HOSPITAL, 720 West Central Avenue, Zip 67042–2144; tel. 316/321–3300; Jim Wilson, President (Total facility includes 23 beds in nursing home-type unit) **A**1 9 10 **F**7 8 19 21 22 23 24 26 28 32 36 37 39 40 44 52 57 64 65 71 73	23	10	87	1695	26	38189	172	13229	6512	205
ELKHART—Morton County										
★ MORTON COUNTY HOSPITAL, 445 Hilltop Street, Zip 67950–0937, Mailing Address: Box 937, Zip 67950–0937; tel. 316/697–2141; Glen Wood, Chief Executive Officer (Total facility includes 60 beds in nursing home-type unit) **A**9 10 **F**7 8 17 19 20 22 26 28 29 30 32 33 35 36 37 39 40 41 44 48 49 51 52 53 54 55 56 57 58 65 71 73 74 **P**6 8	13	10	100	957	75	7702	1	7591	3976	190
ELLINWOOD—Barton County										
★ ELLINWOOD DISTRICT HOSPITAL, 605 North Main Street, Zip 67526; tel. 316/564–2548; Marge Ney R.N., Administrator **A**9 **F**8 19 22 34 35 36 41 49 65 69 71 **S**1535 Great Plains Health Alliance, Inc.	23	10	24	239	13	4842	0	1408	660	31
ELLSWORTH—Ellsworth County										
ELLSWORTH COUNTY HOSPITAL, 300 Kingsley Street, Zip 67439, Mailing Address: Drawer 87, Zip 67439; tel. 913/472–3111; Roger W. Pearson, Administrator **A**9 10 **F**19 21 28 41 45 49 64 65 71	13	10	22	592	9	6834	0	2292	1084	57
★ ST. FRANCIS AT ELLSWORTH, 1655 Avenue K, Zip 67439, Mailing Address: 509 East Elm, Salina Zip 67401; tel. 913/825–0541; Reverend Phillip J. Rapp, President and Chief Executive Officer (Nonreporting)	23	52	26	—		—				—
EMPORIA—Lyon County										
★ NEWMAN MEMORIAL HOSPITAL, 1201 West 12th Avenue, Zip 66801–2597; tel. 316/343–6800; David Christiansen, Chief Executive Officer (Total facility includes 18 beds in nursing home-type unit) **A**1 9 10 **F**3 7 8 11 14 15 16 19 21 22 23 30 31 32 33 34 35 36 37 40 42 44 45 46 49 64 65 67 71 **S**0002 Quorum Health Group/Quorum Health Resources	13	10	152	3609	50	42117	572	22705	10618	381
EUREKA—Greenwood County										
★ GREENWOOD COUNTY HOSPITAL, 100 West 16th Street, Zip 67045; tel. 316/583–7451; Jerry Aldridge, Administrator **A**9 10 **F**7 8 15 17 19 20 22 24 26 31 32 33 34 41 44 49 56 65 71 **S**1535 Great Plains Health Alliance, Inc.	23	10	46	867	16	7819	0	4781	2194	103
FORT LEAVENWORTH—Leavenworth County										
★ MUNSON ARMY COMMUNITY HOSPITAL, Pope and Biddle Avenue, Zip 66027–5400; tel. 913/684–6420; Colonel Arthur Hadley MSC, USA, Executive Officer **A**1 9 **F**3 7 8 11 15 19 20 22 24 31 34 35 37 39 40 44 46 47 51 52 54 55 56 58 65 70 71 73 74 **P**6 **S**9395 Department of the Army	42	10	20	1373	8	161368	0	26100	—	371
FORT RILEY—Geary County										
★ IRWIN ARMY COMMUNITY HOSPITAL, Building 600, Zip 66442; tel. 913/239–7101; Colonel James W. Kirkpatrick, Commanding Officer **A**1 2 9 **F**3 8 11 12 14 15 16 18 19 20 21 22 28 30 31 34 35 37 39 40 41 42 44 45 46 49 51 52 53 54 56 58 65 67 71 73 74 **S**9395 Department of the Army	42	10	97	6909	43	368866	1166	58692	40224	988

Hospitals, U.S. / KANSAS

	Classification Codes		Utilization Data					Expense (thousands) of dollars		
Hospital, Address, Telephone, Administrator, Approval, Facility, and Physician Codes, Health Care System	Control	Service	Beds	Admissions	Census	Outpatient Visits	Births	Total	Payroll	Personnel
FORT SCOTT—Bourbon County ★ MERCY HOSPITALS OF KANSAS, 821 Burke Street, Zip 66701; tel. 316/223–2200; Susan Barrett, President and Chief Executive Officer (Total facility includes 23 beds in nursing home–type unit) **A**1 9 10 **F**7 8 12 15 16 17 19 21 22 23 24 27 28 30 32 33 34 35 37 38 39 40 41 44 48 49 51 64 65 67 71 73 **P**8 **S**5185 Sisters of Mercy Health System–St. Louis	21	10	105	3919	58	27982	280	19378	8736	376
FREDONIA—Wilson County ★ FREDONIA REGIONAL HOSPITAL, 1527 Madison Street, Zip 66736, Mailing Address: Box 579, Zip 66736; tel. 316/378–2121; Terry Deschaine, Administrator **A**9 10 **F**8 14 19 22 32 44 49 58 65 71 **S**1535 Great Plains Health Alliance, Inc.	14	10	42	471	9	12752	0	3304	1532	73
GARDEN CITY—Finney County ★ ST. CATHERINE HOSPITAL, 410 East Walnut, Zip 67846–5672; tel. 316/272–2222; Steven D. Wilkinson, President and Chief Executive Officer **A**1 9 10 **F**7 8 14 15 16 17 19 20 21 22 23 26 28 30 31 33 34 35 36 37 38 39 40 41 42 44 46 49 52 54 55 56 57 58 60 65 69 71 73 **S**5175 Catholic Health Corporation	21	10	99	4615	62	35311	982	27723	11864	434
GARDNER—Johnson County △ MEADOWBROOK HOSPITAL, 427 West Main Street, Zip 66030; tel. 913/884–8711; James H. Brown, Administrator (Total facility includes 21 beds in nursing home–type unit) **A**7 9 10 **F**12 14 19 20 27 35 48 49 54 64 65 67 71 73	33	46	84	229	32	216	0	6895	3120	101
GARNETT—Anderson County ANDERSON COUNTY HOSPITAL, 421 South Maple, Zip 66032, Mailing Address: Box 309, Zip 66032; tel. 913/448–3131; James K. Johnson, Administrator (Total facility includes 32 beds in nursing home–type unit) **A**9 10 **F**8 11 19 22 26 28 32 33 34 35 40 44 49 54 58 65 71	13	10	66	506	39	10615	29	2846	1487	80
GIRARD—Crawford County ★ CRAWFORD COUNTY HOSPITAL DISTRICT ONE, 302 North Hospital Drive, Zip 66743–2000; tel. 316/724–8291; Jerry Hanson, Administrator **A**9 10 **F**7 8 11 19 22 32 37 40 44 49 51 63 71 73	16	10	38	901	9	15928	0	6530	2910	111
GOODLAND—Sherman County NORTHWEST KANSAS REGIONAL MEDICAL CENTER, 220 West Second Street, Zip 67735–0661; tel. 913/899–3625; Jim Chaddic, Chief Executive Officer **A**9 10 **F**3 8 10 11 14 15 16 19 20 21 22 26 28 31 33 34 36 37 39 40 42 44 48 49 58 64 65 67 70 71 73	13	10	49	1152	24	30483	82	4997	2079	99
GREAT BEND—Barton County ★ CENTRAL KANSAS MEDICAL CENTER, (Includes Central Kansas Medical Center–St. Joseph Campus, 923 Carroll Avenue, Larned, Kansas, Zip 67550; tel. 316/285–3161) 3515 Broadway Street, Zip 67530; tel. 316/792–2511; Gary L. Barnett, President and Chief Executive Officer **A**1 9 10 **F**2 3 7 8 15 19 21 22 23 28 32 33 34 35 36 37 39 40 41 42 44 45 49 60 64 65 67 71 73 **S**5175 Catholic Health Corporation	23	10	121	3353	61	121845	404	26480	12182	487
GREENSBURG—Kiowa County ★ KIOWA COUNTY MEMORIAL HOSPITAL, 501 South Walnut Street, Zip 67054; tel. 316/723–3341; Larry V. Gales, Administrator **A**9 10 **F**1 7 15 22 24 32 36 39 40 44 49 64	13	10	38	404	15	6773	23	2996	1538	90
HALSTEAD—Harvey County ★ HALSTEAD HOSPITAL, (Formerly Paracelsus Halstead Hospital) 328 Poplar Street, Zip 67056–2099; tel. 316/835–2651; Jeffrey A. Feeney, President and Chief Executive Officer (Total facility includes 17 beds in nursing home–type unit) **A**1 9 10 **F**4 8 10 11 12 13 14 15 16 17 19 20 21 22 23 24 27 28 29 30 32 33 34 35 36 37 39 41 42 43 44 45 46 49 51 52 54 55 56 57 58 61 63 64 65 67 70 71 72 73 74 **S**5765 Paracelsus Healthcare Corporation	33	10	137	3542	66	22428	0	24874	9951	359
HANOVER—Washington County HANOVER HOSPITAL, (Formerly Washington County Hospital, District 1) 205 South Hanover, Zip 66945, Mailing Address: Box 38, Zip 66945; tel. 913/337–2214; Roger D. Warren M.D., Administrator (Total facility includes 32 beds in nursing home–type unit) **A**9 10 **F**14 28 32 36 44 49 51 70 71	16	10	48	328	25	1071	19	1543	803	61
HARPER—Harper County ★ HOSPITAL DISTRICT NUMBER FIVE OF HARPER COUNTY, 1204 Maple, Zip 67058–1438; tel. 316/896–7324; Vernon Minnis, Administrator **A**9 10 **F**8 12 14 17 19 22 28 32 33 34 36 37 44 49 65 71 73	16	10	30	385	19	3863	1	2674	1321	71
HAYS—Ellis County ★ HAYS MEDICAL CENTER, (Includes Hays Medical Center, 201 East Seventh Street, Hays, Kansas, Zip 67601–4198; tel. 913/623–5000; St. Anthony Hospital, 2220 Canterbury Drive, Zip 67601–2542, Mailing Address: P.O. Box 660, Zip 67601; tel. 913/623–5000) 2220 Canterbury Drive, Zip 67601–2323, Mailing Address: P.O. Box 660, Zip 67601; tel. 913/623–5113; Stephen F. Ronstrom, President and Chief Executive Officer **A**1 2 9 10 **F**7 8 14 15 16 17 19 21 22 26 28 30 32 33 34 35 36 37 38 39 40 41 42 44 46 48 49 51 52 53 54 55 56 57 58 60 64 65 70 71 73 **P**6	23	10	147	4814	81	45494	487	36421	15241	642
HERINGTON—Dickinson County HERINGTON MUNICIPAL HOSPITAL, 100 East Helen Street, Zip 67449; tel. 913/258–2207; William D. Peterson, Administrator (Total facility includes 18 beds in nursing home–type unit) **A**9 10 **F**7 8 11 14 15 16 19 20 22 26 28 32 33 35 40 44 64 71 **P**5	14	10	38	570	14	16306	26	3183	1468	76

© 1995 AHA Guide

Hospitals, U.S. / KANSAS

Hospital, Address, Telephone, Administrator, Approval, Facility, and Physician Codes, Health Care System ★ American Hospital Association (AHA) membership □ Joint Commission on Accreditation of Healthcare Organizations (JCAHO) accreditation + American Osteopathic Hospital Association (AOHA) membership ○ American Osteopathic Association (AOA) accreditation △ Commission on Accreditation of Rehabilitation Facilities (CARF) accreditation Control codes 61, 63, 64, 71, 72 and 73 indicate hospitals listed by AOHA, but not registered by AHA. For definition of numerical codes, see page A6	Classification Codes		Utilization Data					Expense (thousands) of dollars		
	Control	Service	Beds	Admissions	Census	Outpatient Visits	Births	Total	Payroll	Personnel
HIAWATHA—Brown County ★ HIAWATHA COMMUNITY HOSPITAL, 300 Utah Street, Zip 66434; tel. 913/742–2131; J. Michael Frost, Administrator **A** 1 9 10 **F** 3 7 8 14 19 20 22 28 30 32 34 35 36 37 39 40 41 44 49 56 64 65 71 73 74 **P** 8 **S** 0805 Stormont-Vail Health Services Corporation	23	10	29	876	13	24249	87	5868	2621	111
HILL CITY—Graham County ★ GRAHAM COUNTY HOSPITAL, 304 West Prout Street, Zip 67642, Mailing Address: P.O. Box 339, Zip 67642; tel. 913/674–2121; Fred J. Meis, Administrator **A** 9 10 **F** 8 16 22 28 32 33 34 36 44 65 71	13	10	27	805	12	8312	13	3334	1729	84
HILLSBORO—Marion County ★ SALEM HOSPITAL, 701 South Main Street, Zip 67063-9981; tel. 316/947–3114; Ron Thompson, Chief Executive Officer (Total facility includes 60 beds in nursing home–type unit) **A** 9 10 **F** 7 8 15 16 19 22 26 32 33 34 40 41 44 48 49 57 62 65 67 71 **P** 5	21	10	86	432	61	5243	34	4430	2207	131
HOISINGTON—Barton County CLARA BARTON HOSPTIAL, 250 West Ninth Street, Zip 67544; tel. 316/653–2114; James Turnbull, Administrator (Total facility includes 12 beds in nursing home–type unit) **A** 9 10 **F** 2 3 7 8 15 19 20 22 23 24 34 35 36 37 40 44 49 64 71 73	23	10	48	625	14	10440	169	3208	1489	73
HOLTON—Jackson County HOLTON COMMUNITY HOSPITAL, 510 Kansas Avenue, Zip 66436; tel. 913/364–2116; Diane S. Gross, Administrator **A** 9 10 **F** 1 7 8 11 13 15 17 19 22 27 29 30 32 33 34 36 39 40 41 44 45 46 49 64 65 66 68 71 73 **P** 8	14	10	15	379	5	15793	27	2068	1083	55
HORTON—Brown County HORTON COMMUNITY HOSPITAL, 240 West 18th Street, Zip 66439, Mailing Address: P.O. Box 191, Zip 66439; tel. 913/486–2642; Robert Beauvais, Administrator **A** 9 10 **F** 3 19 32 36 41 44 54 56 71	23	10	35	409	18	7961	0	2803	1371	92
HOXIE—Sheridan County SHERIDAN COUNTY HOSPITAL, 826 18th Street, Zip 67740-0167, Mailing Address: P.O. Box 167, Zip 67740-0167; tel. 913/675–3281; Joy Bretz, Administrator (Total facility includes 40 beds in nursing home–type unit) **A** 9 10 **F** 1 19 22 26 32 33 34 36 39 40 44 65 71	13	10	59	323	46	6409	11	2554	1409	95
HUGOTON—Stevens County ★ STEVENS COUNTY HOSPITAL, 1006 South Jackson Street, Zip 67951, Mailing Address: Box 10, Zip 67951; tel. 316/544–8511; P. Greg McGee, Administrator **A** 9 10 **F** 8 15 19 22 24 28 29 30 32 34 44 45 49 64 65 67 71	13	10	17	503	2	7333	0	3530	1501	63
HUTCHINSON—Reno County ★ HUTCHINSON HOSPITAL CORPORATION, 1701 East 23rd Street, Zip 67502-1191; tel. 316/665–2000; Gene E. Schmidt, President (Total facility includes 18 beds in nursing home–type unit) **A** 1 9 10 **F** 3 6 7 10 18 19 21 22 32 33 34 37 40 41 42 44 49 52 53 54 55 56 57 58 59 60 62 64 65 67 68 71 73	23	10	160	6792	114	90780	646	38487	16615	663
INDEPENDENCE—Montgomery County ★ MERCY HOSPITALS OF KANSAS, 800 West Myrtle Street, Zip 67301, Mailing Address: Box 388, Zip 67301-0388; tel. 316/331–2200; Susan Barrett, President and Chief Executive Officer (Total facility includes 18 beds in nursing home–type unit) **A** 1 9 10 **F** 7 8 12 16 19 21 22 27 28 30 31 32 33 35 37 40 44 49 64 69 71 73 **P** 1 **S** 5185 Sisters of Mercy Health System–St. Louis	21	10	58	2410	35	43881	187	13760	5564	216
IOLA—Allen County ★ ALLEN COUNTY HOSPITAL, 101 South First Street, Zip 66749, Mailing Address: P.O. Box 540, Zip 66749-0540; tel. 316/365–3131; Franklin K. Wilson, Administrator **A** 1 9 10 **F** 19 21 22 28 30 31 32 37 40 42 44 64 65 71 72 73 **S** 8815 Health Midwest	23	10	49	1241	15	18713	89	—	—	—
JETMORE—Hodgeman County ★ HODGEMAN COUNTY HEALTH CENTER, 809 Bramley, Zip 67854, Mailing Address: P.O. Box 367, Zip 67854; tel. 316/357–8361; Roger Salisbury, Administrator (Total facility includes 36 beds in nursing home–type unit) **A** 9 10 **F** 7 8 12 14 15 16 19 20 26 33 35 40 44 45 49 51 64 65 71	13	10	52	297	40	2064	18	2585	1310	43
JOHNSON—Stanton County ★ STANTON COUNTY HOSPITAL AND LONG-TERM CARE UNIT, 404 North Chestnut Street, Zip 67855-0779, Mailing Address: Box 779, Zip 67855-0779; tel. 316/492–6250; Ed Finley, Administrator (Total facility includes 28 beds in nursing home–type unit) **A** 9 10 **F** 1 7 8 15 16 22 26 28 30 34 39 40 49 65 66 71	13	10	46	267	24	1704	112	2103	1120	60
JUNCTION CITY—Geary County ★ GEARY COMMUNITY HOSPITAL, Ash and St Mary's Road, Zip 66441, Mailing Address: Box 490, Zip 66441-0490; tel. 913/238–4131; Gaylon C. Lowery, Chief Executive Officer **A** 1 9 10 **F** 3 8 15 16 19 20 21 22 23 31 32 33 34 35 37 39 40 42 44 45 46 49 50 65 67 71 **P** 5	13	10	49	1587	18	56432	135	8580	4285	203
KANSAS CITY—Wyandotte County ★ △ BETHANY MEDICAL CENTER, 51 North 12th Street, Zip 66102-9990; tel. 913/281–8400; John L. Millard, President and Chief Executive Officer (Total facility includes 35 beds in nursing home–type unit) **A** 1 2 3 5 7 9 10 **F** 2 3 4 7 8 10 12 14 15 16 17 19 20 21 22 23 26 27 28 29 30 32 33 34 35 37 39 40 41 42 43 44 45 46 48 49 51 52 53 54 55 56 58 60 64 65 67 71 73 **P** 4 6	23	10	249	9097	156	78671	765	64189	29466	1033
★ PROVIDENCE MEDICAL CENTER, 8929 Parallel Parkway, Zip 66112-0430; tel. 913/596–4000; Sister Ann Marita Loosen, President and Chief Executive Officer (Total facility includes 26 beds in nursing home–type unit) **A** 1 2 9 10 **F** 4 7 8 10 15 16 17 18 19 20 21 22 26 27 28 29 30 31 32 33 34 35 37 39 40 41 42 43 44 45 46 49 52 53 54 55 56 57 58 59 60 63 64 65 66 67 71 73 74 **P** 1 4 5 6 7 8 **S** 5095 Sisters of Charity of Leavenworth Health Services Corporation	21	10	209	7965	141	42698	948	63389	26550	837

Hospitals, U.S. / KANSAS

Hospital, Address, Telephone, Administrator, Approval, Facility, and Physician Codes, Health Care System	Classification Codes		Utilization Data					Expense (thousands) of dollars		
★ American Hospital Association (AHA) membership ☐ Joint Commission on Accreditation of Healthcare Organizations (JCAHO) accreditation + American Osteopathic Hospital Association (AOHA) membership ○ American Osteopathic Association (AOA) accreditation △ Commission on Accreditation of Rehabilitation Facilities (CARF) accreditation Control codes 61, 63, 64, 71, 72 and 73 indicate hospitals listed by AOHA, but not registered by AHA. For definition of numerical codes, see page A6	Control	Service	Beds	Admissions	Census	Outpatient Visits	Births	Total	Payroll	Personnel
★ △ UNIVERSITY OF KANSAS HOSPITAL, 3901 Rainbow Boulevard, Zip 66160–7200; tel. 913/588–1270; Glenn E. Potter, Vice Chancellor **A**1 2 3 5 7 8 9 10 **F**3 4 5 7 8 9 10 11 17 19 21 22 23 24 26 28 29 30 31 32 33 34 35 37 38 39 40 41 42 43 44 46 47 48 49 51 52 53 54 55 56 57 58 60 61 63 65 66 67 69 70 71 73 74 **P**1 3	12	10	456	14402	289	368809	1083	176796	93270	2676
KINGMAN—Kingman County										
★ KINGMAN COMMUNITY HOSPITAL, 750 Avenue D West, Zip 67068; tel. 316/532–3147; Sam J. Allen, Chief Executive Officer **A**9 10 **F**7 8 12 14 15 16 17 19 22 25 27 28 30 32 36 40 42 44 46 49 51 58 65 67 71 73 **P**1 **S**0002 Quorum Health Group/Quorum Health Resources	23	10	49	813	11	15269	52	4126	2040	104
KINSLEY—Edwards County										
EDWARDS COUNTY HOSPITAL AND HEALTHCARE CENTER, 620 West Eighth Street, Zip 67547–2329, Mailing Address: Box 99, Zip 67547–2329; tel. 316/659–3621; Thomas Henton, Administrator and Chief Executive Officer **A**9 10 **F**15 16 22 28 32 33 36 40 44 46 49 51 64 71	13	10	49	417	6	7224	0	2719	1281	69
KIOWA—Barber County										
★ KIOWA DISTRICT HOSPITAL, 810 Drumm Street, Zip 67070; tel. 316/825–4131; Buck McKinney Jr., Chief Executive Officer **A**9 10 **F**8 12 14 15 16 19 22 28 33 44 71	16	10	24	231	3	4386	0	1157	444	38
LA CROSSE—Rush County										
★ RUSH COUNTY MEMORIAL HOSPITAL, Eighth and Locust Streets, Zip 67548, Mailing Address: P.O. Box 520, Zip 67548–0520; tel. 913/222–2545; Ronnie Dean Trible, Administrator (Total facility includes 26 beds in nursing home–type unit) **A**9 10 **F**7 14 15 19 22 32 40 44 71 **P**5	13	10	50	364	30	3701	15	1940	1022	52
LAKIN—Kearny County										
KEARNY COUNTY HOSPITAL, 500 Thorpe Street, Zip 67860, Mailing Address: Box 744, Zip 67860; tel. 316/355–7111; Steven S. Reiner, Administrator **A**9 10 **F**1 3 7 8 13 15 16 17 19 22 28 30 32 33 34 36 37 40 44 49 51 62 65 67 71 **P**6	13	10	20	214	7	6375	28	2255	1102	51
LARNED—Pawnee County										
☐ LARNED STATE HOSPITAL, Mailing Address: Rural Route 3, P.O. Box 89, Zip 67550–9365; tel. 316/285–4360; Mani Lee Ph.D., Superintendent **A**1 9 10 **F**2 7 8 11 19 20 21 22 23 31 35 37 39 40 41 42 44 45 46 47 52 53 56 57 60 65 67 71 72 73 **P**6	12	22	478	1456	467	0	0	32549	22322	942
LAWRENCE—Douglas County										
★ LAWRENCE MEMORIAL HOSPITAL, 325 Maine, Zip 66044–1393; tel. 913/749–6100; Robert B. Ohlen, President and Chief Executive Officer (Total facility includes 18 beds in nursing home–type unit) **A**1 9 10 **F**7 8 10 14 15 16 19 20 21 22 23 28 31 32 33 34 35 36 37 39 40 41 44 46 49 52 64 65 71 73	14	10	149	5777	68	70317	863	36675	17427	585
LEAVENWORTH—Leavenworth County										
☐ CUSHING MEMORIAL HOSPITAL, 711 Marshall Street, Zip 66048; tel. 913/684–1100; Charles L. Rogers, President **A**1 9 10 **F**7 8 17 19 21 22 26 28 30 32 33 34 35 37 40 44 45 46 49 52 57 59 64 65 67 71 73 74	23	10	77	1797	31	15376	183	12467	5888	256
★ DWIGHT D. EISENHOWER VETERANS AFFAIRS MEDICAL CENTER, 4101 S Fourth St Trafficway, Zip 66048–5055; tel. 913/682–2000; Carole Bishop Smith, Director (Total facility includes 111 beds in nursing home–type unit) **A**1 3 5 9 **F**1 2 3 4 6 8 10 16 19 20 21 23 26 27 28 29 30 31 32 33 34 35 37 39 41 42 43 44 45 46 48 49 50 52 54 56 57 58 60 63 64 65 67 69 70 71 73 74 **S**9295 Department of Veterans Affairs	45	10	318	3909	273	108640	0	65071	36267	1041
★ SAINT JOHN HOSPITAL, 3500 South Fourth Street, Zip 66048–5092; tel. 913/682–3721; Frank Creeden, Chief Operating Officer **A**1 9 10 **F**7 8 15 16 17 19 22 30 31 32 34 37 40 41 42 44 49 63 65 67 71 73 74 **P**1 4 5 6 7 8 **S**5095 Sisters of Charity of Leavenworth Health Services Corporation	21	10	30	2063	21	35774	303	12237	5869	242
LENEXA—Johnson County										
☐ CPC COLLEGE MEADOWS HOSPITAL, 14425 College Boulevard, Zip 66215; tel. 913/469–1100; Stephen Chesney, Chief Executive Officer (Nonreporting) **A**1 9 10 **S**0785 Community Psychiatric Centers	33	22	120	—	—	—	—	—	—	—
LEOTI—Wichita County										
★ WICHITA COUNTY HOSPITAL, (Includes Wichita County Hospital Long Term Care, Leoti, Kansas, Mailing Address: P.O. Box 968, Zip 67861) 211 East Earl, Zip 67861–0968, Mailing Address: RR2, Box 38, Zip 67861–0968; tel. 316/375–2233; Beverly Kessler, Administrator (Total facility includes 30 beds in nursing home–type unit) **A**9 10 **F**14 15 16 22 51 64 **P**6	15	10	43	173	26	9890	0	2148	1104	0
LIBERAL—Seward County										
★ SOUTHWEST MEDICAL CENTER, 315 West 15th Street, Zip 67901–1340, Mailing Address: Box 1340, Zip 67905–1340; tel. 316/624–1651; Dave Kindel, President and Chief Executive Officer (Total facility includes 13 beds in nursing home–type unit) **A**1 9 10 **F**7 8 14 15 16 19 21 22 23 28 32 33 34 35 37 39 40 44 49 64 65 71 73	13	10	70	3189	43	95212	759	22448	8298	342
LINCOLN—Lincoln County										
LINCOLN COUNTY HOSPITAL, 624 North Second Street, Zip 67455, Mailing Address: P.O. Box 406, Zip 67455; tel. 913/524–4403; Jolene Yager R.N., Administrator (Total facility includes 20 beds in nursing home–type unit) **A**9 10 **F**8 15 20 22 32 34 36 41 44 65 71 **S**1535 Great Plains Health Alliance, Inc.	13	10	34	468	24	4431	0	2442	1232	65

Hospitals, U.S. / KANSAS

Hospital, Address, Telephone, Administrator, Approval, Facility, and Physician Codes, Health Care System	Classification Codes		Utilization Data					Expense (thousands) of dollars		
★ American Hospital Association (AHA) membership □ Joint Commission on Accreditation of Healthcare Organizations (JCAHO) accreditation + American Osteopathic Hospital Association (AOHA) membership ○ American Osteopathic Association (AOA) accreditation △ Commission on Accreditation of Rehabilitation Facilities (CARF) accreditation Control codes 61, 63, 64, 71, 72 and 73 indicate hospitals listed by AOHA, but not registered by AHA. For definition of numerical codes, see page A6	Control	Service	Beds	Admissions	Census	Outpatient Visits	Births	Total	Payroll	Personnel
LINDSBORG—McPherson County										
★ LINDSBORG COMMUNITY HOSPITAL, 605 West Lincoln Street, Zip 67456–2399; tel. 913/227–3308; John E. Keelan, Administrator and Chief Executive Officer **A**9 10 **F**15 22 24 28 32 34 36 42 44 45 49 64 71 **P**1 3	23	10	12	651	7	23563	0	2786	1428	66
LYONS—Rice County										
★ RICE COUNTY HOSPITAL DISTRICT NUMBER ONE, (Formerly Hospital District Number 1) 619 South Clark Street, Zip 67554, Mailing Address: P.O. Box 828, Zip 67554; tel. 316/257–5173; Robert L. Mullen, Administrator **A**9 10 **F**6 8 12 14 15 16 17 20 26 28 30 31 32 33 36 39 40 44 46 62 71 73	16	10	44	638	21	6297	112	3076	1440	64
MANHATTAN—Riley County										
✠ MEMORIAL HOSPITAL, 1105 Sunset Avenue, Zip 66502, Mailing Address: Box 1208, Zip 66502; tel. 913/776–3300; E. Michael Nunamaker, Chief Executive Officer **A**1 9 10 **F**7 8 15 16 17 19 20 22 23 24 28 29 30 31 32 34 35 36 37 38 39 40 41 42 44 46 48 49 56 60 61 65 67 71 73 74 **S**0805 Stormont–Vail Health Services Corporation	23	10	81	1445	14	14180	522	11007	4482	200
✠ SAINT MARY HOSPITAL, 1823 College Avenue, Zip 66502, Mailing Address: Box 1047, Zip 66502–0041; tel. 913/776–3322; J. H. Seitz, President and Chief Executive Officer **A**1 9 10 **F**7 8 12 15 19 21 22 28 29 30 31 35 37 39 40 41 44 49 52 53 54 55 56 58 59 63 65 67 71 73 74 **S**5435 CSJ Health System of Wichita	21	10	106	2738	39	33725	357	16364	7487	295
MANKATO—Jewell County										
JEWELL COUNTY HOSPITAL, 100 Crest Vue, Zip 66956, Mailing Address: Box 327, Zip 66956; tel. 913/378–3137; Rodney Brockelman, Administrator (Nonreporting) **A**9 10	13	10	57	—	—	—	—	—	—	—
MARION—Marion County										
★ ST. LUKE HOSPITAL, 1014 East Melvin, Zip 66861; tel. 316/382–2179; Craig Hanson, Administrator (Total facility includes 32 beds in nursing home–type unit) **A**9 10 **F**7 8 11 12 14 15 19 20 22 24 30 32 33 34 36 39 40 41 44 45 49 64 71 73 **S**2235 Lutheran Health Systems	23	10	54	482	37	13773	38	3199	1553	75
MARYSVILLE—Marshall County										
★ COMMUNITY MEMORIAL HOSPITAL, 708 North 18th Street, Zip 66508–1399; tel. 913/562–2311; Harley B. Appel, Chief Executive Officer **A**9 10 **F**7 8 12 16 19 22 24 28 29 32 33 34 35 36 40 41 42 44 46 63 65 67 71 73 **P**7	23	10	55	1053	12	16479	71	5500	2413	97
MCPHERSON—McPherson County										
✠ MEMORIAL HOSPITAL, 1000 Hospital Drive, Zip 67460–2321; tel. 316/241–2250; Stan Regehr, President and Chief Executive Officer **A**1 9 10 **F**7 8 14 15 16 17 19 21 22 24 28 31 32 33 35 36 37 39 40 42 44 45 46 49 65 71 73	23	10	45	1696	22	37627	198	8813	4043	162
MEADE—Meade County										
MEADE DISTRICT HOSPITAL, 510 East Carthage Street, Zip 67864–0680, Mailing Address: P.O. Box 680, Zip 67864–0680; tel. 316/873–2141; Michael P. Thomas, Administrator **A**9 10 **F**15 16 22 24 26 28 32 33 40 44 64 65 71	16	10	20	393	7	8820	29	2471	1069	54
MEDICINE LODGE—Barber County										
★ MEDICINE LODGE MEMORIAL HOSPITAL, 710 North Walnut Street, Zip 67104, Mailing Address: P.O. Drawer C, Zip 67104; tel. 316/886–3771; Kevin A. White, Administrator **A**9 10 **F**8 16 20 22 26 34 44 49 71 **S**1535 Great Plains Health Alliance, Inc.	16	10	42	614	10	6837	0	3830	1736	71
MINNEAPOLIS—Ottawa County										
★ OTTAWA COUNTY HOSPITAL, 215 East Eighth, Zip 67467, Mailing Address: Box 209, Zip 67467; tel. 913/392–2122; Joy Reed R.N., Administrator (Total facility includes 23 beds in nursing home–type unit) **A**9 10 **F**17 20 21 22 24 26 32 34 36 45 49 65 71 **S**1535 Great Plains Health Alliance, Inc.	23	10	53	512	47	4463	0	2686	1508	85
MINNEOLA—Clark County										
★ MINNEOLA DISTRICT HOSPITAL, 212 Main Street, Zip 67865; tel. 316/885–4264; Blaine K. Miller, Administrator **A**9 10 **F**1 8 16 22 28 34 41 44 49 56 65 71 **S**1535 Great Plains Health Alliance, Inc.	16	10	15	540	8	3956	47	2079	828	35
MOUNDRIDGE—McPherson County										
★ MERCY HOSPITAL, 218 East Pack Street, Zip 67107, Mailing Address: Box 180, Zip 67107; tel. 316/345–6391; Doyle K. Johnson, Administrator (Total facility includes 6 beds in nursing home–type unit) **A**9 10 **F**15 22 26 40 44 49 64	21	10	22	188	2	2498	0	830	462	27
NEODESHA—Wilson County										
WILSON COUNTY HOSPITAL, 205 Mill Street, Zip 66757, Mailing Address: Box 360, Zip 66757; tel. 316/325–2611; Deanna Pittman, Administrator **A**9 10 **F**1 7 15 17 19 22 28 30 31 32 34 40 41 44 52 57 64 65 67 71 73	13	10	38	579	12	6393	68	3633	1693	69
NESS CITY—Ness County										
★ NESS COUNTY HOSPITAL NUMBER TWO, 312 East Custer Street, Zip 67560; tel. 913/798–2291; Clyde T. McCracken, Administrator (Total facility includes 27 beds in nursing home–type unit) **A**9 10 **F**7 14 15 17 19 28 32 39 40 44 64 71	16	10	52	309	29	2610	10	2403	1234	81
NEWTON—Harvey County										
✠ NEWTON MEDICAL CENTER, Mailing Address: P.O. Box 308, Zip 67114–0308; tel. 316/283–2700; W. Charles Waters, President (Total facility includes 12 beds in nursing home–type unit) **A**1 9 10 **F**7 19 21 22 23 26 28 29 30 31 33 34 35 37 40 44 49 56 64 65 71	23	10	84	3201	48	26163	440	16393	7921	308
□ PRAIRIE VIEW, 1901 East First Street, Zip 67114, Mailing Address: Box 467, Zip 67114–0467; tel. 316/283–2400; Melvin Goering, Chief Executive Officer **A**1 10 **F**14 15 16 52 53 54 55 56 57 58 59	21	22	60	1217	33	50450	0	14784	9489	303

Hospitals, U.S. / KANSAS

Hospital, Address, Telephone, Administrator, Approval, Facility, and Physician Codes, Health Care System	Classification Codes		Utilization Data					Expense (thousands) of dollars		
	Control	Service	Beds	Admissions	Census	Outpatient Visits	Births	Total	Payroll	Personnel

★ American Hospital Association (AHA) membership
☐ Joint Commission on Accreditation of Healthcare Organizations (JCAHO) accreditation
+ American Osteopathic Hospital Association (AOHA) membership
○ American Osteopathic Association (AOA) accreditation
△ Commission on Accreditation of Rehabilitation Facilities (CARF) accreditation
Control codes 61, 63, 64, 71, 72 and 73 indicate hospitals listed by AOHA, but not registered by AHA. For definition of numerical codes, see page A6

Hospital	Control	Service	Beds	Admissions	Census	Outpatient Visits	Births	Total	Payroll	Personnel
NORTON—Norton County ★ NORTON COUNTY HOSPITAL, 102 East Holme, Zip 67654–0250, Mailing Address: P.O. Box 250, Zip 67654–0250; tel. 913/877–3351; Richard Miller, Administrator A9 10 F2 7 8 15 16 17 19 20 21 22 26 28 30 32 33 34 36 39 40 42 44 45 46 49 51 52 53 54 55 56 57 58 65 71 73 P4	13	10	43	580	11	16588	1	3075	1449	77
OAKLEY—Logan County LOGAN COUNTY HOSPITAL, 211 Cherry Street, Zip 67748; tel. 913/672–3211; Rodney Bates, Administrator (Total facility includes 30 beds in nursing home–type unit) A9 10 F6 7 8 15 16 19 21 32 33 34 36 40 44 49 64 65 71 P6	13	10	51	384	31	9148	23	2034	1052	50
OBERLIN—Decatur County ★ DECATUR COUNTY HOSPITAL, 810 West Columbia, Zip 67749, Mailing Address: P.O. Box 268, Zip 67749; tel. 913/475–2208; R. Kim Hardman, Administrator (Total facility includes 50 beds in nursing home–type unit) A9 10 F7 8 12 14 15 16 19 22 26 28 30 32 34 36 37 39 41 42 44 46 49 65 71 S2235 Lutheran Health Systems	23	10	74	855	53	12038	82	3996	2029	103
OLATHE—Johnson County ☐ KANSAS INSTITUTE, 555 East Santa Fe, Zip 66061–3486, Mailing Address: P.O. Box 2230, Zip 66061–2230; tel. 913/782–7000; Steven R. Cleary, Administrator (Nonreporting) A1 9 10	33	22	105	—	—	—	—	—	—	—
★ OLATHE MEDICAL CENTER, 20333 West 151st Street, Zip 66061–5352; tel. 913/791–4200; Frank H. Devocelle, President and Chief Executive Officer A1 2 9 10 F4 7 8 10 12 14 15 16 17 19 21 22 28 30 31 32 33 34 35 37 39 40 41 42 44 46 49 65 67 71 72 73 P6	23	10	130	6601	76	86085	866	50542	20171	598
ONAGA—Pottawatomie County COMMUNITY HOSPITAL ONAGA, 120 West Eighth Street, Zip 66521–0120; tel. 913/889–4272; Joseph T. Engelken, Chief Executive Officer (Total facility includes 50 beds in nursing home–type unit) A9 F1 2 3 4 5 6 7 8 9 10 11 12 13 14 15 16 17 19 20 21 22 23 24 25 26 27 28 30 31 32 33 34 35 37 38 39 40 41 42 43 44 45 46 47 48 49 50 51 52 53 54 55 56 57 58 59 60 61 62 63 64 65 66 67 68 69 70 71 72 73 74 P4 8	23	10	73	854	30	23192	66	6819	3614	230
OSAWATOMIE—Miami County ☐ OSAWATOMIE STATE HOSPITAL, Osawatomie Road & Hospital Drive, Zip 66064–9757, Mailing Address: P.O. Box 500, Zip 66064–9757; tel. 913/755–3151; Stephen H. Feinstein Ph.D., Superintendent A1 9 10 F2 52 53 56 57 65 73 P6	12	22	260	1234	212	0	0	22362	14259	574
OSBORNE—Osborne County ★ OSBORNE COUNTY MEMORIAL HOSPITAL, 424 West New Hampshire Street, Zip 67473–0070, Mailing Address: P.O. Box 70, Zip 67473–0070; tel. 913/346–2121; Patricia Bernard R.N., Administrator A9 F7 8 19 20 22 33 34 44 71 S1535 Great Plains Health Alliance, Inc.	13	10	29	535	6	7835	34	1974	944	67
OTTAWA—Franklin County ★ RANSOM MEMORIAL HOSPITAL, 1301 South Main Street, Zip 66067–3598; tel. 913/242–3344; Robert E. Bregant Jr., Administrator A1 9 10 F7 8 17 19 21 22 26 28 30 33 34 35 37 39 40 41 42 44 45 46 49 61 63 65 67 68 71 73	13	10	36	1659	20	29578	193	9270	4241	164
OVERLAND PARK—Johnson County ★ △ MID-AMERICA REHABILITATION HOSPITAL, 5701 West 110th Street, Zip 66211; tel. 913/491–2400; Richard L. Allen, Chief Executive Officer A1 7 9 10 F1 12 14 15 16 17 19 20 21 25 27 34 35 41 46 48 49 64 65 66 67 71 73 P4	32	46	80	925	58	18406	0	18466	8372	204
★ OVERLAND PARK REGIONAL MEDICAL CENTER, 10500 Quivira Road, Zip 66215–2373, Mailing Address: P.O. Box 15959, Zip 66215; tel. 913/541–5000; Kevin J. Hicks, Chief Executive Officer (Total facility includes 17 beds in nursing home–type unit) A1 9 10 F1 2 3 4 7 8 10 11 14 15 16 17 18 19 20 21 22 24 26 27 28 29 30 31 32 33 34 35 36 37 38 39 40 41 42 43 44 45 46 48 49 52 53 54 55 56 57 58 59 60 61 64 65 67 70 71 72 73 74 S0048 Columbia/HCA Healthcare Corporation	33	10	250	8561	110	49710	1818	61620	25521	844
PAOLA—Miami County ★ MIAMI COUNTY MEDICAL CENTER, 501 South Hospital Drive, Zip 66071–0365, Mailing Address: P.O. Box 365, Zip 66071–0365; tel. 913/294–2327; Ken Huber, Vice President and Chief Operating Officer A9 10 F8 13 16 19 21 22 28 30 31 32 33 34 39 41 42 44 46 49 51 65 66 71 73	23	10	19	544	7	18250	0	5538	2497	93
PARSONS—Labette County ★ + LABETTE COUNTY MEDICAL CENTER, South Highway 59, Zip 67357, Mailing Address: P.O. Box 956, Zip 67357; tel. 316/421–4880; Richard A. Nye, Administrator A1 9 10 F7 8 14 19 21 22 28 29 30 32 34 35 36 37 40 41 42 44 45 49 63 65 70 71 73	13	10	74	2774	37	34850	336	18826	8136	336
PARSONS STATE HOSPITAL AND TRAINING CENTER, 26th And Gabriel Streets, Zip 67357–0738, Mailing Address: Box 738, Zip 67357–0738; tel. 316/421–6550; Gary J. Daniels Ph.D., Superintendent F8 17 19 20 21 22 30 35 37 42 44 48 52 65 71 73	12	62	240	26	233	0	0	18318	12363	499
PHILLIPSBURG—Phillips County ★ PHILLIPS COUNTY HOSPITAL, 1150 State Street, Zip 67661, Mailing Address: Box 607, Zip 67661; tel. 913/543–5226; James L. Giedd, Administrator (Total facility includes 33 beds in nursing home–type unit) A9 10 F7 8 15 17 19 20 22 28 34 42 44 46 49 65 71 73 S1535 Great Plains Health Alliance, Inc.	23	10	62	954	43	9043	57	5342	2296	111

© 1995 AHA Guide

Hospitals, U.S. / KANSAS

Hospital, Address, Telephone, Administrator, Approval, Facility, and Physician Codes, Health Care System	Classification Codes		Utilization Data					Expense (thousands) of dollars		
	Control	Service	Beds	Admissions	Census	Outpatient Visits	Births	Total	Payroll	Personnel

★ American Hospital Association (AHA) membership
☐ Joint Commission on Accreditation of Healthcare Organizations (JCAHO) accreditation
+ American Osteopathic Hospital Association (AOHA) membership
○ American Osteopathic Association (AOA) accreditation
△ Commission on Accreditation of Rehabilitation Facilities (CARF) accreditation
Control codes 61, 63, 64, 71, 72 and 73 indicate hospitals listed by AOHA, but not registered by AHA. For definition of numerical codes, see page A6

PITTSBURG—Crawford County
★ + MOUNT CARMEL MEDICAL CENTER, Centennial and Rouse Streets, Zip 66762–6686; tel. 316/231–6100; Dan Lingor, President **A**1 2 9 10 **F**8 12 15 16 19 21 22 23 27 32 34 35 36 37 39 40 41 44 45 46 49 52 54 55 56 59 60 64 65 66 67 71 73 **P**6 **S**5435 CSJ Health System of Wichita — 23 10 169 4735 71 47647 354 24518 10994 440

PLAINVILLE—Rooks County
  PLAINVILLE RURAL HOSPITAL DISTRICT NUMBER ONE, 304 South Colorado Avenue, Zip 67663; tel. 913/434–4553; Leonard Hernandez, Administrator **A**9 10 **F**7 8 15 16 19 22 26 27 28 30 44 49 66 71 73 **P**5 — 16 10 27 383 7 6135 23 2547 1082 37

PRATT—Pratt County
★ PRATT REGIONAL MEDICAL CENTER, 200 Commodore Street, Zip 67124–3099; tel. 316/672–7451; Susan M. Page, President and Chief Executive Officer (Total facility includes 15 beds in nursing home–type unit) **A**1 9 10 **F**7 8 13 15 16 19 21 22 25 26 28 29 30 31 33 34 35 36 37 39 40 42 44 45 46 49 61 64 65 66 67 71 73 — 23 10 84 1355 15 18561 187 11463 5311 215

QUINTER—Gove County
  GOVE COUNTY MEDICAL CENTER, Fifth and Garfield Streets, Zip 67752; tel. 913/754–3341; Paul Davis, Administrator (Total facility includes 59 beds in nursing home–type unit) **A**9 10 **F**6 7 19 22 27 32 33 35 40 44 65 71 — 13 10 80 689 52 7516 50 3352 1753 99

RANSOM—Ness County
★ GRISELL MEMORIAL HOSPITAL DISTRICT ONE, 210 South Vermont, Zip 67572–0268, Mailing Address: P.O. Box 268, Zip 67572–0268; tel. 913/731–2231; Kristine Ochs R.N., Administrator (Total facility includes 34 beds in nursing home–type unit) **A**9 10 **F**7 8 19 20 22 26 32 33 35 36 41 44 46 49 51 55 65 71 **S**1535 Great Plains Health Alliance, Inc. — 16 10 46 155 33 3672 4 2308 1264 42

RUSSELL—Russell County
★ RUSSELL REGIONAL HOSPITAL, 200 South Main Street, Zip 67665; tel. 913/483–3131; Thomas J. Earley, President and Chief Executive Officer (Total facility includes 23 beds in nursing home–type unit) **A**1 9 10 **F**7 14 15 16 19 21 22 27 28 29 30 32 34 36 37 40 44 45 49 51 64 65 67 71 73 **P**5 — 13 10 57 724 32 14394 9 4972 2392 113

SABETHA—Nemaha County
★ SABETHA COMMUNITY HOSPITAL, 14th And Oregon Streets, Zip 66534, Mailing Address: P.O. Box 229, Zip 66534; tel. 913/284–2121; Rita K. Buurman, Administrator **A**9 10 **F**1 7 8 15 16 17 19 20 22 26 28 30 32 33 34 35 41 42 44 45 49 54 56 58 65 71 **P**6 **S**1535 Great Plains Health Alliance, Inc. — 23 10 27 528 9 14653 43 3541 1762 61

SAINT FRANCIS—Maricopa County
★ CHEYENNE COUNTY HOSPITAL, 210 West First Street, Zip 67756, Mailing Address: P.O. Box 547, Zip 67756–0547; tel. 913/332–2104; Leslie Lacy, Administrator **A**9 10 **F**7 8 15 16 19 20 22 35 44 65 71 **S**1535 Great Plains Health Alliance, Inc. — 23 10 23 176 3 5686 2 1360 575 35

SALINA—Saline County
★ △ ASBURY–SALINA REGIONAL MEDICAL CENTER, 400 South Santa Fe Avenue, Zip 67401, Mailing Address: Box 5080, Zip 67402–5080; tel. 913/827–4411; Clay D. Edmands, President **A**1 2 3 5 7 9 10 **F**7 8 10 15 16 17 19 21 22 23 24 26 27 29 30 31 33 34 35 37 38 39 40 41 42 44 45 46 48 49 52 54 55 56 57 58 64 65 66 67 68 71 73 74 **P**8 — 23 10 189 6726 102 60261 1100 42215 17676 625

★ ST. FRANCIS AT SALINA, 5097 Cloud Street, Zip 67401, Mailing Address: 509 East Elm, Zip 67401; tel. 913/825–0563; Reverend Phillip J. Rapp, President and Chief Executive Officer (Nonreporting) **A**9 — 23 22 26 — — — — — — —

★ ST. JOHN'S REGIONAL HEALTH CENTER, 139 North Penn Street, Zip 67401–3057, Mailing Address: P.O. Box 5201, Zip 67402–5201; tel. 913/827–5591; John R. Broberg, Interim President and Chief Executive Officer (Total facility includes 19 beds in nursing home–type unit) **A**1 2 3 9 10 **F**15 19 21 22 23 26 28 31 32 33 35 36 37 39 42 44 49 56 60 63 64 65 66 71 73 **P**8 **S**5435 CSJ Health System of Wichita — 21 10 120 2499 44 62034 0 22075 9739 429

SATANTA—Haskell County
★ SATANTA DISTRICT HOSPITAL, Cheyenne and Apache, Zip 67870, Mailing Address: P.O. Box 159, Zip 67870–0159; tel. 316/649–2761; T. G. Lee, Administrator (Total facility includes 29 beds in nursing home–type unit) **A**9 10 **F**7 8 15 17 19 22 32 34 35 39 41 44 45 49 65 71 **S**1535 Great Plains Health Alliance, Inc. — 16 10 42 348 26 4031 1 3660 1679 77

SCOTT CITY—Scott County
★ SCOTT COUNTY HOSPITAL, 310 East Third Street, Zip 67871; tel. 316/872–5811; Greg Unruh, Chief Executive Officer **A**9 10 **F**7 8 19 22 28 36 40 44 64 71 73 — 23 10 27 549 6 4774 32 2353 1061 71

SEDAN—Chautauqua County
  SEDAN CITY HOSPITAL, 300 North Street, Zip 67361, Mailing Address: Box C, Zip 67361; tel. 316/725–3115; Samuel Guild, Administrator **A**9 10 **F**8 14 15 16 22 34 57 71 — 14 10 38 317 11 4774 0 1760 943 42

SENECA—Nemaha County
★ NEMAHA VALLEY COMMUNITY HOSPITAL, 1600 Community Drive, Zip 66538; tel. 913/336–6181; Edward E. Riley, Administrator **A**9 10 **F**5 7 8 14 19 22 26 28 30 32 33 34 40 44 49 56 65 66 67 70 71 — 23 10 24 489 6 9427 59 2967 1274 58

SHAWNEE MISSION—Johnson County
★ SHAWNEE MISSION MEDICAL CENTER, 9100 West 74th Street, Zip 66204–4019, Mailing Address: Box 2923, Zip 66201–1323; tel. 913/676–2000; James W. Boyle, President and Chief Executive Officer **A**1 2 9 10 **F**2 3 4 7 8 10 12 15 16 17 19 21 22 23 28 30 31 32 34 35 37 38 39 40 41 42 43 44 45 46 49 52 53 54 55 57 58 59 61 64 65 66 67 71 72 73 74 **P**5 6 7 8 — 21 10 332 15857 196 145200 3242 127481 58886 1649

Hospitals, U.S. / KANSAS

Hospital, Address, Telephone, Administrator, Approval, Facility, and Physician Codes, Health Care System	Classification Codes		Utilization Data					Expense (thousands) of dollars		
★ American Hospital Association (AHA) membership ☐ Joint Commission on Accreditation of Healthcare Organizations (JCAHO) accreditation + American Osteopathic Hospital Association (AOHA) membership ○ American Osteopathic Association (AOA) accreditation △ Commission on Accreditation of Rehabilitation Facilities (CARF) accreditation Control codes 61, 63, 64, 71, 72 and 73 indicate hospitals listed by AOHA, but not registered by AHA. For definition of numerical codes, see page A6	Control	Service	Beds	Admissions	Census	Outpatient Visits	Births	Total	Payroll	Personnel
SMITH CENTER—Smith County ★ SMITH COUNTY MEMORIAL HOSPITAL, 614 South Main Street, Zip 66967–0349, Mailing Address: P.O. Box 349, Zip 66967–0349; tel. 913/282–6845; John Terrill, Administrator (Total facility includes 28 beds in nursing home–type unit) **A**1 9 10 **F**1 7 8 22 34 35 44 49 71 **S**1535 Great Plains Health Alliance, Inc.	23	10	54	724	34	8289	41	3256	1594	68
STAFFORD—Stafford County STAFFORD DISTRICT HOSPITAL NUMBER FOUR, 502 South Buckeye Street, Zip 67578, Mailing Address: Box 190, Zip 67578; tel. 316/234–5221; Douglas Newman, Administrator **A**9 10 **F**8 17 20 22 26 28 29 30 31 33 34 36 42 44 45 46 49 51 56 65 71 73	16	10	25	383	5	4345	0	1681	819	40
SYRACUSE—Hamilton County HAMILTON COUNTY HOSPITAL, East Avenue G and Huser Street, Zip 67878–0909, Mailing Address: Box 909, Zip 67878–0909; tel. 316/384–7461; Teresa L. Deuel, Chief Executive Officer and Administrator (Total facility includes 46 beds in nursing home–type unit) **A**9 10 **F**1 8 14 15 19 22 26 28 32 34 40 44 64 67 71 **P**5	13	10	75	318	42	980	16	3540	1515	77
TOPEKA—Shawnee County ★ C. F. MENNINGER MEMORIAL HOSPITAL, 5800 West Sixth Street, Zip 66606, Mailing Address: Box 829, Zip 66601–0829; tel. 913/273–7500; Edward J. Zoble Ph.D., Administrator **A**1 3 9 10 **F**1 2 3 4 7 8 9 10 11 15 16 19 21 22 23 24 31 32 33 34 35 37 40 42 43 44 52 53 55 56 57 58 59 60 65 71 74 **P**1	23	22	95	847	75	46013	0	27396	11557	487
CHILD AND ADOLESCENT SERVICES OF THE MENNINGER CLINIC, 5800 Southwest Sixth Street, Zip 66606, Mailing Address: Box 829, Zip 66601; tel. 913/273–7500; Charlotte Dultmeier, Administrator (Nonreporting) **A**3 9	23	52	60	—	—	—	—	—	—	—
★ COLMERY–O'NEIL VETERANS AFFAIRS MEDICAL CENTER, 2200 Gage Boulevard, Zip 66622; tel. 913/272–3111; (Total facility includes 104 beds in nursing home–type unit) **A**1 3 5 9 **F**1 2 3 4 5 8 10 12 14 15 16 17 19 20 21 22 23 24 26 27 30 31 32 33 34 35 37 39 42 43 44 45 46 48 49 50 52 54 55 56 57 58 59 60 61 63 64 65 67 69 70 71 73 74 **P**7 **S**9295 Department of Veterans Affairs	45	10	622	4721	434	138433	0	74394	42507	1117
KANSAS NEUROLOGICAL INSTITUTE, 3107 West 21st Street, Zip 66604–3298; tel. 913/296–5301; Bob Day Ph.D., Superintendent **F**20 39 65 73 **P**6	12	62	302	2	292	0	0	25483	16963	765
☐ △ KANSAS REHABILITATION HOSPITAL, 1504 Southwest Eighth, Zip 66606–2714; tel. 913/235–6600; Julie De Jean, Administrator (Total facility includes 17 beds in nursing home–type unit) **A**1 7 9 10 **F**12 14 15 16 19 21 34 35 41 46 48 49 60 64 65 71	33	46	79	622	34	20843	0	11319	4281	149
★ △ ST. FRANCIS HOSPITAL AND MEDICAL CENTER, 1700 West Seventh Street, Zip 66606–1690; tel. 913/295–8000; Sister Loretto Marie Colwell, President **A**1 2 3 7 9 10 **F**2 3 4 7 8 10 11 12 15 19 20 21 22 24 27 28 30 31 32 33 34 35 36 37 40 41 42 43 44 45 46 48 49 51 56 60 63 65 67 71 73 **P**6 8 **S**5095 Sisters of Charity of Leavenworth Health Services Corporation	21	10	320	10821	295	155556	1071	93792	42907	1245
★ STORMONT–VAIL REGIONAL MEDICAL CENTER, 1500 Southwest Tenth Street, Zip 66604–1353; tel. 913/354–6000; Howard M. Chase, President and Chief Executive Officer **A**1 3 5 9 10 **F**4 7 8 10 11 12 14 15 16 17 19 21 22 23 24 26 27 28 29 30 31 32 33 34 35 36 37 38 39 40 41 42 43 44 45 46 47 49 52 53 55 56 57 58 60 65 67 71 73 74 **S**0805 Stormont–Vail Health Services Corporation	23	10	313	10447	189	92541	1830	92984	43136	1493
☐ TOPEKA STATE HOSPITAL, 2700 West Sixth Street, Zip 66606–1898; tel. 913/296–4596; Randy Proctor, Acting Superintendent **A**1 3 9 10 **F**2 3 8 9 10 12 14 15 16 20 22 24 27 30 35 37 39 40 41 46 47 48 49 50 52 53 54 55 57 63 64 65 66 67 71 73 **P**6	12	22	266	888	238	0	0	20914	18518	633
TRIBUNE—Greeley County ★ GREELEY COUNTY HOSPITAL, 506 Third Street, Zip 67879, Mailing Address: Box 338, Zip 67879; tel. 316/376–4221; Thomas A. Keeffer, Administrator (Total facility includes 32 beds in nursing home–type unit) **A**9 10 **F**1 7 8 15 16 20 22 27 36 39 41 44 46 49 56 57 71 **S**1535 Great Plains Health Alliance, Inc.	23	10	50	387	33	5012	63	2129	1001	73
ULYSSES—Grant County ★ BOB WILSON MEMORIAL GRANT COUNTY HOSPITAL, 415 North Main Street, Zip 67880; tel. 316/356–1266; M. Leo Miller, Chief Executive Officer **A**9 10 **F**8 15 16 19 22 24 28 30 32 34 35 37 44 49 57 65 71	13	10	37	644	8	11533	0	4701	1845	79
WAKEENEY—Trego County ★ TREGO COUNTY–LEMKE MEMORIAL HOSPITAL, 320 13th Street, Zip 67672–2099; tel. 913/743–2182; James Wahlmeier, Administrator (Total facility includes 45 beds in nursing home–type unit) **A**9 10 **F**3 7 8 15 16 17 19 20 22 32 33 34 44 45 49 65 71 **S**1535 Great Plains Health Alliance, Inc.	13	10	73	752	58	6066	2	4032	1811	102
WAMEGO—Pottawatomie County WAMEGO CITY HOSPITAL, 711 Genn Drive, Zip 66547; tel. 913/456–2295; Lisa J. Freeborn, Administrator **A**9 10 **F**8 15 17 22 24 27 28 30 31 32 33 34 39 41 44 45 48 49 64 65 71 73 **P**6 **S**0805 Stormont–Vail Health Services Corporation	14	10	18	412	6	10167	0	2676	1257	65
WASHINGTON—Washington County WASHINGTON COUNTY HOSPITAL, 304 East Third Street, Zip 66968–2098; tel. 913/325–2211; Everett Lutjemeier, Administrator **A**9 10 **F**1 7 8 9 12 14 15 22 24 26 28 29 30 33 36 37 39 40 41 44 49 51 64 65 71 **P**5	13	10	27	286	8	3137	12	1654	838	45
WELLINGTON—Sumner County ★ SUMNER REGIONAL MEDICAL CENTER, (Formerly St. Lukes Hospital) 1323 North A Street, Zip 67152–1323; tel. 316/326–7451; Ray Williams III, Chief Executive Officer (Total facility includes 11 beds in nursing home–type unit) **A**9 10 **F**7 14 19 22 32 34 36 40 44 64 71 73	14	10	80	909	15	17166	93	4533	2013	91

© 1995 AHA Guide

Hospitals, U.S. / KANSAS

Hospital, Address, Telephone, Administrator, Approval, Facility, and Physician Codes, Health Care System	Classification Codes		Utilization Data					Expense (thousands) of dollars		
★ American Hospital Association (AHA) membership ☐ Joint Commission on Accreditation of Healthcare Organizations (JCAHO) accreditation + American Osteopathic Hospital Association (AOHA) membership ○ American Osteopathic Association (AOA) accreditation △ Commission on Accreditation of Rehabilitation Facilities (CARF) accreditation Control codes 61, 63, 64, 71, 72 and 73 indicate hospitals listed by AOHA, but not registered by AHA. For definition of numerical codes, see page A6	Control	Service	Beds	Admissions	Census	Outpatient Visits	Births	Total	Payroll	Personnel
WESTMORELAND—Pottawatomie County										
DECHAIRO HOSPITAL, First and North Streets, Zip 66549; tel. 913/457–3311; Donn Demaree, Administrator **A**9 10 **F**8 15 16 21 32 41 44 49 65 70 **S**0805 Stormont-Vail Health Services Corporation	33	10	13	206	3	4550	0	1080	605	28
WICHITA—Sedgwick County										
HEALTHSOUTH REHABILITATION HOSPITAL See Our Lady of Lourdes Rehabilitation Hospital of Wichita										
☐ OUR LADY OF LOURDES REHABILITATION HOSPITAL OF WICHITA, (Formerly Healthsouth Rehabilitation Hospital) 1151 North Rock Road, Zip 67206–1262; tel. 316/634–3400; Jane David, Interim Chief Executive Officer (Nonreporting) **A**1 10	33	46	40	—	—	—	—	—	—	—
+ ○ RIVERSIDE HEALTH SYSTEM, (Formerly Riverside Hospital) 2622 West Central Street, Zip 67203–4999; tel. 316/946–5000; Robert Dixon, President and Chief Executive Officer (Total facility includes 22 beds in nursing home–type unit) **A**9 10 11 12 13 **F**7 8 11 12 13 14 15 16 17 19 20 21 22 26 28 29 30 31 34 35 37 39 40 41 44 45 46 49 54 56 63 64 65 71 73 **P**3 6	23	10	125	3100	50	28724	242	28501	13130	465
★ ST. FRANCIS REGIONAL MEDICAL CENTER, 929 North St Francis Street, Zip 67214–3882; tel. 316/268–5000; Sister M. Sylvia Egan, President and Chief Executive Officer **A**1 2 3 5 9 10 **F**1 2 3 4 5 6 7 8 9 10 11 12 13 14 15 16 17 18 19 20 21 22 23 24 25 26 27 28 29 30 31 32 33 34 35 36 37 38 39 40 41 42 43 44 45 46 47 48 49 51 52 53 54 55 56 57 58 59 60 61 63 64 65 66 67 68 69 70 71 72 73 74 **P**3 7 **S**5305 Sisters of the Sorrowful Mother United States Health System	21	10	681	21250	340	72327	2123	260093	117315	2821
★ △ ST. JOSEPH MEDICAL CENTER, 3600 East Harry Street, Zip 67218–3713; tel. 316/685–1111; LeRoy E. Rheault, President and Chief Executive Officer (Total facility includes 11 beds in nursing home–type unit) **A**1 2 3 5 7 9 10 **F**1 2 3 4 7 8 10 11 12 15 16 19 20 21 22 23 24 26 32 34 35 37 38 39 40 41 42 43 44 47 48 49 50 51 52 53 56 57 58 59 60 63 64 65 66 68 70 71 73 **P**8 **S**5435 CSJ Health System of Wichita	23	10	480	15501	265	222302	1542	126696	64464	1954
★ VETERANS AFFAIRS MEDICAL AND REGIONAL OFFICE CENTER, 5500 East Kellogg, Zip 67218; tel. 316/685–2221; Jerry Mayhall Ph.D., Director (Total facility includes 60 beds in nursing home–type unit) **A**1 3 5 9 **F**2 3 4 8 9 10 12 16 17 18 19 20 21 22 24 27 31 32 34 35 39 40 41 42 46 48 49 52 54 55 56 57 58 59 60 63 64 65 67 70 71 72 73 74 **P**6 **S**9295 Department of Veterans Affairs	45	10	156	3809	95	80213	0	44587	21679	194
★ WESLEY MEDICAL CENTER, 550 North Hillside Avenue, Zip 67214–4976; tel. 316/688–2468; James R. Kelly Jr., Chief Executive Officer **A**1 2 3 5 9 10 **F**4 7 8 10 11 12 15 16 18 19 20 21 22 23 24 26 28 29 30 31 32 33 34 35 37 38 39 40 41 42 43 44 45 46 47 48 49 56 60 61 63 64 65 66 67 69 70 71 73 74 **P**7 **S**0048 Columbia/HCA Healthcare Corporation	33	10	460	23300	351	155161	4507	223560	85740	2989
★ △ WESLEY REHABILITATION HOSPITAL, 8338 West 13th Street North, Zip 67212–2900; tel. 316/729–9999; G. Curt Meyer, Chief Executive Officer (Total facility includes 15 beds in nursing home–type unit) **A**1 7 10 **F**12 14 16 19 21 22 25 27 34 35 45 46 48 49 50 60 63 64 71 73 **P**1 5 **S**1715 Continental Medical Systems, Inc.	33	46	65	791	43	16463	0	12976	5362	163
WINCHESTER—Jefferson County										
JEFFERSON COUNTY MEMORIAL HOSPITAL, (Includes Jefferson County Memorial Hospital and Geriatric Center) 408 Delaware Street, Zip 66097, Mailing Address: Rural Route 1, Box 1, Zip 66097; tel. 913/774–4340; Steven F. Ashcraft, Administrator (Total facility includes 90 beds in nursing home–type unit) **A**9 10 **F**1 7 8 19 22 26 27 30 32 33 34 35 36 39 40 41 44 49 65 71 73 **P**3	23	10	110	225	85	9368	11	3636	1958	75
WINFIELD—Cowley County										
★ WILLIAM NEWTON MEMORIAL HOSPITAL, 1300 East Fifth Street, Zip 67156–2495; tel. 316/221–2300; Richard H. Vaught, Administrator (Total facility includes 14 beds in nursing home–type unit) **A**1 9 10 **F**7 8 13 16 17 19 21 22 27 28 30 32 35 36 37 39 40 41 42 44 45 46 49 52 58 64 65 66 67 71 73	14	10	44	1665	25	34585	234	10832	5551	238
WINFIELD STATE HOSPITAL AND TRAINING CENTER, 1320 North McCabe, Zip 67156–9701; tel. 316/221–1200; William P. Brooks, Superintendent **A**9 **F**20 21 37 41 52 54 65 **P**6	12	62	297	0	310	0	0	27408	18039	822

KENTUCKY

Resident population 3,789 (in thousands)
Resident population in metro areas 48.5%
Birth rate per 1,000 population 14.6
65 years and over 12.7%
Percent of persons without health insurance 13.6%

★ American Hospital Association (AHA) membership
□ Joint Commission on Accreditation of Healthcare Organizations (JCAHO) accreditation
+ American Osteopathic Hospital Association (AOHA) membership
○ American Osteopathic Association (AOA) accreditation
△ Commission on Accreditation of Rehabilitation Facilities (CARF) accreditation
Control codes 61, 63, 64, 71, 72 and 73 indicate hospitals listed by AOHA, but not registered by AHA. For definition of numerical codes, see page A6.

Hospital, Address, Telephone, Administrator, Approval, Facility, and Physician Codes, Health Care System	Classification Codes		Utilization Data					Expense (thousands) of dollars		
	Control	Service	Beds	Admissions	Census	Outpatient Visits	Births	Total	Payroll	Personnel
ALBANY—Clinton County CLINTON COUNTY HOSPITAL, 723 Burkesville Road, Zip 42602; tel. 606/387-6421; Randel Flowers Ph.D., Administrator A9 10 F11 19 22 34 71	23	10	42	2243	29	12270	0	5338	2469	126
ASHLAND—Greenup County ★ △ KING'S DAUGHTERS' MEDICAL CENTER, 2201 Lexington Avenue, Zip 41101, Mailing Address: P.O. Box 151, Zip 41105-0151; tel. 606/327-4000; William C. Parrish, President and Chief Executive Officer (Total facility includes 10 beds in nursing home–type unit) A1 2 7 9 10 F4 7 8 10 12 15 16 17 19 21 22 25 27 28 30 31 32 33 34 35 36 37 38 39 40 41 42 43 44 45 46 48 49 50 52 53 54 55 56 57 58 60 63 64 65 66 67 71 73 74	23	10	323	14154	238	94944	1067	99276	40764	1328
★ OUR LADY OF BELLEFONTE HOSPITAL, St Christopher Drive, Zip 41105-0789, Mailing Address: P.O. Box 789, Zip 41105-0789; tel. 606/833-3333; Robert J. Maher, President A1 9 10 F2 5 8 12 13 14 15 16 19 22 24 28 29 30 32 35 36 37 39 41 42 44 45 46 49 52 60 65 66 67 71 72 73 P8 S1485 Franciscan Sisters of the Poor Health System, Inc.	21	10	189	7564	124	92738	0	53882	21278	759
BARBOURVILLE—Knox County ★ KNOX COUNTY GENERAL HOSPITAL, 321 High Street, Zip 40906, Mailing Address: P.O. Box 160, Zip 40906; tel. 606/546-4175; Craig Morgan, Administrator A1 9 10 F7 19 21 22 37 40 44 65 71 73	13	10	58	1967	27	14685	240	7276	3762	192
BARDSTOWN—Nelson County ★ FLAGET MEMORIAL HOSPITAL, 201 Cathedral Manor, Zip 40004-1299; tel. 502/348-3923; Suzanne Reasbeck, Acting President and Chief Executive Officer (Nonreporting) A1 9 10 S3045 Sisters of Charity of Nazareth Health System	21	10	52	—	—	—	—	—	—	—
BENTON—Marshall County ★ MARSHALL COUNTY HOSPITAL, 503 George McClain Drive, Zip 42025, Mailing Address: P.O. Box 630, Zip 42025; tel. 502/527-4800; David Fuqua, Administrator (Total facility includes 34 beds in nursing home–type unit) A1 9 10 F1 8 11 15 17 19 21 22 28 35 37 44 64 65 67 71 73 P5 S0002 Quorum Health Group/Quorum Health Resources	16	10	80	848	48	13706	0	8287	3240	185
BEREA—Madison County ★ BEREA HOSPITAL, 305 Estill Street, Zip 40403; tel. 606/986-3151; David E. Burgio FACHE, Administrator and Chief Executive Officer (Total facility includes 62 beds in nursing home–type unit) A1 9 10 F14 15 16 17 19 21 22 26 27 28 30 31 34 37 39 41 44 49 64 65 71 73 74	23	10	110	2029	89	32917	0	15107	6418	297
BOWLING GREEN—Warren County ★ GREENVIEW HOSPITAL, 1801 Ashley Circle, Zip 42104, Mailing Address: Box 90024, Zip 42102-9024; tel. 502/793-1000; Mary T. Brasseaux, Chief Executive Officer A1 9 10 F4 7 8 10 11 17 19 21 22 23 29 30 33 34 35 37 42 43 44 45 46 64 65 67 71 73 74 P5 S0048 Columbia/HCA Healthcare Corporation	33	10	211	6529	106	44946	989	—	—	734
★ MEDICAL CENTER AT BOWLING GREEN, 250 Park Street, Zip 42101, Mailing Address: Box 90010, Zip 42102-9010; tel. 502/745-1000; Laurence C. Hinsdale, Chief Executive Officer (Nonreporting) A1 9 10	23	10	350	—	—	—	—	—	—	—
BURKESVILLE—Cumberland County ★ CUMBERLAND COUNTY HOSPITAL, Highway 90 West, Zip 42717-0280, Mailing Address: P.O. Box 280, Zip 42717-0280; tel. 502/864-2511; Mark Thompson, Chief Executive Officer A9 10 F7 8 12 19 22 27 34 44 46 49 65 71 S0002 Quorum Health Group/Quorum Health Resources	23	10	31	1749	19	12317	80	4907	2004	90
CADIZ—Trigg County ★ TRIGG COUNTY HOSPITAL, Highway 68 East, Zip 42211, Mailing Address: Box 312, Zip 42211; tel. 502/522-3215; David M. Goodcase, Chief Executive Officer (Nonreporting) A9 10 S2285 Alliant Health System	23	10	40	—	—	—	—	—	—	—
CALHOUN—McLean County MCLEAN COUNTY GENERAL HOSPITAL, 200 Highway 81 North, Zip 42327; tel. 502/273-5252; Mynette Dennis R.N., Administrator A9 10 F32	13	10	26	46	17	3125	0	—	—	43
CAMPBELLSVILLE—Taylor County ★ TAYLOR COUNTY HOSPITAL, 1700 Old Lebanon Road, Zip 42718; tel. 502/465-3561; David R. Hayes, Chief Executive Officer A1 2 9 10 F7 8 10 19 22 24 26 27 28 30 32 34 35 36 37 40 42 44 45 46 49 63 67 70 71 73	16	10	90	3379	47	33502	332	22404	9021	418
CARLISLE—Nicholas County ★ NICHOLAS COUNTY HOSPITAL, (Includes Johnson–Mathers Nursing Home) 2323 Concrete Road, Zip 40311, Mailing Address: Box 232, Zip 40311; tel. 606/289-7181; James J. Wente, Administrator (Nonreporting) A1 9 10	13	10	83	—	—	—	—	—	—	—
CARROLLTON—Carroll County ★ CARROLL COUNTY MEMORIAL HOSPITAL, 309 11th Street, Zip 41008; tel. 502/732-4321; Roger Williams, Chief Executive Officer A9 10 F8 15 16 19 22 27 31 32 33 37 44 65 71 73 S2285 Alliant Health System	13	10	39	1009	23	25642	0	7083	2797	138

Hospitals, U.S. / KENTUCKY

Hospital, Address, Telephone, Administrator, Approval, Facility, and Physician Codes, Health Care System	Classi-fication Codes		Utilization Data					Expense (thousands) of dollars		
★ American Hospital Association (AHA) membership □ Joint Commission on Accreditation of Healthcare Organizations (JCAHO) accreditation + American Osteopathic Hospital Association (AOHA) membership ○ American Osteopathic Association (AOA) accreditation △ Commission on Accreditation of Rehabilitation Facilities (CARF) accreditation Control codes 61, 63, 64, 71, 72 and 73 indicate hospitals listed by AOHA, but not registered by AHA. For definition of numerical codes, see page A6	Control	Service	Beds	Admissions	Census	Outpatient Visits	Births	Total	Payroll	Personnel
COLUMBIA—Adair County										
□ WESTLAKE CUMBERLAND HOSPITAL, Westlake Drive, Zip 42728, Mailing Address: P.O. Box 468, Zip 42728–0468; tel. 502/384–4753; Rex A. Tungate, Administrator (Nonreporting) **A**1 9 10	16	10	80	—	—	—	—	—	—	—
CORBIN—Whitley County										
★ BAPTIST REGIONAL MEDICAL CENTER, 1 Trillium Way, Zip 40701-8420; tel. 606/528–1212; John S. Henson, President (Nonreporting) **A**1 9 10 **S**0315 Baptist Healthcare System	23	10	263	—	—	—	—	—	—	—
COVINGTON—Kenton County										
□ CHILDREN'S PSYCHIATRIC HOSPITAL OF NORTHERN KENTUCKY, 502 Farrell Drive, Zip 41012–2680, Mailing Address: Box 2680, Zip 41012–2680; tel. 606/578–3200; Gary Goetz, Director (Nonreporting) **A**1 9 10	23	52	28	—	—	—	—	—	—	—
★ ST. ELIZABETH MEDICAL CENTER–NORTH, (Includes St. Elizabeth Medical Center–South, 1 Medical Village Drive, Edgewood, Kentucky, Zip 41017; tel. 606/344–2000) 401 East 20th Street, Zip 41014; tel. 606/292–4000; Joseph W. Gross, President and Chief Executive Officer (Total facility includes 25 beds in nursing home–type unit) **A**1 2 3 5 9 10 **F**2 3 4 7 8 10 11 14 15 17 19 21 22 28 29 30 31 32 33 34 35 37 38 39 40 41 42 43 44 49 52 55 56 58 59 60 64 65 66 67 71 73 74 **P**8	21	10	497	21078	332	253813	2930	169244	76252	2320
CYNTHIANA—Harrison County										
★ HARRISON MEMORIAL HOSPITAL, Mailing Address: P.O. Box 250, Zip 41031–0250; tel. 606/234–2300; James R. Farris, Administrator (Total facility includes 34 beds in nursing home–type unit) **A**1 9 10 **F**7 8 19 21 22 24 26 32 33 34 37 39 40 42 44 46 49 64 65 71 73 **P**5	23	10	99	2074	68	24044	154	11172	5109	201
DANVILLE—Boyle County										
★ EPHRAIM MCDOWELL REGIONAL MEDICAL CENTER, 217 South Third Street, Zip 40422–9983; tel. 606/239–1000; Thomas W. Smith, President and Chief Executive Officer **A**1 5 9 10 **F**7 8 10 12 14 16 19 20 22 25 26 28 29 30 32 33 34 37 38 39 40 41 42 44 45 46 49 52 55 56 57 60 65 66 71 73 74 **P**3 8	23	10	151	6471	100	36916	912	35591	15409	624
EDGEWOOD—Kenton County										
□ △ HEALTHSOUTH REHABILITATION HOSPITAL OF NORTHERN KENTUCKY, (Formerly Northern Kentucky Rehabilitation Hospital) 201 Medical Village Drive, Zip 41017; tel. 606/341–2044; Frank G. Delisi, Chief Executive Officer and Administrator (Nonreporting) **A**1 7 9 10	33	46	40	—	—	—	—	—	—	—
ELIZABETHTOWN—Hardin County										
★ HARDIN MEMORIAL HOSPITAL, 913 North Dixie Highway, Zip 42701–2599; tel. 502/737–1212; Gary Colberg, Administrator **A**1 9 10 **F**7 8 10 11 12 14 16 17 19 21 22 25 28 30 34 35 37 40 42 44 45 46 52 60 65 71 73 **P**6 8 **S**0002 Quorum Health Group/Quorum Health Resources	13	10	276	11014	190	99876	1161	73210	32295	1143
□ △ LAKEVIEW REHABILITATION HOSPITAL, 134 Heartland Drive, Zip 42701; tel. 502/769–3100; James H. Wesp, Administrator **A**1 7 9 10 **F**1 5 12 17 25 27 30 34 39 41 46 48 49 65 66 73	32	46	40	604	30	11027	0	8193	3978	143
FLEMINGSBURG—Fleming County										
★ FLEMING COUNTY HOSPITAL, 920 Elizaville Avenue, Zip 41041, Mailing Address: Box 388, Zip 41041–0388; tel. 606/849–2351; Bobby B. Emmons, Administrator (Nonreporting) **A**1 9 10 **S**0002 Quorum Health Group/Quorum Health Resources	13	10	52	—	—	—	—	—	—	—
FLORENCE—Boone County										
★ ST. LUKE HOSPITAL WEST, 7380 Turfway Road, Zip 41042; tel. 606/525–5200; John D. Hoyle, President and Chief Executive Officer (Total facility includes 16 beds in nursing home–type unit) **A**9 10 **F**3 7 8 10 11 12 14 15 16 17 19 20 21 22 24 26 28 29 30 31 32 34 35 37 39 40 41 42 44 46 49 52 54 55 56 58 59 60 64 65 67 71 73 74 **P**8	23	10	153	6092	87	54553	632	35825	15294	469
FORT CAMPBELL—Christian County										
★ COLONEL FLORENCE A. BLANCHFIELD ARMY COMMUNITY HOSPITAL, Zip 42223–5349; tel. 502/798–8040 **A**1 2 **F**3 8 12 14 15 17 18 19 20 22 25 28 29 30 31 34 35 37 39 40 41 44 46 51 52 53 54 56 57 58 59 65 67 71 73 74 **P**6 **S**9395 Department of the Army	42	10	155	11369	81	916171	1825	46881	18571	1336
FORT KNOX—Hardin County										
★ IRELAND ARMY COMMUNITY HOSPITAL, 851 Ireland Loop, Zip 40121–5520; tel. 502/624–9020; Colonel Edward Burkhalter, Commander **A**1 5 **F**2 3 4 5 6 7 8 9 10 11 12 15 16 17 18 19 20 21 22 23 24 26 27 28 29 30 31 32 33 34 35 37 38 39 40 41 42 43 44 46 47 48 49 50 51 52 53 54 56 57 58 59 60 61 63 64 65 66 67 68 69 70 71 72 73 74 **P**1 **S**9395 Department of the Army	42	10	97	5999	37	—	864	32939	12846	977
FORT THOMAS—Campbell County										
□ ST. LUKE HOSPITALS, 85 North Grand Avenue, Zip 41075–1796; tel. 606/572–3100; John D. Hoyle, President (Total facility includes 26 beds in nursing home–type unit) **A**1 2 9 10 **F**2 3 7 8 10 11 12 14 15 16 17 19 20 21 22 24 26 28 29 30 31 32 34 35 37 39 40 41 42 44 46 49 56 60 64 65 67 71 73 74 **P**8	23	10	244	9409	141	69895	930	57442	23862	814
FRANKFORT—Franklin County										
★ BLUEGRASS REGIONAL MEDICAL CENTER, (Formerly HCA King's Daughters Memorial Hospital) 299 King's Daughters Drive, Zip 40601–4186; tel. 502/875–5240; Ronald T. Tyrer, Chief Executive Officer **A**1 9 10 **F**2 3 7 8 10 11 14 15 16 19 20 21 22 28 29 32 33 34 35 37 39 40 42 44 46 49 52 54 60 63 65 67 71 73 **S**0048 Columbia/HCA Healthcare Corporation	33	10	146	4464	68	41504	543	27337	10865	456

Hospitals, U.S. / KENTUCKY

Hospital, Address, Telephone, Administrator, Approval, Facility, and Physician Codes, Health Care System ★ American Hospital Association (AHA) membership □ Joint Commission on Accreditation of Healthcare Organizations (JCAHO) accreditation + American Osteopathic Hospital Association (AOHA) membership ○ American Osteopathic Association (AOA) accreditation △ Commission on Accreditation of Rehabilitation Facilities (CARF) accreditation Control codes 61, 63, 64, 71, 72 and 73 indicate hospitals listed by AOHA, but not registered by AHA. For definition of numerical codes, see page A6	Classification Codes		Utilization Data					Expense (thousands) of dollars		
	Control	Service	Beds	Admissions	Census	Outpatient Visits	Births	Total	Payroll	Personnel
FRANKLIN—Simpson County ★ FRANKLIN–SIMPSON MEMORIAL HOSPITAL, Brookhaven Road, Zip 42135–2929, Mailing Address: P.O. Box 2929, Zip 42135–2929; tel. 502/586–3253; William P. Macri, Administrator (Total facility includes 6 beds in nursing home–type unit) **A**9 10 **F**8 16 19 22 37 44 64 71 73 **P**1 **S**0002 Quorum Health Group/Quorum Health Resources	13	10	36	931	15	9389	0	4854	1948	85
FULTON—Fulton County □ PARKWAY REGIONAL HOSPITAL, 2000 Holiday Lane, Zip 42041; tel. 502/472–2522; Mary Jo Lewis, Administrator **A**1 9 10 **F**2 3 8 10 12 15 16 17 19 21 22 28 30 32 33 37 44 46 49 61 67 71 73 **P**5 **S**0875 Community Health Systems, Inc.	33	10	80	1949	33	44827	0	10476	4884	200
GEORGETOWN—Scott County ★ SCOTT GENERAL HOSPITAL, 1140 Lexington Road, Zip 40324; tel. 502/868–1100; Kenneth R. Unger, Chief Executive Officer (Total facility includes 10 beds in nursing home–type unit) **A**1 9 10 **F**7 8 10 12 14 16 17 19 20 21 22 26 28 34 35 37 40 41 42 44 49 51 60 64 65 66 71 73 74 **P**1 7 **S**0048 Columbia/HCA Healthcare Corporation	33	10	61	1969	23	31605	371	11721	4559	197
GLASGOW—Barren County ★ T. J. SAMSON COMMUNITY HOSPITAL, 1301 North Race Street, Zip 42141–3483; tel. 502/651–4444; H. Glenn Joiner, Chief Executive Officer (Total facility includes 16 beds in nursing home–type unit) **A**1 9 10 **F**4 7 8 10 15 19 21 22 32 33 37 38 40 41 44 45 46 49 56 64 65 71 73	23	10	196	7366	110	50985	915	36632	16500	715
GREENSBURG—Green County ★ JANE TODD CRAWFORD MEMORIAL HOSPITAL, 202–206 Milby Street, Zip 42743, Mailing Address: P.O. Box 220, Zip 42743; tel. 502/932–4211; Larry Craig, Chief Executive Officer (Total facility includes 12 beds in nursing home–type unit) **A**9 10 **F**2 8 19 28 34 37 44 49 52 64 71 **S**2285 Alliant Health System	13	10	64	1308	34	7474	0	6063	2589	131
GREENVILLE—Muhlenberg County ★ MUHLENBERG COMMUNITY HOSPITAL, 440 Hopkinsville Street, Zip 42345, Mailing Address: P.O. Box 387, Zip 42345; tel. 502/338–8000; Charles D. Lovell Jr., Chief Executive Officer (Total facility includes 45 beds in nursing home–type unit) **A**1 9 10 **F**7 8 15 16 19 21 22 26 28 32 34 44 46 49 50 54 57 59 63 64 65 71 73 **P**8 **S**0002 Quorum Health Group/Quorum Health Resources	23	10	135	2718	74	85698	342	19496	8145	366
HARDINSBURG—Breckinridge County ★ BRECKINRIDGE MEMORIAL HOSPITAL, 1011 Old Highway 60, Zip 40143–9732; tel. 502/756–2124; George Walz CHE, Chief Executive Officer **A**9 10 **F**8 14 19 22 32 33 44 46 64 71 73 **P**5 **S**2285 Alliant Health System	23	10	45	1221	26	23575	0	5412	2336	129
HARLAN—Harlan County □ HARLAN ARH HOSPITAL, 81 Ball Park Road, Zip 40831–1792; tel. 606/573–8100; Vernon L. Rucks, Administrator **A**1 9 10 **F**7 8 14 15 16 19 21 22 23 28 29 32 33 34 35 36 37 40 44 45 52 54 56 57 58 59 65 71 73 **S**0145 Appalachian Regional Healthcare	23	10	125	3383	44	68364	456	19023	—	304
HARRODSBURG—Mercer County ★ JAMES B. HAGGIN MEMORIAL HOSPITAL, 464 Linden Avenue, Zip 40330–1862; tel. 606/734–5441; Earl James Motzer Ph.D., FACHE, Chief Executive Officer (Total facility includes 25 beds in nursing home–type unit) **A**9 10 **F**8 11 14 15 16 17 19 22 28 29 30 33 34 37 39 42 44 49 64 65 67 71 **P**5 **S**2285 Alliant Health System	23	10	59	965	36	18048	0	6243	3028	144
HARTFORD—Ohio County ★ OHIO COUNTY HOSPITAL, 1211 Main Street, Zip 42347; tel. 502/298–7411; Blaine Pieper, Administrator (Nonreporting) **A**1 9 10 **S**0002 Quorum Health Group/Quorum Health Resources	23	10	54	—	—	—	—	—	—	—
HAZARD—Perry County □ ARH REGIONAL MEDICAL CENTER, 100 Medical Center Drive, Zip 41701–1000; tel. 606/439–6610; David R. Lyon, Administrator (Total facility includes 25 beds in nursing home–type unit) **A**1 3 5 9 10 **F**7 8 10 16 19 21 22 25 32 33 34 35 37 40 42 44 49 51 52 54 55 56 58 60 64 65 67 71 72 73 **S**0145 Appalachian Regional Healthcare	23	10	284	8668	200	84928	561	39532	15592	777
HENDERSON—Henderson County ★ COMMUNITY METHODIST HOSPITAL, 1305 North Elm Street, Zip 42420, Mailing Address: Box 48, Zip 42420–0048; tel. 502/827–7700; Bruce D. Begley, Executive Director (Nonreporting) **A**1 9 10	21	10	213	—	—	—	—	—	—	—
HOPKINSVILLE—Christian County □ CUMBERLAND HALL HOSPITAL, 210 West 17th Street, Zip 42240; tel. 502/886–1919; William C. Heard, Administrator and Chief Executive Officer (Nonreporting) **A**1 10	33	22	56	—	—	—	—	—	—	—
□ JENNIE STUART MEDICAL CENTER, 320 West 18th Street, Zip 42240–6315; tel. 502/887–0100; Eric A. Lee, Interim Administrator (Nonreporting) **A**1 9 10	23	10	147	—	—	—	—	—	—	—
□ WESTERN STATE HOSPITAL, Russellville Road, Zip 42241, Mailing Address: Box 2200, Zip 42241; tel. 502/886–4431; Wayne Taylor, Director (Total facility includes 144 beds in nursing home–type unit) **A**1 9 10 **F**20 39 41 45 46 52 56 57 64 65 67 73 **P**6	12	22	355	1079	248	0	0	—	—	478
HORSE CAVE—Hart County ★ CAVERNA MEMORIAL HOSPITAL, 1501 South Dixie Street, Zip 42749, Mailing Address: P.O. Box 120, Zip 42749–0120; tel. 502/786–2191; James J. Kerins Sr., Administrator **A**9 10 **F**8 14 15 19 22 28 30 34 37 44 64 71 **S**2285 Alliant Health System	23	10	28	930	11	11830	99	2847	1363	71

© 1995 AHA Guide

Hospitals, U.S. / KENTUCKY

Hospital, Address, Telephone, Administrator, Approval, Facility, and Physician Codes, Health Care System	Control	Service	Beds	Admissions	Census	Outpatient Visits	Births	Total	Payroll	Personnel
★ American Hospital Association (AHA) membership □ Joint Commission on Accreditation of Healthcare Organizations (JCAHO) accreditation + American Osteopathic Hospital Association (AOHA) membership ○ American Osteopathic Association (AOA) accreditation △ Commission on Accreditation of Rehabilitation Facilities (CARF) accreditation Control codes 61, 63, 64, 71, 72 and 73 indicate hospitals listed by AOHA, but not registered by AHA. For definition of numerical codes, see page A6										
HYDEN—Leslie County MARY BRECKINRIDGE HOSPITAL, Hospital Drive, Zip 41749–0000; tel. 606/672–2901; David W. Southern, Administrator **A**9 10 **F**7 19 22 32 40 44 49 51 65 71 74	23	10	40	1296	16	39849	193	10327	5716	250
IRVINE—Estill County ★ MARCUM AND WALLACE MEMORIAL HOSPITAL, 201 Richmond Avenue, Zip 40336; tel. 606/723–2115; Christopher M. Goddard, Administrator **A**9 10 **F**8 15 16 17 19 22 28 30 34 71 **S**5155 Mercy Health System	21	10	26	541	9	33499	0	3283	1471	65
JENKINS—Letcher County □ JENKINS COMMUNITY HOSPITAL A SUBSIDIARY OF FIRST HEALTH, INC., Main Street, Zip 41537, Mailing Address: P.O. Box 472, Zip 41537; tel. 606/832–2171; Jason Staggs, Administrator **A**1 9 10 **F**16 19 22 28 32 33 34 37 44 46 51 65 71 **S**1275 First Health, Inc.	33	10	60	1516	16	20864	0	3955	2274	128
LA GRANGE—Oldham County ★ TRI COUNTY BAPTIST HOSPITAL, 1025 New Moody Lane, Zip 40031–0559, Mailing Address: P.O. Box 559, Zip 40031–0559; tel. 502/222–5388; David L. Gray, Administrator (Total facility includes 30 beds in nursing home–type unit) **A**1 9 10 **F**2 3 4 7 8 10 11 12 13 14 15 16 17 18 19 21 22 26 28 29 30 31 32 34 35 37 39 40 41 42 43 44 45 46 48 49 52 53 54 55 56 57 58 59 60 61 63 64 65 67 68 71 73 74 **S**0315 Baptist Healthcare System	23	10	120	2568	65	23781	156	20688	8373	252
LANCASTER—Garrard County ★ GARRARD COUNTY MEMORIAL HOSPITAL, 308 West Maple Avenue, Zip 40444–1098; tel. 606/792–6844; W. David MacCool, Administrator (Total facility includes 100 beds in nursing home–type unit) **A**9 10 **F**8 19 22 41 44 49 64 65 71	13	10	131	835	112	13755	0	—	—	149
LEBANON—Marion County ★ SPRING VIEW MEDICAL CENTER, 320 Loretto Road, Zip 40033–0320; tel. 502/692–3161; Russell Goldberg, Chief Executive Officer (Total facility includes 38 beds in nursing home–type unit) **A**1 9 10 **F**14 15 16 19 21 22 25 28 30 34 35 37 39 40 41 42 44 46 49 51 60 61 63 64 65 67 71 73 74 **P**8 **S**0048 Columbia/HCA Healthcare Corporation	33	10	113	2260	63	19212	272	11893	4648	225
LEITCHFIELD—Grayson County ★ TWIN LAKES REGIONAL MEDICAL CENTER, 910 Wallace Avenue, Zip 42754; tel. 502/259–9400; Stephen L. Meredith, Chief Executive Officer **A**9 10 **F**8 12 14 15 16 19 22 32 34 35 37 44 45 46 49 62 71 **P**3 6 **S**2285 Alliant Health System	23	10	75	2586	38	21938	289	12597	5838	246
LEXINGTON—Fayette County ★ △ CARDINAL HILL REHABILITATIOH HOSPITAL, 2050 Versailles Road, Zip 40504–1499; tel. 606/254–5701; Kerry G. Gillihan, President and Chief Executive Officer (Total facility includes 10 beds in nursing home–type unit) **A**3 5 7 9 10 **F**5 12 14 15 16 17 20 22 24 27 28 30 34 41 45 46 48 49 52 54 64 65 66 67 70 71 73 **P**6	23	46	90	1142	61	29921	0	19246	11194	436
★ CENTRAL BAPTIST HOSPITAL, 1740 Nicholasville Road, Zip 40503; tel. 606/275–6100; William G. Sisson, President **A**1 2 3 5 9 10 **F**4 7 8 10 11 12 15 16 19 21 22 29 30 32 34 35 37 38 39 40 42 43 44 45 46 60 61 63 65 71 73 74 **S**0315 Baptist Healthcare System	23	10	324	14035	221	91668	2955	124761	47297	1430
□ CHARTER RIDGE HOSPITAL, 3050 Rio Dosa Drive, Zip 40509–9990; tel. 606/269–2325; Scott W. Kardenetz, Chief Executive Officer **A**1 3 5 9 10 **F**2 3 15 52 53 54 55 56 57 58 59 65 **S**0695 Charter Medical Corporation	33	22	110	1793	68	—	0	—	—	185
□ EASTERN STATE HOSPITAL, 627 West Fourth Street, Zip 40508–9990; tel. 606/246–7000; Daniel J. Luchtefeld, Director **A**1 5 9 10 **F**15 16 20 52 54 55 57 65 73	12	22	255	1575	165	0	0	21815	12175	448
★ GOOD SAMARITAN HOSPITAL, 310 South Limestone Street, Zip 40508–3008; tel. 606/252–6612; Barton A. Hove, Chief Executive Officer (Total facility includes 34 beds in nursing home–type unit) **A**1 2 9 10 **F**7 8 9 10 11 12 14 15 16 18 19 21 22 26 28 29 30 31 32 33 35 36 37 38 39 40 41 42 44 46 47 49 52 53 54 55 56 57 58 59 61 64 65 67 71 73 74 **P**7 8	32	10	200	6509	116	40898	313	50520	17462	709
□ HUMANA HOSPITAL–LEXINGTON, 150 North Eagle Creek Drive, Zip 40509–1807, Mailing Address: P.O. Box 23260, Zip 40523–3260; tel. 606/268–4800; Jeffrey Helton, Executive Director **A**1 5 9 10 **F**4 7 8 10 11 12 17 19 21 22 26 30 31 32 33 37 39 40 41 42 43 44 45 49 56 63 65 66 71 73 **P**6 **S**0052 Jewish Hospital Healthcare Services	33	10	174	5484	74	38291	620	36682	14588	538
★ SHRINERS HOSPITALS FOR CRIPPLED CHILDREN, LEXINGTON UNIT, 1900 Richmond Road, Zip 40502; tel. 606/266–2101; Tony Lewgood, Administrator **A**1 3 5 **F**9 15 16 17 45 49 65 71 73 **P**6 **S**4125 Shriners Hospitals for Crippled Children	23	57	50	1102	27	14060	0	—	—	182
★ ST. JOSEPH HOSPITAL, One St. Joseph Drive, Zip 40504; tel. 606/278–3436; William D. Fuchs, President (Total facility includes 22 beds in nursing home–type unit) **A**1 2 3 5 9 10 **F**2 3 4 8 10 11 12 15 16 17 19 21 22 23 25 26 28 29 30 31 34 35 37 39 41 42 43 44 47 49 51 54 55 56 57 58 59 60 63 64 65 66 67 71 73 74 **P**6 **S**3045 Sisters of Charity of Nazareth Health System	21	10	325	13229	252	58757	0	112834	45861	1626
★ UNIVERSITY OF KENTUCKY HOSPITAL, 800 Rose Street, Zip 40536–0084; tel. 606/323–5000; Frank Butler, Director **A**1 2 3 5 8 9 10 **F**4 7 9 10 11 12 15 16 17 18 19 20 21 22 23 24 25 26 29 30 31 32 33 34 35 37 38 39 40 41 42 43 44 45 46 47 49 51 52 53 54 55 56 57 58 59 60 61 65 66 69 70 71 73 74 **P**1 7 8	12	10	452	19262	365	326556	2414	194552	80467	2781

Hospitals, U.S. / KENTUCKY

Hospital, Address, Telephone, Administrator, Approval, Facility, and Physician Codes, Health Care System	Classification Codes		Utilization Data					Expense (thousands) of dollars		
★ American Hospital Association (AHA) membership ☐ Joint Commission on Accreditation of Healthcare Organizations (JCAHO) accreditation + American Osteopathic Hospital Association (AOHA) membership ○ American Osteopathic Association (AOA) accreditation △ Commission on Accreditation of Rehabilitation Facilities (CARF) accreditation Control codes 61, 63, 64, 71, 72 and 73 indicate hospitals listed by AOHA, but not registered by AHA. For definition of numerical codes, see page A6	Control	Service	Beds	Admissions	Census	Outpatient Visits	Births	Total	Payroll	Personnel
★ VETERANS AFFAIRS MEDICAL CENTER–LEXINGTON, 2250 Leestown Pike, Zip 40511–1093; tel. 606/233–4511; Helen K. Cornish, Director (Total facility includes 76 beds in nursing home–type unit) **A**1 3 5 8 9 **F**2 3 4 8 10 11 12 16 19 20 21 22 24 26 28 31 32 33 34 35 37 39 41 42 43 44 45 46 48 49 51 52 54 56 57 58 59 60 63 64 65 67 71 73 **P**6 **S**9295 Department of Veterans Affairs	45	10	620	8063	520	130061	0	114657	68733	1892
LONDON—Laurel County ★ MARYMOUNT HOSPITAL, 310 East Ninth Street, Zip 40741–1299; tel. 606/878–6520; Lowell Jones, President (Total facility includes 24 beds in nursing home–type unit) **A**1 9 10 **F**7 10 11 12 15 19 21 22 30 34 37 39 40 42 44 46 49 64 71 73 **P**3 7 **S**3045 Sisters of Charity of Nazareth Health System	21	10	95	3656	50	37957	364	18848	8052	291
LOUISA—Lawrence County ☐ THREE RIVERS MEDICAL CENTER, Highway 644, Zip 41230, Mailing Address: Box 769, Zip 41230; tel. 606/638–9451; Kiser Greg, Executive Director **A**1 9 10 **F**7 8 11 15 16 19 21 22 23 26 28 29 30 32 33 35 37 40 44 45 46 52 55 56 57 58 59 60 63 65 71 73 **S**0875 Community Health Systems, Inc.	33	10	90	2393	30	18089	115	—	—	170
LOUISVILLE—Jefferson County ★ ALLIANT HOSPITALS, (Formerly Norton Hospital of Alliant Health) (Includes Alliant Medical Pavilion, 315 East Broadway, Louisville, Kentucky, Zip 40202, Mailing Address: Box 843, Zip 40201–0843; tel. 502/629–2206; Children's Hospital, Louisville, Kentucky, Zip 40202; tel. 502/629–6000; Douglas J. Eighmey, Senior Vice President & Administrator; Kosair Children's Hospital, 982 Eastern Parkway, Louisville, Kentucky, Zip 40217, Mailing Address: Box 37370, Zip 40233; tel. 502/629–6000; Norton Hospital, Louisville, Kentucky, Mailing Address: P.O. Box 35070, Zip 40232–5070; tel. 502/629–8000) 200 East Chestnut Street, Zip 40202, Mailing Address: Box 35070, Zip 40232–5070; tel. 502/629–8000; Shirley B. Powers, Senior Executive Officer (Total facility includes 17 beds in nursing home–type unit) **A**1 2 3 5 9 10 **F**3 4 5 7 8 9 10 11 12 13 15 17 19 20 21 22 23 25 26 28 29 30 31 32 33 34 35 37 38 40 41 42 43 44 45 46 47 49 52 53 54 55 56 57 58 59 60 61 64 65 67 69 70 71 72 73 74 **S**2285 Alliant Health System	23	10	714	29563	466	158444	4567	266671	120180	4003
★ AUDUBON REGIONAL MEDICAL CENTER, One Audubon Plaza Drive, Zip 40217–1397, Mailing Address: Box 17550, Zip 40217–0550; tel. 502/636–7111; Ronald J. Vigus, President and Chief Executive Officer (Nonreporting) **A**1 10 **S**0048 Columbia/HCA Healthcare Corporation	33	10	480	—	—	—	—	—	—	—
★ △ BAPTIST HOSPITAL EAST, 4000 Kresge Way, Zip 40207–4676; tel. 502/897–8100; Susan Stout Tamme, President **A**1 2 7 9 10 **F**1 2 3 4 7 8 10 12 13 14 15 16 17 18 19 21 22 26 28 29 30 31 32 34 35 37 39 40 41 42 43 44 45 46 48 49 52 53 54 55 56 57 58 59 60 61 65 67 68 71 73 74 **S**0315 Baptist Healthcare System	23	10	407	17872	324	109822	2591	127880	57519	2253
★ CARITAS PEACE CENTER, (Formerly Our Lady of Peace Hospital) 2020 Newburg Road, Zip 40232; tel. 502/451–3330; Peter J. Bernard, President and Chief Executive Officer **A**1 9 10 **F**3 15 16 35 52 53 55 56 57 58 59 73 **S**3045 Sisters of Charity of Nazareth Health System	23	22	156	2288	118	19920	0	20277	9137	325
☐ CENTRAL STATE HOSPITAL, 10510 LaGrange Road, Zip 40223–1228; tel. 502/245–4121; Paula Tamme, Chief Executive Officer **A**1 5 10 **F**15 16 20 27 28 39 52 54 55 56 57 65 73	12	22	192	1644	145	—	0	—	—	415
☐ CHARTER HOSPITAL OF LOUISVILLE, 1405 Browns Lane, Zip 40207; tel. 502/896–0495; Todd B. Graybill, Administrator (Nonreporting) **A**1 9 10 **S**0695 Charter Medical Corporation	33	22	66	—	—	—	—	—	—	—
CHILDREN'S HOSPITAL See Alliant Hospitals										
★ △ FRAZIER REHABILITATION CENTER, 220 Abraham Flexner Way, Zip 40202–1887; tel. 502/582–7400; Joanne Berryman, President; David Watkins, Medical Director **A**1 3 5 7 9 10 **F**1 2 3 4 7 8 10 12 15 16 17 18 19 20 22 23 25 26 27 28 29 30 31 32 34 35 37 39 40 41 42 43 44 45 46 48 49 51 52 53 54 55 56 57 58 59 60 63 64 65 67 69 70 71 73 74 **S**0052 Jewish Hospital Healthcare Services	23	46	95	1521	81	65939	0	23475	12286	391
★ JEWISH HOSPITAL, 217 East Chestnut Street, Zip 40202–1886; tel. 502/587–4011; Douglas E. Shaw, President (Total facility includes 3 beds in nursing home–type unit) **A**1 2 3 5 9 10 **F**1 2 3 4 7 8 10 12 15 16 17 19 20 21 22 23 25 26 27 28 29 30 31 32 33 34 35 37 39 41 42 43 44 45 46 48 49 51 52 53 54 55 56 57 58 59 60 61 63 64 65 67 69 70 71 73 74 **S**0052 Jewish Hospital Healthcare Services	23	10	408	16411	327	96041	0	173015	58641	2004
KOSAIR CHILDREN'S HOSPITAL See Alliant Hospitals										
NORTON HOSPITAL See Alliant Hospitals										
NORTON HOSPITAL OF ALLIANT HEALTH See Alliant Hospitals										
OUR LADY OF PEACE HOSPITAL See Caritas Peace Center										
★ SAINTS MARY AND ELIZABETH HOSPITAL, 1850 Bluegrass Avenue, Zip 40215–1199; tel. 502/361–6000; Peter J. Bernard, President and Chief Executive Officer (Total facility includes 20 beds in nursing home–type unit) **A**1 9 10 **F**1 2 3 4 5 6 7 8 9 10 11 12 13 14 15 16 17 18 19 20 21 22 23 24 25 26 27 28 29 30 31 32 33 34 35 36 37 38 39 40 41 42 43 44 45 46 47 48 49 50 51 52 53 54 55 56 57 58 59 60 61 63 64 65 66 67 68 69 70 71 72 73 74 **P**7 **S**3045 Sisters of Charity of Nazareth Health System	21	10	177	7574	125	67271	0	61184	28111	842
★ SOUTHWEST HOSPITAL, 9820 Third Street Road, Zip 40272–9984; tel. 502/933–8100; Jack Wheatley, Chief Executive Officer (Total facility includes 23 beds in nursing home–type unit) **A**1 10 **F**10 19 22 28 30 32 34 37 39 41 44 45 46 54 64 65 71 73 **S**0048 Columbia/HCA Healthcare Corporation	33	10	150	4578	77	32850	0	—	—	470

© 1995 AHA Guide

Hospitals, U.S. / KENTUCKY

Hospital, Address, Telephone, Administrator, Approval, Facility, and Physician Codes, Health Care System	Classification Codes		Utilization Data					Expense (thousands) of dollars		
★ American Hospital Association (AHA) membership □ Joint Commission on Accreditation of Healthcare Organizations (JCAHO) accreditation + American Osteopathic Hospital Association (AOHA) membership ○ American Osteopathic Association (AOA) accreditation △ Commission on Accreditation of Rehabilitation Facilities (CARF) accreditation Control codes 61, 63, 64, 71, 72 and 73 indicate hospitals listed by AOHA, but not registered by AHA. For definition of numerical codes, see page A6	Control	Service	Beds	Admissions	Census	Outpatient Visits	Births	Total	Payroll	Personnel
★ SUBURBAN MEDICAL CENTER, 4001 Dutchmans Lane, Zip 40207; tel. 502/893–1000; Patricia A. Davis, Chief Executive Officer **A**1 10 **F**2 4 5 6 7 8 9 10 11 12 15 16 19 20 21 22 23 28 30 31 32 33 34 35 37 38 39 40 41 42 43 44 45 47 48 49 51 52 53 54 55 56 57 58 59 60 61 65 66 67 69 70 71 73 74 **P**6 **S**0048 Columbia/HCA Healthcare Corporation	33	10	380	12440	186	80989	1933	74774	32706	905
□ TEN BROECK HOSPITAL, 8521 Old LaGrange Road, Zip 40242; tel. 502/426–6380; Don S. McLendon, Executive Director **A**1 10 **F**1 2 3 14 19 21 22 27 34 35 48 52 53 55 56 58 59 65 71 **S**9605 United Medical Corporation	33	22	94	1857	68	1303	0	10710	4465	156
★ UNIVERSITY OF LOUISVILLE HOSPITAL, 530 South Jackson Street, Zip 40202–3611; tel. 502/562–3000; Ronald A. Hytoff, Chief Executive Officer **A**1 2 3 5 8 9 10 **F**4 8 9 10 11 12 15 19 20 21 22 28 29 31 34 35 37 38 40 41 42 43 44 45 46 49 50 56 60 63 65 70 71 73 **S**0048 Columbia/HCA Healthcare Corporation	33	10	315	13551	241	124295	1954	150424	50057	1646
★ VETERANS AFFAIRS MEDICAL CENTER–LOUISVILLE, 800 Zorn Avenue, Zip 40206–1499; tel. 502/895–3401; Larry J. Sander, Director **A**1 2 3 5 8 9 **F**2 3 4 6 8 10 11 17 19 20 21 22 24 26 28 29 31 32 33 34 35 37 39 41 42 44 45 46 49 51 52 54 56 57 58 60 65 67 71 73 74 **P**6 **S**9295 Department of Veterans Affairs	45	10	246	7726	212	156958	0	94988	49467	1362
MADISONVILLE—Hopkins County										
★ REGIONAL MEDICAL CENTER OF HOPKINS COUNTY, 900 Hospital Drive, Zip 42431–1694; tel. 502/825–5100; Bobby H. Dampier, Chief Executive Officer **A**1 2 3 5 9 10 **F**3 4 7 8 10 11 12 15 17 19 20 21 22 23 24 28 30 31 32 34 35 37 38 39 40 41 42 43 44 45 46 47 49 52 53 56 57 58 60 63 65 66 67 71 73 **P**1 4 5	23	10	410	10550	179	60783	822	71077	32358	1154
MANCHESTER—Clay County										
★ MEMORIAL HOSPITAL, 401 Memorial Drive, Zip 40962–9156; tel. 606/598–5104; T. Henry Scoggins FACHE, President (Total facility includes 11 beds in nursing home–type unit) **A**9 10 **F**7 8 15 16 17 19 22 24 28 32 33 34 37 39 40 44 45 46 49 62 64 65 71 73 74 **S**4165 Adventist Health System–Sunbelt Health Care Corporation	21	10	63	2407	26	29192	285	12829	5900	240
MARION—Crittenden County										
★ CRITTENDEN COUNTY HOSPITAL, Highway 60 South, Zip 42064–0386, Mailing Address: Box 386, Zip 42064; tel. 502/965–5281; Rick Napper, Chief Executive Officer (Nonreporting) **A**1 9 10 **S**0002 Quorum Health Group/Quorum Health Resources	23	10	100	—	—	—	—	—	—	—
MARTIN—Floyd County										
★ OUR LADY OF THE WAY HOSPITAL, Route 1428, Main Street, Zip 41649–0910; tel. 606/285–5181; Lowell Jones, Chief Executive Officer **A**1 9 10 **F**8 15 16 17 19 22 39 44 45 50 65 67 68 71 73 **P**5 **S**5115 Sisters of Charity Health Care Systems, Inc.	21	10	35	1800	17	104111	187	7957	3425	128
MAYFIELD—Graves County										
★ + PINELAKE MEDICAL CENTER, 1099 Medical Center Circle, Zip 42066, Mailing Address: P.O. Box 1099, Zip 42066; tel. 502/251–4100; Harry Alvis, Chief Executive Officer (Total facility includes 14 beds in nursing home–type unit) **A**1 9 10 **F**7 8 10 12 14 15 16 19 20 21 28 29 30 32 35 37 40 41 42 44 45 54 63 64 65 66 67 71 74 **P**1 2 3 5 6 7 8 **S**0048 Columbia/HCA Healthcare Corporation	33	10	106	3764	52	75952	419	—	—	376
MAYSVILLE—Mason County										
★ MEADOWVIEW REGIONAL HOSPITAL, 989 Medical Park Drive, Zip 41056; tel. 606/759–5311; Michael L. Graue, Chief Executive Officer **A**1 9 10 **F**7 8 10 11 12 16 19 21 28 30 34 35 37 39 40 44 49 63 64 65 66 71 73 74 **P**1 7 **S**0048 Columbia/HCA Healthcare Corporation	33	10	111	3310	40	28957	1011	15316	6729	258
MCDOWELL—Floyd County										
□ MCDOWELL ARH HOSPITAL, Route 122, Zip 41647, Mailing Address: Box 247, Zip 41647; tel. 606/377–3400; Jerry Haynes, Administrator **A**1 9 10 **F**8 14 15 16 17 19 22 26 28 29 30 32 34 36 37 39 44 49 51 65 71 73 **S**0145 Appalachian Regional Healthcare	23	10	60	1923	20	—	0	8829	—	137
MIDDLESBORO—Bell County										
□ MIDDLESBORO APPALACHIAN REGIONAL HOSPITAL, 3600 West Cumberland Avenue, Zip 40965, Mailing Address: Box 340, Zip 40965–0340; tel. 606/242–1101; Paul V. Miles, Administrator **A**1 9 10 **F**7 8 16 19 22 28 31 32 34 35 37 40 44 49 65 67 70 71 73 **S**0145 Appalachian Regional Healthcare	23	10	96	4502	55	48548	71	18800	7181	298
MONTICELLO—Wayne County										
□ WAYNE COUNTY HOSPITAL, 166 Hospital Street, Zip 42633–2416; tel. 606/348–9343; Eddy R. Stockton, Administrator **A**1 9 10 **F**8 19 21 22 34 44 49 64 65 71 73	23	10	30	967	14	21553	2	5378	1814	95
MOREHEAD—Rowan County										
★ ST. CLAIRE MEDICAL CENTER, 222 Medical Circle, Zip 40351–1180; tel. 606/783–6500; Mark J. Neff, President and Chief Executive Officer **A**1 5 9 10 1 32 33 34 35 37 40 41 42 44 46 49 51 52 53 54 55 56 57 58 60 63 64 65 67 70 71 73 74	21	10	133	5969	76	236720	648	41641	18709	846
MORGANFIELD—Union County										
□ UNION COUNTY METHODIST HOSPITAL, 4604 Highway 60 West, Zip 42437–9570; tel. 502/389–3030; Patrick Donahue, Administrator (Total facility includes 16 beds in nursing home–type unit) **A**1 9 10 **F**15 16 19 20 22 26 28 30 32 33 35 39 44 49 53 56 57 58 71 73 **P**8	21	10	54	701	21	14408	0	4777	2076	89

Hospitals, U.S. / KENTUCKY

Hospital, Address, Telephone, Administrator, Approval, Facility, and Physician Codes, Health Care System	Classification Codes		Utilization Data					Expense (thousands) of dollars		
★ American Hospital Association (AHA) membership ☐ Joint Commission on Accreditation of Healthcare Organizations (JCAHO) accreditation + American Osteopathic Hospital Association (AOHA) membership ○ American Osteopathic Association (AOA) accreditation △ Commission on Accreditation of Rehabilitation Facilities (CARF) accreditation Control codes 61, 63, 64, 71, 72 and 73 indicate hospitals listed by AOHA, but not registered by AHA. For definition of numerical codes, see page A6	Control	Service	Beds	Admissions	Census	Outpatient Visits	Births	Total	Payroll	Personnel
MOUNT STERLING—Montgomery County										
★ GATEWAY REGIONAL HEALTH SYSTEM, Sterling Avenue, Zip 40353–0007, Mailing Address: P.O. Box 7, Zip 40353; tel. 606/498–1220; Jeffrey L. Buckley, President and Chief Executive Officer (Total facility includes 40 beds in nursing home–type unit) **A**1 9 10 **F**7 8 11 14 15 16 17 19 20 21 22 24 28 30 35 37 39 40 41 42 44 46 48 49 56 63 64 65 67 71 73 74 **P**3 6 8	23	10	103	2407	74	55270	655	14887	5669	315
MOUNT VERNON—Rockcastle County										
★ ROCKCASTLE HOSPITAL, 145 Newcomb Avenue, Zip 40456, Mailing Address: P.O. Box 1310, Zip 40456; tel. 606/256–2195; Lee D. Keene, Administrator (Total facility includes 60 beds in nursing home–type unit) **A**9 10 **F**8 19 22 34 44 65 71	23	10	86	1313	70	20972	0	14078	7049	291
MURRAY—Calloway County										
★ MURRAY–CALLOWAY COUNTY HOSPITAL, 803 Poplar Street, Zip 42071–2432; tel. 502/762–1100; Stuart Poston, Administrator (Total facility includes 214 beds in nursing home–type unit) **A**1 9 10 **F**1 7 8 10 19 21 22 32 33 34 35 37 40 41 42 44 46 52 54 55 56 57 60 63 64 65 67 70 71 73 74	15	10	347	5430	307	136781	682	39446	17055	840
OWENSBORO—Daviess County										
★ △ MERCY HOSPITAL, 1006 Ford Avenue, Zip 42301, Mailing Address: P.O. Box 2839, Zip 42302; tel. 502/686–6100; Douglas Borders, President and Chief Executive Officer **A**1 7 9 10 **F**7 8 12 14 15 16 19 21 22 23 28 30 31 37 38 39 40 41 42 44 45 46 48 49 65 71 73 **P**3 7 **S**5155 Mercy Health System	23	10	149	5257	77	55035	524	36016	14270	544
★ OWENSBORO–DAVIESS COUNTY HOSPITAL, 811 East Parrish Avenue, Zip 42303, Mailing Address: P.O. Box 20007, Zip 42304–0007; tel. 502/688–2000; Mark F. Weber, President and Chief Executive Officer **A**1 2 9 10 **F**4 7 8 10 11 12 14 15 16 19 22 23 26 27 32 34 35 37 38 39 40 41 42 43 44 45 46 49 52 55 57 58 60 65 66 71 73 74	23	10	331	12462	188	96468	1187	84945	34767	1253
VALLEY HOSPITAL, (Formerly Valley Institute of Psychiatry) 1000 Industrial Drive, Zip 42301–8715; tel. 502/686–8477; Alvin R. Freedman Ph.D., Administrator **A**9 10 **F**3 12 16 17 20 25 28 52 53 54 55 56 57 58 59 65 **P**8	23	52	77	407	62	2508	0	10000	4282	184
OWENTON—Owen County										
OWEN COUNTY MEMORIAL HOSPITAL, 330 Roland Avenue, Zip 40359; tel. 502/484–3441; Richard D. McLeod, Administrator (Nonreporting) **A**9 10	33	10	50							
PADUCAH—McCracken County										
☐ CHARTER BEHAVIORAL HEALTH SYSTEM OF PADUCAH, (Formerly Charter Hospital of Paducah) 435 Berger Road, Zip 42001, Mailing Address: P.O. Box 7609, Zip 42002–7609; tel. 502/444–0444; Pat Harrod, Chief Executive Officer **A**1 9 10 **F**2 3 12 17 34 52 53 55 58 59 **S**0695 Charter Medical Corporation	33	22	51	582	41	—	0	—	—	55
★ LOURDES HOSPITAL, 1530 Lone Oak Road, Zip 42001, Mailing Address: P.O. Box 7100, Zip 42002–7100; tel. 502/444–2444; Gerald J. Lagesse, President and Chief Executive Officer **A**1 9 10 **F**1 4 7 8 10 11 12 14 15 16 17 19 20 21 22 23 24 26 28 29 30 31 32 33 34 35 36 37 39 40 41 42 43 44 45 46 48 49 52 55 56 65 67 71 73 **P**6 **S**5155 Mercy Health System	21	10	370	10437	194	154377	256	86884	35746	1154
★ WESTERN BAPTIST HOSPITAL, 2501 Kentucky Avenue, Zip 42003; tel. 502/575–2100; Larry O. Barton, President **A**1 9 10 **F**4 7 8 10 11 15 19 21 22 24 28 30 34 35 37 38 39 40 41 42 43 44 46 48 49 60 65 67 71 72 73 74 **S**0315 Baptist Healthcare System	21	10	309	13147	221	93214	1269	100619	40082	1210
PAINTSVILLE—Johnson County										
☐ PAUL B. HALL REGIONAL MEDICAL CENTER, 625 James S Trimble Boulevard, Zip 41240, Mailing Address: P.O. Box 1487, Zip 41240; tel. 606/789–3511; Deborah T. Meadows, Administrator (Nonreporting) **A**1 9 10 **S**1775 Health Management Associates	33	10	72							
PARIS—Bourbon County										
★ BOURBON GENERAL HOSPITAL, 9 Linville Drive, Zip 40361; tel. 606/987–3600; John R. Grant, Chief Executive Officer **A**1 9 10 **F**2 3 8 10 11 14 15 16 19 22 28 30 34 35 37 41 44 46 48 49 52 53 58 64 65 71 **P**7 **S**0048 Columbia/HCA Healthcare Corporation	33	10	58	1875	32	22584	0	9584	3729	159
PIKEVILLE—Pike County										
★ PIKEVILLE UNITED METHODIST HOSPITAL OF KENTUCKY, 911 South Bypass, Zip 41501–1595; tel. 606/437–3500; Martha Chill, Chief Executive Officer (Nonreporting) **A**1 2 9 10	23	10	189	—	—	—	—	—	—	
PINEVILLE—Bell County										
★ PINEVILLE COMMUNITY HOSPITAL ASSOCIATION, Riverview Avenue, Zip 40977–0850; tel. 606/337–3051; J. Milton Brooks III, Administrator (Total facility includes 30 beds in nursing home–type unit) **A**1 9 10 **F**8 14 19 22 26 32 33 34 37 40 44 46 49 64 65 71 73 **P**5	23	10	150	3960	88	23116	378	16878	6621	310
PRESTONSBURG—Floyd County										
★ HIGHLANDS REGIONAL MEDICAL CENTER, 5000 Kentucky Route 321, Zip 41653, Mailing Address: Box 668, Zip 41653–0668; tel. 606/886–8511; Clarence Traum, President and Chief Executive Officer **A**1 2 5 9 10 **F**5 7 8 10 11 14 15 16 19 21 22 25 28 30 34 35 37 40 42 44 45 54 55 56 65 67 70 71 73	23	10	184	6288	84	61874	574	35114	13383	488
PRINCETON—Caldwell County										
★ CALDWELL COUNTY HOSPITAL, 101 Hospital Drive, Zip 42445–0410, Mailing Address: Box 410, Zip 42445–0410; tel. 502/365–0300; John Svoboda, Administrator **A**1 9 10 **F**7 15 16 19 21 22 32 34 40 44 45 46 49 71 73 **S**2285 Alliant Health System	13	10	20	1078	12	18474	91	7598	3076	164

© 1995 AHA Guide

Hospitals, U.S. / KENTUCKY

Hospital, Address, Telephone, Administrator, Approval, Facility, and Physician Codes, Health Care System	Classification Codes		Utilization Data					Expense (thousands) of dollars		Personnel
★ American Hospital Association (AHA) membership □ Joint Commission on Accreditation of Healthcare Organizations (JCAHO) accreditation + American Osteopathic Hospital Association (AOHA) membership ○ American Osteopathic Association (AOA) accreditation △ Commission on Accreditation of Rehabilitation Facilities (CARF) accreditation Control codes 61, 63, 64, 71, 72 and 73 indicate hospitals listed by AOHA, but not registered by AHA. For definition of numerical codes, see page A6	Control	Service	Beds	Admissions	Census	Outpatient Visits	Births	Total	Payroll	
RADCLIFF—Hardin County ★ LINCOLN TRAIL HOSPITAL, 3909 South Wilson Road, Zip 40160–9714, Mailing Address: P.O. Box 369, Zip 40159–0369; tel. 502/351–9444; Melvin E. Modderman, Administrator **A**1 9 10 **F**2 3 15 17 22 52 53 54 55 56 57 58 59 65 **S**0335 Park Healthcare Company	33	22	67	756	33	—	0	5199	2702	94
RICHMOND—Madison County ★ PATTIE A. CLAY HOSPITAL, EKU By–Pass, Zip 40475, Mailing Address: P.O. Box 1600, Zip 40476–2603; tel. 606/623–3131; Richard M. Thomas, Administrator **A**1 9 10 **F**3 7 8 10 11 14 17 19 22 28 30 39 40 41 44 46 49 63 64 65 71 73 **P**5 **S**0052 Jewish Hospital Healthcare Services	23	10	105	3877	45	35785	889	22852	10305	409
RUSSELL SPRINGS—Russell County RUSSELL COUNTY HOSPITAL, Dowell Road, Zip 42642, Mailing Address: P.O. Box 1610, Zip 42642; tel. 502/866–4141; Jon M. See, Administrator **A**9 10 **F**8 11 14 15 16 19 20 22 29 30 34 37 39 44 45 48 49 65 71 73	13	10	45	1327	21	14362	2	7024	3183	147
RUSSELLVILLE—Logan County ★ LOGAN MEMORIAL HOSPITAL, 1625 South Nashville Road, Zip 42276–0010, Mailing Address: P.O. Box 10, Zip 42276; tel. 502/726–4011; Jeffrey Manley, Chief Executive Officer (Total facility includes 8 beds in nursing home–type unit) **A**1 9 10 **F**7 8 15 19 21 22 25 28 30 34 35 37 39 40 44 63 64 65 67 71 73 **P**7 **S**0048 Columbia/HCA Healthcare Corporation	33	10	100	1896	31	30378	94	14197	4917	178
SALEM—Livingston County ★ LIVINGSTON HOSPITAL AND HEALTHCARE SERVICES, (Formerly Livingston County Hospital) 131 Hospital Drive, Zip 42078, Mailing Address: Box 138, Zip 42078; tel. 502/988–2299; Benedict E. Hesen, Executive Director and Chief Executive Officer **A**9 10 **F**8 14 15 16 19 22 28 30 32 33 34 35 42 44 71 73	23	10	26	1493	16	13109	0	7654	3003	131
SCOTTSVILLE—Allen County ★ MEDICAL CENTER AT SCOTTSVILLE, 99 Hillview Drive, Zip 42164–9309; tel. 502/237–3131; Ronald Peeler, Chief Executive Officer (Data for 335 days) **A**9 10 **F**2 8 11 12 14 15 16 19 22 28 30 34 37 38 40 44 49 52 65 71 **P**6 7 8	23	10	47	756	25	9315	8	3201	1484	100
SHELBYVILLE—Shelby County ★ JEWISH HOSPITAL–SHELBYVILLE, 727 Hospital Drive, Zip 40065; tel. 502/647–4301; Timothy L. Jarm, President and Chief Executive Officer (Total facility includes 8 beds in nursing home–type unit) **A**1 9 10 **F**1 2 3 4 7 8 10 12 15 16 17 19 20 21 22 23 25 26 27 28 29 30 31 32 34 35 37 39 40 41 42 43 44 45 46 48 49 50 51 52 53 54 55 56 57 58 59 60 61 63 64 65 67 69 70 71 73 74 **S**0052 Jewish Hospital Healthcare Services	23	10	72	2742	45	26090	239	18145	7477	270
SOMERSET—Pulaski County ★ LAKE CUMBERLAND REGIONAL HOSPITAL, 305 Langdon Street, Zip 42501, Mailing Address: Box 620, Zip 42502–2750; tel. 606/679–7441; Derek W. Cimala, Chief Executive Officer (Nonreporting) **A**1 2 9 10 **S**0048 Columbia/HCA Healthcare Corporation	33	10	227							
SOUTH WILLIAMSON—Pike County □ WILLIAMSON ARH HOSPITAL, 260 Hospital Drive, Zip 41503; tel. 606/237–1700; John A. Grah, Administrator (Total facility includes 50 beds in nursing home–type unit) **A**1 9 10 **F**4 7 8 12 13 14 15 16 17 19 22 25 28 30 32 33 34 35 37 39 40 42 44 49 52 54 56 57 58 60 63 64 65 71 73 **P**2 3 5 6 **S**0145 Appalachian Regional Healthcare	23	10	173	3121	84	41142	0	17470	8301	324
STANFORD—Lincoln County ★ FORT LOGAN HOSPITAL, 124 Portman Avenue, Zip 40484–1200; tel. 606/365–2187; Terry C. Powers, Administrator (Total facility includes 30 beds in nursing home–type unit) **A**1 9 10 **F**7 8 14 16 19 22 26 31 34 39 40 41 44 46 49 64 71	23	10	73	1334	49	12578	115	6291	3013	131
TOMPKINSVILLE—Monroe County ★ MONROE COUNTY MEDICAL CENTER, 529 Capp Harlan Road, Zip 42167; tel. 502/487–9231; John B. Millstead, Chief Executive Officer **A**1 9 10 **F**8 15 19 22 27 32 34 44 46 49 65 70 71 73 **P**8 **S**0002 Quorum Health Group/Quorum Health Resources	23	10	49	2273	33	16089	0	7781	3326	192
VERSAILLES—Woodford County ★ WOODFORD HOSPITAL, 360 Amsden Avenue, Zip 40383–1286; tel. 606/873–3111; Nancy Littrell, Chief Executive Officer (Total facility includes 23 beds in nursing home–type unit) **A**9 10 **F**8 10 14 15 19 21 22 28 29 34 37 40 44 49 53 64 65 71	23	10	73	959	21	9269	0	8050	3469	133
WEST LIBERTY—Morgan County □ MORGAN COUNTY APPALACHIAN REGIONAL HOSPITAL, Wells Hill Road, Zip 41472, Mailing Address: Box 579, Zip 41472–0579; tel. 606/743–3186; Dennis R. Chaney, Administrator (Total facility includes 25 beds in nursing home–type unit) **A**1 9 10 **F**8 15 16 22 32 33 34 40 44 65 71 73 **S**0145 Appalachian Regional Healthcare	23	10	55	955	30	32844	0	7202	2975	118
WHITESBURG—Letcher County □ WHITESBURG APPALACHIAN REGIONAL HOSPITAL, 550 Jenkins Road, Zip 41858; tel. 606/633–3500; Nick Lewis, Administrator **A**1 9 10 **F**7 19 21 22 23 32 35 37 40 44 46 50 65 71 73 **S**0145 Appalachian Regional Healthcare	23	10	71	4347	49	47221	365	14974	5647	223
WILLIAMSTOWN—Grant County ★ ST. ELIZABETH MEDICAL CENTER–GRANT COUNTY, 238 Barnes Road, Zip 41097; tel. 606/823–5051; Chris Carle, Administrator **A**1 9 10 **F**8 14 15 16 19 22 33 34 65 71	21	10	30	539	6	17052	0	3287	1329	63

Hospitals, U.S. / KENTUCKY

Hospital, Address, Telephone, Administrator, Approval, Facility, and Physician Codes, Health Care System	Classi-fication Codes		Utilization Data					Expense (thousands) of dollars		
	Control	Service	Beds	Admissions	Census	Outpatient Visits	Births	Total	Payroll	Personnel

★ American Hospital Association (AHA) membership
☐ Joint Commission on Accreditation of Healthcare Organizations (JCAHO) accreditation
+ American Osteopathic Hospital Association (AOHA) membership
○ American Osteopathic Association (AOA) accreditation
△ Commission on Accreditation of Rehabilitation Facilities (CARF) accreditation
Control codes 61, 63, 64, 71, 72 and 73 indicate hospitals listed by AOHA, but not registered by AHA. For definition of numerical codes, see page A6

WINCHESTER—Clark County

★ CLARK REGIONAL MEDICAL CENTER, West Lexington Avenue, Zip 40391, Mailing Address: P.O. Box 630, Zip 40392–0630; tel. 606/745–3500; Robert D. Fraraccio, Administrator **A**1 9 10 **F**7 8 11 12 19 20 21 22 28 30 31 33 34 37 39 40 41 42 44 48 49 65 67 71 73 74	23	10	78	2442	38	33908	257	15225	6223	237

Hospitals, U.S. / LOUISIANA

LOUISIANA

Resident population 4,295 (in thousands)
Resident population in metro areas 75.0%
Birth rate per 1,000 population 17.0
65 years and over 11.3%
Percent of persons without health insurance 20.8%

Hospital, Address, Telephone, Administrator, Approval, Facility, and Physician Codes, Health Care System

- ★ American Hospital Association (AHA) membership
- ☐ Joint Commission on Accreditation of Healthcare Organizations (JCAHO) accreditation
- + American Osteopathic Hospital Association (AOHA) membership
- ○ American Osteopathic Association (AOA) accreditation
- △ Commission on Accreditation of Rehabilitation Facilities (CARF) accreditation

Control codes 61, 63, 64, 71, 72 and 73 indicate hospitals listed by AOHA, but not registered by AHA. For definition of numerical codes, see page A6

Hospital	Classification Codes		Utilization Data					Expense (thousands) of dollars		
	Control	Service	Beds	Admissions	Census	Outpatient Visits	Births	Total	Payroll	Personnel

ABBEVILLE—Vermilion Parish

★ ABBEVILLE GENERAL HOSPITAL, 118 North Hospital Drive, Zip 70510, Mailing Address: P.O. Box 580, Zip 70511–0580; tel. 318/893–5466; Ray A. Landry, Administrator **A**1 9 10 **F**8 14 15 16 19 21 22 34 37 39 40 52 64 65 71 73 | 16 | 10 | 105 | 3416 | 49 | 26636 | 184 | 18848 | 8748 | 337 |

ALEXANDRIA—Rapides Parish

★ RAPIDES REGIONAL MEDICAL CENTER, 211 Fourth Street, Zip 71301–8421, Mailing Address: 211 Fourth Street, Box 30101; 71301–8421 tel. 318/473–3000; James T. Montgomery, President **A**1 2 9 10 **F**1 2 3 4 5 6 7 8 9 10 11 12 13 14 15 17 18 19 20 21 22 23 24 25 26 27 28 29 30 31 32 33 34 35 36 37 38 39 40 41 42 43 44 45 46 47 48 49 50 51 52 53 54 55 56 57 58 59 60 61 62 63 64 65 66 67 68 69 70 71 72 73 74 **P**8 **S**0048 Columbia/HCA Healthcare Corporation | 23 | 10 | 359 | 14339 | 206 | 189002 | 1622 | 101935 | 42605 | 1578 |

★ ST. FRANCES CABRINI HOSPITAL, 3330 Masonic Drive, Zip 71301; tel. 318/487–1122; L. Rene' Goux, Chief Executive Officer (Total facility includes 20 beds in nursing home–type unit) **A**1 9 10 **F**1 3 4 7 8 10 11 12 14 15 16 17 19 21 22 23 24 26 27 29 30 32 33 34 35 37 38 39 40 41 42 43 44 45 46 48 49 50 53 54 56 57 58 59 60 63 64 65 66 67 68 70 71 73 74 **P**7 8 **S**0605 Sisters of Charity of the Incarnate Word Healthcare System | 23 | 10 | 264 | 8604 | 148 | 65342 | 665 | 79732 | 34111 | 1310 |

★ VETERANS AFFAIRS MEDICAL CENTER, Shreveport Highway, Zip 71301; tel. 318/473–0010; Billy M. Valentine, Director (Total facility includes 198 beds in nursing home–type unit) **A**1 3 5 **F**3 19 20 21 22 25 27 34 42 44 46 49 52 54 56 58 60 64 65 67 71 73 74 **P**6 **S**9295 Department of Veterans Affairs | 45 | 10 | 468 | 4442 | 359 | 84724 | 0 | 71795 | 33591 | 914 |

AMITE—Tangipahoa Parish

★ HOOD MEMORIAL HOSPITAL, 301 West Walnut Street, Zip 70422; tel. 504/748–9485; A. D. Richardson, Administrator (Nonreporting) **A**9 10 | 16 | 10 | 45 | — | — | — | — | — | — | — |

BARKSDALE AIR FORCE BASE—Caddo Parish

U.S. AIR FORCE HOSPITAL See Shreveport

BASTROP—Morehouse Parish

★ MOREHOUSE GENERAL HOSPITAL, 323 West Walnut Street, Zip 71220, Mailing Address: Box 1060, Zip 71221–1060; tel. 318/281–2431; William W. Bing, Administrator (Nonreporting) **A**1 10 | 16 | 10 | 119 | — | — | — | — | — | — | — |

BATON ROUGE—East Baton Rouge Parish

★ BATON ROUGE GENERAL HEALTH CENTER, 8585 Picardy Avenue, Zip 70809, Mailing Address: P.O. Box 84330, Zip 70884–4330; tel. 504/763–4000; Linda Kay Matessino R.N., President and Chief Executive Officer (Nonreporting) **A**10 **S**0775 General Health System | 23 | 10 | 72 | — | — | — | — | — | — | — |

★ BATON ROUGE GENERAL MEDICAL CENTER, 3600 Florida Street, Zip 70806, Mailing Address: P.O. Box 2511, Zip 70821–2511; tel. 504/387–7000; James L. Brexler, President and Chief Executive Officer (Total facility includes 48 beds in nursing home–type unit) **A**1 2 3 5 6 8 9 10 **F**1 2 3 4 7 8 9 10 11 12 13 15 16 17 18 19 21 22 23 24 26 28 29 30 32 34 35 37 38 39 40 41 42 43 44 45 46 47 48 49 52 53 54 55 56 57 58 59 60 61 64 65 67 71 72 73 74 **P**3 4 7 **S**0775 General Health System | 23 | 10 | 389 | 12503 | 258 | 42458 | 0 | 116870 | 52268 | 1389 |

☐ CPC MEADOW WOOD HOSPITAL, 9032 Perkins Road, Zip 70810; tel. 504/766–8553; Charles J. Hooker III, Chief Executive Officer (Nonreporting) **A**1 9 10 **S**0785 Community Psychiatric Centers | 33 | 22 | 85 | — | — | — | — | — | — | — |

★ EARL K. LONG MEDICAL CENTER, 5825 Airline Highway, Zip 70805; tel. 504/358–1000; Steven L. Smith, Administrator (Nonreporting) **A**1 3 5 9 10 **S**0715 Louisiana Health Care Authority | 12 | 10 | 204 | — | — | — | — | — | — | — |

★ MEDICAL CENTER OF BATON ROUGE, 17000 Medical Center Drive, Zip 70816–3224; tel. 504/755–4800; William L. Anderson, Chief Executive Officer (Total facility includes 16 beds in nursing home–type unit) **A**1 9 10 **F**4 7 10 11 12 15 16 19 20 21 22 23 26 34 35 38 39 40 41 42 43 44 46 48 49 52 56 57 60 61 64 65 71 73 74 **P**6 **S**0048 Columbia/HCA Healthcare Corporation | 33 | 10 | 175 | 5716 | 94 | 39951 | 369 | 49910 | 16423 | 564 |

★ △ OUR LADY OF LAKE REGIONAL MEDICAL CENTER, 5000 Hennessy Boulevard, Zip 70808–4350; tel. 504/765–6565; Robert C. Davidge, President and Chief Executive Officer (Total facility includes 45 beds in nursing home–type unit) **A**1 2 5 7 9 10 **F**1 2 3 4 6 8 10 11 15 16 17 18 19 21 22 23 24 25 26 27 28 29 30 31 32 33 34 35 37 41 42 43 44 45 46 47 48 49 50 51 52 53 54 55 56 57 58 59 60 62 63 64 65 66 67 68 69 71 72 73 74 **P**1 4 6 7 **S**1475 Franciscan Missionaries of Our Lady Health System, Inc. | 23 | 10 | 676 | 22557 | 432 | 108582 | 3 | 192561 | 78411 | 2807 |

☐ PARKLAND HOSPITAL, 2414 Bunker Hill Drive, Zip 70808; tel. 504/927–9050; Wayne Dodge, Administrator (Nonreporting) **A**1 9 10 | 33 | 22 | 170 | — | — | — | — | — | — | — |

★ △ REHABILITATION HOSPITAL OF BATON ROUGE, 8595 United Plaza Boulevard, Zip 70809; tel. 504/927–0567; Jeff Henderson, Chief Executive Officer (Nonreporting) **A**1 7 9 10 | 33 | 46 | 80 | — | — | — | — | — | — | — |

★ SOUTH LOUISIANA REHABILITATION HOSPITAL, 4040 North Boulevard, Zip 70806–3829; tel. 504/383–5055; Dan Flanagan, Administrator and Chief Executive Officer (Nonreporting) **A**1 9 10 | 33 | 46 | 40 | — | — | — | — | — | — | — |

Hospitals, U.S. / LOUISIANA

Hospital, Address, Telephone, Administrator, Approval, Facility, and Physician Codes, Health Care System

- ★ American Hospital Association (AHA) membership
- □ Joint Commission on Accreditation of Healthcare Organizations (JCAHO) accreditation
- \+ American Osteopathic Hospital Association (AOHA) membership
- ○ American Osteopathic Association (AOA) accreditation
- △ Commission on Accreditation of Rehabilitation Facilities (CARF) accreditation

Control codes 61, 63, 64, 71, 72 and 73 indicate hospitals listed by AOHA, but not registered by AHA. For definition of numerical codes, see page A6

	Classification Codes		Utilization Data					Expense (thousands) of dollars		
	Control	Service	Beds	Admissions	Census	Outpatient Visits	Births	Total	Payroll	Personnel
★ WOMAN'S HOSPITAL, 9050 Airline Highway, Zip 70815, Mailing Address: Box 95009, Zip 70895–9009; tel. 504/927–1300; Vicki L. Romero, President and Chief Executive Officer **A**1 2 5 9 10 **F**7 8 14 15 16 19 22 24 28 29 32 34 38 39 40 42 44 46 54 55 58 61 65 67 71 73 74 **P**8	23	44	149	10859	110	169468	6255	69445	34416	1035
BERNICE—Union Parish TRI-WARD GENERAL HOSPITAL, 409 First Street, Zip 71222, Mailing Address: P.O. Box 697, Zip 71222–0697; tel. 318/285–9066; Charolette Thompson, Administrator (Nonreporting) **A**9 10	16	10	12	—	—	—	—	—	—	—
BOGALUSA—Washington Parish ★ BOGALUSA COMMUNITY MEDICAL CENTER, 433 Plaza Street, Zip 70429–0940; tel. 504/732–7122; William Joseph Allen, Administrator and Chief Executive Officer **A**1 9 10 **F**11 13 14 15 19 21 22 23 30 32 34 39 40 42 44 45 46 49 51 52 54 56 57 65 71 73 **P**5	23	10	126	3486	65	28702	243	13669	7018	253
★ WASHINGTON–ST. TAMMANY REGIONAL MEDICAL CENTER, 400 Memphis Street, Zip 70427–0040, Mailing Address: Box 40, Zip 70429–0040; tel. 504/735–1322; Larry King, Acting Administrator **A**1 9 10 **F**3 19 22 31 37 41 44 45 49 52 65 71 **S**0715 Louisiana Health Care Authority	12	10	55	1878	35	48052	0	10364	5050	186
BOSSIER CITY—Bossier Parish ★ BOSSIER MEDICAL CENTER, 2105 Airline Drive, Zip 71111; tel. 318/741–6000; Robert J. Turner, Executive Director (Total facility includes 17 beds in nursing home–type unit) **A**1 9 10 **F**4 7 8 10 14 19 22 23 25 27 28 29 30 32 33 34 35 37 39 40 42 43 44 45 49 51 63 64 65 67 71 72 73 **P**6	14	10	172	3967	63	50485	334	38200	16450	573
SOUTHWEST MEDICAL CENTER See Summit Institute for Pulmonary Medicine and Rehabilitation										
□ SUMMIT INSTITUTE FOR PULMONARY MEDICINE AND REHABILITATION, (Formerly Southwest Medical Center) 4900 Medical Drive, Zip 71112, Mailing Address: P.O. Box 8450, Zip 71112–8450; tel. 318/747–9500; Danny Edwards, Administrator (Nonreporting) **A**1 9 10 **S**0905 Summit Medical Management, Inc.	33	22	54	—	—	—	—	—	—	—
BREAUX BRIDGE—St. Martin Parish ★ GARY MEMORIAL HOSPITAL, 210 Champagne Boulevard, Zip 70517–3852, Mailing Address: Box 357, Zip 70517–0357; tel. 318/332–2178; Burton Dupuis, Administrator **A**9 10 **F**3 22 28 29 30 31 32 33 34 39 44 46 49 51 52 54 55 56 57 64 65 71	16	10	12	399	4	17766	0	4054	1341	73
BUNKIE—Avoyelles Parish ★ BUNKIE GENERAL HOSPITAL, Evergreen Highway, Zip 71322, Mailing Address: Box 380, Zip 71322–0380; tel. 318/346–6681; Mary L. Gauthier, Administrator (Nonreporting) **A**9 10	16	10	48	—	—	—	—	—	—	—
CAMERON—Cameron Parish ★ SOUTH CAMERON MEMORIAL HOSPITAL, Route 1, Box 277, Zip 70631; tel. 318/542–4111; Joseph Soileau, Administrator (Nonreporting) **A**9 10	16	10	33	—	—	—	—	—	—	—
CHALMETTE—St. Bernard Parish □ CHALMETTE MEDICAL CENTERS, 9001 Patricia Street, Zip 70043; tel. 504/277–8011; James M. Reilly, Acting Managing Director (Nonreporting) **A**1 9 10 **S**9555 Universal Health Services, Inc.	33	10	196	—	—	—	—	—	—	—
CHURCH POINT—Acadia Parish ACADIA–ST. LANDRY HOSPITAL, 810 South Broadway Street, Zip 70525; tel. 318/684–5435; Alcus Trahan, Administrator **A**9 10 **F**19 21 22 32 34 41 44 49 52 56 65 71 73	23	10	39	521	24	17410	1	5331	1521	72
COLUMBIA—Caldwell Parish CALDWELL MEMORIAL HOSPITAL, 410 Main Street, Zip 71418, Mailing Address: Box 899, Zip 71418; tel. 318/649–6111; Faye Long, Administrator (Nonreporting) **A**9 10	33	10	49	—	—	—	—	—	—	—
COUSHATTA—Red River Parish L. S. HUCKABAY MD MEMORIAL HOSPITAL, Mailing Address: Box 369, Zip 71019; tel. 318/932–5784; (Nonreporting) **A**10	33	10	74	—	—	—	—	—	—	—
COVINGTON—St. Tammany Parish □ GREENBRIER HOSPITAL, 201 Greenbrier Boulevard, Zip 70433; tel. 504/893–2970; Craig B. Koele, Chief Executive Officer (Nonreporting) **A**1 9 10 **S**0405 Ramsay Health Care, Inc.	33	22	61	—	—	—	—	—	—	—
HIGHLAND PARK MEDICAL CENTER See Lakeview Regional Medical Center										
★ LAKEVIEW REGIONAL MEDICAL CENTER, (Formerly Highland Park Medical Center) 95 East Fairway Drive, Zip 70433, Mailing Address: P.O. Box 99, Mandeville Zip 70470; tel. 504/876–3800; James E. Rogers, Chief Executive Officer **A**1 9 10 **F**4 7 8 10 11 12 14 15 17 19 22 23 25 26 28 32 34 35 38 40 41 43 44 45 49 52 55 57 64 71 73 **P**1 7 **S**0048 Columbia/HCA Healthcare Corporation	33	10	163	3091	40	54283	535	30129	11914	—
★ ST. TAMMANY PARISH HOSPITAL, 1202 South Tyler Street, Zip 70433–2394; tel. 504/898–4000; Thomas J. Stone, Administrator **A**1 9 10 **F**4 7 8 10 12 14 15 19 21 22 25 26 30 31 32 33 34 35 36 37 38 39 40 41 42 43 44 46 49 51 61 63 64 65 71 72 73 74 **P**6	16	10	135	5920	85	50091	941	48321	22478	761
CROWLEY—Acadia Parish ★ AMERICAN LEGION HOSPITAL, 1305 Crowley Rayne Highway, Zip 70526–9410; tel. 318/783–3222; Leonard J. Spears, Administrator **A**1 9 10 **F**2 8 15 16 19 21 22 32 35 37 39 40 44 46 52 53 57 65 71 **P**2	23	10	178	3460	50	28868	589	20171	9055	347

© 1995 AHA Guide

Hospitals, U.S. / LOUISIANA

Hospital, Address, Telephone, Administrator, Approval, Facility, and Physician Codes, Health Care System	Classification Codes		Utilization Data					Expense (thousands) of dollars		
★ American Hospital Association (AHA) membership □ Joint Commission on Accreditation of Healthcare Organizations (JCAHO) accreditation + American Osteopathic Hospital Association (AOHA) membership ○ American Osteopathic Association (AOA) accreditation △ Commission on Accreditation of Rehabilitation Facilities (CARF) accreditation Control codes 61, 63, 64, 71, 72 and 73 indicate hospitals listed by AOHA, but not registered by AHA. For definition of numerical codes, see page A6	Control	Service	Beds	Admissions	Census	Outpatient Visits	Births	Total	Payroll	Personnel
CUT OFF—Lafourche Parish										
★ LADY OF THE SEA GENERAL HOSPITAL, 200 West 134th Place, Zip 70345; tel. 504/632–6401; Lane Cheramie, Chief Executive Officer **A**1 9 10 **F**8 12 15 16 19 21 22 23 32 35 41 44 46 52 57 65 67 71 73 **S**0585 Brim, Inc.	16	10	55	1324	16	30944	0	12350	4718	180
DE QUINCY—Calcasieu Parish										
DEQUINCY MEMORIAL HOSPITAL, 110 West Fourth Street, Zip 70633, Mailing Address: Box 1166, Zip 70633; tel. 318/786–1200; Michael Daiken, Administrator (Nonreporting) **A**9 10	14	10	41	—	—	—	—	—	—	—
DE RIDDER—Beauregard Parish										
★ BEAUREGARD MEMORIAL HOSPITAL, 600 South Pine Street, Zip 70634, Mailing Address: P.O. Box 730, Zip 70634–0730; tel. 318/462–7100; Theodore J. Badger Jr., Chief Executive Officer **A**1 9 10 **F**8 19 20 21 22 23 24 28 32 34 37 40 42 44 46 49 63 65 71 73 **P**8	16	10	102	4030	49	25275	753	19878	9465	465
DELHI—Richland Parish										
★ RICHLAND PARISH HOSPITAL–DELHI, 507 Cincinnati Street, Zip 71232; tel. 318/878–5171; Michael W. Carroll, Administrator (Nonreporting) **A**10	16	10	42	—	—	—	—	—	—	—
DONALDSONVILLE—Ascension Parish										
★ PREVOST MEMORIAL HOSPITAL, 301 Memorial Drive, Zip 70346, Mailing Address: Box 186, Zip 70346; tel. 504/473–7931; Vince Cataldo, Administrator **A**1 9 10 **F**2 15 19 22 28 35 44 49 64 65 71 73	16	10	35	383	10	24316	0	2355	—	57
EUNICE—St. Landry Parish										
★ MOOSA MEMORIAL HOSPITAL, Moosa Boulevard, Zip 70535, Mailing Address: Box 1026, Zip 70535; tel. 318/457–5244; Craig A. Ortego, Administrator **A**1 9 10 **F**1 2 7 8 11 14 15 16 19 21 22 23 29 30 32 34 35 37 40 42 44 45 47 48 49 52 54 57 65 71 73 74 **P**5	16	10	62	1664	23	19377	167	11283	4038	180
FARMERVILLE—Union Parish										
UNION GENERAL HOSPITAL, 901 James Avenue, Zip 71241, Mailing Address: P.O. Box 398, Zip 71241; tel. 318/368–9751; Evalyn Ormond, Administrator **A**9 10 **F**22 32 44 51 64 **P**6	23	10	35	741	12	18685	0	—	—	87
FERRIDAY—Concordia Parish										
★ RIVERLAND MEDICAL CENTER, 1700 East E. Wallace Boulevard, Zip 71334, Mailing Address: Box 111, Zip 71334; tel. 318/757–6551; Vernon R. Stevens Jr., Administrator (Nonreporting) **A**9 10	16	10	49	—	—	—	—	—	—	—
FORT POLK—Vernon Parish										
★ BAYNE–JONES ARMY COMMUNITY HOSPITAL, Zip 71459–6000; tel. 318/531–3928; Colonel Joseph Gonzales, Deputy Commander and Administrator **A**1 **F**3 7 8 12 13 14 15 16 18 19 20 22 27 29 31 32 34 35 37 39 40 41 44 45 46 49 51 52 53 54 55 56 58 65 67 71 73 74 **P**6 **S**9395 Department of the Army	42	10	52	5456	39	337811	868	53240	35481	1009
FRANKLIN—St. Mary Parish										
★ FRANKLIN FOUNDATION HOSPITAL, 1501 Hospital Avenue, Zip 70538, Mailing Address: Box 577, Zip 70538–0577; tel. 318/828–0760; A. Dale Morgan, Administrator (Nonreporting) **A**1 9 10 **S**0002 Quorum Health Group/Quorum Health Resources	16	10	43	—	—	—	—	—	—	—
FRANKLINTON—Washington Parish										
★ RIVERSIDE MEDICAL CENTER, Enon Highway, Zip 70438, Mailing Address: Box 528, Zip 70438; tel. 504/839–4431; Craig R. Cudworth, Administrator **A**1 9 10 **F**8 12 19 21 22 28 32 34 37 41 44 48 64 65 71 73 **S**0002 Quorum Health Group/Quorum Health Resources	16	10	48	1447	22	11011	0	8800	3849	162
GONZALES—Ascension Parish										
□ ASCENSION HOSPITAL, 615 East Worthy Road, Zip 70737; tel. 504/647–2891; Michael J. Nolan, Chief Executive Officer (Nonreporting) **A**1 9 10	33	10	112	—	—	—	—	—	—	—
★ RIVERVIEW MEDICAL CENTER, 1125 West Louisiana Highway 30, Zip 70737; tel. 504/647–5000; Glenn L. Craig, Chief Executive Officer (Total facility includes 15 beds in nursing home–type unit) **A**1 9 10 **F**8 15 19 21 22 32 35 37 41 44 49 52 57 59 64 65 71 **S**0048 Columbia/HCA Healthcare Corporation	33	10	104	2819	51	26718	0	19762	7491	208
GREENSBURG—St. Helena Parish										
★ ST. HELENA PARISH HOSPITAL, Highway 43 North, Zip 70441, Mailing Address: Box 337, Zip 70441–0337; tel. 504/222–6111; L. J. Pecot, Administrator (Nonreporting) **A**9 10	16	10	99	—	—	—	—	—	—	—
GREENWELL SPRINGS—East Baton Rouge Parish										
★ GREENWELL SPRINGS HOSPITAL, 23260 Greenwell Springs Road, Zip 70739, Mailing Address: P.O. Box 549, Zip 70739–0549; tel. 504/261–2730; Wilbur A. Smith, Chief Executive Officer (Nonreporting) **A**1 9 10 **S**0047 Louisiana State Hospitals	12	52	79	—	—	—	—	—	—	—
GRETNA—Jefferson Parish										
□ MEADOWCREST HOSPITAL, 2500 Belle Chase Highway, Zip 70056; tel. 504/392–3131; Jaime A. Wesolowski, Chief Executive Officer (Total facility includes 24 beds in nursing home–type unit) **A**1 3 9 10 **F**2 3 4 7 8 10 11 12 14 16 19 21 22 23 24 31 32 35 37 38 40 41 42 43 44 45 46 47 48 49 52 53 54 55 56 57 58 59 61 63 64 65 66 71 73 74 **P**1 5 7 **S**0063 TENET Healthcare Corporation	33	10	161	6836	79	39966	1953	46634	15487	486
HAMMOND—Tangipahoa Parish										
★ NORTH OAKS MEDICAL CENTER, 15790 Medical Center Drive, Zip 70403, Mailing Address: Box 2668, Zip 70404; tel. 504/345–2700; James E. Cathey Jr., Chief Executive Officer **A**1 9 10 **F**1 4 7 8 10 12 15 16 19 22 23 26 28 32 33 34 35 37 38 39 41 42 43 44 45 46 49 52 56 57 58 64 65 66 71 73 74 **S**0002 Quorum Health Group/Quorum Health Resources	16	10	240	9614	151	88502	1717	68273	35231	1354

A172 Hospitals © 1995 AHA Guide

Hospitals, U.S. / LOUISIANA

Hospital, Address, Telephone, Administrator, Approval, Facility, and Physician Codes, Health Care System

- ★ American Hospital Association (AHA) membership
- ☐ Joint Commission on Accreditation of Healthcare Organizations (JCAHO) accreditation
- + American Osteopathic Hospital Association (AOHA) membership
- ○ American Osteopathic Association (AOA) accreditation
- △ Commission on Accreditation of Rehabilitation Facilities (CARF) accreditation

Control codes 61, 63, 64, 71, 72 and 73 indicate hospitals listed by AOHA, but not registered by AHA. For definition of numerical codes, see page A6.

Hospital	Control	Service	Beds	Admissions	Census	Outpatient Visits	Births	Total	Payroll	Personnel
HOMER—Claiborne Parish										
HOMER MEMORIAL HOSPITAL, 620 East College Street, Zip 71040; tel. 318/927–2024; J. Larry Jordan, Administrator (Nonreporting) A9 10	14	10	57	—	—	—	—	—	—	—
HOUMA—Terrebonne Parish										
☐ BAYOU OAKS HOSPITAL, 934 East Main Street, Zip 70360, Mailing Address: P.O. Box 4374, Zip 70361-4374; tel. 504/876–2020; George H. Perry Ph.D., Chief Executive Officer (Nonreporting) A1 9 10 S0405 Ramsay Health Care, Inc.	33	22	88	—	—	—	—	—	—	—
★ LEONARD J. CHABERT MEDICAL CENTER, 1978 Industrial Boulevard, Zip 70363; tel. 504/873-2200; William B. Mohon, Chief Executive Officer A1 3 9 10 F1 3 4 5 6 7 8 10 12 13 14 15 16 17 18 19 20 21 22 23 24 25 26 27 28 29 30 31 32 33 34 35 36 37 38 39 40 41 42 43 44 45 46 48 49 50 51 52 53 54 55 56 57 58 59 60 61 62 63 65 66 67 68 69 70 71 72 73 74 S0715 Louisiana Health Care Authority	12	10	151	7180	96	169878	1401	48086	20436	891
★ TERREBONNE GENERAL MEDICAL CENTER, 936 East Main Street, Zip 70360, Mailing Address: Box 6037, Zip 70361; tel. 504/873–4664; Alex B. Smith Ph.D., Executive Director A1 9 10 F4 6 7 8 10 11 12 13 14 15 17 18 19 20 21 22 28 29 30 34 35 37 39 40 41 42 43 44 45 46 48 49 60 64 65 66 67 68 71 72 73 74	16	10	245	10746	169	64126	816	65378	29325	1068
INDEPENDENCE—St. Helena Parish										
★ LALLIE KEMP MEDICAL CENTER, 900 Highway 51 South, Zip 70443; tel. 504/878–9421; William C. Bankston, Administrator (Nonreporting) A1 9 10 S0715 Louisiana Health Care Authority	12	10	60	—	—	—	—	—	—	—
JACKSON—East Feliciana Parish										
☐ EAST LOUISIANA STATE HOSPITAL, Mailing Address: P.O. Box 498, Zip 70748; tel. 504/634–2651; Fred E. Calcote Jr., Chief Executive Officer (Nonreporting) A1 9 10 S0047 Louisiana State Hospitals	12	22	452	—	—	—	—	—	—	—
★ VILLA FELICIANA CHRONIC DISEASE HOSPITAL AND REHABILITATION CENTER, Mailing Address: P.O. Box 438, Zip 70748; tel. 504/634–4000; John A. London, Director (Total facility includes 284 beds in nursing home–type unit) A10 F20 26 27 65 73	12	48	295	176	259	0	0	14253	8888	423
JEFFERSON—Jefferson Parish										
☐ ELMWOOD MEDICAL CENTER, 1221 South Clearview Parkway, Zip 70121; tel. 504/734–1900; Deborah C. Keel, Acting Administrator (Nonreporting) A1 10 S5765 Paracelsus Healthcare Corporation	33	10	108	—	—	—	—	—	—	—
JENA—La Salle Parish										
★ LA SALLE GENERAL HOSPITAL, Highway 84, Zip 71342–1388, Mailing Address: P.O. Box 1388, Zip 71342; tel. 318/992–8231; Mary M. Denton, Administrator (Total facility includes 10 beds in nursing home–type unit) A9 10 F19 22 28 30 32 44 49 64 71	16	10	67	1786	34	12222	0	8326	3745	164
JENNINGS—Jefferson Davis Parish										
★ JENNINGS AMERICAN LEGION HOSPITAL, 1634 Elton Road, Zip 70546; tel. 318/824–2490; Terry J. Terrebonne, Administrator A1 9 10 F7 8 12 16 17 19 21 22 32 35 37 40 44 45 46 49 64 65 71 73 P8	23	10	49	2590	25	14978	447	10062	4042	188
JONESBORO—Jackson Parish										
JACKSON PARISH HOSPITAL, 600 Beech Springs Road, Zip 71251, Mailing Address: Box 685, Zip 71251; tel. 318/259–4435; Judy Andrews, Acting Administrator (Nonreporting) A10 S0585 Brim, Inc.	16	10	59	—	—	—	—	—	—	—
KAPLAN—Vermilion Parish										
★ ABROM KAPLAN MEMORIAL HOSPITAL, 1310 West Seventh Street, Zip 70548; tel. 318/643–8300; Lyman Trahan, Admnistrator A9 10 F19 21 22 25 32 33 34 35 37 41 44 49 52 57 65 71 73	16	10	60	903	18	32987	0	6019	2242	82
KENNER—Jefferson Parish										
★ KENNER REGIONAL MEDICAL CENTER, (Formerly St. Jude Medical Center) 180 West Esplanade Avenue, Zip 70065; tel. 504/468–8600; Steven J. Greene, Administrator (Nonreporting) A1 9 10 S0063 TENET Healthcare Corporation	33	10	124	—	—	—	—	—	—	—
KINDER—Allen Parish										
★ ALLEN PARISH HOSPITAL, Mailing Address: P.O. Box 1670, Zip 70648; tel. 318/738–2527; Michael E. Geissler, Administrator A9 10 F14 15 16 22 34 52 71	16	10	45	316	10	3013	0	2102	898	93
LAFAYETTE—Lafayette Parish										
ACADIAN OAKS HOSPITAL See Charter Behavioral Health System at Acadian Oaks Hospital										
☐ CHARTER BEHAVIORAL HEALTH SYSTEM AT ACADIAN OAKS HOSPITAL, (Formerly Acadian Oaks Hospital) 310 Youngsville Highway, Zip 70508; tel. 318/837–8787; Joseph A. Dunston, Interim Chief Executive Officer (Nonreporting) A1 9 10 S0695 Charter Medical Corporation	33	10	39	—	—	—	—	—	—	—
★ CYPRESS HOSPITAL, 302 Dulles Drive, Zip 70506; tel. 318/233–9024; James B. Juneau, Chief Executive Officer A1 9 10 F2 3 15 16 52 53 54 58 59 S0048 Columbia/HCA Healthcare Corporation	33	22	116	899	42	1736	0	6390	3385	89
★ △ LAFAYETTE GENERAL MEDICAL CENTER, 1214 Coolidge Avenue, Zip 70503, Mailing Address: Box 52009 OCS, Zip 70505; tel. 318/289–7991; John J. Burdin Jr., President (Total facility includes 12 beds in nursing home–type unit) A1 2 7 9 10 F4 7 8 10 11 12 13 15 17 19 21 22 23 24 25 26 27 28 29 30 31 32 34 35 37 38 39 40 41 42 43 44 45 46 47 48 49 51 52 53 54 55 56 57 58 59 60 61 63 64 65 66 67 70 71 72 73 74 P8	23	10	337	12371	188	53960	1089	106062	46309	1469

© 1995 AHA Guide

Hospitals, U.S. / LOUISIANA

Hospital, Address, Telephone, Administrator, Approval, Facility, and Physician Codes, Health Care System	Classification Codes		Utilization Data					Expense (thousands) of dollars		
	Control	Service	Beds	Admissions	Census	Outpatient Visits	Births	Total	Payroll	Personnel

Symbols:
- ★ American Hospital Association (AHA) membership
- ☐ Joint Commission on Accreditation of Healthcare Organizations (JCAHO) accreditation
- + American Osteopathic Hospital Association (AOHA) membership
- ○ American Osteopathic Association (AOA) accreditation
- △ Commission on Accreditation of Rehabilitation Facilities (CARF) accreditation

Control codes 61, 63, 64, 71, 72 and 73 indicate hospitals listed by AOHA, but not registered by AHA. For definition of numerical codes, see page A6

Hospital	Control	Service	Beds	Admissions	Census	Outpatient Visits	Births	Total	Payroll	Personnel
★ MEDICAL CENTER OF SOUTHWEST LOUISIANA, 2810 Ambassador Caffery Parkway, Zip 70506; tel. 318/981–2949; Gerald A. Fornoff, Chief Executive Officer **A**1 9 10 **F**4 8 10 15 16 19 21 22 28 30 32 34 35 37 41 43 44 45 46 48 49 63 64 65 71 73 **P**7 8 **S**0048 Columbia/HCA Healthcare Corporation	33	10	105	2709	41	67599	0	26048	9191	346
★ △ OUR LADY OF LOURDES REGIONAL MEDICAL CENTER, 611 St. Landry Street, Zip 70506–4697, Mailing Address: Box 4027, Zip 70502–4027; tel. 318/289–2000; Dudley Romero, President and Chief Executive Officer **A**1 7 9 10 **F**4 7 8 10 11 12 14 15 16 17 19 21 22 23 24 26 28 29 30 31 32 33 34 35 37 40 41 42 43 44 45 46 48 49 63 64 65 66 71 73 **P**8 **S**1475 Franciscan Missionaries of Our Lady Health System, Inc.	21	10	317	10513	198	72539	459	94513	38951	1175
★ UNIVERSITY MEDICAL CENTER, 2390 West Congress Street, Zip 70506, Mailing Address: P.O. Box 4016–C, Zip 70502–4016; tel. 318/261–6004; Larry T. Dorsey, Administrator **A**1 2 3 5 9 10 **F**2 8 10 11 19 21 22 25 31 35 37 38 39 40 42 44 46 52 56 57 59 60 61 65 71 73 74 **P**1 **S**0715 Louisiana Health Care Authority	12	10	166	10278	139	141489	1764	—	—	1005
★ VERMILION HOSPITAL, 2520 North University, Zip 70507, Mailing Address: P.O. Box 91526, Zip 70509–1526; tel. 318/234–5614; John Patout, Administrator (Nonreporting) **A**9 10 **S**0775 General Health System	23	22	54	—	—	—	—	—	—	—
★ WOMEN'S AND CHILDREN'S HOSPITAL, 4600 Ambassador Caffery Parkway, Zip 70508, Mailing Address: P.O. Box 81607, Zip 70598–1607; tel. 318/981–9100; Mimi Roberson, Chief Executive Officer **A**1 9 10 **F**7 8 12 15 19 20 28 32 34 40 44 61 65 67 71 73 74 **P**6 7 **S**0048 Columbia/HCA Healthcare Corporation	33	10	93	3161	29	30863	2044	13105	5888	293
LAKE CHARLES—Calcasieu Parish										
☐ CHARTER HOSPITAL OF LAKE CHARLES, 4250 Fifth Avenue South, Zip 70605–3812; tel. 318/474–6133; Peter Lomonte, Chief Executive Officer (Nonreporting) **A**1 9 10 **S**0695 Charter Medical Corporation	33	22	60	—	—	—	—	—	—	—
★ LAKE AREA MEDICAL CENTER, 4200 Nelson Road, Zip 70605; tel. 318/474–6370; James E. Richardson FACHE, Chief Executive Officer **A**1 9 10 **F**7 8 15 16 19 22 25 34 37 38 39 40 44 45 64 65 71 73 74 **S**0048 Columbia/HCA Healthcare Corporation	33	10	80	2107	19	10200	892	12628	5914	205
★ △ LAKE CHARLES MEMORIAL HOSPITAL, 1701 Oak Park Boulevard, Zip 70601, Mailing Address: P.O. Drawer M, Zip 70602; tel. 318/494–3000; Elton L. Williams Jr. CPA, President (Total facility includes 20 beds in nursing home–type unit) **A**1 2 3 7 9 10 **F**1 2 3 4 7 8 10 12 15 17 19 20 21 22 23 28 29 30 32 33 34 35 36 37 38 39 40 41 42 43 44 45 46 48 49 50 52 53 54 55 56 57 60 63 64 65 66 67 70 71 73 74 **P**3 7 8	23	10	303	10892	199	57263	1539	93316	31465	1246
★ △ ST. PATRICK HOSPITAL OF LAKE CHARLES, 524 South Ryan Street, Zip 70601, Mailing Address: P.O. Box 3401, Zip 70602–3401; tel. 318/436–2511; J. William Hankins, Administrator and Chief Executive Officer (Nonreporting) **A**1 2 7 9 10 **S**0605 Sisters of Charity of the Incarnate Word Healthcare System	21	10	298	—	—	—	—	—	—	—
★ WALTER OLIN MOSS REGIONAL MEDICAL CENTER, 1000 Walters Street, Zip 70605; tel. 318/475–8100; Philip H. Rome, Administrator **A**9 10 **F**3 8 10 12 14 15 16 18 19 20 29 30 31 36 37 39 41 42 44 45 46 49 51 52 55 56 57 58 60 65 67 70 71 73 **P**6 **S**0715 Louisiana Health Care Authority	12	10	66	1268	36	64296	0	18525	6936	208
LAKE PROVIDENCE—East Carroll Parish										
EAST CARROLL PARISH HOSPITAL, 226 North Hood Street, Zip 71254; tel. 318/559–2441; LaDonna Englerth, Administrator (Nonreporting) **A**9 10	16	10	29	—	—	—	—	—	—	—
LAPLACE—St. John The Baptist Parish										
☐ RIVER PARISHES HOSPITAL, 500 Rue De Sante, Zip 70068; tel. 504/652–7000; John Lloyd Hummer, Chief Executive Officer and Managing Director (Nonreporting) **A**1 9 **S**9555 Universal Health Services, Inc.	33	10	120	—	—	—	—	—	—	—
LEESVILLE—Vernon Parish										
☐ BYRD REGIONAL HOSPITAL, 1020 Fertitta Boulevard, Zip 71446; tel. 318/239–9041; Robert J. Trautman, Executive Director (Nonreporting) **A**1 9 10 **S**5895 Hallmark Healthcare Corporation	33	10	59	—	—	—	—	—	—	—
LULING—St. Charles Parish										
☐ ST. CHARLES HOSPITAL, Paul Maillard Road, Zip 70070, Mailing Address: Box 87, Zip 70070–0087; tel. 504/785–6242; Fred Martinez Jr., Administrator **A**1 9 10 **F**2 8 11 15 19 22 26 28 29 30 32 34 35 37 39 44 45 49 52 55 56 65 67 71 73	16	10	104	2048	67	14659	3	24029	7929	318
LUTCHER—St. James Parish										
★ ST. JAMES PARISH HOSPITAL, 2471 Louisiana Avenue, Zip 70071; tel. 504/869–5512; Thomas Bickham Jr., Administrator (Nonreporting) **A**1 9 10	16	10	41	—	—	—	—	—	—	—
MAMOU—Evangeline Parish										
★ SAVOY MEDICAL CENTER, 801 Poinciana Avenue, Zip 70554; tel. 318/468–5261; J. E. Richardson, Chief Executive Officer (Total facility includes 103 beds in nursing home–type unit) **A**1 9 10 **F**1 2 3 6 7 8 12 14 15 16 19 21 22 25 26 27 28 29 30 31 32 33 34 37 40 42 44 45 46 48 49 52 57 61 64 65 68 71 73	23	10	298	3848	182	32171	442	34984	16103	710
MANDEVILLE—St. Tammany Parish										
BOWLING GREEN HOSPITAL, 701 Florida Avenue, Zip 70448, Mailing Address: P.O. Box 417, Zip 70448; tel. 504/626–5661; A. Brooks Cagle, Administrator (Nonreporting) **A**9	33	22	44	—	—	—	—	—	—	—
★ SOUTHEAST LOUISIANA HOSPITAL, Mailing Address: P.O. Box 3850, Zip 70470–3850; tel. 504/626–8161; Joseph C. Vinturella B.C.S.W., Chief Executive Officer (Nonreporting) **A**1 9 10 **S**0047 Louisiana State Hospitals	12	22	357	—	—	—	—	—	—	—

Hospitals, U.S. / LOUISIANA

Hospital, Address, Telephone, Administrator, Approval, Facility, and Physician Codes, Health Care System	Classification Codes		Utilization Data					Expense (thousands) of dollars		Personnel
★ American Hospital Association (AHA) membership ☐ Joint Commission on Accreditation of Healthcare Organizations (JCAHO) accreditation + American Osteopathic Hospital Association (AOHA) membership ○ American Osteopathic Association (AOA) accreditation △ Commission on Accreditation of Rehabilitation Facilities (CARF) accreditation Control codes 61, 63, 64, 71, 72 and 73 indicate hospitals listed by AOHA, but not registered by AHA. For definition of numerical codes, see page A6	Control	Service	Beds	Admissions	Census	Outpatient Visits	Births	Total	Payroll	
MANSFIELD—De Soto Parish										
★ DE SOTO GENERAL HOSPITAL, 207 Jefferson Street, Zip 71052, Mailing Address: P.O. Box 672, Zip 71052; tel. 318/872–4610; Robert R. Taylor, President **A**9 10 **F**15 19 22 28 30 32 44 46 71 73 **P**3	23	10	35	1366	21	11226	0	5397	2184	101
MANY—Sabine Parish										
SABINE MEDICAL CENTER, 240 Highland Drive, Zip 71449–3718; tel. 318/256–5691; Frances F. Hopkins, Administrator **A**9 **F**8 12 14 16 19 22 28 30 32 34 37 44 46 49 71 **S**5895 Hallmark Healthcare Corporation	33	10	68	1397	17	12396	0	5369	2384	99
MARKSVILLE—Avoyelles Parish										
★ AVOYELLES HOSPITAL, 4231 Highway 1192, Zip 71351, Mailing Address: Box 255, Zip 71351; tel. 318/253–8611; David Mitchel, Chief Executive Officer **A**1 9 10 **F**3 19 22 26 35 37 44 45 46 49 57 71 73 **P**8 **S**0048 Columbia/HCA Healthcare Corporation	33	10	55	1024	14	15529	0	—	—	124
MARRERO—Jefferson Parish										
★ WEST JEFFERSON MEDICAL CENTER, 1101 Medical Center Boulevard, Zip 70072–3191; tel. 504/347–5511; David M. Smith FACHE, President **A**1 9 10 **F**1 2 4 7 8 10 11 12 14 15 17 19 20 21 22 23 28 30 32 35 37 38 40 41 42 43 44 45 46 47 50 51 52 56 60 63 65 66 67 70 71 73 74	16	10	382	13414	207	70130	1215	106246	48086	1669
MERRYVILLE—Beauregard Parish										
MERRYVILLE GENERAL HOSPITAL, Bryan Street, Zip 70653, Mailing Address: Drawer C, Zip 70653; tel. 318/825–6181; Robert Hicks, Fiscal Administrator (Nonreporting) **A**9 10	16	10	21	—	—	—	—	—	—	—
METAIRIE—Jefferson Parish										
★ DOCTORS HOSPITAL OF JEFFERSON, 4320 Houma Boulevard, Zip 70006–2973; tel. 504/456–5800; Michael D. Snow, Chief Executive Officer **A**1 3 9 10 **F**4 7 8 10 12 15 16 19 21 22 31 35 37 39 40 41 43 44 45 49 53 54 55 57 58 59 61 63 64 65 71 73 **P**1 5 7 **S**0063 TENET Healthcare Corporation	33	10	114	2950	44	18510	0	35703	11183	321
★ △ EAST JEFFERSON GENERAL HOSPITAL, 4200 Houma Boulevard, Zip 70011–9987; tel. 504/454–4000; Peter J. Betts, President and Chief Executive Officer (Total facility includes 17 beds in nursing home–type unit) **A**1 2 3 5 7 9 10 **F**3 4 7 8 10 11 19 20 22 23 27 30 32 33 34 35 37 38 40 41 42 43 44 48 49 52 60 64 65 71 73 74 **P**6 8	16	10	437	16671	322	157322	1558	168646	71359	1962
★ LAKESIDE HOSPITAL, 4700 I–10 Service Road, Zip 70001–1269; tel. 504/885–3333; Hugh D. Wilson, Chief Executive Officer **A**1 9 10 **F**7 8 10 11 12 13 15 16 19 21 22 24 28 29 30 32 34 35 37 38 39 40 42 43 44 45 46 49 61 63 64 65 66 67 71 72 73 74 **P**8 **S**0048 Columbia/HCA Healthcare Corporation	33	44	122	3884	33	19379	2727	28159	9945	377
SHORELINE MEDICAL CENTER, 4700 I–10 Service Road, Zip 70001; tel. 504/456–2031; Martha Schell, Administrator (Nonreporting) **A**9 10	33	22	58	—	—	—	—	—	—	—
MINDEN—Webster Parish										
☐ MINDEN MEDICAL CENTER, 1 Medical Plaza, Zip 71055; tel. 318/377–2321; George E. French III, Administrator **A**1 9 10 **F**7 8 15 16 19 22 28 29 32 34 37 41 44 46 57 65 71 73 74 **S**6525 Ornda Healthcorp	33	10	108	2747	31	21226	614	11001	4860	200
MONROE—Ouachita Parish										
★ E. A. CONWAY MEDICAL CENTER, 4864 Jackson Street, Zip 71201, Mailing Address: P.O. Box 1881, Zip 71210–1881; tel. 318/388–7000; Roy D. Bostick, Director **A**1 3 5 9 10 **F**3 8 15 19 22 28 31 34 35 37 38 39 40 42 43 44 52 56 65 69 71 73 **P**1 **S**0715 Louisiana Health Care Authority	12	10	210	8379	133	137556	1938	43762	21952	873
★ NORTH MONROE HOSPITAL, 3421 Medical Park Drive, Zip 71203; tel. 318/388–1946; George E. Miller, Chief Executive Officer (Nonreporting) **A**1 10 **S**0048 Columbia/HCA Healthcare Corporation	33	10	130	—	—	—	—	—	—	—
★ ST. FRANCIS MEDICAL CENTER, 309 Jackson Street, Zip 71201, Mailing Address: Box 1901, Zip 71210–1901; tel. 318/327–4000; H. Gerald Smith, President and Chief Executive Officer (Nonreporting) **A**1 2 10 **S**1475 Franciscan Missionaries of Our Lady Health System, Inc.	21	10	425	—	—	—	—	—	—	—
MORGAN CITY—St. Mary Parish										
★ LAKEWOOD HOSPITAL, 1125 Marguerite Street, Zip 70380, Mailing Address: Drawer 2308, Zip 70381; tel. 504/384–2200; Joyce Grove Hein, Chief Executive Officer **A**1 9 10 **F**7 8 10 17 19 22 23 26 28 34 35 37 40 44 45 46 52 55 56 57 64 65 71 74 **S**0002 Quorum Health Group/Quorum Health Resources	16	10	99	3857	58	34216	652	20039	8439	332
NAPOLEONVILLE—Assumption Parish										
☐ ASSUMPTION GENERAL HOSPITAL, 135 Highway 402, Zip 70390, Mailing Address: P.O. Drawer 546, Zip 70390; tel. 504/369–7241; Ty Gautreau, Administrator **A**1 9 10 **F**8 12 17 19 22 28 32 34 44 46 52 53 57 58 59 65 71 72 73	15	10	60	618	27	—	0	7688	2969	112
NATCHITOCHES—Natchitoches Parish										
★ NATCHITOCHES PARISH HOSPITAL, 501 Keyser Avenue, Zip 71457, Mailing Address: Box 2009, Zip 71457–2009; tel. 318/352–1200; Eugene Spillman, Executive Director (Nonreporting) **A**1 10	16	10	177	—	—	—	—	—	—	—
NEW IBERIA—Iberia Parish										
★ DAUTERIVE HOSPITAL, 600 North Lewis Street, Zip 70560, Mailing Address: P.O. Box 11210, Zip 70562–1210; tel. 318/365–7311; Kyle J. Viator, Chief Executive Officer (Nonreporting) **A**1 9 10 **S**0048 Columbia/HCA Healthcare Corporation	33	10	113	—	—	—	—	—	—	—
★ IBERIA GENERAL HOSPITAL AND MEDICAL CENTER, 2315 East Main Street, Zip 70560, Mailing Address: P.O. Box 13338, Zip 70562–3338; tel. 318/364–0441; Robert R. Stanley, Chief Executive Officer (Total facility includes 12 beds in nursing home–type unit) **A**1 9 10 **F**7 8 10 14 19 20 21 22 34 35 37 40 44 64 71	16	10	63	2513	31	45778	272	21533	9042	321

© 1995 AHA Guide

Hospitals, U.S. / LOUISIANA

Hospital, Address, Telephone, Administrator, Approval, Facility, and Physician Codes, Health Care System	Classification Codes		Utilization Data					Expense (thousands) of dollars		
	Control	Service	Beds	Admissions	Census	Outpatient Visits	Births	Total	Payroll	Personnel

★ American Hospital Association (AHA) membership
☐ Joint Commission on Accreditation of Healthcare Organizations (JCAHO) accreditation
+ American Osteopathic Hospital Association (AOHA) membership
○ American Osteopathic Association (AOA) accreditation
△ Commission on Accreditation of Rehabilitation Facilities (CARF) accreditation
Control codes 61, 63, 64, 71, 72 and 73 indicate hospitals listed by AOHA, but not registered by AHA. For definition of numerical codes, see page A6

NEW ORLEANS—Orleans Parish

Hospital	Control	Service	Beds	Admissions	Census	Outpatient Visits	Births	Total	Payroll	Personnel
★ △ CHILDREN'S HOSPITAL, 200 Henry Clay Avenue, Zip 70118–5799; tel. 504/899–9511; Steve Worley, Executive Director **A**1 2 3 5 7 8 9 10 **F**4 5 10 12 17 19 20 21 22 31 34 35 38 39 42 43 44 46 47 48 49 53 54 56 58 65 66 67 71 73	23	50	175	7674	125	105181	0	—	—	1279
★ CHRISTIAN HEALTH MINISTRIES, (Includes Mercy Baptist Medical Center, 2700 Napoleon Avenue, New Orleans, Louisiana, Zip 70115-6996; tel. 504/899–9311; Mercy Hospital of New Orleans, 301 North Jefferson Davis Parkway, New Orleans, Louisiana, Zip 70119; tel. 504/483–5000) 2700 Napoleon Avenue, Zip 70115; tel. 504/899–9311; Byron R. Harrell, President (Total facility includes 110 beds in nursing home–type unit) **A**1 2 9 10 **F**4 7 8 10 11 12 14 16 17 19 20 21 22 24 25 26 28 29 30 31 32 33 34 35 37 38 39 40 41 42 43 44 45 46 47 48 49 51 56 60 61 64 65 66 67 69 71 73 74 **P**5 6 8	23	10	634	16023	294	72640	1743	161886	75999	2063
★ CPC COLISEUM MEDICAL CENTER, 3601 Coliseum Street, Zip 70115; tel. 504/897–9700; Darlene Salvant, Chief Executive Officer (Nonreporting) **A**1 9 10 **S**0785 Community Psychiatric Centers	33	22	109	—	—	—	—	—	—	—
☐ CPC EAST LAKE HOSPITAL, 5650 Read Boulevard, Zip 70127–3145; tel. 504/241–0888; Darlene Salvant, Chief Executive Officer **A**1 9 10 **F**1 2 3 4 8 9 10 11 14 15 16 17 18 19 22 25 26 35 37 38 39 40 41 42 43 44 45 47 48 52 53 54 55 56 57 58 59 60 65 67 **P**5 7 8 **S**0785 Community Psychiatric Centers	33	22	72	1022	51	7275	0	5849	3445	148
★ DEPAUL HOSPITAL, 1040 Calhoun Street, Zip 70118; tel. 504/899–8282; David Hoidal, Chief Executive Officer **A**1 9 10 **F**2 3 12 14 15 16 34 39 52 53 56 58 59 65 **S**0048 Columbia/HCA Healthcare Corporation	33	22	102	858	51	3176	0	9991	4742	155
☐ EYE, EAR, NOSE AND THROAT HOSPITAL, 2626 Napoleon Avenue, Zip 70115; tel. 504/896–1100; William F. Finegan, Chief Executive Officer (Nonreporting) **A**1 3 5 9 10	23	45	39	—	—	—	—	—	—	—
F. EDWARD HEBERT HOSPITAL, 1 Sanctuary Drive, Zip 70114; tel. 504/363–2200; Jack J. Magiera, Chief Executive Officer (Nonreporting) **A**9 10	33	46	194	—	—	—	—	—	—	—
☐ JO ELLEN SMITH MEDICAL CENTER, 4444 General Meyer Avenue, Zip 70131; tel. 504/363–7011; Stan Morton, Administrator and Chief Executive Officer **A**1 3 9 10 **F**2 3 4 7 8 10 12 16 17 19 20 22 24 28 29 30 32 33 34 35 37 38 40 41 42 43 44 46 48 49 52 53 54 55 57 58 59 64 65 67 71 73 74 **P**5 7 8 **S**0063 TENET Healthcare Corporation	33	10	186	3283	56	28374	0	31369	12753	416
★ LAKELAND MEDICAL CENTER, 6000 Bullard Avenue, Zip 70128; tel. 504/241–6335; M. P. Gandy Jr., Chief Executive Officer (Total facility includes 20 beds in nursing home–type unit) **A**1 9 10 **F**4 7 8 10 11 12 16 17 19 21 22 24 26 28 29 30 31 32 35 37 40 41 42 43 44 46 48 49 56 61 64 65 67 71 73 74 **S**0048 Columbia/HCA Healthcare Corporation	33	10	150	4600	75	28085	1010	43634	16869	425
★ MEDICAL CENTER OF LOUISIANA, 1532 Tulane Avenue, Zip 70140; tel. 504/568–3201; Jonathan Roberts, Chief Executive Officer **A**1 2 3 5 8 9 10 **F**4 7 8 10 12 15 16 18 19 20 21 22 23 26 31 34 35 37 38 40 42 43 44 46 47 48 49 51 52 53 54 55 56 58 60 61 63 65 67 71 73 **S**0715 Louisiana Health Care Authority	12	10	611	25726	480	492087	3590	241236	94627	5232
★ MEDICAL CENTER OF LOUISIANA–UNIVERSITY HOSPITAL CAMPUS, (Formerly University Hospital) 2021 Perdido Street, Zip 70112–1396, Mailing Address: Box 61262, Zip 70161–1262; tel. 504/588–3000; Robert L. Marier M.D., Chief Administrative Officer (Total facility includes 30 beds in nursing home–type unit) **A**3 5 9 10 **F**4 8 10 11 15 16 19 21 22 23 26 28 30 32 33 34 35 37 42 43 44 45 60 63 64 65 66 67 69 71 73 **S**0715 Louisiana Health Care Authority	12	10	272	6271	128	117009	0	89180	41410	1076
MERCY BAPTIST MEDICAL CENTER See Christian Health Ministries										
MERCY HOSPITAL OF NEW ORLEANS See Christian Health Ministries										
☐ METHODIST PSYCHIATRIC PAVILLION, 5610 Read Boulevard, Zip 70127; tel. 504/244–5661; Daniel Aguillard, Chief Executive Officer (Nonreporting) **A**1 9 10	32	22	34	—	—	—	—	—	—	—
★ MONTELEPRE EXTENDED CARE HOSPITAL, 3125 Canal Street, Zip 70119; tel. 504/822–8222; Robert A. Leonhard Jr., Administrator (Nonreporting) **A**9 10	33	10	40	—	—	—	—	—	—	—
☐ NEW ORLEANS ADOLESCENT HOSPITAL, 210 State Street, Zip 70118; tel. 504/897–3400; (Nonreporting) **A**1 9 10 **S**0047 Louisiana State Hospitals	12	22	104	—	—	—	—	—	—	—
★ OCHSNER FOUNDATION HOSPITAL, 1516 Jefferson Highway, Zip 70121; tel. 504/842–3303; Phillip D. Robinson, Director (Total facility includes 31 beds in nursing home–type unit) **A**1 2 3 5 8 9 10 **F**3 4 7 8 10 11 12 16 17 19 20 21 22 23 24 28 30 31 32 33 34 35 37 38 40 41 42 43 44 46 47 48 49 51 52 53 54 55 56 58 59 60 63 64 65 67 69 71 72 73 **P**3 6	23	10	377	17736	269	256246	1067	235180	88384	3922
★ PENDLETON MEMORIAL METHODIST HOSPITAL, 5620 Read Boulevard, Zip 70127–3154; tel. 504/244–5100; Frederick C. Young Jr., President (Total facility includes 22 beds in nursing home–type unit) **A**1 9 10 **F**2 3 4 8 10 11 15 16 19 21 22 23 31 32 33 34 35 37 38–40 41 42 43 44 45 46 48 49 52 53 54 55 56 58 59 64 65 66 67 71 73 74 **P**7 8	23	10	211	7935	139	64888	1481	87870	35685	992
☐ RIVER OAKS HOSPITAL, 1525 River Oaks Road West, Zip 70123; tel. 504/734–1740; Daryl Sue White R.N., Managing Director (Nonreporting) **A**1 9 10 **S**9555 Universal Health Services, Inc.	33	22	94	—	—	—	—	—	—	—
☐ ST. CHARLES GENERAL HOSPITAL, 3700 St. Charles Avenue, Zip 70115; tel. 504/899–7441; Lynn C. Orfgen, Chief Executive Officer (Total facility includes 18 beds in nursing home–type unit) **A**1 9 10 **F**14 16 17 19 20 22 27 34 35 37 41 44 45 46 49 64 65 67 71 73 **P**1 5 7 **S**0063 TENET Healthcare Corporation	33	10	173	3281	68	7579	0	26016	8758	237

Hospitals, U.S. / LOUISIANA

Hospital, Address, Telephone, Administrator, Approval, Facility, and Physician Codes, Health Care System	Classification Codes		Utilization Data					Expense (thousands) of dollars		
★ American Hospital Association (AHA) membership ☐ Joint Commission on Accreditation of Healthcare Organizations (JCAHO) accreditation + American Osteopathic Hospital Association (AOHA) membership ○ American Osteopathic Association (AOA) accreditation △ Commission on Accreditation of Rehabilitation Facilities (CARF) accreditation Control codes 61, 63, 64, 71, 72 and 73 indicate hospitals listed by AOHA, but not registered by AHA. For definition of numerical codes, see page A6	Control	Service	Beds	Admissions	Census	Outpatient Visits	Births	Total	Payroll	Personnel
★ TOURO INFIRMARY, 1401 Foucher Street, Zip 70115–3593; tel. 504/897–7011; Gary M. Stein, President and Chief Executive Officer **A**1 2 3 5 8 9 10 **F**1 4 7 8 10 11 12 14 16 17 18 19 21 22 23 24 25 26 28 29 30 32 34 35 37 38 39 40 41 42 43 44 45 46 48 49 51 52 54 55 56 57 58 59 60 61 63 65 66 67 70 71 72 73 74 **P**1 3	23	10	332	9265	219	74257	973	100931	45860	1457
★ TULANE UNIVERSITY HOSPITAL AND CLINICS, 1415 Tulane Avenue, Zip 70112–2632; tel. 504/588–5263; Stephen A. Pickett, Administrator and Chief Operating Officer **A**1 3 5 8 9 10 **F**4 7 8 10 11 14 16 19 21 22 23 26 29 31 32 34 35 37 38 39 40 42 43 44 46 47 49 51 52 53 54 56 57 59 63 65 66 69 71 73 **S**0048 Columbia/HCA Healthcare Corporation	23	10	259	9424	194	329576	738	163849	69918	1378
☐ UNITED MEDICAL CENTER NEW ORLEANS, 3419 St. Claude Avenue, Zip 70117; tel. 504/948–8200; Romona Baudy, Executive Director (Nonreporting) **A**1 9 10 **S**9605 United Medical Corporation	33	10	136	—	—	—	—	—	—	—
UNIVERSITY HOSPITAL See Medical Center of Louisiana–University Hospital Campus										
★ VETERANS AFFAIRS MEDICAL CENTER, 1601 Perdido Street, Zip 70146; tel. 504/568–0811; John D. Church Jr., Director **A**1 2 3 5 8 **F**2 3 4 8 10 11 12 14 15 16 17 18 19 20 21 22 26 27 28 29 30 31 32 33 34 37 39 42 43 44 45 46 49 51 52 54 55 56 57 58 59 60 63 65 67 71 73 74 **S**9295 Department of Veterans Affairs	45	10	255	7622	239	250773	0	—	—	1741
NEW ROADS—Pointe Coupee Parish										
★ POINTE COUPEE GENERAL HOSPITAL, 2202 False River Drive, Zip 70760; tel. 504/638–6331; Larry J. Ayres, Administrator and Chief Executive Officer (Nonreporting) **A**9 10	16	10	28	—	—	—	—	—	—	—
OAK GROVE—West Carroll Parish										
WEST CARROLL MEMORIAL HOSPITAL, Ross Street, Zip 71263, Mailing Address: Box 748, Zip 71263; tel. 318/428–3237; Raymond R. Morris, Administrator (Nonreporting) **A**9 10	23	10	87	—	—	—	—	—	—	—
OAKDALE—Allen Parish										
★ OAKDALE COMMUNITY HOSPITAL, 130 North Hospital Drive, Zip 71463, Mailing Address: Box 629, Zip 71463; tel. 318/335–3700; Robert Bauer, Chief Executive Officer **A**1 9 10 **F**2 3 4 7 8 9 10 12 15 16 17 19 21 22 23 24 26 27 28 29 30 31 32 33 34 35 37 39 40 41 42 43 44 45 46 52 54 57 58 59 60 61 65 66 67 70 71 72 73 74 **P**7 8 **S**0048 Columbia/HCA Healthcare Corporation	32	10	60	1787	29	19984	0	8812	4098	134
OLLA—La Salle Parish										
★ HARDTNER MEDICAL CENTER, Mailing Address: P.O. Box 1218, Zip 71465; tel. 318/495–3131; Malcolm L. Barksdale, Administrator **A**9 10 **F**7 19 22 32 34 40 44 46 49 65 71 73	16	10	31	940	12	7052	171	3986	1624	82
OPELOUSAS—St. Landry Parish										
★ DOCTORS' HOSPITAL OF OPELOUSAS, 5101 Highway 167 South, Zip 70570; tel. 318/948–2100; Gregory L. Gibson, Administrator (Nonreporting) **A**1 9 10 **S**0048 Columbia/HCA Healthcare Corporation	32	10	105	—	—	—	—	—	—	—
★ OPELOUSAS GENERAL HOSPITAL, 520 Prudhomme Lane, Zip 70570, Mailing Address: Box 1208, Zip 70571–1208; tel. 318/948–3011; Patrick Brian Carrier, Administrator **A**1 2 9 10 **F**7 10 15 16 17 18 19 21 22 24 28 31 32 35 37 40 42 44 45 49 51 60 63 64 65 71 72 73 **P**1 4 **S**0002 Quorum Health Group/Quorum Health Resources	16	10	131	4683	69	59329	653	32761	12785	551
PINEVILLE—Rapides Parish										
★ CENTRAL LOUISIANA STATE HOSPITAL, 242 West Shamrock Avenue, Zip 71360–6439, Mailing Address: P.O. Box 5031, Zip 71361–5031; tel. 318/484–6200; Gary S. Grand, Chief Executive Officer **A**1 9 10 **F**2 14 15 16 20 27 52 53 55 65 73 **S**0047 Louisiana State Hospitals	12	22	280	342	217	0	0	—	—	525
★ HUEY P. LONG MEDICAL CENTER, 352 Hospital Boulevard, Zip 71360, Mailing Address: Box 5352, Zip 71361–5352; tel. 318/448–0811; James E. Morgan, Director (Nonreporting) **A**1 3 5 9 10 **S**0715 Louisiana Health Care Authority	12	10	123	—	—	—	—	—	—	—
☐ RIVERNORTH HOSPITAL CENTER, 5505 Shreveport Highway, Zip 71360; tel. 318/640–0222; Daniel W. Johnson, Chief Executive Officer (Nonreporting) **A**1 10 **S**5895 Hallmark Healthcare Corporation	33	22	53	—	—	—	—	—	—	—
PLAQUEMINE—Iberville Parish										
☐ RIVER WEST MEDICAL CENTER, 59355 River West Drive, Zip 70764–9543; tel. 504/687–9222; Joseph R. Tucker, Executive Director **A**1 9 10 **F**2 7 8 12 17 19 20 22 28 30 32 34 35 37 39 40 42 44 45 46 49 52 57 60 65 67 71 73	32	10	151	3851	86	24647	869	24835	9163	340
RACELAND—Lafourche Parish										
★ ST. ANNE GENERAL HOSPITAL, Highway 1 and Twin Oaks Drive, Zip 70394, Mailing Address: Box 440, Zip 70394; tel. 504/537–6841; Milton D. Bourgeois Jr., Administrator (Total facility includes 11 beds in nursing home–type unit) **A**1 9 10 **F**8 16 19 21 22 32 37 40 44 46 52 57 58 64 65 71	16	10	90	1986	21	12969	462	15543	5994	272
RAYVILLE—Richland Parish										
RICHARDSON MEDICAL CENTER, Christian Drive at Greer Road, Zip 71269–9985, Mailing Address: Box 388, Zip 71269–9985; tel. 318/728–4181; David D. Kervin, Administrator (Nonreporting) **A**10	16	10	60	—	—	—	—	—	—	—
RUSTON—Lincoln Parish										
★ LINCOLN GENERAL HOSPITAL, 401 East Vaughn Street, Zip 71270, Mailing Address: P.O. Drawer 1368, Zip 71273–1368; tel. 318/254–2100; E. Allen Tuten, Administrator; Clyde Grau, Assistant Administrator (Total facility includes 12 beds in nursing home–type unit) **A**1 10 **F**8 10 12 14 16 17 19 22 23 28 30 32 33 34 35 37 39 40 41 42 44 49 64 65 71 73	16	10	107	5880	84	29801	600	29929	13326	478

© 1995 AHA Guide

Hospitals, U.S. / LOUISIANA

Hospital, Address, Telephone, Administrator, Approval, Facility, and Physician Codes, Health Care System	Classification Codes		Utilization Data					Expense (thousands) of dollars		
	Control	Service	Beds	Admissions	Census	Outpatient Visits	Births	Total	Payroll	Personnel

Symbols:
- ★ American Hospital Association (AHA) membership
- ☐ Joint Commission on Accreditation of Healthcare Organizations (JCAHO) accreditation
- + American Osteopathic Hospital Association (AOHA) membership
- ○ American Osteopathic Association (AOA) accreditation
- △ Commission on Accreditation of Rehabilitation Facilities (CARF) accreditation

Control codes 61, 63, 64, 71, 72 and 73 indicate hospitals listed by AOHA, but not registered by AHA. For definition of numerical codes, see page A6

Hospital	Control	Service	Beds	Admissions	Census	Outpatient Visits	Births	Total	Payroll	Personnel
★ △ NORTH LOUISIANA REHABILITATION HOSPITAL, 1401 Ezell Street, Zip 71270, Mailing Address: P.O. Box 490, Zip 71273-0490; tel. 318/251-5354; Alice M. Prophit, Chief Executive Officer (Nonreporting) A1 7 10	33	46	90	—	—	—	—	—	—	—
SAINT FRANCISVILLE—West Feliciana Parish										
★ WEST FELICIANA PARISH HOSPITAL, Mailing Address: Box 368, Zip 70775-0368; tel. 504/635-3811; John Green, Administrator A9 10 F21 22 28 32 34 65 71 P5	16	10	23	223	3	8410	0	3602	1662	62
SHREVEPORT—Bossier Parish										
★ CHARTER FOREST BEHAVIORAL HEALTH SYSTEM, (Formerly Charter Forest Hospital) 9320 Linwood Avenue, Zip 71106, Mailing Address: P.O. Box 18130, Zip 71138-1130; tel. 318/688-3930; Randy J. Watson, Administrator (Nonreporting) A1 3 5 10 S0695 Charter Medical Corporation	33	22	65	—	—	—	—	—	—	—
CHARTER FOREST HOSPITAL See Charter Forest Behavioral Health System										
★ CPC BRENTWOOD HOSPITAL, 1800 Irving Place, Zip 71101-4698; tel. 318/424-6761; Michael Amador, Chief Executive Officer (Nonreporting) A1 9 10 S0785 Community Psychiatric Centers	33	22	88	—	—	—	—	—	—	—
☐ △ DOCTORS' HOSPITAL OF SHREVEPORT, 1130 Louisiana Avenue, Zip 71165, Mailing Address: Box 1526, Zip 71101; tel. 318/227-1211; Charles E. Boyd, Administrator A1 7 9 10 F2 3 4 8 15 16 19 22 23 27 30 35 37 44 48 65 66 67 71 P6 S9555 Universal Health Services, Inc.	33	10	142	2042	42	20354	0	24013	10923	364
★ HIGHLAND HOSPITAL, 1453 East Bert Kouns Industrial Loop, Zip 71105-6050; tel. 318/798-4300; Ronald J. Elder, Chief Executive Officer A1 9 10 F1 2 3 4 7 8 10 11 12 14 15 16 17 18 19 20 21 22 23 24 26 28 29 30 31 32 33 34 35 37 38 39 40 41 42 43 44 45 46 47 48 49 52 53 54 55 56 57 58 60 63 64 65 66 67 70 71 72 73 74 P1 2 6 S0048 Columbia/HCA Healthcare Corporation	33	10	120	4891	67	55297	346	35797	13341	429
★ LIFECARE HOSPITALS, (Long Term Acute Care/Critically Ill) 1128 Louisiana Avenue, Suite A, Zip 71101, Mailing Address: P.O. Box 4506, Zip 71134-0506; tel. 318/222-2273; David B. LeBlanc, President (Nonreporting) A10	33	49	40	—	—	—	—	—	—	—
☐ LSU MEDICAL CENTER–UNIVERSITY HOSPITAL, 1541 Kings Highway, Zip 71130-3932, Mailing Address: Box 33932, Zip 71130; tel. 318/675-5000; Ingo Angermeier FACHE, Administrator A1 2 3 5 8 9 10 F2 4 5 7 8 9 10 11 14 16 17 19 20 21 22 23 26 30 31 34 35 37 38 39 40 41 42 43 44 46 47 48 49 50 51 52 54 56 58 60 61 63 64 65 67 68 69 70 71 73 74 P1	12	10	448	19414	329	406966	2378	157019	93230	2919
★ OVERTON BROOKS VETERANS AFFAIRS MEDICAL CENTER, 510 East Stoner Avenue, Zip 71101-4295; tel. 318/221-8411; Michael E. Hamilton, Director (Nonreporting) A1 2 3 5 8 S9295 Department of Veterans Affairs	45	10	259	—	—	—	—	—	—	—
★ △ SCHUMPERT MEDICAL CENTER, One St. Mary Place, Zip 71101, Mailing Address: P.O. Box 21976, Zip 71120-1076; tel. 318/227-4500; Arthur A. Gonzalez Dr.P.H., Chief Executive Officer (Nonreporting) A1 2 3 5 7 9 10 S0605 Sisters of Charity of the Incarnate Word Healthcare System	21	10	486	—	—	—	—	—	—	—
★ SHRINERS HOSPITALS FOR CRIPPLED CHILDREN, SHREVEPORT UNIT, 3100 Samford Avenue, Zip 71103; tel. 318/222-5704; Thomas R. Schneider, Administrator A1 3 5 F5 16 19 34 39 49 65 71 73 S4125 Shriners Hospitals for Crippled Children	23	57	45	702	18	9032	0	—	—	121
★ U.S. AIR FORCE HOSPITAL, BARKSDALE AIR FORCE BASE, (Formerly Listed Under Barksdale Air Force Base) Zip 71110-5300; tel. 318/456-6004; Lieutenant Colonel Allen Middleton MSC, USAF, Administrator (Nonreporting) S9495 Department of the Air Force	41	10	25	—	—	—	—	—	—	—
★ △ WILLIS–KNIGHTON MEDICAL CENTER, 2600 Greenwood Road, Zip 71103-2600, Mailing Address: P.O. Box 32600, Zip 71130-2600; tel. 318/632-4600; James K. Elrod, President (Nonreporting) A1 3 5 7 9 10	23	10	426	—	—	—	—	—	—	—
SLIDELL—St. Tammany Parish										
☐ NORTH SHORE PSYCHIATRIC HOSPITAL, 104 Medical Center Drive, Zip 70461; tel. 504/646-5500; Becky Reeves, Administrator A1 9 10 F1 2 3 14 15 16 26 46 52 53 54 55 56 57 58 59 65 67 P5	33	22	58	820	36	2095	0	6884	2516	123
☐ NORTHSHORE REGIONAL MEDICAL CENTER, 100 Medical Center Drive, Zip 70461-8572; tel. 504/649-7070; Nicholas J. Marzocco, Executive Director (Nonreporting) A1 9 10 S0063 TENET Healthcare Corporation	33	10	147	—	—	—	—	—	—	—
★ SLIDELL MEMORIAL HOSPITAL AND MEDICAL CENTER, 1001 Gause Boulevard, Zip 70458-2987; tel. 504/643-2200; Jimmy A. Ledoux, Chief Executive Officer A1 2 9 10 F4 7 8 10 12 15 16 17 19 21 22 23 24 27 28 30 32 33 34 35 37 38 39 40 41 42 43 44 45 46 48 49 60 63 64 65 66 67 71 73 74 P5	16	10	173	6387	105	50274	764	66719	27842	1183
SPRINGHILL—Webster Parish										
★ SPRINGHILL MEDICAL CENTER, 2001 Doctors Drive, Zip 71075, Mailing Address: Box 917, Zip 71075-0917; tel. 318/539-9161; James B. Warren, Chief Executive Officer (Nonreporting) A1 9 10 S0048 Columbia/HCA Healthcare Corporation	33	10	86	—	—	—	—	—	—	—
STERLINGTON—Ouachita Parish										
STERLINGTON HOSPITAL, Highway 2, Zip 71280, Mailing Address: P.O. Box 567, Zip 71280-0567; tel. 318/665-2526; Evalyn Ormond, Administrator A9 10 F19 21 32 35 65 71	23	10	32	870	15	265	0	2918	1279	67
SULPHUR—Calcasieu Parish										
★ WEST CALCASIEU CAMERON HOSPITAL, Cypress Street, Zip 70663, Mailing Address: P.O. Box 2269, Zip 70664-2269; tel. 318/527-4240; Wayne A. Swiniarski, Chief Executive Officer A1 9 10 F2 3 8 13 16 17 19 22 24 27 28 29 30 32 34 35 37 39 40 41 44 45 49 63 65 66 71 73	16	10	120	3291	46	57937	229	30864	13934	516

Hospitals, U.S. / LOUISIANA

Hospital, Address, Telephone, Administrator, Approval, Facility, and Physician Codes, Health Care System	Classification Codes		Utilization Data					Expense (thousands) of dollars		
	Control	Service	Beds	Admissions	Census	Outpatient Visits	Births	Total	Payroll	Personnel

★ American Hospital Association (AHA) membership
☐ Joint Commission on Accreditation of Healthcare Organizations (JCAHO) accreditation
+ American Osteopathic Hospital Association (AOHA) membership
○ American Osteopathic Association (AOA) accreditation
△ Commission on Accreditation of Rehabilitation Facilities (CARF) accreditation
Control codes 61, 63, 64, 71, 72 and 73 indicate hospitals listed by AOHA, but not registered by AHA. For definition of numerical codes, see page A6

Hospital	Control	Service	Beds	Admissions	Census	Outpatient Visits	Births	Total	Payroll	Personnel
TALLULAH—Madison Parish MADISON PARISH HOSPITAL, 900 Johnson Street, Zip 71282, Mailing Address: P.O. Box 1559, Zip 71284–1559; tel. 318/574–2374; Woodrow N. Burke, Administrator (Nonreporting) A9 10	23	10	47	—	—	—	—	—	—	—
THIBODAUX—Lafourche Parish ★ △ THIBODAUX HOSPITAL AND HEALTH CENTERS, 602 North Acadia Road, Zip 70301, Mailing Address: Box 1118, Zip 70302–1118; tel. 504/447–5500; Greg K. Stock, Chief Executive Officer A1 7 9 10 F7 8 10 11 14 15 19 21 22 23 28 29 30 32 35 37 40 42 43 44 45 46 48 49 60 64 65 67 71 73 74 P2 8 S0002 Quorum Health Group/Quorum Health Resources	16	10	100	4783	56	38749	749	33504	13342	539
VILLE PLATTE—Evangeline Parish ★ VILLE PLATTE MEDICAL CENTER, 800 East Main Street, Zip 70586, Mailing Address: Box 349, Zip 70586; tel. 318/363–5684 A1 9 10 F7 8 11 15 16 19 22 32 34 35 37 40 44 57 64 71 P8 S0048 Columbia/HCA Healthcare Corporation	33	10	116	2731	36	12169	216	12979	5590	225
VIVIAN—Caddo Parish ★ NORTH CADDO MEMORIAL HOSPITAL, 1000 South Spruce Street, Zip 71082, Mailing Address: Box 792, Zip 71082; tel. 318/375–3235; Patricia S. Wilkins, Administrator (Nonreporting) A1 9 10	16	10	33	—	—	—	—	—	—	—
WELSH—Jefferson Davis Parish WELSH GENERAL HOSPITAL, 410 South Simmons Street, Zip 70591–5000; tel. 318/734–2555; Doug Landreneau, Administrator (Nonreporting) A9 10	14	10	81	—	—	—	—	—	—	—
WEST MONROE—Ouachita Parish ★ GLENWOOD REGIONAL MEDICAL CENTER, 503 McMillan Road, Zip 71291, Mailing Address: Box 35805, Zip 71294–5805; tel. 318/329–4200; Larry D. Rentfro FACHE, President and Chief Executive Officer (Total facility includes 20 beds in nursing home–type unit) A1 2 10 F7 8 10 11 12 15 16 19 21 22 24 25 29 31 32 33 34 35 36 37 39 40 41 42 44 45 47 49 60 64 65 66 67 71 73 74	23	10	186	8702	114	46574	384	60743	24224	932
☐ WOODLAND HILLS HOSPITAL, 6200 Cypress Street, Zip 71291–9012, Mailing Address: P.O. Box 1436, Zip 71294–1436; tel. 318/396–5900; Don P. Johnson, Administrator (Nonreporting) A1 9 10	33	22	60	—	—	—	—	—	—	—
WINNFIELD—Winn Parish ★ WINN PARISH MEDICAL CENTER, 301 West Boundary Street, Zip 71483, Mailing Address: Box 152, Zip 71483; tel. 318/628–2721; Bobby Jordan, Chief Executive Officer (Nonreporting) A1 9 10 S0048 Columbia/HCA Healthcare Corporation	33	10	103	—	—	—	—	—	—	—
WINNSBORO—Franklin Parish FRANKLIN MEDICAL CENTER, 2106 Loop Road, Zip 71295; tel. 318/435–9411; Ann Netherland, Chief Executive Officer A9 10 F14 15 16 17 19 21 22 27 28 32 37 44 65 71 73	16	10	46	2576	31	9971	0	8355	3475	182
ZACHARY—East Baton Rouge Parish ★ LANE MEMORIAL HOSPITAL, 6300 Main Street, Zip 70791–9990; tel. 504/658–4000; Charlie L. Massey, Administrator (Total facility includes 50 beds in nursing home–type unit) A1 9 10 F7 8 12 17 19 20 21 22 28 29 30 31 32 34 35 37 40 44 45 63 64 65 71 73 P6 S0002 Quorum Health Group/Quorum Health Resources	16	10	136	4598	100	71181	434	29253	14144	509

Hospitals, U.S. / MAINE

MAINE

Resident population 1,239 (in thousands)
Resident population in metro areas 35.7%
Birth rate per 1,000 population 13.6
65 years and over 13.7%
Percent of persons without health insurance 11.1%

Hospital, Address, Telephone, Administrator, Approval, Facility, and Physician Codes, Health Care System	Classi-fication Codes		Utilization Data					Expense (thousands) of dollars		
★ American Hospital Association (AHA) membership □ Joint Commission on Accreditation of Healthcare Organizations (JCAHO) accreditation + American Osteopathic Hospital Association (AOHA) membership ○ American Osteopathic Association (AOA) accreditation △ Commission on Accreditation of Rehabilitation Facilities (CARF) accreditation Control codes 61, 63, 64, 71, 72 and 73 indicate hospitals listed by AOHA, but not registered by AHA. For definition of numerical codes, see page A6	Control	Service	Beds	Admissions	Census	Outpatient Visits	Births	Total	Payroll	Personnel
AUGUSTA—Kennebec County										
□ AUGUSTA MENTAL HEALTH INSTITUTE, Arsenal Street, Zip 04330, Mailing Address: Box 724, Zip 04330; tel. 207/289-7200; Linda Breslin, Superintendent (Nonreporting) **A**1 9 10	12	22	230	—	—	—	—	—	—	—
★ KENNEBEC VALLEY MEDICAL CENTER, 6 East Chestnut Street, Zip 04330-9988; tel. 207/626-1000; Warren C. Kessler, President (Total facility includes 29 beds in nursing home–type unit) **A**1 2 3 5 9 10 **F**1 2 3 7 8 11 14 15 16 17 19 20 21 22 24 25 26 28 30 31 32 33 34 35 37 39 40 41 42 44 46 48 49 51 52 53 54 55 56 57 58 59 60 64 65 66 67 71 73 **P**4 5 8	23	10	124	6060	108	115512	677	44584	21845	756
BANGOR—Penobscot County										
★ ACADIA HOSPITAL, 286 Stillwater Avenue, Zip 04401, Mailing Address: P.O. Box 422, Zip 04402-0422; tel. 207/973-6100; Dennis P. King, President **A**1 10 **F**3 15 34 41 52 53 54 55 56 57 58 59 65 73 **P**1 6 **S**0555 Eastern Maine Healthcare	23	22	72	1131	66	3484	0	17259	9005	288
□ BANGOR MENTAL HEALTH INSTITUTE, 656 State Street, Zip 04402-0926, Mailing Address: P.O. Box 926, Zip 04402-0926; tel. 207/941-4000; N. Lawrence Ventura, Superintendent (Total facility includes 17 beds in nursing home–type unit) **A**1 9 10 **F**1 15 16 26 35 52 56 57 59 65	12	22	242	292	203	6512	0	24044	12519	505
★ EASTERN MAINE MEDICAL CENTER, (Includes Ross Skilled Nursing Facility) 489 State Street, Zip 04401; tel. 207/945-7000; Norman A. Ledwin, President and Chief Executive Officer (Total facility includes 15 beds in nursing home–type unit) **A**1 2 3 5 9 10 12 **F**2 3 4 5 6 7 8 10 11 13 14 15 16 17 18 19 21 22 24 26 28 29 30 31 32 33 34 35 37 38 39 40 41 42 43 44 45 46 47 48 49 51 52 53 54 55 56 57 58 59 60 61 63 64 65 66 67 68 71 72 73 74 **P**4 **S**0555 Eastern Maine Healthcare	23	10	347	15519	266	262274	1638	144698	69905	2018
★ ST. JOSEPH HOSPITAL, 360 Broadway, Zip 04401-3897, Mailing Address: P.O. Box 403, Zip 04402-0403; tel. 207/947-8311; Sister Mary Norberta Malinowski, President **A**1 9 10 **F**3 8 14 16 17 19 21 22 23 28 30 31 32 33 34 35 37 41 42 44 45 46 49 53 54 56 65 67 71 73 74 **P**7	21	10	100	3401	58	46088	0	32776	14914	572
BAR HARBOR—Hancock County										
★ MOUNT DESERT ISLAND HOSPITAL, Wayman Lane, Zip 04609-0008, Mailing Address: P.O. Box 8, Zip 04609-0008; tel. 207/288-5081; Leslie A. Hawkins, Chief Executive Officer **A**1 9 10 **F**3 7 8 15 16 17 19 21 22 28 30 32 34 37 39 40 42 44 45 49 51 54 56 65 71 74 **P**6	23	10	49	1564	21	14380	92	11593	5554	188
BATH—Sagadahoc County										
BATH MEMORIAL HOSPITAL See Mid Coast Hospital										
★ MID COAST HOSPITAL, (Includes Bath Memorial Hospital, Bath, Maine, Mailing Address: 1356 Washington Street, Zip 04530-2897; Herbert Paris, President; Regional Memorial Hospital, 58 Baribeau Drive, Brunswick, Maine, Zip 04011-3286; tel. 207/729-0181; Herbert Paris, President) 1356 Washington Street, Zip 04530-2897; tel. 207/443-5524; Herbert Paris, President (Total facility includes 16 beds in nursing home–type unit) **A**1 9 10 **F**2 3 6 7 8 10 12 15 16 17 19 21 22 26 27 28 29 30 31 32 33 34 35 36 37 39 40 41 42 44 45 46 49 52 54 55 56 57 58 60 62 64 65 67 71 73 **P**1	23	10	115	4340	71	78522	248	27390	13547	329
BELFAST—Waldo County										
□ WALDO COUNTY GENERAL HOSPITAL, Northport Avenue, Zip 04915, Mailing Address: P.O. Box 287, Zip 04915-0287; tel. 207/338-2500; Mark A. Biscone, Executive Director **A**1 9 10 **F**1 3 6 7 8 11 14 15 16 18 19 22 24 28 30 32 33 34 35 37 40 41 42 44 46 49 53 54 55 56 57 58 62 65 66 67 71 73 **P**8	23	10	49	1651	24	53473	181	11471	6040	231
BIDDEFORD—York County										
★ SOUTHERN MAINE MEDICAL CENTER, One Medical Center Drive, Zip 04005, Mailing Address: P.O. Box 626, Zip 04005-0626; tel. 207/283-7000; Edward J. McGeachey, President and Chief Executive Officer **A**1 2 9 10 **F**7 8 14 15 16 18 19 21 22 26 28 29 30 31 34 35 37 39 40 41 42 44 49 52 53 54 55 56 57 59 60 61 65 71 73 74	23	10	150	5030	87	70772	534	36991	18710	633
BLUE HILL—Hancock County										
★ BLUE HILL MEMORIAL HOSPITAL, Water Street, Zip 04614-0823, Mailing Address: P.O. Box 823, Zip 04614-0823; tel. 207/374-2836; Bruce D. Cummings, Chief Executive Officer **A**1 9 10 **F**7 8 15 16 17 19 22 32 34 37 40 42 44 62 65 71 73 **P**3 8	23	10	26	932	11	20879	186	9596	—	140
BOOTHBAY HARBOR—Lincoln County										
★ ST. ANDREWS HOSPITAL, 3 St. Andrews Lane, Zip 04538, Mailing Address: P.O. Box 417, Zip 04538-0417; tel. 207/633-2121; Donald A. Keller, Chief Executive Officer (Total facility includes 30 beds in nursing home–type unit) **A**1 9 10 **F**3 7 8 12 13 14 16 22 29 32 33 34 39 40 41 44 49 65 71 73 74 **P**6 **S**0002 Quorum Health Group/Quorum Health Resources	23	10	52	488	34	10767	25	5870	2888	122
BRIDGTON—Cumberland County										
★ NORTHERN CUMBERLAND MEMORIAL HOSPITAL, South High Street, Zip 04009, Mailing Address: P.O. Box 230, Zip 04009-0230; tel. 207/647-8841; John Wiesendanger, President **A**1 9 10 **F**7 8 11 17 19 21 22 30 33 37 39 40 41 42 44 45 65 67 71 73 **P**4 7 8	23	10	40	1837	25	27354	58	11604	5741	195

Hospitals, U.S. / MAINE

Hospital, Address, Telephone, Administrator, Approval, Facility, and Physician Codes, Health Care System	Classification Codes		Utilization Data					Expense (thousands) of dollars		
★ American Hospital Association (AHA) membership □ Joint Commission on Accreditation of Healthcare Organizations (JCAHO) accreditation + American Osteopathic Hospital Association (AOHA) membership ○ American Osteopathic Association (AOA) accreditation △ Commission on Accreditation of Rehabilitation Facilities (CARF) accreditation Control codes 61, 63, 64, 71, 72 and 73 indicate hospitals listed by AOHA, but not registered by AHA. For definition of numerical codes, see page A6	Control	Service	Beds	Admissions	Census	Outpatient Visits	Births	Total	Payroll	Personnel
BRUNSWICK—Cumberland County										
★ PARKVIEW MEMORIAL HOSPITAL, 329 Maine Street, Zip 04011–3398; tel. 207/729–1641; Norman L. McBride FACHE, President and Chief Executive Officer **A**1 9 10 **F**7 8 15 17 22 26 28 29 30 31 32 33 34 37 39 40 42 44 45 46 49 65 67 71 73 74	21	10	51	2029	23	39863	654	13759	7197	214
REGIONAL MEMORIAL HOSPITAL See Mid Coast Hospital, Bath										
CALAIS—Washington County										
★ CALAIS REGIONAL HOSPITAL, 50 Franklin Street, Zip 04619–1398; tel. 207/454–7521; Ray H. Davis Jr., Chief Executive Officer **A**1 9 10 **F**3 7 8 14 16 19 21 22 34 35 37 40 44 49 60 63 64 65 71 73 **S**0002 Quorum Health Group/Quorum Health Resources	23	10	49	1216	17	34022	128	10164	4666	174
CARIBOU—Aroostook County										
★ CARY MEDICAL CENTER, 37 Van Buren Road, Zip 04736–2599; tel. 207/498–3111; John J. McCormack, Executive Director (Total facility includes 9 beds in nursing home–type unit) **A**1 9 10 **F**7 8 15 19 21 22 25 28 30 34 35 37 39 40 42 44 45 49 54 56 58 65 67 70 71 72 73 **S**0002 Quorum Health Group/Quorum Health Resources	14	10	74	2180	43	57883	222	19513	9113	377
DAMARISCOTTA—Lincoln County										
★ MILES MEMORIAL HOSPITAL, Bristol Road, Zip 04543, Mailing Address: Rural Route 2, Box 4500, Zip 04543; tel. 207/563–1234; Judith Tarr, Chief Executive Officer **A**1 9 10 **F**1 3 7 8 11 14 15 16 17 19 22 26 27 28 32 33 34 36 37 39 40 44 49 53 54 56 57 58 61 62 64 65 67 71 73 74 **P**2	23	10	30	1523	19	35702	123	11565	5105	240
DOVER-FOXCROFT—Piscataquis County										
★ MAYO REGIONAL HOSPITAL, 75 West Main Street, Zip 04426; tel. 207/564–8401; William J. Thompson, Interim Chief Executive Officer **A**1 9 10 **F**1 7 8 17 19 22 28 37 40 42 44 49 65 71 73 74 **P**7 **S**0002 Quorum Health Group/Quorum Health Resources	16	10	48	1636	22	34833	151	11994	5738	227
ELLSWORTH—Hancock County										
★ MAINE COAST MEMORIAL HOSPITAL, 50 Union Street, Zip 04605–1599; tel. 207/667–5311; David L. Hample, President **A**1 9 10 **F**7 8 12 15 16 17 18 19 21 22 24 25 26 28 29 30 33 34 35 37 39 40 41 44 45 46 50 51 53 56 57 58 60 63 65 66 71 73 **P**6 **S**0002 Quorum Health Group/Quorum Health Resources	23	10	55	2151	31	40850	233	15282	6519	249
FARMINGTON—Franklin County										
★ FRANKLIN MEMORIAL HOSPITAL, One Hospital Drive, Zip 04938–9990; tel. 207/778–6031; Richard A. Batt, President and Chief Executive Officer **A**1 9 10 **F**3 7 8 13 14 15 16 17 19 22 24 28 31 33 36 37 39 40 41 42 44 45 49 52 53 54 55 56 58 65 66 67 71 73 **P**6 8	23	10	70	2711	34	65072	391	18529	9059	340
FORT FAIRFIELD—Aroostook County										
COMMUNITY GENERAL HOSPITAL See Aroostook Medical Center, Presque Isle										
FORT KENT—Aroostook County										
★ NORTHERN MAINE MEDICAL CENTER, 143 East Main Street, Zip 04743; tel. 207/834–3155; Martin B. Bernstein, Executive Director (Total facility includes 45 beds in nursing home–type unit) **A**1 9 10 **F**7 8 12 14 15 16 19 21 22 28 32 33 34 35 36 37 39 40 41 42 44 45 46 49 52 53 54 55 56 57 58 63 65 71 **P**6	23	10	81	1146	61	28000	118	9252	4782	198
GREENVILLE—Piscataquis County										
CHARLES A. DEAN MEMORIAL HOSPITAL, Pritham Avenue, Zip 04441–1395, Mailing Address: Box 1129, Zip 04441; tel. 207/695–2223; Andrew Finegan, Administrator (Total facility includes 36 beds in nursing home–type unit) **A**9 10 **F**14 15 16 22 24 40 44 64 65 71	23	10	50	549	41	—	34	3702	2099	97
HOULTON—Aroostook County										
★ HOULTON REGIONAL HOSPITAL, 20 Hartford Street, Zip 04730–9998; tel. 207/532–9471; Bradley C. Bean, Administrator (Total facility includes 28 beds in nursing home–type unit) **A**1 9 10 **F**3 7 8 12 14 15 19 20 21 22 24 28 31 32 33 34 35 36 37 39 40 41 42 44 46 49 54 56 57 63 64 65 71 73 **S**0002 Quorum Health Group/Quorum Health Resources	23	10	77	2041	55	46381	182	13417	7003	231
JACKMAN—Somerset County										
MARIE JOSEPH HOSPITAL See Mid–Maine Medical Center, Waterville										
LEWISTON—Androscoggin County										
★ CENTRAL MAINE MEDICAL CENTER, 300 Main Street, Zip 04240–0305; tel. 207/795–0111; William W. Young Jr., President **A**1 2 3 5 9 10 12 **F**7 8 9 10 11 12 14 15 17 19 21 22 25 28 29 30 31 32 35 37 40 41 42 44 45 46 48 49 51 60 63 64 65 67 69 71 73 **P**6 8	23	10	146	9083	146	130916	1001	72156	29976	954
★ ST. MARY'S REGIONAL MEDICAL CENTER, 45 Golder Street, Zip 04240, Mailing Address: P.O. Box 291, Zip 04243–0291; tel. 207/777–8100; James E. Cassidy, President and Chief Executive Officer **A**1 2 9 10 **F**2 3 6 7 8 9 10 11 12 13 15 16 18 19 21 22 24 26 28 30 31 32 34 35 37 39 40 41 42 44 45 46 48 49 51 52 53 54 55 56 57 58 59 60 61 62 63 64 65 66 67 68 71 73 74 **P**4 5 6 8 **S**5885 Covenant Health Systems, Inc.	23	10	233	5233	104	81592	350	49221	18160	644
LINCOLN—Penobscot County										
★ PENOBSCOT VALLEY HOSPITAL, Transalpine Road, Zip 04457–0368, Mailing Address: P.O. Box 368, Zip 04457–0368; tel. 207/794–3321; Ronald D. Victory, Administrator (Total facility includes 9 beds in nursing home–type unit) **A** 9 10 **F**7 8 15 19 22 27 28 30 31 34 36 37 39 40 41 42 44 45 46 49 64 65 66 71 73 **P**5 **S**0002 Quorum Health Group/Quorum Health Resources	16	10	42	1279	21	33800	95	8808	3426	178

© 1995 AHA Guide

Hospitals, U.S. / MAINE

Hospital, Address, Telephone, Administrator, Approval, Facility, and Physician Codes, Health Care System	Classification Codes		Utilization Data					Expense (thousands) of dollars		Personnel
★ American Hospital Association (AHA) membership ☐ Joint Commission on Accreditation of Healthcare Organizations (JCAHO) accreditation + American Osteopathic Hospital Association (AOHA) membership ○ American Osteopathic Association (AOA) accreditation △ Commission on Accreditation of Rehabilitation Facilities (CARF) accreditation Control codes 61, 63, 64, 71, 72 and 73 indicate hospitals listed by AOHA, but not registered by AHA. For definition of numerical codes, see page A6	Control	Service	Beds	Admissions	Census	Outpatient Visits	Births	Total	Payroll	
MACHIAS—Washington County										
★ DOWN EAST COMMUNITY HOSPITAL, Upper Court Street, Zip 04654, Mailing Address: Rural Route 1, Box 11, Zip 04654; tel. 207/255–3356; George Avery, Administrator **A**1 9 10 **F**3 7 8 14 19 20 22 28 30 40 42 44 45 46 49 54 65 67 71 **S**0002 Quorum Health Group/Quorum Health Resources	23	10	38	1546	20	21516	187	10039	4501	152
MARS HILL—Aroostook County										
AROOSTOOK HEALTH CENTER See Aroostook Medical Center, Presque Isle										
MILLINOCKET—Penobscot County										
★ MILLINOCKET REGIONAL HOSPITAL, 200 Somerset Street, Zip 04462; tel. 207/723–5161; Craig A. Kantos, Chief Executive Officer **A**1 9 10 **F**7 8 17 19 21 22 28 35 37 40 42 44 49 60 **S**0002 Quorum Health Group/Quorum Health Resources	23	10	29	1293	19	24959	75	10730	4834	165
NORWAY—Oxford County										
★ STEPHENS MEMORIAL HOSPITAL, 80 Main Street, Zip 04268–1297; tel. 207/743–5933; Harrison F. Hahn, President **A**1 9 10 **F**1 2 3 6 7 8 13 15 16 17 18 19 20 21 22 23 24 26 27 28 29 32 33 34 35 36 37 38 39 42 44 49 51 52 53 54 55 57 58 60 61 62 64 65 66 67 68 69 71 73	23	10	46	2350	35	81620	251	16767	8915	289
PITTSFIELD—Somerset County										
★ SEBASTICOOK VALLEY HOSPITAL, 99 Grove Street, Zip 04967–1199; tel. 207/487–5141; Ann Morrison R.N., Chief Executive Officer **A**9 10 **F**3 8 15 16 19 22 28 29 30 33 34 37 39 44 45 46 49 56 65 66 67 71 73	23	10	28	1448	16	29756	0	8441	3491	132
PORTLAND—Cumberland County										
☐ + ○ BRIGHTON MEDICAL CENTER, 335 Brighton Avenue, Zip 04102–0602; tel. 207/879–8000; James W. Donovan, President **A**1 9 10 11 12 13 **F**7 8 12 14 15 16 17 19 20 21 22 26 28 30 31 34 35 37 40 41 42 44 45 51 60 61 63 65 66 70 71 73 74	23	10	110	4883	76	71495	482	38541	17925	511
★ MAINE MEDICAL CENTER, 22 Bramhall Street, Zip 04102; tel. 207/871–0111; Donald L. McDowell, President and Chief Executive Officer **A**1 2 3 5 8 9 10 **F**4 8 10 11 14 15 16 17 19 20 21 22 23 25 27 28 29 30 31 34 35 37 38 39 40 41 42 43 44 45 46 48 49 51 52 53 54 55 56 57 58 59 60 61 63 65 69 70 71 73 **P**6 7 8	23	10	598	22723	453	126512	2454	219931	114111	3299
★ MERCY HOSPITAL, 144 State Street, Zip 04101–3795; tel. 207/879–3000; Howard R. Buckley, President **A**1 3 9 10 **F**2 7 8 15 16 17 19 21 22 31 34 35 37 39 40 41 42 44 49 54 63 65 67 71 73 **P**8 **S**3595 Eastern Mercy Health System	21	10	158	7251	115	67348	777	48784	23661	679
☐ △ NEW ENGLAND REHABILITATION HOSPITAL OF PORTLAND, 13 Charles Street, Zip 04102–9924; tel. 207/775–4000; Gregg Stanley, Executive Vice President and Chief Executive Officer **A**1 7 9 10 **F**12 15 16 17 20 25 28 30 32 34 39 41 45 48 65 67 73	33	46	80	918	59	—	0	13705	6652	—
PRESQUE ISLE—Aroostook County										
★ AROOSTOOK MEDICAL CENTER, (Includes Aroostook Health Center, 15 Highland Avenue, Mars Hill, Maine, Zip 04758, Mailing Address: P.O. Box 410, Zip 04758; tel. 207/768–4900; Arthur R. Gould Memorial Hospital, Academy Street, Presque Isle, Maine, Zip 04769, Mailing Address: P.O. Box 151, Zip 04769; tel. 207/768–4000; Community General Hospital, 3 Green Street, Fort Fairfield, Maine, Zip 04742; tel. 207/768–4700; Washburn Regional Health Center, Washburn, Maine, Mailing Address: P.O. Box 510, Zip 04786) Academy Street, Zip 04769, Mailing Address: P.O. Box 151, Zip 04769–0151; tel. 207/768–4000; David A. Peterson, Chief Executive Officer (Total facility includes 96 beds in nursing home–type unit) **A**1 9 10 **F**7 8 15 16 19 21 22 24 25 26 28 30 33 34 35 36 37 39 40 41 42 44 48 49 51 52 53 54 55 56 58 59 60 64 65 67 71 73 74	23	10	212	3011	139	70689	330	32576	14344	490
ARTHUR R. GOULD MEMORIAL HOSPITAL See Aroostook Medical Center										
ROCKPORT—Knox County										
★ PENOBSCOT BAY MEDICAL CENTER, 6 Glen Cove Drive, Zip 04856–4241; tel. 207/596–8200; Gary R. Daniels, President (Total facility includes 57 beds in nursing home–type unit) **A**1 2 9 10 **F**6 7 8 12 14 15 16 17 19 20 21 22 27 28 29 30 31 32 33 34 35 37 39 40 41 42 44 46 49 52 53 54 55 56 57 58 61 64 65 66 68 71 73 74 **P**4	23	10	152	4384	119	71381	411	33675	18404	636
RUMFORD—Oxford County										
★ RUMFORD COMMUNITY HOSPITAL, 420 Franklin Street, Zip 04276; tel. 207/364–4581; John H. Welsh, Chief Executive Officer **A**1 2 9 10 **F**2 3 7 8 11 14 16 19 20 21 22 24 28 30 34 37 40 44 48 49 65 71 73	23	10	50	1343	18	23442	72	11163	4841	146
SANFORD—York County										
★ HENRIETTA D. GOODALL HOSPITAL, 25 June Street, Zip 04073–2645; tel. 207/324–4310; Peter G. Booth, President (Total facility includes 102 beds in nursing home–type unit) **A**1 9 10 **F**7 8 11 15 16 19 22 28 30 34 35 40 41 44 49 64 65 71 73	23	10	170	2320	139	41847	319	21898	10456	389
SKOWHEGAN—Somerset County										
★ REDINGTON–FAIRVIEW GENERAL HOSPITAL, Fairview Avenue, Zip 04976, Mailing Address: Box 468, Zip 04976; tel. 207/474–5121; Richard Willett, Executive Director **A**1 2 9 10 **F**7 8 12 15 16 17 19 21 22 30 32 33 34 35 37 40 41 42 44 45 49 54 56 58 65 66 67 71 73	23	10	72	3422	42	54906	238	18185	9230	312
SOUTH PORTLAND—Cumberland County										
☐ JACKSON BROOK INSTITUTE, 175 Running Hill Road, Zip 04106; tel. 207/761–2200; Vincent Furey, President **A**1 3 9 10 **F**3 12 16 18 19 25 26 32 34 35 39 41 45 46 51 52 53 54 55 56 57 58 59 65 67 **P**5 **S**0215 Community Care Systems, Inc.	33	22	106	2020	90	9087	0	19086	9566	260

Hospitals, U.S. / MAINE

Hospital, Address, Telephone, Administrator, Approval, Facility, and Physician Codes, Health Care System	Classification Codes		Utilization Data					Expense (thousands) of dollars		
★ American Hospital Association (AHA) membership ☐ Joint Commission on Accreditation of Healthcare Organizations (JCAHO) accreditation + American Osteopathic Hospital Association (AOHA) membership ○ American Osteopathic Association (AOA) accreditation △ Commission on Accreditation of Rehabilitation Facilities (CARF) accreditation Control codes 61, 63, 64, 71, 72 and 73 indicate hospitals listed by AOHA, but not registered by AHA. For definition of numerical codes, see page A6	Control	Service	Beds	Admissions	Census	Outpatient Visits	Births	Total	Payroll	Personnel
TOGUS—Kennebec County										
✚ VETERANS AFFAIRS MEDICAL CENTER, Zip 04330; tel. 207/623–8411; John H. Sims Jr., Director (Total facility includes 60 beds in nursing home–type unit) **A**1 2 3 **F**1 2 3 4 5 9 10 12 14 15 16 17 19 20 21 22 24 25 26 27 28 29 30 31 32 33 34 35 37 39 41 42 43 44 46 48 49 51 52 54 55 56 57 58 59 60 61 63 64 65 67 69 71 73 74 **P**6 **S**9295 Department of Veterans Affairs	45	10	315	4305	272	122104	0	53557	35323	1042
WATERVILLE—Kennebec County										
✚ MID–MAINE MEDICAL CENTER, (Includes Marie Joseph Hospital, Jackman, Maine) 30 Chase Avenue, Zip 04901–4974; tel. 207/872–1000; Scott B. Bullock, President (Total facility includes 18 beds in nursing home–type unit) **A**1 2 3 5 9 10 **F**2 3 4 7 8 11 13 15 16 17 19 20 21 22 25 28 30 31 33 34 35 37 39 40 41 42 44 46 48 49 51 52 54 55 56 57 58 59 60 63 65 66 67 69 71 72 73 **P**8	23	10	232	7849	157	77183	722	64945	31582	1044
★ + ○ WATERVILLE OSTEOPATHIC HOSPITAL, Kennedy Memorial Drive, Zip 04901; tel. 207/873–0731; Wilfred J. Addison, Administrator **A**9 10 11 12 13 **F**7 8 15 19 22 24 34 35 37 40 41 42 44 45 49 71 73 **S**0002 Quorum Health Group/Quorum Health Resources	23	10	42	1514	18	57660	229	14437	6846	223
WESTBROOK—Cumberland County										
WESTBROOK COMMUNITY HOSPITAL, 40 Park Road, Zip 04092; tel. 207/854–8464; Joel P. Rogers, Chief Executive Officer (Nonreporting) **A**9 10	23	82	30	—	—	—	—	—	—	—
YORK—York County										
✚ YORK HOSPITAL, 15 Hospital Drive, Zip 03909–1099; tel. 207/363–4321; Jud Knox, President **A**1 9 10 **F**3 4 7 8 10 11 12 15 16 17 19 21 22 23 27 31 32 33 35 37 39 40 42 44 45 49 64 65 67 71 73 **P**8	23	10	79	3357	56	31150	252	22629	11146	362

© 1995 AHA Guide

Hospitals, U.S. / MARYLAND

MARYLAND

Resident population 4,965 (in thousands)
Resident population in metro areas 92.8%
Birth rate per 1,000 population 16.3
65 years and over 11.1%
Percent of persons without health insurance 12.3%

Hospital, Address, Telephone, Administrator, Approval, Facility, and Physician Codes, Health Care System	Classification Codes		Utilization Data					Expense (thousands) of dollars		
★ American Hospital Association (AHA) membership ☐ Joint Commission on Accreditation of Healthcare Organizations (JCAHO) accreditation + American Osteopathic Hospital Association (AOHA) membership ○ American Osteopathic Association (AOA) accreditation △ Commission on Accreditation of Rehabilitation Facilities (CARF) accreditation Control codes 61, 63, 64, 71, 72 and 73 indicate hospitals listed by AOHA, but not registered by AHA. For definition of numerical codes, see page A6	Control	Service	Beds	Admissions	Census	Outpatient Visits	Births	Total	Payroll	Personnel
ANDREWS AIR FORCE BASE—Prince George's County										
★ MALCOLM GROW MEDICAL CENTER, 1050 West Perimeter, Suite A1–9, Zip 20748; Mailing Address: Andrews Air Force Base, Washington, DC Zip 20331–6600; tel. 301/981–3002; Colonel Ray J. Chappelle MSC, USAF, Administrator **A**1 3 5 **F**1 2 3 5 6 7 8 9 10 11 12 13 14 15 17 18 19 20 21 22 23 24 25 26 27 28 29 30 31 32 33 34 35 36 37 38 39 40 41 42 43 44 45 46 47 48 49 50 51 52 53 54 55 56 57 58 59 60 61 62 63 64 65 66 67 68 69 70 71 72 73 74 **S**9495 Department of the Air Force	41	10	185	7680	115	414112	1011	47502	10767	1564
ANNAPOLIS—Anne Arundel County										
★ ANNE ARUNDEL MEDICAL CENTER, Franklin and Cathedral Streets, Zip 21401–2777; tel. 410/267–1000; Martin L. Doordan, President **A**1 2 9 10 **F**2 3 8 10 11 12 14 15 16 17 19 20 22 29 32 33 34 35 37 39 40 42 44 45 46 49 56 60 65 67 71 73 74	23	10	291	15178	169	136608	2816	94625	46069	1524
BALTIMORE—Baltimore City County										
★ BON SECOURS HOSPITAL, 2000 West Baltimore Street, Zip 21223–1597; tel. 410/362–3000; Jane R. Durney, Chief Executive Officer **A**1 9 10 **F**3 8 10 11 12 15 16 17 19 20 21 22 25 26 27 28 30 31 32 33 34 35 37 39 40 42 44 45 46 49 51 54 62 65 67 71 73 **P**1 6 **S**5085 Bon Secours Health System, Inc.	21	10	150	5814	123	52828	0	57056	25538	925
★ △ CHILDREN'S HOSPITAL AND CENTER FOR RECONSTRUCTIVE SURGERY, 3825 Greenspring Avenue, Zip 21211–1398; tel. 410/462–6800; Robert A. Chrzan, President and Chief Executive Officer **A**1 3 5 7 9 10 **F**12 15 19 20 21 24 28 32 34 35 37 39 44 45 46 48 49 65 66 73	23	47	76	1444	21	44230	0	16654	6666	221
★ CHURCH HOSPITAL CORPORATION, 100 North Broadway, Zip 21231–1593; tel. 410/522–8000; James R. Bobb, President (Total facility includes 31 beds in nursing home–type unit) **A**1 9 10 **F**1 2 3 4 8 10 12 14 17 19 20 21 22 25 26 27 28 29 30 31 32 33 34 35 37 39 41 42 44 45 46 48 49 54 55 56 57 58 60 62 63 64 65 67 71 72 73 **S**2355 Helix Health System	23	10	247	6281	118	58732	0	51113	22027	669
★ DEATON SPECIALTY HOSPITAL AND HOME, 611 South Charles Street, Zip 21230; tel. 410/547–8500; Errol G. Newport, President and Chief Executive Officer (Total facility includes 180 beds in nursing home–type unit) **A**1 5 9 10 **F**14 26 31 33 41 64 65 67 73 **P**5	23	48	360	574	339	0	0	30989	13315	449
★ FRANKLIN SQUARE HOSPITAL CENTER, 9000 Franklin Square Drive, Zip 21237; tel. 410/682–7000; Charles D. Mross, President **A**1 3 5 8 9 10 **F**2 3 4 7 8 10 11 12 16 17 18 19 21 22 23 26 28 29 30 31 32 33 34 35 37 38 39 40 41 42 43 44 45 46 47 48 49 51 52 53 54 55 56 57 58 59 60 61 62 63 64 65 66 67 68 70 71 73 74 **P**7 **S**2355 Helix Health System	23	10	405	21424	290	122012	3624	136063	70979	1918
★ △ GOOD SAMARITAN HOSPITAL OF MARYLAND, 5601 Loch Raven Boulevard, Zip 21239–2995; tel. 410/532–8000; Lawrence M. Beck, President **A**1 3 5 7 9 10 **F**3 4 5 6 7 8 10 12 14 15 16 17 18 19 21 22 23 26 27 28 29 30 31 32 33 34 35 37 39 41 42 43 44 45 46 48 49 51 53 54 55 56 57 58 59 60 61 62 63 65 66 67 68 70 71 73 74 **P**3 7 **S**2355 Helix Health System	23	10	273	9717	210	90642	0	89932	42337	1459
★ GREATER BALTIMORE MEDICAL CENTER, 6701 North Charles Street, Zip 21204; tel. 410/828–2000; Robert P. Kowal, President **A**1 3 5 8 9 10 **F**3 7 8 10 11 12 16 17 19 21 22 23 24 25 28 29 30 32 33 34 35 37 38 40 41 42 44 45 46 49 51 53 54 55 56 57 58 59 60 61 65 66 67 69 71 73 74 **P**2 3 4 5 6 7 8	23	10	387	21977	270	113763	4962	171251	80681	2244
☐ GUNDRY–GLASS HOSPITAL, 2 North Wickham Road, Zip 21229, Mailing Address: 1777 Reisterstown Road, Pikesville Zip 21208; tel. 410/484–2700; Elliott Neal White, President **A**1 9 10 **F**3 12 15 17 18 19 21 25 26 27 28 29 34 35 45 46 49 52 53 54 55 56 57 58 59 65 67 71 **P**3 4 5 7 8	33	22	85	2050	71	4765	0	9689	5394	182
★ HARBOR HOSPITAL CENTER, 3001 South Hanover Street, Zip 21225; tel. 410/347–3200; L. Barney Johnson, President and Chief Executive Officer (Nonreporting) **A**1 3 5 6 9 10	23	10	300	—	—	—	—	—	—	—
★ △ JAMES LAWRENCE KERNAN HOSPITAL, 2200 North Forest Park Avenue, Zip 21207–6697; tel. 410/448–2500; James E. Ross, Executive Director **A**1 3 5 7 9 10 **F**12 19 25 26 27 34 35 37 44 45 46 48 49 54 65 66 71 73 **P**1	23	47	76	1646	41	30000	0	20759	8922	313
★ JOHNS HOPKINS BAYVIEW MEDICAL CENTER, 4940 Eastern Avenue, Zip 21224; tel. 410/550–0100; Ronald R. Peterson, President (Total facility includes 302 beds in nursing home–type unit) **A**1 3 5 8 9 10 **F**1 2 3 4 5 7 8 9 10 11 12 13 14 15 16 17 18 19 20 21 22 23 24 25 26 27 28 29 30 31 32 33 34 35 37 38 39 40 41 42 43 44 45 46 47 49 50 51 52 53 54 55 56 57 58 59 60 61 63 64 65 66 67 68 69 70 71 72 73 74 **P**5 6 **S**1015 Johns Hopkins Health System	23	10	667	15556	517	226178	921	139827	54164	2041
★ △ JOHNS HOPKINS HOSPITAL, 600 North Wolfe Street, Zip 21287; tel. 410/955–5000; James A. Block M.D., President and Chief Executive Officer **A**1 2 3 5 7 8 9 10 **F**1 2 3 4 5 7 8 9 10 11 12 15 17 19 20 21 22 23 24 25 26 31 32 34 35 37 38 40 41 42 43 44 45 46 47 49 50 52 53 54 55 56 57 58 59 60 61 63 64 65 66 67 68 69 70 71 73 74 **P**6 **S**1015 Johns Hopkins Health System	23	10	954	39185	758	276483	2701	473581	187134	4605
★ △ KENNEDY KRIEGER INSTITUTE, (Rehabilitation and Special Pediatric) 707 North Broadway, Zip 21205–1890; tel. 410/550–9000; Gary W. Goldstein M.D., President **A**1 7 9 10 **F**6 12 14 15 16 17 19 21 22 32 34 35 39 45 46 48 49 50 53 54 55 58 63 65 67 70 71 73 **P**6	23	59	57	430	45	61767	0	33837	15920	962

Hospitals, U.S. / MARYLAND

Hospital, Address, Telephone, Administrator, Approval, Facility, and Physician Codes, Health Care System	Classification Codes		Utilization Data					Expense (thousands) of dollars		
★ American Hospital Association (AHA) membership ☐ Joint Commission on Accreditation of Healthcare Organizations (JCAHO) accreditation + American Osteopathic Hospital Association (AOHA) membership ○ American Osteopathic Association (AOA) accreditation △ Commission on Accreditation of Rehabilitation Facilities (CARF) accreditation Control codes 61, 63, 64, 71, 72 and 73 indicate hospitals listed by AOHA, but not registered by AHA. For definition of numerical codes, see page A6	Control	Service	Beds	Admissions	Census	Outpatient Visits	Births	Total	Payroll	Personnel
★ △ LEVINDALE HEBREW GERIATRIC CENTER AND HOSPITAL, (Rehabilitation, Hospice, Chronic Medical and Long–term Care) 2434 West Belvedere Avenue, Zip 21215–5299; tel. 410/466–8700; Stanford A. Alliker FACHE, President **A**1 7 9 10 **F**1 12 15 16 19 20 21 26 31 32 33 35 36 45 48 52 54 57 59 64 65 67 73	23	49	288	739	265	20864	0	24923	11116	473
★ LIBERTY MEDICAL CENTER, (Includes Lutheran Hospital of Maryland, 730 Ashburton Street, Baltimore, Maryland, Zip 21216; tel. 301/945–1600; Provident Hospital, Baltimore, Maryland) 2600 Liberty Heights Avenue, Zip 21215; tel. 410/383–4000; Everard O. Rutledge FACHE, President and Chief Executive Officer **A**1 9 10 **F**3 8 12 13 14 15 16 17 18 19 20 21 22 25 26 27 28 30 31 32 34 37 39 42 44 45 46 49 51 52 53 54 55 56 58 59 61 63 65 67 71 73 74 **P**2 3 4 5 7 8 LUTHERAN HOSPITAL OF MARYLAND See Liberty Medical Center	23	10	175	6752	143	56323	0	56641	29608	777
★ △ MARYLAND GENERAL HOSPITAL, 827 Linden Avenue, Zip 21201–4606; tel. 410/225–8000; James R. Wood, Chairman and Chief Executive Officer **A**1 3 5 7 9 10 **F**3 7 8 10 11 12 17 19 21 22 25 26 27 29 30 31 32 34 35 37 39 40 41 42 44 45 48 49 51 52 54 56 57 60 65 71 73 **P**8	23	10	246	8411	174	81496	818	78885	43087	1280
★ MERCY MEDICAL CENTER, 301 St. Paul Place, Zip 21202–2165; tel. 410/332–9000; Sister Helen Amos, President and Chief Executive Officer **A**1 3 5 9 10 **F**2 7 8 10 11 16 17 19 20 21 22 23 24 25 26 29 30 31 32 34 35 37 38 39 40 41 42 44 45 46 49 51 52 53 56 58 60 65 67 71 72 73 74 **P**5 6 **S**6015 Sisters of Mercy of the Americas–Regional Community of Baltimore	21	10	245	11637	170	156045	1852	98959	43047	1849
★ △ MONTEBELLO REHABILITATION HOSPITAL–UNIVERSITY OF MARYLAND MEDICAL SYSTEM, 2201 Argonne Drive, Zip 21218–1698; tel. 410/554–5200; James E. Ross, Executive Director **A**1 5 7 9 10 **F**1 3 4 7 8 10 11 12 13 15 16 17 18 19 20 21 22 25 26 28 30 31 32 34 35 37 38 40 41 42 43 44 46 47 48 49 50 51 52 53 54 55 56 57 58 59 60 61 63 65 66 67 69 70 71 72 73 74 **P**1	23	46	137	928	82	4375	0	20869	11138	406
★ △ MT. WASHINGTON PEDIATRIC HOSPITAL, (Specialty Pediatric and Rehabilitation) 1708 West Rogers Avenue, Zip 21209–4596; tel. 410/578–8600; Francis A. Pommett, President **A**1 5 7 9 10 **F**2 11 12 14 17 19 20 21 22 23 26 27 29 31 32 33 34 35 37 38 39 40 42 45 46 47 48 49 50 51 52 53 54 55 56 57 58 59 60 61 65 67 68 69 70 71 73 74 PROVIDENT HOSPITAL See Liberty Medical Center	23	59	129	416	105	3802	0	22688	—	259
★ SHEPPARD AND ENOCH PRATT HOSPITAL, 6501 North Charles Street, Zip 21204, Mailing Address: P.O. Box 6815, Zip 21285–6815; tel. 410/938–3000; Steven S. Sharfstein, President, Medical Director and Chief Executive Officer **A**1 3 5 9 10 **F**1 3 12 15 16 18 25 26 27 34 46 52 53 54 55 56 57 58 59 65 67 **P**3	23	22	209	3767	176	121136	0	52751	28617	1020
★ △ SINAI HOSPITAL OF BALTIMORE, 2401 West Belvedere Avenue, Zip 21215–5271; tel. 410/578–5678; Warren A. Green, President and Chief Executive Officer **A**1 2 3 5 7 8 9 10 **F**3 4 6 7 8 10 11 13 14 15 17 18 19 20 21 22 23 24 26 27 28 29 30 31 32 33 34 35 36 37 38 39 40 41 42 43 44 45 46 47 48 49 51 52 53 54 55 56 57 58 59 60 61 63 65 67 70 71 73 74 **P**6 8	23	10	431	20627	344	128228	2984	226735	116831	2801
★ ST. AGNES HOSPITAL OF THE CITY OF BALTIMORE, 900 Caton Avenue, Zip 21229–5299; tel. 410/368–6000; Robert E. Pezzoli, President and Chief Executive Officer **A**1 2 3 5 9 10 **F**1 3 7 8 10 11 13 15 16 17 19 21 22 26 28 29 30 32 33 34 35 39 40 41 42 44 45 46 47 49 51 53 54 55 56 58 59 60 61 63 65 67 68 70 71 73 74 **P**6 7 8 **S**1855 Daughters of Charity National Health System ST. JOSEPH HOSPITAL See St. Joseph Medical Center, Towson	23	10	424	18769	270	135665	2063	150249	74739	2180
★ △ UNION MEMORIAL HOSPITAL, 201 East University Parkway, Zip 21218–2391; tel. 410/554–2000; Edward J. Kelly III, President and Chief Executive Officer (Total facility includes 31 beds in nursing home–type unit) **A**1 3 5 6 7 9 10 **F**4 5 7 8 10 11 12 14 15 16 17 18 19 21 22 23 26 27 28 30 32 33 34 35 37 38 40 41 42 43 44 46 48 49 51 52 54 58 59 60 61 63 64 65 66 67 70 71 73 **P**2 3 5 6 7 **S**2355 Helix Health System	23	10	376	16874	306	123914	1270	135231	67998	2234
★ UNIVERSITY OF MARYLAND MEDICAL SYSTEM, 22 South Greene Street, Zip 21201–1595; tel. 410/328–8667; Morton I. Rapoport M.D., President and Chief Executive Officer **A**1 2 3 5 8 9 10 **F**3 4 5 7 8 10 11 12 13 14 15 16 17 19 20 21 22 23 25 26 27 28 29 30 31 32 33 34 35 37 38 39 40 41 42 43 44 45 46 47 48 49 51 52 53 54 55 56 57 58 59 60 61 65 66 67 68 69 70 71 72 73 74 **P**1 7	23	10	633	26233	550	190516	2296	329818	142491	4723
★ VETERANS AFFAIRS MEDICAL CENTER, 10 North Greene Street, Zip 21201–1524; tel. 410/605–7001; Michael B. Phaup, Director **A**1 2 3 5 8 9 **F**1 2 3 8 10 11 12 17 19 20 21 22 26 30 31 32 33 34 35 37 42 43 44 46 48 49 51 52 54 55 56 57 58 59 60 63 64 65 67 71 73 74 **P**6 **S**9295 Department of Veterans Affairs	45	10	236	7048	168	242989	0	—	—	—
BEL AIR—Harford County										
CHARTER BEHAVIORAL HEALTH SYSTEM, (Formerly New Beginnings at Hidden Brook) 522 Thomas Run Road, Zip 21014–7607; tel. 410/879–1919; (Nonreporting) **A**9 **S**0695 Charter Medical Corporation	33	82	48	—	—	—	—	—	—	—
BERLIN—Worcester County										
★ ATLANTIC GENERAL HOSPITAL, 9733 Healthway Drive, Zip 21811; tel. 410/641–1100; William B. Donatelli, President **A**10 **F**8 15 17 19 21 22 25 28 30 33 37 39 41 44 49 51 65 71 **P**6 **S**0002 Quorum Health Group/Quorum Health Resources	23	10	62	1447	29	34513	5	13925	5360	218
BETHESDA—Montgomery County										
★ CLINICAL CENTER, NATIONAL INSTITUTES OF HEALTH, (Biomedical Research) 9000 Rockville Pike, Zip 20892–1504; tel. 301/496–4114; John I. Gallin M.D., Director (Nonreporting) **A**1 3 8 **S**9195 U.S. Public Health Service Indian Health Service	44	49	385	—	—	—	—	—	—	—

© 1995 AHA Guide

Hospitals, U.S. / MARYLAND

Hospital, Address, Telephone, Administrator, Approval, Facility, and Physician Codes, Health Care System

- ★ American Hospital Association (AHA) membership
- ☐ Joint Commission on Accreditation of Healthcare Organizations (JCAHO) accreditation
- + American Osteopathic Hospital Association (AOHA) membership
- ○ American Osteopathic Association (AOA) accreditation
- △ Commission on Accreditation of Rehabilitation Facilities (CARF) accreditation

Control codes 61, 63, 64, 71, 72 and 73 indicate hospitals listed by AOHA, but not registered by AHA. For definition of numerical codes, see page A6.

Hospital	Control	Service	Beds	Admissions	Census	Outpatient Visits	Births	Total	Payroll	Personnel
✣ NATIONAL NAVAL MEDICAL CENTER, Zip 20889-5600; tel. 301/295-5800; Rear Admiral David M. Lichtman MC, USN, Commander (Nonreporting) A1 2 3 5 S9655 Department of Navy	43	10	362	—	—	—	—	—	—	—
✣ SUBURBAN HOSPITAL, 8600 Old Georgetown Road, Zip 20814; tel. 301/530-3100; Brian G. Grissler, President and Chief Executive Officer (Total facility includes 22 beds in nursing home–type unit) A1 2 3 5 10 F2 3 4 6 8 10 11 15 17 19 21 22 25 26 28 29 30 31 32 33 34 35 37 39 41 42 44 46 49 52 53 54 55 56 57 58 59 60 61 63 64 65 67 70 71 73 74 P8	23	10	297	10786	192	74350	0	96767	46230	1350
CAMBRIDGE—Dorchester County										
✣ DORCHESTER GENERAL HOSPITAL, 300 Byrn Street, Zip 21613; tel. 410/228-5511; Kenneth A. Richmond, President and Chief Executive Officer A1 2 9 10 F7 8 17 19 21 22 28 29 30 31 34 35 37 39 40 41 44 45 49 52 53 54 56 58 65 71 73 74 P3	23	10	82	3953	61	37532	305	23582	11637	408
☐ EASTERN SHORE HOSPITAL CENTER, Mailing Address: Box 800, Zip 21613; tel. 410/221-2300; Mary K. Noren, Acting Superintendent A1 10 F14 15 16 28 37 44 46 48 52 54 55 57 58 65 73 P6	12	22	128	240	102	0	0	14930	8831	309
CATONSVILLE—Baltimore County										
☐ SPRING GROVE HOSPITAL CENTER, Wade Avenue, Zip 21228; tel. 410/455-6000; William B. Landis, Acting Superintendent (Total facility includes 70 beds in nursing home–type unit) A1 3 5 10 F15 20 27 45 46 52 55 57 65 73 P6	12	22	567	835	548	0	0	40434	—	840
CHESTERTOWN—Kent County										
✣ KENT AND QUEEN ANNE'S HOSPITAL, 100 Brown Street, Zip 21620-1499; tel. 410/778-3300; William R. Kirk Jr., President and Chief Executive Officer A1 9 10 F7 8 11 12 14 15 16 17 19 21 22 24 28 30 35 37 39 40 44 45 48 49 56 63 67 71 73	23	10	64	3137	41	35838	153	17090	8189	248
CHEVERLY—Prince George's County										
✣ PRINCE GEORGE'S HOSPITAL CENTER, 3001 Hospital Drive, Zip 20785; tel. 301/618-2000; Allan Earl Atzrott, President A1 3 5 10 F4 7 8 10 11 12 13 14 15 16 17 18 19 20 22 25 26 27 28 30 31 32 33 34 35 36 37 39 40 41 42 43 44 46 48 49 51 52 53 54 56 58 60 63 64 65 67 68 70 71 72 73 P6 7 8 S0029 Dimensions Health Corporation	23	10	394	15997	276	107812	3800	123266	65790	1511
CLINTON—Prince George's County										
✣ SOUTHERN MARYLAND HOSPITAL, 7503 Surratts Road, Zip 20735-3395; tel. 301/868-8000; Francis P. Chiaramonte M.D., Chief Executive Officer A1 10 F4 7 8 10 11 12 14 15 16 17 19 21 22 23 24 25 28 30 32 34 35 37 38 40 41 42 44 46 49 52 53 54 55 56 57 60 63 65 67 71 73 74 P8	33	10	356	12345	197	50068	1284	80193	40026	1033
COLUMBIA—Howard County										
✣ HOWARD COUNTY GENERAL HOSPITAL, 5755 Cedar Lane, Zip 21044-2999; tel. 410/740-7890; Victor A. Broccolino, President A1 5 9 10 F7 8 14 15 16 19 21 22 26 28 29 30 32 33 34 35 37 40 42 44 45 46 49 52 56 57 58 59 60 65 67 68 71 73	23	10	200	11961	131	46465	2972	69888	30177	779
CRISFIELD—Somerset County										
☐ EDWARD W. MCCREADY MEMORIAL HOSPITAL, 201 Hall Highway, Zip 21817-1299; tel. 410/968-1200; Dean B. Massey D.D.S., Chief Executive Officer A1 9 10 F8 14 15 16 17 19 22 23 24 26 28 30 34 35 39 41 44 46 49 52 57 61 64 65 71 73 P5	23	10	45	706	27	13521	0	5566	2456	123
CROWNSVILLE—Anne Arundel County										
☐ CROWNSVILLE HOSPITAL CENTER, Zip 21032; tel. 410/987-6200; Barry Rudnick M.D., Acting Clinical Director A1 5 10 F2 14 15 16 20 26 27 29 30 31 41 45 52 53 55 57 65 73	12	22	283	670	248	0	0	28651	17217	626
CUMBERLAND—Allegany County										
✣ MEMORIAL AND MEDICAL CENTER OF CUMBERLAND, 600 Memorial Avenue, Zip 21502-3797; tel. 301/777-4000; Barry P. Ronan, President A1 9 10 F4 5 7 8 10 11 14 15 16 17 19 20 21 22 28 30 31 32 33 34 35 36 37 39 40 41 42 44 45 48 49 54 60 61 65 67 70 71 72 73 74	23	10	222	9231	165	54966	506	62169	27835	899
✣ SACRED HEART HOSPITAL, 900 Seton Drive, Zip 21502; tel. 301/759-4200; Edward M. Dinan, President A1 2 9 10 F1 3 7 8 10 12 14 15 16 18 19 21 22 24 25 26 30 31 32 33 34 35 37 39 40 42 44 45 46 51 52 53 56 57 58 59 60 63 65 71 73 74 P5 S1855 Daughters of Charity National Health System	23	10	240	8473	156	71310	740	56088	27302	776
☐ THOMAS B. FINAN CENTER, Country Club Road, Zip 21501, Mailing Address: Box 1722, Zip 21501-1722; tel. 301/777-2240; Archie T. Wallace, Chief Executive Officer A1 10 F1 3 4 5 6 7 8 9 10 11 12 13 17 18 19 20 21 22 23 24 25 26 27 28 29 30 31 32 33 35 37 38 40 41 42 43 44 45 46 47 50 52 54 55 56 57 60 61 62 63 64 65 66 67 68 69 70 71 72 73 74 P6	12	22	119	306	103	0	0	8204	5882	230
EAST NEW MARKET—Dorchester County										
NEW BEGINNINGS AT WARWICK MANOR, 3680 Warwick Road, Zip 21631; tel. 410/943-8108; Larry Foxwell, Executive Director (Nonreporting) A9	33	82	42	—	—	—	—	—	—	—
EASTON—Talbot County										
✣ MEMORIAL HOSPITAL AT EASTON MARYLAND, 219 South Washington Street, Zip 21601-2996; tel. 410/822-1000; Joseph P. Ross, President and Chief Executive Officer (Total facility includes 31 beds in nursing home–type unit) A1 2 6 10 F1 3 7 8 10 12 14 15 16 19 20 21 22 25 27 28 30 31 32 33 34 35 36 37 39 40 41 42 44 49 52 54 56 57 58 59 60 63 64 65 67 70 71 72 73 P3	23	10	200	8286	143	253490	843	62004	29943	1110

Hospitals, U.S. / MARYLAND

Hospital, Address, Telephone, Administrator, Approval, Facility, and Physician Codes, Health Care System	Classification Codes		Utilization Data					Expense (thousands) of dollars		
	Control	Service	Beds	Admissions	Census	Outpatient Visits	Births	Total	Payroll	Personnel

★ American Hospital Association (AHA) membership
☐ Joint Commission on Accreditation of Healthcare Organizations (JCAHO) accreditation
+ American Osteopathic Hospital Association (AOHA) membership
○ American Osteopathic Association (AOA) accreditation
△ Commission on Accreditation of Rehabilitation Facilities (CARF) accreditation
Control codes 61, 63, 64, 71, 72 and 73 indicate hospitals listed by AOHA, but not registered by AHA. For definition of numerical codes, see page A6

ELKTON—Cecil County
★ UNION HOSPITAL, 106 Bow Street, Zip 21921–5596; tel. 410/398–4000; Robert D. Joplin, Chief Executive Officer **A**1 9 10 **F**1 7 8 12 17 19 21 22 29 31 34 35 37 40 41 44 45 49 54 56 65 66 71 73 **P**8 | 23 | 10 | 111 | 5399 | 65 | 82272 | 569 | 38352 | 18667 | 575

ELLICOTT CITY—Howard County
☐ TAYLOR MANOR HOSPITAL, 4100 College Avenue, Zip 21041–0396, Mailing Address: Box 396, Zip 21041–0396; tel. 410/465–3322; Morris L. Scherr, Executive Vice President **A**1 9 10 **F**2 3 15 16 18 19 20 21 35 46 50 52 53 55 57 58 59 63 65 71 **P**5 | 33 | 22 | 78 | 970 | 47 | 0 | 0 | 9723 | 5787 | 184

EMMITSBURG—Frederick County
MOUNTAIN MANOR TREATMENT CENTER, Route 15, Zip 21727, Mailing Address: Box E, Zip 21727; tel. 301/447–2361; William J. Roby, Executive Director (Nonreporting) | 33 | 82 | 60 | — | — | — | — | — | — | —

FALLSTON—Harford County
★ FALLSTON GENERAL HOSPITAL, 200 Milton Avenue, Zip 21047–2777; tel. 410/877–3700 **A**1 9 10 **F**8 10 15 16 19 21 22 25 27 28 29 30 32 34 35 37 41 44 45 46 49 52 56 63 65 67 71 73 **P**5 6 **S**0038 Upper Chesapeake Health System | 23 | 10 | 148 | 7080 | 102 | 40716 | 0 | 37937 | 17080 | 601

FORT GEORGE G. MEADE—Anne Arundel County
★ KIMBROUGH ARMY COMMUNITY HOSPITAL, Fort George G Meade, Zip 20755; tel. 301/677–4171; Colonel Robert R. McMeekin, Commanding Officer (Nonreporting) **A**1 5 **S**9395 Department of the Army | 42 | 10 | 47 | — | — | — | — | — | — | —

FORT HOWARD—Baltimore County
★ VETERANS AFFAIRS MEDICAL CENTER, (General Medical Long Term Care) 9600 North Point Road, Zip 21052–9989; tel. 410/477–1800; Charles Clark, Director (Total facility includes 47 beds in nursing home–type unit) **A**1 5 9 **F**1 2 3 12 20 22 24 26 28 30 31 32 33 34 37 39 41 45 46 48 49 51 54 55 57 58 64 65 71 73 **P**6 **S**9295 Department of Veterans Affairs | 45 | 49 | 221 | 1780 | 204 | 36559 | 0 | | | 423

FREDERICK—Frederick County
★ FREDERICK MEMORIAL HOSPITAL, 400 West Seventh Street, Zip 21701–4593; tel. 301/698–3300; James K. Kluttz, President and Chief Executive Officer **A**1 2 9 10 **F**7 8 10 12 13 14 15 16 17 18 19 20 21 22 25 28 29 30 31 32 33 34 35 37 40 41 42 44 46 49 52 53 54 55 56 59 60 65 67 71 73 74 **P**5 | 23 | 10 | 153 | 12929 | 158 | 98593 | 1973 | 77200 | 36909 | 1221

GLEN BURNIE—Anne Arundel County
★ NORTH ARUNDEL HOSPITAL, 301 Hospital Drive, Zip 21061–5803; tel. 410/787–4000; James R. Walker, President and Chief Executive Officer **A**1 9 10 **F**10 11 12 17 19 22 29 30 32 34 37 41 42 44 49 51 52 54 56 59 65 67 71 72 73 74 **P**1 5 6 7 | 23 | 10 | 275 | 14005 | 216 | 76278 | 0 | 89103 | 44743 | 1413

HAGERSTOWN—Washington County
☐ BROOK LANE PSYCHIATRIC CENTER, 13218 Brook Lane Drive, Zip 21742–1945, Mailing Address: P.O. Box 1945, Zip 21742–1945; tel. 301/733–0330; R. Lynn Rushing, Chief Executive Officer **A**1 9 10 **F**1 3 14 15 25 26 34 52 53 54 55 56 57 58 59 65 **P**5 | 23 | 22 | 65 | 984 | 38 | 14018 | 0 | 7678 | 4739 | 165
★ WASHINGTON COUNTY HOSPITAL ASSOCIATION, 251 East Antietam Street, Zip 21740–5771; tel. 301/790–8000; Horace W. Murphy, President (Total facility includes 47 beds in nursing home–type unit) **A**1 2 9 10 **F**3 4 7 8 10 11 14 15 16 17 19 21 22 23 25 26 28 29 30 31 32 33 34 35 36 37 39 40 41 42 44 45 46 49 51 52 54 55 56 58 59 60 61 63 64 65 67 70 71 73 74 **P**6 | 23 | 10 | 300 | 14596 | 218 | 158994 | 1555 | 90312 | 48754 | 1511
☐ WESTERN MARYLAND CENTER, 1500 Pennsylvania Avenue, Zip 21742–3194; tel. 301/791–4400; Carl A. Fischer M.D., Director (Nonreporting) **A**1 9 10 | 12 | 48 | 120 | — | — | — | — | — | — | —

HAVRE DE GRACE—Harford County
★ HARFORD MEMORIAL HOSPITAL, 501 South Union Avenue, Zip 21078–3493; tel. 410/939–2400; Linda S. Widra R.N., Ph.D., Senior Vice President and Chief Operating Officer **A**1 9 10 **F**3 7 8 10 11 14 15 16 17 19 20 21 22 24 28 29 30 32 34 35 37 40 41 42 44 45 46 48 54 56 57 58 60 65 67 69 71 73 **P**4 5 **S**0038 Upper Chesapeake Health System | 23 | 10 | 175 | 6837 | 87 | 42346 | 646 | 36341 | 15668 | 543

JESSUP—Anne Arundel County
☐ CLIFTON T. PERKINS HOSPITAL CENTER, 8450 Dorsey Run Road, Zip 20794, Mailing Address: P.O. Box 1000, Zip 20794–1000; tel. 410/792–4022; W. Lawrence Fitch J.D., Acting Superintendent (Nonreporting) **A**1 5 | 12 | 49 | 220 | — | — | — | — | — | — | —

LA PLATA—Charles County
★ PHYSICIANS MEMORIAL HOSPITAL, 701 East Charles Street, Zip 20646, Mailing Address: P.O. Box 1070, Zip 20646; tel. 301/609–4000; Susan L. Hunsaker, President and Chief Executive Officer **A**1 9 10 **F**7 8 11 15 16 17 19 21 22 30 34 35 37 39 40 42 44 49 56 65 67 71 73 74 | 23 | 10 | 108 | 5072 | 72 | 40538 | 617 | 32713 | 14913 | 511

LANHAM—Prince George's County
★ DOCTORS COMMUNITY HOSPITAL, 8118 Good Luck Road, Zip 20706–3596; tel. 301/552–8118; Philip Down, President **A**1 10 **F**8 10 12 15 16 17 19 21 22 23 28 31 32 34 35 37 39 41 42 44 45 49 60 65 67 71 73 | 23 | 10 | 250 | 8963 | 157 | 58475 | 0 | 77127 | 25763 | 762

LAUREL—Prince George's County
★ △ LAUREL REGIONAL HOSPITAL, (Formerly Greater Laurel Beltsville Hospital) 7300 Van Dusen Road, Zip 20707–9266; tel. 301/725–4300; Patrick F. Mutch, President **A**1 7 10 **F**2 3 4 5 7 8 9 10 11 12 15 17 18 19 21 22 25 26 28 29 30 31 32 33 34 35 36 37 38 39 40 41 42 43 44 45 46 47 48 49 51 52 53 54 55 56 57 58 59 60 63 64 65 67 68 69 70 71 72 73 **P**1 6 7 **S**0029 Dimensions Health Corporation | 23 | 10 | 185 | 7263 | 116 | 40762 | 638 | 51554 | 24997 | 615

© 1995 AHA Guide

Hospitals, U.S. / MARYLAND

Hospital, Address, Telephone, Administrator, Approval, Facility, and Physician Codes, Health Care System	Classification Codes		Utilization Data					Expense (thousands) of dollars		
★ American Hospital Association (AHA) membership ☐ Joint Commission on Accreditation of Healthcare Organizations (JCAHO) accreditation + American Osteopathic Hospital Association (AOHA) membership ○ American Osteopathic Association (AOA) accreditation △ Commission on Accreditation of Rehabilitation Facilities (CARF) accreditation Control codes 61, 63, 64, 71, 72 and 73 indicate hospitals listed by AOHA, but not registered by AHA. For definition of numerical codes, see page A6	Control	Service	Beds	Admissions	Census	Outpatient Visits	Births	Total	Payroll	Personnel
LEONARDTOWN—St. Marys County										
☒ ST. MARY'S HOSPITAL, 234 Jefferson Street, Zip 20650, Mailing Address: P.O. Box 527, Zip 20650; tel. 301/475–8981; Christine R. Wray, Chief Executive Officer **A**1 9 10 **F**7 8 14 15 16 17 19 22 27 28 30 33 34 35 37 39 40 41 42 44 49 52 56 65 67 68 71 73 74	23	10	107	5269	71	95985	694	28477	13520	493
OAKLAND—Garrett County										
☒ GARRETT COUNTY MEMORIAL HOSPITAL, 251 North Fourth Street, Zip 21550; tel. 301/334–2155; Benjamin Rosenthal, Chief Executive Officer **A**1 9 10 **F**7 8 11 15 16 17 18 19 20 21 22 30 33 36 39 40 44 45 46 49 52 54 56 65 71 73 **P**3 8	23	10	76	3239	39	54726	326	19391	9398	290
OLNEY—Montgomery County										
☒ MONTGOMERY GENERAL HOSPITAL, 18101 Prince Philip Drive, Zip 20832–9990; tel. 301/774–8882; Peter W. Monge, President **A**1 2 9 10 **F**2 3 7 8 11 15 17 19 21 22 26 28 30 31 32 35 37 40 41 42 44 49 52 53 54 55 56 57 58 59 60 63 65 67 71 73 **P**6 8	23	10	229	8110	122	39485	854	51821	26920	871
PATUXENT RIVER—St. Marys County										
★ NAVAL HOSPITAL, Zip 20670–5370; tel. 301/826–1418 **F**7 12 16 22 27 28 29 30 34 40 44 45 51 54 58 65 71 72 **S**9655 Department of Navy	43	10	20	870	5	88781	245	18492	7568	274
PERRY POINT—Cecil County										
☒ VETERANS AFFAIRS MEDICAL CENTER, Circle Drive, Zip 21902; tel. 410/642–2411; Allan S. Goss, Director (Total facility includes 80 beds in nursing home-type unit) **A**1 5 9 **F**1 2 3 4 5 6 8 9 10 11 12 17 18 19 20 21 22 23 24 25 26 27 28 29 30 31 32 33 34 35 37 39 41 42 43 44 45 46 48 49 50 51 52 54 55 56 57 58 59 60 63 64 65 67 69 70 71 73 74 **P**6 **S**9295 Department of Veterans Affairs	45	22	634	3135	491	93002	0	73174	58079	1332
PRINCE FREDERICK—Calvert County										
☒ CALVERT MEMORIAL HOSPITAL, 100 Hospital Road, Zip 20678; tel. 410/535–4000; James J. Xinis, President **A**1 2 9 10 **F**8 13 14 15 16 17 18 19 22 24 25 28 29 30 33 35 36 37 39 40 41 42 44 45 46 49 52 53 56 59 65 66 67 71 73 74 **P**8	23	10	109	5464	76	49722	695	26708	13100	421
RANDALLSTOWN—Baltimore County										
☒ NORTHWEST HOSPITAL CENTER, 5401 Old Court Road, Zip 21133–5185; tel. 410/521–2200; Robert W. Fischer, President **A**1 9 10 **F**8 10 15 16 17 19 21 22 23 28 29 30 31 32 33 34 35 37 41 42 44 46 49 51 56 60 63 64 65 67 71 72 73 **P**1 6 7	23	10	198	10445	170	47494	0	72296	34355	1042
ROCKVILLE—Montgomery County										
☐ CHARTER BEHAVIORAL HEALTH SYSTEM OF POTOMAC RIDGE, 14901 Broschart Road, Zip 20850; tel. 301/251–4500; Jonathan A. Garber, Administrator and Chief Executive Officer (Nonreporting) **A**1 10 **S**0695 Charter Medical Corporation	33	22	88	—	—	—	—	—	—	—
☒ CHESTNUT LODGE HOSPITAL, 500 West Montgomery Avenue, Zip 20850; tel. 301/424–8300; Dexter M. Bullard Jr. M.D., Medical Director and President (Nonreporting) **A**1 10	33	22	72	—	—	—	—	—	—	—
☐ SHADY GROVE ADVENTIST HOSPITAL, 9901 Medical Center Drive, Zip 20850–3395; tel. 301/279–6000; Bryan L. Breckenridge, President **A**1 10 **F**1 2 4 6 7 8 10 11 15 16 17 19 21 22 26 28 29 30 31 32 33 34 35 36 37 38 39 40 41 42 43 44 45 46 47 49 52 53 54 55 56 57 59 60 61 63 64 65 67 69 71 73 74 **P**4 5 7 8	21	10	253	11399	178	99806	4977	110715	53976	1357
SALISBURY—Wicomico County										
☐ DEER'S HEAD CENTER, Mailing Address: Box 2018, Zip 21802–2018; tel. 410/543–4000; Dorothy A. Bradshaw, Acting Director (Total facility includes 60 beds in nursing home–type unit) **A**1 10 **F**4 8 10 11 15 16 19 20 21 22 26 27 28 29 30 31 33 35 37 42 44 45 46 48 49 52 53 54 55 56 57 58 60 64 65 67 69 71 73 74	12	48	84	93	67	17948	0	12728	5908	263
☒ PENINSULA REGIONAL MEDICAL CENTER, 100 East Carroll Street, Zip 21801–5493; tel. 410/546–6400; Dan H. Akin, President **A**1 2 9 10 **F**2 4 7 8 10 11 15 16 17 19 20 21 22 23 24 25 26 28 30 31 32 34 35 37 40 41 42 43 44 46 51 52 56 60 61 65 67 70 71 73 **P**3	23	10	377	17219	275	271790	2102	108766	50385	1573
SILVER SPRING—Montgomery County										
☒ HOLY CROSS HOSPITAL OF SILVER SPRING, 1500 Forest Glen Road, Zip 20910; tel. 301/905–0100; James P. Hamill, President **A**1 3 5 8 10 **F**1 2 3 4 8 9 10 11 12 13 14 15 16 17 18 19 20 21 22 26 27 28 29 30 31 32 33 34 35 36 37 38 39 40 42 43 44 45 46 47 48 49 51 52 53 54 55 56 57 58 59 60 63 65 67 71 73 74 **P**1 3 **S**5585 Holy Cross Health System Corporation	21	10	366	24310	311	160250	5626	138899	56677	1808
SUITLAND—Prince George's County										
★ SAINT LUKE INSTITUTE, 2420 Brooks Drive, Zip 20746–5294; tel. 301/967–3700; Reverend Canice Connors Ph.D., President and Chief Executive Officer **F**2 3 39 45 46 52 54 55 58	23	22	24	62	24	1588	0	4444	2481	62
SYKESVILLE—Carroll County										
☐ SPRINGFIELD HOSPITAL CENTER, 6655 Sykesville Road, Zip 21784; tel. 410/795–2100; Paula A. Langmead, Superintendent **A**1 5 10 **F**52 54 55 57	12	22	416	1156	417	0	0	—	—	952
TAKOMA PARK—Montgomery County										
☒ WASHINGTON ADVENTIST HOSPITAL, 7600 Carroll Avenue, Zip 20912–6392; tel. 301/891–7600; Kiltie Leach, Chief Operating Officer **A**1 9 10 **F**1 2 3 4 6 7 8 10 11 15 16 17 19 21 22 28 29 30 32 34 35 36 37 38 39 40 41 42 43 44 45 46 47 49 52 53 55 56 57 58 59 60 62 64 65 67 69 71 73 **P**7 8	21	10	300	14433	234	77023	2175	127711	56642	1263
TOWSON—Baltimore County										
☒ ST. JOSEPH MEDICAL CENTER, (Formerly St. Joseph Hospital) 7620 York Road, Zip 21204; tel. 410/337–1000; John S. Prout, President and Chief Executive Officer **A**1 9 10 **F**2 4 5 7 8 10 11 12 13 14 15 16 17 19 21 22 23 25 26 28 29 30 31 32 33 34 35 37 38 39 40 41 42 43 44 45 46 49 51 52 53 55 56 57 60 63 65 67 71 72 73 74 **P**2 5 7 8 **S**5325 Franciscan Health System	21	10	460	19827	276	56533	1832	134096	61766	1690

Hospital, Address, Telephone, Administrator, Approval, Facility, and Physician Codes, Health Care System	Classi- fication Codes		Utilization Data					Expense (thousands) of dollars		
★ American Hospital Association (AHA) membership ☐ Joint Commission on Accreditation of Healthcare Organizations (JCAHO) accreditation + American Osteopathic Hospital Association (AOHA) membership ○ American Osteopathic Association (AOA) accreditation △ Commission on Accreditation of Rehabilitation Facilities (CARF) accreditation Control codes 61, 63, 64, 71, 72 and 73 indicate hospitals listed by AOHA, but not registered by AHA. For definition of numerical codes, see page A6	Control	Service	Beds	Admissions	Census	Outpatient Visits	Births	Total	Payroll	Personnel
WESTMINSTER—Carroll County ★ CARROLL COUNTY GENERAL HOSPITAL, Memorial Avenue, Zip 21157–5799; tel. 410/848–3000; John M. Sernulka, Executive Vice President **A**1 9 10 **F**4 8 10 12 15 16 17 19 21 22 23 30 33 34 35 37 39 40 41 42 44 45 46 49 50 52 53 54 55 56 57 63 65 71 73 **P**5 7	23	10	158	8412	123	75885	736	49081	22877	722

Hospitals, U.S. / MASSACHUSETTS

MASSACHUSETTS

Resident population 6,012 (in thousands)
Resident population in metro areas 96.2%
Birth rate per 1,000 population 14.7
65 years and over 14.0%
Percent of persons without health insurance 10.1%

Hospital, Address, Telephone, Administrator, Approval, Facility, and Physician Codes, Health Care System	Classification Codes		Utilization Data					Expense (thousands) of dollars		
★ American Hospital Association (AHA) membership □ Joint Commission on Accreditation of Healthcare Organizations (JCAHO) accreditation + American Osteopathic Hospital Association (AOHA) membership ○ American Osteopathic Association (AOA) accreditation △ Commission on Accreditation of Rehabilitation Facilities (CARF) accreditation Control codes 61, 63, 64, 71, 72 and 73 indicate hospitals listed by AOHA, but not registered by AHA. For definition of numerical codes, see page A6	Control	Service	Beds	Admissions	Census	Outpatient Visits	Births	Total	Payroll	Personnel
AMHERST—Hampshire County										
UNIVERSITY HEALTH SERVICES, University of Massachusetts, Zip 01003–4310; tel. 413/549–2671; Bernette A. Melby, Executive Director (Nonreporting) **A**3 9 10	12	11	22	—	—	—	—	—	—	—
ANDOVER—Essex County										
ISHAM HEALTH CENTER, (Formerly Isham Infirmary) (Adolescent Medicine) Phillips Academy, Zip 01810; tel. 508/749–4455; Robb Nochimow, Administrator **F**2 4 5 8 9 10 11 13 14 17 18 19 20 21 22 23 24 25 27 28 29 30 31 34 35 37 38 39 41 42 43 45 46 47 48 50 51 52 53 54 55 56 58 59 60 61 63 64 66 67 68 69 70 71 72 73 74 **P**6	23	59	20	289	1	10385	0	—	—	26
ARLINGTON—Middlesex County										
✱ MEDICAL CENTER AT SYMMES, (Formerly Symmes Hospital) Hospital Road, Zip 02174–2199; tel. 617/646–1500; John F. Corridan III, Chief Executive Officer (Data for 306 days) **A**1 9 10 **F**8 11 12 15 16 17 19 21 22 26 28 30 33 34 35 36 37 39 42 44 46 49 56 60 65 67 71 72 73 **P**4 5	23	10	88	2405	57	12663	0	14436	10271	283
ASHBURNHAM—Worcester County										
NAUKEAG HOSPITAL, 216 Lake Road, Zip 01430; tel. 617/827–5115; Geraldine A. McQuoid, Director (Nonreporting) **A**9	33	82	26	—	—	—	—	—	—	—
ATHOL—Worcester County										
✱ ATHOL MEMORIAL HOSPITAL, 2033 Main Street, Zip 01331–3598; tel. 508/249–3511; William DiFederico, President (Nonreporting) **A**1 9 10	23	10	48	—	—	—	—	—	—	—
ATTLEBORO—Bristol County										
✱ STURDY MEMORIAL HOSPITAL, 211 Park Street, Zip 02703, Mailing Address: P.O. Box 2963, Zip 02703; tel. 508/222–5200; Linda Shyavitz, President and Chief Executive Officer **A**1 2 9 10 **F**7 8 10 12 13 15 16 17 18 19 20 21 22 23 25 26 28 29 30 31 34 35 37 38 39 40 41 42 44 46 49 50 51 61 63 65 67 68 71 72 73 74 **P**3 6	23	10	178	5974	79	122376	906	46603	25120	733
AYER—Middlesex County										
✱ DEACONESS–NASHOBA HOSPITAL, 200 Groton Road, Zip 01432; tel. 508/772–0200; Jeffrey R. Kelly, President and Chief Executive Officer **A**1 9 10 **F**2 8 9 11 12 13 14 15 16 17 18 19 20 21 22 26 28 29 30 32 33 35 37 38 41 42 44 45 47 48 49 52 56 58 63 64 65 67 70 71 73 74 **P**5 6 8	23	10	59	2217	32	66008	0	22682	11565	291
BEDFORD—Middlesex County										
✱ EDITH NOURSE ROGERS MEMORIAL VETERANS HOSPITAL, 200 Springs Road, Zip 01730; tel. 617/275–7500; William A. Conte, Director (Total facility includes 265 beds in nursing home–type unit) **A**1 3 5 9 **F**1 2 3 4 5 8 10 11 19 20 21 22 23 26 27 28 29 30 31 32 33 34 35 37 39 41 42 43 44 45 46 49 51 52 54 55 57 58 59 60 64 65 67 69 71 73 74 **P**1 **S**9295 Department of Veterans Affairs	45	22	725	2713	671	142213	0	82887	47958	1188
BELMONT—Middlesex County										
✱ MCLEAN HOSPITAL, 115 Mill Street, Zip 02178–9106; tel. 617/855–2000; Steven M. Mirin M.D., Chief Executive Officer and Psychiatrist in Chief **A**1 3 5 9 10 **F**2 7 8 10 11 12 17 19 22 26 29 30 31 34 35 37 38 40 41 42 43 44 47 48 49 50 51 52 53 54 55 56 57 58 59 60 61 63 64 66 69 70 71 74 **P**5 6 **S**1785 Massachusetts General Hospital Corporation	23	22	205	4397	178	—	0	87339	42940	1131
BEVERLY—Essex County										
✱ BEVERLY HOSPITAL, 85 Herrick Street, Zip 01915–1777; tel. 508/922–3000; Robert R. Fanning Jr., President (Total facility includes 60 beds in nursing home–type unit) **A**1 2 3 9 10 **F**1 2 3 4 5 6 8 10 11 12 13 14 15 16 17 18 19 20 21 22 23 24 26 27 28 29 30 31 32 33 34 35 37 39 40 41 42 43 44 45 46 48 49 51 52 53 54 55 56 57 58 59 60 61 64 65 66 67 68 71 73 74 **P**1 2 3 4 5 6	23	10	257	12657	170	266559	2608	100107	49007	1367
BOSTON—Suffolk County										
□ ARBOUR HOSPITAL, 49 Robinwood Avenue, Zip 02130, Mailing Address: P.O. Box 9, Zip 02130; tel. 617/522–4400; Roy A. Ettlinger, Managing Director (Nonreporting) **A**1 10 **S**9555 Universal Health Services, Inc.	33	22	118	—	—	—	—	—	—	—
✱ BETH ISRAEL HOSPITAL, 330 Brookline Avenue, Zip 02215; tel. 617/667–2000; Mitchell T. Rabkin M.D., President **A**1 2 3 5 8 9 10 **F**4 5 7 8 10 11 12 17 18 19 20 21 22 23 24 25 26 27 28 29 30 31 32 34 35 37 38 39 40 41 42 43 44 45 48 49 51 52 53 54 55 57 58 60 61 63 65 66 67 69 71 72 73 74 **P**3 4 5 6 7 8	23	10	447	24085	341	219895	5412	—	—	4326
□ BOSTON CITY HOSPITAL, 818 Harrison Avenue, Zip 02118; tel. 617/534–5000; Lawrence Dwyer, Commissioner **A**1 2 3 5 9 10 **F**3 7 8 11 12 13 14 15 16 17 18 19 20 21 22 24 25 26 27 28 29 30 31 32 34 35 37 38 39 40 42 44 45 46 47 49 50 51 53 54 56 57 58 60 61 65 66 67 68 70 71 72 73 74 **P**1 3 5 **S**6995 Department of Health and Hospitals	14	10	282	14012	212	220359	1458	182871	80820	2613
✱ BOSTON SPECIALTY AND REHABILITATION HOSPITAL, 249 River Street, Zip 02126; tel. 617/534–2000; Dorothy L. Turner-Small R.N., Administrator **A**1 9 10 **F**1 4 5 7 8 12 14 16 17 19 20 21 22 26 27 28 29 30 31 32 34 35 41 42 46 49 51 54 56 58 60 61 65 68 71 72 73 74 **S**6995 Department of Health and Hospitals	14	48	87	578	72	0	0	—	—	229
✱ BOSTON UNIVERSITY MEDICAL CENTER–UNIVERSITY HOSPITAL, 88 East Newton Street, Zip 02118–2393; tel. 617/638–8000; Elaine S. Ullian, President and Chief Executive Officer **A**1 2 3 5 8 9 10 **F**4 5 8 10 11 12 14 15 16 17 19 22 23 25 26 29 30 31 34 35 37 39 41 42 43 44 45 46 48 49 51 52 56 57 58 59 60 61 63 65 66 69 70 71 72 73 74 **P**6	23	10	311	9649	192	109218	0	178072	80673	1796

A190 Hospitals © 1995 AHA Guide

Hospitals, U.S. / MASSACHUSETTS

Hospital, Address, Telephone, Administrator, Approval, Facility, and Physician Codes, Health Care System	Classification Codes		Utilization Data					Expense (thousands) of dollars		
	Control	Service	Beds	Admissions	Census	Outpatient Visits	Births	Total	Payroll	Personnel

- ★ American Hospital Association (AHA) membership
- ☐ Joint Commission on Accreditation of Healthcare Organizations (JCAHO) accreditation
- + American Osteopathic Hospital Association (AOHA) membership
- ○ American Osteopathic Association (AOA) accreditation
- △ Commission on Accreditation of Rehabilitation Facilities (CARF) accreditation

Control codes 61, 63, 64, 71, 72 and 73 indicate hospitals listed by AOHA, but not registered by AHA. For definition of numerical codes, see page A6.

Hospital	Control	Service	Beds	Admissions	Census	Outpatient Visits	Births	Total	Payroll	Personnel
★ BRIGHAM AND WOMEN'S HOSPITAL, 75 Francis Street, Zip 02115–6195; tel. 617/732–5500; Jeffrey Otten, Chief Executive Officer **A**1 2 3 5 8 10 **F**3 4 5 7 8 9 10 11 12 14 15 16 17 19 20 21 22 23 24 25 26 29 30 31 34 35 37 38 39 40 41 42 43 44 45 46 47 48 49 51 52 53 54 55 56 57 58 59 60 61 65 66 67 68 69 70 71 73 74 **P**3 6	23	10	712	36488	549	604982	8692	609450	236320	6907
★ CARNEY HOSPITAL, 2100 Dorchester Avenue, Zip 02124–5666; tel. 617/296–4000; Matthias D. Maguire, President **A**1 2 3 5 9 10 **F**3 8 10 11 13 14 15 16 17 18 19 21 22 24 25 26 27 28 29 30 31 34 35 37 39 41 42 44 46 49 51 52 54 55 56 58 59 65 67 68 71 72 73 **P**4 5 6 **S**1855 Daughters of Charity National Health System	21	10	221	10297	182	116275	0	98043	51455	1333
★ CHILDREN'S HOSPITAL, 300 Longwood Avenue, Zip 02115; tel. 617/355–6000; David Stephen Weiner, President **A**1 3 5 8 9 10 **F**10 11 12 13 15 16 17 19 20 21 22 25 29 30 31 34 35 38 39 41 42 43 44 45 46 47 49 51 52 53 54 55 56 60 61 63 65 66 67 68 69 70 71 72 73 **P**7	23	50	325	16711	254	260443	0	274975	134323	4098
★ DANA–FARBER CANCER INSTITUTE, 44 Binney Street, Zip 02115–6084; tel. 617/632–3000; Terry C. Bradford, Chief Operating Officer (Nonreporting) **A**1 3 10	23	49	57	—	—	—	—	—	—	—
★ DEACONESS HOSPITAL, (Formerly New England Deaconess Hospital) One Deaconess Road, Zip 02215; tel. 617/632–7000; Albert B. Washko, President (Total facility includes 23 beds in nursing home–type unit) **A**1 2 3 5 8 9 10 **F**1 2 3 4 5 7 8 10 11 15 16 17 18 19 21 22 24 25 26 28 29 30 31 32 33 34 35 37 39 40 41 42 43 44 45 46 49 51 52 53 54 55 56 57 58 59 60 61 63 64 65 66 67 69 71 72 73 74 **P**1 5 6	23	10	314	11835	288	149846	0	232047	94195	2845
★ FAULKNER HOSPITAL, Mailing Address: 1153 Centre Sreet, Zip 02130; tel. 617/983–7000; David J. Trull, President and Chief Executive Officer **A**1 2 3 5 8 9 10 **F**1 2 3 4 8 10 11 12 15 16 17 19 21 22 25 30 31 32 33 34 35 37 39 41 42 44 45 46 49 51 52 54 55 56 57 58 59 65 67 71 72 73 **P**5	23	10	183	6566	116	164659	0	65276	34008	856
☐ △ FRANCISCAN CHILDREN'S HOSPITAL AND REHABILITATION CENTER, (Children's General Medical, Surgical and Rehabilitation) Mailing Address: 30 Warren Street, Zip 02135–3680; tel. 617/254–3800; Paul J. Dellarocco, President and Chief Executive Officer (Nonreporting) **A**1 5 7 9 10	21	59	100	—	—	—	—	—	—	—
★ HEBREW REHABILITATION CENTER FOR AGED, Mailing Address: 1200 Centre Street, Zip 02131–1097; tel. 617/325–8000; Maurice May, President **A**10 **F**1 6 15 16 17 20 24 26 27 28 33 39 46 51 54 57 59 62 65 67 73 **P**6	23	48	725	178	707	0	0	—	—	735
★ JEWISH MEMORIAL HOSPITAL AND REHABILITATION CENTER, (Rehabilitation and Chronic Disease) 59 Townsend Street, Zip 02119–9918; tel. 617/442–8760; Stanley M. Fertel, President **A**1 3 5 9 10 **F**12 15 16 17 19 20 21 22 26 30 31 32 34 35 39 45 48 49 54 57 65 67 71 73 **P**6 8	23	49	207	561	121	1100	0	27795	13983	393
★ LEMUEL SHATTUCK HOSPITAL, 170 Morton Street, Jamaica Plain, Zip 02130–3787; tel. 617/522–8110; Robert Wakefield Jr., Executive Director (Nonreporting) **A**1 3 5 9 10 **S**0013 Massachusetts Department of Mental Health	12	10	230	—	—	—	—	—	—	—
☐ MASSACHUSETTS EYE AND EAR INFIRMARY, 243 Charles Street, Zip 02114–3096; tel. 617/523–7900; F. Curtis Smith, President **A**1 3 5 9 10 **F**15 16 19 22 35 44 46 65 67 70 71 73 **P**8	23	45	65	2849	26	167944	0	77055	26409	1294
★ MASSACHUSETTS GENERAL HOSPITAL, 32 Fruit Street, Zip 02114; tel. 617/726–2000; Richard Crater, Chief Executive Officer **A**1 2 3 5 8 9 10 **F**3 4 5 8 9 10 11 12 14 17 18 19 20 21 22 23 25 26 27 28 30 31 34 35 37 38 39 41 42 43 44 46 47 49 50 51 52 53 54 55 56 57 58 59 60 61 63 65 66 67 68 69 70 71 72 73 74 **P**1 3 4 5 6 7 8 **S**1785 Massachusetts General Hospital Corporation	23	10	899	34992	704	616346	0	713321	262990	7075
★ MASSACHUSETTS MENTAL HEALTH CENTER, 74 Fenwood Road, Zip 02115; tel. 617/734–1300; Catherine Howard, Chief Executive Officer (Nonreporting) **A**3 5 9 **S**0013 Massachusetts Department of Mental Health	12	22	27	—	—	—	—	—	—	—
★ NEW ENGLAND BAPTIST HOSPITAL, 125 Parker Hill Avenue, Zip 02120–3297; tel. 617/738–5800; Raymond C. McAfoose, President and Chief Executive Officer (Total facility includes 20 beds in nursing home–type unit) **A**1 3 5 6 10 **F**5 8 10 15 16 19 20 21 26 35 37 39 41 42 44 45 48 49 54 64 65 66 71 73 **P**5 8	23	10	173	6469	122	69302	0	87854	34922	911
NEW ENGLAND DEACONESS HOSPITAL See Deaconess Hospital										
★ NEW ENGLAND MEDICAL CENTER, 750 Washington Street, Zip 02111–1845; tel. 617/636–5000; Jerome H. Grossman M.D., Chairman and Chief Executive Officer **A**1 2 3 5 8 9 10 **F**1 3 4 5 7 8 9 10 11 12 13 15 16 17 18 19 20 21 22 25 26 27 28 29 30 31 34 35 37 38 39 40 41 42 43 44 45 46 47 49 51 52 54 55 56 57 58 59 60 61 63 65 66 67 68 69 70 71 73 74 **P**5 7	23	10	453	18878	368	406012	1543	362139	148259	4604
★ SHRINERS HOSPITAL FOR CRIPPLED CHILDREN, BURNS INSTITUTE BOSTON UNIT, 51 Blossom Street, Zip 02114–2699; tel. 617/722–3000; Robert F. Bories, Administrator **A**1 5 **F**16 19 21 22 35 45 49 53 65 67 71 73 **S**4125 Shriners Hospitals for Crippled Children	23	59	30	671	20	2968	0	—	—	229
★ △ SPAULDING REHABILITATION HOSPITAL, 125 Nashua Street, Zip 02114; tel. 617/720–6400; Manuel J. Lipson M.D., Chief Executive Officer **A**1 3 7 9 10 **F**2 3 12 17 19 20 21 22 25 26 27 28 29 30 32 35 39 41 45 46 48 49 53 54 55 56 57 58 60 64 65 66 71 73 **S**1785 Massachusetts General Hospital Corporation	23	46	284	3753	261	58742	0	60367	37210	1198
★ ST. ELIZABETH'S MEDICAL CENTER OF BOSTON, 736 Cambridge Street, Zip 02135; tel. 617/789–3000; Michael F. Collins M.D., President **A**1 2 3 5 6 8 9 10 **F**1 2 3 4 7 8 10 11 12 13 14 15 16 17 19 21 22 23 25 26 27 28 30 31 32 33 34 35 37 38 39 40 41 42 43 44 46 49 51 52 53 54 55 57 58 59 60 65 66 67 71 73 74 **P**3 5 7 **S**1125 Caritas Christi Health Care System	21	10	415	13955	283	159048	1825	195987	84228	2428

© 1995 AHA Guide

Hospitals, U.S. / MASSACHUSETTS

	Hospital, Address, Telephone, Administrator, Approval, Facility, and Physician Codes, Health Care System	Classification Codes		Utilization Data					Expense (thousands) of dollars		
		Control	Service	Beds	Admissions	Census	Outpatient Visits	Births	Total	Payroll	Personnel

Approval codes:
- ★ American Hospital Association (AHA) membership
- □ Joint Commission on Accreditation of Healthcare Organizations (JCAHO) accreditation
- + American Osteopathic Hospital Association (AOHA) membership
- ○ American Osteopathic Association (AOA) accreditation
- △ Commission on Accreditation of Rehabilitation Facilities (CARF) accreditation

Control codes 61, 63, 64, 71, 72 and 73 indicate hospitals listed by AOHA, but not registered by AHA. For definition of numerical codes, see page A6

	Hospital	Control	Service	Beds	Admissions	Census	Outpatient Visits	Births	Total	Payroll	Personnel
★	ST. JOHN OF GOD HOSPITAL, Mailing Address: 296 Allston Street, Brighton, Zip 02146; tel. 617/277–5750; William K. Brinkert, President **A**1 9 10 **F**1 2 3 4 7 8 10 11 17 19 22 26 30 31 33 34 35 37 38 40 41 42 43 44 48 49 50 51 52 54 56 57 58 60 61 65 66 71 73 74 **P**8 **S**1125 Caritas Christi Health Care System	21	48	50	285	48	0	0	8905	4850	134
★	VETERANS AFFAIRS MEDICAL CENTER, Mailing Address: 150 South Huntington Avenue, Jamaica Plain Station, Zip 02130–4820; tel. 617/232–9500; Smith Jenkins Jr., Director **A**1 2 3 5 8 **F**1 2 3 5 8 10 11 19 20 21 22 24 25 26 27 31 32 33 34 35 37 39 41 42 44 45 46 48 49 51 52 56 58 60 65 69 71 72 73 74 **S**9295 Department of Veterans Affairs	45	10	448	9156	315	350266	0	181026	109412	2212

BRAINTREE—Norfolk County

	Hospital	Control	Service	Beds	Admissions	Census	Outpatient Visits	Births	Total	Payroll	Personnel
★ △	BRAINTREE HOSPITAL REHABILITATION NETWORK, 250 Pond Street, Zip 02185; tel. 617/848–5353; Ernest J. Broadbent, President and Chief Executive Officer **A**1 3 7 9 10 **F**5 12 13 14 15 16 17 20 24 25 26 27 28 29 30 31 32 33 34 39 41 42 44 45 46 48 49 54 65 66 67 71 73 74 **P**6 **S**1715 Continental Medical Systems, Inc.	33	46	166	2726	156	197081	0	62669	39183	1281
★	MASSACHUSETTS RESPIRATORY HOSPITAL, 2001 Washington Street, Zip 02184; tel. 617/848–2600; Edward F. Kittredge, Chief Executive Officer **A**1 9 10 **F**28 30 34 36 41 45 49 65 67 73 **P**6 **S**0002 Quorum Health Group/Quorum Health Resources	13	33	98	644	79	6513	0	15545	—	209

BRIDGEWATER—Plymouth County

	Hospital	Control	Service	Beds	Admissions	Census	Outpatient Visits	Births	Total	Payroll	Personnel
	BRIDGEWATER STATE HOSPITAL, Administration Road, Zip 02324; tel. 617/697–8161; Kenneth W. Nelson, Superintendent **F**2 11 20 37 52	12	22	350	794	142	0	0	—	—	345

BROCKTON—Plymouth County

	Hospital	Control	Service	Beds	Admissions	Census	Outpatient Visits	Births	Total	Payroll	Personnel
★	BROCKTON HOSPITAL, 680 Centre Street, Zip 02402–3395; tel. 508/941–7000; Norman B. Goodman, President and Chief Executive Officer **A**1 2 3 5 6 9 10 **F**1 3 4 6 7 8 10 11 12 13 15 16 17 19 21 22 26 29 30 31 32 33 34 35 37 39 40 41 42 43 44 45 46 49 51 52 54 55 56 57 58 59 60 61 63 65 67 68 71 72 73 74 **P**6 8	23	10	260	10720	171	107701	1265	89262	45103	1157
★	BROCKTON–WEST ROXBURY VETERANS AFFAIRS MEDICAL CENTER, 940 Belmont Street, Zip 02401; tel. 508/583–4500; Michael E. Lawson, Director (Total facility includes 149 beds in nursing home–type unit) **A**1 3 5 8 **F**2 3 10 19 20 21 22 25 26 27 31 37 42 43 44 46 48 49 51 52 54 55 56 58 59 64 65 67 70 71 73 74 **S**9295 Department of Veterans Affairs	45	10	765	7340	634	249103	0	169603	98686	2378
	GOOD SAMARITAN MEDICAL CENTER–CUSHING CAMPUS See Good Samaritan Medical Center, Stoughton										

BROOKLINE—Norfolk County

	Hospital	Control	Service	Beds	Admissions	Census	Outpatient Visits	Births	Total	Payroll	Personnel
□	BOURNEWOOD HOSPITAL, 300 South Street, Zip 02167–3694; tel. 617/469–0300; Nasir A. Khan M.D., Director (Nonreporting) **A**1 9 10	33	22	76	—	—	—	—	—	—	—
□	H.R.I. HOSPITAL, 227 Babcock Street, Zip 02146; tel. 617/731–3200; Roy A. Ettlinger, Managing Director **A**1 9 10 **F**52 57 58 59 **P**1 **S**9555 Universal Health Services, Inc.	33	22	68	1025	38	14280	0	10011	4433	117

BURLINGTON—Middlesex County

	Hospital	Control	Service	Beds	Admissions	Census	Outpatient Visits	Births	Total	Payroll	Personnel
★	LAHEY HITCHCOCK CLINIC, (Formerly Lahey Clinic) 41 Mall Road, Zip 01805–0001; tel. 617/273–8546; Bruce W. Steinhauer, Chief Executive Officer **A**1 2 3 5 10 **F**4 8 10 11 12 13 14 15 16 17 18 19 21 22 23 26 28 30 31 32 33 34 35 36 37 39 41 42 43 44 45 46 48 49 51 52 53 54 55 56 57 58 59 60 61 63 65 66 67 69 71 73 74 **P**6	23	10	272	12393	220	554235	0	197242	85041	3104

CAMBRIDGE—Middlesex County

	Hospital	Control	Service	Beds	Admissions	Census	Outpatient Visits	Births	Total	Payroll	Personnel
★	CAMBRIDGE HOSPITAL, 1493 Cambridge Street, Zip 02139–1099; tel. 617/498–1000; John G. O'Brien, Chief Executive Officer **A**1 3 5 9 10 **F**1 2 3 4 7 8 10 12 13 14 15 16 17 18 19 20 21 22 25 26 27 28 29 30 31 32 33 34 35 36 37 39 40 41 42 44 45 46 49 51 52 53 54 55 56 57 58 59 61 64 65 66 67 68 71 73 74 **P**6 8	14	10	170	6381	117	231179	778	77532	38366	1085
□	M. I. T. MEDICAL DEPARTMENT, 77 Massachusetts Avenue, Zip 02139; tel. 617/253–4596; Arnold N. Weinberg M.D., Director (Nonreporting) **A**1	23	11	18	—	—	—	—	—	—	—
★	MOUNT AUBURN HOSPITAL, 330 Mount Auburn Street, Zip 02238; tel. 617/492–3500; Francis P. Lynch, President and Chief Executive Officer **A**1 2 3 5 8 9 10 **F**3 4 7 8 10 11 12 14 15 16 17 19 21 22 26 28 29 30 31 32 34 35 37 39 40 41 42 43 44 45 46 49 51 52 54 55 56 57 58 59 60 65 67 70 71 72 73 74 **P**1 3 5 6	23	10	279	11674	173	189884	1742	117434	59999	1548
★	STILLMAN INFIRMARY, HARVARD UNIVERSITY HEALTH SERVICES, 75 Mount Auburn Street, Zip 02138; tel. 617/495–2010; David S. Rosenthal M.D., Director **A**1 9 10 **F**12 13 14 16 17 18 20 25 28 29 30 34 44 45 46 49 51 56 58 65 67 68 71 72 **P**6	23	11	18	702	6	170081	0	25602	12786	231
★ △	YOUVILLE HOSPITAL AND REHABILITATION CENTER, (Rehabilitation and Chronic Disease) 1575 Cambridge Street, Zip 02138–4398; tel. 617/876–4344; T. Richard Quigley, President and Chief Executive Officer (Total facility includes 80 beds in nursing home–type unit) **A**1 7 10 **F**5 12 15 16 17 19 20 26 28 30 31 33 34 35 42 45 48 49 51 54 57 58 64 65 67 71 73 **P**6 **S**5885 Covenant Health Systems, Inc.	21	49	305	1804	207	7815	0	47982	25864	642

CANTON—Norfolk County

	Hospital	Control	Service	Beds	Admissions	Census	Outpatient Visits	Births	Total	Payroll	Personnel
★	MASSACHUSETTS HOSPITAL SCHOOL, 3 Randolph Street, Zip 02021–2397; tel. 617/828–2440; John H. Britt, Chief Executive Officer **A**1 5 10 **F**5 6 12 13 14 15 16 19 20 21 24 27 30 34 37 39 41 44 47 48 49 50 51 53 54 58 61 63 64 65 67 68 71 73 **S**0013 Massachusetts Department of Mental Health	12	56	143	79	61	2375	0	—	—	233

Hospitals, U.S. / MASSACHUSETTS

Hospital, Address, Telephone, Administrator, Approval, Facility, and Physician Codes, Health Care System	Classification Codes		Utilization Data					Expense (thousands) of dollars		
★ American Hospital Association (AHA) membership ☐ Joint Commission on Accreditation of Healthcare Organizations (JCAHO) accreditation + American Osteopathic Hospital Association (AOHA) membership ○ American Osteopathic Association (AOA) accreditation △ Commission on Accreditation of Rehabilitation Facilities (CARF) accreditation Control codes 61, 63, 64, 71, 72 and 73 indicate hospitals listed by AOHA, but not registered by AHA. For definition of numerical codes, see page A6	Control	Service	Beds	Admissions	Census	Outpatient Visits	Births	Total	Payroll	Personnel
CHELSEA—Suffolk County ★ LAWRENCE F. QUIGLEY MEMORIAL HOSPITAL, (General Medical, Surgical and Geriatric) 91 Crest Avenue, Zip 02150–2199; tel. 617/884–5660; William D. Thompson, Chief Executive Officer (Nonreporting) **A**1 10	12	49	159	—	—	—	—	—	—	—
CLINTON—Worcester County ☐ CLINTON HOSPITAL, 201 Highland Street, Zip 01510; tel. 508/368–3000; Steven E. Levitsky, Chief Executive Officer **A**1 9 10 **F**2 8 14 15 16 19 22 26 31 32 33 41 42 44 46 48 49 52 54 55 57 60 61 65 71 73 **P**5	23	10	49	1954	40	58205	0	10570	5386	181
CONCORD—Middlesex County ★ EMERSON HOSPITAL, 133 Old Road to Nine Acre Corner, Zip 01742–9120; tel. 508/369–1400; Geoffrey F. Cole, President and Chief Executive Officer **A**1 2 5 9 10 **F**3 7 8 11 13 15 16 17 19 21 22 28 29 30 31 32 33 34 35 36 37 39 40 42 44 45 46 49 52 53 54 55 56 57 58 59 61 63 65 66 67 68 69 71 73 **P**5 6 8	23	10	170	8349	105	154204	1610	65070	33451	886
EVERETT—Middlesex County ★ WHIDDEN MEMORIAL HOSPITAL, 103 Garland Street, Zip 02149–5095; tel. 617/389–6270; Ross T. France, Executive Vice President and Chief Executive Officer (Nonreporting) **A**1 9 10	23	10	121	—	—	—	—	—	—	—
FALL RIVER—Bristol County ★ △ CHARLTON MEMORIAL HOSPITAL, 363 Highland Avenue, Zip 02720–3794; tel. 508/679–3131; Ronald B. Goodspeed M.D., M.P.H., President **A**1 2 7 9 10 **F**3 7 8 10 11 12 15 16 17 19 21 22 23 24 26 28 29 30 32 33 34 35 37 39 40 41 42 44 45 46 48 49 50 54 56 60 63 64 65 67 71 72 73	23	10	344	13825	280	139289	1759	110494	50301	1302
★ SAINT ANNE'S HOSPITAL, 795 Middle Street, Zip 02721–1798; tel. 508/674–5741; Joseph W. Wilczek, Acting President **A**1 2 9 10 **F**3 8 15 16 17 19 21 22 28 30 31 34 35 37 41 42 44 46 48 49 53 54 56 58 59 60 63 65 67 71 73 **S**1125 Caritas Christi Health Care System	21	10	175	6111	104	—	0	46656	20961	709
FALMOUTH—Barnstable County ★ FALMOUTH HOSPITAL, 100 Ter Heun Drive, Zip 02540–2599; tel. 508/548–5300; Roy A. Hitchings Jr. FACHE, President **A**1 9 10 **F**1 7 8 10 14 15 16 17 19 21 22 25 26 27 28 29 30 31 32 34 35 37 40 41 42 44 46 49 64 65 66 67 71 73 74 **P**5 6 8	23	10	117	5459	77	31239	650	41786	20686	508
FITCHBURG—Worcester County HEALTH ALLIANCE–BURBANK HOSPITAL See Health Alliance Hospital–Leominster, Leominster										
FRAMINGHAM—Middlesex County FRAMINGHAM UNION HOSPITAL See Metrowest Medical Center										
☐ METROWEST MEDICAL CENTER, (Includes Framingham Union Hospital, 115 Lincoln Street, Framingham, Massachusetts, Zip 01701; tel. 508/383–1000; Leonard Morse Hospital, 67 Union Street, Natick, Massachusetts, Zip 01760; tel. 508/650–7000) 115 Lincoln Street, Zip 01701; tel. 508/383–1000; Lawrence Kaplan M.D., Administrator **A**1 2 3 5 6 9 10 **F**1 2 3 4 5 7 8 10 11 12 13 14 15 16 17 19 20 21 22 23 25 26 27 28 29 31 32 33 34 35 36 37 38 39 40 41 42 44 45 49 51 52 53 54 55 56 57 58 59 60 61 62 65 66 67 68 70 71 72 73 74 **P**1 3 4 6	23	10	469	18309	242	108829	2988	136202	63456	1658
GARDNER—Worcester County ☐ HEYWOOD HOSPITAL, 242 Green Street, Zip 01440; tel. 508/632–3420; Daniel P. Moen, President and Chief Executive Officer **A**1 5 9 10 **F**1 3 5 6 7 8 12 14 15 16 17 18 19 21 22 26 28 30 31 32 33 34 35 37 39 40 41 42 44 45 46 49 51 52 53 54 55 56 57 58 59 61 65 66 67 68 71 73 74 **P**1	23	10	126	4147	71	109242	354	28820	14638	445
GEORGETOWN—Essex County BALDPATE HOSPITAL, Baldpate Road, Zip 01833; tel. 617/352–2131; Lucille M. Batal, Administrator (Nonreporting) **A**9 10	33	22	59	—	—	—	—	—	—	—
GLOUCESTER—Essex County ★ ADDISON GILBERT HOSPITAL, 298 Washington Street, Zip 01930–4887; tel. 508/283–4000; Robert L. Shapler, Chief Executive Officer **A**1 2 9 10 **F**3 7 8 12 14 15 16 17 18 19 21 22 26 28 29 30 31 32 33 37 39 40 41 42 44 45 46 49 52 54 56 57 58 59 61 63 64 65 66 67 71 73 74 **P**1 5 6	23	10	97	3622	53	37703	211	28220	12477	391
GREAT BARRINGTON—Berkshire County ★ FAIRVIEW HOSPITAL, 29 Lewis Avenue, Zip 01230–1713; tel. 413/528–0790; Claire L. Bowen, President **A**1 9 10 **F**7 10 12 15 16 17 19 20 21 22 23 25 26 28 29 30 31 32 33 34 35 37 39 40 41 42 44 49 54 55 61 65 66 67 71 73 74 **S**2435 Berkshire Health Systems, Inc.	23	10	40	1649	23	12672	162	15773	6569	189
GREENFIELD—Franklin County ★ FRANKLIN MEDICAL CENTER, 164 High Street, Zip 01301; tel. 413/773–0211; Harlan J. Smith, President **A**1 2 9 10 **F**1 2 3 7 8 12 13 15 16 17 18 19 21 22 26 27 29 30 31 32 33 34 35 37 39 40 41 42 44 49 51 52 53 54 55 56 57 58 59 63 65 67 68 71 73 **P**3 5 6 7 8 **S**1095 Baystate Health Systems, Inc.	23	10	115	4898	70	136279	642	53954	26676	717
HAVERHILL—Essex County ★ HALE HOSPITAL, 140 Lincoln Avenue, Zip 01830; tel. 508/374–2000; John J. Buckley, Chief Executive Officer and Administrator **A**1 9 10 **F**7 8 14 16 19 20 21 22 28 29 30 32 34 35 37 39 40 41 44 49 54 56 58 61 63 65 67 71 73 74 **S**0002 Quorum Health Group/Quorum Health Resources	14	10	153	5660	83	57821	675	37817	17895	513
★ △ WHITTIER REHABILITATION HOSPITAL, 76 Summer Street, Zip 01830; tel. 508/372–8000; Alfred Arcidi M.D., President **A**1 7 10 **F**1 12 15 25 27 32 34 41 48 49 54 57 65 66 73	33	46	122	866	56	10435	0	14310	8699	266

© 1995 AHA Guide

Hospitals, U.S. / MASSACHUSETTS

Hospital, Address, Telephone, Administrator, Approval, Facility, and Physician Codes, Health Care System	Classification Codes		Utilization Data					Expense (thousands) of dollars		
★ American Hospital Association (AHA) membership ☐ Joint Commission on Accreditation of Healthcare Organizations (JCAHO) accreditation + American Osteopathic Hospital Association (AOHA) membership ○ American Osteopathic Association (AOA) accreditation △ Commission on Accreditation of Rehabilitation Facilities (CARF) accreditation Control codes 61, 63, 64, 71, 72 and 73 indicate hospitals listed by AOHA, but not registered by AHA. For definition of numerical codes, see page A6	Control	Service	Beds	Admissions	Census	Outpatient Visits	Births	Total	Payroll	Personnel
HOLYOKE—Hampden County										
★ HOLYOKE HOSPITAL, 575 Beech Street, Zip 01040–2296; tel. 413/534–2500; Hank J. Porten, President (Nonreporting) **A**1 2 9 10	23	10	225	—	—	—	—	—	—	—
★ PROVIDENCE HOSPITAL, 1233 Main Street, Zip 01040–5381; tel. 413/536–5111; Vincent J. McCorkle, President and Chief Executive Officer **A**1 2 9 10 **F**1 2 3 4 5 7 8 10 11 12 15 16 17 18 19 21 22 25 27 28 29 30 31 34 35 37 39 40 41 42 44 45 46 48 49 52 53 54 55 56 57 58 63 64 65 66 67 68 71 73 74 **S**5285 Sisters of Providence Health System	21	10	202	7174	116	139378	1085	45507	18653	557
★ SOLDIERS' HOME IN HOLYOKE, 110 Cherry Street, Zip 01040; tel. 413/532–9475; Rudy Chmura, Superintendent (Total facility includes 309 beds in nursing home–type unit) **A**1 9 10 **F**20 22 41 49 58 64 65 73 **S**0013 Massachusetts Department of Mental Health	12	10	336	150	291	12481	0	—	—	306
HYANNIS—Barnstable County										
★ CAPE COD HOSPITAL, 27 Park Street, Zip 02601; tel. 508/771–1800; James F. Lyons, President **A**1 2 5 9 10 **F**3 4 7 8 10 11 12 13 14 15 16 17 19 21 22 23 26 27 28 30 31 34 35 37 39 40 41 42 44 45 46 49 51 52 53 54 55 56 57 58 59 60 63 64 65 66 67 68 71 72 73 74 **P**5 6	23	10	258	13124	188	168259	1101	110572	53027	1262
LAWRENCE—Essex County										
☐ LAWRENCE GENERAL HOSPITAL, 1 General Street, Zip 01842–0389, Mailing Address: P.O. Box 189, Zip 01842–0389; tel. 508/683–4000; Joseph S. McManus, President and Chief Executive Officer **A**1 2 3 9 10 **F**7 8 10 11 14 15 16 17 19 22 23 25 28 29 30 31 33 34 35 37 40 41 42 44 46 60 61 63 65 67 68 71 72 73 74 **P**1 4 5	23	10	243	10628	153	129912	1757	65272	33605	944
LEOMINSTER—Worcester County										
★ △ HEALTH ALLIANCE HOSPITAL–LEOMINSTER, (Includes Health Alliance–Burbank Hospital, 275 Nichols Road, Fitchburg, Massachusetts, Zip 01420–8209; tel. 508/343–5000) 60 Hospital Road, Zip 01453–8004; tel. 508/537–4811; Francis J. Cronin, President and Chief Executive Officer **A**1 3 5 7 9 10 **F**1 2 3 4 5 7 8 9 10 11 12 14 15 16 17 19 21 22 23 24 26 28 30 31 32 33 34 35 37 38 40 41 42 43 44 46 47 48 49 51 52 53 54 55 56 57 63 64 65 66 67 68 69 70 71 72 73 74 **P**3 5 7 8	23	10	260	9861	149	85006	1984	84557	39762	603
LOWELL—Middlesex County										
H. C. SOLOMON MENTAL HEALTH CENTER, 391 Varnum Avenue, Zip 01854–2199; tel. 508/454–8851; Linda D. Sutter, Superintendent **A**9 10 **F**12 22 34 52 53 54 55 56 57 58 65 **P**6	12	22	16	92	14	6025	0	—	—	110
★ LOWELL GENERAL HOSPITAL, 295 Varnum Avenue, Zip 01854–2195; tel. 508/937–6000; Robert A. Donovan, President **A**1 2 9 10 **F**1 3 7 8 10 12 14 15 16 17 19 21 22 23 25 26 28 29 30 31 34 35 37 39 40 41 42 44 45 46 49 52 54 55 56 57 58 59 60 65 67 70 71 73 **P**5 8	23	10	208	9535	133	124853	2264	62537	30499	939
★ SAINTS MEMORIAL MEDICAL CENTER, (Includes Saints Memorial Medical Center–East Campus, Lowell, Massachusetts; Saints Memorial Medical Center–West Campus, 220 Pawtucket Street, Lowell, Massachusetts, Zip 01854–3071; tel. 508/453–1761) Hospital Drive, Zip 01852, Mailing Address: P.O. Box 30, Zip 01853–0030; tel. 508/458–1411; Thom Clark, Chief Executive Officer (Total facility includes 23 beds in nursing home–type unit) **A**1 2 10 **F**3 7 8 10 15 16 17 19 21 22 23 29 30 31 33 35 37 39 40 41 42 44 45 49 51 53 54 55 56 58 59 63 64 65 67 68 71 72 73 74 **P**4 5 6	23	10	227	9056	161	130920	362	94690	40406	1012
LUDLOW—Hampden County										
☐ LUDLOW HOSPITAL, 14 Chestnut Place, Zip 01056; tel. 413/583–8361; (Nonreporting) **A**1 10	23	10	45	—	—	—	—	—	—	—
★ REHABILITATION HOSPITAL OF WESTERN NEW ENGLAND, 14 Chestnut Place, Zip 01056; tel. 413/589–7581; Barbara A. Rohan, President and Chief Executive Officer (Nonreporting) **A**1 10	33	46	40	—	—	—	—	—	—	—
LYNN—Essex County										
★ ATLANTICARE MEDICAL CENTER, (Includes AtlantiCare Hospital, 212 Boston Street, Lynn, Massachusetts, Zip 01904; tel. 617/598–5100) 500 Lynnfield Street, Zip 01904–1487; tel. 617/581–9200; Andrew J. Riddell, President and Chief Executive Officer **A**1 2 5 9 10 **F**2 3 8 11 12 14 15 16 17 18 19 22 24 25 26 27 28 29 30 31 34 35 37 39 41 42 44 45 46 49 51 52 53 54 55 56 57 58 59 60 65 66 67 70 71 72 73 74 **P**3 5	23	10	318	9757	216	96757	0	85199	45805	1077
MALDEN—Middlesex County										
★ MALDEN HOSPITAL, 100 Hospital Road, Zip 02148–3591; tel. 617/322–7560; Stanley W. Krygowski, President (Total facility includes 23 beds in nursing home–type unit) **A**1 3 5 9 10 **F**4 7 8 10 12 15 16 17 18 19 21 22 26 28 29 30 32 33 34 35 37 39 40 41 42 44 45 49 51 52 54 55 56 57 58 59 60 61 63 64 65 66 67 71 72 73 **P**5	23	10	195	6287	118	76209	1169	58827	26976	780
MARLBOROUGH—Middlesex County										
★ MARLBOROUGH HOSPITAL, 57 Union Street, Zip 01752; tel. 508/485–1121; Thomas E. Cummings, President and Chief Executive Officer **A**1 5 9 10 **F**2 3 8 12 13 15 16 17 19 22 26 29 30 31 34 37 39 41 42 44 46 49 52 53 54 55 56 57 58 59 63 65 67 71 73 74 **P**4 5	23	10	90	3711	54	85756	0	32835	16644	430
MEDFIELD—Norfolk County										
★ MEDFIELD STATE HOSPITAL, 45 Hospital Road, Zip 02052; tel. 508/359–7312; Barbara A. Leadholm, Area Director (Nonreporting) **A**1 9 10 **S**0013 Massachusetts Department of Mental Health	12	22	212	—	—	—	—	—	—	—

Hospitals, U.S. / MASSACHUSETTS

Hospital, Address, Telephone, Administrator, Approval, Facility, and Physician Codes, Health Care System	Classification Codes		Utilization Data					Expense (thousands) of dollars		
	Control	Service	Beds	Admissions	Census	Outpatient Visits	Births	Total	Payroll	Personnel

★ American Hospital Association (AHA) membership
□ Joint Commission on Accreditation of Healthcare Organizations (JCAHO) accreditation
+ American Osteopathic Hospital Association (AOHA) membership
○ American Osteopathic Association (AOA) accreditation
△ Commission on Accreditation of Rehabilitation Facilities (CARF) accreditation
Control codes 61, 63, 64, 71, 72 and 73 indicate hospitals listed by AOHA, but not registered by AHA. For definition of numerical codes, see page A6

MEDFORD—Middlesex County
★ LAWRENCE MEMORIAL HOSPITAL OF MEDFORD, 170 Governors Avenue, Zip 02155; tel. 617/396-9250; Charles F. Johnson, President (Total facility includes 19 beds in nursing home-type unit) **A**1 5 6 9 10 **F**14 15 16 19 21 22 25 26 27 29 30 32 34 35 36 37 39 42 44 49 52 54 57 58 59 60 63 64 65 66 67 71 73 74 **P**5 6 8

| | 23 | 10 | 169 | 5074 | 99 | 117276 | 0 | 42945 | 24432 | 776 |

MELROSE—Middlesex County
★ MELROSE–WAKEFIELD HOSPITAL ASSOCIATION, 585 Lebanon Street, Zip 02176; tel. 617/979-3000; Richard S. Quinlan, President (Total facility includes 21 beds in nursing home-type unit) **A**1 2 9 10 **F**3 4 7 8 10 12 13 14 15 16 17 19 20 21 22 26 27 28 29 30 32 33 34 35 36 37 39 40 41 42 44 45 46 49 51 52 53 54 55 56 57 58 59 60 61 63 64 65 66 67 68 71 73 74 **P**1 4 5 6 7

| | 23 | 10 | 225 | 9427 | 136 | 162025 | 1353 | 69540 | 32784 | 1072 |

METHUEN—Essex County
★ HOLY FAMILY HOSPITAL AND MEDICAL CENTER, 70 East Street, Zip 01844-4597; tel. 508/687-0151; William L. Lane, President **A**1 2 9 10 **F**3 7 8 10 11 12 13 14 15 16 17 18 19 20 21 22 23 25 26 28 29 30 31 32 33 34 35 37 39 40 41 42 44 45 46 49 51 52 53 54 55 56 57 58 59 60 63 65 66 67 68 71 72 73 74 **P**3 5 **S**1125 Caritas Christi Health Care System

| | 21 | 10 | 261 | 8239 | 156 | 75611 | 890 | 62919 | 31611 | 971 |

MIDDLEBOROUGH—Plymouth County
□ CRANBERRY SPECIALITY HOSPITAL OF PLYMOUTH COUNTY, 52 Oak Street, Zip 02346; tel. 508/947-1000; Edward B. Leary, President and Chief Executive Officer (Nonreporting) **A**1 9 10

| | 13 | 46 | 68 | — | — | — | — | — | — | — |

MILFORD—Worcester County
★ MILFORD–WHITINSVILLE REGIONAL HOSPITAL, (Includes Whitinsville Hospital, 18 Granite Street, Whitinsville, Massachusetts, Zip 01588; tel. 508/234-6311; Vitaliano Turci, Administrator) 14 Prospect Street, Zip 01757; tel. 508/473-1190; Francis M. Saba, President and Chief Executive Officer (Nonreporting) **A**1 5 9 10

| | 23 | 10 | 146 | — | — | — | — | — | — | — |

MILTON—Norfolk County
★ MILTON HOSPITAL, 92 Highland Street, Zip 02186-3807; tel. 617/696-4600; George A. Geary, President **A**1 9 10 **F**8 11 12 15 16 17 19 22 28 29 30 34 35 36 37 39 41 44 46 49 63 65 66 71 73 **P**6 8

| | 23 | 10 | 125 | 4717 | 83 | 36900 | 0 | 32669 | 15574 | 465 |

NANTUCKET—Nantucket County
★ NANTUCKET COTTAGE HOSPITAL, 57 Prospect Street, Zip 02554-2799; tel. 508/228-1200; Peter W. Brown, President **A**1 9 10 **F**1 3 7 8 14 16 22 30 31 32 33 36 37 39 40 42 44 65 67 71

| | 23 | 10 | 19 | 733 | 10 | 18588 | 91 | 8214 | 4534 | 107 |

NEEDHAM—Norfolk County
★ DEACONESS–GLOVER HOSPITAL CORPORATION, (Formerly Glover Memorial Hospital) 148 Chestnut Street, Zip 02192-2483; tel. 617/444-5600; John Dalton, President and Chief Executive Officer **A**1 2 9 10 **F**4 8 10 11 12 15 16 17 19 21 22 26 27 28 30 31 32 33 34 35 36 37 39 41 42 43 44 45 46 49 50 53 54 55 56 57 58 59 60 63 65 66 67 69 70 71 72 73 74 **P**5

| | 14 | 10 | 58 | 2357 | 39 | 46166 | 0 | 19558 | 9886 | 279 |

NEW BEDFORD—Bristol County
★ ST. LUKE'S HOSPITAL OF NEW BEDFORD, 101 Page Street, Zip 02740, Mailing Address: P.O. Box H-3000, Zip 02741-3000; tel. 508/997-1515; John B. Day, President and Chief Executive Officer **A**1 2 9 10 **F**4 7 8 10 11 12 15 16 19 20 21 22 26 28 30 31 32 33 34 35 37 40 42 44 46 49 51 52 54 55 56 57 58 60 63 64 65 67 71 73 **P**1

| | 23 | 10 | 390 | 16679 | 282 | 92093 | 1790 | 122070 | 66299 | 1782 |

NEWBURYPORT—Essex County
★ ANNA JAQUES HOSPITAL, 25 Highland Avenue, Zip 01950-3894; tel. 508/463-1000; Allan L. DesRosiers, President **A**1 9 10 **F**7 8 10 11 12 13 14 15 16 17 18 19 21 22 23 29 30 31 32 33 34 35 36 37 39 40 41 42 44 45 46 49 52 53 54 56 58 59 63 65 66 67 71 72 73 **P**5

| | 23 | 10 | 134 | 6578 | 99 | 121606 | 842 | 45449 | 22187 | 509 |

NEWTON—Middlesex County
★ NEWTON–WELLESLEY HOSPITAL, 2014 Washington Street, Zip 02162; tel. 617/243-6000; John P. Bihldorff, President and Chief Executive Officer **A**1 2 3 5 9 10 **F**1 2 3 5 7 8 10 12 15 16 17 19 21 22 25 26 27 28 30 31 32 34 35 36 37 39 40 41 42 44 46 48 49 52 54 55 56 57 58 59 61 63 65 67 71 73 74 **P**5 8

| | 23 | 10 | 291 | 13605 | 175 | 84442 | 4050 | 117941 | 61205 | 1465 |

NORFOLK—Norfolk County
★ SOUTHWOOD COMMUNITY HOSPITAL, 111 Dedham Street, Zip 02056; tel. 508/668-0385; (Nonreporting) **A**1 2 10 **S**3175 Neponset Valley Health System

| | 23 | 10 | 182 | — | — | — | — | — | — | — |

NORTH ADAMS—Berkshire County
★ NORTH ADAMS REGIONAL HOSPITAL, Hospital Avenue, Zip 01247; tel. 413/663-3701; Patrick Muldoon, President and Chief Executive Officer (Total facility includes 20 beds in nursing home-type unit) **A**1 2 9 10 **F**7 8 13 14 15 16 17 19 21 22 28 32 33 35 37 39 40 42 52 54 55 56 57 64 65 71 73

| | 23 | 10 | 136 | 4519 | 70 | 63623 | 403 | 31969 | 16028 | 435 |

NORTHAMPTON—Hampshire County
★ COOLEY DICKINSON HOSPITAL, 30 Locust Street, Zip 01061-5001, Mailing Address: P.O. Box 5001, Zip 01061-5001; tel. 413/582-2000; Craig N. Melin, President and Chief Executive Officer **A**1 2 9 10 **F**3 7 8 12 14 15 16 17 19 20 21 22 27 28 30 31 32 33 34 35 37 39 40 41 42 44 45 46 49 52 54 55 56 57 60 63 65 66 67 68 71 72 73 **P**3 5 6

| | 23 | 10 | 168 | 7083 | 94 | 137266 | 1043 | 53854 | 29186 | 770 |

★ VETERANS AFFAIRS MEDICAL CENTER, Route 9, Zip 01060-1288; tel. 413/584-4040; Gary J. Rossio, Chief Executive Officer (Total facility includes 50 beds in nursing home-type unit) **A**1 **F**1 2 3 6 8 10 12 14 16 17 18 19 20 24 25 26 27 28 29 30 31 32 33 34 37 39 41 44 46 49 51 52 54 55 57 58 60 64 65 67 71 72 73 74 **S**9295 Department of Veterans Affairs

| | 45 | 22 | 379 | 2591 | 284 | 126148 | 0 | — | — | 809 |

© 1995 AHA Guide

Hospitals, U.S. / MASSACHUSETTS

Hospital, Address, Telephone, Administrator, Approval, Facility, and Physician Codes, Health Care System	Classification Codes		Utilization Data					Expense (thousands) of dollars		
★ American Hospital Association (AHA) membership □ Joint Commission on Accreditation of Healthcare Organizations (JCAHO) accreditation + American Osteopathic Hospital Association (AOHA) membership ○ American Osteopathic Association (AOA) accreditation △ Commission on Accreditation of Rehabilitation Facilities (CARF) accreditation Control codes 61, 63, 64, 71, 72 and 73 indicate hospitals listed by AOHA, but not registered by AHA. For definition of numerical codes, see page A6	Control	Service	Beds	Admissions	Census	Outpatient Visits	Births	Total	Payroll	Personnel
NORWOOD—Norfolk County										
★ NORWOOD HOSPITAL, 800 Washington Street, Zip 02062; tel. 617/769-4000; Yolanda Landrau R.N., Ed.D., President **A**1 2 9 10 **F**1 2 3 7 8 10 11 19 21 24 25 26 27 28 29 30 31 32 33 34 35 36 37 39 40 41 42 44 45 46 48 49 51 52 53 54 55 56 57 58 59 60 61 65 66 67 68 71 72 73 74 **P**5 8 **S**3175 Neponset Valley Health System	23	10	201	8304	111	95601	1115	71129	31034	775
OAK BLUFFS—Dukes County										
★ MARTHA'S VINEYARD HOSPITAL, Linton Lane, Zip 02557, Mailing Address: P.O. Box 1477, Zip 02557; tel. 508/693-0410; Abbie Taylor, President and Chief Executive Officer (Total facility includes 81 beds in nursing home–type unit) **A**1 9 10 **F**1 3 6 7 8 12 13 14 15 16 17 18 19 20 22 26 27 28 29 30 31 32 33 34 36 37 39 40 41 42 44 46 49 53 54 55 56 57 58 61 64 65 67 71 73 74 **P**6	23	10	110	1154	53	25360	116	13634	6612	144
PALMER—Hampden County										
★ WING MEMORIAL HOSPITAL AND MEDICAL CENTERS, 40 Wright Street, Zip 01069-1187; tel. 413/283-7651; Richard H. Scheffer, President **A**1 2 9 10 **F**3 8 12 19 21 22 25 28 30 31 32 33 34 37 41 42 44 49 51 52 53 54 55 56 57 58 59 61 65 66 67 71 73 74 **P**6	23	10	51	2073	31	101869	0	21405	11535	351
PEABODY—Essex County										
★ THC – BOSTON, (Formerly Josiah B. Thomas Hospital) 15 King Street, Zip 01960; tel. 508/531-2900; Allan Freeman, Chief Executive Officer (Nonreporting) **A**9 10	14	10	59	—	—	—	—	—	—	—
PEMBROKE—Plymouth County										
□ PEMBROKE HOSPITAL, 199 Oak Street, Zip 02359; tel. 617/826-8161; Sherwin Z. Goodblatt, Chief Executive Officer (Nonreporting) **A**1 9 10	33	22	115	—	—	—	—	—	—	—
PITTSFIELD—Berkshire County										
★ △ BERKSHIRE MEDICAL CENTER, (Includes St. Luke's Hospital, 379 East Street, Pittsfield, Massachusetts, Zip 01201; tel. 413/443-9121) 725 North Street, Zip 01201; tel. 413/447-2000; Kevin E. Nolan, President **A**1 2 3 5 7 8 9 10 **F**7 8 10 11 12 15 16 17 19 20 21 22 23 25 26 28 30 31 32 33 34 35 37 39 40 41 42 44 45 46 48 49 51 52 53 54 55 56 57 58 59 60 61 62 63 65 67 70 71 72 73 74 **P**6 **S**2435 Berkshire Health Systems, Inc.	23	10	330	10867	199	61094	1053	100014	48695	1067
★ HILLCREST HOSPITAL, 165 Tor Court, Zip 01201-3099, Mailing Address: Box 1155, Zip 01202-1155; tel. 413/443-4761; Eugene A. Dellea, President and Chief Executive Officer **A**1 9 10 **F**2 3 8 11 12 13 14 15 16 17 18 19 21 22 25 26 28 29 30 31 37 39 41 42 44 45 46 49 51 54 58 61 62 65 68 71 72 73 74	23	10	116	3063	62	67595	0	21749	12588	431
PLYMOUTH—Plymouth County										
★ JORDAN HOSPITAL, 275 Sandwich Street, Zip 02360-2196; tel. 508/746-2001; Elliot L. Schwartz, Acting President and Chief Executive Officer **A**1 2 9 10 **F**1 2 3 4 7 8 11 12 15 16 17 18 19 21 22 23 27 28 29 31 33 34 35 37 39 40 41 42 44 45 46 48 49 52 53 54 56 60 64 65 66 67 68 71 73 **P**4 5 6 7 8 **S**0002 Quorum Health Group/Quorum Health Resources	23	10	145	6874	92	131752	876	54077	25930	568
POCASSET—Barnstable County										
□ BARNSTABLE COUNTY HOSPITAL, 870 County Road, Zip 02559; tel. 508/563-5941; Edward B. Leary, President (Nonreporting) **A**1 9 10	13	46	39	—	—	—	—	—	—	—
QUINCY—Norfolk County										
★ QUINCY HOSPITAL, 114 Whitwell Street, Zip 02169-1899; tel. 617/773-6100; Ralph Dipisa, Chief Executive Officer (Total facility includes 28 beds in nursing home–type unit) **A**1 9 10 **F**7 8 10 12 15 16 17 19 21 22 26 27 28 29 30 34 35 37 40 41 42 44 45 46 49 52 54 55 56 57 59 60 63 64 65 67 70 71 73 **P**8 **S**0002 Quorum Health Group/Quorum Health Resources	14	10	286	8729	155	65637	955	68213	30893	800
SALEM—Essex County										
NORTH SHORE CHILDREN'S HOSPITAL See Salem Hospital										
★ SALEM HOSPITAL, (Includes North Shore Children's Hospital, Salem, Massachusetts; tel. 508/745-2100) 81 Highland Avenue, Zip 01970; tel. 508/741-1200; Michael J. Geaney Jr., President **A**1 2 3 5 9 10 **F**2 3 7 8 10 11 12 14 15 16 17 18 19 21 22 23 24 25 26 27 28 29 30 31 32 33 34 35 36 37 38 40 41 42 44 45 46 49 51 52 53 54 55 56 57 58 59 60 61 63 65 66 67 68 70 71 72 73 74 **P**4 5 6 8	23	10	322	13341	186	335248	2029	127256	66788	1939
★ △ SHAUGHNESSY-KAPLAN REHABILITATION HOSPITAL, Dove Avenue, Zip 01970; tel. 508/745-9000; Judith Ritchie, President (Total facility includes 40 beds in nursing home–type unit) **A**1 7 9 10 **F**2 3 7 8 10 11 12 14 15 16 17 18 19 20 21 22 23 26 27 28 29 30 31 32 33 34 37 38 39 40 41 42 43 44 45 46 47 48 49 51 52 53 54 56 57 58 59 60 61 63 64 65 66 67 71 72 73 74	23	46	160	2049	128	20630	0	20822	10715	258
SOMERVILLE—Middlesex County										
□ HERITAGE HOSPITAL, 26 Central Street, Zip 02143; tel. 617/625-8900; Jay Mitchell, Administrator **A**1 10 **F**1 2 3 26 52 54 55 56 57 58 59 **S**0075 Cumberland Health Systems, Inc.	33	82	93	2464	41	—	0	—	—	140
★ SOMERVILLE HOSPITAL, 230 Highland Avenue, Zip 02143; tel. 617/666-4400; Carl Zack, President **A**1 3 6 9 10 **F**1 3 4 5 6 7 8 10 12 13 14 15 16 17 18 19 20 21 22 25 26 27 28 29 31 32 33 34 35 36 37 39 40 41 42 43 44 45 46 49 51 52 53 54 55 56 57 58 59 60 61 64 65 66 67 68 69 71 72 73 74 **P**4 5 6 7	23	10	87	2990	60	146084	0	33676	16576	565
SOUTH ATTLEBORO—Bristol County										
□ FULLER MEMORIAL HOSPITAL, 231 Washington Street, Zip 02703-5599; tel. 508/761-8500; Landon Kite, President (Nonreporting) **A**1 9 10	21	22	46	—	—	—	—	—	—	—

Hospitals, U.S. / MASSACHUSETTS

Hospital, Address, Telephone, Administrator, Approval, Facility, and Physician Codes, Health Care System	Classification Codes		Utilization Data					Expense (thousands) of dollars		
	Control	Service	Beds	Admissions	Census	Outpatient Visits	Births	Total	Payroll	Personnel

★ American Hospital Association (AHA) membership
☐ Joint Commission on Accreditation of Healthcare Organizations (JCAHO) accreditation
+ American Osteopathic Hospital Association (AOHA) membership
○ American Osteopathic Association (AOA) accreditation
△ Commission on Accreditation of Rehabilitation Facilities (CARF) accreditation
Control codes 61, 63, 64, 71, 72 and 73 indicate hospitals listed by AOHA, but not registered by AHA. For definition of numerical codes, see page A6

SOUTH WEYMOUTH—Norfolk County

★ SOUTH SHORE HOSPITAL, 55 Fogg Road, Zip 02190–2455; tel. 617/340–8000; David T. Hannan, President **A**1 2 9 10 **F**6 7 11 14 16 19 21 22 23 25 27 29 30 31 32 33 34 35 37 39 40 42 44 46 49 54 56 58 60 61 63 65 67 70 71 73 74 **P**5 6 7 8 — 23 10 247 15061 209 139202 2705 118995 55610 1491

SOUTHBRIDGE—Worcester County

★ HARRINGTON MEMORIAL HOSPITAL, 100 South Street, Zip 01550–4045; tel. 508/765–9771; Richard M. Mangion, President and Chief Executive Officer **A**1 9 10 **F**1 3 4 5 6 7 8 10 11 14 15 16 17 18 19 20 21 22 23 24 25 26 27 28 30 31 32 33 34 35 36 37 39 40 41 42 43 44 45 46 47 49 50 51 52 53 54 55 56 57 58 59 60 61 62 63 65 66 67 68 69 70 71 73 74 **P**8 — 23 10 115 4267 58 164340 451 32321 17008 455

SPRINGFIELD—Hampden County

★ BAYSTATE MEDICAL CENTER, 759 Chestnut Street, Zip 01199–0001; tel. 413/784–0000; Mark R. Tolosky, Chief Executive Officer **A**1 2 3 5 6 8 9 10 **F**4 7 8 10 11 13 14 15 16 17 19 20 21 22 23 24 25 26 28 30 31 32 33 34 35 37 38 39 40 41 42 43 44 45 46 47 49 51 52 53 54 55 56 57 58 59 60 61 63 65 67 68 69 70 71 72 73 74 **P**1 3 5 6 7 **S**1095 Baystate Health Systems, Inc. — 23 10 669 32012 516 296528 5623 294711 136730 4367

★ △ MERCY HOSPITAL, 271 Carew Street, Zip 01104, Mailing Address: P.O. Box 9012, Zip 01102–9012; tel. 413/748–9000; Vincent J. McCorkle, President and Chief Executive Officer **A**1 2 7 9 10 **F**1 3 5 7 8 10 11 12 17 19 20 21 22 25 26 28 29 30 31 34 35 37 39 41 42 44 45 46 48 49 51 53 54 55 56 57 58 59 60 63 65 67 68 71 73 74 **S**5285 Sisters of Providence Health System — 21 10 276 9419 202 96938 0 83508 36182 1174

★ SHRINERS HOSPITALS FOR CRIPPLED CHILDREN, SPRINGFIELD UNIT, 516 Carew Street, Zip 01104–2396; tel. 413/787–2000; Mark L. Niederpruem, Administrator **A**1 3 5 **F**17 49 65 73 **S**4125 Shriners Hospitals for Crippled Children — 23 57 40 837 28 11162 0 — — 206

☐ SPRINGFIELD MUNICIPAL HOSPITAL, 1400 State Street, Zip 01109–2589; tel. 413/787–6700; Theresa M. Theroux, Administrator (Total facility includes 220 beds in nursing home–type unit) **A**1 10 **F**14 16 20 26 27 41 46 52 54 57 64 65 67 73 — 14 48 394 355 264 0 0 24120 11432 221

STOCKBRIDGE—Berkshire County

★ AUSTEN RIGGS CENTER, 25 Main Street, Zip 01262–0962, Mailing Address: P.O. Box 962, Zip 01262–0962; tel. 413/298–5511; Edward R. Shapiro M.D., Medical Director and Chief Executive Officer (Nonreporting) **A**1 3 — 23 22 47 — — — — — — —

STONEHAM—Middlesex County

★ BOSTON REGIONAL MEDICAL CENTER, (Formerly New England Memorial Hospital) 5 Woodland Road, Zip 02180, Mailing Address: P.O. Box 9102, Zip 02180–9102; tel. 617/979–7000; Charles S. Ricks, President and Chief Executive Officer **A**1 2 3 9 10 **F**2 3 5 7 8 10 11 12 14 15 16 17 19 21 22 29 32 35 39 40 41 42 44 45 49 52 53 54 55 56 57 58 59 60 61 65 67 71 73 74 **P**5 6 8 — 21 10 187 6576 105 190150 1044 58630 31387 1141

STOUGHTON—Norfolk County

★ GOOD SAMARITAN MEDICAL CENTER, (Includes Good Samaritan Medical Center – Cushing Campus, 235 North Pearl Street, Brockton, Massachusetts, Zip 02401–1794; tel. 508/588–4000; Good Samaritan Medical Center – Goddard Campus, Stoughton, Massachusetts) 909 Sumner Street, Zip 02072; tel. 617/344–5100; Frank J. Larkin, Chief Executive Officer (Nonreporting) **A**1 2 3 5 9 10 **S**1125 Caritas Christi Health Care System — 22 10 473 — — — — — — —

★ △ NEW ENGLAND SINAI HOSPITAL AND REHABILITATION CENTER, 150 York Street, Zip 02072–1881; tel. 617/364–4850; Donald H. Goldberg, President **A**1 3 7 9 10 **F**1 5 15 16 20 28 33 34 39 42 48 49 54 65 66 67 71 73 — 23 49 212 1190 168 21000 0 36179 19870 558

TAUNTON—Bristol County

★ MORTON HOSPITAL AND MEDICAL CENTER, 88 Washington Street, Zip 02780–2499; tel. 508/824–6911; Thomas C. Porter, President **A**1 9 10 **F**7 8 15 16 19 21 22 23 28 30 34 35 37 38 39 40 41 42 44 46 48 49 65 66 71 73 74 — 23 10 201 7183 122 83835 686 63927 31479 773

TAUNTON STATE HOSPITAL, 60 Hodges Avenue Extension, Zip 02780, Mailing Address: P.O. Box 4007, Zip 02780; tel. 508/824–7551; Gary Phillips, Administrator and Chief Operating Officer **A**9 10 **F**20 45 46 52 53 54 55 57 65 67 73 **P**6 — 12 22 225 424 201 0 0 21500 10800 460

TEWKSBURY—Middlesex County

★ TEWKSBURY HOSPITAL, East Street, Zip 01876–1998; tel. 508/851–7321; Raymond D. Sanzone, Executive Director **A**6 9 10 **F**3 15 16 20 22 27 31 32 39 42 44 46 49 52 54 55 65 67 73 **P**6 **S**0013 Massachusetts Department of Mental Health — 12 48 720 1297 672 0 0 — — 765

WALTHAM—Middlesex County

★ MIDDLESEX HOSPITAL, 775 Trapelo Road, Zip 02254, Mailing Address: P.O. Box 9151, Zip 02254–9151; tel. 617/895–7000; Elaine Noble, Director (Nonreporting) **A**1 9 10 — 13 48 120 — — — — — — —

★ WALTHAMWESTON HOSPITAL & MEDICAL CENTER, (Formerly Walthamweston Hospital and Medical Center) Hope Avenue, Zip 02254–9116; tel. 617/647–6000; James L. Salsbury, President and Chief Executive Officer (Total facility includes 21 beds in nursing home–type unit) **A**1 2 5 9 10 **F**3 7 8 10 12 13 14 15 16 17 18 19 20 21 22 23 26 27 28 30 31 32 33 35 36 39 41 42 43 45 46 49 51 53 54 55 56 57 58 59 60 61 65 66 67 68 69 70 71 72 73 74 **P**5 6 8 — 23 10 206 7076 115 61193 407 55614 28464 675

WARE—Hampshire County

★ MARY LANE HOSPITAL, 85 South Street, Zip 01082; tel. 413/967–6211; Christine Shirtcliff, Executive Vice President **A**1 9 10 **F**1 7 8 12 14 15 16 17 19 21 22 26 28 29 30 31 32 33 34 37 39 40 41 42 44 45 49 54 58 65 71 73 74 **P**3 5 6 8 — 23 10 40 1964 20 51411 245 14812 7901 249

© 1995 AHA Guide

Hospitals, U.S. / MASSACHUSETTS

Hospital, Address, Telephone, Administrator, Approval, Facility, and Physician Codes, Health Care System	Classification Codes		Utilization Data					Expense (thousands) of dollars		
★ American Hospital Association (AHA) membership □ Joint Commission on Accreditation of Healthcare Organizations (JCAHO) accreditation + American Osteopathic Hospital Association (AOHA) membership ○ American Osteopathic Association (AOA) accreditation △ Commission on Accreditation of Rehabilitation Facilities (CARF) accreditation Control codes 61, 63, 64, 71, 72 and 73 indicate hospitals listed by AOHA, but not registered by AHA. For definition of numerical codes, see page A6	Control	Service	Beds	Admissions	Census	Outpatient Visits	Births	Total	Payroll	Personnel
WAREHAM—Plymouth County □ TOBEY HOSPITAL, 43 High Street, Zip 02571; tel. 508/295-0880; John M. Carlson, President **A**1 9 10 **F**4 7 8 14 15 16 17 19 21 22 28 29 30 31 32 33 34 35 37 39 40 41 42 44 46 49 53 54 56 58 65 67 71 73 **P**6	23	10	60	3096	38	23764	406	24739	12738	313
WEBSTER—Worcester County ★ HUBBARD REGIONAL HOSPITAL, 340 Thompson Road, Zip 01570-0608; tel. 508/943-2600; Gerald J. Barbini, Administrator and Chief Executive Officer **A**1 9 10 **F**8 15 16 19 21 22 27 30 34 37 39 41 42 44 45 46 49 56 58 65 71 72 73 74 **P**3 **S**0002 Quorum Health Group/Quorum Health Resources	23	10	37	1656	23	40322	0	14683	6289	209
WELLESLEY—Norfolk County □ CHARLES RIVER HOSPITAL, 203 Grove Street, Zip 02181; tel. 617/235-8400; E. Lorraine Baugh, President and Chief Executive Officer **A**1 3 9 10 **F**14 15 16 27 28 29 30 32 34 39 41 45 46 52 53 54 55 57 58 59 65 67 74 **P**6 **S**0215 Community Care Systems, Inc.	33	22	62	521	17	959	0	7765	4083	103
SIMPSON INFIRMARY, WELLESLEY COLLEGE, Worcester Street, Zip 02181-8277; tel. 617/283-2810; Charlotte K. Sanner M.D., Director Health Service (Data for 304 days) **A**9 **F**25 28 29 30 31 34 45 51 53 54 55 56 58 61 65 67 68 74	23	11	11	149	1	7383	0	—	—	14
WESTBOROUGH—Worcester County WESTBOROUGH STATE HOSPITAL, Mailing Address: P.O. Box 288, Zip 01581; tel. 508/366-4401; Steven Scheibel, Chief Operating Officer (Nonreporting) **A**5 9 10 **S**0013 Massachusetts Department of Mental Health	12	22	267	—	—	—	—	—	—	—
WESTFIELD—Hampden County ★ NOBLE HOSPITAL, 115 West Silver Street, Zip 01086-1634; tel. 413/572-5040; George J. Koller, President and Chief Executive Officer **A**1 2 9 10 **F**8 14 15 16 19 21 22 28 29 30 32 33 35 37 41 42 44 46 48 49 52 54 55 56 58 65 67 71 73 74	23	10	102	3065	63	62792	0	25537	13858	385
WESTWOOD—Norfolk County □ WESTWOOD LODGE HOSPITAL, 45 Clapboardtree Street, Zip 02090; tel. 617/762-7764; Sherwin Z. Goodblatt, Chief Executive Officer (Nonreporting) **A**1 5 9 10	33	22	100	—	—	—	—	—	—	—
WHITINSVILLE—Worcester County WHITINSVILLE HOSPITAL See Milford–Whitinsville Regional Hospital, Milford										
WINCHESTER—Middlesex County ★ WINCHESTER HOSPITAL, 41 Highland Avenue, Zip 01890-9920; tel. 617/729-9000; Stephen R. Laverty, President and Chief Executive Officer **A**1 2 5 9 10 **F**7 8 12 13 14 15 16 17 19 20 21 22 25 26 27 28 29 30 32 34 35 36 37 38 39 40 41 42 44 45 46 49 51 61 63 65 66 67 71 72 73 74 **P**1 5	23	10	183	9095	116	225705	2155	68906	33778	893
WOBURN—Middlesex County ★ CHOATE HEALTH SYSTEMS, 23 Warren Avenue, Zip 01801; tel. 617/933-6700; David Fassler M.D., President (Nonreporting) **A**10	33	22	21	—	—	—	—	—	—	—
□ △ NEW ENGLAND REHABILITATION HOSPITAL, Two Rehabilitation Way, Zip 01801-6098; tel. 617/935-5050; John F. Corridan III, Chief Executive Officer **A**1 7 9 10 **F**8 12 19 21 22 27 28 30 32 35 36 37 39 41 42 44 45 46 48 49 54 55 62 65 66 67 71 **P**6	33	46	198	3121	183	—	0	46047	25886	—
WORCESTER—Worcester County ADCARE HOSPITAL OF WORCESTER, 107 Lincoln Street, Zip 01605-2499; tel. 508/799-9000; David W. Hillis, President (Nonreporting) **A**9 10	33	82	88	—	—	—	—	—	—	—
□ △ FAIRLAWN REHABILITATION HOSPITAL, 189 May Street, Zip 01602-4399; tel. 508/791-6351; Ellen Ferrante, President **A**1 5 7 9 10 **F**12 15 25 26 34 45 46 48 49 65 73	33	46	110	1624	89	8160	0	22594	9661	239
★ MEDICAL CENTER OF CENTRAL MASSACHUSETTS, (Includes Medical Center of Central Massachusetts–Hahnemann, 281 Lincoln Street, Worcester, Massachusetts, Zip 01605; tel. 617/792-8000; Medical Center of Central Massachusetts–Memorial, Worcester, Massachusetts, Zip 01605; tel. 508/793-6611) 119 Belmont Street, Zip 01605-2982; tel. 508/793-6264; Peter H. Levine M.D., President and Chief Executive Officer (Total facility includes 31 beds in nursing home–type unit) **A**1 2 3 5 8 9 10 12 **F**3 7 8 10 11 12 13 15 16 17 19 21 22 23 25 26 28 29 30 31 32 33 34 35 37 38 40 42 44 45 49 51 52 53 54 55 56 57 58 59 60 61 63 64 65 66 67 68 71 72 73 74 **P**3 8	23	10	363	19514	296	321695	3934	179906	86702	2341
★ SAINT VINCENT HOSPITAL, 25 Winthrop Street, Zip 01604-4593; tel. 508/798-1234; Denis J. FitzGerald M.D., President and Chief Executive Officer **A**1 2 3 5 8 9 10 12 **F**3 4 5 7 8 10 11 12 14 15 16 17 19 21 22 26 28 30 31 32 34 36 37 39 40 42 43 44 47 48 49 52 54 55 56 57 58 60 65 70 71 72 73 **P**5 8	23	10	382	18711	295	102116	2453	141290	68100	1903
★ UNIVERSITY OF MASSACHUSETTS MEDICAL CENTER, 55 Lake Avenue North, Zip 01655; tel. 508/856-0011; Anne M. Bourgeois R.N., Interim Director (Nonreporting) **A**1 2 3 5 8 10	12	10	408	—	—	—	—	—	—	—
WORCESTER STATE HOSPITAL, 305 Belmont Street, Zip 01604; tel. 508/752-4681 **A**5 9 10 **F**12 14 20 22 26 27 31 35 39 52 54 55 56 57 58 59 65 67 71 73 **P**4	12	22	200	265	196	0	0	—	—	602

MICHIGAN

Resident population 9,478 (in thousands)
Resident population in metro areas 82.7%
Birth rate per 1,000 population 16.0
65 years and over 12.4%
Percent of persons without health insurance 9.4%

★ American Hospital Association (AHA) membership
☐ Joint Commission on Accreditation of Healthcare Organizations (JCAHO) accreditation
+ American Osteopathic Hospital Association (AOHA) membership
○ American Osteopathic Association (AOA) accreditation
△ Commission on Accreditation of Rehabilitation Facilities (CARF) accreditation
Control codes 61, 63, 64, 71, 72 and 73 indicate hospitals listed by AOHA, but not registered by AHA. For definition of numerical codes, see page A6

Hospital, Address, Telephone, Administrator, Approval, Facility, and Physician Codes, Health Care System	Classification Codes		Utilization Data					Expense (thousands) of dollars		
	Control	Service	Beds	Admissions	Census	Outpatient Visits	Births	Total	Payroll	Personnel
ADDISON—Lenawee County										
ADDISON COMMUNITY HOSPITAL, 421 North Steer Street, Zip 49220; tel. 517/547-6151; Trevor J. Dyksterhouse, Administrator (Nonreporting) A9 10	16	10	24	—	—	—	—	—	—	—
ADRIAN—Lenawee County										
★ BIXBY MEDICAL CENTER, 818 Riverside Avenue, Zip 49221; tel. 517/263-0711; John R. Robertstad, President and Chief Executive Officer A1 2 9 10 F3 8 15 16 19 21 22 28 29 30 33 34 35 37 40 42 44 46 49 52 53 56 57 60 64 67 71 73 P1	23	10	99	3916	51	91182	645	32266	16396	630
ALBION—Calhoun County										
★ ALBION COMMUNITY HOSPITAL, 809 West Erie Street, Zip 49224-1556; tel. 517/629-2191; Michael G. Boff, President A1 9 10 F7 8 10 11 12 14 15 16 17 19 20 21 22 26 27 28 29 30 32 33 34 35 37 39 40 41 42 44 51 53 54 55 56 57 58 59 63 65 71 72 73 P1 5 8	23	10	61	2209	18	40464	167	11571	5415	174
ALLEGAN—Allegan County										
★ ALLEGAN GENERAL HOSPITAL, 555 Linn Street, Zip 49010-1594; tel. 616/673-8424; Jack L. Denton, President A1 9 10 F7 8 14 15 19 21 22 30 34 35 37 39 40 41 42 44 46 49 51 52 55 56 57 58 59 63 65 66 67 71 72 73	23	10	63	1863	26	30985	249	16982	7771	253
ALLEN PARK—Wayne County										
★ VETERANS AFFAIRS MEDICAL CENTER, Southfield and Outer Drive, Zip 48101; tel. 313/562-6000; Carlos B. Lott Jr., Acting Director (Total facility includes 72 beds in nursing home-type unit) A1 2 3 5 8 9 F2 3 4 5 6 8 10 11 12 14 15 16 17 18 19 20 21 22 23 26 27 28 29 30 31 32 33 34 35 37 39 40 41 42 43 44 46 49 50 51 52 54 55 56 58 59 60 61 63 64 65 67 69 70 71 72 73 74 P6 S9295 Department of Veterans Affairs	45	10	464	8580	336	209128	0	113873	62961	1514
ALMA—Gratiot County										
★ GRATIOT COMMUNITY HOSPITAL, 300 Warwick Drive, Zip 48801; tel. 517/463-1101; Bob M. Baker, President A1 9 10 F3 7 8 10 14 16 19 20 21 22 28 30 31 32 33 34 35 37 39 40 41 44 45 46 48 49 52 54 55 56 57 65 67 71 73	23	10	127	4165	60	61317	631	30572	13665	494
ALPENA—Alpena County										
★ ALPENA GENERAL HOSPITAL, 1501 West Chisholm Street, Zip 49707-1498; tel. 517/356-7390; John A. McVeety, Chief Executive Officer A1 2 9 10 F2 3 4 7 8 10 12 15 17 19 21 22 28 29 30 31 32 33 34 35 39 40 41 42 44 45 46 52 53 54 55 56 57 58 63 65 67 71 72 73 74	13	10	176	5222	79	75530	537	41157	18892	552
ANN ARBOR—Washtenaw County										
★ △ CATHERINE MCAULEY HEALTH SYSTEM, (Includes St. Joseph Mercy Hospital, 5301 East Huron River Drive, Ann Arbor, Michigan, Zip 48106, Mailing Address: Box 995, Zip 48106; tel. 313/572-3456) 5305 East Huron River Drive, Zip 48106, Mailing Address: Box 992, Zip 48106-0992; tel. 313/712-3456; Garry C. Faja, President and Chief Executive Officer A1 2 3 5 7 8 9 10 F1 4 7 8 10 11 12 14 15 16 17 18 19 21 22 25 26 29 30 31 32 34 35 36 37 39 40 41 42 43 44 45 46 48 49 51 52 53 54 56 57 58 59 60 65 67 70 71 72 73 74 P4 5 8 S5165 Mercy Health Services	21	10	530	28145	425	175692	4310	323984	134373	3667
ST. JOSEPH MERCY HOSPITAL See Catherine McAuley Health System										
☐ UNIVERSITY OF MICHIGAN HOSPITALS, 1500 East Medical Center Drive, Zip 48109-0827; tel. 313/936-4000; John D. Forsyth, Executive Director A1 2 3 5 8 9 10 F2 3 4 5 7 8 9 10 11 12 13 14 17 18 19 20 21 22 23 24 25 26 28 29 30 31 32 34 35 37 38 39 40 41 42 43 44 45 46 47 48 49 50 51 52 53 54 55 56 57 58 60 61 63 65 66 67 69 70 71 72 73 74	23	10	859	34688	700	855912	2180	581086	259837	7505
★ VETERANS AFFAIRS MEDICAL CENTER, 2215 Fuller Road, Zip 48105; tel. 313/769-7100; Edward L. Gamache, Director (Total facility includes 90 beds in nursing home-type unit) A1 3 5 8 9 F2 3 4 5 8 10 11 14 16 19 20 21 22 23 25 26 27 29 30 31 32 33 34 35 37 39 41 42 43 44 45 46 49 50 51 52 54 55 56 57 58 59 60 64 65 67 69 71 72 73 74 S9295 Department of Veterans Affairs	45	10	311	6623	256	323958	0	102330	58751	1847
AUBURN HILLS—Oakland County										
☐ HAVENWYCK HOSPITAL, 1525 University Drive, Zip 48326-2675; tel. 810/373-9200; Robert A. Kercorian, Chief Executive Officer A1 10 F12 16 18 30 39 46 52 53 54 55 56 57 59 65 67 S0405 Ramsay Health Care, Inc.	33	22	120	1825	73	6383	0	10736	4548	162
BAD AXE—Huron County										
★ HURON MEMORIAL HOSPITAL, 1100 South Van Dyke Road, Zip 48413-9799; tel. 517/269-9521; James B. Gardner, President A1 9 10 F7 8 15 16 19 21 27 28 30 33 34 37 39 40 41 42 44 49 63 65 67 71	23	10	64	1763	21	44544	226	14091	6240	200
BATTLE CREEK—Calhoun County										
☐ BATTLE CREEK ADVENTIST HOSPITAL, 165 North Washington Avenue, Zip 49016; tel. 616/964-7121; Ronald C. Brown, President and Chief Executive Officer (Nonreporting) A1	21	22	86	—	—	—	—	—	—	—
★ BATTLE CREEK HEALTH SYSTEM, (Includes Community Hospital, 183 West Street, Battle Creek, Michigan, Zip 49016; tel. 616/966-8000; Leila Hospital, Battle Creek, Michigan) 300 North Avenue, Zip 49016-3396; tel. 616/966-8000; Stephen L. Abbott, President and Chief Executive Officer (Total facility includes 77 beds in nursing home-type unit) A1 9 10 F3 6 7 8 10 11 12 13 14 15 16 17 19 21 22 26 27 28 29 30 32 34 35 37 39 40 41 42 44 45 46 49 52 53 54 55 56 57 58 59 60 63 64 65 66 67 71 73 74 P8 S5165 Mercy Health Services	23	10	358	11227	155	123445	1231	97470	35747	1392
COMMUNITY HOSPITAL See Battle Creek Health System										
LEILA HOSPITAL See Battle Creek Health System										

© 1995 AHA Guide

Hospitals, U.S. / MICHIGAN

Hospital, Address, Telephone, Administrator, Approval, Facility, and Physician Codes, Health Care System	Classification Codes		Utilization Data					Expense (thousands) of dollars		Personnel
★ American Hospital Association (AHA) membership □ Joint Commission on Accreditation of Healthcare Organizations (JCAHO) accreditation + American Osteopathic Hospital Association (AOHA) membership ○ American Osteopathic Association (AOA) accreditation △ Commission on Accreditation of Rehabilitation Facilities (CARF) accreditation Control codes 61, 63, 64, 71, 72 and 73 indicate hospitals listed by AOHA, but not registered by AHA. For definition of numerical codes, see page A6	Control	Service	Beds	Admissions	Census	Outpatient Visits	Births	Total	Payroll	
★ △ SOUTHWESTERN MICHIGAN REHABILITATION HOSPITAL, 183 West Street, Zip 49017; tel. 616/965-3206; David Mungenast, President **A**7 9 10 **F**14 19 21 27 35 48 49 50 54 65 71	23	46	30	359	14	24699	0	4487	1749	50
☒ VETERANS AFFAIRS MEDICAL CENTER, 5500 Armstrong Road, Zip 49016; tel. 616/966-5600; (Total facility includes 205 beds in nursing home-type unit) **A**1 5 9 **F**1 2 3 4 5 6 7 8 10 12 15 16 17 18 19 20 21 22 23 24 25 26 27 28 29 30 31 32 33 34 35 36 37 39 41 42 43 44 45 46 49 50 51 52 54 55 56 57 58 59 60 63 64 65 67 70 71 72 73 74 **S**9295 Department of Veterans Affairs	45	22	806	4234	669	131373	0	84320	51744	1497
BAY CITY—Bay County										
☒ △ BAY MEDICAL CENTER, (Includes Bay Medical Center-West Campus, 3250 East Midland Road, Bay City, Michigan, Zip 48706; tel. 517/894-6550; Samaritan Health Center, 713 Ninth Street, Bay City, Michigan, Zip 48708; tel. 517/894-3799) 1900 Columbus Avenue, Zip 48708; tel. 517/894-3000; Anthony W. Armstrong, Chief Executive Officer **A**1 2 7 9 10 12 **F**2 3 6 7 8 10 12 14 15 16 17 18 19 20 21 22 26 28 29 30 31 32 33 34 35 36 37 39 40 41 42 44 45 46 48 49 52 54 55 56 58 59 63 65 66 67 70 71 72 73 74 **P**6 8 BAY MEDICAL CENTER-WEST CAMPUS See Bay Medical Center SAMARITAN HEALTH CENTER See Bay Medical Center	23	10	337	16453	239	216661	1289	102656	42727	1601
BERRIEN CENTER—Berrien County										
☒ BERRIEN GENERAL HOSPITAL, 6418 Dean's Hill Road, Zip 49102-9704; tel. 616/471-5610; Linda Wegener, Vice President Operations and Patient Services (Nonreporting) **A**1 9 10 **S**0056 Lakeland Regional Health System, Inc.	13	10	248	—	—	—	—	—	—	—
BIG RAPIDS—Mecosta County										
☒ MECOSTA COUNTY GENERAL HOSPITAL, 405 Winter Avenue, Zip 49307-2099; tel. 616/796-8691; Thomas E. Daugherty, Chief Executive Officer **A**1 9 10 **F**7 11 14 19 22 28 34 36 37 39 40 41 42 44 49 51 65 67 71 73 **S**0002 Quorum Health Group/Quorum Health Resources	13	10	74	2361	25	66663	651	15708	7227	245
BRIGHTON—Livingston County										
★ BRIGHTON HOSPITAL, 12851 East Grand River Avenue, Zip 48116-8596; tel. 313/227-1211; Ivan C. Harner, President and Chief Executive Officer **A**9 10 **F**2 14 16 25	23	82	83	1139	45	8447	0	7115	2864	125
BUCHANAN—Berrien County										
☒ + REHABILITATION INSTITUTE AT TRI-STATE HOSPITAL, 15198 North Main Street, Zip 49107-1331; tel. 616/695-3851; Stephen Vargo, Administrator **A**1 9 10 **F**12 19 27 35 39 41 45 46 48 49 65	33	46	42	215	27	—	0	8438	4152	130
CADILLAC—Wexford County										
☒ MERCY HOSPITAL, 400 Hobart Street, Zip 49601-9596; tel. 616/779-7200; Dennis J. Renander, President and Chief Executive Officer **A**1 9 10 **F**7 8 10 14 15 16 17 19 20 21 22 28 29 30 31 32 33 34 35 37 39 40 41 42 44 45 46 48 49 52 54 55 56 58 63 65 66 67 71 73 **P**1 2 3 4 5 6 7 8 **S**5165 Mercy Health Services	21	10	133	4883	56	32911	574	34731	14479	585
CARO—Tuscola County										
★ CARO COMMUNITY HOSPITAL, 401 North Hooper Street, Zip 48723, Mailing Address: P.O. Box 71, Zip 48723; tel. 517/673-3141; William P. Miller, Chief Executive Officer **A**9 10 **F**8 15 16 19 21 22 25 28 30 34 37 41 42 44 46 49 51 56 65 71 **P**6	15	10	19	853	9	43189	0	7136	3360	106
□ CARO REGIONAL MENTAL HEALTH CENTER, 2000 Wak Road, Zip 48723-0153, Mailing Address: Box A, Zip 48723-0153; tel. 517/673-3191; P. S. Kumar M.D., Medical Director **A**1 9 10 **F**3 4 5 7 8 9 10 11 12 15 16 18 19 20 21 22 23 26 30 31 32 33 35 37 39 40 42 43 44 45 46 47 52 53 54 55 56 57 58 59 60 61 65 67 69 70 71 74	12	22	234	436	213	0	0	71588	23832	543
CARSON CITY—Montcalm County										
+ ○ CARSON CITY HOSPITAL, 406 East Elm Street, Zip 48811-0879, Mailing Address: P.O. Box 879, Zip 48811-0879; tel. 517/584-3131; Bruce L. Traverse, President **A**9 10 11 12 13 **F**7 8 15 17 19 22 28 30 32 34 35 37 40 41 42 44 51 52 54 55 56 58 65 67 71 73 74 **P**6	23	10	76	2708	33	42290	446	18523	8962	437
CASS CITY—Tuscola County										
☒ HILLS AND DALES GENERAL HOSPITAL, 4675 Hill Street, Zip 48726-1099; tel. 517/872-2121; Deborah A. Sopo, President and Chief Executive Officer **A**1 9 10 **F**7 8 19 21 22 24 28 29 30 31 32 33 34 40 41 44 46 49 51 56 65 66 71	23	10	47	869	10	18533	3	7151	3359	121
CHARLEVOIX—Charlevoix County										
☒ CHARLEVOIX AREA HOSPITAL, Lake Shore Drive, Zip 49720-1931; tel. 616/547-4024; Richard L. Krueger, President **A**1 9 10 **F**7 8 15 16 20 22 28 30 37 40 41 44 49 65 66 70 71 73	23	10	33	1412	14	18621	156	8551	4074	156
CHARLOTTE—Eaton County										
☒ HAYES-GREEN-BEACH MEMORIAL HOSPITAL, 321 East Harris Street, Zip 48813; tel. 517/543-1050; Bruce A. Smith, President and Executive Officer **A**1 9 10 **F**7 8 14 15 16 19 21 24 28 29 30 31 32 34 36 39 40 41 42 44 48 49 51 65 66 67 71 73 **P**6	23	10	46	1408	15	60580	187	10955	5561	188
CHEBOYGAN—Cheboygan County										
☒ COMMUNITY MEMORIAL HOSPITAL, 748 South Main Street, Zip 49721-2299, Mailing Address: P.O. Box 419, Zip 49721-0419; tel. 616/627-5601; Howard J. Purcell Jr., President (Total facility includes 50 beds in nursing home-type unit) **A**1 9 10 **F**8 19 20 21 22 32 33 37 40 44 65 71 73	23	10	92	2261	75	44122	207	15204	7148	238

Hospitals, U.S. / MICHIGAN

Hospital, Address, Telephone, Administrator, Approval, Facility, and Physician Codes, Health Care System	Classification Codes		Utilization Data					Expense (thousands) of dollars		Personnel
★ American Hospital Association (AHA) membership ☐ Joint Commission on Accreditation of Healthcare Organizations (JCAHO) accreditation + American Osteopathic Hospital Association (AOHA) membership ○ American Osteopathic Association (AOA) accreditation △ Commission on Accreditation of Rehabilitation Facilities (CARF) accreditation Control codes 61, 63, 64, 71, 72 and 73 indicate hospitals listed by AOHA, but not registered by AHA. For definition of numerical codes, see page A6	Control	Service	Beds	Admissions	Census	Outpatient Visits	Births	Total	Payroll	
CHELSEA—Washtenaw County ☐ △ CHELSEA COMMUNITY HOSPITAL, 775 South Main Street, Zip 48118–1399; tel. 313/475–1311; Willard H. Johnson, President **A**1 3 5 7 9 10 **F**3 4 8 10 14 15 17 19 21 22 24 25 26 27 28 29 30 32 33 34 37 39 41 42 44 45 46 48 49 52 53 54 55 57 58 59 61 65 67 71 72 73 74 **P**3	23	10	107	2981	65	115874	6	35893	18019	597
CLARE—Clare County ★ ○ MIDMICHIGAN REGIONAL MEDICAL CENTER–CLARE, 104 West Sixth Street, Zip 48617–1409; tel. 517/386–9951; Lawrence F. Barco, President **A**9 10 11 **F**7 8 15 17 19 21 22 28 30 32 33 34 35 40 41 42 44 49 63 67 71 72 73 74 **P**6 8 **S**0001 MidMichigan Regional Health System	23	10	64	2191	23	30386	373	14870	6965	203
CLINTON TOWNSHIP—Macomb County ※ ST. JOSEPH'S MERCY HOSPITALS AND HEALTH SERVICES, (Includes St. Joseph's Mercy Hospital–East, 215 North Avenue, Mount Clemens, Michigan, Zip 48043; tel. 810/466–9300; St. Joseph's Mercy Hospital–West, Clinton Township, Michigan, Zip 48038; tel. 810/263–2300; St. Joseph's Mercy–North, 80650 North Van Dyke, Romeo, Michigan, Zip 48065; tel. 810/798–8551) 15855 19 Mile Road, Zip 48038; tel. 810/263–2707; Robert L. Beyer, President and Chief Executive Officer (Total facility includes 475 beds in nursing home–type unit) **A**1 9 10 **F**3 6 7 8 10 12 15 16 17 19 21 22 27 28 29 30 31 32 33 34 35 36 39 40 41 42 44 45 46 48 49 52 54 55 56 58 59 61 64 65 67 71 72 73 74 **P**6 8 **S**5165 Mercy Health Services	23	10	855	15788	697	200261	1957	125242	59709	2004
COLDWATER—Branch County ※ + ○ COMMUNITY HEALTH CENTER OF BRANCH COUNTY, 274 East Chicago Street, Zip 49036–2088; tel. 517/279–5400; Earl Tamar, Chief Executive Officer **A**1 9 10 11 12 **F**3 7 8 10 16 19 21 22 31 32 33 34 35 37 40 41 42 44 49 51 52 54 55 56 57 58 59 65 67 70 71 73 **P**6 **S**0002 Quorum Health Group/Quorum Health Resources	13	10	96	3402	43	72515	438	29351	12517	428
COMMERCE TOWNSHIP—Oakland County ※ HURON VALLEY HOSPITAL, 1601 East Commerce Road, Zip 48382; tel. 810/360–3300; Elliot Joseph, President **A**1 3 5 10 **F**7 8 10 19 21 22 27 28 30 31 33 34 37 39 40 41 42 44 45 46 49 54 65 66 67 71 73 **P**4 6 **S**2145 Detroit Medical Center	23	10	137	7504	99	52007	1689	59028	21880	728
CRYSTAL FALLS—Iron County ※ CRYSTAL FALLS COMMUNITY HOSPITAL, 212 South Third Street, Zip 49920, Mailing Address: P.O. Box 60, Zip 49920–0060; tel. 906/875–6661; H. B. Purdy, Administrator and Chief Executive Officer **A**1 9 10 **F**11 22 34 37 44	14	10	35	428	6	11789	1	2904	1323	52
DEARBORN—Wayne County ※ OAKWOOD HOSPITAL AND MEDICAL CENTER – DEARBORN, (Formerly Oakwood Hospital) 18101 Oakwood Boulevard, Zip 48124, Mailing Address: P.O. Box 2500, Zip 48123–2500; tel. 313/593–7000; Gerald D. Fitzgerald, President **A**1 2 3 5 8 9 10 **F**1 3 4 6 7 8 10 11 12 14 17 18 19 20 21 22 23 25 26 27 28 29 32 33 34 35 37 38 39 40 41 42 43 44 45 46 49 51 52 53 54 55 56 57 58 59 60 61 62 63 65 66 67 68 71 73 74 **P**5 6 **S**1165 Oakwood Healthcare System	23	10	615	23484	441	191146	4222	261154	122426	3578
DECKERVILLE—Sanilac County ※ DECKERVILLE COMMUNITY HOSPITAL, 3559 Pine Street, Zip 48427–0126; tel. 810/376–2835; David M. Simmons, Administrator **A**1 9 10 **F**5 8 15 17 19 22 28 30 32 34 41 42 44 45 46 49 65 67 70 71 72 **S**5165 Mercy Health Services	23	10	17	304	3	13156	0	2627	1287	65
DETROIT—Wayne County ○ AURORA HOSPITAL FOR CHILDREN, 3737 Lawton, Zip 48208; tel. 313/361–7600 **A**10 11 **F**12 16 18 52 53 54 55 58 59 65 67 **S**2055 Michigan Health Care Corporation	23	52	80	1105	58	8505	0	22917	9427	187
※ △ CHILDREN'S HOSPITAL OF MICHIGAN, 3901 Beaubien, Zip 48201–9985; tel. 313/745–0073; Thomas M. Rozek, President **A**1 3 5 7 8 9 10 **F**1 2 3 4 5 7 8 9 10 11 12 14 15 16 17 18 19 20 21 22 23 24 25 26 27 28 30 31 32 33 34 35 37 38 39 40 41 42 43 44 45 46 47 48 49 50 51 52 53 54 55 56 57 58 59 60 61 63 64 65 66 67 69 70 71 72 73 74 **P**4 5 6 8 **S**2145 Detroit Medical Center	23	50	257	13690	177	203047	0	170523	67556	1818
※ DETROIT RECEIVING HOSPITAL AND UNIVERSITY HEALTH CENTER, 4201 St. Antoine Boulevard, Zip 48201–2194; tel. 313/745–3605; Edward S. Thomas, President **A**1 3 5 8 10 **F**4 7 8 9 10 11 12 17 18 19 20 21 22 23 27 28 29 30 31 32 34 35 37 39 41 42 43 44 46 49 50 51 52 54 56 57 58 60 65 67 70 71 72 73 **S**2145 Detroit Medical Center	23	10	310	11639	237	110425	0	161921	60758	1630
※ DETROIT RIVERVIEW HOSPITAL, 7733 East Jefferson Avenue, Zip 48214; tel. 313/499–3000; Richard T. Young, Administrator **A**1 9 10 **F**3 4 10 11 14 15 16 19 21 22 25 26 27 28 29 30 31 32 34 35 37 38 40 41 42 44 45 46 52 54 56 58 59 60 61 63 65 67 68 69 71 73 **P**5 8 **S**0042 Detroit–Macomb Hospital Corporation	23	10	230	10988	179	72064	2002	95691	36728	1248
※ GRACE HOSPITAL, 6071 West Outer Drive, Zip 48235; tel. 313/966–3300; Mark A. Eustis, President **A**1 3 5 8 9 10 12 **F**2 3 4 6 7 8 9 10 11 12 13 19 20 21 22 25 26 28 29 30 31 32 33 34 35 37 38 39 40 41 42 43 44 45 46 47 48 49 50 51 52 53 54 55 56 57 58 59 60 61 63 64 65 66 69 70 71 72 73 74 **P**5 6 7 8 **S**2145 Detroit Medical Center	23	10	476	18550	321	157357	3641	202454	81204	2357
※ HARPER HOSPITAL, 3990 John R, Zip 48201–9027; tel. 313/745–8040; Paul L. Broughton, President **A**1 2 3 5 8 9 10 **F**2 3 4 7 8 9 10 11 12 14 15 16 17 19 20 21 22 23 24 25 26 27 28 29 30 31 32 33 34 35 36 37 38 39 40 41 42 43 44 46 47 48 49 50 51 52 53 54 56 57 58 60 61 63 64 65 66 67 69 70 71 72 73 74 **S**2145 Detroit Medical Center	23	10	549	19090	424	147732	0	291589	103485	2934

© 1995 AHA Guide

Hospitals, U.S. / MICHIGAN

Hospital, Address, Telephone, Administrator, Approval, Facility, and Physician Codes, Health Care System	Classification Codes		Utilization Data					Expense (thousands) of dollars		
★ American Hospital Association (AHA) membership □ Joint Commission on Accreditation of Healthcare Organizations (JCAHO) accreditation + American Osteopathic Hospital Association (AOHA) membership ○ American Osteopathic Association (AOA) accreditation △ Commission on Accreditation of Rehabilitation Facilities (CARF) accreditation Control codes 61, 63, 64, 71, 72 and 73 indicate hospitals listed by AOHA, but not registered by AHA. For definition of numerical codes, see page A6	Control	Service	Beds	Admissions	Census	Outpatient Visits	Births	Total	Payroll	Personnel
★ HENRY FORD HOSPITAL, 2799 West Grand Boulevard, Zip 48202-2689; tel. 313/876-2600; Stephen H. Velick, Group Vice President, Henry Ford Health System and Chief Operating Officer A1 2 3 5 6 8 9 10 F2 3 4 5 6 7 8 9 10 11 12 13 14 15 16 17 18 19 20 21 22 23 25 26 27 28 29 30 31 32 33 34 35 37 38 39 40 41 42 43 44 45 46 47 48 49 51 52 53 54 55 56 57 58 59 60 61 63 64 65 66 67 68 69 70 71 72 73 74 P6 S9505 Henry Ford Health System	23	10	903	36337	601	552891	2235	293029	106242	9737
★ HOLY CROSS HOSPITAL, 4777 East Outer Drive, Zip 48234-0401; tel. 313/369-9100; James E. Koerper, President and Chief Executive Officer A1 9 10 F1 2 3 4 5 6 7 8 9 10 11 12 13 15 16 17 18 19 20 21 22 23 24 25 26 27 28 29 30 31 32 33 34 35 36 37 38 39 40 41 42 43 44 45 46 47 48 49 50 51 52 53 54 55 56 57 58 59 60 61 62 63 64 65 66 67 68 69 70 71 72 73 74 P8 S5375 Franciscan Services Corporation	21	10	214	5333	134	49310	0	49342	24800	604
★ HUTZEL HOSPITAL, 4707 St. Antoine Boulevard, Zip 48201-0154; tel. 313/745-7174; Frank P. Iacobell, President A1 3 5 8 9 10 F1 3 4 5 7 8 9 10 11 12 13 16 17 18 19 20 21 22 23 24 25 26 27 28 29 30 31 32 33 34 35 37 38 39 40 41 42 43 44 45 46 47 48 49 50 51 52 53 54 55 56 57 58 59 60 61 64 65 66 67 69 70 71 72 73 74 S2145 Detroit Medical Center	23	10	296	15676	206	85155	7703	145840	58799	1790
MARGARET W. MONTGOMERY HOSPITAL, 28303 Joy Road, Zip 48185; tel. 313/458-9208; Barbara J. Clark, Vice President and Chief Operating Officer A9 10 F16 52 57 58 59 65 67 S2055 Michigan Health Care Corporation	23	22	60	612	24	7761	0	10956	2966	52
★ MERCY HOSPITAL, 5555 Conner Avenue, Zip 48213-3499; tel. 313/579-4000; Brenita Crawford, President and Chief Executive Officer A1 3 10 F1 2 3 7 8 10 12 13 14 15 16 17 19 22 25 26 27 28 30 31 32 33 34 37 40 41 42 44 45 46 49 51 52 53 54 55 56 57 58 59 64 65 67 71 73 74 P5 8 S5165 Mercy Health Services	21	10	268	8619	190	187326	944	87898	38983	1168
+ ○ MICHIGAN HOSPITAL AND MEDICAL CENTER, 2700 Martin Luther King Jr. Boulevard, Zip 48208; tel. 313/361-8112; Patricia Kennedy-Scott, Vice President and Chief Operating Officer A9 10 11 12 13 F2 7 8 11 12 15 16 19 21 25 27 28 29 30 32 33 34 37 39 40 42 44 46 49 51 52 60 61 63 65 67 71 72 73 74 P6 S2055 Michigan Health Care Corporation	23	10	416	11738	300	33711	980	83038	32478	470
□ NEW CENTER HOSPITAL, 801 Virginia Park, Zip 48202; tel. 313/874-2800; Alfred Moore, Chief Executive Officer (Nonreporting) A1 10	23	10	145	—	—	—	—	—	—	—
★ △ REHABILITATION INSTITUTE OF MICHIGAN, 261 Mack Boulevard, Zip 48201; tel. 313/745-1203; Bruce M. Gans M.D., President A1 3 5 7 9 10 F3 5 7 8 10 11 16 17 19 21 22 23 25 26 28 29 30 31 32 33 34 35 37 38 39 40 41 42 43 44 45 47 48 49 50 51 52 53 54 55 56 57 58 59 60 61 63 64 65 66 67 69 70 71 72 73 74 P5 S2145 Detroit Medical Center	23	46	128	1542	80	84848	0	38439	21068	540
★ △ SARATOGA COMMUNITY HOSPITAL, 15000 Gratiot Avenue, Zip 48205-1999; tel. 313/245-1200; Michael F. Breen, President and Chief Executive Officer A1 7 9 10 F8 12 14 15 16 17 19 22 25 26 27 28 30 31 34 37 39 42 44 45 48 49 63 65 67 71 73 P5 8	23	10	170	5072	111	30562	8	41611	19475	613
★ △ SINAI HOSPITAL, 6767 West Outer Drive, Zip 48235-2899; tel. 313/493-6800; Phillip S. Schaengold J.D., President and Chief Executive Officer A1 3 5 7 8 9 10 F4 7 8 10 11 12 14 15 16 17 18 19 21 22 25 26 27 28 30 31 32 33 34 37 38 39 40 41 42 43 44 46 48 49 51 52 54 55 56 57 58 59 60 61 63 65 67 71 73 74 P4 6 8	23	10	530	20324	401	194466	3624	262053	132651	3169
★ ST. JOHN HOSPITAL AND MEDICAL CENTER, 22101 Moross Road, Zip 48236-2172; tel. 313/343-4000; Timothy J. Grajewski, President and Chief Executive Officer (Data for 364 days) A1 3 5 8 9 10 F1 3 4 7 8 10 11 12 13 14 15 16 17 18 19 20 22 25 26 27 28 29 30 31 32 33 34 35 37 38 39 40 41 42 43 44 46 49 51 52 53 54 55 58 59 60 61 63 65 66 67 68 69 70 71 72 73 74 P5 6 8 S5555 Sisters of St. Joseph Health System	21	10	589	25050	448	190699	3604	259495	125746	4099
DOWAGIAC—Cass County										
★ LEE MEMORIAL HOSPITAL, 420 West High Street, Zip 49047-1907; tel. 616/782-8681; Merrill A. Frank, Chief Executive Officer A1 9 10 F3 7 8 10 15 19 21 22 28 29 30 33 35 37 39 40 42 44 45 49 53 54 55 56 57 58 59 71 73 P6 S5555 Sisters of St. Joseph Health System	21	10	57	1948	26	28060	146	12573	5825	190
EAST CHINA—St. Clair County										
★ RIVER DISTRICT HOSPITAL, 4100 South River Road, Zip 48054; tel. 810/329-7111; John E. Knox, President and Chief Executive Officer A1 9 10 F3 7 8 15 16 19 21 22 30 37 40 41 42 44 46 49 56 58 65 67 71 P1 6 S5555 Sisters of St. Joseph Health System	23	10	68	2646	30	49612	438	20220	9073	290
EATON RAPIDS—Eaton County										
□ EATON RAPIDS COMMUNITY HOSPITAL, 1500 South Main Street, Zip 48827-0130, Mailing Address: P.O. Box 130, Zip 48827-0130; tel. 517/663-2671; Jeffrey S. Allison, Chief Executive Officer A1 9 10 F8 12 15 16 19 22 28 30 34 35 36 39 42 44 45 46 51 56 65 71 72 73 S1515 Michigan Capital Healthcare	23	10	21	681	6	24330	0	5824	2565	113
ESCANABA—Delta County										
★ ST. FRANCIS HOSPITAL, 3401 Ludington Street, Zip 49829; tel. 906/786-3311; Roger M. Burgess, Administrator (Nonreporting) A1 9 10 S5335 OSF Healthcare System	21	10	66	—	—	—	—	—	—	—
FARMINGTON HILLS—Oakland County										
★ + ○ △ BOTSFORD GENERAL HOSPITAL, 28050 Grand River Avenue, Zip 48336-5933; tel. 810/471-8000; Gerson Cooper, President A7 9 10 11 12 13 F3 7 8 10 11 12 14 15 16 17 19 21 22 24 25 26 27 28 29 30 31 32 33 34 35 37 40 41 42 44 45 46 48 49 51 52 54 57 58 62 65 66 67 69 71 72 73 P5 6 7	23	10	321	13228	248	689572	856	141846	67205	1659

Hospitals, U.S. / MICHIGAN

Hospital, Address, Telephone, Administrator, Approval, Facility, and Physician Codes, Health Care System	Classification Codes		Utilization Data					Expense (thousands) of dollars		
	Control	Service	Beds	Admissions	Census	Outpatient Visits	Births	Total	Payroll	Personnel

★ American Hospital Association (AHA) membership
☐ Joint Commission on Accreditation of Healthcare Organizations (JCAHO) accreditation
+ American Osteopathic Hospital Association (AOHA) membership
○ American Osteopathic Association (AOA) accreditation
△ Commission on Accreditation of Rehabilitation Facilities (CARF) accreditation
Control codes 61, 63, 64, 71, 72 and 73 indicate hospitals listed by AOHA, but not registered by AHA. For definition of numerical codes, see page A6.

FERNDALE—Oakland County

☒ KINGSWOOD HOSPITAL, 10300 West Eight Mile Road, Zip 48220; tel. 810/398–3200; Kathleen Emrich Ed.D., R.N., Assistant Vice President **A**1 3 9 10 **F**19 21 22 34 35 41 52 53 54 55 58 59 65 71 **P**4 **S**9505 Henry Ford Health System — 23 22 64 1858 48 31364 0 10082 5143 164

FLINT—Genesee County

+ ○ △ GENESYS REGIONAL MEDICAL CENTER–FLINT OSTEOPATHIC CAMPUS, 3921 Beecher Road, Zip 48532–3699; tel. 810/762–4000; Young S. Suh, President **A**7 9 10 11 12 13 **F**1 3 4 6 7 8 10 11 12 13 15 16 17 18 19 21 22 23 25 26 27 28 29 30 31 32 33 34 35 37 39 40 41 42 43 44 45 46 48 49 51 53 54 56 57 58 60 63 65 67 68 70 71 73 74 **P**1 2 6 7 **S**5555 Sisters of St. Joseph Health System — 21 10 263 11976 172 104802 1516 89675 44037 1153

★ GENESYS REGIONAL MEDICAL CENTER–GENESEE MEMORIAL CAMPUS, 702 South Ballenger Highway, Zip 48532–3899; tel. 810/766–8800; Young S. Suh, President and Chief Executive Officer **A**9 10 **F**1 2 3 4 6 7 8 10 11 12 13 15 16 17 18 19 21 22 23 25 26 27 28 29 30 31 32 33 34 35 37 39 40 41 42 43 46 48 49 51 53 54 56 57 58 60 63 64 65 67 68 70 71 73 74 **P**1 2 6 7 **S**5555 Sisters of St. Joseph Health System — 21 45 40 172 1 11793 0 7842 3108 74

☒ GENESYS REGIONAL MEDICAL CENTER–ST. JOSEPH CAMPUS, 302 Kensington Avenue, Zip 48503–2000; tel. 810/762–8000; Young S. Suh, President **A**1 2 3 5 9 10 **F**1 2 3 4 6 7 8 10 11 12 15 16 17 18 19 21 22 23 25 26 27 28 29 30 31 32 33 34 35 37 39 40 41 42 43 44 45 46 48 49 51 53 54 56 57 58 63 64 65 67 68 70 71 73 74 **P**1 2 6 7 **S**5555 Sisters of St. Joseph Health System — 21 10 337 15463 211 194391 1590 122896 62947 1623

☒ HURLEY MEDICAL CENTER, One Hurley Plaza, Zip 48503–5993; tel. 810/257–9000; Phillip C. Dutcher, President and Chief Executive Officer **A**1 2 3 5 6 8 9 10 **F**3 4 7 8 9 10 11 12 13 14 15 16 17 18 19 20 21 22 24 25 26 27 28 29 30 31 32 33 34 35 37 38 39 40 41 42 43 44 45 46 47 48 49 51 52 53 54 55 56 57 58 59 60 61 63 65 66 67 68 69 70 71 73 **P**3 5 6 — 14 10 543 20112 335 285718 3266 195027 91012 2505

☒ △ MCLAREN REGIONAL MEDICAL CENTER, 401 South Ballenger Highway, Zip 48532–3685; tel. 810/762–2000; Philip A. Incarnati, President and Chief Executive Officer **A**1 2 3 5 7 8 9 10 **F**1 2 3 4 7 8 10 11 12 13 14 15 16 17 18 19 20 21 22 24 25 26 27 28 29 30 31 32 33 34 35 37 39 40 41 42 43 44 45 46 48 49 51 52 53 54 55 56 57 58 59 60 61 63 64 65 66 67 69 71 72 73 74 **P**4 6 — 23 10 436 16733 303 349720 981 163717 75118 1831

FRANKFORT—Benzie County

☒ PAUL OLIVER MEMORIAL HOSPITAL, 224 Park Avenue, Zip 49635; tel. 616/352–9621; James D. Austin, Administrator (Total facility includes 24 beds in nursing home–type unit) **A**1 9 10 **F**8 15 16 17 19 20 22 26 28 32 33 34 44 46 49 64 65 71 73 **P**7 **S**1465 Munson Healthcare — 23 10 48 395 27 19822 1 6020 2027 77

FREMONT—Newaygo County

☒ GERBER MEMORIAL HOSPITAL, 212 South Sullivan Street, Zip 49412; tel. 616/924–3300; Ned B. Hughes Jr., President **A**1 9 10 **F**7 8 14 15 17 19 22 30 32 33 34 37 39 40 41 42 44 45 46 49 52 54 55 56 57 58 71 73 74 — 23 10 73 2352 33 60840 306 20194 9937 368

GARDEN CITY—Wayne County

+ ○ GARDEN CITY HOSPITAL, 6245 North Inkster Road, Zip 48135; tel. 313/421–3300; Gary R. Ley, Chief Executive Officer **A**9 10 11 12 13 **F**2 3 7 8 10 11 12 17 19 22 27 28 29 33 34 35 37 38 39 40 41 42 44 46 48 49 51 60 65 66 67 71 72 73 **P**8 — 23 10 260 10248 198 75483 754 85485 40292 1288

GAYLORD—Otsego County

☒ OTSEGO MEMORIAL HOSPITAL, (Includes McReynolds Hall) 825 North Center Street, Zip 49735; tel. 517/732–2216; John L. MacLeod, Administrator and Chief Executive Officer (Total facility includes 34 beds in nursing home–type unit) **A**1 9 10 **F**8 14 15 16 19 22 24 26 28 29 30 34 35 37 39 40 41 44 45 46 49 51 60 63 64 65 71 73 — 23 10 87 1907 48 36399 231 11804 5339 200

GLADWIN—Gladwin County

☒ MIDMICHIGAN REGIONAL MEDICAL CENTER–GLADWIN, 455 South Quarter Street, Zip 48624; tel. 517/426–9286; Mark E. Bush, Vice President and Controller **A**1 9 10 **F**8 15 19 22 28 30 32 44 45 49 71 **S**0001 MidMichigan Regional Health System — 23 10 42 1410 19 31725 0 7962 3452 149

GOODRICH—Genesee County

☒ GENESYS REGIONAL MEDICAL CENTER–WHEELOCK MEMORIAL CAMPUS, 7280 State Road, Zip 48438; tel. 810/636–2221; Joseph W. Kyle, Vice President **A**1 9 10 **F**1 2 3 4 6 7 8 10 11 12 13 15 16 17 18 19 21 23 25 26 27 28 29 30 31 32 33 34 35 37 39 40 41 42 43 44 45 46 48 49 51 53 54 56 57 58 60 63 64 65 67 68 70 71 73 74 **P**1 2 6 7 **S**5555 Sisters of St. Joseph Health System — 23 10 31 680 8 20719 0 6325 2922 122

GRAND HAVEN—Ottawa County

☒ NORTH OTTAWA COMMUNITY HOSPITAL, 1309 Sheldon Road, Zip 49417–2488; tel. 616/842–3600; Fred Van Bemmelen, Chairman **A**1 9 10 **F**3 7 8 14 19 22 31 32 33 35 36 37 40 41 42 44 49 64 65 66 67 71 72 73 — 16 10 81 2669 28 142066 505 27251 11939 389

GRAND RAPIDS—Kent County

☒ BLODGETT MEMORIAL MEDICAL CENTER, 1840 Wealthy Street S.E., Zip 49506–2921; tel. 616/774–7444; Terrence Michael O'Rourke, President **A**1 2 3 5 8 9 10 **F**4 5 7 8 9 10 11 13 14 15 17 19 21 22 24 25 26 29 30 31 32 33 34 35 37 38 40 42 43 44 49 51 54 56 58 60 61 65 66 67 70 71 72 73 74 **P**1 5 6 — 23 10 328 15996 224 334327 2870 126629 58112 2192

☒ BUTTERWORTH HOSPITAL, 100 Michigan Street N.E., Zip 49503–2551; tel. 616/774–1774; Philip H. McCorkle Jr., Chief Executive Officer **A**1 2 3 5 8 9 10 **F**4 7 8 10 11 13 14 17 19 21 22 25 28 30 32 34 35 37 38 40 41 42 43 44 47 48 49 51 60 61 65 67 69 70 71 72 73 74 **P**6 — 23 10 529 25194 388 485179 5343 232817 111282 3448

Hospitals, U.S. / MICHIGAN

Hospital, Address, Telephone, Administrator, Approval, Facility, and Physician Codes, Health Care System	Classification Codes		Utilization Data					Expense (thousands) of dollars		Personnel
★ American Hospital Association (AHA) membership □ Joint Commission on Accreditation of Healthcare Organizations (JCAHO) accreditation + American Osteopathic Hospital Association (AOHA) membership ○ American Osteopathic Association (AOA) accreditation △ Commission on Accreditation of Rehabilitation Facilities (CARF) accreditation Control codes 61, 63, 64, 71, 72 and 73 indicate hospitals listed by AOHA, but not registered by AHA. For definition of numerical codes, see page A6	Control	Service	Beds	Admissions	Census	Outpatient Visits	Births	Total	Payroll	
★ FERGUSON HOSPITAL, (Diseases of the Colon and Rectum) 72 Sheldon Boulevard S.E., Zip 49503–4294; tel. 616/456–0202; Jack B. Carter, President (Nonreporting) **A**5 9	23	49	54	—	—	—	—	—	—	—
□ FOREST VIEW HOSPITAL, 1055 Medical Park Drive S.E., Zip 49546; tel. 616/942–9610; Gerard Cyranowski, Managing Director **A**1 10 **F**25 52 53 55 56 58 59 65 67 **S**9555 Universal Health Services, Inc.	33	22	62	832	26	4802	0	5690	2434	99
★ KENT COMMUNITY HOSPITAL COMPLEX, (Psychiatric/Chemical Dependency) 750 Fuller Avenue N.E., Zip 49503–1995; tel. 616/336–3300; Lori Portfleet, Executive Director (Total facility includes 294 beds in nursing home–type unit) **A**1 9 10 **F**2 3 14 15 52 58 59 64 65 73	13	49	390	2517	334	—	0	24025	12562	482
★ △ MARY FREE BED HOSPITAL AND REHABILITATION CENTER, 235 Wealthy S.E., Zip 49503–5299; tel. 616/242–0300; William H. Blessing, President **A**1 7 9 10 **F**15 16 25 34 45 48 49 65 67 73	23	46	80	648	52	42824	0	25136	14366	478
+ ○ △ METROPOLITAN HOSPITAL, 1919 Boston Street S.E., Zip 49506, Mailing Address: P.O. Box 158, Zip 49501–0158; tel. 616/247–7200; Michael D. Faas, President **A**7 9 10 11 12 13 **F**1 3 4 7 8 10 12 14 15 16 17 19 21 22 23 24 25 26 28 29 30 31 32 33 34 35 37 39 40 41 42 44 48 49 51 53 54 55 56 57 58 59 60 61 63 65 66 67 71 73 74 **P**3 7	23	10	201	7693	112	118843	962	66258	30915	859
★ PINE REST CHRISTIAN HOSPITAL, 300 68th Street S.E., Zip 49501–0165, Mailing Address: P.O. Box 165, Zip 49501–0165; tel. 616/455–5000; Daniel L. Holwerda, President and Chief Executive Officer **A**1 3 5 9 10 **F**3 12 14 15 16 17 26 32 41 45 52 53 54 55 56 57 58 59 65 67 73 **P**6	23	22	118	1608	67	60748	0	28610	17073	531
★ SAINT MARY'S HEALTH SERVICES, 200 Jefferson Avenue S.E., Zip 49503; tel. 616/774–6399; Nancy Conlee Hart, President and Chief Executive Officer **A**1 2 3 5 9 10 **F**7 8 10 12 14 15 16 17 19 20 21 22 24 25 28 29 30 31 32 34 35 39 40 42 44 45 49 51 52 54 55 56 57 60 63 64 65 66 69 70 71 73 74 **P**3 **S**5165 Mercy Health Services	21	10	250	11241	153	243392	2250	123657	46031	1898
GRAYLING—Crawford County										
★ MERCY HOSPITAL, 1100 Michigan Avenue, Zip 49738–1398; tel. 517/348–5461; Dennis J. Renander, President and Chief Executive Officer (Total facility includes 40 beds in nursing home–type unit) **A**1 9 10 **F**7 8 10 11 15 16 17 19 22 28 29 32 33 34 39 40 44 49 51 64 65 71 73 **P**8 **S**5165 Mercy Health Services	21	10	130	2887	74	47220	276	23155	9084	350
GREENVILLE—Montcalm County										
★ UNITED MEMORIAL HOSPITAL, 615 South Bower Street, Zip 48838–2614, Mailing Address: P.O. Box 430, Zip 48838–0430; tel. 616/754–4691; Michael Mihora, Chief Executive Officer (Total facility includes 40 beds in nursing home–type unit) **A**1 9 10 **F**7 8 14 15 16 19 21 22 25 28 30 31 34 37 40 41 42 44 46 49 63 64 65 71 73 74 **P**6	23	10	83	2139	57	79103	207	16915	6370	282
GROSSE POINTE—Wayne County										
★ BON SECOURS HOSPITAL, 468 Cadieux Road, Zip 48230; tel. 313/343–1000; Henry Devries Jr., Chief Executive Officer **A**1 3 5 9 10 **F**3 7 8 10 15 16 17 18 19 21 22 24 25 26 27 28 29 30 31 32 33 34 35 36 37 39 40 42 44 45 46 52 53 63 65 67 71 73 74 **P**3 **S**5085 Bon Secours Health System, Inc.	21	10	256	10745	177	125499	1533	94476	48474	1155
GROSSE POINTE FARMS—Wayne County										
★ HENRY FORD COTTAGE HOSPITAL, 159 Kercheval Avenue, Zip 48236–3692; tel. 313/884–8600; Gregory J. Vasse, President and Chief Executive Officer **A**1 3 10 **F**1 7 8 14 18 19 22 27 28 29 30 31 33 34 37 39 40 42 44 45 46 48 49 52 54 55 56 57 58 59 63 65 66 67 71 72 73 74 **P**6 **S**9505 Henry Ford Health System	23	10	175	4871	85	76166	570	41438	18662	688
HANCOCK—Houghton County										
★ PORTAGE HOSPITAL, (Formerly Portage View Hospital) 200 Michigan Avenue, Zip 49930; tel. 906/487–8000; James Bogan, Chief Executive Officer (Total facility includes 30 beds in nursing home–type unit) **A**1 9 10 **F**1 7 8 12 13 14 15 16 17 19 22 26 28 30 31 32 33 34 35 36 37 39 40 41 44 45 49 51 54 56 57 58 61 63 65 66 67 71 73 74 **P**6	23	10	74	2179	52	54810	403	14922	7068	233
HARBOR BEACH—Huron County										
★ HARBOR BEACH COMMUNITY HOSPITAL, Broad and First Streets, Zip 48441–1236, Mailing Address: P.O. Box 40, Zip 48441; tel. 517/479–3201; Pauline Siemen R.N., President (Total facility includes 40 beds in nursing home–type unit) **A**9 10 **F**8 14 15 19 22 34 40 44 49 64 71	23	10	67	424	43	14784	30	4477	2537	78
HARRISON TOWNSHIP—Ottawa County										
★ △ ST. JOHN HOSPITAL–MACOMB CENTER, 26755 Ballard Road, Zip 48045–2458; tel. 810/465–5501; David Sessions, Administrator **A**1 7 10 **F**2 3 4 6 7 8 10 11 12 14 15 16 17 18 19 20 21 22 23 25 26 27 28 29 30 31 32 33 34 35 36 37 38 40 41 42 43 44 45 46 47 48 49 51 52 54 55 56 57 58 59 60 63 64 65 66 67 69 70 71 72 73 74 **P**5 8 **S**5555 Sisters of St. Joseph Health System	21	10	65	1311	33	21087	0	14106	7355	267
HASTINGS—Barry County										
□ PENNOCK HOSPITAL, 1009 West Green Street, Zip 49058–1790; tel. 616/945–3451; Daniel Hamilton, Chief Executive Officer **A**1 9 10 **F**6 7 8 10 11 12 14 15 16 19 21 22 24 26 28 29 31 32 33 34 35 37 39 40 41 42 44 45 46 48 49 56 62 63 65 66 67 71 73	23	10	89	2928	43	99206	337	21019	9091	350
HILLSDALE—Hillsdale County										
★ HILLSDALE COMMUNITY HEALTH CENTER, 168 South Howell Street, Zip 49242–2081; tel. 517/437–4451; Charles A. Bianchi, President **A**1 9 10 **F**7 8 12 14 15 16 17 19 21 22 26 27 28 29 30 31 34 35 36 37 39 40 41 44 46 49 51 53 54 56 58 65 66 67 71 72 73 74	14	10	68	2347	26	73210	378	15491	5971	242

Hospitals, U.S. / MICHIGAN

Hospital, Address, Telephone, Administrator, Approval, Facility, and Physician Codes, Health Care System ★ American Hospital Association (AHA) membership ☐ Joint Commission on Accreditation of Healthcare Organizations (JCAHO) accreditation + American Osteopathic Hospital Association (AOHA) membership ○ American Osteopathic Association (AOA) accreditation △ Commission on Accreditation of Rehabilitation Facilities (CARF) accreditation Control codes 61, 63, 64, 71, 72 and 73 indicate hospitals listed by AOHA, but not registered by AHA. For definition of numerical codes, see page A6	Classification Codes		Utilization Data					Expense (thousands) of dollars		
	Control	Service	Beds	Admissions	Census	Outpatient Visits	Births	Total	Payroll	Personnel
HOLLAND—Ottawa County ★ HOLLAND COMMUNITY HOSPITAL, 602 Michigan Avenue, Zip 49423–4999; tel. 616/392–5141; Judeth N. Javorek, President and Chief Executive Officer **A**1 9 10 **F**7 11 14 15 19 20 21 22 28 32 34 35 36 37 40 42 44 45 47 49 52 53 54 55 56 57 58 59 60 63 65 67 71 72 73 **P**8	23	10	177	7394	86	89664	1568	48914	21152	725
HOWELL—Livingston County ★ MCPHERSON HOSPITAL, 620 Byron Road, Zip 48843–1093; tel. 517/545–6000; Robert B. Carbeck M.D., President and Chief Executive Officer **A**1 9 10 **F**3 7 8 12 15 16 17 19 20 22 32 34 37 40 41 44 49 51 58 65 71 72 73 **P**5 **S**5165 Mercy Health Services	21	10	85	3347	37	151813	537	34163	15907	634
HUDSON—Lenawee County ★ THORN HOSPITAL, 458 Cross Street, Zip 49247; tel. 517/448–2371; Rodney M. Nelson, President and Chief Executive Officer **A**9 10 **F**15 37 44 67 71	23	10	22	282	2	2332	0	4561	1892	60
IONIA—Ionia County ★ IONIA COUNTY MEMORIAL HOSPITAL, 479 Lafayette Street, Zip 48846–1834, Mailing Address: Box 1001, Zip 48846–1899; tel. 616/527–4200; Evonne G. Ulmer, Chief Executive Officer **A**1 9 10 **F**3 7 8 11 14 15 17 19 22 26 28 29 30 31 32 33 34 35 37 39 40 41 42 44 45 46 49 51 53 54 55 56 57 58 65 66 67 71 72 73 **P**6	14	10	77	1290	18	62683	187	8732	4303	151
IRON MOUNTAIN—Dickinson County ★ DICKINSON COUNTY MEMORIAL HOSPITAL SYSTEM, (Includes Anderson Memorial Hospital, Main Street, Norway, Michigan, Zip 49870; tel. 906/563–9243) 400 Woodward Avenue, Zip 49801–4696; tel. 906/774–1313; John Schon, Administrator and Chief Executive Officer **A**1 9 10 **F**7 8 15 16 19 21 22 26 28 34 35 37 40 41 42 44 45 46 49 51 58 63 65 66 67 71 72 73 **P**3	13	10	99	4572	55	78920	591	32159	16780	490
★ VETERANS AFFAIRS MEDICAL CENTER, H Street, Zip 49801; tel. 906/774–3300; Glen W. Grippen, Director (Total facility includes 40 beds in nursing home–type unit) **A**1 5 9 **F**2 3 8 10 11 12 17 18 19 20 21 22 23 25 26 27 28 30 31 33 34 35 37 39 41 42 43 44 45 46 48 49 50 51 52 54 55 56 57 58 59 60 64 65 69 71 73 74 **P**6 **S**9295 Department of Veterans Affairs	45	10	160	2432	109	40863	0	28002	14679	394
IRON RIVER—Iron County ★ IRON COUNTY GENERAL HOSPITAL, 1400 West Ice Lake Road, Zip 49935; tel. 906/265–6121; Claude Chatterton, Administrator and Chief Executive Officer **A**1 9 10 **F**8 15 19 22 24 26 30 34 37 42 44 49 51 56 63 65 71 72	13	10	36	814	12	20948	0	6234	2583	103
IRONWOOD—Gogebic County ★ GRAND VIEW HOSPITAL, N10561 Grand View Lane, Zip 49938–9622; tel. 906/932–2525; Wayne P. Hellerstedt, Executive Director **A**1 9 10 **F**7 11 14 15 16 17 19 21 22 27 28 30 32 33 34 35 39 40 41 42 44 45 49 61 65 66 67 71 72 73 74 **P**8	23	10	46	1710	26	45433	229	13667	8050	198
ISHPEMING—Marquette County ☐ BELL MEMORIAL HOSPITAL, 101 South Fourth Street, Zip 49849; tel. 906/486–4431; Kevin P. Calhoun, Chief Executive Officer **A**1 9 10 **F**7 8 11 15 19 21 22 25 28 33 34 40 41 44 49 61 71 72 73	23	10	64	1471	14	41771	166	10908	5316	171
JACKSON—Jackson County ★ + ○ DOCTORS HOSPITAL OF JACKSON, 110 North Elm Avenue, Zip 49202–3595; tel. 517/787–1440; Michael J. Falatko, President and Chief Executive Officer **A**9 10 11 **F**8 14 15 16 19 21 22 26 28 30 31 33 34 35 37 39 41 42 44 45 46 49 51 56 63 65 66 67 71 72 73	23	10	71	1008	12	33612	0	13876	5248	187
★ DUANE L. WATERS HOSPITAL, 3857 Cooper Street, Zip 49201; tel. 517/780–5600; Eric P. Jacobson, Administrator **A**1 **F**4 10 11 18 19 20 21 22 23 24 25 26 30 31 33 34 35 37 40 42 43 44 49 50 52 54 56 57 58 60 63 65 67 71 **P**6	12	11	86	1441	61	—	0	19544	13466	—
☐ W. A. FOOTE MEMORIAL HOSPITAL, 205 North East Avenue, Zip 49201–1789; tel. 517/788–4800; Georgia R. Fojtasek, President **A**1 9 10 **F**2 3 7 8 10 11 12 14 15 16 17 18 19 21 22 24 26 28 29 30 33 34 35 36 37 39 40 41 42 44 45 46 49 51 52 53 54 55 56 57 58 59 63 65 67 71 73	23	10	365	16272	210	306756	1845	98785	48237	1581
KALAMAZOO—Kalamazoo County ★ △ BORGESS MEDICAL CENTER, 1521 Gull Road, Zip 49001–1640; tel. 616/383–7000; R. Timothy Stack FACHE, President **A**1 2 3 5 7 9 10 **F**3 4 5 7 8 10 11 12 13 14 15 16 17 18 19 20 21 22 23 24 26 28 29 30 31 32 33 34 35 37 39 40 41 42 43 44 45 46 48 49 51 52 53 54 55 56 57 58 59 60 63 65 66 67 69 71 72 73 74 **P**3 5 6 **S**5555 Sisters of St. Joseph Health System	21	10	351	15303	229	281812	1479	171715	66545	1879
★ BRONSON METHODIST HOSPITAL, 252 East Lovell Street, Zip 49007–5345; tel. 616/341–6000; Patric E. Ludwig, President **A**1 2 3 5 6 9 10 **F**1 2 3 4 6 7 8 9 10 11 12 13 14 15 16 17 18 19 20 21 22 23 24 25 26 27 28 29 30 31 33 34 35 37 38 39 40 41 42 43 44 45 46 47 48 49 51 52 53 54 55 56 57 58 59 60 62 64 65 66 67 68 70 71 72 73 74 **P**2 5 7 8 **S**0595 Bronson Healthcare Group, Inc.	23	10	312	14510	202	266637	2870	156950	80011	1834
☐ KALAMAZOO REGIONAL PSYCHIATRIC HOSPITAL, 1312 Oakland Drive, Zip 49008; tel. 616/337–3000; James Coleman, Director **A**1 9 10 **F**14 15 16 20 22 24 26 27 30 41 45 46 51 52 53 54 55 56 57 65 73 74 **P**1	12	22	369	1081	264	0	0	47832	24842	696
KALKASKA—Kalkaska County ★ KALKASKA MEMORIAL HEALTH CENTER, 419 Coral Street, Zip 49646, Mailing Address: P.O. Box 249, Zip 49646–0249; tel. 616/258–9142; James D. Austin, Administrator (Total facility includes 68 beds in nursing home–type unit) **A**9 10 **F**8 14 16 19 22 26 28 32 33 34 41 45 49 53 64 65 67 71 72 73 74 **P**5 **S**1465 Munson Healthcare	16	10	81	337	68	28804	0	7092	3090	100

© 1995 AHA Guide

Hospitals, U.S. / MICHIGAN

Hospital, Address, Telephone, Administrator, Approval, Facility, and Physician Codes, Health Care System	Classification Codes		Utilization Data					Expense (thousands) of dollars		
★ American Hospital Association (AHA) membership ☐ Joint Commission on Accreditation of Healthcare Organizations (JCAHO) accreditation + American Osteopathic Hospital Association (AOHA) membership ○ American Osteopathic Association (AOA) accreditation △ Commission on Accreditation of Rehabilitation Facilities (CARF) accreditation Control codes 61, 63, 64, 71, 72 and 73 indicate hospitals listed by AOHA, but not registered by AHA. For definition of numerical codes, see page A6	Control	Service	Beds	Admissions	Census	Outpatient Visits	Births	Total	Payroll	Personnel
L'ANSE—Baraga County										
★ BARAGA COUNTY MEMORIAL HOSPITAL, 770 North Main Street, Zip 49946–1195; tel. 906/524–6166; John P. Tembreull, Administrator (Total facility includes 28 beds in nursing home–type unit) **A**1 9 10 **F**8 15 16 21 22 30 32 42 44 58 64 65 67 71	13	10	52	898	38	16374	0	6852	2895	111
LAKEVIEW—Montcalm County										
☐ KELSEY MEMORIAL HOSPITAL, 418 Washington Avenue, Zip 48850; tel. 517/352–7211; Thomas Hicks, Chief Executive Officer (Total facility includes 42 beds in nursing home–type unit) **A**1 9 10 **F**16 19 20 22 25 33 34 39 40 41 44 48 49 64 65 71 72 74 **P**6	23	10	71	964	53	24055	156	6621	3194	171
LANSING—Eaton County										
INGHAM MEDICAL CENTER See Michigan Affiliated Health System										
LANSING GENERAL HOSPITAL See Michigan Affiliated Health System										
★ △ MICHIGAN AFFILIATED HEALTH SYSTEM, (Includes Ingham Medical Center, Lansing, Michigan, Zip 48910–2819; tel. 517/334–2121; Lansing General Hospital, 2727 South Pennsylvania Avenue, Lansing, Michigan, Zip 48910; tel. 517/372–8220) 401 West Greenlawn Avenue, Zip 48910–2819; tel. 517/334–2121; Edward B. McRee, President **A**1 3 7 8 9 10 **F**2 3 4 6 7 8 9 10 11 12 13 17 18 19 20 21 22 23 24 26 28 29 30 31 32 33 34 35 36 37 38 39 40 41 42 43 44 45 46 47 48 49 51 52 53 54 55 56 57 58 59 60 61 62 63 64 65 66 67 68 70 71 72 73 74 **P**5 8	23	10	369	14508	247	144832	856	175899	79116	2715
★ SPARROW HOSPITAL, 1215 East Michigan Avenue, Zip 48912, Mailing Address: P.O. Box 30480, Zip 48909–7980; tel. 517/483–2700; Joseph F. Damore, President **A**1 2 3 5 9 10 12 **F**2 3 4 6 7 8 9 10 11 12 13 14 15 16 17 18 19 21 22 23 28 29 30 32 33 34 35 36 37 38 39 40 41 42 43 44 46 47 48 49 51 52 53 54 55 56 57 58 59 60 61 63 65 67 68 70 71 72 73 74 **P**1 6	23	10	382	19662	290	191785	4255	180630	90140	2751
★ ○ ST. LAWRENCE HOSPITAL AND HEALTHCARE SERVICES, 1210 West Saginaw Street, Zip 48915–1999; tel. 517/372–3610; Arthur Knueppel, President (Total facility includes 178 beds in nursing home–type unit) **A**1 2 3 5 9 10 11 12 **F**2 3 5 7 8 14 15 16 17 18 19 21 22 24 25 26 28 30 31 32 33 34 35 37 40 41 42 44 49 52 53 54 56 57 58 59 64 65 66 71 73 74 **P**4 5 6 8 **S**5165 Mercy Health Services	21	10	389	7497	295	286342	1255	92662	43146	1425
LAPEER—Lapeer County										
☐ LAPEER REGIONAL HOSPITAL, 1375 North Main Street, Zip 48446; tel. 313/667–5500; Donald C. Kooy, President and Chief Executive Officer **A**1 9 10 **F**2 3 4 7 8 9 10 11 12 13 15 16 17 18 19 20 21 22 24 25 28 30 32 33 34 35 38 40 41 42 44 45 46 47 49 51 52 53 54 55 56 57 58 59 60 63 64 65 66 67 71 72 73 74 **P**4 6	23	10	178	4968	81	191510	625	46004	20693	705
LAURIUM—Houghton County										
★ KEWEENAW MEMORIAL MEDICAL CENTER, (Formerly Calumet Public Hospital) 205 Osceola Street, Zip 49913–2199; tel. 906/337–3100; Rick Wright CPA, FACHE, President and Chief Executive Officer **A**1 9 10 **F**7 8 11 12 16 17 19 20 21 22 31 37 40 44 46 65 71	23	10	48	1230	20	25245	68	8716	4277	152
LINCOLN PARK—Wayne County										
★ OAKWOOD HOSPITAL DOWNRIVER CENTER – LINCOLN PARK, (Formerly Oakwood Downriver Medical Center) 25750 West Outer Drive, Zip 48146–1574; tel. 313/382–6000; Mindy L. Richards, Administrator **A**1 9 10 **F**1 2 3 4 6 7 8 10 11 12 13 15 16 17 18 19 20 21 22 23 24 25 26 27 28 29 30 31 32 33 34 35 37 38 39 40 41 42 43 44 45 46 48 49 50 52 53 54 55 56 57 58 59 60 61 62 63 64 65 66 67 68 69 70 71 72 73 74 **P**4 5 **S**1165 Oakwood Healthcare System	23	10	49	1708	25	58236	3	12011	5722	239
☐ VENCOR HOSPITAL–DETROIT, 26400 West Outer Drive, Zip 48146; tel. 313/594–6000; Joseph R. Gordon, Administrator (Nonreporting) **A**1 9 10 **S**0026 Vencor, Incorporated	23	10	218	—	—	—	—	—	—	—
LIVONIA—Wayne County										
★ ST. MARY HOSPITAL, 36475 Five Mile Road, Zip 48154–1988; tel. 313/464–4800; Sister Mary Modesta, President and Chief Executive Officer **A**1 9 10 **F**2 3 4 5 6 7 8 10 11 12 13 15 17 18 19 20 21 22 23 24 27 28 29 30 31 32 33 34 35 37 38 39 40 41 42 43 44 45 46 47 48 49 50 52 54 55 56 57 58 59 60 63 64 65 67 69 70 71 73 74 **P**4 5	21	10	261	9541	176	134224	433	80497	43364	1234
LUDINGTON—Mason County										
★ MEMORIAL MEDICAL CENTER OF WEST MICHIGAN, One Atkinson Drive, Zip 49431–1999; tel. 616/845–2384; Robert C. Marquardt, President **A**1 9 10 **F**7 8 12 14 15 17 19 21 22 31 32 34 35 37 39 40 41 42 44 45 49 52 54 55 56 57 63 65 66 67 71 73 74	23	10	85	3159	44	58722	378	21531	9869	279
MADISON HEIGHTS—Oakland County										
★ MADISON COMMUNITY HOSPITAL, 30671 Stephenson Highway, Zip 48071; tel. 810/588–8000; Charles Frederick Pinkerman, Administrator **A**1 9 10 **F**8 15 16 19 20 21 26 27 28 30 32 35 37 41 44 46 49 52 56 57 59 65 67 68 71	23	10	56	1261	26	23812	0	9751	4924	152
☐ + ○ OAKLAND GENERAL HEALTH SYSTEM, 27351 Dequindre, Zip 48071; tel. 313/967–7000; Anthony R. Tersigni Ed.D., FACHE, President and Chief Executive Officer **A**1 9 10 11 12 13 **F**3 4 6 7 8 10 12 13 14 15 16 17 18 19 20 21 22 23 24 25 26 27 28 29 30 31 32 33 34 37 43 44 45 46 49 51 52 53 54 55 56 57 58 59 60 63 65 66 67 69 70 71 72 73 74 **P**3 8	23	10	166	5903	123	44249	0	55685	26276	724
MANISTEE—Manistee County										
★ WEST SHORE HOSPITAL, 1465 East Parkdale Avenue, Zip 49660; tel. 616/723–3501; Burton O. Parks III, Administrator **A**1 9 10 **F**7 8 10 13 16 17 18 19 21 22 24 28 30 31 33 34 35 37 39 40 41 42 44 45 51 56 63 65 67 68 71 73 74	13	10	54	1629	25	35727	190	14180	6853	233

Hospitals, U.S. / MICHIGAN

Hospital, Address, Telephone, Administrator, Approval, Facility, and Physician Codes, Health Care System	Classification Codes		Utilization Data					Expense (thousands) of dollars		
★ American Hospital Association (AHA) membership ☐ Joint Commission on Accreditation of Healthcare Organizations (JCAHO) accreditation + American Osteopathic Hospital Association (AOHA) membership ○ American Osteopathic Association (AOA) accreditation △ Commission on Accreditation of Rehabilitation Facilities (CARF) accreditation Control codes 61, 63, 64, 71, 72 and 73 indicate hospitals listed by AOHA, but not registered by AHA. For definition of numerical codes, see page A6	Control	Service	Beds	Admissions	Census	Outpatient Visits	Births	Total	Payroll	Personnel
MANISTIQUE—Schoolcraft County ★ SCHOOLCRAFT MEMORIAL HOSPITAL, 500 Main Street, Zip 49854–0000; tel. 906/341–3200; David B. Jahn, Administrator **A**1 9 10 **F**2 3 4 7 8 9 10 11 15 17 18 19 20 21 22 23 24 26 28 29 30 31 32 33 34 35 37 38 39 40 41 42 43 44 45 46 47 48 49 50 51 52 53 54 55 56 57 58 59 60 63 64 65 66 67 70 71 73 74 **P**4	13	10	38	569	5	16867	144	5904	2700	95
MARLETTE—Sanilac County ★ MARLETTE COMMUNITY HOSPITAL, 2770 Main Street, Zip 48453–0307, Mailing Address: P.O. Box 307, Zip 48453–0307; tel. 517/635–7491; David S. McEwen, Administrator (Total facility includes 43 beds in nursing home–type unit) **A**1 9 10 **F**1 14 15 16 19 21 22 26 30 33 36 37 42 44 45 62 64 65 71 **S**0002 Quorum Health Group/Quorum Health Resources	23	10	71	929	50	25633	0	10475	5128	232
MARQUETTE—Marquette County ★ △ MARQUETTE GENERAL HOSPITAL, 420 West Magnetic Street, Zip 49855; tel. 906/228–9440; Robert C. Neldberg, Chief Executive Officer and Administrator **A** 1 2 3 5 7 9 10 **F**2 3 4 7 8 10 11 13 15 16 17 18 19 21 22 23 24 25 28 29 30 32 34 35 37 38 39 40 41 42 43 44 45 46 48 49 51 52 53 54 55 56 57 58 59 60 63 65 66 67 70 71 72 73 74 **P**6	23	10	320	10462	189	210795	600	118649	60295	1742
MARSHALL—Calhoun County ★ OAKLAWN HOSPITAL, 200 North Madison Street, Zip 49068; tel. 616/781–4271; Rob Covert, Administrator **A**1 9 10 **F**3 4 5 7 8 10 12 15 16 17 19 21 22 24 29 30 31 32 33 34 35 36 37 39 40 41 43 44 45 46 49 52 54 56 58 61 63 65 66 71 73	23	10	94	2445	29	56636	483	18566	9179	307
MIDLAND—Midland County ★ △ MIDMICHIGAN REGIONAL MEDICAL CENTER, 4005 Orchard Drive, Zip 48670; tel. 517/839–3000; David A. Reece, President **A**1 2 3 5 7 10 **F**6 7 8 10 11 12 15 16 19 20 21 22 26 27 28 29 30 31 32 33 34 36 37 39 40 41 42 44 45 46 48 49 51 52 54 55 56 57 58 60 62 64 65 66 67 71 72 73 74 **P**6 8 **S**0001 MidMichigan Regional Health System	23	10	221	9890	153	157463	1255	104677	46247	1369
MONROE—Monroe County ★ MERCY MEMORIAL HOSPITAL, 718 North Macomb Street, Zip 48161–2930, Mailing Address: P.O. Box 67, Zip 48161; tel. 313/241–1700; Richard S. Hiltz, President (Total facility includes 70 beds in nursing home–type unit) **A**1 9 10 **F**1 2 3 4 5 6 7 8 9 10 11 12 13 14 15 16 17 18 19 20 21 22 23 24 25 26 27 28 29 30 31 32 33 34 35 36 37 38 39 40 41 42 43 44 45 46 47 48 49 50 51 52 53 54 55 56 57 58 59 60 61 62 63 64 65 66 67 68 69 70 71 72 73 74	23	10	246	7504	172	75752	846	58997	27652	843
MORENCI—Lenawee County ☐ MORENCI AREA HOSPITAL, 13101 Sims Highway, Zip 49256–1099; tel. 517/458–2236; Cecelia A. Carpenter, Chief Executive Officer and Chief Operating Officer **A**1 9 10 **F**15 16 22 28 30 36 37 39 42 44 46 49 66 71	14	10	16	178	2	9240	0	2041	891	47
MOUNT CLEMENS—Macomb County ★ + ○ MOUNT CLEMENS GENERAL HOSPITAL, 1000 Harrington Boulevard, Zip 48043–2992; tel. 810/466–8000; Ralph J. La Gro, Chief Executive Officer **A**9 10 11 12 13 **F**4 7 8 10 12 13 15 16 17 18 19 20 21 22 24 25 26 27 28 29 30 31 32 33 34 35 37 39 40 41 42 43 44 45 46 49 51 61 65 66 67 68 70 71 72 73 74 **P**6 ST. JOSEPH'S MERCY HOSPITAL–EAST See St. Joseph's Mercy Hospitals and Health Services, Clinton Township	23	10	264	10769	168	113265	1460	123066	59453	1568
MOUNT PLEASANT—Isabella County ★ + ○ CENTRAL MICHIGAN COMMUNITY HOSPITAL, 1221 South Drive, Zip 48858–3234; tel. 517/772–6700; Mark A. Cwiek, President and Chief Executive Officer **A**1 9 10 11 **F**8 14 15 16 19 20 21 22 24 25 28 29 30 31 32 33 34 35 37 39 40 41 44 48 49 52 53 54 55 57 59 67 71 72 73 74 **P**8	23	10	118	3681	46	89404	346	27239	13189	442
MUNISING—Alger County ☐ MUNISING MEMORIAL HOSPITAL, Sand Point Road, Zip 49862, Mailing Address: Route 1, Box 501, Zip 49862; tel. 906/387–4110; Carl J. Velte, Chief Executive Officer (Nonreporting) **A**1 9 10	23	10	40	—	—	—	—	—	—	—
MUSKEGON—Muskegon County ★ HACKLEY HOSPITAL, 1700 Clinton Street, Zip 49443–3302, Mailing Address: P.O. Box 3302, Zip 49443–3302; tel. 616/726–3511; Gordon A. Mudler, President and Chief Executive Officer **A**1 2 9 10 **F**7 8 10 12 14 15 16 19 21 22 26 27 29 30 31 34 35 37 40 41 42 44 46 48 49 51 52 55 56 57 59 60 63 65 66 67 71 72 73 74 **P**4 5 6 MERCY HOSPITAL See Muskegon Mercy Community Healthcare System	23	10	228	8949	138	323042	1425	66851	30657	1051
+ ○ MUSKEGON GENERAL HOSPITAL, 1700 Oak Avenue, Zip 49442; tel. 616/773–3311; Roger Spoelman, President **A**9 10 11 12 13 **F**4 7 8 10 14 15 16 19 21 22 24 25 27 28 29 30 31 32 33 35 37 40 41 44 48 49 51 63 65 66 67 71 73 74 **P**8	23	10	127	3933	50	59897	1002	29393	12621	337
★ MUSKEGON MERCY COMMUNITY HEALTHCARE SYSTEM, (Formerly Mercy Hospital) 1500 East Sherman Boulevard, Zip 49443, Mailing Address: P.O. Box 358, Zip 49443–0358; tel. 616/739–9341; Sandra Bennett Bruce, President and Chief Executive Officer **A**1 9 10 **F**2 3 4 8 10 11 12 14 15 16 17 19 20 21 22 24 26 27 28 29 30 31 32 33 34 35 36 37 39 42 43 44 45 46 48 49 51 54 55 56 57 58 59 60 62 64 65 66 67 68 69 71 72 73 **P**1 5 6 8 **S**5165 Mercy Health Services	23	10	217	5511	95	202725	0	74469	26090	921

© 1995 AHA Guide

Hospitals, U.S. / MICHIGAN

Hospital, Address, Telephone, Administrator, Approval, Facility, and Physician Codes, Health Care System	Classification Codes		Utilization Data					Expense (thousands) of dollars		
★ American Hospital Association (AHA) membership □ Joint Commission on Accreditation of Healthcare Organizations (JCAHO) accreditation + American Osteopathic Hospital Association (AOHA) membership ○ American Osteopathic Association (AOA) accreditation △ Commission on Accreditation of Rehabilitation Facilities (CARF) accreditation Control codes 61, 63, 64, 71, 72 and 73 indicate hospitals listed by AOHA, but not registered by AHA. For definition of numerical codes, see page A6	Control	Service	Beds	Admissions	Census	Outpatient Visits	Births	Total	Payroll	Personnel
NEW BALTIMORE—Macomb County										
★ HARBOR OAKS HOSPITAL, 35031 23 Mile Road, Zip 48047; tel. 810/725–5777; Gary J. La Hood, Administrator and Chief Executive Officer (Nonreporting) A1 9 10	32	22	64	—	—	—	—	—	—	—
NEWBERRY—Luce County										
★ HELEN NEWBERRY JOY HOSPITAL, (Includes Helen Newberry Joy Hospital Annex) 502 West Harrie Street, Zip 49868–0070; tel. 906/293–9200; Bruce C. Huron, Administrator (Nonreporting) A1 9 10	13	10	86	—	—	—	—	—	—	—
NILES—Berrien County										
★ PAWATING HOSPITAL, 31 North St. Joseph Avenue, Zip 49120–2287; tel. 616/683–5510; Gerald W. Dechert, Senior Vice President and Chief Operating Officer A1 9 10 F3 7 8 12 15 16 19 21 22 30 32 33 34 35 36 37 40 41 42 44 49 65 71 73 P8 S0056 Lakeland Regional Health System, Inc.	23	10	106	3465	41	218374	403	26800	12369	392
NORTHPORT—Leelanau County										
★ LEELANAU MEMORIAL HOSPITAL, 215 South High Street, Zip 49670, Mailing Address: P.O. Box 217, Zip 49670; tel. 616/386–5101; James Packard, Administrator (Total facility includes 72 beds in nursing home–type unit) A1 9 10 F1 8 15 17 22 24 26 28 30 33 34 36 39 41 44 49 51 56 64 65 66 71 72 73 P3 5 6 7 8 S1465 Munson Healthcare	23	10	95	286	59	11394	0	4742	2396	82
NORTHVILLE—Wayne County										
□ HAWTHORN CENTER, 18471 Haggerty Road, Zip 48167; tel. 810/349–3000; Hubert A. Carbone M.D., Interim Director A1 3 5 9 F12 14 18 39 52 53 54 55 56 58	12	52	108	102	75	3726	0	17417	11056	266
□ NORTHVILLE REGIONAL PSYCHIATRIC HOSPITAL, 41001 West Seven Mile Road, Zip 48167; tel. 313/349–1800; Richard Fletcher, Administrative Officer (Nonreporting) A1 10	12	22	754	—	—	—	—	—	—	—
NORWAY—Dickinson County										
ANDERSON MEMORIAL HOSPITAL See Dickinson County Memorial Hospital System, Iron Mountain										
ONTONAGON—Ontonagon County										
□ ONTONAGON MEMORIAL HOSPITAL, 601 Seventh Street, Zip 49953; tel. 906/884–4134; Fred Nelson, Administrator (Nonreporting) A1 9 10	14	10	87	—	—	—	—	—	—	—
OWOSSO—Shiawassee County										
★ MEMORIAL HOSPITAL, 826 West King Street, Zip 48867–2198; tel. 517/723–5211; Margaret S. Gulick R.N., Administrator (Total facility includes 16 beds in nursing home–type unit) A1 9 10 F1 7 8 11 12 15 16 19 21 22 27 28 30 32 33 35 36 37 40 41 42 44 45 46 48 49 52 56 58 59 64 65 67 71 72 73 P1 3 5 6	23	10	148	4889	79	127059	537	39791	21667	655
PAW PAW—Van Buren County										
★ LAKE VIEW COMMUNITY HOSPITAL, 408 Hazen Street, Zip 49079, Mailing Address: Box 209, Zip 49079–0209; tel. 616/657–3141; Sue E. Johnson, President and Chief Executive Officer (Total facility includes 120 beds in nursing home–type unit) A1 9 10 F7 8 14 15 16 19 20 22 32 33 34 35 39 40 41 44 45 48 49 52 57 61 64 65 67 71 72 73 P3 4 5 S0002 Quorum Health Group/Quorum Health Resources	16	10	174	1635	146	44936	152	17340	8136	321
PETOSKEY—Emmet County										
★ NORTHERN MICHIGAN HOSPITAL, 416 Connable Avenue, Zip 49770–2297; tel. 616/348–4000; Jeffrey T. Wendling, President A1 2 5 9 10 F3 4 7 8 10 14 15 19 20 21 22 27 28 29 30 31 32 33 34 35 36 37 39 40 41 42 43 44 45 46 49 51 52 53 54 56 58 59 60 61 63 64 65 66 67 71 72 73 P1 4 5 7	23	10	263	9225	148	57503	945	72061	33180	1072
PIGEON—Huron County										
★ SCHEURER HOSPITAL, 170 North Caseville Road, Zip 48755–9704; tel. 517/453–3223; Dwight Gascho, Administrator (Total facility includes 19 beds in nursing home–type unit) A1 9 10 F7 8 15 19 21 22 28 29 30 33 34 36 39 40 41 42 44 45 46 49 51 62 63 65 71 72 P6	23	10	42	605	25	—	14	6443	3041	110
PLAINWELL—Allegan County										
★ PIPP COMMUNITY HOSPITAL, 411 Naomi Street, Zip 49080–9911; tel. 616/685–6811; Fritz Fahrenbacher, Chief Executive Officer A1 9 10 F7 8 10 12 15 16 17 19 20 22 24 30 32 33 35 39 40 41 44 45 46 49 62 65 71 72 P6	23	10	43	899	8	35180	204	10659	4567	183
PONTIAC—Oakland County										
□ CLINTON VALLEY CENTER, 140 Elizabeth Lake Road, Zip 48341–1000; tel. 810/452–8700; Neil Wasserman, Director A1 10 F1 3 4 5 6 7 8 9 10 11 12 17 18 19 20 21 22 23 25 26 29 30 31 34 35 37 39 40 41 42 43 44 45 48 49 50 51 52 54 55 56 57 58 60 61 63 65 66 67 69 70 71 72 73 74 P6	12	22	318	811	382	0	0	39038	24081	656
★ NORTH OAKLAND MEDICAL CENTERS, 461 West Huron Street, Zip 48341–1651; tel. 810/857–7200; James M. Wright, President A1 3 5 9 10 F4 7 8 10 12 14 16 17 18 19 20 21 22 25 26 28 29 30 31 33 34 37 38 39 40 41 42 44 45 46 48 49 51 52 54 55 56 57 58 60 61 63 65 67 68 71 72 73 P3 8	23	10	269	9725	147	138383	1668	97064	44955	1190
+ ○ PONTIAC OSTEOPATHIC HOSPITAL, 50 North Perry Street, Zip 48342; tel. 313/338–5000; Jack H. Whitlow, Executive Director A9 10 11 12 13 F2 3 7 8 10 12 13 15 16 17 18 19 21 22 24 25 28 29 30 31 32 33 34 35 37 39 40 41 42 44 45 49 51 54 55 56 57 61 63 65 66 67 70 71 72 73 74 P4 5 6 8	23	10	185	6790	100	119679	506	72036	35280	1074
★ △ ST. JOSEPH MERCY COMMUNITY HEALTHCARE SYSTEM, 900 Woodward Avenue, Zip 48341–2985; tel. 313/858–3000; John P. Cullen, President and Chief Executive Officer A1 3 5 7 9 10 F2 3 4 6 7 8 10 12 14 15 16 17 19 22 28 30 31 32 33 34 35 36 39 40 42 44 46 48 49 52 53 54 55 56 57 58 59 60 61 62 65 66 67 70 71 72 73 74 P6 8 S5165 Mercy Health Services	21	10	421	18590	309	255889	2618	170866	81493	2311

Hospitals, U.S. / MICHIGAN

Hospital, Address, Telephone, Administrator, Approval, Facility, and Physician Codes, Health Care System	Classification Codes		Utilization Data					Expense (thousands) of dollars		
★ American Hospital Association (AHA) membership □ Joint Commission on Accreditation of Healthcare Organizations (JCAHO) accreditation + American Osteopathic Hospital Association (AOHA) membership ○ American Osteopathic Association (AOA) accreditation △ Commission on Accreditation of Rehabilitation Facilities (CARF) accreditation Control codes 61, 63, 64, 71, 72 and 73 indicate hospitals listed by AOHA, but not registered by AHA. For definition of numerical codes, see page A6	Control	Service	Beds	Admissions	Census	Outpatient Visits	Births	Total	Payroll	Personnel
PORT HURON—St. Clair County ★ △ MERCY HOSPITAL, 2601 Electric Avenue, Zip 48061–6518; tel. 313/985–1510; Mary R. Trimmer, President and Chief Executive Officer **A**1 2 7 9 10 **F**4 8 10 12 14 15 16 17 19 21 22 28 30 31 32 33 34 35 37 39 41 42 43 44 45 46 48 49 60 63 65 67 71 73 **S**5165 Mercy Health Services	21	10	119	4223	72	49366	0	40300	17598	543
★ PORT HURON HOSPITAL, 1001 Kearney Street, Zip 48061–5011; tel. 313/987–5000; Donald C. Fletcher, President **A**1 2 9 10 **F**3 4 7 8 10 11 12 14 15 16 17 19 20 21 22 26 29 30 31 33 34 35 37 40 41 42 43 44 45 46 49 52 54 55 56 57 58 59 63 65 66 67 71 73 74 **S**0053 Blue Water Health Services Corporation	23	10	184	8374	110	135329	1341	59682	27568	915
REED CITY—Osceola County ★ REED CITY HOSPITAL CORPORATION, 7665 Patterson Road, Zip 49677–1122; tel. 616/832–3271; David M. Coates Ph.D., Administrator (Total facility includes 54 beds in nursing home–type unit) **A**1 9 10 **F**8 11 15 19 22 28 30 32 33 37 41 44 48 49 64 65 71 73 **P**5	23	10	89	1503	64	26139	0	10145	4041	209
ROCHESTER—Oakland County ★ CRITTENTON HOSPITAL, 1101 West University Drive, Zip 48307–1831; tel. 810/652–5000; Gordon T. Ridley, President and Chief Executive Officer **A**1 2 9 10 **F**7 8 10 11 19 21 22 24 28 29 30 32 33 34 35 37 39 40 41 42 44 45 46 48 49 52 54 55 56 58 59 63 65 66 67 71 73 74 **P**5	23	10	215	11073	142	134189	1672	86898	40512	1168
ROMEO—Macomb County ST. JOSEPH'S MERCY–NORTH See St. Joseph's Mercy Hospitals and Health Services, Clinton Township										
ROYAL OAK—Oakland County ★ △ WILLIAM BEAUMONT HOSPITAL, 3601 West Thirteen Mile Road, Zip 48073–6769; tel. 810/551–5000; Kenneth J. Matzick, Vice President and Director **A**1 2 3 5 7 8 9 10 **F**4 7 8 10 11 12 14 16 19 21 22 23 24 25 26 28 30 31 32 33 34 35 37 38 39 40 42 43 44 45 46 47 48 49 50 51 52 54 55 56 57 59 60 61 63 64 65 66 67 69 70 71 73 **P**8 **S**9575 William Beaumont Hospital Corporation	23	10	894	40940	707	603000	5188	471736	220487	7011
SAGINAW—Saginaw County ★ △ HEALTHSOURCE SAGINAW, (Formerly Saginaw Community Hospital) (Regional Rehabilitation Center, Behavioral Medicine and Substance and Senior Care) 3340 Hospital Road, Zip 48603, Mailing Address: P.O. Box 6280, Zip 48608–9623; tel. 517/790–7700; Lester Hayboer Jr., President and Chief Executive Officer (Total facility includes 201 beds in nursing home–type unit) **A**1 7 9 10 **F**2 3 20 26 34 39 41 45 46 48 49 52 53 54 55 57 58 64 65 67 73 **P**6	13	49	280	1927	239	13332	0	18307	10232	428
SAGINAW COMMUNITY HOSPITAL See Healthsource Saginaw										
★ SAGINAW GENERAL HOSPITAL, 1447 North Harrison Street, Zip 48602; tel. 517/771–4000; Donald E. Juenemann, President **A**1 3 5 9 10 **F**7 10 11 15 16 17 19 21 22 24 25 26 30 31 32 33 34 35 37 38 39 40 41 42 44 45 46 49 52 53 54 56 58 59 61 65 67 71 73 74 **P**4 5 8	23	10	262	10741	166	95280	3344	88837	38877	1089
★ △ ST. LUKE'S HOSPITAL, 700 Cooper Avenue, Zip 48602; tel. 517/771–6000; Spencer Maidlow, President **A**1 3 5 7 9 10 **F**4 7 8 10 11 14 15 16 19 22 25 27 28 34 35 37 40 42 43 44 45 46 47 48 49 65 66 70 71 72 73 **P**6	23	10	273	12775	192	162427	824	111980	52482	1490
★ ST. MARY'S MEDICAL CENTER, 830 South Jefferson Avenue, Zip 48601–2594; tel. 517/776–8000; Frederic L. Fraizer, President and Chief Executive Officer **A**1 2 3 5 9 10 **F**4 8 9 10 11 16 19 21 22 25 27 28 30 34 35 37 39 42 43 44 46 49 54 56 60 63 65 70 71 73 **P**8 **S**1855 Daughters of Charity National Health System	21	10	268	10159	184	66760	0	98022	42556	1543
★ VETERANS AFFAIRS MEDICAL CENTER, 1500 Weiss Street, Zip 48602; tel. 517/793–2340; Robert H. Sabin, Medical Center Director (Total facility includes 120 beds in nursing home–type unit) **A**1 5 9 **F**3 8 19 20 21 30 31 33 37 44 46 49 58 64 65 67 71 73 74 **S**9295 Department of Veterans Affairs	45	10	215	2539	131	48612	0	33065	17371	479
SAINT IGNACE—Mackinac County MACKINAC STRAITS HOSPITAL AND HEALTH CENTER, 220 Burdette Street, Zip 49781; tel. 906/643–8585; Mary E. Tamlyn, Administrator (Total facility includes 60 beds in nursing home–type unit) **A**9 10 **F**15 22 64 65	16	10	75	61	65	15910	0	3938	2414	—
SAINT JOHNS—Clinton County ★ CLINTON MEMORIAL HOSPITAL, 805 South Oakland Street, Zip 48879–0260; tel. 517/224–6881; Paul E. McNamara, President **A**1 9 10 **F**7 8 15 16 17 19 22 32 33 34 36 40 41 42 44 65 71 72 73 **P**8	23	10	28	996	10	18572	167	13297	4964	167
SAINT JOSEPH—Berrien County ★ △ MERCY–MEMORIAL MEDICAL CENTER, 1234 Napier Avenue, Zip 49085; tel. 616/983–8300; Joseph A. Wasserman, President and Chief Executive Officer **A**1 2 7 9 10 **F**3 4 7 8 10 12 15 16 19 21 22 26 28 29 30 31 32 33 34 35 37 40 41 42 43 44 48 49 51 52 56 59 60 63 65 66 67 71 73 74 **P**8 **S**0056 Lakeland Regional Health System, Inc.	23	10	254	10327	163	208808	1020	99852	40349	1344
SALINE—Washtenaw County ★ SALINE COMMUNITY HOSPITAL, 400 West Russell Street, Zip 48176–1101; tel. 313/429–1500; James F. Harns, Chief Operating Officer **A**1 9 10 **F**2 3 8 14 19 20 21 22 28 30 31 33 37 41 44 49 65 71 73 74 **P**3 **S**5165 Mercy Health Services	21	10	54	1850	26	80498	0	20210	8750	350
SANDUSKY—Sanilac County ★ MCKENZIE MEMORIAL HOSPITAL, 120 Delaware Street, Zip 48471–1087; tel. 810/648–3770; Joseph W. Weiler, Administrator **A**9 10 **F**3 8 12 16 19 21 22 25 26 33 34 37 40 41 42 44 45 46 49 54 56 63 65 69 71 73 **P**6	23	10	25	683	7	14885	102	6930	3265	118

© 1995 AHA Guide

Hospitals, U.S. / MICHIGAN

Hospital, Address, Telephone, Administrator, Approval, Facility, and Physician Codes, Health Care System	Classification Codes		Utilization Data					Expense (thousands) of dollars		
★ American Hospital Association (AHA) membership □ Joint Commission on Accreditation of Healthcare Organizations (JCAHO) accreditation + American Osteopathic Hospital Association (AOHA) membership ○ American Osteopathic Association (AOA) accreditation △ Commission on Accreditation of Rehabilitation Facilities (CARF) accreditation Control codes 61, 63, 64, 71, 72 and 73 indicate hospitals listed by AOHA, but not registered by AHA. For definition of numerical codes, see page A6	Control	Service	Beds	Admissions	Census	Outpatient Visits	Births	Total	Payroll	Personnel
SAULT SAINTE MARIE—Chippewa County ★ CHIPPEWA COUNTY WAR MEMORIAL HOSPITAL, 500 Osborn Boulevard, Zip 49783–4467; tel. 906/635–4460; Jerry Popowski, Chief Executive Officer (Nonreporting) A1 9 10 S0585 Brim, Inc.	23	10	137	—	—	—	—	—	—	—
SHELBY—Oceana County ★ LAKESHORE COMMUNITY HOSPITAL, 72 South State Street, Zip 49455–1299; tel. 616/861–2156; Martin E. Anderson, Administrator A1 9 10 F7 8 14 15 16 17 22 28 39 40 44 71	23	10	32	883	8	32070	153	4634	2342	93
SHERIDAN—Montcalm County + ○ SHERIDAN COMMUNITY HOSPITAL, 301 North Main Street, Zip 48884, Mailing Address: P.O. Box 279, Zip 48884–0279; tel. 517/291–3261; Jack Howey, Administrator A9 10 11 F8 14 15 16 17 19 22 25 28 30 32 37 42 44 46 49 51 71 73	23	10	19	560	6	28714	25	5401	2798	102
SOUTH HAVEN—Van Buren County ★ SOUTH HAVEN COMMUNITY HOSPITAL, 955 South Bailey Avenue, Zip 49090; tel. 616/637–5271; Craig J. Marks, President and Chief Executive Officer A1 9 10 F7 8 11 14 15 16 19 21 22 24 28 31 32 33 35 36 39 40 42 44 45 49 61 65 66 69 71 73 74	23	10	52	1385	12	41258	367	10932	4247	153
SOUTHFIELD—Oakland County ○ △ GREAT LAKES REHABILITATION HOSPITAL, 22401 Foster Winter Drive, Zip 48075; tel. 810/569–1500; Joseph R. Gordon, Chief Executive Officer (Total facility includes 26 beds in nursing home–type unit) (Data for 275 days) A7 9 10 11 F12 14 15 16 34 39 41 45 46 48 49 54 57 64 65 73	31	46	101	521	40	1170	0	5628	3144	163
★ PROVIDENCE HOSPITAL AND MEDICAL CENTERS, 16001 West Nine Mile Road, Zip 48075–4854, Mailing Address: Box 2043, Zip 48037–2043; tel. 810/424–3000; Michael A. Slubowski, Chief Executive Officer A1 2 3 5 8 9 10 F1 2 3 4 7 8 10 11 12 13 14 15 16 17 18 19 21 22 25 26 28 29 30 31 32 33 34 35 37 38 39 40 41 42 43 44 46 48 49 51 52 53 54 55 56 59 60 65 66 67 70 71 72 73 74 P1 5 6 S1855 Daughters of Charity National Health System	21	10	459	20002	333	860417	4532	239743	110420	3062
★ STRAITH HOSPITAL FOR SPECIAL SURGERY, 23901 Lahser Road, Zip 48034–3296; tel. 313/357–3360; Gregory R. Hoose, Chief Executive Officer A1 9 10 F12 15 44 65	23	45	22	848	6	5196	0	9110	3803	112
STANDISH—Arenac County ★ STANDISH COMMUNITY HOSPITAL, 805 West Cedar Street, Zip 48658, Mailing Address: P.O. Box 579, Zip 48658; tel. 517/846–4521; Thomas G. Westhoff, Chief Executive Officer (Total facility includes 44 beds in nursing home–type unit) A1 9 10 F3 5 8 10 11 14 15 16 17 19 20 21 22 30 31 44 45 46 49 53 54 56 58 63 64 66 71 72 73 P6	23	10	65	899	53	23834	0	8849	4388	205
STURGIS—St. Joseph County ★ STURGIS HOSPITAL, 916 Myrtle, Zip 49091–2001; tel. 616/659–4400; David James, Chief Executive Officer A1 9 10 F7 8 10 11 14 15 16 19 21 22 24 30 32 33 34 35 36 37 39 40 41 42 44 49 63 65 67 71 73 P6 S0002 Quorum Health Group/Quorum Health Resources	14	10	53	2141	22	50794	336	17838	7058	213
TAWAS CITY—Iosco County ★ TAWAS ST. JOSEPH HOSPITAL, 200 Hemlock, Zip 48763, Mailing Address: P.O. Box 659, Zip 48764–0659; tel. 517/362–3411; Paul R. Schmidt, President and Chief Executive Officer A1 9 10 F7 8 15 16 17 19 21 22 27 28 30 32 33 37 40 41 42 44 63 65 67 69 71 73 74 S5555 Sisters of St. Joseph Health System	23	10	69	2403	28	82063	329	18646	8386	322
TAYLOR—Wayne County HERITAGE HOSPITAL See Oakwood Hospital–Heritage Center ★ OAKWOOD HOSPITAL–HERITAGE CENTER, (Formerly Heritage Hospital) 10000 Telegraph Road, Zip 48180–3349; tel. 313/295–5232; Thomas E. Johnson, Vice President, Administrator A1 9 10 F1 2 3 4 6 7 8 10 11 12 14 15 16 17 19 21 22 23 26 27 28 29 30 32 33 34 35 37 38 39 40 41 43 44 46 48 49 51 52 54 56 57 59 60 61 62 63 64 65 66 67 71 72 73 P5 S1165 Oakwood Healthcare System	23	10	245	7107	177	47493	0	59357	26963	702
TECUMSEH—Lenawee County ★ ○ HERRICK MEMORIAL HOSPITAL, 500 East Pottawatamie Street, Zip 49286–2097; tel. 517/423–3834; Dan Wakeman, President and Chief Executive Officer (Total facility includes 25 beds in nursing home–type unit) A1 9 10 11 F3 7 8 11 14 15 16 17 19 20 21 22 24 29 30 33 34 39 40 41 44 48 49 52 53 55 58 59 63 65 66 67 71 72 73 74 P7 8	23	10	85	2203	53	33272	261	18809	7898	278
THREE RIVERS—St. Joseph County ★ △ THREE RIVERS AREA HOSPITAL, 1111 West Broadway, Zip 49093–9362; tel. 616/278–1145; Brad Solberg, President and Chief Executive Officer A1 9 10 F7 8 10 12 15 16 17 19 21 22 24 28 31 33 34 35 37 39 40 41 42 44 45 48 49 61 65 71 73 74 S0002 Quorum Health Group/Quorum Health Resources	16	10	60	1734	24	32725	236	15856	6424	219
TRAVERSE CITY—Grand Traverse County □ △ MUNSON MEDICAL CENTER, 1105 Sixth Street, Zip 49684–2386; tel. 616/935–5000; Ralph J. Cerny, President A1 2 7 9 10 F2 3 4 7 8 10 11 12 15 17 18 19 20 21 22 23 24 25 26 27 28 30 31 32 33 34 35 36 37 38 39 40 41 42 43 44 45 46 47 48 49 51 52 54 55 56 57 60 61 64 65 66 70 71 73 74 P5 7	23	10	408	16325	238	260004	1831	142616	65307	2116
TRENTON—Wayne County ★ OAKWOOD HOSPITAL SEAWAY CENTER, (Formerly Seaway Hospital) 5450 Fort Street, Zip 48183; tel. 313/671–3800; Edward E. Freysinger, Vice President and Administrator A1 9 10 F2 3 8 11 12 14 15 16 19 21 22 28 30 32 33 34 35 36 37 40 41 42 44 45 46 48 49 51 52 55 56 57 58 59 60 63 64 65 66 67 68 71 72 73 S1165 Oakwood Healthcare System	23	10	97	2956	40	45455	206	30018	12507	285

Hospitals, U.S. / MICHIGAN

Hospital, Address, Telephone, Administrator, Approval, Facility, and Physician Codes, Health Care System	Classification Codes		Utilization Data					Expense (thousands) of dollars		
★ American Hospital Association (AHA) membership □ Joint Commission on Accreditation of Healthcare Organizations (JCAHO) accreditation + American Osteopathic Hospital Association (AOHA) membership ○ American Osteopathic Association (AOA) accreditation △ Commission on Accreditation of Rehabilitation Facilities (CARF) accreditation Control codes 61, 63, 64, 71, 72 and 73 indicate hospitals listed by AOHA, but not registered by AHA. For definition of numerical codes, see page A6	Control	Service	Beds	Admissions	Census	Outpatient Visits	Births	Total	Payroll	Personnel
+ ○ RIVERSIDE OSTEOPATHIC HOSPITAL, 150 Truax Street, Zip 48183–2151; tel. 313/676–4200; Dennis A. Christen, Vice President and Administrator **A**9 10 11 12 13 **F**7 8 10 12 14 15 16 17 18 19 20 21 22 24 25 26 27 28 29 30 31 32 33 34 35 36 37 39 40 41 42 44 45 46 49 52 54 56 60 61 63 65 66 71 73 74 **S**1035 Horizon Health System SEAWAY HOSPITAL See Oakwood Hospital Seaway Center	23	10	185	5540	89	96131	677	55205	25545	614
TROY—Oakland County ★ WILLIAM BEAUMONT HOSPITAL–TROY, 44201 Dequindre Road, Zip 48098-1198; tel. 810/828–5100; John D. Labriola, Vice President and Director **A**1 3 9 10 **F**4 7 8 10 12 14 16 19 21 22 23 24 26 28 29 30 31 32 33 34 35 37 39 40 41 42 43 44 45 46 49 50 51 54 55 56 57 59 60 61 63 64 65 66 67 69 71 73 **P**8 **S**9575 William Beaumont Hospital Corporation	23	10	189	11599	154	268202	1322	108541	49869	1503
VICKSBURG—Kalamazoo County ★ △ BRONSON VICKSBURG HOSPITAL, 13326 North Boulevard, Zip 49097–1099; tel. 616/649–2321 **A**1 7 9 10 **F**8 12 14 16 19 21 22 26 28 30 34 35 41 44 45 48 49 54 65 71 73 **P**7 **S**0595 Bronson Healthcare Group, Inc.	23	46	41	357	14	29607	0	7338	4853	107
WARREN—Macomb County + ○ △ BI-COUNTY COMMUNITY HOSPITAL, 13355 East Ten Mile Road, Zip 48089–2065; tel. 810/759–7300; Gary W. Popiel, Chief Executive Officer **A**7 9 10 11 12 13 **F**3 7 8 10 12 14 15 16 19 21 22 24 27 28 29 30 31 34 35 37 39 40 41 42 44 45 46 48 49 51 53 54 55 60 61 63 65 66 71 73 **P**5 **S**1035 Horizon Health System	23	10	185	6850	136	142838	542	69068	31547	849
□ CARLYLE CENTER, 6902 Chicago Road, Zip 48092; tel. 313/264–8875; Dennis J. Dishong, Chairman of Board **A**1 9 10 **F**1 16 52 53 54 55 56 57 58 59 **P**8	33	22	100	1205	29	—	0	6318	3005	94
★ KERN HOSPITAL FOR SPECIAL SURGERY, (Podiatry Medical and Surgical) 21230 Dequindre, Zip 48091–2287; tel. 313/759–4520; Dennis P. Markiewicz, Chief Executive Officer **A**1 9 10 **F**2 3 14 44 49 65	23	49	45	649	12	10746	0	7102	3663	140
★ MACOMB HOSPITAL CENTER, 11800 East Twelve Mile Road, Zip 48093; tel. 810/573–5000; George P. Caralis, Administrator **A**1 2 9 10 **F**7 8 10 11 14 16 17 19 21 22 27 28 29 30 32 33 34 35 37 39 40 42 44 45 46 48 49 51 52 54 55 56 57 58 59 60 63 65 67 71 73 **P**4 5 6 8 **S**0042 Detroit–Macomb Hospital Corporation	23	10	288	11751	205	106000	1460	102361	43771	1169
WATERVLIET—Berrien County ★ △ COMMUNITY HOSPITAL, Medical Park Drive, Zip 49098-0158, Mailing Address: Box 158, Zip 49098; tel. 616/463–3111; Douglas L. Rahn, Administrator **A**1 7 9 10 **F**8 10 14 15 16 19 22 26 28 29 30 32 33 34 35 37 39 44 45 46 48 49 64 65 71 73 **P**8 **S**0002 Quorum Health Group/Quorum Health Resources	23	10	54	1579	28	27820	0	11831	5179	204
WAYNE—Wayne County ★ OAKWOOD HOSPITAL ANNAPOLIS CENTER, (Includes Oakwood Hospital Merriman Center–Westland, 2345 Merriman Road, Westland, Michigan, Zip 48185; tel. 313/467–2300) 33155 Annapolis Road, Zip 48184; tel. 313/467–4000; Carla O'Malley, Senior Vice President, Acute Care Services **A**1 9 10 **F**1 2 3 4 6 7 8 10 11 12 14 15 16 19 21 22 26 27 28 29 30 32 33 34 35 37 38 39 40 41 42 43 44 45 46 48 49 52 53 54 55 56 57 58 59 60 61 62 63 64 65 66 67 71 73 74 **P**3 6 **S**1165 Oakwood Healthcare System	23	10	381	11285	231	93813	795	79912	30798	871
WEST BRANCH—Ogemaw County ★ TOLFREE MEMORIAL HOSPITAL, 335 East Houghton Avenue, Zip 48661–1199; tel. 517/345–3660; Douglas E. Pattullo, Chief Executive Officer **A**1 9 10 **F**6 7 8 11 16 19 22 32 33 40 42 44 71 **P**3	14	10	92	3280	45	36712	338	14491	6950	281
WESTLAND—Wayne County □ WALTER P. REUTHER PSYCHIATRIC HOSPITAL, 30901 Palmer Road, Zip 48185–5389; tel. 313/722–4500; Norma C. Josef M.D., Director **A**1 10 **F**14 52 57 65 67 73 OAKWOOD HOSPITAL MERRIMAN CENTER–WESTLAND See Oakwood Hospital Annapolis Center, Wayne	12	22	194	199	226	0	0	25333	14072	377
WYANDOTTE—Wayne County ★ △ WYANDOTTE HOSPITAL AND MEDICAL CENTER, 2333 Biddle Avenue, Zip 48192; tel. 313/284–2400; William R. Alvin, President **A**1 7 9 10 **F**1 8 10 19 22 25 28 30 32 33 34 37 40 41 42 44 46 48 49 52 53 54 56 58 59 65 66 71 73 **S**9505 Henry Ford Health System	23	10	355	12400	244	0	1142	95333	50483	1472
YALE—St. Clair County ★ YALE COMMUNITY HOSPITAL, 420 North Street, Zip 48097, Mailing Address: P.O. Box 129, Zip 48097–0129; tel. 313/387–3211; Joyce Laupichler, Interim Administrator **A**1 9 10 **F**15 22 33 34 44 49 51 65 71	23	10	22	268	3	13295	0	3079	1345	41
YPSILANTI—Washtenaw County ★ OAKWOOD HOSPITAL BEYER CENTER–YPSILANTI, (Formerly Beyer Hospital) 135 South Prospect Street, Zip 48198–5693; tel. 313/484–2200; Mary A. Finn, Vice President and Administrator **A**1 9 10 **F**3 7 8 10 15 16 17 19 21 22 26 28 30 32 34 35 37 40 41 44 45 46 49 56 58 63 65 71 74 **S**1165 Oakwood Healthcare System	23	10	78	3249	45	38110	493	28823	12908	319
ZEELAND—Ottawa County ★ ZEELAND COMMUNITY HOSPITAL, 100 South Pine Street, Zip 49464; tel. 616/772–4644; Henry A. Veenstra, President **A**1 9 10 **F**7 8 11 14 15 16 17 19 21 22 28 30 33 36 39 42 44 45 48 49 52 71 72 73 74	23	10	57	1813	21	40680	352	12550	6079	191

© 1995 AHA Guide

Hospitals, U.S. / MINNESOTA

MINNESOTA

Resident population 4,517 (in thousands)
Resident population in metro areas 69.3%
Birth rate per 1,000 population 15.1
65 years and over 12.6%
Percent of persons without health insurance 8.8%

Hospital, Address, Telephone, Administrator, Approval, Facility, and Physician Codes, Health Care System	Classification Codes		Utilization Data					Expense (thousands) of dollars		
★ American Hospital Association (AHA) membership □ Joint Commission on Accreditation of Healthcare Organizations (JCAHO) accreditation + American Osteopathic Hospital Association (AOHA) membership ○ American Osteopathic Association (AOA) accreditation △ Commission on Accreditation of Rehabilitation Facilities (CARF) accreditation Control codes 61, 63, 64, 71, 72 and 73 indicate hospitals listed by AOHA, but not registered by AHA. For definition of numerical codes, see page A6	Control	Service	Beds	Admissions	Census	Outpatient Visits	Births	Total	Payroll	Personnel
ADA—Norman County ★ ADA MUNICIPAL HOSPITAL, (Includes John Wimmer Memorial Home) 405 East Second Avenue, Zip 56510–0233; tel. 218/784–2561; Kyle Rasmussen, Administrator (Total facility includes 49 beds in nursing home–type unit) **A**9 10 **F**1 11 15 19 21 22 27 34 44 49 64 71 **P**6	14	10	77	283	48	7036	0	4183	2353	90
ADRIAN—Nobles County ARNOLD MEMORIAL HOSPITAL, 601 Louisiana Avenue, Zip 56110–0279, Mailing Address: Box 279, Zip 56110–0279; tel. 507/483–2668; Gerald E. Carl, Administrator (Nonreporting) **A**9 10	14	10	50	—	—	—	—	—	—	—
AITKIN—Aitkin County RIVERWOOD HEALTH CARE CENTER, 301 Minnesota Avenue South, Zip 56431–1626; tel. 218/927–2121; Debra Boardman, Chief Executive Officer (Total facility includes 48 beds in nursing home–type unit) **A**9 10 **F**7 8 11 15 19 22 28 34 35 42 44 49 64 65 71 73	23	10	68	911	54	15795	60	7416	3672	155
ALBANY—Stearns County ★ ALBANY AREA HOSPITAL AND MEDICAL CENTER, 300 Third Avenue, Zip 56307; tel. 612/845–2121; Fred Struzyk, Chief Operating Officer **A**9 10 **F**7 8 12 15 16 17 19 22 32 33 34 44 49 58 71 **P**6 **S**5175 Catholic Health Corporation	21	10	17	379	4	4581	76	3303	1517	60
ALBERT LEA—Freeborn County ★ △ NAEVE HOSPITAL, 404 West Fountain Street, Zip 56007–2473; tel. 507/373–2384; Lawrence W. Pfaff, President and Chief Executive Officer **A**1 7 9 10 **F**2 3 7 15 16 17 19 21 22 24 28 32 33 34 35 36 37 39 40 41 44 46 48 52 54 65 66 67 71 **P**8	23	10	75	2883	35	60539	440	19004	8740	309
ALEXANDRIA—Douglas County ★ DOUGLAS COUNTY HOSPITAL, 111 17th Avenue East, Zip 56308–3798; tel. 612/762–1511; William G. Flaig, Administrator **A**1 9 10 **F**3 7 8 14 15 19 21 22 23 28 29 31 32 33 34 35 36 37 40 41 42 44 45 49 54 55 56 58 59 65 66 67 71 73	13	10	110	3669	42	41578	522	26308	12485	375
ANOKA—Anoka County □ ANOKA–METROPOLITAN REGIONAL TREATMENT CENTER, 3300 Fourth Avenue North, Zip 55303–1119; tel. 612/422–4150; Elaine J. Timmer, Chief Executive Officer (Nonreporting) **A**1 9 10	12	22	337	—	—	—	—	—	—	—
APPLETON—Swift County APPLETON MUNICIPAL HOSPITAL AND NURSING HOME, 30 South Behl Street, Zip 56208–1699; tel. 612/289–2422; Mark E. Paulson, Administrator (Total facility includes 84 beds in nursing home–type unit) **A**9 10 **F**7 14 17 19 22 32 33 34 36 39 41 44 45 49 58 62 63 64 65 71 73 **P**7	14	10	104	367	87	3285	7	3621	2387	104
ARLINGTON—Sibley County ★ ARLINGTON MUNICIPAL HOSPITAL, 601 West Chandler Street, Zip 55307; tel. 612/964–2271; Lynette Froehlich R.N., Administrator **A**1 9 10 **F**1 3 8 15 16 19 20 22 27 30 31 32 33 34 35 42 44 45 46 49 53 62 64 65 66 67 71 72 73 **P**7 8	14	10	17	378	5	3838	0	2367	1077	48
AURORA—St. Louis County ★ WHITE COMMUNITY HOSPITAL, 5211 Highway 110, Zip 55705; tel. 218/229–2211; Cheryl High, Administrator (Total facility includes 69 beds in nursing home–type unit) **A**9 10 **F**7 17 22 26 28 31 34 36 44 49 60 64 65 66 67	23	10	85	399	70	4767	10	3567	2328	94
AUSTIN—Mower County □ AUSTIN MEDICAL CENTER, 300 Northwest Eighth Avenue, Zip 55912; tel. 507/437–4551; Donald R. Brezicka, Executive Vice President **A**1 9 10 **F**2 3 7 10 19 21 22 32 33 34 35 37 40 41 42 44 49 52 53 54 56 57 58 71 73	23	10	108	3132	34	—	406	—	—	—
BAGLEY—Clearwater County ★ CLEARWATER COUNTY MEMORIAL HOSPITAL, 203 Fourth Street N.W., Zip 56621, Mailing Address: Rural Route 3, Box 46, Zip 56621; tel. 218/694–6501; Larry Laudon, Administrator (Total facility includes 70 beds in nursing home–type unit) **A**9 10 **F**1 7 8 19 22 26 39 40 44 49 64 71	13	10	88	536	74	3233	43	5235	2546	127
BAUDETTE—Lake Of The Woods County ★ LAKEWOOD HEALTH CENTER, 600 South Main Avenue, Zip 56623, Mailing Address: Route 1, Box 2120, Zip 56623; tel. 218/634–2120; David A. Nelson, President and Chief Executive Officer (Total facility includes 52 beds in nursing home–type unit) **A**9 10 **F**7 13 14 17 22 27 30 32 34 40 44 64 65 **S**5175 Catholic Health Corporation	21	10	73	493	48	4514	43	4591	2147	95
BEMIDJI—Beltrami County ★ NORTH COUNTRY REGIONAL HOSPITAL, 1100 West 38th Street, Zip 56601–9972; tel. 218/751–5430; Mark D. Richardson, President and Chief Executive Officer (Total facility includes 78 beds in nursing home–type unit) **A**1 9 10 **F**4 7 8 12 14 16 19 22 24 29 30 32 34 35 37 39 40 41 44 48 49 62 64 65 66 67 71 73 **P**6	23	10	176	5465	133	31846	735	33464	15372	378
BENSON—Swift County ★ SWIFT COUNTY–BENSON HOSPITAL, 1815 Wisconsin Avenue, Zip 56215–1653; tel. 612/843–4232; John Stindt, Chief Executive Officer **A**9 10 **F**8 11 14 15 19 22 32 33 34 35 36 39 41 44 54 58 65 71 **S**0585 Brim, Inc.	15	10	31	596	7	7963	30	2790	1240	55

Hospitals, U.S. / MINNESOTA

Hospital, Address, Telephone, Administrator, Approval, Facility, and Physician Codes, Health Care System	Classification Codes		Utilization Data					Expense (thousands) of dollars		Personnel
★ American Hospital Association (AHA) membership ☐ Joint Commission on Accreditation of Healthcare Organizations (JCAHO) accreditation + American Osteopathic Hospital Association (AOHA) membership ○ American Osteopathic Association (AOA) accreditation △ Commission on Accreditation of Rehabilitation Facilities (CARF) accreditation Control codes 61, 63, 64, 71, 72 and 73 indicate hospitals listed by AOHA, but not registered by AHA. For definition of numerical codes, see page A6	Control	Service	Beds	Admissions	Census	Outpatient Visits	Births	Total	Payroll	
BIGFORK—Itasca County ★ NORTHERN ITASCA HEALTH CARE CENTER, 258 Pine Tree Drive, Zip 56628, Mailing Address: P.O. Box 258, Zip 56628–0258; tel. 218/743–3177; Lillian Carr, Administrator (Total facility includes 40 beds in nursing home–type unit) **A**9 10 **F**1 6 7 8 15 16 19 20 22 26 27 32 33 34 40 44 49 64 65 71 **P**5	16	10	60	422	45	10100	31	4200	2195	78
BLUE EARTH—Faribault County ★ UNITED HOSPITAL DISTRICT, 515 South Moore Street, Zip 56013–0160; tel. 507/526–3273; Frank Lawatsch, Administrator **A**1 9 10 **F**7 8 15 16 17 19 22 27 28 30 31 32 33 34 35 36 37 39 40 41 44 49 53 54 55 58 65 71	16	10	43	942	11	30402	48	6012	2544	104
BRAINERD—Crow Wing County ☐ BRAINERD REGIONAL HUMAN SERVICES CENTER, 1777 Highway 18 East, Zip 56401; tel. 218/828–2201; Harvey G. Caldwell, Administrator and Chief Executive Officer (Nonreporting) **A**1 9 10	12	22	337	—	—	—	—	—	—	—
☐ ST. JOSEPH'S MEDICAL CENTER, 523 North Third Street, Zip 56401–3098; tel. 218/829–2861; Thomas K. Prusak, President **A**1 9 10 **F**2 3 7 8 12 15 16 19 21 22 28 29 30 31 32 33 34 35 36 37 39 40 41 42 44 46 48 49 52 53 54 55 56 58 59 65 66 67 71 73 **P**3 5 **S**0515 Benedictine Health System	21	10	162	6013	80	109531	616	39667	16701	477
BRECKENRIDGE—Wilkin County ★ ST. FRANCIS MEDICAL CENTER, 415 Oak Street, Zip 56520; tel. 218/643–3000; Mark C. McNelly, President and Chief Executive Officer (Total facility includes 124 beds in nursing home–type unit) **A**1 5 9 10 **F**1 3 7 8 11 15 17 18 19 20 22 26 28 30 32 33 34 35 36 37 39 40 41 44 45 46 48 49 51 54 55 56 57 58 59 64 66 67 68 71 73 **P**8 **S**5175 Catholic Health Corporation	21	10	171	1877	141	—	307	15021	7275	321
BUFFALO—Wright County ★ BUFFALO HOSPITAL, 303 Catlin Street, Zip 55313–0609, Mailing Address: P.O. Box 609, Zip 55313–0609; tel. 612/682–7180; Mary Ellen Wells, President (Nonreporting) **A**1 9 10 **S**0041 Allina Health System	23	10	43	—	—	—	—	—	—	—
BURNSVILLE—Dakota County ★ FAIRVIEW RIDGES HOSPITAL, 201 East Nicollet Boulevard, Zip 55337–5799; tel. 612/892–2000; Donald C. Berglund, Senior Vice President and Administrator (Nonreporting) **A**1 9 10 **S**1325 Fairview Hospital and Healthcare Services	21	10	123	—	—	—	—	—	—	—
CAMBRIDGE—Isanti County ★ CAMBRIDGE MEDICAL CENTER, (Formerly Cambridge Memorial Hospital) 725 South Dellwood Street, Zip 55008–1920; tel. 612/689–1500; Lowell L. Becker M.D., President **A**1 9 10 **F**2 3 7 8 12 15 16 17 19 20 21 22 24 26 28 29 30 31 32 33 34 35 36 37 39 40 41 42 44 45 46 49 51 58 60 62 65 66 67 70 71 73 **P**8 **S**0041 Allina Health System	23	10	86	2852	30	17557	434	20234	10850	384
CANBY—Yellow Medicine County ★ CANBY COMMUNITY HEALTH SERVICES, (Includes Senior Haven Convalescent Nursing Center) 112 St. Olaf Avenue, Zip 56220–1433; tel. 507/223–7277; Robert J. Salmon, Chief Executive Officer (Total facility includes 75 beds in nursing home–type unit) **A**9 10 **F**7 8 15 17 19 20 21 22 26 27 28 29 30 32 33 34 35 36 37 39 40 41 44 48 49 53 62 64 65 66 71 73 **P**6	23	10	102	480	81	4403	31	4465	2323	123
CANNON FALLS—Goodhue County ★ COMMUNITY HOSPITAL, 1116 West Mill Street, Zip 55009–1898; tel. 507/263–4221; Donald J. Finn, Administrator **A**9 10 **F**1 2 3 4 5 6 7 8 9 10 11 12 13 14 17 18 19 20 21 22 23 24 25 26 27 28 29 30 31 32 33 34 35 36 37 38 39 40 41 42 43 44 45 46 47 48 49 50 51 52 53 54 55 56 57 58 59 61 62 63 64 65 66 67 68 69 70 71 72 73 74 **P**8	16	10	21	526	5	15010	37	3049	1322	54
CASS LAKE—Cass County ★ U.S. PUBLIC HEALTH SERVICE INDIAN HOSPITAL, 7th Street & Grant Utley Ave N.W., Zip 56633; tel. 218/335–2293; Luella Brown, Service Unit Director (Nonreporting) **A**1 5 10 **S**9195 U.S. Public Health Service Indian Health Service	47	10	13	—	—	—	—	—	—	—
CHISAGO CITY—Chisago County ★ CHISAGO HEALTH SERVICES, 11685 Lake Boulevard North, Zip 55013–9540; tel. 612/257–8400; Scott Wordelman, President and Chief Executive Officer (Nonreporting) **A**1 9 10	23	10	89	—	—	—	—	—	—	—
CLOQUET—Carlton County ★ COMMUNITY MEMORIAL HOSPITAL AND CONVALESCENT AND NURSING CARE SECTION, 512 Skyline Boulevard, Zip 55720–1199; tel. 218/879–4641; James J. Carroll, Administrator (Total facility includes 88 beds in nursing home–type unit) **A**9 10 **F**7 8 12 19 22 30 32 34 35 36 37 39 40 41 42 44 45 46 49 51 64 65 67 71 73 **P**3	23	10	124	1403	99	21394	129	10716	5815	207
COOK—St. Louis County ★ COOK HOSPITAL AND CONVALESCENT NURSING CARE UNIT, (Formerly Cook Community Hospital) 10 South Fifth Street East, Zip 55723; tel. 218/666–5945; Allen J. Vogt, Administrator (Total facility includes 41 beds in nursing home–type unit) **A**9 10 **F**1 14 15 16 22 26 33 34 41 49 64 65 71 73	16	10	55	387	45	—	0	3149	1750	59
COONS RAPIDS—Anoka County MERCY HOSPITAL See Unity Hospital, Fridley										
CROOKSTON—Polk County ★ RIVERVIEW HEALTHCARE ASSOCIATION, 323 South Minnesota Street, Zip 56716–1600; tel. 218/281–4682; Thomas C. Lenertz, President and Chief Executive Officer (Total facility includes 162 beds in nursing home–type unit) **A**1 5 9 10 **F**1 2 3 7 8 15 19 20 21 22 26 28 29 30 31 32 33 34 36 37 40 41 44 45 46 49 56 64 65 66 67 71 73 **P**5	23	10	234	1314	171	18357	144	14039	7355	176

© 1995 AHA Guide

Hospitals, U.S. / MINNESOTA

Hospital, Address, Telephone, Administrator, Approval, Facility, and Physician Codes, Health Care System

★ American Hospital Association (AHA) membership
□ Joint Commission on Accreditation of Healthcare Organizations (JCAHO) accreditation
+ American Osteopathic Hospital Association (AOHA) membership
○ American Osteopathic Association (AOA) accreditation
△ Commission on Accreditation of Rehabilitation Facilities (CARF) accreditation
Control codes 61, 63, 64, 71, 72 and 73 indicate hospitals listed by AOHA, but not registered by AHA. For definition of numerical codes, see page A6

Hospital	Classification Codes		Utilization Data					Expense (thousands) of dollars		
	Control	Service	Beds	Admissions	Census	Outpatient Visits	Births	Total	Payroll	Personnel
CROSBY—Crow Wing County										
★ CUYUNA REGIONAL MEDICAL CENTER, 320 East Main Street, Zip 56441; tel. 218/546-7000; Thomas F. Reek, Chief Executive Officer (Total facility includes 130 beds in nursing home-type unit) **A**9 10 **F**7 8 15 16 19 21 22 26 28 30 31 32 33 34 35 37 40 41 42 44 49 64 65 66 71 73 **P**7 8	16	10	160	1213	139	26284	149	13437	6800	256
DAWSON—Lac Qui Parle County										
JOHNSON MEMORIAL HOSPITAL AND HOME, 1282 Walnut Street, Zip 56232; tel. 612/769-4323; Julie A. Gruenenwald, Administrator (Total facility includes 70 beds in nursing home-type unit) **A**9 10 **F**7 8 15 17 19 20 22 26 28 29 30 32 36 44 45 49 63 64 65 71 **P**6	16	10	94	487	74	3659	25	3780	2029	116
DEER RIVER—Itasca County										
★ COMMUNITY MEMORIAL HOSPITAL OF DEER RIVER, 1002 Comstock Drive, Zip 56636; tel. 218/246-2900; Vern Silvernale, Administrator (Nonreporting) **A**9 10	23	10	70	—	—	—	—	—	—	—
DETROIT LAKES—Becker County										
✠ ST. MARY'S REGIONAL HEALTH CENTER, 1027 Washington Avenue, Zip 56501-3598; tel. 218/847-5611; John H. Solheim, Chief Executive Officer (Total facility includes 100 beds in nursing home-type unit) **A**1 9 10 **F**2 3 7 8 10 12 15 16 19 21 22 28 30 32 35 37 40 41 42 44 49 60 64 65 66 69 71 74 **P**3 **S**0515 Benedictine Health System	21	10	165	2570	131	10581	333	13555	6382	236
DULUTH—St. Louis County										
✠ △ MILLER-DWAN MEDICAL CENTER, 502 East Second Street, Zip 55805-1982; tel. 218/727-8762; William H. Palmer, President **A**1 5 7 9 10 **F**2 3 6 9 12 14 15 16 17 18 19 21 26 31 32 34 35 37 39 41 42 44 45 46 48 49 52 53 55 56 57 58 59 60 65 67 71 73 **P**5	14	10	165	3155	80	80581	0	37230	17415	523
✠ ST. LUKE'S HOSPITAL, 915 East First Street, Zip 55805-2193; tel. 218/726-5555; Phillip A. Alioto, President and Chief Executive Officer **A**1 2 3 5 9 10 **F**4 7 8 10 11 14 15 16 19 21 22 23 32 33 35 37 39 40 41 42 52 53 56 58 59 65 67 71 72 73	23	10	258	7443	103	72120	907	65223	32235	949
✠ ST. MARY'S MEDICAL CENTER, 407 East Third Street, Zip 55805-1984; tel. 218/726-4000; Sister Kathleen Hofer, President **A**1 3 5 9 10 **F**1 2 3 4 5 7 8 10 11 13 14 15 16 17 18 19 21 22 23 24 27 28 29 31 32 33 34 35 37 39 40 41 42 43 44 45 46 47 48 49 52 53 54 55 56 57 58 59 60 64 65 66 67 69 71 72 73 74 **S**0515 Benedictine Health System	21	10	283	14744	206	109267	1497	114566	52586	1573
EDINA—Hennepin County										
RIVERSIDE MEDICAL CENTER See Fairview Riverside Medical Center, Minneapolis										
ELBOW LAKE—Grant County										
★ GRANT COUNTY HEALTH CENTER, (Formerly Grant County Hospital) 930 First Street N.E., Zip 56531; tel. 218/685-4461; Chad Cooper, Chief Operating Officer **A**9 10 **F**7 8 14 19 22 26 37 40 44 51 54 71 73 74	23	10	15	334	4	—	8	—	—	49
ELY—St. Louis County										
★ ELY-BLOOMENSON COMMUNITY HOSPITAL, 328 West Conan Street, Zip 55731-1198; tel. 218/365-3271; Larry Ravenberg, Administrator (Total facility includes 99 beds in nursing home-type unit) **A**9 10 **F**1 7 8 11 17 19 21 22 32 33 34 35 36 39 40 44 49 64 65 67 71 72 73 **P**6	23	10	138	641	105	5390	61	7300	3810	160
FAIRMONT—Martin County										
✠ FAIRMONT COMMUNITY HOSPITAL, (Includes Lutz Wing Convalescent and Nursing Care Unit) 835 Johnson Street, Zip 56031-0835, Mailing Address: P.O. Box 835, Zip 56031-0835; tel. 507/238-4254; Gerry Gilbertson, Administrator (Total facility includes 40 beds in nursing home-type unit) **A**1 9 10 **F**6 7 8 11 14 15 16 19 20 21 22 24 28 29 32 40 41 44 45 49 60 61 64 65 66 71 73	23	10	114	1990	60	35499	331	13896	6388	186
FARIBAULT—Rice County										
✠ DISTRICT ONE HOSPITAL, 631 Southeast First Street, Zip 55021-6321; tel. 507/334-6451; James N. Wolf, Executive Director and Chief Executive Officer **A**1 9 10 **F**7 8 10 15 16 19 22 28 30 33 35 36 37 39 40 41 42 44 45 46 67 71 73	16	10	64	2077	20	32774	351	13872	5632	170
FARIBAULT REGIONAL CENTER, 802 Circle Drive, Zip 55021-6399; tel. 507/332-3000; Bridget K. Stroud, Chief Executive Officer **A**9 **F**27 41 46 65 73 **P**6	12	62	263	20	272	0	0	44653	25000	605
□ WILSON CENTER PSYCHIATRIC FACILITY FOR CHILDREN AND ADOLESCENTS, 14th Street N.E., Zip 55021, Mailing Address: P.O. Box 917, Zip 55021; tel. 507/334-5561; Kevin J. Mahoney, President and Chief Executive Officer **A**1 9 **F**16 52 53 54 55 56 58 59 65	33	52	73	163	58	5994	0	11166	6307	222
FARMINGTON—Dakota County										
✠ SOUTH SUBURBAN MEDICAL CENTER, 913 Main Street, Zip 55024-1197; tel. 612/463-7825; Robert D. Johnson, Chief Executive Officer (Total facility includes 65 beds in nursing home-type unit) **A**1 9 10 **F**6 7 8 12 15 17 19 21 22 26 28 30 33 34 40 41 42 44 45 46 48 49 51 54 57 58 62 64 65 67 71 72 **P**3 6	23	10	90	550	69	4762	110	7063	3037	118
FERGUS FALLS—Otter Tail County										
□ FERGUS FALLS REGIONAL TREATMENT CENTER, Fir and Union Avenues, Zip 56537, Mailing Address: Box 157, Zip 56537-0157; tel. 218/739-7200; (Nonreporting) **A**1 9 10	12	22	255	—	—	—	—	—	—	—
✠ LAKE REGION HOSPITAL AND NURSING HOME, 712 South Cascade Street, Zip 56537, Mailing Address: P.O. Box 728, Zip 56538-0728; tel. 218/736-8000; Edward J. Mehl, Chief Executive Officer (Total facility includes 44 beds in nursing home-type unit) **A**1 9 10 **F**7 15 17 19 21 22 32 33 34 35 37 40 41 44 49 52 53 54 55 56 57 64 65 66 67 71 73	23	10	136	3751	90	33207	346	25701	12506	367

Hospitals, U.S. / MINNESOTA

Hospital, Address, Telephone, Administrator, Approval, Facility, and Physician Codes, Health Care System	Classification Codes		Utilization Data					Expense (thousands) of dollars		
★ American Hospital Association (AHA) membership ☐ Joint Commission on Accreditation of Healthcare Organizations (JCAHO) accreditation + American Osteopathic Hospital Association (AOHA) membership ○ American Osteopathic Association (AOA) accreditation △ Commission on Accreditation of Rehabilitation Facilities (CARF) accreditation Control codes 61, 63, 64, 71, 72 and 73 indicate hospitals listed by AOHA, but not registered by AHA. For definition of numerical codes, see page A6	Control	Service	Beds	Admissions	Census	Outpatient Visits	Births	Total	Payroll	Personnel
FOREST LAKE—Washington County ✠ DISTRICT MEMORIAL HOSPITAL, 246 11th Avenue S.E., Zip 55025–1898; tel. 612/464–3341; John F. Lannon, Administrator (Nonreporting) **A**1 9 10	16	10	44	—	—	—	—	—	—	—
FOSSTON—Polk County ★ FIRST CARE MEDICAL SERVICES, 900 South Hilligoss Boulevard East, Zip 56542–1599; tel. 218/435–1133; David Hubbard, Chief Executive Officer (Total facility includes 50 beds in nursing home–type unit) **A**9 10 **F**7 8 14 15 16 19 20 22 26 27 28 30 32 34 36 40 41 42 44 48 49 63 64 65 71 73	23	10	93	693	57	32933	54	5483	2235	134
FRIDLEY—Anoka County ✠ UNITY HOSPITAL, (Includes Mercy Hospital, 4050 Coon Rapids Boulevard, Coon Rapids, Minnesota, Zip 55433–2586; tel. 612/421–8888) 550 Osborne Road N.E., Minneapolis, Zip 55432–2791; tel. 612/421–2222; William T. MacNally, President **A**1 2 9 10 **F**2 3 7 8 10 11 12 14 15 16 17 18 19 21 22 23 25 27 28 29 30 32 33 34 35 37 40 41 42 43 44 45 46 49 52 53 54 55 56 57 58 59 60 63 65 67 68 70 71 72 73 **P**3 4 5 6 7 8 **S**0041 Allina Health System	23	10	462	22024	234	139958	4183	—	—	1791
GLENCOE—Mcleod County ✠ GLENCOE AREA HEALTH CENTER, 705 East 18th Street, Zip 55336–1499; tel. 612/864–3121; Jon D. Braband, Chief Executive Officer (Total facility includes 110 beds in nursing home–type unit) **A**1 9 10 **F**1 6 7 8 11 15 16 19 22 26 28 30 33 34 35 37 40 41 42 44 58 64 65 71 73 **S**1985 HealthSystem Minnesota	14	10	149	1268	121	13128	125	12383	5866	269
GLENWOOD—Pope County ★ GLACIAL RIDGE HOSPITAL, 10 Fourth Avenue S.E., Zip 56334–1898; tel. 612/634–4521; Douglas J. Reker, Administrator and Chief Executive Officer **A**9 10 **F**7 8 14 15 19 21 22 24 32 33 34 35 37 40 41 44 49 53 54 65 70 71 73 **P**6	16	10	34	563	4	7245	56	3882	1921	109
GOLDEN VALLEY—Hennepin County ✠ TRANSITIONAL HOSPITAL CORPORATION OF MINNEAPOLIS, (Long Term Acute Care) 4101 Golden Valley Road, Zip 55422; tel. 612/588–2750; Lee Larson, Chief Executive Officer (Newly Registered) **A**1 10	33	49	49	—	—	—	—	—	—	—
GRACEVILLE—Big Stone County HOLY TRINITY HOSPITAL, 115 West Second Street, Zip 56240–0157; tel. 612/748–7223; Ken Knutson, Chief Executive Officer (Nonreporting) **A**9 10	23	10	92	—	—	—	—	—	—	—
GRAND MARAIS—Cook County COOK COUNTY NORTH SHORE HOSPITAL, Mailing Address: P.O. Box 10, Zip 55604–0010; tel. 218/387–1500; Diane Pearson, Administrator (Total facility includes 47 beds in nursing home–type unit) **A**9 10 **F**7 8 11 15 22 32 33 34 40 49 56 64 65 71	16	10	59	329	46	8971	32	3560	2059	75
GRAND RAPIDS—Itasca County ✠ ITASCA MEDICAL CENTER, 126 First Avenue S.E., Zip 55744–3698; tel. 218/326–3401; Darwin Root, Administrator (Total facility includes 35 beds in nursing home–type unit) **A**1 2 9 10 **F**1 7 8 11 12 15 17 19 21 22 26 31 32 34 35 39 40 41 44 46 49 52 56 57 59 64 65 66 71 73 74 **S**0002 Quorum Health Group/Quorum Health Resources	13	10	112	2712	62	23059	331	19783	9539	223
GRANITE FALLS—Yellow Medicine County ✠ GRANITE FALLS MUNICIPAL HOSPITAL AND MANOR, 345 Tenth Avenue, Zip 56241–1499; tel. 612/564–3111; George Gerlach, Administrator (Total facility includes 64 beds in nursing home–type unit) **A**1 9 10 **F**8 14 15 16 17 19 22 28 30 31 32 33 35 36 40 44 46 49 63 64 65 71 **S**0041 Allina Health System	14	10	94	646	71	7328	46	6073	3008	155
HALLOCK—Kittson County KITTSON MEMORIAL HOSPITAL, 1010 South Birch Street, Zip 56728, Mailing Address: P.O. Box 700, Zip 56728; tel. 218/843–3612; Richard J. Failing, Chief Executive Officer (Total facility includes 95 beds in nursing home–type unit) **A**9 10 **F**8 11 15 19 20 22 28 34 35 39 40 44 49 64 65 71	23	10	116	256	89	5819	16	3924	2025	101
HARMONY—Fillmore County HARMONY COMMUNITY HOSPITAL, 815 South Main Avenue, Zip 55939, Mailing Address: Route 1, Box 173, Zip 55939; tel. 507/886–6544; Greg Braun, Administrator (Total facility includes 45 beds in nursing home–type unit) **A**9 10 **F**1 15 16 17 26 27 28 30 32 33 34 41 54 64 67 72 73 **P**3	23	10	53	179	46	5002	0	1955	1206	53
HASTINGS—Dakota County ✠ REGINA MEDICAL CENTER, 1175 Nininger Road, Zip 55033; tel. 612/437–3121; Lynn W. Olson, Administrator and Chief Executive Officer (Total facility includes 61 beds in nursing home–type unit) **A**1 9 10 **F**6 7 8 11 12 15 17 19 22 24 27 28 29 30 32 34 35 36 39 40 41 44 46 49 51 62 64 65 67 71 73 **P**4	23	10	118	1734	76	19587	329	18214	9350	352
HENDRICKS—Lincoln County ★ HENDRICKS COMMUNITY HOSPITAL, East Lincoln Street, Zip 56136; tel. 507/275–3134; Kirk Stensrud, Administrator (Total facility includes 70 beds in nursing home–type unit) **A**9 10 **F**1 6 7 8 11 12 14 15 16 17 19 20 21 22 24 28 30 31 32 33 34 37 40 44 63 64 65 67 71 73	23	10	82	397	72	4558	39	3557	1911	113
HIBBING—St. Louis County ✠ MESABI REGIONAL MEDICAL CENTER, 750 East 34th Street, Zip 55746; tel. 218/262–4881; Fran Gardeski, Chief Executive Officer **A**1 9 10 **F**1 2 3 7 8 14 15 16 19 20 21 22 26 31 32 33 34 35 36 37 39 40 42 44 49 52 53 54 55 56 57 58 59 65 66 67 70 71 73	23	10	175	3656	56	62804	322	25485	11970	387
HUTCHINSON—McLeod County ✠ HUTCHINSON COMMUNITY HOSPITAL, 1095 Highway 15 South, Zip 55350–3500; tel. 612/234–5000; Philip G. Graves, President (Total facility includes 127 beds in nursing home–type unit) **A**1 9 10 **F**1 3 7 8 11 12 14 15 19 22 26 28 30 32 33 34 35 36 37 40 41 42 44 45 46 48 49 52 53 54 55 56 57 58 59 63 64 65 66 67 71 **S**0041 Allina Health System	14	10	187	2498	147	35346	340	20879	9733	203

© 1995 AHA Guide

Hospitals, U.S. / MINNESOTA

Hospital, Address, Telephone, Administrator, Approval, Facility, and Physician Codes, Health Care System	Classification Codes		Utilization Data					Expense (thousands) of dollars		Personnel
★ American Hospital Association (AHA) membership ☐ Joint Commission on Accreditation of Healthcare Organizations (JCAHO) accreditation + American Osteopathic Hospital Association (AOHA) membership ○ American Osteopathic Association (AOA) accreditation △ Commission on Accreditation of Rehabilitation Facilities (CARF) accreditation Control codes 61, 63, 64, 71, 72 and 73 indicate hospitals listed by AOHA, but not registered by AHA. For definition of numerical codes, see page A6	Control	Service	Beds	Admissions	Census	Outpatient Visits	Births	Total	Payroll	
INTERNATIONAL FALLS—Koochiching County ★ FALLS MEMORIAL HOSPITAL, 1400 Highway 11–71, Zip 56649–2189; tel. 218/283–4481; James F. Hanko, Administrator and Chief Executive Officer **A**9 10 **F**2 8 11 15 17 19 22 28 32 34 35 37 39 40 42 44 46 48 49 71 73 **P**4 **S**0002 Quorum Health Group/Quorum Health Resources	23	10	42	1276	11	24364	127	6789	3116	117
IVANHOE—Lincoln County ★ DIVINE PROVIDENCE HEALTH CENTER, 312 East George Street, Zip 56142–0136, Mailing Address: P.O. Box G, Zip 56142–0136; tel. 507/694–1414; Loren Ellery, Administrator (Nonreporting) **A**9 10	23	10	79	—	—	—	—	—	—	—
JACKSON—Jackson County ★ JACKSON MUNICIPAL HOSPITAL, NURSING HOME AND CLINIC, 1430 North Highway, Zip 56143–1098; tel. 507/847–2420; Charlotte Highcamp, Chief Executive Officer (Total facility includes 21 beds in nursing home–type unit) **A**9 10 **F**19 22 34 40 45 58 64 **P**6	14	10	41	341	23	11617	9	3193	1617	91
KARLSTAD—Kittson County KARLSTAD HEALTH FACILITIES, First and Roosevelt, Zip 56732, Mailing Address: Box I, Zip 56732; tel. 218/436–2141; Kevin M. Quinn, Administrator (Nonreporting) **A**9 10	14	10	90	—	—	—	—	—	—	—
LAKE CITY—Wabasha County ☐ LAKE CITY HOSPITAL, 904 South Lakeshore Drive, Zip 55041; tel. 612/345–3321; Mark Rinehardt, Chief Executive Officer (Total facility includes 115 beds in nursing home–type unit) **A**1 9 10 **F**3 7 8 15 17 19 22 26 32 33 34 40 44 45 49 64 65 71 72 73	14	10	144	674	114	5979	47	6549	3488	160
LE SUEUR—Le Sueur County MINNESOTA VALLEY HEALTH CENTER, (Includes Gardenview Nursing Home) 621 South Fourth Street, Zip 56058–2203; tel. 612/665–3375; Jennifer D. Pfeffer, Interim Administrator (Total facility includes 85 beds in nursing home–type unit) **A**9 10 **F**6 7 8 11 14 15 16 19 22 28 30 33 34 36 40 41 42 44 49 64 65 71 72 74 **P**4	23	10	103	285	83	12016	41	4385	2479	121
LITCHFIELD—Meeker County ★ MEEKER COUNTY MEMORIAL HOSPITAL, 612 South Sibley Avenue, Zip 55355–3398; tel. 612/693–3242; Ronald E. Johnson, Administrator **A**9 10 **F**7 8 15 19 21 22 26 28 29 30 34 35 37 40 42 44 45 49 63 67 71	13	10	38	1189	12	12610	166	6021	2924	100
LITTLE FALLS—Morrison County ☐ ST. GABRIEL'S HOSPITAL, 815 Second Street S.E., Zip 56345–3596; tel. 612/632–5441; Larry A. Schulz, President and Chief Executive Officer (Total facility includes 150 beds in nursing home–type unit) **A**1 9 10 **F**3 7 8 15 16 19 21 22 24 28 31 32 33 34 35 37 40 41 42 44 46 49 50 53 55 56 57 58 63 64 65 66 71 73 **S**5175 Catholic Health Corporation	21	10	205	2336	171	46547	270	25270	10552	414
LONG PRAIRIE—Todd County ☐ LONG PRAIRIE MEMORIAL HOSPITAL AND HOME, 20 Ninth Street S.E., Zip 56347–1225; tel. 612/732–2141; Kevin J. Smith, President (Nonreporting) **A**1 9 10 **S**0041 Allina Health System	23	10	138	—	—	—	—	—	—	—
LUVERNE—Rock County LUVERNE COMMUNITY HOSPITAL, 305 East Luverne Street, Zip 56156, Mailing Address: P.O. Box 1019, Zip 56156; tel. 507/283–2321; Gerald E. Carl, Administrator (Nonreporting) **A**9 10	14	10	38	—	—	—	—	—	—	—
MADELIA—Watonwan County ☐ MADELIA COMMUNITY HOSPITAL, 121 Drew Avenue S.E., Zip 56062; tel. 507/642–3255; Candace Fenske R.N., Administrator **A**1 9 10 **F**7 14 15 16 19 20 21 22 29 32 33 34 36 40 41 44 45 49 65 71	23	10	25	517	6	4875	50	2063	971	46
MADISON—Lac Qui Parle County ★ MADISON HOSPITAL, 820 Third Avenue, Zip 56256, Mailing Address: Box 184, Zip 56256; tel. 612/598–7556; John Fossum, Chief Executive Officer **A**9 10 **F**1 7 8 15 19 21 22 28 30 32 33 34 36 40 44 51 64 65 71	21	10	21	163	1	—	9	1345	565	22
MAHNOMEN—Mahnomen County MAHNOMEN COUNTY AND VILLAGE HOSPITAL, CLINIC AND NURSING CENTER, 414 Jefferson Avenue, Zip 56557, Mailing Address: Box 396, Zip 56557–0396; tel. 218/935–2511; Jeanie L. Hocking, Chief Executive Officer (Total facility includes 48 beds in nursing home–type unit) **A**9 10 **F**1 7 14 16 19 22 34 40 44 49 64 65 71	15	10	66	186	49	6370	0	4256	2268	77
MANKATO—Blue Earth County ☐ IMMANUEL–ST. JOSEPH'S HOSPITAL, 1025 Marsh Street, Zip 56001, Mailing Address: P.O. Box 8673, Zip 56002–8673; tel. 507/625–4031; Jerome A. Crest, President **A**1 2 9 10 **F**2 3 7 8 10 12 14 15 16 17 19 20 21 22 23 29 31 32 33 34 35 37 39 40 41 42 44 45 49 52 53 54 55 56 57 58 59 60 63 65 67 71 73 74 **P**8	23	10	147	7112	94	63050	1003	44333	20491	610
MAPLEWOOD—Ramsey County ☐ HEALTHEAST ST. JOHN'S HOSPITAL, 1575 Beam Avenue, Zip 55109; tel. 612/232–7000; William Knutson, Administrator **A**1 2 3 5 9 10 **F**2 3 4 7 8 10 11 12 14 15 16 17 19 21 22 25 26 27 29 31 32 33 34 35 37 39 40 41 42 43 44 45 46 47 60 63 64 65 70 71 73 **P**2 3 4 5 6 7 8 **S**2185 HealthEast	23	10	179	10199	108	30288	2495	57216	27057	597
MARSHALL—Lyon County ☐ WEINER MEMORIAL MEDICAL CENTER, 300 South Bruce Street, Zip 56258–1616; tel. 507/532–9661; Ronald Jensen, Administrator (Total facility includes 76 beds in nursing home–type unit) **A**1 9 10 **F**7 8 15 16 17 19 20 22 23 24 26 27 28 29 30 31 32 33 35 37 39 40 42 44 49 56 62 63 64 65 67 71 73 **P**3 4	14	10	100	1880	91	—	434	12934	6561	173

Hospitals, U.S. / MINNESOTA

Hospital, Address, Telephone, Administrator, Approval, Facility, and Physician Codes, Health Care System	Classification Codes		Utilization Data					Expense (thousands) of dollars		
	Control	Service	Beds	Admissions	Census	Outpatient Visits	Births	Total	Payroll	Personnel

★ American Hospital Association (AHA) membership
☐ Joint Commission on Accreditation of Healthcare Organizations (JCAHO) accreditation
+ American Osteopathic Hospital Association (AOHA) membership
○ American Osteopathic Association (AOA) accreditation
△ Commission on Accreditation of Rehabilitation Facilities (CARF) accreditation
Control codes 61, 63, 64, 71, 72 and 73 indicate hospitals listed by AOHA, but not registered by AHA. For definition of numerical codes, see page A6

MELROSE—Stearns County

★ MELROSE HOSPITAL AND PINE VILLA NURSING HOME, 11 North Fifth Avenue West, Zip 56352; tel. 612/256-4231; Joan Bangasser, Administrator (Total facility includes 75 beds in nursing home-type unit) A9 10 F1 7 14 15 16 17 19 22 26 27 28 30 32 33 34 35 36 39 40 41 44 49 62 64 65 66 67 71 73 P5	14	10	87	397	80	8035	79	4396	2279	112

MINNEAPOLIS—Hennepin County

★ △ ABBOTT NORTHWESTERN HOSPITAL, (Includes Sister Kenny Institute, Minneapolis, Minnesota) 800 East 28th Street, Zip 55407-3799; tel. 612/863-4000; Robert K. Spinner, President A1 2 3 5 7 9 10 F2 3 4 5 7 8 10 11 12 15 17 19 21 22 23 24 25 26 27 28 29 30 31 32 33 34 35 36 37 39 40 41 42 43 44 45 46 48 49 51 52 53 54 55 56 57 58 59 60 61 63 65 67 69 71 72 73 74 P5 6 8 S0041 Allina Health System	23	10	607	27696	423	170753	2798	295820	130917	3119
☐ CHILDREN'S HEALTH CARE, (Formerly Minneapolis Children's Medical Center) 2525 Chicago Avenue South, Zip 55404-9976; tel. 612/813-6100; Brock D. Nelson, Chief Executive Officer A1 2 3 9 10 F3 4 5 6 7 8 9 10 12 13 14 15 16 17 18 19 20 21 22 23 24 25 27 28 29 30 31 32 33 34 35 38 39 41 42 43 44 45 46 47 49 50 51 53 54 55 56 58 59 60 61 63 65 66 67 68 69 71 72 73 74 P1 3 5	23	50	163	6219	115	—	0	106104	52829	1247
★ FAIRVIEW RIVERSIDE MEDICAL CENTER, (Formerly Riverside Medical Center) (Includes Fairview Riverside Hospital, 2312 South Sixth Street, Minneapolis, Minnesota, Zip 55454; St. Mary's Hospital and Rehabilitation Center, 2414 South Seventh Street, Minneapolis, Minnesota, Zip 55454; tel. 612/338-2229) 2450 Riverside Avenue, Zip 55454-9978; tel. 612/672-6300; Pamela L. Tibbetts, Senior Vice President and Administrator (Nonreporting) A1 2 3 5 9 10 S1325 Fairview Hospital and Healthcare Services	21	10	808	—	—	—	—	—	—	—
★ FAIRVIEW SOUTHDALE HOSPITAL, 6401 France Avenue South, Zip 55435-2199; tel. 612/924-5000; Mark M. Enger, Senior Vice President and Administrator (Nonreporting) A1 2 9 10 S1325 Fairview Hospital and Healthcare Services	23	10	390	—	—	—	—	—	—	—
★ △ HENNEPIN COUNTY MEDICAL CENTER, 701 Park Avenue South, Zip 55415; tel. 612/347-2121; John W. Bluford, Chief Executive Officer A1 2 3 5 7 8 9 10 F3 4 5 7 8 9 10 11 12 13 14 16 17 18 19 20 21 22 23 25 26 27 28 29 30 31 35 37 38 39 40 41 42 43 44 45 46 47 48 49 51 52 53 54 55 56 57 58 60 61 65 66 67 69 70 71 72 73 74 P1	13	10	458	20206	295	375211	2180	256600	120716	3733
MINNEAPOLIS CHILDREN'S MEDICAL CENTER See Children's Health Care										
★ PHILLIPS EYE INSTITUTE, 2215 Park Avenue, Zip 55404; tel. 612/336-6000; Shari E. Levy, President A1 10 F11 14 15 21 22 32 34 37 46 47 65 P3 4 7 8 S0041 Allina Health System	23	49	10	703	2	9872	0	10980	3702	105
★ SHRINERS HOSPITALS FOR CRIPPLED CHILDREN, TWIN CITIES UNIT, 2025 East River Road, Zip 55414-3696; tel. 612/335-5300; Laurence E. Johnson, Administrator A1 3 5 F15 17 19 34 35 39 44 45 46 49 53 65 67 71 73 P6 S4125 Shriners Hospitals for Crippled Children	23	59	40	879	19	8324	0	—	—	129
★ UNIVERSITY OF MINNESOTA HOSPITAL AND CLINIC, Harvard Street at E River Road, Zip 55455-0392; tel. 612/626-3000; Gregory Hart, President (Nonreporting) A1 3 5 8 9 10	12	10	554	—	—	—	—	—	—	—
★ VETERANS AFFAIRS MEDICAL CENTER, One Veterans Drive, Zip 55417-2399; tel. 612/725-2000; Charles A. Milbrandt, Director (Total facility includes 110 beds in nursing home-type unit) A1 2 3 5 8 F1 2 3 4 5 8 10 11 12 15 16 17 18 19 20 21 22 23 24 25 26 27 28 29 30 31 32 33 34 35 37 39 41 42 43 44 45 46 48 49 50 51 52 53 54 55 56 57 58 59 60 63 64 65 67 69 71 72 73 74 P6 S9295 Department of Veterans Affairs	45	10	604	14242	339	311147	0	213630	110520	3178

MONTEVIDEO—Chippewa County

CHIPPEWA COUNTY MONTEVIDEO HOSPITAL, 824 North 11th Street, Zip 56265; tel. 612/269-8878; Fred Knutson, Administrator (Nonreporting) A9 10	15	10	29	—	—	—	—	—	—	—

MONTICELLO—Wright County

★ MONTICELLO-BIG LAKE COMMUNITY HOSPITAL, 1013 Hart Boulevard, Zip 55362-0480, Mailing Address: Box 480, Zip 55362-0480; tel. 612/295-2945; Barbara Schwientek, Director (Total facility includes 91 beds in nursing home-type unit) A1 9 10 F1 3 7 8 11 14 15 19 22 32 33 34 35 36 37 40 42 44 58 64 65 66 71	16	10	120	819	97	39909	173	11193	5353	138

MOOSE LAKE—Carlton County

★ MERCY HOSPITAL & HEALTH CARE CENTER, 710 South Kenwood Avenue, Zip 55767; tel. 218/485-4481; Dianne Mandernach, Administrator (Total facility includes 94 beds in nursing home-type unit) A9 10 F7 8 12 14 15 17 19 22 24 28 30 34 37 39 40 41 44 45 46 49 61 64 65 67 70 71 73	16	10	125	853	100	6286	85	8312	4476	157
☐ MOOSE LAKE REGIONAL TREATMENT CENTER, 1000 Lake Shore Drive, Zip 55767; tel. 218/485-4411; Frank R. Milczark, Chief Executive Officer (Nonreporting) A1 9 10	12	22	480	—	—	—	—	—	—	—

MORA—Kanabec County

★ KANABEC HOSPITAL, 300 Clark Street, Zip 55051; tel. 612/679-1212; John A. Kayfes FACHE, Administrator A1 9 10 F8 16 17 19 21 22 28 30 35 37 40 42 44 45 46 49 65 71 73	13	10	49	1095	11	9787	189	6346	3238	107

MORRIS—Stevens County

★ STEVENS COMMUNITY MEDICAL CENTER, (Formerly Stevens Community Memorial Hospital) 400 East First Street, Zip 56267, Mailing Address: P.O. Box 660, Zip 56267; tel. 612/589-1313; John Rau, President and Chief Executive Officer A1 9 10 F3 7 8 10 14 19 22 27 31 34 35 37 40 42 44 45 49 53 54 55 56 57 58 65 67 71 S0041 Allina Health System	23	10	37	1017	13	6300	80	6855	3185	133

© 1995 AHA Guide

Hospitals, U.S. / MINNESOTA

Hospital, Address, Telephone, Administrator, Approval, Facility, and Physician Codes, Health Care System	Classification Codes		Utilization Data					Expense (thousands) of dollars		
★ American Hospital Association (AHA) membership □ Joint Commission on Accreditation of Healthcare Organizations (JCAHO) accreditation + American Osteopathic Hospital Association (AOHA) membership ○ American Osteopathic Association (AOA) accreditation △ Commission on Accreditation of Rehabilitation Facilities (CARF) accreditation Control codes 61, 63, 64, 71, 72 and 73 indicate hospitals listed by AOHA, but not registered by AHA. For definition of numerical codes, see page A6	Control	Service	Beds	Admissions	Census	Outpatient Visits	Births	Total	Payroll	Personnel
NEW PRAGUE—Le Sueur County										
★ QUEEN OF PEACE HOSPITAL, 301 Second Street N.E., Zip 56071–1799; tel. 612/758–4431; Sister Jean Juenemann, Chief Executive Officer **A**1 9 10 **F**7 8 17 19 20 21 23 24 31 32 33 34 35 37 39 40 41 42 44 45 46 49 50 58 67 71 72 73 **S**0535 Benedictine Sisters	21	10	28	1126	11	49152	168	8684	4002	135
NEW ULM—Brown County										
★ SIOUX VALLEY HOSPITAL, 1324 Fifth Street North, Zip 56073, Mailing Address: Box 577, Zip 56073; tel. 507/354–2111; Robert Stevens, President **A**1 9 10 **F**2 3 7 15 17 18 19 21 22 24 27 28 29 30 32 33 35 36 37 40 41 42 44 49 52 53 54 55 56 57 58 62 66 67 71 72 **P**7 **S**0041 Allina Health System	23	10	85	1991	23	47576	390	14595	6608	231
NORTHFIELD—Rice County										
★ NORTHFIELD HOSPITAL, (Includes H. O. Dilley Skilled Nursing Facility) 801 West First Street, Zip 55057–1697; tel. 507/645–6661; Kendall C. Bank, Chief Executive Officer (Total facility includes 40 beds in nursing home–type unit) **A**1 9 10 **F**7 8 11 14 15 16 19 20 22 26 28 30 32 33 35 36 39 40 41 42 44 45 46 49 61 64 65 66 67 71 73 **S**0041 Allina Health System	14	10	69	1333	46	15990	304	11352	5459	143
OLIVIA—Renville County										
RENVILLE COUNTY HOSPITAL, 611 East Fairview Avenue, Zip 56277–1397; tel. 612/523–1261; Dean G. Slagter, Administrator **A**9 10 **F**7 8 11 15 17 19 21 22 28 30 33 35 36 39 40 44 49 63 65 71 **P**5	13	10	28	574	5	6021	68	2201	1383	59
ONAMIA—Mille Lacs County										
★ MILLE LACS HEALTH SYSTEM, 200 North Elm Street, Zip 56359–0800; tel. 612/532–3154; Frederick W. Haack, Chief Executive Officer (Total facility includes 80 beds in nursing home–type unit) **A**1 9 10 **F**1 2 7 8 15 16 17 19 20 22 26 28 30 32 39 40 41 44 45 48 49 51 64 65 67 71 72 **P**6 **S**0041 Allina Health System	23	10	108	811	86	11791	48	8502	4709	133
ORTONVILLE—Big Stone County										
ORTONVILLE AREA HEALTH SERVICES, 750 Eastvold Avenue, Zip 56278; tel. 612/839–2502; Donald Wee, Administrator (Total facility includes 74 beds in nursing home–type unit) **A**9 10 **F**7 8 15 16 19 21 22 27 30 33 34 35 36 39 42 44 45 46 49 53 54 56 57 58 64 65 67 71 73 **S**2235 Lutheran Health Systems	14	10	105	569	78	9000	73	5157	2256	104
OWATONNA—Steele County										
★ OWATONNA HOSPITAL, 903 South Oak Avenue, Zip 55060–3296; tel. 507/451–3850; Richard G. Slieter, President **A**1 9 10 **F**7 8 12 15 16 19 21 22 28 30 32 33 35 36 37 40 44 49 52 54 55 56 57 58 65 66 67 71 **S**0041 Allina Health System	23	10	65	1929	20	—	433	12704	5205	160
PARK RAPIDS—Hubbard County										
★ ST. JOSEPH'S HOSPITAL, 600 Pleasant Avenue, Zip 56470; tel. 218/732–3311; David R. Hove, President **A**1 9 10 **F**7 8 15 16 19 22 32 33 34 37 40 44 49 65 71 **S**5175 Catholic Health Corporation	21	10	42	1734	22	17373	154	12236	5686	189
PAYNESVILLE—Stearns County										
★ PAYNESVILLE AREA HOSPITAL, 200 First Street West, Zip 56362; tel. 612/243–3767; William M. LaCroix, Administrator (Total facility includes 64 beds in nursing home–type unit) **A**9 10 **F**1 7 8 11 14 15 19 21 22 24 26 27 32 34 35 36 39 40 42 44 46 48 62 64 65 67 71 **P**8	16	10	94	611	69	8584	75	7054	3438	172
PERHAM—Otter Tail County										
★ PERHAM MEMORIAL HOSPITAL AND HOME, 665 Third Street S.W., Zip 56573–1199; tel. 218/346–4500; Ronald Bervig, Administrator (Nonreporting) **A**1 9 10	16	10	131	—	—	—	—	—	—	—
PIPESTONE—Pipestone County										
PIPESTONE COUNTY MEDICAL CENTER, 911 Fifth Avenue S.W., Zip 56164, Mailing Address: P.O. Box 370, Zip 56164; tel. 507/825–5811; Carl P. Vaagenes, Administrator (Nonreporting) **A**9 10	13	10	87	—	—	—	—	—	—	—
PRINCETON—Mille Lacs County										
★ FAIRVIEW NORTHLAND REGIONAL HOSPITAL, 911 Northland Drive, Zip 55371; tel. 612/389–1313; Glenn G. Erickson, Vice President and Administrator **A**1 9 10 **F**3 7 8 15 16 17 19 20 21 22 25 28 29 30 32 33 34 35 36 37 39 40 41 42 44 46 49 65 66 67 71 **S**1325 Fairview Hospital and Healthcare Services	23	10	41	1788	15	26514	290	—	—	179
RED WING—Goodhue County										
★ ST. JOHN'S REGIONAL HEALTH CENTER, 1407 West Fourth Street, Zip 55066–2198; tel. 612/388–6721; John A. Nordwick, President **A**1 9 10 **F**2 3 7 8 11 15 16 17 19 26 28 29 31 32 33 34 35 36 37 39 40 41 42 44 45 46 49 51 65 67 71 73	23	10	84	2204	29	19816	368	—	—	—
REDLAKE—Beltrami County										
★ U.S. PUBLIC HEALTH SERVICE INDIAN HOSPITAL, Zip 56671; tel. 218/679–3912; Essimae Stevens, Service Unit Director (Nonreporting) **A**1 10 **S**9195 U.S. Public Health Service Indian Health Service	47	10	23	—	—	—	—	—	—	—
REDWOOD FALLS—Redwood County										
★ REDWOOD FALLS MUNICIPAL HOSPITAL, 100 Fallwood Road, Zip 56283–1828; tel. 507/637–2907; James E. Schulte, Administrator (Nonreporting) **A**9 10	14	10	35	—	—	—	—	—	—	—
ROBBINSDALE—Hennepin County										
★ △ NORTH MEMORIAL MEDICAL CENTER, 3300 Oakdale Avenue North, Zip 55422–2900; tel. 612/520–5200; Scott R. Anderson, President **A**1 2 3 5 7 9 10 **F**4 7 8 10 11 12 14 15 16 17 19 20 21 22 26 27 28 30 32 33 34 35 36 37 38 39 40 41 42 43 44 46 47 48 49 51 52 54 55 56 57 61 63 65 66 67 71 72 73 74 **P**5	23	10	402	20334	246	621707	3338	196841	97706	2596

Hospitals, U.S. / MINNESOTA

Hospital, Address, Telephone, Administrator, Approval, Facility, and Physician Codes, Health Care System	Classification Codes		Utilization Data					Expense (thousands) of dollars		
★ American Hospital Association (AHA) membership ☐ Joint Commission on Accreditation of Healthcare Organizations (JCAHO) accreditation + American Osteopathic Hospital Association (AOHA) membership ○ American Osteopathic Association (AOA) accreditation △ Commission on Accreditation of Rehabilitation Facilities (CARF) accreditation Control codes 61, 63, 64, 71, 72 and 73 indicate hospitals listed by AOHA, but not registered by AHA. For definition of numerical codes, see page A6	Control	Service	Beds	Admissions	Census	Outpatient Visits	Births	Total	Payroll	Personnel
ROCHESTER—Olmsted County										
★ OLMSTED COMMUNITY HOSPITAL, 1650 Fourth Street S.E., Zip 55904–4700; tel. 507/285–8485; Joseph C. Cartney, Chief Operating Officer **A**1 9 10 **F**7 15 19 20 22 24 36 37 39 40 44 46 71 73	13	10	47	2038	17	18307	877	12763	6112	162
★ ROCHESTER METHODIST HOSPITAL, 201 West Center Street, Zip 55902–3084; tel. 507/266–7890; Stephen C. Waldhoff, Administrator **A**1 3 5 9 10 **F**3 4 5 7 8 10 19 20 21 22 23 24 25 26 29 30 31 32 33 34 35 37 38 39 40 41 42 43 44 45 46 49 50 51 53 54 55 56 57 58 59 60 61 62 63 65 66 67 69 70 71 72 73 **P**6 **S**1875 Mayo Foundation	23	10	350	14761	236	—	1745	108894	44343	1163
★ △ SAINT MARYS HOSPITAL OF ROCHESTER, 1216 Second Street S.W., Zip 55902–1970; tel. 507/255–5123; Gerald T. Mahoney, Administrator **A**1 3 5 7 8 9 10 **F**3 4 5 7 8 10 11 12 18 19 20 21 22 23 24 25 31 32 33 34 35 37 38 40 41 42 43 44 45 46 47 48 49 50 51 52 53 54 55 56 57 58 59 60 61 62 63 65 66 67 69 70 71 72 73 74 **P**6 **S**1875 Mayo Foundation	23	10	903	28709	561	—	0	251284	107629	2883
ROSEAU—Roseau County										
★ ROSEAU AREA HOSPITAL DISTRICT, 715 Delmore Avenue, Zip 56751; tel. 218/463–2500; David F. Hagen, Administrator (Total facility includes 64 beds in nursing home–type unit) **A**1 9 10 **F**8 10 11 19 21 22 30 32 35 44 45 63 64 65 67 71 73 **P**5	16	10	101	1041	77	13975	223	8237	4060	159
RUSH CITY—Chisago County										
RUSH CITY HOSPITAL, 760 West Fourth Street, Zip 55069; tel. 612/358–4708; Lynn Clayton, Administrator **A**9 10 **F**15 19 22 28 30 44 49 71 72 **P**6	14	10	26	247	2	13631	8	2468	1249	49
SAINT CLOUD—Stearns County										
★ ST. CLOUD HOSPITAL, 1406 Sixth Avenue North, Zip 56303–0016; tel. 612/251–2700; John R. Frobenius, President and Chief Executive Officer **A**1 2 9 10 **F**1 2 3 4 6 7 8 10 11 12 13 15 16 17 18 19 20 21 22 23 25 26 27 28 30 31 32 33 34 35 36 37 38 39 40 41 42 43 44 45 46 48 49 51 52 53 55 56 57 58 59 60 61 62 65 66 67 68 70 71 72 73 74 **S**0535 Benedictine Sisters	23	10	335	14242	195	80232	2192	111522	52620	1651
★ VETERANS AFFAIRS MEDICAL CENTER, 4801 Eighth Street North, Zip 56303–2099; tel. 612/252–1670; Thomas A. Holthaus, Director (Total facility includes 207 beds in nursing home–type unit) **A**1 **F**1 2 3 20 22 26 33 34 39 41 44 46 49 52 54 56 57 58 59 64 65 67 73 **P**6 **S**9295 Department of Veterans Affairs	45	22	566	2965	476	87897	0	—	—	886
SAINT JAMES—Watonwan County										
☐ WATONWAN MEMORIAL HOSPITAL, 1207 Sixth Avenue South, Zip 56081; tel. 507/375–3261; Donald Loren Johnson, Administrator **A**1 9 10 **F**7 8 15 16 17 19 20 21 22 28 30 32 39 40 44 45 46 49 51 65 71 **P**6	23	10	27	308	5	13952	32	2362	832	51
SAINT LOUIS PARK—Hennepin County										
★ △ METHODIST HOSPITAL, 6500 Excelsior Boulevard, Zip 55426–4702, Mailing Address: Box 650, Minneapolis Zip 55440–9946; tel. 612/932–5000; Terry S. Finzen, Senior Vice President and Chief Operating Officer (Total facility includes 35 beds in nursing home–type unit) **A**1 2 3 5 7 9 10 **F**3 4 5 6 7 8 10 11 12 14 15 17 18 19 20 22 23 24 25 26 28 29 30 31 32 33 34 35 36 37 39 40 41 42 43 44 45 46 48 49 53 54 55 56 57 58 59 60 61 64 65 66 67 68 69 70 71 72 73 **P**4 6 7 **S**1985 HealthSystem Minnesota	23	10	355	17774	240	200051	2991	146487	68239	1928
SAINT PAUL—Ramsey County										
★ CHILDREN'S HOSPITAL, 345 North Smith Avenue, Zip 55102; tel. 612/220–6000; Brock D. Nelson, President **A**1 3 5 9 10 **F**2 3 4 7 10 13 14 15 16 17 19 20 21 22 23 24 27 31 32 34 35 38 39 41 42 43 44 45 46 47 48 49 51 52 53 54 55 56 58 59 60 61 65 67 68 70 71 73 **P**1	23	50	105	5543	78	73562	0	62928	25971	592
☐ △ GILLETTE CHILDREN'S HOSPITAL, (Neuromuscoskeletal, Pediatrics, Brain Injury, Cerebral Palsy, Chronic Pain, Epilepsy, Myelomeningocele, Orthopedic Surgery, Technology Dependent Rehabilitation) 200 University Avenue East, Zip 55101; tel. 612/291–2848; Margaret Perryman, Chief Executive Officer **A**1 3 5 7 9 10 **F**5 14 16 17 20 34 39 41 44 46 49 65 67 **P**5 6 7	23	59	48	976	20	29973	0	23374	10189	289
★ △ HEALTHEAST BETHESDA LUTHERAN HOSPITAL AND REHABILITATION CENTER, (Long Term Acute Care) 559 Capitol Boulevard, Zip 55103; tel. 612/232–2133; Bonnie Watkins, Administrator (Total facility includes 35 beds in nursing home–type unit) **A**1 7 9 10 **F**1 2 3 4 5 7 8 9 10 11 12 13 14 15 16 17 18 19 20 21 22 25 26 27 28 29 30 31 32 33 34 35 36 37 39 40 41 42 43 44 45 46 48 49 50 51 52 53 54 55 56 57 58 59 60 61 62 63 64 65 66 67 68 70 71 72 73 74 **P**1 3 4 5 6 7 **S**2185 HealthEast	23	49	135	1470	108	4200	0	27296	13290	371
★ HEALTHEAST MIDWAY HOSPITAL, 1700 University Avenue, Zip 55104–2791; tel. 612/232–5000; Douglas P. Cropper, Vice President and Administrator (Total facility includes 37 beds in nursing home–type unit) **A**1 9 10 **F**1 3 4 7 8 10 12 14 15 19 21 22 25 26 27 28 29 31 32 33 34 35 37 38 39 40 41 42 43 44 45 46 49 53 54 55 56 57 58 59 61 63 64 65 66 67 68 71 72 73 **P**1 3 4 5 7 8 **S**2185 HealthEast	23	10	201	7076	99	27942	725	45358	20229	486
★ HEALTHEAST ST. JOSEPH'S HOSPITAL, 69 West Exchange Street, Zip 55102; tel. 612/232–3000; Milton Hertel, Administrator **A**1 2 3 5 10 **F**1 2 3 4 7 8 10 11 12 14 15 16 17 18 19 21 22 23 25 26 27 28 29 35 36 37 38 39 40 41 42 43 44 45 46 47 48 49 51 52 53 54 55 58 60 63 64 65 67 70 71 72 73 74 **S**2185 HealthEast	23	10	297	10663	154	49780	1219	96238	40145	1088
★ △ ST. PAUL–RAMSEY MEDICAL CENTER, 640 Jackson Street, Zip 55101–2595; tel. 612/221–3456; James B. Dixon, President **A**1 2 3 5 7 8 9 10 **F**2 3 4 5 7 8 9 10 11 17 18 19 20 21 22 25 26 29 31 32 33 34 35 38 40 41 42 43 44 47 48 49 51 52 53 54 56 57 58 61 65 70 71 72 73 74 **P**3 5 8	23	10	325	17037	249	340225	1674	177363	91796	2068

© 1995 AHA Guide

Hospitals, U.S. / MINNESOTA

Hospital, Address, Telephone, Administrator, Approval, Facility, and Physician Codes, Health Care System	Classification Codes		Utilization Data					Expense (thousands) of dollars		
★ American Hospital Association (AHA) membership □ Joint Commission on Accreditation of Healthcare Organizations (JCAHO) accreditation + American Osteopathic Hospital Association (AOHA) membership ○ American Osteopathic Association (AOA) accreditation △ Commission on Accreditation of Rehabilitation Facilities (CARF) accreditation Control codes 61, 63, 64, 71, 72 and 73 indicate hospitals listed by AOHA, but not registered by AHA. For definition of numerical codes, see page A6	Control	Service	Beds	Admissions	Census	Outpatient Visits	Births	Total	Payroll	Personnel
★ UNITED HOSPITAL, 333 North Smith Street, Zip 55102–2389; tel. 612/220–8000; David B M. Jones, President **A**1 2 3 5 9 10 **F**3 4 7 8 10 12 14 15 16 17 19 21 22 23 24 27 28 29 30 31 32 33 34 35 37 39 40 41 42 43 44 45 46 48 49 51 52 53 54 55 58 59 60 61 63 65 67 71 73 **S**0041 Allina Health System	23	10	366	21623	299	83472	3970	182006	77320	1573
SAINT PETER—Nicollet County										
COMMUNITY HOSPITAL AND HEALTH CARE CENTER, 618 West Broadway, Zip 56082–1327; tel. 507/931–2200; Jeanne Johnson, Chief Executive Officer (Nonreporting) **A**9 10	14	10	118	—	—	—	—	—	—	—
MINNESOTA SECURITY HOSPITAL See St. Peter Regional Treatment Center										
□ ST. PETER REGIONAL TREATMENT CENTER, (Includes Minnesota Security Hospital, Sheppard Drive, Saint Peter, Minnesota, Zip 56082; tel. 507/931–7100) 100 Freeman Drive, Zip 56082–1599; tel. 507/931–7100; William L. Pedersen, Chief Executive Officer **A**1 10 **F**2 14 15 16 20 46 52 56 57 65 73	12	22	582	965	507	0	0	38824	26666	846
SANDSTONE—Pine County										
NORTH PINE AREA HOSPITAL, 317 Court Street, Zip 55072; tel. 612/245–2212; Clark Graebel, Chief Executive Officer (Total facility includes 86 beds in nursing home–type unit) **A**9 10 **F**8 17 19 21 22 26 30 34 41 44 49 64 65 67 71	16	10	106	370	88	7201	1	4891	2600	112
SAUK CENTRE—Stearns County										
★ ST. MICHAEL'S HOSPITAL, 425 North Elm Street, Zip 56378; tel. 612/352–2221; Del Christianson, Administrator (Nonreporting) **A**9 10	15	10	88	—	—	—	—	—	—	—
SHAKOPEE—Scott County										
★ ST. FRANCIS REGIONAL MEDICAL CENTER, 325 West Fifth Avenue, Zip 55379–1200; tel. 612/445–2322; Donald J. Leivermann, President and Chief Executive Officer **A**1 9 10 **F**7 8 15 17 19 20 21 22 28 30 31 32 33 34 35 36 37 39 40 41 42 44 45 46 49 54 56 63 65 66 67 71 73 **P**5 **S**0041 Allina Health System	21	10	63	2411	20	46578	609	20773	9151	260
SLAYTON—Murray County										
MURRAY COUNTY MEMORIAL HOSPITAL, 2042 Juniper Avenue, Zip 56172; tel. 507/836–6111; Jerry Bobeldyk, Administrator (Nonreporting) **A**9 10	13	10	35	—	—	—	—	—	—	—
SLEEPY EYE—Brown County										
SLEEPY EYE MUNICIPAL HOSPITAL, 400 Fourth Avenue N.W., Zip 56085; tel. 507/794–3571; Scott E. Morin, Administrator **A**9 10 **F**7 8 11 12 15 16 19 22 24 28 29 30 32 33 34 35 36 37 39 40 41 44 45 46 49 62 67 71	14	10	25	483	4	5583	22	2485	1177	52
SPRING GROVE—Houston County										
TWEETEN LUTHERAN HEALTH CARE CENTER, 125 Fifth Avenue S.E., Zip 55974; tel. 507/498–3211; Robert Schmidt, Administrator (Total facility includes 79 beds in nursing home–type unit) **A**9 10 **F**3 15 16 17 20 26 28 29 30 32 33 34 39 41 44 49 64 65 71 73 **P**6	23	10	89	154	76	4387	0	2965	1675	86
SPRING VALLEY—Fillmore County										
COMMUNITY MEMORIAL HOSPITAL AND NURSING HOME, 800 Memorial Drive, Zip 55975; tel. 507/346–7381; David Herder, Administrator (Nonreporting) **A**9 10	23	10	74	—	—	—	—	—	—	—
SPRINGFIELD—Brown County										
□ SPRINGFIELD COMMUNITY HOSPITAL, 625 North Jackson, Zip 56087, Mailing Address: Box 146, Zip 56087; tel. 507/723–6201; Scott Thoreson, Administrator **A**1 9 10 **F**7 8 15 16 19 20 22 28 30 32 40 41 44 48 49 58 64 65 71	14	10	22	427	5	5584	34	2128	905	32
STAPLES—Todd County										
GREATER STAPLES HOSPITAL, 401 East Prairie Avenue, Zip 56479–9415; tel. 218/894–1515; Tim Rice, Administrator (Nonreporting) **A**9 10	16	10	140	—	—	—	—	—	—	—
STARBUCK—Pope County										
★ MINNEWASKA DISTRICT HOSPITAL, 610 West Sixth Street, Zip 56381, Mailing Address: P.O. Box 160, Zip 56381–0610; tel. 612/239–2201; Roxann A. Wellman, Chief Executive Officer **A**9 10 **F**7 8 14 15 19 22 27 28 32 33 34 36 37 40 41 44 62 65 71	16	10	19	456	6	840	11	1906	880	42
STILLWATER—Washington County										
★ LAKEVIEW MEMORIAL HOSPITAL, 927 West Churchill Street, Zip 55082–5930; tel. 612/439–5330; Jeffrey J. Robertson, Administrator **A**1 9 10 **F**7 8 11 15 16 17 19 21 22 28 29 30 32 33 34 35 37 39 40 41 42 44 45 46 65 67 71 73	23	10	48	2503	22	17527	567	19635	8278	273
THIEF RIVER FALLS—Pennington County										
★ NORTHWEST MEDICAL CENTER, 120 LaBree Avenue South, Zip 56701–2819; tel. 218/681–4240; Richard A. Spyhalski, Chief Executive Officer (Total facility includes 90 beds in nursing home–type unit) **A**1 9 10 **F**7 8 11 15 19 21 22 27 28 29 30 33 34 35 36 37 39 40 41 42 44 45 46 49 52 53 54 55 56 57 58 59 63 64 65 66 67 71 73 74	23	10	169	2090	114	18267	218	15278	8502	303
TRACY—Lyon County										
★ TRACY MUNICIPAL HOSPITAL, Fifth Street East, Zip 56175–1536; tel. 507/629–3200; Thomas Quinlivan, Administrator **A**1 9 10 **F**7 8 15 16 17 19 22 26 28 29 30 31 32 33 34 35 37 40 42 44 45 58 62 67 71 **P**6	14	10	37	377	3	10518	8	2096	779	44
TWO HARBORS—Lake County										
LAKE VIEW MEMORIAL HOSPITAL, 325 11th Avenue, Zip 55616–1298; tel. 218/834–7300; Marge Johnson, Interim Administrator (Total facility includes 50 beds in nursing home–type unit) **A**9 10 **F**3 6 7 16 22 28 40 44 49 64 65 71 73	23	10	80	584	55	4484	44	4041	2401	93
TYLER—Lincoln County										
★ A.L. VADHEIM MEMORIAL HOSPITAL, 240 Willow Street, Zip 56178–0280; tel. 507/247–5521; James Rotert, Administrator (Total facility includes 43 beds in nursing home–type unit) **A**10 **F**1 7 8 15 16 19 22 26 33 35 36 40 44 49 64 67 71 **P**5 **S**5255 Presentation Health System	23	10	63	249	46	4998	3	3137	1466	92

Hospitals, U.S. / MINNESOTA

Hospital, Address, Telephone, Administrator, Approval, Facility, and Physician Codes, Health Care System	Classification Codes		Utilization Data					Expense (thousands) of dollars		
★ American Hospital Association (AHA) membership ☐ Joint Commission on Accreditation of Healthcare Organizations (JCAHO) accreditation + American Osteopathic Hospital Association (AOHA) membership ○ American Osteopathic Association (AOA) accreditation △ Commission on Accreditation of Rehabilitation Facilities (CARF) accreditation Control codes 61, 63, 64, 71, 72 and 73 indicate hospitals listed by AOHA, but not registered by AHA. For definition of numerical codes, see page A6	Control	Service	Beds	Admissions	Census	Outpatient Visits	Births	Total	Payroll	Personnel
VIRGINIA—St. Louis County ★ VIRGINIA REGIONAL MEDICAL CENTER, 901 Ninth Street North, Zip 55792–2398; tel. 218/741–3340; Gerald R. Lundberg, Administrator (Total facility includes 116 beds in nursing home–type unit) **A**1 9 10 **F**7 8 14 17 19 20 21 22 23 26 30 32 34 35 37 40 44 48 49 65 71 73 **S**0002 Quorum Health Group/Quorum Health Resources	14	10	199	2720	146	21029	262	23253	11015	330
WABASHA—Wabasha County ★ ST. ELIZABETH HOSPITAL, 1200 Fifth Grand Boulevard W., Zip 55981; tel. 612/565–4531; Thomas Crowley, President (Total facility includes 167 beds in nursing home–type unit) **A**1 9 10 **F**1 2 3 4 5 6 7 8 9 10 11 12 13 14 15 16 17 18 19 20 21 22 23 24 25 26 27 28 29 30 31 32 33 34 35 36 37 38 39 40 41 42 43 44 45 46 47 48 49 50 51 52 53 54 55 56 57 58 59 60 61 62 63 64 65 66 67 68 69 70 71 72 73 74 **P**1 2 3 4 5 6 7 8 **S**5305 Sisters of the Sorrowful Mother United States Health System	21	10	198	614	145	13473	75	8336	4301	—
WACONIA—Carver County ★ RIDGEVIEW MEDICAL CENTER, 500 South Maple Street, Zip 55387; tel. 612/442–2191; John P. Devins, President and Chief Executive Officer **A**1 9 10 **F**7 8 11 14 15 17 18 19 20 21 22 28 29 30 32 33 34 35 37 39 40 41 42 44 49 65 66 67 70 71 72 73 74 **P**4 5	14	10	102	4515	44	50271	912	33113	16920	510
WADENA—Wadena County ★ TRI–COUNTY HOSPITAL, 415 Jefferson Street North, Zip 56482; tel. 218/631–3510; (Nonreporting) **A**1 9 10	23	10	24	—	—	—	—	—	—	—
WARREN—Marshall County ★ NORTH VALLEY HEALTH CENTER, (Formerly Warren Community Hospital) 109 South Minnesota Street, Zip 56762–1499; tel. 218/745–4211; Everett A. Butler, Administrator **A**9 10 **F**7 8 11 13 15 17 19 22 28 30 32 33 34 35 37 40 41 44 45 48 65 66 71 72 73 **P**4	23	10	31	426	3	11735	24	2663	1328	53
WASECA—Waseca County ★ WASECA AREA MEMORIAL HOSPITAL, 100 Fifth Avenue N.W., Zip 56093–2422; tel. 507/835–1210; Dennis C. Miley, Executive Vice–President **A**1 9 10 **F**3 7 8 11 14 15 16 17 22 24 30 32 34 36 39 40 41 44 46 48 49 65 66 71 72 **P**1	23	10	26	384	5	24734	101	5968	3050	83
WESTBROOK—Cottonwood County DR. HENRY SCHMIDT MEMORIAL HOSPITAL, 920 Bell Avenue, Zip 56183, Mailing Address: P.O. Box 188, Zip 56183–0188; tel. 507/274–6121; Judy Lichty, Administrator (Nonreporting) **A**9 10	23	10	8	—	—	—	—	—	—	—
WHEATON—Traverse County WHEATON COMMUNITY HOSPITAL, 401 12th Street North, Zip 56296–1099; tel. 612/563–8226; James J. Talley, Administrator **A**9 10 **F**7 8 19 21 22 27 31 32 34 35 40 44 48 49 64 71	14	10	35	585	9	11493	25	2861	1186	50
WILLMAR—Kandiyohi County ★ RICE MEMORIAL HOSPITAL, 301 Becker Avenue S.W., Zip 56201–3395; tel. 612/231–4227; Lawrence J. Massa, Chief Executive Officer **A**1 2 9 10 **F**7 8 15 17 19 21 22 23 26 30 32 33 34 35 37 40 42 44 45 49 52 53 54 55 56 57 58 59 60 63 65 66 67 71 73	14	10	118	4880	58	40576	730	34917	16531	479
☐ WILLMAR REGIONAL TREATMENT CENTER, North Highway 71, Zip 56201–1128, Mailing Address: Box 1128, Zip 56201–1128; tel. 612/231–5100; Gregory G. Spartz, Chief Executive Officer **A**1 9 10 **F**1 2 3 12 15 16 17 18 19 20 21 22 26 27 29 34 35 41 44 45 46 52 53 54 55 56 57 58 65 67 71 73 **P**6	12	22	402	1110	332	0	0	28795	20069	559
WINDOM—Cottonwood County WINDOM AREA HOSPITAL, Highways 60 and 71 North, Zip 56101, Mailing Address: Box 339, Zip 56101; tel. 507/831–2400; Loretta Ulferts, Administrator **A**9 10 **F**7 8 16 17 19 20 22 28 30 34 35 40 44 49 65 67 71 73 **P**6	14	10	35	806	9	11128	138	3447	1430	59
WINONA—Winona County ★ COMMUNITY MEMORIAL HOSPITAL AND CONVALESCENT AND REHABILITATION UNIT, 855 Mankato Avenue, Zip 55987–4894, Mailing Address: P.O. Box 5600, Zip 55987–0600; tel. 507/454–3650; Roger L. Metz, Administrator (Total facility includes 104 beds in nursing home–type unit) **A**1 9 10 **F**1 2 3 6 7 8 10 11 15 16 17 19 21 22 23 26 28 30 32 33 37 39 40 41 44 45 46 49 51 52 53 54 55 56 57 58 60 63 64 65 66 67 71 73	23	10	203	3260	130	42316	431	21668	11861	431
WORTHINGTON—Nobles County ☐ WORTHINGTON REGIONAL HOSPITAL, 1018 Sixth Ave, Zip 56187, Mailing Address: P.O. Box 997, Zip 56187; tel. 507/372–2941; Melvin J. Platt, Administrator (Total facility includes 5 beds in nursing home–type unit) **A**1 9 10 **F**12 14 15 16 19 22 32 33 34 35 36 37 39 40 44 45 49 52 53 55 56 57 64 65 70 71 73	14	10	93	2467	26	13648	341	10762	5568	168
ZUMBROTA—Goodhue County ★ ZUMBROTA HEALTH CARE, 383 West Fifth Street, Zip 55992; tel. 507/732–5131; Daniel Will, Administrator (Nonreporting) **A**1 9 10	23	10	19	—	—	—	—	—	—	—

© 1995 AHA Guide

Hospitals, U.S. / MISSISSIPPI

MISSISSIPPI

Resident population 2,643 (in thousands)
Resident population in metro areas 30.7%
Birth rate per 1,000 population 16.7
65 years and over 12.5%
Percent of persons without health insurance 19.3%

- ★ American Hospital Association (AHA) membership
- □ Joint Commission on Accreditation of Healthcare Organizations (JCAHO) accreditation
- + American Osteopathic Hospital Association (AOHA) membership
- ○ American Osteopathic Association (AOA) accreditation
- △ Commission on Accreditation of Rehabilitation Facilities (CARF) accreditation
  Control codes 61, 63, 64, 71, 72 and 73 indicate hospitals listed by AOHA, but not registered by AHA. For definition of numerical codes, see page A6

Hospital, Address, Telephone, Administrator, Approval, Facility, and Physician Codes, Health Care System	Classification Codes		Utilization Data					Expense (thousands) of dollars		
	Control	Service	Beds	Admissions	Census	Outpatient Visits	Births	Total	Payroll	Personnel
ABERDEEN—Monroe County ABERDEEN–MONROE COUNTY HOSPITAL, 400 South Chestnut Street, Zip 39730, Mailing Address: Box 747, Zip 39730; tel. 601/369-2455; Victor M. Ribeiro, Administrator **A**9 10 **F**8 26 30 37 51 62 64 70 71 73	15	10	27	731	14	7803	0	—	—	71
ACKERMAN—Choctaw County CHOCTAW COUNTY MEDICAL CENTER, 148 West Cherry Street, Zip 39735–0417, Mailing Address: P.O. Box 417, Zip 39735–0417; tel. 601/285-6235; Mack Martin, Administrator (Total facility includes 60 beds in nursing home–type unit) **A**9 10 **F**2 3 16 22 31 32 34 53 64 65 71	13	10	88	497	68	3203	0	—	—	103
AMORY—Monroe County ★ GILMORE MEMORIAL HOSPITAL, 1105 Earl Frye Boulevard, Zip 38821, Mailing Address: P.O. Box 459, Zip 38821–0459; tel. 601/256-7111; Charles L. Stewart, President and Chief Executive Officer **A**1 9 10 **F**7 8 11 12 15 16 19 22 28 37 38 40 41 44 47 49 65 71 73 74 **P**8	23	10	95	3703	46	23741	928	17148	8091	307
BATESVILLE—Panola County SOUTH PANOLA COMMUNITY HOSPITAL, Hospital Drive, Zip 38606, Mailing Address: Box 433, Zip 38606; tel. 601/563-5611; Richard W. Manning, Administrator **A**9 10 **F**19 22 28 30 44 65 67 71 73	13	10	70	1702	31	13834	0	7430	2595	147
BAY SPRINGS—Jasper County JASPER GENERAL HOSPITAL, (Includes Jasper County Nursing Home) Sixth Street, Zip 39422, Mailing Address: Box 527, Zip 39422; tel. 601/764-2101; M. Kenneth Posey FACHE, Administrator (Total facility includes 94 beds in nursing home–type unit) **A**9 10 **F**64 65 71	13	10	114	439	102	—	0	—	—	147
BAY SAINT LOUIS—Hancock County ★ HANCOCK MEDICAL CENTER, 149 Drinkwater Boulevard, Zip 39520, Mailing Address: P.O. Box 2790, Zip 39521; tel. 601/467-9081; Donald G. Henderson, Administrator **A**1 9 10 **F**7 8 11 12 14 15 16 17 19 22 28 30 33 34 35 37 44 46 49 56 65 71 73 **P**1 **S**0002 Quorum Health Group/Quorum Health Resources	13	10	66	2656	34	32339	149	15673	5443	234
BELZONI—Humphreys County ★ HUMPHREYS COUNTY MEMORIAL HOSPITAL, 500 CCC Road, Zip 39038, Mailing Address: P.O. Box 510, Zip 39038; tel. 601/247-3831; Debra L. Griffin, Administrator **A**9 10 **F**7 17 20 24 31 64 65 71	13	10	28	943	10	4432	10	—	—	54
BILOXI—Harrison County □ BILOXI REGIONAL MEDICAL CENTER, 150 Reynoir Street, Zip 39530, Mailing Address: Box 128, Zip 39533; tel. 601/432-1571; James D. Baker, Executive Director **A**1 2 9 10 **F**7 8 11 12 14 15 16 17 19 20 21 22 25 28 31 32 34 37 38 39 40 42 44 45 46 47 48 49 52 59 60 62 63 65 71 73 74 **P**2 5 7 8 **S**1775 Health Management Associates	33	10	153	6652	104	114795	600	—	—	493
□ GULF COAST MEDICAL CENTER, 180–A Debuys Road, Zip 39531–4405, Mailing Address: Box 4518, Zip 39531–4518; tel. 601/388-6711; C. L. Smith, Chief Executive Officer **A**1 9 10 **F**2 3 8 12 15 16 19 21 22 26 27 28 30 31 34 35 37 41 44 46 52 53 54 55 56 57 58 59 64 65 67 71 73 **P**4 5 **S**6525 Ornda Healthcorp	33	10	189	3202	67	23813	0	32508	11374	440
GULF OAKS HOSPITAL, 180–C Debuys Road, Zip 39531; tel. 601/388-0600; Hugh S. Simcoe III, Administrator (Nonreporting) **A**9 **S**6525 Ornda Healthcorp	33	22	45	—						
★ VETERANS AFFAIRS MEDICAL CENTER, (Includes Veterans Affairs Medical Center, Gulfport Division, East Beach Street, Gulfport, Mississippi, Zip 39501; tel. 601/863-1972) 400 Veterans Avenue, Zip 39531–2410; tel. 601/388-5541; George Rodman, Director (Total facility includes 320 beds in nursing home–type unit) **A**1 2 3 5 **F**3 11 12 16 17 19 20 21 22 26 27 28 29 30 31 32 33 34 35 37 39 41 42 44 45 46 49 52 54 55 56 57 58 60 61 64 65 67 71 72 73 74 **P**6 **S**9295 Department of Veterans Affairs	45	10	510	5734	172	—	0	—	—	
BOONEVILLE—Prentiss County ★ BAPTIST MEMORIAL HOSPITAL–BOONEVILLE, 100 Hospital Street, Zip 38829; tel. 601/728-5331; William A. Tuttle, Administrator **A**1 9 10 **F**11 14 16 17 19 20 21 22 31 37 40 44 46 65 71 73 **P**4 5 **S**1625 Baptist Memorial Health Care System, Inc.	21	10	78	2167	31	18319	0	9475	4547	168
BRANDON—Rankin County ★ RANKIN MEDICAL CENTER, 350 Crossgates Boulevard, Zip 39042; tel. 601/825-2811; Thomas Wiman, Administrator **A**1 2 9 10 **F**8 11 19 21 22 24 26 30 31 32 33 34 37 39 41 42 44 45 46 49 63 64 65 71 73 **P**1	13	10	90	2927	47	43371	0	20855	9788	363
BROOKHAVEN—Lincoln County ★ KING'S DAUGHTERS HOSPITAL, Highway 51 North, Zip 39601, Mailing Address: P.O. Box 948, Zip 39601; tel. 601/833-6011; Wallace Cooper, Chief Executive Officer **A**1 9 10 **F**6 7 8 12 15 16 17 19 20 22 23 24 25 28 30 32 33 34 35 37 40 41 44 45 49 51 62 65 67 71 73 **P**3 **S**0002 Quorum Health Group/Quorum Health Resources	23	10	95	3261	47	30730	564	18920	8104	316

Hospitals, U.S. / MISSISSIPPI

Hospital, Address, Telephone, Administrator, Approval, Facility, and Physician Codes, Health Care System	Classification Codes		Utilization Data					Expense (thousands) of dollars		
★ American Hospital Association (AHA) membership ☐ Joint Commission on Accreditation of Healthcare Organizations (JCAHO) accreditation + American Osteopathic Hospital Association (AOHA) membership ○ American Osteopathic Association (AOA) accreditation △ Commission on Accreditation of Rehabilitation Facilities (CARF) accreditation Control codes 61, 63, 64, 71, 72 and 73 indicate hospitals listed by AOHA, but not registered by AHA. For definition of numerical codes, see page A6	Control	Service	Beds	Admissions	Census	Outpatient Visits	Births	Total	Payroll	Personnel
BRUCE—Calhoun County BRUCE HOSPITAL, (Includes Bruce Hospital Long-Term Care Facility) Highway 9 South, Zip 38915, Mailing Address: Box 429, Zip 38915-0429; tel. 601/983-5100; Robert M. Perry, Administrator (Total facility includes 22 beds in nursing home-type unit) **F**18 19 20 22 26 28 30 34 44 46 48 49 60 64 65 71 73 **S**1275 First Health, Inc.	23	10	47	394	5	1867	0	—	—	97
CALHOUN CITY—Calhoun County HILLCREST HOSPITAL, 140 Burke-Calhoun City Road, Zip 38916-0770, Mailing Address: Route 2, Box 226-A, Burke Road, Zip 38916; tel. 601/628-6611; Charles R. Daugherty, Administrator **A**9 10 **F**19 22 44 65 71	14	10	30	734	12	5831	0	2578	1169	44
CANTON—Madison County MADISON GENERAL HOSPITAL, Highway 16 East, Zip 39046, Mailing Address: P.O. Box 1607, Zip 39046; tel. 601/859-1331; G. Wayne Schuler, Executive Director (Total facility includes 60 beds in nursing home-type unit) **A**9 10 **F**3 8 12 15 16 19 22 26 37 40 49 54 57 59 64 65 71 **P**8	13	10	127	1584	95	27635	394	—	—	219
CARTHAGE—Leake County LEAKE MEMORIAL HOSPITAL, 300 Ellis Street, Zip 39051-0557, Mailing Address: P.O. Box 557, Zip 39051-0557; tel. 601/267-4511; Ted C. Lorenz Jr., Administrator (Total facility includes 44 beds in nursing home-type unit) **A**9 10 **F**19 22 31 64 65 71 73	23	10	76	1062	63	6626	3	—	—	135
CENTREVILLE—Wilkinson County ★ FIELD MEMORIAL COMMUNITY HOSPITAL, 270 West Main Street, Zip 39631, Mailing Address: Box 639, Zip 39631-0639; tel. 601/645-5221; Brock A. Slabach, Administrator **A**1 9 10 **F**8 12 17 19 21 22 26 28 34 40 44 46 48 49 51 64 65 70 71 **S**0002 Quorum Health Group/Quorum Health Resources	13	10	66	1734	23	8184	159	6081	2586	109
CHARLESTON—Tallahatchie County TALLAHATCHIE GENERAL HOSPITAL, 201 South Market, Zip 38921, Mailing Address: P.O. Box 230, Zip 38921-0230; tel. 601/647-5535; F. W. Ergle Jr., Administrator (Total facility includes 61 beds in nursing home-type unit) **A**9 10 **F**15 16 22 27 34 44 46 64 65 71 72 **P**5	13	10	77	346	67	2930	1	3235	1673	125
CLARKSDALE—Coahoma County ★ NORTHWEST MISSISSIPPI REGIONAL MEDICAL CENTER, 1970 Hospital Drive, Zip 38614, Mailing Address: Box 1218, Zip 38614; tel. 601/624-3401; Clifford L. Johnson Jr., Executive Director (Total facility includes 20 beds in nursing home-type unit) **A**1 9 10 **F**11 17 19 21 22 31 32 37 38 40 44 45 64 65 71 73	13	10	195	7057	123	45191	1365	31360	16628	634
CLEVELAND—Bolivar County ★ BOLIVAR COUNTY HOSPITAL, Highway 8 East, Zip 38732, Mailing Address: P.O. Box 1380, Zip 38732; tel. 601/846-0061; Robert L. Hawley Jr., Chief Executive Officer (Total facility includes 34 beds in nursing home-type unit) **A**1 9 10 **F**7 8 12 15 17 19 20 22 24 26 27 28 34 37 40 42 44 45 46 49 65 67 71 73 **S**0002 Quorum Health Group/Quorum Health Resources	13	10	143	4689	106	24631	654	—	—	434
COLLINS—Covington County ☐ COVINGTON COUNTY HOSPITAL, Sixth and Holly Streets, Zip 39428, Mailing Address: P.O. Box 1149, Zip 39428-1149; tel. 601/765-6711; Irving Hitt, Administrator **A**1 9 10 **F**7 11 14 15 19 20 21 22 32 34 37 40 44 48 49 61 65 71 73	13	10	82	1526	27	15925	238	5224	2716	129
COLUMBIA—Marion County METHODIST HOSPITAL OF MARION COUNTY, 1560 Sumrall Road, Zip 39429, Mailing Address: Box 630, Zip 39429; tel. 601/736-6303; Jerry M. Howell, Chief Operating Officer **A**9 10 **F**11 17 19 20 21 22 26 31 32 34 37 44 45 46 47 48 49 65 66 71 73	13	10	90	1815	33	22913	0	9322	4560	192
COLUMBUS—Lowndes County ★ BAPTIST MEMORIAL HOSPITAL–GOLDEN TRIANGLE, 2520 Fifth Street North, Zip 39703-2095, Mailing Address: P.O. Box 1307, Zip 39701-1307; tel. 601/243-1000; J. Stuart Mitchell III, Administrator **A**1 9 10 **F**6 7 8 9 11 12 13 17 18 19 20 21 22 24 26 27 28 30 31 33 34 38 39 40 41 43 44 45 46 47 49 52 54 56 58 59 64 65 67 68 71 72 73 **S**1625 Baptist Memorial Health Care System, Inc.	21	10	328	8999	130	46746	1122	—	—	885
★ U.S. AIR FORCE HOSPITAL, 201 Independence, Ste 101, Zip 39701-5300; tel. 601/434-2297; Lieutenant Colonel Karen A. Bradway USAF, MSC, Administrator (Nonreporting) **S**9495 Department of the Air Force	41	10	7	—	—	—	—	—	—	—
CORINTH—Alcorn County ★ MAGNOLIA REGIONAL HEALTH CENTER, (Formerly Magnolia Hospital) 611 Alcorn Drive, Zip 38834; tel. 601/286-6961; Rohn J. Butterfield, Chief Executive Officer **A**1 9 10 **F**7 10 11 12 14 15 16 17 19 21 24 26 28 30 32 33 34 35 37 40 41 42 44 45 46 49 52 60 61 63 64 65 67 71 72 73 74 **S**0002 Quorum Health Group/Quorum Health Resources	15	10	150	4920	97	45733	402	39240	15950	632
DE KALB—Kemper County KEMPER COMMUNITY HOSPITAL, Highway 39 & 16 Intersection, Zip 39328, Mailing Address: Box 246, Zip 39328; tel. 601/743-5851; Franklin K. Parker, Administrator (Total facility includes 19 beds in nursing home-type unit) **A**9 10 **F**25 26 48 51 64	13	10	24	78	19	0	0	—	—	29
DURANT—Holmes County DISTRICT TWO COMMUNITY HOSPITAL, 603 North West Avenue, Zip 39063, Mailing Address: P.O. Box 312, Zip 39063; tel. 601/653-3081; Tina Peirce, Administrator **A**9 10 **F**19 20 27 33 35 41 49 64 65 71 73 **P**3	13	10	29	622	14	4884	0	1926	855	62
ELLISVILLE—Jones County ELLISVILLE MUNICIPAL HOSPITAL See South Central Regional Medical Center, Laurel										

Hospitals, U.S. / MISSISSIPPI

Hospital, Address, Telephone, Administrator, Approval, Facility, and Physician Codes, Health Care System	Classification Codes		Utilization Data					Expense (thousands) of dollars		
★ American Hospital Association (AHA) membership □ Joint Commission on Accreditation of Healthcare Organizations (JCAHO) accreditation + American Osteopathic Hospital Association (AOHA) membership ○ American Osteopathic Association (AOA) accreditation △ Commission on Accreditation of Rehabilitation Facilities (CARF) accreditation Control codes 61, 63, 64, 71, 72 and 73 indicate hospitals listed by AOHA, but not registered by AHA. For definition of numerical codes, see page A6	Control	Service	Beds	Admissions	Census	Outpatient Visits	Births	Total	Payroll	Personnel
EUPORA—Webster County										
WEBSTER HEALTH SERVICES, 500 Highway 9 South, Zip 39744; tel. 601/258–6221; Harold H. Whitaker Sr., Administrator (Total facility includes 30 beds in nursing home–type unit) **A**9 10 **F**17 19 20 21 22 24 33 44 45 46 48 60 64 65 71 **S**0032 North Mississippi Health Services, Inc.	23	10	76	1189	46	9630	0	4963	2497	141
FAYETTE—Jefferson County										
JEFFERSON COUNTY HOSPITAL, 809 South Main Street, Zip 39069, Mailing Address: Box 577, Zip 39069; tel. 601/786–3401; Maurice Kilpatrick, Administrator **A**9 10 **F**20 22 26 31 35 45 49 71	23	10	30	973	10	3346	0	2022	944	54
FOREST—Scott County										
LACKEY MEMORIAL HOSPITAL, 330 North Broad Street, Zip 39074–0428, Mailing Address: Box 428, Zip 39074–0428; tel. 601/469–4151; George Posey, Administrator (Total facility includes 30 beds in nursing home–type unit) **A**9 10 **F**19 22 27 44 49 64 71 73 **P**5	23	10	74	1185	33	14000	0	—	—	114
GREENVILLE—Washington County										
★ DELTA REGIONAL MEDICAL CENTER, 1400 East Union Street, Zip 38703–3246, Mailing Address: Box 5247, Zip 38704–5247; tel. 601/378–3783; E. Berton Whitaker, Administrator and Chief Executive Officer **A**1 9 10 **F**2 3 7 8 9 10 13 14 15 16 17 19 21 22 23 28 29 30 31 32 33 34 35 37 40 41 42 44 45 46 49 52 59 60 63 65 67 71 73 **P**5 8 **S**0002 Quorum Health Group/Quorum Health Resources	13	10	150	5082	95	29864	495	32399	13927	651
★ KING'S DAUGHTERS HOSPITAL, 300 Washington Avenue, Zip 38701, Mailing Address: Box 1857, Zip 38702–1857; tel. 601/378–2020; Donald Joe Fisher, Administrator **A**1 9 10 **F**7 9 11 14 16 17 19 20 21 22 29 31 37 40 44 45 46 62 63 65 71	23	10	137	3728	51	29658	755	20293	7466	351
GREENWOOD—Leflore County										
□ GREENWOOD LEFLORE HOSPITAL, 1401 River Road, Zip 38930–1410, Mailing Address: Drawer 1410, Zip 38930–1410; tel. 601/459–7000; Terrell M. Cobb, Executive Director **A**1 9 10 **F**2 7 17 19 20 21 22 31 34 37 40 44 45 46 48 49 65 70 71 73 74	15	10	187	6717	108	83407	707	—	—	696
GRENADA—Grenada County										
★ GRENADA LAKE MEDICAL CENTER, 960 Avent Drive, Zip 38901–5094; tel. 601/226–8111; Donald L. Ray, Executive Director **A**1 9 10 **F**2 3 7 8 11 19 21 22 24 26 30 32 33 38 40 44 46 47 63 69 71 73	13	10	118	4833	84	27553	774	20407	9096	431
GULFPORT—Harrison County										
□ CPC SAND HILL HOSPITAL, 11150 Highway 49 North, Zip 39503–4110; tel. 601/831–1700; Michael A. Zieman, Chief Executive Officer **A**1 9 10 **F**2 3 8 9 11 12 17 22 31 37 43 44 45 47 52 53 54 55 56 65 **S**0785 Community Psychiatric Centers	33	22	60	790	43	0	0	—	—	107
★ GARDEN PARK COMMUNITY HOSPITAL, 1520 Broad Avenue, Zip 39501, Mailing Address: P.O. Box 1240, Zip 39502; tel. 601/864–4210; William E. Peaks, Executive Director **A**1 9 10 **F**7 11 17 19 20 21 22 31 34 35 37 40 44 45 46 49 65 66 71 **S**0048 Columbia/HCA Healthcare Corporation	33	10	120	2111	39	20730	0	—	—	310
★ △ MEMORIAL HOSPITAL AT GULFPORT, 4500 13th Street, Zip 39501, Mailing Address: Box 1810, Zip 39502–1810; tel. 601/867–4000; W. R. Burton, Administrator **A**1 7 9 10 **F**4 7 8 10 14 15 16 19 21 22 23 24 33 35 37 40 41 42 43 44 46 48 49 52 54 55 56 58 60 63 64 65 66 67 71 73 74 **P**1 3 8	15	10	302	13343	214	173578	2057	101295	42717	1514
VETERANS AFFAIRS MEDICAL CENTER, GULFPORT DIVISION See Biloxi										
HATTIESBURG—Forrest County										
★ FORREST GENERAL HOSPITAL, 400 South 28th Avenue, Zip 39401, Mailing Address: P.O. Box 16389, Zip 39404–6389; tel. 601/288–7000; Lowery A. Woodall, Executive Director **A**1 2 9 10 **F**2 3 4 6 7 8 10 11 12 14 15 16 17 19 20 21 22 23 24 25 28 29 30 31 32 33 34 35 37 38 39 40 41 42 43 44 45 46 48 49 51 52 53 54 55 56 58 59 60 65 66 67 68 71 72 73 74 **P**8	13	10	471	21000	343	102349	3120	122436	52167	2175
★ METHODIST HOSPITAL OF HATTIESBURG, 5001 Hardy Street, Zip 39402, Mailing Address: Box 16509, Zip 39404–6509; tel. 601/268–8000; William K. Ray, President and Chief Executive Officer **A**1 9 10 **F**8 14 15 16 17 19 21 22 23 24 28 30 32 34 35 37 39 41 44 46 49 50 63 64 65 66 67 71 73 **P**7	23	10	201	6929	110	54053	0	48165	17605	841
HAZLEHURST—Copiah County										
★ HARDY WILSON MEMORIAL HOSPITAL, 233 Magnolia Street, Zip 39083, Mailing Address: P.O. Box 889, Zip 39083–0889; tel. 601/894–4541; L. Pat Moreland, Administrator **A**9 10 **F**15 22 28 30 44 64 65 71 **P**5	13	10	49	1665	25	9222	265	—	—	137
HOLLY SPRINGS—Marshall County										
HOLLY SPRINGS MEMORIAL HOSPITAL, 1430 East Salem, Zip 38635, Mailing Address: P.O. Box 6000, Zip 38634–6000; tel. 601/252–1212; Bill Renick, Administrator **A**9 10 **F**15 19 21 23 29 31 32 36 44 51 65 70 71 **P**5	23	10	40	823	11	14301	1	—	—	77
HOUSTON—Chickasaw County										
□ TRACE REGIONAL HOSPITAL, Highway 8 East, Zip 38851, Mailing Address: P.O. Box 626, Zip 38851; tel. 601/456–3700; Bristol Messer, Chief Executive Officer **A**1 9 10 **F**2 11 17 19 21 22 24 31 34 37 44 45 46 49 60 62 63 65 71	33	10	84	2018	29	11830	0	—	—	199
INDIANOLA—Sunflower County										
★ SOUTH SUNFLOWER COUNTY HOSPITAL, 121 East Baker Street, Zip 38751; tel. 601/887–5235; H. J. Blessitt, Administrator **A**1 9 10 **F**7 15 19 22 27 37 44 49 65 71	13	10	69	2365	30	11243	454	8593	3180	142

Hospitals, U.S. / MISSISSIPPI

Hospital, Address, Telephone, Administrator, Approval, Facility, and Physician Codes, Health Care System	Classification Codes		Utilization Data					Expense (thousands) of dollars		
★ American Hospital Association (AHA) membership ☐ Joint Commission on Accreditation of Healthcare Organizations (JCAHO) accreditation + American Osteopathic Hospital Association (AOHA) membership ○ American Osteopathic Association (AOA) accreditation △ Commission on Accreditation of Rehabilitation Facilities (CARF) accreditation Control codes 61, 63, 64, 71, 72 and 73 indicate hospitals listed by AOHA, but not registered by AHA. For definition of numerical codes, see page A6	Control	Service	Beds	Admissions	Census	Outpatient Visits	Births	Total	Payroll	Personnel
IUKA—Tishomingo County										
☐ IUKA HOSPITAL & NURSING FACILITY, 1410 West Quitman, Zip 38852, Mailing Address: P.O. Box 860, Zip 38852; tel. 601/423-6051; Glendon Spigner, Administrator (Total facility includes 36 beds in nursing home–type unit) A1 9 10 F2 11 19 21 31 37 44 45 52 64 65 70 71 P3 5 S0032 North Mississippi Health Services, Inc.	23	10	88	1709	62	17891	0	8291	3741	152
JACKSON—Hinds County										
☐ CHARTER HOSPITAL OF JACKSON, 3531 Lakeland Drive, Zip 39208, Mailing Address: Box 4297, Zip 39296; tel. 601/939-9030; Jim R. Johnson, Administrator A1 9 10 F3 52 53 56 59 65 S0695 Charter Medical Corporation	33	22	111	1919	94	3896	0	—	—	203
★ METHODIST MEDICAL CENTER, 1850 Chadwick Drive, Zip 39204-3479, Mailing Address: P.O. Box 59001, Zip 39204-9001; tel. 601/376-1000; Thomas L. Harper, President and Chief Executive Officer A1 2 5 9 10 F3 7 8 10 11 12 15 16 17 20 22 23 26 28 29 30 32 33 34 37 38 39 40 41 42 43 49 52 60 P8 S9345 Methodist Health Systems, Inc.	23	10	277	11330	213	60195	1635	—	—	1220
★ MISSISSIPPI BAPTIST MEDICAL CENTER, 1225 North State Street, Zip 39202-2002; tel. 601/968-1000; M. Kent Strum, Executive Director A1 2 5 9 10 F2 3 7 10 11 14 16 17 19 20 21 22 23 24 31 33 34 35 37 38 40 41 43 44 45 46 47 49 54 60 64 65 66 71 73 74 P1 3 7 8	21	10	594	21664	376	93029	1521	143483	66293	2575
★ △ MISSISSIPPI METHODIST HOSPITAL AND REHABILITATION CENTER, 1350 Woodrow Wilson Drive, Zip 39216; tel. 601/364-3462; Mark A. Adams, President and Chief Executive Officer A1 7 10 F1 3 4 5 7 8 12 14 15 16 17 19 20 22 23 24 26 28 30 31 32 33 34 35 36 39 41 42 43 44 45 46 48 49 64 65 70 71 73 P7	23	46	116	1299	79	3978	0	—	—	586
☐ RIVER OAKS EAST–WOMAN'S PAVILION, (Formerly Woman's Hospital) 1026 North Flowood Drive, Zip 39208-9599, Mailing Address: P.O. Box 4546, Zip 39296-4546; tel. 601/932-1000; Carl Etter, Executive Director A1 9 10 F7 8 12 15 16 19 21 26 28 30 34 35 38 40 44 45 65 71 73 P7	33	44	84	3284	28	1911	2044	—	—	248
★ RIVER OAKS HOSPITAL, 1030 River Oaks Drive, Zip 39208, Mailing Address: P.O. Box 5100, Zip 39296-5100; tel. 601/932-1030; Albert A. Brust III, President and Chief Executive Officer A10 F4 7 8 14 17 19 20 21 22 29 30 33 35 37 40 41 42 44 45 46 49 61 65 67 71 73 74	33	10	100	5352	73	28109	1	41409	14256	557
★ ST. DOMINIC–JACKSON MEMORIAL HOSPITAL, 969 Lakeland Drive, Zip 39216-4699; tel. 601/982-0121; Claude W. Harbarger, President A1 2 5 9 10 F2 4 8 10 11 12 14 15 16 17 19 20 21 22 23 24 28 30 31 32 34 35 37 39 42 43 44 45 49 52 54 55 56 57 58 59 62 63 64 65 71 73 P8 S1295 Dominican Sisters of Springfield	23	10	571	12031	296	124055	0	80747	35403	1464
★ UNIVERSITY HOSPITALS AND CLINICS, UNIVERSITY OF MISSISSIPPI MEDICAL CENTER, 2500 North State Street, Zip 39216-4505; tel. 601/984-1000; Frederick Woodrell, Director A1 2 3 5 8 9 10 F3 9 10 11 17 19 20 21 22 23 26 27 31 33 34 35 37 38 40 41 43 44 45 46 47 48 49 52 53 54 55 58 60 64 65 66 69 71 73 S0002 Quorum Health Group/Quorum Health Resources	12	10	485	21053	384	171137	3688	134071	66621	2773
★ VETERANS AFFAIRS MEDICAL CENTER, 1500 East Woodrow Wilson Drive, Zip 39216-5199; tel. 601/364-1201; Richard P. Miller, Director (Total facility includes 120 beds in nursing home–type unit) A1 2 3 5 8 F2 3 4 8 10 11 12 19 20 21 22 24 26 27 29 30 31 32 33 34 35 37 39 41 42 43 44 45 46 49 51 52 54 55 56 58 60 61 64 65 67 69 71 72 73 74 S9295 Department of Veterans Affairs	45	10	492	8935	399	—	0	—	—	1520
WOMAN'S HOSPITAL See River Oaks East–Woman's Pavilion										
KEESLER AIR FORCE BASE—Dawson County										
★ U.S. AIR FORCE MEDICAL CENTER KEESLER, 301 Fisher Street, Suite 101, Zip 39534-2519; tel. 601/377-6510; Brigadier General Pedro N. Rivera MC, USAF, Commander A1 2 3 5 F2 3 4 7 8 10 11 12 13 14 15 16 19 20 21 22 25 28 34 35 37 38 40 41 42 43 44 45 46 48 49 50 51 52 53 54 55 56 57 58 59 60 61 63 64 65 67 71 73 P8 S9495 Department of the Air Force	41	10	270	11465	172	428142	905	56000	—	2061
KILMICHAEL—Montgomery County										
KILMICHAEL HOSPITAL, 301 Lamar Avenue, Zip 39747-0188, Mailing Address: P.O. Box 188, Zip 39747-0188; tel. 601/262-4311; Clint Gee III, Chief Executive Officer A9 10 F6 8 11 12 13 15 17 18 19 20 22 26 27 28 29 30 31 34 38 51 55 60 61 65 69 71 72	13	10	19	708	15	3517	0	—	—	44
KOSCIUSKO—Attala County										
MONTFORT JONES MEMORIAL HOSPITAL, Highway 12 West, Zip 39090-3209, Mailing Address: Box 677, Zip 39090-0677; tel. 601/289-4311; Thomas Bland, Administrator A9 10 F8 11 15 19 22 27 28 33 37 40 41 44 49 64 65 71	13	10	72	1865	39	18900	223	9117	3267	154
LAUREL—Jones County										
★ SOUTH CENTRAL REGIONAL MEDICAL CENTER, (Includes Ellisville Municipal Hospital, Ivy Street, Ellisville, Mississippi, Zip 39437; tel. 601/477-9381) 1220 Jefferson, Zip 39441, Mailing Address: P.O. Box 607, Zip 39441; tel. 601/426-4000; G. Douglas Higginbotham, Executive Director A1 9 10 F2 7 8 11 17 19 20 21 22 23 24 28 29 31 32 33 34 35 40 41 44 45 46 48 49 60 64 65 66 67 71 73 74	13	10	285	8322	130	57414	1124	48366	21502	963
LEXINGTON—Holmes County										
★ METHODIST HOSPITAL OF MIDDLE MISSISSIPPI, 1 Bowling Green Street, Zip 39095, Mailing Address: Box 641, Zip 39095; tel. 601/834-1321; Joe Dan Edwards, Administrator A1 9 10 F19 21 22 27 44 49 65 71 S9345 Methodist Health Systems, Inc.	23	10	84	2040	35	18097	126	—	—	139

© 1995 AHA Guide

Hospitals, U.S. / MISSISSIPPI

Hospital, Address, Telephone, Administrator, Approval, Facility, and Physician Codes, Health Care System

- ★ American Hospital Association (AHA) membership
- □ Joint Commission on Accreditation of Healthcare Organizations (JCAHO) accreditation
- + American Osteopathic Hospital Association (AOHA) membership
- ○ American Osteopathic Association (AOA) accreditation
- △ Commission on Accreditation of Rehabilitation Facilities (CARF) accreditation

Control codes 61, 63, 64, 71, 72 and 73 indicate hospitals listed by AOHA, but not registered by AHA. For definition of numerical codes, see page A6

	Classification Codes		Utilization Data					Expense (thousands) of dollars		
	Control	Service	Beds	Admissions	Census	Outpatient Visits	Births	Total	Payroll	Personnel

LOUISVILLE—Winston County

□ WINSTON COUNTY COMMUNITY HOSPITAL AND NURSING HOME, Highway 14 East, Zip 39339, Mailing Address: Box 967, Zip 39339; tel. 601/773–6211; W. Dale Saulters, Administrator (Total facility includes 120 beds in nursing home–type unit) **A**1 9 10 **F**15 22 37 44 64 71 — 23 10 185 1039 130 15227 1 — — 217

LUCEDALE—George County

GEORGE COUNTY HOSPITAL, 305 South Winter Street, Zip 39452, Mailing Address: P.O. Box 607, Zip 39452; tel. 601/947–3161; Paul A. Gardner CPA, Administrator **A**9 10 **F**8 11 12 19 20 21 22 26 27 28 29 30 31 34 35 36 37 39 44 51 60 61 62 63 65 67 68 69 71 72 — 13 10 53 1932 25 23436 0 — — 165

LUMBERTON—Lamar County

LUMBERTON CITIZENS HOSPITAL, 600 11th Avenue, Zip 39455, Mailing Address: Box 193, Zip 39455; tel. 601/796–2681; Howard Beall, Administrator **A**9 10 **F**28 51 — 14 10 23 330 6 962 0 1203 642 47

MACON—Noxubee County

★ NOXUBEE GENERAL HOSPITAL, 606 North Jefferson Street, Zip 39341, Mailing Address: Box 480, Zip 39341; tel. 601/726–4231; Arthur Nester Jr., Administrator (Total facility includes 60 beds in nursing home–type unit) **A**9 10 **F**20 21 22 26 34 44 64 65 **P**8 — 13 10 109 975 74 6120 0 4685 2256 123

MAGEE—Simpson County

MAGEE GENERAL HOSPITAL, 300 Southeast Third Avenue, Zip 39111; tel. 601/849–5070; Lester R. Terrell, Administrator **A**9 10 **F**15 19 44 71 73 — 23 10 64 2559 43 23921 4 7621 3017 167

MAGNOLIA—Pike County

BEACHAM MEMORIAL HOSPITAL, North Cherry Street, Zip 39652–0351; tel. 601/783–2351; Marilyn Speed, Administrator **A**9 10 **F**7 19 20 22 40 44 54 60 65 71 — 15 10 34 835 14 3523 0 — 1002 76

MARKS—Quitman County

QUITMAN COUNTY HOSPITAL AND NURSING HOME, 340 Getwell Drive, Zip 38646–9785; tel. 601/326–8031; Richard E. Waller M.D., Interim Administrator (Total facility includes 60 beds in nursing home–type unit) **A**9 10 **F**15 16 19 22 46 49 64 65 71 73 — 33 10 96 1138 76 7597 3 4857 2316 134

MCCOMB—Clearwater County

★ SOUTHWEST MISSISSIPPI REGIONAL MEDICAL CENTER, 215 Marion Avenue, Zip 39648–2798, Mailing Address: P.O. Box 1307, Zip 39648–1307; tel. 601/249–5500; Norman M. Price FACHE, Administrator **A**1 9 10 **F**7 8 15 16 17 19 20 22 28 29 32 35 37 40 41 44 49 64 65 67 70 71 74 — 15 10 112 5942 76 40991 938 35268 15910 516

MEADVILLE—Franklin County

FRANKLIN COUNTY MEMORIAL HOSPITAL, Highway 84, Zip 39653, Mailing Address: Box 636, Zip 39653–0636; tel. 601/384–5801; Semmes Ross Jr., Administrator **A**9 10 **F**2 3 19 21 22 34 35 37 49 64 65 70 71 73 — 13 10 53 506 15 3106 0 — — 87

MENDENHALL—Simpson County

SIMPSON GENERAL HOSPITAL, 931 Jackson Avenue, Zip 39114; tel. 601/847–2221; Wayne Harris, Administrator **A**9 10 **F**15 16 17 19 20 21 22 28 30 32 34 44 45 46 49 60 65 71 73 **P**5 — 13 10 49 1488 31 11305 6 6629 2760 141

MERIDIAN—Lauderdale County

EAST MISSISSIPPI STATE HOSPITAL, 4555 Highland Park Drive, Zip 39307, Mailing Address: Box 4128, West Station, Zip 39304–4128; tel. 601/482–6186; Ramiro J. Martinez M.D., Director (Total facility includes 250 beds in nursing home–type unit) **F**2 6 12 20 26 33 46 52 53 54 55 57 64 65 73 **S**0017 Mississippi State Department of Mental Health — 12 22 657 1523 589 0 0 26812 16161 920

★ JEFF ANDERSON REGIONAL MEDICAL CENTER, 2124 14th Street, Zip 39301; tel. 601/483–8811; Mark D. McPhail, Chief Executive Officer **A**1 9 10 **F**4 7 8 10 11 14 15 16 19 21 22 23 24 35 37 38 40 41 42 43 44 45 46 49 50 60 63 65 66 67 71 73 **P**8 — 23 10 260 8371 132 44754 1142 — — 722

□ LAUREL WOOD CENTER, 5000 Highway 39 North, Zip 39303; tel. 601/483–6211; Barbara Friday, Administrator **A**1 10 **F**2 3 46 52 53 54 57 59 65 67 **P**6 — 33 22 79 980 39 0 0 — — 168

★ RILEY MEMORIAL HOSPITAL, 1102 21st Avenue, Zip 39302–1810, Mailing Address: Box 1810, Zip 39302–1810; tel. 601/484–3590; Eric E. Weis FACHE, Chief Executive Officer **A**1 9 10 **F**4 7 8 10 11 13 15 17 19 21 22 23 24 25 28 29 30 32 34 35 37 39 40 41 42 44 46 49 60 61 63 64 65 67 71 73 74 **P**7 8 — 23 10 180 7124 119 29506 0 42862 18704 697

★ RUSH FOUNDATION HOSPITAL, 1314 19th Avenue, Zip 39301; tel. 601/483–0011; Wallace Strickland, Administrator **A**1 9 10 **F**4 6 7 8 10 11 12 14 15 16 17 18 19 21 22 23 28 30 32 33 34 37 38 39 40 41 42 44 45 46 49 51 54 60 63 64 65 66 67 71 72 73 74 **P**1 3 7 — 23 10 189 9187 129 — 1196 44917 21296 1015

MONTICELLO—Lawrence County

LAWRENCE COUNTY HOSPITAL, Highway 84 East, Zip 39654–0788, Mailing Address: Box 788, Zip 39654; tel. 601/587–4051; C. W. Nelson, Administrator **A**9 10 **F**11 16 19 21 32 65 71 — 13 10 53 1212 20 6079 0 3416 2243 116

NATCHEZ—Adams County

□ NATCHEZ COMMUNITY HOSPITAL, 129 Jefferson Davis Boulevard, Zip 39120, Mailing Address: Box 1203, Zip 39121; tel. 601/445–6200; Raymond Bane, Executive Director **A**1 9 10 **F**7 8 14 17 19 21 22 23 35 37 40 44 46 65 67 68 71 73 **S**1775 Health Management Associates — 33 10 101 2582 35 20187 559 — — 252

★ NATCHEZ REGIONAL MEDICAL CENTER, Seargent S Prentiss Drive, Zip 39120, Mailing Address: Box 1488, Zip 39121–1488; tel. 601/443–2100; Jonathan F. Godfrey FACHE, Chief Executive Officer **A**1 9 10 **F**7 11 16 18 21 22 35 36 37 38 40 44 45 49 51 65 71 **S**0002 Quorum Health Group/Quorum Health Resources — 13 10 137 3928 62 50406 441 24795 11613 395

Hospitals, U.S. / MISSISSIPPI

Hospital, Address, Telephone, Administrator, Approval, Facility, and Physician Codes, Health Care System	Classification Codes		Utilization Data					Expense (thousands) of dollars		
	Control	Service	Beds	Admissions	Census	Outpatient Visits	Births	Total	Payroll	Personnel

★ American Hospital Association (AHA) membership
☐ Joint Commission on Accreditation of Healthcare Organizations (JCAHO) accreditation
+ American Osteopathic Hospital Association (AOHA) membership
○ American Osteopathic Association (AOA) accreditation
△ Commission on Accreditation of Rehabilitation Facilities (CARF) accreditation
Control codes 61, 63, 64, 71, 72 and 73 indicate hospitals listed by AOHA, but not registered by AHA. For definition of numerical codes, see page A6

NEW ALBANY—Union County
★ BAPTIST MEMORIAL HOSPITAL–UNION COUNTY, Highway 30 West, Zip 38652-3197; tel. 601/538-7631; John Tompkins, Administrator A1 9 10 F7 8 14 15 19 22 28 30 35 37 39 40 42 44 45 46 65 67 71 73 74 P3 S1625 Baptist Memorial Health Care System, Inc.

| | 21 | 10 | 153 | 6702 | 72 | 34595 | 1144 | — | — | 356 |

OCEAN SPRINGS—Jackson County
☐ OCEAN SPRINGS HOSPITAL, 3109 Bienville Boulevard, Zip 39564; tel. 601/872-1111; Dwight Rimes, Administrator A1 9 10 F7 8 12 13 14 15 16 17 18 19 20 21 22 27 28 30 32 33 34 35 37 39 40 41 42 44 45 49 63 65 67 71 74 P3 8 S0067 Singing River Hospital System

| | 13 | 10 | 124 | 4576 | 66 | 61084 | 445 | — | — | 391 |

OKOLONA—Chickasaw County
★ OKOLONA COMMUNITY HOSPITAL, (Includes Shearer–Richardson Memorial Nursing Home) Rockwell Drive, Zip 38860-0420, Mailing Address: P.O. Box 420, Zip 38860-0420; tel. 601/447-3311; Allen Lockhart, Administrator (Total facility includes 66 beds in nursing home–type unit) A9 10 F64 65

| | 13 | 10 | 76 | 226 | 71 | — | 0 | — | — | 75 |

OLIVE BRANCH—De Soto County
☐ PARKWOOD HOSPITAL, 8135 Goodman Road, Zip 38654-2199; tel. 601/895-4900; Thomas I. Hayes Jr., Administrator A1 9 10 F2 3 52 53 56 58 59 65 S0875 Community Health Systems, Inc.

| | 33 | 22 | 66 | 1204 | 47 | — | 0 | — | — | 140 |

OXFORD—Lafayette County
★ BAPTIST MEMORIAL HOSPITAL–NORTH MISSISSIPPI, 2301 South Lamar Boulevard, Zip 38655, Mailing Address: Box 946, Zip 38655; tel. 601/232-8100; Stephen L. Mansfield, Administrator A1 9 10 F4 7 8 10 11 12 15 17 19 21 22 24 28 30 31 32 34 35 37 39 40 41 42 43 44 45 46 47 48 52 63 65 66 67 68 71 73 74 S1625 Baptist Memorial Health Care System, Inc.

| | 23 | 10 | 150 | 7438 | 106 | 35295 | 634 | 36485 | 11417 | 557 |

PASCAGOULA—Jackson County
★ SINGING RIVER HOSPITAL, 2809 Denny Avenue, Zip 39581; tel. 601/938-5000; James S. Kaigler FACHE, Administrator A1 2 9 10 F2 3 4 7 8 10 12 13 14 15 16 17 18 19 20 21 22 23 27 28 30 32 33 34 35 37 39 40 41 42 43 44 45 49 52 53 55 57 60 63 65 67 71 74 P3 8 S0067 Singing River Hospital System

| | 13 | 10 | 322 | 11903 | 196 | 135380 | 1042 | 111039 | 50847 | 1282 |

PHILADELPHIA—Neshoba County
★ CHOCTAW HEALTH CENTER, Hospital Street, Zip 39350, Mailing Address: Route 7, Box R-50, Zip 39350; tel. 601/656-2211; Jim Wallace, Executive Director (Nonreporting) A1 10 S9195 U.S. Public Health Service Indian Health Service

| | 47 | 10 | 35 | — | — | — | — | — | — | — |

NESHOBA COUNTY GENERAL HOSPITAL, Highway 19 South, Zip 39350, Mailing Address: P.O. Box 648, Zip 39350; tel. 601/656-2121; Lawrence Graeber, Administrator (Total facility includes 120 beds in nursing home–type unit) A9 10 F19 22 31 40 44 64 65 71

| | 13 | 10 | 174 | 1429 | 137 | 23150 | 3 | — | — | 244 |

PICAYUNE—Pearl River County
CROSBY MEMORIAL HOSPITAL, 801 Goodyear Boulevard, Zip 39466, Mailing Address: Box 909, Zip 39466; tel. 601/798-4711; Glenn E. Lowery, Administrator A9 10 F7 8 19 21 22 24 28 32 33 36 37 40 44 48 49 65 67 71

| | 23 | 10 | 61 | 2089 | 25 | 27131 | 381 | 10398 | 3966 | 185 |

PONTOTOC—Pontotoc County
PONTOTOC HOSPITAL AND EXTENDED CARE FACILITY, 176 South Main Street, Zip 38863, Mailing Address: P.O. Box C, Zip 38863; tel. 601/489-5510; Fred B. Hood, Administrator (Total facility includes 44 beds in nursing home–type unit) A9 10 F3 7 8 10 12 17 19 22 23 24 27 28 30 31 35 37 38 45 49 51 60 64 65 66 67 71 73 74 S0032 North Mississippi Health Services, Inc.

| | 23 | 10 | 61 | 577 | 57 | 17852 | 0 | — | — | 97 |

POPLARVILLE—Pearl River County
PEARL RIVER COUNTY HOSPITAL, West Moody Street, Zip 39470, Mailing Address: Box 392, Zip 39470; tel. 601/795-4543; Paul Majors, Administrator (Total facility includes 60 beds in nursing home–type unit) A9 10 F52 60 64 65 71

| | 33 | 10 | 84 | 706 | 68 | 5100 | 0 | — | — | 74 |

PORT GIBSON—Claiborne County
★ CLAIBORNE COUNTY HOSPITAL, 123 McComb Avenue, Zip 39150, Mailing Address: P.O. Box 1004, Zip 39150; tel. 601/437-5141; Wanda C. Fleming, Administrator A9 10 F12 16 17 19 22 28 30 40 45 49 51 71

| | 13 | 10 | 27 | 693 | 11 | 8614 | 49 | 3363 | 1141 | 74 |

PRENTISS—Jefferson Davis County
JEFFERSON DAVIS COUNTY HOSPITAL, Berry Street, Zip 39474, Mailing Address: P.O. Box 1288, Zip 39474; tel. 601/792-4276; Paul W. Strode Jr., Administrator (Total facility includes 60 beds in nursing home–type unit) A9 10 F11 17 22 30 34 45 49 62 64 71

| | 13 | 10 | 101 | 638 | 69 | 8664 | 0 | 4171 | 1882 | 133 |

QUITMAN—Clarke County
★ H.C. WATKINS MEMORIAL HOSPITAL, 605 South Archusa Avenue, Zip 39355-2398; tel. 601/776-6925; Thomas G. Bartlett, President and Chief Executive Officer (Total facility includes 10 beds in nursing home–type unit) A9 10 F7 11 19 37 38 44 45 64 65 70 71 S0002 Quorum Health Group/Quorum Health Resources

| | 23 | 10 | 42 | 1073 | 34 | 6076 | 0 | — | — | 120 |

RICHTON—Perry County
★ PERRY COUNTY GENERAL HOSPITAL, 206 Bay Street, Zip 39476, Mailing Address: Drawer Y, Zip 39476; tel. 601/788-6316; Elaine F. Brannan, Administrator (Total facility includes 60 beds in nursing home–type unit) A9 10 F22 32 44 64 71

| | 13 | 10 | 82 | 403 | 66 | 7295 | 1 | — | — | 107 |

RIPLEY—Tippah County
★ TIPPAH COUNTY HOSPITAL, 1005 City Avenue North, Zip 38663-0499; tel. 601/837-9221; Jerry Green, Administrator (Total facility includes 36 beds in nursing home–type unit) A1 9 10 F8 11 16 19 21 22 26 28 30 44 64 65 71 S1625 Baptist Memorial Health Care System, Inc.

| | 13 | 10 | 106 | 1917 | 61 | 14843 | 0 | 7277 | 3283 | 190 |

© 1995 AHA Guide

Hospitals, U.S. / MISSISSIPPI

Hospital, Address, Telephone, Administrator, Approval, Facility, and Physician Codes, Health Care System	Classification Codes		Utilization Data					Expense (thousands) of dollars		
★ American Hospital Association (AHA) membership □ Joint Commission on Accreditation of Healthcare Organizations (JCAHO) accreditation + American Osteopathic Hospital Association (AOHA) membership ○ American Osteopathic Association (AOA) accreditation △ Commission on Accreditation of Rehabilitation Facilities (CARF) accreditation Control codes 61, 63, 64, 71, 72 and 73 indicate hospitals listed by AOHA, but not registered by AHA. For definition of numerical codes, see page A6	Control	Service	Beds	Admissions	Census	Outpatient Visits	Births	Total	Payroll	Personnel
RULEVILLE—Sunflower County NORTH SUNFLOWER COUNTY HOSPITAL, 840 North Oak Avenue, Zip 38771–0369, Mailing Address: P.O. Box 369, Zip 38771–0369; tel. 601/756–2711; Robert Crook, Acting Administrator (Total facility includes 42 beds in nursing home–type unit) **A**9 10 **F**2 3 22 32 33 40 41 44 54 64 71	13	10	86	1248	66	5980	31	5986	3002	155
SENATOBIA—Tate County □ SENATOBIA COMMUNITY HOSPITAL, 401 Getwell Drive, Zip 38668, Mailing Address: P.O. Box 648, Zip 38668; tel. 601/562–3100; James D. Tesar, Administrator **A**1 9 10 **F**7 8 12 15 16 19 20 28 31 33 34 44 46 60 61 65 70 71 **P**5 **S**5765 Paracelsus Healthcare Corporation	33	10	52	1189	13	14440	175	6732	2477	118
SOUTHAVEN—De Soto County ★ △ BAPTIST MEMORIAL HOSPITAL–DESOTO, 7601 Southcrest Parkway, Zip 38671; tel. 601/349–4000; Melvin E. Walker, Administrator **A**1 7 9 10 **F**3 7 8 10 12 16 18 19 20 21 22 24 25 26 27 28 30 31 32 34 35 37 39 40 41 42 43 44 45 46 48 49 54 55 56 57 58 59 60 65 66 67 69 71 72 73 74 **P**3 7 8 **S**1625 Baptist Memorial Health Care System, Inc.	23	10	130	5168	72	32286	865	26279	9028	359
STARKVILLE—Oktibbeha County ★ OKTIBBEHA COUNTY HOSPITAL, 400 Hospital Road, Zip 39759, Mailing Address: Drawer 1506, Zip 39759; tel. 601/323–4320; Arthur C. Kelly, Administrator and Chief Executive Officer **A**1 9 10 **F**7 8 11 14 15 16 17 19 21 22 24 28 30 35 37 39 40 44 46 49 65 66 67 71 73	13	10	96	3746	42	46091	1101	19114	8840	408
TUPELO—Lee County □ △ NORTH MISSISSIPPI MEDICAL CENTER, 830 South Gloster Street, Zip 38801–4934; tel. 601/841–3000; Jeffrey B. Barber Ph.D., Dr.P.H., President and Chief Executive Officer (Data for 361 days) **A**1 2 5 7 9 10 **F**2 3 4 7 8 10 11 12 13 14 15 16 17 18 19 21 22 23 24 25 26 28 29 30 31 33 34 35 37 38 39 40 41 42 43 44 45 46 48 49 50 51 52 53 54 55 56 57 58 59 60 63 64 65 66 67 68 71 72 73 74 **P**3 6 7 **S**0032 North Mississippi Health Services, Inc.	23	10	610	24455	423	100397	2216	177804	76175	3042
TYLERTOWN—Walthall County WALTHALL COUNTY GENERAL HOSPITAL, 100 Hospital Drive, Zip 39667; tel. 601/876–2122; Jimmy Graves, Administrator **A**9 10 **F**8 15 19 22 24 28 31 44 45 60 70 71 73	13	10	49	1604	27	13251	0	5753	2630	100
UNION—Newton County LAIRD HOSPITAL, 108 Highway 15 By-Pass North, Zip 39365; tel. 601/774–8214; James P. Franklin, Executive Director **A**9 10 **F**19 20 21 22 24 31 32 33 34 35 37 41 45 46 65 71 73	33	10	50	2427	35	16244	5	—	—	437
VICKSBURG—Warren County ★ PARKVIEW REGIONAL MEDICAL CENTER, 100 McAuley Drive, Zip 39180–2897, Mailing Address: P.O. Box 590, Zip 39181–0590; tel. 601/631–2131; Lewis T. Peeples, Administrator and Chief Executive Officer (Total facility includes 14 beds in nursing home–type unit) **A**1 2 9 10 **F**2 3 7 8 12 15 16 17 19 22 23 24 26 28 29 30 32 34 35 37 40 41 42 44 45 46 49 52 57 60 64 65 67 71 72 73 **P**1 2 7 **S**0002 Quorum Health Group/Quorum Health Resources	33	10	189	5460	117	66496	1193	—	—	498
★ VICKSBURG MEDICAL CENTER, 1111 Frontage Road, Zip 39181–5298; tel. 601/636–2611; G. Thomas Usher, Administrator **A**1 9 10 **F**7 8 12 16 17 19 20 21 22 23 26 28 29 30 31 34 35 37 39 40 42 44 46 51 52 57 61 64 65 66 71 73 **P**7 **S**0048 Columbia/HCA Healthcare Corporation	33	10	154	4378	79	35856	302	28678	10318	377
WATER VALLEY—Yalobusha County YALOBUSHA GENERAL HOSPITAL, Highway 7 South, Zip 38965, Mailing Address: Box 728, Zip 38965–0728; tel. 601/473–1411; James R. Carter Jr., Administrator (Total facility includes 59 beds in nursing home–type unit) **A**9 10 **F**14 19 20 28 30 34 44 45 51 64 71	13	10	85	825	75	3600	0	—	—	124
WAYNESBORO—Wayne County WAYNE GENERAL HOSPITAL, 950 Matthew Drive, Zip 39367, Mailing Address: Box 1249, Zip 39367; tel. 601/735–5151; Donald Hemeter, Administrator **A**9 10 **F**7 11 19 20 21 31 33 34 35 37 40 44 45 48 60 61 65 71	13	10	77	3198	43	25161	245	—	—	208
WEST POINT—Clay County CLAY COUNTY MEDICAL CENTER, 835 Medical Center Drive, Zip 39773; tel. 601/495–2300; David M. Reid, Administrator **A**9 10 **F**7 8 11 15 17 19 20 21 22 24 25 28 29 30 33 34 37 40 42 44 45 46 61 65 67 71 73 74 **P**3 8 **S**0032 North Mississippi Health Services, Inc.	23	10	60	2181	31	21157	345	10745	5088	163
WHITFIELD—Rankin County ★ MISSISSIPPI STATE HOSPITAL, Mailing Address: P.O. Box 157-A, Zip 39193–0157; tel. 601/351–8000; James G. Chastain, Director (Total facility includes 457 beds in nursing home–type unit) **A**3 5 9 **F**2 3 6 7 8 9 10 11 12 15 17 18 19 20 22 23 26 27 28 29 30 31 34 37 38 44 48 51 52 55 60 61 62 64 65 67 73 **S**0017 Mississippi State Department of Mental Health	12	22	1293	1834	1227	2290	0	62375	38627	2089
□ WHITFIELD MEDICAL SURGICAL HOSPITAL, Zip 39193; tel. 601/351–8000; James I. Morton FACHE, Administrator **A**1 9 10 **F**3 4 5 8 10 11 12 19 20 21 22 27 31 34 35 37 41 42 44 51 52 53 54 55 56 57 58 60 64 65 70 71	12	10	43	391	11	3925	0	—	—	84
WINONA—Montgomery County TYLER HOLMES MEMORIAL HOSPITAL, Tyler Holmes Drive, Zip 38967–1599; tel. 601/283–4114; Gary C. Morse, Administrator **A**9 10 **F**17 19 22 31 40 44 45 65 71	13	10	49	1874	30	16140	58	—	—	133

Hospitals, U.S. / MISSISSIPPI

Hospital, Address, Telephone, Administrator, Approval, Facility, and Physician Codes, Health Care System	Classification Codes		Utilization Data					Expense (thousands) of dollars		
★ American Hospital Association (AHA) membership □ Joint Commission on Accreditation of Healthcare Organizations (JCAHO) accreditation + American Osteopathic Hospital Association (AOHA) membership ○ American Osteopathic Association (AOA) accreditation △ Commission on Accreditation of Rehabilitation Facilities (CARF) accreditation Control codes 61, 63, 64, 71, 72 and 73 indicate hospitals listed by AOHA, but not registered by AHA. For definition of numerical codes, see page A6	Control	Service	Beds	Admissions	Census	Outpatient Visits	Births	Total	Payroll	Personnel
YAZOO CITY—Yazoo County KING'S DAUGHTERS HOSPITAL, 823 Grand Avenue, Zip 39194–0329, Mailing Address: Box 329, Zip 39194–0329; tel. 601/746–2261; Noel W. Hart, Administrator **A**9 10 **F**8 11 19 22 28 44 46 49 64 65 71 73 **P**3	23	10	54	1833	33	32540	9	8583	3012	167

© 1995 AHA Guide

Hospitals, U.S. / MISSOURI

MISSOURI

Resident population 5,234 (in thousands)
Resident population in metro areas 68.3%
Birth rate per 1,000 population 15.3
65 years and over 14.2%
Percent of persons without health insurance 13.1%

Hospital, Address, Telephone, Administrator, Approval, Facility, and Physician Codes, Health Care System	Classification Codes		Utilization Data					Expense (thousands) of dollars		Personnel
	Control	Service	Beds	Admissions	Census	Outpatient Visits	Births	Total	Payroll	

★ American Hospital Association (AHA) membership
□ Joint Commission on Accreditation of Healthcare Organizations (JCAHO) accreditation
+ American Osteopathic Hospital Association (AOHA) membership
○ American Osteopathic Association (AOA) accreditation
△ Commission on Accreditation of Rehabilitation Facilities (CARF) accreditation
Control codes 61, 63, 64, 71, 72 and 73 indicate hospitals listed by AOHA, but not registered by AHA. For definition of numerical codes, see page A6

Hospital	Control	Service	Beds	Admissions	Census	Outpatient Visits	Births	Total	Payroll	Personnel
ALBANY—Gentry County ★ GENTRY COUNTY MEMORIAL HOSPITAL, Clark and College Streets, Zip 64402–1499; tel. 816/726–3941; John W. Richmond, President (Total facility includes 10 beds in nursing home–type unit) A9 10 F8 11 12 14 15 16 17 19 22 26 27 28 29 30 31 32 33 34 37 39 40 41 42 44 46 48 49 51 63 64 65 66 67 71 73 74 P5	23	10	35	791	15	8106	0	4823	2406	100
APPLETON CITY—St. Clair County ELLETT MEMORIAL HOSPITAL, 610 North Ohio Avenue, Zip 64724; tel. 816/476–2111; Sandy Morlan, Administrator A9 10 F19 22 64 P5	16	10	25	357	5	1757	0	1702	787	42
AURORA—Lawrence County AURORA COMMUNITY HOSPITAL, 500 Porter Street, Zip 65605; tel. 417/678–2122; Don Buchanan, Chief Operating Officer A9 10 F7 8 11 12 14 17 19 22 24 26 27 28 29 30 32 34 36 37 39 40 41 44 45 46 49 51 65 71 73	14	10	38	1331	14	16355	137	6855	3586	156
BELTON—Cass County ★ RESEARCH BELTON HOSPITAL, 17065 South 71 Highway, Zip 64012–0487; tel. 816/348–1200; Daniel F. Sheehan, Administrator A9 F1 2 3 4 5 6 7 8 9 10 11 12 13 14 15 16 17 18 19 20 22 24 26 28 29 30 31 32 33 34 35 37 38 40 41 42 43 44 46 47 48 49 52 53 54 55 56 57 58 59 60 61 63 64 65 69 70 71 73 74 P1 S8815 Health Midwest	23	10	40	1249	17	21041	0	12531	4544	110
BETHANY—Harrison County ★ HARRISON COUNTY COMMUNITY HOSPITAL, Highway 69 and 136, Zip 64424, Mailing Address: P.O. Box 428, Zip 64424–0428; tel. 816/425–2211; William H. Koellner, Administrator A9 10 F8 13 14 15 19 20 22 28 29 30 32 33 34 36 37 39 41 44 46 62 64 65 71	16	10	23	591	8	15215	0	3330	1384	73
BLUE SPRINGS—Jackson County ★ △ ST. MARY'S HOSPITAL OF BLUE SPRINGS, 201 West R D Mize Road, Zip 64014; tel. 816/228–5900; N. Gary Wages, President A1 7 9 10 F7 8 10 12 15 19 22 24 26 28 30 31 32 33 34 35 37 39 40 41 42 44 48 49 60 63 65 67 71 73 P6 S5945 Carondelet Health System	23	10	110	4091	57	39193	828	40402	17485	485
BOLIVAR—Polk County ★ CITIZENS MEMORIAL HOSPITAL, 1500 North Oakland, Zip 65613–3099; tel. 417/326–6000; Donald J. Babb, Chief Executive Officer A1 9 10 F7 8 14 15 16 17 19 22 26 28 30 31 32 33 34 37 39 40 42 44 46 48 49 52 56 57 58 64 65 70 71 73 74	16	10	74	2708	37	29711	349	21900	11511	375
BONNE TERRE—St. Francois County BONNE TERRE HOSPITAL See Parkland Health Center, Farmington										
BOONVILLE—Cooper County ★ COOPER COUNTY MEMORIAL HOSPITAL, 17651 B Highway, Zip 65233, Mailing Address: P.O. Box 88, Zip 65233; tel. 816/882–7461; Wilbert E. Meyer, Administrator (Total facility includes 24 beds in nursing home–type unit) A1 9 10 F8 12 15 16 17 19 20 22 24 28 30 32 34 40 49 64 65 71 73	13	10	49	587	27	14626	0	5931	2824	153
BRANSON—Taney County ★ SKAGGS COMMUNITY HOSPITAL, Cahill Road, Zip 65616–2035, Mailing Address: P.O. Box 650, Zip 65616–0650; tel. 417/335–7000; Russ Russell, Administrator (Total facility includes 14 beds in nursing home–type unit) A1 9 10 F7 8 15 17 19 22 26 27 28 30 31 32 33 34 37 39 40 41 42 44 51 64 65 67 70 71 72 73	23	10	87	3825	55	193774	366	26831	11393	504
BRIDGETON—St. Louis County ST. VINCENT'S PSYCHIATRIC DIVISION See DePaul Health Center, Saint Louis										
BROOKFIELD—Linn County □ GENERAL JOHN J. PERSHING MEMORIAL HOSPITAL, 130 East Lockling Avenue, Zip 64628–0130, Mailing Address: P.O. Box 408, Zip 64628–0408; tel. 816/258–2222; Don L. Sipes, Chief Executive Officer A1 9 10 F7 8 12 14 17 19 22 28 30 31 32 33 37 39 40 42 44 46 49 51 65 71 73	23	10	34	1404	15	42042	73	9773	4975	160
BUTLER—Bates County BATES COUNTY MEMORIAL HOSPITAL, 615 West Nursery Street, Zip 64730–0370; tel. 816/679–4381; James W. Baldwin Jr., Administrator (Total facility includes 9 beds in nursing home–type unit) A9 10 F7 8 14 19 22 29 30 32 33 34 37 39 40 41 42 44 46 54 64 65 67 71	13	10	31	1522	27	15066	36	7892	3419	151
CAMERON—Clinton County CAMERON COMMUNITY HOSPITAL, 1015 West Fourth Street, Zip 64429–1498; tel. 816/632–2101; Joseph F. Abrutz Jr., Administrator A9 10 F8 11 12 14 15 16 19 20 22 24 26 27 28 29 30 31 32 33 34 37 39 40 42 44 49 58 64 64 67 71 73 P6	23	10	38	1096	14	20003	0	9462	4295	167
CAPE GIRARDEAU—Cape Girardeau County ★ SAINT FRANCIS MEDICAL CENTER, 211 St. Francis Drive, Zip 63701–8399; tel. 314/335–1251; John E. Fidler, President (Total facility includes 26 beds in nursing home–type unit) A1 2 9 10 F2 3 4 5 8 10 11 12 13 14 15 16 17 18 19 22 23 28 29 30 31 32 33 34 35 37 39 40 41 42 43 44 48 49 63 64 65 71 73 74	23	10	264	7298	144	67286	0	71487	28949	1103
★ SOUTHEAST MISSOURI HOSPITAL, 1701 Lacey Street, Zip 63701; tel. 314/334–4822; James W. Wente CPA, CHE, Administrator (Total facility includes 10 beds in nursing home–type unit) A1 2 6 9 10 F2 3 4 5 7 8 10 11 12 13 14 15 16 17 19 22 23 24 25 28 29 30 31 32 33 35 36 37 38 39 40 41 42 43 44 46 47 48 49 52 54 55 56 57 60 63 64 65 67 68 71 73 74 P8	23	10	258	8783	134	74719	1526	71668	28983	1177

Hospitals, U.S. / MISSOURI

Hospital, Address, Telephone, Administrator, Approval, Facility, and Physician Codes, Health Care System	Classification Codes		Utilization Data					Expense (thousands) of dollars		Personnel
★ American Hospital Association (AHA) membership □ Joint Commission on Accreditation of Healthcare Organizations (JCAHO) accreditation + American Osteopathic Hospital Association (AOHA) membership ○ American Osteopathic Association (AOA) accreditation △ Commission on Accreditation of Rehabilitation Facilities (CARF) accreditation Control codes 61, 63, 64, 71, 72 and 73 indicate hospitals listed by AOHA, but not registered by AHA. For definition of numerical codes, see page A6	Control	Service	Beds	Admissions	Census	Outpatient Visits	Births	Total	Payroll	
CARROLLTON—Carroll County CARROLL COUNTY MEMORIAL HOSPITAL, 1502 North Jefferson Street, Zip 64633; tel. 816/542–1695; Jack L. Tindle, Chief Executive Officer **A**9 10 **F**8 15 16 19 22 32 33 34 40 41 42 44 46 49 64 65 71	23	10	52	505	37	15107	0	2786	1350	72
CARTHAGE—Jasper County ★ MCCUNE–BROOKS HOSPITAL, 627 West Centennial Avenue, Zip 64836–0677; tel. 417/358–8121; James W. McPheeters III, Chief Executive Officer (Total facility includes 7 beds in nursing home–type unit) **A**9 10 **F**8 11 19 22 28 30 32 33 35 36 37 39 40 44 49 52 57 64 65 66 67 71	14	10	70	1934	38	51200	0	14662	6319	313
CASSVILLE—Barry County SOUTH BARRY COUNTY MEMORIAL HOSPITAL, 87 Gravel Street, Zip 65625; tel. 417/847–4115; Deborah Stubbs, Chief Executive Officer **A**9 10 **F**8 19 22 24 28 30 32 33 34 39 41 44 49 51 64 71 **P**5	16	10	18	685	9	23447	0	4544	1815	104
CHESTERFIELD—St. Louis County ★ ST. LUKE'S HOSPITAL, 232 South Woods Mill Road, Zip 63017–3480; tel. 314/434–1500; George Tucker M.D., Acting President and Chief Executive Officer (Total facility includes 126 beds in nursing home–type unit) **A**1 2 3 5 9 10 **F**3 4 5 6 7 8 10 11 12 13 14 15 16 17 18 19 20 22 23 24 25 26 27 28 29 30 31 32 33 34 35 36 37 39 40 41 42 43 44 46 48 49 52 54 55 56 57 58 59 60 61 62 63 64 65 66 67 69 71 72 73 74 **P**8	23	10	495	17306	334	166914	2737	149645	81477	2339
CHILLICOTHE—Livingston County ★ HEDRICK MEDICAL CENTER, 100 Central Avenue, Zip 64601–1599; tel. 816/646–1480; Richard L. Conklin, President and Senior Executive Officer **A**9 10 **F**8 12 18 19 22 31 32 33 34 35 36 37 40 41 42 44 46 55 71 73 **S**0051 BJC Health System	23	10	64	2185	35	15968	519	14252	5962	227
CLINTON—Henry County ★ GOLDEN VALLEY MEMORIAL HOSPITAL, 1600 North Second Street, Zip 64735–1197; tel. 816/885–5511; Randy S. Wertz, Administrator (Total facility includes 12 beds in nursing home–type unit) **A**1 9 10 **F**7 8 14 15 17 19 22 28 30 31 32 33 35 37 39 40 41 42 44 49 52 53 54 55 56 57 58 59 63 64 65 66 67 71 72 73 74	16	10	108	4069	67	10463	390	20783	9481	390
COLUMBIA—Boone County AMI COLUMBIA REGIONAL HOSPITAL See Columbia Regional Hospital										
★ BOONE HOSPITAL CENTER, 1600 East Broadway, Zip 65201; tel. 314/875–4545; Michael Shirk, President (Total facility includes 19 beds in nursing home–type unit) **A**1 2 3 5 9 10 **F**3 4 7 8 10 12 14 15 17 19 22 23 24 25 26 28 29 30 31 34 35 37 38 39 40 41 42 43 44 45 46 49 52 54 55 56 57 58 59 60 63 64 65 66 67 69 70 71 72 73 74 **P**3 5 8 **S**0051 BJC Health System	23	10	303	10837	180	68634	1292	99858	42108	1260
★ △ COLUMBIA REGIONAL HOSPITAL, (Formerly AMI Columbia Regional Hospital) 404 Keene Street, Zip 65201; tel. 314/875–9000; Richard A. Royer, Chief Executive Officer (Total facility includes 30 beds in nursing home–type unit) **A**1 2 3 5 7 9 10 **F**1 4 8 10 12 14 15 16 18 19 20 22 23 26 28 30 31 32 33 34 35 37 39 41 42 44 46 48 49 50 52 54 55 56 57 58 59 60 64 65 66 67 69 71 73 74 **P**4 **S**0063 TENET Healthcare Corporation	33	10	274	5522	129	55652	0	64281	22628	826
ELLIS FISCHEL CANCER CENTER, 115 Business Loop 70 West, Zip 65203; tel. 314/882–5460; Patsy J. Hart, Director (Nonreporting) **A**2 9	12	49	48	—	—	—	—	—	—	—
★ HARRY S. TRUMAN MEMORIAL VETERANS HOSPITAL, 800 Hospital Drive, Zip 65201–5297; tel. 314/443–2511; John T. Carson, Director (Total facility includes 81 beds in nursing home–type unit) **A**1 3 5 8 **F**1 2 3 4 5 8 10 11 19 20 22 26 29 30 31 32 33 34 35 37 39 41 42 43 44 46 48 49 52 54 55 56 57 58 60 63 64 65 67 71 73 74 **P**6 **S**9295 Department of Veterans Affairs	45	10	291	7542	248	84648	0	74106	42027	1061
□ MID MISSOURI MENTAL HEALTH CENTER, 3 Hospital Drive, Zip 65201; tel. 314/449–2511; Mark Stansberry, Superintendent **A**1 3 5 10 **F**14 15 17 22 52 53 54 55 56 57 58 59 65 70 **P**6	12	22	69	1306	66	6319	0	11906	6378	261
□ △ UNIVERSITY AND CHILDRENS HOSPITALS, One Hospital Drive, Zip 65212; tel. 314/882–8000; Thomas J. Murray, Director **A**1 3 5 7 8 9 10 **F**2 4 5 7 8 9 10 11 12 13 17 18 19 20 22 23 24 25 26 28 29 30 31 34 35 37 38 39 40 41 42 43 44 45 46 47 48 49 51 52 53 54 55 56 57 58 59 60 61 63 65 66 67 69 70 71 72 73 74 **P**1	12	10	437	13409	280	349097	1861	194161	86609	2954
CRYSTAL CITY—Jefferson County ★ JEFFERSON MEMORIAL HOSPITAL, Highway 61 South, Zip 63019, Mailing Address: P.O. Box 350, Zip 63019–0350; tel. 314/933–1000; Bill M. Seek, Chief Executive Officer (Total facility includes 20 beds in nursing home–type unit) **A**1 9 10 **F**2 3 7 8 10 12 15 16 17 19 22 25 27 28 29 30 31 32 33 34 35 37 39 40 41 44 46 48 49 52 53 54 55 56 57 58 63 64 65 66 67 70 71 73	23	10	228	6239	124	62118	647	52839	23410	811
DEXTER—Stoddard County □ DEXTER MEMORIAL HOSPITAL, 1200 North One Mile Road, Zip 63841–1099; tel. 314/624–5566; Win Coburn, Chief Executive Officer **A**1 9 10 **F**8 14 15 19 20 22 25 26 28 29 30 31 32 33 34 37 40 44 45 48 49 51 63 64 65 71 73 **P**8	23	10	50	1069	14	27515	0	8435	3943	148
DONIPHAN—Ripley County RIPLEY COUNTY MEMORIAL HOSPITAL, Grand and Plum Streets, Zip 63935; tel. 314/996–2141; Charles Ray Freeman, Administrator **A**9 10 **F**15 19 22 28 32 34 44 46 51 65 71 73	15	10	30	513	18	5846	0	—	—	68

Hospitals, U.S. / MISSOURI

Hospital, Address, Telephone, Administrator, Approval, Facility, and Physician Codes, Health Care System	Classification Codes		Utilization Data					Expense (thousands) of dollars		
★ American Hospital Association (AHA) membership ☐ Joint Commission on Accreditation of Healthcare Organizations (JCAHO) accreditation + American Osteopathic Hospital Association (AOHA) membership ○ American Osteopathic Association (AOA) accreditation △ Commission on Accreditation of Rehabilitation Facilities (CARF) accreditation Control codes 61, 63, 64, 71, 72 and 73 indicate hospitals listed by AOHA, but not registered by AHA. For definition of numerical codes, see page A6	Control	Service	Beds	Admissions	Census	Outpatient Visits	Births	Total	Payroll	Personnel
EL DORADO SPRINGS—Cedar County										
CEDAR COUNTY MEMORIAL HOSPITAL, 1401 South Park Street, Zip 64744; tel. 417/876–2511; Jackie Boyles, Administrator **A**9 10 **F**7 8 12 13 15 16 17 18 19 22 26 28 29 30 31 32 34 39 40 41 44 48 49 64 65 71 **P**4 5	13	10	34	791	11	15614	96	3989	1963	87
ELLINGTON—Reynolds County										
REYNOLDS COUNTY GENERAL MEMORIAL HOSPITAL, Highway 21 South, Zip 63638, Mailing Address: P.O. Box 520, Zip 63638; tel. 314/663–2511; David McNail, Acting Administrator **A**9 10 **F**8 19 20 22 25 26 28 29 30 31 32 34 40 48 49 51 65 67 71	16	10	29	332	3	8302	17	2192	922	47
EXCELSIOR SPRINGS—Clay County										
☐ EXCELSIOR SPRINGS MEDICAL CENTER, 1700 Rainbow Drive, Zip 64024–1190; tel. 816/630–6081; Sally S. Pannell, Chief Executive Officer (Total facility includes 60 beds in nursing home–type unit) **A**1 9 10 **F**8 12 14 15 17 19 20 22 26 27 28 30 32 33 34 36 37 39 42 44 46 49 51 64 65 67 71 73	14	10	85	853	67	16691	0	8829	4571	196
FAIRFAX—Atchison County										
COMMUNITY HOSPITAL, Highway 59, Zip 64446–0107; tel. 816/686–2211; Larry S. Goodloe, Administrator **A**9 10 **F**7 8 11 15 19 20 22 30 32 34 35 37 40 42 44 46 49 64 71	23	10	49	822	19	7950	79	4644	2131	99
FARMINGTON—St. Francois County										
+ ○ MINERAL AREA REGIONAL MEDICAL CENTER, 1212 Weber Road, Zip 63640; tel. 314/756–4581; Kenneth West, Administrator **A**9 10 11 **F**1 2 3 7 8 16 19 20 22 28 30 32 35 37 39 40 42 44 46 49 51 53 54 58 59 65 70 71 73	23	10	129	3599	46	52484	447	22917	10584	456
★ PARKLAND HEALTH CENTER, (Includes Bonne Terre Hospital, 10 Lake Drive, Bonne Terre, Missouri, Zip 63628–1899; tel. 314/358–2211) 1101 West Liberty Street, Zip 63640–1997; tel. 314/756–6451; William D. Blair, President and Senior Executive Officer **A**1 9 **F**1 2 3 4 5 6 7 8 9 10 11 12 13 14 15 16 17 18 19 20 22 23 24 25 26 27 28 29 30 31 32 33 34 35 36 37 38 39 40 41 42 43 44 45 46 47 48 49 50 51 52 53 54 55 56 57 58 59 60 61 62 63 64 65 66 67 68 69 70 71 72 73 74 **P**1 2 3 4 5 6 7 8 **S**0051 BJC Health System	23	10	87	3265	39	48864	341	25116	10977	427
☐ SOUTHEAST MISSOURI MENTAL HEALTH CENTER, 1010 West Columbia, Zip 63640–2997; tel. 314/756–6792; Donald L. Barton, Superintendent **A**1 10 **F**2 3 4 5 6 12 15 16 17 19 20 22 24 28 34 35 39 46 49 52 56 58 65 67 70 73	12	22	196	1294	172	7256	0	20464	13722	617
FAYETTE—Howard County										
AMI KELLER MEMORIAL HOSPITAL, 600 West Morrison Street, Zip 65248; tel. 816/248–2261; Curtis Baylor, Administrator (Total facility includes 30 beds in nursing home–type unit) **A**9 10 **F**15 19 22 35 41 46 49 65 71 73 **P**6	33	10	64	359	49	1872	0	3881	1645	79
FLORISSANT—St. Louis County										
CHRISTIAN HOSPITAL NORTHWEST See Christian Hospital Northeast–Northwest, Saint Louis										
FORT LEONARD WOOD—Pulaski County										
★ GENERAL LEONARD WOOD ARMY COMMUNITY HOSPITAL, Zip 65473; tel. 314/596–0414; Colonel Dennis Dohanos, Administrator **A**1 2 **F**7 8 12 13 14 15 16 17 18 19 20 22 25 28 29 30 31 34 35 37 39 40 41 44 45 46 49 51 52 53 54 55 56 58 59 65 71 73 **S**9395 Department of the Army	42	10	88	5425	43	417018	458	65363	33283	1036
FREDERICKTOWN—Madison County										
MADISON MEMORIAL HOSPITAL, 100 South Wood At West College, Zip 63645, Mailing Address: P.O. Box 431, Zip 63645–0431; tel. 314/783–3341; Floyd Bounds, Administrator (Total facility includes 123 beds in nursing home–type unit) **A**9 10 **F**8 15 16 17 19 22 28 30 32 34 37 40 41 44 46 49 51 64 65 71	13	10	151	708	122	12925	94	7679	3881	129
FULTON—Callaway County										
☐ CALLAWAY COMMUNITY HOSPITAL, 10 South Hospital Drive, Zip 65251; tel. 314/642–3376; Gerald M. Torba, Chief Executive Officer **A**1 9 10 **F**7 8 13 14 15 16 19 22 26 30 32 34 37 39 40 41 44 46 49 51 61 64 71	23	10	36	897	11	17042	124	7335	2597	127
☐ FULTON STATE HOSPITAL, 600 East Fifth Street, Zip 65251; tel. 314/592–4100; Stephen C. Reeves, Superintendent **A**1 10 **F**2 3 20 26 27 28 39 41 45 46 49 52 65 67 73 **P**6	12	22	519	722	469	0	0	41129	25904	1198
HANNIBAL—Marion County										
☐ + HANNIBAL REGIONAL HOSPITAL, Highway 36 West, Zip 63401, Mailing Address: P.O. Box 551, Zip 63401–0551; tel. 314/248–1300; John Grossmeier, President and Chief Executive Officer **A**1 2 9 10 **F**7 8 10 14 15 16 17 18 19 22 23 25 27 28 29 30 31 32 33 34 35 37 39 40 41 42 44 46 49 51 52 53 54 55 56 57 58 59 61 65 66 67 68 71 73 74 **P**6	23	10	105	4030	57	78128	472	29906	11255	499
HARRISONVILLE—Cass County										
★ CASS MEDICAL CENTER, 1800 East Mechanic Street, Zip 64701; tel. 816/884–3291; David G. Couser, Administrator **A**1 9 10 **F**8 12 14 15 16 19 20 22 29 30 33 34 37 39 41 42 44 45 46 49 51 53 54 55 56 57 58 60 65 66 71 73 **P**6 7 **S**8815 Health Midwest	13	10	42	1092	14	14737	0	10141	3477	132
HAYTI—Pemiscot County										
PEMISCOT MEMORIAL HEALTH SYSTEM, Highway 61 and Reed, Zip 63851, Mailing Address: P.O. Box 489, Zip 63851; tel. 314/359–1372; Glenn D. Haynes, Administrator (Total facility includes 153 beds in nursing home–type unit) **A**9 10 **F**8 11 15 19 20 22 25 26 27 28 29 30 31 32 33 34 35 36 37 39 40 44 49 51 64 65 69 71 73 **P**6	13	10	199	2057	137	26916	165	15024	7586	424

Hospitals, U.S. / MISSOURI

Hospital, Address, Telephone, Administrator, Approval, Facility, and Physician Codes, Health Care System	Classification Codes		Utilization Data					Expense (thousands) of dollars		
★ American Hospital Association (AHA) membership □ Joint Commission on Accreditation of Healthcare Organizations (JCAHO) accreditation + American Osteopathic Hospital Association (AOHA) membership ○ American Osteopathic Association (AOA) accreditation △ Commission on Accreditation of Rehabilitation Facilities (CARF) accreditation Control codes 61, 63, 64, 71, 72 and 73 indicate hospitals listed by AOHA, but not registered by AHA. For definition of numerical codes, see page A6	Control	Service	Beds	Admissions	Census	Outpatient Visits	Births	Total	Payroll	Personnel
HERMANN—Gasconade County										
★ HERMANN AREA DISTRICT HOSPITAL, Mailing Address: P.O. Box 470, Zip 65041–0470; tel. 314/486–2191; Dan McKinney, Administrator **A**9 10 **F**8 12 15 19 28 30 32 33 34 36 39 40 42 44 46 49 64 65 71 73	16	10	41	441	24	8059	43	4416	1980	103
HOUSTON—Texas County										
TEXAS COUNTY MEMORIAL HOSPITAL, 1333 Sam Houston Boulevard, Zip 65483–2046; tel. 417/967–3311; Beverly Derrickson, Administrator **A**9 10 **F**8 14 16 19 20 22 24 25 28 29 30 31 32 33 34 36 37 39 40 41 44 46 49 51 61 64 65 71 73 **P**4 5	13	10	53	2466	28	11149	319	8842	4295	215
INDEPENDENCE—Jackson County										
★ INDEPENDENCE REGIONAL HEALTH CENTER, 1509 West Truman Road, Zip 64050; tel. 816/836–8100; Paul F. Herzog, Chief Executive Officer (Total facility includes 71 beds in nursing home–type unit) **A**1 2 5 9 10 **F**1 2 3 4 5 6 7 8 9 10 12 13 14 15 16 17 18 19 20 22 23 24 26 27 28 29 30 31 32 33 34 35 36 37 38 40 41 42 43 44 45 46 47 48 49 50 51 52 53 54 55 56 57 58 59 60 61 63 64 65 66 67 70 71 72 73 74 **P**5 6 **S**0048 Columbia/HCA Healthcare Corporation	33	10	335	7662	166	213628	301	63448	30452	1180
★ MEDICAL CENTER OF INDEPENDENCE, 17203 East 23rd Street, Zip 64057; tel. 816/478–5000; Mike Chappelow, President and Chief Executive Officer **A**1 9 10 **F**1 2 3 4 5 7 8 9 10 11 12 13 14 15 16 17 18 19 20 22 23 24 25 26 27 28 29 30 31 32 33 34 35 36 37 38 39 40 41 42 43 44 45 46 47 48 49 51 52 53 54 55 56 57 58 59 60 61 63 64 65 66 67 68 69 71 73 74 **P**1 5 6 **S**8815 Health Midwest	23	10	133	3685	45	33735	747	27351	12239	402
JEFFERSON CITY—Cole County										
★ + ○ △ CAPITAL REGION MEDICAL CENTER–STILL CAMPUS, (Formerly Still Regional Medical Center) 1125 Madison Street, Zip 65101–5227, Mailing Address: P.O. Box 1128, Zip 65102–1128; tel. 314/635–7141; Edward F. Farnsworth, President (Total facility includes 18 beds in nursing home–type unit) **A**1 7 9 10 11 12 13 **F**1 3 7 8 10 12 13 14 15 16 17 18 19 20 22 23 26 28 29 30 31 32 33 34 35 36 37 39 40 41 42 44 45 46 48 49 51 60 63 64 65 66 67 70 71 73 **P**6 8	23	10	122	3564	64	54459	261	33059	14669	572
CAPITAL REGION MEDICAL CENTER–MEMORIAL CAMPUS, (Formerly Memorial Community Hospital) 1432 Southwest Boulevard, Zip 65109–4420, Mailing Address: P.O. Box 104420, Zip 65110–4420; tel. 314/635–6811; Gordon H. Butler, Vice President and Administrator **A**1 9 10 **F**1 3 8 10 13 15 16 17 18 19 22 23 24 25 26 28 29 30 31 32 33 34 35 36 37 40 41 42 43 44 46 48 49 52 53 54 55 57 58 59 60 63 64 65 66 67 70 71 72 73 **P**6 8	23	10	84	2799	45	68166	0	31444	13826	497
MEMORIAL COMMUNITY HOSPITAL See Capital Region Medical Center–Memorial Campus										
★ ST. MARYS HEALTH CENTER, 100 St Marys Medical Plaza, Zip 65101; tel. 314/761–7151; John S. Dubis, President (Total facility includes 120 beds in nursing home–type unit) **A**1 9 10 **F**4 7 8 10 12 13 14 15 16 17 18 19 20 22 28 30 31 32 34 35 37 39 40 41 42 43 44 46 49 52 54 55 56 57 58 59 63 64 65 67 70 71 72 73 **P**1 **S**5455 SSM Health Care System	23	10	263	6816	199	165488	1043	62566	24930	809
STILL REGIONAL MEDICAL CENTER See Capital Region Medical Center–Still Campus										
JOPLIN—Newton County										
★ FREEMAN HOSPITAL, 1102 West 32nd Street, Zip 64804–3599; tel. 417/625–6601; Kelby K. Krabbenhoft, President and Chief Executive Officer (Total facility includes 18 beds in nursing home–type unit) **A**1 9 10 **F**4 5 7 8 10 12 13 15 17 19 20 22 23 26 28 29 30 31 32 33 34 35 36 37 38 39 40 41 42 43 44 49 51 61 64 65 66 67 70 71 72 73 74 **P**6 7 8	23	10	186	6991	93	97300	1951	65681	26121	1001
+ ○ OAK HILL HOSPITAL, 932 East 34th Street, Zip 64804–3999; tel. 417/623–4640; Michael R. Miller, President (Total facility includes 14 beds in nursing home–type unit) **A**9 10 11 12 **F**4 7 8 10 14 15 16 19 20 22 29 30 31 32 34 35 37 39 40 41 43 44 45 46 49 54 56 63 64 65 67 70 71 73 **P**4 6	23	10	89	3491	53	47894	796	29897	10695	366
★ △ ST. JOHN'S REGIONAL MEDICAL CENTER, 2727 McClelland Boulevard, Zip 64804; tel. 417/781–2727; Robert G. Brueckner, President and Chief Executive Officer **A**1 2 7 9 10 **F**4 8 10 11 12 14 15 16 17 18 19 20 22 23 24 25 28 29 30 31 32 33 34 35 36 37 39 40 41 42 43 44 48 49 51 52 54 56 57 58 59 60 65 66 67 69 70 71 72 73 **P**1 **S**5175 Catholic Health Corporation	23	10	331	11510	207	129293	0	100036	35071	1585
KANSAS CITY—Jackson County										
★ BAPTIST MEDICAL CENTER, 6601 Rockhill Road, Zip 64131–1197; tel. 816/276–7000; Dan H. Anderson, President and Chief Executive Officer (Total facility includes 23 beds in nursing home–type unit) **A**1 2 3 5 9 10 **F**2 3 4 5 7 8 9 10 11 12 13 14 15 16 17 18 19 22 23 24 25 26 27 28 29 30 31 32 33 34 35 36 37 38 39 40 41 42 43 44 45 46 47 48 49 51 52 53 54 55 56 57 58 59 60 61 63 64 65 66 67 68 69 71 73 74 **P**1 5 6 **S**8815 Health Midwest	23	10	315	7604	154	49574	557	84332	36553	1116
★ CHILDREN'S MERCY HOSPITAL, (Includes Childrens Cardiac Center, 4052 Warwick Boulevard, Kansas City, Missouri, Zip 64111) 2401 Gillham Road, Zip 64108–9898; tel. 816/234–3000; Randall L. O'Donnell Ph.D., President and Chief Executive Officer **A**1 2 3 5 8 9 10 **F**4 5 9 10 11 12 13 15 16 17 19 20 22 25 29 31 32 34 35 37 38 39 40 41 42 43 44 46 47 48 49 51 54 58 60 65 67 68 69 70 71 72 73 **P**6	23	50	159	6884	111	205957	0	130554	69766	1892
CHILDRENS CARDIAC CENTER See Children's Mercy Hospital										
CRITTENTON, 10918 Elm Avenue, Zip 64134–4199; tel. 816/765–6600; Robert D. Gray, Chief Executive Officer **A**9 10 **F**12 16 17 18 22 29 39 41 45 46 52 53 55 56 58 59 67 68 73 **P**6 7 8	23	52	28	512	16	16275	0	8375	4687	138

© 1995 AHA Guide

Hospitals, U.S. / MISSOURI

Hospital, Address, Telephone, Administrator, Approval, Facility, and Physician Codes, Health Care System	Classi-fication Codes		Utilization Data					Expense (thousands) of dollars		
	Control	Service	Beds	Admissions	Census	Outpatient Visits	Births	Total	Payroll	Personnel

- ★ American Hospital Association (AHA) membership
- □ Joint Commission on Accreditation of Healthcare Organizations (JCAHO) accreditation
- + American Osteopathic Hospital Association (AOHA) membership
- ○ American Osteopathic Association (AOA) accreditation
- △ Commission on Accreditation of Rehabilitation Facilities (CARF) accreditation
- Control codes 61, 63, 64, 71, 72 and 73 indicate hospitals listed by AOHA, but not registered by AHA. For definition of numerical codes, see page A6

Hospital	Control	Service	Beds	Admissions	Census	Outpatient Visits	Births	Total	Payroll	Personnel
★ MENORAH MEDICAL CENTER, 4949 Rockhill Road, Zip 64110–2298; tel. 816/276–8000; Roy A. Powell, President (Total facility includes 21 beds in nursing home–type unit) A1 2 3 5 9 10 F1 2 3 4 5 7 8 9 10 11 12 13 14 15 16 17 18 19 22 23 24 25 26 27 28 29 30 31 32 33 34 35 36 37 38 39 40 41 42 43 44 45 46 47 48 49 51 52 53 54 55 56 57 58 59 60 61 63 64 65 66 67 68 69 71 72 73 74 P1 5 6 S8815 Health Midwest	23	10	259	8979	138	44064	1658	75473	28585	800
□ NORTH HILLS HOSPITAL OF KANSAS CITY, 4800 Northwest 88th Street, Zip 64154; tel. 816/436–3900; John De Lamare, Administrator A1 9 10 F12 15 16 17 18 19 22 26 27 35 39 41 52 53 54 55 56 57 59 65 71	33	22	76	275	12	—	0	4174	2010	74
□ + ○ PARK LANE MEDICAL CENTER, 5151 Raytown Road, Zip 64133; tel. 816/358–8000; Derell Taloney, President (Total facility includes 15 beds in nursing home–type unit) A1 9 10 11 12 F2 3 8 12 15 16 17 18 19 20 22 26 27 28 29 30 31 32 34 35 36 37 39 40 41 42 44 46 49 51 52 54 55 56 57 58 63 64 65 71 73	23	10	94	2276	43	16170	0	23034	10149	375
△ REHABILITATION INSTITUTE, 3011 Baltimore, Zip 64108–3465; tel. 816/756–2250; John H. Parker, President A7 9 10 F1 2 3 4 5 6 7 8 9 10 11 12 13 14 15 16 17 18 20 22 23 24 25 26 27 28 29 30 31 32 33 34 35 36 37 38 39 40 41 42 43 44 45 46 47 48 49 51 52 53 54 55 56 57 58 59 60 61 64 65 66 67 68 69 71 72 73 74 P2 5 8 S8815 Health Midwest	23	46	20	290	19	17500	0	10049	5324	196
★ RESEARCH MEDICAL CENTER, 2316 East Meyer Boulevard, Zip 64132–1199; tel. 816/276–4000; Dan H. Anderson, President and Chief Executive Officer (Total facility includes 35 beds in nursing home–type unit) A1 2 5 9 10 F1 2 3 4 5 7 8 9 10 11 12 13 14 15 16 17 18 19 22 23 24 25 26 27 28 29 30 31 32 33 34 35 36 37 38 39 40 41 42 43 44 45 46 47 48 49 50 51 52 53 54 55 56 57 58 59 60 61 63 64 65 66 67 68 69 70 71 72 73 74 P5 7 8 S8815 Health Midwest	23	10	480	15138	311	77969	1525	174618	74661	2036
★ RESEARCH PSYCHIATRIC CENTER, 2323 East 63rd Street, Zip 64130; tel. 816/444–8161; Steven R. Newton, Administrator and Chief Executive Officer A1 9 10 F3 4 5 6 7 8 10 12 13 15 16 17 18 20 22 23 24 26 27 28 29 30 31 32 33 34 35 39 41 42 43 44 45 46 49 51 52 53 54 55 56 57 58 59 60 61 62 65 66 67 68 69 70 72 73 74 P4 5 8 S0048 Columbia/HCA Healthcare Corporation	33	22	100	1699	56	3367	0	11106	4393	142
★ SAINT JOSEPH HEALTH CENTER, 1000 Carondelet Drive, Zip 64114–4673; tel. 816/942–4400; Richard M. Abell, President A1 2 9 10 F1 4 5 7 8 10 12 13 16 19 22 24 28 29 30 31 32 33 34 35 37 38 39 40 41 42 43 44 45 46 47 48 49 63 64 65 67 70 71 72 73 P3 4 5 6 7 S5945 Carondelet Health System	23	10	254	9987	152	63758	1700	98797	37842	1226
SAINT LUKE'S NORTHLAND HOSPITAL – BARRY ROAD CAMPUS, 5830 N.W. Barry Road, Zip 64154–9988; tel. 816/891–6000; James M. Brophy, Chief Executive Officer F4 5 7 8 10 11 14 15 16 17 19 22 24 25 26 27 28 29 30 31 32 33 34 35 37 38 39 40 41 42 43 44 45 46 47 48 51 52 53 54 55 56 57 58 59 60 61 63 64 65 66 67 69 70 71 73 74 P6 8	23	10	55	2435	25	26968	633	18693	7946	209
★ ST. LUKE'S HOSPITAL, 4400 Wornall Road, Zip 64111–3238, Mailing Address: P.O. Box 119000, Zip 64171–9000; tel. 816/932–2000; G. Richard Hastings, Chief Executive Officer (Total facility includes 30 beds in nursing home–type unit) A1 2 3 5 8 9 10 F4 5 7 8 10 11 12 14 15 16 17 18 19 22 24 25 26 27 28 29 30 31 32 33 34 35 37 38 39 40 41 42 43 44 45 46 48 49 52 53 54 55 56 57 58 59 60 61 63 64 65 66 67 69 70 71 73 74 P6 8	23	10	531	17743	320	85514	2620	208458	92143	2504
★ TRINITY LUTHERAN HOSPITAL, (Includes St. Mary's Hospital, 101 Memorial Drive, Kansas City, Missouri, Zip 64108; tel. 816/751–4600) 3030 Baltimore Avenue, Zip 64108–3404; tel. 816/751–4600; Ronald A. Ommen, President (Total facility includes 30 beds in nursing home–type unit) A1 2 3 5 9 10 F1 2 3 4 5 7 8 9 10 11 12 13 14 15 16 17 18 19 20 22 23 24 25 26 27 28 29 30 31 32 33 34 35 36 37 38 39 40 41 42 43 44 45 46 47 48 49 51 52 53 54 55 56 57 58 59 60 61 64 65 66 67 68 69 70 71 72 73 74 P1 5 6 S8815 Health Midwest	23	10	358	7326	185	171391	0	79611	37199	1220
★ △ TRUMAN MEDICAL CENTER–EAST, 7900 Lee's Summit Road, Zip 64139–1241; tel. 816/373–4415; Ross P. Marine, Administrator and Chief Executive Officer (Total facility includes 212 beds in nursing home–type unit) A1 3 5 7 9 10 F3 7 8 10 11 12 13 14 15 16 17 19 20 22 26 27 28 29 30 31 32 34 35 37 38 39 40 41 42 44 45 46 48 49 51 52 54 56 57 58 61 65 66 70 71 73 74 S9255 Truman Medical Center	23	10	300	3845	264	95643	1060	38677	18917	741
★ TRUMAN MEDICAL CENTER–WEST, 2301 Holmes Street, Zip 64108; tel. 816/556–3000; Rosa L. Miller R.N., Administrator A1 3 5 8 9 10 F3 4 7 8 10 14 16 17 19 20 22 26 31 34 35 37 38 40 41 42 43 44 45 46 48 49 51 52 53 54 55 56 57 58 59 60 61 63 64 65 66 70 71 73 74 S9255 Truman Medical Center	23	10	225	10261	179	312295	2399	97305	49817	1422
□ TWO RIVERS PSYCHIATRIC HOSPITAL, 5121 Raytown Road, Zip 64133–2141; tel. 816/356–5688; Craig Nuckles, Administrator A1 9 10 F14 17 39 45 52 53 54 55 57 59 65 67 68 P1 2 3 4 5 6 7 8 S9555 Universal Health Services, Inc.	33	22	80	1081	42	804	0	8810	3421	115
□ VENCOR HOSPITAL–KANSAS CITY, 8701 Troost Avenue, Zip 64131; tel. 816/995–2000; Suzanne R. Wilsey R.N., Administrator (Total facility includes 16 beds in nursing home–type unit) A1 9 F10 12 15 16 19 22 27 35 37 39 40 41 42 46 47 50 52 54 57 63 64 65 67 70 71 73 P5 S0026 Vencor, Incorporated	33	10	167	460	60	—	0	—	—	164
★ VETERANS AFFAIRS MEDICAL CENTER, 4801 Linwood Boulevard, Zip 64128–2295; tel. 816/922–2048; Hugh F. Doran, Director A1 2 3 5 8 F2 3 4 9 10 11 16 17 19 20 22 23 24 25 26 27 28 30 31 32 34 35 37 39 40 41 42 43 44 46 48 49 50 51 52 54 55 56 57 58 59 60 61 63 64 65 67 71 72 73 74 S9295 Department of Veterans Affairs	45	10	273	7644	226	165720	0	—	—	1342

Hospitals, U.S. / MISSOURI

Hospital, Address, Telephone, Administrator, Approval, Facility, and Physician Codes, Health Care System	Classification Codes		Utilization Data					Expense (thousands) of dollars		
Approval key: ★ American Hospital Association (AHA) membership; □ Joint Commission on Accreditation of Healthcare Organizations (JCAHO) accreditation; + American Osteopathic Hospital Association (AOHA) membership; ○ American Osteopathic Association (AOA) accreditation; △ Commission on Accreditation of Rehabilitation Facilities (CARF) accreditation. Control codes 61, 63, 64, 71, 72 and 73 indicate hospitals listed by AOHA, but not registered by AHA. For definition of numerical codes, see page A6	Control	Service	Beds	Admissions	Census	Outpatient Visits	Births	Total	Payroll	Personnel
□ WESTERN MISSOURI MENTAL HEALTH CENTER, 600 East 22nd Street, Zip 64108; tel. 816/471-3000; Gloria Joseph MSW, Superintendent **A**1 3 5 10 **F**15 19 22 24 27 34 35 39 41 46 52 53 54 55 56 57 63 65 67 71 73 **P**7	12	22	110	2612	95	4747	0	23315	12828	562
KENNETT—Dunklin County										
□ TWIN RIVERS REGIONAL MEDICAL CENTER, 1301 First Street, Zip 63857; tel. 314/888-4522; Cliff Yeager, Chief Executive Officer (Total facility includes 10 beds in nursing home-type unit) **A**1 9 10 **F**8 12 14 15 16 19 20 22 23 24 27 28 30 32 34 35 37 39 40 41 42 44 49 64 65 66 71 73 **P**6 **S**6525 Ornda Healthcorp	33	10	116	3050	39	43886	352	18990	6802	328
KIRKSVILLE—Adair County										
□ GRIM-SMITH HOSPITAL AND CLINIC, 112 East Patterson Avenue, Zip 63501; tel. 816/665-7241; Steven E. Clark, Administrator (Total facility includes 13 beds in nursing home-type unit) **A**1 9 10 **F**4 7 8 14 15 16 17 18 19 20 22 24 28 29 30 31 32 34 35 37 39 40 41 44 46 49 54 58 59 64 65 67 70 71 74 **P**5 8	33	10	68	2632	31	19145	316	18515	7420	334
+ ○ KIRKSVILLE OSTEOPATHIC MEDICAL CENTER, 800 West Jefferson Street, Zip 63501-1497; tel. 816/626-2121; Herbert F. Dorsett, Chief Executive Officer (Nonreporting) **A**5 9 10 11 12 13 **S**0063 TENET Healthcare Corporation	33	22	238	—	—	—	—	—	—	—
LAKE SAINT LOUIS—St. Charles County										
★ ST. JOSEPH HOSPITAL WEST, 100 Medical Plaza, Zip 63367-1395; tel. 314/625-5200; Kevin F. Kast, President (Total facility includes 11 beds in nursing home-type unit) **A**10 **F**3 4 5 7 8 10 12 13 14 15 16 17 18 20 22 23 24 25 26 28 29 30 31 32 33 34 35 37 39 40 41 42 43 44 46 49 51 53 54 55 56 57 58 59 60 61 63 64 65 66 67 68 69 70 71 72 73 74 **P**1 2 4 5 6 7 8 **S**5455 SSM Health Care System	23	10	100	2920	31	20017	425	19975	8738	199
LAMAR—Barton County										
★ BARTON COUNTY MEMORIAL HOSPITAL, Second and Gulf Streets, Zip 64759-0626; tel. 417/682-6081; Keith Adams, Interim Administrator (Total facility includes 12 beds in nursing home-type unit) **A**9 10 **F**7 8 11 19 20 22 28 30 32 34 35 37 39 40 41 44 46 48 49 64 65 71	13	10	44	1183	17	17056	98	7062	3284	159
LEBANON—Laclede County										
★ BREECH MEDICAL CENTER, 325 Harwood Avenue, Zip 65536, Mailing Address: P.O. Box N, Zip 65536; tel. 417/532-2136; Gary W. Pulsipher, Chief Executive Officer (Total facility includes 7 beds in nursing home-type unit) **A**1 9 10 **F**8 11 19 22 27 28 30 32 33 34 37 40 44 49 64 65 71 **S**0002 Quorum Health Group/Quorum Health Resources	23	10	42	692	9	27278	5	9430	4235	205
LEES SUMMIT—Jackson County										
★ LEE'S SUMMIT HOSPITAL, 530 North Murray Road, Zip 64081-1497; tel. 816/251-7000; John L. Jacobson, President and Chief Executive Officer **A**1 9 10 **F**8 12 14 15 16 17 18 19 22 27 28 29 30 34 35 36 37 39 40 41 42 44 45 46 49 63 65 66 67 71 72 73 **P**1 5 7 8 **S**8815 Health Midwest	23	10	77	2664	35	25218	0	21896	9147	242
LEXINGTON—Lafayette County										
★ LAFAYETTE REGIONAL HEALTH CENTER, 1500 State Street, Zip 64067-1199; tel. 816/259-2203; Michael S. McCoy, Administrator **A**1 9 10 **F**7 8 16 19 22 25 27 29 30 32 34 37 39 40 41 42 45 46 49 51 64 65 71 73 74 **P**4 **S**8815 Health Midwest	23	10	37	1498	17	41523	179	10390	4025	174
LIBERTY—Clay County										
★ LIBERTY HOSPITAL, 2525 Glenn Hendren Drive, Zip 64068-9625; tel. 816/781-7200; Joseph Crossett, Administrator (Total facility includes 20 beds in nursing home-type unit) **A**1 9 10 **F**5 7 8 9 10 15 16 17 19 22 23 26 27 28 30 32 33 34 35 36 37 38 39 40 41 42 43 44 48 49 60 64 65 67 70 71 73 **P**3	16	10	173	6802	103	52164	856	50338	22279	725
LOUISIANA—Pike County										
★ PIKE COUNTY MEMORIAL HOSPITAL, 2305 West Georgia Street, Zip 63353-0020; tel. 314/754-5531; Thomas E. Lefebvre, President **A**1 9 10 **F**3 7 8 14 15 16 19 22 27 28 30 34 35 39 40 44 49 54 55 58 65 67 68 71 73 **P**8 **S**5455 SSM Health Care System	13	10	25	1167	12	13327	69	6467	2851	123
MACON—Macon County										
SAMARITAN MEMORIAL HOSPITAL, North Jackson Street, Zip 63552, Mailing Address: P.O. Box 217, Zip 63552; tel. 816/385-3151; Bernard A. Orman Jr., Administrator **A**9 10 **F**1 3 7 8 12 14 15 16 17 18 19 22 26 27 28 29 30 31 32 33 34 35 36 39 40 41 42 44 45 46 49 52 56 57 58 59 64 65 67 69 71 73 74	13	10	35	980	17	11270	17	6026	2503	125
MARSHALL—Saline County										
★ FITZGIBBON HOSPITAL, 2305 South 65 Highway, Zip 65340-0250, Mailing Address: P.O. Box 250, Zip 65340-0250; tel. 816/886-7431; Ronald A. Ott, Chief Executive Officer (Total facility includes 13 beds in nursing home-type unit) **A**9 10 **F**7 8 15 17 19 22 27 28 30 32 33 34 35 37 39 40 41 44 46 49 53 54 57 58 59 64 65 66 71 74	23	10	56	2081	28	57012	255	14219	5640	297
MARYVILLE—Nodaway County										
★ ST. FRANCIS HOSPITAL, 2016 South Main Street, Zip 64468-2693; tel. 816/562-2600; Ray Brazier, President **A**1 9 10 **F**3 7 8 12 14 15 16 18 19 20 22 25 27 29 30 31 32 33 34 35 39 40 41 42 44 46 49 51 52 54 55 56 57 58 59 64 65 71 73 **P**1 6 7 8 **S**5455 SSM Health Care System	23	10	55	1644	21	28622	291	12838	6224	286
MEMPHIS—Scotland County										
○ SCOTLAND COUNTY MEMORIAL HOSPITAL, Sigler Avenue, Zip 63555, Mailing Address: Route 1, Box 53, Zip 63555; tel. 816/465-8511; Marcia R. Dial, Administrator **A**9 10 11 **F**5 7 8 15 16 17 19 20 22 26 28 29 30 33 34 36 37 39 40 42 44 45 49 51 64 71	16	10	27	438	8	8584	30	2390	1098	63

© 1995 AHA Guide

Hospitals, U.S. / MISSOURI

Hospital, Address, Telephone, Administrator, Approval, Facility, and Physician Codes, Health Care System	Classification Codes		Utilization Data					Expense (thousands) of dollars		
	Control	Service	Beds	Admissions	Census	Outpatient Visits	Births	Total	Payroll	Personnel

★ American Hospital Association (AHA) membership
☐ Joint Commission on Accreditation of Healthcare Organizations (JCAHO) accreditation
+ American Osteopathic Hospital Association (AOHA) membership
○ American Osteopathic Association (AOA) accreditation
△ Commission on Accreditation of Rehabilitation Facilities (CARF) accreditation
Control codes 61, 63, 64, 71, 72 and 73 indicate hospitals listed by AOHA, but not registered by AHA. For definition of numerical codes, see page A6

Hospital	Control	Service	Beds	Admissions	Census	Outpatient Visits	Births	Total	Payroll	Personnel
MEXICO—Audrain County ★ + AUDRAIN MEDICAL CENTER, 620 East Monroe Street, Zip 65265–0858; tel. 314/581-1760; Charles P. Jansen, Administrator (Total facility includes 51 beds in nursing home–type unit) **A**1 9 10 **F**1 3 7 8 10 12 14 15 17 18 19 20 22 23 25 26 29 30 32 33 34 35 37 39 40 41 42 44 45 46 49 51 52 53 54 55 56 57 58 59 63 64 65 66 67 68 71 73 74 **P**6	23	10	176	4631	101	119781	328	39936	18438	682
MILAN—Sullivan County ★ SULLIVAN COUNTY MEMORIAL HOSPITAL, 630 West Third Street, Zip 63556; tel. 816/265-4212; Nancy Bauman, Chief Executive Officer (Total facility includes 12 beds in nursing home–type unit) **A**9 10 **F**17 19 20 22 28 30 32 34 36 44 49 64 65 71 **S**0585 Brim, Inc.	13	10	47	291	26	7893	0	2860	1174	65
MOBERLY—Randolph County ★ + MOBERLY REGIONAL MEDICAL CENTER, 1515 Union Avenue, Zip 65270–9449, Mailing Address: P.O. Box 3000, Zip 65270–3000; tel. 816/263-8400; Jack P. Nyiri, Executive Director (Total facility includes 21 beds in nursing home–type unit) **A**1 5 9 10 **F**7 8 12 19 22 24 26 27 28 29 30 32 33 34 37 39 40 41 44 46 49 52 54 57 64 65 66 67 70 71 73 **P**6 **S**0875 Community Health Systems, Inc.	33	10	101	2237	33	43061	350	15716	5311	208
MONETT—Barry County ★ COX–MONETT HOSPITAL, 801 Lincoln Avenue, Zip 65708–1698; tel. 417/235-3144; Donald C. Lamkins, Administrator **A**9 10 **F**8 12 14 15 16 17 19 22 26 27 28 29 30 31 32 34 37 39 41 44 46 49 51 64 65 67 71 73 **P**1 3	23	10	53	933	14	39157	0	6981	3032	149
MOUNT VERNON—Lawrence County ☐ △ MISSOURI REHABILITATION CENTER, 600 North Main, Zip 65712–1099; tel. 417/466-3711; Charles Drewel, Director **A**1 7 10 **F**3 6 15 16 19 26 27 29 30 31 33 34 37 39 41 42 46 48 49 65 67 71 73 **P**6	12	10	136	563	73	16525	0	16821	8607	430
MOUNTAIN VIEW—Howell County ★ ST. FRANCIS HOSPITAL, Highway 60, Zip 65548, Mailing Address: P.O. Box 82, Zip 65548–0082; tel. 417/934-2246; Sister M. Cornelia Blasko, Administrator **A**1 9 10 **F**8 14 15 19 22 32 34 39 44 46 49 64 65 71	23	10	20	427	6	14325	0	3156	1368	77
NEOSHO—Newton County FREEMAN NEOSHO HOSPITAL, 113 West Hickory Street, Zip 64850–1799; tel. 417/451-1234; Phil Willcoxon, Administrator **A**9 10 **F**5 7 8 10 14 15 16 19 22 26 32 33 34 35 37 39 40 41 42 44 46 48 49 51 61 64 65 66 71 73 **P**4 8	23	10	54	1957	45	76652	0	—	—	251
NEVADA—Vernon County ☐ HEARTLAND HOSPITAL, 1500 West Ashland, Zip 64772; tel. 417/667-2666; Eugene Hastings, Administrator **A**1 9 10 **F**1 2 3 8 12 15 16 18 25 39 41 52 53 54 55 56 57 58 59 65 73 **P**1 **S**0405 Ramsay Health Care, Inc.	33	22	60	408	17	6000	0	10085	4943	64
★ NEVADA REGIONAL MEDICAL CENTER, 800 South Ash Street, Zip 64772; tel. 417/667-3355; Michael L. Mullins, President (Total facility includes 10 beds in nursing home–type unit) **A**1 10 **F**7 8 15 17 19 22 27 28 30 31 32 33 34 36 37 39 40 41 42 44 59 60 64 65 71 73 **P**1 2 3 4 5 6 7 8 **S**0002 Quorum Health Group/Quorum Health Resources	14	10	97	2244	28	23541	274	12368	5093	243
NORTH KANSAS CITY—Clay County ★ NORTH KANSAS CITY HOSPITAL, 2800 Clay Edwards Drive, Zip 64116–3281; tel. 816/691-2000; Michael E. Payne, President (Total facility includes 39 beds in nursing home–type unit) **A**1 9 10 **F**2 3 4 6 7 8 10 11 15 16 17 18 19 20 22 23 28 30 32 33 34 35 37 39 40 41 42 43 44 48 49 52 54 55 56 57 58 59 60 63 64 65 67 70 71 73 **P**6	14	10	348	10925	193	66792	1051	97293	41766	1199
OSAGE BEACH—Camden County ★ LAKE OF THE OZARKS GENERAL HOSPITAL, 54 Hospital Drive, Zip 65065; tel. 314/348-8000; Michael E. Henze, Chief Executive Officer (Total facility includes 14 beds in nursing home–type unit) **A**1 9 10 **F**7 8 15 16 19 22 23 28 29 30 34 35 37 39 40 41 42 44 46 49 63 64 65 67 71 73	23	10	91	3003	42	41931	579	24685	9582	420
OSCEOLA—St. Clair County ★ SAC–OSAGE HOSPITAL, Junction Hwys 13 & Business 13, Zip 64776, Mailing Address: P.O. Box 426, Zip 64776–0426; tel. 417/646-8181; Terry E. Erwine, Administrator **A**1 9 10 **F**7 8 15 16 19 22 28 29 30 31 34 37 39 40 41 42 44 45 46 64 65 67 71 73	16	10	47	1225	20	5695	60	5054	2412	117
PERRYVILLE—Perry County ☐ PERRY COUNTY MEMORIAL HOSPITAL, 434 North West Street, Zip 63775–1398; tel. 314/547-2536; Patrick G. Bira, Administrator **A**1 9 10 **F**1 7 8 12 14 15 16 17 19 22 23 24 26 27 28 29 30 32 33 34 35 37 39 40 41 42 44 45 67 68 71 73 **P**8	13	10	55	1272	17	20729	149	9552	3879	192
PILOT KNOB—Iron County ★ ARCADIA VALLEY HOSPITAL, Highway 21, Zip 63663, Mailing Address: P.O. Box 548, Zip 63663–0548; tel. 314/546-3924; H. Clark Duncan, Administrator (Total facility includes 24 beds in nursing home–type unit) **A**1 9 10 **F**8 12 15 17 19 22 25 26 28 30 31 32 33 34 37 39 40 41 44 46 64 65 71 73 **P**8 **S**5455 SSM Health Care System	23	10	50	841	36	17139	0	7044	3214	148
POPLAR BLUFF—Butler County AMI LUCY LEE HOSPITAL See Lucy Lee Hospital										
☐ DOCTORS REGIONAL MEDICAL CENTER, 621 Pine Boulevard, Zip 63901; tel. 314/686-4111; Daniel R. Kelly, Chief Executive Officer **A**1 2 9 10 **F**2 3 7 8 12 14 15 16 17 18 19 20 22 23 25 26 28 29 30 31 32 34 35 37 39 40 41 42 44 45 46 48 49 51 52 53 54 55 58 59 65 66 67 70 71 72 73 74	33	10	182	6875	106	52225	492	41237	13171	669

Hospitals, U.S. / MISSOURI

Hospital, Address, Telephone, Administrator, Approval, Facility, and Physician Codes, Health Care System	Classification Codes		Utilization Data					Expense (thousands) of dollars		Personnel
★ American Hospital Association (AHA) membership ☐ Joint Commission on Accreditation of Healthcare Organizations (JCAHO) accreditation + American Osteopathic Hospital Association (AOHA) membership ○ American Osteopathic Association (AOA) accreditation △ Commission on Accreditation of Rehabilitation Facilities (CARF) accreditation Control codes 61, 63, 64, 71, 72 and 73 indicate hospitals listed by AOHA, but not registered by AHA. For definition of numerical codes, see page A6	Control	Service	Beds	Admissions	Census	Outpatient Visits	Births	Total	Payroll	
★ JOHN J. PERSHING VETERANS AFFAIRS MEDICAL CENTER, 1500 North Westwood Boulevard, Zip 63901; tel. 314/686–4151; (Total facility includes 49 beds in nursing home–type unit) **A**1 **F**2 3 4 5 8 10 15 16 20 22 23 24 25 27 28 29 30 31 32 34 37 39 41 42 43 44 45 46 48 49 50 51 52 54 56 57 58 64 65 67 69 71 73 74 **P**6 **S**9295 Department of Veterans Affairs	45	10	174	3281	139	46323	0	28213	14506	390
★ △ LUCY LEE HOSPITAL, (Formerly AMI Lucy Lee Hospitals) 2620 North Westwood Boulevard, Zip 63901–2341; tel. 314/785–7721; David L. Archer, Chief Executive Officer (Total facility includes 24 beds in nursing home–type unit) **A**1 2 7 9 10 **F**3 5 7 8 11 12 17 19 22 24 25 26 28 29 30 31 32 33 34 35 37 39 40 41 42 44 45 46 48 49 51 52 53 54 55 56 57 58 59 60 61 64 65 66 67 71 72 73 74 **P**1 7 **S**0063 TENET Healthcare Corporation	33	10	189	6069	102	161318	984	42076	12209	820
POTOSI—Washington County										
WASHINGTON COUNTY MEMORIAL HOSPITAL, 300 Health Way, Zip 63664–1499; tel. 314/438–5451; William Schwarten, Administrator **A**9 10 **F**8 14 15 16 19 22 25 28 29 30 32 34 37 39 40 41 44 46 48 49 60 65 67 71 74	13	10	42	559	9	21695	0	5494	2094	117
RICHMOND—Ray County										
RAY COUNTY MEMORIAL HOSPITAL, 904 Wollard Boulevard, Zip 64085–2243; tel. 816/776–5432; Tommy L. Hicks, Administrator (Total facility includes 11 beds in nursing home–type unit) **A**10 **F**8 14 15 19 22 30 34 35 37 39 41 42 44 49 51 54 58 64 65 66 71 73	13	10	50	1240	21	7976	0	8823	3998	177
ROLLA—Phelps County										
★ ○ PHELPS COUNTY REGIONAL MEDICAL CENTER, 1000 West Tenth Street, Zip 65401; tel. 314/364–3100; Dan Smigelski, Chief Executive Officer (Total facility includes 38 beds in nursing home–type unit) **A**1 9 10 11 12 **F**7 8 14 15 16 17 18 19 21 23 28 29 30 31 33 34 35 37 39 40 41 42 46 48 49 52 54 55 56 57 58 59 60 64 65 66 67 70 71 73 74 **P**1 3 **S**0002 Quorum Health Group/Quorum Health Resources	13	10	245	7660	130	44989	972	43065	17053	644
SAINT CHARLES—St. Charles County										
☐ CPC SPIRIT OF ST. LOUIS HOSPITAL, 5931 Highway 94 South, Saint Charles, Zip 63304–5601; tel. 314/441–7300 **A**1 9 10 **F**2 3 12 15 16 18 20 22 27 34 52 53 54 55 56 57 58 59 65 67 **S**0785 Community Psychiatric Centers	33	22	104	709	57	—	0	6575	3174	98
★ ST. JOSEPH HEALTH CENTER, 300 First Capitol Drive, Saint Charles, Zip 63301–2835; tel. 314/947–5000; Kevin F. Kast, President (Total facility includes 24 beds in nursing home–type unit) **A**1 2 9 10 **F**3 4 5 7 8 10 12 13 14 15 16 17 18 19 20 22 23 24 25 26 28 29 30 31 32 33 34 35 37 39 40 41 42 43 44 45 46 48 49 51 52 53 54 55 56 57 58 59 60 61 63 64 65 66 67 68 69 70 71 72 73 74 **P**1 2 4 5 6 7 8 **S**5455 SSM Health Care System	23	10	362	12254	183	45098	1183	89110	36356	1040
SAINT JOSEPH—Andrew County										
★ HEARTLAND HOSPITAL EAST, 5325 Faraon Street, Saint Joseph, Zip 64506; tel. 816/271–6000; Lowell C. Kruse, President **A**1 9 10 **F**4 5 7 8 10 11 12 14 15 16 17 18 19 22 25 27 28 30 32 33 34 35 37 39 40 41 42 43 44 46 48 49 51 52 54 55 56 57 60 64 65 66 67 70 71 73 74 **S**2485 Heartland Health System	23	10	205	7768	135	68389	0	—	—	—
★ △ HEARTLAND HOSPITAL WEST, 801 Faraon Street, Saint Joseph, Zip 64501; tel. 816/271–7111; Lowell C. Kruse, President (Total facility includes 196 beds in nursing home–type unit) **A**1 2 7 9 10 **F**4 5 7 8 10 11 12 14 15 16 17 18 19 22 23 25 27 28 30 32 33 34 35 37 39 40 41 42 43 44 46 48 49 51 52 54 55 56 57 60 64 65 66 70 71 73 74 **S**2485 Heartland Health System	23	10	341	6667	253	123292	1576	128283	57887	1883
☐ ST. JOSEPH STATE HOSPITAL, 3400 Frederick Avenue, Saint Joseph, Zip 64506; tel. 816/387–2300; Ron Dittemore Ed.D., Superintendent **A**1 9 10 **F**15 52 56 65 73	12	22	128	133	73	131	0	17006	10576	464
SAINT LOUIS—St. Louis County										
☐ ALEXIAN BROTHERS HOSPITAL, 3933 South Broadway, Saint Louis, Zip 63118–9984; tel. 314/865–3333; Deno E. Fabbre, President and Chief Executive Officer (Total facility includes 40 beds in nursing home–type unit) **A**1 9 10 **F**2 3 5 6 8 10 12 15 16 17 19 22 25 26 27 28 30 31 32 33 34 35 36 37 39 41 42 44 46 49 52 54 55 56 57 59 62 63 64 65 67 71 72 73 **P**5 6 8 **S**0065 Alexian Brothers Health System, Inc.	23	10	182	5162	122	33285	0	38552	17737	670
★ BARNES HOSPITAL, (Includes Queeny Tower; Rand–Johnson; The Pavilion) One Barnes Hospital Plaza, Saint Louis, Zip 63110–1094; tel. 314/362–5000; John J. Finan, President and Senior Executive Officer (Total facility includes 120 beds in nursing home–type unit) **A**1 2 3 5 8 9 10 **F**2 3 4 5 6 7 8 9 10 11 12 13 14 15 16 17 19 20 22 23 24 25 26 27 28 29 30 31 32 33 34 35 36 37 38 39 40 41 42 43 44 46 47 48 49 50 51 52 53 54 55 56 57 58 59 60 61 62 63 64 65 66 67 68 69 70 71 72 73 74 **P**1 5 6 7 8 **S**0051 BJC Health System	23	10	1088	33784	707	277590	2237	432503	190186	6002
★ BARNES WEST COUNTY HOSPITAL, 12634 Olive Street Road, Saint Louis, Zip 63141–6354; tel. 314/434–0600; Gregory T. Wozniak, Administrator (Total facility includes 10 beds in nursing home–type unit) **A**1 9 10 **F**1 2 3 4 5 6 7 8 9 10 11 12 13 14 15 16 17 18 19 20 22 23 24 25 26 27 28 29 30 31 32 33 34 35 36 37 38 39 40 41 42 43 44 45 46 47 48 49 50 51 52 53 54 55 56 57 58 59 60 61 62 63 64 65 66 67 68 69 70 71 72 73 74 **P**1 5 7 8 **S**0051 BJC Health System	23	10	87	1807	32	32557	0	24824	7605	242
★ △ BETHESDA GENERAL HOSPITAL, 3655 Vista Avenue, Saint Louis, Zip 63110; tel. 314/772–9200; John F. Norwood, President (Total facility includes 28 beds in nursing home–type unit) **A**1 5 7 9 10 **F**1 4 8 10 12 14 17 19 22 23 26 27 28 30 31 32 33 34 35 36 37 39 41 42 43 44 46 48 49 50 52 57 60 62 63 64 65 67 69 71 73	23	10	118	1205	49	2709	0	15083	6523	272

© 1995 AHA Guide

Hospitals, U.S. / MISSOURI

Hospital, Address, Telephone, Administrator, Approval, Facility, and Physician Codes, Health Care System	Classification Codes		Utilization Data					Expense (thousands) of dollars		
	Control	Service	Beds	Admissions	Census	Outpatient Visits	Births	Total	Payroll	Personnel
★ CARDINAL GLENNON CHILDREN'S HOSPITAL, 1465 South Grand Boulevard, Saint Louis, Zip 63104–1095; tel. 314/577–5600; Douglas A. Ries, President **A**1 3 5 9 10 **F**2 3 4 5 6 9 10 12 13 14 15 16 17 18 19 20 22 23 25 26 27 28 29 30 31 32 33 34 35 38 39 40 41 42 43 44 45 46 47 48 49 50 51 52 53 54 55 56 58 59 60 63 65 66 67 68 69 70 71 72 73 74 **P**1 2 6 8 **S**5455 SSM Health Care System	23	50	190	8351	130	139719	0	100334	43041	1236
★ △ CHRISTIAN HOSPITAL NORTHEAST–NORTHWEST, (Includes Christian Hospital Northwest, 1225 Graham Road, Florissant, Missouri, Zip 63031; tel. 314/839–3800) 11133 Dunn Road, Saint Louis, Zip 63136–6192; tel. 314/653–5729; W. R. Van Bokkelen, President and Senior Executive Officer (Total facility includes 16 beds in nursing home–type unit) **A**1 2 7 9 10 **F**1 2 3 4 5 6 7 8 9 10 11 12 13 14 15 16 17 18 19 20 21 22 23 24 25 26 27 28 29 30 31 32 33 34 35 37 38 39 40 41 42 43 44 45 46 47 48 49 50 52 53 54 55 56 57 58 59 60 63 64 65 66 67 68 69 70 71 73 74 **P**5 6 7 8 **S**0051 BJC Health System	23	10	575	23574	383	161061	1762	202164	93799	2715
★ DEACONESS HEALTH SYSTEM, 6150 Oakland Avenue, Saint Louis, Zip 63139–3297; tel. 314/768–3000; Jerry W. Paul, President **A**1 2 3 5 9 10 **F**3 4 7 8 10 11 12 14 15 16 17 19 20 22 25 27 28 30 31 32 33 34 35 37 39 40 41 42 43 44 48 49 51 52 54 55 56 57 58 59 60 61 62 65 66 67 71 72 73 74 **P**6	23	10	362	13194	240	108773	2636	147222	74294	2079
+ ○ DEACONESS MEDICAL CENTER–WEST CAMPUS, (Includes Metropolitan Medical Center–West, 530 Des Peres Road, Saint Louis, Missouri, Zip 63131; tel. 314/821–5850) 8225 Florissant Road, Saint Louis, Zip 63121–2204, Mailing Address: 530 Des Peres Road, Zip 63131–2203; tel. 314/966–9108; Joan D'Ambrose, Executive Vice President and Chief Operating Officer **A**10 11 12 13 **F**2 3 4 7 8 10 11 12 13 16 17 19 20 22 23 27 28 30 31 32 33 34 35 37 39 40 41 42 43 44 45 48 49 51 52 54 55 56 57 58 59 60 61 62 63 65 67 71 72 73 74 **P**6	23	10	110	3178	50	23750	0	38652	14941	561
★ △ DEPAUL HEALTH CENTER, (Includes St. Anne's Skilled Nursing Division; DePaul Hospital, Bridgeton, Missouri; St. Vincent's Psychiatric Division, Bridgeton, Missouri) 12303 DePaul Drive, Saint Louis, Zip 63044–2588; tel. 314/344–6000; Robert J. Henkel, President and Chief Executive Officer (Total facility includes 94 beds in nursing home–type unit) **A**1 5 7 9 10 **F**2 3 4 7 8 9 10 11 12 14 15 16 17 18 19 22 24 25 27 28 29 30 31 32 33 34 35 36 37 38 39 40 41 42 43 44 45 46 47 48 49 51 52 53 54 55 56 57 58 59 60 63 64 65 66 67 69 70 71 73 74 **P**1 4 6 **S**1855 Daughters of Charity National Health System	21	10	466	13432	275	97980	1148	122282	52747	1572
★ INCARNATE WORD HOSPITAL, 3545 Lafayette Avenue, Saint Louis, Zip 63104–9984; tel. 314/865–6500; Linda M. Allin, President and Chief Executive Officer (Total facility includes 86 beds in nursing home–type unit) **A**1 9 10 **F**4 6 8 10 11 12 14 15 16 17 19 22 26 27 28 29 30 31 32 33 34 35 37 39 41 42 44 45 48 49 52 54 55 56 57 60 62 63 64 65 67 71 73 74 **P**8 **S**5565 Incarnate Word Health Services	21	10	296	6152	164	36882	0	53910	26312	777
★ △ JEWISH HOSPITAL OF ST. LOUIS, 216 S Kingshighway Boulevard, Saint Louis, Zip 63110; tel. 314/454–7000; Wayne M. Lerner Dr.P.H., President **A**1 2 3 5 6 7 8 9 10 **F**1 2 3 4 5 6 7 8 9 10 11 12 13 14 16 17 18 19 20 22 23 24 25 26 27 28 29 30 31 32 33 34 35 37 38 39 40 41 42 43 44 45 46 47 48 49 50 51 52 53 54 55 56 57 58 59 60 61 62 64 65 66 67 68 69 70 71 72 73 74 **P**5 6 7 **S**0051 BJC Health System	23	10	358	14618	258	203911	1803	171571	76238	2596
□ LUTHERAN MEDICAL CENTER, 2639 Miami Street, Saint Louis, Zip 63118–3999; tel. 314/772–1456; William T. Moore, Chief Executive Officer (Total facility includes 20 beds in nursing home–type unit) **A**1 6 9 10 **F**2 3 7 8 10 12 14 16 18 19 22 27 30 31 32 33 34 35 37 39 40 41 42 44 46 48 49 51 52 53 54 55 56 57 58 59 60 63 64 65 66 67 71 73 74 **P**4 5 6 8 **S**0063 TENET Healthcare Corporation	33	10	294	5316	139	114881	754	50676	20964	590
□ MALCOLM BLISS MENTAL HEALTH CENTER, 5400 Arsenal, Saint Louis, Zip 63139; tel. 314/644–7800; Gregory L. Dale, Superintendent **A**1 3 5 9 10 **F**1 2 3 6 12 17 20 22 28 39 46 52 53 55 56 57 58 59 65 67 70 73	12	22	111	1583	92	5447	0	19530	8699	309
METROPOLITAN MEDICAL CENTER–WEST See Deaconess Medical Center–West Campus										
MISSOURI BAPTIST MEDICAL CENTER See Town and Country										
QUEENY TOWER See Barnes Hospital										
RAND–JOHNSON See Barnes Hospital										
★ SAINT LOUIS UNIVERSITY HOSPITAL, 3635 Vista At Grand Boulevard, Saint Louis, Zip 63110–0250, Mailing Address: P.O. Box 15250, Zip 63110–0250; tel. 314/577–8000; Herbert B. Schneiderman, Chief Executive Officer **A**1 3 5 8 9 10 **F**4 5 8 10 11 14 19 20 22 23 26 28 30 31 32 34 35 37 39 41 42 43 44 46 49 50 52 53 54 55 57 58 59 60 61 63 65 66 67 69 70 71 73	23	10	319	12142	258	137289	0	181074	64216	2052
★ SHRINERS HOSPITALS FOR CRIPPLED CHILDREN, ST. LOUIS UNIT, 2001 South Lindbergh Boulevard, Saint Louis, Zip 63131–3597; tel. 314/432–3600; Patricia E. Carey FACHE, Administrator **A**1 3 **F**12 15 19 27 28 29 30 34 35 41 46 49 51 53 54 55 58 63 65 66 67 68 71 73 **S**4125 Shriners Hospitals for Crippled Children	23	57	80	1927	30	11676	0	—	—	230
★ △ SSM REHABILITATION INSTITUTE, 555 N New Ballas Rd, Ste 150, Saint Louis, Zip 63141–6827; tel. 314/994–0157; Carla S. Baum, President (Nonreporting) **A**1 7 9 10 **S**5455 SSM Health Care System	21	46	100							
★ ST. ANTHONY'S MEDICAL CENTER, 10010 Kennerly Road, Saint Louis, Zip 63128; tel. 314/525–1000; Richard Grisham, President and Chief Executive Officer (Total facility includes 96 beds in nursing home–type unit) **A**1 2 9 10 **F**1 2 3 4 5 6 7 8 9 10 11 12 13 14 15 16 17 18 19 20 22 23 24 25 27 28 29 30 31 32 33 34 35 36 37 38 39 40 41 42 43 44 45 46 47 48 49 51 52 53 54 55 56 57 58 59 60 62 64 65 66 67 68 69 70 71 72 73 74 **P**8	23	10	862	23429	530	152057	1219	164380	75290	2824

Hospitals, U.S. / MISSOURI

Hospital, Address, Telephone, Administrator, Approval, Facility, and Physician Codes, Health Care System	Classification Codes		Utilization Data					Expense (thousands) of dollars		
★ American Hospital Association (AHA) membership ☐ Joint Commission on Accreditation of Healthcare Organizations (JCAHO) accreditation + American Osteopathic Hospital Association (AOHA) membership ○ American Osteopathic Association (AOA) accreditation △ Commission on Accreditation of Rehabilitation Facilities (CARF) accreditation Control codes 61, 63, 64, 71, 72 and 73 indicate hospitals listed by AOHA, but not registered by AHA. For definition of numerical codes, see page A6	Control	Service	Beds	Admissions	Census	Outpatient Visits	Births	Total	Payroll	Personnel
★ △ ST. JOHN'S MERCY MEDICAL CENTER, (Includes St. John's Mercy Hospital, 200 Madison Avenue, Washington, Missouri, Zip 63090; tel. 314/239–8000) 615 South New Ballas Road, Saint Louis, Zip 63141–8277; tel. 314/239–8000; Charles Thoele, Chief Executive Officer (Total facility includes 140 beds in nursing home–type unit) **A**1 2 3 5 7 8 9 10 **F**2 3 4 5 7 8 9 10 11 12 13 14 15 16 17 18 19 20 21 22 23 25 26 27 28 29 30 31 32 33 34 35 36 37 38 40 44 45 46 47 48 49 50 51 52 53 54 55 56 57 58 59 61 63 64 65 66 67 68 69 70 71 72 73 74 **P**1 4 6 7 **S**5185 Sisters of Mercy Health System–St. Louis	21	10	867	34853	920	360949	6586	298112	148862	4531
★ ST. JOSEPH HOSPITAL, 525 Couch Avenue, Saint Louis, Zip 63122–5594; tel. 314/966–1500; Michael E. Zilm, President (Total facility includes 34 beds in nursing home–type unit) **A**1 9 10 **F**4 7 8 10 12 14 15 16 17 18 19 20 22 26 28 29 30 32 33 34 35 36 37 39 40 41 42 43 44 45 46 49 50 60 63 64 65 66 67 71 73 74 **P**1 4 7 **S**5455 SSM Health Care System	23	10	240	6733	116	96940	901	54901	25531	846
★ ST. LOUIS CHILDREN'S HOSPITAL, One Children's Place, Saint Louis, Zip 63110–1077; tel. 314/454–6000; Alan W. Brass, President **A**1 3 5 8 9 10 **F**1 2 3 4 5 6 7 8 9 10 11 12 13 14 15 16 17 18 19 20 22 23 24 25 26 27 28 29 30 31 32 33 34 35 36 37 38 39 40 41 42 43 44 45 46 47 48 49 50 51 52 53 54 55 56 57 58 59 60 61 62 63 64 65 66 67 68 69 70 71 72 73 74 **P**3 4 5 6 7 8 **S**0051 BJC Health System	23	50	235	12299	168	110112	0	149212	65645	1735
★ ST. LOUIS REGIONAL MEDICAL CENTER, 5535 Delmar Boulevard, Saint Louis, Zip 63112–3095; tel. 314/361–1212; Sherman P. McCoy, President **A**1 3 5 9 10 1 32 34 36 37 38 39 40 41 42 44 45 46 49 51 53 54 58 60 61 63 65 66 67 68 71 72 73 74 **P**6	23	10	229	9363	146	318533	2650	94827	40592	1584
☐ ST. LOUIS STATE HOSPITAL, 5400 Arsenal Street, Saint Louis, Zip 63139–1494; tel. 314/644–8000; John M. Twiehaus Ph.D., Superintendent **A**1 10 **F**8 12 20 39 52 54 55 65 67 73 **P**6	12	22	215	65	205	—	0	28990	16824	668
★ △ ST. MARY'S HEALTH CENTER, 6420 Clayton Road, Saint Louis, Zip 63117–1811; tel. 314/768–8000; Ronald J. Levy, President (Total facility includes 40 beds in nursing home–type unit) **A**1 2 3 5 7 9 10 **F**2 3 4 5 7 8 10 11 12 13 15 17 18 19 20 22 23 25 26 27 28 29 30 31 32 33 34 35 36 37 38 39 40 41 42 43 44 45 46 48 49 51 52 53 54 55 56 57 58 59 60 61 63 64 65 66 68 70 71 72 73 74 **P**2 6 7 8 **S**5455 SSM Health Care System	23	10	515	16933	314	173374	2889	145586	60739	1853
THE PAVILION See Barnes Hospital										
★ VETERANS AFFAIRS MEDICAL CENTER, Saint Louis, Zip 63125; tel. 314/894–6661; Donald L. Ziegenhorn, Director (Total facility includes 129 beds in nursing home–type unit) **A**1 2 3 5 8 **F**2 3 4 5 8 10 12 18 19 22 24 26 31 32 34 35 37 41 46 49 50 52 54 56 57 58 59 60 63 64 65 69 71 73 **S**9295 Department of Veterans Affairs	45	10	629	12942	543	282220	0	—	—	2127
SAINT PETERS—St. Charles County										
★ BARNES ST. PETERS HOSPITAL, 10 Hospital Drive, Saint Peters, Zip 63376–1659; tel. 314/447–6600; John Gloss, President and Chief Executive Officer **A**1 9 10 **F**2 3 7 8 10 14 15 16 17 19 22 26 28 29 30 31 32 33 34 35 37 39 40 41 42 44 49 52 53 54 55 56 57 58 59 63 65 66 67 71 72 73 74 **P**5 6 8 **S**0051 BJC Health System	23	10	103	3638	40	60662	639	30945	12433	377
SALEM—Dent County										
SALEM MEMORIAL DISTRICT HOSPITAL, Highway 72 North, Zip 65560, Mailing Address: P.O. Box 774, Zip 65560; tel. 314/729–6626; Dennis Pryor, Administrator (Total facility includes 18 beds in nursing home–type unit) **A**9 10 **F**14 15 16 19 22 27 28 30 32 34 39 41 44 46 49 65 71	16	10	43	667	32	12668	0	6281	2665	155
SEDALIA—Pettis County										
★ BOTHWELL REGIONAL HEALTH CENTER, 601 East 14th Street, Zip 65301–1706, Mailing Address: P.O. Box 1706, Zip 65302–1706; tel. 816/826–8833; James T. Rank, Administrator **A**1 9 10 **F**4 7 8 15 16 19 20 22 23 30 32 33 34 35 37 39 40 41 42 44 49 52 53 56 57 60 65 66 67 71	14	10	158	5701	87	34345	548	35611	15673	621
SIKESTON—Scott County										
★ MISSOURI DELTA MEDICAL CENTER, 1008 North Main Street, Zip 63801–5099; tel. 314/471–1600; Charles D. Ancell, President (Total facility includes 14 beds in nursing home–type unit) **A**1 9 10 **F**3 4 5 6 7 8 10 12 14 15 16 17 18 19 20 22 23 24 25 26 27 28 29 30 32 33 34 35 36 37 39 40 41 42 43 44 45 46 48 49 51 53 54 55 56 57 58 59 60 61 62 63 64 65 66 67 69 71 72 73 74	23	10	148	4598	83	37452	505	29620	14272	588
SMITHVILLE—Clay County										
★ SAINT LUKE'S NORTHLAND HOSPITAL–SMITHVILLE CAMPUS, 601 South 169 Highway, Zip 64089; tel. 816/891–6090; James M. Brophy, Chief Executive Officer (Total facility includes 16 beds in nursing home–type unit) **A**1 10 **F**4 5 7 8 10 14 15 16 17 19 22 24 25 26 27 28 29 30 31 32 33 34 35 37 39 40 41 42 43 44 45 48 49 51 52 53 54 55 56 57 58 59 60 61 63 64 65 66 69 70 71 73 74 **P**6 8	23	10	82	1880	39	10144	0	15612	7332	241
SPRINGFIELD—Greene County										
○ DOCTORS HOSPITAL OF SPRINGFIELD, 2828 North National Street, Zip 65801, Mailing Address: Box 783, Jewell Station, Zip 65801–0783; tel. 417/869–5571; Charles M. Boughton, Administrator and Chief Executive Officer (Total facility includes 19 beds in nursing home–type unit) **A**9 10 11 **F**2 3 7 8 15 19 20 22 27 30 31 32 33 34 37 39 40 41 42 44 46 49 51 54 56 57 58 59 61 64 65 71 73	33	10	120	2355	51	28623	201	16225	7633	357
☐ LAKELAND REGIONAL HOSPITAL, 440 South Market Street, Zip 65806; tel. 417/865–5581; John William Thompson Ph.D., Administrator and Chief Executive Officer **A**1 9 10 **F**12 17 18 19 22 26 34 35 41 45 52 53 54 55 56 57 58 59 65 67 71 **P**5 6	33	22	114	1797	86	3068	0	11040	4524	209

© 1995 AHA Guide

Hospitals, U.S. / MISSOURI

	Classification Codes		Utilization Data					Expense (thousands) of dollars		
Hospital, Address, Telephone, Administrator, Approval, Facility, and Physician Codes, Health Care System	Control	Service	Beds	Admissions	Census	Outpatient Visits	Births	Total	Payroll	Personnel

★ American Hospital Association (AHA) membership
☐ Joint Commission on Accreditation of Healthcare Organizations (JCAHO) accreditation
+ American Osteopathic Hospital Association (AOHA) membership
○ American Osteopathic Association (AOA) accreditation
△ Commission on Accreditation of Rehabilitation Facilities (CARF) accreditation
Control codes 61, 63, 64, 71, 72 and 73 indicate hospitals listed by AOHA, but not registered by AHA. For definition of numerical codes, see page A6

Hospital	Control	Service	Beds	Admissions	Census	Outpatient Visits	Births	Total	Payroll	Personnel
★ LESTER E. COX HEALTH SYSTEMS, (Includes Lester E. Cox Medical Center North, 1423 North Jefferson Street, Zip 65802; tel. 417/296–3000; Lester E. Cox Medical Center South, 3801 South National Avenue, Zip 65807; tel. 417/885–6000) 1423 North Jefferson Street, Zip 65802–1988; tel. 417/296–3000; Larry D. Wallis, Chief Executive Officer and Executive Administrator (Total facility includes 26 beds in nursing home–type unit) **A**1 2 3 6 10 **F**1 2 3 4 5 6 8 10 11 12 16 17 19 20 21 22 23 24 26 27 28 29 30 31 32 33 34 36 37 38 39 40 41 42 43 44 46 47 48 49 50 51 52 53 54 55 56 57 58 59 60 61 63 64 65 66 67 68 71 73 74 **P**8	21	10	638	20583	342	883828	3362	194587	88688	3194
★ SPRINGFIELD COMMUNITY HOSPITAL, 3535 South National Avenue, Zip 65807; tel. 417/882–4700; Fred Woody, Chief Executive Officer (Total facility includes 19 beds in nursing home–type unit) **A**1 9 10 **F**8 12 14 15 16 19 22 26 28 32 34 37 39 44 48 49 52 54 56 57 58 64 65 71 **P**2 7 8 **S**0048 Columbia/HCA Healthcare Corporation	33	10	114	2432	48	80338	0	32582	11861	421
★ △ ST. JOHN'S REGIONAL HEALTH CENTER, 1235 East Cherokee Street, Zip 65804–2263; tel. 417/885–2000; Allen L. Shockley, President and Chief Executive Officer (Total facility includes 52 beds in nursing home–type unit) **A**1 2 6 7 10 **F**3 4 5 7 8 9 10 11 12 13 14 15 16 17 18 19 20 22 23 24 25 26 27 28 29 30 31 32 33 34 35 37 38 39 40 41 42 43 44 45 46 47 48 49 52 53 54 55 56 57 58 60 63 64 65 66 67 68 69 70 71 72 73 74 **P**6 **S**5185 Sisters of Mercy Health System–St. Louis	23	10	866	29375	535	225051	2164	204221	94676	3391
☐ U.S. MEDICAL CENTER FOR FEDERAL PRISONERS, 1900 West Sunshine Street, Zip 65808, Mailing Address: P.O. Box 4000, Zip 65808; tel. 417/862–7041; R. H. Rison, Warden **A**1 **F**3 4 5 12 18 19 20 24 25 26 31 33 34 35 41 42 44 46 49 52 55 56 57 58 59 60 65 69 71 73	48	11	587	1226	589	—	0	—	—	686

SAINTE GENEVIEVE—Sainte Genevieve County

Hospital	Control	Service	Beds	Admissions	Census	Outpatient Visits	Births	Total	Payroll	Personnel
STE. GENEVIEVE COUNTY MEMORIAL HOSPITAL, Highways 61 and 32, Sainte Genevieve, Zip 63670–0468; tel. 314/883–2751; Joseph Moss, Administrator **A**9 10 **F**7 8 14 15 17 18 19 20 22 23 26 28 29 30 32 34 35 37 39 40 41 42 44 45 65 67 68 71 73	13	10	38	802	11	13873	76	7910	3664	174

SULLIVAN—Crawford County

Hospital	Control	Service	Beds	Admissions	Census	Outpatient Visits	Births	Total	Payroll	Personnel
★ MISSOURI BAPTIST HOSPITAL OF SULLIVAN, 751 Sappington Bridge Road, Zip 63080, Mailing Address: P.O. Box 190, Zip 63080; tel. 314/468–4186; Davis D. Skinner, Administrator (Total facility includes 6 beds in nursing home–type unit) **A**1 9 10 **F**7 8 12 14 15 16 17 18 19 20 22 26 27 28 30 31 32 33 34 35 37 39 40 41 42 44 46 49 64 65 66 71 73 **P**5 **S**0051 BJC Health System	23	10	58	1493	19	55759	131	11682	4974	168

TOWN AND COUNTRY—Adair County

Hospital	Control	Service	Beds	Admissions	Census	Outpatient Visits	Births	Total	Payroll	Personnel
★ MISSOURI BAPTIST MEDICAL CENTER, 3015 North Ballas Road, Zip 63131–2374; tel. 314/432–1212; Fred R. Mills, President **A**1 6 9 10 **F**2 3 4 5 6 7 8 9 10 11 12 13 15 16 17 18 19 20 22 23 24 25 26 27 28 29 30 31 32 33 34 35 37 38 39 40 41 42 43 44 45 46 47 48 49 50 52 53 54 55 56 57 58 59 60 61 62 63 64 65 66 67 68 69 71 72 73 74 **P**3 4 5 6 7 8 **S**0051 BJC Health System	23	10	331	10572	190	148478	576	123427	50385	1674

TRENTON—Grundy County

Hospital	Control	Service	Beds	Admissions	Census	Outpatient Visits	Births	Total	Payroll	Personnel
★ WRIGHT MEMORIAL HOSPITAL, 701 East First Street, Zip 64683–0648, Mailing Address: P.O. Box 628, Zip 64683–0628; tel. 816/359–5621; Johnnye L. Dennis, Interim Administrator and Chief Executive Officer **A**1 10 **F**8 15 19 20 22 26 27 32 33 34 37 39 40 41 42 43 44 48 49 51 64 65 67 71 73 **P**8	23	10	50	788	12	20329	1	6521	3041	121

TROY—Lincoln County

Hospital	Control	Service	Beds	Admissions	Census	Outpatient Visits	Births	Total	Payroll	Personnel
☐ LINCOLN COUNTY MEMORIAL HOSPITAL, 1000 East Cherry, Zip 63379; tel. 314/528–8551; Floyd B. Dowell Jr., Administrator (Total facility includes 8 beds in nursing home–type unit) **A**1 9 10 **F**8 11 12 15 16 17 19 20 22 25 28 29 30 32 33 34 37 39 40 41 42 43 44 45 46 49 64 65 67 70 71 **P**1 7 8	13	10	36	1578	22	24758	133	12845	5758	215

WARRENSBURG—Johnson County

Hospital	Control	Service	Beds	Admissions	Census	Outpatient Visits	Births	Total	Payroll	Personnel
☐ WESTERN MISSOURI MEDICAL CENTER, 403 Burkarth Road, Zip 64093–3101; tel. 816/747–2500; Gregory B. Vinardi, President (Total facility includes 15 beds in nursing home–type unit) **A**1 10 **F**7 8 12 13 14 15 16 19 20 22 23 24 27 28 29 30 31 32 33 34 35 36 37 39 40 41 42 44 45 46 61 62 64 65 66 67 68 71 72 73	13	10	72	2491	34	29696	276	14334	6575	271

WASHINGTON—Franklin County

ST. JOHN'S MERCY HOSPITAL See St. John's Mercy Medical Center, Saint Louis

WENTZVILLE—St. Charles County

Hospital	Control	Service	Beds	Admissions	Census	Outpatient Visits	Births	Total	Payroll	Personnel
☐ DOCTORS HOSPITAL–WENTZVILLE, 500 Medical Drive, Zip 63385–0711; tel. 314/327–1000; Daniel J. Rothery, Administrator (Total facility includes 27 beds in nursing home–type unit) **A**1 9 10 **F**7 8 14 15 16 19 22 23 28 29 30 32 33 35 37 39 40 41 42 44 46 49 53 54 55 56 57 58 59 60 63 64 65 66 67 70 71 73	32	10	94	1341	18	160690	122	15032	5717	197

WEST PLAINS—Howell County

Hospital	Control	Service	Beds	Admissions	Census	Outpatient Visits	Births	Total	Payroll	Personnel
★ OZARKS MEDICAL CENTER, 1100 Kentucky Avenue, Zip 65775, Mailing Address: P.O. Box 1100, Zip 65775–1100; tel. 417/256–9111; Charles R. Brackney, President and Chief Executive Officer (Total facility includes 16 beds in nursing home–type unit) **A**9 10 **F**7 8 10 12 16 19 20 22 28 30 31 32 33 34 37 39 40 42 44 46 52 53 54 55 56 57 58 60 64 65 67 70 71 73 **P**8	23	10	120	5471	73	61962	730	37098	18183	735

WHITEMAN AIR FORCE BASE—Johnson County

Hospital	Control	Service	Beds	Admissions	Census	Outpatient Visits	Births	Total	Payroll	Personnel
★ U.S. AIR FORCE HOSPITAL WHITEMAN, Zip 65305–5001; tel. 816/687–2109; Major Thomas E. Fewell, Administrator **F**1 2 3 4 5 6 7 8 9 10 11 12 13 14 15 16 17 18 19 20 21 22 23 24 25 26 27 28 29 30 31 32 33 34 35 36 37 38 39 40 41 42 43 44 45 46 47 48 49 50 51 52 53 54 55 56 57 58 59 60 61 62 63 64 65 66 67 68 69 70 71 72 73 74 **S**9495 Department of the Air Force	41	10	22	1504	6	92406	283	—	—	255

Hospitals, U.S. / MONTANA

MONTANA

Resident population 839 (in thousands)
Resident population in metro areas 24.0%
Birth rate per 1,000 population 14.2
65 years and over 13.4%
Percent of persons without health insurance 12.0%

★ American Hospital Association (AHA) membership
☐ Joint Commission on Accreditation of Healthcare Organizations (JCAHO) accreditation
+ American Osteopathic Hospital Association (AOHA) membership
○ American Osteopathic Association (AOA) accreditation
△ Commission on Accreditation of Rehabilitation Facilities (CARF) accreditation
Control codes 61, 63, 64, 71, 72 and 73 indicate hospitals listed by AOHA, but not registered by AHA. For definition of numerical codes, see page A6

Hospital, Address, Telephone, Administrator, Approval, Facility, and Physician Codes, Health Care System	Classi-fication Codes		Utilization Data					Expense (thousands) of dollars		
	Control	Service	Beds	Admissions	Census	Outpatient Visits	Births	Total	Payroll	Personnel
ANACONDA—Deer Lodge County ★ COMMUNITY HOSPITAL OF ANACONDA, 401 West Pennsylvania Avenue, Zip 59711; tel. 406/563-5261; James J. Cliborne Jr., Interim Administrator (Total facility includes 67 beds in nursing home–type unit) **A**9 10 **F**19 22 27 33 44 64 65 71 **S**0002 Quorum Health Group/Quorum Health Resources	23	10	102	951	75	—	57	8016	3627	78
BAKER—Fallon County ★ FALLON MEDICAL COMPLEX, 320 Hospital Drive, Zip 59313-0820, Mailing Address: Box 820, Zip 59313-0820; tel. 406/778-3331; (Total facility includes 40 beds in nursing home–type unit) **A**9 10 **F**7 8 11 15 16 19 20 22 28 32 34 35 36 62 64 65 71 73 **P**2	23	10	52	473	38	5549	30	6671	—	60
BIG SANDY—Chouteau County BIG SANDY MEDICAL CENTER, Mailing Address: P.O. Box 530, Zip 59520-0530; tel. 406/378-2188; Harry Bold, Chief Executive Officer (Total facility includes 22 beds in nursing home–type unit) **A**9 10 **F**15 16 22 34 49 64	23	10	30	41	23	2409	0	965	532	28
BILLINGS—Yellowstone County ✠ DEACONESS MEDICAL CENTER, 2800 10th Avenue North, Zip 59101-0799, Mailing Address: P.O. Box 37000, Zip 59107-7001; tel. 406/657-4000; Lane W. Basso, President **A**1 9 10 **F**3 4 6 8 10 12 15 16 17 18 19 21 22 23 26 28 29 31 34 35 37 39 41 42 43 44 45 46 49 51 52 53 54 55 56 58 59 60 65 66 70 71 72 73 74 **P**3 6	23	10	238	8754	166	30658	0	86397	34306	1143
✠ △ SAINT VINCENT HOSPITAL AND HEALTH CENTER, 1233 North 30th Street, Zip 59101, Mailing Address: P.O. Box 35200, Zip 59107-5200; tel. 406/657-7000; James T. Paquette, President and Chief Executive Officer **A**1 7 9 10 **F**4 7 8 10 12 15 16 17 18 19 21 22 24 28 29 30 31 35 37 38 40 41 42 43 44 45 46 48 49 60 61 64 65 66 67 71 73 74 **S**5095 Sisters of Charity of Leavenworth Health Services Corporation	21	10	285	14924	241	89437	1975	92443	36972	1195
BOZEMAN—Gallatin County ★ BOZEMAN DEACONESS HOSPITAL, 915 Highland Boulevard, Zip 59715-6999; tel. 406/585-5000; Gordon L. Davidson, Acting Administrator **A**9 10 **F**7 14 19 20 22 29 32 33 34 35 37 39 40 42 44 45 49 54 58 60 62 65 71 73 **P**3	23	10	86	4035	37	42829	657	20860	8042	281
BROWNING—Glacier County ✠ U.S. PUBLIC HEALTH SERVICE INDIAN HOSPITAL, Mailing Address: P.O. Box 7, Zip 59417-0760; tel. 406/338-6100; Mary Ellen Lafromboise, Service Unit Director **A**1 10 **F**8 13 17 19 20 22 27 35 40 44 49 51 71 **S**9195 U.S. Public Health Service Indian Health Service	47	10	25	1475	13	84163	197	—	—	—
BUTTE—Silver Bow County ✠ ST. JAMES COMMUNITY HOSPITAL, 400 South Clark Street, Zip 59701, Mailing Address: P.O. Box 3300, Zip 59702; tel. 406/782-8361; Thomas R. Hochwalt, Chief Executive Officer **A**1 9 10 **F**12 15 17 19 20 21 22 23 26 29 30 33 34 35 37 38 40 42 44 45 46 49 58 63 64 65 66 67 70 71 73 **S**5095 Sisters of Charity of Leavenworth Health Services Corporation	23	10	103	4609	65	37606	522	35104	15106	488
CHESTER—Liberty County ★ LIBERTY COUNTY HOSPITAL AND NURSING HOME, Mailing Address: P.O. Box 705, Zip 59522-0705; tel. 406/759-5181; Danna J. Miller, Administrator (Total facility includes 45 beds in nursing home–type unit) **A**9 10 **F**7 8 11 22 32 34 37 40 44 49 64 65 71	13	10	56	424	40	5408	19	2535	1207	74
CHOTEAU—Teton County TETON MEDICAL CENTER, 915 Fourth Street Northwest, Zip 59422; tel. 406/466-5763; Jay Pottenger, Administrator (Total facility includes 35 beds in nursing home–type unit) **A**9 10 **F**8 11 21 22 28 33 34 41 44 49 64 65 67 73 **P**5	16	10	46	193	39	3464	0	2490	1051	53
CIRCLE—McCone County MCCONE COUNTY MEDICAL ASSISTANCE FACILITY, Mailing Address: Box 47, Zip 59215-0047; tel. 406/485-3381; Doug Faus, Administrator (Total facility includes 38 beds in nursing home–type unit) **A**9 10 **F**1 8 12 16 20 22 26 27 28 29 30 32 34 36 44 45 46 48 64	23	10	40	47	37	1919	0	1244	578	39
COLUMBUS—Stillwater County STILLWATER COMMUNITY HOSPITAL, 44 West Fourth Avenue North, Zip 59019, Mailing Address: Box 959, Zip 59019-0959; tel. 406/322-5316; Tim Russell, Administrator (Total facility includes 9 beds in nursing home–type unit) **A**9 10 **F**7 12 13 15 17 22 28 30 32 33 34 37 39 40 44 49 62 64 65 70 71	23	10	23	187	10	5855	32	1674	867	36
CONRAD—Pondera County ★ PONDERA MEDICAL CENTER, 805 Sunset Boulevard, Zip 59425; tel. 406/278-3211; L. Carl Hanson, Administrator (Total facility includes 67 beds in nursing home–type unit) **A**9 10 **F**7 8 13 15 16 20 22 27 30 32 33 36 39 41 44 49 62 64 71 72	23	10	94	717	68	6775	19	5039	2624	115
CROW AGENCY—Big Horn County ✠ U.S. PUBLIC HEALTH SERVICE INDIAN HOSPITAL, Mailing Address: Box 9, Zip 59022; tel. 406/638-2626; Tennyson Doney, Service Unit Director (Nonreporting) **A**1 10 **S**9195 U.S. Public Health Service Indian Health Service	47	10	34	—	—	—	—	—	—	—

© 1995 AHA Guide

Hospitals, U.S. / MONTANA

Hospital, Address, Telephone, Administrator, Approval, Facility, and Physician Codes, Health Care System

- ★ American Hospital Association (AHA) membership
- □ Joint Commission on Accreditation of Healthcare Organizations (JCAHO) accreditation
- + American Osteopathic Hospital Association (AOHA) membership
- ○ American Osteopathic Association (AOA) accreditation
- △ Commission on Accreditation of Rehabilitation Facilities (CARF) accreditation

Control codes 61, 63, 64, 71, 72 and 73 indicate hospitals listed by AOHA, but not registered by AHA. For definition of numerical codes, see page A6.

Hospital	Control	Service	Beds	Admissions	Census	Outpatient Visits	Births	Total	Payroll	Personnel
CULBERTSON—Roosevelt County										
★ ROOSEVELT MEMORIAL MEDICAL CENTER, (Formerly Roosevelt Memorial Hospital and Nursing Home) Mailing Address: P.O. Box 419, Zip 59218; tel. 406/787–6281; Walter Busch, Administrator (Total facility includes 44 beds in nursing home–type unit) **A**9 10 **F**1 8 13 15 17 22 26 27 28 30 32 34 36 39 41 44 46 49 51 64 65 66 71 73 **P**6	23	10	54	212	37	34	0	1861	1282	72
CUT BANK—Glacier County										
GLACIER COUNTY MEDICAL CENTER, 802 Second Street S.E., Zip 59427; tel. 406/873–2251; Michael D. Billing, Chief Executive Officer (Total facility includes 39 beds in nursing home–type unit) **A**9 10 **F**7 8 11 14 15 16 19 20 22 30 32 34 37 40 44 51 56 64 71	13	10	59	461	43	9006	40	3881	1958	91
DEER LODGE—Powell County										
★ POWELL COUNTY MEMORIAL HOSPITAL, 1101 Texas Avenue, Zip 59722–1828; tel. 406/846–2212; Tony Pfaff, Chief Executive Officer (Total facility includes 16 beds in nursing home–type unit) **A**9 10 **F**7 11 22 28 32 34 36 40 44 64 70 71 **P**7 **S**0585 Brim, Inc.	23	10	35	247	17	6226	16	2600	1113	50
DILLON—Beaverhead County										
★ BARRETT MEMORIAL HOSPITAL, 1260 South Atlantic Street, Zip 59725; tel. 406/683–2324; Jim D. Le Brun, Chief Executive Officer **A**9 10 **F**7 8 14 15 16 17 19 22 28 30 32 34 37 40 41 44 46 49 51 61 65 66 71 73 **P**5 **S**0585 Brim, Inc.	16	10	31	931	8	17217	83	3228	2163	96
ENNIS—Madison County										
MADISON VALLEY HOSPITAL, 217 North Main Street, Zip 59729–0397, Mailing Address: P.O. Box 397, Zip 59729–0397; tel. 406/682–4222; Geri Wilson, Administrator **A**9 10 **F**11 15 22 25 32 44 49 51 71	16	10	9	181	1	4705	0	1162	—	22
FORSYTH—Rosebud County										
★ ROSEBUD HEALTH CARE CENTER, 383 North 17th Avenue, Zip 59327–0268; tel. 406/356–2161; John M. Chioutsis, Chief Executive Officer (Total facility includes 55 beds in nursing home–type unit) **A**9 10 **F**11 26 28 34 64 67 73 **S**0585 Brim, Inc.	23	10	75	353	63	8100	0	2964	1525	86
FORT BENTON—Chouteau County										
★ MISSOURI RIVER MEDICAL CENTER, 1501 St. Charles Street, Zip 59442–0249, Mailing Address: Box 249, Zip 59442–0249; tel. 406/622–3331; Steve Krautscheid, Administrator (Total facility includes 41 beds in nursing home–type unit) **A**9 10 **F**6 8 21 22 25 31 32 33 34 64 65 **P**6	16	10	52	272	37	7386	0	2474		88
FORT HARRISON—Lewis And Clark County										
✣ VETERANS AFFAIRS HOSPITAL, Zip 59636; tel. 406/442–6410; Joe Underkofler, Director **A**1 **F**2 3 8 9 19 20 21 22 24 26 27 30 31 32 33 37 39 42 44 45 46 49 52 54 55 57 58 64 65 71 73 **S**9295 Department of Veterans Affairs	45	10	113	3460	75	43207	0	27984	13555	341
GLASGOW—Valley County										
✣ FRANCES MAHON DEACONESS HOSPITAL, 621 Third Street South, Zip 59230; tel. 406/228–4351; Douglas A. McMillan, Administrator (Total facility includes 6 beds in nursing home–type unit) **A**1 9 10 **F**3 7 8 11 19 21 22 24 26 28 31 32 34 35 42 44 45 46 49 50 54 63 64 71 **P**3	23	10	36	1017	10	17719	123	10223	4455	181
GLENDIVE—Dawson County										
✣ GLENDIVE MEDICAL CENTER, 202 Prospect Drive, Zip 59330; tel. 406/365–3306; Paul Hanson, Chief Executive Officer (Total facility includes 75 beds in nursing home–type unit) **A**1 9 10 **F**2 7 8 12 14 17 18 19 20 21 22 24 26 27 28 30 31 32 33 34 35 36 37 39 40 41 42 44 46 48 49 52 58 60 64 65 67 71 73 **P**3 4	23	10	115	1065	90	10259	31	8468	3942	128
GREAT FALLS—Cascade County										
✣ △ COLUMBUS HOSPITAL, 500 15th Avenue South, Zip 59403, Mailing Address: Box 5013, Zip 59403–5013; tel. 406/727–3333; Daniel W. Boatman, Executive Vice President and Chief Operating Officer **A**1 2 7 9 10 **F**4 5 7 8 10 14 15 19 21 22 23 24 27 28 29 30 31 32 33 34 35 37 40 41 42 44 48 49 56 60 65 67 69 71 72 73 74 **S**5265 Providence Services	21	10	145	5224	84	81485	524	46583	21372	770
✣ △ MONTANA DEACONESS MEDICAL CENTER, 1101 26th Street South, Zip 59405–5193; tel. 406/761–1200; Kirk G. Wilson, President (Total facility includes 124 beds in nursing home–type unit) **A**1 7 9 10 **F**1 2 3 4 8 10 11 12 15 17 19 21 23 24 26 27 28 29 30 31 32 33 34 35 36 37 38 39 40 41 42 43 44 45 46 47 48 49 52 53 54 55 56 57 58 59 60 63 64 65 66 70 71 73 74	23	10	339	7971	248	79600	962	61372	31407	956
HAMILTON—Ravalli County										
★ MARCUS DALY MEMORIAL HOSPITAL, 1200 Westwood Drive, Zip 59840–2395; tel. 406/363–2211; John M. Bartos, Administrator **A**9 10 **F**7 8 14 15 16 19 22 28 30 32 33 34 37 40 42 44 49 56 65 67 71 73 **P**8	23	10	48	1339	13	49384	181	11107	5657	225
HARDIN—Big Horn County										
★ BIG HORN COUNTY MEMORIAL HOSPITAL, 17 North Miles Street, Zip 59034, Mailing Address: P.O. Box 430, Zip 59034; tel. 406/665–2310; Raymond T. Hino, Chief Executive Officer (Total facility includes 37 beds in nursing home–type unit) **A**9 10 **F**7 8 22 34 40 44 45 49 64 65 71 73 **S**0585 Brim, Inc.	23	10	53	609	38	5234	78	3038	1463	84
HARLEM—Blaine County										
✣ U.S. PUBLIC HEALTH SERVICE INDIAN HOSPITAL, Rural Route 1, Box 67, Zip 59526; tel. 406/353–2651; Charles D. Plumage, Director **A**1 10 **F**2 3 4 7 8 9 10 11 12 13 14 15 16 17 18 19 20 21 22 24 25 28 29 30 32 34 35 36 37 38 39 40 42 43 44 45 46 47 48 49 50 52 53 56 58 60 61 63 64 65 66 67 69 70 71 74 **S**9195 U.S. Public Health Service Indian Health Service	47	10	12	493	3	39958	0	—	—	76

Hospitals, U.S. / MONTANA

Hospital, Address, Telephone, Administrator, Approval, Facility, and Physician Codes, Health Care System	Classification Codes		Utilization Data					Expense (thousands) of dollars		
★ American Hospital Association (AHA) membership ☐ Joint Commission on Accreditation of Healthcare Organizations (JCAHO) accreditation + American Osteopathic Hospital Association (AOHA) membership ○ American Osteopathic Association (AOA) accreditation △ Commission on Accreditation of Rehabilitation Facilities (CARF) accreditation Control codes 61, 63, 64, 71, 72 and 73 indicate hospitals listed by AOHA, but not registered by AHA. For definition of numerical codes, see page A6	Control	Service	Beds	Admissions	Census	Outpatient Visits	Births	Total	Payroll	Personnel
HARLOWTON—Wheatland County ★ WHEATLAND MEMORIAL HOSPITAL, 530 Third Street N.W., Zip 59036, Mailing Address: Box 287, Zip 59036; tel. 406/632–4351; Diane Jones, Administrator (Total facility includes 33 beds in nursing home–type unit) **A**9 10 **F**11 14 15 17 20 22 25 26 27 28 29 30 31 32 33 41 42 44 45 46 51 57 58 61 64 65 66 67 68 71 72 73 **P**5	13	10	56	185	38	11952	0	2482	1164	66
HAVRE—Hill County ★ NORTHERN MONTANA HOSPITAL, 30 13th Street, Zip 59501, Mailing Address: Box 1231, Zip 59501; tel. 406/265–2211; David Henry, President and Chief Executive Officer (Total facility includes 33 beds in nursing home–type unit) **A**1 9 10 **F**3 7 8 11 12 15 16 19 21 22 26 28 34 35 39 40 41 44 46 56 60 64 65 66 71 73	23	10	131	3480	65	36955	74	17574	8495	323
HELENA—Lewis And Clark County ★ SHODAIR CHILDREN'S HOSPITAL, 840 Helena Avenue, Zip 59601, Mailing Address: P.O. Box 5539, Zip 59604; tel. 406/444–7500; Jack Casey, Administrator **A**1 9 10 **F**15 16 52 53 55 58 59 61 65	23	52	66	163	38	6952	0	7781	4426	179
★ ST. PETER'S COMMUNITY HOSPITAL, 2475 Broadway, Zip 59601; tel. 406/442–2480; Robert W. Ladenburger, Chief Executive Officer **A**1 9 10 **F**7 8 10 12 14 15 16 17 19 21 22 25 27 28 29 30 31 32 33 34 35 36 37 38 39 40 41 42 44 45 46 49 50 52 53 54 56 57 58 59 60 63 65 67 71 73 **P**5	23	10	80	5064	49	50325	703	36319	16870	616
KALISPELL—Flathead County ★ △ KALISPELL REGIONAL HOSPITAL, 310 Sunnyview Lane, Zip 59901–3199; tel. 406/752–5111; William F. Diers, President and Chief Executive Officer **A**1 7 9 10 **F**1 2 3 4 7 8 10 12 13 14 15 16 17 18 19 20 21 22 23 24 26 27 28 29 30 32 33 34 35 37 39 40 41 42 44 45 46 48 49 51 52 53 54 55 56 57 58 59 60 63 64 65 66 67 68 71 73 **P**7 8	23	10	150	5777	65	91124	747	40862	17812	556
LEWISTOWN—Fergus County ★ CENTRAL MONTANA MEDICAL CENTER, 408 Wendell Avenue, Zip 59457, Mailing Address: Box 580, Zip 59457; tel. 406/538–6201; Kyle Hopstad, Administrator and Chief Executive Officer (Total facility includes 85 beds in nursing home–type unit) **A**9 10 **F**1 7 8 11 12 19 21 22 28 32 33 34 35 37 39 40 44 49 64 65 67 71 **S**0002 Quorum Health Group/Quorum Health Resources	23	10	126	1584	100	28722	169	11436	5327	215
LIBBY—Lincoln County ★ ST. JOHN'S LUTHERAN HOSPITAL, 350 Louisiana Avenue, Zip 59923; tel. 406/293–7761; Richard L. Palagi, Chief Executive Officer **A**9 10 **F**7 8 19 22 30 32 39 40 41 44 48 49 66 71 72 **S**0585 Brim, Inc.	23	10	26	1122	14	19229	134	6851	2836	122
LIVINGSTON—Park County ★ LIVINGSTON MEMORIAL HOSPITAL, 504 South 13th Street, Zip 59047–0986; tel. 406/222–3541; Richard V. Brown, Chief Executive Officer **A**9 10 **F**7 8 11 15 17 19 21 22 28 29 30 32 33 37 40 42 44 49 63 71	23	10	35	1254	13	18637	166	6877	3146	116
MALTA—Phillips County PHILLIPS COUNTY HOSPITAL, 417 South Fourth Street East, Zip 59538, Mailing Address: Box 640, Zip 59538–0640; tel. 406/654–1100; Larry E. Putnam, Administrator **A**9 10 **F**7 8 12 15 16 22 28 32 39 44 49 51 66 71 73 **P**3	23	10	21	196	2	4323	3	1779	921	46
MILES CITY—Custer County ★ HOLY ROSARY HOSPITAL, 2101 Clark Street, Zip 59301–2796; tel. 406/232–2540; H. Ray Gibbons, President and Chief Executive Officer (Total facility includes 103 beds in nursing home–type unit) **A**1 9 10 **F**2 3 7 8 11 12 13 14 15 16 17 19 21 22 24 27 28 30 32 35 36 37 39 40 42 44 48 49 52 53 54 55 56 57 58 63 64 65 67 71 73 **P**5 **S**5255 Presentation Health System	21	10	146	1854	111	13736	281	13806	6211	177
★ VETERANS AFFAIRS MEDICAL CENTER, 210 South Winchester Avenue, Zip 59301–4798; tel. 406/232–3060; Richard J. Stanley, Director (Total facility includes 26 beds in nursing home–type unit) **A**1 **F**12 15 20 30 37 44 46 49 51 58 64 65 71 73 74 **S**9295 Department of Veterans Affairs	45	10	41	945	45	26663	0	—	—	176
MISSOULA—Missoula County ★ △ COMMUNITY MEDICAL CENTER, 2827 Fort Missoula Road, Zip 59801–7493; tel. 406/728–4100; Grant M. Winn, President **A**1 7 9 10 **F**7 8 12 19 20 22 30 37 38 39 40 41 42 44 48 49 65 71 73 **P**6 **S**0585 Brim, Inc.	23	10	123	5001	66	136030	1410	45747	23013	611
★ ST. PATRICK HOSPITAL, 500 West Broadway, Zip 59802–4096, Mailing Address: Box 4587, Zip 59806–4587; tel. 406/543–7271; Lawrence L. White Jr., President **A**1 9 10 **F**2 3 4 8 10 11 12 14 15 16 17 19 21 22 23 24 27 29 30 31 32 33 34 35 36 37 39 41 42 43 44 45 47 49 52 53 54 55 56 57 59 60 63 65 67 68 69 71 73 **P**7 **S**5265 Providence Services	21	10	213	8242	113	98162	0	66677	26127	857
PHILIPSBURG—Granite County GRANITE COUNTY MEMORIAL HOSPITAL AND NURSING HOME, Mailing Address: Box 729, Zip 59858–0729; tel. 406/859–3271; Doris White, Acting Administrator (Total facility includes 28 beds in nursing home–type unit) **A**9 10 **F**1 15 22 30 32 33 34 49 51 64 71 **P**5	13	10	59	51	19	1397	0	904	528	27
PLAINS—Sanders County ★ CLARK FORK VALLEY HOSPITAL, Mailing Address: P.O. Box 768, Zip 59859–0768; tel. 406/826–3601; Tom Mitchell, Chief Executive Officer (Total facility includes 28 beds in nursing home–type unit) **A**9 10 **F**3 4 5 7 8 10 11 14 15 16 22 23 26 28 29 30 31 32 33 34 37 39 41 42 43 44 49 64 67 71 73 **S**0585 Brim, Inc.	23	10	44	561	34	19699	0	4991	2283	110

© 1995 AHA Guide

Hospitals, U.S. / MONTANA

Hospital, Address, Telephone, Administrator, Approval, Facility, and Physician Codes, Health Care System	Classification Codes		Utilization Data					Expense (thousands) of dollars		
★ American Hospital Association (AHA) membership □ Joint Commission on Accreditation of Healthcare Organizations (JCAHO) accreditation + American Osteopathic Hospital Association (AOHA) membership ○ American Osteopathic Association (AOA) accreditation △ Commission on Accreditation of Rehabilitation Facilities (CARF) accreditation Control codes 61, 63, 64, 71, 72 and 73 indicate hospitals listed by AOHA, but not registered by AHA. For definition of numerical codes, see page A6	Control	Service	Beds	Admissions	Census	Outpatient Visits	Births	Total	Payroll	Personnel
PLENTYWOOD—Sheridan County										
SHERIDAN MEMORIAL HOSPITAL, 440 West Laurel Avenue, Zip 59254–1596; tel. 406/765–1420; Tom Nordwick, Administrator (Total facility includes 78 beds in nursing home–type unit) **A**9 10 **F**7 8 12 15 16 19 22 28 30 31 32 34 37 39 40 41 44 46 49 51 64 65 67 71 73 **P**3	23	10	97	607	86	—	39	4605	2168	131
POLSON—Lake County										
✠ ST. JOSEPH HOSPITAL, Skyline Drive & 14th Avenue, Zip 59860, Mailing Address: Box 1010, Zip 59860–1010; tel. 406/883–5377; John W. Glueckert, President **A**1 9 10 **F**7 8 15 22 32 40 44 65 71 73 **S**5265 Providence Services	21	10	22	737	5	17521	94	3782	1875	82
POPLAR—Roosevelt County										
COMMUNITY HOSPITAL, H and Court Avenue, Zip 59255, Mailing Address: P.O. Box 38, Zip 59255; tel. 406/768–3452; Margaret Norgaard, Administrator (Total facility includes 22 beds in nursing home–type unit) **A**9 10 **F**1 7 14 15 16 22 32 36 40 44 64 71	23	10	44	597	24	6514	35	3105	1638	71
RED LODGE—Carbon County										
★ CARBON COUNTY MEMORIAL HOSPITAL AND NURSING HOME, 600 West 20th Street, Zip 59068, Mailing Address: P.O. Box 590, Zip 59068–0590; tel. 406/446–2345; Kelley Going, Administrator (Total facility includes 30 beds in nursing home–type unit) **A**9 10 **F**7 8 11 16 17 22 28 32 34 37 40 44 64 65 71 73 **P**3	23	10	52	582	34	2669	32	2610	1320	68
RONAN—Lake County										
★ ST. LUKE COMMUNITY HOSPITAL, 107 Sixth Avenue S.W., Zip 59864; tel. 406/676–4441; Shane Roberts, Chief Executive Officer (Total facility includes 68 beds in nursing home–type unit) **A**9 10 **F**7 8 14 15 16 22 24 31 34 44 64 71 **P**6	23	10	92	858	73	23896	94	7353	3985	191
ROUNDUP—Musselshell County										
★ ROUNDUP MEMORIAL HOSPITAL, 1202 Third Street West, Zip 59072, Mailing Address: P.O. Box 627, Zip 59072–0627; tel. 406/323–2302; Donna Beane, Administrator (Total facility includes 37 beds in nursing home–type unit) **A**9 10 **F**1 8 14 15 16 17 22 28 29 30 34 36 49 64 65 71 74 **P**2 **S**0585 Brim, Inc.	23	10	54	146	43	4439	0	2515	1184	65
SCOBEY—Daniels County										
DANIELS MEMORIAL HOSPITAL, 105 Fifth Avenue East, Zip 59263, Mailing Address: Box 400, Zip 59263–0400; tel. 406/487–2296; Gregory Maurer, Administrator (Total facility includes 48 beds in nursing home–type unit) **A**9 10 **F**1 7 8 11 13 15 16 17 21 22 28 30 32 36 40 41 49 64 65 67 71 73 **P**3 8	23	10	54	105	38	5619	8	1704	940	58
SHELBY—Toole County										
TOOLE COUNTY HOSPITAL AND NURSING HOME, 640 Park Drive, Zip 59474, Mailing Address: P.O. Box 915, Zip 59474; tel. 406/434–5536; Jerry Morasko, Administrator (Total facility includes 63 beds in nursing home–type unit) **A**9 **F**7 8 11 14 19 22 28 30 32 37 39 40 44 46 64 65 67 71 73	13	10	83	884	67	6976	91	—	—	213
SHERIDAN—Madison County										
★ RUBY VALLEY HOSPITAL, 220 East Crofoot Street, Zip 59749, Mailing Address: Box 336, Zip 59749–0336; tel. 406/842–5453; Steve Lang, Administrator **A**9 10 **F**7 22 32 71	16	10	14	195	2	2646	10	937	519	19
SIDNEY—Richland County										
★ COMMUNITY MEMORIAL HOSPITAL, 216 14th Avenue S.W., Zip 59270, Mailing Address: Box 1690, Zip 59270–1690; tel. 406/482–2120; Donald J. Rush, Chief Executive Officer **A**9 10 **F**1 3 8 12 15 19 21 22 24 30 32 33 34 35 36 37 40 42 44 49 51 63 65 66 67 70 71 73	23	10	42	1585	20	27569	151	11907	5042	217
SUPERIOR—Mineral County										
★ MINERAL COMMUNITY HOSPITAL, Roosevelt and Brooklyn, Zip 59872, Mailing Address: Box 66, Zip 59872–0066; tel. 406/822–4841; Madelyn Faller, Executive Director (Total facility includes 20 beds in nursing home–type unit) **A**9 10 **F**7 8 11 15 21 26 28 29 37 40 44 49 64 70 71 **S**0585 Brim, Inc.	23	10	30	310	23	5283	10	2317	1314	59
TERRY—Prairie County										
★ PRAIRIE COMMUNITY MEDICAL ASSISTANCE FACILITY, 312 South Adams Avenue, Zip 59349–0156, Mailing Address: Box 156, Zip 59349–0156; tel. 406/637–5511; James R. Mantz, Administrator (Total facility includes 19 beds in nursing home–type unit) **A**10 **F**8 13 15 22 26 28 36 51 64	16	10	21	27	19	914	0	909	530	30
TOWNSEND—Broadwater County										
BROADWATER HEALTH CENTER, 110 North Oak Street, Zip 59644, Mailing Address: P.O. Box 519, Zip 59644; tel. 406/266–3186; Gerald E. Hughes, Chief Executive Officer (Total facility includes 32 beds in nursing home–type unit) **A**9 10 **F**1 7 14 15 16 19 20 21 22 26 27 28 30 31 32 33 35 36 37 39 40 41 42 44 46 49 50 51 53 54 55 58 59 60 61 62 63 64 65 66 67 69 71 73 74 **P**5	23	10	42	237	38	5645	4	2940	1428	62
WARM SPRINGS—Deer Lodge County										
MONTANA STATE HOSPITAL, Zip 59756; tel. 406/693–7000; Carl Keener M.D., Medical Director (Nonreporting)	12	10	32	—	—	—	—	—	—	—
WHITE SULPHUR SPRINGS—Madison County										
MOUNTAINVIEW MEMORIAL HOSPITAL, 16 West Main, Zip 59645, Mailing Address: P.O. Box Q, White Sulphur Spgs Zip 59645; tel. 406/547–3321; Brad Robinson, Administrator (Total facility includes 31 beds in nursing home–type unit) **A**9 10 **F**13 20 26 28 39 49 64 71	23	10	37	146	30	—	9	2164	1116	68
WHITEFISH—Flathead County										
★ NORTH VALLEY HOSPITAL, 6575 Highway 93 South, Zip 59937–2990; tel. 406/863–2501; Kenneth E S Platou, Chief Executive Officer (Total facility includes 56 beds in nursing home–type unit) **A**9 10 **F**1 7 8 16 17 19 21 22 26 30 31 32 35 37 40 41 44 48 49 54 55 56 58 64 65 66 71 73 **S**0002 Quorum Health Group/Quorum Health Resources	23	10	100	1627	72	23435	192	10302	4726	129

Hospitals, U.S. / MONTANA

Hospital, Address, Telephone, Administrator, Approval, Facility, and Physician Codes, Health Care System	Classi-fication Codes		Utilization Data					Expense (thousands) of dollars		
	Control	Service	Beds	Admissions	Census	Outpatient Visits	Births	Total	Payroll	Personnel

★ American Hospital Association (AHA) membership
☐ Joint Commission on Accreditation of Healthcare Organizations (JCAHO) accreditation
+ American Osteopathic Hospital Association (AOHA) membership
○ American Osteopathic Association (AOA) accreditation
△ Commission on Accreditation of Rehabilitation Facilities (CARF) accreditation
Control codes 61, 63, 64, 71, 72 and 73 indicate hospitals listed by AOHA, but not registered by AHA. For definition of numerical codes, see page A6

WOLF POINT—Roosevelt County

★ TRINITY HOSPITAL, 315 Knapp Street, Zip 59201-1898; tel. 406/653-2100; Earl N. Sheehy, President (Total facility includes 60 beds in nursing home–type unit) **A**9 10 **F**1 6 7 8 15 16 22 27 28 30 32 36 40 44 46 49 62 64 71 **P**6	23	10	84	650	65	6477	129	5185	2570	137

Hospitals, U.S. / NEBRASKA

NEBRASKA

Resident population 1,607 (in thousands)
Resident population in metro areas 50.6%
Birth rate per 1,000 population 15.1
65 years and over 14.2%
Percent of persons without health insurance 8.7%

★ American Hospital Association (AHA) membership
□ Joint Commission on Accreditation of Healthcare Organizations (JCAHO) accreditation
+ American Osteopathic Hospital Association (AOHA) membership
○ American Osteopathic Association (AOA) accreditation
△ Commission on Accreditation of Rehabilitation Facilities (CARF) accreditation
Control codes 61, 63, 64, 71, 72 and 73 indicate hospitals listed by AOHA, but not registered by AHA. For definition of numerical codes, see page A6

Hospital, Address, Telephone, Administrator, Approval, Facility, and Physician Codes, Health Care System	Classification Codes		Utilization Data					Expense (thousands) of dollars		
	Control	Service	Beds	Admissions	Census	Outpatient Visits	Births	Total	Payroll	Personnel
AINSWORTH—Brown County BROWN COUNTY HOSPITAL, 945 East Zero, Zip 69210; tel. 402/387–2800; Richard W. Martin, Administrator (Nonreporting) **A**9 10	13	10	23	—	—	—	—	—	—	—
ALBION—Boone County ★ BOONE COUNTY HEALTH CENTER, 723 West Fairview Street, Zip 68620, Mailing Address: P.O. Box 151, Zip 68620–0151; tel. 402/395–2191; Gayle E. Primrose, Administrator **A**9 10 **F**1 2 3 6 7 8 15 16 19 22 24 25 26 31 32 33 34 35 37 39 40 42 44 45 48 49 52 53 54 55 57 58 65 66 67 71 73 **P**3 6	13	10	34	606	8	54913	75	4517	2452	115
ALLIANCE—Box Butte County □ BOX BUTTE GENERAL HOSPITAL, 2101 Box Butte Avenue, Zip 69301–0810, Mailing Address: P.O. Box 810, Zip 69301–0810; tel. 308/762–6660; Terrance J. Padden, Administrator **A**1 9 10 **F**7 8 12 15 16 17 19 22 28 29 30 31 32 33 34 37 39 41 42 44 46 49 56 65 66 67 71 73 **P**5	13	10	44	764	7	15390	159	5309	2346	89
ALMA—Harlan County ★ HARLAN COUNTY HOSPITAL, 717 North Brown, Zip 68920, Mailing Address: P.O. Box 836, Zip 68920; tel. 308/928–2151; Allen Van Driel, Administrator **A**9 10 **F**8 22 31 32 33 34 44 49 71 **P**6 **S**1535 Great Plains Health Alliance, Inc.	13	10	25	207	8	5017	0	1961	906	35
ATKINSON—Holt County WEST HOLT MEMORIAL HOSPITAL, 406 Legion Street, Zip 68713, Mailing Address: Rural Route 1, Box 200, Zip 68713; tel. 402/925–2811; Mel Snow, Administrator **A**9 10 **F**8 11 14 15 16 19 22 28 32 34 37 40 44 49 65 71 **P**3	23	10	18	384	3	8857	35	—	—	49
AUBURN—Nemaha County ★ NEMAHA COUNTY HOSPITAL, 2022 13th Street, Zip 68305–1799; tel. 402/274–4366; Glen Krueger, Administrator **A**9 10 **F**8 12 15 19 22 28 34 35 37 40 42 44 49 64 65 71	13	10	33	655	13	15394	53	2845	1421	68
AURORA—Hamilton County MEMORIAL HOSPITAL, 1423 Seventh Street, Zip 68818–1197; tel. 402/694–3171; Eldon A. Wall, Administrator (Total facility includes 53 beds in nursing home–type unit) **A**9 10 **F**7 8 11 14 15 22 28 30 32 33 34 36 37 40 41 42 44 49 65 66 71 **P**6	23	10	78	819	57	14046	102	5936	3327	90
BASSETT—Rock County ROCK COUNTY HOSPITAL, Mailing Address: P.O. Box 100, Zip 68714–0100; tel. 402/684–3366; Don Hall, Administrator (Total facility includes 30 beds in nursing home–type unit) **A**9 10 **F**19 22 40 44 64 69 71	13	10	42	160	31	3487	0	1868	976	65
BEATRICE—Gage County ★ BEATRICE COMMUNITY HOSPITAL AND HEALTH CENTER, 1110 North Tenth Street, Zip 68310, Mailing Address: P.O. Box 278, Zip 68310–0278; tel. 402/228–3344; Kenneth J. Zimmerman, Administrator (Total facility includes 87 beds in nursing home–type unit) **A**1 9 10 **F**8 10 11 15 16 17 19 20 21 22 23 26 28 30 31 32 33 34 36 37 40 41 42 44 45 46 49 54 62 64 65 66 67 71 73 **P**5	23	10	143	1271	95	34077	187	13001	6942	301
BENKELMAN—Dundy County DUNDY COUNTY HOSPITAL, North Cheyenne Street, Zip 69021, Mailing Address: P.O. Box 626, Zip 69021–0626; tel. 308/423–2204; Clyde E. Bolton, Administrator **A**9 10 **F**8 17 19 22 24 28 30 34 39 42 44 49 51 61 71 73 **P**3	13	10	14	191	2	10701	3	2102	949	57
BLAIR—Washington County ★ MEMORIAL COMMUNITY HOSPITAL, 810 North 22nd Street, Zip 68008–1199; tel. 402/426–2182; Dianne Runnestrand, Chief Executive Officer **A**1 9 10 **F**7 8 14 16 17 18 19 22 28 30 32 33 34 35 36 37 39 41 42 44 45 65 67 71 73	23	10	44	935	11	8456	119	6758	3794	147
BRIDGEPORT—Morrill County MORRILL COUNTY COMMUNITY HOSPITAL, 1313 South Street, Zip 69336, Mailing Address: P.O. Box 579, Zip 69336; tel. 308/262–1616; Julia Morrow, Administrator (Nonreporting) **A**9 10	13	10	20	—	—	—	—	—	—	—
BROKEN BOW—Custer County JENNIE M. MELHAM MEMORIAL MEDICAL CENTER, 145 Memorial Drive, Zip 68822, Mailing Address: P.O. Box 250, Zip 68822–0250; tel. 308/872–6891; Michael J. Steckler, Chief Executive Officer (Total facility includes 77 beds in nursing home–type unit) **A**9 10 **F**6 7 8 19 22 32 33 34 35 44 50 62 67 71	23	10	116	766	84	11490	103	6150	2815	84
CALLAWAY—Custer County ★ CALLAWAY DISTRICT HOSPITAL, 211 Kimball, Zip 68825, Mailing Address: P.O. Box 100, Zip 68825; tel. 308/836–2228; Marvin Neth, Administrator **A**9 10 **F**11 15 16 19 22 33 37 40 44 71 **P**3	16	10	12	311	3	6157	11	1085	484	27
CAMBRIDGE—Furnas County ★ CAMBRIDGE MEMORIAL HOSPITAL, West Highway 6 and 34, Zip 69022, Mailing Address: P.O. Box 488, Zip 69022; tel. 308/697–3329; James D. Naeve, Chief Executive Officer and Administrator (Nonreporting) **A**9 10	23	10	71	—	—	—	—	—	—	—
CENTRAL CITY—Merrick County LITZENBERG MEMORIAL COUNTY HOSPITAL, 1715 26th Street, Zip 68826, Mailing Address: Route 2, Box 1, Zip 68826; tel. 308/946–3015; Mike Bowman, Administrator (Total facility includes 46 beds in nursing home–type unit) **A**9 10 **F**6 7 8 11 19 22 26 27 28 33 34 35 40 44 48 49 57 58 64 65 71	13	10	71	699	60	6041	69	3915	1856	62

Hospitals, U.S. / NEBRASKA

Hospital, Address, Telephone, Administrator, Approval, Facility, and Physician Codes, Health Care System	Classification Codes		Utilization Data					Expense (thousands) of dollars		
★ American Hospital Association (AHA) membership □ Joint Commission on Accreditation of Healthcare Organizations (JCAHO) accreditation + American Osteopathic Hospital Association (AOHA) membership ○ American Osteopathic Association (AOA) accreditation △ Commission on Accreditation of Rehabilitation Facilities (CARF) accreditation Control codes 61, 63, 64, 71, 72 and 73 indicate hospitals listed by AOHA, but not registered by AHA. For definition of numerical codes, see page A6	Control	Service	Beds	Admissions	Census	Outpatient Visits	Births	Total	Payroll	Personnel
CHADRON—Dawes County										
CHADRON COMMUNITY HOSPITAL, 821 Morehead Street, Zip 69337–2599; tel. 308/432–5586; Harold L. Krueger Jr., Administrator **A**9 10 **F**7 8 13 14 15 16 17 19 22 28 32 33 37 39 40 44 45 49 56 65 71 73 **P**3 8	23	10	42	708	9	5365	121	3812	1738	85
COLUMBUS—Platte County										
⊞ COLUMBUS COMMUNITY HOSPITAL, 3111 19th Street, Zip 68602, Mailing Address: P.O. Box 819, Zip 68602; tel. 402/564–7118; Donald H. Zornes, Administrator (Total facility includes 19 beds in nursing home–type unit) **A**1 9 10 **F**7 8 10 11 12 15 16 17 19 20 21 22 28 30 32 34 35 36 37 38 39 40 41 42 44 45 46 49 64 65 67 71 73	23	10	54	2118	41	39128	514	12997	5823	209
COZAD—Dawson County										
COZAD COMMUNITY HOSPITAL, 300 East 12th, Zip 69130, Mailing Address: P.O. Box 108, Zip 69130–0108; tel. 308/784–2261; Lyle Davis, Administrator **A**9 10 **F**19 22 32 33 34 36 37 44 49 71 **P**6	16	10	30	253	5	3945	37	2500	1232	74
CRAWFORD—Dawes County										
LEGEND BUTTES HEALTH SERVICES, 11 Paddock Street, Zip 69339, Mailing Address: P.O. Box 272, Zip 69339; tel. 308/665–1770; Dale Grant, Chief Executive Officer **A**9 10 **F**3 8 19 22 32 34 44 61 64 65 **P**6	14	10	20	109	1	1696	1	672	507	26
CREIGHTON—Knox County										
LUNDBERG MEMORIAL HOSPITAL, 1503 Main Street, Zip 68729, Mailing Address: P.O. Box 186, Zip 68729; tel. 402/358–3322; Paul Hurd, Administrator (Total facility includes 47 beds in nursing home–type unit) **A**9 10 **F**1 7 8 15 16 17 19 22 27 30 32 34 35 37 40 42 44 64 65 67 71	14	10	77	488	57	5880	26	2787	1451	88
CRETE—Saline County										
★ CRETE MUNICIPAL HOSPITAL, 1540 Grove Streets, Zip 68333, Mailing Address: P.O. Box 220, Zip 68333; tel. 402/826–2154; Tony Staynings, Chief Executive Officer (Total facility includes 22 beds in nursing home–type unit) **A**9 10 **F**7 8 11 12 17 19 20 22 26 28 29 30 32 33 34 37 40 42 44 45 46 48 49 64 65 67 71 73 **S**0002 Quorum Health Group/Quorum Health Resources	14	10	57	604	48	10811	52	3799	1867	99
DAVID CITY—Butler County										
★ BUTLER COUNTY HEALTH CARE CENTER, 372 South Ninth Street, Zip 68632; tel. 402/367–3115 **A**9 10 **F**7 8 15 21 24 28 32 40 44 71	13	10	31	616	12	17695	89	3494	1818	77
FAIRBURY—Jefferson County										
⊞ JEFFERSON COMMUNITY HEALTH CENTER, (Formerly Jefferson County Memorial Hospital) Mailing Address: P.O. Box 277, Zip 68352–0277; tel. 402/729–3351; Bill Welch, Administrator (Total facility includes 41 beds in nursing home–type unit) **A**1 9 10 **F**7 8 11 15 19 24 28 32 34 40 42 44 46 49 61 64 67 71	23	10	72	675	46	15261	62	3886	1684	100
FALLS CITY—Richardson County										
★ COMMUNITY HOSPITAL, 2307 Barada Street, Zip 68355–1599; tel. 402/245–2428; Victor Lee, Chief Executive Officer and Administrator **A**9 10 **F**7 8 15 16 17 19 21 22 26 28 30 34 35 42 44 49 71 **S**1535 Great Plains Health Alliance, Inc.	23	10	49	852	11	14656	95	4300	1949	98
FRANKLIN—Franklin County										
★ FRANKLIN COUNTY MEMORIAL HOSPITAL, 1406 Q Street, Zip 68939–0127, Mailing Address: P.O. Box 127, Zip 68939–0127; tel. 308/425–6221; Jerrell F. Gerdes, Administrator **A**9 10 **F**7 8 11 14 15 16 19 22 27 28 30 32 33 40 44 51 71 **P**6 8	13	10	20	298	4	4930	14	1744	880	52
FREMONT—Dodge County										
⊞ MEMORIAL HOSPITAL OF DODGE COUNTY, 450 East 23rd Street, Zip 68025–2387; tel. 402/721–1610; Vincent J. O'Connor Jr., President (Total facility includes 162 beds in nursing home–type unit) **A**1 9 10 **F**1 7 8 11 15 17 19 21 22 26 27 28 29 30 31 32 33 34 35 37 39 40 41 42 44 45 46 48 49 60 63 64 65 66 67 71 73	13	10	262	3965	201	53702	427	31771	15945	599
FRIEND—Saline County										
WARREN MEMORIAL HOSPITAL, 905 Second Street, Zip 68359; tel. 402/947–2541; John Ramsey, Administrator (Nonreporting) **A**9 10	14	10	73	—						
GENEVA—Fillmore County										
FILLMORE COUNTY HOSPITAL, 1325 H Street, Zip 68361–1325, Mailing Address: P.O. Box 193, Zip 68361; tel. 402/759–3167; L. L. Eichelberger, Administrator (Total facility includes 20 beds in nursing home–type unit) **A**9 10 **F**7 8 15 19 22 24 26 27 28 29 30 31 32 33 34 35 36 37 39 41 42 44 45 46 49 51 61 65 66 67 68 71 73	13	10	53	360	28	7760	41	3055	1368	61
GENOA—Nance County										
GENOA COMMUNITY HOSPITAL, 706 Ewing Avenue, Zip 68640; tel. 402/993–2283; Sue Cromwell, Acting Administrator (Total facility includes 59 beds in nursing home–type unit) **A**9 10 **F**7 11 14 15 16 19 21 22 27 28 29 30 32 35 37 39 40 41 44 65 71 73 **P**6	14	10	79	129	55	2643	1	—	—	84
GORDON—Sheridan County										
★ GORDON MEMORIAL HOSPITAL DISTRICT, 300 East Eighth Street, Zip 69343–9990; tel. 308/282–0401; Gladys Phemister, Administrator **A**9 10 **F**3 8 16 17 19 22 28 30 32 40 44 71	16	10	40	820	12	12590	87	3638	1751	86
GOTHENBURG—Dawson County										
GOTHENBURG MEMORIAL HOSPITAL, 910 20th Street, Zip 69138, Mailing Address: P.O. Box 469, Zip 69138–0469; tel. 308/537–3661; Roger Heidebrink, Administrator (Nonreporting) **A**9 10	16	10	45	—						

Hospitals, U.S. / NEBRASKA

Hospital, Address, Telephone, Administrator, Approval, Facility, and Physician Codes, Health Care System	Classification Codes		Utilization Data					Expense (thousands) of dollars		
★ American Hospital Association (AHA) membership □ Joint Commission on Accreditation of Healthcare Organizations (JCAHO) accreditation + American Osteopathic Hospital Association (AOHA) membership ○ American Osteopathic Association (AOA) accreditation △ Commission on Accreditation of Rehabilitation Facilities (CARF) accreditation Control codes 61, 63, 64, 71, 72 and 73 indicate hospitals listed by AOHA, but not registered by AHA. For definition of numerical codes, see page A6	Control	Service	Beds	Admissions	Census	Outpatient Visits	Births	Total	Payroll	Personnel

GRAND ISLAND—Hall County

★ SAINT FRANCIS MEDICAL CENTER, (Includes Saint Francis Memorial Health Center, 2116 West Faidley Avenue, Grand Island, Nebraska, Zip 68802, Mailing Address: P.O. Box 9804, Zip 68802; tel. 308/384–4600) 2620 West Faidley Avenue, Zip 68803–, Mailing Address: Box 9804, Zip 68802–9804; tel. 308/384–4600; Michael R. Gloor, President and Chief Executive Officer (Total facility includes 36 beds in nursing home–type unit) **A**1 2 3 5 9 10 **F**2 3 7 8 10 11 12 15 16 17 19 20 21 22 23 27 28 30 32 33 34 35 37 38 40 41 42 44 48 49 60 64 65 66 67 71 73 **P**1 **S**5115 Sisters of Charity Health Care Systems, Inc. | 23 | 10 | 165 | 5877 | 85 | 57430 | 897 | 44960 | 17751 | 727

★ VETERANS AFFAIRS MEDICAL CENTER, 2201 North Broadwell Avenue, Zip 68803–2196; tel. 308/382–3660; (Total facility includes 76 beds in nursing home–type unit) **A**1 **F**1 2 3 8 10 20 21 22 27 28 30 31 32 33 34 37 41 42 44 46 49 51 54 57 58 64 65 67 71 73 74 **S**9295 Department of Veterans Affairs | 45 | 10 | 154 | 1459 | 107 | 31746 | 0 | 26020 | 14321 | 318

GRANT—Perkins County

PERKINS COUNTY HEALTH SERVICES, (Formerly Perkins County Community Hospital) (Includes GOLDEN OURS CONVALESCENT HOME) 900 Lincoln Avenue, Zip 69140, Mailing Address: Rural Route 1, Box 26, Zip 69140; tel. 308/352–7200; Paul L. Kellogg, Chief Executive Officer (Total facility includes 56 beds in nursing home–type unit) **A**9 10 **F**7 8 11 14 15 17 19 22 28 30 32 34 37 39 40 44 64 65 67 71 | 16 | 10 | 76 | 565 | 59 | 4924 | 48 | 3408 | 1749 | 99

HASTINGS—Adams County

□ HASTINGS REGIONAL CENTER, (Psychiatric, Alcoholism and Other Chemical Dependency) Mailing Address: Box 579, Zip 68902–0579; tel. 402/463–2471; Michael J. Sheehan, Facility Administrator (Nonreporting) **A**1 9 10 | 12 | 49 | 232 | — | — | — | — | — | — | —

★ MARY LANNING MEMORIAL HOSPITAL, 715 North St Joseph Avenue, Zip 68901–4497; tel. 402/461–5108; W. Michael Kearney, Administrator **A**1 2 9 10 **F**2 3 7 8 10 13 15 16 17 19 20 21 22 23 24 28 31 32 33 34 35 36 37 39 40 41 42 44 45 46 51 52 53 54 55 56 57 58 59 60 62 65 66 67 70 71 73 74 **P**6 | 23 | 10 | 194 | 4245 | 56 | 67284 | 630 | 30398 | 15057 | 579

HEBRON—Thayer County

★ THAYER COUNTY MEMORIAL HOSPITAL, 120 Park Avenue, Zip 68370, Mailing Address: P.O. Box 49, Zip 68370; tel. 402/768–6041; Larry E. Leaming, Administrator **A**9 10 **F**7 8 13 17 19 22 24 27 28 29 30 32 33 34 36 37 40 42 44 49 51 58 64 65 66 67 71 **P**6 | 13 | 10 | 22 | 367 | 4 | 10251 | 32 | 2612 | 1223 | 58

HENDERSON—York County

HENDERSON COMMUNITY HOSPITAL, 1621 Front Street, Zip 68371–0217, Mailing Address: P.O. Box 217, Zip 68371–0217; tel. 402/723–4512; Michael Boyles, Chief Executive Officer (Total facility includes 42 beds in nursing home–type unit) **A**9 10 **F**1 7 8 11 15 16 22 25 26 27 33 36 39 40 44 49 64 65 67 71 **P**8 | 23 | 10 | 55 | 154 | 44 | 4893 | 13 | — | — | 74

HOLDREGE—Phelps County

★ PHELPS MEMORIAL HEALTH CENTER, 1220 Miller Street, Zip 68949, Mailing Address: P.O. Box 828, Zip 68949–0828; tel. 308/995–2211; Jerome Jr Seigfreid, Chief Executive Officer **A**1 9 10 **F**7 8 10 14 15 16 19 20 22 26 27 28 30 32 33 35 36 37 44 45 65 66 67 69 71 73 **P**3 8 **S**0002 Quorum Health Group/Quorum Health Resources | 23 | 10 | 55 | 1486 | 17 | 12207 | 171 | 6941 | 3343 | 139

HUMBOLDT—Richardson County

COMMUNITY MEMORIAL HOSPITAL, 1128 Grand Avenue, Zip 68376, Mailing Address: P.O. Box 626, Zip 68376; tel. 402/862–2231; Marlyn Reinitz, Administrator (Nonreporting) **A**9 10 | 23 | 10 | 20 | — | — | — | — | — | — | —

IMPERIAL—Chase County

CHASE COUNTY COMMUNITY HOSPITAL, 600 West 12th Street, Zip 69033; tel. 308/882–7111; Jim O'Neal, Administrator **A**9 10 **F**7 8 10 19 21 22 28 34 35 37 40 42 44 49 71 73 | 13 | 10 | 21 | 754 | 8 | 10180 | 65 | 2727 | 1245 | 62

KEARNEY—Buffalo County

★ △ GOOD SAMARITAN HEALTH SYSTEMS, (Formerly Good Samaritan Hospital) (Includes Richard H. Young Psychiatric Hospital, 4600 17th Avenue, Kearney, Nebraska, Zip 68847, Mailing Address: P.O. Box 1750, Zip 68848–1705; tel. 308/236–2000; James Gallagher, Chief Operating Officer) 10 East 31st Street, Zip 68847–2926, Mailing Address: P.O. Box 1990, Zip 68848–1990; tel. 308/236–8511; William Wilson Hendrickson, President (Total facility includes 22 beds in nursing home–type unit) **A**1 2 3 5 7 9 10 **F**1 2 3 4 7 8 9 10 11 12 14 15 16 17 19 21 22 28 29 30 32 33 34 35 36 37 38 39 40 41 42 43 44 45 46 48 49 52 53 54 59 60 64 65 67 68 71 73 **P**8 **S**5115 Sisters of Charity Health Care Systems, Inc. | 21 | 10 | 267 | 7687 | 166 | 58099 | 882 | 65686 | 28697 | 1021

RICHARD H. YOUNG PSYCHIATRIC HOSPITAL See Good Samaritan Health Systems

KIMBALL—Kimball County

KIMBALL COUNTY HOSPITAL, 505 South Burg Street, Zip 69145; tel. 308/235–3621; Dennis W. Marshall, Administrator **A**9 10 **F**19 22 28 32 40 44 64 71 73 | 13 | 10 | 24 | 306 | 4 | 3378 | 35 | 1806 | 878 | 43

LEXINGTON—Dawson County

★ TRI-COUNTY AREA HOSPITAL, 13th and Erie Streets, Zip 68850–0980, Mailing Address: P.O. Box 980, Zip 68850–0980; tel. 308/324–5651; Calvin A. Hiner, Administrator **A**1 9 10 **F**8 10 11 15 16 19 22 28 30 32 33 35 37 39 40 42 44 45 49 62 65 66 71 | 16 | 10 | 40 | 1308 | 13 | 20649 | 248 | 5337 | 2644 | 125

LINCOLN—Lancaster County

★ BRYAN MEMORIAL HOSPITAL, 1600 South 48th Street, Zip 68506–1299; tel. 402/489–0200; R. Lynn Wilson, President **A**1 2 3 5 6 9 10 **F**4 7 8 10 11 12 14 15 16 19 21 22 23 28 30 31 32 34 35 40 42 43 44 52 54 57 63 65 67 69 71 73 | 23 | 10 | 316 | 11473 | 172 | 148821 | 911 | 113189 | 45192 | 1501

Hospitals, U.S. / NEBRASKA

Hospital, Address, Telephone, Administrator, Approval, Facility, and Physician Codes, Health Care System	Classification Codes		Utilization Data					Expense (thousands) of dollars		
	Control	Service	Beds	Admissions	Census	Outpatient Visits	Births	Total	Payroll	Personnel

★ American Hospital Association (AHA) membership
☐ Joint Commission on Accreditation of Healthcare Organizations (JCAHO) accreditation
+ American Osteopathic Hospital Association (AOHA) membership
○ American Osteopathic Association (AOA) accreditation
△ Commission on Accreditation of Rehabilitation Facilities (CARF) accreditation
Control codes 61, 63, 64, 71, 72 and 73 indicate hospitals listed by AOHA, but not registered by AHA. For definition of numerical codes, see page A6.

Hospital	Control	Service	Beds	Admissions	Census	Outpatient Visits	Births	Total	Payroll	Personnel
★ LINCOLN GENERAL HOSPITAL, 2300 South 16th Street, Zip 68502-3781; tel. 402/475-1011; Arlan L. Stromberg, Administrator **A**1 2 3 5 9 10 **F**2 3 7 8 14 15 16 22 23 26 29 34 37 40 42 44 46 52 53 56 58 59 60 65 67 70 71 73 **P**7 8	14	10	226	6604	106	78377	767	58781	23005	867
☐ LINCOLN REGIONAL CENTER, Folsom and Van Dorn Streets, Zip 68509, Mailing Address: P.O. Box 94949, Zip 68509-4949; tel. 402/471-4444; Bill H. Zinn, Chief Executive Officer **A**1 9 10 **F**20 52 53 55 59 65 73	12	22	246	318	218	—	0	19272	10164	408
★ △ MADONNA REHABILITATION HOSPITAL, 5401 South Street, Zip 68506-2134; tel. 402/489-7102; Marsha Lommel Halpern, President and Chief Executive Officer (Total facility includes 192 beds in nursing home-type unit) **A**7 10 **F**1 12 14 15 16 17 19 24 26 27 28 29 30 32 34 35 39 41 45 46 48 49 58 64 65 67 71 73 **P**6	21	46	252	1446	229	—	0	25832	15035	1088
★ ST. ELIZABETH COMMUNITY HEALTH CENTER, 555 South 70th Street, Zip 68510-2494; tel. 402/489-7181; Robert J. Lanik, President **A**1 2 3 5 9 10 **F**7 8 9 10 14 19 22 23 28 30 31 32 33 35 37 38 40 41 42 44 46 49 65 66 73 **P**3 7 **S**5115 Sisters of Charity Health Care Systems, Inc.	21	10	177	6815	90	56541	1983	58984	23751	956
★ VETERANS AFFAIRS MEDICAL CENTER, 600 South 70th Street, Zip 68510-2493; tel. 402/489-3802 **A**1 3 5 **F**2 3 4 8 10 11 14 15 16 19 20 21 22 23 31 34 37 39 41 42 43 44 45 46 49 52 54 58 65 71 73 74 **S**9295 Department of Veterans Affairs	45	10	113	3009	74	49579	0	—	—	420
LYNCH—Boyd County										
NIOBRARA VALLEY HOSPITAL, Mailing Address: P.O. Box 118, Zip 68746; tel. 402/569-2451; E. R. Testerman, Administrator **A**9 10 **F**7 8 19 22 26 28 32 34 39 40 44 45 49 61 64 71 **P**5	23	10	29	790	10	886	6	1711	—	43
MCCOOK—Red Willow County										
★ COMMUNITY HOSPITAL, 1301 East H Street, Zip 69001-1328, Mailing Address: P.O. Box 1328, Zip 69001-1328; tel. 308/345-2650; Gary Bieganski, President **A**1 9 10 **F**7 8 11 14 15 17 19 21 22 28 30 35 37 40 44 45 49 65 71 73 74	23	10	44	1065	13	35575	117	6845	2941	125
MINDEN—Kearney County										
★ KEARNEY COUNTY COMMUNITY HOSPITAL, 727 East First Street, Zip 68959; tel. 308/832-1440; Marcia Shannon, Administrator (Total facility includes 50 beds in nursing home-type unit) **A**9 10 **F**7 8 20 22 26 28 30 32 33 37 40 44 49 65 71 **P**6	15	10	80	250	52	4770	24	2936	1575	92
NEBRASKA CITY—Otoe County										
★ ST. MARY'S HOSPITAL, 1314 Third Avenue, Zip 68410; tel. 402/873-3321; Richard W. Waller, Interim Administrator **A**1 9 10 **F**3 7 8 15 16 19 21 22 32 35 36 39 42 63 65 71 73 **S**5115 Sisters of Charity Health Care Systems, Inc.	21	10	28	631	12	19784	68	4360	1800	91
NELIGH—Antelope County										
★ ANTELOPE MEMORIAL HOSPITAL, 102 West Ninth Street, Zip 68756-0229, Mailing Address: P.O. Box 229, Zip 68756-0229; tel. 402/887-4151; Jack W. Green, Administrator **A**9 10 **F**7 8 15 17 19 20 22 24 32 34 40 42 44 45 46 49 65 71	23	10	49	760	16	7185	56	3473	1917	80
NORFOLK—Madison County										
★ LUTHERAN COMMUNITY HOSPITAL, 2700 Norfolk Avenue, Zip 68701, Mailing Address: Box 869, Zip 68702-0869; tel. 402/371-4880; Daryl Mackender, Administrator **A**1 9 10 **F**3 7 8 15 19 22 23 28 30 32 33 34 35 37 40 41 42 44 49 60 65 67 71	23	10	85	3011	30	27583	526	20807	9047	379
☐ NORFOLK REGIONAL CENTER, 1700 North Victory Road, Zip 68701, Mailing Address: Box 1209, Zip 68702-1209; tel. 402/370-3400; Lisa Ulrich Walters, Administrator **A**1 9 10 **F**12 17 18 27 52 54 55 56 57 58 59 65 73	12	22	174	457	170	0	0	11662	7683	320
★ OUR LADY OF LOURDES HOSPITAL, 1500 Koenigstein Avenue, Zip 68701-3698; tel. 402/371-3402; Randall Richards, President and Chief Executive Officer **A**1 9 10 **F**7 8 12 14 15 17 19 21 22 23 24 28 29 30 32 34 35 36 37 39 40 41 42 44 45 46 49 52 56 59 61 65 66 67 68 71 73 **P**7 **S**2855 Missionary Benedictine Sisters American Province	21	10	76	2060	24	40827	319	15093	6251	251
NORTH PLATTE—Lincoln County										
★ GREAT PLAINS REGIONAL MEDICAL CENTER, 601 West Leota Street, Zip 69101, Mailing Address: Box 1167, Zip 69103; tel. 308/534-9310; Lucinda A. Bradley, President **A**1 9 10 **F**7 8 10 11 15 16 17 19 21 22 24 28 29 30 31 32 33 34 35 37 38 40 41 42 44 45 46 47 48 49 52 57 60 61 65 66 67 69 71 73 74 **P**3 8 **S**0002 Quorum Health Group/Quorum Health Resources	23	10	113	3445	55	76751	470	29866	12789	447
O'NEILL—Holt County										
★ ST. ANTHONY'S HOSPITAL, Second and Adams Streets, Zip 68763-1597; tel. 402/336-2611; Ronald J. Cork, President and Chief Executive Officer **A**1 9 10 **F**7 8 12 15 16 17 18 19 20 22 28 29 30 31 32 34 35 39 40 42 44 49 54 61 63 65 66 67 71 **P**3	21	10	29	911	12	11994	98	4606	1852	79
OAKLAND—Burt County										
★ OAKLAND MEMORIAL HOSPITAL, 601 East Second Street, Zip 68045; tel. 402/685-5601; Karen Vlach, Acting Administrator **A**9 10 **F**7 8 12 15 16 19 22 28 32 33 34 36 39 44 51 65 67 71 **P**5	23	10	23	298	5	4006	2	1356	677	32
OFFUTT AIR FORCE BASE—Sarpy County										
★ EHRLING BERGQUIST HOSPITAL, 2501 Capehart Road, Zip 68113-2160; tel. 402/294-7312; Colonel Gary J. Seitz MSC, USAF, Administrator **A**1 3 5 **F**3 4 7 8 10 12 15 16 18 19 20 22 24 25 28 29 34 35 37 39 40 41 43 45 46 49 51 52 58 61 65 71 73 **S**9495 Department of the Air Force	41	10	50	4360	32	292632	724	—	—	838
OGALLALA—Keith County										
★ OGALLALA COMMUNITY HOSPITAL, 300 East Tenth Street, Zip 69153; tel. 308/284-4011; Linda Morris, Administrator **A**9 10 **F**7 8 12 13 15 17 19 22 25 28 32 34 35 40 44 49 65 67 71 **P**6 **S**2235 Lutheran Health Systems	23	10	41	639	7	18981	103	3905	1991	80

© 1995 AHA Guide

Hospitals, U.S. / NEBRASKA

Hospital, Address, Telephone, Administrator, Approval, Facility, and Physician Codes, Health Care System	Classification Codes		Utilization Data					Expense (thousands) of dollars		
★ American Hospital Association (AHA) membership □ Joint Commission on Accreditation of Healthcare Organizations (JCAHO) accreditation + American Osteopathic Hospital Association (AOHA) membership ○ American Osteopathic Association (AOA) accreditation △ Commission on Accreditation of Rehabilitation Facilities (CARF) accreditation Control codes 61, 63, 64, 71, 72 and 73 indicate hospitals listed by AOHA, but not registered by AHA. For definition of numerical codes, see page A6	Control	Service	Beds	Admissions	Census	Outpatient Visits	Births	Total	Payroll	Personnel

OMAHA—Douglas County
AMI ST. JOSEPH CENTER FOR MENTAL HEALTH See St. Joseph Center for Mental Health
ARCHBISHOP BERGAN MERCY CENTER See Bergan Mercy Medical Center

★ BERGAN MERCY MEDICAL CENTER, (Formerly Archbishop Bergan Mercy Center) 7500 Mercy Road, Zip 68124; tel. 402/398–6060; Richard A. Hachten II, President (Total facility includes 255 beds in nursing home–type unit) **A**1 2 3 5 9 10 **F**1 2 3 4 6 7 8 10 11 12 14 15 16 17 18 19 20 21 22 23 24 25 26 27 28 29 30 31 32 33 34 35 36 37 38 39 40 41 42 43 44 45 46 48 49 51 52 53 54 55 56 57 58 59 60 61 62 63 64 65 66 67 68 70 71 72 73 74 **P**6 8 **S**5175 Catholic Health Corporation	21	10	607	14290	420	108195	2480	125107	55264	1695
★ BISHOP CLARKSON MEMORIAL HOSPITAL, 44th And Dewey Avenue, Zip 68105–1018, Mailing Address: P.O. Box 3328, Zip 68103–0329; tel. 402/552–2000; Louis Burgher M.D., Ph.D., President and Chief Executive Officer (Data for 364 days) **A**1 2 3 5 9 10 **F**4 7 8 10 11 12 14 15 16 19 21 22 23 25 26 30 31 32 34 35 39 40 41 42 43 44 45 49 51 60 63 64 65 66 67 69 71 72 73 74 **P**5 7 8	23	10	231	7762	129	119573	730	107268	—	1415
□ BOYS TOWN NATIONAL RESEARCH HOSPITAL, 555 North 30th Street, Zip 68131; tel. 402/498–6511; John K. Arch, Administrator **A**1 3 9 10 **F**16 17 25 34 44 45 46 51 73 **P**6	23	50	12	1086	3	81180	0	—	—	346
★ CHILDRENS MEMORIAL HOSPITAL, 8301 Dodge Street, Zip 68114–4199; tel. 402/390–5400; Gary A. Perkins, President and Chief Executive Officer **A**1 3 5 9 10 **F**10 17 19 21 22 23 29 32 34 35 38 39 42 43 44 47 60 63 65 67 71 73 **P**7	23	50	100	4708	67	37771	0	47562	20106	658
DOUGLAS COUNTY HOSPITAL, 4102 Woolworth Avenue, Zip 68105–1899; tel. 402/444–7000; James C. Tourville, Administrator (Nonreporting) **A**5 9 10	13	49	329	—	—	—	—	—	—	—
★ △ IMMANUEL MEDICAL CENTER, 6901 North 72nd Street, Zip 68122–1799; tel. 402/572–2121; Charles J. Marr, President (Total facility includes 200 beds in nursing home–type unit) **A**1 2 7 9 10 **F**1 2 3 4 5 7 8 10 11 12 14 15 16 17 18 19 20 21 22 24 25 26 27 28 29 30 31 32 33 34 35 36 37 38 39 40 41 42 43 44 45 46 48 49 50 51 52 53 54 55 56 57 58 59 60 61 62 63 64 65 66 67 68 69 70 71 72 73 74 **P**6 7 8	23	10	532	10038	384	161147	797	129035	52676	1949
★ METHODIST RICHARD YOUNG, (Includes Richard H. Young Memorial Hospital, 402 South 26th Street, Omaha, Nebraska, Zip 68131, Mailing Address: P.O. Box 3434, Zip 68103) 515 South 26th Street, Zip 68105–4119; tel. 402/536–6600; Sandra C. Carson FACHE, President and Chief Executive Officer **A**1 9 10 **F**1 2 3 4 7 8 10 11 12 13 17 19 20 21 22 23 25 26 27 28 29 30 31 32 33 34 35 36 37 38 39 40 41 42 43 44 45 46 47 48 49 51 52 53 54 55 56 57 58 59 60 61 64 65 66 67 68 69 70 71 72 73 74 **P**1 4 7	21	22	157	1818	122	28095	0	22410	12531	458
★ △ NEBRASKA METHODIST HOSPITAL, 8303 Dodge Street, Zip 68114–4199; tel. 402/390–4000; Stephen D. Long, President and Executive Officer **A**1 2 3 7 10 **F**2 3 4 7 8 10 11 15 16 17 19 21 22 23 24 25 26 27 28 29 30 31 32 33 34 35 37 39 40 41 42 43 44 45 48 49 51 52 53 54 55 56 57 58 59 60 61 63 65 66 67 70 71 73 74 **P**1 4 7	23	10	250	12020	163	70861	2780	122242	53481	1729
RICHARD H. YOUNG MEMORIAL HOSPITAL See Methodist Richard Young										
★ SAINT JOSEPH CENTER FOR MENTAL HEALTH, (Formerly AMI St. Joseph Center for Mental Health) 819 Dorcas, Zip 68108–1137; tel. 402/449–4653; Johanna M. Anderson, Chief Executive Officer (Nonreporting) **A**3 5 9	33	22	171							
★ SAINT JOSEPH HOSPITAL, (Formerly AMI Saint Joseph Hospital) 601 North 30th Street, Zip 68131–2197; tel. 402/449–5021; Matthew A. Kurs, President and Chief Executive Officer (Nonreporting) **A**1 2 3 5 8 9 10 **S**0063 TENET Healthcare Corporation	33	10	299	—	—	—	—	—	—	—
★ UNIVERSITY OF NEBRASKA MEDICAL CENTER, 600 South 42nd Street, Zip 68198–4085; tel. 402/559–7400; C. Edward Schwartz, Chief Executive Officer (Total facility includes 30 beds in nursing home–type unit) **A**1 2 3 5 8 9 10 **F**4 5 6 7 8 10 12 13 15 17 18 19 20 21 22 23 24 26 27 28 29 30 31 33 34 35 36 37 38 39 40 41 42 43 44 45 46 47 49 51 52 54 55 56 57 58 59 60 61 63 64 65 66 69 70 71 72 73 **P**1 4 6 7	12	10	342	11744	237	96470	978	163797	60954	2070
★ VETERANS AFFAIRS MEDICAL CENTER, 4101 Woolworth Avenue, Zip 68105–1873; tel. 402/449–0600; John J. Phillips, Director **A**1 3 5 8 **F**1 2 3 4 5 8 10 12 17 19 20 21 22 23 26 28 30 31 33 34 35 37 39 41 42 43 44 45 46 49 50 51 52 54 56 57 58 60 63 65 67 69 71 73 74 **P**1 **S**9295 Department of Veterans Affairs	45	10	226	5886	175	108272	0	68307	35525	1060

ORD—Valley County

★ VALLEY COUNTY HOSPITAL, 217 Westridge Drive, Zip 68862; tel. 308/728–3211; (Total facility includes 78 beds in nursing home–type unit) **A**9 10 **F**7 8 11 14 15 16 19 20 22 24 27 28 32 33 34 40 41 44 64 65 66 71	13	10	96	455	71	12375	47	4439	2433	121

OSCEOLA—Polk County

ANNIE JEFFREY MEMORIAL COUNTY HOSPITAL, Mailing Address: P.O. Box 428, Zip 68651; tel. 402/747–2031; Curt Koesterer, Administrator **A**9 10 **F**7 14 15 16 17 19 20 22 24 26 28 29 30 31 32 33 34 36 39 44 45 49 65 71 73 **P**4 5 6 7 8	13	10	21	625	9	9391	32	2333	1026	53

OSHKOSH—Garden County

GARDEN COUNTY HOSPITAL, Mailing Address: P.O. Box 320, Zip 69154; tel. 308/772–3283; Keith Hillman, Administrator (Total facility includes 36 beds in nursing home–type unit) **A**9 10 **F**1 8 11 15 17 22 25 26 27 28 34 37 39 44 49 51 64 71 73 **P**5	13	10	56	220	34	2312	0	1980	1025	61

Hospitals, U.S. / NEBRASKA

Hospital, Address, Telephone, Administrator, Approval, Facility, and Physician Codes, Health Care System	Classification Codes		Utilization Data					Expense (thousands) of dollars		
	Control	Service	Beds	Admissions	Census	Outpatient Visits	Births	Total	Payroll	Personnel

- ★ American Hospital Association (AHA) membership
- □ Joint Commission on Accreditation of Healthcare Organizations (JCAHO) accreditation
- + American Osteopathic Hospital Association (AOHA) membership
- ○ American Osteopathic Association (AOA) accreditation
- △ Commission on Accreditation of Rehabilitation Facilities (CARF) accreditation

Control codes 61, 63, 64, 71, 72 and 73 indicate hospitals listed by AOHA, but not registered by AHA. For definition of numerical codes, see page A6.

Hospital	Control	Service	Beds	Admissions	Census	Outpatient Visits	Births	Total	Payroll	Personnel
OSMOND—Pierce County ★ OSMOND GENERAL HOSPITAL, 5th and Maple Street, Zip 68765-0429; tel. 402/748-3393; Leonard R. Frodyma, Administrator A9 10 F8 15 19 20 22 28 30 32 33 35 44 49 65 71 P6	23	10	30	413	7	4857	0	2296	1275	57
PAPILLION—Sarpy County ✴ MIDLANDS COMMUNITY HOSPITAL, 11111 South 84th Street, Zip 68046; tel. 402/593-3000; Don M. Chase, Administrator A1 9 10 F2 3 7 8 19 21 22 28 31 35 37 40 41 42 44 45 52 53 54 55 56 59 60 63 65 66 70 71 72 S0002 Quorum Health Group/Quorum Health Resources	23	10	160	2823	44	29019	389	26937	10673	355
PAWNEE CITY—Pawnee County PAWNEE COUNTY MEMORIAL HOSPITAL, 600 I Street, Zip 68420; tel. 402/852-2231; James A. Kubik, Administrator A9 10 F7 14 19 21 22 30 32 33 34 36 44 51 71 P6	13	10	21	217	3	6467	9	1776	—	52
PENDER—Thurston County ★ PENDER COMMUNITY HOSPITAL, 603 Earl Street, Zip 68047-0100, Mailing Address: Box 100, Zip 68047-0100; tel. 402/385-3083; Ryan Baldwin, Administrator A9 10 F7 8 11 17 19 22 37 40 42 44 64 71 P3 S5165 Mercy Health Services	16	10	24	718	9	7414	70	2642	1201	—
PLAINVIEW—Pierce County PLAINVIEW PUBLIC HOSPITAL, Mailing Address: P.O. Box 489, Zip 68769; tel. 402/582-4245; Michael K. Loftis, Administrator A9 10 F14 15 16 19 37 44 45 49 51 P6	14	10	19	216	3	2994	0	1966	1055	41
RED CLOUD—Webster County WEBSTER COUNTY COMMUNITY HOSPITAL, Sixth Avenue and Franklin St, Zip 68970-0465; tel. 402/746-2291; Terry Hoffart, Administrator A9 10 F8 19 28 30 31 32 37 44 49 66 71 73 P3 8	13	10	26	262	3	597	0	1394	646	34
SAINT PAUL—Howard County ★ HOWARD COUNTY COMMUNITY HOSPITAL, 1102 Kendall Street, Zip 68873, Mailing Address: Box 374, Zip 68873; tel. 308/754-4421; Russell W. Swigart, Administrator A9 10 F8 14 19 22 30 33 35 40 44 45 49 64 65 67 71 73 P3	13	10	36	532	20	5291	52	2232	1097	66
SARGENT—Custer County SARGENT DISTRICT HOSPITAL, 1201 West Main, Zip 68874; tel. 308/527-3414; Douglas W. Ellis, Administrator (Nonreporting) A9 10	16	10	18	—	—	—	—	—	—	—
SCHUYLER—Colfax County ★ MEMORIAL HOSPITAL, 104 West 17th Street, Zip 68661; tel. 402/352-2441; James L. Clough, Administrator (Total facility includes 31 beds in nursing home–type unit) A9 10 F8 15 17 19 21 22 30 32 34 36 40 42 44 48 49 51 64 65 71 P3	23	10	49	492	33	24014	62	3902	1855	93
SCOTTSBLUFF—Scotts Bluff County ✴ REGIONAL WEST MEDICAL CENTER, 4021 Avenue B, Zip 69361-4695; tel. 308/635-3711; David M. Nitschke, President and Chief Executive Officer (Total facility includes 22 beds in nursing home–type unit) A1 2 9 10 F2 3 4 7 8 10 19 21 22 24 27 28 30 32 33 35 36 37 38 39 40 41 42 44 45 46 49 52 53 54 55 56 57 58 59 60 64 65 66 67 71 73 74	23	10	265	6015	85	33782	670	45448	18684	686
SEWARD—Seward County MEMORIAL HEALTH CARE SYSTEM, 300 North Columbia Avenue, Zip 68434-9907; tel. 402/643-2971; Ronald D. Waltz, Chief Executive Officer (Total facility includes 119 beds in nursing home–type unit) A9 10 F1 8 15 17 19 22 28 32 33 34 35 36 39 41 44 46 49 62 64 71	23	10	153	658	140	15682	95	8880	4744	219
SIDNEY—Cheyenne County ★ MEMORIAL HEALTH CENTER, 645 Osage Street, Zip 69162; tel. 308/254-5825; Rex D. Walk, Administrator (Total facility includes 70 beds in nursing home–type unit) A9 10 F3 7 8 10 11 12 19 22 26 28 29 30 31 32 34 35 36 37 39 40 41 42 44 45 46 49 58 64 65 66 67 71 73 P3	23	10	133	787	79	12560	110	7173	3593	154
SUPERIOR—Nuckolls County ★ BRODSTONE MEMORIAL HOSPITAL, 520 East Tenth, Zip 68978, Mailing Address: P.O. Box 187, Zip 68978-0187; tel. 402/879-3281; Ronald D. Waggoner, Administrator and Chief Executive Officer A10 F7 8 19 20 22 26 28 32 34 36 37 40 42 44 45 49 64 65 71	23	10	49	815	12	—	61	3779	1621	103
SYRACUSE—Otoe County COMMUNITY MEMORIAL HOSPITAL, 1579 Midland Street, Zip 68446, Mailing Address: Box N, Zip 68446; tel. 402/269-2011; Ron Anderson, Administrator A9 10 F7 8 11 19 22 32 33 37 44 71	16	10	18	359	4	5979	34	1853	770	37
TECUMSEH—Johnson County ★ JOHNSON COUNTY HOSPITAL, 202 High Street, Zip 68450-0599; tel. 402/335-3361; Lavonne M. Rowe, Administrator A9 10 F1 7 8 14 15 16 17 19 22 28 30 32 34 37 40 41 42 44 49 56 58 71	13	10	30	505	7	4377	35	2133	929	50
TILDEN—Antelope County TILDEN COMMUNITY HOSPITAL, Mailing Address: Box 340, Zip 68781; tel. 402/368-5343; Douglas W. Ellis, Administrator (Nonreporting) A9 10	23	10	20	—	—	—	—	—	—	—
VALENTINE—Cherry County CHERRY COUNTY HOSPITAL, Highway 12 & Green Street, Zip 69201-0410; tel. 402/376-2525; Brent Peterson, Administrator A9 10 F8 14 15 16 17 19 22 28 29 30 32 37 44 46 71	13	10	27	386	5	6099	126	2527	1148	61

© 1995 AHA Guide

Hospitals, U.S. / NEBRASKA

Hospital, Address, Telephone, Administrator, Approval, Facility, and Physician Codes, Health Care System	Classification Codes		Utilization Data					Expense (thousands) of dollars		Personnel
	Control	Service	Beds	Admissions	Census	Outpatient Visits	Births	Total	Payroll	

★ American Hospital Association (AHA) membership
☐ Joint Commission on Accreditation of Healthcare Organizations (JCAHO) accreditation
+ American Osteopathic Hospital Association (AOHA) membership
○ American Osteopathic Association (AOA) accreditation
△ Commission on Accreditation of Rehabilitation Facilities (CARF) accreditation
Control codes 61, 63, 64, 71, 72 and 73 indicate hospitals listed by AOHA, but not registered by AHA. For definition of numerical codes, see page A6

Hospital	Control	Service	Beds	Admissions	Census	Outpatient Visits	Births	Total	Payroll	Personnel
WAHOO—Saunders County SAUNDERS COUNTY HEALTH SERVICE, 805 West Tenth Street, Zip 68066, Mailing Address: P.O. Box 185, Zip 68066; tel. 402/443-4191; Michael Brown, Administrator (Total facility includes 73 beds in nursing home-type unit) **A**9 10 **F**8 16 17 22 28 29 30 32 33 34 44 45 49 51 54 61 64 65 71 **P**6	13	10	103	290	82	10250	0	4700	2554	119
WAYNE—Wayne County PROVIDENCE MEDICAL CENTER, 1200 Providence Road, Zip 68787; tel. 402/375-3800; Marcile Thomas, Administrator **A**9 10 **F**7 14 15 16 19 22 24 32 33 35 44 49 65 66 71 **S**2855 Missionary Benedictine Sisters American Province	21	10	34	791	12	6439	129	3628	1577	65
WEST POINT—Cuming County ★ ST. FRANCIS MEMORIAL HOSPITAL, 430 North Monitor Street, Zip 68788-1595; tel. 402/372-2404; Sister Helena Young, President **A**9 10 **F**7 14 16 19 22 24 30 32 44 65 66 71 73 **S**1455 Franciscan Sisters of Christian Charity Healthcare Ministry, Inc	21	10	32	663	8	21546	101	4483	2043	94
WINNEBAGO—Thurston County ✠ U.S. PUBLIC HEALTH SERVICE INDIAN HOSPITAL, Zip 68071; tel. 402/878-2231; Wehnona St. Cyr, Service Unit Director **A**1 10 **F**2 4 5 7 8 10 14 15 16 18 19 20 21 22 23 24 26 27 28 30 31 32 33 34 35 36 39 41 42 43 44 45 46 49 50 51 53 54 55 56 58 59 60 62 63 65 66 67 68 69 70 71 73 **P**6 **S**9195 U.S. Public Health Service Indian Health Service	47	10	30	621	17	33273	1	6471	3145	104
YORK—York County ★ YORK GENERAL HOSPITAL, 2222 Lincoln Avenue, Zip 68467-1095; tel. 402/362-6671 **A**9 10 **F**7 11 19 24 32 33 34 35 37 39 40 42 44 49 65 67 71 74	23	10	48	895	9	25956	147	6126	2740	121

NEVADA

Resident population 1,389 (in thousands)
Resident population in metro areas 84.8%
Birth rate per 1,000 population 17.2
65 years and over 11.1%
Percent of persons without health insurance 19.3%

Hospitals, U.S. / NEVADA

- ★ American Hospital Association (AHA) membership
- □ Joint Commission on Accreditation of Healthcare Organizations (JCAHO) accreditation
- + American Osteopathic Hospital Association (AOHA) membership
- ○ American Osteopathic Association (AOA) accreditation
- △ Commission on Accreditation of Rehabilitation Facilities (CARF) accreditation

Control codes 61, 63, 64, 71, 72 and 73 indicate hospitals listed by AOHA, but not registered by AHA. For definition of numerical codes, see page A6

Hospital, Address, Telephone, Administrator, Approval, Facility, and Physician Codes, Health Care System	Classification Codes		Utilization Data					Expense (thousands) of dollars		Personnel
	Control	Service	Beds	Admissions	Census	Outpatient Visits	Births	Total	Payroll	
BATTLE MOUNTAIN—Lander County										
BATTLE MOUNTAIN GENERAL HOSPITAL, 535 West Humboldt Street, Zip 89820–1994; tel. 702/635–2550; Kathy Ancho, Administrator (Nonreporting) **A**10	16	10	14	—	—	—	—	—	—	—
BOULDER CITY—Clark County										
★ BOULDER CITY HOSPITAL, 901 Adams Boulevard, Zip 89005; tel. 702/293–4111; Ray Bernardi, Administrator (Total facility includes 47 beds in nursing home–type unit) **A**9 10 **F**8 11 14 15 16 19 20 21 22 26 32 35 37 41 44 59 64 65 71 72 73 **P**4 5	23	10	67	1141	49	13205	0	8812	4060	150
CARSON CITY—Carson City County										
★ CARSON TAHOE HOSPITAL, 775 Fleischmann Way, Zip 89701, Mailing Address: P.O. Box 2168, Zip 89702–2168; tel. 702/882–1361; Steve Smith, Administrator **A**1 9 10 **F**1 2 3 8 10 14 15 17 19 21 22 25 26 28 30 32 33 34 35 37 39 40 41 42 44 46 49 52 54 55 56 57 58 59 60 63 65 67 71 72 73 74 **P**5	15	10	124	7330	88	84932	789	41103	18165	576
ELKO—Elko County										
★ ELKO GENERAL HOSPITAL, 1297 College Avenue, Zip 89801–3499; tel. 702/753–1999; Anne Ruger R.N., Administrator **A**1 10 **F**7 8 14 17 19 22 28 30 35 39 40 44 46 49 65 71 73 **P**5	13	10	50	2166	17	28762	629	15400	7600	228
ELY—White Pine County										
★ WILLIAM BEE RIRIE HOSPITAL, 1500 Avenue H, Zip 89301–2699; tel. 702/289–3001; Jack T. Wood, Administrator (Nonreporting) **A**1 10	13	10	40	—	—	—	—	—	—	—
FALLON—Churchill County										
★ CHURCHILL COMMUNITY HOSPTIAL, 155 North Taylor Street, Zip 89406–2797; tel. 702/423–3151; Jeffrey Feike, Administrator and Chief Executive Officer (Nonreporting) **A**9 10 **S**2235 Lutheran Health Systems	23	10	40	—	—	—	—	—	—	—
HAWTHORNE—Mineral County										
MOUNT GRANT GENERAL HOSPITAL, First and A Street, Zip 89415, Mailing Address: P.O. Box 1510, Zip 89415; tel. 702/945–2461; Richard Munger, Administrator (Nonreporting) **A**10	16	10	35	—	—	—	—	—	—	—
HENDERSON—Clark County										
★ ST. ROSE DOMINICAN HOSPITAL, 102 Lake Mead Drive, Zip 89015; tel. 702/564–2622; Rod A. Davis, President and Chief Executive Officer **A**1 9 10 **F**2 3 7 8 10 12 14 15 19 21 22 25 28 31 32 34 35 37 40 41 42 44 45 48 49 52 56 57 58 59 60 65 71 73 **P**3 5 8 **S**5205 Catholic Healthcare West	21	10	117	5155	56	50052	1306	39000	15061	600
LAS VEGAS—Clark County										
□ CHARTER BEHAVIORAL HEALTH SYSTEM OF NEVADA, 7000 W Spring Mountain Road, Zip 89117; tel. 702/876–4357; Gerald A. Greene, Chief Executive Officer (Nonreporting) **A**1 9 10 **S**0695 Charter Medical Corporation	33	22	84	—	—	—	—	—	—	—
★ DESERT SPRINGS HOSPITAL, 2075 East Flamingo Road, Zip 89119, Mailing Address: P.O. Box 19204, Zip 89132; tel. 702/733–8800; Catherine M. Pelley, Chief Executive Officer **A**1 10 **F**8 10 12 15 16 17 19 21 22 25 26 27 28 29 30 31 32 34 35 37 42 43 44 46 49 56 63 65 67 71 72 73 **P**4 5 6 7	33	10	225	11298	177	109196	0	78927	28751	774
□ MONTEVISTA HOSPITAL, 5900 West Rochelle Avenue, Zip 89103; tel. 702/364–1111; R. Dale Reynolds, Administrator **A**1 10 **F**2 3 11 14 15 16 19 22 26 29 35 37 45 52 53 54 55 56 57 58 59 65 70 **S**0069 Behavioral Healthcare Corporation	33	22	80	1840	48	7509	0	8547	4111	121
★ NELLIS FEDERAL HOSPITAL, (Formerly U.S. Air Force Hospital) Nellis AFB, Zip 89191–7007; tel. 702/653–2000; Lieutenant Colonel D. Creager Brown MSC, USAF, Administrator (Nonreporting) **A**1 **S**9495 Department of the Air Force	41	10	35	—	—	—	—	—	—	—
★ △ SUNRISE HOSPITAL AND MEDICAL CENTER, 3186 Maryland Parkway, Zip 89109–2306, Mailing Address: P.O. Box 98530, Zip 89193–8530; tel. 702/731–8000; A. Allan Stipe, President and Chief Executive Officer (Nonreporting) **A**1 2 7 9 10 **S**0048 Columbia/HCA Healthcare Corporation	33	10	688	—	—	—	—	—	—	—
U.S. AIR FORCE HOSPITAL See Nellis Federal Hospital										
□ UNIVERSITY MEDICAL CENTER, 1800 West Charleston Boulevard, Zip 89102; tel. 702/383–2000; William R. Hale, Chief Executive Officer (Nonreporting) **A**1 2 3 5 10	13	10	506	—	—	—	—	—	—	—
□ VALLEY HOSPITAL MEDICAL CENTER, 620 Shadow Lane, Zip 89106; tel. 702/388–4000; Claus Eggers, Managing Director (Total facility includes 10 beds in nursing home–type unit) **A**1 9 10 **F**4 7 8 10 11 14 15 17 19 20 21 22 25 26 28 29 30 31 34 35 37 40 41 42 43 44 45 46 49 50 60 61 62 63 64 71 73 74 **S**9555 Universal Health Services, Inc.	33	10	390	17936	262	61434	2482	118137	41338	937
WOMENS HOSPITAL, 2025 East Sahara Avenue, Zip 89104; tel. 702/735–7106; Len Merryman, Administrator (Nonreporting) **A**3 9	33	44	82	—	—	—	—	—	—	—
LOVELOCK—Pershing County										
PERSHING GENERAL HOSPITAL, 855 Sixth Street, Zip 89419, Mailing Address: P.O. Box 661, Zip 89419; tel. 702/273–2621; John Schaper, Administrator (Nonreporting) **A**10 **S**2235 Lutheran Health Systems	16	10	34	—	—	—	—	—	—	—

© 1995 AHA Guide

Hospitals, U.S. / NEVADA

Hospital, Address, Telephone, Administrator, Approval, Facility, and Physician Codes, Health Care System	Classification Codes		Utilization Data					Expense (thousands) of dollars		
★ American Hospital Association (AHA) membership □ Joint Commission on Accreditation of Healthcare Organizations (JCAHO) accreditation + American Osteopathic Hospital Association (AOHA) membership ○ American Osteopathic Association (AOA) accreditation △ Commission on Accreditation of Rehabilitation Facilities (CARF) accreditation Control codes 61, 63, 64, 71, 72 and 73 indicate hospitals listed by AOHA, but not registered by AHA. For definition of numerical codes, see page A6	Control	Service	Beds	Admissions	Census	Outpatient Visits	Births	Total	Payroll	Personnel
NORTH LAS VEGAS—Clark County										
□ LAKE MEAD HOSPITAL MEDICAL CENTER, 1409 East Lake Mead Boulevard, Zip 89030; tel. 702/649–7711; Ernest Libman, Administrator and Chief Executive Officer (Nonreporting) **A**1 9 10 **S**6525 Ornda Healthcorp	33	10	140	—	—	—	—	—	—	—
OWYHEE—Elko County										
★ U.S. PUBLIC HEALTH SERVICE OWYHEE COMMUNITY HEALTH FACILITY, Mailing Address: P.O. Box 130, Zip 89832–0130; tel. 702/757–2415; Kay C. Jewett, Acting Service Unit Director **A**1 10 **F**1 2 3 4 5 7 8 9 10 11 12 13 14 15 16 17 18 19 20 21 22 23 25 27 28 29 30 31 32 33 34 35 36 37 38 39 40 41 42 43 44 45 47 48 49 50 51 52 53 54 55 56 57 58 59 60 61 63 64 65 66 68 69 70 71 73 74 **P**1 **S**9195 U.S. Public Health Service Indian Health Service	47	10	15	126	2	12715	0	3291	1968	58
RENO—Washoe County										
★ IOANNIS A. LOUGARIS VETERANS AFFAIRS MEDICAL CENTER, 1000 Locust Street, Zip 89520–0100; tel. 702/786–7200; Gary R. Whitfield, Director (Total facility includes 60 beds in nursing home–type unit) **A**1 3 5 **F**1 3 8 10 12 15 17 18 19 20 21 22 24 26 27 28 29 30 31 32 33 34 35 37 41 42 44 45 46 49 52 54 56 57 58 59 60 63 64 65 67 71 72 73 74 **P**6 **S**9295 Department of Veterans Affairs	45	10	167	3797	74	122044	0	53914	29416	691
★ △ ST. MARY'S REGIONAL MEDICAL CENTER, 235 West Sixth Street, Zip 89520; tel. 702/323–2041; Jeff K. Bills, President (Total facility includes 16 beds in nursing home–type unit) **A**1 7 10 **F**2 3 4 7 8 10 11 12 13 16 17 19 20 21 22 23 25 27 28 29 30 32 33 34 35 37 38 39 40 41 42 43 44 45 46 48 49 61 63 64 65 67 71 72 73 74 **P**3 5 6 8 **S**1195 Dominican Sisters Congregation of the Most Holy Name	21	10	341	12128	192	132242	1884	124259	52175	1477
★ WASHOE MEDICAL CENTER, 77 Pringle Way, Zip 89520–0109; tel. 702/328–4100; Robert B. Burn Jr., President and Chief Executive Officer (Nonreporting) **A**1 2 3 5 9 10	23	10	573	—	—	—	—	—	—	—
□ WEST HILLS HOSPITAL, 1240 East Ninth Street, Zip 89512, Mailing Address: P.O. Box 30012, Zip 89520; tel. 702/323–0478; Neal Cury, Chief Executive Officer (Nonreporting) **A**1 3 5 9 10 **S**0069 Behavioral Healthcare Corporation	33	22	95	—	—	—	—	—	—	—
WILLOW SPRINGS CENTER FOR CHILDREN AND ADOLESCENTS, 690 Edison Way, Zip 89502, Mailing Address: P.O. Box 30012, Zip 89520; tel. 702/858–3303; Robert Bartlett, Administrator (Nonreporting) **S**0069 Behavioral Healthcare Corporation	33	22	74	—	—	—	—	—	—	—
SPARKS—Washoe County										
□ NEVADA MENTAL HEALTH INSTITUTE, 480 Galletti Way, Zip 89431–5574; tel. 702/688–2001; Richard Rahe M.D., Director **A**1 3 5 10 **F**1 6 12 34 52 56 57 58 59 65 **P**6	12	22	52	865	38	52050	0	16546	7234	174
□ NORTHERN NEVADA MEDICAL CENTER, (Formerly Sparks Family Hospital) 2375 East Prater Way, Zip 89434–9645; tel. 702/331–7000; Michael Callahan, Chief Executive Officer **A**1 9 10 **F**1 7 8 11 12 14 15 16 19 21 22 23 25 28 32 34 35 37 40 41 42 43 44 46 48 52 57 59 65 71 73 **S**9555 Universal Health Services, Inc.	33	10	138	2188	27	35963	194	23175	9399	286
SPARKS FAMILY HOSPITAL See Northern Nevada Medical Center										
TONOPAH—Esmeralda County										
NYE REGIONAL MEDICAL CENTER, 825 Erie Main, Zip 89049, Mailing Address: Box 391, Zip 89049; tel. 702/482–6233; Janet Slay, Administrator (Nonreporting) **A**9 10	13	10	45	—	—	—	—	—	—	—
WINNEMUCCA—Humboldt County										
★ HUMBOLDT GENERAL HOSPITAL, 118 East Haskell Street, Zip 89445; tel. 702/623–5222; Byron Quinton, Administrator (Total facility includes 10 beds in nursing home–type unit) **A**9 **F**3 7 8 14 15 19 22 35 37 40 44 64 65 67 71 73	16	10	28	661	17	16320	272	7107	3565	94
YERINGTON—Lyon County										
★ SOUTH LYON MEDICAL CENTER, Surprise At Whitacre Avenue, Zip 89447, Mailing Address: P.O. Box 940, Zip 89447–0940; tel. 702/463–2301; Joan S. Hall R.N., Administrator (Total facility includes 30 beds in nursing home–type unit) **A**9 10 **F**8 11 22 28 34 44 49 64	23	10	44	331	31	23616	0	4447	2666	100

NEW HAMPSHIRE

Resident population 1,125 (in thousands)
Resident population in metro areas 59.4%
Birth rate per 1,000 population 14.8
65 years and over 11.9%
Percent of persons without health insurance 10.9%

Hospital, Address, Telephone, Administrator, Approval, Facility, and Physician Codes, Health Care System	Classification Codes		Utilization Data					Expense (thousands) of dollars		
	Control	Service	Beds	Admissions	Census	Outpatient Visits	Births	Total	Payroll	Personnel

- ★ American Hospital Association (AHA) membership
- □ Joint Commission on Accreditation of Healthcare Organizations (JCAHO) accreditation
- + American Osteopathic Hospital Association (AOHA) membership
- ○ American Osteopathic Association (AOA) accreditation
- △ Commission on Accreditation of Rehabilitation Facilities (CARF) accreditation
  Control codes 61, 63, 64, 71, 72 and 73 indicate hospitals listed by AOHA, but not registered by AHA. For definition of numerical codes, see page A6

BERLIN—Coos County

★ ANDROSCOGGIN VALLEY HOSPITAL, 59 Page Hill Road, Zip 03570–3531; tel. 603/752–2200; Donald F. Saunders, President **A**1 9 10 **F**7 8 12 14 19 21 22 26 28 29 30 31 32 34 35 37 40 41 42 44 48 49 52 55 56 57 58 59 64 65 70 71 73	23	10	82	2430	48	43497	117	17612	7791	247

CLAREMONT—Sullivan County

★ VALLEY REGIONAL HOSPITAL, 243 Elm Street, Zip 03743–2099; tel. 603/542–7771; Donald R. Holl, President **A**1 9 10 **F**1 7 8 11 12 13 15 16 17 18 19 21 22 23 24 25 26 28 29 30 31 32 33 34 35 39 40 41 42 44 45 46 49 51 52 53 54 55 56 57 58 59 63 64 65 67 68 70 71 72 73 74 **P**6 7	23	10	71	1993	26	49987	310	19394	7677	308

COLEBROOK—Coos County

★ UPPER CONNECTICUT VALLEY HOSPITAL, Corliss Lane, Zip 03576, Mailing Address: RFD 2, Box 13, Zip 03576; tel. 603/237–4971; Deanna S. Howard, Chief Executive Officer **A**1 9 10 **F**7 8 13 15 16 17 19 22 28 30 32 34 37 40 42 44 56 65 71 73	23	10	20	540	10	15260	45	4322	1878	109

CONCORD—Merrimack County

★ CONCORD HOSPITAL, 250 Pleasant Street, Zip 03301–2598; tel. 603/225–2711; Michael B. Green, President **A**1 2 5 10 **F**7 8 10 11 12 13 14 15 19 21 22 23 24 29 30 31 32 33 34 35 37 39 40 41 42 44 45 49 51 52 53 54 55 56 57 59 63 65 67 69 70 71 72 73 74 **P**6 7	23	10	187	8521	144	86643	1357	72967	32369	992
★ HEALTHSOUTH REHABILITATION HOSPITAL, 254 Pleasant Street, Zip 03301; tel. 603/226–9800; (Nonreporting) **A**9 10 12 **S**0023 Healthsouth Corporation	33	46	53	—						
□ NEW HAMPSHIRE HOSPITAL, 105 Pleasant Street, Zip 03301–3861; tel. 603/271–5200; Paul G. Gorman Ed.D., Superintendent (Total facility includes 145 beds in nursing home–type unit) **A**1 3 9 10 **F**14 16 20 26 28 31 39 41 45 46 52 53 54 55 57 65 67 73 **P**4 6	12	22	317	1218	259	0	0	38464	23264	929

DERRY—Rockingham County

★ PARKLAND MEDICAL CENTER, One Parkland Drive, Zip 03038; tel. 603/432–1500; Steven R. Gordon, Chief Executive Officer **A**1 9 10 **F**4 8 10 11 13 14 15 16 17 19 21 22 23 25 26 27 28 29 30 34 35 37 39 40 41 42 43 44 45 49 52 57 65 67 68 71 72 73 74 **P**1 6 7 **S**0048 Columbia/HCA Healthcare Corporation	33	10	86	3096	43	53428	585	—	—	350

DOVER—Strafford County

SEABORNE HOSPITAL, Seaborne Drive, Zip 03820; tel. 603/742–9300; Ray McGarty, Executive Director (Nonreporting) **A**9	33	82	86							
★ WENTWORTH–DOUGLASS HOSPITAL, 789 Central Avenue, Zip 03820–2589; tel. 603/742–5252; Ralph Gabarro, President **A**1 2 9 10 **F**5 7 8 10 12 14 15 16 17 19 21 22 23 24 29 30 32 33 34 35 37 39 40 41 42 44 45 46 49 54 56 57 60 61 63 65 67 70 71 73 74 **P**5 8	23	10	112	4553	62	87569	800	44326	19792	645

DUBLIN—Cheshire County

BEECH HILL HOSPITAL, New Harrisville Road, Zip 03444, Mailing Address: Box 254, Zip 03444; tel. 603/563–8511; Barbara R. Duckett, President **A**9 **F**2 3 15 16 **P**6	23	82	70	1100	48	—	0	5610	3388	122

EXETER—Rockingham County

★ EXETER HOSPITAL, 10 Buzell Avenue, Zip 03833–2515; tel. 603/778–7311; Kevin J. Callahan, President and Chief Executive Officer (Total facility includes 115 beds in nursing home–type unit) **A**1 2 9 10 **F**4 7 8 10 13 14 15 17 19 21 22 23 25 27 29 30 31 32 33 35 37 39 40 41 42 44 49 53 54 55 56 57 58 59 60 61 63 64 65 66 67 70 71 73 74 **P**6 7 8	23	10	215	4314	161	66164	781	46934	19555	622

FRANKLIN—Merrimack County

★ FRANKLIN REGIONAL HOSPITAL, 15 Aiken Avenue, Zip 03235–1299; tel. 603/934–2060; Walter A. Strauch, Executive Director **A**1 9 10 **F**7 8 14 15 16 17 19 22 28 29 30 32 33 34 37 40 41 44 45 46 49 64 65 67 68 71 73 74 **P**6	23	10	49	1674	30	27572	133	12122	5612	200

GREENFIELD—Hillsborough County

CROTCHED MOUNTAIN REHABILITATION CENTER, 1 Verney Drive, Zip 03047–0010; tel. 603/547–3311; Major W. Wheelock, President (Total facility includes 62 beds in nursing home–type unit) **A**9 **F**12 20 48 49 53 64 65 **P**3	23	46	142	55	106	27	0	15759	10551	460

HAMPSTEAD—Rockingham County

□ HAMPSTEAD HOSPITAL, East Road, Zip 03841–2228; tel. 603/329–5311; Phillip Kubiak, President **A**1 9 10 **F**2 16 19 35 52 53 54 55 56 57 59 65 67 71 **P**1	33	22	85	1466	47	0	0	9715	5511	140

HANOVER—Grafton County

★ DARTMOUTH COLLEGE HEALTH SERVICE, (Formerly Dick Hall's House) 7 Rope Ferry Road, Zip 03755–1421; tel. 603/650–1400; John Turco M.D., Director (Data for 320 days) **A**9 **F**3 12 15 16 17 18 27 28 29 30 31 34 39 41 45 51 54 55 56 58 59 61 65 66 67 74	23	11	10	445	3	17875	0	2983	1506	43

KEENE—Cheshire County

★ △ CHESHIRE MEDICAL CENTER, 580 Court Street, Zip 03431–1718; tel. 603/352–4111; Robert J. Langlais, President **A**1 2 7 9 10 **F**7 8 11 12 14 15 16 17 18 19 20 21 22 23 24 28 29 30 31 34 35 37 39 40 41 42 44 45 46 48 49 52 53 54 55 56 57 58 60 63 65 66 67 70 71 73	23	10	162	4847	99	50300	453	39278	18382	646

Hospitals, U.S. / NEW HAMPSHIRE

Hospital, Address, Telephone, Administrator, Approval, Facility, and Physician Codes, Health Care System	Classification Codes		Utilization Data					Expense (thousands) of dollars		
★ American Hospital Association (AHA) membership □ Joint Commission on Accreditation of Healthcare Organizations (JCAHO) accreditation + American Osteopathic Hospital Association (AOHA) membership ○ American Osteopathic Association (AOA) accreditation △ Commission on Accreditation of Rehabilitation Facilities (CARF) accreditation Control codes 61, 63, 64, 71, 72 and 73 indicate hospitals listed by AOHA, but not registered by AHA. For definition of numerical codes, see page A6	Control	Service	Beds	Admissions	Census	Outpatient Visits	Births	Total	Payroll	Personnel
LACONIA—Belknap County										
★ LAKES REGION GENERAL HOSPITAL, Highland Street, Zip 03246–3298; tel. 603/524–3211; Thomas Clairmont, President **A**1 2 9 10 **F**3 4 7 8 10 12 13 14 15 16 17 19 20 22 23 26 28 30 31 33 34 35 37 40 41 42 44 45 49 52 53 54 55 56 57 63 65 67 70 71 72 73 74 **P**6	23	10	117	5008	75	36361	568	42745	20556	616
LANCASTER—Coos County										
★ WEEKS MEMORIAL HOSPITAL, Middle Street, Zip 03584, Mailing Address: Rural Route 1, Box 8, Zip 03584–9702; tel. 603/788–4911; Patsy Pilgrim, Chief Executive Officer **A**1 9 10 **F**7 8 12 14 15 16 17 19 21 22 26 28 29 30 31 34 37 39 40 41 42 44 46 49 56 65 66 67 71 73 74 **P**6	23	10	49	1188	22	58157	107	12256	5156	216
LEBANON—Grafton County										
★ ALICE PECK DAY MEMORIAL HOSPITAL, 125 Mascoma Street, Zip 03766; tel. 603/448–3121; Robert Mesropian, President (Total facility includes 50 beds in nursing home–type unit) **A**1 9 10 **F**6 7 8 14 15 17 19 22 25 28 30 34 39 40 41 42 44 46 48 49 51 64 65 71 72 73 **P**1	23	10	72	769	55	66839	276	11057	5245	150
★ MARY HITCHCOCK MEMORIAL HOSPITAL, One Medical Center Drive, Zip 03756–0001; tel. 603/650–5000; James W. Varnum, President **A**1 2 3 5 8 9 10 **F**4 7 8 10 11 12 15 16 17 19 20 21 22 23 27 28 29 30 31 34 35 37 38 40 41 42 43 44 45 46 47 49 50 51 52 53 54 56 57 58 59 60 61 63 65 66 67 69 71 72 73 74 **P**4	23	10	403	17807	319	279572	1023	214935	78989	2648
LITTLETON—Grafton County										
★ LITTLETON REGIONAL HOSPITAL, 107 Cottage Street, Zip 03561; tel. 603/444–7731; Robert S. Pearson, Administrator **A**1 2 9 10 **F**7 8 15 16 17 19 21 22 28 30 34 35 37 39 40 41 42 44 46 49 60 65 66 71 73 **S**0002 Quorum Health Group/Quorum Health Resources	23	10	54	1291	18	26903	276	13510	5227	173
MANCHESTER—Hillsborough County										
★ △ CATHOLIC MEDICAL CENTER, 100 McGregor Street, Zip 03102–3770; tel. 603/668–3545; William N. Sirak, Acting Chief Operating Officer **A**1 2 7 9 10 **F**2 3 4 5 6 7 8 10 11 15 17 18 19 21 22 23 24 25 26 27 28 29 31 32 33 34 35 36 37 39 40 41 42 43 44 45 46 48 49 52 54 56 59 60 61 62 65 66 67 69 71 72 73 74 **P**1	23	10	255	9703	180	79516	637	101676	—	1284
★ ELLIOT HOSPITAL, One Elliot Way, Zip 03103; tel. 603/669–5300; Robert G. Cholette, Chief Executive Officer **A**1 2 9 10 **F**1 3 7 8 10 11 12 15 16 17 19 21 22 23 25 26 27 29 30 31 32 33 34 35 37 40 41 42 43 44 46 47 49 52 54 55 56 57 60 61 62 63 65 67 70 71 72 73 74 **P**8	23	10	218	7034	106	83443	1464	63625	—	1246
★ VETERANS AFFAIRS MEDICAL CENTER, 718 Smyth Road, Zip 03104–4098; tel. 603/624–4366; Eugene L. Ochocki, Director (Total facility includes 120 beds in nursing home–type unit) **A**1 2 3 5 9 **F**1 2 3 4 5 6 8 10 12 16 17 18 19 20 21 22 24 25 26 27 28 29 30 31 32 33 34 35 36 37 39 41 42 43 44 45 46 49 50 51 54 55 56 57 58 59 60 61 63 64 65 67 69 70 71 72 73 74 **P**6 **S**9295 Department of Veterans Affairs	45	10	228	2858	186	82004	0	44043	23397	541
NASHUA—Hillsborough County										
□ CHARTER BROOKSIDE BEHAVIORAL HEALTH SYSTEM OF NEW ENGLAND, (Formerly Nashua Brookside Hospital) 29 Northwest Boulevard, Zip 03063; tel. 603/886–5000; Joel Rosenhaus, Administrator (Nonreporting) **A**1 9 10 **S**0695 Charter Medical Corporation	33	22	100	—	—	—	—	—	—	—
NASHUA BROOKSIDE HOSPITAL See Charter Brookside Behavioral Health System of New England										
NASHUA MEMORIAL HOSPITAL See Southern New Hampshire Regional Medical Center										
★ SOUTHERN NEW HAMPSHIRE REGIONAL MEDICAL CENTER, (Formerly Nashua Memorial Hospital) 8 Prospect Street, Zip 03060, Mailing Address: Box 2014, Zip 03061–2014; tel. 603/577–2000; Thomas E. Wilhelmsen Jr., President **A**1 2 9 10 **F**3 7 8 10 12 14 15 16 18 19 22 23 28 29 30 34 35 37 38 40 41 42 44 45 46 49 52 53 56 57 58 59 63 65 67 71 73 74 **P**3 4 6 7 8	23	10	154	6212	85	108157	1442	51969	25254	822
★ △ ST. JOSEPH HOSPITAL AND TRAUMA CENTER, 172 Kinsley Street, Zip 03061, Mailing Address: Caller Service 2013, Zip 03061; tel. 603/882–3000; Peter B. Davis, President and Chief Executive Officer **A**1 2 6 7 9 10 **F**1 2 3 7 8 10 11 12 13 14 15 16 17 18 19 20 21 22 23 24 25 26 27 29 30 31 32 33 34 35 36 37 39 40 41 42 44 46 48 49 51 52 54 55 56 58 60 61 63 65 66 67 70 71 72 73 74 **P**6 8 **S**5885 Covenant Health Systems, Inc.	21	10	208	6250	111	114438	1102	64198	30424	813
NEW LONDON—Merrimack County										
★ NEW LONDON HOSPITAL, 270 County Road, Zip 03257; tel. 603/526–2911; Alyson R. Pitman, President and Chief Executive Officer (Total facility includes 54 beds in nursing home–type unit) **A**1 9 10 **F**7 8 15 16 17 19 20 22 28 30 34 35 36 37 39 40 41 42 44 45 49 51 61 64 65 67 71 73 **P**8	23	10	89	1220	71	31365	162	13679	7039	182
NORTH CONWAY—Carroll County										
□ MEMORIAL HOSPITAL, 3073 Main Street, Zip 03860–5001, Mailing Address: P.O. Box 5001, Zip 03860–5001; tel. 603/356–5461; Gary R. Poquette FACHE, Executive Director (Total facility includes 45 beds in nursing home–type unit) **A**1 9 10 **F**7 8 11 14 15 16 17 19 21 22 29 30 33 34 35 37 40 41 42 44 45 49 56 59 64 65 66 71 73 **P**3	23	10	80	1217	94	27451	215	13076	5233	176
PETERBOROUGH—Hillsborough County										
★ MONADNOCK COMMUNITY HOSPITAL, 452 Old Street Road, Zip 03458; tel. 603/924–7191; Frank A. Niro, Chief Executive Officer **A**1 9 10 **F**1 7 8 13 17 18 19 22 28 30 32 33 34 36 39 40 41 42 44 45 46 48 49 51 52 54 55 56 57 58 59 63 65 67 69 71 73 74 **P**3 **S**0002 Quorum Health Group/Quorum Health Resources	23	10	62	1808	27	45479	410	14795	5912	218

Hospitals, U.S. / NEW HAMPSHIRE

Hospital, Address, Telephone, Administrator, Approval, Facility, and Physician Codes, Health Care System	Classification Codes		Utilization Data					Expense (thousands) of dollars		
★ American Hospital Association (AHA) membership ☐ Joint Commission on Accreditation of Healthcare Organizations (JCAHO) accreditation + American Osteopathic Hospital Association (AOHA) membership ○ American Osteopathic Association (AOA) accreditation △ Commission on Accreditation of Rehabilitation Facilities (CARF) accreditation Control codes 61, 63, 64, 71, 72 and 73 indicate hospitals listed by AOHA, but not registered by AHA. For definition of numerical codes, see page A6	Control	Service	Beds	Admissions	Census	Outpatient Visits	Births	Total	Payroll	Personnel
PLYMOUTH—Grafton County ★ SPEARE MEMORIAL HOSPITAL, Hospital Road, Zip 03264–1199; tel. 603/536–1120; David L. Pearse, Executive Director **A**1 9 10 **F**7 8 11 12 14 15 17 19 21 22 28 30 33 37 39 40 41 42 44 49 54 56 65 66 67 71 73	23	10	47	1180	16	39552	101	8518	4226	140
PORTSMOUTH—Rockingham County PORTSMOUTH PAVILION See Portsmouth Regional Hospital ★ PORTSMOUTH REGIONAL HOSPITAL, (Includes Portsmouth Pavilion, Portsmouth, New Hampshire) 333 Borthwick Avenue, Zip 03802–7004; tel. 603/436–5110; William J. Schuler, Chief Executive Officer (Total facility includes 65 beds in nursing home–type unit) **A**1 10 **F**4 7 8 10 17 19 21 22 23 28 30 35 37 40 41 42 44 49 52 53 54 55 56 57 59 63 65 71 72 73 **P**1 8 **S**0048 Columbia/HCA Healthcare Corporation	33	10	181	5967	99	77604	818	—	—	604
ROCHESTER—Strafford County ★ FRISBIE MEMORIAL HOSPITAL, 11 Whitehall Road, Zip 03867–3297; tel. 603/332–5211; Alvin D. Felgar, President and Chief Executive Officer **A**1 2 9 10 **F**2 3 7 8 10 11 15 17 18 19 21 22 26 30 31 33 34 35 37 39 40 41 42 44 49 52 54 55 56 57 58 63 65 66 67 71 73 **P**1 3 5	23	10	88	3134	54	43108	512	27634	12389	389
SALEM—Rockingham County ☐ △ NORTHEAST REHABILITATION HOSPITAL, 70 Butler Street, Zip 03079; tel. 603/893–2900; John F. Prochilo, Chief Executive Officer and Administrator **A**1 7 9 10 **F**12 14 15 16 17 25 32 34 39 41 42 46 48 49 58 65 66 67 71 74	33	46	102	1113	65	45184	0	19357	9525	278
WOLFEBORO—Carroll County ★ HUGGINS HOSPITAL, 240 South Main Street, Zip 03894, Mailing Address: Box 912, Zip 03894–0912; tel. 603/569–2150; Leslie N H. MacLeod, President (Total facility includes 21 beds in nursing home–type unit) **A**1 9 10 **F**1 7 8 15 16 19 21 22 31 35 37 40 41 44 45 46 49 53 54 55 56 57 58 64 65 71 73 **P**6	23	10	82	1743	43	33989	106	11921	4582	215
WOODSVILLE—Grafton County ★ COTTAGE HOSPITAL, Swiftwater Road, Zip 03785–2001, Mailing Address: P.O. Box 2001, Zip 03785; tel. 603/747–2761; Reginald J. Lavoie, Administrator **A**1 2 9 10 **F**7 8 15 16 19 22 36 37 40 42 44 54 65 67 71 72 73 74	23	10	38	837	13	28622	60	7314	3372	120

Hospitals, U.S. / NEW JERSEY

NEW JERSEY

Resident population 7,879 (in thousands)
Resident population in metro areas 100.0%
Birth rate per 1,000 population 15.6
65 years and over 13.6%
Percent of persons without health insurance 11.3%

Hospital, Address, Telephone, Administrator, Approval, Facility, and Physician Codes, Health Care System	Classification Codes		Utilization Data					Expense (thousands) of dollars		
★ American Hospital Association (AHA) membership □ Joint Commission on Accreditation of Healthcare Organizations (JCAHO) accreditation + American Osteopathic Hospital Association (AOHA) membership ○ American Osteopathic Association (AOA) accreditation △ Commission on Accreditation of Rehabilitation Facilities (CARF) accreditation Control codes 61, 63, 64, 71, 72 and 73 indicate hospitals listed by AOHA, but not registered by AHA. For definition of numerical codes, see page A6	Control	Service	Beds	Admissions	Census	Outpatient Visits	Births	Total	Payroll	Personnel
ATLANTIC CITY—Atlantic County										
✠ ATLANTIC CITY MEDICAL CENTER, 1925 Pacific Avenue, Zip 08401–6713; tel. 609/344–4081; David P. Tilton, President **A**1 2 3 5 9 10 12 **F**2 3 5 7 8 10 11 15 16 17 18 19 21 22 25 26 28 30 31 33 34 35 37 38 40 41 42 44 46 49 51 52 53 54 55 56 57 58 59 60 61 63 65 67 68 70 71 72 73 74 **P**6	23	10	472	25630	404	194584	2526	173614	70596	2106
BAYONNE—Hudson County										
✠ BAYONNE HOSPITAL, 29th Street At Avenue E, Zip 07002; tel. 201/858–5000; Michael R. D'Agnes, President and Chief Executive Officer **A**1 2 6 9 10 **F**1 2 3 7 8 14 16 17 19 21 22 26 27 28 29 30 33 34 37 40 42 44 46 49 52 56 60 63 65 67 71 73	23	10	299	9100	236	33337	531	77054	35769	1034
BELLE MEAD—Somerset County										
✠ CARRIER FOUNDATION, County Rt 601, P.O. Box 147, Zip 08502; tel. 908/281–1000; Stanley J. Birch Jr. CPA, President and Chief Executive Officer **A**1 5 9 10 **F**2 3 16 17 19 21 34 35 50 52 53 54 55 56 57 58 59 63 65 67 68 71 73 74 **P**6	23	22	176	2432	113	36218	0	28354	16828	511
BELLEVILLE—Essex County										
✠ CLARA MAASS HEALTH SYSTEM, (Formerly Clara Maass Medical Center) One Clara Maass Drive, Zip 07109; tel. 201/450–2000; Robert S. Curtis, President (Total facility includes 120 beds in nursing home–type unit) **A**1 2 9 10 **F**1 6 7 8 12 13 14 15 16 17 19 21 22 26 27 28 29 31 32 33 34 37 39 40 41 42 45 46 49 51 52 53 54 55 57 60 61 63 64 65 67 71 72 73 74 **P**5 8	23	10	595	11471	378	123933	1078	93898	50558	1470
BERKELEY HEIGHTS—Union County										
★ RUNNELLS SPECIALIZED HOSPITAL, (Long Term Care, Psychiatric, Physical Medicine and Rehabilitation) 40 Watchung Way, Zip 07922–2618; tel. 908/771–5700; Joseph W. Sharp, Administrator (Total facility includes 300 beds in nursing home–type unit) **A**9 10 **F**20 27 42 48 49 52 65 67 73 **P**6	13	49	345	784	328	0	0	30241	16813	553
BERLIN—Camden County										
✠ WEST JERSEY HOSPITAL–BERLIN, 100 Townsend Avenue, Zip 08009; tel. 609/768–6006; Martin B. Idler, Executive Director **A**1 9 10 **F**2 5 7 8 14 16 17 19 22 26 28 30 31 32 34 35 37 39 42 44 45 46 49 60 65 67 71 73 74 **P**3 4 7 **S**6725 West Jersey Health System	23	10	95	3163	71	24378	0	—	—	293
BOONTON TOWNSHIP—Morris County										
ST. CLARES RIVERSIDE–BOONTON TOWNSHIP See Northwest Covenant Medical Center, Denville										
BLACKWOOD—Camden County										
□ CAMDEN COUNTY HEALTH SERVICES CENTER, (Long–Term Nursing Care) Collier Drive, Zip 08012–2799, Mailing Address: P.O. Box 1639, Zip 08012–2799; tel. 609/757–3434; Anthony Peters, Chief Executive Officer (Total facility includes 275 beds in nursing home–type unit) **A**1 3 10 **F**14 15 19 20 26 27 39 45 46 52 56 57 64 65 73 **P**4	13	49	422	868	398	0	0	34289	16985	454
BRIDGETON—Cumberland County										
BRIDGETON DIVISION See South Jersey Hospital System										
✠ SOUTH JERSEY HOSPITAL SYSTEM, (Includes Bridgeton Division, 333 Irving Avenue, Bridgeton, New Jersey, Zip 08302; tel. 609/451–6600; Millville Division, 1200 North High, Millville, New Jersey, Zip 08332–2586; tel. 609/825–3500; South Jersey Hospital System–Elmer Division, West Front Street, Elmer, New Jersey, Zip 08318–0516, Mailing Address: P.O. Box 1090, Zip 08318–1090; tel. 609/358–2341) 333 Irving Avenue, Zip 08302–2100; tel. 609/451–6600; Paul S. Cooper, President and Chief Executive Officer **A**1 2 9 10 **F**3 7 8 11 12 14 15 16 17 18 19 20 21 22 24 25 27 28 29 30 32 33 34 36 37 39 40 41 42 44 45 49 52 53 54 55 56 57 58 59 60 65 66 67 68 69 71 73 **P**3 8	23	10	376	12654	239	148442	872	99051	44551	1336
BROWNS MILLS—Burlington County										
✠ DEBORAH HEART AND LUNG CENTER, 200 Trenton Road, Zip 08015; tel. 609/893–6611; John R. Ernst, Executive Director **A**1 3 5 9 10 **F**4 10 14 19 21 28 29 30 34 37 43 45 50 54 63 65 67 71 73	23	49	161	5355	119	26019	0	109965	59036	1723
CAMDEN—Camden County										
✠ COOPER HOSPITAL–UNIVERSITY MEDICAL CENTER, One Cooper Plaza, Zip 08103–1489; tel. 609/342–2000; Kevin G. Halpern, President and Chief Executive Officer **A**1 2 3 5 8 9 10 **F**4 7 8 10 11 15 17 19 21 22 24 26 28 29 30 31 32 34 35 37 38 40 41 42 43 44 45 46 47 49 51 52 53 54 55 56 57 58 60 61 63 65 67 69 70 71 73 74 **P**4 6	23	10	422	19024	351	459137	1932	267169	145458	3394
✠ △ OUR LADY OF LOURDES MEDICAL CENTER, 1600 Haddon Avenue, Zip 08103; tel. 609/757–3500; Alexander J. Hatala, Chief Executive Officer **A**1 3 5 7 9 10 **F**4 7 8 10 11 12 13 15 16 17 18 19 20 21 22 23 25 26 28 29 31 32 33 34 35 37 38 39 40 41 42 43 44 45 46 48 49 51 52 53 54 55 58 59 60 63 65 67 68 69 70 71 73 74 **P**5 7 8 **S**1385 Allegany Health System	23	10	327	12985	296	178548	1447	127347	61528	1817
✠ WEST JERSEY HOSPITAL–CAMDEN, 1000 Atlantic Avenue, Zip 08104–1595; tel. 609/342–4000; Joan T. Meyers R.N., Executive Director **A**1 2 3 9 10 **F**2 3 5 14 15 16 17 19 21 22 26 28 29 30 31 32 33 34 35 37 39 42 44 45 46 49 51 60 63 65 67 71 73 **P**3 4 7 **S**6725 West Jersey Health System	23	10	222	9125	127	46049	0	225985	115529	1153

Hospitals, U.S. / NEW JERSEY

Hospital, Address, Telephone, Administrator, Approval, Facility, and Physician Codes, Health Care System	Classification Codes		Utilization Data					Expense (thousands) of dollars		
★ American Hospital Association (AHA) membership □ Joint Commission on Accreditation of Healthcare Organizations (JCAHO) accreditation + American Osteopathic Hospital Association (AOHA) membership ○ American Osteopathic Association (AOA) accreditation △ Commission on Accreditation of Rehabilitation Facilities (CARF) accreditation Control codes 61, 63, 64, 71, 72 and 73 indicate hospitals listed by AOHA, but not registered by AHA. For definition of numerical codes, see page A6	Control	Service	Beds	Admissions	Census	Outpatient Visits	Births	Total	Payroll	Personnel
CAPE MAY COURT HOUSE—Cape May County ★ BURDETTE TOMLIN MEMORIAL HOSPITAL, Stone Harbor Boulevard, Zip 08210–9990; tel. 609/463-2000; Thomas L. Scott FACHE, President and Chief Executive Officer **A**1 9 10 **F**2 7 8 11 14 15 16 17 19 22 28 29 30 31 33 34 35 40 41 42 44 46 49 54 56 63 65 67 71 73 **P**1 4 5 8	23	10	234	9273	180	82896	775	63879	28718	871
CEDAR GROVE—Essex County □ ESSEX COUNTY HOSPITAL CENTER, 125 Fairview Avenue, Zip 07009; tel. 201/228-8200; Robert P. Arnold, Director **A**1 10 **F**4 8 10 11 15 16 19 20 21 22 35 37 39 43 44 46 50 52 60 65 67 70 71 73 **P**6	13	22	400	522	360	0	0	41758	31028	763
CHERRY HILL—Camden County ★ + ○ KENNEDY MEMORIAL HOSPITALS–UNIVERSITY MEDICAL CENTER, (Includes Kennedy Memorial Hospital, 18 East Laurel Road, Stratford, New Jersey, Zip 08084; tel. 609/346-6000; C. Barry Dykes, Associate Vice President and Administrator; Kennedy Memorial Hospital, 435 Hurffville–Cross Keys Road, Turnersville, New Jersey, Zip 08012; tel. 609/582-2500; Ann Witkowski, Associate Vice President and Administrator; Kennedy Memorial Hospitals–University Medical Center, 2201 Chapel Avenue West, Cherry Hill, New Jersey, Zip 08002-2048; tel. 609/488-6500; Michael Dennis, Associate Vice President and Administrator) 500 Marlboro Avenue, Zip 08034-5087, Mailing Address: P.O. Box 5087, Zip 08034-5087; tel. 609/661-5100; Richard E. Murray, President and Chief Executive Officer **A**9 10 11 12 13 **F**2 3 4 5 7 8 10 11 12 13 16 17 18 19 20 21 22 23 24 25 26 27 28 29 30 31 32 33 34 35 36 37 38 39 40 41 42 43 44 45 46 49 51 52 53 54 55 56 57 58 59 61 63 64 65 66 67 68 69 71 73 74 **P**2 7	23	10	604	21043	357	147780	2142	161835	69981	2238
CHESTER—Morris County ★ △ WELKIND REHABILITATION HOSPITAL, Pleasant Hill Road, Zip 07930; tel. 201/584-8145; Kenneth W. Aitchison, President and Chief Executive Officer **A**1 7 10 **F**12 17 25 28 30 32 34 45 48 49 65 67 73	23	46	72	984	52	13891	0	12907	7238	154
DENVILLE—Morris County ★ NORTHWEST COVENANT MEDICAL CENTER, (Formerly St. Clares–Riverside Medical Center) (Includes Dover General–Dover Campus, Jardine Street, Dover, New Jersey, Zip 07801-3311; tel. 201/989-3000; St. Clares Riverside Boonton Township Campus, 130 Powerville Road, Boonton Township, New Jersey, Zip 07005; tel. 201/625-6000; St. Clares–Riverside Medical Center–Sussex Campus, 20 Walnut Street, Sussex, New Jersey, Zip 07461; tel. 201/702-2200; St. Clares Riverside Hospital–Denville Campus, 25 Pocono Road, Denville, New Jersey, Zip 07834; tel. 201/625-6000) 25 Pocono Road, Zip 07834-2995; tel. 201/625-6000; Joseph A. Trunfio Ph.D., President and Chief Executive Officer (Total facility includes 17 beds in nursing home–type unit) **A**1 2 5 9 10 **F**1 2 3 6 7 8 12 13 14 15 16 17 18 19 20 21 22 23 24 25 26 27 28 29 30 31 32 33 34 35 36 39 41 42 43 44 45 46 49 51 52 53 54 55 56 57 58 59 60 62 63 65 66 67 69 71 72 73 74 **P**1 4 5 6 7 **S**5305 Sisters of the Sorrowful Mother United States Health System	21	10	804	24624	489	247240	2085	206995	97721	2693
DOVER—Morris County DOVER GENERAL HOSPITAL AND MEDICAL CENTER See Northwest Covenant Medical Center, Denville										
EAST ORANGE—Essex County ★ EAST ORANGE GENERAL HOSPITAL, 300 Central Avenue, Zip 07019-2819; tel. 201/672-8400; Mark Chastang, President and Chief Executive Officer **A**1 9 10 **F**2 3 8 12 14 15 16 17 18 19 21 22 25 26 27 28 29 30 31 32 34 37 39 41 42 44 45 46 49 51 52 53 54 56 57 58 59 65 67 71 73 **P**1	23	10	238	7144	196	125038	0	63670	31729	1123
★ VETERANS AFFAIRS MEDICAL CENTER, 385 Tremont Avenue, Zip 07018-1095; tel. 201/676-1000; Kenneth H. Mizrach, Director (Total facility includes 60 beds in nursing home–type unit) **A**1 2 3 5 8 9 **F**2 3 4 8 10 11 12 19 20 21 22 23 24 25 26 28 30 31 32 34 35 37 39 41 42 44 45 46 48 49 51 52 54 56 58 59 60 63 65 67 69 71 73 74 **P**6 **S**9295 Department of Veterans Affairs	45	10	602	9223	471	233188	0	162632	92737	2089
EDISON—Middlesex County ★ △ JFK JOHNSON REHABILITATION INSTITUTE, 65 James Street, Zip 08818-3059; tel. 908/321-7050; Scott Gebhard, Administrator **A**1 3 7 9 10 **F**1 3 6 7 8 11 12 13 14 15 16 17 18 19 20 21 22 24 26 27 28 30 31 32 33 36 37 39 40 41 42 44 45 46 48 49 53 54 55 56 57 58 60 63 65 66 71 73 74 **P**8 **S**8855 JFK Health Systems, Inc.	23	46	90	1370	77	—	0	31829	20258	419
★ JFK MEDICAL CENTER, 65 James Street, Zip 08818-3059; tel. 908/321-7000; John P. McGee, President and Chief Executive Officer **A**1 2 3 5 9 **F**1 3 6 7 8 10 11 12 13 14 15 16 17 18 19 20 21 22 24 25 26 27 28 29 30 31 32 33 34 35 36 37 39 40 41 42 43 44 45 46 48 49 51 53 54 55 56 57 58 60 63 64 65 66 67 68 71 73 74 **P**1 3 5 7 8 **S**8855 JFK Health Systems, Inc.	23	10	417	15301	321	161505	1915	127428	62929	1717
★ ROOSEVELT HOSPITAL, Parsonage Road, Zip 08837, Mailing Address: P.O. Box 151, CN 4003, Metuchen Zip 08840-0151; tel. 908/321-6800; Thomas J. Romeo, Superintendent and Chief Executive Officer (Total facility includes 536 beds in nursing home–type unit) **A**9 10 **F**19 20 21 26 27 33 34 35 41 45 46 54 60 64 65 71 73 **P**6	13	10	564	632	511	5618	0	36500	23397	878
ELIZABETH—Union County ★ ELIZABETH GENERAL MEDICAL CENTER, (Includes Elizabeth General Medical Center–East, 655 East Jersey Street, Elizabeth, New Jersey, Zip 07206; tel. 201/351-9000; Elizabeth General Medical Center–West, Elizabeth, New Jersey) 925 East Jersey Street, Zip 07201-2728; tel. 908/289-8600; David A. Fletcher, President and Chief Executive Officer (Total facility includes 120 beds in nursing home–type unit) **A**1 2 3 5 6 9 10 **F**1 3 7 8 12 14 15 16 17 18 19 20 21 22 26 28 29 30 31 33 37 39 40 41 42 44 45 49 51 52 53 54 55 56 57 58 59 60 64 65 67 71 73 74 **P**6 8	23	10	537	15776	417	223354	1322	136219	70225	2114

© 1995 AHA Guide

Hospitals, U.S. / NEW JERSEY

Hospital, Address, Telephone, Administrator, Approval, Facility, and Physician Codes, Health Care System	Classification Codes		Utilization Data					Expense (thousands) of dollars		
	Control	Service	Beds	Admissions	Census	Outpatient Visits	Births	Total	Payroll	Personnel

★ American Hospital Association (AHA) membership
☐ Joint Commission on Accreditation of Healthcare Organizations (JCAHO) accreditation
+ American Osteopathic Hospital Association (AOHA) membership
○ American Osteopathic Association (AOA) accreditation
△ Commission on Accreditation of Rehabilitation Facilities (CARF) accreditation
Control codes 61, 63, 64, 71, 72 and 73 indicate hospitals listed by AOHA, but not registered by AHA. For definition of numerical codes, see page A6

Hospital	Control	Service	Beds	Admissions	Census	Outpatient Visits	Births	Total	Payroll	Personnel
★ ST. ELIZABETH HOSPITAL, 225 Williamson Street, Zip 07207–3600; tel. 908/527–5122; Sister Elizabeth Ann Maloney, President and Chief Executive Officer **A**1 2 3 9 10 **F**2 3 7 8 10 12 14 15 16 17 19 21 22 24 26 27 28 30 31 33 34 35 37 39 40 41 42 44 45 49 54 60 63 65 68 71 73 74 **P**5 6	21	10	304	12845	240	84755	1079	89072	42108	1293
ELMER—Salem County										
SOUTH JERSEY HOSPITAL SYSTEM–ELMER DIVISION See South Jersey Hospital System, Bridgeton										
ENGLEWOOD—Bergen County										
★ ENGLEWOOD HOSPITAL AND MEDICAL CENTER, (Formerly Englewood Hospital) 350 Engle Street, Zip 07631; tel. 201/894–3000; Daniel A. Kane, President and Chief Executive Officer **A**1 2 3 5 6 9 10 **F**3 4 7 8 10 11 13 15 16 17 19 20 21 22 23 28 29 30 31 32 33 34 35 36 37 39 40 41 42 44 45 46 49 51 52 54 55 56 57 58 59 60 61 63 65 66 67 68 71 73 74 **P**5 8	23	10	520	15259	291	341082	2218	148042	76878	1781
FLEMINGTON—Hunterdon County										
★ HUNTERDON MEDICAL CENTER, 2100 Wescott Drive, Zip 08822–4604; tel. 908/788–6100; Robert P. Wise, President and Chief Executive Officer **A**1 3 5 9 10 **F**1 3 7 8 12 14 15 16 17 18 19 22 25 26 28 29 30 31 32 33 34 35 37 39 40 41 42 44 45 46 49 52 53 54 55 56 57 58 59 61 65 67 68 71 72 73 74 **P**5 6	23	10	176	7384	116	126476	1212	62798	30368	978
FORT MONMOUTH—Monmouth County										
★ PATTERSON ARMY COMMUNITY HOSPITAL, Zip 07703–5607; tel. 908/532–1266; Colonel Royal C. Hudson Jr., Commander **A**1 **F**1 2 3 4 5 6 7 8 9 10 11 12 13 16 17 18 19 20 21 22 23 24 25 26 27 28 29 30 31 32 33 34 37 38 39 41 42 43 44 46 47 48 49 50 51 52 53 54 55 56 57 58 59 60 61 62 63 64 65 66 67 68 69 70 71 72 73 74 **P**5 **S**9395 Department of the Army	42	10	35	1052	7	138010	0	33300	—	495
FREEHOLD—Monmouth County										
★ CENTRASTATE MEDICAL CENTER, 901 West Main Street, Zip 07728–2549; tel. 908/431–2000; Thomas H. Litz, President and Chief Executive Officer **A**1 9 10 **F**7 8 11 13 14 15 16 17 19 20 22 23 25 26 28 29 30 31 32 33 34 35 37 39 40 41 42 44 45 46 49 51 52 54 55 56 58 61 62 64 65 67 68 71 72 73 74 **P**5	23	10	244	13736	192	121441	1237	81917	39562	1077
GLEN GARDNER—Hunterdon County										
☐ SENATOR GARRET T. W. HAGEDORN GERO PSYCHIATRIC HOSPITAL, (Formerly Senator Garret W Hagedorn Center for Geriatrics) 200 Sanitorium Road, Zip 08826–9752; tel. 908/537–2141; Edna Volpe-Way, Chief Executive Officer (Nonreporting) **A**1 10 **S**0010 Division of Mental Health Services, Department of Human Services, State of New Jersey	12	22	181	—	—	—	—	—	—	—
GREYSTONE PARK—Morris County										
★ GREYSTONE PARK PSYCHIATRIC HOSPITAL, Central Avenue, Zip 07950, Mailing Address: P.O. Box A, Zip 07950; tel. 201/538–1800; George A. Waters Jr. FACHE, Chief Executive Officer **A**1 9 10 **F**2 3 8 11 12 15 16 19 20 21 22 23 26 27 28 31 34 35 37 39 40 42 43 44 46 48 49 50 52 54 55 56 57 60 61 63 65 67 70 71 73 **P**6 **S**0010 Division of Mental Health Services, Department of Human Services, State of New Jersey	12	22	607	457	572	0	0	—	—	1240
HACKENSACK—Bergen County										
★ HACKENSACK MEDICAL CENTER, (Includes Hasbrouck Heights Facilities Clinic, 214 Terrace Avenue, Hasbrouck Heights, New Jersey, Zip 07604; tel. 201/393–7474) 30 Prospect Avenue, Zip 07601–1991; tel. 201/996–2002; John P. Ferguson, President and Chief Executive Officer **A**1 2 3 5 8 9 10 **F**3 4 5 7 8 9 10 11 13 14 15 16 17 18 19 20 21 23 24 25 26 27 28 29 30 31 32 33 34 35 36 37 38 39 40 41 42 43 44 45 46 47 49 51 52 53 54 55 56 57 58 59 60 61 63 65 66 67 68 69 70 71 72 73 74 **P**1 5	23	10	566	35231	488	778245	2965	294178	144310	3738
HACKETTSTOWN—Warren County										
★ HACKETTSTOWN COMMUNITY HOSPITAL, 651 Willow Grove Street, Zip 07840–1798; tel. 908/852–5100; Gene C. Milton, President and Chief Executive Officer **A**1 2 9 10 **F**3 7 8 12 15 16 19 20 22 28 30 32 34 35 36 37 39 40 41 42 44 45 46 49 65 67 71 73	21	10	106	4016	57	36667	520	25183	11677	377
HAMILTON—Mercer County										
☐ ROBERT WOOD JOHNSON UNIVERSITY HOSPITAL AT HAMILTON, (Formerly Hamilton Hospital) One Hamilton Health Place, Zip 08690; tel. 609/586–7900; W. Michael Bryant, President and Chief Executive Officer **A**1 9 10 **F**1 3 8 11 12 14 15 16 17 19 20 21 22 26 27 28 29 30 31 32 33 34 35 36 37 39 41 42 44 45 46 49 51 63 65 67 71 72 73 **P**1 3	23	10	166	5631	113	50143	0	36295	15728	498
HAMMONTON—Atlantic County										
☐ ANCORA PSYCHIATRIC HOSPITAL, 202 Spring Garden Road, Zip 08037–9699; tel. 609/561–1700; William J. Camarota, Chief Executive Officer (Nonreporting) **A**1 10 **S**0010 Division of Mental Health Services, Department of Human Services, State of New Jersey	12	22	626	—	—	—	—	—	—	—
★ WILLIAM B. KESSLER MEMORIAL HOSPITAL, 600 South White Horse Pike, Zip 08037–2099; tel. 609/561–6700; Warren E. Gager, Chief Executive Officer **A**1 9 10 **F**8 11 14 15 16 19 20 21 22 28 30 32 34 37 41 44 45 46 63 65 67 71 73 **P**6	23	10	130	3403	71	62768	0	30814	15316	466
HOBOKEN—Hudson County										
★ ST. MARY HOSPITAL, 308 Willow Avenue, Zip 07030–3889; tel. 201/418–1000; Ulrich J. Rosa, President and Chief Executive Officer **A**1 3 9 10 **F**3 4 7 8 11 12 13 15 16 17 18 19 20 21 23 26 27 28 30 31 34 35 37 39 40 41 42 44 45 46 49 51 52 53 54 55 56 57 58 59 60 61 65 67 68 69 70 71 73 **P**8 **S**1485 Franciscan Sisters of the Poor Health System, Inc.	23	10	328	9299	206	78713	1155	77912	33931	1093

Hospitals, U.S. / NEW JERSEY

Hospital, Address, Telephone, Administrator, Approval, Facility, and Physician Codes, Health Care System	Classification Codes		Utilization Data					Expense (thousands) of dollars		
★ American Hospital Association (AHA) membership □ Joint Commission on Accreditation of Healthcare Organizations (JCAHO) accreditation + American Osteopathic Hospital Association (AOHA) membership ○ American Osteopathic Association (AOA) accreditation △ Commission on Accreditation of Rehabilitation Facilities (CARF) accreditation Control codes 61, 63, 64, 71, 72 and 73 indicate hospitals listed by AOHA, but not registered by AHA. For definition of numerical codes, see page A6	Control	Service	Beds	Admissions	Census	Outpatient Visits	Births	Total	Payroll	Personnel
HOLMDEL—Monmouth County										
★ BAYSHORE COMMUNITY HOSPITAL, 727 North Beers Street, Zip 07733; tel. 908/739–5900; Thomas Goldman, President **A**1 9 10 **F**1 3 4 6 7 8 10 11 12 13 14 15 16 17 18 19 20 21 22 23 24 25 26 27 28 29 30 31 32 33 34 35 36 37 39 41 42 43 44 45 46 49 50 51 52 53 54 55 56 57 58 59 60 61 63 65 66 67 68 69 70 71 72 73 74 **P**5 7	23	10	225	7273	182	68497	0	54354	26218	662
IRVINGTON—Essex County										
□ IRVINGTON GENERAL HOSPITAL, 832 Chancellor Avenue, Zip 07111–0709; tel. 201/399–6006; Gerry Goodrich, President and Chief Executive Officer (Nonreporting) **A**1 9 10	23	10	157	—	—	—	—	—	—	—
JERSEY CITY—Hudson County										
★ CHRIST HOSPITAL, 176 Palisade Avenue, Zip 07306–1196, Mailing Address: P.O. Box BX J–1, Zip 07306–1196; tel. 201/795–8400; Paul A. Hoyt, President and Chief Executive Officer **A**1 2 6 9 10 **F**2 3 7 11 12 15 17 20 21 22 26 27 30 31 32 33 37 40 41 42 44 46 49 51 52 53 54 55 56 57 58 59 60 63 65 67 71 73 74 **P**5 8	23	10	402	15930	305	411947	1096	105707	57866	1148
□ GREENVILLE HOSPITAL, 1825 Kennedy Boulevard, Zip 07305; tel. 201/547–6100; Jonathan M. Metsch Dr.P.H., President and Chief Executive Officer **A**1 9 10 **F**2 3 4 7 8 10 11 12 13 15 16 17 18 19 20 21 22 25 26 27 28 30 31 34 35 37 38 40 41 42 44 46 47 49 52 53 54 55 56 57 58 61 63 65 66 67 68 70 71 73 74 **P**3 6	23	10	86	2873	70	16997	0	19099	9378	266
★ JERSEY CITY MEDICAL CENTER, 50 Baldwin Avenue, Zip 07304–3199; tel. 201/915–2000; Jonathan M. Metsch Dr.P.H., President and Chief Executive Officer **A**1 3 5 9 10 **F**3 9 10 11 16 20 22 26 28 34 37 38 40 44 46 47 52 53 56 58 59 65 70 **P**6	23	10	487	18522	362	234003	2878	192479	89926	2275
★ ST. FRANCIS HOSPITAL, 25 McWilliams Place, Zip 07302–1698; tel. 201/418–1000; Ulrich J. Rosa, President and Chief Executive Officer **A**1 6 9 10 **F**3 4 8 11 12 15 16 17 18 19 20 21 22 23 24 26 27 28 31 32 35 37 41 42 43 44 45 46 49 51 52 53 54 55 56 57 58 59 60 61 65 67 68 69 70 71 73 **P**8 **S**1485 Franciscan Sisters of the Poor Health System, Inc.	23	10	243	5964	153	33340	0	54951	24616	738
KEARNY—Hudson County										
★ WEST HUDSON HOSPITAL, 206 Bergen Avenue, Zip 07032; tel. 201/955–7051; Carmen Bruce Alecci, Chief Executive Officer (Nonreporting) **A**1 9 10	23	10	214	—	—	—	—	—	—	—
LAKEWOOD—Ocean County										
★ KIMBALL MEDICAL CENTER, 600 River Avenue, Zip 08701–5281; tel. 908/363–1900; Angela Melillo, Chief Operating Officer **A**1 9 10 **F**1 2 3 7 8 10 11 12 13 14 15 16 17 18 19 20 21 22 24 25 26 27 28 29 30 31 32 34 35 37 38 39 40 41 42 44 45 46 49 51 52 53 54 55 56 57 58 60 63 64 65 67 68 71 72 73 74 **P**5 6 7 8	23	10	352	11417	230	98510	875	94351	47276	1506
LAWRENCEVILLE—Mercer County										
★ △ ST. LAWRENCE REHABILITATION CENTER, 2381 Lawrenceville Road, Zip 08648; tel. 609/896–9500; Charles L. Brennan, Chief Executive Officer (Nonreporting) **A**1 7 10	21	46	116	—	—	—	—	—	—	—
LIVINGSTON—Essex County										
★ SAINT BARNABAS MEDICAL CENTER, 94 Old Short Hills Road, Zip 07039; tel. 201/533–5000; Ronald Del Mauro, Chairman and Chief Executive Officer **A**1 2 3 5 8 9 10 **F**1 2 3 4 5 7 8 9 10 11 12 13 14 15 16 17 18 19 20 21 22 23 25 26 27 28 30 31 32 33 34 35 36 37 38 39 40 41 42 44 45 46 47 49 50 51 52 56 57 58 60 61 63 64 65 66 67 68 69 70 71 72 73 74 **P**4 5 8	23	10	594	32087	451	200000	5352	245731	101927	2347
LONG BRANCH—Monmouth County										
★ MONMOUTH MEDICAL CENTER, 300 Second Avenue, Zip 07740–6303; tel. 908/222–5200; Christopher M. Dadlez, President and Chief Executive Officer **A**1 2 3 5 8 9 10 **F**1 3 7 8 11 12 15 16 17 19 20 21 22 26 27 29 30 31 37 38 39 40 41 42 44 45 46 49 52 53 54 55 56 57 58 59 60 61 65 67 71 72 73 74 **P**5 7 8	23	10	433	16156	303	259481	3432	163882	80080	2178
LYONS—Somerset County										
★ VETERANS AFFAIRS MEDICAL CENTER, 151 Knollcroft Road, Zip 07939–9998; tel. 908/647–0180; A. Paul Kidd FACHE, Director (Total facility includes 240 beds in nursing home–type unit) **A**1 3 5 9 **F**1 3 8 12 19 20 22 26 28 30 31 34 35 37 39 41 42 44 45 46 48 49 51 52 54 55 56 57 58 60 63 64 65 67 71 73 74 **S**9295 Department of Veterans Affairs	45	22	937	3192	843	73689	0	—	—	1722
MANAHAWKIN—Ocean County										
□ SOUTHERN OCEAN COUNTY HOSPITAL, 1140 Route 72 West; Zip 08050; tel. 609/597–6011; Steven G. Littleson, President and Chief Executive Officer **A**1 9 10 **F**3 8 13 14 15 17 19 21 22 25 28 29 30 32 33 34 37 42 44 45 46 49 56 63 65 66 67 71 73 **P**5 8	23	10	134	4720	92	54067	0	33226	15034	519
MARLBORO—Monmouth County										
★ MARLBORO PSYCHIATRIC HOSPITAL, 546 County Road 520, Zip 07746–1099; tel. 908/946–8100; Michael Ross Ph.D., Chief Executive Officer **A**1 9 10 **F**19 20 21 35 46 50 52 54 56 57 59 63 65 71 73 **S**0010 Division of Mental Health Services, Department of Human Services, State of New Jersey	12	22	869	1693	766	0	0	56576	—	1298
MARLTON—Burlington County										
★ WEST JERSEY HOSPITAL–MARLTON, Route 73 and Brick Road, Zip 08053; tel. 609/596–3500; Kevin M. Manley, Executive Director **A**1 9 10 **F**2 5 8 15 17 19 21 22 26 28 29 30 32 35 37 39 42 44 45 46 49 60 65 67 71 73 **P**3 4 7 **S**6725 West Jersey Health System	23	10	202	13096	149	33227	0	—	—	746
MILLVILLE—Cumberland County										
MILLVILLE DIVISION See South Jersey Hospital System, Bridgeton										

Hospitals, U.S. / NEW JERSEY

Hospital, Address, Telephone, Administrator, Approval, Facility, and Physician Codes, Health Care System	Classification Codes		Utilization Data					Expense (thousands) of dollars		
★ American Hospital Association (AHA) membership ☐ Joint Commission on Accreditation of Healthcare Organizations (JCAHO) accreditation + American Osteopathic Hospital Association (AOHA) membership ○ American Osteopathic Association (AOA) accreditation △ Commission on Accreditation of Rehabilitation Facilities (CARF) accreditation Control codes 61, 63, 64, 71, 72 and 73 indicate hospitals listed by AOHA, but not registered by AHA. For definition of numerical codes, see page A6	Control	Service	Beds	Admissions	Census	Outpatient Visits	Births	Total	Payroll	Personnel

MONTCLAIR—Essex County
★ MONTCLAIR COMMUNITY HOSPITAL, 120 Harrison Avenue, Zip 07042–2498; tel. 201/744–7300; Emilie M. Murphy R.N., Director **A**1 9 10 **F**2 3 11 19 21 22 28 30 33 37 41 44 45 46 48 49 52 53 54 55 56 57 58 59 65 66 71 73 — 23 10 100 2562 41 9412 0 16072 9024 244

★ MOUNTAINSIDE HOSPITAL, Bay and Highland Avenues, Zip 07042–4898; tel. 201/429–6000; Robert A. Silver, President and Chief Executive Officer **A**1 2 3 5 6 9 10 **F**3 7 8 10 11 12 13 15 16 17 18 19 20 21 22 24 26 30 31 32 33 34 35 37 39 40 41 42 44 46 49 52 54 55 56 57 58 59 60 61 63 65 66 67 71 73 74 **P**3 8 — 23 10 396 12541 241 91439 947 111015 55229 1502

MORRISTOWN—Morris County
★ MORRISTOWN MEMORIAL HOSPITAL, (Includes Rehabilitation Institute at the Mount Kemble Division) 100 Madison Avenue, Zip 07962–1956; tel. 201/971–5000; Richard P. Oths, President and Chief Executive Officer **A**1 2 3 5 8 9 10 **F**2 3 4 7 8 10 11 12 13 15 16 17 19 20 21 22 26 27 28 29 30 31 32 33 34 35 36 37 38 39 40 41 42 43 44 45 46 48 49 51 52 53 54 55 56 58 59 60 63 64 65 67 68 70 71 73 **P**6 8 — 23 10 637 23820 463 233907 3366 249528 117574 2466

MOUNT HOLLY—Burlington County
★ MEMORIAL HOSPITAL OF BURLINGTON COUNTY, 175 Madison Avenue, Zip 08060–2099; tel. 609/261–7011; Chester B. Kaletkowski, President and Chief Executive Officer **A**1 2 3 5 9 10 **F**1 3 5 7 8 11 12 15 18 19 21 22 23 25 26 28 30 31 32 33 35 36 37 40 41 42 44 45 46 49 52 54 55 56 57 58 60 61 65 67 69 71 73 74 **P**2 4 5 7 8 — 23 10 346 15743 247 107966 1735 104349 49490 1639

MOUNTAINSIDE—Union County
★ △ CHILDREN'S SPECIALIZED HOSPITAL, (Includes Children's Specialized Hospital, 94 Stevens Rd., Tom River, New Jersey, Zip 08755; tel. 908/914–1100) 150 New Providence Road, Zip 07091–2590; tel. 908/233–3720; Richard B. Ahlfeld, President (Total facility includes 39 beds in nursing home–type unit) **A**1 7 10 **F**12 15 17 20 25 27 28 29 30 34 39 45 46 48 49 54 64 65 67 73 **P**6 — 23 56 115 356 92 94013 0 33428 18902 496

NEPTUNE—Monmouth County
★ JERSEY SHORE MEDICAL CENTER, 1945 Route 33, Zip 07754–0397; tel. 908/775–5500; John K. Lloyd, President **A**1 2 3 5 6 8 9 10 **F**3 4 7 8 10 11 12 15 16 18 19 20 21 22 24 25 30 31 32 33 34 35 37 38 40 41 42 43 44 46 47 49 51 52 53 54 55 56 57 58 59 60 61 63 65 66 67 70 71 73 **P**7 8 — 23 10 492 18148 375 229899 1559 179177 87865 2085

NEW BRUNSWICK—Middlesex County
HURTADO HEALTH CENTER, 11 Bishop Place, Zip 08903–5069; tel. 908/932–7401; Robert H. Bierman M.D., Director (Nonreporting) — 12 11 27 — — — — — — —

★ ROBERT WOOD JOHNSON UNIVERSITY HOSPITAL, 1 Robert Wood Johnson Place, Zip 08903–2601; tel. 908/828–3000; Harvey A. Holzberg, President and Chief Executive Officer **A**1 2 3 5 8 9 10 **F**4 7 8 10 11 12 15 16 17 19 20 21 22 23 24 25 26 28 29 30 31 32 33 34 35 37 40 41 42 43 44 45 46 47 49 51 61 65 67 70 71 72 73 74 **P**5 8 — 23 10 409 16585 328 127498 1188 197495 85084 2415

★ ST. PETER'S MEDICAL CENTER, 254 Easton Avenue, Zip 08901, Mailing Address: P.O. Box 591, Zip 08903–0591; tel. 908/745–8600; John E. Matuska, President and Chief Executive Officer **A**1 2 3 5 9 10 **F**1 2 3 7 8 10 11 12 13 14 15 16 17 19 20 21 22 23 26 28 30 31 32 33 34 35 36 37 38 39 40 41 42 44 45 46 48 49 51 52 53 54 56 57 58 60 61 63 64 65 66 67 68 71 73 74 **P**7 — 23 10 416 29843 378 122241 6577 167839 79139 2208

NEWARK—Essex County
☐ COLUMBUS HOSPITAL, 495 North 13th Street, Zip 07107–1397; tel. 201/268–1400; John G. Magliaro, Administrator **A**1 9 10 **F**7 8 12 14 15 19 21 22 28 29 30 31 35 37 39 40 41 42 44 46 49 51 60 61 67 71 73 74 **P**1 — 23 10 190 7054 140 46011 1022 50563 27012 736

★ ○ NEWARK BETH ISRAEL MEDICAL CENTER, 201 Lyons Avenue, Zip 07112–2027; tel. 201/926–7000; Lester M. Bornstein, President **A**1 2 3 5 8 9 10 11 **F**1 4 7 8 10 11 12 13 17 19 20 21 22 25 26 30 31 33 34 35 37 38 39 40 42 43 44 46 47 49 51 52 53 54 55 56 58 59 60 61 65 67 69 71 72 73 74 **P**4 5 6 8 — 23 10 558 20263 452 314671 2492 207574 106262 2944

NEWARK EYE AND EAR INFIRMARY See United Hospitals Medical Center
ORTHOPEDIC UNIT See United Hospitals Medical Center
PRESBYTERIAN UNIT See United Hospitals Medical Center

★ SAINT JAMES HOSPITAL OF NEWARK, 155 Jefferson Street, Zip 07105; tel. 201/589–1300; Dominick R. Calgi, Administrator **A**1 3 9 10 **F**2 4 7 8 9 10 16 17 18 19 20 21 22 23 25 26 27 28 29 30 31 32 33 34 35 37 38 39 40 41 42 43 44 45 46 47 48 49 54 60 64 65 66 67 69 70 71 73 74 **S**6545 Cathedral Healthcare System, Inc. — 21 10 189 5007 108 23622 510 169518 83381 419

★ SAINT MICHAEL'S MEDICAL CENTER, 268 Dr. Martin Luther King Jr. Boulevard, Zip 07102–2094; tel. 201/877–5000; Dominick R. Calgi, Administrator **A**1 3 5 9 10 12 **F**4 7 8 10 11 13 14 17 19 21 22 30 31 34 35 37 38 39 40 41 42 43 44 46 48 49 50 63 65 66 71 73 74 **P**5 **S**6545 Cathedral Healthcare System, Inc. — 21 10 419 10475 244 71864 1040 169518 83381 1968

☐ UNITED HOSPITALS MEDICAL CENTER, (Includes Children's Hospital of New Jersey; Newark Eye and Ear Infirmary; Orthopedic Unit; Presbyterian Unit) 15 S. Ninth St., Zip 07107; tel. 201/268–8000; John Dandridge Jr., President **A**1 3 5 9 10 — — — — 9756 — — — — — —

★ UNIVERSITY OF MEDICINE AND DENTISTRY OF NEW JERSEY–UNIVERSITY HOSPITAL, 150 Bergen Street, Zip 07103–2406; tel. 201/982–4300; William L. Vazquez, Vice President and Chief Executive Officer **A**1 2 3 5 8 9 10 **F**3 4 7 8 10 11 12 15 16 17 19 20 21 22 23 24 26 27 28 30 31 33 34 35 37 38 39 40 41 42 43 44 46 47 49 51 52 53 54 56 58 59 60 61 65 66 67 68 69 70 71 73 74 **P**7 — 12 10 518 17485 404 252167 2744 329824 181570 3182

Hospitals, U.S. / NEW JERSEY

Hospital, Address, Telephone, Administrator, Approval, Facility, and Physician Codes, Health Care System	Classification Codes		Utilization Data					Expense (thousands) of dollars		Personnel
★ American Hospital Association (AHA) membership □ Joint Commission on Accreditation of Healthcare Organizations (JCAHO) accreditation + American Osteopathic Hospital Association (AOHA) membership ○ American Osteopathic Association (AOA) accreditation △ Commission on Accreditation of Rehabilitation Facilities (CARF) accreditation Control codes 61, 63, 64, 71, 72 and 73 indicate hospitals listed by AOHA, but not registered by AHA. For definition of numerical codes, see page A6	Control	Service	Beds	Admissions	Census	Outpatient Visits	Births	Total	Payroll	
NEWTON—Sussex County										
★ △ NEWTON MEMORIAL HOSPITAL, 175 High Street, Zip 07860–1004; tel. 201/383–2121; Dennis H. Collette, President and Chief Executive Officer **A**1 2 7 9 10 **F**2 3 8 11 12 14 15 16 17 18 19 21 22 30 31 34 35 37 39 40 41 42 44 45 46 48 49 52 53 54 55 56 57 58 59 63 65 67 71 73	23	10	165	8349	103	140810	962	45788	22005	592
NORTH BERGEN—Hudson County										
★ PALISADES GENERAL HOSPITAL, 7600 River Road, Zip 07047–6217; tel. 201/854–5000; Bruce J. Markowitz, President and Chief Executive Officer **A**1 9 10 **F**3 7 8 15 16 17 19 22 28 30 34 37 39 40 42 44 45 49 56 58 65 71 73 74 **P**5	23	10	202	7185	165	40308	1262	56507	25958	607
OLD BRIDGE—Middlesex County										
OLD BRIDGE DIVISION See Raritan Bay Medical Center, Perth Amboy										
ORANGE—Essex County										
★ HOSPITAL CENTER AT ORANGE, (Includes New Jersey Orthopedic Hospital Unit, Orange, New Jersey; Orange Memorial Hospital Unit, Orange, New Jersey) 188 South Essex Avenue, Zip 07051; tel. 201/266–2200; Ronald Wayne Weitz, Chief Executive Officer **A**1 2 3 5 6 9 10 **F**1 3 7 8 11 12 14 15 16 17 18 19 20 21 22 23 25 26 27 28 30 31 32 33 34 35 36 37 39 40 41 42 44 45 46 49 53 54 55 56 57 58 59 60 63 65 66 67 71 72 73 74 **P**3 5	23	10	290	10905	220	117000	484	83835	39230	999
PARAMUS—Bergen County										
★ BERGEN PINES COUNTY HOSPITAL, 230 East Ridgewood Avenue, Zip 07652–4131; tel. 201/967–4000; Edward M. Lewis, Chief Executive Officer (Total facility includes 610 beds in nursing home–type unit) **A**1 3 5 6 9 10 **F**1 3 12 14 15 16 17 18 19 20 21 22 25 26 27 28 30 34 37 39 41 44 49 52 53 54 55 56 57 58 59 64 65 67 71 73 74 **P**6	13	10	1075	8372	965	46466	0	103655	69943	1949
PASSAIC—Passaic County										
★ BETH ISRAEL HOSPITAL, 70 Parker Avenue, Zip 07055; tel. 201/365–5000; Jeffrey S. Moll, President and Chief Executive Officer **A**1 2 9 10 **F**3 15 17 19 21 22 26 31 32 33 34 36 37 41 42 44 45 46 49 60 61 63 65 71 73 74	23	10	223	6213	132	233528	0	49595	25322	832
★ GENERAL HOSPITAL CENTER AT PASSAIC, 350 Boulevard, Zip 07055–2800; tel. 201/365–4300; Daniel L. Marcantuono FACHE, President and Chief Executive Officer **A**1 2 9 10 **F**4 7 8 10 12 13 14 17 19 21 22 23 24 27 28 30 31 32 34 35 37 39 40 41 42 43 44 46 49 65 67 71 73 **P**7	23	10	303	15159	235	73890	1500	103546	50455	1282
★ ST. MARY'S HOSPITAL, 211 Pennington Avenue, Zip 07055; tel. 201/470–3000; Patricia Peterson, President and Chief Executive Officer **A**1 9 10 **F**4 7 8 11 12 13 15 16 17 18 19 21 22 26 27 28 29 30 31 32 34 35 37 40 42 44 45 49 51 52 53 54 55 56 57 58 59 60 61 65 67 68 69 71 73 74 **P**4 5	21	10	229	5262	126	60654	709	48475	23708	764
PATERSON—Passaic County										
★ BARNERT HOSPITAL, 680 Broadway, Zip 07514; tel. 201/977–6600; Fred L. Lang, President and Chief Executive Officer **A**1 9 10 **F**1 3 7 8 11 14 15 16 17 19 21 22 24 26 30 31 34 35 36 37 40 41 42 44 45 46 49 52 63 65 71 73 **P**5 8	23	10	256	9676	207	111002	1174	65537	32755	886
★ ST. JOSEPH'S HOSPITAL AND MEDICAL CENTER, 703 Main Street, Zip 07503–2691; tel. 201/754–2100; Sister Jane Frances Brady, President (Total facility includes 141 beds in nursing home–type unit) **A**1 2 3 5 8 9 10 **F**1 3 4 5 7 8 9 10 11 12 13 14 15 16 17 18 19 20 21 22 24 25 26 27 28 29 30 31 32 33 34 35 36 37 38 39 40 41 42 43 44 45 46 47 49 50 51 52 53 54 55 56 57 58 59 60 61 63 64 65 66 67 69 70 71 72 73 74 **P**1 3 5	21	10	792	22240	497	315607	2611	250092	131991	3286
PEAPACK—Somerset County										
★ △ MATHENY SCHOOL AND HOSPITAL, (Children's Cerebral Palsy) Main Street, Zip 07977; tel. 908/234–0011; Robert Schonhorn, President **A**7 10 **F**41 64 65 73	23	59	93	12	83	0	0	12158	7363	266
PERTH AMBOY—Middlesex County										
★ RARITAN BAY MEDICAL CENTER, (Includes Old Bridge Division, One Hospital Plaza, Old Bridge, New Jersey, Zip 08857; tel. 908/360–1000; Perth Amboy Division, Perth Amboy, New Jersey) 530 New Brunswick Avenue, Zip 08861; tel. 908/442–3700; Keith H. McLaughlin, President and Chief Executive Officer **A**1 3 5 6 9 10 **F**2 3 6 7 8 11 12 14 15 16 17 18 19 21 22 23 27 28 29 30 31 32 33 34 35 36 37 39 40 41 42 44 49 52 54 55 56 58 63 65 67 68 71 73 **P**1 5	23	10	461	15058	349	194684	1075	129747	69154	1747
PHILLIPSBURG—Warren County										
★ WARREN HOSPITAL, 185 Roseberry Street, Zip 08865–9955; tel. 908/859–6700; John A. DeMarrais, President and Chief Executive Officer **A**1 2 3 5 9 10 12 13 **F**1 2 3 4 7 8 9 10 11 12 14 15 16 17 18 19 20 21 22 25 26 27 29 30 31 32 33 34 35 36 37 38 39 40 41 42 43 44 45 46 47 48 49 51 52 53 54 56 57 58 59 60 64 65 67 69 70 71 73 **P**5	23	10	214	8270	150	45240	401	51049	24953	800
PISCATAWAY—Middlesex County										
UNIVERSITY OF MEDICINE AND DENTISTRY OF NEW JERSEY, COMMUNITY MENTAL HEALTH CENTER AT PISCATWAY, 671 Hoes Lane, Zip 08854–5633, Mailing Address: P.O. Box 1392, Zip 08855–1392; tel. 908/235–5500; Gary W. Lamson, Vice President and Chef Executive Officer Mental Health Services (Nonreporting) **A**3 5 10	12	22	64	—	—	—	—	—	—	—
PLAINFIELD—Union County										
★ MUHLENBERG REGIONAL MEDICAL CENTER, Park Avenue and Randolph Road, Zip 07061; tel. 908/668–2000; John R. Kopicki, President and Chief Executive Officer **A**1 3 5 6 9 10 **F**1 3 7 8 10 11 12 16 17 19 22 25 26 28 29 30 31 32 33 34 35 37 39 40 41 42 44 45 46 49 50 51 52 53 55 56 57 58 59 63 65 67 70 71 72 73 74 **P**5 7 8	23	10	328	14129	254	189046	2024	113070	57044	1693

© 1995 AHA Guide

Hospitals, U.S. / NEW JERSEY

Hospital, Address, Telephone, Administrator, Approval, Facility, and Physician Codes, Health Care System	Classification Codes		Utilization Data					Expense (thousands) of dollars		
★ American Hospital Association (AHA) membership ☐ Joint Commission on Accreditation of Healthcare Organizations (JCAHO) accreditation + American Osteopathic Hospital Association (AOHA) membership ○ American Osteopathic Association (AOA) accreditation △ Commission on Accreditation of Rehabilitation Facilities (CARF) accreditation Control codes 61, 63, 64, 71, 72 and 73 indicate hospitals listed by AOHA, but not registered by AHA. For definition of numerical codes, see page A6	Control	Service	Beds	Admissions	Census	Outpatient Visits	Births	Total	Payroll	Personnel
POINT PLEASANT—Ocean County ★ MEDICAL CENTER OF OCEAN COUNTY, (Includes Brick Hospital Division, 425 Jack Martin Boulevard, Brick Township, New Jersey, Zip 08724; tel. 908/840–2200; Point Pleasant Hospital Division, 2121 Edgewater Place, Point Pleasant, New Jersey, Zip 08742; tel. 908/892–1100) 2121 Edgewater Place, Zip 08742–2290; tel. 908/892–1100; John T. Gribbin, President and Chief Executive Officer **A**1 2 9 10 **F**1 3 5 7 8 11 12 13 14 15 16 17 18 19 21 22 24 25 26 27 28 29 30 31 32 33 34 35 36 37 38 39 40 41 42 44 45 46 49 54 55 57 58 60 61 63 65 66 67 68 71 73 74 **P**1 4 5 7 POINT PLEASANT HOSPITAL DIVISION See Medical Center of Ocean County	23	10	357	15323	279	103109	1494	115294	52845	1754
POMONA—Atlantic County ★ △ BETTY BACHARACH REHABILITATION HOSPITAL, 61 West Jim Leeds Road, Zip 08240–0723; tel. 609/652–7000; Richard J. Kathrins, Administrator **A**1 7 10 **F**5 12 15 16 20 25 28 30 34 45 46 48 49 65 66 67 73	23	46	80	1340	73	34070	0	19400	11918	352
POMPTON PLAINS—Morris County ★ CHILTON MEMORIAL HOSPITAL, 97 West Parkway, Zip 07444–1696; tel. 201/831–5000; James J. Doyle Jr., President and Chief Executive Officer **A**1 9 10 **F**7 8 12 13 15 16 17 19 20 21 22 25 26 27 28 29 30 31 32 33 34 35 37 38 39 40 41 42 44 45 47 49 51 52 55 56 57 60 63 65 66 67 69 70 71 72 73 **P**7 8	23	10	270	13922	168	75923	1519	68895	34242	927
PRINCETON—Mercer County ★ MEDICAL CENTER AT PRINCETON, (Includes Acute General Hospital, Merwick Unit–Extended Care and Rehabilitation, Princeton House Unit–Community Mental Health and Substance Abuse) 253 Witherspoon Street, Zip 08540–3213; tel. 609/497–4000; Dennis W. Doody, President and Chief Executive Officer (Total facility includes 93 beds in nursing home–type unit) **A**1 2 3 5 9 10 **F**2 3 7 8 10 11 12 15 18 19 20 21 22 26 28 29 30 31 32 33 34 35 37 39 40 41 42 44 48 49 52 54 55 56 57 58 59 60 63 64 65 71 73 **P**7 8	23	10	457	14934	331	121514	1709	108418	52726	1406
PRINCETON UNIVERSITY HEALTH SERVICES, MCCOSH HEALTH CENTER, Washington Road, Zip 08544–1004; tel. 609/258–3129; Pamela Bowen, Director (Nonreporting)	23	11	21	—	—	—	—	—	—	—
RAHWAY—Union County ★ RAHWAY HOSPITAL, 865 Stone Street, Zip 07065; tel. 908/381–4200; Kirk C. Tice, President (Total facility includes 16 beds in nursing home–type unit) **A**1 9 10 **F**7 8 11 12 14 15 16 17 18 19 20 21 22 23 26 27 28 29 30 33 34 35 37 39 40 41 42 44 45 46 49 51 54 55 56 57 58 59 60 64 65 67 68 71 72 73 74 **P**5 8	23	10	305	14133	249	59830	999	80915	38955	1030
RED BANK—Monmouth County ★ △ RIVERVIEW MEDICAL CENTER, 1 Riverview Plaza, Zip 07701–9982; tel. 908/741–2700; Laurence M. Merlis, President and Chief Executive Officer **A**1 2 7 9 10 **F**2 3 7 8 11 12 14 15 16 17 18 19 21 22 26 27 28 29 30 31 33 34 37 39 40 41 43 44 46 48 49 51 52 54 55 56 58 59 60 61 63 65 67 71 73 74 **P**5	23	10	420	15020	292	113587	2435	114864	53297	1713
RIDGEWOOD—Bergen County ★ VALLEY HOSPITAL, 223 North Van Dien Avenue, Zip 07450–9982; tel. 201/447–8000; Michael W. Azzara, President **A**1 2 9 10 **F**2 3 4 7 8 10 11 12 15 16 17 19 20 21 22 26 28 29 30 31 32 33 34 35 37 38 39 40 41 42 43 44 45 46 49 51 52 53 54 55 56 57 58 59 60 61 63 65 66 67 68 71 73 74 **P**1 5	23	10	421	33412	397	133514	3235	165234	86097	2061
RIVERSIDE—Burlington County ☐ ZURBRUGG MEMORIAL HOSPITAL, Hospital Plaza, Zip 08075; tel. 609/461–6700; Garry L. Scheib, President **A**1 9 10 **F**1 8 15 16 17 19 20 21 22 26 28 29 30 32 33 35 37 39 41 42 44 59 63 65 67 71 73 74 **S**0006 Graduate Health System	23	10	54	1888	44	54857	0	20760	9433	358
SALEM—Salem County ★ MEMORIAL HOSPITAL OF SALEM COUNTY, Salem Woodstown Road, Zip 08079–2080; tel. 609/935–1000; Joseph Michael Galvin Jr., President and Chief Executive Officer **A**1 2 9 10 **F**3 7 8 10 12 14 16 25 26 28 29 30 31 32 33 35 36 37 39 40 42 44 45 46 49 53 54 55 56 57 58 59 60 65 66 71 73	23	10	152	5845	88	75007	496	48487	23358	720
SECAUCUS—Hudson County ★ MEADOWLANDS HOSPITAL MEDICAL CENTER, Meadowland Parkway, Zip 07096–1580; tel. 201/392–3100; Paul V. Cavalli M.D., President (Nonreporting) **A**1 9 10	23	10	200	—	—	—	—	—	—	—
SOMERS POINT—Atlantic County ★ SHORE MEMORIAL HOSPITAL, 1 East New York Avenue, Zip 08244–2387; tel. 609/653–3500; Richard A. Pitman, President **A**1 2 9 10 **F**1 2 7 8 12 15 16 19 21 26 28 29 30 31 32 33 34 35 37 39 40 42 44 45 46 60 63 65 67 71 73 74	23	10	268	11973	219	72620	1244	90492	42118	1277
SOMERVILLE—Somerset County ★ SOMERSET MEDICAL CENTER, 110 Rehill Avenue, Zip 08876–2598; tel. 908/685–2200; William J. Monagle, President and Chief Executive Officer **A**1 2 3 5 9 10 **F**3 4 7 8 11 12 14 15 16 17 19 21 22 26 28 29 30 31 33 34 35 37 39 40 41 42 44 46 49 50 51 52 57 58 59 63 65 67 71 73 74 **P**5	23	10	312	11771	210	121316	647	91069	46538	1304
SOUTH AMBOY—Middlesex County ★ MEMORIAL MEDICAL CENTER AT SOUTH AMBOY, (Formerly South Amboy Memorial Hospital) 540 Bordentown Avenue, Zip 08879; tel. 908/721–1000; Irv J. Diamond, Chief Executive Officer **A**1 9 10 **F**3 8 12 16 17 18 19 20 21 22 28 29 30 35 36 37 42 44 46 49 52 53 54 55 56 57 58 59 65 67 71 73	23	10	161	3970	108	61824	0	33541	18300	557
STRATFORD—Camden County STRATFORD DIVISION See Kennedy Memorial Hospital, University Medical Center, Cherry Hill										

Hospitals, U.S. / NEW JERSEY

Hospital, Address, Telephone, Administrator, Approval, Facility, and Physician Codes, Health Care System	Classification Codes		Utilization Data					Expense (thousands) of dollars		
	Control	Service	Beds	Admissions	Census	Outpatient Visits	Births	Total	Payroll	Personnel

★ American Hospital Association (AHA) membership
☐ Joint Commission on Accreditation of Healthcare Organizations (JCAHO) accreditation
+ American Osteopathic Hospital Association (AOHA) membership
○ American Osteopathic Association (AOA) accreditation
△ Commission on Accreditation of Rehabilitation Facilities (CARF) accreditation
Control codes 61, 63, 64, 71, 72 and 73 indicate hospitals listed by AOHA, but not registered by AHA. For definition of numerical codes, see page A6

Hospital	Control	Service	Beds	Admissions	Census	Outpatient Visits	Births	Total	Payroll	Personnel
SUMMIT—Union County										
☐ CHARTER BEHAVIORAL HEALTH SYSTEM OF NEW JERSEY–SUMMIT, (Formerly Fair Oaks Hospital) 19 Prospect Street, Zip 07902–0100; tel. 908/522–7000 **A**1 9 10 **F**2 3 18 25 26 34 52 53 54 55 56 57 58 59 65 **P**1 **S**0695 Charter Medical Corporation	33	22	80	1712	65	15000	0	2675	1914	—
FAIR OAKS HOSPITAL See Charter Behavioral Health System of New Jersey–Summit										
★ OVERLOOK HOSPITAL, 99 Beauvoir Avenue, Zip 07902–0220; tel. 908/522–2000; Michael J. Sniffen, President and Chief Executive Officer (Total facility includes 410 beds in nursing home–type unit) **A**1 2 3 5 8 9 10 **F**1 3 4 5 6 7 8 10 11 12 13 14 15 16 17 18 19 20 21 22 23 24 25 26 28 29 30 31 32 33 34 35 36 37 38 39 40 41 42 43 44 45 46 49 50 51 52 53 54 55 56 57 58 59 60 61 63 65 67 68 69 71 72 73 74 **P**6 8	23	10	464	18495	332	375715	2775	188834	95486	2654
SUSSEX—Sussex County										
ST. CLARES–RIVERSIDE MEDICAL CENTER–SUSSEX CAMPUS See Northwest Covenant Medical Center, Denville										
TEANECK—Bergen County										
★ HOLY NAME HOSPITAL, 718 Teaneck Road, Zip 07666; tel. 201/833–3000; Sister Patricia A. Lynch, President and Chief Executive Officer **A**1 2 3 6 9 10 **F**1 3 5 7 8 12 13 15 16 17 19 20 21 22 26 27 28 29 30 32 33 34 35 37 39 40 41 42 44 45 46 49 51 52 53 54 55 56 57 58 65 67 71 73 74 **P**8	23	10	342	15177	257	135106	1754	112090	57375	1546
TOMS RIVER—Ocean County										
CHILDREN'S SPECIALIZED HOSPITAL See Children's Specialized Hospital, Mountainside										
★ COMMUNITY MEDICAL CENTER, 99 Highway 37 West, Zip 08755–6423; tel. 908/240–8000; Mark D. Pilla, President and Chief Executive Officer **A**1 2 9 10 **F**2 3 4 7 8 10 11 12 13 14 15 16 17 18 19 20 21 22 23 24 25 26 27 28 29 30 31 32 33 34 35 36 37 39 40 41 42 44 45 46 49 51 52 53 54 55 56 57 58 59 60 61 64 65 66 67 68 69 71 72 73 74 **P**5 7	23	10	596	20156	412	266878	2019	169075	78618	2445
☐ △ HEALTHSOUTH REHABILITATION HOSPITAL OF NEW JERSEY, (Formerly Healthsouth Garden State Rehabilitation Hospital) 14 Hospital Drive, Zip 08755; tel. 908/244–3100; David Coluzzi, Administrator and Chief Executive Officer (Nonreporting) **A**1 7 10 **S**0023 Healthsouth Corporation	33	46	119	—	—	—	—	—	—	—
TRENTON—Mercer County										
★ HELENE FULD MEDICAL CENTER, 750 Brunswick Avenue, Zip 08638; tel. 609/394–6000; Ira G. Shimp, President and Chief Executive Officer **A**1 3 5 6 9 10 **F**2 3 7 8 11 12 13 14 15 16 17 18 19 20 21 22 23 27 28 29 30 31 32 33 34 35 36 37 38 39 40 41 42 44 45 46 49 52 53 54 55 56 57 58 59 61 63 65 66 67 69 71 73 **P**6 8	23	10	340	9799	203	185943	1003	92953	49080	1295
★ MERCER MEDICAL CENTER, 446 Bellevue Avenue, Zip 08618, Mailing Address: Box 1658, Zip 08607; tel. 609/394–4000; Charles E. Baer, President **A**1 2 6 9 10 **F**1 7 8 11 15 16 17 19 21 22 26 30 31 34 35 37 38 40 42 44 46 49 60 61 63 65 66 71 73 **P**5 7 8	23	10	340	13055	192	171971	2617	101154	48385	1461
★ ST. FRANCIS MEDICAL CENTER, 601 Hamilton Avenue, Zip 08629–1986; tel. 609/599–5000; Patrick F. Roche, President **A**1 2 3 5 6 9 10 **F**3 7 8 10 11 12 15 16 17 19 21 22 23 26 27 28 30 31 32 33 34 35 37 40 42 44 45 46 49 51 52 54 55 56 58 59 63 65 67 68 71 72 73 74 **P**5 6 7 **S**5325 Franciscan Health System	21	10	344	10892	207	127363	598	90105	45266	1089
★ TRENTON PSYCHIATRIC HOSPITAL, Sullivan Way, Station A, Zip 08625, Mailing Address: P.O. Box 7500, West Trenton Zip 08628; tel. 609/633–1500; Joseph Jupin Jr., Chief Executive Officer **A**1 3 9 10 **F**4 5 8 9 10 11 14 15 16 19 20 21 22 23 26 27 28 30 31 35 37 39 41 42 43 44 45 46 48 49 50 52 55 56 57 58 59 60 61 63 65 66 67 69 71 73 74 **S**0010 Division of Mental Health Services, Department of Human Services, State of New Jersey	12	22	379	416	324	0	0	37966	—	816
TURNERSVILL—Gloucester County										
KENNEDY MEMORIAL HOSPITAL See Kennedy Memorial Hospitals–University Medical Center, Cherry Hill										
UNION—Union County										
★ + ○ UNION HOSPITAL, 1000 Galloping Hill Road, Zip 07083–7951; tel. 908/687–1900; Patricia A. Polansky R.N., Executive Vice President **A**1 2 9 10 11 12 13 **F**1 2 3 4 7 8 9 10 12 14 15 17 18 19 20 21 22 25 26 27 28 29 30 31 32 34 35 37 38 39 40 41 42 44 45 46 47 48 49 52 60 61 63 64 65 66 69 70 71 72 73 74 **P**4 5	23	10	201	6596	143	74650	0	67049	29578	955
VINELAND—Camden County										
★ NEWCOMB MEDICAL CENTER, 65 South State Street, Zip 08360; tel. 609/691–9000; Joseph A. Ierardi, President and Chief Executive Officer **A**1 2 9 10 **F**3 7 8 11 12 13 16 17 19 21 22 26 27 28 29 30 31 32 33 34 35 37 38 39 40 41 42 44 45 46 49 51 54 56 60 61 65 66 71 73 74 **P**5 8	23	10	191	6707	98	96220	1222	57182	27840	798
☐ VINELAND DEVELOPMENT CENTER HOSPITAL, 1676 East Landis Avenue, Zip 08360; tel. 609/696–6200; Shishir Vidwans M.D., Chief of Staff **A**1 10 **F**8 19 20 21 22 23 27 34 35 37 42 45 54 56 57 58 59 60 65 71 **P**6	12	12	100	627	49	6191	0	—	—	244
VOORHEES—Camden County										
★ WEST JERSEY HOSPITAL–VOORHEES, 101 Carnie Boulevard, Zip 08043–1597; tel. 609/772–5000; James R. Shedno, Executive Director **A**1 3 5 9 10 **F**2 3 4 5 7 8 10 14 15 16 17 19 20 21 26 27 28 29 30 31 32 33 34 35 37 38 39 40 41 42 44 45 46 49 51 55 60 61 63 65 67 71 73 74 **P**3 4 5 7 **S**6725 West Jersey Health System	23	10	262	15135	199	73570	4731	—	—	1181

© 1995 AHA Guide

Hospitals, U.S. / NEW JERSEY

Hospital, Address, Telephone, Administrator, Approval, Facility, and Physician Codes, Health Care System	Classification Codes		Utilization Data					Expense (thousands) of dollars		
★ American Hospital Association (AHA) membership ☐ Joint Commission on Accreditation of Healthcare Organizations (JCAHO) accreditation + American Osteopathic Hospital Association (AOHA) membership ○ American Osteopathic Association (AOA) accreditation △ Commission on Accreditation of Rehabilitation Facilities (CARF) accreditation Control codes 61, 63, 64, 71, 72 and 73 indicate hospitals listed by AOHA, but not registered by AHA. For definition of numerical codes, see page A6	Control	Service	Beds	Admissions	Census	Outpatient Visits	Births	Total	Payroll	Personnel
WAYNE—Passaic County										
★ WAYNE GENERAL HOSPITAL, 224 Hamburg Turnpike, Zip 07470–2161; tel. 201/942–6900; Justin E. Doheny, President and Chief Executive Officer **A**1 9 10 **F**3 7 8 11 15 19 21 22 23 25 26 28 30 31 32 33 34 35 37 40 41 42 44 45 46 49 51 53 54 55 56 57 58 59 60 63 65 67 71 73 **P**5 8	23	10	219	7821	175	104071	959	66743	34719	967
WEST ORANGE—Essex County										
★ △ KESSLER INSTITUTE FOR REHABILITATION, (Includes East Orange Facility, West Orange Facility and Saddle Brook Facility) 1199 Pleasant Valley Way, Zip 07052–1419; tel. 201/243–6801; Kenneth W. Aitchison, President and Chief Executive Officer **A**1 3 5 7 10 **F**15 16 32 48 49 **P**6	23	46	246	3493	218	85765	0	59269	37435	839
WESTAMPTON TOWNSHIP—Burlington County										
★ HAMPTON HOSPITAL, Rancocas Road, Zip 08073, Mailing Address: P.O. Box 7000, Zip 08073; tel. 609/267–7000; Michael Terwilliger, Acting Chief Executive Officer **A**1 9 10 **F**3 14 15 52 53 55 57 58 59 **P**1 **S**0455 Hospital Group of America	33	22	100	1357	56	3031	0	16196	6335	158
WESTWOOD—Bergen County										
★ PASCACK VALLEY HOSPITAL, Old Hook Road, Zip 07675–3181; tel. 201/358–3000; Louis R. Ycre Jr., President and Chief Executive Officer **A**1 2 9 10 **F**3 4 7 8 9 11 12 13 14 15 16 17 19 21 22 26 27 28 29 30 32 33 35 36 37 38 39 40 41 42 44 45 46 47 48 49 51 60 61 65 66 67 69 71 73 74 **P**1 5 7	23	10	291	15609	181	99583	1292	88498	42402	1168
WILLINGBORO—Burlington County										
☐ RANCOCAS HOSPITAL, 218–A Sunset Road, Zip 08046–1162; tel. 609/835–2900; Garry L. Scheib, President **A**1 2 10 **F**1 7 8 11 14 15 16 17 19 20 21 22 26 28 29 30 31 32 33 35 37 39 40 41 42 44 46 49 52 54 56 57 59 65 66 67 71 73 74 **S**0006 Graduate Health System	23	10	246	9305	148	85059	1556	63327	30267	930
WOODBRIDGE—Middlesex County										
WOODBRIDGE DEVELOPMENT CENTER, Rahway Avenue, Zip 07095, Mailing Address: P.O. Box 189, Zip 07095; tel. 201/499–5673; Amy R. Bailon M.D., Medical Director (Nonreporting)	12	12	125	—	—	—	—	—	—	—
WOODBURY—Gloucester County										
★ UNDERWOOD–MEMORIAL HOSPITAL, 509 North Broad Street, Zip 08096–7359, Mailing Address: P.O. Box 359, Zip 08096; tel. 609/845–0100; William D. Thompson, President **A**1 3 5 10 **F**7 8 11 12 16 17 18 19 20 21 22 23 26 28 30 31 34 35 37 40 41 42 44 45 46 49 51 52 54 56 57 65 67 68 71 73	23	10	325	11721	241	101842	1317	78551	37631	1103
WYCKOFF—Bergen County										
★ RAMAPO RIDGE PSYCHIATRIC HOSPITAL, 301 Sicomac Avenue, Zip 07481–2194; tel. 201/848–5200; Joan P. Craper, Executive Vice President and Administrator **A**1 10 **F**14 15 16 19 20 21 22 27 35 41 45 50 52 53 54 55 56 57 58 59 63 65 67 71 73 **P**6	23	22	80	577	58	5106	0	—	—	133

Hospitals, U.S. / NEW MEXICO

NEW MEXICO

Resident population 1,616 (in thousands)
Resident population in metro areas 56.0%
Birth rate per 1,000 population 18.0
65 years and over 11.0%
Percent of persons without health insurance 21.0%

Hospital, Address, Telephone, Administrator, Approval, Facility, and Physician Codes, Health Care System	Classification Codes		Utilization Data					Expense (thousands) of dollars		
	Control	Service	Beds	Admissions	Census	Outpatient Visits	Births	Total	Payroll	Personnel

★ American Hospital Association (AHA) membership
□ Joint Commission on Accreditation of Healthcare Organizations (JCAHO) accreditation
+ American Osteopathic Hospital Association (AOHA) membership
○ American Osteopathic Association (AOA) accreditation
△ Commission on Accreditation of Rehabilitation Facilities (CARF) accreditation
Control codes 61, 63, 64, 71, 72 and 73 indicate hospitals listed by AOHA, but not registered by AHA. For definition of numerical codes, see page A6.

ALAMOGORDO—Otero County

Hospital	Control	Service	Beds	Admissions	Census	Outpatient Visits	Births	Total	Payroll	Personnel
★ GERALD CHAMPION MEMORIAL HOSPITAL, 1209 Ninth Street, Zip 88310–0597; Mailing Address: P.O. Box 597, Zip 88311–0597; tel. 505/439–2100; Carl W. Mantey, Chief Executive Officer **A**1 9 10 **F**7 8 14 15 16 19 21 22 24 28 30 33 34 35 37 40 42 44 65 66 67 71 73 **P**5 **S**0002 Quorum Health Group/Quorum Health Resources	23	10	74	3363	39	24966	769	17946	6461	230

ALBUQUERQUE—Bernalillo County

Hospital	Control	Service	Beds	Admissions	Census	Outpatient Visits	Births	Total	Payroll	Personnel
★ CARRIE TINGLEY HOSPITAL, 1127 University Boulevard N.E., Zip 87102–1715; tel. 505/272–5200; James C. Drennan M.S.H.A., M.D., Medical Director and Chief Executive Officer **A**3 5 9 10 **F**15 16 17 19 20 21 29 32 35 37 41 44 45 46 47 48 49 50 53 54 55 61 63 65 71 73 **P**3 6 **S**0021 University of New Mexico	23	57	18	463	6	12430	0	8088	3890	128
□ CHARTER HOSPITAL OF ALBUQUERQUE, 5901 Zuni Road S.E., Zip 87108; tel. 505/265–8800; Joel A. Hart FACHE, Chief Executive Officer **A**1 9 10 **F**1 2 3 15 16 22 25 52 53 54 55 56 57 58 59 **P**4 **S**0695 Charter Medical Corporation	33	22	80	1123	61	5109	0	14180	4867	135
□ △ HEALTHSOUTH REHABILITATION HOSPITAL, 7000 Jefferson N.E., Zip 87109; tel. 505/344–9478; Darby Brockette, Administrator (Nonreporting) **A**1 7 9 10 **S**0023 Healthsouth Corporation	33	46	60	—	—	—	—	—	—	—
★ HEIGHTS PSYCHIATRIC HOSPITAL, 103 Hospital Loop N.E., Zip 87109; tel. 505/883–8777; Andrea Brightwell, Chief Executive Officer **A**1 9 10 **F**3 12 21 22 27 46 52 53 54 55 56 57 58 59 65 67 **S**0048 Columbia/HCA Healthcare Corporation	33	22	92	1236	49	0	0	8988	4305	135
□ LOVELACE MEDICAL CENTER, 5400 Gibson Boulevard S.E., Zip 87108; tel. 505/262–7000; John L. Lucas M.D., Chief Executive Officer **A**1 2 3 5 9 10 **F**1 2 3 4 6 7 8 10 11 12 13 14 15 16 17 18 19 20 21 22 23 24 25 28 29 30 31 32 33 34 35 37 38 39 40 41 42 43 44 45 46 47 48 49 51 52 60 61 64 65 67 68 69 70 71 72 73 74 **P**1 3 5 6	33	10	235	6016	115	987846	2023	281965	—	3385
□ MEMORIAL HOSPITAL, THE PSYCHIATRIC CENTER OF ALBUQUERQUE, 806 Central Avenue S.E., Zip 87102, Mailing Address: P.O. Box 26568, Zip 87125–6568; tel. 505/247–0220; R. G. Lingenfelser, Administrator **A**1 10 **F**1 2 3 15 16 34 52 53 54 55 57 58 59	32	22	58	630	31	4420	0	5533	3537	128
★ PRESBYTERIAN HOSPITAL, 1100 Central Avenue S.E., Zip 87102, Mailing Address: P.O. Box 26666, Zip 87125–6666; tel. 505/841–1234; James Hinton, Vice President Operations **A**1 2 5 9 10 **F**2 3 4 5 7 8 9 10 11 12 13 14 16 17 18 19 21 22 23 24 25 26 30 32 33 34 35 36 37 38 40 41 42 43 44 46 47 49 51 52 53 54 55 56 57 58 59 60 61 63 64 65 66 67 69 70 71 72 73 74 **P**1 4 5 6 7 **S**3505 Presbyterian Healthcare Services	23	10	433	25701	303	0	4004	—	—	—
★ PRESBYTERIAN KASEMAN HOSPITAL, 8300 Constitution Avenue N.E., Zip 87110; tel. 505/291–2000; Jim Purdy, Administrative Director **A**9 10 **F**2 3 4 5 7 8 9 10 11 12 13 14 16 17 18 19 21 22 23 24 25 26 30 32 33 34 35 36 37 38 39 40 41 42 43 44 46 47 49 51 52 53 54 55 56 57 58 59 60 61 63 64 65 66 67 69 70 71 72 73 74 **P**1 4 5 6 7 **S**3505 Presbyterian Healthcare Services	23	10	120	5447	75	39449	0	—	—	361
★ PUBLIC HEALTH SERVICE INDIAN HOSPITAL, 801 Vassar Drive N.E., Zip 87106–2799; tel. 505/256–4000; Raymond L. Rodgers, Administrator **A**1 10 **F**12 14 15 16 17 19 20 25 30 31 34 37 39 51 54 58 65 71 72 **S**9195 U.S. Public Health Service Indian Health Service	47	10	28	670	10	70889	0	10170	5839	275
★ ST. JOSEPH MEDICAL CENTER, 601 Martin Luther King Dr N.E., Zip 87102, Mailing Address: P.O. Box 25555, Zip 87125; tel. 505/244–8000; Ray H. Barton III, President and Chief Executive Officer (Total facility includes 22 beds in nursing home–type unit) **A**1 2 9 10 **F**2 3 4 7 8 10 11 12 19 21 22 23 27 28 30 32 33 34 35 36 37 39 40 41 42 43 44 45 46 48 49 51 52 54 56 57 58 60 61 63 64 65 67 68 70 71 72 73 74 **P**5 6 7 **S**5115 Sisters of Charity Health Care Systems, Inc.	21	10	275	8562	138	36602	0	71708	28822	976
★ ST. JOSEPH NORTHEAST HEIGHTS HOSPITAL, 4701 Montgomery N.E., Zip 87109, Mailing Address: P.O. Box 25555, Zip 87125–0555; tel. 505/888–7800; C. Vincent Townsend Jr., Vice President **A**1 9 10 **F**4 7 8 10 11 12 19 21 22 23 27 30 32 33 34 35 36 37 39 40 42 43 44 46 49 51 54 56 57 58 60 61 63 65 67 68 71 72 73 74 **P**5 6 7 **S**5115 Sisters of Charity Health Care Systems, Inc.	21	10	112	3303	35	18115	828	16612	7291	215
★ △ ST. JOSEPH REHABILITATION HOSPITAL AND OUTPATIENT CENTER, 505 Elm Street N.E., Zip 87102, Mailing Address: P.O. Box 25555, Zip 87125–2500; tel. 505/244–4700; Mary Lou Coors, Administrator **A**7 9 10 **F**3 4 7 8 10 11 12 19 21 22 27 28 30 32 33 34 35 36 37 38 39 40 41 42 43 44 45 46 48 49 51 54 56 57 58 60 61 63 64 65 67 68 70 71 72 73 74 **P**5 6 7 **S**5115 Sisters of Charity Health Care Systems, Inc.	21	46	63	744	45	3006	0	12644	7282	227
□ ST. JOSEPH WEST MESA HOSPITAL, 10501 Golf Course Road N.W., Zip 87114, Mailing Address: P.O. Box 25555, Zip 87125–0555; tel. 505/893–2003; C. Vincent Townsend Jr., Vice President (Total facility includes 22 beds in nursing home–type unit) **A**1 9 10 **F**3 4 7 8 10 12 19 21 22 23 27 30 32 33 34 35 36 37 39 40 42 43 44 46 49 51 54 56 57 58 61 63 64 65 67 68 71 72 73 74 **P**5 6 7 **S**5115 Sisters of Charity Health Care Systems, Inc.	21	10	128	2830	42	15727	527	17890	7692	234

© 1995 AHA Guide

Hospitals, U.S. / NEW MEXICO

Hospital, Address, Telephone, Administrator, Approval, Facility, and Physician Codes, Health Care System	Classification Codes		Utilization Data					Expense (thousands) of dollars		Personnel
★ American Hospital Association (AHA) membership ☐ Joint Commission on Accreditation of Healthcare Organizations (JCAHO) accreditation + American Osteopathic Hospital Association (AOHA) membership ○ American Osteopathic Association (AOA) accreditation △ Commission on Accreditation of Rehabilitation Facilities (CARF) accreditation Control codes 61, 63, 64, 71, 72 and 73 indicate hospitals listed by AOHA, but not registered by AHA. For definition of numerical codes, see page A6	Control	Service	Beds	Admissions	Census	Outpatient Visits	Births	Total	Payroll	
THC – ALBUQUERQUE, 700 High Street N.E., Zip 87102; tel. 505/242–4444; (Nonreporting) A10	33	48	61	—	—	—	—	—	—	—
☒ UNIVERSITY HOSPITAL, 2211 Lomas Boulevard N.E., Zip 87106; tel. 505/843–2121; William H. Johnson Jr., Chief Executive Officer A1 2 3 5 8 9 10 F3 4 5 7 8 9 10 14 15 16 17 19 21 22 23 24 26 28 29 30 31 32 33 34 35 37 38 40 41 42 43 44 45 46 47 49 54 55 60 61 63 65 66 67 68 69 70 71 72 73 74 S0021 University of New Mexico	12	10	318	18270	252	302524	3532	154267	—	2349
★ UNIVERSITY OF NEW MEXICO CHILDREN'S PSYCHIATRIC HOSPITAL, 1001 Yale Boulevard N.E., Zip 87131; tel. 505/843–2945; Christina B. Gunn, Chief Executive Officer A3 5 9 F19 21 35 41 52 53 54 55 56 65 71 S0021 University of New Mexico	12	52	53	122	50	0	0	7073	4689	204
★ UNIVERSITY OF NEW MEXICO MENTAL HEALTH CENTER, 2600 Marble N.E., Zip 87131–2600; tel. 505/843–2870; Christina B. Gunn, Chief Executive Officer A3 5 9 F2 3 14 15 16 17 18 31 39 52 53 54 55 56 57 58 59 S0021 University of New Mexico	13	22	60	1397	48	99923	0	18328	11590	405
☒ VETERANS AFFAIRS MEDICAL CENTER, 2100 Ridgecrest Drive S.E., Zip 87108; tel. 505/265–1711; Bruce A. Gordon, Acting Director (Total facility includes 47 beds in nursing home–type unit) A1 2 3 5 8 F1 2 3 4 5 8 10 12 17 18 19 20 21 22 23 26 27 30 31 32 33 34 35 37 39 41 42 43 44 45 46 48 49 52 54 55 56 58 59 60 61 63 64 65 71 72 73 74 S9295 Department of Veterans Affairs	45	10	468	9519	305	225447	0	134127	64528	1843
ARTESIA—Eddy County										
☒ ARTESIA GENERAL HOSPITAL, 702 North 13th Street, Zip 88210; tel. 505/748–3333; William D. Haddock FACHE, Administrator A1 9 10 F7 8 14 15 17 19 28 30 32 33 34 36 40 44 49 71 S3505 Presbyterian Healthcare Services	16	10	38	725	8	20201	130	6692	—	—
CANNON AIR FORCE BASE—Curry County										
☒ U.S. AIR FORCE HOSPITAL, Zip 88103–5300; tel. 505/784–4582; Lieutenant Colonel James E. Tart USAF, MSC, Administrator A1 F1 2 3 4 5 6 7 8 9 10 11 12 13 14 15 16 17 18 19 20 21 22 23 24 25 26 27 28 29 30 31 32 33 34 35 36 37 38 39 40 41 42 43 44 45 46 47 48 49 50 51 52 53 54 55 56 57 58 59 60 61 62 63 64 65 66 67 68 69 70 71 72 73 74 P6 S9495 Department of the Air Force	41	10	29	1064	7	107437	308	—	—	290
CARLSBAD—Eddy County										
☒ GUADALUPE MEDICAL CENTER, 2430 West Pierce Street, Zip 88220–3597; tel. 505/887–4100; Thomas H. Steel, Chief Executive Officer A1 9 10 F3 6 8 11 12 13 17 19 21 22 23 28 30 31 32 33 35 36 37 40 42 44 49 52 56 58 59 60 63 64 65 71 73 P1 S0048 Columbia/HCA Healthcare Corporation	33	10	115	4510	55	50877	621	26981	10291	416
CLAYTON—Union County										
★ UNION COUNTY GENERAL HOSPITAL, 301 Harding Street, Zip 88415, Mailing Address: P.O. Box 489, Zip 88415–0489; tel. 505/374–2585; Carrell R. Blakely, Administrator A9 10 F7 8 12 14 15 16 21 22 27 28 32 33 44 71 S2235 Lutheran Health Systems	23	10	28	520	5	10445	49	2457	968	42
CLOVIS—Curry County										
☒ PLAINS REGIONAL MEDICAL CENTER – CLOVIS, 2100 North Thomas Street, Zip 88101, Mailing Address: P.O. Box 1688, Zip 88101–1688; tel. 505/769–2141; Grant H. Nelson, Administrator (Nonreporting) A1 9 10 S3505 Presbyterian Healthcare Services	23	10	106	—	—	—	—	—	—	—
CROWNPOINT—McKinley County										
☒ U.S. PUBLIC HEALTH SERVICE INDIAN HOSPITAL, Mailing Address: Box 358, Zip 87313–0358; tel. 505/786–5291; Anita Muneta, Chief Executive Officer A1 10 F3 4 7 8 9 10 11 12 13 14 15 16 17 18 19 20 21 22 23 24 25 26 27 28 29 30 31 32 34 35 37 38 40 42 43 44 45 46 47 48 49 51 53 54 55 56 58 60 61 64 65 67 68 69 70 71 72 74 S9195 U.S. Public Health Service Indian Health Service	47	10	32	1019	11	51329	186	16688	7924	255
DEMING—Luna County										
MIMBRES MEMORIAL HOSPITAL, 900 West Ash Street, Zip 88030; tel. 505/546–2761; Michael Christensen, Administrator and Chief Executive Officer (Nonreporting) A9 10	13	10	119	—	—	—	—	—	—	—
ESPANOLA—Rio Arriba County										
☒ ESPANOLA HOSPITAL, 1010 Spruce Street, Zip 87532; tel. 505/753–7111; Marcella A. Romero, Administrator A1 9 10 F7 8 12 14 15 16 19 22 28 32 33 34 35 37 40 44 46 51 65 71 73 P3 5 S3505 Presbyterian Healthcare Services	23	10	61	2174	19	34221	249	13901	7175	209
FARMINGTON—San Juan County										
DESERT HILLS HOSPITAL, 5310 Siquoia Road, Zip 87401; tel. 505/836–7330; Marcia Hille, Administrator and Chief Executive Officer (Nonreporting)	33	22	35	—	—	—	—	—	—	—
☒ SAN JUAN REGIONAL MEDICAL CENTER, 801 West Maple Street, Zip 87401; tel. 505/325–5011; Donald R. Carlson, President and Chief Executive Officer (Total facility includes 15 beds in nursing home–type unit) A1 2 9 10 F7 8 14 15 16 17 19 22 23 27 28 29 30 34 35 37 40 41 42 44 46 48 49 56 58 60 64 65 67 70 71 72 73 P5 8	23	10	143	6246	74	56936	1119	51361	21738	746
SUN CREST HOSPITAL, 1101 West Murray Drive, Zip 87401; tel. 505/326–9151; Jo Martinez, Administrator (Nonreporting) A9 10	33	22	54	—	—	—	—	—	—	—
FORT BAYARD—Grant County										
★ FORT BAYARD MEDICAL CENTER, Calle Centro, Zip 88036, Mailing Address: P.O. Box 36219, Zip 88036; tel. 505/537–3302; Marquita George, Administrator (Nonreporting)	12	82	230	—	—	—	—	—	—	—

Hospitals, U.S. / NEW MEXICO

Hospital, Address, Telephone, Administrator, Approval, Facility, and Physician Codes, Health Care System	Classification Codes		Utilization Data					Expense (thousands) of dollars		Personnel
	Control	Service	Beds	Admissions	Census	Outpatient Visits	Births	Total	Payroll	

★ American Hospital Association (AHA) membership
☐ Joint Commission on Accreditation of Healthcare Organizations (JCAHO) accreditation
+ American Osteopathic Hospital Association (AOHA) membership
○ American Osteopathic Association (AOA) accreditation
△ Commission on Accreditation of Rehabilitation Facilities (CARF) accreditation
Control codes 61, 63, 64, 71, 72 and 73 indicate hospitals listed by AOHA, but not registered by AHA. For definition of numerical codes, see page A6

Hospital	Control	Service	Beds	Admissions	Census	Outpatient Visits	Births	Total	Payroll	Personnel
FORT SUMNER—De Baca County ★ DEBACA GENERAL HOSPITAL, Mailing Address: P.O. Box 349, Zip 88119; tel. 505/355-2414; Kay Stark, Administrator (Nonreporting) A9 10	13	10	25	—	—	—	—	—	—	—
GALLUP—McKinley County ★ GALLUP INDIAN MEDICAL CENTER, 516 East Nizhoni Boulevard, Zip 87301-1334, Mailing Address: Box 1337, Zip 87301-1344; tel. 505/722-1000; Timothy G. Fleming M.D., Chief Executive Officer A1 10 F3 7 8 12 14 15 16 17 19 20 21 22 25 27 28 29 34 35 37 39 40 44 45 46 49 53 54 56 58 65 68 71 74 S9195 U.S. Public Health Service Indian Health Service	47	10	107	5188	58	184926	1088	52750	27190	734
★ REHOBOTH MCKINLEY CHRISTIAN HOSPITAL, 1901 Red Rock Drive, Zip 87301-1901; tel. 505/863-7000; David J. Baltzer R.N., President A1 9 10 F2 3 7 8 14 16 19 21 22 28 31 32 33 34 37 40 41 44 45 46 49 51 52 53 56 58 65 71 73 74 P3 5 8	23	10	138	3144	67	53850	413	21738	8558	330
GRANTS—Cibola County ★ CIBOLA GENERAL HOSPITAL, 1212 Bonita Avenue, Zip 87020; tel. 505/287-4446; Polly Pine, Administrator A1 9 10 F7 8 11 19 22 37 40 44 71 73 S0002 Quorum Health Group/Quorum Health Resources	23	10	43	1042	9	8785	204	5041	2518	93
HOBBS—Lea County ★ LEA REGIONAL HOSPITAL, Lovington Highway 18, Zip 88240, Mailing Address: P.O. Box 3000, Zip 88240; tel. 505/392-6581; R. Gordon Taylor, Chief Executive Officer (Nonreporting) A1 10 S0048 Columbia/HCA Healthcare Corporation	33	10	250	—	—	—	—	—	—	—
HOLLOMAN AIR FORCE BASE—Otero County ★ U.S. AIR FORCE HOSPITAL, 280 First Street, Zip 88330-8273; tel. 505/475-5587; Colonel Willy I. Huyghe MSC, Commander A1 F15 18 20 22 28 29 30 34 39 41 44 45 46 49 51 53 54 55 56 58 71 S9495 Department of the Air Force	41	10	8	1037	5	118287	0	—	—	295
KIRTLAND AIR FORCE BASE—Bernalillo County ★ U.S. AIR FORCE HOSPITAL-KIRTLAND, Zip 87117-5559; tel. 505/846-3547; Colonel George Seignious MSC, USAF, Commander A1 3 5 F4 7 8 10 12 14 19 20 22 24 29 34 35 41 42 43 44 46 49 51 58 59 60 61 63 65 66 69 71 72 74 S9495 Department of the Air Force	41	10	35	2801	14	215456	0	—	—	490
LAS CRUCES—Dona Ana County ★ MEMORIAL MEDICAL CENTER, 2450 South Telshor Boulevard, Zip 88011-5076; tel. 505/522-8641 A1 5 9 10 F4 7 8 10 15 19 21 22 23 35 37 40 42 43 44 49 52 56 60 64 65 70 71 72 73 74	15	10	221	10873	143	89987	2834	69683	26818	1120
☐ MESILLA VALLEY HOSPITAL, 3751 Del Rey Boulevard, Zip 88012-7710, Mailing Address: P.O. Box 429, Zip 88004; tel. 505/382-3500; Thomas Rourke, Administrator (Nonreporting) A1 9 10	32	22	85	—	—	—	—	—	—	—
LAS VEGAS—San Miguel County ☐ LAS VEGAS MEDICAL CENTER, Hot Springs Boulevard, Zip 87701, Mailing Address: P.O. Box 1388, Zip 87701; tel. 505/454-2100; Pablo Hernandez M.D., Administrator (Nonreporting) A1 9	12	22	397	—	—	—	—	—	—	—
★ NORTHEASTERN REGIONAL HOSPITAL, 1235 Eighth Street, Zip 87701, Mailing Address: P.O. Box 238, Zip 87701-0238; tel. 505/425-6751; Richard L. Mendoza, Chief Executive Officer (Nonreporting) A1 9 10 S0585 Brim, Inc.	23	10	62	—	—	—	—	—	—	—
LOS ALAMOS—Los Alamos County ★ LOS ALAMOS MEDICAL CENTER, 3917 West Road, Zip 87544; tel. 505/662-4201; Paul J. Wilson, Administrator A1 9 10 F7 12 14 15 16 17 19 21 22 28 30 32 33 34 35 36 37 39 40 42 44 45 46 49 51 65 71 72 73 74 P3 5 8 S2235 Lutheran Health Systems	23	10	53	1742	15	34770	317	16204	6348	228
LOS LUNAS—Cibola County LOS LUNAS HOSPITAL AND TRAINING SCHOOL, Mailing Address: P.O. Box 1269, Zip 87031; tel. 505/865-9611; Matthew McCue, Administrator (Nonreporting)	12	62	357	—	—	—	—	—	—	—
LOVINGTON—Lea County ★ NOR-LEA GENERAL HOSPITAL, 1600 North Main, Zip 88260; tel. 505/396-6611; David J. Parker, Administrator (Nonreporting) A1 9 10	16	10	28	—	—	—	—	—	—	—
MESCALERO—Otero County ★ U.S. PUBLIC HEALTH SERVICE INDIAN HOSPITAL, Mailing Address: Box 210, Zip 88340-0210; tel. 505/671-4441; Joe Wahnee Jr., Service Unit Director (Nonreporting) A1 10 S9195 U.S. Public Health Service Indian Health Service	47	10	13	—	—	—	—	—	—	—
PORTALES—Roosevelt County ☐ PLAINS REGIONAL MEDICAL CENTER–PORTALES, 1700 South Avenue O, Zip 88130, Mailing Address: P.O. Drawer 60, Zip 88130; tel. 505/356-4411; Grant H. Nelson, Administrator (Nonreporting) A1 9 10 S3505 Presbyterian Healthcare Services	33	10	103	—	—	—	—	—	—	—
RATON—Colfax County ★ MINERS' COLFAX MEDICAL CENTER, (Includes Miners' Hospital of New Mexico, Raton, New Mexico; tel. 505/445-2741) 200 Hospital Drive, Zip 87740-2099; tel. 505/445-3661; David Antle, Chief Executive Officer (Nonreporting) A9 10	13	10	68	—	—	—	—	—	—	—
ROSWELL—Chaves County ★ EASTERN NEW MEXICO MEDICAL CENTER, 405 West Country Club Road, Zip 88201-9981; tel. 505/622-8170; Ronald J. Shafer, President and Chief Executive Officer (Nonreporting) A1 9 10	13	10	194	—	—	—	—	—	—	—
☐ △ NEW MEXICO REHABILITATION CENTER, 31 Gail Harris Avenue, Riac, Zip 88201; tel. 505/347-5491; Harvey J. Featherstone M.D., Administrator A1 7 9 10 F2 48 49 65 P6	12	46	39	483	28	1811	0	5436	2681	115

© 1995 AHA Guide

Hospitals, U.S. / NEW MEXICO

Hospital, Address, Telephone, Administrator, Approval, Facility, and Physician Codes, Health Care System

- ★ American Hospital Association (AHA) membership
- ☐ Joint Commission on Accreditation of Healthcare Organizations (JCAHO) accreditation
- + American Osteopathic Hospital Association (AOHA) membership
- ○ American Osteopathic Association (AOA) accreditation
- △ Commission on Accreditation of Rehabilitation Facilities (CARF) accreditation

Control codes 61, 63, 64, 71, 72 and 73 indicate hospitals listed by AOHA, but not registered by AHA. For definition of numerical codes, see page A6.

Hospital	Control	Service	Beds	Admissions	Census	Outpatient Visits	Births	Total	Payroll	Personnel
RUIDOSO—Lincoln County										
✠ LINCOLN COUNTY MEDICAL CENTER, 211 Sudderth Drive, Zip 88345, Mailing Address: P.O. Drawer 3C/D, Hollywood Station, Zip 88345; tel. 505/257-7381; Valerie Miller, Administrator **A**1 9 10 **F**7 8 15 16 17 19 20 22 25 28 30 37 40 41 42 44 46 49 71 73 **P**2 8 **S**3505 Presbyterian Healthcare Services	23	10	38	1034	9	26370	254	8894	3928	138
SAN FIDEL—Cibola County										
✠ ACOMA-CANONCITO-LAGUNA HOSPITAL, Mailing Address: P.O. Box 130, Zip 87049; tel. 505/552-6634; Richard L. Zephier Ph.D., Service Unit Director (Nonreporting) **A**1 10 **S**9195 U.S. Public Health Service Indian Health Service	47	10	25	—	—	—	—	—	—	—
SANTA FE—Santa Fe County										
✠ PHS SANTA FE INDIAN HOSPITAL, 1700 Cerrillos Road, Zip 87505; tel. 505/988-9821; Lawrence A. Jordan, Director (Nonreporting) **A**1 10 **S**9195 U.S. Public Health Service Indian Health Service	47	10	39	—	—	—	—	—	—	—
☐ PINON HILLS HOSPITAL, 313 Camino Alire, Zip 87501; tel. 505/988-8003; Jerry Smith, Administrator **A**1 9 10 **F**2 3 14 15 16 17 52 53 54 55 56 59 68	33	22	36	485	21	1248	0	—	—	33
✠ △ ST. VINCENT HOSPITAL, 455 St Michael's Drive, Zip 87505, Mailing Address: P.O. Box 2107, Zip 87504-2107; tel. 505/983-3361; Ronald C. Winger, President and Chief Executive Officer (Nonreporting) **A**1 2 5 7 9 10	23	10	268	—	—	—	—	—	—	—
SANTA TERESA—Dona Ana County										
☐ ALLIANCE HOSPITAL OF SANTA TERESA, 100 Laura Court, Zip 88008, Mailing Address: P.O. Box 6, Zip 88008; tel. 505/589-0033; Frank M. Braden, Administrator (Nonreporting) **A**1 9 10	33	22	72	—	—	—	—	—	—	—
SHIPROCK—San Juan County										
✠ SHIPROCK INDIAN HOSPITAL, Mailing Address: Box 160, Zip 87420; tel. 505/368-4971; Dee Hutchison, Chief Executive Officer **A**1 10 **F**2 3 4 7 8 9 10 11 12 13 15 16 17 18 19 20 22 23 25 28 29 30 31 32 33 34 36 37 38 39 40 42 43 44 46 47 48 49 51 52 53 54 57 58 64 65 66 68 69 70 71 74 **S**9195 U.S. Public Health Service Indian Health Service	47	10	50	2945	29	113891	753	34607	19805	597
SILVER CITY—Grant County										
✠ GILA REGIONAL MEDICAL CENTER, 1313 East 32nd Street, Zip 88061; tel. 505/538-4000; Steve Jacobson, Administrator (Nonreporting) **A**1 9 10 **S**0002 Quorum Health Group/Quorum Health Resources	13	10	68	—	—	—	—	—	—	—
SOCORRO—Socorro County										
✠ SOCORRO GENERAL HOSPITAL, 1202 Highway 60 West, Zip 87801, Mailing Address: P.O. Box 1009, Zip 87801-1009; tel. 505/835-1140; Jeff Dye, Administrator **A**1 9 10 **F**7 8 15 22 26 28 30 32 40 44 49 65 67 68 71 **S**3505 Presbyterian Healthcare Services	23	10	30	1388	12	16005	210	6058	2222	104
TAOS—Taos County										
★ HOLY CROSS HOSPITAL, 630 Paseo De Pueblo Sur, Zip 87571, Mailing Address: P.O. Box Dd, Zip 87571; tel. 505/751-2234; Rita Campbell, Administrator (Nonreporting) **A**9 10 **S**0002 Quorum Health Group/Quorum Health Resources	23	10	29	—	—	—	—	—	—	—
TRUTH OR CONSEQUENCES—Bernalillo County										
✠ SIERRA VISTA HOSPITAL, 800 East Ninth Avenue, Zip 87901; tel. 505/894-2111; Amy Clithero, Interim Assistant Administrator (Total facility includes 11 beds in nursing home-type unit) **A**1 9 10 **F**7 8 12 13 14 17 19 20 22 27 28 30 32 34 35 36 39 44 46 49 53 54 55 56 57 58 61 62 64 65 67 71 73 **P**5	21	10	43	467	9	10011	21	—	—	—
TUCUMCARI—Quay County										
★ DR DAN C. TRIGG MEMORIAL HOSPITAL, 301 East Miel De Luna Avenue, Zip 88401, Mailing Address: P.O. Box 608, Zip 88401; tel. 505/461-0141; Dan Noteware, Administrator **A**9 10 **F**7 14 15 16 19 22 32 34 40 44 71 **S**3505 Presbyterian Healthcare Services	23	10	29	875	9	27511	99	5319	1936	72
ZUNI—McKinley County										
✠ U.S. PUBLIC HEALTH SERVICE INDIAN HOSPITAL, Mailing Address: P.O. Box 467, Zip 87327; tel. 505/782-4431; Jean Othole, Service Unit Director (Nonreporting) **A**1 10 **S**9195 U.S. Public Health Service Indian Health Service	47	10	37	—	—	—	—	—	—	—

NEW YORK

Resident population 18,197 (in thousands)
Resident population in metro areas 91.7%
Birth rate per 1,000 population 16.2
65 years and over 13.1%
Percent of persons without health insurance 12.6%

★ American Hospital Association (AHA) membership
□ Joint Commission on Accreditation of Healthcare Organizations (JCAHO) accreditation
+ American Osteopathic Hospital Association (AOHA) membership
○ American Osteopathic Association (AOA) accreditation
△ Commission on Accreditation of Rehabilitation Facilities (CARF) accreditation
Control codes 61, 63, 64, 71, 72 and 73 indicate hospitals listed by AOHA, but not registered by AHA. For definition of numerical codes, see page A6

Hospital, Address, Telephone, Administrator, Approval, Facility, and Physician Codes, Health Care System	Control	Service	Beds	Admissions	Census	Outpatient Visits	Births	Total	Payroll	Personnel
ALBANY—Albany County										
★ ALBANY MEDICAL CENTER HOSPITAL, 43 New Scotland Avenue, Zip 12208; tel. 518/262-3125; James J. Barba, President and Chief Executive Officer A1 2 3 5 8 9 10 12 F4 7 8 10 11 12 16 17 19 20 21 22 23 25 26 30 31 32 34 35 37 38 39 40 41 42 43 44 45 46 47 48 49 51 52 53 54 55 56 57 58 59 60 61 63 65 66 67 69 70 71 72 73 74	23	10	594	22662	499	400855	2686	244148	97240	3100
★ CAPITAL DISTRICT PSYCHIATRIC CENTER, 75 New Scotland Avenue, Zip 12208; tel. 518/447-9611; Jesse Nixon Jr. Ph.D., Director (Nonreporting) A1 3 5 10 S0009 New York State Department of Mental Health	12	22	225	—	—	—	—	—	—	—
★ CHILD'S HOSPITAL, 25 Hackett Boulevard, Zip 12208; tel. 518/487-7200; Stephen J. Lauko, Chief Executive Officer (Nonreporting) A1 3 5 9 10	23	45	20	—	—	—	—	—	—	—
★ MEMORIAL HOSPITAL, 600 Northern Boulevard, Zip 12204-1083; tel. 518/471-3221; Bernard Shapiro, President and Chief Executive Officer A1 6 9 10 F4 8 11 12 14 19 21 22 23 25 31 33 34 37 42 44 49 51 61 63 65 71 72 73	23	10	212	6738	143	128689	0	56922	30535	795
★ ST. PETER'S HOSPITAL, 315 South Manning Boulevard, Zip 12208-1789; tel. 518/454-1550; Steven P. Boyle, President and Chief Executive Officer A1 2 3 5 9 10 F2 3 4 7 8 10 11 12 13 14 15 16 17 18 19 20 21 22 25 26 28 29 30 32 33 34 35 36 37 38 39 40 41 42 43 44 45 46 48 49 51 54 60 63 65 67 70 71 73 74 P5 7 8 S3595 Eastern Mercy Health System	23	10	437	18881	371	328575	2216	141670	66410	2409
★ VETERANS AFFAIRS MEDICAL CENTER, 113 Holland Avenue, Zip 12208-3473; tel. 518/462-3311; Frederick L. Malphurs, Director (Total facility includes 67 beds in nursing home-type unit) A1 2 3 5 8 F1 2 3 4 8 10 11 12 15 16 17 18 19 20 21 22 23 25 26 27 28 29 30 31 32 33 34 35 37 39 41 42 43 44 45 46 48 49 51 52 54 55 56 57 58 59 60 63 64 65 67 69 71 72 73 74 S9295 Department of Veterans Affairs	45	10	406	6458	314	187069	0	117146	78108	1616
ALEXANDRIA BAY—Jefferson County										
□ E. J. NOBLE HOSPITAL OF ALEXANDRIA BAY, 19 Fuller Street, Zip 13607; tel. 315/482-2511; William P. Koughan, President (Nonreporting) A1 9 10	23	10	52	—	—	—	—	—	—	—
AMITYVILLE—Suffolk County										
★ BRUNSWICK GENERAL HOSPITAL, (Includes Brunswick Hall, 80 Louden Avenue, Amityville, New York, Zip 11701-2735; tel. 516/789-7100; Brunswick Nursing Home, Amityville, New York; Brunswick Physical Medicine & Rehabilitation Hospital, 366 Broadway, Amityville, New York, Zip 11701) 366 Broadway, Zip 11701-9820; tel. 516/789-7000; Benjamin M. Stein M.D., President; Harold A. Levine, Administrator (Total facility includes 94 beds in nursing home-type unit) A1 9 10 F3 8 11 15 16 17 19 21 22 26 27 28 30 31 32 33 35 37 42 44 46 48 49 52 53 54 56 57 58 60 64 65 67 69 71 73	33	10	474	6787	368	130970	0	72972	39416	1286
□ SOUTH OAKS HOSPITAL, 400 Sunrise Highway, Zip 11701; tel. 516/264-4000; Jean P. Smith, Chief Executive Officer (Nonreporting) A1 9 10	33	22	334	—	—	—	—	—	—	—
AMSTERDAM—Montgomery County										
★ AMSTERDAM MEMORIAL HOSPITAL, 4988 State Highway 30, Zip 12010-1699; tel. 518/842-3100; Charles E. Rice, President and Chief Executive Officer (Total facility includes 160 beds in nursing home-type unit) A1 9 10 F1 8 12 14 15 16 17 19 21 22 26 27 28 29 30 31 33 34 35 37 39 42 44 45 46 49 51 54 61 64 65 66 67 70 71 73 74 P5	23	10	242	2711	209	49609	0	30679	13702	548
★ ST. MARY'S HOSPITAL, 427 Guy Park Avenue, Zip 12010-1095; tel. 518/842-1900; Peter E. Capobianco, President and Chief Executive Officer A1 9 10 F1 2 3 7 8 14 15 16 17 18 19 21 22 25 26 27 28 29 30 32 33 34 35 37 39 40 41 42 44 45 46 49 51 52 53 54 55 56 57 58 59 61 63 65 67 71 73 74 P5 6 S5945 Carondelet Health System	23	10	143	4737	105	144890	709	38760	20725	705
AUBURN—Cayuga County										
★ AUBURN MEMORIAL HOSPITAL, Lansing Street, Zip 13021; tel. 315/255-7011; Christopher J. Rogers, Administrator A1 5 9 10 F7 8 11 16 19 21 22 25 34 37 40 44 49 52 54 63 64 65 67 71 72 73	23	10	266	8135	226	80238	635	47925	26741	1004
BATAVIA—Genesee County										
★ GENESEE MEMORIAL HOSPITAL, 127 North Street, Zip 14020-1697; tel. 716/343-6030; Douglas T. Jones, President and Chief Executive Officer A1 9 10 F7 8 12 14 15 16 17 19 21 22 25 28 29 30 31 33 34 36 37 39 40 41 42 44 46 49 51 61 63 65 66 67 71 73 74	23	10	70	3383	55	65446	553	20596	9772	454
★ ST. JEROME HOSPITAL, 16 Bank Street, Zip 14020-2260; tel. 716/343-3131; Charles W. Smith Jr., Chief Executive Officer A1 9 10 F2 8 11 12 15 16 17 18 19 22 28 29 30 32 33 34 35 37 41 44 45 51 62 65 66 71 73 S3595 Eastern Mercy Health System	21	10	96	2837	65	65947	0	19631	9172	375
★ VETERANS AFFAIRS MEDICAL CENTER, 222 Richmond Avenue, Zip 14020; tel. 716/343-7500; Paul J. McCool, Director (Total facility includes 70 beds in nursing home-type unit) A1 5 9 F2 3 4 5 8 10 14 15 16 19 20 21 22 25 26 27 29 30 32 33 34 35 37 39 41 42 43 44 45 46 48 49 50 51 52 54 55 57 58 60 63 64 65 67 71 73 74 P6 S9295 Department of Veterans Affairs	45	10	158	987	131	70143	0	31471	15261	428

Hospitals, U.S. / NEW YORK

Hospital, Address, Telephone, Administrator, Approval, Facility, and Physician Codes, Health Care System	Classification Codes		Utilization Data					Expense (thousands) of dollars		
	Control	Service	Beds	Admissions	Census	Outpatient Visits	Births	Total	Payroll	Personnel

★ American Hospital Association (AHA) membership
□ Joint Commission on Accreditation of Healthcare Organizations (JCAHO) accreditation
+ American Osteopathic Hospital Association (AOHA) membership
○ American Osteopathic Association (AOA) accreditation
△ Commission on Accreditation of Rehabilitation Facilities (CARF) accreditation
Control codes 61, 63, 64, 71, 72 and 73 indicate hospitals listed by AOHA, but not registered by AHA. For definition of numerical codes, see page A6.

BATH—Steuben County

★ IRA DAVENPORT MEMORIAL HOSPITAL, 7571 State Route 54, Zip 14810; tel. 607/776-2141; Timothy F. Reardon, Chief Executive Officer (Total facility includes 120 beds in nursing home–type unit) **A**1 9 10 **F**1 7 8 16 17 19 22 26 30 31 33 34 37 40 42 44 49 51 64 65 71 73 — 23 10 186 2268 152 9003 251 15911 7496 328

★ VETERANS AFFAIRS MEDICAL CENTER, 76 Veterans Avenue, Zip 14810-0842; tel. 607/776-2111; Mel A. Gores FACHE, Director (Total facility includes 642 beds in nursing home–type unit) **A**1 **F**3 8 10 17 19 20 24 26 27 28 31 32 33 34 35 37 39 41 42 45 46 49 52 56 58 64 65 67 71 73 74 **S**9295 Department of Veterans Affairs — 45 10 850 2137 685 59647 0 39838 24053 658

BAY SHORE—Suffolk County

★ SOUTHSIDE HOSPITAL, 301 East Main Street, Zip 11706-8458; tel. 516/968-3000; Theodore A. Jospe, President **A**1 3 5 9 10 **F**2 3 4 7 8 10 11 12 13 14 15 16 17 18 19 20 21 22 25 28 29 30 31 32 33 34 37 38 39 40 41 42 43 44 46 48 49 51 52 53 54 56 58 60 63 65 66 67 68 70 71 73 74 — 23 10 451 15452 306 80715 2648 107223 57661 1335

BEACON—Dutchess County

★ CRAIG HOUSE HOSPITAL, Howland Avenue, Zip 12508; tel. 914/831-1200; Paul S. Hochenberg, President and Chief Executive Officer **A**1 10 **F**2 16 52 53 55 **P**1 — 33 22 61 538 31 0 0 — — 77

SAINT FRANCIS HOSPITAL See Saint Francis Hospital, Poughkeepsie

BELLEROSE—Queens County, See New York City

BETHPAGE—Nassau County

□ MID-ISLAND HOSPITAL, 4295 Hempstead Turnpike, Zip 11714-5769; tel. 516/579-6000; Robert J. Reed, President (Nonreporting) **A**1 9 10 — 33 10 223 — — — — — — —

BINGHAMTON—Broome County

BINGHAMTON GENERAL HOSPITAL See United Health Services Hospitals–Binghamton

★ BINGHAMTON PSYCHIATRIC CENTER, 425 Robinson Street, Zip 13901; tel. 607/773-4022; David J. Woodlock, Acting Executive Director **A**1 10 **F**15 16 20 25 39 45 46 52 53 55 57 58 65 73 **S**0009 New York State Department of Mental Health — 12 22 250 212 260 45542 0 — — 661

MEDICENTER See United Health Services Hospitals–Binghamton

★ OUR LADY OF LOURDES MEMORIAL HOSPITAL, 169 Riverside Drive, Zip 13905-4198; tel. 607/798-5111; Michael G. Guley, President and Chief Executive Officer **A**1 2 9 10 **F**5 7 8 9 12 14 15 16 17 19 22 24 25 26 27 28 29 30 31 32 33 34 35 37 38 39 40 41 42 44 45 46 48 49 51 52 56 60 63 65 66 67 71 73 74 **P**5 7 **S**1855 Daughters of Charity National Health System — 21 10 202 9257 169 426415 1407 76065 34259 1104

★ ○ UNITED HEALTH SERVICES HOSPITALS–BINGHAMTON, (Includes Binghamton General Hospital, Binghamton, New York; Medicenter, 600 High Avenue, Endicott, New York, Zip 13760; tel. 607/754-7171; Wilson Memorial Regional Medical Center, 33-57 Harrison Street, Johnson City, New York, Zip 13790; tel. 607/763-6000) 10-42 Mitchell Avenue, Zip 13903; tel. 607/763-6000; Matthew J. Salanger, President and Chief Executive Officer **A**1 2 3 5 8 10 11 12 13 **F**2 3 4 6 7 8 10 11 12 13 14 15 16 17 18 19 21 22 26 27 28 29 30 31 32 34 35 37 38 39 40 41 42 43 44 45 46 48 49 51 52 53 54 55 56 57 58 60 61 63 64 65 66 67 68 69 70 71 72 73 74 **P**1 7 — 23 10 511 20094 422 129023 1766 164684 71680 2276

BROCKPORT—Monroe County

★ LAKESIDE MEMORIAL HOSPITAL, 156 West Avenue, Zip 14420-1286; tel. 716/637-3131; Robert W. Harris, President (Nonreporting) **A**1 9 10 — 23 10 61 — — — — — — —

BRONX–Bronx County, See New York City

BRONXVILLE—Westchester County

★ LAWRENCE HOSPITAL, 55 Palmer Avenue, Zip 10708-3491; tel. 914/787-1000; Roger G. Dvorak, President **A**1 2 9 10 **F**7 8 11 16 17 19 21 22 26 28 30 32 33 34 35 36 37 39 40 42 44 45 48 49 54 56 63 65 66 67 71 73 **P**5 8 — 23 10 280 9094 206 29947 1480 64460 34774 891

BROOKLYN–Kings County, See New York City

BUFFALO—Erie County

□ BRYLIN HOSPITALS, 1263 Delaware Avenue, Zip 14209; tel. 716/886-8200; Leonard Pleskow, Chairman and Chief Executive Officer **A**1 9 10 **F**1 2 3 52 53 54 55 56 57 58 59 **P**6 — 33 22 150 2890 91 24643 0 — — 292

★ BUFFALO COLUMBUS HOSPITAL, 300 Niagara Street, Zip 14201; tel. 716/845-4300; Andres Garcia, President and Chief Executive Officer (Nonreporting) **A**9 10 — 23 10 46 — — — — — — —

★ BUFFALO GENERAL HOSPITAL, (Includes Deaconess Center, 1001 Humboldt Parkway, Zip 14208; tel. 716/886-4400) 100 High Street, Zip 14203-1154; tel. 716/845-5600; John E. Friedlander, President and Chief Executive Officer (Total facility includes 242 beds in nursing home–type unit) **A**1 3 5 8 9 10 **F**3 4 5 7 8 10 11 12 14 15 16 19 20 21 22 23 26 29 30 31 32 33 34 35 37 40 41 42 43 44 46 48 49 50 51 52 53 54 55 56 57 58 60 61 62 64 65 69 71 72 73 74 **P**5 7 — 23 10 984 26275 852 238746 1987 251361 125616 3605

★ BUFFALO PSYCHIATRIC CENTER, 400 Forest Avenue, Zip 14213-1298; tel. 716/885-2261; George Molnar M.D., Executive Director **A**1 10 **F**1 2 3 4 5 6 7 8 9 10 12 15 16 17 18 19 20 21 22 23 25 26 27 30 31 35 39 40 41 42 43 44 45 46 48 49 50 51 52 54 55 56 57 58 59 60 61 63 65 67 69 70 71 73 **P**1 **S**0009 New York State Department of Mental Health — 12 22 436 532 443 59018 0 60264 40238 1274

□ CHILDREN'S HOSPITAL, (Children's General Medical, Surgical and Maternity) 219 Bryant Street, Zip 14222-2099; tel. 716/878-7000; Joseph A. Ruffolo, President and Chief Executive Officer (Nonreporting) **A**1 3 5 9 10 — 23 59 313 — — — — — — —

Hospitals, U.S. / NEW YORK

Hospital, Address, Telephone, Administrator, Approval, Facility, and Physician Codes, Health Care System	Classification Codes		Utilization Data					Expense (thousands) of dollars		
★ American Hospital Association (AHA) membership □ Joint Commission on Accreditation of Healthcare Organizations (JCAHO) accreditation + American Osteopathic Hospital Association (AOHA) membership ○ American Osteopathic Association (AOA) accreditation △ Commission on Accreditation of Rehabilitation Facilities (CARF) accreditation Control codes 61, 63, 64, 71, 72 and 73 indicate hospitals listed by AOHA, but not registered by AHA. For definition of numerical codes, see page A6	Control	Service	Beds	Admissions	Census	Outpatient Visits	Births	Total	Payroll	Personnel
□ ERIE COUNTY MEDICAL CENTER, 462 Grider Street, Zip 14215; tel. 716/898–3000; Paul J. Candino, Chief Executive Officer (Nonreporting) **A**1 3 5 9 10	13	10	675	—	—	—	—	—	—	—
★ MERCY HOSPITAL, 565 Abbott Road, Zip 14220; tel. 716/828–2001; Sister Kathi Sweeney, Chief Executive Officer (Total facility includes 74 beds in nursing home–type unit) **A**1 3 5 9 10 **F**7 10 11 12 14 19 20 21 22 25 26 30 32 33 34 35 37 39 40 42 44 46 48 49 63 64 65 66 67 71 72 73 **P**6 8 **S**3595 Eastern Mercy Health System	21	10	423	13850	370	217592	2244	93389	47405	1795
★ MILLARD FILLMORE HEALTH SYSTEM, (Formerly Millard Fillmore Hospitals) (Includes Millard Fillmore Suburban Hospital, 1540 Maple Road, Williamsville, New York, Zip 14221; tel. 716/688–3100; Evelyn G. Brown, Chief Executive Officer) 3 Gates Circle, Zip 14209–9986; tel. 716/887–4600; Charles B. Van Vorst, President and Chief Executive Officer (Total facility includes 75 beds in nursing home–type unit) **A**1 3 5 6 8 9 10 **F**4 7 8 10 11 12 13 15 16 17 18 19 20 21 22 25 26 28 29 31 32 33 34 35 37 40 41 42 43 44 45 46 49 50 51 60 61 63 64 65 71 73 74 **P**7 8	23	10	560	21921	520	228525	3108	209207	85152	2867
□ ROSWELL PARK CANCER INSTITUTE, (Cancer Research) Elm and Carlton Streets, Zip 14263–0001; tel. 716/845–2300; Thomas B. Tomasi M.D., Ph.D., President and Chief Executive Officer **A**1 2 3 5 9 10 **F**8 15 16 17 19 20 21 25 28 29 30 31 33 34 35 37 39 41 42 44 45 46 49 50 53 54 60 63 65 67 69 71 73 74 **P**6	12	49	124	4894	102	94575	0	138603	61407	1940
□ SHEEHAN MEMORIAL HOSPITAL, 425 Michigan Avenue, Zip 14203–2297; tel. 716/848–2000; Ruben A. Medina, President and Chief Executive Officer (Nonreporting) **A**1 9 10	23	10	109	—	—	—	—	—	—	—
★ SISTERS OF CHARITY HOSPITAL OF BUFFALO, 2157 Main Street, Zip 14214–2692; tel. 716/862–2000; John J. Maher, President and Chief Executive Officer (Total facility includes 80 beds in nursing home–type unit) **A**1 3 5 6 9 10 12 13 **F**2 3 7 8 11 12 14 15 16 17 18 19 20 21 22 25 26 29 30 32 33 34 35 37 38 39 40 41 42 44 45 46 48 49 51 60 61 64 65 67 71 72 73 74 **P**3 7 **S**1855 Daughters of Charity National Health System	21	10	493	13706	363	208125	3257	97730	47141	1701
★ VETERANS AFFAIRS MEDICAL CENTER, 3495 Bailey Avenue, Zip 14215–1129; tel. 716/834–9200; Richard S. Droske, Director; Dennis Tepper, Chief Operating Officer (Total facility includes 96 beds in nursing home–type unit) **A**1 2 3 5 8 9 **F**1 2 3 4 8 10 11 12 17 18 19 20 21 22 26 27 28 29 30 31 32 33 34 37 39 41 42 43 44 45 46 48 49 50 51 52 54 55 56 57 58 59 60 63 64 65 67 69 71 73 74 **S**9295 Department of Veterans Affairs	45	10	472	8054	368	195494	0	119806	71524	1682
CAMBRIDGE—Washington County										
□ MARY MCCLELLAN HOSPITAL, One Myrtle Avenue, Zip 12816; tel. 518/677–2611; Alan J. Burgess, President and Chief Executive Officer (Nonreporting) **A**1 9 10	23	10	113	—	—	—	—	—	—	—
CANANDAIGUA—Ontario County										
★ F. F. THOMPSON HEALTH SYSTEM, 350 Parrish Street, Zip 14424–1793; tel. 716/396–6535; Linda Janczak, President and Chief Executive Officer (Total facility includes 148 beds in nursing home–type unit) **A**1 3 9 10 **F**1 7 8 13 14 15 16 17 19 21 22 25 26 27 28 29 30 32 33 34 35 37 39 40 41 42 44 45 46 49 51 63 64 65 66 67 69 71 72 73 74 **P**8	23	10	261	4656	215	—	630	39030	20014	728
★ VETERANS AFFAIRS MEDICAL CENTER, (Includes Long–term Medical and Psychiatric) 400 Fort Hill Avenue, Zip 14424–1197; tel. 716/396–3601; Stuart C. Collyer, Director; Dennis Tepper, Chief Operating Officer (Total facility includes 100 beds in nursing home–type unit) **A**1 **F**2 3 12 17 20 22 26 27 28 30 31 33 37 41 44 46 49 51 52 54 55 56 57 58 59 64 65 67 71 73 74 **P**6 **S**9295 Department of Veterans Affairs	45	49	661	1779	579	75000	0	59611	40322	1186
CARMEL—Putnam County										
ARMS ACRES, Seminary Hill Road, Zip 10512, Mailing Address: P.O. Box X, Zip 10512; tel. 914/225–3400; Mark Schottinger, Director (Nonreporting)	33	82	129	—	—	—	—	—	—	—
★ PUTNAM HOSPITAL CENTER, Stoneleigh Avenue, Zip 10512–9948; tel. 914/279–5711; William R. Wedral, President **A**1 9 10 **F**2 3 4 7 8 9 10 11 12 14 15 16 17 18 19 21 22 26 28 29 30 32 33 34 35 36 37 38 39 40 41 42 43 44 45 46 47 48 49 52 53 54 55 56 57 58 59 63 64 65 67 69 71 73 74 **P**3 5 7 8	23	10	164	6465	117	45507	613	46957	22861	626
CARTHAGE—Jefferson County										
★ CARTHAGE AREA HOSPITAL, 1001 West Street, Zip 13619–9703; tel. 315/493–1000; Kenn C. Rishel, Supervising Administrator and Chief Executive Officer (Total facility includes 30 beds in nursing home–type unit) **A**1 9 10 **F**7 8 14 15 16 19 20 21 22 28 32 33 35 36 40 41 44 49 54 58 61 64 65 71 73 **P**3	23	10	78	1861	55	43544	392	12751	6702	192
CASTLE POINT—Dutchess County										
★ VETERANS AFFAIRS MEDICAL CENTER, Zip 12511–9999; tel. 914/831–2000; Ronald F. Lipp, Director (Total facility includes 113 beds in nursing home–type unit) **A**1 3 **F**2 3 4 8 10 11 12 17 18 19 20 22 23 24 25 26 27 28 31 32 33 34 35 37 39 40 42 43 44 46 48 49 51 52 54 56 57 58 60 61 63 65 67 71 72 73 **S**9295 Department of Veterans Affairs	45	10	235	2181	211	56728	0	46222	26988	677
CENTRAL ISLIP—Suffolk County										
★ CENTRAL ISLIP PSYCHIATRIC CENTER, Carleton Avenue, Zip 11722–4598; tel. 516/234–6262; James E. Ramseur, Exeuctive Director (Nonreporting) **A**1 10 **S**0009 New York State Department of Mental Health	12	22	375	—	—	—	—	—	—	—
CHEEKTOWAGA—Erie County										
★ ST. JOSEPH HOSPITAL, 2605 Harlem Road, Zip 14225–4097; tel. 716/891–2400; Patrick J. Wiles, Chief Executive Officer **A**1 9 10 **F**4 7 8 10 11 12 15 16 17 19 22 23 25 28 29 30 31 32 33 34 35 37 41 42 43 44 45 46 49 50 51 60 63 65 69 70 71 73 74 **P**6	21	10	184	5603	156	110609	0	42336	20521	710

Hospitals, U.S. / NEW YORK

Hospital, Address, Telephone, Administrator, Approval, Facility, and Physician Codes, Health Care System	Classification Codes		Utilization Data					Expense (thousands) of dollars		
	Control	Service	Beds	Admissions	Census	Outpatient Visits	Births	Total	Payroll	Personnel

★ American Hospital Association (AHA) membership
□ Joint Commission on Accreditation of Healthcare Organizations (JCAHO) accreditation
+ American Osteopathic Hospital Association (AOHA) membership
○ American Osteopathic Association (AOA) accreditation
△ Commission on Accreditation of Rehabilitation Facilities (CARF) accreditation
Control codes 61, 63, 64, 71, 72 and 73 indicate hospitals listed by AOHA, but not registered by AHA. For definition of numerical codes, see page A6

CLIFTON SPRINGS—Ontario County

★ CLIFTON SPRINGS HOSPITAL AND CLINIC, 2 Coulter Road, Zip 14432–1189; tel. 315/462–1311; John P. Galati, President and Chief Executive Officer (Total facility includes 108 beds in nursing home–type unit) **A**1 9 10 **F**2 3 4 8 10 14 15 16 17 19 21 22 25 26 27 28 29 30 33 34 35 37 39 41 42 44 45 46 49 51 52 54 56 57 58 60 64 65 66 67 71 73 **P**7	23	10	262	3422	157	103550	0	29583	15950	616

COBLESKILL—Schoharie County

BASSETT HOSPITAL OF SCHOHARIE COUNTY, (Formerly Community Hospital of Schoharie County) 41 Grandview Drive, Zip 12043–1331; tel. 518/234–2511; James J. Morrissey Jr., Administrator (Data for 92 days) **A**9 10 **F**8 16 19 21 22 33 34 41 42 44 49 51 65 71 73 74 **P**6	23	10	40	226	21	—	0	334	306	111

COOPERSTOWN—Otsego County

★ MARY IMOGENE BASSETT HOSPITAL, (Includes Mary Imogene Bassett Hospital, Andes Road, Route 28, Delhi, New York, Zip 13753; tel. 607/746–2371; Margaret Warden, Administrative Director) One Atwell Road, Zip 13326–1394; tel. 607/547–3100; William F. Streck M.D., President and Chief Executive Officer **A**1 2 3 5 8 9 10 **F**7 8 10 12 14 15 16 19 20 21 22 25 29 30 31 34 35 37 39 40 41 42 44 45 46 49 51 52 53 54 55 56 58 59 60 61 63 65 67 70 71 73 **P**6	23	10	208	8892	140	378719	757	110366	64047	1875

CORNING—Steuben County

★ CORNING HOSPITAL, 176 Denison Parkway East, Zip 14830; tel. 607/937–7200; John E. Pignatore, President and Chief Executive Officer (Total facility includes 120 beds in nursing home–type unit) **A**1 9 10 **F**7 8 14 15 16 19 21 22 30 31 34 35 37 40 42 44 49 64 65 66 67 71 73	23	10	274	5305	213	95186	527	34040	14583	556

CORNWALL—Orange County

★ CORNWALL HOSPITAL, Laurel Avenue, Zip 12518–1499; tel. 914/534–7711; Val S. Gray, Executive Director **A**1 9 10 **F**14 15 16 17 19 20 22 28 29 30 34 35 37 44 49 52 54 56 63 65 67 71 73	23	10	125	4043	90	39098	0	26697	13621	403

CORTLAND—Cortland County

★ CORTLAND MEMORIAL HOSPITAL, 134 Homer Avenue, Zip 13045–0960; tel. 607/756–3500; Robert M. Lovell, President and Chief Executive Officer (Total facility includes 82 beds in nursing home–type unit) **A**1 10 **F**1 7 8 15 19 21 22 24 26 28 30 31 32 34 35 37 40 41 44 45 46 49 52 56 63 64 65 66 67 71 73	23	10	259	5609	147	97116	716	30259	15191	662

CUBA—Allegany County

□ CUBA MEMORIAL HOSPITAL, 140 West Main Street, Zip 14727–1398; tel. 716/968–2000; Marc A. Subject, Chief Executive Officer (Total facility includes 61 beds in nursing home–type unit) **A**1 3 9 10 **F**2 3 7 8 9 11 12 13 14 15 16 17 18 19 20 21 22 26 27 28 29 30 31 32 33 34 35 36 37 39 40 41 44 45 47 49 50 51 52 53 54 55 56 57 58 59 60 61 63 64 65 66 67 68 69 70 71 72 73 74 **P**1 5	23	10	87	762	129	39871	0	8383	4352	214

DANSVILLE—Livingston County

★ NICHOLAS H. NOYES MEMORIAL HOSPITAL, 111 Clara Barton Street, Zip 14437–9527; tel. 716/335–6001; Richard S. Warren, President and Chief Executive Officer **A**1 9 10 **F**7 8 15 17 19 21 22 28 29 32 34 36 37 40 42 44 49 58 63 65 68 71 73	23	10	72	2896	45	58099	325	17038	8228	337

DIX HILLS—Suffolk County

★ SAGAMORE CHILDREN'S PSYCHIATRIC CENTER, 197 Half Hollow Road, Zip 11746; tel. 516/673–7700; Robert Schweitzer Ed.D., Executive Director **A**1 **F**12 14 15 16 19 21 22 32 35 39 45 46 52 53 54 55 56 58 65 71 73 **S**0009 New York State Department of Mental Health	12	52	69	200	72	22407	0	—	—	244

DELHI—Delaware County

MARY IMOGENE BASSETT HOSPITAL See Mary Imogene Bassett Hospital, Cooperstown

DOBBS FERRY—Westchester County

□ COMMUNITY HOSPITAL AT DOBBS FERRY, 128 Ashford Avenue, Zip 10522; tel. 914/693–0700; Thomas E. Green, President and Chief Executive Officer (Nonreporting) **A**1 9 10	23	10	50	—	—	—	—	—	—	—

DUNKIRK—Chautauqua County

★ BROOKS MEMORIAL HOSPITAL, 529 Central Avenue, Zip 14048–2599; tel. 716/366–1111; Richard H. Ketcham, President **A**1 9 10 **F**7 8 17 19 21 22 25 26 28 29 30 32 33 35 36 37 40 41 42 44 46 49 60 65 71 73	23	10	133	3489	65	78242	471	23388	10425	380

EAST MEADOW—Nassau County

★ NASSAU COUNTY MEDICAL CENTER, 2201 Hempstead Turnpike, Zip 11554–1854; tel. 516/572–0123; Joseph R. Erazo, Chief Executive Officer (Nonreporting) **A**1 2 3 5 8 9 10	13	10	1384	—	—	—	—	—	—	—

ELIZABETHTOWN—Essex County

★ ELIZABETHTOWN COMMUNITY HOSPITAL, Park Street, Zip 12932–0277; tel. 518/873–6377 **A**1 9 10 **F**8 11 13 15 16 17 22 28 34 39 44 45 46 51 65 67 68 71 73	23	10	25	488	18	21843	0	4180	2480	85

ELLENVILLE—Ulster County

□ ELLENVILLE COMMUNITY HOSPITAL, Route 209, Zip 12428–0668, Mailing Address: P.O. Box 668, Zip 12428–0668; tel. 914/647–6400; Richard F. Spreer, Executive Vice President (Nonreporting) **A**1 9 10	23	10	51	—	—	—	—	—	—	—

ELMHURST—Queens County, See New York City

ELMIRA—Chemung County

★ ARNOT OGDEN MEDICAL CENTER, 600 Roe Avenue, Zip 14905–1629; tel. 607/737–4100; Anthony J. Cooper, President and Chief Executive Officer (Total facility includes 40 beds in nursing home–type unit) **A**1 2 6 9 10 **F**4 7 8 10 11 14 15 16 17 19 21 22 28 29 30 31 33 34 35 37 38 40 41 42 43 44 46 49 51 60 63 64 65 67 68 70 71 73 74 **P**6	23	10	271	7824	191	160979	1420	76254	32368	1130

Hospitals, U.S. / NEW YORK

Hospital, Address, Telephone, Administrator, Approval, Facility, and Physician Codes, Health Care System	Classification Codes		Utilization Data					Expense (thousands) of dollars		
★ American Hospital Association (AHA) membership □ Joint Commission on Accreditation of Healthcare Organizations (JCAHO) accreditation + American Osteopathic Hospital Association (AOHA) membership ○ American Osteopathic Association (AOA) accreditation △ Commission on Accreditation of Rehabilitation Facilities (CARF) accreditation Control codes 61, 63, 64, 71, 72 and 73 indicate hospitals listed by AOHA, but not registered by AHA. For definition of numerical codes, see page A6	Control	Service	Beds	Admissions	Census	Outpatient Visits	Births	Total	Payroll	Personnel
★ ELMIRA PSYCHIATRIC CENTER, 100 Washington Street, Zip 14902–1527; tel. 607/737–4739; Bert W. Pyle Jr., Director **A**1 10 **F**1 3 4 5 6 7 8 10 12 13 17 18 19 20 21 22 23 25 26 27 28 29 30 31 32 33 34 35 36 39 41 42 43 44 45 46 49 50 51 52 53 54 55 56 57 58 59 60 61 62 63 65 66 67 68 69 71 72 73 74 **S**0009 New York State Department of Mental Health	12	22	122	420	129	15956	0	21090	14409	362
★ ST. JOSEPH'S HOSPITAL, (Includes Twin Tiers Rehabilitation Center) 555 East Market Street, Zip 14902–1512; tel. 607/733–6541; Sister Marie Castagnaro, President and Chief Executive Officer (Total facility includes 31 beds in nursing home–type unit) **A**1 2 9 10 **F**2 3 8 9 11 12 14 15 16 17 18 19 21 22 23 28 30 33 34 35 37 41 42 44 46 48 49 51 52 54 55 56 57 58 62 64 65 66 67 69 70 71 73 **P**6 7	21	10	255	5432	168	100476	0	—	—	756
FAR ROCKAWAY–Queens County, See New York City										
FLUSHING–Queens County, See New York City										
FOREST HILLS–Queens County, See New York City										
FREEPORT—Nassau County FREEPORT HOSPITAL, 267 South Ocean Avenue, Zip 11520; tel. 516/378–0800; Frank Herzlin M.D., Chief Executive Officer (Nonreporting) **A**9	32	82	52							
FULTON—Oswego County ★ ALBERT LINDLEY LEE MEMORIAL HOSPITAL, 510 South Fourth Street, Zip 13069–2994; tel. 315/592–2224; Dennis A. Casey, Executive Director **A**1 9 10 **F**3 4 8 10 16 19 20 21 22 25 28 29 30 31 32 34 37 41 42 44 45 50 54 55 56 57 58 59 63 65 66 69 71 73	23	10	67	2449	55	50448	0	17556	8212	299
GENEVA—Ontario County ★ GENEVA GENERAL HOSPITAL, 196 North Street, Zip 14456–1694; tel. 315/787–4025; James J. Dooley, President (Total facility includes 305 beds in nursing home–type unit) **A**1 6 9 10 **F**1 2 4 7 8 10 12 14 15 16 17 19 21 22 25 26 27 28 29 30 31 32 33 34 35 36 37 39 40 41 42 44 45 46 49 54 56 62 64 65 67 68 69 71 72 73 74	23	10	443	4947	387	253922	692	50702	22912	892
GLEN COVE—Nassau County ★ NORTH SHORE UNIVERSITY HOSPITAL AT GLEN COVE, St Andrews Lane, Zip 11542; tel. 516/676–5000; John S. T. Gallagher, President **A**1 2 3 5 9 10 **F**3 7 8 11 12 15 16 17 19 20 21 22 26 28 30 34 36 37 40 42 44 48 49 51 52 57 58 60 65 67 71 73 74 **P**5 6 7 8 **S**0062 North Shore Health System	23	10	265	8642	210	66961	709	80591	46716	—
GLEN OAKS–Queens County, See New York City										
GLENS FALLS—Warren County ★ GLENS FALLS HOSPITAL, 100 Park Street, Zip 12801–9898; tel. 518/792–3151; David G. Kruczlnicki, President and Chief Executive Officer **A**1 2 5 9 10 **F**3 7 8 11 14 15 16 17 19 20 21 22 24 25 28 30 31 32 33 34 35 37 39 40 41 42 44 46 49 52 53 54 55 56 57 58 60 65 67 70 71 72 73 **P**5	23	10	442	12567	266	341072	1680	96280	47291	1627
GLENVILLE—New York County CONIFER PARK, (Formerly Listed Under Scotia) 79 Glenridge Road, Zip 12302; tel. 518/399–6446; Mr. Gail Harkness, Executive Director **A**9 **F**2 3 16 65 67 74 **P**6	33	82	225	2852	151	—	0	—	—	244
GLOVERSVILLE—Fulton County □ NATHAN LITTAUER HOSPITAL AND NURSING HOME, 99 East State Street, Zip 12078; tel. 518/725–8621; Thomas J. Dowd, Executive Director (Total facility includes 84 beds in nursing home–type unit) **A**1 5 9 10 **F**3 4 8 10 12 14 15 16 17 18 19 20 21 22 25 26 28 29 30 31 32 33 34 35 37 39 40 41 42 44 45 46 49 51 53 54 55 56 57 58 61 64 65 67 71 73 74 **P**5 6	23	10	208	4572	167	84873	475	34514	18547	586
GOSHEN—Orange County ★ ARDEN HILL HOSPITAL, 4 Harriman Drive, Zip 10924–2499; tel. 914/294–5441; A. Gordon McAleer, President **A**1 9 10 **F**3 7 8 15 16 19 20 22 28 31 33 34 35 37 40 41 42 44 52 53 54 55 56 57 58 59 63 65 67 71 73	23	10	176	6595	151	55539	560	38174	18891	582
GOUVERNEUR—St. Lawrence County EDWARD JOHN NOBLE HOSPITAL OF GOUVERNEUR, 77 West Barney Street, Zip 13642; tel. 315/287–1000; Charles P. Conole FACHE, Administrator **A**9 10 **F**7 8 9 12 13 14 15 16 17 18 19 21 22 26 28 30 33 34 35 36 37 38 39 40 44 46 47 48 49 52 53 54 56 57 60 61 64 65 71 74 **P**2	23	10	47	1516	26	24206	114	8389	4225	208
GOWANDA—Cattaraugus County □ TRI–COUNTY MEMORIAL HOSPITAL, 100 Memorial Drive, Zip 14070–1194; tel. 716/532–3377; John P. Davanzo, Chief Executive Officer (Nonreporting) **A**1 9 10	23	10	60	—	—	—				
GREENPORT—Suffolk County □ EASTERN LONG ISLAND HOSPITAL, 201 Manor Place, Zip 11944–1298; tel. 516/477–1000; Thomas B. Doolan, President and Chief Executive Officer **A**1 9 10 **F**2 3 8 11 14 15 16 17 19 21 22 25 26 27 30 31 32 33 34 35 37 44 45 46 47 52 54 56 65 67 71 73	23	10	80	2228	61	19155	0	17579	—	256
HAMILTON—Madison County ★ COMMUNITY MEMORIAL HOSPITAL, Broad Street, Zip 13346–9518; tel. 315/824–1100; David Felton, Administrator (Nonreporting) **A**1 9 10	23	10	84	—	—	—				
HARRIS—Sullivan County □ COMMUNITY GENERAL HOSPITAL OF SULLIVAN COUNTY, Bushville Road, Zip 12742, Mailing Address: P.O. Box 800, Zip 12742–0800; tel. 914/794–3300; Martin Richman, Executive Director (Total facility includes 40 beds in nursing home–type unit) **A**1 9 10 **F**1 2 5 7 8 11 12 15 17 21 22 25 26 28 30 31 32 33 34 35 37 40 42 44 45 46 48 49 52 53 54 56 64 65 67 70 71 73 **P**6	23	10	284	7203	179	105060	535	52545	25768	688
HARRISON—Westchester County ST. VINCENT'S HOSPITAL See St. Vincent's Hospital and Medical Center, New York City										

© 1995 AHA Guide

Hospitals, U.S. / NEW YORK

Hospital, Address, Telephone, Administrator, Approval, Facility, and Physician Codes, Health Care System	Classification Codes		Utilization Data					Expense (thousands) of dollars		
★ American Hospital Association (AHA) membership □ Joint Commission on Accreditation of Healthcare Organizations (JCAHO) accreditation + American Osteopathic Hospital Association (AOHA) membership ○ American Osteopathic Association (AOA) accreditation △ Commission on Accreditation of Rehabilitation Facilities (CARF) accreditation Control codes 61, 63, 64, 71, 72 and 73 indicate hospitals listed by AOHA, but not registered by AHA. For definition of numerical codes, see page A6	Control	Service	Beds	Admissions	Census	Outpatient Visits	Births	Total	Payroll	Personnel
HEMPSTEAD—Nassau County										
□ HEMPSTEAD GENERAL HOSPITAL MEDICAL CENTER, 800 Front Street, Zip 11550–4600; tel. 516/560–1200; Robert Emerman, Chief Executive Officer (Total facility includes 251 beds in nursing home–type unit) **A**1 9 10 **F**2 8 9 11 15 16 17 19 21 22 26 28 30 31 33 34 35 37 40 42 44 46 47 48 49 50 52 54 56 57 64 65 67 71 73	32	10	464	4501	375	18150	0	54198	26722	576
HOLLISWOOD–Queens County, See New York City										
HORNELL—Steuben County										
★ ST. JAMES MERCY HOSPITAL, 411 Canisteo Street, Zip 14843–2197; tel. 607/324–8000; Paul E. Shephard, President and Chief Executive Officer (Total facility includes 55 beds in nursing home–type unit) **A**1 6 9 10 **F**1 2 3 7 8 9 11 15 17 19 20 21 22 25 26 27 28 29 30 31 32 33 34 35 37 39 40 41 42 44 46 49 51 52 53 54 55 56 57 58 60 64 65 67 70 71 72 73 74 **P**6 **S**3595 Eastern Mercy Health System	23	10	220	4585	149	126752	375	33926	16867	786
HUDSON—Columbia County										
★ COLUMBIA MEMORIAL HOSPITAL, (Formerly Columbia–Greene Medical Center, Catskill) 71 Prospect Avenue, Zip 12534; tel. 518/828–8244; Jane Ehrlich, President and Chief Executive Officer (Nonreporting) **A**1 9 10	23	10	267	—	—	—	—	—	—	—
HUNTINGTON—Suffolk County										
★ HUNTINGTON HOSPITAL, 270 Park Avenue, Zip 11743–2799; tel. 516/351–2000; J. Ronald Gaudreault, President and Chief Executive Officer **A**1 5 9 10 **F**8 11 14 15 19 21 22 26 28 30 34 35 36 37 39 40 42 44 46 49 52 54 60 61 63 65 67 71 73 74 **S**0062 North Shore Health System	23	10	314	12132	250	—	1679	95769	50729	1238
ILION—Herkimer County										
MOHAWK VALLEY DIVISION See St. Luke's Memorial Hospital Center, Utica										
IRVING—Chautauqua County										
★ LAKE SHORE HOSPITAL, 845 Route 5 and 20, Zip 14081–9716; tel. 716/934–2654; James B. Foster, Chief Executive Officer (Total facility includes 120 beds in nursing home–type unit) **A**9 10 **F**1 19 22 32 33 34 37 41 44 49 52 54 56 64 65 71 73 **P**3	23	10	184	1738	164	35274	0	18435	8496	282
ITHACA—Tompkins County										
★ TOMPKINS COMMUNITY HOSPITAL, 101 Dates Drive, Zip 14850–1383; tel. 607/274–4011; Bonnie H. Howell, President and Chief Executive Officer **A**1 2 9 10 **F**4 7 8 12 14 15 17 19 21 22 24 25 28 30 32 33 34 35 36 37 39 40 41 42 44 45 49 52 54 56 57 60 65 66 67 71 72 73	23	10	204	6939	125	137533	1079	38655	17916	609
JACKSON HEIGHTS–Queens County, See New York City										
JAMAICA–Queens County, See New York City										
JAMESTOWN—Chautauqua County										
★ WOMAN'S CHRISTIAN ASSOCIATION HOSPITAL, 207 Foote Avenue, Zip 14702–9975; tel. 716/487–0141; Mark E. Celmer, President and Chief Executive Officer **A**1 2 9 10 **F**2 3 7 8 13 15 16 18 19 20 21 22 25 29 30 31 33 34 35 37 40 41 42 44 48 49 51 52 53 54 55 56 58 59 60 65 66 67 69 70 71 73 74	23	10	342	10005	232	153952	869	57158	28542	1353
JOHNSON CITY—Broome County										
WILSON MEMORIAL REGIONAL MEDICAL CENTER See United Health Services Hospitals–Binghamton, Binghamton										
KATONAH—Westchester County										
★ FOUR WINDS HOSPITAL, 800 Cross River Road, Zip 10536; tel. 914/763–8151; Samuel C. Klagsbrun M.D., Director **A**1 9 10 **F**3 15 16 34 52 53 54 58 59 65 **P**7	31	22	115	1272	109	—	0	—	—	492
KENMORE—Erie County										
★ KENMORE MERCY HOSPITAL, 2950 Elmwood Avenue, Zip 14217–1390; tel. 716/879–6100; Sister Mary Joel Schimscheiner, Chief Executive Officer **A**1 9 10 **F**5 8 11 12 14 15 16 17 18 19 22 25 26 28 29 30 32 33 34 35 36 37 41 42 44 45 46 49 51 61 65 71 73 74 **P**8 **S**3595 Eastern Mercy Health System	21	10	219	7436	168	33090	0	54726	28259	947
KINGS PARK—Suffolk County										
★ KINGS PARK PSYCHIATRIC CENTER, Mailing Address: Box 9000, Zip 11754–9000; tel. 516/544–2957; Alan M. Weinstock MS, M.P.A., Chief Executive Officer **A**1 10 **F**4 7 8 9 10 11 12 14 15 16 18 19 20 21 22 23 25 27 31 34 35 37 39 40 42 43 44 48 50 51 52 54 55 56 58 60 63 65 69 70 71 73 **P**6 **S**0009 New York State Department of Mental Health	12	22	990	1592	1003	124415	0	105336	74609	1797
KINGSTON—Ulster County										
★ BENEDICTINE HOSPITAL, 105 Marys Avenue, Zip 12401–5894; tel. 914/338–2500; Sister Louise Garley, President **A**1 3 5 9 10 **F**7 8 11 14 15 16 17 19 21 22 27 30 34 37 40 42 44 46 49 51 52 56 57 63 65 67 71 73 74	21	10	222	7517	167	46037	1219	45357	23897	711
□ KINGSTON HOSPITAL, 396 Broadway, Zip 12401; tel. 914/331–3131; Anthony P. Marmo, Chief Executive Officer (Nonreporting) **A**1 3 5 9 10	23	10	140	—	—	—	—	—	—	—
LACKAWANNA—Erie County										
★ OUR LADY OF VICTORY HOSPITAL, 55 Melroy at Ridge Road, Zip 14218–1687; tel. 716/825–8000; Albert L. Condino, President and Chief Executive Officer (Total facility includes 10 beds in nursing home–type unit) **A**1 9 10 **F**8 11 12 16 17 19 20 21 22 25 27 28 30 32 33 35 37 39 41 42 44 45 48 51 60 64 65 71 73	21	10	242	6246	200	67774	0	49477	21734	694
LAKE PLACID—Franklin County										
ADIRONDACK MEDICAL CENTER–LAKE PLACID SITE See Adirondack Medical Center, Saranac Lake										

Hospitals, U.S. / NEW YORK

Hospital, Address, Telephone, Administrator, Approval, Facility, and Physician Codes, Health Care System	Classification Codes		Utilization Data					Expense (thousands) of dollars		
★ American Hospital Association (AHA) membership □ Joint Commission on Accreditation of Healthcare Organizations (JCAHO) accreditation + American Osteopathic Hospital Association (AOHA) membership ○ American Osteopathic Association (AOA) accreditation △ Commission on Accreditation of Rehabilitation Facilities (CARF) accreditation Control codes 61, 63, 64, 71, 72 and 73 indicate hospitals listed by AOHA, but not registered by AHA. For definition of numerical codes, see page A6	Control	Service	Beds	Admissions	Census	Outpatient Visits	Births	Total	Payroll	Personnel
LEWISTON—Niagara County ★ MOUNT ST. MARY'S HOSPITAL OF NIAGARA FALLS, 5300 Military Road, Zip 14092-1997; tel. 716/297-4800; Henry G. Lobl, President and Chief Executive Officer **A**1 10 **F**2 3 7 8 11 14 15 16 19 20 21 22 25 30 31 33 34 35 37 39 40 44 46 49 51 56 59 61 65 67 71 73 **P**1	21	10	179	5573	127	128808	281	36733	17607	651
LITTLE FALLS—Herkimer County ★ LITTLE FALLS HOSPITAL, 140 Burwell Street, Zip 13365-1725; tel. 315/823-1000; David S. Armstrong Jr., Administrator (Total facility includes 34 beds in nursing home–type unit) **A**1 9 10 **F**7 14 15 19 21 22 33 34 37 40 44 49 54 61 64 65 69 71 73	23	10	134	3621	101	63631	370	16654	9399	388
LITTLE NECK–Queens County, See New York City										
LOCKPORT—Niagara County ★ LOCKPORT MEMORIAL HOSPITAL, 521 East Avenue, Zip 14094-3299; tel. 716/434-9111; Richard W. Petersen, President **A**1 9 10 **F**2 8 17 19 21 22 25 28 29 30 32 33 34 37 40 41 42 44 45 49 65 66 71 73 **P**5	23	10	121	4435	94	91546	365	31366	13494	459
LONG BEACH—Nassau County ★ LONG BEACH MEDICAL CENTER, (Formerly Long Beach Memorial Hospital and Nursing Home) 455 East Bay Drive, Zip 11561-2300, Mailing Address: P.O. Box 300, Zip 11561-2300; tel. 516/897-1000; Martin F. Nester Jr., Chief Executive Officer (Total facility includes 200 beds in nursing home–type unit) **A**1 9 10 12 13 **F**3 4 5 8 11 12 14 15 16 17 18 19 20 21 22 26 28 29 30 31 32 34 37 42 44 45 46 48 49 51 52 53 54 56 57 58 63 64 65 66 67 71 73 **P**1	23	10	395	5636	366	206500	0	68106	35440	922
LONG ISLAND CITY–Queens County, See New York City										
LOWVILLE—Herkimer County ★ LEWIS COUNTY GENERAL HOSPITAL, 7785 North State Street, Zip 13367-1297; tel. 315/376-5200; G. William Udovich, Chief Executive Officer and Administrator (Nonreporting) **A**1 9 10 **S**0585 Brim, Inc.	13	10	214	—	—	—	—	—	—	—
MALONE—Franklin County ★ ALICE HYDE HOSPITAL ASSOCIATION, 115 Park Street, Zip 12953-0729, Mailing Address: P.O. Box 729, Zip 12953-0729; tel. 518/483-3000; John W. Johnson, President **A**1 9 10 **F**3 7 8 12 13 15 18 19 20 22 26 28 30 32 33 35 36 37 39 40 41 42 44 46 53 54 56 57 58 60 64 65 67 71 73	23	10	155	3693	135	48273	368	21379	11352	409
MANHASSET—Nassau County MANHASSET AMBULATORY CARE PAVILION See Long Island Jewish Medical Center, New York										
★ NORTH SHORE UNIVERSITY HOSPITAL, 300 Community Drive, Zip 11030; tel. 516/562-0100; John S T. Gallagher, President (Total facility includes 253 beds in nursing home–type unit) **A**1 2 3 5 8 9 10 **F**3 4 7 8 10 11 12 13 15 16 17 19 20 21 22 23 25 26 27 28 30 31 32 34 35 36 37 38 39 40 42 43 44 46 47 49 50 51 52 53 54 55 56 57 58 60 61 63 64 65 66 67 68 70 71 72 73 74 **P**5 6 7 8	23	10	958	37366	911	278427	5414	503940	276547	—
MANHATTAN–New York County, See New York City										
MARGARETVILLE—Delaware County ★ MARGARETVILLE MEMORIAL HOSPITAL, Route 28, Zip 12455, Mailing Address: P.O. Box 200, Zip 12455; tel. 914/586-2631; Christine Wasyl, Chief Executive Officer (Nonreporting) **A**1 9 10	23	10	53	—	—	—	—	—	—	—
MASSENA—St. Lawrence County □ MASSENA MEMORIAL HOSPITAL, One Hospital Drive, Zip 13662; tel. 315/764-1711; James B. Watson, Chief Executive Officer **A**1 9 10 **F**7 8 11 12 13 14 15 16 17 19 22 23 26 28 29 30 32 33 34 35 36 37 39 40 41 42 44 45 46 48 49 51 65 71 73 74 **P**3	14	10	40	2496	36	60318	312	15206	7122	263
MEDINA—Orleans County ★ MEDINA MEMORIAL HOSPITAL, 200 Ohio Street, Zip 14103; tel. 716/798-2000; Walter S. Becker, Administrator (Total facility includes 30 beds in nursing home–type unit) **A**1 9 10 **F**7 14 15 16 17 19 21 22 25 30 33 34 37 40 41 44 46 64 71 **P**5	23	10	101	2685	70	51329	304	17111	7496	316
MIDDLETOWN—Orange County ★ △ HORTON MEDICAL CENTER, 60 Prospect Avenue, Zip 10940-4133; tel. 914/343-2424; Paul Dell Uomo, President and Chief Executive Officer **A**1 7 9 10 **F**3 7 8 11 12 16 19 21 22 23 26 27 28 30 32 33 34 35 37 39 40 42 44 46 48 49 56 60 61 63 65 67 71 73	23	10	286	10059	166	99173	1746	64856	33182	871
★ MIDDLETOWN PSYCHIATRIC CENTER, 141 Monhagen Avenue, Zip 10940-6198, Mailing Address: Box 1453, Zip 10940; tel. 914/342-5511; James Bopp, Executive Director **A**1 3 10 **F**2 3 4 8 9 11 12 15 16 18 19 20 21 22 25 27 30 31 35 37 39 40 41 42 43 44 45 46 48 52 55 56 57 58 59 64 65 67 70 71 73 **P**6 **S**0009 New York State Department of Mental Health	12	22	423	454	459	41070	0	—	—	—
MINEOLA—Nassau County ★ WINTHROP–UNIVERSITY HOSPITAL, 259 First Street, Zip 11501; tel. 516/663-0333; Martin J. Delaney, President and Chief Executive Officer (Nonreporting) **A**1 2 3 5 8 9 10	23	10	591	—	—	—	—	—	—	—
MONTOUR FALLS—Schuyler County ★ SCHUYLER HOSPITAL, 220 Steuben Street, Zip 14865-9709; tel. 607/535-7121; Robert M. Swinnerton, President and Chief Executive Officer (Total facility includes 120 beds in nursing home–type unit) **A**1 9 10 **F**3 7 8 14 15 16 19 22 26 28 31 34 36 37 39 40 44 45 46 49 51 64 65 70 71 72 73	23	10	169	1446	136	51616	208	16466	8734	362

© 1995 AHA Guide

Hospitals, U.S. / NEW YORK

Hospital, Address, Telephone, Administrator, Approval, Facility, and Physician Codes, Health Care System	Classification Codes		Utilization Data					Expense (thousands) of dollars		
★ American Hospital Association (AHA) membership ☐ Joint Commission on Accreditation of Healthcare Organizations (JCAHO) accreditation + American Osteopathic Hospital Association (AOHA) membership ○ American Osteopathic Association (AOA) accreditation △ Commission on Accreditation of Rehabilitation Facilities (CARF) accreditation Control codes 61, 63, 64, 71, 72 and 73 indicate hospitals listed by AOHA, but not registered by AHA. For definition of numerical codes, see page A6	Control	Service	Beds	Admissions	Census	Outpatient Visits	Births	Total	Payroll	Personnel
MONTROSE—Westchester County										
★ FRANKLIN DELANO ROOSEVELT VETERANS AFFAIRS HOSPITAL, Route 9A, Zip 10548, Mailing Address: P.O. Box 100, Zip 10548; tel. 914/737-4400; Lee J. Kauper, Director (Total facility includes 122 beds in nursing home-type unit) **A**1 3 5 **F**1 2 3 4 5 6 7 8 9 10 11 12 15 16 17 18 19 20 21 22 23 24 26 28 29 30 31 33 34 35 37 39 40 41 42 43 44 45 46 48 49 50 51 52 54 55 56 57 58 59 60 61 63 64 65 67 69 70 71 73 74 **P**6 **S**9295 Department of Veterans Affairs	45	22	698	3335	633	69438	0	85899	52032	1406
MOUNT KISCO—Westchester County										
★ NORTHERN WESTCHESTER HOSPITAL CENTER, 400 Main Street, Zip 10549; tel. 914/666-1200; Donald W. Davis, President (Nonreporting) **A**1 2 9 10	23	10	259	—	—	—	—	—	—	—
MOUNT VERNON—Westchester County										
☐ MOUNT VERNON HOSPITAL, 12 North Seventh Avenue, Zip 10550; tel. 914/664-8000; Richard L. Petrillo M.D., Executive Director **A**1 3 5 9 10 **F**2 7 8 10 11 12 14 15 16 17 18 19 22 23 27 28 29 30 32 33 34 35 37 39 40 41 42 44 49 52 54 56 58 59 60 65 67 69 70 71 73 74	23	10	245	7374	169	156484	1010	59754	34515	936
NEW HYDE PARK—Queens County, See New York City										
NEW ROCHELLE—Westchester County										
★ NEW ROCHELLE HOSPITAL MEDICAL CENTER, 16 Guion Place, Zip 10802; tel. 914/632-5000; John R. Spicer, President and Chief Executive Officer **A**1 2 3 5 9 10 **F**3 7 8 9 11 13 14 15 16 17 18 19 20 21 22 26 28 29 30 31 32 33 34 35 36 37 38 39 40 41 42 44 45 46 48 49 51 52 53 54 56 57 58 60 61 63 64 65 67 68 69 70 71 72 73 **P**6 8	23	10	253	9409	201	173661	1047	96431	45779	1239
NEW YORK CITY (Includes all hospitals located within the five boroughs) **BRONX** – Bronx County (Mailing Address – Bronx) **BROOKLYN** – Kings County (Mailing Address – Brooklyn) **MANHATTAN** – New York County (Mailing Address – New York) **QUEENS** – Queens County (Mailing Addresses – Bellerose, Elmhurst, Far Rockaway, Flushing, Forest Hills, Glen Oaks, Holliswood, Jackson Heights, Jamaica, Little Neck, Long Island City, New Hyde Park, and Queens Village) **RICHMOND VALLEY** – Richmond County (Mailing Address – Staten Island) ABRAHAM JACOBI GENERAL CARE HOSPITAL AND PSYCHIATRIC UNITS See Bronx Municipal Hospital Center										
★ BAYLEY SETON HOSPITAL, 75 Vanderbilt Avenue, Staten Island, Zip 10304-3850; tel. 718/390-6000; John N. Kastanis FACHE, Executive Vice President **A**1 2 3 5 9 10 **F**2 3 7 8 10 11 12 14 15 16 17 19 20 21 26 27 28 29 30 31 32 33 34 36 37 38 40 42 44 46 47 48 49 51 52 53 54 55 56 57 58 59 61 64 65 67 70 71 73 74 **P**6 **S**6095 Sisters of Charity Health Care System Corporation	21	10	191	7231	160	149346	0	103560	41193	853
★ BELLEVUE HOSPITAL CENTER, First Avenue and 27th Street, Zip 10016; tel. 212/562-4141; Howard C. Cohen, Acting Executive Director **A**1 2 3 5 9 10 **F**1 2 3 4 5 7 8 10 11 12 13 14 15 16 17 18 19 20 21 22 23 26 28 29 30 31 34 35 37 38 39 40 41 42 43 44 45 46 47 48 49 51 52 53 54 55 56 57 58 59 60 61 65 66 67 68 70 71 72 73 74 **P**6 **S**3075 New York City Health and Hospitals Corporation	14	10	1150	25657	940	554841	2214	409720	245243	5617
★ BETH ISRAEL MEDICAL CENTER, (Includes Beth Israel Medical Center–North Division, 170 East End Avenue, New York, New York, Zip 10128; tel. 212/870-9000) First Avenue and 16th Street, Zip 10003-3803; tel. 212/420-2000; Robert G. Newman M.D., President **A**1 3 5 6 8 9 10 **F**2 3 4 5 7 8 10 11 12 13 14 15 16 17 18 19 20 21 22 23 25 26 27 28 29 30 31 32 33 34 35 37 38 39 40 41 42 43 44 45 46 48 49 50 51 52 53 54 55 56 57 58 59 60 61 63 65 66 67 68 69 71 73 74 **P**6	23	10	1165	47164	1061	325643	5289	652021	321194	6613
★ BRONX CHILDREN'S PSYCHIATRIC CENTER, 1000 Waters Place, Bronx, Zip 10461-2799; tel. 718/892-0808; E. Richard Feinberg M.D., Executive Director (Nonreporting) **A**1 3 **S**0009 New York State Department of Mental Health	12	52	75	—	—	—	—	—	—	—
★ BRONX MUNICIPAL HOSPITAL CENTER, (Includes Abraham Jacobi General Care Hospital and Psychiatric Units, Bronx; Van Etten Hospitals, Bronx) Pelham Parkway S. & Eastchester Road, Bronx, Zip 10461; tel. 718/918-6000; Lorraine C. Tregde, Executive Director (Nonreporting) **A**1 3 5 8 10 **S**3075 New York City Health and Hospitals Corporation	14	10	725	—	—	—	—	—	—	—
★ BRONX PSYCHIATRIC CENTER, 1500 Waters Place, Bronx, Zip 10461; tel. 718/931-0600; Marlene Lopez, Executive Director (Nonreporting) **A**1 3 5 10 **S**0009 New York State Department of Mental Health	12	22	658	—	—	—	—	—	—	—
★ BRONX–LEBANON HOSPITAL CENTER, (Includes Bronx–Lebanon Hospital Center, 1650 Grand Concourse, Bronx, Zip 10457; tel. 212/590-1800) 1276 Fulton Avenue, Bronx, Zip 10456; tel. 718/590-1800; Miguel A. Fuentes, President and Chief Executive Officer **A**1 2 3 5 8 9 10 **F**1 2 3 4 8 10 11 12 13 14 16 17 18 19 20 21 22 25 26 28 29 30 31 33 34 37 38 40 42 44 46 48 49 51 52 53 54 55 56 57 58 60 61 65 66 67 68 71 73 **P**6	23	10	674	22834	598	544680	3181	292156	159248	3848
☐ BROOKDALE HOSPITAL MEDICAL CENTER, Linden Boulevard at Brookdale Plaza, Brooklyn, Zip 11212-3198; tel. 718/240-5000; Frank J. Maddalena, President and Chief Executive Officer **A**1 2 3 5 8 9 10 12 **F**4 7 8 10 11 12 15 16 17 19 20 21 22 23 25 26 28 30 31 32 34 37 38 40 41 42 44 46 47 49 51 52 53 54 55 56 57 58 59 60 61 64 65 66 67 68 70 71 73 **P**5	23	10	719	25295	625	309612	2551	286037	165252	4528
★ BROOKLYN HOSPITAL CENTER, (Includes Downtown Campus, 121 DeKalb Avenue, Brooklyn, New York, Zip 11201; tel. 718/250-8000; Caledonian Campus, 100 Parkside Avenue, Brooklyn, New York, Zip 11226; tel. 718/940-2000) 121 Dekalb Avenue, Brooklyn, Zip 11201-5493; tel. 718/250-8000; Frederick D. Alley, President and Chief Executive Officer **A**1 2 3 5 8 9 10 **F**1 4 7 8 10 12 13 14 15 16 17 19 20 21 22 25 26 27 28 29 30 31 32 33 34 35 37 38 39 40 41 42 43 44 46 51 54 60 61 63 65 67 68 69 70 71 73 74	23	10	653	26663	526	225958	5194	254743	141226	3287

Hospitals, U.S. / NEW YORK

Hospital, Address, Telephone, Administrator, Approval, Facility, and Physician Codes, Health Care System	Classification Codes		Utilization Data					Expense (thousands) of dollars		
★ American Hospital Association (AHA) membership □ Joint Commission on Accreditation of Healthcare Organizations (JCAHO) accreditation + American Osteopathic Hospital Association (AOHA) membership ○ American Osteopathic Association (AOA) accreditation △ Commission on Accreditation of Rehabilitation Facilities (CARF) accreditation Control codes 61, 63, 64, 71, 72 and 73 indicate hospitals listed by AOHA, but not registered by AHA. For definition of numerical codes, see page A6	Control	Service	Beds	Admissions	Census	Outpatient Visits	Births	Total	Payroll	Personnel
★ CABRINI MEDICAL CENTER, 227 East 19th Street, Zip 10003–2600; tel. 212/995–6000; Jeffrey Frerichs, President and Chief Executive Officer A1 2 3 5 8 9 10 F3 4 5 7 8 10 11 12 13 14 15 16 17 19 20 21 22 23 25 26 27 28 29 30 31 32 33 34 35 37 38 39 40 41 42 43 44 45 46 47 48 49 51 52 53 54 55 56 57 58 59 60 61 63 64 65 66 67 69 70 71 73 P5 6 8	23	10	493	10956	375	62027	0	156068	80603	1750
CALEDONIAN CAMPUS See Brooklyn Hospital Center										
★ CALVARY HOSPITAL, (Advanced Cancer) 1740 Eastchester Road, Bronx, Zip 10461–2392; tel. 718/863–6900; Frank A. Calamari, President and Chief Executive Officer A1 9 10 F8 16 19 20 21 22 32 34 39 41 42 45 46 48 60 65 67 73	21	49	200	2240	180	21107	0	52449	30942	736
★ CATHOLIC MEDICAL CENTER OF BROOKLYN AND QUEENS, (Includes Holy Family Home, 1740 84th Street, Brooklyn, New York, Zip 11214; tel. 718/232–3666; Ann C. Carroll, Administrator; Mary Immaculate Hospital, 152–11 89th Avenue, Jamaica, New York, Zip 11432; tel. 718/291–3300; Ann Allen–Ryan, Executive Director; Monsignor James H Fitzpatrick Pavilion for Skilled Nursing Care, 152–11 89th Avenue, Jamaica, New York, Zip 11432; tel. 718/291–4300; Gregory R. Bradley, Administrator; St. John's Queens Hospital, New York; tel. 718/457–1300; Sister Helen Faulds, Executive Director; St. Joseph's Hospital, 158–40 79th Avenue, Flushing, New York, Zip 11366; tel. 212/591–1000; Katherine Dolan, Executive Director; St. Mary's Hospital, 170 Buffalo Avenue, Brooklyn, New York, Zip 11213; tel. 718/774–3600; Bernard M. McCaffrey, Director) 88–25 153rd Street, Jamaica, Zip 11432–3731; tel. 718/657–6800; Mark L. Lane, Acting President (Total facility includes 303 beds in nursing home–type unit) A1 2 3 5 6 8 9 10 F1 2 3 4 5 7 8 9 10 11 12 13 14 15 16 17 18 19 20 21 22 23 25 26 27 28 30 31 32 33 34 35 37 38 39 40 41 42 43 44 46 47 48 49 51 52 53 54 55 56 57 58 59 60 64 65 66 67 68 69 70 71 72 73 74 P8	21	10	1407	42053	1203	462328	5803	525794	272454	5829
★ COLER MEMORIAL HOSPITAL, Franklin D. Roosevelt Island, Zip 10044; tel. 212/848–6000; Mark J. Kator, Executive Director (Total facility includes 775 beds in nursing home–type unit) A1 10 F1 2 3 4 5 8 9 10 11 12 15 17 18 19 20 21 22 23 24 25 26 27 28 29 30 31 32 33 34 36 37 38 39 40 41 43 44 45 46 47 48 49 51 52 53 54 55 56 57 58 59 60 61 64 65 66 67 68 70 71 72 73 74 P6 S3075 New York City Health and Hospitals Corporation	14	48	1025	852	1003	0	0	98187	61997	1781
COMMUNITY HOSPITAL OF BROOKLYN See The New York Community Hospital of Brooklyn										
★ CONEY ISLAND HOSPITAL, 2601 Ocean Parkway, Brooklyn, Zip 11235–7795; tel. 718/615–4000; Howard C. Cohen, Executive Director A1 2 3 5 9 10 12 F3 4 5 7 8 10 11 12 14 15 16 18 19 20 21 22 23 25 26 27 28 30 31 34 37 40 41 42 44 46 48 49 51 52 53 54 55 56 57 58 59 65 67 71 73 74 P6 S3075 New York City Health and Hospitals Corporation	14	82	462	14543	407	404903	1871	216573	131642	2953
CORNERSTONE OF MEDICAL ARTS CENTER HOSPITAL, (Formerly Medical Arts Center Hospital) 57 West 57th Street, Zip 10019; tel. 212/755–0200; Norman J. Sokolow, President A9 F2 3 16 65 P6	33	82	74	3375	68	5703	0	10188	4871	109
★ CREEDMOOR PSYCHIATRIC CENTER, Jamaica, Mailing Address: 80–45 Winchester Boulevard, Queens Village, Zip 11427; tel. 718/264–3300; Charlotte Seltzer, Chief Executive Officer A1 3 10 F2 3 4 6 8 9 10 11 12 17 18 19 20 21 22 24 25 27 30 31 32 33 34 35 37 39 40 41 42 43 44 45 46 48 49 51 52 55 56 58 60 64 65 67 71 73 P6 S0009 New York State Department of Mental Health	12	22	955	1893	925	110347	0	—	—	1791
★ DOCTORS' HOSPITAL OF STATEN ISLAND, 1050 Targee Street, Staten Island, Zip 10304; tel. 718/390–1400; Stephen N. F. Anderson, Director A1 9 10 F4 7 10 14 15 16 19 21 22 28 29 30 31 32 35 36 37 39 42 43 44 45 46 49 50 54 60 63 65 71 73	33	10	117	3749	81	31670	0	24141	10887	339
★ △ ELMHURST HOSPITAL CENTER, 79–01 Broadway, Elmhurst, Zip 11373; tel. 718/334–4000; Pete Velez, Executive Director A1 2 3 5 7 8 9 10 F2 3 4 5 7 8 9 10 11 12 13 14 15 16 17 18 19 20 21 22 23 25 26 27 28 29 30 31 32 34 35 37 38 39 40 41 42 43 44 45 46 47 48 49 50 51 52 53 54 55 56 57 58 59 60 61 63 65 67 68 69 70 71 73 74 P6 S3075 New York City Health and Hospitals Corporation	14	10	574	19726	505	522187	4742	271054	165585	3913
□ FLUSHING HOSPITAL MEDICAL CENTER, 45th Avenue at Parsons Boulevard, Flushing, Zip 11355; tel. 718/670–5000; Charles J. Pendola, President and Chief Executive Officer (Nonreporting) A1 3 5 9 10	23	10	415	—	—	—	—	—	—	—
★ △ GOLDWATER MEMORIAL HOSPITAL, Franklin D Roosevelt Island, Zip 10044; tel. 212/318–8000; Samuel Lehrfeld, Executive Director (Total facility includes 510 beds in nursing home–type unit) A1 3 5 7 10 F19 20 31 41 45 46 48 64 65 73 P6 S3075 New York City Health and Hospitals Corporation	14	48	952	1130	912	0	0	100655	63923	1685
★ GRACIE SQUARE HOSPITAL, 420 East 76th Street, Zip 10021–3104; tel. 212/988–4400; Frank Bruno, Chief Executive Officer A1 9 10 F3 22 39 46 52 57 65 P1 5 7	23	22	100	2403	109	37802	0	24386	12178	335
★ △ HARLEM HOSPITAL CENTER, (Includes Harlem General Care Unit and Harlem Psychiatric Unit) 506 Lenox Avenue, Zip 10037–1894; tel. 212/939–1340; Bruce Goldman, Executive Director (Nonreporting) A1 2 3 5 7 8 9 10 S3075 New York City Health and Hospitals Corporation	14	10	688	—	—	—	—	—	—	—
HILLSIDE HOSPITAL See Long Island Jewish Medical Center										
★ HOLLISWOOD HOSPITAL, 87–37 Palermo Street, Holliswood, Zip 11423; tel. 718/776–8181; Alan D. Barry Ph.D., Chief Executive Officer A1 9 10 F14 15 16 52 59	33	22	100	1974	90	0	0	—	—	180

© 1995 AHA Guide

Hospitals, U.S. / NEW YORK

Hospital, Address, Telephone, Administrator, Approval, Facility, and Physician Codes, Health Care System	Classification Codes		Utilization Data					Expense (thousands) of dollars		
	Control	Service	Beds	Admissions	Census	Outpatient Visits	Births	Total	Payroll	Personnel

★ American Hospital Association (AHA) membership
□ Joint Commission on Accreditation of Healthcare Organizations (JCAHO) accreditation
+ American Osteopathic Hospital Association (AOHA) membership
○ American Osteopathic Association (AOA) accreditation
△ Commission on Accreditation of Rehabilitation Facilities (CARF) accreditation
Control codes 61, 63, 64, 71, 72 and 73 indicate hospitals listed by AOHA, but not registered by AHA. For definition of numerical codes, see page A6

Hospital	Control	Service	Beds	Admissions	Census	Outpatient Visits	Births	Total	Payroll	Personnel
★ △ HOSPITAL FOR JOINT DISEASES ORTHOPEDIC INSTITUTE, 301 East 17th Street, Zip 10003–3890; tel. 212/598–6000; Victor H. Frankel M.D., President and Chief Executive Officer; Reuven Savitz, Executive Vice President and Co–Chief Executive Officer A1 3 5 7 8 9 10 F5 12 14 15 16 17 18 19 21 24 25 26 30 34 35 39 41 42 44 45 46 48 49 51 54 63 65 66 71 72 73	23	49	220	6206	153	54712	0	133813	55799	1159
★ HOSPITAL FOR SPECIAL SURGERY, 535 East 70th Street, Zip 10021–4898; tel. 212/606–1000; John R. Ahearn, President A1 3 5 6 8 9 10 F1 2 3 4 5 6 7 8 9 10 11 12 13 14 15 16 17 18 19 20 21 22 23 24 25 26 27 28 29 30 31 32 33 34 35 36 37 38 39 40 41 43 44 45 46 47 48 49 50 51 52 53 54 55 56 57 58 59 60 61 63 65 66 67 68 69 70 71 72 73 74 P5 8	23	47	160	6196	106	147021	0	139400	62431	1157
□ INTERFAITH MEDICAL CENTER, (Includes Brooklyn Jewish Division, 555 Prospect Place, Brooklyn, New York, Zip 11238; tel. 718/935–7000; St. John's Episcopal Hospital Division, 1545 Atlantic Avenue, Brooklyn, New York, Zip 11213; tel. 718/604–6000) 555 Prospect Place, Brooklyn, Zip 11238–4299; tel. 718/935–7000; Corbett A. Price, Chief Executive Officer A1 3 5 6 9 10 F2 3 7 8 10 11 12 15 16 17 19 20 21 22 25 28 30 31 32 34 35 37 38 40 42 44 46 47 49 52 56 58 59 60 63 65 69 71 73 P3	23	10	543	14043	468	251271	1737	174500	100107	2411
★ JAMAICA HOSPITAL MEDICAL CENTER, (Formerly Jamaica Hospital) 8900 Van Wyck Expressway, Jamaica, Zip 11418–2832; tel. 718/206–6000; David P. Rosen, President A1 3 5 9 10 12 F8 10 11 13 15 16 17 18 19 20 21 22 25 26 28 29 30 32 34 35 37 40 41 42 44 45 48 49 51 54 61 65 68 70 71 72 73	23	10	315	13668	268	166555	2717	147550	75406	1874
★ KINGS COUNTY HOSPITAL CENTER, 451 Clarkson Avenue, Brooklyn, Zip 11203–2097; tel. 718/245–3131; Jean G. Leon R.N., M.P.A., Interim Executive Director A1 2 3 5 9 10 F1 2 3 4 5 7 8 11 12 13 15 17 18 19 20 21 22 23 24 25 26 27 28 29 30 31 32 33 34 35 36 37 38 39 40 41 42 43 44 45 46 47 48 49 50 51 52 53 54 55 56 57 58 59 60 61 62 63 65 66 67 68 69 70 71 72 73 74 P6 S3075 New York City Health and Hospitals Corporation	14	10	1150	28823	893	798330	3321	469571	270053	6906
□ KINGS HIGHWAY HOSPITAL CENTER, 3201 Kings Highway, Brooklyn, Zip 11234; tel. 718/252–3000; Samuel Berson M.D., Executive Director (Nonreporting) A1 9 10	33	10	212	—	—	—	—	—	—	—
★ KINGSBORO PSYCHIATRIC CENTER, 681 Clarkson Avenue, Brooklyn, Zip 11203; tel. 718/221–7395; Colga B. Hylton MS, Acting Executive Director A1 5 10 F1 3 4 5 8 10 12 15 16 17 18 19 20 21 22 23 25 26 29 30 31 32 33 34 35 39 41 42 43 44 45 46 49 50 51 52 53 54 55 56 57 58 59 60 61 65 67 69 70 71 73 74 S0009 New York State Department of Mental Health	12	22	526	1828	559	67376	0	5028	—	1179
★ △ KINGSBROOK JEWISH MEDICAL CENTER, 585 Schenectady Avenue, Brooklyn, Zip 11203–1891; tel. 718/604–5000; Milton M. Gutman, Chief Executive Officer (Total facility includes 538 beds in nursing home–type unit) A1 3 5 7 9 10 F1 8 11 14 15 16 17 19 20 21 22 25 26 27 28 29 31 32 34 35 37 41 42 44 45 46 48 49 51 53 54 55 56 57 58 60 63 64 65 66 68 71 73 P3 5 8	23	10	881	7688	831	78294	0	150380	80177	2123
★ LA GUARDIA HOSPITAL, Flushing, Mailing Address: 102–01 66th Road, Forest Hills, Zip 11375; tel. 718/830–4000; Michael N. Dreisiger, President A1 2 3 5 9 10 F7 8 11 12 13 14 15 16 17 18 19 21 22 26 29 30 31 32 37 39 40 41 42 44 45 46 49 61 65 67 71 72 73 74	23	10	231	9412	183	48139	2109	88157	43088	945
★ LENOX HILL HOSPITAL, 100 East 77th Street, Zip 10021–1883; tel. 212/434–2000; Gladys George, President A1 3 5 8 9 10 F5 8 10 11 12 14 15 16 18 19 21 22 25 28 29 30 31 32 34 35 37 38 40 41 42 43 44 45 46 49 51 52 53 54 55 56 57 58 60 61 63 65 66 67 70 71 73 74 P8	23	10	652	24722	557	229039	3874	284066	142712	3036
★ LINCOLN MEDICAL AND MENTAL HEALTH CENTER, 234 East 149th Street, Bronx, Zip 10451–9998; tel. 718/579–5700; Roberto Rodriguez, Executive Director A1 3 5 9 10 F1 3 7 8 11 14 15 16 17 19 20 21 28 29 30 31 32 37 38 40 41 42 44 46 47 49 51 52 54 56 58 60 61 71 73 74 S3075 New York City Health and Hospitals Corporation	14	10	554	21821	510	504843	4227	335306	172116	4428
LITTLE NECK COMMUNITY HOSPITAL, 55–15 Little Neck Parkway, Little Neck, Zip 11362; tel. 718/428–3000; Michael Marigliano, Administrator (Nonreporting) A9 10	32	10	195	—	—	—	—	—	—	—
□ LONG ISLAND COLLEGE HOSPITAL, 340 Henry Street, Brooklyn, Zip 11201; tel. 718/780–1000; Harold L. Light, President and Chief Executive Officer A1 2 3 5 8 9 10 F2 3 7 10 11 15 16 19 20 21 22 23 27 31 32 34 35 37 38 40 41 42 44 45 46 47 48 49 52 53 54 55 57 60 61 65 71 73 74 P5	23	10	601	19792	493	458379	3944	271043	139286	3171
LONG ISLAND JEWISH HOSPITAL See Long Island Jewish Medical Center										
★ LONG ISLAND JEWISH MEDICAL CENTER, (Includes Hillside Hospital, 75–59 263rd Street, Glen Oaks, New York, Zip 11004; tel. 718/470–8000; Henry Hoffman, Administrator; Long Island Jewish Hospital, 270–05 76th Avenue, New Hyde Park, New York, Zip 11040; tel. 718/470–7000; Stephen Grabel, Administrator; Manhasset Ambulatory Care Pavilion, 1554 Northern Boulevard, Manhasset, New York, Zip 11030; tel. 516/365–2070; Schneider Children's Hospital, New Hyde Park, New York, Mailing Address: 270–05 76th Avenue, Zip 11040; tel. 718/470–3000; Larry L. Levine, Administrator) 270–05 76th Avenue, New Hyde Park, Zip 11040; tel. 718/470–7000; David R. Dantzker M.D., President A1 2 3 5 8 9 10 F1 3 4 5 6 7 8 10 11 12 13 14 15 16 17 18 19 20 21 22 23 25 26 27 28 29 30 31 32 34 35 37 38 39 40 41 43 44 45 46 47 49 50 51 52 53 54 55 57 58 59 60 61 63 65 66 67 68 69 71 72 73 74 P5	23	10	829	31183	758	488895	4371	458503	243181	6128
★ LUTHERAN MEDICAL CENTER, 150 55th Street, Brooklyn, Zip 11220–2570; tel. 718/630–7000; George Adams, President and Chief Executive Officer A1 3 5 9 10 12 F1 2 3 7 8 11 12 13 14 15 16 17 19 20 21 22 25 26 27 28 29 30 31 32 34 35 36 37 38 39 40 41 42 44 45 46 48 49 51 53 54 55 56 57 58 60 61 62 63 65 67 68 69 71 72 73 74	23	10	520	17632	404	381819	3034	191257	101460	2509

Hospitals, U.S. / NEW YORK

Hospital, Address, Telephone, Administrator, Approval, Facility, and Physician Codes, Health Care System	Classification Codes		Utilization Data					Expense (thousands) of dollars		
★ American Hospital Association (AHA) membership ☐ Joint Commission on Accreditation of Healthcare Organizations (JCAHO) accreditation + American Osteopathic Hospital Association (AOHA) membership ○ American Osteopathic Association (AOA) accreditation △ Commission on Accreditation of Rehabilitation Facilities (CARF) accreditation Control codes 61, 63, 64, 71, 72 and 73 indicate hospitals listed by AOHA, but not registered by AHA. For definition of numerical codes, see page A6	Control	Service	Beds	Admissions	Census	Outpatient Visits	Births	Total	Payroll	Personnel
★ MAIMONIDES MEDICAL CENTER, 4802 Tenth Avenue, Brooklyn, Zip 11219–2916; tel. 718/283–6000; Stanley Brezenoff, President **A**1 3 5 8 9 10 **F**1 4 7 8 10 11 12 13 14 15 16 17 18 19 20 21 22 25 26 27 28 30 31 32 34 35 37 38 39 40 41 42 43 44 46 49 51 52 53 54 56 57 58 59 60 61 63 65 66 67 68 71 72 73 74 **P**5 6	23	10	705	23934	620	148406	3879	319297	183905	3817
★ MANHATTAN EYE, EAR AND THROAT HOSPITAL, 210 East 64th Street, Zip 10021–9885; tel. 212/838–9200; George A. Sarkar J.D., Executive Director **A**1 3 5 10 **F**14 15 16 22 27 28 30 34 44 45 65 67 69 73 **P**5	23	45	30	3520	16	86418	0	41105	18948	453
★ MANHATTAN PSYCHIATRIC CENTER–WARD'S ISLAND, 600 East 125th Street, Zip 10035–9998; tel. 212/369–0500; Michael H. Ford M.D., Executive Director **A**1 3 5 10 **F**3 4 5 7 8 12 19 20 21 22 23 24 25 31 32 33 34 35 42 43 44 46 50 52 54 55 56 57 58 59 60 63 65 70 71 73 **S**0009 New York State Department of Mental Health	12	22	875	615	916	12776	0	—	—	1507
MEDICAL ARTS CENTER HOSPITAL See Cornerstone of Medical Arts Center Hospital										
★ MEMORIAL HOSPITAL FOR CANCER AND ALLIED DISEASES, 1275 York Avenue, Zip 10021; tel. 212/639–2000; John R. Gunn, Executive Vice President **A**1 2 3 5 8 9 10 **F**8 14 15 16 17 19 20 21 22 25 28 29 31 32 33 34 35 37 39 42 44 45 46 49 50 54 60 63 65 67 69 71 72 73 **P**6	23	49	480	20510	438	250451	0	493456	222212	3631
★ METROPOLITAN HOSPITAL CENTER, (Includes Metropolitan General Care Unit, Metropolitan Drug Detoxification and Metropolitan Psychiatric Unit) 1901 First Avenue, Zip 10029; tel. 212/230–6262; Lorraine C. Tregde, Acting Executive Director **A**1 3 5 8 9 10 **F**2 3 7 8 10 11 12 13 14 15 16 17 18 19 20 21 22 25 27 28 29 30 31 32 34 35 37 38 39 40 41 42 43 44 45 46 47 48 49 51 52 53 54 56 58 59 60 61 63 65 71 73 74 **S**3075 New York City Health and Hospitals Corporation	14	10	607	15841	511	352269	2100	231121	139342	3767
★ MONTEFIORE MEDICAL CENTER, (Includes Jack D. Weiler Hospital of Albert Einstein College of Medicine, 1825 Eastchester Road, Bronx, New York, Zip 10461–2373; tel. 718/904–2000; Patrick R. Wardell, Vice President Operations; Loeb Center Nursing Rehabilitation, 111 East 210th Street, Bronx, New York, Zip 10467–2490; tel. 718/920–4321) 111 East 210th Street, Bronx, Zip 10467–2490; tel. 718/920–4321; Spencer Foreman M.D., President (Total facility includes 80 beds in nursing home–type unit) **A**1 2 3 5 8 9 10 **F**4 8 10 11 12 15 16 17 18 19 20 21 22 23 25 26 28 30 31 32 34 35 37 38 39 40 41 42 43 44 45 46 47 48 49 51 52 55 60 61 63 64 65 66 67 69 71 73 74 **P**5 6 7	23	10	1141	42069	982	1137090	3635	962393	381510	9058
★ MOUNT SINAI MEDICAL CENTER, One Gustave L. Levy Place, Zip 10029–6574; tel. 212/241–8888; John W. Rowe M.D., President **A**1 3 5 8 9 10 **F**1 2 3 4 5 6 7 8 10 11 12 14 15 16 17 19 21 22 23 25 26 28 29 30 31 32 33 34 35 37 38 39 40 41 42 43 44 45 46 47 48 49 50 51 52 53 54 55 56 57 58 59 60 61 63 64 65 66 67 68 69 71 73 74 **P**5	23	10	1171	38868	987	351938	5342	686527	335891	9030
☐ NEW YORK DOWNTOWN HOSPITAL, 170 William Street, Zip 10038; tel. 212/312–5000; Alan H. Channing, President and Chief Executive Officer **A**1 3 5 9 10 **F**3 4 8 10 11 12 13 14 15 16 17 19 20 21 22 26 29 30 31 32 34 35 37 39 40 41 42 43 44 46 48 49 51 52 60 61 65 66 69 70 71 73 74 **P**5 6 7	23	10	213	8158	167	117025	1737	94181	49381	1295
★ NEW YORK EYE AND EAR INFIRMARY, 310 East 14th Street, Zip 10003–4201; tel. 212/979–4000; Joseph P. Corcoran, President **A**1 3 5 9 10 **F**20 25 28 30 34 44 60 65 69 70 71 73	23	45	103	5303	30	159269	0	50063	25523	538
NEW YORK HOSPITAL See Society of the New York Hospital										
★ NEW YORK HOSPITAL MEDICAL CENTER OF QUEENS, 56–45 Main Street, Flushing, Zip 11355; tel. 718/670–1231; Stephen S. Mills, President and Chief Executive Officer (Nonreporting) **A**1 2 3 5 9 10	23	10	487	—	—	—	—	—	—	—
★ NEW YORK METHODIST HOSPITAL, 506 Sixth Street, Brooklyn, Zip 11215; tel. 718/780–3000; Mark J. Mundy, President and Chief Executive Officer **A**1 2 3 5 8 9 10 12 **F**1 2 3 4 5 7 8 9 10 11 12 13 14 15 16 17 19 20 21 22 23 24 25 26 27 28 29 30 31 32 33 34 35 36 37 38 39 40 41 42 43 44 45 46 47 48 49 50 52 53 54 55 56 57 58 59 60 61 63 64 65 66 67 68 69 70 71 72 73 74 **P**5 6 7	23	10	560	21405	532	156634	3073	197663	104223	2286
★ NEW YORK STATE PSYCHIATRIC INSTITUTE, 722 West 168th Street, Zip 10032; tel. 212/960–2200; John M. Oldham M.D., Director **A**1 3 5 10 **F**14 15 16 52 53 55 57 58 **S**0009 New York State Department of Mental Health	12	22	70	340	58	54311	0	—	—	640
★ △ NEW YORK UNIVERSITY MEDICAL CENTER, (Includes Rusk Institute) 550 First Avenue, Zip 10016–4576; tel. 212/263–7300; Theresa Bischoff, Deputy Provost and Executive Vice President **A**1 3 5 7 8 9 10 **F**3 4 7 8 10 11 12 13 15 16 17 18 19 20 21 22 23 24 26 27 28 29 30 31 32 33 34 35 36 37 38 39 40 41 42 43 44 45 46 47 48 49 50 51 52 53 54 55 56 57 58 59 60 61 63 65 66 67 68 69 70 71 72 73 74 **P**5	23	10	879	27476	757	71064	2319	445704	223162	4303
★ NORTH CENTRAL BRONX HOSPITAL, 3424 Kossuth Avenue, Bronx, Zip 10467; tel. 718/519–3500; Lorraine C. Tregde, Acting Executive Director **A**1 3 5 9 10 **F**3 4 7 8 10 12 13 14 15 16 17 18 19 20 21 22 28 29 30 31 34 35 37 38 39 40 41 42 44 45 46 48 49 51 52 53 54 56 58 60 61 63 65 68 71 73 74 **S**3075 New York City Health and Hospitals Corporation	14	10	403	12250	288	251039	2977	184000	106574	—
★ NORTH GENERAL HOSPITAL, 1879 Madison Avenue, Zip 10035–2745; tel. 212/423–4000; Eugene McCabe, President (Nonreporting) **A**1 3 5 6 9 10	23	10	240	—	—	—	—	—	—	—
★ OUR LADY OF MERCY MEDICAL CENTER, (Includes Florence D'Urso Pavilion, 1870 Pelham Parkway South, Bronx, New York, Zip 10461; tel. 212/430–6000) 600 East 233rd Street, Bronx, Zip 10466; tel. 718/920–9000; Gary S. Horan, President and Chief Executive Officer **A**1 2 3 5 8 9 10 **F**2 3 4 7 8 10 11 13 15 16 17 19 20 21 22 23 26 27 28 29 30 31 32 33 34 35 36 37 38 39 40 41 42 43 44 45 46 47 48 49 51 52 54 56 57 58 59 60 63 64 65 66 67 68 71 72 73 74 **P**6 8	21	10	526	17654	434	208649	3367	167297	95271	2102

© 1995 AHA Guide

Hospitals, U.S. / NEW YORK

Hospital, Address, Telephone, Administrator, Approval, Facility, and Physician Codes, Health Care System	Classification Codes		Utilization Data					Expense (thousands) of dollars		
★ American Hospital Association (AHA) membership □ Joint Commission on Accreditation of Healthcare Organizations (JCAHO) accreditation + American Osteopathic Hospital Association (AOHA) membership ○ American Osteopathic Association (AOA) accreditation △ Commission on Accreditation of Rehabilitation Facilities (CARF) accreditation Control codes 61, 63, 64, 71, 72 and 73 indicate hospitals listed by AOHA, but not registered by AHA. For definition of numerical codes, see page A6	Control	Service	Beds	Admissions	Census	Outpatient Visits	Births	Total	Payroll	Personnel
★ PARKWAY HOSPITAL, 70-35 113th Street, Flushing, Zip 11375; tel. 718/990-4100; Paul E. Svensson, Chief Executive Officer **A**1 9 10 **F**4 8 10 11 14 15 16 19 20 21 22 26 28 30 33 35 37 39 42 43 44 46 48 52 56 60 63 65 67 71 73 **P**3 8	33	10	251	8073	227	8211	0	69035	35634	618
PAYNE WHITNEY PSYCHIATRIC CLINIC See Society of the New York Hospital										
□ ○ PENINSULA HOSPITAL CENTER, 51-15 Beach Channel Drive, Far Rockaway, Zip 11691-1074; tel. 718/945-7100; Paul S. Cohen, Chief Executive Officer **A**1 9 10 11 12 13 **F**8 11 15 16 17 19 20 21 22 23 32 34 35 37 42 44 46 49 60 67 70 71 73	23	10	241	5467	218	72208	0	69467	38848	973
★ △ PRESBYTERIAN HOSPITAL IN THE CITY OF NEW YORK, Columbia-Presbyterian Medical Center, Zip 10032-3784; tel. 212/305-2500; William T. Speck M.D., President and Chief Executive Officer **A**1 3 5 7 8 9 10 **F**4 7 8 10 11 12 13 14 15 16 17 18 19 20 21 22 25 26 27 28 29 30 31 32 34 35 37 38 39 40 41 42 43 44 46 47 48 49 50 51 52 53 54 56 58 60 63 65 66 67 68 69 71 72 73 74 **P**7 8	23	10	1198	47808	1134	820006	5598	669547	327040	7367
★ QUEENS CHILDREN'S PSYCHIATRIC CENTER, 74-03 Commonwealth Boulevard, Bellerose, Zip 11426; tel. 718/264-4506; Gloria Faretra M.D., Executive Director (Nonreporting) **A**1 **S**0009 New York State Department of Mental Health	12	52	70	—	—	—	—	—	—	—
★ QUEENS HOSPITAL CENTER, 82-68 164 Street, Jamaica, Zip 11432; tel. 718/883-3000; Arnoline W. Jones, Executive Director **A**1 2 3 5 9 10 **F**2 3 4 7 8 10 12 13 14 16 17 19 20 21 22 25 26 31 32 34 35 37 38 40 42 43 44 46 48 49 51 52 53 54 56 57 58 59 60 63 65 67 68 71 73 74 **P**6 **S**3075 New York City Health and Hospitals Corporation	14	10	483	14364	390	329908	2328	229894	137554	3200
□ ROCKEFELLER UNIVERSITY HOSPITAL, (General Medical and Clinical Research) 1230 York Avenue, Zip 10021-6399; tel. 212/327-8000; (Nonreporting) **A**1 3 9 10	23	49	30	—	—	—	—	—	—	—
SCHNEIDER CHILDREN'S HOSPITAL See Long Island Jewish Medical Center										
★ SOCIETY OF THE NEW YORK HOSPITAL, (Includes New York Hospital, New York, New York; New York Hospital, Westchester Division, White Plains, New York; Payne Whitney Psychiatric Clinic, New York, New York) 525 East 68th Street, Zip 10021; tel. 212/746-5454; David B. Skinner M.D., President and Chief Executive Officer (Nonreporting) **A**1 2 3 5 8 10	23	10	1310	—	—	—	—	—	—	—
★ SOUTH BEACH PSYCHIATRIC CENTER, 777 Seaview Avenue, Staten Island, Zip 10305; tel. 718/667-2300; Lucy Sarkis M.D., Executive Director (Nonreporting) **A**1 10 **S**0009 New York State Department of Mental Health	12	22	342	—	—	—	—	—	—	—
□ ○ ST. BARNABAS HOSPITAL, 183rd Street and Third Avenue, Bronx, Zip 10457-9998; tel. 718/960-9000; Ronald Gade M.D., President (Nonreporting) **A**1 3 5 9 10 11 12 13	23	10	458	—	—	—	—	—	—	—
□ ST. CLARE'S HOSPITAL AND HEALTH CENTER, 415 West 51st Street, Zip 10019; tel. 212/586-1500; Richard N. Yezzo, President **A**1 9 10 12 **F**3 4 7 8 10 12 16 19 20 21 22 26 28 31 32 33 34 35 37 39 42 43 44 45 46 49 52 54 57 58 60 65 67 69 70 71 73	21	10	233	4772	191	61960	0	75376	42809	911
ST. JOHN'S EPISCOPAL HOSPITAL DIVISION See Interfaith Medical Center										
★ ST. JOHN'S EPISCOPAL HOSPITAL-SOUTH SHORE, 327 Beach 19th Street, Far Rockaway, Zip 11691-4424; tel. 718/868-7000; Paul J. Connor III, Administrator (Data for 356 days) **A**1 3 5 9 **F**1 2 3 4 7 8 10 11 12 13 14 15 16 17 18 19 20 21 22 24 25 26 27 28 29 30 31 32 33 34 35 37 39 40 41 42 43 44 45 46 48 49 51 52 53 54 55 56 57 58 59 61 63 64 65 67 68 69 71 73 **P**6 **S**0735 Episcopal Health Services Inc.	21	10	314	10168	286	141419	1245	102841	59987	1246
★ ST. LUKE'S-ROOSEVELT HOSPITAL CENTER, (Includes Roosevelt Hospital, 1000 Tenth Avenue, New York, New York, Zip 10019; tel. 212/523-4000; St. Luke's Hospital Center, 1111 Amsterdam Avenue, New York, New York, Zip 10025; tel. 212/523-4000) 1111 Amsterdam Avenue, Zip 10025; tel. 212/523-4295; Gary Gambuti, President and Chief Executive Officer **A**1 3 5 8 9 10 **F**1 2 3 4 7 8 10 11 12 14 15 16 17 18 19 20 21 22 26 27 28 29 30 31 32 34 35 37 38 39 40 43 44 45 46 48 49 51 52 53 54 55 56 57 58 59 60 61 65 66 67 68 69 70 71 73 74 **P**1	23	10	1032	39542	932	645048	4840	—	—	6597
★ ST. VINCENT'S HOSPITAL AND MEDICAL CENTER OF NEW YORK, (Includes St. Vincent's Hospital, 275 North Street, Harrison, New York, Zip 10528; tel. 914/967-6500) 153 West 11th Street, Zip 10011-8397; tel. 212/604-7000; Karl P. Adler M.D., President and Chief Executive Officer **A**1 2 3 5 6 8 9 10 **F**1 2 3 4 7 8 10 11 14 15 16 17 18 19 21 22 24 25 26 27 28 29 30 31 32 33 34 35 36 37 38 39 40 41 42 43 44 45 46 48 49 52 53 54 55 56 57 58 59 60 61 63 65 67 69 70 71 73 **S**5995 Sisters of Charity Center	21	10	978	25034	794	358431	2229	378412	191181	3976
★ ST. VINCENT'S MEDICAL CENTER OF RICHMOND, 355 Bard Avenue, Staten Island, Zip 10310-1699; tel. 718/876-1234; Dominick M. Stanzione, Executive Vice President **A**1 2 3 5 6 9 10 **F**1 3 7 8 10 11 12 14 15 16 17 18 19 20 21 22 26 28 29 30 31 32 33 34 35 37 38 39 40 42 43 44 46 47 49 52 53 54 56 57 58 59 60 61 62 63 65 67 69 70 71 72 73 74 **P**5 8 **S**6095 Sisters of Charity Health Care System Corporation	21	10	440	17280	378	186826	3064	150598	81751	2034
□ △ STATEN ISLAND UNIVERSITY HOSPITAL, 475 Seaview Avenue, Staten Island, Zip 10305-9998; tel. 718/226-9000; Rick J. Varone, President (Nonreporting) **A**1 2 3 5 7 9 10	23	10	617	—	—	—	—	—	—	—
★ THE NEW YORK COMMUNITY HOSPITAL OF BROOKLYN, (Formerly Community Hospital of Brooklyn) 2525 Kings Highway, Brooklyn, Zip 11229-1798; tel. 718/692-5300; Louise Kane, President and Chief Executive Officer (Nonreporting) **A**1 9 10	23	10	134	—	—	—	—	—	—	—

Hospitals, U.S. / NEW YORK

Hospital, Address, Telephone, Administrator, Approval, Facility, and Physician Codes, Health Care System	Classification Codes		Utilization Data					Expense (thousands) of dollars		
★ American Hospital Association (AHA) membership □ Joint Commission on Accreditation of Healthcare Organizations (JCAHO) accreditation + American Osteopathic Hospital Association (AOHA) membership ○ American Osteopathic Association (AOA) accreditation △ Commission on Accreditation of Rehabilitation Facilities (CARF) accreditation Control codes 61, 63, 64, 71, 72 and 73 indicate hospitals listed by AOHA, but not registered by AHA. For definition of numerical codes, see page A6	Control	Service	Beds	Admissions	Census	Outpatient Visits	Births	Total	Payroll	Personnel
□ UNION HOSPITAL OF THE BRONX, 260 East 188th Street, Bronx, Zip 10458; tel. 718/220-2020; Ronald Gade M.D., President (Nonreporting) **A**1 9 10	23	10	197	—	—	—	—	—	—	—
★ UNIVERSITY HOSPITAL OF BROOKLYN–STATE UNIVERSITY OF NEW YORK HEALTH SCIENCE CENTER AT BROOKLYN, 445 Lenox Road, Brooklyn, Zip 11203-2098; tel. 718/270-2404; Percy Allen, Vice President Hospital Affairs and Executive Director (Nonreporting) **A**1 2 3 5 8 9 10	12	10	376	—	—	—	—	—	—	—
VAN ETTEN HOSPITALS See Bronx Municipal Hospital Center										
★ VETERANS AFFAIRS MEDICAL CENTER, 800 Poly Place, Brooklyn, Zip 11209; tel. 718/630-3500; James J. Farsetta FACHE, Director (Total facility includes 268 beds in nursing home–type unit) **A**1 3 5 8 **F**1 2 3 4 8 10 11 14 15 16 17 19 20 21 22 25 26 27 28 29 30 31 32 34 35 37 39 41 42 43 44 46 48 49 51 52 56 58 59 60 64 65 69 71 72 73 74 **S**9295 Department of Veterans Affairs	45	10	886	9002	764	379527	0	189584	110922	2019
★ VETERANS AFFAIRS MEDICAL CENTER, 130 West Kingsbridge Road, Bronx, Zip 10468-7511; tel. 718/584-9000; Maryann Musumeci, Director (Total facility includes 120 beds in nursing home–type unit) **A**1 2 3 5 8 **F**1 2 3 4 8 10 11 12 14 15 16 17 18 19 20 21 22 23 25 26 27 28 29 30 31 32 33 34 35 37 39 41 42 44 45 46 48 49 51 52 56 57 58 59 60 61 62 63 65 67 71 73 74 **P**6 **S**9295 Department of Veterans Affairs	45	10	620	5995	461	236775	0	—	—	2012
★ VETERANS AFFAIRS MEDICAL CENTER, 423 East 23rd Street, Zip 10010-0070; tel. 212/686-7500; John J. Donnellan Jr., Director **A**1 2 3 5 8 **F**1 2 3 4 8 10 11 12 16 19 20 22 26 30 31 33 34 35 37 39 42 43 44 45 46 48 49 51 52 54 56 57 58 65 71 73 74 **S**9295 Department of Veterans Affairs	45	10	492	7437	407	313120	0	174180	95945	2130
□ VICTORY MEMORIAL HOSPITAL, 9036 Seventh Avenue, Brooklyn, Zip 11228-3625; tel. 718/630-1234; Krishin L. Bhatia, Administrator (Nonreporting) **A**1 9 10	23	10	404	—	—	—	—	—	—	—
□ WESTCHESTER SQUARE MEDICAL CENTER, 2475 St. Raymond Avenue, Bronx, Zip 10461; tel. 718/430-7300; Alan Kopman, President and Chief Executive Officer **A**1 9 10 **F**11 19 22 34 35 37 39 42 44 49 65 71 73 **P**5	33	10	205	6698	183	39563	0	53698	26189	819
□ WESTERN QUEENS COMMUNITY HOSPITAL, Long Island City, Mailing Address: 25-10 30th Avenue, Astoria Station, Zip 11102-2495; tel. 718/932-1000; Elliot J. Simon FACHE, Chief Operating Officer (Nonreporting) **A**1 9 10	33	10	235	—	—	—	—	—	—	—
★ WOODHULL MEDICAL AND MENTAL HEALTH CENTER, 760 Broadway, Brooklyn, Zip 11206; tel. 718/963-8101; Norma Noriega, Executive Director **A**1 3 9 10 **F**2 3 7 8 11 12 14 15 16 17 18 19 20 21 22 25 26 27 28 29 30 31 34 37 39 40 41 42 44 45 46 48 49 51 52 53 54 55 56 57 58 60 61 63 65 67 68 71 73 74 **P**6 **S**3075 New York City Health and Hospitals Corporation	14	10	558	17377	489	234742	2009	240446	143705	2923
□ ○ WYCKOFF HEIGHTS MEDICAL CENTER, 374 Stockholm Street, Brooklyn, Zip 11237-4099; tel. 718/963-7102; Charles J. Pendola, President (Nonreporting) **A**1 3 5 9 10 11 12 13	23	10	395	—	—	—	—	—	—	—
NEWARK—Wayne County										
★ NEWARK–WAYNE COMMUNITY HOSPITAL, Driving Park Avenue, Zip 14513, Mailing Address: P.O. Box 111, Zip 14513-0111; tel. 315/332-2022; L. J. Danehy, President (Total facility includes 160 beds in nursing home–type unit) **A**1 9 10 **F**1 7 8 12 15 19 21 22 24 26 31 35 40 41 42 44 45 46 52 56 61 64 65 71 73 74 **P**4 5 **S**0046 Greater Rochester Health System, Inc.	23	10	280	3942	184	55621	378	32358	14001	715
NEWBURGH—Orange County										
★ ST. LUKE'S HOSPITAL, 70 Dubois Street, Zip 12550-4898, Mailing Address: P.O. Box 631, Zip 12550; tel. 914/561-4400; Arthur E. Santilli, President and Chief Executive Officer (Nonreporting) **A**1 9 10	23	10	205	—	—	—	—	—	—	—
NEWFANE—Niagara County										
□ INTER–COMMUNITY MEMORIAL HOSPITAL, 2600 William Street, Zip 14108; tel. 716/778-5111; Clare A. Haar, Chief Executive Officer **A**1 9 10 **F**8 15 19 20 22 25 30 33 34 37 40 41 44 45 49 65 71 73	23	10	71	2426	40	40694	215	12565	5406	267
NIAGARA FALLS—Niagara County										
★ NIAGARA FALLS MEMORIAL MEDICAL CENTER, 621 Tenth Street, Zip 14302-0708, Mailing Address: P.O. Box 708, Zip 14302-0708; tel. 716/278-4000; Timothy J. Finan FACHE, President **A**1 3 9 10 **F**3 7 8 12 13 14 15 16 17 18 19 20 21 22 25 26 27 28 29 30 31 32 33 34 35 37 39 40 41 42 44 45 46 49 51 52 53 55 56 58 60 65 67 68 71 72 73 74 **P**7	23	10	288	8260	193	225153	847	57876	30134	1111
NORTH TARRYTOWN—Westchester County										
★ PHELPS MEMORIAL HOSPITAL CENTER, 701 North Broadway, Zip 10591-1096; tel. 914/366-1000; Keith F. Safian, President and Chief Executive Officer **A**1 9 10 **F**3 7 8 9 11 12 14 15 16 17 19 20 21 22 26 27 28 29 30 32 33 34 35 36 37 38 39 40 41 42 44 45 46 47 48 49 51 52 54 55 56 57 58 61 63 64 65 66 67 68 70 71 72 73 74 **P**5 8	23	10	215	7787	150	107100	798	59062	30177	851
NORTH TONAWANDA—Niagara County										
□ DE GRAFF MEMORIAL HOSPITAL, 445 Tremont Street, Zip 14120-0750; tel. 716/694-4500; Thomas F. Schifferli, President and Chief Executive Officer (Nonreporting) **A**1 9 10	23	10	235	—	—	—	—	—	—	—
NORTHPORT—Suffolk County										
★ VETERANS AFFAIRS MEDICAL CENTER, 79 Middleville Road, Zip 11768-2293; tel. 516/261-4400; E. M. Travers M.D., Medical Center Director (Total facility includes 190 beds in nursing home–type unit) **A**1 2 3 5 8 **F**2 3 4 8 10 11 14 19 20 21 22 23 25 26 27 28 29 31 32 33 34 35 37 39 41 42 43 44 45 46 48 49 51 52 54 55 56 57 58 59 60 61 63 64 65 67 69 71 72 73 74 **P**6 **S**9295 Department of Veterans Affairs	45	10	698	6056	587	239683	0	139237	100956	1939

© 1995 AHA Guide

Hospitals, U.S. / NEW YORK

Hospital, Address, Telephone, Administrator, Approval, Facility, and Physician Codes, Health Care System	Classification Codes		Utilization Data					Expense (thousands) of dollars		
★ American Hospital Association (AHA) membership ☐ Joint Commission on Accreditation of Healthcare Organizations (JCAHO) accreditation + American Osteopathic Hospital Association (AOHA) membership ○ American Osteopathic Association (AOA) accreditation △ Commission on Accreditation of Rehabilitation Facilities (CARF) accreditation Control codes 61, 63, 64, 71, 72 and 73 indicate hospitals listed by AOHA, but not registered by AHA. For definition of numerical codes, see page A6	Control	Service	Beds	Admissions	Census	Outpatient Visits	Births	Total	Payroll	Personnel
NORWICH—Chenango County										
☐ CHENANGO MEMORIAL HOSPITAL, 179 North Broad Street, Zip 13815; tel. 607/335–4111; Frank W. Mirabito, President (Total facility includes 80 beds in nursing home–type unit) **A**1 9 10 **F**7 8 12 19 20 21 22 25 26 28 30 31 32 33 34 36 37 39 40 41 42 44 45 46 48 51 63 64 65 67 73 **P**5	23	10	138	2181	104	91880	417	21619	10828	362
NYACK—Rockland County										
★ NYACK HOSPITAL, North Midland Avenue, Zip 10960–1998; tel. 914/348–2000; Greger C. Anderson, President and Chief Executive Officer **A**1 2 5 9 10 **F**2 9 11 12 14 15 16 17 18 19 21 22 30 31 32 34 35 37 39 40 41 42 44 45 46 48 49 50 51 52 54 65 69 70 71 73 74 **P**1	23	10	375	12896	239	146717	1894	106947	36198	1417
OCEANSIDE—Nassau County										
★ SOUTH NASSAU COMMUNITIES HOSPITAL, 2445 Oceanside Road, Zip 11572–1500; tel. 516/763–2030; Michael Rodzenko, Executive Director **A**1 2 3 5 9 10 **F**5 7 8 10 11 15 16 19 21 22 26 28 29 30 31 32 34 35 37 40 41 42 44 45 46 49 51 52 53 54 55 56 57 58 60 63 65 67 68 70 71 73	23	10	429	11952	320	80038	1298	92505	49477	1304
OGDENSBURG—St. Lawrence County										
A. BARTON HEPBURN HOSPITAL See Hepburn Medical Center										
★ HEPBURN MEDICAL CENTER, (Formerly A Barton Hepburn Hospital) 214 King Street, Zip 13669–1192; tel. 315/393–3600; Donald C. Lewis, President and Chief Executive Officer (Total facility includes 29 beds in nursing home–type unit) **A**1 9 10 **F**4 7 8 14 15 16 17 18 19 21 22 23 24 26 28 29 30 33 34 35 39 40 41 42 44 45 46 49 51 52 54 55 56 60 63 64 65 67 71 73 74 **P**7	23	10	149	4470	106	83581	449	28743	14343	491
★ ST. LAWRENCE PSYCHIATRIC CENTER, Mailing Address: Station A, Zip 13669; tel. 315/393–3000; John R. Scott, Acting Director (Nonreporting) **A**1 10 **S**0009 New York State Department of Mental Health	12	22	418	—	—	—	—	—	—	—
OLEAN—Cattaraugus County										
★ OLEAN GENERAL HOSPITAL, (Includes Olean General West, 2221 West State Street, Zip 14760–1984; tel. 716/372–5300) 515 Main Street, Zip 14760–9912; tel. 716/373–2600; Robert A. Catalano M.D., President and Chief Executive Officer **A**1 3 6 9 10 **F**7 8 9 11 12 13 15 16 17 19 22 23 28 30 31 34 35 37 38 39 40 44 45 46 47 52 56 59 63 65 67 71 73	23	10	217	7785	128	91298	678	43282	20061	773
ONEIDA—Madison County										
★ ONEIDA CITY HOSPITAL, 321 Genesee Street, Zip 13421–0321; tel. 315/363–6000; Richard G. Smith, Administrator (Total facility includes 160 beds in nursing home–type unit) **A**1 9 10 **F**7 8 11 14 15 16 19 21 22 28 32 34 36 37 39 40 41 44 45 46 49 51 64 65 71 73 **P**6	14	10	261	3492	215	74719	489	33102	16216	765
ONEONTA—Otsego County										
★ AURELIA OSBORN FOX MEMORIAL HOSPITAL, 1 Norton Avenue, Zip 13820–2697; tel. 607/432–2000; John R. Remillard, President (Total facility includes 131 beds in nursing home–type unit) **A**1 9 10 **F**1 7 8 11 15 17 18 19 21 22 23 25 26 28 30 32 33 34 35 36 39 40 41 42 44 45 46 49 51 52 54 56 57 58 63 64 65 71 73 **P**5	23	10	259	4693	223	97316	381	42364	19665	617
ORANGEBURG—Rockland County										
★ ROCKLAND CHILDREN'S PSYCHIATRIC CENTER, Convent Road, Zip 10962; tel. 914/359–7400; James McDermott, Administrator (Nonreporting) **A**3 **S**0009 New York State Department of Mental Health	12	52	69	—	—	—	—	—	—	—
★ ROCKLAND PSYCHIATRIC CENTER, 140 Old Orangeburg Road, Zip 10962–0071; tel. 914/359–1000; Stephen N. Lawrence Ph.D., M.P.A., Chief Executive Officer (Nonreporting) **A**1 5 10 **S**0009 New York State Department of Mental Health	12	22	902	—	—	—	—	—	—	—
OSSINING—Westchester County										
OSSINING CORRECTIONAL FACILITIES HOSPITAL, 354 Hunter Street, Zip 10562; tel. 914/941–0108; Benjamin Dyett M.D., Director (Nonreporting)	12	11	25	—	—	—	—	—	—	—
☐ STONY LODGE HOSPITAL, 40 Croton Dam Road, Zip 10562, Mailing Address: Box 1250, Briarcliff Manor Zip 10510; tel. 914/941–7400; Jeffrey Loker, Executive Director (Nonreporting) **A**1	33	22	61	—	—	—	—	—	—	—
OSWEGO—Oswego County										
★ OSWEGO HOSPITAL, 110 West Sixth Street, Zip 13126–9985; tel. 315/349–5511; Corte J. Spencer, Chief Executive Officer (Total facility includes 38 beds in nursing home–type unit) **A**1 9 10 **F**3 7 8 12 13 14 15 16 17 18 19 21 22 28 29 30 31 32 33 34 35 37 40 41 42 44 45 49 51 52 53 54 56 58 59 63 64 65 71 72 73 74	23	10	202	4809	132	157699	871	31294	16337	574
PATCHOGUE—Suffolk County										
★ BROOKHAVEN MEMORIAL HOSPITAL MEDICAL CENTER, 101 Hospital Road, Zip 11772–9998; tel. 516/654–7100; Thomas Ockers, President **A**1 3 9 10 **F**3 7 8 11 14 15 16 17 19 21 22 24 25 28 30 31 32 33 34 35 36 37 39 40 41 42 44 45 46 51 54 56 58 61 65 67 70 71 73 **P**7	23	10	321	10399	231	167572	1088	89973	48033	1229
PEEKSKILL—Westchester County										
★ HUDSON VALLEY HOSPITAL CENTER, 1980 Crompond Road, Zip 10566–4182; tel. 914/737–9000; John C. Federspiel, President and Chief Executive Officer **A**1 9 10 **F**1 2 3 4 5 6 7 8 9 10 11 12 13 15 16 17 18 19 20 21 22 23 24 25 26 27 28 29 30 31 32 33 34 35 36 37 38 39 40 41 42 43 44 45 46 47 48 49 50 51 52 53 54 55 56 57 58 59 60 61 62 63 64 65 66 67 68 69 70 71 72 73 74 **P**1 5 6 8	23	10	114	5901	95	80039	1079	38637	19243	518
PENN YAN—Yates County										
★ SOLDIERS AND SAILORS MEMORIAL HOSPITAL OF YATES COUNTY, 418 North Main Street, Zip 14527–1085; tel. 315/536–4431; Scott Murray, Chief Executive Officer (Nonreporting) **A**1 9 10	23	10	145	—	—	—	—	—	—	—

Hospitals, U.S. / NEW YORK

Hospital, Address, Telephone, Administrator, Approval, Facility, and Physician Codes, Health Care System	Classification Codes		Utilization Data					Expense (thousands) of dollars		
★ American Hospital Association (AHA) membership ☐ Joint Commission on Accreditation of Healthcare Organizations (JCAHO) accreditation + American Osteopathic Hospital Association (AOHA) membership ○ American Osteopathic Association (AOA) accreditation △ Commission on Accreditation of Rehabilitation Facilities (CARF) accreditation Control codes 61, 63, 64, 71, 72 and 73 indicate hospitals listed by AOHA, but not registered by AHA. For definition of numerical codes, see page A6	Control	Service	Beds	Admissions	Census	Outpatient Visits	Births	Total	Payroll	Personnel
PLAINVIEW—Nassau County										
★ NORTH SHORE UNIVERSITY HOSPITAL AT PLAINVIEW, (Formerly Central General Hospital) 888 Old Country Road, Zip 11803-4978; tel. 516/681-8900; Glenn S. Hirsch, Administrator (Data for 356 days) **A**1 2 9 10 **F**2 3 7 8 11 15 16 19 22 28 30 36 37 40 42 44 46 52 57 60 65 67 71 73 **P**1 **S**0062 North Shore Health System	33	10	279	8996	183	25476	806	59117	30054	691
PLATTSBURGH—Clinton County										
★ CHAMPLAIN VALLEY PHYSICIANS HOSPITAL MEDICAL CENTER, 75 Beekman Street, Zip 12901-1493; tel. 518/561-2000; Kevin J. Carroll, President (Total facility includes 54 beds in nursing home-type unit) **A**1 2 5 9 10 **F**7 8 10 11 15 16 19 20 21 22 24 28 30 31 33 34 35 37 40 41 42 44 46 49 52 56 60 64 65 70 71 73 74	23	10	346	11205	262	257728	1349	80788	41304	1292
★ U.S. AIR FORCE HOSPITAL, Plattsburgh AFB, Zip 12903; tel. 518/565-7414; Steven C. Mirick, Administrator (Nonreporting) **S**9495 Department of the Air Force	41	10	5	—	—	—	—	—	—	—
POMONA—Rockland County										
☐ DOCTOR ROBERT L. YEAGER HEALTH CENTER, (Long Term Geriatric) (Includes Summit Park Hospital–Rockland County Infirmary) Sanatorium Road, Zip 10970; tel. 914/364-2000; George T. Giacobbe, Commissioner (Total facility includes 300 beds in nursing home-type unit) **A**1 10 **F**1 2 3 12 15 16 17 18 20 21 26 27 31 33 34 45 46 48 52 53 56 58 59 64 65 67 71 73	13	49	408	1710	387	0	0	62963	34154	—
PORT CHESTER—Westchester County										
★ HIGH POINT HOSPITAL, 1104 Upper King Street, Zip 10573; tel. 914/939-4420; Wali Mohammad M.D., Medical Director **A**1 10 **F**14 15 19 21 22 35 45 52 53 55 65 71 **P**6	31	22	45	50	40	0	0	—	—	72
★ UNITED HOSPITAL MEDICAL CENTER, 406 Boston Post Road, Zip 10573; tel. 914/939-7000; Kevin Dahill, President and Chief Executive Officer (Total facility includes 40 beds in nursing home-type unit) **A**1 9 10 **F**2 3 7 8 12 15 16 17 19 21 22 26 28 30 31 32 33 34 35 36 37 39 40 41 42 44 46 49 51 52 53 54 55 56 57 58 61 63 64 65 67 69 71 73 **P**5 8	23	10	280	7346	209	—	685	70220	34375	1011
PORT JEFFERSON—Suffolk County										
★ JOHN T. MATHER MEMORIAL HOSPITAL, 75 North Country Road, Zip 11777-2190; tel. 516/473-1320; Kenneth D. Roberts, President **A**1 2 9 10 **F**1 2 3 4 8 10 11 14 15 16 19 20 21 22 26 31 32 33 34 36 37 39 41 42 43 44 45 46 49 52 53 54 55 56 57 58 60 61 63 65 67 69 70 71 73	23	10	248	9183	200	69750	0	73252	36005	1007
★ ST. CHARLES HOSPITAL AND REHABILITATION CENTER, 200 Belle Terre Road, Zip 11777; tel. 516/474-6000; Barry T. Zeman, President and Chief Executive Officer **A**1 2 5 9 10 **F**2 3 4 5 6 7 8 10 14 15 16 17 19 20 21 22 23 24 25 26 27 28 29 30 31 32 33 34 35 36 37 39 40 41 42 43 44 45 46 48 49 50 51 53 54 55 56 57 58 59 60 61 62 63 65 66 67 68 69 70 71 72 73 74 **P**5 8	21	10	235	8600	202	85272	2050	70333	36859	860
PORT JERVIS—Orange County										
★ MERCY COMMUNITY HOSPITAL, (Includes Mercy Community Hospital, 160 Hammond Street, Zip 12771; tel. 914/856-5351) 160 East Main Street, Zip 12771-0268, Mailing Address: P.O. Box 1014, Zip 12771; tel. 914/856-5351; Thomas J. Moakler, President and Chief Executive Officer (Total facility includes 40 beds in nursing home-type unit) **A**1 2 9 10 **F**2 7 8 11 14 19 20 22 30 32 33 35 39 40 42 46 49 52 56 64 65 67 71 73 **S**5165 Mercy Health Services	21	10	180	3930	117	56328	248	30000	13026	540
POTSDAM—St. Lawrence County										
★ CANTON–POTSDAM HOSPITAL, 50 Leroy Street, Zip 13676; tel. 315/265-3300; Bruce C. Potter, President **A**1 9 10 **F**2 7 8 14 16 19 21 22 28 30 35 37 39 40 42 44 46 49 65 70 71 73	23	10	94	3582	70	73252	308	—	—	415
POUGHKEEPSIE—Dutchess County										
★ HUDSON RIVER PSYCHIATRIC CENTER, Branch B, Zip 12601-1197; tel. 914/452-8000; Wendy P. Acrish M.P.S., Executive Director (Nonreporting) **A**1 10 **S**0009 New York State Department of Mental Health	12	22	1258	—	—	—	—	—	—	—
★ △ SAINT FRANCIS HOSPITAL, (Includes Saint Francis Hospital–Beacon, 60 Delavan Avenue, Beacon, New York, Zip 12508; tel. 914/831-3500) North Road, Zip 12601-1399; tel. 914/431-8116; Sister M. Ann Elizabeth, President **A**1 3 7 9 10 **F**2 3 8 11 14 15 16 17 19 21 22 23 26 27 28 29 30 31 32 34 35 36 37 39 41 42 44 45 46 48 49 52 53 54 55 56 57 58 63 65 66 70 71 72 73	21	10	358	10957	298	195000	0	88251	45592	1326
★ VASSAR BROTHERS HOSPITAL, Reade Place, Zip 12601; tel. 914/454-8500; Ronald T. Mullahey, President **A**1 2 9 10 **F**3 7 8 10 11 15 16 17 18 19 20 21 22 23 27 28 30 31 32 33 35 37 38 40 41 42 44 45 49 51 53 54 55 56 58 59 60 61 63 65 66 67 68 70 71 73 74 **P**5	23	10	279	12514	219	130692	2430	77761	37139	955
QUEENS–Queens County, See New York City										
QUEENS VILLAGE–Queens County, See New York City										
RHINEBECK—Dutchess County										
★ NORTHERN DUTCHESS HOSPITAL, 10 Springbrook Avenue, Zip 12572-1602, Mailing Address: P.O. Box 5002, Zip 12572; tel. 914/876-3001; Michael C. Mazzarella, Chief Executive Officer (Total facility includes 50 beds in nursing home-type unit) **A**1 9 10 **F**7 8 14 15 16 19 20 21 22 24 25 26 28 30 31 32 33 35 37 39 40 42 44 45 46 49 51 54 56 62 64 65 67 69 71 73 **P**5	23	10	121	2912	54	52962	670	18874	8353	301
RICHMOND VALLEY–Richmond County, See New York City										
RIVERHEAD—Suffolk County										
★ CENTRAL SUFFOLK HOSPITAL, 1300 Roanoke Avenue, Zip 11901-2028; tel. 516/548-6000; Joseph F. Turner, President (Total facility includes 60 beds in nursing home-type unit) **A**1 9 10 **F**4 7 8 14 15 16 19 21 22 28 29 30 32 34 35 37 40 42 44 45 49 64 65 67 71 73	23	10	214	5150	184	35521	143	47671	22724	540

© 1995 AHA Guide

Hospitals, U.S. / NEW YORK

Hospital, Address, Telephone, Administrator, Approval, Facility, and Physician Codes, Health Care System

- ★ American Hospital Association (AHA) membership
- □ Joint Commission on Accreditation of Healthcare Organizations (JCAHO) accreditation
- + American Osteopathic Hospital Association (AOHA) membership
- ○ American Osteopathic Association (AOA) accreditation
- △ Commission on Accreditation of Rehabilitation Facilities (CARF) accreditation

Control codes 61, 63, 64, 71, 72 and 73 indicate hospitals listed by AOHA, but not registered by AHA. For definition of numerical codes, see page A6.

Hospital	Control	Service	Beds	Admissions	Census	Outpatient Visits	Births	Total	Payroll	Personnel
ROCHESTER—Monroe County										
★ GENESEE HOSPITAL, 224 Alexander Street, Zip 14607-4055; tel. 716/263-6000; Joseph J. DeSilva FACHE, President and Chief Executive Officer (Total facility includes 40 beds in nursing home–type unit) A1 2 3 5 8 9 10 F1 3 4 5 6 7 8 10 11 12 13 15 16 17 18 19 20 21 22 23 24 25 26 27 28 29 30 31 32 33 34 35 36 37 39 40 41 42 43 44 45 46 49 50 51 52 53 54 56 57 58 59 60 61 62 64 65 66 67 68 69 71 72 73 74 S0046 Greater Rochester Health System, Inc.	23	10	385	14823	327	648748	2552	143099	79717	2326
★ HIGHLAND HOSPITAL OF ROCHESTER, 1000 South Avenue, Zip 14620; tel. 716/473-2200; Michael J. Weidner, President A1 2 3 5 9 10 F4 6 7 8 12 14 15 16 19 20 21 22 26 28 29 30 31 32 34 37 39 40 42 44 45 46 49 51 54 60 62 65 67 70 71 73 74	23	10	272	10540	167	138300	2769	81900	43172	1570
□ MONROE COMMUNITY HOSPITAL, (Treatment of the Aged and Chronically Ill) 435 East Henrietta Road, Zip 14620-4684; tel. 716/274-7100; Frank Tripodi, Executive Director (Nonreporting) A1 3 5 9 10	13	49	605	—	—	—	—	—	—	—
★ PARK RIDGE HOSPITAL, 1555 Long Pond Road, Zip 14626-4182; tel. 716/723-7000; Timothy R. McCormick, President A1 2 9 10 F1 2 3 4 6 10 12 14 15 16 17 18 19 21 22 26 30 32 33 34 35 37 39 41 42 43 44 45 46 48 49 51 52 53 54 55 56 57 58 59 60 62 64 65 66 67 68 69 70 71 72 73 P7	23	10	259	8831	220	204391	0	75459	36310	1249
★ ROCHESTER GENERAL HOSPITAL, 1425 Portland Avenue, Zip 14621-3099; tel. 716/338-4000; Steven I. Goldstein, President and Chief Executive Officer A1 2 3 5 6 8 9 10 F1 4 6 7 8 10 12 13 15 16 17 19 20 21 22 26 28 29 30 31 32 34 37 38 40 41 42 43 44 45 46 49 51 52 56 58 59 60 61 62 64 65 67 68 70 71 73 74 P3 6 S0046 Greater Rochester Health System, Inc.	23	10	526	21927	438	617960	2184	202538	97701	3323
★ ROCHESTER PSYCHIATRIC CENTER, 1111 Elmwood Avenue, Zip 14620-3005; tel. 716/473-3230; Martin H. Vonholden, Executive Director A1 3 5 10 F1 2 3 4 5 6 7 8 9 10 11 12 13 14 15 16 17 18 19 20 21 22 23 24 25 26 27 28 29 30 31 32 33 34 35 36 37 38 39 40 41 42 43 44 45 46 47 48 49 50 51 52 53 54 55 56 57 58 59 60 61 62 63 64 65 66 67 68 69 70 71 72 73 74 S0009 New York State Department of Mental Health	12	22	345	207	350	106785	0	43212	30175	797
★ ST. MARY'S HOSPITAL, 89 Genesee Street, Zip 14611-3285; tel. 716/464-3000; Patrick Madden, President A1 2 3 5 9 10 F7 8 10 11 12 13 14 15 16 17 19 20 21 22 24 25 26 28 30 31 34 35 37 39 40 41 42 44 45 46 48 49 51 53 54 55 57 58 61 65 68 71 72 73 P5 6 S1855 Daughters of Charity National Health System	21	10	227	7897	182	397274	1121	87472	46103	1507
★ △ STRONG MEMORIAL HOSPITAL OF THE UNIVERSITY OF ROCHESTER, 601 Elmwood Avenue, Zip 14642; tel. 716/275-2100; Leo P. Brideau, General Director and Chief Executive Director A1 3 5 7 8 9 10 F3 4 5 7 8 9 10 11 12 13 17 18 19 20 21 22 23 26 30 31 32 33 34 35 37 38 39 40 41 42 43 46 47 48 49 51 52 53 54 55 56 57 58 59 60 61 63 65 66 67 68 69 70 71 72 73 74	23	10	715	29307	669	261840	4267	319839	156823	4664
ROCKVILLE CENTRE—Nassau County										
★ MERCY MEDICAL CENTER, 1000 North Village Avenue, Zip 11570-1098; tel. 516/255-0111; John C. Johnson, President and Chief Executive Officer A1 2 3 9 10 F3 4 7 8 9 10 11 12 14 15 16 17 19 21 23 26 28 30 31 32 33 34 35 37 38 40 41 42 43 44 49 52 54 55 56 57 58 59 60 63 64 65 66 67 69 71 73 74 P8	21	10	387	13460	297	120205	2045	106551	55250	1668
ROME—Oneida County										
★ ROME MEMORIAL HOSPITAL, (Formerly Rome Hospital and Murphy Memorial Hospital) 1500 North James Street, Zip 13440-2898; tel. 315/338-7000; Alvin C. White, President and Chief Executive Officer (Total facility includes 40 beds in nursing home–type unit) A1 9 10 F3 7 8 14 15 16 19 22 28 30 31 34 37 39 40 41 44 45 49 64 65 71 73 74	14	10	184	5430	122	164625	562	29982	15077	558
★ U.S. AIR FORCE HOSPITAL, Griffiss AFB, Zip 13441; tel. 315/330-7711; Thomas A. Rupp, Administrator F17 19 20 28 29 30 35 40 44 46 49 51 53 54 55 58 65 71 72 S9495 Department of the Air Force	41	10	30	1189	7	100104	279	—	—	273
ROSLYN—Nassau County										
★ ST. FRANCIS HOSPITAL, (Cardiovascular Specialty) 100 Port Washington Boulevard, Zip 11576-1348; tel. 516/562-6000; Robert F. Vizza Ph.D., President and Chief Executive Officer A1 9 10 F3 4 8 10 11 17 19 20 21 22 24 28 34 36 37 39 43 44 45 46 47 49 54 56 65 69 71 73	23	49	247	11393	280	69009	0	136408	61776	1455
RYE—Westchester County										
★ RYE HOSPITAL CENTER, 754 Boston Post Road, Zip 10580; tel. 914/967-4567; Jack C. Schoenholtz M.D., Medical Director and Administrator A1 10 F19 20 21 22 27 35 48 50 52 53 55 57 63 65 67 71 73	33	22	34	150	34	0	0	5051	1930	63
SARANAC LAKE—Franklin County										
★ ADIRONDACK MEDICAL CENTER, (Includes Adirondack Medical Center–Lake Placid Site, Church Street, Lake Placid, New York, Zip 12946; tel. 518/523-3311) Lake Colby Drive, Zip 12983, Mailing Address: P.O. Box 471, Zip 12983; tel. 518/891-4141; Chandler M. Ralph, President and Chief Executive Officer A1 9 10 F7 8 11 14 15 16 19 20 21 22 23 28 33 34 35 36 37 40 41 42 44 63 65 66 70 71 73 S0585 Brim, Inc.	23	10	100	3722	68	85123	339	26508	12953	451
SARATOGA SPRINGS—Saratoga County										
★ SARATOGA HOSPITAL, 211 Church Street, Zip 12866-1003; tel. 518/587-3222; David Andersen, President & Chief Executive Officer (Total facility includes 72 beds in nursing home–type unit) A1 5 9 10 F7 8 16 19 21 22 27 28 30 31 33 35 37 40 41 42 44 46 49 52 54 56 58 64 65 67 71 72 73	23	10	231	6505	194	109005	821	44150	21096	738

Hospitals, U.S. / NEW YORK

Hospital, Address, Telephone, Administrator, Approval, Facility, and Physician Codes, Health Care System	Classi-fication Codes		Utilization Data					Expense (thousands) of dollars		
	Control	Service	Beds	Admissions	Census	Outpatient Visits	Births	Total	Payroll	Personnel

★ American Hospital Association (AHA) membership
☐ Joint Commission on Accreditation of Healthcare Organizations (JCAHO) accreditation
+ American Osteopathic Hospital Association (AOHA) membership
○ American Osteopathic Association (AOA) accreditation
△ Commission on Accreditation of Rehabilitation Facilities (CARF) accreditation
Control codes 61, 63, 64, 71, 72 and 73 indicate hospitals listed by AOHA, but not registered by AHA. For definition of numerical codes, see page A6

SCHENECTADY—Schenectady County

Hospital	Control	Service	Beds	Admissions	Census	Outpatient Visits	Births	Total	Payroll	Personnel
★ BELLEVUE – THE WOMAN'S HOSPITAL, 2210 Troy Road, Zip 12309-4797; tel. 518/346-9400; Michael A. Mangini, Administrator and Chief Executive Officer (Nonreporting) **A**1 9 10	33	44	55	—	—	—	—	—	—	—
★ ELLIS HOSPITAL, 1101 Nott Street, Zip 12308-2487; tel. 518/382-4124; G. B. Serrill, President and Chief Executive Officer (Total facility includes 82 beds in nursing home–type unit) **A**1 2 3 5 9 10 **F**4 7 8 10 11 12 13 14 15 16 17 18 19 20 21 22 26 28 29 30 31 34 35 37 39 40 41 42 43 44 45 46 49 51 52 54 55 56 58 59 60 61 63 64 65 66 67 70 71 73 **S**0002 Quorum Health Group/Quorum Health Resources	23	10	434	11506	333	218437	551	106724	50314	1594
★ ST. CLARE'S HOSPITAL OF SCHENECTADY, 600 McClellan Street, Zip 12304; tel. 518/382-2000; Jerome G. Stewart, President **A**1 3 5 9 10 12 **F**7 8 11 14 15 16 17 19 20 21 22 24 26 28 30 31 32 33 34 35 37 38 39 40 42 44 46 47 48 49 51 56 57 65 71 73 **P**3	21	10	201	7662	145	143874	755	58895	29996	1064
★ △ SUNNYVIEW HOSPITAL AND REHABILITATION CENTER, 1270 Belmont Avenue, Zip 12308-2104; tel. 518/382-4500; Bradford M. Goodwin, President **A**1 3 5 7 9 10 **F**15 19 21 22 26 34 35 45 48 49 54 55 56 65 71 73 **P**5 6	23	46	101	1674	82	—	0	19848	12880	392

SCOTIA—Schenectady County
CONIFER PARK See Glenville

SEAFORD—Nassau County

Hospital	Control	Service	Beds	Admissions	Census	Outpatient Visits	Births	Total	Payroll	Personnel
+ ○ MASSAPEQUA GENERAL HOSPITAL, 750 Hicksville Road, Zip 11783, Mailing Address: Box 20, Zip 11783; tel. 516/520-6000; John P. Breen, Chief Executive Officer (Nonreporting) **A**9 10 11 12	33	10	122	—	—	—	—	—	—	—

SIDNEY—Delaware County

Hospital	Control	Service	Beds	Admissions	Census	Outpatient Visits	Births	Total	Payroll	Personnel
★ THE HOSPITAL, Pearl Street, Zip 13838; tel. 607/563-3512; Thomas J. Graham, Chief Executive Officer (Total facility includes 40 beds in nursing home–type unit) **A**1 9 10 **F**7 8 12 19 22 25 30 31 33 34 37 39 40 41 44 49 51 64 65 71 **S**0585 Brim, Inc.	14	10	87	2206	66	28606	136	11287	5487	214

SMITHTOWN—Suffolk County

Hospital	Control	Service	Beds	Admissions	Census	Outpatient Visits	Births	Total	Payroll	Personnel
☐ COMMUNITY HOSPITAL OF WESTERN SUFFOLK, 498 Smithtown By-Pass, Zip 11787-5018; tel. 516/979-9800; David G. Hay, Administrator (Data for 136 days) **A**1 9 10 **F**2 3 7 8 10 11 14 15 16 19 22 28 36 37 40 42 44 49 52 64 65 67 70 71 73 **P**5	21	10	112	1165	66	—	160	12595	6997	590
★ ST. JOHN'S EPISCOPAL HOSPITAL-SMITHTOWN, 50 Route 25-A, Zip 11787-1398; tel. 516/862-3000; Laura Righter, Administrator **A**1 9 **F**3 4 7 8 10 14 15 16 17 19 20 21 22 23 26 27 28 30 31 32 33 34 35 37 39 40 41 42 43 44 45 46 49 51 52 53 54 55 56 57 58 59 60 61 62 63 65 67 69 70 71 73 **P**5 7 8 **S**0735 Episcopal Health Services Inc.	21	10	366	11786	243	56949	1182	88374	46083	—

SODUS—Wayne County

Hospital	Control	Service	Beds	Admissions	Census	Outpatient Visits	Births	Total	Payroll	Personnel
★ MYERS COMMUNITY HOSPITAL, 6600 Middle Road, Zip 14551-0310; tel. 315/483-3000; Terrance M. Bedient, President and Chief Executive Officer **A**1 9 10 **F**7 8 11 14 15 16 19 22 28 30 37 40 41 44 49 71	23	10	54	1966	32	48754	242	12019	5250	193

SOUTHAMPTON—Suffolk County

Hospital	Control	Service	Beds	Admissions	Census	Outpatient Visits	Births	Total	Payroll	Personnel
★ SOUTHAMPTON HOSPITAL, 240 Meeting House Lane, Zip 11968-5090; tel. 516/726-8555; John J. Ferry Jr. M.D., President and Chief Executive Officer **A**1 9 10 **F**2 3 7 8 9 10 11 14 15 16 17 18 19 20 21 22 23 24 25 26 28 29 30 31 32 33 34 35 37 38 39 40 41 42 44 45 46 47 48 49 52 54 60 63 64 65 66 67 70 71 73 74	23	10	194	5215	89	144760	817	47619	22994	573

SPRINGVILLE—Erie County

Hospital	Control	Service	Beds	Admissions	Census	Outpatient Visits	Births	Total	Payroll	Personnel
BERTRAND CHAFFEE HOSPITAL, 224 East Main Street, Zip 14141-1497; tel. 716/592-2871; Roger A. Ford, Administrator (Nonreporting) **A**9 10	23	10	49	—	—	—	—	—	—	—

STAR LAKE—St. Lawrence County

Hospital	Control	Service	Beds	Admissions	Census	Outpatient Visits	Births	Total	Payroll	Personnel
★ CLIFTON-FINE HOSPITAL, Oswegatchie Trail, Zip 13690, Mailing Address: Box 10, Zip 13690-0010; tel. 315/848-3351; Rodney C. Boula, Administrator **A**9 10 **F**16 19 20 22 27 28 33 34 49 53 54 55 56 57 58 59 71 72	16	10	20	467	5	9588	0	2218	1280	50

STATEN ISLAND–Richmond County, See New York City

STONY BROOK—Suffolk County

Hospital	Control	Service	Beds	Admissions	Census	Outpatient Visits	Births	Total	Payroll	Personnel
★ UNIVERSITY HOSPITAL, State University of New York, Zip 11794-8410; tel. 516/689-8333; Michael A. Maffetone, Director and Chief Executive Officer **A**1 2 3 5 8 9 10 **F**4 5 7 8 10 11 12 13 15 16 17 18 19 20 21 22 23 25 26 28 29 30 31 34 35 37 38 39 40 41 42 43 44 45 46 47 49 51 52 53 54 55 56 57 58 59 60 61 63 65 66 67 68 69 70 71 72 73 74 **P**1 4 6 7	12	10	504	22317	405	549647	3241	289941	138203	3493

SUFFERN—Rockland County

Hospital	Control	Service	Beds	Admissions	Census	Outpatient Visits	Births	Total	Payroll	Personnel
★ GOOD SAMARITAN HOSPITAL, 255 Lafayette Avenue, Zip 10901-4869; tel. 914/368-5000; Joan Regan, President and Chief Executive Officer **A**1 9 10 **F**1 2 3 4 5 7 8 9 10 11 12 15 16 17 19 20 21 22 25 28 30 31 32 33 34 35 36 37 38 40 41 42 44 45 46 47 48 49 51 52 53 54 55 56 57 58 60 63 64 65 67 69 70 71 73 **P**8	21	10	370	11992	232	271080	2040	111835	48768	1179

SYOSSET—Nassau County

Hospital	Control	Service	Beds	Admissions	Census	Outpatient Visits	Births	Total	Payroll	Personnel
★ SYOSSET COMMUNITY HOSPITAL, 221 Jericho Turnpike, Zip 11791-4567; tel. 516/496-6400; Andrew J. Mitchell, Chief Executive Officer **A**1 3 9 10 **F**4 7 8 9 10 12 14 15 16 17 19 21 22 30 31 33 35 36 37 39 40 41 42 44 45 46 52 56 58 59 65 67 71 73	23	10	186	7191	143	22892	1687	64903	31093	704

Hospitals, U.S. / NEW YORK

Hospital, Address, Telephone, Administrator, Approval, Facility, and Physician Codes, Health Care System

- ★ American Hospital Association (AHA) membership
- ☐ Joint Commission on Accreditation of Healthcare Organizations (JCAHO) accreditation
- + American Osteopathic Hospital Association (AOHA) membership
- ○ American Osteopathic Association (AOA) accreditation
- △ Commission on Accreditation of Rehabilitation Facilities (CARF) accreditation

Control codes 61, 63, 64, 71, 72 and 73 indicate hospitals listed by AOHA, but not registered by AHA. For definition of numerical codes, see page A6

Hospital	Control	Service	Beds	Admissions	Census	Outpatient Visits	Births	Total	Payroll	Personnel
SYRACUSE—Onondaga County										
☐ BENJAMIN RUSH CENTER, 650 South Salina Street, Zip 13202-3524; tel. 315/476-2161; Robert C. Long, Administrator and Chief Executive Officer (Nonreporting) A1 9 10	31	22	129	—	—	—	—	—	—	—
★ COMMUNITY-GENERAL HOSPITAL OF GREATER SYRACUSE, Broad Road, Zip 13215; tel. 315/492-5011; Kent A. Arnold, President (Total facility includes 50 beds in nursing home–type unit) A1 3 5 9 10 F4 7 8 12 14 16 19 21 22 25 26 28 29 30 31 34 37 39 40 41 42 44 52 54 55 56 64 65 73 P8	23	10	356	12321	291	143221	1911	74025	38997	1318
★ CROUSE IRVING MEMORIAL HOSPITAL, 736 Irving Avenue, Zip 13210-1690; tel. 315/470-7111; James W. Maher, President A1 3 5 6 9 10 F2 3 4 7 8 10 11 12 15 16 17 19 22 24 26 29 31 32 33 34 35 37 38 40 42 44 48 49 54 58 60 65 67 69 70 71 73 P1	23	10	513	21974	433	166123	4102	163426	68544	2245
★ RICHARD H. HUTCHINGS PSYCHIATRIC CENTER, 620 Madison Street, Zip 13210-2319; tel. 315/473-4980; Bryan F. Rudes, Executive Director (Nonreporting) A1 3 5 10 S0009 New York State Department of Mental Health	12	22	184	—	—	—	—	—	—	—
☐ ST. JOSEPH'S HOSPITAL HEALTH CENTER, 301 Prospect Avenue, Zip 13203; tel. 315/448-5111; William J. Watt, President (Nonreporting) A1 3 5 6 9 10 S5955 Sisters of the 3rd Franciscan Order	21	10	431	—	—	—	—	—	—	—
★ UNIVERSITY HOSPITAL-SUNY HEALTH SCIENCE CENTER AT SYRACUSE, 750 East Adams Street, Zip 13210; tel. 315/464-5540; Ben Moore III, Executive Director A1 2 3 5 8 9 10 F4 8 9 10 11 17 19 20 21 22 23 26 28 31 34 35 37 41 42 43 44 46 47 48 49 52 53 54 55 56 57 58 59 60 61 65 69 70 71 73 74	12	10	350	11082	283	266917	0	182670	87371	2669
★ VETERANS AFFAIRS MEDICAL CENTER, 800 Irving Avenue, Zip 13210; tel. 315/476-7461; Philip P. Thomas, Associate Director (Nonreporting) A1 3 5 8 S9295 Department of Veterans Affairs	45	10	255	—	—	—	—	—	—	—
TICONDEROGA—Essex County										
☐ MOSES LUDINGTON HOSPITAL, Wicker Street, Zip 12883-1097; tel. 518/585-2831; H. Rudolph Wirth, Chief Executive Officer A1 9 10 F3 7 8 14 15 16 17 22 28 29 30 32 33 34 39 40 44 45 46 49 65 67 71 73 P5	23	10	39	832	20	32572	60	6574	3198	149
TROY—Rensselaer County										
LEONARD HOSPITAL See Seton Health System										
☐ SAMARITAN HOSPITAL, 2215 Burdett Avenue, Zip 12180; tel. 518/271-3300; David A. Kadish, President (Nonreporting) A1 5 6 9 10	23	10	272	—	—	—	—	—	—	—
★ SETON HEALTH SYSTEM, (Includes Leonard Hospital, 74 New Turnpike Road, Troy, New York, Zip 12182-1498; tel. 518/235-0310; St. Mary's Hospital, 1300 Massachusetts Avenue, Troy, New York, Zip 12180) 1300 Massachusetts Avenue, Zip 12180; tel. 518/272-5000; Edward G. Murphy M.D., President and Chief Executive Officer (Nonreporting) A1 5 9 10 S1855 Daughters of Charity National Health System	21	10	444	—	—	—	—	—	—	—
ST. MARY'S HOSPITAL See Seton Health System										
UTICA—Oneida County										
★ FAXTON HOSPITAL, 1676 Sunset Avenue, Zip 13502; tel. 315/738-6200; Keith A. Fenstemacher, President and Chief Executive Officer A1 2 9 10 F1 7 8 10 15 17 19 20 21 22 23 25 26 28 29 30 32 33 34 35 36 37 38 40 41 42 44 45 48 49 52 60 64 65 67 69 71 73 74 P3 8	23	10	170	5536	136	107139	0	42795	19240	741
★ MOHAWK VALLEY PSYCHIATRIC CENTER, 1400 Noyes at York, Zip 13502-3803; tel. 315/797-6800; Sarah F. Rudes, Executive Director (Nonreporting) A1 10 S0009 New York State Department of Mental Health	12	22	614	—	—	—	—	—	—	—
★ ST. ELIZABETH HOSPITAL, 2209 Genesee Street, Zip 13501-5999; tel. 315/798-8100; Sister Rose Vincent, President and Chief Executive Officer A1 3 5 6 9 10 12 F7 8 10 14 15 16 18 19 21 22 28 29 30 31 34 35 37 40 42 44 45 49 51 52 56 63 65 66 70 71 73 74 S5955 Sisters of the 3rd Franciscan Order	21	10	217	8159	161	221398	591	60271	30302	998
★ ST. LUKE'S MEMORIAL HOSPITAL CENTER, (Includes Allen-Calder Skilled Nursing Facility; Mohawk Valley Division, 295 West Main Street, Ilion, New York, Zip 13357-1599; tel. 315/895-7474; Pearl T. Gentile, Acting Administrator) Mailing Address: P.O. Box 479, Zip 13503-0479; tel. 315/798-6000; Andrew E. Peterson, Executive Director (Total facility includes 124 beds in nursing home–type unit) A1 10 F1 7 8 10 11 14 15 16 19 20 21 22 23 26 28 29 30 31 32 33 35 37 40 41 42 44 46 49 51 52 61 63 64 65 67 71 73 74	23	10	414	11566	371	246011	1851	76583	36818	1117
VALHALLA—Westchester County										
★ BLYTHEDALE CHILDREN'S HOSPITAL, Bradhurst Avenue, Zip 10595-1697; tel. 914/592-7555; Robert Stone, President A1 10 F14 15 16 20 28 29 30 32 34 41 45 46 48 49 53 54 55 58 65 67 71 73 P6	23	56	92	287	83	22656	0	18994	11703	332
☐ WESTCHESTER COUNTY MEDICAL CENTER, Valhalla Campus, Zip 10595; tel. 914/285-7000; Edward A. Stolcenberg, Commissioner (Nonreporting) A1 2 3 5 8 9 10	13	10	638	—	—	—	—	—	—	—
VALLEY STREAM—Nassau County										
★ FRANKLIN HOSPITAL MEDICAL CENTER, 900 Franklin Avenue, Zip 11580-2190; tel. 516/256-6000; Albert Dicker, Executive Vice President (Total facility includes 120 beds in nursing home–type unit) A1 2 9 10 F1 3 4 7 8 10 11 12 16 19 20 21 22 25 26 27 28 30 32 35 37 40 41 42 43 44 46 52 53 54 55 56 57 58 60 61 64 65 70 71 73 P5	23	10	405	8251	347	294077	638	73235	37604	1100

Hospitals, U.S. / NEW YORK

Hospital, Address, Telephone, Administrator, Approval, Facility, and Physician Codes, Health Care System	Classification Codes		Utilization Data					Expense (thousands) of dollars		
★ American Hospital Association (AHA) membership □ Joint Commission on Accreditation of Healthcare Organizations (JCAHO) accreditation + American Osteopathic Hospital Association (AOHA) membership ○ American Osteopathic Association (AOA) accreditation △ Commission on Accreditation of Rehabilitation Facilities (CARF) accreditation Control codes 61, 63, 64, 71, 72 and 73 indicate hospitals listed by AOHA, but not registered by AHA. For definition of numerical codes, see page A6	Control	Service	Beds	Admissions	Census	Outpatient Visits	Births	Total	Payroll	Personnel
WALTON—Delaware County □ DELAWARE VALLEY HOSPITAL, 1 Titus Place, Zip 13856; tel. 607/865-4101; David J. Polge, President and Chief Executive Officer **A**1 9 10 **F**2 7 8 15 17 19 21 22 25 26 27 28 30 32 33 34 37 39 40 42 44 49 61 63 65 67 71 73 74 **P**6	23	10	42	1610	26	33676	137	10076	5174	193
WARSAW—Wyoming County □ WYOMING COUNTY COMMUNITY HOSPITAL, 400 North Main Street, Zip 14569; tel. 716/786-2233; Joseph E. Matthews, Interim Administrator (Total facility includes 160 beds in nursing home–type unit) **A**1 9 10 **F**7 8 15 16 19 22 25 33 34 35 37 40 42 44 49 52 60 64 71 73 74	13	10	262	3434	219	22040	455	27793	13099	521
WARWICK—Orange County ★ ST. ANTHONY COMMUNITY HOSPITAL, 15-19 Maple Avenue, Zip 10990; tel. 914/986-2276; F. Dennis Harrington, President **A**1 9 10 **F**7 11 16 19 22 34 36 37 40 44 65 71 73 **S**1485 Franciscan Sisters of the Poor Health System, Inc.	21	10	73	2936	55	31605	478	17587	7920	242
WATERTOWN—Jefferson County □ SAMARITAN MEDICAL CENTER, (Formerly House of the Good Samaritan) 830 Washington Street, Zip 13601, Mailing Address: P.O. Box 517, Zip 13601-0517; tel. 315/785-4000; William P. Koughan, President and Chief Executive Officer (Nonreporting) **A**1 9 10	23	10	234	—						
WELLSVILLE—Allegany County ★ JONES MEMORIAL HOSPITAL, 191 North Main Street, Zip 14895, Mailing Address: P.O. Box 72, Zip 14895; tel. 716/593-1100; William M. Diberardino FACHE, President **A**1 9 10 **F**7 8 9 11 12 15 16 17 19 22 30 33 34 35 36 37 38 40 41 42 44 49 51 65 66 67 69 71 73	23	10	90	3606	48	55344	487	19645	8493	335
WEST BRENTWOOD—Suffolk County ★ PILGRIM PSYCHIATRIC CENTER, Crooked Hill Road, Zip 11717, Mailing Address: Box A, Zip 11717; tel. 516/434-7500; Peggy O'Neill R.N., Executive Director (Nonreporting) **A**1 10 **S**0009 New York State Department of Mental Health	12	22	1478	—	—	—	—	—	—	—
WEST HAVERSTRAW—Rockland County ★ HELEN HAYES HOSPITAL, Route 9W, Zip 10993-1195; tel. 914/947-3000; Magdalena Ramirez, Director **A**1 3 5 9 10 **F**15 19 20 28 30 34 35 37 44 45 46 48 54 57 65 67 71 73 **P**6	12	46	155	1712	128	—	0	53856	21862	758
WEST ISLIP—Suffolk County ★ GOOD SAMARITAN HOSPITAL MEDICAL CENTER, 1000 Montauk Highway, Zip 11795-4958; tel. 516/376-3000; Daniel P. Walsh, President (Total facility includes 100 beds in nursing home–type unit) **A**1 9 10 **F**7 8 10 11 12 14 15 16 17 19 21 22 23 25 26 28 29 30 31 32 33 34 35 36 37 38 39 40 42 44 45 46 49 50 51 54 56 57 60 63 64 65 66 67 69 70 71 73 74 **P**5 7 8	21	10	525	19134	467	235345	2982	134522	67925	1407
WEST POINT—Orange County ★ KELLER ARMY COMMUNITY HOSPITAL, U.S. Military Academy, Zip 10996-1197; tel. 914/938-3305; Livio F. Pardi MC, Commander **A**1 3 **F**3 15 19 20 22 34 35 37 40 44 46 49 51 54 56 58 65 66 71 **S**9395 Department of the Army	42	10	65	3029	21	149244	174	—	—	472
WEST SENECA—Erie County ★ WESTERN NEW YORK CHILDREN'S PSYCHIATRIC CENTER, 1010 East and West Road, Zip 14224; tel. 716/674-9730; Allen R. Morganstein M.D., Clinical Director (Nonreporting) **A**1 3 **S**0009 New York State Department of Mental Health	12	52	46	—	—	—	—	—	—	—
WESTFIELD—Chautauqua County ★ WESTFIELD MEMORIAL HOSPITAL, 189 East Main Street, Zip 14787-1195; tel. 716/326-4921; Barbara A. Malinowski, Administrator **A**9 10 **F**7 8 15 16 17 19 22 33 34 40 44 65 67 71 73 74 **P**6	23	10	32	1465	17	31544	232	7307	4077	161
WHITE PLAINS—Westchester County ★ BURKE REHABILITATION HOSPITAL, 785 Mamaroneck Avenue, Zip 10605; tel. 914/948-0050; Fletcher H. McDowell M.D., Executive Director (Nonreporting) **A**1 9 10	23	46	150							
NEW YORK HOSPITAL, WESTCHESTER DIVISION See Society of the New York Hospital, New York City										
□ ST. AGNES HOSPITAL, (Includes Children's Rehabilitation Center) 305 North Street, Zip 10605; tel. 914/681-4500; Edward Alan Stolzenberg, President and Chief Executive Officer (Nonreporting) **A**1 5 10	21	10	191	—						
★ WHITE PLAINS HOSPITAL CENTER, Davis Avenue at East Post Road, Zip 10601-4699; tel. 914/681-0600; Jon B. Schandler, President and Chief Executive Officer (Nonreporting) **A**1 5 9 10	23	10	301	—						
WILLIAMSVILLE—Erie County MILLARD FILLMORE SUBURBAN HOSPITAL See Millard Fillmore Health System, Buffalo										
YONKERS—Westchester County ★ ST. JOHN'S RIVERSIDE HOSPITAL, 967 North Broadway, Zip 10701; tel. 914/964-4444; James Foy, President and Chief Executive Officer **A**1 6 9 10 **F**3 7 8 10 14 15 16 17 19 21 22 24 27 28 29 30 31 32 33 34 35 37 39 40 41 42 43 44 49 56 60 65 66 67 69 71 73 74 **P**7 8	23	10	273	10284	192	69300	1729	80698	34915	979
★ ST. JOSEPH'S MEDICAL CENTER, 127 South Broadway, Zip 10701-4080; tel. 914/378-7000; Sister Mary Linehan, President (Total facility includes 200 beds in nursing home–type unit) **A**1 3 5 9 10 **F**1 3 4 8 9 13 16 17 18 19 20 21 22 25 26 28 30 32 34 35 36 37 38 39 40 41 42 44 45 46 48 49 51 52 53 54 55 56 57 58 59 60 63 64 65 67 69 71 72 73 **P**1 **S**5995 Sisters of Charity Center	23	10	394	6159	355	223600	0	72917	35144	913

© 1995 AHA Guide

Hospitals, U.S. / NEW YORK

Hospital, Address, Telephone, Administrator, Approval, Facility, and Physician Codes, Health Care System	Classi-fication Codes		Utilization Data					Expense (thousands) of dollars		
	Control	Service	Beds	Admissions	Census	Outpatient Visits	Births	Total	Payroll	Personnel

★ American Hospital Association (AHA) membership
☐ Joint Commission on Accreditation of Healthcare Organizations (JCAHO) accreditation
+ American Osteopathic Hospital Association (AOHA) membership
○ American Osteopathic Association (AOA) accreditation
△ Commission on Accreditation of Rehabilitation Facilities (CARF) accreditation
Control codes 61, 63, 64, 71, 72 and 73 indicate hospitals listed by AOHA, but not registered by AHA. For definition of numerical codes, see page A6

✠ YONKERS GENERAL HOSPITAL, Two Park Avenue, Zip 10703–3497; tel. 914/964–7300; B. J. Oppenheimer M.D., Administrator and Chief Executive Officer **A**1 9 10 **F**2 3 8 14 15 16 17 18 19 21 22 31 34 37 41 42 44 45 46 54 60 63 65 70 71 73	23	10	190	5602	138	145287	0	42463	26633	767

Hospitals, U.S. / NORTH CAROLINA

NORTH CAROLINA

Resident population 6,945 (in thousands)
Resident population in metro areas 66.3%
Birth rate per 1,000 population 15.2
65 years and over 12.5%
Percent of persons without health insurance 14.2%

Hospital, Address, Telephone, Administrator, Approval, Facility, and Physician Codes, Health Care System	Classification Codes		Utilization Data					Expense (thousands) of dollars		Personnel
★ American Hospital Association (AHA) membership ☐ Joint Commission on Accreditation of Healthcare Organizations (JCAHO) accreditation + American Osteopathic Hospital Association (AOHA) membership ○ American Osteopathic Association (AOA) accreditation △ Commission on Accreditation of Rehabilitation Facilities (CARF) accreditation Control codes 61, 63, 64, 71, 72 and 73 indicate hospitals listed by AOHA, but not registered by AHA. For definition of numerical codes, see page A6	Control	Service	Beds	Admissions	Census	Outpatient Visits	Births	Total	Payroll	
AHOSKIE—Hertford County ★ ROANOKE–CHOWAN HOSPITAL, Academy Street, Zip 27910, Mailing Address: Box 1385, Zip 27910; tel. 919/332–8121; Peter N. Geilich, President **A**1 3 9 10 **F**7 8 12 19 20 21 22 28 30 32 33 34 35 37 40 41 42 44 46 49 51 52 54 56 57 58 65 71 73 **P**7	23	10	124	4807	79	167798	578	21762	12316	533
ALBEMARLE—Stanly County ★ STANLY MEMORIAL HOSPITAL, 301 Yadkin Street, Zip 28001, Mailing Address: Box 1489, Zip 28002; tel. 704/983–5111 **A**1 9 10 **F**1 7 8 10 11 12 15 19 20 22 23 26 31 32 34 35 36 37 39 40 41 42 44 45 46 48 49 52 53 55 56 57 64 65 66 67 71 73	23	10	110	3815	52	72596	470	23765	10141	318
ANDREWS—Cherokee County DISTRICT MEMORIAL HOSPITAL, 71 Whitaker Lane, Zip 28901; tel. 704/321–1291; Daniel C. White, Chief Executive Officer **A**9 10 **F**8 15 16 17 19 22 34 35 37 41 44 49 65 71 73	23	10	29	1231	37	17049	0	6582	3449	135
ASHEBORO—Randolph County ★ RANDOLPH HOSPITAL, 364 White Oak Street, Zip 27203, Mailing Address: Box 1048, Zip 27203–1048; tel. 910/625–5151; Robert E. Morrison, President **A**1 9 10 **F**7 8 14 15 19 21 22 28 34 35 37 39 40 42 44 49 65 71 73	23	10	101	4296	54	61565	623	28797	11839	471
ASHEVILLE—Buncombe County CHARTER ASHEVILLE, (Formerly Highland Hall) 60 Caledonia Road, Zip 28803, Mailing Address: P.O. Box 5534, Zip 28813; tel. 704/253–3681; Jay Cutspec, Chief Executive Officer **A**10 **F**2 3 12 14 16 18 19 21 25 34 35 46 50 52 53 54 55 56 57 58 59 63 65 71 **S**0695 Charter Medical Corporation	33	22	100	1270	52	2700	0	8440	5340	101
HIGHLAND HALL See Charter Asheville										
★ MEMORIAL MISSION MEDICAL CENTER, 509 Biltmore Avenue, Zip 28801–4690; tel. 704/255–4000; Robert F. Burgin, President **A**1 2 3 5 9 10 **F**4 7 8 10 11 12 13 14 15 16 17 19 20 21 22 25 27 30 31 32 34 35 37 38 39 40 41 42 43 44 45 47 49 56 60 63 65 66 67 70 71 73 74 **P**8	23	10	418	17970	272	147324	3084	163077	68089	2439
★ ST. JOSEPH'S HOSPITAL, 428 Biltmore Avenue, Zip 28801–4502; tel. 704/255–3100; J. Lewis Daniels, President and Chief Executive Officer (Total facility includes 30 beds in nursing home–type unit) **A**1 2 9 10 **F**3 10 11 14 15 16 19 22 23 24 25 27 29 31 32 33 34 35 37 39 41 42 44 45 49 52 56 57 59 60 63 64 65 71 72 73 **S**5985 Sisters of Mercy	21	10	292	14347	214	96006	0	81530	37004	1131
★ △ THOMS REHABILITATION HOSPITAL, 68 Sweeten Creek Road, Zip 28803–1599, Mailing Address: P.O. Box 15025, Zip 28813–0025; tel. 704/274–2400; Charles D. Norvell, President **A**7 9 10 **F**12 14 15 16 26 34 41 48 49 64 65 73	23	46	80	770	50	29604	0	14359	9223	284
★ VETERANS AFFAIRS MEDICAL CENTER, 1100 Tunnel Road, Zip 28805–2087; tel. 704/298–7911; James A. Christian, Director (Total facility includes 64 beds in nursing home–type unit) **A**1 3 5 9 **F**1 2 3 4 8 10 11 12 15 19 20 21 23 26 27 28 30 31 32 33 34 35 37 39 42 43 45 46 49 51 52 54 55 56 57 58 59 60 61 64 65 67 69 71 73 74 **P**6 **S**9295 Department of Veterans Affairs	45	10	358	6265	299	86907	0	63444	37281	778
BANNER ELK—Avery County ☐ CHARLES A. CANNON JR. MEMORIAL HOSPITAL, Highway 184, Zip 28604, Mailing Address: P.O. Box 8, Zip 28604–0008; tel. 704/898–5111; Edward C. Greene Jr., Administrator **A**1 9 10 **F**7 8 11 12 19 22 28 30 33 35 37 40 42 44 52 56 57 64 65 71 73 **P**3	23	10	79	1819	36	18828	68	10550	4814	229
BELHAVEN—Beaufort County PUNGO DISTRICT HOSPITAL, Front Street, Zip 27810–9998; tel. 919/943–2111; Thomas O. Miller, Administrator (Nonreporting) **A**9 10	23	10	49	—	—	—	—	—	—	—
BLACK MOUNTAIN—Buncombe County ALCOHOL AND DRUG ABUSE TREATMENT CENTER, 301 Tabernacle Road, Zip 28711; tel. 704/669–3402; William A. Rafter, Director **A**9 **F**2 3 12 18 25 26 27 31 45 46 73 74 **P**6	12	82	110	1279	94	0	0	4833	2929	99
BLOWING ROCK—Watauga County ★ BLOWING ROCK HOSPITAL, (Includes Dr. Charles Davant Rehabilitation and Extended Care Center) Chestnut Street, Zip 28605–0148, Mailing Address: Box 148, Zip 28605–0148; tel. 704/295–3136; Patricia Gray, Administrator and Chief Executive Officer (Total facility includes 72 beds in nursing home–type unit) **A**1 9 10 **F**1 14 15 16 19 22 26 27 28 29 30 32 34 41 44 45 46 49 56 57 64 65 67 71 73	23	10	100	391	83	10264	0	4610	2718	138
BOILING SPRINGS—Cleveland County CRAWLEY MEMORIAL HOSPITAL, 315 West College Avenue, Zip 28017, Mailing Address: Box 996, Zip 28017; tel. 704/434–9466; Daphne Bridges, President (Nonreporting) **A**9 10	23	10	51	—	—	—	—	—	—	—
BOONE—Watauga County ★ WATAUGA MEDICAL CENTER, Deerfield Road, Zip 28607–2600, Mailing Address: P.O. Box 2600, Zip 28607–2600; tel. 704/262–4100; Richard G. Sparks, President **A**1 9 10 **F**7 8 14 15 16 17 19 20 21 22 24 28 29 30 32 34 35 37 38 40 42 44 45 49 60 64 65 67 71 73 **P**3 8	13	10	105	4669	58	39653	587	26874	11955	442

© 1995 AHA Guide

Hospitals, U.S. / NORTH CAROLINA

Hospital, Address, Telephone, Administrator, Approval, Facility, and Physician Codes, Health Care System	Classification Codes		Utilization Data					Expense (thousands) of dollars		
★ American Hospital Association (AHA) membership □ Joint Commission on Accreditation of Healthcare Organizations (JCAHO) accreditation + American Osteopathic Hospital Association (AOHA) membership ○ American Osteopathic Association (AOA) accreditation △ Commission on Accreditation of Rehabilitation Facilities (CARF) accreditation Control codes 61, 63, 64, 71, 72 and 73 indicate hospitals listed by AOHA, but not registered by AHA. For definition of numerical codes, see page A6	Control	Service	Beds	Admissions	Census	Outpatient Visits	Births	Total	Payroll	Personnel
BREVARD—Transylvania County ★ TRANSYLVANIA COMMUNITY HOSPITAL, Hospital Drive, Zip 28712–9998, Mailing Address: Box 1116, Zip 28712; tel. 704/884–9111; Ray C. Brees, Administrator **A**1 9 10 **F**2 7 8 11 12 14 15 16 17 19 22 29 30 32 33 34 36 37 40 42 44 45 49 63 65 67 71 **P**5 8	23	10	90	2377	52	25677	170	20328	10298	359
BRYSON CITY—Swain County □ SWAIN COUNTY HOSPITAL, 45 Plateau Street, Zip 28713; tel. 704/488–2155; W. Joseph Seel, Administrator **A**1 9 10 **F**3 8 15 16 17 19 20 22 28 30 33 42 44 48 49 56 65 70 71 73	23	10	42	800	11	12500	0	5104	2272	127
BURGAW—Pender County PENDER MEMORIAL HOSPITAL, 507 Freemont Street, Zip 28425, Mailing Address: Box 835, Zip 28425; tel. 910/259–5451; Floyd A. Oathout, Administrator (Total facility includes 23 beds in nursing home–type unit) **A**9 10 **F**11 15 16 19 22 30 33 35 39 41 44 46 49 64 65 71 73	13	10	66	1522	43	24380	0	8476	4203	176
BURLINGTON—Alamance County ★ ALAMANCE REGIONAL MEDICAL CENTER, (Includes Alamance County Hospital, Burlington, North Carolina, Zip 27216; tel. 910/570–4000; Alamance Memorial Hospital, Burlington, North Carolina, Zip 27216; tel. 910/570–5000) North Graham Road, Zip 27216–0202, Mailing Address: P.O. Box 202, Zip 27216–0202; tel. 910/570–4000; Thomas E. Ryan, President (Nonreporting) **A**1 2 10	23	10	332	—	—	—	—	—	—	—
BUTNER—Granville County ALCOHOL AND DRUG ABUSE TREATMENT CENTER, 205 West E Street, Zip 27509; tel. 919/575–7928; Johnny O. Rodgers, Director **F**2 19 20 30 35 37 45 46 54 56 67 71 73 74 **P**6	12	82	80	960	57	0	0	3873	2655	91
□ JOHN UMSTEAD HOSPITAL, 1003 12th Street, Zip 27509–1626; tel. 919/575–7211; Patricia L. Christian R.N., Ph.D., Director **A**1 3 5 9 10 **F**52 53 54 56 57 58	12	22	611	3016	480	4103	0	56200	39857	1326
CAMP LEJEUNE—Onslow County ★ NAVAL HOSPITAL, Zip 28547–0100; tel. 910/451–4300; Captain Michael L. Cowan MC, USN, Commanding Officer **A**1 9 **F**2 4 8 10 15 16 17 19 22 25 27 29 30 31 32 34 35 36 37 39 40 41 42 44 45 46 49 51 52 56 58 59 61 65 66 67 71 72 73 74 **P**5 **S**9655 Department of Navy	43	10	176	7549	71	520764	1213	—	—	184
CHAPEL HILL—Orange County ★ UNIVERSITY OF NORTH CAROLINA HOSPITALS, (Includes North Carolina Children's Hospital; North Carolina Neurosciences Hospital, Chapel Hill, North Carolina) 101 Manning Drive, Zip 27514; tel. 919/966–4131; Eric B. Munson, Executive Director **A**1 2 3 5 8 9 10 **F**2 4 5 7 8 9 10 11 12 13 14 15 16 19 20 21 22 23 26 30 31 32 33 34 35 37 38 39 40 41 42 43 44 45 46 47 48 49 50 51 52 53 54 55 56 57 58 60 61 63 64 65 66 67 69 70 71 73 74 **P**1	12	10	659	23685	486	577473	2077	309728	148371	4398
CHARLOTTE—Mecklenburg County AMETHYST, 1715 Sharon Road West, Zip 28210, Mailing Address: P.O. Box 240516, Zip 28224–0516; tel. 704/554–8373; William Kyle Brown, Vice President and Administrator **F**2 3 4 5 7 8 9 10 11 13 16 19 20 21 22 27 32 33 34 35 36 37 38 39 40 41 42 43 44 45 46 47 48 49 50 51 52 53 54 55 56 57 58 59 60 61 63 64 65 66 69 70 71 72 73 74 **P**3	16	82	94	644	33	3558	0	—	—	76
★ CAROLINAS MEDICAL CENTER, 1000 Blythe Boulevard, Zip 28203, Mailing Address: P.O. Box 32861, Zip 28232–2861; tel. 704/355–2000; Harry A. Nurkin Ph.D., President **A**1 2 3 5 8 9 10 **F**1 2 3 4 5 6 7 8 10 11 12 13 14 15 17 18 19 20 21 22 24 25 27 28 30 31 32 33 34 35 37 38 40 41 42 43 44 45 46 47 48 49 50 51 52 53 54 55 56 57 58 59 60 61 62 63 64 65 66 67 68 69 70 71 72 73 74 **P**6 **S**0705 Charlotte–Mecklenburg Hospital Authority	16	10	843	33464	614	310250	5605	—	—	5440
★ △ CHARLOTTE INSTITUTE OF REHABILITATION, 1100 Blythe Boulevard, Zip 28203; tel. 704/355–4300; Hollis Hamilton, Administrator **A**1 3 7 9 10 **F**2 3 4 5 7 8 9 10 11 12 19 20 21 22 24 27 30 32 34 35 37 38 40 41 42 43 44 45 46 47 48 49 50 52 53 54 55 56 57 58 59 60 61 64 65 66 67 69 70 71 72 73 74 **S**0705 Charlotte–Mecklenburg Hospital Authority	16	46	114	1344	92	121583	0	28319	15968	429
□ CHARTER PINES HOSPITAL, 3621 Randolph Road, Zip 28211, Mailing Address: P.O. Box 221709, Zip 28222–1709; tel. 704/365–5368; Edward Payton, Chief Executive Officer (Nonreporting) **A**1 9 10 **S**0695 Charter Medical Corporation	33	22	60	—	—	—	—	—	—	—
★ △ MERCY HOSPITAL, 2001 Vail Avenue, Zip 28207; tel. 704/379–5000; C. Curtis Copenhaver, President **A**1 6 7 9 10 **F**1 2 3 4 7 8 10 11 12 14 16 19 21 22 30 31 32 34 35 37 38 39 40 41 43 44 48 49 63 65 71 73 **P**6 **S**5985 Sisters of Mercy	21	10	276	8848	159	94241	933	87595	40191	1144
★ PRESBYTERIAN HOSPITAL, 200 Hawthorne Lane, Zip 28204, Mailing Address: Box 33549, Zip 28233–3549; tel. 704/384–4000; Paul F. Betzold, President and Chief Executive Officer **A**1 2 6 9 10 **F**4 7 8 10 11 12 13 15 16 17 18 19 21 22 23 24 25 26 27 28 29 30 31 32 33 34 35 37 38 39 40 41 42 43 44 45 46 47 49 50 51 52 53 54 56 57 58 59 60 61 65 67 68 71 72 73 74 **P**1 6	23	10	537	27675	444	143529	4485	241425	93622	3349
★ PRESBYTERIAN SPECIALTY HOSPITAL, 1600 East Third Street, Zip 28204, Mailing Address: P.O. Box 34425, Zip 28234–4425; tel. 704/384–6000; Chip Day, Chief Operating Officer **A**9 10 **F**12 19 23 28 34 35 41 44 49 65 67 69 **P**1 3 7 8	23	45	15	301	5	7842	0	9730	3718	99
★ PRESBYTERIAN–ORTHOPAEDIC HOSPITAL, 1901 Randolph Road, Zip 28207; tel. 704/375–6792; Tom Pemberton, President (Nonreporting) **A**1 3 9 10 **S**0048 Columbia/HCA Healthcare Corporation	33	47	166	—	—	—	—	—	—	—

Hospitals, U.S. / NORTH CAROLINA

Hospital, Address, Telephone, Administrator, Approval, Facility, and Physician Codes, Health Care System	Classi-fication Codes		Utilization Data					Expense (thousands) of dollars		
★ American Hospital Association (AHA) membership □ Joint Commission on Accreditation of Healthcare Organizations (JCAHO) accreditation + American Osteopathic Hospital Association (AOHA) membership ○ American Osteopathic Association (AOA) accreditation △ Commission on Accreditation of Rehabilitation Facilities (CARF) accreditation Control codes 61, 63, 64, 71, 72 and 73 indicate hospitals listed by AOHA, but not registered by AHA. For definition of numerical codes, see page A6	Control	Service	Beds	Admissions	Census	Outpatient Visits	Births	Total	Payroll	Personnel
□ UNIVERSITY HOSPITAL, 8800 North Tryon Street, Zip 28262, Mailing Address: P.O. Box 560727, Zip 28256; tel. 704/548–6000; W. Spencer Lilly, Administrator **A**1 9 10 **F**2 4 6 7 8 9 10 11 14 16 19 20 21 22 24 28 29 30 31 32 34 35 37 38 39 40 41 42 43 44 47 48 49 50 51 52 53 54 55 56 57 58 59 60 61 63 64 65 66 67 69 70 71 72 73 74 **P**3 6 8 **S**0705 Charlotte–Mecklenburg Hospital Authority	16	10	107	3922	49	54743	776	31502	12989	381
CHEROKEE—Swain County ⊞ U.S. PUBLIC HEALTH SERVICE INDIAN HOSPITAL, Hospital Road, Zip 28719; tel. 704/497–9163; G. E. Graning M.D., Administrator **A**1 10 **F**2 3 16 20 22 30 33 34 39 51 58 65 68 71 74 **S**9195 U.S. Public Health Service Indian Health Service	47	10	30	902	13	92929	0	10787	—	143
CHERRY POINT—Craven County ⊞ NAVAL HOSPITAL, Zip 28533–5008; tel. 919/466–3620; Captain V. Peters MSC, USN, Commanding Officer (Nonreporting) **A**1 9 **S**9655 Department of Navy	43	10	43	—	—	—	—	—	—	—
CLINTON—Sampson County ⊞ SAMPSON COUNTY MEMORIAL HOSPITAL, 607 Beaman Street, Zip 28328, Mailing Address: Drawer 258, Zip 28328; tel. 910/592–8511; Lee Pridgen Jr., Administrator (Total facility includes 30 beds in nursing home–type unit) **A**1 9 10 **F**7 8 11 12 15 16 17 19 20 21 22 23 26 28 30 32 34 35 39 40 44 49 63 64 65 71 73	13	10	146	3812	78	39600	459	24481	12296	469
CLYDE—Haywood County ⊞ HAYWOOD COUNTY HOSPITAL, 90 Hospital Drive, Zip 28721–9434; tel. 704/456–7311; David O. Rice, President (Total facility includes 20 beds in nursing home–type unit) **A**1 9 10 **F**7 8 14 15 16 19 21 22 23 24 28 29 30 32 33 34 35 37 41 42 44 45 49 54 60 64 65 66 71 73 74 **P**3	13	10	150	5212	74	46056	289	30501	14867	604
COLUMBUS—Polk County □ ST. LUKE'S HOSPITAL, 220 Hospital Drive, Zip 28722; tel. 704/894–3311; C. Cameron Highsmith Jr., President and Chief Executive Officer **A**1 9 10 **F**8 12 14 15 16 19 21 22 27 28 29 30 32 33 37 39 44 49 51 65 67 71 73 **P**7	23	10	55	1067	13	23289	0	8334	3901	237
CONCORD—Cabarrus County ⊞ CABARRUS MEMORIAL HOSPITAL, 920 Church Street North, Zip 28025–2983; tel. 704/783–3000; Thomas R. Revels, President **A**1 5 6 9 10 **F**4 7 8 10 11 14 15 16 19 21 22 24 32 33 34 35 36 37 40 42 43 44 48 60 65 74 **P**3	23	10	327	12390	229	216782	1371	109275	53518	1668
CROSSNORE—Avery County ⊞ SLOOP MEMORIAL HOSPITAL, One Crossnore Drive, Zip 28616, Mailing Address: Drawer 470, Zip 28616; tel. 704/733–9231; Frederick L. Blair, President **A**1 9 10 **F**7 8 15 16 19 22 30 36 40 44 65 71 73 **P**3	23	10	38	1588	19	23159	105	8407	4433	296
DANBURY—Stokes County ⊞ STOKES–REYNOLDS MEMORIAL HOSPITAL, Mailing Address: Box 10, Zip 27016–0010; tel. 910/593–2831; Sandra D. Priddy, President (Total facility includes 40 beds in nursing home–type unit) **A**1 9 10 **F**8 17 19 20 22 25 28 30 33 34 37 44 64 65 71 72 73 **P**3 7	21	10	93	993	74	21087	0	9277	4381	234
DUNN—Harnett County □ BETSY JOHNSON MEMORIAL HOSPITAL, 800 Tilghman Drive, Zip 28334, Mailing Address: Box 1706, Zip 28335; tel. 910/892–7161; Shannon D. Brown, Administrator **A**1 9 10 **F**7 8 14 15 19 22 28 30 34 35 37 40 44 46 63 65 71 73 **P**5	14	10	88	3317	38	40987	494	17841	9034	350
DURHAM—Durham County DUKE UNIVERSITY HOSPITAL See Duke University Medical Center										
⊞ DUKE UNIVERSITY MEDICAL CENTER, (Includes Duke University Hospital, Durham, North Carolina) Irwin Road, Zip 27710, Mailing Address: Box 3708, Zip 27710; tel. 919/684–8111; Mark C. Rogers M.D., Executive Director, Chief Executive Officer, and Vice Chancellor **A**1 2 3 5 8 9 10 **F**3 4 7 8 9 10 11 12 13 15 16 17 18 19 20 21 22 23 26 27 28 29 30 31 34 35 37 38 39 40 41 42 43 44 45 46 47 48 49 50 51 52 53 55 56 57 58 60 61 63 65 66 67 69 70 71 73 74 **P**1	23	10	958	35495	762	576488	2124	562256	220250	6407
⊞ DURHAM REGIONAL HOSPITAL, 3643 North Roxboro Road, Zip 27704–2763; tel. 919/470–4000; Richard L. Myers, President **A**1 3 5 6 9 10 **F**3 4 7 8 10 11 12 15 16 17 19 21 22 23 25 26 27 28 30 31 32 34 35 37 39 40 41 42 43 44 45 46 49 51 52 53 54 55 56 57 58 59 61 63 65 67 71 72 73 74 **P**1	13	10	244	15506	232	84307	2841	117749	59070	1836
★ NORTH CAROLINA EYE AND EAR HOSPITAL, 1110 West Main Street, Zip 27701; tel. 919/682–9341; H. Ed Jones, Chief Executive Officer (Nonreporting) **A**5 9 10	33	45	24	—	—	—	—	—	—	—
⊞ VETERANS AFFAIRS MEDICAL CENTER, 508 Fulton Street, Zip 27705; tel. 919/286–0411; Barbara A. Small, Director (Total facility includes 120 beds in nursing home–type unit) **A**1 3 5 8 9 **F**3 4 8 10 11 15 16 19 20 21 22 26 27 28 29 30 31 32 34 35 37 39 41 42 43 44 45 46 49 51 52 54 55 56 57 58 60 63 64 65 67 69 71 73 74 **S**9295 Department of Veterans Affairs	45	10	376	8330	311	132268	0	113948	61417	1530
EDEN—Rockingham County ⊞ MOREHEAD MEMORIAL HOSPITAL, 117 East King's Highway, Zip 27288–5299; tel. 910/623–9711; Robert Enders, President (Total facility includes 121 beds in nursing home–type unit) **A**1 9 10 **F**7 8 12 13 15 16 17 19 21 22 23 26 28 30 33 34 35 36 37 39 40 41 42 44 45 46 49 60 63 64 65 66 67 68 71 73 74 **S**0002 Quorum Health Group/Quorum Health Resources	23	10	213	4705	103	82119	677	26928	11844	406
EDENTON—Chowan County ⊞ CHOWAN HOSPITAL, 211 Virginia Road, Zip 27932–0629, Mailing Address: P.O. Box 629, Zip 27932–0629; tel. 919/482–8451; Barbara R. Cale, Administrator (Total facility includes 40 beds in nursing home–type unit) **A**1 9 10 **F**7 8 12 14 15 16 17 19 20 21 22 28 30 31 32 34 37 39 40 42 44 45 49 52 54 56 58 59 64 65 67 71 73 **P**3	13	10	110	2237	73	18064	395	14712	7236	306

© 1995 AHA Guide

Hospitals, U.S. / NORTH CAROLINA

Hospital, Address, Telephone, Administrator, Approval, Facility, and Physician Codes, Health Care System	Classification Codes		Utilization Data				Expense (thousands) of dollars		
★ American Hospital Association (AHA) membership ☐ Joint Commission on Accreditation of Healthcare Organizations (JCAHO) accreditation + American Osteopathic Hospital Association (AOHA) membership ○ American Osteopathic Association (AOA) accreditation △ Commission on Accreditation of Rehabilitation Facilities (CARF) accreditation Control codes 61, 63, 64, 71, 72 and 73 indicate hospitals listed by AOHA, but not registered by AHA. For definition of numerical codes, see page A6	Control	Service	Beds	Admissions	Census	Outpatient Visits	Births	Total	Payroll	Personnel
ELIZABETH CITY—Pasquotank County										
★ ALBEMARLE HOSPITAL, 1144 North Road Street, Zip 27909, Mailing Address: Box 1587, Zip 27906–1587; tel. 919/335–0531; Douglas L. Fairfax, Chief Executive Officer **A**1 9 10 **F**7 8 10 11 12 15 19 20 21 22 23 28 29 30 34 35 37 39 40 41 42 44 45 46 49 60 65 71 73	13	10	130	5950	115	65192	720	40453	18777	682
ELIZABETHTOWN—Bladen County										
★ BLADEN COUNTY HOSPITAL, Clarkton Road, Zip 28337–0398, Mailing Address: Box 398, Zip 28337–0398; tel. 910/862–5100; Leo A. Petit Jr., Chief Executive Officer (Total facility includes 10 beds in nursing home–type unit) **A**1 9 10 **F**7 8 11 15 16 17 19 21 22 25 28 29 32 33 34 35 37 39 40 44 45 49 64 65 67 71 72 73 **P**6 7 8	13	10	62	2083	27	27083	254	12610	5648	264
ELKIN—Surry County										
★ HUGH CHATHAM MEMORIAL HOSPITAL, Parkwood Drive, Zip 28621–0560, Mailing Address: P.O. Box 560, Zip 28621–0560; tel. 910/835–3722; Richard D. Osmus, Chief Executive Officer (Total facility includes 79 beds in nursing home–type unit) **A**1 9 10 **F**2 3 4 7 8 9 10 12 14 17 19 20 21 22 28 30 31 32 33 34 35 36 37 38 40 41 42 44 45 47 49 52 53 54 55 56 57 58 59 60 61 62 63 64 65 66 67 69 70 71 73 74 **S**0002 Quorum Health Group/Quorum Health Resources	23	10	160	3529	132	31337	247	18863	9817	346
ERWIN—Harnett County										
☐ GOOD HOPE HOSPITAL, 410 Denim Drive, Zip 28339–0668, Mailing Address: P.O. Box 668, Zip 28339–0668; tel. 910/897–6151; David L. Boucher, Chief Executive Officer **A**1 9 10 **F**11 16 17 19 21 22 28 29 30 32 33 34 35 44 49 51 52 54 55 56 57 65 66 67 71 73 **P**6	23	10	72	1477	21	17954	0	6887	4000	192
FAYETTEVILLE—Cumberland County										
★ △ CAPE FEAR VALLEY MEDICAL CENTER, 1638 Owen Drive, Zip 28304, Mailing Address: Box 2000, Zip 28302–2000; tel. 910/609–4000; John T. Carlisle, Chief Executive Officer **A**1 2 3 5 7 9 10 **F**3 4 7 8 10 11 12 14 15 16 17 19 21 22 28 31 32 33 34 35 37 38 40 41 42 43 44 45 46 48 49 52 53 54 56 57 58 59 60 65 67 71 73 74 **P**6	13	10	453	17964	322	246129	4722	152566	65963	2524
CUMBERLAND HOSPITAL, 3425 Melrose Road, Zip 28304; tel. 910/609–3000; Edward J. Whitehouse, Administrator **A**9 10 **F**1 2 3 4 7 8 10 11 12 14 15 16 17 19 20 21 22 23 25 26 28 29 30 31 32 33 34 35 37 38 39 40 41 42 43 44 45 46 48 49 52 53 54 55 56 57 58 59 60 63 65 67 71 73 **P**6	13	22	100	1109	61	17500	0	10265	5313	260
★ HIGHSMITH–RAINEY MEMORIAL HOSPITAL, 150 Robeson Street, Zip 28301–5570; tel. 910/609–1000; William A. Adams, Chief Executive Officer **A**1 9 10 **F**8 12 14 15 16 19 21 22 32 33 34 35 37 42 44 46 54 63 65 71 73 **S**0048 Columbia/HCA Healthcare Corporation	33	10	150	3890	73	40201	0	—	—	492
★ VETERANS AFFAIRS MEDICAL CENTER, 2300 Ramsey Street, Zip 28301–3899; tel. 919/822–7059; Jerome Calhoun, Director (Total facility includes 39 beds in nursing home–type unit) **A**1 9 **F**2 3 6 8 12 15 16 17 19 20 21 22 23 24 26 27 28 30 31 32 33 34 35 37 39 41 44 45 46 49 52 54 55 56 57 58 61 64 65 67 71 73 74 **S**9295 Department of Veterans Affairs	45	10	220	4256	221	100447	0	46730	32450	724
FLETCHER—Henderson County										
★ PARK RIDGE HOSPITAL, Naples Road, Zip 28732, Mailing Address: P.O. Box 1569, Zip 28732–1569; tel. 704/684–8501; Robert W. Burchard, President **A**1 9 10 **F**7 8 10 11 14 15 19 21 22 23 25 30 32 33 35 37 40 41 44 45 46 52 53 56 58 59 65 71 73 **P**6 **S**4165 Adventist Health System–Sunbelt Health Care Corporation	23	10	87	2565	49	32715	447	24071	10475	392
FORT BRAGG—Cumberland County										
★ WOMACK ARMY MEDICAL CENTER, Zip 28307–5000; tel. 919/432–4802; Colonel Harold L. Timboe, Commander **A**1 3 5 9 **F**7 8 12 13 14 19 20 21 22 34 35 37 39 40 41 42 44 46 49 51 52 53 54 55 56 57 58 59 60 65 71 73 **P**1 **S**9395 Department of the Army	42	10	264	18513	148	1089065	2013	—	—	2010
FRANKLIN—Macon County										
★ ANGEL COMMUNITY HOSPITAL, Riverview & White Oak Streets, Zip 28734, Mailing Address: P.O. Box 1209, Zip 28734–1209; tel. 704/524–8411; Michael E. Zuliani, Administrator **A**1 9 10 **F**7 8 12 15 17 19 22 32 34 35 37 42 44 45 46 49 61 65 71 73 74 **S**0002 Quorum Health Group/Quorum Health Resources	23	10	59	2122	32	31126	8	15117	6760	270
GASTONIA—Gaston County										
★ GASTON MEMORIAL HOSPITAL, 2525 Court Drive, Zip 28054, Mailing Address: Box 1747, Zip 28053–1747; tel. 704/834–2000; Wayne F. Shovelin, President and Chief Executive Officer **A**1 2 9 10 **F**7 8 10 15 16 17 18 19 21 22 23 30 34 37 39 40 41 42 44 45 46 49 52 53 54 55 56 57 58 59 60 63 65 67 70 71 73 74	23	10	404	14918	285	98342	2163	105508	49791	1708
GOLDSBORO—Wayne County										
☐ CHERRY HOSPITAL, Steven Mill Road, Zip 27533–8000, Mailing Address: Caller Box 8000, Zip 27533–8000; tel. 919/731–3200; J. Field Montgomery Jr., Director (Total facility includes 201 beds in nursing home–type unit) **A**1 3 5 9 10 **F**12 20 46 52 53 57 64 65 73 **P**6	12	22	690	2513	577	0	0	50917	32721	1182
★ WAYNE MEMORIAL HOSPITAL, 2700 Wayne Memorial Drive, Zip 27534–8001, Mailing Address: P.O. Box 8001, Zip 27533–8001; tel. 919/736–1110; James W. Hubbell, President and Chief Executive Officer (Data for 364 days) **A**1 9 10 **F**7 8 10 14 17 19 21 22 23 26 29 30 31 32 33 34 35 37 42 44 45 46 49 50 52 53 54 55 56 57 60 63 65 66 71 73	23	10	267	11183	200	74920	1215	67726	28520	1057
GREENSBORO—Guilford County										
☐ CHARTER GREENSBORO BEHAVIORAL HEALTH SYSTEM, (Formerly Charter Hospital of Greensboro) 700 Walter Reed Drive, Zip 27403–1129, Mailing Address: P.O. Box 10399, Zip 27404–0399; tel. 910/852–4821; Joe Crabtree, Chief Executive Officer (Nonreporting) **A**1 9 10 **S**0695 Charter Medical Corporation	33	22	68	—	—	—	—	—	—	—

Hospitals, U.S. / NORTH CAROLINA

Hospital, Address, Telephone, Administrator, Approval, Facility, and Physician Codes, Health Care System	Classification Codes		Utilization Data					Expense (thousands) of dollars		
★ American Hospital Association (AHA) membership □ Joint Commission on Accreditation of Healthcare Organizations (JCAHO) accreditation + American Osteopathic Hospital Association (AOHA) membership ○ American Osteopathic Association (AOA) accreditation △ Commission on Accreditation of Rehabilitation Facilities (CARF) accreditation Control codes 61, 63, 64, 71, 72 and 73 indicate hospitals listed by AOHA, but not registered by AHA. For definition of numerical codes, see page A6	Control	Service	Beds	Admissions	Census	Outpatient Visits	Births	Total	Payroll	Personnel
MEMORIAL HOSPITAL OF GREENSBORO, 2401 Southside Boulevard, Zip 27406, Mailing Address: P.O. Drawer 16167, Zip 27406; tel. 919/275–9741; Ronald E. Burrell, Chief Executive Officer (Total facility includes 41 beds in nursing home–type unit) **A**9 10 **F**12 19 20 21 22 27 35 37 39 41 45 49 54 55 57 64 65 67 71 73 **P**4 5	33	10	71	160	78	4	0	6980	3535	78
★ △ MOSES CONE HEALTH SYSTEM, (Includes Moses H. Cone Memorial Hospital, 1200 North Elm Street, Greensboro, North Carolina, Zip 27401; tel. 910/574–7000; David McCombs, Executive Vice–President; Women's Hospital of Greensboro, 801 Green Valley Road, Greensboro, North Carolina, Zip 27408; tel. 910/574–6500; James R. Whiting, Executive Vice–President) 1200 North Elm Street, Zip 27401–1020; tel. 910/574–7000; Dennis R. Barry, President (Total facility includes 150 beds in nursing home–type unit) **A**1 2 3 5 7 8 9 10 **F**4 7 8 10 11 12 14 15 16 17 19 20 21 22 23 25 26 28 29 30 31 32 33 34 35 37 38 39 40 41 42 43 44 45 46 48 49 52 54 55 57 60 61 63 65 66 67 70 71 73 74	23	10	796	25913	652	219486	3831	209424	110329	3364
MOSES H. CONE MEMORIAL HOSPITAL See Moses Cone Health System										
★ WESLEY LONG COMMUNITY HOSPITAL, 501 North Elam Avenue, Zip 27403, Mailing Address: P.O. Box 2747, Zip 27402; tel. 910/854–6100; Gary L. Park, President **A**1 9 10 **F**4 7 8 10 12 14 15 16 17 19 22 28 29 30 31 34 35 37 39 40 41 42 44 45 46 48 49 61 63 65 67 71 72 73 74 **P**7 8	23	10	199	8633	132	84059	983	66226	28829	852
WOMEN'S HOSPITAL OF GREENSBORO See Moses Cone Health System										
□ YOUTH FOCUS PSYCHIATRIC HOSPITAL, 1601 Huffine Mill Road, Zip 27405–5509; tel. 910/375–8333; David Coleman, Director (Nonreporting) **A**1 9	23	52	12	—	—	—	—	—	—	—
GREENVILLE—Pitt County										
★ △ PITT COUNTY MEMORIAL HOSPITAL–UNIVERSITY MEDICAL CENTER OF EASTERN CAROLINA–PITT COUNTY, 2100 Stantonsburg Road, Zip 27835–6028, Mailing Address: Box 6028, Zip 27835–6028; tel. 919/816–4451; Dave C. McRae, President and Chief Executive Officer **A**1 2 3 5 7 8 9 10 **F**4 7 8 10 11 12 15 16 17 19 20 21 22 23 24 27 30 31 34 35 37 38 40 41 42 43 44 45 46 47 48 49 52 53 54 55 56 57 60 61 65 69 70 71 73 74 **P**5	13	10	669	29392	532	103529	2988	252495	123401	3906
WALTER B. JONES ALCOHOL AND DRUG ABUSE TREATMENT CENTER, 2577 West Fifth Street, Zip 27834; tel. 919/830–3426; Phillip A. Mooring, Director (Nonreporting) **A**9	12	82	76	—	—	—	—	—	—	—
HAMLET—Richmond County										
□ HAMLET HOSPITAL, Rice and Vance Streets, Zip 28345, Mailing Address: Box 1109, Zip 28345; tel. 910/582–3611; Page Vaughan, Administrator **A**1 9 10 **F**8 15 17 19 22 26 27 28 29 30 33 34 35 37 39 41 44 45 46 49 52 54 55 56 57 65 66 67 71 73 **S**1775 Health Management Associates	33	10	64	2535	37	20000	0	—	—	140
HENDERSON—Vance County										
★ MARIA PARHAM HOSPITAL, 1805 Ruin Creek Road, Zip 27536–2957; tel. 919/438–4143; Philip S. Lakernick, President and Chief Executive Officer **A**1 9 10 **F**5 7 8 10 14 15 16 17 19 20 21 22 24 26 28 29 30 31 33 34 35 37 40 41 42 44 45 46 48 49 56 65 66 67 71 72 73 74	23	10	95	3863	47	44855	662	21007	8680	387
HENDERSONVILLE—Henderson County										
★ MARGARET R. PARDEE MEMORIAL HOSPITAL, 715 Fleming Street, Zip 28739–2563; tel. 704/696–1000; Frank J. Aaron Jr., Chief Executive Officer (Total facility includes 40 beds in nursing home–type unit) (Data for 363 days) **A**1 9 10 **F**1 7 8 12 13 14 15 16 17 19 20 21 22 23 26 28 29 30 32 34 35 37 40 41 42 44 45 49 52 54 55 56 57 59 60 63 64 65 67 71 72 73 74 **P**5 7	13	10	201	7148	139	63519	355	43278	20454	808
HICKORY—Catawba County										
AMI FRYE REGIONAL MEDICAL CENTER See Frye Regional Medical Center										
★ CATAWBA MEMORIAL HOSPITAL, 810 Fairgrove Church Road S.E., Zip 28602; tel. 704/326–3000; J. Anthony Rose, President and Chief Executive Officer **A**1 9 10 **F**4 7 8 10 14 15 16 17 19 20 21 22 23 24 26 28 30 31 32 33 34 35 37 40 41 42 43 44 46 49 52 53 54 55 56 57 58 60 61 65 66 67 71 73 74 **P**8	13	10	187	7206	103	173832	1379	64140	29203	942
★ △ FRYE REGIONAL MEDICAL CENTER, (Formerly AMI Frye Regional Medical Center) (Includes Frye Regional Medical Center–South Campus, One Third Avenue N.W., Hickory, North Carolina, Zip 28601, Mailing Address: P.O. Box 369, Zip 28603; tel. 704/328–2226) 420 North Center Street, Zip 28601; tel. 704/322–6070; Dennis Phillips, Chief Executive Officer **A**1 7 9 10 **F**2 3 4 7 8 10 11 12 14 19 20 21 22 28 32 34 35 37 38 40 41 42 43 44 48 49 52 53 54 56 57 64 65 71 73 **P**7 8 **S**0063 TENET Healthcare Corporation	33	10	314	10182	181	76078	797	71892	26973	1050
FRYE REGIONAL MEDICAL CENTER–SOUTH CAMPUS See Frye Regional Medical Center										
HIGH POINT—Guilford County										
★ HIGH POINT REGIONAL HOSPITAL, 601 North Elm Street, Zip 27262, Mailing Address: P.O. Box HP-5, Zip 27261; tel. 910/884–8400; Jeffrey S. Miller, President (Total facility includes 30 beds in nursing home–type unit) **A**1 9 10 **F**2 3 4 7 8 10 11 12 14 15 16 17 19 20 21 22 23 24 26 28 29 30 31 32 33 34 35 37 39 40 41 42 43 44 45 46 49 52 54 55 56 57 58 59 60 64 65 66 67 71 73 74 **P**7 8	23	10	321	14589	235	71804	1853	90749	39851	1431
HIGHLANDS—Macon County										
★ HIGHLANDS–CASHIERS HOSPITAL, Hospital Drive, Zip 28741, Mailing Address: P.O. Drawer 190, Zip 28741; tel. 704/526–1200; Alton T. Byers, President and Chief Executive Officer (Total facility includes 80 beds in nursing home–type unit) **A**1 9 10 **F**6 8 13 15 16 17 19 22 28 30 34 44 49 62 64 65 71 72 **P**3	23	10	104	565	46	10208	0	5855	2767	95

© 1995 AHA Guide

Hospitals, U.S. / NORTH CAROLINA

Hospital, Address, Telephone, Administrator, Approval, Facility, and Physician Codes, Health Care System	Classification Codes		Utilization Data					Expense (thousands) of dollars		
★ American Hospital Association (AHA) membership □ Joint Commission on Accreditation of Healthcare Organizations (JCAHO) accreditation + American Osteopathic Hospital Association (AOHA) membership ○ American Osteopathic Association (AOA) accreditation △ Commission on Accreditation of Rehabilitation Facilities (CARF) accreditation Control codes 61, 63, 64, 71, 72 and 73 indicate hospitals listed by AOHA, but not registered by AHA. For definition of numerical codes, see page A6	Control	Service	Beds	Admissions	Census	Outpatient Visits	Births	Total	Payroll	Personnel
JACKSONVILLE—Onslow County										
□ BRYNN MARR HOSPITAL, 192 Village Drive, Zip 28546; tel. 919/577-1400; Dale Armstrong, Administrator (Nonreporting) **A**1 9 10 **S**0405 Ramsay Health Care, Inc.	33	22	76	—	—	—	—	—	—	—
★ ONSLOW MEMORIAL HOSPITAL, 317 Western Boulevard, Zip 28540, Mailing Address: Box 1358, Zip 28540; tel. 919/577-2281; Douglas Kramer, Chief Executive Officer **A**1 9 10 **F**10 15 16 19 21 22 34 35 37 40 42 44 63 71 73 **P**8	16	10	133	9119	80	59928	1885	36315	15472	568
JEFFERSON—Ashe County										
★ ASHE MEMORIAL HOSPITAL, 200 Hospital Avenue, Zip 28640-0008, Mailing Address: P.O. Box 8, Zip 28640-0008; tel. 910/246-7101; R. D. Williams, Administrator (Total facility includes 60 beds in nursing home-type unit) **A**1 9 10 **F**1 7 8 14 16 19 20 21 22 24 28 29 30 34 35 39 40 41 44 45 49 64 65 67 71 73 **P**5 **S**0002 Quorum Health Group/Quorum Health Resources	23	10	115	2250	90	27748	76	11985	5276	216
KENANSVILLE—Duplin County										
★ DUPLIN GENERAL HOSPITAL, 401 North Main Street, Zip 28349-0278, Mailing Address: P.O. Box 278, Zip 28349-0278; tel. 910/296-0941; Richard E. Harrell, President (Total facility includes 20 beds in nursing home-type unit) **A**1 9 10 **F**7 8 14 15 16 19 21 22 26 31 34 37 40 44 49 51 52 55 56 57 64 65 71 73 74	23	10	80	2425	53	19642	446	11752	5909	240
KINGS MOUNTAIN—Cleveland County										
★ KINGS MOUNTAIN HOSPITAL, 706 West King Street, Zip 28086, Mailing Address: P.O. Box 339, Zip 28086; tel. 704/739-3601; Hank Neal, Administrator (Total facility includes 10 beds in nursing home-type unit) **A**9 10 **F**8 19 22 34 37 44 47 52 65 71 73	23	10	102	1660	48	17548	0	10690	5106	214
KINSTON—Lenoir County										
CASWELL CENTER, 2415 West Vernon Avenue, Zip 28501; tel. 919/559-5222; Jim S. Woodall, Director **A**9 **F**11 15 16 19 20 27 31 35 37 39 41 42 46 48 65 71 73	12	62	813	64	722	—	0	57501	39360	1717
★ LENOIR MEMORIAL HOSPITAL, 100 Airport Road, Zip 28501-0678, Mailing Address: P.O. Drawer 1678, Zip 28501-1678; tel. 919/522-7171; Gary E. Black, President and Chief Executive Officer (Total facility includes 26 beds in nursing home-type unit) **A**1 9 10 **F**7 10 11 12 14 15 19 20 21 22 24 28 30 31 32 33 34 35 37 39 40 41 42 44 45 46 48 49 56 64 65 70 71 73	13	10	266	9658	185	60510	800	58935	28393	1064
LAURINBURG—Scotland County										
★ SCOTLAND MEMORIAL HOSPITAL, 500 Lauchwood Drive, Zip 28352, Mailing Address: P.O. Box 8000, Zip 28353; tel. 910/276-2121; Gregory C. Wood, Chief Executive Officer (Total facility includes 40 beds in nursing home-type unit) **A**1 9 10 **F**1 2 3 6 7 8 10 19 20 21 22 23 25 27 28 30 31 32 33 34 35 36 37 39 40 41 42 44 46 49 51 60 61 62 64 65 67 68 71 72 73 74	23	10	164	4937	114	56491	724	30354	18088	541
LENOIR—Caldwell County										
★ CALDWELL MEMORIAL HOSPITAL, 321 Mulberry Street S.W., Zip 28645, Mailing Address: P.O. Box 1890, Zip 28645; tel. 704/757-5100; Frederick L. Soule, President and Chief Executive Officer (Total facility includes 10 beds in nursing home-type unit) **A**1 9 10 **F**7 8 10 12 15 17 19 21 22 30 31 32 34 35 37 40 44 49 54 64 65 67 71 73 **P**3 7 8	23	10	110	4852	68	56127	521	30893	14941	588
LEXINGTON—Davidson County										
★ LEXINGTON MEMORIAL HOSPITAL, Old Salisbury Road, Zip 27292, Mailing Address: Box 1817, Zip 27293-1817; tel. 704/246-5161; John H. Frank, President **A**1 9 10 **F**7 8 11 14 15 17 19 20 22 28 30 32 33 34 35 37 39 40 42 44 46 48 49 52 56 63 65 71 73 **P**3	23	10	86	4165	55	62087	713	24660	11771	415
LINCOLNTON—Lincoln County										
□ LINCOLN COUNTY HOSPITAL, Gamble Drive, Zip 28092-0677, Mailing Address: Box 677, Zip 28093-0677; tel. 704/735-3071; Peter W. Acker, Chief Executive Officer **A**1 9 10 **F**7 10 14 15 17 19 21 22 23 26 27 30 34 35 36 37 40 44 49 65 67 71 73	13	10	75	3278	43	31329	467	20871	9654	335
LOUISBURG—Franklin County										
□ FRANKLIN REGIONAL MEDICAL CENTER, 100 Hospital Drive, Zip 27549, Mailing Address: Box 609, Zip 27549; tel. 919/496-5131; Mike H. McNair, Administrator (Nonreporting) **A**1 9 10 **S**1775 Health Management Associates	33	10	85	—	—	—	—	—	—	—
LUMBERTON—Robeson County										
★ SOUTHEASTERN REGIONAL MEDICAL CENTER, 300 West 27th Street, Zip 28358, Mailing Address: Box 1408, Zip 28359-1408; tel. 910/671-5000; Donald C. Hiscott, President and Chief Executive Officer **A**1 9 10 **F**1 2 3 7 8 10 14 15 16 17 19 20 21 22 23 24 28 29 30 31 32 33 34 35 37 38 39 40 41 42 44 45 46 49 51 52 53 56 57 65 66 67 71 73	23	10	281	11114	205	196443	1305	69650	32852	1484
MARION—McDowell County										
★ MCDOWELL HOSPITAL, 100 Rankin Drive, Zip 28752, Mailing Address: P.O. Box 730, Zip 28752; tel. 704/659-5000; Jeffrey M. Judd, President and Chief Executive Officer **A**1 9 10 **F**7 8 14 17 19 21 22 23 24 30 37 40 42 44 45 46 49 63 65 67 71 73 74	23	10	65	2468	35	36617	296	15922	6945	270
MCCAIN—Hoke County										
MCCAIN CORRECTIONAL HOSPITAL, Mailing Address: P.O. Box 5118, Zip 28361-5118; tel. 910/944-2351; F. D. Hubbard, Superintendent (Nonreporting)	12	11	81	—	—	—	—	—	—	—
MOCKSVILLE—Davie County										
★ DAVIE COUNTY HOSPITAL, 223 Hospital Street, Zip 27028, Mailing Address: Box 908, Zip 27028; tel. 704/634-8100; Mike Kimel, Administrator **A**1 9 10 **F**8 15 16 19 28 32 35 37 41 44 45 48 49 65 70 71 73 **P**1 6 7 8	23	10	46	1405	24	15209	0	10107	5571	135

Hospitals, U.S. / NORTH CAROLINA

Hospital, Address, Telephone, Administrator, Approval, Facility, and Physician Codes, Health Care System	Classification Codes		Utilization Data					Expense (thousands) of dollars		
★ American Hospital Association (AHA) membership ☐ Joint Commission on Accreditation of Healthcare Organizations (JCAHO) accreditation + American Osteopathic Hospital Association (AOHA) membership ○ American Osteopathic Association (AOA) accreditation △ Commission on Accreditation of Rehabilitation Facilities (CARF) accreditation Control codes 61, 63, 64, 71, 72 and 73 indicate hospitals listed by AOHA, but not registered by AHA. For definition of numerical codes, see page A6	Control	Service	Beds	Admissions	Census	Outpatient Visits	Births	Total	Payroll	Personnel
MONROE—Union County ★ UNION MEMORIAL HOSPITAL, 600 Hospital Drive, Zip 28110–0510, Mailing Address: P.O. Box 5003, Zip 28111; tel. 704/283–3100; J. Larry Bishop, President and Chief Executive Officer (Total facility includes 66 beds in nursing home–type unit) **A**1 9 10 **F**2 3 7 8 10 11 19 21 22 23 25 26 30 32 34 35 37 40 44 45 46 49 64 65 71 73 **P**6	23	10	185	5281	134	54927	937	33792	15166	599
MOORESVILLE—Iredell County ☐ LAKE NORMAN REGIONAL MEDICAL CENTER, 610 East Center Avenue, Zip 28115, Mailing Address: Box 360, Zip 28115; tel. 704/663–1113; David L. Miller, Executive Director **A**1 9 10 **F**7 8 10 14 15 16 17 19 22 23 25 26 27 30 35 37 40 42 44 46 49 65 67 71 73 74 **P**8 **S**1775 Health Management Associates	33	10	100	3477	42	28010	223	—	—	251
MOREHEAD CITY—Carteret County ★ CARTERET GENERAL HOSPITAL, 3500 Arendell Street, Zip 28557–1619, Mailing Address: P.O. Box 1619, Zip 28557; tel. 919/247–1616; F. A. Odell III FACHE, President (Total facility includes 108 beds in nursing home–type unit) **A**1 9 10 **F**7 8 11 15 16 17 19 21 22 23 25 28 30 39 40 41 42 44 45 46 49 53 54 56 63 64 65 67 71 72 73 **P**4	13	10	225	5470	176	55688	499	35005	16121	619
MORGANTON—Burke County ☐ BROUGHTON HOSPITAL, 1000 South Sterling Street, Zip 28655–3999; tel. 704/433–2111; Millard F. Hall Jr., Director **A**1 9 10 **F**19 20 21 26 35 46 52 53 57 60 64 65 71 73 **P**6	12	22	725	4137	604	0	0	55685	37375	1418
★ GRACE HOSPITAL, 2201 South Sterling Street, Zip 28655–4058; tel. 704/438–2000; V. Otis Wilson Jr., President **A**1 9 10 **F**7 8 10 15 19 21 22 23 24 32 34 35 37 39 40 41 42 44 49 52 59 60 62 65 71 73 74 **P**7	23	10	149	6512	92	60764	809	38939	15194	658
MOUNT AIRY—Surry County ★ NORTHERN HOSPITAL OF SURRY COUNTY, 830 Rockford Street, Zip 27030, Mailing Address: Box 1101, Zip 27030–1101; tel. 910/719–7000; Charles K. Van Sluyter, President and Chief Executive Officer (Total facility includes 13 beds in nursing home–type unit) **A**1 9 10 **F**7 8 11 12 15 17 19 20 22 28 29 30 32 33 34 35 37 40 41 42 44 45 52 56 59 64 65 70 71 73 **S**0002 Quorum Health Group/Quorum Health Resources	16	10	129	4176	64	70050	559	29706	15196	568
MURPHY—Cherokee County ★ MURPHY MEDICAL CENTER, 2002 U.S. Highway 64 East, Zip 28906; tel. 704/837–8161; Mike Stevenson, Administrator (Total facility includes 120 beds in nursing home–type unit) **A**1 9 10 **F**7 8 15 19 21 22 24 27 28 37 41 44 49 63 64 65 71 73	23	10	170	1798	136	13271	170	13835	6629	250
NEW BERN—Craven County ★ CRAVEN REGIONAL MEDICAL AUTHORITY, 2000 Neuse Boulevard, Zip 28560, Mailing Address: Box 12157, Zip 28561; tel. 919/633–8111; Gary L. White, President and Chief Executive Officer **A**1 2 9 10 **F**4 7 8 10 11 12 14 19 21 22 23 27 28 29 30 31 32 34 35 37 39 40 41 42 43 44 45 48 49 52 54 55 56 57 58 59 60 63 65 66 71 73 74	16	10	276	10246	183	84365	1183	75517	30139	1169
NORTH WILKESBORO—Wilkes County ★ WILKES REGIONAL MEDICAL CENTER, 1370 West D Street, Zip 28659, Mailing Address: Box 609, Zip 28659–0609; tel. 910/651–8100; David L. Henson, Chief Executive Officer (Nonreporting) **A**1 9 10	15	10	137	—	—	—	—	—	—	—
OXFORD—Granville County ★ GRANVILLE MEDICAL CENTER, 1010 College Street, Zip 27565–2507, Mailing Address: Box 947, Zip 27565–0947; tel. 919/690–3000; Andrew Mannich, Administrator (Nonreporting) **A**1 9 10 **S**0002 Quorum Health Group/Quorum Health Resources	13	10	146	—	—	—	—	—	—	—
PINEHURST—Moore County ★ MOORE REGIONAL HOSPITAL, Page Road, Zip 28374, Mailing Address: P.O. Box 3000, Zip 28374–3000; tel. 910/215–1000; Charles T. Frock, President and Chief Executive Officer **A**1 9 10 **F**2 3 4 7 8 10 11 12 15 16 17 19 20 21 22 23 24 26 27 29 31 34 35 37 40 41 42 43 44 46 48 49 52 53 54 55 56 57 58 59 60 63 65 66 67 71 73 **P**7	23	10	326	13392	251	84627	1242	93573	44681	1441
PINEVILLE—Mecklenburg County ☐ CPC CEDAR SPRING HOSPITAL, 9600 Pineville–Matthews Road, Zip 28134–7548; tel. 704/541–6676; David G. Blackburn, Chief Executive Officer (Nonreporting) **A**1 9 10 **S**0785 Community Psychiatric Centers	33	22	70	—	—	—	—	—	—	—
PLYMOUTH—Washington County ★ WASHINGTON COUNTY HOSPITAL, 1 Medical Plaza, Zip 27962; tel. 919/793–4135; Jack Floyd, Interim Administrator **A**9 10 **F**14 15 16 19 21 22 42 44 49 51 65 71 **S**0002 Quorum Health Group/Quorum Health Resources	13	10	49	726	16	13796	0	5301	2394	121
RALEIGH—Wake County CENTRAL PRISON HOSPITAL, 1300 Western Boulevard, Zip 27606–2148; tel. 919/733–0800; Carl V. Strayhorn Jr., Administrator **F**19 20 22 27 31 34 35 59 71 **P**6	12	11	86	2023	49	35400	0	—	—	95
☐ DOROTHEA DIX HOSPITAL, 820 South Boylan Avenue, Zip 27603–2176; tel. 919/733–5324; Walter Stelle Ph.D., Director **A**1 3 5 9 10 **F**4 8 9 10 11 14 15 16 19 20 21 26 27 28 30 31 35 37 39 41 42 45 46 48 52 53 54 55 57 58 60 63 65 71 73	12	22	460	3815	462	0	0	165522	38537	1282
★ HOLLY HILL MENTAL HEALTH SERVICES, (Formerly Holly Hill Hospital) 3019 Falstaff Road, Zip 27610; tel. 919/250–7000; Grayce M. Crockett, Chief Executive Officer **A**1 9 10 **F**1 2 3 14 16 19 21 35 52 54 56 57 58 59 65 73 **P**1 2 7 8 **S**0048 Columbia/HCA Healthcare Corporation	33	22	70	1569	47	2962	0	—	—	103

© 1995 AHA Guide

Hospitals, U.S. / NORTH CAROLINA

Hospital, Address, Telephone, Administrator, Approval, Facility, and Physician Codes, Health Care System	Classification Codes		Utilization Data					Expense (thousands) of dollars		
	Control	Service	Beds	Admissions	Census	Outpatient Visits	Births	Total	Payroll	Personnel

★ American Hospital Association (AHA) membership
☐ Joint Commission on Accreditation of Healthcare Organizations (JCAHO) accreditation
+ American Osteopathic Hospital Association (AOHA) membership
○ American Osteopathic Association (AOA) accreditation
△ Commission on Accreditation of Rehabilitation Facilities (CARF) accreditation
Control codes 61, 63, 64, 71, 72 and 73 indicate hospitals listed by AOHA, but not registered by AHA. For definition of numerical codes, see page A6

Hospital	Control	Service	Beds	Admissions	Census	Outpatient Visits	Births	Total	Payroll	Personnel
★ RALEIGH COMMUNITY HOSPITAL, 3400 Wake Forest Road, Zip 27609-7373, Mailing Address: P.O. Box 28280, Zip 27611; tel. 919/954-3000; G. Michael Girone, Chief Executive Officer **A**1 9 10 **F**7 8 12 14 15 19 21 22 23 24 28 30 31 32 34 35 37 39 40 41 42 44 45 49 52 55 59 65 66 71 73 **S**0048 Columbia/HCA Healthcare Corporation	33	10	162	6378	92	55724	719	—	—	650
★ REX HOSPITAL, 4420 Lake Boone Trail, Zip 27607-6599; tel. 919/783-3100; James W. Albright, President and Chief Executive Officer (Total facility includes 140 beds in nursing home-type unit) **A**1 2 9 10 **F**4 6 7 8 10 11 12 14 16 17 19 21 22 23 24 28 30 31 32 33 35 37 38 39 40 41 42 43 44 46 49 54 60 63 64 65 66 67 70 71 73 **P**5 6	23	10	534	22540	415	255380	4557	152405	73115	2125
WAKE COUNTY ALCOHOLISM TREATMENT CENTER, 3000 Falstaff Road, Zip 27610-1897; tel. 919/250-1500; Roy Nickell, Director Acute Services **A**9 10 **F**2 3 12 16 27 54 56 58 59 65 67 **P**5	13	82	34	901	28	8995	0	5182	2808	131
★ WAKE MEDICAL CENTER, (Includes Eastern Wake Hospital, 320 Hospital Road, Zebulon, North Carolina, Zip 27597; tel. 919/269-7406; William J. Mountford Jr., Director; Northern Wake Hospital, Allen Road, Wake Forest, North Carolina, Zip 27587, Mailing Address: P.O. Box 152, Zip 27587; tel. 919/556-5151; Diane Long, Administrator; Southern Wake Hospital, 400 West Ranson Street, Fuquay-Varina, North Carolina, Zip 27526; tel. 919/552-2206; William J. Mountford Jr., Director; Western Wake Hospital, 763 Hunter Street, Apex, North Carolina, Zip 27502; tel. 919/362-8321; Diane Long R.N., Director) 3000 New Bern Avenue, Zip 27610; tel. 919/250-8000; Raymond L. Champ, President (Total facility includes 24 beds in nursing home-type unit) **A**1 3 5 9 10 **F**4 5 7 8 10 11 13 15 16 17 19 21 22 23 24 25 28 30 31 34 35 37 38 40 41 42 43 44 45 46 47 48 49 51 63 64 65 66 67 70 71 73 74 **P**3	13	10	671	28132	529	214231	3387	232721	104245	3086
REIDSVILLE—Rockingham County										
★ ANNIE PENN HOSPITAL, 618 South Main Street, Zip 27320-5094; tel. 910/634-1010; Susan H. Fitzgibbon, President and Chief Executive Officer (Total facility includes 42 beds in nursing home-type unit) **A**1 9 10 **F**5 7 8 13 14 15 16 19 20 21 22 23 26 28 29 30 31 32 33 34 35 37 40 41 42 44 45 46 49 54 56 59 64 65 67 68 71 73 74	23	10	152	3837	103	58286	362	28471	11357	438
ROANOKE RAPIDS—Halifax County										
★ HALIFAX MEMORIAL HOSPITAL, 250 Smith Church Road, Zip 27870, Mailing Address: P.O. Box 1089, Zip 27870-1089; tel. 919/535-8011; M. E. Gilstrap, President and Chief Executive Officer **A**1 9 10 **F**7 8 11 12 14 19 21 22 23 28 30 32 34 35 36 40 44 45 46 49 51 52 53 55 56 57 58 60 63 65 67 71 73 74	23	10	172	7061	134	69379	924	42528	18106	722
ROCKINGHAM—Richmond County										
★ RICHMOND MEMORIAL HOSPITAL, 925 Long Drive, Zip 28379-1928, Mailing Address: Box 1928, Zip 28379-1928; tel. 910/417-3000; David G. Hohl, Chief Executive Officer (Total facility includes 45 beds in nursing home-type unit) **A**1 9 10 **F**7 8 10 12 14 15 17 19 22 23 28 30 32 33 35 37 39 40 41 42 44 46 51 64 65 67 71	23	10	129	3769	87	34742	563	24281	11008	444
ROCKY MOUNT—Nash County										
☐ COMMUNITY HOSPITAL OF ROCKY MOUNT, 1031 Noell Lane, Zip 27804; tel. 919/937-5100; Roger L. Hall, Administrator (Nonreporting) **A**1 9 10 **S**0875 Community Health Systems, Inc.	33	10	50	—	—	—	—	—	—	—
★ NASH GENERAL HOSPITAL, 2460 Curtis Ellis Drive, Zip 27804-2297; tel. 919/443-8000; Bryant T. Aldridge, President and Chief Executive Officer **A**1 9 10 **F**3 4 7 8 10 11 17 18 19 21 22 23 25 30 33 34 35 37 40 41 42 44 45 46 49 52 53 54 55 56 57 58 60 63 65 66 67 71 73 74 **P**7	13	10	330	9347	157	42061	1411	64127	30998	1270
ROXBORO—Person County										
★ PERSON COUNTY MEMORIAL HOSPITAL, 615 Ridge Road, Zip 27573-4630; tel. 910/599-2121; H. James Graham, Administrator (Total facility includes 43 beds in nursing home-type unit) **A**1 9 10 **F**3 8 12 16 19 20 22 28 30 34 35 37 41 42 44 49 54 56 58 59 64 71 73 **S**0002 Quorum Health Group/Quorum Health Resources	23	10	85	1384	57	27820	0	9986	4525	218
RUTHERFORDTON—Rutherford County										
★ RUTHERFORD HOSPITAL, 308 South Ridgecrest Avenue, Zip 28139-3097; tel. 704/286-5000; Larry H. Chewning III, President (Total facility includes 150 beds in nursing home-type unit) **A**1 9 10 **F**1 7 8 10 14 16 19 21 22 23 28 30 32 34 35 37 44 46 49 52 54 56 59 64 65 67 71 73 74 **S**0002 Quorum Health Group/Quorum Health Resources	23	10	260	4511	214	57707	774	30378	13440	485
SALISBURY—Rowan County										
★ ROWAN MEMORIAL HOSPITAL, 612 Mocksville Avenue, Zip 28144-2799; tel. 704/638-1000; James M. Freeman, Chief Executive Officer **A**1 9 10 **F**2 3 7 8 10 11 14 16 19 21 22 23 26 30 31 34 35 37 39 40 42 43 44 45 46 49 52 53 54 56 57 58 63 65 67 69 71 73 74	23	10	223	9535	139	55600	952	52887	26099	901
★ VETERANS AFFAIRS MEDICAL CENTER, 1601 Brenner Avenue, Zip 28144; tel. 704/638-9000; R. Eugene Konik, Director (Total facility includes 93 beds in nursing home-type unit) **A**1 9 **F**2 3 4 10 12 14 15 17 18 19 20 21 22 23 24 25 26 28 30 31 32 33 34 35 37 39 41 42 44 45 46 49 51 52 54 56 57 58 60 61 63 64 65 67 70 71 73 74 **S**9295 Department of Veterans Affairs	45	22	695	3457	523	94230	0	90638	48766	1528
SANFORD—Lee County										
★ CENTRAL CAROLINA HOSPITAL, (Formerly AMI Central Carolina Hospital) 1135 Carthage Street, Zip 27330; tel. 919/774-2100; James E. Lathren, Executive Director **A**1 9 10 **F**7 8 10 12 19 21 22 23 31 32 33 34 35 36 37 39 40 41 42 44 46 52 65 71 73 **P**8 **S**0063 TENET Healthcare Corporation	33	10	137	5599	72	41892	876	24725	10882	469

Hospitals, U.S. / NORTH CAROLINA

Hospital, Address, Telephone, Administrator, Approval, Facility, and Physician Codes, Health Care System	Classification Codes		Utilization Data					Expense (thousands) of dollars		
★ American Hospital Association (AHA) membership □ Joint Commission on Accreditation of Healthcare Organizations (JCAHO) accreditation + American Osteopathic Hospital Association (AOHA) membership ○ American Osteopathic Association (AOA) accreditation △ Commission on Accreditation of Rehabilitation Facilities (CARF) accreditation Control codes 61, 63, 64, 71, 72 and 73 indicate hospitals listed by AOHA, but not registered by AHA. For definition of numerical codes, see page A6	Control	Service	Beds	Admissions	Census	Outpatient Visits	Births	Total	Payroll	Personnel
SCOTLAND NECK—Halifax County OUR COMMUNITY HOSPITAL, 921 Junior High Road, Zip 27874–0405, Mailing Address: Box 405, Zip 27874–0405; tel. 919/826–4144; T. K. Majure, Administrator (Total facility includes 80 beds in nursing home–type unit) **A**9 10 **F**14 15 16 22 26 36 51 64 65 71 73	23	10	100	154	57	1904	0	—	—	83
SEYMOUR JOHNSON AIR FORCE BASE—Wayne County ★ U.S. AIR FORCE HOSPITAL SEYMOUR JOHNSON, 1050 Curtiss Avenue, Zip 27531–5300; tel. 919/736–5201; Colonel David G. Young USAF, MC, Commander (Nonreporting) **A**1 5 9 **S**9495 Department of the Air Force	41	10	15	—	—	—	—	—	—	—
SHELBY—Cleveland County ★ CLEVELAND MEMORIAL HOSPITAL, 201 Grover Street, Zip 28150; tel. 704/487–3000; Austin Letson, President (Total facility includes 120 beds in nursing home–type unit) **A**1 2 9 10 **F**7 8 10 11 12 13 17 19 20 21 22 23 25 26 28 29 30 31 32 33 34 35 37 38 39 40 42 44 45 46 47 48 49 51 54 56 60 64 65 67 69 70 71 73	13	10	285	6995	218	67968	1250	50875	21687	831
SILER CITY—Chatham County ★ CHATHAM HOSPITAL, West Third Street & Ivy Avenue, Zip 27344–2343, Mailing Address: P.O. Box 649, Zip 27344; tel. 919/663–2113; Ted G. Chapin, Chief Executive Officer **A**1 5 9 10 **F**8 15 19 22 28 35 39 44 49 65 71 73 **S**0002 Quorum Health Group/Quorum Health Resources	23	10	42	1016	18	11953	0	6458	2910	137
SMITHFIELD—Johnston County ★ JOHNSTON MEMORIAL HOSPITAL, 509 North Bright Leaf Boulevard, Zip 27577–1376, Mailing Address: P.O. Box 1376, Zip 27577–1376; tel. 919/934–8171; Leland E. Farnell, President **A**1 9 10 **F**7 8 10 14 15 16 19 20 21 22 23 25 27 28 30 31 32 33 35 36 37 40 42 44 51 52 54 56 57 65 68 69 71 73 **S**0002 Quorum Health Group/Quorum Health Resources	13	10	127	4720	71	64113	587	29523	14038	566
SOUTHPORT—Brunswick County ★ J. ARTHUR DOSHER MEMORIAL HOSPITAL, 924 Howe Street, Zip 28461; tel. 910/457–5271; Edgar Haywood III, Administrator **A**9 10 **F**8 15 17 19 22 26 28 30 33 34 35 39 41 44 48 49 51 65 67 71 73	16	10	40	1314	16	25095	0	8580	3482	143
SPARTA—Alleghany County ★ ALLEGHANY MEMORIAL HOSPITAL, 617 Doctor's Street, Zip 28675–0009, Mailing Address: P.O. Box 9, Zip 28675–0009; tel. 910/372–5511; James Yarborough, Chief Executive Officer **A**1 9 10 **F**7 8 14 15 19 21 32 34 35 44 46 49 51 63 65 71 73 **S**0002 Quorum Health Group/Quorum Health Resources	23	10	46	1359	26	13763	37	5666	2934	150
SPRUCE PINE—Mitchell County □ SPRUCE PINE COMMUNITY HOSPITAL, 125 Hospital Drive, Zip 28777, Mailing Address: P.O. Drawer 9, Zip 28777; tel. 704/765–4201; Charles H. Aldridge, Administrator and President **A**1 9 10 **F**7 8 11 14 15 19 21 22 28 31 33 34 39 41 42 44 65 71 73 74 **P**3	23	10	42	1804	21	29920	178	9146	4397	183
STATESVILLE—Iredell County ★ DAVIS COMMUNITY HOSPITAL, Old Mocksville Road, Zip 28677, Mailing Address: P.O. Box 1800, Zip 28677; tel. 704/873–0281; Stephen J. Aragon, Chief Executive Officer (Nonreporting) **A**1 9 10 **S**0048 Columbia/HCA Healthcare Corporation	33	10	149	—	—	—	—	—	—	—
★ IREDELL MEMORIAL HOSPITAL, 557 Brookdale Drive, Zip 28677–1828, Mailing Address: P.O. Box 1828, Zip 28687–1828; tel. 704/873–5661; S. Arnold Nunnery, President and Chief Executive Officer (Total facility includes 18 beds in nursing home–type unit) **A**1 2 9 10 **F**7 8 10 11 14 15 16 17 19 21 22 28 29 30 32 33 35 37 40 41 42 44 45 46 49 51 53 54 55 56 57 58 60 63 64 65 67 71 73 74	23	10	201	7525	144	76800	844	58522	28317	947
SUPPLY—Brunswick County ★ BRUNSWICK HOSPITAL, 1 Medical Center Drive, Zip 28462, Mailing Address: P.O. Box 139, Zip 28462; tel. 910/754–8121; C. Mark Gregson, Chief Executive Officer **A**1 9 10 **F**7 8 14 15 16 17 19 20 22 25 28 30 32 33 34 35 37 40 44 46 52 53 58 59 65 71 73 **P**8 **S**0048 Columbia/HCA Healthcare Corporation	33	10	60	1837	24	19038	204	10392	4417	194
SYLVA—Jackson County ★ HARRIS REGIONAL HOSPITAL, (Formerly C. J. Harris Community Hospital) 59 Hospital Road, Zip 28779–2795; tel. 704/586–7000; Isaac S. Coe, President (Total facility includes 60 beds in nursing home–type unit) **A**1 9 10 **F**7 8 15 16 17 19 21 22 23 28 32 33 34 35 37 39 40 41 42 44 45 46 49 54 60 63 64 65 67 71 73 74	23	10	146	4142	111	82524	834	29136	13464	476
TARBORO—Edgecombe County ★ HERITAGE HOSPITAL, 111 Hospital Drive, Zip 27886; tel. 919/641–7700; James Raynor, Chief Executive Officer (Total facility includes 10 beds in nursing home–type unit) **A**1 9 10 **F**7 8 10 12 19 21 22 23 34 37 40 44 46 48 49 63 64 71 73 **P**8 **S**0048 Columbia/HCA Healthcare Corporation	33	10	127	3694	56	22311	805	19585	7623	212
TAYLORSVILLE—Alexander County ★ ALEXANDER COMMUNITY HOSPITAL, 326 Third Street S.W., Zip 28681–3096; tel. 704/632–4282; Robert D. Jones, Administrator **A**1 9 10 **F**8 10 17 19 22 30 34 37 44 46 49 51 65 71 73 **P**6 **S**0002 Quorum Health Group/Quorum Health Resources	23	10	36	1218	25	10756	0	6685	2641	130
THOMASVILLE—Davidson County ★ COMMUNITY GENERAL HOSPITAL OF THOMASVILLE, 207 Old Lexington Road, Zip 27360, Mailing Address: Box 789, Zip 27361; tel. 910/476–2526; Perry T. Jones, President (Total facility includes 15 beds in nursing home–type unit) **A**1 9 10 **F**7 8 10 11 14 15 16 19 21 22 28 31 34 36 37 39 40 42 44 45 46 52 56 57 63 64 65 67 68 71 73 74	23	10	123	4396	73	92385	572	22297	11495	451

Hospitals, U.S. / NORTH CAROLINA

Hospital, Address, Telephone, Administrator, Approval, Facility, and Physician Codes, Health Care System	Classification Codes		Utilization Data					Expense (thousands) of dollars		
★ American Hospital Association (AHA) membership □ Joint Commission on Accreditation of Healthcare Organizations (JCAHO) accreditation + American Osteopathic Hospital Association (AOHA) membership ○ American Osteopathic Association (AOA) accreditation △ Commission on Accreditation of Rehabilitation Facilities (CARF) accreditation Control codes 61, 63, 64, 71, 72 and 73 indicate hospitals listed by AOHA, but not registered by AHA. For definition of numerical codes, see page A6	Control	Service	Beds	Admissions	Census	Outpatient Visits	Births	Total	Payroll	Personnel
TROY—Caswell County □ MONTGOMERY MEMORIAL HOSPITAL, 520 Allen Street, Zip 27371, Mailing Address: Box 486, Zip 27371–0486; tel. 910/572–1301; Kerry A. Anderson R.N., Administrator (Total facility includes 51 beds in nursing home–type unit) **A**1 9 10 **F**15 19 22 40 44 64 71 73	23	10	83	1390	55	16756	192	7698	3955	150
VALDESE—Burke County ★ VALDESE GENERAL HOSPITAL, Mailing Address: Box 700, Zip 28690–0700; tel. 704/874–2251; Lloyd E. Wallace, President and Chief Executive Officer **A**1 2 9 10 **F**7 8 10 11 14 15 16 17 19 21 22 23 26 28 30 32 34 35 37 40 41 42 44 45 46 48 49 60 62 63 64 65 70 71 73 **P**8	23	10	79	2948	41	25069	358	23571	10810	418
WADESBORO—Anson County ★ ANSON COUNTY HOSPITAL AND SKILLED NURSING FACILITY, 500 Morven Road, Zip 28170; tel. 704/694–5131; Frederick G. Thompson, Administrator and Chief Executive Officer (Total facility includes 95 beds in nursing home–type unit) **A**1 9 10 **F**8 12 14 17 19 21 22 26 27 29 30 32 33 34 42 44 46 49 63 64 65 67 71	13	10	125	1387	111	19591	0	12399	4863	231
WASHINGTON—Beaufort County ★ BEAUFORT COUNTY HOSPITAL, 628 East 12th Street, Zip 27889–3498; tel. 919/975–4100; Kenneth E. Ragland, Administrator **A**1 9 10 **F**3 4 7 8 10 11 12 14 15 16 18 19 20 21 22 24 27 28 29 30 32 33 34 35 36 39 41 42 43 44 45 46 49 51 53 54 55 56 57 58 59 60 62 65 66 67 68 69 70 71 72 73 74 **P**3 5	23	10	98	3173	46	39068	287	20157	10081	406
WHITEVILLE—Columbus County ★ COLUMBUS COUNTY HOSPITAL, 500 Jefferson Street, Zip 28472–9987; tel. 910/642–8011; William S. Clark, Chief Executive Officer **A**9 10 **F**7 10 11 12 14 15 16 17 19 22 23 28 30 34 35 36 37 39 40 44 45 48 49 51 65 66 71 73 **S**0002 Quorum Health Group/Quorum Health Resources	23	10	136	5643	82	46400	553	29055	13019	504
WILLIAMSTON—Martin County ★ MARTIN GENERAL HOSPITAL, 310 South McCaskey Road, Zip 27892, Mailing Address: P.O. Box 1128, Zip 27892; tel. 919/792–2186; George H. Brandt Jr., Administrator **A**1 3 9 10 **F**7 8 15 19 20 22 35 37 40 44 54 65 67 71	13	10	49	1664	22	23600	177	10289	4868	220
WILMINGTON—New Hanover County ★ CAPE FEAR MEMORIAL HOSPITAL, 5301 Wrightsville Avenue, Zip 28403, Mailing Address: P.O. Box 4549, Zip 28406–6599; tel. 910/452–8100; Joseph L. Soto, President **A**1 9 10 **F**7 8 14 15 16 17 19 21 22 26 28 30 34 35 37 39 40 41 44 45 46 49 66 71 73 74 **P**3 5 6	23	10	83	4079	63	80031	403	41522	17552	579
★ NEW HANOVER REGIONAL MEDICAL CENTER, 2131 South 17th Street, Zip 28401, Mailing Address: Box 9000, Zip 28402–9000; tel. 910/343–7000; Jim R. Hobbs, President and Chief Executive Officer **A**1 3 5 9 10 **F**4 8 10 11 12 15 17 19 22 25 26 28 30 32 35 37 38 39 40 42 43 44 45 46 49 52 53 54 55 60 65 67 70 71 73 74	13	10	568	21160	373	—	2620	160683	—	2346
WILSON—Wilson County ★ WILSON MEMORIAL HOSPITAL, 1705 South Tarboro Street, Zip 27893–3428; tel. 919/399–8040; Christopher T. Durrer, President and Chief Executive Officer **A**1 9 10 **F**3 7 8 10 14 15 16 19 20 22 23 28 29 30 32 34 35 36 37 39 40 42 44 45 46 49 52 53 54 55 56 57 58 59 65 67 71 73	23	10	317	7985	142	106487	1081	57895	22772	765
WINDSOR—Bertie County ★ BERTIE COUNTY MEMORIAL HOSPITAL, 401 Sterlingworth Street, Zip 27983–1726, Mailing Address: P.O. Box 40, Zip 27983–1726; tel. 919/794–3141; Anthony F. Mullen, Administrator **A**9 10 **F**8 15 19 22 32 33 34 44 71 **S**0585 Brim, Inc.	23	10	49	654	34	12269	0	3771	1950	90
WINSTON-SALEM—Forsyth County AMOS COTTAGE REHABILITATION HOSPITAL, 3325 Silas Creek Parkway, Zip 27103; tel. 910/765–9916; Douglas M. Cody, Administrator **A**9 10 **F**12 17 34 41 46 48 49 65 67	23	56	41	96	27	1593	0	3432	2287	127
□ CHARTER HOSPITAL OF WINSTON–SALEM, 3637 Old Vineyard Road, Zip 27104; tel. 910/768–7710; Marina Cecchini, Chief Executive Officer (Nonreporting) **A**1 9 10 **S**0695 Charter Medical Corporation	33	22	99							
★ △ FORSYTH MEMORIAL HOSPITAL, 3333 Silas Creek Parkway, Zip 27103–3090; tel. 910/718–5000; Paul M. Wiles, President **A**1 2 3 5 7 9 10 **F**3 4 7 8 10 11 12 14 15 16 17 19 20 21 22 23 24 26 28 29 30 31 32 33 34 35 37 38 39 40 41 42 43 44 45 46 48 49 51 52 56 57 58 59 60 61 63 65 66 67 71 73 74 **P**1 6	23	10	747	30583	600	90104	5622	202375	96784	3094
★ MEDICAL PARK HOSPITAL, 1950 South Hawthorne Road, Zip 27103–3993, Mailing Address: P.O. Box 24728, Zip 27114–4728; tel. 910/768–7680; Eduard R. Koehler, Administrator **A**1 2 9 10 **F**3 4 7 8 10 11 12 14 15 16 19 20 21 22 24 26 27 28 29 30 31 32 33 34 35 37 38 39 40 41 43 44 45 46 49 51 54 55 56 57 58 59 60 63 65 66 67 71 73 74 **P**6	23	10	101	2794	29	13595	0	25099	10365	302
★ △ NORTH CAROLINA BAPTIST HOSPITAL, Medical Center Boulevard, Zip 27157; tel. 910/716–2011; Len B. Preslar Jr., President and Chief Executive Officer (Total facility includes 170 beds in nursing home–type unit) **A**1 2 3 5 7 8 9 10 **F**2 3 4 7 8 9 10 11 12 13 15 16 17 19 20 21 22 23 26 28 29 30 31 32 34 35 37 38 40 41 42 43 44 45 46 47 48 49 50 51 52 53 54 55 56 57 58 59 60 61 63 64 65 66 67 69 70 71 73 **P**1 3 4 7	23	10	756	25719	560	93282	1	324171	152759	5132
YADKINVILLE—Yadkin County ★ HOOTS MEMORIAL HOSPITAL, 624 West Main Street, Zip 27055, Mailing Address: P.O. Box 68, Zip 27055; tel. 910/679–2041; Lance C. Labine, President (Data for 181 days) **A**1 9 10 **F**7 8 15 16 19 22 28 30 32 33 34 35 37 44 49 51 54 63 65 66 71 73 **P**7	13	10	46	342	6	4336	3	2618	1110	102

Hospitals, U.S. / NORTH CAROLINA

Hospital, Address, Telephone, Administrator, Approval, Facility, and Physician Codes, Health Care System	Classification Codes		Utilization Data					Expense (thousands) of dollars		
★ American Hospital Association (AHA) membership □ Joint Commission on Accreditation of Healthcare Organizations (JCAHO) accreditation + American Osteopathic Hospital Association (AOHA) membership ○ American Osteopathic Association (AOA) accreditation △ Commission on Accreditation of Rehabilitation Facilities (CARF) accreditation Control codes 61, 63, 64, 71, 72 and 73 indicate hospitals listed by AOHA, but not registered by AHA. For definition of numerical codes, see page A6	Control	Service	Beds	Admissions	Census	Outpatient Visits	Births	Total	Payroll	Personnel

ZEBULON—Wake County
   EASTERN WAKE HOSPITAL See Wake Medical Center, Raleigh

Hospitals, U.S. / NORTH DAKOTA

NORTH DAKOTA

Resident population 635 (in thousands)
Resident population in metro areas 41.6%
Birth rate per 1,000 population 14.0
65 years and over 14.8%
Percent of persons without health insurance 7.4%

Hospital, Address, Telephone, Administrator, Approval, Facility, and Physician Codes, Health Care System	Classification Codes		Utilization Data					Expense (thousands) of dollars		
	Control	Service	Beds	Admissions	Census	Outpatient Visits	Births	Total	Payroll	Personnel

★ American Hospital Association (AHA) membership
☐ Joint Commission on Accreditation of Healthcare Organizations (JCAHO) accreditation
+ American Osteopathic Hospital Association (AOHA) membership
○ American Osteopathic Association (AOA) accreditation
△ Commission on Accreditation of Rehabilitation Facilities (CARF) accreditation
Control codes 61, 63, 64, 71, 72 and 73 indicate hospitals listed by AOHA, but not registered by AHA. For definition of numerical codes, see page A6

Hospital	Control	Service	Beds	Admissions	Census	Outpatient Visits	Births	Total	Payroll	Personnel
ASHLEY—McIntosh County										
★ ASHLEY MEDICAL CENTER, 612 North Center Avenue, Zip 58413–0556; tel. 701/288–3433; Stephen H. Johnson, Administrator (Total facility includes 44 beds in nursing home–type unit) **A**9 10 **F**7 8 11 14 15 16 19 22 24 27 30 31 32 33 34 37 39 40 44 45 46 64 65 71 73	23	10	70	237	51	1625	0	3172	1592	119
BELCOURT—Rolette County										
✠ U.S. PUBLIC HEALTH SERVICE INDIAN HOSPITAL, Mailing Address: P.O. Box 130, Zip 58316–0130; tel. 701/477–6111; Clarence Frederick, Director (Nonreporting) **A**1 5 10 **S**9195 U.S. Public Health Service Indian Health Service	47	10	42	—	—	—	—	—	—	—
BISMARCK—Burleigh County										
✠ △ MEDCENTER ONE, 300 North Seventh Street, Zip 58501–4439, Mailing Address: P.O. Box 5525, Zip 58501–5525; tel. 701/224–6000; Terrance G. Brosseau, President **A**1 2 3 5 7 9 10 **F**1 4 7 8 10 11 12 13 14 17 19 21 22 23 24 25 26 27 28 29 30 31 32 33 34 35 36 37 38 39 40 41 42 43 44 45 46 47 48 49 51 52 53 54 56 57 58 59 60 64 65 66 67 69 70 71 73 74 **P**1 3 6	23	10	204	6731	122	93974	595	91450	45140	1475
✠ △ ST. ALEXIUS MEDICAL CENTER, 900 East Broadway, Zip 58501, Mailing Address: P.O. Box 5510, Zip 58506–5510; tel. 701/224–7000; Richard A. Tschider FACHE, Administrator and Chief Executive Officer **A**1 2 3 5 7 9 10 **F**3 4 5 7 8 10 12 13 14 15 16 17 18 19 20 21 22 23 24 25 26 27 28 29 30 31 32 33 34 35 37 38 39 40 41 42 43 44 45 47 48 49 51 52 53 54 55 56 57 58 59 61 64 65 66 67 70 71 72 73 74 **P**1 7 **S**0545 Benedictine Sisters of the Annunciation	21	10	291	8781	157	80677	962	80935	35609	1189
BOTTINEAU—Bottineau County										
ST. ANDREW'S HEALTH CENTER, (Formerly St. Andrew's Medical Center) 316 Ohmer Street, Zip 58318–1018; tel. 701/228–2255; Keith Korman, President (Total facility includes 32 beds in nursing home–type unit) **A**5 9 10 **F**6 7 8 15 16 19 22 26 28 30 32 34 36 39 40 49 53 54 55 57 62 64 65 66 70 71 73 **P**3 **S**5805 Sisters of Mary of the Presentation Health Corporation	23	10	67	483	39	5000	21	3004	1471	82
BOWMAN—Bowman County										
★ ST. LUKE'S TRI–STATE HOSPITAL, 202 Sixth Avenue S.W., Zip 58623–0009, Mailing Address: Drawer C, Zip 58623; tel. 701/523–5265; Jim Opdahl, Administrator (Nonreporting) **A**5 9 10	23	10	36	—	—	—	—	—	—	—
CANDO—Towner County										
★ TOWNER COUNTY MEMORIAL HOSPITAL, Mailing Address: P.O. Box 688, Zip 58324–0688; tel. 701/968–4411; Timothy J. Tracy, Administrator (Total facility includes 10 beds in nursing home–type unit) **A**5 9 10 **F**6 8 13 14 17 19 22 26 28 30 31 32 34 35 40 42 44 45 46 51 64 65 71 74 **P**6	23	10	32	451	18	5102	25	2465	1180	55
CARRINGTON—Foster County										
★ CARRINGTON HEALTH CENTER, 800 North Fourth Street, Zip 58421; tel. 701/652–3141; Michael A. Baumgartner, President (Total facility includes 40 beds in nursing home–type unit) **A**5 9 10 **F**7 8 15 16 19 22 25 26 29 31 33 44 49 64 65 67 71 73 **P**4 **S**5175 Catholic Health Corporation	21	10	70	845	47	23579	50	8270	3098	95
CAVALIER—Pembina County										
★ PEMBINA COUNTY MEMORIAL HOSPITAL AND WEDGEWOOD MANOR, 205 East Third Avenue, Zip 58220, Mailing Address: Box M, Zip 58220; tel. 701/265–8461; Glen Gray, Chief Executive Officer (Total facility includes 60 beds in nursing home–type unit) **A**5 9 10 **F**6 7 8 11 12 13 15 16 17 19 20 21 22 25 27 28 30 32 33 34 36 37 39 40 41 44 46 48 49 64 65 67 71 73 **P**5 **S**2235 Lutheran Health Systems	23	10	89	837	71	9762	55	5263	2561	123
COOPERSTOWN—Griggs County										
GRIGGS COUNTY HOSPITAL AND NURSING HOME, 1200 Roberts Avenue, Zip 58425, Mailing Address: Box 728, Zip 58425; tel. 701/797–2221; Patrick J. Rafferty, Administrator (Total facility includes 58 beds in nursing home–type unit) **A**9 10 **F**7 8 14 15 16 17 19 20 22 24 26 28 30 32 34 36 39 42 46 49 56 58 64 65 67 70 71 73 **P**3 5	23	10	69	200	60	4804	10	2457	1379	83
CROSBY—Divide County										
ST. LUKE'S HOSPITAL, 702 First Street Southwest, Zip 58730–0010; tel. 701/965–6384; Leslie O. Urvand, Administrator **A**9 10 **F**8 11 14 19 22 28 29 34 36 40 44 46 49 71	23	10	29	305	12	1089	6	1470	722	38
DEVILS LAKE—Ramsey County										
✠ MERCY HOSPITAL, 1031 Seventh Street, Zip 58301–2798; tel. 701/662–2131; Marlene Krein, President and Chief Executive Officer **A**1 5 9 10 **F**7 11 14 15 16 17 19 21 22 28 29 30 31 32 33 35 39 40 42 44 45 46 49 65 67 68 71 73 **P**5 **S**5175 Catholic Health Corporation	21	10	55	1822	23	12577	291	10143	5165	178
DICKINSON—Stark County										
✠ ST. JOSEPH'S HOSPITAL AND HEALTH CENTER, 30 Seventh Street West, Zip 58601; tel. 701/225–7200; John S. Studsrud, President **A**1 5 9 10 **F**7 8 15 16 17 19 21 22 24 30 32 33 34 35 36 37 40 41 44 46 49 52 53 55 56 57 58 59 63 65 66 67 71 73 **P**3 **S**5175 Catholic Health Corporation	21	10	85	2717	35	25891	424	20593	9057	344

Hospitals, U.S. / NORTH DAKOTA

Hospital, Address, Telephone, Administrator, Approval, Facility, and Physician Codes, Health Care System	Classification Codes		Utilization Data				Expense (thousands) of dollars		
★ American Hospital Association (AHA) membership □ Joint Commission on Accreditation of Healthcare Organizations (JCAHO) accreditation + American Osteopathic Hospital Association (AOHA) membership ○ American Osteopathic Association (AOA) accreditation △ Commission on Accreditation of Rehabilitation Facilities (CARF) accreditation Control codes 61, 63, 64, 71, 72 and 73 indicate hospitals listed by AOHA, but not registered by AHA. For definition of numerical codes, see page A6	Control	Service	Beds	Admissions	Census	Outpatient Visits	Births	Total	Payroll	Personnel
ELGIN—Grant County										
JACOBSON MEMORIAL HOSPITAL CARE CENTER, 601 East Street North, Zip 58533–0376; tel. 701/584–2792; Jacqueline Seibel, Administrator (Nonreporting) **A**9 10	23	10	50	—	—	—	—	—	—	—
FARGO—Cass County										
★ △ DAKOTA HOSPITAL, 1720 South University Drive, Zip 58103, Mailing Address: P.O. Box 6014, Zip 58108–6014; tel. 701/280–4100; Peter W. Thoreen, President and Chief Executive Officer **A**1 2 3 5 7 9 10 **F**3 4 5 6 7 8 10 11 12 13 14 15 16 17 18 19 20 21 22 24 27 28 29 30 31 32 33 34 35 37 38 40 41 42 43 44 45 46 48 49 51 54 56 58 60 61 65 66 67 69 71 72 73 74 **P**8	23	10	160	6541	93	33261	672	57829	21118	788
□ HEARTLAND MEDICAL CENTER, 510 Fourth Street South, Zip 58103; tel. 701/232–3331; Peter W. Thoreen, President and Chief Executive Officer **A**1 2 5 9 10 **F**1 3 7 8 14 15 16 17 19 21 22 24 29 31 32 33 34 35 37 40 41 42 44 45 46 49 52 53 54 55 56 57 58 59 61 65 71 72 73 **P**8	33	10	113	4100	58	78884	631	30476	11888	377
★ △ MERITCARE MEDICAL CENTER, 720 Fourth Street North, Zip 58122; tel. 701/234–6000; Roger Gilbertson M.D., President (Nonreporting) **A**1 2 3 5 7 9 10	23	10	378	—	—	—	—	—	—	—
★ VETERANS AFFAIRS MEDICAL AND REGIONAL OFFICE CENTER, 2101 Elm Street, Zip 58102–2498; tel. 701/232–3241; Douglas M. Kenyon, Director (Total facility includes 50 beds in nursing home–type unit) **A**1 3 5 **F**2 3 8 15 16 17 19 20 21 27 28 30 31 32 33 34 35 37 39 41 42 44 45 46 48 49 51 52 56 58 60 64 65 67 71 73 74 **S**9295 Department of Veterans Affairs	45	10	163	3663	123	54280	0	41104	21065	522
FORT YATES—Sioux County										
★ U.S. PUBLIC HEALTH SERVICE INDIAN HOSPITAL, Mailing Address: P.O. Box J, Zip 58538; tel. 701/854–3831; Terry Pourier, Service Unit Director (Nonreporting) **A**1 5 10 **S**9195 U.S. Public Health Service Indian Health Service	47	10	16	—	—	—	—	—	—	—
GARRISON—Mclean County										
★ GARRISON MEMORIAL HOSPITAL, 407 Third Avenue S.E., Zip 58540–0039; tel. 701/463–2275; Richard Spilovoy, Administrator (Nonreporting) **A**5 9 10 **S**0545 Benedictine Sisters of the Annunciation	21	10	49	—	—	—	—	—	—	—
GRAFTON—Walsh County										
★ UNITY MEDICAL CENTER, 164 West 13th Street, Zip 58237; tel. 701/352–1620; Steve Feltman, Chief Executive Officer **A**1 5 9 10 **F**7 8 15 16 17 19 22 28 29 30 32 34 37 40 41 42 44 49 51 54 65 67 71 73 **P**6	23	10	27	608	9	35793	66	4827	2790	99
GRAND FORKS—Grand Forks County										
★ △ MEDICAL CENTER REHABILITATION HOSPITAL, (Formerly University of North Dakota–Medical Center Rehabilitation Hospital) 1300 South Columbia Road, Zip 58201, Mailing Address: P.O. Box 9017, Zip 58202; tel. 701/780–2311; Jack A. Carroll Ph.D., Executive Director **A**7 9 10 **F**12 13 14 15 16 24 27 48 49 65 66 67 73 **P**3	12	46	42	783	26	33345	0	11099	6282	226
★ UNITED HEALTH SERVICES, 1200 South Columbia Road, Zip 58201; tel. 701/780–5000; Rosemary Jacobson, President and Chief Executive Officer **A**1 2 3 5 9 10 **F**2 3 4 6 7 10 11 12 15 16 17 19 20 21 22 23 28 30 31 32 33 34 35 36 37 39 40 41 42 43 44 45 46 49 50 51 52 53 54 55 56 57 58 59 60 61 62 63 65 66 67 71 73 **P**2 7	23	10	287	11273	172	62723	1336	94893	43395	1310
UNIVERSITY OF NORTH DAKOTA–MEDICAL CENTER REHABILITATION HOSPITAL See Medical Center Rehabilitation Hospital										
GRAND FORKS AIR FORCE BASE—Grand Forks County										
★ U.S. AIR FORCE HOSPITAL, Grand Forks SAC, Zip 58205–6332; tel. 701/747–5391; Major Norman J. Latini MSC, USAF, Administrator (Nonreporting) **A**5 **S**9495 Department of the Air Force	41	10	15	—	—	—	—	—	—	—
HARVEY—Wells County										
★ ST. ALOISIUS MEDICAL CENTER, 325 East Brewster Street, Zip 58341–1605; tel. 701/324–4651; Ronald J. Volk, President (Total facility includes 116 beds in nursing home–type unit) **A**5 9 10 **F**7 8 19 22 27 28 30 32 35 37 40 42 44 49 53 58 62 64 65 67 71 73 **S**5805 Sisters of Mary of the Presentation Health Corporation	21	10	165	589	127	6882	31	5980	3075	123
HAZEN—Mercer County										
★ SAKAKAWEA MEDICAL CENTER, 510 Eighth Avenue N.E., Zip 58545–4637; tel. 701/748–2225; Dan Howell, Chief Executive Officer **A**5 9 10 **F**3 7 8 11 15 16 19 26 28 30 32 35 37 39 40 44 45 70 71 73 **P**3 6	23	10	32	875	12	7870	67	4552	2059	76
HETTINGER—Adams County										
□ WEST RIVER REGIONAL MEDICAL CENTER, Mailing Address: Rural Route 2, Box 124, Zip 58639–0124; tel. 701/567–4561; Jim K. Long CPA, Administrator and Chief Executive Officer **A**1 5 9 10 **F**7 8 12 13 15 18 19 20 21 22 25 27 30 32 34 35 37 39 40 41 42 44 46 49 51 58 63 65 66 67 70 71 73 74 **P**3	23	10	45	1595	21	56454	161	12102	4436	194
HILLSBORO—Traill County										
★ HILLSBORO COMMUNITY HOSPITAL, 12 Third Street S.E., Zip 58045, Mailing Address: P.O. Box 609, Zip 58045–0609; tel. 701/436–4501; Bruce D. Bowersox, Administrator (Nonreporting) **A**5 9 10	23	10	74	—	—	—	—	—	—	—
JAMESTOWN—Stutsman County										
★ JAMESTOWN HOSPITAL, 419 Fifth Street N.E., Zip 58401–3360; tel. 701/252–1050; Richard W. Hall, President **A**1 5 9 10 **F**7 8 15 16 19 21 22 30 31 32 34 35 37 39 40 41 44 45 46 56 61 63 65 67 71 73	23	10	56	2134	24	39760	330	11755	6071	201

Hospitals, U.S. / NORTH DAKOTA

Hospital, Address, Telephone, Administrator, Approval, Facility, and Physician Codes, Health Care System	Classification Codes		Utilization Data					Expense (thousands) of dollars		
★ American Hospital Association (AHA) membership ☐ Joint Commission on Accreditation of Healthcare Organizations (JCAHO) accreditation + American Osteopathic Hospital Association (AOHA) membership ○ American Osteopathic Association (AOA) accreditation △ Commission on Accreditation of Rehabilitation Facilities (CARF) accreditation Control codes 61, 63, 64, 71, 72 and 73 indicate hospitals listed by AOHA, but not registered by AHA. For definition of numerical codes, see page A6	Control	Service	Beds	Admissions	Census	Outpatient Visits	Births	Total	Payroll	Personnel
☒ NORTH DAKOTA STATE HOSPITAL, Mailing Address: Box 476, Zip 58402–0476; tel. 701/253–3650; Mary Anne Perleberg, Administrator **A**1 5 9 10 **F**2 20 28 29 30 41 45 46 48 52 53 54 55 56 57 59 65 67 73 **P**6	12	22	301	1610	225	0	0	23637	15067	569
KENMARE—Ward County KENMARE COMMUNITY HOSPITAL, (General Medical/Long Term Care) 317 First Avenue N.W., Zip 58746, Mailing Address: P.O. Box 337, Zip 58746–0337; tel. 701/385–4296; Doris Goettle R.N., President and Chief Executive Officer (Total facility includes 12 beds in nursing home–type unit) **A**9 10 **F**15 16 17 19 26 28 30 32 33 36 49 53 54 55 57 58 64 65 70 71 73 74 **P**5	21	49	42	37	1	658	1	1655	871	54
LANGDON—Cavalier County ★ CAVALIER COUNTY MEMORIAL HOSPITAL, 909 Second Street, Zip 58249; tel. 701/256–6180; Daryl J. Wilkens, Administrator **A**5 9 10 **F**8 11 17 19 22 28 29 30 32 34 37 40 41 44 49 71	23	10	28	479	7	7372	41	2280	1258	65
LINTON—Emmons County ★ LINTON HOSPITAL, 518 North Broadway, Zip 58552, Mailing Address: P.O. Box 850, Zip 58552; tel. 701/254–4511; Richard Albrecht, Administrator **A**5 9 10 **F**7 8 15 19 22 25 32 36 37 40 44 70 71 74	23	10	25	508	5	6316	45	2720	1622	78
LISBON—Ransom County ★ COMMUNITY MEMORIAL HOSPITAL, 905 Main, Zip 58054–0353; tel. 701/683–5241; Deb J. Krmpotic R.N., Administrator (Nonreporting) **A**5 9 10 **S**2235 Lutheran Health Systems	23	10	70	—	—	—	—	—	—	—
MANDAN—Morton County ★ MEDCENTER ONE MANDAN, 1000 18th Street N.W., Zip 58554–1698; tel. 701/663–6471; James R. Hubbard, Administrator (Total facility includes 120 beds in nursing home–type unit) **A**5 9 10 **F**1 2 4 7 8 10 11 14 15 16 17 19 21 22 23 24 26 27 30 31 32 33 34 35 37 38 39 40 41 42 43 44 47 48 49 51 52 53 54 55 56 57 58 60 61 64 65 66 67 69 71 73 74 **P**3	23	10	162	596	143	3716	0	6277	3471	179
MAYVILLE—Traill County ★ UNION HOSPITAL, 42 Sixth Avenue S.E., Zip 58257–1598; tel. 701/786–3800; James MacKay Jr., Chief Executive Officer **A**5 9 10 **F**7 8 15 16 19 22 24 26 32 33 34 40 44 49 65 71 73 **P**5	23	10	30	673	10	10233	38	2706	1286	53
MCVILLE—Nelson County ★ COMMUNITY HOSPITAL IN NELSON COUNTY, Main Street, Zip 58254, Mailing Address: P.O. Box H, Zip 58254–0787; tel. 701/322–4328; C. Gary Kopp, Administrator **A**9 10 **F**17 19 26 28 30 32 64 65 71 **P**3	23	10	14	195	4	11574	0	1532	805	37
MINOT—Ward County ST. JOSEPH'S HOSPITAL See UniMed Medical Center										
☒ △ TRINITY MEDICAL CENTER, Burdick Expressway at Main Street, Zip 58701–5020, Mailing Address: P.O. Box 5020, Zip 58702–5020; tel. 701/857–5000; Terry G. Hoff, President (Total facility includes 294 beds in nursing home–type unit) **A**1 3 5 7 9 10 **F**1 4 7 8 10 11 12 13 14 15 16 17 19 21 22 23 24 25 26 28 30 31 32 33 34 35 37 38 39 40 41 43 44 45 46 48 49 51 62 63 64 65 66 67 68 70 71 72 73 74 **P**1 3 4 5 6	23	10	468	6009	394	20955	636	74672	33644	1112
☒ U.S. AIR FORCE REGIONAL HOSPITAL, 10 Missle Avenue, Zip 58705–5024; tel. 701/723–5103; Lieutenant Colonel David Houglum MC, Chief of Medical Staff (Nonreporting) **A**1 5 **S**9495 Department of the Air Force	41	10	47	—	—	—	—	—	—	—
☒ UNIMED MEDICAL CENTER, (Formerly St. Joseph's Hospital) Third Street & Burdick Expressway S.E., Zip 58702–5001; tel. 701/857–2000; Dean Mattern, President **A**1 2 3 5 9 10 **F**2 3 4 7 8 10 12 13 17 19 20 21 22 26 27 28 29 30 31 32 33 34 35 37 39 40 41 42 43 44 45 46 49 52 53 55 56 57 58 59 60 65 67 71 73 74 **P**7	21	10	173	5127	88	27924	265	37473	15980	651
NORTHWOOD—Grand Forks County ★ NORTHWOOD DEACONESS HEALTH CENTER, 4 North Park Street, Zip 58267–0190; tel. 701/587–6060; Larry E. Feickert, Chief Administrative Officer (Total facility includes 112 beds in nursing home–type unit) **A**5 9 10 **F**6 7 11 15 17 19 20 22 26 27 28 30 34 35 36 37 39 40 44 45 46 49 51 59 60 64 65 71 72 73 74 **P**5	21	10	124	355	107	2314	7	4268	2298	118
OAKES—Dickey County ☒ OAKES COMMUNITY HOSPITAL, 314 South Eighth Street, Zip 58474–2099; tel. 701/742–3291; Sister Mary Jane Reiber, Administrator **A**1 9 10 **F**7 11 14 15 19 22 32 40 70 71 **P**4	21	10	30	741	10	16024	38	3165	1837	70
PARK RIVER—Walsh County ★ ST. ANSGAR'S HOSPITAL, 115 Vivian Street, Zip 58270–9998; tel. 701/284–7500; Michael D. Mahrer, President **A**9 10 **F**7 8 15 16 19 22 26 28 31 32 34 35 40 41 44 45 61 65 71 **P**5 **S**5175 Catholic Health Corporation	21	10	20	395	11	8392	19	2546	1268	65
RICHARDTON—Stark County RICHARDTON HEALTH CENTER, Mailing Address: P.O. Box H, Zip 58652; tel. 701/974–3304; Jeanne Messmer R.N., Administrator (Nonreporting) **A**9 10	23	10	26	—	—	—	—	—	—	—
ROLLA—Rolette County PRESENTATION MEDICAL CENTER, 213 Second Avenue N.E., Zip 58367, Mailing Address: P.O. Box 759, Zip 58367–0759; tel. 701/477–3161; Kimber Wraalstad, Chief Executive Officer (Total facility includes 48 beds in nursing home–type unit) **A**5 9 10 **F**7 8 19 20 22 28 30 32 34 36 37 40 41 42 44 45 49 53 54 57 58 64 65 71 **P**6 **S**5805 Sisters of Mary of the Presentation Health Corporation	23	10	102	1041	56	6256	201	6362	3377	145

Hospitals, U.S. / NORTH DAKOTA

Hospital, Address, Telephone, Administrator, Approval, Facility, and Physician Codes, Health Care System	Classification Codes		Utilization Data					Expense (thousands) of dollars		
★ American Hospital Association (AHA) membership ☐ Joint Commission on Accreditation of Healthcare Organizations (JCAHO) accreditation + American Osteopathic Hospital Association (AOHA) membership ○ American Osteopathic Association (AOA) accreditation △ Commission on Accreditation of Rehabilitation Facilities (CARF) accreditation Control codes 61, 63, 64, 71, 72 and 73 indicate hospitals listed by AOHA, but not registered by AHA. For definition of numerical codes, see page A6	Control	Service	Beds	Admissions	Census	Outpatient Visits	Births	Total	Payroll	Personnel
RUGBY—Pierce County ✠ HEART OF AMERICA MEDICAL CENTER, Rugby Heights, Zip 58368, Mailing Address: P.O. Box 197, Zip 58368; tel. 701/776–5261; Jerry E. Jurena, Executive Director (Total facility includes 198 beds in nursing home–type unit) **A**1 5 9 10 **F**3 7 19 21 22 26 28 31 32 33 34 35 36 37 40 44 64 65 66 71 73	23	10	236	1208	219	8161	94	9650	4838	160
STANLEY—Mountrail County ★ STANLEY COMMUNITY HOSPITAL, 502 Third Street S.E., Zip 58784, Mailing Address: Box 399, Zip 58784–0399; tel. 701/628–2424; David Sandberg, Administrator **A**9 10 **F**7 8 19 22 36 44 64 70 71 **P**8	23	10	25	272	5	—	12	1401	746	40
TIOGA—Williams County ★ TIOGA MEDICAL CENTER, 810 North Welo Street, Zip 58852–0159, Mailing Address: P.O. Box 159, Zip 58852–0159; tel. 701/664–3305; Lowell D. Herfindahl, President and Chief Executive Officer (Total facility includes 30 beds in nursing home–type unit) **A**5 9 10 **F**7 8 11 12 19 20 21 22 26 27 30 32 40 42 44 45 46 49 56 57 64 65 70 71 **P**4	23	10	59	672	37	4692	18	2335	1381	45
TURTLE LAKE—Mclean County COMMUNITY MEMORIAL HOSPITAL, 220 Fifth Avenue, Zip 58575, Mailing Address: P.O. Box 280, Zip 58575; tel. 701/448–2331; Richard Spilovoy, Administrator **A**9 10 **F**14 15 16 19 20 22 32 37 40 44 49 51 65 71	21	10	35	419	6	—	5	1114	671	50
VALLEY CITY—Barnes County ✠ MERCY HOSPITAL, 570 Chautauqua Boulevard, Zip 58072–3199; tel. 701/845–0440; Greg Hanson, President **A**1 5 9 10 **F**1 7 8 11 15 19 22 26 28 29 30 32 34 35 37 39 40 44 49 65 66 71 **S**5175 Catholic Health Corporation	21	10	50	1059	35	14318	107	6062	3332	143
WATFORD CITY—McKenzie County ★ MCKENZIE COUNTY MEMORIAL HOSPITAL, 508 North Main Street, Zip 58854, Mailing Address: P.O. Box 548, Zip 58854–0548; tel. 701/842–3000; Tim Gullingsrud, Administrator **A**9 10 **F**1 8 14 15 16 19 20 21 22 24 28 29 30 34 39 40 41 44 45 48 49 51 60 61 71	23	10	24	359	6	5959	22	1624	—	28
WILLISTON—Williams County ✠ MERCY MEDICAL CENTER, 1301 15th Avenue West, Zip 58801–3896; tel. 701/774–7400; Duane D. Jerde, President and Chief Executive Officer **A**1 9 10 **F**2 3 7 8 12 15 19 20 21 22 23 26 32 33 34 35 37 39 40 41 42 44 46 49 52 53 58 64 65 66 67 71 73 **S**5175 Catholic Health Corporation	21	10	113	2772	57	25330	341	21338	9680	360
WISHEK—Mcintosh County ★ WISHEK COMMUNITY HOSPITAL, 1007 Fourth Avenue South, Zip 58495, Mailing Address: P.O. Box 647, Zip 58495; tel. 701/452–2326; George A. Rohrich, Administrator **A**5 9 10 **F**8 12 15 16 19 28 29 30 32 33 44 45 50 65 70 71 73 **P**6	23	10	24	676	7	11143	2	3658	1826	99

© 1995 AHA Guide

Hospitals, U.S. / OHIO

OHIO

Resident population 11,091 (in thousands)
Resident population in metro areas 81.3%
Birth rate per 1,000 population 15.2
65 years and over 13.3%
Percent of persons without health insurance 10.5%

Hospital, Address, Telephone, Administrator, Approval, Facility, and Physician Codes, Health Care System	Classification Codes		Utilization Data					Expense (thousands) of dollars		
★ American Hospital Association (AHA) membership □ Joint Commission on Accreditation of Healthcare Organizations (JCAHO) accreditation + American Osteopathic Hospital Association (AOHA) membership ○ American Osteopathic Association (AOA) accreditation △ Commission on Accreditation of Rehabilitation Facilities (CARF) accreditation Control codes 61, 63, 64, 71, 72 and 73 indicate hospitals listed by AOHA, but not registered by AHA. For definition of numerical codes, see page A6	Control	Service	Beds	Admissions	Census	Outpatient Visits	Births	Total	Payroll	Personnel
AKRON—Summit County										
AKRON CITY HOSPITAL See Summa Health System										
★ AKRON GENERAL MEDICAL CENTER, 400 Wabash Avenue, Zip 44307-2433; tel. 216/384-6000; Michael A. West, President **A**1 2 3 5 9 10 **F**4 7 8 10 11 12 14 16 19 21 22 23 26 28 29 30 31 32 35 37 40 41 42 43 44 45 46 49 51 52 54 56 58 59 60 61 63 65 66 67 69 71 72 73 74 **P**7 8	23	10	495	20818	371	218575	2480	193875	90206	2354
★ CHILDREN'S HOSPITAL MEDICAL CENTER OF AKRON, One Perkins Square, Zip 44308-1062; tel. 216/379-8200; William H. Considine, President **A**1 3 5 8 9 10 **F**9 10 14 15 16 17 19 20 21 22 29 30 31 32 34 35 38 39 41 42 44 45 46 47 49 51 52 53 54 55 56 58 65 66 67 68 69 71 73	23	50	253	8107	136	216307	0	110503	52392	1487
★ △ EDWIN SHAW HOSPITAL, 1621 Flickinger Road, Zip 44312-4495; tel. 216/784-1271; Daniel K. Church Ph.D., President (Total facility includes 49 beds in nursing home–type unit) **A**1 5 7 9 10 **F**2 3 6 12 14 15 16 17 20 26 27 34 39 41 46 48 49 64 65 67 68 73	13	46	231	2547	158	0	0	23226	11447	422
SAINT THOMAS HOSPITAL See Summa Health System										
★ SUMMA HEALTH SYSTEM, (Includes Akron City Hospital, 525 East Market Street, Akron, Ohio, Zip 44309-2090, Mailing Address: P.O. Box 2090, Zip 44309-2090; tel. 216/375-3000; Saint Thomas Hospital, 444 North Main Street, Akron, Ohio, Zip 44310; tel. 216/375-3000) 525 East Market Street, Zip 44304, Mailing Address: P.O. Box 2090, Zip 44309-2090; tel. 216/375-3000; Albert F. Gilbert Ph.D., President and Chief Executive Officer **A**1 2 3 5 6 8 9 10 **F**2 3 4 5 7 8 10 11 12 15 16 19 21 22 23 24 26 27 28 29 30 31 32 33 34 35 36 37 39 40 41 42 43 44 46 48 49 51 52 54 55 56 57 58 59 60 61 65 66 67 69 70 71 73 74 **P**1 2	23	10	632	32430	538	438881	4074	328566	143779	4380
ALLIANCE—Stark County										
□ △ ALLIANCE COMMUNITY HOSPITAL, 264 East Rice Street, Zip 44601; tel. 216/829-4000; James A. Bingham, Chief Executive Officer (Total facility includes 78 beds in nursing home–type unit) **A**1 7 9 10 **F**7 8 10 14 15 17 19 21 22 25 28 30 32 33 34 35 36 37 39 40 41 42 44 45 46 48 49 51 64 65 66 67 71 72 73	23	10	234	5750	138	60916	668	38620	18408	712
AMHERST—Lorain County										
★ ○ AMHERST HOSPITAL, 254 Cleveland Avenue, Zip 44001-1699; tel. 216/988-2831; Bradley P. Smith, President and Chief Executive Officer **A**1 9 10 11 **F**1 2 3 4 5 6 7 8 10 11 12 13 14 15 16 17 18 19 20 21 22 23 24 25 26 27 28 29 30 31 32 33 34 35 36 37 38 39 40 41 42 43 44 45 46 47 48 49 50 51 52 53 54 55 56 57 58 59 60 61 62 63 64 65 66 67 68 69 70 71 72 73 74 **P**4 5 7 **S**0002 Quorum Health Group/Quorum Health Resources	23	10	71	1347	15	25542	264	12959	6809	226
ASHLAND—Ashland County										
★ SAMARITAN HOSPITAL, 1025 Center Street, Zip 44805-4098; tel. 419/289-0491; William C. Kelley Jr. FACHE, President and Chief Executive Officer (Nonreporting) **A**1 9 10	23	10	65	—	—	—	—	—	—	—
ASHTABULA—Ashtabula County										
★ ASHTABULA COUNTY MEDICAL CENTER, 2420 Lake Avenue, Zip 44004-4993; tel. 216/997-2262; R. D. Richardson, President and Chief Executive Officer **A**1 9 10 **F**7 8 14 15 16 19 21 22 27 31 32 33 34 35 37 40 41 42 44 45 46 49 52 53 54 55 56 57 58 59 63 65 66 71 73 **P**4	23	10	148	5635	71	129338	773	40506	17277	584
ATHENS—Athens County										
★ + O'BLENESS MEMORIAL HOSPITAL, 55 Hospital Drive, Zip 45701-2302; tel. 614/593-5551; Richard F. Castrop, President **A**1 9 10 12 13 **F**7 8 14 19 21 22 26 28 30 31 34 35 37 39 40 42 44 45 46 48 49 56 63 65 67 71 73	23	10	75	2747	31	50464	594	19136	8481	295
□ SOUTHEAST PSYCHIATRIC CENTER, 100 Hospital Drive, Zip 45701; tel. 614/594-5000; Donald D. Gold Jr. M.D., Chief Medical Director (Nonreporting) **A**1 9 10	12	22	60	—	—	—	—	—	—	—
BARBERTON—Summit County										
★ BARBERTON CITIZENS HOSPITAL, 155 Fifth Street N.E., Zip 44203; tel. 216/745-1611; Mike A. Bernatovicz, President (Total facility includes 46 beds in nursing home–type unit) **A**1 2 3 5 9 10 **F**2 3 6 7 8 10 11 17 19 21 22 23 26 29 30 31 34 35 37 40 41 42 44 45 46 47 49 52 53 54 55 56 57 58 59 60 63 64 65 66 67 69 70 71 73 74 **P**7 8	23	10	275	9384	190	126557	1021	72402	35733	1093
BARNESVILLE—Belmont County										
★ BARNESVILLE HOSPITAL ASSOCIATION, 639 West Main Street, Zip 43713-1096; tel. 614/425-3941; Richard L. Doan, Chief Executive Officer **A**1 5 9 10 **F**8 13 15 17 19 21 22 27 30 31 32 33 34 36 37 44 45 46 49 54 56 65 67 71 73	23	10	66	2183	33	29727	1	10605	5432	264
BATAVIA—Clermont County										
★ CLERMONT MERCY HOSPITAL, 3000 Hospital Drive, Zip 45103-1998; tel. 513/732-8200; Karen S. Ehrat Ph.D., President and Chief Executive Officer **A**1 9 10 **F**8 14 15 16 19 21 22 30 31 32 33 35 37 41 42 44 46 49 51 52 53 54 59 60 65 71 72 73 **P**6 7 8 **S**5155 Mercy Health System	21	10	151	4944	70	140836	0	41417	19907	862

Hospitals, U.S. / OHIO

Hospital, Address, Telephone, Administrator, Approval, Facility, and Physician Codes, Health Care System	Classification Codes		Utilization Data					Expense (thousands) of dollars		
★ American Hospital Association (AHA) membership □ Joint Commission on Accreditation of Healthcare Organizations (JCAHO) accreditation + American Osteopathic Hospital Association (AOHA) membership ○ American Osteopathic Association (AOA) accreditation △ Commission on Accreditation of Rehabilitation Facilities (CARF) accreditation Control codes 61, 63, 64, 71, 72 and 73 indicate hospitals listed by AOHA, but not registered by AHA. For definition of numerical codes, see page A6	Control	Service	Beds	Admissions	Census	Outpatient Visits	Births	Total	Payroll	Personnel
BEDFORD—Cuyahoga County										
★ UNIVERSITY HOSPITALS HEALTH SYSTEM BEDFORD MEDICAL CENTER, 44 Blaine Avenue, Zip 44146–2799; tel. 216/439–2000; Gerald M. Szkotnicki, President **A**1 9 10 **F**3 7 8 11 12 16 17 19 20 21 22 27 28 29 30 32 33 34 35 36 37 39 40 41 42 44 45 46 49 61 63 65 66 71 72 73 74 **P**1 5 6 7	23	10	110	3376	54	116203	185	25687	11089	365
BELLAIRE—Belmont County										
★ CITY HOSPITAL, 4697 Harrison Street, Zip 43906–0719, Mailing Address: Box 653, Zip 43906; tel. 614/671–1200; John J. Yeager, Chief Executive Officer **A**1 9 10 **F**7 8 11 19 22 33 34 37 40 44 45 49 52 53 54 55 56 58 59 65 71 73	23	10	83	2439	41	35323	268	14373	7274	270
BELLEFONTAINE—Logan County										
★ MARY RUTAN HOSPITAL, 205 Palmer Avenue, Zip 43311; tel. 513/592–4015; Ewing H. Crawfis, President (Nonreporting) **A**1 5 9 10	23	10	72	—	—	—	—	—	—	—
BELLEVUE—Huron County										
★ BELLEVUE HOSPITAL, 811 Northwest Street, Zip 44811, Mailing Address: Box 8004, Zip 44811; tel. 419/483–4040; Michael K. Winthrop, President **A**1 2 9 10 **F**2 7 8 15 19 21 22 26 27 30 31 32 33 34 35 37 40 41 42 44 45 49 54 57 58 59 64 65 66 67 71 73 **P**3	23	10	62	2507	26	32968	445	15886	6859	254
BLUFFTON—Allen County										
★ BLUFFTON COMMUNITY HOSPITAL, 139 Garau Street, Zip 45817–0048, Mailing Address: P.O. Box 48, Zip 45817–0048; tel. 419/358–9010; Clifford K. Harmon, Administrator **A**9 10 **F**7 15 22 34 40 44 71	23	10	42	1048	8	16924	292	6354	2647	91
BOWLING GREEN—Wood County										
★ WOOD COUNTY HOSPITAL, 950 West Wooster Street, Zip 43402–2699; tel. 419/354–8900; Michael A. Miesle, Administrator **A**1 9 10 **F**7 8 10 14 19 22 28 31 34 35 36 37 39 40 41 42 43 44 53 54 55 56 57 58 59 63 65 66 71 73 **P**8	23	10	98	3970	50	70416	544	24031	10880	404
BUCYRUS—Crawford County										
★ BUCYRUS COMMUNITY HOSPITAL, 629 North Sandusky Avenue, Zip 44820–0627, Mailing Address: Box 627, Zip 44820–0627; tel. 419/562–4677; V. Richard Stelzer, Administrator and Chief Executive Officer (Nonreporting) **A**1 9 10 **S**9095 U.S. Health Corporation	23	10	55	—	—	—	—	—	—	—
CADIZ—Harrison County										
★ HARRISON COMMUNITY HOSPITAL, 951 East Market Street, Zip 43907; tel. 614/942–4631; Terry Carson, Chief Executive Officer **A**1 9 10 **F**8 13 14 19 22 24 28 29 30 32 34 35 37 41 44 45 49 65 67 69 71 73 74	23	10	48	717	28	15677	0	5750	2805	142
CAMBRIDGE—Guernsey County										
□ CAMBRIDGE PSYCHIATRIC HOSPITAL, 66737 Old 21 Road, Zip 43725–9298; tel. 614/439–1371; Prabha R. Tripathi M.D., Chief Clinical Officer **A**1 9 10 **F**14 15 16 39 52 56 57 65 67 73	12	22	164	373	136	0	0	—	—	395
GUERNSEY MEMORIAL HOSPITAL See Southeastern Ohio Regional Medical Center										
★ SOUTHEASTERN OHIO REGIONAL MEDICAL CENTER, (Formerly Guernsey Memorial Hospital) 1341 North Clark Street, Zip 43725–0610, Mailing Address: P.O. Box 610, Zip 43725–0610; tel. 614/439–3561; Philip E. Hearing, President and Chief Executive Officer (Total facility includes 20 beds in nursing home–type unit) **A**1 2 9 10 **F**7 8 12 15 16 17 19 21 22 28 30 32 33 34 35 36 37 39 40 41 42 44 46 49 64 65 66 67 68 71 73 74	23	10	140	5313	91	62700	468	34284	14449	559
CANTON—Stark County										
★ AULTMAN HOSPITAL, 2600 Sixth Street S.W., Zip 44710; tel. 216/452–9911; Richard J. Pryce, President (Data for 364 days) **A**1 2 3 5 6 9 10 **F**4 7 8 10 11 12 14 15 16 19 21 22 23 24 25 26 27 28 29 30 31 32 33 34 35 37 38 40 41 42 43 44 45 46 49 51 52 54 56 57 59 60 61 65 66 67 69 70 71 73 74	23	10	682	19970	346	282451	2594	—	—	2206
□ △ TIMKEN MERCY MEDICAL CENTER, 1320 Timken Mercy Drive N.W., Zip 44708–2641; tel. 216/489–1000; Jack W. Topoleski, President and Chief Executive Officer **A**1 2 3 5 7 9 10 **F**2 3 4 7 9 11 14 15 16 17 19 21 22 24 26 27 28 30 32 34 35 37 38 39 40 41 42 43 44 45 46 48 49 50 52 53 54 55 56 57 58 59 60 63 65 66 68 69 70 71 72 73 74 **S**5125 Sisters of Charity of St. Augustine Health System	21	10	416	14362	270	206259	1626	113615	49553	1697
CHAGRIN FALLS—Cuyahoga County										
★ WINDSOR HOSPITAL, 115 East Summit Street, Zip 44022; tel. 216/247–5300; Stewart Powers, Administrator **A**1 9 10 **F**16 19 46 52 53 54 55 57 58 59 65 **P**8	33	22	51	1082	32	0	0	6462	2942	97
CHARDON—Geauga County										
★ GEAUGA HOSPITAL, 13207 Ravenna Road, Zip 44024–0249, Mailing Address: Box 249, Zip 44024–0249; tel. 216/269–6000; Richard J. Frenchie, President **A**1 2 9 10 **F**7 8 14 15 19 21 22 23 27 28 30 33 35 37 39 40 41 42 44 46 49 51 63 65 66 67 71 73 **P**1	23	10	101	3566	42	56064	746	31226	13398	357
□ △ HEATHER HILL REHABILITATION HOSPITAL, (Long–term Care Hospital) 12340 Bass Lake Road, Zip 44024; tel. 216/942–6424; Robert Glenn Harr, President (Total facility includes 194 beds in nursing home–type unit) **A**1 7 9 10 **F**1 12 14 15 17 19 21 26 27 30 32 33 34 35 39 41 45 48 49 57 58 64 65 66 67 71 73	23	49	250	1105	217	900	0	18435	9232	390
CHILLICOTHE—Ross County										
★ MEDICAL CENTER HOSPITAL, 272 Hospital Road, Zip 45601–0708; tel. 614/772–7500; Allen V. Rupiper, President **A**1 5 10 **F**7 8 10 11 14 15 16 17 19 21 22 25 26 28 30 31 32 33 34 35 37 39 40 41 42 44 48 49 52 54 55 56 57 58 59 60 63 65 67 68 71 73 74 **P**8	23	10	171	7516	87	108287	997	54060	23339	748

Hospitals, U.S. / OHIO

Hospital, Address, Telephone, Administrator, Approval, Facility, and Physician Codes, Health Care System	Classification Codes		Utilization Data					Expense (thousands) of dollars		
★ American Hospital Association (AHA) membership ☐ Joint Commission on Accreditation of Healthcare Organizations (JCAHO) accreditation + American Osteopathic Hospital Association (AOHA) membership ○ American Osteopathic Association (AOA) accreditation △ Commission on Accreditation of Rehabilitation Facilities (CARF) accreditation Control codes 61, 63, 64, 71, 72 and 73 indicate hospitals listed by AOHA, but not registered by AHA. For definition of numerical codes, see page A6	Control	Service	Beds	Admissions	Census	Outpatient Visits	Births	Total	Payroll	Personnel
★ VETERANS AFFAIRS MEDICAL CENTER, 17273 State Route 104, Zip 45601–0999; tel. 614/773–1141; Michael W. Walton, Director (Total facility includes 212 beds in nursing home–type unit) **A**1 5 9 **F**2 3 4 8 12 15 16 19 20 21 22 26 27 28 30 31 32 33 34 35 37 41 42 44 46 49 51 52 54 55 56 57 58 64 65 67 71 73 74 **S**9295 Department of Veterans Affairs	45	22	587	6294	518	86045	0	73415	42707	1268
CINCINNATI—Hamilton County										
★ BETHESDA NORTH HOSPITAL, 10500 Montgomery Road, Zip 45242; tel. 513/745–1111; William F. Groneman, Executive Vice President and System Leader (Data for 364 days) **A**1 9 10 **F**1 2 3 6 7 8 10 12 13 14 17 18 19 21 22 23 24 25 26 27 29 30 31 32 33 34 35 37 39 40 41 42 44 45 46 48 49 51 52 53 54 55 56 58 59 60 61 62 63 64 65 67 71 72 73 74 **P**6 **S**0415 Bethesda Hospital, Inc.	23	10	244	14020	169	142027	2154	—	—	1168
★ △ BETHESDA OAK HOSPITAL, 619 Oak Street, Zip 45206–1690; tel. 513/569–6111; William F. Groneman, Executive Vice President and System Leader (Data for 364 days) **A**1 2 3 5 7 9 10 **F**1 2 3 6 7 8 10 12 13 14 17 18 19 21 22 23 24 25 26 27 30 31 32 33 34 35 37 39 40 41 42 44 45 46 48 49 51 52 53 54 55 56 58 59 60 61 62 63 64 65 67 71 72 73 74 **P**6 **S**0415 Bethesda Hospital, Inc.	23	10	310	12615	123	85555	3442	—	—	1665
CAREUNIT HOSPITAL OF CINCINNATI, 3156 Glenmore Avenue, Zip 45211–6696; tel. 513/481–8822; Daniel A. Kidd, Administrator and Vice President (Nonreporting) **A**10	33	82	128	—	—	—	—	—	—	—
CHILDREN'S HOSPITAL See Children's Hospital Medical Center										
★ CHILDREN'S HOSPITAL MEDICAL CENTER, (Includes Division of Adolescent Medicine, Cincinnati Center for Developmental Disorders, and Convalescent Hospital for Children; Children's Hospital, Cincinnati, Ohio) 3333 Burnet Avenue, Zip 45229–3039; tel. 513/559–4200; William K. Schubert M.D., President and Chief Executive Officer **A**1 2 3 5 8 9 10 **F**4 5 10 15 16 19 20 21 22 23 25 28 29 30 31 34 35 38 39 41 42 43 44 45 46 47 48 49 51 52 53 54 55 56 58 59 60 63 65 66 67 69 70 71 72 73 **P**6	23	50	335	15172	207	296864	0	188845	76119	2781
★ △ CHRIST HOSPITAL, 2139 Auburn Avenue, Zip 45219–2989; tel. 513/369–2000; Jack M. Cook, President and Chief Executive Officer (Total facility includes 20 beds in nursing home–type unit) **A**1 2 3 5 6 7 9 10 **F**3 4 8 10 11 14 19 21 22 23 31 32 33 34 35 37 40 41 42 43 44 45 46 48 49 50 52 57 58 59 60 61 64 65 69 71 73 74 **P**1 5 6	23	10	550	21347	314	160469	3796	200040	88353	2140
★ DEACONESS HOSPITAL, 311 Straight Street, Zip 45219–1099; tel. 513/559–2100; E. Anthony Woods, President (Total facility includes 20 beds in nursing home–type unit) **A**1 9 10 **F**1 2 3 4 5 8 10 11 12 14 15 16 17 18 19 20 21 22 24 25 26 27 28 29 30 32 33 34 35 37 39 41 42 43 44 45 46 48 49 51 52 54 55 56 57 58 59 64 65 66 67 69 71 73 74 **P**6 7	23	10	265	6087	118	—	0	72577	32213	1070
★ △ DRAKE CENTER, 151 West Galbraith Road, Zip 45216–1096; tel. 513/948–2500; Earl Gilreath, President and Chief Executive Officer (Total facility includes 213 beds in nursing home–type unit) **A**1 3 5 7 9 10 **F**12 14 15 16 17 19 20 27 28 29 31 34 35 39 48 49 50 64 65 67 71 73 **P**6	23	46	273	592	220	4359	0	38611	18619	647
★ △ GOOD SAMARITAN HOSPITAL, 375 Dixmyth Avenue, Zip 45220–2489; tel. 513/872–1400; Sister Myra James Bradley, Chairman of the Executive Board and Chief Executive Officer **A**1 2 3 5 6 7 8 9 10 **F**4 7 8 10 11 15 16 17 19 21 22 25 26 28 30 31 32 35 37 38 39 40 41 42 43 44 45 46 48 49 51 52 53 54 55 56 57 58 59 60 65 67 69 70 71 73 **P**6 **S**5115 Sisters of Charity Health Care Systems, Inc.	21	10	479	20976	297	133506	5187	183812	80612	2322
☐ + ○ JEWISH HOSPITAL KENWOOD, 8000 Kenwood Road, Zip 45236–2891; tel. 513/745–2200; M. Aurora Lambert, Executive Vice President **A**1 9 10 11 **F**1 2 3 4 6 7 8 10 11 12 14 15 16 17 18 19 20 21 22 24 25 26 27 28 29 30 31 32 33 34 35 36 37 38 39 40 41 42 43 44 45 46 48 49 51 52 53 54 55 56 57 58 59 60 61 63 64 65 66 67 68 69 71 72 73 74 **P**1 6 7 **S**2415 Jewish Health Systems, Inc.	23	10	60	1322	19	—	0	12207	4919	163
★ △ JEWISH HOSPITAL OF CINCINNATI, 3200 Burnet Avenue, Zip 45229–3099; tel. 513/569–2000; Warren C. Falberg, President and Chief Executive Officer (Total facility includes 20 beds in nursing home–type unit) **A**1 2 3 5 7 9 10 **F**1 2 3 4 6 7 8 10 11 12 14 15 16 17 18 19 20 21 22 24 25 26 27 28 29 30 31 32 33 34 35 36 37 38 39 40 41 42 43 44 45 46 48 49 51 52 53 54 55 56 57 58 59 60 61 63 64 65 66 67 68 69 71 72 73 74 **P**1 6 7 **S**2415 Jewish Health Systems, Inc.	23	10	489	12608	214	94431	951	138235	62253	1852
★ MERCY HOSPITAL ANDERSON, 7500 State Road, Zip 45255–2492; tel. 513/624–4500; Karen S. Ehrat Ph.D., President and Chief Executive Officer **A**1 2 9 10 **F**1 6 7 8 10 12 15 16 17 19 21 22 28 30 32 33 34 35 37 39 40 41 42 44 45 46 49 52 53 54 55 56 57 58 59 60 62 63 64 65 66 67 71 72 73 74 **P**6 8 **S**5155 Mercy Health System	21	10	186	8409	100	77265	1655	61794	21088	709
☐ PAULINE WARFIELD LEWIS CENTER, 1101 Summit Road, Zip 45237; tel. 513/948–3600; Anthony E. Thompson, Chief Executive Officer (Nonreporting) **A**1 9 10	12	22	357							
★ PROVIDENCE HOSPITAL, 2446 Kipling Avenue, Zip 45239–6695; tel. 513/853–5000; R. Christopher West, President and Chief Executive Officer **A**1 2 3 5 9 10 **F**2 3 4 6 8 10 12 14 15 16 17 19 21 22 24 27 28 29 30 31 32 34 35 36 37 41 42 44 46 48 49 51 52 53 54 55 56 57 58 59 62 63 64 65 66 67 71 72 73 74 **P**4 7 **S**1485 Franciscan Sisters of the Poor Health System, Inc.	21	10	238	7834	122	90126	0	62573	27714	—
★ SHRINERS HOSPITALS FOR CRIPPLED CHILDREN, CINCINNATI BURNS INSTITUTE, 3229 Burnet Avenue, Zip 45229–3095; tel. 513/872–6000; Ronald R. Hitzler, Administrator **A**1 **F**9 12 19 21 34 35 41 44 46 49 50 54 56 63 65 67 69 71 73 **S**4125 Shriners Hospitals for Crippled Children	23	59	30	838	18	4182	0	—	—	315

Hospitals, U.S. / OHIO

Hospital, Address, Telephone, Administrator, Approval, Facility, and Physician Codes, Health Care System	Classification Codes		Utilization Data					Expense (thousands) of dollars		
	Control	Service	Beds	Admissions	Census	Outpatient Visits	Births	Total	Payroll	Personnel

★ American Hospital Association (AHA) membership
☐ Joint Commission on Accreditation of Healthcare Organizations (JCAHO) accreditation
+ American Osteopathic Hospital Association (AOHA) membership
○ American Osteopathic Association (AOA) accreditation
△ Commission on Accreditation of Rehabilitation Facilities (CARF) accreditation
Control codes 61, 63, 64, 71, 72 and 73 indicate hospitals listed by AOHA, but not registered by AHA. For definition of numerical codes, see page A6

Hospital	Control	Service	Beds	Admissions	Census	Outpatient Visits	Births	Total	Payroll	Personnel
★ △ ST. FRANCIS–ST. GEORGE HOSPITAL, 3131 Queen City Avenue, Zip 45238–2396; tel. 513/389–5000; R. Christopher West, President **A**1 2 7 9 10 **F**2 3 4 6 8 10 12 14 15 16 17 19 21 22 24 25 26 27 28 29 30 31 32 34 35 36 37 41 42 44 46 48 49 51 52 53 54 55 56 57 58 59 62 63 64 65 66 67 71 72 73 74 **P**4 7 **S**1485 Franciscan Sisters of the Poor Health System, Inc.	21	10	229	8475	155	77904	0	61816	27532	—
★ △ UNIVERSITY OF CINCINNATI HOSPITAL, 234 Goodman Street, Zip 45267–0700; tel. 513/558–1000; Jack M. Cook, President and Chief Executive Officer **A**1 2 3 5 7 8 9 10 **F**4 5 7 8 9 10 11 12 14 15 16 17 18 19 20 21 22 24 26 27 28 30 31 32 33 34 35 37 38 40 41 42 43 44 46 49 50 51 52 53 54 55 56 57 58 60 61 63 65 66 67 68 69 70 71 73 74 **P**8	12	10	520	21666	377	254885	2539	300688	125506	3590
★ VETERANS AFFAIRS MEDICAL CENTER, 3200 Vine Street, Zip 45220–2288; tel. 513/861–3100; Gary N. Nugent, Medical Director (Total facility includes 64 beds in nursing home–type unit) **A**1 3 5 8 9 **F**1 2 3 4 8 10 11 12 17 18 19 20 21 22 26 27 28 29 31 32 33 35 36 37 39 41 42 43 44 45 46 48 49 51 52 54 56 57 58 60 61 63 64 65 67 69 71 73 74 **S**9295 Department of Veterans Affairs	45	10	352	6673	294	159337	0	91719	47407	1392
CIRCLEVILLE—Pickaway County										
★ BERGER HOSPITAL, 600 North Pickaway Street, Zip 43113–1499; tel. 614/474–2126; Brian R. Colfack, Chief Executive Officer and Administrator **A**1 9 10 **F**8 12 14 15 17 19 20 21 22 27 28 29 30 32 33 34 35 37 39 41 42 44 45 46 49 63 65 66 67 71 72 73 74	15	10	56	1626	23	42688	5	17222	5887	211
CLEVELAND—Cuyahoga County										
★ CLEVELAND CLINIC HOSPITAL, 9500 Euclid Avenue, Zip 44195–5108; tel. 216/444–2200; Frank L. Lordeman, Chief Operating Officer **A**1 2 3 5 8 9 10 **F**2 3 4 5 7 8 10 11 12 14 15 16 17 19 20 21 22 23 24 25 26 27 28 29 30 31 32 33 34 35 37 38 39 40 41 42 43 44 45 46 47 48 49 50 51 52 53 54 55 56 57 58 59 60 61 63 64 65 66 67 69 71 73 74 **P**3	23	10	945	39439	707	871604	0	505419	223900	—
☐ CLEVELAND PSYCHIATRIC INSTITUTE, 1708 Southpoint Drive, Zip 44109; tel. 216/787–0500; Sandra Rahe, Chief Executive Officer **A**1 3 10 **F**1 2 3 4 5 6 7 8 9 10 11 12 14 15 16 17 18 19 20 21 22 23 24 25 26 27 28 29 30 31 32 33 34 35 36 37 39 40 41 42 43 44 45 46 48 49 50 51 52 53 54 55 56 57 58 59 60 61 62 63 64 65 66 67 68 69 70 71 72 73 74 **P**6 8	12	22	175	3530	128	0	0	19463	12054	349
★ DEACONESS HOSPITAL OF CLEVELAND, 4229 Pearl Road, Zip 44109; tel. 216/459–6300; William D. Myers, President and Chief Executive Officer (Nonreporting) **A**1 2 9 10	23	10	197							
★ FAIRVIEW GENERAL HOSPITAL, 18101 Lorain Avenue, Zip 44111–5656; tel. 216/476–4040; Thomas M. LaMotte, President and Chief Executive Officer (Total facility includes 20 beds in nursing home–type unit) **A**1 3 5 6 9 10 **F**1 4 5 7 8 10 11 17 19 21 22 25 26 27 28 30 31 32 33 34 35 37 38 39 40 41 42 43 44 45 46 48 49 51 52 54 57 58 59 60 64 65 66 67 70 71 72 73 74 **P**1 6 **S**2515 Fairview Health System	23	10	453	21546	273	308244	4161	129536	67709	1902
GLENBEIGH HOSPITAL OF CLEVELAND, 18120 Puritas Avenue, Zip 44135; tel. 216/476–0222; John Sajan R.N., Executive Director (Nonreporting) **A**9 10 **S**0645 Glenbeigh, Inc.	33	82	50	—	—	—	—	—	—	—
★ GRACE HOSPITAL, 2307 West 14th Street, Zip 44113–3698; tel. 216/687–1500; Robert P. Range, President and Chief Executive Officer (Nonreporting) **A**1 9 10	23	10	48							
★ HEALTH HILL HOSPITAL FOR CHILDREN, Mailing Address: 2801 Martin Luther King Jr Drive, Zip 44104–3865; tel. 216/721–5400; Thomas A. Rathbone, President and Chief Executive Officer **A**1 9 10 **F**12 14 34 39 41 45 49 53 54 65 73	23	56	46	282	36	2226	0	13228	7149	192
★ LUTHERAN MEDICAL CENTER, 2609 Franklin Boulevard, Zip 44113–2992; tel. 216/696–4300; Thomas M. LaMotte, President and Chief Executive Officer (Total facility includes 35 beds in nursing home–type unit) **A**1 3 9 10 **F**1 4 5 7 8 10 11 17 19 21 22 25 26 27 28 30 31 32 33 34 35 37 38 39 40 41 42 43 44 45 46 48 49 52 57 58 59 60 63 64 65 66 67 70 71 72 73 **P**1 6 **S**2515 Fairview Health System	23	10	174	5142	114	116361	0	61654	—	823
★ MERIDIA HILLCREST HURON HOSPITAL, 13951 Terrace Road, Zip 44112; tel. 216/761–3300; Charles B. Miner, President and Chief Operating Officer (Total facility includes 20 beds in nursing home–type unit) **A**1 2 3 5 6 9 10 **F**2 3 4 7 8 10 11 12 13 14 15 16 17 19 21 22 24 25 26 27 28 29 30 31 32 33 34 35 36 37 38 39 40 41 42 43 44 45 46 48 49 50 52 54 55 56 57 58 59 60 61 63 64 65 66 67 68 70 71 72 73 74 **P**1 4 8 **S**8835 Meridia Health System	23	10	289	7334	153	51365	0	73520	26711	926
★ △ METROHEALTH MEDICAL CENTER, 2500 Metrohealth Drive, Zip 44109–1998; tel. 216/398–6000; Terry R. White, President and Chief Executive Officer (Total facility includes 320 beds in nursing home–type unit) **A**1 3 5 6 7 8 9 10 **F**3 4 5 7 8 9 10 11 12 14 15 16 17 19 20 21 22 23 25 26 27 28 29 30 31 32 33 35 37 38 39 40 41 42 43 44 45 46 47 48 49 51 52 53 54 55 56 57 58 59 60 61 63 64 65 70 71 72 73 74 **P**1 6 8 **S**8285 Metrohealth System	13	10	1000	23416	704	566514	4048	337073	172233	4551
★ MT. SINAI MEDICAL CENTER, One Mt. Sinai Drive, Zip 44106–4198; tel. 216/421–4000; Robert J. Shakno, President **A**1 2 3 5 8 9 10 **F**2 3 4 5 7 8 9 10 11 12 13 14 15 16 17 19 20 21 22 24 26 28 30 31 32 33 34 35 37 38 39 40 41 42 43 44 45 46 49 51 52 53 54 55 56 57 58 59 60 61 65 66 67 69 70 71 73 74 **P**1 5 7 8	23	10	344	16601	270	306105	2323	186622	87440	2262
★ + ○ RICHMOND HEIGHTS GENERAL HOSPITAL, 27100 Chardon Road, Zip 44143; tel. 216/585–6500; Keith J. Petersen, Chief Executive Officer (Nonreporting) **A**9 10 11 12 13	23	10	138	—	—	—	—	—	—	—

© 1995 AHA Guide

Hospitals, U.S. / OHIO

Hospital, Address, Telephone, Administrator, Approval, Facility, and Physician Codes, Health Care System	Classification Codes		Utilization Data					Expense (thousands) of dollars		Personnel
★ American Hospital Association (AHA) membership □ Joint Commission on Accreditation of Healthcare Organizations (JCAHO) accreditation + American Osteopathic Hospital Association (AOHA) membership ○ American Osteopathic Association (AOA) accreditation △ Commission on Accreditation of Rehabilitation Facilities (CARF) accreditation Control codes 61, 63, 64, 71, 72 and 73 indicate hospitals listed by AOHA, but not registered by AHA. For definition of numerical codes, see page A6	Control	Service	Beds	Admissions	Census	Outpatient Visits	Births	Total	Payroll	
★ SAINT LUKE'S MEDICAL CENTER, 11311 Shaker Boulevard, Zip 44104–9989; tel. 216/368–7000; Samuel R. Huston, President and Chief Executive Officer **A**1 3 5 8 9 10 **F**1 4 5 7 8 10 11 12 14 16 17 19 20 21 22 26 31 32 34 35 36 37 38 39 40 42 43 44 49 52 53 54 55 56 58 59 60 65 67 69 70 71 73 74 **P**1	23	10	254	10624	175	143415	1905	101533	52223	1374
★ ST. ALEXIS HOSPITAL MEDICAL CENTER, 5163 Broadway, Zip 44127–1593; tel. 216/429–8000; William P. Lawrence, President and Chief Executive Officer (Nonreporting) **A**1 2 9 10	21	10	188	—	—	—	—	—	—	—
□ ST. VINCENT CHARITY HOSPITAL, 2351 East 22nd Street, Zip 44115; tel. 216/861–6200; Samuel H. Turner, President (Nonreporting) **A**1 2 3 5 9 10 **S**5125 Sisters of Charity of St. Augustine Health System	21	10	266	—	—	—	—	—	—	—
★ △ UNIVERSITY HOSPITALS OF CLEVELAND, (Includes Alfred and Norma Lerner Tower, Bolwell Health Center, Hanna Pavilion, Lakeside Hospital, Rainbow Babies and Childrens Hospital, Samuel Mather Pavilion, University MacDonald Women's Hospital; MacDonald Hospital for Women; Rainbow Babies and Children's Hospital) 11100 Euclid Avenue, Zip 44106–5000; tel. 216/844–1000; Farah M. Walters, President and Chief Executive Officer **A**1 2 3 5 7 8 9 10 **F**3 4 5 7 8 10 11 13 14 16 17 18 19 20 21 22 23 24 25 26 27 28 29 30 31 32 33 34 35 37 38 39 40 41 42 43 44 45 46 47 49 50 51 52 53 54 55 56 57 58 59 60 61 63 65 66 67 68 69 70 71 72 73 74 **P**3 5 6 7	23	10	677	31768	528	421600	4238	—	—	5393
★ VETERANS AFFAIRS MEDICAL CENTER, 10701 East Boulevard, Zip 44106; tel. 216/791–3800; Krista Ludenia Ph.D., Director (Nonreporting) **A**1 3 5 8 9 **S**9295 Department of Veterans Affairs	45	10	914	—	—	—	—	—	—	—
COLDWATER—Mercer County										
★ MERCER COUNTY JOINT TOWNSHIP COMMUNITY HOSPITAL, 800 West Main Street, Zip 45828–1698; tel. 419/678–2341; James W. Isaacs, Chief Executive Officer **A**1 9 10 **F**7 8 19 21 22 25 26 28 30 31 32 33 34 35 37 40 41 42 44 45 46 65 66 67 71 72 73	16	10	93	2548	30	60336	497	19294	8165	289
COLUMBUS—Franklin County										
★ ARTHUR G. JAMES CANCER HOSPITAL AND RESEARCH INSTITUTE, 300 West Tenth Avenue, Zip 43210; tel. 614/293–5485; Dennis J. Smith, Director **A**1 2 3 5 9 10 **F**3 4 5 8 9 10 11 12 14 15 16 17 19 20 21 22 23 25 26 28 29 30 31 32 34 35 37 38 39 41 42 43 44 45 46 48 49 51 52 53 54 55 56 57 58 59 60 61 63 65 66 67 69 70 71 72 73 74 **P**5	12	10	125	4790	99	67318	0	81578	20941	588
□ CENTRAL OHIO PSYCHIATRIC HOSPITAL, 1960 West Broad Street, Zip 43223–1295; tel. 614/752–0333; James Ignelzi, Chief Executive Officer **A**1 9 10 **F**12 14 15 16 41 52 58 65 73 **P**6	12	22	214	716	191	0	0	29023	15477	491
★ △ CHILDREN'S HOSPITAL, 700 Children's Drive, Zip 43205–2696; tel. 614/722–2000; Stuart W. Williams, Chief Executive Officer **A**1 2 3 5 7 9 10 **F**4 9 10 12 13 17 19 20 21 22 25 27 28 29 31 32 33 34 35 38 39 42 43 44 45 47 48 49 51 53 54 55 56 58 65 67 68 69 70 71 72 73 **P**8	23	50	281	10914	181	361583	0	145474	101113	—
COLUMBUS COMMUNITY HOSPITAL, 1430 South High Street, Zip 43207; tel. 614/445–5000; Bobby Meadows, President and Chief Executive Officer (Nonreporting) **A**9 10	32	10	90	—	—	—	—	—	—	—
★ + ○ △ DOCTORS HOSPITAL, (Includes Doctors Hospital West, 5100 West Broad Street, Columbus, Ohio, Zip 43228; tel. 614/297–5000) 1087 Dennison Avenue, Zip 43201; tel. 614/297–4000; Richard A. Vincent, President **A**1 5 7 9 10 11 12 13 **F**3 4 7 8 10 12 14 15 16 17 19 20 21 22 23 25 26 27 28 30 31 32 33 34 35 37 38 39 40 41 42 43 44 45 46 48 49 51 52 54 55 56 57 60 61 63 65 66 67 71 73 74 **P**3 7 8 **S**1045 Doctors Hospital	23	10	407	12817	211	148402	814	129627	52215	927
★ GRANT MEDICAL CENTER, 111 South Grant Avenue, Zip 43215–1898; tel. 614/461–3232; David Paul Blom, President and Chief Executive Officer **A**1 2 3 5 8 9 10 **F**1 2 3 4 7 8 10 11 12 13 15 16 17 18 19 20 21 22 24 25 26 27 28 29 30 31 32 33 34 35 37 38 39 40 41 42 43 44 45 46 49 50 51 52 53 54 55 56 57 58 59 60 61 63 64 65 66 67 68 69 70 71 72 73 74 **P**3 5 6 7 **S**9095 U.S. Health Corporation	23	10	439	19393	291	0	3094	182003	74083	2759
★ MOUNT CARMEL HEALTH, (Includes Mount Carmel East Hospital, 6001 East Broad Street, Columbus, Ohio, Zip 43213; tel. 614/234–6000; Mount Carmel Medical Center, 793 West State Street, Columbus, Ohio, Zip 43222; tel. 614/234–5000) 793 West State Street, Zip 43222–9988; tel. 614/225–5000; Dale St. Arnold, President and Chief Executive Officer **A**1 2 3 5 9 10 **F**7 8 10 11 12 14 15 16 17 19 21 22 23 26 27 28 29 30 31 32 33 34 35 36 37 38 39 40 41 42 43 44 45 46 48 49 50 51 52 54 55 56 57 58 59 60 65 67 70 71 72 73 74 **P**1 2 3 5 6 7 **S**5585 Holy Cross Health System Corporation	21	10	749	32621	502	244665	3885	272676	107371	3125
★ △ OHIO STATE UNIVERSITY MEDICAL CENTER, 450 West 10th Avenue, Zip 43210–1228; tel. 614/293–8000; R. Reed Fraley, Associate Vice President for Health Sciences and Chief Executive Officer **A**1 3 5 7 8 9 10 **F**3 4 5 8 9 10 11 12 14 15 16 17 19 20 21 22 23 25 26 28 29 30 31 32 34 35 37 38 39 40 41 42 43 44 45 46 48 49 51 52 53 54 55 56 57 58 59 60 61 63 65 66 67 69 70 71 72 73 74 **P**5	12	10	643	25224	489	277775	3479	317151	126924	4077
★ PARK MEDICAL CENTER, 1492 East Broad Street, Zip 43205–1546; tel. 614/251–3000; Neil Serle, Chief Executive Officer (Total facility includes 20 beds in nursing home–type unit) **A**1 2 3 9 10 **F**2 3 4 6 8 10 12 14 16 19 21 22 23 24 26 27 28 30 31 32 33 35 37 41 42 44 45 46 49 51 60 64 65 67 71 73 **P**7	33	10	175	6513	107	37106	0	—	—	223
★ RIVERSIDE METHODIST HOSPITALS, 3535 Olentangy River Road, Zip 43214; tel. 614/566–5000; Nancy M. Schlichting, President and Chief Executive Officer **A**1 2 3 5 8 9 10 **F**1 2 3 4 7 8 10 11 12 14 15 16 17 18 19 20 21 22 24 25 26 27 28 29 30 31 32 33 34 35 37 38 39 40 41 42 43 44 45 46 49 50 51 52 53 54 55 56 57 58 59 60 61 63 64 65 66 67 68 70 71 72 73 74 **P**3 **S**9095 U.S. Health Corporation	21	10	884	37591	583	290839	6098	358921	168933	4451

Hospitals, U.S. / OHIO

Hospital, Address, Telephone, Administrator, Approval, Facility, and Physician Codes, Health Care System	Classification Codes		Utilization Data					Expense (thousands) of dollars		
★ American Hospital Association (AHA) membership □ Joint Commission on Accreditation of Healthcare Organizations (JCAHO) accreditation + American Osteopathic Hospital Association (AOHA) membership ○ American Osteopathic Association (AOA) accreditation △ Commission on Accreditation of Rehabilitation Facilities (CARF) accreditation Control codes 61, 63, 64, 71, 72 and 73 indicate hospitals listed by AOHA, but not registered by AHA. For definition of numerical codes, see page A6	Control	Service	Beds	Admissions	Census	Outpatient Visits	Births	Total	Payroll	Personnel
CONNEAUT—Ashtabula County										
★ BROWN MEMORIAL HOSPITAL, 158 West Main Road, Zip 44030, Mailing Address: P.O. Box 648, Zip 44030; tel. 216/593–1131; C. Thomas Moore, Chief Executive Officer (Nonreporting) A1 9 10	23	10	70	—	—	—	—	—	—	—
COSHOCTON—Coshocton County										
★ COSHOCTON COUNTY MEMORIAL HOSPITAL, 1460 Orange Street, Zip 43812–6330, Mailing Address: P.O. Box 1330, Zip 43812–6330; tel. 614/622–6411; Gregory M. Nowak, Administrator (Nonreporting) A1 9 10	23	10	151	—	—	—	—	—	—	—
CRESTLINE—Crawford County										
★ CRESTLINE MEMORIAL HOSPITAL, 291 Heiser Court, Zip 44827, Mailing Address: P.O. Box 350, Zip 44827; tel. 419/683–1212; Robert E. Wirtz Jr., President and Chief Executive Officer A1 9 10 F2 3 15 16 19 22 27 28 29 30 32 33 34 41 44 48 49 64 65 67 73	23	10	40	837	21	11422	0	6911	3191	170
CUYAHOGA FALLS—Summit County										
+ ○ CUYAHOGA FALLS GENERAL HOSPITAL, 1900 23rd Street, Zip 44223–1499; tel. 216/971–7000; Fred Anthony, President and Chief Executive Officer A9 10 11 12 13 F7 8 12 14 15 16 19 21 22 28 29 30 32 34 35 37 40 41 42 44 45 46 48 49 51 52 55 56 59 63 65 67 71 73 P3 8	23	10	257	4182	69	67890	605	41564	18766	573
□ FALLSVIEW PSYCHIATRIC HOSPITAL, 330 Broadway East, Zip 44221–3398; tel. 216/929–8301; Hem Sharma M.D., Medical Director (Nonreporting) A1 5 10	12	22	96	—	—	—	—	—	—	—
DAYTON—Montgomery County										
★ CHILDREN'S MEDICAL CENTER, One Children's Plaza, Zip 45404–1815; tel. 513/226–8300; Laurence P. Harkness, President and Chief Executive Officer A1 3 5 8 9 10 F9 10 13 14 15 16 17 19 20 21 22 25 28 31 32 34 35 38 39 41 42 44 45 46 47 49 51 53 54 55 58 65 67 71 72 73 P6	23	50	155	6349	98	113595	0	70249	33150	1060
□ DARTMOUTH HOSPITAL, 5350 Lamme Road, Zip 45439; tel. 513/299–9511; Judy Wortham, Chief Executive Officer (Nonreporting) A1 9 10	33	22	98	—	—	—	—	—	—	—
□ DAYTON MENTAL HEALTH CENTER, 2611 Wayne Avenue, Zip 45420–1800; tel. 513/258–0440; Patricia A. Torvik Ph.D., Chief Executive Officer A1 9 10 F19 20 35 39 41 45 46 52 56 57 65 67 71 73 P6	12	22	290	565	234	0	0	26812	16738	502
★ GOOD SAMARITAN HOSPITAL AND HEALTH CENTER, 2222 Philadelphia Drive, Zip 45406–1891; tel. 513/278–2612; K. Douglas Deck, President and Chief Executive Officer A1 2 3 5 9 10 F2 3 4 7 8 10 11 12 14 15 16 17 18 19 20 21 22 25 28 29 30 31 34 35 37 40 42 43 44 45 46 49 51 52 53 54 55 56 57 58 59 60 65 66 67 71 73 74 P2 S5115 Sisters of Charity Health Care Systems, Inc.	21	10	560	17485	290	199466	1805	146702	65731	2135
★ ○ GRANDVIEW HOSPITAL AND MEDICAL CENTER, (Includes Southview Hospital and Family Health Center, 1997 Miamisburg–Centerville Rd, Dayton, Ohio, Zip 45459–3800; tel. 513/439–6000) 405 Grand Avenue, Zip 45405–4796; tel. 513/226–3200; Richard J. Minor, President A9 10 11 12 13 F2 3 4 7 8 10 11 12 13 14 15 16 17 18 19 21 22 23 25 26 27 28 29 30 31 32 33 34 35 36 37 39 40 41 42 43 44 45 46 47 51 52 54 55 56 57 58 60 61 65 66 67 68 69 71 72 73 74 P5 6 8	23	10	320	10506	175	93116	378	116550	49997	1241
★ △ MIAMI VALLEY HOSPITAL, One Wyoming Street, Zip 45409–2793; tel. 513/223–6192; Thomas G. Breitenbach, President and Chief Executive Officer A1 2 3 5 7 8 9 10 F1 2 3 4 7 8 9 10 11 12 14 15 16 17 18 19 20 21 22 23 24 25 26 27 28 29 30 31 32 34 35 36 37 38 39 40 41 42 43 44 46 48 49 51 52 54 55 56 57 58 59 60 61 63 65 66 67 68 69 70 71 72 73 74 P5 6	23	10	757	25026	463	402820	5376	240350	102971	3090
★ △ ST. ELIZABETH MEDICAL CENTER, 601 Edwin C Moses Boulevard, Zip 45408–1498; tel. 513/229–6000; James M. Strieby, President and Chief Executive Officer (Total facility includes 30 beds in nursing home–type unit) A1 2 3 5 7 9 10 F1 4 6 7 8 10 11 12 14 15 16 17 19 20 21 22 26 27 28 30 31 32 34 35 37 39 40 41 42 43 44 45 48 49 51 52 53 54 55 56 58 59 60 62 64 65 66 67 70 71 72 73 74 P4 6 8 S1485 Franciscan Sisters of the Poor Health System, Inc.	21	10	379	15843	285	288918	1302	139011	66661	2057
★ VETERANS AFFAIRS MEDICAL CENTER, 4100 West Third Street, Zip 45428–1002; tel. 513/268–6511; Ed Thorsland Jr., Director (Total facility includes 726 beds in nursing home–type unit) A1 3 5 8 9 F1 2 3 4 8 9 10 12 14 15 16 17 19 20 21 22 23 24 26 27 28 30 31 32 33 34 35 37 41 42 43 44 45 46 48 49 51 52 54 58 60 63 64 65 69 71 73 74 P6 S9295 Department of Veterans Affairs	45	10	991	6508	844	193272	0	115888	74799	1833
DEFIANCE—Defiance County										
★ DEFIANCE HOSPITAL, 1206 East Second Street, Zip 43512–2495; tel. 419/783–6955; Richard C. Sommer, Administrator A1 9 10 F3 7 8 15 17 19 20 21 22 27 28 29 30 31 32 33 35 36 37 40 41 42 44 52 59 63 65 71 73 S0002 Quorum Health Group/Quorum Health Resources	23	10	96	2707	30	27309	426	19193	7658	258
DELAWARE—Delaware County										
★ GRADY MEMORIAL HOSPITAL, 561 West Central Avenue, Zip 43015; tel. 614/369–8711; Everett P. Weber Jr., President and Chief Executive Officer A1 2 9 10 F7 8 14 15 16 19 21 22 23 26 28 29 30 32 33 34 35 36 37 39 40 41 42 44 45 49 53 54 55 56 58 59 65 66 67 70 71 72 73 P6 7 8	23	10	69	2762	31	107974	322	28547	11538	407
DENNISON—Tuscarawas County										
★ TWIN CITY HOSPITAL, 819 North First Street, Zip 44621–1098; tel. 614/922–2800; Robert A. Victor, Chief Executive Officer A1 9 10 F8 11 12 14 19 21 22 29 30 32 33 34 37 39 41 42 44 45 46 48 49 51 63 64 65 71 73	23	10	53	918	11	45673	0	6092	2861	119

© 1995 AHA Guide

Hospitals, U.S. / OHIO

Hospital, Address, Telephone, Administrator, Approval, Facility, and Physician Codes, Health Care System	Classification Codes		Utilization Data					Expense (thousands) of dollars		
	Control	Service	Beds	Admissions	Census	Outpatient Visits	Births	Total	Payroll	Personnel

★ American Hospital Association (AHA) membership
☐ Joint Commission on Accreditation of Healthcare Organizations (JCAHO) accreditation
+ American Osteopathic Hospital Association (AOHA) membership
○ American Osteopathic Association (AOA) accreditation
△ Commission on Accreditation of Rehabilitation Facilities (CARF) accreditation
Control codes 61, 63, 64, 71, 72 and 73 indicate hospitals listed by AOHA, but not registered by AHA. For definition of numerical codes, see page A6

DOVER—Tuscarawas County

★ UNION HOSPITAL, 659 Boulevard, Zip 44622-2077; tel. 216/343-3311; William W. Harding, President and Chief Executive Officer **A**1 9 10 **F**7 8 15 16 19 21 22 30 32 33 34 35 36 37 39 40 44 49 55 58 63 65 66 67 71 73 — 23 10 122 4573 55 108579 724 30822 13953 501

EAST LIVERPOOL—Columbiana County

★ EAST LIVERPOOL CITY HOSPITAL, 425 West Fifth Street, Zip 43920-2498; tel. 216/385-7200; Melvin R. Creeley, President (Total facility includes 20 beds in nursing home-type unit) **A**1 9 10 **F**7 8 13 15 16 19 20 21 22 27 28 30 31 32 35 37 39 40 42 44 49 52 54 56 58 64 65 67 71 73 **P**7 — 23 10 186 6531 101 255432 434 35684 16308 594

POTTERS MEDICAL CENTER, 332 West Sixth Street, Zip 43920-2804; tel. 216/386-5003; Betty Woodward, Interim Administrator (Nonreporting) **A**9 10 — 33 10 43 — — — — — — —

ELYRIA—Lorain County

★ EMH REGIONAL MEDICAL CENTER, 630 East River Street, Zip 44035-5981; tel. 216/329-7500; James L. Keegan, President and Chief Executive Officer **A**1 2 9 10 **F**4 7 8 10 11 14 15 16 19 21 22 23 28 30 32 33 34 35 37 38 39 40 42 43 44 49 51 52 56 57 59 63 65 67 69 71 73 74 **P**7 8 — 23 10 280 10290 136 156648 1265 77713 33028 1098

EUCLID—Cuyahoga County

★ △ MERIDIA EUCLID HOSPITAL, 18901 Lake Shore Boulevard, Zip 44119-1090; tel. 216/531-9000; Fred L. Jackson, President (Total facility includes 20 beds in nursing home-type unit) **A**1 2 7 9 10 **F**2 3 4 7 8 10 11 12 13 14 15 16 17 19 21 22 24 25 26 27 28 30 31 32 33 34 35 36 37 38 39 40 41 42 43 44 45 46 48 49 50 52 54 55 56 57 58 59 60 61 63 64 65 66 67 68 70 71 72 73 74 **P**1 4 8 **S**8835 Meridia Health System — 23 10 224 7961 162 44352 1009 63498 26976 743

FAIRFIELD—Butler County

MERCY HOSPITAL OF FAIRFIELD See Mercy Hospital, Hamilton

FINDLAY—Hancock County

★ BLANCHARD VALLEY HOSPITAL, 145 West Wallace Street, Zip 45840-1299; tel. 419/423-4500; William E. Ruse FACHE, President **A**1 9 10 **F**1 6 7 8 10 11 12 13 15 16 17 19 21 22 25 28 29 30 32 33 34 35 40 41 42 44 52 60 62 65 66 67 71 73 **P**6 — 23 10 150 6943 85 94127 1005 44006 20074 740

FOSTORIA—Seneca County

★ FOSTORIA COMMUNITY HOSPITAL, 501 Van Buren Street, Zip 44830; tel. 419/435-7734; Brad A. Higgins M.H.S.A., Administrator and Chief Executive Officer **A**1 9 10 **F**7 8 11 14 15 17 19 22 24 27 28 29 30 31 32 36 37 39 40 41 42 44 45 46 65 71 73 — 23 10 50 1491 14 34532 222 11125 4677 181

FREMONT—Sandusky County

★ MEMORIAL HOSPITAL, 715 South Taft Avenue, Zip 43420-3296; tel. 419/332-7321; John A. Gorman, Chief Executive Officer **A**1 9 10 **F**7 8 15 17 19 21 22 29 30 32 33 35 36 37 40 41 42 44 45 46 49 52 54 55 57 58 65 71 73 **P**8 **S**0002 Quorum Health Group/Quorum Health Resources — 23 10 132 3403 37 — 500 45522 11841 396

GALION—Crawford County

★ GALION COMMUNITY HOSPITAL, Portland Way South, Zip 44833; tel. 419/468-4841; Mark E. Marley, Chief Executive Officer (Total facility includes 29 beds in nursing home-type unit) **A**1 9 10 **F**7 8 14 15 16 19 21 22 28 36 37 40 41 42 44 64 65 67 71 73 **P**4 7 **S**9095 U.S. Health Corporation — 23 10 120 3420 48 32075 283 22711 10337 388

GALLIPOLIS—Gallia County

★ △ HOLZER MEDICAL CENTER, 100 Jackson Pike, Zip 45631-1563; tel. 614/446-5000; Charles Adkins Jr., President **A**1 2 5 7 9 10 **F**7 8 11 12 17 19 21 22 24 25 26 28 29 30 32 33 35 37 40 41 42 44 46 48 49 58 60 63 64 65 67 69 71 73 74 **P**5 — 23 10 269 7898 110 35022 859 39365 17038 712

GARFIELD HEIGHTS—Cuyahoga County

★ MARYMOUNT HOSPITAL, 12300 McCracken Road, Zip 44125-2975; tel. 216/581-0500; Thomas J. Trudell, President and Chief Executive Officer **A**1 2 6 9 10 **F**3 5 6 7 8 10 12 14 15 16 18 19 21 22 23 25 27 28 30 31 32 34 35 36 37 39 40 41 42 44 46 49 52 53 54 55 56 57 58 59 62 63 65 66 69 71 72 73 74 **P**3 7 8 — 21 10 218 9061 156 78729 1188 71786 32097 1047

GENEVA—Ashtabula County

★ MEMORIAL HOSPITAL OF GENEVA, 870 West Main Street, Zip 44041; tel. 216/466-1141; Gerard D. Klein, Chief Executive Officer **A**1 9 10 **F**8 12 19 22 28 29 30 32 33 34 37 41 44 46 63 65 71 **S**0002 Quorum Health Group/Quorum Health Resources — 23 10 46 1209 16 31592 0 10145 4216 168

GEORGETOWN—Brown County

★ BROWN COUNTY GENERAL HOSPITAL, 425 Home Street, Zip 45121-1449; tel. 513/378-6121; Diana D. Fisher, President and Chief Executive Officer **A**1 9 10 **F**3 7 8 14 19 21 22 28 32 33 35 37 40 41 42 44 45 46 53 54 55 56 57 58 59 65 67 69 71 73 **P**6 — 13 10 53 1796 19 42810 467 14522 6703 244

GREEN SPRINGS—Seneca County

★ △ ST. FRANCIS HEALTH CARE CENTRE, 401 North Broadway, Zip 44836-9638; tel. 419/639-2626; Gregory T. Storer, Chief Executive Officer (Nonreporting) **A**1 7 9 10 — 21 46 186 — — — — — — —

GREENFIELD—Highland County

★ GREENFIELD AREA MEDICAL CENTER, 545 South Street, Zip 45123-0545; tel. 513/981-2116; Mark E. Marchetti, Chief Executive Officer **A**1 9 10 **F**8 15 16 17 19 22 27 28 29 30 32 35 41 42 44 46 48 49 65 71 73 **S**0002 Quorum Health Group/Quorum Health Resources — 23 10 36 1175 21 24312 0 8034 3141 118

Hospitals, U.S. / OHIO

Hospital, Address, Telephone, Administrator, Approval, Facility, and Physician Codes, Health Care System	Classification Codes		Utilization Data					Expense (thousands) of dollars		
	Control	Service	Beds	Admissions	Census	Outpatient Visits	Births	Total	Payroll	Personnel

★ American Hospital Association (AHA) membership
☐ Joint Commission on Accreditation of Healthcare Organizations (JCAHO) accreditation
+ American Osteopathic Hospital Association (AOHA) membership
○ American Osteopathic Association (AOA) accreditation
△ Commission on Accreditation of Rehabilitation Facilities (CARF) accreditation
Control codes 61, 63, 64, 71, 72 and 73 indicate hospitals listed by AOHA, but not registered by AHA. For definition of numerical codes, see page A6

GREENVILLE—Darke County

☐ WAYNE HOSPITAL, 835 Sweitzer Street, Zip 45331–1077; tel. 513/548–1141; Raymond E. Laughlin Jr., President and Chief Executive Officer **A**1 9 10 **F**7 11 15 17 19 21 22 32 33 34 35 40 44 45 49 65 67 71 73 — 23 10 92 2662 34 54285 413 16828 7652 358

HAMILTON—Butler County

★ FORT HAMILTON–HUGHES MEMORIAL HOSPITAL, 630 Eaton Avenue, Zip 45013; tel. 513/867–2000; James A. Kingsbury, President and Chief Executive Officer **A**1 2 9 10 **F**2 3 7 8 10 13 14 15 16 17 19 21 22 25 26 28 29 30 31 32 33 34 35 36 37 39 40 41 42 44 45 46 49 52 54 55 56 57 60 62 63 65 67 68 71 72 73 74 **P**7 8 — 23 10 209 7503 107 78250 1378 52142 22651 763

★ MERCY HOSPITAL, (Includes Mercy Hospital of Fairfield, 3000 Mack Road, Fairfield, Ohio; Mercy Hospital of Hamilton, 100 Riverfront Plaza, Hamilton, Ohio) 100 River Front Plaza, Zip 45012, Mailing Address: P.O. Box 418, Zip 45012–0418; tel. 513/870–7080; Thomas S. Urban, President and Chief Executive Officer (Total facility includes 53 beds in nursing home–type unit) **A**1 9 10 **F**4 8 10 12 14 15 16 17 19 21 22 24 25 26 27 28 29 30 31 32 33 34 35 37 39 41 42 43 44 45 46 48 49 53 54 55 56 57 58 60 63 64 65 67 71 72 73 **P**3 4 5 7 8 **S**5155 Mercy Health System — 21 10 260 8383 143 167524 0 73127 30547 976

HICKSVILLE—Defiance County

★ COMMUNITY MEMORIAL HOSPITAL, 208 North Columbus Street, Zip 43526–1299; tel. 419/542–6692; Major Deryl E. Gulliford, Administrator **A**9 10 **F**7 8 14 15 16 17 19 22 24 26 28 30 31 32 34 35 36 39 40 41 44 45 49 51 66 71 72 73 — 16 10 30 658 6 6054 95 4403 1708 81

HILLSBORO—Highland County

★ HIGHLAND DISTRICT HOSPITAL, 1275 North High Street, Zip 45133–8571; tel. 513/393–6100; Eloise Moran, Administrator **A**1 9 10 **F**7 8 14 15 17 19 21 22 32 33 34 35 40 42 44 46 49 65 66 71 73 — 16 10 44 1819 20 101286 308 13823 5493 222

IRONTON—Lawrence County

☐ LAWRENCE COUNTY MEDICAL CENTER, 2228 South Ninth Street, Zip 45638–2592; tel. 614/532–3231; Terry L. Vanderhoof, President (Nonreporting) **A**1 5 9 10 — 13 10 181 — — — — — — —

KENTON—Hardin County

★ HARDIN MEMORIAL HOSPITAL, 921 East Franklin Street, Zip 43326–2099, Mailing Address: P.O. Box 710, Zip 43326–0710; tel. 419/673–0761; Don J. Sabol, Administrator **A**1 9 10 **F**1 3 4 5 7 8 10 12 13 14 15 16 17 18 19 20 21 22 23 26 28 29 30 31 32 33 34 35 36 37 39 40 41 42 43 44 45 46 49 50 51 53 54 55 56 57 58 59 60 61 63 65 66 67 69 70 71 73 74 **P**3 5 7 8 **S**9095 U.S. Health Corporation — 23 10 51 2069 27 40883 217 12867 4762 164

KETTERING—Montgomery County

CHARLES F. KETTERING MEMORIAL HOSPITAL See Kettering Medical Center

★ KETTERING MEDICAL CENTER, (Includes Charles F. Kettering Memorial Hospital, 3535 Southern Boulevard, Kettering, Ohio, Zip 45429; tel. 513/298–4331; Sycamore Hospital, 2150 Leiter Road, Miamisburg, Ohio, Zip 45342; tel. 513/866–0551) 3535 Southern Boulevard, Zip 45429–1298; tel. 513/298–4331; Frank J. Perez, President and Chief Executive Officer **A**1 2 3 5 8 9 10 **F**2 3 4 6 7 8 10 11 12 17 19 21 22 26 30 32 34 35 37 38 40 41 42 43 44 45 46 49 50 51 52 53 56 58 59 60 62 63 64 65 66 67 70 71 73 74 **P**8 — 21 10 569 17466 269 192199 2019 186228 79440 2680

LAKEWOOD—Cuyahoga County

★ LAKEWOOD HOSPITAL, 14519 Detroit Avenue, Zip 44107–4383; tel. 216/521–4200; Jules W. Bouthillet, President and Chief Executive Officer (Total facility includes 45 beds in nursing home–type unit) **A**1 2 9 10 **F**1 3 4 7 8 10 11 12 13 14 15 16 17 19 21 22 25 26 28 29 30 31 32 33 34 35 36 37 39 40 41 42 43 44 45 46 49 52 53 54 55 56 57 58 60 63 64 65 67 70 71 73 74 **P**3 5 7 — 23 10 334 10642 228 134136 526 84098 36673 1127

LANCASTER—Fairfield County

★ FAIRFIELD MEDICAL CENTER, 401 North Ewing Street, Zip 43130–3371; tel. 614/687–8000; Joseph D. McKelvey, President (Total facility includes 24 beds in nursing home–type unit) **A**9 10 **F**7 8 14 16 17 18 19 21 22 24 25 26 28 29 30 32 33 34 35 37 39 40 41 42 44 46 49 52 54 55 56 57 58 59 60 64 65 66 71 72 73 74 — 23 10 195 8706 101 176811 1232 60312 24874 835

LIMA—Allen County

★ LIMA MEMORIAL HOSPITAL, 1001 Bellefontaine Avenue, Zip 45804–2895; tel. 419/228–3335; John B. White, President and Chief Executive Officer **A**1 9 10 **F**8 10 11 15 19 21 22 26 28 32 34 35 36 37 39 41 42 44 45 49 60 64 65 66 67 71 73 74 **P**3 4 7 — 23 10 241 6927 109 148524 0 67895 29510 1024

OAKWOOD FORENSIC CENTER, 3200 North West Street, Zip 45801; tel. 419/225–8052; John S. Allen, Chief Executive Officer (Nonreporting) **A**9 — 12 22 82 — — — — — — —

★ △ ST. RITA'S MEDICAL CENTER, 730 West Market Street, Zip 45801–4667; tel. 419/227–3361; James P. Reber, President **A**1 2 7 9 10 **F**2 3 7 8 9 10 11 12 13 14 15 16 17 18 19 20 21 22 24 25 26 27 28 29 30 31 32 33 34 35 37 38 39 40 41 42 44 45 46 47 48 49 52 54 55 56 57 58 59 60 63 64 65 66 67 71 72 73 **P**7 **S**5155 Mercy Health System — 21 10 360 13262 177 195513 2336 103217 48657 1705

LODI—Medina County

★ LODI COMMUNITY HOSPITAL, 225 Elyria Street, Zip 44254–1031; tel. 216/948–1222; Thomas L. Lockard, President and Chief Executive Officer (Total facility includes 7 beds in nursing home–type unit) **A**1 5 9 10 **F**17 19 21 22 28 29 30 32 35 36 39 41 42 44 49 64 65 71 73 — 23 10 25 659 11 32692 0 5776 2878 109

© 1995 AHA Guide

Hospitals, U.S. / OHIO

Hospital, Address, Telephone, Administrator, Approval, Facility, and Physician Codes, Health Care System	Classification Codes		Utilization Data					Expense (thousands) of dollars		Personnel
★ American Hospital Association (AHA) membership □ Joint Commission on Accreditation of Healthcare Organizations (JCAHO) accreditation + American Osteopathic Hospital Association (AOHA) membership ○ American Osteopathic Association (AOA) accreditation △ Commission on Accreditation of Rehabilitation Facilities (CARF) accreditation Control codes 61, 63, 64, 71, 72 and 73 indicate hospitals listed by AOHA, but not registered by AHA. For definition of numerical codes, see page A6	Control	Service	Beds	Admissions	Census	Outpatient Visits	Births	Total	Payroll	
LOGAN—Hocking County ★ HOCKING VALLEY COMMUNITY HOSPITAL, Route 2, State Route 664, Zip 43138, Mailing Address: Box 966, Zip 43138; tel. 614/385–5631; Larry Willard, Administrator (Total facility includes 30 beds in nursing home–type unit) **A**1 9 10 **F**7 14 15 16 19 22 28 29 30 34 35 37 40 41 44 45 49 51 64 65 66 67 71 73 **P**3	13	10	92	1721	46	17727	161	13506	5569	243
LONDON—Madison County ★ MADISON COUNTY HOSPITAL, 210 North Main Street, Zip 43140–1115; tel. 614/852–1372; Gary J. Lehman, President (Total facility includes 11 beds in nursing home–type unit) **A**1 9 10 **F**1 3 7 8 11 14 15 16 17 19 22 24 26 28 29 30 31 32 33 34 36 37 39 40 41 42 44 45 49 52 53 54 58 59 64 65 66 67 68 71 73 74	23	10	86	2036	43	29534	271	16895	7573	260
LORAIN—Lorain County ★ △ LORAIN COMMUNITY/ST. JOSEPH REGIONAL HEALTH CENTER, (Includes Lorain Community/St. Joseph Regional Health Center–West Campus, (Formerly Lorain Community Hospital); Lorain Community/St. Joseph Health Center—East Campus, 205 West 20th Street, Lorain, Ohio, Zip 44052–3794; tel. 216/233–1000) 3700 Kolbe Road, Zip 44053–1697; tel. 216/960–3000; Paul C. Balcom, President and Chief Executive Officer (Nonreporting) **A**1 2 7 9 10 **S**5645 Humility of Mary Health Care Corporation	21	10	484	—	—	—	—	—	—	—
LOUISVILLE—Stark County ★ MOLLY STARK HOSPITAL, 7900 Columbus Road N.E., Zip 44641–9748; tel. 216/875–5531; Linda Scherger, Executive Director **A**9 10 **F**20 21 39 46 65	13	62	54	33	63	0	0	—	—	120
MANSFIELD—Richland County ★ MANSFIELD GENERAL HOSPITAL, 335 Glessner Avenue, Zip 44903–2265; tel. 419/526–8000; James E. Meyer, President **A**1 2 6 9 10 **F**7 8 10 11 12 17 19 20 21 22 29 30 31 32 33 34 35 37 39 40 41 42 44 45 46 48 49 52 53 54 55 56 57 58 60 63 65 66 67 70 71 73 74 **P**5 8	23	10	319	9685	169	100143	1265	75733	36848	1171
★ PEOPLES HOSPITAL, 597 Park Avenue East, Zip 44905–2898; tel. 419/526–7300; Philip R. Dever, Chief Executive Officer **A**9 10 **F**8 19 21 30 33 34 35 37 39 44 46 49 65 71 72 73	23	10	47	1381	23	39938	0	9710	3811	173
★ RICHLAND HOSPITAL, 1451 Lucas Road, Zip 44901–0637, Mailing Address: Box 637, Zip 44901–0637; tel. 419/589–5511; S. J. Cocuzza, Administrator (Nonreporting) **A**1 9 10	23	22	92	—	—	—	—	—	—	—
MARIETTA—Washington County ★ MARIETTA MEMORIAL HOSPITAL, 401 Matthew Street, Zip 45750–1699; tel. 614/374–1400; Larry J. Unroe, President **A**1 9 10 **F**2 3 7 8 14 15 16 17 19 21 22 24 30 31 32 33 35 39 40 41 42 44 45 46 48 52 54 55 56 58 59 65 67 71 73 74	23	10	204	6283	77	108562	935	40560	18670	715
★ + ○ SELBY GENERAL HOSPITAL, 1106 Colgate Drive, Zip 45750–1323; tel. 614/373–0582; William M. Greene, Chief Executive Officer **A**9 10 11 12 **F**7 8 15 16 19 21 22 30 31 32 34 35 36 37 39 40 41 42 44 61 65 66 67 71 72 73 74 **S**0002 Quorum Health Group/Quorum Health Resources	23	10	75	1569	20	23504	37	11376	4090	166
MARION—Marion County ★ MARION GENERAL HOSPITAL, McKinley Park Drive, Zip 43302–6397; tel. 614/383–8400; Frank V. Swinehart, President and Chief Executive Officer **A**1 2 9 10 **F**1 7 8 10 12 14 16 17 19 21 22 28 30 31 32 33 35 37 39 40 41 42 44 45 49 52 53 54 55 58 59 60 65 67 71 73 74 **S**9095 U.S. Health Corporation	23	10	151	6468	87	74479	1000	46580	20325	708
□ MEDCENTER HOSPITAL, 1050 Delaware Avenue, Zip 43302; tel. 614/383–7706; Philip W. Smith Jr., President **A**1 9 10 **F**1 3 10 12 14 15 16 19 21 22 30 32 34 35 37 41 42 44 45 48 54 55 56 58 60 63 65 67 71 73 74	23	10	85	3237	46	39290	0	23428	8965	356
MARTINS FERRY—Belmont County □ EAST OHIO REGIONAL HOSPITAL, 90 North Fourth Street, Zip 43935; tel. 614/633–1100; Brian K. Felici, Vice President and Administrator (Total facility includes 94 beds in nursing home–type unit) **A**1 9 10 **F**2 3 5 7 8 10 11 12 14 15 16 17 18 19 21 22 23 24 26 27 28 29 30 31 32 34 35 37 39 41 42 44 45 46 47 48 49 51 52 53 54 55 56 57 58 59 60 61 63 64 65 66 70 71 73 74 **P**6 8 **S**2305 Allegheny Health, Education and Research Foundation	23	10	201	4464	152	100048	0	33222	13787	561
MARYSVILLE—Union County ★ MEMORIAL HOSPITAL, 500 London Avenue, Zip 43040–1594; tel. 513/644–6115; Danny L. Boggs, Administrator **A**1 9 10 **F**7 8 12 14 15 16 19 21 22 24 25 27 28 30 31 32 34 35 36 37 39 40 41 42 44 51 53 54 55 56 57 58 59 63 65 66 71 72 73 **P**6	13	10	56	2341	23	157251	466	28516	11748	404
MASSILLON—Stark County + ○ DOCTORS HOSPITAL OF STARK COUNTY, 400 Austin Avenue N.W., Zip 44646; tel. 216/837–7200; Thomas E. Cecconi, President and Chief Executive Officer **A**2 9 10 11 12 13 **F**7 8 10 14 15 16 19 21 22 23 26 27 28 30 31 32 34 35 37 39 40 41 42 44 45 49 51 54 60 61 63 65 67 68 71 73	23	10	162	5786	74	56282	514	43195	19386	714
★ △ MASSILLON COMMUNITY HOSPITAL, 875 Eighth Street N.E., Zip 44646–9983, Mailing Address: P.O. Box 805, Zip 44648–9983; tel. 216/832–8761; Mervin F. Strine, President (Total facility includes 20 beds in nursing home–type unit) **A**1 7 9 10 **F**2 3 4 7 8 10 12 15 16 17 19 20 21 22 23 26 28 29 30 31 32 34 35 37 39 40 41 42 44 45 46 48 49 60 63 64 65 67 71 73 **P**3	23	10	179	5438	89	95399	297	39486	15043	693
□ MASSILLON PSYCHIATRIC CENTER, 3000 Erie Street, Zip 44646–7993, Mailing Address: Box 540, Zip 44648–7993; tel. 216/833–3135; Frank D. Fleischer, Chief Executive Officer **A**1 5 10 **F**4 7 8 10 12 14 15 16 19 20 22 26 34 35 41 42 43 44 45 46 50 52 55 56 57 60 63 65 71 73 **P**6	12	22	204	1030	166	0	0	26932	—	391

Hospitals, U.S. / OHIO

Hospital, Address, Telephone, Administrator, Approval, Facility, and Physician Codes, Health Care System	Classi-fication Codes		Utilization Data					Expense (thousands) of dollars		
★ American Hospital Association (AHA) membership □ Joint Commission on Accreditation of Healthcare Organizations (JCAHO) accreditation + American Osteopathic Hospital Association (AOHA) membership ○ American Osteopathic Association (AOA) accreditation △ Commission on Accreditation of Rehabilitation Facilities (CARF) accreditation Control codes 61, 63, 64, 71, 72 and 73 indicate hospitals listed by AOHA, but not registered by AHA. For definition of numerical codes, see page A6	Control	Service	Beds	Admissions	Census	Outpatient Visits	Births	Total	Payroll	Personnel
MAUMEE—Lucas County										
★ CHARTER HOSPITAL OF TOLEDO, 1725 Timber Line Road, Zip 43537–4015; tel. 419/891–9333; Michael Cornelison, Chief Executive Officer (Nonreporting) A1 9 10 S0695 Charter Medical Corporation	33	52	38	—	—	—	—	—	—	—
★ ST. LUKE'S HOSPITAL, 5901 Monclova Road, Zip 43537–1899; tel. 419/893–5911; Frank J. Bartell III, President and Chief Executive Officer (Total facility includes 26 beds in nursing home–type unit) A1 9 10 F8 10 12 15 17 19 21 22 23 27 28 30 32 34 35 36 37 41 42 44 45 46 49 54 63 64 65 66 67 71 73 P8	23	10	240	8925	142	87680	0	62563	28310	822
MAYFIELD HEIGHTS—Cuyahoga County										
★ MERIDIA HILLCREST HOSPITAL, 6780 Mayfield Road, Zip 44124–2294; tel. 216/449–4500; Charles B. Miner, President A1 2 3 9 10 F2 3 4 7 8 10 11 12 13 14 15 16 17 19 21 22 24 25 26 27 28 29 30 31 33 34 35 36 37 38 39 40 41 42 43 44 45 46 48 49 50 52 54 55 56 57 58 59 60 61 63 64 65 66 67 68 70 71 72 73 74 P1 4 8 S8835 Meridia Health System	23	10	263	14319	175	105089	3042	106846	37524	1200
MEDINA—Medina County										
★ MEDINA GENERAL HOSPITAL, 1000 East Washington Street, Zip 44256, Mailing Address: P.O. Box 427, Zip 44258–0427; tel. 216/725–1000; Gary D. Hallman, President (Nonreporting) A1 2 9 10	23	10	118	—	—	—	—	—	—	—
MIAMISBURG—Montgomery County										
SYCAMORE HOSPITAL See Kettering Medical Center, Kettering										
MIDDLEBURG HEIGHTS—Cuyahoga County										
★ SOUTHWEST COMMUNITY HEALTH SYSTEM AND HOSPITAL, 18697 Bagley Road, Zip 44130–3497; tel. 216/826–8000; L. Jon Schurmeier, President and Chief Executive Officer A1 2 9 10 F2 3 7 8 10 11 12 13 14 15 16 17 18 19 20 21 22 23 24 25 26 27 28 29 30 31 32 33 34 35 37 38 39 40 41 42 44 45 46 48 49 51 52 53 54 55 56 58 59 60 63 64 65 66 67 70 71 72 73 74 P6 7	23	10	306	12326	184	224947	1556	95938	45546	1721
MIDDLETOWN—Butler County										
★ MIDDLETOWN REGIONAL HOSPITAL, 105 McKnight Drive, Zip 45044–4898; tel. 513/424–2111; Douglas W. McNeill FACHE, President and Chief Executive Officer A1 2 9 10 F2 3 7 8 10 11 15 16 19 21 22 33 34 35 36 37 40 41 42 44 46 48 49 52 53 54 55 56 57 58 61 63 65 66 71 73 74 P8	23	10	251	8902	117	115010	1042	64256	29152	787
MILLERSBURG—Holmes County										
□ JOEL POMERENE MEMORIAL HOSPITAL, 981 Wooster Road, Zip 44654–1094; tel. 216/674–1015; Peter Tuerpitz, Administrator and Chief Executive Officer A1 9 10 F7 8 11 12 19 20 21 22 32 35 37 40 41 44 49 65 71 73	13	10	44	1791	16	23257	531	9663	4120	159
MONTPELIER—Williams County										
□ COMMUNITY HOSPITALS OF WILLIAMS COUNTY, (Includes Bryan Hospital, 433 West High Street, Bryan, Ohio, Zip 43506; tel. 419/636–1131; Montpelier Hospital, Snyder and Lincoln Avenue, Montpelier, Ohio, Zip 43543; tel. 419/485–3154) 909 Snyder Avenue, Zip 43543; tel. 419/636–1131; Rusty O. Brunicardi, President (Nonreporting) A1 9 10	23	10	121	—	—	—	—	—	—	—
MONTPELIER HOSPITAL See Community Hospitals of Williams County										
MOUNT GILEAD—Morrow County										
★ MORROW COUNTY HOSPITAL, 651 West Marion Road, Zip 43338; tel. 419/946–5015; Alan C. Pauley, Administrator (Total facility includes 10 beds in nursing home–type unit) A1 9 10 F7 8 15 17 19 21 22 28 30 35 36 37 39 40 42 44 49 51 64 65 71 73 S9095 U.S. Health Corporation	13	10	56	993	29	20497	225	8763	3229	123
MOUNT VERNON—Knox County										
★ KNOX COMMUNITY HOSPITAL, 1330 Coshocton Road, Zip 43050; tel. 614/393–9000; Robert G. Polahar, Chief Executive Officer A1 5 9 10 F7 19 21 22 32 34 35 36 37 40 42 44 46 52 63 65 71 73 S0002 Quorum Health Group/Quorum Health Resources	23	10	117	4340	56	43156	488	30579	11212	392
NAPOLEON—Henry County										
★ HENRY COUNTY HOSPITAL, 11–600 State Road 424, Zip 43545–9399; tel. 419/592–4015; Robert J. Coholich, Chief Executive Officer A9 10 F3 7 8 11 12 15 16 17 18 19 20 21 22 24 26 28 29 30 31 32 33 34 35 36 37 39 40 41 42 44 45 46 48 49 58 64 65 66 67 71 73 74	23	10	50	899	8	—	160	7988	2635	126
NELSONVILLE—Athens County										
+ ○ DOCTORS HOSPITAL OF NELSONVILLE, 1950 Mount Saint Mary Drive, Zip 45764; tel. 614/753–1931; Mark R. Seckinger, Administrator (Total facility includes 45 beds in nursing home–type unit) A9 10 11 F8 11 19 22 30 34 42 44 56 71 S1045 Doctors Hospital	23	10	77	1079	54	20539	0	—	—	—
NEWARK—Licking County										
★ LICKING MEMORIAL HOSPITAL, 1320 West Main Street, Zip 43055–3699; tel. 614/344–0331; William J. Andrews, President A1 9 10 F7 8 10 11 12 14 15 16 17 19 21 22 28 31 32 37 40 41 42 44 45 46 52 53 54 56 57 58 59 60 63 65 67 71 73	23	10	185	6969	89	152036	1098	49984	25713	1055
NORTHFIELD—Summit County										
□ WESTERN RESERVE PSYCHIATRIC HOSPITAL, 1756 Sagamore Road, Zip 44067, Mailing Address: Box 305, Zip 44067; tel. 216/467–7131; George P. Gintoli, Chief Executive Officer A1 10 F12 27 52 55 65 67 73 P6	12	22	250	35	274	0	0	—	—	588
NORWALK—Huron County										
★ + ○ FISHER–TITUS MEDICAL CENTER, 272 Benedict Avenue, Zip 44857; tel. 419/668–8101; Richard C. Westhofen, President (Total facility includes 54 beds in nursing home–type unit) A1 2 9 10 11 F7 8 19 21 22 23 26 32 33 34 35 37 40 41 42 44 46 49 53 54 55 56 57 58 59 60 61 63 64 65 66 71 73 74	23	10	166	3437	90	47926	576	28816	12707	425

© 1995 AHA Guide

Hospitals, U.S. / OHIO

Hospital, Address, Telephone, Administrator, Approval, Facility, and Physician Codes, Health Care System

- ★ American Hospital Association (AHA) membership
- ☐ Joint Commission on Accreditation of Healthcare Organizations (JCAHO) accreditation
- \+ American Osteopathic Hospital Association (AOHA) membership
- ○ American Osteopathic Association (AOA) accreditation
- △ Commission on Accreditation of Rehabilitation Facilities (CARF) accreditation

Control codes 61, 63, 64, 71, 72 and 73 indicate hospitals listed by AOHA, but not registered by AHA. For definition of numerical codes, see page A6

Hospital	Classification Codes		Utilization Data					Expense (thousands) of dollars		
	Control	Service	Beds	Admissions	Census	Outpatient Visits	Births	Total	Payroll	Personnel
OAK HILL—Jackson County										
★ OAK HILL COMMUNITY MEDICAL CENTER, 350 Charlotte Avenue, Zip 45656-0175; tel. 614/682-7717; Robert A. Bowers, Chief Executive Officer (Nonreporting) **A**1 9 10	23	10	68	—	—	—	—	—	—	—
OBERLIN—Lorain County										
★ ALLEN MEMORIAL HOSPITAL, 200 West Lorain Street, Zip 44074-1077; tel. 216/775-1211; James H. Schaum, President and Chief Executive Officer (Total facility includes 16 beds in nursing home-type unit) **A**1 9 10 **F**7 8 14 19 20 21 22 30 31 32 33 34 35 36 37 39 40 41 42 44 45 49 60 61 64 65 71 72 73	23	10	91	2032	30	17278	498	12784	6119	202
OREGON—Lucas County										
★ ST. CHARLES HOSPITAL, 2600 Navarre Avenue, Zip 43616-3297; tel. 419/698-7200; Randall D. Kordash, President **A**1 2 9 10 **F**3 4 7 8 10 11 12 15 17 19 21 22 23 24 26 27 28 30 31 33 34 35 36 37 38 40 41 42 43 44 46 49 51 52 53 56 57 58 59 60 62 63 65 66 67 71 73 74 **P**3 4 6 8 **S**5155 Mercy Health System	21	10	234	9576	186	115063	782	81547	37264	1264
ORRVILLE—Wayne County										
★ DUNLAP MEMORIAL HOSPITAL, 832 South Main Street, Zip 44667; tel. 216/682-3010; Robert A. Reed, President and Chief Executive Officer **A**1 9 10 **F**7 8 12 17 19 21 22 27 28 29 30 35 39 40 41 42 44 45 46 49 59 63 65 71 73	23	10	38	854	8	13873	282	7934	3091	137
OXFORD—Butler County										
★ MCCULLOUGH-HYDE MEMORIAL HOSPITAL, 110 North Poplar Street, Zip 45056-1292; tel. 513/523-2111; Richard A. Daniels, President and Chief Executive Officer **A**1 9 10 **F**7 8 12 15 16 17 19 21 22 27 28 30 33 34 35 36 37 39 40 42 44 49 63 65 71 73 **P**3	23	10	60	2821	26	46492	573	20721	8960	310
PAINESVILLE—Lake County										
★ LAKE HOSPITAL SYSTEM, Washington At Liberty, Zip 44077-3472; tel. 216/354-2400; Ralph Sorrell, President and Chief Executive Officer **A**1 9 10 **F**4 7 8 10 12 13 14 15 16 17 18 19 20 21 22 23 25 26 27 28 29 30 31 32 33 34 35 36 37 39 40 41 42 43 44 45 46 49 60 63 64 65 66 67 69 71 72 73 74 **P**1 7	23	10	359	12181	172	225415	1337	96390	44498	1448
PARMA—Cuyahoga County										
★ △ PARMA COMMUNITY GENERAL HOSPITAL, 7007 Powers Boulevard, Zip 44129-5495; tel. 216/888-1800; Thomas A. Selden, President and Chief Executive Officer **A**1 2 7 9 10 **F**1 7 8 10 11 12 13 14 16 17 19 21 22 24 27 28 29 30 31 32 33 34 37 39 40 41 42 44 45 46 48 49 54 63 64 65 66 67 71 73 **P**1 7	23	10	171	9341	172	114818	564	77313	36055	1133
PAULDING—Paulding County										
★ PAULDING COUNTY HOSPITAL, 11558 S R 111, Zip 45879-9605; tel. 419/399-4080; Joseph M. Dorko, Chief Executive Officer **A**9 10 **F**7 8 21 22 32 34 35 36 40 44 49 71 73 **S**0002 Quorum Health Group/Quorum Health Resources	13	10	51	703	6	33582	120	7598	3344	134
PIQUA—Miami County										
★ PIQUA MEMORIAL MEDICAL CENTER, 624 Park Avenue, Zip 45356-2098; tel. 513/778-6500; Michael J. Maiberger, Administrator **A**1 2 9 10 **F**3 7 8 10 12 13 15 16 17 18 19 21 22 25 27 28 29 30 31 32 34 35 36 37 39 40 41 42 44 45 46 48 49 52 53 54 55 56 57 58 59 60 62 64 65 66 67 68 71 72 73 74 **P**2 6 **S**1965 Upper Valley Medical Centers	23	10	149	3690	57	44025	477	40480	16745	659
POMEROY—Meigs County										
★ VETERANS MEMORIAL HOSPITAL OF MEIGS COUNTY, 115 East Memorial Drive, Zip 45769-9572; tel. 614/992-2104; Walter S. Lucas, Administrator (Total facility includes 40 beds in nursing home-type unit) **A**1 9 10 **F**19 22 28 32 37 41 42 44 45 64 71 72 73	23	10	69	630	48	25991	0	7541	3237	145
PORT CLINTON—Ottawa County										
☐ H. B. MAGRUDER MEMORIAL HOSPITAL, 615 Fulton Street, Zip 43452-2097; tel. 419/734-3131; David R. Norwine, President and Chief Executive Officer **A**1 9 10 **F**8 12 14 17 19 21 22 28 30 34 36 37 39 42 44 45 46 54 65 66 67 71 **P**6	23	10	41	1736	19	43083	0	13276	5460	209
PORTSMOUTH—Scioto County										
MERCY HOSPITAL See Southern Ohio Medical Center										
☐ PORTSMOUTH RECEIVING HOSPITAL, 25th Street and Elmwood Drive, Zip 45662; tel. 614/354-2804; Rick E. Harlow, Chief Executive Officer **A**1 10 **F**15 52 55 65 73	12	22	30	280	19	0	0	—	—	—
SCIOTO MEMORIAL HOSPITAL See Southern Ohio Medical Center										
★ SOUTHERN OHIO MEDICAL CENTER, (Includes Mercy Hospital, 1248 Kinneys Lane, Portsmouth, Ohio, Zip 45662; Scioto Memorial Hospital, 1805 27th Street, Portsmouth, Ohio, Zip 45662) 1805 27th Street, Zip 45662-2654; tel. 614/354-5000; Randal M. Arnett, President and Chief Executive Officer **A**1 9 10 **F**7 8 15 19 21 22 24 26 28 30 31 32 33 34 35 36 37 39 40 41 42 44 45 46 48 49 51 54 56 58 60 62 63 65 66 67 71 73 74 **P**3 **S**9095 U.S. Health Corporation	23	10	281	11053	169	147831	1560	87605	38259	1516
RAVENNA—Portage County										
★ ROBINSON MEMORIAL HOSPITAL, 6847 North Chestnut Street, Zip 44266-1204, Mailing Address: P.O. Box 1204, Zip 44266; tel. 216/297-0811; Stephen Colecchi, President and Chief Executive Officer **A**1 2 5 9 10 **F**7 8 10 11 12 13 15 16 17 19 20 21 22 25 26 28 29 30 31 34 35 37 39 40 41 42 44 45 46 49 51 52 54 55 56 61 63 65 66 67 71 72 73 74 **P**1	13	10	285	7326	101	100654	971	63586	28300	955
ROCK CREEK—Ashtabula County										
GLENBEIGH HOSPITAL OF ROCK CREEK, Route 45, Zip 44084, Mailing Address: Route 45, P.O. Box 298, Zip 44084; tel. 216/563-3400; Patricia Weston-Hall, Executive Director **A**9 10 **F**2 3 15 16 **P**5 **S**0645 Glenbeigh, Inc.	33	82	80	735	20	5878	0	—	—	57

Hospitals, U.S. / OHIO

Hospital, Address, Telephone, Administrator, Approval, Facility, and Physician Codes, Health Care System	Classification Codes		Utilization Data					Expense (thousands) of dollars		
	Control	Service	Beds	Admissions	Census	Outpatient Visits	Births	Total	Payroll	Personnel

★ American Hospital Association (AHA) membership
☐ Joint Commission on Accreditation of Healthcare Organizations (JCAHO) accreditation
+ American Osteopathic Hospital Association (AOHA) membership
○ American Osteopathic Association (AOA) accreditation
△ Commission on Accreditation of Rehabilitation Facilities (CARF) accreditation
Control codes 61, 63, 64, 71, 72 and 73 indicate hospitals listed by AOHA, but not registered by AHA. For definition of numerical codes, see page A6

SAINT CLAIRSVILLE—Belmont County

☐ FOX RUN HOSPITAL, 67670 Traco Drive, Zip 43950; tel. 614/695–2131; Garrett O. McGrath, Administrator **A**1 10 **F**14 15 16 52 53 58 59	33	52	65	448	31	1453	0	—	—	143

SAINT MARYS—Auglaize County

★ JOINT TOWNSHIP DISTRICT MEMORIAL HOSPITAL, 200 St. Clair Street, Zip 45885–2400; tel. 419/394–3387; James R. Chick, President (Total facility includes 19 beds in nursing home–type unit) **A**1 9 10 **F**7 8 17 19 21 22 25 27 28 30 32 33 34 35 37 39 40 41 44 46 49 51 64 65 67 71 73	23	10	87	4058	55	55143	401	26201	11417	381

SALEM—Columbiana County

★ SALEM COMMUNITY HOSPITAL, 1995 East State Street, Zip 44460–0121; tel. 216/332–1551; Eugene Zentko, Administrator and Chief Executive Officer (Total facility includes 15 beds in nursing home–type unit) **A**1 5 9 10 **F**2 3 4 7 8 9 10 11 12 14 15 19 20 21 22 28 30 32 33 34 35 36 37 38 39 40 41 42 44 45 47 49 51 52 60 63 64 65 67 70 71 73	23	10	159	5839	85	69823	254	40309	18904	647

SANDUSKY—Erie County

★ + ○ △ FIRELANDS COMMUNITY HOSPITAL, (Includes Firelands Community Hospital–Decatur Street, Sandusky, Ohio; Firelands Community Hospital–Hayes Avenue, 2020 Hayes Avenue, Sandusky, Ohio, Zip 44870–8005; tel. 419/626–7400) 1101 Decatur Street, Zip 44870–8005; tel. 419/626–7795; Nelson Alward, President and Chief Executive Officer **A**1 2 7 9 10 11 12 13 **F**2 3 7 8 12 14 15 16 17 18 19 20 21 22 27 28 29 30 31 32 33 34 35 36 37 39 40 41 42 44 45 46 48 49 51 52 53 54 55 56 57 58 59 60 65 66 67 71 73 74	23	10	222	6816	102	178832	1110	58787	22700	788
FIRELANDS COMMUNITY HOSPITAL–DECATUR STREET See Firelands Community Hospital										
FIRELANDS COMMUNITY HOSPITAL–HAYES AVENUE See Firelands Community Hospital										
★ PROVIDENCE HOSPITAL, 1912 Hayes Avenue, Zip 44870–4788; tel. 419/621–7000; Sister Nancy Linenkugel FACHE, President and Chief Executive Officer (Total facility includes 46 beds in nursing home–type unit) **A**1 2 6 9 10 **F**2 3 8 10 11 12 14 15 16 17 19 20 21 22 25 26 27 28 29 30 31 32 33 34 35 37 39 41 42 45 46 49 53 54 55 56 57 58 60 63 64 65 67 71 73 74 **S**5375 Franciscan Services Corporation	21	10	261	3581	100	44734	0	37266	14723	768

SHELBY—Richland County

★ SHELBY MEMORIAL HOSPITAL, Morris Road, Zip 44875–0608, Mailing Address: Box 608, Zip 44875; tel. 419/342–5015; Ron Distl, President **A**1 9 10 **F**7 8 15 17 19 22 28 30 31 32 34 35 36 37 40 42 44 45 49 63 65 71 73	23	10	37	1223	13	23034	188	11009	4417	177

SIDNEY—Shelby County

★ WILSON MEMORIAL HOSPITAL, 915 West Michigan Street, Zip 45365–3501; tel. 513/498–2311; Michael T. Moore, President and Chief Executive Officer **A**1 9 10 **F**7 8 14 15 19 21 22 28 29 30 32 33 34 35 36 37 40 41 44 45 46 51 65 67 71 73	23	10	106	3817	47	83059	453	30248	13071	520

SPRINGFIELD—Clark County

★ COMMUNITY HOSPITAL, 2615 East High Street, Zip 45501–1228, Mailing Address: Box 1228, Zip 45501; tel. 513/325–0531; Neal E. Kresheck, President (Total facility includes 41 beds in nursing home–type unit) **A**1 6 9 10 **F**2 3 7 8 10 11 12 13 14 15 16 17 19 21 22 24 25 27 28 29 30 31 32 33 34 35 36 37 39 40 41 42 44 45 46 49 53 60 63 64 65 67 71 73 74	23	10	232	9123	139	128196	1995	73964	30880	1168
★ △ MERCY MEDICAL CENTER, 1343 North Fountain Boulevard, Zip 45501–1380; tel. 513/390–5000; David C. Hunter, Administrator (Total facility includes 20 beds in nursing home–type unit) **A**1 5 7 9 10 **F**1 6 8 10 11 12 13 14 15 16 17 19 21 22 26 27 28 29 30 31 32 33 34 35 36 37 39 41 42 46 48 49 60 62 64 65 66 67 71 73 74 **P**5 8 **S**5155 Mercy Health System	21	10	218	7470	107	93689	0	64748	25680	1069

STEUBENVILLE—Jefferson County

☐ OHIO VALLEY HOSPITAL, One Ross Park, Zip 43952–2699; tel. 614/283–7000; Fred B. Brower, President (Nonreporting) **A**1 2 6 9 10	23	10	272	—	—	—	—	—	—	—
★ ST. JOHN MEDICAL CENTER, St. John Heights, Zip 43952–2393; tel. 614/264–8000; Angelo G. Calbone, President and Chief Executive Officer **A**1 9 10 **F**2 3 8 10 12 16 19 20 21 22 25 26 27 28 30 31 32 34 35 37 39 41 42 44 45 46 49 52 53 54 55 56 57 58 59 60 63 65 66 67 71 73 74 **P**6 7 8 **S**5375 Franciscan Services Corporation	21	10	161	4540	86	49506	0	39220	16358	579

SYLVANIA—Lucas County

★ △ FLOWER HOSPITAL, 5200 Harroun Road, Zip 43560; tel. 419/824–1444; William W. Glover, President and Chief Executive Officer (Total facility includes 226 beds in nursing home–type unit) **A**1 2 3 5 7 9 10 **F**2 4 6 7 8 9 10 11 12 15 16 19 21 22 23 26 27 28 29 30 31 34 35 37 38 40 42 43 44 45 46 47 48 49 51 52 53 56 57 58 60 61 62 63 64 65 66 67 70 71 72 73 74 **P**3	23	10	373	7763	333	—	962	75275	34101	1382

TIFFIN—Seneca County

★ MERCY HOSPITAL, 485 West Market Street, Zip 44883, Mailing Address: Box 727, Zip 44883–0727; tel. 419/447–3130; Mark David Shugarman, President **A**1 9 10 **F**7 8 11 15 19 22 28 29 30 31 32 34 35 36 40 41 42 44 46 49 56 65 71 73 **P**8 **S**5155 Mercy Health System	21	10	70	2729	30	54848	425	22942	9584	364

TOLEDO—Lucas County

★ △ MEDICAL COLLEGE OF OHIO HOSPITAL, 3000 Arlington Avenue, Zip 43614–2598, Mailing Address: P.O. Box 10008, Zip 43699–0008; tel. 419/381–4172; Debora M. Less, Administrator and Chief Operating Officer **A**1 2 3 5 7 8 10 **F**4 8 10 11 12 19 20 21 22 24 25 26 30 31 35 37 39 41 42 43 44 45 46 47 48 49 52 53 54 55 59 60 61 63 65 66 67 68 69 70 71 73	12	10	261	8655	186	217079	0	127593	52975	2965

© 1995 AHA Guide

Hospitals, U.S. / OHIO

Hospital, Address, Telephone, Administrator, Approval, Facility, and Physician Codes, Health Care System	Classification Codes		Utilization Data					Expense (thousands) of dollars		
	Control	Service	Beds	Admissions	Census	Outpatient Visits	Births	Total	Payroll	Personnel

★ American Hospital Association (AHA) membership
☐ Joint Commission on Accreditation of Healthcare Organizations (JCAHO) accreditation
+ American Osteopathic Hospital Association (AOHA) membership
○ American Osteopathic Association (AOA) accreditation
△ Commission on Accreditation of Rehabilitation Facilities (CARF) accreditation
Control codes 61, 63, 64, 71, 72 and 73 indicate hospitals listed by AOHA, but not registered by AHA. For definition of numerical codes, see page A6

Hospital	Control	Service	Beds	Admissions	Census	Outpatient Visits	Births	Total	Payroll	Personnel
★ MERCY HOSPITAL, 2200 Jefferson Avenue, Zip 43624–9988; tel. 419/259–1500; Randall D. Kordash, President and Chief Executive Officer (Total facility includes 20 beds in nursing home–type unit) **A**1 3 5 9 10 **F**2 3 7 8 10 11 12 13 14 15 16 17 19 20 21 22 23 26 27 28 30 31 32 33 34 35 37 39 40 41 42 44 45 46 47 48 49 51 52 54 56 57 59 60 62 63 64 65 67 70 71 73 74 **P**3 5 6 8 **S**5155 Mercy Health System	21	10	170	5465	109	74900	154	53230	26100	900
★ RIVERSIDE HOSPITAL, 1600 North Superior Street, Zip 43604; tel. 419/729–6000; Scott E. Shook, President (Total facility includes 12 beds in nursing home–type unit) **A**1 2 9 10 **F**7 8 10 11 12 16 17 19 21 22 23 24 25 26 29 30 31 32 33 34 35 36 37 38 39 40 41 42 44 45 46 49 51 52 54 57 58 59 62 63 64 65 66 67 71 72 73 **P**5 6 7 8	23	10	259	6962	120	—	916	67192	27222	939
★ ST. VINCENT MEDICAL CENTER, 2213 Cherry Street, Zip 43608–2691; tel. 419/321–3232; Darryl R. Lippman, President **A**1 2 3 5 6 9 10 **F**2 3 4 7 8 9 10 11 15 16 17 19 21 22 23 25 26 28 29 30 31 32 33 34 35 37 38 39 40 41 42 43 44 46 47 48 49 51 52 53 54 55 56 57 58 59 60 63 65 67 68 69 70 71 73 74 **P**7 8 **S**5885 Covenant Health Systems, Inc.	21	10	472	17966	285	185714	2197	221021	95813	2983
★ THE TOLEDO HOSPITAL, 2142 North Cove Boulevard, Zip 43606; tel. 419/471–4000; Daniel J. Rissing, President and Chief Executive Officer **A**1 2 3 5 8 9 10 **F**2 3 4 5 7 8 10 11 12 15 16 19 21 22 30 32 35 37 38 40 41 42 43 44 46 47 49 50 51 52 53 54 56 57 58 59 60 61 63 65 66 68 71 73 74 **P**3 7 8	23	10	605	24973	413	234622	4568	274401	123614	3821
☐ TOLEDO MENTAL HEALTH CENTER, 930 South Detroit Avenue, Zip 43614–2701; tel. 419/381–1881; G. Terrence Smith, Chief Executive Officer **A**1 3 5 9 10 **F**14 15 16 46 52 55 57 65 73	12	22	140	620	126	0	0	—	—	318
TROY—Miami County										
★ DETTMER HOSPITAL, (Psychiatric, Chemical Dependency, Transitional and Residential Care) 3130 North Dixie Highway, Zip 45373–1039; tel. 513/332–7500; Michael J. Maiberger, Vice President and Chief Operating Officer (Total facility includes 16 beds in nursing home–type unit) **A**1 9 10 **F**2 3 4 7 8 10 11 12 13 14 15 16 17 18 19 20 21 22 23 24 25 26 27 28 29 30 32 34 35 36 37 39 40 41 42 43 45 46 48 49 52 53 54 55 56 57 58 59 60 62 63 64 65 66 67 68 70 71 72 73 74 **P**5 6 7 **S**1965 Upper Valley Medical Centers	23	49	105	1393	42	484	0	14552	7229	233
★ △ STOUDER MEMORIAL HOSPITAL, 920 Summit Avenue, Zip 45373; tel. 513/332–8500; Michael J. Maiberger, Vice President and Chief Operating Officer **A**1 2 7 9 10 **F**1 3 7 8 10 11 13 14 15 16 19 20 21 22 24 25 26 27 28 29 30 31 32 33 34 35 36 37 39 40 41 42 44 45 46 48 49 53 54 55 56 57 58 59 60 62 63 65 66 67 71 72 73 **P**2 6 **S**1965 Upper Valley Medical Centers	23	10	138	4124	63	72574	573	42378	17638	512
UPPER SANDUSKY—Wyandot County										
★ WYANDOT MEMORIAL HOSPITAL, 885 North Sandusky Avenue, Zip 43351–1098; tel. 419/294–4991; Joseph A. D'Ettorre, Administrator **A**5 9 10 **F**7 8 11 12 19 22 33 34 35 37 40 41 42 44 46 56 71 73	16	10	31	1056	12	27645	164	8457	3311	138
URBANA—Champaign County										
★ MERCY MEMORIAL HOSPITAL, 904 Scioto Street, Zip 43078–2200; tel. 513/653–5231; David C. Hunter, Administrator **A**1 9 10 **F**3 8 12 13 14 15 16 17 19 21 22 28 30 32 33 34 37 39 41 44 46 49 61 64 65 68 71 73 **P**5 8 **S**5155 Mercy Health System	21	10	43	1337	15	202658	0	20784	7465	313
VAN WERT—Van Wert County										
★ VAN WERT COUNTY HOSPITAL, 1250 South Washington Street, Zip 45891–2599; tel. 419/238–2390; Mark J. Minick, President and Chief Executive Officer **A**1 9 10 **F**7 8 11 13 14 15 16 17 18 19 22 26 28 29 30 35 37 39 40 41 42 44 46 63 65 66 71 73 **P**1 7 8	23	10	100	1990	22	74269	270	18289	7949	269
WADSWORTH—Medina County										
★ WADSWORTH–RITTMAN HOSPITAL, 195 Wadsworth Road, Zip 44281–9505; tel. 216/334–1504; James W. Brumlow Jr., President and Chief Executive Officer **A**1 5 9 10 **F**7 8 19 22 34 37 40 41 42 44 49 63 65 67 71 73	23	10	81	1963	24	41140	217	15054	6836	225
WARREN—Trumbull County										
★ △ HILLSIDE REHABILITATION HOSPITAL, 8747 Squires Lane N.E., Zip 44484–1697; tel. 216/841–3700; William O'Connor, Chief Executive Officer **A**1 5 7 9 10 **F**2 3 12 14 16 30 41 48 49 65 73 **P**6	13	46	93	1257	71	21116	0	20500	8731	265
★ ST. JOSEPH RIVERSIDE HOSPITAL, 1400 Tod Avenue N.W., Zip 44485; tel. 216/841–4000; Sister Mildred Ely, President and Chief Executive Officer (Total facility includes 11 beds in nursing home–type unit) **A**1 9 10 **F**2 3 4 5 7 8 10 11 14 15 19 21 22 25 28 29 30 31 32 33 35 36 37 39 40 41 42 44 45 52 54 56 58 59 60 63 64 65 66 69 71 73 74 **P**5 8 **S**5645 Humility of Mary Health Care Corporation	21	10	203	6274	84	67616	720	48941	20491	621
★ TRUMBULL MEMORIAL HOSPITAL, 1350 East Market Street, Zip 44482–1269; tel. 216/841–9011; Charles A. Johns, President **A**1 2 5 9 10 **F**7 10 11 13 14 15 16 19 21 22 24 28 29 31 33 34 35 37 39 40 41 42 44 45 49 52 56 57 59 60 63 65 66 71 73	23	10	338	15375	211	202537	1038	106288	47869	1617
★ ○ WARREN GENERAL HOSPITAL, 667 Eastland Avenue S.E., Zip 44484–0128; tel. 216/373–9000; Kevin R. Andrews, Chief Executive Officer (Nonreporting) **A**9 10 11 12 13 **S**0002 Quorum Health Group/Quorum Health Resources	23	10	139	—	—	—	—	—	—	—
WARRENSVILLE HEIGHTS—Cuyahoga County										
★ + ○ MERIDIA SOUTH POINTE, 4110 Warrensville Center Road, Zip 44122–7099; tel. 216/283–2900; Thomas J. Strauss, President and Chief Operating Officer (Data for 291 days) **A**9 10 11 12 13 **F**8 14 15 16 19 21 22 25 28 31 34 35 37 41 42 44 45 55 63 65 67 71 73 74 **S**8835 Meridia Health System	23	10	152	2578	54	66374	0	29841	12931	399

Hospitals, U.S. / OHIO

Hospital, Address, Telephone, Administrator, Approval, Facility, and Physician Codes, Health Care System	Classification Codes		Utilization Data					Expense (thousands) of dollars		Personnel
★ American Hospital Association (AHA) membership ☐ Joint Commission on Accreditation of Healthcare Organizations (JCAHO) accreditation + American Osteopathic Hospital Association (AOHA) membership ○ American Osteopathic Association (AOA) accreditation △ Commission on Accreditation of Rehabilitation Facilities (CARF) accreditation Control codes 61, 63, 64, 71, 72 and 73 indicate hospitals listed by AOHA, but not registered by AHA. For definition of numerical codes, see page A6	Control	Service	Beds	Admissions	Census	Outpatient Visits	Births	Total	Payroll	
★ MERIDIA SOUTH POINTE HOSPITAL, 4180 Warrensville Center Road, Zip 44122–7098; tel. 216/491–6000; Thomas J. Strauss, President and Chief Operating Officer **A**1 2 9 10 **F**2 3 4 7 8 10 11 12 13 14 15 16 17 19 21 22 24 25 26 27 28 29 30 31 32 33 34 35 36 37 38 39 40 41 42 43 44 45 46 48 49 50 52 54 55 56 57 58 59 60 61 63 64 65 66 67 68 70 71 72 73 74 **P**1 4 8 **S**8835 Meridia Health System	23	10	291	5482	91	67944	0	51557	20153	917
WASHINGTON COURT HOUSE—Pickaway County										
★ FAYETTE COUNTY MEMORIAL HOSPITAL, 1430 Columbus Avenue, Zip 43160–1791; tel. 614/333–2705; Francis G. Albarano, Administrator **A**1 5 9 10 **F**7 8 14 19 21 22 28 32 33 34 35 36 37 40 41 42 44 46 49 56 65 66 71 73 **S**0002 Quorum Health Group/Quorum Health Resources	13	10	35	1434	15	44570	277	13498	5682	188
WAUSEON—Fulton County										
★ FULTON COUNTY HEALTH CENTER, 725 South Shoop Avenue, Zip 43567–1701; tel. 419/335–2015; E. Dean Beck, Administrator **A**1 2 9 10 **F**7 8 14 15 19 21 22 23 28 30 33 35 36 37 40 42 44 49 52 55 56 58 59 65 66 67 71 73	23	10	86	2242	25	76494	357	17271	7925	282
WAVERLY—Pike County										
☐ PIKE COMMUNITY HOSPITAL, 100 Dawn Lane, Zip 45690; tel. 614/947–2186; Richard E. Sobota, President and Chief Executive Officer (Nonreporting) **A**1 9 10	23	10	40	—	—	—	—	—	—	—
WEST UNION—Adams County										
☐ ADAMS COUNTY HOSPITAL, 210 North Wilson Drive, Zip 45693–1574; tel. 513/544–5571; Philip S. Hanna, Administrator (Total facility includes 18 beds in nursing home–type unit) **A**1 9 10 **F**15 16 19 22 34 35 44 48 49 64 65 71 **P**5	13	10	49	1199	34	42988	0	11183	5035	164
WESTERVILLE—Franklin County										
★ ST. ANN'S HOSPITAL OF COLUMBUS, 500 South Cleveland Avenue, Zip 43081–8998; tel. 614/898–4000; John B. Sandman, President (Total facility includes 14 beds in nursing home–type unit) **A**1 3 5 9 10 **F**7 10 12 14 15 16 19 21 22 28 30 32 34 35 37 38 40 41 44 45 46 49 63 64 65 66 70 71 73 **P**1	23	10	164	9882	114	85352	3406	70497	29281	911
WESTLAKE—Cuyahoga County										
☐ + ○ ST. JOHN WEST SHORE HOSPITAL, 29000 Center Ridge Road, Zip 44145–5294; tel. 216/835–8000; Fred M. Degrandis, President (Nonreporting) **A**1 9 10 11 **S**5125 Sisters of Charity of St. Augustine Health System	21	10	183	—	—	—	—	—	—	—
WILLARD—Huron County										
★ MERCY HOSPITAL–WILLARD, 110 East Howard Street, Zip 44890–1699; tel. 419/933–2931; James O. Detwiler, President **A**1 9 10 **F**7 8 15 16 19 22 23 28 29 30 32 33 34 35 36 37 40 41 42 44 49 58 63 65 66 67 71 73 **P**3 8 **S**5155 Mercy Health System	21	10	30	988	8	22840	228	10160	4038	115
WILLOUGHBY—Lake County										
★ LAURELWOOD HOSPITAL, 35900 Euclid Avenue, Zip 44094; tel. 216/951–1177; Farshid Afsarifard, Executive Director **A**1 9 10 **F**2 3 4 8 9 10 11 12 13 14 15 16 17 18 19 20 21 22 25 26 27 28 29 30 31 32 34 35 37 38 39 40 41 42 43 44 45 46 48 49 50 51 52 53 54 55 56 57 58 59 60 61 64 65 66 67 68 69 70 71 73 74 **P**8	23	22	160	2311	68	10053	0	12735	6620	191
WILMINGTON—Clinton County										
★ CLINTON MEMORIAL HOSPITAL, 610 West Main Street, Zip 45177–2194; tel. 513/382–6611; Thomas F. Kurtz Jr., President and Chief Executive Officer **A**1 9 10 **F**4 7 8 16 17 19 20 21 22 24 25 26 30 31 32 34 35 36 37 39 40 41 42 44 45 46 49 54 58 60 65 66 67 71 73 74 **P**6	13	10	81	3642	30	74437	406	28599	13368	405
WOOSTER—Wayne County										
★ WOOSTER COMMUNITY HOSPITAL, 1761 Beall Avenue, Zip 44691; tel. 216/263–8100; William E. Sheron, Chief Executive Officer **A**1 2 9 10 **F**7 8 12 15 16 17 19 21 22 28 30 31 32 33 34 35 36 37 39 40 41 42 44 45 46 49 63 65 67 71 73 **P**3 **S**0002 Quorum Health Group/Quorum Health Resources	14	10	90	4431	48	51195	773	28117	13885	505
WORTHINGTON—Franklin County										
☐ HARDING HOSPITAL, 445 East Granville Road, Zip 43085–3195; tel. 614/885–5381; S. R. Thorward M.D., Chief Executive Officer (Nonreporting) **A**1 3 5 9 10	23	22	79	—	—	—	—	—	—	—
WRIGHT-PATTERSON AIR FORCE BASE—Montgomery County										
★ U.S. AIR FORCE MEDICAL CENTER WRIGHT-PATTERSON, 4881 Sugar Maple Drive, Zip 45433–5529; tel. 513/257–9133; Colonel Timothy J. Elders, Administrator **A**1 2 3 5 **F**2 4 5 7 8 9 10 11 12 14 16 19 20 21 22 24 28 29 30 31 34 35 37 38 39 40 41 42 43 44 45 46 47 48 49 51 52 53 54 56 58 60 61 64 65 66 67 68 71 72 73 74 **S**9495 Department of the Air Force	41	10	165	9262	118	535180	780	—	—	1916
XENIA—Greene County										
★ GREENE MEMORIAL HOSPITAL, 1141 North Monroe Drive, Zip 45385; tel. 513/372–8011; Michael R. Stephens, President (Total facility includes 12 beds in nursing home–type unit) **A**1 2 5 9 10 **F**2 3 6 7 8 10 12 15 17 19 22 26 28 30 32 34 35 36 37 39 40 41 42 44 45 46 48 49 51 52 53 54 55 56 57 58 59 60 62 63 64 65 66 67 71 72 73 **P**1 6 7	23	10	150	5098	87	83055	508	40982	16656	621
YOUNGSTOWN—Mahoning County										
★ BELMONT PINES HOSPITAL, 615 Churchill–Hubbard Road, Zip 44505; tel. 216/759–2700; Al Scott Ed.D., Administrator **A**1 9 10 **F**3 12 13 14 15 16 17 18 28 30 52 53 54 55 56 58 59 65 67 68 **P**6	33	52	77	606	37	0	0	6387	2045	85
NORTHSIDE MEDICAL CENTER See Western Reserve Care System										
SOUTHSIDE MEDICAL CENTER See Western Reserve Care System										
★ ST. ELIZABETH HOSPITAL MEDICAL CENTER, 1044 Belmont Avenue, Zip 44501–1790, Mailing Address: Box 1790, Zip 44501–1790; tel. 216/746–7211; Andrew W. Allen, President and Chief Executive Officer **A**1 2 3 5 6 8 9 10 **F**1 2 3 4 7 8 10 11 12 14 15 16 17 19 20 21 22 24 25 26 27 28 30 31 32 34 35 37 38 39 40 41 42 43 44 48 49 51 52 54 55 56 57 58 59 60 61 63 64 65 67 69 70 71 72 73 74 **P**1 **S**5645 Humility of Mary Health Care Corporation	21	10	430	18647	351	229806	2240	196180	90171	2465
TOD CHILDREN'S HOSPITAL See Western Reserve Care System										

Hospitals, U.S. / OHIO

Hospital, Address, Telephone, Administrator, Approval, Facility, and Physician Codes, Health Care System	Classification Codes		Utilization Data					Expense (thousands) of dollars		
	Control	Service	Beds	Admissions	Census	Outpatient Visits	Births	Total	Payroll	Personnel

★ American Hospital Association (AHA) membership
☐ Joint Commission on Accreditation of Healthcare Organizations (JCAHO) accreditation
+ American Osteopathic Hospital Association (AOHA) membership
○ American Osteopathic Association (AOA) accreditation
△ Commission on Accreditation of Rehabilitation Facilities (CARF) accreditation
Control codes 61, 63, 64, 71, 72 and 73 indicate hospitals listed by AOHA, but not registered by AHA. For definition of numerical codes, see page A6

Hospital	Control	Service	Beds	Admissions	Census	Outpatient Visits	Births	Total	Payroll	Personnel
★ △ WESTERN RESERVE CARE SYSTEM, (Includes Northside Medical Center, 500 Gypsy Lane, Youngstown, Ohio, Zip 44501-0240; tel. 216/747-1444; Southside Medical Center, 345 Oak Hill Avenue, Youngstown, Ohio, Zip 44501-0990; tel. 216/747-0777; Tod Children's Hospital, 500 Gypsy Lane, Youngstown, Ohio, Zip 44501-0240; tel. 216/747-6700) 345 Oak Hill Avenue, Zip 44501-0990; Mailing Address: P.O. Box 990, Zip 44501-0990; tel. 216/747-0777; Gary E. Kaatz, President and Chief Executive Officer (Total facility includes 26 beds in nursing home–type unit) A1 2 3 5 7 8 9 10 F2 3 4 6 7 8 10 12 13 14 15 16 17 18 19 20 21 22 23 25 26 28 30 31 32 33 34 35 36 37 38 39 40 41 42 43 44 46 47 48 49 51 52 53 54 55 56 57 58 59 60 61 63 64 65 67 68 71 72 73 74	23	10	616	21365	385	197841	1859	—	—	1627
☐ WOODSIDE HOSPITAL, 800 East Indianola Avenue, Zip 44502-2396; tel. 216/788-8712; Barbara K. Yates, Chief Executive Officer A1 5 9 10 F12 14 15 16 52 56 65 73	12	22	86	1179	55	0	0	9176	—	128
+ ○ YOUNGSTOWN OSTEOPATHIC HOSPITAL, 1319 Florencedale Avenue, Zip 44501-1258, Mailing Address: Box 1258, Zip 44501; tel. 216/744-9200; David A. Folker FACHE, Chief Executive Officer (Nonreporting) A9 10 11 12 13	23	10	175	—	—	—	—	—	—	—
ZANESVILLE—Muskingum County										
★ BETHESDA HOSPITAL, 2951 Maple Avenue, Zip 43701-0551; tel. 614/454-4000; Thomas L. Sieber, President and Chief Executive Officer (Total facility includes 17 beds in nursing home–type unit) A1 2 5 9 10 F1 7 8 10 11 14 15 16 19 21 22 24 28 29 30 32 33 34 35 37 39 40 41 42 44 45 46 52 53 54 55 56 57 58 59 60 64 65 66 71 73 74	23	10	214	8744	122	116678	1082	75461	35424	1312
★ △ GOOD SAMARITAN MEDICAL AND REHABILITATION CENTER, 800 Forest Avenue, Zip 43701; tel. 614/454-5000; Thomas A. Barone, President (Total facility includes 27 beds in nursing home–type unit) A1 2 5 7 9 10 F2 3 7 8 10 12 14 15 16 17 19 21 22 24 25 26 27 28 29 30 31 32 33 34 35 36 37 39 40 41 42 44 45 46 48 49 51 53 54 55 56 57 58 59 60 61 64 65 67 71 72 73 74 S1455 Franciscan Sisters of Christian Charity Healthcare Ministry, Inc	21	10	281	7510	134	149385	915	69063	29902	1095

Hospitals, U.S. / OKLAHOMA

OKLAHOMA

Resident population 3,231 (in thousands)
Resident population in metro areas 60.1%
Birth rate per 1,000 population 15.1
65 years and over 13.6%
Percent of persons without health insurance 19.5%

Hospital, Address, Telephone, Administrator, Approval, Facility, and Physician Codes, Health Care System	Classification Codes		Utilization Data					Expense (thousands) of dollars		
	Control	Service	Beds	Admissions	Census	Outpatient Visits	Births	Total	Payroll	Personnel

★ American Hospital Association (AHA) membership
☐ Joint Commission on Accreditation of Healthcare Organizations (JCAHO) accreditation
+ American Osteopathic Hospital Association (AOHA) membership
○ American Osteopathic Association (AOA) accreditation
△ Commission on Accreditation of Rehabilitation Facilities (CARF) accreditation
Control codes 61, 63, 64, 71, 72 and 73 indicate hospitals listed by AOHA, but not registered by AHA. For definition of numerical codes, see page A6

ADA—Pontotoc County

Hospital	Control	Service	Beds	Admissions	Census	Outpatient Visits	Births	Total	Payroll	Personnel
★ CARL ALBERT INDIAN HEALTH FACILITY, 1001 North Country Club Road, Zip 74820–2847; tel. 405/436–3980; Catherine E. Hanley FACHE, Director, Chickasaw Nation Health System (Nonreporting) **A**1 10 **S**9195 U.S. Public Health Service Indian Health Service	47	10	53	—	—	—	—	—	—	—
★ ROLLING HILLS HOSPITAL, 1000 Rolling Hills Lane, Zip 74820, Mailing Address: P.O. Box 1927, Zip 74821–1927; tel. 405/436–3600; Sherri Owen–Calaway CPA, Executive Director **A**1 10 **F**2 3 12 14 15 16 19 21 22 27 31 34 35 52 53 54 55 56 57 58 59 65 67 71	33	22	40	471	26	0	0	5298	2280	112
★ △ VALLEY VIEW REGIONAL HOSPITAL, 430 North Monta Vista, Zip 74820–4610; tel. 405/332–2323; Philip Fisher, President (Nonreporting) **A**1 2 7 9 10	23	10	148	—	—	—	—	—	—	—

ALTUS—Jackson County

Hospital	Control	Service	Beds	Admissions	Census	Outpatient Visits	Births	Total	Payroll	Personnel
★ JACKSON COUNTY MEMORIAL HOSPITAL, 1200 East Pecan Street, Zip 73521–6192, Mailing Address: Box 8190, Zip 73523–8190; tel. 405/482–4781; William G. Wilson, President and Chief Executive Officer (Total facility includes 25 beds in nursing home–type unit) **A**1 9 10 **F**1 7 8 15 16 17 19 21 22 28 30 32 33 34 35 36 37 39 40 41 42 44 45 46 49 56 58 59 64 65 66 67 70 71 73	16	10	128	3834	61	26419	363	27793	10979	493
★ U.S. AIR FORCE HOSPITAL ALTUS, Altus AFB, Zip 73523–5005; tel. 405/481–5205; Colonel Jack A. Gupton MSC, USAF, Commander (Nonreporting) **S**9495 Department of the Air Force	41	10	28	—	—	—	—	—	—	—

ALVA—Woods County

Hospital	Control	Service	Beds	Admissions	Census	Outpatient Visits	Births	Total	Payroll	Personnel
★ SHARE MEDICAL CENTER, 800 Share Drive, Zip 73717, Mailing Address: P.O. Box 727, Zip 73717–0727; tel. 405/327–2800; Michael McCoy, Chief Executive Officer (Total facility includes 80 beds in nursing home–type unit) **A**9 10 **F**7 8 14 19 22 31 32 34 36 40 42 44 64 71 **S**0002 Quorum Health Group/Quorum Health Resources	16	10	120	814	82	12137	94	3571	1540	116

ANADARKO—Caddo County

Hospital	Control	Service	Beds	Admissions	Census	Outpatient Visits	Births	Total	Payroll	Personnel
ANADARKO MUNICIPAL HOSPITAL, 1002 Central Boulevard East, Zip 73005–4496; tel. 405/247–2551; Nancy Allen, Acting Administrator **A**9 10 **F**7 19 22 40 44 71 73	14	10	49	508	6	3669	61	1737	916	52

ANTLERS—Pushmataha County

Hospital	Control	Service	Beds	Admissions	Census	Outpatient Visits	Births	Total	Payroll	Personnel
PUSHMATAHA COUNTY–TOWN OF ANTLERS HOSPITAL AUTHORITY, 510 East Main Street, Zip 74523, Mailing Address: Box 518, Zip 74523; tel. 405/298–3342; Les Alexander, Administrator (Nonreporting) **A**9 10	15	10	47	—	—	—	—	—	—	—

ARDMORE—Carter County

Hospital	Control	Service	Beds	Admissions	Census	Outpatient Visits	Births	Total	Payroll	Personnel
★ MEMORIAL HOSPITAL OF SOUTHERN OKLAHOMA, 1011 14th Street N.W., Zip 73401–1889; tel. 405/223–5400; Joseph H. Neely, President and Chief Executive Officer (Nonreporting) **A**1 9 10	23	10	178	—	—	—	—	—	—	—

ATOKA—Atoka County

Hospital	Control	Service	Beds	Admissions	Census	Outpatient Visits	Births	Total	Payroll	Personnel
★ ATOKA MEMORIAL HOSPITAL, 1501 South Virginia, Zip 74525; tel. 405/889–3333; J. R. Caton, Administrator **A**9 10 **F**19 22 28 32 34 41 71 **P**6 **S**0002 Quorum Health Group/Quorum Health Resources	13	10	37	627	11	20942	1	3529	2013	126

BARTLESVILLE—Washington County

Hospital	Control	Service	Beds	Admissions	Census	Outpatient Visits	Births	Total	Payroll	Personnel
★ JANE PHILLIPS MEDICAL CENTER, (Formerly Jane Phillips–Episcopal Memorial Medical Center) 3500 East Frank Phillips Boulevard, Zip 74006–2409; tel. 918/333–7200; Larry Minden, Chief Executive Officer (Total facility includes 54 beds in nursing home–type unit) **A**1 2 5 9 10 **F**7 8 10 11 12 14 15 16 17 19 21 22 23 24 26 28 30 32 33 34 35 37 40 41 42 44 45 46 48 49 52 54 56 57 60 63 64 65 66 71 73	23	10	233	6167	147	49393	756	46262	19714	744

BEAVER—Beaver County

Hospital	Control	Service	Beds	Admissions	Census	Outpatient Visits	Births	Total	Payroll	Personnel
BEAVER COUNTY MEMORIAL HOSPITAL, 212 East Eighth Street, Zip 73932, Mailing Address: Box 640, Zip 73932–0640; tel. 405/625–4551; La Vern Melton, Administrator (Nonreporting) **A**9 10	16	10	24	—	—	—	—	—	—	—

BETHANY—Oklahoma County

Hospital	Control	Service	Beds	Admissions	Census	Outpatient Visits	Births	Total	Payroll	Personnel
☐ BETHANY HEALTH CENTER, 7600 N.W. 23rd Street, Zip 73008; tel. 405/787–3450; David Lundquist, Administrator and Chief Executive Officer **A**1 9 10 **F**10 19 22 32 33 37 44 52 53 57 58 59 71 73 **P**3	33	10	75	1744	39	13688	0	13634	6565	302

BLACKWELL—Kay County

Hospital	Control	Service	Beds	Admissions	Census	Outpatient Visits	Births	Total	Payroll	Personnel
★ BLACKWELL REGIONAL HOSPITAL, 710 South 13th Street, Zip 74631; tel. 405/363–2311; Greg Martin, Administrator (Nonreporting) **A**9 10 **S**0305 Oklahoma Health System	23	10	34	—	—	—	—	—	—	—

BOISE CITY—Cimarron County

Hospital	Control	Service	Beds	Admissions	Census	Outpatient Visits	Births	Total	Payroll	Personnel
CIMARRON MEMORIAL HOSPITAL, 100 South Ellis, Zip 73933; tel. 405/544–2501; Ronny Lathrop, Chief Executive Officer and Administrator (Nonreporting) **A**9 10	13	10	64	—	—	—	—	—	—	—

BRISTOW—Creek County

Hospital	Control	Service	Beds	Admissions	Census	Outpatient Visits	Births	Total	Payroll	Personnel
★ BRISTOW MEMORIAL HOSPITAL, Seventh and Spruce Streets, Zip 74010, Mailing Address: Box 780, Zip 74010; tel. 918/367–2215; William L. Legate, Administrator **A**9 10 **F**13 15 16 19 20 30 32 37 44 49 51 65 71 **P**6 **S**0305 Oklahoma Health System	23	10	32	501	5	9452	1	2929	1288	54

© 1995 AHA Guide

Hospitals, U.S. / OKLAHOMA

Hospital, Address, Telephone, Administrator, Approval, Facility, and Physician Codes, Health Care System	Classification Codes		Utilization Data					Expense (thousands) of dollars		
	Control	Service	Beds	Admissions	Census	Outpatient Visits	Births	Total	Payroll	Personnel
★ American Hospital Association (AHA) membership □ Joint Commission on Accreditation of Healthcare Organizations (JCAHO) accreditation + American Osteopathic Hospital Association (AOHA) membership ○ American Osteopathic Association (AOA) accreditation △ Commission on Accreditation of Rehabilitation Facilities (CARF) accreditation Control codes 61, 63, 64, 71, 72 and 73 indicate hospitals listed by AOHA, but not registered by AHA. For definition of numerical codes, see page A6										
BROKEN ARROW—Tulsa County										
□ △ BROKEN ARROW MEDICAL CENTER, 3000 South Elm Place, Zip 74012; tel. 918/455-3535; Bruce Switzer, Administrator **A**1 7 9 10 **F**1 3 4 5 6 7 8 10 12 13 14 16 17 18 19 20 21 22 23 24 25 26 27 28 29 30 31 32 33 34 35 36 37 39 41 42 43 44 45 46 48 49 50 51 53 54 55 56 57 58 59 60 61 63 65 66 67 68 69 70 71 72 73 74 **P**6	23	10	66	1729	32	25000	0	15427	7745	303
BUFFALO—Harper County										
HARPER COUNTY COMMUNITY HOSPITAL, Highway 64 North, Zip 73834, Mailing Address: Box 60, Zip 73834; tel. 405/735-2555; Jane McDowell, Chief Executive Officer **A**9 10 **F**11 15 17 22 30 33 34 36 39 40 44 46 64 71	13	10	25	264	4	1202	19	1246	635	49
CARNEGIE—Caddo County										
★ CARNEGIE TRI-COUNTY MUNICIPAL HOSPITAL, 102 North Broadway, Zip 73015, Mailing Address: Box 97, Zip 73015; tel. 405/654-1050; Patti Davis, Administrator (Nonreporting) **A**9 10	14	10	28	—	—	—	—	—	—	—
CHEYENNE—Roger Mills County										
★ ROGER MILLS MEMORIAL HOSPITAL, Fifth and L. L. Males Avenue, Zip 73628, Mailing Address: Box 219, Zip 73628; tel. 405/497-3336; James Hale, Interim Administrator (Nonreporting) **A**9 10	16	10	15	—	—	—	—	—	—	—
CHICKASHA—Grady County										
★ GRADY MEMORIAL HOSPITAL, 2220 Iowa, Zip 73018; tel. 405/224-2300; Roger R. Boid, Administrator **A**1 2 9 10 **F**11 19 21 22 32 33 37 40 44 49 56 65 67 71 73 **P**5	16	10	156	3248	48	14609	417	19406	8689	345
CLAREMORE—Rogers County										
★ CLAREMORE REGIONAL HOSPITAL, 1202 North Muskogee Place, Zip 74017; tel. 918/341-2556; Ken Seidel, Executive Director (Nonreporting) **A**1 9 10 **S**0048 Columbia/HCA Healthcare Corporation	33	10	74	—	—	—	—	—	—	—
★ U.S. PUBLIC HEALTH SERVICE COMPREHENSIVE INDIAN HEALTH FACILITY, 101 South Moore Avenue, Zip 74017-5091; tel. 918/341-8430; John Daugherty Jr., Service Unit Director **A**1 5 10 **F**3 12 13 15 16 20 22 28 31 37 38 40 44 49 51 61 65 71 **P**6 **S**9195 U.S. Public Health Service Indian Health Service	47	10	50	2402	28	142867	828	14870	9477	349
CLEVELAND—Pawnee County										
CLEVELAND AREA HOSPITAL, 1401 West Pawnee Street, Zip 74020-3019; tel. 918/358-2501; Stacy D. Holland, Administrator **A**9 10 **F**28 30 32 36 70 71 73	16	10	25	288	5	7409	0	2897	1710	97
CLINTON—Custer County										
★ CLINTON REGIONAL HOSPITAL, 100 North 30th Street, Zip 73601, Mailing Address: Box 1569, Zip 73601; tel. 405/323-2363; George H. Dashner, President and Chief Executive Officer **A**1 9 10 **F**7 8 12 14 15 16 17 19 20 21 22 28 30 32 33 34 35 37 39 40 42 44 49 54 60 65 71 73	14	10	50	2068	26	13287	289	9220	4332	201
★ U.S. PUBLIC HEALTH SERVICE INDIAN HOSPITAL, Mailing Address: P.O. Box 279, Zip 73601; tel. 405/323-2884; Thedis V. Mitchell, Director **A**1 10 **F**2 4 8 9 11 12 13 14 16 17 18 19 20 22 25 27 28 29 30 31 34 35 38 40 42 43 44 46 47 53 54 56 58 59 65 69 70 71 72 74 **P**6 **S**9195 U.S. Public Health Service Indian Health Service	47	10	11	253	3	15853	0	3632	2294	—
COALGATE—Coal County										
MARY HURLEY HOSPITAL, 6 North Covington Street, Zip 74538-2002; tel. 405/927-2327; C. Dan Phares, Chief Executive Officer (Total facility includes 70 beds in nursing home-type unit) **A**9 10 **F**14 15 17 19 21 22 26 27 28 30 32 44 45 46 70 71 73 **P**5	23	10	90	570	9	4176	0	1971	1003	64
CORDELL—Washita County										
★ CORDELL MEMORIAL HOSPITAL, 1220 North Glenn English Street, Zip 73632; tel. 405/832-3339; Charles H. Greene Jr., Administrator **A**9 10 **F**15 22 28 30 44 71	14	10	28	521	7	3868	0	1698	779	40
CUSHING—Payne County										
★ CUSHING REGIONAL HOSPITAL, 1027 East Cherry, Zip 74023, Mailing Address: Box 1409, Zip 74023-1409; tel. 918/225-2915; Ron Cackler, Chief Executive Officer **A**1 9 10 **F**1 3 7 8 11 12 15 17 19 20 21 22 25 26 28 29 30 32 33 34 36 40 41 42 44 45 46 49 52 54 55 56 57 58 59 64 65 66 67 71 73 **P**8 **S**0002 Quorum Health Group/Quorum Health Resources	14	10	75	2961	54	10891	425	13377	5112	243
DRUMRIGHT—Creek County										
★ DRUMRIGHT MEMORIAL HOSPITAL, 501 South Lou Allard Drive, Zip 74030-4899; tel. 918/352-2525; Jerry Jones, Administrator **A**9 10 **F**8 15 19 22 28 30 32 34 35 37 44 71 73 **P**3 **S**0305 Oklahoma Health System	33	10	43	751	11	6576	0	3142	1608	79
DUNCAN—Stephens County										
★ DUNCAN REGIONAL HOSPITAL, 1407 Whisenant Drive, Zip 73533, Mailing Address: P.O. Box 2000, Zip 73534-2000; tel. 405/252-5300; David Robertson, Chief Executive Officer (Total facility includes 12 beds in nursing home-type unit) **A**1 9 10 **F**7 8 11 13 15 16 17 19 20 21 22 28 30 32 33 34 35 37 39 40 41 42 44 45 64 65 66 71 73 **P**8	23	10	100	3488	48	35628	401	20715	8887	462
DURANT—Bryan County										
□ MEDICAL CENTER OF SOUTHEASTERN OKLAHOMA, 1800 University, Zip 74701, Mailing Address: P.O. Box 1207, Zip 74702; tel. 405/924-3080; Gary D. Newsome, Chief Executive Director **A**1 10 **F**7 8 12 14 17 19 21 22 23 28 30 32 33 34 35 37 44 49 61 63 65 67 70 71 73 74 **P**8 **S**1775 Health Management Associates	33	10	103	3940	47	23228	467	14545	6310	252

Hospitals, U.S. / OKLAHOMA

Hospital, Address, Telephone, Administrator, Approval, Facility, and Physician Codes, Health Care System	Classification Codes		Utilization Data					Expense (thousands) of dollars		
★ American Hospital Association (AHA) membership ☐ Joint Commission on Accreditation of Healthcare Organizations (JCAHO) accreditation + American Osteopathic Hospital Association (AOHA) membership ○ American Osteopathic Association (AOA) accreditation △ Commission on Accreditation of Rehabilitation Facilities (CARF) accreditation Control codes 61, 63, 64, 71, 72 and 73 indicate hospitals listed by AOHA, but not registered by AHA. For definition of numerical codes, see page A6	Control	Service	Beds	Admissions	Census	Outpatient Visits	Births	Total	Payroll	Personnel
EDMOND—Oklahoma County										
★ EDMOND REGIONAL MEDICAL CENTER, 1 South Bryant Street, Zip 73034–4798; tel. 405/359–5530; Stanley D. Tatum, Chief Executive Officer (Nonreporting) A1 9 10 S0048 Columbia/HCA Healthcare Corporation	33	10	79	—	—	—	—	—	—	—
EL RENO—Canadian County										
★ PARK VIEW HOSPITAL, 2115 Parkview Drive, Zip 73036, Mailing Address: P.O. Box 129, Zip 73036–0129; tel. 405/262–2640; Lex Smith, Administrator A9 10 F7 14 22 28 29 30 32 33 34 39 40 44 45 46 49 56 58 65 67 71 73 P6	16	10	54	2054	28	41905	174	11289	5554	299
ELK CITY—Beckham County										
★ GREAT PLAINS REGIONAL MEDICAL CENTER, 1705 West Second Street, Zip 73644, Mailing Address: P.O. Box 2339, Zip 73648–2339; tel. 405/225–2511; Tim Francis, Chief Executive Officer A1 9 10 F8 11 12 14 17 19 21 22 24 28 29 30 32 35 37 40 42 44 45 46 49 51 60 63 65 71 73	23	10	78	1684	22	22008	188	11954	5186	274
ENID—Garfield County										
★ BASS MEMORIAL BAPTIST HOSPITAL, 600 South Monroe, Zip 73701, Mailing Address: Box 3168, Zip 73702; tel. 405/233–2300; W. Eugene Baxter Dr.P.H., Administrator A1 3 5 9 10 F7 8 10 12 15 19 21 22 24 26 28 29 30 31 32 33 34 35 36 37 39 40 41 42 44 46 52 60 64 67 71 73 74 P6 7 S0305 Oklahoma Health System	23	10	119	3884	71	26941	603	28161	12051	527
+ ○ ENID REGIONAL HOSPITAL, 401 South Third, Zip 73701, Mailing Address: Box 3467, Zip 73702; tel. 405/234–3371; John E. Walker, Administrator A9 10 11 12 F1 2 3 7 8 11 12 14 15 16 19 20 21 22 25 26 30 32 34 37 39 40 44 45 46 49 52 53 54 55 56 57 58 59 63 64 65 67 71 73 P6 S0875 Community Health Systems, Inc.	33	10	109	1665	25	11634	71	—	—	198
☐ MEADOWLAKE HOSPITAL, 2216 South Van Buren, Zip 73703, Mailing Address: P.O. Box 5409, Zip 73702; tel. 405/234–2220; Dave Lamerton, Chief Executive Officer (Nonreporting) A1 10 S0405 Ramsay Health Care, Inc.	33	22	50	—	—	—	—	—	—	—
★ △ ST. MARY'S MEDICAL CENTER, (Formerly St. Mary's Hospital) 305 South Fifth Street, Zip 73701–5899, Mailing Address: Box 232, Zip 73702–0232; tel. 405/233–6100; Jim O'Loughlin, Chief Executive Officer (Nonreporting) A1 2 3 5 7 9 10 S0048 Columbia/HCA Healthcare Corporation	33	10	177	—	—	—	—	—	—	—
EUFAULA—McIntosh County										
COMMUNITY HOSPITAL–LAKEVIEW, 1 Hospital Drive, Zip 74432, Mailing Address: P.O. Box 629, Zip 74432; tel. 918/689–2535; Sharon J. Steward, Administrator (Nonreporting) A9 10	33	10	33	—	—	—	—	—	—	—
FAIRFAX—Osage County										
★ FAIRFAX MEMORIAL HOSPITAL, Taft Avenue and Highway 18, Zip 74637, Mailing Address: Box 219, Zip 74637; tel. 918/642–3291; Annabeth Murray, Administrator A9 10 F19 20 22 26 28 32 33 35 44 46 71	14	10	21	401	6	1289	0	2211	978	52
FAIRVIEW—Major County										
★ FAIRVIEW HOSPITAL, 523 East State Road, Zip 73737; tel. 405/227–3721; Arthur H. Frable, Administrator (Nonreporting) A9 10	14	10	24	—	—	—	—	—	—	—
FORT SILL—Comanche County										
★ REYNOLDS ARMY COMMUNITY HOSPITAL, 4700 Hartell Boulevard, Zip 73503–6300; tel. 405/458–2000; Colonel Joseph Andronaco, Administrator A1 F3 7 8 13 17 18 19 20 21 22 24 25 28 29 30 34 35 37 39 40 41 42 44 45 46 49 51 54 56 58 60 63 65 67 71 72 73 P6 S9395 Department of the Army	42	10	116	6443	46	446923	938	—	—	1837
FORT SUPPLY—Woodward County										
☐ WESTERN STATE PSYCHIATRIC CENTER, (Formerly Western State Hospital) Mailing Address: P.O. Box 1, Zip 73841–0001; tel. 405/766–2311; Steve Norwood, Director A1 10 F2 3 12 16 20 41 52 53 54 55 56 57 58 59 65 73 P6 S0018 Oklahoma State Department of Mental Health and Substance Abuse Services	12	22	178	1237	157	28796	0	10279	5462	276
FREDERICK—Tillman County										
MEMORIAL HOSPITAL, 319 East Josephine, Zip 73542–2299; tel. 405/335–7565; Doug Weaver, Chief Executive Officer (Total facility includes 30 beds in nursing home–type unit) A9 10 F3 4 8 10 11 12 17 18 19 20 21 22 23 26 28 30 32 33 34 35 36 40 41 42 43 44 46 49 50 53 54 55 56 57 58 59 60 63 64 65 66 67 68 69 71 73 74	15	10	66	882	43	—	21	5016	2202	96
GROVE—Delaware County										
★ GROVE GENERAL HOSPITAL, 1310 South Main Street, Zip 74344–1310, Mailing Address: Box 1348, Zip 74344–1348; tel. 918/786–2243; Randy DuBois, Administrator A1 9 10 F2 3 4 5 6 7 8 9 10 11 13 15 16 17 18 19 20 21 22 23 25 26 27 28 30 31 32 33 34 35 36 37 38 40 41 42 43 44 47 48 49 50 51 52 53 54 55 56 57 58 59 60 61 62 63 64 65 66 67 68 69 70 71 72 73 74 S0305 Oklahoma Health System	23	10	62	2809	35	25587	154	13915	5758	308
GUTHRIE—Logan County										
★ LOGAN HOSPITAL AND MEDICAL CENTER, Highway 33 West at Academy Road, Zip 73044, Mailing Address: P.O. Box 1017, Zip 73044; tel. 405/282–6700; (Nonreporting) A9 10 S0305 Oklahoma Health System	16	10	50	—	—	—	—	—	—	—
GUYMON—Texas County										
★ MEMORIAL HOSPITAL OF TEXAS COUNTY, 520 Medical Drive, Zip 73942–4438; tel. 405/338–6515; Lu Ann Weldon, Administrator A9 10 F7 8 12 16 19 20 21 22 28 29 30 31 32 34 36 37 40 41 44 45 46 49 51 65 66 68 71 73 S0305 Oklahoma Health System	13	10	27	1569	18	6688	152	7551	2695	124

© 1995 AHA Guide

Hospitals, U.S. / OKLAHOMA

Hospital, Address, Telephone, Administrator, Approval, Facility, and Physician Codes, Health Care System	Classification Codes		Utilization Data					Expense (thousands) of dollars		
★ American Hospital Association (AHA) membership □ Joint Commission on Accreditation of Healthcare Organizations (JCAHO) accreditation + American Osteopathic Hospital Association (AOHA) membership ○ American Osteopathic Association (AOA) accreditation △ Commission on Accreditation of Rehabilitation Facilities (CARF) accreditation Control codes 61, 63, 64, 71, 72 and 73 indicate hospitals listed by AOHA, but not registered by AHA. For definition of numerical codes, see page A6	Control	Service	Beds	Admissions	Census	Outpatient Visits	Births	Total	Payroll	Personnel
HEALDTON—Carter County HEALDTON MUNICIPAL HOSPITAL, 918 S.W. Eighth Street, Zip 73438, Mailing Address: Box 928, Zip 73438; tel. 405/229-0701; Zeb Wright, Administrator (Nonreporting)	14	10	28	—	—	—	—	—	—	—
HENRYETTA—Okmulgee County ★ HENRYETTA MEDICAL CENTER, Dewey Bartlett & Main Streets, Zip 74437, Mailing Address: P.O. Box 1269, Zip 74437-1269; tel. 918/652-4463; James P. Bailey, Administrator and Chief Executive Officer **A**1 9 10 **F**7 8 14 19 22 26 32 34 40 44 49 52 57 64 71 **P**5 **S**0002 Quorum Health Group/Quorum Health Resources	16	10	52	587	13	7660	9	5447	2489	112
HOBART—Kiowa County ★ ELKVIEW GENERAL HOSPITAL, 429 West Elm Street, Zip 73651-1699; tel. 405/726-3324; J. W. Finch, Administrator **A**9 10 **F**7 8 11 15 16 19 21 22 32 42 44 45 49 56 71 **P**5	16	10	41	1150	17	6305	89	4132	1910	95
HOLDENVILLE—Hughes County ★ HOLDENVILLE GENERAL HOSPITAL, 100 Crestview Drive, Zip 74848-9700; tel. 405/379-6631; Charles M. Smith, Administrator **A**9 10 **F**8 19 20 22 28 32 42 44 46 49 71 **P**1 2 **S**0002 Quorum Health Group/Quorum Health Resources	14	10	27	871	11	—	0	4042	1682	82
HOLLIS—Harmon County ★ HARMON MEMORIAL HOSPITAL, 400 East Chestnut Street, Zip 73550, Mailing Address: P.O. Box 791, Zip 73550; tel. 405/688-3363; Calvin Castleman, Interim Administrator (Nonreporting) **A**9 10	13	10	20	—	—	—	—	—	—	—
HUGO—Choctaw County ★ CHOCTAW MEMORIAL HOSPITAL, 1405 East Kirk Road, Zip 74743; tel. 405/326-6414; Michael R. Morel, Administrator (Nonreporting) **A**9 10 **S**0305 Oklahoma Health System	16	10	52	—	—	—	—	—	—	—
IDABEL—Mccurtain County ★ MCCURTAIN MEMORIAL HOSPITAL, 1301 Lincoln, Zip 74745; tel. 405/286-7623; Ronald Campbell, Administrator (Nonreporting) **A**9 10	23	10	89	—	—	—	—	—	—	—
KINGFISHER—Kingfisher County ★ KINGFISHER REGIONAL HOSPITAL, 500 South Ninth Street, Zip 73750, Mailing Address: Box 59, Zip 73750-0059; tel. 405/375-3342; Steven G. Daniel, Administrator (Nonreporting) **A**9 10 **S**0002 Quorum Health Group/Quorum Health Resources	23	10	24	—	—	—	—	—	—	—
LAWTON—Comanche County ★ COMANCHE COUNTY MEMORIAL HOSPITAL, 3401 Gore Boulevard, Zip 73505-0129, Mailing Address: Box 129, Zip 73502-0129; tel. 405/355-8620; Randy Curry, President **A**1 9 10 **F**2 3 4 6 7 8 10 11 14 15 16 17 19 20 21 22 28 29 30 31 32 34 35 37 40 41 42 43 44 45 46 48 49 52 53 54 55 56 58 60 63 64 65 66 67 70 71 72 73 **P**6	16	10	289	8546	163	76651	723	88038	34327	1787
GREAT PLAINS HOSPITAL See Southwestern Psychiatric Center										
★ SOUTHWESTERN MEDICAL CENTER, 5602 S.W. Lee Boulevard, Zip 73505-9635, Mailing Address: P.O. Box 7290, Zip 73506-7290; tel. 405/531-4700; Ben White, Executive Director (Nonreporting) **A**1 2 9 10 **S**0048 Columbia/HCA Healthcare Corporation	33	10	110	—	—	—	—	—	—	—
SOUTHWESTERN PSYCHIATRIC CENTER, (Formerly Great Plains Hospital) 1602 S.W. 82nd Street, Zip 73505; tel. 405/536-0077; Jerry Cole, Administrator and Chief Executive Officer (Nonreporting) **A**10 **S**0054 Healthtrust, Inc	33	22	99	—	—	—	—	—	—	—
★ U.S. PUBLIC HEALTH SERVICE INDIAN HOSPITAL, 1515 Lawrie Tatum Road, Zip 73507; tel. 405/353-0350; George F. Howell, Chief Executive Officer (Nonreporting) **A**1 10 **S**9195 U.S. Public Health Service Indian Health Service	47	10	42	—	—	—	—	—	—	—
LINDSAY—Garvin County LINDSAY MUNICIPAL HOSPITAL, Highway 19 West, Zip 73052, Mailing Address: Box 888, Zip 73052; tel. 405/756-4321; Jim Standridge, Administrator **A**9 10 **F**19 22 32 44 71	16	10	25	711	10	2016	1	3691	1547	87
MADILL—Marshall County MARSHALL MEMORIAL HOSPITAL, 1 Hospital Drive, Zip 73446, Mailing Address: P.O. Box 827, Zip 73446; tel. 405/795-3384; Norma Howard, Administrator **A**9 10 **F**14 15 16 19 20 22 28 30 31 32 34 35 44 49 71 73 **S**0305 Oklahoma Health System	13	10	25	644	10	9849	1	3193	1683	83
MANGUM—Greer County MANGUM CITY HOSPITAL, One Wickersham Drive, Zip 73554, Mailing Address: Box 280, Zip 73554; tel. 405/782-3353; Kent A. Rader, Chief Executive Officer (Nonreporting) **A**9 10	14	10	40	—	—	—	—	—	—	—
MARIETTA—Love County ★ LOVE COUNTY HEALTH CENTER, 300 Wanda Street, Zip 73448; tel. 405/276-3347; Richard Barker, Administrator (Nonreporting) **A**9 10	13	10	30	—	—	—	—	—	—	—
MCALESTER—Caddo County ★ MCALESTER REGIONAL HEALTH CENTER, One Clark Bass Boulevard, Zip 74501-4267, Mailing Address: P.O. Box 1228, Zip 74502-1228; tel. 918/426-1800; Ed Majors, Chief Executive Officer **A**1 9 10 **F**7 8 10 19 21 22 31 32 33 34 35 36 37 39 40 41 42 44 48 49 63 64 65 71 73	16	10	198	5259	90	30569	702	26119	10681	515
MIAMI—Ottawa County ★ BAPTIST REGIONAL HEALTH CENTER, 200 Second Street S.W., Zip 74354, Mailing Address: Box 1207, Zip 74355-1207; tel. 918/542-6611; Randy DuBois, Administrator **A**1 9 10 **F**8 12 14 15 16 17 19 21 22 26 28 30 32 35 36 37 39 40 42 44 45 46 52 57 63 64 65 66 67 71 73 **P**2 4 6 7 8 **S**0305 Oklahoma Health System	23	10	124	4519	73	29277	276	25425	11342	455

Hospitals, U.S. / OKLAHOMA

Hospital, Address, Telephone, Administrator, Approval, Facility, and Physician Codes, Health Care System	Classification Codes		Utilization Data					Expense (thousands) of dollars		
★ American Hospital Association (AHA) membership □ Joint Commission on Accreditation of Healthcare Organizations (JCAHO) accreditation + American Osteopathic Hospital Association (AOHA) membership ○ American Osteopathic Association (AOA) accreditation △ Commission on Accreditation of Rehabilitation Facilities (CARF) accreditation Control codes 61, 63, 64, 71, 72 and 73 indicate hospitals listed by AOHA, but not registered by AHA. For definition of numerical codes, see page A6	Control	Service	Beds	Admissions	Census	Outpatient Visits	Births	Total	Payroll	Personnel
□ WILLOW CREST HOSPITAL, 130 A Street S.W., Zip 74354; tel. 918/542-1836; Kenneth O'Rourke, Administrator and Chief Executive Officer (Nonreporting) **A**1 9 10 **S**0044 Sterling Healthcare Corporation	33	22	50	—	—	—	—	—	—	—
MIDWEST CITY—Oklahoma County										
★ MIDWEST CITY REGIONAL HOSPITAL, 2825 Parklawn Drive, Zip 73110-4258; tel. 405/737-4411; Karl Weinmeister, President **A**1 2 9 10 **F**4 7 8 10 12 19 21 22 27 32 33 34 35 36 37 39 40 41 42 43 44 45 46 49 52 57 63 64 65 70 71 73 74 **P**5 8	16	10	206	7575	116	48097	563	58371	22788	878
MUSKOGEE—Muskogee County										
★ △ MUSKOGEE REGIONAL MEDICAL CENTER, 300 Edna M. Rockefeller Drive, Zip 74401; tel. 918/682-5501; Bill R. Kennedy, President and Chief Executive Officer **A**1 2 7 9 10 **F**7 8 10 12 15 16 17 19 20 21 22 23 30 32 34 35 37 40 42 44 46 48 52 60 65 67 71 72 73	16	10	225	8705	138	—	1048	54955	24249	929
★ VETERANS AFFAIRS MEDICAL CENTER, Honor Heights Drive, Zip 74401-1399; tel. 918/683-3261 **A**1 3 5 **F**1 3 4 8 10 12 19 20 21 22 23 24 25 26 27 29 31 32 34 35 37 39 41 42 43 44 45 46 49 50 51 54 56 58 59 60 61 65 67 69 71 72 73 74 **P**6 **S**9295 Department of Veterans Affairs	45	10	140	4285	82	126915	0	59177	29521	645
NORMAN—Cleveland County										
□ GRIFFIN MEMORIAL HOSPITAL, 900 East Main Street, Zip 73070-0101, Mailing Address: Box 151, Zip 73070; tel. 405/321-4880; Stand LaBoon, Superintendent **A**1 3 5 10 **F**4 8 19 20 21 22 35 39 44 46 50 52 54 55 56 65 71 73 **P**6 **S**0018 Oklahoma State Department of Mental Health and Substance Abuse Services	12	22	215	2216	186	5979	0	22514	14857	572
□ J. D. MCCARTY CENTER FOR CHILDREN WITH DEVELOPMENTAL DISABILITIES, 1125 East Alameda, Zip 73071-5264; tel. 405/321-4830; Curtis A. Peters, Chief Executive Officer **A**1 10 **F**20 34 39 48 49 54 65 73 **P**6	12	56	36	131	23	845	0	3491	2153	99
★ NORMAN REGIONAL HOSPITAL, 901 North Porter Street, Zip 73071, Mailing Address: Box 1308, Zip 73070-1308; tel. 405/321-1700; Craig W. Jones, President and Chief Executive Officer (Nonreporting) **A**1 2 9 10	16	10	236							
NOWATA—Nowata County										
★ JANE PHILLIPS NOWATA HEALTH CENTER, 237 South Locust Street, Zip 74048-0426, Mailing Address: P.O. Box 426, Zip 74048-0426; tel. 918/273-3102; Maggie Blevins, Administrator (Nonreporting) **A**9 10	23	10	24	—	—	—	—	—	—	—
OKEENE—Blaine County										
OKEENE MUNICIPAL HOSPITAL, 207 East F Street, Zip 73763, Mailing Address: P.O. Box 489, Zip 73763; tel. 405/822-4417; Patty Lamle, Administrator (Total facility includes 44 beds in nursing home–type unit) **A**9 10 **F**19 22 26 28 29 30 31 32 34 36 39 41 44 49 **P**5	14	10	74	558	42	1850	101	2244	1413	103
OKLAHOMA CITY—Oklahoma County										
★ △ BAPTIST MEDICAL CENTER OF OKLAHOMA, 3300 N.W. Expressway, Zip 73112-4481; tel. 405/949-3011; Stanley F. Hupfeld, President **A**1 2 3 5 7 9 10 **F**4 7 8 9 10 11 12 14 15 16 17 19 21 22 24 25 26 30 31 33 34 35 38 39 41 42 43 44 46 47 48 49 54 55 56 57 60 61 65 67 68 69 71 72 73 74 **P**1 2 5 6 7 8 **S**0305 Oklahoma Health System	23	10	529	22546	366	38910	2320	202333	77365	3321
★ BONE AND JOINT HOSPITAL, 1111 North Dewey Avenue, Zip 73103-2615; tel. 405/272-9671; James A. Hyde, Administrator **A**1 3 5 9 10 **F**5 14 17 19 21 22 34 35 44 45 65 71	23	47	67	2700	19	2540	0	17792	6980	258
★ DEACONESS HOSPITAL, 5501 North Portland Avenue, Zip 73112-2097; tel. 405/946-5581; John P. Ellis, Administrator **A**1 2 9 10 **F**4 7 8 10 11 12 16 19 21 22 23 24 26 28 31 32 33 34 35 37 38 40 41 42 43 44 46 49 52 54 57 58 60 63 64 65 71 73 74 **P**8	23	10	206	7335	131	46752	1204	49703	25171	825
□ △ HEALTHSOUTH REHABILITATION HOSPITAL, 700 N.W. Seventh Street, Zip 73102-1295; tel. 405/236-3131; Ronald J. Castagnl FACHE, Chief Executive Officer (Nonreporting) **A**1 7 10 **S**0023 Healthsouth Corporation	33	46	46	—	—	—	—	—	—	—
★ HIGH POINTE, 6501 N.E. 50th Street, Zip 73141-9613; tel. 405/424-3383; Charlene Arnett, Chief Executive Officer (Nonreporting) **A**10 **S**0665 Century Healthcare Corporation	33	22	68							
★ + ○ HILLCREST HEALTH CENTER, 2129 S.W. 59th Street, Zip 73119-7001; tel. 405/680-2105; John E. Barrett Jr., Chief Executive Officer (Nonreporting) **A**9 10 11 12 13	23	10	186							
★ MERCY HEALTH CENTER, 4300 West Memorial Road, Zip 73120-8362; tel. 405/755-1515; Bruce Forrest Buchanan FACHE, President and Chief Executive Officer **A**1 2 9 10 **F**1 4 7 8 10 11 12 14 15 16 17 18 19 21 22 24 25 26 27 28 29 30 31 32 33 34 35 36 37 38 39 40 41 42 43 44 45 47 48 49 51 52 53 54 55 56 58 59 60 64 65 67 71 73 74 **P**1 4 **S**5185 Sisters of Mercy Health System–St. Louis	21	10	385	11257	195	85625	1763	102771	46754	1510
★ PRESBYTERIAN HOSPITAL, 700 N.E. 13th Street, Zip 73104-5070; tel. 405/271-5100; David L. Dunlap, Chief Executive Officer (Nonreporting) **A**1 2 3 5 9 10 **S**0048 Columbia/HCA Healthcare Corporation	33	10	354							
★ △ SOUTHWEST MEDICAL CENTER OF OKLAHOMA, 4401 South Western, Zip 73109-3413; tel. 405/636-7000; Bob Phillips, President and Chief Executive Officer **A**1 2 7 9 10 **F**4 7 8 10 11 12 14 15 16 17 19 21 22 24 26 27 28 30 31 32 33 36 37 39 40 41 42 43 44 48 49 51 54 55 56 58 59 60 64 65 66 67 69 71 73 74 **P**1 3 **S**0305 Oklahoma Health System	23	10	298	10640	210	129577	902	93162	35214	1435
★ △ ST. ANTHONY HOSPITAL, 1000 North Lee Street, Zip 73102, Mailing Address: Box 205, Zip 73101-0205; tel. 405/272-7000; Steven L. Hunter, President **A**1 2 3 5 7 9 10 **F**1 2 3 4 7 8 10 11 12 14 15 16 17 19 20 21 22 24 25 26 28 29 30 31 32 34 35 37 39 40 41 42 43 44 48 49 51 52 53 54 55 56 57 58 59 60 61 63 65 66 67 69 71 73 **P**1 7 **S**5455 SSM Health Care System	21	10	247	13084	256	103278	1101	116845	60677	1598

© 1995 AHA Guide

Hospitals, U.S. / OKLAHOMA

Hospital, Address, Telephone, Administrator, Approval, Facility, and Physician Codes, Health Care System	Classification Codes		Utilization Data					Expense (thousands) of dollars		
	Control	Service	Beds	Admissions	Census	Outpatient Visits	Births	Total	Payroll	Personnel
★ △ UNIVERSITY HOSPITALS, (Includes Children's Hospital of Oklahoma, 940 N.E. 13th Street, Oklahoma City, Oklahoma, Zip 73104, Mailing Address: P.O. Box 26307, Zip 73126; tel. 405/271–6165; Mike Noel, Administrator; O'Donoghue Rehabilitation Institute, 1122 N.E. 13th Street, Oklahoma City, Oklahoma, Zip 73104, Mailing Address: P.O. Box 26307, Zip 73126; tel. 405/271–6955; Karen Mumina, Administrator; Oklahoma Memorial Hospital, 800 N.E. 13th Street, Oklahoma City, Oklahoma, Zip 73104, Mailing Address: Box 26307, Zip 73126; tel. 405/271–6644) 800 N.E. 13th Street, Zip 73104–5068, Mailing Address: P.O. Box 26307, Zip 73126; tel. 405/271–5911; R. Timothy Coussons M.D., Chief Executive Officer (Nonreporting) **A**1 2 3 5 7 8 9 10	12	10	420	—	—	—	—	—	—	—
★ VETERANS AFFAIRS MEDICAL CENTER, 921 N.E. 13th Street, Zip 73104–5028; tel. 405/270–0501; Steven J. Gentling, Director **A**1 3 5 8 **F**2 3 11 15 16 22 34 37 44 48 52 **P**6 **S**9295 Department of Veterans Affairs	45	10	297	8569	213	215812	0	118680	53408	1681
OKMULGEE—Okmulgee County										
GEORGE NIGH REHABILITATION INSTITUTE, 900 East Airport Road, Zip 74447, Mailing Address: P.O. Box 1118, Zip 74447; tel. 918/756–9211; Mitchell Townsend, Administrator **A**10 **F**19 21 32 35 41 45 46 48 49 50 54 60 63 65 71 73	12	46	48	230	15	0	0	3202	1816	74
★ OMH MEDICAL CENTER, 1401 Morris Drive, Zip 74447, Mailing Address: Box 1038, Zip 74447; tel. 918/756–4233; David D. Rasmussen, Administrator **A**1 9 10 **F**8 15 19 20 22 26 44 52 57 65 71 73 **P**5	23	10	66	2624	34	—	461	11700	5188	199
PAULS VALLEY—Garvin County										
☐ PAULS VALLEY GENERAL HOSPITAL, 100 Valley Drive, Zip 73075–0368, Mailing Address: Box 368, Zip 73075–0368; tel. 405/238–5501; Charles Johnston, Administrator (Total facility includes 8 beds in nursing home–type unit) **A**1 9 10 **F**7 8 12 19 20 22 28 32 33 34 37 40 44 46 49 64 65 71	14	10	42	1604	23	13558	108	7405	3235	110
PAWHUSKA—Osage County										
★ PAWHUSKA HOSPITAL, 1101 East 15th Street, Zip 74056; tel. 918/287–3232; Samuel T. Guild, Administrator (Nonreporting) **A**9 10	23	10	25							
PAWNEE—Pawnee County										
★ PAWNEE MUNICIPAL HOSPITAL, 1212 Fourth Street, Zip 74058, Mailing Address: Box 467, Zip 74058; tel. 918/762–2577; Dan A. Clements, Administrator (Nonreporting) **A**9 10 **S**0305 Oklahoma Health System	33	10	40	—	—	—	—	—	—	—
PERRY—Noble County										
★ PERRY MEMORIAL HOSPITAL, 501 14th Street, Zip 73077–5099; tel. 405/336–3541; Judith K. Feuquay, Chief Executive Officer **A**1 9 10 **F**8 12 15 16 19 21 22 29 32 33 34 44 71 73 **P**5 8 **S**0002 Quorum Health Group/Quorum Health Resources	16	10	28	847	11	11688	30	3919	1623	76
PONCA CITY—Kay County										
★ ST. JOSEPH REGIONAL MEDICAL CENTER OF NORTHERN OKLAHOMA, 14th Street & Hartford Avenue, Zip 74601–2035, Mailing Address: Box 1270, Zip 74602–1270; tel. 405/765–3321; Garry L. England, President and Chief Executive Officer **A**1 9 10 **F**4 7 8 11 12 14 15 16 19 21 22 23 24 27 28 30 31 32 34 35 36 37 39 40 44 49 52 54 56 59 60 63 65 67 71 73 **S**5435 CSJ Health System of Wichita	21	10	75	3760	50	43398	615	24319	10211	364
POTEAU—Le Flore County										
★ EASTERN OKLAHOMA MEDICAL CENTER, 105 Wall Street, Zip 74953, Mailing Address: P.O. Box 1148, Zip 74953; tel. 918/647–8161; Bobby D. Cox, Chief Executive Officer **A**1 9 10 **F**7 8 11 14 15 16 19 22 23 28 32 33 34 37 40 42 44 65 70 71 73	16	10	84	3154	36	21036	400	14150	6091	318
PRYOR—Mayes County										
★ MAYES COUNTY MEDICAL CENTER, (Formerly Grand Valley Hospital) 129 North Kentucky, Zip 74361, Mailing Address: Box 278, Zip 74362–0278; tel. 918/825–1600; Charles Jordan, Administrator (Nonreporting) **A**1 9 10 **S**0305 Oklahoma Health System	23	10	43	—	—	—	—	—	—	—
PURCELL—McClain County										
★ PURCELL MUNICIPAL HOSPITAL, 1500 North Green Avenue, Zip 73080, Mailing Address: P.O. Box 511, Zip 73080–0511; tel. 405/527–6524; Joe Duerr, Administrator **A**9 10 **F**7 17 19 22 25 28 30 33 39 40 44 71 73 **P**5 **S**0002 Quorum Health Group/Quorum Health Resources	14	10	36	1432	18	20146	108	5483	2181	140
SALLISAW—Sequoyah County										
SEQUOYAH MEMORIAL HOSPITAL, 213 East Redwood Street, Zip 74955, Mailing Address: Box 505, Zip 74955–0505; tel. 918/775–4483; Ruth Ann Roark, Administrator (Nonreporting) **A**9 10	15	10	50	—	—	—	—	—	—	—
SAPULPA—Creek County										
☐ BARTLETT MEMORIAL MEDICAL CENTER, 519 South Division Street, Zip 74066, Mailing Address: Box 1368, Zip 74067–1368; tel. 918/224–4280; Barbara Benedict, Chief Executive Officer (Nonreporting) **A**1 9 10	23	10	113							
SAYRE—Beckham County										
★ SAYRE MEMORIAL HOSPITAL, 501 East Washington Street, Zip 73662, Mailing Address: Box 680, Zip 73662; tel. 405/928–5541; Larry Anderson, Administrator (Nonreporting) **A**9 10	23	10	46							
SEILING—Dewey County										
SEILING HOSPITAL, Highway 60 N.E., Zip 73663, Mailing Address: P.O. Box 720, Zip 73663–0720; tel. 405/922–7361; Winnetta Marsh, Administrator (Data for 315 days) **A**9 10 **F**15 19 22 32 44 71 73	14	10	18	413	6	2183	0	1022	538	38

Hospitals, U.S. / OKLAHOMA

Hospital, Address, Telephone, Administrator, Approval, Facility, and Physician Codes, Health Care System	Classification Codes		Utilization Data					Expense (thousands) of dollars		
★ American Hospital Association (AHA) membership □ Joint Commission on Accreditation of Healthcare Organizations (JCAHO) accreditation + American Osteopathic Hospital Association (AOHA) membership ○ American Osteopathic Association (AOA) accreditation △ Commission on Accreditation of Rehabilitation Facilities (CARF) accreditation Control codes 61, 63, 64, 71, 72 and 73 indicate hospitals listed by AOHA, but not registered by AHA. For definition of numerical codes, see page A6	Control	Service	Beds	Admissions	Census	Outpatient Visits	Births	Total	Payroll	Personnel
SEMINOLE—Seminole County										
★ SEMINOLE MUNICIPAL HOSPITAL, 606 West Evans Street, Zip 74868, Mailing Address: P.O. Box 2130, Zip 74818–2130; tel. 405/382–0600; Bruce A. Bennett, President and Chief Executive Officer (Nonreporting) **A**9 10 **S**0002 Quorum Health Group/Quorum Health Resources	14	10	39	—	—	—	—	—	—	—
SHATTUCK—Ellis County										
★ NEWMAN MEMORIAL HOSPITAL, 905 South Main Street, Zip 73858–9602, Mailing Address: Box 279, Zip 73858–0279; tel. 405/938–2551; Gary W. Mitchell, Chief Executive Officer **A**1 9 10 **F**7 8 14 15 16 19 21 22 24 30 32 34 36 37 40 44 49 65 66 71 73 **P**5	23	10	54	919	11	47850	110	5527	2578	126
SHAWNEE—Pottawatomie County										
★ MISSION HILL MEMORIAL HOSPITAL, 1900 Gordon Cooper Drive, Zip 74801; tel. 405/273–2240; Thomas G. Honaker III, Administrator **A**1 9 10 **F**7 8 10 19 22 25 30 32 33 35 37 39 40 44 51 65 71 73 **P**4 8 **S**0585 Brim, Inc.	16	10	78	1698	21	—	0	7505	3326	174
□ OAK CREST HOSPITAL, 1601 Gordon Cooper Drive, Zip 74801; tel. 405/275–9610; Rodger Hopkins, Administrator **A**1 10 **F**2 52 **P**6 **S**0044 Sterling Healthcare Corporation	33	22	50	565	20	14835	0	6402	2908	112
★ SHAWNEE REGIONAL HOSPITAL, 1102 West MacArthur, Zip 74801, Mailing Address: Box 909, Zip 74801; tel. 405/273–2270; Robert F. Maynard, Chief Executive Officer **A**1 9 10 **F**7 8 16 17 19 21 22 26 28 30 32 33 34 35 37 40 42 44 49 60 65 66 71 73	23	10	106	3782	43	66452	901	22259	9320	369
SPENCER—Oklahoma County										
★ WILLOW VIEW MENTAL HEALTH SYSTEM, 2601 Spencer Road, Zip 73084–3699, Mailing Address: P.O. Box 11137, Oklahoma City Zip 73136–0137; tel. 405/427–2441; Gary L. Watson, Chief Executive Officer **A**1 10 **F**3 12 26 34 52 53 54 55 56 57 58 59 65 **P**6 **S**0002 Quorum Health Group/Quorum Health Resources	23	22	74	699	38	25090	0	8276	4776	150
STIGLER—Haskell County										
★ HASKELL COUNTY HOSPITAL, 401 N.W. H Street, Zip 74462; tel. 918/967–4682; John C. Neal, Administrator and Chief Executive Officer **A**9 10 **F**8 15 16 21 22 28 32 33 34 37 41 42 44 64 65 71 73	13	10	31	706	10	6854	1	3775	2034	120
STILLWATER—Payne County										
★ STILLWATER MEDICAL CENTER, 1323 West Sixth Avenue, Zip 74074, Mailing Address: Box 2408, Zip 74076–2408; tel. 405/372–1480; Jerry G. Moeller, President and Chief Executive Officer (Total facility includes 18 beds in nursing home-type unit) **A**1 9 10 **F**8 10 14 15 16 19 21 22 23 31 32 33 34 35 36 37 40 41 44 46 49 56 60 63 64 65 71 73 **P**8	16	10	107	4201	54	50240	774	30244	12206	515
STROUD—Lincoln County										
★ STROUD MUNICIPAL HOSPITAL, Highway 66 West, Zip 74079, Mailing Address: P.O. Box 530, Zip 74079; tel. 918/968–3571; Jerrell J. Horton, Chief Executive Officer **A**9 10 **F**8 15 16 21 22 28 29 32 33 37 44 46 65 71 73 **S**0305 Oklahoma Health System	23	10	30	524	8	5269	34	—	—	73
SULPHUR—Murray County										
ARBUCKLE MEMORIAL HOSPITAL, 2011 West Broadway, Zip 73086, Mailing Address: Box 411, Zip 73086; tel. 405/622–2161; Marvin R. Hyde, Administrator (Nonreporting) **A**9 10	13	10	58	—	—	—	—	—	—	—
TAHLEQUAH—Cherokee County										
★ TAHLEQUAH CITY HOSPITAL, 1400 East Downing Street, Zip 74464, Mailing Address: Box 1008, Zip 74465–1008; tel. 918/456–0641; L. Gene Matthews, Chief Executive Officer **A**1 9 10 **F**8 15 16 19 21 22 28 30 32 33 34 35 37 39 40 44 45 49 71 73 **S**0002 Quorum Health Group/Quorum Health Resources	16	10	65	2208	27	54191	271	14653	6205	269
★ WILLIAM W. HASTINGS INDIAN HOSPITAL, 100 South Bliss Avenue, Zip 74464–3399; tel. 918/458–3100; John A. Boren, Acting Administrator **A**1 10 **F**7 8 12 13 15 17 19 20 22 28 31 32 34 37 39 40 44 52 53 54 55 56 57 58 65 71 73 **P**6 **S**9195 U.S. Public Health Service Indian Health Service	47	10	60	3210	32	167077	1041	30921	13179	411
TALIHINA—Latimer County										
★ CHOCTAW NATION INDIAN HOSPITAL, Route 2, Box 1725, Zip 74571; tel. 918/567–2211; Bat Shunatona, Administrator (Nonreporting) **A**1 10 **S**9195 U.S. Public Health Service Indian Health Service	47	10	52	—	—	—	—	—	—	—
TINKER AIR FORCE BASE—De Kalb County										
★ U.S. AIR FORCE HOSPITAL TINKER, 5700 Arnold Street, Zip 73145; tel. 405/734–8211; Colonel David D. Bissell USAF, MC, Commander **A**1 **F**3 7 8 12 14 16 19 20 22 28 30 35 39 40 41 44 45 49 51 58 71 **S**9495 Department of the Air Force	41	10	25	3576	21	253000	600	—	—	589
TISHOMINGO—Johnston County										
JOHNSTON MEMORIAL HOSPITAL, 1101 South Byrd Street, Zip 73460–3299; tel. 405/371–2327; Garry D. Crain, Administrator and Chief Executive Officer (Nonreporting) **A**9 10	13	10	33	—	—	—	—	—	—	—
TULSA—Tulsa County										
□ BROOKHAVEN HOSPITAL, 201 South Garnett Road, Zip 74128; tel. 918/438–4257; Lance Beard, Chief Executive Officer and Administrator (Nonreporting) **A**1 9 10	31	22	40	—	—	—	—	—	—	—
★ CHILDREN'S MEDICAL CENTER, 5300 East Skelly Drive, Zip 74135–6599, Mailing Address: Box 35648, Zip 74153–0648; tel. 918/664–6600; Gerard J. Rothlein Jr., President and Chief Executive Officer (Nonreporting) **A**1 3 5 9 10	23	52	108	—	—	—	—	—	—	—

© 1995 AHA Guide

Hospitals, U.S. / OKLAHOMA

Hospital, Address, Telephone, Administrator, Approval, Facility, and Physician Codes, Health Care System	Classification Codes		Utilization Data					Expense (thousands) of dollars		
★ American Hospital Association (AHA) membership □ Joint Commission on Accreditation of Healthcare Organizations (JCAHO) accreditation + American Osteopathic Hospital Association (AOHA) membership ○ American Osteopathic Association (AOA) accreditation △ Commission on Accreditation of Rehabilitation Facilities (CARF) accreditation Control codes 61, 63, 64, 71, 72 and 73 indicate hospitals listed by AOHA, but not registered by AHA. For definition of numerical codes, see page A6	Control	Service	Beds	Admissions	Census	Outpatient Visits	Births	Total	Payroll	Personnel
★ DOCTORS' HOSPITAL, 2323 South Harvard Avenue, Zip 74114-3370; tel. 918/744-4000; Anthony R. Young, President and Chief Executive Officer (Data for 335 days) **A**1 9 10 **F**7 19 21 22 26 29 31 32 35 37 40 41 44 49 52 57 59 64 65 71 73 **P**1 7 **S**0048 Columbia/HCA Healthcare Corporation	33	10	148	3151	60	24885	905	21115	9642	525
★ △ HILLCREST MEDICAL CENTER, 1120 South Utica, Zip 74104-4090; tel. 918/579-1000; Donald A. Lorack Jr., President and Chief Executive Officer (Total facility includes 32 beds in nursing home–type unit) **A**1 2 3 5 7 9 10 **F**4 5 7 8 9 10 11 12 15 17 18 19 20 21 22 23 24 25 26 27 28 29 30 31 32 34 35 37 38 39 40 41 42 43 44 45 46 48 49 52 54 55 56 57 58 59 60 61 64 65 66 67 69 71 72 73 74 **P**3	23	10	446	16939	278	74856	3528	132526	47942	1693
★ LAUREATE PSYCHIATRIC CLINIC AND HOSPITAL, 6655 South Yale, Zip 74136; tel. 918/481-4000; James R. Hardman FACHE, Chief Executive Officer **A**1 3 5 10 **F**3 12 16 17 18 19 21 22 27 30 35 39 41 52 53 54 55 56 57 58 59 63 65 68 70 71 73 **P**6	23	22	75	1116	28	15012	0	11387	6996	206
□ MEMORIAL MEDICAL CENTER, 8181 South Lewis, Zip 74137; tel. 918/496-5000; Joseph A. Gagliardi, President (Nonreporting) **A**1 10	33	10	71	—	—	—	—	—	—	—
PARKSIDE HOSPITAL, 1620 East 12th Street, Zip 74120-5499; tel. 918/582-2131; Quentin Henley, Chief Executive Officer (Nonreporting) **A**3 5 10	23	22	20	—	—	—	—	—	—	—
★ SAINT FRANCIS HOSPITAL, 6161 South Yale Avenue, Zip 74136-1992; tel. 918/494-2200; James R. Hardman FACHE, Chief Executive Officer **A**1 2 3 5 8 9 10 **F**2 3 4 7 8 10 11 12 15 16 17 18 19 20 21 22 23 24 25 28 29 30 31 32 33 34 35 37 38 39 40 41 42 43 44 45 46 47 48 49 51 52 53 54 55 56 57 58 59 60 63 64 65 66 67 68 69 70 71 72 73 74 **P**1 4 5 6	21	10	621	26097	434	231346	2784	213936	93471	3162
□ SHADOW MOUNTAIN HOSPITAL, (Formerly Shadow Mountain Institute) 6262 South Sheridan Road, Zip 74133-4099; tel. 918/492-8200; Mark M. Jackson, Chief Executive Officer (Nonreporting) **A**1 9	33	52	40	—	—	—	—	—	—	—
★ △ ST. JOHN MEDICAL CENTER, 1923 South Utica Avenue, Zip 74104-5445; tel. 918/744-2345; Sister M. Therese Gottschalk, President **A**1 2 3 5 7 9 10 **F**1 2 3 4 7 8 10 11 12 14 15 16 17 18 19 20 21 22 23 24 26 28 29 30 31 32 33 34 35 37 38 39 40 41 42 43 45 47 48 49 51 52 53 54 55 56 57 58 59 60 41 62 65 66 67 68 69 70 71 73 74 **P**5 7 **S**5305 Sisters of the Sorrowful Mother United States Health System	21	10	597	19302	378	81659	1737	175326	68388	3112
★ + ○ △ TULSA REGIONAL MEDICAL CENTER, 744 West Ninth Street, Zip 74127-9990; tel. 918/599-5900; James M. MacCallum, President and Chief Executive Officer **A**7 9 10 11 12 13 **F**3 4 7 8 10 11 12 15 16 19 21 22 23 26 28 29 30 31 32 34 35 37 39 40 41 42 43 44 45 46 48 49 50 52 53 54 55 56 57 58 59 60 61 63 64 65 66 67 68 69 70 71 73 **P**3 4 8	23	10	345	10763	204	118476	946	93929	39957	1388
VINITA—Craig County										
★ CRAIG GENERAL HOSPITAL, 735 North Foreman Street, Zip 74301-1418, Mailing Address: Box 326, Zip 74301-0326; tel. 918/256-7551; B. Joe Gunn FACHE, Administrator and Chief Executive Officer **A**1 9 10 **F**8 11 14 15 16 19 22 28 30 32 34 37 39 40 44 45 46 49 65 71 73 **P**8	13	10	34	1111	12	15037	108	6202	2792	119
□ EASTERN STATE HOSPITAL, 720 North Brown, Zip 74301, Mailing Address: P.O. Box 69, Zip 74301; tel. 918/256-7841; Jerald Goodner FACHE, Acting Superintendent **A**1 10 **F**20 26 31 45 46 52 55 56 65 73 **P**6	12	22	324	2219	277	0	0	27089	15550	597
WAGONER—Wagoner County										
★ WAGONER COMMUNITY HOSPITAL, 1200 West Cherokee, Zip 74467-4681, Mailing Address: Box 407, Zip 74477-0407; tel. 918/485-5514; John W. Crawford, Chief Executive Officer **A**1 9 10 **F**2 3 8 12 15 16 17 19 22 24 28 29 30 31 34 37 41 44 45 46 49 52 55 56 57 58 65 71 73 74 **P**7 8 **S**0048 Columbia/HCA Healthcare Corporation	33	10	100	2320	51	12521	0	11423	4499	242
WATONGA—Blaine County										
★ WATONGA MUNICIPAL HOSPITAL, 500 North Nash Boulevard, Zip 73772-0370, Mailing Address: Box 370, Zip 73772-0370; tel. 405/623-7211; Frank D. Loveless, Administrator (Nonreporting) **A**9 10 **S**0305 Oklahoma Health System	14	10	25	—	—	—	—	—	—	—
WAURIKA—Jefferson County										
★ JEFFERSON COUNTY HOSPITAL, Mailing Address: P.O. Box 90, Zip 73573-0090; tel. 405/228-2344; Curtis R. Pryor, Administrator (Nonreporting) **A**9 10	13	10	31	—	—	—	—	—	—	—
WEATHERFORD—Custer County										
★ SOUTHWESTERN MEMORIAL HOSPITAL, 215 North Kansas Street, Zip 73096-5499; tel. 405/772-5551; Ronnie D. Walker, President **A**9 10 **F**7 19 28 44 71	16	10	60	858	8	11578	189	3797	1923	75
WETUMKA—Hughes County										
□ WETUMKA GENERAL HOSPITAL, 325 South Washita, Zip 74883-5500; tel. 405/452-3276; Carolyn Keesee, Administrator (Nonreporting) **A**1 9 10	14	10	34	—	—	—	—	—	—	—
WILBURTON—Latimer County										
LATIMER COUNTY GENERAL HOSPITAL, 806 Highway 2 North, Zip 74578; tel. 918/465-2391; Hershel Earp, Administrator (Nonreporting) **A**9 10	13	10	33	—	—	—	—	—	—	—
WOODWARD—Harper County										
★ WOODWARD HOSPITAL AND HEALTH CENTER, 900 17th Street, Zip 73801; tel. 405/256-5511; Warren K. Spellman, Administrator **A**1 9 10 **F**7 8 11 13 17 19 21 22 26 28 30 31 32 33 36 37 39 40 41 42 44 49 52 57 61 62 64 65 66 67 71 72 73 **P**4 5 8 **S**0002 Quorum Health Group/Quorum Health Resources	23	10	68	1725	29	19375	258	12490	5142	237

OREGON

Resident population 3,032 (in thousands)
Resident population in metro areas 70.0%
Birth rate per 1,000 population 14.5
65 years and over 13.8%
Percent of persons without health insurance 13.3%

- ★ American Hospital Association (AHA) membership
- ☐ Joint Commission on Accreditation of Healthcare Organizations (JCAHO) accreditation
- + American Osteopathic Hospital Association (AOHA) membership
- ○ American Osteopathic Association (AOA) accreditation
- △ Commission on Accreditation of Rehabilitation Facilities (CARF) accreditation

Control codes 61, 63, 64, 71, 72 and 73 indicate hospitals listed by AOHA, but not registered by AHA. For definition of numerical codes, see page A6

Hospital, Address, Telephone, Administrator, Approval, Facility, and Physician Codes, Health Care System	Classification Codes		Utilization Data					Expense (thousands) of dollars		
	Control	Service	Beds	Admissions	Census	Outpatient Visits	Births	Total	Payroll	Personnel
ALBANY—Linn County ★ ALBANY GENERAL HOSPITAL, 1046 West Sixth Avenue, Zip 97321–1999; tel. 503/926–2244; Richard J. Delano, President **A**1 2 9 10 **F**7 8 10 12 17 19 21 22 28 29 30 32 33 34 35 37 39 40 41 42 44 46 49 56 59 60 65 67 68 70 71 72 73 **P**5 6	23	10	71	3467	32	41770	600	24916	11494	247
ASHLAND—Jackson County ☐ ASHLAND COMMUNITY HOSPITAL, 280 Maple Street, Zip 97520, Mailing Address: Box 98, Zip 97520; tel. 503/482–2441; James R. Watson, Administrator **A**1 9 10 **F**7 8 15 16 19 22 28 30 32 34 36 37 40 44 45 46 64 65 70 71 **P**5	14	10	37	1541	14	24910	287	11608	5162	193
ASTORIA—Clatsop County ★ COLUMBIA MEMORIAL HOSPITAL, 2111 Exchange Street, Zip 97103; tel. 503/338–7505; Terry O. Finklein, Chief Executive Officer **A**1 9 10 **F**7 8 14 19 21 22 28 32 33 37 39 40 41 42 44 46 49 65 70 71 73 **P**5	23	10	37	1782	16	37750	397	13867	6229	222
BAKER CITY—Baker County ☐ ST. ELIZABETH HEALTH SERVICES, (Formerly St. Elizabeth Hospital and Medical Center) 3325 Pocahontas Road, Zip 97814; tel. 503/523–6461; Rod Barton, President and Chief Operating Officer (Total facility includes 112 beds in nursing home–type unit) **A**1 9 10 **F**7 8 14 19 22 26 28 30 32 34 35 37 40 41 44 49 64 67 70 71 **P**5 **S**5325 Franciscan Health System	21	10	154	1208	95	25424	117	12670	5530	153
BANDON—Coos County ★ SOUTHERN COOS GENERAL HOSPITAL, 640 West Fourth, Zip 97411; tel. 503/347–2426; Daniel L. Smith HRM, Administrator **A**9 10 **F**14 22 34 44 49	16	10	18	175	2	5366	0	1612	747	35
BEND—Deschutes County ★ ST. CHARLES MEDICAL CENTER, 2500 N.E. Neff Road, Zip 97701–6015; tel. 503/382–4321 **A**1 2 3 9 10 **F**4 7 10 12 14 15 16 19 21 22 23 25 28 30 32 35 37 38 40 41 42 43 44 45 48 49 52 54 60 63 65 67 70 71 73 **P**5	23	10	181	9034	97	55369	1286	65628	29424	868
BURNS—Harney County HARNEY DISTRICT HOSPITAL, 557 West Washington Street, Zip 97720–1497; tel. 503/573–7281; David L. Harman, Administrator **A**9 10 **F**7 14 15 16 17 34 37 40 44 70 71 **P**8	16	10	44	383	4	26762	57	3597	1547	52
CLACKAMAS—Clackamas County ★ KAISER FOUNDATION HOSPITAL, 10200 S.E. Sunnyside Road, Zip 97015–9303; tel. 503/652–2880; Alide Chase, Administrator **A**1 2 10 **F**3 4 7 8 10 16 19 21 22 23 29 30 31 32 33 34 35 37 40 41 42 43 44 45 49 53 54 55 56 57 61 65 66 69 71 72 73 **P**6 **S**2105 Kaiser Foundation Hospitals	23	10	177	12350	133	231728	1715	—	—	1291
COOS BAY—Coos County ★ BAY AREA HOSPITAL, 1775 Thompson Road, Zip 97420–2198; tel. 503/269–8111; Colleen A. Chapp R.N., Interim Chief Executive Officer **A**1 2 9 10 **F**7 11 12 14 16 17 19 21 22 23 31 32 33 34 35 37 40 41 44 45 46 49 52 53 54 56 58 59 60 65 67 70 71 72 73 **P**5	16	10	129	6632	76	43442	622	45021	22653	624
COQUILLE—Coos County COQUILLE VALLEY HOSPITAL, 940 East Fifth Street, Zip 97423; tel. 503/396–3101; Edna J. Cotner, Administrator **A**9 10 **F**7 22 32 34 40 44 71	16	10	30	331	2	6314	56	2636	1133	49
CORVALLIS—Benton County ★ GOOD SAMARITAN HOSPITAL CORVALLIS, 3600 N.W. Samaritan Drive, Zip 97330, Mailing Address: Box 1068, Zip 97339; tel. 503/757–5111; Larry A. Mullins, President and Chief Executive Officer **A**1 2 9 10 **F**4 7 8 10 12 14 15 16 17 19 20 21 22 23 30 31 32 33 34 35 37 39 40 41 42 44 45 49 51 52 54 55 56 57 60 63 65 67 70 71 73 74 **P**6	23	10	124	5788	66	107524	988	48125	25083	640
COTTAGE GROVE—Lane County ★ COTTAGE GROVE HOSPITAL, 1340 Birch Avenue, Zip 97424; tel. 503/942–0511; William N. Wilber, Chief Executive Officer (Total facility includes 40 beds in nursing home–type unit) **A**1 9 10 **F**7 8 12 14 19 20 22 26 28 29 30 31 32 33 34 37 40 41 44 45 46 48 49 51 52 57 64 65 67 70 71 73 74 **P**6 **S**0585 Brim, Inc.	23	10	71	966	46	86282	153	9540	5592	383
DALLAS—Polk County ☐ VALLEY COMMUNITY HOSPITAL, 550 S.E. Clay Street, Zip 97338, Mailing Address: P.O. Box 378, Zip 97338; tel. 503/623–8301; Stephen A. Bowles, President **A**1 9 10 **F**1 2 3 7 8 12 14 15 16 17 19 21 22 23 28 29 30 34 35 37 40 41 44 45 46 49 65 66 67 70 71 73 **P**5	23	10	44	1304	11	22160	207	10466	5085	131
ENTERPRISE—Wallowa County ★ WALLOWA MEMORIAL HOSPITAL, 401 East First Street, Zip 97828, Mailing Address: Box 460, Zip 97828; tel. 503/426–3111; (Total facility includes 32 beds in nursing home–type unit) **A**9 10 **F**7 8 11 17 19 22 27 30 32 33 34 40 42 44 52 59 64 67 70 71 73 **P**5	16	10	55	458	35	11205	47	2939	1725	110
EUGENE—Lane County ★ △ SACRED HEART MEDICAL CENTER, (Formerly Sacred Heart General Hospital) 1255 Hilyard Street, Zip 97401, Mailing Address: Box 10905, Zip 97440; tel. 503/686–7300; Andrew R. McCulloch, Administrator **A**1 2 7 9 10 **F**3 4 7 10 14 15 16 17 19 22 24 28 31 33 35 37 38 42 43 44 48 49 52 53 54 55 56 58 59 60 61 65 66 67 70 71 73 74 **P**7 **S**5415 PeaceHealth	21	10	396	18723	245	243423	2473	172548	65572	1859

© 1995 AHA Guide

Hospitals, U.S. / OREGON

Hospital, Address, Telephone, Administrator, Approval, Facility, and Physician Codes, Health Care System	Classification Codes		Utilization Data					Expense (thousands) of dollars		
★ American Hospital Association (AHA) membership ☐ Joint Commission on Accreditation of Healthcare Organizations (JCAHO) accreditation + American Osteopathic Hospital Association (AOHA) membership ○ American Osteopathic Association (AOA) accreditation △ Commission on Accreditation of Rehabilitation Facilities (CARF) accreditation Control codes 61, 63, 64, 71, 72 and 73 indicate hospitals listed by AOHA, but not registered by AHA. For definition of numerical codes, see page A6	Control	Service	Beds	Admissions	Census	Outpatient Visits	Births	Total	Payroll	Personnel
SERENITY LANE, 616 East 16th, Zip 97401; tel. 503/687–1110; Neil H. McNaughton, Executive Director **F**2 3 12 14 15 17 18 67 **P**5	23	82	55	746	32	0	0	—	—	—
FLORENCE—Lane County										
✠ PEACE HARBOR HOSPITAL, 400 Ninth Street, Zip 97439, Mailing Address: Box 580, Zip 97439; tel. 503/997–8412; James Barnhart, Administrator **A**1 9 10 **F**7 8 14 15 16 19 21 22 30 32 35 37 40 44 45 49 56 65 70 71 73 **P**6 **S**5415 PeaceHealth	21	10	21	1093	11	14824	99	9602	4587	111
FOREST GROVE—Washington County										
✠ TUALITY FOREST GROVE HOSPITAL, 1809 Maple Street, Zip 97116–1995; tel. 503/357–2173; Barbara J. Saylor, Administrator **A**1 9 10 **F**2 3 7 8 10 13 14 17 19 21 22 23 24 25 26 27 28 29 30 32 33 34 35 37 39 40 41 42 44 45 49 64 65 66 67 71 72 73 74 **P**1 4 7	23	10	48	1092	13	37562	245	9306	3637	123
GOLD BEACH—Curry County										
★ CURRY GENERAL HOSPITAL, 220 East Fourth Street, Zip 97444–9990; tel. 503/247–6621; Gordon Ensley, Administrator (Nonreporting) **A**9 10	16	10	26	—	—	—	—	—	—	—
GRANTS PASS—Josephine County										
✠ THREE RIVERS COMMUNITY HOSPITAL, 715 N.W. Dimmick Street, Zip 97526–1596; tel. 503/476–6831; John F. Bringhurst, Executive Vice President and Administrator **A**1 9 10 **F**7 8 11 15 16 19 21 22 23 32 35 37 40 44 46 49 65 70 71 72 73	23	10	87	3016	25	65567	651	18414	8005	317
☐ THREE RIVERS COMMUNITY HOSPITAL AND HEALTH CENTER, 1505 N.W. Washington Boulevard, Zip 97526; tel. 503/479–7531 **A**1 9 10 **F**7 8 11 15 16 19 21 22 23 24 28 30 32 33 35 36 37 40 41 42 44 46 49 51 54 56 58 65 67 70 71 72 73	23	10	63	2482	29	65102	0	17500	10368	230
GRESHAM—Multnomah County										
✠ LEGACY MOUNT HOOD MEDICAL CENTER, 24800 S.E. Stark, Zip 97030–3399; tel. 503/667–1122; Barbara A. Zappas, President **A**1 10 **F**3 8 9 11 12 14 15 16 17 19 21 22 26 28 30 32 33 34 35 37 38 39 40 41 42 43 44 47 48 49 52 53 54 55 56 57 58 59 60 64 65 67 71 72 73 74 **P**5 **S**2755 Legacy Health System	23	10	97	2992	36	45350	0	24812	10632	305
HEPPNER—Linn County										
PIONEER MEMORIAL HOSPITAL, 564 East Pioneer Drive, Zip 97836, Mailing Address: P.O. Box 9, Zip 97836; tel. 503/676–9133; Kevin R. Erich, Administrator (Nonreporting) **A**9 10 **S**0235 Adventist Health System/West	13	10	32							
HERMISTON—Umatilla County										
✠ GOOD SHEPHERD COMMUNITY HOSPITAL, 610 N.W. 11th Street, Zip 97838–9696; tel. 503/567–6483; Dennis E. Burke, Chief Executive Officer **A**1 9 10 **F**7 8 19 22 28 30 32 34 35 37 39 40 44 45 46 65 70 71 73 **P**5 8	23	10	45	1978	20	35719	425	14744	6269	216
HILLSBORO—Washington County										
✠ TUALITY COMMUNITY HOSPITAL, 335 S.E. Eighth Avenue, Zip 97123, Mailing Address: P.O. Box 309, Zip 97123; tel. 503/681–1111; Richard Vincent Stenson, Administrator (Total facility includes 22 beds in nursing home–type unit) **A**1 9 10 **F**2 3 7 8 10 13 14 17 19 21 22 23 24 25 26 27 28 29 30 32 33 34 35 37 39 40 41 42 44 45 49 64 65 66 67 71 72 73 74 **P**1 4 7	23	10	129	6517	77	109373	1148	50886	14823	483
HOOD RIVER—Hood River County										
★ HOOD RIVER MEMORIAL HOSPITAL, 13th and May Streets, Zip 97031, Mailing Address: P.O. Box 149, Zip 97031; tel. 503/386–3911; Tim Simmons, Administrator **A**9 10 **F**3 7 8 11 15 16 19 22 29 31 32 33 34 35 37 40 42 44 45 62 65 70 71 73	23	10	21	1308	10	25677	357	11199	4638	219
JOHN DAY—Grant County										
★ BLUE MOUNTAIN HOSPITAL, 170 Ford Road, Zip 97845; tel. 503/575–1311; David G. Triebes, Administrator (Total facility includes 52 beds in nursing home–type unit) **A**9 10 **F**1 7 8 17 19 22 28 30 32 34 37 40 44 45 48 49 56 64 65 66 67 68 70 71 **P**5 8 **S**0585 Brim, Inc.	16	10	68	532	54	10382	66	5513	2823	—
KLAMATH FALLS—Klamath County										
✠ MERLE WEST MEDICAL CENTER, 2865 Daggett Street, Zip 97601–1180; tel. 503/882–6311; Paul R. Stewart, President (Total facility includes 120 beds in nursing home–type unit) **A**1 2 3 9 10 **F**4 7 8 10 11 12 15 19 20 21 22 23 28 30 31 32 34 35 40 41 42 44 49 51 52 56 57 60 61 63 65 66 67 70 71 72 73 **P**5 8	23	10	251	6598	144	123754	884	—	—	325
LA GRANDE—Union County										
✠ GRANDE RONDE HOSPITAL, 900 Sunset Drive, Zip 97850, Mailing Address: Box 3290, Zip 97850; tel. 503/963–8421; James A. Mattes, President (Total facility includes 20 beds in nursing home–type unit) **A**1 9 10 **F**7 8 11 15 16 17 19 21 22 23 26 28 30 32 33 34 35 39 40 44 45 46 49 53 54 55 56 57 58 59 63 64 65 67 71 73 **P**3 5	23	10	69	2006	19	39168	352	17658	8313	292
LAKEVIEW—Lake County										
LAKE DISTRICT HOSPITAL, 700 South J Street, Zip 97630–1679; tel. 503/947–2114; Richard T. Moore, Chief Executive Officer (Total facility includes 47 beds in nursing home–type unit) **A**9 10 **F**2 7 8 11 14 15 16 22 37 40 41 44 49 56 61 64 70 71 73 **P**5	16	10	68	420	33	11515	73	4461	2174	82
LEBANON—Linn County										
✠ LEBANON COMMUNITY HOSPITAL, 525 North Santiam Highway, Zip 97355, Mailing Address: P.O. Box 739, Zip 97355–0739; tel. 503/258–2101; Alan R. Yordy, Chief Executive Officer **A**1 9 10 **F**7 8 15 17 19 22 32 33 37 40 41 44 49 64 65 67 71 73 **P**3 4 6	23	10	49	3324	27	60492	351	19498	10439	362
LINCOLN CITY—Lincoln County										
✠ NORTH LINCOLN HOSPITAL, 3043 N.E. 28th Street, Zip 97367–4523, Mailing Address: Box 767, Zip 97367–0767; tel. 503/994–3661; Eric Buckland, Administrator **A**1 9 10 **F**7 8 17 19 21 22 23 32 33 35 37 40 41 44 49 65 67 70 71 73 **P**6	16	10	26	1231	11	42110	178	12874	6254	225

Hospitals, U.S. / OREGON

Hospital, Address, Telephone, Administrator, Approval, Facility, and Physician Codes, Health Care System	Classification Codes		Utilization Data					Expense (thousands) of dollars		
★ American Hospital Association (AHA) membership ☐ Joint Commission on Accreditation of Healthcare Organizations (JCAHO) accreditation + American Osteopathic Hospital Association (AOHA) membership ○ American Osteopathic Association (AOA) accreditation △ Commission on Accreditation of Rehabilitation Facilities (CARF) accreditation Control codes 61, 63, 64, 71, 72 and 73 indicate hospitals listed by AOHA, but not registered by AHA. For definition of numerical codes, see page A6	Control	Service	Beds	Admissions	Census	Outpatient Visits	Births	Total	Payroll	Personnel
MADRAS—Jefferson County										
★ MOUNTAIN VIEW HOSPITAL DISTRICT, 470 N.E. A Street, Zip 97741; tel. 503/475–3882; Ronald W. Barnes, Executive Director (Total facility includes 68 beds in nursing home–type unit) **A**9 10 **F**1 7 14 15 16 19 21 22 28 30 31 32 33 35 37 40 41 44 51 64 70 71 **P**5 **S**0585 Brim, Inc.	16	10	102	1254	71	14800	154	8646	4445	162
MCMINNVILLE—Yamhill County										
★ MCMINNVILLE COMMUNITY HOSPITAL, 603 South Baker Street, Zip 97128–6498; tel. 503/472–6131 **A**1 9 10 **F**7 8 10 12 15 16 18 19 21 22 23 30 32 33 34 35 37 39 40 41 44 45 46 49 54 56 65 70 71 73 **P**5 8 **S**0048 Columbia/HCA Healthcare Corporation	33	10	67	2712	24	31496	489	15182	7086	221
MEDFORD—Jackson County										
★ PROVIDENCE MEDFORD MEDICAL CENTER, 1111 Crater Lake Avenue, Zip 97504–6241; tel. 503/773–6611; Andrea Y. Coleman, Chief Executive, Southern Oregon Service Area and Administrator **A**1 2 9 10 **F**1 4 8 10 12 14 15 16 19 22 23 26 27 28 29 30 31 32 33 34 35 37 39 41 42 44 45 46 48 49 51 56 65 67 70 71 73 **P**4 5 6 **S**5275 Sisters of Providence Health System	21	10	118	4281	58	222177	0	39593	19034	585
★ ROGUE VALLEY MEDICAL CENTER, 2825 Barnett Road, Zip 97504–8332; tel. 503/773–4900; Jon Keith Mitchell, President and Chief Executive Officer **A**1 2 9 10 **F**1 2 3 4 7 8 10 11 14 15 16 17 19 21 22 24 26 27 28 29 30 32 33 34 35 37 38 39 40 41 42 43 44 45 46 47 49 51 52 54 56 57 60 63 64 65 67 70 71 73 **P**6	23	10	246	9993	124	200619	1838	98355	47677	1353
MILWAUKIE—Clackamas County										
★ PROVIDENCE MILWAUKIE HOSPITAL, 10150 S.E. 32nd Avenue, Zip 97222–6593; tel. 503/652–8300; Sister Betsy Mickel, Chief Operating Officer **A**1 2 9 10 **F**1 2 3 4 5 7 8 9 10 11 15 16 17 19 20 22 23 24 26 29 32 33 34 35 37 38 39 40 41 42 43 44 47 48 49 51 52 53 57 58 60 64 55 66 67 69 70 71 72 73 74 **P**3 5 **S**5275 Sisters of Providence Health System	21	10	56	2804	23	150765	461	23553	10564	288
NEWBERG—Yamhill County										
★ PROVIDENCE NEWBERG HOSPITAL, 501 Villa Road, Zip 97132; tel. 503/537–1555; Mark W. Meinert CHE, Chief Executive, Yamhill Service Area **A**1 9 10 **F**7 15 16 19 21 22 32 34 37 40 44 70 71 72 **P**3 **S**5275 Sisters of Providence Health System	14	10	35	1243	11	47126	282	12337	5828	180
NEWPORT—Lincoln County										
★ PACIFIC COMMUNITIES HOSPITAL, 930 S.W. Abbey Street, Zip 97365–4820; tel. 503/265–2244; Michael Fraser, Administrator **A**1 9 10 **F**7 8 11 14 19 21 22 23 32 33 34 35 39 40 41 44 49 65 70 71 73 **P**5	16	10	42	1552	15	61252	172	15117	7227	230
ONTARIO—Malheur County										
★ HOLY ROSARY MEDICAL CENTER, 351 S.W. Ninth Street, Zip 97914–2693; tel. 503/889–5331; Bruce Jensen, President and Chief Executive Officer **A**1 9 10 **F**7 8 11 15 16 19 21 22 30 31 32 35 40 44 45 46 49 56 63 65 70 71 **P**5 **S**5175 Catholic Health Corporation	23	10	74	3491	37	62123	644	23588	9880	272
OREGON CITY—Clackamas County										
★ WILLAMETTE FALLS HOSPITAL, 1500 Division Street, Zip 97045–1597; tel. 503/656–1631; Robert A. Steed, Administrator **A**1 2 9 10 **F**7 8 12 19 21 22 26 30 32 33 34 37 39 40 41 42 44 45 49 51 60 65 71 72 73 **P**5 8	23	10	96	5207	40	41122	992	37840	18185	475
PENDLETON—Umatilla County										
EASTERN OREGON PSYCHIATRIC CENTER, 2575 Westgate, Zip 97801; tel. 503/276–4511; Evelyn Jenson, Superintendent **A**9 10 **F**20 52 65	12	22	60	235	55	0	0	4003	2275	66
★ ST. ANTHONY HOSPITAL, 1601 S.E. Court Avenue, Zip 97801–3297; tel. 503/276–5121; Jeffrey S. Drop, President **A**1 2 9 10 **F**7 8 12 19 21 22 23 24 28 30 31 32 33 35 37 39 40 42 44 49 65 70 71 73 **S**5325 Franciscan Health System	23	10	49	1854	17	20037	438	17533	6943	252
PORTLAND—Multnomah County										
★ BESS KAISER MEDICAL CENTER, 5055 North Greeley Avenue, Zip 97217–3591; tel. 503/285–9321; Alide Chase, Administrator (Nonreporting) **A**1 5 10 **S**2105 Kaiser Foundation Hospitals	23	10	216	—	—	—	—	—	—	—
DOERNBECHER CHILDREN'S HOSPITAL See University Hospital										
○ EASTMORELAND HOSPITAL, 2900 S.E. Steele Street, Zip 97202; tel. 503/234–0411; Ken Giles, Administrator (Nonreporting) **A**9 10 11 12 13 **S**6525 Ornda Healthcorp	33	10	77	—	—	—	—	—	—	—
EMANUEL HOSPITAL AND HEALTH CENTER See Legacy Emanuel Hospital and Health Center										
GOOD SAMARITAN HOSPITAL AND MEDICAL CENTER See Legacy Good Samaritan Hospital and Health Center										
HOLLADAY PARK MEDICAL CENTER See Legacy Emanuel Hospital and Health Center										
★ △ LEGACY EMANUEL HOSPITAL AND HEALTH CENTER, (Formerly Emanuel Hospital and Health Center) (Includes Holladay Park Medical Center, 1225 N.E. Second Avenue, Portland, Oregon, Zip 97232; tel. 503/233–4567) 2801 North Gantenbein Avenue, Zip 97227–1674; tel. 503/280–3200; James E. May, President (Total facility includes 36 beds in nursing home–type unit) **A**1 3 5 7 9 10 **F**1 2 3 4 7 8 9 10 11 12 13 14 15 16 17 19 21 22 23 24 25 26 28 29 30 31 32 33 34 35 37 38 39 40 41 42 43 44 45 46 47 48 49 51 52 53 54 55 56 57 58 59 60 61 63 64 65 66 67 69 70 71 72 73 74 **S**2755 Legacy Health System	23	10	346	15251	232	157090	2084	163105	72039	1867
★ LEGACY GOOD SAMARITAN HOSPITAL AND HEALTH CENTER, (Includes Good Samaritan Hospital and Medical Center, Portland, Oregon; Rehabilitation Institute of Oregon, Portland, Oregon) 1015 N.W. 22nd Avenue, Zip 97210; tel. 503/229–7711; James E. May, President (Total facility includes 106 beds in nursing home–type unit) **A**1 2 3 5 9 10 **F**1 2 3 4 7 8 9 10 11 12 13 14 15 16 17 19 21 22 23 24 25 26 28 29 30 31 32 33 34 35 37 38 39 40 41 42 43 44 45 46 47 48 49 51 52 53 54 55 56 57 58 59 60 61 63 64 65 66 67 69 70 71 72 73 74 **S**2755 Legacy Health System	23	10	393	9523	236	197321	2018	141470	61199	1487

Hospitals, U.S. / OREGON

Hospital, Address, Telephone, Administrator, Approval, Facility, and Physician Codes, Health Care System	Classification Codes		Utilization Data					Expense (thousands) of dollars		
★ American Hospital Association (AHA) membership ☐ Joint Commission on Accreditation of Healthcare Organizations (JCAHO) accreditation + American Osteopathic Hospital Association (AOHA) membership ○ American Osteopathic Association (AOA) accreditation △ Commission on Accreditation of Rehabilitation Facilities (CARF) accreditation Control codes 61, 63, 64, 71, 72 and 73 indicate hospitals listed by AOHA, but not registered by AHA. For definition of numerical codes, see page A6	Control	Service	Beds	Admissions	Census	Outpatient Visits	Births	Total	Payroll	Personnel
☐ PACIFIC GATEWAY HOSPITAL AND COUNSELING CENTER, 1345 S.E. Harney, Zip 97202; tel. 503/234–5353; George B. Rex, Administrator (Nonreporting) **A**1 9 10	33	22	66	—	—	—	—	—	—	—
★ PORTLAND ADVENTIST MEDICAL CENTER, 10123 S.E. Market, Zip 97216–9966; tel. 503/257–2500; Larry D. Dodds, President **A**1 2 5 9 10 **F**1 3 4 7 8 10 12 15 16 17 19 21 22 23 24 26 28 29 30 32 33 34 35 37 39 40 41 42 44 45 46 49 52 53 54 55 56 57 58 59 60 61 65 66 67 71 72 73 74 **P**5 6 7 **S**0235 Adventist Health System/West	21	10	270	9018	96	94731	1852	89664	40408	1419
★ △ PROVIDENCE PORTLAND MEDICAL CENTER, 4805 N.E. Glisan Street, Zip 97213–2967; tel. 503/230–1111; Marvin O'Quinn, Chief Operating Officer (Total facility includes 20 beds in nursing home–type unit) **A**1 2 3 5 7 9 10 **F**2 5 7 10 11 12 14 15 16 19 21 22 24 25 31 32 33 34 35 37 38 40 41 42 43 44 45 48 49 51 52 53 54 55 56 57 58 59 60 61 64 65 66 69 71 72 73 74 **P**5 **S**5275 Sisters of Providence Health System	21	10	449	15632	265	471487	1595	171815	71411	2141
★ PROVIDENCE ST. VINCENT MEDICAL CENTER, (Formerly St. Vincent Hospital and Medical Center) 9205 S.W. Barnes Road, Zip 97225–6661; tel. 503/297–4411; Donald Elsom, Chief Operating Officer **A**1 2 3 5 9 10 **F**1 2 3 4 7 8 10 11 12 14 15 16 17 18 19 22 24 30 32 33 34 35 37 38 39 40 41 42 43 44 45 48 49 51 52 53 56 58 59 60 64 65 66 69 71 72 73 74 **P**5 6 **S**5275 Sisters of Providence Health System	21	10	275	18565	225	454842	2896	192071	76283	2210
REHABILITATION INSTITUTE OF OREGON See Legacy Good Samaritan Hospital and Health Center										
★ SHRINERS HOSPITALS FOR CRIPPLED CHILDREN, PORTLAND UNIT, 3101 S.W. Sam Jackson Park Road, Zip 97201; tel. 503/241–5090; Patricia J. Sadowski, Administrator **A**1 3 5 **F**17 30 49 65 **S**4125 Shriners Hospitals for Crippled Children	23	57	40	1119	16	9553	0	—	—	228
ST. VINCENT HOSPITAL AND MEDICAL CENTER See Providence St. Vincent Medical Center										
★ UNIVERSITY HOSPITAL, (Includes Doernbecher Children's Hospital, Portland, Oregon) 3181 S.W. Sam Jackson Park Road, Zip 97201–3098; tel. 503/494–8311; Timothy M. Goldfarb, Director **A**1 2 3 5 8 9 10 **F**4 7 8 10 11 12 13 16 17 19 20 21 22 24 25 26 27 28 30 31 32 33 35 37 38 40 41 42 43 44 46 47 49 51 52 53 54 55 56 57 58 59 60 61 65 66 67 69 70 71 72 73 74 **P**7	12	10	350	17287	274	275576	2312	252307	106971	2763
★ VETERANS AFFAIRS MEDICAL CENTER, 3710 S.W. U.S. Veterans Hospital Road, Zip 97201; tel. 503/220–8262; Barry L. Bell, Director (Total facility includes 120 beds in nursing home–type unit) **A**1 2 3 5 8 **F**1 2 3 4 8 10 11 19 20 21 22 23 24 25 26 29 31 32 34 35 37 41 42 43 44 45 46 48 49 51 52 54 56 57 58 60 63 64 65 67 69 71 73 74 **S**9295 Department of Veterans Affairs	45	10	622	10851	444	238739	0	164176	91353	2512
☐ WOODLAND PARK HOSPITAL, 10300 N.E. Hancock, Zip 97220; tel. 503/257–5500; William E. Price, Chief Executive Officer (Nonreporting) **A**1 9 10 **S**6525 Ornda Healthcorp	33	10	123	—	—	—	—	—	—	—
PRINEVILLE—Crook County PIONEER MEMORIAL HOSPITAL, 1201 North Elm Street, Zip 97754; tel. 503/447–6254; Roger W. Strobel, President and Chief Executive Officer (Nonreporting) **A**9 10 **S**0235 Adventist Health System/West	23	10	25	—	—	—	—	—	—	—
REDMOND—Deschutes County ★ CENTRAL OREGON DISTRICT HOSPITAL, 1253 North Canal Boulevard, Zip 97756–1395; tel. 503/548–8131; James A. Diegel, Executive Director **A**1 9 10 **F**7 8 12 15 17 19 21 22 28 29 30 32 34 37 39 40 44 45 65 67 70 71 73 74 **P**1 5 **S**2235 Lutheran Health Systems	16	10	47	1505	12	20158	255	11540	5669	190
REEDSPORT—Douglas County LOWER UMPQUA HOSPITAL DISTRICT, 600 Ranch Road, Zip 97467–1795; tel. 503/271–2171; Sandra Reese, Administrator (Total facility includes 22 beds in nursing home–type unit) **A**9 10 **F**7 8 11 15 19 22 28 32 33 37 40 44 49 64 65 67 70 71 73 **P**3	16	10	40	442	29	7973	59	5180	2724	107
ROSEBURG—Douglas County ★ + △ DOUGLAS COMMUNITY HOSPITAL, 738 West Harvard Boulevard, Zip 97470–2996; tel. 503/673–6641; Christopher L. Boyd, Chief Executive Officer (Nonreporting) **A**1 2 7 9 10 **S**0048 Columbia/HCA Healthcare Corporation	33	10	118	—	—	—	—	—	—	—
★ MERCY MEDICAL CENTER, 2700 Stewart Parkway, Zip 97470; tel. 503/673–0611; Jacquetta Taylor, President and Chief Executive Officer **A**1 2 9 10 **F**1 6 7 8 10 12 14 15 16 17 19 21 22 23 24 28 29 30 32 33 34 35 37 40 41 42 44 45 49 51 52 53 56 57 59 60 62 65 67 71 72 73 74 **P**3 4 5 7 **S**5175 Catholic Health Corporation	21	10	96	6088	60	130054	686	36783	15368	487
★ VETERANS AFFAIRS MEDICAL CENTER, 913 N.W. Garden Valley Boulevard, Zip 97470–6513; tel. 503/440–1000; Alan S. Perry, Medical Center Director (Nonreporting) **A**1 **S**9295 Department of Veterans Affairs	45	10	272	—	—	—	—	—	—	—
SALEM—Marion County ☐ OREGON STATE HOSPITAL, 2600 Center Street N.E., Zip 97310–0530; tel. 503/945–2870; Stanley F. Mazur-Hart Ph.D., Superintendent (Nonreporting) **A**1 5 9 10	12	22	759	—	—	—	—	—	—	—
PSYCHIATRIC MEDICINE CENTER See Salem Hospital REGIONAL REHABILITATION CENTER See Salem Hospital										
★ SALEM HOSPITAL, (Includes Psychiatric Medicine Center, 1127 Oak Street S.E., Salem, Oregon, Zip 97301; Regional Rehabilitation Center, 2561 Center Street N.E., Salem, Oregon, Zip 97301; tel. 503/370–5986) 665 Winter Street S.E., Zip 97301, Mailing Address: Box 14001, Zip 97309–5014; tel. 503/370–5200; Dennis Noonan, President (Total facility includes 69 beds in nursing home–type unit) **A**1 2 9 10 **F**3 4 7 8 10 11 12 14 15 16 17 19 21 22 24 26 27 28 29 30 31 32 33 34 35 37 39 40 41 42 43 44 45 46 48 49 52 54 56 57 58 59 60 61 64 65 66 67 69 70 71 72 73	23	10	428	16916	268	126744	3362	131419	71009	1995

Hospital, Address, Telephone, Administrator, Approval, Facility, and Physician Codes, Health Care System	Classification Codes		Utilization Data					Expense (thousands) of dollars		
★ American Hospital Association (AHA) membership □ Joint Commission on Accreditation of Healthcare Organizations (JCAHO) accreditation + American Osteopathic Hospital Association (AOHA) membership ○ American Osteopathic Association (AOA) accreditation △ Commission on Accreditation of Rehabilitation Facilities (CARF) accreditation Control codes 61, 63, 64, 71, 72 and 73 indicate hospitals listed by AOHA, but not registered by AHA. For definition of numerical codes, see page A6	Control	Service	Beds	Admissions	Census	Outpatient Visits	Births	Total	Payroll	Personnel
SEASIDE—Clatsop County ★ PROVIDENCE SEASIDE HOSPITAL, 725 South Wahanna Road, Zip 97138, Mailing Address: Box 740, Zip 97138-0740; tel. 503/738-8463; Ronald Swanson, Administrator **A**1 9 10 **F**7 8 17 19 22 30 32 34 37 39 40 42 44 45 46 49 51 66 67 71 73 **P**5 6 **S**5275 Sisters of Providence Health System	21	10	29	910	8	50244	71	8445	4217	127
SILVERTON—Marion County ★ SILVERTON HOSPITAL, 342 Fairview Street, Zip 97381; tel. 503/873-1500; William E. Winter, Administrative Director **A**9 10 **F**7 8 17 19 22 25 27 28 29 30 34 37 40 41 44 45 46 67 68 70 71 73	23	10	38	1809	16	28440	561	9393	4475	165
SPRINGFIELD—Lane County ★ MCKENZIE-WILLAMETTE HOSPITAL, 1460 G Street, Zip 97477-4197; tel. 503/726-4400; Roy J. Orr, President and Chief Executive Officer (Data for 364 days) **A**1 9 10 **F**1 2 3 4 6 7 8 9 10 11 12 13 14 15 16 17 18 19 20 21 22 23 24 26 27 28 29 30 31 32 33 34 35 36 37 38 39 40 41 42 43 44 45 48 49 52 53 54 56 58 60 61 62 63 64 65 67 70 71 72 73 74 **P**1	23	10	105	4596	48	38556	771	42793	20341	567
STAYTON—Marion County ★ SANTIAM MEMORIAL HOSPITAL, 1401 North 10th Avenue, Zip 97383; tel. 503/769-2175; Terry L. Fletchall, Chief Executive Officer **A**1 9 10 **F**7 14 15 16 19 20 34 40 44 64 71	23	10	40	698	7	15183	101	4501	2201	68
THE DALLES—Wasco County ★ + MID-COLUMBIA MEDICAL CENTER, 1700 East 19th Street, Zip 97058-3316; tel. 503/296-1111; Mark D. Scott, President (Nonreporting) **A**1 9 10	23	10	49	—	—	—	—	—	—	—
TILLAMOOK—Tillamook County □ TILLAMOOK COUNTY GENERAL HOSPITAL, 1000 Third Street, Zip 97141-3430; tel. 503/842-4444; Wendell Hesseltine, President **A**1 9 10 **F**7 8 14 15 16 19 22 28 32 33 34 35 37 40 44 52 65 70 71 73 **S**0235 Adventist Health System/West	21	10	20	1426	13	34910	128	13546	6315	233
TUALATIN—Washington County ★ LEGACY MERIDIAN PARK HOSPITAL, (Formerly Meridian Park Hospital) 19300 S.W. 65th Avenue, Zip 97062-9741; tel. 503/692-1212; Jane C. Cummins, President and Chief Executive Officer **A**1 2 9 10 **F**2 3 4 7 8 9 10 11 12 14 17 18 19 21 22 23 24 25 26 27 28 29 30 32 33 34 35 37 39 40 41 42 43 44 45 46 47 48 49 52 53 54 55 56 57 58 59 60 63 64 65 67 70 71 72 73 74 **P**4 5 **S**2755 Legacy Health System	23	10	108	6321	60	55732	722	42275	17012	461
WILSONVILLE—Clackamas County □ DAMMASCH STATE HOSPITAL, 28801 S.W. 110th Street, Zip 97070, Mailing Address: Box 38, Zip 97070-38; tel. 503/682-3111; Marvin Fickle M.D., Superintendent (Nonreporting) **A**1 5 9	12	22	272	—	—	—	—	—	—	—

Hospitals, U.S. / PENNSYLVANIA

PENNSYLVANIA

Resident population 12,048 (in thousands)
Resident population in metro areas 84.8%
Birth rate per 1,000 population 14.1
65 years and over 15.8%
Percent of persons without health insurance 8.8%

Hospital, Address, Telephone, Administrator, Approval, Facility, and Physician Codes, Health Care System	Classification Codes		Utilization Data					Expense (thousands) of dollars		
★ American Hospital Association (AHA) membership □ Joint Commission on Accreditation of Healthcare Organizations (JCAHO) accreditation + American Osteopathic Hospital Association (AOHA) membership ○ American Osteopathic Association (AOA) accreditation △ Commission on Accreditation of Rehabilitation Facilities (CARF) accreditation Control codes 61, 63, 64, 71, 72 and 73 indicate hospitals listed by AOHA, but not registered by AHA. For definition of numerical codes, see page A6	Control	Service	Beds	Admissions	Census	Outpatient Visits	Births	Total	Payroll	Personnel
ABINGTON—Montgomery County										
★ △ ABINGTON MEMORIAL HOSPITAL, 1200 Old York Road, Zip 19001-3788; tel. 215/576-2000; Felix M. Pilla, President and Chief Executive Officer **A**1 2 3 5 6 7 9 10 **F**1 3 7 8 10 11 15 16 17 19 20 21 22 23 24 25 26 27 30 31 32 33 34 35 36 37 38 39 40 41 42 44 46 47 48 49 51 52 53 56 57 58 59 60 61 65 67 68 70 71 73 74	23	10	456	20125	346	—	3174	194666	96740	2557
ALIQUIPPA—Beaver County										
★ ALIQUIPPA HOSPITAL, 2500 Hospital Drive, Zip 15001-2191; tel. 412/857-1212; Charles Lonchar, President and Chief Executive Officer (Total facility includes 16 beds in nursing home-type unit) **A**1 9 10 **F**3 11 15 19 21 22 26 28 32 33 34 35 39 41 42 44 49 52 53 54 55 56 57 58 59 64 65 71 **P**7 **S**0002 Quorum Health Group/Quorum Health Resources	23	10	183	5720	111	49668	0	39680	18984	611
ALLENTOWN—Lehigh County										
+ ○ ALLENTOWN OSTEOPATHIC MEDICAL CENTER, 1736 Hamilton Street, Zip 18104-9990; tel. 610/770-8300; John M. Sherwood FACHE, President and Chief Executive Officer **A**9 10 11 12 13 **F**2 3 4 7 8 10 14 15 16 19 21 22 23 30 32 34 35 37 39 40 42 44 45 46 49 51 63 65 67 71 73	23	10	150	4866	78	68546	561	35017	16051	522
□ ALLENTOWN STATE HOSPITAL, 1600 Hanover Avenue, Zip 18103; tel. 610/740-3200; David W. Jay, Superintendent **A**1 9 10 **F**4 5 6 8 9 10 11 12 19 20 21 22 23 24 26 27 28 31 35 37 39 40 41 42 43 44 45 46 48 50 52 55 56 57 60 63 65 67 70 71 73 **P**6	12	22	415	231	445	—	0	32162	20372	598
□ △ GOOD SHEPHERD REHABILITATION HOSPITAL, 543 St. John Street, Zip 18103-3279; tel. 610/776-3120; Reverend Dale Sandstrom, President **A**1 7 9 10 **F**5 12 14 15 16 17 22 45 48 49 54 65 67 73 **P**6	23	46	75	1401	63	50132	0	24551	19583	448
★ LEHIGH VALLEY HOSPITAL, Cedar Crest Boulevard & I-78, Zip 18103, Mailing Address: P.O. Box 689, Zip 18105-1556; tel. 610/402-8000; Elliot J. Sussman M.D., President and Chief Executive Officer **A**1 2 3 5 8 9 10 12 **F**1 4 5 6 7 9 10 11 12 13 14 15 16 17 18 19 20 21 22 23 24 28 29 30 31 32 33 34 35 37 38 39 40 41 42 43 44 45 46 49 50 51 52 53 54 55 56 57 58 59 60 61 63 65 66 67 68 69 70 71 73 74 **P**5 7 8	23	10	692	28212	568	233663	3195	286503	139190	4091
★ SACRED HEART HOSPITAL, Fourth and Chew Streets, Zip 18102-3490; tel. 610/776-4500; Joseph M. Cimerola FACHE, President and Chief Executive Officer (Total facility includes 22 beds in nursing home-type unit) **A**1 2 3 5 9 10 **F**4 7 8 10 11 12 13 14 15 16 17 18 19 20 21 22 25 28 29 30 31 32 33 34 35 37 38 39 40 41 42 43 44 45 46 49 51 54 55 56 57 58 60 63 64 65 67 68 69 71 72 73 74 **P**1 6	23	10	245	7705	151	161769	631	60709	26065	834
ALTOONA—Blair County										
ALTOONA CENTER, 1515 Fourth Street, Zip 16601; tel. 814/946-6900; Barry C. Benford, Director (Nonreporting)	12	62	130	—	—	—	—	—	—	—
★ ○ ALTOONA HOSPITAL, 620 Howard Avenue, Zip 16601-4899; tel. 814/946-2011; James W. Barner, President and Chief Executive Officer; Warren Rhyner, Vice President Professional Services **A**1 2 3 5 6 9 10 11 12 **F**2 3 4 7 8 10 11 14 15 16 18 19 22 23 26 30 33 34 35 37 39 40 41 42 43 44 46 49 52 53 54 56 57 58 60 65 67 71 73 74 **P**1	23	10	331	13215	212	229825	1324	105415	51725	1453
□ △ HEALTHSOUTH REHABILITATION HOSPITAL OF ALTOONA, 2005 Valley View Boulevard, Zip 16602; tel. 814/944-3535; Felix Mariani, Administrator (Nonreporting) **A**1 7 10 **S**0023 Healthsouth Corporation	33	46	66	—	—	—	—	—	—	—
★ JAMES E. VAN ZANDT VETERANS AFFAIRS MEDICAL CENTER, 2907 Pleasant Valley Boulevard, Zip 16602-4377; tel. 814/943-8164; Gerald L. Williams, Director (Total facility includes 33 beds in nursing home-type unit) **A**1 **F**3 8 12 15 17 19 20 22 26 27 29 30 31 33 34 37 39 44 45 46 49 51 54 58 61 65 67 71 73 74 **P**6 **S**9295 Department of Veterans Affairs	45	10	135	2357	105	43699	0	25912	13999	385
★ MERCY REGIONAL HEALTH SYSTEM, 2500 Seventh Avenue, Zip 16602; tel. 814/944-1681; David J. Davies, Chief Executive Officer **A**1 2 9 10 **F**7 8 14 15 16 17 19 21 22 27 28 30 31 33 34 35 37 40 41 42 44 45 46 48 49 52 54 57 60 65 66 67 71 73 **P**1 5 7 8	23	10	153	5835	114	108847	542	45927	20138	680
AMBLER—Montgomery County										
□ HORSHAM CLINIC, 722 East Butler Pike, Zip 19002; tel. 215/643-7800; David A. Baron D.O., Medical Director; Mark A. Benz, Administrator (Nonreporting) **A**1 5 9 10 **S**2635 First Hospital Corporation	33	22	138	—	—	—	—	—	—	—
ASHLAND—Schuylkill County										
□ ASHLAND REGIONAL MEDICAL CENTER, Route 61, Zip 17921-2198; tel. 717/875-2000; Michael J. Callan Sr., Chief Executive Officer (Total facility includes 20 beds in nursing home-type unit) **A**1 9 10 **F**8 19 20 21 22 28 34 37 39 42 44 49 64 65 67 71 73 74	23	10	85	2578	53	31878	0	16540	7785	242
BALA CYNWYD—Montgomery County										
★ △ MERCY HEALTH CORPORATION OF SOUTHEASTERN PENNSYLVANIA, (Includes Fitzgerald Mercy Hospital, 1500 South Lansdowne Avenue, Darby, Pennsylvania, Zip 19023; tel. 215/237-4020; J. Douglas MacBride, Senior Vice President; Mercy Catholic Medical Center, 54th Street and Cedar Avenue, Philadelphia, Pennsylvania, Zip 19143; tel. 215/748-9000; Wesley K. McGavock, Senior Vice President) One Bala Plaza, Suite 402, Zip 19004; tel. 215/237-4000; Plato A. Marinakos, President and Chief Executive Officer (Total facility includes 22 beds in nursing home-type unit) **A**1 2 3 5 7 8 9 10 **F**2 4 7 8 10 11 12 13 14 15 16 17 18 19 20 21 22 23 25 28 29 30 31 32 33 34 35 36 37 38 39 40 41 42 44 46 48 49 52 55 56 57 58 60 63 64 65 71 73 74 **P**6 7 8 **S**3595 Eastern Mercy Health System	21	10	530	22293	399	172048	1749	178666	88804	2289

Hospitals, U.S. / PENNSYLVANIA

Hospital, Address, Telephone, Administrator, Approval, Facility, and Physician Codes, Health Care System	Classification Codes		Utilization Data					Expense (thousands) of dollars		
★ American Hospital Association (AHA) membership □ Joint Commission on Accreditation of Healthcare Organizations (JCAHO) accreditation + American Osteopathic Hospital Association (AOHA) membership ○ American Osteopathic Association (AOA) accreditation △ Commission on Accreditation of Rehabilitation Facilities (CARF) accreditation Control codes 61, 63, 64, 71, 72 and 73 indicate hospitals listed by AOHA, but not registered by AHA. For definition of numerical codes, see page A6	Control	Service	Beds	Admissions	Census	Outpatient Visits	Births	Total	Payroll	Personnel
BEAVER—Beaver County ★ THE MEDICAL CENTER, 1000 Dutch Ridge Road, Zip 15009–9700; tel. 412/728–7000; Larry A. Crowell, President and Chief Executive Officer (Total facility includes 31 beds in nursing home–type unit) **A**1 2 3 5 9 10 **F**4 5 7 8 10 15 16 17 19 20 21 22 23 26 28 29 30 31 32 33 34 35 37 39 40 41 42 43 44 45 46 49 51 52 54 56 57 60 61 63 64 65 67 71 73 74	23	10	470	16121	280	463604	1584	122679	58256	1857
BENSALEM—Bucks County LIVENGRIN FOUNDATION, 4833 Hulmeville Road, Zip 19020; tel. 215/638–5200; Richard M. Pine, Executive Director and Chief Executive Officer (Nonreporting)	23	82	76	—	—	—	—	—	—	—
BERWICK—Columbia County ★ BERWICK HOSPITAL CENTER, 701 East 16th Street, Zip 18603–2397; tel. 717/759–5000; Thomas R. Sphatt, President and Chief Executive Officer (Total facility includes 240 beds in nursing home–type unit) **A**1 9 10 **F**2 3 7 8 14 15 17 19 20 21 22 25 26 27 29 30 32 34 35 37 39 40 41 44 46 49 51 58 61 64 65 66 67 71 73 **P**1 **S**0002 Quorum Health Group/Quorum Health Resources	23	10	409	3979	173	70998	226	26102	12134	546
BETHLEHEM—Northampton County ★ MUHLENBERG HOSPITAL CENTER, 2545 Schoenersville Road, Zip 18017–7384; tel. 610/861–2200; William R. Mason, President **A**1 9 10 **F**8 10 12 14 15 16 17 19 20 21 22 28 29 30 34 37 41 44 45 46 49 52 56 57 58 59 63 65 71 73	23	10	148	5803	111	76995	0	41301	17974	593
□ ST. LUKE'S HOSPITAL, 801 Ostrum Street, Zip 18015–1014; tel. 610/954–4000; Richard A. Anderson, President **A**1 2 3 5 6 9 10 12 **F**3 4 7 8 10 11 12 13 14 15 16 17 19 21 22 23 25 26 28 29 30 31 32 34 35 37 38 39 41 42 43 44 45 49 51 52 54 60 61 65 67 71 72 73 74 **P**8	23	10	402	17630	308	257195	2282	132465	65674	1745
BLOOMSBURG—Columbia County ★ BLOOMSBURG HOSPITAL, 549 East Fair Street, Zip 17815–0340; tel. 717/387–2100; Robert J. Spinelli, Administrator **A**1 9 10 **F**2 3 7 8 14 15 17 19 21 22 28 29 30 34 35 37 40 41 42 44 46 52 54 56 58 59 63 65 67 71 73 **P**3	23	10	125	3938	47	70112	655	23609	10317	430
BRADDOCK—Allegheny County □ BRADDOCK MEDICAL CENTER, 400 Holland Avenue, Zip 15104–1599; tel. 412/636–5000; Richard Wilson Benfer, President **A**1 9 10 **F**8 11 15 16 17 19 21 22 23 28 29 30 31 34 35 36 37 42 44 49 52 54 56 57 63 65 67 71 73	23	10	234	8614	163	77946	0	41662	20144	620
BRADFORD—McKean County ★ BRADFORD REGIONAL MEDICAL CENTER, 116 Interstate Parkway, Zip 16701–0218; tel. 814/368–4143; George E. Leonhardt, President and Chief Executive Officer (Total facility includes 95 beds in nursing home–type unit) **A**1 9 10 **F**7 8 14 17 19 21 22 23 24 25 26 27 28 30 31 32 33 34 35 37 39 40 41 44 45 46 49 51 52 53 54 55 56 57 58 60 63 64 65 66 67 71 73	23	10	216	4897	180	117073	306	35306	15406	534
BRIDGEVILLE—Allegheny County □ MAYVIEW STATE HOSPITAL, 1601 Mayview Road, Zip 15017–1599; tel. 412/257–6500; F. V. Forkus, Superintendent (Total facility includes 92 beds in nursing home–type unit) **A**1 5 10 **F**20 26 27 31 39 46 52 53 57 60 64 65 73 **P**6	12	22	826	667	645	0	0	74463	43118	1446
BRISTOL—Bucks County ★ LOWER BUCKS HOSPITAL, 501 Bath Road, Zip 19007–3190; tel. 215/785–9200; Dennis J. Kain, Chief Executive Officer **A**1 3 5 9 10 **F**4 7 8 10 11 14 15 16 17 18 19 21 22 23 24 27 28 29 30 32 33 34 35 37 38 40 41 42 43 44 45 46 49 51 52 54 55 56 57 58 60 61 63 65 66 67 68 69 71 73 **P**5 8	23	10	198	9057	149	134373	1400	66222	33703	1043
BROOKVILLE—Jefferson County ★ BROOKVILLE HOSPITAL, 100 Hospital Road, Zip 15825–1363; tel. 814/849–1461; Warren J. Bassett FACHE, President **A**1 9 10 **F**7 8 11 14 15 16 17 19 20 21 22 23 28 30 32 39 40 41 42 44 45 49 63 65 66 69 71 **P**5	23	10	73	2802	36	40143	157	19949	8503	344
BROWNSVILLE—Fayette County ★ BROWNSVILLE GENERAL HOSPITAL, 125 Simpson Road, Zip 15417; tel. 412/785–7200; Alvin W. Allison Jr., Interim Chief Executive Officer (Nonreporting) **A**1 9 10 **S**0002 Quorum Health Group/Quorum Health Resources	23	10	115	—	—	—	—	—	—	—
BRYN MAWR—Delaware County BRYN MAWR COLLEGE INFIRMARY, Bryn Mawr College Campus, Zip 19010; tel. 610/526–7360; Kay Kerr M.D., Medical Director (Nonreporting)	23	11	7	—	—	—	—	—	—	—
★ BRYN MAWR HOSPITAL, 130 South Bryn Mawr Avenue, Zip 19010–3160; tel. 610/526–3000; Kenneth Hanover, President and Chief Executive Officer **A**1 2 3 5 9 10 **F**4 5 7 8 10 11 12 13 14 15 16 17 19 20 22 28 30 37 38 40 41 42 43 44 49 51 52 53 60 61 65 67 71 73 74 **S**7775 Main Line Health	23	10	281	14077	219	115763	1898	139634	59959	1577
BUTLER—Butler County ★ BUTLER MEMORIAL HOSPITAL, 911 East Brady Street, Zip 16001–4697; tel. 412/283–6666; Scott A. Becker, President and Chief Executive Officer (Total facility includes 19 beds in nursing home–type unit) **A**1 9 10 **F**2 3 5 7 8 10 11 13 14 15 16 19 21 22 23 24 25 27 28 32 33 35 37 40 44 46 49 52 53 54 56 57 63 64 65 67 71 72 **P**4	23	10	286	10336	188	128538	1085	68167	31308	1037
★ VETERANS AFFAIRS MEDICAL CENTER, (Extended and Primary Medical Care) 325 New Castle Road, Zip 16001–2480; tel. 412/287–4781; P. Stajduhar M.D., Director (Total facility includes 172 beds in nursing home–type unit) **A**1 **F**1 2 3 4 8 10 12 17 18 19 20 21 22 23 24 26 27 28 30 31 32 34 35 37 42 43 44 45 46 48 49 51 54 56 58 59 60 65 67 69 71 73 74 **P**6 **S**9295 Department of Veterans Affairs	45	49	333	2425	275	54919	0	37421	22154	557

Hospitals, U.S. / PENNSYLVANIA

Hospital, Address, Telephone, Administrator, Approval, Facility, and Physician Codes, Health Care System	Classification Codes		Utilization Data					Expense (thousands) of dollars		
★ American Hospital Association (AHA) membership ☐ Joint Commission on Accreditation of Healthcare Organizations (JCAHO) accreditation + American Osteopathic Hospital Association (AOHA) membership ○ American Osteopathic Association (AOA) accreditation △ Commission on Accreditation of Rehabilitation Facilities (CARF) accreditation Control codes 61, 63, 64, 71, 72 and 73 indicate hospitals listed by AOHA, but not registered by AHA. For definition of numerical codes, see page A6	Control	Service	Beds	Admissions	Census	Outpatient Visits	Births	Total	Payroll	Personnel
CAMP HILL—Cumberland County										
★ HOLY SPIRIT HOSPITAL, 503 North 21st Street, Zip 17011–2288; tel. 717/763–2111; Sister Romaine Niemeyer, President and Chief Executive Officer **A**1 5 9 10 **F**2 3 4 7 8 10 12 15 18 19 21 22 23 27 28 29 30 31 32 34 35 37 39 40 41 42 44 46 51 52 53 54 55 56 57 58 59 60 63 65 67 68 69 71 73 **P**8	21	10	317	11475	208	177534	538	75371	39933	1293
STATE CORRECTIONAL INSTITUTION AT CAMP HILL, 2500 Lisbon Road, Zip 17011, Mailing Address: Box 200, Zip 17011; tel. 717/737–4531; Kathy Montag, Administrator Health Care (Nonreporting)	12	49	34	—	—	—	—	—	—	—
CANONSBURG—Washington County										
★ CANONSBURG GENERAL HOSPITAL, 100 Medical Boulevard, Zip 15317; tel. 412/745–6100; Robert R. Tracht, President and Chief Executive Officer; Barbara A. Bensaia, Executive Vice President (Total facility includes 23 beds in nursing home–type unit) **A**1 9 10 **F**8 10 12 14 17 19 21 22 28 30 32 34 35 37 39 41 44 49 63 64 65 67 73 **S**0002 Quorum Health Group/Quorum Health Resources	23	10	120	3975	84	56240	0	29768	12554	372
CARBONDALE—Lackawanna County										
★ MARIAN COMMUNITY HOSPITAL, 100 Lincoln Avenue, Zip 18407; tel. 717/281–1000; Sister Jean Coughlin, President **A**1 9 10 **F**1 8 12 14 15 16 17 19 21 22 28 29 30 31 34 37 42 44 45 49 52 56 65 67 69 71 73 **P**3 8	21	10	99	3740	69	48077	0	23491	9675	399
CARLISLE—Cumberland County										
★ CARLISLE HOSPITAL, 246 Parker Street, Zip 17013–0310; tel. 717/249–1212; Michael J. Halstead, Interim President and Chief Executive Officer **A**1 9 10 **F**7 8 12 15 17 18 19 21 22 23 28 29 30 32 33 34 35 37 39 40 42 44 45 46 49 52 53 56 57 60 62 63 65 67 68 70 71 72 73 **S**0002 Quorum Health Group/Quorum Health Resources	23	10	183	6369	98	336813	773	42085	20722	631
CENTRE HALL—Centre County										
☐ MEADOWS PSYCHIATRIC CENTER, Mailing Address: Rural Delivery 1, Box 259, Zip 16828; tel. 814/364–2161; Joseph Barszczewski, Chief Executive Officer **A**1 9 10 **F**1 12 15 16 22 45 52 53 54 55 56 57 59 65 70 **P**6 **S**2635 First Hospital Corporation	33	22	101	1628	64	1667	0	8957	4346	180
CHAMBERSBURG—Franklin County										
★ △ CHAMBERSBURG HOSPITAL, 112 North Seventh Street, Zip 17201–0187, Mailing Address: P.O. Box 187, Zip 17201–0187; tel. 717/264–5171; Norman B. Epstein, President **A**1 7 9 10 **F**2 7 8 9 10 11 14 15 16 18 19 20 22 23 25 26 28 29 30 31 32 33 34 35 37 39 40 41 42 44 45 46 48 49 52 54 56 57 58 59 60 63 65 67 71 73 **P**6 8	23	10	224	8930	148	144053	1081	60614	29861	990
CHESTER—Delaware County										
COMMUNITY HOSPITAL–CHESTER See Crozer–Chester Medical Center, Upland										
KEYSTONE CENTER, 2001 Providence Avenue, Zip 19013–5504; tel. 610/876–9000; Daniel A. Kidd, Chief Executive Officer and Managing Director (Nonreporting) **S**9555 Universal Health Services, Inc.	33	82	76	—	—	—	—	—	—	—
CLARION—Clarion County										
★ + ○ CLARION HOSPITAL, One Hospital Drive, Zip 16214; tel. 814/226–9500; John J. Shepard, President and Chief Executive Officer **A**9 10 11 12 13 **F**7 8 19 20 21 22 33 34 35 40 41 42 44 49 63 71 73 **P**3 **S**0002 Quorum Health Group/Quorum Health Resources	23	10	88	3465	44	71684	257	22704	8263	364
☐ CLARION PSYCHIATRIC CENTER, 2 Hospital Drive, RD 3, Zip 16214; tel. 814/226–9545; Michael R. Keefer, Administrator and Chief Executive Officer (Nonreporting) **A**1 10 **S**2635 First Hospital Corporation	33	22	52							
CLARKS SUMMIT—Lackawanna County										
☐ CLARKS SUMMIT STATE HOSPITAL, 1451 Hillside Drive, Zip 18411; tel. 717/586–2011; Robert G. McAnderew, Superintendent (Total facility includes 167 beds in nursing home–type unit) **A**1 10 **F**1 4 8 10 12 14 16 17 18 19 20 21 22 23 26 27 28 30 31 35 39 42 44 45 46 50 52 54 55 57 60 61 63 64 65 67 70 71 73 **P**6	12	22	512	168	433	0	0	12681	—	516
CLEARFIELD—Clearfield County										
★ CLEARFIELD HOSPITAL, 809 Turnpike Avenue, Zip 16830, Mailing Address: Box 992, Zip 16830; tel. 814/765–5341; John A. Ireland, President and Chief Executive Officer **A**1 5 9 10 **F**7 8 10 12 14 16 19 21 22 23 25 30 32 33 34 35 37 40 41 42 43 44 45 56 63 65 66 71 **P**5	23	10	105	5112	66	212570	557	39547	19071	629
COAL TOWNSHIP—Northumberland County										
★ SHAMOKIN AREA COMMUNITY HOSPITAL, 4200 Hospital Road, Zip 17866–9697; tel. 717/644–4200; Harold C. Warman Jr., President and Chief Executive Officer **A**9 10 **F**8 14 15 16 17 19 21 22 26 28 30 31 33 35 37 41 44 45 46 49 61 63 65 66 71 73 **P**8	23	10	45	1776	27	53572	0	12415	5239	183
COALDALE—Schuylkill County										
☐ MINER'S MEMORIAL MEDICAL CENTER, Seventh Street, Zip 18218; tel. 717/645–2131; Gerald D. Neal, Chief Executive Officer and Administrator (Total facility includes 48 beds in nursing home–type unit) **A**1 9 10 **F**8 14 15 16 19 21 22 26 30 32 34 35 37 42 44 56 59 64 65 71 73	23	10	110	2671	86	29841	0	20668	9638	348
COATESVILLE—Chester County										
★ BRANDYWINE HOSPITAL, 201 Reeceville Road, Zip 19320–1536; tel. 215/383–8000; James H. Thorton, President and Chief Executive Officer **A**1 2 6 9 10 **F**4 5 7 8 10 13 14 17 19 20 21 22 24 25 26 28 29 30 31 32 33 34 35 36 37 39 40 41 42 44 45 46 49 52 53 56 60 61 65 66 67 70 71 72 73 74 **P**8	23	10	190	7501	126	75196	818	63291	27496	919

Hospitals, U.S. / PENNSYLVANIA

Hospital, Address, Telephone, Administrator, Approval, Facility, and Physician Codes, Health Care System	Classification Codes		Utilization Data					Expense (thousands) of dollars		
★ American Hospital Association (AHA) membership ☐ Joint Commission on Accreditation of Healthcare Organizations (JCAHO) accreditation + American Osteopathic Hospital Association (AOHA) membership ○ American Osteopathic Association (AOA) accreditation △ Commission on Accreditation of Rehabilitation Facilities (CARF) accreditation Control codes 61, 63, 64, 71, 72 and 73 indicate hospitals listed by AOHA, but not registered by AHA. For definition of numerical codes, see page A6	Control	Service	Beds	Admissions	Census	Outpatient Visits	Births	Total	Payroll	Personnel
★ VETERANS AFFAIRS MEDICAL CENTER, Black Horse Hill Road, Zip 19320–9985; tel. 610/380–4303; Gary W. Devansky, Director (Total facility includes 208 beds in nursing home–type unit) A1 5 9 F1 2 3 6 8 12 15 16 18 19 20 21 24 26 27 30 31 32 34 35 37 39 41 44 45 46 49 51 52 54 56 57 58 64 65 67 71 73 74 P6 S9295 Department of Veterans Affairs	45	22	792	3100	748	73972	0	—	—	1440
COLUMBIA—Lancaster County ★ LANCASTER GENERAL HOSPITAL – SUSQUEHANNA DIVISION, (Formerly Columbia Hospital) 631 Poplar Street, Zip 17512, Mailing Address: P.O. Box 926, Zip 17512–0926; tel. 717/684–2841; Scott A. Berlucchi, President and Chief Executive Officer A1 9 10 F2 3 7 8 14 15 16 17 19 22 30 33 39 40 41 44 45 46 49 63 65 67 71 73	23	10	81	1578	43	52647	51	8233	4484	173
CONNELLSVILLE—Fayette County ★ HIGHLANDS HOSPITAL, 401 East Murphy Avenue, Zip 15425–2797; tel. 412/628–1500; Michael J. Evans, Executive Director A1 9 10 F3 8 10 12 15 16 17 18 19 20 21 22 23 26 28 29 30 31 32 33 35 37 39 41 42 44 46 49 52 53 54 55 56 57 58 60 63 65 67 71 73 P8	23	10	92	3420	65	48838	0	18526	8613	301
CORRY—Erie County ☐ CORRY MEMORIAL HOSPITAL, 612 West Smith Street, Zip 16407–1196; tel. 814/664–4641; Joseph T. Hodges, President A1 9 10 F8 11 14 15 19 21 22 27 32 34 37 40 41 44 49 65 69 71 73 P7	23	10	82	2290	27	32866	336	11779	4970	211
COUDERSPORT—Potter County ★ CHARLES COLE MEMORIAL HOSPITAL, Rural Route 1, Box 205, Zip 16915; tel. 814/274–9300; Benjamin L. Stimaker, Chief Executive Officer (Total facility includes 50 beds in nursing home–type unit) A1 9 10 F3 6 7 8 12 16 19 21 22 24 25 28 30 32 33 35 37 39 40 41 44 46 49 53 54 55 58 63 64 65 66 71 73 P6 7	23	10	104	2796	85	67605	354	22547	9505	367
DANVILLE—Montour County ☐ DANVILLE STATE HOSPITAL, Zip 17821–0700; tel. 717/275–7011; Elizabeth A. Williams R.N., Superintendent (Total facility includes 119 beds in nursing home–type unit) A1 9 10 F1 2 3 4 5 6 7 8 9 10 11 12 13 17 18 19 20 21 22 23 24 25 26 27 28 29 30 31 32 33 34 35 36 37 38 39 40 41 42 43 44 45 46 47 48 49 50 51 52 53 54 55 56 57 58 59 60 61 62 63 64 65 66 67 68 69 70 71 72 73 74 P6	12	22	408	154	397	0	0	31295	18616	575
★ GEISINGER MEDICAL CENTER, 100 North Academy Avenue, Zip 17822–2201; tel. 717/271–6168; Stuart Heydt, Chief Executive Officer (Nonreporting) A1 2 3 5 6 8 9 10 S5570 Geisinger Health Care System	23	10	577	—	—	—	—	—	—	—
DARBY—Montgomery County FITZGERALD MERCY HOSPITAL See Mercy Health Corporation of Souteastern Pennsylvania, Bala Cynwyd										
DEVON—Chester County DEVEREUX FOUNDATION–FRENCH CENTER, 119 Old Lancaster Road, Zip 19333, Mailing Address: Box 400, Zip 19333; tel. 215/964–3214; Howard D. Margolis, Executive Director (Nonreporting)	23	59	110	—	—	—	—	—	—	—
DOWNINGTOWN—Chester County ★ VILLA ST. JOHN VIANNEY HOSPITAL, Lincoln Highway at Woodbine Road, Zip 19335–0219; tel. 610/269–2600; Louis D. Horvath, Administrator F15 34 52 58 P5	21	22	54	81	41	0	0	4796	2801	79
DOYLESTOWN—Bucks County ☐ DELAWARE VALLEY MENTAL HEALTH FOUNDATION, 833 East Butler Avenue, Zip 18901; tel. 215/345–0444; William P. Miller, Chief Executive Officer (Nonreporting) A1 10	23	22	45	—	—	—	—	—	—	—
★ △ DOYLESTOWN HOSPITAL, 595 West State Street, Zip 18901; tel. 215/345–2200; Richard Reif, President and Chief Executive Officer (Total facility includes 536 beds in nursing home–type unit) A1 5 7 9 10 F6 7 8 10 12 15 16 17 18 19 21 22 23 26 27 28 30 31 32 33 34 35 37 39 40 41 42 44 45 46 48 49 52 54 55 56 57 58 59 61 62 64 65 67 71 73 P8	23	10	749	8450	687	148259	976	84271	41170	1001
DREXEL HILL—Delaware County ★ DELAWARE COUNTY MEMORIAL HOSPITAL, 501 North Lansdowne Avenue, Zip 19026–1186; tel. 610/284–8100; Dante Caruso Jr., President and Chief Executive Officer A1 2 3 5 9 10 F2 3 4 5 7 8 9 10 11 12 13 14 15 16 17 19 21 22 24 28 29 30 32 33 34 35 37 38 39 40 41 42 43 44 45 46 48 49 50 52 54 59 60 61 63 64 66 67 70 71 72 73 74 P3 5 7 S0008 Crozer–Keystone Health System	23	10	285	11153	190	70738	1228	82345	35668	1072
DUBOIS—Clearfield County ☐ DUBOIS REGIONAL MEDICAL CENTER, 100 Hospital Avenue, Zip 15801, Mailing Address: P.O. Box 447, Zip 15801–0447; tel. 814/371–2200; Raymond A. Graeca, President and Chief Executive Officer (Total facility includes 14 beds in nursing home–type unit) A1 2 9 10 F2 3 7 8 10 15 16 17 19 21 22 23 25 26 27 28 29 30 32 33 34 35 37 38 39 40 41 42 44 46 49 51 52 53 54 55 56 57 58 60 61 63 64 65 66 67 71 73 P6	23	10	194	8277	127	185544	790	51940	25710	892
EAGLEVILLE—Montgomery County ★ EAGLEVILLE HOSPITAL, 100 Eagleville Road, Zip 19403–1800; tel. 610/539–6000; Frederick M. Carey, Chief Executive Officer A9 10 F2 14 15 20 22 28 29 39 45 54 55 56 59 65 67 73 74	23	82	159	2564	142	0	0	18151	10408	334
EAST STROUDSBURG—Monroe County ★ POCONO MEDICAL CENTER, 206 East Brown Street, Zip 18301; tel. 717/421–4000; Marilyn R. Rettaliata, President A1 2 9 10 F7 8 11 15 19 22 25 28 30 31 34 35 37 40 41 42 44 45 46 49 52 56 60 63 65 67 71 73 74	23	10	228	10056	156	135957	1046	60487	27982	897

Hospitals, U.S. / PENNSYLVANIA

Hospital, Address, Telephone, Administrator, Approval, Facility, and Physician Codes, Health Care System	Classification Codes		Utilization Data					Expense (thousands) of dollars		
★ American Hospital Association (AHA) membership ☐ Joint Commission on Accreditation of Healthcare Organizations (JCAHO) accreditation + American Osteopathic Hospital Association (AOHA) membership ○ American Osteopathic Association (AOA) accreditation △ Commission on Accreditation of Rehabilitation Facilities (CARF) accreditation Control codes 61, 63, 64, 71, 72 and 73 indicate hospitals listed by AOHA, but not registered by AHA. For definition of numerical codes, see page A6	Control	Service	Beds	Admissions	Census	Outpatient Visits	Births	Total	Payroll	Personnel
EASTON—Northampton County										
★ EASTON HOSPITAL, 250 South 21st Street, Zip 18042-3892; tel. 610/250-4000; Donna Mulholland, President **A**1 2 3 5 9 10 **F**4 7 8 10 14 15 16 17 19 21 22 28 29 30 31 34 36 37 38 40 41 42 43 44 45 46 48 49 54 56 57 59 60 63 65 67 71 73 74 **P**8	23	10	296	12589	246	207369	888	92020	44028	1589
ELKINS PARK—Montgomery County										
☐ MEDICAL COLLEGE HOSPITALS – ELKINS PARK CAMPUS, 60 East Township Line Road, Zip 19117; tel. 215/663-6000; Margaret M. McGoldrick, Executive Director and Chief Executive Officer (Nonreporting) **A**1 3 9 10 **S**2305 Allegheny Health, Education and Research Foundation	23	10	217	—	—	—	—	—	—	—
ELLWOOD CITY—Lawrence County										
ELLWOOD CITY HOSPITAL, 724 Pershing Street, Zip 16117-1499; tel. 412/752-0081; Herbert S. Skuba, President (Nonreporting) **A**9 10	23	10	118	—	—	—	—	—	—	—
EPHRATA—Lancaster County										
☐ EPHRATA COMMUNITY HOSPITAL, 169 Martin Avenue, Zip 17522-1002, Mailing Address: P.O. Box 1002, Zip 17522-1002; tel. 717/733-0311; John M. Porter Jr., President **A**1 9 10 **F**7 8 14 15 16 19 21 22 30 31 32 33 34 35 36 37 39 40 41 42 44 45 46 49 51 52 53 54 56 57 58 59 63 65 67 71 73 74 **P**8	23	10	134	5031	67	60458	517	33572	17406	526
ERIE—Erie County										
★ HAMOT MEDICAL CENTER, 201 State Street, Zip 16550-0001; tel. 814/877-6000; John T. Malone, President and Chief Executive Officer (Total facility includes 20 beds in nursing home-type unit) **A**1 2 3 5 8 9 10 **F**2 3 4 5 6 7 8 10 14 15 16 17 18 19 21 22 23 24 25 26 27 28 29 30 31 32 33 34 35 36 37 38 39 40 41 42 43 44 46 49 50 51 52 53 54 55 56 57 58 59 60 61 62 63 64 65 66 67 68 70 71 72 73 74 **P**6	23	10	526	15344	265	137556	1539	138712	59915	2212
☐ △ HEALTHSOUTH GREAT LAKES REHABILITATION HOSPITAL, 143 East Second Street, Zip 16507; tel. 814/878-1200; William R. Fox, Chief Executive Officer **A**1 7 9 10 **F**5 12 14 16 19 22 27 34 35 41 45 46 48 49 65 67 73 **P**6 **S**0023 Healthsouth Corporation	33	46	108	979	62	17469	0	14572	7560	200
☐ △ HEALTHSOUTH LAKE ERIE INSTITUTE OF REHABILITATION, 137 West Second Street, Zip 16507-1403; tel. 814/453-5602; William R. Fox, Chief Executive Officer (Nonreporting) **A**1 7 9 10 **S**0023 Healthsouth Corporation	33	46	99	—	—	—	—	—	—	—
★ ○ METRO HEALTH CENTER, 252 West 11th Street, Zip 16501; tel. 814/870-3400; J. B. Frith, Chief Executive Officer **A**10 11 12 13 **F**7 8 14 15 16 19 21 22 30 34 35 37 40 41 44 49 51 63 65 71 72 73 **P**8 **S**0002 Quorum Health Group/Quorum Health Resources	23	10	101	3590	52	41661	296	20979	7773	298
+ ○ MILLCREEK COMMUNITY HOSPITAL, 5515 Peach Street, Zip 16509-2695; tel. 814/864-4031; Mary L. Eckert, Executive Director **A**9 10 11 12 13 **F**7 8 15 16 19 22 28 30 35 37 40 42 44 51 65 71 72 73	23	10	101	3447	46	44243	179	16762	6870	268
☐ SAINT VINCENT HOSPITAL, 232 West 25th Street, Zip 16544; tel. 814/452-5000; Sister Catherine Manning, President and Chief Executive Officer **A**1 3 5 6 9 10 **F**3 4 7 8 10 11 12 13 14 15 16 17 18 19 20 21 22 24 25 28 29 30 32 33 34 35 37 38 39 40 41 42 43 44 45 46 48 49 51 52 53 54 56 57 58 59 60 61 63 65 67 70 71 72 73 74 **P**6	23	10	469	15841	282	142212	1934	134558	61080	2053
★ SHRINERS HOSPITALS FOR CRIPPLED CHILDREN, ERIE UNIT, 1645 West 8th Street, Zip 16505; tel. 814/875-8700; Richard W. Brzuz, Administrator **A**1 3 **F**5 14 15 16 17 25 34 39 45 46 48 49 65 71 73 **S**4125 Shriners Hospitals for Crippled Children	23	57	30	702	13	8738	0	—	—	102
★ VETERANS AFFAIRS MEDICAL CENTER, 135 East 38th Street, Zip 16504-1596; tel. 814/868-6210; Stephen M. Lucas, Director (Total facility includes 40 beds in nursing home-type unit) **A**1 **F**1 2 3 12 15 16 18 19 20 22 26 27 29 30 31 33 37 39 41 42 44 45 46 48 49 51 52 54 55 56 57 58 64 65 67 71 73 74 **P**6 **S**9295 Department of Veterans Affairs	45	10	159	1957	98	63070	0	32361	15481	440
EVERETT—Bedford County										
★ MEMORIAL HOSPITAL OF BEDFORD COUNTY, Rural Delivery 1, Box 80, Zip 15537-9513; tel. 814/623-6161; James C. Vreeland FACHE, President and Chief Executive Officer **A**1 9 10 **F**1 3 4 6 7 8 10 12 13 14 15 16 17 18 19 20 21 22 23 24 26 27 28 29 30 31 32 33 34 35 36 37 39 40 41 42 43 44 49 51 53 54 55 56 57 58 59 60 63 65 67 69 70 71 73 **P**8	23	10	78	2988	32	60163	259	18770	8100	317
FARRELL—Mercer County										
SHENANGO VALLEY MEDICAL CENTER See Horizon Hospital System, Greenville										
FORT WASHINGTON—Montgomery County										
☐ NORTHWESTERN INSTITUTE, 450 Bethlehem Pike, Zip 19034-0209; tel. 215/641-5300; Richard Jensen, Administrator **A**1 3 9 10 **F**1 3 19 22 26 35 46 52 53 54 55 56 57 58 59 65 **P**5 **S**0455 Hospital Group of America	33	22	146	2423	119	312	0	—	—	382
FRANKLIN—Venango County										
☐ NORTHWEST MEDICAL CENTER, (Includes Northwest Medical Center–Franklin Campus, Franklin, Pennsylvania; Northwest Medical Center–Oil City Campus, 174 East Bissell Avenue, Oil City, Pennsylvania, Zip 16301-0568, Mailing Address: Box 1068, Zip 16301-0568; tel. 814/677-1711) 1 Spruce Street, Zip 16323, Mailing Address: 1 Spruce Street, Zip 16323; tel. 814/437-7000; Neil E. Todhunter, Chief Executive Officer **A**1 2 9 10 **F**3 4 7 8 13 19 21 22 23 28 30 34 35 36 37 39 40 41 42 44 45 48 49 51 52 54 55 56 57 58 59 60 63 65 66 71 72	23	10	173	9546	150	173891	541	61843	26962	843

Hospitals, U.S. / PENNSYLVANIA

Hospital, Address, Telephone, Administrator, Approval, Facility, and Physician Codes, Health Care System	Classification Codes		Utilization Data					Expense (thousands) of dollars		Personnel
	Control	Service	Beds	Admissions	Census	Outpatient Visits	Births	Total	Payroll	

★ American Hospital Association (AHA) membership
□ Joint Commission on Accreditation of Healthcare Organizations (JCAHO) accreditation
+ American Osteopathic Hospital Association (AOHA) membership
○ American Osteopathic Association (AOA) accreditation
△ Commission on Accreditation of Rehabilitation Facilities (CARF) accreditation
Control codes 61, 63, 64, 71, 72 and 73 indicate hospitals listed by AOHA, but not registered by AHA. For definition of numerical codes, see page A6

Hospital	Control	Service	Beds	Admissions	Census	Outpatient Visits	Births	Total	Payroll	Personnel
GETTYSBURG—Adams County ★ GETTYSBURG HOSPITAL, 147 Gettys Street, Zip 17325–9978; tel. 717/334–2121; Steven W. Renner, President; Richard A. Harley, Vice President Finance **A**1 9 10 **F**3 4 7 8 14 15 16 19 21 22 23 28 30 32 33 34 35 37 39 40 42 44 46 49 56 65 67 71 73 **P**8	23	10	102	4555	59	94312	681	34205	16179	502
GREENSBURG—Westmoreland County ★ WESTMORELAND REGIONAL HOSPITAL, 532 West Pittsburgh Street, Zip 15601–2282; tel. 412/832–4000; Joseph J. Peluso, President and Chief Executive Officer **A**1 2 3 9 10 **F**2 3 4 7 8 10 11 13 14 16 17 19 20 21 22 23 25 26 27 28 29 30 31 32 33 34 35 37 39 40 41 42 43 44 45 46 48 49 52 53 54 55 56 57 58 59 60 61 63 65 67 68 71 72 73 74 **P**8	23	10	321	12826	250	144625	751	98635	44915	1293
GREENVILLE—Mercer County HORIZON HOSPITAL SYSTEM, (Formerly Listed Under Hermitage) (Includes Greenville Regional Hospital, 110 North Main Street, Greenville, Pennsylvania, Zip 16125–1795; tel. 412/588–2100; Shenango Valley Medical Center, 2200 Memorial Drive, Farrell, Pennsylvania, Zip 16121–1398; tel. 412/981–3500) 110 North Main Street, Zip 16125; tel. 412/346–3557; J. Larry Heinike, President (Total facility includes 28 beds in nursing home–type unit) **A**2 10 **F**2 3 5 7 8 10 12 13 14 15 16 17 19 20 21 22 23 24 25 26 27 28 29 30 32 33 34 35 37 39 40 41 42 43 44 45 46 48 49 54 55 56 57 58 60 63 64 65 66 67 68 71 72 73 74 **P**4 8	23	10	319	11963	186	—	691	79461	34059	1101
GROVE CITY—Mercer County ★ + ○ UNITED COMMUNITY HOSPITAL, 631 North Broad Street Extension, Zip 16127–9703; tel. 412/458–5442; William J. Grego Jr., Administrator **A**1 9 10 11 **F**3 7 8 11 15 16 19 20 21 22 27 28 30 32 33 34 35 39 40 42 44 45 46 49 56 58 60 63 66 67 70 71 73 **P**8	23	10	99	3407	49	63931	290	21940	9378	337
HANOVER—York County ★ HANOVER GENERAL HOSPITAL, 300 Highland Avenue, Zip 17331–2297; tel. 717/637–3711; William R. Walb, President and Chief Executive Officer **A**1 5 9 10 **F**4 7 8 11 15 16 17 18 19 20 21 22 25 28 30 31 33 34 35 37 39 40 41 42 44 45 49 52 53 57 63 65 67 71 73 **P**4 8	23	10	154	6227	103	89124	670	41855	18875	691
HARRISBURG—Dauphin County + ○ COMMUNITY GENERAL OSTEOPATHIC HOSPITAL, 4300 Londonderry Road, Zip 17109, Mailing Address: P.O. Box 3000, Zip 17105–3000; tel. 717/652–3000; George R. Strohl Jr., President **A**9 10 11 12 13 **F**8 11 14 15 16 19 21 22 25 30 33 34 39 41 42 44 45 49 65 67 71 73 **P**6	23	10	115	4817	82	111501	0	43677	18833	545
□ EDGEWATER PSYCHIATRIC CENTER, 1829 North Front Street, Zip 17102–2299; tel. 717/238–8666; Michael J. Dalesio Ph.D., Acting Executive Director **A**1 9 10 **F**14 52 58 59	23	22	26	449	21	0	0	4660	1896	116
★ HARRISBURG HOSPITAL, 111 South Front Street, Zip 17101–2099; tel. 717/782–3131; Susan Edwards, Senior Vice President and Chief Operating Officer **A**1 3 5 9 10 **F**3 4 6 7 8 10 11 12 13 15 16 17 19 21 22 23 24 27 28 29 30 31 32 33 34 35 37 38 39 40 41 42 43 44 46 49 51 53 54 57 58 59 60 61 64 65 67 68 69 71 72 73 74 **P**7 **S**2135 Capital Health System	23	10	398	15169	242	218050	2990	138618	57059	1616
□ HARRISBURG STATE HOSPITAL, Cameron and Maclay Streets, Zip 17105–1300, Mailing Address: Pouch A, Zip 17105–1300; tel. 717/772–7600; Bruce Darney, Superintendent (Nonreporting) **A**1 9 10	12	22	455	—						
★ POLYCLINIC MEDICAL CENTER OF HARRISBURG, 2601 North Third Street, Zip 17110–2098; tel. 717/782–4141; Stephen H. Franklin, President (Total facility includes 88 beds in nursing home–type unit) **A**1 2 3 5 9 10 **F**1 2 3 4 5 6 7 8 10 11 12 13 14 15 16 17 18 19 20 21 22 23 25 26 27 28 29 31 32 33 34 35 37 38 39 40 41 42 43 44 45 46 48 49 51 52 53 54 55 56 57 58 59 60 61 63 64 65 67 68 71 72 73 74 **P**6 8	23	10	453	15056	347	359761	2187	—	—	1847
HAVERFORD—Delaware County □ HAVERFORD STATE HOSPITAL, 3500 Darby Road, Zip 19041–1098; tel. 610/525–9620; Aidan Altenor Ph.D., Superintendent (Total facility includes 60 beds in nursing home–type unit) **A**1 9 10 **F**15 20 52 64 65 73	12	22	400	93	361	0	0	33086	18056	518
HAVERTOWN—Delaware County ★ MERCY HAVERFORD HOSPITAL, 2000 Old West Chester Pike, Zip 19083; tel. 610/645–3600; Andrew E. Harris, Chief Executive Director **A**1 9 10 **F**2 8 16 17 19 21 22 28 30 31 37 39 41 42 44 46 49 63 65 71 73 **P**5 **S**3595 Eastern Mercy Health System	21	10	107	3630	49	30492	0	21876	10538	459
HAZLETON—Luzerne County ★ HAZLETON GENERAL HOSPITAL, 700 East Broad Street, Zip 18201–6897; tel. 717/450–4357; E. Richard Moore, President **A**1 9 10 **F**1 3 4 5 6 7 8 10 12 13 14 15 16 17 18 19 20 21 22 23 24 25 26 27 28 29 30 31 32 33 34 35 36 37 39 41 42 43 44 45 46 49 50 51 52 53 54 56 57 58 59 60 61 62 63 65 66 67 68 69 70 71 72 73 74 **P**8	23	10	152	4799	108	37620	0	27849	11627	510
★ HAZLETON–ST. JOSEPH MEDICAL CENTER, 687 North Church Street, Zip 18201–3198; tel. 717/459–4444; Bernard C. Rudegeair, President and Chief Executive Officer **A**1 9 10 **F**1 3 4 5 7 8 10 15 17 19 21 22 23 24 25 26 28 30 31 32 33 34 35 36 37 39 40 41 42 43 44 50 51 54 55 56 57 60 63 65 66 67 69 70 71 72 73 74 **P**5	21	10	124	4331	78	148657	521	29143	13643	516
HERMITAGE—Mercer County HORIZON HOSPITAL SYSTEM See Greenville										

Hospitals, U.S. / PENNSYLVANIA

Hospital, Address, Telephone, Administrator, Approval, Facility, and Physician Codes, Health Care System	Classi- fication Codes		Utilization Data					Expense (thousands) of dollars		
★ American Hospital Association (AHA) membership □ Joint Commission on Accreditation of Healthcare Organizations (JCAHO) accreditation + American Osteopathic Hospital Association (AOHA) membership ○ American Osteopathic Association (AOA) accreditation △ Commission on Accreditation of Rehabilitation Facilities (CARF) accreditation Control codes 61, 63, 64, 71, 72 and 73 indicate hospitals listed by AOHA, but not registered by AHA. For definition of numerical codes, see page A6	Control	Service	Beds	Admissions	Census	Outpatient Visits	Births	Total	Payroll	Personnel
HERSHEY—Dauphin County										
★ △ PENN STATE UNIVERSITY HOSPITAL – MILTON S. HERSHEY MEDICAL CENTER, 500 University Drive, Zip 17033, Mailing Address: P.O. Box 850, Zip 17033–0850; tel. 717/531–8521; Allan C. Anderson, Director **A**1 2 3 5 7 8 9 10 **F**3 4 7 8 10 14 15 16 17 19 21 22 23 24 25 28 29 30 31 34 35 37 38 39 40 41 42 43 44 45 46 47 48 49 51 52 53 54 56 57 58 59 60 61 63 65 66 67 69 70 71 73 **P**6	23	10	465	17785	370	265049	1052	230743	110564	3547
HONESDALE—Wayne County										
★ WAYNE MEMORIAL HOSPITAL, 601 Park Street, Zip 18431–1498; tel. 717/253–8100; Richard Garman, Executive Director (Total facility includes 28 beds in nursing home–type unit) **A**1 9 10 **F**7 8 11 15 17 19 21 22 24 28 30 31 32 33 34 35 37 40 41 42 44 45 49 52 53 55 56 57 58 59 60 64 65 66 67 71 73 **P**5	23	10	119	3471	95	80000	440	25476	11929	439
HUNTINGDON—Huntingdon County										
★ J.C. BLAIR MEMORIAL HOSPITAL, Warm Springs Avenue, Zip 16652; tel. 814/643–2290; Stephen Schoaps, Chief Executive Officer **A**1 9 10 **F**3 5 7 14 15 16 19 21 22 23 28 32 33 34 35 37 40 41 42 44 46 49 52 54 56 58 59 65 66 70 71 73 **S**0002 Quorum Health Group/Quorum Health Resources	23	10	104	3509	53	57045	300	24876	10084	393
INDIANA—Indiana County										
★ INDIANA HOSPITAL, Hospital Road, Zip 15701, Mailing Address: P.O. Box 788, Zip 15701; tel. 412/357–7000; Donald D. Sandoval FACHE, President and Chief Executive Officer **A**1 9 10 **F**7 8 14 15 16 19 21 22 23 28 29 30 31 32 33 35 37 39 40 41 42 44 45 49 60 65 67 71 73	23	10	145	6927	100	153916	710	51234	22970	858
JEANNETTE—Westmoreland County										
□ JEANNETTE DISTRICT MEMORIAL HOSPITAL, 600 Jefferson Avenue, Zip 15644; tel. 412/527–3551; Robert J. Bulger, President and Chief Executive Officer (Total facility includes 11 beds in nursing home–type unit) **A**1 9 10 **F**7 8 11 14 15 16 19 21 22 25 28 35 37 40 44 45 48 49 64 65 71 72 73 **P**8	23	10	175	6318	109	95762	460	36268	17713	627
□ MONSOUR MEDICAL CENTER, 70 Lincoln Way East, Zip 15644; tel. 412/527–1511; Jerry Joseph, Chief Executive Officer **A**1 9 10 **F**2 7 8 10 11 12 14 15 16 18 19 22 28 30 31 32 35 37 39 40 42 44 53 65 69 71 **S**0985 Amerihealth, Inc.	23	10	151	2605	53	37873	128	21376	9238	332
JERSEY SHORE—Lycoming County										
★ JERSEY SHORE HOSPITAL, 1020 Thompson Street, Zip 17740–0689; tel. 717/398–0100; Louis A. Ditzel Jr., President and Chief Executive Officer **A**1 9 10 **F**8 14 15 16 17 19 21 22 28 29 30 32 37 41 44 45 49 63 65 66 71 73 **P**6 7 **S**0002 Quorum Health Group/Quorum Health Resources	23	10	55	1568	17	35898	0	9961	4397	182
JOHNSTOWN—Cambria County										
★ GOOD SAMARITAN MEDICAL CENTER, 1020 Franklin Street, Zip 15905–4186; tel. 814/533–1000; Timothy J. Karnes FACHE, President and Chief Executive Officer (Total facility includes 73 beds in nursing home–type unit) **A**1 9 10 **F**3 8 14 15 16 17 19 21 22 24 25 29 30 32 33 34 35 37 39 40 41 44 45 46 49 50 51 52 53 54 55 56 63 64 65 66 67 71 72 73 **P**6	23	10	240	4987	138	91306	410	36380	12811	613
★ LEE HOSPITAL, 320 Main Street, Zip 15901–1694; tel. 814/533–0123; John W. Ungar, President and Chief Executive Officer **A**1 2 9 10 **F**6 7 8 10 11 12 14 15 16 19 21 22 26 27 28 29 30 32 33 34 35 37 39 40 41 42 44 48 49 56 60 64 65 67 71 72 73 **P**8	23	10	237	8935	172	91867	442	67395	32316	1157
★ MEMORIAL MEDICAL CENTER, 1086 Franklin Street, Zip 15905–4398; tel. 814/533–9000; William F. Casey, Chief Executive Officer **A**1 2 3 5 6 9 10 12 **F**4 7 8 10 11 14 15 16 19 20 21 22 23 24 25 26 27 28 29 30 31 32 34 35 37 38 39 40 41 42 43 44 45 46 49 51 52 54 57 58 60 63 64 65 67 70 71 72 73	23	10	352	13902	246	267359	784	122049	51312	1973
KANE—McKean County										
□ COMMUNITY HOSPITAL, North Fraley Street, Zip 16735; tel. 814/837–8585; Patricia J. Stubber, Chief Executive Officer (Nonreporting) **A**1 9 10	23	10	53	—	—	—	—	—	—	—
KINGSTON—Luzerne County										
NESBITT MEMORIAL HOSPITAL See Wyoming Valley Health Care System										
★ WYOMING VALLEY HEALTH CARE SYSTEM, (Formerly Listed Under Wilkes–Barre) (Includes Nesbitt Memorial Hospital, 562 Wyoming Avenue, Kingston, Pennsylvania, Zip 18704–3784; tel. 717/283–7000; Wilkes–Barre General Hospital, North River and Auburn Streets, Wilkes–Barre, Pennsylvania, Zip 18764; tel. 717/829–8111) 562 Wyoming Avenue, Zip 18704–3764; tel. 717/283–7000; Ron Stern, President and Chief Executive Officer **A**1 2 3 5 9 10 **F**2 3 4 7 8 10 11 14 15 16 17 18 19 21 22 24 25 27 28 30 32 33 34 35 37 39 40 41 42 43 44 46 49 52 53 54 55 56 57 58 59 60 64 65 66 67 71 73 74 **P**6 8	23	10	661	23974	479	383721	2152	162549	67480	2608
KITTANNING—Armstrong County										
★ ARMSTRONG COUNTY MEMORIAL HOSPITAL, One Nolte Drive, Zip 16201–8808; tel. 412/543–8500; George D. Harnett, Acting President and Chief Executive Officer (Total facility includes 17 beds in nursing home–type unit) **A**1 9 10 **F**7 8 10 11 12 14 15 17 19 21 22 28 29 32 34 35 37 39 40 41 42 44 46 49 50 51 52 53 54 55 56 57 60 63 64 65 66 67 71 73 **P**4 5	23	10	217	7164	136	132007	536	45623	23089	736
LAFAYETTE HILL—Montgomery County										
□ EUGENIA HOSPITAL, 660 Thomas Road, Zip 19444–1199; tel. 215/836–7700; John P. Ash FACHE, President and Chief Executive Officer (Nonreporting) **A**1 9 10	33	22	126	—	—	—	—	—	—	—
LANCASTER—Lancaster County										
+ ○ COMMUNITY HOSPITAL OF LANCASTER, 1100 East Orange Street, Zip 17602–3218, Mailing Address: Box 3002, Zip 17604–3002; tel. 717/397–3711; Mark C. Barabas, President **A**9 10 11 12 13 **F**7 8 10 12 15 16 17 19 20 21 22 23 25 28 29 30 31 32 33 34 35 37 39 40 41 42 44 48 49 51 52 54 55 56 58 63 65 67 71 73 74 **P**3 6 8	23	10	140	5415	72	65855	997	39111	18126	606

Hospitals, U.S. / PENNSYLVANIA

Hospital, Address, Telephone, Administrator, Approval, Facility, and Physician Codes, Health Care System	Classification Codes		Utilization Data					Expense (thousands) of dollars		
	Control	Service	Beds	Admissions	Census	Outpatient Visits	Births	Total	Payroll	Personnel

★ American Hospital Association (AHA) membership
☐ Joint Commission on Accreditation of Healthcare Organizations (JCAHO) accreditation
+ American Osteopathic Hospital Association (AOHA) membership
○ American Osteopathic Association (AOA) accreditation
△ Commission on Accreditation of Rehabilitation Facilities (CARF) accreditation
Control codes 61, 63, 64, 71, 72 and 73 indicate hospitals listed by AOHA, but not registered by AHA. For definition of numerical codes, see page A6

Hospital	Control	Service	Beds	Admissions	Census	Outpatient Visits	Births	Total	Payroll	Personnel
☐ △ LANCASTER GENERAL HOSPITAL, 555 North Duke Street, Zip 17602, Mailing Address: Box 3555, Zip 17604–3555; tel. 717/290–5511; Michael A. Young, President and Chief Executive Officer **A**1 2 3 5 6 7 9 10 **F**3 4 5 7 8 10 11 12 13 14 15 16 17 19 20 21 22 23 25 26 28 29 30 31 32 33 34 35 37 38 39 40 41 42 43 44 45 46 48 49 51 52 53 54 55 56 57 58 59 60 61 65 66 67 68 69 70 71 72 73 74 **P**3 4 5 6 7 8	23	10	517	22595	328	288846	2778	176642	97604	2598
★ △ ST. JOSEPH HOSPITAL, 250 College Avenue, Zip 17604; tel. 717/291–8211; John Kerr Tolmie, Interim President and Chief Executive Officer **A**1 2 6 7 9 10 **F**1 2 3 4 7 8 10 11 12 14 15 16 19 21 22 23 26 28 29 30 31 32 33 34 35 37 38 39 40 41 42 43 44 45 46 48 49 51 52 53 54 56 57 58 59 60 61 63 65 67 69 71 73 74 **P**5 6 7 8 **S**5325 Franciscan Health System	21	10	246	10521	151	146923	1415	74932	31996	861
LANGHORNE—Bucks County										
+ ○ DELAWARE VALLEY MEDICAL CENTER, 200 Oxford Valley Road, Zip 19047; tel. 215/949–5100; Carl E. Brown, President **A**10 11 12 13 **F**2 8 10 11 14 15 16 17 19 21 22 23 29 30 31 32 34 35 37 39 41 42 44 45 46 49 52 53 56 57 61 63 65 66 69 71 73 74	23	10	173	6577	113	66610	0	51306	21567	675
★ △ ST. MARY MEDICAL CENTER, Langhorne–Newtown Road, Zip 19047–1295; tel. 215/750–2000; Sister Clare Carty, President (Nonreporting) **A**1 2 7 9 10 **S**5325 Franciscan Health System	21	10	287	—	—	—	—	—	—	—
LANSDALE—Montgomery County										
★ NORTH PENN HOSPITAL, 100 Medical Campus Drive, Zip 19446–1200; tel. 215/368–2100; Robert H. McKay, President **A**1 2 9 10 **F**7 8 14 19 21 22 28 30 37 40 41 42 44 46 49 61 63 65 67 71 73 **P**3 5 7 8	23	10	150	5785	82	92069	897	41193	19615	612
LATROBE—Westmoreland County										
★ LATROBE AREA HOSPITAL, 121 West Second Avenue, Zip 15650–1096; tel. 412/537–1000; Douglas A. Clark, Executive Director **A**1 2 3 5 9 10 **F**5 7 8 10 11 12 15 16 19 21 22 24 25 26 27 28 29 30 31 32 33 34 35 37 39 40 41 42 44 45 49 51 52 53 54 55 56 58 59 60 61 65 67 68 71 73	23	10	252	12577	202	139423	875	84745	45233	1274
LEBANON—Lebanon County										
★ GOOD SAMARITAN HOSPITAL, Fourth and Walnut Streets, Zip 17042, Mailing Address: P.O. Box 1281, Zip 17042–1281; tel. 717/270–7500; Robert J. Longo, President and Chief Executive Officer **A**1 3 5 9 10 **F**7 8 10 12 14 15 16 17 19 21 22 27 28 30 31 32 33 34 35 37 40 41 42 44 45 46 48 49 51 54 55 56 63 65 66 67 71 73 74 **P**8	23	10	190	9189	135	—	1167	59399	27423	941
★ VETERANS AFFAIRS MEDICAL CENTER, 1700 South Lincoln Avenue, Zip 17042–7597; tel. 717/272–6621; Leonard Washington Jr., Director (Total facility includes 177 beds in nursing home–type unit) **A**1 3 5 9 **F**2 3 4 8 10 15 17 19 20 21 22 25 26 27 28 30 31 33 34 35 37 39 41 42 43 44 45 46 48 49 50 51 52 54 56 57 58 59 63 64 65 67 71 72 73 74 **P**6 **S**9295 Department of Veterans Affairs	45	10	646	3548	531	89176	0	76557	42967	1306
LEHIGHTON—Carbon County										
★ GNADEN HUETTEN MEMORIAL HOSPITAL, 211 North 12th Street, Zip 18235; tel. 610/377–1300; Robert J. Clark FACHE, President and Chief Executive Officer (Total facility includes 91 beds in nursing home–type unit) **A**1 9 10 **F**7 8 17 19 20 21 22 26 27 28 30 32 33 35 36 37 39 40 41 42 44 45 46 49 51 52 53 54 55 56 57 58 59 61 63 64 65 67 71 73 74 **P**1 7	23	10	200	4180	156	95904	391	31633	13945	477
LEWISBURG—Union County										
EVANGELICAL COMMUNITY HOSPITAL, One Hospital Drive, Zip 17837–9390; tel. 717/522–2000; Michael Daniloff, President (Nonreporting) **A**9 10	23	10	155	—	—	—	—	—	—	—
U.S. PENITENTIARY HOSPITAL, Route 3, Zip 17837; tel. 717/523–1251; Ronald D. Hillwig, Administrator (Nonreporting)	48	11	17	—	—	—	—	—	—	—
LEWISTOWN—Mifflin County										
★ ○ LEWISTOWN HOSPITAL, 400 Highland Avenue, Zip 17044–1198; tel. 717/248–5411; John R. Whitcomb, President and Chief Executive Officer **A**1 2 9 10 11 **F**2 3 7 8 11 14 16 17 19 20 21 22 26 30 31 32 33 34 35 37 39 40 41 42 44 48 49 52 53 54 55 56 57 58 60 63 65 66 67 69 71 73 **P**2 3	23	10	198	8259	133	—	770	44953	21086	834
LOCK HAVEN—Clinton County										
★ LOCK HAVEN HOSPITAL, 24 Cree Drive, Zip 17745; tel. 717/893–5000; Gary R. Rhoads, President and Chief Executive Officer (Total facility includes 120 beds in nursing home–type unit) **A**1 9 10 **F**7 8 15 19 20 21 22 25 26 27 32 33 34 35 37 39 40 41 44 45 46 49 53 54 55 56 57 58 59 63 64 65 71 73 74 **P**6 **S**0002 Quorum Health Group/Quorum Health Resources	23	10	250	3295	153	36506	311	20100	8732	480
MALVERN—Chester County										
★ △ BRYN MAWR REHABILITATION HOSPITAL, 414 Paoli Pike, Zip 19355–3300, Mailing Address: P.O. Box 3007, Zip 19355–3007; tel. 610/251–5400; Barry S. Rabner, President and Chief Executive Officer **A**1 7 9 10 **F**4 7 8 10 11 12 15 16 19 22 28 32 34 35 37 38 40 41 42 43 44 46 47 48 49 50 60 65 67 71 73 74 **P**5 8 **S**7775 Main Line Health	23	46	131	2324	101	29368	0	27621	16815	497
★ DEVEREUX MAPLETON PSYCHIATRIC INSTITUTE–MAPLETON CENTER, 655 Sugartown Road, Zip 19355–0297, Mailing Address: Box 297, Zip 19355–0297; tel. 610/296–6923; Kenneth Tenley, Director (Nonreporting) **S**0845 Devereux Foundation	23	52	24	—	—	—	—	—	—	—
MALVERN INSTITUTE, 940 King Road, Zip 19355–2058; tel. 610/647–0330; Valerie Craig, Administrator and Chief Executive Officer **A**9 **F**1 2 3 4 5 6 7 8 9 10 11 12 13 16 17 18 19 20 21 22 23 24 25 26 28 29 30 31 32 33 34 35 36 37 38 39 40 41 42 43 44 45 46 47 48 49 50 51 52 53 54 55 57 58 59 60 61 62 63 64 65 66 67 68 69 70 71 72 73 74 **S**0455 Hospital Group of America	33	82	36	675	27	906	0	2708	1465	48

© 1995 AHA Guide

Hospitals, U.S. / PENNSYLVANIA

Hospital, Address, Telephone, Administrator, Approval, Facility, and Physician Codes, Health Care System	Classification Codes		Utilization Data					Expense (thousands) of dollars		
★ American Hospital Association (AHA) membership □ Joint Commission on Accreditation of Healthcare Organizations (JCAHO) accreditation + American Osteopathic Hospital Association (AOHA) membership ○ American Osteopathic Association (AOA) accreditation △ Commission on Accreditation of Rehabilitation Facilities (CARF) accreditation Control codes 61, 63, 64, 71, 72 and 73 indicate hospitals listed by AOHA, but not registered by AHA. For definition of numerical codes, see page A6	Control	Service	Beds	Admissions	Census	Outpatient Visits	Births	Total	Payroll	Personnel
MCCONNELLSBURG—Fulton County										
★ FULTON COUNTY MEDICAL CENTER, 216 South First Street, Zip 17233–1399; tel. 717/485–3155; Robert E. Swadley, Interim President and Chief Executive Officer (Total facility includes 57 beds in nursing home–type unit) **A**9 10 **F**8 11 15 19 22 34 35 40 44 64 65 71	23	10	96	1034	70	96090	125	9417	4389	191
MCKEES ROCKS—Allegheny County										
★ OHIO VALLEY GENERAL HOSPITAL, 25 Heckel Road, Zip 15136–1694; tel. 412/777–6161; William Provenzano, President **A**1 6 9 10 **F**4 7 8 10 13 14 15 16 17 18 19 20 21 22 23 24 25 26 28 29 30 32 33 34 35 36 37 39 40 41 42 44 45 49 60 61 65 67 71 73 **P**5 **S**0002 Quorum Health Group/Quorum Health Resources	23	10	135	5471	93	93232	521	42966	16458	531
MCKEESPORT—Allegheny County										
★ MCKEESPORT HOSPITAL, 1500 Fifth Avenue, Zip 15132–2482; tel. 412/664–2000; Ronald H. Ott, President and Chief Executive Officer (Total facility includes 32 beds in nursing home–type unit) **A**1 3 5 9 10 **F**7 8 10 11 12 13 15 16 17 19 21 22 25 26 28 29 30 31 32 33 34 37 39 40 41 42 44 45 46 48 49 51 52 54 55 56 57 60 61 64 65 67 71 73 74 **P**8	23	10	339	11766	238	132562	483	89282	44818	1269
MEADOWBROOK—Montgomery County										
★ HOLY REDEEMER HOSPITAL AND MEDICAL CENTER, 1648 Huntingdon Pike, Zip 19046–8099; tel. 215/947–3000; Mark T. Jones, President (Nonreporting) **A**1 5 9 10	23	10	272	—	—	—	—	—	—	—
MEADVILLE—Crawford County										
★ MEADVILLE MEDICAL CENTER, (Includes Meadville City Hospital, 751 Liberty Street, Meadville, Pennsylvania, Zip 16335; tel. 814/333–5000; Spencer Hospital, 1034 Grove Street, Meadville, Pennsylvania, Zip 16335) 751 Liberty Street, Zip 16335; tel. 814/333–5000; Anthony J. DeFail, President (Total facility includes 24 beds in nursing home–type unit) **A**1 2 9 10 **F**2 3 7 8 15 18 19 21 22 30 32 33 34 35 37 39 40 41 42 44 48 49 51 52 53 54 55 56 57 58 59 61 64 71 73 74 **P**1 7	23	10	234	8855	163	107618	666	56694	23317	839
SPENCER HOSPITAL See Meadville Medical Center										
MECHANICSBURG—Cumberland County										
□ △ HEALTHSOUTH REHABILITATION OF MECHANICSBURG, 175 Lancaster Boulevard, Zip 17055–2016, Mailing Address: P.O. Box 2016, Zip 17055–2016; tel. 717/691–3700; Glen R. Davis, Administrator and Chief Executive Officer **A**1 7 9 10 **F**5 9 12 24 25 26 32 41 42 48 49 64 66 73 **S**0023 Healthsouth Corporation	33	46	103	1649	78	39210	0	18894	10211	271
★ SEIDLE MEMORIAL HOSPITAL, 120 South Filbert Street, Zip 17055–6591; tel. 717/795–6760; Susan Edwards, Senior Vice President and Chief Operating Officer (Total facility includes 35 beds in nursing home–type unit) **A**1 9 10 **F**3 4 6 7 8 10 11 12 13 15 16 17 19 21 22 23 24 27 28 29 30 31 33 34 35 37 38 39 40 41 42 43 44 46 49 51 53 54 57 58 59 60 61 64 65 67 68 69 71 72 73 74 **P**7 **S**2135 Capital Health System	23	10	52	32	38	113987	0	9432	4194	135
MEDIA—Delaware County										
★ RIDDLE MEMORIAL HOSPITAL, 1068 West Baltimore Pike, Zip 19063–5177; tel. 610/566–9400; Donald L. Laughlin, President (Total facility includes 22 beds in nursing home–type unit) **A**1 2 9 10 **F**7 8 10 12 13 15 19 21 22 24 26 30 31 32 34 35 37 38 39 40 41 42 44 45 46 49 64 65 66 67 71 73 74 **P**5	23	10	198	9003	157	73790	847	60157	29268	916
MEYERSDALE—Somerset County										
★ MEYERSDALE MEDICAL CENTER, (Formerly Meyersdale Community Hospital) 200 Hospital Drive, Zip 15552–1247; tel. 814/634–5911; Kenneth N. Wenrich, Executive Director **A**1 9 10 **F**15 16 19 22 28 34 37 44 65 71 73	23	10	43	732	12	17131	0	5037	2403	106
MONONGAHELA—Washington County										
★ MONONGAHELA VALLEY HOSPITAL, Country Club Road, Route 88, Zip 15063–1095; tel. 412/258–1000; Anthony M. Lombardi, President and Chief Executive Officer **A**1 2 9 10 **F**2 5 7 8 10 11 13 14 15 16 17 19 20 21 22 23 26 28 29 30 31 32 33 34 35 37 39 40 41 42 44 46 49 52 53 54 56 57 60 61 65 66 67 68 71 73 74	23	10	283	11553	226	188430	498	67889	32409	1047
MONROEVILLE—Allegheny County										
★ FORBES REGIONAL HOSPITAL, 2570 Haymaker Road, Zip 15146–3592; tel. 412/858–2000; Dana W. Ramish, Senior Vice President Operations **A**1 2 3 5 9 10 **F**4 7 8 10 12 14 16 17 19 22 24 26 28 29 30 32 33 34 35 36 37 39 40 41 42 44 45 46 49 51 52 54 56 57 60 63 65 67 71 72 73 **P**1 3 5 **S**1355 Forbes Health System	23	10	353	16675	270	73929	1422	97496	36545	1200
□ △ HEALTHSOUTH GREATER PITTSBURGH REHAB HOSPITAL, 2380 McGinley Road, Zip 15146; tel. 412/856–2400; Faith A. Deigan, Administrator **A**1 7 9 10 **F**5 12 14 15 16 17 19 20 21 25 28 29 30 34 35 39 41 45 46 48 49 50 54 63 65 67 71 73 **S**0023 Healthsouth Corporation	33	46	89	1325	76	33811	0	20523	10449	259
MONTROSE—Susquehanna County										
MONTROSE GENERAL HOSPITAL, 1 Grow Avenue, Zip 18801–1199; tel. 717/278–3801; Rex Catlin, Administrator **A**9 10 **F**8 13 14 15 19 21 22 30 33 34 35 37 44 49 60 65 71 **P**4	33	10	34	951	12	29126	0	5144	2269	96
MOUNT GRETNA—Lebanon County										
★ PHILHAVEN, (Formerly Philhaven Hospital) 283 South Butler Road, Zip 17064, Mailing Address: P.O. Box 550, Zip 17064–0550; tel. 717/273–8871; LaVern J. Yutzy, Chief Executive Officer **A**1 9 10 **F**15 52 53 54 55 56 57 58 59 65 73 **P**1	21	22	106	2096	92	43154	0	21518	13381	477
MOUNT PLEASANT—Westmoreland County										
★ FRICK HOSPITAL AND COMMUNITY HEALTH CENTER, 508 South Church Street, Zip 15666–1790; tel. 412/547–1500; Rodney L. Gunderson, Executive Director **A**1 9 10 **F**7 8 10 11 12 14 15 16 17 18 19 20 21 22 25 28 29 30 31 32 34 35 37 39 40 41 42 44 45 46 49 53 54 55 56 57 58 59 60 63 65 67 69 71 73	23	10	179	6830	108	98274	655	40417	19778	617

Hospitals, U.S. / PENNSYLVANIA

Hospital, Address, Telephone, Administrator, Approval, Facility, and Physician Codes, Health Care System	Classification Codes		Utilization Data					Expense (thousands) of dollars		
★ American Hospital Association (AHA) membership ☐ Joint Commission on Accreditation of Healthcare Organizations (JCAHO) accreditation + American Osteopathic Hospital Association (AOHA) membership ○ American Osteopathic Association (AOA) accreditation △ Commission on Accreditation of Rehabilitation Facilities (CARF) accreditation Control codes 61, 63, 64, 71, 72 and 73 indicate hospitals listed by AOHA, but not registered by AHA. For definition of numerical codes, see page A6	Control	Service	Beds	Admissions	Census	Outpatient Visits	Births	Total	Payroll	Personnel
MUNCY—Lycoming County										
★ MUNCY VALLEY HOSPITAL, 215 East Water Street, Zip 17756–8700; tel. 717/546–8282; Diane M. Burfeindt, Assistant Administrator (Total facility includes 69 beds in nursing home–type unit) **A**1 9 10 **F**1 8 14 15 16 17 19 20 22 26 28 29 30 31 32 33 34 35 37 39 41 42 44 46 49 58 64 65 66 67 71 73 **P**4 6 8 **S**0066 Susquehanna Health System	23	10	120	2044	98	65661	0	13044	6309	263
NANTICOKE—Luzerne County										
★ MERCY HOSPITAL OF NANTICOKE, (Acute Long Term Care) 128 West Washington Street, Zip 18634; tel. 717/735–5000; Robert D. Williams, Administrator (Nonreporting) **A**9 10 **S**5155 Mercy Health System	12	49	18	—	—	—	—	—	—	—
NATRONA HEIGHTS—Allegheny County										
★ ALLEGHENY VALLEY HOSPITAL, 1301 Carlisle Street, Zip 15065–1192; tel. 412/224–5100; John R. England, President and Chief Executive Officer **A**1 2 9 10 **F**3 7 8 10 11 14 16 17 19 21 22 28 30 31 32 33 34 35 37 39 40 41 42 44 45 49 52 54 55 56 60 63 65 66 67 71 73	23	10	278	9827	188	136366	655	70864	32506	1005
NEW CASTLE—Lawrence County										
★ △ JAMESON MEMORIAL HOSPITAL, 1211 Wilmington Avenue, Zip 16105–2595; tel. 412/658–9001; Thomas White, President (Total facility includes 18 beds in nursing home–type unit) **A**1 2 6 7 9 10 **F**1 7 8 11 12 13 14 15 16 17 19 20 21 22 23 26 28 29 30 32 34 35 37 39 40 41 42 44 45 48 49 54 56 60 61 63 64 65 67 71 72 73 74 **P**3 8	23	10	220	8335	142	185837	613	56260	25672	1041
★ ST. FRANCIS HOSPITAL OF NEW CASTLE, 1000 South Mercer Street, Zip 16101–4673; tel. 412/658–3511; Sister Donna Zwigart, Chief Executive Officer (Total facility includes 45 beds in nursing home–type unit) **A**1 6 9 10 **F**2 3 5 7 8 11 12 13 14 15 16 17 18 19 20 21 22 23 28 29 30 31 32 33 35 36 39 40 41 42 44 45 46 48 49 52 53 54 55 56 57 58 59 60 61 62 63 64 65 67 71 73 74 **P**8 **S**2255 St. Francis Health System	23	10	193	4136	112	68083	0	28283	13015	479
NEW KENSINGTON—Westmoreland County										
☐ CITIZENS GENERAL HOSPITAL, 651 Fourth Avenue, Zip 15068–6591; tel. 412/337–3541; Robert E. Marino, Executive Director (Total facility includes 20 beds in nursing home–type unit) **A**1 6 9 10 **F**3 7 8 11 13 14 15 16 18 19 21 22 23 28 29 30 31 32 34 35 37 39 40 41 42 44 45 49 60 63 64 65 67 71 73	23	10	143	6152	104	79915	368	43716	19837	619
NORRISTOWN—Montgomery County										
☐ MONTGOMERY COUNTY EMERGENCY SERVICE, 50 Beech Drive, Zip 19401, Mailing Address: Caller Box 3005, Zip 19404–3005; tel. 610/279–6100; Rocio Nell M.D., Medical and Executive Director **A**1 9 10 **F**3 15 17 18 52 53 54 55 56 57 58 65 **P**6	23	22	53	1839	48	1466	0	7897	5417	181
☐ MONTGOMERY HOSPITAL, 1301 Powell Street, Zip 19401, Mailing Address: P.O. Box 992, Zip 19404–0992; tel. 610/270–2000; Timothy M. Casey, President (Total facility includes 17 beds in nursing home–type unit) **A**1 2 7 8 10 11 12 14 15 16 19 21 22 23 25 27 30 32 33 37 38 40 42 44 46 49 51 52 53 57 60 64 65 67 71 73 74	23	10	291	8509	141	129472	627	66396	—	1190
☐ NORRISTOWN STATE HOSPITAL, 1001 Sterigere Street, Zip 19401–5399; tel. 215/270–1000; Albert R. Di Dario, Superintendent **A**1 3 5 9 10 **F**14 20 52 57 65 73	12	22	681	498	637	0	0	73170	42351	1121
+ ○ SUBURBAN GENERAL HOSPITAL, 2701 De Kalb Pike, Zip 19401; tel. 610/278–2000; Edward R. Solvibile, President **A**9 10 11 12 13 **F**7 8 10 16 18 19 22 26 27 28 29 30 31 32 33 34 35 37 39 40 41 42 44 45 46 49 60 61 62 65 66 67 70 71 73 74	23	10	118	4464	63	69575	361	35227	16598	580
★ VALLEY FORGE MEDICAL CENTER AND HOSPITAL, 1033 West Germantown Pike, Zip 19403–3998; tel. 610/539–8500; Marian W. Colcher, President (Nonreporting) **A**1 9 10	33	10	70	—	—	—	—	—	—	—
NORTH WARREN—Warren County										
☐ WARREN STATE HOSPITAL, 33 Main Drive, Zip 16365–5099; tel. 814/723–5500; Carmen N. Ferranto, Superintendent **A**1 10 **F**7 8 11 16 19 20 21 33 35 37 40 41 42 44 46 48 52 57 60 65 70 71 73	12	22	424	316	382	0	0	36495	21796	703
OIL CITY—Venango County										
NORTHWEST MEDICAL CENTER–OIL CITY CAMPUS See Northwest Medical Center, Franklin										
PALMERTON—Carbon County										
☐ PALMERTON HOSPITAL, 135 Lafayette Avenue, Zip 18071–9990; tel. 610/826–3141; Peter L. Kern, President and Chief Executive Officer **A**1 9 10 **F**7 8 11 15 19 22 30 33 40 44 45 46 65 67 71	23	10	70	2623	39	34825	189	15699	7266	271
PAOLI—Chester County										
★ PAOLI MEMORIAL HOSPITAL, 255 West Lancaster Avenue, Zip 19301–1792; tel. 610/648–1201; Leland White, President **A**1 2 5 9 10 **F**3 4 8 10 11 14 15 16 17 19 20 21 22 26 28 30 31 32 33 35 37 41 42 44 46 49 52 53 54 55 56 57 58 59 60 61 65 67 71 73 **P**3 5 7 **S**7775 Main Line Health	23	10	146	7272	101	136093	0	57526	24450	671
PECKVILLE—Lackawanna County										
★ MID-VALLEY HOSPITAL, 1400 Main Street, Zip 18452; tel. 717/383–5500; Gerard H. Warner Jr., Administrator (Nonreporting) **A**9 10	23	10	57	—	—	—	—	—	—	—
PHILADELPHIA—Philadelphia County										
★ ALBERT EINSTEIN MEDICAL CENTER, (Includes Moss Rehabilitation Hospital, 1200 West Tabor Road, Philadelphia, Pennsylvania, Zip 19141–3099; tel. 215/456–9070) 5501 Old York Road, Zip 19141–3098; tel. 215/456–7890; Martin Goldsmith, President (Total facility includes 102 beds in nursing home–type unit) **A**1 2 3 5 8 9 10 13 **F**1 2 3 4 5 7 8 10 11 14 15 17 18 19 20 21 22 25 26 28 29 30 31 33 34 35 37 38 39 40 41 42 44 45 46 47 48 49 51 52 53 54 55 56 57 58 59 60 61 63 64 65 67 69 70 71 73 **P**3 6 7 **S**1685 Albert Einstein Healthcare Network	23	10	767	23594	605	271158	1666	285043	122819	3707

© 1995 AHA Guide

Hospitals, U.S. / PENNSYLVANIA

Hospital, Address, Telephone, Administrator, Approval, Facility, and Physician Codes, Health Care System	Classification Codes		Utilization Data					Expense (thousands) of dollars		
★ American Hospital Association (AHA) membership □ Joint Commission on Accreditation of Healthcare Organizations (JCAHO) accreditation + American Osteopathic Hospital Association (AOHA) membership ○ American Osteopathic Association (AOA) accreditation △ Commission on Accreditation of Rehabilitation Facilities (CARF) accreditation Control codes 61, 63, 64, 71, 72 and 73 indicate hospitals listed by AOHA, but not registered by AHA. For definition of numerical codes, see page A6	Control	Service	Beds	Admissions	Census	Outpatient Visits	Births	Total	Payroll	Personnel
□ BELMONT CENTER FOR COMPREHENSIVE TREATMENT, 4200 Monument Road, Zip 19131–1689; tel. 215/877–2000; Jack H. Dembow, General Director **A**1 3 5 9 **F**1 3 12 18 27 34 46 52 53 56 57 58 59 65 73 74 **P**6 **S**1685 Albert Einstein Healthcare Network	23	22	146	3092	125	34048	0	24192	12609	403
□ CHARTER FAIRMOUNT INSTITUTE, 561 Fairthorne Avenue, Zip 19128–2499; tel. 215/487–4000; Paul B. Henry, Administrator (Nonreporting) **A**1 9 10 **S**0695 Charter Medical Corporation	33	22	146	—	—	—	—	—	—	—
★ CHESTNUT HILL HOSPITAL, 8835 Germantown Avenue, Zip 19118–2767; tel. 215/248–8200; Cary F. Leptuck, President and Chief Executive Officer **A**1 3 5 9 10 **F**1 4 6 7 8 11 14 15 16 17 19 21 22 25 26 27 28 30 31 32 33 34 35 36 37 39 40 42 44 45 46 49 60 62 63 65 67 71 73 **P**2 5 7 8	23	10	190	8914	129	87083	1430	56234	28474	846
★ CHILDREN'S HOSPITAL OF PHILADELPHIA, 34th Street & Civic Center Boulevard, Zip 19104–4399; tel. 215/590–1000; Edmond F. Notebaert, President and Chief Executive Officer **A**1 2 3 5 8 9 10 **F**5 10 12 13 14 15 16 17 18 19 20 21 22 25 28 29 30 31 32 34 35 38 39 42 43 44 45 46 47 48 49 51 52 53 54 55 56 57 58 59 60 65 67 69 70 71 73	23	50	294	15627	237	215418	0	212685	100074	2702
★ CHILDREN'S REHABILITATION HOSPITAL, 3905 Ford Road, Zip 19131; tel. 215/578–3408; Robert J. Moylan, Administrator; Stephen McGeady, Medical Director **A**1 9 10 **F**15 16 19 21 34 41 48 49 54 65 71 **P**6	23	56	40	223	28	5658	0	9036	4324	89
□ CHILDREN'S SEASHORE HOUSE, 3405 Civic Center Boulevard, Zip 19104–4388; tel. 215/895–3600; Richard W. Shepherd, President **A**1 3 5 9 10 **F**5 12 15 17 25 28 34 45 48 49 53 65 73 **P**5	23	56	70	544	65	25245	0	30814	14619	454
★ EPISCOPAL HOSPITAL, (Includes George L. Harrison Memorial House) 100 East Lehigh Avenue, Zip 19125–1098; tel. 215/427–7000; Mark T. Bateman, President and Chief Executive Officer (Total facility includes 35 beds in nursing home–type unit) **A**1 2 3 5 6 8 9 10 **F**2 4 7 8 10 12 14 16 17 19 20 21 22 26 27 28 29 30 31 32 34 35 37 38 39 40 41 42 43 44 45 46 49 51 54 63 64 65 67 71 73 74 **P**3 7	23	10	236	9187	194	56371	1522	84335	47362	1076
★ FOX CHASE CANCER CENTER–AMERICAN ONCOLOGIC HOSPITAL, 7701 Burholme Avenue, Zip 19111; tel. 215/728–6900; Robert C. Young M.D., President **A**1 2 3 5 9 10 **F**8 12 14 15 16 17 18 19 20 21 28 29 30 32 33 34 35 37 39 41 42 44 45 46 49 54 60 67 69 73 **P**6	23	49	82	3980	63	35910	0	58690	19877	564
FRANKFORD CAMPUS See Frankford Hospital of the City of Philadelphia										
★ FRANKFORD HOSPITAL OF THE CITY OF PHILADELPHIA, (Includes Frankford Campus, Frankford Avenue & Wakeling Street, Philadelphia, Pennsylvania, Zip 19124; tel. 215/831–2000; Torresdale Campus, Philadelphia, Pennsylvania) Knights and Red Lion Roads, Zip 19114–1486; tel. 215/612–4000; John B. Neff, President **A**1 3 5 6 8 9 10 **F**2 3 7 8 11 13 14 15 16 17 19 21 22 23 24 25 26 27 28 29 30 31 32 34 35 37 38 39 40 41 42 44 45 46 48 49 51 54 60 61 65 67 70 71 73 74 **P**7	23	10	387	17427	312	208599	2089	145638	68203	1859
FRIEDMAN HOSPITAL OF THE HOME FOR THE JEWISH AGED, (Geriatric) 5301 Old York Road, Zip 19141–2996; tel. 215/456–2900; Frank Podietz, President (Nonreporting) **A**10	23	49	28	—	—	—	—	—	—	—
★ FRIENDS HOSPITAL, 4641 Roosevelt Boulevard, Zip 19124–2399; tel. 215/831–4600; Gary L. Gottlieb M.D., Chief Executive Officer **A**1 3 5 9 10 **F**1 3 12 14 15 17 26 32 34 41 45 46 52 53 54 55 57 58 59 65 73 **P**1 7	23	22	192	2691	150	6542	0	34257	19989	602
★ GERMANTOWN HOSPITAL AND MEDICAL CENTER, One Penn Boulevard, Zip 19144–1498; tel. 215/951–8000; David A. Ricci, President (Total facility includes 20 beds in nursing home–type unit) **A**1 3 5 6 8 9 10 **F**7 8 11 12 15 16 17 19 21 22 26 27 28 29 30 32 33 34 35 37 38 39 40 41 42 44 46 47 49 51 60 63 64 65 67 69 71 73 74 **P**8	23	10	184	7137	136	80572	465	65256	31018	739
GIRARD MEDICAL CENTER See North Philadelphia Health System										
+ ○ GRADUATE HEALTH SYSTEM–CITY AVENUE HOSPITAL, 4150 City Avenue, Zip 19131–1696; tel. 215/871–1000; Melvyn E. Smith, Executive Director and Chief Executive Officer **A**9 10 11 12 13 **F**2 4 7 8 10 11 12 16 19 20 21 22 23 26 28 30 31 32 33 34 35 37 38 40 41 42 43 44 46 48 49 50 51 52 54 56 57 58 59 60 63 64 65 67 71 73 74 **P**3 5 **S**0006 Graduate Health System	23	10	190	7351	126	42212	1263	65924	27224	726
○ GRADUATE HEALTH SYSTEM–PARKVIEW HOSPITAL, 1331 East Wyoming Avenue, Zip 19124; tel. 215/537–7400; Bernadette M. Mangan, President (Total facility includes 19 beds in nursing home–type unit) (Data for 345 days) **A**9 11 12 13 **F**4 7 8 10 11 12 14 15 16 17 19 20 21 22 23 24 27 28 30 31 32 33 34 35 37 40 41 42 43 44 45 46 49 51 52 54 56 60 63 64 65 66 67 71 73 74 **P**1 5 6 7 **S**0006 Graduate Health System	23	10	181	5169	88	34449	804	39474	17593	684
□ GRADUATE HOSPITAL, One Graduate Plaza, Zip 19146–1497; tel. 215/893–2000; Samuel H. Steinberg, President **A**1 2 3 5 8 9 10 **F**1 2 3 4 5 8 10 11 12 19 20 21 22 25 26 28 30 31 32 33 34 35 37 41 42 43 44 45 46 48 49 51 52 53 54 55 56 57 58 59 60 61 63 64 65 66 71 73 74 **P**1 3 **S**0006 Graduate Health System	23	10	306	11609	227	152602	0	169759	64653	1641
□ HAHNEMANN UNIVERSITY HOSPITAL, Broad and Vine Streets, Zip 19102–1192; tel. 215/762–1650; Shelley Gebar, Executive Director and Chief Executive Officer (Nonreporting) **A**1 2 3 5 8 9 10 **S**2305 Allegheny Health, Education and Research Foundation	23	10	618	—	—	—	—	—	—	—
★ △ HOSPITAL OF THE UNIVERSITY OF PENNSYLVANIA, 3400 Spruce Street, Zip 19104–4283; tel. 215/662–4000; Donald F. Snell, Interim Executive Director **A**1 3 5 8 9 10 **F**4 5 7 8 10 11 12 14 15 16 17 19 20 21 22 23 25 26 28 29 30 32 35 37 38 39 40 41 42 43 44 45 46 49 50 51 52 54 55 56 57 58 60 61 63 65 66 69 70 71 73 74 **P**1 6 7	23	10	671	27373	556	91050	2719	411522	163451	5394
INSTITUTE OF PENNSYLVANIA HOSPITAL See Pennsylvania Hospital										

Hospitals, U.S. / PENNSYLVANIA

Hospital, Address, Telephone, Administrator, Approval, Facility, and Physician Codes, Health Care System	Classification Codes		Utilization Data					Expense (thousands) of dollars		
	Control	Service	Beds	Admissions	Census	Outpatient Visits	Births	Total	Payroll	Personnel

★ American Hospital Association (AHA) membership
☐ Joint Commission on Accreditation of Healthcare Organizations (JCAHO) accreditation
+ American Osteopathic Hospital Association (AOHA) membership
○ American Osteopathic Association (AOA) accreditation
△ Commission on Accreditation of Rehabilitation Facilities (CARF) accreditation
Control codes 61, 63, 64, 71, 72 and 73 indicate hospitals listed by AOHA, but not registered by AHA. For definition of numerical codes, see page A6

Hospital	Control	Service	Beds	Admissions	Census	Outpatient Visits	Births	Total	Payroll	Personnel
☐ PASSANT HOSPITAL, (Formerly North Hills Passavant Hospital) 9100 Babcock Boulevard, Zip 15237–5842; tel. 412/367–6700; Ralph T. Destefano, President (Nonreporting) **A**1 9 10	23	10	292	—	—	—	—	—	—	—
★ PODIATRY HOSPITAL OF PITTSBURGH, 215 South Negley Avenue, Zip 15206–3594; tel. 412/661–0814; Jack Decerce, Chief Executive Officer **A**9 10 **F**44	23	49	13	206	1	9931	0	6186	2761	92
PRESBYTERIAN UNIVERSITY HOSPITAL See University of Pittsburgh Medical Center										
★ △ REHABILITATION INSTITUTE, 6301 Northumberland Street, Zip 15217–1396; tel. 412/521–9000; John A. Wilson, President and Chief Executive Officer **A**1 7 10 **F**5 12 14 15 16 17 26 32 34 41 46 48 49 53 59 65 66 73	23	46	97	878	49	62055	0	20549	12379	430
★ SHADYSIDE HOSPITAL, 5230 Centre Avenue, Zip 15232–1304; tel. 412/623–2121; Henry A. Mordoh, President (Nonreporting) **A**1 2 3 5 6 8 9 10	23	10	603	—	—	—	—	—	—	—
★ SOUTH HILLS HEALTH SYSTEM, Coal Valley Road, Zip 15236–0119, Mailing Address: Box 18119, Zip 15236–0119; tel. 412/469–5000; William R. Jennings, President (Total facility includes 74 beds in nursing home–type unit) **A**1 9 10 **F**2 3 8 10 12 13 14 15 16 17 18 19 20 21 22 24 26 28 29 30 31 32 33 34 35 37 39 41 42 44 45 46 48 49 51 52 54 55 56 57 58 60 64 65 66 67 71 73 **P**4 8	23	10	466	16020	343	165467	0	124000	57808	1460
☐ SOUTH SIDE HOSPITAL OF PITTSBURGH, 2000 Mary Street, Zip 15203–2095; tel. 412/488–5550; George J. Korbakes, President **A**1 9 10 **F**4 8 10 11 12 14 15 16 19 20 21 22 26 27 28 29 30 31 32 34 35 37 39 41 42 44 45 46 48 49 52 54 55 56 57 65 71 72 73	23	10	169	6162	143	60262	0	42027	19195	611
☐ SOUTHWOOD PSYCHIATRIC HOSPITAL, 2575 Boyce Plaza Road, Zip 15241–3925; tel. 412/257–2290; Alan A. Axelson M.D., Chief Executive Officer **A**1 **F**3 52 53 58 59 **P**4 **S**2635 First Hospital Corporation	33	52	50	994	30	0	0	6570	—	110
★ ST. CLAIR HOSPITAL, 1000 Bower Hill Road, Zip 15243; tel. 412/561–4900; Benjamin E. Snead, President **A**1 9 10 **F**1 3 4 5 6 7 8 10 11 12 13 14 15 17 18 19 20 21 22 23 24 25 26 27 28 29 30 31 32 33 34 35 37 38 39 40 41 42 43 44 45 46 47 48 49 51 52 53 54 55 56 57 58 59 60 61 63 64 65 66 67 68 69 71 72 73 74 **P**5	23	10	337	12296	216	112823	1046	86387	42113	1293
★ ST. FRANCIS CENTRAL HOSPITAL, 1200 Centre Avenue, Zip 15219–3594; tel. 412/562–3000; Kenneth F. Sample, Chief Executive Officer **A**1 9 10 12 **F**2 3 4 5 7 8 10 11 12 14 15 16 17 19 20 21 22 23 24 25 26 27 28 29 30 31 32 34 35 37 39 40 41 42 43 44 45 46 48 49 51 52 53 54 55 56 57 58 59 60 61 63 64 65 67 68 69 71 72 73 74 **P**6 **S**2255 St. Francis Health System	23	10	143	4631	77	62308	0	41229	18766	510
★ △ ST. FRANCIS MEDICAL CENTER, 400 45th Street, Zip 15201–1198; tel. 412/622–4343; Sister Florence Brandt, Chief Executive Officer (Total facility includes 300 beds in nursing home–type unit) **A**1 2 3 5 6 7 8 9 10 **F**2 3 4 5 7 8 10 11 12 14 15 16 19 20 21 22 23 24 25 26 27 28 30 31 32 34 35 37 39 40 41 42 43 44 45 46 48 49 51 52 53 54 55 56 57 58 59 60 63 64 65 66 67 68 69 71 72 73 74 **S**2255 St. Francis Health System	23	10	965	15757	441	162854	810	189740	85641	2538
★ ST. MARGARET MEMORIAL HOSPITAL, 815 Freeport Road, Zip 15215–3399; tel. 412/784–4000; Stanley J. Kevish, President **A**1 3 5 6 9 10 **F**5 8 10 15 16 17 19 21 22 25 26 28 29 30 31 32 34 35 37 39 41 42 44 45 46 48 49 53 54 56 57 58 60 62 65 66 67 68 71 73 **P**8	23	10	267	9421	167	117445	0	90163	37865	1126
STATE CORRECTIONAL INSTITUTION HOSPITAL, Doerr Street, Zip 15233, Mailing Address: Box 99901, Zip 15233; tel. 412/761–1955; Joseph Morrash, Administrator (Nonreporting)	12	11	27	—	—	—	—	—	—	—
☐ SUBURBAN GENERAL HOSPITAL, 100 South Jackson Avenue, Zip 15202–3499; tel. 412/734–6000; Thomas H. Prickett, President and Chief Executive Officer (Total facility includes 25 beds in nursing home–type unit) **A**1 9 10 **F**11 14 19 22 32 35 37 41 44 48 49 64 65 71 73	23	10	146	4526	99	56892	0	30878	15121	514
TORRESDALE CAMPUS See Frankford Hospital of the City of Philadelphia										
★ UNIVERSITY OF PITTSBURGH MEDICAL CENTER, (Includes Eye and Ear Hospital of Pittsburgh, 230 Lothrop Street, Pittsburgh, Pennsylvania, Zip 15213–2592; tel. 412/647–2014; Montefiore Hospital, 3459 Fifth Avenue, Pittsburgh, Pennsylvania, Zip 15213; tel. 412/648–6000; Frank Rubenstein, Chairman; Presbyterian University Hospital, Pittsburgh, Pennsylvania; John W. Paul, Executive Vice President; University of Pittsburgh Western Psychiatric Institute and Clinic, 3811 O'Hara Street, Pittsburgh, Pennsylvania, Zip 15213–2593; tel. 412/624–2100; Thomas Detre M.D., Director and Chief Executive Officer) 200 Lothrop Street, Zip 15213; tel. 412/647–3000; Jeffrey A. Romoff, President **A**1 2 3 5 **F**1 2 3 4 5 6 8 10 11 12 14 16 17 18 19 20 21 22 23 25 26 29 30 31 32 34 35 37 39 41 42 43 44 45 46 48 49 50 51 52 53 54 55 56 57 58 59 60 62 64 65 66 67 68 69 70 71 73 74 **P**5	23	10	1107	34013	893	393097	0	734801	268012	8518
UNIVERSITY OF PITTSBURGH WESTERN PSYCHIATRIC INSTITUTE AND CLINIC See University of Pittsburgh Medical Center										
★ VETERANS AFFAIRS MEDICAL CENTER, 7180 Highland Drive, Zip 15206–1297; tel. 412/365–4900; Laura Miller, Director **A**1 **F**1 2 3 4 5 6 8 10 11 12 16 17 18 19 20 21 22 24 26 27 28 29 30 31 32 33 34 35 37 39 41 42 43 44 45 46 48 49 50 51 52 54 55 56 57 58 59 60 61 63 65 67 69 70 71 72 73 74 **P**1 **S**9295 Department of Veterans Affairs	45	22	574	2898	459	101929	0	—	—	1147
★ VETERANS AFFAIRS MEDICAL CENTER, University Drive C, Zip 15240–1001; tel. 412/692–3200; Thomas A. Cappello, Director (Total facility includes 240 beds in nursing home–type unit) **A**1 3 5 8 **F**1 3 4 6 10 11 12 14 17 19 20 21 22 26 28 30 31 32 34 37 41 42 43 45 46 48 49 50 51 57 60 64 65 67 69 71 73 74 **S**9295 Department of Veterans Affairs	45	10	698	7771	571	133298	0	136269	85000	1822

© 1995 AHA Guide

Hospitals, U.S. / PENNSYLVANIA

Hospital, Address, Telephone, Administrator, Approval, Facility, and Physician Codes, Health Care System	Classification Codes		Utilization Data					Expense (thousands) of dollars		
★ American Hospital Association (AHA) membership ☐ Joint Commission on Accreditation of Healthcare Organizations (JCAHO) accreditation + American Osteopathic Hospital Association (AOHA) membership ○ American Osteopathic Association (AOA) accreditation △ Commission on Accreditation of Rehabilitation Facilities (CARF) accreditation Control codes 61, 63, 64, 71, 72 and 73 indicate hospitals listed by AOHA, but not registered by AHA. For definition of numerical codes, see page A6	Control	Service	Beds	Admissions	Census	Outpatient Visits	Births	Total	Payroll	Personnel
★ WESTERN PENNSYLVANIA HOSPITAL, 4800 Friendship Avenue, Zip 15224; tel. 412/578–5000; Charles M. O'Brien Jr., President and Chief Executive Officer **A**1 2 3 5 6 8 9 10 **F**4 7 8 9 10 11 12 14 15 16 17 19 20 21 22 26 27 28 30 31 32 33 34 35 37 38 40 41 42 43 44 45 46 49 50 51 52 54 55 57 60 61 63 65 67 68 69 71 73 74 **P**1 5 6 7	23	10	488	19698	374	167058	2002	211485	97796	2707
PLEASANT GAP—Centre County										
☐ △ HEALTHSOUTH NITTANY VALLEY REHABILITATION HOSPITAL, 550 West College Avenue, Zip 16823–8808; tel. 814/359–3421; Mary Jane Hawkins, Administrator and Chief Executive Officer (Nonreporting) **A**1 7 9 10 **S**0023 Healthsouth Corporation	33	46	88	—	—	—	—	—	—	—
POTTSTOWN—Chester County										
★ POTTSTOWN MEMORIAL MEDICAL CENTER, 1600 East High Street, Zip 19464–5008; tel. 215/327–7000; Neal R. Fegely, Acting President and Chief Executive Officer **A**1 2 9 10 **F**4 7 8 10 11 13 14 15 16 17 19 21 22 24 25 28 29 30 31 34 35 36 37 39 40 41 42 44 45 46 49 51 52 56 60 63 65 66 71 73 74	23	10	212	8319	129	80565	803	62564	27785	830
POTTSVILLE—Schuylkill County										
★ GOOD SAMARITAN REGIONAL MEDICAL CENTER, 700 East Norwegian Street, Zip 17901–2798; tel. 717/621–4000; Gino J. Pazzaglini, President and Chief Executive Officer **A**1 2 5 9 10 **F**3 4 7 8 11 12 14 15 16 19 22 26 28 30 31 32 33 34 35 36 37 39 40 41 42 44 45 46 60 65 67 71 73 74 **S**1855 Daughters of Charity National Health System	21	10	221	8121	161	140516	508	47909	21512	740
★ △ POTTSVILLE HOSPITAL AND WARNE CLINIC, 420 South Jackson Street, Zip 17901–3692; tel. 717/621–5000; Donald R. Gintzig, President and Chief Executive Officer **A**1 2 6 7 9 10 **F**7 8 14 15 16 17 19 20 21 22 26 28 30 31 32 33 34 35 37 40 41 42 44 45 48 49 52 53 56 57 58 60 61 65 66 71 73 **P**5 **S**0002 Quorum Health Group/Quorum Health Resources	23	10	195	5715	142	52278	389	39848	17911	702
PUNXSUTAWNEY—Jefferson County										
☐ PUNXSUTAWNEY AREA HOSPITAL, 81 Hillcrest Drive, Zip 15767–2616; tel. 814/938–1800; Daniel D. Blough Jr., Administrator (Total facility includes 14 beds in nursing home–type unit) **A**1 9 10 **F**7 8 15 16 19 21 22 28 30 31 32 34 37 40 44 49 64 65 68 71	23	10	69	2429	36	72610	213	14612	5554	236
QUAKERTOWN—Bucks County										
★ QUAKERTOWN COMMUNITY HOSPITAL, 1021 Park Avenue, Zip 18951; tel. 215/538–4500; Roger B. Hiser, Administrator and Chief Executive Officer (Nonreporting) **A**1 2 9 10	23	10	89	—	—	—	—	—	—	—
READING—Berks County										
☐ COMMUNITY GENERAL HOSPITAL, 145 North Sixth Street, Zip 19601, Mailing Address: P.O. Box 1728, Zip 19603–1728; tel. 610/376–2100; S. Michael Francis, President and Chief Executive Officer (Total facility includes 25 beds in nursing home–type unit) **A**1 2 9 10 12 13 **F**7 8 10 12 13 14 15 16 17 18 19 20 21 22 25 26 27 28 29 30 31 33 34 35 37 39 40 41 42 44 45 46 49 51 52 57 60 61 63 64 65 66 67 71 73 74 **P**1 2 5 **S**0006 Graduate Health System	23	10	161	4809	84	141463	769	37290	15807	500
★ △ READING REHABILITATION HOSPITAL, 1623 Morgantown Road, Zip 19607–9727; tel. 610/796–6000; Clint Kreitner, President and Chief Executive Officer (Total facility includes 19 beds in nursing home–type unit) **A**1 3 5 7 10 **F**12 15 16 17 24 27 34 39 41 48 49 64 65 67 73	21	46	95	1258	66	31337	0	17468	9813	336
★ ST. JOSEPH MEDICAL CENTER, Twelfth & Walnut Streets, Zip 19603–0316, Mailing Address: P.O. Box 316, Zip 19603–0316; tel. 610/378–2000; David A. Ferrell, President and Chief Executive Officer **A**1 2 3 5 9 10 **F**2 3 4 7 8 10 19 20 21 22 23 24 25 30 31 32 33 34 35 37 39 40 41 42 43 44 46 49 51 52 53 54 55 56 60 62 65 66 69 71 73 74 **P**8 **S**5325 Franciscan Health System	21	10	257	9510	147	173852	972	70806	32560	1064
RENOVO—Clinton County										
BUCKTAIL MEDICAL CENTER, 1001 Pine Street, Zip 17764–1620; tel. 717/923–1000; Daniel Wolfberg, Administrator (Nonreporting) **A**9 10	23	10	50	—	—	—	—	—	—	—
RIDGWAY—Elk County										
★ ELK COUNTY REGIONAL MEDICAL CENTER, 94 Hospital Street, Zip 15853; tel. 814/776–6111; J. Allan Bickling, Chief Executive Officer **A**9 10 **F**8 14 15 16 17 19 22 23 28 29 30 33 36 37 39 40 41 42 44 46 52 55 56 57 61 65 71 73 74	23	10	63	2506	33	18000	0	8214	3461	181
RIDLEY PARK—Delaware County										
☐ TAYLOR HOSPITAL, 175 East Chester Pike, Zip 19078; tel. 215/595–6000; William Michael Tomlinson, President and Chief Executive Officer (Total facility includes 23 beds in nursing home–type unit) **A**1 2 9 10 **F**8 10 12 14 15 16 17 19 20 21 22 30 32 33 34 35 36 37 39 41 42 44 45 46 48 49 54 64 65 66 67 71 73 74 **P**3 7 8	23	10	213	7235	136	39152	0	59760	27384	663
ROARING SPRING—Blair County										
★ NASON HOSPITAL, 105 Nason Drive, Zip 16673–1201; tel. 814/224–2141; John P. Kinney, President and Chief Executive Officer **A**1 5 9 10 **F**7 8 19 21 22 28 29 32 33 34 35 37 40 44 45 49 63 65 67 71 73	23	10	50	2014	28	38842	203	12976	5570	221
SAINT MARYS—Elk County										
★ ST. MARYS REGIONAL MEDICAL CENTER, 763 Johnsonburg Road, Zip 15857–3417; tel. 814/781–7500; John N. Christenson, President (Total facility includes 138 beds in nursing home–type unit) **A**1 9 10 **F**7 8 12 14 19 21 22 28 29 30 35 37 40 41 44 45 46 49 62 64 65 66 71 73 74	23	10	233	3625	168	52246	450	25650	12025	557
SAYRE—Bradford County										
★ ROBERT PACKER HOSPITAL, Guthrie Square, Zip 18840; tel. 717/888–6666; Russell M. Knight, President **A**1 2 3 5 9 10 **F**1 4 7 8 10 11 12 13 14 15 16 17 18 19 21 22 23 24 26 27 28 29 30 31 32 33 34 35 36 37 39 40 42 43 44 45 46 49 52 53 54 55 56 57 59 60 61 63 64 65 66 67 68 70 71 72 73 74 **S**0675 Guthrie Healthcare System	23	10	366	12555	210	166659	808	102604	40482	1375

Hospitals, U.S. / PENNSYLVANIA

Hospital, Address, Telephone, Administrator, Approval, Facility, and Physician Codes, Health Care System	Classification Codes		Utilization Data					Expense (thousands) of dollars		
★ American Hospital Association (AHA) membership ☐ Joint Commission on Accreditation of Healthcare Organizations (JCAHO) accreditation + American Osteopathic Hospital Association (AOHA) membership ○ American Osteopathic Association (AOA) accreditation △ Commission on Accreditation of Rehabilitation Facilities (CARF) accreditation Control codes 61, 63, 64, 71, 72 and 73 indicate hospitals listed by AOHA, but not registered by AHA. For definition of numerical codes, see page A6	Control	Service	Beds	Admissions	Census	Outpatient Visits	Births	Total	Payroll	Personnel
SCRANTON—Lackawanna County ★ △ ALLIED SERVICES REHABILITATION HOSPITAL, 475 Morgan Highway, Zip 18508; tel. 717/348-1300; James L. Brady, President (Nonreporting) **A**1 7 9 10	23	46	98	—	—	—	—	—	—	—
★ COMMUNITY MEDICAL CENTER, 1822 Mulberry Street, Zip 18510; tel. 717/969-8000; Gene K. Miyamoto, President and Chief Executive Officer **A**1 3 9 10 **F**3 4 6 7 8 10 14 15 16 17 18 19 21 22 23 26 27 30 32 33 34 35 37 38 40 42 43 44 46 49 52 53 54 55 56 57 58 59 60 63 64 65 67 68 70 71 72 73 74 **P**8	23	10	327	12262	229	205121	2043	91218	40988	1200
★ MERCY HOSPITAL OF SCRANTON, 746 Jefferson Avenue, Zip 18501-0994; tel. 717/348-7100; John L. Nespoli, President and Chief Executive Officer (Total facility includes 14 beds in nursing home-type unit) **A**1 2 3 5 9 10 **F**4 7 8 10 11 12 16 17 19 21 22 23 33 34 35 36 37 39 40 42 43 44 60 64 65 67 71 73 74 **P**8 **S**5155 Mercy Health System	21	10	293	11256	226	147467	907	88044	37977	1191
★ MOSES TAYLOR HOSPITAL, 700 Quincy Avenue, Zip 18510-1724; tel. 717/963-2100; Harold E. Anderson, Chief Executive Officer (Total facility includes 32 beds in nursing home-type unit) **A**1 3 5 9 10 **F**1 8 19 21 22 23 26 32 33 34 35 37 39 41 42 44 46 49 57 64 65 71 73 **P**8	23	10	202	7023	167	84199	0	57637	21433	738
SELLERSVILLE—Bucks County ★ GRAND VIEW HOSPITAL, 700 Lawn Avenue, Zip 18960-1581; tel. 215/453-4000; Stuart H. Fine, Chief Executive Officer (Total facility includes 20 beds in nursing home-type unit) **A**1 2 5 9 10 **F**2 3 7 8 11 12 13 15 16 17 18 19 21 22 23 24 26 28 29 30 31 32 33 34 35 36 37 40 41 42 44 45 46 48 49 52 53 54 55 56 57 58 59 60 63 64 65 67 71 73 74 **P**1 3 5 7	23	10	241	8011	140	123211	1078	73482	35505	1064
SEWICKLEY—Allegheny County ★ △ D.T. WATSON REHABILITATION HOSPITAL, Camp Meeting Road, Zip 15143-8545; tel. 412/741-9500; Francis W. Finley Jr., Interim Chief Executive Officer **A**1 7 9 10 **F**12 14 15 16 34 41 48 49 58 65 67 73 **P**4 6	23	46	40	354	18	23041	0	9931	4794	150
★ SEWICKLEY VALLEY HOSPITAL, 720 Blackburn Road, Zip 15143-1498; tel. 412/741-6600; Donald W. Spalding, President **A**1 6 9 10 **F**4 7 8 10 12 15 19 21 22 26 28 29 30 31 32 33 34 36 37 40 41 42 44 48 49 52 53 54 55 57 58 59 60 65 67 71 73 74 **P**6 8	23	10	183	9228	135	172997	952	84662	37119	1169
SHARON—Mercer County ★ SHARON REGIONAL HEALTH SYSTEM, 740 East State Street, Zip 16146-7001; tel. 412/983-3911; Wayne W. Johnston, President and Chief Executive Officer (Total facility includes 40 beds in nursing home-type unit) **A**1 6 9 10 **F**3 7 8 10 11 13 14 15 16 17 19 21 22 23 25 26 28 29 30 32 33 34 35 37 39 40 41 42 44 45 48 49 51 52 53 54 55 56 57 58 59 60 63 64 65 66 67 71 72 73 74 **P**6 8	23	10	234	8397	169	235565	750	57333	26928	1022
SHICKSHINNY—Luzerne County CLEAR BROOK LODGE, Bethel Road, Zip 18655, Mailing Address: Rural Delivery 2, Box 2166, Zip 18655; tel. 717/864-3116; Dave Lombard, President and Chief Executive Officer (Nonreporting)	23	82	65	—	—	—	—	—	—	—
SOMERSET—Somerset County ★ SOMERSET HOSPITAL CENTER FOR HEALTH, 225 South Center Avenue, Zip 15501-2088; tel. 814/443-5000; Michael J. Farrell, Chief Executive Officer (Total facility includes 14 beds in nursing home-type unit) **A**1 9 10 **F**1 3 7 8 11 13 14 15 16 19 21 22 23 26 28 29 30 32 33 34 35 39 40 41 42 44 45 46 49 52 53 54 55 56 57 58 59 61 64 65 66 67 68 71 73 74 **P**6	23	10	104	5180	78	74388	518	33155	14505	599
☐ SOMERSET STATE HOSPITAL, Route 5, Zip 15501, Mailing Address: Box 631, Zip 15501-0631; tel. 814/445-6501; Richard A. Stillwagon, Superintendent **A**1 10 **F**1 2 3 4 5 6 7 8 9 10 11 12 13 15 16 17 18 19 20 21 22 23 24 25 26 27 28 29 30 31 32 33 34 35 36 37 38 39 40 41 42 43 44 45 46 47 48 49 50 51 52 53 54 56 57 58 59 60 61 62 63 64 65 66 67 68 69 70 71 72 73 74 **P**6	12	22	244	189	222	0	0	19103	11101	351
SPANGLER—Cambria County ★ MINERS HOSPITAL NORTHERN CAMBRIA, 2205 Crawford Avenue, Zip 15775, Mailing Address: P.O. Box 490, Zip 15775; tel. 814/948-7171; Roger P. Winn, Administrator **A**1 9 10 **F**8 15 19 21 22 23 26 28 30 33 34 35 37 39 41 42 44 49 56 65 71 **S**0002 Quorum Health Group/Quorum Health Resources	23	10	40	2341	28	45808	0	12505	4944	180
SPRINGFIELD—Delaware County ★ ○ SPRINGFIELD HOSPITAL, 190 West Sproul Road, Zip 19064-2097; tel. 215/328-8700; Stephen A. Robbins, Executive Director **A**1 9 10 11 12 13 **F**2 3 4 8 9 10 11 12 13 14 15 16 17 19 21 22 24 26 28 29 30 32 33 35 37 38 39 40 41 42 43 44 45 48 49 50 54 58 59 60 63 64 65 66 67 70 71 72 73 74 **P**7 **S**0008 Crozer-Keystone Health System	23	10	32	1906	36	48620	0	19204	7308	176
STATE COLLEGE—Centre County ★ CENTRE COMMUNITY HOSPITAL, 1800 East Park Avenue, Zip 16803-6797; tel. 814/231-7000; Lance H. Rose FACHE, President **A**1 2 5 9 10 **F**7 8 14 15 16 19 21 22 23 28 32 33 34 35 37 38 39 40 41 46 52 56 60 63 65 71 73	23	10	177	7384	112	94298	1139	54993	25412	716
SUNBURY—Northumberland County ★ SUNBURY COMMUNITY HOSPITAL, 350 North Eleventh Street, Zip 17801-0737; tel. 717/286-3333; Nicholas A. Prisco, Chief Executive Officer (Total facility includes 29 beds in nursing home-type unit) **A**1 9 10 **F**7 8 10 11 12 14 15 16 17 19 20 21 22 23 24 26 28 30 31 33 34 35 36 39 40 44 49 54 59 60 64 65 66 67 68 71 73 74	23	10	135	3001	86	74356	88	20414	9986	393
SUSQUEHANNA—Susquehanna County ★ BARNES-KASSON COUNTY HOSPITAL, 400 Turnpike Street, Zip 18847-1699; tel. 717/853-3135; Sara C. Iveson, Executive Director (Total facility includes 58 beds in nursing home-type unit) **A**9 10 **F**7 8 12 16 17 19 20 22 27 30 32 34 35 36 37 40 42 44 45 49 54 63 64 65 71 73	23	10	105	1822	84	33560	165	11084	5181	197

© 1995 AHA Guide

Hospitals, U.S. / PENNSYLVANIA

Hospital, Address, Telephone, Administrator, Approval, Facility, and Physician Codes, Health Care System	Classification Codes		Utilization Data					Expense (thousands) of dollars		
	Control	Service	Beds	Admissions	Census	Outpatient Visits	Births	Total	Payroll	Personnel

- ★ American Hospital Association (AHA) membership
- ☐ Joint Commission on Accreditation of Healthcare Organizations (JCAHO) accreditation
- + American Osteopathic Hospital Association (AOHA) membership
- ○ American Osteopathic Association (AOA) accreditation
- △ Commission on Accreditation of Rehabilitation Facilities (CARF) accreditation

Control codes 61, 63, 64, 71, 72 and 73 indicate hospitals listed by AOHA, but not registered by AHA. For definition of numerical codes, see page A6

Hospital	Control	Service	Beds	Admissions	Census	Outpatient Visits	Births	Total	Payroll	Personnel
TITUSVILLE—Crawford County ★ TITUSVILLE AREA HOSPITAL, 406 West Oak Street, Zip 16354; tel. 814/827–1851; Anthony J. Nasralla FACHE, President and Chief Executive Officer (Nonreporting) **A**1 9 10	23	10	99	—	—	—	—	—	—	—
TORRANCE—Westmoreland County ☐ TORRANCE STATE HOSPITAL, Torrance Road, Zip 15779–0111; tel. 412/459–8000; R. E. Bullard Jr. M.D., Superintendent (Total facility includes 55 beds in nursing home-type unit) **A**1 10 **F**8 11 14 15 16 19 20 22 35 37 52 57 64 73	12	22	375	158	318	0	0	32318	17703	563
TOWANDA—Bradford County ★ MEMORIAL HOSPITAL, One Hospital Drive, Zip 18848–9767; tel. 717/265–2191; Gary A. Baker, President (Total facility includes 44 beds in nursing home-type unit) **A**1 9 10 **F**7 8 11 12 14 15 19 20 22 28 29 30 32 33 35 36 39 40 44 45 49 64 65 66 71 73 **S**0002 Quorum Health Group/Quorum Health Resources	23	10	104	2153	70	22622	345	13335	6430	233
TREVOSE—Bucks County ☐ EASTERN STATE SCHOOL AND HOSPITAL, 3740 Lincoln Highway, Zip 19047; tel. 215/953–6001 **A**1 5 9 10 **F**12 13 14 16 19 20 22 30 35 39 41 45 46 52 53 65 73 **P**6	12	52	159	135	116	0	0	19097	12027	381
TROY—Bradford County ★ ○ TROY COMMUNITY HOSPITAL, 100 John Street, Zip 16947; tel. 717/297–2121; Mark A. Webster, President **A**9 10 11 **F**1 4 7 8 10 11 14 15 16 19 20 21 22 23 24 27 30 32 33 34 35 36 37 40 41 42 43 44 45 46 47 49 50 52 54 55 58 59 60 63 64 65 66 67 70 71 73 74 **S**0675 Guthrie Healthcare System	23	10	35	463	28	32064	0	6715	3329	149
TUNKHANNOCK—Wyoming County ★ TYLER MEMORIAL HOSPITAL, Rural Delivery 1, Zip 18657–9765, Mailing Address: Rural Delivery 1, Box 273, Zip 18657–9765; tel. 717/836–2161; William M. Milligan Jr., President and Chief Executive Officer **A**1 2 9 10 **F**7 8 11 14 15 16 17 19 22 28 30 32 35 37 40 42 44 45 46 49 65 71 73	23	10	63	3012	41	42793	246	15388	7105	255
TYRONE—Blair County ★ TYRONE HOSPITAL, One Hospital Drive, Zip 16686–1898; tel. 814/684–1255; Philip J. Stoner, Chief Executive Officer (Nonreporting) **A**1 9 10 **S**0002 Quorum Health Group/Quorum Health Resources	23	10	59	—	—	—	—	—	—	—
UNION CITY—Erie County ★ UNION CITY MEMORIAL HOSPITAL, 130 North Main Street, Zip 16438, Mailing Address: P.O. Box 111, Zip 16438; tel. 814/438–1000; Thomas McLoughlin, President **A**1 9 10 **F**7 8 12 13 14 15 16 19 22 25 30 32 33 34 37 39 40 41 44 46 49 65 67 71 73	23	10	25	1007	11	16183	74	5359	2386	89
UNIONTOWN—Fayette County ★ UNIONTOWN HOSPITAL, 500 West Berkeley Street, Zip 15401–5596; tel. 412/430–5000; Paul Bacharach, President and Chief Executive Officer **A**1 2 9 10 **F**7 8 15 16 19 21 22 23 30 32 33 34 35 37 39 40 42 44 46 49 60 62 63 65 67 71 73	23	10	230	9680	159	133141	805	59820	26808	830
UPLAND—Delaware County ★ CROZER–CHESTER MEDICAL CENTER, (Includes Community Hospital–Chester, 2600 West Ninth Street, Chester, Pennsylvania, Zip 19013; tel. 610/494–0700; Peter Guzzetti, Executive Director) One Medical Center Boulevard, Zip 19013–3995; tel. 215/447–2000; Gerald Miller, President **A**1 2 3 5 8 9 10 **F**1 2 3 4 6 7 8 9 10 11 12 13 14 15 17 18 19 21 22 23 24 26 28 29 30 31 32 33 34 35 37 38 39 40 41 42 43 44 45 46 48 49 51 52 53 54 55 56 57 58 59 60 61 64 65 66 67 68 70 71 73 74 **P**1 5 6 7 8 **S**0008 Crozer–Keystone Health System	23	10	478	16901	315	280459	2887	190042	84413	2475
WARMINSTER—Bucks County ☐ BUCKS COUNTY HOSPITAL, 225 Newtown Road, Zip 18974; tel. 215/441–6600; Margaret M. McGoldrick, Executive Director and Chief Executive Officer (Nonreporting) **A**1 10 **S**2305 Allegheny Health, Education and Research Foundation	23	10	166	—	—	—	—	—	—	—
WARREN—Warren County ☐ WARREN GENERAL HOSPITAL, 2 Crescent Park West, Zip 16365; tel. 814/723–3300; Alton M. Schadt, Executive Director **A**1 9 10 **F**2 3 7 8 15 19 21 22 23 28 29 30 32 33 35 37 40 42 44 46 49 52 53 54 55 56 57 58 59 60 65 66 71 73 **P**3 8	23	10	105	3977	63	92352	437	28299	13248	492
WARREN STATE HOSPITAL See North Warren										
WASHINGTON—Washington County ★ WASHINGTON HOSPITAL, 155 Wilson Avenue, Zip 15301–9986; tel. 412/225–7000; Telford W. Thomas, President and Chief Executive Officer **A**1 3 5 6 9 10 **F**4 7 8 10 11 12 13 15 16 17 19 20 21 22 23 25 26 28 29 30 31 32 34 35 37 39 40 41 42 43 44 45 49 51 52 54 56 60 61 65 66 67 68 71 73 **P**1	23	10	312	13208	217	296637	1049	99767	50370	1457
WAYMART—Wayne County FARVIEW STATE HOSPITAL, Mailing Address: Box 128, Zip 18472; tel. 717/488–6111; Thomas Glacken MSW, Superintendent **A**10 **F**11 14 16 19 20 21 22 31 35 37 42 44 46 48 50 51 52 60 65 67 71 73 **P**6	12	22	160	367	133	0	0	17601	11872	322
WAYNESBORO—Franklin County ★ + WAYNESBORO HOSPITAL, 501 East Main Street, Zip 17268–2394; tel. 717/765–4000; William G. George, President **A**1 5 9 10 **F**1 7 8 14 15 16 17 19 21 22 28 29 30 33 34 37 39 40 41 42 44 45 46 60 65 67 68 71 73 74 **P**8	23	10	69	3234	46	47453	480	20537	9856	312

Hospitals, U.S. / PENNSYLVANIA

Hospital, Address, Telephone, Administrator, Approval, Facility, and Physician Codes, Health Care System	Classification Codes		Utilization Data					Expense (thousands) of dollars		
★ American Hospital Association (AHA) membership ☐ Joint Commission on Accreditation of Healthcare Organizations (JCAHO) accreditation + American Osteopathic Hospital Association (AOHA) membership ○ American Osteopathic Association (AOA) accreditation △ Commission on Accreditation of Rehabilitation Facilities (CARF) accreditation Control codes 61, 63, 64, 71, 72 and 73 indicate hospitals listed by AOHA, but not registered by AHA. For definition of numerical codes, see page A6	Control	Service	Beds	Admissions	Census	Outpatient Visits	Births	Total	Payroll	Personnel
WAYNESBURG—Greene County ★ GREENE COUNTY MEMORIAL HOSPITAL, Seventh Street and Bonar Avenue, Zip 15370; tel. 412/627-3101; Raoul Walsh, Chief Executive Officer (Total facility includes 18 beds in nursing home–type unit) **A**1 9 10 **F**8 14 15 16 19 21 22 23 26 28 30 31 32 34 35 37 41 42 44 45 46 49 64 65 67 71 73 74 **P**1 **S**0002 Quorum Health Group/Quorum Health Resources	23	10	78	3319	58	41241	0	24455	10111	310
WELLSBORO—Tioga County ★ SOLDIERS AND SAILORS MEMORIAL HOSPITAL, 32–36 Central Avenue, Zip 16901–1899; tel. 717/723–7764; Ronald J. Butler, Executive Director **A**1 9 10 **F**1 7 8 11 14 15 16 17 19 20 21 22 23 25 26 28 30 32 33 34 35 36 37 39 40 41 44 46 49 52 53 54 56 57 58 59 61 62 65 66 68 71 73	23	10	103	3755	51	88883	372	19937	9467	385
WERNERSVILLE—Berks County ☐ WERNERSVILLE STATE HOSPITAL, Route 422, Zip 19565–0300, Mailing Address: P.O. Box 300, Zip 19565–0300; tel. 610/678–3411; Thomas V. Sellars, Superintendent (Total facility includes 67 beds in nursing home–type unit) **A**1 9 10 **F**3 4 8 10 19 20 21 31 35 42 43 44 45 46 49 52 57 60 64 65 71 73	12	22	465	292	435	0	0	—	—	562
WEST CHESTER—Chester County ★ CHESTER COUNTY HOSPITAL, 701 East Marshall Street, Zip 19380–4412; tel. 610/431–5000; H. L. Perry Pepper, President **A**1 2 6 9 10 **F**7 8 10 11 13 14 15 16 17 19 21 22 24 28 29 30 32 34 35 36 37 39 40 41 42 44 45 46 49 51 56 60 63 65 67 71 73 74 **P**8	23	10	200	11064	160	210347	1998	83112	39376	1068
WEST GROVE—Chester County ★ SOUTHERN CHESTER COUNTY MEDICAL CENTER, 1015 West Baltimore Pike, Zip 19390–9499; tel. 610/869–1000; Larry K. Spaid, President **A**1 9 10 **F**3 8 15 16 17 18 19 21 22 29 30 31 32 33 34 35 37 39 41 42 44 49 51 56 58 65 67 71 73 **P**1	23	10	67	2619	42	41871	0	23680	9706	370
WEST READING—Berks County ★ READING HOSPITAL AND MEDICAL CENTER, Sixth Avenue and Spruce Street, Zip 19611, Mailing Address: P.O. Box 16052, Reading Zip 19612–6052; tel. 610/378–6000; Charles Sullivan, President and Chief Executive Officer **A**1 2 3 5 6 9 10 **F**3 4 7 8 10 11 14 15 16 17 18 19 20 21 22 23 25 26 28 29 30 31 33 34 35 37 38 40 42 43 44 45 46 49 51 52 53 54 55 56 57 58 59 60 61 62 63 65 67 68 69 71 72 73 74 **P**8	23	10	494	22534	367	—	2520	167795	79328	2531
WILKES–BARRE—Luzerne County CLEAR BROOK MANOR, RD 10 East Northampton Street, Zip 18702; tel. 717/823–1171; Donald Noll, Director (Nonreporting)	23	82	50	—	—	—	—	—	—	—
☐ FIRST HOSPITAL WYOMING VALLEY, 149 Dana Street, Zip 18702; tel. 717/829–7900; John Kasenchak, Administrator (Nonreporting) **A**1 9 10 **S**2635 First Hospital Corporation	33	22	96	—	—	—	—	—	—	—
★ GEISINGER WYOMING VALLEY MEDICAL CENTER, 1000 East Mountain Drive, Zip 18711–0025; tel. 717/826–7300; Conrad W. Schintz, Senior Vice President Operations **A**1 9 10 **F**3 7 8 11 14 15 16 19 21 22 28 29 30 34 35 37 39 40 41 42 44 45 46 48 49 54 56 60 65 66 67 70 71 73 **P**1 6 **S**5570 Geisinger Health Care System	23	10	195	7393	136	97293	693	54936	21833	799
★ △ JOHN HEINZ INSTITUTE OF REHABILITATION MEDICINE, 150 Mundy Street, Zip 18702–6883; tel. 717/826–3800; Thomas E. Pugh, Vice President Rehabilitation Services **A**1 7 9 10 **F**12 14 15 16 17 27 28 34 39 41 45 46 48 49 65 67 73	23	46	103	1612	90	43472	0	16996	8013	337
★ MERCY HOSPITAL OF WILKES–BARRE, 25 Church Street, Zip 18765, Mailing Address: Box 658, Zip 18765; tel. 717/826–3100; Robert P. Goodwin, President and Chief Executive Officer **A**1 9 10 **F**4 7 8 10 11 12 14 15 16 17 19 21 22 23 28 29 30 32 33 34 35 37 39 40 41 42 43 44 45 49 51 52 53 56 57 60 65 66 67 68 71 73 **P**8 **S**5155 Mercy Health System	23	10	226	8093	153	87655	373	50572	22955	706
★ VETERANS AFFAIRS MEDICAL CENTER, 1111 East End Boulevard, Zip 18711–0026; tel. 717/824–3521; Reedes Hurt, Director (Total facility includes 180 beds in nursing home–type unit) **A**1 2 3 5 9 **F**1 2 3 4 5 6 8 10 11 12 14 15 16 17 18 19 20 21 22 23 24 25 26 27 30 31 32 33 34 35 37 39 41 42 43 44 45 46 48 49 50 51 52 54 56 57 58 59 60 63 64 65 67 69 71 73 74 **S**9295 Department of Veterans Affairs WILKES–BARRE GENERAL HOSPITAL See Wyoming Valley Health Care System, Kingston WYOMING VALLEY HEALTH CARE SYSTEM See Kingston	45	10	517	5212	437	153993	0	77632	44109	1219
WILLIAMSBURG—Blair County CHARTER BEHAVIORAL HEALTH SYSTEM AT COVE FORGE, (Formerly New Beginnings at Cove Forge) Route 1, Box 79, Zip 16693, Mailing Address: P.O. Box B, Zip 16693; tel. 814/832–2121; Jonathan Wolf, Chief Executive Officer (Nonreporting) **S**0695 Charter Medical Corporation	33	82	100	—	—	—	—	—	—	—
WILLIAMSPORT—Lycoming County ★ DIVINE PROVIDENCE HOSPITAL, 1100 Grampian Boulevard, Zip 17701–1995; tel. 717/326–8181; Kirby O. Smith, President **A**1 2 5 9 10 **F**7 8 10 14 15 16 17 19 21 22 24 26 28 30 31 32 33 34 35 37 39 40 41 42 44 45 48 49 52 53 54 57 58 59 60 65 67 71 72 73 **P**6 7 8 **S**0066 Susquehanna Health System	23	10	194	5929	100	108419	530	48746	20716	825
★ △ WILLIAMSPORT HOSPITAL AND MEDICAL CENTER, 777 Rural Avenue, Zip 17701–3198; tel. 717/321–1000; Steven P. Johnson, Senior Vice President and Chief Operating Officer **A**1 2 3 5 7 9 10 **F**3 4 5 7 8 10 11 13 14 15 16 17 19 21 22 23 24 27 29 30 31 32 33 34 35 37 39 40 41 42 43 44 45 48 49 52 53 54 55 56 57 58 59 60 61 63 65 66 67 68 71 72 73 74 **P**3 6 7 8 **S**0066 Susquehanna Health System	23	10	252	9665	152	227892	1151	71825	33637	1244

Hospitals, U.S. / PENNSYLVANIA

Hospital, Address, Telephone, Administrator, Approval, Facility, and Physician Codes, Health Care System

★ American Hospital Association (AHA) membership
□ Joint Commission on Accreditation of Healthcare Organizations (JCAHO) accreditation
+ American Osteopathic Hospital Association (AOHA) membership
○ American Osteopathic Association (AOA) accreditation
△ Commission on Accreditation of Rehabilitation Facilities (CARF) accreditation
Control codes 61, 63, 64, 71, 72 and 73 indicate hospitals listed by AOHA, but not registered by AHA. For definition of numerical codes, see page A6

Hospital	Classification Codes		Utilization Data					Expense (thousands) of dollars		
	Control	Service	Beds	Admissions	Census	Outpatient Visits	Births	Total	Payroll	Personnel
WILLOW GROVE—Montgomery County										
□ HUNTINGTON HOSPITAL, 240 Fitzwatertown Road, Zip 19090–2399; tel. 215/657–4010; John P. Ash FACHE, President and Chief Executive Officer (Nonreporting) **A**1 9 10	23	22	31	—	—	—	—	—	—	—
WINDBER—Somerset County										
★ WINDBER HOSPITAL, 600 Somerset Avenue, Zip 15963–1397; tel. 814/467–6611; Timothy A. Churchill, Chief Executive Officer **A**1 10 **F**7 14 16 19 21 22 32 33 34 35 37 40 41 42 44 48 65 67 71 73 74	23	10	67	2202	30	26498	196	14863	5944	283
WYNDMOOR—Philadelphia County										
★ △ CHESTNUT HILL REHABILITATION HOSPITAL, 8601 Stenton Avenue, Zip 19038; tel. 215/233–6200; James B. McCaslin, Director (Total facility includes 31 beds in nursing home–type unit) **A**1 7 10 **F**1 4 5 6 7 8 11 12 13 14 15 16 17 19 20 21 22 26 28 29 30 32 33 34 35 36 37 40 41 44 45 46 48 49 51 60 61 62 64 65 66 67 71 73 74 **P**3 4 5 7	23	46	88	1305	73	5724	0	13033	5842	248
WYNNEWOOD—Montgomery County										
★ LANKENAU HOSPITAL, 100 Lancaster Avenue, Zip 19096; tel. 610/645–2000; Kenneth Hanover, President and Chief Executive Officer **A**1 3 5 9 10 **F**4 7 8 10 12 15 16 17 19 20 21 22 28 31 32 33 34 35 37 38 40 42 43 44 45 46 48 49 51 52 54 57 59 60 61 63 65 66 69 71 73 **P**7 **S**7775 Main Line Health	23	10	350	14830	272	194838	1935	150972	69011	1957
YORK—York County										
□ △ HEALTHSOUTH REHABILITATION HOSPITAL OF YORK, 1850 Normandie Drive, Zip 17404–1534; tel. 717/767–6941; Patricia McMurry, Administrator **A**1 7 9 10 **F**12 14 15 16 17 25 28 30 34 41 42 48 49 71 73 **S**0023 Healthsouth Corporation	33	46	88	1459	67	23825	0	15890	9807	301
★ + ○ MEMORIAL HOSPITAL, 325 South Belmont Street, Zip 17403–2609, Mailing Address: P.O. Box 15118, Zip 17405–5118; tel. 717/843–8623; Dennis P. Heinle, President and Chief Executive Officer (Nonreporting) **A**9 10 11 12 13	23	10	150	—	—	—	—	—	—	—
★ YORK HOSPITAL, 1001 South George Street, Zip 17405–3676; tel. 717/851–2345; Bruce M. Bartels, President **A**1 2 3 5 8 9 10 **F**2 3 4 7 8 10 12 14 15 16 17 18 19 20 21 22 23 25 26 28 29 30 31 32 34 35 37 38 39 40 41 42 43 44 45 46 49 51 52 53 54 56 57 58 59 60 61 63 65 67 69 70 71 73 74 **P**4 **S**0068 York Health System	23	10	428	22551	376	398490	2948	181877	93757	2972

RHODE ISLAND

Resident population 1,000 (in thousands)
Resident population in metro areas 93.6%
Birth rate per 1,000 population 14.7
65 years and over 15.5%
Percent of persons without health insurance 10.2%

Hospital, Address, Telephone, Administrator, Approval, Facility, and Physician Codes, Health Care System

- ★ American Hospital Association (AHA) membership
- □ Joint Commission on Accreditation of Healthcare Organizations (JCAHO) accreditation
- + American Osteopathic Hospital Association (AOHA) membership
- ○ American Osteopathic Association (AOA) accreditation
- △ Commission on Accreditation of Rehabilitation Facilities (CARF) accreditation

Control codes 61, 63, 64, 71, 72 and 73 indicate hospitals listed by AOHA, but not registered by AHA. For definition of numerical codes, see page A6

Hospital	Classification Codes		Utilization Data					Expense (thousands) of dollars		Personnel
	Control	Service	Beds	Admissions	Census	Outpatient Visits	Births	Total	Payroll	

CRANSTON—Providence County

★ ELEANOR SLATER HOSPITAL, (Includes Eleanor Slater Hospital (Formerly Dr. U. E. Zambarano Hospital), 2090 Wallum Lake Road, Pascoag, Zip 02859–1813; tel. 401/568–2551; Rhode Island Medical Center, Mailing Address: P.O. Box 8269, Zip 02920; tel. 401/464–3085) A. Kathryn Powers, Director **A**1 10 **F**19 20 21 26 31 35 48 52 71 73 **P**6 — 12 48 800 436 445 0 0 66297 34725 1238

RHODE ISLAND MEDICAL CENTER See Eleanor Slater Hospital

EAST PROVIDENCE—Providence County

★ EMMA PENDLETON BRADLEY HOSPITAL, 1011 Veterans Memorial Parkway, Zip 02915–5099; tel. 401/434–3400; Daniel J. Wall, President and Chief Operating Officer (Nonreporting) **A**1 3 5 9 10 — 23 52 60 — — — — — — —

HOWARD—Providence County

□ INSTITUTE OF MENTAL HEALTH–RHODE ISLAND MEDICAL CENTER, Howard Avenue, Zip 02920, Mailing Address: Box 8281, Cranston Zip 02920–0281; tel. 401/464–2495; Betty A. Fielder, Clinical Administrative Officer (Nonreporting) **A**1 10 — 12 22 71 — — — — — — —

NEWPORT—Newport County

★ △ NEWPORT HOSPITAL, 11 Friendship Street, Zip 02840–2299; tel. 401/846–6400; Arthur J. Sampson, President and Chief Executive Officer **A**1 2 7 9 10 **F**7 8 12 17 18 19 21 22 24 25 26 28 29 30 31 34 35 36 37 39 40 41 44 46 48 49 52 54 56 57 65 66 67 71 73 **P**4 — 23 10 168 6378 99 88521 791 46068 23677 693

NORTH PROVIDENCE—Providence County

OUR LADY OF FATIMA HOSPITAL See St. Joseph Health Services of Rhode Island

★ △ ST. JOSEPH HEALTH SERVICES OF RHODE ISLAND, (Includes Our Lady of Fatima Hospital, 200 High Service Avenue, North Providence, Rhode Island, Zip 02904; St. Joseph Hospital, 21 Peace Street, Providence, Rhode Island, Zip 02907; tel. 401/456–3000) 200 High Service Avenue, Zip 02904; tel. 401/456–3000; H. John Keimig, President and Chief Executive Officer **A**1 6 7 9 10 **F**4 6 7 8 11 12 13 16 17 19 20 21 22 23 32 34 35 36 37 38 39 40 41 42 44 46 47 48 49 51 52 54 55 56 57 58 60 65 67 70 71 72 73 **P**7 — 21 10 340 12174 254 134270 635 100948 58377 1591

NORTH SMITHFIELD—Providence County

LANDMARK MEDICAL CENTER, FOGARTY UNIT See Landmark Medical Center, Woonsocket

PASCOAG—Providence County

DR U. E. ZAMBARANO MEM HOSPITAL See Eleanor Slater Hospital–Zambarano Unit, Cranston

PAWTUCKET—Providence County

★ △ MEMORIAL HOSPITAL OF RHODE ISLAND, 111 Brewster Street, Zip 02860–4499; tel. 401/729–2000; Francis R. Dietz, President **A**1 2 3 5 7 8 9 10 **F**1 2 3 4 5 6 7 8 9 10 11 12 13 15 16 17 18 19 20 21 22 25 26 27 28 29 30 31 32 33 34 35 36 37 38 39 40 41 42 43 44 45 46 47 48 49 51 52 53 54 56 57 58 59 60 62 63 65 66 67 68 70 71 72 73 74 **P**6 7 8 — 23 10 201 8817 150 73128 755 86560 47365 1288

PROVIDENCE—Providence County

★ BUTLER HOSPITAL, 345 Blackstone Boulevard, Zip 02906–4829; tel. 401/455–6200; Frank A. Delmonico, President and Chief Executive Officer (Nonreporting) **A**1 3 5 9 10 — 23 22 108 — — — — — — —

★ MIRIAM HOSPITAL, 164 Summit Avenue, Zip 02906–2895; tel. 401/331–8500; Steven D. Baron, President and Chief Executive Officer **A**1 2 3 5 8 9 10 **F**4 5 8 10 11 12 13 15 16 17 18 19 20 21 22 23 24 26 28 29 30 31 32 34 35 37 39 41 42 43 44 45 47 48 49 51 52 53 54 55 56 57 58 60 63 65 66 67 69 70 71 73 74 **P**3 4 5 7 **S**0060 Lifespan Corporation — 23 10 247 11056 202 127024 0 106421 47119 1445

★ RHODE ISLAND HOSPITAL, 593 Eddy Street, Zip 02903; tel. 401/444–4000; Steven D. Baron, President and Chief Executive Officer **A**1 2 3 5 8 9 10 **F**4 5 8 10 11 12 13 14 15 16 17 18 19 20 21 22 23 24 26 28 29 30 31 34 35 37 39 41 42 43 44 45 47 48 49 51 52 53 54 55 56 57 58 60 63 65 66 67 69 70 71 73 74 **P**3 4 5 6 8 **S**0060 Lifespan Corporation — 23 10 655 31281 539 364763 0 310673 147860 4366

★ ROGER WILLIAMS MEDICAL CENTER, 825 Chalkstone Avenue, Zip 02908; tel. 401/456–2000; Robert A. Urciuoli, President and Chief Executive Officer **A**1 2 3 5 8 9 10 **F**3 8 10 12 15 16 19 21 22 25 26 28 29 30 32 33 34 35 37 39 42 44 46 49 54 58 60 63 65 69 71 73 **P**5 8 — 23 10 150 6740 127 67490 0 76370 41342 1163

ST. JOSEPH HOSPITAL See St. Joseph Health Services of Rhode Island, North Providence

★ VETERANS AFFAIRS MEDICAL CENTER, 830 Chalkstone Avenue, Zip 02908–4799; tel. 401/457–3042; Edward H. Seiler, Director **A**1 3 5 9 **F**1 3 4 8 10 11 16 17 18 19 20 21 22 25 26 27 28 30 31 32 34 35 37 41 42 43 44 46 49 51 52 54 56 57 58 59 60 61 63 65 69 71 73 74 **S**9295 Department of Veterans Affairs — 45 10 136 4236 117 172721 0 68067 34609 966

★ WOMEN & INFANTS HOSPITAL OF RHODE ISLAND, 101 Dudley Street, Zip 02905–2499; tel. 401/274–1100; Thomas G. Parris Jr., President **A**1 3 5 8 9 10 **F**2 3 4 7 8 10 11 12 13 14 15 16 17 18 19 20 23 24 26 27 28 29 30 31 32 34 35 37 38 39 40 41 42 43 44 45 46 47 48 49 51 52 53 54 56 57 58 59 60 61 65 66 67 68 70 71 73 74 **P**5 6 8 — 23 44 197 14150 173 58062 9200 113936 57596 1502

Hospitals, U.S. / RHODE ISLAND

Hospital, Address, Telephone, Administrator, Approval, Facility, and Physician Codes, Health Care System	Classification Codes		Utilization Data					Expense (thousands) of dollars		
★ American Hospital Association (AHA) membership □ Joint Commission on Accreditation of Healthcare Organizations (JCAHO) accreditation + American Osteopathic Hospital Association (AOHA) membership ○ American Osteopathic Association (AOA) accreditation △ Commission on Accreditation of Rehabilitation Facilities (CARF) accreditation Control codes 61, 63, 64, 71, 72 and 73 indicate hospitals listed by AOHA, but not registered by AHA. For definition of numerical codes, see page A6	Control	Service	Beds	Admissions	Census	Outpatient Visits	Births	Total	Payroll	Personnel
RIVERSIDE—Providence County EMMA PENDLETON BRADLEY HOSPITAL See East Providence										
WAKEFIELD—Washington County □ SOUTH COUNTY HOSPITAL, 100 Kenyon Avenue, Zip 02879; tel. 401/782–8000; Ralph L. Misto Jr., President **A**1 9 10 **F**1 3 7 8 11 12 13 14 15 16 17 18 19 20 21 22 24 26 28 29 30 31 33 35 36 37 39 40 41 42 44 45 46 49 51 53 54 55 56 57 58 59 62 63 65 66 67 71 72 73 74 **P**2 4 5 7 8	23	10	100	4616	55	81528	598	34274	16440	515
WARWICK—Kent County ★ KENT COUNTY MEMORIAL HOSPITAL, 455 Tollgate Road, Zip 02886–2770; tel. 401/737–7000; John J. Hynes, President and Chief Executive Officer **A**1 2 9 10 **F**7 10 15 16 19 21 22 23 28 29 30 31 32 34 35 37 39 40 41 42 44 45 46 49 52 54 65 71 73 **P**1	23	10	359	14657	258	156616	1245	107805	55822	1500
WESTERLY—Washington County ★ WESTERLY HOSPITAL, 25 Wells Street, Zip 02891–2934; tel. 401/596–6000; Michael K. Lally, President and Chief Executive Officer **A**1 9 10 **F**3 7 8 17 19 21 22 23 26 30 34 35 36 37 39 40 41 42 44 45 46 48 49 61 65 66 67 68 71 72 73 74 **P**7 8	23	10	80	4082	59	33169	554	37538	18723	355
WOONSOCKET—Providence County ★ LANDMARK MEDICAL CENTER, (Includes Landmark Medical Center–Fogarty Unit, Eddie Dowling Highway, North Smithfield, Rhode Island, Zip 02896; tel. 401/769–4100; Landmark Medical Center–Woonsocket Unit, 115 Cass Avenue, Woonsocket, Rhode Island, Zip 02895; tel. 401/769–4100) 115 Cass Avenue, Zip 02895–4731; tel. 401/769–4100; Robert D. Walker, President and Chief Executive Officer **A**1 9 10 **F**7 8 11 15 16 17 19 21 22 26 28 29 30 32 33 34 35 37 39 40 41 42 44 45 48 49 52 53 54 55 56 57 58 59 63 65 67 71 72 73 **P**1 6 7	23	10	233	7906	140	123422	687	68080	32254	768

Hospitals, U.S. / SOUTH CAROLINA

SOUTH CAROLINA

Resident population 3,643 (in thousands)
Resident population in metro areas 69.8%
Birth rate per 1,000 population 16.2
65 years and over 11.7%
Percent of persons without health insurance 15.4%

Hospital, Address, Telephone, Administrator, Approval, Facility, and Physician Codes, Health Care System	Classi- fication Codes		Utilization Data					Expense (thousands) of dollars		
	Control	Service	Beds	Admissions	Census	Outpatient Visits	Births	Total	Payroll	Personnel

★ American Hospital Association (AHA) membership
☐ Joint Commission on Accreditation of Healthcare Organizations (JCAHO) accreditation
+ American Osteopathic Hospital Association (AOHA) membership
○ American Osteopathic Association (AOA) accreditation
△ Commission on Accreditation of Rehabilitation Facilities (CARF) accreditation
Control codes 61, 63, 64, 71, 72 and 73 indicate hospitals listed by AOHA, but not registered by AHA. For definition of numerical codes, see page A6

Hospital	Control	Service	Beds	Admissions	Census	Outpatient Visits	Births	Total	Payroll	Personnel
ABBEVILLE—Abbeville County ABBEVILLE COUNTY MEMORIAL HOSPITAL, Highway 72, Zip 29620-0887, Mailing Address: P.O. Box 887, Zip 29620; tel. 803/459-5011; Bruce P. Bailey, Administrator **A**9 10 **F**7 8 11 16 17 19 22 26 27 28 29 30 32 33 34 36 37 40 41 44 45 48 49 53 54 56 57 58 62 63 65 67 71 73 74	13	10	48	1259	14	20288	175	7155	3825	163
AIKEN—Aiken County ★ AIKEN REGIONAL MEDICAL CENTERS, (Includes Aurora Pavilion, 655 Medical Park Drive, Aiken, South Carolina, Zip 29801, Mailing Address: P.O. Box 1073, Zip 29802; tel. 803/641-5900) 202 University Parkway, Zip 29801-2757, Mailing Address: P.O. Box 1117, Zip 29802-1117; tel. 803/641-5000; Richard H. Satcher, Interim Chief Executive Officer (Nonreporting) **A**1 2 9 10 **S**0048 Columbia/HCA Healthcare Corporation	33	10	233	—	—	—	—	—	—	—
ANDERSON—Anderson County ★ ANDERSON AREA MEDICAL CENTER, 800 North Fant Street, Zip 29621-5793; tel. 803/261-1000; D. K. Oglesby Jr., President **A**1 2 3 5 9 10 **F**2 3 7 8 9 10 11 14 15 16 17 19 20 21 22 23 24 25 26 27 28 29 30 31 32 33 34 35 37 38 40 41 42 44 45 46 47 48 49 51 52 53 54 55 56 57 58 59 60 61 63 65 66 67 70 71 73 74 **P**5 6	23	10	445	17631	287	258689	1941	119643	53667	2166
BAMBERG—Bamberg County ★ BAMBERG COUNTY MEMORIAL HOSPITAL AND NURSING CENTER, North and McGee Streets, Zip 29003-0507, Mailing Address: P.O. Box 507, Zip 29003-0507; tel. 803/245-4321; Warren E. Hammett, Administrator (Total facility includes 44 beds in nursing home-type unit) **A**9 10 **F**7 8 19 22 40 44 65 71 74	13	10	84	1219	62	9786	107	8269	3618	179
BARNWELL—Barnwell County ★ BARNWELL COUNTY HOSPITAL, Reynolds and Wren Streets, Zip 29812, Mailing Address: Box 588, Zip 29812-0588; tel. 803/259-1000; Meredith Smith, Administrator **A**9 10 **F**15 17 19 21 22 26 28 29 30 31 37 44 45 48 71 73 74 **P**5	13	10	35	850	16	29154	0	6557	2855	115
BEAUFORT—Beaufort County ★ BEAUFORT MEMORIAL HOSPITAL, 121 South Ribaut Road, Zip 29902, Mailing Address: P.O. Box 1068, Zip 29901-1068; tel. 803/522-5200; Charles W. Elliott Jr., Chief Executive Officer **A**1 9 10 **F**7 8 14 15 16 17 19 21 22 24 28 29 30 31 34 35 37 39 40 44 45 46 52 54 55 56 57 63 65 66 71 73 74 **S**0002 Quorum Health Group/Quorum Health Resources	13	10	141	4859	57	75193	1060	30304	12570	496
★ NAVAL HOSPITAL, 1 Pinckney Boulevard, Zip 29902-6148; tel. 803/525-5301; Captain Mark V. Brown MC, USN, Commanding Officer (Nonreporting) **A**1 9 **S**9655 Department of Navy	43	10	49	—	—	—	—	—	—	—
BENNETTSVILLE—Marlboro County ★ MARLBORO PARK HOSPITAL, 1138 Cheraw Highway, Zip 29512-0738, Mailing Address: Box 738, Zip 29512-0738; tel. 803/479-2881; James W. White, Chief Executive Officer **A**1 9 10 **F**7 8 11 17 19 21 22 23 28 29 30 31 33 35 37 39 40 44 45 46 49 65 71 73 74 **P**1 5 **S**0048 Columbia/HCA Healthcare Corporation	33	10	101	2067	29	13698	329	14301	5184	216
CAMDEN—Kershaw County ★ KERSHAW COUNTY MEDICAL CENTER, (Formerly Kershaw County Memorial Hospital) Haile and Roberts Streets, Zip 29020-7003, Mailing Address: P.O. Box 7003, Zip 29020-7003; tel. 803/425-6228; Dennis A. Lofe FACHE, President (Total facility includes 110 beds in nursing home-type unit) **A**1 9 10 **F**1 2 3 4 6 7 8 9 10 11 13 14 15 16 17 18 19 20 21 22 26 27 28 29 30 31 32 33 34 35 36 37 38 39 40 41 42 43 44 45 46 47 48 49 51 52 53 54 55 56 57 58 59 60 61 62 63 65 67 68 70 71 73 74 **P**6	13	10	220	4095	128	58359	355	30843	12826	502
CHARLESTON—Charleston County BAKER HOSPITAL See Roper Hospital North										
★ BON SECOURS-ST. FRANCIS XAVIER HOSPITAL, 135 Rutledge Avenue, Zip 29401-1399; tel. 803/577-1000; Creighton E. Likes Jr., Chief Executive Officer (Total facility includes 24 beds in nursing home-type unit) **A**1 9 10 **F**2 3 7 8 10 11 14 15 16 17 19 21 22 25 26 27 28 30 31 32 33 34 35 36 37 38 39 40 41 44 45 46 49 52 54 55 56 57 58 59 60 61 65 71 73 74 **S**5085 Bon Secours Health System, Inc.	21	10	214	7601	142	50684	1085	58942	26348	877
★ CHARLESTON MEMORIAL HOSPITAL, 326 Calhoun Street, Zip 29401-1189; tel. 803/577-0600; Agnes E. Arnold R.N., B.S.N., Director Operations **A**1 3 5 9 10 **F**4 7 8 10 11 14 17 19 22 23 31 32 35 37 40 44 45 46 52 54 56 57 60 65 71 73 74 **P**5	13	10	141	4470	72	48790	886	41269	17304	521
☐ CHARTER HOSPITAL OF CHARLESTON, 2777 Speissegger Drive, Zip 29405-8299; tel. 803/747-5830; James E. Ledbetter Ph.D., Administrator **A**1 10 **F**17 28 45 52 53 54 55 56 57 58 59 65 **P**5 **S**0695 Charter Medical Corporation	33	22	102	1136	54	5159	0	9719	3490	125
★ △ MUSC MEDICAL CENTER OF MEDICAL UNIVERSITY OF SOUTH CAROLINA, 171 Ashley Avenue, Zip 29425-0950; tel. 803/792-2300; Charlene G. Stuart, Executive Director **A**1 2 3 5 7 8 9 10 **F**1 2 3 4 6 7 8 9 10 11 13 14 15 16 17 18 19 20 21 22 23 24 25 26 27 28 29 30 31 32 33 34 35 36 37 38 39 40 41 42 43 44 45 46 47 48 49 50 51 52 53 54 55 56 57 58 59 60 61 62 63 65 66 67 68 69 70 71 73 74 **P**3 5 8	12	10	582	19513	402	316596	1180	426289	134816	4886

© 1995 AHA Guide

Hospitals, U.S. / SOUTH CAROLINA

Hospital, Address, Telephone, Administrator, Approval, Facility, and Physician Codes, Health Care System	Classification Codes		Utilization Data					Expense (thousands) of dollars		
★ American Hospital Association (AHA) membership ☐ Joint Commission on Accreditation of Healthcare Organizations (JCAHO) accreditation + American Osteopathic Hospital Association (AOHA) membership ○ American Osteopathic Association (AOA) accreditation △ Commission on Accreditation of Rehabilitation Facilities (CARF) accreditation Control codes 61, 63, 64, 71, 72 and 73 indicate hospitals listed by AOHA, but not registered by AHA. For definition of numerical codes, see page A6	Control	Service	Beds	Admissions	Census	Outpatient Visits	Births	Total	Payroll	Personnel
★ NAVAL HOSPITAL, Zip 29405; tel. 803/743–7000; Captain H. B. Etienne MC, Commanding Officer (Nonreporting) A1 3 5 9 S9655 Department of Navy	43	10	160	—	—	—	—	—	—	—
★ ROPER HOSPITAL, 316 Calhoun Street, Zip 29401–1125; tel. 803/724–2000; James H. Rogers FACHE, President and Chief Executive Officer A1 5 9 10 F4 7 8 10 11 14 15 16 17 19 20 21 22 23 28 29 30 31 32 33 35 37 40 41 42 43 44 45 46 48 49 54 60 63 65 70 71 73 74 P5	23	10	400	15253	280	48938	1538	139723	57284	1937
★ ROPER HOSPITAL NORTH, (Formerly Baker Hospital) 2750 Speissegger Drive, Zip 29405–8294; tel. 803/744–2110; John C. Hales, President and Chief Executive Officer A1 9 10 F1 2 3 4 5 6 8 9 10 11 13 17 18 19 20 21 22 23 24 25 26 27 28 29 30 31 32 33 34 35 36 37 38 39 40 41 42 43 44 45 46 47 48 49 50 51 52 53 54 55 56 57 58 59 60 61 62 63 65 66 67 68 69 70 71 73 74	23	10	104	1660	42	36803	0	18345	6473	—
★ TRIDENT REGIONAL MEDICAL CENTER, 9330 Medical Plaza Drive, Zip 29406–9195; tel. 803/797–7000; Frank B. Murphy, President and Chief Executive Officer A1 9 10 F2 3 4 7 8 10 11 13 16 17 19 21 22 23 24 25 28 29 30 31 32 34 35 37 38 39 40 41 42 43 44 45 46 49 52 53 55 56 57 58 59 60 63 65 66 67 70 71 73 74 P2 4 5 6 7 S0048 Columbia/HCA Healthcare Corporation	33	10	282	12154	192	129344	2016	73900	44902	1235
★ VETERANS AFFAIRS MEDICAL CENTER, 109 Bee Street, Zip 29401–5799; tel. 803/577–5011; Dean S. Billik, Director A1 3 5 8 9 F2 3 4 8 10 11 17 19 20 21 22 26 28 30 31 32 33 34 35 37 41 42 43 44 45 46 48 49 51 52 54 55 57 58 60 63 65 71 73 74 P5 S9295 Department of Veterans Affairs	45	10	265	6081	182	114129	0	73578	50378	1054
CHERAW—Chesterfield County										
★ CHESTERFIELD GENERAL HOSPITAL, Highway 9, Zip 29520, Mailing Address: Box 151, Zip 29520-0151; tel. 803/537–7881; Steve Dean, Chief Executive Officer (Nonreporting) A1 9 10 S0048 Columbia/HCA Healthcare Corporation	33	10	66	—	—	—	—	—	—	—
CHESTER—Chester County										
☐ CHESTER COUNTY HOSPITAL AND NURSING CENTER, Great Falls Road, Zip 29706–9799; tel. 803/581–3151; Ronald V. Hunter, Administrator (Total facility includes 100 beds in nursing home–type unit) A1 9 10 F2 3 7 8 9 11 13 17 18 19 20 21 22 26 28 29 31 32 34 36 37 38 39 40 44 45 47 51 52 62 65 67 68 71 73 74	13	10	163	3184	142	15677	302	19749	9350	358
CLINTON—Laurens County										
★ LAURENS COUNTY HEALTHCARE SYSTEM, (Includes Laurens County Hospital, Clinton, South Carolina, Mailing Address: P.O. Box 976, Zip 29325; tel. 803/833–9100) Highway 76 West, Zip 29325, Mailing Address: P.O. Box 976, Zip 29325–0976; tel. 803/833–9100; Randall M. Olson, Chief Executive Officer (Nonreporting) A1 9 10 S0002 Quorum Health Group/Quorum Health Resources	16	10	203	—	—	—	—	—	—	—
WHITTEN CENTER HOSPITAL, Whitten Center, Zip 29325, Mailing Address: Drawer 239, Zip 29325; tel. 803/833–2733; (Nonreporting) A9 10	12	12	26	—	—	—	—	—	—	—
COLUMBIA—Richland County										
★ BAPTIST MEDICAL CENTER–COLUMBIA, Taylor at Marion Street, Zip 29220; tel. 803/771–5010; Charles D. Beaman Jr., President and Chief Executive Officer A1 2 9 10 F2 3 4 7 8 10 11 14 15 16 17 19 21 22 23 25 26 28 29 30 31 32 33 34 35 37 38 39 40 41 42 43 44 45 46 47 48 49 52 53 54 55 56 57 58 59 60 63 65 67 71 73 74 P5 6 7 S4155 Baptist Health Care System of South Carolina	21	10	411	17757	293	168707	3649	150263	63867	2180
CRAFTS–FARROW STATE HOSPITAL, 7901 Farrow Road, Zip 29203–3299; tel. 803/935–7173; Samuel J. Boyd, Administrator (Nonreporting) A9 10	12	22	550	—	—	—	—	—	—	—
★ △ HEALTHSOUTH REHABILITATION HOSPITAL, 2935 Colonial Drive, Zip 29203; tel. 803/254–7777; Mark J. Stepanik, Administrator (Nonreporting) A1 7 10 S0023 Healthsouth Corporation	33	46	89	—	—	—	—	—	—	—
MIDLANDS CENTER, 8301 Farrow Road, Zip 29203–3294; tel. 803/935–7508; Ronald P. Childs FACHE, Health Services Administrator (Nonreporting) A10	12	12	34	—	—	—	—	—	—	—
☐ PROVIDENCE HOSPITAL, 2435 Forest Drive, Zip 29204–2098; tel. 803/256–5313; M. John Heydel, President and Chief Executive Officer A1 9 10 F4 8 10 11 14 15 16 17 19 20 21 22 23 25 28 29 30 31 32 33 34 35 37 38 40 42 43 44 45 46 48 49 52 53 54 55 56 57 58 59 60 63 65 67 69 71 73 74 P5 S5125 Sisters of Charity of St. Augustine Health System	21	10	211	8780	170	56715	0	87481	32329	895
★ RICHLAND MEMORIAL HOSPITAL, Five Richland Medical Park, Zip 29203–6897; tel. 803/434–7000; Kester S. Freeman Jr., President and Chief Executive Officer A1 2 3 5 8 9 10 F1 2 3 4 6 7 8 9 10 11 15 16 17 18 19 20 21 22 24 25 26 28 30 31 32 33 34 35 37 38 40 41 42 43 44 45 46 47 48 49 51 52 53 54 55 56 57 58 59 60 63 65 66 68 69 70 71 73 74 P5	13	10	583	25161	467	224249	2529	248712	108385	3310
☐ SOUTH CAROLINA STATE HOSPITAL, 2100 Bull Street, Zip 29202, Mailing Address: Box 119, Zip 29202–0119; tel. 803/734–6520; Jaime E. Condom M.D., Director A1 F1 2 3 4 5 6 8 9 10 11 13 17 18 19 20 21 22 23 24 25 26 27 28 29 30 31 32 33 34 35 36 37 38 39 40 41 42 43 44 45 46 47 48 49 50 51 52 53 54 55 56 57 58 59 60 61 62 63 65 66 67 68 70 71 73 74	12	22	365	167	370	0	0	—	—	618
★ WILLIAM JENNINGS BRYAN DORN VETERANS HOSPITAL, 6439 Garners Ferry Road, Zip 29201; tel. 803/776–4000; Robert M. Athey, Director A1 2 3 5 9 F1 2 3 6 8 10 11 17 19 20 22 25 26 30 31 34 35 37 42 44 45 46 48 49 51 52 54 55 56 57 58 59 60 63 65 71 73 74 P5 S9295 Department of Veterans Affairs	45	10	370	7075	286	945	0	94892	48603	1283
★ WILLIAM S. HALL PSYCHIATRIC INSTITUTE, 1800 Colonial Drive, Zip 29203, Mailing Address: Box 202, Zip 29202–0202; tel. 803/734–7113; Larry R. Faulkner M.D., Director A1 3 5 9 10 F34 52 53 54 55 56 57 58 59 73 P5	12	22	149	1332	98	0	0	22362	—	502

Hospitals, U.S. / SOUTH CAROLINA

Hospital, Address, Telephone, Administrator, Approval, Facility, and Physician Codes, Health Care System	Classification Codes		Utilization Data					Expense (thousands) of dollars		
★ American Hospital Association (AHA) membership ☐ Joint Commission on Accreditation of Healthcare Organizations (JCAHO) accreditation + American Osteopathic Hospital Association (AOHA) membership ○ American Osteopathic Association (AOA) accreditation △ Commission on Accreditation of Rehabilitation Facilities (CARF) accreditation Control codes 61, 63, 64, 71, 72 and 73 indicate hospitals listed by AOHA, but not registered by AHA. For definition of numerical codes, see page A6	Control	Service	Beds	Admissions	Census	Outpatient Visits	Births	Total	Payroll	Personnel
CONWAY—Horry County ☐ COASTAL CAROLINA HOSPITAL, 152 Waccamaw Medical Park Drive, Zip 29526; tel. 803/347-7156; Shawn J. O'Connor, Administrator and Chief Executive Officer **A1** 10 **F2** 3 14 15 16 17 25 28 30 41 45 52 53 54 55 56 57 58 59 65 67 **P5 S**0405 Ramsay Health Care, Inc.	33	22	80	655	33	5502	0	—	—	106
★ CONWAY HOSPITAL, 300 Singleton Ridge Road, Zip 29526, Mailing Address: Box 829, Zip 29526; tel. 803/347-7111; Philip A. Clayton, President and Chief Executive Officer **A1** 9 10 **F**7 8 11 15 16 17 19 21 22 23 28 30 31 32 34 35 37 38 39 40 44 45 46 48 49 65 70 71 73 74	23	10	142	6429	88	66819	795	38367	15200	588
DARLINGTON—Darlington County WILSON MEDICAL CENTER See McLeod Regional Medical Center, Florence										
DILLON—Dillon County ★ SAINT EUGENE COMMUNITY HOSPITAL, 301 East Jackson Street, Zip 29536-2509; tel. 803/774-4111; Ronald W. Webb, President **A1** 9 10 **F**7 8 10 11 14 15 16 17 19 21 22 24 25 28 30 31 33 35 37 40 44 45 46 47 48 49 63 65 66 67 71 73 74 **S**5455 SSM Health Care System	21	10	85	3906	46	24796	315	18577	7373	251
EASLEY—Pickens County ★ BAPTIST MEDICAL CENTER EASLEY, 200 Fleetwood Drive, Zip 29640, Mailing Address: P.O. Box 2129, Zip 29641-2129; tel. 803/855-7603; Roddey E. Gettys III, Executive Vice President **A1** 9 10 **F**7 8 11 13 14 15 16 17 19 21 22 23 24 26 28 29 30 31 34 35 37 39 40 41 44 45 46 48 49 65 66 67 71 73 74 **P5** 8 **S**4155 Baptist Health Care System of South Carolina	21	10	90	3505	61	19824	648	29991	13658	486
EDGEFIELD—Edgefield County ☐ EDGEFIELD COUNTY HOSPITAL, Bausket Street, Zip 29824, Mailing Address: Box 590, Zip 29824-0590; tel. 803/637-3174; Robert J. Welsh, Administrator (Nonreporting) **A1** 9 10	13	10	40	—	—	—	—	—	—	—
FAIRFAX—Allendale County ★ ALLENDALE COUNTY HOSPITAL, Highway 278 West, Zip 29827-0278, Mailing Address: Box 218, Zip 29827-0218; tel. 803/632-3311; M. K. Hiatt, Administrator (Total facility includes 44 beds in nursing home–type unit) **A**9 10 **F**7 8 19 22 31 40 65 71 74	13	10	78	1133	53	20068	140	5793	2259	122
FLORENCE—Florence County ★ BRUCE HOSPITAL SYSTEM, 121 East Cedar Street, Zip 29501, Mailing Address: P.O. Box 100549, Zip 29501-0549; tel. 803/661-3000; H. Arnold Green, President (Nonreporting) **A1** 9 10	23	10	193	—	—	—	—	—	—	—
FLORENCE GENERAL HOSPITAL, 512 South Irby Street, Zip 29501-5210; tel. 803/667-3200; Robert F. Letson, President (Total facility includes 44 beds in nursing home–type unit) **A**9 10 **F**8 14 15 16 17 19 21 22 23 28 31 32 34 37 41 44 45 48 52 56 57 64 65 71 74 **P**5	23	10	179	6061	143	29310	0	38864	16182	628
★ MCLEOD REGIONAL MEDICAL CENTER, (Includes Wilson Medical Center (Formerly Wilson Clinic & Hospital)), 701 Cashua Ferry Road, Darlington, South Carolina, Zip 29532, Mailing Address: Box 1859, Zip 29532; tel. 803/395-1100; Debbie Locklair, Administrator) 555 East Cheves Street, Zip 29506-2617, Mailing Address: P.O. Box 100551, Zip 29501-0551; tel. 803/667-2000; J. Bruce Barragan, President and Chief Executive Officer (Nonreporting) **A1** 2 3 5 9 10	23	10	331	—	—	—	—	—	—	—
FORT JACKSON—Richland County ★ MONCRIEF ARMY COMMUNITY HOSPITAL, Mailing Address: P.O. Box 500, Zip 29207-5720; tel. 803/751-2648; Colonel Robert T. Hawkins MSC, Deputy Commander Administration **A1** 2 5 9 **F**3 7 8 10 12 15 16 17 18 19 20 21 22 25 28 30 31 34 37 40 41 42 44 46 49 51 52 54 56 58 65 71 73 **S**9395 Department of the Army	42	10	90	8483	82	384994	0	68892	29537	1006
GAFFNEY—Cherokee County ☐ UPSTATE CAROLINA MEDICAL CENTER, 1530 North Limestone Street, Zip 29340; tel. 803/487-4271; Steve Midkiff, Executive Director (Nonreporting) **A1** 9 10 **S**1775 Health Management Associates	33	10	125	—	—	—	—	—	—	—
GEORGETOWN—Georgetown County ★ GEORGETOWN MEMORIAL HOSPITAL, 606 Black River Road, Zip 29440, Mailing Address: Drawer 1718, Zip 29442-1718; tel. 803/527-7000; Paul D. Gatens Sr., Administrator **A1** 9 10 **F**2 3 5 7 8 9 10 11 16 17 18 19 20 21 22 23 24 25 26 28 29 30 31 33 34 35 37 39 40 41 42 44 45 46 47 48 49 51 52 54 55 56 58 59 61 63 65 66 70 71 73 74 **P5 S**0002 Quorum Health Group/Quorum Health Resources	23	10	141	7431	96	72452	757	38559	14171	508
GREENVILLE—Greenville County ★ GREENVILLE GENERAL HOSPITAL, 100 Mallard Street, Zip 29601-4211, Mailing Address: 701 Grove Road, Zip 29605-4295; tel. 803/455-8609; William W. Heizer, Administrator **A**2 3 5 9 10 **F**2 3 4 8 10 11 13 14 15 16 17 18 19 20 21 22 24 25 26 28 29 30 31 32 33 34 35 37 38 40 41 42 43 45 47 48 51 52 53 54 55 56 57 58 59 60 61 63 65 66 67 70 71 73 74 **P**1 6 **S**1555 Greenville Hospital System	23	46	14	76	3	11935	0	2686	1171	21
★ GREENVILLE MEMORIAL HOSPITAL, 701 Grove Road, Zip 29605-4295; tel. 803/455-7000; J. Bland Burkhardt Jr., Senior Vice President and Administrator **A**1 2 5 8 9 10 **F**2 3 4 8 7 8 10 11 13 17 18 19 21 22 24 25 28 29 30 31 32 33 34 35 37 38 40 41 42 43 44 45 46 47 48 49 51 52 53 54 55 56 57 58 59 60 61 63 65 66 67 70 71 73 74 **P**5 **S**1555 Greenville Hospital System	23	10	843	29493	594	395840	4411	304676	124963	3271
★ MARSHALL I. PICKENS HOSPITAL, 701 Grove Road, Zip 29605-4295; tel. 803/455-7836; Ryan D. Beaty, Administrator (Nonreporting) **A**1 5 9 10 **S**1555 Greenville Hospital System	23	22	106	—	—	—	—	—	—	—

© 1995 AHA Guide

Hospitals, U.S. / SOUTH CAROLINA

Hospital, Address, Telephone, Administrator, Approval, Facility, and Physician Codes, Health Care System	Classification Codes		Utilization Data					Expense (thousands) of dollars		
★ American Hospital Association (AHA) membership ☐ Joint Commission on Accreditation of Healthcare Organizations (JCAHO) accreditation + American Osteopathic Hospital Association (AOHA) membership ○ American Osteopathic Association (AOA) accreditation △ Commission on Accreditation of Rehabilitation Facilities (CARF) accreditation Control codes 61, 63, 64, 71, 72 and 73 indicate hospitals listed by AOHA, but not registered by AHA. For definition of numerical codes, see page A6	Control	Service	Beds	Admissions	Census	Outpatient Visits	Births	Total	Payroll	Personnel
★ △ ROGER C. PEACE REHABILITATION HOSPITAL, 701 Grove Road, Zip 29605-4295; tel. 803/455-7000; (Nonreporting) A1 5 7 9 10 S1555 Greenville Hospital System	23	46	50	—	—	—	—	—	—	—
★ SHRINERS HOSPITALS FOR CRIPPLED CHILDREN, GREENVILLE UNIT, 950 West Faris Road, Zip 29605-4277; tel. 803/271-3444; Gary F. Fraley, Administrator A1 3 5 F11 19 21 22 31 34 35 38 39 40 41 45 47 48 49 52 53 54 60 65 70 71 73 P6 S4125 Shriners Hospitals for Crippled Children	23	57	60	986	19	11486	0	—	—	197
★ △ ST. FRANCIS HEALTH SYSTEM, (Formerly St. Francis Hospital) One St. Francis Drive, Zip 29601-3207; tel. 803/255-1000; Richard C. Neugent, President A1 7 9 10 F2 3 4 8 10 11 15 16 17 19 21 22 23 24 25 28 29 30 31 32 33 34 35 37 38 39 40 41 42 43 44 45 46 48 49 52 53 55 57 58 59 60 63 65 66 67 71 73 74 P2 6 7 S1485 Franciscan Sisters of the Poor Health System, Inc.	23	10	237	7549	163	78363	0	72637	33337	1189
W. J. BARGE MEMORIAL HOSPITAL, Wade Hampton Boulevard, Zip 29614; tel. 803/242-5100; William Brown, Administrator (Nonreporting) A9	23	11	79	—	—	—	—	—	—	—
GREENWOOD—Greenwood County										
★ SELF MEMORIAL HOSPITAL, 1325 Spring Street, Zip 29646-3860; tel. 803/227-4111; J. L. Dozier Jr. FACHE, President A1 2 3 5 9 10 F2 3 7 8 10 11 13 15 16 17 18 19 20 21 22 23 24 26 28 29 30 31 32 33 34 35 37 38 39 40 41 42 44 45 46 47 49 51 52 53 54 55 56 57 58 60 63 65 66 67 68 70 71 73 74 P5	23	10	355	11382	203	127978	1682	75584	37216	1357
GREER—Greenville County										
★ ALLEN BENNETT HOSPITAL, (Includes Roger Huntington Nursing Center) Mailing Address: Box 1149, Zip 29652-1149; tel. 803/848-8130; Michael W. Massey, Administrator (Total facility includes 88 beds in nursing home-type unit) A1 9 10 F2 3 4 7 8 10 11 13 14 15 16 17 18 19 20 21 22 24 25 26 28 29 30 31 32 33 34 35 36 37 38 39 40 41 42 43 44 45 46 47 48 49 51 52 53 54 55 56 57 58 59 60 61 63 65 66 67 70 71 73 74 P1 5 6 S1555 Greenville Hospital System	23	10	158	2077	122	48356	30	22540	8434	283
☐ CHARTER HOSPITAL OF GREENVILLE, 2700 East Phillips Road, Zip 29650; tel. 803/879-3402; Louis R. Joseph III, Administrator A1 9 10 F2 3 15 16 17 19 21 28 29 34 35 45 46 52 53 54 55 56 57 58 59 65 67 71 P5 S0695 Charter Medical Corporation	33	22	60	1748	51	314	0	7028	3888	111
HARTSVILLE—Darlington County										
★ BYERLY HOSPITAL, 413 East Carolina Avenue, Zip 29550-4309; tel. 803/339-2100 A1 9 10 F7 8 11 16 17 19 21 22 28 30 31 32 33 36 37 40 44 45 63 65 67 68 71 74 S0002 Quorum Health Group/Quorum Health Resources	23	10	100	4050	57	33921	582	21072	7963	309
HILTON HEAD ISLAND—Beaufort County										
★ HILTON HEAD HOSPITAL, Mailing Address: P.O. Box 21117, Zip 29925-1117; tel. 803/681-6122; Dennis Ray Bruns, President and Chief Executive Officer A1 9 10 F3 4 7 8 9 10 11 15 16 17 19 20 21 22 24 25 26 28 29 30 31 32 33 34 36 37 38 40 41 42 44 45 47 48 49 51 52 53 54 56 57 65 66 69 70 71 73 74 S0063 TENET Healthcare Corporation	23	10	68	3948	40	49621	324	29570	11111	363
KINGSTREE—Williamsburg County										
☐ WILLIAMSBURG COUNTY MEMORIAL HOSPITAL, 500 Nelson Boulevard, Zip 29556, Mailing Address: P.O. Drawer 568, Zip 29556-0568; tel. 803/354-9661; Harold H. Hunter Jr., Administrator A1 9 10 F8 11 17 19 21 22 28 31 33 34 37 44 45 49 65 71 73 74	13	10	48	1316	17	21754	0	8106	3394	150
LAKE CITY—Florence County										
LAKE CITY COMMUNITY HOSPITAL, U.S. Highway 52 North, Zip 29560-1035, Mailing Address: Box 1035, Zip 29560-1035; tel. 803/394-2036; Richard Gamber, Administrator A9 10 F8 17 19 22 28 29 31 34 36 39 44 45 65 71 73 74	16	10	34	1213	13	29807	0	8162	3218	152
LANCASTER—Lancaster County										
★ △ SPRINGS MEMORIAL HOSPITAL, (Formerly Elliott White Springs Memorial Hospital) 800 West Meeting Street, Zip 29720; tel. 803/286-1214; Dace W. Jones Jr., President A1 7 9 10 F2 3 7 8 11 17 19 21 22 28 31 32 33 34 37 40 41 44 45 48 49 65 71 73 74 P8	23	10	166	5507	105	45504	683	—	—	511
LOCKHART—Union County										
★ HOPE HOSPITAL, 102 Hope Drive, Zip 29364, Mailing Address: Box 280, Zip 29364-0280; tel. 803/545-6500; Mildred W. Purvis, Administrator A9 F17 28 45 74	13	10	10	165	3	0	0	611	336	12
LORIS—Horry County										
★ LORIS COMMUNITY HOSPITAL, 3655 Mitchell Street, Zip 29569-2827; tel. 803/756-4011; J. Curtiss Gore, Chief Executive Officer (Total facility includes 88 beds in nursing home-type unit) A1 9 10 F7 8 11 14 15 16 17 19 21 22 28 30 31 34 35 37 40 44 45 46 63 64 65 70 71 74	16	10	193	3083	125	37541	304	22021	8353	409
MANNING—Clarendon County										
★ CLARENDON MEMORIAL HOSPITAL, 10 Hospital Street, Zip 29102, Mailing Address: Box 550, Zip 29102-0550; tel. 803/435-8463; Edward R. Frye Jr., Administrator A1 9 10 F7 8 11 14 15 16 17 18 19 20 21 22 26 27 29 30 31 32 33 36 37 39 40 44 45 48 51 54 62 65 67 68 71 73 74	16	10	56	1891	32	38579	314	11546	4939	204
MARION—Marion County										
★ MARION MEMORIAL HOSPITAL, (Formerly Marion County Hospital District) 1108 North Main Street, Zip 29571, Mailing Address: Box 1150, Zip 29571-1150; tel. 803/423-3210; Thomas E. Fuller, Administrator (Total facility includes 44 beds in nursing home-type unit) A1 9 10 F7 8 11 14 15 16 17 19 21 22 28 31 34 37 40 41 44 45 65 71 73 74	16	10	68	3727	36	15894	637	15095	6222	324

Hospitals, U.S. / SOUTH CAROLINA

Hospital, Address, Telephone, Administrator, Approval, Facility, and Physician Codes, Health Care System	Classification Codes		Utilization Data					Expense (thousands) of dollars		
★ American Hospital Association (AHA) membership □ Joint Commission on Accreditation of Healthcare Organizations (JCAHO) accreditation + American Osteopathic Hospital Association (AOHA) membership ○ American Osteopathic Association (AOA) accreditation △ Commission on Accreditation of Rehabilitation Facilities (CARF) accreditation Control codes 61, 63, 64, 71, 72 and 73 indicate hospitals listed by AOHA, but not registered by AHA. For definition of numerical codes, see page A6	Control	Service	Beds	Admissions	Census	Outpatient Visits	Births	Total	Payroll	Personnel
MOUNT PLEASANT—Charleston County ★ EAST COOPER COMMUNITY HOSPITAL, (Formerly East Cooper Community Hospital) 1200 Johnnie Dodds Boulevard, Zip 29464; tel. 803/881–0100; John Holland, Executive Director **A**9 10 **F**7 8 9 10 11 14 15 16 17 19 22 26 30 31 33 34 35 37 40 44 45 46 47 49 51 56 61 65 70 71 73 74 **P**1 4 **S**0063 TENET Healthcare Corporation	33	10	100	3432	41	31555	941	23170	7137	296
MULLINS—Marion County ★ MULLINS HOSPITAL, 518 South Main Street, Zip 29574, Mailing Address: Drawer 849, Zip 29574–0849; tel. 803/464–8211; Donald H. Lloyd II, Administrator **A**1 9 10 **F**1 2 3 4 6 8 10 11 13 14 15 16 17 18 19 20 21 22 23 24 25 26 27 28 29 30 31 32 33 34 35 36 37 38 39 40 41 42 43 44 45 46 47 48 49 51 52 53 54 55 56 57 58 59 60 63 65 66 67 68 70 71 73 74 **P**2 3 4 7 8	16	10	80	3474	54	11494	0	16404	6266	260
MYRTLE BEACH—Horry County ★ GRAND STRAND REGIONAL MEDICAL CENTER, (Formerly Grand Strand General Hospital) 809 82nd Parkway, Zip 29572–1413; tel. 803/449–4411; Doug White, Chief Executive Officer **A**1 9 10 **F**3 7 8 10 11 14 15 16 17 19 21 22 23 25 28 29 30 31 32 33 34 35 37 40 41 44 45 46 52 60 63 65 70 71 73 74 **S**0048 Columbia/HCA Healthcare Corporation	33	10	151	7955	96	90326	783	30458	—	597
NEWBERRY—Newberry County ★ NEWBERRY COUNTY MEMORIAL HOSPITAL, 2669 Kinard Street, Zip 29108–0497, Mailing Address: P.O. Box 497, Zip 29108–0497; tel. 803/276–7570; Lynn W. Beasley, President and Chief Executive Officer **A**1 9 10 **F**7 8 11 15 16 17 19 21 22 28 29 30 31 37 39 40 41 44 45 47 49 65 71 73 74 **S**0002 Quorum Health Group/Quorum Health Resources	13	10	64	1941	31	15688	193	13545	5503	242
ORANGEBURG—Orangeburg County ★ REGIONAL MEDICAL CENTER OF ORANGEBURG AND CALHOUN COUNTIES, 3000 St. Matthews Road, Zip 29115–1498; tel. 803/533–2200; Thomas C. Dandridge, President **A**1 2 9 10 **F**1 2 3 4 5 6 7 8 9 10 11 13 14 16 17 18 19 20 21 22 23 24 25 26 27 28 29 30 31 32 33 34 35 36 37 38 39 40 41 42 43 44 45 46 47 48 49 50 51 52 53 54 55 56 57 58 61 62 63 65 66 67 68 71 73 74 **P**8 **S**0002 Quorum Health Group/Quorum Health Resources	13	10	295	9235	167	40140	1501	59480	24600	931
PICKENS—Pickens County ★ CANNON MEMORIAL HOSPITAL, 123 Medical Park Drive, Zip 29671, Mailing Address: Box 188, Zip 29671–0188; tel. 803/878–4791; Norman G. Rentz, President **A**1 9 **F**8 11 13 16 17 19 20 22 28 29 30 31 33 34 36 37 44 45 65 71 74 **P**8	23	10	42	1215	19	20879	0	7967	3838	148
RIDGELAND—Beaufort County LOW COUNTRY GENERAL HOSPITAL, Highway 278, Zip 29936, Mailing Address: Drawer 400, Zip 29936–0400; tel. 803/726–8111; Mark Greenberg, Chief Executive Officer (Nonreporting) **A**9 10	13	10	31	—	—	—	—	—	—	—
ROCK HILL—York County ★ PIEDMONT MEDICAL CENTER, (Formerly AMI Piedmont Medical Center) 222 Herlong Avenue, Zip 29732; tel. 803/329–1234; Paul A. Walker, President **A**1 9 10 **F**7 8 10 11 15 16 17 19 21 22 23 28 31 33 34 35 37 40 44 45 46 51 52 53 54 55 56 58 59 65 70 71 73 74 **S**0063 TENET Healthcare Corporation	33	10	276	11073	162	82170	1558	69511	24384	861
SENECA—Oconee County ★ OCONEE MEMORIAL HOSPITAL, (Includes Lila Doyle Nursing Care Facility) 298 Memorial Drive, Zip 29678, Mailing Address: P.O. Box 858, Zip 29679–0858; tel. 803/882–3351; W. H. Hudson, President (Total facility includes 79 beds in nursing home–type unit) **A**1 9 10 **F**7 11 14 15 16 17 19 21 22 23 28 30 31 35 37 40 41 44 45 46 65 71 73 74 **P**1	23	10	195	5799	165	66640	531	38671	16675	616
SHAW AIR FORCE BASE—Red River County ★ U.S. AIR FORCE HOSPITAL SHAW, 431 Meadowlark Street, Zip 29152–5300; tel. 803/668–2639; Lieutenant Colonel William R. Renwick MSC, USAF, Administrator **A**1 9 **F**7 17 18 20 22 28 30 34 39 40 41 45 46 51 53 54 55 56 58 59 65 67 71 73 **S**9495 Department of the Air Force	41	10	25	2235	17	145143	444	—	—	440
SIMPSONVILLE—Greenville County ★ HILLCREST HOSPITAL, 729 Southeast Main Street, Zip 29681, Mailing Address: Box 279, Zip 29681–0279; tel. 803/967–6100; James Dover, Administrator **A**1 9 10 **F**2 3 4 8 10 11 13 14 15 16 17 18 19 20 21 22 24 25 26 28 29 30 31 32 33 34 35 36 37 38 39 40 41 42 43 44 45 46 47 48 49 51 52 53 54 55 56 57 58 59 60 61 63 65 66 67 70 71 73 74 **P**1 6 **S**1555 Greenville Hospital System	23	10	46	1215	20	34667	0	14950	5078	139
SPARTANBURG—Spartanburg County ★ MARY BLACK MEMORIAL HOSPITAL, 1700 Skylyn Drive, Zip 29307, Mailing Address: Box 3217, Zip 29304–3217; tel. 803/573–3000; Gerald W. Landis, President **A**1 9 10 **F**7 8 10 11 14 15 16 17 19 21 22 23 25 28 29 30 31 33 34 35 37 38 40 41 42 44 45 46 48 49 52 63 65 69 71 73 74 **P**1 8 **S**0002 Quorum Health Group/Quorum Health Resources	23	10	201	8529	144	153406	1466	57496	24797	819
★ SPARTANBURG REGIONAL MEDICAL CENTER, 101 East Wood Street, Zip 29303–3016; tel. 803/560–6000; Joseph Michael Oddis, President **A**1 2 3 5 9 10 **F**4 7 8 10 11 16 17 19 21 22 25 26 28 30 31 32 33 34 35 37 38 40 41 42 43 44 45 46 47 51 52 53 54 55 56 57 58 59 60 62 63 65 67 70 71 73 74 **P**2 4 5 6 **S**4195 Spartanburg Hospital System	13	10	448	17466	347	206420	2026	156904	71045	2684
SUMMERVILLE—Dorchester County ★ SUMMERVILLE MEDICAL CENTER, 295 Midland Parkway, Zip 29485; tel. 803/875–3993; James G. Thaw, President and Chief Executive Officer (Nonreporting) **S**0048 Columbia/HCA Healthcare Corporation	33	10	80	—	—	—	—	—	—	—

© 1995 AHA Guide

Hospitals, U.S. / SOUTH CAROLINA

Hospital, Address, Telephone, Administrator, Approval, Facility, and Physician Codes, Health Care System	Classification Codes		Utilization Data					Expense (thousands) of dollars		Personnel
	Control	Service	Beds	Admissions	Census	Outpatient Visits	Births	Total	Payroll	

★ American Hospital Association (AHA) membership
□ Joint Commission on Accreditation of Healthcare Organizations (JCAHO) accreditation
+ American Osteopathic Hospital Association (AOHA) membership
○ American Osteopathic Association (AOA) accreditation
△ Commission on Accreditation of Rehabilitation Facilities (CARF) accreditation
Control codes 61, 63, 64, 71, 72 and 73 indicate hospitals listed by AOHA, but not registered by AHA. For definition of numerical codes, see page A6

Hospital	Control	Service	Beds	Admissions	Census	Outpatient Visits	Births	Total	Payroll	Personnel
SUMTER—Sumter County										
★ TUOMEY REGIONAL MEDICAL CENTER, 129 North Washington Street, Zip 29150–4983; tel. 803/778–9000; Jay Cox, President and Chief Executive Officer **A**1 9 10 **F**2 4 7 8 10 11 14 17 19 20 21 22 23 24 25 28 29 30 31 33 34 35 37 38 40 42 43 44 45 46 47 48 49 51 52 53 56 57 60 63 65 66 67 70 71 73 74 **S**0002 Quorum Health Group/Quorum Health Resources	23	10	230	8644	187	59553	1642	68579	30127	1084
TRAVELERS REST—Greenville County										
★ NORTH GREENVILLE HOSPITAL, 807 North Main Street, Zip 29690–0628; tel. 803/834–5131; Ryan D. Beaty, Administrator (Nonreporting) **A**1 5 9 10 **S**1555 Greenville Hospital System	23	82	53	—	—	—	—	—	—	—
UNION—Union County										
★ WALLACE THOMSON HOSPITAL, 322 West South Street, Zip 29379–0789, Mailing Address: Box 789, Zip 29379; tel. 803/429–2600; Mark H. Petermann, Chief Executive Officer **A**1 9 10 **F**4 8 14 16 17 19 22 23 27 28 30 32 34 35 36 37 39 40 44 45 46 63 65 71 73 74 **P**3 **S**0002 Quorum Health Group/Quorum Health Resources	16	10	107	3137	50	36023	213	19377	8101	315
VARNVILLE—Hampton County										
★ HAMPTON GENERAL HOSPITAL, 503 Carolina Avenue West, Zip 29944, Mailing Address: P.O. Box 338, Zip 29944–0338; tel. 803/943–2771; Dave H. Hamill, President and Chief Executive Officer **A**9 10 **F**8 14 15 16 17 19 22 28 29 30 34 44 45 51 65 71 73 74 **P**5	13	10	36	281	3	17462	0	3352	1151	66
WALTERBORO—Colleton County										
★ COLLETON REGIONAL HOSPITAL, 501 Robertson Boulevard, Zip 29488; tel. 803/549–6371; Michael H. Greene, Chief Executive Officer (Total facility includes 15 beds in nursing home–type unit) **A**1 9 10 **F**2 3 4 7 8 9 10 11 15 16 17 18 19 20 21 22 23 25 28 30 31 33 35 37 38 40 41 43 44 45 46 47 48 49 51 52 53 54 55 56 57 58 59 65 67 70 71 73 74 **S**0048 Columbia/HCA Healthcare Corporation	33	10	116	4210	72	54775	440	19352	—	320
WEST COLUMBIA—Lexington County										
□ CHARTER RIVERS HOSPITAL, 2900 Sunset Boulevard, Zip 29169, Mailing Address: P.O. Box 4116, Zip 29171–4116; tel. 803/796–9911; Janet N. Chubb, Chief Executive Officer **A**1 9 10 **F**1 2 3 6 14 15 16 17 25 26 28 34 45 52 53 54 55 56 57 58 59 65 73 **P**5 **S**0695 Charter Medical Corporation	33	22	80	1352	41	0	0	9054	2925	112
★ LEXINGTON MEDICAL CENTER, 2720 Sunset Boulevard, Zip 29169–4816; tel. 803/791–2000; Kenneth A. Shull, President **A**1 9 10 **F**1 2 3 4 6 7 8 10 11 13 14 15 16 17 18 19 20 21 22 23 24 25 26 27 28 29 30 31 33 34 35 37 38 39 40 41 42 43 44 45 46 47 48 49 50 51 52 53 54 55 56 57 58 59 60 62 63 65 66 67 70 71 73 74	16	10	287	12694	200	111664	2175	90080	39129	1347
WINNSBORO—Fairfield County										
★ FAIRFIELD MEMORIAL HOSPITAL, 321 By-Pass, Zip 29180, Mailing Address: Box 620, Zip 29180–0620; tel. 803/635–5548; Brent R. Lammers, Administrator **A**1 5 9 10 **F**2 3 8 13 17 18 19 20 22 27 28 29 34 36 39 44 45 51 62 65 67 68 71 73 74	13	10	41	1110	18	20977	0	8106	3485	152
WOODRUFF—Spartanburg County										
★ B.J. WORKMAN MEMORIAL HOSPITAL, 751 East Georgia Street, Zip 29388, Mailing Address: P.O. Box 699, Zip 29388–0699; tel. 803/476–8122; G. Curtis Walker R.N., Administrator **A**9 **F**16 21 22 34 35 44 46 71 74 **P**2 4 5 6 **S**4195 Spartanburg Hospital System	13	10	32	668	9	14025	0	4883	2075	87

Hospitals, U.S. / SOUTH DAKOTA

SOUTH DAKOTA

Resident population 715 (in thousands)
Resident population in metro areas 32.6%
Birth rate per 1,000 population 15.6
65 years and over 14.7%
Percent of persons without health insurance 12.2%

★ American Hospital Association (AHA) membership
☐ Joint Commission on Accreditation of Healthcare Organizations (JCAHO) accreditation
+ American Osteopathic Hospital Association (AOHA) membership
○ American Osteopathic Association (AOA) accreditation
△ Commission on Accreditation of Rehabilitation Facilities (CARF) accreditation
Control codes 61, 63, 64, 71, 72 and 73 indicate hospitals listed by AOHA, but not registered by AHA. For definition of numerical codes, see page A6

Hospital, Address, Telephone, Administrator, Approval, Facility, and Physician Codes, Health Care System	Classification Codes		Utilization Data					Expense (thousands) of dollars		
	Control	Service	Beds	Admissions	Census	Outpatient Visits	Births	Total	Payroll	Personnel
ABERDEEN—Brown County ★ △ ST. LUKE'S MIDLAND REGIONAL MEDICAL CENTER, 305 South State Street, Zip 57402–4450; tel. 605/622–5000; Dale J. Stein, President and Chief Executive Officer **A**1 2 7 9 10 **F**2 3 7 8 12 14 15 16 17 19 21 22 23 27 28 30 31 32 33 34 35 36 37 39 40 41 42 44 45 46 48 49 52 53 54 55 56 57 58 59 60 61 65 66 67 71 73 **P**8 **S**5255 Presentation Health System	21	10	225	7436	107	114959	742	57118	25167	860
ARMOUR—Douglas County DOUGLAS COUNTY MEMORIAL HOSPITAL, Mailing Address: Box 26, Zip 57313–0160; tel. 605/724–2159; Steve J. Simonin, Administrator **A**9 10 **F**8 16 19 20 22 32 44 49 63 71	23	10	9	252	3	3765	16	1254	585	34
BELLE FOURCHE—Butte County ★ BELLE FOURCHE HEALTH CARE CENTER, 2200 13th Avenue, Zip 57717; tel. 605/892–3331; Stephen G. Carlson, Administrator (Nonreporting) **A**9 10 **S**2235 Lutheran Health Systems	23	10	128	—	—	—	—	—	—	—
BOWDLE—Edmunds County ★ BOWDLE HOSPITAL, 9051 West Fifth, Zip 57428–0566; tel. 605/285–6146; Ken Senger, Administrator (Total facility includes 38 beds in nursing home–type unit) **A**9 10 **F**8 14 15 19 20 22 33 34 40 44 64 65 71	14	10	58	508	44	7724	18	2542	1280	30
BRITTON—Marshall County MARSHALL COUNTY MEMORIAL HOSPITAL, 413 Ninth Street, Zip 57430–0230, Mailing Address: Box 230, Zip 57430–0230; tel. 605/448–2253; Jeff R. Dorn, Administrator **A**9 10 **F**15 16 19 22 28 30 32 44 71 **P**5 **S**5255 Presentation Health System	23	10	38	526	8	4061	0	1680	642	—
BROOKINGS—Brookings County ★ BROOKINGS HOSPITAL, 300 22nd Avenue, Zip 57006–2496; tel. 605/692–6351; David B. Johnson, Administrator (Total facility includes 79 beds in nursing home–type unit) **A**1 3 9 10 **F**7 12 16 17 19 20 22 26 27 32 33 35 36 37 39 40 44 45 46 64 65 71 73	14	10	140	1926	100	33049	270	11594	6406	229
BURKE—Gregory County COMMUNITY MEMORIAL HOSPITAL, Mailing Address: Box 319, Zip 57523; tel. 605/775–2621; Robert L. Sheckler, Administrator **A**9 10 **F**1 7 8 11 14 15 16 17 19 22 26 32 33 35 40 46 71 73 **P**5	23	10	23	192	13	4101	17	1206	643	45
CANTON—Lincoln County ★ CANTON–INWOOD MEMORIAL HOSPITAL, Hiawatha Drive, Zip 57013–9404, Mailing Address: Rural Route 3, Box 7, Zip 57013; tel. 605/987–2621; John Devick, Chief Executive Officer **A**9 10 **F**7 8 11 15 16 19 21 22 23 24 31 33 35 37 40 44 49 50 60 63 70 71	23	10	25	619	7	8095	42	2446	1180	61
CHAMBERLAIN—Brule County ★ MID DAKOTA HOSPITAL, 300 South Byron Boulevard, Zip 57325; tel. 605/734–5511; Mick Penticoff, Administrator **A**9 10 **F**8 11 15 16 17 19 22 26 28 30 37 40 42 44 65 71 **P**5 **S**0002 Quorum Health Group/Quorum Health Resources	23	10	54	1689	25	6113	12	6139	2563	82
CLEAR LAKE—Deuel County DEUEL COUNTY MEMORIAL HOSPITAL, 701 Third Avenue South, Zip 57226–1037, Mailing Address: P.O. Box 1037, Zip 57226–1037; tel. 605/874–2141 **A**9 10 **F**8 14 15 16 17 19 20 22 24 26 28 30 32 33 34 39 41 44 49 65 71 **S**5255 Presentation Health System	23	10	20	179	5	4110	0	1267	480	33
CUSTER—Custer County CUSTER COMMUNITY HOSPITAL, 1039 Montgomery Street, Zip 57730; tel. 605/673–2229; Steve Pautler, Administrator (Nonreporting) **A**9 10	23	10	16	—	—	—	—	—	—	—
DE SMET—Kingsbury County DE SMET MEMORIAL HOSPITAL, 306 Prairie Avenue S.W., Zip 57231–9499; tel. 605/854–3329; Gloria Kruger, Administrator (Nonreporting) **A**9 10	14	10	17	—	—	—	—	—	—	—
DEADWOOD—Lawrence County ★ NORTHERN HILLS GENERAL HOSPITAL, 61 Charles Street, Zip 57732; tel. 605/578–2313; Charles K. Schulz, Chief Executive Officer **A**1 9 10 **F**2 3 7 8 11 15 19 20 22 32 33 35 36 40 44 49 53 54 55 56 66 71	23	10	29	749	6	31875	67	5345	2767	110
DELL RAPIDS—Minnehaha County DELL RAPIDS COMMUNITY HOSPITAL, 909 North Iowa Street, Zip 57022; tel. 605/428–5431; Tamara Miller, Administrator **A**9 10 **F**7 8 11 15 17 19 20 22 24 27 32 33 34 35 39 40 41 44 49 71 73	23	10	29	515	5	5399	47	2167	1168	62
EAGLE BUTTE—Dewey County ★ U.S. PUBLIC HEALTH SERVICE INDIAN HOSPITAL, Mailing Address: P.O. Box 1012, Zip 57625–1012; tel. 605/964–7030; Terry Pourier, Administrator **A**1 10 **F**1 2 3 4 5 6 7 8 9 10 11 12 14 15 17 18 19 20 21 22 23 24 25 26 27 28 29 30 31 32 33 34 35 36 37 38 39 40 41 42 43 44 45 46 47 48 49 50 51 52 53 54 55 56 57 58 59 60 61 62 63 64 65 66 67 68 69 70 71 72 73 74 **S**9195 U.S. Public Health Service Indian Health Service	47	10	27	891	8	27302	91	—	—	76

© 1995 AHA Guide

Hospitals A361

Hospitals, U.S. / SOUTH DAKOTA

Hospital, Address, Telephone, Administrator, Approval, Facility, and Physician Codes, Health Care System	Classification Codes		Utilization Data					Expense (thousands) of dollars		
	Control	Service	Beds	Admissions	Census	Outpatient Visits	Births	Total	Payroll	Personnel
ELLSWORTH AIR FORCE BASE—Meade County ★ U.S. AIR FORCE HOSPITAL, Zip 57706; tel. 605/385–3201; Colonel Ted J. W. Rodgers, Administrator (Nonreporting) **A**1 **S**9495 Department of the Air Force	41	10	38	—	—	—	—	—	—	—
EUREKA—McPherson County EUREKA COMMUNITY HOSPITAL, 410 Ninth Street, Zip 57437–0517; tel. 605/284–2661; Robert A. Dockter, Administrator (Nonreporting) **A**9 10	23	10	25	—	—	—	—	—	—	—
FAULKTON—Faulk County FAULK COUNTY MEMORIAL HOSPITAL, Mailing Address: P.O. Box 100, Zip 57438; tel. 605/598–6263; Karen Collins, Administrator **A**9 10 **F**15 16 19 22 71 **P**6	23	10	12	140	2	6268	0	1315	667	25
FLANDREAU—Moody County ★ FLANDREAU MUNICIPAL HOSPITAL, 214 North Prairie Avenue, Zip 57028–1243; tel. 605/997–2433; Kent Olson, Administrator **A**9 10 **F**7 19 22 32 33 41 44 49 71 **P**5 **S**5255 Presentation Health System	14	10	20	348	6	4702	14	1776	684	37
FORT MEADE—Meade County ★ VETERANS AFFAIRS MEDICAL CENTER, 113 Comanche Road, Zip 57741–1099; tel. 605/347–2511; Peter P. Henry, Director (Total facility includes 115 beds in nursing home–type unit) **A**1 5 9 **F**2 3 4 7 8 10 16 19 20 22 26 27 30 31 33 35 37 39 41 42 43 46 49 51 52 54 55 56 57 58 64 65 67 71 73 74 **S**9295 Department of Veterans Affairs	45	10	260	2786	214	53380	0	44011	20858	592
FREEMAN—Hutchinson County ★ FREEMAN COMMUNITY HOSPITAL, 510 East Eighth Street, Zip 57029–0510, Mailing Address: P.O. Box 370, Zip 57029–0370; tel. 605/925–4231; James M. Krehbiel, Chief Executive Officer (Total facility includes 59 beds in nursing home–type unit) **A**9 10 **F**1 7 8 11 14 15 16 17 19 22 26 28 30 32 34 36 37 39 40 41 44 45 49 63 64 65 67 71 73 **P**4	23	10	85	383	64	7370	35	3512	1945	94
GETTYSBURG—Potter County ★ GETTYSBURG MEDICAL CENTER, 606 East Garfield, Zip 57442; tel. 605/765–2488; Brian J. McDermott, Administrator (Nonreporting) **A**9 10 **S**5175 Catholic Health Corporation	23	10	12	—	—	—	—	—	—	—
GREGORY—Gregory County ★ GREGORY COMMUNITY HOSPITAL, 400 Park Street, Zip 57533–0400, Mailing Address: Box 408, Zip 57533–0408; tel. 605/835–8394; Carol A. Varland, Administrator (Total facility includes 58 beds in nursing home–type unit) **A**9 10 **F**1 12 14 15 16 17 19 20 21 22 26 28 29 30 32 35 37 40 42 44 46 58 64 65 66 67 68 71 **S**2235 Lutheran Health Systems	23	10	90	744	67	16009	29	4956	2219	103
HOT SPRINGS—Fall River County ★ SOUTHERN HILLS GENERAL HOSPITAL, (Includes Castle Manor) 209 North 16th Street, Zip 57747–1375; tel. 605/745–3159; Linda Iverson, Administrator (Total facility includes 48 beds in nursing home–type unit) **A**9 10 **F**7 11 14 15 19 22 28 30 32 34 35 40 44 45 46 49 64 65 71 72 **S**2235 Lutheran Health Systems	23	10	74	336	51	14851	24	3684	1746	91
★ VETERANS AFFAIRS MEDICAL CENTER, 500 North Fifth, Zip 57747; tel. 605/745–2052; Daniel L. Marsh, Director (Total facility includes 32 beds in nursing home–type unit) **A**1 9 **F**2 3 4 5 8 10 11 12 15 16 17 19 20 21 22 23 26 28 30 31 33 34 36 37 39 41 42 43 44 46 48 49 51 52 54 57 58 60 65 67 69 71 73 74 **P**6 **S**9295 Department of Veterans Affairs	45	10	148	2382	84	75838	0	—	—	460
HOVEN—Potter County ★ HOLY INFANT HOSPITAL, Main Street, Zip 57450–1696, Mailing Address: P.O. Box 158, Zip 57450–0158; tel. 605/948–2262; Gavin Hjerleid, Administrator (Nonreporting) **A**9 10	23	10	22	—	—	—	—	—	—	—
HURON—Beadle County ★ HURON REGIONAL MEDICAL CENTER, 172 Fourth Street S.E., Zip 57350–2590; tel. 605/353–6200; John L. Single, Chief Executive Officer **A**1 9 10 **F**1 7 8 14 19 21 22 24 32 33 35 37 39 40 41 44 49 56 65 66 71 73 74 **P**3 **S**0002 Quorum Health Group/Quorum Health Resources	23	10	91	2795	33	43409	288	16515	7105	245
LEMMON—Perkins County FIVE COUNTIES HOSPITAL, 401 Sixth Avenue West, Zip 57638, Mailing Address: Box 479, Zip 57638; tel. 605/374–3871; Helen S. Lindquist, Administrator (Total facility includes 52 beds in nursing home–type unit) **A**9 10 **F**22 64	23	10	56	46	50	3625	0	1638	806	64
MADISON—Lake County ★ MADISON COMMUNITY HOSPITAL, 917 North Washington Avenue, Zip 57042; tel. 605/256–6551; Dick Soukup, Administrator **A**1 9 10 **F**7 8 14 15 17 19 22 27 28 30 32 33 35 36 37 39 40 41 44 49 65 67 71 73 **P**5	23	10	49	1051	18	13711	95	4423	2163	101
MARTIN—Bennett County BENNETT COUNTY COMMUNITY HOSPITAL, Merriman Star Route, Zip 57551, Mailing Address: P.O. Box 70D, Zip 57551; tel. 605/685–6622; Shirley May, Administrator (Total facility includes 48 beds in nursing home–type unit) **A**9 10 **F**7 8 15 22 32 40 64 73	13	10	68	566	51	1691	16	2787	1504	90
MILBANK—Grant County ☐ ST. BERNARD'S PROVIDENCE HOSPITAL, (Includes St. William Home for the Aged) 901 East Virgil Avenue, Zip 57252, Mailing Address: Box 432, Zip 57252; tel. 605/432–4538; Sister Genevieve Karels, Administrator (Total facility includes 82 beds in nursing home–type unit) **A**1 9 10 **F**6 14 15 16 19 22 32 34 37 39 40 42 44 49 65 71	23	10	117	560	87	6439	37	4312	1993	130

Hospitals, U.S. / SOUTH DAKOTA

Approval codes (key):
- ★ American Hospital Association (AHA) membership
- □ Joint Commission on Accreditation of Healthcare Organizations (JCAHO) accreditation
- \+ American Osteopathic Hospital Association (AOHA) membership
- ○ American Osteopathic Association (AOA) accreditation
- △ Commission on Accreditation of Rehabilitation Facilities (CARF) accreditation

Control codes 61, 63, 64, 71, 72 and 73 indicate hospitals listed by AOHA, but not registered by AHA. For definition of numerical codes, see page A6.

Hospital, Address, Telephone, Administrator, Approval, Facility, and Physician Codes, Health Care System	Classification Codes		Utilization Data					Expense (thousands of dollars)		
	Control	Service	Beds	Admissions	Census	Outpatient Visits	Births	Total	Payroll	Personnel
MILLER—Hand County										
★ HAND COUNTY MEMORIAL HOSPITAL, 300 West Fifth Street, Zip 57362; tel. 605/853–2421; Clarence A. Lee, Administrator A9 10 F3 8 11 12 14 16 17 19 20 21 22 26 27 28 29 30 31 32 34 36 37 39 41 42 44 45 46 48 49 53 54 55 56 57 58 63 65 66 67 68 69 70 71 P1 3 4 5 6 7 8 S5255 Presentation Health System	23	10	30	513	6	4053	1	2117	977	59
MITCHELL—Davison County										
★ QUEEN OF PEACE HOSPITAL, 525 North Foster, Zip 57301–2999; tel. 605/995–2000; Ronald L. Jacobson, President and Chief Executive Officer A1 9 10 F7 8 12 14 15 16 17 19 22 23 24 26 28 30 32 33 34 35 36 37 39 40 41 42 44 45 49 56 65 66 67 71 73 74 P3 6 S5255 Presentation Health System	21	10	99	4627	67	65869	476	25959	11847	390
MOBRIDGE—Walworth County										
★ MOBRIDGE REGIONAL HOSPITAL, Mailing Address: P.O. Box 580, Zip 57601–0580; tel. 605/845–3693; Rodney Kosters, Interim Administrator A9 10 F8 14 15 16 19 22 24 26 28 29 30 31 34 37 40 44 45 56 57 67 71 P5	23	10	48	957	10	6485	53	3661	1955	87
PARKSTON—Hutchinson County										
★ ST. BENEDICT HEALTH CENTER, Glynn Drive, Zip 57366, Mailing Address: P.O. Box B, Zip 57366; tel. 605/928–3311; Gale Walker, Administrator (Nonreporting) A9 10 S5175 Catholic Health Corporation	21	10	105	—	—	—	—	—	—	—
PHILIP—Haakon County										
HANS P. PETERSON MEMORIAL HOSPITAL, 603 West Pine, Zip 57567, Mailing Address: P.O. Box 790, Zip 57567; tel. 605/859–2511; David Dick, Administrator (Total facility includes 30 beds in nursing home–type unit) A9 10 F14 15 16 21 22 36 64 65	23	10	50	276	41	2622	8	1611	868	77
PIERRE—Hughes County										
★ ST. MARY'S HOSPITAL, 800 East Dakota Avenue, Zip 57501–3313; tel. 605/224–3100; James D. M. Russell, Chief Executive Officer (Total facility includes 105 beds in nursing home–type unit) A1 9 10 F8 11 14 15 16 19 22 32 33 35 36 40 41 42 44 49 62 64 65 71 P5 S5175 Catholic Health Corporation	23	10	191	2748	124	17747	405	16729	8032	246
PINE RIDGE—Shannon County										
★ U.S. PUBLIC HEALTH SERVICE INDIAN HOSPITAL, Zip 57770–1201; tel. 605/867–5131; George E. Howell, Unit Director (Nonreporting) A1 10 S9195 U.S. Public Health Service Indian Health Service	47	10	46	—	—	—	—	—	—	—
PLATTE—Charles Mix County										
★ PLATTE COMMUNITY MEMORIAL HOSPITAL, 609 East Seventh, Zip 57369, Mailing Address: P.O. Box 200, Zip 57369–0200; tel. 605/337–3364; John Jacobs, Chief Executive Officer (Total facility includes 48 beds in nursing home–type unit) A9 10 F1 7 8 11 14 15 16 17 19 22 24 32 34 36 41 44 45 49 64 71	23	10	67	340	56	6876	32	3111	1906	47
RAPID CITY—Pennington County										
BLACK HILLS REHABILITATION HOSPITAL See Rapid City Regional Hospital										
★ INDIAN HEALTH SERVICE–SIOUX SAN HOSPITAL, 3200 Canyon Lake Drive, Zip 57702; tel. 605/355–2280; James Cournoyer, Director A1 10 F2 3 8 9 11 13 15 16 19 20 21 22 23 24 25 26 27 28 29 30 31 32 34 35 36 37 38 39 40 41 42 43 44 45 46 47 48 49 50 51 52 53 54 56 57 58 59 60 61 62 63 64 65 66 67 68 69 70 71 72 73 74 S9195 U.S. Public Health Service Indian Health Service	47	10	32	669	12	50168	0	5064	2799	153
★ △ RAPID CITY REGIONAL HOSPITAL, (Includes Black Hills Rehabilitation Hospital, 2908 Fifth Street, Rapid City, South Dakota, Zip 57701; tel. 605/399–1101; Nan L. Hoffman R.N., Vice President) 353 Fairmont Boulevard, Zip 57701–7393, Mailing Address: P.O. Box 6000, Zip 57709–6000; tel. 605/341–1000; Adil M. Ameer, President and Chief Executive Officer A1 2 5 7 9 10 F2 3 4 7 8 10 14 16 19 20 21 22 23 26 27 28 30 31 32 33 34 35 37 38 39 40 41 42 43 44 45 46 47 48 49 52 53 54 55 56 57 58 60 63 65 66 67 71 73 P6	23	10	360	14383	232	96817	1810	117479	51079	1541
REDFIELD—Spink County										
★ COMMUNITY MEMORIAL HOSPITAL, 110 West Tenth Avenue, Zip 57469–0420, Mailing Address: P.O. Box 420, Zip 57469–0420; tel. 605/472–1111; Larry D. Carlson, Administrator A9 10 F8 11 19 32 34 36 44 49	14	10	35	576	10	7461	0	3876	1824	77
ROSEBUD—Todd County										
★ U.S. PUBLIC HEALTH SERVICE INDIAN HOSPITAL, Zip 57570; tel. 605/747–2231; Gayla J. Twiss, Service Unit Director A1 10 F7 12 13 14 15 16 20 22 27 29 30 31 34 39 40 44 45 46 61 66 71 74 S9195 U.S. Public Health Service Indian Health Service	47	10	35	1450	12	70008	149	—	—	240
SCOTLAND—Bon Homme County										
★ LANDMANN–JUNGMAN MEMORIAL HOSPITAL, 600 Billars Street, Zip 57059, Mailing Address: P.O. Box 307, Zip 57059–0307; tel. 605/583–2226; Steve J. Simonin, Administrator A9 10 F1 8 14 15 16 19 20 22 24 28 32 33 34 36 39 44 46 49 51 62 65 71 73	23	10	19	366	9	1895	8	1896	1007	50
SIOUX FALLS—Minnehaha County										
□ CHARTER SIOUX FALLS BEHAVIORAL HEALTH SYSTEM, (Formerly Charter Hospital of Sioux Falls) 2812 South Louise Avenue, Zip 57106; tel. 605/361–8111; John N. Olson, Administrator A1 3 9 10 F1 2 3 19 22 26 35 52 53 54 55 56 57 58 59 65 67 71 S0695 Charter Medical Corporation	33	22	60	773	27	0	0	—	—	69
CHILDRENS CARE HOSPITAL AND SCHOOL, 2501 West 26th Street, Zip 57105–2498; tel. 605/336–1840; Charisse S. Oland, President and Chief Executive Officer F12 17 25 34 49 65 73 P8	23	56	96	58	68	—	0	8984	5562	173

Hospitals, U.S. / SOUTH DAKOTA

Hospital, Address, Telephone, Administrator, Approval, Facility, and Physician Codes, Health Care System	Classi-fication Codes		Utilization Data					Expense (thousands) of dollars		
★ American Hospital Association (AHA) membership □ Joint Commission on Accreditation of Healthcare Organizations (JCAHO) accreditation + American Osteopathic Hospital Association (AOHA) membership ○ American Osteopathic Association (AOA) accreditation △ Commission on Accreditation of Rehabilitation Facilities (CARF) accreditation Control codes 61, 63, 64, 71, 72 and 73 indicate hospitals listed by AOHA, but not registered by AHA. For definition of numerical codes, see page A6	Control	Service	Beds	Admissions	Census	Outpatient Visits	Births	Total	Payroll	Personnel
★ △ MCKENNAN HOSPITAL, 800 East 21st Street, Zip 57105, Mailing Address: P.O. Box 5045, Zip 57117–5045; tel. 605/339–8000; Fredrick Slunecka, President and Chief Executive Officer **A**1 2 3 5 7 9 10 **F**2 3 4 5 6 7 8 9 10 11 12 13 14 15 16 17 18 19 21 22 23 24 26 27 28 29 30 31 32 33 34 35 37 38 39 40 41 42 43 44 45 46 47 48 49 51 52 53 54 55 56 57 58 59 60 62 63 65 66 67 68 69 70 71 73 74 **P**6 7 **S**5255 Presentation Health System	21	10	429	14645	228	116478	1223	118804	49253	1853
ROYAL C. JOHNSON VETERANS MEMORIAL HOSPITAL, 2501 West 22nd Street, Zip 57105, Mailing Address: P.O. Box 5046, Zip 57117–5046; tel. 605/336–3230; R. Vincent Crawford, Director (Total facility includes 42 beds in nursing home-type unit) **A**1 3 5 9 **F**2 3 4 8 10 11 14 15 16 19 20 21 22 23 26 28 30 31 33 35 37 41 42 43 44 46 48 49 51 52 54 55 56 57 58 60 64 65 67 69 71 73 74 **P**6 **S**9295 Department of Veterans Affairs	45	10	217	3516	178	64675	0	49310	29714	760
★ △ SIOUX VALLEY HOSPITAL, 1100 South Euclid Avenue, Zip 57105–0496, Mailing Address: P.O. Box 5039, Zip 57117–5039; tel. 605/333–1000; Lyle E. Schroeder, President **A**1 2 3 5 7 9 10 **F**4 7 8 10 11 12 13 14 15 16 17 18 19 20 21 22 24 25 26 27 28 29 30 31 32 33 34 35 37 38 39 40 41 42 43 44 45 46 47 48 49 51 52 53 55 56 58 61 65 66 67 70 71 72 73 74 **P**6	23	10	477	16894	281	97053	1826	—	—	—
SISSETON—Roberts County										
★ COTEAU DES PRAIRIES HOSPITAL, 205 Orchard Drive, Zip 57262; tel. 605/698–7647; Bill Nelson, Administrator **A**9 10 **F**7 8 11 16 17 19 20 21 22 27 28 30 32 33 34 37 40 44 48 49 71	23	10	31	675	6	13646	112	2248	1080	52
★ U.S. PUBLIC HEALTH SERVICE INDIAN HOSPITAL, Chestnut Street, Zip 57262, Mailing Address: P.O. Box 189, Zip 57262; tel. 605/698–7606; Richard Huff, Administrator **A**1 10 **F**2 3 4 7 8 9 10 11 12 13 15 16 17 18 19 20 21 22 23 27 28 29 30 31 32 33 34 35 36 37 38 39 40 42 43 44 45 46 47 48 49 50 51 52 53 54 55 56 57 58 59 60 61 63 64 65 66 67 68 69 70 71 73 74 **P**6 **S**9195 U.S. Public Health Service Indian Health Service	47	10	18	432	4	—	0	—	—	66
SPEARFISH—Lawrence County										
★ LOOKOUT MEMORIAL HOSPITAL, 1440 North Main Street, Zip 57783–1504; tel. 605/642–2617; Stephen G. Carlson, Administrator **A**9 10 **F**1 7 8 12 14 15 16 19 21 22 27 28 30 32 33 34 35 36 37 39 44 45 46 49 61 62 63 65 66 67 68 71 73 74 **P**6 7 **S**2235 Lutheran Health Systems	23	10	34	1587	15	37985	293	7796	3563	139
STURGIS—Meade County										
★ STURGIS COMMUNITY HEALTH CARE CENTER, 949 Harmon Street, Zip 57785–0279, Mailing Address: P.O. Box 279, Zip 57785–0279; tel. 605/347–2536; Roger R. Heidt, Administrator (Total facility includes 84 beds in nursing home-type unit) **A**9 10 **F**7 8 12 14 15 16 19 22 28 32 35 36 40 44 63 64 65 67 71 **S**2235 Lutheran Health Systems	23	10	114	1255	100	7284	91	8617	3710	100
VERMILLION—Clay County										
★ DAKOTA HOSPITAL, 20 South Plum Street, Zip 57069; tel. 605/624–2611; Larry W. Veitz, Chief Executive Officer (Total facility includes 66 beds in nursing home-type unit) **A**9 10 **F**7 8 11 14 17 19 20 22 27 28 29 30 32 33 34 35 37 39 40 42 44 45 46 51 60 64 65 66 67 73 **P**3	23	10	95	814	74	8764	51	5353	2574	74
VIBORG—Turner County										
★ PIONEER MEMORIAL HOSPITAL, Washington Street, Zip 57070, Mailing Address: P.O. Box 368, Zip 57070–0368; tel. 605/326–5161; Georgia Pokorney, Chief Executive Officer (Total facility includes 52 beds in nursing home-type unit) **A**9 10 **F**1 3 4 7 8 10 11 19 20 21 22 24 26 28 32 33 34 36 37 38 39 40 42 43 44 45 47 51 65 67 71 **P**5	23	10	77	438	56	6729	10	2857	1327	53
WAGNER—Charles Mix County										
★ WAGNER COMMUNITY MEMORIAL HOSPITAL, Third and Walnut, Zip 57380, Mailing Address: P.O. Box 280, Zip 57380–0280; tel. 605/384–3611; Arlene C. Bich, Administrator **A**9 10 **F**8 11 15 16 19 20 26 32 33 34 37 40 44 49 62 70 71	23	10	20	754	8	9136	26	2699	1205	48
WATERTOWN—Codington County										
★ + PRAIRIE LAKES HOSPITAL AND CARE CENTER, (Formerly Prairie Lakes Health Care Center) 400 Tenth Avenue N.W., Zip 57201, Mailing Address: P.O. Box 1210, Zip 57201–1210; tel. 605/882–7000; Edmond L. Weiland, Administrator (Total facility includes 51 beds in nursing home-type unit) **A**1 2 3 9 10 **F**7 8 17 19 22 29 32 33 34 35 37 39 40 41 42 44 45 46 49 56 59 64 65 71 73 **S**0041 Allina Health System	23	10	119	3204	89	35469	647	22483	9642	380
WEBSTER—Day County										
★ LAKE AREA HOSPITAL, North First Street, Zip 57274, Mailing Address: P.O. Box 489, Zip 57274–0489; tel. 605/345–3336; Gilbert DeSpiegler, Administrator **A**9 10 **F**7 11 19 21 22 30 31 34 41 44 46 49 71 **P**3	23	10	30	695	11	5389	25	2899	1590	68
WESSINGTON SPRINGS—Jerauld County										
WESKOTA MEMORIAL MEDICAL CENTER, 609 First Street N.E., Zip 57382; tel. 605/539–1201; Thomas V. Richter, Administrator **A**9 10 **F**7 15 19 22 32 44 49 71	23	10	28	427	9	3174	20	1362	650	38
WINNER—Tripp County										
★ WINNER REGIONAL HEALTHCARE CENTER, 745 East Eighth Street, Zip 57580–2677, Mailing Address: Box 745, Zip 57580–0745; tel. 605/842–2110; Robert Houser, Chief Executive Officer (Total facility includes 81 beds in nursing home-type unit) **A**9 10 **F**3 7 8 14 15 17 19 21 22 28 29 30 31 32 33 34 35 36 37 39 40 44 45 49 50 63 64 67 69 71	23	10	121	940	88	7593	152	6576	3489	107

Hospitals, U.S. / SOUTH DAKOTA

Hospital, Address, Telephone, Administrator, Approval, Facility, and Physician Codes, Health Care System	Classi-fication Codes		Utilization Data					Expense (thousands) of dollars		
★ American Hospital Association (AHA) membership ☐ Joint Commission on Accreditation of Healthcare Organizations (JCAHO) accreditation + American Osteopathic Hospital Association (AOHA) membership ○ American Osteopathic Association (AOA) accreditation △ Commission on Accreditation of Rehabilitation Facilities (CARF) accreditation Control codes 61, 63, 64, 71, 72 and 73 indicate hospitals listed by AOHA, but not registered by AHA. For definition of numerical codes, see page A6	Control	Service	Beds	Admissions	Census	Outpatient Visits	Births	Total	Payroll	Personnel
YANKTON—Yankton County ★ △ SACRED HEART HEALTH SERVICES, (Formerly Sacred Heart Hospital) 501 Summit, Zip 57078-3899; tel. 605/665-9371; Dennis A. Sokol, President and Chief Executive Officer (Total facility includes 113 beds in nursing home–type unit) **A**1 2 5 7 9 10 **F**1 7 8 10 11 12 14 15 16 17 19 21 22 23 24 26 27 29 30 32 33 34 35 36 37 38 39 40 41 42 44 45 46 48 49 60 63 64 65 67 71 73 **P**3 **S**5175 Catholic Health Corporation	21	10	257	5076	182	22487	630	29169	12458	414

© 1995 AHA Guide

Hospitals, U.S. / TENNESSEE

TENNESSEE

Resident population 5,099 (in thousands)
Resident population in metro areas 67.7%
Birth rate per 1,000 population 15.0
65 years and over 12.8%
Percent of persons without health insurance 13.6%

Hospital, Address, Telephone, Administrator, Approval, Facility, and Physician Codes, Health Care System

★ American Hospital Association (AHA) membership
☐ Joint Commission on Accreditation of Healthcare Organizations (JCAHO) accreditation
+ American Osteopathic Hospital Association (AOHA) membership
○ American Osteopathic Association (AOA) accreditation
△ Commission on Accreditation of Rehabilitation Facilities (CARF) accreditation
Control codes 61, 63, 64, 71, 72 and 73 indicate hospitals listed by AOHA, but not registered by AHA. For definition of numerical codes, see page A6

Hospital	Classification Codes		Utilization Data					Expense (thousands of dollars)		
	Control	Service	Beds	Admissions	Census	Outpatient Visits	Births	Total	Payroll	Personnel
ASHLAND CITY—Cheatham County										
★ CHEATHAM MEDICAL CENTER, 313 North Main Street, Zip 37015, Mailing Address: P.O. Box 599, Zip 37015; tel. 615/792-3030; Pegg Miller R.N., Acting Administrator **A**9 10 **F**8 15 16 19 22 28 39 41 44 49 51 71 73	23	10	29	1332	15	18159	0	5571	2514	92
ATHENS—McMinn County										
★ ATHENS COMMUNITY HOSPITAL, 1114 West Madison Avenue, Zip 37303, Mailing Address: Box 250, Zip 37371-0250; tel. 615/745-1411; Brenda M. Waltz, Administrator **A**1 9 10 **F**3 4 7 8 14 15 16 17 19 21 22 23 26 29 30 31 35 37 39 40 41 42 44 45 46 49 50 53 54 55 56 57 58 59 61 63 65 67 71 73 74 **P**1 **S**0048 Columbia/HCA Healthcare Corporation	33	10	97	2539	28	45313	181	14539	5871	228
BOLIVAR—Hardeman County										
★ BOLIVAR COMMUNITY HOSPITAL, 650 Nuckolls Road, Zip 38008; tel. 901/658-3100; George L. Austin, Chief Executive Officer **A**1 9 10 **F**2 3 15 19 22 26 32 33 34 44 49 52 57 71 73 **S**0002 Quorum Health Group/Quorum Health Resources	23	10	47	711	14	9805	0	5801	2796	151
BRISTOL—Sullivan County										
★ BRISTOL REGIONAL MEDICAL CENTER, 1 Medical Park Boulevard, Zip 37620; tel. 615/844-4200; Eddie A. George, President **A**1 2 3 5 9 10 **F**4 7 8 10 11 12 14 15 16 17 19 20 21 22 23 24 25 26 28 29 30 31 32 33 34 35 36 37 39 40 41 42 43 44 46 49 51 52 55 56 57 58 59 60 63 64 65 66 67 70 71 72 73 74 **P**2 5 6 7 8 **S**0002 Quorum Health Group/Quorum Health Resources	23	10	336	12166	200	116168	486	104023	43326	1353
BROWNSVILLE—Haywood County										
★ METHODIST–HAYWOOD PARK HOSPITAL, 2545 North Washington Avenue, Zip 38012; tel. 901/772-4110; H. Lee Kirk Jr., Administrator **A**1 9 10 **F**7 14 15 16 17 19 22 27 28 29 30 39 40 44 45 46 49 71 73 74 **P**3 7 8 **S**9345 Methodist Health Systems, Inc.	33	10	44	1177	16	13439	70	5097	2044	118
CAMDEN—Benton County										
★ VALLEY REGIONAL HOSPITAL, Hospital Street, Zip 38320, Mailing Address: P.O. Box 468, Zip 38320-1696; tel. 901/584-6135; Alfred P. Taylor, Administrator and Chief Executive Officer **A**9 10 **F**8 15 16 19 21 22 30 34 44 46 51 67 71 **S**0004 West Tennessee Healthcare, Inc.	23	10	45	727	10	8783	1	4688	2059	117
CARTHAGE—Smith County										
★ CARTHAGE GENERAL HOSPITAL, Highway 70 North, Zip 37030, Mailing Address: P.O. Box 319, Zip 37030-0319; tel. 615/735-9815; Wayne Winfree, Administrator **A**1 9 10 **F**7 8 12 15 19 22 28 32 44 65 71	23	10	29	1524	20	10668	41	4559	2331	131
★ SMITH COUNTY MEMORIAL HOSPITAL, 158 Hospital Drive, Zip 37030-1096; tel. 615/735-1560; Jerry H. Futrell, Chief Executive Officer **A**1 9 10 **F**7 8 12 14 15 16 17 19 21 22 26 28 29 30 32 35 40 44 49 52 57 64 65 66 71 73 **P**7 8 **S**0048 Columbia/HCA Healthcare Corporation	33	10	63	1317	15	16547	84	7105	2475	110
CELINA—Clay County										
CLAY COUNTY HOSPITAL, McArthur Street, Zip 38551, Mailing Address: Box 427, Zip 38551; tel. 615/243-3581; Donald E. Downey, Administrator (Nonreporting) **A**9 10 **S**5765 Paracelsus Healthcare Corporation	33	10	36	—	—	—	—	—	—	—
CENTERVILLE—Hickman County										
☐ HICKMAN COUNTY HEALTH SERVICES, 135 East Swan Street, Zip 37033-1499; tel. 615/729-4271; Jack M. Keller, Administrator (Total facility includes 40 beds in nursing home–type unit) **A**1 9 10 **F**8 14 15 16 19 22 30 32 33 34 41 44 49 63 65 71	13	10	68	486	46	8446	0	4605	2918	—
CHATTANOOGA—Hamilton County										
☐ CHATTANOOGA REHABILITATION HOSPITAL, 2412 McCallie Avenue, Zip 37404; tel. 615/698-0221; Jim Henson, Administrator and Chief Executive Officer (Nonreporting) **A**1 10	33	46	50	—	—	—	—	—	—	—
☐ ERLANGER MEDICAL CENTER, (Includes Erlanger North Hospital, 632 Morrison Springs Road, Chattanooga, Tennessee, Zip 37415; tel. 615/778-3300; T. C. Thompson Children's Hospital, 910 Blackford Street, Chattanooga, Tennessee, Zip 37403; tel. 615/778-6011; Willie D. Miller Eye Center, Chattanooga, Tennessee) 975 East Third Street, Zip 37403; tel. 615/778-7000; Sylvester L. Reeder III, President and Chief Executive Officer (Nonreporting) **A**1 2 3 5 9 10	16	10	587	—	—	—	—	—	—	—
ERLANGER NORTH HOSPITAL See Erlanger Medical Center										
★ MEMORIAL HOSPITAL, 2525 De Sales Avenue, Zip 37404-3322; tel. 615/495-2525; L. Clark Taylor Jr., President and Chief Executive Officer **A**1 2 9 10 **F**1 2 3 4 5 7 8 10 12 13 15 17 18 19 21 22 23 25 26 27 28 29 30 32 33 34 35 37 39 41 42 43 44 45 46 49 51 52 54 55 56 57 58 59 60 63 64 65 66 67 71 72 73 74 **P**1 3 7 **S**3045 Sisters of Charity of Nazareth Health System	21	10	296	12355	206	102092	0	107933	43561	1536
☐ MOCCASIN BEND MENTAL HEALTH INSTITUTE, 100 Moccasin Bend Road, Zip 37405; tel. 615/265-2271; Russell K. Vatter, Superintendent **A**1 10 **F**14 16 31 52 53 54 55 56	12	22	200	1799	205	0	0	16589	10596	485

Hospitals, U.S. / TENNESSEE

Hospital, Address, Telephone, Administrator, Approval, Facility, and Physician Codes, Health Care System	Classification Codes		Utilization Data					Expense (thousands) of dollars		
★ American Hospital Association (AHA) membership ☐ Joint Commission on Accreditation of Healthcare Organizations (JCAHO) accreditation + American Osteopathic Hospital Association (AOHA) membership ○ American Osteopathic Association (AOA) accreditation △ Commission on Accreditation of Rehabilitation Facilities (CARF) accreditation Control codes 61, 63, 64, 71, 72 and 73 indicate hospitals listed by AOHA, but not registered by AHA. For definition of numerical codes, see page A6	Control	Service	Beds	Admissions	Census	Outpatient Visits	Births	Total	Payroll	Personnel
★ NORTH PARK HOSPITAL, 2051 Hamill Road, Zip 37343–4096; tel. 615/870–1300; Roger W. Glass, Administrator **A**1 9 10 **F**8 10 12 14 15 16 17 19 20 21 22 28 32 34 35 37 39 41 44 45 46 49 63 65 71 73 **S**2795 Healthcorp of Tennessee, Inc.	23	10	83	3194	41	28344	0	26922	8919	345
★ PARKRIDGE MEDICAL CENTER, 2333 McCallie Avenue, Zip 37404–3285; tel. 615/698–6061; Kelly E. McBryde, Chief Executive Officer (Total facility includes 28 beds in nursing home–type unit) **A**1 9 10 **F**2 3 4 8 10 12 14 16 19 20 21 22 23 24 26 28 30 31 32 33 34 35 37 38 39 40 41 42 43 44 45 46 49 52 53 54 55 56 57 58 59 60 61 64 65 67 71 72 73 74 **P**8 **S**0048 Columbia/HCA Healthcare Corporation	33	10	271	7414	154	40467	0	54298	21006	655
★ △ SISKIN HOSPITAL FOR PHYSICAL REHABILITATION, One Siskin Plaza, Zip 37403; tel. 615/634–1200; Robert P. Main, President and Chief Executive Officer **A**1 7 9 10 **F**2 5 9 11 12 14 15 16 17 19 20 22 30 34 35 37 41 42 44 45 47 48 49 52 54 60 64 65 66 67 70 73 **P**1 5	23	46	72	658	60	18928	0	19679	9422	285
T. C. THOMPSON CHILDREN'S HOSPITAL See Erlanger Medical Center										
★ VALLEY PSYCHIATRIC HOSPITAL, 2200 Morris Hill Road, Zip 37421; tel. 615/894–4220; Mary Palmer, Chief Executive Officer **A**1 10 **F**3 14 15 16 52 53 54 55 56 57 58 59 65 **S**0048 Columbia/HCA Healthcare Corporation	33	22	118	1382	60	581	0	8370	3903	134
☐ VENCOR HOSPITAL–CHATTANOOGA, (Longterm Acute Care) 709 Walnut Street, Zip 37402; tel. 615/266–7721; Doug Sundlof, Administrator **A**1 9 10 **F**19 21 22 35 37 65 69 71 **S**0026 Vencor, Incorporated	33	10	49	128	15	6	0	6229	2891	86
WILLIE D. MILLER EYE CENTER See Erlanger Medical Center										
CLARKSVILLE—Montgomery County										
★ CLARKSVILLE MEMORIAL HOSPITAL, 1771 Madison Street, Zip 37043, Mailing Address: Box 3160, Zip 37043–3160; tel. 615/552–6622; James Lee Decker, President and Chief Executive Officer **A**1 9 10 **F**7 8 10 13 14 15 16 19 21 22 23 26 28 30 31 32 33 34 35 37 40 41 42 44 45 46 49 51 52 56 57 58 59 60 65 67 71 73 74 **P**8	16	10	180	8658	113	71609	1135	52067	22741	869
CLEVELAND—Bradley County										
★ BRADLEY MEMORIAL HOSPITAL, 2305 Chambliss Avenue N.W., Zip 37311, Mailing Address: Box 3060, Zip 37320–3060; tel. 615/559–6000; Jim Whitlock, Administrator **A**1 9 10 **F**7 8 10 12 14 15 16 17 19 20 21 22 23 25 28 30 32 33 35 37 40 41 42 44 45 46 49 52 53 54 56 58 59 65 67 71 73 74	13	10	196	8997	104	188936	1083	56180	22537	774
☐ CLEVELAND COMMUNITY HOSPITAL, 2800 Westside Drive N.W., Zip 37312; tel. 615/339–4100; Stanley G. Hilliard, Administrator (Nonreporting) **A**1 9 10 **S**5895 Hallmark Healthcare Corporation	33	10	70	—	—	—	—	—	—	—
COLUMBIA—Maury County										
★ MAURY REGIONAL HOSPITAL, 1224 Trotwood Avenue, Zip 38401; tel. 615/381–1111; William R. Walter, Administrator **A**1 9 10 **F**3 7 8 10 11 14 19 20 21 22 23 25 28 31 32 33 34 35 37 39 40 41 42 44 45 49 51 52 54 56 57 58 59 60 65 71 73 **P**8	13	10	275	11413	137	114514	1331	69459	29538	1035
COOKEVILLE—Putnam County										
★ COOKEVILLE GENERAL HOSPITAL, 142 West Fifth Street, Zip 38501, Mailing Address: P.O. Box 340, Zip 38503–0340; tel. 615/528–2541; Mike Mayes FACHE, Administrator and Chief Executive Officer **A**1 9 10 **F**2 4 7 8 11 14 16 17 19 21 22 23 28 30 32 33 34 35 37 38 39 40 41 44 45 46 49 52 55 56 57 63 65 67 71 73 74	14	10	157	5351	66	79944	985	34300	12585	581
COPPERHILL—Polk County										
☐ COPPER BASIN MEDICAL CENTER, State Highway 68, Zip 37317, Mailing Address: P.O. Box 990, Zip 37317; tel. 615/496–5511; Grady Scott, Administrator **A**1 9 10 **F**14 19 22 27 28 49 71	23	10	44	1076	11	11219	0	3239	1825	87
COVINGTON—Tipton County										
★ BAPTIST MEMORIAL HOSPITAL–TIPTON, 1995 Highway 51 South, Zip 38019; tel. 901/476–2621; William T. Moorer, Administrator **A**1 9 10 **F**2 3 7 8 11 14 16 19 20 22 24 28 35 37 39 40 44 46 51 63 65 71 **P**3 **S**1625 Baptist Memorial Health Care System, Inc.	21	10	100	2753	38	27409	282	15017	4514	284
CROSSVILLE—Cumberland County										
★ CUMBERLAND MEDICAL CENTER, 811 South Main Street, Zip 38555; tel. 615/484–9511; Edwin S. Anderson, President **A**1 9 10 **F**7 8 11 14 15 16 19 22 28 29 30 31 32 33 34 35 37 39 40 41 44 49 65 67 71 73	23	10	160	6514	78	43747	445	24252	13472	604
DAYTON—Rhea County										
★ RHEA MEDICAL CENTER, 7900 Rhea County Highway, Zip 37321; tel. 615/775–1121; Kennedy L. Croom Jr., Administrator and Chief Executive Officer (Total facility includes 89 beds in nursing home–type unit) **A**9 10 **F**14 15 19 22 35 37 44 65 71 73 **S**0002 Quorum Health Group/Quorum Health Resources	13	10	125	1330	102	24378	0	10012	4638	151
DICKSON—Dickson County										
★ GOODLARK REGIONAL MEDICAL CENTER, 111 Highway 70 East, Zip 37055–2079; tel. 615/446–0446; Rick Wallace, Administrator **A**1 9 10 **F**2 7 8 10 15 16 19 21 22 28 32 33 35 39 40 41 42 44 46 49 51 52 53 56 71 73	23	10	114	5370	89	59264	421	26090	12659	475
DYERSBURG—Dyer County										
★ METHODIST HOSPITAL OF DYERSBURG, 400 Tickle Street, Zip 38024–3182; tel. 901/285–2410; Richard McCormick, Administrator **A**1 9 10 **F**7 8 12 14 15 19 20 21 22 28 30 32 33 34 35 37 40 44 46 49 65 71 73 **S**9345 Methodist Health Systems, Inc.	23	10	125	3462	52	43741	715	24604	9801	337

© 1995 AHA Guide

Hospitals, U.S. / TENNESSEE

Hospital, Address, Telephone, Administrator, Approval, Facility, and Physician Codes, Health Care System	Classification Codes		Utilization Data					Expense (thousands) of dollars		
★ American Hospital Association (AHA) membership ☐ Joint Commission on Accreditation of Healthcare Organizations (JCAHO) accreditation + American Osteopathic Hospital Association (AOHA) membership ○ American Osteopathic Association (AOA) accreditation △ Commission on Accreditation of Rehabilitation Facilities (CARF) accreditation Control codes 61, 63, 64, 71, 72 and 73 indicate hospitals listed by AOHA, but not registered by AHA. For definition of numerical codes, see page A6	Control	Service	Beds	Admissions	Census	Outpatient Visits	Births	Total	Payroll	Personnel
EAST RIDGE—Hamilton County										
★ EAST RIDGE HOSPITAL, 941 Spring Creek Road, Zip 37412, Mailing Address: P.O. Box 91229, Zip 37412-6229; tel. 615/894-7870; William M. Donohoo FACHE, Chief Executive Officer **A**1 9 10 **F**2 3 4 7 8 10 11 14 16 18 19 20 21 22 23 24 28 29 30 32 35 37 38 40 42 43 44 45 46 49 51 52 53 54 55 56 57 58 59 60 61 64 65 66 67 71 72 73 74 **P**4 **S**0048 Columbia/HCA Healthcare Corporation	33	10	128	5317	56	29464	2404	31123	12288	512
ELIZABETHTON—Carter County										
★ SYCAMORE SHOALS HOSPITAL, 1501 West Elk Avenue, Zip 37643-1368; tel. 615/542-1300; Larry R. Jeter, Chief Executive Officer (Total facility includes 12 beds in nursing home-type unit) **A**1 9 10 **F**7 8 11 12 14 16 19 22 24 26 28 29 30 32 34 35 37 38 40 44 46 47 49 64 65 71 73 74 **P**1 7 **S**0048 Columbia/HCA Healthcare Corporation	33	10	112	2481	32	38011	410	15357	6423	250
ERIN—Houston County										
★ TRINITY HOSPITAL, 353 Main Street, Zip 37061, Mailing Address: P.O. Box 489, Zip 37061-0489; tel. 615/289-4211; Jack S. Buck, Chief Executive Officer **A**1 9 10 **F**8 16 19 22 32 44 45 49 71 **P**8 **S**0048 Columbia/HCA Healthcare Corporation	33	10	35	1070	11	8941	0	4259	2005	81
ERWIN—Unicoi County										
★ UNICOI COUNTY MEMORIAL HOSPITAL, Greenway Circle, Zip 37650-2196; tel. 615/743-3141; James L. McMackin, Chief Executive Officer (Total facility includes 46 beds in nursing home-type unit) **A**1 9 10 **F**4 7 8 10 12 14 15 17 19 20 21 22 24 28 30 32 33 34 35 37 41 42 43 44 45 49 60 64 65 66 69 70 71 73 **P**5	16	10	94	1282	80	20617	0	8284	3627	169
ETOWAH—McMinn County										
★ WOODS MEMORIAL HOSPITAL DISTRICT, Highway 411 North, Zip 37331, Mailing Address: Box 410, Zip 37331; tel. 615/263-3600; Phil Campbell, Administrator (Nonreporting) **A**1 9 10	13	10	160	—	—	—	—	—	—	—
FAYETTEVILLE—Lincoln County										
★ LINCOLN REGIONAL HOSPITAL, 700 West Maple Street, Zip 37334; tel. 615/438-1111; George Repa, Chief Executive Officer **A**1 9 10 **F**2 3 7 8 14 15 16 17 19 21 22 24 26 27 28 30 31 32 33 34 35 37 40 41 44 46 49 65 70 71 73 **S**0002 Quorum Health Group/Quorum Health Resources	13	10	63	2287	29	44394	210	—	—	273
FRANKLIN—Williamson County										
★ WILLIAMSON MEDICAL CENTER, 2021 Carothers Road, Zip 37068, Mailing Address: P.O. Box 681600, Zip 37068-1600; tel. 615/791-0500; Ronald G. Joyner, Chief Executive Officer **A**1 9 10 **F**3 7 8 10 19 21 22 23 28 30 33 34 35 37 40 41 42 44 46 49 54 56 63 65 66 67 71 73	13	10	108	4853	72	69752	507	39345	15933	525
GAINESBORO—Jackson County										
☐ JACKSON COUNTY HOSPITAL, 620 Hospital Drive, Zip 38562, Mailing Address: Box 36, Zip 38562-0036; tel. 615/268-0211; Tim Tapp, Administrator (Nonreporting) **A**1 9 10	33	10	30	—	—	—	—	—	—	—
GALLATIN—Sumner County										
★ △ SUMNER REGIONAL MEDICAL CENTER, 555 Hartsville Pike, Zip 37066, Mailing Address: P.O. Box 1558, Zip 37066-1558; tel. 615/452-4210; William T. Sugg, President and Chief Executive Officer **A**1 7 9 10 **F**2 3 4 5 7 8 9 10 11 12 13 14 15 17 19 20 21 22 23 24 25 26 28 29 30 31 32 33 34 35 37 38 39 40 41 42 43 44 45 46 47 48 49 50 51 52 53 54 55 56 57 58 59 60 61 63 65 66 67 68 69 70 71 72 73 74	23	10	148	4430	72	53531	556	36073	13234	451
GERMANTOWN—Shelby County										
★ REHABILITATION HOSPITAL-MIDSOUTH, (Formerly Baptist Memorial Hospital-Germantown) 2100 Exeter Road, Zip 38138; tel. 901/757-1350; B. Richard Moseley, Chief Executive Officer (Nonreporting) **A**9 10 **S**1715 Continental Medical Systems, Inc.	21	46	50	—	—	—	—	—	—	—
GREENEVILLE—Greene County										
★ LAUGHLIN MEMORIAL HOSPITAL, 1420 Tusculum Boulevard, Zip 37743-5099; tel. 615/787-5000; Jack G. Wilson, Administrator (Total facility includes 90 beds in nursing home-type unit) **A**1 9 10 **F**7 8 15 16 19 21 22 28 30 32 33 34 35 37 40 41 42 44 49 60 64 65 71 74 **P**5	23	10	267	5717	161	38718	475	22631	10112	425
★ TAKOMA ADVENTIST HOSPITAL, 401 Takoma Avenue, Zip 37743; tel. 615/639-3151; Paul Michael Norman, President (Total facility includes 12 beds in nursing home-type unit) **A**1 9 10 **F**7 8 12 14 15 16 17 18 19 20 21 22 26 28 30 31 32 35 37 40 41 44 45 46 49 50 52 54 55 56 57 58 59 63 64 65 67 71 73 74 **P**8 **S**4165 Adventist Health System-Sunbelt Health Care Corporation	21	10	116	2964	47	39731	294	15950	6744	249
HARRIMAN—Roane County										
★ HARRIMAN CITY HOSPITAL, 412 Devonia Street, Zip 37748-0489, Mailing Address: P.O. Box 489, Zip 37748-0489; tel. 615/882-1323; Jim Gann, Administrator (Nonreporting) **A**1 9 10	14	10	84	—	—	—	—	—	—	—
HARTSVILLE—Trousdale County										
HARTSVILLE MEDICAL CENTER, 500 Church Street, Zip 37074; tel. 615/374-2221; Jim Marshall, Administrator (Nonreporting) **A**9 10	33	10	34	—	—	—	—	—	—	—
HENDERSONVILLE—Sumner County										
★ HENDERSONVILLE HOSPITAL, 355 New Shackle Island Road, Zip 37075-2393; tel. 615/264-4000; Lawrence H. Kloess,III, Chief Executive Officer (Total facility includes 10 beds in nursing home-type unit) **A**1 9 10 **F**7 8 10 12 14 15 19 21 22 26 28 30 32 34 35 37 40 42 44 49 50 64 65 67 71 72 73 **P**7 8 **S**0048 Columbia/HCA Healthcare Corporation	33	10	63	2399	28	49684	527	—	—	322

Hospitals, U.S. / TENNESSEE

Hospital, Address, Telephone, Administrator, Approval, Facility, and Physician Codes, Health Care System	Classification Codes		Utilization Data					Expense (thousands) of dollars		
	Control	Service	Beds	Admissions	Census	Outpatient Visits	Births	Total	Payroll	Personnel

★ American Hospital Association (AHA) membership
☐ Joint Commission on Accreditation of Healthcare Organizations (JCAHO) accreditation
+ American Osteopathic Hospital Association (AOHA) membership
○ American Osteopathic Association (AOA) accreditation
△ Commission on Accreditation of Rehabilitation Facilities (CARF) accreditation
Control codes 61, 63, 64, 71, 72 and 73 indicate hospitals listed by AOHA, but not registered by AHA. For definition of numerical codes, see page A6

Hospital	Control	Service	Beds	Admissions	Census	Outpatient Visits	Births	Total	Payroll	Personnel
HERMITAGE—Davidson County										
★ SUMMIT MEDICAL CENTER, (Formerly Donelson Hospital) 5655 Frist Boulevard, Zip 37076; tel. 615/316–3000; Bryan Dearing, Chief Executive Officer **A**1 9 10 **F**2 3 4 7 8 10 12 13 14 15 16 17 18 19 20 21 22 23 26 28 29 30 31 32 34 35 37 38 39 40 41 42 43 44 45 46 49 51 52 53 54 55 56 57 58 59 60 61 63 64 65 66 67 71 72 73 74 **P**5 7 8 **S**0048 Columbia/HCA Healthcare Corporation	33	10	204	7237	92	45421	855	42397	18010	525
HOHENWALD—Lewis County										
LEWIS COMMUNITY HOSPITAL, 617 West Main, Zip 38462, Mailing Address: P.O. Box 879, Zip 38462; tel. 615/796–4901; Stephen Chapman, Chief Executive Officer (Nonreporting) **A**9 **S**0075 Cumberland Health Systems, Inc.	23	10	52	—	—	—	—	—	—	—
HUMBOLDT—Gibson County										
★ HUMBOLDT GENERAL HOSPITAL, 3525 Chere Carol Road, Zip 38343–3699; tel. 901/784–0301; Billy Alred, Administrator **A**1 9 10 **F**7 8 14 19 22 28 32 33 44 49 65 71 73 **P**3 **S**0004 West Tennessee Healthcare, Inc.	16	10	42	1488	21	17461	185	5998	2674	112
HUNTINGDON—Carroll County										
★ BAPTIST MEMORIAL HOSPITAL–HUNTINGDON, 631 R. B. Wilson Drive, Zip 38344; tel. 901/986–4461; Jamie Townsend, Administrator **A**1 9 10 **F**8 10 12 15 16 19 22 24 27 28 29 30 31 32 33 37 39 41 44 46 49 58 63 65 71 73 **P**3 7 **S**1625 Baptist Memorial Health Care System, Inc.	21	10	70	1800	29	13206	0	6882	2699	159
JACKSON—Madison County										
★ JACKSON–MADISON COUNTY GENERAL HOSPITAL, 708 West Forest Avenue, Zip 38301–3855; tel. 901/425–5000; James T. Moss, President (Total facility includes 78 beds in nursing home–type unit) **A**1 2 3 5 9 10 **F**3 4 7 8 10 11 12 14 15 16 17 18 19 20 21 22 23 27 28 29 30 31 32 33 34 35 37 38 39 40 41 42 43 44 45 46 48 49 51 53 54 55 56 57 58 59 60 64 65 66 67 71 73 74 **P**5 **S**0004 West Tennessee Healthcare, Inc.	16	10	636	19406	404	90598	2893	161344	66265	2309
★ REGIONAL HOSPITAL OF JACKSON, 367 Hospital Boulevard, Zip 38305–4518, Mailing Address: P.O. Box 3310, Zip 38303–0310; tel. 901/661–2000; Donald H. Wilkerson, Chief Executive Officer **A**1 9 10 **F**4 7 8 10 11 14 17 19 20 21 22 23 26 30 31 34 35 37 40 42 44 45 46 49 65 66 71 73 74 **S**0048 Columbia/HCA Healthcare Corporation	33	10	139	4564	71	29488	8	32463	12974	479
WEST TENNESSEE BEHAVIORAL CENTER, 238 Summar Drive, Zip 38301; tel. 901/935–8200 **A**10 **F**1 3 14 15 16 18 25 52 54 55 56 57 58 59 65 **S**0004 West Tennessee Healthcare, Inc.	16	22	25	813	15	67413	0	—	—	176
JAMESTOWN—Fentress County										
☐ FENTRESS COUNTY GENERAL HOSPITAL, Highway 52–W, Zip 38556, Mailing Address: P.O. Box 1500, Zip 38556; tel. 615/879–8171; Curtis B. Courtney, Administrator (Total facility includes 13 beds in nursing home–type unit) **A**1 9 10 **F**2 3 7 8 12 14 15 16 17 19 22 26 28 29 30 32 44 46 49 64 65 67 68 71 73 **S**5765 Paracelsus Healthcare Corporation	33	10	73	3486	42	37360	167	—	—	426
JEFFERSON CITY—Jefferson County										
★ JEFFERSON MEMORIAL HOSPITAL, 1800 Bishop Avenue, Zip 37760, Mailing Address: P.O. Box 560, Zip 37760–0560; tel. 615/475–2091; Robert H. Foster, Administrator **A**1 9 10 **F**8 15 16 19 21 22 28 30 31 33 34 37 39 44 45 46 49 51 65 71 73	15	10	67	1981	27	35483	0	10351	4512	196
JELLICO—Campbell County										
★ JELLICO COMMUNITY HOSPITAL, Mailing Address: Route 1, Box 197, Zip 37762; tel. 615/784–7252; Kenneth R. Mattison, President **A**1 9 10 **F**7 10 11 14 15 16 19 21 22 32 35 37 40 41 44 46 49 65 71 **S**4165 Adventist Health System–Sunbelt Health Care Corporation	23	10	54	2486	24	28393	260	10747	4851	223
JOHNSON CITY—Washington County										
★ △ JOHNSON CITY MEDICAL CENTER HOSPITAL, 400 North State of Franklin Road, Zip 37604–6094; tel. 615/461–6111; Dennis Vonderfecht, Administrator and Chief Executive Officer **A**1 2 3 5 7 9 10 **F**2 3 4 7 8 10 12 14 16 17 19 21 22 23 24 26 27 28 29 30 32 33 34 35 37 38 39 40 41 42 43 44 45 46 47 48 49 51 52 53 54 55 56 57 58 59 60 63 65 66 67 68 69 70 71 72 73 74 **P**3 8	23	10	407	15027	258	90885	1244	139891	52011	1961
★ JOHNSON CITY SPECIALTY HOSPITAL, 203 East Watauga Avenue, Zip 37601; tel. 615/926–1111; Lori Caudell Fatherree, Chief Executive Officer **A**1 9 10 **F**2 3 4 7 8 10 11 15 16 19 22 23 24 26 28 30 32 35 37 38 39 40 42 43 44 48 49 52 56 58 64 65 66 69 71 72 73 74 **P**5 7 8 **S**0048 Columbia/HCA Healthcare Corporation	33	10	49	1102	8	9833	612	8952	3529	133
★ NORTH SIDE HOSPITAL, 401 Princeton Road, Zip 37601, Mailing Address: P.O. Box 4900, Zip 37602; tel. 615/854–5900; John B. Crysel, Chief Executive Officer **A**1 9 10 **F**2 3 4 7 8 9 10 11 12 14 15 16 18 19 21 22 23 24 26 27 28 29 30 31 32 33 34 35 37 38 39 40 41 42 43 44 45 46 47 48 49 51 52 54 55 56 58 59 60 61 64 65 66 67 68 69 70 71 72 73 74 **P**7 8 **S**0048 Columbia/HCA Healthcare Corporation	33	10	127	3395	51	42245	0	27418	8896	310
WOODRIDGE HOSPITAL, 403 State of Franklin Road, Zip 37604; tel. 615/928–7111; Thomas J. De Martini, Administrator **A**3 5 9 10 **F**1 2 3 12 14 15 18 25 26 31 45 52 53 54 55 56 57 58 59 65 **P**6	23	22	65	2178	46	82313	0	12167	6613	166
KINGSPORT—Sullivan County										
★ HOLSTON VALLEY HOSPITAL AND MEDICAL CENTER, West Ravine Street, Zip 37662–0224, Mailing Address: Box 238, Zip 37662–0224; tel. 615/224–5001; Randall Hoover, President and Chief Executive Officer (Total facility includes 21 beds in nursing home–type unit) **A**1 2 3 5 9 10 **F**4 7 8 10 11 12 14 15 16 17 19 21 22 23 26 28 30 31 32 33 35 37 38 40 41 42 43 44 46 47 48 49 50 52 53 54 55 56 57 58 59 60 63 64 65 66 69 70 71 73 74 **P**4 5 7	23	10	383	14391	240	111187	1403	135980	56781	1760

© 1995 AHA Guide

Hospitals, U.S. / TENNESSEE

Hospital, Address, Telephone, Administrator, Approval, Facility, and Physician Codes, Health Care System	Classification Codes		Utilization Data					Expense (thousands) of dollars		
★ American Hospital Association (AHA) membership ☐ Joint Commission on Accreditation of Healthcare Organizations (JCAHO) accreditation + American Osteopathic Hospital Association (AOHA) membership ○ American Osteopathic Association (AOA) accreditation △ Commission on Accreditation of Rehabilitation Facilities (CARF) accreditation Control codes 61, 63, 64, 71, 72 and 73 indicate hospitals listed by AOHA, but not registered by AHA. For definition of numerical codes, see page A6	Control	Service	Beds	Admissions	Census	Outpatient Visits	Births	Total	Payroll	Personnel
★ INDIAN PATH MEDICAL CENTER, 2000 Brookside Drive, Zip 37660-4604; tel. 615/392-7000; Robert Benson, Chief Executive Officer **A**1 9 10 **F**3 4 7 8 10 12 14 15 16 19 21 22 23 26 27 30 31 32 34 35 37 40 41 42 43 44 49 54 55 56 57 58 59 61 63 65 66 71 74 **P**1 5 6 8 **S**0048 Columbia/HCA Healthcare Corporation	33	10	140	4854	71	51288	548	45160	16618	901
★ INDIAN PATH PAVILION, 2300 Pavilion Drive, Zip 37660-4672; tel. 615/378-7500; Robert Benson, Chief Executive Officer (Nonreporting) **A**1 10 **S**0048 Columbia/HCA Healthcare Corporation	33	22	61	—	—	—	—	—	—	—
KNOXVILLE—Knox County										
★ △ BAPTIST HOSPITAL OF EAST TENNESSEE, 137 Blount Avenue S.E., Zip 37920, Mailing Address: Box 1788, Zip 37901-1788; tel. 615/632-5011; Michael Williams, President and Chief Operating Officer **A**1 2 7 9 10 **F**3 4 8 10 11 12 15 16 17 18 19 20 21 22 26 27 28 29 30 31 32 33 34 35 37 39 41 42 43 44 46 48 49 52 54 56 57 58 59 60 61 63 65 67 69 71 73 74 **S**2155 Baptist Health System of Tennessee	21	10	345	12297	226	99452	0	113751	44488	1550
☐ EAST TENNESSEE CHILDREN'S HOSPITAL, 2018 Clinch Avenue, Zip 37916, Mailing Address: P.O. Box 15010, Zip 37901-5010; tel. 615/541-8000; Robert F. Koppel, President and Chief Executive Officer **A**1 9 10 **F**9 10 13 15 17 19 20 21 22 23 24 25 27 28 31 32 34 35 38 39 40 41 42 43 44 45 46 47 48 49 51 52 53 54 55 56 58 59 60 64 65 66 67 70 71 73 **P**5	23	50	103	4282	63	69044	0	37623	18075	636
★ △ FORT SANDERS REGIONAL MEDICAL CENTER, 1901 Clinch Avenue S.W., Zip 37916-2394; tel. 615/541-1111; James R. Burkhart, Administrator (Total facility includes 22 beds in nursing home-type unit) **A**1 2 6 7 9 10 **F**3 4 7 8 10 11 12 14 15 16 17 19 21 22 23 24 25 28 30 31 32 33 34 35 37 40 41 42 43 44 45 46 48 49 53 54 55 56 57 58 59 60 61 64 65 66 67 71 73 74 **P**4 6 7	23	10	394	14766	256	68497	1908	125515	47752	2097
★ FORT SANDERS–PARKWEST MEDICAL CENTER, 9352 Park West Boulevard, Zip 37923, Mailing Address: P.O. Box 22993, Zip 37933-0993; tel. 615/694-5700; James R. Burkhart, Administrator **A**1 9 10 **F**1 2 3 4 5 6 7 8 9 10 11 12 13 14 15 16 17 18 19 20 21 22 23 24 25 26 27 28 29 30 31 32 33 34 35 36 37 38 39 40 41 42 43 44 45 46 47 48 49 50 51 52 53 54 55 56 57 58 59 60 61 62 63 64 65 66 67 68 69 70 71 72 73 74 **P**1 3 7 8	23	10	267	10798	160	77212	637	83646	27711	956
☐ LAKESHORE MENTAL HEALTH INSTITUTE, 5908 Lyons View Drive, Zip 37919; tel. 615/584-1561; Richard Lee Thomas, Superintendent **A**1 10 **F**1 4 5 6 8 10 12 19 20 21 22 25 27 31 35 43 44 46 49 50 52 53 54 55 56 57 58 60 63 65 67 69 71 73 **P**6	12	22	277	2420	256	0	0	—	—	663
☐ OAKWOOD MEDICAL CENTER, 5310 Ball Camp, Zip 37921; tel. 615/584-9191; Steve Petty, Administrator (Nonreporting) **A**1 9 10 **S**0075 Cumberland Health Systems, Inc.	33	22	23	—	—	—	—	—	—	—
★ △ ST. MARY'S HEALTH SYSTEM, (Formerly St. Mary's Medical Center) 900 East Oak Hill Avenue, Zip 37917-4556; tel. 615/545-8000; Richard C. Williams, President and Chief Executive Officer **A**1 2 3 7 9 10 **F**1 4 5 7 10 11 12 14 15 16 17 19 21 22 23 25 26 28 29 30 32 33 34 35 37 39 40 41 42 43 44 45 46 48 49 52 53 54 55 56 58 59 60 65 67 70 71 72 73 74 **P**1 5 6 7 **S**5155 Mercy Health System	21	10	377	16416	261	187310	1971	132977	49223	1899
★ UNIVERSITY OF TENNESSEE MEMORIAL HOSPITAL, 1924 Alcoa Highway, Zip 37920; tel. 615/544-9000; Gene Hall, Administrator (Nonreporting) **A**1 2 3 9 10	23	10	542	—	—	—	—	—	—	—
LA FOLLETTE—Campbell County										
★ LA FOLLETTE MEDICAL CENTER, East Avenue, Zip 37766, Mailing Address: Box 1301, Zip 37766-1301; tel. 615/562-2211; J. B. Wright, Administrator (Nonreporting) **A**1 9 10	14	10	165	—	—	—	—	—	—	—
LAFAYETTE—Macon County										
★ MACON COUNTY GENERAL HOSPITAL, 204 Medical Drive, Zip 37083, Mailing Address: P.O. Box 378, Zip 37083; tel. 615/666-2147; Dennis Wolford, Administrator **A**1 9 10 **F**14 15 16 19 22 28 30 44 51 65 71 **S**0002 Quorum Health Group/Quorum Health Resources	23	10	43	1141	16	9857	0	3795	1519	74
LAWRENCEBURG—Lawrence County										
★ CROCKETT HOSPITAL, U.S. Highway 43 South, Zip 38464-0847, Mailing Address: Box 847, Zip 38464-0847; tel. 615/762-6571; John A. Marshall, Chief Executive Officer **A**1 9 10 **F**7 8 12 15 16 19 22 26 28 30 34 35 37 39 40 41 44 45 46 49 51 65 66 67 71 **P**7 8 **S**0048 Columbia/HCA Healthcare Corporation	33	10	83	3284	35	40226	334	14844	6144	243
LEBANON—Wilson County										
MCFARLAND SPECIALTY HOSPITAL See University Medical Center										
☐ UNIVERSITY MEDICAL CENTER, (Includes McFarland Specialty Hospital, 500 Park Avenue, Lebanon, Tennessee, Zip 37087-3720; tel. 615/449-0500) 1411 Baddour Parkway, Zip 37087; tel. 615/444-8262; Larry W. Keller, Chief Executive Officer **A**1 9 10 **F**2 3 7 8 10 12 19 20 21 22 26 28 30 34 35 37 39 40 41 42 44 46 48 49 52 54 56 57 59 64 65 66 71 73 74 **S**0063 TENET Healthcare Corporation	33	10	260	7961	131	46682	787	—	—	566
LEWISBURG—Marshall County										
☐ MARSHALL MEDICAL CENTER, (Formerly Lewisburg Community Hospital) 1080 North Ellington Parkway, Zip 37091, Mailing Address: P.O. Box 1609, Zip 37091; tel. 615/359-6241; Woody Gilliland, Administrator **A**1 9 10 **F**8 12 14 15 16 19 22 37 40 44 47 48 49 65 71 73	33	10	112	1767	21	27137	116	11376	4160	142
LEXINGTON—Henderson County										
★ METHODIST HOSPITAL OF LEXINGTON, 200 West Church Street, Zip 38351, Mailing Address: Box 160, Zip 38351; tel. 901/968-3646; Gene Ragghianti, Administrator (Nonreporting) **A**1 9 10 **S**9345 Methodist Health Systems, Inc.	21	10	35	—	—	—	—	—	—	—

Hospitals, U.S. / TENNESSEE

Hospital, Address, Telephone, Administrator, Approval, Facility, and Physician Codes, Health Care System	Classification Codes		Utilization Data					Expense (thousands) of dollars		
★ American Hospital Association (AHA) membership ☐ Joint Commission on Accreditation of Healthcare Organizations (JCAHO) accreditation + American Osteopathic Hospital Association (AOHA) membership ○ American Osteopathic Association (AOA) accreditation △ Commission on Accreditation of Rehabilitation Facilities (CARF) accreditation Control codes 61, 63, 64, 71, 72 and 73 indicate hospitals listed by AOHA, but not registered by AHA. For definition of numerical codes, see page A6	Control	Service	Beds	Admissions	Census	Outpatient Visits	Births	Total	Payroll	Personnel
LINDEN—Perry County ☐ PERRY MEMORIAL HOSPITAL, Highway 13 South, Zip 37096, Mailing Address: Route 10, Box 8, Zip 37096; tel. 615/589–2121; Judy G. Eads R.N., Administrator (Nonreporting) **A**1 9 10 **S**0075 Cumberland Health Systems, Inc.	23	10	53	—	—	—	—	—	—	—
LIVINGSTON—Overton County ★ LIVINGSTON REGIONAL HOSPITAL, 315 Oak Street, Zip 38570, Mailing Address: P.O. Box 550, Zip 38570; tel. 615/823–5611; Timothy W. McGill, Chief Executive Officer (Total facility includes 15 beds in nursing home–type unit) **A**1 9 10 **F**7 8 11 12 14 15 16 19 20 22 26 28 30 35 40 44 64 65 66 71 73 **P**7 8 **S**0048 Columbia/HCA Healthcare Corporation	33	10	111	3546	50	28843	220	12607	5426	227
LOUDON—Loudon County ★ FORT SANDERS LOUDON MEDICAL CENTER, 1125 Grove Street, Zip 37774, Mailing Address: Box 217, Zip 37774–0217; tel. 615/458–8222; Keith Altshuler, Administrator **A**1 9 10 **F**1 7 8 14 15 16 19 22 27 28 32 33 34 35 37 39 40 41 42 44 48 49 63 65 66 71 73 **P**7	23	10	50	1622	16	32779	235	8095	4105	239
LOUISVILLE—Blount County ☐ PENINSULA HOSPITAL, Jones Bend Road, Zip 37777, Mailing Address: P.O. Box 2000, Zip 37777; tel. 615/970–9800; Anthony L. Spezia, Administrator (Nonreporting) **A**1 9 10	33	22	155	—	—	—	—	—	—	—
MADISON—Davidson County ★ NASHVILLE MEMORIAL HOSPITAL, 612 West Due West Avenue, Zip 37115–4474; tel. 615/865–3511; Thomas R. Pentz, Chief Executive Officer **A**1 2 9 10 **F**4 7 8 10 11 12 16 17 19 20 21 22 24 26 28 29 30 31 32 33 34 35 37 39 40 41 42 43 44 45 46 49 52 56 58 60 61 63 65 67 71 72 73 74 **P**7 8 **S**0048 Columbia/HCA Healthcare Corporation	33	10	250	9449	158	97474	264	69626	32498	965
★ △ TENNESSEE CHRISTIAN MEDICAL CENTER, 500 Hospital Drive, Zip 37115; tel. 615/865–2373; Milton R. Siepman, President and Chief Executive Officer (Total facility includes 50 beds in nursing home–type unit) **A**1 7 9 10 **F**2 3 4 7 8 12 16 19 21 22 24 26 27 28 29 30 32 34 35 37 39 40 41 42 44 48 49 52 53 54 55 56 57 58 59 60 63 64 65 67 71 72 73 **P**1 3 **S**4165 Adventist Health System–Sunbelt Health Care Corporation	21	10	289	6573	164	32459	294	46887	22019	775
MANCHESTER—Coffee County ★ COFFEE MEDICAL CENTER, 1001 McArthur Drive, Zip 37355, Mailing Address: P.O. Box 1079, Zip 37355; tel. 615/728–3586; Keith Heuser, Administrator (Nonreporting) **A**9 10 **S**0002 Quorum Health Group/Quorum Health Resources	16	10	106	—	—	—	—	—	—	—
○ MEDICAL CENTER OF MANCHESTER, 481 Interstate Drive, Zip 37355, Mailing Address: P.O. Box 1409, Zip 37355; tel. 615/728–6354; Anthony N. Brock, Administrator (Nonreporting) **A**9 10 11	33	10	40	—	—	—	—	—	—	—
MARTIN—Weakley County ★ VOLUNTEER GENERAL HOSPITAL, 161 Mount Pelia Road, Zip 38237, Mailing Address: Box 967, Zip 38237; tel. 901/587–4261; Donald E. Annis, Chief Executive Officer **A**1 9 10 **F**7 8 16 19 21 22 23 24 28 30 34 35 37 42 44 49 65 71 73 **P**8 **S**0048 Columbia/HCA Healthcare Corporation	33	10	65	2655	39	16693	102	14209	5206	239
MARYVILLE—Blount County ★ BLOUNT MEMORIAL HOSPITAL, 907 East Lamar Alexander Parkway, Zip 37804–5193; tel. 615/983–7211; Joseph M. Dawson, Administrator **A**1 9 10 **F**2 3 4 7 8 10 11 14 15 16 17 19 21 22 23 24 31 32 33 34 35 37 40 41 42 44 49 52 53 54 55 56 58 59 60 63 65 67 70 71 73	13	10	204	7999	120	435675	807	54788	25258	985
MCKENZIE—Carroll County ★ METHODIST HOSPITAL OF MCKENZIE, 161 Hospital Drive, Zip 38201; tel. 901/352–4170; Randal E. Carson, Administrator **A**1 9 10 **F**7 8 19 22 24 28 32 40 41 44 49 65 66 71 73 **P**5 **S**9345 Methodist Health Systems, Inc.	23	10	27	1304	11	18810	524	7403	3367	152
MCMINNVILLE—Warren County ★ RIVER PARK HOSPITAL, 1560 Sparta Road, Zip 37110; tel. 615/473–8411; William Russell Spray, Chief Executive Officer **A**1 9 10 **F**7 8 11 12 13 14 15 17 18 19 21 22 23 26 28 29 30 32 35 37 39 40 41 44 45 46 48 49 51 52 54 56 57 59 63 65 66 71 72 73 **P**5 7 8 **S**0048 Columbia/HCA Healthcare Corporation	33	10	90	4674	55	52867	489	20114	8116	348
MEMPHIS—Shelby County ★ △ BAPTIST MEMORIAL HOSPITAL, (Includes Baptist Memorial Hospital East, 6019 Walnut Grove Road, Memphis, Tennessee, Zip 38119; tel. 901/227–2727; Baptist Memorial Hospital Rehabilitation Center, Memphis, Tennessee) 899 Madison Avenue, Zip 38146; tel. 901/227–2727; Stephen Curtis Reynolds, President and Chief Executive Officer (Total facility includes 48 beds in nursing home–type unit) **A**1 2 3 5 6 7 9 10 **F**2 3 4 7 8 10 11 12 14 15 16 17 19 21 22 23 24 25 30 32 34 35 37 38 39 40 41 42 43 44 46 48 49 52 54 55 57 58 59 60 63 64 65 66 69 70 71 72 73 74 **P**3 7 8 **S**1625 Baptist Memorial Health Care System, Inc. BAPTIST MEMORIAL HOSPITAL EAST See Baptist Memorial Hospital BAPTIST MEMORIAL HOSPITAL REHABILITATION CENTER See Baptist Memorial Center	21	10	1261	44957	882	188284	5743	428486	160965	5569
☐ CHARTER LAKESIDE HOSPITAL, 2911 Brunswick Road, Zip 38133, Mailing Address: P.O. Box 341308, Zip 38134; tel. 901/377–4700; Sherry C. Thornton, Chief Executive Officer (Nonreporting) **A**1 9 10 **S**0695 Charter Medical Corporation	33	22	174	—	—	—	—	—	—	—
☐ EASTWOOD MEDICAL CENTER, 3000 Getwell Road, Zip 38118; tel. 901/369–8500; Lee A. Simpson Jr., President and Chief Executive Officer **A**1 9 10 **F**2 3 8 10 17 19 21 22 26 27 28 29 30 34 35 37 39 42 44 49 52 56 57 58 59 65 67 71 73	33	10	209	3872	98	24116	0	32256	12033	463

© 1995 AHA Guide

Hospitals, U.S. / TENNESSEE

Hospital, Address, Telephone, Administrator, Approval, Facility, and Physician Codes, Health Care System	Classification Codes		Utilization Data					Expense (thousands) of dollars		
★ American Hospital Association (AHA) membership □ Joint Commission on Accreditation of Healthcare Organizations (JCAHO) accreditation + American Osteopathic Hospital Association (AOHA) membership ○ American Osteopathic Association (AOA) accreditation △ Commission on Accreditation of Rehabilitation Facilities (CARF) accreditation Control codes 61, 63, 64, 71, 72 and 73 indicate hospitals listed by AOHA, but not registered by AHA. For definition of numerical codes, see page A6	Control	Service	Beds	Admissions	Census	Outpatient Visits	Births	Total	Payroll	Personnel
□ LE BONHEUR CHILDREN'S MEDICAL CENTER, One Children's Plaza, Zip 38103-2893; tel. 901/572-3000; Eugene K. Cashman Jr., President (Nonreporting) **A**1 3 5 9 10	23	50	208	—	—	—	—	—	—	—
□ MEMPHIS MENTAL HEALTH INSTITUTE, 865 Poplar Avenue, Zip 38105, Mailing Address: P.O. Box 40966, Zip 38174-0966; tel. 901/524-1201; Elisabeth Banks, Superintendent **A**1 5 9 10 **F**2 15 16 46 52 54 55 56 57 65 67 73	12	22	98	1242	91	0	0	11542	7360	294
★ METHODIST HOSPITALS OF MEMPHIS, (Includes Methodist Hospitals of Memphis-Central, Memphis, Tennessee; Methodist Hospitals of Memphis-South Unit, 1300 Wesley Drive, Memphis, Tennessee, Zip 38116; tel. 901/346-3700; Cecelia Wilson, Administrator; Methodist North-J. Harris Hospital, 3960 New Covington Pike, Memphis, Tennessee, Zip 38128; tel. 901/372-5200; Tim Deaton, Administrator) 1265 Union Avenue, Zip 38104-3499; tel. 901/726-7000; Gary S. Shorb, President (Total facility includes 24 beds in nursing home-type unit) **A**1 2 3 5 6 9 10 **F**2 3 4 7 8 10 11 12 15 16 17 19 21 22 23 25 26 27 28 29 30 31 32 33 34 35 37 38 39 40 41 42 43 44 45 46 48 49 51 52 53 54 55 57 58 59 60 63 64 65 66 67 69 70 71 72 73 74 **P**5 6 7 **S**9345 Methodist Health Systems, Inc.	23	10	1051	36599	656	209753	5194	302484	126429	4301
METHODIST HOSPITALS OF MEMPHIS-CENTRAL See Methodist Hospitals of Memphis										
METHODIST NORTH-J. HARRIS HOSPITAL See Methodist Hospitals of Memphis										
□ MIDSOUTH HOSPITAL, 135 North Pauline Street, Zip 38105; tel. 901/527-5211; Stephen Wilensky, Administrator **A**1 9 10 **F**2 3 12 14 19 21 35 50 52 53 54 55 56 57 58 59 63 71	33	22	134	946	55	1726	0	8634	3742	81
□ REGIONAL MEDICAL CENTER AT MEMPHIS, 877 Jefferson Avenue, Zip 38103; tel. 901/545-7100; Burton W. Waller Jr., President and Chief Executive Officer **A**1 2 3 5 8 9 10 **F**7 8 9 11 12 14 15 16 17 19 20 21 22 28 30 31 34 37 38 39 40 41 42 44 46 49 51 56 60 61 65 68 69 70 71 72 73 74	23	10	529	20392	372	221288	6248	210506	84336	2459
★ ST. FRANCIS HOSPITAL, 5959 Park Avenue, Zip 38119-5198, Mailing Address: P.O. Box 171808, Zip 38187-1808; tel. 901/765-1000; Jake Henry Jr., President (Total facility includes 197 beds in nursing home-type unit) **A**1 2 3 5 9 10 **F**2 3 4 7 8 10 12 14 15 16 17 19 20 21 22 23 24 25 26 28 29 30 31 32 33 34 35 37 39 40 41 42 43 44 45 46 48 49 51 52 53 54 55 56 57 58 59 60 61 64 65 66 67 70 73 74 **P**5 7 8 **S**0063 TENET Healthcare Corporation	33	10	609	17595	511	118388	1495	163141	59932	1671
★ △ ST. JOSEPH HOSPITAL AND HEALTH CENTERS, 220 Overton Avenue, Zip 38105-2789; tel. 901/577-2700; Joan M. Carlson, President and Chief Executive Officer **A**1 3 6 7 9 10 **F**2 3 4 8 10 12 16 17 18 19 20 21 22 24 26 28 29 30 31 32 34 35 37 39 41 42 43 44 45 46 48 49 52 53 54 55 56 57 58 59 60 63 65 67 71 73 **P**4 8 **S**5345 Sisters of St. Francis Health Services, Inc.	21	10	372	8608	233	50168	0	63409	26588	976
★ ST. JUDE CHILDREN'S RESEARCH HOSPITAL, (Pediatric Catastrophic Diseases) 332 North Lauderdale Street, Zip 38105-2794, Mailing Address: Box 318, Zip 38101-0318; tel. 901/522-0300; Arthur W. Nienhuis M.D., Director **A**1 2 3 5 9 10 **F**16 19 20 21 31 34 35 39 42 44 45 46 47 48 49 54 60 63 65 67 69 71 73 **P**6	23	59	48	1932	35	34990	0	114981	53239	1488
□ UNIVERSITY OF TENNESSEE BOWLD HOSPITAL, (Formerly University of Tennessee Medical Center) 951 Court Avenue, Zip 38103-2898; tel. 901/448-4000; Jeffrey R. Woodside M.D., Executive Director **A**1 2 3 5 9 10 **F**4 10 19 21 22 23 26 31 34 35 37 39 42 43 44 45 46 60 61 65 69 71	12	10	113	3490	70	48124	0	39792	13718	489
★ VETERANS AFFAIRS MEDICAL CENTER, 1030 Jefferson Avenue, Zip 38104-2193; tel. 901/523-8990; K. L. Mulholland Jr., Director (Total facility includes 120 beds in nursing home-type unit) **A**1 2 3 5 8 **F**2 3 4 8 10 11 12 14 15 16 17 19 20 21 22 23 24 25 26 27 30 31 32 33 34 35 37 39 41 42 43 44 45 46 49 51 52 54 55 57 58 59 60 63 64 65 67 71 73 74 **P**6 **S**9295 Department of Veterans Affairs	45	10	684	10124	381	216104	0	134885	75112	2402
MILAN—Gibson County										
★ CITY OF MILAN HOSPITAL, 4039 South Highland, Zip 38358; tel. 901/686-1591; Mark D. Le Neave, Chief Executive Officer **A**1 9 10 **F**8 16 19 22 44 52 57 65 **S**0002 Quorum Health Group/Quorum Health Resources	14	10	61	1300	22	15502	1	7048	2595	109
MILLINGTON—Shelby County										
★ NAVAL HOSPITAL, Zip 38054-5201; tel. 901/873-5804; Captain Michael Kilpatrick MSC, USN, Commanding Officer **A**1 **F**14 15 20 21 22 25 28 34 39 41 44 46 49 51 52 54 58 65 67 71 72 73 **P**1 **S**9655 Department of Navy	43	10	36	2799	26	141479	267	42578	—	780
MORRISTOWN—Hamblen County										
□ LAKEWAY REGIONAL HOSPITAL, 726 McFarland Street, Zip 37814-3990; tel. 615/586-2302; Stephen L. Taylor, Executive Director **A**1 9 10 **F**8 12 14 15 19 21 22 26 35 37 44 45 46 48 49 52 54 55 57 65 71 73 **P**8 **S**0875 Community Health Systems, Inc.	33	10	135	2541	43	17544	0	14082	4542	202
★ MORRISTOWN-HAMBLEN HOSPITAL, 908 West Fourth North Street, Zip 37814-1178; tel. 615/586-4231; Richard L. Clark, Administrator and Chief Executive Officer (Nonreporting) **A**1 9 10	23	10	143	—	—	—	—	—	—	—
MOUNTAIN HOME—Washington County										
★ VETERANS AFFAIRS MEDICAL CENTER, Zip 37684; tel. 615/926-1171; Carl J. Gerber M.D., Ph.D., Director (Total facility includes 120 beds in nursing home-type unit) **A**1 2 3 5 8 **F**2 3 4 5 6 8 10 11 12 14 16 17 18 19 20 21 22 23 24 26 27 28 29 30 31 32 33 34 35 36 37 39 41 42 43 44 45 46 49 50 51 52 54 55 56 57 58 63 64 65 66 67 69 70 71 73 74 **P**6 **S**9295 Department of Veterans Affairs	45	10	994	6737	297	176213	0	89455	52229	1522
MURFREESBORO—Rutherford County										
★ ALVIN C. YORK VETERANS AFFAIRS MEDICAL CENTER, 3400 Lebanon Road, Zip 37129; tel. 615/893-1360; Brian Heckert, Director (Total facility includes 166 beds in nursing home-type unit) **A**1 3 5 **F**1 2 3 4 8 10 16 17 19 20 21 22 25 26 27 28 29 30 31 32 33 34 35 36 37 39 41 42 44 45 46 49 51 52 54 55 57 58 59 60 64 65 67 71 73 74 **P**6 **S**9295 Department of Veterans Affairs	45	10	676	4515	582	77485	0	77014	47146	1314

Hospitals, U.S. / TENNESSEE

Hospital, Address, Telephone, Administrator, Approval, Facility, and Physician Codes, Health Care System	Classification Codes		Utilization Data					Expense (thousands) of dollars		
★ American Hospital Association (AHA) membership □ Joint Commission on Accreditation of Healthcare Organizations (JCAHO) accreditation + American Osteopathic Hospital Association (AOHA) membership ○ American Osteopathic Association (AOA) accreditation △ Commission on Accreditation of Rehabilitation Facilities (CARF) accreditation Control codes 61, 63, 64, 71, 72 and 73 indicate hospitals listed by AOHA, but not registered by AHA. For definition of numerical codes, see page A6	Control	Service	Beds	Admissions	Census	Outpatient Visits	Births	Total	Payroll	Personnel
★ MIDDLE TENNESSEE MEDICAL CENTER, 400 North Highland Avenue, Zip 37130–3854, Mailing Address: P.O. Box 1178, Zip 37133–1178; tel. 615/849–4100; Arthur W. Hastings, President and Chief Executive Officer **A**1 9 10 **F**7 8 10 11 14 15 16 19 21 22 23 24 31 32 33 34 35 37 39 40 42 44 45 49 54 56 60 65 66 71 73 74	21	10	194	10708	141	70861	1742	67036	24334	894
NASHVILLE—Davidson County										
★ BAPTIST HOSPITAL, 2000 Church Street, Zip 37236–0002; tel. 615/329–5555; C. David Stringfield, President **A**1 3 5 9 10 **F**2 3 4 5 7 8 10 11 12 14 16 17 19 22 23 24 25 26 28 30 31 32 33 34 35 37 38 39 40 41 42 43 44 45 46 48 49 52 56 58 59 60 61 65 66 69 71 72 73 74 **P**3 7	23	10	649	30043	441	239899	5252	241063	99407	3309
★ △ CENTENNIAL MEDICAL CENTER, 2300 Patterson Street, Zip 37203; tel. 615/342–1000; William Paul Rutledge, President and Chief Executive Officer (Nonreporting) **A**1 2 7 9 10 **S**0048 Columbia/HCA Healthcare Corporation	33	10	680	—	—	—	—	—	—	—
□ GEORGE W. HUBBARD HOSPITAL OF MEHARRY MEDICAL COLLEGE, 1005 D B. Todd Boulevard, Zip 37208–3599; tel. 615/327–5831; Andre L. Lee, Executive Director (Nonreporting) **A**1 3 5 8 9 10	23	10	215							
★ METROPOLITAN NASHVILLE GENERAL HOSPITAL, 72 Hermitage Avenue, Zip 37210–2110; tel. 615/862–4490; John M. Stone, Director **A**1 2 3 5 9 10 **F**4 7 8 10 13 14 15 17 19 22 23 27 30 31 32 33 34 35 38 39 40 42 43 44 46 49 51 53 54 55 56 57 58 59 60 61 65 71 73 **S**0022 Metropolitan Nashville General Hospital	15	10	105	5483	78	134804	666	53612	21636	776
□ MIDDLE TENNESSEE MENTAL HEALTH INSTITUTE, 1501 Murfreesboro Road, Zip 37217; tel. 615/366–2322; Joseph W. Carobene, Superintendent (Total facility includes 60 beds in nursing home–type unit) **A**1 3 10 **F**14 15 16 20 21 41 45 46 52 53 54 55 56 57 65 73	12	22	337	1401	270	0	0	29410	18795	803
★ NASHVILLE METROPOLITAN BORDEAUX HOSPITAL, 1414 County Hospital Road, Zip 37218–3001; tel. 615/862–7000; Wayne Hayes, Administrator (Total facility includes 525 beds in nursing home–type unit) **A**10 **F**15 20 26 27 28 41 46 64 65 67 73 **P**1 **S**0022 Metropolitan Nashville General Hospital	15	48	555	539	492	0	0	32300	15575	586
★ NASHVILLE REHABILITATION HOSPITAL, 610 Gallatin Road, Zip 37206; tel. 615/226–4330; Edward Giannotti Jr., Administrator and Chief Executive Officer (Nonreporting) **A**1 9 10	33	46	46							
★ PSYCHIATRIC HOSPITAL AT VANDERBILT, 1601 23rd Avenue South, Zip 37212; tel. 615/320–7770; Robert England, Administrator and Chief Executive Officer **A**1 3 10 **F**2 15 16 17 19 21 35 50 52 53 54 55 56 59 65 70 71 **P**7 **S**0048 Columbia/HCA Healthcare Corporation	32	22	80	1043	49	2362	0	9941	4829	145
★ SOUTHERN HILLS MEDICAL CENTER, 391 Wallace Road, Zip 37211; tel. 615/781–4100; Lawrence L. Pieretti, Chief Executive Officer **A**1 9 10 **F**1 2 3 4 5 6 7 8 9 10 11 12 13 14 15 16 17 18 19 20 21 22 23 24 25 26 27 29 30 31 32 33 34 35 37 38 39 40 42 43 44 45 46 47 48 49 50 51 52 53 54 55 56 57 58 59 60 61 63 64 65 66 67 68 69 71 72 73 74 **P**6 7 8 **S**0048 Columbia/HCA Healthcare Corporation	33	10	146	5888	74	50570	817	44835	16561	462
★ ST. THOMAS HOSPITAL, 4220 Harding Road, Zip 37205, Mailing Address: Box 380, Zip 37202; tel. 615/222–2111; John F. Tighe, President and Chief Executive Officer **A**1 3 5 9 10 **F**4 8 10 12 14 15 16 17 18 19 21 22 24 27 30 31 32 34 35 37 39 41 42 43 44 45 46 49 51 52 54 57 60 63 65 66 67 69 70 71 73 **P**5 6 7 8	21	10	571	23884	422	42580	0	214383	92266	3275
★ VANDERBILT UNIVERSITY HOSPITAL, (Formerly Vanderbilt University Hospital and Clinic) 1161 21st Avenue South, Zip 37232–2102; tel. 615/322–5000; Norman B. Urmy, Executive Director (Nonreporting) **A**1 2 3 5 8 9 10	23	10	646	—	—	—	—	—	—	—
★ VETERANS AFFAIRS MEDICAL CENTER, 1310 24th Avenue South, Zip 37212–2637; tel. 615/327–4751; Larry E. Deters, Director (Nonreporting) **A**1 3 5 8 **S**9295 Department of Veterans Affairs	45	10	334	—	—	—	—	—	—	—
NEWPORT—Cocke County										
BAPTIST HOSPITAL OF COCKE COUNTY, 435 Second Street, Zip 37821; tel. 615/625–2200; Wayne Buckner, Administrator (Total facility includes 56 beds in nursing home–type unit) **A**9 10 **F**7 8 15 19 20 21 22 26 28 29 30 32 34 39 40 41 42 44 45 46 48 49 61 65 71 73 **S**2155 Baptist Health System of Tennessee	21	10	109	2790	85	27982	309	17554	7082	292
OAK RIDGE—Anderson County										
□ METHODIST MEDICAL CENTER OF OAK RIDGE, 990 Oak Ridge Turnpike, Zip 37830, Mailing Address: P.O. Box 2529, Zip 37831–2529; tel. 615/481–1000; Marshall Whisnant, President **A**1 2 9 10 **F**2 3 4 7 8 10 11 12 16 19 21 22 28 29 30 31 32 33 35 37 40 41 42 43 44 46 49 51 52 53 54 56 57 59 60 63 65 66 67 71 72 73 74 **P**7	21	10	285	11052	186	100551	943	80082	33059	1012
□ RIDGEVIEW PSYCHIATRIC HOSPITAL AND CENTER, 240 West Tyrone Road, Zip 37830; tel. 615/482–1076; Robert J. Benning MSW, Chief Executive Officer **A**1 10 **F**3 12 52 53 54 55 56 57 58 59 65 **P**6	23	22	20	375	8	53284	0	6479	4273	168
ONEIDA—Scott County										
□ SCOTT COUNTY HOSPITAL, U.S. Highway 27, Zip 37841–4939, Mailing Address: Box 4939, Zip 37841–4939; tel. 615/569–8521; Doug Dailey, Administrator **A**1 9 10 **F**3 7 15 16 19 21 22 28 37 40 44 49 52 59 65 71 73 **S**0875 Community Health Systems, Inc.	33	10	77	3231	46	19052	16	9987	4324	218

© 1995 AHA Guide

Hospitals, U.S. / TENNESSEE

Hospital, Address, Telephone, Administrator, Approval, Facility, and Physician Codes, Health Care System	Classification Codes		Utilization Data					Expense (thousands) of dollars		
★ American Hospital Association (AHA) membership ☐ Joint Commission on Accreditation of Healthcare Organizations (JCAHO) accreditation + American Osteopathic Hospital Association (AOHA) membership ○ American Osteopathic Association (AOA) accreditation △ Commission on Accreditation of Rehabilitation Facilities (CARF) accreditation Control codes 61, 63, 64, 71, 72 and 73 indicate hospitals listed by AOHA, but not registered by AHA. For definition of numerical codes, see page A6	Control	Service	Beds	Admissions	Census	Outpatient Visits	Births	Total	Payroll	Personnel
PARIS—Henry County ★ HENRY COUNTY MEDICAL CENTER, Tyson Avenue, Zip 38242–4544, Mailing Address: Box 1030, Zip 38242–1030; tel. 901/644–8537; Thomas H. Gee, Administrator (Total facility includes 172 beds in nursing home–type unit) **A**1 9 10 **F**7 8 19 21 22 23 28 30 31 32 33 34 35 37 39 40 42 44 46 49 52 53 54 55 56 57 59 60 65 67 69 71 73	13	10	267	3883	226	38645	292	18360	8241	348
PARSONS—Decatur County DECATUR COUNTY GENERAL HOSPITAL, 1200 Tennessee Avenue South, Zip 38363–0250, Mailing Address: Box 250, Zip 38363–0250; tel. 901/847–3031; Larry N. Lindsey, Administrator (Nonreporting) **A**9 10	13	10	40	—	—	—	—	—	—	—
PIKEVILLE—Bledsoe County ☐ BLEDSOE COUNTY GENERAL HOSPITAL, Mailing Address: P.O. Box 428, Zip 37367–0428; tel. 615/447–2112; Gary Burton, Administrator (Nonreporting) **A**1 9 10 **S**5765 Paracelsus Healthcare Corporation	33	10	32	—	—	—	—	—	—	—
PULASKI—Giles County ☐ HILLSIDE HOSPITAL, 1265 East College Street, Zip 38478; tel. 615/363–7531; Rex Macklin, Chief Executive Officer and Administrator (Nonreporting) **A**1 9 10 **S**0875 Community Health Systems, Inc.	33	10	95	—	—	—	—	—	—	—
RIPLEY—Lauderdale County ★ BAPTIST MEMORIAL HOSPITAL–LAUDERDALE, 326 Asbury Road, Zip 38063–9701; tel. 901/635–1331; W. Tate Moorer, Administrator **A**1 9 10 **F**2 3 8 15 16 19 22 32 34 39 41 44 46 49 54 58 65 71 73 **P**3 7 **S**1625 Baptist Memorial Health Care System, Inc.	21	10	70	1117	18	15108	0	6526	2366	127
ROCKWOOD—Roane County ★ BAPTIST HOSPITAL OF ROANE COUNTY, 241 South Chamberlain Avenue, Zip 37854, Mailing Address: P.O. Box 388, Zip 37854; tel. 615/354–1121; William E. Torrence Jr., Chief Executive Officer **A**1 9 10 **F**2 3 4 7 8 10 11 15 16 17 19 22 26 28 30 31 32 33 34 35 37 39 41 42 43 44 45 46 56 61 65 70 71 **S**2155 Baptist Health System of Tennessee	23	10	66	2384	34	24059	88	12159	4780	147
ROGERSVILLE—Hawkins County ★ HAWKINS COUNTY MEMORIAL HOSPITAL, Locust Street, Zip 37857; tel. 615/272–2671; R. Frank Testerman, Administrator **A**1 9 10 **F**7 8 17 19 22 28 30 31 34 35 40 41 44 45 49 64 65 71 73	13	10	55	1608	22	37708	0	6793	2681	142
SAVANNAH—Hardin County HARDIN COUNTY GENERAL HOSPITAL, 2006 Wayne Road, Zip 38372; tel. 901/925–4954; Charlotte Burns, Acting Administrator (Nonreporting) **A**9 10	13	10	121	—	—	—	—	—	—	—
SELMER—McNairy County ★ MCNAIRY COUNTY GENERAL HOSPITAL, 705 East Poplar Avenue, Zip 38375–1748; tel. 901/645–3221; Rosamond M. Tyler, Administrator **A**1 9 10 **F**7 8 19 21 22 27 28 29 30 33 34 40 44 45 49 54 65 71 73	13	10	86	1543	17	23637	295	6574	3077	150
SEVIERVILLE—Sevier County ★ FORT SANDERS–SEVIER MEDICAL CENTER, 709 Middle Creek Road, Zip 37862, Mailing Address: P.O. Box 8005, Zip 37864–8005; tel. 615/429–6617; Ralph T. Williams, Administrator (Total facility includes 54 beds in nursing home–type unit) **A**1 9 10 **F**7 8 10 12 15 19 21 22 28 30 31 32 34 35 37 40 41 44 45 49 63 67 71 73 **P**7	23	10	100	2052	75	55911	464	15538	6461	273
SEWANEE—Franklin County EMERALD–HODGSON HOSPITAL See Southern Tennessee Medical Center, Winchester										
SHELBYVILLE—Bedford County ☐ BEDFORD COUNTY GENERAL HOSPITAL, 845 Union Street, Zip 37160–9971; tel. 615/685–5433; Richard L. Graham, Administrator (Total facility includes 107 beds in nursing home–type unit) **A**1 9 10 **F**7 8 12 13 14 15 16 19 22 28 30 32 34 37 39 40 41 44 49 64 65 68 69 71 73	13	10	182	2158	131	62332	144	14039	6288	218
SMITHVILLE—DeKalb County ☐ DEKALB GENERAL HOSPITAL, 520 West Main Street, Zip 37166, Mailing Address: P.O. Box 640, Zip 37166–0640; tel. 615/597–7171; Alan Markowitz Ph.D., FACHE, Administrator **A**1 9 10 **F**7 8 10 12 17 19 21 22 24 25 26 28 30 34 35 37 40 42 44 45 46 49 65 66 71 73 **P**5	32	10	58	2105	21	5888	88	7604	3426	130
SOMERVILLE—Fayette County ★ METHODIST HOSPITAL OF FAYETTE, 214 Lakeview Road, Zip 38068–0001, Mailing Address: Box 909, Zip 38068–0001; tel. 901/465–3594; Stan Caummisar, Administrator (Nonreporting) **A**1 9 10 **S**9345 Methodist Health Systems, Inc.	21	10	38	—	—	—	—	—	—	—
SOUTH PITTSBURG—Marion County ★ SOUTH PITTSBURG MUNICIPLE HOSPITAL, 210 West 12th Street, Zip 37380, Mailing Address: P.O. Box 349, Zip 37380–0349; tel. 615/837–6781; Greg Griffith, Chief Executive Officer (Nonreporting) **A**1 9 10 **S**0048 Columbia/HCA Healthcare Corporation	33	10	47	—	—	—	—	—	—	—
SPARTA—White County ☐ WHITE COUNTY COMMUNITY HOSPITAL, 401 Sewell Road, Zip 38583; tel. 615/738–9211; Raymond W. Acker, Administrator (Nonreporting) **A**1 9 10 **S**5895 Hallmark Healthcare Corporation	33	10	60	—	—	—	—	—	—	—
SPRINGFIELD—Robertson County ★ JESSE HOLMAN JONES HOSPITAL, 509 Brown Street, Zip 37172–2984; tel. 615/384–2411; John M. Faulkner FACHE, President and Chief Executive Officer **A**1 9 10 **F**7 8 10 15 16 19 21 22 28 30 32 33 34 35 37 39 40 41 42 44 45 46 49 52 54 55 56 57 58 65 71 73	23	10	115	3688	48	40971	526	22537	9926	360

Hospitals, U.S. / TENNESSEE

Hospital, Address, Telephone, Administrator, Approval, Facility, and Physician Codes, Health Care System	Classification Codes		Utilization Data					Expense (thousands) of dollars		
	Control	Service	Beds	Admissions	Census	Outpatient Visits	Births	Total	Payroll	Personnel

★ American Hospital Association (AHA) membership
☐ Joint Commission on Accreditation of Healthcare Organizations (JCAHO) accreditation
+ American Osteopathic Hospital Association (AOHA) membership
○ American Osteopathic Association (AOA) accreditation
△ Commission on Accreditation of Rehabilitation Facilities (CARF) accreditation
Control codes 61, 63, 64, 71, 72 and 73 indicate hospitals listed by AOHA, but not registered by AHA. For definition of numerical codes, see page A6

Hospital	Control	Service	Beds	Admissions	Census	Outpatient Visits	Births	Total	Payroll	Personnel
SWEETWATER—Monroe County ★ SWEETWATER HOSPITAL, 304 Wright Street, Zip 37874; tel. 615/337–6171; Scott Bowman, Administrator (Nonreporting) **A**9 10	23	10	59	—	—	—	—	—	—	—
TAZEWELL—Claiborne County ★ CLAIBORNE COUNTY HOSPITAL, 1850 Old Knoxville Road, Zip 37879, Mailing Address: Box 219, Zip 37879; tel. 615/626–4211; Richard Welch, Administrator (Total facility includes 50 beds in nursing home–type unit) **A**1 9 10 **F**8 16 17 19 22 26 28 32 33 34 41 44 45 46 49 65 71	13	10	110	3214	90	38083	2	13341	6508	295
TRENTON—Gibson County ☐ GIBSON GENERAL HOSPITAL, 200 Hosptial Drive, Zip 38382, Mailing Address: Box 488, Zip 38382; tel. 901/855–2551; David Alred, Administrator (Nonreporting) **A**1 9 10	33	10	83	—	—	—	—	—	—	—
TULLAHOMA—Coffee County ☐ HARTON REGIONAL MEDICAL CENTER, 1801 North Jackson Street, Zip 37388, Mailing Address: P.O. Box 460, Zip 37388; tel. 615/393–3000; Brian T. Flynn, Administrator and Chief Executive Officer (Nonreporting) **A**1 9 10 **S**0063 TENET Healthcare Corporation	16	10	137	—	—	—	—	—	—	—
UNION CITY—Obion County ★ BAPTIST MEMORIAL HOSPITAL–UNION CITY, 1201 Bishop Street, Zip 38261, Mailing Address: Box 310, Zip 38281–0310; tel. 901/884–8601; Mike Perryman, Administrator **A**1 9 10 **F**2 3 7 8 10 12 15 16 17 19 22 25 28 30 31 32 35 37 39 40 42 44 46 49 52 54 56 58 59 60 65 67 71 73 **P**3 **S**1625 Baptist Memorial Health Care System, Inc.	21	10	95	4793	65	29819	534	20820	7871	352
WAVERLY—Humphreys County THREE RIVERS COMMUNITY HOSPITAL, 451 Highway 13 South, Zip 37185–2149, Mailing Address: P.O. Box 437, Zip 37185–2149; tel. 615/296–4203; Samuel R. Heflin Jr., Administrator (Total facility includes 10 beds in nursing home–type unit) **A**9 10 **F**19 22 28 30 32 41 44 46 48 51 64 65 71 73	32	10	52	875	12	19300	0	4689	1809	87
WAYNESBORO—Wayne County ☐ WAYNE COUNTY GENERAL HOSPITAL, Highway 64 East, Zip 38485, Mailing Address: P.O. Box 580, Zip 38485–0580; tel. 615/722–5411; Donald H. Polk D.O., President (Nonreporting) **A**1 9 10	33	10	70	—	—	—	—	—	—	—
WESTERN INSTITUTE—Hardeman County ☐ WESTERN MENTAL HEALTH INSTITUTE, Highway 64 West, Zip 38074; tel. 901/658–5141; James M. Flynn, Superintendent (Nonreporting) **A**1 10	12	22	267	—	—	—	—	—	—	—
WINCHESTER—Franklin County ★ SOUTHERN TENNESSEE MEDICAL CENTER, (Includes Emerald–Hodgson Hospital, University Avenue, Sewanee, Tennessee, Zip 37375; tel. 615/598–5691; Renaye Smith, Administrator) 185 Hospital Road, Zip 37398; tel. 615/967–8200; Michael W. Garfield, Administrator (Total facility includes 71 beds in nursing home–type unit) **A**1 9 10 **F**7 8 12 14 15 16 19 21 22 26 27 28 29 30 32 34 35 37 39 40 41 42 44 45 46 49 51 63 64 65 66 71 73 74 **P**7 8 **S**0048 Columbia/HCA Healthcare Corporation	33	10	216	4512	102	47581	315	25119	11803	391
WOODBURY—Cannon County ★ STONES RIVER HOSPITAL, Doolittle Road, Zip 37190, Mailing Address: P.O. Box 458, Zip 37190–0458; tel. 615/563–4001; Ron Walker, Chief Executive Officer **A**1 9 10 **F**8 12 14 15 17 19 21 22 26 28 29 30 32 35 39 41 44 46 49 51 52 57 63 65 71 73 **P**5 7 8 **S**0048 Columbia/HCA Healthcare Corporation	33	10	55	1464	20	9875	0	6205	2486	101

Hospitals, U.S. / TEXAS

TEXAS

Resident population 18,031 (in thousands)
Resident population in metro areas 83.9%
Birth rate per 1,000 population 18.3
65 years and over 10.2%
Percent of persons without health insurance 21.9%

Hospital, Address, Telephone, Administrator, Approval, Facility, and Physician Codes, Health Care System	Classification Codes		Utilization Data					Expense (thousands) of dollars		
★ American Hospital Association (AHA) membership ☐ Joint Commission on Accreditation of Healthcare Organizations (JCAHO) accreditation + American Osteopathic Hospital Association (AOHA) membership ○ American Osteopathic Association (AOA) accreditation △ Commission on Accreditation of Rehabilitation Facilities (CARF) accreditation Control codes 61, 63, 64, 71, 72 and 73 indicate hospitals listed by AOHA, but not registered by AHA. For definition of numerical codes, see page A6	Control	Service	Beds	Admissions	Census	Outpatient Visits	Births	Total	Payroll	Personnel
ABILENE—Taylor County										
★ ABILENE REGIONAL MEDICAL CENTER, 6250 Highway 83–84 at Antilley Road, Zip 79606; tel. 915/695–9900; David M. Collins, President and Chief Executive Officer **A**1 9 10 **F**4 7 10 12 15 16 17 19 22 24 25 26 27 28 29 30 34 35 37 38 39 40 43 44 45 46 49 51 65 68 71 73 74 **P**7 8 **S**0002 Quorum Health Group/Quorum Health Resources	33	10	145	6112	107	34905	394	58984	21530	676
★ △ HENDRICK MEDICAL CENTER, 1242 North 19th Street, Zip 79601–2316; tel. 915/670–2000; Michael C. Waters, President (Total facility includes 21 beds in nursing home–type unit) **A**1 7 9 10 **F**2 3 4 6 7 8 10 15 16 17 18 19 21 22 23 26 28 29 30 31 32 33 34 35 37 39 40 41 42 43 44 45 46 47 48 49 54 55 56 57 58 59 60 62 64 65 67 71 73 74 **P**7	21	10	371	11513	173	89566	2009	109772	49903	1955
★ U.S. AIR FORCE HOSPITAL, Dyess AFB, Zip 79607–1367; tel. 915/696–5427; Colonel Robert Blum MSC, Administrator **F**7 8 14 15 16 19 20 22 40 44 58 61 65 71 **S**9495 Department of the Air Force	41	10	15	1337	8	138201	401	—	—	343
★ WOODS PSYCHIATRIC INSTITUTE, 1302 Petroleum Drive, Zip 79602, Mailing Address: P.O. Box 5749, Zip 79608; tel. 915/698–2320; Everett E. Woods, Chief Executive Officer **A**1 9 10 **F**2 16 22 31 52 53 54 56 57 58 59 65	33	22	72	449	31	3997	0	6103	3450	164
ALBANY—Shackelford County										
SHACKELFORD COUNTY HOSPITAL DISTRICT, 840 Greer Street, Zip 76430, Mailing Address: P.O. Box 1507, Zip 76430; tel. 915/762–3313; David R. Jordan, Administrator **A**9 10 **F**14 15 16 22 34 71	16	10	24	115	1	720	0	833	455	18
ALICE—Jim Wells County										
★ ALICE PHYSICIANS AND SURGEONS HOSPITAL, 300 East Third Street, Zip 78332–4794; tel. 512/664–4376; Earl S. Whiteley CHE, Chief Executive Officer (Total facility includes 17 beds in nursing home–type unit) **A**1 9 10 **F**7 8 11 12 14 15 16 18 19 20 21 22 26 28 29 30 31 32 33 34 37 38 40 41 44 45 46 47 49 50 51 52 55 57 63 64 65 67 71 73 **P**6 7 8 **S**0048 Columbia/HCA Healthcare Corporation	33	10	118	3456	44	26507	341	20982	8264	375
ALPINE—Brewster County										
BIG BEND REGIONAL MEDICAL CENTER, 801 East Brown Street, Zip 79830; tel. 915/837–3447; Richard D. Arnold, Administrator **A**9 10 **F**7 13 14 15 16 17 18 20 21 22 26 28 31 32 33 34 36 39 40 42 44 45 46 51 64 65 71 73	16	10	34	1299	12	25247	277	—	—	163
ALVIN—Brazoria County										
★ ALVIN COMMUNITY HOSPITAL, 301 Medic Lane, Zip 77511; tel. 713/331–6141; Betsy Postlethwait, Executive Director (Total facility includes 14 beds in nursing home–type unit) (Data for 335 days) **A**1 9 10 **F**8 12 14 15 16 19 22 34 35 36 37 39 41 44 49 64 66 71 73 **P**8 **S**0048 Columbia/HCA Healthcare Corporation	33	10	41	1694	28	17366	2	12750	5424	170
AMARILLO—Potter County										
★ AMARILLO HOSPITAL DISTRICT, (Includes Northwest Texas Hospital, 1501 South Coulter, Amarillo, Texas, Zip 79106; Psychiatric Pavilion, 7201 Evans, Amarillo, Texas, Zip 79106) Mailing Address: P.O. Box 1110, Zip 79175–1110); tel. 806/354–1000; William W. Webster, President and Chief Executive Officer **A**1 3 5 10 **F**2 3 4 7 8 10 11 12 13 14 15 16 17 18 19 20 21 22 23 24 25 26 29 30 31 32 33 34 35 37 38 39 40 41 42 43 44 45 46 47 48 49 51 52 53 54 55 56 57 58 59 60 61 63 64 65 66 67 71 73 74 **P**3 6 7	16	10	350	13531	215	209002	2824	121204	51589	1857
○ FAMILY HOSPITAL CENTER, 2828 West 27th Street, Zip 79109, Mailing Address: Box 7408, Zip 79114–7408; tel. 806/358–3131; Jerry S. Hogue, Administrator **A**9 10 11 **F**15 19 22 26 30 33 34 37 44 71 73	23	10	50	283	6	—	0	3134	1541	—
★ △ HIGH PLAINS BAPTIST HEALTH SYSTEM, 1600 Wallace Boulevard, Zip 79106; tel. 806/358–5800; T. H. Holloway FACHE, President and Chief Executive Officer (Total facility includes 31 beds in nursing home–type unit) **A**1 2 5 7 9 10 **F**4 5 6 7 8 10 11 12 15 16 19 21 22 23 24 25 26 32 33 35 36 37 39 40 41 42 43 44 45 46 48 49 60 62 64 66 67 69 71 72 73 74 **P**5 7	21	10	328	11573	177	78129	1066	98210	41099	1341
NORTHWEST TEXAS HOSPITAL See Amarillo Hospital District										
PSYCHIATRIC PAVILION See Amarillo Hospital District										
★ ST. ANTHONY'S HOSPITAL, 200 Northwest Seventh, Zip 79107–9872, Mailing Address: Box 950, Zip 79176–0950; tel. 806/376–4411; John D. Koobs, President and Chief Executive Officer (Total facility includes 27 beds in nursing home–type unit) **A**1 2 3 5 9 10 **F**8 10 11 12 14 15 16 17 19 21 22 24 26 28 30 32 33 35 37 41 42 43 44 45 48 49 52 54 55 56 57 58 59 60 63 64 65 66 71 72 73 **S**5565 Incarnate Word Health Services	21	10	290	7869	141	47995	3	69850	26262	751
★ VETERANS AFFAIRS MEDICAL CENTER, 6010 Amarillo Boulevard West, Zip 79106; tel. 806/355–9703; Y. C. Parris, Director (Total facility includes 120 beds in nursing home–type unit) **A**1 2 3 5 **F**1 2 3 4 10 12 18 19 20 21 22 26 27 28 30 31 33 35 37 42 43 44 45 46 49 51 54 55 56 57 58 59 60 63 64 65 67 69 71 72 73 74 **S**9295 Department of Veterans Affairs	45	10	246	4190	183	88066	0	51494	25411	686
ANAHUAC—Chambers County										
★ BAYSIDE COMMUNITY HOSPITAL, 200 Hospital Drive, Zip 77514, Mailing Address: Box 398, Zip 77514; tel. 409/267–3143; John Henry Luff, Executive Director **A**9 10 **F**22 36 44 **P**6	16	10	289	4	5121	1	2010	940	44	

Hospitals, U.S. / TEXAS

Hospital, Address, Telephone, Administrator, Approval, Facility, and Physician Codes, Health Care System	Classification Codes		Utilization Data					Expense (thousands) of dollars		
★ American Hospital Association (AHA) membership ☐ Joint Commission on Accreditation of Healthcare Organizations (JCAHO) accreditation + American Osteopathic Hospital Association (AOHA) membership ○ American Osteopathic Association (AOA) accreditation △ Commission on Accreditation of Rehabilitation Facilities (CARF) accreditation Control codes 61, 63, 64, 71, 72 and 73 indicate hospitals listed by AOHA, but not registered by AHA. For definition of numerical codes, see page A6	Control	Service	Beds	Admissions	Census	Outpatient Visits	Births	Total	Payroll	Personnel
ANDREWS—Andrews County ★ PERMIAN GENERAL HOSPITAL, Northeast By-Pass, Zip 79714, Mailing Address: Box 2108, Zip 79714; tel. 915/523-2200; Terry R. Andris CHE, Chief Executive Officer (Total facility includes 16 beds in nursing home–type unit) **A**1 9 10 **F**7 8 14 15 16 19 22 24 28 29 30 31 32 33 34 37 38 40 44 45 46 48 49 64 65 70 71 73 **S**0036 Lubbock Methodist Hospital System	13	10	76	1572	17	18801	310	9679	4333	152
ANGLETON—Brazoria County ★ ANGLETON-DANBURY GENERAL HOSPITAL, 132 Hospital Drive, Zip 77515; tel. 409/849-7721; David A. Bleakney, Administrator **A**1 9 10 **F**7 8 10 12 14 15 16 19 21 22 24 28 29 30 31 33 34 35 37 40 44 45 46 49 65 66 70 71 73 **P**8 **S**2645 Memorial Healthcare System	16	10	64	2495	21	23309	661	17736	6769	121
ANSON—Jones County ★ ANSON GENERAL HOSPITAL, 101 Avenue J, Zip 79501; tel. 915/823-3231; Dudley R. White, Administrator **A**9 10 **F**19 22 32 33 34 44 49 71 73 **P**3 8	14	10	35	661	15	31686	1	4649	2034	110
ARANSAS PASS—San Patricio County ★ COASTAL BEND HOSPITAL, 1711 West Wheeler Street, Zip 78336; tel. 512/758-8585; Shirley Gallagher, Chief Executive Officer **A**1 9 10 **F**7 8 12 16 17 19 22 24 26 28 29 30 32 34 37 40 41 44 49 51 52 57 65 66 71 73 **P**5 **S**0048 Columbia/HCA Healthcare Corporation	33	10	68	1997	33	35021	255	16984	5601	254
ARLINGTON—Tarrant County ★ ARLINGTON MEDICAL CENTER, 3301 Matlock Road, Zip 76015; tel. 817/465-3241; Michael S. Spurlock, Chief Executive Officer **A**1 9 10 **F**2 3 4 7 8 10 11 12 14 15 16 19 22 23 32 34 35 37 40 41 42 43 44 46 48 49 50 52 56 58 59 60 63 65 71 73 **P**3 5 7 **S**0048 Columbia/HCA Healthcare Corporation	33	10	223	6691	81	50394	1743	41684	14750	550
★ ARLINGTON MEMORIAL HOSPITAL, 800 West Randol Mill Road, Zip 76012; tel. 817/548-6100; Rex C. McRae, President **A**1 9 10 **F**4 7 8 10 11 12 14 15 17 19 21 22 23 24 32 34 35 37 38 39 40 41 42 43 44 45 49 60 65 71 73 74 **P**1	23	10	314	14502	201	77293	2382	105001	40906	1461
☐ CPC MILLWOOD HOSPITAL, 1011 North Cooper Street, Zip 76011; tel. 817/261-3121; Wayne Hallford, Chief Executive Officer **A**1 9 10 **F**2 3 15 16 18 19 21 22 28 30 35 41 46 52 53 54 55 56 57 58 59 65 67 71 **P**5 **S**0785 Community Psychiatric Centers	33	22	98	719	26	4098	0	5777	3346	109
☐ △ REHABILITATION HOSPITAL OF NORTH TEXAS, 3200 Matlock Road, Zip 76015-2911; tel. 817/468-4000; Malcolm Berry, Administrator (Total facility includes 18 beds in nursing home–type unit) **A**1 7 9 10 **F**5 12 26 34 48 49 64 65 73	33	46	60	556	33	3985	0	9662	4108	143
☐ WILLOW CREEK HOSPITAL, 7000 Highway 287 South, Zip 76017-2805; tel. 817/561-1600; Donald K. Sykes Jr., Chief Executive Officer **A**1 9 **F**2 3 14 15 17 18 52 53 54 55 56 57 58 59 67 73 **S**4165 Adventist Health System–Sunbelt Health Care Corporation	21	22	92	963	40	—	0	5820	2306	89
ASPERMONT—Stonewall County ★ STONEWALL MEMORIAL HOSPITAL, U.S. Highway 380 & 83 North, Zip 79502, Mailing Address: Drawer C, Zip 79502; tel. 817/989-3551; Bob Rutherford, Administration **A**9 10 **F**12 15 16 17 19 21 22 34 35 41 44 50 60 63 71	16	10	16	126	2	1934	0	1445	794	42
ATHENS—Henderson County ★ EAST TEXAS MEDICAL CENTER ATHENS, 2000 South Palestine, Zip 75751; tel. 903/675-2216; Patrick L. Wallace, Administrator **A**1 9 10 **F**8 15 19 22 23 28 32 35 37 40 42 44 49 63 65 71 **P**7 **S**1895 East Texas Medical Center Regional Healthcare System	23	10	108	4832	58	65813	646	28419	9755	348
ATLANTA—Cass County ★ ATLANTA MEMORIAL HOSPITAL, Highway 77 at South Williams, Zip 75551, Mailing Address: Box 1049, Zip 75551-1049; tel. 903/796-4151; Tom Crow, Administrator **A**9 10 **F**7 8 15 17 22 28 30 32 34 37 40 44 45 65 71 73	16	10	53	1408	17	10140	201	5197	2974	—
BROOKS HOSPITAL, Louise Street, Zip 75551, Mailing Address: P.O. Box 1069, Zip 75551; tel. 903/796-2873; Jesse Brooks M.D., Administrator **A**9 10 **F**1 3 4 5 6 7 8 10 12 13 17 18 19 20 21 22 23 24 25 26 27 28 29 30 31 32 33 34 35 36 39 41 42 43 44 45 46 49 50 51 53 54 55 56 57 58 59 60 61 62 63 65 66 67 68 69 70 71 72 73 74 **P**1 2 3 4 5 6 7 8	33	10	22	538	5	176	0	—	—	52
AUSTIN—Travis County ☐ AUSTIN STATE HOSPITAL, 4110 Guadalupe Street, Zip 78751-4296; tel. 512/452-0381; Kenny Dudley, Superintendent **A**1 3 9 10 **F**12 52 53 54 55 56 57 58 73	12	22	324	1596	324	0	0	43717	26863	—
☐ BRACKENRIDGE HOSPITAL, (Includes Children's Hospital of Austin) 601 East 15th Street, Zip 78701; tel. 512/476-6461; Keith R. Poisson, Chief Executive Officer **A**1 3 9 10 **F**4 7 8 10 11 12 13 14 15 16 17 19 21 22 27 28 29 30 31 34 37 38 39 40 41 42 43 44 47 49 53 56 61 63 65 69 71 73 74	14	10	328	17203	233	115178	3754	149077	61235	1407
☐ CHARTER BEHAVIORAL HEALTH SYSTEM OF AUSTIN, 8402 Cross Park Drive, Zip 78754, Mailing Address: P.O. Box 140585, Zip 78714-0585; tel. 512/837-1800; Trish Mitchell, Network Chief Executive Officer **A**1 9 10 **F**2 3 14 15 16 19 22 27 35 48 51 52 53 54 55 56 57 58 59 60 65 **S**0695 Charter Medical Corporation	33	22	70	1048	23	5311	0	6767	2144	71
CHRISTOPHER HOUSE, (HIV, Aids) 2820 East Martin Luther King, Zip 78702; tel. 512/370-8500; Carol Cody, Administrator (Data for 292 days) **A**10 **F**12 14 15 16 31 65 73 **P**8	23	49	15	221	8	0	0	2003	890	42

© 1995 AHA Guide

Hospitals, U.S. / TEXAS

Hospital, Address, Telephone, Administrator, Approval, Facility, and Physician Codes, Health Care System	Classification Codes		Utilization Data					Expense (thousands) of dollars		
	Control	Service	Beds	Admissions	Census	Outpatient Visits	Births	Total	Payroll	Personnel

★ American Hospital Association (AHA) membership
☐ Joint Commission on Accreditation of Healthcare Organizations (JCAHO) accreditation
+ American Osteopathic Hospital Association (AOHA) membership
○ American Osteopathic Association (AOA) accreditation
△ Commission on Accreditation of Rehabilitation Facilities (CARF) accreditation
Control codes 61, 63, 64, 71, 72 and 73 indicate hospitals listed by AOHA, but not registered by AHA. For definition of numerical codes, see page A6

Hospital	Control	Service	Beds	Admissions	Census	Outpatient Visits	Births	Total	Payroll	Personnel
☐ CPC CAPITAL HOSPITAL, 12151 Hunters Chase Drive, Zip 78729; tel. 512/250–8667; Kevin E. Blackwell, Chief Executive Officer **A**1 9 10 **F**2 3 12 14 15 22 25 27 28 30 34 52 53 54 55 56 58 59 74 **S**0785 Community Psychiatric Centers	33	22	86	646	31	3565	0	6722	3237	113
☐ HEALTHCARE REHABILITATION CENTER, 1106 West Dittmar, Zip 78745–9990, Mailing Address: P.O. Box 43148, Zip 78745–9990; tel. 512/444–4835; Cindy McLendon, Administrator (Nonreporting) **A**1 **S**0395 Healthcare International, Inc.	33	46	149	—	—	—	—	—	—	—
★ △ HEALTHSOUTH REHABILITATION HOSPITAL OF AUSTIN, 1215 Red River Street, Zip 78701, Mailing Address: P.O. Box 13366, Zip 78711–3366; tel. 512/474–5700; Mike Munnerlyn, Chief Executive Officer **A**1 7 9 10 **F**12 19 34 35 48 49 73 **S**0023 Healthsouth Corporation	33	46	80	813	40	13083	0	12663	6535	193
MERIDELL ACHIEVEMENT CENTER, Mailing Address: Box 203638, Zip 78720–3638; tel. 512/259–5107; Mark Snow, Managing Director (Nonreporting) **S**9555 Universal Health Services, Inc.	33	52	78	—	—	—	—	—	—	—
☐ OAKS TREATMENT CENTER, 1407 West Stassney Lane, Zip 78745; tel. 512/444–9561; Richard R. Hardin, Executive Director **A**1 **F**1 6 12 15 19 20 21 22 35 50 52 53 55 57 58 59 63 71 **P**1 6 8 **S**0395 Healthcare International, Inc.	33	52	98	209	39	349	0	5770	3472	94
★ SETON MEDICAL CENTER, 1201 West 38th Street, Zip 78705–1056; tel. 512/323–1000; Charles J. Barnett, President **A**1 2 9 10 **F**4 7 8 10 11 12 15 16 17 19 21 22 23 25 28 29 30 31 32 34 35 37 38 40 41 42 43 44 46 49 60 65 66 67 69 71 73 **P**7 8 **S**1855 Daughters of Charity National Health System	21	10	532	25027	330	205693	4501	166480	71255	1907
☐ SHOAL CREEK HOSPITAL, 3501 Mills Avenue, Zip 78731; tel. 512/452–0361; Gail M. Oberta, Administrator and Chief Executive Officer **A**1 9 10 **F**2 3 15 16 26 34 52 53 54 55 56 57 58 59 **P**8 **S**0069 Behavioral Healthcare Corporation	33	22	118	1795	35	9421	0	8121	3867	94
★ SOUTH AUSTIN MEDICAL CENTER, 901 West Ben White Boulevard, Zip 78704–6903; tel. 512/447–2211; Richard W. Klusmann, Chief Executive Officer **A**1 9 10 **F**4 7 8 10 11 12 15 17 19 21 22 23 28 30 33 34 35 37 40 42 43 44 49 60 65 67 69 71 73 74 **P**1 7 **S**0048 Columbia/HCA Healthcare Corporation	33	10	150	5848	78	47261	805	39210	15648	550
SPECIALTY HOSPITAL OF AUSTIN, 4207 Burnet Road, Zip 78756; tel. 512/706–1900; I. Lynn Jeane, Administrator and Chief Executive Officer **A**10 **F**4 10 12 19 20 21 22 26 27 35 42 44 50 60 63 65 67 71	33	10	104	195	18	0	0	5538	2586	190
★ ST. DAVID'S HEALTH CARE SYSTEM, 919 East 32nd Street, Zip 78705, Mailing Address: Box 4039, Zip 78765–4039; tel. 512/476–7111; Jack L. Campbell, President **A**1 2 9 10 **F**1 2 3 4 5 7 8 10 11 12 14 15 16 17 18 19 21 22 23 24 25 26 27 28 29 30 31 32 34 35 36 37 38 39 40 41 42 43 44 45 46 48 49 52 53 54 55 57 58 59 60 61 63 64 65 66 67 68 69 71 72 73 74 **P**1 6 7 8 **S**0003 St. David's Health Care System	23	10	296	19055	190	108850	4253	99100	43234	1315
★ ST. DAVID'S PAVILION, 1025 East 32nd Street, Zip 78765; tel. 512/867–5800; Deborah L. Ryle, Administrator **A**1 9 10 **F**1 2 3 4 7 8 10 11 12 14 15 16 18 19 21 22 24 25 26 27 28 29 30 31 32 34 35 36 37 38 39 40 41 42 43 44 45 46 48 49 52 53 54 55 57 58 59 61 63 64 65 66 69 71 72 73 74 **P**1 6 7 8 **S**0003 St. David's Health Care System	23	22	38	960	24	4916	0	8060	2502	82
★ △ ST. DAVID'S REHABILITATION CENTER, 1005 East 32nd Street, Zip 78705, Mailing Address: P.O. Box 4270, Zip 78765–4270; tel. 512/867–5100; Deborah L. Ryle, Administrator (Total facility includes 37 beds in nursing home–type unit) **A**1 7 9 10 **F**1 2 3 4 7 8 10 11 12 14 15 16 17 18 19 21 22 23 28 30 31 32 34 35 36 37 38 39 40 41 42 43 44 45 46 48 49 52 53 54 55 57 58 59 61 63 64 65 67 69 71 72 73 74 **P**6 7 8 **S**0003 St. David's Health Care System	23	46	103	1761	81	136498	0	19882	8835	273
AZLE—Parker County										
★ HARRIS METHODIST–NORTHWEST, 108 Denver Trail, Zip 76020; tel. 817/444–8600; Larry Thompson, Vice President and Administrator **A**1 9 10 **F**1 2 3 4 5 7 8 10 11 12 13 14 15 16 17 18 19 21 22 23 24 25 26 27 28 29 30 31 32 33 34 35 37 38 39 40 41 42 43 44 45 46 48 49 50 52 53 55 56 58 59 60 61 63 64 65 66 67 69 70 71 72 73 74 **P**2 3 4 **S**2345 Harris Methodist Health System	21	10	38	1092	11	17892	1	10154	3824	156
BALLINGER—Runnels County										
BALLINGER MEMORIAL HOSPITAL, 608 Avenue B, Zip 76821–2499; tel. 915/365–2531; Robert E. Vernor, Administrator **A**9 10 **F**15 16 22 24 31 71 73	16	10	16	287	5	5500	1	1813	701	46
BAY CITY—Matagorda County										
★ MATAGORDA GENERAL HOSPITAL, 1115 Avenue G, Zip 77414–3544; tel. 409/245–6383; Wendell H. Baker Jr., Chief Executive Officer **A**1 9 10 **F**4 7 8 12 16 19 20 21 22 23 24 26 30 31 32 34 35 37 40 44 49 52 56 57 65 67 71 73 **P**5 8	16	10	65	2303	29	25033	424	18428	6902	270
BAYTOWN—Harris County										
BAYCOAST MEDICAL CENTER, (Includes Gulf Coast Hospital, 2800 Garth Road, Baytown, Texas, Zip 77521; tel. 713/425–9100) 1700 James Bowie Drive, Zip 77520, Mailing Address: P.O. Box 1451, Zip 77520; tel. 713/420–6100; Jeff Webster, Administrator **A**10 **F**7 8 10 11 12 14 19 20 21 22 23 28 30 32 33 34 35 37 39 40 41 44 46 48 49 61 63 64 65 71 72 73 74 **P**5 7 8	33	10	191	3776	55	43615	631	35442	12312	379
GULF COAST HOSPITAL See Baycoast Medical Center										
★ SAN JACINTO METHODIST HOSPITAL, 4401 Garth Road, Zip 77521; tel. 713/420–8600; Rod Seidel, President and Chief Executive Officer (Total facility includes 35 beds in nursing home–type unit) **A**1 3 5 9 10 **F**2 3 7 8 10 15 19 21 22 23 24 26 28 30 31 32 34 35 37 39 40 41 42 44 46 48 49 51 52 53 54 55 56 58 59 60 61 64 65 71 73 **P**8 **S**7235 Methodist Hospital System	21	10	266	8817	165	113515	1239	63636	27607	892

Hospitals, U.S. / TEXAS

Hospital, Address, Telephone, Administrator, Approval, Facility, and Physician Codes, Health Care System	Classification Codes		Utilization Data					Expense (thousands) of dollars		
★ American Hospital Association (AHA) membership ☐ Joint Commission on Accreditation of Healthcare Organizations (JCAHO) accreditation + American Osteopathic Hospital Association (AOHA) membership ○ American Osteopathic Association (AOA) accreditation △ Commission on Accreditation of Rehabilitation Facilities (CARF) accreditation Control codes 61, 63, 64, 71, 72 and 73 indicate hospitals listed by AOHA, but not registered by AHA. For definition of numerical codes, see page A6	Control	Service	Beds	Admissions	Census	Outpatient Visits	Births	Total	Payroll	Personnel
BEAUMONT—Jefferson County										
★ BAPTIST HOSPITAL OF SOUTHEAST TEXAS, College and 11th Streets, Zip 77701, Mailing Address: Drawer 1591, Zip 77704–1491; tel. 409/835–3781; David N. Parmer, President and Chief Executive Officer **A**1 9 10 **F**2 3 4 8 10 11 12 14 15 16 17 19 20 21 22 23 27 28 30 32 33 34 35 37 41 42 43 44 45 46 47 48 49 52 53 54 55 56 57 58 59 60 64 65 67 71 72 73 74 **P**3 5 8 BEAUMONT NEUROLOGICAL HOSPITAL See Beaumont Regional Medical Center	21	10	222	6209	120	82082	0	57456	23852	874
★ BEAUMONT REGIONAL MEDICAL CENTER, (Formerly Beaumont Neurological Hospital) (Includes Fannin Pavilion of Beaumont Regional Medical Center, 3250 Fannin Street, Beaumont, Texas, Zip 77701; tel. 409/833–1411) 3080 College, Zip 77701, Mailing Address: P.O. Box 5817, Zip 77726–5817; tel. 409/833–1411; Michael S. Miller, Chief Executive Officer **A**1 9 10 **F**2 3 7 8 12 15 16 17 19 20 21 22 26 27 28 29 30 31 32 35 37 38 40 42 44 45 46 52 53 54 55 56 57 58 59 64 65 67 71 73 74 **P**3 5 7 8 **S**0048 Columbia/HCA Healthcare Corporation FANNIN PAVILION OF BEAUMONT REGIONAL MEDICAL CENTER See Beaumont Regional Medical Center	33	10	362	8442	152	—	1669	53417	23490	869
★ △ SOUTHEAST TEXAS REHABILITATION HOSPITAL, 3340 Plaza 10 Boulevard, Zip 77707; tel. 409/835–0835; David J. Holly, Chief Executive Officer (Total facility includes 12 beds in nursing home–type unit) **A**1 7 9 10 **F**5 12 14 16 19 20 24 25 27 28 34 35 41 48 49 63 64 65 66 67 71 73 **P**7 **S**1715 Continental Medical Systems, Inc.	33	46	60	766	40	18465	0	13198	5480	148
★ △ ST. ELIZABETH HOSPITAL, 2830 Calder Avenue, Zip 77702, Mailing Address: P.O. Box 5405, Zip 77726–5405; tel. 409/892–7171; Sister M. Fatima McCarthy, Administrator (Total facility includes 20 beds in nursing home–type unit) **A**1 2 7 9 10 **F**4 5 7 8 10 11 12 14 15 16 17 19 20 21 22 23 26 27 28 29 30 31 32 33 34 35 37 38 39 40 41 42 43 44 45 46 47 48 49 51 60 64 65 67 71 73 **P**2 3 4 5 6 7 8 **S**0605 Sisters of Charity of the Incarnate Word Healthcare System	21	10	483	19773	350	266959	2272	160851	70002	2432
BEDFORD—Tarrant County										
★ HARRIS METHODIST–HEB, (Includes Harris Methodist–Springwood, 1608 Hospital Parkway, Bedford, Texas, Zip 76022; tel. 817/355–7700; Raymond L. Ford, Senior Vice President and Administrator) 1600 Hospital Parkway, Zip 76022–6913, Mailing Address: P.O. Box 669, Zip 76095; tel. 817/685–4000; (Nonreporting) **A**1 2 9 10 **S**2345 Harris Methodist Health System	21	10	177	—	—	—	—	—	—	—
★ ○ NORTHEAST COMMUNITY HOSPITAL, 1301 Airport Freeway, Zip 76021–5698; tel. 817/868–5600; Ernie Meier, Chief Executive Officer (Total facility includes 12 beds in nursing home–type unit) **A**1 9 10 11 12 13 **F**7 8 10 11 12 14 15 16 19 20 21 22 23 24 28 30 31 32 33 34 35 37 39 40 41 42 44 45 46 48 49 63 64 65 66 71 73 **P**7 **S**0048 Columbia/HCA Healthcare Corporation	33	10	122	3641	53	67947	893	38505	12358	418
BEEVILLE—Bee County										
☐ BEE COUNTY REGIONAL MEDICAL CENTER, 1500 East Houston Street, Zip 78102; tel. 512/358–5431; Andrew E. Anderson Jr., Administrator **A**1 9 10 **F**8 15 17 19 21 22 28 34 37 44 45 46 49 65 71 73 74	13	10	59	2833	32	26711	377	12107	5657	274
BELLVILLE—Austin County										
☐ BELLVILLE GENERAL HOSPITAL, 44 North Cummings, Zip 77418–0148, Mailing Address: Box 977, Zip 77418; tel. 409/865–3141; John W. Araiza, Administrator **A**1 9 10 **F**8 19 21 22 26 28 30 32 34 44 49 71 73 **P**3	16	10	32	775	8	8610	119	4129	1844	78
BIG LAKE—Reagan County										
REAGAN MEMORIAL HOSPITAL, 805 North Main Street, Zip 76932; tel. 915/884–2561; Ron Galloway, Administrator (Total facility includes 48 beds in nursing home–type unit) **A**9 **F**22 24 26 49 66	16	10	66	62	38	7792	3	—	—	48
BIG SPRING—Howard County										
☐ BIG SPRING STATE HOSPITAL, Lamesa Highway, Zip 79720, Mailing Address: P.O. Box 231, Zip 79721–0231; tel. 915/267–8216; Robert Von Rosenberg, Superintendent **A**1 9 10 **F**12 15 52 53 54 55 56 57 58	12	22	270	969	270	—	0	32513	20522	979
☐ SCENIC MOUNTAIN MEDICAL CENTER, 1601 West 11th Place, Zip 79720; tel. 915/263–1211; Kenneth W. Randall, Administrator **A**1 9 10 **F**12 16 19 21 22 23 27 28 31 32 34 35 37 40 44 46 49 52 57 63 65 71 **P**5 7 8 **S**5895 Hallmark Healthcare Corporation	33	10	153	4155	63	21634	325	24149	8168	284
★ VETERANS AFFAIRS MEDICAL CENTER, 300 Veterans Boulevard, Zip 79720–5500; tel. 915/263–7361; Cary D. Brown, Director (Total facility includes 40 beds in nursing home–type unit) **A**1 2 3 5 **F**2 3 4 5 8 9 10 11 16 19 20 21 22 23 27 31 33 34 35 37 39 40 41 42 43 44 45 46 48 49 50 51 52 58 60 64 65 69 71 72 73 **S**9295 Department of Veterans Affairs	45	10	249	2890	137	37540	0	—	—	414
BONHAM—Fannin County										
☐ NORTHEAST MEDICAL CENTER, 504 Lipscomb Boulevard, Zip 75418–4096, Mailing Address: P.O. Drawer C, Zip 75418; tel. 903/583–8585 **A**1 9 10 **F**8 12 19 22 27 28 30 32 34 35 37 44 46 65 71 73 **P**1 **S**1775 Health Management Associates	32	10	65	1220	16	—	0	10211	4118	145
★ SAM RAYBURN MEMORIAL VETERANS CENTER, (General Medical/Long Term Care) 1201 East Ninth Street, Zip 75418; tel. 903/583–2111; Charles C. Freeman, Director (Total facility includes 100 beds in nursing home–type unit) **A**1 **F**15 20 26 30 32 33 34 37 39 41 45 49 51 57 58 64 65 67 73 **S**9295 Department of Veterans Affairs	45	49	391	3033	323	49554	0	—	—	427

© 1995 AHA Guide

Hospitals, U.S. / TEXAS

Hospital, Address, Telephone, Administrator, Approval, Facility, and Physician Codes, Health Care System	Control	Service	Beds	Admissions	Census	Outpatient Visits	Births	Total	Payroll	Personnel
★ American Hospital Association (AHA) membership ☐ Joint Commission on Accreditation of Healthcare Organizations (JCAHO) accreditation + American Osteopathic Hospital Association (AOHA) membership ○ American Osteopathic Association (AOA) accreditation △ Commission on Accreditation of Rehabilitation Facilities (CARF) accreditation Control codes 61, 63, 64, 71, 72 and 73 indicate hospitals listed by AOHA, but not registered by AHA. For definition of numerical codes, see page A6										
BORGER—Hutchinson County ★ GOLDEN PLAINS COMMUNITY HOSPITAL, 200 South McGee Street, Zip 79007; tel. 806/273–1100; Larry J. Lehner, Chief Executive Officer **A**1 9 10 **F**7 8 12 19 22 23 28 33 34 35 36 40 44 46 50 63 65 67 70 71 73 **S**0585 Brim, Inc.	16	10	55	1472	14	16029	182	4909	3476	163
BOWIE—Montague County ★ BOWIE MEMORIAL HOSPITAL, 1000 Lamb Street, Zip 76230; tel. 817/872–1126; Joseph F. Sloan CHE, Chief Executive Officer **A**9 10 **F**14 15 16 19 22 28 32 33 35 37 44 49 65 71	16	10	44	1139	16	27367	0	5837	2940	139
BRADY—Mcculloch County HEART OF TEXAS MEMORIAL HOSPITAL, Nine Road, Zip 76825–1150, Mailing Address: P.O. Box 1150, Zip 76825–1150; tel. 915/597–2901; Windell M. McCord, Administrator **A**9 10 **F**11 19 24 32 34 41 44 49 64 70 71 73	16	10	27	611	7	8135	0	3656	1848	79
BRECKENRIDGE—Stephens County STEPHENS MEMORIAL HOSPITAL, 200 South Geneva Street, Zip 76424; tel. 817/559–2241; James Reese, Administrator **A**9 10 **F**7 8 19 22 26 30 32 34 40 44 49 64 65 71 73	13	10	33	1064	14	8651	43	4215	1711	99
BRENHAM—Washington County ★ TRINITY COMMUNITY MEDICAL CENTER OF BRENHAM, 700 Medical Parkway, Zip 77833; tel. 409/836–6173; John L. Simms, President **A**1 9 10 **F**7 11 14 15 19 22 23 28 30 32 37 40 44 48 49 65 71 **P**7 **S**5375 Franciscan Services Corporation	21	10	60	2030	27	17350	341	14074	5887	221
BROWNFIELD—Terry County ★ BROWNFIELD REGIONAL MEDICAL CENTER, 705 East Felt, Zip 79316–3439; tel. 806/637–3551; Mike Click, Administrator **A**1 9 10 **F**7 8 14 15 16 17 19 21 22 24 28 29 30 31 32 34 40 44 46 49 65 69 70 71 73	16	10	42	794	10	30028	139	6535	2474	124
BROWNSVILLE—Cameron County AMI BROWNSVILLE MEDICAL CENTER See Brownsville Medical Center ★ BROWNSVILLE MEDICAL CENTER, (Formerly AMI Brownsville Medical Center) 1040 West Jefferson Street, Zip 78520–5829, Mailing Address: Box 3590, Zip 78523–3590; tel. 210/544–1400; Robert Collette, Executive Director (Nonreporting) **A**1 9 10 **S**0063 TENET Healthcare Corporation	32	10	168	—	—	—	—	—	—	—
★ VALLEY REGIONAL MEDICAL CENTER, 1 Ted Hunt Boulevard, Zip 78521, Mailing Address: Box 3710, Zip 78521; tel. 210/831–9611; David Butler, Interim Chief Executive Officer (Total facility includes 13 beds in nursing home–type unit) **A**1 10 **F**4 7 8 10 12 14 15 16 19 21 22 24 25 28 30 32 34 35 37 38 39 40 41 43 44 48 63 64 65 67 71 72 73 74 **P**5 **S**0048 Columbia/HCA Healthcare Corporation	33	10	167	6782	89	30309	2337	41240	14247	463
BROWNWOOD—Brown County ★ BROWNWOOD REGIONAL MEDICAL CENTER, 1501 Burnet Drive, Zip 76801, Mailing Address: Box 760, Zip 76804; tel. 915/646–8541; Art Layne, Administrator and Chief Executive Officer (Total facility includes 20 beds in nursing home–type unit) **A**1 9 10 **F**7 8 10 12 14 15 16 17 19 21 22 23 24 25 26 28 30 32 34 35 36 37 39 40 41 42 44 45 46 48 49 51 52 54 57 58 59 60 63 64 65 67 71 73 74 **P**7 **S**0048 Columbia/HCA Healthcare Corporation	33	10	164	6427	106	94171	724	40113	14264	531
BRYAN—Brazos County ★ ST. JOSEPH REGIONAL HEALTH CENTER, 2801 Franciscan Drive, Zip 77802; tel. 409/776–3777; Sister Gretchen Kunz, President (Total facility includes 19 beds in nursing home–type unit) **A**1 9 10 **F**4 7 8 10 11 12 14 15 16 17 19 21 22 23 25 28 30 32 33 34 35 37 39 40 41 42 43 44 49 63 64 65 67 71 73 **P**7 8 **S**5375 Franciscan Services Corporation	21	10	172	9069	115	74469	1557	72544	28550	915
BURNET—Burnet County ☐ HIGHLAND LAKES MEDICAL CENTER, Highway 281 South, Zip 78611, Mailing Address: P.O. Box 840, Zip 78611; tel. 512/756–6000; Harrell L. Connelly, Administrator **A**1 9 10 **F**19 22 32 33 44 71	16	10	42	1070	11	17296	0	7170	2733	156
CAMERON—Milam County CENTRAL TEXAS HOSPITAL, 806 North Crockett, Zip 76520; tel. 817/697–6591; Louis West, President **A**9 10 **F**8 14 15 16 19 22 27 28 34 37 41 44 49 64 71	23	10	33	472	7	11946	40	3588	1457	61
CANADIAN—Hemphill County HEMPHILL COUNTY HOSPITAL, 1020 South Fourth Street, Zip 79014; tel. 806/323–6422; Robert Ezzell, Administrator **A**9 10 **F**8 15 16 22 26 27 28 32 33 36 39 44 45 46 49 51 64 65 71	16	10	19	228	4	9720	1	2702	1257	68
CANYON—Randall County ★ PALO DURO HOSPITAL, 2 Hospital Drive, Zip 79015–3199; tel. 806/655–7751; Tommye Wilhite R.N., Administrator **A**1 9 10 **F**2 3 7 8 15 16 17 19 22 26 31 32 33 34 36 39 40 44 45 49 54 56 58 65 67 71	16	10	49	1810	16	41003	124	8287	4026	165
CARRIZO SPRINGS—Dimmit County DIMMIT COUNTY MEMORIAL HOSPITAL, 704 Hospital Drive, Zip 78834; tel. 210/876–2424; Ernest Flores Jr., Administrator **A**9 10 **F**7 15 16 19 22 32 34 44 61 71	13	10	26	774	8	11767	16	4256	1959	109
CARROLLTON—Denton County ☐ TRINITY MEDICAL CENTER, 4343 North Josey Lane, Zip 75010; tel. 214/492–1010; Thomas E. Casaday, Chief Executive Officer **A**1 9 10 **F**4 7 8 10 11 12 15 16 19 21 22 23 26 28 30 32 33 34 35 37 38 39 40 41 42 44 45 49 61 63 65 66 67 71 72 73 74 **P**3 **S**0063 TENET Healthcare Corporation	33	10	125	4559	42	51164	1613	28163	11454	394

Hospitals, U.S. / TEXAS

Hospital, Address, Telephone, Administrator, Approval, Facility, and Physician Codes, Health Care System	Classi-fication Codes		Utilization Data					Expense (thousands) of dollars		
★ American Hospital Association (AHA) membership □ Joint Commission on Accreditation of Healthcare Organizations (JCAHO) accreditation + American Osteopathic Hospital Association (AOHA) membership ○ American Osteopathic Association (AOA) accreditation △ Commission on Accreditation of Rehabilitation Facilities (CARF) accreditation Control codes 61, 63, 64, 71, 72 and 73 indicate hospitals listed by AOHA, but not registered by AHA. For definition of numerical codes, see page A6	Control	Service	Beds	Admissions	Census	Outpatient Visits	Births	Total	Payroll	Personnel
CARTHAGE—Panola County □ PANOLA GENERAL HOSPITAL, 409 Cottage Road, Zip 75633, Mailing Address: Box 549, Zip 75633-0549; tel. 903/693-3841; Gary Mikeal Hudson, Administrator **A**1 9 10 **F**8 12 16 19 21 22 28 32 37 44 46 49 65 71 73	13	10	30	954	13	21507	0	7213	3421	148
CENTER—Shelby County □ MEMORIAL HOSPITAL, 602 Hurst Street, Zip 75935, Mailing Address: Box 1749, Zip 75935; tel. 409/598-2781; Anton P. Zurbrugg CHE, Administrator and Chief Executive Officer **A**1 9 10 **F**8 12 16 19 22 28 30 32 33 40 44 49 65 70 71 **S**0335 Park Healthcare Company	33	10	42	1429	13	22440	148	7244	3236	143
CENTER POINT—Kerr County ★ STARLITE VILLAGE HOSPITAL, Elm Pass Road, Zip 78010, Mailing Address: Box 317, Zip 78010-0317; tel. 210/634-2212; David L. Howard, Administrator **A**1 9 10 **F**2 3 19 21 35 56 58 59 65 71 **P**5	33	10	42	735	23	167	0	2877	1411	56
CHANNELVIEW—Harris County SUN BELT REGIONAL MEDICAL CENTER EAST See Sun Belt Regional Medical Center, Houston										
CHILDRESS—Childress County □ CHILDRESS REGIONAL MEDICAL CENTER, Highway 83 North, Zip 79201, Mailing Address: Box 1030, Zip 79201; tel. 817/937-6371; Frances T. Smith, Administrator **A**1 9 10 **F**15 16 19 21 22 27 30 31 32 34 39 40 44 45 46 49 65 70 71 73	16	10	35	908	10	29150	169	6089	2998	146
CHILLICOTHE—Hardeman County CHILLICOTHE HOSPITAL DISTRICT, 303 Avenue I, Zip 79225, Mailing Address: Box 370, Zip 79225; tel. 817/852-5131; Linda Hall, Administrator **A**9 10 **F**15 16 19 22 32 70	16	10	21	74	1	648	0	1010	503	26
CLARKSVILLE—Red River County ★ RED RIVER GENERAL HOSPITAL, Highway 82 West, Zip 75426, Mailing Address: Box 1270, Zip 75426; tel. 903/427-3851; James D. Luft, Executive Director **A**1 9 10 **F**11 14 15 19 21 22 28 29 32 44 45 46 65 71 73	16	10	36	1576	17	12860	0	5566	2332	122
CLEBURNE—Johnson County ★ WALLS REGIONAL HOSPITAL, 201 Walls Drive, Zip 76031; tel. 817/641-2551; Brent D. Magers, Administrator **A**1 9 10 **F**2 3 4 7 8 10 11 12 13 14 15 16 17 18 19 21 22 23 24 26 27 28 29 30 31 32 33 34 35 37 38 39 40 41 42 43 44 45 46 48 49 50 52 53 54 55 56 58 59 60 61 63 64 65 66 67 69 70 71 72 73 74 **P**2 3 4 **S**2345 Harris Methodist Health System	21	10	102	3403	29	64232	782	22886	7516	302
CLEVELAND—Liberty County □ CLEVELAND REGIONAL MEDICAL CENTER, 300 East Crockett Street, Zip 77327, Mailing Address: Box 1688, Zip 77328; tel. 713/593-1811; A. C. Buchanon, Administrator **A**1 9 10 **F**7 8 16 19 22 25 34 35 37 39 40 42 44 49 71 **P**5 7 8	32	10	104	2735	34	23711	92	21891	7188	260
CLIFTON—Bosque County ★ GOODALL-WITCHER HOSPITAL, 101 South Avenue T, Zip 76634, Mailing Address: Box 549, Zip 76634; tel. 817/675-8322; Jim B. Smith, Administrator (Total facility includes 13 beds in nursing home–type unit) **A**9 10 **F**15 19 21 22 28 30 32 33 34 37 40 44 49 51 64 65 70 71 73 **P**3	23	10	59	1455	25	5275	191	9214	3791	168
COLEMAN—Coleman County COLEMAN COUNTY MEDICAL CENTER, 310 South Pecos Street, Zip 76834; tel. 915/625-2135; John Stevens, Administrator **A**9 10 **F**14 15 16 19 22 34 36 49 71 73 **P**5	16	10	22	602	7	7461	0	2203	1185	56
COLLEGE STATION—Brazos County ★ BRAZOS VALLEY MEDICAL CENTER, 1604 Rock Prairie Road, Zip 77845, Mailing Address: P.O. Box 10000, Zip 77842-3500; tel. 409/764-5100; Steve Koran, Interim Chief Executive Officer **A**1 9 10 **F**7 8 19 21 22 23 24 26 30 31 32 35 37 40 44 63 65 71 **P**1 **S**0048 Columbia/HCA Healthcare Corporation	33	10	100	4252	42	38526	1361	22540	9793	279
COLORADO CITY—Mitchell County ★ MITCHELL COUNTY HOSPITAL, 1543 Chestnut Street, Zip 79512-3998; tel. 915/728-3431; Wendell Alford, Administrator **A**9 10 **F**14 15 16 19 22 32 34 44 64 65 71 73 **P**6 **S**0036 Lubbock Methodist Hospital System	16	10	33	682	9	32245	76	6451	2747	178
COLUMBUS—Colorado County □ COLUMBUS COMMUNITY HOSPITAL, 110 Shult Drive, Zip 78934, Mailing Address: Box 865, Zip 78934; tel. 409/732-2371; Robert Thomas, Administrator **A**1 9 10 **F**7 8 15 16 19 22 28 32 34 44 49 71	23	10	36	563	6	21094	91	4951	1951	95
COMANCHE—Comanche County COMANCHE COMMUNITY HOSPITAL, 211 South Austin Street, Zip 76442; tel. 915/356-5241; Don Hopkins, Administrator **A**9 10 **F**19 21 24 32 40 44 71	16	10	19	459	6	6463	5	3849	2086	84
COMMERCE—Hunt County PRESBYTERIAN HOSPITAL OF COMMERCE See Hunt Memorial Hospital District, Greenville										
CONROE—Montgomery County ★ DOCTORS HOSPITAL, 3205 West Davis, Zip 77304, Mailing Address: Box 1349, Zip 77305; tel. 409/756-0631; Duane K. Rossmann, Chief Executive Officer (Total facility includes 12 beds in nursing home–type unit) **A**1 10 **F**4 7 8 10 12 16 19 20 21 22 23 31 32 33 34 35 37 40 42 43 44 49 52 57 60 63 64 65 71 73 **P**8 **S**0048 Columbia/HCA Healthcare Corporation	33	10	84	2938	36	40204	689	19305	7991	226
★ MEDICAL CENTER HOSPITAL, 504 Medical Center Boulevard, Zip 77304, Mailing Address: Box 1538, Zip 77305-1538; tel. 409/539-1111; Duane K. Rossmann, Chief Executive Officer **A**1 3 9 10 **F**4 7 8 10 11 12 19 20 21 22 23 31 33 34 35 37 38 40 42 43 44 49 57 60 63 65 71 73 **P**8 **S**0048 Columbia/HCA Healthcare Corporation	33	10	178	7150	105	54084	1324	54696	21320	580

© 1995 AHA Guide

Hospitals, U.S. / TEXAS

Hospital, Address, Telephone, Administrator, Approval, Facility, and Physician Codes, Health Care System	Classification Codes		Utilization Data					Expense (thousands) of dollars		
★ American Hospital Association (AHA) membership ☐ Joint Commission on Accreditation of Healthcare Organizations (JCAHO) accreditation + American Osteopathic Hospital Association (AOHA) membership ○ American Osteopathic Association (AOA) accreditation △ Commission on Accreditation of Rehabilitation Facilities (CARF) accreditation Control codes 61, 63, 64, 71, 72 and 73 indicate hospitals listed by AOHA, but not registered by AHA. For definition of numerical codes, see page A6	Control	Service	Beds	Admissions	Census	Outpatient Visits	Births	Total	Payroll	Personnel
CORPUS CHRISTI—Nueces County										
★ BAY AREA MEDICAL CENTER, 7101 South Padre Island Drive, Zip 78412; tel. 512/985–1200; Stephen M. Erixon, Chief Executive Officer (Total facility includes 10 beds in nursing home–type unit) **A**9 10 **F**2 3 4 7 8 9 10 11 12 15 16 19 21 22 26 28 30 31 32 34 35 37 38 39 40 42 43 44 47 48 49 52 53 54 55 56 57 58 59 64 65 67 69 70 71 73 74 **P**1 **S**0048 Columbia/HCA Healthcare Corporation	32	10	149	5166	64	19807	1417	23502	14600	466
✠ BAYVIEW HOSPITAL, 6629 Wooldridge Road, Zip 78414; tel. 512/993–9700; Janie L. Harwood, Chief Executive Officer (Nonreporting) **A**1 9 10 **S**0048 Columbia/HCA Healthcare Corporation	33	22	68	—	—	—	—	—	—	—
☐ CHARTER BEHAVIORAL HEALTH SYSTEM–CORPUS CHRISTI, (Formerly Charter Hospital of Corpus Christi) 3126 Rodd Field Road, Zip 78414; tel. 512/993–8893; Steve Kamber, Administrator **A**1 9 10 **F**1 3 4 5 6 7 8 9 10 11 12 13 14 15 17 18 19 20 21 22 23 24 25 26 27 28 29 30 31 32 33 34 35 36 37 38 39 40 41 42 43 44 45 46 47 48 49 50 51 52 53 54 55 56 57 58 59 60 61 62 63 64 65 66 67 68 69 70 71 72 73 74 **P**1 **S**0695 Charter Medical Corporation	33	22	80	1309	47	12921	0	9784	3640	110
CHARTER HOSPITAL OF CORPUS CHRISTI See Charter Behavioral Health System–Corpus Christi										
✠ DOCTORS REGIONAL MEDICAL CENTER, 3315 South Alameda, Zip 78411, Mailing Address: P.O. Box 3828, Zip 78463–3828; tel. 512/857–1501; Steven Woerner, Chief Executive Officer **A**1 9 10 **F**2 3 4 7 10 12 15 16 19 20 21 22 23 25 26 27 28 29 30 31 32 34 35 37 38 39 40 41 42 43 44 45 46 49 52 53 54 55 56 57 58 59 64 65 69 70 71 73 74 **P**8 **S**0048 Columbia/HCA Healthcare Corporation	32	10	270	9273	121	27282	2835	52077	17795	622
✠ DRISCOLL CHILDREN'S HOSPITAL, 3533 South Alameda Street, Zip 78411, Mailing Address: Box 6530, Zip 78466–6530; tel. 512/850–5000; J. E. Ted Stibbards Ph.D., President and Chief Executive Officer **A**1 3 5 9 10 **F**4 5 10 12 14 15 16 17 19 20 21 22 25 27 28 29 30 31 32 33 34 35 38 39 42 43 44 47 49 51 60 63 65 66 67 68 69 71 72 73 74	23	50	166	7095	122	80249	0	53232	24144	1014
✠ MEMORIAL MEDICAL CENTER, 2606 Hospital Boulevard, Zip 78405–1818; tel. 512/881–4000; David S. Lopez FACHE, President and Chief Executive Officer (Total facility includes 35 beds in nursing home–type unit) **A**1 3 9 10 12 13 **F**2 4 5 7 8 9 10 11 12 14 15 16 17 18 19 20 21 22 25 26 27 28 29 30 31 32 34 35 37 39 40 41 42 43 44 45 46 48 50 51 52 53 54 55 56 57 58 59 60 63 64 65 69 71 72 73 **P**5 7	16	10	307	10316	191	141863	1067	89601	36957	1348
✠ NAVAL HOSPITAL, Zip 78419–5200; tel. 512/939–2685; Captain F. G. Barina Jr., Commanding Officer **A**1 **F**15 22 27 28 29 30 34 41 44 45 46 49 51 58 65 71 74 **S**9655 Department of Navy	43	10	25	2122	23	121580	0	34589	20987	506
✠ △ REHABILITATION HOSPITAL OF SOUTH TEXAS, 6226 Saratoga Boulevard, Zip 78414–3499; tel. 512/991–9690; Jonny F. Hipp, Chief Executive Officer **A**1 7 9 10 **F**2 3 4 7 8 10 12 15 16 19 20 21 22 25 26 27 28 29 31 32 34 35 37 38 39 40 41 42 43 44 45 46 48 49 52 53 54 55 56 57 58 59 64 65 69 71 73 74 **P**5 8 **S**0048 Columbia/HCA Healthcare Corporation	32	46	80	480	27	9951	0	9177	5119	163
✠ RIVERSIDE COMMUNITY HOSPITAL, 13725 Farm Road 624, Zip 78410; tel. 512/767–4300; Winston Borland, Chief Executive Officer (Total facility includes 7 beds in nursing home–type unit) **A**1 9 10 **F**7 8 15 19 20 21 22 24 25 28 31 32 34 37 40 41 44 48 49 63 64 65 66 71 **S**0048 Columbia/HCA Healthcare Corporation	33	10	81	2322	38	44285	110	18919	7363	312
✠ △ SPOHN HEALTH SYSTEM, 600 Elizabeth Street, Zip 78404–2235; tel. 512/881–3000; Sister Kathleen Coughlin, President **A**1 2 7 9 10 **F**1 4 7 8 10 11 12 14 15 17 19 21 22 24 26 28 29 30 31 32 33 34 35 37 39 40 41 42 43 44 45 46 48 60 63 65 66 67 70 71 73 74 **P**1 6 **S**5565 Incarnate Word Health Services	21	10	428	17028	287	88676	1722	151525	61090	1872
CORSICANA—Navarro County										
✠ NAVARRO REGIONAL HOSPITAL, 3201 West Highway 22, Zip 75110; tel. 903/872–4861; Harvey L. Fishero, Administrator **A**1 9 10 **F**7 8 10 11 14 15 16 19 20 22 23 28 30 31 35 37 40 41 42 44 48 49 64 65 71 73 **S**0048 Columbia/HCA Healthcare Corporation	33	10	148	4619	67	36439	446	25587	9548	364
CRANE—Crane County										
★ CRANE MEMORIAL HOSPITAL, 1310 South Alford, Zip 79731; tel. 915/558–3555; Jerry Varnado, Administrator **A**9 10 **F**14 16 22 34 44 71	13	10	28	99	1	6654	0	2981	1317	39
CROCKETT—Houston County										
✠ HOUSTON COUNTY HOSPITAL, 1100 Loop 304 East, Zip 75835–1810; tel. 409/544–2002; Kathleen S. Wegener, Administrator and Chief Executive Officer **A**1 9 10 **F**19 21 22 31 34 37 40 44 46 51 61 63 65 71 **S**0002 Quorum Health Group/Quorum Health Resources	16	10	50	1636	20	14689	153	7691	3221	146
CROSBYTON—Crosby County										
★ CROSBYTON CLINIC HOSPITAL, 710 West Main Street, Zip 79322; tel. 806/675–2382; Michael Johnson, Administrator and Chief Executive Officer **A**9 10 **F**8 15 16 19 22 24 29 30 32 45 46 49 69 71 **S**5425 St. Joseph Health System	23	10	35	998	15	20154	0	4515	2341	205
CUERO—De Witt County										
✠ CUERO COMMUNITY HOSPITAL, 2550N Esplanade at Hospital Dr, Zip 77954–0807, Mailing Address: P.O. Box 807, Zip 77954–0807; tel. 512/275–6191; Larry D. Krupala, Administrator **A**1 9 10 **F**7 8 14 15 19 21 22 28 30 31 32 34 37 39 40 41 44 45 49 65 66 71 73	16	10	49	2431	35	64701	179	11912	6008	302
DALHART—Dallam County										
✠ COON MEMORIAL HOSPITAL AND HOME, 1411 Denver Avenue, Zip 79022; tel. 806/249–4571; Larry Baggett, Chief Executive Officer **A**9 10 **F**7 8 14 15 17 18 19 21 22 26 28 29 30 34 36 39 40 44 45 49 53 60 65 70 71 73 **P**5	16	10	23	481	5	0	83	4118	1507	60

Hospitals, U.S. / TEXAS

Hospital, Address, Telephone, Administrator, Approval, Facility, and Physician Codes, Health Care System	Classification Codes		Utilization Data					Expense (thousands) of dollars		Personnel
★ American Hospital Association (AHA) membership □ Joint Commission on Accreditation of Healthcare Organizations (JCAHO) accreditation + American Osteopathic Hospital Association (AOHA) membership ○ American Osteopathic Association (AOA) accreditation △ Commission on Accreditation of Rehabilitation Facilities (CARF) accreditation Control codes 61, 63, 64, 71, 72 and 73 indicate hospitals listed by AOHA, but not registered by AHA. For definition of numerical codes, see page A6	Control	Service	Beds	Admissions	Census	Outpatient Visits	Births	Total	Payroll	Personnel

DALLAS—Dallas County

A. WEBB ROBERTS HOSPITAL See Baylor University Medical Center

★ BAYLOR CENTER FOR RESTORATIVE CARE, 3504 Swiss Avenue, Zip 75204; tel. 214/823–1684; Gerry Brueckner R.N., Administrator **A**9 10 **F**3 4 5 7 8 10 11 12 13 17 19 21 22 23 24 25 26 28 29 30 31 32 33 34 35 37 38 40 41 42 43 44 45 46 47 48 49 50 52 53 54 56 57 58 59 60 61 63 64 65 66 67 69 70 71 73 74 **P**3 5 7 8 **S**0095 Baylor Health Care System
 — 21 10 74 670 60 0 0 9384 4765 129

★ △ BAYLOR INSTITUTE FOR REHABILITATION, 3505 Gaston Avenue, Zip 75246–2018; tel. 214/826–7030; Judith C. Waterston, Administrator **A**3 7 10 **F**2 3 4 5 7 8 9 10 11 12 15 16 17 19 21 22 23 24 25 26 27 28 29 30 31 32 33 34 35 37 38 39 40 41 42 43 44 45 46 47 48 49 51 52 53 56 57 58 60 61 64 65 66 67 69 70 71 73 74 **P**5 7 **S**0095 Baylor Health Care System
 — 21 46 75 1098 67 8234 0 19989 9900 291

🌟 BAYLOR UNIVERSITY MEDICAL CENTER, (Includes A. Webb Roberts Hospital, Dallas, Texas; Carr P. Collins Hospital, Dallas, Texas; Erik and Margaret Jonsson Hospital, Dallas, Texas; George W. Truett Memorial Hospital, Dallas, Texas; Karl and Esther Hoblitzelle Memorial Hospital, Dallas, Texas) 3500 Gaston Avenue, Zip 75246–2088; tel. 214/820–0111; Boone Powell Jr., President **A**1 2 3 5 8 9 10 **F**2 4 5 6 7 9 10 11 15 17 18 19 21 22 23 24 26 28 29 30 31 32 33 34 35 36 37 38 39 40 41 42 43 44 46 47 48 49 52 53 54 55 56 58 59 60 61 63 64 65 66 67 69 70 71 73 74 **P**7 **S**0095 Baylor Health Care System
 — 21 10 922 34319 575 436969 3727 383930 155930 4878

CARR P. COLLINS HOSPITAL See Baylor University Medical Center

🌟 CHARLTON METHODIST HOSPITAL, 3500 West Wheatland Road, Zip 75237–3460, Mailing Address: Box 225357, Zip 75222–5357; tel. 214/296–2511; Kim N. Hollon, Executive Director and Senior Vice President **A**1 9 10 **F**3 4 7 8 10 14 15 17 19 21 22 23 24 28 30 31 34 35 37 39 40 41 42 43 44 49 51 54 55 56 60 63 65 67 69 70 71 73 74 **P**1 8 **S**2735 Methodist Hospitals of Dallas
 — 23 10 105 6704 86 76181 1026 39923 16970 538

🌟 CHILDREN'S MEDICAL CENTER OF DALLAS, 1935 Motor Street, Zip 75235; tel. 214/640–2000; George D. Farr, President and Chief Executive Officer **A**1 3 5 9 10 **F**4 10 13 15 16 17 19 20 21 22 25 27 28 30 31 32 34 35 39 41 42 43 44 45 46 47 49 51 52 53 54 55 56 58 59 63 65 66 67 69 70 71 73
 — 23 50 214 8742 131 152608 0 153872 75168 1984

🌟 DALLAS COUNTY HOSPITAL DISTRICT–PARKLAND MEMORIAL HOSPITAL, 5201 Harry Hines Boulevard, Zip 75235–7731; tel. 214/590–8000; Ron J. Anderson M.D., President and Chief Executive Officer **A**1 2 3 5 8 9 10 **F**4 5 7 8 9 10 11 12 15 16 17 18 19 20 21 22 23 25 26 27 28 30 31 34 35 37 38 39 40 41 42 43 45 46 47 48 49 51 52 54 55 56 57 58 60 61 63 65 68 69 70 71 73 74
 — 16 10 901 41529 643 812896 14268 429852 183673 6185

○ DALLAS FAMILY HOSPITAL, 2929 South Hampton Road, Zip 75224; tel. 214/330–4611; Gary A. Saff, Administrator **A**9 10 11 12 13 **F**3 4 7 8 10 11 12 17 19 20 21 22 23 28 30 31 32 33 35 37 39 40 41 42 43 44 45 46 48 49 52 53 54 55 56 57 58 59 60 61 64 65 66 67 69 71 73 74 **P**5 **S**9555 Universal Health Services, Inc.
 — 33 10 104 2172 32 35678 0 23098 9122 267

DALLAS SPECIALTY HOSPITAL See Healthsouth Medical Center

□ DOCTORS HOSPITAL OF DALLAS, 9440 Poppy Drive, Zip 75218; tel. 214/324–6100; C. E. Ward, Administrator (Total facility includes 18 beds in nursing home–type unit) **A**1 9 10 **F**3 4 8 10 12 14 15 16 19 21 23 27 28 29 30 31 32 33 34 35 37 40 42 43 44 45 46 49 52 54 55 56 57 63 64 65 67 70 71 73 **P**5 **S**0063 TENET Healthcare Corporation
 — 33 10 231 7668 127 39968 626 59771 22035 737

ERIK AND MARGARET JONSSON HOSPITAL See University Medical Center
GEORGE W. TRUETT MEMORIAL HOSPITAL See University Medical Center

□ GREEN OAKS HOSPITAL, 7808 Clodus Fields Drive, Zip 75251; tel. 214/991–9504; Thomas M. Collins, Administrator **A**1 9 10 **F**2 3 12 15 32 45 46 52 53 54 55 56 58 59 65 67 **P**5 **S**0395 Healthcare International, Inc.
 — 32 22 106 1096 31 6253 0 10161 3843 —

□ △ HEALTHSOUTH DALLAS REHABILITATION INSTITUTE, 9713 Harry Hines Boulevard, Zip 75220–5441; tel. 214/358–6000; Phillip L. Coppage, Administrator **A**1 3 7 9 10 **F**5 6 12 16 19 21 22 27 34 35 37 44 46 48 49 65 67 71 **S**0023 Healthsouth Corporation
 — 33 46 126 887 51 11647 0 21925 10317 266

HEALTHSOUTH MEDICAL CENTER, (Formerly Dallas Specialty Hospital) 2124 Research Row, Zip 75235; tel. 214/904–6100; (Data for 263 days) **A**10 **F**1 5 12 14 15 19 25 34 35 41 44 48 49 64 66 **P**5 8 **S**0023 Healthsouth Corporation
 — 33 10 96 419 9 3379 0 6613 1416 96

KARL AND ESTHER HOBLITZELLE MEMORIAL HOSPITAL See University Medical Center

★ MARY SHIELS HOSPITAL, 3515 Howell Street, Zip 75204; tel. 214/443–3000; Rob Shiels, Administrator **A**9 10 **F**34 44 45 46 49
 — 33 10 15 676 3 2836 0 5993 2775 75

🌟 MEDICAL ARTS HOSPITAL, 6161 Harry Hines Boulevard, Zip 75235; tel. 214/688–1111; Thomas Permetti, Chief Executive Officer **A**1 9 10 **F**12 16 19 22 27 34 35 39 44 46 49 65 **S**0048 Columbia/HCA Healthcare Corporation
 — 33 10 32 442 7 8933 0 10892 3552 144

🌟 △ MEDICAL CITY DALLAS HOSPITAL, 7777 Forest Lane, Zip 75230–2598; tel. 214/661–7000; C. W. Smith, Chief Operating Officer **A**1 2 7 9 10 **F**3 4 7 8 9 10 11 12 14 17 18 19 20 21 22 23 26 27 28 29 30 31 32 34 35 37 38 39 40 41 42 43 44 45 47 48 49 50 51 53 54 55 56 57 58 59 60 61 63 64 65 66 69 71 73 74 **P**5 **S**0048 Columbia/HCA Healthcare Corporation
 — 33 10 491 20410 273 94823 4097 195666 62220 1877

🌟 METHODIST MEDICAL CENTER, 1441 North Beckley Avenue, Zip 75203, Mailing Address: Box 655999, Zip 75265–5999; tel. 214/947–8181; John W. Carver FACHE, Executive Director **A**1 2 3 8 10 **F**4 7 8 10 11 14 15 17 19 21 22 24 28 30 31 33 34 35 37 38 39 40 41 43 44 45 46 48 49 51 60 61 63 65 67 69 70 71 73 74 **P**1 7 **S**2735 Methodist Hospitals of Dallas
 — 23 10 362 14262 270 126149 2029 127604 51596 1617

© 1995 AHA Guide

Hospitals, U.S. / TEXAS

Hospital, Address, Telephone, Administrator, Approval, Facility, and Physician Codes, Health Care System	Control	Service	Beds	Admissions	Census	Outpatient Visits	Births	Total	Payroll	Personnel
★ American Hospital Association (AHA) membership ☐ Joint Commission on Accreditation of Healthcare Organizations (JCAHO) accreditation + American Osteopathic Hospital Association (AOHA) membership ○ American Osteopathic Association (AOA) accreditation △ Commission on Accreditation of Rehabilitation Facilities (CARF) accreditation Control codes 61, 63, 64, 71, 72 and 73 indicate hospitals listed by AOHA, but not registered by AHA. For definition of numerical codes, see page A6										
☐ NORTH DALLAS REHABILITATION HOSPITAL, (Formerly Spring Creek Rehabilitation Hospital) 8383 Meadow Road, Zip 75231; tel. 214/891-0880; Carol T. Holguin, Administrator and Chief Executive Officer **A**1 9 10 **F**16 34 49	33	46	36	161	9	—	0	4249	1703	71
PEDIATRIC CENTER FOR RESTORATIVE CARE, 3301 Swiss Avenue, Zip 75204; tel. 214/828-4747; Geraldine Brueckner, Administrator (Data for 183 days) **A**10 **F**2 3 4 8 9 10 11 12 13 17 19 21 22 24 25 27 28 29 30 31 32 33 34 35 37 38 40 41 42 43 44 45 46 47 48 49 50 52 53 54 55 56 58 59 60 61 63 64 65 66 67 68 69 70 71 73 **P**1 3 4 5 7	21	50	26	31	2	3100	0	1639	783	—
★ △ PRESBYTERIAN HOSPITAL OF DALLAS, 8200 Walnut Hill Lane, Zip 75231-4402; tel. 214/345-6789; Mark H. Merrill, Executive Director (Total facility includes 52 beds in nursing home-type unit) **A**1 2 3 5 7 9 10 **F**2 3 4 5 6 7 8 10 11 12 15 16 17 19 21 22 23 24 25 26 28 29 30 31 32 33 34 35 37 38 40 41 42 43 44 46 48 49 51 52 54 55 56 57 58 59 60 61 62 64 65 71 73 74 **P**1 **S**1130 Presbyterian Healthcare System	23	10	558	20167	321	138181	3475	231671	82570	2850
☐ RHD MEMORIAL MEDICAL CENTER, Seven Medical Parkway, Zip 75234, Mailing Address: P.O. Box 819094, Zip 75381-9094; tel. 214/247-1000; James R. Shafer, Executive Director **A**1 10 **F**4 7 8 10 12 14 15 16 17 19 21 22 26 28 30 31 32 33 34 35 37 38 39 40 41 42 43 44 45 46 49 60 61 64 65 71 73 74 **P**1 3 5 7 8 **S**0063 TENET Healthcare Corporation	33	10	136	4986	75	56926	352	—	—	478
SPRING CREEK REHABILITATION HOSPITAL See North Dallas Rehabilitation Hospital										
★ ST. PAUL MEDICAL CENTER, 5909 Harry Hines Boulevard, Zip 75235; tel. 214/879-1000; Anthony L. Bunker, President **A**1 2 3 5 8 9 10 **F**2 3 4 5 7 8 10 11 12 13 15 16 17 19 21 22 23 24 25 27 28 29 30 31 32 33 34 35 37 38 40 41 42 43 44 45 49 51 52 53 54 55 56 57 58 59 60 61 64 65 67 69 71 73 74 **P**7 **S**1855 Daughters of Charity National Health System	21	10	383	14355	242	146074	2577	146231	63028	1892
★ TEXAS SCOTTISH RITE HOSPITAL FOR CHILDREN, (Pediatric Orthopedic and Pediatric Learning Disabilities) 2222 Welborn Street, Zip 75219-0567, Mailing Address: Box 190567, Zip 75219-0567; tel. 214/521-3168; J. C. Montgomery Jr., President **A**1 3 5 9 **F**5 17 19 20 24 28 34 41 45 65 71 73 **P**6	23	59	64	1952	24	36683	0	35468	—	506
★ TIMBERLAWN PSYCHIATRIC HOSPITAL, 4600 Samuell Boulevard, Zip 75228, Mailing Address: Box 151489, Zip 75315-1489; tel. 214/381-7181; Sheryl Howard, Executive Director **A**1 3 5 9 10 **F**2 3 15 16 34 52 53 54 55 56 57 58 59 65 **P**1	33	22	117	1455	66	46132	0	17624	9210	292
★ ○ TRI-CITY HEALTH CENTRE, 7525 Scyene Road, Zip 75227; tel. 214/381-7171; Danny Morten, Administrator **A**1 10 11 12 13 **F**7 8 10 14 15 16 17 19 21 22 25 26 27 32 33 34 35 37 40 42 44 46 49 57 58 63 65 71 73 **P**1 4	23	10	137	3016	39	49058	735	32926	12571	469
☐ VENCOR HOSPITAL – DALLAS, 1600 Abrams Road, Zip 75214-4499; tel. 214/818-2401 **A**1 10 **F**19 22 35 37 65 71 **S**0026 Vencor, Incorporated	33	10	55	273	45	0	0	9430	5129	174
★ VETERANS AFFAIRS MEDICAL CENTER, 4500 South Lancaster Road, Zip 75216-7167; tel. 214/376-5451; Alan G. Harper, Director (Nonreporting) **A**1 2 3 5 8 **S**9295 Department of Veterans Affairs	45	10	644	—	—	—	—	—	—	—
☐ ZALE LIPSHY UNIVERSITY HOSPITAL, 5151 Harry Hines Boulevard, Zip 75235-7786; tel. 214/590-3000; Robert B. Smith, President and Chief Executive Officer **A**1 3 5 8 9 10 **F**4 8 10 12 15 16 19 21 22 32 35 37 41 42 43 44 45 46 48 52 54 55 56 57 59 60 61 65 67 71 73 **P**7	23	10	119	4515	78	5991	0	59581	19790	447
DE LEON—Comanche County										
★ DE LEON HOSPITAL, 407 South Texas Avenue, Zip 76444, Mailing Address: Box 319, Zip 76444; tel. 817/893-2011; Michael K. Hare, Administrator **A**1 9 10 **F**7 8 14 16 19 21 22 28 34 35 37 40 44 46 49 65 70 71 73	16	10	18	1050	16	21229	78	5380	2465	105
DE SOTO—Dallas County										
☐ CEDARS HOSPITAL, 2000 North Old Hickory Trail, Zip 75115; tel. 214/298-7323; David E. Brown, Administrator **A**1 9 10 **F**2 3 26 34 41 45 52 53 54 55 56 57 58 59 65	33	22	66	850	32	2205	0	9743	3357	76
☐ HAVEN HOSPITAL, 800 Kirnwood Drive, Zip 75115-2092; tel. 214/709-3700; Dan Aranda, Chief Executive Officer **A**1 9 10 **F**2 3 12 14 15 16 26 52 53 54 55 57 58 59 65 67 **S**0405 Ramsay Health Care, Inc.	33	22	46	547	19	2668	0	5568	—	133
DECATUR—Wise County										
★ DECATUR COMMUNITY HOSPITAL, 2000 South FM 51, Zip 76234-9295; tel. 817/627-5921; Steve Summers, Administrator **A**1 9 10 **F**7 14 15 16 19 22 26 28 30 32 34 37 39 40 44 45 49 51 65 67 71 73 **P**5	14	10	50	1972	19	33722	313	9766	4560	202
DEL RIO—Val Verde County										
★ VAL VERDE MEMORIAL HOSPITAL, 801 Bedell Avenue, Zip 78840, Mailing Address: P.O. Box 1527, Zip 78840; tel. 210/775-8566; Scott D. Evans FACHE, Administrator **A**1 9 10 **F**7 8 15 16 19 21 22 27 32 33 34 35 36 37 40 44 45 46 65 71 73 **P**5 **S**2645 Memorial Healthcare System	16	10	78	3150	38	34588	854	14373	7631	307
DENISON—Grayson County										
★ TEXOMA MEDICAL CENTER, (Includes Texoma Medical Center, 401 East Hull Street, Denison, Texas, Zip 75020; tel. 903/465-5128) 1000 Memorial Drive, Zip 75020, Mailing Address: Box 890, Zip 75021-9988; tel. 903/465-2313; Arthur L. Hohenberger FACHE, President and Chief Executive Officer **A**1 9 10 **F**2 3 4 7 8 10 11 12 14 15 16 17 19 21 22 23 30 32 33 34 35 37 39 40 41 42 43 44 46 49 52 54 56 57 58 59 60 64 65 66 67 71 73 74 **P**1	23	10	156	5643	87	42102	427	49828	20551	706
DENTON—Denton County										
★ DENTON COMMUNITY HOSPITAL, (Formerly HCA Denton Community Hospital) 207 North Bonnie Brae, Zip 76201; tel. 817/898-7000; Scott Koenig, Chief Executive Officer **A**1 10 **F**4 7 8 10 14 19 21 22 23 28 30 31 32 33 35 37 40 42 44 49 56 63 65 66 67 71 73 **P**5 **S**0048 Columbia/HCA Healthcare Corporation	33	10	110	4553	56	26818	850	30127	10939	395

Hospitals, U.S. / TEXAS

Hospital, Address, Telephone, Administrator, Approval, Facility, and Physician Codes, Health Care System	Classification Codes		Utilization Data					Expense (thousands) of dollars		
★ American Hospital Association (AHA) membership □ Joint Commission on Accreditation of Healthcare Organizations (JCAHO) accreditation + American Osteopathic Hospital Association (AOHA) membership ○ American Osteopathic Association (AOA) accreditation △ Commission on Accreditation of Rehabilitation Facilities (CARF) accreditation Control codes 61, 63, 64, 71, 72 and 73 indicate hospitals listed by AOHA, but not registered by AHA. For definition of numerical codes, see page A6	Control	Service	Beds	Admissions	Census	Outpatient Visits	Births	Total	Payroll	Personnel
★ DENTON REGIONAL MEDICAL CENTER, 4405 North Interstate 35, Zip 76207; tel. 817/566–4000; Bob J. Haley, Executive Director **A**1 9 10 **F**4 7 8 10 11 12 15 16 17 19 20 21 22 23 25 28 30 32 33 35 36 40 42 43 44 48 49 52 57 59 60 64 65 70 71 73 74 **P**5 7 **S**0048 Columbia/HCA Healthcare Corporation HCA DENTON COMMUNITY HOSPITAL See Denton Community Hospital	33	10	297	4788	77	—	562	51824	16766	811
DENVER CITY—Yoakum County ★ YOAKUM COUNTY HOSPITAL, 412 Mustang Avenue, Zip 79323, Mailing Address: P.O. Drawer 1130, Zip 79323; tel. 806/592–5484; Edward Rodgers, Chief Executive Officer **A**9 10 **F**7 8 14 15 16 22 28 30 37 40 44 71	13	10	24	470	4	4702	65	—	—	60
DIMMITT—Castro County PLAINS MEMORIAL HOSPITAL, 310 West Halsell Street, Zip 79027, Mailing Address: Box 278, Zip 79027; tel. 806/647–2191; Stephen M. Goode, Administrator **A**9 10 **F**19 22 25 28 32 33 34 36 37 40 44 49 71	16	10	30	740	7	3616	84	3259	1549	86
DUMAS—Moore County ★ MEMORIAL HOSPITAL, 224 East Second Street, Zip 79029; tel. 806/935–7171; David D. Clark CHE, Administrator and Chief Executive Officer (Total facility includes 60 beds in nursing home–type unit) **A**1 9 10 **F**7 8 15 16 19 20 21 22 23 26 28 32 33 34 37 40 44 45 46 49 64 65 67 69 71 73	16	10	112	1794	77	30709	382	8820	3632	194
EAGLE LAKE—Colorado County ★ EAGLE LAKE COMMUNITY HOSPITAL, 600 South Austin Road, Zip 77434–3298, Mailing Address: P.O. Box 277, Zip 77434–0277; tel. 409/234–5571; James E. Buckner, Administrator **A**1 9 10 **F**7 8 14 15 16 19 22 28 30 32 40 70 71 73 **P**6	23	10	47	741	6	14325	152	4048	1819	90
EAGLE PASS—Maverick County ★ FORT DUNCAN MEDICAL CENTER, 350 South Adams Street, Zip 78852; tel. 210/757–7501; Don Spaulding, Administrator and Chief Executive Officer **A**9 10 **F**7 8 12 15 17 18 19 20 22 25 28 31 32 36 37 39 40 44 46 49 51 53 54 58 65 71 73 **S**0002 Quorum Health Group/Quorum Health Resources	16	10	57	3819	49	17032	1264	17270	7156	287
EASTLAND—Eastland County EASTLAND MEMORIAL HOSPITAL, 304 South Daugherty Street, Zip 76448, Mailing Address: Box 897, Zip 76448; tel. 817/629–2601; Marcia Carr, Administrator **A**9 10 **F**19 40 44 71	16	10	38	1403	14	13036	157	4320	2236	113
EDEN—Concho County CONCHO COUNTY HOSPITAL, Eaker and Burleson Streets, Zip 76837, Mailing Address: Box L, Zip 76837; tel. 915/869–5911; Albert M. Everett Jr., Administrator **A**9 10 **F**14 15 16 22 26 28 30 32 71 **P**1 2 3 4 5 6 7 8	16	10	20	367	5	1710	0	1382	672	34
EDINBURG—Hidalgo County ★ EDINBURG HOSPITAL, 333 West Freddy Gonzalez Drive, Zip 78539–6199; tel. 210/383–6211; Leon J. Belila, Administrator **A**1 9 10 **F**8 14 15 16 17 19 21 22 28 30 34 37 40 44 48 49 65 70 71 73 **P**5 **S**9555 Universal Health Services, Inc.	16	10	112	3795	50	31397	1210	24786	10033	342
EDNA—Jackson County ★ JACKSON COUNTY HOSPITAL, 1013 South Wells Street, Zip 77957, Mailing Address: P.O. Box 670, Zip 77957; tel. 512/782–5241; Bill Johnson, District Administrator **A**9 10 **F**8 15 16 19 22 32 34 44 69 71 73	16	10	31	610	6	17144	0	4602	1882	89
EL CAMPO—Wharton County ★ EL CAMPO MEMORIAL HOSPITAL, 303 Sandy Corner Road, Zip 77437; tel. 409/543–6251; Corinne L. Maib, Interim Administrator **A**1 9 10 **F**8 12 19 21 22 33 34 37 44 51 71 73 **S**0048 Columbia/HCA Healthcare Corporation	33	10	60	817	10	21856	0	5576	2219	93
EL PASO—El Paso County ★ COLUMBIA BEHAVIORAL CENTER, 1155 Idaho Street, Zip 79902–1699; tel. 915/544–4000; David M. Polunas, Administrator **A**9 10 **F**1 2 3 4 7 8 9 10 11 12 15 16 17 18 19 20 21 22 23 24 25 26 27 28 30 31 32 34 35 37 38 39 40 41 42 43 44 46 48 49 52 53 54 55 56 57 58 59 60 63 64 65 66 67 68 71 73 74 **P**1 **S**0048 Columbia/HCA Healthcare Corporation	33	22	117	1437	42	9349	0	10502	5535	130
★ COLUMBIA MEDICAL CENTER–EAST, 10301 Gateway West, Zip 79925–7798, Mailing Address: P.O. Box 937003, Zip 79937–1690; tel. 915/595–9000; Douglas A. Matney, Chief Executive Officer **A**1 9 10 **F**2 3 4 7 8 9 10 11 12 16 18 19 20 21 22 23 24 25 26 27 28 29 30 31 32 33 34 35 37 38 39 40 41 42 43 44 45 46 48 49 52 53 54 55 56 57 58 59 60 63 64 65 66 67 68 71 73 74 **P**8 **S**0048 Columbia/HCA Healthcare Corporation	32	10	266	9246	167	85009	1397	75340	30891	967
★ COLUMBIA MEDICAL CENTER–WEST, 1801 North Oregon Street, Zip 79902; tel. 915/521–1200; Ray Fusco, Chief Executive Officer (Total facility includes 18 beds in nursing home–type unit) **A**1 9 10 **F**2 3 4 7 8 9 10 11 12 15 16 18 19 20 21 22 23 24 25 26 27 28 30 31 32 34 35 37 38 39 40 41 42 43 44 45 46 48 49 52 53 54 55 56 57 58 59 60 63 64 65 66 67 68 71 73 74 **P**1 **S**0048 Columbia/HCA Healthcare Corporation	32	10	212	6770	127	50608	365	79717	27103	1156
★ COLUMBIA REHABILITATION HOSPITAL, 300 Waymore, Zip 77902; tel. 915/577–2600; William G. Collins, Chief Executive Officer (Nonreporting) **S**0048 Columbia/HCA Healthcare Corporation	33	46	40	—	—	—	—	—	—	—
★ PROVIDENCE MEMORIAL HOSPITAL, 2001 North Oregon Street, Zip 79902; tel. 915/577–6011; David P. Buchmueller, President and Chief Executive Officer **A**1 2 5 10 **F**4 7 8 10 11 12 14 15 16 17 19 21 22 25 28 29 30 31 32 33 34 35 37 38 40 41 42 43 44 47 48 49 61 63 64 65 68 69 71 73 74 **P**5 7 8	23	10	383	16840	260	107880	3860	145571	57633	1944
□ R. E. THOMASON GENERAL HOSPITAL, 4815 Alameda Avenue, Zip 79905, Mailing Address: Box 20009, Zip 79998; tel. 915/544–1200; Pete Duarte, Chief Executive Officer **A**1 2 3 5 9 10 **F**3 4 8 10 11 14 15 16 17 19 20 21 22 27 28 33 35 37 38 39 40 41 42 43 44 45 46 47 49 52 53 54 55 56 57 58 59 60 61 65 68 70 71 73	16	10	299	14878	217	281869	6790	102617	38740	1336

© 1995 AHA Guide

Hospitals, U.S. / TEXAS

Hospital, Address, Telephone, Administrator, Approval, Facility, and Physician Codes, Health Care System	Classi-fication Codes		Utilization Data					Expense (thousands) of dollars		
★ American Hospital Association (AHA) membership ☐ Joint Commission on Accreditation of Healthcare Organizations (JCAHO) accreditation + American Osteopathic Hospital Association (AOHA) membership ○ American Osteopathic Association (AOA) accreditation △ Commission on Accreditation of Rehabilitation Facilities (CARF) accreditation Control codes 61, 63, 64, 71, 72 and 73 indicate hospitals listed by AOHA, but not registered by AHA. For definition of numerical codes, see page A6	Control	Service	Beds	Admissions	Census	Outpatient Visits	Births	Total	Payroll	Personnel
☒ △ RIO VISTA REHABILITATION HOSPITAL, 1740 Curie Drive, Zip 79902; tel. 915/543–6826; Patsy A. Parker, Administrator and Chief Executive Officer **A**1 7 9 10 **F**4 7 8 10 11 12 15 16 19 20 21 22 28 29 30 31 32 35 37 38 40 44 45 46 47 48 49 60 63 65 66 67 69 71 73 74	33	46	100	965	69	22633	0	23745	11727	318
☐ SIERRA MEDICAL CENTER, 1625 Medical Center Drive, Zip 79902–5044; tel. 915/747–4000; L. Marcus Fry Jr., Chief Executive Officer **A**1 2 9 10 **F**4 7 8 10 11 12 15 16 19 20 21 22 28 29 30 31 32 34 35 36 37 38 39 40 41 42 43 44 45 46 47 48 49 60 63 65 66 67 69 71 73 74 **P**7 8 **S**0063 TENET Healthcare Corporation	33	10	365	12212	185	82850	2532	125393	37008	1169
☐ SOUTHWESTERN GENERAL HOSPITAL, 1221 North Cotton, Zip 79902-3096; tel. 915/533–9361; Stephen J. Campbell, Administrator **A**1 10 **F**7 15 16 17 19 22 28 31 34 37 40 44 46 49 65 71 74	32	10	102	2269	23	14588	153	12691	5476	186
☒ WILLIAM BEAUMONT ARMY MEDICAL CENTER, Zip 79920–5001; tel. 915/569–2121; Colonel Thomas J. Scully, Medical Corps Commanding **A**1 2 3 5 **F**2 3 8 10 11 12 13 14 15 16 19 20 21 22 24 25 29 31 35 37 38 39 40 42 44 45 46 49 51 52 53 54 55 56 58 60 61 65 70 71 73 74 **S**9395 Department of the Army	42	10	320	13167	173	606509	1520	—	—	2585
ELDORADO—Schleicher County										
SCHLEICHER COUNTY MEDICAL CENTER, 305 Mertzon Highway, Zip 76936, Mailing Address: Box V, Zip 76936; tel. 915/853–2507; James G. Blum, Administrator **A**9 10 **F**1 22 28 45 49 65 73 **P**6	16	10	16	73	9	4756	0	1243	578	41
ELECTRA—Wichita County										
ELECTRA MEMORIAL HOSPITAL, 1207 South Bailey Street, Zip 76360, Mailing Address: Box 1112, Zip 76360-1112; tel. 817/495–3981; Jan A. Reed CPA, Administrator **A**9 10 **F**15 16 22 26 28 30 31 32 34 39 41 44 45 49 65 71 73	16	10	23	290	4	13247	0	2255	961	54
ENNIS—Ellis County										
BAYLOR MEDICAL CENTER–ELLIS COUNTY See Baylor Medical Center–Ellis County, Waxahachie										
FAIRFIELD—Freestone County										
FAIRFIELD MEMORIAL HOSPITAL, 125 Newman Street, Zip 75840; tel. 903/389–2121; Milton W. Meadows, Administrator **A**9 10 **F**15 16 19 22 25 28 30 33 34 37 44 71	16	10	15	353	6	4919	0	2546	1157	55
FALFURRIAS—Brooks County										
★ BROOKS COUNTY HOSPITAL, 1400 South St. Mary's Street, Zip 78355; tel. 512/325–2511; Iris Almendarez, Chief Executive Officer **A**9 10 **F**11 14 15 30 34 40 71	13	10	31	415	5	8154	1	3023	1319	72
FLORESVILLE—Wilson County										
WILSON MEMORIAL HOSPITAL, 1301 Hospital Boulevard, Zip 78114; tel. 210/393–3122; Harry McClain, Administrator **A**9 10 **F**8 19 21 22 32 33 44 46 49 65 71 73	16	10	30	479	8	28860	0	4133	1785	80
FORT HOOD—Bell County										
☒ DARNALL ARMY COMMUNITY HOSPITAL, Zip 76544-5063; tel. 817/288–8000; Colonel William F. Hughes MC, USA, Commander **A**1 2 3 5 **F**1 3 4 7 8 9 10 11 12 13 14 15 16 18 19 20 21 22 23 25 26 28 29 30 31 32 33 34 35 37 38 39 40 41 42 43 44 46 48 49 51 52 53 54 56 58 59 60 61 65 66 67 69 70 71 73 74 **P**6 **S**9395 Department of the Army	42	10	220	14126	98	823218	3461	67437	—	1546
FORT STOCKTON—Pecos County										
☒ PECOS COUNTY MEMORIAL HOSPITAL, Sanderson Highway, Zip 79735, Mailing Address: Box 1648, Zip 79735; tel. 915/336–2241; George N. Miller Jr., Administrator and Chief Executive Officer **A**1 9 10 **F**7 10 12 13 14 15 16 17 19 22 24 27 28 29 30 32 34 39 40 44 45 46 49 65 70 71 72 73 74	13	10	28	1065	11	14262	219	7801	3281	172
FORT WORTH—Tarrant County										
☒ ALL SAINTS EPISCOPAL HOSPITAL OF FORT WORTH, 1400 Eighth Avenue, Zip 76104, Mailing Address: P.O. Box 31, Zip 76101; tel. 817/926–2544; James P. Schuessler, President and Chief Executive Officer (Total facility includes 32 beds in nursing home–type unit) **A**1 9 10 **F**2 3 4 7 8 10 11 12 14 15 16 17 18 19 22 24 25 26 27 28 29 30 32 33 34 35 37 38 39 40 41 42 43 44 45 46 48 49 52 53 54 55 56 57 58 59 60 61 64 65 66 67 71 72 73 74 **P**3 4 5 7 8	23	10	336	12695	201	46662	1973	107324	48645	1580
★ ALL SAINTS HOSPITAL–CITYVIEW, 7100 Oakmont Boulevard, Zip 76132; tel. 817/346–5870; Marcia Swinson, Administrator (Nonreporting)	23	10	43	—	—	—	—	—	—	—
☐ CAREUNIT HOSPITAL OF DALLAS–FORT WORTH, 1066 West Magnolia Avenue, Zip 76104; tel. 817/336–2828; Dorothy Grasty, Administrator (Nonreporting) **A**1 9 10	33	22	83	—	—	—	—	—	—	—
☐ CHARTER BEHAVIORAL HEALTH SYSTEM, 6201 Overton Ridge Boulevard, Zip 76132-3699; tel. 817/292–6844; Liam J. Mulvaney, Chief Executive Officer **A**1 9 10 **F**3 12 14 15 16 34 45 46 52 53 54 55 57 58 59 65 67 **P**7 **S**0695 Charter Medical Corporation	33	22	80	1250	32	6186	0	6750	3114	92
☐ COOK–FORT WORTH CHILDREN'S MEDICAL CENTER, 801 Seventh Avenue, Zip 76104-2796; tel. 817/885–4000; Russell K. Tolman, President **A**1 3 10 **F**10 12 13 15 16 17 18 19 20 21 22 25 27 28 29 30 31 32 33 34 35 38 39 41 42 43 44 45 46 47 48 49 51 52 53 55 56 58 59 60 63 65 66 67 68 69 70 71 73 **P**3 4	23	50	181	6719	122	99776	0	101084	43608	1296
☒ △ FORT WORTH REHABILITATION HOSPITAL, 6701 Oakmont Boulevard, Zip 76132; tel. 817/370–4700; Joseph F. Pitingolo Jr., Chief Executive Officer (Total facility includes 12 beds in nursing home–type unit) **A**1 7 9 10 **F**5 12 14 16 19 21 22 27 28 35 41 45 46 48 49 50 63 64 65 71	33	46	60	728	48	8401	0	13259	5664	155

Hospitals, U.S. / TEXAS

Hospital, Address, Telephone, Administrator, Approval, Facility, and Physician Codes, Health Care System	Classification Codes		Utilization Data					Expense (thousands) of dollars		
★ American Hospital Association (AHA) membership □ Joint Commission on Accreditation of Healthcare Organizations (JCAHO) accreditation + American Osteopathic Hospital Association (AOHA) membership ○ American Osteopathic Association (AOA) accreditation △ Commission on Accreditation of Rehabilitation Facilities (CARF) accreditation Control codes 61, 63, 64, 71, 72 and 73 indicate hospitals listed by AOHA, but not registered by AHA. For definition of numerical codes, see page A6	Control	Service	Beds	Admissions	Census	Outpatient Visits	Births	Total	Payroll	Personnel
★ △ HARRIS CONTINUED CARE HOSPITAL, (Long Term Subacute Care) 1301 Pennsylvania Avenue, 4th Fl, Zip 76104, Mailing Address: P.O. Box 3471, Zip 76113; tel. 817/878–5500; Karen Van Wagner Ph.D., Administrator A1 7 10 F2 3 4 7 8 10 11 12 13 16 17 18 19 21 22 23 24 26 27 28 29 30 31 32 33 34 35 37 38 39 40 41 42 43 44 45 46 47 48 49 50 52 53 54 55 56 57 58 59 60 61 63 64 65 66 67 69 70 71 72 73 74 P2 3 4 S2345 Harris Methodist Health System	21	49	10	63	5	0	0	3659	1171	44
★ HARRIS METHODIST FORT WORTH, 1301 Pennsylvania Avenue, Zip 76104–2895; tel. 817/882–2000; Barclay E. Berdan, Administrator A1 2 3 7 9 10 F2 3 4 7 8 10 11 12 13 14 15 16 17 18 19 21 22 23 24 26 27 28 29 30 31 32 33 34 35 37 38 39 40 41 42 43 44 45 46 47 48 49 50 52 53 54 55 56 58 59 60 61 63 64 65 66 67 69 70 71 72 73 74 P2 3 4 S2345 Harris Methodist Health System	21	10	581	22303	320	84194	4302	195121	69792	2602
★ HARRIS METHODIST SOUTHWEST, 6100 Harris Parkway, Zip 76132; tel. 817/346–5050; Kim Callanan, Senior Vice President and Administrator A1 9 10 F2 3 4 7 8 10 11 12 13 14 15 16 17 18 19 21 22 23 24 26 27 28 29 30 31 32 33 34 35 37 38 39 40 41 42 43 44 45 46 47 48 49 50 51 52 53 54 55 56 58 59 60 61 63 64 65 66 67 69 70 71 72 73 74 P2 3 4 S2345 Harris Methodist Health System	21	10	58	3421	25	46429	1412	26792	8933	360
□ △ HEALTHSOUTH REHABILITATION HOSPITAL, 1212 West Lancaster, Zip 76102; tel. 817/870–2336; Laura J. Lycan, Administrator (Total facility includes 15 beds in nursing home–type unit) A1 7 9 10 F5 14 16 34 48 49 64 S0023 Healthsouth Corporation	33	46	60	409	26	3697	0	7782	3690	111
★ HUGULEY MEMORIAL MEDICAL CENTER, 11801 South Freeway, Zip 76115, Mailing Address: Box 6337, Zip 76115–0337; tel. 817/293–9110; A. David Jimenez, President and Chief Executive Officer (Total facility includes 33 beds in nursing home–type unit) A1 9 10 F2 3 7 8 10 11 12 13 14 15 16 17 19 22 23 24 25 26 28 29 30 32 33 34 35 37 38 39 40 41 42 44 45 46 47 49 51 52 53 54 55 56 57 58 59 60 63 64 65 67 71 73 74 P1 3 7 S4165 Adventist Health System–Sunbelt Health Care Corporation	21	10	213	5800	81	—	1005	59444	22261	892
JOHN PETER SMITH HOSPITAL See Tarrant County Hospital District										
□ + ○ OSTEOPATHIC MEDICAL CENTER OF TEXAS, 1000 Montgomery Street, Zip 76107; tel. 817/731–4311; Jay E. Sandelin, Chief Executive Officer (Total facility includes 19 beds in nursing home–type unit) A1 9 10 11 12 13 F4 7 8 10 11 12 13 14 15 16 17 19 21 22 24 26 27 28 30 31 32 33 34 35 37 39 40 41 42 43 44 46 48 49 52 53 54 55 56 57 61 64 65 71 73 P1 3 5 7	23	10	182	6766	120	59707	936	80137	26624	813
★ △ PLAZA MEDICAL CENTER–EAST, (Formerly Saint Joseph Hospital) 1401 South Main Street, Zip 76104–4945; tel. 817/347–4700; Wayne S. Heatherly, President and Chief Executive Officer (Nonreporting) A1 7 9 10 S0048 Columbia/HCA Healthcare Corporation	21	10	228	—	—	—	—	—	—	—
★ PLAZA MEDICAL CENTER–WEST, 900 Eighth Avenue, Zip 76104–3986; tel. 817/336–2100; Wayne S. Heatherly, Chief Executive Officer A1 9 10 F1 2 3 4 5 6 7 8 9 10 11 12 13 15 17 18 19 20 21 22 23 24 25 26 27 28 29 30 31 32 33 34 35 36 37 38 39 40 41 42 43 44 45 46 47 48 49 50 51 52 54 55 56 57 58 59 60 61 62 63 64 65 66 67 68 69 70 71 72 73 74 P4 5 7 8 S0048 Columbia/HCA Healthcare Corporation	33	10	599	8046	140	18155	292	66340	27742	1256
SAINT JOSEPH HOSPITAL See Plaza Medical Center–East										
★ TARRANT COUNTY HOSPITAL DISTRICT, (Includes John Peter Smith Hospital, Fort Worth, Texas) 1500 South Main Street, Zip 76104–4941; tel. 817/921–3431; Marion Timothy Philpot, President and Chief Executive Officer A1 3 5 9 10 F4 7 8 10 12 16 17 19 20 21 22 23 25 27 28 30 31 32 33 34 35 37 38 40 41 42 43 44 46 51 52 53 54 55 56 58 59 60 61 63 65 67 68 71 73 74 P5 S0039 Tarrant County Hospital District	16	10	360	13832	261	394481	4618	178034	69411	2729
TARRANT COUNTY PSYCHIATRIC CENTER, 1527 Hemphill Street, Zip 76104; tel. 817/923–6467; Connie Oliverson Perra, Director (Nonreporting) A10	16	22	39	—	—	—	—	—	—	—
★ TRINITY SPRINGS PAVILION–EAST, 1500 South Main Street, Zip 76104–4917; tel. 817/927–3636; Robert Bourassa, Executive Director (Nonreporting) S0039 Tarrant County Hospital District	16	52	39	—	—	—	—	—	—	—
TWIN OAKS MEDICAL CENTER, 2919 Markum Drive, Zip 76117–0729, Mailing Address: Box 14729, Zip 76117–0729; tel. 817/831–0311; Lawrence Wedekind, Administrator (Nonreporting) A9 10	33	10	34	—	—	—	—	—	—	—
VENCOR HOSPITAL–FORT WORTH SOUTH See Vencor Hospital–Fort Worth, Mansfield										
FREDERICKSBURG—Gillespie County										
★ HILL COUNTRY MEMORIAL HOSPITAL, 1020 Kerrville Road, Zip 78624, Mailing Address: Box 835, Zip 78624–0835; tel. 210/997–4353; Jerry L. Durr, Administrator A1 9 10 F7 8 15 16 19 21 22 23 24 29 30 32 33 34 35 37 40 42 44 46 49 63 65 70 71 P8	23	10	58	2904	32	32995	391	15654	7160	308
FRIONA—Parmer County										
PARMER COUNTY COMMUNITY HOSPITAL, 1307 Cleveland Street, Zip 79035; tel. 806/247–2754; Bill J. Neely, Administrator A9 10 F8 15 19 22 30 32 33 34 36 71	23	10	26	330	4	10497	0	3153	1148	59
GAINESVILLE—Cooke County										
GAINESVILLE MEMORIAL HOSPITAL, 1016 Ritchey Street, Zip 76240–3539; tel. 817/665–1751; Gerald Culwell, Administrator (Total facility includes 22 beds in nursing home–type unit) A9 10 F17 19 22 31 32 35 37 44 45 64 71 73	16	10	50	2186	29	—	283	11195	5839	269

© 1995 AHA Guide

Hospitals, U.S. / TEXAS

Hospital, Address, Telephone, Administrator, Approval, Facility, and Physician Codes, Health Care System	Classification Codes		Utilization Data					Expense (thousands) of dollars		Personnel
★ American Hospital Association (AHA) membership □ Joint Commission on Accreditation of Healthcare Organizations (JCAHO) accreditation + American Osteopathic Hospital Association (AOHA) membership ○ American Osteopathic Association (AOA) accreditation △ Commission on Accreditation of Rehabilitation Facilities (CARF) accreditation Control codes 61, 63, 64, 71, 72 and 73 indicate hospitals listed by AOHA, but not registered by AHA. For definition of numerical codes, see page A6	Control	Service	Beds	Admissions	Census	Outpatient Visits	Births	Total	Payroll	
GALVESTON—Galveston County										
★ SHRINERS HOSPITALS FOR CRIPPLED CHILDREN, GALVESTON BURNS INSTITUTE, 815 Market Street, Zip 77550–2725; tel. 409/770–6600; John A. Swartwout, Administrator **A**1 3 5 **F**9 12 19 34 35 46 54 65 71 73 **S**4125 Shriners Hospitals for Crippled Children	23	59	30	780	19	3241	0	—	—	284
★ ST. MARY'S HOSPITAL, 404 St. Mary's Boulevard, Zip 77550; tel. 409/763–5301; James E. Gardner Jr., Administrator (Total facility includes 21 beds in nursing home–type unit) **A**1 9 10 **F**2 3 7 8 12 15 17 18 19 20 21 22 32 34 35 37 40 41 42 44 46 49 52 56 58 59 63 64 65 70 71 73 74 **P**3 5 6 7 8 **S**0605 Sisters of Charity of the Incarnate Word Healthcare System	21	10	235	3513	65	28877	226	36314	15595	387
★ UNIVERSITY OF TEXAS MEDICAL BRANCH HOSPITALS, 301 University Boulevard, Zip 77555–0138; tel. 409/772–1011; James F. Arens M.D., Vice President Clinical Affairs and Chief Executive Officer **A**1 2 3 5 8 9 10 **F**1 3 4 7 8 9 10 11 12 15 16 17 19 20 21 22 23 24 26 27 28 30 31 32 33 34 35 37 39 40 41 42 43 44 46 47 48 49 51 52 53 54 55 56 57 58 59 60 61 63 65 69 70 71 73 74 **P**5 6 **S**0033 University of Texas Hospitals	12	10	860	29934	593	437178	4218	373904	170964	5551
GARLAND—Dallas County										
★ BAYLOR MEDICAL CENTER AT GARLAND, 2300 Marie Curie Boulevard, Zip 75042–5706; tel. 214/487–5000; Gary D. Brock, Executive Director (Total facility includes 13 beds in nursing home–type unit) **A**1 9 10 **F**4 7 8 10 11 12 15 16 19 20 21 22 24 25 26 27 28 29 30 32 34 35 37 38 39 40 41 42 43 44 45 46 47 48 49 51 52 53 54 55 56 58 60 61 64 65 66 67 69 70 71 73 74 **P**6 7 8 **S**0095 Baylor Health Care System	23	10	159	6274	82	62824	1112	46437	20109	660
□ GARLAND COMMUNITY HOSPITAL, 2696 West Walnut Street, Zip 75042; tel. 214/276–7116; Gary L. Stokes, Administrator and Chief Executive Officer **A**1 9 10 **F**2 3 8 10 16 19 21 22 26 27 28 30 32 33 35 37 39 41 44 49 53 54 55 56 57 58 59 63 64 65 71 73 **S**6525 Ornda Healthcorp	32	10	113	2198	39	62104	0	26312	10382	362
GATESVILLE—Coryell County										
★ CORYELL MEMORIAL HOSPITAL, 1507 West Main Street, Zip 76528, Mailing Address: P.O. Box 659, Zip 76528; tel. 817/865–8251; Matt Maxfield, Administrator **A**1 9 10 **F**15 16 19 22 32 37 44 51 65 71 73 **P**6	16	10	44	815	13	—	0	7781	3895	261
GEORGETOWN—Williamson County										
★ GEORGETOWN HOSPITAL, 2000 Scenic Drive, Zip 78626; tel. 512/863–6531; Kenneth W. Poteete, President and Chief Executive Officer **A**1 9 10 **F**2 7 8 14 15 16 19 21 22 28 30 32 34 37 39 40 41 42 44 49 60 64 65 67 71 73	16	10	98	2631	29	27387	566	15260	7354	409
GILMER—Upshur County										
★ GILMER MEDICAL CENTER, 712 North Wood Street, Zip 75644; tel. 903/843–5611; Al Chapa, Administrator **A**1 9 10 **F**8 10 11 15 19 22 24 28 30 32 34 35 37 38 40 44 45 47 48 49 52 57 66 71 72 73 **P**7 8 **S**0048 Columbia/HCA Healthcare Corporation	33	10	40	1186	22	27283	0	8302	3133	128
GLEN ROSE—Somervell County										
★ GLEN ROSE MEDICAL CENTER, 1021 Holden Street, Zip 76043, Mailing Address: Box 2099, Zip 76043; tel. 817/897–2215; Gary A. Marks, Administrator (Total facility includes 42 beds in nursing home–type unit) (Data for 273 days) **A**1 9 10 **F**14 16 19 21 22 26 28 31 32 33 35 44 46 49 64 65 70 71	13	10	58	425	76	6509	0	4151	1690	43
GOLIAD—Goliad County										
GOLIAD COUNTY HOSPITAL, 303 West Franklin Street, Zip 77963, Mailing Address: P.O. Drawer 938, Zip 77963; tel. 512/645–8221; Bob Lively, Administrator **A**9 10 **F**19 22 34 44 71	13	10	20	113	1	1304	0	—	—	40
GONZALES—Gonzales County										
MEMORIAL HOSPITAL, Highway 90 A By–Pass, Zip 78629, Mailing Address: Box 587, Zip 78629; tel. 210/672–7581; Douglas Langley, Administrator **A**9 10 **F**8 14 15 16 19 22 28 32 33 34 37 39 40 44 46 49 65 66 71 73	16	10	34	886	10	11605	103	5855	2403	88
★ △ WARM SPRINGS REHABILITATION HOSPITAL, Mailing Address: P.O. Box 58, Zip 78629; tel. 210/672–6592; Judi H. Guthrie, Administrator **A**1 7 9 10 **F**12 14 15 16 19 21 32 34 35 39 41 45 48 49 65 67 73 **P**5	23	46	52	528	39	6755	0	8230	4020	168
GRAHAM—Young County										
GRAHAM GENERAL HOSPITAL, 1301 Montgomery Road, Zip 76450, Mailing Address: Box 1390, Zip 76450; tel. 817/549–3400; Frank Beaman, Administrator **A**9 10 **F**7 8 10 11 15 19 21 22 26 28 31 32 33 36 37 39 40 44 45 48 49 71	14	10	37	1761	18	55573	177	8758	3872	194
GRANBURY—Hood County										
★ HOOD GENERAL HOSPITAL, 1310 Paluxy Road, Zip 76048; tel. 817/573–2683; Michael A. Kozar, Administrator **A**1 9 10 **F**4 7 8 9 10 11 12 15 16 19 21 22 24 27 28 35 36 37 38 40 42 44 45 47 48 49 63 64 65 67 69 70 71 73 **P**3 5 **S**0002 Quorum Health Group/Quorum Health Resources	16	10	56	1711	23	22755	132	13541	5404	181
GRAND PRAIRIE—Dallas County										
★ + ○ DALLAS–FORT WORTH MEDICAL CENTER, 2709 Hospital Boulevard, Zip 75051–1083; tel. 214/641–5000; Timothy Baylor, Chief Executive Officer (Total facility includes 11 beds in nursing home–type unit) **A**1 9 10 11 12 13 **F**4 7 8 10 11 12 13 15 16 17 19 22 23 24 28 32 33 37 40 41 42 44 47 52 57 64 65 71 73 74 **P**5 **S**0002 Quorum Health Group/Quorum Health Resources	23	10	124	4172	60	81965	1040	42235	17927	385
GRAND SALINE—Van Zandt County										
COZBY–GERMANY HOSPITAL, 707 North Waldrip Street, Zip 75140; tel. 903/962–4242; William Rowton, Chief Executive Officer **A**9 10 **F**8 15 19 22 26 32 34 44 58 71	23	10	26	382	4	5831	0	2642	1540	65

Hospitals, U.S. / TEXAS

Hospital, Address, Telephone, Administrator, Approval, Facility, and Physician Codes, Health Care System	Classification Codes		Utilization Data					Expense (thousands) of dollars		
★ American Hospital Association (AHA) membership ☐ Joint Commission on Accreditation of Healthcare Organizations (JCAHO) accreditation + American Osteopathic Hospital Association (AOHA) membership ○ American Osteopathic Association (AOA) accreditation △ Commission on Accreditation of Rehabilitation Facilities (CARF) accreditation Control codes 61, 63, 64, 71, 72 and 73 indicate hospitals listed by AOHA, but not registered by AHA. For definition of numerical codes, see page A6	Control	Service	Beds	Admissions	Census	Outpatient Visits	Births	Total	Payroll	Personnel
GRAPEVINE—Tarrant County										
★ BAYLOR MEDICAL CENTER AT GRAPEVINE, 1650 West College Street, Zip 76051–1650; tel. 817/329–2500; Mark C. Hood, Director (Total facility includes 9 beds in nursing home–type unit) **A**1 9 10 **F**1 2 3 4 5 7 8 9 10 11 12 13 15 16 17 18 19 20 21 22 23 24 25 26 27 28 29 30 31 32 33 34 35 36 37 38 39 40 41 42 43 44 45 46 47 48 49 50 51 52 53 54 55 56 57 58 59 60 61 63 64 65 66 67 69 70 71 73 74 **P**3 5 7 8 **S**0095 Baylor Health Care System	21	10	58	2960	30	30478	522	23119	8788	239
☐ CHARTER GRAPEVINE BEHAVIORAL HEALTH SYSTEM, 2300 William D. Tate Avenue, Zip 76051–9964; tel. 817/481–1900; Richard C. Gibson, Chief Executive Officer **A**1 9 10 **F**2 14 15 16 32 34 39 45 46 52 53 54 55 56 57 58 59 65 67 **P**7 **S**0695 Charter Medical Corporation	33	22	80	1630	40	13139	0	9100	3668	123
GREENVILLE—Hunt County										
☐ GLEN OAKS HOSPITAL, 301 East Division, Zip 75401; tel. 903/454–6000; Jerry W. Echols, Administrator **A**1 9 10 **F**1 2 3 19 22 35 52 53 54 55 56 57 58 59 65 71 **P**6 **S**9555 Universal Health Services, Inc.	33	22	54	794	21	1840	0	5223	2298	97
★ HUNT MEMORIAL HOSPITAL DISTRICT, (Includes Presbyterian Hospital of Commerce, 2900 Sterling Hart Drive, Commerce, Texas, Zip 75428; tel. 903/886–3161; Presbyterian Hospital of Greenville, Greenville, Texas) Mailing Address: P.O. Drawer 1059, Zip 75403–1059; tel. 903/408–5000; Patrick A. Hite, District Administrator and Chief Executive Officer **A**1 9 10 **F**7 8 12 14 15 16 19 21 22 28 30 32 34 35 37 40 41 42 44 45 49 65 67 71 73 **P**8	16	10	127	4974	59	62500	800	28952	12543	480
GROESBECK—Limestone County										
LIMESTONE MEDICAL CENTER, 900 North Ellis Street, Zip 76642; tel. 817/729–3281; Joe Wright, Administrator **A**9 10 **F**15 16 19 21 22 28 32 34 39 44 46 51 71 73	16	10	38	439	4	13081	1	4035	1870	93
GROVES—Jefferson County										
★ + ○ DOCTORS HOSPITAL, 5500 39th Street, Zip 77619–9805; tel. 409/962–5733; John Isbell, Chief Executive Officer **A**9 10 11 12 **F**3 4 7 8 10 11 12 14 15 19 21 22 26 28 30 32 34 35 37 41 42 43 44 46 49 51 52 53 57 60 63 65 66 70 71 73 **P**1 **S**0002 Quorum Health Group/Quorum Health Resources	23	10	84	2129	29	12570	0	—	—	178
HALE CENTER—Hale County										
★ HI-PLAINS HOSPITAL, 203 West Fourth Street, Zip 79041, Mailing Address: Box H, Zip 79041; tel. 806/839–2471; Michael J. Keller, Administrator (Total facility includes 44 beds in nursing home–type unit) **A**1 9 10 **F**7 15 16 17 19 21 24 26 28 30 31 32 34 40 44 45 49 65 66 70 71 73 74	23	10	84	732	48	5565	71	3229	2318	64
HALLETTSVILLE—Lavaca County										
LAVACA MEDICAL CENTER, 1400 North Texana Street, Zip 77964; tel. 512/798–3671; James Vanek, Administrator **A**9 10 **F**8 19 22 33 34 44 71	16	10	30	844	10	—	1	6195	2278	97
HAMLIN—Jones County										
★ HAMLIN MEMORIAL HOSPITAL, 632 Northwest Second Street, Zip 79520, Mailing Address: P.O. Box 400, Zip 79520; tel. 915/576–3646; Charley C. Latham, Administrator **A**9 10 **F**11 19 34 36 44 71 **P**5	16	10	25	408	6	1522	2	1828	888	45
HARLINGEN—Cameron County										
RIO GRANDE STATE CENTER, 1401 Rangerville Road, Zip 78550; tel. 210/425–8900; Sonia Hernandez, Director **A**9 **F**2 3 6 12 16 17 18 20 22 25 29 30 31 46 48 52 53 54 55 56 57 58 60 64 65 73 **P**6	12	22	190	1130	107	0	0	15608	10091	501
★ SOUTH TEXAS HOSPITAL, 1301 Rangerville Road, Zip 78552–7609, Mailing Address: P.O. Box 592, Zip 78551–0592; tel. 210/423–3420; James N. Elkins FACHE, Director **A**1 10 **F**8 12 14 15 16 19 20 21 27 28 29 30 31 34 35 39 41 44 45 46 49 51 65 71 73 74 **P**6 **S**0020 Texas Department of Health	12	10	85	680	43	26747	0	11264	5307	261
★ VALLEY BAPTIST MEDICAL CENTER, 2101 Pease Street, Zip 78550, Mailing Address: P.O. Drawer 2588, Zip 78551–2588; tel. 210/421–1100; Ben M. McKibbens, President (Total facility includes 60 beds in nursing home–type unit) **A**1 2 10 **F**7 8 10 11 12 13 15 16 17 18 19 21 22 23 26 28 29 30 32 33 35 37 38 39 40 41 42 43 44 45 46 47 49 52 53 54 55 57 58 59 60 61 63 64 65 67 71 73 74 **P**8	21	10	456	19330	254	74476	3980	128381	58322	1991
HASKELL—Haskell County										
HASKELL MEMORIAL HOSPITAL, 1 North Avenue N, Zip 79521, Mailing Address: P.O. Box 1117, Zip 79521; tel. 817/864–2621; Bill Nemir, Administrator **A**9 10 **F**9 11 14 15 16 19 20 22 27 28 29 32 33 37 38 44 46 47 49 66 71 73 **P**1	16	10	30	432	5	—	0	2159	1020	50
HEMPHILL—Sabine County										
★ SABINE COUNTY HOSPITAL, Highway 83 West, Zip 75948, Mailing Address: P.O. Box 750, Zip 75948; tel. 409/787–3300; Edith McCauley, Administrator **A**9 10 **F**19 20 22 28 32 34 40 41 44 49 71	16	10	36	509	6	5960	29	2486	1083	60
HENDERSON—Rusk County										
★ HENDERSON MEMORIAL HOSPITAL, 300 Wilson Street, Zip 75652; tel. 903/657–7541; George T. Roberts Jr., Chief Executive Officer (Total facility includes 16 beds in nursing home–type unit) **A**1 10 **F**4 7 8 10 12 15 16 19 20 22 28 29 30 31 32 34 35 37 39 40 44 45 46 49 63 64 65 71 **P**8 **S**0002 Quorum Health Group/Quorum Health Resources	23	10	96	2917	40	40418	536	15098	6835	280
HENRIETTA—Clay County										
CLAY COUNTY MEMORIAL HOSPITAL, 310 West South Street, Zip 76365–3399; tel. 817/538–5621; Edward E. Browning, Administrator **A**9 10 **F**19 21 22 27 30 32 34 37 44 71 **P**8	13	10	32	290	4	5609	0	1982	837	49

© 1995 AHA Guide

Hospitals, U.S. / TEXAS

Hospital, Address, Telephone, Administrator, Approval, Facility, and Physician Codes, Health Care System

- ★ American Hospital Association (AHA) membership
- □ Joint Commission on Accreditation of Healthcare Organizations (JCAHO) accreditation
- + American Osteopathic Hospital Association (AOHA) membership
- ○ American Osteopathic Association (AOA) accreditation
- △ Commission on Accreditation of Rehabilitation Facilities (CARF) accreditation

Control codes 61, 63, 64, 71, 72 and 73 indicate hospitals listed by AOHA, but not registered by AHA. For definition of numerical codes, see page A6.

Hospital	Classification Codes		Utilization Data					Expense (thousands) of dollars		Personnel
	Control	Service	Beds	Admissions	Census	Outpatient Visits	Births	Total	Payroll	
HEREFORD—Deaf Smith County										
★ HEREFORD REGIONAL MEDICAL CENTER, 801 East Third Street, Zip 79045, Mailing Address: Box 1858, Zip 79045; tel. 806/364–2141; James M. Robinson Sr., Administrator **A**1 9 10 **F**8 11 15 16 19 21 22 28 32 33 37 40 44 46 71 **P**4 **S**0036 Lubbock Methodist Hospital System	16	10	40	1525	14	17255	267	9560	4130	180
HILLSBORO—Hill County										
□ HILL REGIONAL HOSPITAL, 101 Circle Drive, Zip 76645; tel. 817/582–8425; Jan McClure, Chief Executive Officer (Total facility includes 23 beds in nursing home–type unit) **A**1 9 10 **F**7 12 14 15 16 19 22 26 30 34 37 41 44 45 46 52 57 64 71 73 **S**5895 Hallmark Healthcare Corporation	33	10	92	1309	19	13405	211	8214	2983	103
HONDO—Medina County										
MEDINA COMMUNITY HOSPITAL, Highway 462, Zip 78861; tel. 210/426–5363; Ernest Parisi, Administrator **A**9 10 **F**7 15 19 21 22 28 29 32 33 34 35 40 44 46 71 **P**4	15	10	32	891	9	61374	171	8768	4009	216
HOUSTON—Harris County										
AMI PARK PLAZA HOSPITAL See Tenet Park Plaza Hospital										
AMI TWELVE OAKS HOSPITAL See Twelve Oaks Hospital										
★ BELLAIRE HOSPITAL, 5314 Dashwood Street, Zip 77081–4689; tel. 713/669–4000; Thomas M. Keefe, Chief Executive Officer (Total facility includes 15 beds in nursing home–type unit) **A**1 9 10 **F**2 3 7 8 12 14 15 16 17 19 21 22 28 30 32 35 37 40 41 42 44 46 49 52 53 55 56 58 59 64 65 67 71 73 74 **P**5 7 8 **S**0048 Columbia/HCA Healthcare Corporation	33	10	191	5195	96	16073	1337	46530	16153	576
BEN TAUB GENERAL HOSPITAL See Harris County Hospital District										
★ CASA, A SPECIAL HOSPITAL, (Special Hospital Subacute/Medical) 1803 Old Spanish Trail, Zip 77054–2001; tel. 713/796–2272; Gretchen Thorp R.N., Administrator **F**6 12 15 22 31 32 42 64 65 73	33	49	40	317	19	0	0	2798	1021	38
CYPRESS CREEK HOSPITAL, 17750 Cali Drive, Zip 77090–2700; tel. 713/586–7600; Dan R. Riley, Administrator **A**9 10 **F**2 3 52 53 54 55 56 57 58 59 65 67 **S**0395 Healthcare International, Inc.	33	22	78	857	32	4545	0	7395	3322	127
★ CYPRESS FAIRBANKS MEDICAL CENTER, 10655 Steepletop Drive, Zip 77065; tel. 713/890–4285; Bill Klier, President and Chief Executive Officer (Total facility includes 14 beds in nursing home–type unit) **A**1 9 10 **F**2 7 8 10 12 14 16 19 21 22 28 29 30 31 34 35 37 40 41 44 46 48 49 50 52 63 64 65 67 71 73 74 **P**1	32	10	144	5875	66	51150	800	38987	16018	579
★ DIAGNOSTIC CENTER HOSPITAL, 6447 Main Street, Zip 77030; tel. 713/790–0790; William A. Gregory, Chief Executive Officer (Total facility includes 25 beds in nursing home–type unit) **A**1 3 9 10 **F**2 4 7 9 10 11 12 17 19 20 21 22 23 24 26 27 28 30 31 32 34 35 37 38 39 40 41 42 43 44 45 46 47 48 49 50 52 54 55 57 58 60 61 63 64 65 66 67 69 71 73 **P**1 **S**7235 Methodist Hospital System	23	10	145	3688	73	12524	0	32684	11936	415
□ DOCTORS HOSPITAL, 5815 Airline Drive, Zip 77076; tel. 713/695–6041; Lee Brown, Administrator **A**1 9 10 12 13 **F**7 8 10 15 19 22 32 34 35 37 40 44 48 64 65 67 71 **P**5 8	32	10	114	6029	74	38070	1093	27480	12492	378
□ DOCTORS HOSPITAL EAST LOOP, 9339 North Loop East, Zip 77029, Mailing Address: Box 24216, Zip 77229; tel. 713/675–3241; John Styles Jr., Administrator **A**1 9 10 **F**8 12 15 19 20 21 22 23 26 30 31 32 33 34 35 37 39 41 42 44 45 49 51 56 64 65 66 67 71 **P**1	32	10	150	3377	66	19828	0	26093	8890	285
FOREST SPRINGS HOSPITAL, 1120 Cypress Station, Zip 77090–3031; tel. 713/893–7200; Rose K. Gantner Ed.D., Administrator **A**1 9 10 **F**3 18 52 53 55 56 58 59 65 **P**8	33	22	36	465	17	1778	0	—	—	47
★ GULF PINES BEHAVIORAL HEALTH SERVICES, 205 Hollow Tree Lane, Zip 77090; tel. 713/537–0700; Lawrence Story, Chief Executive Officer and Administrator (Data for 273 days) **A**1 9 10 **F**2 12 46 52 53 54 55 56 57 59	33	22	140	535	23	0	0	4860	1798	56
□ HARRIS COUNTY HOSPITAL DISTRICT, (Includes Ben Taub General Hospital, 1504 Taub Loop, Houston, Texas, Zip 77030; tel. 713/793–2300; Michael R. Bullard, Senior Vice President; Lyndon B. Johnson General Hospital, 5656 Kelley, Houston, Texas, Zip 77026; tel. 713/636–5000; Margo Hilliard M.D., Senior Vice President; Quentin Mease Hospital, 3601 North MacGregor, Houston, Texas, Zip 77004; tel. 713/528–1499; Michael R. Bullard, Senior Vice President) 2525 Holly Hall, Zip 77054, Mailing Address: Box 66769, Zip 77266–6769; tel. 713/746–6403; Lois Jean Moore, President and Chief Executive Officer **A**1 2 3 5 8 9 10 **F**3 4 7 8 10 11 12 14 15 17 18 19 20 21 22 23 25 26 27 30 31 32 34 35 37 38 40 42 43 44 47 48 49 52 56 58 59 60 61 63 65 67 68 70 71 73 **P**6	16	10	852	42929	701	810747	12544	389447	160459	5725
★ HARRIS COUNTY PSYCHIATRIC CENTER, 2800 South MacGregor, Zip 77021, Mailing Address: P.O. Box 20249, Zip 77225–0249; tel. 713/741–5000; Robert W. Guynn M.D., Executive Director (Nonreporting) **A**1 3 5 10	12	22	250	—	—	—	—	—	—	—
★ △ HEIGHTS HOSPITAL, 1917 Ashland Street, Zip 77008–3994, Mailing Address: P.O. Box 7497, Zip 77248; tel. 713/861–6161; Charles D. Schuetz, Chief Executive Officer (Nonreporting) **A**1 7 9 10	32	10	209	—	—	—	—	—	—	—
★ HERMANN HOSPITAL, 6411 Fannin, Zip 77030–1501; tel. 713/704–3711; David R. Page, President and Chief Executive Officer (Total facility includes 15 beds in nursing home–type unit) **A**1 3 5 8 10 **F**4 7 8 9 10 11 12 14 15 16 17 19 20 21 22 23 24 25 26 27 28 31 32 34 35 37 38 39 40 41 42 43 44 45 46 47 48 49 50 51 56 60 61 63 64 65 66 67 68 69 70 71 72 73 74 **P**1 7	23	10	654	26856	463	155596	4143	374348	168013	4247
★ HOUSTON NORTHWEST MEDICAL CENTER, 710 FM 1960 West, Zip 77090–3496; tel. 713/440–1000; J. Barry Shevchuk FACHE, Chief Executive Officer (Total facility includes 20 beds in nursing home–type unit) **A**1 9 10 **F**3 4 7 8 10 12 15 16 19 20 21 22 23 24 28 29 30 31 32 33 34 35 37 40 41 42 43 44 45 46 48 49 52 53 54 55 56 58 59 60 61 64 65 67 70 71 72 73 74 **P**1 5 7	33	10	389	15786	197	141075	3315	143386	44885	1234

Hospitals, U.S. / TEXAS

Hospital, Address, Telephone, Administrator, Approval, Facility, and Physician Codes, Health Care System	Classification Codes		Utilization Data					Expense (thousands) of dollars		
	Control	Service	Beds	Admissions	Census	Outpatient Visits	Births	Total	Payroll	Personnel

★ American Hospital Association (AHA) membership
☐ Joint Commission on Accreditation of Healthcare Organizations (JCAHO) accreditation
+ American Osteopathic Hospital Association (AOHA) membership
○ American Osteopathic Association (AOA) accreditation
△ Commission on Accreditation of Rehabilitation Facilities (CARF) accreditation
Control codes 61, 63, 64, 71, 72 and 73 indicate hospitals listed by AOHA, but not registered by AHA. For definition of numerical codes, see page A6

Hospital	Control	Service	Beds	Admissions	Census	Outpatient Visits	Births	Total	Payroll	Personnel
★ △ HOUSTON REHABILITATION INSTITUTE, 17506 Red Oak Drive, Zip 77090, Mailing Address: P.O. Box 73684, Zip 77273–7721; tel. 713/580–1212; Anne R. Leon, Chief Executive Officer **A**1 7 9 10 **F**12 14 19 21 27 34 35 48 49 64 65 67 71 73	32	46	80	747	52	11605	0	15251	6734	182
☐ INTRACARE MEDICAL CENTER HOSPITAL, 7601 Fannin, Zip 77054; tel. 713/790–0949; David Harrod, Administrator **A**1 9 10 **F**2 3 19 21 22 35 52 53 54 55 56 58 59 65	33	22	50	979	36	0	0	4979	—	77
LYNDON B. JOHNSON GENERAL HOSPITAL See Harris County Hospital District										
★ △ MEDICAL CENTER HOSPITAL, 8081 Greenbriar, Zip 77054–1900; tel. 713/790–8100; Edward W. Myers, Chief Executive Officer **A**1 7 9 10 **F**2 3 4 7 8 9 10 11 12 14 15 16 19 20 22 23 24 25 26 27 28 30 31 32 34 35 37 38 39 40 41 42 43 44 46 47 48 49 52 53 55 56 57 59 63 64 65 66 67 71 73 74 **P**5 7 8 **S**0048 Columbia/HCA Healthcare Corporation	33	10	165	1883	50	—	0	31499	13210	342
★ MEMORIAL HOSPITAL – MEMORIAL CITY, 920 Frostwood Drive, Zip 77024–9173; tel. 713/932–3055; Gerel T. Humphrey, Vice President and Chief Executive Officer (Total facility includes 24 beds in nursing home–type unit) **A**1 9 10 **F**2 3 4 6 7 8 10 11 12 15 16 17 18 19 21 22 25 26 28 29 30 31 32 33 34 35 37 38 39 40 41 42 43 44 45 46 48 49 52 53 54 55 56 57 58 59 60 61 62 63 64 65 66 67 68 71 72 73 74 **P**1 3 7 **S**2645 Memorial Healthcare System	23	10	340	12209	154	—	2338	—	—	1049
MEMORIAL HOSPITAL NORTHWEST See Memorial Hospital System										
MEMORIAL HOSPITAL SOUTHEAST See Memorial Hospital System										
MEMORIAL HOSPITAL SOUTHWEST See Memorial Hospital System										
MEMORIAL REHABILITATION HOSPITAL See Memorial Hospital System										
★ MEMORIAL HOSPITAL SYSTEM, (Includes Memorial Hospital Northwest, 1635 North Loop West, Houston, Texas, Zip 77008; Jerel T. Humphrey, Vice President and Chief Executive Officer; Memorial Hospital Southeast, 11800 Astoria, Houston, Texas, Zip 77089; tel. 713/929–6100; Daniel W. Martin, Vice President; Memorial Hospital Southwest, 7600 Beechnut, Houston, Texas, Zip 77074; tel. 713/776–5000; Memorial Rehabilitation Hospital, 3042 Gessner, Houston, Texas, Zip 77080; tel. 713/462–2515; Rick Truskoloski, Vice President and Chief Executive Officer) 7600 Beechnut, Zip 77074–1850; tel. 713/776–5111; Dan S. Wilford, President and Chief Executive Officer (Total facility includes 84 beds in nursing home–type unit) **A**1 2 3 5 10 **F**2 3 4 6 7 8 10 11 12 15 16 17 18 19 21 22 25 26 28 29 30 31 32 33 34 35 37 38 39 40 41 42 43 44 45 46 48 49 52 53 54 55 56 57 58 59 60 61 62 63 64 65 66 67 68 71 72 73 74 **P**1 3 7 **S**2645 Memorial Healthcare System	23	10	1480	52564	811	—	8619	383887	128760	9521
★ MEMORIAL SPRING SHADOWS GLEN, 2801 Gessner, Zip 77080–2599; tel. 713/462–4000; G. Jerry Mueck, Vice President and Chief Executive Officer **A**1 9 **F**2 3 4 6 7 8 10 11 12 14 15 16 17 18 19 21 22 25 26 28 29 30 31 32 33 34 35 37 38 39 40 41 42 43 44 45 46 48 49 52 53 54 55 56 57 58 59 60 61 62 63 64 65 66 67 68 71 72 73 74 **P**1 3 7 **S**2645 Memorial Healthcare System	23	22	104	1335	51	0	0	—	—	172
NORTHSIDE GENERAL HOSPITAL, 2807 Little York Road, Zip 77093–3495; tel. 713/697–7777; J. James Raymond, President and Chief Executive Officer **A**9 10 **F**19 21 22 26 32 34 35 37 44 49 71	33	10	39	635	8	2222	0	—	—	19
★ PARKWAY HOSPITAL, 233 West Parker Road, Zip 77076; tel. 713/697–2831; Mel Bishop, Chief Executive Officer (Total facility includes 21 beds in nursing home–type unit) **A**1 9 10 **F**3 7 8 10 14 15 16 19 21 22 27 32 33 37 40 41 44 46 48 49 52 57 58 59 64 65 71 73 **S**0048 Columbia/HCA Healthcare Corporation	33	10	197	6434	115	32000	1390	37471	13288	524
☐ RIVERSIDE GENERAL HOSPITAL, 3204 Ennis, Zip 77004; tel. 713/526–2441; Earnest Gibson III, Administrator **A**1 9 10 **F**2 3 7 14 15 16 26 30 34 37 39 40 44 52 53 56 58 61 65 71 73 74	23	10	98	614	16	1714	11	5241	2302	201
QUENTIN MEASE HOSPITAL See Harris County Hospital District										
★ △ ROSEWOOD MEDICAL CENTER, 9200 Westheimer Road, Zip 77063; tel. 713/780–7900; Pat Currie, Chief Executive Officer (Total facility includes 14 beds in nursing home–type unit) **A**1 7 9 10 **F**2 3 4 5 7 8 10 12 14 16 18 19 20 21 22 23 24 26 27 28 30 31 32 33 34 35 37 39 40 41 42 43 44 48 49 51 52 53 54 55 56 57 59 60 64 65 66 67 71 73 74 **P**5 7 8 **S**0048 Columbia/HCA Healthcare Corporation	32	10	184	5041	83	35617	405	35168	15698	505
SAM HOUSTON MEMORIAL HOSPITAL See Spring Branch Medical Center										
☐ SHARPSTOWN GENERAL HOSPITAL, 6700 Bellaire at Tarnef, Zip 77074–4999, Mailing Address: P.O. Box 740389, Zip 77274–0389; tel. 713/774–7611; J. O. Lewis, Administrator **A**1 9 10 **F**2 7 8 12 14 15 16 17 19 20 21 22 27 28 30 32 34 37 40 41 44 47 52 53 57 59 65 67 71 **P**5 7 8 **S**6525 Ornda Healthcorp	33	10	53	2132	17	13774	1014	14875	6525	179
★ SHRINERS HOSPITALS FOR CRIPPLED CHILDREN, HOUSTON UNIT, 1402 North MacGregor Drive, Zip 77030–1695; tel. 713/797–1616; Steven B. Reiter, Administrator **A**1 3 5 **F**5 9 12 19 28 34 35 39 44 45 49 50 54 65 67 71 73 **P**6 **S**4125 Shriners Hospitals for Crippled Children	23	57	40	672	20	9746	0	—	—	140
★ SPECIALTY HOSPITAL OF HOUSTON, 5556 Gasmer, Zip 77035; tel. 713/551–5300; Nona Fain, Chief Executive Officer and Administrator **A**1 10 **F**1 3 4 7 8 10 12 14 17 19 20 21 22 27 28 30 31 32 34 35 37 42 43 44 47 50 65 67 71 73	33	10	33	158	12	0	0	3652	1204	53
★ SPRING BRANCH MEDICAL CENTER, (Includes Sam Houston Memorial Hospital, 1615 Hillendahl, Houston, Texas, Zip 77055; tel. 713/932–5500) 8850 Long Point Road, Zip 77055; tel. 713/467–6555; Stephen L. Royal, President and Chief Executive Officer **A**1 2 9 10 **F**3 4 7 8 10 12 14 15 16 17 19 21 22 23 25 26 27 28 29 30 31 32 34 35 37 38 39 40 41 42 43 44 45 46 48 49 51 52 53 54 55 56 57 58 59 60 61 64 65 66 67 68 69 71 73 74 **P**5 8 **S**0048 Columbia/HCA Healthcare Corporation	33	10	331	9366	142	86648	1255	104945	31762	1307

© 1995 AHA Guide

Hospitals, U.S. / TEXAS

Hospital, Address, Telephone, Administrator, Approval, Facility, and Physician Codes, Health Care System	Classification Codes		Utilization Data					Expense (thousands) of dollars		Personnel
	Control	Service	Beds	Admissions	Census	Outpatient Visits	Births	Total	Payroll	

*American Hospital Association (AHA) membership
□ Joint Commission on Accreditation of Healthcare Organizations (JCAHO) accreditation
+ American Osteopathic Hospital Association (AOHA) membership
○ American Osteopathic Association (AOA) accreditation
△ Commission on Accreditation of Rehabilitation Facilities (CARF) accreditation
Control codes 61, 63, 64, 71, 72 and 73 indicate hospitals listed by AOHA, but not registered by AHA. For definition of numerical codes, see page A6

Hospital	Control	Service	Beds	Admissions	Census	Outpatient Visits	Births	Total	Payroll	Personnel
★ ST. JOSEPH HOSPITAL, 1919 LaBranch Street, Zip 77002; tel. 713/757-1000; Raymond J. Khoury, Administrator (Total facility includes 15 beds in nursing home-type unit) A1 2 3 5 9 10 F2 3 4 7 8 9 10 11 12 13 14 15 16 17 18 19 21 22 23 24 28 29 30 31 32 34 35 37 38 39 40 41 42 43 44 45 46 48 49 51 52 53 54 55 56 57 59 60 61 63 64 65 66 67 68 69 71 72 73 74 P3 8 S0605 Sisters of Charity of the Incarnate Word Healthcare System	21	10	611	18285	301	141548	3947	173367	78151	2497
★ ST. LUKE'S EPISCOPAL HOSPITAL, 6720 Bertner Avenue, Zip 77030-2697, Mailing Address: Box 20269, Zip 77225-0269; tel. 713/791-2011; Michael K. Jhin, President and Chief Executive Officer A1 3 5 8 9 10 F4 7 8 10 11 12 14 15 19 21 22 28 29 30 32 34 35 37 39 40 41 42 43 44 45 46 48 49 54 56 61 63 65 67 69 71 73 74 P5 7 8	21	10	591	28595	449	158789	3638	330554	128799	3593
★ SUN BELT REGIONAL MEDICAL CENTER, (Includes Sun Belt Regional Medical Center East, 15101 East Freeway, Channelview, Texas, Zip 77530; tel. 713/452-1511) 13111 East Freeway, Zip 77015; tel. 713/455-6911; John Smithhisler, Chief Executive Officer (Total facility includes 9 beds in nursing home-type unit) A1 9 10 F7 8 10 11 14 15 16 17 19 21 22 26 28 30 31 32 35 37 40 41 44 45 46 48 52 57 59 63 64 65 71 73 74 P5 S0048 Columbia/HCA Healthcare Corporation	33	10	136	4652	51	54601	1260	29442	11089	461
★ TENET PARK PLAZA HOSPITAL, (Formerly AMI Park Plaza Hospital) 1313 Hermann Drive, Zip 77004; tel. 713/527-5000; Judith Novak, President and Chief Executive Officer (Total facility includes 40 beds in nursing home-type unit) A1 2 9 10 F4 7 8 10 12 17 19 21 22 28 30 31 32 34 35 37 40 41 42 44 45 46 48 49 60 61 63 64 65 71 73 P3 5 6 7 S0063 TENET Healthcare Corporation	32	10	382	8752	193	21876	786	86847	31965	968
★ TEXAS CHILDREN'S HOSPITAL, 6621 Fannin Street, Zip 77030-2399, Mailing Address: Box 300630, Zip 77230-0630; tel. 713/770-1000; Mark A. Wallace, Executive Director A1 3 5 8 9 10 F4 5 10 12 13 14 15 16 17 19 20 21 22 24 25 29 30 31 32 34 35 38 39 41 42 43 44 45 46 47 49 50 51 54 55 58 60 63 65 66 67 68 69 70 71 72 73 P5	23	50	360	16777	298	295901	0	256009	114965	2955
★ TEXAS ORTHOPEDIC HOSPITAL, 7401 South Main Street, Zip 77030; tel. 713/799-8600; Kathy Sunderland, Administrative Assistant (Nonreporting) S0048 Columbia/HCA Healthcare Corporation	33	47	46	—	—	—	—	—	—	—
★ △ THE INSTITUTE FOR REHABILITATION AND RESEARCH, 1333 Moursund, Zip 77030-3405; tel. 713/799-5000; Charles C. Beall Jr., President A1 3 5 7 9 10 F12 14 15 16 19 20 21 22 29 34 35 41 44 45 46 48 49 65 66 67 71 73 P1 5	23	46	92	731	54	32358	0	35454	15119	460
★ △ THE METHODIST HOSPITAL, 6565 Fannin, Zip 77030; tel. 713/790-3311; Larry L. Mathis FACHE, President and Chief Executive Officer (Total facility includes 25 beds in nursing home-type unit) A1 2 3 5 7 8 9 10 F1 2 3 4 5 7 8 10 11 12 15 16 17 19 20 21 22 23 26 27 28 30 31 32 33 34 35 37 39 40 41 42 43 44 45 46 48 49 52 54 55 56 57 58 59 60 63 64 65 66 67 69 71 73 74 P5 S7235 Methodist Hospital System	23	10	845	28024	576	323139	1999	435851	162047	4108
★ TWELVE OAKS HOSPITAL, (Formerly AMI Twelve Oaks Hospital) 4200 Portsmouth Street, Zip 77027; tel. 713/623-2500; Walter J. Ornsteen, Executive Director A1 9 10 F2 3 4 8 10 11 12 16 17 19 21 22 28 30 31 35 37 41 42 43 44 46 48 49 52 54 55 56 58 59 64 65 67 71 73 P5 7 S0063 TENET Healthcare Corporation	32	10	336	4868	117	6983	0	—	—	481
★ UNIVERSITY OF TEXAS M. D. ANDERSON CANCER CENTER, (Diagnosis and Treatment of Cancer) 1515 Holcombe Boulevard, Zip 77030-4096; tel. 713/792-6170; Donna K. Sollenberger, Vice President A1 2 3 5 8 9 10 F8 15 16 17 19 20 21 22 25 27 29 30 34 35 37 39 41 42 44 45 46 47 49 50 53 54 55 56 58 59 60 63 65 67 69 71 73 P6 S0033 University of Texas Hospitals	12	49	467	17449	350	353122	0	467372	230398	7988
★ VENCOR HOSPITAL-HOUSTON, 6441 Main Street, Zip 77030; tel. 713/790-0500; Darrell L. Pile, Administrator A1 10 F12 16 19 21 22 31 35 65 67 71 S0026 Vencor, Incorporated	32	10	94	403	67	0	0	16716	8169	218
★ VETERANS AFFAIRS MEDICAL CENTER, 2002 Holcombe Boulevard, Zip 77030-4298; tel. 713/791-1414; Robert F. Stott, Director (Total facility includes 155 beds in nursing home-type unit) A1 3 5 8 F2 3 4 5 8 10 11 15 16 17 18 19 20 21 22 23 25 26 27 31 32 33 34 35 37 39 41 42 43 44 46 48 49 52 54 56 57 58 60 64 65 67 71 73 74 P6 S9295 Department of Veterans Affairs	45	10	899	16603	615	338146	0	204273	118353	2880
★ WEST HOUSTON MEDICAL CENTER, 12141 Richmond Avenue, Zip 77082-2499; tel. 713/558-3444; Janie R. Kauffman, Chief Executive Officer (Total facility includes 18 beds in nursing home-type unit) A1 10 F4 7 8 10 12 16 19 21 22 32 34 35 37 38 40 42 43 44 46 49 52 57 61 64 65 71 73 P1 2 5 7 8 S0048 Columbia/HCA Healthcare Corporation	33	10	169	4662	75	28352	928	42975	14740	363
□ WEST OAKS HOSPITAL, 6500 Hornwood, Zip 77074, Mailing Address: Box 741389, Zip 77274; tel. 713/995-0909; Margo Bonner, Administrator A1 9 10 F2 3 12 18 35 39 52 53 55 56 58 59 65 P4 5 7 S0395 Healthcare International, Inc.	33	22	150	1777	49	9378	0	8560	4271	172
★ WESTBURY HOSPITAL, 5556 Gasmer Road, Zip 77035-4598; tel. 713/729-1111; Larry C. Andrews, Chief Executive Officer (Total facility includes 10 beds in nursing home-type unit) A1 9 10 F11 12 19 21 22 34 35 44 45 52 57 63 64 65 69 71 73 P8 S0048 Columbia/HCA Healthcare Corporation	33	10	100	1203	31	11206	0	16854	7114	238
★ WOMAN'S HOSPITAL OF TEXAS, 7600 Fannin Street, Zip 77054-1900; tel. 713/790-1234; Linda B. Russell, Chief Executive Officer A1 5 9 10 F2 3 4 7 8 9 10 11 12 19 21 22 23 24 25 26 27 30 31 32 34 35 37 38 39 40 41 42 43 44 45 46 47 48 49 51 52 53 54 55 56 57 58 59 60 64 65 66 67 68 71 73 74 P8 S0048 Columbia/HCA Healthcare Corporation	33	44	138	5865	50	23680	3761	38429	15396	442

Hospitals, U.S. / TEXAS

Hospital, Address, Telephone, Administrator, Approval, Facility, and Physician Codes, Health Care System	Classification Codes		Utilization Data					Expense (thousands) of dollars		
★ American Hospital Association (AHA) membership □ Joint Commission on Accreditation of Healthcare Organizations (JCAHO) accreditation + American Osteopathic Hospital Association (AOHA) membership ○ American Osteopathic Association (AOA) accreditation △ Commission on Accreditation of Rehabilitation Facilities (CARF) accreditation Control codes 61, 63, 64, 71, 72 and 73 indicate hospitals listed by AOHA, but not registered by AHA. For definition of numerical codes, see page A6	Control	Service	Beds	Admissions	Census	Outpatient Visits	Births	Total	Payroll	Personnel
★ YALE CLINIC AND HOSPITAL, 510 West Tidwell Road, Zip 77091; tel. 713/691–1111; Charles Veldekens, Chief Executive Officer (Nonreporting) **A**1 9	31	10	68	—	—	—	—	—	—	—
HUMBLE—Harris County										
□ △ HEALTHSOUTH REHABILITATION HOSPITAL, 19002 McKay Drive, Zip 77338; tel. 713/446–6148; Jessica A. Nantz, Chief Executive Officer (Total facility includes 10 beds in nursing home–type unit) **A**1 7 9 10 **F**5 12 14 15 16 19 20 22 25 26 27 35 39 41 45 46 48 49 54 57 64 65 66 67 71 **S**0023 Healthsouth Corporation	33	46	69	434	29	4112	0	7620	4092	110
★ NORTHEAST MEDICAL CENTER HOSPITAL, 18951 Memorial North, Zip 77338–4297; tel. 713/540–7700; Fred J. Mery, Administrator (Total facility includes 16 beds in nursing home–type unit) **A**1 2 10 **F**7 8 10 11 12 15 16 17 19 21 22 25 26 27 28 29 30 31 32 33 34 35 37 39 40 42 44 46 49 51 60 63 64 65 67 68 71 72 73 74 **P**3 8	16	10	175	7619	111	82008	1170	61364	23433	724
HUNT—Kerr County										
LA HACIENDA TREATMENT CENTER, FM 1340, Zip 78024, Mailing Address: Box 1, Zip 78024–0001; tel. 210/238–4222; Frank Sadlack Ph.D., Executive Director **A**9 **F**2 3 12 16 19 20 21 22 24 25 30 31 39 41 45 46 49 54 56 **P**1	32	82	88	572	24	0	0	4740	2168	85
HUNTSVILLE—Walker County										
★ HUNTSVILLE MEMORIAL HOSPITAL, 3000 I–45, Zip 77340, Mailing Address: P.O. Box 4001, Zip 77342–4001; tel. 409/291–3411; Ralph E. Beaty, Administrator **A**1 9 10 **F**7 8 13 14 17 19 22 28 29 30 33 34 35 37 39 40 44 45 49 65 67 71 73 74 **P**1 **S**0002 Quorum Health Group/Quorum Health Resources	23	10	119	3606	38	43980	508	21627	8992	323
IRAAN—Pecos County										
□ PECOS COUNTY GENERAL HOSPITAL, (Formerly General Hospital) 305 West Fifth Street, Zip 79744, Mailing Address: Box 665, Zip 79744; tel. 915/639–2871; Debbie Parker, Administrator **A**1 9 10 **F**14 15 16 22 25 32 40 44 71 **P**5	13	10	8	104	1	2695	0	1811	726	31
IRVING—Dallas County										
★ AMERICAN TRANSITIONAL CARE HOSPITAL–DALLAS/FORT WORTH, (Long Term Acute Care) 1745 West Irving Boulevard, Zip 75061; tel. 214/251–2824; Louis P. Bradley Jr., Administrator and Chief Executive Officer **A**1 10 **F**12 33 34 39 49 65	33	49	43	249	22	16	0	5764	2467	141
★ IRVING HEALTHCARE SYSTEM, 1901 North MacArthur Boulevard, Zip 75061; tel. 214/579–8100; Michael F. O'Keefe FACHE, President (Total facility includes 18 beds in nursing home–type unit) **A**1 2 10 **F**1 4 7 8 10 11 12 15 16 19 21 22 24 26 27 28 30 31 32 33 34 35 37 39 40 41 42 43 44 46 48 49 60 64 65 67 71 73 74 **P**1 7	16	10	221	10926	148	146743	1909	89401	37329	1404
JACKSBORO—Jack County										
FAITH COMMUNITY HOSPITAL, 717 Magnolia Street, Zip 76458; tel. 817/567–6633; Ronald G. Ammons, Administrator **A**10 **F**19 21 32 33 44 65 70 71 **P**6	16	10	21	554	5	3863	0	4021	1534	61
JACKSONVILLE—Cherokee County										
★ NAN TRAVIS MEMORIAL HOSPITAL, 501 South Ragsdale Street, Zip 75766; tel. 903/586–3000; Steve Bowen, President (Total facility includes 18 beds in nursing home–type unit) **A**1 9 10 **F**7 8 14 16 17 19 22 23 24 28 30 34 35 37 40 42 44 46 49 62 64 65 66 71 73 74 **P**4 6	23	10	123	3444	68	38107	193	22927	10184	304
JASPER—Jasper County										
★ JASPER MEMORIAL HOSPITAL, 1275 Marvin Hancock Drive, Zip 75951; tel. 409/384–5461; Imogene Weber R.N., Acting Administrator **A**1 9 10 **F**7 8 19 22 28 32 37 40 44 46 65 71 73	16	10	50	2267	22	15760	380	—	—	275
MARY E. DICKERSON MEMORIAL HOSPITAL, 1001 Dickerson Drive, Zip 75951, Mailing Address: P.O. Box 1990, Zip 75951; tel. 409/384–2575; Spencer Guimarin, Administrator **A**9 10 **F**7 8 19 32 34 40 44 65 70 71 73	32	10	35	1198	16	13080	82	6408	3147	147
JOURDANTON—Atascosa County										
□ TRI-CITY COMMUNITY HOSPITAL, Highway 97 East, Zip 78026, Mailing Address: Box 189, Zip 78026; tel. 512/769–3515; Stephen B. Hill, Administrator **A**1 9 10 **F**8 16 19 20 22 32 34 35 41 42 44 49 51 65 66 71 72 **P**5	32	10	30	1330	17	63777	0	10648	4631	210
JUNCTION—Kimble County										
★ KIMBLE HOSPITAL, 2101 Main Street, Zip 76849–2101; tel. 915/446–3321; Ben Snead, Administrator **A**9 10 **F**22 32 34 44 71	16	10	18	369	4	4731	0	2636	1286	64
KATY—Harris County										
★ KATY MEDICAL CENTER, 5602 Medical Center Drive, Zip 77494; tel. 713/392–1111; Brian S. Barbe, Executive Director **A**1 9 10 **F**7 8 10 12 16 19 20 21 22 23 28 29 30 31 32 33 34 35 36 37 40 41 43 44 52 53 54 55 56 57 58 59 60 61 64 65 66 69 70 71 73 74 **P**8 **S**0048 Columbia/HCA Healthcare Corporation	33	10	73	3370	31	51617	731	23687	9093	311
KAUFMAN—Kaufman County										
★ PRESBYTERIAN HOSPITAL OF KAUFMAN, Highway 243 West at Highway 175, Zip 75142–9998, Mailing Address: Box 310, Zip 75142; tel. 214/932–7200; Argus D. Forrest, Executive Vice President and Executive Director (Total facility includes 10 beds in nursing home–type unit) **A**1 9 10 **F**8 15 19 21 22 26 28 30 34 37 40 41 42 44 49 63 64 65 71 73 **S**1130 Presbyterian Healthcare System	23	10	72	2749	25	21338	386	8844	5787	185
KENEDY—Karnes County										
OTTO KAISER MEMORIAL HOSPITAL, Highway 181 North, Zip 78119, Mailing Address: Route 1, Box 450, Zip 78119–9718; tel. 210/583–3401; Harold L. Boening, Administrator **A**9 10 **F**19 22 32 37 44 49 71	16	10	34	419	7	20702	0	3343	1442	74
KERMIT—Winkler County										
★ MEMORIAL HOSPITAL, 821 Jeffee Drive, Zip 79745, Mailing Address: Drawer H, Zip 79745; tel. 915/586–5864; Walt Haislip, Administrator **A**9 10 **F**22 34 44 51 71	13	10	16	410	5	7706	0	3150	1721	71

© 1995 AHA Guide

Hospitals, U.S. / TEXAS

Hospital, Address, Telephone, Administrator, Approval, Facility, and Physician Codes, Health Care System	Classification Codes		Utilization Data					Expense (thousands) of dollars		
★ American Hospital Association (AHA) membership □ Joint Commission on Accreditation of Healthcare Organizations (JCAHO) accreditation + American Osteopathic Hospital Association (AOHA) membership ○ American Osteopathic Association (AOA) accreditation △ Commission on Accreditation of Rehabilitation Facilities (CARF) accreditation Control codes 61, 63, 64, 71, 72 and 73 indicate hospitals listed by AOHA, but not registered by AHA. For definition of numerical codes, see page A6	Control	Service	Beds	Admissions	Census	Outpatient Visits	Births	Total	Payroll	Personnel
KERRVILLE—Kerr County										
□ KERRVILLE STATE HOSPITAL, 721 Thompson Drive, Zip 78028–5199; tel. 210/896–2211; Gloria P. Olsen Ph.D., Superintendent **A**1 9 10 **F**12 52 53 54 55 56 57 58 73	12	22	179	479	179	—	0	28500	17684	832
★ SID PETERSON MEMORIAL HOSPITAL, 710 Water Street, Zip 78028–5398; tel. 210/896–4200; F. W. Hall Jr., Administrator (Total facility includes 30 beds in nursing home–type unit) **A**1 9 10 **F**4 7 8 11 12 14 15 16 19 21 22 23 28 30 32 34 37 41 42 44 45 46 47 48 49 62 64 65 71 73 74 **P**8	23	10	123	3847	57	65338	359	26483	12938	461
★ VETERANS AFFAIRS MEDICAL CENTER, 3600 Memorial Boulevard, Zip 78028; tel. 210/896–2020; Arnold E. Mouish, Director (Total facility includes 154 beds in nursing home–type unit) **A**1 **F**2 3 4 8 10 18 19 20 25 26 30 31 32 33 34 35 37 39 41 42 43 44 46 48 49 51 54 58 64 65 67 71 72 73 74 **S**9295 Department of Veterans Affairs	45	10	345	3395	270	41757	0	33661	19854	560
KILGORE—Gregg County										
★ ROY H. LAIRD MEMORIAL HOSPITAL, 1612 South Henderson Boulevard, Zip 75662; tel. 903/984–3505; Roderick G. La Grone, President **A**1 9 10 **F**7 8 19 22 26 32 34 37 40 44 65 71 73 74	14	10	51	1718	17	19078	181	10663	4663	176
KILLEEN—Bell County										
★ METROPLEX HOSPITAL, 2201 South Clear Creek Road, Zip 76542–9305; tel. 817/526–7523; Ernie W. Sadau, President and Chief Executive Officer (Total facility includes 10 beds in nursing home–type unit) **A**1 9 10 **F**7 8 14 15 17 18 19 21 22 28 29 30 32 34 35 37 39 40 42 44 45 46 50 52 53 54 56 57 59 63 64 65 71 73 **P**8 **S**4165 Adventist Health System–Sunbelt Health Care Corporation	21	10	198	4694	73	50336	657	36644	12675	512
KINGSVILLE—Kleberg County										
★ SPOHN KLEBERG MEMORIAL HOSPITAL, 1300 General Cavazos Boulevard, Zip 78363, Mailing Address: P.O. Box 1197, Zip 78363–1197; tel. 512/595–1661; Andrew M. Harris, Administrator **A**1 9 10 **F**7 8 14 15 16 17 19 21 22 25 29 30 31 32 33 34 37 39 40 44 45 46 49 64 65 67 68 70 71 73 **P**1 **S**5565 Incarnate Word Health Services	21	10	100	4669	56	26464	515	21835	10062	335
KINGWOOD—Harris County										
□ CHARTER BEHAVIORAL HEALTH SYSTEM, (Formerly Charter Hospital of Kingwood) 2001 Ladbrook Drive, Zip 77339–3004; tel. 713/358–4501; Mark Micheletti, Chief Executive Officer **A**1 9 10 **F**2 3 18 22 26 27 34 41 45 52 53 54 55 56 57 58 59 65 67 **S**0695 Charter Medical Corporation	33	22	80	884	24	—	0	8209	2442	81
CHARTER HOSPITAL OF KINGWOOD See Charter Behavioral Health System										
□ PLAZA REHABILITATION HOSPITAL AT KINGWOOD, 22999 U.S. Highway 59, Ste 244, Zip 77325–6009; tel. 713/359–1313; Randy E. Johnson, Administrator (Total facility includes 16 beds in nursing home–type unit) **A**1 10 **F**7 8 10 12 14 15 16 19 20 21 22 23 28 30 32 35 37 40 41 44 49 63 64 65 67 70 71 73 74 **P**1 5	32	10	117	6096	82	32795	684	24942	14238	525
LA GRANGE—Fayette County										
★ FAYETTE MEMORIAL HOSPITAL, 543 North Jackson Street, Zip 78945–2040; tel. 409/968–3166; Marvin E. Cole, President and Chief Executive Officer **A**1 9 10 **F**7 8 12 14 15 16 19 21 22 28 29 30 32 40 41 42 44 45 49 64 65 71 73 74 **P**1 5	23	10	43	1450	26	21151	216	8389	3267	171
LACKLAND AIR FORCE BASE—Bexar County										
★ WILFORD HALL U.S. AIR FORCE MEDICAL CENTER, Zip 78236–5300; tel. 210/670–7100; James T. Vande Hey, Administrator (Nonreporting) **A**1 2 3 5 **S**9495 Department of the Air Force	41	10	747	—	—	—	—	—	—	—
LAKE JACKSON—Brazoria County										
★ BRAZOSPORT MEMORIAL HOSPITAL, 100 Medical Drive, Zip 77566–9983; tel. 409/297–4411; Wesley W. Oswald, Chief Executive Officer **A**1 9 10 **F**2 7 8 10 15 19 21 22 23 32 35 36 37 40 41 42 44 45 46 48 49 52 56 59 60 65 67 71 73 74 **P**8 **S**0002 Quorum Health Group/Quorum Health Resources	23	10	134	5506	64	69508	698	34975	13931	469
LAMESA—Dawson County										
★ MEDICAL ARTS HOSPITAL, 1600 North Bryan Avenue, Zip 79331; tel. 806/872–2183; Arla Jeffcoat, Administrator **A**1 9 10 **F**7 8 15 19 22 30 32 34 40 44 46 49 65 70 71 73	13	10	38	871	10	15481	134	6356	3461	180
LANCASTER—Dallas County										
★ MIDWAY PARK MEDICAL CENTER, 2600 West Pleasant Run Road, Zip 75146–1199; tel. 214/223–9600; Douglas P. DeGraaf, Chief Executive Officer (Total facility includes 10 beds in nursing home–type unit) **A**1 9 10 **F**1 4 7 8 9 10 11 12 16 17 19 21 22 23 24 25 26 28 29 32 34 35 37 38 39 40 41 42 43 44 45 46 47 48 49 52 54 55 56 57 60 61 63 64 65 66 69 70 71 72 73 74 **P**1 4 5 7 **S**0048 Columbia/HCA Healthcare Corporation	33	10	87	2563	42	34335	248	—	—	233
LAREDO—Webb County										
★ DOCTORS HOSPITAL OF LAREDO, 500 East Mann Road, Zip 78041; tel. 210/723–1131; David Hodgson, Chief Executive Officer (Total facility includes 6 beds in nursing home–type unit) **A**1 9 10 **F**8 10 11 15 16 19 20 21 22 23 27 28 30 32 34 35 37 40 42 44 49 60 63 64 65 71 72 **P**8 **S**0048 Columbia/HCA Healthcare Corporation	32	10	90	4333	52	33057	1634	27477	8545	347
★ MERCY REGIONAL MEDICAL CENTER, 1515 Logan Avenue, Zip 78040, Mailing Address: Drawer 2068, Zip 78044–2068; tel. 210/718–6230; Michael L. Morgan, President and Chief Executive Officer (Total facility includes 18 beds in nursing home–type unit) **A**1 9 10 **F**4 7 8 10 11 12 13 15 16 17 19 21 22 23 25 27 28 30 31 32 34 35 37 38 39 40 44 45 47 49 63 64 65 71 72 73 74 **P**8 **S**5185 Sisters of Mercy Health System–St. Louis	21	10	309	12894	210	123428	3589	75709	30826	1453

Hospitals, U.S. / TEXAS

Hospital, Address, Telephone, Administrator, Approval, Facility, and Physician Codes, Health Care System	Classification Codes		Utilization Data					Expense (thousands) of dollars		
★ American Hospital Association (AHA) membership □ Joint Commission on Accreditation of Healthcare Organizations (JCAHO) accreditation + American Osteopathic Hospital Association (AOHA) membership ○ American Osteopathic Association (AOA) accreditation △ Commission on Accreditation of Rehabilitation Facilities (CARF) accreditation Control codes 61, 63, 64, 71, 72 and 73 indicate hospitals listed by AOHA, but not registered by AHA. For definition of numerical codes, see page A6	Control	Service	Beds	Admissions	Census	Outpatient Visits	Births	Total	Payroll	Personnel
LAUGHLIN AIR FORCE BASE—Taylor County ★ U.S. AIR FORCE HOSPITAL, 590 Mitchell Boulevard, Zip 78843–5200; tel. 210/298–6311; Major Roy J. Ruff MSC, Administrator (Nonreporting) S9495 Department of the Air Force	41	10	7	—	—	—	—	—	—	—
LEAGUE CITY—Galveston County □ DEVEREUX TEXAS TREATMENT NETWORK, 1150 Devereux Drive, Zip 77573; tel. 713/335–1000; Gail Atkinson, Executive Director A1 9 10 F3 12 13 15 16 17 18 25 30 34 39 45 46 52 53 54 55 56 57 58 59 65 67 68 P6 S0845 Devereux Foundation	23	22	88	387	27	466	0	7161	4224	122
LEVELLAND—Hockley County ★ METHODIST HOSPITAL–LEVELLAND, 1900 South College Avenue, Zip 79336; tel. 806/894–4963; Jerry Osburn, Administrator A1 9 10 F3 7 8 14 15 16 17 19 20 21 22 28 29 30 31 32 33 34 36 39 40 43 44 45 46 49 51 53 54 55 56 57 58 59 65 71 73 P7 S0036 Lubbock Methodist Hospital System	21	10	44	1771	19	15784	267	10492	3670	186
LEWISVILLE—Denton County ★ LEWISVILLE MEDICAL CENTER HOSPITAL, (Formerly Lewisville Hospital) 500 West Main, Zip 75057–3699; tel. 214/420–1000; Raymond M. Dunning Jr., Chief Executive Officer A1 9 10 F4 7 8 19 22 32 33 35 37 40 41 42 44 49 64 65 66 67 71 73 74 S0048 Columbia/HCA Healthcare Corporation	33	10	105	5012	51	42165	1051	35546	13366	440
LIBERTY—Liberty County BAPTIST HOSPITAL LIBERTY, 1353 North Travis Street, Zip 77575–1353; tel. 409/336–7316; Daniel F. Sheehan, Interim Administrator A9 10 F15 19 22 44 49 65 71	21	10	29	555	4	14507	0	5565	2370	136
LINDEN—Cass County LINDEN MUNICIPAL HOSPITAL, North Kaufman Street, Zip 75563, Mailing Address: Box 32, Zip 75563; tel. 903/756–5561; Fred Wilbanks, Administrators A9 10 F8 11 16 19 20 22 26 32 34 37 44 46 48 49 65 71	16	10	39	890	14	—	0	4503	2645	120
LITTLEFIELD—Lamb County ★ LAMB HEALTHCARE CENTER, 1500 South Sunset, Zip 79339; tel. 806/385–6411; Randall A. Young, Administrator A1 10 F15 16 19 22 28 30 34 36 39 44 45 46 65 71 S0036 Lubbock Methodist Hospital System	13	10	41	475	9	5189	3	3289	1238	65
LIVINGSTON—Polk County POLK COUNTY MEMORIAL HOSPITAL, 602 East Church Street, Zip 77351–1257, Mailing Address: P.O. Box 1257, Zip 77351–1257; tel. 409/327–4381; Troy A. Dean, Interim Administrator A9 10 F14 15 16 19 22 28 30 33 34 40 44 51 71 73 P3	13	10	24	942	8	—	252	6405	2382	141
LLANO—Llano County ★ LLANO MEMORIAL HOSPITAL, 200 West Ollie Street, Zip 78643–2628; tel. 915/247–5040; Diane M. G. Gage R.N., Administrator A9 10 F8 15 16 17 19 21 22 28 32 33 34 42 44 65 71 73	13	10	27	1244	13	21139	187	6008	2956	132
LOCKNEY—Floyd County W. J. MANGOLD MEMORIAL HOSPITAL, 320 North Main Street, Zip 79241–0037, Mailing Address: Box 37, Zip 79241–0037; tel. 806/652–3373; Robin Satterwhite, Administrator A9 10 F7 22 25 28 33 34 40 44 61 71	16	10	27	622	7	21797	139	2677	1373	64
LONGVIEW—Gregg County ★ △ GOOD SHEPHERD MEDICAL CENTER, 700 East Marshall Avenue, Zip 75601–5571; tel. 903/236–2000; Jerry D. Adair, President and Chief Executive Officer (Total facility includes 26 beds in nursing home–type unit) A1 7 9 10 F4 7 8 10 12 14 15 16 17 19 20 21 22 23 25 26 27 28 29 30 31 32 34 35 37 39 40 41 42 43 44 45 46 48 51 56 60 63 64 65 66 69 70 71 73 74 P1	23	10	297	13195	222	149914	1453	103852	42108	1586
★ LONGVIEW REGIONAL HOSPITAL, 2901 North Fourth Street, Zip 75601–1903, Mailing Address: P.O. Box 15000, Zip 75607–5000; tel. 903/758–1818; Velinda Stevens, Administrator and Chief Executive Officer A1 9 10 F4 7 8 10 12 15 16 19 20 21 22 23 24 28 29 30 31 32 34 35 37 40 41 42 43 44 45 46 48 49 63 65 66 67 70 71 73 P7 8 S0048 Columbia/HCA Healthcare Corporation	33	10	95	3546	44	34390	634	31909	11120	369
LUBBOCK—Lubbock County □ CHARTER BEHAVIORAL HEALTH SYSTEM, 801 North Quaker, Zip 79416, Mailing Address: P.O. Box 10560, Zip 79408; tel. 806/744–5505; Liam J. Mulvaney, Chief Executive Officer and Administrator A1 9 10 F2 3 12 30 34 46 52 53 54 56 57 58 59 65 S0695 Charter Medical Corporation	33	22	72	1073	35	4520	0	8100	2652	85
□ HIGHLAND MEDICAL CENTER, 2412 50th Street, Zip 79412; tel. 806/795–8251; David Conejo, Administrator A1 2 9 10 F7 8 11 12 15 16 19 20 21 22 26 29 30 32 33 34 35 37 38 39 40 41 42 44 45 46 48 49 64 65 69 71 72 73 74 S0875 Community Health Systems, Inc.	33	10	76	2162	32	21270	0	16956	5982	176
HORIZON SPECIALTY HOSPITAL, 1409 9th Street, Zip 79401; tel. 806/767–9133; Bruce W. Reinhardt, Administrator (Newly Registered) A9 10	33	46	30	—	—	—	—	—	—	—
★ METHODIST CHILDREN'S HOSPITAL, 3610 21st Street, Zip 79410; tel. 806/784–5040; William D. Poteet III FACHE, President and Chief Executive Officer A9 10 F4 7 8 10 15 16 19 21 22 23 24 26 30 31 32 35 38 41 42 43 44 45 47 49 60 65 69 70 71 P7 S0036 Lubbock Methodist Hospital System	21	50	50	2069	29	19200	0	14879	2239	72
★ △ METHODIST HOSPITAL, 3615 19th Street, Zip 79410–1201, Mailing Address: Box 1201, Zip 79408–1201; tel. 806/792–1011; William D. Poteet III FACHE, President and Chief Executive Officer A1 2 6 7 9 10 F4 7 8 10 11 15 16 17 19 21 22 23 24 26 30 31 34 35 37 38 39 40 41 42 43 44 45 47 48 49 60 64 65 66 67 69 70 71 73 74 P7 S0036 Lubbock Methodist Hospital System	21	10	635	21015	497	199694	1333	217418	84567	3210

© 1995 AHA Guide

Hospitals, U.S. / TEXAS

Hospital, Address, Telephone, Administrator, Approval, Facility, and Physician Codes, Health Care System	Control	Service	Beds	Admissions	Census	Outpatient Visits	Births	Total	Payroll	Personnel
☐ SOUTH PARK HOSPITAL, 6610 Quaker Avenue, Zip 79413-5938; tel. 806/791-8000; Steve Rowley, Chief Executive Officer A1 10 F2 4 7 8 9 10 11 13 15 17 19 20 21 22 24 27 28 30 31 32 34 35 37 38 39 40 42 43 44 45 46 47 50 51 52 63 64 65 66 71 73 74 P7 S6525 Ornda Healthcorp	33	10	61	2000	22	19793	482	23825	5727	203
✣ ST. MARY OF THE PLAINS HOSPITAL, 4000 24th Street, Zip 79410; tel. 806/796-6000; Charley O. Trimble, President and Chief Executive Officer; Anthony W. Heep, Executive Vice President and Chief Operating Officer A1 2 3 5 9 10 F2 3 4 7 8 10 11 15 16 17 19 20 21 22 29 30 31 32 35 37 38 40 41 42 43 44 45 46 47 48 52 56 59 60 64 65 67 71 73 74 P3 5 6 7 S5425 St. Joseph Health System	21	10	410	12324	294	51038	917	99579	34497	1619
✣ UNIVERSITY MEDICAL CENTER, 602 Indiana Avenue, Zip 79415, Mailing Address: P.O. Box 5980, Zip 79408-5980; tel. 806/743-3111; James P. Courtney, President and Chief Executive Officer A1 2 3 5 10 F2 4 7 8 9 10 11 12 17 19 21 22 23 28 29 30 31 32 35 37 38 40 42 43 44 46 47 48 49 52 54 56 60 63 64 65 66 67 69 70 71 73 74	16	10	277	14776	192	159284	2040	110153	39450	1470
LUFKIN—Angelina County										
✣ MEMORIAL HEALTH SYSTEM OF EAST TEXAS, (Formerly Memorial Medical Center of East Texas) 1201 Frank Street, Zip 75901, Mailing Address: P.O. Box 1447, Zip 75902-1447; tel. 409/634-8111; Gary Lex Whatley, President and Chief Executive Officer (Total facility includes 30 beds in nursing home-type unit) A1 9 10 F7 8 10 11 12 16 17 18 19 21 22 23 26 27 28 29 30 31 32 33 34 35 37 39 40 41 42 44 45 46 48 49 51 52 54 55 56 57 58 59 60 64 65 67 71 72 73 74 P5 7	23	10	252	7759	131	58444	557	53539	22060	988
PINEYWOODS HOSPITAL, 1201 Frank Street, Zip 75901, Mailing Address: P.O. Box 1447, Zip 75901; tel. 409/639-7590; Joseph W. McCulley, Administrator A10 F1 3 12 17 18 22 52 53 55 56 58 65 P6	13	22	16	462	9	0	0	1367	667	50
✣ WOODLAND HEIGHTS MEDICAL CENTER, 500 Gaslight Boulevard, Zip 75901, Mailing Address: Box 150610, Zip 75915-0610; tel. 409/634-8311; Don H. McBride, Chief Executive Officer (Total facility includes 16 beds in nursing home-type unit) A1 9 10 F4 7 8 10 11 12 14 15 16 17 19 20 21 22 28 29 30 31 32 34 35 37 39 40 41 43 44 45 49 63 64 65 66 67 71 73 74 P1 4 5 7 8 S0048 Columbia/HCA Healthcare Corporation	33	10	116	4866	73	29503	444	31432	10828	379
LULING—Caldwell County										
★ EDGAR B. DAVIS MEMORIAL HOSPITAL, 130 Hays Street, Zip 78648, Mailing Address: P.O. Box 510, Zip 78648-0510; tel. 210/875-5643; Robert Haynes, Administrator (Total facility includes 6 beds in nursing home-type unit) A9 10 F8 15 16 19 22 32 34 44 53 64 65 71 73 P8	14	10	21	1012	12	15093	117	3987	1755	100
MADISONVILLE—Madison County										
☐ MADISON COUNTY HOSPITAL, 100 West Cross Street, Zip 77864-0698, Mailing Address: Box 698, Zip 77864-0698; tel. 409/348-2631; James P. Gibson, Administrator A1 9 10 F14 15 16 21 22 25 28 31 32 34 44 49 65 71 73 P5 6	13	10	28	750	13	14703	23	6929	3472	134
MANSFIELD—Tarrant County										
☐ VENCOR HOSPITAL–FORT WORTH SOUTH, (Acute Care Long-term) (Includes Vencor Hospital–Fort Worth West, 815 Eighth Avenue, Fort Worth, Texas, Zip 76104; tel. 817/332-4812) 1802 Highway 157 North, Zip 76063-9555; tel. 817/473-6101; James L. Ashbaugh, Administrator A1 9 10 F14 16 19 21 22 35 37 39 65 71 73 S0026 Vencor, Incorporated	33	49	94	284	39	321	0	9380	4669	166
MARLIN—Falls County										
FALLS COMMUNITY HOSPITAL AND CLINIC, 322 Coleman Street, Zip 76661-2358, Mailing Address: Box 60, Zip 76661-0060; tel. 817/883-3561; Billy Don York, Administrator A9 10 F8 15 19 20 22 25 28 29 30 34 39 49 71	23	10	29	743	8	41450	0	4299	1869	82
✣ VETERANS AFFAIRS MEDICAL CENTER, 1016 Ward Street, Zip 76661-2162; tel. 817/883-3511; Melvin E. Baker, Director A1 F2 3 8 9 11 12 19 20 21 22 23 26 28 30 31 34 35 37 39 41 42 44 45 46 48 49 51 52 54 55 56 57 58 60 65 71 72 74 P6 S9295 Department of Veterans Affairs	45	10	134	1486	86	18065	0	—	—	332
MARSHALL—Harrison County										
✣ MARSHALL MEMORIAL HOSPITAL, 811 South Washington, Zip 75670, Mailing Address: Box 1599, Zip 75671-1599; tel. 903/927-6000; Robert L. Driewer, Chief Executive Officer (Total facility includes 10 beds in nursing home-type unit) A1 9 10 F7 8 15 17 19 22 28 30 31 32 34 35 37 39 40 41 42 44 48 49 64 65 70 71 73 P8	23	10	103	2929	38	31512	560	17089	7909	343
MCALLEN—Hidalgo County										
☐ CHARTER BEHAVIORAL HEALTH SYSTEM, (Formerly Charter Palms Hospital) 1421 East Jackson Avenue, Zip 78501, Mailing Address: P.O. Box 5239, Zip 78502; tel. 512/631-5421; Leslie B. Hedfelt, Chief Executive Officer A1 9 10 F2 3 16 34 52 53 56 57 58 59 S0695 Charter Medical Corporation	33	22	72	946	28	3941	0	6985	2368	90
CHARTER PALMS HOSPITAL See Charter Behavioral Health System										
☐ MCALLEN MEDICAL CENTER, 301 West Expressway 83, Zip 78503; tel. 210/632-4000; John L. Mims, Executive Director A1 3 9 10 F2 4 7 8 10 11 15 16 19 20 21 22 23 24 29 30 34 35 37 38 39 40 41 42 43 44 46 47 48 49 51 52 53 55 56 57 58 60 61 64 65 66 70 71 73 74 P8 S9555 Universal Health Services, Inc.	33	10	408	21125	330	100890	6137	117035	48485	1456
✣ RIO GRANDE REGIONAL HOSPITAL, 101 East Ridge Road, Zip 78503; tel. 210/632-6000; Randall M. Everts, Chief Executive Officer A1 9 10 F4 7 8 10 11 12 14 15 16 17 19 21 22 23 25 28 30 31 32 33 34 35 37 38 39 40 41 42 43 44 46 49 54 56 60 64 65 67 71 73 74 P8 S0048 Columbia/HCA Healthcare Corporation	33	10	198	8451	126	31545	1012	46790	17966	620

Hospitals, U.S. / TEXAS

Hospital, Address, Telephone, Administrator, Approval, Facility, and Physician Codes, Health Care System	Classification Codes		Utilization Data					Expense (thousands) of dollars		
★ American Hospital Association (AHA) membership □ Joint Commission on Accreditation of Healthcare Organizations (JCAHO) accreditation + American Osteopathic Hospital Association (AOHA) membership ○ American Osteopathic Association (AOA) accreditation △ Commission on Accreditation of Rehabilitation Facilities (CARF) accreditation Control codes 61, 63, 64, 71, 72 and 73 indicate hospitals listed by AOHA, but not registered by AHA. For definition of numerical codes, see page A6	Control	Service	Beds	Admissions	Census	Outpatient Visits	Births	Total	Payroll	Personnel
MCCAMEY—Upton County MCCAMEY HOSPITAL, Highway 305 South, Zip 79752, Mailing Address: Box 1200, Zip 79752–1200; tel. 915/652–8626; Bill Boswell, Chief Executive Officer (Total facility includes 30 beds in nursing home–type unit) **A**9 10 **F**15 22 32 34 44 65 **P**5	16	10	46	91	30	9985	0	3923	1670	87
MCKINNEY—Collin County ★ NORTH TEXAS MEDICAL CENTER, (Includes North Texas Medical Center–Westpark Campus, 130 South Central Expressway, McKinney, Texas, Zip 75070; tel. 214/548–5300; Don S. Ciulla, Executive Director) 1800 North Graves Street, Zip 75069; tel. 214/548–3000; Don S. Ciulla, Chief Executive Officer **A**1 9 10 **F**7 8 11 12 16 19 21 22 23 24 25 26 27 28 31 32 33 34 35 37 39 40 42 44 46 48 49 52 54 56 57 58 59 64 65 67 71 72 73 74 **P**7 **S**0048 Columbia/HCA Healthcare Corporation	32	10	172	4995	70	39006	918	41704	14334	532
MEMPHIS—Hall County HALL COUNTY HOSPITAL, 1800 North Boykin Drive, Zip 79245; tel. 806/259–3504; Jody Dixon, Administrator **A**9 10 **F**8 19 22 32 33 39 49 71	16	10	28	318	4	4462	1	1826	854	54
MESQUITE—Dallas County □ MEDICAL CENTER OF MESQUITE, 1011 North Galloway Avenue, Zip 75149; tel. 214/320–7000; Terry J. Fontenot, Administrator **A**1 9 10 **F**4 8 10 11 12 14 15 16 17 19 20 21 22 25 28 29 30 31 32 33 34 35 37 39 41 42 43 44 45 48 49 52 53 54 55 56 63 64 65 71 73 74 **P**5 7 8 **S**5765 Paracelsus Healthcare Corporation	33	10	152	3866	60	42220	0	37556	12448	418
★ MESQUITE COMMUNITY HOSPITAL, 3500 I–30 at Motley, Zip 75150–2696; tel. 214/270–3300; Raymond P. De Blasi, Chief Executive Officer (Nonreporting) **A**1 10	33	10	117	—	—	—	—	—	—	—
MEXIA—Limestone County ★ PARKVIEW REGIONAL HOSPITAL, 312 East Glendale Street, Zip 76667–3699; tel. 817/562–5332; Karl R. Stinson, Administrator **A**1 9 10 **F**1 3 4 5 6 7 8 10 11 12 13 15 17 18 19 20 21 22 23 24 25 26 27 28 29 30 31 32 33 34 35 36 37 39 40 41 42 43 44 45 46 49 50 51 52 53 54 55 56 57 58 59 60 61 62 63 65 66 67 68 69 70 71 72 73 74 **S**0585 Brim, Inc.	23	10	36	1059	10	18191	127	7374	2906	130
MIDLAND—Midland County ★ △ MEMORIAL HOSPITAL AND MEDICAL CENTER, (Includes Memorial Rehabilitation Hospital, Midland, Texas, Mailing Address: P.O. Box 4757, Zip 79704; tel. 915/697–5200; Harold Rubin, President) 2200 West Illinois Avenue, Zip 79701–9980; tel. 915/685–1111; Harold Rubin, President and Chief Executive Officer (Total facility includes 17 beds in nursing home–type unit) **A**1 2 5 7 9 10 **F**4 7 8 10 12 13 14 15 16 17 18 19 20 21 22 23 25 29 30 33 34 35 37 39 40 41 42 43 44 45 46 48 49 50 51 52 53 54 55 56 57 58 59 60 63 64 65 67 71 72 73 **P**3 7 8	16	10	270	9162	165	143617	1779	101377	36991	1166
PHYSICIANS AND SURGEONS HOSPITAL, 3201 Sage Street, Zip 79705; tel. 915/683–2273; Michael S. Potter, President and Chief Executive Officer **A**9 10 **F**8 12 15 16 28 31 32 37 44 46 49 66 71 **P**7	33	10	42	1609	23	15756	0	11577	4952	160
MINERAL WELLS—Palo Pinto County ★ PALO PINTO GENERAL HOSPITAL, 400 Southwest 25th Avenue, Zip 76067–9685; tel. 817/325–7891; Guy Hazlett II FACHE, Chief Executive Officer **A**1 9 10 **F**4 7 8 14 15 16 19 21 22 29 30 32 35 37 40 44 45 51 65 66 71 73 74	16	10	44	2629	37	22948	345	17795	8669	334
MISSION—Hidalgo County ★ MISSION HOSPITAL, 900 South Bryan Road, Zip 78572; tel. 210/580–9000; Thomas B. Symonds, Administrator **A**1 9 10 **F**7 15 19 22 29 34 35 37 40 41 42 44 46 65 67 71 73 **P**8 **S**0002 Quorum Health Group/Quorum Health Resources	23	10	110	5259	67	26442	1301	27446	10343	414
MISSOURI CITY—Fort Bend County ★ FORT BEND HOSPITAL, 3803 FM 1092 at Highway 6, Zip 77459; tel. 713/499–4800; Wilson J. Weber, Executive Director (Total facility includes 12 beds in nursing home–type unit) **A**1 9 10 **F**3 4 7 8 10 12 14 15 16 17 19 22 23 24 25 26 28 29 30 31 32 33 34 35 37 39 40 41 42 43 44 45 49 53 54 55 56 57 58 59 60 63 64 65 66 71 73 74 **P**6 8 **S**0048 Columbia/HCA Healthcare Corporation	33	10	64	2427	26	10468	475	15694	6076	248
MONAHANS—Ward County ★ WARD MEMORIAL HOSPITAL, 406 South Gary Street, Zip 79756; tel. 915/943–2511 **A**1 9 10 **F**7 15 17 19 22 26 27 28 29 30 32 37 40 41 44 45 49 65 71 73	13	10	41	541	7	12943	46	6152	2482	97
MORTON—Cochran County ★ COCHRAN MEMORIAL HOSPITAL, 201 East Grant Street, Zip 79346; tel. 806/266–5565; Geneva Hunter, Administrator **A**9 10 **F**13 19 25 34 44 71 **P**5	16	10	30	219	2	2158	1	1949	—	44
MOUNT PLEASANT—Franklin County ★ TITUS REGIONAL MEDICAL CENTER, 2001 North Jefferson, Zip 75455; tel. 903/577–6000; Wayne L. Ogburn FACHE, Chief Executive Officer and Administrator **A**1 9 10 **F**8 15 19 21 22 23 26 34 35 39 40 44 51 64 65 70 71 73 **P**5 8 **S**0002 Quorum Health Group/Quorum Health Resources	16	10	165	5058	58	19319	966	29248	11775	523
MOUNT VERNON—Franklin County ★ EAST TEXAS MEDICAL CENTER–MOUNT VERNON, Highway 37 South, Zip 75457, Mailing Address: Box 477, Zip 75457–0477; tel. 903/537–4552; Perry Henderson, Administrator **A**1 9 10 **F**8 12 15 17 19 20 21 22 26 27 29 30 32 34 44 49 51 65 71 72 **P**1 **S**1895 East Texas Medical Center Regional Healthcare System	23	10	30	868	10	—	0	5321	2500	101
MUENSTER—Cooke County MUENSTER MEMORIAL HOSPITAL, 605 North Maple Street, Zip 76252, Mailing Address: Box 370, Zip 76252; tel. 817/759–2271; Jack R. Endres, Administrator **A**9 10 **F**8 19 20 22 28 32 33 34 42 44 49 65 67 71	16	10	18	291	3	5875	0	2094	991	46

© 1995 AHA Guide

Hospitals, U.S. / TEXAS

Hospital, Address, Telephone, Administrator, Approval, Facility, and Physician Codes, Health Care System	Classification Codes		Utilization Data					Expense (thousands) of dollars		
★ American Hospital Association (AHA) membership ☐ Joint Commission on Accreditation of Healthcare Organizations (JCAHO) accreditation + American Osteopathic Hospital Association (AOHA) membership ○ American Osteopathic Association (AOA) accreditation △ Commission on Accreditation of Rehabilitation Facilities (CARF) accreditation Control codes 61, 63, 64, 71, 72 and 73 indicate hospitals listed by AOHA, but not registered by AHA. For definition of numerical codes, see page A6	Control	Service	Beds	Admissions	Census	Outpatient Visits	Births	Total	Payroll	Personnel
MULESHOE—Bailey County										
★ MULESHOE AREA MEDICAL CENTER, 708 South First Street, Zip 79347; tel. 806/272–4524; Richard Murphy, Administrator **A**9 10 **F**7 14 19 22 28 32 44 49 71 **S**0036 Lubbock Methodist Hospital System	16	10	31	653	6	11357	45	4555	2016	110
NACOGDOCHES—Nacogdoches County										
AMI NACOGDOCHES MEDICAL CENTER See Nacogdoches Medical Center										
✠ NACOGDOCHES MEDICAL CENTER, (Formerly AMI Nacogdoches Medical Center) 4920 Northeast Stallings, Zip 75961, Mailing Address: Box 631604, Zip 75963–1604; tel. 409/569–9481; Bryant H. Krenek Jr., Director **A**1 9 10 **F**7 8 10 15 16 19 21 22 23 32 34 35 37 40 42 44 46 51 60 65 67 71 73 **S**0063 TENET Healthcare Corporation	33	10	142	4974	59	—	590	25729	10244	335
✠ △ NACOGDOCHES MEMORIAL HOSPITAL, 1204 Mound Street, Zip 75961–9987; tel. 409/568–8521; Robert V. Deen, Administrator **A**1 7 9 10 **F**4 7 8 10 15 19 21 22 28 30 31 32 33 34 35 37 40 41 42 43 44 48 61 65 71 73 **P**8	16	10	155	5767	97	38024	726	44717	17921	734
☐ PINELANDS HOSPITAL, 4632 Northeast Stallings Drive, Zip 75961, Mailing Address: P.O. Box 1004, Zip 79563–1004; tel. 409/560–5900; Jerry Wilson, Administrator **A**1 9 10 **F**12 15 17 18 22 26 52 53 54 55 56 57 58 59 65 67 **P**1 5 7 **S**0455 Hospital Group of America	33	22	38	477	19	362	0	3887	1641	46
NASSAU BAY—Harris County										
✠ ST. JOHN HOSPITAL, 2050 Space Park Drive, Zip 77058; tel. 713/333–5503 **A**1 9 10 **F**2 3 4 5 7 8 9 10 11 12 14 15 16 17 18 19 20 21 22 24 26 28 29 30 31 32 33 34 35 36 37 38 39 40 41 42 43 44 45 46 47 48 49 50 51 52 53 54 55 56 57 58 59 60 61 63 64 65 66 67 69 71 72 73 74 **P**3 7 8 **S**0605 Sisters of Charity of the Incarnate Word Healthcare System	23	10	133	6872	70	91790	1331	53500	23950	648
NAVASOTA—Grimes County										
CLC-NAVASOTA REGIONAL HOSPITAL, 210 South Judson Street, Zip 77868, Mailing Address: P.O. Box 1390, Zip 77868–1390; tel. 409/825–6585; Molly Hurst, Administrator **A**9 10 **F**14 15 16 19 22 34 35 44 71 73	33	10	18	599	8	4698	0	2468	1013	50
NEDERLAND—Jefferson County										
✠ MID–JEFFERSON HOSPITAL, (Formerly AMI Mid–Jefferson Hospital) Highway 365 and 27th Street, Zip 77627, Mailing Address: P.O. Box 1917, Zip 77627–1917; tel. 409/727–2321; Luis G. Silva, Chief Executive Officer (Total facility includes 18 beds in nursing home–type unit) **A**1 9 10 **F**7 8 12 13 15 16 17 19 21 22 23 28 29 30 31 32 34 35 37 40 44 45 46 51 64 65 71 73 74 **P**3 **S**0063 TENET Healthcare Corporation	32	10	138	3425	41	56987	662	19450	8112	312
NEW BRAUNFELS—Comal County										
✠ MCKENNA MEMORIAL HOSPITAL, 143 East Garza Street, Zip 78130–4191; tel. 210/606–9111; Marion P. Johnson FACHE, Administrator and Chief Executive Officer **A**1 9 10 **F**7 8 11 15 16 19 21 22 26 28 30 34 35 37 40 41 42 44 45 46 49 65 71 73 74 **P**8	23	10	77	4313	43	46216	660	24623	11158	435
NOCONA—Montague County										
★ NOCONA GENERAL HOSPITAL, 100 Park Street, Zip 76255; tel. 817/825–3235; Wanda Billings, Administrator **A**9 10 **F**8 12 15 16 22 26 28 40 42 44 49 65 71 73 **P**5	16	10	32	994	11	19322	119	4666	2205	111
NORTH RICHLAND HILLS—Tarrant County										
✠ NORTH HILLS HOSPITAL, 4401 Booth Calloway Road, Zip 76180–7399; tel. 817/284–1431; Randy Moresi, Chief Executive Officer **A**1 9 10 **F**4 7 8 10 11 12 15 16 19 21 22 23 24 28 29 30 33 34 35 37 38 39 40 41 42 43 44 45 46 48 49 52 64 65 67 71 73 74 **P**5 **S**0048 Columbia/HCA Healthcare Corporation	33	10	151	4048	55	29106	500	28910	11993	383
☐ RICHLAND HOSPITAL, 7501 Glenview Drive, Zip 76180; tel. 817/595–5000; Darryl S. Dubroca, Administrator and Chief Executive Officer **A**1 9 10 **F**2 3 18 22 52 53 54 55 56 57 58 59 65 67 68 **S**0069 Behavioral Healthcare Corporation	33	22	77	616	17	4932	0	6263	2782	93
ODESSA—Ector County										
AMI ODESSA WOMEN'S AND CHILDREN'S HOSPITAL See Odessa Regional Hospital										
✠ MEDICAL CENTER HOSPITAL, 500 West Fourth Street, Zip 79761–5059, Mailing Address: P.O. Drawer 7239, Zip 79760; tel. 915/333–7111; J. Michael Stephans, Administrator (Total facility includes 25 beds in nursing home–type unit) **A**1 2 3 5 9 10 **F**4 7 8 10 11 16 17 19 21 22 23 25 30 33 34 35 37 38 40 42 43 44 46 49 50 51 60 63 64 65 71 73 74 **P**8	16	10	301	10911	211	107513	1534	95359	38244	1408
✠ ODESSA REGIONAL HOSPITAL, (Formerly AMI Odessa Women's and Children's Hospital) 520 East Sixth Street, Zip 79761, Mailing Address: Box 4859, Zip 79760; tel. 915/334–8200; Lex A. Guinn, Chief Executive Officer **A**1 9 10 **F**7 8 14 15 16 19 27 28 29 30 34 36 37 38 39 40 44 45 46 65 71 73 74 **P**7 **S**0063 TENET Healthcare Corporation	32	44	100	3241	37	16823	1295	22616	7144	241
OLNEY—Young County										
★ HAMILTON HOSPITAL, 903 West Hamilton Street, Zip 76374, Mailing Address: Box 158, Zip 76374; tel. 817/564–5521; William R. Smith, Administrator **A**9 10 **F**7 19 22 28 32 33 37 40 44 45 71 73 **P**5	16	10	46	945	14	38309	35	4480	2066	91
ORANGE—Orange County										
☐ BAPTIST HOSPITAL–ORANGE, 608 Strickland, Zip 77630, Mailing Address: P.O. Box 7800, Zip 77631–7800; tel. 409/883–9361; Sammy E. Davis, Administrator **A**1 9 10 **F**2 3 7 8 12 15 17 19 21 22 26 27 28 30 31 34 35 37 40 41 44 48 49 65 67 71 72 73 **P**8	21	10	136	3926	58	36021	286	28138	10142	386

Hospitals, U.S. / TEXAS

Hospital, Address, Telephone, Administrator, Approval, Facility, and Physician Codes, Health Care System	Classification Codes		Utilization Data					Expense (thousands) of dollars		
★ American Hospital Association (AHA) membership ☐ Joint Commission on Accreditation of Healthcare Organizations (JCAHO) accreditation + American Osteopathic Hospital Association (AOHA) membership ○ American Osteopathic Association (AOA) accreditation △ Commission on Accreditation of Rehabilitation Facilities (CARF) accreditation Control codes 61, 63, 64, 71, 72 and 73 indicate hospitals listed by AOHA, but not registered by AHA. For definition of numerical codes, see page A6	Control	Service	Beds	Admissions	Census	Outpatient Visits	Births	Total	Payroll	Personnel
OZONA—Crockett County CROCKETT COUNTY HOSPITAL AND CARE CENTER, Avenue H and First Street, Zip 76943, Mailing Address: Box 640, Zip 76943–0640; tel. 915/392–2671; Gerard Phillips, Administrator A9 F14 15 16 22 P8	13	10	20	9	0	3289	0	1597	675	35
PALACIOS—Matagorda County ★ WAGNER GENERAL HOSPITAL, 310 Green Street, Zip 77465, Mailing Address: Box 859, Zip 77465; tel. 512/972–2511; Helen Dolezal, Director A9 10 F8 15 19 22 30 32 34 65 71 P5	16	10	6	113	1	6524	0	1770	832	21
PALESTINE—Anderson County ★ MEMORIAL HOSPITAL, 900 South Sycamore Street, Zip 75801, Mailing Address: Box 4070, Zip 75802; tel. 903/729–6981; Bob Charron, Administrator A1 9 10 F8 10 19 21 22 27 28 30 32 34 35 37 39 44 45 46 63 65 66 71 P5 8	23	10	84	3778	44	39544	0	23088	8332	405
☐ TRINITY VALLEY MEDICAL CENTER, 2900 South Loop 256, Zip 75801; tel. 903/731–1000; Larry C. Bozeman, Chief Executive Officer (Total facility includes 12 beds in nursing home–type unit) A1 10 F7 10 15 16 19 21 22 23 28 29 30 32 34 35 37 40 41 44 45 46 48 49 52 55 56 63 64 65 67 71 73 74 S6525 Ornda Healthcorp	33	10	126	3817	54	39233	863	27459	9766	411
PAMPA—Gray County ★ CORONADO HOSPITAL, One Medical Plaza, Zip 79065; tel. 806/665–3721; H. Douglas Garner, Chief Executive Officer (Total facility includes 14 beds in nursing home–type unit) A1 9 10 F7 8 10 12 15 16 19 21 22 23 28 30 32 34 35 37 40 41 44 46 48 49 61 64 65 67 71 73 P8 S0048 Columbia/HCA Healthcare Corporation	33	10	96	2270	33	19255	360	18926	6424	290
PARIS—Lamar County ★ MCCUISTION REGIONAL MEDICAL CENTER, 865 Deshong Drive, Zip 75462, Mailing Address: P.O. Box 160, Zip 75461–0160; tel. 903/737–1111; Anthony A. Daigle, Administrator A1 9 10 F7 8 10 12 14 15 16 17 19 21 22 23 24 26 28 29 30 31 32 33 34 35 37 40 41 42 44 45 46 49 52 54 55 56 57 60 65 66 71 73 74 P5 8	23	10	157	6345	75	41720	722	30673	12356	504
★ ST. JOSEPH'S HOSPITAL AND HEALTH CENTER, 820 Clarksville Street, Zip 75460–9070, Mailing Address: P.O. Box 9070, Zip 75461–9070; tel. 903/785–4521; Monty E. McLaurin, President A1 9 10 F3 4 8 10 11 12 14 15 16 19 21 22 23 24 26 28 29 30 31 32 33 34 35 37 39 41 42 43 44 46 48 49 52 54 55 56 57 58 59 60 65 66 70 71 73 P7 8 S5565 Incarnate Word Health Services	21	10	177	6616	113	50349	0	46357	19522	645
PASADENA—Harris County ★ BAYSHORE MEDICAL CENTER, 4000 Spencer Highway, Zip 77504–1294; tel. 713/944–6666; Karen Poole, Chief Executive Officer (Total facility includes 29 beds in nursing home–type unit) A1 2 9 10 F2 3 4 7 8 10 11 12 15 16 17 18 19 20 21 22 23 25 26 28 30 32 33 34 35 37 38 39 40 41 42 43 44 45 46 48 49 52 53 54 55 56 58 59 60 64 65 67 68 71 72 73 74 P1 8 S0048 Columbia/HCA Healthcare Corporation	33	10	352	12120	180	92352	1690	63084	24802	947
☐ PASADENA GENERAL HOSPITAL, 1004 Seymour Street, Zip 77506; tel. 713/473–1771; Elizabeth A. Primeaux, Administrator (Nonreporting) A1 9 10	33	10	146	—	—	—	—	—	—	—
☐ SOUTHMORE MEDICAL CENTER, 906 East Southmore Avenue, Zip 77502–1124, Mailing Address: Box 1879, Zip 77502; tel. 713/477–0411; Dennis M. Knox, President and Chief Executive Officer (Total facility includes 21 beds in nursing home–type unit) A1 9 10 F7 8 10 11 15 19 20 21 22 23 26 28 30 31 32 34 35 37 39 40 41 42 44 45 46 49 52 53 54 55 56 57 64 65 70 71 73 74 P7 8	32	10	172	4898	86	27325	1226	37368	12827	489
PEARSALL—Frio County FRIO HOSPITAL, 320 Berry Ranch Road, Zip 78061; tel. 210/334–3617; Alan D. Holmes, Chief Executive Officer A9 10 F7 8 15 16 22 32 44 71	23	10	22	874	8	12372	229	4205	2055	92
PECOS—Reeves County ★ REEVES COUNTY HOSPITAL, 2323 Texas Street, Zip 79772; tel. 915/447–3551; Bruce K. Brichell, Administrator A10 F7 14 19 22 28 31 37 40 44 46 65 69 71 73 S0002 Quorum Health Group/Quorum Health Resources	16	10	46	985	10	10952	139	6803	2661	105
PERRYTON—Ochiltree County OCHILTREE GENERAL HOSPITAL, 3101 Garrett Drive, Zip 79070–5393; tel. 806/435–3606; Wallace N. Boyd, Administrator A9 10 F7 8 15 19 21 22 28 29 32 33 34 36 37 40 44 49 64 65 67 71 73	16	10	45	1023	13	—	179	5132	2539	110
PITTSBURG—Camp County ★ EAST TEXAS MEDICAL CENTER PITTSBURG, 414 Quitman Street, Zip 75686–1032; tel. 903/856–6663; Charles N. Butts, Administrator A1 9 10 F1 8 19 20 21 22 25 26 32 44 65 71 P3 S1895 East Texas Medical Center Regional Healthcare System	23	10	42	1168	21	93442	0	10266	4815	220
PLAINVIEW—Hale County ★ METHODIST HOSPITAL PLAINVIEW, 2601 Dimmitt Road, Zip 79072–1833; tel. 806/296–5531; Donald W. Shouse, Administrator A1 9 10 F2 3 7 8 12 14 15 16 17 18 19 20 21 22 23 25 28 30 31 32 34 35 36 37 39 40 42 44 45 46 49 51 52 53 54 55 56 57 58 59 64 65 66 70 71 73 P3 7 8 S0036 Lubbock Methodist Hospital System	21	10	90	2556	35	40650	422	17925	6164	254
PLANO—Collin County ★ MEDICAL CENTER OF PLANO, 3901 West 15th Street, Zip 75075–7799; tel. 214/596–6800; Allyn Harris, President and Chief Executive Officer A1 2 9 10 F4 7 8 10 11 12 16 17 18 19 21 22 24 25 28 30 31 32 33 34 35 37 38 40 41 42 43 44 45 46 49 60 65 66 67 70 71 73 74 P8 S0048 Columbia/HCA Healthcare Corporation	33	10	233	12139	134	76661	3376	78046	33250	1004

© 1995 AHA Guide

Hospitals, U.S. / TEXAS

Hospital, Address, Telephone, Administrator, Approval, Facility, and Physician Codes, Health Care System	Classi-fication Codes		Utilization Data					Expense (thousands) of dollars		
★ American Hospital Association (AHA) membership □ Joint Commission on Accreditation of Healthcare Organizations (JCAHO) accreditation + American Osteopathic Hospital Association (AOHA) membership ○ American Osteopathic Association (AOA) accreditation △ Commission on Accreditation of Rehabilitation Facilities (CARF) accreditation Control codes 61, 63, 64, 71, 72 and 73 indicate hospitals listed by AOHA, but not registered by AHA. For definition of numerical codes, see page A6	Control	Service	Beds	Admissions	Census	Outpatient Visits	Births	Total	Payroll	Personnel
★ △ PLANO REHABILITATION HOSPITAL, 2800 West 15th Street, Zip 75075; tel. 214/612–9000; Laurence J. Frayne, Chief Executive Officer (Total facility includes 8 beds in nursing home–type unit) **A**1 7 9 10 **F**1 5 12 15 16 19 21 22 24 27 32 34 35 39 41 48 49 50 54 58 63 64 65 71 73 74 **P**5	33	46	60	902	51	10236	0	13161	5639	170
★ PRESBYTERIAN HOSPITAL OF PLANO, 6200 West Parker Road, Zip 75093–7914; tel. 214/608–8000; Philip M. Wentworth FACHE, President and Chief Executive Officer **A**1 9 10 **F**2 3 7 8 12 14 15 16 17 19 21 22 23 27 28 29 30 32 33 34 35 37 39 40 44 46 49 52 53 54 55 56 58 59 63 65 66 71 73 74 **P**7 8 **S**1130 Presbyterian Healthcare System	23	10	87	3709	33	19839	755	38702	10762	450
PORT ARTHUR—Jefferson County AMI PARK PLACE MEDICAL CENTER See Park Place Medical Center										
★ PARK PLACE MEDICAL CENTER, (Formerly AMI Park Place Medical Center) 3050 39th Street, Zip 77642, Mailing Address: Box 1648, Zip 77641; tel. 409/983–4951; Luis G. Silva, Chief Executive Officer (Total facility includes 21 beds in nursing home–type unit) **A**1 9 10 **F**4 7 8 10 12 15 16 17 19 21 22 23 28 29 30 31 34 35 37 40 42 43 44 45 46 48 51 60 64 65 71 72 73 74 **P**3 7 **S**0063 TENET Healthcare Corporation	32	10	233	5123	92	24005	639	32510	13298	545
★ ST. MARY HOSPITAL, 3600 Gates Boulevard, Zip 77642–3601, Mailing Address: P.O. Box 3696, Zip 77643–3696; tel. 409/985–7431; John K. Barto Jr., Administrator (Total facility includes 19 beds in nursing home–type unit) **A**1 3 5 9 10 **F**4 7 8 10 12 17 19 20 21 22 24 25 32 35 37 40 42 43 44 46 49 52 54 56 57 59 60 64 65 71 73 74 **P**1 3 4 5 6 7 8 **S**0605 Sisters of Charity of the Incarnate Word Healthcare System	21	10	226	8556	156	98817	1027	69357	29220	1017
PORT LAVACA—Calhoun County ★ MEMORIAL MEDICAL CENTER, 815 North Virginia Street, Zip 77979, Mailing Address: P.O. Box 25, Zip 77979; tel. 512/552–6713; Bob L. Bybee, Administrator **A**1 9 10 **F**7 8 13 14 15 16 19 20 21 22 28 30 31 32 37 38 39 40 41 44 45 49 65 67 71 73	13	10	48	1535	16	9535	282	10087	4532	212
POST—Garza County ★ GARZA MEMORIAL HOSPITAL, 608 West Sixth Street, Zip 79356–3699; tel. 806/495–2828; Maritta Reed, Administrator **A**9 10 **F**8 22 33 44 65 71 **P**6 **S**0036 Lubbock Methodist Hospital System	16	10	13	155	2	4857	0	1524	753	34
QUANAH—Hardeman County HARDEMAN COUNTY MEMORIAL HOSPITAL, 402 Mercer Street, Zip 79252, Mailing Address: Box 90, Zip 79252; tel. 817/663–2795; Charles Hurt, Administrator **A**9 10 **F**8 16 19 22 32 35 44 70 71 73 **P**8	16	10	23	279	4	6222	0	1515	781	45
QUITMAN—Wood County WOOD COUNTY CENTRAL HOSPITAL DISTRICT, 117 Winnsboro Street, Zip 75783, Mailing Address: P.O. Box 1000, Zip 75783–1000; tel. 903/763–4505; Marion W. Stanberry, Administrator **A**9 10 **F**7 19 22 30 34 40 44 49 70 73	16	10	28	1108	13	8436	162	5026	2227	109
RANKIN—Upton County RANKIN HOSPITAL DISTRICT, 1105 Elizabeth Street, Zip 79778, Mailing Address: Box 327, Zip 79778; tel. 915/693–2443; John Paul Loyless, Administrator **A**9 10 **F**14 15 16 17 22 33 34 39 40 44 46 51 71 73	16	10	20	135	1	550	43	1522	767	23
REESE AIR FORCE BASE—Lubbock County ★ U.S. AIR FORCE HOSPITAL, 250 13th Street, Zip 79489–5008; tel. 806/885–3542; Major Randy Borg MSC, USAF, Administrator (Nonreporting) **A**3 5 **S**9495 Department of the Air Force	41	10	10	—	—	—	—	—	—	—
REFUGIO—Refugio County ★ REFUGIO COUNTY MEMORIAL HOSPITAL, 107 Swift Street, Zip 78377; tel. 512/526–2321; Haskell G. Silkwood, Administrator **A**1 9 10 **F**14 15 16 17 19 22 25 30 31 34 36 39 44 45 46 49 51 65 66 67 71 73 **P**6	16	10	20	369	4	7907	0	4145	1689	77
RICHARDSON—Dallas County □ BAYLOR RICHARDSON MEDICAL CENTER, (Formerly Richardson Medical Center) 401 West Campbell Road, Zip 75080; tel. 214/498–4000; Ronald L. Boring, President and Chief Executive Officer **A**1 9 10 **F**2 3 4 7 8 10 11 12 17 19 22 23 26 28 30 31 32 33 34 35 37 40 43 44 45 46 48 49 51 52 53 54 55 56 57 58 59 60 61 64 66 71 73 **P**3 5 6 7 8 **S**0095 Baylor Health Care System	16	10	163	3802	54	30258	458	35300	15006	534
RICHMOND—Fort Bend County ★ POLLY RYON MEMORIAL HOSPITAL, 1705 Jackson Street, Zip 77469–3289; tel. 713/342–2811; Sam L. Steffee, Executive Director and Chief Executive Officer (Total facility includes 36 beds in nursing home–type unit) **A**1 9 10 **F**7 8 14 19 21 22 31 32 33 34 35 37 40 41 44 64 65 66 67 70 71 73 **P**5 8	16	10	145	3229	55	28057	654	22782	10404	343
RIO GRANDE CITY—Starr County ★ STARR COUNTY MEMORIAL HOSPITAL, Route 1, Zip 78582, Mailing Address: P.O. Box 78, Zip 78582; tel. 210/487–5561; Thalia H. Munoz, Administrator **A**9 10 **F**7 8 14 15 16 19 22 34 37 39 40 44 65 71 73	16	10	44	2165	21	55220	900	7547	3350	168
ROCKDALE—Milam County RICHARDS MEMORIAL HOSPITAL, 1700 Brazos Street, Zip 76567–2517, Mailing Address: Drawer 1010, Zip 76567–1010; tel. 512/446–2513; Edward F. Lynch, Administrator **A**9 10 **F**15 19 21 22 28 32 44 64 71	14	10	47	491	6	9502	0	3854	1599	51
ROTAN—Fisher County FISHER COUNTY HOSPITAL DISTRICT, Roby Highway, Zip 79546, Mailing Address: Drawer F, Zip 79546; tel. 915/735–2256; Ella Raye Helms, Administrator **A**9 10 **F**8 14 15 16 17 19 20 28 30 32 34 36 39 44 45 51 65 70 71 73 **P**5 6 **S**0036 Lubbock Methodist Hospital System	16	10	30	386	4	28257	2	3427	1643	71

Hospitals, U.S. / TEXAS

Hospital, Address, Telephone, Administrator, Approval, Facility, and Physician Codes, Health Care System	Classification Codes		Utilization Data					Expense (thousands) of dollars		
	Control	Service	Beds	Admissions	Census	Outpatient Visits	Births	Total	Payroll	Personnel

★ American Hospital Association (AHA) membership
☐ Joint Commission on Accreditation of Healthcare Organizations (JCAHO) accreditation
+ American Osteopathic Hospital Association (AOHA) membership
○ American Osteopathic Association (AOA) accreditation
△ Commission on Accreditation of Rehabilitation Facilities (CARF) accreditation
Control codes 61, 63, 64, 71, 72 and 73 indicate hospitals listed by AOHA, but not registered by AHA. For definition of numerical codes, see page A6

ROUND ROCK—Williamson County

★ ROUND ROCK HOSPITAL, 2400 Round Rock Avenue, Zip 78681; tel. 512/255–6066; Larry M. Graham, Administrator (Total facility includes 9 beds in nursing home–type unit) **A**1 9 10 **F**7 15 19 22 28 29 30 34 37 40 44 64 65 71 73 74 **P**7 8 **S**0048 Columbia/HCA Healthcare Corporation | 33 | 10 | 75 | 3318 | 32 | 35204 | 762 | 17171 | 7049 | 301

ROWLETT—Rockwall County

☐ LAKE POINTE MEDICAL CENTER, 6800 Scenic Drive, Zip 75088–1550, Mailing Address: P.O. Box 1550, Zip 75030–1500; tel. 214/412–2273; Kenneth R. Teel, Administrator **A**1 9 10 **F**7 8 11 16 19 22 24 28 31 32 33 34 35 40 41 42 44 45 49 64 65 67 71 73 **S**6525 Ornda Healthcorp | 33 | 10 | 92 | 3726 | 31 | 43624 | 308 | 23418 | 9262 | 328

RUSK—Cherokee County

★ EAST TEXAS MEDICAL CENTER RUSK, Copeland and Bonner Streets, Zip 75785, Mailing Address: P.O. Box 317, Zip 75785; tel. 903/683–2273; Donna S. Gunter B.S.N., R.N., C.P.H.Q., Administrator **A**1 9 10 **F**14 15 19 22 28 32 44 65 71 **P**7 **S**1895 East Texas Medical Center Regional Healthcare System | 23 | 10 | 25 | 674 | 7 | 4719 | 0 | 5378 | 2503 | 87

☐ RUSK STATE HOSPITAL, Jacksonville Highway North, Zip 75785, Mailing Address: P.O. Box 318, Zip 75785–0318; tel. 903/683–3421; Harold R. Parrish, Superintendent **A**1 10 **F**12 52 53 54 55 56 57 58 73 | 12 | 22 | 394 | 1407 | 394 | — | 0 | 33241 | 21911 | 1153

SAN ANGELO—Tom Green County

★ ANGELO COMMUNITY HOSPITAL, 3501 Knickerbocker Road, Zip 76904–7698; tel. 915/949–9511; Robert E. Butler, President **A**1 2 9 10 **F**4 5 7 8 10 19 21 22 23 24 26 30 31 32 33 34 35 37 40 41 42 44 45 46 48 49 60 63 65 66 71 72 73 74 **P**1 | 23 | 10 | 137 | 6751 | 77 | — | 813 | 36229 | 13748 | 550

★ CONCHO VALLEY REGIONAL HOSPITAL, 2018 Pulliam Street, Zip 76905–5197; tel. 915/659–7100; Samuel G. Feazell, Chief Executive Officer **A**1 9 10 **F**2 3 8 10 12 16 19 21 22 23 25 27 28 30 32 34 35 37 39 41 42 44 46 49 52 53 54 55 56 57 58 59 64 65 66 67 71 72 73 **P**8 | 33 | 10 | 121 | 2926 | 49 | 31981 | 0 | 24470 | 8954 | 357

☐ RIVER CREST HOSPITAL, 1636 Hunters Glen Road, Zip 76901–5016; tel. 915/949–5722 **A**1 9 10 **F**2 3 12 15 16 19 22 41 52 53 55 56 57 59 65 71 **S**9555 Universal Health Services, Inc. | 33 | 22 | 80 | 552 | 16 | 974 | 0 | 3667 | 1900 | 66

★ △ SHANNON MEDICAL CENTER, 120 East Harris Street, Zip 76903, Mailing Address: Box 1879, Zip 76902; tel. 915/653–6741; (Total facility includes 13 beds in nursing home–type unit) **A**1 7 9 10 **F**4 7 10 12 15 16 17 19 21 22 24 25 28 32 34 35 37 40 41 42 43 44 45 46 48 49 56 60 64 65 67 71 72 73 74 | 23 | 10 | 220 | 8670 | 162 | 73497 | 1102 | 65202 | 28249 | 1045

SAN ANTONIO—Bexar County

★ AUDIE L. MURPHY MEMORIAL VETERANS HOSPITAL, 7400 Merton Minter Boulevard, Zip 78284–5799; tel. 210/617–5140; Jose R. Coronado FACHE, Director (Total facility includes 120 beds in nursing home–type unit) **A**1 2 3 5 8 **F**1 2 3 4 8 10 11 14 15 16 19 20 21 22 26 27 31 32 33 34 35 37 41 42 43 44 46 48 49 51 52 54 55 56 57 58 59 64 65 69 70 71 73 **S**9295 Department of Veterans Affairs | 45 | 10 | 732 | 12596 | 409 | 318919 | 0 | 182861 | 105731 | 2569

★ BAPTIST MEDICAL CENTER, 111 Dallas Street, Zip 78205–1230; tel. 210/222–8431; William L. Chessher, Administrator (Total facility includes 30 beds in nursing home–type unit) **A**1 2 3 6 9 10 **F**2 3 4 7 8 9 10 11 12 14 15 16 17 19 20 21 22 23 26 28 29 30 31 33 34 35 37 38 39 40 41 42 43 44 45 46 48 49 52 54 55 56 57 59 60 63 64 65 67 69 70 71 73 **P**8 **S**0265 Baptist Memorial Hospital System | 21 | 10 | 483 | 15415 | 290 | 59434 | 2184 | 113885 | 60943 | 2118

★ BEXAR COUNTY HOSPITAL DISTRICT, (Includes University Center for Community Health, 4502 Medical Drive, Zip 78229–4493; tel. 210/431–7400; Theresa De La Haya, Administrator; University Health Center–Downtown (Formerly Brady Green Community Health Center), 4502 Medical Drive, Zip 78229–4493; tel. 210/270–3400; Stephen L. Enders, Administrator; University Family Health Centers–Southeast, Southwest, Basse and La Clinica Amistad, 4502 Medical Drive, Zip 78229–4493; tel. 210/270–3400; Stephen L. Enders, Administrator; University Hospital (Formerly Medical Center Hospital), 4502 Medical Drive, Zip 78229–4493; tel. 210/616–4000; Jeff Turner, Senior Executive Vice President and Chief Operating Officer) 4502 Medical Drive, Zip 78229–4493; tel. 210/616–4000; John A. Guest, President and Chief Executive Officer **A**1 2 3 8 9 10 **F**1 4 7 8 9 10 11 12 13 14 15 16 17 18 19 20 21 22 23 26 27 28 29 30 31 32 34 35 37 38 39 40 41 42 43 44 45 46 47 48 49 50 51 52 53 54 55 56 57 58 59 60 61 63 65 66 67 68 69 70 71 72 73 74 | 16 | 10 | 563 | 19208 | 304 | 362513 | 4009 | 221630 | 101596 | 3729

BRADY–GREEN COMMUNITY HEALTH CENTER See Bexar County Hospital District

★ BROOKE ARMY MEDICAL CENTER, Fort Sam Houston, Zip 78234–6213; tel. 210/916–8225; Colonel Herbert K. Reamey III, Chief of Staff **A**1 2 3 5 **F**3 4 7 8 9 10 11 12 15 16 19 21 22 28 30 31 34 35 37 38 39 40 41 42 43 44 46 49 51 52 53 54 56 58 60 61 63 65 67 69 70 71 73 **P**6 **S**9395 Department of the Army | 42 | 10 | 464 | 19388 | 292 | 707257 | 824 | — | — | 3322

☐ CHARTER BEHAVIORAL HEALTH SYSTEM, 8550 Huebner Road, Zip 78240, Mailing Address: P.O. Box 380157, Zip 78280; tel. 210/699–8585; Michael Lee, Administrator **A**1 9 10 **F**1 2 3 12 14 16 19 21 27 31 32 34 35 39 41 46 50 52 53 54 55 56 57 58 59 63 65 67 71 **S**0695 Charter Medical Corporation | 33 | 22 | 96 | 1710 | 55 | 12008 | 0 | 12676 | 4050 | 142

☐ △ HEALTHSOUTH REHABILITATION INSTITUTE OF SAN ANTONIO, 9119 Cinnamon Hill, Zip 78240; tel. 210/691–0737; Diane B. Lampe R.N., Administrator and Chief Executive Officer **A**1 7 10 **F**5 12 14 15 16 17 19 21 25 26 27 32 35 41 42 44 46 48 49 50 63 65 66 67 71 73 **S**0023 Healthsouth Corporation | 33 | 46 | 108 | 1094 | 64 | 12098 | 0 | 19806 | 8879 | 310

HORIZON SPECIALTY HOSPITAL, 7310 Oak Manor Drive, Zip 78229; tel. 210/308–0261; Wendy Paulen Hill, Administrator **A**10 **F**12 14 15 16 65 | 33 | 48 | 30 | 201 | 16 | 0 | 0 | 4743 | 1515 | 56

MEDICAL CENTER HOSPITAL See Bexar County Hospital District

© 1995 AHA Guide

Hospitals, U.S. / TEXAS

Hospital, Address, Telephone, Administrator, Approval, Facility, and Physician Codes, Health Care System	Classification Codes		Utilization Data					Expense (thousands) of dollars		
★ American Hospital Association (AHA) membership ☐ Joint Commission on Accreditation of Healthcare Organizations (JCAHO) accreditation + American Osteopathic Hospital Association (AOHA) membership ○ American Osteopathic Association (AOA) accreditation △ Commission on Accreditation of Rehabilitation Facilities (CARF) accreditation Control codes 61, 63, 64, 71, 72 and 73 indicate hospitals listed by AOHA, but not registered by AHA. For definition of numerical codes, see page A6	Control	Service	Beds	Admissions	Census	Outpatient Visits	Births	Total	Payroll	Personnel
★ METROPOLITAN HOSPITAL, 1310 McCullough Avenue, Zip 78212–2617; tel. 210/208–2900; John Hanshaw, Chief Executive Officer **A**1 9 10 **F**2 4 7 8 10 11 17 19 20 21 22 23 24 27 28 29 30 31 32 33 35 37 38 40 41 42 43 44 47 48 49 50 52 56 57 59 60 61 63 64 65 67 69 70 71 72 73 74 **P**7 **S**0048 Columbia/HCA Healthcare Corporation	32	10	263	9869	129	36511	2507	50633	22977	751
☐ MISSION VISTA HOSPITAL, 14747 Jones Maltsberger, Zip 78247–3713; tel. 210/490–0000; Dan Aranda, Chief Executive Officer **A**1 9 10 **F**3 15 16 18 52 53 54 56 58 59 **S**0405 Ramsay Health Care, Inc.	33	22	48	489	17	2814	0	5166	2541	81
☐ NIX HEALTH CARE SYSTEM, (Formerly Nix Medical Center) 414 Navarro Street, Zip 78205–2522; tel. 210/271–1800; John F. Strieby, President and Chief Executive Officer (Total facility includes 17 beds in nursing home–type unit) **A**1 3 9 10 **F**4 7 8 10 16 19 21 28 30 32 34 35 37 39 40 41 42 43 44 45 46 49 52 57 59 60 64 65 66 67 69 71 74 **P**1 5 7	33	10	123	3010	50	30769	595	28946	9681	377
NORTHEAST BAPTIST HOSPITAL, 8811 Village Drive, Zip 78217; tel. 210/653–2330; Morris R. Harris Jr., Administrator **F**3 4 7 8 10 11 12 14 15 16 17 19 20 21 22 23 26 28 29 30 31 33 34 35 37 38 39 40 41 42 43 44 45 46 48 49 54 55 56 57 59 60 61 63 65 67 69 70 71 73 **P**8 **S**0265 Baptist Memorial Hospital System	21	10	208	9612	143	37074	1736	68513	27522	977
★ SAN ANTONIO REGIONAL HOSPITAL, 8026 Floyd Curl Drive, Zip 78229–3915; tel. 210/692–8110; Earl H. Denning, Chief Executive Officer (Total facility includes 22 beds in nursing home–type unit) **A**1 3 5 9 10 **F**2 3 4 8 10 11 12 14 15 16 19 20 21 22 23 34 35 37 41 42 43 44 45 48 49 52 54 55 56 57 58 59 60 64 65 67 69 71 73 **P**7 **S**0048 Columbia/HCA Healthcare Corporation	33	10	297	6779	116	36830	0	64825	23221	696
SAN ANTONIO STATE CHEST HOSPITAL See Texas Center for Infectious Desease										
☐ SAN ANTONIO STATE HOSPITAL, 6711 South New Braunfels, Zip 78223, Mailing Address: Box 23991 Highland Hills Station, Zip 78223–0991; tel. 210/532–8811; Robert C. Arizpe, Superintendent **A**1 9 10 **F**12 52 53 54 55 56 57 58 73	12	22	446	2358	447	—	0	49444	32060	1494
★ △ SAN ANTONIO WARM SPRINGS REHABILITATION HOSPITAL, 5101 Medical Drive, Zip 78229–6098; tel. 210/616–0100; Richard G. Allison, Administrator **A**1 3 7 9 10 **F**12 15 16 19 21 34 35 48 49 54 56 65 71 73 **P**8	23	46	60	926	55	7794	0	15065	6584	204
★ △ SANTA ROSA HEALTH CARE CORPORATION, 519 West Houston Street, Zip 78207–3108, Mailing Address: Box 7330, Station A, Zip 78207–3108; tel. 210/704–2011; Robert J. Nolan, President and Chief Executive Officer **A**1 2 3 5 7 9 10 **F**2 3 4 5 7 8 10 11 12 14 15 16 17 19 20 21 22 25 26 27 28 29 30 31 32 33 34 35 37 38 39 40 41 42 43 44 45 46 47 48 49 51 52 53 54 55 56 58 59 60 63 65 66 67 68 69 71 73 74 **P**1 5 7 **S**5565 Incarnate Word Health Services	21	10	702	21822	389	145167	2801	191410	80546	2614
SOUTHEAST BAPTIST HOSPITAL, 4214 East Southcross, Zip 78222; tel. 210/337–6900; Harry E. Smith, Administrator **F**2 3 4 7 8 9 10 11 12 14 15 16 17 19 20 21 23 26 28 29 30 31 33 34 35 37 38 39 40 41 42 43 44 45 46 48 49 52 54 55 56 57 59 60 63 64 65 67 69 70 71 73 **P**8 **S**0265 Baptist Memorial Hospital System	21	10	153	5703	91	42297	492	39659	18060	667
☐ SOUTHWEST GENERAL HOSPITAL, 7400 Barlite Boulevard, Zip 78224–1399; tel. 210/921–2000; Mark L. Bernard, Chief Executive Officer (Total facility includes 31 beds in nursing home–type unit) **A**1 10 **F**8 12 15 16 17 19 21 22 26 27 28 32 33 34 35 37 39 41 42 44 46 48 49 52 57 59 60 63 64 65 71 73 **P**7 **S**6525 Ornda Healthcorp	33	10	199	5151	129	63051	0	38287	17369	652
SOUTHWEST NEUROPSYCHIATRIC INSTITUTE, 8535 Tom Slick, Zip 78229–3363; tel. 210/616–0300; Sharon M. Stanush, President **A**3 5 9 **F**12 15 18 19 20 22 28 29 34 35 46 52 53 54 55 56 58 59 65 **P**8	23	52	92	76	45	98	0	4325	2366	96
★ SOUTHWEST TEXAS METHODIST HOSPITAL, 7700 Floyd Curl Drive, Zip 78229–3993; tel. 210/692–4000; James C. Scoggin Jr., Chief Executive Officer **A**1 2 3 9 10 **F**4 7 8 10 11 15 16 19 21 22 23 28 29 30 31 34 35 37 38 39 40 42 43 44 45 46 47 60 63 65 66 67 69 70 71 73 74 **P**3 8 **S**0048 Columbia/HCA Healthcare Corporation	23	10	553	22331	328	81138	4321	188187	76740	2598
ST. LUKE'S LUTHERAN HOSPITAL See St. Luke's Baptist Hospital										
★ ST. LUKE'S BAPTIST HOSPITAL, (Formerly St. Luke's Lutheran Hospital) 7930 Floyd Curl Drive, Zip 78229–0100, Mailing Address: Box 29100, Zip 78229–0100; tel. 210/692–8703; Peggy W. Brown, Administrator (Total facility includes 29 beds in nursing home–type unit) **A**1 3 5 9 **F**2 3 4 8 9 10 11 12 14 15 16 17 19 20 21 22 28 29 30 31 33 34 35 37 38 39 40 41 42 43 44 45 46 48 49 52 60 63 64 65 67 70 71 73 **P**8 **S**0265 Baptist Memorial Hospital System	21	10	225	7151	114	21179	0	66098	23742	762
★ TEXAS CENTER FOR INFECTIOUS DESEASE, (Formerly San Antonio State Chest Hospital) 2303 Southeast Military Drive, Zip 78223–2334, Mailing Address: Box 23340, Zip 78223–2334; tel. 210/534–8857; Hugh N. Keel, Chief Administrative Officer **A**1 9 **F**14 19 20 34 37 44 65 71 73 **P**6 **S**0020 Texas Department of Health	12	33	129	549	78	9634	0	12430	7453	285
UNIVERSITY CENTER FOR COMMUNITY HEALTH See Bexar County Hospital District										
UNIVERSITY FAMILY HEALTH CENTERS–SOUTHEAST, SOUTHWEST, BASSE AND LA CLINICA AMISTAD See Bexar County Hospital District										
UNIVERSITY HEALTH CENTER–DOWNTOWN See Bexar County Hospital District										
UNIVERSITY HOSPITAL See Bexar County Hospital District										
★ VILLAGE OAKS MEDICAL CENTER, 12412 Judson Road, Zip 78233, Mailing Address: P.O. Box 659510, Zip 78265–9510; tel. 210/650–4949; John R. Nickens III, Chief Executive Officer **A**1 9 10 **F**3 4 7 8 10 12 14 15 19 20 21 22 23 25 26 27 28 29 30 31 34 35 37 41 42 43 44 45 48 49 53 54 55 56 57 58 59 60 61 63 64 65 66 67 69 71 72 73 74 **P**5 7 **S**0048 Columbia/HCA Healthcare Corporation	33	10	100	2752	46	40348	2	23579	9354	361

Hospitals, U.S. / TEXAS

Hospital, Address, Telephone, Administrator, Approval, Facility, and Physician Codes, Health Care System	Classification Codes		Utilization Data					Expense (thousands) of dollars		Personnel
★ American Hospital Association (AHA) membership □ Joint Commission on Accreditation of Healthcare Organizations (JCAHO) accreditation + American Osteopathic Hospital Association (AOHA) membership ○ American Osteopathic Association (AOA) accreditation △ Commission on Accreditation of Rehabilitation Facilities (CARF) accreditation Control codes 61, 63, 64, 71, 72 and 73 indicate hospitals listed by AOHA, but not registered by AHA. For definition of numerical codes, see page A6	Control	Service	Beds	Admissions	Census	Outpatient Visits	Births	Total	Payroll	
★ WOMEN'S AND CHILDREN'S HOSPITAL, 8109 Fredericksburg Road, Zip 78229–3383; tel. 210/692–5000; Angeline M. Marano, Chief Executive Officer **A**1 9 10 **F**2 3 4 7 8 10 11 12 14 15 16 17 19 22 23 24 25 27 28 29 34 35 37 38 39 40 41 42 43 44 45 46 47 48 49 51 52 57 58 59 60 61 64 65 66 69 71 73 74 **P**2 8 **S**0048 Columbia/HCA Healthcare Corporation	33	44	150	7129	65	34160	4125	37023	16928	532
SAN AUGUSTINE—San Augustine County SAN AUGUSTINE MEMORIAL HOSPITAL, 511 Hospital Street, Zip 75972, Mailing Address: Box 658, Zip 75972; tel. 409/275–3446; Carolyn Ladner, Administrator **A**9 10 **F**15 16 17 22 25 28 30 32 33 44 46 49 64 65 71	16	10	22	458	5	18684	2	2581	1193	63
SAN BENITO—Cameron County ★ DOLLY VINSANT MEMORIAL HOSPITAL, 400 East Highway 77, Zip 78586, Mailing Address: Box 42, Zip 78586; tel. 210/399–1313; R. William Warren, Chairman and Chief Executive Officer **A**1 10 **F**19 21 22 28 34 39 44 45 71 73	33	10	49	1307	17	10988	0	4408	2999	137
SAN MARCOS—Hays County ★ CENTRAL TEXAS MEDICAL CENTER, 1301 Wonder World Drive, Zip 78666, Mailing Address: Box 1169, Zip 78667; tel. 512/353–8979; Joel W. Hass, President and Chief Executive Officer (Total facility includes 9 beds in nursing home–type unit) **A**1 9 10 **F**7 8 11 12 14 15 16 17 19 21 22 23 24 27 28 30 32 33 35 37 39 40 41 42 44 45 46 49 64 65 66 67 71 73 74 **P**4 7 8 **S**4165 Adventist Health System–Sunbelt Health Care Corporation	21	10	109	3635	38	50197	846	29461	9895	396
□ SAN MARCOS TREATMENT CENTER, Mailing Address: P.O. Box 768, Zip 78667–0768; tel. 512/396–8500; Armin Steege, Administrator **A**1 **F**52 53 **P**1 **S**0395 Healthcare International, Inc.	33	22	152	220	86	7	0	16258	5598	190
SEGUIN—Guadalupe County ★ GUADALUPE VALLEY HOSPITAL, 1215 East Court Street, Zip 78155–5189; tel. 210/379–2411; Don L. Richey, Administrator **A**1 9 10 **F**3 7 8 12 15 16 18 19 21 22 23 26 28 31 32 33 34 35 37 39 40 44 45 46 49 58 61 63 65 66 70 71 73 **P**3 8	15	10	77	3497	43	68000	730	23049	11287	491
SEMINOLE—Gaines County ★ MEMORIAL HOSPITAL, 209 Northwest Eighth Street, Zip 79360; tel. 915/758–5811; Kirk Cristy, Administrator **A**9 10 **F**3 4 5 6 7 8 10 12 13 14 17 18 19 20 21 22 23 24 26 27 28 29 30 31 32 33 34 35 36 39 40 41 42 43 44 45 46 49 50 51 53 54 55 56 57 58 59 60 61 62 63 64 65 66 67 69 70 71 72 73 74	16	10	33	934	8	18214	167	6424	3271	186
SEYMOUR—Baylor County ★ SEYMOUR HOSPITAL, 200 Stadium Drive, Zip 76380; tel. 817/888–5572; Leroy Schaffner, Administrator **A**9 10 **F**7 19 21 28 32 33 37 40 44 65 71 73	16	10	39	1097	19	11150	62	4135	1610	93
SHAMROCK—Wheeler County SHAMROCK GENERAL HOSPITAL, 1000 South Main Street, Zip 79079; tel. 806/256–2114; Allen R. Alberty, Chief Executive Officer (Total facility includes 11 beds in nursing home–type unit) **A**9 10 **F**7 12 14 22 40 44 71 73	16	10	43	347	11	11100	14	1804	889	47
SHEPPARD AIR FORCE BASE—Wichita County ★ U.S. AIR FORCE REGIONAL HOSPITAL–SHEPPARD, 149 Hart Street, Suite 1, Zip 76311–3478; tel. 817/676–2010; Lieutenant Colonel James J. Hooper III MC, USAF, Director Base Medical Services (Nonreporting) **A**1 **S**9495 Department of the Air Force	41	10	115	—	—	—	—	—	—	—
SHERMAN—Grayson County ★ MEDICAL PLAZA HOSPITAL, 1111 Gallagher Road, Zip 75090; tel. 903/870–7000; J. F. Adams, Chief Executive Officer (Total facility includes 22 beds in nursing home–type unit) **A**1 9 10 **F**7 8 12 15 19 21 22 26 28 29 30 31 32 33 34 35 37 40 41 42 44 46 48 49 52 57 63 64 65 67 71 73 74 **P**1 7 **S**0048 Columbia/HCA Healthcare Corporation	33	10	162	2722	53	19153	277	24375	10460	335
★ WILSON N. JONES MEMORIAL HOSPITAL, 500 North Highland Avenue, Zip 75092, Mailing Address: Box 1258, Zip 75091–1258; tel. 903/870–4611; Harry F. Barnes FACHE, President and Chief Executive Officer **A**1 9 10 **F**2 3 7 8 10 12 14 15 16 19 21 22 23 24 25 28 31 32 33 34 35 37 40 41 42 44 46 49 52 53 56 57 60 63 64 65 67 71 73 74 **P**1 6	23	10	195	7280	122	50471	776	53602	20525	750
SILSBEE—Hardin County ★ SILSBEE DOCTORS HOSPITAL, Highway 418, Zip 77656, Mailing Address: Box 1208, Zip 77656; tel. 409/385–5531; David Cottey, Chief Executive Officer (Total facility includes 13 beds in nursing home–type unit) **A**9 10 **F**8 15 16 19 21 22 27 30 32 37 44 46 64 71 73 **S**0048 Columbia/HCA Healthcare Corporation	33	10	57	2198	37	86587	0	17509	7227	286
SMITHVILLE—Bastrop County SMITHVILLE HOSPITAL, Ninth and Mills Streets, Zip 78957, Mailing Address: Box 359, Zip 78957; tel. 512/237–3214; James W. Langford, Administrator **A**9 10 **F**7 8 19 22 31 34 40 44 71	16	10	25	822	9	6107	50	5074	2147	123
SNYDER—Scurry County ★ D. M. COGDELL MEMORIAL HOSPITAL, 1700 Cogdell Boulevard, Zip 79549–6198; tel. 915/573–6374; Jeff Reecer, Chief Executive Officer **A**1 9 10 **F**3 7 8 11 12 13 15 19 20 21 22 24 26 28 30 32 34 37 40 44 45 46 49 65 67 70 71 73 **P**6 **S**5425 St. Joseph Health System	13	10	72	1223	46	23859	170	11039	4728	252
SONORA—Sutton County LILLIAN M. HUDSPETH MEMORIAL HOSPITAL, 308 Hudspeth Avenue, Zip 76950, Mailing Address: Box 455, Zip 76950–0455; tel. 915/387–2521; Ann Fagan–Cook, Administrator (Total facility includes 39 beds in nursing home–type unit) **A**9 10 **F**22	16	10	52	268	32	3725	1	2277	1135	57

© 1995 AHA Guide

Hospitals, U.S. / TEXAS

Hospital, Address, Telephone, Administrator, Approval, Facility, and Physician Codes, Health Care System	Classi-fication Codes		Utilization Data					Expense (thousands) of dollars		
★ American Hospital Association (AHA) membership ☐ Joint Commission on Accreditation of Healthcare Organizations (JCAHO) accreditation + American Osteopathic Hospital Association (AOHA) membership ○ American Osteopathic Association (AOA) accreditation △ Commission on Accreditation of Rehabilitation Facilities (CARF) accreditation Control codes 61, 63, 64, 71, 72 and 73 indicate hospitals listed by AOHA, but not registered by AHA. For definition of numerical codes, see page A6	Control	Service	Beds	Admissions	Census	Outpatient Visits	Births	Total	Payroll	Personnel
SPEARMAN—Hansford County										
★ HANSFORD HOSPITAL, 707 South Roland Street, Zip 79081; tel. 806/659-2535; Anne Snow, Administrator (Total facility includes 84 beds in nursing home–type unit) **A**9 10 **F**8 14 15 16 17 22 26 28 32 33 36 42 45 49 64 65 71 73	16	10	112	319	77	2683	0	4974	1963	137
STAMFORD—Jones County										
STAMFORD MEMORIAL HOSPITAL, Highway 6 East, Zip 79553, Mailing Address: Box 911, Zip 79553; tel. 915/773-2725; Craig Haterius, Administrator **A**9 10 **F**12 13 14 15 16 17 18 19 24 25 26 27 30 34 44 51 56 60 70 71 73	16	10	35	133	2	—	0	2312	1046	34
STANTON—Martin County										
MARTIN COUNTY HOSPITAL DISTRICT, 610 North St. Peter Street, Zip 79782, Mailing Address: Box 640, Zip 79782; tel. 915/756-3345; Rick Jacobus, Administrator **A**9 10 **F**15 16 22 40 44 71 **P**5	16	10	26	141	2	3111	46	1993	1050	36
STEPHENVILLE—Erath County										
★ HARRIS METHODIST–ERATH COUNTY, 411 North Belknap Street, Zip 76401-1399, Mailing Address: Box 1399, Zip 76401; tel. 817/965-1500; Michael D. Murphy, Administrator **A**1 9 10 **F**2 3 4 7 8 10 11 12 13 15 16 17 18 19 21 22 23 24 26 27 28 29 30 31 32 33 34 35 37 38 39 40 41 42 43 44 45 46 48 49 50 52 53 54 55 56 58 59 60 61 63 64 65 66 67 69 70 71 72 73 74 **P**2 3 4 **S**2345 Harris Methodist Health System	21	10	72	3086	35	40560	316	17754	6524	273
SULPHUR SPRINGS—Hopkins County										
★ HOPKINS COUNTY MEMORIAL HOSPITAL, 115 Airport Road, Zip 75482-0115, Mailing Address: Box 275, Zip 75483-0275; tel. 903/885-7671; Donald R. Magee, Chief Executive Officer **A**1 9 10 **F**14 15 16 19 22 28 30 32 34 35 37 40 41 42 44 46 49 64 65 71 73	16	10	66	3522	37	—	848	13900	7182	303
SWEENY—Brazoria County										
☐ SWEENY COMMUNITY HOSPITAL, 305 North McKinney Street, Zip 77480, Mailing Address: Box 1000, Zip 77480; tel. 409/548-3311; Herbert Anthony Turk FACHE, Administrator **A**1 9 10 **F**19 22 37 44 49 65 71 73	16	10	29	328	4	5865	0	4610	1926	69
SWEETWATER—Nolan County										
☐ ROLLING PLAINS MEMORIAL HOSPITAL, 200 East Arizona Street, Zip 79556, Mailing Address: P.O. Box 690, Zip 79556; tel. 915/235-1701; Thomas F. Kennedy, Administrator **A**1 9 10 **F**7 8 14 15 16 19 20 22 28 31 32 33 35 37 40 44 49 65 71 73	16	10	54	1652	26	19740	115	9260	3946	165
TAHOKA—Lynn County										
LYNN COUNTY HOSPITAL DISTRICT, Brownfield Highway, Zip 79373-1310, Mailing Address: Box 1310, Zip 79373-1310; tel. 806/998-4533; Louise Landers, Administrator **A**9 10 **F**6 8 15 19 22 32 35 44 49 51 70 71 73 **P**8	16	10	24	258	6	4740	30	2656	981	54
TAYLOR—Williamson County										
☐ JOHNS COMMUNITY HOSPITAL, 305 Mallard Lane, Zip 76574-1208; tel. 512/352-7611; Ernest Balla, Administrator **A**1 9 10 **F**8 11 15 19 21 22 28 30 32 34 37 44 49 64 65 71	23	10	49	1209	30	10608	0	6917	3643	126
TEMPLE—Bell County										
★ KING'S DAUGHTERS HOSPITAL, 1901 Southwest H K Dodgen Loop, Zip 76502-1896; tel. 817/771-8600; Tucker Bonner, President (Total facility includes 8 beds in nursing home–type unit) **A**1 10 **F**7 14 15 16 19 21 22 23 28 30 31 32 33 34 35 37 40 41 42 44 45 49 63 64 65 67 71 73 **P**8	23	10	106	2933	40	18644	368	21842	9310	367
★ OLIN E. TEAGUE VETERANS' CENTER, 1901 South First Street, Zip 76504; tel. 817/778-4811; (Nonreporting) **A**1 2 3 5 **S**9295 Department of Veterans Affairs	45	10	914	—	—	—	—	—	—	—
★ △ SCOTT AND WHITE MEMORIAL HOSPITAL, 2401 South 31st Street, Zip 76508; tel. 817/724-2111; Dick Sweeden, Administrator (Total facility includes 34 beds in nursing home–type unit) **A**1 2 3 5 7 8 9 10 **F**1 2 3 4 7 8 10 11 12 14 15 16 17 19 20 21 22 23 24 25 26 27 28 29 30 31 32 33 34 35 37 38 40 41 42 43 44 45 46 47 48 49 52 53 54 56 57 58 59 60 61 64 65 66 67 71 72 73 74 **P**3	23	10	424	17367	294	63325	2337	205811	78158	5201
TERRELL—Kaufman County										
★ TERRELL COMMUNITY HOSPITAL, 1551 Highway 34 South, Zip 75160-4833; tel. 214/563-7611; I. Douglas Streckert, Chief Executive Officer (Total facility includes 18 beds in nursing home–type unit) **A**1 9 10 **F**7 8 12 19 21 22 29 32 34 35 37 39 40 41 44 45 46 48 64 65 71 73 **P**1 **S**0048 Columbia/HCA Healthcare Corporation	33	10	101	3984	56	27724	284	25222	7685	289
☐ TERRELL STATE HOSPITAL, Brin Street, Zip 75160, Mailing Address: Box 70, Zip 75160-0070; tel. 214/563-6452; Beatrice Butler, Superintendent **A**1 3 5 9 10 **F**12 52 53 54 55 56 57 58 73	12	22	332	1713	333	0	0	41729	25229	1147
TEXARKANA—Bowie County										
★ HEALTHSOUTH REHABILITATION HOSPITAL OF TEXARKANA, 515 West 12th Street, Zip 75501; tel. 903/793-0088; Hank Ross, Chief Executive Officer **A**9 10 **F**14 15 16 46 48 49 65 66 **S**0023 Healthsouth Corporation	33	46	60	486	32	9637	0	8898	5361	136
★ MEDICAL ARTS HOSPITAL, 2501 College Drive, Zip 75501-2703, Mailing Address: P.O. Box 6045, Zip 75505-6045; tel. 903/798-5100; Jerry Kincade, Chief Executive Officer (Data for 335 days) **A**9 10 **F**8 11 12 16 19 21 22 28 30 32 34 35 37 39 42 44 45 46 49 51 65 66 71 73 **P**7 8 **S**0048 Columbia/HCA Healthcare Corporation	33	10	76	1356	24	23219	0	16663	5758	233
★ ST. MICHAEL HEALTH CARE CENTER, 2600 St. Michael Drive, Zip 75503; tel. 903/614-1000; Stephen F. Wright, Interim Administrator and Chief Executive Officer (Newly Registered) **A**1 9 10 **S**0605 Sisters of Charity of the Incarnate Word Healthcare System	21	10	239	—	—	—	—	—	—	—

Hospitals, U.S. / TEXAS

Hospital, Address, Telephone, Administrator, Approval, Facility, and Physician Codes, Health Care System ★ American Hospital Association (AHA) membership □ Joint Commission on Accreditation of Healthcare Organizations (JCAHO) accreditation + American Osteopathic Hospital Association (AOHA) membership ○ American Osteopathic Association (AOA) accreditation △ Commission on Accreditation of Rehabilitation Facilities (CARF) accreditation Control codes 61, 63, 64, 71, 72 and 73 indicate hospitals listed by AOHA, but not registered by AHA. For definition of numerical codes, see page A6	Classification Codes		Utilization Data					Expense (thousands) of dollars		
	Control	Service	Beds	Admissions	Census	Outpatient Visits	Births	Total	Payroll	Personnel
★ ST. MICHAEL REHABILITATION HOSPITAL, 2400 St. Michael Drive, Zip 75503; tel. 903/614–4000; Freeman P. Lockhart, Administrator **A**1 10 **F**12 15 16 19 21 22 24 28 32 33 34 35 37 42 44 48 49 60 64 73 **P**1 3 5 7 **S**0605 Sisters of Charity of the Incarnate Word Healthcare System	21	46	80	370	19	0	0	3942	—	181
★ WADLEY REGIONAL MEDICAL CENTER, 1000 Pine Street, Zip 75501–5170, Mailing Address: Box 1878, Zip 75504–1878; tel. 903/798–8000; Hugh R. Hallgren, President and Chief Executive Officer **A**1 2 9 10 **F**1 3 7 8 10 12 15 16 19 21 22 23 27 28 29 30 31 32 33 34 35 37 39 40 41 42 43 44 45 46 49 50 52 53 54 55 56 57 58 59 60 63 64 65 70 71 72 73 74 **P**3 8	23	10	382	13979	198	75970	2134	91228	35126	1280
TEXAS CITY—Galveston County ★ △ MAINLAND CENTER HOSPITAL, 6801 E F Lowry Expressway, Zip 77591; tel. 409/938–5000; Sally E. Jeffcoat, Chief Executive Officer (Total facility includes 31 beds in nursing home–type unit) **A**1 7 9 10 **F**2 3 7 8 10 11 12 14 15 16 18 19 21 22 24 27 28 29 30 32 33 34 35 37 39 40 41 42 44 45 46 48 49 51 52 53 54 55 56 57 58 59 63 64 65 66 67 71 73 74 **P**7 8 **S**0048 Columbia/HCA Healthcare Corporation	33	10	277	6492	114	56496	471	41268	20619	564
THE WOODLANDS—Montgomery County ★ MEMORIAL HOSPITAL–THE WOODLANDS, 9250 Pinecroft, Zip 77380; tel. 713/364–2300; Steve Sanders, Vice President and Chief Executive Officer **A**1 9 10 **F**2 3 4 6 7 8 10 11 12 15 16 17 18 19 21 22 25 26 29 30 32 33 34 35 37 38 39 40 41 42 43 44 45 46 48 49 52 53 54 55 56 57 58 60 61 62 63 64 65 66 67 68 71 72 73 74 **P**1 3 7 **S**2645 Memorial Healthcare System	23	10	68	3270	35	—	1208	21516	7830	218
THROCKMORTON—Throckmorton County THROCKMORTON COUNTY MEMORIAL HOSPITAL, Seymour Highway, Zip 76483, Mailing Address: P.O. Box 729, Zip 76483; tel. 817/849–2151 **A**9 10 **F**19 22 44 71	13	10	20	177	2	1350	0	883	462	21
TOMBALL—Harris County ★ △ TOMBALL REGIONAL HOSPITAL, 605 Holderrieth Street, Zip 77375–0889, Mailing Address: Box 889, Zip 77377–0889; tel. 713/351–1623; Robert F. Schaper, President and Chief Executive Officer (Total facility includes 18 beds in nursing home–type unit) **A**1 7 9 10 **F**4 7 8 10 11 12 15 16 19 21 22 23 24 28 29 30 32 34 35 37 39 40 42 43 44 45 46 49 52 54 56 57 58 59 60 64 65 66 67 71 73 **P**8	16	10	207	6080	105	37869	517	49020	16003	612
TRINITY—Trinity County TRINITY MEMORIAL HOSPITAL, 900 Prospect Drive, Zip 75862–0471, Mailing Address: Box 471, Zip 75862; tel. 409/594–3541; Terry Cutler, Administrator **A**10 **F**8 22 32 34 44 73	16	10	22	545	7	12707	0	2804	1502	64
TULIA—Swisher County SWISHER MEMORIAL HOSPITAL DISTRICT, 539 Southeast Second, Zip 79088; tel. 806/995–3581; Ted Strote, Interim Administrator **A**9 10 **F**15 19 22 32 33 34 44 51 65 70 71	16	10	30	188	5	0	0	2339	783	51
TYLER—Smith County + DOCTORS MEMORIAL HOSPITAL, 1400 West Southwest Loop 323, Zip 75701; tel. 903/561–3771; Olie E. Clem, Chief Executive Officer **A**9 10 **F**4 8 10 11 15 19 22 26 28 32 35 37 40 42 43 44 46 47 48 49 52 60 70 71 **P**7 8	23	10	46	1602	22	5411	192	5637	2422	142
★ △ EAST TEXAS MEDICAL CENTER, (Includes East Texas Medical Center–Psychiatric Unit, 4101 University Boulevard, Tyler, Texas, Zip 75701–6600; tel. 903/566–8668) 1000 South Beckham Street, Zip 75701–1996, Mailing Address: Box 6400, Zip 75711–6400; tel. 903/597–0351; (Total facility includes 20 beds in nursing home–type unit) **A**1 2 7 9 10 **F**4 7 8 10 11 12 14 16 19 21 22 23 28 30 32 33 34 35 37 39 40 41 42 43 44 46 48 49 52 54 55 56 57 58 59 60 63 64 65 66 69 70 71 73 **P**6 7 8	23	10	341	10147	191	110098	87	119798	44698	1772
EAST TEXAS MEDICAL CENTER–PSYCHIATRIC UNIT See East Texas Medical Center										
★ MOTHER FRANCES HOSPITAL REGIONAL HEALTHCARE CENTER, 800 East Dawson, Zip 75701–2093; tel. 903/593–8441; J. Lindsey Bradley Jr. FACHE, President **A**1 3 9 10 **F**2 3 4 7 8 10 11 12 13 15 16 17 18 19 20 21 22 24 25 26 28 29 30 31 32 33 34 35 37 38 39 40 41 42 43 44 45 46 49 52 53 54 55 56 57 58 59 60 63 65 66 67 70 71 73 74 **P**5 6 7 8	23	10	287	17356	210	148345	2543	121380	43520	1440
□ △ TYLER REHABILITATION HOSPITAL, 3131 Troup Highway, Zip 75701; tel. 903/510–7000; Thomas J. Cook, Chief Executive Officer (Total facility includes 15 beds in nursing home–type unit) **A**1 7 10 **F**12 14 15 16 19 21 27 28 30 34 35 39 41 46 48 49 64 66 67 71 73	32	46	60	649	38	4695	0	10404	—	104
★ UNIVERSITY OF TEXAS HEALTH CENTER AT TYLER, (Pulmonary and Heart Disease) Gladewater Highway, Zip 75708, Mailing Address: Box 2003, Zip 75710–2003; tel. 903/877–7750; George A. Hurst M.D., Director **A**1 3 5 9 10 **F**4 5 7 8 9 10 11 12 13 14 15 16 17 19 21 22 23 24 25 26 28 29 30 31 32 33 34 35 36 37 38 39 40 41 42 43 44 45 47 48 49 51 54 58 60 64 65 66 67 70 71 72 73 74 **P**3 5 **S**0033 University of Texas Hospitals	12	49	146	3134	82	91097	0	67858	37079	1101
UVALDE—Uvalde County UVALDE MEMORIAL HOSPITAL, Garner Field Road, Zip 78801–1025; tel. 210/278–6251; Ben M. Durr, Administrator **A**9 10 **F**1 8 15 16 19 21 25 28 34 35 37 40 44 45 49 70 71 73	16	10	52	2691	32	114734	642	11198	5307	227
VAN HORN—Culberson County CULBERSON HOSPITAL DISTRICT, Eisenhower–Farm Market Roads 2185, Zip 79855, Mailing Address: Box 609, Zip 79855–0609; tel. 915/283–2760; Richard Lee, Administrator **A**9 10 **F**7 8 14 15 16 22 28 39 40 44 71 **P**5	16	10	25	126	1	—	51	1684	764	36

© 1995 AHA Guide

Hospitals, U.S. / TEXAS

Hospital, Address, Telephone, Administrator, Approval, Facility, and Physician Codes, Health Care System	Classification Codes		Utilization Data					Expense (thousands) of dollars		
★ American Hospital Association (AHA) membership □ Joint Commission on Accreditation of Healthcare Organizations (JCAHO) accreditation + American Osteopathic Hospital Association (AOHA) membership ○ American Osteopathic Association (AOA) accreditation △ Commission on Accreditation of Rehabilitation Facilities (CARF) accreditation Control codes 61, 63, 64, 71, 72 and 73 indicate hospitals listed by AOHA, but not registered by AHA. For definition of numerical codes, see page A6	Control	Service	Beds	Admissions	Census	Outpatient Visits	Births	Total	Payroll	Personnel
VERNON—Wilbarger County										
□ WILBARGER GENERAL HOSPITAL, 920 Hillcrest Drive, Zip 76384; tel. 817/552-9351; Larry Parsons, Administrator **A**1 9 10 **F**14 15 16 19 21 22 28 32 34 40 44 45 46 49 54 65 67 70 71	16	10	52	1746	25	104066	99	6757	3378	170
VICTORIA—Victoria County										
★ CITIZENS MEDICAL CENTER, 2701 Hospital Drive, Zip 77901-5749; tel. 512/573-9181; David P. Brown, Administrator (Total facility includes 20 beds in nursing home–type unit) **A**1 2 9 10 **F**4 8 10 12 15 16 17 18 19 20 21 22 23 25 26 28 29 30 31 32 33 34 35 37 39 41 42 43 44 45 46 47 49 50 52 54 55 56 57 60 63 64 65 67 71 73 **P**8	13	10	233	6933	126	51275	0	50074	21310	714
★ DETAR HOSPITAL, 506 East San Antonio Street, Zip 77901-6060, Mailing Address: Box 2089, Zip 77902-2089; tel. 512/575-7441; William R. Blanchard, Chief Executive Officer (Total facility includes 20 beds in nursing home–type unit) **A**1 9 10 **F**7 8 10 12 13 14 16 17 19 20 21 22 24 26 28 29 30 31 32 33 34 35 37 38 39 40 41 42 44 45 46 47 48 49 56 60 63 64 65 67 71 73 74 **P**3 **S**0048 Columbia/HCA Healthcare Corporation	33	10	224	7003	96	83604	1478	38770	15124	611
★ DEVEREUX–VICTORIA, 120 David Wade Drive, Zip 77902-2666; tel. 512/575-8271; L. Gail Atkinson, Executive Director **A**9 **F**1 3 12 15 16 17 25 45 46 52 53 54 55 56 58 59 65 **P**4 **S**0845 Devereux Foundation	23	52	84	63	40	0	0	4403	1079	29
□ VICTORIA REGIONAL MEDICAL CENTER, 101 Medical Drive, Zip 77904; tel. 512/573-6100; J. Michael Mastej, Chief Executive Officer and Managing Director **A**1 9 10 **F**3 7 8 12 14 15 16 19 21 22 28 29 30 31 34 37 40 41 44 45 46 49 52 53 54 55 56 57 58 59 65 67 71 73 **S**9555 Universal Health Services, Inc.	33	10	105	3179	48	12736	378	24211	8292	247
WACO—McLennan County										
★ △ HILLCREST BAPTIST MEDICAL CENTER, 3000 Herring Avenue, Zip 76708-3299, Mailing Address: Box 5100, Zip 76708-0100; tel. 817/756-8011; Richard E. Scott, President **A**1 2 3 7 9 10 **F**1 4 5 7 8 10 11 12 13 15 16 17 19 20 21 22 23 24 26 27 28 29 30 31 32 33 34 35 37 38 39 40 41 42 43 44 45 46 48 49 56 60 63 65 66 67 71 73 74 **P**3 7 8	21	10	282	12929	175	91673	3317	88871	34699	1274
★ PROVIDENCE HEALTH CENTER, 6901 Medical Parkway, Zip 76712, Mailing Address: P.O. Box 2589, Zip 76702-2589; tel. 817/751-4000; Kent A. Keahey, President (Nonreporting) **A**1 2 3 9 10 **S**1855 Daughters of Charity National Health System	21	10	415	—	—	—	—	—	—	—
★ VETERANS AFFAIRS MEDICAL CENTER, 4800 Memorial Drive, Zip 76711-1397; tel. 817/752-6581; Wallace M. Hopkins FACHE, Director (Total facility includes 160 beds in nursing home–type unit) **A**1 **F**15 20 25 26 28 29 30 33 39 41 45 46 48 49 51 52 57 58 64 65 73 74 **S**9295 Department of Veterans Affairs	45	48	804	3527	666	90196	0	73455	54676	1329
WAXAHACHIE—Ellis County										
★ BAYLOR MEDICAL CENTER – ELLIS COUNTY, (Includes Baylor Medical Center – Ellis County, 803 West Lampasas Street, Ennis, Texas, Zip 75119; tel. 214/875-9071) 1405 West Jefferson Street, Zip 75165; tel. 214/923-7000; J. Michael Lee, Executive Director **A**1 9 10 **F**7 8 11 15 19 22 24 28 30 32 35 36 37 39 40 42 44 46 49 64 65 66 71 73 **P**5 7 8 **S**0095 Baylor Health Care System	21	10	73	4457	50	47506	852	33241	14710	620
WEATHERFORD—Parker County										
★ CAMPBELL MEMORIAL HOSPITAL, 713 East Anderson Street, Zip 76086-9971; tel. 817/596-8751; Carolyn Hamilton, Acting Administrator **A**1 9 10 **F**7 8 14 15 16 17 19 22 23 24 28 30 31 33 34 35 36 37 39 40 41 42 44 49 65 67 71 73	16	10	83	3433	35	47443	561	18916	8939	332
WEBSTER—Harris County										
BAYWOOD BEHAVIORAL HEALTH SYSTEM See Charter Behavioral Health System of Clear Lake										
□ CHARTER BEHAVIORAL HEALTH SYSTEM OF CLEAR LAKE, (Formerly Baywood Behavioral Health System) 709 Medical Center Boulevard, Zip 77598; tel. 713/332-9550; Chris Duello, Administrator and Chief Executive Officer **A**1 9 10 **F**3 12 17 18 30 34 39 46 52 53 55 56 57 58 59 65 67 **S**0695 Charter Medical Corporation	33	22	84	869	23	1957	0	—	—	111
★ CLEAR LAKE REGIONAL MEDICAL CENTER, 500 Medical Center Boulevard, Zip 77598; tel. 713/332-2511; Donald A. Shaffett, Chief Executive Officer (Total facility includes 25 beds in nursing home–type unit) **A**1 9 10 **F**4 7 8 10 11 14 15 16 19 21 22 23 30 33 34 35 37 38 40 42 43 44 49 57 60 64 71 73 **P**7 **S**0048 Columbia/HCA Healthcare Corporation	33	10	431	10918	141	86630	1968	69703	26848	965
WEIMAR—Colorado County										
COLORADO–FAYETTE MEDICAL CENTER, 400 Youens Drive, Zip 78962-9561; tel. 409/725-9531; Randy Bacus, Administrator (Total facility includes 12 beds in nursing home–type unit) **A**9 10 **F**8 19 22 28 29 32 34 41 44 49 64	23	10	37	1221	21	18617	0	6778	2826	124
WELLINGTON—Collingsworth County										
COLLINGSWORTH GENERAL HOSPITAL, 1014 15th Street, Zip 79095; tel. 806/447-2521; Travis W. Roderick, Administrator and Chief Executive Officer **A**9 10 **F**8 12 14 15 16 19 22 26 28 30 32 33 34 46 49 51 64 71 **P**6	16	10	17	195	4	3483	0	2252	998	56
WESLACO—Hidalgo County										
★ KNAPP MEDICAL CENTER, 1401 East Eighth Street, Zip 78596, Mailing Address: Box 1110, Zip 78599; tel. 210/968-8567; Robert W. VanderVeer, Administrator **A**1 9 10 **F**7 8 15 16 19 21 22 23 26 27 30 31 32 34 35 37 39 40 42 44 45 46 49 63 65 70 71 73 74	23	10	180	9183	122	45131	1758	48106	19900	707

Hospitals, U.S. / TEXAS

Hospital, Address, Telephone, Administrator, Approval, Facility, and Physician Codes, Health Care System	Classification Codes		Utilization Data					Expense (thousands) of dollars		Personnel
★ American Hospital Association (AHA) membership ☐ Joint Commission on Accreditation of Healthcare Organizations (JCAHO) accreditation + American Osteopathic Hospital Association (AOHA) membership ○ American Osteopathic Association (AOA) accreditation △ Commission on Accreditation of Rehabilitation Facilities (CARF) accreditation Control codes 61, 63, 64, 71, 72 and 73 indicate hospitals listed by AOHA, but not registered by AHA. For definition of numerical codes, see page A6	Control	Service	Beds	Admissions	Census	Outpatient Visits	Births	Total	Payroll	
WEST—Mclennan County ☐ WEST COMMUNITY HOSPITAL, 501 Meadow Drive, Zip 76691, Mailing Address: Box 478, Zip 76691; tel. 817/826–7000; Betty York, Executive Director **A**1 9 10 **F**14 15 16 19 22 32 44 46 51 71 73 **P**8	16	10	23	656	10	6339	7	2982	1491	78
WHARTON—Wharton County ★ △ GULF COAST MEDICAL CENTER, 1400 Highway 59, Zip 77488–3004, Mailing Address: P.O. Box 3004, Zip 77488–3004; tel. 409/532–2500; Craig B. Watson, Chief Executive Officer (Total facility includes 17 beds in nursing home–type unit) **A**1 2 7 9 10 **F**7 10 12 15 16 19 21 22 23 30 32 33 34 35 37 40 42 44 45 46 48 49 52 56 57 60 63 64 65 67 71 73 74 **S**0048 Columbia/HCA Healthcare Corporation	33	10	161	3828	64	49352	578	29072	11483	445
WHEELER—Wheeler County PARKVIEW HOSPITAL, 1000 Sweetwater Street, Zip 79096, Mailing Address: Box 1030, Zip 79096; tel. 806/826–5581; B. W. Robertson, Administrator **A**9 10 **F**8 14 15 16 17 19 22 32 46 71	16	10	20	426	7	834	0	2365	1067	57
WHITNEY—Hill County LAKE WHITNEY MEMORIAL HOSPITAL, 201 North San Jacinto Street, Zip 76692, Mailing Address: Box 458, Zip 76692; tel. 817/694–3165; Joe M. Stevens, Administrator **A**9 10 **F**2 3 4 6 7 8 9 10 11 12 13 17 18 19 20 21 22 23 24 25 26 27 28 29 30 31 32 33 34 35 36 37 38 40 41 42 43 44 47 49 50 52 53 54 55 56 57 58 60 61 63 64 65 66 67 69 70 71 72 73	16	10	56	495	16	1141	0	2651	1051	77
WICHITA FALLS—Wichita County ★ BETHANIA REGIONAL HEALTH CARE CENTER, 1600 11th Street, Zip 76301–9988; tel. 817/723–4111; David D. Whitaker, President and Chief Executive Officer **A**1 3 9 10 **F**4 7 8 10 11 12 14 15 16 17 19 20 22 23 26 27 28 30 31 32 33 34 35 37 39 40 41 42 43 44 46 49 63 65 67 71 73 74 **P**8	21	10	164	7104	123	32106	0	59883	26369	882
☐ RED RIVER HOSPITAL, 1505 Eighth Street, Zip 76301–3106; tel. 817/322–3171; Ricky Powell, Administrator **A**1 9 10 **F**2 3 12 19 20 22 52 53 54 55 56 57 59 65	33	22	50	700	21	664	0	4917	2051	71
☐ WICHITA FALLS STATE HOSPITAL, 6515 Lake Road, Zip 76308–5419, Mailing Address: Box 300, Zip 76307–0300; tel. 817/692–1220; Richard M. Bruner, Superintendent **A**1 9 10 **F**12 52 53 54 55 56 57 58 73	12	22	352	1280	352	—	0	39401	25612	1292
★ WICHITA GENERAL HOSPITAL, 1600 Eighth Street, Zip 76301; tel. 817/723–1461; Jeffrey E. Hausler, President and Chief Executive Officer **A**1 2 3 5 9 10 **F**7 8 10 11 13 14 15 16 17 19 20 21 22 23 28 29 30 31 32 34 35 37 39 40 41 42 44 46 56 60 61 64 65 67 68 69 71 73 74 **P**7	23	10	222	8064	112	70913	1950	49543	21758	840
WINNIE—Chambers County ☐ MEDICAL CENTER OF WINNIE, Broadway at Campbell Road, Zip 77665, Mailing Address: Box 208, Zip 77665; tel. 409/296–2131; J. L. Flotte', Chief Executive Officer (Total facility includes 14 beds in nursing home–type unit) **A**1 9 10 **F**10 17 19 20 22 30 32 44 64 65 71 73 **P**8	23	10	44	813	15	31386	0	6986	3020	135
WINNSBORO—Wood County ★ PRESBYTERIAN HOSPITAL OF WINNSBORO, 719 West Coke Road, Zip 75494–3098, Mailing Address: P.O. Box 628, Zip 75494–0628; tel. 903/342–5227; Jerry Hopper, Vice President and Executive Director (Total facility includes 8 beds in nursing home–type unit) **A**1 9 10 **F**8 15 16 17 19 22 27 28 29 30 37 42 44 46 49 64 65 67 71 73 **P**1 4 7 8 **S**1130 Presbyterian Healthcare System	23	10	50	969	16	15782	1	8432	2989	107
WINTERS—Runnels County NORTH RUNNELS HOSPITAL, East Highway 53, Zip 79567, Mailing Address: Box 185, Zip 79567; tel. 915/754–4553; Larry Suit, Administrator **A**9 10 **F**16 19 22 28 30 32 33 41 44 71	16	10	21	404	4	4683	1	1733	786	54
WOODVILLE—Tyler County TYLER COUNTY HOSPITAL, 1100 West Bluff Street, Zip 75979, Mailing Address: P.O. Box 549, Zip 75979; tel. 409/283–8141; James W. Gainey, Administrator **A**9 10 **F**19 22 28 30 32 33 34 44 49 71	16	10	36	1385	16	17118	68	5137	2395	111
WYLIE—Dallas County ☐ PHYSICIANS REGIONAL HOSPITAL, 801 South Highway 78, Zip 75098, Mailing Address: P.O. Box 1500, Zip 75098; tel. 214/442–5414; Kathryn P. Sukkar, Administrator **A**1 9 10 **F**7 8 14 15 16 19 22 24 26 27 28 29 30 32 33 34 39 40 41 44 49 52 54 57 65 66 67 71 73	33	10	34	904	10	11866	181	7149	3141	118
YOAKUM—Lavaca County ★ YOAKUM COMMUNITY HOSPITAL, 303 Hubbard Street, Zip 77995, Mailing Address: Box 753, Zip 77995–0753; tel. 512/293–2321; Elwood E. Currier Jr., Chief Executive Officer **A**1 9 10 **F**7 8 12 14 16 17 19 20 22 26 32 33 34 35 39 41 44 45 49 51 57 59 65 66 67 71 73	23	10	25	779	9	13048	152	5782	2815	103

Hospitals, U.S. / UTAH

UTAH

Resident population 1,860 (in thousands)
Resident population in metro areas 77.5%
Birth rate per 1,000 population 20.4
65 years and over 8.9%
Percent of persons without health insurance 11.5%

Hospital, Address, Telephone, Administrator, Approval, Facility, and Physician Codes, Health Care System	Classification Codes		Utilization Data					Expense (thousands) of dollars		
★ American Hospital Association (AHA) membership □ Joint Commission on Accreditation of Healthcare Organizations (JCAHO) accreditation + American Osteopathic Hospital Association (AOHA) membership ○ American Osteopathic Association (AOA) accreditation △ Commission on Accreditation of Rehabilitation Facilities (CARF) accreditation Control codes 61, 63, 64, 71, 72 and 73 indicate hospitals listed by AOHA, but not registered by AHA. For definition of numerical codes, see page A6	Control	Service	Beds	Admissions	Census	Outpatient Visits	Births	Total	Payroll	Personnel
AMERICAN FORK—Utah County ★ AMERICAN FORK HOSPITAL, 1100 East 170 North, Zip 84003-9787; tel. 801/763-3300; Craig M. Smedley, Administrator (Total facility includes 12 beds in nursing home–type unit) A1 9 10 F4 7 8 12 14 17 19 21 22 26 28 30 32 33 36 37 39 40 41 44 49 64 65 70 71 73 74 P5 S1815 Intermountain Health Care, Inc.	23	10	67	4440	33	55651	1755	19179	8856	220
BEAVER—Beaver County BEAVER VALLEY HOSPITAL, 85 North 400 East, Zip 84713, Mailing Address: P.O. Box 1670, Zip 84713; tel. 801/438-2531; Craig Val Davidson, Administrator (Total facility includes 24 beds in nursing home–type unit) A9 10 F7 14 15 16 22 30 32 44 46 48 49 64 65 71 73 P3	14	10	36	578	29	5430	97	2852	1659	50
BOUNTIFUL—Davis County ★ LAKEVIEW HOSPITAL, 630 East Medical Drive, Zip 84010-4996; tel. 801/299-2500; Kay Matsumura, Chief Executive Officer A1 9 10 F2 3 4 7 8 10 12 15 16 17 18 19 21 22 26 27 28 30 32 35 37 38 40 41 42 44 49 52 53 54 55 56 58 59 63 64 65 66 67 69 71 72 73 74 P5 7 8 S0048 Columbia/HCA Healthcare Corporation	33	10	128	4205	45	45963	819	27936	10106	435
BRIGHAM CITY—Box Elder County ★ BRIGHAM CITY COMMUNITY HOSPITAL, 950 South 500 West, Zip 84302; tel. 801/734-9471; Robert H. Parker Jr., Chief Executive Officer A1 9 10 F2 3 7 8 11 12 14 17 18 19 21 22 23 24 27 28 29 30 32 35 37 39 40 41 42 44 45 46 48 49 52 53 54 55 56 57 58 59 61 65 66 67 71 72 73 74 P7 8 S0048 Columbia/HCA Healthcare Corporation	33	10	53	1721	13	20665	474	9746	3982	163
CEDAR CITY—Iron County ★ VALLEY VIEW MEDICAL CENTER, 595 South 75 East, Zip 84720; tel. 801/586-6587; Margaret Holm, Administrator A1 9 10 F7 8 15 16 19 21 22 30 32 34 37 40 44 49 51 64 65 71 73 P6 S1815 Intermountain Health Care, Inc.	23	10	36	1495	10	46257	430	9803	4548	152
DELTA—Millard County ★ DELTA COMMUNITY MEDICAL CENTER, 126 South White Sage Avenue, Zip 84624; tel. 801/864-5591; James E. Beckstrand, Administrator A9 10 F1 3 6 7 8 14 17 18 22 26 28 29 30 32 33 34 39 40 44 45 46 48 49 53 54 55 56 57 58 64 65 66 71 73 74 P6 7 S1815 Intermountain Health Care, Inc.	23	10	20	322	5	11185	100	2753	1037	43
FILLMORE—Millard County ★ FILLMORE COMMUNITY MEDICAL CENTER, 674 South Highway 99, Zip 84631; tel. 801/743-5591; James E. Beckstrand, Administrator A9 10 F7 8 14 22 28 29 30 32 34 44 45 46 49 65 71 73 S1815 Intermountain Health Care, Inc.	23	10	20	288	14	28303	56	3253	1210	63
GUNNISON—Sanpete County GUNNISON VALLEY HOSPITAL, Zip 84634; tel. 801/528-7246; Mark R. Stoddard, Administrator A9 10 F3 7 8 13 15 19 21 25 27 28 29 30 32 34 40 44 48 49 51 64 67 71 72	16	10	21	629	8	—	144	3710	1571	78
HEBER CITY—Wasatch County ★ WASATCH COUNTY HOSPITAL, 55 South Fifth East, Zip 84032-1848; tel. 801/654-2500; Randall K. Probst, Administrator A9 10 F7 8 14 15 16 20 21 22 28 30 32 34 36 40 44 45 64 65 67 71 73 P5 S1815 Intermountain Health Care, Inc.	23	10	40	428	4	8921	105	3240	1351	61
HILL AIR FORCE BASE—Davis County ★ U.S. AIR FORCE HOSPITAL, 7321 11th Street, Zip 84056-5012; tel. 801/777-5457; Colonel George P. Taylor Jr., Commander A1 F7 8 22 30 34 40 44 45 46 51 58 71 S9495 Department of the Air Force	41	10	25	2509	14	171603	296	—	—	384
KANAB—Kane County ★ KANE COUNTY HOSPITAL, 220 West 300 North, Zip 84741; tel. 801/644-5811; Mike Sinclair, Administrator A9 10 F7 15 19 22 32 34 40 44 73	16	10	33	429	15	5749	68	2463	1208	49
LAYTON—Davis County ★ DAVIS HOSPITAL AND MEDICAL CENTER, 1600 West Antelope Drive, Zip 84041-1142; tel. 801/825-9561; Floyd D. Morgan, Chief Executive Officer A1 9 10 F4 7 8 10 12 14 15 16 17 19 21 22 24 26 28 29 30 34 35 37 38 40 41 44 45 46 49 52 57 63 64 65 66 71 73 74 S0048 Columbia/HCA Healthcare Corporation	33	10	120	4549	41	55003	1108	24535	9549	308
LOGAN—Cache County ★ LOGAN REGIONAL HOSPITAL, 1400 North 500 East, Zip 84321-2499; tel. 801/752-2050; Richard Smith, Administrator A1 9 10 F2 3 8 10 11 12 15 16 19 21 22 24 28 29 30 32 33 34 35 39 40 41 42 44 45 49 51 52 54 56 58 59 64 65 67 71 72 73 74 P6 S1815 Intermountain Health Care, Inc.	23	10	133	6380	57	79200	1848	37125	15571	507
MIDVALE—Salt Lake County □ CHARTER CANYON TREATMENT CANTER, 175 West 7200 South, Zip 84047; tel. 801/561-8181; Larry W. Carter, Administrator (Nonreporting) A1 10	33	22	62	—	—	—	—	—	—	—
MILFORD—Beaver County ★ MILFORD VALLEY MEMORIAL HOSPITAL, 451 North Main Street, Zip 84751-0640, Mailing Address: Box 640, Zip 84751-0640; tel. 801/387-2411; John E. Gledhill, Administrator (Total facility includes 24 beds in nursing home–type unit) A9 10 F1 6 7 15 16 22 26 28 29 30 32 33 40 44 46 49 51 58 64 70 73 P8	16	10	34	296	17	2654	16	2048	917	60

Hospitals, U.S. / UTAH

Hospital, Address, Telephone, Administrator, Approval, Facility, and Physician Codes, Health Care System	Classification Codes		Utilization Data					Expense (thousands) of dollars		Personnel
★ American Hospital Association (AHA) membership □ Joint Commission on Accreditation of Healthcare Organizations (JCAHO) accreditation + American Osteopathic Hospital Association (AOHA) membership ○ American Osteopathic Association (AOA) accreditation △ Commission on Accreditation of Rehabilitation Facilities (CARF) accreditation Control codes 61, 63, 64, 71, 72 and 73 indicate hospitals listed by AOHA, but not registered by AHA. For definition of numerical codes, see page A6	Control	Service	Beds	Admissions	Census	Outpatient Visits	Births	Total	Payroll	
MOAB—Grand County ★ ALLEN MEMORIAL HOSPITAL, 719 West 400 North Street, Zip 84532, Mailing Address: Box 998, Zip 84532; tel. 801/259-7191; Charles A. Davis, Administrator (Total facility includes 19 beds in nursing home-type unit) **A**9 10 **F**2 3 7 8 11 12 13 14 15 17 18 20 22 27 28 29 30 31 32 33 34 36 39 40 41 44 45 46 51 52 53 54 55 56 57 58 61 62 64 65 67 68 70 71 73 74 **S**0048 Columbia/HCA Healthcare Corporation	13	10	38	265	23	8221	29	3389	1479	17
MONTICELLO—San Juan County ⚕ SAN JUAN HOSPITAL, 364 West First North, Zip 84535, Mailing Address: Box 308, Zip 84535-0308; tel. 801/587-2116; Dana K. Barnett, Executive Director **A**1 9 10 **F**7 8 16 17 22 28 30 31 36 40 44 49 65 71 72 73 **P**6 **S**2235 Lutheran Health Systems	16	10	33	702	10	5980	212	3874	1540	62
MONUMENT VALLEY—San Juan County ★ MONUMENT VALLEY HOSPITAL, 4 Rock Door Canyon, Zip 84536, Mailing Address: P.O. Box 360004, Zip 84536; tel. 801/727-3241; Raymond T. Carney, Chief Executive Officer (Nonreporting) **A**9 10 **S**0235 Adventist Health System/West	21	10	20	—	—	—	—	—	—	—
MOUNT PLEASANT—Sanpete County ★ SANPETE VALLEY HOSPITAL, 1100 South Medical Drive, Zip 84647; tel. 801/462-2441; George Winn, Administrator **A**9 10 **F**7 8 12 17 28 30 32 33 44 46 48 49 54 56 64 65 71 **P**6 **S**1815 Intermountain Health Care, Inc.	23	10	20	475	10	70871	78	5887	1741	85
MURRAY—Salt Lake County ⚕ COTTONWOOD HOSPITAL MEDICAL CENTER, 5770 South 300 East, Zip 84107; tel. 801/262-3461; Douglas R. Fonnesbeck, Administrator **A**1 2 9 10 **F**2 3 4 7 8 10 11 12 13 14 17 19 21 22 24 26 29 30 31 32 33 34 35 37 38 40 41 42 43 44 45 46 47 48 49 51 52 53 54 55 56 57 58 59 60 61 63 64 65 66 67 69 70 71 72 73 74 **P**4 6 **S**1815 Intermountain Health Care, Inc.	23	10	163	9488	78	181182	2944	71651	27489	997
NEPHI—Juab County ★ CENTRAL VALLEY MEDICAL CENTER, 549 North 400 East, Zip 84648; tel. 801/623-1242; Mark R. Stoddard, Administrator **A**9 10 **F**8 13 14 15 16 17 19 22 26 28 30 32 34 39 40 44 45 46 49 51 64 65 71 **P**6	23	10	22	509	4	—	55	4881	2525	81
OGDEN—Weber County ⚕ △ MCKAY-DEE HOSPITAL CENTER, 3939 Harrison Boulevard, Zip 84409-2386, Mailing Address: Box 9370, Zip 84409-0370; tel. 801/627-2800; Thomas Hanrahan, Administrator and Chief Executive Officer **A**1 2 3 5 7 9 10 **F**2 3 4 7 8 10 11 12 14 15 17 18 19 21 22 24 25 26 28 29 30 31 32 33 34 35 37 38 39 40 41 42 43 44 45 48 49 51 52 53 54 55 56 57 58 59 61 64 65 66 67 69 70 71 72 73 74 **P**3 6 **S**1815 Intermountain Health Care, Inc.	23	10	340	12472	155	120528	2377	116034	46848	1635
⚕ OGDEN REGIONAL MEDICAL CENTER, (Formerly St. Benedict's Hospital) 5475 South 500 East, Zip 84405-6978; tel. 801/479-2111; Les Beard, Chief Executive Officer **A**1 2 9 10 **F**2 3 4 7 8 9 10 11 12 13 14 15 16 17 18 19 21 22 24 28 29 30 31 32 34 35 37 38 39 40 41 42 43 44 45 46 47 49 52 53 54 55 57 58 59 60 65 67 68 70 71 73 74 **P**4 8 **S**0048 Columbia/HCA Healthcare Corporation	21	10	151	7214	82	120291	1960	59069	20053	863
ST. BENEDICT'S HOSPITAL See Ogden Regional Medical Center										
OREM—Utah County ★ OREM COMMUNITY HOSPITAL, 331 North 400 West, Zip 84057; tel. 801/224-4080; Mark F. Dalley, Administrator and Chief Operating Officer **A**9 10 **F**2 3 4 7 8 9 10 11 12 14 15 16 17 19 21 22 24 25 28 29 30 31 32 35 37 38 40 41 42 43 44 47 48 49 52 53 54 55 56 57 58 59 60 63 64 65 66 69 70 71 73 74 **S**1815 Intermountain Health Care, Inc.	23	10	20	1068	5	31451	752	—	—	125
PANGUITCH—Garfield County ★ GARFIELD MEMORIAL HOSPITAL AND CLINICS, 200 North Fourth East, Zip 84759, Mailing Address: P.O. Box 389, Zip 84759-0389; tel. 801/676-8811; Wayne R. Ross, Administrator **A**9 10 **F**7 12 22 25 28 30 40 44 56 65 71 **P**3 6 **S**1815 Intermountain Health Care, Inc.	23	10	20	515	3	5200	44	2745	1109	48
PAYSON—Utah County ⚕ MOUNTAIN VIEW HOSPITAL, 1000 East Highway 6, Zip 84651-1690; tel. 801/465-7101; Don Larsen, Chief Executive Officer (Total facility includes 18 beds in nursing home-type unit) **A**1 5 9 10 **F**4 7 8 10 11 12 19 21 22 26 28 30 32 34 35 39 40 41 44 45 46 52 53 54 55 56 57 58 59 64 65 70 71 73 74 **P**8 **S**0048 Columbia/HCA Healthcare Corporation	33	10	121	4150	44	25547	1224	—	—	366
PRICE—Carbon County ⚕ CASTLEVIEW HOSPITAL, 300 North Hospital Drive, Zip 84501; tel. 801/637-4800; R. Alan Larson, Administrator and Chief Executive Officer (Total facility includes 10 beds in nursing home-type unit) **A**1 9 10 **F**3 7 8 11 14 15 16 19 21 22 24 27 28 29 34 35 37 38 39 40 41 44 46 47 51 61 63 64 65 71 73 74 **P**7 8 **S**0048 Columbia/HCA Healthcare Corporation	33	10	84	2144	22	50688	346	15345	6621	280
PROVO—Utah County □ UTAH STATE HOSPITAL, 1300 East Center Street, Zip 84606, Mailing Address: Box 270, Zip 84603-0270; tel. 801/344-4400; Mark I. Payne, Superintendent **A**1 9 10 **F**14 15 16 20 22 52 53 54 55 56 57 58 65 73	12	22	343	368	322	0	0	24936	14531	633
⚕ UTAH VALLEY REGIONAL MEDICAL CENTER, 1034 North 500 West, Zip 84605-0390; tel. 801/373-7850; Larry R. Dursteler, Administrator and Chief Operating Officer (Total facility includes 14 beds in nursing home-type unit) **A**1 2 9 10 **F**4 7 8 10 11 12 14 15 16 17 18 19 20 21 22 24 25 27 28 29 30 31 32 33 34 35 36 37 38 39 40 41 42 43 44 45 46 47 48 49 52 53 54 55 56 57 58 59 60 63 64 65 67 68 70 71 72 73 74 **P**5 6 **S**1815 Intermountain Health Care, Inc.	23	10	343	16764	220	286143	3936	129436	53850	1762

Hospitals, U.S. / UTAH

Hospital, Address, Telephone, Administrator, Approval, Facility, and Physician Codes, Health Care System	Classification Codes		Utilization Data					Expense (thousands) of dollars		
★ American Hospital Association (AHA) membership ☐ Joint Commission on Accreditation of Healthcare Organizations (JCAHO) accreditation + American Osteopathic Hospital Association (AOHA) membership ○ American Osteopathic Association (AOA) accreditation △ Commission on Accreditation of Rehabilitation Facilities (CARF) accreditation Control codes 61, 63, 64, 71, 72 and 73 indicate hospitals listed by AOHA, but not registered by AHA. For definition of numerical codes, see page A6	Control	Service	Beds	Admissions	Census	Outpatient Visits	Births	Total	Payroll	Personnel
RICHFIELD—Sevier County										
★ SEVIER VALLEY HOSPITAL, 1100 North Main Street, Zip 84701; tel. 801/896–8271; Gary E. Beck, Administrator A1 9 10 F7 8 14 15 16 19 21 22 28 32 33 34 40 44 49 65 71 73 P5 6 S1815 Intermountain Health Care, Inc.	23	10	42	1234	9	54583	191	8640	2847	112
ROOSEVELT—Duchesne County										
★ UINTAH BASIN MEDICAL CENTER, 250 West 300 North, 75–2, Zip 84066–2399; tel. 801/722–6163; Bradley D. LeBaron, Administrator A9 10 F7 8 11 14 15 16 19 21 22 27 28 30 32 34 35 37 40 44 49 51 70 71 73 P7	13	10	42	1839	15	25526	408	14198	5276	253
SAINT GEORGE—Washington County										
★ DIXIE REGIONAL MEDICAL CENTER, 544 South 400 East, Zip 84770; tel. 801/634–4000; L. Steven Wilson, Administrator A1 2 9 10 F7 8 10 11 15 16 17 19 21 22 23 27 28 30 32 33 34 35 37 39 40 41 42 44 45 46 49 50 51 52 54 58 60 61 63 65 66 67 69 71 73 74 P5 6 8 S1815 Intermountain Health Care, Inc.	23	10	137	7037	67	77049	1379	40489	16063	505
SALT LAKE CITY—Salt Lake County										
☐ CPC OLYMPUS VIEW HOSPITAL, 1430 East 4500 South, Zip 84117–4208; tel. 801/272–8000; Susan Kosta, Administrator A1 9 10 F1 2 3 14 15 16 22 34 52 53 54 55 56 57 58 59 65 P5 6 S0785 Community Psychiatric Centers	33	22	102	774	49	0	0	—	—	100
HIGHLAND RIDGE HOSPITAL, 4578 Highland Drive, Zip 84117; tel. 801/272–9851; Michael Dusoc, Administrator (Nonreporting) A9	33	82	32	—	—	—	—	—	—	—
HOLY CROSS HOSPITAL See Salt Lake Regional Medical Center										
★ △ LDS HOSPITAL, Eighth Avenue and C Street, Zip 84143; tel. 801/321–1100; Richard M. Cagen, Administrator (Total facility includes 32 beds in nursing home–type unit) A1 2 3 5 7 9 10 F2 3 4 7 8 10 11 12 14 15 16 17 18 19 21 22 24 25 26 28 30 31 32 34 35 37 38 40 41 42 43 44 45 46 47 48 49 51 52 53 54 55 56 57 58 59 60 61 63 64 65 66 67 69 70 71 72 73 74 P2 4 6 S1815 Intermountain Health Care, Inc.	23	10	440	17608	225	372775	3669	206944	82261	2498
★ PRIMARY CHILDREN'S MEDICAL CENTER, (Pediatric Medical/Surgical, Psychiatric and Rehabilitation) 100 North Medical Drive, Zip 84113–1100; tel. 801/588–2000; Joseph R. Horton, Chief Executive Officer and Administrator (Total facility includes 36 beds in nursing home–type unit) A1 3 5 9 10 F2 3 4 7 8 10 11 12 13 14 15 17 19 20 21 22 26 30 31 32 34 35 37 38 39 40 41 42 43 44 45 46 47 48 49 51 52 53 54 55 56 58 59 60 61 63 64 65 66 67 69 70 71 72 73 74 S1815 Intermountain Health Care, Inc.	23	59	208	9219	143	154364	0	113839	53224	1328
★ SALT LAKE REGIONAL MEDICAL CENTER, (Formerly Holy Cross Hospital) 1050 East South Temple, Zip 84102–1599; tel. 801/350–4111; David L. Jones, Chief Executive Officer A1 2 3 5 9 10 F4 7 8 10 14 15 16 17 18 19 21 22 23 24 31 32 33 34 35 37 38 40 41 42 43 44 45 46 48 49 54 55 56 57 58 63 65 67 71 73 74 P2 4 5 8 S0048 Columbia/HCA Healthcare Corporation	21	10	200	8410	95	126493	2124	70083	21773	792
★ SHRINERS HOSPITALS FOR CRIPPLED CHILDREN, INTERMOUNTAIN UNIT, Fairfax Road & Virginia Street, Zip 84103–4399; tel. 801/532–5307; Douglas P. Schweikhart, Administrator A1 3 5 F12 19 34 35 39 41 47 49 54 65 67 71 73 S4125 Shriners Hospitals for Crippled Children	23	57	40	755	21	3614	0	—	—	120
★ ST. MARK'S HOSPITAL, 1200 East 3900 South, Zip 84124; tel. 801/268–7000; Larry Hancock, Chief Executive Officer (Total facility includes 18 beds in nursing home–type unit) A1 2 3 9 10 F4 7 8 10 11 14 15 16 18 19 21 22 23 25 26 28 29 30 32 33 34 37 40 42 43 44 45 46 49 60 64 67 71 73 74 P5 S0048 Columbia/HCA Healthcare Corporation	33	10	223	9830	110	93079	1928	70735	23845	789
★ △ UNIVERSITY OF UTAH HOSPITALS AND CLINICS, 50 North Medical Drive, Zip 84132; tel. 801/581–2121; Christine St. Andre, Executive Director A1 2 3 5 7 8 9 10 F4 6 7 8 9 10 14 15 16 17 18 19 20 21 22 23 25 26 28 29 30 31 32 34 35 37 38 40 41 42 43 44 45 46 48 49 51 52 53 54 55 56 57 58 59 60 61 65 66 67 68 69 70 71 72 73 74 P5	12	10	395	15319	301	262251	2235	224857	76421	3163
☐ UNIVERSITY OF UTAH NEUROPSYCHIATRIC INSTITUTE, (Formerly Utah Neuropsychiatric Institute) 501 Chipeta Way, Zip 84108–1225; tel. 801/583–2500; Ross Van Vranken, Chief Executive Officer (Data for 108 days) A1 3 5 10 F1 2 3 12 14 16 19 21 26 35 45 46 53 54 55 56 57 58 59 65 67 68 P5 8	23	22	90	1402	185	7378	0	11130	5227	216
★ VETERANS AFFAIRS MEDICAL CENTER, 500 Foothill Drive, Zip 84148; tel. 801/582–1565; William L. Hodson, Administrator A1 2 3 5 8 9 F2 3 4 8 10 15 16 17 18 19 20 21 22 23 25 26 27 28 29 30 31 32 34 35 37 39 41 42 43 44 45 46 48 49 51 52 54 55 56 58 59 60 63 65 67 69 71 73 74 S9295 Department of Veterans Affairs	45	10	294	7563	217	153300	0	107451	52941	1580
★ WASATCH CANYONS HOSPITAL, 5770 South 1500 West, Zip 84123; tel. 801/262–6199; Jill Green, Administrator A1 9 10 F2 3 14 52 54 55 56 57 58 59 67 P6 S1815 Intermountain Health Care, Inc.	23	22	44	662	13	3314	0	5577	2854	0
SANDY—Salt Lake County										
★ ALTA VIEW HOSPITAL, 9660 South 1300 East, Zip 84094; tel. 801/576–2600; Wes Thompson, Administrator A1 9 10 F2 3 4 7 8 10 11 12 13 14 15 16 17 19 21 24 26 28 30 31 32 33 34 35 38 40 41 42 44 45 46 47 48 49 51 52 53 54 55 56 57 58 59 60 61 63 64 65 66 67 68 69 71 72 73 74 P4 6 S1815 Intermountain Health Care, Inc.	23	10	70	4064	26	58662	1563	27547	10084	337
☐ △ HEALTHSOUTH REHABILITATION HOSPITAL OF UTAH, (Formerly Healthsouth Western Rehabilitation Institute) 8074 South 1300 East, Zip 84094; tel. 801/561–3400; Robert Cash, Administrator and Chief Executive Officer (Total facility includes 36 beds in nursing home–type unit) A1 7 9 10 F5 12 24 25 27 28 30 32 34 39 41 45 46 48 49 64 65 66 67 73 P4 S0023 Healthsouth Corporation	33	46	73	727	36	8432	0	9864	5501	185

Hospitals, U.S. / UTAH

Hospital, Address, Telephone, Administrator, Approval, Facility, and Physician Codes, Health Care System	Classification Codes		Utilization Data					Expense (thousands) of dollars		
★ American Hospital Association (AHA) membership □ Joint Commission on Accreditation of Healthcare Organizations (JCAHO) accreditation + American Osteopathic Hospital Association (AOHA) membership ○ American Osteopathic Association (AOA) accreditation △ Commission on Accreditation of Rehabilitation Facilities (CARF) accreditation Control codes 61, 63, 64, 71, 72 and 73 indicate hospitals listed by AOHA, but not registered by AHA. For definition of numerical codes, see page A6	Control	Service	Beds	Admissions	Census	Outpatient Visits	Births	Total	Payroll	Personnel
TOOELE—Tooele County ★ TOOELE VALLEY REGIONAL MEDICAL CENTER, 211 South 100 East, Zip 84074–2794; tel. 801/882–1697; Matthew Chambers, Chief Executive Officer (Total facility includes 84 beds in nursing home–type unit) **A**1 9 10 **F**7 8 14 15 16 19 21 22 28 30 32 34 39 40 41 44 46 49 64 71 73 74 **P**5 **S**0002 Quorum Health Group/Quorum Health Resources	16	10	107	571	80	16004	86	9107	3971	255
TREMONTON—Box Elder County ★ BEAR RIVER VALLEY HOSPITAL, 440 West 600 North, Zip 84337; tel. 801/257–7441; Robert F. Jex, Administrator (Total facility includes 19 beds in nursing home–type unit) **A**9 10 **F**7 12 14 15 17 20 22 32 33 40 44 46 64 71 73 **P**3 **S**1815 Intermountain Health Care, Inc.	23	10	20	315	2	5595	55	2135	1099	28
VERNAL—Uintah County ★ ASHLEY VALLEY MEDICAL CENTER, 151 West 200 North, Zip 84078; tel. 801/789–3342; Ronald J. Perry, Chief Executive Officer **A**9 10 **F**7 8 11 12 14 15 19 22 26 28 29 30 32 35 37 39 40 41 44 45 46 51 64 65 71 73 **P**7 8 **S**0048 Columbia/HCA Healthcare Corporation	33	10	29	1270	10	36202	261	9431	4000	156
WEST JORDAN—Salt Lake County HOLY CROSS JORDAN VALLEY HOSPITAL See Jordan Valley Hospital										
★ JORDAN VALLEY HOSPITAL, (Formerly Holy Cross Jordan Valley Hospital) 3580 West 9000 South, Zip 84088–8811; tel. 801/561–8888; Keith Alexander, Chief Executive Officer (Data for 181 days) **A**10 **F**7 8 14 15 16 19 21 22 23 28 30 32 34 37 40 44 46 63 65 71 73 74 **P**2 6 7 8 **S**0048 Columbia/HCA Healthcare Corporation	33	10	50	1156	17	25678	453	—	—	337
RIVENDELL PSYCHIATRIC CENTER, 5899 West Rivendell Drive, Zip 84088, Mailing Address: P.O. Box 459, Zip 84084; tel. 801/561–3377; John T. Young, Chief Executive Officer **A**10 **F**16 52 53 58 59 **P**5	33	52	80	288	50	491	0	5686	2827	80
WEST VALLEY CITY—Salt Lake County ★ PIONEER VALLEY HOSPITAL, 3460 South Pioneer Parkway, Zip 84120; tel. 801/964–3100; Steven B. Bateman, Chief Executive Officer **A**1 2 9 10 **F**2 3 7 8 10 11 12 14 15 16 17 18 19 20 21 22 24 28 30 32 34 35 37 39 40 41 42 44 45 46 49 52 54 55 56 57 58 59 63 64 65 66 67 69 71 73 74 **P**1 7 **S**0048 Columbia/HCA Healthcare Corporation	33	10	127	3862	42	89492	795	33023	11948	360
WOODS CROSS—Davis County □ BENCHMARK REGIONAL HOSPITAL, 592 West 1350 South, Zip 84087–1665; tel. 801/299–5300; Richard O. Hurt Jr., Chief Executive Officer **A**1 9 10 **F**2 3 14 15 16 22 52 53 56 57 58 59 65 67 **P**6 8 **S**0405 Ramsay Health Care, Inc.	33	22	68	792	41	2273	0	7187	3055	143

© 1995 AHA Guide

Hospitals, U.S. / VERMONT

VERMONT

Resident population 576 (in thousands)
Resident population in metro areas 27.0%
Birth rate per 1,000 population 14.0
65 years and over 12.0%
Percent of persons without health insurance 10.6%

Hospital, Address, Telephone, Administrator, Approval, Facility, and Physician Codes, Health Care System	Control	Service	Beds	Admissions	Census	Outpatient Visits	Births	Total	Payroll	Personnel
★ American Hospital Association (AHA) membership
□ Joint Commission on Accreditation of Healthcare Organizations (JCAHO) accreditation
+ American Osteopathic Hospital Association (AOHA) membership
○ American Osteopathic Association (AOA) accreditation
△ Commission on Accreditation of Rehabilitation Facilities (CARF) accreditation
Control codes 61, 63, 64, 71, 72 and 73 indicate hospitals listed by AOHA, but not registered by AHA. For definition of numerical codes, see page A6										
BARRE—Washington County
★ CENTRAL VERMONT MEDICAL CENTER, Fisher Road, Zip 05641, Mailing Address: P.O. Box 547, Zip 05641–0547; tel. 802/371-4100; Philo D. Hall, President (Total facility includes 153 beds in nursing home–type unit) **A**1 9 10 **F**3 7 8 15 17 19 21 22 23 28 30 31 32 33 34 35 37 39 40 41 42 44 45 46 49 51 52 53 54 56 57 58 60 61 64 65 66 71 73 74 **P**6 8	23	10	275	4640	224	140323	727	36284	26320	511
BENNINGTON—Bennington County
★ SOUTHWESTERN VERMONT MEDICAL CENTER, 100 Hospital Drive East, Zip 05201–5013; tel. 802/442-6361; Harvey M. Yorke, President **A**1 2 9 10 **F**2 3 7 8 11 15 16 17 19 21 22 24 27 28 30 32 33 34 37 39 40 41 42 44 45 46 49 52 54 55 56 57 58 59 63 64 65 67 70 71 73 74 **P**8	23	10	140	5108	72	83277	425	34099	15481	233
BRATTLEBORO—Windham County
★ BRATTLEBORO MEMORIAL HOSPITAL, 9 Belmont Avenue, Zip 05301; tel. 802/257-0341; Brian R. Mitteer, President **A**1 9 10 **F**7 8 11 14 15 16 17 19 21 22 24 28 30 31 34 37 39 40 41 42 44 46 49 63 67 71 73	23	10	61	2601	35	46077	388	18895	9147	329
★ BRATTLEBORO RETREAT, 75 Linden Street, Zip 05301–0803, Mailing Address: P.O. Box 803, Zip 05302; tel. 802/257-7785; C. Richard Sarle, Chief Executive Officer (Nonreporting) **A**1 3 5 10	23	22	199	—	—	—	—	—	—	—
BURLINGTON—Chittenden County
★ FLETCHER ALLEN HEALTH CARE, Colchester Avenue, Zip 05401; tel. 802/656-2345; John W. Frymoyer M.D., Chief Executive Officer (Nonreporting) **A**1 2 3 5 8 9 10	23	10	499	—	—	—	—	—	—	—
COLCHESTER—Chittenden County
★ FANNY ALLEN HOSPITAL, 101 College Parkway, Zip 05446–3035; tel. 802/655-1234 **A**1 2 3 5 9 10 **F**4 8 10 17 19 21 22 26 28 29 30 31 32 33 34 35 37 39 41 42 44 46 49 65 71 72 73	21	10	83	2395	32	43518	0	22545	10882	367
MIDDLEBURY—Addison County
★ PORTER HOSPITAL, South Street, Zip 05753–8606; tel. 802/388-4741; James L. Daily, President (Total facility includes 118 beds in nursing home–type unit) **A**1 9 10 **F**7 8 12 17 20 21 22 26 30 37 39 40 44 45 46 49 54 64 65 67 71 73	23	10	163	1784	135	47607	384	20497	9014	388
MORRISVILLE—Lamoille County
★ COPLEY HOSPITAL, Washington Highway, Zip 05661–9209; tel. 802/888-4231; Carolyn C. Roberts, President **A**1 9 10 **F**7 8 11 16 17 19 21 30 33 34 37 39 40 42 44 46 48 49 53 56 58 64 65 66 67 71 73 **P**8	23	10	33	1757	24	43186	280	13748	6326	219
NEWPORT—Orleans County
★ NORTH COUNTRY HOSPITAL AND HEALTH CENTER, Prouty Drive, Zip 05855; tel. 802/334-7331; Sidney A. Toll, President **A**1 9 10 **F**7 8 14 15 16 17 19 21 22 34 37 39 40 41 42 44 46 49 56 65 67 71 73 74 **P**6	23	10	42	2549	30	39182	230	17062	8876	303
RANDOLPH—Orange County
★ GIFFORD MEDICAL CENTER, 44 South Main Street, Zip 05060, Mailing Address: Box 2000, Zip 05060; tel. 802/728-4441; Thomas S. Wingardner, President (Total facility includes 51 beds in nursing home–type unit) **A**1 2 9 10 **F**3 6 7 8 11 12 13 14 15 16 17 18 19 21 22 25 26 27 28 29 30 31 32 33 34 36 37 39 40 41 42 44 45 46 49 51 53 54 55 56 57 58 60 61 64 65 66 67 68 71 72 73 74 **P**6	23	10	92	1613	61	50156	276	14142	7517	183
RUTLAND—Rutland County
★ RUTLAND REGIONAL MEDICAL CENTER, 160 Allen Street, Zip 05701–4595; tel. 802/775-7111; James T. Bowse, President **A**1 2 9 10 **F**4 6 7 8 14 15 16 19 20 21 22 23 28 30 31 32 33 34 35 37 40 41 42 44 45 46 48 49 52 54 55 56 58 59 60 63 65 66 67 70 71 72 73 **P**1 5	23	10	188	7276	125	94697	730	57694	28203	772
SAINT ALBANS—Windsor County
★ NORTHWESTERN MEDICAL CENTER, Fairfield Street, Zip 05478–1004, Mailing Address: Box 1370, Zip 05478; tel. 802/524-5911; Peter A. Hofstetter, Chief Executive Officer **A**1 2 9 10 **F**7 8 11 12 14 15 16 19 22 28 29 30 32 33 34 39 40 42 44 45 49 51 61 65 67 71 73 74 **P**8 **S**0002 Quorum Health Group/Quorum Health Resources	23	10	70	2579	37	20817	388	19153	8919	318
SAINT JOHNSBURY—Denton County
★ NORTHEASTERN VERMONT REGIONAL HOSPITAL, Hospital Drive, Zip 05819–9962; tel. 802/748-8141; Paul R. Bengtson, Chief Executive Officer **A**1 9 10 **F**3 7 8 11 14 15 16 17 19 21 22 29 31 33 37 39 40 41 42 44 49 53 54 56 63 65 66 67 71 73 74 **S**0002 Quorum Health Group/Quorum Health Resources	23	10	72	2228	36	47538	284	18218	7983	311
SPRINGFIELD—Windsor County
★ SPRINGFIELD HOSPITAL, 25 Ridgewood Road, Zip 05156, Mailing Address: P.O. Box 2003, Zip 05156–3057; tel. 802/885-2151; David J. Pagniucci, Chief Executive Officer **A**1 9 10 **F**3 7 8 12 15 19 21 22 25 26 28 31 33 34 35 37 40 41 42 44 52 54 56 58 63 65 66 67 71 72 73 **P**4 7	23	10	69	2335	29	34785	210	18743	6861	255
TOWNSHEND—Windham County
★ GRACE COTTAGE HOSPITAL, (Includes Stratton House Nursing Home) Route 35, Zip 05353, Mailing Address: P.O. Box 216, Zip 05353–0126; tel. 802/365-7357; Albert La Rochelle, Administrator (Total facility includes 30 beds in nursing home–type unit) **A**9 10 **F**1 7 16 22 27 33 36 40 41 44 49 64 65 73	23	10	45	338	33	8845	17	2935	1805	72

Hospitals, U.S. / VERMONT

Hospital, Address, Telephone, Administrator, Approval, Facility, and Physician Codes, Health Care System	Classification Codes		Utilization Data					Expense (thousands) of dollars		Personnel
	Control	Service	Beds	Admissions	Census	Outpatient Visits	Births	Total	Payroll	
★ American Hospital Association (AHA) membership
☐ Joint Commission on Accreditation of Healthcare Organizations (JCAHO) accreditation
+ American Osteopathic Hospital Association (AOHA) membership
○ American Osteopathic Association (AOA) accreditation
△ Commission on Accreditation of Rehabilitation Facilities (CARF) accreditation
Control codes 61, 63, 64, 71, 72 and 73 indicate hospitals listed by AOHA, but not registered by AHA. For definition of numerical codes, see page A6										
WATERBURY—Washington County
VERMONT STATE HOSPITAL, 103 South Main Street, Zip 05671–2501; tel. 802/241–3100; Claudia P. Stone, Executive Director (Total facility includes 20 beds in nursing home–type unit) **A**9 10 **F**20 52 56 57 64 65 73 **P**5	12	22	70	306	83	0	0	10996	7627	198
WHITE RIVER JUNCTION—Windsor County
★ VETERANS AFFAIRS MEDICAL CENTER, North Hartland Road, Zip 05009–0001; tel. 802/295–9363; Gary M. De Gasta, Director (Total facility includes 30 beds in nursing home–type unit) **A**1 3 5 8 9 **F**1 2 3 4 5 6 8 10 11 12 16 17 18 19 20 21 22 24 25 26 27 28 29 30 31 32 33 34 35 37 39 41 42 43 44 45 46 48 49 51 52 53 54 55 56 57 58 60 61 62 64 65 67 69 71 73 74 **P**6 **S**9295 Department of Veterans Affairs	45	10	150	3613	114	82653	0	54454	24542	882
WINDSOR—Windsor County
★ MOUNT ASCUTNEY HOSPITAL AND HEALTH CENTER, Rural Route 1, Box 6, Zip 05089–9702; tel. 802/674–6711; Richard Slusky, Administrator (Total facility includes 66 beds in nursing home–type unit) **A**1 9 10 **F**12 15 16 17 22 26 27 30 31 32 33 34 36 37 39 41 44 48 49 51 54 55 56 58 64 65 71 73 74 **P**4 6	23	10	99	800	82	12514	0	9609	4969	206

© 1995 AHA Guide

VIRGINIA

Resident population 6,491 (in thousands)
Resident population in metro areas 77.5%
Birth rate per 1,000 population 15.5
65 years and over 11.0%
Percent of persons without health insurance 15.5%

Hospital, Address, Telephone, Administrator, Approval, Facility, and Physician Codes, Health Care System	Classification Codes		Utilization Data					Expense (thousands) of dollars		
★ American Hospital Association (AHA) membership ☐ Joint Commission on Accreditation of Healthcare Organizations (JCAHO) accreditation + American Osteopathic Hospital Association (AOHA) membership ○ American Osteopathic Association (AOA) accreditation △ Commission on Accreditation of Rehabilitation Facilities (CARF) accreditation Control codes 61, 63, 64, 71, 72 and 73 indicate hospitals listed by AOHA, but not registered by AHA. For definition of numerical codes, see page A6	Control	Service	Beds	Admissions	Census	Outpatient Visits	Births	Total	Payroll	Personnel
ABINGDON—Washington County										
★ JOHNSTON MEMORIAL HOSPITAL, 351 North Court Street, Zip 24210–2921; tel. 703/676–7000; Clark R. Beil, Chief Executive Officer **A**1 2 9 10 **F**7 8 12 14 15 16 19 22 24 26 28 31 34 37 38 39 40 41 44 46 49 65 66 67 71 73 **P**6 8	23	10	135	4857	73	58469	977	29987	12556	513
ALEXANDRIA—Independent City										
★ ALEXANDRIA HOSPITAL, 4320 Seminary Road, Zip 22304–1594; tel. 703/504–3000; H. Patrick Walters, President **A**1 2 3 5 9 10 **F**4 7 8 10 11 12 15 16 19 21 22 26 28 30 31 32 33 34 35 37 38 39 40 41 42 43 44 45 46 49 52 54 56 59 60 61 63 65 67 70 71 73 74 **P**4 5 7 8	23	10	321	15161	226	105728	3309	105658	54376	1481
★ △ MOUNT VERNON HOSPITAL, 2501 Parker's Lane, Zip 22306–3209; tel. 703/664–7000; Joanne Carrocino, Administrator **A**1 2 3 7 10 **F**1 2 3 4 6 7 8 9 10 11 12 13 14 15 16 17 19 21 22 23 24 25 26 27 28 29 30 31 32 33 34 35 36 37 38 39 40 41 42 43 44 45 46 47 48 49 51 52 53 54 55 56 57 58 59 60 61 63 64 65 66 67 68 69 70 71 72 73 74 **P**1 3 6 7 8 **S**1305 Inova Health System	23	10	229	7158	141	56569	0	70571	31395	798
ARLINGTON—Arlington County										
★ ARLINGTON HOSPITAL, 1701 North George Mason Drive, Zip 22205–3698; tel. 703/558–5000; James B. Cole, Acting President and Chief Executive Officer **A**1 2 3 5 9 10 **F**3 4 6 7 8 10 11 12 15 19 21 22 28 30 31 32 33 34 35 37 38 40 42 43 44 46 49 52 56 58 59 60 62 63 64 65 67 71 73 74 **P**1 5 7	23	10	322	14454	212	113748	3260	102765	47628	1262
☐ HOSPICE OF NORTHERN VIRGINIA, 4715 North 15th Street, Zip 22205; tel. 703/525–7070; Karen Price Woods R.N., Acting Administrator (Nonreporting) **A**1 10	23	49	15	—	—	—	—	—	—	—
★ NATIONAL HOSPITAL FOR ORTHOPAEDICS AND REHABILITATION, 2455 Army Navy Drive, Zip 22206; tel. 703/920–6700; Edward J. Jenkins, President **A**1 5 9 10 **F**14 15 16 19 21 22 27 28 30 34 35 37 41 44 46 49 63 65 66 71 72 73 **P**4 5	23	10	61	1765	40	24367	0	28158	13574	343
★ NORTHERN VIRGINIA DOCTORS' HOSPITAL, 601 South Carlin Springs Road, Zip 22204–1096; tel. 703/671–1200; (Nonreporting) **A**1 5 9 10 **S**0048 Columbia/HCA Healthcare Corporation	33	10	211							
BEDFORD—Bedford City										
★ BEDFORD COUNTY MEMORIAL HOSPITAL, Oakwood Street, Zip 24523–0688, Mailing Address: P.O. Box 688, Zip 24523–0688; tel. 703/586–2441; John H. Fretz, Administrator (Nonreporting) **A**1 9 10 **S**0070 Carilion Health System	23	10	166							
BIG STONE GAP—Wise County										
★ LONESOME PINE HOSPITAL, 1990 Holton Avenue East, Zip 24219–0230, Mailing Address: Drawer I, Zip 24219; tel. 703/523–8609; John L. Thorsten, Administrator **A**1 9 10 **F**7 8 14 15 16 17 19 21 22 23 28 30 32 34 35 37 39 40 44 46 49 63 65 68 71 73 **S**0070 Carilion Health System	23	10	60	1978	25	26505	236	12026	4827	215
BLACKSBURG—Montgomery County										
★ MONTGOMERY REGIONAL HOSPITAL, 3700 South Main Street, Zip 24060, Mailing Address: P.O. Box 90004, Zip 24062–9004; tel. 703/953–5101; Gene B. Wright, Chief Executive Officer (Nonreporting) **A**1 9 10 **S**0048 Columbia/HCA Healthcare Corporation	33	10	146							
BURKEVILLE—Nottoway County										
★ PIEDMONT GERIATRIC HOSPITAL, (Geriatric and Psychiatric) Highway 460/360, Zip 23922–9999; tel. 804/767–4401; Willard R. Pierce Jr., Director **A**1 9 10 **F**19 20 22 26 27 35 41 46 52 55 57 60 65 67 71 73 **S**0012 Virginia Department of Mental Health	12	49	210	148	198	0	0	15099	9139	405
CATAWBA—Roanoke County										
☐ CATAWBA HOSPITAL, Mailing Address: P.O. Box 200, Zip 24070; tel. 703/375–4200; R. Michael Marsh Ph.D., Director **A**1 9 10 **F**14 15 16 19 20 26 35 45 46 52 57 65 73 **P**6	12	22	218	364	180	0	0	15515	8695	362
CHARLOTTESVILLE—Independent City										
☐ CHARTER BEHAVIORAL HEALTH SYSTEM OF CHARLOTTESVILLE, (Formerly Charter Hospital Charlottesville) 2101 Arlington Boulevard, Zip 22903–1593; tel. 804/977–1120; David W. Pedrick, Chief Executive Officer **A**1 9 10 **F**2 3 15 52 53 54 55 56 57 58 59 65 **S**0695 Charter Medical Corporation	33	22	75	983	21	2970	0	—	—	77
★ MARTHA JEFFERSON HOSPITAL, 459 Locust Avenue, Zip 22902–9940; tel. 804/982–7000; James E. Haden, President and Chief Executive Officer **A**1 2 9 10 **F**7 8 12 14 16 17 19 20 21 22 23 24 25 26 27 28 29 30 31 32 33 34 35 37 39 40 41 42 44 45 46 49 51 60 63 65 66 67 68 71 73 74 **P**7 8	23	10	156	9232	109	89814	1182	60508	27448	970
★ UNIVERSITY OF VIRGINIA MEDICAL CENTER, Jefferson Park Avenue, Zip 22908, Mailing Address: Box 148, Medical Center, Zip 22908–0002; tel. 804/924–0211; Michael J. Halseth, Executive Director **A**1 2 3 5 8 9 10 **F**1 2 3 4 5 6 7 8 9 10 11 12 13 14 15 16 17 19 20 21 22 23 24 25 28 29 30 31 32 33 34 35 36 37 38 39 40 41 42 43 44 45 46 47 48 49 50 51 52 53 54 55 56 57 58 59 60 61 62 63 64 65 66 67 68 69 70 71 73 74 **P**3	12	10	658	27252	485	411667	1768	366061	140948	4531

Hospitals, U.S. / VIRGINIA

Hospital, Address, Telephone, Administrator, Approval, Facility, and Physician Codes, Health Care System	Classification Codes		Utilization Data					Expense (thousands) of dollars		
★ American Hospital Association (AHA) membership ☐ Joint Commission on Accreditation of Healthcare Organizations (JCAHO) accreditation + American Osteopathic Hospital Association (AOHA) membership ○ American Osteopathic Association (AOA) accreditation △ Commission on Accreditation of Rehabilitation Facilities (CARF) accreditation Control codes 61, 63, 64, 71, 72 and 73 indicate hospitals listed by AOHA, but not registered by AHA. For definition of numerical codes, see page A6	Control	Service	Beds	Admissions	Census	Outpatient Visits	Births	Total	Payroll	Personnel
CHESAPEAKE—Independent City										
★ CHESAPEAKE GENERAL HOSPITAL, 736 Battlefield Boulevard North, Zip 23320–4941, Mailing Address: P.O. Box 2028, Zip 23327–2028; tel. 804/547–8121; Donald S. Buckley FACHE, President **A**1 2 9 10 **F**4 6 7 8 10 12 14 15 16 17 18 19 21 22 23 24 26 27 28 29 30 31 32 35 36 37 39 40 41 42 44 45 46 49 52 54 55 56 57 59 61 63 65 67 71 73 74	16	10	260	12589	190	117543	2698	84587	37809	1335
CLINTWOOD—Dickenson County										
DICKENSON COUNTY MEDICAL CENTER, Hospital Drive, Zip 24228, Mailing Address: Box 1390, Zip 24228–1390; tel. 703/926–0300; John F. Davis FACHE, Interim Administrator **A**9 10 **F**14 19 22 26 28 30 32 34 35 37 44 51 63 67 71 73 74 **P**6 **S**0075 Cumberland Health Systems, Inc.	23	10	50	1223	14	15432	0	8317	3012	136
CULPEPER—Culpeper County										
★ CULPEPER MEMORIAL HOSPITAL, 501 Sunset Lane, Zip 22701–3917, Mailing Address: Box 592, Zip 22701–0592; tel. 703/829–4100; William A. Gravely Jr., President **A**1 9 10 **F**2 7 8 12 14 15 17 19 20 22 23 28 29 30 32 33 34 35 37 40 41 44 46 48 49 52 54 55 56 57 58 59 60 63 65 67 71 **P**7 8	23	10	78	3005	34	29783	300	17999	8738	358
DANVILLE—Independent City										
★ DANVILLE REGIONAL MEDICAL CENTER, 142 South Main Street, Zip 24541–2987; tel. 804/799–2100; Larry T. DePriest, President (Total facility includes 36 beds in nursing home–type unit) **A**1 2 3 5 6 9 10 **F**2 3 7 8 10 11 12 14 19 21 22 28 29 30 31 32 34 35 37 39 40 42 44 45 46 48 49 51 52 55 56 58 59 60 61 62 63 64 65 67 71 72 73 74 **P**6	23	10	336	11968	217	82836	1251	78454	37708	1239
☐ SOUTHERN VIRGINIA MENTAL HEALTH INSTITUTE, 382 Taylor Drive, Zip 24541–4023; tel. 804/799–6220; Constance N. Fletcher Ph.D., Director (Nonreporting) **A**1 9 10 **S**0012 Virginia Department of Mental Health	12	22	96	—	—	—	—	—	—	—
EMPORIA—Emporia City										
★ GREENSVILLE MEMORIAL HOSPITAL, 214 Weaver Avenue, Zip 23847–1288; tel. 804/348–2000; Charles Mitchener Jr., Chief Executive Officer (Total facility includes 65 beds in nursing home–type unit) **A**1 9 10 **F**7 8 14 19 21 22 30 32 33 34 35 36 37 40 44 45 46 49 63 64 65 71 73 **S**0002 Quorum Health Group/Quorum Health Resources	23	10	182	3349	113	29179	179	17351	8304	328
FAIRFAX—Independent City										
★ FAIR OAKS HOSPITAL, 3600 Joseph Siewick Drive, Zip 22033; tel. 703/391–3600; Steven E. Brown, Administrator **A**1 2 5 9 10 **F**1 2 3 4 7 8 9 10 12 13 15 16 17 19 20 22 28 29 30 31 32 33 34 35 38 40 42 43 44 46 47 48 49 52 53 56 57 58 60 61 63 64 65 67 69 70 71 72 73 74 **P**7 8 **S**1305 Inova Health System	23	10	136	9242	95	48354	2050	58084	27048	731
FALLS CHURCH—Independent City										
★ DOMINION HOSPITAL, 2960 Sleepy Hollow Road, Zip 22044–2001; tel. 703/536–2000; Barbara D. S. Hekimian, Chief Executive Officer **A**1 9 10 **F**14 19 35 52 53 54 55 56 57 58 59 65 67 **S**0048 Columbia/HCA Healthcare Corporation	33	22	100	2143	64	3833	0	12908	5674	147
★ FAIRFAX HOSPITAL, 3300 Gallows Road, Zip 22046–3300; tel. 703/698–3372; Jolene Tornabeni, Administrator **A**1 2 3 5 8 9 10 **F**1 2 3 4 6 7 8 10 11 12 13 16 17 19 21 22 25 28 29 30 31 32 33 34 35 36 37 39 40 41 42 43 44 45 46 47 48 49 51 52 53 54 55 56 57 58 59 60 61 63 64 65 66 67 68 69 70 71 72 73 74 **P**1 2 3 4 6 7 8 **S**1305 Inova Health System	23	10	656	43882	554	149972	9643	328984	148328	3332
★ NORTHERN VIRGINIA MENTAL HEALTH INSTITUTE, 3302 Gallows Road, Zip 22042–3398; tel. 703/207–7111; David A. Rosenquist M.H.A., Acting Facility Director (Nonreporting) **A**1 9 10 **S**0012 Virginia Department of Mental Health	12	22	114	—	—	—	—	—	—	—
FARMVILLE—Prince Edward County										
★ SOUTHSIDE COMMUNITY HOSPITAL, 800 Oak Street, Zip 23901–1199; tel. 804/392–8811; Robert E. Huch, President (Total facility includes 20 beds in nursing home–type unit) **A**1 9 10 **F**7 8 14 15 19 22 32 37 40 42 44 45 65 71 73 **S**0070 Carilion Health System	23	10	136	3760	46	41238	393	21584	9398	389
FISHERSVILLE—Augusta County										
☐ AUGUSTA MEDICAL CENTER, (Includes King's Daughters' Hospital, 1410 North Augusta Street, Staunton, Virginia, Zip 24401; tel. 703/332–4000; Waynesboro Community Hospital, 501 Oak Avenue, Waynesboro, Virginia, Zip 22980; tel. 703/942–2273) Mailing Address: P.O. Box 1000, Zip 22939; tel. 703/942–6325; Richard H. Graham, President **A**1 9 10 **F**2 3 7 8 10 12 14 16 17 19 21 22 23 24 26 27 28 29 30 31 32 33 34 35 36 37 39 40 41 42 44 45 46 48 49 51 52 54 55 56 57 58 59 61 63 64 65 66 71 73 74 **P**8	23	10	255	10324	142	189167	895	63959	30082	1117
☐ WOODROW WILSON REHABILITATION CENTER–HOSPITAL, Zip 22939–0100; tel. 703/332–7214; David J. Schwemer, Administrator **A**1 9 10 **F**3 12 19 22 27 34 35 45 48 49 50 65 67 71 73	12	46	30	182	16	1225	0	—	—	162
FORT BELVOIR—Fairfax County										
★ DEWITT ARMY COMMUNITY HOSPITAL, Zip 22060–5901; tel. 703/805–0510; Colonel Warren A. Todd Jr. MSC, Commander **A**1 3 5 **F**3 8 13 15 17 19 22 25 27 30 34 37 39 40 41 44 45 46 51 53 54 58 65 66 71 73 74 **S**9395 Department of the Army	42	10	68	6152	40	390715	1044	—	—	866
FORT LEE—Dinwiddie County										
★ KENNER ARMY COMMUNITY HOSPITAL, Zip 23801–5260; tel. 804/734–9256; Colonel Charles M. Ellis Jr. MSC, Commanding Officer **A**1 5 **F**3 8 12 14 15 16 17 18 20 22 25 28 29 30 31 34 37 39 41 44 45 46 49 51 53 54 55 56 58 61 65 67 71 74 **P**6 **S**9395 Department of the Army	42	10	48	2540	15	220962	0	18268	6542	508

Hospitals, U.S. / VIRGINIA

Hospital, Address, Telephone, Administrator, Approval, Facility, and Physician Codes, Health Care System	Classification Codes		Utilization Data					Expense (thousands) of dollars		
★ American Hospital Association (AHA) membership □ Joint Commission on Accreditation of Healthcare Organizations (JCAHO) accreditation + American Osteopathic Hospital Association (AOHA) membership ○ American Osteopathic Association (AOA) accreditation △ Commission on Accreditation of Rehabilitation Facilities (CARF) accreditation Control codes 61, 63, 64, 71, 72 and 73 indicate hospitals listed by AOHA, but not registered by AHA. For definition of numerical codes, see page A6	Control	Service	Beds	Admissions	Census	Outpatient Visits	Births	Total	Payroll	Personnel
★ MEDICAL COLLEGE OF VIRGINIA HOSPITALS, VIRGINIA COMMONWEALTH UNIVERSITY, 401 North 12th Street, Zip 23219–0510, Mailing Address: P.O. Box 980510, Zip 23298–0510; tel. 804/828–9000; Carl R. Fischer, Associate Vice President and Chief Executive Officer A1 2 3 5 8 9 10 F3 4 7 8 9 10 11 12 14 16 19 20 21 22 23 25 26 27 29 30 31 32 34 35 37 38 40 41 42 43 44 45 46 47 48 49 51 52 53 54 56 57 58 59 60 61 65 66 67 69 70 71 72 73 74	12	10	804	30278	562	293808	3243	361892	177448	5002
□ METROPOLITAN HOSPITAL, 701 West Grace Street, Zip 23220; tel. 804/775–4100 A1 9 10 F14 15 16 19 21 22 31 34 41 44 52 54 56 57 63 65 66 71 S0985 Amerihealth, Inc.	32	10	180	3606	95	25868	0	20109	8672	382
PSYCHIATRIC INSTITUTE OF RICHMOND, 12800 West Creek Parkway, Zip 23238; tel. 804/784–2200; Mark S. Roth, Chief Executive Officer (Nonreporting) A9 10 S0695 Charter Medical Corporation	33	22	84	—	—	—	—	—	—	—
★ RETREAT HOSPITAL, 2621 Grove Avenue, Zip 23220–4308; tel. 804/254–5100; W. Trent Crable, President and Chief Executive Officer A1 9 10 F4 8 10 11 12 17 19 22 25 26 27 28 30 32 33 34 35 37 39 41 42 43 44 45 46 49 51 63 65 71 73 74 P2 6 8 S0048 Columbia/HCA Healthcare Corporation	23	10	227	4223	75	49100	0	—	—	476
★ RICHMOND COMMUNITY HOSPITAL, 1500 North 28th Street, Zip 23223–5396, Mailing Address: Box 27184, Zip 23261–7184; tel. 804/225–1700; Samuel F. Lillard, Executive Director A1 9 10 F2 3 8 10 15 16 17 19 30 34 35 37 44 45 46 49 52 54 63 65 71 73	23	10	88	2177	42	—	0	11316	4623	201
★ RICHMOND EYE AND EAR HOSPITAL, 1001 East Marshall Street, Zip 23219; tel. 804/775–4500; Karen A. Fiducia, Chief Executive Officer A1 9 10 F14 15 16 28 30 44 46 65 69 P1 S0002 Quorum Health Group/Quorum Health Resources	23	45	33	870	4	6369	0	8008	2867	101
★ RICHMOND MEMORIAL HOSPITAL, 1300 Westwood Avenue, Zip 23227–4699, Mailing Address: Box 26783, Zip 23261–6783; tel. 804/254–6000; (Total facility includes 20 beds in nursing home–type unit) A1 2 5 6 9 10 F4 7 8 10 11 12 14 15 17 19 21 22 25 26 28 29 30 31 32 33 34 35 37 38 39 40 41 42 43 44 45 46 49 52 56 57 61 62 63 64 65 71 73 P6	23	10	261	9539	181	50773	1158	90686	34321	1150
□ △ SHELTERING ARMS REHABILITATION HOSPITAL, 1311 Palmyra Avenue, Zip 23227–4418; tel. 804/342–4100; Richard C. Craven, President A1 5 7 9 10 F4 7 8 10 11 12 15 17 19 21 22 25 26 28 29 30 31 32 33 34 35 37 38 40 41 42 43 44 46 47 48 49 52 57 58 59 60 62 65 66 67 71 72 73 74 P6	23	46	40	607	36	42386	0	17156	9936	280
★ ST. MARY'S HOSPITAL, 5801 Bremo Road, Zip 23226–1900; tel. 804/285–2011; Christopher M. Carney, Chief Executive Officer A1 2 3 5 9 10 F3 4 7 8 10 11 12 15 16 17 19 21 22 23 26 30 31 32 33 34 35 37 38 40 41 42 43 44 45 46 47 49 51 52 53 54 56 57 58 59 60 65 68 71 73 74 P6 8 S5085 Bon Secours Health System, Inc.	21	10	391	17975	246	111795	3014	122833	50391	1876
ROANOKE—Independent City										
★ COMMUNITY HOSPITAL OF ROANOKE VALLEY, 101 Elm Avenue S.E., Zip 24013, Mailing Address: P.O. Box 12946, Zip 24029; tel. 703/985–8000; Dorman Fawley, President and Chief Executive Officer A1 2 3 5 9 10 F2 3 4 7 8 10 11 12 14 15 16 17 18 19 20 21 22 23 24 25 28 29 30 31 32 33 34 35 37 38 39 40 41 42 43 44 45 46 47 48 49 50 51 52 53 54 55 56 57 58 59 60 61 63 65 66 67 68 69 70 71 72 73 74 P4 5 6 7 8 S0070 Carilion Health System	23	10	232	13292	196	113624	3001	95865	47305	1536
★ GILL MEMORIAL EYE, EAR, NOSE AND THROAT HOSPITAL, 711 South Jefferson Street, Zip 24016–5103, Mailing Address: P.O. Box 1560, Zip 24007–1560; tel. 703/343–3368; Donald J. Love, Administrator (Data for 254 days) A9 10 F14 15 34 44 45 P4 5 6 7 8 S0070 Carilion Health System	23	45	12	62	1	2351	0	2686	1015	25
★ △ ROANOKE MEMORIAL HOSPITALS, (Includes Roanoke Memorial Rehabilitation Center, South Jefferson and McClanahan Streets, Roanoke, Virginia, Zip 24014, Mailing Address: P.O. Box 13367, Zip 24033) Belleview at Jefferson Street, Zip 24014, Mailing Address: P.O. Box 13367, Zip 24033–3367; tel. 703/981–7000; Houston L. Bell Jr., President and Chief Executive Officer A1 2 3 5 7 8 9 10 F3 4 7 8 10 11 12 13 14 15 16 17 18 19 20 21 22 24 25 26 27 28 29 30 31 32 33 34 35 36 37 38 39 40 41 42 43 44 45 46 47 48 49 52 53 54 55 56 57 58 60 61 62 63 64 65 66 67 68 69 70 71 72 73 74 P4 8 S0070 Carilion Health System	23	10	454	18059	351	229157	0	180378	72968	2525
ROCKY MOUNT—Franklin County										
★ FRANKLIN MEMORIAL HOSPITAL, 124 Floyd Avenue S.W., Zip 24151–1389; tel. 703/483–5277; Rayburn A. Thompson Jr., Administrator A1 9 10 F7 8 11 15 16 17 19 22 30 32 33 34 40 41 42 44 49 65 67 71 P2 7 8 S0070 Carilion Health System	23	10	37	2273	21	72077	262	13050	5740	246
SALEM—Roanoke County										
★ △ LEWIS–GALE HOSPITAL, 1900 Electric Road, Zip 24153; tel. 703/776–4000; Karl N. Miller, Chief Executive Officer A1 2 7 9 10 F1 2 3 4 5 6 7 8 9 10 11 12 13 14 15 17 18 19 20 21 22 24 25 27 28 29 30 31 32 33 34 35 37 38 39 40 41 42 43 44 45 46 47 48 49 51 52 53 54 55 56 57 58 59 60 64 65 66 67 68 69 71 72 73 74 P1 2 S0048 Columbia/HCA Healthcare Corporation	33	10	376	10961	190	128746	897	—	—	1061
★ LEWIS–GALE PSYCHIATRIC CENTER, 1902 Braeburn Drive, Zip 24153–7391; tel. 703/772–2800; James Sholes, Chief Executive Officer A1 10 F3 14 15 16 25 26 34 52 53 56 57 58 59 65 P1 5 S0048 Columbia/HCA Healthcare Corporation	33	22	144	2284	57	4806	0	8489	4584	153
MOUNT REGIS CENTER, 405 Kimball Avenue, Zip 24153; tel. 703/389–4761; Mark Cowell, Administrator (Nonreporting)	33	82	25	—	—	—	—	—	—	—
★ VETERANS AFFAIRS MEDICAL CENTER, 1970 Roanoke Boulevard, Zip 24153; tel. 703/982–2463; John M. Presley Ph.D., Director (Total facility includes 90 beds in nursing home–type unit) A1 2 3 5 8 F1 2 3 8 10 12 14 15 16 17 19 20 21 22 23 25 26 27 28 29 30 31 32 33 34 35 37 39 41 42 43 44 45 46 48 49 50 51 52 54 55 56 57 58 59 60 63 64 65 67 69 71 73 74 S9295 Department of Veterans Affairs	45	10	500	6932	379	174608	0	98978	55536	1636

© 1995 AHA Guide

Hospitals, U.S. / VIRGINIA

Hospital, Address, Telephone, Administrator, Approval, Facility, and Physician Codes, Health Care System	Classification Codes		Utilization Data					Expense (thousands) of dollars		Personnel
★ American Hospital Association (AHA) membership ☐ Joint Commission on Accreditation of Healthcare Organizations (JCAHO) accreditation + American Osteopathic Hospital Association (AOHA) membership ○ American Osteopathic Association (AOA) accreditation △ Commission on Accreditation of Rehabilitation Facilities (CARF) accreditation Control codes 61, 63, 64, 71, 72 and 73 indicate hospitals listed by AOHA, but not registered by AHA. For definition of numerical codes, see page A6	Control	Service	Beds	Admissions	Census	Outpatient Visits	Births	Total	Payroll	
SOUTH BOSTON—Halifax County ★ HALIFAX REGIONAL HOSPITAL, 2204 Wilborn Avenue, Zip 24592; tel. 804/575-3100; Chris A. Lumsden, Administrator (Total facility includes 19 beds in nursing home–type unit) **A**1 9 10 **F**7 8 10 11 12 14 15 16 17 19 20 21 22 28 29 30 31 32 34 35 37 40 41 44 45 46 48 49 56 63 64 65 71 73 **P**7 8 **S**0002 Quorum Health Group/Quorum Health Resources	23	10	192	5518	101	39853	664	31211	12892	548
SOUTH HILL—Mecklenburg County ★ COMMUNITY MEMORIAL HEALTHCENTER, 125 Buena Vista Circle, Zip 23970-0090, Mailing Address: P.O. Box 90, Zip 23970-0090; tel. 804/447-3151; Steve Kelly, President (Total facility includes 155 beds in nursing home–type unit) **A**1 9 10 **F**2 7 8 11 12 13 14 15 16 17 19 21 22 26 27 28 30 31 32 33 34 35 36 37 39 40 41 42 44 45 46 49 52 54 56 57 59 63 64 65 67 71 73	23	10	270	4008	205	42466	193	28270	12536	642
STAUNTON—Staunton City ★ DE JARNETTE CENTER, 1290 Richmond Road, Zip 24401-1091, Mailing Address: Box 2309, Zip 24402-2309; tel. 703/332-8800; Andrea C. Newsome FACHE, Director **A**3 **F**2 14 16 20 22 37 45 46 47 52 53 54 55 56 59 65 73 **P**6 **S**0012 Virginia Department of Mental Health	12	52	60	402	44	0	0	5062	3569	125
KING'S DAUGHTER HOSPITAL See Augusta Medical Center, Fishersville										
★ WESTERN STATE HOSPITAL, 1301 Richmond Avenue, Zip 24401, Mailing Address: Box 2500, Zip 24402-2500; tel. 703/332-8000; L. F. Harding, Director **A**1 9 10 **F**2 4 5 8 9 10 11 12 19 20 21 22 23 26 27 30 31 35 37 39 40 41 42 43 44 48 49 50 52 57 60 63 65 67 69 71 73 **S**0012 Virginia Department of Mental Health	12	22	460	1127	474	0	0	37723	24569	990
STUART—Patrick County ★ R. J. REYNOLDS–PATRICK COUNTY MEMORIAL HOSPITAL, Mailing Address: Route 2, Box 71, Zip 24171-9512; tel. 703/694-3151; Alan W. Adkins, Administrator (Total facility includes 25 beds in nursing home–type unit) **A**1 9 10 **F**7 8 14 15 16 17 19 21 22 28 30 32 33 34 36 37 40 44 63 64 65 71 73	23	10	59	1361	40	37042	138	8383	4723	191
SUFFOLK—Accomack County ★ LOUISE OBICI MEMORIAL HOSPITAL, 1900 North Main Street, Zip 23434, Mailing Address: P.O. Box 1100, Zip 23439; tel. 804/934-4000; William C. Giermak, President and Chief Executive Officer **A**1 2 5 6 9 10 **F**7 8 10 12 14 15 17 19 22 23 30 32 34 35 36 37 40 41 42 44 45 46 48 49 52 60 65 67 71 73 74 **P**3	23	10	176	7273	115	76555	794	50489	23416	723
TAPPAHANNOCK—Essex County ☐ RIVERSIDE TAPPAHANNOCK HOSPITAL, Mailing Address: Route 2, Box 612, Zip 22560; tel. 804/443-3311; Glenn D. Waters, Administrator (Nonreporting) **A**1 9 10 **S**4810 Riverside Health System	23	10	100	—	—	—	—	—	—	—
TAZEWELL—Tazewell County ★ TAZEWELL COMMUNITY HOSPITAL, 141 Ben Bolt Avenue, Zip 24651; tel. 703/988-2506; John H. Greer, Administrator **A**1 9 10 **F**8 14 15 16 19 22 30 32 34 35 37 44 46 71 73 **P**8 **S**0070 Carilion Health System	23	10	56	1070	15	16347	0	7393	3098	128
VIRGINIA BEACH—Independent City ★ SENTARA BAYSIDE HOSPITAL, 800 Independence Boulevard, Zip 23455-6076; tel. 804/363-6100; Edward L. Berdick, President **A**1 9 10 **F**4 6 7 8 9 10 11 12 13 14 15 16 17 18 19 20 22 23 25 26 27 28 29 30 31 32 33 34 35 37 38 39 40 41 42 43 44 45 46 47 48 49 51 52 56 60 61 63 64 65 66 67 69 70 71 72 73 74 **P**4 5 6 **S**2565 Sentara Health System	23	10	170	6376	83	61505	1579	42320	16237	616
☐ TIDEWATER PSYCHIATRIC INSTITUTE, 1701 Will-O-Wisp Drive, Zip 23454; tel. 804/481-1211; Richard Warden, Chief Executive Officer (Nonreporting) **A**1 5 9 10 **S**0695 Charter Medical Corporation	33	22	65	—	—	—	—	—	—	—
★ VIRGINIA BEACH GENERAL HOSPITAL, 1060 First Colonial Road, Zip 23454-9000; tel. 804/481-8000; Robert L. Graves, Administrator **A**1 2 3 5 9 10 **F**4 7 8 10 11 14 16 17 19 21 22 23 24 25 28 29 30 31 32 34 35 37 38 39 40 41 42 43 44 45 49 60 61 63 65 66 67 69 70 71 72 73 **P**6 **S**2205 Tidewater Health Care, Inc.	23	10	274	12754	163	122756	2777	81027	32845	1009
WARRENTON—Fauquier County ★ FAUQUIER HOSPITAL, 500 Hospital Drive, Zip 22186-3099; tel. 703/347-2550; Rodger H. Baker, President and Chief Executive Officer **A**1 9 10 **F**7 8 12 14 15 16 19 21 22 26 28 29 30 32 33 34 35 37 39 40 41 42 44 45 46 49 63 65 67 71 73 **P**2	23	10	106	4099	51	47558	448	27179	13450	501
WAYNESBORO—Augusta County WAYNESBORO COMMUNITY HOSPITAL See Augusta Medical Center, Fishersville										
WILLIAMSBURG—Williamsburg City ★ EASTERN STATE HOSPITAL, Mailing Address: P.O. Box 8791, Zip 23187-8791; tel. 804/253-5161; John M. Favret, Director (Total facility includes 310 beds in nursing home–type unit) **A**1 5 9 10 **F**7 14 19 20 21 24 26 35 41 42 45 46 49 52 54 55 56 57 60 64 65 71 73 **S**0012 Virginia Department of Mental Health	12	22	727	2252	645	—	0	60855	36051	1447
★ WILLIAMSBURG COMMUNITY HOSPITAL, 301 Monticello Avenue, Zip 23187-8700, Mailing Address: Box 8700, Zip 23187-8700; tel. 804/259-6000; Les A. Donahue, President and Chief Executive Officer **A**1 5 9 10 **F**2 3 4 6 7 8 10 12 14 15 16 17 18 19 20 21 22 23 28 29 30 31 32 34 35 36 37 39 40 41 42 44 45 46 49 54 56 63 65 66 67 71 73	23	10	139	5825	61	64577	921	44982	17098	625
WINCHESTER—Frederick County ★ WINCHESTER MEDICAL CENTER, 1840 Amherst Street, Zip 22601-2540, Mailing Address: P.O. Box 3340, Zip 22604-3340; tel. 703/722-8000; George B. Caley, President **A**1 2 9 10 **F**4 7 8 10 11 12 14 15 16 19 21 22 27 32 33 34 35 36 37 38 39 40 41 42 43 44 46 48 49 52 53 58 59 60 63 65 71 72 73 **P**5	23	10	401	17937	263	168131	1672	117111	49985	1756

© 1995 AHA Guide

Hospitals, U.S. / VIRGINIA

Hospital, Address, Telephone, Administrator, Approval, Facility, and Physician Codes, Health Care System	Classification Codes		Utilization Data					Expense (thousands) of dollars		
★ American Hospital Association (AHA) membership ☐ Joint Commission on Accreditation of Healthcare Organizations (JCAHO) accreditation + American Osteopathic Hospital Association (AOHA) membership ○ American Osteopathic Association (AOA) accreditation △ Commission on Accreditation of Rehabilitation Facilities (CARF) accreditation Control codes 61, 63, 64, 71, 72 and 73 indicate hospitals listed by AOHA, but not registered by AHA. For definition of numerical codes, see page A6	Control	Service	Beds	Admissions	Census	Outpatient Visits	Births	Total	Payroll	Personnel
WISE—Wise County ☐ WISE ARH HOSPITAL, Mailing Address: P.O. Box 3267, Zip 24293–3267; tel. 703/328–2511; Dan Fitzpatrick, Administrator **A**1 9 10 **F**8 11 14 15 17 19 21 22 28 30 32 34 35 37 39 40 44 46 65 71 73 **P**6 **S**0145 Appalachian Regional Healthcare	23	10	67	2397	31	28000	91	10074	5170	166
WOODBRIDGE—Prince William County ★ POTOMAC HOSPITAL, 2300 Opitz Boulevard, Zip 22191–3399; tel. 703/670–1313; William Mason Moss, President **A**1 9 10 **F**7 8 10 12 14 15 16 17 19 21 22 25 28 29 30 31 32 33 34 35 37 40 42 44 46 49 51 52 53 56 57 60 62 63 65 66 67 71 72 73 **P**1	23	10	153	7328	77	81761	1783	53298	24607	632
WOODSTOCK—Shenandoah County ★ SHENANDOAH MEMORIAL HOSPITAL, 755 South Main Street, Zip 22664; tel. 703/459–4021; Edwin E. Hurysz, President and Chief Executive Officer (Total facility includes 34 beds in nursing home–type unit) **A**1 9 10 **F**3 4 7 8 10 12 14 19 21 22 23 27 30 32 35 37 39 40 41 44 45 46 49 50 52 53 54 55 56 57 58 59 60 63 65 69 70 71 73	23	10	129	2521	66	35355	242	17681	8702	349
WYTHEVILLE—Wythe County ★ WYTHE COUNTY COMMUNITY HOSPITAL, 600 West Ridge Road, Zip 24382; tel. 703/228–0200; Howard Newman Ainsley, Chief Executive Officer (Total facility includes 8 beds in nursing home–type unit) **A**1 9 10 **F**2 3 4 7 8 10 11 12 14 15 16 17 19 20 21 22 23 26 27 28 29 30 31 32 33 34 35 37 38 39 40 41 42 43 44 45 46 47 48 49 52 53 54 55 57 58 59 60 61 63 64 65 66 67 69 70 71 73 **P**8 **S**0070 Carilion Health System	23	10	90	3039	44	35930	315	18719	8645	348

WASHINGTON

Resident population 5,255 (in thousands)
Resident population in metro areas 83.0%
Birth rate per 1,000 population 15.9
65 years and over 11.6%
Percent of persons without health insurance 10.7%

★ American Hospital Association (AHA) membership
☐ Joint Commission on Accreditation of Healthcare Organizations (JCAHO) accreditation
+ American Osteopathic Hospital Association (AOHA) membership
○ American Osteopathic Association (AOA) accreditation
△ Commission on Accreditation of Rehabilitation Facilities (CARF) accreditation
Control codes 61, 63, 64, 71, 72 and 73 indicate hospitals listed by AOHA, but not registered by AHA. For definition of numerical codes, see page A6

Hospital, Address, Telephone, Administrator, Approval, Facility, and Physician Codes, Health Care System	Classification Codes		Utilization Data					Expense (thousands) of dollars		
	Control	Service	Beds	Admissions	Census	Outpatient Visits	Births	Total	Payroll	Personnel
ABERDEEN—Grays Harbor County ★ GRAYS HARBOR COMMUNITY HOSPITAL, 915 Anderson Drive, Zip 98520; tel. 360/532-8330; Michael J. Madden, Administrator (Total facility includes 60 beds in nursing home–type unit) **A**1 9 10 **F**2 3 7 12 16 19 21 22 23 25 32 35 37 40 42 44 45 49 54 56 64 65 71 73 **P**8	23	10	172	3905	120	88369	534	32324	15345	418
ANACORTES—Skagit County ★ ISLAND HOSPITAL, 1211 24th Street, Zip 98221-2590; tel. 360/293-3181; C. Philip Sandifer, Administrator (Nonreporting) **A**1 2 9 10	16	10	43	—	—	—	—	—	—	—
ARLINGTON—Snohomish County ★ SNOHOMISH COUNTY PUBLIC HOSPITAL DISTRICT THREE, CASCADE VALLEY HOSPITAL, 330 South Stillaguamish Street, Zip 98223-1642; tel. 360/435-2133; Robert Campbell Jr., Administrator **A**9 10 **F**7 8 11 15 16 19 21 22 35 37 40 44 64 65 70 71 73 **P**8	16	10	36	1670	16	25197	308	15899	7324	230
AUBURN—King County ☐ AUBURN GENERAL HOSPITAL, 20 Second Street N.E., Zip 98002-0000; tel. 206/833-7711; Michael M. Gherardini, Managing Director (Nonreporting) **A**1 2 9 10 **S**9555 Universal Health Services, Inc.	33	10	100	—	—	—	—	—	—	—
BELLEVUE—King County ★ OVERLAKE HOSPITAL MEDICAL CENTER, 1035 116th Avenue N.E., Zip 98004; tel. 206/688-5000; Kenneth D. Graham, President and Chief Executive Officer **A**1 2 9 10 **F**1 4 7 8 10 11 12 14 15 16 17 19 21 22 27 28 29 30 31 32 34 35 37 38 39 40 41 42 43 44 45 46 48 49 52 53 54 56 57 59 60 61 63 65 66 67 70 71 72 73 74	23	10	225	12586	130	66252	2633	100476	45720	961
BELLINGHAM—Whatcom County ★ ST. JOSEPH HOSPITAL, 2901 Squalicum Parkway, Zip 98225-1898; tel. 206/734-5400; John Hayward, Administrator **A**1 2 9 10 **F**1 2 3 4 7 10 14 15 16 17 19 21 22 23 26 27 35 37 40 41 42 43 44 45 46 48 49 52 53 56 59 60 63 65 70 71 73 **P**8 **S**5415 PeaceHealth	23	10	195	10512	108	145410	1806	76621	33928	924
BREMERTON—Kitsap County ★ HARRISON MEMORIAL HOSPITAL, 2520 Cherry Street, Zip 98310-4270; tel. 360/377-3911; David W. Gitch, President and Chief Executive Officer **A**1 2 9 10 **F**4 7 10 12 14 15 16 17 19 21 22 23 25 26 27 28 30 31 32 33 34 35 37 39 40 42 44 45 46 49 52 53 54 55 56 57 58 60 61 65 67 70 71 73 74 **P**5 8	23	10	252	12976	157	75718	1858	72408	36049	903
★ NAVAL HOSPITAL, Boone Road, Zip 98312-1898; tel. 206/479-9344; Captain Richard A. Mayo MSC, Commanding Officer (Nonreporting) **A**1 3 5 **S**9655 Department of Navy	43	10	106	—	—	—	—	—	—	—
BREWSTER—Okanogan County ★ OKANOGAN-DOUGLAS COUNTY HOSPITAL, 703 Northwest Second, Zip 98812, Mailing Address: P.O. Box 577, Zip 98812; tel. 509/689-2517; Howard M. Gamble, Administrator **A**9 10 **F**7 8 11 16 19 21 22 25 26 28 29 30 34 37 40 44 47 65 66 70 71 73	16	10	43	1113	10	23258	154	6043	3044	117
BURIEN—Thurston County ★ △ HIGHLINE COMMUNITY HOSPTIAL, (Formerly Listed Under Seattle) (Includes Highline Specialty Center, 12844 Military Road Fork, Tukwila, Zip 98168; Mark Benedum, Administrator) 16251 Sylvester Road S.W., Zip 98166; tel. 206/244-9970; Paul Tucker, Administrator (Nonreporting) **A**1 2 7 9 10	23	10	249	—	—	—	—	—	—	—
CENTRALIA—Lewis County ★ PROVIDENCE CENTRALIA HOSPITAL, (Formerly Providence Hospital) 1820 Cooks Hill Road, Zip 98531; tel. 360/736-2803; Sister Maureen Comer, Administrator (Nonreporting) **A**1 9 10 **S**5275 Sisters of Providence Health System	21	10	149	—	—	—	—	—	—	—
CHELAN—Chelan County LAKE CHELAN COMMUNITY HOSPITAL, 503 East Highland Avenue, Zip 98816, Mailing Address: Box 908, Zip 98816; tel. 509/682-2531; Moe Chaudry, Administrator **A**9 10 **F**2 7 8 12 15 17 18 19 22 24 28 32 33 34 36 37 39 40 41 44 46 49 52 56 58 71 72 73 **P**5 7	16	10	34	697	12	16799	92	4859	2830	104
CHEWELAH—Stevens County ★ ST. JOSEPH'S HOSPITAL, 500 East Webster Street, Zip 99109, Mailing Address: P.O. Box 197, Zip 99109; tel. 509/935-8211; Gary V. Peck, Chief Executive Officer (Total facility includes 40 beds in nursing home–type unit) **A**9 10 **F**7 15 16 21 22 24 28 29 30 34 40 41 44 46 49 51 56 64 65 66 67 71 73 **P**5 8 **S**5265 Providence Services	21	10	65	857	46	11256	73	5748	2621	104
CLARKSTON—Asotin County ☐ TRI-STATE MEMORIAL HOSPITAL, 1221 Highland Avenue, Zip 99403-0189, Mailing Address: P.O. Box 189, Zip 99403-0189; tel. 509/758-5511; Joseph K. Lillard, Administrator **A**1 9 10 **F**6 8 11 14 15 17 19 21 22 28 30 32 33 34 35 37 44 46 60 62 65 67 69 71 73 **P**8	23	10	38	1135	14	24665	0	10717	4208	156

© 1995 AHA Guide

Hospitals, U.S. / WASHINGTON

Hospital, Address, Telephone, Administrator, Approval, Facility, and Physician Codes, Health Care System	Classification Codes		Utilization Data					Expense (thousands) of dollars		
★ American Hospital Association (AHA) membership □ Joint Commission on Accreditation of Healthcare Organizations (JCAHO) accreditation + American Osteopathic Hospital Association (AOHA) membership ○ American Osteopathic Association (AOA) accreditation △ Commission on Accreditation of Rehabilitation Facilities (CARF) accreditation Control codes 61, 63, 64, 71, 72 and 73 indicate hospitals listed by AOHA, but not registered by AHA. For definition of numerical codes, see page A6	Control	Service	Beds	Admissions	Census	Outpatient Visits	Births	Total	Payroll	Personnel
COLFAX—Whitman County										
★ WHITMAN HOSPITAL AND MEDICAL CENTER, 1200 Almota Road, Zip 99111–5252; tel. 509/397–3435; Gordon C. McLean, Administrator (Nonreporting) **A**9 10	13	10	32	—	—	—	—	—	—	—
COLVILLE—Stevens County										
✣ MOUNT CARMEL HOSPITAL, 982 East Columbia Street, Zip 99114–0351, Mailing Address: Box 351, Zip 99114–0351; tel. 509/684–2561; Gloria Cooper, Chief Executive Officer **A**1 9 10 **F**7 8 12 14 15 16 19 22 34 37 40 41 44 45 46 49 56 71 **P**8 **S**5265 Providence Services	21	10	33	1384	11	16695	252	8591	3881	109
COUPEVILLE—Island County										
✣ WHIDBEY GENERAL HOSPITAL, 101 North Main Street, Zip 98239–0400, Mailing Address: Box 400, Zip 98239–0400; tel. 360/678–5151; Robert Zylstra, Administrator (Nonreporting) **A**1 2 9 10	16	10	51	—	—	—	—	—	—	—
DAVENPORT—Lincoln County										
★ LINCOLN HOSPITAL, 10 Nicholls Street, Zip 99122; tel. 509/725–7101; Thomas J. Martin, Chief Executive Officer (Total facility includes 71 beds in nursing home–type unit) **A**9 10 **F**1 7 8 11 12 14 15 16 17 19 20 22 27 28 29 30 34 37 39 40 42 44 45 49 51 64 65 67 70 71 73 **P**7 8	16	10	95	409	72	9758	32	—	—	134
DAYTON—Columbia County										
DAYTON GENERAL HOSPITAL, 1012 South Third Street, Zip 99328; tel. 509/382–2531; Oral R. Compson, Administrator (Nonreporting) **A**9 10	16	10	18	—	—	—	—	—	—	—
EDMONDS—Snohomish County										
✣ STEVENS HOSPITAL, (Formerly Stevens Memorial Hospital) 21601 76th Avenue West, Zip 98026–7506; tel. 206/640–4000; Steve C. McCary, President and Chief Executive Officer **A**1 2 9 10 **F**4 7 8 10 11 12 13 14 15 17 18 19 21 22 23 28 29 30 33 34 35 37 40 41 42 44 45 46 49 51 52 54 55 56 58 59 60 63 65 71 73 **P**6	16	10	184	8637	99	115856	1478	69770	31312	822
ELLENSBURG—Kittitas County										
KITTITAS VALLEY COMMUNITY HOSPITAL, 603 South Chestnut Street, Zip 98926; tel. 509/962–9841; Robert Schwartz, Administrator **A**9 10 **F**7 8 11 14 15 16 17 19 22 32 33 35 36 37 40 44 48 65 67 69 71 73 **P**3	16	10	36	1319	13	31962	237	11778	5680	160
ENUMCLAW—King County										
COMMUNITY MEMORIAL HOSPITAL, 2125 C Street, Zip 98022, Mailing Address: P.O. Box 218, Zip 98022–0218; tel. 360/825–2505; Dennis A. Popp, Administrator **A**10 **F**11 19 21 22 34 35 37 40 44 63 71 73 **P**1	23	10	28	1220	10	20403	307	10520	4592	131
EPHRATA—Grant County										
★ COLUMBIA BASIN HOSPITAL, 200 Southeast Boulevard, Zip 98823–1997; tel. 509/754–4631; Jerry Hawley, Administrator (Nonreporting) **A**9 10	16	10	58	—	—	—	—	—	—	—
EVERETT—Snohomish County										
✣ △ PROVIDENCE GENERAL MEDICAL CENTER, (Includes Providence General Medical Center – Colby Campus, 14th and Colby Avenue, Everett, Washington, Zip 98201, Mailing Address: P.O. Box 1147, Zip 98206; tel. 206/258–6300; Providence General Medical Center – Pacific Campus, Pacific and Nassau Streets, Everett, Washington, Zip 98201, Mailing Address: Box 1067, Zip 98206–1067; tel. 206/258–7123) Pacific and Nassau Streets, Zip 98201, Mailing Address: P.O. Box 1067, Zip 98206–1067; tel. 206/258–7267; John P. Rinset, President and Chief Executive Officer (Total facility includes 12 beds in nursing home–type unit) **A**1 2 7 9 10 **F**2 3 4 7 8 10 11 12 14 15 16 17 19 21 22 23 24 25 26 28 29 30 31 32 33 34 35 37 39 40 41 42 43 44 45 46 48 49 50 51 53 56 60 63 64 65 66 67 68 71 73 74 **P**6 8 **S**5275 Sisters of Providence Health System	23	10	327	16918	188	363620	3120	153988	65663	1741
FAIRCHILD AIR FORCE BASE—Erie County										
✣ U.S. AIR FORCE HOSPITAL, 701 Hospital Loop, Zip 99011–8701; tel. 509/247–5216; Colonel Gary L. Mueller M.D., MSC, Commander **A**1 **F**8 12 13 14 17 18 20 27 28 29 30 34 37 39 40 41 45 46 51 54 55 58 61 65 66 67 69 71 73 74 **S**9495 Department of the Air Force	41	10	35	2076	14	139283	218	—	—	417
FEDERAL WAY—King County										
✣ ST. FRANCIS HOSPITAL, (Formerly St. Francis Community Hospital) 34515 Ninth Avenue South, Zip 98003–9710; tel. 206/838–9700; Craig L. Hendrickson, Chief Operating Officer **A**1 2 9 10 **F**4 7 8 10 12 13 15 17 18 19 21 22 23 28 30 32 33 34 35 37 39 40 41 42 43 44 49 52 53 55 56 57 63 65 67 68 71 72 73 74 **P**3 5 8 **S**5325 Franciscan Health System	21	10	67	6188	45	52864	1802	42831	17492	447
FORKS—Clallam County										
FORKS COMMUNITY HOSPITAL, 530 Bogachiel Way, Zip 98331–9699; tel. 360/374–6271; Eric Jensen, Administrator (Total facility includes 36 beds in nursing home–type unit) **A**9 10 **F**3 7 8 13 17 18 22 28 29 30 31 34 40 44 53 54 55 56 57 58 64 65 71	16	10	53	481	24	20598	50	6969	3691	115
FORT STEILACOOM—Pierce County										
□ WESTERN STATE HOSPITAL, Zip 98494; tel. 206/756–2525; John Reynolds, Superintendent (Nonreporting) **A**1 9 10	12	22	1035	—	—	—	—	—	—	—
GOLDENDALE—Klickitat County										
★ KLICKITAT VALLEY HOSPITAL, 310 South Roosevelt, Zip 98620, Mailing Address: P.O. Box 5, Zip 98620; tel. 509/773–4022; Merlin L. Traylor, Administrator **A**9 10 **F**7 19 22 28 32 33 34 35 41 44 51 65 69 71	16	10	31	496	4	16063	68	3767	1902	67
GRAND COULEE—Grant County										
★ COULEE COMMUNITY HOSPITAL, 411 Fortuyn Road, Zip 99133–0840, Mailing Address: P.O. Box H, Zip 99133; tel. 509/633–1753; Michael C. Wiltermood, Chief Executive Officer (Total facility includes 29 beds in nursing home–type unit) **A**10 **F**14 15 16 19 21 22 34 40 44 51 64 71 **S**0585 Brim, Inc.	16	10	48	428	31	10467	1	4622	2500	98

Hospitals, U.S. / WASHINGTON

Hospital, Address, Telephone, Administrator, Approval, Facility, and Physician Codes, Health Care System	Classi-fication Codes		Utilization Data					Expense (thousands) of dollars		
	Control	Service	Beds	Admissions	Census	Outpatient Visits	Births	Total	Payroll	Personnel
ILWACO—Pacific County										
★ OCEAN BEACH HOSPITAL, Mailing Address: Drawer H, Zip 98624; tel. 360/642–3181; Ronald Bender, Administrator (Nonreporting) **A**9 10	16	10	19	—	—	—	—	—	—	—
KENNEWICK—Benton County										
★ KENNEWICK GENERAL HOSPITAL, 900 South Auburn Street, Zip 99336–0128, Mailing Address: Box 6128, Zip 99336; tel. 509/586–6111; Michael J. Tuohy, Administrator **A**1 2 9 10 **F**7 8 10 12 15 17 19 20 21 22 28 29 32 34 35 37 39 40 41 42 44 45 46 49 51 65 66 71 72 73 74 **P**3	16	10	70	3713	32	57289	1018	29346	13296	340
KIRKLAND—King County										
CAREUNIT HOSPITAL OF KIRKLAND, 10322 N.E. 132nd, Zip 98034–2898; tel. 206/821–1122; John Thompson, Administrator **A**9 10 **F**2 3 15 37 52 54 55 57 58 59	33	82	25	604	14	7470	0	2819	1324	46
□ CPC FAIRFAX HOSPITAL, 10200 Northeast 132nd Street, Zip 98034; tel. 206/821–2000; Robert C. Hails, Chief Executive Officer (Nonreporting) **A**1 9 10 **S**0785 Community Psychiatric Centers	33	22	133	—	—	—	—	—	—	—
★ EVERGREEN HOSPITAL MEDICAL CENTER, 12040 Northeast 128th Street, Zip 98034; tel. 206/899–1000; Andrew Fallat FACHE, Chief Executive Officer **A**1 2 5 9 10 **F**4 7 8 10 12 14 15 16 17 19 21 22 23 24 26 27 29 30 31 32 33 34 35 37 39 40 42 44 45 46 60 63 65 67 70 71 73 **P**7	16	10	149	9162	81	114474	2590	78647	35704	943
LONGVIEW—Cowlitz County										
★ ST. JOHN'S MEDICAL CENTER, (Includes Monticello Medical Center, 600 Broadway, Longview, Washington, Zip 98632, Mailing Address: P.O. Box 3002, Zip 98632; St. John's Hospital, 1614 East Kessler Boulevard, Longview, Washington, Zip 98632, Mailing Address: P.O. Box 3002, Zip 98632; tel. 206/423–1530; Margaret M. Chuman, Interim Chief Executive Officer) 1614 East Kessler Boulevard, Zip 98632, Mailing Address: P.O. Box 3002, Zip 98632–0302; tel. 206/423–1530; Mark E. McGourty, Regional Chief Executive Officer **A**1 2 9 10 **F**2 3 7 8 10 11 12 14 15 16 19 22 31 38 40 41 42 44 45 52 53 54 55 57 58 60 65 70 71 73 **P**4 **S**5415 PeaceHealth	23	10	200	10318	112	96157	1353	66427	31031	872
MCCLEARY—Grays Harbor County										
MARK REED HOSPITAL, 322 South Birch Street, Zip 98557, Mailing Address: P.O. Box 1300, Zip 98557–1300; tel. 360/495–3244; Jean E. Roberts, Administrator (Nonreporting) **A**9 10 **S**5275 Sisters of Providence Health System	16	10	8	—	—	—	—	—	—	—
MEDICAL LAKE—Spokane County										
□ EASTERN STATE HOSPITAL, Mailing Address: P.O. Box A, Zip 99022–0045; tel. 509/299–4351; Harold E. Wilson, Acting Superintendent **A**1 9 10 **F**14 15 16 20 27 45 46 52 54 55 56 57 65 73 **P**6	12	22	332	1009	311	0	0	35904	24022	652
MONROE—Snohomish County										
★ VALLEY GENERAL HOSPITAL, 14701 179th S.E., Zip 98272, Mailing Address: P.O. Box 646, Zip 98272–0646; tel. 360/794–7497; Lane A. Savitch, Administrator **A**1 9 10 **F**2 3 7 8 11 14 15 16 19 21 22 24 28 30 31 33 34 37 40 44 46 49 56 65 66 67 68 71 73	16	10	71	1832	26	17117	328	16099	7431	166
MORTON—Lewis County										
MORTON GENERAL HOSPITAL, 521 Adams Street, Zip 98356, Mailing Address: Drawer C, Zip 98356; tel. 360/496–5112; (Nonreporting) **A**9 10 **S**5275 Sisters of Providence Health System	16	10	46	—	—	—	—	—	—	—
MOSES LAKE—Grant County										
★ SAMARITAN HOSPITAL, 801 East Wheeler Road, Zip 98837–1899; tel. 509/765–5606; Keith J. Baldwin, Administrator **A**1 9 10 **F**7 16 17 19 21 22 28 29 30 34 35 37 39 40 44 45 46 49 51 65 66 70 71 73 **P**8	16	10	50	2540	19	28312	787	18706	8067	252
MOUNT VERNON—Skagit County										
★ AFFILIATED HEALTH SERVICES, (Includes Skagit Valley Hospital, 1415 Kincaid Street, Mount Vernon, Washington, Zip 98273, Mailing Address: P.O. Box 1376, Zip 98273–1376; tel. 360/424–4111; Gregg A. Davidson, Associate Administrator; United General Hospital, 1971 Highway 20, Sedro Woolley, Washington, Zip 98284, Mailing Address: P.O. Box 1376, Zip 98273; tel. 360/856–6021) 1415 Kincaid Street, Zip 98273, Mailing Address: P.O. Box 1376, Zip 98273–1376; tel. 360/424–4111; Patrick R. Mahoney, Administrator and Chief Executive Officer **A**1 2 9 10 **F**7 8 10 11 12 15 16 17 19 22 23 29 30 32 33 34 35 36 37 39 40 42 44 49 52 54 55 56 58 60 63 65 67 70 71 72 73 74 **P**5 8	16	10	140	7491	68	80790	1248	57763	25327	666
NEWPORT—Pend Oreille County										
★ NEWPORT COMMUNITY HOSPITAL, 714 West Pine, Zip 99156; tel. 509/447–2441; Dave McIvor, Administrator (Nonreporting) **A**9 10	16	10	65	—	—	—	—	—	—	—
OAK HARBOR—Island County										
★ NAVAL HOSPITAL, 3475 North Saratoga Street, Zip 98278–8800; tel. 360/257–9500 **A**1 **F**8 22 27 34 40 51 58 65 71 **P**1 **S**9655 Department of Navy	43	10	27	2188	11	121717	506	—	—	318
ODESSA—Lincoln County										
★ ODESSA MEMORIAL HOSPITAL, 502 East Amende, Zip 99159, Mailing Address: Box 368, Zip 99159–0368; tel. 509/982–2611; Carol Schott, Administrator (Total facility includes 23 beds in nursing home–type unit) **A**9 10 **F**15 16 17 22 30 32 49 51 64 65 66 67 73 **P**6 8	16	10	44	98	27	3104	0	1711	1236	55
OLYMPIA—Thurston County										
★ CAPITAL MEDICAL CENTER, 3900 Capital Mall Drive S.W., Zip 98502–8654, Mailing Address: P.O. Box 19002, Zip 98507–0013; tel. 360/754–5858; Kelly H. Adams, Chief Executive Officer **A**1 2 9 10 **F**4 7 8 10 12 19 21 22 23 27 32 33 34 35 37 40 41 42 44 49 60 71 73 74 **P**5 **S**0048 Columbia/HCA Healthcare Corporation	33	10	110	3551	35	37962	487	32636	12183	346

© 1995 AHA Guide

Hospitals, U.S. / WASHINGTON

Hospital, Address, Telephone, Administrator, Approval, Facility, and Physician Codes, Health Care System	Classification Codes		Utilization Data					Expense (thousands) of dollars		
★ American Hospital Association (AHA) membership □ Joint Commission on Accreditation of Healthcare Organizations (JCAHO) accreditation + American Osteopathic Hospital Association (AOHA) membership ○ American Osteopathic Association (AOA) accreditation △ Commission on Accreditation of Rehabilitation Facilities (CARF) accreditation Control codes 61, 63, 64, 71, 72 and 73 indicate hospitals listed by AOHA, but not registered by AHA. For definition of numerical codes, see page A6	Control	Service	Beds	Admissions	Census	Outpatient Visits	Births	Total	Payroll	Personnel
※ △ PROVIDENCE ST. PETER HOSPITAL, (Formerly St. Peter Hospital) 413 Lilly Road N.E., Zip 98506–5166; tel. 206/491–9480; C. Scott Bond, Administrator (Nonreporting) **A**1 2 3 5 7 9 10 **S**5275 Sisters of Providence Health System ST. PETER HOSPITAL See Providence St. Peter Hospital	21	10	327	—	—	—	—	—	—	—
OMAK—Okanogan County										
★ MID–VALLEY HOSPITAL, 810 Valley Way Road, Zip 98841, Mailing Address: Box 793, Zip 98841; tel. 509/826–1760; Ralph Paulding, Administrator (Nonreporting) **A**9 10	16	10	29	—	—	—	—	—	—	—
OTHELLO—Adams County										
★ OTHELLO COMMUNITY HOSPITAL, 315 North 14th Street, Zip 99344; tel. 509/488–2636; Jerry Lane, Administrator **A**9 10 **F**7 8 19 22 27 28 30 36 39 44 46 49 56 71 **P**1	16	10	38	1000	6	15672	409	—	—	69
PASCO—Franklin County										
※ OUR LADY OF LOURDES HEALTH CENTER, 520 North Fourth Avenue, Zip 99301, Mailing Address: P.O. Box 2568, Zip 99302; tel. 509/547–7704; Thomas Corley, Administrator (Total facility includes 21 beds in nursing home–type unit) **A**1 2 9 10 **F**2 3 7 8 15 16 19 21 22 32 33 35 37 40 41 42 44 45 48 49 52 54 55 56 58 59 64 65 66 67 71 73 **P**1 5 6 7 8 **S**5945 Carondelet Health System	21	10	132	3861	59	39365	642	28378	13503	453
POMEROY—Garfield County										
GARFIELD COUNTY MEMORIAL HOSPITAL, 66th North Sixth Street, Zip 99347–0880, Mailing Address: P.O. Box 880, Zip 99347; tel. 509/843–1591; Arnie Seim, Administrator (Total facility includes 40 beds in nursing home–type unit) **A**9 10 **F**1 13 15 26 28 30 49 51 64 65	16	10	54	69	42	2485	0	1908	1156	64
PORT ANGELES—Clallam County										
□ OLYMPIC MEMORIAL HOSPITAL, 939 Caroline Street, Zip 98362–3997; tel. 360/417–7000; Tom Stegbauer, Administrator (Nonreporting) **A**1 2 9 10	16	10	126	—	—	—	—	—	—	—
PORT TOWNSEND—Jefferson County										
★ JEFFERSON GENERAL HOSPITAL, 834 Sheridan, Zip 98368; tel. 360/385–2200; Victor J. Dirksen, Administrator **A**9 10 **F**7 19 22 31 32 33 34 41 44 49 71 **P**8	15	10	31	1408	11	—	115	10701	5443	158
PROSSER—Benton County										
★ PROSSER MEMORIAL HOSPITAL, 723 Memorial Street, Zip 99350–1593; tel. 509/786–2222; John E. Rohrer, Administrator (Total facility includes 26 beds in nursing home–type unit) **A**9 10 **F**7 8 22 26 40 44 64 65 71	16	10	57	847	28	14429	500	6484	3259	118
PULLMAN—Whitman County										
※ PULLMAN MEMORIAL HOSPITAL, N.E. 1125 Washington Avenue, Zip 99163–4742; tel. 509/332–2541; Scott K. Adams, Administrator **A**1 9 10 **F**1 2 3 4 5 6 7 8 9 10 11 12 14 15 16 17 18 19 20 21 22 23 24 25 26 27 28 29 30 31 32 33 34 35 36 37 38 39 40 41 42 43 44 45 46 47 48 49 50 51 52 53 54 55 56 57 58 59 60 61 62 63 64 65 66 67 68 69 70 71 72 73 74 **P**8 **S**0585 Brim, Inc.	16	10	36	1438	8	29955	326	10600	4693	180
PUYALLUP—Pierce County										
※ △ GOOD SAMARITAN COMMUNITY HEALTHCARE, 407 14th Avenue S.E., Zip 98372–0192, Mailing Address: Box 1247, Zip 98371–0192; tel. 206/848–6661; David K. Hamry, President **A**1 2 7 9 10 **F**1 6 7 11 12 14 15 16 17 18 19 21 22 24 25 26 29 30 32 34 37 39 40 41 42 44 45 46 48 49 53 54 55 56 57 58 59 63 65 66 67 68 70 71 73 **P**1 6 7	21	10	207	8868	115	257624	1352	91565	52623	1523
QUINCY—Grant County										
QUINCY VALLEY HOSPITAL, 908 Tenth Avenue S.W., Zip 98848; tel. 509/787–3531; Jerry Hawley, Administrator (Nonreporting) **A**9 10	13	10	38	—	—	—	—	—	—	—
REDMOND—King County										
★ THE EASTSIDE HOSPITAL, (Formerly Group Health Eastside Hospital) 2700 152nd Avenue N.E., Zip 98052–5560; tel. 206/883–5151; Janice Jones, East Region Vice President (Nonreporting) **S**9995 Group Health Cooperative of Puget Sound	23	10	142	—	—	—	—	—	—	—
RENTON—King County										
※ VALLEY MEDICAL CENTER, 400 South 43rd Street, Zip 98055–9987; tel. 206/228–3450; Richard D. Roodman, Administrator (Total facility includes 39 beds in nursing home–type unit) **A**1 2 3 5 9 10 **F**3 7 8 10 12 13 14 15 16 17 18 19 21 22 24 28 29 30 31 35 37 39 40 41 42 44 45 46 49 51 52 54 56 58 60 64 65 67 71 73 **P**6	16	10	204	14828	134	167099	2841	107909	48168	1257
REPUBLIC—Ferry County										
FERRY COUNTY MEMORIAL HOSPITAL, 470 North Klondike Road, Zip 99166, Mailing Address: P.O. Box 365, Zip 99166; tel. 509/775–3333; Nancy McIntyre, Administrator (Total facility includes 14 beds in nursing home–type unit) **A**9 10 **F**1 3 7 8 12 13 15 16 17 18 19 20 26 27 29 30 31 32 33 34 36 37 39 40 41 44 45 46 49 51 53 54 55 56 57 58 59 61 62 64 65 66 67 68 69 70 71 73 74	16	10	25	423	16	5707	19	2568	1175	43
RICHLAND—Benton County										
★ CARONDELET PSYCHIATRIC CARE CENTER, 1175 Carondelet Drive, Zip 99352–1175; tel. 509/943–9104; Jacquelyn Perry, Executive Director (Nonreporting) **A**9 10	21	22	32	—	—	—	—	—	—	—
※ KADLEC MEDICAL CENTER, 888 Swift Boulevard, Zip 99352–9974; tel. 509/946–4611; Marcel Loh, Chief Executive Officer **A**1 2 9 10 **F**1 7 8 10 12 15 17 19 21 22 32 35 37 38 39 40 41 42 44 45 46 48 49 51 65 71 73 **S**0002 Quorum Health Group/Quorum Health Resources	23	10	135	5628	65	126413	1156	50678	22161	560
RITZVILLE—Adams County										
EAST ADAMS RURAL HOSPITAL, 903 South Adams Street, Zip 99169–2298; tel. 509/659–1200; James G. Parrish, Administrator (Nonreporting) **A**9 10	16	10	17	—	—	—	—	—	—	—

Hospitals, U.S. / WASHINGTON

Hospital, Address, Telephone, Administrator, Approval, Facility, and Physician Codes, Health Care System ★ American Hospital Association (AHA) membership □ Joint Commission on Accreditation of Healthcare Organizations (JCAHO) accreditation + American Osteopathic Hospital Association (AOHA) membership ○ American Osteopathic Association (AOA) accreditation △ Commission on Accreditation of Rehabilitation Facilities (CARF) accreditation Control codes 61, 63, 64, 71, 72 and 73 indicate hospitals listed by AOHA, but not registered by AHA. For definition of numerical codes, see page A6	Classification Codes		Utilization Data					Expense (thousands) of dollars		
	Control	Service	Beds	Admissions	Census	Outpatient Visits	Births	Total	Payroll	Personnel
SEATTLE—King County										
★ CHILDREN'S HOSPITAL AND MEDICAL CENTER, 4800 Sand Point Way N.E., Zip 98105, Mailing Address: Box 5371, Zip 98105–0371; tel. 206/526–2000; Treuman Katz, President and Chief Executive Officer **A**1 2 3 5 8 9 10 **F**5 10 12 13 14 15 16 17 19 20 21 22 28 31 32 34 35 38 39 42 43 44 45 47 48 49 51 52 53 54 55 58 59 60 65 66 67 68 69 70 71 72 73 **P**6 8	23	50	208	9379	136	103613	0	121780	53554	1427
FIFTH AVENUE HOSPITAL See THC–Seattle Hospital										
★ GROUP HEALTH COOPERATIVE CENTRAL HOSPITAL, 201 16th Avenue East, Zip 98112–5298; tel. 206/326–3000; Sue Hennessy, Regional Vice President (Nonreporting) **A**1 2 3 5 10 **S**9995 Group Health Cooperative of Puget Sound	23	10	222	—	—	—	—	—	—	—
★ HARBORVIEW MEDICAL CENTER, 325 Ninth Avenue, Zip 98104–2499; tel. 206/223–3000; David E. Jaffe, Executive Director and Chief Executive Officer **A**1 3 5 8 9 10 **F**2 3 4 5 7 8 9 10 11 12 13 15 16 17 18 19 20 21 22 23 25 26 27 28 31 32 33 34 35 37 38 39 40 41 42 43 44 45 46 47 48 49 50 51 52 53 54 55 56 57 58 59 60 65 66 67 68 69 70 71 72 73 74 **P**3	13	10	326	11936	253	226952	0	183761	91606	2568
★ △ NORTHWEST HOSPITAL, 1550 North 115th Street, Zip 98133–8498; tel. 206/364–0500; James D. Hart, President and Chief Executive Officer (Total facility includes 42 beds in nursing home–type unit) **A**1 3 7 9 10 **F**4 7 8 10 11 12 14 15 16 17 19 20 21 22 23 24 25 26 29 30 31 32 33 34 35 37 38 39 40 41 42 44 45 46 48 49 51 52 54 55 56 57 58 59 60 61 63 64 65 66 67 71 73 74 **P**6 8	23	10	229	10857	150	269140	1720	85967	39939	1062
★ △ PROVIDENCE SEATTLE MEDICAL CENTER, 500 17th Avenue, Zip 98122, Mailing Address: P.O. Box 34008, Zip 98124–1008; tel. 206/320–2000; Nancy A. Giunto, Administrator **A**1 2 3 5 7 9 10 **F**1 4 6 7 8 10 11 12 14 15 16 17 19 20 21 22 24 25 26 27 28 29 30 31 32 33 34 35 37 39 40 41 42 43 44 45 46 48 49 51 52 56 57 59 60 62 63 64 65 66 67 68 71 72 73 74 **P**6 **S**5275 Sisters of Providence Health System	21	10	334	16249	208	94447	1938	140769	62832	1979
□ SCHICK SHADEL HOSPITAL, 12101 Ambaum Boulevard S.W., Zip 98146–2699, Mailing Address: Box 48149, Zip 98148–0149; tel. 206/244–8100; Mary Ellen Stewart, Administrator (Nonreporting) **A**1 9 10 **S**0575 Schick Laboratories, Inc.	33	82	63	—	—	—	—	—	—	—
★ SWEDISH HEALTH SERVICES–SEATTLE, (Formerly Swedish Medical Center–Seattle) 747 Broadway Avenue, Zip 98114–0999, Mailing Address: P.O. Box 14999, Zip 98114–0999; tel. 206/386–6000; Richard H. Peterson, President and Chief Executive Officer **A**1 2 3 5 9 10 **F**2 3 4 7 8 10 11 12 13 14 15 16 19 21 22 23 24 25 27 28 29 30 31 32 33 34 35 37 38 39 40 41 42 43 44 45 46 48 49 51 52 60 61 63 64 65 67 69 70 71 73 **P**4 5 6 7	23	10	558	25815	373	514813	4056	311423	130935	3798
★ SWEDISH MEDICAL CENTER–BALLARD, Northwest Market and Barnes, Zip 98107–1507, Mailing Address: Box 70707, Zip 98107; tel. 206/782–2700; Elvira S. Fife, Chief Operating Officer (Nonreporting) **A**9	23	10	149	—	—	—	—	—	—	—
★ ○ THC–SEATTLE HOSPITAL, (Formerly Fifth Avenue Hospital) 10560 Fifth Avenue N.E., Zip 98125–0977; tel. 206/364–2050; Gregory S. Fritz, Chief Executive Officer (Nonreporting) **A**9 10 11	33	10	55	—	—	—	—	—	—	—
★ UNIVERSITY OF WASHINGTON MEDICAL CENTER, 1959 Northeast Pacific Street, Zip 98195–0001; tel. 206/548–3300; Robert H. Muilenburg, Executive Director **A**1 3 5 8 9 10 **F**4 5 6 7 8 10 11 12 14 15 16 19 20 21 22 23 24 25 26 28 29 30 31 32 33 34 35 37 38 39 40 41 42 43 44 45 46 48 49 50 51 52 54 55 56 57 58 59 60 61 63 65 66 67 69 70 71 72 73 74	12	10	377	14310	258	242753	1475	222949	96213	2503
★ VETERANS AFFAIRS MEDICAL CENTER, 1660 South Columbian Way, Zip 98108–1597; tel. 206/762–1010; Timothy B. Williams, Director (Total facility includes 56 beds in nursing home–type unit) **A**1 3 5 8 **F**1 2 3 4 8 10 11 12 14 19 20 21 22 26 27 28 31 33 34 35 37 41 42 43 44 45 46 48 49 51 52 54 56 57 58 60 64 65 67 69 71 73 74 **P**2 **S**9295 Department of Veterans Affairs	45	10	408	8913	311	223156	0	164110	78090	1780
★ VIRGINIA MASON MEDICAL CENTER, 1100 Ninth Avenue, Zip 98111–0900, Mailing Address: P.O. Box 900, Zip 98111–0900; tel. 206/223–6600; J. Michael Rona, Executive Administrator (Total facility includes 35 beds in nursing home–type unit) **A**1 2 3 5 9 10 **F**1 3 4 5 7 8 10 14 15 16 17 19 21 22 23 25 26 30 31 32 34 35 37 40 41 42 43 44 45 46 48 49 51 53 54 58 60 61 64 65 66 67 69 71 72 73 74 **P**6	23	10	231	10905	183	728199	1155	278751	140422	3021
HIGHLINE COMMUNITY HOSPITAL See Burien										
SEDRO WOOLLEY—Skagit County										
UNITED GENERAL HOSPITAL See Affiliated Health Services, Mount Vernon										
SHELTON—Mason County										
□ MASON GENERAL HOSPITAL, 901 Mountainview Drive, Zip 98584, Mailing Address: P.O. Box 1668, Zip 98584; tel. 206/426–1611; G. Robert Appel, Administrator (Nonreporting) **A**1 9 10	16	10	68	—	—	—	—	—	—	—
SNOQUALMIE—Klickitat County										
SNOQUALMIE VALLEY HOSPITAL, 1505 Meadowbrook Way S.E., Zip 98065–2011; tel. 206/831–2300; Carol L. Johnson, Administrator (Newly Registered) **A**9 10	13	10	28	—	—	—	—	—	—	—
SOUTH BEND—Pacific County										
WILLAPA HARBOR HOSPITAL, Alder and Cedar Streets, Zip 98586–0438, Mailing Address: Box 438, Zip 98586–0438; tel. 206/875–5526; Victor Vander Does, Administrator (Nonreporting) **A**9 10	16	10	18	—	—	—	—	—	—	—
SPOKANE—Spokane County										
□ DEACONESS MEDICAL CENTER–SPOKANE, 800 West Fifth Avenue, Zip 99204, Mailing Address: P.O. Box 248, Zip 99210–0248; tel. 509/458–5800; Thomas J. Zellers, Chief Operating Officer (Nonreporting) **A**1 2 3 5 9 10 **S**0945 Empire Health Centers Group	23	10	326	—	—	—	—	—	—	—

© 1995 AHA Guide

Hospitals, U.S. / WASHINGTON

Hospital, Address, Telephone, Administrator, Approval, Facility, and Physician Codes, Health Care System

- ★ American Hospital Association (AHA) membership
- ☐ Joint Commission on Accreditation of Healthcare Organizations (JCAHO) accreditation
- + American Osteopathic Hospital Association (AOHA) membership
- ○ American Osteopathic Association (AOA) accreditation
- △ Commission on Accreditation of Rehabilitation Facilities (CARF) accreditation

Control codes 61, 63, 64, 71, 72 and 73 indicate hospitals listed by AOHA, but not registered by AHA. For definition of numerical codes, see page A6

Hospital	Control	Service	Beds	Admissions	Census	Outpatient Visits	Births	Total	Payroll	Personnel
★ HOLY FAMILY HOSPITAL, North 5633 Lidgerwood Avenue, Zip 99220; tel. 509/482-0111; Ronald J. Schurra, Chief Executive Officer **A**1 2 9 10 **F**2 7 8 9 10 14 15 16 17 19 21 22 26 28 29 30 34 35 37 38 39 40 41 42 44 46 47 48 49 50 52 53 54 55 56 57 58 59 60 63 65 67 68 69 70 71 72 73 74 **P**3 7 8 **S**5265 Providence Services	21	10	190	8557	97	69083	1265	53754	24986	662
MOUNTAINVIEW HOSPITAL OF SPOKANE, 628 South Cowley, Zip 99202; tel. 509/624-3226; Ben Camp, Administrator (Nonreporting) **A**9	33	82	34	—	—	—	—	—	—	—
★ SACRED HEART MEDICAL CENTER, West 101 Eighth Avenue, Zip 99220, Mailing Address: P.O. Box 2555, Zip 99220-2555; tel. 509/455-3040; Gerald P. Leahy, President **A**1 2 3 5 9 10 **F**1 4 7 8 10 11 12 13 14 15 17 19 20 21 22 23 24 25 26 27 28 29 30 31 32 33 34 35 37 38 39 40 42 43 44 45 46 47 48 49 50 51 52 53 54 55 56 57 59 60 63 64 65 67 69 71 73 74 **S**5265 Providence Services	21	10	623	25183	411	—	2193	234036	123046	2673
★ SHRINERS HOSPITALS FOR CRIPPLED CHILDREN–SPOKANE UNIT, 911 West Fifth Avenue, Zip 99204-2901, Mailing Address: P.O. Box 2472, Zip 99210-2472; tel. 509/455-7844; Charles R. Young, Administrator **A**1 3 **F**12 15 17 20 34 47 49 65 73 **S**4125 Shriners Hospitals for Crippled Children	23	57	30	730	16	6596	0	—	—	114
△ ST. LUKES REHABILITATION INSTITUTE, 711 South Cowley Street, Zip 99202, Mailing Address: P.O. Box 288, Zip 99210-0288; tel. 509/838-4771; Debra D. Hanks, Administrator (Nonreporting) **A**7 9 10 **S**0945 Empire Health Centers Group	23	10	87	—	—	—	—	—	—	—
☐ VALLEY HOSPITAL AND MEDICAL CENTER, 12606 East Mission Avenue, Zip 99216-9969; tel. 509/924-6650; Michael T. Liepman, Chief Operating Officer (Nonreporting) **A**1 9 10 **S**0945 Empire Health Centers Group	23	10	117	—	—	—	—	—	—	—
★ VETERANS AFFAIRS MEDICAL CENTER, North 4815 Assembly Street, Zip 99205-6197; tel. 509/328-4521; Joseph M. Manley, Director (Nonreporting) **A**1 **S**9295 Department of Veterans Affairs	45	10	192	—	—	—	—	—	—	—
SUNNYSIDE—Yakima County										
★ + ○ SUNNYSIDE COMMUNITY HOSPITAL, 10th and Tacoma Avenue, Zip 98944, Mailing Address: P.O. Box 719, Zip 98944-0719; tel. 509/837-1500; Jon D. Smiley, Chief Executive Officer **A**9 10 11 **F**7 8 11 19 20 21 22 30 32 33 34 39 40 44 45 46 65 67 70 71 73 **S**0585 Brim, Inc.	23	10	38	1717	16	39997	409	13731	6242	215
TACOMA—Pierce County										
☐ ALLENMORE HOSPITAL, South 19th and Union Streets, Zip 98405, Mailing Address: P.O. Box 11414, Zip 98411-0414; tel. 206/572-2323; Charles Hoffman, Administrator (Nonreporting) **A**1 9 10 **S**6555 Multicare Health System	23	10	82	—	—	—	—	—	—	—
★ MADIGAN ARMY MEDICAL CENTER, Zip 98431-5000; tel. 206/968-1110; Major General James B. Peake M.D., MSC, USA, Commanding General **A**1 2 3 5 **F**3 4 7 8 10 11 12 13 14 16 19 20 21 22 24 25 28 29 30 31 32 34 35 37 38 39 40 41 42 43 44 45 46 47 51 54 58 60 61 65 67 71 73 74 **S**9395 Department of the Army	42	10	334	19083	197	1051012	2234	204648	134416	3248
☐ MARY BRIDGE CHILDREN'S HOSPITAL AND HEALTH CENTER, 317 Martin Luther King Jr Way, Zip 98405, Mailing Address: Box 5299, Zip 98405-0299; tel. 206/552-1400; William B. Connoley, President and Chief Executive Officer (Nonreporting) **A**1 3 5 10 **S**6555 Multicare Health System	23	50	72	—	—	—	—	—	—	—
☐ PUGET SOUND HOSPITAL, 215 South 36th Street, Zip 98408, Mailing Address: P.O. Box 11412, Zip 98411-0412; tel. 206/474-0561; Bruce Brandler, Administrator (Nonreporting) **A**1 9 10 **S**6525 Ornda Healthcorp	33	10	146	—	—	—	—	—	—	—
★ ST. CLARE HOSPITAL, 11315 Bridgeport Way S.W., Zip 98499-0998, Mailing Address: P.O. Box 99998, Zip 98499-0998; tel. 206/588-1711; Craig L. Hendrickson, President (Nonreporting) **A**1 9 10 **S**5325 Franciscan Health System	23	10	60	—	—	—	—	—	—	—
★ △ ST. JOSEPH MEDICAL CENTER, 1717 South J Street, Zip 98405, Mailing Address: P.O. Box 2197, Zip 98401-2197; tel. 206/627-4101; Philip G. Dionne, President and Chief Operating Officer **A**1 2 7 9 10 **F**2 4 6 7 8 9 10 11 12 13 17 18 19 20 21 22 23 24 25 26 28 29 30 31 32 33 34 35 36 37 38 39 40 41 42 43 44 45 46 47 48 49 51 52 54 56 57 58 59 60 61 63 64 65 67 68 69 71 72 73 74 **P**5 6 8 **S**5325 Franciscan Health System	21	10	271	13042	167	150248	2274	138746	61672	1519
★ TACOMA GENERAL HOSPITAL, 315 South K Street, Zip 98405, Mailing Address: P.O. Box 5299, Zip 98405-0299; tel. 206/552-1000; William B. Connoley, President and Chief Executive Officer (Nonreporting) **A**1 2 3 5 9 10 **S**6555 Multicare Health System	23	10	306	—	—	—	—	—	—	—
★ VETERANS AFFAIRS MEDICAL CENTER, Zip 98493; tel. 206/582-8440; Frank Taylor, Director (Total facility includes 76 beds in nursing home-type unit) **A**1 3 **F**2 3 4 8 9 10 12 14 17 18 19 20 21 22 26 27 31 32 33 35 37 39 41 42 43 44 45 46 48 49 51 52 54 55 56 57 58 60 64 65 69 70 71 73 74 **P**1 **S**9295 Department of Veterans Affairs	45	10	339	1183	270	141202	0	—	—	827
TONASKET—Okanogan County										
NORTH VALLEY HOSPITAL, Second and Western, Zip 98855, Mailing Address: P.O. Box 488, Zip 98855; tel. 509/486-2151; Donald W. James, Administrator (Nonreporting) **A**9 10	16	10	92	—	—	—	—	—	—	—
TOPPENISH—Yakima County										
★ PROVIDENCE TOPPENISH HOSPITAL, (Formerly Providence Hospital) 504 West Fourth Avenue, Zip 98948, Mailing Address: P.O. Box 672, Zip 98948-0672; tel. 509/865-3105; Roy W. Holmes, Administrator **A**1 9 10 **F**14 15 16 19 21 32 33 34 37 40 41 44 46 51 65 71 73 **P**3 **S**5275 Sisters of Providence Health System	21	10	48	2016	19	47224	730	12165	5665	154

Hospitals, U.S. / WASHINGTON

Hospital, Address, Telephone, Administrator, Approval, Facility, and Physician Codes, Health Care System	Classification Codes		Utilization Data					Expense (thousands) of dollars		
★ American Hospital Association (AHA) membership ☐ Joint Commission on Accreditation of Healthcare Organizations (JCAHO) accreditation + American Osteopathic Hospital Association (AOHA) membership ○ American Osteopathic Association (AOA) accreditation △ Commission on Accreditation of Rehabilitation Facilities (CARF) accreditation Control codes 61, 63, 64, 71, 72 and 73 indicate hospitals listed by AOHA, but not registered by AHA. For definition of numerical codes, see page A6	Control	Service	Beds	Admissions	Census	Outpatient Visits	Births	Total	Payroll	Personnel
VANCOUVER—Clark County										
★ SOUTHWEST WASHINGTON MEDICAL CENTER, (Includes St. Joseph Community Hospital, 600 N.E. 92nd Avenue, Vancouver, Washington, Zip 98664; tel. 206/256–2000; Vancouver Memorial Hospital, 3400 Main Street, Vancouver, Washington, Zip 98663; tel. 206/696–5000) 400 Northeast Mother Joseph Place, Zip 98664, Mailing Address: P.O. Box 1600, Zip 98668; tel. 206/256–2000; Jeffrey D. Selberg, President **A**1 2 9 10 **F**2 3 4 7 8 10 15 19 21 22 23 24 28 30 32 33 34 35 37 40 41 42 43 44 45 46 48 49 52 54 55 56 57 58 59 60 65 70 71 73 **P**1	23	10	310	14022	171	141747	2651	111918	54578	1506
WALLA WALLA—Walla Walla County										
★ △ ST. MARY MEDICAL CENTER, 401 West Poplar Street, Zip 99362, Mailing Address: Box 1477, Zip 99362–0312; tel. 509/525–3320; John A. Isely, President **A**1 2 7 9 10 **F**7 8 14 19 22 28 30 31 32 33 34 35 37 38 39 40 41 42 44 48 49 52 56 58 60 65 70 71 73 74 **P**7 **S**5265 Providence Services	21	10	120	3736	48	56301	352	35722	16423	507
STATE PENITENTIARY HOSPITAL, Mailing Address: Box 520, Zip 99362; tel. 509/525–3610; Barbara Croft, Health Care Manager (Nonreporting)	12	11	31	—	—	—	—	—	—	—
★ VETERANS AFFAIRS MEDICAL CENTER, 77 Wainwright Drive, Zip 99362–3975; tel. 509/525–5200; George Marnell, Director (Total facility includes 30 beds in nursing home–type unit) **A**1 **F**2 3 15 17 19 20 22 27 31 33 34 37 41 44 45 46 48 49 51 52 54 55 56 58 59 64 65 67 71 73 74 **P**6 **S**9295 Department of Veterans Affairs	45	10	132	1844	72	36121	0	23660	12393	329
☐ WALLA WALLA GENERAL HOSPITAL, 1025 South Second Avenue, Zip 99362, Mailing Address: Box 1398, Zip 99362; tel. 509/525–0480; Rodney T. Applegate, President (Nonreporting) **A**1 2 9 10 **S**0235 Adventist Health System/West	21	10	72	—	—	—	—	—	—	—
WENATCHEE—Chelan County										
★ CENTRAL WASHINGTON HOSPITAL, 1300 Fuller Street, Zip 98801–1948, Mailing Address: Box 1887, Zip 98807–1887; tel. 509/662–1511; Thomas J. Troy, President (Nonreporting) **A**1 2 9 10	23	10	176	—	—	—	—	—	—	—
WHITE SALMON—Klickitat County										
SKYLINE HOSPITAL, 211 Skyline Drive, Zip 98672–0099, Mailing Address: Box 99, Zip 98672–0099; tel. 509/493–1101; Lynn Milnes, Administrator **A**9 10 **F**7 8 11 12 14 15 22 28 33 34 37 40 42 44 46 49 51 56 64 67 70 71 72 73 **P**5	16	10	22	792	6	11541	112	4330	2525	96
YAKIMA—Yakima County										
★ PROVIDENCE YAKIMA MEDICAL CENTER, 110 South Ninth Avenue, Zip 98902–3397; tel. 509/575–5000; Barbara A. Hood, Acting Administrator (Total facility includes 12 beds in nursing home–type unit) **A**1 2 3 9 10 **F**4 7 8 10 11 15 16 19 22 27 28 29 30 32 33 34 37 40 41 42 43 44 45 46 48 49 64 65 67 71 72 73 74 **P**4 5 **S**5275 Sisters of Providence Health System	21	10	184	6609	102	204159	457	63354	27764	723
★ YAKIMA VALLEY MEMORIAL HOSPITAL, 2811 Tieton Drive, Zip 98902–3799; tel. 509/575–8000; Richard W. Linneweh Jr., President **A**1 2 3 9 10 **F**7 8 10 11 12 13 14 15 16 17 19 21 22 23 28 29 30 32 34 35 37 38 39 40 41 42 43 44 45 49 52 54 56 58 59 60 63 65 66 71 73 74	23	10	200	10002	109	105952	2542	70512	30316	878

Hospitals, U.S. / WEST VIRGINIA

WEST VIRGINIA

Resident population 1,820 (in thousands)
Resident population in metro areas 41.8%
Birth rate per 1,000 population 12.5
65 years and over 15.3%
Percent of persons without health insurance 15.0%

Hospital, Address, Telephone, Administrator, Approval, Facility, and Physician Codes, Health Care System	Classification Codes		Utilization Data					Expense (thousands) of dollars		
	Control	Service	Beds	Admissions	Census	Outpatient Visits	Births	Total	Payroll	Personnel

★ American Hospital Association (AHA) membership
□ Joint Commission on Accreditation of Healthcare Organizations (JCAHO) accreditation
+ American Osteopathic Hospital Association (AOHA) membership
○ American Osteopathic Association (AOA) accreditation
△ Commission on Accreditation of Rehabilitation Facilities (CARF) accreditation
Control codes 61, 63, 64, 71, 72 and 73 indicate hospitals listed by AOHA, but not registered by AHA. For definition of numerical codes, see page A6

BECKLEY—Raleigh County

□ BECKLEY APPALACHIAN REGIONAL HOSPITAL, 306 Stanaford Road, Zip 25801; tel. 304/255-3000; Wilbur D. Crosley, Administrator A1 9 10 F1 8 11 12 15 16 19 21 22 26 28 29 30 31 32 35 37 39 42 44 45 49 52 53 54 55 56 57 59 65 71 73 S0145 Appalachian Regional Healthcare	23	10	173	5066	113	—	0	23299	11040	446
BECKLEY HOSPITAL, 1007 South Oakwood Avenue, Zip 25801; tel. 304/256-1200; Albert M. Tieche Jr., Administrator A9 10 F8 15 17 19 21 22 32 33 34 35 37 42 44 52 56 60 65 71 73	33	10	57	2355	47	26689	0	14363	5984	288
★ RALEIGH GENERAL HOSPITAL, 1710 Harper Road, Zip 25801-3397; tel. 304/256-4100; Kenneth M. Holt, Chief Executive Officer A1 9 10 F7 8 10 11 12 14 15 16 19 20 21 22 23 24 28 29 30 31 34 35 37 38 39 40 41 42 44 45 46 49 52 56 65 66 67 71 73 74 S0048 Columbia/HCA Healthcare Corporation	33	10	293	9546	154	48882	1662	51518	19497	702
★ VETERANS AFFAIRS MEDICAL CENTER, 200 Veterans Avenue, Zip 25801-6499; tel. 304/255-2121; G. P. Husson, Director A1 12 F3 19 20 21 22 26 27 28 30 31 32 34 35 37 39 42 44 45 46 49 51 54 55 56 57 58 60 64 65 71 73 74 S9295 Department of Veterans Affairs	45	10	186	2949	116	40502	0	29909	15826	430

BERKELEY SPRINGS—Morgan County

★ MORGAN COUNTY WAR MEMORIAL HOSPITAL, 1124 Fairfax Street, Zip 25411-1718; tel. 304/258-1234; David A. Sweeney, Administrator (Total facility includes 16 beds in nursing home-type unit) A9 10 F8 15 16 20 22 27 30 32 33 34 39 44 45 46 49 64 65 71 73 P5 8	13	10	44	735	32	12984	0	4897	2077	90

BLUEFIELD—Mercer County

★ BLUEFIELD REGIONAL MEDICAL CENTER, 500 Cherry Street, Zip 24701-3390; tel. 304/327-1100; Eugene P. Pawlinski, President A1 9 10 F7 8 10 11 13 14 16 19 21 22 24 30 33 34 35 37 39 40 41 42 44 45 49 50 60 63 65 71 72 73 P3 8	23	10	265	7902	134	90095	661	52066	22708	850
★ ST. LUKE'S HOSPITAL, 1333 Southview Drive, Zip 24701, Mailing Address: P.O. Box 1190, Zip 24701; tel. 304/327-2900; Barry A. Papania, Chief Executive Officer A1 9 10 12 F8 12 14 15 16 19 21 22 23 26 35 37 44 48 49 54 56 63 65 71 73 S0048 Columbia/HCA Healthcare Corporation	33	10	79	1911	31	21140	0	16586	5737	198

BUCKHANNON—Upshur County

★ ST. JOSEPH'S HOSPITAL, Amalia Drive, Zip 26201-2222; tel. 304/473-2000; Ralph G. Horton, Chief Executive Officer (Total facility includes 16 beds in nursing home-type unit) A1 9 10 F7 8 12 14 15 16 17 19 22 32 33 34 35 37 40 42 44 46 49 52 54 55 56 57 64 65 67 71 73 P7 8	23	10	95	2541	46	21504	338	16123	6468	283

CHARLESTON—Kanawha County

★ △ CHARLESTON AREA MEDICAL CENTER, (Includes General Division, 501 Morris Street, Charleston, West Virginia, Zip 25301, Mailing Address: Box 1393, Zip 25325; tel. 304/348-5432; Memorial Division, 3200 Maccorkle Avenue S.E., Charleston, West Virginia, Zip 25304; tel. 304/348-5432; Women and Children's Hospital, 800 Pennsylvania Avenue, Charleston, West Virginia, Zip 25302; tel. 304/348-5432) 501 Morris Street, Zip 25301, Mailing Address: Box 1547, Zip 25326; tel. 304/348-5432; Phillip H. Goodwin, President and Chief Executive Officer A1 2 3 5 7 8 9 10 12 F3 4 5 7 8 10 11 12 15 16 17 19 20 21 22 23 24 25 26 27 28 29 30 31 32 33 34 35 37 38 39 40 41 42 43 44 45 46 47 48 49 51 52 54 55 56 57 58 59 60 61 63 65 66 67 68 69 70 71 72 73 74 P2 6 7 S0955 Camcare, Inc.	23	10	776	33611	580	343928	3659	328686	129081	4434
★ EYE AND EAR CLINIC OF CHARLESTON, 1306 Kanawha Boulevard East, Zip 25301, Mailing Address: Box 2271, Zip 25328-2271; tel. 304/343-4371; W. Allen Shelton II, Administrator A1 9 10 F34 44	33	45	26	123	1	6855	0	5922	2153	85
GENERAL DIVISION See Charleston Area Medical Center										
★ HIGHLAND HOSPITAL, 300 56th Street S.E., Zip 25304, Mailing Address: P.O. Box 4107, Zip 25364-4107; tel. 304/926-1600; David M. McWatters, Administrator A1 9 10 F2 3 12 16 18 52 53 54 55 56 57 58 59 65 67 P6	23	22	58	773	34	15	0	6249	3306	153
MEMORIAL DIVISION See Charleston Area Medical Center										
★ SAINT FRANCIS HOSPITAL, 333 Laidley Street, Zip 25301, Mailing Address: Box 471, Zip 25322; tel. 304/347-6500; David R. Sirk, President and Chief Executive Officer (Total facility includes 20 beds in nursing home-type unit) A1 9 10 F10 16 19 21 22 25 34 36 37 39 41 44 45 46 49 51 60 64 65 66 71 73 S0048 Columbia/HCA Healthcare Corporation	21	10	145	5495	104	35669	0	54157	19606	554
WOMEN AND CHILDREN'S HOSPITAL See Charleston Area Medical Center										

CLARKSBURG—Harrison County

★ LOUIS A. JOHNSON VETERANS AFFAIRS MEDICAL CENTER, Zip 26301-4199; tel. 304/623-3461; Michael W. Neusch FACHE, Director A1 2 3 5 F1 2 3 4 5 6 8 9 10 11 12 17 18 19 20 21 22 23 24 25 27 29 30 31 32 33 34 35 37 39 42 43 44 45 46 48 49 51 52 54 55 56 57 58 59 60 63 64 65 67 69 70 71 73 74 S9295 Department of Veterans Affairs	45	10	160	3541	112	75098	0	42131	20964	606
★ UNITED HOSPITAL CENTER, U.S. Route 19 South, Zip 26301, Mailing Address: Box 1680, Zip 26302-1680; tel. 304/624-2121; Bruce C. Carter, President (Total facility includes 32 beds in nursing home-type unit) A1 2 3 5 9 10 F7 8 10 11 12 14 15 19 20 21 23 25 28 29 30 32 33 34 35 37 40 42 44 45 46 49 51 52 54 56 57 58 60 63 64 65 67 71 72 73	23	10	312	10177	176	150110	896	76784	31584	1206

Hospitals, U.S. / WEST VIRGINIA

Hospital, Address, Telephone, Administrator, Approval, Facility, and Physician Codes, Health Care System

★ American Hospital Association (AHA) membership
☐ Joint Commission on Accreditation of Healthcare Organizations (JCAHO) accreditation
+ American Osteopathic Hospital Association (AOHA) membership
○ American Osteopathic Association (AOA) accreditation
△ Commission on Accreditation of Rehabilitation Facilities (CARF) accreditation
Control codes 61, 63, 64, 71, 72 and 73 indicate hospitals listed by AOHA, but not registered by AHA. For definition of numerical codes, see page A6

Hospital	Classification Codes		Utilization Data					Expense (thousands) of dollars		
	Control	Service	Beds	Admissions	Census	Outpatient Visits	Births	Total	Payroll	Personnel
ELKINS—Randolph County										
★ DAVIS MEMORIAL HOSPITAL, Gorman Avenue and Reed Street, Zip 26241, Mailing Address: Box 1484, Zip 26241; tel. 304/636–3300; Robert L. Hammer II, Chief Executive Officer **A**1 9 10 **F**2 3 4 6 7 8 9 10 11 16 19 21 22 23 28 30 31 32 33 34 35 36 37 38 39 40 42 43 44 46 47 48 49 50 52 53 54 55 56 57 58 59 60 63 64 65 70 71 73 **P**8	23	10	115	6690	78	113994	461	35550	14787	517
FAIRMONT—Marion County										
★ FAIRMONT GENERAL HOSPITAL, 1325 Locust Avenue, Zip 26554–0000; tel. 304/367–7100; Richard W. Graham FACHE, President (Total facility includes 44 beds in nursing home–type unit) **A**1 9 10 **F**2 3 7 8 10 14 15 16 17 19 21 22 23 28 29 30 35 36 37 39 40 41 42 44 46 49 52 53 54 55 56 57 58 63 64 65 66 67 71 73 74 **P**7 8 **S**0002 Quorum Health Group/Quorum Health Resources	23	10	238	6695	160	122984	572	46783	20685	719
GASSAWAY—Braxton County										
★ BRAXTON COUNTY MEMORIAL HOSPITAL, 100 Hoylman Drive, Zip 26624–9308; tel. 304/364–5156; Tony E. Atkins, Administrator (Nonreporting) **A**9 10 **S**0955 Camcare, Inc.	23	10	30	—	—	—	—	—	—	—
GLEN DALE—Marshall County										
★ REYNOLDS MEMORIAL HOSPITAL, 800 Wheeling Avenue, Zip 26038–1697; tel. 304/845–3211; John Sicurella, Chief Executive Officer (Total facility includes 20 beds in nursing home–type unit) **A**1 9 10 **F**1 3 7 8 15 16 19 22 23 24 28 29 30 32 33 35 37 39 40 42 44 45 46 49 53 54 55 56 57 58 59 63 64 65 66 70 71 73	23	10	140	3679	69	45324	269	28703	12347	456
GRAFTON—Taylor County										
☐ GRAFTON CITY HOSPITAL, 500 Market Street, Zip 26354; tel. 304/265–6401; Randall L. Roberts, Administrator (Total facility includes 77 beds in nursing home–type unit) **A**1 9 10 **F**8 11 14 15 16 19 20 21 24 26 27 28 29 30 31 33 34 36 37 39 42 44 45 46 49 56 64 65 69 70 71 73 74	23	10	136	1132	77	84949	0	4466	3190	225
GRANTSVILLE—Calhoun County										
★ CALHOUN GENERAL HOSPITAL, High Street, Zip 26147, Mailing Address: Box 490, Zip 26147; tel. 304/354–6121; J. Douglas Yarbrough, Administrator **A**1 9 10 **F**15 16 19 21 22 28 34 44 46 51 66 71 73	23	10	20	444	5	9727	0	3683	1643	82
HINTON—Summers County										
SUMMERS COUNTY APPALACHIAN REGIONAL HOSPITAL, (Formerly Appalachian Regional Hospital–Summers County) Terrace Street, Zip 25951, Mailing Address: Drawer 940, Zip 25951–0940; tel. 304/466–1000; Scot Mitchell, Administrator (Total facility includes 24 beds in nursing home–type unit) **A**9 10 **F**8 14 15 16 17 19 22 28 30 32 34 35 37 44 51 64 65 71 73 **S**0145 Appalachian Regional Healthcare	23	10	95	1030	43	18947	0	7576	3843	161
HUNTINGTON—Cabell County										
★ + CABELL HUNTINGTON HOSPITAL, 1340 Hal Greer Boulevard, Zip 25701–0195; tel. 304/526–2000; W. Don Smith II, President and Chief Executive Officer (Total facility includes 15 beds in nursing home–type unit) **A**1 3 5 9 10 **F**4 7 8 9 14 15 16 19 20 21 22 23 28 29 30 31 32 33 34 35 37 38 39 40 41 42 44 45 46 47 48 49 51 60 61 63 64 65 67 69 70 71 73 74 **P**5 8	23	10	293	12139	181	129058	2543	87456	40309	1267
★ △ HUNTINGTON REHABILITATION HOSPITAL, 6900 West Country Club Drive, Zip 25705; tel. 304/733–1060; William R. Wright, Administrator **A**1 7 10 **F**12 15 41 48 49 65 67 73	33	46	40	645	36	—	0	7346	3342	116
★ RIVER PARK HOSPITAL, 1230 Sixth Avenue, Zip 25701, Mailing Address: Box 1875, Zip 25719; tel. 304/526–9111; Ronald E. Yates, Chief Executive Officer **A**1 9 10 **F**1 2 3 14 19 27 35 52 53 54 55 56 57 58 59 **S**0048 Columbia/HCA Healthcare Corporation	33	22	165	2098	98	6513	0	16086	6472	247
★ ST. MARY'S HOSPITAL, 2900 First Avenue, Zip 25702–1271; tel. 304/526–1234; J. Thomas Jones, Executive Director (Total facility includes 20 beds in nursing home–type unit) **A**1 2 3 5 6 9 10 **F**2 4 7 8 10 11 12 15 16 17 19 21 22 23 26 28 29 30 31 32 33 34 35 37 39 40 41 42 43 44 45 49 52 53 54 55 56 57 59 60 63 64 65 67 70 71 73 74 **P**8	21	10	440	14212	265	87441	600	104736	47372	1597
★ VETERANS AFFAIRS MEDICAL CENTER, 1540 Spring Valley Drive, Zip 25704; tel. 304/429–6741; Philip S. Elkins, Director (Nonreporting) **A**1 3 5 **S**9295 Department of Veterans Affairs	45	10	159	—	—	—	—	—	—	—
HURRICANE—Putnam County										
★ PUTNAM GENERAL HOSPITAL, 1400 Hospital Drive, Zip 25526–9210, Mailing Address: P.O. Box 900, Zip 25526–0900; tel. 304/757–1700; Stephens M. Mundy, Chief Executive Officer (Nonreporting) **A**1 9 10 **S**0048 Columbia/HCA Healthcare Corporation	33	10	55	—	—	—	—	—	—	—
KEYSER—Mineral County										
☐ POTOMAC VALLEY HOSPITAL, South Mineral Street, Zip 26726; tel. 304/788–3141; James F. Heitzenrater, Administrator (Nonreporting) **A**1 9 10	33	10	42	—	—	—	—	—	—	—
KINGWOOD—Preston County										
★ PRESTON MEMORIAL HOSPITAL, 300 South Price Street, Zip 26537–1495; tel. 304/329–1400; Raymond E. Wood, President and Chief Executive Officer **A**1 9 10 **F**2 3 7 8 12 13 15 16 17 19 22 24 28 31 32 34 37 39 40 41 44 45 46 49 65 66 67 68 71 72 73 74 **P**1 8	23	10	58	1385	17	63631	196	10848	4659	191
LOGAN—Logan County										
★ GUYAN VALLEY HOSPITAL, 396 Dingess Street, Zip 25601; tel. 304/792–1700; Linda Saunders, Administrator **A**10 **F**14 15 16 22 31 32 34 65	23	10	43	218	7	51842	0	3605	1764	85

© 1995 AHA Guide

Hospitals, U.S. / WEST VIRGINIA

Hospital, Address, Telephone, Administrator, Approval, Facility, and Physician Codes, Health Care System	Classification Codes		Utilization Data					Expense (thousands) of dollars		
	Control	Service	Beds	Admissions	Census	Outpatient Visits	Births	Total	Payroll	Personnel

★ American Hospital Association (AHA) membership
☐ Joint Commission on Accreditation of Healthcare Organizations (JCAHO) accreditation
+ American Osteopathic Hospital Association (AOHA) membership
○ American Osteopathic Association (AOA) accreditation
△ Commission on Accreditation of Rehabilitation Facilities (CARF) accreditation
Control codes 61, 63, 64, 71, 72 and 73 indicate hospitals listed by AOHA, but not registered by AHA. For definition of numerical codes, see page A6

Hospital	Control	Service	Beds	Admissions	Census	Outpatient Visits	Births	Total	Payroll	Personnel
★ LOGAN GENERAL HOSPITAL, 20 Hospital Drive, Zip 25601; tel. 304/792–1101; C. David Morrison, President **A**1 10 12 **F**8 11 15 16 19 20 21 22 34 37 40 41 42 44 49 54 55 56 58 65 71 **P**6	23	10	132	7508	100	164070	635	61567	32573	877
MADISON—Boone County										
★ BOONE MEMORIAL HOSPITAL, 701 Madison Avenue, Zip 25130; tel. 304/369–1230; Tommy H. Mullins, Administrator **A**1 9 10 **F**15 16 19 22 24 32 34 44 45 49 65 71 73	13	10	38	843	17	38171	0	3968	2333	111
MAN—Logan County										
☐ MAN ARH HOSPITAL, 700 East McDonald Avenue, Zip 25635–1011; tel. 304/583–8421; Adrian Farmer, Administrator **A**1 9 10 **F**3 4 7 8 10 11 12 13 14 15 16 17 19 21 22 25 28 29 30 31 32 34 35 36 37 38 39 40 43 44 45 46 47 49 52 56 58 60 64 65 69 70 71 73 74 **P**4 5 **S**0145 Appalachian Regional Healthcare	23	10	42	1469	15	18549	0	9632	4423	136
MARLINTON—Pocahontas County										
★ POCAHONTAS MEMORIAL HOSPITAL, 103 Eighth Street, Zip 24954–9999; tel. 304/799–7400; Al Lawson, Administrator **A**9 10 **F**1 14 15 16 21 22 26 28 29 30 32 33 34 41 44 45 46 48 49 51 64 65 71 72 73	13	10	40	686	12	10247	0	3113	1359	79
MARTINSBURG—Berkeley County										
★ CITY HOSPITAL, Dry Run Road, Zip 25401, Mailing Address: P.O. Box 1418, Zip 25401–1418; tel. 304/264–1000; Peter L. Mulford, Administrator **A**1 2 9 10 **F**1 3 7 8 11 12 15 17 19 21 22 23 24 28 30 32 33 34 35 37 39 40 41 42 44 45 46 48 49 52 54 57 58 59 65 66 71 73 74 **P**3 **S**0002 Quorum Health Group/Quorum Health Resources	23	10	182	7068	112	81841	747	41047	16610	656
★ VETERANS AFFAIRS MEDICAL CENTER, Charles Town Road, Zip 25401–0205; tel. 304/263–0811; Richard Pell Jr., Director (Total facility includes 150 beds in nursing home–type unit) **A**1 3 5 **F**2 3 4 5 8 10 14 15 16 19 20 21 22 25 26 28 31 33 34 35 37 41 42 44 45 46 49 50 51 52 54 56 57 58 60 63 64 65 70 71 72 73 74 **S**9295 Department of Veterans Affairs	45	10	771	4959	693	135016	0	77625	45217	1268
MONTGOMERY—Fayette County										
★ MONTGOMERY GENERAL HOSPITAL, 401 Sixth Avenue, Zip 25136–0270, Mailing Address: P.O. Box 270, Zip 25136–0270; tel. 304/442–5151; Kenneth R. Fultz, President (Total facility includes 44 beds in nursing home–type unit) **A**1 9 10 **F**14 15 16 19 22 34 44 63 64 65	23	10	90	1849	68	92155	0	17857	7178	273
MORGANTOWN—Monongalia County										
☐ CHESTNUT RIDGE HOSPITAL, 930 Chestnut Ridge Road, Zip 26505; tel. 304/293–4000; Lawrence J. Drake, Chief Executive Officer (Nonreporting) **A**1 9 10 **S**0405 Ramsay Health Care, Inc.	33	22	62	—	—	—	—	—	—	—
★ MONONGALIA GENERAL HOSPITAL, 1200 J. D. Anderson Drive, Zip 26505; tel. 304/598–1200; Thomas J. Senker, President and Chief Executive Officer **A**1 3 5 9 10 **F**4 7 8 10 11 12 14 15 16 17 19 22 23 25 28 30 31 32 33 34 35 37 40 42 43 44 46 49 54 61 63 65 66 67 71 73 74 **P**3 7	23	10	198	8307	133	85249	492	64253	27612	888
★ WEST VIRGINIA UNIVERSITY HOSPITALS, Medical Center Drive, Zip 26506–4749; tel. 304/598–4000; Bernard G. Westfall, President **A**1 2 3 5 8 9 10 **F**2 3 4 7 8 10 11 17 19 20 21 22 23 25 26 28 29 30 31 32 33 34 35 37 38 40 41 42 43 44 45 46 47 49 50 51 52 53 54 55 56 57 58 59 60 61 63 64 65 66 69 70 71 73 **P**6	23	10	330	15056	254	320054	1540	164851	62555	2204
NEW MARTINSVILLE—Wetzel County										
★ WETZEL COUNTY HOSPITAL, 3 East Benjamin Drive, Zip 26155; tel. 304/455–8000; Daniel C. Dunmyer, Chief Executive Officer **A**1 9 10 **F**7 8 13 14 15 16 17 19 21 22 24 28 30 32 33 34 37 40 44 45 46 65 67 70 71 73 **P**4	13	10	55	2146	26	42393	171	14387	5349	270
OAK HILL—Fayette County										
☐ PLATEAU MEDICAL CENTER, 430 Main Street, Zip 25901; tel. 304/469–8600; Albert H. Michaels, Administrator **A**1 9 10 **F**8 10 14 15 16 19 22 26 32 33 34 37 44 45 49 63 65 71 73 **S**6525 Ornda Healthcorp	33	10	80	2719	53	21730	0	15388	5431	253
PARKERSBURG—Wood County										
★ CAMDEN–CLARK MEMORIAL HOSPITAL, 800 Garfield Avenue, Zip 26101, Mailing Address: P.O. Box 718, Zip 26102–0718; tel. 304/424–2111; Thomas J. Corder, President and Chief Executive Officer **A**1 2 9 10 **F**7 8 11 12 14 15 17 19 21 22 23 24 25 28 30 35 37 40 41 42 44 45 46 49 60 63 65 67 71 73 74 **P**7	14	10	214	10272	155	136624	894	68795	28878	1063
★ ST. JOSEPH'S HOSPITAL, 1824 Murdoch Avenue, Zip 26101, Mailing Address: Box 327, Zip 26102–0327; tel. 304/424–4382; Arthur A. Maher, President and Chief Executive Officer (Total facility includes 20 beds in nursing home–type unit) **A**1 10 **F**7 8 10 11 15 16 17 19 21 22 23 24 27 28 29 30 31 32 34 35 37 39 40 41 42 44 46 49 52 53 54 55 56 57 64 65 66 67 71 73 74 **P**5	21	10	294	9553	155	131732	470	61407	27002	1090
☐ △ WESTERN HILLS REHABILITATION HOSPITAL, 3 Western Hills Drive, Zip 26101, Mailing Address: P.O. Box 1428, Zip 26102–1428; tel. 304/420–1300; Claudia A. Eisenmann, Chief Executive Officer **A**1 7 9 10 **F**12 14 15 16 27 48 49 65 66 67 73	33	46	40	615	36	4629	0	8916	4124	130
PETERSBURG—Grant County										
★ GRANT MEMORIAL HOSPITAL, Mailing Address: Box 1019, Zip 26847; tel. 304/257–1026; Robert L. Harman, Administrator (Total facility includes 10 beds in nursing home–type unit) **A**9 10 **F**8 12 13 15 17 19 21 22 26 28 29 30 32 33 34 37 40 42 44 58 64 65 71 74	13	10	65	2665	40	64008	355	13808	6028	307
PHILIPPI—Barbour County										
BROADDUS HOSPITAL, College Hill, Zip 26416; tel. 304/457–1760; Susannah Higgins, Administrator (Nonreporting) **A**9 10	23	10	12	—	—	—	—	—	—	—

Hospitals, U.S. / WEST VIRGINIA

Hospital, Address, Telephone, Administrator, Approval, Facility, and Physician Codes, Health Care System	Classification Codes		Utilization Data					Expense (thousands) of dollars		
	Control	Service	Beds	Admissions	Census	Outpatient Visits	Births	Total	Payroll	Personnel

★ American Hospital Association (AHA) membership
□ Joint Commission on Accreditation of Healthcare Organizations (JCAHO) accreditation
+ American Osteopathic Hospital Association (AOHA) membership
○ American Osteopathic Association (AOA) accreditation
△ Commission on Accreditation of Rehabilitation Facilities (CARF) accreditation
Control codes 61, 63, 64, 71, 72 and 73 indicate hospitals listed by AOHA, but not registered by AHA. For definition of numerical codes, see page A6

POINT PLEASANT—Mason County										
★ PLEASANT VALLEY HOSPITAL, 2520 Valley Drive, Zip 25550–2083; tel. 304/675–4340; Michael G. Sellards, Executive Director (Total facility includes 100 beds in nursing home–type unit) **A**1 9 10 **F**7 8 17 19 21 22 23 24 31 32 34 35 37 40 42 44 49 63 64 65 67 71 73 **P**8	23	10	208	4173	152	45847	213	32224	14163	573
PRINCETON—Mercer County										
★ PRINCETON COMMUNITY HOSPITAL, 12th Street, Zip 24740–1369, Mailing Address: P.O. Box 1369, Zip 24740–1369; tel. 304/487–7000; William L. Sheppard, Chief Executive Officer (Total facility includes 23 beds in nursing home–type unit) **A**1 9 10 **F**3 4 7 8 11 14 15 16 17 19 20 21 22 23 26 28 30 31 32 33 34 35 37 39 40 41 42 44 45 46 49 51 52 53 54 55 56 57 58 59 60 63 64 65 66 69 71 72 73 **P**3 8	14	10	211	8674	146	92295	547	51840	24583	994
★ △ SOUTHERN HILLS REGIONAL REHABILITATION HOSPITAL, 120 Twelfth Street, Zip 24740; tel. 304/487–8000; Glenn R. Sago, Administrator **A**1 7 9 10 **F**12 15 16 27 34 48 49 65 66 67 **P**6	33	46	40	669	35	7666	0	10323	4688	147
RANSON—Jefferson County										
★ JEFFERSON MEMORIAL HOSPITAL, 300 South Preston Street, Zip 25438–1699; tel. 304/725–3411; Jon D. Applebaum, Administrator **A**1 9 10 **F**7 8 15 16 17 19 21 22 24 27 28 30 32 33 34 35 37 39 40 41 42 44 45 46 54 65 66 67 71 73	23	10	56	2759	30	35584	228	17777	8114	341
RICHWOOD—Nicholas County										
RICHWOOD AREA MEDICAL CENTER, Riverside Addition, Zip 26261, Mailing Address: Box 511, Zip 26261; tel. 304/846–2573; Enrico C. Tonelli, Administrator **A**10 **F**22 44 69 71 73	33	10	30	497	6	8401	0	3208	1085	51
RIPLEY—Jackson County										
★ JACKSON GENERAL HOSPITAL, Pinnell Street, Zip 25271, Mailing Address: P.O. Box 720, Zip 25271; tel. 304/372–2731; William S. Chapman, President **A**1 9 10 **F**7 8 11 16 19 21 22 28 34 35 37 40 44 49 65 66 71 **P**3	23	10	82	2880	29	38639	140	16003	7003	308
ROMNEY—Hampshire County										
HAMPSHIRE MEMORIAL HOSPITAL, 549 Center Avenue, Zip 26757–1199; tel. 304/822–4561; Roberta D. McCauley, Chief Executive Officer (Nonreporting) **A**9 10	33	10	47	—	—	—	—	—	—	—
RONCEVERTE—Greenbrier County										
★ GREENBRIER VALLEY MEDICAL CENTER, 202 Maplewood Avenue, Zip 24970–0497, Mailing Address: P.O. Box 497, Zip 24970–0497; tel. 304/647–4411; James B. Wood, Chief Executive Officer **A**1 9 10 12 **F**4 7 8 12 16 19 20 21 22 23 30 32 33 34 35 37 40 42 44 46 49 63 65 66 71 73 **S**0048 Columbia/HCA Healthcare Corporation	33	10	122	4300	59	32278	362	22700	9600	331
SISTERSVILLE—Tyler County										
SISTERSVILLE GENERAL HOSPITAL, 314 South Wells Street, Zip 26175; tel. 304/652–2611; (Nonreporting) **A**9 10	14	10	15	—	—	—	—	—	—	—
SOUTH CHARLESTON—Kanawha County										
★ THOMAS MEMORIAL HOSPITAL, 4605 MacCorkle Avenue S.W., Zip 25309–1398; tel. 304/766–3600; Stephen P. Dexter, Chief Executive Officer **A**1 5 9 10 **F**2 3 7 8 11 15 16 17 19 21 22 24 26 27 28 29 30 32 33 34 35 36 37 39 40 41 42 44 45 49 52 53 54 55 56 57 58 59 60 63 64 65 67 71 72 73 74 **P**1 7	23	10	216	7779	134	131130	438	60049	24482	739
SPENCER—Roane County										
★ ROANE GENERAL HOSPITAL, 200 Hospital Drive, Zip 25276; tel. 304/927–6200; Andrew Mazon, Administrator (Total facility includes 9 beds in nursing home–type unit) **A**1 9 10 **F**1 7 8 17 19 21 22 28 30 32 34 40 44 45 64 65 71 73	23	10	40	1890	24	23923	142	11294	5118	224
SUMMERSVILLE—Nicholas County										
★ SUMMERSVILLE MEMORIAL HOSPITAL, 400 Fairview Heights Road, Zip 26651–0400; tel. 304/872–2891; Gregory D. Johnson, Administrator (Total facility includes 52 beds in nursing home–type unit) **A**9 10 **F**7 8 11 16 19 22 25 26 28 30 34 35 37 40 42 44 49 51 64 65 71 72	14	10	109	2269	79	41379	296	14912	6607	306
WEBSTER SPRINGS—Webster County										
★ WEBSTER COUNTY MEMORIAL HOSPITAL, (Rural Primary Care Hospital) 324 Miller Mountain Drive, Zip 26288; tel. 304/847–5682; Stephen M. Gavalchik, Administrator **A**9 **F**2 4 7 8 9 10 11 15 16 17 19 21 22 25 26 28 29 30 33 34 35 37 38 40 41 42 44 45 46 47 48 49 51 52 54 58 60 64 65 66 67 70 71 72 73	13	49	6	208	2	10609	0	2210	1364	45
WEIRTON—Brooke County										
★ WEIRTON MEDICAL CENTER, 601 Colliers Way, Zip 26062–5091; tel. 304/797–6000; Donald Muhlenthaler FACHE, President and Chief Executive Officer (Total facility includes 23 beds in nursing home–type unit) **A**1 9 10 **F**7 8 10 11 13 14 15 16 17 19 20 21 22 24 25 26 27 28 29 30 31 32 33 34 35 37 39 40 41 42 44 45 49 52 53 55 56 57 58 59 60 63 64 65 66 67 69 70 71 73 **P**1 2	23	10	260	7360	115	76003	266	39560	18028	654
WESTON—Lewis County										
SHARPE HOSPITAL, (Formerly Weston Hospital) U.S. 33 West, Zip 26452, Mailing Address: Drawer 1127, Zip 26452; tel. 304/269–1210; Michael Todt Ph.D., Administrator **F**14 15 20 26 27 45 52 55 57 65 73 **P**6	12	22	150	1378	158	0	0	18500	8500	475
★ STONEWALL JACKSON MEMORIAL HOSPITAL, Route 4, Zip 26452, Mailing Address: Route 4, Box 10, Zip 26452; tel. 304/269–8000; David D. Shaffer, Chief Executive Officer (Total facility includes 10 beds in nursing home–type unit) **A**1 9 10 **F**7 8 19 20 21 22 35 37 40 42 44 45 64 65 71 **P**8	23	10	70	2648	29	44966	240	13744	6503	221
WESTON HOSPITAL See Sharpe Hospital										

© 1995 AHA Guide

Hospitals, U.S. / WEST VIRGINIA

Hospital, Address, Telephone, Administrator, Approval, Facility, and Physician Codes, Health Care System ★ American Hospital Association (AHA) membership ☐ Joint Commission on Accreditation of Healthcare Organizations (JCAHO) accreditation + American Osteopathic Hospital Association (AOHA) membership ○ American Osteopathic Association (AOA) accreditation △ Commission on Accreditation of Rehabilitation Facilities (CARF) accreditation Control codes 61, 63, 64, 71, 72 and 73 indicate hospitals listed by AOHA, but not registered by AHA. For definition of numerical codes, see page A6	Classification Codes		Utilization Data					Expense (thousands) of dollars		
	Control	Service	Beds	Admissions	Census	Outpatient Visits	Births	Total	Payroll	Personnel
WHEELING—Ohio County										
☐ OHIO VALLEY MEDICAL CENTER, 2000 Eoff Street, Zip 26003; tel. 304/234-0123; Thomas P. Galinski, President and Chief Executive Officer (Total facility includes 172 beds in nursing home–type unit) **A**1 2 3 5 9 10 12 **F**3 5 7 8 10 11 12 14 15 16 17 18,19 21 22 23 24 26 27 28 29 30 31 32 34 35 37 39 40 41 42 44 45 47 48 49 51 52 54 55 56 57 58 59 60 61 63 64 65 66 67 71 73 74 **P**6 8 **S**2305 Allegheny Health, Education and Research Foundation	23	10	417	6833	264	69644	414	59995	24131	883
★ WHEELING HOSPITAL, Medical Park, Zip 26003-0708; tel. 304/243-3000; Donald H. Hofreuter M.D., Administrator and Chief Executive Officer **A**1 2 3 5 9 10 **F**3 4 7 8 10 11 13 15 16 17 19 20 21 22 23 24 26 27 28 29 30 31 32 34 35 37 39 40 41 42 43 44 45 46 49 51 54 55 56 58 59 60 65 66 67 70 71 72 73 74 **P**8	23	10	276	11283	169	193501	1163	81820	36929	1315
WILLIAMSON—Mingo County										
☐ WILLIAMSON MEMORIAL HOSPITAL, 859 Alderson Street, Zip 25661, Mailing Address: P.O. Box 1980, Zip 25661; tel. 304/235-2500; Roger C. LeDoux, Administrator **A**1 9 10 **F**7 8 12 16 19 21 22 28 30 31 34 37 39 44 45 46 63 65 70 71 **P**1 8 **S**1775 Health Management Associates	33	10	76	3510	48	26012	322	15922	5621	229

WISCONSIN

Resident population 5,038 (in thousands)
Resident population in metro areas 68.1%
Birth rate per 1,000 population 14.5
65 years and over 13.4%
Percent of persons without health insurance 7.9%

Hospital, Address, Telephone, Administrator, Approval, Facility, and Physician Codes, Health Care System	Classification Codes		Utilization Data					Expense (thousands) of dollars		
	Control	Service	Beds	Admissions	Census	Outpatient Visits	Births	Total	Payroll	Personnel

★ American Hospital Association (AHA) membership
☐ Joint Commission on Accreditation of Healthcare Organizations (JCAHO) accreditation
+ American Osteopathic Hospital Association (AOHA) membership
○ American Osteopathic Association (AOA) accreditation
△ Commission on Accreditation of Rehabilitation Facilities (CARF) accreditation
Control codes 61, 63, 64, 71, 72 and 73 indicate hospitals listed by AOHA, but not registered by AHA. For definition of numerical codes, see page A6

Hospital	Control	Service	Beds	Admissions	Census	Outpatient Visits	Births	Total	Payroll	Personnel
AMERY—Polk County ★ APPLE RIVER HOSPITAL, 230 Deronda Street, Zip 54001-1412; tel. 715/268-7151; Michael Karuschak Jr., Administrator **A**1 9 10 **F**7 8 11 17 19 21 22 27 33 35 36 37 39 40 42 44 48 49 65 71 73 **S**0002 Quorum Health Group/Quorum Health Resources	23	10	13	958	9	11337	127	6286	2638	104
ANTIGO—Langlade County ☐ LANGLADE MEMORIAL HOSPITAL, 112 East Fifth Avenue, Zip 54409-2796; tel. 715/623-2331; David R. Schneider, Executive Director **A**1 9 10 **F**1 2 3 7 8 10 19 21 22 28 32 33 35 36 40 42 44 45 49 52 62 63 65 67 71 73	21	10	49	1937	27	27038	274	14175	6612	254
APPLETON—Outagamie County ★ APPLETON MEDICAL CENTER, 1818 North Meade Street, Zip 54911; tel. 414/731-4101; Walter L. Edwards, President **A**1 2 3 5 9 10 **F**3 4 6 7 8 10 12 13 17 18 19 21 22 23 26 28 30 32 34 35 37 39 40 41 43 44 45 51 60 61 62 65 66 67 68 69 71 72 **S**2445 United Health Group	23	10	161	6802	94	64541	1130	62345	25753	734
★ △ ST. ELIZABETH HOSPITAL, 1506 South Oneida Street, Zip 54915-1397; tel. 414/738-2000; Otto L. Cox, President **A**1 2 3 5 7 10 **F**3 5 6 7 8 10 12 13 17 19 21 23 25 26 27 28 29 30 31 32 33 35 36 39 40 41 42 43 44 45 48 49 51 52 53 57 58 60 61 62 65 66 67 68 69 70 71 72 74 **S**6745 Wheaton Franciscan Services, Inc.	21	10	218	7953	124	185413	1312	67939	30856	940
ARCADIA—Trempealeau County ★ ST. JOSEPH'S HOSPITAL, 464 South St Joseph Avenue, Zip 54612-1401; tel. 608/323-3341; Eugene E. Molitor, Chief Administrative Officer (Total facility includes 75 beds in nursing home–type unit) **A**1 9 10 **F**7 8 12 19 22 26 28 29 30 31 32 33 34 37 40 41 42 44 45 46 49 51 61 63 64 65 66 67 71 **S**9650 Franciscan Health System, Inc.	21	10	101	416	76	11929	83	3808	1932	144
ASHLAND—Ashland County ★ MEMORIAL MEDICAL CENTER, 1615 Maple Lane, Zip 54806-3689; tel. 715/682-4563; Daniel J. Hymans, President **A**1 9 10 **F**2 3 7 8 19 20 21 22 28 33 34 35 37 39 40 41 42 44 49 52 53 56 58 63 65 66 71 73	23	10	101	3400	48	30791	319	21133	10808	354
BALDWIN—St. Croix County ★ BALDWIN HOSPITAL, (Formerly Baldwin Community Memorial Hospital) 730 10th Avenue, Zip 54002-0045; tel. 715/684-3311; Richard L. Range, Administrator **A**9 10 **F**7 8 11 17 19 22 26 28 30 32 34 35 36 37 39 40 41 42 44 45 48 49 56 64 65 66 67 70 71	23	10	27	720	7	16217	69	4949	2499	77
BARABOO—Sauk County ★ ST. CLARE HOSPITAL AND HEALTH SERVICES, 707 14th Street, Zip 53913-1597; tel. 608/356-5561; Thomas R. Warwick, President **A**1 9 10 **F**2 3 7 8 19 22 26 30 31 34 35 36 37 39 40 41 44 45 46 49 65 66 67 71 73 **S**5455 SSM Health Care System	21	10	78	2535	30	34874	274	15787	7021	276
BARRON—Barron County ☐ BARRON MEMORIAL MEDICAL CENTER, 1222 Woodland Avenue, Zip 54812; tel. 715/537-3186; Mark D. Wilson, Administrator (Total facility includes 50 beds in nursing home–type unit) **A**1 9 10 **F**7 8 17 19 22 28 34 37 39 40 41 44 45 46 49 56 62 64 65 66 67 70 71 73	23	10	92	1217	63	23002	64	7302	3628	—
BEAVER DAM—Dodge County ★ BEAVER DAM COMMUNITY HOSPITALS, 707 South University Avenue, Zip 53916-3089; tel. 414/887-7181; John R. Landdeck, President (Total facility includes 123 beds in nursing home–type unit) **A**1 9 10 **F**2 6 8 19 22 27 28 30 32 33 35 36 37 39 40 42 44 45 62 64 67	23	10	216	3462	146	42628	323	21833	11092	431
BELOIT—Rock County ☐ △ BELOIT MEMORIAL HOSPITAL, 1969 West Hart Road, Zip 53511-2299; tel. 608/364-5011; Gregory K. Britton, President and Chief Executive Officer **A**1 7 9 10 **F**5 7 8 10 12 19 20 21 22 23 25 26 27 28 30 34 35 37 39 40 41 42 44 45 46 48 49 51 53 55 57 58 60 63 65 66 67 69 71 72 73 74	23	10	148	5281	76	104115	807	38289	17561	630
BERLIN—Green Lake County ☐ COMMUNITY HEALTH NETWORK, (Includes Berlin Memorial Hospital, Juliette Manor Nursing Home, Community Clinics) 225 Memorial Drive, Zip 54923-1295; tel. 414/361-5580; Craig W C. Schmidt, President and Chief Executive Officer (Total facility includes 102 beds in nursing home–type unit) **A**1 9 10 **F**3 7 8 10 15 19 21 28 30 32 33 35 36 37 39 40 41 42 44 45 51 53 54 55 56 57 58 59 60 62 63 64 65 67 70 71 72	23	10	163	2249	122	33963	232	19145	8302	298
BLACK RIVER FALLS—Jackson County ★ BLACK RIVER MEMORIAL HOSPITAL, 711 West Adams Street, Zip 54615-9113; tel. 715/284-5361; Stanley J. Gaynor, Chief Executive Officer **A**1 10 **F**7 12 17 19 22 28 30 35 36 40 41 44 49 65 67 71 73	23	10	38	1193	13	7519	178	6165	2738	106
BLOOMER—Chippewa County ★ BLOOMER COMMUNITY MEMORIAL HOSPITAL AND SKILLED NURSING FALILITY, 1501 Thompson Street, Zip 54724; tel. 715/568-2000; John Perushek, Administrator (Total facility includes 75 beds in nursing home–type unit) **A**1 9 10 **F**7 8 17 18 19 20 21 22 26 28 30 31 32 33 34 37 40 44 48 49 51 53 54 56 57 58 61 62 64 65 66 67 71 73 74	23	10	104	587	78	8923	65	4797	2560	132

© 1995 AHA Guide

Hospitals, U.S. / WISCONSIN

Hospital, Address, Telephone, Administrator, Approval, Facility, and Physician Codes, Health Care System	Classi-fication Codes		Utilization Data					Expense (thousands) of dollars		
★ American Hospital Association (AHA) membership □ Joint Commission on Accreditation of Healthcare Organizations (JCAHO) accreditation + American Osteopathic Hospital Association (AOHA) membership ○ American Osteopathic Association (AOA) accreditation △ Commission on Accreditation of Rehabilitation Facilities (CARF) accreditation Control codes 61, 63, 64, 71, 72 and 73 indicate hospitals listed by AOHA, but not registered by AHA. For definition of numerical codes, see page A6	Control	Service	Beds	Admissions	Census	Outpatient Visits	Births	Total	Payroll	Personnel
BOSCOBEL—Grant County BOSCOBEL AREA HEALTH CARE, 205 Parker Street, Zip 53805; tel. 608/375–4112; (Total facility includes 88 beds in nursing home–type unit) **A**9 10 **F**7 8 17 18 19 22 26 28 29 30 41 44 45 52 56 58 59 65 67 70 72	23	10	132	1183	90	9804	72	—	—	—
BROOKFIELD—Waukesha County ★ △ ELMBROOK MEMORIAL HOSPITAL, 19333 West North Avenue, Zip 53045–4198; tel. 414/785–2000; Kimry A. Johnsrud, President **A**1 7 9 10 **F**2 3 7 8 10 19 21 23 25 26 32 34 35 37 38 39 40 41 42 44 45 48 49 53 54 55 56 57 58 59 60 61 63 65 66 70 71 74 **S**6745 Wheaton Franciscan Services, Inc.	21	10	136	4939	62	53147	895	37725	15653	450
BURLINGTON—Racine County ★ MEMORIAL HOSPITAL, 252 McHenry Street, Zip 53105–1828; tel. 414/763–2411; Paul A. Miller, President and Chief Executive Officer **A**1 9 10 **F**8 10 19 21 22 26 34 35 37 40 41 44 45 46 65 71 73 74	23	10	87	3398	38	50016	584	29754	12056	361
CHILTON—Calumet County ★ CALUMET MEDICAL CENTER, 614 Memorial Drive, Zip 53014; tel. 414/849–2386; Joseph L. Schumacher, Administrator **A**9 10 **F**8 12 17 19 20 22 30 32 34 36 37 39 42 44 46 49 65 71 73	23	10	53	841	11	28352	0	8575	3698	144
CHIPPEWA FALLS—Chippewa County ★ ST. JOSEPH'S HOSPITAL, 2661 County Road I, Zip 54729–1498; tel. 715/723–1811; David B. Fish, Executive Vice President **A**1 9 10 **F**2 3 7 8 17 19 21 22 28 29 30 32 33 37 39 40 41 42 44 45 46 65 71 73 **S**5355 Hospital Sisters Health System	21	10	127	3487	61	47389	379	22642	10943	373
COLUMBUS—Columbia County ★ COLUMBUS COMMUNITY HOSPITAL, 1515 Park Avenue, Zip 53925; tel. 414/623–2200; Miles Meyer, Administrator **A**1 9 10 **F**7 8 17 19 22 25 26 30 32 37 40 41 44 46 49 51 63 65 71 72 74	23	10	53	1571	21	24384	123	9193	4125	137
CUBA CITY—Grant County CUBA CITY MEDICAL CENTER See Southwest Health Center, Platteville										
CUDAHY—Milwaukee County ★ △ TRINITY MEMORIAL HOSPITAL, 5900 South Lake Drive, Zip 53110–8903; tel. 414/769–9000; Terrance E. Wilson, Interim Chief Operating Officer (Nonreporting) **A**1 2 7 9 10 **S**5175 Catholic Health Corporation	21	10	178	—	—	—	—	—	—	—
CUMBERLAND—Barron County □ CUMBERLAND MEMORIAL HOSPITAL, 1110 Seventh Avenue, Zip 54829, Mailing Address: Box 37, Zip 54829–0037; tel. 715/822–2741; James M. O'Keefe, Administrator (Total facility includes 51 beds in nursing home–type unit) **A**1 9 10 **F**1 7 8 18 22 26 27 30 34 40 41 42 44 49 52 56 57 58 62 64 65 66 67 71 73	23	10	91	1506	68	7110	102	7367	3653	149
DARLINGTON—Lafayette County MEMORIAL HOSPITAL OF LAFAYETTE COUNTY, 800 Clay Street, Zip 53530, Mailing Address: P.O. Box 70, Zip 53530; tel. 608/776–4466; Don Easley, Administrator **A**9 10 **F**7 8 17 19 28 30 33 35 40 44 65 71	13	10	28	660	5	13746	78	3289	1216	50
DODGEVILLE—Iowa County ★ MEMORIAL HOSPITAL OF IOWA COUNTY, 825 South Iowa Street, Zip 53533–1999; tel. 608/935–2711; Ray Marmorstone, Administrator (Total facility includes 44 beds in nursing home–type unit) **A**1 9 10 **F**7 8 12 13 15 17 19 22 32 33 35 37 39 40 42 44 45 49 64 65 66 67 71 72 **S**0585 Brim, Inc.	23	10	82	1398	53	27386	203	10316	4643	200
DURAND—Pepin County ★ CHIPPEWA VALLEY HOSPITAL AND OAKVIEW CARE CENTER, 1220 Third Avenue West, Zip 54736, Mailing Address: P.O. Box 224, Zip 54736–0224; tel. 715/672–4211; Malcolm P. Cole, President (Total facility includes 60 beds in nursing home–type unit) **A**9 10 **F**7 8 17 19 21 22 26 28 34 36 39 40 41 44 45 64 65 71 72	21	10	90	713	67	8879	68	5451	2310	102
EAGLE RIVER—Vilas County ★ EAGLE RIVER MEMORIAL HOSPITAL, Mailing Address: P.O. Box 129, Zip 54521–0129; tel. 715/479–7411; Patricia Richardson, President **A**9 10 **F**3 6 8 21 22 27 28 32 33 34 36 40 44 49 64 71	23	10	8	675	8	12740	31	4758	2169	98
EAU CLAIRE—Eau Claire County ★ LUTHER HOSPITAL, 1221 Whipple Street, Zip 54702–4105; tel. 715/839–3311; William Rupp M.D., President and Chief Executive Officer **A**1 2 3 5 9 10 **F**2 3 4 7 8 9 10 11 12 17 19 21 22 23 29 32 33 34 35 37 38 39 40 41 42 43 44 45 46 47 48 52 53 54 55 56 57 58 59 60 61 63 65 66 67 69 70 71 73 74 **S**1875 Mayo Foundation	23	10	207	7376	104	86519	872	54217	25203	763
★ SACRED HEART HOSPITAL, 900 West Clairemont Avenue, Zip 54701–5105; tel. 715/839–4121; Matthew W. Hubler, Executive Vice President **A**1 2 3 5 9 10 **F**7 8 12 15 17 19 21 23 24 25 26 27 28 29 30 31 32 33 34 35 36 37 38 39 40 41 42 44 45 46 47 48 49 51 52 53 54 55 56 57 58 59 60 61 62 63 65 66 67 68 70 71 72 73 74 **S**5355 Hospital Sisters Health System	21	10	301	6923	100	83221	816	46847	21693	736
EDGERTON—Rock County MEMORIAL COMMUNITY HOSPITAL, 313 Stoughton Road, Zip 53534–1198; tel. 608/884–3441; John P. Kosanovich, Chief Executive Officer (Total facility includes 61 beds in nursing home–type unit) **A**9 10 **F**8 19 22 26 32 33 34 35 37 39 41 44 45 49 63 64 65 66 71 74	23	10	101	950	76	15500	0	—	—	—

Hospitals, U.S. / WISCONSIN

Hospital, Address, Telephone, Administrator, Approval, Facility, and Physician Codes, Health Care System	Classification Codes		Utilization Data					Expense (thousands) of dollars		Personnel
	Control	Service	Beds	Admissions	Census	Outpatient Visits	Births	Total	Payroll	

★ American Hospital Association (AHA) membership
□ Joint Commission on Accreditation of Healthcare Organizations (JCAHO) accreditation
+ American Osteopathic Hospital Association (AOHA) membership
○ American Osteopathic Association (AOA) accreditation
△ Commission on Accreditation of Rehabilitation Facilities (CARF) accreditation
Control codes 61, 63, 64, 71, 72 and 73 indicate hospitals listed by AOHA, but not registered by AHA. For definition of numerical codes, see page A6

Hospital Entry	Control	Service	Beds	Admissions	Census	Outpatient Visits	Births	Total	Payroll	Personnel
ELKHORN—Walworth County ★ △ LAKELAND MEDICAL CENTER, Highway NN, Zip 53121-1002, Mailing Address: Box 1002, Zip 53121-1002; tel. 414/741-2000; Loren J. Anderson, Administrator and Chief Executive Officer **A**1 7 9 10 **F**3 7 8 10 19 21 22 28 30 32 33 34 35 37 40 41 42 44 45 49 53 54 56 57 59 60 63 65 66 67 71 73 74	13	10	88	3371	43	45762	375	28637	11977	385
FOND DU LAC—Fond Du Lac County ★ △ ST. AGNES HOSPITAL, 430 East Division Street, Zip 54936-0385; tel. 414/929-2300; James J. Sexton, President and Chief Executive Officer **A**1 2 7 9 10 **F**1 3 5 7 8 10 17 18 19 21 22 23 26 28 29 30 31 32 33 34 35 36 37 39 40 41 42 44 45 48 49 52 53 54 55 56 57 58 59 60 63 65 66 67 68 71 73 74 **S**5695 Congregation of St. Agnes	21	10	161	6603	98	204526	1039	57554	27657	776
FORT ATKINSON—Jefferson County ★ FORT ATKINSON MEMORIAL HEALTH SERVICES, 611 East Sherman Avenue, Zip 53538-1998; tel. 414/568-5000; John C. Albaugh, President **A**1 9 10 **F**2 3 7 8 12 19 22 27 28 30 32 33 34 35 37 39 40 41 44 45 46 48 49 51 63 65 66 67 71 72 74	23	10	96	4163	48	94041	396	28102	13224	400
FRIENDSHIP—Adams County □ ADAMS COUNTY MEMORIAL HOSPITAL AND NURSING CARE UNIT, 402 West Lake Street, Zip 53934, Mailing Address: P.O. Box 40, Zip 53934; tel. 608/339-3331; Allen Teal, Administrator (Total facility includes 18 beds in nursing home–type unit) **A**1 9 10 **F**1 8 17 19 22 25 26 27 28 29 30 32 34 35 41 42 44 49 56 62 64 65 67 71 73	23	10	58	665	27	21401	0	6770	3378	150
GRANTSBURG—Burnett County BURNETT GENERAL HOSPITAL, 257 West St. George Avenue, Zip 54840-7827; tel. 715/463-5353; Thomas R. Lemon, Chief Executive Officer (Total facility includes 53 beds in nursing home–type unit) **A**9 10 **F**1 7 8 12 17 19 21 22 26 30 34 35 40 41 42 44 45 46 49 51 64 65 67 71	23	10	84	640	54	9196	52	3617	1967	96
GREEN BAY—Brown County ★ BELLIN MEMORIAL HOSPITAL, 725 South Webster Avenue, Zip 54301, Mailing Address: P.O. Box 23400, Zip 54305-3400; tel. 414/433-3500; George Kerwin, President **A**1 9 10 **F**4 6 7 8 10 11 17 19 21 23 24 27 28 29 30 32 33 34 35 39 40 41 42 43 44 45 46 49 51 63 65 66 67 71 72 73	21	10	167	7021	86	76941	1531	71575	31729	1113
□ BELLIN PSYCHIATRIC CENTER, 301 East St. Joseph Street, Zip 54301, Mailing Address: P.O. Box 23725, Zip 54305-3725; tel. 414/433-3630; Robert W. Fry, President **A**1 10 **F**2 3 4 7 8 10 11 17 19 21 24 26 30 32 33 34 35 37 40 41 43 44 46 48 49 50 52 53 55 56 57 58 59 63 65 66 72 73	21	22	60	1693	44	11672	0	8290	3743	120
□ BROWN COUNTY MENTAL HEALTH CENTER, 2900 St. Anthony Drive, Zip 54311; tel. 414/468-1136; Mark Quam, Executive Director **A**1 10 **F**2 3 22 52 53 54 55 56 57 58 65 73	13	22	77	1751	61	30507	0	9772	5611	202
★ ST. MARY'S HOSPITAL MEDICAL CENTER, 1726 Shawano Avenue, Zip 54303-3282; tel. 414/498-4200; James G. Coller, Executive Vice President and Administrator **A**1 9 10 **F**7 8 19 21 22 24 28 29 30 34 36 37 39 40 42 44 45 49 56 61 63 65 70 71 72 **S**5355 Hospital Sisters Health System	21	10	120	4979	62	75338	717	39032	17265	516
★ △ ST. VINCENT HOSPITAL, 835 South Van Buren Street, Zip 54301, Mailing Address: P.O. Box 13508, Zip 54307-3508; tel. 414/433-0111; Joseph J. Neidenbach, Administrator and Executive Vice President **A**1 2 7 9 10 **F**4 7 8 10 11 12 17 19 20 21 22 23 25 29 30 32 33 34 35 36 37 38 39 40 41 42 43 44 45 46 48 49 65 67 68 71 72 73 **S**5355 Hospital Sisters Health System	21	10	349	13256	211	99371	1744	111110	52775	1595
GREENFIELD—Milwaukee County CPC GREENBRIAR BEHAVIORAL HEALTH CENTER See Milwaukee										
HARTFORD—Washington County ★ HARTFORD MEMORIAL HOSPITAL, 1032 East Sumner Street, Zip 53027; tel. 414/673-2300; Mark Schwartz, President **A**1 9 10 **F**1 7 8 10 11 12 17 19 20 21 22 24 26 27 30 31 32 33 34 35 36 37 39 40 41 42 43 44 45 46 49 50 51 53 54 55 56 57 58 59 60 61 63 65 66 67 68 69 70 71 72 73 74	23	10	58	1601	29	28444	219	15168	7078	248
HAYWARD—Sawyer County ★ HAYWARD AREA MEMORIAL HOSPITAL AND NURSING HOME, Mailing Address: Route 3, Box 3999, Zip 54843; tel. 715/634-8911; Barbara A. Peickert R.N., Chief Executive Officer (Total facility includes 76 beds in nursing home–type unit) **A**1 9 10 **F**7 8 17 19 21 22 26 28 30 33 40 42 44 49 50 64 65 66 71 73	23	10	117	970	91	24708	82	7120	3479	111
HAZEL GREEN—Grant County HAZEL GREEN HOSPITAL See Southwest Health Center, Platteville										
HILLSBORO—Vernon County ★ ST. JOSEPH'S MEMORIAL HOSPITAL AND NURSING HOME, 400 Water Avenue, Zip 54634-0527, Mailing Address: P.O. Box 527, Zip 54634-0527; tel. 608/489-2211; Jacqueline Pavelski, Chief Executive Officer (Total facility includes 65 beds in nursing home–type unit) **A**1 9 10 **F**7 8 19 21 22 39 40 41 44 45 49 54 56 57 64 **S**0585 Brim, Inc.	21	10	85	510	64	18930	55	4270	2199	119
HUDSON—St. Croix County □ HUDSON MEDICAL CENTER, 400 Wisconsin Street, Zip 54016-1600; tel. 715/386-9321; John W. Marnell, Chief Executive Officer **A**1 9 10 **F**1 2 3 7 8 19 22 27 28 30 32 33 35 36 37 39 40 41 44 49 65 66 67 71 73	23	10	49	1255	23	17432	166	8155	4139	163

© 1995 AHA Guide

Hospitals, U.S. / WISCONSIN

Hospital, Address, Telephone, Administrator, Approval, Facility, and Physician Codes, Health Care System	Classification Codes		Utilization Data					Expense (thousands) of dollars		
	Control	Service	Beds	Admissions	Census	Outpatient Visits	Births	Total	Payroll	Personnel

★ American Hospital Association (AHA) membership
☐ Joint Commission on Accreditation of Healthcare Organizations (JCAHO) accreditation
+ American Osteopathic Hospital Association (AOHA) membership
○ American Osteopathic Association (AOA) accreditation
△ Commission on Accreditation of Rehabilitation Facilities (CARF) accreditation
Control codes 61, 63, 64, 71, 72 and 73 indicate hospitals listed by AOHA, but not registered by AHA. For definition of numerical codes, see page A6

JANESVILLE—Rock County

★ MERCY HEALTH SYSTEM, (Formerly Mercy Hospital of Janesville) (Includes Parkside Lodge of Wisconsin, 320 Lincoln Street, Zip 53547, Mailing Address: Box 749, Zip 53547-0749; tel. 608/754-2264; Ron Del Ciello, Executive Director) 1000 Mineral Point Avenue, Zip 53545-5003, Mailing Address: P.O. Box 5003, Zip 53547-5003; tel. 608/756-6000; Javon R. Bea, President and Chief Executive Officer **A**1 3 9 10 **F**1 2 3 4 5 6 7 8 9 10 12 13 17 18 19 21 22 23 24 25 26 28 29 30 32 33 34 35 36 37 39 40 41 42 43 44 45 46 48 49 51 52 53 54 55 56 57 58 59 60 61 62 63 64 65 66 67 70 71 72 73 74	23	10	241	9351	132	316701	1352	90145	42992	1065

KAUKAUNA—Outagamie County

★ KAUKAUNA COMMUNITY HOSPITAL, 308 East 14th Street, Zip 54130; tel. 414/766-4211; Gregory S. Holub, President and Chief Executive Officer **A**1 9 10 **F**3 5 6 7 8 10 12 13 17 19 21 25 26 27 28 29 30 31 32 34 35 36 39 40 41 42 44 45 46 51 53 57 58 60 61 62 67 68 69 70 71 72 74 **S**6745 Wheaton Franciscan Services, Inc.	21	10	40	708	15	13963	119	5056	2047	58

KENOSHA—Kenosha County

★ KENOSHA HOSPITAL AND MEDICAL CENTER, 6308 Eighth Avenue, Zip 53143; tel. 414/656-2011; Richard O. Schmidt Jr., President and Chief Executive Officer **A**1 9 10 **F**3 4 5 7 8 10 19 21 22 23 24 26 28 29 30 31 32 33 34 35 36 37 39 40 41 42 43 44 49 51 53 54 55 56 57 58 63 65 66 67 71 72 73 74 **S**0027 Horizon Healthcare, Inc.	23	10	128	5508	64	86784	738	47204	21851	626
★ ST. CATHERINE'S HOSPITAL, 3556 Seventh Avenue, Zip 53140-2595; tel. 414/656-3011; Bruce Rampage, President and Chief Executive Officer **A**1 3 5 9 10 **F**3 7 8 10 12 17 19 20 21 22 23 24 25 26 28 29 30 31 32 33 34 35 36 37 39 40 41 42 43 44 46 48 49 52 54 55 56 57 58 60 63 65 66 69 70 71 73 74 **S**5175 Catholic Health Corporation	21	10	170	7471	100	121724	859	45404	20986	647

KEWAUNEE—Kewaunee County

☐ ST. MARY'S KEWAUNEE AREA MEMORIAL HOSPITAL, First and Lincoln Streets, Zip 54216; tel. 414/388-2210; Dennis Mack, President and Chief Executive Officer **A**1 9 10 **F**7 21 22 25 32 33 34 40 41 44 46 49 51 65 71 72	23	10	17	284	4	10643	32	2650	1274	60

LA CROSSE—La Crosse County

★ △ LUTHERAN HOSPITAL–LA CROSSE, 1910 South Avenue, Zip 54601-9980; tel. 608/785-0530; Jack Schwem, President and Chief Executive Officer (Data for 364 days) **A**1 2 5 7 9 10 **F**3 6 7 8 11 12 13 15 17 18 19 20 21 22 26 27 28 29 30 31 35 36 37 38 39 40 42 44 47 48 51 52 53 54 55 56 57 58 59 60 61 62 63 67 68 69 70 72	23	10	313	14308	204	115927	1521	114745	52870	1736
★ ST. FRANCIS MEDICAL CENTER, 700 West Avenue South, Zip 54601-4783; tel. 608/785-0940; Ronald R. Paczkowski, Chief Executive Officer **A**1 2 3 9 10 **F**2 3 4 6 7 8 10 11 12 17 18 19 20 21 22 23 24 25 26 27 28 29 30 32 33 34 35 36 37 38 39 40 41 42 43 44 45 46 47 48 49 51 52 53 54 55 56 57 58 59 60 61 62 64 65 66 67 70 71 72 73 **S**9650 Franciscan Health System, Inc.	21	10	226	8294	132	65526	845	53858	24832	732

LADYSMITH—Rusk County

RUSK COUNTY MEMORIAL HOSPITAL AND NURSING HOME, 900 College Avenue West, Zip 54848-2116; tel. 715/532-5561; J. Michael Shaw, Administrator (Total facility includes 107 beds in nursing home-type unit) **A**9 10 **F**2 3 7 8 9 19 21 22 26 30 34 35 37 38 40 41 44 45 48 49 51 52 53 54 55 56 57 58 59 61 64 65 67 71 73	13	10	142	1210	109	21705	163	8850	3887	173

LANCASTER—Grant County

★ LANCASTER MEMORIAL HOSPITAL, 507 South Monroe Street, Zip 53813; tel. 608/723-2143; Gregory E. Patten, Administrator **A**1 9 10 **F**3 7 8 19 21 25 26 33 34 35 40 41 42 44 45 46 49 61 65 66 70 71 **S**0585 Brim, Inc.	14	10	31	994	10	25664	134	5542	2247	96

MADISON—Dane County

☐ MENDOTA MENTAL HEALTH INSTITUTE, 301 Troy Drive, Zip 53704; tel. 608/243-2500; Steve Watters, Chief Executive Officer **A**1 3 5 10 **F**25 26 30 31 39 52 55 56 57 58 65	12	22	295	798	243	9975	0	32751	20634	635
★ △ MERITER HOSPITAL, (Includes Meriter–Methodist Hospital, 309 West Washington Avenue, Madison, Wisconsin, Zip 53703; tel. 608/251-2371; Meriter/Park Hospital, 202 South Park Street, Madison, Wisconsin, Zip 53715; tel. 608/267-6000) 202 South Park Street, Zip 53715-1599; tel. 608/267-6000; Terri L. Potter, President and Chief Executive Officer **A**1 2 3 5 7 9 10 **F**1 2 3 4 5 7 8 9 10 11 12 13 17 18 19 20 21 22 23 24 25 26 27 28 29 30 31 32 33 34 35 36 37 38 39 40 41 42 43 44 45 46 47 48 49 51 52 53 54 55 56 57 58 59 60 61 62 65 66 67 71 73 74 MERITER–METHODIST HOSPITAL See Meriter Hospital MERITER/PARK HOSPITAL See Meriter Hospital	23	10	415	16644	243	130832	3210	132599	61238	1721
★ ST. MARYS HOSPITAL MEDICAL CENTER, 707 South Mills Street, Zip 53715-0450; tel. 608/251-6100; Gerald W. Lefert, President **A**1 3 5 9 10 **F**1 4 7 8 10 11 17 19 21 22 23 32 33 35 36 37 38 40 42 43 44 45 46 47 52 53 54 55 56 57 59 65 71 73 **S**5455 SSM Health Care System	23	10	340	17399	244	38830	3007	112039	49379	1295
★ △ UNIVERSITY OF WISCONSIN HOSPITAL AND CLINICS, (Includes University of Wisconsin CHildren's Hospital) 600 Highland Avenue, Zip 53792; tel. 608/263-6400; Gordon M. Derzon, Superintendent **A**1 3 5 7 8 9 10 **F**3 4 5 8 9 10 11 12 13 17 18 19 20 21 22 23 24 25 26 27 28 29 30 31 32 33 34 35 42 43 44 45 46 47 48 49 50 51 52 53 54 55 56 57 58 60 61 63 65 66 68 69 70 71 73 74	12	10	503	17698	362	382269	0	259665	110901	3424
★ WILLIAM S. MIDDLETON MEMORIAL VETERANS HOSPITAL, 2500 Overlook Terrace, Zip 53705-2286; tel. 608/256-1901; Nathan L. Geraths, Director **A**1 3 5 **F**3 8 10 11 12 17 19 27 30 31 32 35 37 39 41 42 43 44 45 50 51 52 54 55 56 57 58 60 61 63 65 67 69 72 74 **S**9295 Department of Veterans Affairs	45	10	200	5174	143	74145	0	72077	42969	786

Hospitals, U.S. / WISCONSIN

Hospital, Address, Telephone, Administrator, Approval, Facility, and Physician Codes, Health Care System	Classification Codes		Utilization Data					Expense (thousands) of dollars		Personnel
	Control	Service	Beds	Admissions	Census	Outpatient Visits	Births	Total	Payroll	

★ American Hospital Association (AHA) membership
□ Joint Commission on Accreditation of Healthcare Organizations (JCAHO) accreditation
+ American Osteopathic Hospital Association (AOHA) membership
○ American Osteopathic Association (AOA) accreditation
△ Commission on Accreditation of Rehabilitation Facilities (CARF) accreditation
Control codes 61, 63, 64, 71, 72 and 73 indicate hospitals listed by AOHA, but not registered by AHA. For definition of numerical codes, see page A6

Hospital	Control	Service	Beds	Admissions	Census	Outpatient Visits	Births	Total	Payroll	Personnel
MANITOWOC—Manitowoc County ★ △ HOLY FAMILY MEMORIAL MEDICAL CENTER, 2300 Western Avenue, Zip 54220, Mailing Address: P.O. Box 1450, Zip 54221–1450; tel. 414/684–2011; Daniel B. McGinty, President and Chief Operating Officer **A**1 7 9 10 **F**2 3 7 8 12 19 20 21 22 23 27 28 30 32 33 34 35 37 39 40 41 42 44 48 49 50 51 52 55 56 58 59 60 63 65 66 67 71 73 **S**1455 Franciscan Sisters of Christian Charity Healthcare Ministry, Inc	21	10	216	5766	94	87794	462	41528	18231	630
MARINETTE—Marinette County ★ BAY AREA MEDICAL CENTER, 3100 Shore Drive, Zip 54143–4297; tel. 715/735–6621; Rick Ament, Chief Executive Officer **A**1 9 10 **F**3 7 8 12 19 21 22 25 26 27 28 29 32 34 35 36 39 40 44 45 52 54 55 57 60 65 66 68 71 **S**0002 Quorum Health Group/Quorum Health Resources	23	10	115	4135	57	42809	413	29458	13725	391
MARSHFIELD—Wood County NORWOOD HEALTH CENTER, 1600 North Chestnut Avenue, Zip 54449–1499; tel. 715/384–2188; Randy Bestul, Administrator **A**10 **F**52 53 57 65	13	22	19	478	9	0	0	1367	812	43
★ △ SAINT JOSEPH'S HOSPITAL, 611 St. Joseph Avenue, Zip 54449–1898; tel. 715/387–1713; Michael A. Schmidt, President and Chief Executive Officer **A**1 2 3 5 7 9 10 **F**2 3 7 8 10 11 17 19 21 22 25 27 28 31 32 33 34 35 36 37 38 39 40 41 42 43 44 45 46 47 48 49 50 52 53 54 55 56 57 58 59 61 63 65 66 67 68 69 70 71 72 73 74 **S**5305 Sisters of the Sorrowful Mother United States Health System	21	10	524	17006	305	88032	1241	134278	54022	1555
MAUSTON—Juneau County □ MILE BLUFF MEDICAL CENTER, (Formerly Hess Memorial Hospital) 1050 Division Street, Zip 53948; tel. 608/847–6161; Daniel N. Manders, President and Chief Executive Officer (Total facility includes 60 beds in nursing home–type unit) **A**1 9 10 **F**7 8 12 13 17 19 22 28 30 32 35 40 44 46 49 51 62 64 65 67 71 73	23	10	95	2134	80	43179	229	—	—	184
MEDFORD—Taylor County ★ MEMORIAL HOSPITAL OF TAYLOR COUNTY, (Includes Memorial Nursing Home) 135 South Gibson Street, Zip 54451–1696; tel. 715/748–8100; Eugene W. Arnett, President (Total facility includes 104 beds in nursing home–type unit) **A**1 9 10 **F**1 6 7 8 11 12 17 19 21 22 28 29 30 33 34 40 42 44 45 46 48 49 51 62 63 64 65 67 71	23	10	153	1227	118	21608	190	11288	6217	211
MENOMONEE FALLS—Waukesha County ★ △ COMMUNITY MEMORIAL HOSPITAL, W180 N8085 Town Hall Road, Zip 53051, Mailing Address: P.O. Box 408, Zip 53052–0408; tel. 414/251–1000; Robert Eugene Drisner, President and Chief Executive Officer **A**1 2 7 9 10 **F**3 4 5 7 8 10 12 17 18 19 20 21 22 23 24 26 28 29 30 32 33 34 35 36 37 39 40 41 42 43 44 45 46 48 49 52 53 54 55 56 57 58 59 60 65 66 67 69 70 71 73 74 **S**0027 Horizon Healthcare, Inc.	23	10	153	6442	89	32776	979	45311	20537	702
MENOMONIE—Dunn County □ MYRTLE WERTH MEDICAL CENTER, 2321 Stout Road, Zip 54751; tel. 715/235–5531; Thomas Miller III, Chief Executive Officer **A**1 9 10 **F**1 7 8 11 37 39 40 44 45 67 70	23	10	55	1534	14	26204	317	7797	3664	153
MEQUON—Ozaukee County ★ ST. MARY'S HOSPITAL OZAUKEE, 13111 N Port Washington Road, Zip 53097–2416; tel. 414/243–7300; Sister Renee Rose, President and Chief Executive Officer **A**1 9 10 **F**3 4 7 8 9 10 11 12 13 17 18 19 22 25 26 27 29 30 31 32 33 34 35 37 38 39 40 41 42 43 44 46 48 49 52 53 57 58 59 60 65 66 67 68 69 71 72 73 74 **S**1855 Daughters of Charity National Health System	21	10	82	2421	33	110437	231	22286	10951	362
MERRILL—Lincoln County ★ GOOD SAMARITAN HEALTH CENTER OF MERRILL, 601 Center Avenue South, Zip 54452; tel. 715/536–5511; Michael Hammer, President and Chief Executive Officer **A**1 9 10 **F**1 7 8 17 19 22 23 28 30 35 36 37 40 41 44 45 46 49 65 70 71 73 74 **S**5175 Catholic Health Corporation	21	10	63	1407	16	35810	153	9699	4342	169
MILWAUKEE—Milwaukee County CHARTER HOSPITAL OF MILWAUKEE, 11101 West Lincoln Avenue, Zip 53227; tel. 414/327–3000; Gary M. Gilberti, Chief Executive Officer **A**10 **F**2 3 25 26 34 52 53 54 55 56 57 58 59 65 **S**0695 Charter Medical Corporation	33	22	80	976	39	8013	0	9606	2990	65
★ CHILDREN'S HOSPITAL OF WISCONSIN, 9000 West Wisconsin Avenue, Zip 53226, Mailing Address: Box 1997, Zip 53201–1997; tel. 414/266–2000; Jon E. Vice, President and Chief Executive Officer **A**1 3 5 8 9 10 **F**9 10 12 13 17 19 20 21 22 25 27 29 31 32 33 35 38 41 42 43 45 46 47 48 49 51 53 54 56 58 60 65 66 67 69 70 71 72 73	23	50	222	16953	174	176007	0	127564	49967	1427
★ CLEMENT J. ZABLOCKI VETERANS AFFAIRS MEDICAL CENTER, 5000 West National Avenue, Zip 53295–1000; tel. 414/384–2000; R. E. Struble, Director (Total facility includes 196 beds in nursing home–type unit) **A**1 2 3 5 8 **F**1 2 3 4 5 8 10 17 19 20 21 22 23 24 25 26 27 28 29 30 31 32 33 35 37 41 42 43 44 45 46 48 49 51 52 54 55 57 58 59 60 63 64 65 67 69 71 72 73 74 **S**9295 Department of Veterans Affairs	45	10	566	8107	435	250598	0	—	—	2357
★ △ COLUMBIA HOSPITAL, 2025 East Newport Avenue, Zip 53211–2990; tel. 414/961–3300; John F. Schuler, President **A**1 2 3 5 7 9 10 **F**2 3 4 5 7 8 9 10 11 12 17 19 21 22 23 26 30 31 32 33 34 35 37 38 39 40 41 42 43 44 45 46 47 48 49 50 51 52 53 54 55 56 57 58 59 60 61 63 64 65 66 67 68 69 70 71 73 74 **S**0027 Horizon Healthcare, Inc.	23	10	339	11586	212	155618	1124	111648	49034	1482

© 1995 AHA Guide

Hospitals, U.S. / WISCONSIN

Symbols:
- ★ American Hospital Association (AHA) membership
- □ Joint Commission on Accreditation of Healthcare Organizations (JCAHO) accreditation
- + American Osteopathic Hospital Association (AOHA) membership
- ○ American Osteopathic Association (AOA) accreditation
- △ Commission on Accreditation of Rehabilitation Facilities (CARF) accreditation

Control codes 61, 63, 64, 71, 72 and 73 indicate hospitals listed by AOHA, but not registered by AHA. For definition of numerical codes, see page A6

Hospital, Address, Telephone, Administrator, Approval, Facility, and Physician Codes, Health Care System	Classification Codes		Utilization Data					Expense (thousands) of dollars		
	Control	Service	Beds	Admissions	Census	Outpatient Visits	Births	Total	Payroll	Personnel
□ CPC GREENBRIAR BEHAVIORAL HEALTH CENTER, (Formerly Listed Under Greenfield) 5015 South 110th Street, Zip 53228–3134; tel. 414/425–8000; Jeff Bergren, Chief Executive Officer and Administrator A1 10 F1 2 3 12 25 26 52 53 54 55 56 57 58 59 65 S0785 Community Psychiatric Centers	33	22	44	1043	23	692	0	5448	2250	76
DE PAUL HOSPITAL, 4143 South 13th Street, Zip 53221–1756; tel. 414/281–4400; N. Lee Carroll, Administrator A9 10 F2 3 41 52 53 58	23	82	40	857	19	33865	0	9014	4311	137
★ △ FROEDTERT MEMORIAL LUTHERAN HOSPITAL, 9200 West Wisconsin Avenue, Zip 53226–3596; tel. 414/259–3000; William D. Petasnick, President A1 3 5 7 8 9 10 F2 3 7 10 11 19 21 22 23 26 32 33 34 35 37 38 40 41 42 44 45 46 47 48 49 52 57 60 61 63 65 66 69 71 74 S0027 Horizon Healthcare, Inc.	23	10	241	9597	187	59201	0	129328	38590	1227
★ JOHN L. DOYNE HOSPITAL, (Includes Regional Eye Institute) 8700 West Wisconsin Avenue, Zip 53226; tel. 414/257–7996; Thomas Brophy, Interim Administrator A1 2 3 5 6 9 10 F2 3 4 5 7 8 9 10 11 12 13 17 18 19 20 21 22 23 25 26 27 29 30 31 32 33 34 35 37 38 39 40 41 42 43 44 45 46 47 48 49 51 52 53 54 55 56 57 58 59 60 61 63 65 66 67 68 69 70 71 72 73 S3775 Milwaukee County Board of Supervisors	13	10	339	12741	271	210989	704	183685	53014	1712
★ △ MILWAUKEE COUNTY MENTAL HEALTH COMPLEX, 9455 Watertown Plank Road, Zip 53226–3559; tel. 414/257–6995; M. Kathleen Eilers, Administrator (Total facility includes 436 beds in nursing home–type unit) A1 3 5 7 10 F2 3 4 5 6 7 8 9 10 11 12 13 17 18 19 20 21 22 23 25 26 27 31 32 34 35 36 37 38 39 40 41 42 43 44 45 46 47 48 49 51 52 53 54 55 56 57 58 59 60 61 63 64 65 67 68 69 70 71 72 73 S3775 Milwaukee County Board of Supervisors	13	22	726	4837	652	107931	0	92371	47424	1472
MILWAUKEE PSYCHIATRIC HOSPITAL See Wauwatosa										
○ NORTHWEST GENERAL HOSPITAL, 5310 West Capitol Drive, Zip 53216–2299; tel. 414/447–8543; C. Dennis Barr, President and Chief Executive Officer A9 10 11 F2 3 8 11 12 13 15 17 19 22 27 28 29 30 35 37 39 41 42 44 48 49 65 71 72	23	10	95	2227	39	25880	0	12268	6167	202
★ △ SACRED HEART REHABILITATION HOSPITAL, 1545 South Layton Boulevard, Zip 53215–1924; tel. 414/383–4490; William H. Lange, President and Chief Executive Officer A1 5 7 9 10 F12 17 26 30 41 46 48 49 65 67 73	21	46	118	1201	74	13864	0	20361	12705	337
★ △ SINAI SAMARITAN MEDICAL CENTER, (Includes Sinai Samaritan Medical Center–East Campus, 945 North 12th Street, Milwaukee, Wisconsin, Zip 53233; Sinai Samaritan Medical Center–West Campus, 2000 West Kilbourn Avenue, Milwaukee, Wisconsin, Zip 53233) 945 North 12th Street, Zip 53233, Mailing Address: P.O. Box 342, Zip 53201–0342; tel. 414/345–3400; William I. Jenkins, President and Chief Executive Officer A1 2 3 5 7 8 9 10 F1 2 3 4 5 7 8 10 11 12 13 15 17 18 19 21 22 23 24 25 26 29 30 31 32 33 34 35 37 38 39 40 41 42 43 44 45 46 47 48 49 50 51 52 53 54 55 56 57 58 59 60 61 63 65 66 67 68 69 70 71 72 73 74 S2215 Aurora Health Care, Inc.	23	10	209	17340	255	243415	4721	163507	62363	1915
SINAI SAMARITAN MEDICAL CENTER–EAST CAMPUS See Sinai Samaritan Medical Center										
SINAI SAMARITAN MEDICAL CENTER–WEST CAMPUS See Sinai Samaritan Medical Center										
★ ST. FRANCIS HOSPITAL, 3237 South 16th Street, Zip 53215–4592; tel. 414/647–5000; Gregory A. Banaszynski, President A1 2 5 9 10 F2 3 4 5 6 7 8 10 11 12 13 17 18 19 20 21 22 23 24 25 26 27 28 29 30 31 32 33 34 35 37 38 39 40 41 42 43 44 45 46 48 49 50 51 52 53 54 55 56 57 58 59 60 63 64 65 66 67 68 70 71 73 74 S6745 Wheaton Franciscan Services, Inc.	23	10	279	11723	172	102556	1348	78905	35792	1243
★ △ ST. JOSEPH'S HOSPITAL, 5000 West Chambers Street, Zip 53210–9988; tel. 414/447–2000; Jon L. Wachs, President and Chief Operating Officer A1 2 3 5 7 9 10 F1 2 3 4 5 6 7 8 10 11 12 13 17 18 19 21 22 23 24 25 26 27 28 29 30 31 32 33 34 35 36 37 38 39 40 41 42 43 44 45 46 48 49 50 51 52 53 54 55 56 57 58 59 60 61 63 64 65 66 67 69 70 71 73 74 S6745 Wheaton Franciscan Services, Inc.	21	10	495	21152	371	123380	4195	156783	64145	2014
★ △ ST. LUKE'S MEDICAL CENTER, 2900 West Oklahoma Avenue, Zip 53215, Mailing Address: P.O. Box 2901, Zip 53201; tel. 414/649–6000; Mark R. Ambrosius, President A1 2 3 5 7 8 9 10 F1 2 3 4 5 7 8 10 11 12 13 15 17 18 19 21 22 23 24 25 26 29 30 31 32 33 34 35 37 38 39 40 41 42 43 44 45 46 47 48 49 50 51 52 53 54 55 56 57 58 59 60 61 63 65 66 67 69 70 71 72 73 74 S2215 Aurora Health Care, Inc.	23	10	368	23764	468	290950	1105	267916	96423	2991
★ ST. MARY'S HILL HOSPITAL, 2350 North Lake Drive, Zip 53211–4581; tel. 414/291–1650; Sister Renee Rose, President and Chief Executive Officer A1 5 9 10 F3 12 17 52 53 54 55 56 57 58 59 65 S1855 Daughters of Charity National Health System	21	22	20	635	20	10787	0	5932	3651	86
★ ST. MARY'S HOSPITAL, 2323 North Lake Drive, Zip 53211–9682, Mailing Address: Box 503, Zip 53201–0503; tel. 414/291–1000; Sister Renee Rose, President and Chief Executive Officer A1 2 3 5 9 10 F2 3 4 7 8 9 10 11 12 17 18 19 21 22 23 25 26 27 28 30 31 32 33 34 35 37 38 39 40 41 42 43 44 48 49 50 52 53 54 56 57 58 59 60 61 64 65 66 69 71 72 73 74 S1855 Daughters of Charity National Health System	21	10	331	14155	181	227042	2138	123162	54572	1553
★ △ ST. MICHAEL HOSPITAL, 2400 West Villard Avenue, Zip 53209; tel. 414/527–8000; Stephen R. Young, President and Chief Executive Officer A1 3 5 7 9 10 F2 3 4 7 8 10 12 15 17 19 21 22 23 24 26 27 28 29 30 31 32 35 37 39 40 41 44 46 49 51 52 53 54 55 56 57 58 59 60 63 67 68 70 71 72 73 74 S6745 Wheaton Franciscan Services, Inc.	21	10	168	9579	157	130384	1152	80846	34780	1089

Hospitals, U.S. / WISCONSIN

Hospital, Address, Telephone, Administrator, Approval, Facility, and Physician Codes, Health Care System	Classification Codes		Utilization Data					Expense (thousands) of dollars		
	Control	Service	Beds	Admissions	Census	Outpatient Visits	Births	Total	Payroll	Personnel
★ American Hospital Association (AHA) membership □ Joint Commission on Accreditation of Healthcare Organizations (JCAHO) accreditation + American Osteopathic Hospital Association (AOHA) membership ○ American Osteopathic Association (AOA) accreditation △ Commission on Accreditation of Rehabilitation Facilities (CARF) accreditation Control codes 61, 63, 64, 71, 72 and 73 indicate hospitals listed by AOHA, but not registered by AHA. For definition of numerical codes, see page A6										
MONROE—Green County										
□ THE MONROE CLINIC, (Formerly Monroe Clinic Hospital) 515 22nd Avenue, Zip 53566–1598; tel. 608/324–1000; James D. Beyers, President (Nonreporting) **A**1 2 9 10 **S**5695 Congregation of St. Agnes	21	10	139	—	—	—	—	—	—	—
NEENAH—Winnebago County										
★ △ THEDA CLARK REGIONAL MEDICAL CENTER, 130 Second Street, Zip 54956, Mailing Address: P.O. Box 2021, Zip 54957–2021; tel. 414/729–3100; Paul E. Macek, President **A**1 7 9 10 **F**2 3 4 6 7 8 10 12 13 17 18 19 21 22 23 26 28 30 34 35 37 38 39 40 41 43 44 45 48 51 52 53 55 56 57 58 59 60 62 63 65 66 67 68 72 73 74 **S**2445 United Health Group	23	10	223	8654	138	58248	1331	65942	30418	1129
NEILLSVILLE—Clark County										
MEMORIAL MEDICAL CENTER, (Includes Neillsville Memorial Home) 216 Sunset Place, Zip 54456; tel. 715/743–3101; Glen E. Grady, Administrator (Total facility includes 170 beds in nursing home–type unit) **A**9 10 **F**7 8 12 13 17 18 19 20 21 22 25 26 27 28 29 30 31 32 33 34 35 40 41 44 45 46 49 51 61 62 65 66 67 71 73 74	23	10	202	1049	160	34410	41	8581	4821	229
NEW LONDON—Outagamie County										
★ NEW LONDON FAMILY MEDICAL CENTER, 1405 Mill Street, Zip 54961; tel. 414/982–5330 **A**1 9 10 **F**10 19 22 34 37 40 41 44 49 71 73	23	10	52	1576	18	27560	166	8609	3999	134
NEW RICHMOND—St. Croix County										
★ HOLY FAMILY HOSPITAL, 535 Hospital Road, Zip 54017; tel. 715/246–2101; Jean M. Needham, President **A**9 10 **F**7 8 17 19 22 28 29 30 35 36 39 40 41 42 44 45 46 49 51 63 65 67 71 73	21	10	18	1133	14	11167	134	5595	2702	93
OCONOMOWOC—Waukesha County										
★ △ MEMORIAL HOSPITAL AT OCONOMOWOC, 791 Summit Avenue, Zip 53066–3896; tel. 414/569–0201; Douglas Guy, President and Chief Executive Officer **A**1 7 9 10 **F**1 3 7 8 12 13 17 19 21 22 24 25 26 27 28 29 30 31 32 33 34 35 36 37 39 40 41 42 44 45 46 48 49 60 61 63 65 67 70 71 72 73 74	23	10	69	2909	31	71442	439	27136	12603	369
★ ROGERS MEMORIAL HOSPITAL, 34700 Valley Road, Zip 53066–4599; tel. 414/646–4411; David Moulthrop Ph.D., President and Chief Executive Officer **A**1 9 10 **F**52 53 55 56 57 59	23	22	90	668	33	1587	0	5977	2914	131
OCONTO—Oconto County										
★ OCONTO MEMORIAL HOSPITAL, 405 First Street, Zip 54153; tel. 414/834–8800; Steve Dewoody, Chief Executive Officer **A**9 10 **F**7 8 12 17 19 21 26 27 28 29 30 31 32 33 34 35 41 44 45 46 49 51 65 67 70 71 72 73 **S**0002 Quorum Health Group/Quorum Health Resources	23	10	25	421	5	21244	31	4198	2157	72
OCONTO FALLS—Oconto County										
COMMUNITY MEMORIAL HOSPITAL, 855 South Main Street, Zip 54154; tel. 414/846–3444; Richard Cayer, Administrator **A**9 10 **F**3 8 19 21 22 26 30 32 34 37 39 41 44 49 51 65 67 71 74	23	10	24	792	13	17111	0	6426	3165	118
OSCEOLA—Polk County										
OSCEOLA MEDICAL CENTER, 301 River Street, Zip 54020, Mailing Address: P.O. Box 218, Zip 54020; tel. 715/294–2111; Bobbe Teigen, Chief Executive Officer (Total facility includes 40 beds in nursing home–type unit) **A**9 10 **F**7 8 15 17 19 22 26 28 30 31 32 33 39 40 41 42 44 45 49 61 64 65 67 71 73	23	10	63	654	46	13397	38	3727	2024	96
OSHKOSH—Winnebago County										
★ △ MERCY MEDICAL CENTER, 631 Hazel Street, Zip 54902, Mailing Address: Box 1100, Zip 54902–1100; tel. 414/236–2000; Otto L. Cox, President **A**1 2 3 7 9 10 **F**3 4 5 7 8 10 13 17 19 21 22 23 25 28 29 30 32 33 34 35 36 37 39 40 41 42 43 44 45 46 48 49 52 53 54 55 56 57 58 59 60 63 65 66 67 70 71 72 73 **S**5305 Sisters of the Sorrowful Mother United States Health System	21	10	236	7837	128	331613	702	66357	30736	972
OSSEO—Trempealeau County										
OSSEO AREA MUNICIPAL HOSPITAL AND NURSING HOME, 674 Eighth Street, Zip 54758, Mailing Address: P.O. Box 70, Zip 54758; tel. 715/597–3121; James G. Sokup, Administrator (Total facility includes 83 beds in nursing home–type unit) **A**10 **F**6 8 11 17 19 26 32 33 34 37 41 44 45 46 48 49 51 64 65 70 71	14	10	99	197	73	16001	0	3429	1773	105
PARK FALLS—Price County										
★ FLAMBEAU MEDICAL CENTER, 98 Sherry Avenue, Zip 54552, Mailing Address: Box 310, Zip 54552; tel. 715/762–2484; Curtis A. Johnson, Administrator **A**1 9 10 **F**7 8 12 17 19 21 22 28 30 32 34 37 39 40 42 44 46 49 51 65 66 67 71 72 73	23	10	42	1005	13	16576	119	6631	3369	134
PHELPS—Vilas County										
NORTHWOODS HOSPITAL, Mailing Address: P.O. Box 126, Zip 54554; tel. 715/545–2313; (Total facility includes 81 beds in nursing home–type unit) **A**9 10 **F**8 15 20 26 27 28 30 32 36 39 51 60 62 68 72	23	10	99	248	72	13910	0	4823	2355	101
PLATTEVILLE—Grant County										
★ SOUTHWEST HEALTH CENTER, (Includes Cuba City Medical Center, 808 South Washington Street, Cuba City, Wisconsin, Zip 53807; tel. 608/744–2161; Hazel Green Hospital, 2110 Church Street, Hazel Green, Wisconsin, Zip 53811; tel. 608/854–2231) 1100 Fifth Avenue, Zip 53818; tel. 608/348–2331; Anne K. Klawiter, Chief Executive Officer (Total facility includes 86 beds in nursing home–type unit) **A**1 9 10 **F**7 8 19 22 27 34 35 36 39 40 41 44 64 65 71 **S**0585 Brim, Inc.	23	10	100	1240	95	17495	142	9855	3628	143
PLYMOUTH—Sheboygan County										
★ VALLEY VIEW MEDICAL CENTER, 901 Reed Street, Zip 53073–2409; tel. 414/893–1771; Patrick J. Trotter, President (Total facility includes 60 beds in nursing home–type unit) **A**1 9 10 **F**3 7 8 11 19 22 30 32 33 34 35 36 37 39 40 41 42 44 49 53 56 58 62 63 64 65 71 72 74 **S**2215 Aurora Health Care, Inc.	23	10	98	1119	70	17120	160	8993	3953	194

© 1995 AHA Guide

Hospitals, U.S. / WISCONSIN

Hospital, Address, Telephone, Administrator, Approval, Facility, and Physician Codes, Health Care System	Classification Codes		Utilization Data					Expense (thousands) of dollars		
★ American Hospital Association (AHA) membership □ Joint Commission on Accreditation of Healthcare Organizations (JCAHO) accreditation + American Osteopathic Hospital Association (AOHA) membership ○ American Osteopathic Association (AOA) accreditation △ Commission on Accreditation of Rehabilitation Facilities (CARF) accreditation Control codes 61, 63, 64, 71, 72 and 73 indicate hospitals listed by AOHA, but not registered by AHA. For definition of numerical codes, see page A6	Control	Service	Beds	Admissions	Census	Outpatient Visits	Births	Total	Payroll	Personnel
PORT WASHINGTON—Ozaukee County ST. MARY'S HOSPITAL OZAUKEE See Mequon										
PORTAGE—Columbia County ★ DIVINE SAVIOR HOSPITAL AND NURSING HOME, 1015 West Pleasant Street, Zip 53901–9987, Mailing Address: P.O. Box 387, Zip 53901; tel. 608/742–4131; Delmar Medill, Chief Executive Officer (Total facility includes 111 beds in nursing home–type unit) **A**1 9 10 **F**3 7 8 17 19 21 22 26 28 30 33 34 35 36 37 39 40 41 42 44 49 56 63 64 65 66 67 70 71 73 **S**0585 Brim, Inc.	21	10	160	1932	128	46116	209	16701	7294	332
PRAIRIE DU CHIEN—Crawford County ★ PRAIRIE DU CHIEN MEMORIAL HOSPITAL, 705 East Taylor Street, Zip 53821; tel. 608/326–2431; Harold W. Brown, Chief Executive Officer **A**1 9 10 **F**3 7 8 19 26 32 33 34 35 37 39 40 41 42 45 49 53 54 56 58 59 70 71	23	10	44	1598	31	15762	144	8697	4320	171
PRAIRIE DU SAC—Sauk County ★ SAUK PRAIRIE MEMORIAL HOSPITAL, 80 First Street, Zip 53578–1550; tel. 608/643–3311; Wilbur C. Beach, Administrator **A**1 9 10 **F**1 2 3 4 5 6 7 8 9 10 11 12 13 17 18 19 20 21 22 23 24 25 26 27 28 29 30 31 32 33 34 35 36 37 38 39 40 41 42 43 44 45 46 47 48 49 50 51 52 53 54 55 56 57 58 59 60 61 62 63 64 65 66 67 68 69 70 71 72 73 74	23	10	36	1991	24	33622	227	17705	8050	277
RACINE—Racine County ★ △ SAINT MARY'S MEDICAL CENTER, 3801 Spring Street, Zip 53405; tel. 414/636–4011; Edward P. Demeulenaere, President and Chief Executive Officer **A**1 7 9 10 **F**3 4 7 8 10 13 15 17 19 21 23 24 26 28 29 30 32 33 34 35 37 39 41 42 43 44 45 46 48 49 51 53 54 55 56 57 58 59 60 61 65 66 67 70 71 72 73 74 **S**6745 Wheaton Franciscan Services, Inc. ST. LUKE'S HOSPITAL See St. Luke's Memorial Hospital	21	10	226	7978	134	75008	0	89169	42630	1501
★ ST. LUKE'S MEMORIAL HOSPITAL, (Includes St. Luke's Hospital, Racine, Wisconsin) 1320 Wisconsin Avenue, Zip 53403–1987; tel. 414/636–2011; Ray Di Iulio, President and Chief Executive Officer **A**1 2 5 9 10 **F**2 3 4 7 8 10 15 17 19 21 22 23 24 26 28 29 30 32 33 34 37 38 39 40 41 42 43 44 45 46 49 51 52 53 54 55 56 57 58 59 60 61 65 66 67 71 72 74 **S**6745 Wheaton Franciscan Services, Inc.	23	10	238	6711	111	58081	2139	45041	20069	711
REEDSBURG—Sauk County □ REEDSBURG AREA MEDICAL CENTER, 2000 North Dewey Street, Zip 53959; tel. 608/524–6487; George L. Johnson, President (Total facility includes 50 beds in nursing home–type unit) **A**1 9 10 **F**7 19 20 22 26 34 36 37 40 44 45 49 62 64 65 71 73	23	10	72	1657	68	27825	195	12268	5570	177
RHINELANDER—Oneida County ★ SACRED HEART–ST. MARY'S HOSPITALS, (Includes Sacred Heart Hospital, 216 North Seventh Street, Tomahawk, Wisconsin, Zip 54487; tel. 715/453–7700; St. Mary's Hospital, 1044 Kabel Avenue, Rhinelander, Wisconsin, Zip 54501; tel. 715/369–6600) 1044 Kabel Avenue, Zip 54501–3998, Mailing Address: P.O. Box 20, Zip 54501; tel. 715/369–6600; Kevin J. O'Donnell, President and Chief Executive Officer **A**1 9 10 **F**2 3 7 8 12 17 19 21 22 23 24 28 32 33 34 35 36 37 40 41 42 44 45 52 53 54 55 56 57 58 60 63 65 66 71 **S**5305 Sisters of the Sorrowful Mother United States Health System ST. MARY'S HOSPITAL See Sacred Heart–St. Mary's Hospitals	21	10	62	4670	62	46040	475	31017	14995	531
RICE LAKE—Barron County ★ LAKEVIEW MEDICAL CENTER, 1100 North Main Street, Zip 54868–1238; tel. 715/234–1515; Edward H. Wolf, President **A**1 9 10 **F**7 11 19 21 22 24 32 35 36 37 39 40 41 44 45 49 65 71 73	23	10	69	2826	33	22911	440	16076	8024	246
RICHLAND CENTER—Richland County □ RICHLAND HOSPITAL, 431 North Park Street, Zip 53581; tel. 608/647–6321; Thomas J. Werner, Administrator **A**1 9 10 **F**2 3 7 8 10 19 21 22 30 32 33 34 35 36 39 40 41 44 49 52 54 55 56 58 65 71 72	23	10	38	1434	17	12941	182	9617	4947	186
RIPON—Fond Du Lac County ★ RIPON MEDICAL CENTER, 933 Newbury Street, Zip 54971, Mailing Address: P.O. Box 390, Zip 54971–0390; tel. 414/748–3101; Jon W. Baker, Administrator and Chief Executive Officer **A**1 9 10 **F**7 8 11 19 21 22 28 30 33 35 37 39 40 41 42 44 46 47 49 63 65 66 67 70 71 74 **S**0585 Brim, Inc.	23	10	29	1141	12	23432	90	8279	3221	112
RIVER FALLS—St. Croix County ★ RIVER FALLS AREA HOSPITAL, 1629 East Division Street, Zip 54022; tel. 715/425–6155; Sharon Whelan, President **A**1 9 10 **F**7 8 12 13 17 19 21 22 28 30 32 33 34 35 36 37 39 40 44 45 46 49 54 56 58 65 66 67 71 73 **S**0041 Allina Health System	23	10	36	1022	9	10625	224	9569	3632	109
SAINT CROIX FALLS—Outagamie County ★ ST. CROIX VALLEY MEMORIAL HOSPITAL, 204 South Adams Street, Zip 54024; tel. 715/483–3261; Steve L. Urosevich, Chief Executive Officer **A**1 9 10 **F**2 3 7 8 10 17 18 19 21 24 27 28 29 30 32 33 34 35 39 40 41 42 44 45 49 50 53 54 56 57 58 63 65 66 67 70 71 73 74	23	10	69	2303	25	24918	308	13128	6503	185
SHAWANO—Shawano County ★ SHAWANO MEDICAL CENTER, 309 North Bartlette Street, Zip 54166–2199; tel. 715/526–2111; John J. Kestly, Administrator **A**1 9 10 **F**7 8 10 19 21 22 32 33 35 37 39 40 44 56 71 **S**0585 Brim, Inc.	23	10	53	2646	27	32914	338	11296	5186	190

Hospitals, U.S. / WISCONSIN

Hospital, Address, Telephone, Administrator, Approval, Facility, and Physician Codes, Health Care System	Classification Codes		Utilization Data					Expense (thousands) of dollars		
★ American Hospital Association (AHA) membership ☐ Joint Commission on Accreditation of Healthcare Organizations (JCAHO) accreditation + American Osteopathic Hospital Association (AOHA) membership ○ American Osteopathic Association (AOA) accreditation △ Commission on Accreditation of Rehabilitation Facilities (CARF) accreditation Control codes 61, 63, 64, 71, 72 and 73 indicate hospitals listed by AOHA, but not registered by AHA. For definition of numerical codes, see page A6	Control	Service	Beds	Admissions	Census	Outpatient Visits	Births	Total	Payroll	Personnel
SHEBOYGAN—Sheboygan County										
★ △ SHEBOYGAN MEMORIAL MEDICAL CENTER, 2629 North Seventh Street, Zip 53083–4998; tel. 414/451–5000; Patrick J. Trotter, President **A**1 2 7 9 10 **F**2 3 6 7 8 10 17 19 21 22 23 27 28 30 31 32 33 34 35 37 40 41 42 44 45 46 49 51 52 53 54 55 56 57 58 61 63 65 67 70 71 73 74 **S**2215 Aurora Health Care, Inc.	23	10	138	4651	60	37938	685	30116	13186	495
★ ST. NICHOLAS HOSPITAL, 1601 North Taylor Drive, Zip 53081–2496; tel. 414/459–8300; Thomas W. Laux, Executive Vice President and Administrator **A**1 2 9 10 **F**4 7 8 10 11 12 17 18 19 20 21 22 24 25 26 27 28 29 30 31 32 33 34 35 36 37 39 40 41 42 44 45 46 49 56 60 63 65 67 69 70 71 72 73 **S**5355 Hospital Sisters Health System	21	10	112	3441	44	116998	487	29312	11193	348
SHELL LAKE—Washburn County										
☐ INDIANHEAD MEDICAL CENTER, 215 Fourth Avenue West, Zip 54871; tel. 715/468–7833; Larry Abrams, Administrator **A**1 9 10 **F**7 8 19 26 34 35 37 40 42 44 45 61 65 70 71	33	10	49	811	9	10110	56	4119	1650	57
SPARTA—Monroe County										
★ ST. MARY'S HOSPITAL, West Main and K Streets, Zip 54656, Mailing Address: P.O. Box 529, Zip 54656; tel. 608/269–2132; Bill Sexton, Chief Executive Officer and Administrator (Total facility includes 30 beds in nursing home–type unit) **A**1 9 10 **F**7 8 12 15 19 21 33 34 35 36 39 40 41 44 45 46 49 53 65 70 71 72 74 **S**9650 Franciscan Health System, Inc.	21	10	60	793	23	38473	139	—	—	—
SPOONER—Washburn County										
★ COMMUNITY MEMORIAL HOSPITAL AND NURSING HOME, 819 Ash Street, Zip 54801; tel. 715/635–2111; Michael Schafer, Administrator (Total facility includes 90 beds in nursing home–type unit) **A**1 9 10 **F**2 7 8 11 12 22 26 28 29 30 32 34 37 39 40 41 42 44 45 49 64 65 67 71 **S**0585 Brim, Inc.	23	10	136	988	97	14585	115	6704	3304	147
STANLEY—Chippewa County										
★ VICTORY MEDICAL CENTER, 230 East Fourth Avenue, Zip 54768; tel. 715/644–5571; David Olson, Interim Administrator (Total facility includes 86 beds in nursing home–type unit) **A**1 9 10 **F**1 8 19 22 32 34 40 41 44 49 64 65 70 71	23	10	127	591	89	16676	25	7329	3785	161
STEVENS POINT—Portage County										
★ SAINT MICHAEL'S HOSPITAL, 900 Illinois Avenue, Zip 54481; tel. 715/346–5000; Jeffrey L. Martin, President and Chief Executive Officer **A**1 9 10 **F**7 8 17 19 21 22 23 25 28 30 35 37 40 41 42 44 46 49 52 53 54 55 56 57 63 65 66 67 71 73 **S**5305 Sisters of the Sorrowful Mother United States Health System	21	10	115	4338	53	39393	783	32192	13400	418
STOUGHTON—Dane County										
☐ STOUGHTON HOSPITAL ASSOCIATION, 900 Ridge Street, Zip 53589–1896; tel. 608/873–6611; Terrence Brenny, President **A**1 9 10 **F**1 2 3 8 17 19 22 26 30 31 32 33 34 37 41 44 45 49 63 65 71 72 73	23	10	41	1350	20	32231	0	9901	4858	194
STURGEON BAY—Door County										
★ DOOR COUNTY MEMORIAL HOSPITAL, 330 South 16th Place, Zip 54235–1495; tel. 414/746–3701; Gerald M. Worrick, Administrator (Total facility includes 30 beds in nursing home–type unit) **A**1 9 10 **F**1 7 8 10 19 21 22 26 28 30 31 32 34 35 37 40 41 42 43 44 49 53 54 55 61 64 65 67 69 71 73	23	10	77	2208	59	25432	185	19254	9257	288
SUPERIOR—Douglas County										
☐ SUPERIOR MEMORIAL HOSPITAL, 3500 Tower Avenue, Zip 54880–5395; tel. 715/392–8281; Paul E. Gurgel, Chief Executive Officer **A**1 9 10 **F**11 19 21 22 27 29 34 35 39 41 44 45 49 65 71 73 **S**0585 Brim, Inc.	23	10	42	1672	19	56865	0	11200	4835	146
TOMAH—Monroe County										
☐ TOMAH MEMORIAL HOSPITAL, 321 Butts Avenue, Zip 54660, Mailing Address: Box 548, Zip 54660–0548; tel. 608/372–2181; Philip Stuart, Administrator **A**1 9 10 **F**3 7 12 15 17 18 19 21 26 28 30 33 36 39 40 41 44 45 49 65 67 70 71	23	10	45	1074	11	18372	170	6145	2989	99
★ VETERANS AFFAIRS MEDICAL CENTER, 500 East Veterans Street, Zip 54660–9225; tel. 608/372–3971; Stan Johnson, Director (Total facility includes 100 beds in nursing home–type unit) **A**1 **F**1 2 3 4 8 9 10 11 17 18 19 20 21 22 23 24 25 26 27 28 30 31 32 33 34 35 37 39 41 42 43 44 45 46 48 49 50 51 52 54 55 56 57 58 59 60 61 63 65 67 69 71 73 74 **S**9295 Department of Veterans Affairs	45	22	601	2385	523	56753	0	54937	34241	928
TOMAHAWK—Lincoln County										
SACRED HEART HOSPITAL See Sacred Heart–St. Mary's Hospitals, Rhinelander										
TWO RIVERS—Manitowoc County										
★ TWO RIVERS COMMUNITY HOSPITAL AND HAMILTON MEMORIAL HOME, 2500 Garfield Street, Zip 54241; tel. 414/793–1178; Steven H. Spencer, President and Chief Executive Officer (Nonreporting) **A**1 9 10	23	10	138	—	—	—	—	—	—	—
VIROQUA—Vernon County										
VERNON MEMORIAL HOSPITAL, 507 South Main Street, Zip 54665; tel. 608/637–2101; Garith W. Steiner, Chief Executive Officer **A**9 10 **F**2 3 7 8 13 17 19 24 26 28 30 32 33 34 36 39 41 44 45 49 54 55 56 57 58 65 66 67 69 70 71	23	10	14	1623	18	15210	188	8268	4470	174
WATERTOWN—Dodge County										
★ WATERTOWN MEMORIAL HOSPITAL, 125 Hospital Drive, Zip 53098; tel. 414/261–4210; Leo C. Bargielski, President **A**1 9 10 **F**3 7 8 10 12 19 21 22 28 30 32 33 34 35 36 37 39 40 41 42 44 45 49 53 54 58 63 65 66 67 69 71 73	23	10	88	2170	24	57570	419	18602	8769	277
WAUKESHA—Waukesha County										
★ △ WAUKESHA MEMORIAL HOSPITAL, 725 American Avenue, Zip 53188–5099; tel. 414/544–2011; Rexford W. Titus III, President and Chief Executive Officer **A**1 2 3 5 7 9 10 **F**2 6 7 8 10 12 17 18 19 21 22 23 25 26 27 30 32 33 34 35 36 37 38 39 40 41 42 43 44 45 46 48 49 51 52 53 54 55 56 57 58 59 60 61 62 63 64 65 66 67 70 71 72 73 74	23	10	319	12235	184	181143	1884	108780	42538	1109

© 1995 AHA Guide

Hospitals, U.S. / WISCONSIN

Hospital, Address, Telephone, Administrator, Approval, Facility, and Physician Codes, Health Care System	Classification Codes		Utilization Data					Expense (thousands) of dollars		
★ American Hospital Association (AHA) membership □ Joint Commission on Accreditation of Healthcare Organizations (JCAHO) accreditation + American Osteopathic Hospital Association (AOHA) membership ○ American Osteopathic Association (AOA) accreditation △ Commission on Accreditation of Rehabilitation Facilities (CARF) accreditation Control codes 61, 63, 64, 71, 72 and 73 indicate hospitals listed by AOHA, but not registered by AHA. For definition of numerical codes, see page A6	Control	Service	Beds	Admissions	Census	Outpatient Visits	Births	Total	Payroll	Personnel
WAUPACA—Waupaca County										
★ RIVERSIDE MEDICAL CENTER, 800 Riverside Drive, Zip 54981–1999; tel. 715/258–1000; Jan V. Carrell, Administrator **A**1 9 10 **F**7 8 10 17 19 20 21 23 26 28 30 31 33 34 35 37 40 41 42 44 45 46 49 50 51 61 63 65 66 67 70 71 73 **S**0002 Quorum Health Group/Quorum Health Resources	23	10	40	1809	19	41850	230	13025	5886	194
WAUPUN—Fond Du Lac County										
★ WAUPUN MEMORIAL HOSPITAL, 620 West Brown Street, Zip 53963–1799; tel. 414/324–5581; James J. Sexton, President and Chief Executive Officer **A**1 9 10 **F**7 8 19 22 23 28 30 32 33 35 36 37 40 41 44 49 65 66 71 73 **S**5695 Congregation of St. Agnes	21	10	49	1289	17	30167	149	10546	4581	155
WAUSAU—Marathon County										
NORTH CENTRAL HEALTH CARE FACILITIES, 1100 Lakeview Drive, Zip 54403–6799; tel. 715/848–4600; Peter Desantis, Chief Executive Officer (Total facility includes 382 beds in nursing home–type unit) **A**9 10 **F**3 12 26 33 46 49 52 53 54 55 56 57 58 64 65 73	13	22	432	1501	400	83192	0	33770	17706	566
★ △ WAUSAU HOSPITAL, 333 Pine Ridge Boulevard, Zip 54401; tel. 715/847–2121; Paul A. Spaude, President and Chief Executive Officer **A**1 2 3 5 7 9 10 **F**1 3 4 6 8 10 18 19 20 21 22 23 26 28 29 30 31 32 33 34 35 36 37 39 40 41 42 43 44 45 46 48 49 51 52 53 54 56 57 58 59 60 63 65 67 69 70 71 73 74	23	10	257	10514	152	69732	1494	94530	36686	1142
WAUWATOSA—Milwaukee County										
+ ○ LAKEVIEW HOSPITAL, 10010 West Blue Mound Road, Zip 53226; tel. 414/259–7200; J. E. Race, Administrator and Chief Executive Officer **A**9 10 11 12 13 **F**8 11 19 21 30 34 37 39 41 44 63 65 71 72 73	23	10	72	1039	20	14875	0	11660	6217	233
★ MILWAUKEE PSYCHIATRIC HOSPITAL, (Formerly Listed Under Milwaukee) 1220 Dewey Avenue, Zip 53213–2598; tel. 414/454–6600; Gerald E. Schley, President **A**1 3 5 9 10 **F**1 2 3 4 5 7 8 9 11 12 13 17 18 19 21 22 23 24 25 26 27 28 29 30 31 32 33 34 35 36 37 38 39 40 41 42 43 44 45 46 47 48 49 50 51 52 53 54 55 56 57 58 59 60 61 63 65 66 67 68 69 70 71 72 73 74	23	22	95	1511	45	28805	0	13072	6380	185
WEST ALLIS—Milwaukee County										
★ WEST ALLIS MEMORIAL HOSPITAL, 8901 West Lincoln Avenue, Zip 53227–0901, Mailing Address: P.O. Box 27901, Zip 53227–0901; tel. 414/328–6000; Peter S. Fine, President (Data for 364 days) **A**1 2 9 10 **F**5 7 8 11 17 19 21 22 26 27 28 29 30 34 35 36 37 39 40 41 42 44 46 49 60 61 63 65 66 67 70 71 73	23	10	236	10301	154	170160	1583	84940	41330	1129
WEST BEND—Washington County										
★ ST. JOSEPH'S COMMUNITY HOSPITAL OF WEST BEND, 551 South Silverbrook Drive, Zip 53095–3898; tel. 414/334–5533; Gregory T. Burns, Executive Director **A**1 9 10 **F**7 8 15 19 21 30 35 36 37 39 40 42 44 45 52 54 57 63 65 67 70 71	23	10	121	4742	60	39135	672	24442	11953	382
WHITEHALL—Trempealeau County										
TRI-COUNTY MEMORIAL HOSPITAL, 1801 Lincoln Street, Zip 54773–0065, Mailing Address: Box 65, Zip 54773–0065; tel. 715/538–4361; Ronald B. Fields, President (Total facility includes 68 beds in nursing home–type unit) **A**9 10 **F**5 7 8 10 13 15 17 18 19 21 26 28 30 31 35 36 37 39 44 45 50 51 53 54 55 56 57 58 59 61 63 64 65 69 70 72 74	23	10	98	654	77	9263	2	5484	2848	135
WILD ROSE—Waushara County										
WILD ROSE COMMUNITY MEMORIAL HOSPITAL, Mailing Address: Box 243, Zip 54984–0243; tel. 414/622–3257; Donald Caves, President **A**9 10 **F**3 8 19 26 32 33 34 37 40 41 45 49 56 61 65 70 71	23	10	26	468	6	11273	32	2725	1360	71
WINNEBAGO—Winnebago County										
□ WINNEBAGO MENTAL HEALTH INSTITUTE, Mailing Address: Box 9, Zip 54985; tel. 414/235–4910; Stanley York, Director **A**1 3 10 **F**2 20 22 24 28 31 41 52 53 55 56 65 67 73	12	22	330	811	239	275	0	29413	18556	668
WISCONSIN RAPIDS—Wood County										
★ RIVERVIEW HOSPITAL ASSOCIATION, (Includes Riverview Manor) 410 Dewey Street, Zip 54494, Mailing Address: P.O. Box 8080, Zip 54495–8080; tel. 715/423–6060; Celse A. Berard, President (Total facility includes 116 beds in nursing home–type unit) **A**1 9 10 **F**7 8 19 21 22 28 30 33 34 35 36 37 39 40 41 42 44 49 62 63 64 65 71	23	10	194	3372	136	27089	602	25155	11449	379
WOODRUFF—Oneida County										
★ HOWARD YOUNG MEDICAL CENTER, 240 Maple, Zip 54568, Mailing Address: Box 470, Zip 54568–0470; tel. 715/356–8000; Douglas O. Rosenberg, President and Chief Executive Officer **A**1 9 10 **F**3 6 7 8 9 10 11 12 13 17 18 19 21 22 24 26 27 28 32 33 35 37 40 41 42 44 45 47 48 49 56 58 63 65 66 67 71 73	23	10	65	3869	46	30016	246	27991	11627	462

WYOMING

Resident population 470 (in thousands)
Resident population in metro areas 29.7%
Birth rate per 1,000 population 14.6
65 years and over 10.9%
Percent of persons without health insurance 11.9%

Hospital, Address, Telephone, Administrator, Approval, Facility, and Physician Codes, Health Care System	Classification Codes		Utilization Data					Expense (thousands) of dollars		
	Control	Service	Beds	Admissions	Census	Outpatient Visits	Births	Total	Payroll	Personnel

★ American Hospital Association (AHA) membership
☐ Joint Commission on Accreditation of Healthcare Organizations (JCAHO) accreditation
+ American Osteopathic Hospital Association (AOHA) membership
○ American Osteopathic Association (AOA) accreditation
△ Commission on Accreditation of Rehabilitation Facilities (CARF) accreditation
Control codes 61, 63, 64, 71, 72 and 73 indicate hospitals listed by AOHA, but not registered by AHA. For definition of numerical codes, see page A6

AFTON—Lincoln County
- ★ STAR VALLEY HOSPITAL, 110 Hospital Lane, Zip 83110, Mailing Address: P.O. Box 579, Zip 83110; tel. 307/886–3841; Carolyne Jo Allen, Chief Executive Officer **A**9 10 **F**7 8 12 14 17 22 28 30 32 34 40 44 51 64 71 **P**6 **S**1815 Intermountain Health Care, Inc.
  16 10 15 474 5 8391 90 2846 1080 42

BUFFALO—Johnson County
- ☐ JOHNSON COUNTY MEMORIAL HOSPITAL, 497 West Lott Street, Zip 82834; tel. 307/684–5521; Sandy Ward, Administrator (Total facility includes 54 beds in nursing home–type unit) **A**1 9 10 **F**19 22 28 32 33 35 37 40 44 49 65 71
  16 10 83 616 37 13421 92 4691 — 89

CASPER—Natrona County
- ★ △ WYOMING MEDICAL CENTER, 1233 East Second Street, Zip 82601; tel. 307/577–7201; Lin Carriger, President **A**1 3 7 9 10 **F**3 4 7 8 10 12 13 14 15 17 19 20 21 22 23 25 27 30 32 34 35 37 39 40 41 42 43 44 46 48 49 52 53 54 55 56 57 58 60 61 63 65 67 71 72 73 74 **P**3 5
  23 10 221 7186 93 48844 993 64886 29304 974

CHEYENNE—Laramie County
- MEMORIAL HOSPITAL HOSPITAL OF LARAMIE COUNTY See United Medical Center
- ★ U.S. AIR FORCE HOSPITAL, Francis E Warren AFB, Zip 82005–3913; tel. 307/775–2045; Major Gary S. Forthman MSC, Administrator **F**7 8 12 18 20 22 24 25 27 28 29 30 34 39 40 41 44 45 46 48 49 51 54 58 64 65 67 68 71 **P**7 8 **S**9495 Department of the Air Force
  41 10 15 1515 9 100823 282 — — 199
- ★ UNITED MEDICAL CENTER, (Formerly Memorial Hospital Hospital of Laramie County) (Includes De Paul Hospital, 2600 East 18th Street, Cheyenne, Wyoming, Zip 82001–5511; tel. 307/632–6411) 300 East 23rd Street, Zip 82001–3790; tel. 307/634–2273; Jon M. Gates, Chief Executive Officer **A**1 2 3 9 10 **F**3 4 7 8 10 11 12 17 19 20 21 22 23 24 28 30 31 32 33 34 35 37 38 40 41 42 43 44 45 46 48 49 52 53 54 55 56 57 58 60 63 64 65 66 67 71 73
  13 10 231 7546 101 126738 870 52047 22374 582
- ★ VETERANS AFFAIRS CENTER, 2360 East Pershing Boulevard, Zip 82001–5392; tel. 307/778–7550; Frank Drake, Director (Total facility includes 50 beds in nursing home–type unit) **A**1 **F**2 3 8 12 16 17 18 19 20 21 22 26 28 30 31 32 33 37 41 44 46 49 51 54 56 57 58 64 65 67 71 73 74 **P**6 **S**9295 Department of Veterans Affairs
  45 10 125 1744 91 43800 0 26602 13478 386

CODY—Park County
- ★ WEST PARK HOSPITAL, 707 Sheridan Avenue, Zip 82414; tel. 307/527–7501; Gary Bishop, Administrator (Total facility includes 140 beds in nursing home–type unit) **A**1 10 **F**2 3 7 8 15 16 19 21 22 28 32 33 34 35 37 40 44 48 49 52 56 58 64 67 71 **S**0002 Quorum Health Group/Quorum Health Resources
  16 10 202 2214 130 9996 225 13764 5062 280

DOUGLAS—Converse County
- ★ CONVERSE COUNTY MEMORIAL HOSPITAL, 111 South Fifth Street, Zip 82633; tel. 307/358–2122; Fred F. Schroeder, Administrator **A**9 10 **F**1 8 12 14 16 17 19 22 27 28 29 30 32 33 34 35 40 41 44 45 46 48 49 64 65 66 67 71 73 **P**3
  13 10 44 491 7 19452 78 5100 2990 218

EVANSTON—Uinta County
- ★ IHC EVANSTON REGIONAL HOSPITAL, 190 Arrowhead Drive, Zip 82930; tel. 307/789–3636; Robert W. Allen, Administrator **A**9 10 **F**7 8 12 15 16 17 19 20 22 28 29 30 32 34 35 37 39 40 44 46 49 65 67 70 71 73 **S**1815 Intermountain Health Care, Inc.
  23 10 42 1074 9 22201 200 9582 3083 126
- WYOMING STATE HOSPITAL, Highway 150, Zip 82931, Mailing Address: P.O. Box 177, Zip 82931–0177; tel. 307/789–3464; Leon C. Pruett, Superintendent **A**9 10 **F**46 52 53 57 65 73 **P**6
  12 22 196 481 129 0 0 16318 9844 452

GILLETTE—Campbell County
- ★ CAMPBELL COUNTY MEMORIAL HOSPITAL, 501 South Burma Avenue, Zip 82716, Mailing Address: Box 3011, Zip 82717; tel. 307/682–8811; Jack F. Houghton, Chief Executive Officer **A**1 9 10 **F**2 3 7 8 11 12 15 16 17 19 20 21 22 24 28 30 32 34 35 36 37 38 39 40 41 42 44 46 49 52 53 54 56 58 63 65 67 71 72 73 74 **P**3 **S**0002 Quorum Health Group/Quorum Health Resources
  16 10 119 2203 25 60789 408 28027 11849 368

JACKSON—Teton County
- ★ ST. JOHN'S HOSPITAL AND NURSING HOME, 625 East Broadway, Zip 83001, Mailing Address: P.O. Box 428, Zip 83001–0428; tel. 307/733–3636; Pamala L. Maples, Administrator (Total facility includes 60 beds in nursing home–type unit) **A**1 9 10 **F**7 8 12 15 16 17 19 21 22 24 25 26 28 30 31 32 33 34 35 37 40 41 42 44 46 49 51 56 64 65 66 67 71 73
  16 10 104 2179 74 16754 274 20385 8098 358

KEMMERER—Lincoln County
- ★ SOUTH LINCOLN MEDICAL CENTER, Moose and Onyx Streets, Zip 83101, Mailing Address: Box 390, Zip 83101–0390; tel. 307/877–4401; Marla Shelby, Administrator and Chief Executive Officer **A**9 10 **F**7 8 11 15 22 28 32 34 40 41 44 49 71 **P**2
  16 10 18 218 2 20164 49 3532 1430 64

LANDER—Fremont County
- ☐ LANDER VALLEY MEDICAL CENTER, 1320 Bishop Randall Drive, Zip 82520; tel. 307/332–4420; Andrew Gramlich, Chief Executive Officer (Nonreporting) **A**1 9 10 **S**6525 Ornda Healthcorp
  33 10 102 — — — — — — —

Hospitals, U.S. / WYOMING

Hospital, Address, Telephone, Administrator, Approval, Facility, and Physician Codes, Health Care System	Classification Codes		Utilization Data					Expense (thousands) of dollars		
	Control	Service	Beds	Admissions	Census	Outpatient Visits	Births	Total	Payroll	Personnel

★ American Hospital Association (AHA) membership
☐ Joint Commission on Accreditation of Healthcare Organizations (JCAHO) accreditation
+ American Osteopathic Hospital Association (AOHA) membership
○ American Osteopathic Association (AOA) accreditation
△ Commission on Accreditation of Rehabilitation Facilities (CARF) accreditation
Control codes 61, 63, 64, 71, 72 and 73 indicate hospitals listed by AOHA, but not registered by AHA. For definition of numerical codes, see page A6

Hospital	Control	Service	Beds	Admissions	Census	Outpatient Visits	Births	Total	Payroll	Personnel
LARAMIE—Albany County ★ IVINSON MEMORIAL HOSPITAL, 255 North 30th Street, Zip 82070–5195; tel. 307/742–2141; Thomas A. Nord FACHE, President and Chief Executive Officer (Total facility includes 12 beds in nursing home–type unit) **A**1 10 **F**2 3 7 8 10 14 15 16 17 19 20 21 22 23 24 28 30 34 35 37 40 41 44 48 49 52 53 54 55 56 57 58 59 63 64 65 67 71 73 74	16	10	111	3038	32	32087	562	24009	10422	373
LOVELL—Big Horn County ★ NORTH BIG HORN HOSPITAL, 1115 Lane 12, Zip 82431, Mailing Address: P.O. Box 518, Zip 82431; tel. 307/548–2771; Kent Kellersberger, Chief Executive Officer (Total facility includes 90 beds in nursing home–type unit) **A**9 10 **F**1 7 8 11 12 14 15 16 17 22 24 26 29 30 31 32 34 37 39 40 41 44 45 46 49 51 64 65 66 67 69 71 73	16	10	110	544	88	5921	8	6287	3087	151
LUSK—Niobrara County ★ NIOBRARA COUNTY HOSPITAL DISTRICT, 900 Ballencee Avenue, Zip 82225, Mailing Address: Box 780, Zip 82225; tel. 307/334–2711; Jeff Struble, Administrator (Total facility includes 36 beds in nursing home–type unit) **A**9 10 **F**14 19 21 22 28 35 44 48 49 64 **P**6	16	10	52	144	3	6156	0	2314	1081	67
NEWCASTLE—Weston County ★ WESTON COUNTY MEMORIAL HOSPITAL, 1124 Washington Street, Zip 82701–2996; tel. 307/746–4491; F. Ann Snow, Administrator (Total facility includes 51 beds in nursing home–type unit) **A**9 10 **F**1 7 8 12 15 17 19 22 28 31 32 34 35 39 40 44 45 49 56 63 64 66 71	13	10	75	534	54	9812	61	3023	1309	114
POWELL—Park County ★ POWELL HOSPITAL, 777 Avenue H, Zip 82435; tel. 307/754–2267; Greg Roraff, Chief Executive Officer (Total facility includes 98 beds in nursing home–type unit) **A**1 9 10 **F**6 7 8 12 15 16 19 20 21 22 26 27 28 30 34 35 37 39 40 44 46 49 51 64 65 66 67 69 71 73 **P**3 8 **S**0585 Brim, Inc.	23	10	138	1035	106	21724	173	8538	4118	202
RAWLINS—Carbon County ★ MEMORIAL HOSPITAL OF CARBON COUNTY, 2221 West Elm, Zip 82301; tel. 307/324–2221; Patricia L. Carter, Acting Chief Executive Officer (Total facility includes 10 beds in nursing home–type unit) **A**1 9 10 **F**11 15 19 22 24 28 30 35 37 44 45 49 66 71	13	10	35	1401	22	32000	0	11442	5179	173
RIVERTON—Fremont County ★ RIVERTON MEMORIAL HOSPITAL, 2100 West Sunset Drive, Zip 82501; tel. 307/856–4161; Kenneth H. Armstrong, Chief Executive Officer **A**1 9 10 **F**7 8 11 15 19 21 22 23 28 30 31 32 33 34 35 39 40 44 45 46 49 65 71 73 **P**5 **S**0048 Columbia/HCA Healthcare Corporation	33	10	70	1835	17	42826	235	11764	4713	206
ROCK SPRINGS—Sweetwater County ★ MEMORIAL HOSPITAL OF SWEETWATER COUNTY, 1200 College Drive, Zip 82901–5868, Mailing Address: Box 1359, Zip 82902–1359; tel. 307/362–3711; John M. Ferry, Executive Director **A**1 9 10 **F**7 8 17 19 20 21 22 23 26 28 29 30 31 34 35 37 39 40 42 44 45 46 49 51 56 65 71 73	13	10	99	2433	26	71949	595	20162	8793	326
SHERIDAN—Sheridan County ☐ MEMORIAL HOSPITAL OF SHERIDAN COUNTY, 1401 West Fifth Street, Zip 82801–2799; tel. 307/672–1000; T. Marvin Goldman, Administrator **A**1 9 10 **F**7 8 11 14 15 19 21 22 23 28 32 37 40 42 44 46 56 65 67 71 73 **P**5	13	10	59	2677	27	—	288	15797	8301	316
★ VETERANS AFFAIRS MEDICAL CENTER, Zip 82801; tel. 307/672–3473; J. A. Brinkers, Director (Total facility includes 50 beds in nursing home–type unit) **A**1 **F**1 2 3 8 11 15 16 19 20 21 22 26 27 28 30 33 34 35 39 41 42 44 45 46 49 50 51 52 54 56 57 58 60 63 64 65 67 71 73 74 **S**9295 Department of Veterans Affairs	45	22	292	1721	162	27376	0	—	—	585
SUNDANCE—Crook County CROOK COUNTY MEDICAL SERVICES DISTRICT, (Formerly Crook County Medical Systems District) 713 Oak Street, Zip 82729, Mailing Address: Box 517, Zip 82729–0517; tel. 307/283–3501; Don A. Nelson, Administrator (Total facility includes 32 beds in nursing home–type unit) **A**9 10 **F**1 14 15 16 22 28 33 34 45 46 49 64 65 71 **P**6	16	10	48	229	36	6171	0	2905	1238	72
THERMOPOLIS—Hot Springs County ★ HOT SPRINGS COUNTY MEMORIAL HOSPITAL, 150 East Arapahoe, Zip 82443; tel. 307/864–3121; Edward G. Leake, Administrator **A**1 9 10 **F**7 8 11 14 15 16 19 20 21 22 28 32 35 37 40 44 45 48 54 63 65 70 71 **P**3	13	10	49	1079	12	13788	67	5651	2244	98
TORRINGTON—Goshen County ★ COMMUNITY HOSPITAL, 2000 Campbell Drive, Zip 82240; tel. 307/532–4181; Charles Myers, Administrator (Nonreporting) **A**1 9 10 **S**2235 Lutheran Health Systems	23	10	36	—	—	—	—	—	—	—
WHEATLAND—Platte County ★ PLATTE COUNTY MEMORIAL HOSPITAL, 201 14th Street, Zip 82201, Mailing Address: P.O. Box 848, Zip 82201; tel. 307/322–3636; Jon Frantsvog, Administrator (Total facility includes 43 beds in nursing home–type unit) **A**1 9 10 **F**7 8 12 14 15 16 19 22 28 32 34 37 40 44 65 71 73 **P**5 **S**2235 Lutheran Health Systems	23	10	86	1065	66	25712	103	4558	2191	97
WORLAND—Washakie County ★ WASHAKIE MEMORIAL HOSPITAL, 400 South 15th Street, Zip 82401, Mailing Address: Box 700, Zip 82401; tel. 307/347–3221; John Johnson, Administrator **A**1 9 10 **F**7 8 12 14 15 16 17 19 20 21 22 28 29 30 31 32 35 39 40 44 46 49 65 67 71 73 **S**2235 Lutheran Health Systems	23	10	30	798	8	29497	61	5014	2394	100

Hospitals in Areas Associated with the United States, by Area

Hospital, Address, Telephone, Administrator, Approval, Facility, and Physician Codes, Health Care System	Classification Codes		Utilization Data					Expense (thousands) of dollars		Personnel
	Control	Service	Beds	Admissions	Census	Outpatient Visits	Births	Total	Payroll	

★ American Hospital Association (AHA) membership
☐ Joint Commission on Accreditation of Healthcare Organizations (JCAHO) accreditation
+ American Osteopathic Hospital Association (AOHA) membership
○ American Osteopathic Association (AOA) accreditation
△ Commission on Accreditation of Rehabilitation Facilities (CARF) accreditation
Control codes 61, 63, 64, 71, 72 and 73 indicate hospitals listed by AOHA, but not registered by AHA. For definition of numerical codes, see page A6

AMERICAN SAMOA

Hospital	Control	Service	Beds	Admissions	Census	Outpatient Visits	Births	Total	Payroll	Personnel
PAGO PAGO—American Samoa County LYNDON B. JOHNSON TROPICAL MEDICAL CENTER, Zip 96799; tel. 684/633-1222; Bob E. Park, Chief Executive Officer and Administrator (Nonreporting) A10	16	10	130	—	—	—	—	—	—	—

GUAM

Hospital	Control	Service	Beds	Admissions	Census	Outpatient Visits	Births	Total	Payroll	Personnel
AGANA—Guam County ☒ U.S. NAVAL HOSPITAL, Mailing Address: Box 7607, FPO, AP Zip 96538-1600; tel. 671/344-9340; J. M. Ricciardi, Commanding Officer (Nonreporting) A1 S9655 Department of Navy	43	10	55	—	—	—	—	—	—	—
TAMUNING—Guam County ☒ GUAM MEMORIAL HOSPITAL AUTHORITY, 850 Governor Carlos G Camacho Road, Zip 96911; tel. 671/646-6711; Helen B. Ripple, Administrator (Total facility includes 32 beds in nursing home-type unit) A10 F7 8 15 16 19 20 22 31 34 37 38 39 40 42 44 45 46 47 48 49 54 56 63 64 65 71 73	16	10	188	11816	138	—	3588	52818	30278	834

MARSHALL ISLANDS

Hospital	Control	Service	Beds	Admissions	Census	Outpatient Visits	Births	Total	Payroll	Personnel
KWAJALEIN ISLAND—Marshall Islands County USAKA HOSPITAL, Mailing Address: Box 1702, APO, AP Zip 96555-5000; tel. 805/238-7994; Mike Mathews, Administrator F7 8 11 12 13 20 22 25 29 30 34 37 38 40 44 45 47 49 51 71 P1 S9395 Department of the Army	42	10	14	221	3	14192	20	—	—	73

PUERTO RICO

Hospital	Control	Service	Beds	Admissions	Census	Outpatient Visits	Births	Total	Payroll	Personnel
AGUADILLA—Aguadilla County ☒ AGUADILLA GENERAL HOSPITAL, Carr Aguadilla San Juan, Zip 00605, Mailing Address: P.O. Box 3968, Zip 00605; tel. 809/891-3000; Luis Acevedo, Executive Director (Nonreporting) A1 9 10 S0011 Puerto Rico Department of Health	12	10	104	—	—	—	—	—	—	—
AIBONITO—Aibonito County ★ MENNONITE GENERAL HOSPITAL, Mailing Address: Box 1379, Zip 00705; tel. 809/735-8001; Domingo Torres Zayas, Executive Director A9 10 F19 22 33 34 39 42 44 49 56 58 65 70 71 73	23	10	102	6932	88	47918	980	16058	6502	460
ARECIBO—Arecibo County ★ ARECIBO REGIONAL HOSPITAL, San Luis Avenue, Zip 00612, Mailing Address: Call Box 1500, Zip 00612; tel. 809/878-7272; Jose L. Mirauda M.D., Executive Director (Nonreporting) A9 10 S0011 Puerto Rico Department of Health	12	10	183	—	—	—	—	—	—	—
HOSPITAL DR. SUSONI, 55 Nicomedes Rivera Street, Zip 00612; tel. 809/878-1010; Hector Barreto M.D., Director (Nonreporting) A9 10	33	10	138	—	—	—	—	—	—	—
ARROYO—San Juan County ★ LAFAYETTE HOSPITAL, Central Lafayette, Zip 00714, Mailing Address: Box 207, Zip 00714; tel. 809/839-3232; Luis Martin-Jimenez, Administrator A9 10 F14 15 16 44 51 65 71	33	10	30	1726	19	21092	41	3357	1025	189
BAYAMON—Bayamon County ☒ HOSPITAL HERMANOS MELENDEZ, Route 2, KM 11-7, Zip 00960, Mailing Address: P.O. Box 306, Zip 00960; tel. 809/785-9784; Tomas Martinez M.H.S.A., Administrator A1 9 10 F8 10 19 22 37 44 49 65 67 71 73 P5	33	10	211	14296	170	43032	—	30029	7891	624

Hospitals, U.S. / PUERTO RICO

Hospital, Address, Telephone, Administrator, Approval, Facility, and Physician Codes, Health Care System	Classification Codes		Utilization Data					Expense (thousands) of dollars		
★ American Hospital Association (AHA) membership □ Joint Commission on Accreditation of Healthcare Organizations (JCAHO) accreditation + American Osteopathic Hospital Association (AOHA) membership ○ American Osteopathic Association (AOA) accreditation △ Commission on Accreditation of Rehabilitation Facilities (CARF) accreditation Control codes 61, 63, 64, 71, 72 and 73 indicate hospitals listed by AOHA, but not registered by AHA. For definition of numerical codes, see page A6	Control	Service	Beds	Admissions	Census	Outpatient Visits	Births	Total	Payroll	Personnel
HOSPITAL MATILDE BRENES, Extension Hermanas Davila, Zip 00960, Mailing Address: Box 2957, Zip 00960; tel. 809/786–6315; Manuel J. Vazquez, Administrator (Nonreporting) **A**9 10	33	10	97	—	—	—	—	—	—	—
★ HOSPITAL SAN PABLO, Calle San Cruz 70, Zip 00961, Mailing Address: Box 236, Zip 00960; tel. 809/740–4747; Jorge De Jesus, Executive Director **A**1 3 5 9 10 **F**4 7 8 10 11 19 22 23 34 37 39 40 42 43 44 61 65 71 73	33	10	335	18366	262	295729	1942	62506	18641	1271
★ HOSPITAL UNIVERSITARIO DR. RAMON RUIZ ARNAU, Avenue Laurel, Santa Juanita, Zip 00956; tel. 809/787–5151; Ivan Millon, Executive Director **A**1 3 5 10 **F**5 7 11 13 15 16 19 20 22 27 31 34 37 38 39 40 41 42 44 46 47 49 51 65 71 **P**6 **S**0011 Puerto Rico Department of Health	12	10	340	14847	259	122279	5426	39687	16033	558
★ MEPSI CENTER, Carretera Numero 2 K 8–2, Zip 00959-6089, Mailing Address: Call Box 60–89, Zip 00960-6089; tel. 809/793–3030; Manuel G. Mendez, Operating Trustee **A**1 10 **F**2 14 15 16 20 35 41 46 49 52 55 56 57 65	33	22	426	2498	137	0	0	11230	4710	320
CAGUAS—Caguas County										
★ CAGUAS REGIONAL HOSPITAL, Carretera Caguas A Cidra, Zip 00725, Mailing Address: Box 5729, Zip 00726; tel. 809/744–2500; Noemi Davis Marte M.D., Medical Director (Nonreporting) **A**1 3 5 9 10	12	10	251	—	—	—	—	—	—	—
□ HOSPITAL INTERAMERICANO DE MEDICINA AVANZADA, Avenida Luis Munoz Marin, Zip 00726, Mailing Address: Apartado 4980, Zip 00726; tel. 809/743–3434; Carlos M. Pineiro, Executive Vice President (Nonreporting) **A**1 10	32	10	300	—	—	—	—	—	—	—
CAROLINA—Carolina County										
★ HOSPITAL DR. FEDERICO TRILLA, 65th Infanteria, KM 8 3, Zip 00984, Mailing Address: P.O. Box 3869, Zip 00984; tel. 809/757–1800; (Nonreporting) **A**1 3 9 10	33	10	220	—	—	—	—	—	—	—
CASTANER—Lares County										
★ CASTANER GENERAL HOSPITAL, KM 64–2, Route 135, Zip 00631, Mailing Address: Box 1003, Zip 00631; tel. 809/829–5010; Domingo Monroig, Administrator **A**9 10 **F**12 13 14 15 16 20 22 30 31 34 37 39 40 44 45 51 65 **P**6	23	10	33	729	9	5701	37	2157	1331	113
CAYEY—McKean County										
HOSPITAL MENONITA DE CAYEY, 4 H Mendoza Street, Zip 00737, Mailing Address: Box 967, Zip 00737; tel. 809/738–2181; Domingo Torres-Zayas, Executive Director (Nonreporting) **A**9 10	23	10	50	—	—	—	—	—	—	—
CIDRA—Cidra County										
★ FIRST HOSPITAL PANAMERICANO, State Road 787 KM 1 5, Zip 00739, Mailing Address: P.O. Box 1398, Zip 00739; tel. 809/739–5555; Marina Diaz, Administrator (Nonreporting) **A**1 5 10 **S**2635 First Hospital Corporation	33	22	165	—	—	—	—	—	—	—
FAJARDO—Fajardo County										
★ DOCTORS GUBERN'S HOSPITAL, (Includes Dr. Gubern's Hospital, General Valero Avenida 267 & 261, Fajardo, Puerto Rico, Zip 00738, Mailing Address: Box 846, Zip 00738; tel. 809/792–3495; Antonio R. Barcelo, Director) 110 Antonio R Barcelo, Zip 00738, Mailing Address: Box 846, Zip 00738; tel. 809/863–0924; Montserrat G. De Garcia, Executive Director (Nonreporting) **A**9 10	33	10	51	—	—	—	—	—	—	—
★ DR. JOSE RAMOS LEBRON HOSPITAL, General Valero Avenida, 194, Zip 00738, Mailing Address: P.O. Box 1283, Zip 00738-1283; tel. 809/863–0505; Domingo Velez M.H.S.A., Executive Administrator (Nonreporting) **A**1 9 10 **S**0011 Puerto Rico Department of Health	33	10	180	—	—	—	—	—	—	—
GUAYAMA—Guayama County										
★ DR. ALEJANDRO BUITRAGO–GUAYAMA AREA HOSPITAL, Urb La Hacienda, Zip 00785; tel. 809/864–4300; Carlos Rodriguez Mateo M.D., Medical Director (Nonreporting) **A**1 10	12	10	155	—	—	—	—	—	—	—
★ HOSPITAL SANTA ROSA, Aveterans Avenue, Zip 00784, Mailing Address: Box 988, Zip 00785; tel. 809/864–0101; Humberto M. Monserrate, Administrator **A**10 **F**7 8 16 19 22 32 33 35 37 40 71 **P**8	23	10	89	5125	54	40529	330	7162	2478	244
HUMACAO—Humacao County										
★ FONT MARTELO HOSPITAL, 3 Font Martelo Street, Zip 00792, Mailing Address: Box 639, Zip 00792-0639; tel. 809/852–2424; Julio A. Ortiz M.D., Chairman **A**1 9 10 **F**8 15 19 22 27 31 37 39 40 44 45 49 65	33	10	64	3168	44	31235	61	6598	2646	202
HOSPITAL DR. DOMINGUEZ, 300 Font Martelo Street, Zip 00791, Mailing Address: Box 699, Zip 00792; tel. 809/852–0505; Rogelio Diaz-Reyes, Administrator (Nonreporting) **A**9 10	33	10	54	—	—	—	—	—	—	—
★ HOSPITAL SUB–REGIONAL DR. VICTOR R. NUNEZ, Avenida Tejas, Expreso Cruz Ortiz Stella, Zip 00791; tel. 809/852–2727; Luis R. Emanuelli, Administrator **F**2 3 4 5 8 9 10 11 14 15 16 19 20 21 22 23 30 31 32 33 34 35 37 38 40 42 43 47 48 49 50 52 53 54 55 56 57 58 59 60 61 63 64 65 69 70 71 73 **P**5	12	10	74	4781	50	68024	1666	13680	5505	387
★ RYDER MEMORIAL HOSPITAL, Mailing Address: P.O. Box 859, Zip 00792; tel. 809/852–0768; Saturnino Pena Flores, Executive Director (Total facility includes 62 beds in nursing home–type unit) **A**9 10 **F**1 5 6 8 11 12 13 14 15 16 17 19 20 21 22 24 25 26 27 28 29 30 31 32 34 35 37 38 39 40 41 42 44 45 46 49 51 54 56 58 60 61 62 63 64 65 71 73 **P**8	23	10	208	9192	135	167302	626	—	—	943
MAYAGUEZ—Mayaguez County										
★ BELLA VISTA HOSPITAL, State Road 349, Zip 00680, Mailing Address: P.O. Box 1750, Zip 00681; tel. 809/834–6000; Nemuel O. Artiles, Executive Director **A**1 9 10 **F**8 10 12 17 19 20 21 22 25 28 30 31 34 37 39 40 42 44 46 49 54 65 67 68 71 73 **P**1 6	21	10	157	8379	111	21152	1010	20143	7638	588
CLINICA DOCTOR PEREA See Hospital Perea										

Hospitals, U.S. / PUERTO RICO

Hospital, Address, Telephone, Administrator, Approval, Facility, and Physician Codes, Health Care System	Classification Codes		Utilization Data					Expense (thousands) of dollars		
★ American Hospital Association (AHA) membership □ Joint Commission on Accreditation of Healthcare Organizations (JCAHO) accreditation + American Osteopathic Hospital Association (AOHA) membership ○ American Osteopathic Association (AOA) accreditation △ Commission on Accreditation of Rehabilitation Facilities (CARF) accreditation Control codes 61, 63, 64, 71, 72 and 73 indicate hospitals listed by AOHA, but not registered by AHA. For definition of numerical codes, see page A6	Control	Service	Beds	Admissions	Census	Outpatient Visits	Births	Total	Payroll	Personnel
CLINICA ESPANOLA, Bo La Quinta, Zip 00680; tel. 809/832–0442; Emigdio Inigo-Agostini M.D., Board President (Nonreporting) A9 10	33	10	69	—	—	—	—	—	—	—
★ DR. RAMON E. BETANCES HOSPITAL–MAYAGUEZ MEDICAL CENTER BRANCH, Zip 00680; tel. 809/834–8686; Miguel A. Sepulvida, Administrator A3 5 10 F7 8 11 13 16 19 20 22 34 37 38 40 42 44 45 47 49 54 60 65 71	12	10	253	11287	160	108689	2659	—	—	1253
★ HOSPITAL PEREA, (Formerly Clinica Doctor Perea) 15 Basora Street, Zip 00681, Mailing Address: Box 170, Zip 00681; tel. 809/834–0101; Jaime F. Maestre, Executive Administrator (Nonreporting) A10	33	10	82	—	—	—	—	—	—	—
PONCE—Ponce County										
□ DR. PILA'S HOSPITAL, Avenida Las Americas, Zip 00731, Mailing Address: Box 1910, Zip 00733–1910; tel. 809/848–5600; Jose Cora, Executive Director A1 3 5 9 10 F7 8 10 15 16 19 20 22 26 31 32 33 34 37 40 44 49 65	23	10	174	9933	132	150665	633	28573	9181	586
★ HOSPITAL DE DAMAS, Ponce By Pass, Zip 00731; tel. 809/840–8686; Roberto A. Rentas, Administrator (Nonreporting) A1 2 3 5 8 9 10	23	10	334	—	—	—	—	—	—	—
★ HOSPITAL EPISCOPAL SAN LUCAS, (Formerly Hospital San Lucas) Guadalupe Street, Zip 00731, Mailing Address: Box 2027, Zip 00733; tel. 809/840–4545; Pedro Brull-Joy, Executive Director A1 3 5 10 F4 7 8 10 11 15 16 19 22 31 34 37 38 40 43 44 65 71	21	10	160	9206	142	22059	739	24618	7471	508
★ HOSPITAL ONCOLOGICO ANDRES GRILLASCA, (Cancer) Centro Medico De Ponce, Zip 00733, Mailing Address: Box 1324, Zip 00733; tel. 809/848–0800; Angel M. Franceschi, Administrator A1 2 3 9 10 F8 15 19 21 31 33 34 35 42 44 45 49 50 54 60 63 65 70 71 73 P3 5 6	23	49	59	1766	34	19017	0	5312	1731	183
★ PONCE REGIONAL HOSPITAL, Barrio Machuelo, Zip 00731; tel. 809/844–2080; Jose Toro Font M.D., Medical Director (Nonreporting) A1 3 5 9 10 S0011 Puerto Rico Department of Health	12	10	407	—	—	—	—	—	—	—
SAN GERMAN—San German County										
★ HOSPITAL DE LA CONCEPCION, 41 Luna Street, Zip 00683, Mailing Address: Box 285, Zip 00683; tel. 809/892–1860; Herson E. Morales, Administrator A1 2 3 5 9 10 F8 15 16 19 21 22 37 40 42 44 49 63 65 71	21	10	167	6016	91	87836	388	18095	6528	515
SAN JUAN—San Juan County										
★ ASHFORD PRESBYTERIAN COMMUNITY HOSPITAL, 1451 Ashford Avenue Condado, Zip 00907, Mailing Address: Box 32, Zip 00902–0032; tel. 809/721–2160; Ivan E. Colon, Executive Director (Nonreporting) A1 9 10	23	10	180	—	—	—	—	—	—	—
★ AUXILIO MUTUO HOSPITAL, Ponce De Leon Avenue, Zip 00919, Mailing Address: Box 191227, Zip 00919–1227; tel. 809/758–2000; Jose Luis Suarez Fonseca, Administrator (Nonreporting) A1 3 9 10	23	10	386	—	—	—	—	—	—	—
□ CPC HOSPITAL SAN JUAN CAPESTRANO, Rio Piedras, Mailing Address: Rural Route 2, Box 11, Zip 00928; tel. 809/760–0222; Laura Vargas, Administrator (Nonreporting) A1 10 S0785 Community Psychiatric Centers	33	22	88	—	—	—	—	—	—	—
DOCTORS HOSPITAL, 1395 San Rafael Street, Zip 00910, Mailing Address: Box 11338, Santurce Station, Zip 00910; tel. 809/723–2950; Nilda E. Diaz, Executive Director (Nonreporting) A9 10	33	10	96	—	—	—	—	—	—	—
★ FUNDACION HOSPITAL METROPOLITAN, Caparra, Mailing Address: P.O. Box 11981, Zip 00922; tel. 809/793–6200; Milton Maldonado, Administrator (Nonreporting) A9	23	10	119	—	—	—	—	—	—	—
HATO REY COMMUNITY HOSPITAL, Mailing Address: 435 Ponce De Leon, Hato Rey, Zip 00917; tel. 809/754–0909; Nilda E. Diaz, Executive Director (Nonreporting) A9 10	33	10	167	—	—	—	—	—	—	—
HOSPITAL DE DIEGO, 310 De Diego Avenue Stop 22, Zip 00923, Mailing Address: Box 41268, Santurce, Zip 00940; tel. 809/721–8181; Eduardo Artau, Administrator (Nonreporting) A9	33	10	84	—	—	—	—	—	—	—
★ HOSPITAL DEL MAESTRO, Domenech Avenue, Zip 00918, Mailing Address: P.O. Box 364708, Zip 00936–4708; tel. 809/758–8383; Maria M. Rivera M.H.S.A., Administrator A1 10 F8 10 11 15 19 22 40 42 44 49 63 65 67 71 73	23	10	249	10721	170	110169	895	23751	7989	548
□ HOSPITAL PAVIA, 1462 Asia Street, Zip 00909, Mailing Address: Box 11137, Santurce Station, Zip 00910; tel. 809/727–6060; Alfredo E. Volckers, Executive Director (Nonreporting) A1 9 10 S9605 United Medical Corporation	33	10	165	—	—	—	—	—	—	—
★ HOSPITAL SAN FRANCISCO, 371 De Diego Avenue, Zip 00929, Mailing Address: P.O. Box 29025, Zip 00929–0025; tel. 809/767–2528; Domingo Nevarez, Executive Director A10 F14 15 16 19 22 35 44 49 65 71 73	33	10	154	6668	108	46082	0	—	—	412
★ I. GONZALEZ MARTINEZ ONCOLOGIC HOSPITAL, (Oncology) Puerto Rico Medical Center, Hato Rey, Zip 00935, Mailing Address: Box 191811, Zip 00919–1811; tel. 809/765–2382; Celia Molano, Executive Director A1 2 5 9 10 F11 19 20 21 29 34 35 37 40 42 44 60 65 71	23	49	80	2174	43	32256	0	9534	4823	320
★ INDUSTRIAL HOSPITAL, Puerto Rico Medical Center, Zip 00936, Mailing Address: Box 5028, Zip 00936; tel. 809/764–3660; Evelyn Vargas-Torres, Administrator A3 5 F4 9 11 11 19 21 22 27 34 35 37 39 41 43 44 48 49 63 65 67 69 70 71 72 P5	12	10	125	3269	77	180602	0	—	—	753
SAN CARLOS GENERAL HOSPITAL, 1822 Ponce De Leon Avenue, Zip 00919, Mailing Address: Call Box 8410, Zip 00910–8410; tel. 809/727–5858; Marilyn Perez De Vazquez, Executive Director (Nonreporting) A9 10	33	10	66	—	—	—	—	—	—	—
SAN JORGE CHILDREN'S HOSPITAL, 258 San Jorge Avenue, Zip 00912; tel. 809/727–1000; Domingo Cruz Vivaldi, Administrator (Nonreporting) A9 S9605 United Medical Corporation	33	50	85	—	—	—	—	—	—	—

© 1995 AHA Guide

Hospitals, U.S. / PUERTO RICO

Hospital, Address, Telephone, Administrator, Approval, Facility, and Physician Codes, Health Care System	Classification Codes		Utilization Data					Expense (thousands) of dollars		
	Control	Service	Beds	Admissions	Census	Outpatient Visits	Births	Total	Payroll	Personnel

★ American Hospital Association (AHA) membership
☐ Joint Commission on Accreditation of Healthcare Organizations (JCAHO) accreditation
+ American Osteopathic Hospital Association (AOHA) membership
○ American Osteopathic Association (AOA) accreditation
△ Commission on Accreditation of Rehabilitation Facilities (CARF) accreditation
Control codes 61, 63, 64, 71, 72 and 73 indicate hospitals listed by AOHA, but not registered by AHA. For definition of numerical codes, see page A6

Hospital	Control	Service	Beds	Admissions	Census	Outpatient Visits	Births	Total	Payroll	Personnel
★ SAN JUAN CITY HOSPITAL, Puerto Rico Medical Center, Zip 00928, Mailing Address: Apartado 21405, Rio Piedras, Zip 00928; tel. 809/766–2222; Efrain Rodriguez Vigil M.D., Medical Services Director **A**1 3 5 10 **F**4 8 10 11 13 19 20 22 31 32 35 37 38 40 42 43 44 45 46 47 49 50 51 54 60 63 65 70 71 73	14	10	267	13251	224	112413	4167	51947	15806	1192
★ STATE PSYCHIATRIC HOSPITAL, Mailing Address: Call Box 2100, Caparra Heights Station, Zip 00922–2100; tel. 809/766–4646; Judy Fernandez M.D., Medical Director (Nonreporting) **A**3 **S**0011 Puerto Rico Department of Health	12	22	425	—	—	—	—	—	—	—
★ U.S. NAVAL HOSPITAL, Roosevelt Roads, Mailing Address: Box 3007, FPO, AA Zip 34051–8100; tel. 809/865–6171; M. G. Ashamalla, Commanding Officer **A**1 **F**7 8 12 13 20 22 28 29 34 39 40 41 44 45 46 49 51 54 56 57 58 65 71 **S**9655 Department of Navy	43	10	35	1454	12	85906	208	—	—	419
★ UNIVERSITY HOSPITAL, Puerto Rico Medical Center, Rio Piedras Station, Zip 00935; tel. 809/754–3654; Gorye Sanchez M.D., Director (Nonreporting) **A**1 2 3 5 8 9 10 **S**0011 Puerto Rico Department of Health	12	10	297	—	—	—	—	—	—	—
★ UNIVERSITY PEDIATRIC HOSPITAL, Mailing Address: GPO Box 365067, Zip 00910–1079; tel. 809/767–3182; Sylvia Mercado M.H.S.A., Chief Executive Officer (Nonreporting) **A**1 3 5 9 10	12	50	135	—	—	—	—	—	—	—
★ VETERANS AFFAIRS MEDICAL CENTER, One Veterans Plaza, Zip 00927–5800; tel. 809/766–5665; Edward Valenzuela, Director (Total facility includes 120 beds in nursing home–type unit) **A**1 2 3 5 8 **F**1 3 10 11 15 16 17 19 20 21 22 26 28 29 30 31 32 33 34 35 37 39 41 42 43 44 46 48 49 51 52 54 55 56 57 58 59 60 63 65 67 71 73 **S**9295 Department of Veterans Affairs	45	10	728	11481	538	369114	0	—	—	1253

SANTURCE—Ponce County
HOSPITAL ONCOLOGICO ANDRES GRILLASCA See Ponce

VEGA BAJA—Vega Alta County

Hospital	Control	Service	Beds	Admissions	Census	Outpatient Visits	Births	Total	Payroll	Personnel
★ WILMA N. VAZQUEZ MEDICAL CENTER, KM 395 Road 2, Call Box 7001, Zip 00694; tel. 809/858–1580; Ramon J. Vilar, Administrator (Nonreporting) **A**9 10	33	10	150	—	—	—	—	—	—	—

YAUCO—Yauco County

Hospital	Control	Service	Beds	Admissions	Census	Outpatient Visits	Births	Total	Payroll	Personnel
★ HOSPITAL DE AREA DE YAUCO, Carretera 128 KM 1 0, Zip 00698, Mailing Address: Box 68, Zip 00698; tel. 809/856–2105; William Rosas Couret, Administrator (Nonreporting) **A**5 10	12	10	124	—	—	—	—	—	—	—

VIRGIN ISLANDS

CHARLOTTE AMALIE—Bayamon County
ST. THOMAS HOSPITAL AND COMMUNITY HEALTH SERVICE See Saint Thomas

CHRISTIANSTED—St. Croix County

Hospital	Control	Service	Beds	Admissions	Census	Outpatient Visits	Births	Total	Payroll	Personnel
★ ST. CROIX HOSPITAL, 4007 Estate Diamond Ruby, Zip 00820–4421; tel. 809/778–6311; George H. McCoy, Chief Executive Officer (Nonreporting)	12	10	87	—	—	—	—	—	—	—

SAINT THOMAS—Bayamon County

Hospital	Control	Service	Beds	Admissions	Census	Outpatient Visits	Births	Total	Payroll	Personnel
ST. THOMAS HOSPITAL AND COMMUNITY HEALTH SERVICE, 48 Sugar Estate, Zip 00802; tel. 809/774–1300; (Nonreporting) **A**10	12	10	120	—	—	—	—	—	—	—

U.S. Government Hospitals
Outside the United States, by Area

BELGIUM

Shape: ★ U.S. Army Hospital, APO, AE 09705

CUBA

Guantanamo Bay: ★ Naval Regional Medical Center, FPO, AE 09593

GERMANY

Augsburg: ★ U.S. Army Hospital, APO, AE 09178
Heidelberg: ★ U.S. Army Hospital, APO, AE 09014
Landstuhl: ★ Landstuhl Army Regional Medical Center, APO, AE 09180
Wurzburg: ★ U.S. Army Hospital, APO, Usameddac Wurzburg, AE 09244

ICELAND

Keflavilk: ★ U.S. Naval Hospital, FPO, Box 8, AE 09728

ITALY

Naples: ★ U.S. Naval Hospital, FPO, AE 09619
Vicenza: ★ U.S. Army Hospital, APO, AE 09630

JAPAN

Yokosuka: ★ U.S. Naval Hospital, FPO, Box 1487, AP 96350

KOREA

Seoul: ★ U.S. Army Community Hospital Seoul, APO, AP 96205

PANAMA

Ancon: ★ Gorgas Army Hospital, APO, AA 34004

SPAIN

Rota: ★ U.S. Naval Hospital, FPO, Box 18, AE 09645

TAIWAN

Taipei: U.S. Naval Hospital Taipei, Taipei, No 300 Shin–Pai Road, Sec 2

★Indicates membership in the American Hospital Association

All U.S. Hospitals Alphabetically

This section is an index of all U.S. hospitals in alphabetical order by hospital name, followed by the city, state and page reference to the hospital's listing in Section A.

A

A. G. HOLLEY STATE HOSPITAL, LANTANA, FL, p. A 88
A.L. VADHEIM MEMORIAL HOSPITAL, TYLER, MN, p. A220
ABBEVILLE COUNTY MEMORIAL HOSPITAL, ABBEVILLE, SC, p. A355
ABBEVILLE GENERAL HOSPITAL, ABBEVILLE, LA, p. A170
ABBOTT NORTHWESTERN HOSPITAL, MINNEAPOLIS, MN, p. A217
ABERDEEN–MONROE COUNTY HOSPITAL, ABERDEEN, MS, p. A222
ABILENE REGIONAL MEDICAL CENTER, ABILENE, TX, p. A376
ABINGTON MEMORIAL HOSPITAL, ABINGTON, PA, p. A334
ABRAHAM LINCOLN MEMORIAL HOSPITAL, LINCOLN, IL, p. A126
ABROM KAPLAN MEMORIAL HOSPITAL, KAPLAN, LA, p. A173
ACADIA–ST. LANDRY HOSPITAL, CHURCH POINT, LA, p. A171
ACADIA HOSPITAL, BANGOR, ME, p. A180
ACOMA–CANONCITO–LAGUNA HOSPITAL, SAN FIDEL, NM, p. A270
ADA MUNICIPAL HOSPITAL, ADA, MN, p. A212
ADAIR COUNTY MEMORIAL HOSPITAL, GREENFIELD, IA, p. A145
ADAMS COUNTY HOSPITAL, WEST UNION, OH, p. A319
ADAMS COUNTY MEMORIAL HOSPITAL, DECATUR, IN, p. A134
ADAMS COUNTY MEMORIAL HOSPITAL AND NURSING CARE UNIT, FRIENDSHIP, WI, p. A437
ADCARE HOSPITAL OF WORCESTER, WORCESTER, MA, p. A198
ADDISON COMMUNITY HOSPITAL, ADDISON, MI, p. A199
ADDISON GILBERT HOSPITAL, GLOUCESTER, MA, p. A193
ADIRONDACK MEDICAL CENTER, SARANAC LAKE, NY, p. A286
ADOLF MEYER MENTAL HEALTH CENTER, DECATUR, IL, p. A121
AFFILIATED HEALTH SERVICES, MOUNT VERNON, WA, p. A425
AGUADILLA GENERAL HOSPITAL, AGUADILLA, PR, p. A447
AIKEN REGIONAL MEDICAL CENTERS, AIKEN, SC, p. A355
AKRON GENERAL MEDICAL CENTER, AKRON, OH, p. A306
ALACHUA GENERAL HOSPITAL, GAINESVILLE, FL, p. A 85
ALAMANCE REGIONAL MEDICAL CENTER, BURLINGTON, NC, p. A292
ALAMAR HOSPITAL, SANTA BARBARA, CA, p. A 62
ALAMEDA HOSPITAL, ALAMEDA, CA, p. A 36
ALASKA PSYCHIATRIC HOSPITAL, ANCHORAGE, AK, p. A 21
ALASKA REGIONAL HOSPITAL, ANCHORAGE, AK, p. A 21
ALBANY AREA HOSPITAL AND MEDICAL CENTER, ALBANY, MN, p. A212
ALBANY GENERAL HOSPITAL, ALBANY, OR, p. A329
ALBANY MEDICAL CENTER HOSPITAL, ALBANY, NY, p. A271
ALBEMARLE HOSPITAL, ELIZABETH CITY, NC, p. A294
ALBERT EINSTEIN MEDICAL CENTER, PHILADELPHIA, PA, p. A343
ALBERT LINDLEY LEE MEMORIAL HOSPITAL, FULTON, NY, p. A275
ALBION COMMUNITY HOSPITAL, ALBION, MI, p. A199
ALCOHOL AND DRUG ABUSE TREATMENT CENTER, BLACK MOUNTAIN, NC, p. A291
ALCOHOL AND DRUG ABUSE TREATMENT CENTER, BUTNER, NC, p. A292
ALCOHOLISM TREATMENT CENTER, WINFIELD, IL, p. A132
ALEXANDER COMMUNITY HOSPITAL, TAYLORSVILLE, NC, p. A299
ALEXANDRIA HOSPITAL, ALEXANDRIA, VA, p. A414
ALEXIAN BROTHERS HOSPITAL, SAN JOSE, CA, p. A 61
ALEXIAN BROTHERS HOSPITAL, SAINT LOUIS, MO, p. A237
ALEXIAN BROTHERS MEDICAL CENTER, ELK GROVE VILLAGE, IL, p. A122
ALFRED I. DUPONT INSTITUTE, WILMINGTON, DE, p. A 78
ALHAMBRA HOSPITAL, ALHAMBRA, CA, p. A 36
ALICE HYDE HOSPITAL ASSOCIATION, MALONE, NY, p. A277
ALICE PECK DAY MEMORIAL HOSPITAL, LEBANON, NH, p. A256
ALICE PHYSICIANS AND SURGEONS HOSPITAL, ALICE, TX, p. A376

ALIQUIPPA HOSPITAL, ALIQUIPPA, PA, p. A334
ALL CHILDREN'S HOSPITAL, SAINT PETERSBURG, FL, p. A 94
ALL SAINTS EPISCOPAL HOSPITAL OF FORT WORTH, FORT WORTH, TX, p. A386
ALL SAINTS HOSPITAL–CITYVIEW, FORT WORTH, TX, p. A386
ALLEGAN GENERAL HOSPITAL, ALLEGAN, MI, p. A199
ALLEGHANY MEMORIAL HOSPITAL, SPARTA, NC, p. A299
ALLEGHANY REGIONAL HOSPITAL, LOW MOOR, VA, p. A417
ALLEGHENY GENERAL HOSPITAL, PITTSBURGH, PA, p. A346
ALLEGHENY VALLEY HOSPITAL, NATRONA HEIGHTS, PA, p. A343
ALLEN BENNETT HOSPITAL, GREER, SC, p. A358
ALLEN COUNTY HOSPITAL, IOLA, KS, p. A154
ALLEN MEMORIAL HOSPITAL, WATERLOO, IA, p. A150
ALLEN MEMORIAL HOSPITAL, OBERLIN, OH, p. A316
ALLEN MEMORIAL HOSPITAL, MOAB, UT, p. A409
ALLEN PARISH HOSPITAL, KINDER, LA, p. A173
ALLENDALE COUNTY HOSPITAL, FAIRFAX, SC, p. A357
ALLENMORE HOSPITAL, TACOMA, WA, p. A428
ALLENTOWN OSTEOPATHIC MEDICAL CENTER, ALLENTOWN, PA, p. A334
ALLENTOWN STATE HOSPITAL, ALLENTOWN, PA, p. A334
ALLIANCE COMMUNITY HOSPITAL, ALLIANCE, OH, p. A306
ALLIANCE HOSPITAL OF SANTA TERESA, SANTA TERESA, NM, p. A270
ALLIANT HOSPITALS, LOUISVILLE, KY, p. A165
ALLIED SERVICES REHABILITATION HOSPITAL, SCRANTON, PA, p. A349
ALPENA GENERAL HOSPITAL, ALPENA, MI, p. A199
ALTA BATES MEDICAL CENTER–ASHBY CAMPUS, BERKELEY, CA, p. A 38
ALTA DISTRICT HOSPITAL, DINUBA, CA, p. A 41
ALTA VIEW HOSPITAL, SANDY, UT, p. A410
ALTON MEMORIAL HOSPITAL, ALTON, IL, p. A116
ALTON MENTAL HEALTH CENTER, ALTON, IL, p. A116
ALTOONA CENTER, ALTOONA, PA, p. A334
ALTOONA HOSPITAL, ALTOONA, PA, p. A334
ALVARADO HOSPITAL MEDICAL CENTER, SAN DIEGO, CA, p. A 59
ALVIN C. YORK VETERANS AFFAIRS MEDICAL CENTER, MURFREESBORO, TN, p. A372
ALVIN COMMUNITY HOSPITAL, ALVIN, TX, p. A376
AMARILLO HOSPITAL DISTRICT, AMARILLO, TX, p. A376
AMERICAN FORK HOSPITAL, AMERICAN FORK, UT, p. A408
AMERICAN LEGION HOSPITAL, CROWLEY, LA, p. A171
AMERICAN TRANSITIONAL CARE HOSPITAL–DALLAS/FORT WORTH, IRVING, TX, p. A393
AMETHYST, CHARLOTTE, NC, p. A292
AMHERST HOSPITAL, AMHERST, OH, p. A306
AMI KELLER MEMORIAL HOSPITAL, FAYETTE, MO, p. A232
AMOS COTTAGE REHABILITATION HOSPITAL, WINSTON–SALEM, NC, p. A300
AMSTERDAM MEMORIAL HOSPITAL, AMSTERDAM, NY, p. A271
ANACAPA HOSPITAL, PORT HUENEME, CA, p. A 56
ANADARKO MUNICIPAL HOSPITAL, ANADARKO, OK, p. A321
ANAHEIM GENERAL HOSPITAL, ANAHEIM, CA, p. A 36
ANAHEIM MEMORIAL HOSPITAL, ANAHEIM, CA, p. A 36
ANAMOSA COMMUNITY HOSPITAL, ANAMOSA, IA, p. A142
ANCHOR HOSPITAL, ATLANTA, GA, p. A 98
ANCORA PSYCHIATRIC HOSPITAL, HAMMONTON, NJ, p. A260
ANDALUSIA HOSPITAL, ANDALUSIA, AL, p. A 13
ANDERSON AREA MEDICAL CENTER, ANDERSON, SC, p. A355
ANDERSON COUNTY HOSPITAL, GARNETT, KS, p. A153
ANDERSON HOSPITAL, MARYVILLE, IL, p. A126
ANDREW MCFARLAND MENTAL HEALTH CENTER, SPRINGFIELD, IL, p. A130
ANDROSCOGGIN VALLEY HOSPITAL, BERLIN, NH, p. A255
ANGEL COMMUNITY HOSPITAL, FRANKLIN, NC, p. A294
ANGELO COMMUNITY HOSPITAL, SAN ANGELO, TX, p. A401
ANGLETON–DANBURY GENERAL HOSPITAL, ANGLETON, TX, p. A377
ANNA JAQUES HOSPITAL, NEWBURYPORT, MA, p. A195
ANNE ARUNDEL MEDICAL CENTER, ANNAPOLIS, MD, p. A184
ANNIE JEFFREY MEMORIAL COUNTY HOSPITAL, OSCEOLA, NE, p. A250
ANNIE PENN HOSPITAL, REIDSVILLE, NC, p. A298
ANOKA–METROPOLITAN REGIONAL TREATMENT CENTER, ANOKA, MN, p. A212

ANSON COUNTY HOSPITAL AND SKILLED NURSING FACILITY, WADESBORO, NC, p. A300
ANSON GENERAL HOSPITAL, ANSON, TX, p. A377
ANTELOPE MEMORIAL HOSPITAL, NELIGH, NE, p. A249
ANTELOPE VALLEY HOSPITAL MEDICAL CENTER, LANCASTER, CA, p. A 47
APPLE RIVER HOSPITAL, AMERY, WI, p. A435
APPLETON MEDICAL CENTER, APPLETON, WI, p. A435
APPLETON MUNICIPAL HOSPITAL AND NURSING HOME, APPLETON, MN, p. A212
APPLING GENERAL HOSPITAL, BAXLEY, GA, p. A100
ARBOUR HOSPITAL, BOSTON, MA, p. A190
ARBUCKLE MEMORIAL HOSPITAL, SULPHUR, OK, p. A327
ARCADIA VALLEY HOSPITAL, PILOT KNOB, MO, p. A236
ARDEN HILL HOSPITAL, GOSHEN, NY, p. A275
ARECIBO REGIONAL HOSPITAL, ARECIBO, PR, p. A447
ARH REGIONAL MEDICAL CENTER, HAZARD, KY, p. A163
ARIZONA STATE HOSPITAL, PHOENIX, AZ, p. A 25
ARKANSAS CHILDREN'S HOSPITAL, LITTLE ROCK, AR, p. A 32
ARKANSAS CITY MEMORIAL HOSPITAL, ARKANSAS CITY, KS, p. A151
ARKANSAS METHODIST HOSPITAL, PARAGOULD, AR, p. A 33
ARKANSAS STATE HOSPITAL, LITTLE ROCK, AR, p. A 32
ARKANSAS VALLEY REGIONAL MEDICAL CENTER, LA JUNTA, CO, p. A 71
ARLINGTON HOSPITAL, ARLINGTON, VA, p. A414
ARLINGTON MEDICAL CENTER, ARLINGTON, TX, p. A377
ARLINGTON MEMORIAL HOSPITAL, ARLINGTON, TX, p. A377
ARLINGTON MUNICIPAL HOSPITAL, ARLINGTON, MN, p. A212
ARMS ACRES, CARMEL, NY, p. A273
ARMSTRONG COUNTY MEMORIAL HOSPITAL, KITTANNING, PA, p. A340
ARNOLD MEMORIAL HOSPITAL, ADRIAN, MN, p. A212
ARNOT OGDEN MEDICAL CENTER, ELMIRA, NY, p. A274
AROOSTOOK MEDICAL CENTER, PRESQUE ISLE, ME, p. A182
ARROWHEAD COMMUNITY HOSPITAL AND MEDICAL CENTER, GLENDALE, AZ, p. A 24
ARROYO GRANDE COMMUNITY HOSPITAL, ARROYO GRANDE, CA, p. A 36
ARTESIA GENERAL HOSPITAL, ARTESIA, NM, p. A268
ARTHUR G. JAMES CANCER HOSPITAL AND RESEARCH INSTITUTE, COLUMBUS, OH, p. A310
ASBURY–SALINA REGIONAL MEDICAL CENTER, SALINA, KS, p. A158
ASCENSION HOSPITAL, GONZALES, LA, p. A172
ASHE MEMORIAL HOSPITAL, JEFFERSON, NC, p. A296
ASHFORD PRESBYTERIAN COMMUNITY HOSPITAL, SAN JUAN, PR, p. A449
ASHLAND COMMUNITY HOSPITAL, ASHLAND, OR, p. A329
ASHLAND DISTRICT HOSPITAL, ASHLAND, KS, p. A151
ASHLAND REGIONAL MEDICAL CENTER, ASHLAND, PA, p. A334
ASHLEY MEDICAL CENTER, ASHLEY, ND, p. A302
ASHLEY MEMORIAL HOSPITAL, CROSSETT, AR, p. A 30
ASHLEY VALLEY MEDICAL CENTER, VERNAL, UT, p. A411
ASHTABULA COUNTY MEDICAL CENTER, ASHTABULA, OH, p. A306
ASPEN HILL HOSPITAL, FLAGSTAFF, AZ, p. A 23
ASPEN VALLEY HOSPITAL DISTRICT, ASPEN, CO, p. A 68
ASSUMPTION GENERAL HOSPITAL, NAPOLEONVILLE, LA, p. A175
ATASCADERO STATE HOSPITAL, ATASCADERO, CA, p. A 37
ATCHISON HOSPITAL, ATCHISON, KS, p. A151
ATHENS–LIMESTONE HOSPITAL, ATHENS, AL, p. A 13
ATHENS COMMUNITY HOSPITAL, ATHENS, TN, p. A366
ATHENS REGIONAL MEDICAL CENTER, ATHENS, GA, p. A 98
ATHOL MEMORIAL HOSPITAL, ATHOL, MA, p. A190
ATLANTA MEMORIAL HOSPITAL, ATLANTA, TX, p. A377
ATLANTIC CITY MEDICAL CENTER, ATLANTIC CITY, NJ, p. A258
ATLANTIC GENERAL HOSPITAL, BERLIN, MD, p. A185
ATLANTICARE MEDICAL CENTER, LYNN, MA, p. A194
ATMORE COMMUNITY HOSPITAL, ATMORE, AL, p. A 13
ATOKA MEMORIAL HOSPITAL, ATOKA, OK, p. A321
AUBURN FAITH COMMUNITY HOSPITAL, AUBURN, CA, p. A 37
AUBURN GENERAL HOSPITAL, AUBURN, WA, p. A423
AUBURN MEMORIAL HOSPITAL, AUBURN, NY, p. A271

Hospitals, Alphabetically / Bessemer Carraway Medical Center

AUDIE L. MURPHY MEMORIAL VETERANS HOSPITAL, SAN ANTONIO, TX, p. A401
AUDRAIN MEDICAL CENTER, MEXICO, MO, p. A236
AUDUBON COUNTY MEMORIAL HOSPITAL, AUDUBON, IA, p. A142
AUDUBON REGIONAL MEDICAL CENTER, LOUISVILLE, KY, p. A165
AUGUSTA MEDICAL CENTER, FISHERSVILLE, VA, p. A415
AUGUSTA MEDICAL COMPLEX, AUGUSTA, KS, p. A151
AUGUSTA MENTAL HEALTH INSTITUTE, AUGUSTA, ME, p. A180
AUGUSTA REGIONAL MEDICAL CENTER, AUGUSTA, GA, p. A99
AULTMAN HOSPITAL, CANTON, OH, p. A307
AURELIA OSBORN FOX MEMORIAL HOSPITAL, ONEONTA, NY, p. A284
AURORA COMMUNITY HOSPITAL, AURORA, MO, p. A230
AURORA HOSPITAL FOR CHILDREN, DETROIT, MI, p. A201
AURORA PRESBYTERIAN HOSPITAL, AURORA, CO, p. A68
AURORA REGIONAL MEDICAL CENTER, AURORA, CO, p. A68
AUSTEN RIGGS CENTER, STOCKBRIDGE, MA, p. A197
AUSTIN MEDICAL CENTER, AUSTIN, MN, p. A212
AUSTIN STATE HOSPITAL, AUSTIN, TX, p. A377
AUTAUGA MEDICAL CENTER, PRATTVILLE, AL, p. A19
AUXILIO MUTUO HOSPITAL, SAN JUAN, PR, p. A449
AVALON MUNICIPAL HOSPITAL AND CLINIC, AVALON, CA, p. A37
AVENTURA HOSPITAL AND MEDICAL CENTER, MIAMI, FL, p. A89
AVISTA HOSPITAL, LOUISVILLE, CO, p. A72
AVOYELLES HOSPITAL, MARKSVILLE, LA, p. A175

B

B.J. WORKMAN MEMORIAL HOSPITAL, WOODRUFF, SC, p. A360
B.J.C. MEDICAL CENTER, COMMERCE, GA, p. A102
BACON COUNTY HOSPITAL, ALMA, GA, p. A98
BAKERSFIELD MEMORIAL HOSPITAL, BAKERSFIELD, CA, p. A37
BALDPATE HOSPITAL, GEORGETOWN, MA, p. A193
BALDWIN HOSPITAL, BALDWIN, WI, p. A435
BALL MEMORIAL HOSPITAL, MUNCIE, IN, p. A139
BALLINGER MEMORIAL HOSPITAL, BALLINGER, TX, p. A378
BAMBERG COUNTY MEMORIAL HOSPITAL AND NURSING CENTER, BAMBERG, SC, p. A355
BANGOR MENTAL HEALTH INSTITUTE, BANGOR, ME, p. A180
BANNOCK REGIONAL MEDICAL CENTER, POCATELLO, ID, p. A114
BAPTIST HOSPITAL–ORANGE, ORANGE, TX, p. A398
BAPTIST HOSPITAL, PENSACOLA, FL, p. A92
BAPTIST HOSPITAL, NASHVILLE, TN, p. A373
BAPTIST HOSPITAL EAST, LOUISVILLE, KY, p. A165
BAPTIST HOSPITAL LIBERTY, LIBERTY, TX, p. A395
BAPTIST HOSPITAL OF COCKE COUNTY, NEWPORT, TN, p. A373
BAPTIST HOSPITAL OF EAST TENNESSEE, KNOXVILLE, TN, p. A370
BAPTIST HOSPITAL OF MIAMI, MIAMI, FL, p. A89
BAPTIST HOSPITAL OF ROANE COUNTY, ROCKWOOD, TN, p. A374
BAPTIST HOSPITAL OF SOUTHEAST TEXAS, BEAUMONT, TX, p. A379
BAPTIST MEDICAL CENTER–BEACHES, JACKSONVILLE BEACH, FL, p. A86
BAPTIST MEDICAL CENTER–COLUMBIA, COLUMBIA, SC, p. A356
BAPTIST MEDICAL CENTER–NASSAU, FERNANDINA BEACH, FL, p. A84
BAPTIST MEDICAL CENTER, MONTGOMERY, AL, p. A18
BAPTIST MEDICAL CENTER, LITTLE ROCK, AR, p. A32
BAPTIST MEDICAL CENTER, JACKSONVILLE, FL, p. A86
BAPTIST MEDICAL CENTER, KANSAS CITY, MO, p. A233
BAPTIST MEDICAL CENTER, SAN ANTONIO, TX, p. A401
BAPTIST MEDICAL CENTER ARKADELPHIA, ARKADELPHIA, AR, p. A29
BAPTIST MEDICAL CENTER EASLEY, EASLEY, SC, p. A357
BAPTIST MEDICAL CENTER OF OKLAHOMA, OKLAHOMA CITY, OK, p. A325
BAPTIST MEMORIAL HOSPITAL–BLYTHEVILLE, BLYTHEVILLE, AR, p. A29
BAPTIST MEMORIAL HOSPITAL–BOONEVILLE, BOONEVILLE, MS, p. A222
BAPTIST MEMORIAL HOSPITAL–DESOTO, SOUTHAVEN, MS, p. A228

BAPTIST MEMORIAL HOSPITAL–EASTERN OZARKS, CHEROKEE VILLAGE, AR, p. A29
BAPTIST MEMORIAL HOSPITAL–FORREST CITY, FORREST CITY, AR, p. A30
BAPTIST MEMORIAL HOSPITAL–GOLDEN TRIANGLE, COLUMBUS, MS, p. A223
BAPTIST MEMORIAL HOSPITAL–HUNTINGDON, HUNTINGDON, TN, p. A369
BAPTIST MEMORIAL HOSPITAL–LAUDERDALE, RIPLEY, TN, p. A374
BAPTIST MEMORIAL HOSPITAL–NORTH MISSISSIPPI, OXFORD, MS, p. A227
BAPTIST MEMORIAL HOSPITAL–OSCEOLA, OSCEOLA, AR, p. A33
BAPTIST MEMORIAL HOSPITAL–TIPTON, COVINGTON, TN, p. A367
BAPTIST MEMORIAL HOSPITAL–UNION CITY, UNION CITY, TN, p. A375
BAPTIST MEMORIAL HOSPITAL–UNION COUNTY, NEW ALBANY, MS, p. A227
BAPTIST MEMORIAL HOSPITAL, MEMPHIS, TN, p. A371
BAPTIST MEMORIAL MEDICAL CENTER, NORTH LITTLE ROCK, AR, p. A33
BAPTIST NORTH HOSPITAL, CUMMING, GA, p. A102
BAPTIST REGIONAL HEALTH CENTER, MIAMI, OK, p. A324
BAPTIST REGIONAL MEDICAL CENTER, CORBIN, KY, p. A162
BAPTIST REHABILITATION INSTITUTE OF ARKANSAS, LITTLE ROCK, AR, p. A32
BARAGA COUNTY MEMORIAL HOSPITAL, L'ANSE, MI, p. A206
BARBERTON CITIZENS HOSPITAL, BARBERTON, OH, p. A306
BARLOW RESPIRATORY HOSPITAL, LOS ANGELES, CA, p. A48
BARNERT HOSPITAL, PATERSON, NJ, p. A263
BARNES-KASSON COUNTY HOSPITAL, SUSQUEHANNA, PA, p. A349
BARNES HOSPITAL, SAINT LOUIS, MO, p. A237
BARNES ST. PETERS HOSPITAL, SAINT PETERS, MO, p. A239
BARNES WEST COUNTY HOSPITAL, SAINT LOUIS, MO, p. A237
BARNESVILLE HOSPITAL ASSOCIATION, BARNESVILLE, OH, p. A306
BARNSTABLE COUNTY HOSPITAL, POCASSET, MA, p. A196
BARNWELL COUNTY HOSPITAL, BARNWELL, SC, p. A355
BARRETT MEMORIAL HOSPITAL, DILLON, MT, p. A242
BARRON MEMORIAL MEDICAL CENTER, BARRON, WI, p. A435
BARROW MEDICAL CENTER, WINDER, GA, p. A109
BARSTOW COMMUNITY HOSPITAL, BARSTOW, CA, p. A37
BARTLETT MEMORIAL HOSPITAL, JUNEAU, AK, p. A21
BARTLETT MEMORIAL MEDICAL CENTER, SAPULPA, OK, p. A326
BARTON COUNTY MEMORIAL HOSPITAL, LAMAR, MO, p. A235
BARTON MEMORIAL HOSPITAL, SOUTH LAKE TAHOE, CA, p. A64
BARTOW MEMORIAL HOSPITAL, BARTOW, FL, p. A81
BASCOM PALMER EYE INSTITUTE–ANNE BATES LEACH EYE HOSPITAL, MIAMI, FL, p. A89
BASS MEMORIAL BAPTIST HOSPITAL, ENID, OK, p. A323
BASSETT ARMY COMMUNITY HOSPITAL, FAIRBANKS, AK, p. A21
BASSETT HOSPITAL OF SCHOHARIE COUNTY, COBLESKILL, NY, p. A274
BATES COUNTY MEMORIAL HOSPITAL, BUTLER, MO, p. A230
BATES MEDICAL CENTER, BENTONVILLE, AR, p. A29
BATH COUNTY COMMUNITY HOSPITAL, HOT SPRINGS, VA, p. A416
BATON ROUGE GENERAL HEALTH CENTER, BATON ROUGE, LA, p. A170
BATON ROUGE GENERAL MEDICAL CENTER, BATON ROUGE, LA, p. A170
BATTLE CREEK ADVENTIST HOSPITAL, BATTLE CREEK, MI, p. A199
BATTLE CREEK HEALTH SYSTEM, BATTLE CREEK, MI, p. A199
BATTLE MOUNTAIN GENERAL HOSPITAL, BATTLE MOUNTAIN, NV, p. A253
BAUM HARMON MEMORIAL HOSPITAL, PRIMGHAR, IA, p. A149
BAXTER COUNTY REGIONAL HOSPITAL, MOUNTAIN HOME, AR, p. A33
BAY AREA HOSPITAL, COOS BAY, OR, p. A329
BAY AREA MEDICAL CENTER, CORPUS CHRISTI, TX, p. A382
BAY AREA MEDICAL CENTER, MARINETTE, WI, p. A439
BAY HARBOR HOSPITAL, LOS ANGELES, CA, p. A48
BAY MEDICAL CENTER, PANAMA CITY, FL, p. A92
BAY MEDICAL CENTER, BAY CITY, MI, p. A200
BAYCOAST MEDICAL CENTER, BAYTOWN, TX, p. A378
BAYFRONT MEDICAL CENTER, SAINT PETERSBURG, FL, p. A94
BAYLEY SETON HOSPITAL, NEW YORK CITY, NY, p. A278
BAYLOR CENTER FOR RESTORATIVE CARE, DALLAS, TX, p. A383
BAYLOR INSTITUTE FOR REHABILITATION, DALLAS, TX, p. A383

BAYLOR MEDICAL CENTER – ELLIS COUNTY, WAXAHACHIE, TX, p. A406
BAYLOR MEDICAL CENTER AT GARLAND, GARLAND, TX, p. A388
BAYLOR MEDICAL CENTER AT GRAPEVINE, GRAPEVINE, TX, p. A389
BAYLOR RICHARDSON MEDICAL CENTER, RICHARDSON, TX, p. A400
BAYLOR UNIVERSITY MEDICAL CENTER, DALLAS, TX, p. A383
BAYNE-JONES ARMY COMMUNITY HOSPITAL, FORT POLK, LA, p. A172
BAYONNE HOSPITAL, BAYONNE, NJ, p. A258
BAYOU OAKS HOSPITAL, HOUMA, LA, p. A173
BAYSHORE COMMUNITY HOSPITAL, HOLMDEL, NJ, p. A261
BAYSHORE MEDICAL CENTER, PASADENA, TX, p. A399
BAYSIDE COMMUNITY HOSPITAL, ANAHUAC, TX, p. A376
BAYSTATE MEDICAL CENTER, SPRINGFIELD, MA, p. A197
BAYVIEW HOSPITAL, CHULA VISTA, CA, p. A39
BAYVIEW HOSPITAL, CORPUS CHRISTI, TX, p. A382
BEACHAM MEMORIAL HOSPITAL, MAGNOLIA, MS, p. A226
BEAR LAKE MEMORIAL HOSPITAL, MONTPELIER, ID, p. A113
BEAR RIVER VALLEY HOSPITAL, TREMONTON, UT, p. A411
BEAR VALLEY COMMUNITY HOSPITAL, BIG BEAR LAKE, CA, p. A38
BEATRICE COMMUNITY HOSPITAL AND HEALTH CENTER, BEATRICE, NE, p. A246
BEAUFORT COUNTY HOSPITAL, WASHINGTON, NC, p. A300
BEAUFORT MEMORIAL HOSPITAL, BEAUFORT, SC, p. A355
BEAUMONT REGIONAL MEDICAL CENTER, BEAUMONT, TX, p. A379
BEAUREGARD MEMORIAL HOSPITAL, DE RIDDER, LA, p. A172
BEAVER COUNTY MEMORIAL HOSPITAL, BEAVER, OK, p. A321
BEAVER DAM COMMUNITY HOSPITALS, BEAVER DAM, WI, p. A435
BEAVER VALLEY HOSPITAL, BEAVER, UT, p. A408
BECKLEY APPALACHIAN REGIONAL HOSPITAL, BECKLEY, WV, p. A430
BECKLEY HOSPITAL, BECKLEY, WV, p. A430
BEDFORD COUNTY GENERAL HOSPITAL, SHELBYVILLE, TN, p. A374
BEDFORD COUNTY MEMORIAL HOSPITAL, BEDFORD, VA, p. A414
BEDFORD REGIONAL MEDICAL CENTER, BEDFORD, IN, p. A133
BEE COUNTY REGIONAL MEDICAL CENTER, BEEVILLE, TX, p. A379
BEEBE MEDICAL CENTER, LEWES, DE, p. A78
BEECH HILL HOSPITAL, DUBLIN, NH, p. A255
BELL MEMORIAL HOSPITAL, ISHPEMING, MI, p. A205
BELLA VISTA HOSPITAL, MAYAGUEZ, PR, p. A448
BELLAIRE HOSPITAL, HOUSTON, TX, p. A390
BELLE FOURCHE HEALTH CARE CENTER, BELLE FOURCHE, SD, p. A361
BELLEVUE – THE WOMAN'S HOSPITAL, SCHENECTADY, NY, p. A287
BELLEVUE HOSPITAL, BELLEVUE, OH, p. A307
BELLEVUE HOSPITAL CENTER, NEW YORK CITY, NY, p. A278
BELLFLOWER MEDICAL CENTER, BELLFLOWER, CA, p. A37
BELLIN MEMORIAL HOSPITAL, GREEN BAY, WI, p. A437
BELLIN PSYCHIATRIC CENTER, GREEN BAY, WI, p. A437
BELLVILLE GENERAL HOSPITAL, BELLVILLE, TX, p. A379
BELLWOOD GENERAL HOSPITAL, BELLFLOWER, CA, p. A37
BELMOND COMMUNITY HOSPITAL, BELMOND, IA, p. A142
BELMONT CENTER FOR COMPREHENSIVE TREATMENT, PHILADELPHIA, PA, p. A344
BELMONT PINES HOSPITAL, YOUNGSTOWN, OH, p. A319
BELOIT MEMORIAL HOSPITAL, BELOIT, WI, p. A435
BENCHMARK REGIONAL HOSPITAL, WOODS CROSS, UT, p. A411
BENEDICTINE HOSPITAL, KINGSTON, NY, p. A276
BENEWAH COMMUNITY HOSPITAL, SAINT MARIES, ID, p. A114
BENJAMIN RUSH CENTER, SYRACUSE, NY, p. A288
BENNETT COUNTY COMMUNITY HOSPITAL, MARTIN, SD, p. A362
BENSON HOSPITAL, BENSON, AZ, p. A23
BEREA HOSPITAL, BEREA, KY, p. A161
BERGAN MERCY MEDICAL CENTER, OMAHA, NE, p. A250
BERGEN PINES COUNTY HOSPITAL, PARAMUS, NJ, p. A263
BERGER HOSPITAL, CIRCLEVILLE, OH, p. A309
BERKSHIRE MEDICAL CENTER, PITTSFIELD, MA, p. A196
BERRIEN COUNTY HOSPITAL, NASHVILLE, GA, p. A106
BERRIEN GENERAL HOSPITAL, BERRIEN CENTER, MI, p. A200
BERT FISH MEDICAL CENTER, NEW SMYRNA BEACH, FL, p. A91
BERTIE COUNTY MEMORIAL HOSPITAL, WINDSOR, NC, p. A300
BERTRAND CHAFFEE HOSPITAL, SPRINGVILLE, NY, p. A287
BERWICK HOSPITAL CENTER, BERWICK, PA, p. A335
BESS KAISER MEDICAL CENTER, PORTLAND, OR, p. A331
BESSEMER CARRAWAY MEDICAL CENTER, BESSEMER, AL, p. A13

Hospitals, Alphabetically / Beth Israel Hospital

BETH ISRAEL HOSPITAL, BOSTON, MA, p. A190
BETH ISRAEL HOSPITAL, PASSAIC, NJ, p. A263
BETH ISRAEL MEDICAL CENTER, NEW YORK CITY, NY, p. A278
BETHANIA REGIONAL HEALTH CARE CENTER, WICHITA FALLS, TX, p. A407
BETHANY HEALTH CENTER, BETHANY, OK, p. A321
BETHANY HOSPITAL, CHICAGO, IL, p. A118
BETHANY MEDICAL CENTER, KANSAS CITY, KS, p. A154
BETHESDA GENERAL HOSPITAL, SAINT LOUIS, MO, p. A237
BETHESDA HOSPITAL, ZANESVILLE, OH, p. A320
BETHESDA MEMORIAL HOSPITAL, BOYNTON BEACH, FL, p. A 82
BETHESDA NORTH HOSPITAL, CINCINNATI, OH, p. A308
BETHESDA OAK HOSPITAL, CINCINNATI, OH, p. A308
BETSY JOHNSON MEMORIAL HOSPITAL, DUNN, NC, p. A293
BETTY BACHARACH REHABILITATION HOSPITAL, POMONA, NJ, p. A264
BEVERLY HOSPITAL, MONTEBELLO, CA, p. A 53
BEVERLY HOSPITAL, BEVERLY, MA, p. A190
BEXAR COUNTY HOSPITAL DISTRICT, SAN ANTONIO, TX, p. A401
BI-COUNTY COMMUNITY HOSPITAL, WARREN, MI, p. A211
BIBB MEDICAL CENTER, CENTREVILLE, AL, p. A 14
BIG BEND REGIONAL MEDICAL CENTER, ALPINE, TX, p. A376
BIG HORN COUNTY MEMORIAL HOSPITAL, HARDIN, MT, p. A242
BIG SANDY MEDICAL CENTER, BIG SANDY, MT, p. A241
BIG SPRING STATE HOSPITAL, BIG SPRING, TX, p. A379
BIGGS–GRIDLEY MEMORIAL HOSPITAL, GRIDLEY, CA, p. A 44
BILOXI REGIONAL MEDICAL CENTER, BILOXI, MS, p. A222
BINGHAM MEMORIAL HOSPITAL, BLACKFOOT, ID, p. A112
BINGHAMTON PSYCHIATRIC CENTER, BINGHAMTON, NY, p. A272
BIRMINGHAM BAPTIST MEDICAL CENTER–MONTCLAIR CAMPUS, BIRMINGHAM, AL, p. A 13
BIRMINGHAM BAPTIST MEDICAL CENTER–PRINCETON, BIRMINGHAM, AL, p. A 13
BISHOP CLARKSON MEMORIAL HOSPITAL, OMAHA, NE, p. A250
BIXBY MEDICAL CENTER, ADRIAN, MI, p. A199
BLACK RIVER MEMORIAL HOSPITAL, BLACK RIVER FALLS, WI, p. A435
BLACKFORD COUNTY HOSPITAL, HARTFORD CITY, IN, p. A136
BLACKWELL REGIONAL HOSPITAL, BLACKWELL, OK, p. A321
BLADEN COUNTY HOSPITAL, ELIZABETHTOWN, NC, p. A294
BLANCHARD VALLEY HOSPITAL, FINDLAY, OH, p. A312
BLECKLEY MEMORIAL HOSPITAL, COCHRAN, GA, p. A101
BLEDSOE COUNTY GENERAL HOSPITAL, PIKEVILLE, TN, p. A374
BLESSING HOSPITAL, QUINCY, IL, p. A129
BLODGETT MEMORIAL MEDICAL CENTER, GRAND RAPIDS, MI, p. A203
BLOOMER COMMUNITY MEMORIAL HOSPITAL AND SKILLED NURSING FALILITY, BLOOMER, WI, p. A435
BLOOMINGTON HOSPITAL, BLOOMINGTON, IN, p. A133
BLOOMSBURG HOSPITAL, BLOOMSBURG, PA, p. A335
BLOSS MEMORIAL HOSPITAL DISTRICT, ATWATER, CA, p. A 37
BLOUNT MEMORIAL HOSPITAL, ONEONTA, AL, p. A 19
BLOUNT MEMORIAL HOSPITAL, MARYVILLE, TN, p. A371
BLOWING ROCK HOSPITAL, BLOWING ROCK, NC, p. A291
BLUE HILL MEMORIAL HOSPITAL, BLUE HILL, ME, p. A180
BLUE MOUNTAIN HOSPITAL, JOHN DAY, OR, p. A330
BLUEFIELD REGIONAL MEDICAL CENTER, BLUEFIELD, WV, p. A430
BLUEGRASS REGIONAL MEDICAL CENTER, FRANKFORT, KY, p. A162
BLUFFTON COMMUNITY HOSPITAL, BLUFFTON, OH, p. A307
BLYTHEDALE CHILDREN'S HOSPITAL, VALHALLA, NY, p. A288
BOAZ-ALBERTVILLE MEDICAL CENTER, BOAZ, AL, p. A 14
BOB WILSON MEMORIAL GRANT COUNTY HOSPITAL, ULYSSES, KS, p. A159
BOCA RATON COMMUNITY HOSPITAL, BOCA RATON, FL, p. A 81
BOGALUSA COMMUNITY MEDICAL CENTER, BOGALUSA, LA, p. A171
BOLIVAR COMMUNITY HOSPITAL, BOLIVAR, TN, p. A366
BOLIVAR COUNTY HOSPITAL, CLEVELAND, MS, p. A223
BON SECOURS–MARYVIEW MEDICAL CENTER, PORTSMOUTH, VA, p. A419
BON SECOURS–ST. FRANCIS XAVIER HOSPITAL, CHARLESTON, SC, p. A355
BON SECOURS–ST. JOSEPH HOSPITAL, PORT CHARLOTTE, FL, p. A 93
BON SECOURS–STUART CIRCLE, RICHMOND, VA, p. A419
BON SECOURS HOSPITAL, BALTIMORE, MD, p. A184
BON SECOURS HOSPITAL, GROSSE POINTE, MI, p. A204
BONE AND JOINT HOSPITAL, OKLAHOMA CITY, OK, p. A325
BONNER GENERAL HOSPITAL, SANDPOINT, ID, p. A114
BOONE COUNTY HEALTH CENTER, ALBION, NE, p. A246

BOONE COUNTY HOSPITAL, BOONE, IA, p. A142
BOONE HOSPITAL CENTER, COLUMBIA, MO, p. A231
BOONE MEMORIAL HOSPITAL, MADISON, WV, p. A432
BOONEVILLE COMMUNITY HOSPITAL, BOONEVILLE, AR, p. A 29
BORGESS MEDICAL CENTER, KALAMAZOO, MI, p. A205
BOSCOBEL AREA HEALTH CARE, BOSCOBEL, WI, p. A436
BOSSIER MEDICAL CENTER, BOSSIER CITY, LA, p. A171
BOSTON CITY HOSPITAL, BOSTON, MA, p. A190
BOSTON REGIONAL MEDICAL CENTER, STONEHAM, MA, p. A197
BOSTON SPECIALTY AND REHABILITATION HOSPITAL, BOSTON, MA, p. A190
BOSTON UNIVERSITY MEDICAL CENTER–UNIVERSITY HOSPITAL, BOSTON, MA, p. A190
BOTHWELL REGIONAL HEALTH CENTER, SEDALIA, MO, p. A239
BOTSFORD GENERAL HOSPITAL, FARMINGTON HILLS, MI, p. A202
BOULDER CITY HOSPITAL, BOULDER CITY, NV, p. A253
BOULDER COMMUNITY HOSPITAL, BOULDER, CO, p. A 68
BOURBON GENERAL HOSPITAL, PARIS, KY, p. A167
BOURNEWOOD HOSPITAL, BROOKLINE, MA, p. A192
BOWDLE HOSPITAL, BOWDLE, SD, p. A361
BOWDON AREA HOSPITAL, BOWDON, GA, p. A100
BOWIE MEMORIAL HOSPITAL, BOWIE, TX, p. A380
BOWLING GREEN HOSPITAL, MANDEVILLE, LA, p. A174
BOX BUTTE GENERAL HOSPITAL, ALLIANCE, NE, p. A246
BOYS TOWN NATIONAL RESEARCH HOSPITAL, OMAHA, NE, p. A250
BOZEMAN DEACONESS HOSPITAL, BOZEMAN, MT, p. A241
BRACKENRIDGE HOSPITAL, AUSTIN, TX, p. A377
BRADDOCK MEDICAL CENTER, BRADDOCK, PA, p. A335
BRADFORD–PARKSIDE ADOLESCENT AT OAK MOUNTAIN, PELHAM, AL, p. A 19
BRADFORD HOSPITAL, STARKE, FL, p. A 95
BRADFORD PARKSIDE AT BIRMINGHAM, BIRMINGHAM, AL, p. A 13
BRADFORD PARKSIDE AT MADISON, MADISON, AL, p. A 17
BRADFORD REGIONAL MEDICAL CENTER, BRADFORD, PA, p. A335
BRADLEY CENTER, COLUMBUS, GA, p. A101
BRADLEY COUNTY MEMORIAL HOSPITAL, WARREN, AR, p. A 34
BRADLEY MEMORIAL HOSPITAL, CLEVELAND, TN, p. A367
BRADLEY MEMORIAL HOSPITAL AND HEALTH CENTER, SOUTHINGTON, CT, p. A 76
BRAINERD REGIONAL HUMAN SERVICES CENTER, BRAINERD, MN, p. A213
BRAINTREE HOSPITAL REHABILITATION NETWORK, BRAINTREE, MA, p. A192
BRANDON HOSPITAL, BRANDON, FL, p. A 82
BRANDYWINE HOSPITAL, COATESVILLE, PA, p. A336
BRATTLEBORO MEMORIAL HOSPITAL, BRATTLEBORO, VT, p. A412
BRATTLEBORO RETREAT, BRATTLEBORO, VT, p. A412
BRAWNER NORTH, SMYRNA, GA, p. A108
BRAXTON COUNTY MEMORIAL HOSPITAL, GASSAWAY, WV, p. A431
BRAZOS VALLEY MEDICAL CENTER, COLLEGE STATION, TX, p. A381
BRAZOSPORT MEMORIAL HOSPITAL, LAKE JACKSON, TX, p. A394
BREA COMMUNITY HOSPITAL, BREA, CA, p. A 38
BRECKINRIDGE MEMORIAL HOSPITAL, HARDINSBURG, KY, p. A163
BREECH MEDICAL CENTER, LEBANON, MO, p. A235
BRIDGEPORT HOSPITAL, BRIDGEPORT, CT, p. A 74
BRIDGEWATER STATE HOSPITAL, BRIDGEWATER, MA, p. A192
BRIDGEWAY, NORTH LITTLE ROCK, AR, p. A 33
BRIGHAM AND WOMEN'S HOSPITAL, BOSTON, MA, p. A191
BRIGHAM CITY COMMUNITY HOSPITAL, BRIGAM CITY, UT, p. A408
BRIGHTON HOSPITAL, BRIGHTON, MI, p. A200
BRIGHTON MEDICAL CENTER, PORTLAND, ME, p. A182
BRISTOL HOSPITAL, BRISTOL, CT, p. A 74
BRISTOL REGIONAL MEDICAL CENTER, BRISTOL, TN, p. A366
BRISTOW MEMORIAL HOSPITAL, BRISTOW, OK, p. A321
BROADDUS HOSPITAL, PHILIPPI, WV, p. A432
BROADLAWNS MEDICAL CENTER, DES MOINES, IA, p. A144
BROADWATER HEALTH CENTER, TOWNSEND, MT, p. A244
BROCKTON–WEST ROXBURY VETERANS AFFAIRS MEDICAL CENTER, BROCKTON, MA, p. A192
BROCKTON HOSPITAL, BROCKTON, MA, p. A192
BRODSTONE MEMORIAL HOSPITAL, SUPERIOR, NE, p. A251
BROKEN ARROW MEDICAL CENTER, BROKEN ARROW, OK, p. A322
BROMENN HEALTHCARE, NORMAL, IL, p. A127
BRONSON METHODIST HOSPITAL, KALAMAZOO, MI, p. A205

BRONSON VICKSBURG HOSPITAL, VICKSBURG, MI, p. A211
BRONX–LEBANON HOSPITAL CENTER, NEW YORK CITY, NY, p. A278
BRONX CHILDREN'S PSYCHIATRIC CENTER, NEW YORK CITY, NY, p. A278
BRONX MUNICIPAL HOSPITAL CENTER, NEW YORK CITY, NY, p. A278
BRONX PSYCHIATRIC CENTER, NEW YORK CITY, NY, p. A278
BROOK LANE PSYCHIATRIC CENTER, HAGERSTOWN, MD, p. A187
BROOKDALE HOSPITAL MEDICAL CENTER, NEW YORK CITY, NY, p. A278
BROOKE ARMY MEDICAL CENTER, SAN ANTONIO, TX, p. A401
BROOKHAVEN HOSPITAL, TULSA, OK, p. A327
BROOKHAVEN MEMORIAL HOSPITAL MEDICAL CENTER, PATCHOGUE, NY, p. A284
BROOKINGS HOSPITAL, BROOKINGS, SD, p. A361
BROOKLYN HOSPITAL CENTER, NEW YORK CITY, NY, p. A278
BROOKS COUNTY HOSPITAL, QUITMAN, GA, p. A107
BROOKS COUNTY HOSPITAL, FALFURRIAS, TX, p. A386
BROOKS HOSPITAL, ATLANTA, TX, p. A377
BROOKS MEMORIAL HOSPITAL, DUNKIRK, NY, p. A274
BROOKSIDE HOSPITAL, SAN PABLO, CA, p. A 62
BROOKSVILLE REGIONAL HOSPITAL, BROOKSVILLE, FL, p. A 82
BROOKVILLE HOSPITAL, BROOKVILLE, PA, p. A335
BROOKWOOD MEDICAL CENTER, BIRMINGHAM, AL, p. A 13
BROTMAN MEDICAL CENTER, CULVER CITY, CA, p. A 41
BROUGHTON HOSPITAL, MORGANTON, NC, p. A297
BROWARD GENERAL MEDICAL CENTER, FORT LAUDERDALE, FL, p. A 84
BROWN COUNTY GENERAL HOSPITAL, GEORGETOWN, OH, p. A312
BROWN COUNTY HOSPITAL, AINSWORTH, NE, p. A246
BROWN COUNTY MENTAL HEALTH CENTER, GREEN BAY, WI, p. A437
BROWN MEMORIAL HOSPITAL, CONNEAUT, OH, p. A311
BROWNFIELD REGIONAL MEDICAL CENTER, BROWNFIELD, TX, p. A380
BROWNSVILLE GENERAL HOSPITAL, BROWNSVILLE, PA, p. A335
BROWNSVILLE MEDICAL CENTER, BROWNSVILLE, TX, p. A380
BROWNWOOD REGIONAL MEDICAL CENTER, BROWNWOOD, TX, p. A380
BRUCE HOSPITAL, BRUCE, MS, p. A223
BRUCE HOSPITAL SYSTEM, FLORENCE, SC, p. A357
BRUNSWICK GENERAL HOSPITAL, AMITYVILLE, NY, p. A271
BRUNSWICK HOSPITAL, SUPPLY, NC, p. A299
BRYAN MEMORIAL HOSPITAL, LINCOLN, NE, p. A248
BRYAN W. WHITFIELD MEMORIAL HOSPITAL, DEMOPOLIS, AL, p. A 15
BRYCE HOSPITAL, TUSCALOOSA, AL, p. A 20
BRYLIN HOSPITALS, BUFFALO, NY, p. A272
BRYN MAWR COLLEGE INFIRMARY, BRYN MAWR, PA, p. A335
BRYN MAWR HOSPITAL, BRYN MAWR, PA, p. A335
BRYN MAWR REHABILITATION HOSPITAL, MALVERN, PA, p. A341
BRYNN MARR HOSPITAL, JACKSONVILLE, NC, p. A296
BUCHANAN GENERAL HOSPITAL, GRUNDY, , p. A416
BUCKS COUNTY HOSPITAL, WARMINSTER, PA, p. A350
BUCKTAIL MEDICAL CENTER, RENOVO, PA, p. A348
BUCYRUS COMMUNITY HOSPITAL, BUCYRUS, OH, p. A307
BUENA PARK MEDICAL CENTER, BUENA PARK, CA, p. A 38
BUENA VISTA COUNTY HOSPITAL, STORM LAKE, IA, p. A150
BUFFALO COLUMBUS HOSPITAL, BUFFALO, NY, p. A272
BUFFALO GENERAL HOSPITAL, BUFFALO, NY, p. A272
BUFFALO HOSPITAL, BUFFALO, MN, p. A213
BUFFALO PSYCHIATRIC CENTER, BUFFALO, NY, p. A272
BULLHEAD COMMUNITY HOSPITAL, BULLHEAD CITY, AZ, p. A 23
BULLOCH MEMORIAL HOSPITAL, STATESBORO, GA, p. A108
BULLOCK COUNTY HOSPITAL, UNION SPRINGS, AL, p. A 20
BUNKIE GENERAL HOSPITAL, BUNKIE, LA, p. A171
BURDETTE TOMLIN MEMORIAL HOSPITAL, CAPE MAY COURT HOUSE, NJ, p. A259
BURDICK–WEST MEMORIAL HOSPITAL, HALEYVILLE, AL, p. A 17
BURGESS MEMORIAL HOSPITAL, ONAWA, IA, p. A148
BURKE COUNTY HOSPITAL, WAYNESBORO, GA, p. A109
BURKE REHABILITATION HOSPITAL, WHITE PLAINS, NY, p. A289
BURLINGTON MEDICAL CENTER, BURLINGTON, IA, p. A142
BURNETT GENERAL HOSPITAL, GRANTSBURG, WI, p. A437
BUTLER COUNTY HEALTH CARE CENTER, DAVID CITY, NE, p. A247
BUTLER HOSPITAL, PROVIDENCE, RI, p. A353
BUTLER MEMORIAL HOSPITAL, BUTLER, PA, p. A335
BUTTERWORTH HOSPITAL, GRAND RAPIDS, MI, p. A203
BYERLY HOSPITAL, HARTSVILLE, SC, p. A358

BYRD REGIONAL HOSPITAL, LEESVILLE, LA, p. A174

C

C. F. MENNINGER MEMORIAL HOSPITAL, TOPEKA, KS, p. A159
CABARRUS MEMORIAL HOSPITAL, CONCORD, NC, p. A293
CABELL HUNTINGTON HOSPITAL, HUNTINGTON, WV, p. A431
CABRINI MEDICAL CENTER, NEW YORK CITY, NY, p. A279
CAGUAS REGIONAL HOSPITAL, CAGUAS, PR, p. A448
CALAIS REGIONAL HOSPITAL, CALAIS, ME, p. A181
CALDWELL COUNTY HOSPITAL, PRINCETON, KY, p. A167
CALDWELL MEMORIAL HOSPITAL, COLUMBIA, LA, p. A171
CALDWELL MEMORIAL HOSPITAL, LENOIR, NC, p. A296
CALEXICO HOSPITAL, CALEXICO, CA, p. A 38
CALHOUN–LIBERTY HOSPITAL, BLOUNTSTOWN, FL, p. A 81
CALHOUN GENERAL HOSPITAL, GRANTSVILLE, WV, p. A431
CALHOUN MEMORIAL HOSPITAL, ARLINGTON, GA, p. A 98
CALIFORNIA HOSPITAL MEDICAL CENTER, LOS ANGELES, CA, p. A 48
CALIFORNIA MEDICAL FACILITY, VACAVILLE, CA, p. A 66
CALIFORNIA MENS COLONY HOSPITAL, SAN LUIS OBISPO, CA, p. A 61
CALIFORNIA PACIFIC MEDICAL CENTER, SAN FRANCISCO, CA, p. A 60
CALLAWAY COMMUNITY HOSPITAL, FULTON, MO, p. A232
CALLAWAY DISTRICT HOSPITAL, CALLAWAY, NE, p. A246
CALUMET MEDICAL CENTER, CHILTON, WI, p. A436
CALVARY HOSPITAL, NEW YORK CITY, NY, p. A279
CALVERT MEMORIAL HOSPITAL, PRINCE FREDERICK, MD, p. A188
CAMARILLO STATE HOSPITAL AND DEVELOPMENT CENTER, CAMARILLO, CA, p. A 38
CAMBRIDGE HOSPITAL, CAMBRIDGE, MA, p. A192
CAMBRIDGE MEDICAL CENTER, CAMBRIDGE, MN, p. A213
CAMBRIDGE MEMORIAL HOSPITAL, CAMBRIDGE, NE, p. A246
CAMBRIDGE PSYCHIATRIC HOSPITAL, CAMBRIDGE, OH, p. A307
CAMDEN–CLARK MEMORIAL HOSPITAL, PARKERSBURG, WV, p. A432
CAMDEN COUNTY HEALTH SERVICES CENTER, BLACKWOOD, NJ, p. A258
CAMDEN MEDICAL CENTER, SAINT MARYS, GA, p. A107
CAMERON COMMUNITY HOSPITAL, CAMERON, MO, p. A230
CAMERON MEMORIAL COMMUNITY HOSPITAL, ANGOLA, IN, p. A133
CAMINO HEALTHCARE, MOUNTAIN VIEW, CA, p. A 53
CAMPBELL COUNTY MEMORIAL HOSPITAL, GILLETTE, WY, p. A445
CAMPBELL MEMORIAL HOSPITAL, WEATHERFORD, TX, p. A406
CAMPBELLTON GRACEVILLE HOSPITAL, GRACEVILLE, FL, p. A 85
CANBY COMMUNITY HEALTH SERVICES, CANBY, MN, p. A213
CANDLER COUNTY HOSPITAL, METTER, GA, p. A106
CANDLER HOSPITAL, SAVANNAH, GA, p. A107
CANNON MEMORIAL HOSPITAL, PICKENS, SC, p. A359
CANONSBURG GENERAL HOSPITAL, CANONSBURG, PA, p. A336
CANTON–INWOOD MEMORIAL HOSPITAL, CANTON, SD, p. A361
CANTON–POTSDAM HOSPITAL, POTSDAM, NY, p. A285
CANYON RIDGE HOSPITAL, CHINO, CA, p. A 39
CANYON SPRINGS HOSPITAL, CATHEDRAL CITY, CA, p. A 39
CAPE CANAVERAL HOSPITAL, COCOA BEACH, FL, p. A 82
CAPE COD HOSPITAL, HYANNIS, MA, p. A194
CAPE CORAL HOSPITAL, CAPE CORAL, FL, p. A 82
CAPE FEAR MEMORIAL HOSPITAL, WILMINGTON, NC, p. A300
CAPE FEAR VALLEY MEDICAL CENTER, FAYETTEVILLE, NC, p. A294
CAPISTRANO BY THE SEA HOSPITAL, DANA POINT, CA, p. A 41
CAPITAL DISTRICT PSYCHIATRIC CENTER, ALBANY, NY, p. A271
CAPITAL MEDICAL CENTER, OLYMPIA, WA, p. A425
CAPITAL REGION MEDICAL CENTER–MEMORIAL CAMPUS, JEFFERSON CITY, MO, p. A233
CAPITAL REGION MEDICAL CENTER–STILL CAMPUS, JEFFERSON CITY, MO, p. A233
CARBON COUNTY MEMORIAL HOSPITAL AND NURSING HOME, RED LODGE, MT, p. A244
CARDINAL GLENNON CHILDREN'S HOSPITAL, SAINT LOUIS, MO, p. A238
CARDINAL HILL REHABILITATIOH HOSPITAL, LEXINGTON, KY, p. A164
CAREUNIT HOSPITAL OF CINCINNATI, CINCINNATI, OH, p. A308

CAREUNIT HOSPITAL OF DALLAS–FORT WORTH, FORT WORTH, TX, p. A386
CAREUNIT HOSPITAL OF KIRKLAND, KIRKLAND, WA, p. A425
CARIBOU MEMORIAL HOSPITAL AND NURSING HOME, SODA SPRINGS, ID, p. A114
CARITAS PEACE CENTER, LOUISVILLE, KY, p. A165
CARL ALBERT INDIAN HEALTH FACILITY, ADA, OK, p. A321
CARL T. HAYDEN VETERANS AFFAIRS MEDICAL CENTER, PHOENIX, AZ, p. A 25
CARLE FOUNDATION HOSPITAL, URBANA, IL, p. A131
CARLINVILLE AREA HOSPITAL, CARLINVILLE, IL, p. A117
CARLISLE HOSPITAL, CARLISLE, PA, p. A336
CARLYLE CENTER, WARREN, MI, p. A211
CARNEGIE TRI–COUNTY MUNICIPAL HOSPITAL, CARNEGIE, OK, p. A322
CARNEY HOSPITAL, BOSTON, MA, p. A191
CARO COMMUNITY HOSPITAL, CARO, MI, p. A200
CARO REGIONAL MENTAL HEALTH CENTER, CARO, MI, p. A200
CAROLINAS MEDICAL CENTER, CHARLOTTE, NC, p. A292
CARONDELET PSYCHIATRIC CARE CENTER, RICHLAND, WA, p. A426
CARONDELET ST. JOSEPH'S HOSPITAL, TUCSON, AZ, p. A 27
CARONDELET ST. MARY'S HOSPITAL, TUCSON, AZ, p. A 27
CARONDOLET HOLY CROSS HOSPITAL, NOGALES, AZ, p. A 25
CARRAWAY METHODIST MEDICAL CENTER, BIRMINGHAM, AL, p. A 13
CARRAWAY NORTHWEST MEDICAL CENTER, WINFIELD, AL, p. A 20
CARRIE TINGLEY HOSPITAL, ALBUQUERQUE, NM, p. A267
CARRIER FOUNDATION, BELLE MEAD, NJ, p. A258
CARRINGTON HEALTH CENTER, CARRINGTON, ND, p. A302
CARROLL COUNTY GENERAL HOSPITAL, WESTMINSTER, MD, p. A189
CARROLL COUNTY MEMORIAL HOSPITAL, CARROLLTON, KY, p. A161
CARROLL COUNTY MEMORIAL HOSPITAL, CARROLLTON, MO, p. A231
CARROLL REGIONAL MEDICAL CENTER, BERRYVILLE, AR, p. A 29
CARSON CITY HOSPITAL, CARSON CITY, MI, p. A200
CARSON TAHOE HOSPITAL, CARSON CITY, NV, p. A253
CARTERET GENERAL HOSPITAL, MOREHEAD CITY, NC, p. A297
CARTERSVILLE MEDICAL CENTER, CARTERSVILLE, GA, p. A101
CARTHAGE AREA HOSPITAL, CARTHAGE, NY, p. A273
CARTHAGE GENERAL HOSPITAL, CARTHAGE, TN, p. A366
CARY MEDICAL CENTER, CARIBOU, ME, p. A181
CASA COLINA HOSPITAL FOR REHABILITATIVE MEDICINE, POMONA, CA, p. A 56
CASA GRANDE REGIONAL MEDICAL CENTER, CASA GRANDE, AZ, p. A 23
CASA, A SPECIAL HOSPITAL, HOUSTON, TX, p. A390
CASS COUNTY MEMORIAL HOSPITAL, ATLANTIC, IA, p. A142
CASS MEDICAL CENTER, HARRISONVILLE, MO, p. A232
CASSIA REGIONAL MEDICAL CENTER, BURLEY, ID, p. A112
CASTANER GENERAL HOSPITAL, CASTANER, PR, p. A448
CASTLE MEDICAL CENTER, KAILUA, HI, p. A110
CASTLEVIEW HOSPITAL, PRICE, UT, p. A409
CASWELL CENTER, KINSTON, NC, p. A296
CATAWBA HOSPITAL, CATAWBA, VA, p. A414
CATAWBA MEMORIAL HOSPITAL, HICKORY, NC, p. A295
CATHERINE MCAULEY HEALTH SYSTEM, ANN ARBOR, MI, p. A199
CATHOLIC MEDICAL CENTER, MANCHESTER, NH, p. A256
CATHOLIC MEDICAL CENTER OF BROOKLYN AND QUEENS, NEW YORK CITY, NY, p. A279
CAVALIER COUNTY MEMORIAL HOSPITAL, LANGDON, ND, p. A304
CAVERNA MEMORIAL HOSPITAL, HORSE CAVE, KY, p. A163
CAYLOR–NICKEL MEDICAL CENTER, BLUFFTON, IN, p. A133
CEDAR COUNTY MEMORIAL HOSPITAL, EL DORADO SPRINGS, MO, p. A232
CEDAR SPRINGS PSYCHIATRIC HOSPITAL, COLORADO SPRINGS, CO, p. A 68
CEDAR VALE REGIONAL HOSPITAL, CEDAR VALE, KS, p. A151
CEDAR VISTA HOSPITAL PSYCHIATRIC SERVICES, FRESNO, CA, p. A 43
CEDARCREST REGIONAL HOSPITAL, NEWINGTON, CT, p. A 76
CEDARS–SINAI MEDICAL CENTER, LOS ANGELES, CA, p. A 48
CEDARS HOSPITAL, DE SOTO, TX, p. A384
CEDARS MEDICAL CENTER, MIAMI, FL, p. A 89
CENTENNIAL MEDICAL CENTER, NASHVILLE, TN, p. A373
CENTINELA HOSPITAL MEDICAL CENTER, INGLEWOOD, CA, p. A 45
CENTRAL ARIZONA MEDICAL CENTER, FLORENCE, AZ, p. A 23
CENTRAL ARKANSAS HOSPITAL, SEARCY, AR, p. A 34
CENTRAL ARKANSAS REHABILITATION HOSPITAL, SHERWOOD, AR, p. A 34

CENTRAL BAPTIST HOSPITAL, LEXINGTON, KY, p. A164
CENTRAL CAROLINA HOSPITAL, SANFORD, NC, p. A298
CENTRAL COMMUNITY HOSPITAL, CLIFTON, IL, p. A121
CENTRAL COMMUNITY HOSPITAL, ELKADER, IA, p. A145
CENTRAL DUPAGE HOSPITAL, WINFIELD, IL, p. A132
CENTRAL FLORIDA REGIONAL HOSPITAL, SANFORD, FL, p. A 95
CENTRAL ISLIP PSYCHIATRIC CENTER, CENTRAL ISLIP, NY, p. A273
CENTRAL KANSAS MEDICAL CENTER, GREAT BEND, KS, p. A153
CENTRAL LOUISIANA STATE HOSPITAL, PINEVILLE, LA, p. A177
CENTRAL MAINE MEDICAL CENTER, LEWISTON, ME, p. A181
CENTRAL MICHIGAN COMMUNITY HOSPITAL, MOUNT PLEASANT, MI, p. A207
CENTRAL MONTANA MEDICAL CENTER, LEWISTOWN, MT, p. A243
CENTRAL OHIO PSYCHIATRIC HOSPITAL, COLUMBUS, OH, p. A310
CENTRAL OREGON DISTRICT HOSPITAL, REDMOND, OR, p. A332
CENTRAL PENINSULA GENERAL HOSPITAL, SOLDOTNA, AK, p. A 22
CENTRAL PRISON HOSPITAL, RALEIGH, NC, p. A297
CENTRAL STATE HOSPITAL, MILLEDGEVILLE, GA, p. A106
CENTRAL STATE HOSPITAL, LOUISVILLE, KY, p. A165
CENTRAL STATE HOSPITAL, PETERSBURG, VA, p. A418
CENTRAL SUFFOLK HOSPITAL, RIVERHEAD, NY, p. A285
CENTRAL TEXAS HOSPITAL, CAMERON, TX, p. A380
CENTRAL TEXAS MEDICAL CENTER, SAN MARCOS, TX, p. A403
CENTRAL VALLEY GENERAL HOSPITAL, HANFORD, CA, p. A 44
CENTRAL VALLEY MEDICAL CENTER, NEPHI, UT, p. A409
CENTRAL VERMONT MEDICAL CENTER, BARRE, VT, p. A412
CENTRAL VIRGINIA TRAINING CENTER, MADISON HEIGHTS, VA, p. A417
CENTRAL WASHINGTON HOSPITAL, WENATCHEE, WA, p. A429
CENTRASTATE MEDICAL CENTER, FREEHOLD, NJ, p. A260
CENTRE COMMUNITY HOSPITAL, STATE COLLEGE, PA, p. A349
CENTURY CITY HOSPITAL, LOS ANGELES, CA, p. A 48
CGH MEDICAL CENTER, STERLING, IL, p. A131
CHADRON COMMUNITY HOSPITAL, CHADRON, NE, p. A247
CHALMETTE MEDICAL CENTERS, CHALMETTE, LA, p. A171
CHAMBERS MEMORIAL HOSPITAL, DANVILLE, AR, p. A 30
CHAMBERSBURG HOSPITAL, CHAMBERSBURG, PA, p. A336
CHAMPLAIN VALLEY PHYSICIANS HOSPITAL MEDICAL CENTER, PLATTSBURGH, NY, p. A285
CHANDLER REGIONAL HOSPITAL, CHANDLER, AZ, p. A 23
CHAPMAN GENERAL HOSPITAL, ORANGE, CA, p. A 55
CHARLES A. CANNON JR. MEMORIAL HOSPITAL, BANNER ELK, NC, p. A291
CHARLES A. DEAN MEMORIAL HOSPITAL, GREENVILLE, ME, p. A181
CHARLES COLE MEMORIAL HOSPITAL, COUDERSPORT, PA, p. A337
CHARLES RIVER HOSPITAL, WELLESLEY, MA, p. A198
CHARLESTON AREA MEDICAL CENTER, CHARLESTON, WV, p. A430
CHARLESTON MEMORIAL HOSPITAL, CHARLESTON, SC, p. A355
CHARLEVOIX AREA HOSPITAL, CHARLEVOIX, MI, p. A200
CHARLOTTE HUNGERFORD HOSPITAL, TORRINGTON, CT, p. A 77
CHARLOTTE INSTITUTE OF REHABILITATION, CHARLOTTE, NC, p. A292
CHARLOTTE REGIONAL MEDICAL CENTER, PUNTA GORDA, FL, p. A 94
CHARLTON MEMORIAL HOSPITAL, FOLKSTON, GA, p. A103
CHARLTON MEMORIAL HOSPITAL, FALL RIVER, MA, p. A193
CHARLTON METHODIST HOSPITAL, DALLAS, TX, p. A383
CHARTER ASHEVILLE, ASHEVILLE, NC, p. A291
CHARTER BARCLAY HOSPITAL, CHICAGO, IL, p. A118
CHARTER BEACON, FORT WAYNE, IN, p. A135
CHARTER BEHAVIORAL HEALTH SYSTEM–CORPUS CHRISTI, CORPUS CHRISTI, TX, p. A382
CHARTER BEHAVIORAL HEALTH SYSTEM–TUCSON, TUCSON, AZ, p. A 27
CHARTER BEHAVIORAL HEALTH SYSTEM, CHANDLER, AZ, p. A 23
CHARTER BEHAVIORAL HEALTH SYSTEM, GLENDALE, AZ, p. A 24
CHARTER BEHAVIORAL HEALTH SYSTEM, BEL AIR, MD, p. A185
CHARTER BEHAVIORAL HEALTH SYSTEM, FORT WORTH, TX, p. A386
CHARTER BEHAVIORAL HEALTH SYSTEM, KINGWOOD, TX, p. A394

Hospitals, Alphabetically / Charter Behavioral Health System

CHARTER BEHAVIORAL HEALTH SYSTEM, LUBBOCK, TX, p. A395
CHARTER BEHAVIORAL HEALTH SYSTEM, MCALLEN, TX, p. A396
CHARTER BEHAVIORAL HEALTH SYSTEM, SAN ANTONIO, TX, p. A401
CHARTER BEHAVIORAL HEALTH SYSTEM AT ACADIAN OAKS HOSPITAL, LAFAYETTE, LA, p. A173
CHARTER BEHAVIORAL HEALTH SYSTEM AT CENTENNIAL PEAKS, LOUISVILLE, CO, p. A 72
CHARTER BEHAVIORAL HEALTH SYSTEM AT COVE FORGE, WILLIAMSBURG, PA, p. A351
CHARTER BEHAVIORAL HEALTH SYSTEM AT MEDFIELD, LARGO, FL, p. A 88
CHARTER BEHAVIORAL HEALTH SYSTEM AT SPRINGWOOD, LEESBURG, VA, p. A416
CHARTER BEHAVIORAL HEALTH SYSTEM OF AUSTIN, AUSTIN, TX, p. A377
CHARTER BEHAVIORAL HEALTH SYSTEM OF CHARLOTTESVILLE, CHARLOTTESVILLE, VA, p. A414
CHARTER BEHAVIORAL HEALTH SYSTEM OF CLEAR LAKE, WEBSTER, TX, p. A406
CHARTER BEHAVIORAL HEALTH SYSTEM OF MICHIGAN CITY, MICHIGAN CITY, IN, p. A139
CHARTER BEHAVIORAL HEALTH SYSTEM OF NEVADA, LAS VEGAS, NV, p. A253
CHARTER BEHAVIORAL HEALTH SYSTEM OF NEW JERSEY–SUMMIT, SUMMIT, NJ, p. A265
CHARTER BEHAVIORAL HEALTH SYSTEM OF NORTHWEST INDIANA, HOBART, IN, p. A136
CHARTER BEHAVIORAL HEALTH SYSTEM OF PADUCAH, PADUCAH, KY, p. A167
CHARTER BEHAVIORAL HEALTH SYSTEM OF POTOMAC RIDGE, ROCKVILLE, MD, p. A188
CHARTER BEHAVIORAL HEALTH SYSTEM OF SOUTHERN CALIFORNIA–CHARTER OAK, COVINA, CA, p. A 40
CHARTER BEHAVIORAL HEALTH SYSTEM OF SOUTHERN CALIFORNIA–LONG BEACH, LONG BEACH, CA, p. A 48
CHARTER BEHAVIORAL HEALTH SYSTEM OF SOUTHERN CALIFORNIA–LOS ALTOS, LONG BEACH, CA, p. A 48
CHARTER BEHAVIORAL HEALTH SYSTEM OF SOUTHERN CALIFORNIA–THOUSAND OAKS, THOUSAND OAKS, CA, p. A 65
CHARTER BEHAVIORAL HEALTH SYSTEM OF THE INLAND EMPIRE, CORONA, CA, p. A 40
CHARTER BEHAVIORAL HEALTH SYSTEMS, LAFAYETTE, IN, p. A138
CHARTER BROOKSIDE BEHAVIORAL HEALTH SYSTEM OF NEW ENGLAND, NASHUA, NH, p. A256
CHARTER BY-THE-SEA HOSPITAL, SAINT SIMONS ISLAND, GA, p. A107
CHARTER CANYON TREATMENT CANTER, MIDVALE, UT, p. A408
CHARTER COMMUNITY HOSPITAL, HAWAIIAN GARDENS, CA, p. A 45
CHARTER FAIRMOUNT INSTITUTE, PHILADELPHIA, PA, p. A344
CHARTER FOREST BEHAVIORAL HEALTH SYSTEM, SHREVEPORT, LA, p. A178
CHARTER GLADE BEHAVIORAL HEALTH SYSTEM, FORT MYERS, FL, p. A 84
CHARTER GRAPEVINE BEHAVIORAL HEALTH SYSTEM, GRAPEVINE, TX, p. A389
CHARTER GREENSBORO BEHAVIORAL HEALTH SYSTEM, GREENSBORO, NC, p. A294
CHARTER HOSPITAL OF ALBUQUERQUE, ALBUQUERQUE, NM, p. A267
CHARTER HOSPITAL OF CHARLESTON, CHARLESTON, SC, p. A355
CHARTER HOSPITAL OF GREENVILLE, GREER, SC, p. A358
CHARTER HOSPITAL OF JACKSON, JACKSON, MS, p. A225
CHARTER HOSPITAL OF JACKSONVILLE, JACKSONVILLE, FL, p. A 86
CHARTER HOSPITAL OF LAKE CHARLES, LAKE CHARLES, LA, p. A174
CHARTER HOSPITAL OF LITTLE ROCK, MAUMELLE, AR, p. A 32
CHARTER HOSPITAL OF LOUISVILLE, LOUISVILLE, KY, p. A165
CHARTER HOSPITAL OF MIAMI, MIAMI, FL, p. A 89
CHARTER HOSPITAL OF MILWAUKEE, MILWAUKEE, WI, p. A439
CHARTER HOSPITAL OF MISSION VIEJO, MISSION VIEJO, CA, p. A 52
CHARTER HOSPITAL OF MOBILE, MOBILE, AL, p. A 18
CHARTER HOSPITAL OF PASCO, LUTZ, FL, p. A 88
CHARTER HOSPITAL OF TAMPA BAY, TAMPA, FL, p. A 96
CHARTER HOSPITAL OF TOLEDO, MAUMEE, OH, p. A315
CHARTER HOSPITAL OF WINSTON–SALEM, WINSTON–SALEM, NC, p. A300
CHARTER HOSPITAL ORLANDO SOUTH, KISSIMMEE, FL, p. A 87
CHARTER INDIANAPOLIS BEHAVIORAL HEALTH SYSTEM, INDIANAPOLIS, IN, p. A136

CHARTER LAKE HOSPITAL, MACON, GA, p. A105
CHARTER LAKESIDE HOSPITAL, MEMPHIS, TN, p. A371
CHARTER NORTH HOSPITAL, ANCHORAGE, AK, p. A 21
CHARTER PEACHFORD HOSPITAL, ATLANTA, GA, p. A 98
CHARTER PINES HOSPITAL, CHARLOTTE, NC, p. A292
CHARTER RIDGE HOSPITAL, LEXINGTON, KY, p. A164
CHARTER RIVERS HOSPITAL, WEST COLUMBIA, SC, p. A360
CHARTER SAVANNAH BEHAVIORAL HEALTH SYSTEM, SAVANNAH, GA, p. A107
CHARTER SIOUX FALLS BEHAVIORAL HEALTH SYSTEM, SIOUX FALLS, SD, p. A363
CHARTER SPRINGS HOSPITAL, OCALA, FL, p. A 91
CHARTER VISTA HOSPITAL, FAYETTEVILLE, AR, p. A 30
CHARTER WESTBROOK BEHAVIORAL HEALTH SYSTEM, RICHMOND, VA, p. A419
CHARTER WINDS HOSPITAL, ATHENS, GA, p. A 98
CHARTER WOODS BEHAVIORAL HEALTH SYSTEM, DOTHAN, AL, p. A 15
CHASE COUNTY COMMUNITY HOSPITAL, IMPERIAL, NE, p. A248
CHATHAM HOSPITAL, SILER CITY, NC, p. A299
CHATTANOOGA REHABILITATION HOSPITAL, CHATTANOOGA, TN, p. A366
CHATTOOGA COUNTY HOSPITAL, SUMMERVILLE, GA, p. A108
CHATUGE REGIONAL HOSPITAL AND NURSING HOME, HIAWASSEE, GA, p. A104
CHEATHAM MEDICAL CENTER, ASHLAND CITY, TN, p. A366
CHELSEA COMMUNITY HOSPITAL, CHELSEA, MI, p. A201
CHEMICAL DEPENDENCY INSTITUTE OF NORTHERN CALIFORNIA, CAMPBELL, CA, p. A 39
CHENANGO MEMORIAL HOSPITAL, NORWICH, NY, p. A284
CHEROKEE BAPTIST MEDICAL CENTER, CENTRE, AL, p. A 14
CHERRY COUNTY HOSPITAL, VALENTINE, NE, p. A251
CHERRY HOSPITAL, GOLDSBORO, NC, p. A294
CHESAPEAKE GENERAL HOSPITAL, CHESAPEAKE, VA, p. A415
CHESHIRE MEDICAL CENTER, KEENE, NH, p. A255
CHESTER COUNTY HOSPITAL, WEST CHESTER, PA, p. A351
CHESTER COUNTY HOSPITAL AND NURSING CENTER, CHESTER, SC, p. A356
CHESTER MENTAL HEALTH CENTER, CHESTER, IL, p. A118
CHESTERFIELD GENERAL HOSPITAL, CHERAW, SC, p. A356
CHESTNUT HILL HOSPITAL, PHILADELPHIA, PA, p. A344
CHESTNUT HILL REHABILITATION HOSPITAL, WYNDMOOR, PA, p. A352
CHESTNUT LODGE HOSPITAL, ROCKVILLE, MD, p. A188
CHESTNUT RIDGE HOSPITAL, MORGANTOWN, WV, p. A432
CHEYENNE COUNTY HOSPITAL, SAINT FRANCIS, KS, p. A158
CHICAGO-READ MENTAL HEALTH CENTER, CHICAGO, IL, p. A118
CHICAGO LAKESHORE HOSPITAL, CHICAGO, IL, p. A118
CHICAGO OSTEOPATHIC HOSPITAL AND MEDICAL CENTERS, CHICAGO, IL, p. A118
CHICO COMMUNITY HOSPITAL, CHICO, CA, p. A 39
CHICOT MEMORIAL HOSPITAL, LAKE VILLAGE, AR, p. A 32
CHILD AND ADOLESCENT SERVICES OF THE MENNINGER CLINIC, TOPEKA, KS, p. A159
CHILD'S HOSPITAL, ALBANY, NY, p. A271
CHILDREN'S HEALTH CARE, MINNEAPOLIS, MN, p. A217
CHILDREN'S HOME OF PITTSBURGH, PITTSBURGH, PA, p. A346
CHILDREN'S HOSPITAL – OAKLAND, OAKLAND, CA, p. A 54
CHILDREN'S HOSPITAL, DENVER, CO, p. A 69
CHILDREN'S HOSPITAL, NEW ORLEANS, LA, p. A176
CHILDREN'S HOSPITAL, BOSTON, MA, p. A191
CHILDREN'S HOSPITAL, SAINT PAUL, MN, p. A219
CHILDREN'S HOSPITAL, BUFFALO, NY, p. A272
CHILDREN'S HOSPITAL, COLUMBUS, OH, p. A310
CHILDREN'S HOSPITAL, RICHMOND, VA, p. A419
CHILDREN'S HOSPITAL AND CENTER FOR RECONSTRUCTIVE SURGERY, BALTIMORE, MD, p. A184
CHILDREN'S HOSPITAL AND HEALTH CENTER, SAN DIEGO, CA, p. A 59
CHILDREN'S HOSPITAL AND MEDICAL CENTER, SEATTLE, WA, p. A427
CHILDREN'S HOSPITAL MEDICAL CENTER, CINCINNATI, OH, p. A308
CHILDREN'S HOSPITAL MEDICAL CENTER OF AKRON, AKRON, OH, p. A306
CHILDREN'S HOSPITAL OF ALABAMA, BIRMINGHAM, AL, p. A 14
CHILDREN'S HOSPITAL OF MICHIGAN, DETROIT, MI, p. A201
CHILDREN'S HOSPITAL OF ORANGE COUNTY, ORANGE, CA, p. A 55
CHILDREN'S HOSPITAL OF PHILADELPHIA, PHILADELPHIA, PA, p. A344
CHILDREN'S HOSPITAL OF PITTSBURGH, PITTSBURGH, PA, p. A346
CHILDREN'S HOSPITAL OF THE KING'S DAUGHTERS, NORFOLK, VA, p. A418

CHILDREN'S HOSPITAL OF WISCONSIN, MILWAUKEE, WI, p. A439
CHILDREN'S MEDICAL CENTER, DAYTON, OH, p. A311
CHILDREN'S MEDICAL CENTER, TULSA, OK, p. A327
CHILDREN'S MEDICAL CENTER OF DALLAS, DALLAS, TX, p. A383
CHILDREN'S MEMORIAL HOSPITAL, CHICAGO, IL, p. A118
CHILDREN'S MERCY HOSPITAL, KANSAS CITY, MO, p. A233
CHILDREN'S NATIONAL MEDICAL CENTER, WASHINGTON, DC, p. A 79
CHILDREN'S PSYCHIATRIC HOSPITAL OF NORTHERN KENTUCKY, COVINGTON, KY, p. A162
CHILDREN'S REHABILITATION HOSPITAL, PHILADELPHIA, PA, p. A344
CHILDREN'S SEASHORE HOUSE, PHILADELPHIA, PA, p. A344
CHILDREN'S SPECIALIZED HOSPITAL, MOUNTAINSIDE, NJ, p. A262
CHILDRENS CARE HOSPITAL AND SCHOOL, SIOUX FALLS, SD, p. A363
CHILDRENS HOSPITAL OF LOS ANGELES, LOS ANGELES, CA, p. A 49
CHILDRENS MEMORIAL HOSPITAL, OMAHA, NE, p. A250
CHILDRESS REGIONAL MEDICAL CENTER, CHILDRESS, TX, p. A381
CHILLICOTHE HOSPITAL DISTRICT, CHILLICOTHE, TX, p. A381
CHILTON MEMORIAL HOSPITAL, POMPTON PLAINS, NJ, p. A264
CHINESE HOSPITAL, SAN FRANCISCO, CA, p. A 60
CHINLE COMPREHENSIVE HEALTH CARE FACILITY, CHINLE, AZ, p. A 23
CHINO VALLEY MEDICAL CENTER, CHINO, CA, p. A 39
CHIPPENHAM MEDICAL CENTER, RICHMOND, VA, p. A419
CHIPPEWA COUNTY MONTEVIDEO HOSPITAL, MONTEVIDEO, MN, p. A217
CHIPPEWA COUNTY WAR MEMORIAL HOSPITAL, SAULT SAINTE MARIE, MI, p. A210
CHIPPEWA VALLEY HOSPITAL AND OAKVIEW CARE CENTER, DURAND, WI, p. A436
CHISAGO HEALTH SERVICES, CHISAGO CITY, MN, p. A213
CHOATE HEALTH SYSTEMS, WOBURN, MA, p. A198
CHOATE MENTAL HEALTH AND DEVELOPMENTAL CENTER, ANNA, IL, p. A116
CHOCTAW COUNTY MEDICAL CENTER, ACKERMAN, MS, p. A222
CHOCTAW HEALTH CENTER, PHILADELPHIA, MS, p. A227
CHOCTAW MEMORIAL HOSPITAL, HUGO, OK, p. A324
CHOCTAW NATION INDIAN HOSPITAL, TALIHINA, OK, p. A327
CHOWAN HOSPITAL, EDENTON, NC, p. A293
CHOWCHILLA DISTRICT MEMORIAL HOSPITAL, CHOWCHILLA, CA, p. A 39
CHRIST HOSPITAL, JERSEY CITY, NJ, p. A261
CHRIST HOSPITAL, CINCINNATI, OH, p. A308
CHRIST HOSPITAL AND MEDICAL CENTER, OAK LAWN, IL, p. A128
CHRISTIAN HEALTH MINISTRIES, NEW ORLEANS, LA, p. A176
CHRISTIAN HOSPITAL NORTHEAST–NORTHWEST, SAINT LOUIS, MO, p. A238
CHRISTOPHER HOUSE, AUSTIN, TX, p. A377
CHURCH HOSPITAL CORPORATION, BALTIMORE, MD, p. A184
CHURCHILL COMMUNITY HOSPTIAL, FALLON, NV, p. A253
CIBOLA GENERAL HOSPITAL, GRANTS, NM, p. A269
CIMARRON MEMORIAL HOSPITAL, BOISE CITY, OK, p. A321
CIRCLES OF CARE, MELBOURNE, FL, p. A 89
CITIZENS BAPTIST MEDICAL CENTER, TALLADEGA, AL, p. A 20
CITIZENS GENERAL HOSPITAL, NEW KENSINGTON, PA, p. A343
CITIZENS MEDICAL CENTER, COLBY, KS, p. A152
CITIZENS MEDICAL CENTER, VICTORIA, TX, p. A406
CITIZENS MEMORIAL HOSPITAL, BOLIVAR, MO, p. A230
CITRUS MEMORIAL HOSPITAL, INVERNESS, FL, p. A 86
CITY HOSPITAL, BELLAIRE, OH, p. A307
CITY HOSPITAL, MARTINSBURG, WV, p. A432
CITY OF HOPE NATIONAL MEDICAL CENTER, DUARTE, CA, p. A 41
CITY OF MILAN HOSPITAL, MILAN, TN, p. A372
CLAGETT MEMORIAL HOSPITAL, RIFLE, CO, p. A 72
CLAIBORNE COUNTY HOSPITAL, PORT GIBSON, MS, p. A227
CLAIBORNE COUNTY HOSPITAL, TAZEWELL, TN, p. A375
CLARA BARTON HOSPTIAL, HOISINGTON, KS, p. A154
CLARA MAASS HEALTH SYSTEM, BELLEVILLE, NJ, p. A258
CLAREMORE REGIONAL HOSPITAL, CLAREMORE, OK, p. A322
CLARENDON MEMORIAL HOSPITAL, MANNING, SC, p. A358
CLARINDA MUNICIPAL HOSPITAL, CLARINDA, IA, p. A143
CLARION HOSPITAL, CLARION, PA, p. A336
CLARION PSYCHIATRIC CENTER, CLARION, PA, p. A336
CLARK FORK VALLEY HOSPITAL, PLAINS, MT, p. A243
CLARK MEMORIAL HOSPITAL, JEFFERSONVILLE, IN, p. A137
CLARK REGIONAL MEDICAL CENTER, WINCHESTER, KY, p. A169

Hospitals, Alphabetically / Cooper Hospital–University Medical Center

CLARKE COUNTY HOSPITAL, OSCEOLA, IA, p. A148
CLARKS SUMMIT STATE HOSPITAL, CLARKS SUMMIT, PA, p. A336
CLARKSVILLE MEMORIAL HOSPITAL, CLARKSVILLE, TN, p. A367
CLAY COUNTY HOSPITAL, FLORA, IL, p. A123
CLAY COUNTY HOSPITAL, BRAZIL, IN, p. A133
CLAY COUNTY HOSPITAL, CLAY CENTER, KS, p. A151
CLAY COUNTY HOSPITAL, CELINA, TN, p. A366
CLAY COUNTY HOSPITAL AND NURSING HOME, ASHLAND, AL, p. A 13
CLAY COUNTY MEDICAL CENTER, WEST POINT, MS, p. A228
CLAY COUNTY MEMORIAL HOSPITAL, HENRIETTA, TX, p. A389
CLC–NAVASOTA REGIONAL HOSPITAL, NAVASOTA, TX, p. A398
CLEAR BROOK LODGE, SHICKSHINNY, PA, p. A349
CLEAR BROOK MANOR, WILKES–BARRE, PA, p. A351
CLEAR LAKE REGIONAL MEDICAL CENTER, WEBSTER, TX, p. A406
CLEARFIELD HOSPITAL, CLEARFIELD, PA, p. A336
CLEARWATER COMMUNITY HOSPITAL, CLEARWATER, FL, p. A 82
CLEARWATER COUNTY MEMORIAL HOSPITAL, BAGLEY, MN, p. A212
CLEARWATER VALLEY HOSPITAL, OROFINO, ID, p. A114
CLEBURNE MEMORIAL HOSPITAL, HEBER SPRINGS, AR, p. A 31
CLEMENT J. ZABLOCKI VETERANS AFFAIRS MEDICAL CENTER, MILWAUKEE, WI, p. A439
CLEO WALLACE CENTER HOSPITAL, WESTMINSTER, CO, p. A 73
CLERMONT MERCY HOSPITAL, BATAVIA, OH, p. A306
CLEVELAND AREA HOSPITAL, CLEVELAND, OK, p. A322
CLEVELAND CLINIC HOSPITAL, FORT LAUDERDALE, FL, p. A 84
CLEVELAND CLINIC HOSPITAL, CLEVELAND, OH, p. A309
CLEVELAND COMMUNITY HOSPITAL, CLEVELAND, TN, p. A367
CLEVELAND MEMORIAL HOSPITAL, SHELBY, NC, p. A299
CLEVELAND PSYCHIATRIC INSTITUTE, CLEVELAND, OH, p. A309
CLEVELAND REGIONAL MEDICAL CENTER, CLEVELAND, TX, p. A381
CLIFTON–FINE HOSPITAL, STAR LAKE, NY, p. A287
CLIFTON SPRINGS HOSPITAL AND CLINIC, CLIFTON SPRINGS, NY, p. A274
CLIFTON T. PERKINS HOSPITAL CENTER, JESSUP, MD, p. A187
CLINCH MEMORIAL HOSPITAL, HOMERVILLE, GA, p. A104
CLINCH VALLEY MEDICAL CENTER, RICHLANDS, VA, p. A419
CLINICA ESPANOLA, MAYAGUEZ, PR, p. A449
CLINICAL CENTER, NATIONAL INSTITUTES OF HEALTH, BETHESDA, MD, p. A185
CLINTON COUNTY HOSPITAL, FRANKFORT, IN, p. A135
CLINTON COUNTY HOSPITAL, ALBANY, KY, p. A161
CLINTON HOSPITAL, CLINTON, MA, p. A193
CLINTON MEMORIAL HOSPITAL, SAINT JOHNS, MI, p. A209
CLINTON MEMORIAL HOSPITAL, WILMINGTON, OH, p. A319
CLINTON REGIONAL HOSPITAL, CLINTON, OK, p. A322
CLINTON VALLEY CENTER, PONTIAC, MI, p. A208
CLOVIS COMMUNITY HOSPITAL, CLOVIS, CA, p. A 40
COALINGA REGIONAL MEDICAL CENTER, COALINGA, CA, p. A 40
COAST PLAZA DOCTORS HOSPITAL, NORWALK, CA, p. A 54
COASTAL BEND HOSPITAL, ARANSAS PASS, TX, p. A377
COASTAL CAROLINA HOSPITAL, CONWAY, SC, p. A357
COASTAL COMMUNITIES HOSPITAL, SANTA ANA, CA, p. A 62
COBB HOSPITAL AND MEDICAL CENTER, AUSTELL, GA, p. A100
COBB MEMORIAL HOSPITAL, ROYSTON, GA, p. A107
COBRE VALLEY COMMUNITY HOSPIAL, CLAYPOOL, AZ, p. A 23
COCHRAN MEMORIAL HOSPITAL, MORTON, TX, p. A397
COFFEE MEDICAL CENTER, MANCHESTER, TN, p. A371
COFFEE REGIONAL MEDICAL CENTER, DOUGLAS, GA, p. A103
COFFEY COUNTY HOSPITAL, BURLINGTON, KS, p. A151
COFFEYVILLE REGIONAL MEDICAL CENTER, COFFEYVILLE, KS, p. A151
COLEMAN COUNTY MEDICAL CENTER, COLEMAN, TX, p. A381
COLER MEMORIAL HOSPITAL, NEW YORK CITY, NY, p. A279
COLISEUM MEDICAL CENTERS, MACON, GA, p. A105
COLISEUM PSYCHIATRIC HOSPITAL, MACON, GA, p. A105
COLLEGE HOSPITAL, CERRITOS, CA, p. A 39
COLLEGE HOSPITAL COSTA MESA, COSTA MESA, CA, p. A 40
COLLETON REGIONAL HOSPITAL, WALTERBORO, SC, p. A360
COLLINGSWORTH GENERAL HOSPITAL, WELLINGTON, TX, p. A406
COLMERY–O'NEIL VETERANS AFFAIRS MEDICAL CENTER, TOPEKA, KS, p. A159
COLONEL FLORENCE A. BLANCHFIELD ARMY COMMUNITY HOSPITAL, FORT CAMPBELL, KY, p. A162

COLORADO–FAYETTE MEDICAL CENTER, WEIMAR, TX, p. A406
COLORADO MENTAL HEALTH INSTITUTE AT FORT LOGAN, DENVER, CO, p. A 69
COLORADO MENTAL HEALTH INSTITUTE AT PUEBLO, PUEBLO, CO, p. A 72
COLORADO PLAINS MEDICAL CENTER, FORT MORGAN, CO, p. A 70
COLQUITT REGIONAL MEDICAL CENTER, MOULTRIE, GA, p. A106
COLUMBIA BASIN HOSPITAL, EPHRATA, WA, p. A424
COLUMBIA BEHAVIORAL CENTER, EL PASO, TX, p. A385
COLUMBIA DOCTORS HOSPITAL, LITTLE ROCK, AR, p. A 32
COLUMBIA HOSPITAL, WEST PALM BEACH, FL, p. A 97
COLUMBIA HOSPITAL, MILWAUKEE, WI, p. A439
COLUMBIA HOSPITAL FOR WOMEN MEDICAL CENTER, WASHINGTON, DC, p. A 79
COLUMBIA MEDICAL CENTER–EAST, EL PASO, TX, p. A385
COLUMBIA MEDICAL CENTER–WEST, EL PASO, TX, p. A385
COLUMBIA MEMORIAL HOSPITAL, HUDSON, NY, p. A276
COLUMBIA MEMORIAL HOSPITAL, ASTORIA, OR, p. A329
COLUMBIA PARK MEDICAL CENTER, ORLANDO, FL, p. A 91
COLUMBIA REGIONAL HOSPITAL, COLUMBIA, MO, p. A231
COLUMBIA REGIONAL MEDICAL CENTER AT BAYONET POINT, HUDSON, FL, p. A 86
COLUMBIA REHABILITATION HOSPITAL, EL PASO, TX, p. A385
COLUMBINE PSYCHIATRIC CENTER, LITTLETON, CO, p. A 71
COLUMBUS COMMUNITY HOSPITAL, COLUMBUS, NE, p. A247
COLUMBUS COMMUNITY HOSPITAL, COLUMBUS, OH, p. A310
COLUMBUS COMMUNITY HOSPITAL, COLUMBUS, TX, p. A381
COLUMBUS COMMUNITY HOSPITAL, COLUMBUS, WI, p. A436
COLUMBUS COUNTY HOSPITAL, WHITEVILLE, NC, p. A300
COLUMBUS HOSPITAL, CHICAGO, IL, p. A118
COLUMBUS HOSPITAL, GREAT FALLS, MT, p. A242
COLUMBUS HOSPITAL, NEWARK, NJ, p. A262
COLUMBUS REGIONAL HOSPITAL, COLUMBUS, IN, p. A134
COLUSA COMMUNITY HOSPITAL, COLUSA, CA, p. A 40
COMANCHE COMMUNITY HOSPITAL, COMANCHE, TX, p. A381
COMANCHE COUNTY HOSPITAL, COLDWATER, KS, p. A152
COMANCHE COUNTY MEMORIAL HOSPITAL, LAWTON, OK, p. A324
COMMMUNITY HOSPITAL OF SAN BERNARDINO, SAN BERNARDINO, CA, p. A 59
COMMUNITY–GENERAL HOSPITAL OF GREATER SYRACUSE, SYRACUSE, NY, p. A288
COMMUNITY AND MISSION HOSPITALS OF HUNTINGTON, HUNTINGTON PARK, CA, p. A 45
COMMUNITY GENERAL HOSPITAL, READING, PA, p. A348
COMMUNITY GENERAL HOSPITAL OF SULLIVAN COUNTY, HARRIS, NY, p. A275
COMMUNITY GENERAL HOSPITAL OF THOMASVILLE, THOMASVILLE, NC, p. A299
COMMUNITY GENERAL OSTEOPATHIC HOSPITAL, HARRISBURG, PA, p. A339
COMMUNITY HEALTH CENTER OF BRANCH COUNTY, COLDWATER, MI, p. A201
COMMUNITY HEALTH NETWORK, BERLIN, WI, p. A435
COMMUNITY HOSPITAL–LAKEVIEW, EUFAULA, OK, p. A323
COMMUNITY HOSPITAL, TALLASSEE, AL, p. A 20
COMMUNITY HOSPITAL, SANTA ROSA, CA, p. A 63
COMMUNITY HOSPITAL, GRAND JUNCTION, CO, p. A 70
COMMUNITY HOSPITAL, BONNERS FERRY, ID, p. A112
COMMUNITY HOSPITAL, MUNSTER, IN, p. A139
COMMUNITY HOSPITAL, WILLIAMSPORT, IN, p. A141
COMMUNITY HOSPITAL, WATERVLIET, MI, p. A211
COMMUNITY HOSPITAL, CANNON FALLS, MN, p. A213
COMMUNITY HOSPITAL, FAIRFAX, MO, p. A232
COMMUNITY HOSPITAL, POPLAR, MT, p. A244
COMMUNITY HOSPITAL, FALLS CITY, NE, p. A247
COMMUNITY HOSPITAL, MCCOOK, NE, p. A249
COMMUNITY HOSPITAL, SPRINGFIELD, OH, p. A317
COMMUNITY HOSPITAL, KANE, PA, p. A340
COMMUNITY HOSPITAL, TORRINGTON, WY, p. A446
COMMUNITY HOSPITAL AND HEALTH CARE CENTER, SAINT PETER, MN, p. A220
COMMUNITY HOSPITAL AND REHABILITATION CENTER OF LOS GATOS–SARATOGA, LOS GATOS, CA, p. A 51
COMMUNITY HOSPITAL AT DOBBS FERRY, DOBBS FERRY, NY, p. A274
COMMUNITY HOSPITAL IN NELSON COUNTY, MCVILLE, ND, p. A304
COMMUNITY HOSPITAL MEDICAL CENTER, PHOENIX, AZ, p. A 25
COMMUNITY HOSPITAL OF ANACONDA, ANACONDA, MT, p. A241
COMMUNITY HOSPITAL OF ANDERSON AND MADISON COUNTY, ANDERSON, IN, p. A133
COMMUNITY HOSPITAL OF BREMEN, BREMEN, IN, p. A134
COMMUNITY HOSPITAL OF GARDENA, GARDENA, CA, p. A 44
COMMUNITY HOSPITAL OF LANCASTER, LANCASTER, PA, p. A340

COMMUNITY HOSPITAL OF OTTAWA, OTTAWA, IL, p. A128
COMMUNITY HOSPITAL OF ROANOKE VALLEY, ROANOKE, VA, p. A420
COMMUNITY HOSPITAL OF ROCKY MOUNT, ROCKY MOUNT, NC, p. A298
COMMUNITY HOSPITAL OF THE MONTEREY PENINSULA, MONTEREY, CA, p. A 53
COMMUNITY HOSPITAL OF WESTERN SUFFOLK, SMITHTOWN, NY, p. A287
COMMUNITY HOSPITAL ONAGA, ONAGA, KS, p. A157
COMMUNITY HOSPITALS OF INDIANAPOLIS, INDIANAPOLIS, IN, p. A136
COMMUNITY HOSPITALS OF WILLIAMS COUNTY, MONTPELIER, OH, p. A315
COMMUNITY MEDICAL CENTER, MISSOULA, MT, p. A243
COMMUNITY MEDICAL CENTER, TOMS RIVER, NJ, p. A265
COMMUNITY MEDICAL CENTER, SCRANTON, PA, p. A349
COMMUNITY MEMORIAL HEALTHCENTER, SOUTH HILL, VA, p. A421
COMMUNITY MEMORIAL HOSPITAL, MONMOUTH, IL, p. A127
COMMUNITY MEMORIAL HOSPITAL, STAUNTON, IL, p. A131
COMMUNITY MEMORIAL HOSPITAL, CLARION, IA, p. A143
COMMUNITY MEMORIAL HOSPITAL, MISSOURI VALLEY, IA, p. A147
COMMUNITY MEMORIAL HOSPITAL, SUMNER, IA, p. A150
COMMUNITY MEMORIAL HOSPITAL, MARYSVILLE, KS, p. A156
COMMUNITY MEMORIAL HOSPITAL, CHEBOYGAN, MI, p. A200
COMMUNITY MEMORIAL HOSPITAL, SIDNEY, MT, p. A244
COMMUNITY MEMORIAL HOSPITAL, HUMBOLDT, NE, p. A248
COMMUNITY MEMORIAL HOSPITAL, SYRACUSE, NE, p. A251
COMMUNITY MEMORIAL HOSPITAL, HAMILTON, NY, p. A275
COMMUNITY MEMORIAL HOSPITAL, LISBON, ND, p. A304
COMMUNITY MEMORIAL HOSPITAL, TURTLE LAKE, ND, p. A305
COMMUNITY MEMORIAL HOSPITAL, HICKSVILLE, OH, p. A313
COMMUNITY MEMORIAL HOSPITAL, BURKE, SD, p. A361
COMMUNITY MEMORIAL HOSPITAL, REDFIELD, SD, p. A363
COMMUNITY MEMORIAL HOSPITAL, ENUMCLAW, WA, p. A424
COMMUNITY MEMORIAL HOSPITAL, MENOMONEE FALLS, WI, p. A439
COMMUNITY MEMORIAL HOSPITAL, OCONTO FALLS, WI, p. A441
COMMUNITY MEMORIAL HOSPITAL AND CONVALESCENT AND NURSING CARE SECTION, CLOQUET, MN, p. A213
COMMUNITY MEMORIAL HOSPITAL AND CONVALESCENT AND REHABILITATION UNIT, WINONA, MN, p. A221
COMMUNITY MEMORIAL HOSPITAL AND NURSING HOME, SPRING VALLEY, MN, p. A220
COMMUNITY MEMORIAL HOSPITAL AND NURSING HOME, SPOONER, WI, p. A443
COMMUNITY MEMORIAL HOSPITAL OF DEER RIVER, DEER RIVER, MN, p. A214
COMMUNITY MEMORIAL HOSPITAL OF SAN BUENAVENTURA, VENTURA, CA, p. A 66
COMMUNITY METHODIST HOSPITAL, HENDERSON, KY, p. A163
CONCHO COUNTY HOSPITAL, EDEN, TX, p. A385
CONCHO VALLEY REGIONAL HOSPITAL, SAN ANGELO, TX, p. A401
CONCORD HOSPITAL, CONCORD, NH, p. A255
CONDELL MEDICAL CENTER, LIBERTYVILLE, IL, p. A126
CONEJOS COUNTY HOSPITAL, LA JARA, CO, p. A 71
CONEY ISLAND HOSPITAL, NEW YORK CITY, NY, p. A279
CONIFER PARK, GLENVILLE, NY, p. A275
CONNECTICUT DEPARTMENT OF CORRECTION'S HOSPITAL, SOMERS, CT, p. A 76
CONNECTICUT MENTAL HEALTH CENTER, NEW HAVEN, CT, p. A 75
CONNECTICUT VALLEY HOSPITAL, MIDDLETOWN, CT, p. A 75
CONVERSE COUNTY MEMORIAL HOSPITAL, DOUGLAS, WY, p. A445
CONWAY COUNTY HOSPITAL, MORRILTON, AR, p. A 33
CONWAY HOSPITAL, CONWAY, SC, p. A357
CONWAY REGIONAL MEDICAL CENTER, CONWAY, AR, p. A 29
COOK–FORT WORTH CHILDREN'S MEDICAL CENTER, FORT WORTH, TX, p. A386
COOK COUNTY HOSPITAL, CHICAGO, IL, p. A118
COOK COUNTY NORTH SHORE HOSPITAL, GRAND MARAIS, MN, p. A215
COOK HOSPITAL AND CONVALESCENT NURSING CARE UNIT, COOK, MN, p. A213
COOKEVILLE GENERAL HOSPITAL, COOKEVILLE, TN, p. A367
COOLEY DICKINSON HOSPITAL, NORTHAMPTON, MA, p. A195
COON MEMORIAL HOSPITAL AND HOME, DALHART, TX, p. A382
COOPER COUNTY MEMORIAL HOSPITAL, BOONVILLE, MO, p. A230
COOPER GREEN HOSPITAL, BIRMINGHAM, AL, p. A 14
COOPER HOSPITAL–UNIVERSITY MEDICAL CENTER, CAMDEN, NJ, p. A258

Hospitals A457

© 1995 AHA Guide

Hospitals, Alphabetically / Coosa Valley Baptist Medical Center

COOSA VALLEY BAPTIST MEDICAL CENTER, SYLACAUGA, AL, p. A 20
COPLEY HOSPITAL, MORRISVILLE, VT, p. A412
COPLEY MEMORIAL HOSPITAL, AURORA, IL, p. A116
COPPER BASIN MEDICAL CENTER, COPPERHILL, TN, p. A367
COPPER QUEEN COMMUNITY HOSPITAL, BISBEE, AZ, p. A 23
COQUILLE VALLEY HOSPITAL, COQUILLE, OR, p. A329
CORAL GABLES HOSPITAL, CORAL GABLES, FL, p. A 83
CORAL RIDGE PSYCHIATRIC HOSPITAL, FORT LAUDERDALE, FL, p. A 84
CORAL SPRINGS MEDICAL CENTER, CORAL SPRINGS, FL, p. A 83
CORCORAN DISTRICT HOSPITAL, CORCORAN, CA, p. A 40
CORDELL MEMORIAL HOSPITAL, CORDELL, OK, p. A322
CORDOVA COMMUNITY HOSPITAL, CORDOVA, AK, p. A 21
CORNERSTONE OF MEDICAL ARTS CENTER HOSPITAL, NEW YORK CITY, NY, p. A279
CORNING HOSPITAL, CORNING, NY, p. A274
CORNWALL HOSPITAL, CORNWALL, NY, p. A274
CORONA REGIONAL MEDICAL CENTER, CORONA, CA, p. A 40
CORONADO HOSPITAL, CORONADO, CA, p. A 40
CORONADO HOSPITAL, PAMPA, TX, p. A399
CORRY MEMORIAL HOSPITAL, CORRY, PA, p. A337
CORTLAND MEMORIAL HOSPITAL, CORTLAND, NY, p. A274
CORYELL MEMORIAL HOSPITAL, GATESVILLE, TX, p. A388
COSHOCTON COUNTY MEMORIAL HOSPITAL, COSHOCTON, OH, p. A311
COTEAU DES PRAIRIES HOSPITAL, SISSETON, SD, p. A364
COTTAGE GROVE HOSPITAL, COTTAGE GROVE, OR, p. A329
COTTAGE HOSPITAL, WOODSVILLE, NH, p. A257
COTTONWOOD HOSPITAL MEDICAL CENTER, MURRAY, UT, p. A409
COULEE COMMUNITY HOSPITAL, GRAND COULEE, WA, p. A424
COUNCIL COMMUNITY HOSPITAL AND NURSING HOME, COUNCIL, ID, p. A113
COVENANT MEDICAL CENTER, URBANA, IL, p. A131
COVENANT MEDICAL CENTER, WATERLOO, IA, p. A150
COVINA VALLEY COMMUNITY HOSPITAL, WEST COVINA, CA, p. A 67
COVINGTON COUNTY HOSPITAL, COLLINS, MS, p. A223
COX–MONETT HOSPITAL, MONETT, MO, p. A236
COZAD COMMUNITY HOSPITAL, COZAD, NE, p. A247
COZBY–GERMANY HOSPITAL, GRAND SALINE, TX, p. A388
CPC ALHAMBRA HOSPITAL, ROSEMEAD, CA, p. A 58
CPC BELMONT HILLS HOSPITAL, BELMONT, CA, p. A 38
CPC BRENTWOOD HOSPITAL, SHREVEPORT, LA, p. A178
CPC CAPITAL HOSPITAL, AUSTIN, TX, p. A378
CPC CEDAR SPRING HOSPITAL, PINEVILLE, NC, p. A297
CPC COLISEUM MEDICAL CENTER, NEW ORLEANS, LA, p. A176
CPC COLLEGE MEADOWS HOSPITAL, LENEXA, KS, p. A155
CPC EAST LAKE HOSPITAL, NEW ORLEANS, LA, p. A176
CPC FAIRFAX HOSPITAL, KIRKLAND, WA, p. A425
CPC FORT LAUDERDALE HOSPITAL, FORT LAUDERDALE, FL, p. A 84
CPC FREMONT HOSPITAL, FREMONT, CA, p. A 43
CPC GREENBRIAR BEHAVIORAL HEALTH CENTER, MILWAUKEE, WI, p. A440
CPC HERITAGE OAKS HOSPITAL, SACRAMENTO, CA, p. A 58
CPC HOSPITAL SAN JUAN CAPESTRANO, SAN JUAN, PR, p. A449
CPC INTERMOUNTAIN HOSPITAL OF BOISE, BOISE, ID, p. A112
CPC MEADOW WOOD HOSPITAL, BATON ROUGE, LA, p. A170
CPC MILLWOOD HOSPITAL, ARLINGTON, TX, p. A377
CPC OLD ORCHARD HOSPITAL, SKOKIE, IL, p. A130
CPC OLYMPUS VIEW HOSPITAL, SALT LAKE CITY, UT, p. A410
CPC PALM BAY HOSPITAL, PALM BAY, FL, p. A 92
CPC PARKWOOD HOSPITAL, ATLANTA, GA, p. A 98
CPC PINNACLE POINTE HOSPITAL, LITTLE ROCK, AR, p. A 32
CPC RANCHO LINDO HOSPITAL, FONTANA, CA, p. A 42
CPC SAN LUIS REY HOSPITAL, ENCINITAS, CA, p. A 42
CPC SAND HILL HOSPITAL, GULFPORT, MS, p. A224
CPC SANTA ANA HOSPITAL, SANTA ANA, CA, p. A 62
CPC SIERRA VISTA HOSPITAL, SACRAMENTO, CA, p. A 58
CPC SPIRIT OF ST. LOUIS HOSPITAL, SAINT CHARLES, MO, p. A237
CPC ST. JOHNS RIVER HOSPITAL, JACKSONVILLE, FL, p. A 86
CPC STREAMWOOD HOSPITAL, STREAMWOOD, IL, p. A131
CPC VALLE VISTA HOSPITAL, GREENWOOD, IN, p. A136
CPC VISTA DEL MAR HOSPITAL, VENTURA, CA, p. A 66
CPC WALNUT CREEK HOSPITAL, WALNUT CREEK, CA, p. A 66
CRAFTS–FARROW STATE HOSPITAL, COLUMBIA, SC, p. A356
CRAIG GENERAL HOSPITAL, VINITA, OK, p. A328
CRAIG HOSPITAL, ENGLEWOOD, CO, p. A 70
CRAIG HOUSE HOSPITAL, BEACON, NY, p. A272
CRANBERRY SPECIALITY HOSPITAL OF PLYMOUTH COUNTY, MIDDLEBOROUGH, MA, p. A195
CRANE MEMORIAL HOSPITAL, CRANE, TX, p. A382

CRAVEN REGIONAL MEDICAL AUTHORITY, NEW BERN, NC, p. A297
CRAWFORD COUNTY HOSPITAL DISTRICT ONE, GIRARD, KS, p. A153
CRAWFORD COUNTY MEMORIAL HOSPITAL, DENISON, IA, p. A144
CRAWFORD LONG HOSPITAL OF EMORY UNIVERSITY, ATLANTA, GA, p. A 98
CRAWFORD MEMORIAL HOSPITAL, VAN BUREN, AR, p. A 34
CRAWFORD MEMORIAL HOSPITAL, ROBINSON, IL, p. A129
CRAWLEY MEMORIAL HOSPITAL, BOILING SPRINGS, NC, p. A291
CREEDMOOR PSYCHIATRIC CENTER, NEW YORK CITY, NY, p. A279
CRENSHAW BAPTIST HOSPITAL, LUVERNE, AL, p. A 17
CRESTLINE MEMORIAL HOSPITAL, CRESTLINE, OH, p. A311
CRESTWOOD HOSPITAL, HUNTSVILLE, AL, p. A 17
CRETE MUNICIPAL HOSPITAL, CRETE, NE, p. A247
CRISP REGIONAL HOSPITAL, CORDELE, GA, p. A102
CRITTENDEN COUNTY HOSPITAL, MARION, KY, p. A166
CRITTENDEN MEMORIAL HOSPITAL, WEST MEMPHIS, AR, p. A 34
CRITTENTON, KANSAS CITY, MO, p. A233
CRITTENTON HOSPITAL, ROCHESTER, MI, p. A209
CROCKETT COUNTY HOSPITAL AND CARE CENTER, OZONA, TX, p. A399
CROCKETT HOSPITAL, LAWRENCEBURG, TN, p. A370
CROOK COUNTY MEDICAL SERVICES DISTRICT, SUNDANCE, WY, p. A446
CROSBY MEMORIAL HOSPITAL, PICAYUNE, MS, p. A227
CROSBYTON CLINIC HOSPITAL, CROSBYTON, TX, p. A382
CROSS COUNTY HOSPITAL, WYNNE, AR, p. A 35
CROSSROADS COMMUNITY HOSPITAL, MOUNT VERNON, IL, p. A127
CROTCHED MOUNTAIN REHABILITATION CENTER, GREENFIELD, NH, p. A255
CROUSE IRVING MEMORIAL HOSPITAL, SYRACUSE, NY, p. A288
CROWNSVILLE HOSPITAL CENTER, CROWNSVILLE, MD, p. A186
CROZER–CHESTER MEDICAL CENTER, UPLAND, PA, p. A350
CRYSTAL FALLS COMMUNITY HOSPITAL, CRYSTAL FALLS, MI, p. A201
CUBA MEMORIAL HOSPITAL, CUBA, NY, p. A274
CUERO COMMUNITY HOSPITAL, CUERO, TX, p. A382
CULBERSON HOSPITAL DISTRICT, VAN HORN, TX, p. A405
CULLMAN REGIONAL MEDICAL CENTER, CULLMAN, AL, p. A 15
CULPEPER MEMORIAL HOSPITAL, CULPEPER, VA, p. A415
CULVER UNION HOSPITAL, CRAWFORDSVILLE, IN, p. A134
CUMBERLAND COUNTY HOSPITAL, BURKESVILLE, KY, p. A161
CUMBERLAND HALL HOSPITAL, HOPKINSVILLE, KY, p. A163
CUMBERLAND HOSPITAL, FAYETTEVILLE, NC, p. A294
CUMBERLAND HOSPITAL FOR CHILDREN AND ADOLESCENTS, NEW KENT, VA, p. A417
CUMBERLAND MEDICAL CENTER, CROSSVILLE, TN, p. A367
CUMBERLAND MEMORIAL HOSPITAL, CUMBERLAND, WI, p. A436
CURRY GENERAL HOSPITAL, GOLD BEACH, OR, p. A330
CUSHING MEMORIAL HOSPITAL, LEAVENWORTH, KS, p. A155
CUSHING REGIONAL HOSPITAL, CUSHING, OK, p. A322
CUSTER COMMUNITY HOSPITAL, CUSTER, SD, p. A361
CUYAHOGA FALLS GENERAL HOSPITAL, CUYAHOGA FALLS, OH, p. A311
CUYUNA REGIONAL MEDICAL CENTER, CROSBY, MN, p. A214
CYPRESS CREEK HOSPITAL, HOUSTON, TX, p. A390
CYPRESS FAIRBANKS MEDICAL CENTER, HOUSTON, TX, p. A390
CYPRESS HOSPITAL, LAFAYETTE, LA, p. A173

D

D. M. COGDELL MEMORIAL HOSPITAL, SNYDER, TX, p. A403
D. W. MCMILLAN MEMORIAL HOSPITAL, BREWTON, AL, p. A 14
D.T. WATSON REHABILITATION HOSPITAL, SEWICKLEY, PA, p. A349
DADE CITY HOSPITAL, DADE CITY, FL, p. A 83
DAKOTA HOSPITAL, FARGO, ND, p. A303
DAKOTA HOSPITAL, VERMILLION, SD, p. A364
DALE MEDICAL CENTER, OZARK, AL, p. A 19
DALLAS–FORT WORTH MEDICAL CENTER, GRAND PRAIRIE, TX, p. A388
DALLAS COUNTY HOSPITAL, FORDYCE, AR, p. A 30
DALLAS COUNTY HOSPITAL, PERRY, IA, p. A149

DALLAS COUNTY HOSPITAL DISTRICT–PARKLAND MEMORIAL HOSPITAL, DALLAS, TX, p. A383
DALLAS FAMILY HOSPITAL, DALLAS, TX, p. A383
DAMERON HOSPITAL, STOCKTON, CA, p. A 64
DAMMASCH STATE HOSPITAL, WILSONVILLE, OR, p. A333
DANA–FARBER CANCER INSTITUTE, BOSTON, MA, p. A191
DANBURY HOSPITAL, DANBURY, CT, p. A 74
DANIEL FREEMAN MARINA HOSPITAL, MARINA DEL REY, CA, p. A 52
DANIEL FREEMAN MEMORIAL HOSPITAL, INGLEWOOD, CA, p. A 46
DANIELS MEMORIAL HOSPITAL, SCOBEY, MT, p. A244
DANVILLE REGIONAL MEDICAL CENTER, DANVILLE, VA, p. A415
DANVILLE STATE HOSPITAL, DANVILLE, PA, p. A337
DARDANELLE HOSPITAL, DARDANELLE, AR, p. A 30
DARNALL ARMY COMMUNITY HOSPITAL, FORT HOOD, TX, p. A386
DARTMOUTH COLLEGE HEALTH SERVICE, HANOVER, NH, p. A255
DARTMOUTH HOSPITAL, DAYTON, OH, p. A311
DAUTERIVE HOSPITAL, NEW IBERIA, LA, p. A175
DAVENPORT MEDICAL CENTER, DAVENPORT, IA, p. A144
DAVID GRANT MEDICAL CENTER, TRAVIS AIR FORCE BASE, CA, p. A 65
DAVIE COUNTY HOSPITAL, MOCKSVILLE, NC, p. A296
DAVIES MEDICAL CENTER, SAN FRANCISCO, CA, p. A 60
DAVIESS COUNTY HOSPITAL, WASHINGTON, IN, p. A141
DAVIS COMMUNITY HOSPITAL, STATESVILLE, NC, p. A299
DAVIS COUNTY HOSPITAL, BLOOMFIELD, IA, p. A142
DAVIS HOSPITAL AND MEDICAL CENTER, LAYTON, UT, p. A408
DAVIS MEMORIAL HOSPITAL, ELKINS, WV, p. A431
DAY KIMBALL HOSPITAL, PUTNAM, CT, p. A 76
DAYTON GENERAL HOSPITAL, DAYTON, WA, p. A424
DAYTON MENTAL HEALTH CENTER, DAYTON, OH, p. A311
DAYTONA MEDICAL CENTER, DAYTONA BEACH, FL, p. A 83
DCH REGIONAL MEDICAL CENTER, TUSCALOOSA, AL, p. A 20
DCH REHABILITATION PAVILION, TUSCALOOSA, AL, p. A 20
DE GRAFF MEMORIAL HOSPITAL, NORTH TONAWANDA, NY, p. A283
DE JARNETTE CENTER, STAUNTON, VA, p. A421
DE LEON HOSPITAL, DE LEON, TX, p. A384
DE PAUL HOSPITAL, MILWAUKEE, WI, p. A440
DE QUEEN REGIONAL MEDICAL CENTER, DE QUEEN, AR, p. A 30
DE SMET MEMORIAL HOSPITAL, DE SMET, SD, p. A361
DE SOTO GENERAL HOSPITAL, MANSFIELD, LA, p. A175
DEACONESS–GLOVER HOSPITAL CORPORATION, NEEDHAM, MA, p. A195
DEACONESS–NASHOBA HOSPITAL, AYER, MA, p. A190
DEACONESS HEALTH SYSTEM, SAINT LOUIS, MO, p. A238
DEACONESS HOSPITAL, EVANSVILLE, IN, p. A135
DEACONESS HOSPITAL, BOSTON, MA, p. A191
DEACONESS HOSPITAL, CINCINNATI, OH, p. A308
DEACONESS HOSPITAL, OKLAHOMA CITY, OK, p. A325
DEACONESS HOSPITAL OF CLEVELAND, CLEVELAND, OH, p. A309
DEACONESS MEDICAL CENTER–SPOKANE, SPOKANE, WA, p. A427
DEACONESS MEDICAL CENTER–WEST CAMPUS, SAINT LOUIS, MO, p. A238
DEACONESS MEDICAL CENTER, BILLINGS, MT, p. A241
DEARBORN COUNTY HOSPITAL, LAWRENCEBURG, IN, p. A138
DEATON SPECIALTY HOSPITAL AND HOME, BALTIMORE, MD, p. A184
DEBACA GENERAL HOSPITAL, FORT SUMNER, NM, p. A269
DEBORAH HEART AND LUNG CENTER, BROWNS MILLS, NJ, p. A258
DECATUR COMMUNITY HOSPITAL, DECATUR, TX, p. A384
DECATUR COUNTY GENERAL HOSPITAL, PARSONS, TN, p. A374
DECATUR COUNTY HOSPITAL, LEON, IA, p. A147
DECATUR COUNTY HOSPITAL, OBERLIN, KS, p. A157
DECATUR COUNTY MEMORIAL HOSPITAL, GREENSBURG, IN, p. A136
DECATUR GENERAL HOSPITAL–WEST, DECATUR, AL, p. A 15
DECATUR GENERAL HOSPITAL, DECATUR, AL, p. A 15
DECATUR HOSPITAL, DECATUR, GA, p. A102
DECATUR MEMORIAL HOSPITAL, DECATUR, IL, p. A121
DECHAIRO HOSPITAL, WESTMORELAND, KS, p. A160
DECKERVILLE COMMUNITY HOSPITAL, DECKERVILLE, MI, p. A201
DEER'S HEAD CENTER, SALISBURY, MD, p. A188
DEERING HOSPITAL, MIAMI, FL, p. A 89
DEFIANCE HOSPITAL, DEFIANCE, OH, p. A311
DEKALB BAPTIST MEDICAL CENTER, FORT PAYNE, AL, p. A 16
DEKALB GENERAL HOSPITAL, SMITHVILLE, TN, p. A374
DEKALB MEDICAL CENTER, DECATUR, GA, p. A102

Hospitals, Alphabetically / Eden Hospital Medical Center

DEKALB MEMORIAL HOSPITAL, AUBURN, IN, p. A133
DEL AMO HOSPITAL, TORRANCE, CA, p. A 65
DEL E. WEBB MEMORIAL HOSPITAL, SUN CITY WEST, AZ, p. A 27
DEL PUERTO HOSPITAL, PATTERSON, CA, p. A 56
DELANO REGIONAL MEDICAL CENTER, DELANO, CA, p. A 41
DELAWARE COUNTY MEMORIAL HOSPITAL, MANCHESTER, IA, p. A147
DELAWARE COUNTY MEMORIAL HOSPITAL, DREXEL HILL, PA, p. A337
DELAWARE STATE HOSPITAL, NEW CASTLE, DE, p. A 78
DELAWARE VALLEY HOSPITAL, WALTON, NY, p. A289
DELAWARE VALLEY MEDICAL CENTER, LANGHORNE, PA, p. A341
DELAWARE VALLEY MENTAL HEALTH FOUNDATION, DOYLESTOWN, PA, p. A337
DELL RAPIDS COMMUNITY HOSPITAL, DELL RAPIDS, SD, p. A361
DELNOR–COMMUNITY HOSPITAL, GENEVA, IL, p. A123
DELRAY COMMUNITY HOSPITAL, DELRAY BEACH, FL, p. A 83
DELTA COMMUNITY MEDICAL CENTER, DELTA, UT, p. A408
DELTA COUNTY MEMORIAL HOSPITAL, DELTA, CO, p. A 69
DELTA MEMORIAL HOSPITAL, DUMAS, AR, p. A 30
DELTA MEMORIAL HOSPITAL, ANTIOCH, CA, p. A 36
DELTA REGIONAL MEDICAL CENTER, GREENVILLE, MS, p. A224
DENTON COMMUNITY HOSPITAL, DENTON, TX, p. A384
DENTON REGIONAL MEDICAL CENTER, DENTON, TX, p. A385
DENVER HEALTH AND HOSPITALS, DENVER, CO, p. A 69
DEPAUL HEALTH CENTER, SAINT LOUIS, MO, p. A238
DEPAUL HOSPITAL, NEW ORLEANS, LA, p. A176
DEPAUL MEDICAL CENTER, NORFOLK, VA, p. A418
DEQUINCY MEMORIAL HOSPITAL, DE QUINCY, LA, p. A172
DES MOINES GENERAL HOSPITAL, DES MOINES, IA, p. A144
DESERT HILLS CENTER FOR YOUTH AND FAMILIES, TUCSON, AZ, p. A 27
DESERT HILLS HOSPITAL, FARMINGTON, NM, p. A268
DESERT HOSPITAL, PALM SPRINGS, CA, p. A 55
DESERT PALMS COMMUNITY HOSPITAL, PALMDALE, CA, p. A 55
DESERT SAMARITAN MEDICAL CENTER, MESA, AZ, p. A 24
DESERT SPRINGS HOSPITAL, LAS VEGAS, NV, p. A253
DESERT VISTA HOSPITAL, MESA, AZ, p. A 24
DESOTO MEMORIAL HOSPITAL, ARCADIA, FL, p. A 81
DETAR HOSPITAL, VICTORIA, TX, p. A406
DETROIT RECEIVING HOSPITAL AND UNIVERSITY HEALTH CENTER, DETROIT, MI, p. A201
DETROIT RIVERVIEW HOSPITAL, DETROIT, MI, p. A201
DETTMER HOSPITAL, TROY, OH, p. A318
DEUEL COUNTY MEMORIAL HOSPITAL, CLEAR LAKE, SD, p. A361
DEVEREUX–VICTORIA, VICTORIA, TX, p. A406
DEVEREUX CENTER–GEORGIA, KENNESAW, GA, p. A105
DEVEREUX FOUNDATION–FRENCH CENTER, DEVON, PA, p. A337
DEVEREUX HOSPITAL AND CHILDREN'S CENTER OF FLORIDA, MELBOURNE, FL, p. A 89
DEVEREUX MAPLETON PSYCHIATRIC INSTITUTE–MAPLETON CENTER, MALVERN, PA, p. A341
DEVEREUX TEXAS TREATMENT NETWORK, LEAGUE CITY, TX, p. A395
DEWITT ARMY COMMUNITY HOSPITAL, FORT BELVOIR, VA, p. A415
DEWITT CITY HOSPITAL, DE WITT, AR, p. A 30
DEWITT COMMUNITY HOSPITAL, DEWITT, IA, p. A144
DEXTER MEMORIAL HOSPITAL, DEXTER, MO, p. A231
DIAGNOSTIC CENTER HOSPITAL, HOUSTON, TX, p. A390
DICKENSON COUNTY MEDICAL CENTER, CLINTWOOD, VA, p. A415
DICKINSON COUNTY MEMORIAL HOSPITAL, SPIRIT LAKE, IA, p. A150
DICKINSON COUNTY MEMORIAL HOSPITAL SYSTEM, IRON MOUNTAIN, MI, p. A205
DIMMIT COUNTY MEMORIAL HOSPITAL, CARRIZO SPRINGS, TX, p. A380
DISTRICT MEMORIAL HOSPITAL, FOREST LAKE, MN, p. A215
DISTRICT MEMORIAL HOSPITAL, ANDREWS, NC, p. A291
DISTRICT OF COLUMBIA GENERAL HOSPITAL, WASHINGTON, DC, p. A 79
DISTRICT ONE HOSPITAL, FARIBAULT, MN, p. A214
DISTRICT TWO COMMUNITY HOSPITAL, DURANT, MS, p. A223
DIVINE PROVIDENCE HEALTH CENTER, IVANHOE, MN, p. A216
DIVINE PROVIDENCE HOSPITAL, WILLIAMSPORT, PA, p. A351
DIVINE SAVIOR HOSPITAL AND NURSING HOME, PORTAGE, WI, p. A442
DIXIE REGIONAL MEDICAL CENTER, SAINT GEORGE, UT, p. A410
DOCTOR ROBERT L. YEAGER HEALTH CENTER, POMONA, NY, p. A285

DOCTOR'S MEMORIAL HOSPITAL, PERRY, FL, p. A 93
DOCTORS COMMUNITY HOSPITAL, LANHAM, MD, p. A187
DOCTORS GUBERN'S HOSPITAL, FAJARDO, PR, p. A448
DOCTORS HOSPITAL–WENTZVILLE, WENTZVILLE, MO, p. A240
DOCTORS HOSPITAL, COLUMBUS, GA, p. A101
DOCTORS HOSPITAL, SPRINGFIELD, IL, p. A130
DOCTORS HOSPITAL, COLUMBUS, OH, p. A310
DOCTORS HOSPITAL, SAN JUAN, PR, p. A449
DOCTORS HOSPITAL, CONROE, TX, p. A381
DOCTORS HOSPITAL, GROVES, TX, p. A389
DOCTORS HOSPITAL, HOUSTON, TX, p. A390
DOCTORS HOSPITAL EAST LOOP, HOUSTON, TX, p. A390
DOCTORS HOSPITAL OF DALLAS, DALLAS, TX, p. A383
DOCTORS HOSPITAL OF HYDE PARK, CHICAGO, IL, p. A118
DOCTORS HOSPITAL OF JACKSON, JACKSON, MI, p. A205
DOCTORS HOSPITAL OF JEFFERSON, METAIRIE, LA, p. A175
DOCTORS HOSPITAL OF LAREDO, LAREDO, TX, p. A394
DOCTORS HOSPITAL OF MANTECA, MANTECA, CA, p. A 52
DOCTORS HOSPITAL OF NELSONVILLE, NELSONVILLE, OH, p. A315
DOCTORS HOSPITAL OF PINOLE, PINOLE, CA, p. A 56
DOCTORS HOSPITAL OF SANTA ANA, SANTA ANA, CA, p. A 62
DOCTORS HOSPITAL OF SARASOTA, SARASOTA, FL, p. A 95
DOCTORS HOSPITAL OF SPRINGFIELD, SPRINGFIELD, MO, p. A239
DOCTORS HOSPITAL OF STARK COUNTY, MASSILLON, OH, p. A314
DOCTORS HOSPITAL OF WEST COVINA, WEST COVINA, CA, p. A 67
DOCTORS MEDICAL CENTER, MODESTO, CA, p. A 52
DOCTORS MEMORIAL HOSPITAL, BONIFAY, FL, p. A 81
DOCTORS MEMORIAL HOSPITAL, TYLER, TX, p. A405
DOCTORS REGIONAL MEDICAL CENTER, POPLAR BLUFF, MO, p. A236
DOCTORS REGIONAL MEDICAL CENTER, CORPUS CHRISTI, TX, p. A382
DOCTORS' HOSPITAL, TULSA, OK, p. A328
DOCTORS' HOSPITAL OF MONTCLAIR, MONTCLAIR, CA, p. A 53
DOCTORS' HOSPITAL OF OPELOUSAS, OPELOUSAS, LA, p. A177
DOCTORS' HOSPITAL OF SHREVEPORT, SHREVEPORT, LA, p. A178
DOCTORS' HOSPITAL OF STATEN ISLAND, NEW YORK CITY, NY, p. A279
DODGE COUNTY HOSPITAL, EASTMAN, GA, p. A103
DOHENY EYE INSTITUTE, LOS ANGELES, CA, p. A 49
DOLLY VINSANT MEMORIAL HOSPITAL, SAN BENITO, TX, p. A403
DOMINICAN SANTA CRUZ HOSPITAL, SANTA CRUZ, CA, p. A 63
DOMINION HOSPITAL, FALLS CHURCH, VA, p. A415
DONALSONVILLE HOSPITAL, DONALSONVILLE, GA, p. A102
DOOLY MEDICAL CENTER, VIENNA, GA, p. A109
DOOR COUNTY MEMORIAL HOSPITAL, STURGEON BAY, WI, p. A443
DORCHESTER GENERAL HOSPITAL, CAMBRIDGE, MD, p. A186
DORMINY MEDICAL CENTER, FITZGERALD, GA, p. A103
DOROTHEA DIX HOSPITAL, RALEIGH, NC, p. A297
DOS PALOS MEMORIAL HOSPITAL, DOS PALOS, CA, p. A 41
DOUGLAS COMMUNITY HOSPITAL, ROSEBURG, OR, p. A332
DOUGLAS COUNTY HOSPITAL, ALEXANDRIA, MN, p. A212
DOUGLAS COUNTY HOSPITAL, OMAHA, NE, p. A250
DOUGLAS COUNTY MEMORIAL HOSPITAL, ARMOUR, SD, p. A361
DOWN EAST COMMUNITY HOSPITAL, MACHIAS, ME, p. A182
DOWNEY COMMUNITY HOSPITAL FOUNDATION, DOWNEY, CA, p. A 41
DOYLESTOWN HOSPITAL, DOYLESTOWN, PA, p. A337
DR DAN C. TRIGG MEMORIAL HOSPITAL, TUCUMCARI, NM, p. A270
DR. ALEJANDRO BUITRAGO–GUAYAMA AREA HOSPITAL, GUAYAMA, PR, p. A448
DR. HENRY SCHMIDT MEMORIAL HOSPITAL, WESTBROOK, MN, p. A221
DR. JOHN WARNER HOSPITAL, CLINTON, IL, p. A121
DR. JOSE RAMOS LEBRON HOSPITAL, FAJARDO, PR, p. A448
DR. PILA'S HOSPITAL, PONCE, PR, p. A449
DR. RAMON E. BETANCES HOSPITAL–MAYAGUEZ MEDICAL CENTER BRANCH, MAYAGUEZ, PR, p. A449
DRAKE CENTER, CINCINNATI, OH, p. A308
DREW MEMORIAL HOSPITAL, MONTICELLO, AR, p. A 33
DRISCOLL CHILDREN'S HOSPITAL, CORPUS CHRISTI, TX, p. A382
DRUMRIGHT MEMORIAL HOSPITAL, DRUMRIGHT, OK, p. A322
DUANE L. WATERS HOSPITAL, JACKSON, MI, p. A205
DUBOIS REGIONAL MEDICAL CENTER, DUBOIS, PA, p. A337
DUKE UNIVERSITY MEDICAL CENTER, DURHAM, NC, p. A293
DUKES MEMORIAL HOSPITAL, PERU, IN, p. A139

DUNCAN REGIONAL HOSPITAL, DUNCAN, OK, p. A322
DUNDY COUNTY HOSPITAL, BENKELMAN, NE, p. A246
DUNLAP MEMORIAL HOSPITAL, ORRVILLE, OH, p. A316
DUNN MEMORIAL HOSPITAL, BEDFORD, IN, p. A133
DUNWOODY MEDICAL CENTER, ATLANTA, GA, p. A 98
DUPLIN GENERAL HOSPITAL, KENANSVILLE, NC, p. A296
DURHAM REGIONAL HOSPITAL, DURHAM, NC, p. A293
DWIGHT D. EISENHOWER VETERANS AFFAIRS MEDICAL CENTER, LEAVENWORTH, KS, p. A155
DWIGHT DAVID EISENHOWER ARMY MEDICAL CENTER, FORT GORDON, GA, p. A103

E

E. A. CONWAY MEDICAL CENTER, MONROE, LA, p. A175
E. J. NOBLE HOSPITAL OF ALEXANDRIA BAY, ALEXANDRIA BAY, NY, p. A271
EAGLE LAKE COMMUNITY HOSPITAL, EAGLE LAKE, TX, p. A385
EAGLE RIVER MEMORIAL HOSPITAL, EAGLE RIVER, WI, p. A436
EAGLEVILLE HOSPITAL, EAGLEVILLE, PA, p. A337
EARL K. LONG MEDICAL CENTER, BATON ROUGE, LA, p. A170
EARLY MEMORIAL HOSPITAL, BLAKELY, GA, p. A100
EAST ADAMS RURAL HOSPITAL, RITZVILLE, WA, p. A426
EAST ALABAMA MEDICAL CENTER, OPELIKA, AL, p. A 19
EAST BAY HOSPITAL, RICHMOND, CA, p. A 57
EAST CARROLL PARISH HOSPITAL, LAKE PROVIDENCE, LA, p. A174
EAST COOPER COMMUNITY HOSPITAL, MOUNT PLEASANT, SC, p. A359
EAST JEFFERSON GENERAL HOSPITAL, METAIRIE, LA, p. A175
EAST LIVERPOOL CITY HOSPITAL, EAST LIVERPOOL, OH, p. A312
EAST LOS ANGELES DOCTORS HOSPITAL, LOS ANGELES, CA, p. A 49
EAST LOUISIANA STATE HOSPITAL, JACKSON, LA, p. A173
EAST MISSISSIPPI STATE HOSPITAL, MERIDIAN, MS, p. A226
EAST MONTGOMERY MEDICAL CENTER, MONTGOMERY, AL, p. A 18
EAST MORGAN COUNTY HOSPITAL, BRUSH, CO, p. A 68
EAST OHIO REGIONAL HOSPITAL, MARTINS FERRY, OH, p. A314
EAST ORANGE GENERAL HOSPITAL, EAST ORANGE, NJ, p. A259
EAST PASCO MEDICAL CENTER, ZEPHYRHILLS, FL, p. A 97
EAST POINTE HOSPITAL, LEHIGH ACRES, FL, p. A 88
EAST RIDGE HOSPITAL, EAST RIDGE, TN, p. A368
EAST TENNESSEE CHILDREN'S HOSPITAL, KNOXVILLE, TN, p. A370
EAST TEXAS MEDICAL CENTER–MOUNT VERNON, MOUNT VERNON, TX, p. A397
EAST TEXAS MEDICAL CENTER, TYLER, TX, p. A405
EAST TEXAS MEDICAL CENTER ATHENS, ATHENS, TX, p. A377
EAST TEXAS MEDICAL CENTER PITTSBURG, PITTSBURG, TX, p. A399
EAST TEXAS MEDICAL CENTER RUSK, RUSK, TX, p. A401
EASTERN IDAHO REGIONAL MEDICAL CENTER, IDAHO FALLS, ID, p. A113
EASTERN LONG ISLAND HOSPITAL, GREENPORT, NY, p. A275
EASTERN MAINE MEDICAL CENTER, BANGOR, ME, p. A180
EASTERN NEW MEXICO MEDICAL CENTER, ROSWELL, NM, p. A269
EASTERN OKLAHOMA MEDICAL CENTER, POTEAU, OK, p. A326
EASTERN OREGON PSYCHIATRIC CENTER, PENDLETON, OR, p. A331
EASTERN PLUMAS DISTRICT HOSPITAL, PORTOLA, CA, p. A 56
EASTERN SHORE HOSPITAL CENTER, CAMBRIDGE, MD, p. A186
EASTERN STATE HOSPITAL, LEXINGTON, KY, p. A164
EASTERN STATE HOSPITAL, VINITA, OK, p. A328
EASTERN STATE HOSPITAL, WILLIAMSBURG, VA, p. A421
EASTERN STATE HOSPITAL, MEDICAL LAKE, WA, p. A425
EASTERN STATE SCHOOL AND HOSPITAL, TREVOSE, PA, p. A350
EASTLAND MEMORIAL HOSPITAL, EASTLAND, TX, p. A385
EASTMORELAND HOSPITAL, PORTLAND, OR, p. A331
EASTON HOSPITAL, EASTON, PA, p. A338
EASTSIDE MEDICAL CENTER, SNELLVILLE, GA, p. A108
EASTWOOD MEDICAL CENTER, MEMPHIS, TN, p. A371
EATON RAPIDS COMMUNITY HOSPITAL, EATON RAPIDS, MI, p. A202
ED FRASER MEMORIAL HOSPITAL, MACCLENNY, FL, p. A 88
EDEN HOSPITAL MEDICAL CENTER, CASTRO VALLEY, CA, p. A 39

Hospitals, Alphabetically / Edgar B. Davis Memorial Hospital

EDGAR B. DAVIS MEMORIAL HOSPITAL, LULING, TX, p. A396
EDGE REGIONAL MEDICAL CENTER, TROY, AL, p. A 20
EDGEFIELD COUNTY HOSPITAL, EDGEFIELD, SC, p. A357
EDGEMONT HOSPITAL, LOS ANGELES, CA, p. A 49
EDGEWATER MEDICAL CENTER, CHICAGO, IL, p. A118
EDGEWATER PSYCHIATRIC HOSPITAL, HARRISBURG, PA, p. A339
EDINBURG HOSPITAL, EDINBURG, TX, p. A385
EDITH NOURSE ROGERS MEMORIAL VETERANS HOSPITAL, BEDFORD, MA, p. A190
EDMOND REGIONAL MEDICAL CENTER, EDMOND, OK, p. A323
EDWARD A. UTLAUT MEMORIAL HOSPITAL, GREENVILLE, IL, p. A124
EDWARD HOSPITAL, NAPERVILLE, IL, p. A127
EDWARD JOHN NOBLE HOSPITAL OF GOUVERNEUR, GOUVERNEUR, NY, p. A275
EDWARD W. MCCREADY MEMORIAL HOSPITAL, CRISFIELD, MD, p. A186
EDWARD WHITE HOSPITAL, SAINT PETERSBURG, FL, p. A 94
EDWARDS COUNTY HOSPITAL AND HEALTHCARE CENTER, KINSLEY, KS, p. A155
EDWIN SHAW HOSPITAL, AKRON, OH, p. A306
EFFINGHAM HOSPITAL, SPRINGFIELD, GA, p. A108
EGLESTON CHILDREN'S HOSPITAL AT EMORY UNIVERSITY, ATLANTA, GA, p. A 98
EHRLING BERGQUIST HOSPITAL, OFFUTT AIR FORCE BASE, NE, p. A249
EISENHOWER MEMORIAL HOSPITAL AT EISENHOWER MEDICAL CENTER, RANCHO MIRAGE, CA, p. A 57
EL CAMPO MEMORIAL HOSPITAL, EL CAMPO, TX, p. A385
EL CENTRO REGIONAL MEDICAL CENTER, EL CENTRO, CA, p. A 42
EL DORADO HOSPITAL AND MEDICAL CENTER, TUCSON, AZ, p. A 27
ELBA GENERAL HOSPITAL, ELBA, AL, p. A 15
ELBERT MEMORIAL HOSPITAL, ELBERTON, GA, p. A103
ELDORA REGIONAL MEDICAL CENTER, ELDORA, IA, p. A145
ELEANOR SLATER HOSPITAL, CRANSTON, , p. A353
ELECTRA MEMORIAL HOSPITAL, ELECTRA, TX, p. A386
ELGIN MENTAL HEALTH CENTER, ELGIN, IL, p. A122
ELIZA COFFEE MEMORIAL HOSPITAL, FLORENCE, AL, p. A 16
ELIZABETH GENERAL MEDICAL CENTER, ELIZABETH, NJ, p. A259
ELIZABETHTOWN COMMUNITY HOSPITAL, ELIZABETHTOWN, NY, p. A274
ELK COUNTY REGIONAL MEDICAL CENTER, RIDGWAY, PA, p. A348
ELKHART GENERAL HOSPITAL, ELKHART, IN, p. A134
ELKO GENERAL HOSPITAL, ELKO, NV, p. A253
ELKVIEW GENERAL HOSPITAL, HOBART, OK, p. A324
ELLENVILLE COMMUNITY HOSPITAL, ELLENVILLE, NY, p. A274
ELLETT MEMORIAL HOSPITAL, APPLETON CITY, MO, p. A230
ELLINWOOD DISTRICT HOSPITAL, ELLINWOOD, KS, p. A152
ELLIOT HOSPITAL, MANCHESTER, NH, p. A256
ELLIS FISCHEL CANCER CENTER, COLUMBIA, MO, p. A231
ELLIS HOSPITAL, SCHENECTADY, NY, p. A287
ELLSWORTH COUNTY HOSPITAL, ELLSWORTH, KS, p. A152
ELLSWORTH MUNICIPAL HOSPITAL, IOWA FALLS, IA, p. A146
ELLWOOD CITY HOSPITAL, ELLWOOD CITY, PA, p. A338
ELMBROOK MEMORIAL HOSPITAL, BROOKFIELD, WI, p. A436
ELMCREST PSYCHIATRIC INSTITUTE, PORTLAND, CT, p. A 76
ELMHURST HOSPITAL CENTER, NEW YORK CITY, NY, p. A279
ELMHURST MEMORIAL HOSPITAL, ELMHURST, IL, p. A122
ELMIRA PSYCHIATRIC CENTER, ELMIRA, NY, p. A275
ELMORE COMMUNITY HOSPITAL, WETUMPKA, AL, p. A 20
ELMORE MEDICAL CENTER, MOUNTAIN HOME, ID, p. A113
ELMWOOD MEDICAL CENTER, JEFFERSON, LA, p. A173
ELY–BLOOMENSON COMMUNITY HOSPITAL, ELY, MN, p. A214
EMANUEL COUNTY HOSPITAL, SWAINSBORO, GA, p. A108
EMANUEL MEDICAL CENTER, TURLOCK, CA, p. A 65
EMERALD COAST HOSPITAL, APALACHICOLA, FL, p. A 81
EMERSON HOSPITAL, CONCORD, MA, p. A193
EMH REGIONAL MEDICAL CENTER, ELYRIA, OH, p. A312
EMMA PENDLETON BRADLEY HOSPITAL, EAST PROVIDENCE, RI, p. A353
EMORY UNIVERSITY HOSPITAL, ATLANTA, GA, p. A 98
ENCINO–TARZANA REGIONAL MEDICAL CENTER, LOS ANGELES, CA, p. A 49
ENGLEWOOD COMMUNITY HOSPITAL, ENGLEWOOD, FL, p. A 84
ENGLEWOOD HOSPITAL AND MEDICAL CENTER, ENGLEWOOD, NJ, p. A260
ENID REGIONAL HOSPITAL, ENID, OK, p. A323
EPHRAIM MCDOWELL REGIONAL MEDICAL CENTER, DANVILLE, KY, p. A162
EPHRATA COMMUNITY HOSPITAL, EPHRATA, PA, p. A338
EPISCOPAL HOSPITAL, PHILADELPHIA, PA, p. A344
ERIE COUNTY MEDICAL CENTER, BUFFALO, NY, p. A273
ERLANGER MEDICAL CENTER, CHATTANOOGA, TN, p. A366
ESPANOLA HOSPITAL, ESPANOLA, NM, p. A268

ESSEX COUNTY HOSPITAL CENTER, CEDAR GROVE, NJ, p. A259
ESTES PARK MEDICAL CENTER, ESTES PARK, CO, p. A 70
EUGENIA HOSPITAL, LAFAYETTE HILL, PA, p. A340
EUREKA COMMUNITY HOSPITAL, EUREKA, SD, p. A362
EUREKA SPRINGS HOSPITAL, EUREKA SPRINGS, AR, p. A 30
EVANGELICAL COMMUNITY HOSPITAL, LEWISBURG, PA, p. A341
EVANS MEMORIAL HOSPITAL, CLAXTON, GA, p. A101
EVANS U.S. ARMY COMMUNITY HOSPITAL, FORT CARSON, CO, p. A 70
EVANSTON HOSPITAL, EVANSTON, IL, p. A123
EVANSVILLE STATE HOSPITAL, EVANSVILLE, IN, p. A135
EVERGLADES REGIONAL MEDICAL CENTER, PAHOKEE, FL, p. A 92
EVERGREEN HOSPITAL MEDICAL CENTER, KIRKLAND, WA, p. A425
EXCELSIOR SPRINGS MEDICAL CENTER, EXCELSIOR SPRINGS, MO, p. A232
EXETER HOSPITAL, EXETER, NH, p. A255
EYE AND EAR CLINIC OF CHARLESTON, CHARLESTON, WV, p. A430
EYE FOUNDATION HOSPITAL, BIRMINGHAM, AL, p. A 14
EYE, EAR, NOSE AND THROAT HOSPITAL, NEW ORLEANS, LA, p. A176

F

F. EDWARD HEBERT HOSPITAL, NEW ORLEANS, LA, p. A176
F. F. THOMPSON HEALTH SYSTEM, CANANDAIGUA, NY, p. A273
FAIR OAKS HOSPITAL, FAIRFAX, VA, p. A415
FAIR OAKS HOSPITAL AT BOCA DELRAY, DELRAY BEACH, FL, p. A 83
FAIRBANKS HOSPITAL, INDIANAPOLIS, IN, p. A136
FAIRBANKS MEMORIAL HOSPITAL, FAIRBANKS, AK, p. A 21
FAIRBURY HOSPITAL, FAIRBURY, IL, p. A123
FAIRFAX HOSPITAL, FALLS CHURCH, VA, p. A415
FAIRFAX MEMORIAL HOSPITAL, FAIRFAX, OK, p. A323
FAIRFIELD HILLS HOSPITAL, NEWTOWN, CT, p. A 76
FAIRFIELD MEDICAL CENTER, LANCASTER, OH, p. A313
FAIRFIELD MEMORIAL HOSPITAL, FAIRFIELD, IL, p. A123
FAIRFIELD MEMORIAL HOSPITAL, WINNSBORO, SC, p. A360
FAIRFIELD MEMORIAL HOSPITAL, FAIRFIELD, TX, p. A386
FAIRLAWN REHABILITATION HOSPITAL, WORCESTER, MA, p. A198
FAIRMONT COMMUNITY HOSPITAL, FAIRMONT, MN, p. A214
FAIRMONT GENERAL HOSPITAL, FAIRMONT, WV, p. A431
FAIRMONT HOSPITAL, SAN LEANDRO, CA, p. A 61
FAIRVIEW GENERAL HOSPITAL, CLEVELAND, OH, p. A309
FAIRVIEW HOSPITAL, GREAT BARRINGTON, MA, p. A193
FAIRVIEW HOSPITAL, FAIRVIEW, OK, p. A323
FAIRVIEW NORTHLAND REGIONAL HOSPITAL, PRINCETON, MN, p. A218
FAIRVIEW PARK HOSPITAL, DUBLIN, GA, p. A103
FAIRVIEW RIDGES HOSPITAL, BURNSVILLE, MN, p. A213
FAIRVIEW RIVERSIDE MEDICAL CENTER, MINNEAPOLIS, MN, p. A217
FAIRVIEW SOUTHDALE HOSPITAL, MINNEAPOLIS, MN, p. A217
FAITH COMMUNITY HOSPITAL, JACKSBORO, TX, p. A393
FALLBROOK HOSPITAL DISTRICT, FALLBROOK, CA, p. A 42
FALLON MEDICAL COMPLEX, BAKER, MT, p. A241
FALLS COMMUNITY HOSPITAL AND CLINIC, MARLIN, TX, p. A396
FALLS MEMORIAL HOSPITAL, INTERNATIONAL FALLS, MN, p. A216
FALLSTON GENERAL HOSPITAL, FALLSTON, MD, p. A187
FALLSVIEW PSYCHIATRIC HOSPITAL, CUYAHOGA FALLS, OH, p. A311
FALMOUTH HOSPITAL, FALMOUTH, MA, p. A193
FAMILY HEALTH WEST, FRUITA, CO, p. A 70
FAMILY HOSPITAL, AMARILLO, TX, p. A376
FANNIN REGIONAL HOSPITAL, BLUE RIDGE, GA, p. A100
FANNY ALLEN HOSPITAL, COLCHESTER, VT, p. A412
FARIBAULT REGIONAL CENTER, FARIBAULT, MN, p. A214
FARVIEW STATE HOSPITAL, WAYMART, PA, p. A350
FAULK COUNTY MEMORIAL HOSPITAL, FAULKTON, SD, p. A362
FAULKNER HOSPITAL, BOSTON, MA, p. A191
FAUQUIER HOSPITAL, WARRENTON, VA, p. A421
FAWCETT MEMORIAL HOSPITAL, PORT CHARLOTTE, FL, p. A 93
FAXTON HOSPITAL, UTICA, NY, p. A288
FAYETTE COUNTY HOSPITAL, VANDALIA, IL, p. A131

FAYETTE COUNTY HOSPITAL AND NURSING HOME, FAYETTE, AL, p. A 16
FAYETTE COUNTY MEMORIAL HOSPITAL, WASHINGTON COURT HOUSE, OH, p. A319
FAYETTE MEMORIAL HOSPITAL, CONNERSVILLE, IN, p. A134
FAYETTE MEMORIAL HOSPITAL, LA GRANGE, TX, p. A394
FAYETTEVILLE CITY HOSPITAL, FAYETTEVILLE, AR, p. A 30
FEATHER RIVER HOSPITAL, PARADISE, CA, p. A 55
FENTRESS COUNTY GENERAL HOSPITAL, JAMESTOWN, TN, p. A369
FERGUS FALLS REGIONAL TREATMENT CENTER, FERGUS FALLS, MN, p. A214
FERGUSON HOSPITAL, GRAND RAPIDS, MI, p. A204
FERRELL HOSPITAL, ELDORADO, IL, p. A122
FERRY COUNTY MEMORIAL HOSPITAL, REPUBLIC, WA, p. A426
FHP HOSPITAL – FOUNTAIN VALLEY, FOUNTAIN VALLEY, CA, p. A 43
FIELD MEMORIAL COMMUNITY HOSPITAL, CENTREVILLE, MS, p. A223
FILLMORE COMMUNITY MEDICAL CENTER, FILLMORE, UT, p. A408
FILLMORE COUNTY HOSPITAL, GENEVA, NE, p. A247
FINLEY HOSPITAL, DUBUQUE, IA, p. A145
FIRELANDS COMMUNITY HOSPITAL, SANDUSKY, OH, p. A317
FIRST CARE MEDICAL SERVICES, FOSSTON, MN, p. A215
FIRST HOSPITAL PANAMERICANO, CIDRA, PR, p. A448
FIRST HOSPITAL VALLEJO, VALLEJO, CA, p. A 66
FIRST HOSPITAL WYOMING VALLEY, WILKES-BARRE, PA, p. A351
FISHER–TITUS MEDICAL CENTER, NORWALK, OH, p. A315
FISHER COUNTY HOSPITAL DISTRICT, ROTAN, TX, p. A400
FISHERMEN'S HOSPITAL, MARATHON, FL, p. A 88
FITZGIBBON HOSPITAL, MARSHALL, MO, p. A235
FITZSIMONS ARMY MEDICAL CENTER, AURORA, CO, p. A 68
FIVE COUNTIES HOSPITAL, LEMMON, SD, p. A362
FLAGET MEMORIAL HOSPITAL, BARDSTOWN, KY, p. A161
FLAGLER HOSPITAL, SAINT AUGUSTINE, FL, p. A 94
FLAGSTAFF MEDICAL CENTER, FLAGSTAFF, AZ, p. A 23
FLAMBEAU MEDICAL CENTER, PARK FALLS, WI, p. A441
FLANDREAU MUNICIPAL HOSPITAL, FLANDREAU, SD, p. A362
FLEMING COUNTY HOSPITAL, FLEMINGSBURG, KY, p. A162
FLETCHER ALLEN HEALTH CARE, BURLINGTON, VT, p. A412
FLINT RIVER COMMUNITY HOSPITAL, MONTEZUMA, GA, p. A106
FLORALA MEMORIAL HOSPITAL, FLORALA, AL, p. A 16
FLORENCE GENERAL HOSPITAL, FLORENCE, SC, p. A357
FLORENCE HOSPITAL, FLORENCE, AL, p. A 16
FLORIDA CENTER FOR ADDICTIONS AND DUAL DISORDERS, AVON PARK, FL, p. A 81
FLORIDA HOSPITAL–WALKER, AVON PARK, FL, p. A 81
FLORIDA HOSPITAL–WATERMAN, EUSTIS, FL, p. A 84
FLORIDA HOSPITAL KISSIMMEE, KISSIMMEE, FL, p. A 87
FLORIDA HOSPITAL MEDICAL CENTER, ORLANDO, FL, p. A 91
FLORIDA MEDICAL CENTER HOSPITAL, FORT LAUDERDALE, FL, p. A 84
FLORIDA STATE HOSPITAL, CHATTAHOOCHEE, FL, p. A 82
FLOWER HOSPITAL, SYLVANIA, OH, p. A317
FLOWERS HOSPITAL, DOTHAN, AL, p. A 15
FLOYD COUNTY MEMORIAL HOSPITAL, CHARLES CITY, IA, p. A143
FLOYD MEDICAL CENTER, ROME, GA, p. A107
FLOYD MEMORIAL HOSPITAL AND HEALTHCARE SERVICES, NEW ALBANY, IN, p. A139
FLOYD VALLEY HOSPITAL, LE MARS, IA, p. A147
FLUSHING HOSPITAL MEDICAL CENTER, NEW YORK CITY, NY, p. A279
FONT MARTELO HOSPITAL, HUMACAO, PR, p. A448
FOOTHILL PRESBYTERIAN HOSPITAL–MORRIS L. JOHNSTON MEMORIAL, GLENDORA, CA, p. A 44
FORBES METROPOLITAN HOSPITAL, PITTSBURGH, PA, p. A346
FORBES REGIONAL HOSPITAL, MONROEVILLE, PA, p. A342
FOREST HOSPITAL, DES PLAINES, IL, p. A122
FOREST SPRINGS HOSPITAL, HOUSTON, TX, p. A390
FOREST VIEW HOSPITAL, GRAND RAPIDS, MI, p. A204
FORKS COMMUNITY HOSPITAL, FORKS, WA, p. A424
FORREST GENERAL HOSPITAL, HATTIESBURG, MS, p. A224
FORSYTH MEMORIAL HOSPITAL, WINSTON–SALEM, NC, p. A300
FORT ATKINSON MEMORIAL HEALTH SERVICES, FORT ATKINSON, WI, p. A437
FORT BAYARD MEDICAL CENTER, FORT BAYARD, NM, p. A268
FORT BEND HOSPITAL, MISSOURI CITY, TX, p. A397
FORT DUNCAN MEDICAL CENTER, EAGLE PASS, TX, p. A385
FORT HAMILTON–HUGHES MEMORIAL HOSPITAL, HAMILTON, OH, p. A313
FORT LOGAN HOSPITAL, STANFORD, KY, p. A168
FORT MADISON COMMUNITY HOSPITAL, FORT MADISON, IA, p. A145
FORT SANDERS–PARKWEST MEDICAL CENTER, KNOXVILLE, TN, p. A370

Hospitals, Alphabetically / Good Samaritan Medical Center

FORT SANDERS–SEVIER MEDICAL CENTER, SEVIERVILLE, TN, p. A374
FORT SANDERS LOUDON MEDICAL CENTER, LOUDON, TN, p. A371
FORT SANDERS REGIONAL MEDICAL CENTER, KNOXVILLE, TN, p. A370
FORT WALTON BEACH MEDICAL CENTER, FORT WALTON BEACH, FL, p. A 85
FORT WORTH REHABILITATION HOSPITAL, FORT WORTH, TX, p. A386
45TH STREET MENTAL HEALTH CENTER, WEST PALM BEACH, FL, p. A 97
FOSTORIA COMMUNITY HOSPITAL, FOSTORIA, OH, p. A312
FOUNTAIN VALLEY REGIONAL HOSPITAL AND MEDICAL CENTER, FOUNTAIN VALLEY, CA, p. A 43
FOUR RIVERS MEDICAL CENTER, SELMA, AL, p. A 19
FOUR WINDS HOSPITAL, KATONAH, NY, p. A276
FOX ARMY COMMUNITY HOSPITAL, REDSTONE ARSENAL, AL, p. A 19
FOX CHASE CANCER CENTER–AMERICAN ONCOLOGIC HOSPITAL, PHILADELPHIA, PA, p. A344
FOX RUN HOSPITAL, SAINT CLAIRSVILLE, OH, p. A317
FRANCES MAHON DEACONESS HOSPITAL, GLASGOW, MT, p. A242
FRANCISCAN CHILDREN'S HOSPITAL AND REHABILITATION CENTER, BOSTON, MA, p. A191
FRANK R. HOWARD MEMORIAL HOSPITAL, WILLITS, CA, p. A 67
FRANKFORD HOSPITAL OF THE CITY OF PHILADELPHIA, PHILADELPHIA, PA, p. A344
FRANKLIN–SIMPSON MEMORIAL HOSPITAL, FRANKLIN, KY, p. A163
FRANKLIN COUNTY MEDICAL CENTER, PRESTON, ID, p. A114
FRANKLIN COUNTY MEMORIAL HOSPITAL, MEADVILLE, MS, p. A226
FRANKLIN COUNTY MEMORIAL HOSPITAL, FRANKLIN, NE, p. A247
FRANKLIN DELANO ROOSEVELT VETERANS AFFAIRS HOSPITAL, MONTROSE, NY, p. A278
FRANKLIN FOUNDATION HOSPITAL, FRANKLIN, LA, p. A172
FRANKLIN GENERAL HOSPITAL, HAMPTON, IA, p. A146
FRANKLIN HOSPITAL AND SKILLED NURSING CARE UNIT, BENTON, IL, p. A117
FRANKLIN HOSPITAL MEDICAL CENTER, VALLEY STREAM, NY, p. A288
FRANKLIN MEDICAL CENTER, WINNSBORO, LA, p. A179
FRANKLIN MEDICAL CENTER, GREENFIELD, MA, p. A193
FRANKLIN MEMORIAL HOSPITAL, FARMINGTON, ME, p. A181
FRANKLIN MEMORIAL HOSPITAL, ROCKY MOUNT, VA, p. A420
FRANKLIN REGIONAL HOSPITAL, FRANKLIN, NH, p. A255
FRANKLIN REGIONAL MEDICAL CENTER, LOUISBURG, NC, p. A296
FRANKLIN SQUARE HOSPITAL CENTER, BALTIMORE, MD, p. A184
FRAZIER REHABILITATION CENTER, LOUISVILLE, KY, p. A165
FREDERICK MEMORIAL HOSPITAL, FREDERICK, MD, p. A187
FREDONIA REGIONAL HOSPITAL, FREDONIA, KS, p. A153
FREEMAN COMMUNITY HOSPITAL, FREEMAN, SD, p. A362
FREEMAN HOSPITAL, JOPLIN, MO, p. A233
FREEMAN NEOSHO HOSPITAL, NEOSHO, MO, p. A236
FREEPORT HOSPITAL, FREEPORT, NY, p. A275
FREEPORT MEMORIAL HOSPITAL, FREEPORT, IL, p. A123
FREMONT MEDICAL CENTER, YUBA CITY, CA, p. A 67
FRENCH HOSPITAL MEDICAL CENTER, SAN LUIS OBISPO, CA, p. A 62
FRESNO COMMUNITY HOSPITAL AND MEDICAL CENTER, FRESNO, CA, p. A 43
FRICK HOSPITAL AND COMMUNITY HEALTH CENTER, MOUNT PLEASANT, PA, p. A342
FRIEDMAN HOSPITAL OF THE HOME FOR THE JEWISH AGED, PHILADELPHIA, PA, p. A344
FRIENDLY HILLS REGIONAL MEDICAL CENTER, LA HABRA, CA, p. A 46
FRIENDS HOSPITAL, PHILADELPHIA, PA, p. A344
FRIO HOSPITAL, PEARSALL, TX, p. A399
FRISBIE MEMORIAL HOSPITAL, ROCHESTER, NH, p. A257
FROEDTERT MEMORIAL LUTHERAN HOSPITAL, MILWAUKEE, WI, p. A440
FRYE REGIONAL MEDICAL CENTER, HICKORY, NC, p. A295
FULLER MEMORIAL HOSPITAL, SOUTH ATTLEBORO, MA, p. A196
FULTON COUNTY HEALTH CENTER, WAUSEON, OH, p. A319
FULTON COUNTY HOSPITAL, SALEM, AR, p. A 34
FULTON COUNTY MEDICAL CENTER, MCCONNELLSBURG, PA, p. A342
FULTON STATE HOSPITAL, FULTON, MO, p. A232
FUNDACION HOSPITAL METROPOLITAN, SAN JUAN, PR, p. A449

G

G. PIERCE WOOD MEMORIAL HOSPITAL, ARCADIA, FL, p. A 81
GADSDEN MEMORIAL HOSPITAL, QUINCY, FL, p. A 94
GADSDEN REGIONAL MEDICAL CENTER, GADSDEN, AL, p. A 16
GAINESVILLE MEMORIAL HOSPITAL, GAINESVILLE, TX, p. A387
GALENA–STAUSS HOSPITAL, GALENA, IL, p. A123
GALESBURG COTTAGE HOSPITAL, GALESBURG, IL, p. A123
GALION COMMUNITY HOSPITAL, GALION, OH, p. A312
GALLUP INDIAN MEDICAL CENTER, GALLUP, NM, p. A269
GARDEN CITY HOSPITAL, GARDEN CITY, MI, p. A203
GARDEN COUNTY HOSPITAL, OSHKOSH, NE, p. A250
GARDEN GROVE HOSPITAL AND MEDICAL CENTER, GARDEN GROVE, CA, p. A 44
GARDEN PARK COMMUNITY HOSPITAL, GULFPORT, MS, p. A224
GARFIELD COUNTY MEMORIAL HOSPITAL, POMEROY, WA, p. A426
GARFIELD MEDICAL CENTER, MONTEREY PARK, CA, p. A 53
GARFIELD MEMORIAL HOSPITAL AND CLINICS, PANGUITCH, UT, p. A409
GARLAND COMMUNITY HOSPITAL, GARLAND, TX, p. A388
GARRARD COUNTY MEMORIAL HOSPITAL, LANCASTER, KY, p. A164
GARRETT COUNTY MEMORIAL HOSPITAL, OAKLAND, MD, p. A188
GARRISON MEMORIAL HOSPITAL, GARRISON, ND, p. A303
GARY MEMORIAL HOSPITAL, BREAUX BRIDGE, LA, p. A171
GARZA MEMORIAL HOSPITAL, POST, TX, p. A400
GASTON MEMORIAL HOSPITAL, GASTONIA, NC, p. A294
GATEWAY REGIONAL HEALTH SYSTEM, MOUNT STERLING, KY, p. A167
GATEWAYS HOSPITAL AND MENTAL HEALTH CENTER, LOS ANGELES, CA, p. A 49
GAYLORD HOSPITAL, WALLINGFORD, CT, p. A 77
GEARY COMMUNITY HOSPITAL, JUNCTION CITY, KS, p. A154
GEAUGA HOSPITAL, CHARDON, OH, p. A307
GEISINGER MEDICAL CENTER, DANVILLE, PA, p. A337
GEISINGER WYOMING VALLEY MEDICAL CENTER, WILKES–BARRE, PA, p. A351
GENERAL HOSPITAL, EUREKA, CA, p. A 42
GENERAL HOSPITAL CENTER AT PASSAIC, PASSAIC, NJ, p. A263
GENERAL JOHN J. PERSHING MEMORIAL HOSPITAL, BROOKFIELD, MO, p. A230
GENERAL LEONARD WOOD ARMY COMMUNITY HOSPITAL, FORT LEONARD WOOD, MO, p. A232
GENESEE HOSPITAL, ROCHESTER, NY, p. A286
GENESEE MEMORIAL HOSPITAL, BATAVIA, NY, p. A271
GENESIS MEDICAL CENTER, DAVENPORT, IA, p. A144
GENESYS REGIONAL MEDICAL CENTER–FLINT OSTEOPATHIC CAMPUS, FLINT, MI, p. A203
GENESYS REGIONAL MEDICAL CENTER–GENESEE MEMORIAL CAMPUS, FLINT, MI, p. A203
GENESYS REGIONAL MEDICAL CENTER–ST. JOSEPH CAMPUS, FLINT, MI, p. A203
GENESYS REGIONAL MEDICAL CENTER–WHEELOCK MEMORIAL CAMPUS, GOODRICH, MI, p. A203
GENEVA GENERAL HOSPITAL, GENEVA, NY, p. A275
GENOA COMMUNITY HOSPITAL, GENOA, NE, p. A247
GENTRY COUNTY MEMORIAL HOSPITAL, ALBANY, MO, p. A230
GEORGE A. ZELLER MENTAL HEALTH CENTER, PEORIA, IL, p. A128
GEORGE COUNTY HOSPITAL, LUCEDALE, MS, p. A226
GEORGE H. LANIER MEMORIAL HOSPITAL AND NURSING HOME, VALLEY, AL, p. A 20
GEORGE L. MEE MEMORIAL HOSPITAL, KING CITY, CA, p. A 46
GEORGE NIGH REHABILITATION INSTITUTE, OKMULGEE, OK, p. A326
GEORGE W. HUBBARD HOSPITAL OF MEHARRY MEDICAL COLLEGE, NASHVILLE, TN, p. A373
GEORGE WASHINGTON UNIVERSITY HOSPITAL, WASHINGTON, DC, p. A 79
GEORGETOWN HOSPITAL, GEORGETOWN, TX, p. A388
GEORGETOWN MEMORIAL HOSPITAL, GEORGETOWN, SC, p. A357
GEORGETOWN UNIVERSITY HOSPITAL, WASHINGTON, DC, p. A 79
GEORGIA BAPTIST MEDICAL CENTER, ATLANTA, GA, p. A 99
GEORGIA MENTAL HEALTH INSTITUTE, ATLANTA, GA, p. A 99
GEORGIA REGIONAL HOSPITAL AT ATLANTA, DECATUR, GA, p. A102
GEORGIA REGIONAL HOSPITAL AT AUGUSTA, AUGUSTA, GA, p. A100

GEORGIA REGIONAL HOSPITAL AT SAVANNAH, SAVANNAH, GA, p. A108
GEORGIANA DOCTORS HOSPITAL, GEORGIANA, AL, p. A 16
GERALD CHAMPION MEMORIAL HOSPITAL, ALAMOGORDO, NM, p. A267
GERBER MEMORIAL HOSPITAL, FREMONT, MI, p. A203
GERMANTOWN HOSPITAL AND MEDICAL CENTER, PHILADELPHIA, PA, p. A344
GETTYSBURG HOSPITAL, GETTYSBURG, PA, p. A339
GETTYSBURG MEDICAL CENTER, GETTYSBURG, SD, p. A362
GIBSON COMMUNITY HOSPITAL, GIBSON CITY, IL, p. A123
GIBSON GENERAL HOSPITAL, PRINCETON, IN, p. A140
GIBSON GENERAL HOSPITAL, TRENTON, TN, p. A375
GIFFORD MEDICAL CENTER, RANDOLPH, VT, p. A412
GILA REGIONAL MEDICAL CENTER, SILVER CITY, NM, p. A270
GILES MEMORIAL HOSPITAL, PEARISBURG, VA, p. A418
GILL MEMORIAL EYE, EAR, NOSE AND THROAT HOSPITAL, ROANOKE, VA, p. A420
GILLETTE CHILDREN'S HOSPITAL, SAINT PAUL, MN, p. A219
GILMER MEDICAL CENTER, GILMER, TX, p. A388
GILMORE MEMORIAL HOSPITAL, AMORY, MS, p. A222
GLACIAL RIDGE HOSPITAL, GLENWOOD, MN, p. A215
GLACIER COUNTY MEDICAL CENTER, CUT BANK, MT, p. A242
GLADES GENERAL HOSPITAL, BELLE GLADE, FL, p. A 81
GLEN OAKS HOSPITAL, GREENVILLE, TX, p. A389
GLEN ROSE MEDICAL CENTER, GLEN ROSE, TX, p. A388
GLENBEIGH HOSPITAL OF CLEVELAND, CLEVELAND, OH, p. A309
GLENBEIGH HOSPITAL OF ROCK CREEK, ROCK CREEK, OH, p. A316
GLENCOE AREA HEALTH CENTER, GLENCOE, MN, p. A215
GLENDALE ADVENTIST MEDICAL CENTER, GLENDALE, CA, p. A 44
GLENDALE MEMORIAL HOSPITAL AND HEALTH CENTER, GLENDALE, CA, p. A 44
GLENDIVE MEDICAL CENTER, GLENDIVE, MT, p. A242
GLENN GENERAL HOSPITAL, WILLOWS, CA, p. A 67
GLENOAKS HOSPITAL AND MEDICAL CENTER, GLENDALE HEIGHTS, IL, p. A124
GLENS FALLS HOSPITAL, GLENS FALLS, NY, p. A275
GLENWOOD REGIONAL MEDICAL CENTER, WEST MONROE, LA, p. A179
GLENWOOD STATE HOSPITAL SCHOOL, GLENWOOD, IA, p. A145
GNADEN HUETTEN MEMORIAL HOSPITAL, LEHIGHTON, PA, p. A341
GOLDEN GLADES REGIONAL MEDICAL CENTER, MIAMI, FL, p. A 89
GOLDEN PLAINS COMMUNITY HOSPITAL, BORGER, TX, p. A380
GOLDEN VALLEY MEMORIAL HOSPITAL, CLINTON, MO, p. A231
GOLDWATER MEMORIAL HOSPITAL, NEW YORK CITY, NY, p. A279
GOLETA VALLEY COMMUNITY HOSPITAL, SANTA BARBARA, CA, p. A 62
GOLIAD COUNTY HOSPITAL, GOLIAD, TX, p. A388
GOOD HOPE HOSPITAL, ERWIN, NC, p. A294
GOOD SAMARITAN COMMUNITY HEALTHCARE, PUYALLUP, WA, p. A426
GOOD SAMARITAN HEALTH CENTER OF MERRILL, MERRILL, WI, p. A439
GOOD SAMARITAN HEALTH SYSTEMS, KEARNEY, NE, p. A248
GOOD SAMARITAN HOSPITAL–MISSION OAKS, LOS GATOS, CA, p. A 51
GOOD SAMARITAN HOSPITAL, BAKERSFIELD, CA, p. A 37
GOOD SAMARITAN HOSPITAL, DOWNERS GROVE, IL, p. A122
GOOD SAMARITAN HOSPITAL, VINCENNES, IN, p. A141
GOOD SAMARITAN HOSPITAL, LEXINGTON, KY, p. A164
GOOD SAMARITAN HOSPITAL, SUFFERN, NY, p. A287
GOOD SAMARITAN HOSPITAL, CINCINNATI, OH, p. A308
GOOD SAMARITAN HOSPITAL, LEBANON, PA, p. A341
GOOD SAMARITAN HOSPITAL AND HEALTH CENTER, DAYTON, OH, p. A311
GOOD SAMARITAN HOSPITAL CORVALLIS, CORVALLIS, OR, p. A329
GOOD SAMARITAN HOSPITAL MEDICAL CENTER, WEST ISLIP, NY, p. A289
GOOD SAMARITAN HOSPITAL OF MARYLAND, BALTIMORE, MD, p. A184
GOOD SAMARITAN HOSPITAL OF SANTA CLARA VALLEY, SAN JOSE, CA, p. A 61
GOOD SAMARITAN MEDICAL AND REHABILITATION CENTER, ZANESVILLE, OH, p. A320
GOOD SAMARITAN MEDICAL CENTER, WEST PALM BEACH, FL, p. A 97
GOOD SAMARITAN MEDICAL CENTER, STOUGHTON, MA, p. A197
GOOD SAMARITAN MEDICAL CENTER, JOHNSTOWN, PA, p. A340

Hospitals A461

© 1995 AHA Guide

GOOD SAMARITAN REGIONAL HEALTH CENTER, MOUNT VERNON, IL, p. A127
GOOD SAMARITAN REGIONAL MEDICAL CENTER, PHOENIX, AZ, p. A 25
GOOD SAMARITAN REGIONAL MEDICAL CENTER, POTTSVILLE, PA, p. A348
GOOD SHEPHERD COMMUNITY HOSPITAL, HERMISTON, OR, p. A330
GOOD SHEPHERD HOSPITAL, BARRINGTON, IL, p. A116
GOOD SHEPHERD MEDICAL CENTER, LONGVIEW, TX, p. A395
GOOD SHEPHERD REHABILITATION HOSPITAL, ALLENTOWN, PA, p. A334
GOODALL–WITCHER HOSPITAL, CLIFTON, TX, p. A381
GOODING COUNTY MEMORIAL HOSPITAL, GOODING, ID, p. A113
GOODLARK REGIONAL MEDICAL CENTER, DICKSON, TN, p. A367
GORDON HOSPITAL, CALHOUN, GA, p. A100
GORDON MEMORIAL HOSPITAL DISTRICT, GORDON, NE, p. A247
GOSHEN GENERAL HOSPITAL, GOSHEN, IN, p. A135
GOTHENBURG MEMORIAL HOSPITAL, GOTHENBURG, NE, p. A247
GOTTLIEB MEMORIAL HOSPITAL, MELROSE PARK, IL, p. A126
GOVE COUNTY MEDICAL CENTER, QUINTER, KS, p. A158
GRACE COTTAGE HOSPITAL, TOWNSHEND, VT, p. A412
GRACE HOSPITAL, DETROIT, MI, p. A201
GRACE HOSPITAL, MORGANTON, NC, p. A297
GRACE HOSPITAL, CLEVELAND, OH, p. A309
GRACEWOOD STATE SCHOOL AND HOSPITAL, GRACEWOOD, GA, p. A104
GRACIE SQUARE HOSPITAL, NEW YORK CITY, NY, p. A279
GRADUATE HEALTH SYSTEM–CITY AVENUE HOSPITAL, PHILADELPHIA, PA, p. A344
GRADUATE HEALTH SYSTEM–PARKVIEW HOSPITAL, PHILADELPHIA, PA, p. A344
GRADUATE HOSPITAL, PHILADELPHIA, PA, p. A344
GRADY GENERAL HOSPITAL, CAIRO, GA, p. A100
GRADY MEMORIAL HOSPITAL, ATLANTA, GA, p. A 99
GRADY MEMORIAL HOSPITAL, DELAWARE, OH, p. A311
GRADY MEMORIAL HOSPITAL, CHICKASHA, OK, p. A322
GRAFTON CITY HOSPITAL, GRAFTON, WV, p. A431
GRAHAM COUNTY HOSPITAL, HILL CITY, KS, p. A154
GRAHAM GENERAL HOSPITAL, GRAHAM, TX, p. A388
GRAHAM HOSPITAL, CANTON, IL, p. A117
GRANADA HILLS COMMUNITY HOSPITAL, LOS ANGELES, CA, p. A 49
GRAND STRAND REGIONAL MEDICAL CENTER, MYRTLE BEACH, SC, p. A359
GRAND VIEW HOSPITAL, IRONWOOD, MI, p. A205
GRAND VIEW HOSPITAL, SELLERSVILLE, PA, p. A349
GRANDE RONDE HOSPITAL, LA GRANDE, OR, p. A330
GRANDVIEW HOSPITAL AND MEDICAL CENTER, DAYTON, OH, p. A311
GRANITE COUNTY MEMORIAL HOSPITAL AND NURSING HOME, PHILIPSBURG, MT, p. A243
GRANITE FALLS MUNICIPAL HOSPITAL AND MANOR, GRANITE FALLS, MN, p. A215
GRANT CENTER OF DEERING HOSPITAL, MIAMI, FL, p. A 89
GRANT COUNTY HEALTH CENTER, ELBOW LAKE, MN, p. A214
GRANT HOSPITAL, CHICAGO, IL, p. A118
GRANT MEDICAL CENTER, COLUMBUS, OH, p. A310
GRANT MEMORIAL HOSPITAL, PETERSBURG, WV, p. A432
GRANVILLE MEDICAL CENTER, OXFORD, NC, p. A297
GRAPE COMMUNITY HOSPITAL, HAMBURG, IA, p. A146
GRATIOT COMMUNITY HOSPITAL, ALMA, MI, p. A199
GRAVETTE MEDICAL CENTER HOSPITAL, GRAVETTE, AR, p. A 31
GRAYDON MANOR, LEESBURG, VA, p. A416
GRAYS HARBOR COMMUNITY HOSPITAL, ABERDEEN, WA, p. A423
GREAT LAKES REHABILITATION HOSPITAL, SOUTHFIELD, MI, p. A210
GREAT PLAINS REGIONAL MEDICAL CENTER, NORTH PLATTE, NE, p. A249
GREAT PLAINS REGIONAL MEDICAL CENTER, ELK CITY, OK, p. A323
GREATER BALTIMORE MEDICAL CENTER, BALTIMORE, MD, p. A184
GREATER BRIDGEPORT COMMUNITY MENTAL HEALTH CENTER, BRIDGEPORT, CT, p. A 74
GREATER COMMUNITY HOSPITAL, CRESTON, IA, p. A144
GREATER EL MONTE COMMUNITY HOSPITAL, SOUTH EL MONTE, CA, p. A 64
GREATER SOUTHEAST COMMUNITY HOSPITAL, WASHINGTON, DC, p. A 79
GREATER STAPLES HOSPITAL, STAPLES, MN, p. A220
GREELEY COUNTY HOSPITAL, TRIBUNE, KS, p. A159
GREEN HOSPITAL OF SCRIPPS CLINIC, LA JOLLA, CA, p. A 46

GREEN OAKS HOSPITAL, DALLAS, TX, p. A383
GREENBRIER HOSPITAL, COVINGTON, LA, p. A171
GREENBRIER VALLEY MEDICAL CENTER, RONCEVERTE, WV, p. A433
GREENE COUNTY GENERAL HOSPITAL, LINTON, IN, p. A138
GREENE COUNTY HOSPITAL, EUTAW, AL, p. A 16
GREENE COUNTY MEDICAL CENTER, JEFFERSON, IA, p. A146
GREENE COUNTY MEMORIAL HOSPITAL, WAYNESBURG, PA, p. A351
GREENE MEMORIAL HOSPITAL, XENIA, OH, p. A319
GREENFIELD AREA MEDICAL CENTER, GREENFIELD, OH, p. A312
GREENLEAF CENTER, JONESBORO, AR, p. A 31
GREENLEAF CENTER, FORT OGLETHORPE, GA, p. A103
GREENLEAF CENTER, VALDOSTA, GA, p. A109
GREENSVILLE MEMORIAL HOSPITAL, EMPORIA, VA, p. A415
GREENVIEW HOSPITAL, BOWLING GREEN, KY, p. A161
GREENVILLE GENERAL HOSPITAL, GREENVILLE, SC, p. A357
GREENVILLE HOSPITAL, JERSEY CITY, NJ, p. A261
GREENVILLE MEMORIAL HOSPITAL, GREENVILLE, SC, p. A357
GREENWELL SPRINGS HOSPITAL, GREENWELL SPRINGS, LA, p. A172
GREENWICH HOSPITAL, GREENWICH, CT, p. A 74
GREENWOOD COUNTY HOSPITAL, EUREKA, KS, p. A152
GREENWOOD LEFLORE HOSPITAL, GREENWOOD, MS, p. A224
GREGORY COMMUNITY HOSPITAL, GREGORY, SD, p. A362
GRENADA LAKE MEDICAL CENTER, GRENADA, MS, p. A224
GREYSTONE PARK PSYCHIATRIC HOSPITAL, GREYSTONE PARK, NJ, p. A260
GRIFFIN HOSPITAL, DERBY, CT, p. A 74
GRIFFIN MEMORIAL HOSPITAL, NORMAN, OK, p. A325
GRIGGS COUNTY HOSPITAL AND NURSING HOME, COOPERSTOWN, ND, p. A302
GRIM–SMITH HOSPITAL AND CLINIC, KIRKSVILLE, MO, p. A235
GRINNELL REGIONAL MEDICAL CENTER, GRINNELL, IA, p. A145
GRISELL MEMORIAL HOSPITAL DISTRICT ONE, RANSOM, KS, p. A158
GRITMAN MEDICAL CENTER, MOSCOW, ID, p. A113
GROSSMONT HOSPITAL, LA MESA, CA, p. A 46
GROUP HEALTH COOPERATIVE CENTRAL HOSPITAL, SEATTLE, WA, p. A427
GROVE GENERAL HOSPITAL, GROVE, OK, p. A323
GROVE HILL MEMORIAL HOSPITAL, GROVE HILL, AL, p. A 17
GRUNDY COUNTY MEMORIAL HOSPITAL, GRUNDY CENTER, IA, p. A145
GUADALUPE MEDICAL CENTER, CARLSBAD, NM, p. A268
GUADALUPE VALLEY HOSPITAL, SEGUIN, TX, p. A403
GUAM MEMORIAL HOSPITAL AUTHORITY, TAMUNING, GU, p. A447
GULF BREEZE HOSPITAL, GULF BREEZE, FL, p. A 85
GULF COAST HOSPITAL, FORT MYERS, FL, p. A 84
GULF COAST HOSPITAL, PANAMA CITY, FL, p. A 92
GULF COAST MEDICAL CENTER, BILOXI, MS, p. A222
GULF COAST MEDICAL CENTER, WHARTON, TX, p. A407
GULF OAKS HOSPITAL, BILOXI, MS, p. A222
GULF PINES BEHAVIORAL HEALTH SERVICES, HOUSTON, TX, p. A390
GULF PINES HOSPITAL, PORT SAINT JOE, FL, p. A 93
GUNDRY–GLASS HOSPITAL, BALTIMORE, MD, p. A184
GUNNISON VALLEY HOSPITAL, GUNNISON, CO, p. A 71
GUNNISON VALLEY HOSPITAL, GUNNISON, UT, p. A408
GUNTERSVILLE–ARAB MEDICAL CENTER, GUNTERSVILLE, AL, p. A 17
GUTHRIE COUNTY HOSPITAL, GUTHRIE CENTER, IA, p. A145
GUTTENBERG MUNICIPAL HOSPITAL, GUTTENBERG, IA, p. A146
GUYAN VALLEY HOSPITAL, LOGAN, WV, p. A431

H

H. B. MAGRUDER MEMORIAL HOSPITAL, PORT CLINTON, OH, p. A316
H. C. SOLOMON MENTAL HEALTH CENTER, LOWELL, MA, p. A194
H. DOUGLAS SINGER MENTAL HEALTH AND DEVELOPMENTAL CENTER, ROCKFORD, IL, p. A129
H. LEE MOFFITT CANCER CENTER, TAMPA, FL, p. A 96
H.C. WATKINS MEMORIAL HOSPITAL, QUITMAN, MS, p. A227
H.R.I. HOSPITAL, BROOKLINE, MA, p. A192
HABERSHAM COUNTY MEDICAL CENTER, DEMOREST, GA, p. A102
HACKENSACK MEDICAL CENTER, HACKENSACK, NJ, p. A260
HACKETTSTOWN COMMUNITY HOSPITAL, HACKETTSTOWN, NJ, p. A260

HACKLEY HOSPITAL, MUSKEGON, MI, p. A207
HADLEY MEMORIAL HOSPITAL, WASHINGTON, DC, p. A 79
HAHNEMANN UNIVERSITY HOSPITAL, PHILADELPHIA, PA, p. A344
HALE COUNTY HOSPITAL, GREENSBORO, AL, p. A 17
HALE HOSPITAL, HAVERHILL, MA, p. A193
HALIFAX MEDICAL CENTER, DAYTONA BEACH, FL, p. A 83
HALIFAX MEMORIAL HOSPITAL, ROANOKE RAPIDS, NC, p. A298
HALIFAX REGIONAL HOSPITAL, SOUTH BOSTON, VA, p. A421
HALL–BROOKE HOSPITAL, A DIVISION OF HALL–BROOKE FOUNDATION, WESTPORT, CT, p. A 77
HALL COUNTY HOSPITAL, MEMPHIS, TX, p. A397
HALSTEAD HOSPITAL, HALSTEAD, KS, p. A153
HAMILTON CENTER, TERRE HAUTE, IN, p. A141
HAMILTON COUNTY HOSPITAL, SYRACUSE, KS, p. A159
HAMILTON COUNTY PUBLIC HOSPITAL, WEBSTER CITY, IA, p. A150
HAMILTON HOSPITAL, OLNEY, TX, p. A398
HAMILTON MEDICAL CENTER, DALTON, GA, p. A102
HAMILTON MEMORIAL HOSPITAL, JASPER, FL, p. A 87
HAMILTON MEMORIAL HOSPITAL DISTRICT, MCLEANSBORO, IL, p. A126
HAMLET HOSPITAL, HAMLET, NC, p. A295
HAMLIN MEMORIAL HOSPITAL, HAMLIN, TX, p. A389
HAMMOND–HENRY HOSPITAL, GENESEO, IL, p. A123
HAMOT MEDICAL CENTER, ERIE, PA, p. A338
HAMPSHIRE MEMORIAL HOSPITAL, ROMNEY, WV, p. A433
HAMPSTEAD HOSPITAL, HAMPSTEAD, NH, p. A255
HAMPTON GENERAL HOSPITAL, VARNVILLE, SC, p. A360
HAMPTON HOSPITAL, WESTAMPTON TOWNSHIP, NJ, p. A266
HANCOCK COUNTY MEMORIAL HOSPITAL, BRITT, IA, p. A142
HANCOCK MEDICAL CENTER, BAY SAINT LOUIS, MS, p. A222
HANCOCK MEMORIAL HOSPITAL, SPARTA, GA, p. A108
HANCOCK MEMORIAL HOSPITAL, GREENFIELD, IN, p. A136
HAND COUNTY MEMORIAL HOSPITAL, MILLER, SD, p. A363
HANFORD COMMUNITY MEDICAL CENTER, HANFORD, CA, p. A 44
HANNIBAL REGIONAL HOSPITAL, HANNIBAL, MO, p. A232
HANOVER GENERAL HOSPITAL, HANOVER, PA, p. A339
HANOVER HOSPITAL, HANOVER, KS, p. A153
HANS P. PETERSON MEMORIAL HOSPITAL, PHILIP, SD, p. A363
HANSFORD HOSPITAL, SPEARMAN, TX, p. A404
HARBOR BEACH COMMUNITY HOSPITAL, HARBOR BEACH, MI, p. A204
HARBOR HOSPITAL CENTER, BALTIMORE, MD, p. A184
HARBOR OAKS HOSPITAL, FORT WALTON BEACH, FL, p. A 85
HARBOR OAKS HOSPITAL, NEW BALTIMORE, MI, p. A208
HARBOR VIEW, MIAMI, FL, p. A 89
HARBOR VIEW MEDICAL CENTER, SAN DIEGO, CA, p. A 59
HARBOR VIEW MERCY HOSPITAL, FORT SMITH, AR, p. A 30
HARBORVIEW MEDICAL CENTER, SEATTLE, WA, p. A427
HARDEMAN COUNTY MEMORIAL HOSPITAL, QUANAH, TX, p. A400
HARDIN COUNTY GENERAL HOSPITAL, ROSICLARE, IL, p. A130
HARDIN COUNTY GENERAL HOSPITAL, SAVANNAH, TN, p. A374
HARDIN MEMORIAL HOSPITAL, ELIZABETHTOWN, KY, p. A162
HARDIN MEMORIAL HOSPITAL, KENTON, OH, p. A313
HARDING HOSPITAL, WORTHINGTON, OH, p. A319
HARDTNER MEDICAL CENTER, OLLA, LA, p. A177
HARDY WILSON MEMORIAL HOSPITAL, HAZLEHURST, MS, p. A224
HARFORD MEMORIAL HOSPITAL, HAVRE DE GRACE, MD, p. A187
HARLAN ARH HOSPITAL, HARLAN, KY, p. A163
HARLAN COUNTY HOSPITAL, ALMA, NE, p. A246
HARLEM HOSPITAL CENTER, NEW YORK CITY, NY, p. A279
HARMARVILLE REHABILITATION CENTER, PITTSBURGH, PA, p. A346
HARMON MEMORIAL HOSPITAL, HOLLIS, OK, p. A324
HARMONY COMMUNITY HOSPITAL, HARMONY, MN, p. A215
HARMS MEMORIAL HOSPITAL DISTRICT, AMERICAN FALLS, ID, p. A112
HARNEY DISTRICT HOSPITAL, BURNS, OR, p. A329
HARPER COUNTY COMMUNITY HOSPITAL, BUFFALO, OK, p. A322
HARPER HOSPITAL, DETROIT, MI, p. A201
HARRIMAN CITY HOSPITAL, HARRIMAN, TN, p. A368
HARRINGTON MEMORIAL HOSPITAL, SOUTHBRIDGE, MA, p. A197
HARRIS CONTINUED CARE HOSPITAL, FORT WORTH, TX, p. A387
HARRIS COUNTY HOSPITAL DISTRICT, HOUSTON, TX, p. A390
HARRIS COUNTY PSYCHIATRIC CENTER, HOUSTON, TX, p. A390
HARRIS HOSPITAL, NEWPORT, AR, p. A 33
HARRIS METHODIST–ERATH COUNTY, STEPHENVILLE, TX, p. A404

Hospitals, Alphabetically / Hodgeman County Health Center

HARRIS METHODIST-HEB, BEDFORD, TX, p. A379
HARRIS METHODIST-NORTHWEST, AZLE, TX, p. A378
HARRIS METHODIST FORT WORTH, FORT WORTH, TX, p. A387
HARRIS METHODIST SOUTHWEST, FORT WORTH, TX, p. A387
HARRIS REGIONAL HOSPITAL, SYLVA, NC, p. A299
HARRISBURG HOSPITAL, HARRISBURG, PA, p. A339
HARRISBURG MEDICAL CENTER, HARRISBURG, IL, p. A124
HARRISBURG STATE HOSPITAL, HARRISBURG, PA, p. A339
HARRISON COMMUNITY HOSPITAL, CADIZ, OH, p. A307
HARRISON COUNTY COMMUNITY HOSPITAL, BETHANY, MO, p. A230
HARRISON COUNTY HOSPITAL, CORYDON, IN, p. A134
HARRISON MEMORIAL HOSPITAL, CYNTHIANA, KY, p. A162
HARRISON MEMORIAL HOSPITAL, BREMERTON, WA, p. A423
HARRY S. TRUMAN MEMORIAL VETERANS HOSPITAL, COLUMBIA, MO, p. A231
HART COUNTY HOSPITAL, HARTWELL, GA, p. A104
HARTFORD HOSPITAL, HARTFORD, CT, p. A 74
HARTFORD MEMORIAL HOSPITAL, HARTFORD, WI, p. A437
HARTGROVE HOSPITAL, CHICAGO, IL, p. A118
HARTON REGIONAL MEDICAL CENTER, TULLAHOMA, TN, p. A375
HARTSELLE MEDICAL CENTER, HARTSELLE, AL, p. A 17
HARTSVILLE MEDICAL CENTER, HARTSVILLE, TN, p. A368
HARVARD COMMUNITY MEMORIAL HOSPITAL, HARVARD, IL, p. A124
HASKELL COUNTY HOSPITAL, STIGLER, OK, p. A327
HASKELL MEMORIAL HOSPITAL, HASKELL, TX, p. A389
HASTINGS REGIONAL CENTER, HASTINGS, NE, p. A248
HATO REY COMMUNITY HOSPITAL, SAN JUAN, PR, p. A449
HAVASU SAMARITAN REGIONAL HOSPITAL, LAKE HAVASU CITY, AZ, p. A 24
HAVEN HOSPITAL, DE SOTO, TX, p. A384
HAVENWYCK HOSPITAL, AUBURN HILLS, MI, p. A199
HAVERFORD STATE HOSPITAL, HAVERFORD, PA, p. A339
HAWAII STATE HOSPITAL, KANEOHE, HI, p. A111
HAWARDEN COMMUNITY HOSPITAL, HAWARDEN, IA, p. A146
HAWKINS COUNTY MEMORIAL HOSPITAL, ROGERSVILLE, TN, p. A374
HAWLEY U.S. ARMY COMMUNITY HOSPITAL, INDIANAPOLIS, IN, p. A136
HAWTHORN CENTER, NORTHVILLE, MI, p. A208
HAWTHORNE HOSPITAL, HAWTHORNE, CA, p. A 45
HAXTUN HOSPITAL DISTRICT, HAXTUN, CO, p. A 71
HAYES-GREEN-BEACH MEMORIAL HOSPITAL, CHARLOTTE, MI, p. A200
HAYS MEDICAL CENTER, HAYS, KS, p. A153
HAYWARD AREA MEMORIAL HOSPITAL AND NURSING HOME, HAYWARD, WI, p. A437
HAYWOOD COUNTY HOSPITAL, CLYDE, NC, p. A293
HAZLETON-ST. JOSEPH MEDICAL CENTER, HAZLETON, PA, p. A339
HAZLETON GENERAL HOSPITAL, HAZLETON, PA, p. A339
HEALDSBURG GENERAL HOSPITAL, HEALDSBURG, CA, p. A 45
HEALDTON MUNICIPAL HOSPITAL, HEALDTON, OK, p. A324
HEALTH ALLIANCE HOSPITAL-LEOMINSTER, LEOMINSTER, MA, p. A194
HEALTH CENTRAL, OCOEE, FL, p. A 91
HEALTH HILL HOSPITAL FOR CHILDREN, CLEVELAND, OH, p. A309
HEALTHCARE REHABILITATION CENTER, AUSTIN, TX, p. A378
HEALTHEAST BETHESDA LUTHERAN HOSPITAL AND REHABILITATION CENTER, SAINT PAUL, MN, p. A219
HEALTHEAST MIDWAY HOSPITAL, SAINT PAUL, MN, p. A219
HEALTHEAST ST. JOHN'S HOSPITAL, MAPLEWOOD, MN, p. A216
HEALTHEAST ST. JOSEPH'S HOSPITAL, SAINT PAUL, MN, p. A219
HEALTHONE-BEHAVIORAL HEALTH SERVICES, BETHESDA CAMPUS, DENVER, CO, p. A 69
HEALTHSOURCE SAGINAW, SAGINAW, MI, p. A209
HEALTHSOUTH DALLAS REHABILITATION INSTITUTE, DALLAS, TX, p. A383
HEALTHSOUTH DOCTORS' HOSPITAL, CORAL GABLES, FL, p. A 83
HEALTHSOUTH GREAT LAKES REHABILITATION HOSPITAL, ERIE, PA, p. A338
HEALTHSOUTH GREATER PITTSBURGH REHAB HOSPITAL, MONROEVILLE, PA, p. A342
HEALTHSOUTH LAKE ERIE INSTITUTE OF REHABILITATION, ERIE, PA, p. A338
HEALTHSOUTH LARKIN HOSPITAL, SOUTH MIAMI, FL, p. A 95
HEALTHSOUTH MEDICAL CENTER, BIRMINGHAM, AL, p. A 14
HEALTHSOUTH MEDICAL CENTER, DALLAS, TX, p. A383
HEALTHSOUTH MEDICAL CENTER, RICHMOND, VA, p. A419
HEALTHSOUTH NITTANY VALLEY REHABILITATION HOSPITAL, PLEASANT GAP, PA, p. A348
HEALTHSOUTH REHABILITATION HOSPITAL, LARGO, FL, p. A 88

HEALTHSOUTH REHABILITATION HOSPITAL, CONCORD, NH, p. A255
HEALTHSOUTH REHABILITATION HOSPITAL, ALBUQUERQUE, NM, p. A267
HEALTHSOUTH REHABILITATION HOSPITAL, OKLAHOMA CITY, OK, p. A325
HEALTHSOUTH REHABILITATION HOSPITAL, COLUMBIA, SC, p. A356
HEALTHSOUTH REHABILITATION HOSPITAL, FORT WORTH, TX, p. A387
HEALTHSOUTH REHABILITATION HOSPITAL, HUMBLE, TX, p. A393
HEALTHSOUTH REHABILITATION HOSPITAL OF ALTOONA, ALTOONA, PA, p. A334
HEALTHSOUTH REHABILITATION HOSPITAL OF AUSTIN, AUSTIN, TX, p. A378
HEALTHSOUTH REHABILITATION HOSPITAL OF FORT SMITH, FORT SMITH, AR, p. A 30
HEALTHSOUTH REHABILITATION HOSPITAL OF MONTGOMERY, MONTGOMERY, AL, p. A 18
HEALTHSOUTH REHABILITATION HOSPITAL OF NEW JERSEY, TOMS RIVER, NJ, p. A265
HEALTHSOUTH REHABILITATION HOSPITAL OF NORTHERN KENTUCKY, EDGEWOOD, KY, p. A162
HEALTHSOUTH REHABILITATION HOSPITAL OF TALLAHASSEE, TALLAHASSEE, FL, p. A 95
HEALTHSOUTH REHABILITATION HOSPITAL OF TEXARKANA, TEXARKANA, TX, p. A404
HEALTHSOUTH REHABILITATION HOSPITAL OF UTAH, SANDY, UT, p. A410
HEALTHSOUTH REHABILITATION HOSPITAL OF YORK, YORK, PA, p. A352
HEALTHSOUTH REHABILITATION INSTITUTE OF SAN ANTONIO, SAN ANTONIO, TX, p. A401
HEALTHSOUTH REHABILITATION INSTITUTE OF SARASOTA, SARASOTA, FL, p. A 95
HEALTHSOUTH REHABILITATION OF MECHANICSBURG, MECHANICSBURG, PA, p. A342
HEALTHSOUTH SEA PINES REHABILITATION HOSPITAL, MELBOURNE, FL, p. A 89
HEALTHSOUTH SUNRISE REHABILITATION HOSPITAL, FORT LAUDERDALE, FL, p. A 84
HEALTHSOUTH TREASURE COAST REHABILITATION HOSPITAL, VERO BEACH, FL, p. A 97
HEALTHWEST REGIONAL MEDICAL CENTER, PHOENIX, AZ, p. A 25
HEALTHWIN HOSPITAL, SOUTH BEND, IN, p. A140
HEART OF AMERICA MEDICAL CENTER, RUGBY, ND, p. A305
HEART OF FLORIDA HOSPITAL, HAINES CITY, FL, p. A 85
HEART OF TEXAS MEMORIAL HOSPITAL, BRADY, TX, p. A380
HEART OF THE ROCKIES REGIONAL MEDICAL CENTER, SALIDA, CO, p. A 72
HEARTLAND HOSPITAL, NEVADA, MO, p. A236
HEARTLAND HOSPITAL EAST, SAINT JOSEPH, MO, p. A237
HEARTLAND HOSPITAL WEST, SAINT JOSEPH, MO, p. A237
HEARTLAND MEDICAL CENTER, FARGO, ND, p. A303
HEATHER HILL REHABILITATION HOSPITAL, CHARDON, OH, p. A307
HEBREW HOME AND HOSPITAL, WEST HARTFORD, CT, p. A 77
HEBREW REHABILITATION CENTER FOR AGED, BOSTON, MA, p. A191
HEDRICK MEDICAL CENTER, CHILLICOTHE, MO, p. A231
HEGG MEMORIAL HEALTH CENTER, ROCK VALLEY, IA, p. A149
HEIGHTS HOSPITAL, HOUSTON, TX, p. A390
HEIGHTS PSYCHIATRIC HOSPITAL, ALBUQUERQUE, NM, p. A267
HELEN ELLIS MEMORIAL HOSPITAL, TARPON SPRINGS, FL, p. A 96
HELEN HAYES HOSPITAL, WEST HAVERSTRAW, NY, p. A289
HELEN KELLER HOSPITAL, SHEFFIELD, AL, p. A 20
HELEN NEWBERRY JOY HOSPITAL, NEWBERRY, MI, p. A208
HELENA REGIONAL MEDICAL CENTER, HELENA, AR, p. A 31
HELENE FULD MEDICAL CENTER, TRENTON, NJ, p. A265
HEMET VALLEY MEDICAL CENTER, HEMET, CA, p. A 45
HEMPHILL COUNTY HOSPITAL, CANADIAN, TX, p. A380
HEMPSTEAD GENERAL HOSPITAL MEDICAL CENTER, HEMPSTEAD, NY, p. A276
HENDERSON COMMUNITY HOSPITAL, HENDERSON, NE, p. A248
HENDERSON MEMORIAL HOSPITAL, HENDERSON, TX, p. A389
HENDERSONVILLE HOSPITAL, HENDERSONVILLE, TN, p. A368
HENDRICK MEDICAL CENTER, ABILENE, TX, p. A376
HENDRICKS COMMUNITY HOSPITAL, DANVILLE, IN, p. A134
HENDRICKS COMMUNITY HOSPITAL, HENDRICKS, MN, p. A215
HENDRY GENERAL HOSPITAL, CLEWISTON, FL, p. A 82
HENNEPIN COUNTY MEDICAL CENTER, MINNEAPOLIS, MN, p. A217
HENRICO DOCTOR'S HOSPITAL, RICHMOND, VA, p. A419
HENRIETTA D. GOODALL HOSPITAL, SANFORD, ME, p. A182

HENRY COUNTY HEALTH CENTER, MOUNT PLEASANT, IA, p. A147
HENRY COUNTY HOSPITAL, NAPOLEON, OH, p. A315
HENRY COUNTY MEDICAL CENTER, PARIS, TN, p. A374
HENRY COUNTY MEMORIAL HOSPITAL, NEW CASTLE, IN, p. A139
HENRY D. ALTOBELLO CHILDREN AND YOUTH CENTER, MERIDEN, CT, p. A 75
HENRY FORD COTTAGE HOSPITAL, GROSSE POINTE FARMS, MI, p. A204
HENRY FORD HOSPITAL, DETROIT, MI, p. A202
HENRY GENERAL HOSPITAL, STOCKBRIDGE, GA, p. A108
HENRY MAYO NEWHALL MEMORIAL HOSPITAL, VALENCIA, CA, p. A 66
HENRYETTA MEDICAL CENTER, HENRYETTA, OK, p. A324
HEPBURN MEDICAL CENTER, OGDENSBURG, NY, p. A284
HEREFORD REGIONAL MEDICAL CENTER, HEREFORD, TX, p. A390
HERINGTON MUNICIPAL HOSPITAL, HERINGTON, KS, p. A153
HERITAGE BEVERLY HILLS HOSPITAL, LECANTO, FL, p. A 88
HERITAGE HOSPITAL, SOMERVILLE, MA, p. A196
HERITAGE HOSPITAL, TARBORO, NC, p. A299
HERMANN AREA DISTRICT HOSPITAL, HERMANN, MO, p. A233
HERMANN HOSPITAL, HOUSTON, TX, p. A390
HERRICK MEMORIAL HOSPITAL, TECUMSEH, MI, p. A210
HERRIN HOSPITAL, HERRIN, IL, p. A124
HEYWOOD HOSPITAL, GARDNER, MA, p. A193
HI-DESERT MEDICAL CENTER, JOSHUA TREE, CA, p. A 46
HI-PLAINS HOSPITAL, HALE CENTER, TX, p. A389
HIALEAH HOSPITAL, HIALEAH, FL, p. A 85
HIAWATHA COMMUNITY HOSPITAL, HIAWATHA, KS, p. A154
HICKMAN COUNTY HEALTH SERVICES, CENTERVILLE, TN, p. A366
HIGGINS GENERAL HOSPITAL, BREMEN, GA, p. A100
HIGH PLAINS BAPTIST HEALTH SYSTEM, AMARILLO, TX, p. A376
HIGH POINT HOSPITAL, PORT CHESTER, NY, p. A285
HIGH POINT REGIONAL HOSPITAL, HIGH POINT, NC, p. A295
HIGH POINTE, OKLAHOMA CITY, OK, p. A325
HIGHLAND DISTRICT HOSPITAL, HILLSBORO, OH, p. A313
HIGHLAND GENERAL HOSPITAL, OAKLAND, CA, p. A 54
HIGHLAND HOSPITAL, BELVIDERE, IL, p. A116
HIGHLAND HOSPITAL, SHREVEPORT, LA, p. A178
HIGHLAND HOSPITAL, CHARLESTON, WV, p. A430
HIGHLAND HOSPITAL OF ROCHESTER, ROCHESTER, NY, p. A286
HIGHLAND LAKES MEDICAL CENTER, BURNET, TX, p. A380
HIGHLAND MEDICAL CENTER, LUBBOCK, TX, p. A395
HIGHLAND PARK HOSPITAL, HIGHLAND PARK, IL, p. A124
HIGHLAND RIDGE HOSPITAL, SALT LAKE CITY, UT, p. A410
HIGHLANDS-CASHIERS HOSPITAL, HIGHLANDS, NC, p. A295
HIGHLANDS HOSPITAL, CONNELLSVILLE, PA, p. A337
HIGHLANDS REGIONAL MEDICAL CENTER, SEBRING, FL, p. A 95
HIGHLANDS REGIONAL MEDICAL CENTER, PRESTONSBURG, KY, p. A167
HIGHLINE COMMUNITY HOSPTIAL, BURIEN, WA, p. A423
HIGHSMITH-RAINEY MEMORIAL HOSPITAL, FAYETTEVILLE, NC, p. A294
HILL COUNTRY MEMORIAL HOSPITAL, FREDERICKSBURG, TX, p. A387
HILL CREST BEHAVIORAL HEALTH SERVICES, BIRMINGHAM, AL, p. A 14
HILL REGIONAL HOSPITAL, HILLSBORO, TX, p. A390
HILLCREST BAPTIST MEDICAL CENTER, WACO, TX, p. A406
HILLCREST HEALTH CENTER, OKLAHOMA CITY, OK, p. A325
HILLCREST HOSPITAL, PITTSFIELD, MA, p. A196
HILLCREST HOSPITAL, CALHOUN CITY, MS, p. A223
HILLCREST HOSPITAL, SIMPSONVILLE, SC, p. A359
HILLCREST MEDICAL CENTER, TULSA, OK, p. A328
HILLS AND DALES GENERAL HOSPITAL, CASS CITY, MI, p. A200
HILLSBORO AREA HOSPITAL, HILLSBORO, IL, p. A124
HILLSBORO COMMUNITY HOSPITAL, HILLSBORO, ND, p. A303
HILLSDALE COMMUNITY HEALTH CENTER, HILLSDALE, MI, p. A204
HILLSIDE HOSPITAL, ATLANTA, GA, p. A 99
HILLSIDE HOSPITAL, PULASKI, TN, p. A374
HILLSIDE REHABILITATION HOSPITAL, WARREN, OH, p. A318
HILLTOP REHABILITATION CENTER, GRAND JUNCTION, CO, p. A 70
HILO MEDICAL CENTER, HILO, HI, p. A110
HILTON HEAD HOSPITAL, HILTON HEAD ISLAND, SC, p. A358
HINSDALE HOSPITAL, HINSDALE, IL, p. A125
HOAG MEMORIAL HOSPITAL PRESBYTERIAN, NEWPORT BEACH, CA, p. A 54
HOCKING VALLEY COMMUNITY HOSPITAL, LOGAN, OH, p. A314
HODGEMAN COUNTY HEALTH CENTER, JETMORE, KS, p. A154

© 1995 AHA Guide

Hospitals A463

HOFFMAN ESTATES MEDICAL CENTER, HOFFMAN ESTATES, IL, p. A125
HOLDENVILLE GENERAL HOSPITAL, HOLDENVILLE, OK, p. A324
HOLLAND COMMUNITY HOSPITAL, HOLLAND, MI, p. A205
HOLLISWOOD HOSPITAL, NEW YORK CITY, NY, p. A279
HOLLY HILL MENTAL HEALTH SERVICES, RALEIGH, NC, p. A297
HOLLY SPRINGS MEMORIAL HOSPITAL, HOLLY SPRINGS, MS, p. A224
HOLLYWOOD COMMUNITY HOSPITAL OF HOLLYWOOD, LOS ANGELES, CA, p. A 49
HOLLYWOOD COMMUNITY HOSPITAL OF VAN NUYS, LOS ANGELES, CA, p. A 49
HOLLYWOOD MEDICAL CENTER, HOLLYWOOD, FL, p. A 85
HOLLYWOOD PAVILION, HOLLYWOOD, FL, p. A 85
HOLMES REGIONAL MEDICAL CENTER, MELBOURNE, FL, p. A 89
HOLSTON VALLEY HOSPITAL AND MEDICAL CENTER, KINGSPORT, TN, p. A369
HOLTON COMMUNITY HOSPITAL, HOLTON, KS, p. A154
HOLY CROSS HOSPITAL, FORT LAUDERDALE, FL, p. A 84
HOLY CROSS HOSPITAL, CHICAGO, IL, p. A118
HOLY CROSS HOSPITAL, DETROIT, MI, p. A202
HOLY CROSS HOSPITAL, TAOS, NM, p. A270
HOLY CROSS HOSPITAL OF SILVER SPRING, SILVER SPRING, MD, p. A188
HOLY CROSS MEDICAL CENTER, LOS ANGELES, CA, p. A 49
HOLY FAMILY HOSPITAL, ESTHERVILLE, IA, p. A145
HOLY FAMILY HOSPITAL, SPOKANE, WA, p. A428
HOLY FAMILY HOSPITAL, NEW RICHMOND, WI, p. A441
HOLY FAMILY HOSPITAL AND MEDICAL CENTER, METHUEN, MA, p. A195
HOLY FAMILY MEDICAL CENTER, DES PLAINES, IL, p. A122
HOLY FAMILY MEMORIAL MEDICAL CENTER, MANITOWOC, WI, p. A439
HOLY INFANT HOSPITAL, HOVEN, SD, p. A362
HOLY NAME HOSPITAL, TEANECK, NJ, p. A265
HOLY REDEEMER HOSPITAL AND MEDICAL CENTER, MEADOWBROOK, PA, p. A342
HOLY ROSARY HOSPITAL, MILES CITY, MT, p. A243
HOLY ROSARY MEDICAL CENTER, ONTARIO, OR, p. A331
HOLY SPIRIT HOSPITAL, CAMP HILL, PA, p. A336
HOLY TRINITY HOSPITAL, GRACEVILLE, MN, p. A215
HOLYOKE HOSPITAL, HOLYOKE, MA, p. A194
HOLZER MEDICAL CENTER, GALLIPOLIS, OH, p. A312
HOMER MEMORIAL HOSPITAL, HOMER, LA, p. A173
HONOKAA HOSPITAL, HONOKAA, HI, p. A110
HOOD GENERAL HOSPITAL, GRANBURY, TX, p. A388
HOOD MEMORIAL HOSPITAL, AMITE, LA, p. A170
HOOD RIVER MEMORIAL HOSPITAL, HOOD RIVER, OR, p. A330
HOOPESTON COMMUNITY MEMORIAL HOSPITAL, HOOPESTON, IL, p. A125
HOOTS MEMORIAL HOSPITAL, YADKINVILLE, NC, p. A300
HOPE HOSPITAL, LOCKHART, SC, p. A358
HOPEDALE MEDICAL COMPLEX, HOPEDALE, IL, p. A125
HOPKINS COUNTY MEMORIAL HOSPITAL, SULPHUR SPRINGS, TX, p. A404
HORIZON HOSPITAL, CLEARWATER, FL, p. A 82
HORIZON HOSPITAL SYSTEM, GREENVILLE, PA, p. A339
HORIZON SPECIALTY HOSPITAL, LUBBOCK, TX, p. A395
HORIZON SPECIALTY HOSPITAL, SAN ANTONIO, TX, p. A401
HORN MEMORIAL HOSPITAL, IDA GROVE, IA, p. A146
HORSHAM CLINIC, AMBLER, PA, p. A334
HORTON COMMUNITY HOSPITAL, HORTON, KS, p. A154
HORTON MEDICAL CENTER, MIDDLETOWN, NY, p. A277
HOSPICE OF NORTHERN VIRGINIA, ARLINGTON, VA, p. A414
HOSPICE OF PALM BEACH COUNTY, WEST PALM BEACH, FL, p. A 97
HOSPITAL CENTER AT ORANGE, ORANGE, NJ, p. A263
HOSPITAL DE AREA DE YAUCO, YAUCO, PR, p. A450
HOSPITAL DE DAMAS, PONCE, PR, p. A449
HOSPITAL DE DIEGO, SAN JUAN, PR, p. A449
HOSPITAL DE LA CONCEPCION, SAN GERMAN, PR, p. A449
HOSPITAL DEL MAESTRO, SAN JUAN, PR, p. A449
HOSPITAL DISTRICT NUMBER FIVE OF HARPER COUNTY, HARPER, KS, p. A153
HOSPITAL DISTRICT NUMBER SIX OF HARPER COUNTY, ANTHONY, KS, p. A151
HOSPITAL DR. DOMINGUEZ, HUMACAO, PR, p. A448
HOSPITAL DR. FEDERICO TRILLA, CAROLINA, PR, p. A448
HOSPITAL DR. SUSONI, ARECIBO, PR, p. A447
HOSPITAL EPISCOPAL SAN LUCAS, PONCE, PR, p. A449
HOSPITAL FOR JOINT DISEASES ORTHOPEDIC INSTITUTE, NEW YORK CITY, NY, p. A280
HOSPITAL FOR SICK CHILDREN, WASHINGTON, DC, p. A 79
HOSPITAL FOR SPECIAL CARE, NEW BRITAIN, CT, p. A 75
HOSPITAL FOR SPECIAL SURGERY, NEW YORK CITY, NY, p. A280
HOSPITAL HERMANOS MELENDEZ, BAYAMON, PR, p. A447
HOSPITAL INTERAMERICANO DE MEDICINA AVANZADA, CAGUAS, PR, p. A448
HOSPITAL MATILDE BRENES, BAYAMON, PR, p. A448
HOSPITAL MENONITA DE CAYEY, CAYEY, PR, p. A448
HOSPITAL OF SAINT RAPHAEL, NEW HAVEN, CT, p. A 75
HOSPITAL OF THE CALIFORNIA INSTITUTION FOR MEN, CHINO, CA, p. A 39
HOSPITAL OF THE GOOD SAMARITAN, LOS ANGELES, CA, p. A 49
HOSPITAL OF THE UNIVERSITY OF PENNSYLVANIA, PHILADELPHIA, PA, p. A344
HOSPITAL ONCOLOGICO ANDRES GRILLASCA, PONCE, PR, p. A449
HOSPITAL PAVIA, SAN JUAN, PR, p. A449
HOSPITAL PEREA, MAYAGUEZ, PR, p. A449
HOSPITAL SAN FRANCISCO, SAN JUAN, PR, p. A449
HOSPITAL SAN PABLO, BAYAMON, PR, p. A448
HOSPITAL SANTA ROSA, GUAYAMA, PR, p. A448
HOSPITAL SUB-REGIONAL DR. VICTOR R. NUNEZ, HUMACAO, PR, p. A448
HOSPITAL UNIVERSITARIO DR. RAMON RUIZ ARNAU, BAYAMON, PR, p. A448
HOT SPRING COUNTY MEMORIAL HOSPITAL, MALVERN, AR, p. A 32
HOT SPRINGS COUNTY MEMORIAL HOSPITAL, THERMOPOLIS, WY, p. A446
HOULTON REGIONAL HOSPITAL, HOULTON, ME, p. A181
HOUSATONIC ADOLESCENT HOSPITAL, NEWTOWN, CT, p. A 76
HOUSTON COUNTY HOSPITAL, CROCKETT, TX, p. A382
HOUSTON MEDICAL CENTER, WARNER ROBINS, GA, p. A109
HOUSTON NORTHWEST MEDICAL CENTER, HOUSTON, TX, p. A390
HOUSTON REHABILITATION INSTITUTE, HOUSTON, TX, p. A391
HOWARD COMMUNITY HOSPITAL, KOKOMO, IN, p. A137
HOWARD COUNTY COMMUNITY HOSPITAL, SAINT PAUL, NE, p. A251
HOWARD COUNTY GENERAL HOSPITAL, COLUMBIA, MD, p. A186
HOWARD COUNTY HOSPITAL, CRESCO, IA, p. A144
HOWARD MEMORIAL HOSPITAL, NASHVILLE, AR, p. A 33
HOWARD UNIVERSITY HOSPITAL, WASHINGTON, DC, p. A 79
HOWARD YOUNG MEDICAL CENTER, WOODRUFF, WI, p. A444
HUBBARD REGIONAL HOSPITAL, WEBSTER, MA, p. A198
HUDSON MEDICAL CENTER, HUDSON, WI, p. A437
HUDSON RIVER PSYCHIATRIC CENTER, POUGHKEEPSIE, NY, p. A285
HUDSON VALLEY HOSPITAL CENTER, PEEKSKILL, NY, p. A284
HUERFANO MEDICAL CENTER, WALSENBURG, CO, p. A 73
HUEY P. LONG MEDICAL CENTER, PINEVILLE, LA, p. A177
HUGGINS HOSPITAL, WOLFEBORO, NH, p. A257
HUGH CHATHAM MEMORIAL HOSPITAL, ELKIN, NC, p. A294
HUGHSTON SPORTS MEDICINE HOSPITAL, COLUMBUS, GA, p. A101
HUGULEY MEMORIAL MEDICAL CENTER, FORT WORTH, TX, p. A387
HUHUKAM MEMORIAL HOSPITAL, SACATON, AZ, p. A 26
HUMANA HOSPITAL–LEXINGTON, LEXINGTON, KY, p. A164
HUMBOLDT COUNTY MEMORIAL HOSPITAL, HUMBOLDT, IA, p. A146
HUMBOLDT GENERAL HOSPITAL, WINNEMUCCA, NV, p. A254
HUMBOLDT GENERAL HOSPITAL, HUMBOLDT, TN, p. A369
HUMPHREYS COUNTY MEMORIAL HOSPITAL, BELZONI, MS, p. A222
HUNT MEMORIAL HOSPITAL DISTRICT, GREENVILLE, TX, p. A389
HUNTER HOLMES McGUIRE VETERANS AFFAIRS MEDICAL CENTER, RICHMOND, VA, p. A419
HUNTERDON MEDICAL CENTER, FLEMINGTON, NJ, p. A260
HUNTINGTON BEACH HOSPITAL AND MEDICAL CENTER, HUNTINGTON BEACH, CA, p. A 45
HUNTINGTON EAST VALLEY HOSPITAL, GLENDORA, CA, p. A 44
HUNTINGTON HOSPITAL, HUNTINGTON, NY, p. A276
HUNTINGTON HOSPITAL, WILLOW GROVE, PA, p. A352
HUNTINGTON MEMORIAL HOSPITAL, PASADENA, CA, p. A 55
HUNTINGTON MEMORIAL HOSPITAL, HUNTINGTON, IN, p. A136
HUNTINGTON REHABILITATION HOSPITAL, HUNTINGTON, WV, p. A431
HUNTSVILLE HOSPITAL, HUNTSVILLE, AL, p. A 17
HUNTSVILLE HOSPITAL EAST, HUNTSVILLE, AL, p. A 17
HUNTSVILLE MEMORIAL HOSPITAL, HUNTSVILLE, TX, p. A393
HURLEY MEDICAL CENTER, FLINT, MI, p. A203
HURON MEMORIAL HOSPITAL, BAD AXE, MI, p. A199
HURON REGIONAL MEDICAL CENTER, HURON, SD, p. A362
HURON VALLEY HOSPITAL, COMMERCE TOWNSHIP, MI, p. A201
HURTADO HEALTH CENTER, NEW BRUNSWICK, NJ, p. A262
HUTCHESON MEDICAL CENTER, FORT OGLETHORPE, GA, p. A104
HUTCHINSON COMMUNITY HOSPITAL, HUTCHINSON, MN, p. A215
HUTCHINSON HOSPITAL CORPORATION, HUTCHINSON, KS, p. A154
HUTZEL HOSPITAL, DETROIT, MI, p. A202

I

I. GONZALEZ MARTINEZ ONCOLOGIC HOSPITAL, SAN JUAN, PR, p. A449
IBERIA GENERAL HOSPITAL AND MEDICAL CENTER, NEW IBERIA, LA, p. A175
IDAHO ELKS REHABILITATION HOSPITAL, BOISE, ID, p. A112
IHC EVANSTON REGIONAL HOSPITAL, EVANSTON, WY, p. A445
ILLINI COMMUNITY HOSPITAL, PITTSFIELD, IL, p. A129
ILLINI HOSPITAL, SILVIS, IL, p. A130
ILLINOIS MASONIC MEDICAL CENTER, CHICAGO, IL, p. A118
ILLINOIS STATE PSYCHIATRIC INSTITUTE, CHICAGO, IL, p. A118
ILLINOIS VALLEY COMMUNITY HOSPITAL, PERU, IL, p. A129
IMMANUEL-ST. JOSEPH'S HOSPITAL, MANKATO, MN, p. A216
IMMANUEL MEDICAL CENTER, OMAHA, NE, p. A250
IMPACT DRUG AND ALCOHOL TREATMENT CENTER, PASADENA, CA, p. A 56
IMPERIAL POINT MEDICAL CENTER, FORT LAUDERDALE, FL, p. A 84
INCARNATE WORD HOSPITAL, SAINT LOUIS, MO, p. A238
INDEPENDENCE REGIONAL HEALTH CENTER, INDEPENDENCE, MO, p. A233
INDIAN HEALTH SERVICE–SIOUX SAN HOSPITAL, RAPID CITY, SD, p. A363
INDIAN PATH MEDICAL CENTER, KINGSPORT, TN, p. A370
INDIAN PATH PAVILION, KINGSPORT, TN, p. A370
INDIAN RIVER MEMORIAL HOSPITAL, VERO BEACH, FL, p. A 97
INDIAN VALLEY HOSPITAL DISTRICT, GREENVILLE, CA, p. A 44
INDIANA HOSPITAL, INDIANA, PA, p. A340
INDIANA UNIVERSITY MEDICAL CENTER, INDIANAPOLIS, IN, p. A136
INDIANHEAD MEDICAL CENTER, SHELL LAKE, WI, p. A443
INDUSTRIAL HOSPITAL, SAN JUAN, PR, p. A449
INGALLS MEMORIAL HOSPITAL, HARVEY, IL, p. A124
INGLESIDE HOSPITAL, ROSEMEAD, CA, p. A 58
INLAND VALLEY REGIONAL MEDICAL CENTER, WILDOMAR, CA, p. A 67
INNER HARBOUR HOSPITALS, DOUGLASVILLE, GA, p. A103
INSTITUTE OF LIVING, HARTFORD, CT, p. A 74
INSTITUTE OF MENTAL HEALTH–RHODE ISLAND MEDICAL CENTER, HOWARD, RI, p. A353
INTER–COMMUNITY MEDICAL CENTER, COVINA, CA, p. A 40
INTER–COMMUNITY MEMORIAL HOSPITAL, NEWFANE, NY, p. A283
INTERFAITH MEDICAL CENTER, NEW YORK CITY, NY, p. A280
INTRACARE MEDICAL CENTER, HOUSTON, TX, p. A391
IOANNIS A. LOUGARIS VETERANS AFFAIRS MEDICAL CENTER, RENO, NV, p. A254
IONIA COUNTY MEMORIAL HOSPITAL, IONIA, MI, p. A205
IOWA LUTHERAN HOSPITAL, DES MOINES, IA, p. A144
IOWA MEDICAL AND CLASSIFICATION CENTER, OAKDALE, IA, p. A148
IOWA METHODIST MEDICAL CENTER, DES MOINES, IA, p. A144
IRA DAVENPORT MEMORIAL HOSPITAL, BATH, NY, p. A272
IREDELL MEMORIAL HOSPITAL, STATESVILLE, NC, p. A299
IRELAND ARMY COMMUNITY HOSPITAL, FORT KNOX, KY, p. A162
IRON COUNTY GENERAL HOSPITAL, IRON RIVER, MI, p. A205
IROQUOIS MEMORIAL HOSPITAL AND RESIDENT HOME, WATSEKA, IL, p. A131
IRVINE MEDICAL CENTER, IRVINE, CA, p. A 46
IRVING HEALTHCARE SYSTEM, IRVING, TX, p. A393
IRVINGTON GENERAL HOSPITAL, IRVINGTON, NJ, p. A261
IRWIN ARMY COMMUNITY HOSPITAL, FORT RILEY, KS, p. A152
IRWIN COUNTY HOSPITAL, OCILLA, GA, p. A106
ISHAM HEALTH CENTER, ANDOVER, MA, p. A190
ISLAND HOSPITAL, ANACORTES, WA, p. A423
ITASCA MEDICAL CENTER, GRAND RAPIDS, MN, p. A215
IUKA HOSPITAL & NURSING FACILITY, IUKA, MS, p. A225
IVINSON MEMORIAL HOSPITAL, LARAMIE, WY, p. A446

Hospitals, Alphabetically / Kern Valley Hospital District

Section A Index

J

J. ARTHUR DOSHER MEMORIAL HOSPITAL, SOUTHPORT, NC, p. A299
J. D. MCCARTY CENTER FOR CHILDREN WITH DEVELOPMENTAL DISABILITIES, NORMAN, OK, p. A325
J. PAUL JONES HOSPITAL, CAMDEN, AL, p. A 14
J.C. BLAIR MEMORIAL HOSPITAL, HUNTINGDON, PA, p. A340
JACKSON–MADISON COUNTY GENERAL HOSPITAL, JACKSON, TN, p. A369
JACKSON BROOK INSTITUTE, SOUTH PORTLAND, ME, p. A182
JACKSON COUNTY HOSPITAL, SCOTTSBORO, AL, p. A 19
JACKSON COUNTY HOSPITAL, GAINESBORO, TN, p. A368
JACKSON COUNTY HOSPITAL, EDNA, TX, p. A385
JACKSON COUNTY MEMORIAL HOSPITAL, ALTUS, OK, p. A321
JACKSON COUNTY PUBLIC HOSPITAL, MAQUOKETA, IA, p. A147
JACKSON GENERAL HOSPITAL, RIPLEY, WV, p. A433
JACKSON HOSPITAL, MARIANNA, FL, p. A 89
JACKSON HOSPITAL AND CLINIC, MONTGOMERY, AL, p. A 18
JACKSON MEMORIAL HOSPITAL, MIAMI, FL, p. A 89
JACKSON MUNICIPAL HOSPITAL, NURSING HOME AND CLINIC, JACKSON, MN, p. A216
JACKSON PARISH HOSPITAL, JONESBORO, LA, p. A173
JACKSON PARK HOSPITAL, CHICAGO, IL, p. A119
JACKSONVILLE HOSPITAL, JACKSONVILLE, AL, p. A 17
JACOBSON MEMORIAL HOSPITAL CARE CENTER, ELGIN, ND, p. A303
JAMAICA HOSPITAL MEDICAL CENTER, NEW YORK CITY, NY, p. A280
JAMES A. HALEY VETERANS HOSPITAL, TAMPA, FL, p. A 96
JAMES B. HAGGIN MEMORIAL HOSPITAL, HARRODSBURG, KY, p. A163
JAMES E. VAN ZANDT VETERANS AFFAIRS MEDICAL CENTER, ALTOONA, PA, p. A334
JAMES LAWRENCE KERNAN HOSPITAL, BALTIMORE, MD, p. A184
JAMESON MEMORIAL HOSPITAL, NEW CASTLE, PA, p. A343
JAMESTOWN HOSPITAL, JAMESTOWN, ND, p. A303
JANE PHILLIPS MEDICAL CENTER, BARTLESVILLE, OK, p. A321
JANE PHILLIPS NOWATA HEALTH CENTER, NOWATA, OK, p. A325
JANE TODD CRAWFORD MEMORIAL HOSPITAL, GREENSBURG, KY, p. A163
JASPER COUNTY HOSPITAL, RENSSELAER, IN, p. A140
JASPER GENERAL HOSPITAL, BAY SPRINGS, MS, p. A222
JASPER MEMORIAL HOSPITAL, MONTICELLO, GA, p. A106
JASPER MEMORIAL HOSPITAL, JASPER, TX, p. A393
JAY COUNTY HOSPITAL, PORTLAND, IN, p. A140
JAY HOSPITAL, JAY, FL, p. A 87
JEANES HOSPITAL, PHILADELPHIA, PA, p. A345
JEANNETTE DISTRICT MEMORIAL HOSPITAL, JEANNETTE, PA, p. A340
JEFF ANDERSON REGIONAL MEDICAL CENTER, MERIDIAN, MS, p. A226
JEFF DAVIS HOSPITAL, HAZLEHURST, GA, p. A104
JEFFERSON COMMUNITY HEALTH CENTER, FAIRBURY, NE, p. A247
JEFFERSON COUNTY HOSPITAL, FAIRFIELD, IA, p. A145
JEFFERSON COUNTY HOSPITAL, FAYETTE, MS, p. A224
JEFFERSON COUNTY HOSPITAL, WAURIKA, OK, p. A328
JEFFERSON COUNTY MEMORIAL HOSPITAL, WINCHESTER, KS, p. A160
JEFFERSON DAVIS COUNTY HOSPITAL, PRENTISS, MS, p. A227
JEFFERSON GENERAL HOSPITAL, PORT TOWNSEND, WA, p. A426
JEFFERSON HOSPITAL, LOUISVILLE, GA, p. A105
JEFFERSON MEMORIAL HOSPITAL, CRYSTAL CITY, MO, p. A231
JEFFERSON MEMORIAL HOSPITAL, JEFFERSON CITY, TN, p. A369
JEFFERSON MEMORIAL HOSPITAL, RANSON, WV, p. A433
JEFFERSON REGIONAL MEDICAL CENTER, PINE BLUFF, AR, p. A 33
JELLICO COMMUNITY HOSPITAL, JELLICO, TN, p. A369
JENKINS COMMUNITY HOSPITAL A SUBSIDIARY OF FIRST HEALTH, INC., JENKINS, KY, p. A164
JENKINS COUNTY HOSPITAL, MILLEN, GA, p. A106
JENNIE EDMUNDSON MEMORIAL HOSPITAL, COUNCIL BLUFFS, IA, p. A143
JENNIE M. MELHAM MEMORIAL MEDICAL CENTER, BROKEN BOW, NE, p. A246
JENNIE STUART MEDICAL CENTER, HOPKINSVILLE, KY, p. A163

JENNINGS AMERICAN LEGION HOSPITAL, JENNINGS, LA, p. A173
JENNINGS COMMUNITY HOSPITAL, NORTH VERNON, IN, p. A139
JERRY L. PETTIS MEMORIAL VETERANS HOSPITAL, LOMA LINDA, CA, p. A 47
JERSEY CITY MEDICAL CENTER, JERSEY CITY, NJ, p. A261
JERSEY COMMUNITY HOSPITAL, JERSEYVILLE, IL, p. A125
JERSEY SHORE HOSPITAL, JERSEY SHORE, PA, p. A340
JERSEY SHORE MEDICAL CENTER, NEPTUNE, NJ, p. A262
JESSE HOLMAN JONES HOSPITAL, SPRINGFIELD, TN, p. A374
JEWELL COUNTY HOSPITAL, MANKATO, KS, p. A156
JEWISH HOSPITAL–SHELBYVILLE, SHELBYVILLE, KY, p. A168
JEWISH HOSPITAL, LOUISVILLE, KY, p. A165
JEWISH HOSPITAL KENWOOD, CINCINNATI, OH, p. A308
JEWISH HOSPITAL OF CINCINNATI, CINCINNATI, OH, p. A308
JEWISH HOSPITAL OF ST. LOUIS, SAINT LOUIS, MO, p. A238
JEWISH MEMORIAL HOSPITAL AND REHABILITATION CENTER, BOSTON, MA, p. A191
JFK JOHNSON REHABILITATION INSTITUTE, EDISON, NJ, p. A259
JFK MEDICAL CENTER, ATLANTIS, FL, p. A 81
JFK MEDICAL CENTER, EDISON, NJ, p. A259
JO ELLEN SMITH MEDICAL CENTER, NEW ORLEANS, LA, p. A176
JOEL POMERENE MEMORIAL HOSPITAL, MILLERSBURG, OH, p. A315
JOHN AND MARY KIRBY HOSPITAL, MONTICELLO, IL, p. A127
JOHN C. FREMONT HEALTHCARE DISTRICT, MARIPOSA, CA, p. A 52
JOHN C. LINCOLN HOSPITAL AND HEALTH CENTER, PHOENIX, AZ, p. A 25
JOHN D. ARCHBOLD MEMORIAL HOSPITAL, THOMASVILLE, GA, p. A108
JOHN F. KENNEDY MEMORIAL HOSPITAL, INDIO, CA, p. A 45
JOHN F. KENNEDY MEMORIAL HOSPITAL, PHILADELPHIA, PA, p. A345
JOHN HEINZ INSTITUTE OF REHABILITATION MEDICINE, WILKES–BARRE, PA, p. A351
JOHN J. MADDEN MENTAL HEALTH CENTER, HINES, IL, p. A124
JOHN J. PERSHING VETERANS AFFAIRS MEDICAL CENTER, POPLAR BLUFF, MO, p. A237
JOHN L. DOYNE HOSPITAL, MILWAUKEE, WI, p. A440
JOHN MUIR MEDICAL CENTER, WALNUT CREEK, CA, p. A 66
JOHN RANDOLPH MEDICAL CENTER, HOPEWELL, VA, p. A416
JOHN T. MATHER MEMORIAL HOSPITAL, PORT JEFFERSON, NY, p. A285
JOHN UMSTEAD HOSPITAL, BUTNER, NC, p. A292
JOHNS COMMUNITY HOSPITAL, TAYLOR, TX, p. A404
JOHNS HOPKINS BAYVIEW MEDICAL CENTER, BALTIMORE, MD, p. A184
JOHNS HOPKINS HOSPITAL, BALTIMORE, MD, p. A184
JOHNSON CITY MEDICAL CENTER HOSPITAL, JOHNSON CITY, TN, p. A369
JOHNSON CITY SPECIALTY HOSPITAL, JOHNSON CITY, TN, p. A369
JOHNSON COUNTY HOSPITAL, TECUMSEH, NE, p. A251
JOHNSON COUNTY HOSPITAL, BUFFALO, WY, p. A445
JOHNSON COUNTY REGIONAL HOSPITAL, CLARKSVILLE, AR, p. A 29
JOHNSON MEMORIAL HOSPITAL, STAFFORD SPRINGS, CT, p. A 77
JOHNSON MEMORIAL HOSPITAL, FRANKLIN, IN, p. A135
JOHNSON MEMORIAL HOSPITAL AND HOME, DAWSON, MN, p. A214
JOHNSTON–WILLIS HOSPITAL, RICHMOND, VA, p. A419
JOHNSTON MEMORIAL HOSPITAL, SMITHFIELD, NC, p. A299
JOHNSTON MEMORIAL HOSPITAL, TISHOMINGO, OK, p. A327
JOHNSTON MEMORIAL HOSPITAL, ABINGDON, VA, p. A414
JOINT TOWNSHIP DISTRICT MEMORIAL HOSPITAL, SAINT MARYS, OH, p. A317
JONES MEMORIAL HOSPITAL, WELLSVILLE, NY, p. A289
JORDAN HOSPITAL, PLYMOUTH, MA, p. A196
JORDAN VALLEY HOSPITAL, WEST JORDAN, UT, p. A411
JOSEPH B. WHITEHEAD MEMORIAL INFIRMARY, GEORGIA INSTITUTE OF TECHNOLOGY, ATLANTA, GA, p. A 99
JUPITER MEDICAL CENTER, JUPITER, FL, p. A 87

K

KADLEC MEDICAL CENTER, RICHLAND, WA, p. A426
KAHUKU HOSPITAL, KAHUKU, HI, p. A110

KAISER FOUNDATION HOSPITAL–RIVERSIDE, RIVERSIDE, CA, p. A 57
KAISER FOUNDATION HOSPITAL–WEST LOS ANGELES, LOS ANGELES, CA, p. A 49
KAISER FOUNDATION HOSPITAL, ANAHEIM, CA, p. A 36
KAISER FOUNDATION HOSPITAL, BELLFLOWER, CA, p. A 37
KAISER FOUNDATION HOSPITAL, FONTANA, CA, p. A 42
KAISER FOUNDATION HOSPITAL, FRESNO, CA, p. A 43
KAISER FOUNDATION HOSPITAL, HAYWARD, CA, p. A 45
KAISER FOUNDATION HOSPITAL, LOS ANGELES, CA, p. A 49
KAISER FOUNDATION HOSPITAL, LOS ANGELES, CA, p. A 49
KAISER FOUNDATION HOSPITAL, LOS ANGELES, CA, p. A 49
KAISER FOUNDATION HOSPITAL, LOS ANGELES, CA, p. A 49
KAISER FOUNDATION HOSPITAL, MARTINEZ, CA, p. A 52
KAISER FOUNDATION HOSPITAL, OAKLAND, CA, p. A 54
KAISER FOUNDATION HOSPITAL, REDWOOD CITY, CA, p. A 57
KAISER FOUNDATION HOSPITAL, RICHMOND, CA, p. A 57
KAISER FOUNDATION HOSPITAL, SACRAMENTO, CA, p. A 58
KAISER FOUNDATION HOSPITAL, SACRAMENTO, CA, p. A 58
KAISER FOUNDATION HOSPITAL, SAN DIEGO, CA, p. A 59
KAISER FOUNDATION HOSPITAL, SAN FRANCISCO, CA, p. A 60
KAISER FOUNDATION HOSPITAL, SAN RAFAEL, CA, p. A 62
KAISER FOUNDATION HOSPITAL, SANTA CLARA, CA, p. A 63
KAISER FOUNDATION HOSPITAL, SANTA ROSA, CA, p. A 63
KAISER FOUNDATION HOSPITAL, SOUTH SAN FRANCISCO, CA, p. A 64
KAISER FOUNDATION HOSPITAL, WALNUT CREEK, CA, p. A 66
KAISER FOUNDATION HOSPITAL,*HONOLULU, HI, p. A110
KAISER FOUNDATION HOSPITAL, CLACKAMAS, OR, p. A329
KAISER FOUNDATION HOSPITAL AND REHABILITATION CENTER, VALLEJO, CA, p. A 66
KALAMAZOO REGIONAL PSYCHIATRIC HOSPITAL, KALAMAZOO, MI, p. A205
KALISPELL REGIONAL HOSPITAL, KALISPELL, MT, p. A243
KALKASKA MEMORIAL HEALTH CENTER, KALKASKA, MI, p. A205
KANABEC HOSPITAL, MORA, MN, p. A217
KANAKANAK HOSPITAL, DILLINGHAM, AK, p. A 21
KANE COUNTY HOSPITAL, KANAB, UT, p. A408
KANSAS INSTITUTE, OLATHE, KS, p. A157
KANSAS NEUROLOGICAL INSTITUTE, TOPEKA, KS, p. A159
KANSAS REHABILITATION HOSPITAL, TOPEKA, KS, p. A159
KAPIOLANI MEDICAL CENTER FOR WOMEN AND CHILDREN, HONOLULU, HI, p. A110
KARLSTAD HEALTH FACILITIES, KARLSTAD, MN, p. A216
KATHERINE SHAW BETHEA HOSPITAL, DIXON, IL, p. A122
KATY MEDICAL CENTER, KATY, TX, p. A393
KAU HOSPITAL, PAHALA, HI, p. A111
KAUAI VETERANS MEMORIAL HOSPITAL, WAIMEA, HI, p. A111
KAUKAUNA COMMUNITY HOSPITAL, KAUKAUNA, WI, p. A438
KAWEAH DELTA HEALTHCARE DISTRICT, VISALIA, CA, p. A 66
KEARNEY COUNTY COMMUNITY HOSPITAL, MINDEN, NE, p. A249
KEARNY COUNTY HOSPITAL, LAKIN, KS, p. A155
KEEFE MEMORIAL HOSPITAL, CHEYENNE WELLS, CO, p. A 68
KELLER ARMY COMMUNITY HOSPITAL, WEST POINT, NY, p. A289
KELSEY MEMORIAL HOSPITAL, LAKEVIEW, MI, p. A206
KEMPER COMMUNITY HOSPITAL, DE KALB, MS, p. A223
KENDALL REGIONAL MEDICAL CENTER, MIAMI, FL, p. A 90
KENDRICK MEMORIAL HOSPITAL, MOORESVILLE, IN, p. A139
KENMARE COMMUNITY HOSPITAL, KENMARE, ND, p. A304
KENMORE MERCY HOSPITAL, KENMORE, NY, p. A276
KENNEBEC VALLEY MEDICAL CENTER, AUGUSTA, ME, p. A180
KENNEDY KRIEGER INSTITUTE, BALTIMORE, MD, p. A184
KENNEDY MEMORIAL HOSPITALS–UNIVERSITY MEDICAL CENTER, CHERRY HILL, NJ, p. A259
KENNER ARMY COMMUNITY HOSPITAL, FORT LEE, VA, p. A415
KENNER REGIONAL MEDICAL CENTER, KENNER, LA, p. A173
KENNESTONE HOSPITAL, MARIETTA, GA, p. A105
KENNEWICK GENERAL HOSPITAL, KENNEWICK, WA, p. A425
KENOSHA HOSPITAL AND MEDICAL CENTER, KENOSHA, WI, p. A438
KENSINGTON HOSPITAL, PHILADELPHIA, PA, p. A345
KENT AND QUEEN ANNE'S HOSPITAL, CHESTERTOWN, MD, p. A186
KENT COMMUNITY HOSPITAL COMPLEX, GRAND RAPIDS, MI, p. A204
KENT COUNTY MEMORIAL HOSPITAL, WARWICK, RI, p. A354
KENT GENERAL HOSPITAL, DOVER, DE, p. A 78
KENTFIELD REHABILITATION HOSPITAL, KENTFIELD, CA, p. A 46
KEOKUK AREA HOSPITAL, KEOKUK, IA, p. A146
KEOKUK COUNTY HEALTH CENTER, SIGOURNEY, IA, p. A149
KERN HOSPITAL FOR SPECIAL SURGERY, WARREN, MI, p. A211
KERN MEDICAL CENTER, BAKERSFIELD, CA, p. A 37
KERN VALLEY HOSPITAL DISTRICT, LAKE ISABELLA, CA, p. A 46

Hospitals A465

© 1995 AHA Guide

Hospitals, Alphabetically / Kerrville State Hospital

KERRVILLE STATE HOSPITAL, KERRVILLE, TX, p. A394
KERSHAW COUNTY MEDICAL CENTER, CAMDEN, SC, p. A355
KESSLER INSTITUTE FOR REHABILITATION, WEST ORANGE, NJ, p. A266
KETCHIKAN GENERAL HOSPITAL, KETCHIKAN, AK, p. A 21
KETTERING MEDICAL CENTER, KETTERING, OH, p. A313
KEWANEE HOSPITAL, KEWANEE, IL, p. A125
KEWEENAW MEMORIAL MEDICAL CENTER, LAURIUM, MI, p. A206
KEYSTONE CENTER, CHESTER, PA, p. A336
KILMICHAEL HOSPITAL, KILMICHAEL, MS, p. A225
KIMBALL COUNTY HOSPITAL, KIMBALL, NE, p. A248
KIMBALL MEDICAL CENTER, LAKEWOOD, NJ, p. A261
KIMBLE HOSPITAL, JUNCTION, TX, p. A393
KIMBROUGH ARMY COMMUNITY HOSPITAL, FORT GEORGE G. MEADE, MD, p. A187
KING'S DAUGHTERS HOSPITAL, BROOKHAVEN, MS, p. A222
KING'S DAUGHTERS HOSPITAL, GREENVILLE, MS, p. A224
KING'S DAUGHTERS HOSPITAL, YAZOO CITY, MS, p. A229
KING'S DAUGHTERS HOSPITAL, TEMPLE, TX, p. A404
KING'S DAUGHTERS' HOSPITAL, MADISON, IN, p. A138
KING'S DAUGHTERS' MEDICAL CENTER, ASHLAND, KY, p. A161
KINGFISHER REGIONAL HOSPITAL, KINGFISHER, OK, p. A324
KINGMAN COMMUNITY HOSPITAL, KINGMAN, KS, p. A155
KINGMAN REGIONAL MEDICAL CENTER, KINGMAN, AZ, p. A 24
KINGS COUNTY HOSPITAL CENTER, NEW YORK CITY, NY, p. A280
KINGS HIGHWAY HOSPITAL CENTER, NEW YORK CITY, NY, p. A280
KINGS MOUNTAIN HOSPITAL, KINGS MOUNTAIN, NC, p. A296
KINGS PARK PSYCHIATRIC CENTER, KINGS PARK, NY, p. A276
KINGSBORO PSYCHIATRIC CENTER, NEW YORK CITY, NY, p. A280
KINGSBROOK JEWISH MEDICAL CENTER, NEW YORK CITY, NY, p. A280
KINGSBURG DISTRICT HOSPITAL, KINGSBURG, CA, p. A 46
KINGSTON HOSPITAL, KINGSTON, NY, p. A276
KINGSWOOD HOSPITAL, FERNDALE, MI, p. A203
KINO COMMUNITY HOSPITAL, TUCSON, AZ, p. A 27
KIOWA COUNTY MEMORIAL HOSPITAL, GREENSBURG, KS, p. A153
KIOWA DISTRICT HOSPITAL, KIOWA, KS, p. A155
KIRKSVILLE OSTEOPATHIC MEDICAL CENTER, KIRKSVILLE, MO, p. A235
KISHWAUKEE COMMUNITY HOSPITAL, DE KALB, IL, p. A121
KIT CARSON COUNTY MEMORIAL HOSPITAL, BURLINGTON, CO, p. A 68
KITTITAS VALLEY COMMUNITY HOSPITAL, ELLENSBURG, WA, p. A424
KITTSON MEMORIAL HOSPITAL, HALLOCK, MN, p. A215
KLICKITAT VALLEY HOSPITAL, GOLDENDALE, WA, p. A424
KNAPP MEDICAL CENTER, WESLACO, TX, p. A406
KNOX COMMUNITY HOSPITAL, MOUNT VERNON, OH, p. A315
KNOX COUNTY GENERAL HOSPITAL, BARBOURVILLE, KY, p. A161
KNOXVILLE AREA COMMUNITY HOSPITAL, KNOXVILLE, IA, p. A147
KOALA HOSPITAL AND COUNSELING CENTER, COLUMBUS, IN, p. A134
KOALA HOSPITAL AND COUNSELING CENTER, PLYMOUTH, IN, p. A139
KODIAK ISLAND HOSPITAL AND CARE CENTER, KODIAK, AK, p. A 22
KOHALA HOSPITAL, KOHALA, HI, p. A111
KOKOMO REHABILITATION HOSPITAL, KOKOMO, IN, p. A138
KONA COMMUNITY HOSPITAL, KEALAKEKUA, HI, p. A111
KOOTENAI MEDICAL CENTER, COEUR D'ALENE, ID, p. A112
KOSCIUSKO COMMUNITY HOSPITAL, WARSAW, IN, p. A141
KOSSUTH COUNTY HOSPITAL, ALGONA, IA, p. A142
KREMMLING MEMORIAL HOSPITAL, KREMMLING, CO, p. A 71
KUAKINI MEDICAL CENTER, HONOLULU, HI, p. A110
KULA HOSPITAL, KULA, HI, p. A111

L

L. S. HUCKABAY MD MEMORIAL HOSPITAL, COUSHATTA, LA, p. A171
L. V. STABLER MEMORIAL HOSPITAL, GREENVILLE, AL, p. A 17
L. W. BLAKE HOSPITAL, BRADENTON, FL, p. A 82
LA FOLLETTE MEDICAL CENTER, LA FOLLETTE, TN, p. A370
LA GRANGE MEMORIAL HOSPITAL, LA GRANGE, IL, p. A125
LA GUARDIA HOSPITAL, NEW YORK CITY, NY, p. A280
LA HACIENDA TREATMENT CENTER, HUNT, TX, p. A393
LA PALMA INTERCOMMUNITY HOSPITAL, LA PALMA, CA, p. A 46
LA PORTE HOSPITAL, LA PORTE, IN, p. A138
LA SALLE GENERAL HOSPITAL, JENA, LA, p. A173
LABETTE COUNTY MEDICAL CENTER, PARSONS, KS, p.157
LAC–HARBOR–UNIVERSITY OF CALIFORNIA AT LOS ANGELES MEDICAL CENTER, TORRANCE, CA, p. A 65
LAC–HIGH DESERT HOSPITAL, LANCASTER, CA, p. A 47
LAC–KING–DREW MEDICAL CENTER, LOS ANGELES, CA, p. A 50
LAC–RANCHO LOS AMIGOS MEDICAL CENTER, DOWNEY, CA, p. A 41
LAC UNIVERSITY OF SOUTHERN CALIFORNIA MEDICAL CENTER, LOS ANGELES, CA, p. A 49
LACKEY MEMORIAL HOSPITAL, FOREST, MS, p. A224
LADY OF THE SEA GENERAL HOSPITAL, CUT OFF, LA, p. A172
LAFAYETTE GENERAL MEDICAL CENTER, LAFAYETTE, LA, p. A173
LAFAYETTE HOME HOSPITAL, LAFAYETTE, IN, p. A138
LAFAYETTE HOSPITAL, ARROYO, PR, p. A447
LAFAYETTE REGIONAL HEALTH CENTER, LEXINGTON, MO, p. A235
LAGUNA HILLS HOSPITAL AND MENTAL HEALTH CENTER, LAGUNA BEACH, CA, p. A 46
LAGUNA HONDA HOSPITAL AND REHABILITATION CENTER, SAN FRANCISCO, CA, p. A 60
LAHEY HITCHCOCK CLINIC, BURLINGTON, MA, p. A192
LAIRD HOSPITAL, UNION, MS, p. A228
LAKE AREA HOSPITAL, WEBSTER, SD, p. A364
LAKE AREA MEDICAL CENTER, LAKE CHARLES, LA, p. A174
LAKE CHARLES MEMORIAL HOSPITAL, LAKE CHARLES, LA, p. A174
LAKE CHELAN COMMUNITY HOSPITAL, CHELAN, WA, p. A423
LAKE CITY COMMUNITY HOSPITAL, LAKE CITY, SC, p. A358
LAKE CITY HOSPITAL, LAKE CITY, MN, p. A216
LAKE CITY MEDICAL CENTER, LAKE CITY, FL, p. A 87
LAKE CUMBERLAND REGIONAL HOSPITAL, SOMERSET, KY, p. A168
LAKE DISTRICT HOSPITAL, LAKEVIEW, OR, p. A330
LAKE FOREST HOSPITAL, LAKE FOREST, IL, p. A126
LAKE HOSPITAL SYSTEM, PAINESVILLE, OH, p. A316
LAKE MEAD HOSPITAL MEDICAL CENTER, NORTH LAS VEGAS, NV, p. A254
LAKE NORMAN REGIONAL MEDICAL CENTER, MOORESVILLE, NC, p. A297
LAKE OF THE OZARKS GENERAL HOSPITAL, OSAGE BEACH, MO, p. A236
LAKE POINTE MEDICAL CENTER, ROWLETT, TX, p. A401
LAKE REGION HOSPITAL AND NURSING HOME, FERGUS FALLS, MN, p. A214
LAKE SHORE HOSPITAL, LAKE CITY, FL, p. A 87
LAKE SHORE HOSPITAL, IRVING, NY, p. A276
LAKE TAYLOR HOSPITAL, NORFOLK, VA, p. A418
LAKE VIEW COMMUNITY HOSPITAL, PAW PAW, MI, p. A208
LAKE VIEW MEMORIAL HOSPITAL, TWO HARBORS, MN, p. A220
LAKE WALES MEDICAL CENTERS, LAKE WALES, FL, p. A 87
LAKE WHITNEY MEMORIAL HOSPITAL, WHITNEY, TX, p. A407
LAKELAND MEDICAL CENTER, NEW ORLEANS, LA, p. A176
LAKELAND MEDICAL CENTER, ELKHORN, WI, p. A437
LAKELAND REGIONAL HOSPITAL, SPRINGFIELD, MO, p. A239
LAKELAND REGIONAL MEDICAL CENTER, LAKELAND, FL, p. A 87
LAKES REGION GENERAL HOSPITAL, LACONIA, NH, p. A256
LAKESHORE COMMUNITY HOSPITAL, DADEVILLE, AL, p. A 15
LAKESHORE COMMUNITY HOSPITAL, SHELBY, MI, p. A210
LAKESHORE HOSPITAL, BIRMINGHAM, AL, p. A 14
LAKESHORE MENTAL HEALTH INSTITUTE, KNOXVILLE, TN, p. A370
LAKESIDE HOSPITAL, METAIRIE, LA, p. A175
LAKESIDE MEMORIAL HOSPITAL, BROCKPORT, NY, p. A272
LAKEVIEW COMMUNITY HOSPITAL, EUFAULA, AL, p. A 15
LAKEVIEW HOSPITAL, BOUNTIFUL, UT, p. A408
LAKEVIEW HOSPITAL, WAUWATOSA, WI, p. A444
LAKEVIEW MEDICAL CENTER, RICE LAKE, WI, p. A442
LAKEVIEW MEMORIAL HOSPITAL, STILLWATER, MN, p. A220
LAKEVIEW REGIONAL MEDICAL CENTER, COVINGTON, LA, p. A171
LAKEVIEW REHABILITATION HOSPITAL, ELIZABETHTOWN, KY, p. A162
LAKEWAY REGIONAL HOSPITAL, MORRISTOWN, TN, p. A372
LAKEWOOD HEALTH CENTER, BAUDETTE, MN, p. A212
LAKEWOOD HOSPITAL, MORGAN CITY, LA, p. A175
LAKEWOOD HOSPITAL, LAKEWOOD, OH, p. A313
LAKEWOOD REGIONAL MEDICAL CENTER, LAKEWOOD, CA, p. A 47
LALLIE KEMP MEDICAL CENTER, INDEPENDENCE, LA, p. A173
LAMAR COMMUNITY HOSPITAL, VERNON, AL, p. A 20
LAMB HEALTHCARE CENTER, LITTLEFIELD, TX, p. A395
LANAI COMMUNITY HOSPITAL, LANAI CITY, HI, p. A111
LANCASTER COMMUNITY HOSPITAL, LANCASTER, CA, p. A 47
LANCASTER GENERAL HOSPITAL – SUSQUEHANNA DIVISION, COLUMBIA, PA, p. A337
LANCASTER GENERAL HOSPITAL, LANCASTER, PA, p. A341
LANCASTER MEMORIAL HOSPITAL, LANCASTER, WI, p. A438
LANDER VALLEY MEDICAL CENTER, LANDER, WY, p. A445
LANDMANN–JUNGMAN MEMORIAL HOSPITAL, SCOTLAND, SD, p. A363
LANDMARK MEDICAL CENTER, WOONSOCKET, RI, p. A354
LANE COUNTY HOSPITAL, DIGHTON, KS, p. A152
LANE MEMORIAL HOSPITAL, ZACHARY, LA, p. A179
LANGLADE MEMORIAL HOSPITAL, ANTIGO, WI, p. A435
LANIER PARK REGIONAL HOSPITAL, GAINESVILLE, GA, p. A104
LANKENAU HOSPITAL, WYNNEWOOD, PA, p. A352
LANTERMAN DEVELOPMENTAL CENTER, POMONA, CA, p. A 56
LAPEER REGIONAL HOSPITAL, LAPEER, MI, p. A206
LARABIDA CHILDREN'S HOSPITAL AND RESEARCH CENTER, CHICAGO, IL, p. A119
LARGO MEDICAL CENTER, LARGO, FL, p. A 88
LARNED STATE HOSPITAL, LARNED, KS, p. A155
LARUE D. CARTER MEMORIAL HOSPITAL, INDIANAPOLIS, IN, p. A136
LAS ENCINAS HOSPITAL, PASADENA, CA, p. A 56
LAS VEGAS MEDICAL CENTER, LAS VEGAS, NM, p. A269
LASSEN COMMUNITY HOSPITAL, SUSANVILLE, CA, p. A 64
LATIMER COUNTY GENERAL HOSPITAL, WILBURTON, OK, p. A328
LATROBE AREA HOSPITAL, LATROBE, PA, p. A341
LAUGHLIN MEMORIAL HOSPITAL, GREENEVILLE, TN, p. A368
LAUREATE PSYCHIATRIC CLINIC AND HOSPITAL, TULSA, OK, p. A328
LAUREL OAKS HOSPITAL, ORLANDO, FL, p. A 91
LAUREL REGIONAL HOSPITAL, LAUREL, MD, p. A187
LAUREL WOOD CENTER, MERIDIAN, MS, p. A226
LAURELWOOD HOSPITAL, WILLOUGHBY, OH, p. A319
LAURENS COUNTY HEALTHCARE SYSTEM, CLINTON, SC, p. A356
LAVACA MEDICAL CENTER, HALLETTSVILLE, TX, p. A389
LAWNWOOD REGIONAL MEDICAL CENTER, FORT PIERCE, FL, p. A 84
LAWRENCE AND MEMORIAL HOSPITAL, NEW LONDON, CT, p. A 76
LAWRENCE BAPTIST MEDICAL CENTER, MOULTON, AL, p. A 18
LAWRENCE COUNTY HOSPITAL, MONTICELLO, MS, p. A226
LAWRENCE COUNTY MEDICAL CENTER, IRONTON, OH, p. A313
LAWRENCE COUNTY MEMORIAL HOSPITAL, LAWRENCEVILLE, IL, p. A126
LAWRENCE F. QUIGLEY MEMORIAL HOSPITAL, CHELSEA, MA, p. A193
LAWRENCE GENERAL HOSPITAL, LAWRENCE, MA, p. A194
LAWRENCE HOSPITAL, BRONXVILLE, NY, p. A272
LAWRENCE MEMORIAL HOSPITAL, WALNUT RIDGE, AR, p. A 34
LAWRENCE MEMORIAL HOSPITAL, LAWRENCE, KS, p. A155
LAWRENCE MEMORIAL HOSPITAL OF MEDFORD, MEDFORD, MA, p. A195
LDS HOSPITAL, SALT LAKE CITY, UT, p. A410
LE BONHEUR CHILDREN'S MEDICAL CENTER, MEMPHIS, TN, p. A372
LEA REGIONAL HOSPITAL, HOBBS, NM, p. A269
LEAHI HOSPITAL, HONOLULU, HI, p. A110
LEAKE MEMORIAL HOSPITAL, CARTHAGE, MS, p. A223
LEBANON COMMUNITY HOSPITAL, LEBANON, OR, p. A330
LEE COUNTY COMMUNITY HOSPITAL, PENNINGTON GAP, VA, p. A418
LEE HOSPITAL, JOHNSTOWN, PA, p. A340
LEE MEMORIAL HOSPITAL, FORT MYERS, FL, p. A 84
LEE MEMORIAL HOSPITAL, DOWAGIAC, MI, p. A202
LEE'S SUMMIT HOSPITAL, LEES SUMMIT, MO, p. A235
LEELANAU MEMORIAL HOSPITAL, NORTHPORT, MI, p. A208
LEESBURG REGIONAL MEDICAL CENTER, LEESBURG, FL, p. A 88
LEGACY EMANUEL HOSPITAL AND HEALTH CENTER, PORTLAND, OR, p. A331
LEGACY GOOD SAMARITAN HOSPITAL AND HEALTH CENTER, PORTLAND, OR, p. A331
LEGACY MERIDIAN PARK HOSPITAL, TUALATIN, OR, p. A333
LEGACY MOUNT HOOD MEDICAL CENTER, GRESHAM, OR, p. A330
LEGEND BUTTES HEALTH SERVICES, CRAWFORD, NE, p. A247
LEHIGH VALLEY HOSPITAL, ALLENTOWN, PA, p. A334
LEMUEL SHATTUCK HOSPITAL, BOSTON, MA, p. A191
LENOIR MEMORIAL HOSPITAL, KINSTON, NC, p. A296
LENOX HILL HOSPITAL, NEW YORK CITY, NY, p. A280
LEONARD J. CHABERT MEDICAL CENTER, HOUMA, LA, p. A173
LESTER E. COX HEALTH SYSTEMS, SPRINGFIELD, MO, p. A240

Hospitals, Alphabetically / Marion Memorial Hospital

LEVI HOSPITAL, HOT SPRINGS NATIONAL PARK, AR, p. A 31
LEVINDALE HEBREW GERIATRIC CENTER AND HOSPITAL, BALTIMORE, MD, p. A185
LEWIS-GALE HOSPITAL, SALEM, VA, p. A420
LEWIS-GALE PSYCHIATRIC CENTER, SALEM, VA, p. A420
LEWIS COMMUNITY HOSPITAL, HOHENWALD, TN, p. A369
LEWIS COUNTY GENERAL HOSPITAL, LOWVILLE, NY, p. A277
LEWISTOWN HOSPITAL, LEWISTOWN, PA, p. A341
LEWISVILLE MEDICAL CENTER HOSPITAL, LEWISVILLE, TX, p. A395
LEXINGTON MEDICAL CENTER, WEST COLUMBIA, SC, p. A360
LEXINGTON MEMORIAL HOSPITAL, LEXINGTON, NC, p. A296
LIBERTY COUNTY HOSPITAL AND NURSING HOME, CHESTER, MT, p. A241
LIBERTY HOSPITAL, LIBERTY, MO, p. A235
LIBERTY MEDICAL CENTER, BALTIMORE, MD, p. A185
LIBERTY REGIONAL MEDICAL CENTER, HINESVILLE, GA, p. A104
LICKING MEMORIAL HOSPITAL, NEWARK, OH, p. A315
LIFECARE HOSPITALS, SHREVEPORT, LA, p. A178
LILLIAN M. HUDSPETH MEMORIAL HOSPITAL, SONORA, TX, p. A403
LIMA MEMORIAL HOSPITAL, LIMA, OH, p. A313
LIMESTONE MEDICAL CENTER, GROESBECK, TX, p. A389
LINCOLN COMMUNITY HOSPITAL AND NURSING HOME, HUGO, CO, p. A 71
LINCOLN COUNTY HOSPITAL, LINCOLN, KS, p. A155
LINCOLN COUNTY HOSPITAL, LINCOLNTON, NC, p. A296
LINCOLN COUNTY MEDICAL CENTER, RUIDOSO, NM, p. A270
LINCOLN COUNTY MEMORIAL HOSPITAL, TROY, MO, p. A240
LINCOLN DEVELOPMENTAL CENTER, LINCOLN, IL, p. A126
LINCOLN GENERAL HOSPITAL, RUSTON, LA, p. A177
LINCOLN GENERAL HOSPITAL, LINCOLN, NE, p. A249
LINCOLN HOSPITAL, DAVENPORT, WA, p. A424
LINCOLN HOSPITAL MEDICAL CENTER, LOS ANGELES, CA, p. A 50
LINCOLN MEDICAL AND MENTAL HEALTH CENTER, NEW YORK CITY, NY, p. A280
LINCOLN REGIONAL CENTER, LINCOLN, NE, p. A249
LINCOLN REGIONAL HOSPITAL, FAYETTEVILLE, TN, p. A368
LINCOLN TRAIL HOSPITAL, RADCLIFF, KY, p. A168
LINDEN MUNICIPAL HOSPITAL, LINDEN, TX, p. A395
LINDSAY HOSPITAL MEDICAL CENTER, LINDSAY, CA, p. A 47
LINDSAY MUNICIPAL HOSPITAL, LINDSAY, OK, p. A324
LINDSBORG COMMUNITY HOSPITAL, LINDSBORG, KS, p. A156
LINTON HOSPITAL, LINTON, ND, p. A304
LITTLE COMPANY OF MARY HEALTH SERVICES, TORRANCE, CA, p. A 65
LITTLE COMPANY OF MARY HOSPITAL AND HEALTH CARE CENTERS, EVERGREEN PARK, IL, p. A123
LITTLE FALLS HOSPITAL, LITTLE FALLS, NY, p. A277
LITTLE NECK COMMUNITY HOSPITAL, NEW YORK CITY, NY, p. A280
LITTLE RIVER MEMORIAL HOSPITAL, ASHDOWN, AR, p. A 29
LITTLETON REGIONAL HOSPITAL, LITTLETON, NH, p. A256
LITZENBERG MEMORIAL COUNTY HOSPITAL, CENTRAL CITY, NE, p. A246
LIVENGRIN FOUNDATION, BENSALEM, PA, p. A335
LIVINGSTON HOSPITAL AND HEALTHCARE SERVICES, SALEM, KY, p. A168
LIVINGSTON MEMORIAL HOSPITAL, LIVINGSTON, MT, p. A243
LIVINGSTON REGIONAL HOSPITAL, LIVINGSTON, TN, p. A371
LLANO MEMORIAL HOSPITAL, LLANO, TX, p. A395
LLOYD NOLAND HOSPITAL AND AMBULATORY CENTER, BIRMINGHAM, AL, p. A 14
LOCK HAVEN HOSPITAL, LOCK HAVEN, PA, p. A341
LOCKPORT MEMORIAL HOSPITAL, LOCKPORT, NY, p. A277
LODI COMMUNITY HOSPITAL, LODI, OH, p. A313
LODI MEMORIAL HOSPITAL, LODI, CA, p. A 47
LOGAN COUNTY HOSPITAL, OAKLEY, KS, p. A157
LOGAN GENERAL HOSPITAL, LOGAN, WV, p. A432
LOGAN HOSPITAL AND MEDICAL CENTER, GUTHRIE, OK, p. A323
LOGAN MEMORIAL HOSPITAL, RUSSELLVILLE, KY, p. A168
LOGAN REGIONAL HOSPITAL, LOGAN, UT, p. A408
LOGANSPORT STATE HOSPITAL, LOGANSPORT, IN, p. A138
LOMA LINDA UNIVERSITY BEHAVIORAL MEDICINE CENTER, REDLANDS, CA, p. A 57
LOMA LINDA UNIVERSITY COMMUNITY MEDICAL CENTER, LOMA LINDA, CA, p. A 47
LOMPOC DISTRICT HOSPITAL, LOMPOC, CA, p. A 47
LONESOME PINE HOSPITAL, BIG STONE GAP, VA, p. A414
LONG BEACH COMMUNITY HOSPITAL AND MEDICAL CENTER, LONG BEACH, CA, p. A 48
LONG BEACH DOCTORS HOSPITAL, LONG BEACH, CA, p. A 48
LONG BEACH MEDICAL CENTER, LONG BEACH, NY, p. A277
LONG BEACH MEMORIAL MEDICAL CENTER, LONG BEACH, CA, p. A 48
LONG ISLAND COLLEGE HOSPITAL, NEW YORK CITY, NY, p. A280

LONG ISLAND JEWISH MEDICAL CENTER, NEW YORK CITY, NY, p. A280
LONG PRAIRIE MEMORIAL HOSPITAL AND HOME, LONG PRAIRIE, MN, p. A216
LONGMONT UNITED HOSPITAL, LONGMONT, CO, p. A 72
LONGVIEW GENERAL HOSPITAL, GRAYSVILLE, AL, p. A 17
LONGVIEW REGIONAL HOSPITAL, LONGVIEW, TX, p. A395
LOOKOUT MEMORIAL HOSPITAL, SPEARFISH, SD, p. A364
LORAIN COMMUNITY/ST. JOSEPH REGIONAL HEALTH CENTER, LORAIN, OH, p. A314
LORETTO HOSPITAL, CHICAGO, IL, p. A119
LORING HOSPITAL, SAC CITY, IA, p. A149
LORIS COMMUNITY HOSPITAL, LORIS, SC, p. A358
LOS ALAMITOS MEDICAL CENTER, LOS ALAMITOS, CA, p. A 48
LOS ALAMOS MEDICAL CENTER, LOS ALAMOS, NM, p. A269
LOS ANGELES COMMUNITY HOSPITAL, LOS ANGELES, CA, p. A 50
LOS ANGELES COMMUNITY HOSPITAL OF NORWALK, NORWALK, CA, p. A 54
LOS ANGELES COUNTY CENTRAL JAIL HOSPITAL, LOS ANGELES, CA, p. A 50
LOS ANGELES METROPOLITAN MEDICAL CENTER, LOS ANGELES, CA, p. A 50
LOS BANOS COMMUNITY HOSPITAL, LOS BANOS, CA, p. A 51
LOS LUNAS HOSPITAL AND TRAINING SCHOOL, LOS LUNAS, NM, p. A269
LOS MEDANOS COMMUNITY HOSPITAL, PITTSBURG, CA, p. A 56
LOS ROBLES REGIONAL MEDICAL CENTER, THOUSAND OAKS, CA, p. A 65
LOST RIVERS DISTRICT HOSPITAL, ARCO, ID, p. A112
LOUDOUN HOSPITAL CENTER, LEESBURG, VA, p. A417
LOUIS A. JOHNSON VETERANS AFFAIRS MEDICAL CENTER, CLARKSBURG, WV, p. A430
LOUIS A. WEISS MEMORIAL HOSPITAL, CHICAGO, IL, p. A119
LOUIS SMITH MEMORIAL HOSPITAL, LAKELAND, GA, p. A105
LOUISE OBICI MEMORIAL HOSPITAL, SUFFOLK, VA, p. A421
LOURDES HOSPITAL, PADUCAH, KY, p. A167
LOVE COUNTY HEALTH CENTER, MARIETTA, OK, p. A324
LOVELACE MEDICAL CENTER, ALBUQUERQUE, NM, p. A267
LOW COUNTRY GENERAL HOSPITAL, RIDGELAND, SC, p. A359
LOWELL GENERAL HOSPITAL, LOWELL, MA, p. A194
LOWER BUCKS HOSPITAL, BRISTOL, PA, p. A335
LOWER FLORIDA KEYS HEALTH SYSTEM, KEY WEST, FL, p. A 87
LOWER UMPQUA HOSPITAL DISTRICT, REEDSPORT, OR, p. A332
LOYOLA UNIVERSITY MEDICAL CENTER, MAYWOOD, IL, p. A126
LSU MEDICAL CENTER-UNIVERSITY HOSPITAL, SHREVEPORT, LA, p. A178
LUCAS COUNTY HEALTH CENTER, CHARITON, IA, p. A143
LUCILE SALTER PACKARD CHILDREN'S HOSPITAL AT STANFORD, PALO ALTO, CA, p. A 55
LUCY LEE HOSPITAL, POPLAR BLUFF, MO, p. A237
LUDLOW HOSPITAL, LUDLOW, MA, p. A194
LUMBERTON CITIZENS HOSPITAL, LUMBERTON, MS, p. A226
LUNDBERG MEMORIAL HOSPITAL, CREIGHTON, NE, p. A247
LUTHER HOSPITAL, EAU CLAIRE, WI, p. A436
LUTHERAN COMMUNITY HOSPITAL, NORFOLK, NE, p. A249
LUTHERAN GENERAL HOSPITAL, PARK RIDGE, IL, p. A128
LUTHERAN HOSPITAL-LA CROSSE, LA CROSSE, WI, p. A438
LUTHERAN HOSPITAL OF INDIANA, FORT WAYNE, IN, p. A135
LUTHERAN MEDICAL CENTER, WHEAT RIDGE, CO, p. A 73
LUTHERAN MEDICAL CENTER, SAINT LOUIS, MO, p. A238
LUTHERAN MEDICAL CENTER, NEW YORK CITY, NY, p. A280
LUTHERAN MEDICAL CENTER, CLEVELAND, OH, p. A309
LUVERNE COMMUNITY HOSPITAL, LUVERNE, MN, p. A216
LYNCHBURG GENERAL HOSPITAL, LYNCHBURG, VA, p. A417
LYNDON B. JOHNSON TROPICAL MEDICAL CENTER, PAGO PAGO, AS, p. A447
LYNN COUNTY HOSPITAL DISTRICT, TAHOKA, TX, p. A404
LYSTER U.S. ARMY COMMUNITY HOSPITAL, FORT RUCKER, AL, p. A 16

M

M. I. T. MEDICAL DEPARTMENT, CAMBRIDGE, MA, p. A192
MACKINAC STRAITS HOSPITAL AND HEALTH CENTER, SAINT IGNACE, MI, p. A209
MACNEAL HOSPITAL, BERWYN, IL, p. A117
MACOMB HOSPITAL CENTER, WARREN, MI, p. A211
MACON COUNTY GENERAL HOSPITAL, LAFAYETTE, TN, p. A370

MACON NORTHSIDE HOSPITAL, MACON, GA, p. A105
MAD RIVER COMMUNITY HOSPITAL, ARCATA, CA, p. A 36
MADELIA COMMUNITY HOSPITAL, MADELIA, MN, p. A216
MADERA COMMUNITY HOSPITAL, MADERA, CA, p. A 52
MADIGAN ARMY MEDICAL CENTER, TACOMA, WA, p. A428
MADISON COMMUNITY HOSPITAL, MADISON HEIGHTS, MI, p. A206
MADISON COMMUNITY HOSPITAL, MADISON, SD, p. A362
MADISON COUNTY HOSPITAL, LONDON, OH, p. A314
MADISON COUNTY HOSPITAL, MADISONVILLE, TX, p. A396
MADISON COUNTY MEMORIAL HOSPITAL, MADISON, FL, p. A 88
MADISON COUNTY MEMORIAL HOSPITAL, WINTERSET, IA, p. A150
MADISON GENERAL HOSPITAL, CANTON, MS, p. A223
MADISON HOSPITAL, MADISON, MN, p. A216
MADISON MEMORIAL HOSPITAL, REXBURG, ID, p. A114
MADISON MEMORIAL HOSPITAL, FREDERICKTOWN, MO, p. A232
MADISON PARISH HOSPITAL, TALLULAH, LA, p. A179
MADISON STATE HOSPITAL, MADISON, IN, p. A138
MADISON VALLEY HOSPITAL, ENNIS, MT, p. A242
MADONNA REHABILITATION HOSPITAL, LINCOLN, NE, p. A249
MAGEE-WOMENS HOSPITAL, PITTSBURGH, PA, p. A346
MAGEE GENERAL HOSPITAL, MAGEE, MS, p. A226
MAGEE REHABILITATION HOSPITAL, PHILADELPHIA, PA, p. A345
MAGIC VALLEY REGIONAL MEDICAL CENTER, TWIN FALLS, ID, p. A114
MAGNOLIA HOSPITAL, MAGNOLIA, AR, p. A 32
MAGNOLIA REGIONAL HEALTH CENTER, CORINTH, MS, p. A223
MAHASKA COUNTY HOSPITAL, OSKALOOSA, IA, p. A148
MAHNOMEN COUNTY AND VILLAGE HOSPITAL, CLINIC AND NURSING CENTER, MAHNOMEN, MN, p. A216
MAIMONIDES MEDICAL CENTER, NEW YORK CITY, NY, p. A281
MAINE COAST MEMORIAL HOSPITAL, ELLSWORTH, ME, p. A181
MAINE MEDICAL CENTER, PORTLAND, ME, p. A182
MAINLAND CENTER HOSPITAL, TEXAS CITY, TX, p. A405
MAJOR HOSPITAL, SHELBYVILLE, IN, p. A140
MALCOLM BLISS MENTAL HEALTH CENTER, SAINT LOUIS, MO, p. A238
MALCOLM GROW MEDICAL CENTER, ANDREWS AIR FORCE BASE, MD, p. A184
MALDEN HOSPITAL, MALDEN, MA, p. A194
MALVERN INSTITUTE, MALVERN, PA, p. A341
MAMMOTH HOSPITAL, MAMMOTH LAKES, CA, p. A 52
MAN ARH HOSPITAL, MAN, WV, p. A432
MANATEE MEMORIAL HOSPITAL, BRADENTON, FL, p. A 82
MANCHESTER MEMORIAL HOSPITAL, MANCHESTER, CT, p. A 75
MANGUM CITY HOSPITAL, MANGUM, OK, p. A324
MANHATTAN EYE, EAR AND THROAT HOSPITAL, NEW YORK CITY, NY, p. A281
MANHATTAN PSYCHIATRIC CENTER-WARD'S ISLAND, NEW YORK CITY, NY, p. A281
MANIILAQ HEALTH CENTER, KOTZEBUE, AK, p. A 22
MANNING GENERAL HOSPITAL, MANNING, IA, p. A147
MANSFIELD GENERAL HOSPITAL, MANSFIELD, OH, p. A314
MARCUM AND WALLACE MEMORIAL HOSPITAL, IRVINE, KY, p. A164
MARCUS DALY MEMORIAL HOSPITAL, HAMILTON, MT, p. A242
MARCUS J. LAWRENCE MEDICAL CENTER, COTTONWOOD, AZ, p. A 23
MARENGO MEMORIAL HOSPITAL, MARENGO, IA, p. A147
MARGARET MARY COMMUNITY HOSPITAL, BATESVILLE, IN, p. A133
MARGARET R. PARDEE MEMORIAL HOSPITAL, HENDERSONVILLE, NC, p. A295
MARGARET W. MONTGOMERY HOSPITAL, DETROIT, MI, p. A202
MARGARETVILLE MEMORIAL HOSPITAL, MARGARETVILLE, NY, p. A277
MARIA PARHAM HOSPITAL, HENDERSON, NC, p. A295
MARIAN COMMUNITY HOSPITAL, CARBONDALE, PA, p. A336
MARIAN HEALTH CENTER, SIOUX CITY, IA, p. A149
MARIAN MEDICAL CENTER, SANTA MARIA, CA, p. A 63
MARIANJOY REHABILITATION HOSPITAL AND CLINICS, WHEATON, IL, p. A132
MARICOPA MEDICAL CENTER, PHOENIX, AZ, p. A 25
MARIETTA MEMORIAL HOSPITAL, MARIETTA, OH, p. A314
MARIN GENERAL HOSPITAL, GREENBRAE, CA, p. A 44
MARINERS HOSPITAL, TAVERNIER, FL, p. A 97
MARION BAPTIST MEDICAL CENTER, HAMILTON, AL, p. A 17
MARION COMMUNITY HOSPITAL, OCALA, FL, p. A 91
MARION GENERAL HOSPITAL, MARION, IN, p. A138
MARION GENERAL HOSPITAL, MARION, OH, p. A314
MARION MEMORIAL HOSPITAL, MARION, IL, p. A126

Hospitals, Alphabetically / Marion Memorial Hospital

MARION MEMORIAL HOSPITAL, MARION, SC, p. A358
MARK REED HOSPITAL, MCCLEARY, WA, p. A425
MARK TWAIN ST. JOSEPH'S HOSPITAL, SAN ANDREAS, CA, p. A 58
MARLBORO PARK HOSPITAL, BENNETTSVILLE, SC, p. A355
MARLBORO PSYCHIATRIC HOSPITAL, MARLBORO, NJ, p. A261
MARLBOROUGH HOSPITAL, MARLBOROUGH, MA, p. A194
MARLETTE COMMUNITY HOSPITAL, MARLETTE, MI, p. A207
MARQUETTE GENERAL HOSPITAL, MARQUETTE, MI, p. A207
MARSHALL BROWNING HOSPITAL, DU QUOIN, IL, p. A122
MARSHALL COUNTY HOSPITAL, BENTON, KY, p. A161
MARSHALL COUNTY MEMORIAL HOSPITAL, BRITTON, SD, p. A361
MARSHALL HOSPITAL, PLACERVILLE, CA, p. A 56
MARSHALL I. PICKENS HOSPITAL, GREENVILLE, SC, p. A357
MARSHALL MEDICAL CENTER, LEWISBURG, TN, p. A370
MARSHALL MEMORIAL HOSPITAL, MADILL, OK, p. A324
MARSHALL MEMORIAL HOSPITAL, MARSHALL, TX, p. A396
MARSHALLTOWN MEDICAL AND SURGICAL CENTER, MARSHALLTOWN, IA, p. A147
MARTHA JEFFERSON HOSPITAL, CHARLOTTESVILLE, VA, p. A414
MARTHA'S VINEYARD HOSPITAL, OAK BLUFFS, MA, p. A196
MARTIN ARMY COMMUNITY HOSPITAL, FORT BENNING, GA, p. A103
MARTIN COUNTY HOSPITAL DISTRICT, STANTON, TX, p. A404
MARTIN GENERAL HOSPITAL, WILLIAMSTON, NC, p. A300
MARTIN LUTHER HOSPITAL– ANEHEIM, ANAHEIM, CA, p. A 36
MARTIN MEMORIAL MEDICAL CENTER, STUART, FL, p. A 95
MARY BLACK MEMORIAL HOSPITAL, SPARTANBURG, SC, p. A359
MARY BRECKINRIDGE HOSPITAL, HYDEN, KY, p. A164
MARY BRIDGE CHILDREN'S HOSPITAL AND HEALTH CENTER, TACOMA, WA, p. A428
MARY E. DICKERSON MEMORIAL HOSPITAL, JASPER, TX, p. A393
MARY FREE BED HOSPITAL AND REHABILITATION CENTER, GRAND RAPIDS, MI, p. A204
MARY GREELEY MEDICAL CENTER, AMES, IA, p. A142
MARY HITCHCOCK MEMORIAL HOSPITAL, LEBANON, NH, p. A256
MARY HURLEY HOSPITAL, COALGATE, OK, p. A322
MARY IMMACULATE HOSPITAL, NEWPORT NEWS, VA, p. A417
MARY IMOGENE BASSETT HOSPITAL, COOPERSTOWN, NY, p. A274
MARY LANE HOSPITAL, WARE, MA, p. A197
MARY LANNING MEMORIAL HOSPITAL, HASTINGS, NE, p. A248
MARY MCCLELLAN HOSPITAL, CAMBRIDGE, NY, p. A273
MARY RUTAN HOSPITAL, BELLEFONTAINE, OH, p. A307
MARY SHERMAN HOSPITAL, SULLIVAN, IN, p. A141
MARY SHIELS HOSPITAL, DALLAS, TX, p. A383
MARY WASHINGTON HOSPITAL, FREDERICKSBURG, VA, p. A416
MARYLAND GENERAL HOSPITAL, BALTIMORE, MD, p. A185
MARYMOUNT HOSPITAL, LONDON, KY, p. A165
MARYMOUNT HOSPITAL, GARFIELD HEIGHTS, OH, p. A312
MARYVALE SAMARITAN MEDICAL CENTER, PHOENIX, AZ, p. A 25
MASON DISTRICT HOSPITAL, HAVANA, IL, p. A124
MASON GENERAL HOSPITAL, SHELTON, WA, p. A427
MASONIC HOME AND HOSPITAL, WALLINGFORD, CT, p. A 77
MASSAC MEMORIAL HOSPITAL, METROPOLIS, IL, p. A127
MASSACHUSETTS EYE AND EAR INFIRMARY, BOSTON, MA, p. A191
MASSACHUSETTS GENERAL HOSPITAL, BOSTON, MA, p. A191
MASSACHUSETTS HOSPITAL SCHOOL, CANTON, MA, p. A192
MASSACHUSETTS MENTAL HEALTH CENTER, BOSTON, MA, p. A191
MASSACHUSETTS RESPIRATORY HOSPITAL, BRAINTREE, MA, p. A192
MASSAPEQUA GENERAL HOSPITAL, SEAFORD, NY, p. A287
MASSENA MEMORIAL HOSPITAL, MASSENA, NY, p. A277
MASSILLON COMMUNITY HOSPITAL, MASSILLON, OH, p. A314
MASSILLON PSYCHIATRIC CENTER, MASSILLON, OH, p. A314
MATAGORDA GENERAL HOSPITAL, BAY CITY, TX, p. A378
MATHENY SCHOOL AND HOSPITAL, PEAPACK, NJ, p. A263
MAUDE NORTON MEMORIAL CITY HOSPITAL, COLUMBUS, KS, p. A152
MAUI MEMORIAL HOSPITAL, WAILUKU, HI, p. A111
MAURY REGIONAL HOSPITAL, COLUMBIA, TN, p. A367
MAXWELL HOSPITAL, MONTGOMERY, AL, p. A 18
MAYERS MEMORIAL HOSPITAL DISTRICT, FALL RIVER MILLS, CA, p. A 42
MAYES COUNTY MEDICAL CENTER, PRYOR, OK, p. A326
MAYO REGIONAL HOSPITAL, DOVER-FOXCROFT, ME, p. A181
MAYVIEW STATE HOSPITAL, BRIDGEVILLE, PA, p. A335
MCALESTER REGIONAL HEALTH CENTER, MCALESTER, OK, p. A324
MCALLEN MEDICAL CENTER, MCALLEN, TX, p. A396

MCCAIN CORRECTIONAL HOSPITAL, MCCAIN, NC, p. A296
MCCALL MEMORIAL HOSPITAL, MCCALL, ID, p. A113
MCCAMEY HOSPITAL, MCCAMEY, TX, p. A397
MCCONE COUNTY MEDICAL ASSISTANCE FACILITY, CIRCLE, MT, p. A241
MCCRAY MEMORIAL HOSPITAL, KENDALLVILLE, IN, p. A137
MCCUISTION REGIONAL MEDICAL CENTER, PARIS, TX, p. A399
MCCULLOUGH-HYDE MEMORIAL HOSPITAL, OXFORD, OH, p. A316
MCCUNE-BROOKS HOSPITAL, CARTHAGE, MO, p. A231
MCCURTAIN MEMORIAL HOSPITAL, IDABEL, OK, p. A323
MCDONALD ARMY COMMUNITY HOSPITAL, NEWPORT NEWS, VA, p. A417
MCDONOUGH DISTRICT HOSPITAL, MACOMB, IL, p. A126
MCDOWELL ARH HOSPITAL, MCDOWELL, KY, p. A166
MCDOWELL HOSPITAL, MARION, NC, p. A296
MCDUFFIE COUNTY HOSPITAL, THOMSON, GA, p. A109
MCGEHEE-DESHA COUNTY HOSPITAL, MCGEHEE, AR, p. A 32
MCKAY-DEE HOSPITAL CENTER, OGDEN, UT, p. A409
MCKEE MEDICAL CENTER, LOVELAND, CO, p. A 72
MCKEESPORT HOSPITAL, MCKEESPORT, PA, p. A342
MCKENNA MEMORIAL HOSPITAL, NEW BRAUNFELS, TX, p. A398
MCKENNAN HOSPITAL, SIOUX FALLS, SD, p. A364
MCKENZIE–WILLAMETTE HOSPITAL, SPRINGFIELD, OR, p. A333
MCKENZIE COUNTY MEMORIAL HOSPITAL, WATFORD CITY, ND, p. A305
MCKENZIE MEMORIAL HOSPITAL, SANDUSKY, MI, p. A209
MCLAREN REGIONAL MEDICAL CENTER, FLINT, MI, p. A203
MCLEAN COUNTY GENERAL HOSPITAL, CALHOUN, KY, p. A161
MCLEAN HOSPITAL, BELMONT, MA, p. A190
MCLEOD REGIONAL MEDICAL CENTER, FLORENCE, SC, p. A357
MCMINNVILLE COMMUNITY HOSPITAL, MCMINNVILLE, OR, p. A331
MCNAIRY COUNTY GENERAL HOSPITAL, SELMER, TN, p. A374
MCPHERSON HOSPITAL, HOWELL, MI, p. A205
MEADE DISTRICT HOSPITAL, MEADE, KS, p. A156
MEADOW WOOD HOSPITAL, NEW CASTLE, DE, p. A 78
MEADOWBROOK HOSPITAL, GARDNER, KS, p. A153
MEADOWCREST HOSPITAL, GRETNA, LA, p. A172
MEADOWLAKE HOSPITAL, ENID, OK, p. A323
MEADOWLANDS HOSPITAL MEDICAL CENTER, SECAUCUS, NJ, p. A264
MEADOWS PSYCHIATRIC CENTER, CENTRE HALL, PA, p. A336
MEADOWS REGIONAL MEDICAL CENTER, VIDALIA, GA, p. A109
MEADOWVIEW REGIONAL HOSPITAL, MAYSVILLE, KY, p. A166
MEADVILLE MEDICAL CENTER, MEADVILLE, PA, p. A342
MEASE COUNTRYSIDE HOSPITAL, SAFETY HARBOR, FL, p. A 94
MEASE HOSPITAL DUNEDIN, DUNEDIN, FL, p. A 83
MECOSTA COUNTY GENERAL HOSPITAL, BIG RAPIDS, MI, p. A200
MEDCENTER HOSPITAL, MARION, OH, p. A314
MEDCENTER ONE, BISMARCK, ND, p. A302
MEDCENTER ONE MANDAN, MANDAN, ND, p. A304
MEDFIELD STATE HOSPITAL, MEDFIELD, MA, p. A194
MEDICAL ARTS HOSPITAL, DALLAS, TX, p. A383
MEDICAL ARTS HOSPITAL, LAMESA, TX, p. A394
MEDICAL ARTS HOSPITAL, TEXARKANA, TX, p. A404
MEDICAL CENTER AT BOWLING GREEN, BOWLING GREEN, KY, p. A161
MEDICAL CENTER AT PRINCETON, PRINCETON, NJ, p. A264
MEDICAL CENTER AT SCOTTSVILLE, SCOTTSVILLE, KY, p. A168
MEDICAL CENTER AT SYMMES, ARLINGTON, MA, p. A190
MEDICAL CENTER EAST, BIRMINGHAM, AL, p. A 14
MEDICAL CENTER ENTERPRISE, ENTERPRISE, AL, p. A 15
MEDICAL CENTER HOSPITAL, CHILLICOTHE, OH, p. A307
MEDICAL CENTER HOSPITAL, CONROE, TX, p. A381
MEDICAL CENTER HOSPITAL, HOUSTON, TX, p. A391
MEDICAL CENTER HOSPITAL, ODESSA, TX, p. A398
MEDICAL CENTER OF BATON ROUGE, BATON ROUGE, LA, p. A170
MEDICAL CENTER OF CALICO ROCK, CALICO ROCK, AR, p. A 29
MEDICAL CENTER OF CENTRAL GEORGIA, MACON, GA, p. A105
MEDICAL CENTER OF CENTRAL MASSACHUSETTS, WORCESTER, MA, p. A198
MEDICAL CENTER OF DELAWARE, WILMINGTON, DE, p. A 78
MEDICAL CENTER OF INDEPENDENCE, INDEPENDENCE, MO, p. A233
MEDICAL CENTER OF LOUISIANA–UNIVERSITY HOSPITAL CAMPUS, NEW ORLEANS, LA, p. A176
MEDICAL CENTER OF LOUISIANA, NEW ORLEANS, LA, p. A176
MEDICAL CENTER OF MANCHESTER, MANCHESTER, TN, p. A371

MEDICAL CENTER OF MESQUITE, MESQUITE, TX, p. A397
MEDICAL CENTER OF NORTH HOLLYWOOD, LOS ANGELES, CA, p. A 50
MEDICAL CENTER OF OCEAN COUNTY, POINT PLEASANT, NJ, p. A264
MEDICAL CENTER OF PLANO, PLANO, TX, p. A399
MEDICAL CENTER OF PORT ST. LUCIE, PORT SAINT LUCIE, FL, p. A 94
MEDICAL CENTER OF SOUTH ARKANSAS, EL DORADO, AR, p. A 30
MEDICAL CENTER OF SOUTHEASTERN OKLAHOMA, DURANT, OK, p. A322
MEDICAL CENTER OF SOUTHERN INDIANA, CHARLESTOWN, IN, p. A134
MEDICAL CENTER OF SOUTHWEST LOUISIANA, LAFAYETTE, LA, p. A174
MEDICAL CENTER OF WINNIE, WINNIE, TX, p. A407
MEDICAL CENTER REHABILITATION HOSPITAL, GRAND FORKS, ND, p. A303
MEDICAL CENTER SHOALS, MUSCLE SHOALS, AL, p. A 19
MEDICAL CITY DALLAS HOSPITAL, DALLAS, TX, p. A383
MEDICAL COLLEGE HOSPITALS – ELKINS PARK CAMPUS, ELKINS PARK, PA, p. A338
MEDICAL COLLEGE HOSPITALS, MAIN CLINICAL CAMPUS, PHILADELPHIA, PA, p. A345
MEDICAL COLLEGE OF GEORGIA HOSPITAL AND CLINICS, AUGUSTA, GA, p. A100
MEDICAL COLLEGE OF OHIO HOSPITAL, TOLEDO, OH, p. A317
MEDICAL COLLEGE OF VIRGINIA HOSPITALS, VIRGINIA COMMONWEALTH UNIVERSITY, RICHMOND, VA, p. A420
MEDICAL PARK HOSPITAL, HOPE, AR, p. A 31
MEDICAL PARK HOSPITAL, WINSTON-SALEM, NC, p. A300
MEDICAL PLAZA HOSPITAL, SHERMAN, TX, p. A403
MEDICINE LODGE MEMORIAL HOSPITAL, MEDICINE LODGE, KS, p. A156
MEDINA COMMUNITY HOSPITAL, HONDO, TX, p. A390
MEDINA GENERAL HOSPITAL, MEDINA, OH, p. A315
MEDINA MEMORIAL HOSPITAL, MEDINA, NY, p. A277
MEDIPLEX REHABILITATION–DENVER, THORNTON, CO, p. A 73
MEEKER COUNTY MEMORIAL HOSPITAL, LITCHFIELD, MN, p. A216
MELISSA MEMORIAL HOSPITAL, HOLYOKE, CO, p. A 71
MELROSE-WAKEFIELD HOSPITAL ASSOCIATION, MELROSE, MA, p. A195
MELROSE HOSPITAL AND PINE VILLA NURSING HOME, MELROSE, MN, p. A217
MEMORIAL CENTER, BAKERSFIELD, CA, p. A 37
MEMORIAL COMMUNITY HOSPITAL, BLAIR, NE, p. A246
MEMORIAL COMMUNITY HOSPITAL, EDGERTON, WI, p. A436
MEMORIAL HEALTH CARE SYSTEM, SEWARD, NE, p. A251
MEMORIAL HEALTH CENTER, SIDNEY, NE, p. A251
MEMORIAL HEALTH SYSTEM OF EAST TEXAS, LUFKIN, TX, p. A396
MEMORIAL HOSPITAL–FLAGLER, BUNNELL, FL, p. A 82
MEMORIAL HOSPITAL–ORMOND BEACH, ORMOND BEACH, FL, p. A 92
MEMORIAL HOSPITAL–THE WOODLANDS, THE WOODLANDS, TX, p. A405
MEMORIAL HOSPITAL–WEST VOLUSIA, DE LAND, FL, p. A 83
MEMORIAL HOSPITAL – MEMORIAL CITY, HOUSTON, TX, p. A391
MEMORIAL HOSPITAL, SILOAM SPRINGS, AR, p. A 34
MEMORIAL HOSPITAL, COLORADO SPRINGS, CO, p. A 68
MEMORIAL HOSPITAL, CRAIG, CO, p. A 69
MEMORIAL HOSPITAL, HOLLYWOOD, FL, p. A 85
MEMORIAL HOSPITAL, WEISER, ID, p. A115
MEMORIAL HOSPITAL, BELLEVILLE, IL, p. A116
MEMORIAL HOSPITAL, CARTHAGE, IL, p. A117
MEMORIAL HOSPITAL, CHESTER, IL, p. A118
MEMORIAL HOSPITAL, LOGANSPORT, IN, p. A138
MEMORIAL HOSPITAL, SEYMOUR, IN, p. A140
MEMORIAL HOSPITAL, ABILENE, KS, p. A151
MEMORIAL HOSPITAL, MANHATTAN, KS, p. A156
MEMORIAL HOSPITAL, MCPHERSON, KS, p. A156
MEMORIAL HOSPITAL, MANCHESTER, KY, p. A166
MEMORIAL HOSPITAL, OWOSSO, MI, p. A208
MEMORIAL HOSPITAL, AURORA, NE, p. A246
MEMORIAL HOSPITAL, SCHUYLER, NE, p. A251
MEMORIAL HOSPITAL, NORTH CONWAY, NH, p. A256
MEMORIAL HOSPITAL, ALBANY, NY, p. A271
MEMORIAL HOSPITAL, FREMONT, OH, p. A312
MEMORIAL HOSPITAL, MARYSVILLE, OH, p. A314
MEMORIAL HOSPITAL, FREDERICK, OK, p. A323
MEMORIAL HOSPITAL, TOWANDA, PA, p. A350
MEMORIAL HOSPITAL, YORK, PA, p. A352
MEMORIAL HOSPITAL, CHATTANOOGA, TN, p. A366
MEMORIAL HOSPITAL, CENTER, TX, p. A381
MEMORIAL HOSPITAL, DUMAS, TX, p. A385
MEMORIAL HOSPITAL, GONZALES, TX, p. A388

MEMORIAL HOSPITAL, KERMIT, TX, p. A393
MEMORIAL HOSPITAL, PALESTINE, TX, p. A399
MEMORIAL HOSPITAL, SEMINOLE, TX, p. A403
MEMORIAL HOSPITAL, BURLINGTON, WI, p. A436
MEMORIAL HOSPITAL AND HEALTH CARE CENTER, JASPER, IN, p. A137
MEMORIAL HOSPITAL AND MANOR, BAINBRIDGE, GA, p. A100
MEMORIAL HOSPITAL AND MEDICAL CENTER, MIDLAND, TX, p. A397
MEMORIAL HOSPITAL AND MEDICAL CENTER OF CUMBERLAND, CUMBERLAND, MD, p. A186
MEMORIAL HOSPITAL AT EASTON MARYLAND, EASTON, MD, p. A186
MEMORIAL HOSPITAL AT EXETER, EXETER, CA, p. A 42
MEMORIAL HOSPITAL AT GULFPORT, GULFPORT, MS, p. A224
MEMORIAL HOSPITAL AT OCONOMOWOC, OCONOMOWOC, WI, p. A441
MEMORIAL HOSPITAL FOR CANCER AND ALLIED DISEASES, NEW YORK CITY, NY, p. A281
MEMORIAL HOSPITAL JACKSONVILLE, JACKSONVILLE, FL, p. A 86
MEMORIAL HOSPITAL OF ADEL, ADEL, GA, p. A 98
MEMORIAL HOSPITAL OF BEDFORD COUNTY, EVERETT, PA, p. A338
MEMORIAL HOSPITAL OF BURLINGTON COUNTY, MOUNT HOLLY, NJ, p. A262
MEMORIAL HOSPITAL OF CARBON COUNTY, RAWLINS, WY, p. A446
MEMORIAL HOSPITAL OF CARBONDALE, CARBONDALE, IL, p. A117
MEMORIAL HOSPITAL OF DODGE COUNTY, FREMONT, NE, p. A247
MEMORIAL HOSPITAL OF GARDENA, GARDENA, CA, p. A 44
MEMORIAL HOSPITAL OF GENEVA, GENEVA, OH, p. A312
MEMORIAL HOSPITAL OF GREENSBORO, GREENSBORO, NC, p. A295
MEMORIAL HOSPITAL OF IOWA COUNTY, DODGEVILLE, WI, p. A436
MEMORIAL HOSPITAL OF LAFAYETTE COUNTY, DARLINGTON, WI, p. A436
MEMORIAL HOSPITAL OF MARTINSVILLE AND HENRY COUNTY, MARTINSVILLE, VA, p. A417
MEMORIAL HOSPITAL OF MICHIGAN CITY, MICHIGAN CITY, IN, p. A139
MEMORIAL HOSPITAL OF RHODE ISLAND, PAWTUCKET, RI, p. A353
MEMORIAL HOSPITAL OF SALEM COUNTY, SALEM, NJ, p. A264
MEMORIAL HOSPITAL OF SHERIDAN COUNTY, SHERIDAN, WY, p. A446
MEMORIAL HOSPITAL OF SOUTH BEND, SOUTH BEND, IN, p. A140
MEMORIAL HOSPITAL OF SOUTHERN OKLAHOMA, ARDMORE, OK, p. A321
MEMORIAL HOSPITAL OF SWEETWATER COUNTY, ROCK SPRINGS, WY, p. A446
MEMORIAL HOSPITAL OF TAMPA, TAMPA, FL, p. A 96
MEMORIAL HOSPITAL OF TAYLOR COUNTY, MEDFORD, WI, p. A439
MEMORIAL HOSPITAL OF TEXAS COUNTY, GUYMON, OK, p. A323
MEMORIAL HOSPITAL OF WASHINGTON COUNTY, SANDERSVILLE, GA, p. A107
MEMORIAL HOSPITAL PEMBROKE, PEMBROKE PINES, FL, p. A 92
MEMORIAL HOSPITAL SYSTEM, HOUSTON, TX, p. A391
MEMORIAL HOSPITAL WEST, PEMBROKE PINES, FL, p. A 92
MEMORIAL HOSPITAL, THE PSYCHIATRIC CENTER OF ALBUQUERQUE, ALBUQUERQUE, NM, p. A267
MEMORIAL HOSPITALS ASSOCIATION, MODESTO, CA, p. A 52
MEMORIAL MEDICAL CENTER, SAVANNAH, GA, p. A108
MEMORIAL MEDICAL CENTER, SPRINGFIELD, IL, p. A130
MEMORIAL MEDICAL CENTER, WOODSTOCK, IL, p. A132
MEMORIAL MEDICAL CENTER, LAS CRUCES, NM, p. A269
MEMORIAL MEDICAL CENTER, TULSA, OK, p. A328
MEMORIAL MEDICAL CENTER, JOHNSTOWN, PA, p. A340
MEMORIAL MEDICAL CENTER, CORPUS CHRISTI, TX, p. A382
MEMORIAL MEDICAL CENTER, PORT LAVACA, TX, p. A400
MEMORIAL MEDICAL CENTER, ASHLAND, WI, p. A435
MEMORIAL MEDICAL CENTER, NEILLSVILLE, WI, p. A441
MEMORIAL MEDICAL CENTER AT SOUTH AMBOY, SOUTH AMBOY, NJ, p. A264
MEMORIAL MEDICAL CENTER OF WEST MICHIGAN, LUDINGTON, MI, p. A206
MEMORIAL MISSION MEDICAL CENTER, ASHEVILLE, NC, p. A291
MEMORIAL REHABILITATION HOSPITAL, JACKSONVILLE, FL, p. A 86
MEMORIAL SPRING SHADOWS GLEN, HOUSTON, TX, p. A391

MEMPHIS MENTAL HEALTH INSTITUTE, MEMPHIS, TN, p. A372
MENA MEDICAL CENTER, MENA, AR, p. A 32
MENDOCINO COAST DISTRICT HOSPITAL, FORT BRAGG, CA, p. A 42
MENDOTA COMMUNITY HOSPITAL, MENDOTA, IL, p. A127
MENDOTA MENTAL HEALTH INSTITUTE, MADISON, WI, p. A438
MENIFEE VALLEY MEDICAL CENTER, SUN CITY, CA, p. A 64
MENNONITE GENERAL HOSPITAL, AIBONITO, PR, p. A447
MENORAH MEDICAL CENTER, KANSAS CITY, MO, p. A234
MENTAL HEALTH INSTITUTE, CHEROKEE, IA, p. A143
MENTAL HEALTH INSTITUTE, CLARINDA, IA, p. A143
MENTAL HEALTH INSTITUTE, INDEPENDENCE, IA, p. A146
MENTAL HEALTH INSTITUTE, MOUNT PLEASANT, IA, p. A148
MEPSI CENTER, BAYAMON, PR, p. A448
MERCED COMMUNITY MEDICAL CENTER, MERCED, CA, p. A 52
MERCER COUNTY HOSPITAL, ALEDO, IL, p. A116
MERCER COUNTY JOINT TOWNSHIP COMMUNITY HOSPITAL, COLDWATER, OH, p. A310
MERCER MEDICAL CENTER, TRENTON, NJ, p. A265
MERCY–MEMORIAL MEDICAL CENTER, SAINT JOSEPH, MI, p. A209
MERCY BEHAVIORAL HEALTH, DURANGO, CO, p. A 70
MERCY CENTER FOR HEALTH CARE SERVICES, AURORA, IL, p. A116
MERCY COMMUNITY HOSPITAL, PORT JERVIS, NY, p. A285
MERCY GENERAL HOSPITAL, SACRAMENTO, CA, p. A 58
MERCY HAVERFORD HOSPITAL, HAVERTOWN, PA, p. A339
MERCY HEALTH CENTER, DUBUQUE, IA, p. A145
MERCY HEALTH CENTER, OKLAHOMA CITY, OK, p. A325
MERCY HEALTH CORPORATION OF SOUTHEASTERN PENNSYLVANIA, BALA CYNWYD, PA, p. A334
MERCY HEALTH SYSTEM, JANESVILLE, WI, p. A438
MERCY HEALTHCARE SACRAMENTO, CARMICHAEL, CA, p. A 39
MERCY HOSPITAL–TURNER MEMORIAL, OZARK, AR, p. A 33
MERCY HOSPITAL–WILLARD, WILLARD, OH, p. A319
MERCY HOSPITAL, BAKERSFIELD, CA, p. A 37
MERCY HOSPITAL, MIAMI, FL, p. A 90
MERCY HOSPITAL, CORNING, IA, p. A143
MERCY HOSPITAL, COUNCIL BLUFFS, IA, p. A144
MERCY HOSPITAL, IOWA CITY, IA, p. A146
MERCY HOSPITAL, MOUNDRIDGE, KS, p. A156
MERCY HOSPITAL, OWENSBORO, KY, p. A167
MERCY HOSPITAL, PORTLAND, ME, p. A182
MERCY HOSPITAL, SPRINGFIELD, MA, p. A197
MERCY HOSPITAL, CADILLAC, MI, p. A200
MERCY HOSPITAL, DETROIT, MI, p. A202
MERCY HOSPITAL, GRAYLING, MI, p. A204
MERCY HOSPITAL, PORT HURON, MI, p. A209
MERCY HOSPITAL, BUFFALO, NY, p. A273
MERCY HOSPITAL, CHARLOTTE, NC, p. A292
MERCY HOSPITAL, DEVILS LAKE, ND, p. A302
MERCY HOSPITAL, VALLEY CITY, ND, p. A305
MERCY HOSPITAL, HAMILTON, OH, p. A313
MERCY HOSPITAL, TIFFIN, OH, p. A317
MERCY HOSPITAL, TOLEDO, OH, p. A318
MERCY HOSPITAL & HEALTH CARE CENTER, MOOSE LAKE, MN, p. A217
MERCY HOSPITAL AND HEALTH SERVICES, MERCED, CA, p. A 52
MERCY HOSPITAL AND MEDICAL CENTER, SAN DIEGO, CA, p. A 59
MERCY HOSPITAL AND MEDICAL CENTER, CHICAGO, IL, p. A119
MERCY HOSPITAL ANDERSON, CINCINNATI, OH, p. A308
MERCY HOSPITAL MEDICAL CENTER, DES MOINES, IA, p. A144
MERCY HOSPITAL OF FOLSOM, FOLSOM, CA, p. A 42
MERCY HOSPITAL OF FRANCISCAN SISTERS, OELWEIN, IA, p. A148
MERCY HOSPITAL OF NANTICOKE, NANTICOKE, PA, p. A343
MERCY HOSPITAL OF PITTSBURGH, PITTSBURGH, PA, p. A346
MERCY HOSPITAL OF SCOTT COUNTY, WALDRON, AR, p. A 34
MERCY HOSPITAL OF SCRANTON, SCRANTON, PA, p. A349
MERCY HOSPITAL OF WILKES–BARRE, WILKES–BARRE, PA, p. A351
MERCY HOSPITALS OF KANSAS, FORT SCOTT, KS, p. A153
MERCY HOSPITALS OF KANSAS, INDEPENDENCE, KS, p. A154
MERCY MEDICAL, DAPHNE, AL, p. A 15
MERCY MEDICAL CENTER, REDDING, CA, p. A 57
MERCY MEDICAL CENTER, DURANGO, CO, p. A 70
MERCY MEDICAL CENTER, NAMPA, ID, p. A114
MERCY MEDICAL CENTER, CEDAR RAPIDS, IA, p. A143
MERCY MEDICAL CENTER, BALTIMORE, MD, p. A185
MERCY MEDICAL CENTER, ROCKVILLE CENTRE, NY, p. A286
MERCY MEDICAL CENTER, WILLISTON, ND, p. A305
MERCY MEDICAL CENTER, SPRINGFIELD, OH, p. A317
MERCY MEDICAL CENTER, ROSEBURG, OR, p. A332

MERCY MEDICAL CENTER, OSHKOSH, WI, p. A441
MERCY MEDICAL CENTER MOUNT SHASTA, MOUNT SHASTA, CA, p. A 53
MERCY MEMORIAL HOSPITAL, MONROE, MI, p. A207
MERCY MEMORIAL HOSPITAL, URBANA, OH, p. A318
MERCY PROVIDENCE HOSPITAL, PITTSBURGH, PA, p. A346
MERCY PSYCHIATRIC INSTITUTE, PITTSBURGH, PA, p. A346
MERCY REGIONAL HEALTH SYSTEM, ALTOONA, PA, p. A334
MERCY REGIONAL MEDICAL CENTER, LAREDO, TX, p. A394
MERIDELL ACHIEVEMENT CENTER, AUSTIN, TX, p. A378
MERIDIA EUCLID HOSPITAL, EUCLID, OH, p. A312
MERIDIA HILLCREST HOSPITAL, MAYFIELD HEIGHTS, OH, p. A315
MERIDIA HILLCREST HURON HOSPITAL, CLEVELAND, OH, p. A309
MERIDIA SOUTH POINTE, WARRENSVILLE HEIGHTS, OH, p. A318
MERIDIA SOUTH POINTE HOSPITAL, WARRENSVILLE HEIGHTS, OH, p. A319
MERITCARE MEDICAL CENTER, FARGO, ND, p. A303
MERITER HOSPITAL, MADISON, WI, p. A438
MERIWETHER MEMORIAL HOSPITAL, WARM SPRINGS, GA, p. A109
MERLE WEST MEDICAL CENTER, KLAMATH FALLS, OR, p. A330
MERRILL PIONEER COMMUNITY HOSPITAL, ROCK RAPIDS, IA, p. A149
MERRITHEW MEMORIAL HOSPITAL, MARTINEZ, CA, p. A 52
MERRYVILLE GENERAL HOSPITAL, MERRYVILLE, LA, p. A175
MESA GENERAL HOSPITAL MEDICAL CENTER, MESA, AZ, p. A 24
MESA LUTHERAN HOSPITAL, MESA, AZ, p. A 24
MESA VISTA HOSPITAL, SAN DIEGO, CA, p. A 59
MESABI REGIONAL MEDICAL CENTER, HIBBING, MN, p. A215
MESILLA VALLEY HOSPITAL, LAS CRUCES, NM, p. A269
MESQUITE COMMUNITY HOSPITAL, MESQUITE, TX, p. A397
METHODIST–HAYWOOD PARK HOSPITAL, BROWNSVILLE, TN, p. A366
METHODIST CHILDREN'S HOSPITAL, LUBBOCK, TX, p. A395
METHODIST HOSPITAL–LEVELLAND, LEVELLAND, TX, p. A395
METHODIST HOSPITAL, SACRAMENTO, CA, p. A 58
METHODIST HOSPITAL, SAINT LOUIS PARK, MN, p. A219
METHODIST HOSPITAL, PHILADELPHIA, PA, p. A345
METHODIST HOSPITAL, LUBBOCK, TX, p. A395
METHODIST HOSPITAL OF CHICAGO, CHICAGO, IL, p. A119
METHODIST HOSPITAL OF DYERSBURG, DYERSBURG, TN, p. A367
METHODIST HOSPITAL OF FAYETTE, SOMERVILLE, TN, p. A374
METHODIST HOSPITAL OF HATTIESBURG, HATTIESBURG, MS, p. A224
METHODIST HOSPITAL OF INDIANA, INDIANAPOLIS, IN, p. A137
METHODIST HOSPITAL OF JONESBORO, JONESBORO, AR, p. A 31
METHODIST HOSPITAL OF LEXINGTON, LEXINGTON, TN, p. A370
METHODIST HOSPITAL OF MARION COUNTY, COLUMBIA, MS, p. A223
METHODIST HOSPITAL OF MCKENZIE, MCKENZIE, TN, p. A371
METHODIST HOSPITAL OF MIDDLE MISSISSIPPI, LEXINGTON, MS, p. A225
METHODIST HOSPITAL OF SOUTHERN CALIFORNIA, ARCADIA, CA, p. A 36
METHODIST HOSPITAL PLAINVIEW, PLAINVIEW, TX, p. A399
METHODIST HOSPITALS, GARY, IN, p. A135
METHODIST HOSPITALS OF MEMPHIS, MEMPHIS, TN, p. A372
METHODIST MEDICAL CENTER, JACKSONVILLE, FL, p. A 86
METHODIST MEDICAL CENTER, JACKSON, MS, p. A225
METHODIST MEDICAL CENTER, DALLAS, TX, p. A383
METHODIST MEDICAL CENTER OF ILLINOIS, PEORIA, IL, p. A129
METHODIST MEDICAL CENTER OF OAK RIDGE, OAK RIDGE, TN, p. A373
METHODIST PATHWAY CENTER, JACKSONVILLE, FL, p. A 86
METHODIST PSYCHIATRIC PAVILLION, NEW ORLEANS, LA, p. A176
METHODIST RICHARD YOUNG, OMAHA, NE, p. A250
METRO HEALTH CENTER, ERIE, PA, p. A338
METROHEALTH MEDICAL CENTER, CLEVELAND, OH, p. A309
METROPLEX HOSPITAL, KILLEEN, TX, p. A394
METROPOLITAN HOSPITAL, ATLANTA, GA, p. A 99
METROPOLITAN HOSPITAL, GRAND RAPIDS, MI, p. A204
METROPOLITAN HOSPITAL, SAN ANTONIO, TX, p. A402
METROPOLITAN HOSPITAL, RICHMOND, VA, p. A420
METROPOLITAN HOSPITAL CENTER, NEW YORK CITY, NY, p. A281
METROPOLITAN NASHVILLE GENERAL HOSPITAL, NASHVILLE, TN, p. A373
METROPOLITAN STATE HOSPITAL, NORWALK, CA, p. A 54
METROWEST MEDICAL CENTER, FRAMINGHAM, MA, p. A193

Hospitals, Alphabetically / Meyersdale Medical Center

MEYERSDALE MEDICAL CENTER, MEYERSDALE, PA, p. A342
MIAMI CHILDREN'S HOSPITAL, MIAMI, FL, p. A 90
MIAMI COUNTY MEDICAL CENTER, PAOLA, KS, p. A157
MIAMI HEART INSTITUTE, MIAMI, FL, p. A 90
MIAMI JEWISH HOME AND HOSPITAL FOR AGED, MIAMI, FL, p. A 90
MIAMI VALLEY HOSPITAL, DAYTON, OH, p. A311
MICHAEL REESE HOSPITAL AND MEDICAL CENTER, CHICAGO, IL, p. A119
MICHIANA COMMUNITY HOSPITAL, SOUTH BEND, IN, p. A140
MICHIGAN AFFILIATED HEALTH SYSTEM, LANSING, MI, p. A206
MICHIGAN HOSPITAL AND MEDICAL CENTER, DETROIT, MI, p. A202
MID-AMERICA REHABILITATION HOSPITAL, OVERLAND PARK, KS, p. A157
MID-COLUMBIA MEDICAL CENTER, THE DALLES, OR, p. A333
MID-ISLAND HOSPITAL, BETHPAGE, NY, p. A272
MID-JEFFERSON HOSPITAL, NEDERLAND, TX, p. A398
MID-MAINE MEDICAL CENTER, WATERVILLE, ME, p. A183
MID-VALLEY HOSPITAL, PECKVILLE, PA, p. A343
MID-VALLEY HOSPITAL, OMAK, WA, p. A426
MID COAST HOSPITAL, BATH, ME, p. A180
MID DAKOTA HOSPITAL, CHAMBERLAIN, SD, p. A361
MID MISSOURI MENTAL HEALTH CENTER, COLUMBIA, MO, p. A231
MIDDLE GEORGIA HOSPITAL, MACON, GA, p. A105
MIDDLE TENNESSEE MEDICAL CENTER, MURFREESBORO, TN, p. A373
MIDDLE TENNESSEE MENTAL HEALTH INSTITUTE, NASHVILLE, TN, p. A373
MIDDLESBORO APPALACHIAN REGIONAL HOSPITAL, MIDDLESBORO, KY, p. A166
MIDDLESEX HOSPITAL, MIDDLETOWN, CT, p. A 75
MIDDLESEX HOSPITAL, WALTHAM, MA, p. A197
MIDDLETOWN PSYCHIATRIC CENTER, MIDDLETOWN, NY, p. A277
MIDDLETOWN REGIONAL HOSPITAL, MIDDLETOWN, OH, p. A315
MIDLANDS CENTER, COLUMBIA, SC, p. A356
MIDLANDS COMMUNITY HOSPITAL, PAPILLION, NE, p. A251
MIDMICHIGAN REGIONAL MEDICAL CENTER-CLARE, CLARE, MI, p. A201
MIDMICHIGAN REGIONAL MEDICAL CENTER-GLADWIN, GLADWIN, MI, p. A203
MIDMICHIGAN REGIONAL MEDICAL CENTER, MIDLAND, MI, p. A207
MIDSOUTH HOSPITAL, MEMPHIS, TN, p. A372
MIDWAY HOSPITAL MEDICAL CENTER, LOS ANGELES, CA, p. A 50
MIDWAY PARK MEDICAL CENTER, LANCASTER, TX, p. A394
MIDWEST CITY REGIONAL HOSPITAL, MIDWEST CITY, OK, p. A325
MIDWESTERN REGIONAL MEDICAL CENTER, ZION, IL, p. A132
MILE BLUFF MEDICAL CENTER, MAUSTON, WI, p. A439
MILES MEMORIAL HOSPITAL, DAMARISCOTTA, ME, p. A181
MILFORD-WHITINSVILLE REGIONAL HOSPITAL, MILFORD, MA, p. A195
MILFORD HOSPITAL, MILFORD, CT, p. A 75
MILFORD MEMORIAL HOSPITAL, MILFORD, DE, p. A 78
MILFORD VALLEY MEMORIAL HOSPITAL, MILFORD, UT, p. A408
MILLARD FILLMORE HEALTH SYSTEM, BUFFALO, NY, p. A273
MILLCREEK COMMUNITY HOSPITAL, ERIE, PA, p. A338
MILLE LACS HEALTH SYSTEM, ONAMIA, MN, p. A218
MILLER-DWAN MEDICAL CENTER, DULUTH, MN, p. A214
MILLER COUNTY HOSPITAL, COLQUITT, GA, p. A101
MILLINOCKET REGIONAL HOSPITAL, MILLINOCKET, ME, p. A182
MILLS-PENINSULA HOSPITALS, BURLINGAME, CA, p. A 38
MILTON HOSPITAL, MILTON, MA, p. A195
MILWAUKEE COUNTY MENTAL HEALTH COMPLEX, MILWAUKEE, WI, p. A440
MILWAUKEE PSYCHIATRIC HOSPITAL, WAUWATOSA, WI, p. A444
MIMBRES MEMORIAL HOSPITAL, DEMING, NM, p. A268
MINDEN MEDICAL CENTER, MINDEN, LA, p. A175
MINER'S MEMORIAL MEDICAL CENTER, COALDALE, PA, p. A336
MINERAL AREA REGIONAL MEDICAL CENTER, FARMINGTON, MO, p. A232
MINERAL COMMUNITY HOSPITAL, SUPERIOR, MT, p. A244
MINERS HOSPITAL NORTHERN CAMBRIA, SPANGLER, PA, p. A349
MINERS' COLFAX MEDICAL CENTER, RATON, NM, p. A269
MINIDOKA MEMORIAL HOSPITAL AND EXTENDED CARE FACILITY, RUPERT, ID, p. A114
MINNEOLA DISTRICT HOSPITAL, MINNEOLA, KS, p. A156
MINNESOTA VALLEY HEALTH CENTER, LE SUEUR, MN, p. A216
MINNEWASKA DISTRICT HOSPITAL, STARBUCK, MN, p. A220

MINNIE G. BOSWELL MEMORIAL HOSPITAL, GREENSBORO, GA, p. A104
MIRIAM HOSPITAL, PROVIDENCE, RI, p. A353
MISSION BAY MEMORIAL HOSPITAL, SAN DIEGO, CA, p. A 59
MISSION COMMUNITY HOSPITAL-SAN FERNANDO CAMPUS, SAN FERNANDO, CA, p. A 60
MISSION HILL MEMORIAL HOSPITAL, SHAWNEE, OK, p. A327
MISSION HOSPITAL, MISSION, TX, p. A397
MISSION HOSPITAL REGIONAL MEDICAL CENTER, MISSION VIEJO, CA, p. A 52
MISSION VISTA HOSPITAL, SAN ANTONIO, TX, p. A402
MISSISSIPPI BAPTIST MEDICAL CENTER, JACKSON, MS, p. A225
MISSISSIPPI METHODIST HOSPITAL AND REHABILITATION CENTER, JACKSON, MS, p. A225
MISSISSIPPI STATE HOSPITAL, WHITFIELD, MS, p. A228
MISSOURI BAPTIST HOSPITAL OF SULLIVAN, SULLIVAN, MO, p. A240
MISSOURI BAPTIST MEDICAL CENTER, TOWN AND COUNTRY, MO, p. A240
MISSOURI DELTA MEDICAL CENTER, SIKESTON, MO, p. A239
MISSOURI REHABILITATION CENTER, MOUNT VERNON, MO, p. A236
MISSOURI RIVER MEDICAL CENTER, FORT BENTON, MT, p. A242
MITCHELL COUNTY COMMUNITY HOSPITAL, BELOIT, KS, p. A151
MITCHELL COUNTY HOSPITAL, CAMILLA, GA, p. A101
MITCHELL COUNTY HOSPITAL, COLORADO CITY, TX, p. A381
MITCHELL COUNTY REGIONAL HEALTH CENTER, OSAGE, IA, p. A148
MIZELL MEMORIAL HOSPITAL, OPP, AL, p. A 19
MOBERLY REGIONAL MEDICAL CENTER, MOBERLY, MO, p. A236
MOBILE INFIRMARY MEDICAL CENTER, MOBILE, AL, p. A 18
MOBRIDGE REGIONAL HOSPITAL, MOBRIDGE, SD, p. A363
MOCCASIN BEND MENTAL HEALTH INSTITUTE, CHATTANOOGA, TN, p. A366
MODOC MEDICAL CENTER, ALTURAS, CA, p. A 36
MOHAVE VALLEY HOSPITAL AND MEDICAL CENTER, BULLHEAD CITY, AZ, p. A 23
MOHAWK VALLEY PSYCHIATRIC CENTER, UTICA, NY, p. A288
MOLLY STARK HOSPITAL, LOUISVILLE, OH, p. A314
MOLOKAI GENERAL HOSPITAL, KAUNAKAKAI, HI, p. A111
MONADNOCK COMMUNITY HOSPITAL, PETERBOROUGH, NH, p. A256
MONCRIEF ARMY COMMUNITY HOSPITAL, FORT JACKSON, SC, p. A357
MONMOUTH MEDICAL CENTER, LONG BRANCH, NJ, p. A261
MONONGAHELA VALLEY HOSPITAL, MONONGAHELA, PA, p. A342
MONONGALIA GENERAL HOSPITAL, MORGANTOWN, WV, p. A432
MONROE COMMUNITY HOSPITAL, ROCHESTER, NY, p. A286
MONROE COUNTY HOSPITAL, MONROEVILLE, AL, p. A 18
MONROE COUNTY HOSPITAL, FORSYTH, GA, p. A103
MONROE COUNTY HOSPITAL, ALBIA, IA, p. A142
MONROE COUNTY MEDICAL CENTER, TOMPKINSVILLE, KY, p. A168
MONROVIA COMMUNITY HOSPITAL, MONROVIA, CA, p. A 53
MONSOUR MEDICAL CENTER, JEANNETTE, PA, p. A340
MONTANA DEACONESS MEDICAL CENTER, GREAT FALLS, MT, p. A242
MONTANA STATE HOSPITAL, WARM SPRINGS, MT, p. A244
MONTCLAIR COMMUNITY HOSPITAL, MONTCLAIR, NJ, p. A262
MONTEBELLO REHABILITATION HOSPITAL-UNIVERSITY OF MARYLAND MEDICAL SYSTEM, BALTIMORE, MD, p. A185
MONTEFIORE MEDICAL CENTER, NEW YORK CITY, NY, p. A281
MONTELEPRE EXTENDED CARE HOSPITAL, NEW ORLEANS, LA, p. A176
MONTEREY PARK HOSPITAL, MONTEREY PARK, CA, p. A 53
MONTEVISTA HOSPITAL, LAS VEGAS, NV, p. A253
MONTEZUMA COUNTY HOSPITAL DISTRICT, CORTEZ, CO, p. A 69
MONTFORT JONES MEMORIAL HOSPITAL, KOSCIUSKO, MS, p. A225
MONTGOMERY COUNTY EMERGENCY SERVICE, NORRISTOWN, PA, p. A343
MONTGOMERY COUNTY MEMORIAL HOSPITAL, RED OAK, IA, p. A149
MONTGOMERY GENERAL HOSPITAL, OLNEY, MD, p. A188
MONTGOMERY GENERAL HOSPITAL, MONTGOMERY, WV, p. A432
MONTGOMERY HOSPITAL, NORRISTOWN, PA, p. A343
MONTGOMERY MEMORIAL HOSPITAL, TROY, NC, p. A300
MONTGOMERY REGIONAL HOSPITAL, BLACKSBURG, VA, p. A414
MONTGOMERY REGIONAL MEDICAL CENTER, MONTGOMERY, AL, p. A 18

MONTICELLO-BIG LAKE COMMUNITY HOSPITAL, MONTICELLO, MN, p. A217
MONTROSE GENERAL HOSPITAL, MONTROSE, PA, p. A342
MONTROSE MEMORIAL HOSPITAL, MONTROSE, CO, p. A 72
MONUMENT VALLEY HOSPITAL, MONUMENT VALLEY, UT, p. A409
MOORE REGIONAL HOSPITAL, PINEHURST, NC, p. A297
MOOSA MEMORIAL HOSPITAL, EUNICE, LA, p. A172
MOOSE LAKE REGIONAL TREATMENT CENTER, MOOSE LAKE, MN, p. A217
MOREHEAD MEMORIAL HOSPITAL, EDEN, NC, p. A293
MOREHOUSE GENERAL HOSPITAL, BASTROP, LA, p. A170
MORENCI AREA HOSPITAL, MORENCI, MI, p. A207
MORENO VALLEY COMMUNITY HOSPITAL, MORENO VALLEY, CA, p. A 53
MORGAN COUNTY APPALACHIAN REGIONAL HOSPITAL, WEST LIBERTY, KY, p. A168
MORGAN COUNTY MEMORIAL HOSPITAL, MARTINSVILLE, IN, p. A138
MORGAN COUNTY WAR MEMORIAL HOSPITAL, BERKELEY SPRINGS, WV, p. A430
MORGAN MEMORIAL HOSPITAL, MADISON, GA, p. A105
MORRILL COUNTY COMMUNITY HOSPITAL, BRIDGEPORT, NE, p. A246
MORRIS COUNTY HOSPITAL, COUNCIL GROVE, KS, p. A152
MORRIS HOSPITAL, MORRIS, IL, p. A127
MORRISON COMMUNITY HOSPITAL, MORRISON, IL, p. A127
MORRISTOWN-HAMBLEN HOSPITAL, MORRISTOWN, TN, p. A372
MORRISTOWN MEMORIAL HOSPITAL, MORRISTOWN, NJ, p. A262
MORROW COUNTY HOSPITAL, MOUNT GILEAD, OH, p. A315
MORTON COUNTY HOSPITAL, ELKHART, KS, p. A152
MORTON GENERAL HOSPITAL, MORTON, WA, p. A425
MORTON HOSPITAL AND MEDICAL CENTER, TAUNTON, MA, p. A197
MORTON PLANT HOSPITAL, CLEARWATER, FL, p. A 82
MOSES CONE HEALTH SYSTEM, GREENSBORO, NC, p. A295
MOSES LUDINGTON HOSPITAL, TICONDEROGA, NY, p. A288
MOSES TAYLOR HOSPITAL, SCRANTON, PA, p. A349
MOTHER FRANCES HOSPITAL REGIONAL HEALTHCARE CENTER, TYLER, TX, p. A405
MOTION PICTURE AND TELEVISION FUND HOSPITAL AND RESIDENTIAL SERVICES, LOS ANGELES, CA, p. A 50
MOUNT ASCUTNEY HOSPITAL AND HEALTH CENTER, WINDSOR, VT, p. A413
MOUNT AUBURN HOSPITAL, CAMBRIDGE, MA, p. A192
MOUNT CARMEL HEALTH, COLUMBUS, OH, p. A310
MOUNT CARMEL HOSPITAL, COLVILLE, WA, p. A424
MOUNT CARMEL MEDICAL CENTER, PITTSBURG, KS, p. A158
MOUNT CLEMENS GENERAL HOSPITAL, MOUNT CLEMENS, MI, p. A207
MOUNT DESERT ISLAND HOSPITAL, BAR HARBOR, ME, p. A180
MOUNT DIABLO MEDICAL CENTER, CONCORD, CA, p. A 40
MOUNT GRAHAM COMMUNITY HOSPITAL, SAFFORD, AZ, p. A 26
MOUNT GRANT GENERAL HOSPITAL, HAWTHORNE, NV, p. A253
MOUNT REGIS CENTER, SALEM, VA, p. A420
MOUNT SAN RAFAEL HOSPITAL, TRINIDAD, CO, p. A 73
MOUNT SINAI HOSPITAL, HARTFORD, CT, p. A 74
MOUNT SINAI HOSPITAL MEDICAL CENTER OF CHICAGO, CHICAGO, IL, p. A119
MOUNT SINAI MEDICAL CENTER, MIAMI BEACH, FL, p. A 90
MOUNT SINAI MEDICAL CENTER, NEW YORK CITY, NY, p. A281
MOUNT ST. MARY'S HOSPITAL OF NIAGARA FALLS, LEWISTON, NY, p. A277
MOUNT VERNON HOSPITAL, MOUNT VERNON, NY, p. A278
MOUNT VERNON HOSPITAL, ALEXANDRIA, VA, p. A414
MOUNT ZION MEDICAL CENTER OF UNIVERSITY OF CALIFORNIA-SAN FRANCISCO, SAN FRANCISCO, CA, p. A 60
MOUNTAIN CREST HOSPITAL, FORT COLLINS, CO, p. A 70
MOUNTAIN MANOR TREATMENT CENTER, EMMITSBURG, MD, p. A187
MOUNTAIN VIEW HOSPITAL, GADSDEN, AL, p. A 16
MOUNTAIN VIEW HOSPITAL, PAYSON, UT, p. A409
MOUNTAIN VIEW HOSPITAL DISTRICT, MADRAS, OR, p. A331
MOUNTAINS COMMUNITY HOSPITAL, LAKE ARROWHEAD, CA, p. A 46
MOUNTAINSIDE HOSPITAL, MONTCLAIR, NJ, p. A262
MOUNTAINVIEW HOSPITAL OF SPOKANE, SPOKANE, WA, p. A428
MOUNTAINVIEW MEMORIAL HOSPITAL, WHITE SULPHUR SPRINGS, MT, p. A244
MT. SINAI HOSPITAL, PHILADELPHIA, PA, p. A345
MT. SINAI MEDICAL CENTER, CLEVELAND, OH, p. A309
MT. WASHINGTON PEDIATRIC HOSPITAL, BALTIMORE, MD, p. A185

MUENSTER MEMORIAL HOSPITAL, MUENSTER, TX, p. A397
MUHLENBERG COMMUNITY HOSPITAL, GREENVILLE, KY, p. A163
MUHLENBERG HOSPITAL CENTER, BETHLEHEM, PA, p. A335
MUHLENBERG REGIONAL MEDICAL CENTER, PLAINFIELD, NJ, p. A263
MULESHOE AREA MEDICAL CENTER, MULESHOE, TX, p. A398
MULLINS HOSPITAL, MULLINS, SC, p. A359
MUNCY VALLEY HOSPITAL, MUNCY, PA, p. A343
MUNISING MEMORIAL HOSPITAL, MUNISING, MI, p. A207
MUNROE REGIONAL MEDICAL CENTER, OCALA, FL, p. A 91
MUNSON ARMY COMMUNITY HOSPITAL, FORT LEAVENWORTH, KS, p. A152
MUNSON MEDICAL CENTER, TRAVERSE CITY, MI, p. A210
MURPHY MEDICAL CENTER, MURPHY, NC, p. A297
MURRAY–CALLOWAY COUNTY HOSPITAL, MURRAY, KY, p. A167
MURRAY COUNTY MEMORIAL HOSPITAL, SLAYTON, MN, p. A220
MURRAY MEDICAL CENTER, CHATSWORTH, GA, p. A101
MUSC MEDICAL CENTER OF MEDICAL UNIVERSITY OF SOUTH CAROLINA, CHARLESTON, SC, p. A355
MUSCATINE GENERAL HOSPITAL, MUSCATINE, IA, p. A148
MUSKEGON GENERAL HOSPITAL, MUSKEGON, MI, p. A207
MUSKEGON MERCY COMMUNITY HEALTHCARE SYSTEM, MUSKEGON, MI, p. A207
MUSKOGEE REGIONAL MEDICAL CENTER, MUSKOGEE, OK, p. A325
MYERS COMMUNITY HOSPITAL, SODUS, NY, p. A287
MYRTLE WERTH MEDICAL CENTER, MENOMONIE, WI, p. A439
MYRTUE MEMORIAL HOSPITAL, HARLAN, IA, p. A146

N

N. T. ENLOE MEMORIAL HOSPITAL, CHICO, CA, p. A 39
NACOGDOCHES MEDICAL CENTER, NACOGDOCHES, TX, p. A398
NACOGDOCHES MEMORIAL HOSPITAL, NACOGDOCHES, TX, p. A398
NAEVE HOSPITAL, ALBERT LEA, MN, p. A212
NAN TRAVIS MEMORIAL HOSPITAL, JACKSONVILLE, TX, p. A393
NANTICOKE MEMORIAL HOSPITAL, SEAFORD, DE, p. A 78
NANTUCKET COTTAGE HOSPITAL, NANTUCKET, MA, p. A195
NAPA STATE HOSPITAL, NAPA, CA, p. A 53
NAPLES COMMUNITY HOSPITAL, NAPLES, FL, p. A 90
NASH GENERAL HOSPITAL, ROCKY MOUNT, NC, p. A298
NASHVILLE MEMORIAL HOSPITAL, MADISON, TN, p. A371
NASHVILLE METROPOLITAN BORDEAUX HOSPITAL, NASHVILLE, TN, p. A373
NASHVILLE REHABILITATION HOSPITAL, NASHVILLE, TN, p. A373
NASON HOSPITAL, ROARING SPRING, PA, p. A348
NASSAU COUNTY MEDICAL CENTER, EAST MEADOW, NY, p. A274
NATCHAUG HOSPITAL, MANSFIELD CENTER, CT, p. A 75
NATCHEZ COMMUNITY HOSPITAL, NATCHEZ, MS, p. A226
NATCHEZ REGIONAL MEDICAL CENTER, NATCHEZ, MS, p. A226
NATCHITOCHES PARISH HOSPITAL, NATCHITOCHES, LA, p. A175
NATHAN LITTAUER HOSPITAL AND NURSING HOME, GLOVERSVILLE, NY, p. A275
NATIONAL HOSPITAL FOR ORTHOPAEDICS AND REHABILITATION, ARLINGTON, VA, p. A414
NATIONAL JEWISH CENTER FOR IMMUNOLOGY AND RESPIRATORY MEDICINE, DENVER, CO, p. A 69
NATIONAL NAVAL MEDICAL CENTER, BETHESDA, MD, p. A186
NATIONAL PARK MEDICAL CENTER, HOT SPRINGS, AR, p. A 31
NATIONAL REHABILITATION HOSPITAL, WASHINGTON, DC, p. A 79
NATIVIDAD MEDICAL CENTER, SALINAS, CA, p. A 58
NATURE COAST REGIONAL HOSPITAL, WILLISTON, FL, p. A 97
NAUKEAG HOSPITAL, ASHBURNHAM, MA, p. A190
NAVAL HOSPITAL, CAMP PENDLETON, CA, p. A 38
NAVAL HOSPITAL, LEMOORE, CA, p. A 47
NAVAL HOSPITAL, OAKLAND, CA, p. A 54
NAVAL HOSPITAL, TWENTYNINE PALMS, CA, p. A 65
NAVAL HOSPITAL, GROTON, CT, p. A 74
NAVAL HOSPITAL, JACKSONVILLE, FL, p. A 86
NAVAL HOSPITAL, ORLANDO, FL, p. A 91
NAVAL HOSPITAL, PENSACOLA, FL, p. A 92
NAVAL HOSPITAL, GREAT LAKES, IL, p. A124
NAVAL HOSPITAL, PATUXENT RIVER, MD, p. A188
NAVAL HOSPITAL, CAMP LEJEUNE, NC, p. A292
NAVAL HOSPITAL, CHERRY POINT, NC, p. A293
NAVAL HOSPITAL, BEAUFORT, SC, p. A355
NAVAL HOSPITAL, CHARLESTON, SC, p. A356
NAVAL HOSPITAL, MILLINGTON, TN, p. A372
NAVAL HOSPITAL, CORPUS CHRISTI, TX, p. A382
NAVAL HOSPITAL, BREMERTON, WA, p. A423
NAVAL HOSPITAL, OAK HARBOR, WA, p. A425
NAVAL MEDICAL CENTER, SAN DIEGO, CA, p. A 59
NAVAL MEDICAL CENTER, PORTSMOUTH, VA, p. A419
NAVAPACHE REGIONAL MEDICAL CENTER, SHOW LOW, AZ, p. A 27
NAVARRO REGIONAL HOSPITAL, CORSICANA, TX, p. A382
NAZARETH HOSPITAL, PHILADELPHIA, PA, p. A345
NEBRASKA METHODIST HOSPITAL, OMAHA, NE, p. A250
NEEDLES–DESERT COMMUNITIES HOSPITAL, NEEDLES, CA, p. A 54
NELLIS FEDERAL HOSPITAL, LAS VEGAS, NV, p. A253
NEMAHA COUNTY HOSPITAL, AUBURN, NE, p. A246
NEMAHA VALLEY COMMUNITY HOSPITAL, SENECA, KS, p. A158
NEOSHO MEMORIAL REGIONAL MEDICAL CENTER, CHANUTE, KS, p. A151
NESHOBA COUNTY GENERAL HOSPITAL, PHILADELPHIA, MS, p. A227
NESS COUNTY HOSPITAL NUMBER TWO, NESS CITY, KS, p. A156
NEUMANN MEDICAL CENTER, PHILADELPHIA, PA, p. A345
NEVADA COUNTY HOSPITAL, PRESCOTT, AR, p. A 34
NEVADA MENTAL HEALTH INSTITUTE, SPARKS, NV, p. A254
NEVADA REGIONAL MEDICAL CENTER, NEVADA, MO, p. A236
NEW BEGINNINGS AT WARWICK MANOR, EAST NEW MARKET, MD, p. A186
NEW BRITAIN GENERAL HOSPITAL, NEW BRITAIN, CT, p. A 75
NEW CENTER HOSPITAL, DETROIT, MI, p. A202
NEW ENGLAND BAPTIST HOSPITAL, BOSTON, MA, p. A191
NEW ENGLAND MEDICAL CENTER, BOSTON, MA, p. A191
NEW ENGLAND REHABILITATION HOSPITAL, WOBURN, MA, p. A198
NEW ENGLAND REHABILITATION HOSPITAL OF PORTLAND, PORTLAND, ME, p. A182
NEW ENGLAND SINAI HOSPITAL AND REHABILITATION CENTER, STOUGHTON, MA, p. A197
NEW HAMPSHIRE HOSPITAL, CONCORD, NH, p. A255
NEW HANOVER REGIONAL MEDICAL CENTER, WILMINGTON, NC, p. A300
NEW LONDON FAMILY MEDICAL CENTER, NEW LONDON, WI, p. A441
NEW LONDON HOSPITAL, NEW LONDON, NH, p. A256
NEW MEXICO REHABILITATION CENTER, ROSWELL, NM, p. A269
NEW MILFORD HOSPITAL, NEW MILFORD, CT, p. A 76
NEW ORLEANS ADOLESCENT HOSPITAL, NEW ORLEANS, LA, p. A176
NEW PORT RICHEY HOSPITAL, NEW PORT RICHEY, FL, p. A 90
NEW ROCHELLE HOSPITAL MEDICAL CENTER, NEW ROCHELLE, NY, p. A278
NEW YORK DOWNTOWN HOSPITAL, NEW YORK CITY, NY, p. A281
NEW YORK EYE AND EAR INFIRMARY, NEW YORK CITY, NY, p. A281
NEW YORK HOSPITAL MEDICAL CENTER OF QUEENS, NEW YORK CITY, NY, p. A281
NEW YORK METHODIST HOSPITAL, NEW YORK CITY, NY, p. A281
NEW YORK STATE PSYCHIATRIC INSTITUTE, NEW YORK CITY, NY, p. A281
NEW YORK UNIVERSITY MEDICAL CENTER, NEW YORK CITY, NY, p. A281
NEWARK–WAYNE COMMUNITY HOSPITAL, NEWARK, NY, p. A283
NEWARK BETH ISRAEL MEDICAL CENTER, NEWARK, NJ, p. A262
NEWBERRY COUNTY MEMORIAL HOSPITAL, NEWBERRY, SC, p. A359
NEWCOMB MEDICAL CENTER, VINELAND, NJ, p. A265
NEWHALL COMMUNITY HOSPITAL, NEWHALL, CA, p. A 54
NEWINGTON CHILDREN'S HOSPITAL, NEWINGTON, CT, p. A 76
NEWMAN MEMORIAL HOSPITAL, EMPORIA, KS, p. A152
NEWMAN MEMORIAL HOSPITAL, SHATTUCK, OK, p. A327
NEWNAN HOSPITAL, NEWNAN, GA, p. A106
NEWPORT COMMUNITY HOSPITAL, NEWPORT, WA, p. A425
NEWPORT HOSPITAL, NEWPORT, RI, p. A353
NEWPORT HOSPITAL AND CLINIC, NEWPORT, AR, p. A 33
NEWPORT NEWS GENERAL HOSPITAL, NEWPORT NEWS, VA, p. A418
NEWTON–WELLESLEY HOSPITAL, NEWTON, MA, p. A195
NEWTON GENERAL HOSPITAL, COVINGTON, GA, p. A102
NEWTON MEDICAL CENTER, NEWTON, KS, p. A156
NEWTON MEMORIAL HOSPITAL, NEWTON, NJ, p. A263
NIAGARA FALLS MEMORIAL MEDICAL CENTER, NIAGARA FALLS, NY, p. A283
NICHOLAS COUNTY HOSPITAL, CARLISLE, KY, p. A161
NICHOLAS H. NOYES MEMORIAL HOSPITAL, DANSVILLE, NY, p. A274
NIOBRARA COUNTY HOSPITAL DISTRICT, LUSK, WY, p. A446
NIOBRARA VALLEY HOSPITAL, LYNCH, NE, p. A249
NIX HEALTH CARE SYSTEM, SAN ANTONIO, TX, p. A402
NOBLE ARMY COMMUNITY HOSPITAL, FORT MCCLELLAN, AL, p. A 16
NOBLE HOSPITAL, WESTFIELD, MA, p. A198
NOCONA GENERAL HOSPITAL, NOCONA, TX, p. A398
NOR–LEA GENERAL HOSPITAL, LOVINGTON, NM, p. A269
NORFOLK COMMUNITY HOSPITAL, NORFOLK, VA, p. A418
NORFOLK PSYCHIATRIC CENTER, NORFOLK, VA, p. A418
NORFOLK REGIONAL CENTER, NORFOLK, NE, p. A249
NORMAN REGIONAL HOSPITAL, NORMAN, OK, p. A325
NORRISTOWN STATE HOSPITAL, NORRISTOWN, PA, p. A343
NORTH ADAMS REGIONAL HOSPITAL, NORTH ADAMS, MA, p. A195
NORTH ALABAMA REHABILITATION HOSPITAL, HUNTSVILLE, AL, p. A 17
NORTH ARKANSAS MEDICAL CENTER, HARRISON, AR, p. A 31
NORTH ARUNDEL HOSPITAL, GLEN BURNIE, MD, p. A187
NORTH BALDWIN HOSPITAL, BAY MINETTE, AL, p. A 13
NORTH BAY MEDICAL CENTER, NEW PORT RICHEY, FL, p. A 91
NORTH BIG HORN HOSPITAL, LOVELL, WY, p. A446
NORTH BROWARD MEDICAL CENTER, POMPANO BEACH, FL, p. A 93
NORTH CADDO MEMORIAL HOSPITAL, VIVIAN, LA, p. A179
NORTH CAROLINA BAPTIST HOSPITAL, WINSTON–SALEM, NC, p. A300
NORTH CAROLINA EYE AND EAR HOSPITAL, DURHAM, NC, p. A293
NORTH CENTRAL BRONX HOSPITAL, NEW YORK CITY, NY, p. A281
NORTH CENTRAL HEALTH CARE FACILITIES, WAUSAU, WI, p. A444
NORTH COAST REHABILITATION CENTER, SANTA ROSA, CA, p. A 63
NORTH COLORADO MEDICAL CENTER, GREELEY, CO, p. A 71
NORTH COUNTRY HOSPITAL AND HEALTH CENTER, NEWPORT, VT, p. A412
NORTH COUNTRY REGIONAL HOSPITAL, BEMIDJI, MN, p. A212
NORTH DAKOTA STATE HOSPITAL, JAMESTOWN, ND, p. A304
NORTH DALLAS REHABILITATION HOSPITAL, DALLAS, TX, p. A384
NORTH FLORIDA RECEPTION CENTER HOSPITAL, LAKE BUTLER, FL, p. A 87
NORTH FLORIDA REGIONAL MEDICAL CENTER, GAINESVILLE, FL, p. A 85
NORTH FULTON REGIONAL HOSPITAL, ROSWELL, GA, p. A107
NORTH GENERAL HOSPITAL, NEW YORK CITY, NY, p. A281
NORTH GEORGIA MEDICAL CENTER AND GILMER NURSING HOME, ELLIJAY, GA, p. A103
NORTH GREENVILLE HOSPITAL, TRAVELERS REST, SC, p. A360
NORTH HILLS HOSPITAL, NORTH RICHLAND HILLS, TX, p. A398
NORTH HILLS HOSPITAL OF KANSAS CITY, KANSAS CITY, MO, p. A234
NORTH IOWA MERCY HEALTH CENTER, MASON CITY, IA, p. A147
NORTH JACKSON HOSPITAL, BRIDGEPORT, AL, p. A 14
NORTH KANSAS CITY HOSPITAL, NORTH KANSAS CITY, MO, p. A236
NORTH LINCOLN HOSPITAL, LINCOLN CITY, OR, p. A330
NORTH LOGAN MERCY HOSPITAL, PARIS, AR, p. A 33
NORTH LOUISIANA REHABILITATION HOSPITAL, RUSTON, LA, p. A178
NORTH MEMORIAL MEDICAL CENTER, ROBBINSDALE, MN, p. A218
NORTH MISSISSIPPI MEDICAL CENTER, TUPELO, MS, p. A228
NORTH MONROE HOSPITAL, MONROE, LA, p. A175
NORTH OAKLAND MEDICAL CENTERS, PONTIAC, MI, p. A208
NORTH OAKS MEDICAL CENTER, HAMMOND, LA, p. A172
NORTH OKALOOSA MEDICAL CENTER, CRESTVIEW, FL, p. A 83
NORTH OTTAWA COMMUNITY HOSPITAL, GRAND HAVEN, MI, p. A203
NORTH PARK HOSPITAL, CHATTANOOGA, TN, p. A367
NORTH PENN HOSPITAL, LANSDALE, PA, p. A341
NORTH PHILADELPHIA HEALTH SYSTEM, PHILADELPHIA, PA, p. A345
NORTH PINE AREA HOSPITAL, SANDSTONE, MN, p. A220
NORTH RIDGE MEDICAL CENTER, FORT LAUDERDALE, FL, p. A 84
NORTH RUNNELS HOSPITAL, WINTERS, TX, p. A407

Hospitals, Alphabetically / North Shore Medical Center

NORTH SHORE MEDICAL CENTER, MIAMI, FL, p. A 90
NORTH SHORE PSYCHIATRIC HOSPITAL, SLIDELL, LA, p. A178
NORTH SHORE UNIVERSITY HOSPITAL, MANHASSET, NY, p. A277
NORTH SHORE UNIVERSITY HOSPITAL AT GLEN COVE, GLEN COVE, NY, p. A275
NORTH SHORE UNIVERSITY HOSPITAL AT PLAINVIEW, PLAINVIEW, NY, p. A285
NORTH SIDE HOSPITAL, JOHNSON CITY, TN, p. A369
NORTH STAR HOSPITAL AND COUNSELING CENTER, ANCHORAGE, AK, p. A 21
NORTH SUBURBAN MEDICAL CENTER, THORNTON, CO, p. A 73
NORTH SUNFLOWER COUNTY HOSPITAL, RULEVILLE, MS, p. A228
NORTH TEXAS MEDICAL CENTER, MCKINNEY, TX, p. A397
NORTH VALLEY HEALTH CENTER, WARREN, MN, p. A221
NORTH VALLEY HOSPITAL, WHITEFISH, MT, p. A244
NORTH VALLEY HOSPITAL, TONASKET, WA, p. A428
NORTHAMPTON–ACCOMACK MEMORIAL HOSPITAL, NASSAWADOX, VA, p. A417
NORTHBAY MEDICAL CENTER, FAIRFIELD, CA, p. A 42
NORTHEAST ALABAMA REGIONAL MEDICAL CENTER, ANNISTON, AL, p. A 13
NORTHEAST ARKANSAS REHABILITATION HOSPITAL, JONESBORO, AR, p. A 31
NORTHEAST BAPTIST HOSPITAL, SAN ANTONIO, TX, p. A402
NORTHEAST COMMUNITY HOSPITAL, BEDFORD, TX, p. A379
NORTHEAST GEORGIA MEDICAL CENTER, GAINESVILLE, GA, p. A104
NORTHEAST MEDICAL CENTER, BONHAM, TX, p. A379
NORTHEAST MEDICAL CENTER HOSPITAL, HUMBLE, TX, p. A393
NORTHEAST REHABILITATION HOSPITAL, SALEM, NH, p. A257
NORTHEASTERN HOSPITAL OF PHILADELPHIA, PHILADELPHIA, PA, p. A345
NORTHEASTERN REGIONAL HOSPITAL, LAS VEGAS, NM, p. A269
NORTHEASTERN VERMONT REGIONAL HOSPITAL, SAINT JOHNSBURY, VT, p. A412
NORTHERN COCHISE COMMUNITY HOSPITAL, WILLCOX, AZ, p. A 28
NORTHERN CUMBERLAND MEMORIAL HOSPITAL, BRIDGTON, ME, p. A180
NORTHERN DUTCHESS HOSPITAL, RHINEBECK, NY, p. A285
NORTHERN HILLS GENERAL HOSPITAL, DEADWOOD, SD, p. A361
NORTHERN HOSPITAL OF SURRY COUNTY, MOUNT AIRY, NC, p. A297
NORTHERN ILLINOIS MEDICAL CENTER, MCHENRY, IL, p. A126
NORTHERN INYO HOSPITAL, BISHOP, CA, p. A 38
NORTHERN ITASCA HEALTH CARE CENTER, BIGFORK, MN, p. A213
NORTHERN MAINE MEDICAL CENTER, FORT KENT, ME, p. A181
NORTHERN MICHIGAN HOSPITAL, PETOSKEY, MI, p. A208
NORTHERN MONTANA HOSPITAL, HAVRE, MT, p. A243
NORTHERN NEVADA MEDICAL CENTER, SPARKS, NV, p. A254
NORTHERN VIRGINIA DOCTORS' HOSPITAL, ARLINGTON, VA, p. A414
NORTHERN VIRGINIA MENTAL HEALTH INSTITUTE, FALLS CHURCH, VA, p. A415
NORTHERN WESTCHESTER HOSPITAL CENTER, MOUNT KISCO, NY, p. A278
NORTHFIELD HOSPITAL, NORTHFIELD, MN, p. A218
NORTHLAKE REGIONAL MEDICAL CENTER, ATLANTA, GA, p. A 99
NORTHPORT HOSPITAL-DCH, NORTHPORT, AL, p. A 19
NORTHRIDGE HOSPITAL MEDICAL CENTER, LOS ANGELES, CA, p. A 50
NORTHSHORE REGIONAL MEDICAL CENTER, SLIDELL, LA, p. A178
NORTHSIDE GENERAL HOSPITAL, HOUSTON, TX, p. A391
NORTHSIDE HOSPITAL, SAINT PETERSBURG, FL, p. A 94
NORTHSIDE HOSPITAL, ATLANTA, GA, p. A 99
NORTHVILLE REGIONAL PSYCHIATRIC HOSPITAL, NORTHVILLE, MI, p. A208
NORTHWEST ARKANSAS REHABILITATION HOSPITAL, FAYETTEVILLE, AR, p. A 30
NORTHWEST COMMUNITY HOSPITAL, ARLINGTON HEIGHTS, IL, p. A116
NORTHWEST COVENANT MEDICAL CENTER, DENVILLE, NJ, p. A259
NORTHWEST FAMILY HOSPITAL, GARY, IN, p. A135
NORTHWEST FLORIDA COMMUNITY HOSPITAL, CHIPLEY, FL, p. A 82
NORTHWEST GENERAL HOSPITAL, MILWAUKEE, WI, p. A440
NORTHWEST GEORGIA REGIONAL HOSPITAL, ROME, GA, p. A107

NORTHWEST HOSPITAL, TUCSON, AZ, p. A 28
NORTHWEST HOSPITAL, SEATTLE, WA, p. A427
NORTHWEST HOSPITAL CENTER, RANDALLSTOWN, MD, p. A188
NORTHWEST IOWA HEALTH CENTER, SHELDON, IA, p. A149
NORTHWEST KANSAS REGIONAL MEDICAL CENTER, GOODLAND, KS, p. A153
NORTHWEST MEDICAL CENTER, RUSSELLVILLE, AL, p. A 19
NORTHWEST MEDICAL CENTER, SPRINGDALE, AR, p. A 34
NORTHWEST MEDICAL CENTER, MARGATE, FL, p. A 89
NORTHWEST MEDICAL CENTER, THIEF RIVER FALLS, MN, p. A220
NORTHWEST MEDICAL CENTER, FRANKLIN, PA, p. A338
NORTHWEST MISSISSIPPI REGIONAL MEDICAL CENTER, CLARKSDALE, MS, p. A223
NORTHWESTERN INSTITUTE, FORT WASHINGTON, PA, p. A338
NORTHWESTERN MEDICAL CENTER, SAINT ALBANS, VT, p. A412
NORTHWESTERN MEMORIAL HOSPITAL, CHICAGO, , p. A119
NORTHWESTERN UNIVERSITY STUDENT HEALTH SERVICE HOSPITAL, EVANSTON, IL, p. A123
NORTHWOOD DEACONESS HEALTH CENTER, NORTHWOOD, ND, p. A304
NORTHWOODS HOSPITAL, PHELPS, WI, p. A441
NORTON COMMUNITY HOSPITAL, NORTON, VA, p. A418
NORTON COUNTY HOSPITAL, NORTON, KS, p. A157
NORTON SOUND REGIONAL HOSPITAL, NOME, AK, p. A 22
NORWALK HOSPITAL, NORWALK, CT, p. A 76
NORWEGIAN–AMERICAN HOSPITAL, CHICAGO, IL, p. A119
NORWICH HOSPITAL, NORWICH, CT, p. A 76
NORWOOD HEALTH CENTER, MARSHFIELD, WI, p. A439
NORWOOD HOSPITAL, NORWOOD, MA, p. A196
NOVACARE MERIDIAN POINT REHABILITATION HOSPITAL, SCOTTSDALE, AZ, p. A 26
NOVACARE VALLEY OF THE SUN REHABILITATION HOSPITAL, GLENDALE, AZ, p. A 24
NOVATO COMMUNITY HOSPITAL, NOVATO, CA, p. A 54
NOXUBEE GENERAL HOSPITAL, MACON, MS, p. A226
NYACK HOSPITAL, NYACK, NY, p. A284
NYE REGIONAL MEDICAL CENTER, TONOPAH, NV, p. A254

O

O'BLENESS MEMORIAL HOSPITAL, ATHENS, OH, p. A306
O'CONNOR HOSPITAL, SAN JOSE, CA, p. A 61
OAK CREST HOSPITAL, SHAWNEE, OK, p. A327
OAK FOREST HOSPITAL OF COOK COUNTY, OAK FOREST, IL, p. A128
OAK HILL COMMUNITY MEDICAL CENTER, OAK HILL, OH, p. A316
OAK HILL HOSPITAL, SPRING HILL, FL, p. A 95
OAK HILL HOSPITAL, JOPLIN, MO, p. A233
OAK PARK HOSPITAL, OAK PARK, IL, p. A128
OAK VALLEY DISTRICT HOSPITAL, OAKDALE, CA, p. A 54
OAKDALE COMMUNITY HOSPITAL, OAKDALE, LA, p. A177
OAKES COMMUNITY HOSPITAL, OAKES, ND, p. A304
OAKLAND GENERAL HEALTH SYSTEM, MADISON HEIGHTS, MI, p. A206
OAKLAND MEMORIAL HOSPITAL, OAKLAND, NE, p. A249
OAKLAWN HOSPITAL, MARSHALL, MI, p. A207
OAKLAWN PSYCHIATRIC CENTER, INC., GOSHEN, IN, p. A136
OAKS TREATMENT CENTER, AUSTIN, TX, p. A378
OAKWOOD FORENSIC CENTER, LIMA, OH, p. A313
OAKWOOD HOSPITAL–HERITAGE CENTER, TAYLOR, MI, p. A210
OAKWOOD HOSPITAL AND MEDICAL CENTER – DEARBORN, DEARBORN, MI, p. A201
OAKWOOD HOSPITAL ANNAPOLIS CENTER, WAYNE, MI, p. A211
OAKWOOD HOSPITAL BEYER CENTER–YPSILANTI, YPSILANTI, MI, p. A211
OAKWOOD HOSPITAL DOWNRIVER CENTER – LINCOLN PARK, LINCOLN PARK, MI, p. A206
OAKWOOD HOSPITAL SEAWAY CENTER, TRENTON, MI, p. A210
OAKWOOD MEDICAL CENTER, KNOXVILLE, TN, p. A370
OCEAN BEACH HOSPITAL, ILWACO, WA, p. A425
OCEAN SPRINGS HOSPITAL, OCEAN SPRINGS, MS, p. A227
OCHILTREE GENERAL HOSPITAL, PERRYTON, TX, p. A399
OCHSNER FOUNDATION HOSPITAL, NEW ORLEANS, LA, p. A176
OCONEE MEMORIAL HOSPITAL, SENECA, SC, p. A359
OCONEE REGIONAL MEDICAL CENTER, MILLEDGEVILLE, GA, p. A106

OCONTO MEMORIAL HOSPITAL, OCONTO, WI, p. A441
ODESSA MEMORIAL HOSPITAL, ODESSA, WA, p. A425
ODESSA REGIONAL HOSPITAL, ODESSA, TX, p. A398
OGALLALA COMMUNITY HOSPITAL, OGALLALA, NE, p. A249
OGDEN REGIONAL MEDICAL CENTER, OGDEN, UT, p. A409
OHIO COUNTY HOSPITAL, HARTFORD, KY, p. A163
OHIO STATE UNIVERSITY MEDICAL CENTER, COLUMBUS, OH, p. A310
OHIO VALLEY GENERAL HOSPITAL, MCKEES ROCKS, PA, p. A342
OHIO VALLEY HOSPITAL, STEUBENVILLE, OH, p. A317
OHIO VALLEY MEDICAL CENTER, WHEELING, WV, p. A434
OJAI VALLEY COMMUNITY HOSPITAL, OJAI, CA, p. A 55
OKANOGAN–DOUGLAS COUNTY HOSPITAL, BREWSTER, WA, p. A423
OKEENE MUNICIPAL HOSPITAL, OKEENE, OK, p. A325
OKOLONA COMMUNITY HOSPITAL, OKOLONA, MS, p. A227
OKTIBBEHA COUNTY HOSPITAL, STARKVILLE, MS, p. A228
OLATHE MEDICAL CENTER, OLATHE, KS, p. A157
OLEAN GENERAL HOSPITAL, OLEAN, NY, p. A284
OLIN E. TEAGUE VETERANS' CENTER, TEMPLE, TX, p. A404
OLIVE VIEW MEDICAL CENTER, LOS ANGELES, CA, p. A 50
OLMSTED COMMUNITY HOSPITAL, ROCHESTER, MN, p. A219
OLYMPIA FIELDS HOSPITAL AND MEDICAL CENTER, OLYMPIA FIELDS, IL, p. A128
OLYMPIC MEMORIAL HOSPITAL, PORT ANGELES, WA, p. A426
OMH MEDICAL CENTER, OKMULGEE, OK, p. A326
ONEIDA CITY HOSPITAL, ONEIDA, NY, p. A284
ONEIDA COUNTY HOSPITAL, MALAD CITY, ID, p. A113
ONSLOW MEMORIAL HOSPITAL, JACKSONVILLE, NC, p. A296
ONTARIO COMMUNITY HOSPITAL, ONTARIO, CA, p. A 55
ONTONAGON MEMORIAL HOSPITAL, ONTONAGON, MI, p. A208
OPELOUSAS GENERAL HOSPITAL, OPELOUSAS, LA, p. A177
ORANGE CITY MUNICIPAL HOSPITAL, ORANGE CITY, IA, p. A148
ORANGE COUNTY COMMUNITY HOSPITAL OF BUENA PARK, BUENA PARK, CA, p. A 38
ORANGE COUNTY HOSPITAL, PAOLI, IN, p. A139
ORANGE PARK MEDICAL CENTER, ORANGE PARK, FL, p. A 91
OREGON STATE HOSPITAL, SALEM, OR, p. A332
OREM COMMUNITY HOSPITAL, OREM, UT, p. A409
ORLANDO REGIONAL MEDICAL CENTER, ORLANDO, FL, p. A 91
OROVILLE HOSPITAL, OROVILLE, CA, p. A 55
ORTHOPAEDIC HOSPITAL, LOS ANGELES, CA, p. A 50
ORTONVILLE AREA HEALTH SERVICES, ORTONVILLE, MN, p. A218
OSAWATOMIE STATE HOSPITAL, OSAWATOMIE, KS, p. A157
OSBORNE COUNTY MEMORIAL HOSPITAL, OSBORNE, KS, p. A157
OSCEOLA COMMUNITY HOSPITAL, SIBLEY, IA, p. A149
OSCEOLA MEDICAL CENTER, OSCEOLA, WI, p. A441
OSCEOLA REGIONAL MEDICAL CENTER, KISSIMMEE, FL, p. A 87
OSMOND GENERAL HOSPITAL, OSMOND, NE, p. A251
OSSEO AREA MUNICIPAL HOSPITAL AND NURSING HOME, OSSEO, WI, p. A441
OSSINING CORRECTIONAL FACILITIES HOSPITAL, OSSINING, NY, p. A284
OSTEOPATHIC MEDICAL CENTER OF TEXAS, FORT WORTH, TX, p. A387
OSWEGO HOSPITAL, OSWEGO, NY, p. A284
OTHELLO COMMUNITY HOSPITAL, OTHELLO, WA, p. A426
OTSEGO MEMORIAL HOSPITAL, GAYLORD, MI, p. A203
OTTAWA COUNTY HOSPITAL, MINNEAPOLIS, KS, p. A156
OTTO KAISER MEMORIAL HOSPITAL, KENEDY, TX, p. A393
OTTUMWA REGIONAL HEALTH CENTER, OTTUMWA, IA, p. A148
OUACHITA MEDICAL CENTER, CAMDEN, AR, p. A 29
OUR COMMUNITY HOSPITAL, SCOTLAND NECK, NC, p. A299
OUR LADY OF BELLEFONTE HOSPITAL, ASHLAND, KY, p. A161
OUR LADY OF LAKE REGIONAL MEDICAL CENTER, BATON ROUGE, LA, p. A170
OUR LADY OF LOURDES HEALTH CENTER, PASCO, WA, p. A426
OUR LADY OF LOURDES HOSPITAL, NORFOLK, NE, p. A249
OUR LADY OF LOURDES MEDICAL CENTER, CAMDEN, NJ, p. A258
OUR LADY OF LOURDES MEMORIAL HOSPITAL, BINGHAMTON, NY, p. A272
OUR LADY OF LOURDES REGIONAL MEDICAL CENTER, LAFAYETTE, LA, p. A174
OUR LADY OF LOURDES REHABILITATION HOSPITAL OF WICHITA, WICHITA, KS, p. A160
OUR LADY OF MERCY MEDICAL CENTER, NEW YORK CITY, NY, p. A281
OUR LADY OF THE RESURRECTION MEDICAL CENTER, CHICAGO, IL, p. A119
OUR LADY OF THE WAY HOSPITAL, MARTIN, KY, p. A166
OUR LADY OF VICTORY HOSPITAL, LACKAWANNA, NY, p. A276
OVERLAKE HOSPITAL MEDICAL CENTER, BELLEVUE, WA, p. A423

Hospitals, Alphabetically / Pocahontas Community Hospital

OVERLAND PARK REGIONAL MEDICAL CENTER, OVERLAND PARK, KS, p. A157
OVERLOOK HOSPITAL, SUMMIT, NJ, p. A265
OVERTON BROOKS VETERANS AFFAIRS MEDICAL CENTER, SHREVEPORT, LA, p. A178
OWATONNA HOSPITAL, OWATONNA, MN, p. A218
OWEN COUNTY MEMORIAL HOSPITAL, OWENTON, KY, p. A167
OWENSBORO–DAVIESS COUNTY HOSPITAL, OWENSBORO, KY, p. A167
OZARKS MEDICAL CENTER, WEST PLAINS, MO, p. A240

P

PACIFIC ALLIANCE MEDICAL CENTER, LOS ANGELES, CA, p. A 50
PACIFIC COAST HOSPITAL, SAN FRANCISCO, CA, p. A 60
PACIFIC COMMUNITIES HOSPITAL, NEWPORT, OR, p. A331
PACIFIC GATEWAY HOSPITAL AND COUNSELING CENTER, PORTLAND, OR, p. A332
PACIFIC HOSPITAL OF LONG BEACH, LONG BEACH, CA, p. A 48
PACIFICA HOSPITAL, HUNTINGTON BEACH, CA, p. A 45
PACIFICA HOSPITAL OF THE VALLEY, LOS ANGELES, CA, p. A 50
PAGE HOSPITAL, PAGE, AZ, p. A 25
PAGE MEMORIAL HOSPITAL, LURAY, VA, p. A417
PALISADES GENERAL HOSPITAL, NORTH BERGEN, NJ, p. A263
PALM BEACH GARDENS MEDICAL CENTER, PALM BEACH GARDENS, FL, p. A 92
PALM BEACH REGIONAL HOSPITAL, LAKE WORTH, FL, p. A 87
PALM DRIVE HOSPITAL, SEBASTOPOL, CA, p. A 63
PALM SPRINGS GENERAL HOSPITAL, HIALEAH, FL, p. A 85
PALMER LUTHERAN HEALTH CENTER, WEST UNION, IA, p. A150
PALMERTON HOSPITAL, PALMERTON, PA, p. A343
PALMETTO GENERAL HOSPITAL, HIALEAH, FL, p. A 85
PALMS OF PASADENA HOSPITAL, SAINT PETERSBURG, FL, p. A 94
PALMS WEST HOSPITAL, LOXAHATCHEE, FL, p. A 88
PALMVIEW HOSPITAL, LAKELAND, FL, p. A 87
PALMYRA MEDICAL CENTERS, ALBANY, GA, p. A 98
PALO ALTO COUNTY HOSPITAL, EMMETSBURG, IA, p. A145
PALO DURO HOSPITAL, CANYON, TX, p. A380
PALO PINTO GENERAL HOSPITAL, MINERAL WELLS, TX, p. A397
PALO VERDE HOSPITAL, BLYTHE, CA, p. A 38
PALOMAR MEDICAL CENTER, ESCONDIDO, CA, p. A 42
PALOS COMMUNITY HOSPITAL, PALOS HEIGHTS, IL, p. A128
PAN AMERICAN HOSPITAL, MIAMI, FL, p. A 90
PANA COMMUNITY HOSPITAL, PANA, IL, p. A128
PANOLA GENERAL HOSPITAL, CARTHAGE, TX, p. A381
PAOLI MEMORIAL HOSPITAL, PAOLI, PA, p. A343
PARADISE VALLEY HOSPITAL, PHOENIX, AZ, p. A 25
PARADISE VALLEY HOSPITAL, NATIONAL CITY, CA, p. A 54
PARIS COMMUNITY HOSPITAL, PARIS, IL, p. A128
PARK LANE MEDICAL CENTER, KANSAS CITY, MO, p. A234
PARK MEDICAL CENTER, COLUMBUS, OH, p. A310
PARK PLACE MEDICAL CENTER, PORT ARTHUR, TX, p. A400
PARK RIDGE HOSPITAL, ROCHESTER, NY, p. A286
PARK RIDGE HOSPITAL, FLETCHER, NC, p. A294
PARK VIEW HOSPITAL, EL RENO, OK, p. A323
PARKER COMMUNITY HOSPITAL, PARKER, AZ, p. A 25
PARKLAND HEALTH CENTER, FARMINGTON, MO, p. A232
PARKLAND HOSPITAL, BATON ROUGE, LA, p. A170
PARKLAND MEDICAL CENTER, DERRY, NH, p. A255
PARKRIDGE MEDICAL CENTER, CHATTANOOGA, TN, p. A367
PARKSIDE HOSPITAL, TULSA, OK, p. A328
PARKVIEW COMMUNITY HOSPITAL MEDICAL CENTER, RIVERSIDE, CA, p. A 57
PARKVIEW EPISCOPAL MEDICAL CENTER, PUEBLO, CO, p. A 72
PARKVIEW HOSPITAL, WHEELER, TX, p. A407
PARKVIEW MEMORIAL HOSPITAL, FORT WAYNE, IN, p. A135
PARKVIEW MEMORIAL HOSPITAL, BRUNSWICK, ME, p. A181
PARKVIEW REGIONAL HOSPITAL, MEXIA, TX, p. A397
PARKVIEW REGIONAL MEDICAL CENTER, VICKSBURG, MS, p. A228
PARKWAY HOSPITAL, NEW YORK CITY, NY, p. A282
PARKWAY HOSPITAL, HOUSTON, TX, p. A391
PARKWAY MEDICAL CENTER, LITHIA SPRINGS, GA, p. A105
PARKWAY MEDICAL CENTER HOSPITAL, DECATUR, AL, p. A 15
PARKWAY REGIONAL HOSPITAL, FULTON, KY, p. A163
PARKWAY REGIONAL MEDICAL CENTER, NORTH MIAMI BEACH, FL, p. A 91

PARKWOOD HOSPITAL, OLIVE BRANCH, MS, p. A227
PARMA COMMUNITY GENERAL HOSPITAL, PARMA, OH, p. A316
PARMER COUNTY COMMUNITY HOSPITAL, FRIONA, TX, p. A387
PARRISH MEDICAL CENTER, TITUSVILLE, FL, p. A 97
PARSONS STATE HOSPITAL AND TRAINING CENTER, PARSONS, KS, p. A157
PASADENA GENERAL HOSPITAL, PASADENA, TX, p. A399
PASCACK VALLEY HOSPITAL, WESTWOOD, NJ, p. A266
PASSAVANT AREA HOSPITAL, JACKSONVILLE, IL, p. A125
PASSAVANT HOSPITAL, PITTSBURGH, PA, p. A347
PATTERSON ARMY COMMUNITY HOSPITAL, FORT MONMOUTH, NJ, p. A260
PATTERSON HOSPITAL, CUTHBERT, GA, p. A102
PATTIE A. CLAY HOSPITAL, RICHMOND, KY, p. A168
PATTON STATE HOSPITAL, PATTON, CA, p. A 56
PAUL B. HALL REGIONAL MEDICAL CENTER, PAINTSVILLE, KY, p. A167
PAUL OLIVER MEMORIAL HOSPITAL, FRANKFORT, MI, p. A203
PAULDING COUNTY HOSPITAL, PAULDING, OH, p. A316
PAULINE WARFIELD LEWIS CENTER, CINCINNATI, OH, p. A308
PAULS VALLEY GENERAL HOSPITAL, PAULS VALLEY, OK, p. A326
PAWATING HOSPITAL, NILES, MI, p. A208
PAWHUSKA HOSPITAL, PAWHUSKA, OK, p. A326
PAWNEE COUNTY MEMORIAL HOSPITAL, PAWNEE CITY, NE, p. A251
PAWNEE MUNICIPAL HOSPITAL, PAWNEE, OK, p. A326
PAYNESVILLE AREA HOSPITAL, PAYNESVILLE, MN, p. A218
PAYSON REGIONAL MEDICAL CENTER, PAYSON, AZ, p. A 25
PEACE HARBOR HOSPITAL, FLORENCE, OR, p. A330
PEACH COUNTY HOSPITAL, FORT VALLEY, GA, p. A104
PEACHTREE REGIONAL HOSPITAL, NEWNAN, GA, p. A106
PEARL RIVER COUNTY HOSPITAL, POPLARVILLE, MS, p. A227
PECOS COUNTY GENERAL HOSPITAL, IRAAN, TX, p. A393
PECOS COUNTY MEMORIAL HOSPITAL, FORT STOCKTON, TX, p. A386
PEDIATRIC CENTER FOR RESTORATIVE CARE, DALLAS, TX, p. A384
PEKIN HOSPITAL, PEKIN, IL, p. A128
PELLA COMMUNITY HOSPITAL, PELLA, IA, p. A148
PEMBINA COUNTY MEMORIAL HOSPITAL AND WEDGEWOOD MANOR, CAVALIER, ND, p. A302
PEMBROKE HOSPITAL, PEMBROKE, MA, p. A196
PEMISCOT MEMORIAL HEALTH SYSTEM, HAYTI, MO, p. A232
PENDER COMMUNITY HOSPITAL, PENDER, NE, p. A251
PENDER MEMORIAL HOSPITAL, BURGAW, NC, p. A292
PENDLETON MEMORIAL METHODIST HOSPITAL, NEW ORLEANS, LA, p. A176
PENINSULA HOSPITAL, LOUISVILLE, TN, p. A371
PENINSULA HOSPITAL CENTER, NEW YORK CITY, NY, p. A282
PENINSULA MEDICAL CENTER, ORMOND BEACH, FL, p. A 92
PENINSULA PSYCHIATRIC HOSPITAL, HAMPTON, VA, p. A416
PENINSULA REGIONAL MEDICAL CENTER, SALISBURY, MD, p. A188
PENN STATE UNIVERSITY HOSPITAL – MILTON S. HERSHEY MEDICAL CENTER, HERSHEY, PA, p. A340
PENNOCK HOSPITAL, HASTINGS, MI, p. A204
PENNSYLVANIA HOSPITAL, PHILADELPHIA, PA, p. A345
PENOBSCOT BAY MEDICAL CENTER, ROCKPORT, ME, p. A182
PENOBSCOT VALLEY HOSPITAL, LINCOLN, ME, p. A181
PENROSE–ST. FRANCIS HEALTHCARE SYSTEM, COLORADO SPRINGS, , p. A 68
PEOPLE'S MEMORIAL HOSPITAL, INDEPENDENCE, IA, p. A146
PEOPLES HOSPITAL, MANSFIELD, OH, p. A314
PERHAM MEMORIAL HOSPITAL AND HOME, PERHAM, MN, p. A218
PERKINS COUNTY HEALTH SERVICES, GRANT, NE, p. A248
PERMIAN GENERAL HOSPITAL, ANDREWS, TX, p. A377
PERRY COUNTY GENERAL HOSPITAL, RICHTON, MS, p. A227
PERRY COUNTY MEMORIAL HOSPITAL, TELL CITY, IN, p. A141
PERRY COUNTY MEMORIAL HOSPITAL, PERRYVILLE, MO, p. A236
PERRY HOSPITAL, PERRY, GA, p. A107
PERRY MEMORIAL HOSPITAL, PRINCETON, IL, p. A129
PERRY MEMORIAL HOSPITAL, PERRY, OK, p. A326
PERRY MEMORIAL HOSPITAL, LINDEN, TN, p. A371
PERSHING GENERAL HOSPITAL, LOVELOCK, NV, p. A253
PERSON COUNTY MEMORIAL HOSPITAL, ROXBORO, NC, p. A298
PETALUMA VALLEY HOSPITAL, PETALUMA, CA, p. A 56
PETERSBURG MEDICAL CENTER, PETERSBURG, AK, p. A 22
PHELPS COUNTY REGIONAL MEDICAL CENTER, ROLLA, MO, p. A237
PHELPS MEMORIAL HEALTH CENTER, HOLDREGE, NE, p. A248
PHELPS MEMORIAL HOSPITAL CENTER, NORTH TARRYTOWN, NY, p. A283
PHENIX REGIONAL HOSPITAL, PHENIX CITY, AL, p. A 19

PHILHAVEN, MOUNT GRETNA, PA, p. A342
PHILLIPS COUNTY HOSPITAL, PHILLIPSBURG, KS, p. A157
PHILLIPS COUNTY HOSPITAL, MALTA, MT, p. A243
PHILLIPS EYE INSTITUTE, MINNEAPOLIS, MN, p. A217
PHOEBE PUTNEY MEMORIAL HOSPITAL, ALBANY, GA, p. A 98
PHOENIX BAPTIST HOSPITAL AND MEDICAL CENTER, PHOENIX, AZ, p. A 25
PHOENIX CHILDREN'S HOSPITAL, PHOENIX, AZ, p. A 26
PHOENIX GENERAL HOSPITAL AND MEDICAL CENTER, PHOENIX, AZ, p. A 26
PHOENIXVILLE HOSPITAL, PHOENIXVILLE, PA, p. A346
PHS SANTA FE INDIAN HOSPITAL, SANTA FE, NM, p. A270
PHYSICIANS AND SURGEONS HOSPITAL, MIDLAND, TX, p. A397
PHYSICIANS COMMUNITY HOSPITAL, SAINT PETERSBURG, FL, p. A 94
PHYSICIANS MEMORIAL HOSPITAL, LA PLATA, MD, p. A187
PHYSICIANS REGIONAL HOSPITAL, WYLIE, TX, p. A407
PICKENS COUNTY MEDICAL CENTER, CARROLLTON, AL, p. A 14
PIEDMONT GERIATRIC HOSPITAL, BURKEVILLE, VA, p. A414
PIEDMONT HOSPITAL, ATLANTA, GA, p. A 99
PIEDMONT MEDICAL CENTER, ROCK HILL, SC, p. A359
PIGGOTT COMMUNITY HOSPITAL, PIGGOTT, AR, p. A 33
PIKE COMMUNITY HOSPITAL, WAVERLY, OH, p. A319
PIKE COUNTY MEMORIAL HOSPITAL, MURFREESBORO, AR, p. A 33
PIKE COUNTY MEMORIAL HOSPITAL, LOUISIANA, MO, p. A235
PIKEVILLE UNITED METHODIST HOSPITAL OF KENTUCKY, PIKEVILLE, KY, p. A167
PILGRIM PSYCHIATRIC CENTER, WEST BRENTWOOD, NY, p. A289
PINCKNEYVILLE COMMUNITY HOSPITAL, PINCKNEYVILLE, IL, p. A129
PINE CREST HOSPITAL AND COUNSELING CENTER, COEUR D'ALENE, ID, p. A113
PINE GROVE HOSPITAL AND MENTAL HEALTH CENTER, LOS ANGELES, CA, p. A 50
PINE REST CHRISTIAN HOSPITAL, GRAND RAPIDS, MI, p. A204
PINECREST REHABILITATION HOSPITAL, DELRAY, FL, p. A 83
PINELAKE MEDICAL CENTER, MAYFIELD, KY, p. A166
PINELANDS HOSPITAL, NACOGDOCHES, TX, p. A398
PINELLAS COMMUNITY HOSPITAL, PINELLAS PARK, FL, p. A 93
PINEVILLE COMMUNITY HOSPITAL ASSOCIATION, PINEVILLE, KY, p. A167
PINEYWOODS HOSPITAL, LUFKIN, TX, p. A396
PINON HILLS HOSPITAL, SANTA FE, NM, p. A270
PIONEER HOSPITAL, ARTESIA, CA, p. A 37
PIONEER MEMORIAL HOSPITAL, HEPPNER, OR, p. A330
PIONEER MEMORIAL HOSPITAL, PRINEVILLE, OR, p. A332
PIONEER MEMORIAL HOSPITAL, VIBORG, SD, p. A364
PIONEER VALLEY HOSPITAL, WEST VALLEY CITY, UT, p. A411
PIONEERS HOSPITAL OF RIO BLANCO COUNTY, MEEKER, CO, p. A 72
PIONEERS MEMORIAL HOSPITAL, BRAWLEY, CA, p. A 38
PIPESTONE COUNTY MEDICAL CENTER, PIPESTONE, MN, p. A218
PIPP COMMUNITY HOSPITAL, PLAINWELL, MI, p. A208
PIQUA MEMORIAL MEDICAL CENTER, PIQUA, OH, p. A316
PITT COUNTY MEMORIAL HOSPITAL–UNIVERSITY MEDICAL CENTER OF EASTERN CAROLINA–PITT COUNTY, GREENVILLE, NC, p. A295
PLACENTIA–LINDA COMMUNITY HOSPITAL, PLACENTIA, CA, p. A 56
PLAINS MEMORIAL HOSPITAL, DIMMITT, TX, p. A385
PLAINS REGIONAL MEDICAL CENTER–PORTALES, PORTALES, NM, p. A269
PLAINS REGIONAL MEDICAL CENTER – CLOVIS, CLOVIS, NM, p. A268
PLAINVIEW PUBLIC HOSPITAL, PLAINVIEW, NE, p. A251
PLAINVILLE RURAL HOSPITAL DISTRICT NUMBER ONE, PLAINVILLE, KS, p. A158
PLANO REHABILITATION HOSPITAL, PLANO, TX, p. A400
PLANTATION GENERAL HOSPITAL, PLANTATION, FL, p. A 93
PLATEAU MEDICAL CENTER, OAK HILL, WV, p. A432
PLATTE COMMUNITY MEMORIAL HOSPITAL, PLATTE, SD, p. A363
PLATTE COUNTY MEMORIAL HOSPITAL, WHEATLAND, WY, p. A446
PLATTE VALLEY MEDICAL CENTER, BRIGHTON, CO, p. A 68
PLAZA MEDICAL CENTER–EAST, FORT WORTH, TX, p. A387
PLAZA MEDICAL CENTER–WEST, FORT WORTH, TX, p. A387
PLAZA REHABILITATION HOSPITAL AT KINGWOOD, KINGWOOD, TX, p. A394
PLEASANT VALLEY HOSPITAL, POINT PLEASANT, WV, p. A433
PLUMAS DISTRICT HOSPITAL, QUINCY, CA, p. A 57
PMH HEALTH SERVICES NETWORK, PHOENIX, AZ, p. A 26
POCAHONTAS COMMUNITY HOSPITAL, POCAHONTAS, IA, p. A149

© 1995 AHA Guide Hospitals A473

Hospitals, Alphabetically / Pocahontas Memorial Hospital

POCAHONTAS MEMORIAL HOSPITAL, MARLINTON, WV, p. A432
POCATELLO REGIONAL MEDICAL CENTER, POCATELLO, ID, p. A114
POCONO MEDICAL CENTER, EAST STROUDSBURG, PA, p. A337
PODIATRY HOSPITAL OF PITTSBURGH, PITTSBURGH, PA, p. A347
POINTE COUPEE GENERAL HOSPITAL, NEW ROADS, LA, p. A177
POLK COUNTY MEMORIAL HOSPITAL, LIVINGSTON, TX, p. A395
POLK GENERAL HOSPITAL, BARTOW, FL, p. A 81
POLK GENERAL HOSPITAL, CEDARTOWN, GA, p. A101
POLLY RYON MEMORIAL HOSPITAL, RICHMOND, TX, p. A400
POLYCLINIC MEDICAL CENTER OF HARRISBURG, HARRISBURG, PA, p. A339
POMERADO HOSPITAL, POWAY, CA, p. A 56
POMONA VALLEY HOSPITAL MEDICAL CENTER, POMONA, CA, p. A 56
POMPANO BEACH MEDICAL CENTER, POMPANO BEACH, FL, p. A 93
PONCE REGIONAL HOSPITAL, PONCE, PR, p. A449
PONDERA MEDICAL CENTER, CONRAD, MT, p. A241
PONTIAC OSTEOPATHIC HOSPITAL, PONTIAC, MI, p. A208
PONTOTOC HOSPITAL AND EXTENDED CARE FACILITY, PONTOTOC, MS, p. A227
POPLAR SPRINGS HOSPITAL, PETERSBURG, VA, p. A418
PORT HURON HOSPITAL, PORT HURON, MI, p. A209
PORTAGE HOSPITAL, HANCOCK, MI, p. A204
PORTER CARE HOSPITAL–LITTLETON, LITTLETON, CO, p. A 71
PORTER CARE HOSPITAL, DENVER, CO, p. A 69
PORTER HOSPITAL, MIDDLEBURY, VT, p. A412
PORTER MEMORIAL HOSPITAL, VALPARAISO, IN, p. A141
PORTERVILLE DEVELOPMENTAL CENTER, PORTERVILLE, CA, p. A 56
PORTLAND ADVENTIST MEDICAL CENTER, PORTLAND, OR, p. A332
PORTSMOUTH GENERAL HOSPITAL, PORTSMOUTH, VA, p. A419
PORTSMOUTH RECEIVING HOSPITAL, PORTSMOUTH, OH, p. A316
PORTSMOUTH REGIONAL HOSPITAL, PORTSMOUTH, NH, p. A257
POTOMAC HOSPITAL, WOODBRIDGE, VA, p. A422
POTOMAC VALLEY HOSPITAL, KEYSER, WV, p. A431
POTTERS MEDICAL CENTER, EAST LIVERPOOL, OH, p. A312
POTTSTOWN MEMORIAL MEDICAL CENTER, POTTSTOWN, PA, p. A348
POTTSVILLE HOSPITAL AND WARNE CLINIC, POTTSVILLE, PA, p. A348
POUDRE VALLEY HOSPITAL, FORT COLLINS, CO, p. A 70
POWELL COUNTY MEMORIAL HOSPITAL, DEER LODGE, MT, p. A242
POWELL HOSPITAL, POWELL, WY, p. A446
PRAIRIE COMMUNITY MEDICAL ASSISTANCE FACILITY, TERRY, MT, p. A244
PRAIRIE DU CHIEN MEMORIAL HOSPITAL, PRAIRIE DU CHIEN, WI, p. A442
PRAIRIE LAKES HOSPITAL AND CARE CENTER, WATERTOWN, SD, p. A364
PRAIRIE VIEW, NEWTON, KS, p. A156
PRATT REGIONAL MEDICAL CENTER, PRATT, KS, p. A158
PRESBYTERIAN–ORTHOPAEDIC HOSPITAL, CHARLOTTE, NC, p. A292
PRESBYTERIAN–ST. LUKE'S MEDICAL CENTER, DENVER, CO, p. A 69
PRESBYTERIAN HOSPITAL, ALBUQUERQUE, NM, p. A267
PRESBYTERIAN HOSPITAL, CHARLOTTE, NC, p. A292
PRESBYTERIAN HOSPITAL, OKLAHOMA CITY, OK, p. A325
PRESBYTERIAN HOSPITAL IN THE CITY OF NEW YORK, NEW YORK CITY, NY, p. A282
PRESBYTERIAN HOSPITAL OF DALLAS, DALLAS, TX, p. A384
PRESBYTERIAN HOSPITAL OF KAUFMAN, KAUFMAN, TX, p. A393
PRESBYTERIAN HOSPITAL OF PLANO, PLANO, TX, p. A400
PRESBYTERIAN HOSPITAL OF WINNSBORO, WINNSBORO, TX, p. A407
PRESBYTERIAN INTERCOMMUNITY HOSPITAL, WHITTIER, CA, p. A 67
PRESBYTERIAN KASEMAN HOSPITAL, ALBUQUERQUE, NM, p. A267
PRESBYTERIAN MEDICAL CENTER OF PHILADELPHIA, PHILADELPHIA, PA, p. A345
PRESBYTERIAN SPECIALTY HOSPITAL, CHARLOTTE, NC, p. A292
PRESENTATION MEDICAL CENTER, ROLLA, ND, p. A304
PRESTON MEMORIAL HOSPITAL, KINGWOOD, WV, p. A431
PREVOST MEMORIAL HOSPITAL, DONALDSONVILLE, LA, p. A172

PRIMARY CHILDREN'S MEDICAL CENTER, SALT LAKE CITY, UT, p. A410
PRINCE GEORGE'S HOSPITAL CENTER, CHEVERLY, MD, p. A186
PRINCE WILLIAM HOSPITAL, MANASSAS, VA, p. A417
PRINCETON COMMUNITY HOSPITAL, PRINCETON, WV, p. A433
PRINCETON HOSPITAL, ORLANDO, FL, p. A 92
PRINCETON UNIVERSITY HEALTH SERVICES, MCCOSH HEALTH CENTER, PRINCETON, NJ, p. A264
PROCTOR HOSPITAL, PEORIA, IL, p. A129
PROMINA DOUGLAS HOSPITAL, DOUGLASVILLE, GA, p. A103
PROMINA GWINNETT HOSPITAL SYSTEM, LAWRENCEVILLE, GA, p. A105
PROMINA PAULDING MEMORIAL MEDICAL CENTER, DALLAS, GA, p. A102
PROMINA R. T. JONES HOSPITAL, CANTON, GA, p. A101
PROMINA WINDY HILL HOSPITAL, MARIETTA, GA, p. A106
PROSSER MEMORIAL HOSPITAL, PROSSER, WA, p. A426
PROVENANT ST. ANTHONY HOSPITAL CENTRAL, DENVER, CO, p. A 69
PROVENANT ST. ANTHONY HOSPITAL NORTH, WESTMINSTER, CO, p. A 73
PROVIDENCE ALASKA MEDICAL CENTER, ANCHORAGE, AK, p. A 21
PROVIDENCE CENTRALIA HOSPITAL, CENTRALIA, WA, p. A423
PROVIDENCE GENERAL MEDICAL CENTER, EVERETT, WA, p. A424
PROVIDENCE HEALTH CENTER, WACO, TX, p. A406
PROVIDENCE HOSPITAL, MOBILE, AL, p. A 18
PROVIDENCE HOSPITAL, WASHINGTON, DC, p. A 79
PROVIDENCE HOSPITAL, HOLYOKE, MA, p. A194
PROVIDENCE HOSPITAL, CINCINNATI, OH, p. A308
PROVIDENCE HOSPITAL, SANDUSKY, OH, p. A317
PROVIDENCE HOSPITAL, COLUMBIA, SC, p. A356
PROVIDENCE HOSPITAL AND MEDICAL CENTERS, SOUTHFIELD, MI, p. A210
PROVIDENCE MEDFORD MEDICAL CENTER, MEDFORD, OR, p. A331
PROVIDENCE MEDICAL CENTER, KANSAS CITY, KS, p. A154
PROVIDENCE MEDICAL CENTER, WAYNE, NE, p. A252
PROVIDENCE MEMORIAL HOSPITAL, EL PASO, TX, p. A385
PROVIDENCE MILWAUKIE HOSPITAL, MILWAUKIE, OR, p. A331
PROVIDENCE NEWBERG HOSPITAL, NEWBERG, OR, p. A331
PROVIDENCE PORTLAND MEDICAL CENTER, PORTLAND, OR, p. A332
PROVIDENCE SEASIDE HOSPITAL, SEASIDE, OR, p. A333
PROVIDENCE SEATTLE MEDICAL CENTER, SEATTLE, WA, p. A427
PROVIDENCE ST. PETER HOSPITAL, OLYMPIA, WA, p. A426
PROVIDENCE ST. VINCENT MEDICAL CENTER, PORTLAND, OR, p. A332
PROVIDENCE TOPPENISH HOSPITAL, TOPPENISH, WA, p. A428
PROVIDENCE YAKIMA MEDICAL CENTER, YAKIMA, WA, p. A429
PROVIDENT HOSPITAL OF COOK COUNTY, CHICAGO, IL, p. A119
PROWERS MEDICAL CENTER, LAMAR, CO, p. A 71
PSYCHIATRIC HOSPITAL AT VANDERBILT, NASHVILLE, TN, p. A373
PSYCHIATRIC INSTITUTE OF ATLANTA, ATLANTA, GA, p. A 99
PSYCHIATRIC INSTITUTE OF RICHMOND, RICHMOND, VA, p. A420
PSYCHIATRIC INSTITUTE OF WASHINGTON, WASHINGTON, DC, p. A 79
PUBLIC HEALTH SERVICE INDIAN HOSPITAL, ALBUQUERQUE, NM, p. A267
PUBLIC HOSPITAL OF THE TOWN OF SALEM, SALEM, IL, p. A130
PUGET SOUND HOSPITAL, TACOMA, WA, p. A428
PULASKI COMMUNITY HOSPITAL, PULASKI, VA, p. A419
PULASKI MEMORIAL HOSPITAL, WINAMAC, IN, p. A141
PULLMAN MEMORIAL HOSPITAL, PULLMAN, WA, p. A426
PUNGO DISTRICT HOSPITAL, BELHAVEN, NC, p. A291
PUNXSUTAWNEY AREA HOSPITAL, PUNXSUTAWNEY, PA, p. A348
PURCELL MUNICIPAL HOSPITAL, PURCELL, OK, p. A326
PUSHMATAHA COUNTY–TOWN OF ANTLERS HOSPITAL AUTHORITY, ANTLERS, OK, p. A321
PUTNAM COMMUNITY HOSPITAL, PALATKA, FL, p. A 92
PUTNAM COUNTY HOSPITAL, GREENCASTLE, IN, p. A136
PUTNAM GENERAL HOSPITAL, EATONTON, GA, p. A103
PUTNAM GENERAL HOSPITAL, HURRICANE, WV, p. A431
PUTNAM HOSPITAL CENTER, CARMEL, NY, p. A273

Q

QUAKERTOWN COMMUNITY HOSPITAL, QUAKERTOWN, PA, p. A348
QUEEN OF ANGELS–HOLLYWOOD PRESBYTERIAN MEDICAL CENTER, LOS ANGELES, CA, p. A 50
QUEEN OF PEACE HOSPITAL, NEW PRAGUE, MN, p. A218
QUEEN OF PEACE HOSPITAL, MITCHELL, SD, p. A363
QUEEN OF THE VALLEY HOSPITAL, NAPA, CA, p. A 53
QUEEN OF THE VALLEY HOSPITAL, WEST COVINA, CA, p. A 67
QUEEN'S MEDICAL CENTER, HONOLULU, HI, p. A110
QUEENS CHILDREN'S PSYCHIATRIC CENTER, NEW YORK CITY, NY, p. A282
QUEENS HOSPITAL CENTER, NEW YORK CITY, NY, p. A282
QUINCY HOSPITAL, QUINCY, MA, p. A196
QUINCY VALLEY HOSPITAL, QUINCY, WA, p. A426
QUITMAN COUNTY HOSPITAL AND NURSING HOME, MARKS, MS, p. A226

R

R. E. THOMASON GENERAL HOSPITAL, EL PASO, TX, p. A385
R. J. REYNOLDS–PATRICK COUNTY MEMORIAL HOSPITAL, STUART, VA, p. A421
RABUN COUNTY MEMORIAL HOSPITAL, CLAYTON, GA, p. A101
RADFORD COMMUNITY HOSPITAL, RADFORD, VA, p. A419
RAHWAY HOSPITAL, RAHWAY, NJ, p. A264
RALEIGH COMMUNITY HOSPITAL, RALEIGH, NC, p. A298
RALEIGH GENERAL HOSPITAL, BECKLEY, WV, p. A430
RAMAPO RIDGE PSYCHIATRIC HOSPITAL, WYCKOFF, NJ, p. A266
RANCOCAS HOSPITAL, WILLINGBORO, NJ, p. A266
RANDOLPH COUNTY HOSPITAL, ROANOKE, AL, p. A 19
RANDOLPH COUNTY HOSPITAL, WINCHESTER, IN, p. A141
RANDOLPH COUNTY MEDICAL CENTER, POCAHONTAS, AR, p. A 34
RANDOLPH HOSPITAL, ASHEBORO, NC, p. A291
RANGELY DISTRICT HOSPITAL, RANGELY, CO, p. A 72
RANKIN HOSPITAL DISTRICT, RANKIN, TX, p. A400
RANKIN MEDICAL CENTER, BRANDON, MS, p. A222
RANSOM MEMORIAL HOSPITAL, OTTAWA, KS, p. A157
RAPID CITY REGIONAL HOSPITAL, RAPID CITY, SD, p. A363
RAPIDES REGIONAL MEDICAL CENTER, ALEXANDRIA, LA, p. A170
RAPPAHANNOCK GENERAL HOSPITAL, KILMARNOCK, VA, p. A416
RARITAN BAY MEDICAL CENTER, PERTH AMBOY, NJ, p. A263
RAULERSON HOSPITAL, OKEECHOBEE, FL, p. A 91
RAVENSWOOD HOSPITAL MEDICAL CENTER, CHICAGO, IL, p. A119
RAWLINS COUNTY HOSPITAL, ATWOOD, KS, p. A151
RAY COUNTY MEMORIAL HOSPITAL, RICHMOND, MO, p. A237
RAYMOND W. BLISS ARMY COMMUNITY HOSPITAL, FORT HUACHUCA, AZ, p. A 24
READING HOSPITAL AND MEDICAL CENTER, WEST READING, PA, p. A351
READING REHABILITATION HOSPITAL, READING, PA, p. A348
REAGAN MEMORIAL HOSPITAL, BIG LAKE, TX, p. A379
REBSAMEN REGIONAL MEDICAL CENTER, JACKSONVILLE, AR, p. A 31
RED BAY HOSPITAL, RED BAY, AL, p. A 19
RED RIVER GENERAL HOSPITAL, CLARKSVILLE, TX, p. A381
RED RIVER HOSPITAL, WICHITA FALLS, TX, p. A407
REDBUD COMMUNITY HOSPITAL, CLEARLAKE, CA, p. A 40
REDDING MEDICAL CENTER, REDDING, CA, p. A 57
REDGATE MEMORIAL HOSPITAL, LONG BEACH, CA, p. A 48
REDINGTON–FAIRVIEW GENERAL HOSPITAL, SKOWHEGAN, ME, p. A182
REDLANDS COMMUNITY HOSPITAL, REDLANDS, CA, p. A 57
REDMOND REGIONAL MEDICAL CENTER, ROME, GA, p. A107
REDWOOD FALLS MUNICIPAL HOSPITAL, REDWOOD FALLS, MN, p. A218
REDWOOD MEMORIAL HOSPITAL, FORTUNA, CA, p. A 43
REED CITY HOSPITAL CORPORATION, REED CITY, MI, p. A209
REEDSBURG AREA MEDICAL CENTER, REEDSBURG, WI, p. A442
REEVES COUNTY HOSPITAL, PECOS, TX, p. A399
REFUGIO COUNTY MEMORIAL HOSPITAL, REFUGIO, TX, p. A400
REGINA MEDICAL CENTER, HASTINGS, MN, p. A215
REGIONAL HOSPITAL OF JACKSON, JACKSON, TN, p. A369

Hospitals, Alphabetically / Sage Memorial Hospital

REGIONAL MEDICAL CENTER AT MEMPHIS, MEMPHIS, TN, p. A372
REGIONAL MEDICAL CENTER OF HOPKINS COUNTY, MADISONVILLE, KY, p. A166
REGIONAL MEDICAL CENTER OF ORANGEBURG AND CALHOUN COUNTIES, ORANGEBURG, SC, p. A359
REGIONAL WEST MEDICAL CENTER, SCOTTSBLUFF, NE, p. A251
REHABILITATION HOSPITAL–MIDSOUTH, GERMANTOWN, TN, p. A368
REHABILITATION HOSPITAL OF BATON ROUGE, BATON ROUGE, LA, p. A170
REHABILITATION HOSPITAL OF INDIANA, INDIANAPOLIS, IN, p. A137
REHABILITATION HOSPITAL OF NORTH TEXAS, ARLINGTON, TX, p. A377
REHABILITATION HOSPITAL OF SOUTH TEXAS, CORPUS CHRISTI, TX, p. A382
REHABILITATION HOSPITAL OF THE PACIFIC, HONOLULU, HI, p. A110
REHABILITATION HOSPITAL OF WESTERN NEW ENGLAND, LUDLOW, MA, p. A194
REHABILITATION INSTITUTE, KANSAS CITY, MO, p. A234
REHABILITATION INSTITUTE, PITTSBURGH, PA, p. A347
REHABILITATION INSTITUTE AT SANTA BARBARA, SANTA BARBARA, CA, p. A 62
REHABILITATION INSTITUTE AT TRI-STATE HOSPITAL, BUCHANAN, MI, p. A200
REHABILITATION INSTITUTE OF CHICAGO, CHICAGO, IL, p. A119
REHABILITATION INSTITUTE OF MICHIGAN, DETROIT, MI, p. A202
REHOBOTH MCKINLEY CHRISTIAN HOSPITAL, GALLUP, NM, p. A269
REID HOSPITAL AND HEALTH CARE SERVICES, RICHMOND, IN, p. A140
RENVILLE COUNTY HOSPITAL, OLIVIA, MN, p. A218
REPUBLIC COUNTY HOSPITAL, BELLEVILLE, KS, p. A151
RESEARCH BELTON HOSPITAL, BELTON, MO, p. A230
RESEARCH MEDICAL CENTER, KANSAS CITY, MO, p. A234
RESEARCH PSYCHIATRIC CENTER, KANSAS CITY, MO, p. A234
RESTON HOSPITAL CENTER, RESTON, VA, p. A419
RESURRECTION MEDICAL CENTER, CHICAGO, IL, p. A120
RETREAT HOSPITAL, RICHMOND, VA, p. A420
REX HOSPITAL, RALEIGH, NC, p. A298
REYNOLDS ARMY COMMUNITY HOSPITAL, FORT SILL, OK, p. A323
REYNOLDS COUNTY GENERAL MEMORIAL HOSPITAL, ELLINGTON, MO, p. A232
REYNOLDS MEMORIAL HOSPITAL, GLEN DALE, WV, p. A431
RHD MEMORIAL MEDICAL CENTER, DALLAS, TX, p. A384
RHEA MEDICAL CENTER, DAYTON, TN, p. A367
RHODE ISLAND HOSPITAL, PROVIDENCE, RI, p. A353
RICE COUNTY HOSPITAL DISTRICT NUMBER ONE, LYONS, KS, p. A156
RICE MEMORIAL HOSPITAL, WILLMAR, MN, p. A221
RICHARD H. HUTCHINGS PSYCHIATRIC CENTER, SYRACUSE, NY, p. A288
RICHARD L. ROUDEBUSH VETERANS AFFAIRS MEDICAL CENTER, INDIANAPOLIS, IN, p. A137
RICHARDS MEMORIAL HOSPITAL, ROCKDALE, TX, p. A400
RICHARDSON MEDICAL CENTER, RAYVILLE, LA, p. A177
RICHARDTON HEALTH CENTER, RICHARDTON, ND, p. A304
RICHLAND HOSPITAL, MANSFIELD, OH, p. A314
RICHLAND HOSPITAL, NORTH RICHLAND HILLS, TX, p. A398
RICHLAND HOSPITAL, RICHLAND CENTER, WI, p. A442
RICHLAND MEMORIAL HOSPITAL, OLNEY, IL, p. A128
RICHLAND MEMORIAL HOSPITAL, COLUMBIA, SC, p. A356
RICHLAND PARISH HOSPITAL–DELHI, DELHI, LA, p. A172
RICHMOND COMMUNITY HOSPITAL, RICHMOND, VA, p. A420
RICHMOND EYE AND EAR HOSPITAL, RICHMOND, VA, p. A420
RICHMOND HEIGHTS GENERAL HOSPITAL, CLEVELAND, OH, p. A309
RICHMOND MEMORIAL HOSPITAL, ROCKINGHAM, NC, p. A298
RICHMOND MEMORIAL HOSPITAL, RICHMOND, VA, p. A420
RICHMOND STATE HOSPITAL, RICHMOND, IN, p. A140
RICHWOOD AREA MEDICAL CENTER, RICHWOOD, WV, p. A433
RIDDLE MEMORIAL HOSPITAL, MEDIA, PA, p. A342
RIDEOUT MEMORIAL HOSPITAL, MARYSVILLE, CA, p. A 52
RIDGECREST COMMUNITY HOSPITAL, RIDGECREST, CA, p. A 57
RIDGECREST HOSPITAL, CLAYTON, GA, p. A101
RIDGEVIEW INSTITUTE, SMYRNA, GA, p. A108
RIDGEVIEW MEDICAL CENTER, WACONIA, MN, p. A221
RIDGEVIEW PSYCHIATRIC HOSPITAL AND CENTER, OAK RIDGE, TN, p. A373
RILEY MEMORIAL HOSPITAL, MERIDIAN, MS, p. A226
RINGGOLD COUNTY HOSPITAL, MOUNT AYR, IA, p. A147
RIO GRANDE REGIONAL HOSPITAL, MCALLEN, TX, p. A396

RIO GRANDE STATE CENTER, HARLINGEN, TX, p. A389
RIO VISTA REHABILITATION HOSPITAL, EL PASO, TX, p. A386
RIPLEY COUNTY MEMORIAL HOSPITAL, DONIPHAN, MO, p. A231
RIPON MEDICAL CENTER, RIPON, WI, p. A442
RIVENDELL PSYCHIATRIC CENTER, BENTON, AR, p. A 29
RIVENDELL PSYCHIATRIC CENTER, WEST JORDAN, UT, p. A411
RIVER CREST HOSPITAL, SAN ANGELO, TX, p. A401
RIVER DISTRICT HOSPITAL, EAST CHINA, MI, p. A202
RIVER FALLS AREA HOSPITAL, RIVER FALLS, WI, p. A442
RIVER OAKS EAST–WOMAN'S PAVILION, JACKSON, MS, p. A225
RIVER OAKS HOSPITAL, NEW ORLEANS, LA, p. A176
RIVER OAKS HOSPITAL, JACKSON, MS, p. A225
RIVER PARISHES HOSPITAL, LAPLACE, LA, p. A174
RIVER PARK HOSPITAL, MCMINNVILLE, TN, p. A371
RIVER PARK HOSPITAL, HUNTINGTON, WV, p. A431
RIVER WEST MEDICAL CENTER, PLAQUEMINE, LA, p. A177
RIVEREDGE HOSPITAL, FOREST PARK, IL, p. A123
RIVERLAND MEDICAL CENTER, FERRIDAY, LA, p. A172
RIVERNORTH HOSPITAL CENTER, PINEVILLE, LA, p. A177
RIVERSIDE COMMUNITY HOSPITAL, RIVERSIDE, CA, p. A 57
RIVERSIDE COMMUNITY HOSPITAL, CORPUS CHRISTI, TX, p. A382
RIVERSIDE GENERAL HOSPITAL–UNIVERSITY MEDICAL CENTER, RIVERSIDE, CA, p. A 58
RIVERSIDE GENERAL HOSPITAL, HOUSTON, TX, p. A391
RIVERSIDE HEALTH SYSTEM, WICHITA, KS, p. A160
RIVERSIDE HOSPITAL, WILMINGTON, DE, p. A 78
RIVERSIDE HOSPITAL, JACKSONVILLE, FL, p. A 86
RIVERSIDE HOSPITAL, TOLEDO, OH, p. A318
RIVERSIDE MEDICAL CENTER, JACKSON, AL, p. A 17
RIVERSIDE MEDICAL CENTER, KANKAKEE, IL, p. A125
RIVERSIDE MEDICAL CENTER, FRANKLINTON, LA, p. A172
RIVERSIDE MEDICAL CENTER, WAUPACA, WI, p. A444
RIVERSIDE METHODIST HOSPITALS, COLUMBUS, OH, p. A310
RIVERSIDE OSTEOPATHIC HOSPITAL, TRENTON, MI, p. A211
RIVERSIDE REGIONAL MEDICAL CENTER, NEWPORT NEWS, VA, p. A418
RIVERSIDE TAPPAHANNOCK HOSPITAL, TAPPAHANNOCK, VA, p. A421
RIVERSIDE WALTER REED HOSPITAL, GLOUCESTER, VA, p. A416
RIVERTON MEMORIAL HOSPITAL, RIVERTON, WY, p. A446
RIVERVIEW HEALTHCARE ASSOCIATION, CROOKSTON, MN, p. A213
RIVERVIEW HOSPITAL, NOBLESVILLE, IN, p. A139
RIVERVIEW HOSPITAL ASSOCIATION, WISCONSIN RAPIDS, WI, p. A444
RIVERVIEW HOSPITAL FOR CHILDREN, MIDDLETOWN, CT, p. A 75
RIVERVIEW MEDICAL CENTER, GONZALES, LA, p. A172
RIVERVIEW MEDICAL CENTER, RED BANK, NJ, p. A264
RIVERVIEW REGIONAL MEDICAL CENTER, GADSDEN, AL, p. A 16
RIVERWOOD HEALTH CARE CENTER, AITKIN, MN, p. A212
ROANE GENERAL HOSPITAL, SPENCER, WV, p. A433
ROANOKE–CHOWAN HOSPITAL, AHOSKIE, NC, p. A291
ROANOKE MEMORIAL HOSPITALS, ROANOKE, VA, p. A420
ROBERT F. KENNEDY MEDICAL CENTER, HAWTHORNE, CA, p. A 45
ROBERT PACKER HOSPITAL, SAYRE, PA, p. A348
ROBERT WOOD JOHNSON UNIVERSITY HOSPITAL, NEW BRUNSWICK, NJ, p. A262
ROBERT WOOD JOHNSON UNIVERSITY HOSPITAL AT HAMILTON, HAMILTON, NJ, p. A260
ROBINSON MEMORIAL HOSPITAL, RAVENNA, OH, p. A316
ROCHELLE COMMUNITY HOSPITAL, ROCHELLE, IL, p. A129
ROCHESTER GENERAL HOSPITAL, ROCHESTER, NY, p. A286
ROCHESTER METHODIST HOSPITAL, ROCHESTER, MN, p. A219
ROCHESTER PSYCHIATRIC CENTER, ROCHESTER, NY, p. A286
ROCK COUNTY HOSPITAL, BASSETT, NE, p. A246
ROCKCASTLE HOSPITAL, MOUNT VERNON, KY, p. A167
ROCKDALE HOSPITAL, CONYERS, GA, p. A102
ROCKEFELLER UNIVERSITY HOSPITAL, NEW YORK CITY, NY, p. A282
ROCKFORD CENTER, NEWARK, DE, p. A 78
ROCKFORD MEMORIAL HOSPITAL, ROCKFORD, IL, p. A130
ROCKINGHAM MEMORIAL HOSPITAL, HARRISONBURG, VA, p. A416
ROCKLAND CHILDREN'S PSYCHIATRIC CENTER, ORANGEBURG, NY, p. A284
ROCKLAND PSYCHIATRIC CENTER, ORANGEBURG, NY, p. A284
ROCKVILLE GENERAL HOSPITAL, VERNON ROCKVILLE, CT, p. A 77
ROCKY MOUNTAIN REHABILITATION INSTITUTE, AURORA, CO, p. A 68

ROGER C. PEACE REHABILITATION HOSPITAL, GREENVILLE, SC, p. A358
ROGER MILLS MEMORIAL HOSPITAL, CHEYENNE, OK, p. A322
ROGER WILLIAMS MEDICAL CENTER, PROVIDENCE, RI, p. A353
ROGERS MEMORIAL HOSPITAL, OCONOMOWOC, WI, p. A441
ROGUE VALLEY MEDICAL CENTER, MEDFORD, OR, p. A331
ROLLING HILLS HOSPITAL, ADA, OK, p. A321
ROLLING PLAINS MEMORIAL HOSPITAL, SWEETWATER, TX, p. A404
ROME MEMORIAL HOSPITAL, ROME, NY, p. A286
ROOSEVELT HOSPITAL, EDISON, NJ, p. A259
ROOSEVELT MEMORIAL MEDICAL CENTER, CULBERTSON, MT, p. A242
ROOSEVELT WARM SPRINGS INSTITUTE FOR REHABILITATION, WARM SPRINGS, GA, p. A109
ROPER HOSPITAL, CHARLESTON, SC, p. A356
ROPER HOSPITAL NORTH, CHARLESTON, SC, p. A356
ROSE MEDICAL CENTER, DENVER, CO, p. A 69
ROSEAU AREA HOSPITAL DISTRICT, ROSEAU, MN, p. A219
ROSEBUD HEALTH CARE CENTER, FORSYTH, MT, p. A242
ROSELAND COMMUNITY HOSPITAL, CHICAGO, IL, p. A120
ROSEVILLE HOSPITAL, ROSEVILLE, CA, p. A 58
ROSEWOOD MEDICAL CENTER, HOUSTON, TX, p. A391
ROSS HOSPITAL, KENTFIELD, CA, p. A 46
ROSWELL PARK CANCER INSTITUTE, BUFFALO, NY, p. A273
ROUND ROCK HOSPITAL, ROUND ROCK, TX, p. A401
ROUNDUP MEMORIAL HOSPITAL, ROUNDUP, MT, p. A244
ROUTT MEMORIAL HOSPITAL, STEAMBOAT SPRINGS, CO, p. A 72
ROWAN MEMORIAL HOSPITAL, SALISBURY, NC, p. A298
ROXBOROUGH MEMORIAL HOSPITAL, PHILADELPHIA, PA, p. A345
ROY H. LAIRD MEMORIAL HOSPITAL, KILGORE, TX, p. A394
ROYAL C. JOHNSON VETERANS MEMORIAL HOSPITAL, SIOUX FALLS, SD, p. A364
RUBY VALLEY HOSPITAL, SHERIDAN, MT, p. A244
RUMFORD COMMUNITY HOSPITAL, RUMFORD, ME, p. A182
RUNNELLS SPECIALIZED HOSPITAL, BERKELEY HEIGHTS, NJ, p. A258
RUSH–PRESBYTERIAN–ST. LUKE'S MEDICAL CENTER, CHICAGO, IL, p. A120
RUSH CITY HOSPITAL, RUSH CITY, MN, p. A219
RUSH COUNTY MEMORIAL HOSPITAL, LA CROSSE, KS, p. A155
RUSH FOUNDATION HOSPITAL, MERIDIAN, MS, p. A226
RUSH MEMORIAL HOSPITAL, RUSHVILLE, IN, p. A140
RUSH NORTH SHORE MEDICAL CENTER, SKOKIE, IL, p. A130
RUSK COUNTY MEMORIAL HOSPITAL AND NURSING HOME, LADYSMITH, WI, p. A438
RUSK STATE HOSPITAL, RUSK, TX, p. A401
RUSSELL COUNTY HOSPITAL, RUSSELL SPRINGS, KY, p. A168
RUSSELL COUNTY MEDICAL CENTER, LEBANON, VA, p. A416
RUSSELL HOSPITAL, ALEXANDER CITY, AL, p. A 13
RUSSELL REGIONAL HOSPITAL, RUSSELL, KS, p. A158
RUTHERFORD HOSPITAL, RUTHERFORDTON, NC, p. A298
RUTLAND REGIONAL MEDICAL CENTER, RUTLAND, VT, p. A412
RYDER MEMORIAL HOSPITAL, HUMACAO, PR, p. A448
RYE HOSPITAL CENTER, RYE, NY, p. A286

S

SABETHA COMMUNITY HOSPITAL, SABETHA, KS, p. A158
SABINE COUNTY HOSPITAL, HEMPHILL, TX, p. A389
SABINE MEDICAL CENTER, MANY, LA, p. A175
SAC-OSAGE HOSPITAL, OSCEOLA, MO, p. A236
SACRED HEART–ST. MARY'S HOSPITALS, RHINELANDER, WI, p. A442
SACRED HEART HEALTH SERVICES, YANKTON, SD, p. A365
SACRED HEART HOSPITAL, CHICAGO, IL, p. A120
SACRED HEART HOSPITAL, CUMBERLAND, MD, p. A186
SACRED HEART HOSPITAL, ALLENTOWN, PA, p. A334
SACRED HEART HOSPITAL, EAU CLAIRE, WI, p. A436
SACRED HEART HOSPITAL OF PENSACOLA, PENSACOLA, FL, p. A 93
SACRED HEART MEDICAL CENTER, EUGENE, OR, p. A329
SACRED HEART MEDICAL CENTER, SPOKANE, WA, p. A428
SACRED HEART REHABILITATION HOSPITAL, MILWAUKEE, WI, p. A440
SADDLEBACK MEMORIAL MEDICAL CENTER, LAGUNA HILLS, CA, p. A 46
SAGAMORE CHILDREN'S PSYCHIATRIC CENTER, DIX HILLS, NY, p. A274
SAGE MEMORIAL HOSPITAL, GANADO, AZ, p. A 24

Hospitals, Alphabetically / Saginaw General Hospital

SAGINAW GENERAL HOSPITAL, SAGINAW, MI, p. A209
SAINT ALPHONSUS REGIONAL MEDICAL CENTER, BOISE, ID, p. A112
SAINT ANNE'S HOSPITAL, FALL RIVER, MA, p. A193
SAINT ANTHONY HOSPITAL, CHICAGO, IL, p. A120
SAINT ANTHONY HOSPITAL AND HEALTH CENTERS, MICHIGAN CITY, IN, p. A139
SAINT ANTHONY MEDICAL CENTER, ROCKFORD, IL, p. A130
SAINT ANTHONY'S HEALTH CENTER, ALTON, IL, p. A116
SAINT BARNABAS MEDICAL CENTER, LIVINGSTON, NJ, p. A261
SAINT CABRINI HOSPITAL, CHICAGO, IL, p. A120
SAINT EUGENE COMMUNITY HOSPITAL, DILLON, SC, p. A357
SAINT FRANCIS HOSPITAL, POUGHKEEPSIE, NY, p. A285
SAINT FRANCIS HOSPITAL, TULSA, OK, p. A328
SAINT FRANCIS HOSPITAL, CHARLESTON, WV, p. A430
SAINT FRANCIS HOSPITAL AND MEDICAL CENTER, HARTFORD, CT, p. A 75
SAINT FRANCIS MEDICAL CENTER, PEORIA, IL, p. A129
SAINT FRANCIS MEDICAL CENTER, CAPE GIRARDEAU, MO, p. A230
SAINT FRANCIS MEDICAL CENTER, GRAND ISLAND, NE, p. A248
SAINT FRANCIS MEMORIAL HOSPITAL, SAN FRANCISCO, CA, p. A 60
SAINT JAMES HOSPITAL, PONTIAC, IL, p. A129
SAINT JAMES HOSPITAL OF NEWARK, NEWARK, NJ, p. A262
SAINT JOHN HOSPITAL, LEAVENWORTH, KS, p. A155
SAINT JOHN'S HEALTH SYSTEM, ANDERSON, IN, p. A133
SAINT JOHN'S HOSPITAL AND HEALTH CENTER, SANTA MONICA, CA, p. A 63
SAINT JOSEPH CENTER FOR MENTAL HEALTH, OMAHA, NE, p. A250
SAINT JOSEPH COMMUNITY HOSPITAL, NEW HAMPTON, IA, p. A148
SAINT JOSEPH HEALTH CENTER, KANSAS CITY, MO, p. A234
SAINT JOSEPH HOSPITAL, DENVER, CO, p. A 69
SAINT JOSEPH HOSPITAL, BELVIDERE, IL, p. A116
SAINT JOSEPH HOSPITAL, ELGIN, IL, p. A122
SAINT JOSEPH HOSPITAL, OMAHA, NE, p. A250
SAINT JOSEPH HOSPITAL AND HEALTH CENTER, KOKOMO, IN, p. A138
SAINT JOSEPH MEDICAL CENTER, BURBANK, CA, p. A 38
SAINT JOSEPH MEDICAL CENTER, JOLIET, IL, p. A125
SAINT JOSEPH'S HOSPITAL, MARSHFIELD, WI, p. A439
SAINT JOSEPH'S HOSPITAL OF ATLANTA, ATLANTA, GA, p. A 99
SAINT JOSEPH'S HOSPITAL OF DAHLONEGA, DAHLONEGA, GA, p. A102
SAINT LOUIS UNIVERSITY HOSPITAL, SAINT LOUIS, MO, p. A238
SAINT LOUISE HOSPITAL, MORGAN HILL, CA, p. A 53
SAINT LUKE INSTITUTE, SUITLAND, MD, p. A188
SAINT LUKE'S MEDICAL CENTER, CLEVELAND, OH, p. A310
SAINT LUKE'S NORTHLAND HOSPITAL–SMITHVILLE CAMPUS, SMITHVILLE, MO, p. A239
SAINT LUKE'S NORTHLAND HOSPITAL – BARRY ROAD CAMPUS, KANSAS CITY, MO, p. A234
SAINT MARGARET MERCY HEALTHCARE CENTERS, HAMMOND, IN, p. A136
SAINT MARY HOSPITAL, MANHATTAN, KS, p. A156
SAINT MARY OF NAZARETH HOSPITAL CENTER, CHICAGO, IL, p. A120
SAINT MARY'S HEALTH SERVICES, GRAND RAPIDS, MI, p. A204
SAINT MARY'S MEDICAL CENTER, RACINE, WI, p. A442
SAINT MARYS HOSPITAL OF ROCHESTER, ROCHESTER, MN, p. A219
SAINT MICHAEL'S HOSPITAL, STEVENS POINT, WI, p. A443
SAINT MICHAEL'S MEDICAL CENTER, NEWARK, NJ, p. A262
SAINT THERESE MEDICAL CENTER, WAUKEGAN, IL, p. A131
SAINT VINCENT HOSPITAL, WORCESTER, MA, p. A198
SAINT VINCENT HOSPITAL, ERIE, PA, p. A338
SAINT VINCENT HOSPITAL AND HEALTH CENTER, BILLINGS, MT, p. A241
SAINTS MARY AND ELIZABETH HOSPITAL, LOUISVILLE, KY, p. A165
SAINTS MEMORIAL MEDICAL CENTER, LOWELL, MA, p. A194
SAKAKAWEA MEDICAL CENTER, HAZEN, ND, p. A303
SALEM COMMUNITY HOSPITAL, SALEM, OH, p. A317
SALEM HOSPITAL, HILLSBORO, KS, p. A154
SALEM HOSPITAL, SALEM, MA, p. A196
SALEM HOSPITAL, SALEM, OR, p. A332
SALEM MEMORIAL DISTRICT HOSPITAL, SALEM, MO, p. A239
SALINAS VALLEY MEMORIAL HOSPITAL, SALINAS, CA, p. A 58
SALINE COMMUNITY HOSPITAL, SALINE, MI, p. A209
SALINE MEMORIAL HOSPITAL, BENTON, AR, p. A 29
SALT LAKE REGIONAL MEDICAL CENTER, SALT LAKE CITY, UT, p. A410
SAM RAYBURN MEMORIAL VETERANS CENTER, BONHAM, TX, p. A379

SAMARITAN–WENDY PAINE O'BRIEN TREATMENT CENTER, PHOENIX, AZ, p. A 26
SAMARITAN BEHAVIORAL HEALTH CENTER – DESERT SAMARITAN CAMPUS, MESA, AZ, p. A 25
SAMARITAN BEHAVIORAL HEALTH CENTER – SCOTTSDALE, SCOTTSDALE, AZ, p. A 26
SAMARITAN HEALTH SYSTEM, CLINTON, IA, p. A143
SAMARITAN HOSPITAL, TROY, NY, p. A288
SAMARITAN HOSPITAL, ASHLAND, OH, p. A306
SAMARITAN HOSPITAL, MOSES LAKE, WA, p. A425
SAMARITAN MEDICAL CENTER, WATERTOWN, NY, p. A289
SAMARITAN MEDICAL CENTER SAN CLEMENTE, SAN CLEMENTE, CA, p. A 59
SAMARITAN MEMORIAL HOSPITAL, MACON, MO, p. A235
SAMPSON COUNTY MEMORIAL HOSPITAL, CLINTON, NC, p. A293
SAMUEL MAHELONA MEMORIAL HOSPITAL, KAPAA, HI, p. A111
SAN ANTONIO COMMUNITY HOSPITAL, UPLAND, CA, p. A 65
SAN ANTONIO REGIONAL HOSPITAL, SAN ANTONIO, TX, p. A402
SAN ANTONIO STATE HOSPITAL, SAN ANTONIO, TX, p. A402
SAN ANTONIO WARM SPRINGS REHABILITATION HOSPITAL, SAN ANTONIO, TX, p. A402
SAN AUGUSTINE MEMORIAL HOSPITAL, SAN AUGUSTINE, TX, p. A403
SAN BENITO HOSPITAL DISTRICT, HOLLISTER, CA, p. A 45
SAN BERNARDINO COUNTY MEDICAL CENTER, SAN BERNARDINO, CA, p. A 59
SAN CARLOS GENERAL HOSPITAL, SAN JUAN, PR, p. A449
SAN DIEGO COUNTY LOMA PORTAL MENTAL HEALTH FACILITY, SAN DIEGO, CA, p. A 59
SAN DIEGO COUNTY PSYCHIATRIC HOSPITAL, SAN DIEGO, CA, p. A 59
SAN DIEGO HOSPICE, SAN DIEGO, CA, p. A 59
SAN DIMAS COMMUNITY HOSPITAL, SAN DIMAS, CA, p. A 60
SAN FRANCISCO GENERAL HOSPITAL MEDICAL CENTER, SAN FRANCISCO, CA, p. A 60
SAN GABRIEL VALLEY MEDICAL CENTER, SAN GABRIEL, CA, p. A 61
SAN GORGONIO MEMORIAL HOSPITAL, BANNING, CA, p. A 37
SAN JACINTO METHODIST HOSPITAL, BAYTOWN, TX, p. A378
SAN JOAQUIN COMMUNITY HOSPITAL, BAKERSFIELD, CA, p. A 37
SAN JOAQUIN GENERAL HOSPITAL, FRENCH CAMP, CA, p. A 43
SAN JORGE CHILDREN'S HOSPITAL, SAN JUAN, PR, p. A449
SAN JOSE MEDICAL CENTER, SAN JOSE, CA, p. A 61
SAN JUAN CITY HOSPITAL, SAN JUAN, PR, p. A450
SAN JUAN HOSPITAL, MONTICELLO, UT, p. A409
SAN JUAN REGIONAL MEDICAL CENTER, FARMINGTON, NM, p. A268
SAN LEANDRO HOSPITAL, SAN LEANDRO, CA, p. A 61
SAN LUIS OBISPO GENERAL HOSPITAL, SAN LUIS OBISPO, CA, p. A 62
SAN LUIS VALLEY REGIONAL MEDICAL CENTER, ALAMOSA, CO, p. A 68
SAN MARCOS TREATMENT CENTER, SAN MARCOS, TX, p. A403
SAN MATEO COUNTY GENERAL HOSPITAL, SAN MATEO, CA, p. A 62
SAN PEDRO PENINSULA HOSPITAL, LOS ANGELES, CA, p. A 50
SAN RAMON REGIONAL MEDICAL CENTER, SAN RAMON, CA, p. A 62
SANDWICH COMMUNITY HOSPITAL, SANDWICH, IL, p. A130
SANDYPINES, TEQUESTA, FL, p. A 97
SANGER GENERAL HOSPITAL, SANGER, CA, p. A 62
SANPETE VALLEY HOSPITAL, MOUNT PLEASANT, UT, p. A409
SANTA ANA HOSPITAL MEDICAL CENTER, SANTA ANA, CA, p. A 62
SANTA BARBARA COTTAGE HOSPITAL, SANTA BARBARA, CA, p. A 62
SANTA CLARA VALLEY MEDICAL CENTER, SAN JOSE, CA, p. A 61
SANTA MARTA HOSPITAL, LOS ANGELES, CA, p. A 50
SANTA MONICA HOSPITAL MEDICAL CENTER, SANTA MONICA, CA, p. A 63
SANTA PAULA MEMORIAL HOSPITAL, SANTA PAULA, CA, p. A 63
SANTA ROSA HEALTH CARE CORPORATION, SAN ANTONIO, TX, p. A402
SANTA ROSA MEDICAL CENTER, MILTON, FL, p. A 90
SANTA ROSA MEMORIAL HOSPITAL, SANTA ROSA, CA, p. A 63
SANTA TERESA COMMUNITY HOSPITAL, SAN JOSE, CA, p. A 61
SANTA TERESITA HOSPITAL, DUARTE, CA, p. A 41
SANTA YNEZ VALLEY HOSPITAL, SOLVANG, CA, p. A 63
SANTIAM MEMORIAL HOSPITAL, STAYTON, OR, p. A333

SARAH BUSH LINCOLN HEALTH SYSTEM, MATTOON, IL, p. A126
SARAH D. CULBERTSON MEMORIAL HOSPITAL, RUSHVILLE, IL, p. A130
SARASOTA MEMORIAL HOSPITAL, SARASOTA, FL, p. A 95
SARATOGA COMMUNITY HOSPITAL, DETROIT, MI, p. A202
SARATOGA HOSPITAL, SARATOGA SPRINGS, NY, p. A286
SARGENT DISTRICT HOSPITAL, SARGENT, NE, p. A251
SARTORI MEMORIAL HOSPITAL, CEDAR FALLS, IA, p. A142
SATANTA DISTRICT HOSPITAL, SATANTA, KS, p. A158
SATILLA REGIONAL MEDICAL CENTER, WAYCROSS, GA, p. A109
SAUK PRAIRIE MEMORIAL HOSPITAL, PRAIRIE DU SAC, WI, p. A442
SAUNDERS COUNTY HEALTH SERVICE, WAHOO, NE, p. A252
SAVANNAS HOSPITAL, PORT SAINT LUCIE, FL, p. A 94
SAVOY MEDICAL CENTER, MAMOU, LA, p. A174
SAYRE MEMORIAL HOSPITAL, SAYRE, OK, p. A326
SCENIC MOUNTAIN MEDICAL CENTER, BIG SPRING, TX, p. A379
SCHEURER HOSPITAL, PIGEON, MI, p. A208
SCHICK SHADEL HOSPITAL, SEATTLE, WA, p. A427
SCHLEICHER COUNTY MEDICAL CENTER, ELDORADO, TX, p. A386
SCHOOLCRAFT MEMORIAL HOSPITAL, MANISTIQUE, MI, p. A207
SCHUMPERT MEDICAL CENTER, SHREVEPORT, LA, p. A178
SCHUYLER HOSPITAL, MONTOUR FALLS, NY, p. A277
SCHWAB REHABILITATION HOSPITAL AND CARE NETWORK, CHICAGO, IL, p. A120
SCOTLAND COUNTY MEMORIAL HOSPITAL, MEMPHIS, MO, p. A235
SCOTLAND MEMORIAL HOSPITAL, LAURINBURG, NC, p. A296
SCOTT AND WHITE MEMORIAL HOSPITAL, TEMPLE, TX, p. A404
SCOTT COUNTY HOSPITAL, SCOTT CITY, KS, p. A158
SCOTT COUNTY HOSPITAL, ONEIDA, TN, p. A373
SCOTT GENERAL HOSPITAL, GEORGETOWN, KY, p. A163
SCOTT MEDICAL CENTER, SCOTT AIR FORCE BASE, IL, p. A130
SCOTT MEMORIAL HOSPITAL, SCOTTSBURG, IN, p. A140
SCOTTISH RITE CHILDREN'S MEDICAL CENTER, ATLANTA, GA, p. A 99
SCOTTSDALE MEMORIAL HOSPITAL–NORTH, SCOTTSDALE, AZ, p. A 27
SCOTTSDALE MEMORIAL HOSPITAL, SCOTTSDALE, AZ, p. A 26
SCREVEN COUNTY HOSPITAL, SYLVANIA, GA, p. A108
SCRIPPS HOSPITAL–EAST COUNTY, EL CAJON, CA, p. A 41
SCRIPPS MEMORIAL HOSPITAL–CHULA VISTA, CHULA VISTA, CA, p. A 39
SCRIPPS MEMORIAL HOSPITAL–ENCINITAS, ENCINITAS, CA, p. A 42
SCRIPPS MEMORIAL HOSPITAL – LA JOLLA, LA JOLLA, CA, p. A 46
SEABORNE HOSPITAL, DOVER, NH, p. A255
SEARCY HOSPITAL, MOUNT VERNON, AL, p. A 18
SEARHC MOUNTAIN EDGECUMBE HOSPITAL, SITKA, AK, p. A 22
SEBASTIAN RIVER MEDICAL CENTER, SEBASTIAN, FL, p. A 95
SEBASTICOOK VALLEY HOSPITAL, PITTSFIELD, ME, p. A182
SEDAN CITY HOSPITAL, SEDAN, KS, p. A158
SEDGWICK COUNTY MEMORIAL HOSPITAL, JULESBURG, CO, p. A 71
SEIDLE MEMORIAL HOSPITAL, MECHANICSBURG, PA, p. A342
SEILING HOSPITAL, SEILING, OK, p. A326
SELBY GENERAL HOSPITAL, MARIETTA, OH, p. A314
SELF MEMORIAL HOSPITAL, GREENWOOD, SC, p. A358
SELMA DISTRICT HOSPITAL, SELMA, CA, p. A 63
SEMINOLE MUNICIPAL HOSPITAL, SEMINOLE, OK, p. A327
SENATOBIA COMMUNITY HOSPITAL, SENATOBIA, MS, p. A228
SENATOR GARRET T. W. HAGEDORN GERO PSYCHIATRIC HOSPITAL, GLEN GARDNER, NJ, p. A260
SENECA DISTRICT HOSPITAL, CHESTER, CA, p. A 39
SENTARA BAYSIDE HOSPITAL, VIRGINIA BEACH, VA, p. A421
SENTARA HAMPTON GENERAL HOSPITAL, HAMPTON, VA, p. A416
SENTARA LEIGH HOSPITAL, NORFOLK, VA, p. A418
SENTARA NORFOLK GENERAL HOSPITAL, NORFOLK, VA, p. A418
SEQUOIA HOSPITAL DISTRICT, REDWOOD CITY, CA, p. A 57
SEQUOYAH MEMORIAL HOSPITAL, SALLISAW, OK, p. A326
SERENITY LANE, EUGENE, OR, p. A330
SETON HEALTH SYSTEM, TROY, NY, p. A288
SETON MEDICAL CENTER, DALY CITY, CA, p. A 41
SETON MEDICAL CENTER, AUSTIN, TX, p. A378
SETON MEDICAL CENTER COASTSIDE, MOSS BEACH, CA, p. A 53
SEVEN RIVERS COMMUNITY HOSPITAL, CRYSTAL RIVER, FL, p. A 83

Hospitals, Alphabetically / Southern New Hampshire Regional Medical Center

SEVIER VALLEY HOSPITAL, RICHFIELD, UT, p. A410
SEWARD GENERAL HOSPITAL, SEWARD, AK, p. A 22
SEWICKLEY VALLEY HOSPITAL, SEWICKLEY, PA, p. A349
SEYMOUR HOSPITAL, SEYMOUR, TX, p. A403
SHACKELFORD COUNTY HOSPITAL DISTRICT, ALBANY, TX, p. A376
SHADOW MOUNTAIN HOSPITAL, TULSA, OK, p. A328
SHADY GROVE ADVENTIST HOSPITAL, ROCKVILLE, MD, p. A188
SHADYSIDE HOSPITAL, PITTSBURGH, PA, p. A347
SHAMOKIN AREA COMMUNITY HOSPITAL, COAL TOWNSHIP, PA, p. A336
SHAMROCK GENERAL HOSPITAL, SHAMROCK, TX, p. A403
SHANDS HOSPITAL AT THE UNIVERSITY OF FLORIDA, GAINESVILLE, FL, p. A 85
SHANNON MEDICAL CENTER, SAN ANGELO, TX, p. A401
SHARE MEDICAL CENTER, ALVA, OK, p. A321
SHARON HOSPITAL, SHARON, CT, p. A 76
SHARON REGIONAL HEALTH SYSTEM, SHARON, PA, p. A349
SHARP CABRILLO HOSPITAL, SAN DIEGO, CA, p. A 59
SHARP CHULA VISTA MEDICAL CENTER, CHULA VISTA, CA, p. A 40
SHARP HEALTHCARE MURRIETA, MURRIETA, CA, p. A 53
SHARP MEMORIAL HOSPITAL, SAN DIEGO, CA, p. A 59
SHARPE HOSPITAL, WESTON, WV, p. A433
SHARPSTOWN GENERAL HOSPITAL, HOUSTON, TX, p. A391
SHAUGHNESSY–KAPLAN REHABILITATION HOSPITAL, SALEM, MA, p. A196
SHAWANO MEDICAL CENTER, SHAWANO, WI, p. A442
SHAWNEE MISSION MEDICAL CENTER, SHAWNEE MISSION, KS, p. A158
SHAWNEE REGIONAL HOSPITAL, SHAWNEE, OK, p. A327
SHEBOYGAN MEMORIAL MEDICAL CENTER, SHEBOYGAN, WI, p. A443
SHEEHAN MEMORIAL HOSPITAL, BUFFALO, NY, p. A273
SHELBY MEDICAL CENTER, ALABASTER, AL, p. A 13
SHELBY MEMORIAL HOSPITAL, SHELBYVILLE, IL, p. A130
SHELBY MEMORIAL HOSPITAL, SHELBY, OH, p. A317
SHELTERING ARMS REHABILITATION HOSPITAL, RICHMOND, VA, p. A420
SHENANDOAH MEMORIAL HOSPITAL, SHENANDOAH, IA, p. A149
SHENANDOAH MEMORIAL HOSPITAL, WOODSTOCK, VA, p. A422
SHEPHERD CENTER, ATLANTA, GA, p. A 99
SHEPPARD AND ENOCH PRATT HOSPITAL, BALTIMORE, MD, p. A185
SHERIDAN COMMUNITY HOSPITAL, SHERIDAN, MI, p. A210
SHERIDAN COUNTY HOSPITAL, HOXIE, KS, p. A154
SHERIDAN MEMORIAL HOSPITAL, PLENTYWOOD, MT, p. A244
SHERMAN HOSPITAL, ELGIN, IL, p. A122
SHERMAN OAKS HOSPITAL AND HEALTH CENTER, LOS ANGELES, CA, p. A 50
SHIPROCK INDIAN HOSPITAL, SHIPROCK, NM, p. A270
SHOAL CREEK HOSPITAL, AUSTIN, TX, p. A378
SHODAIR CHILDREN'S HOSPITAL, HELENA, MT, p. A243
SHORE MEMORIAL HOSPITAL, SOMERS POINT, NJ, p. A264
SHORELINE MEDICAL CENTER, METAIRIE, LA, p. A175
SHOSHONE MEDICAL CENTER, KELLOGG, ID, p. A113
SHRINERS HOSPITAL FOR CRIPPLED CHILDREN, BURNS INSTITUTE BOSTON UNIT, BOSTON, MA, p. A191
SHRINERS HOSPITALS FOR CRIPPLED CHILDREN–SPOKANE UNIT, SPOKANE, WA, p. A428
SHRINERS HOSPITALS FOR CRIPPLED CHILDREN, CHICAGO UNIT, CHICAGO, IL, p. A120
SHRINERS HOSPITALS FOR CRIPPLED CHILDREN, CINCINNATI BURNS INSTITUTE, CINCINNATI, OH, p. A308
SHRINERS HOSPITALS FOR CRIPPLED CHILDREN, ERIE UNIT, ERIE, PA, p. A338
SHRINERS HOSPITALS FOR CRIPPLED CHILDREN, GALVESTON BURNS INSTITUTE, GALVESTON, TX, p. A388
SHRINERS HOSPITALS FOR CRIPPLED CHILDREN, GREENVILLE UNIT, GREENVILLE, SC, p. A358
SHRINERS HOSPITALS FOR CRIPPLED CHILDREN, HONOLULU UNIT, HONOLULU, HI, p. A110
SHRINERS HOSPITALS FOR CRIPPLED CHILDREN, HOUSTON UNIT, HOUSTON, TX, p. A391
SHRINERS HOSPITALS FOR CRIPPLED CHILDREN, INTERMOUNTAIN UNIT, SALT LAKE CITY, UT, p. A410
SHRINERS HOSPITALS FOR CRIPPLED CHILDREN, LEXINGTON UNIT, LEXINGTON, KY, p. A164
SHRINERS HOSPITALS FOR CRIPPLED CHILDREN, LOS ANGELES UNIT, LOS ANGELES, CA, p. A 50
SHRINERS HOSPITALS FOR CRIPPLED CHILDREN, PHILADELPHIA UNIT, PHILADELPHIA, PA, p. A345
SHRINERS HOSPITALS FOR CRIPPLED CHILDREN, PORTLAND UNIT, PORTLAND, OR, p. A332
SHRINERS HOSPITALS FOR CRIPPLED CHILDREN, SAN FRANCISCO UNIT, SAN FRANCISCO, CA, p. A 60
SHRINERS HOSPITALS FOR CRIPPLED CHILDREN, SHREVEPORT UNIT, SHREVEPORT, LA, p. A178
SHRINERS HOSPITALS FOR CRIPPLED CHILDREN, SPRINGFIELD UNIT, SPRINGFIELD, MA, p. A197
SHRINERS HOSPITALS FOR CRIPPLED CHILDREN, ST. LOUIS UNIT, SAINT LOUIS, MO, p. A238
SHRINERS HOSPITALS FOR CRIPPLED CHILDREN, TAMPA UNIT, TAMPA, FL, p. A 96
SHRINERS HOSPITALS FOR CRIPPLED CHILDREN, TWIN CITIES UNIT, MINNEAPOLIS, MN, p. A217
SIBLEY MEMORIAL HOSPITAL, WASHINGTON, DC, p. A 79
SID PETERSON MEMORIAL HOSPITAL, KERRVILLE, TX, p. A394
SIERRA–KINGS DISTRICT HOSPITAL, REEDLEY, CA, p. A 57
SIERRA COMMUNITY HOSPITAL, FRESNO, CA, p. A 43
SIERRA MEDICAL CENTER, EL PASO, TX, p. A386
SIERRA NEVADA MEMORIAL HOSPITAL, GRASS VALLEY, CA, p. A 44
SIERRA TUCSON, TUCSON, AZ, p. A 28
SIERRA VALLEY DISTRICT HOSPITAL, LOYALTON, CA, p. A 51
SIERRA VIEW DISTRICT HOSPITAL, PORTERVILLE, CA, p. A 56
SIERRA VISTA COMMUNITY HOSPITAL, SIERRA VISTA, AZ, p. A 27
SIERRA VISTA HOSPITAL, TRUTH OR CONSEQUENCES, NM, p. A270
SILSBEE DOCTORS HOSPITAL, SILSBEE, TX, p. A403
SILVER CROSS HOSPITAL, JOLIET, IL, p. A125
SILVER HILL HOSPITAL, NEW CANAAN, CT, p. A 75
SILVERTON HOSPITAL, SILVERTON, OR, p. A333
SIMI VALLEY HOSPITAL AND HEALTH CARE SERVICES, SIMI VALLEY, CA, p. A 63
SIMPSON GENERAL HOSPITAL, MENDENHALL, MS, p. A226
SIMPSON INFIRMARY, WELLESLEY COLLEGE, WELLESLEY, MA, p. A198
SINAI HOSPITAL, DETROIT, MI, p. A202
SINAI HOSPITAL OF BALTIMORE, BALTIMORE, MD, p. A185
SINAI SAMARITAN MEDICAL CENTER, MILWAUKEE, WI, p. A440
SINGING RIVER HOSPITAL, PASCAGOULA, MS, p. A227
SIOUX CENTER COMMUNITY HOSPITAL, SIOUX CENTER, IA, p. A149
SIOUX VALLEY HOSPITAL, NEW ULM, MN, p. A218
SIOUX VALLEY HOSPITAL, SIOUX FALLS, SD, p. A364
SIOUX VALLEY MEMORIAL HOSPITAL, CHEROKEE, IA, p. A143
SISKIN HOSPITAL FOR PHYSICAL REHABILITATION, CHATTANOOGA, TN, p. A367
SISKIYOU GENERAL HOSPITAL, YREKA, CA, p. A 67
SISTERS OF CHARITY HOSPITAL OF BUFFALO, BUFFALO, NY, p. A273
SISTERSVILLE GENERAL HOSPITAL, SISTERSVILLE, WV, p. A433
SITKA COMMUNITY HOSPITAL, SITKA, AK, p. A 22
SKAGGS COMMUNITY HOSPITAL, BRANSON, MO, p. A230
SKIFF MEDICAL CENTER, NEWTON, IA, p. A148
SKYLINE HOSPITAL, WHITE SALMON, WA, p. A429
SLEEPY EYE MUNICIPAL HOSPITAL, SLEEPY EYE, MN, p. A220
SLIDELL MEMORIAL HOSPITAL AND MEDICAL CENTER, SLIDELL, LA, p. A178
SLOOP MEMORIAL HOSPITAL, CROSSNORE, NC, p. A293
SMH HOMESTEAD HOSPITAL, HOMESTEAD, FL, p. A 86
SMITH COUNTY MEMORIAL HOSPITAL, SMITH CENTER, KS, p. A159
SMITH COUNTY MEMORIAL HOSPITAL, CARTHAGE, TN, p. A366
SMITH HOSPITAL, HAHIRA, GA, p. A104
SMITHVILLE HOSPITAL, SMITHVILLE, TX, p. A403
SMYRNA HOSPITAL, SMYRNA, GA, p. A108
SMYTH COUNTY COMMUNITY HOSPITAL, MARION, VA, p. A417
SNOHOMISH COUNTY PUBLIC HOSPITAL DISTRICT THREE, CASCADE VALLEY HOSPITAL, ARLINGTON, WA, p. A423
SNOQUALMIE VALLEY HOSPITAL, SNOQUALMIE, WA, p. A427
SOCIETY OF THE NEW YORK HOSPITAL, NEW YORK CITY, NY, p. A282
SOCORRO GENERAL HOSPITAL, SOCORRO, NM, p. A270
SOLDIERS AND SAILORS MEMORIAL HOSPITAL, WELLSBORO, PA, p. A351
SOLDIERS AND SAILORS MEMORIAL HOSPITAL OF YATES COUNTY, PENN YAN, NY, p. A284
SOLDIERS' HOME IN HOLYOKE, HOLYOKE, MA, p. A194
SOMERSET HOSPITAL CENTER FOR HEALTH, SOMERSET, PA, p. A349
SOMERSET MEDICAL CENTER, SOMERVILLE, NJ, p. A264
SOMERSET STATE HOSPITAL, SOMERSET, PA, p. A349
SOMERVILLE HOSPITAL, SOMERVILLE, MA, p. A196
SONOMA DEVELOPMENTAL CENTER, ELDRIDGE, CA, p. A 42
SONOMA VALLEY HOSPITAL, SONOMA, CA, p. A 64
SONORA COMMUNITY HOSPITAL, SONORA, CA, p. A 64
SOUTH AUSTIN MEDICAL CENTER, AUSTIN, TX, p. A378
SOUTH BALDWIN HOSPITAL, FOLEY, AL, p. A 16
SOUTH BARRY COUNTY MEMORIAL HOSPITAL, CASSVILLE, MO, p. A231
SOUTH BAY HOSPITAL, SUN CITY CENTER, FL, p. A 95
SOUTH BAY MEDICAL CENTER, REDONDO BEACH, CA, p. A 57
SOUTH BEACH PSYCHIATRIC CENTER, NEW YORK CITY, NY, p. A282
SOUTH CAMERON MEMORIAL HOSPITAL, CAMERON, LA, p. A171
SOUTH CAROLINA STATE HOSPITAL, COLUMBIA, SC, p. A356
SOUTH CENTRAL REGIONAL MEDICAL CENTER, LAUREL, MS, p. A225
SOUTH COAST MEDICAL CENTER, SOUTH LAGUNA, CA, p. A 64
SOUTH COUNTY HOSPITAL, WAKEFIELD, RI, p. A354
SOUTH FLORIDA BAPTIST HOSPITAL, PLANT CITY, FL, p. A 93
SOUTH FLORIDA STATE HOSPITAL, PEMBROKE PINES, FL, p. A 92
SOUTH FULTON MEDICAL CENTER, EAST POINT, GA, p. A103
SOUTH GEORGIA MEDICAL CENTER, VALDOSTA, GA, p. A109
SOUTH HAVEN COMMUNITY HOSPITAL, SOUTH HAVEN, MI, p. A210
SOUTH HILLS HEALTH SYSTEM, PITTSBURGH, PA, p. A347
SOUTH JERSEY HOSPITAL SYSTEM, BRIDGETON, NJ, p. A258
SOUTH LAKE MEMORIAL HOSPITAL, CLERMONT, FL, p. A 82
SOUTH LINCOLN MEDICAL CENTER, KEMMERER, WY, p. A445
SOUTH LOUISIANA REHABILITATION HOSPITAL, BATON ROUGE, LA, p. A170
SOUTH LYON MEDICAL CENTER, YERINGTON, NV, p. A254
SOUTH MIAMI HOSPITAL, MIAMI, FL, p. A 90
SOUTH NASSAU COMMUNITIES HOSPITAL, OCEANSIDE, NY, p. A284
SOUTH OAKS HOSPITAL, AMITYVILLE, NY, p. A271
SOUTH PANOLA COMMUNITY HOSPITAL, BATESVILLE, MS, p. A222
SOUTH PARK HOSPITAL, LUBBOCK, TX, p. A396
SOUTH PENINSULA HOSPITAL, HOMER, AK, p. A 21
SOUTH PITTSBURG MUNICIPLE HOSPITAL, SOUTH PITTSBURG, TN, p. A374
SOUTH SEMINOLE HOSPITAL, LONGWOOD, FL, p. A 88
SOUTH SHORE HOSPITAL, CHICAGO, IL, p. A120
SOUTH SHORE HOSPITAL, SOUTH WEYMOUTH, MA, p. A197
SOUTH SHORE HOSPITAL AND MEDICAL CENTER, MIAMI BEACH, FL, p. A 90
SOUTH SIDE HOSPITAL OF PITTSBURGH, PITTSBURGH, PA, p. A347
SOUTH SUBURBAN HOSPITAL, HAZEL CREST, IL, p. A124
SOUTH SUBURBAN MEDICAL CENTER, FARMINGTON, MN, p. A214
SOUTH SUNFLOWER COUNTY HOSPITAL, INDIANOLA, MS, p. A224
SOUTH TEXAS HOSPITAL, HARLINGEN, TX, p. A389
SOUTH VALLEY HOSPITAL, GILROY, CA, p. A 44
SOUTHAMPTON HOSPITAL, SOUTHAMPTON, NY, p. A287
SOUTHAMPTON MEMORIAL HOSPITAL, FRANKLIN, VA, p. A416
SOUTHEAST ALABAMA MEDICAL CENTER, DOTHAN, AL, p. A 15
SOUTHEAST ARIZONA MEDICAL CENTER, DOUGLAS, AZ, p. A 23
SOUTHEAST BAPTIST HOSPITAL, SAN ANTONIO, TX, p. A402
SOUTHEAST COLORADO HOSPITAL AND LONG TERM CARE, SPRINGFIELD, CO, p. A 72
SOUTHEAST GEORGIA REGIONAL MEDICAL CENTER, BRUNSWICK, GA, p. A100
SOUTHEAST LOUISIANA HOSPITAL, MANDEVILLE, LA, p. A174
SOUTHEAST MISSOURI HOSPITAL, CAPE GIRARDEAU, MO, p. A230
SOUTHEAST MISSOURI MENTAL HEALTH CENTER, FARMINGTON, MO, p. A232
SOUTHEAST PSYCHIATRIC CENTER, ATHENS, OH, p. A306
SOUTHEAST TEXAS REHABILITATION HOSPITAL, BEAUMONT, TX, p. A379
SOUTHEASTERN OHIO REGIONAL MEDICAL CENTER, CAMBRIDGE, OH, p. A307
SOUTHEASTERN REGIONAL MEDICAL CENTER, LUMBERTON, NC, p. A296
SOUTHERN CHESTER COUNTY MEDICAL CENTER, WEST GROVE, PA, p. A351
SOUTHERN COOS GENERAL HOSPITAL, BANDON, OR, p. A329
SOUTHERN HILLS GENERAL HOSPITAL, HOT SPRINGS, SD, p. A362
SOUTHERN HILLS MEDICAL CENTER, NASHVILLE, TN, p. A373
SOUTHERN HILLS REGIONAL REHABILITATION HOSPITAL, PRINCETON, WV, p. A433
SOUTHERN HUMBOLDT COMMUNITY HOSPITAL DISTRICT, GARBERVILLE, CA, p. A 44
SOUTHERN INYO HOSPITAL, LONE PINE, CA, p. A 47
SOUTHERN MAINE MEDICAL CENTER, BIDDEFORD, ME, p. A180
SOUTHERN MARYLAND HOSPITAL, CLINTON, MD, p. A186
SOUTHERN NEW HAMPSHIRE REGIONAL MEDICAL CENTER, NASHUA, NH, p. A256

Hospitals, Alphabetically / Southern Ocean County Hospital

SOUTHERN OCEAN COUNTY HOSPITAL, MANAHAWKIN, NJ, p. A261
SOUTHERN OHIO MEDICAL CENTER, PORTSMOUTH, OH, p. A316
SOUTHERN REGIONAL MEDICAL CENTER, RIVERDALE, GA, p. A107
SOUTHERN TENNESSEE MEDICAL CENTER, WINCHESTER, TN, p. A375
SOUTHERN VIRGINIA MENTAL HEALTH INSTITUTE, DANVILLE, VA, p. A415
SOUTHERN WINDS HOSPITAL, HIALEAH, FL, p. A 85
SOUTHMORE MEDICAL CENTER, PASADENA, TX, p. A399
SOUTHSIDE COMMUNITY HOSPITAL, FARMVILLE, VA, p. A415
SOUTHSIDE HOSPITAL, BAY SHORE, NY, p. A272
SOUTHSIDE REGIONAL MEDICAL CENTER, PETERSBURG, VA, p. A418
SOUTHWEST COMMUNITY HEALTH SYSTEM AND HOSPITAL, MIDDLEBURG HEIGHTS, OH, p. A315
SOUTHWEST FLORIDA REGIONAL MEDICAL CENTER, FORT MYERS, FL, p. A 84
SOUTHWEST GENERAL HOSPITAL, SAN ANTONIO, TX, p. A402
SOUTHWEST HEALTH CENTER, PLATTEVILLE, WI, p. A441
SOUTHWEST HOSPITAL, LITTLE ROCK, AR, p. A 32
SOUTHWEST HOSPITAL, LOUISVILLE, KY, p. A165
SOUTHWEST HOSPITAL AND MEDICAL CENTER, ATLANTA, GA, p. A 99
SOUTHWEST MEDICAL CENTER, LIBERAL, KS, p. A155
SOUTHWEST MEDICAL CENTER OF OKLAHOMA, OKLAHOMA CITY, OK, p. A325
SOUTHWEST MISSISSIPPI REGIONAL MEDICAL CENTER, MCCOMB, MS, p. A226
SOUTHWEST NEUROPSYCHIATRIC INSTITUTE, SAN ANTONIO, TX, p. A402
SOUTHWEST TEXAS METHODIST HOSPITAL, SAN ANTONIO, TX, p. A402
SOUTHWEST WASHINGTON MEDICAL CENTER, VANCOUVER, WA, p. A429
SOUTHWESTERN GENERAL HOSPITAL, EL PASO, TX, p. A386
SOUTHWESTERN MEDICAL CENTER, LAWTON, OK, p. A324
SOUTHWESTERN MEMORIAL HOSPITAL, WEATHERFORD, OK, p. A328
SOUTHWESTERN MICHIGAN REHABILITATION HOSPITAL, BATTLE CREEK, MI, p. A200
SOUTHWESTERN PSYCHIATRIC CENTER, LAWTON, OK, p. A324
SOUTHWESTERN VERMONT MEDICAL CENTER, BENNINGTON, VT, p. A412
SOUTHWESTERN VIRGINIA MENTAL HEALTH INSTITUTE, MARION, VA, p. A417
SOUTHWOOD COMMUNITY HOSPITAL, NORFOLK, MA, p. A195
SOUTHWOOD PSYCHIATRIC HOSPITAL, PITTSBURGH, PA, p. A347
SPALDING REGIONAL HOSPITAL, GRIFFIN, GA, p. A104
SPALDING REHABILITATION HOSPITAL, DENVER, CO, p. A 69
SPARKS REGIONAL MEDICAL CENTER, FORT SMITH, AR, p. A 31
SPARROW HOSPITAL, LANSING, MI, p. A206
SPARTA COMMUNITY HOSPITAL, SPARTA, IL, p. A130
SPARTANBURG REGIONAL MEDICAL CENTER, SPARTANBURG, SC, p. A359
SPAULDING REHABILITATION HOSPITAL, BOSTON, MA, p. A191
SPEARE MEMORIAL HOSPITAL, PLYMOUTH, NH, p. A257
SPECIALTY HOSPITAL JACKSONVILLE, JACKSONVILLE, FL, p. A 86
SPECIALTY HOSPITAL OF AUSTIN, AUSTIN, TX, p. A378
SPECIALTY HOSPITAL OF HOUSTON, HOUSTON, TX, p. A391
SPENCER MUNICIPAL HOSPITAL, SPENCER, IA, p. A149
SPOHN HEALTH SYSTEM, CORPUS CHRISTI, TX, p. A382
SPOHN KLEBERG MEMORIAL HOSPITAL, KINGSVILLE, TX, p. A394
SPRING BRANCH MEDICAL CENTER, HOUSTON, TX, p. A391
SPRING GROVE HOSPITAL CENTER, CATONSVILLE, MD, p. A186
SPRING HILL REGIONAL HOSPITAL, SPRING HILL, FL, p. A 95
SPRING VIEW MEDICAL CENTER, LEBANON, KY, p. A164
SPRINGFIELD COMMUNITY HOSPITAL, SPRINGFIELD, MN, p. A220
SPRINGFIELD COMMUNITY HOSPITAL, SPRINGFIELD, MO, p. A240
SPRINGFIELD HOSPITAL, SPRINGFIELD, PA, p. A349
SPRINGFIELD HOSPITAL, SPRINGFIELD, VT, p. A412
SPRINGFIELD HOSPITAL CENTER, SYKESVILLE, MD, p. A188
SPRINGFIELD MUNICIPAL HOSPITAL, SPRINGFIELD, MA, p. A197
SPRINGHILL MEDICAL CENTER, SPRINGHILL, LA, p. A178
SPRINGHILL MEMORIAL HOSPITAL, MOBILE, AL, p. A 18
SPRINGS MEMORIAL HOSPITAL, LANCASTER, SC, p. A358
SPRUCE PINE COMMUNITY HOSPITAL, SPRUCE PINE, NC, p. A299

SSM REHABILITATION INSTITUTE, SAINT LOUIS, MO, p. A238
ST. ELIZABETHS HOSPITAL, WASHINGTON, DC, p. A 79
ST. AGNES HOSPITAL, WHITE PLAINS, NY, p. A289
ST. AGNES HOSPITAL, FOND DU LAC, WI, p. A437
ST. AGNES HOSPITAL OF THE CITY OF BALTIMORE, BALTIMORE, MD, p. A185
ST. AGNES MEDICAL CENTER, FRESNO, CA, p. A 43
ST. AGNES MEDICAL CENTER, PHILADELPHIA, PA, p. A345
ST. ALBANS PSYCHIATRIC HOSPITAL, RADFORD, VA, p. A419
ST. ALEXIS HOSPITAL MEDICAL CENTER, CLEVELAND, OH, p. A310
ST. ALEXIUS MEDICAL CENTER, BISMARCK, ND, p. A302
ST. ALOISIUS MEDICAL CENTER, HARVEY, ND, p. A303
ST. ANDREW'S HEALTH CENTER, BOTTINEAU, ND, p. A302
ST. ANDREWS HOSPITAL, BOOTHBAY HARBOR, ME, p. A180
ST. ANN'S HOSPITAL OF COLUMBUS, WESTERVILLE, OH, p. A319
ST. ANNE GENERAL HOSPITAL, RACELAND, LA, p. A177
ST. ANSGAR'S HOSPITAL, PARK RIVER, ND, p. A304
ST. ANTHONY COMMUNITY HOSPITAL, WARWICK, NY, p. A289
ST. ANTHONY HOSPITAL, OKLAHOMA CITY, OK, p. A325
ST. ANTHONY HOSPITAL, PENDLETON, OR, p. A331
ST. ANTHONY MEDICAL CENTER, CROWN POINT, IN, p. A134
ST. ANTHONY REGIONAL HOSPITAL, CARROLL, IA, p. A142
ST. ANTHONY'S HOSPITAL, SAINT PETERSBURG, FL, p. A 94
ST. ANTHONY'S HOSPITAL, O'NEILL, NE, p. A249
ST. ANTHONY'S HOSPITAL, AMARILLO, TX, p. A376
ST. ANTHONY'S MEDICAL CENTER, SAINT LOUIS, MO, p. A238
ST. ANTHONY'S MEMORIAL HOSPITAL, EFFINGHAM, IL, p. A122
ST. AUGUSTINE PSYCHIATRIC CENTER, SAINT AUGUSTINE, FL, p. A 94
ST. BARNABAS HOSPITAL, NEW YORK CITY, NY, p. A282
ST. BENEDICT HEALTH CENTER, PARKSTON, SD, p. A363
ST. BENEDICTS FAMILY MEDICAL CENTER, JEROME, ID, p. A113
ST. BERNARD HOSPITAL, CHICAGO, IL, p. A120
ST. BERNARD'S PROVIDENCE HOSPITAL, MILBANK, SD, p. A362
ST. BERNARDINE MEDICAL CENTER, SAN BERNARDINO, CA, p. A 59
ST. BERNARDS REGIONAL MEDICAL CENTER, JONESBORO, AR, p. A 31
ST. CATHERINE HOSPITAL, EAST CHICAGO, IN, p. A134
ST. CATHERINE HOSPITAL, GARDEN CITY, KS, p. A153
ST. CATHERINE'S HOSPITAL, KENOSHA, WI, p. A438
ST. CHARLES GENERAL HOSPITAL, NEW ORLEANS, LA, p. A176
ST. CHARLES HOSPITAL, LULING, LA, p. A174
ST. CHARLES HOSPITAL, OREGON, OH, p. A316
ST. CHARLES HOSPITAL AND REHABILITATION CENTER, PORT JEFFERSON, NY, p. A285
ST. CHARLES MEDICAL CENTER, BEND, OR, p. A329
ST. CHRISTOPHER'S HOSPITAL FOR CHILDREN, PHILADELPHIA, PA, p. A345
ST. CLAIR HOSPITAL, PITTSBURGH, PA, p. A347
ST. CLAIR REGIONAL HOSPITAL, PELL CITY, AL, p. A 19
ST. CLAIRE MEDICAL CENTER, MOREHEAD, KY, p. A166
ST. CLARE HOSPITAL, TACOMA, WA, p. A428
ST. CLARE HOSPITAL AND HEALTH SERVICES, BARABOO, WI, p. A435
ST. CLARE'S HOSPITAL AND HEALTH CENTER, NEW YORK CITY, NY, p. A282
ST. CLARE'S HOSPITAL OF SCHENECTADY, SCHENECTADY, NY, p. A287
ST. CLEMENT HOSPITAL, RED BUD, IL, p. A129
ST. CLOUD HOSPITAL, SAINT CLOUD, MN, p. A219
ST. CLOUD HOSPITAL, A DIVISION OF ORLANDO REGIONAL HEALTHCARE SYSTEM, SAINT CLOUD, FL, p. A 94
ST. CROIX HOSPITAL, CHRISTIANSTED, VI, p. A450
ST. CROIX VALLEY MEMORIAL HOSPITAL, SAINT CROIX FALLS, WI, p. A442
ST. DAVID'S HEALTH CARE SYSTEM, AUSTIN, TX, p. A378
ST. DAVID'S PAVILION, AUSTIN, TX, p. A378
ST. DAVID'S REHABILITATION CENTER, AUSTIN, TX, p. A378
ST. DOMINIC-JACKSON MEMORIAL HOSPITAL, JACKSON, MS, p. A225
ST. EDWARD MERCY MEDICAL CENTER, FORT SMITH, AR, p. A 31
ST. ELIZABETH COMMUNITY HEALTH CENTER, LINCOLN, NE, p. A249
ST. ELIZABETH COMMUNITY HOSPITAL, RED BLUFF, CA, p. A 57
ST. ELIZABETH HEALTH SERVICES, BAKER CITY, OR, p. A329
ST. ELIZABETH HOSPITAL, WABASHA, MN, p. A221
ST. ELIZABETH HOSPITAL, ELIZABETH, NJ, p. A260
ST. ELIZABETH HOSPITAL, UTICA, NY, p. A288
ST. ELIZABETH HOSPITAL, BEAUMONT, TX, p. A379
ST. ELIZABETH HOSPITAL, APPLETON, WI, p. A435

ST. ELIZABETH HOSPITAL MEDICAL CENTER, LAFAYETTE, IN, p. A138
ST. ELIZABETH HOSPITAL MEDICAL CENTER, YOUNGSTOWN, OH, p. A319
ST. ELIZABETH MEDICAL CENTER–GRANT COUNTY, WILLIAMSTOWN, KY, p. A168
ST. ELIZABETH MEDICAL CENTER–NORTH, COVINGTON, KY, p. A162
ST. ELIZABETH MEDICAL CENTER, GRANITE CITY, IL, p. A124
ST. ELIZABETH MEDICAL CENTER, DAYTON, OH, p. A311
ST. ELIZABETH'S HOSPITAL, BELLEVILLE, IL, p. A116
ST. ELIZABETH'S HOSPITAL, CHICAGO, IL, p. A120
ST. ELIZABETH'S MEDICAL CENTER OF BOSTON, BOSTON, MA, p. A191
ST. FRANCES CABRINI HOSPITAL, ALEXANDRIA, LA, p. A170
ST. FRANCIS–ST. GEORGE HOSPITAL, CINCINNATI, OH, p. A309
ST. FRANCIS AT ELLSWORTH, ELLSWORTH, KS, p. A152
ST. FRANCIS AT SALINA, SALINA, KS, p. A158
ST. FRANCIS CENTRAL HOSPITAL, PITTSBURGH, PA, p. A347
ST. FRANCIS HEALTH CARE CENTRE, GREEN SPRINGS, OH, p. A312
ST. FRANCIS HEALTH SYSTEM, GREENVILLE, SC, p. A358
ST. FRANCIS HOSPITAL, WILMINGTON, DE, p. A 78
ST. FRANCIS HOSPITAL, COLUMBUS, GA, p. A101
ST. FRANCIS HOSPITAL, EVANSTON, IL, p. A123
ST. FRANCIS HOSPITAL, LITCHFIELD, IL, p. A126
ST. FRANCIS HOSPITAL, ESCANABA, MI, p. A202
ST. FRANCIS HOSPITAL, MARYVILLE, MO, p. A235
ST. FRANCIS HOSPITAL, MOUNTAIN VIEW, MO, p. A236
ST. FRANCIS HOSPITAL, JERSEY CITY, NJ, p. A261
ST. FRANCIS HOSPITAL, ROSLYN, NY, p. A286
ST. FRANCIS HOSPITAL, MEMPHIS, TN, p. A372
ST. FRANCIS HOSPITAL, FEDERAL WAY, WA, p. A424
ST. FRANCIS HOSPITAL, MILWAUKEE, WI, p. A440
ST. FRANCIS HOSPITAL AND HEALTH CENTER, BLUE ISLAND, IL, p. A117
ST. FRANCIS HOSPITAL AND HEALTH CENTERS, BEECH GROVE, IN, p. A133
ST. FRANCIS HOSPITAL AND MEDICAL CENTER, TOPEKA, KS, p. A159
ST. FRANCIS HOSPITAL OF NEW CASTLE, NEW CASTLE, PA, p. A343
ST. FRANCIS MEDICAL CENTER, LYNWOOD, CA, p. A 51
ST. FRANCIS MEDICAL CENTER, HONOLULU, HI, p. A110
ST. FRANCIS MEDICAL CENTER, MONROE, LA, p. A175
ST. FRANCIS MEDICAL CENTER, BRECKENRIDGE, MN, p. A213
ST. FRANCIS MEDICAL CENTER, TRENTON, NJ, p. A265
ST. FRANCIS MEDICAL CENTER, PITTSBURGH, PA, p. A347
ST. FRANCIS MEDICAL CENTER, LA CROSSE, WI, p. A438
ST. FRANCIS MEDICAL CENTER OF SANTA BARBARA, SANTA BARBARA, CA, p. A 62
ST. FRANCIS MEMORIAL HOSPITAL, WEST POINT, NE, p. A252
ST. FRANCIS REGIONAL MEDICAL CENTER, WICHITA, KS, p. A160
ST. FRANCIS REGIONAL MEDICAL CENTER, SHAKOPEE, MN, p. A220
ST. GABRIEL'S HOSPITAL, LITTLE FALLS, MN, p. A216
ST. HELENA HOSPITAL, DEER PARK, CA, p. A 41
ST. HELENA PARISH HOSPITAL, GREENSBURG, LA, p. A172
ST. JAMES COMMUNITY HOSPITAL, BUTTE, MT, p. A241
ST. JAMES HOSPITAL AND HEALTH CENTERS, CHICAGO HEIGHTS, IL, p. A121
ST. JAMES MERCY HOSPITAL, HORNELL, NY, p. A276
ST. JAMES PARISH HOSPITAL, LUTCHER, LA, p. A174
ST. JEROME HOSPITAL, BATAVIA, NY, p. A271
ST. JOHN HOSPITAL–MACOMB CENTER, HARRISON TOWNSHIP, MI, p. A204
ST. JOHN HOSPITAL, NASSAU BAY, TX, p. A398
ST. JOHN HOSPITAL AND MEDICAL CENTER, DETROIT, MI, p. A202
ST. JOHN MEDICAL CENTER, STEUBENVILLE, OH, p. A317
ST. JOHN MEDICAL CENTER, TULSA, OK, p. A328
ST. JOHN OF GOD HOSPITAL, BOSTON, MA, p. A192
ST. JOHN WEST SHORE HOSPITAL, WESTLAKE, OH, p. A319
ST. JOHN'S EPISCOPAL HOSPITAL–SMITHTOWN, SMITHTOWN, NY, p. A287
ST. JOHN'S EPISCOPAL HOSPITAL–SOUTH SHORE, NEW YORK CITY, NY, p. A282
ST. JOHN'S HOSPITAL, SPRINGFIELD, IL, p. A131
ST. JOHN'S HOSPITAL AND NURSING HOME, JACKSON, WY, p. A445
ST. JOHN'S LUTHERAN HOSPITAL, LIBBY, MT, p. A243
ST. JOHN'S MEDICAL CENTER, LONGVIEW, WA, p. A425
ST. JOHN'S MERCY MEDICAL CENTER, SAINT LOUIS, MO, p. A239
ST. JOHN'S PLEASANT VALLEY HOSPITAL, CAMARILLO, CA, p. A 38
ST. JOHN'S REGIONAL HEALTH CENTER, SALINA, KS, p. A158

ST. JOHN'S REGIONAL HEALTH CENTER, RED WING, MN, p. A218
ST. JOHN'S REGIONAL HEALTH CENTER, SPRINGFIELD, MO, p. A240
ST. JOHN'S REGIONAL MEDICAL CENTER, OXNARD, CA, p. A 55
ST. JOHN'S REGIONAL MEDICAL CENTER, JOPLIN, MO, p. A233
ST. JOHN'S RIVERSIDE HOSPITAL, YONKERS, NY, p. A289
ST. JOSEPH HEALTH CENTER, SAINT CHARLES, MO, p. A237
ST. JOSEPH HEALTH CENTERS AND HOSPITAL, CHICAGO, IL, p. A120
ST. JOSEPH HEALTH SERVICES OF RHODE ISLAND, NORTH PROVIDENCE, RI, p. A353
ST. JOSEPH HOSPITAL, EUREKA, CA, p. A 42
ST. JOSEPH HOSPITAL, ORANGE, CA, p. A 55
ST. JOSEPH HOSPITAL, AUGUSTA, GA, p. A100
ST. JOSEPH HOSPITAL, MISHAWAKA, IN, p. A139
ST. JOSEPH HOSPITAL, CONCORDIA, KS, p. A152
ST. JOSEPH HOSPITAL, LEXINGTON, KY, p. A164
ST. JOSEPH HOSPITAL, BANGOR, ME, p. A180
ST. JOSEPH HOSPITAL, SAINT LOUIS, MO, p. A239
ST. JOSEPH HOSPITAL, POLSON, MT, p. A244
ST. JOSEPH HOSPITAL, CHEEKTOWAGA, NY, p. A273
ST. JOSEPH HOSPITAL, LANCASTER, PA, p. A341
ST. JOSEPH HOSPITAL, HOUSTON, TX, p. A392
ST. JOSEPH HOSPITAL, BELLINGHAM, WA, p. A423
ST. JOSEPH HOSPITAL AND HEALTH CENTERS, MEMPHIS, TN, p. A372
ST. JOSEPH HOSPITAL AND TRAUMA CENTER, NASHUA, NH, p. A256
ST. JOSEPH HOSPITAL WEST, LAKE SAINT LOUIS, MO, p. A235
ST. JOSEPH MEDICAL CENTER, STAMFORD, CT, p. A 77
ST. JOSEPH MEDICAL CENTER, BLOOMINGTON, IL, p. A117
ST. JOSEPH MEDICAL CENTER, WICHITA, KS, p. A160
ST. JOSEPH MEDICAL CENTER, TOWSON, MD, p. A188
ST. JOSEPH MEDICAL CENTER, ALBUQUERQUE, NM, p. A267
ST. JOSEPH MEDICAL CENTER, READING, PA, p. A348
ST. JOSEPH MEDICAL CENTER, TACOMA, WA, p. A428
ST. JOSEPH MEDICAL CENTER OF FORT WAYNE, FORT WAYNE, IN, p. A135
ST. JOSEPH MEMORIAL HOSPITAL, MURPHYSBORO, IL, p. A127
ST. JOSEPH MERCY COMMUNITY HEALTHCARE SYSTEM, PONTIAC, MI, p. A208
ST. JOSEPH NORTHEAST HEIGHTS HOSPITAL, ALBUQUERQUE, NM, p. A267
ST. JOSEPH REGIONAL HEALTH CENTER, BRYAN, TX, p. A380
ST. JOSEPH REGIONAL MEDICAL CENTER, LEWISTON, ID, p. A113
ST. JOSEPH REGIONAL MEDICAL CENTER OF NORTHERN OKLAHOMA, PONCA CITY, OK, p. A326
ST. JOSEPH REHABILITATION HOSPITAL AND OUTPATIENT CENTER, ALBUQUERQUE, NM, p. A267
ST. JOSEPH RIVERSIDE HOSPITAL, WARREN, OH, p. A318
ST. JOSEPH STATE HOSPITAL, SAINT JOSEPH, MO, p. A237
ST. JOSEPH WEST MESA HOSPITAL, ALBUQUERQUE, NM, p. A267
ST. JOSEPH'S BEHAVIORAL HEALTH CENTER, STOCKTON, CA, p. A 64
ST. JOSEPH'S COMMUNITY HOSPITAL OF WEST BEND, WEST BEND, WI, p. A444
ST. JOSEPH'S HOSPITAL, SAVANNAH, GA, p. A108
ST. JOSEPH'S HOSPITAL, BREESE, IL, p. A117
ST. JOSEPH'S HOSPITAL, HIGHLAND, IL, p. A124
ST. JOSEPH'S HOSPITAL, HUNTINGBURG, IN, p. A136
ST. JOSEPH'S HOSPITAL, PARK RAPIDS, MN, p. A218
ST. JOSEPH'S HOSPITAL, ELMIRA, NY, p. A275
ST. JOSEPH'S HOSPITAL, ASHEVILLE, NC, p. A291
ST. JOSEPH'S HOSPITAL, CHEWELAH, WA, p. A423
ST. JOSEPH'S HOSPITAL, BUCKHANNON, WV, p. A430
ST. JOSEPH'S HOSPITAL, PARKERSBURG, WV, p. A432
ST. JOSEPH'S HOSPITAL, ARCADIA, WI, p. A435
ST. JOSEPH'S HOSPITAL, CHIPPEWA FALLS, WI, p. A436
ST. JOSEPH'S HOSPITAL, MILWAUKEE, WI, p. A440
ST. JOSEPH'S HOSPITAL AND HEALTH CENTER, DICKINSON, ND, p. A302
ST. JOSEPH'S HOSPITAL AND HEALTH CENTER, PARIS, TX, p. A399
ST. JOSEPH'S HOSPITAL AND MEDICAL CENTER, PHOENIX, AZ, p. A 26
ST. JOSEPH'S HOSPITAL AND MEDICAL CENTER, PATERSON, NJ, p. A263
ST. JOSEPH'S HOSPITAL HEALTH CENTER, SYRACUSE, NY, p. A288
ST. JOSEPH'S HOSPITAL OF MARSHALL COUNTY, PLYMOUTH, IN, p. A140
ST. JOSEPH'S HOSPITALS, TAMPA, FL, p. A 96

ST. JOSEPH'S MEDICAL CENTER, STOCKTON, CA, p. A 64
ST. JOSEPH'S MEDICAL CENTER, SOUTH BEND, IN, p. A140
ST. JOSEPH'S MEDICAL CENTER, BRAINERD, MN, p. A213
ST. JOSEPH'S MEDICAL CENTER, YONKERS, NY, p. A289
ST. JOSEPH'S MEMORIAL HOSPITAL AND NURSING HOME, HILLSBORO, WI, p. A437
ST. JOSEPH'S MERCY HOSPITAL, CENTERVILLE, IA, p. A143
ST. JOSEPH'S MERCY HOSPITALS AND HEALTH SERVICES, CLINTON TOWNSHIP, MI, p. A201
ST. JOSEPH'S REGIONAL HEALTH CENTER, HOT SPRINGS, AR, p. A 31
ST. JUDE CHILDREN'S RESEARCH HOSPITAL, MEMPHIS, TN, p. A372
ST. JUDE MEDICAL CENTER, FULLERTON, CA, p. A 43
ST. LAWRENCE HOSPITAL AND HEALTHCARE SERVICES, LANSING, MI, p. A206
ST. LAWRENCE PSYCHIATRIC CENTER, OGDENSBURG, NY, p. A284
ST. LAWRENCE REHABILITATION CENTER, LAWRENCEVILLE, NJ, p. A261
ST. LOUIS CHILDREN'S HOSPITAL, SAINT LOUIS, MO, p. A239
ST. LOUIS REGIONAL MEDICAL CENTER, SAINT LOUIS, MO, p. A239
ST. LOUIS STATE HOSPITAL, SAINT LOUIS, MO, p. A239
ST. LUKE COMMUNITY HOSPITAL, RONAN, MT, p. A244
ST. LUKE HOSPITAL, MARION, KS, p. A156
ST. LUKE HOSPITAL WEST, FLORENCE, KY, p. A162
ST. LUKE HOSPITALS, FORT THOMAS, KY, p. A162
ST. LUKE MEDICAL CENTER, PASADENA, CA, p. A 56
ST. LUKE'S-ROOSEVELT HOSPITAL CENTER, NEW YORK CITY, NY, p. A282
ST. LUKE'S BAPTIST HOSPITAL, SAN ANTONIO, TX, p. A402
ST. LUKE'S BEHAVIORAL HEALTH CENTER, PHOENIX, AZ, p. A 26
ST. LUKE'S EPISCOPAL HOSPITAL, HOUSTON, TX, p. A392
ST. LUKE'S HOSPITAL, SAN FRANCISCO, CA, p. A 61
ST. LUKE'S HOSPITAL, JACKSONVILLE, FL, p. A 86
ST. LUKE'S HOSPITAL, CEDAR RAPIDS, IA, p. A143
ST. LUKE'S HOSPITAL, SAGINAW, MI, p. A209
ST. LUKE'S HOSPITAL, DULUTH, MN, p. A214
ST. LUKE'S HOSPITAL, CHESTERFIELD, MO, p. A231
ST. LUKE'S HOSPITAL, KANSAS CITY, MO, p. A234
ST. LUKE'S HOSPITAL, NEWBURGH, NY, p. A283
ST. LUKE'S HOSPITAL, COLUMBUS, NC, p. A293
ST. LUKE'S HOSPITAL, CROSBY, ND, p. A302
ST. LUKE'S HOSPITAL, MAUMEE, OH, p. A315
ST. LUKE'S HOSPITAL, BETHLEHEM, PA, p. A335
ST. LUKE'S HOSPITAL, BLUEFIELD, WV, p. A430
ST. LUKE'S HOSPITAL OF NEW BEDFORD, NEW BEDFORD, MA, p. A195
ST. LUKE'S MEDICAL CENTER, PHOENIX, AZ, p. A 26
ST. LUKE'S MEDICAL CENTER, MILWAUKEE, WI, p. A440
ST. LUKE'S MEMORIAL HOSPITAL, RACINE, WI, p. A442
ST. LUKE'S MEMORIAL HOSPITAL CENTER, UTICA, NY, p. A288
ST. LUKE'S MIDLAND REGIONAL MEDICAL CENTER, ABERDEEN, SD, p. A361
ST. LUKE'S REGIONAL MEDICAL CENTER, BOISE, ID, p. A112
ST. LUKE'S REGIONAL MEDICAL CENTER, SIOUX CITY, IA, p. A149
ST. LUKE'S TRI-STATE HOSPITAL, BOWMAN, ND, p. A302
ST. LUKES REHABILITATION INSTITUTE, SPOKANE, WA, p. A428
ST. MARGARET MEMORIAL HOSPITAL, PITTSBURGH, PA, p. A347
ST. MARGARET'S HOSPITAL, SPRING VALLEY, IL, p. A130
ST. MARK'S HOSPITAL, SALT LAKE CITY, UT, p. A410
ST. MARY-CORWIN REGIONAL MEDICAL CENTER, PUEBLO, CO, p. A 72
ST. MARY-ROGERS MEMORIAL HOSPITAL, ROGERS, AR, p. A 34
ST. MARY DESERT VALLEY HOSPITAL, APPLE VALLEY, CA, p. A 36
ST. MARY HOSPITAL, LIVONIA, MI, p. A206
ST. MARY HOSPITAL, HOBOKEN, NJ, p. A260
ST. MARY HOSPITAL, PORT ARTHUR, TX, p. A400
ST. MARY MEDICAL CENTER, LONG BEACH, CA, p. A 48
ST. MARY MEDICAL CENTER, GALESBURG, IL, p. A123
ST. MARY MEDICAL CENTER, HOBART, IN, p. A136
ST. MARY MEDICAL CENTER, LANGHORNE, PA, p. A341
ST. MARY MEDICAL CENTER, WALLA WALLA, WA, p. A429
ST. MARY OF THE PLAINS HOSPITAL, LUBBOCK, TX, p. A396
ST. MARY'S HEALTH CARE SYSTEM, ATHENS, GA, p. A 98
ST. MARY'S HEALTH CENTER, SAINT LOUIS, MO, p. A239
ST. MARY'S HEALTH SYSTEM, KNOXVILLE, TN, p. A370
ST. MARY'S HILL HOSPITAL, MILWAUKEE, WI, p. A440
ST. MARY'S HOSPITAL, WATERBURY, CT, p. A 77
ST. MARY'S HOSPITAL, WEST PALM BEACH, FL, p. A 97
ST. MARY'S HOSPITAL, COTTONWOOD, ID, p. A113
ST. MARY'S HOSPITAL, CENTRALIA, IL, p. A117

ST. MARY'S HOSPITAL, DECATUR, IL, p. A122
ST. MARY'S HOSPITAL, EAST SAINT LOUIS, IL, p. A122
ST. MARY'S HOSPITAL, STREATOR, IL, p. A131
ST. MARY'S HOSPITAL, LEONARDTOWN, MD, p. A188
ST. MARY'S HOSPITAL, NEBRASKA CITY, NE, p. A249
ST. MARY'S HOSPITAL, PASSAIC, NJ, p. A263
ST. MARY'S HOSPITAL, AMSTERDAM, NY, p. A271
ST. MARY'S HOSPITAL, ROCHESTER, NY, p. A286
ST. MARY'S HOSPITAL, PIERRE, SD, p. A363
ST. MARY'S HOSPITAL, GALVESTON, TX, p. A388
ST. MARY'S HOSPITAL, NORTON, VA, p. A418
ST. MARY'S HOSPITAL, RICHMOND, VA, p. A420
ST. MARY'S HOSPITAL, HUNTINGTON, WV, p. A431
ST. MARY'S HOSPITAL, MILWAUKEE, WI, p. A440
ST. MARY'S HOSPITAL, SPARTA, WI, p. A443
ST. MARY'S HOSPITAL AND MEDICAL CENTER, GRAND JUNCTION, CO, p. A 71
ST. MARY'S HOSPITAL MEDICAL CENTER, GREEN BAY, WI, p. A437
ST. MARY'S HOSPITAL OF BLUE SPRINGS, BLUE SPRINGS, MO, p. A230
ST. MARY'S HOSPITAL OF KANKAKEE, KANKAKEE, IL, p. A125
ST. MARY'S HOSPITAL OZAUKEE, MEQUON, WI, p. A439
ST. MARY'S KEWAUNEE AREA MEMORIAL HOSPITAL, KEWAUNEE, WI, p. A438
ST. MARY'S MEDICAL CENTER, SAN FRANCISCO, CA, p. A 61
ST. MARY'S MEDICAL CENTER, SAGINAW, MI, p. A209
ST. MARY'S MEDICAL CENTER, DULUTH, MN, p. A214
ST. MARY'S MEDICAL CENTER, ENID, OK, p. A323
ST. MARY'S MEDICAL CENTER OF EVANSVILLE, EVANSVILLE, IN, p. A135
ST. MARY'S REGIONAL HEALTH CENTER, DETROIT LAKES, MN, p. A214
ST. MARY'S REGIONAL MEDICAL CENTER, RUSSELLVILLE, AR, p. A 34
ST. MARY'S REGIONAL MEDICAL CENTER, LEWISTON, ME, p. A181
ST. MARY'S REGIONAL MEDICAL CENTER, RENO, NV, p. A254
ST. MARYS HEALTH CENTER, JEFFERSON CITY, MO, p. A233
ST. MARYS HOSPITAL MEDICAL CENTER, MADISON, WI, p. A438
ST. MARYS REGIONAL MEDICAL CENTER, SAINT MARYS, PA, p. A348
ST. MICHAEL HEALTH CARE CENTER, TEXARKANA, TX, p. A404
ST. MICHAEL HOSPITAL, MILWAUKEE, WI, p. A440
ST. MICHAEL REHABILITATION HOSPITAL, TEXARKANA, TX, p. A405
ST. MICHAEL'S HOSPITAL, SAUK CENTRE, MN, p. A220
ST. NICHOLAS HOSPITAL, SHEBOYGAN, WI, p. A443
ST. PATRICK HOSPITAL, MISSOULA, MT, p. A243
ST. PATRICK HOSPITAL OF LAKE CHARLES, LAKE CHARLES, LA, p. A174
ST. PAUL-RAMSEY MEDICAL CENTER, SAINT PAUL, MN, p. A219
ST. PAUL MEDICAL CENTER, DALLAS, TX, p. A384
ST. PETER REGIONAL TREATMENT CENTER, SAINT PETER, MN, p. A220
ST. PETER'S COMMUNITY HOSPITAL, HELENA, MT, p. A243
ST. PETER'S HOSPITAL, ALBANY, NY, p. A271
ST. PETER'S MEDICAL CENTER, NEW BRUNSWICK, NJ, p. A262
ST. PETERSBURG GENERAL HOSPITAL, SAINT PETERSBURG, FL, p. A 95
ST. RITA'S MEDICAL CENTER, LIMA, OH, p. A313
ST. ROSE DOMINICAN HOSPITAL, HENDERSON, NV, p. A253
ST. ROSE HOSPITAL, HAYWARD, CA, p. A 45
ST. TAMMANY PARISH HOSPITAL, COVINGTON, LA, p. A171
ST. THOMAS HOSPITAL, NASHVILLE, TN, p. A373
ST. THOMAS HOSPITAL AND COMMUNITY HEALTH SERVICE, SAINT THOMAS, VI, p. A450
ST. THOMAS MORE HOSPITAL AND PROGRESSIVE CARE CENTER, CANON CITY, CO, p. A 68
ST. VINCENT CHARITY HOSPITAL, CLEVELAND, OH, p. A310
ST. VINCENT GENERAL HOSPITAL, LEADVILLE, CO, p. A 71
ST. VINCENT HOSPITAL, SANTA FE, NM, p. A270
ST. VINCENT HOSPITAL, GREEN BAY, WI, p. A437
ST. VINCENT HOSPITAL AND HEALTH CARE CENTER, INDIANAPOLIS, IN, p. A137
ST. VINCENT INFIRMARY MEDICAL CENTER, LITTLE ROCK, AR, p. A 32
ST. VINCENT MEDICAL CENTER, LOS ANGELES, CA, p. A 51
ST. VINCENT MEDICAL CENTER, TOLEDO, OH, p. A318
ST. VINCENT MEMORIAL HOSPITAL, TAYLORVILLE, IL, p. A131
ST. VINCENT MERCY HOSPITAL, ELWOOD, IN, p. A135
ST. VINCENT'S HOSPITAL, BIRMINGHAM, AL, p. A 14
ST. VINCENT'S HOSPITAL AND MEDICAL CENTER OF NEW YORK, NEW YORK CITY, NY, p. A282
ST. VINCENT'S MEDICAL CENTER, BRIDGEPORT, CT, p. A 74

ST. VINCENT'S MEDICAL CENTER, JACKSONVILLE, FL, p. A 86
ST. VINCENT'S MEDICAL CENTER OF RICHMOND, NEW YORK CITY, NY, p. A282
STAFFORD DISTRICT HOSPITAL NUMBER FOUR, STAFFORD, KS, p. A159
STAMFORD HOSPITAL, STAMFORD, CT, p. A 77
STAMFORD MEMORIAL HOSPITAL, STAMFORD, TX, p. A404
STANDISH COMMUNITY HOSPITAL, STANDISH, MI, p. A210
STANFORD UNIVERSITY HOSPITAL, STANFORD, CA, p. A 64
STANISLAUS BEHAVIORAL HEALTH CENTER, MODESTO, CA, p. A 53
STANISLAUS MEDICAL CENTER, MODESTO, CA, p. A 53
STANLEY COMMUNITY HOSPITAL, STANLEY, ND, p. A305
STANLY MEMORIAL HOSPITAL, ALBEMARLE, NC, p. A291
STANTON COUNTY HOSPITAL AND LONG-TERM CARE UNIT, JOHNSON, KS, p. A154
STAR VALLEY HOSPITAL, AFTON, WY, p. A445
STARKE MEMORIAL HOSPITAL, KNOX, IN, p. A137
STARLITE VILLAGE HOSPITAL, CENTER POINT, TX, p. A381
STARR COUNTY MEMORIAL HOSPITAL, RIO GRANDE CITY, TX, p. A400
STATE CORRECTIONAL INSTITUTION AT CAMP HILL, CAMP HILL, PA, p. A336
STATE CORRECTIONAL INSTITUTION HOSPITAL, PITTSBURGH, PA, p. A347
STATE HOSPITAL NORTH, OROFINO, ID, p. A114
STATE HOSPITAL SOUTH, BLACKFOOT, ID, p. A112
STATE PENITENTIARY HOSPITAL, WALLA WALLA, WA, p. A429
STATE PSYCHIATRIC HOSPITAL, SAN JUAN, PR, p. A450
STATEN ISLAND UNIVERSITY HOSPITAL, NEW YORK CITY, NY, p. A282
STE. GENEVIEVE COUNTY MEMORIAL HOSPITAL, SAINTE GENEVIEVE, MO, p. A240
STEELE MEMORIAL HOSPITAL, SALMON, ID, p. A114
STEPHENS COUNTY HOSPITAL, TOCCOA, GA, p. A109
STEPHENS MEMORIAL HOSPITAL, NORWAY, ME, p. A182
STEPHENS MEMORIAL HOSPITAL, BRECKENRIDGE, TX, p. A380
STERLING REGIONAL MEDCENTER, STERLING, CO, p. A 72
STERLINGTON HOSPITAL, STERLINGTON, LA, p. A178
STEVENS COMMUNITY MEDICAL CENTER, MORRIS, MN, p. A217
STEVENS COUNTY HOSPITAL, HUGOTON, KS, p. A154
STEVENS HOSPITAL, EDMONDS, WA, p. A424
STEWART–WEBSTER HOSPITAL, RICHLAND, GA, p. A107
STEWART MEMORIAL COMMUNITY HOSPITAL, LAKE CITY, IA, p. A147
STILLMAN INFIRMARY, HARVARD UNIVERSITY HEALTH SERVICES, CAMBRIDGE, MA, p. A192
STILLWATER COMMUNITY HOSPITAL, COLUMBUS, MT, p. A241
STILLWATER MEDICAL CENTER, STILLWATER, OK, p. A327
STOKES–REYNOLDS MEMORIAL HOSPITAL, DANBURY, NC, p. A293
STONE COUNTY MEDICAL CENTER, MOUNTAIN VIEW, AR, p. A 33
STONES RIVER HOSPITAL, WOODBURY, TN, p. A375
STONEWALL JACKSON HOSPITAL, LEXINGTON, VA, p. A417
STONEWALL JACKSON MEMORIAL HOSPITAL, WESTON, WV, p. A433
STONEWALL MEMORIAL HOSPITAL, ASPERMONT, TX, p. A377
STONY LODGE HOSPITAL, OSSINING, NY, p. A284
STORMONT-VAIL REGIONAL MEDICAL CENTER, TOPEKA, KS, p. A159
STORY CITY MEMORIAL HOSPITAL, STORY CITY, IA, p. A150
STORY COUNTY HOSPITAL AND LONG TERM CARE FACILITY, NEVADA, IA, p. A148
STOUDER MEMORIAL HOSPITAL, TROY, OH, p. A318
STOUGHTON HOSPITAL ASSOCIATION, STOUGHTON, WI, p. A443
STRAITH HOSPITAL FOR SPECIAL SURGERY, SOUTHFIELD, MI, p. A210
STRAUB CLINIC AND HOSPITAL, HONOLULU, HI, p. A110
STRINGFELLOW MEMORIAL HOSPITAL, ANNISTON, AL, p. A 13
STRONG MEMORIAL HOSPITAL OF THE UNIVERSITY OF ROCHESTER, ROCHESTER, NY, p. A286
STROUD MUNICIPAL HOSPITAL, STROUD, OK, p. A327
STURDY MEMORIAL HOSPITAL, ATTLEBORO, MA, p. A190
STURGIS COMMUNITY HEALTH CARE CENTER, STURGIS, SD, p. A364
STURGIS HOSPITAL, STURGIS, MI, p. A210
STUTTGART MEMORIAL HOSPITAL, STUTTGART, AR, p. A 34
SUBURBAN GENERAL HOSPITAL, NORRISTOWN, PA, p. A343
SUBURBAN GENERAL HOSPITAL, PITTSBURGH, PA, p. A347
SUBURBAN HOSPITAL, HINSDALE, IL, p. A125
SUBURBAN HOSPITAL, BETHESDA, MD, p. A186
SUBURBAN MEDICAL CENTER, PARAMOUNT, CA, p. A 55
SUBURBAN MEDICAL CENTER, LOUISVILLE, KY, p. A166
SULLIVAN COUNTY MEMORIAL HOSPITAL, MILAN, MO, p. A236
SUMMA HEALTH SYSTEM, AKRON, OH, p. A306

SUMMERS COUNTY APPALACHIAN REGIONAL HOSPITAL, HINTON, WV, p. A431
SUMMERSVILLE MEMORIAL HOSPITAL, SUMMERSVILLE, WV, p. A433
SUMMERVILLE MEDICAL CENTER, SUMMERVILLE, SC, p. A359
SUMMIT INSTITUTE FOR PULMONARY MEDICINE AND REHABILITATION, BOSSIER CITY, LA, p. A171
SUMMIT MEDICAL CENTER, OAKLAND, CA, p. A 54
SUMMIT MEDICAL CENTER, HERMITAGE, TN, p. A369
SUMNER COUNTY HOSPITAL DISTRICT ONE, CALDWELL, KS, p. A151
SUMNER REGIONAL MEDICAL CENTER, WELLINGTON, KS, p. A159
SUMNER REGIONAL MEDICAL CENTER, GALLATIN, TN, p. A368
SUMTER REGIONAL HOSPITAL, AMERICUS, GA, p. A 98
SUN BELT REGIONAL MEDICAL CENTER, HOUSTON, TX, p. A392
SUN COAST HOSPITAL, LARGO, FL, p. A 88
SUN CREST HOSPITAL, FARMINGTON, NM, p. A268
SUNBURY COMMUNITY HOSPITAL, SUNBURY, PA, p. A349
SUNNYSIDE COMMUNITY HOSPITAL, SUNNYSIDE, WA, p. A428
SUNNYVIEW HOSPITAL AND REHABILITATION CENTER, SCHENECTADY, NY, p. A287
SUNRISE HOSPITAL AND MEDICAL CENTER, LAS VEGAS, NV, p. A253
SUPERIOR MEMORIAL HOSPITAL, SUPERIOR, WI, p. A443
SURPRISE VALLEY COMMUNITY HOSPITAL, CEDARVILLE, CA, p. A 39
SUSAN B. ALLEN MEMORIAL HOSPITAL, EL DORADO, KS, p. A152
SUTTER AMADOR HOSPITAL, JACKSON, CA, p. A 46
SUTTER CENTER FOR PSYCHIATRY, SACRAMENTO, CA, p. A 58
SUTTER COAST HOSPITAL, CRESCENT CITY, CA, p. A 40
SUTTER DAVIS HOSPITAL, DAVIS, CA, p. A 41
SUTTER GENERAL HOSPITAL, SACRAMENTO, CA, p. A 58
SUTTER LAKESIDE HOSPITAL, LAKEPORT, CA, p. A 47
SUTTER MEMORIAL HOSPITAL, SACRAMENTO, CA, p. A 58
SUTTER SOLANO MEDICAL CENTER, VALLEJO, CA, p. A 66
SUWANNEE HOSPITAL, LIVE OAK, FL, p. A 88
SWAIN COUNTY HOSPITAL, BRYSON CITY, NC, p. A292
SWEDISH COVENANT HOSPITAL, CHICAGO, IL, p. A120
SWEDISH HEALTH SERVICES–SEATTLE, SEATTLE, WA, p. A427
SWEDISH MEDICAL CENTER–BALLARD, SEATTLE, WA, p. A427
SWEDISH MEDICAL CENTER, ENGLEWOOD, CO, p. A 70
SWEDISHAMERICAN HOSPITAL, ROCKFORD, IL, p. A130
SWEENY COMMUNITY HOSPITAL, SWEENY, TX, p. A404
SWEETWATER HOSPITAL, SWEETWATER, TN, p. A375
SWIFT COUNTY–BENSON HOSPITAL, BENSON, MN, p. A212
SWISHER MEMORIAL HOSPITAL DISTRICT, TULIA, TX, p. A405
SYCAMORE SHOALS HOSPITAL, ELIZABETHTON, TN, p. A368
SYLVAN GROVE HOSPITAL, JACKSON, GA, p. A104
SYOSSET COMMUNITY HOSPITAL, SYOSSET, NY, p. A287
SYRINGA GENERAL HOSPITAL, GRANGEVILLE, ID, p. A113

T

T. J. SAMSON COMMUNITY HOSPITAL, GLASGOW, KY, p. A163
TACOMA GENERAL HOSPITAL, TACOMA, WA, p. A428
TAHLEQUAH CITY HOSPITAL, TAHLEQUAH, OK, p. A327
TAHOE FOREST HOSPITAL DISTRICT, TRUCKEE, CA, p. A 65
TAKOMA ADVENTIST HOSPITAL, GREENEVILLE, TN, p. A368
TALLAHASSEE COMMUNITY HOSPITAL, TALLAHASSEE, FL, p. A 95
TALLAHASSEE MEMORIAL REGIONAL MEDICAL CENTER, TALLAHASSEE, FL, p. A 96
TALLAHATCHIE GENERAL HOSPITAL, CHARLESTON, MS, p. A223
TAMPA GENERAL HEALTHCARE, TAMPA, FL, p. A 96
TANNER MEDICAL CENTER–VILLA RICA, VILLA RICA, GA, p. A109
TANNER MEDICAL CENTER, CARROLLTON, GA, p. A101
TARRANT COUNTY HOSPITAL DISTRICT, FORT WORTH, TX, p. A387
TARRANT COUNTY PSYCHIATRIC CENTER, FORT WORTH, TX, p. A387
TATTNALL MEMORIAL HOSPITAL, REIDSVILLE, GA, p. A107
TAUNTON STATE HOSPITAL, TAUNTON, MA, p. A197
TAWAS ST. JOSEPH HOSPITAL, TAWAS CITY, MI, p. A210
TAYLOR COUNTY HOSPITAL, CAMPBELLSVILLE, KY, p. A161
TAYLOR HOSPITAL, RIDLEY PARK, PA, p. A348
TAYLOR MANOR HOSPITAL, ELLICOTT CITY, MD, p. A187
TAYLOR REGIONAL HOSPITAL, HAWKINSVILLE, GA, p. A104
TAZEWELL COMMUNITY HOSPITAL, TAZEWELL, VA, p. A421

TEHACHAPI HOSPITAL, TEHACHAPI, CA, p. A 64
TELFAIR COUNTY HOSPITAL, MCRAE, GA, p. A106
TEMPE ST. LUKE'S HOSPITAL, TEMPE, AZ, p. A 27
TEMPLE COMMUNITY HOSPITAL, LOS ANGELES, CA, p. A 51
TEMPLE UNIVERSITY HOSPITAL, PHILADELPHIA, PA, p. A346
TEN BROECK HOSPITAL, LOUISVILLE, KY, p. A166
TENET PARK PLAZA HOSPITAL, HOUSTON, TX, p. A392
TENET SIERRA VISTA REGIONAL MEDICAL CENTER, SAN LUIS OBISPO, CA, p. A 62
TENNESSEE CHRISTIAN MEDICAL CENTER, MADISON, TN, p. A371
TERRE HAUTE REGIONAL HOSPITAL, TERRE HAUTE, IN, p. A141
TERREBONNE GENERAL MEDICAL CENTER, HOUMA, LA, p. A173
TERRELL COMMUNITY HOSPITAL, TERRELL, TX, p. A404
TERRELL STATE HOSPITAL, TERRELL, TX, p. A404
TETON MEDICAL CENTER, CHOTEAU, MT, p. A241
TETON VALLEY HOSPITAL, DRIGGS, ID, p. A113
TEWKSBURY HOSPITAL, TEWKSBURY, MA, p. A197
TEXAS CENTER FOR INFECTIOUS DESEASE, SAN ANTONIO, TX, p. A402
TEXAS CHILDREN'S HOSPITAL, HOUSTON, TX, p. A392
TEXAS COUNTY MEMORIAL HOSPITAL, HOUSTON, MO, p. A233
TEXAS ORTHOPEDIC HOSPITAL, HOUSTON, TX, p. A392
TEXAS SCOTTISH RITE HOSPITAL FOR CHILDREN, DALLAS, TX, p. A384
TEXOMA MEDICAL CENTER, DENISON, TX, p. A384
THAYER COUNTY MEMORIAL HOSPITAL, HEBRON, NE, p. A248
THC–CHICAGO, CHICAGO, IL, p. A120
THC–SEATTLE HOSPITAL, SEATTLE, WA, p. A427
THC – ALBUQUERQUE, ALBUQUERQUE, NM, p. A268
THC – BOSTON, PEABODY, MA, p. A196
THE EASTSIDE HOSPITAL, REDMOND, WA, p. A426
THE FRIARY OF BAPTIST HEALTH CENTER, GULF BREEZE, FL, p. A 85
THE HOSPITAL, SIDNEY, NY, p. A287
THE INSTITUTE FOR REHABILITATION AND RESEARCH, HOUSTON, TX, p. A392
THE MANORS, TARPON SPRINGS, FL, p. A 97
THE MEDICAL CENTER, COLUMBUS, GA, p. A101
THE MEDICAL CENTER, BEAVER, PA, p. A335
THE METHODIST HOSPITAL, HOUSTON, TX, p. A392
THE MONROE CLINIC, MONROE, WI, p. A441
THE NEW YORK COMMUNITY HOSPITAL OF BROOKLYN, NEW YORK CITY, NY, p. A282
THE PAVILION, CHAMPAIGN, IL, p. A117
THE TOLEDO HOSPITAL, TOLEDO, OH, p. A318
THEDA CLARK REGIONAL MEDICAL CENTER, NEENAH, WI, p. A441
THIBODAUX HOSPITAL AND HEALTH CENTERS, THIBODAUX, LA, p. A179
THOMAS B. FINAN CENTER, CUMBERLAND, MD, p. A186
THOMAS H. BOYD MEMORIAL HOSPITAL, CARROLLTON, IL, p. A117
THOMAS HOSPITAL, FAIRHOPE, AL, p. A 16
THOMAS JEFFERSON UNIVERSITY HOSPITAL–FORD ROAD CAMPUS, PHILADELPHIA, PA, p. A346
THOMAS JEFFERSON UNIVERSITY HOSPITAL, PHILADELPHIA, PA, p. A346
THOMAS MEMORIAL HOSPITAL, SOUTH CHARLESTON, WV, p. A433
THOMASVILLE HOSPITAL, THOMASVILLE, AL, p. A 20
THOMPSON MEMORIAL MEDICAL CENTER, BURBANK, CA, p. A 38
THOMS REHABILITATION HOSPITAL, ASHEVILLE, NC, p. A291
THOREK HOSPITAL AND MEDICAL CENTER, CHICAGO, IL, p. A120
THORN HOSPITAL, HUDSON, MI, p. A205
THREE RIVERS AREA HOSPITAL, THREE RIVERS, MI, p. A210
THREE RIVERS COMMUNITY HOSPITAL, GRANTS PASS, OR, p. A330
THREE RIVERS COMMUNITY HOSPITAL, WAVERLY, TN, p. A375
THREE RIVERS COMMUNITY HOSPITAL AND HEALTH CENTER, GRANTS PASS, OR, p. A330
THREE RIVERS MEDICAL CENTER, LOUISA, KY, p. A165
THROCKMORTON COUNTY MEMORIAL HOSPITAL, THROCKMORTON, TX, p. A405
THUNDERBIRD SAMARITAN MEDICAL CENTER, GLENDALE, AZ, p. A 24
TIDEWATER PSYCHIATRIC INSTITUTE–NORFOLK, NORFOLK, VA, p. A418
TIDEWATER PSYCHIATRIC INSTITUTE, VIRGINIA BEACH, VA, p. A421
TIFT GENERAL HOSPITAL, TIFTON, GA, p. A109
TILDEN COMMUNITY HOSPITAL, TILDEN, NE, p. A251
TILLAMOOK COUNTY GENERAL HOSPITAL, TILLAMOOK, OR, p. A333

Hospitals, Alphabetically / Union County Methodist Hospital

TIMBERLAWN PSYCHIATRIC HOSPITAL, DALLAS, TX, p. A384
TIMKEN MERCY MEDICAL CENTER, CANTON, OH, p. A307
TINLEY PARK MENTAL HEALTH CENTER, TINLEY PARK, IL, p. A131
TIOGA MEDICAL CENTER, TIOGA, ND, p. A305
TIPPAH COUNTY HOSPITAL, RIPLEY, MS, p. A227
TIPTON COUNTY MEMORIAL HOSPITAL, TIPTON, IN, p. A141
TITUS REGIONAL MEDICAL CENTER, MOUNT PLEASANT, TX, p. A397
TITUSVILLE AREA HOSPITAL, TITUSVILLE, PA, p. A350
TOBEY HOSPITAL, WAREHAM, MA, p. A198
TOLEDO MENTAL HEALTH CENTER, TOLEDO, OH, p. A318
TOLFREE MEMORIAL HOSPITAL, WEST BRANCH, MI, p. A211
TOMAH MEMORIAL HOSPITAL, TOMAH, WI, p. A443
TOMBALL REGIONAL HOSPITAL, TOMBALL, TX, p. A405
TOMPKINS COMMUNITY HOSPITAL, ITHACA, NY, p. A276
TOOELE VALLEY REGIONAL MEDICAL CENTER, TOOELE, UT, p. A411
TOOLE COUNTY HOSPITAL AND NURSING HOME, SHELBY, MT, p. A244
TOPEKA STATE HOSPITAL, TOPEKA, KS, p. A159
TORRANCE MEMORIAL MEDICAL CENTER, TORRANCE, CA, p. A65
TORRANCE STATE HOSPITAL, TORRANCE, PA, p. A350
TOUCHETTE REGIONAL HOSPITAL, CENTREVILLE, IL, p. A117
TOURO INFIRMARY, NEW ORLEANS, LA, p. A177
TOWN AND COUNTRY HOSPITAL, TAMPA, FL, p. A96
TOWNER COUNTY MEMORIAL HOSPITAL, CANDO, ND, p. A302
TRACE REGIONAL HOSPITAL, HOUSTON, MS, p. A224
TRACY COMMUNITY MEMORIAL HOSPITAL, TRACY, CA, p. A65
TRACY MUNICIPAL HOSPITAL, TRACY, MN, p. A220
TRANSITIONAL HOSPITAL CORPORATION OF MINNEAPOLIS, GOLDEN VALLEY, MN, p. A215
TRANSYLVANIA COMMUNITY HOSPITAL, BREVARD, NC, p. A292
TREGO COUNTY-LEMKE MEMORIAL HOSPITAL, WAKEENEY, KS, p. A159
TRENTON PSYCHIATRIC HOSPITAL, TRENTON, NJ, p. A265
TRI-CITY COMMUNITY HOSPITAL, JOURDANTON, TX, p. A393
TRI-CITY HEALTH CENTRE, DALLAS, TX, p. A384
TRI-CITY MEDICAL CENTER, OCEANSIDE, CA, p. A54
TRI-COUNTY AREA HOSPITAL, LEXINGTON, NE, p. A248
TRI-COUNTY HOSPITAL, WADENA, MN, p. A221
TRI-COUNTY MEMORIAL HOSPITAL, GOWANDA, NY, p. A275
TRI-COUNTY MEMORIAL HOSPITAL, WHITEHALL, WI, p. A444
TRI-STATE MEMORIAL HOSPITAL, CLARKSTON, WA, p. A423
TRI-STATE REGIONAL REHABILITATION HOSPITAL, EVANSVILLE, IN, p. A135
TRI-WARD GENERAL HOSPITAL, BERNICE, LA, p. A171
TRI COUNTY BAPTIST HOSPITAL, LA GRANGE, KY, p. A164
TRIDENT REGIONAL MEDICAL CENTER, CHARLESTON, SC, p. A356
TRIGG COUNTY HOSPITAL, CADIZ, KY, p. A161
TRINITY COMMUNITY MEDICAL CENTER OF BRENHAM, BRENHAM, TX, p. A380
TRINITY HOSPITAL, WEAVERVILLE, CA, p. A67
TRINITY HOSPITAL, CHICAGO, IL, p. A120
TRINITY HOSPITAL, WOLF POINT, MT, p. A245
TRINITY HOSPITAL, ERIN, TN, p. A368
TRINITY LUTHERAN HOSPITAL, KANSAS CITY, MO, p. A234
TRINITY MEDICAL CENTER-WEST CAMPUS, ROCK ISLAND, IL, p. A129
TRINITY MEDICAL CENTER, MINOT, ND, p. A304
TRINITY MEDICAL CENTER, CARROLLTON, TX, p. A380
TRINITY MEMORIAL HOSPITAL, TRINITY, TX, p. A405
TRINITY MEMORIAL HOSPITAL, CUDAHY, WI, p. A436
TRINITY REGIONAL HOSPITAL, FORT DODGE, IA, p. A145
TRINITY SPRINGS PAVILION-EAST, FORT WORTH, TX, p. A387
TRINITY VALLEY MEDICAL CENTER, PALESTINE, TX, p. A399
TRIPLER ARMY MEDICAL CENTER, HONOLULU, HI, p. A110
TROY COMMUNITY HOSPITAL, TROY, PA, p. A350
TRUMAN MEDICAL CENTER-EAST, KANSAS CITY, MO, p. A234
TRUMAN MEDICAL CENTER-WEST, KANSAS CITY, MO, p. A234
TRUMBULL MEMORIAL HOSPITAL, WARREN, OH, p. A318
TUALITY COMMUNITY HOSPITAL, HILLSBORO, OR, p. A330
TUALITY FOREST GROVE HOSPITAL, FOREST GROVE, OR, p. A330
TUBA CITY INDIAN MEDICAL CENTER, TUBA CITY, AZ, p. A27
TUCSON GENERAL HOSPITAL, TUCSON, AZ, p. A28
TUCSON MEDICAL CENTER, TUCSON, AZ, p. A28
TULANE UNIVERSITY HOSPITAL AND CLINICS, NEW ORLEANS, LA, p. A177
TULARE DISTRICT HOSPITAL, TULARE, CA, p. A65
TULSA REGIONAL MEDICAL CENTER, TULSA, OK, p. A328
TUOLUMNE-GENERAL HOSPITAL, SONORA, CA, p. A64
TUOMEY REGIONAL MEDICAL CENTER, SUMTER, SC, p. A360
TURNING POINT HOSPITAL, MOULTRIE, GA, p. A106
TUSTIN HOSPITAL, TUSTIN, CA, p. A65
TUSTIN REHABILITATION HOSPITAL, TUSTIN, CA, p. A65

TWEETEN LUTHERAN HEALTH CARE CENTER, SPRING GROVE, MN, p. A220
TWELVE OAKS HOSPITAL, HOUSTON, TX, p. A392
TWIN CITIES COMMUNITY HOSPITAL, TEMPLETON, CA, p. A64
TWIN CITIES HOSPITAL, NICEVILLE, FL, p. A91
TWIN CITY HOSPITAL, DENNISON, OH, p. A311
TWIN COUNTY REGIONAL HOSPITAL, GALAX, VA, p. A416
TWIN FALLS CLINIC HOSPITAL, TWIN FALLS, ID, p. A114
TWIN LAKES REGIONAL MEDICAL CENTER, LEITCHFIELD, KY, p. A164
TWIN OAKS MEDICAL CENTER, FORT WORTH, TX, p. A387
TWIN RIVERS REGIONAL MEDICAL CENTER, KENNETT, MO, p. A235
TWO RIVERS COMMUNITY HOSPITAL AND HAMILTON MEMORIAL HOME, TWO RIVERS, WI, p. A443
TWO RIVERS PSYCHIATRIC HOSPITAL, KANSAS CITY, MO, p. A234
TYLER COUNTY HOSPITAL, WOODVILLE, TX, p. A407
TYLER HOLMES MEMORIAL HOSPITAL, WINONA, MS, p. A228
TYLER MEMORIAL HOSPITAL, TUNKHANNOCK, PA, p. A350
TYLER REHABILITATION HOSPITAL, TYLER, TX, p. A405
TYRONE HOSPITAL, TYRONE, PA, p. A350

U

U.S. AIR FORCE HOSPITAL MOODY, MOODY AIR FORCE BASE, GA, p. A106
U.S. PUBLIC HEALTH SERVICE INDIAN HOSPITAL, ZUNI, NM, p. A270
U.S. AIR FORCE ACADEMY HOSPITAL, USAF ACADEMY, CO, p. A73
U.S. AIR FORCE HOSPITAL-KIRTLAND, KIRTLAND AIR FORCE BASE, NM, p. A269
U.S. AIR FORCE HOSPITAL, DAVIS-MONTHAN AIR FORCE BASE, AZ, p. A23
U.S. AIR FORCE HOSPITAL, BEALE AIR FORCE BASE, CA, p. A37
U.S. AIR FORCE HOSPITAL, EDWARDS AIR FORCE BASE, CA, p. A41
U.S. AIR FORCE HOSPITAL, MATHER AIR FORCE BASE, CA, p. A52
U.S. AIR FORCE HOSPITAL, VANDENBERG AIR FORCE BASE, CA, p. A66
U.S. AIR FORCE HOSPITAL, MACDILL AIR FORCE BASE, FL, p. A88
U.S. AIR FORCE HOSPITAL, PANAMA CITY, FL, p. A92
U.S. AIR FORCE HOSPITAL, PATRICK AIR FORCE BASE, FL, p. A92
U.S. AIR FORCE HOSPITAL, COLUMBUS, MS, p. A223
U.S. AIR FORCE HOSPITAL, HOLLOMAN AIR FORCE BASE, NM, p. A269
U.S. AIR FORCE HOSPITAL, PLATTSBURGH, NY, p. A285
U.S. AIR FORCE HOSPITAL, ROME, NY, p. A286
U.S. AIR FORCE HOSPITAL, GRAND FORKS AIR FORCE BASE, ND, p. A303
U.S. AIR FORCE HOSPITAL, ELLSWORTH AIR FORCE BASE, SD, p. A362
U.S. AIR FORCE HOSPITAL, ABILENE, TX, p. A376
U.S. AIR FORCE HOSPITAL, LAUGHLIN AIR FORCE BASE, TX, p. A395
U.S. AIR FORCE HOSPITAL, REESE AIR FORCE BASE, TX, p. A400
U.S. AIR FORCE HOSPITAL, HILL AIR FORCE BASE, UT, p. A408
U.S. AIR FORCE HOSPITAL, FAIRCHILD AIR FORCE BASE, WA, p. A424
U.S. AIR FORCE HOSPITAL, CHEYENNE, WY, p. A445
U.S. AIR FORCE HOSPITAL DOVER, DOVER AIR FORCE BASE, DE, p. A78
U.S. AIR FORCE HOSPITAL LITTLE ROCK, JACKSONVILLE, AR, p. A31
U.S. AIR FORCE HOSPITAL LUKE, GLENDALE, AZ, p. A24
U.S. AIR FORCE HOSPITAL MOUNTAIN HOME, MOUNTAIN HOME AIR FORCE BASE, ID, p. A114
U.S. AIR FORCE HOSPITAL ROBINS, ROBINS AIR FORCE BASE, GA, p. A107
U.S. AIR FORCE HOSPITAL SEYMOUR JOHNSON, SEYMOUR JOHNSON AIR FORCE BASE, NC, p. A299
U.S. AIR FORCE HOSPITAL SHAW, SHAW AIR FORCE BASE, SC, p. A359
U.S. AIR FORCE HOSPITAL TINKER, TINKER AIR FORCE BASE, OK, p. A327
U.S. AIR FORCE HOSPITAL WHITEMAN, WHITEMAN AIR FORCE BASE, MO, p. A240
U.S. AIR FORCE HOSPITAL, BARKSDALE AIR FORCE BASE, SHREVEPORT, LA, p. A178

U.S. AIR FORCE MEDICAL CENTER KEESLER, KEESLER AIR FORCE BASE, MS, p. A225
U.S. AIR FORCE MEDICAL CENTER WRIGHT-PATTERSON, WRIGHT-PATTERSON AIR FORCE BASE, OH, p. A319
U.S. AIR FORCE REGIONAL HOSPITAL-SHEPPARD, SHEPPARD AIR FORCE BASE, TX, p. A403
U.S. AIR FORCE REGIONAL HOSPITAL, ELMENDORF AIR FORCE BASE, AK, p. A21
U.S. AIR FORCE REGIONAL HOSPITAL, MARCH AIR FORCE BASE, CA, p. A52
U.S. AIR FORCE REGIONAL HOSPITAL, EGLIN AIR FORCE BASE, FL, p. A83
U.S. AIR FORCE REGIONAL HOSPITAL, MINOT, ND, p. A304
U.S. MEDICAL CENTER FOR FEDERAL PRISONERS, SPRINGFIELD, MO, p. A240
U.S. NAVAL HOSPITAL, AGANA, GU, p. A447
U.S. NAVAL HOSPITAL, SAN JUAN, PR, p. A450
U.S. PENITENTIARY HOSPITAL, LEWISBURG, PA, p. A341
U.S. PUBLIC HEALTH SERVICE ALASKA NATIVE HOSPITAL, BARROW, AK, p. A21
U.S. PUBLIC HEALTH SERVICE ALASKA NATIVE MEDICAL CENTER, ANCHORAGE, AK, p. A21
U.S. PUBLIC HEALTH SERVICE COMPREHENSIVE INDIAN HEALTH FACILITY, CLAREMORE, OK, p. A322
U.S. PUBLIC HEALTH SERVICE FORT DEFIANCE INDIAN HEALTH SERVICE HOSPITAL, FORT DEFIANCE, AZ, p. A24
U.S. PUBLIC HEALTH SERVICE INDIAN HOSPITAL, PARKER, AZ, p. A25
U.S. PUBLIC HEALTH SERVICE INDIAN HOSPITAL, SELLS, AZ, p. A27
U.S. PUBLIC HEALTH SERVICE INDIAN HOSPITAL, WHITERIVER, AZ, p. A28
U.S. PUBLIC HEALTH SERVICE INDIAN HOSPITAL, WINTERHAVEN, CA, p. A67
U.S. PUBLIC HEALTH SERVICE INDIAN HOSPITAL, BROWNING, MT, p. A241
U.S. PUBLIC HEALTH SERVICE INDIAN HOSPITAL, CROW AGENCY, MT, p. A241
U.S. PUBLIC HEALTH SERVICE INDIAN HOSPITAL, HARLEM, MT, p. A242
U.S. PUBLIC HEALTH SERVICE INDIAN HOSPITAL, WINNEBAGO, NE, p. A252
U.S. PUBLIC HEALTH SERVICE INDIAN HOSPITAL, MESCALERO, NM, p. A269
U.S. PUBLIC HEALTH SERVICE INDIAN HOSPITAL, CHEROKEE, NC, p. A293
U.S. PUBLIC HEALTH SERVICE INDIAN HOSPITAL, BELCOURT, ND, p. A302
U.S. PUBLIC HEALTH SERVICE INDIAN HOSPITAL, FORT YATES, ND, p. A303
U.S. PUBLIC HEALTH SERVICE INDIAN HOSPITAL, CLINTON, OK, p. A322
U.S. PUBLIC HEALTH SERVICE INDIAN HOSPITAL, LAWTON, OK, p. A324
U.S. PUBLIC HEALTH SERVICE INDIAN HOSPITAL, EAGLE BUTTE, SD, p. A361
U.S. PUBLIC HEALTH SERVICE INDIAN HOSPITAL, PINE RIDGE, SD, p. A363
U.S. PUBLIC HEALTH SERVICE INDIAN HOSPITAL, ROSEBUD, SD, p. A363
U.S. PUBLIC HEALTH SERVICE INDIAN HOSPITAL, SISSETON, SD, p. A364
U.S. PUBLIC HEALTH SERVICE OWYHEE COMMUNITY HEALTH FACILITY, OWYHEE, NV, p. A254
U.S. PUBLIC HEALTH SERVICE PHOENIX INDIAN MEDICAL CENTER, PHOENIX, AZ, p. A26
U.S. PUBLIC HEALTH SERVICES INDIAN HOSPITAL, KEAMS CANYON, AZ, p. A24
U.S. AIR FORCE HOSPITAL, CANNON AIR FORCE BASE, NM, p. A268
U.S. AIR FORCE HOSPITAL, HAMPTON, VA, p. A416
U.S. AIR FORCE HOSPITAL ALTUS, ALTUS, OK, p. A321
U.S. PUBLIC HEALTH SERVICE INDIAN HOSPITAL, CASS LAKE, MN, p. A213
U.S. PUBLIC HEALTH SERVICE INDIAN HOSPITAL, REDLAKE, MN, p. A218
U.S. PUBLIC HEALTH SERVICE INDIAN HOSPITAL, CROWNPOINT, NM, p. A268
UINTAH BASIN MEDICAL CENTER, ROOSEVELT, UT, p. A410
UKIAH VALLEY MEDICAL CENTER, UKIAH, CA, p. A65
UNCAS ON THAMES HOSPITAL, NORWICH, CT, p. A76
UNDERWOOD-MEMORIAL HOSPITAL, WOODBURY, NJ, p. A266
UNICOI COUNTY MEMORIAL HOSPITAL, ERWIN, TN, p. A368
UNIMED MEDICAL CENTER, MINOT, ND, p. A304
UNION CITY MEMORIAL HOSPITAL, UNION CITY, PA, p. A350
UNION COUNTY GENERAL HOSPITAL, CLAYTON, NM, p. A268
UNION COUNTY HOSPITAL DISTRICT, ANNA, IL, p. A116
UNION COUNTY METHODIST HOSPITAL, MORGANFIELD, KY, p. A166

Hospitals, Alphabetically / Union General Hospital

UNION GENERAL HOSPITAL, BLAIRSVILLE, GA, p. A100
UNION GENERAL HOSPITAL, FARMERVILLE, LA, p. A172
UNION HOSPITAL, TERRE HAUTE, IN, p. A141
UNION HOSPITAL, ELKTON, MD, p. A187
UNION HOSPITAL, UNION, NJ, p. A265
UNION HOSPITAL, MAYVILLE, ND, p. A304
UNION HOSPITAL, DOVER, OH, p. A312
UNION HOSPITAL OF THE BRONX, NEW YORK CITY, NY, p. A283
UNION MEMORIAL HOSPITAL, BALTIMORE, MD, p. A185
UNION MEMORIAL HOSPITAL, MONROE, NC, p. A297
UNIONTOWN HOSPITAL, UNIONTOWN, PA, p. A350
UNITED COMMUNITY HOSPITAL, GROVE CITY, PA, p. A339
UNITED HEALTH SERVICES, GRAND FORKS, ND, p. A303
UNITED HEALTH SERVICES HOSPITALS–BINGHAMTON, BINGHAMTON, NY, p. A272
UNITED HOSPITAL, SAINT PAUL, MN, p. A220
UNITED HOSPITAL CENTER, CLARKSBURG, WV, p. A430
UNITED HOSPITAL DISTRICT, BLUE EARTH, MN, p. A213
UNITED HOSPITAL MEDICAL CENTER, PORT CHESTER, NY, p. A285
UNITED HOSPITALS MEDICAL CENTER, NEWARK, NJ, p. A262
UNITED MEDICAL CENTER, CHEYENNE, WY, p. A445
UNITED MEDICAL CENTER NEW ORLEANS, NEW ORLEANS, LA, p. A177
UNITED MEMORIAL HOSPITAL, GREENVILLE, MI, p. A204
UNITED SAMARITANS MEDICAL CENTER, DANVILLE, IL, p. A121
UNITY HOSPITAL, FRIDLEY, MN, p. A215
UNITY MEDICAL CENTER, GRAFTON, ND, p. A303
UNIVERSAL MEDICAL CENTER, PLANTATION, FL, p. A 93
UNIVERSITY AND CHILDRENS HOSPITALS, COLUMBIA, MO, p. A231
UNIVERSITY COMMUNITY HOSPITAL – CARROLLWOOD, TAMPA, FL, p. A 96
UNIVERSITY COMMUNITY HOSPITAL, TAMPA, FL, p. A 96
UNIVERSITY GENERAL HOSPITAL, SEMINOLE, FL, p. A 95
UNIVERSITY HEALTH SERVICES, AMHERST, MA, p. A190
UNIVERSITY HOSPITAL–SUNY HEALTH SCIENCE CENTER AT SYRACUSE, SYRACUSE, NY, p. A288
UNIVERSITY HOSPITAL, DENVER, CO, p. A 69
UNIVERSITY HOSPITAL, TAMARAC, FL, p. A 96
UNIVERSITY HOSPITAL, AUGUSTA, GA, p. A100
UNIVERSITY HOSPITAL, CHICAGO, IL, p. A121
UNIVERSITY HOSPITAL, ALBUQUERQUE, NM, p. A268
UNIVERSITY HOSPITAL, STONY BROOK, NY, p. A287
UNIVERSITY HOSPITAL, CHARLOTTE, NC, p. A293
UNIVERSITY HOSPITAL, PORTLAND, OR, p. A332
UNIVERSITY HOSPITAL, SAN JUAN, PR, p. A450
UNIVERSITY HOSPITAL OF ARKANSAS, LITTLE ROCK, AR, p. A 32
UNIVERSITY HOSPITAL OF BROOKLYN–STATE UNIVERSITY OF NEW YORK HEALTH SCIENCE CENTER AT BROOKLYN, NEW YORK CITY, NY, p. A283
UNIVERSITY HOSPITAL, OKLAHOMA CITY, OK, p. A326
UNIVERSITY HOSPITALS AND CLINICS, UNIVERSITY OF MISSISSIPPI MEDICAL CENTER, JACKSON, MS, p. A225
UNIVERSITY HOSPITALS HEALTH SYSTEM BEDFORD MEDICAL CENTER, BEDFORD, OH, p. A307
UNIVERSITY HOSPITALS OF CLEVELAND, CLEVELAND, OH, p. A310
UNIVERSITY MEDICAL CENTER, TUCSON, AZ, p. A 28
UNIVERSITY MEDICAL CENTER, JACKSONVILLE, FL, p. A 86
UNIVERSITY MEDICAL CENTER, LAFAYETTE, LA, p. A174
UNIVERSITY MEDICAL CENTER, LAS VEGAS, NV, p. A253
UNIVERSITY MEDICAL CENTER, LEBANON, TN, p. A370
UNIVERSITY MEDICAL CENTER, LUBBOCK, TX, p. A396
UNIVERSITY OF ALABAMA HOSPITAL, BIRMINGHAM, AL, p. A 14
UNIVERSITY OF CALIFORNIA LOS ANGELES MEDICAL CENTER, LOS ANGELES, CA, p. A 51
UNIVERSITY OF CALIFORNIA LOS ANGELES NEUROPSYCHIATRIC HOSPITAL, LOS ANGELES, CA, p. A 51
UNIVERSITY OF CALIFORNIA SAN DIEGO MEDICAL CENTER, SAN DIEGO, CA, p. A 60
UNIVERSITY OF CALIFORNIA SAN FRANCISCO MEDICAL CENTER, SAN FRANCISCO, CA, p. A 61
UNIVERSITY OF CALIFORNIA, DAVIS MEDICAL CENTER, SACRAMENTO, CA, p. A 58
UNIVERSITY OF CALIFORNIA, IRVINE MEDICAL CENTER, ORANGE, CA, p. A 55
UNIVERSITY OF CHICAGO HOSPITALS, CHICAGO, IL, p. A121
UNIVERSITY OF CINCINNATI HOSPITAL, CINCINNATI, OH, p. A309
UNIVERSITY OF CONNECTICUT HEALTH CENTER, JOHN DEMPSEY HOSPITAL, FARMINGTON, CT, p. A 74
UNIVERSITY OF ILLINOIS AT CHICAGO MEDICAL CENTER, CHICAGO, IL, p. A121
UNIVERSITY OF IOWA HOSPITALS AND CLINICS, IOWA CITY, IA, p. A146

UNIVERSITY OF KANSAS HOSPITAL, KANSAS CITY, KS, p. A155
UNIVERSITY OF KENTUCKY HOSPITAL, LEXINGTON, KY, p. A164
UNIVERSITY OF LOUISVILLE HOSPITAL, LOUISVILLE, KY, p. A166
UNIVERSITY OF MARYLAND MEDICAL SYSTEM, BALTIMORE, MD, p. A185
UNIVERSITY OF MASSACHUSETTS MEDICAL CENTER, WORCESTER, MA, p. A198
UNIVERSITY OF MEDICINE AND DENTISTRY OF NEW JERSEY–UNIVERSITY HOSPITAL, NEWARK, NJ, p. A262
UNIVERSITY OF MEDICINE AND DENTISTRY OF NEW JERSEY, COMMUNITY MENTAL HEALTH CENTER AT PISCATAWAY, PISCATAWAY, NJ, p. A263
UNIVERSITY OF MIAMI HOSPITAL AND CLINICS, MIAMI, FL, p. A 90
UNIVERSITY OF MICHIGAN HOSPITALS, ANN ARBOR, MI, p. A199
UNIVERSITY OF MINNESOTA HOSPITAL AND CLINIC, MINNEAPOLIS, MN, p. A217
UNIVERSITY OF NEBRASKA MEDICAL CENTER, OMAHA, NE, p. A250
UNIVERSITY OF NEW MEXICO CHILDREN'S PSYCHIATRIC HOSPITAL, ALBUQUERQUE, NM, p. A268
UNIVERSITY OF NEW MEXICO MENTAL HEALTH CENTER, ALBUQUERQUE, NM, p. A268
UNIVERSITY OF NORTH CAROLINA HOSPITALS, CHAPEL HILL, NC, p. A292
UNIVERSITY OF PITTSBURGH MEDICAL CENTER, PITTSBURGH, PA, p. A347
UNIVERSITY OF SOUTH ALABAMA DOCTORS HOSPITAL, MOBILE, AL, p. A 18
UNIVERSITY OF SOUTH ALABAMA KNOLLWOOD PARK HOSPITAL, MOBILE, AL, p. A 18
UNIVERSITY OF SOUTH ALABAMA MEDICAL CENTER, MOBILE, AL, p. A 18
UNIVERSITY OF SOUTHERN CALIFORNIA–KENNETH NORRIS JR. CANCER HOSPITAL, LOS ANGELES, CA, p. A 51
UNIVERSITY OF TENNESSEE BOWLD HOSPITAL, MEMPHIS, TN, p. A372
UNIVERSITY OF TENNESSEE MEMORIAL HOSPITAL, KNOXVILLE, TN, p. A370
UNIVERSITY OF TEXAS HEALTH CENTER AT TYLER, TYLER, TX, p. A405
UNIVERSITY OF TEXAS M. D. ANDERSON CANCER CENTER, HOUSTON, TX, p. A392
UNIVERSITY OF TEXAS MEDICAL BRANCH HOSPITALS, GALVESTON, TX, p. A388
UNIVERSITY OF UTAH HOSPITALS AND CLINICS, SALT LAKE CITY, UT, p. A410
UNIVERSITY OF UTAH NEUROPSYCHIATRIC INSTITUTE, SALT LAKE CITY, UT, p. A410
UNIVERSITY OF VIRGINIA MEDICAL CENTER, CHARLOTTESVILLE, VA, p. A414
UNIVERSITY OF WASHINGTON MEDICAL CENTER, SEATTLE, WA, p. A427
UNIVERSITY OF WISCONSIN HOSPITAL AND CLINICS, MADISON, WI, p. A438
UNIVERSITY PEDIATRIC HOSPITAL, SAN JUAN, PR, p. A450
UPPER CONNECTICUT VALLEY HOSPITAL, COLEBROOK, NH, p. A255
UPREACH REHABILITATION HOSPITAL, GAINESVILLE, FL, p. A 85
UPSON REGIONAL MEDICAL CENTER, THOMASTON, GA, p. A108
UPSTATE CAROLINA MEDICAL CENTER, GAFFNEY, SC, p. A357
USAKA HOSPITAL, KWAJALEIN ISLAND, MH, p. A447
UTAH STATE HOSPITAL, PROVO, UT, p. A409
UTAH VALLEY REGIONAL MEDICAL CENTER, PROVO, UT, p. A409
UVALDE MEMORIAL HOSPITAL, UVALDE, TX, p. A405

V

VACAVALLEY HOSPITAL, VACAVILLE, CA, p. A 66
VAIL VALLEY MEDICAL CENTER, VAIL, CO, p. A 73
VAL VERDE MEMORIAL HOSPITAL, DEL RIO, TX, p. A384
VALDESE GENERAL HOSPITAL, VALDESE, NC, p. A300
VALDEZ COMMUNITY HOSPITAL, VALDEZ, AK, p. A 22
VALLEY BAPTIST MEDICAL CENTER, HARLINGEN, TX, p. A389
VALLEY CHILDREN'S HOSPITAL, FRESNO, CA, p. A 43
VALLEY COMMUNITY HOSPITAL, SANTA MARIA, CA, p. A 63
VALLEY COMMUNITY HOSPITAL, DALLAS, OR, p. A329

VALLEY COUNTY HOSPITAL, CASCADE, ID, p. A112
VALLEY COUNTY HOSPITAL, ORD, NE, p. A250
VALLEY FORGE MEDICAL CENTER AND HOSPITAL, NORRISTOWN, PA, p. A343
VALLEY GENERAL HOSPITAL, MONROE, WA, p. A425
VALLEY HOSPITAL, PALMER, AK, p. A 22
VALLEY HOSPITAL, OWENSBORO, KY, p. A167
VALLEY HOSPITAL, RIDGEWOOD, NJ, p. A264
VALLEY HOSPITAL AND MEDICAL CENTER, SPOKANE, WA, p. A428
VALLEY HOSPITAL MEDICAL CENTER, LOS ANGELES, CA, p. A 51
VALLEY HOSPITAL MEDICAL CENTER, LAS VEGAS, NV, p. A253
VALLEY LUTHERAN HOSPITAL, MESA, AZ, p. A 25
VALLEY MEDICAL CENTER, RENTON, WA, p. A426
VALLEY MEDICAL CENTER OF FRESNO, FRESNO, CA, p. A 43
VALLEY MEMORIAL HOSPITAL, LIVERMORE, CA, p. A 47
VALLEY PRESBYTERIAN HOSPITAL, LOS ANGELES, CA, p. A 51
VALLEY PSYCHIATRIC HOSPITAL, CHATTANOOGA, TN, p. A367
VALLEY REGIONAL HOSPITAL, CLAREMONT, NH, p. A255
VALLEY REGIONAL HOSPITAL, CAMDEN, TN, p. A366
VALLEY REGIONAL MEDICAL CENTER, BROWNSVILLE, TX, p. A380
VALLEY VIEW HOSPITAL, GLENWOOD SPRINGS, CO, p. A 70
VALLEY VIEW MEDICAL CENTER, CEDAR CITY, UT, p. A408
VALLEY VIEW MEDICAL CENTER, PLYMOUTH, WI, p. A441
VALLEY VIEW REGIONAL HOSPITAL, ADA, OK, p. A321
VAN BUREN COUNTY HOSPITAL, KEOSAUQUA, IA, p. A147
VAN BUREN COUNTY MEMORIAL HOSPITAL, CLINTON, AR, p. A 29
VAN NUYS HOSPITAL, LOS ANGELES, CA, p. A 51
VAN WERT COUNTY HOSPITAL, VAN WERT, OH, p. A318
VANDERBILT UNIVERSITY HOSPITAL, NASHVILLE, TN, p. A373
VASSAR BROTHERS HOSPITAL, POUGHKEEPSIE, NY, p. A285
VAUGHAN CHILTON MEDICAL CENTER, CLANTON, AL, p. A 15
VAUGHAN PERRY HOSPITAL, MARION, AL, p. A 17
VAUGHAN REGIONAL MEDICAL CENTER, SELMA, AL, p. A 19
VENCOR HOSPITAL–ATLANTA, ATLANTA, GA, p. A 99
VENCOR HOSPITAL–CHATTANOOGA, CHATTANOOGA, TN, p. A367
VENCOR HOSPITAL–CHICAGO NORTH, CHICAGO, IL, p. A121
VENCOR HOSPITAL–CORAL GABLES, CORAL GABLES, FL, p. A 83
VENCOR HOSPITAL–DETROIT, LINCOLN PARK, MI, p. A206
VENCOR HOSPITAL–FORT LAUDERDALE, FORT LAUDERDALE, FL, p. A 84
VENCOR HOSPITAL–FORT WORTH SOUTH, MANSFIELD, TX, p. A396
VENCOR HOSPITAL–HOUSTON, HOUSTON, TX, p. A392
VENCOR HOSPITAL–KANSAS CITY, KANSAS CITY, MO, p. A234
VENCOR HOSPITAL–LAGRANGE, LAGRANGE, IN, p. A138
VENCOR HOSPITAL–SACRAMENTO, FOLSOM, CA, p. A 42
VENCOR HOSPITAL–SAN DIEGO, SAN DIEGO, CA, p. A 60
VENCOR HOSPITAL–SAN LEANDRO, SAN LEANDRO, CA, p. A 61
VENCOR HOSPITAL–SYCAMORE, SYCAMORE, IL, p. A131
VENCOR HOSPITAL – DALLAS, DALLAS, TX, p. A384
VENCOR HOSPITAL – PHOENIX, PHOENIX, AZ, p. A 26
VENCOR HOSPITAL – TAMPA, TAMPA, FL, p. A 96
VENICE HOSPITAL, VENICE, FL, p. A 97
VENTURA COUNTY MEDICAL CENTER, VENTURA, CA, p. A 66
VERDUGO HILLS HOSPITAL, GLENDALE, CA, p. A 44
VERMILION HOSPITAL, LAFAYETTE, LA, p. A174
VERMILLION COUNTY HOSPITAL, CLINTON, IN, p. A134
VERMONT STATE HOSPITAL, WATERBURY, VT, p. A413
VERNON MEMORIAL HOSPITAL, VIROQUA, WI, p. A443
VETERANS AFFAIRS CENTER, CHEYENNE, WY, p. A445
VETERANS AFFAIRS EDWARD HINES, JR. HOSPITAL, HINES, IL, p. A125
VETERANS AFFAIRS HOSPITAL, FORT HARRISON, MT, p. A242
VETERANS AFFAIRS LAKESIDE MEDICAL CENTER, CHICAGO, IL, p. A121
VETERANS AFFAIRS MEDICAL AND REGIONAL OFFICE CENTER, WICHITA, KS, p. A160
VETERANS AFFAIRS MEDICAL AND REGIONAL OFFICE CENTER, FARGO, ND, p. A303
VETERANS AFFAIRS MEDICAL CENTER–LEXINGTON, LEXINGTON, KY, p. A165
VETERANS AFFAIRS MEDICAL CENTER–LOUISVILLE, LOUISVILLE, KY, p. A166
VETERANS AFFAIRS MEDICAL CENTER–WEST LOS ANGELES, LOS ANGELES, CA, p. A 51
VETERANS AFFAIRS MEDICAL CENTER, BIRMINGHAM, AL, p. A 14
VETERANS AFFAIRS MEDICAL CENTER, MONTGOMERY, AL, p. A 18
VETERANS AFFAIRS MEDICAL CENTER, TUSCALOOSA, AL, p. A 20
VETERANS AFFAIRS MEDICAL CENTER, TUSKEGEE, AL, p. A 20

Hospitals, Alphabetically / Walter O. Boswell Memorial Hospital

VETERANS AFFAIRS MEDICAL CENTER, PRESCOTT, AZ, p. A 26
VETERANS AFFAIRS MEDICAL CENTER, TUCSON, AZ, p. A 28
VETERANS AFFAIRS MEDICAL CENTER, FAYETTEVILLE, AR, p. A 30
VETERANS AFFAIRS MEDICAL CENTER, LITTLE ROCK, AR, p. A 32
VETERANS AFFAIRS MEDICAL CENTER, FRESNO, CA, p. A 43
VETERANS AFFAIRS MEDICAL CENTER, LIVERMORE, CA, p. A 47
VETERANS AFFAIRS MEDICAL CENTER, LONG BEACH, CA, p. A 48
VETERANS AFFAIRS MEDICAL CENTER, PALO ALTO, CA, p. A 55
VETERANS AFFAIRS MEDICAL CENTER, SAN DIEGO, CA, p. A 60
VETERANS AFFAIRS MEDICAL CENTER, SAN FRANCISCO, CA, p. A 61
VETERANS AFFAIRS MEDICAL CENTER, DENVER, CO, p. A 70
VETERANS AFFAIRS MEDICAL CENTER, FORT LYON, CO, p. A 70
VETERANS AFFAIRS MEDICAL CENTER, GRAND JUNCTION, CO, p. A 71
VETERANS AFFAIRS MEDICAL CENTER, NEWINGTON, CT, p. A 76
VETERANS AFFAIRS MEDICAL CENTER, WEST HAVEN, CT, p. A 77
VETERANS AFFAIRS MEDICAL CENTER, WILMINGTON, DE, p. A 78
VETERANS AFFAIRS MEDICAL CENTER, WASHINGTON, DC, p. A 79
VETERANS AFFAIRS MEDICAL CENTER, BAY PINES, FL, p. A 81
VETERANS AFFAIRS MEDICAL CENTER, GAINESVILLE, FL, p. A 85
VETERANS AFFAIRS MEDICAL CENTER, LAKE CITY, FL, p. A 87
VETERANS AFFAIRS MEDICAL CENTER, MIAMI, FL, p. A 90
VETERANS AFFAIRS MEDICAL CENTER, AUGUSTA, GA, p. A100
VETERANS AFFAIRS MEDICAL CENTER, DECATUR, GA, p. A102
VETERANS AFFAIRS MEDICAL CENTER, DUBLIN, GA, p. A103
VETERANS AFFAIRS MEDICAL CENTER, BOISE, ID, p. A112
VETERANS AFFAIRS MEDICAL CENTER, DANVILLE, IL, p. A121
VETERANS AFFAIRS MEDICAL CENTER, MARION, IL, p. A126
VETERANS AFFAIRS MEDICAL CENTER, NORTH CHICAGO, IL, p. A128
VETERANS AFFAIRS MEDICAL CENTER, FORT WAYNE, IN, p. A135
VETERANS AFFAIRS MEDICAL CENTER, MARION, IN, p. A138
VETERANS AFFAIRS MEDICAL CENTER, DES MOINES, IA, p. A145
VETERANS AFFAIRS MEDICAL CENTER, IOWA CITY, IA, p. A146
VETERANS AFFAIRS MEDICAL CENTER, KNOXVILLE, IA, p. A147
VETERANS AFFAIRS MEDICAL CENTER, ALEXANDRIA, LA, p. A170
VETERANS AFFAIRS MEDICAL CENTER, NEW ORLEANS, LA, p. A177
VETERANS AFFAIRS MEDICAL CENTER, TOGUS, ME, p. A183
VETERANS AFFAIRS MEDICAL CENTER, BALTIMORE, MD, p. A185
VETERANS AFFAIRS MEDICAL CENTER, FORT HOWARD, MD, p. A187
VETERANS AFFAIRS MEDICAL CENTER, PERRY POINT, MD, p. A188
VETERANS AFFAIRS MEDICAL CENTER, BOSTON, MA, p. A192
VETERANS AFFAIRS MEDICAL CENTER, NORTHAMPTON, MA, p. A195
VETERANS AFFAIRS MEDICAL CENTER, ALLEN PARK, MI, p. A199
VETERANS AFFAIRS MEDICAL CENTER, ANN ARBOR, MI, p. A199
VETERANS AFFAIRS MEDICAL CENTER, BATTLE CREEK, MI, p. A200
VETERANS AFFAIRS MEDICAL CENTER, IRON MOUNTAIN, MI, p. A205
VETERANS AFFAIRS MEDICAL CENTER, SAGINAW, MI, p. A209
VETERANS AFFAIRS MEDICAL CENTER, MINNEAPOLIS, MN, p. A217
VETERANS AFFAIRS MEDICAL CENTER, SAINT CLOUD, MN, p. A219
VETERANS AFFAIRS MEDICAL CENTER, BILOXI, MS, p. A222
VETERANS AFFAIRS MEDICAL CENTER, JACKSON, MS, p. A225
VETERANS AFFAIRS MEDICAL CENTER, KANSAS CITY, MO, p. A234
VETERANS AFFAIRS MEDICAL CENTER, SAINT LOUIS, MO, p. A239
VETERANS AFFAIRS MEDICAL CENTER, MILES CITY, MT, p. A243
VETERANS AFFAIRS MEDICAL CENTER, GRAND ISLAND, NE, p. A248
VETERANS AFFAIRS MEDICAL CENTER, LINCOLN, NE, p. A249

VETERANS AFFAIRS MEDICAL CENTER, OMAHA, NE, p. A250
VETERANS AFFAIRS MEDICAL CENTER, MANCHESTER, NH, p. A256
VETERANS AFFAIRS MEDICAL CENTER, EAST ORANGE, NJ, p. A259
VETERANS AFFAIRS MEDICAL CENTER, LYONS, NJ, p. A261
VETERANS AFFAIRS MEDICAL CENTER, ALBUQUERQUE, NM, p. A268
VETERANS AFFAIRS MEDICAL CENTER, ALBANY, NY, p. A271
VETERANS AFFAIRS MEDICAL CENTER, BATAVIA, NY, p. A271
VETERANS AFFAIRS MEDICAL CENTER, BATH, NY, p. A272
VETERANS AFFAIRS MEDICAL CENTER, BUFFALO, NY, p. A273
VETERANS AFFAIRS MEDICAL CENTER, CANANDAIGUA, NY, p. A273
VETERANS AFFAIRS MEDICAL CENTER, CASTLE POINT, NY, p. A273
VETERANS AFFAIRS MEDICAL CENTER, NEW YORK CITY, NY, p. A283
VETERANS AFFAIRS MEDICAL CENTER, NEW YORK CITY, NY, p. A283
VETERANS AFFAIRS MEDICAL CENTER, NEW YORK CITY, NY, p. A283
VETERANS AFFAIRS MEDICAL CENTER, NORTHPORT, NY, p. A283
VETERANS AFFAIRS MEDICAL CENTER, SYRACUSE, NY, p. A288
VETERANS AFFAIRS MEDICAL CENTER, ASHEVILLE, NC, p. A291
VETERANS AFFAIRS MEDICAL CENTER, DURHAM, NC, p. A293
VETERANS AFFAIRS MEDICAL CENTER, FAYETTEVILLE, NC, p. A294
VETERANS AFFAIRS MEDICAL CENTER, SALISBURY, NC, p. A298
VETERANS AFFAIRS MEDICAL CENTER, CHILLICOTHE, OH, p. A308
VETERANS AFFAIRS MEDICAL CENTER, CINCINNATI, OH, p. A309
VETERANS AFFAIRS MEDICAL CENTER, CLEVELAND, OH, p. A310
VETERANS AFFAIRS MEDICAL CENTER, DAYTON, OH, p. A311
VETERANS AFFAIRS MEDICAL CENTER, MUSKOGEE, OK, p. A325
VETERANS AFFAIRS MEDICAL CENTER, OKLAHOMA CITY, OK, p. A326
VETERANS AFFAIRS MEDICAL CENTER, PORTLAND, OR, p. A332
VETERANS AFFAIRS MEDICAL CENTER, ROSEBURG, OR, p. A332
VETERANS AFFAIRS MEDICAL CENTER, BUTLER, PA, p. A335
VETERANS AFFAIRS MEDICAL CENTER, COATESVILLE, PA, p. A337
VETERANS AFFAIRS MEDICAL CENTER, ERIE, PA, p. A338
VETERANS AFFAIRS MEDICAL CENTER, LEBANON, PA, p. A341
VETERANS AFFAIRS MEDICAL CENTER, PHILADELPHIA, PA, p. A346
VETERANS AFFAIRS MEDICAL CENTER, PITTSBURGH, PA, p. A347
VETERANS AFFAIRS MEDICAL CENTER, PITTSBURGH, PA, p. A347
VETERANS AFFAIRS MEDICAL CENTER, WILKES-BARRE, PA, p. A351
VETERANS AFFAIRS MEDICAL CENTER, SAN JUAN, PR, p. A450
VETERANS AFFAIRS MEDICAL CENTER, PROVIDENCE, RI, p. A353
VETERANS AFFAIRS MEDICAL CENTER, CHARLESTON, SC, p. A356
VETERANS AFFAIRS MEDICAL CENTER, FORT MEADE, SD, p. A362
VETERANS AFFAIRS MEDICAL CENTER, HOT SPRINGS, SD, p. A362
VETERANS AFFAIRS MEDICAL CENTER, MEMPHIS, TN, p. A372
VETERANS AFFAIRS MEDICAL CENTER, MOUNTAIN HOME, TN, p. A372
VETERANS AFFAIRS MEDICAL CENTER, NASHVILLE, TN, p. A373
VETERANS AFFAIRS MEDICAL CENTER, AMARILLO, TX, p. A376
VETERANS AFFAIRS MEDICAL CENTER, BIG SPRING, TX, p. A379
VETERANS AFFAIRS MEDICAL CENTER, DALLAS, TX, p. A384
VETERANS AFFAIRS MEDICAL CENTER, HOUSTON, TX, p. A392
VETERANS AFFAIRS MEDICAL CENTER, KERRVILLE, TX, p. A394
VETERANS AFFAIRS MEDICAL CENTER, MARLIN, TX, p. A396
VETERANS AFFAIRS MEDICAL CENTER, WACO, TX, p. A406
VETERANS AFFAIRS MEDICAL CENTER, SALT LAKE CITY, UT, p. A410
VETERANS AFFAIRS MEDICAL CENTER, WHITE RIVER JUNCTION, VT, p. A413

VETERANS AFFAIRS MEDICAL CENTER, HAMPTON, VA, p. A416
VETERANS AFFAIRS MEDICAL CENTER, SALEM, VA, p. A420
VETERANS AFFAIRS MEDICAL CENTER, SEATTLE, WA, p. A427
VETERANS AFFAIRS MEDICAL CENTER, SPOKANE, WA, p. A428
VETERANS AFFAIRS MEDICAL CENTER, TACOMA, WA, p. A428
VETERANS AFFAIRS MEDICAL CENTER, WALLA WALLA, WA, p. A429
VETERANS AFFAIRS MEDICAL CENTER, BECKLEY, WV, p. A430
VETERANS AFFAIRS MEDICAL CENTER, HUNTINGTON, WV, p. A431
VETERANS AFFAIRS MEDICAL CENTER, MARTINSBURG, WV, p. A432
VETERANS AFFAIRS MEDICAL CENTER, TOMAH, WI, p. A443
VETERANS AFFAIRS MEDICAL CENTER, SHERIDAN, WY, p. A446
VETERANS AFFAIRS WEST SIDE MEDICAL CENTER, CHICAGO, IL, p. A121
VETERANS HOME AND HOSPITAL, ROCKY HILL, CT, p. A 76
VETERANS HOME OF CALIFORNIA, YOUNTVILLE, CA, p. A 67
VETERANS MEMORIAL HOSPITAL, WAUKON, IA, p. A150
VETERANS MEMORIAL HOSPITAL OF MEIGS COUNTY, POMEROY, OH, p. A316
VETERANS MEMORIAL MEDICAL CENTER, MERIDEN, CT, p. A 75
VICKSBURG MEDICAL CENTER, VICKSBURG, MS, p. A228
VICTOR VALLEY COMMUNITY HOSPITAL, VICTORVILLE, CA, p. A 66
VICTORIA REGIONAL MEDICAL CENTER, VICTORIA, TX, p. A406
VICTORY MEDICAL CENTER, STANLEY, WI, p. A443
VICTORY MEMORIAL HOSPITAL, WAUKEGAN, IL, p. A131
VICTORY MEMORIAL HOSPITAL, NEW YORK CITY, NY, p. A283
VILLA FELICIANA CHRONIC DISEASE HOSPITAL AND REHABILITATION CENTER, JACKSON, LA, p. A173
VILLA MARIA NURSING AND REHABILITATION CENTER, NORTH MIAMI, FL, p. A 91
VILLA ST. JOHN VIANNEY HOSPITAL, DOWNINGTOWN, PA, p. A337
VILLAGE OAKS MEDICAL CENTER, SAN ANTONIO, TX, p. A402
VILLAVIEW COMMUNITY HOSPITAL, SAN DIEGO, CA, p. A 60
VILLE PLATTE MEDICAL CENTER, VILLE PLATTE, LA, p. A179
VINELAND DEVELOPMENT CENTER HOSPITAL, VINELAND, NJ, p. A265
VIRGINIA BAPTIST HOSPITAL, LYNCHBURG, VA, p. A417
VIRGINIA BEACH GENERAL HOSPITAL, VIRGINIA BEACH, VA, p. A421
VIRGINIA GAY HOSPITAL, VINTON, IA, p. A150
VIRGINIA MASON MEDICAL CENTER, SEATTLE, WA, p. A427
VIRGINIA REGIONAL MEDICAL CENTER, VIRGINIA, MN, p. A221
VISALIA COMMUNITY HOSPITAL, VISALIA, CA, p. A 66
VISTA HILL HOSPITAL, CHULA VISTA, CA, p. A 40
VOLUNTEER GENERAL HOSPITAL, MARTIN, TN, p. A371

W

W. A. FOOTE MEMORIAL HOSPITAL, JACKSON, MI, p. A205
W. J. BARGE MEMORIAL HOSPITAL, GREENVILLE, SC, p. A358
W. J. MANGOLD MEMORIAL HOSPITAL, LOCKNEY, TX, p. A395
WABASH COUNTY HOSPITAL, WABASH, IN, p. A141
WABASH GENERAL HOSPITAL DISTRICT, MOUNT CARMEL, IL, p. A127
WABASH VALLEY HOSPITAL, WEST LAFAYETTE, IN, p. A141
WADLEY REGIONAL MEDICAL CENTER, TEXARKANA, TX, p. A405
WADSWORTH-RITTMAN HOSPITAL, WADSWORTH, OH, p. A318
WAGNER COMMUNITY MEMORIAL HOSPITAL, WAGNER, SD, p. A364
WAGNER GENERAL HOSPITAL, PALACIOS, TX, p. A399
WAGONER COMMUNITY HOSPITAL, WAGONER, OK, p. A328
WAHIAWA GENERAL HOSPITAL, WAHIAWA, HI, p. A111
WAKE COUNTY ALCOHOLISM TREATMENT CENTER, RALEIGH, NC, p. A298
WAKE MEDICAL CENTER, RALEIGH, NC, p. A298
WALDO COUNTY GENERAL HOSPITAL, BELFAST, ME, p. A180
WALKER BAPTIST MEDICAL CENTER, JASPER, AL, p. A 17
WALKER CENTER, GOODING, ID, p. A113
WALLA WALLA GENERAL HOSPITAL, WALLA WALLA, WA, p. A429
WALLACE THOMSON HOSPITAL, UNION, SC, p. A360
WALLOWA MEMORIAL HOSPITAL, ENTERPRISE, OR, p. A329
WALLS REGIONAL HOSPITAL, CLEBURNE, TX, p. A381
WALTER B. JONES ALCOHOL AND DRUG ABUSE TREATMENT CENTER, GREENVILLE, NC, p. A295
WALTER KNOX MEMORIAL HOSPITAL, EMMETT, ID, p. A113
WALTER O. BOSWELL MEMORIAL HOSPITAL, SUN CITY, AZ, p. A 27

Hospitals, Alphabetically / Walter Olin Moss Regional Medical Center

WALTER OLIN MOSS REGIONAL MEDICAL CENTER, LAKE CHARLES, LA, p. A174
WALTER P. REUTHER PSYCHIATRIC HOSPITAL, WESTLAND, MI, p. A211
WALTER REED ARMY MEDICAL CENTER, WASHINGTON, DC, p. A79
WALTHALL COUNTY GENERAL HOSPITAL, TYLERTOWN, MS, p. A228
WALTHAMWESTON HOSPITAL & MEDICAL CENTER, WALTHAM, MA, p. A197
WALTON MEDICAL CENTER, MONROE, GA, p. A106
WALTON REGIONAL HOSPITAL, DE FUNIAK SPRINGS, FL, p. A83
WALTON REHABILITATION HOSPITAL, AUGUSTA, GA, p. A100
WAMEGO CITY HOSPITAL, WAMEGO, KS, p. A159
WARD MEMORIAL HOSPITAL, MONAHANS, TX, p. A397
WARM SPRINGS REHABILITATION HOSPITAL, GONZALES, TX, p. A388
WARRACK MEDICAL CENTER HOSPITAL, SANTA ROSA, CA, p. A63
WARREN GENERAL HOSPITAL, WARREN, OH, p. A318
WARREN GENERAL HOSPITAL, WARREN, PA, p. A350
WARREN HOSPITAL, PHILLIPSBURG, NJ, p. A263
WARREN MEMORIAL HOSPITAL, FRIEND, NE, p. A247
WARREN MEMORIAL HOSPITAL, FRONT ROYAL, VA, p. A416
WARREN STATE HOSPITAL, NORTH WARREN, PA, p. A343
WARRICK HOSPITAL, BOONVILLE, IN, p. A133
WASATCH CANYONS HOSPITAL, SALT LAKE CITY, UT, p. A410
WASATCH COUNTY HOSPITAL, HEBER CITY, UT, p. A408
WASECA AREA MEMORIAL HOSPITAL, WASECA, MN, p. A221
WASHAKIE MEMORIAL HOSPITAL, WORLAND, WY, p. A446
WASHINGTON–ST. TAMMANY REGIONAL MEDICAL CENTER, BOGALUSA, LA, p. A171
WASHINGTON ADVENTIST HOSPITAL, TAKOMA PARK, MD, p. A188
WASHINGTON COUNTY HOSPITAL, NASHVILLE, IL, p. A127
WASHINGTON COUNTY HOSPITAL, WASHINGTON, IA, p. A150
WASHINGTON COUNTY HOSPITAL, WASHINGTON, KS, p. A159
WASHINGTON COUNTY HOSPITAL, PLYMOUTH, NC, p. A297
WASHINGTON COUNTY HOSPITAL ASSOCIATION, HAGERSTOWN, MD, p. A187
WASHINGTON COUNTY INFIRMARY AND NURSING HOME, CHATOM, AL, p. A15
WASHINGTON COUNTY MEMORIAL HOSPITAL, SALEM, IN, p. A140
WASHINGTON COUNTY MEMORIAL HOSPITAL, POTOSI, MO, p. A237
WASHINGTON HOSPITAL, FREMONT, CA, p. A43
WASHINGTON HOSPITAL, WASHINGTON, PA, p. A350
WASHINGTON HOSPITAL CENTER, WASHINGTON, DC, p. A80
WASHINGTON MEDICAL CENTER, CULVER CITY, CA, p. A41
WASHINGTON REGIONAL MEDICAL CENTER, FAYETTEVILLE, AR, p. A30
WASHOE MEDICAL CENTER, RENO, NV, p. A254
WATAUGA MEDICAL CENTER, BOONE, NC, p. A291
WATERBURY HOSPITAL, WATERBURY, CT, p. A77
WATERTOWN MEMORIAL HOSPITAL, WATERTOWN, WI, p. A443
WATERVILLE OSTEOPATHIC HOSPITAL, WATERVILLE, ME, p. A183
WATONGA MUNICIPAL HOSPITAL, WATONGA, OK, p. A328
WATONWAN MEMORIAL HOSPITAL, SAINT JAMES, MN, p. A219
WATSONVILLE COMMUNITY HOSPITAL, WATSONVILLE, CA, p. A66
WAUKESHA MEMORIAL HOSPITAL, WAUKESHA, WI, p. A443
WAUPUN MEMORIAL HOSPITAL, WAUPUN, WI, p. A444
WAUSAU HOSPITAL, WAUSAU, WI, p. A444
WAVERLY MUNICIPAL HOSPITAL, WAVERLY, IA, p. A150
WAYNE COUNTY GENERAL HOSPITAL, WAYNESBORO, TN, p. A375
WAYNE COUNTY HOSPITAL, CORYDON, IA, p. A143
WAYNE COUNTY HOSPITAL, MONTICELLO, KY, p. A166
WAYNE GENERAL HOSPITAL, WAYNESBORO, MS, p. A228
WAYNE GENERAL HOSPITAL, WAYNE, NJ, p. A266
WAYNE HOSPITAL, GREENVILLE, OH, p. A313
WAYNE MEMORIAL HOSPITAL, JESUP, GA, p. A105
WAYNE MEMORIAL HOSPITAL, GOLDSBORO, NC, p. A294
WAYNE MEMORIAL HOSPITAL, HONESDALE, PA, p. A340
WAYNESBORO HOSPITAL, WAYNESBORO, PA, p. A350
WEBSTER COUNTY COMMUNITY HOSPITAL, RED CLOUD, NE, p. A251
WEBSTER COUNTY MEMORIAL HOSPITAL, WEBSTER SPRINGS, WV, p. A433
WEBSTER HEALTH SERVICES, EUPORA, MS, p. A224
WEDOWEE HOSPITAL, WEDOWEE, AL, p. A20
WEED ARMY COMMUNITY HOSPITAL, FORT IRWIN, CA, p. A43
WEEKS MEMORIAL HOSPITAL, LANCASTER, NH, p. A256
WEINER MEMORIAL MEDICAL CENTER, MARSHALL, MN, p. A216
WEIRTON MEDICAL CENTER, WEIRTON, WV, p. A433

WEISBROD MEMORIAL HOSPITAL, EADS, CO, p. A70
WELBORN MEMORIAL BAPTIST HOSPITAL, EVANSVILLE, IN, p. A135
WELKIND REHABILITATION HOSPITAL, CHESTER, NJ, p. A259
WELLINGTON REGIONAL MEDICAL CENTER, WEST PALM BEACH, FL, p. A97
WELLS COMMUNITY HOSPITAL, BLUFFTON, IN, p. A133
WELLSPRING FOUNDATION, BETHLEHEM, CT, p. A74
WELSH GENERAL HOSPITAL, WELSH, LA, p. A179
WENTWORTH–DOUGLASS HOSPITAL, DOVER, NH, p. A255
WERNERSVILLE STATE HOSPITAL, WERNERSVILLE, PA, p. A351
WESKOTA MEMORIAL MEDICAL CENTER, WESSINGTON SPRINGS, SD, p. A364
WESLEY LONG COMMUNITY HOSPITAL, GREENSBORO, NC, p. A295
WESLEY MEDICAL CENTER, WICHITA, KS, p. A160
WESLEY REHABILITATION HOSPITAL, WICHITA, KS, p. A160
WESLEY WOODS GERIATRIC HOSPITAL, ATLANTA, GA, p. A99
WEST ALLIS MEMORIAL HOSPITAL, WEST ALLIS, WI, p. A444
WEST ANAHEIM MEDICAL CENTER, ANAHEIM, CA, p. A36
WEST BOCA MEDICAL CENTER, BOCA RATON, FL, p. A81
WEST CALCASIEU CAMERON HOSPITAL, SULPHUR, LA, p. A178
WEST CARROLL MEMORIAL HOSPITAL, OAK GROVE, LA, p. A177
WEST COMMUNITY HOSPITAL, WEST, TX, p. A407
WEST FELICIANA PARISH HOSPITAL, SAINT FRANCISVILLE, LA, p. A178
WEST FLORIDA REGIONAL MEDICAL CENTER, PENSACOLA, FL, p. A93
WEST FRANKFORT UNITED MINE WORKERS OF AMERICA UNION HOSPITAL, WEST FRANKFORT, IL, p. A131
WEST GEORGIA MEDICAL CENTER, LA GRANGE, GA, p. A105
WEST HILLS HOSPITAL, RENO, NV, p. A254
WEST HILLS REGIONAL MEDICAL CENTER, LOS ANGELES, CA, p. A51
WEST HOLT MEMORIAL HOSPITAL, ATKINSON, NE, p. A246
WEST HOUSTON MEDICAL CENTER, HOUSTON, TX, p. A392
WEST HUDSON HOSPITAL, KEARNY, NJ, p. A261
WEST JEFFERSON MEDICAL CENTER, MARRERO, LA, p. A175
WEST JERSEY HOSPITAL–BERLIN, BERLIN, NJ, p. A258
WEST JERSEY HOSPITAL–CAMDEN, CAMDEN, NJ, p. A258
WEST JERSEY HOSPITAL–MARLTON, MARLTON, NJ, p. A261
WEST JERSEY HOSPITAL–VOORHEES, VOORHEES, NJ, p. A265
WEST OAKS HOSPITAL, HOUSTON, TX, p. A392
WEST PACES MEDICAL CENTER, ATLANTA, GA, p. A99
WEST PARK HOSPITAL, CODY, WY, p. A445
WEST PINES AT LUTHERAN MEDICAL CENTER, WHEAT RIDGE, CO, p. A73
WEST RIVER REGIONAL MEDICAL CENTER, HETTINGER, ND, p. A303
WEST SHORE HOSPITAL, MANISTEE, MI, p. A206
WEST SIDE DISTRICT HOSPITAL, TAFT, CA, p. A64
WEST SUBURBAN HOSPITAL MEDICAL CENTER, OAK PARK, IL, p. A128
WEST TENNESSEE BEHAVIORAL CENTER, JACKSON, TN, p. A369
WEST VALLEY MEDICAL CENTER, CALDWELL, ID, p. A112
WEST VIRGINIA UNIVERSITY HOSPITALS, MORGANTOWN, WV, p. A432
WESTBOROUGH STATE HOSPITAL, WESTBOROUGH, MA, p. A198
WESTBRIDGE TREATMENT CENTER – NORTH CAMPUS, PHOENIX, AZ, p. A26
WESTBRIDGE TREATMENT CENTER, PHOENIX, AZ, p. A26
WESTBROOK COMMUNITY HOSPITAL, WESTBROOK, ME, p. A183
WESTBURY HOSPITAL, HOUSTON, TX, p. A392
WESTCHESTER COUNTY MEDICAL CENTER, VALHALLA, NY, p. A288
WESTCHESTER GENERAL HOSPITAL, MIAMI, FL, p. A90
WESTCHESTER SQUARE MEDICAL CENTER, NEW YORK CITY, NY, p. A283
WESTERLY HOSPITAL, WESTERLY, RI, p. A354
WESTERN BAPTIST HOSPITAL, PADUCAH, KY, p. A167
WESTERN HILLS REHABILITATION HOSPITAL, PARKERSBURG, WV, p. A432
WESTERN MARYLAND CENTER, HAGERSTOWN, MD, p. A187
WESTERN MEDICAL CENTER–SANTA ANA, SANTA ANA, CA, p. A62
WESTERN MEDICAL CENTER HOSPITAL ANAHEIM, ANAHEIM, CA, p. A36
WESTERN MENTAL HEALTH INSTITUTE, WESTERN INSTITUTE, TN, p. A375
WESTERN MISSOURI MEDICAL CENTER, WARRENSBURG, MO, p. A240
WESTERN MISSOURI MENTAL HEALTH CENTER, KANSAS CITY, MO, p. A235

WESTERN NEW YORK CHILDREN'S PSYCHIATRIC CENTER, WEST SENECA, NY, p. A289
WESTERN PENNSYLVANIA HOSPITAL, PITTSBURGH, PA, p. A348
WESTERN PLAINS REGIONAL HOSPITAL, DODGE CITY, KS, p. A152
WESTERN QUEENS COMMUNITY HOSPITAL, NEW YORK CITY, NY, p. A283
WESTERN RESERVE CARE SYSTEM, YOUNGSTOWN, OH, p. A320
WESTERN RESERVE PSYCHIATRIC HOSPITAL, NORTHFIELD, OH, p. A315
WESTERN STATE HOSPITAL, HOPKINSVILLE, KY, p. A163
WESTERN STATE HOSPITAL, STAUNTON, VA, p. A421
WESTERN STATE HOSPITAL, FORT STEILACOOM, WA, p. A424
WESTERN STATE PSYCHIATRIC CENTER, FORT SUPPLY, OK, p. A323
WESTFIELD MEMORIAL HOSPITAL, WESTFIELD, NY, p. A289
WESTLAKE COMMUNITY HOSPITAL, MELROSE PARK, IL, p. A127
WESTLAKE CUMBERLAND HOSPITAL, COLUMBIA, KY, p. A162
WESTLAKE MEDICAL CENTER, WESTLAKE VILLAGE, CA, p. A67
WESTMORELAND REGIONAL HOSPITAL, GREENSBURG, PA, p. A339
WESTON COUNTY MEMORIAL HOSPITAL, NEWCASTLE, WY, p. A446
WESTSIDE HOSPITAL, LOS ANGELES, CA, p. A51
WESTSIDE REGIONAL MEDICAL CENTER, PLANTATION, FL, p. A93
WESTVIEW HOSPITAL, INDIANAPOLIS, IN, p. A137
WESTWOOD LODGE HOSPITAL, WESTWOOD, MA, p. A198
WETUMKA GENERAL HOSPITAL, WETUMKA, OK, p. A328
WETZEL COUNTY HOSPITAL, NEW MARTINSVILLE, WV, p. A432
WHEATLAND MEMORIAL HOSPITAL, HARLOWTON, MT, p. A243
WHEATON COMMUNITY HOSPITAL, WHEATON, MN, p. A221
WHEELER COUNTY HOSPITAL, GLENWOOD, GA, p. A104
WHEELING HOSPITAL, WHEELING, WV, p. A434
WHIDBEY GENERAL HOSPITAL, COUPEVILLE, WA, p. A424
WHIDDEN MEMORIAL HOSPITAL, EVERETT, MA, p. A193
WHITE COMMUNITY HOSPITAL, AURORA, MN, p. A212
WHITE COUNTY COMMUNITY HOSPITAL, SPARTA, TN, p. A374
WHITE COUNTY HOSPITAL, CARMI, IL, p. A117
WHITE COUNTY MEMORIAL HOSPITAL, SEARCY, AR, p. A34
WHITE COUNTY MEMORIAL HOSPITAL, MONTICELLO, IN, p. A139
WHITE MEMORIAL MEDICAL CENTER, LOS ANGELES, CA, p. A51
WHITE MOUNTAIN COMMUNITIES HOSPITAL, SPRINGERVILLE, AZ, p. A27
WHITE PLAINS HOSPITAL CENTER, WHITE PLAINS, NY, p. A289
WHITE RIVER MEDICAL CENTER, BATESVILLE, AR, p. A29
WHITESBURG APPALACHIAN REGIONAL HOSPITAL, WHITESBURG, KY, p. A168
WHITFIELD MEDICAL SURGICAL HOSPITAL, WHITFIELD, MS, p. A228
WHITING FORENSIC INSTITUTE, MIDDLETOWN, CT, p. A75
WHITLEY COUNTY MEMORIAL HOSPITAL, COLUMBIA CITY, IN, p. A134
WHITMAN HOSPITAL AND MEDICAL CENTER, COLFAX, WA, p. A424
WHITTEN CENTER HOSPITAL, CLINTON, SC, p. A356
WHITTIER HOSPITAL MEDICAL CENTER, WHITTIER, CA, p. A67
WHITTIER REHABILITATION HOSPITAL, HAVERHILL, MA, p. A193
WICHITA COUNTY HOSPITAL, LEOTI, KS, p. A155
WICHITA FALLS STATE HOSPITAL, WICHITA FALLS, TX, p. A407
WICHITA GENERAL HOSPITAL, WICHITA FALLS, TX, p. A407
WICKENBURG COMMUNITY HOSPITAL, WICKENBURG, AZ, p. A28
WILBARGER GENERAL HOSPITAL, VERNON, TX, p. A406
WILCOX MEMORIAL HOSPITAL, LIHUE, HI, p. A111
WILD ROSE COMMUNITY MEMORIAL HOSPITAL, WILD ROSE, WI, p. A444
WILDWOOD LIFESTYLE CENTER AND HOSPITAL, WILDWOOD, GA, p. A109
WILFORD HALL U.S. AIR FORCE MEDICAL CENTER, LACKLAND AIR FORCE BASE, TX, p. A394
WILKES REGIONAL MEDICAL CENTER, NORTH WILKESBORO, NC, p. A297
WILLAMETTE FALLS HOSPITAL, OREGON CITY, OR, p. A331
WILLAPA HARBOR HOSPITAL, SOUTH BEND, WA, p. A427
WILLIAM B. KESSLER MEMORIAL HOSPITAL, HAMMONTON, NJ, p. A260
WILLIAM BEAUMONT ARMY MEDICAL CENTER, EL PASO, TX, p. A386
WILLIAM BEAUMONT HOSPITAL–TROY, TROY, MI, p. A211
WILLIAM BEAUMONT HOSPITAL, ROYAL OAK, MI, p. A209
WILLIAM BEE RIRIE HOSPITAL, ELY, NV, p. A253

WILLIAM JENNINGS BRYAN DORN VETERANS HOSPITAL, COLUMBIA, SC, p. A356
WILLIAM N. WISHARD MEMORIAL HOSPITAL, INDIANAPOLIS, IN, p. A137
WILLIAM NEWTON MEMORIAL HOSPITAL, WINFIELD, KS, p. A160
WILLIAM S. HALL PSYCHIATRIC INSTITUTE, COLUMBIA, SC, p. A356
WILLIAM S. MIDDLETON MEMORIAL VETERANS HOSPITAL, MADISON, WI, p. A438
WILLIAM W. BACKUS HOSPITAL, NORWICH, CT, p. A 76
WILLIAM W. HASTINGS INDIAN HOSPITAL, TAHLEQUAH, OK, p. A327
WILLIAMSBURG COMMUNITY HOSPITAL, WILLIAMSBURG, VA, p. A421
WILLIAMSBURG COUNTY MEMORIAL HOSPITAL, KINGSTREE, SC, p. A358
WILLIAMSON ARH HOSPITAL, SOUTH WILLIAMSON, KY, p. A168
WILLIAMSON MEDICAL CENTER, FRANKLIN, TN, p. A368
WILLIAMSON MEMORIAL HOSPITAL, WILLIAMSON, WV, p. A434
WILLIAMSPORT HOSPITAL AND MEDICAL CENTER, WILLIAMSPORT, PA, p. A351
WILLINGWAY HOSPITAL, STATESBORO, GA, p. A108
WILLIS-KNIGHTON MEDICAL CENTER, SHREVEPORT, LA, p. A178
WILLMAR REGIONAL TREATMENT CENTER, WILLMAR, MN, p. A221
WILLOUGH AT NAPLES, NAPLES, FL, p. A 90
WILLOW CREEK HOSPITAL, ARLINGTON, TX, p. A377
WILLOW CREST HOSPITAL, MIAMI, OK, p. A325
WILLOW SPRINGS CENTER FOR CHILDREN AND ADOLESCENTS, RENO, NV, p. A254
WILLOW VIEW MENTAL HEALTH SYSTEM, SPENCER, OK, p. A327
WILLS EYE HOSPITAL, PHILADELPHIA, PA, p. A346
WILLS MEMORIAL HOSPITAL, WASHINGTON, GA, p. A109
WILMA N. VAZQUEZ MEDICAL CENTER, VEGA BAJA, PR, p. A450
WILSON CENTER PSYCHIATRIC FACILITY FOR CHILDREN AND ADOLESCENTS, FARIBAULT, MN, p. A214
WILSON COUNTY HOSPITAL, NEODESHA, KS, p. A156
WILSON MEMORIAL HOSPITAL, WILSON, NC, p. A300
WILSON MEMORIAL HOSPITAL, SIDNEY, OH, p. A317
WILSON MEMORIAL HOSPITAL, FLORESVILLE, TX, p. A386
WILSON N. JONES MEMORIAL HOSPITAL, SHERMAN, TX, p. A403
WINCHESTER HOSPITAL, WINCHESTER, MA, p. A198
WINCHESTER MEDICAL CENTER, WINCHESTER, VA, p. A421
WINDBER HOSPITAL, WINDBER, PA, p. A352
WINDHAM COMMUNITY MEMORIAL HOSPITAL, WILLIMANTIC, CT, p. A 77
WINDOM AREA HOSPITAL, WINDOM, MN, p. A221
WINDSOR HOSPITAL, CHAGRIN FALLS, OH, p. A307
WINFIELD STATE HOSPITAL AND TRAINING CENTER, WINFIELD, KS, p. A160
WING MEMORIAL HOSPITAL AND MEDICAL CENTERS, PALMER, MA, p. A196
WINN ARMY COMMUNITY HOSPITAL, FORT STEWART, GA, p. A104
WINN PARISH MEDICAL CENTER, WINNFIELD, LA, p. A179
WINNEBAGO MENTAL HEALTH INSTITUTE, WINNEBAGO, WI, p. A444
WINNER REGIONAL HEALTHCARE CENTER, WINNER, SD, p. A364
WINNESHIEK COUNTY MEMORIAL HOSPITAL, DECORAH, IA, p. A144
WINONA MEMORIAL HOSPITAL, INDIANAPOLIS, IN, p. A137
WINSLOW MEMORIAL HOSPITAL, WINSLOW, AZ, p. A 28
WINSTED MEMORIAL HOSPITAL, WINSTED, CT, p. A 77
WINSTON COUNTY COMMUNITY HOSPITAL AND NURSING HOME, LOUISVILLE, MS, p. A226
WINTER HAVEN HOSPITAL, WINTER HAVEN, FL, p. A 97
WINTER PARK MEMORIAL HOSPITAL, WINTER PARK, FL, p. A 97
WINTHROP-UNIVERSITY HOSPITAL, MINEOLA, NY, p. A277
WIREGRASS HOSPITAL, GENEVA, AL, p. A 16
WIRTH OSTEOPATHIC HOSPITAL, OAKLAND CITY, IN, p. A139
WISE ARH HOSPITAL, WISE, VA, p. A422
WISHEK COMMUNITY HOSPITAL, WISHEK, ND, p. A305
WITHAM MEMORIAL HOSPITAL, LEBANON, IN, p. A138
WOMACK ARMY MEDICAL CENTER, FORT BRAGG, NC, p. A294
WOMAN'S CHRISTIAN ASSOCIATION HOSPITAL, JAMESTOWN, NY, p. A276
WOMAN'S HOSPITAL, BATON ROUGE, LA, p. A171
WOMAN'S HOSPITAL OF TEXAS, HOUSTON, TX, p. A392
WOMEN & INFANTS HOSPITAL OF RHODE ISLAND, PROVIDENCE, RI, p. A353
WOMEN'S AND CHILDREN'S HOSPITAL, LAFAYETTE, LA, p. A174
WOMEN'S AND CHILDREN'S HOSPITAL, SAN ANTONIO, TX, p. A403
WOMEN'S HOSPITAL-INDIANAPOLIS, INDIANAPOLIS, IN, p. A137
WOMEN'S HOSPITAL AND MEDICAL CENTER, SEMINOLE, FL, p. A 95
WOMENS HOSPITAL, LAS VEGAS, NV, p. A253
WOOD COUNTY CENTRAL HOSPITAL DISTRICT, QUITMAN, TX, p. A400
WOOD COUNTY HOSPITAL, BOWLING GREEN, OH, p. A307
WOOD RIVER MEDICAL CENTER, SUN VALLEY, ID, p. A114
WOOD RIVER TOWNSHIP HOSPITAL, WOOD RIVER, IL, p. A132
WOODBRIDGE DEVELOPMENT CENTER, WOODBRIDGE, NJ, p. A266
WOODFORD HOSPITAL, VERSAILLES, KY, p. A168
WOODHULL MEDICAL AND MENTAL HEALTH CENTER, NEW YORK CITY, NY, p. A283
WOODLAND COMMUNITY HOSPITAL, CULLMAN, AL, p. A 15
WOODLAND HEIGHTS MEDICAL CENTER, LUFKIN, TX, p. A396
WOODLAND HILLS HOSPITAL, WEST MONROE, LA, p. A179
WOODLAND HOSPITAL, HOFFMAN ESTATES, IL, p. A125
WOODLAND MEMORIAL HOSPITAL, WOODLAND, CA, p. A 67
WOODLAND PARK HOSPITAL, PORTLAND, OR, p. A332
WOODLAWN HOSPITAL, ROCHESTER, IN, p. A140
WOODRIDGE HOSPITAL, CLAYTON, GA, p. A101
WOODRIDGE HOSPITAL, JOHNSON CITY, TN, p. A369
WOODROW WILSON REHABILITATION CENTER-HOSPITAL, FISHERSVILLE, VA, p. A415
WOODRUFF COMMUNITY HOSPITAL, LONG BEACH, CA, p. A 48
WOODS MEMORIAL HOSPITAL DISTRICT, ETOWAH, TN, p. A368
WOODS PSYCHIATRIC INSTITUTE, ABILENE, TX, p. A376
WOODSIDE HOSPITAL, YOUNGSTOWN, OH, p. A320
WOODWARD HOSPITAL AND HEALTH CENTER, WOODWARD, OK, p. A328
WOODWARD STATE HOSPITAL-SCHOOL, WOODWARD, IA, p. A150
WOOSTER COMMUNITY HOSPITAL, WOOSTER, OH, p. A319
WORCESTER STATE HOSPITAL, WORCESTER, MA, p. A198
WORTH COUNTY HOSPITAL, SYLVESTER, GA, p. A108
WORTHINGTON REGIONAL HOSPITAL, WORTHINGTON, MN, p. A221
WRANGELL GENERAL HOSPITAL AND LONG TERM CARE FACILITY, WRANGELL, AK, p. A 22
WRAY COMMUNITY DISTRICT HOSPITAL, WRAY, CO, p. A 73
WRIGHT MEMORIAL HOSPITAL, TRENTON, MO, p. A240
WUESTHOFF HOSPITAL, ROCKLEDGE, FL, p. A 94
WYANDOT MEMORIAL HOSPITAL, UPPER SANDUSKY, OH, p. A318
WYANDOTTE HOSPITAL AND MEDICAL CENTER, WYANDOTTE, MI, p. A211
WYCKOFF HEIGHTS MEDICAL CENTER, NEW YORK CITY, NY, p. A283
WYOMING COUNTY COMMUNITY HOSPITAL, WARSAW, NY, p. A289
WYOMING MEDICAL CENTER, CASPER, WY, p. A445
WYOMING STATE HOSPITAL, EVANSTON, WY, p. A445
WYOMING VALLEY HEALTH CARE SYSTEM, KINGSTON, PA, p. A340
WYTHE COUNTY COMMUNITY HOSPITAL, WYTHEVILLE, VA, p. A422

Y

YAKIMA VALLEY MEMORIAL HOSPITAL, YAKIMA, WA, p. A429
YALE-NEW HAVEN HOSPITAL, NEW HAVEN, CT, p. A 75
YALE CLINIC AND HOSPITAL, HOUSTON, TX, p. A393
YALE COMMUNITY HOSPITAL, YALE, MI, p. A211
YALE PSYCHIATRIC INSTITUTE, NEW HAVEN, CT, p. A 75
YALOBUSHA GENERAL HOSPITAL, WATER VALLEY, MS, p. A228
YAVAPAI REGIONAL MEDICAL CENTER, PRESCOTT, AZ, p. A 26
YOAKUM COMMUNITY HOSPITAL, YOAKUM, TX, p. A407
YOAKUM COUNTY HOSPITAL, DENVER CITY, TX, p. A385
YONKERS GENERAL HOSPITAL, YONKERS, NY, p. A290
YORK GENERAL HOSPITAL, YORK, NE, p. A252
YORK HOSPITAL, YORK, ME, p. A183
YORK HOSPITAL, YORK, PA, p. A352
YOUNGSTOWN OSTEOPATHIC HOSPITAL, YOUNGSTOWN, OH, p. A320
YOUTH FOCUS PSYCHIATRIC HOSPITAL, GREENSBORO, NC, p. A295
YOUVILLE HOSPITAL AND REHABILITATION CENTER, CAMBRIDGE, MA, p. A192
YUKON-KUSKOKWIM DELTA REGIONAL HOSPITAL, BETHEL, AK, p. A 21
YUMA DISTRICT HOSPITAL, YUMA, CO, p. A 73
YUMA REGIONAL MEDICAL CENTER, YUMA, AZ, p. A 28

Z

ZALE LIPSHY UNIVERSITY HOSPITAL, DALLAS, TX, p. A384
ZEELAND COMMUNITY HOSPITAL, ZEELAND, MI, p. A211
ZUMBROTA HEALTH CARE, ZUMBROTA, MN, p. A221
ZURBRUGG MEMORIAL HOSPITAL, RIVERSIDE, NJ, p. A264

AHA Membership Categories

The American Hospital Association is primarily an organization of hospitals and related institutions. its object, according to its bylaws, is "to promote high–quality health care and health services for all the people through leadership in the development of public policy, leadership in the representation and advocacy of hospital and health care organization interests, and leadership in the provision of services to assist hospitals and health care organizations in meeting the health care needs of their communities."

The major source of income for the AHA is its membership dues, which are established by the membership trough the House of Delegates. The types of membership and the basis for dues for each type are described in the following paragraphs.

Institutional Members

Type I–A and I–B, Hospitals
General and special hospitals that care for patients with conditions requiring a comparatively short stay. Type I–A includes short–term hospitals that are freestanding or which are operating units of health care systems not holding type III membership. Type I–B are short–term hospitals that are operating units of health care systems holding type III membership.

Type II–A and II–B, Hospitals
All other hospitals that provide inpatient care. Type II–A includes long–term hospitals that are freestanding or which are operating units of helath care systems not holding type III membership. type II–B includes longer–term hospitals that are operating unites of health care systems holding type III membership.

Type III, Health Care Systems
Only those organizations (corporate headquarters, or similar entity) operating two or more hospitals or a single hospital owning, leasing, or sponsoring at least three operating entities of nonhospital preacute and postacute health care organizations can be classified as type III institutions. Headquarters of health care systems are eligible for type III membership when 90 percent of their owned, leased, managed, or sponsored hospitals are AHA members.

Membership dues are computed individually for each hospital and are based on total reported operating expenses for the most recent 12–month period. Type III members pay no dues other than those dues paid by their type B member units.

Type IV, Nonhospital Preacute and Postacute Health Care Organizations
Type IV–A, and IV–B organizations are defined as nonhospital preacute and postacute organizations that are responsible for delivery or delivery and financing of health care services. Health care delivery, for purposes of this definition, is the availability of professional health care staff during all hours of the organization's operations. Type IV–C members shall be limited to educational organizations.

Professional Members
Hospitals that are in the planning or construction stage and that, on completion, will be eligible for institutional membership type I or type II. Provisional membership may also be granted to applicant institutions that cannot, at present, meet the requirements of type I or type II membership.

Government Institution Group Members
Groups of government hospitals operated by the same unit of government may obtain institutional membership under a group plan. Membership dues are based on a special schedule set forth in the bylaws of the AHA.

Contracting Hospitals

The AHA also provides membership services to certain hospitals that are prevented from holding membership because of legal or other restrictions.

Contracting hospitals pay dues on the same basis as if they were classified as type I or II members.

Associate Members

Associate members are organizations interested in the objectives of the AHA but not eligible for institution membership. Membership dues are a fixed annual sum, depending on the location (inside or outside the United States and Canada) of the organization.

Institutional Members

Types I and II
Hospitals

U.S. hospitals and hospitals in areas associated with the U.S that are type I (short–term) or type II (long–term) members of the American Hospital Association are included in the list of hospitals in section A. Canadian types I and II members of the American Hospital Association are listed below.

Canada

Alberta
Calgary: CALGARY GENERAL HOSPITAL, 841 Centre Avenue East, Zip T2E 0A1; tel. 403/268–9838; Marlene Meyers, President
Edmonton: CAPITAL HEALTH AUTHORITY, 8440 112 Street, Zip T6G 2B7; tel. 403/492–8822; Donald P. Schurman, President
  MISERICORDIA HOSPITAL, 16940 87th Avenue, Zip T5R 4H5; tel. 403/488–0921; G. P. Hiebert, President
  ROYAL ALEXANDRA HOSPITAL, 10240 Kingsway, Zip T5H 3V9; tel. 403/477–4111; Thomas Noseworthy, President
Lamont: LAMONT HEALTH CARE CENTRE, Zip T0B 2R0; tel. 403/895–2211; Harold James, Executive Director
Saint Albert: STURGEON GENERAL HOSPITAL, Zip T8N 1L9; tel. 403/460–6200; C. Brian Spooner, Director
Stony Plain: STONY PLAIN MUNICIPAL HOSPITAL, 4800 55th Avenue, Zip T7Z 1P9; tel. 403/963–2241; Thomas J. Novak, Chief Executive Officer

British Columbia
Langley: LANGLEY MEMORIAL HOSPITAL, 22051 Fraser Highway, Zip V3A 4H4; tel. 604/534–4121; Pat E. Zanon, President and Chief Executive Officer
North Vancouver: LIONS GATE HOSPITAL, 231 East 15th Street, Zip V7L 2L7; tel. 604/988–3131; Robert J. Smith, President
Vancouver: CHILDREN'S HOSPITAL, 4480 Oak Street, Zip V6H 3V4; tel. 604/875–2345; John H. Tegenfeldt, President

Manitoba
Portage La Prarie: PORTAGE DISTRICT GENERAL HOSPITAL, 524 Fifth Street S.E., Zip R1N 3A8; tel. 204/239–2211; Garry C. Mattin, Executive Director
Winnipeg: RIVERVIEW HEALTH CENTRE, 1 Morley Avenue East, tel. 204/452–3411; Norman R. Kasian, Executive Director
  ST. BONIFACE GENERAL HOSPITAL, 409 Tache Avenue, Zip R2H 2A6; tel. 204/237–2330; Peter M. Liba, President and Chief Executive Officer
  VICTORIA GENERAL HOSPITAL, 2340 Pembina Highway, Zip R3T 2E8; tel. 204/269–3570; Marion Suski, President and Chief Executive Officer

Nova Scotia
North Sydney: NORTHSIDE HARBOR VIEW HOSPITAL, tel. 902/794–4725; J. Higgins, Executive Director
Sydney: CAPE BRETON REGIONAL HOSPITAL, 1482 George Street, Zip B1P 1P3; tel. 902/567–8000; Mary S. MacIsaac, Chief Executive Officer

Ontario
Brantford: ST. JOSEPH'S HOSPITAL, 63 Park Road North, Zip N3S 6T6; tel. 519/753–8641; Romeo Cercone, President and Chief Executive Officer
Brockville: ST. VINCENT DE PAUL HOSPITAL, 42 Garden Street, Zip K6V 2C3; tel. 613/342–4461; Thomas P. Harrington, Administrator
Chatham: PUBLIC GENERAL HOSPITAL, 106 Emma Street, Zip N7L 1A8; tel. 519/352–6400; H. David Vigar, Executive Director
Etobicoke: QUEENSWAY GENERAL HOSPITAL, 150 Sherway Drive, Zip M9C 1A5; tel. 416/259–6671; John J. Penaligon, President
Guelph: HOMEWOOD HEALTH CENTER, 150 Delhi Street, Zip N1E 6K9; tel. 519/824–1010; Ronald Pond, Executive Director
London: ST. MARYS' HOSPITAL, P.O. Box 5777, Zip N6A 1Y6; tel. 613/646–6000; Philip Hassen, President
North York: BAYCREST CENTRE–GERIATRIC CARE, 3560 Bathurst Street, Zip M6A 2E1; tel. 416/789–5131; Stephen W. Herbert, President
  NORTH YORK BRANSON HOSPITAL, 555 Finch Avenue West, Zip M2R 1N5; tel. 416/633–9420; J. A. Bruce, President
Ottawa: ROYAL OTTAWA HOSPITAL, 1145 Carling Avenue, Zip K1Z 7K4; tel. 613/722–6521; George F. Langill, Executive Director
Parry Sound: PARRY SOUND GENERAL HOSPITAL, 10 James Street, Zip P2A 1T3; tel. 705/746–9321; Norman Maciver, Chief Executive Officer
Renfrew: RENFREW VICTORIA HOSPITAL, 499 Raglan Street North, Zip K7V 1P6; tel. 613/432–4851; Randy Penney, Executive Director
Sarnia: ST. JOSEPH'S HOSPITAL, 89 Norman Street, Zip NYT 6S3; tel. 519/336–6121; Don McDermott, Executive Director
Strathroy: STRATHROY MIDDLESEX GENERAL HOSPITAL, 395 Carrie Street, Zip N7G 3C9; tel. 519/245–1550; Thomas M. Enright, Executive Director
Sudbury: SUDBURY MEMORIAL HOSPITAL, 865 Regent Street South, Zip P3E 3Y9; tel. 705/671–1000; Esko J. Vainio, Executive Director
Thornhill: SHOULDICE HOSPITAL, Box 370, Zip C3T 4A3; tel. 416/889–1125; Alan O'Dell, Administrator
Toronto: CENTRAL HOSPITAL, 333 Sherbourne Street, Zip M5A 2F5; tel. 416/969–4111; William Louth, Executive Director
  DOCTORS HOSPITAL, 45 Brunswick Avenue, Zip M5S 2M1; tel. 416/923–5411; Brian McFarle, President
  MOUNT SINAI HOSPITAL, 600 University Avenue, Zip M5G 1X5; tel. 416/366–7361; Theodore J. Freedman, President and Chief Executive Officer
  QUEEN ELIZABETH HOSPITAL, 550 University Avenue, Zip M5G 2A2; tel. 416/537–2411; Clifford A. Nordal, President
  ST. JOSEPH'S HEALTH CENTRE, 30 the Queensway, Zip M6R 1B5; tel. 416/534–9531; Leo N. Steven, President and Chief Executive Officer
  WOMEN'S COLLEGE HOSPITAL, 76 Grenville Street, Zip M5S 1B2; tel. 416/966–7111; S. Bruce Goss, Vice President Administration and Finance

Quebec
Laval: JEWISH REHABILITATION HOSPITAL, 3205 Alton Goldbloom Street, Zip H7V 1R2; tel. 514/688–9550; Henry Coopersmith, Executive Director
Montreal: JEWISH GENERAL HOSPITAL, 3755 Cote St–Catherine Road, Zip H3T 1E2; tel. 514/340–8222; Henri Elbaz, Executive Director
  JEWISH HOSPITAL OF HOPE, 5725 Victoria Avenue, Zip H3W 3H6; tel. 514/738–4500; Isaac Katofsky, Executive Director
  MONTREAL CHILDREN'S HOSPITAL, 2300 Tupper Street, Zip H3H 1P3; tel. 514/934–4400; Nicholas Steinnetz, Executive Director
  MOUNT SINAI HOSPITAL CENTER, 5690 Cavendish Cote St–Luc', Zip H4W 1S7; tel. 514/369–2222; Joseph Rothbart, Executive Director
  NOTRE DAME HOSPITAL, 1560 East Sherbrooke, Zip H2L 4ML; tel. 514/876–6421; David Levine, Director General
  REDDY MEMORIAL HOSPITAL, 4039 Tupper Street, Zip H3Z 1T5; tel. 514/933–7511; Rejean Plante, Director General
  ROYAL VICTORIA HOSPITAL, 687 Pine Avenue, Zip H3A 1A1; tel. 514/842–1251; Phillip P. Aspinall, President and Chief Executive Officer
Sherbrooke: SHERBROOKE HOSPITAL, 375 Argyle Street, Zip J1J 3H5; tel. 819/569–3661; Marie Trousdell, Director General

Type III
Health Care Systems

Health Care Systems that are type III members of the American Hospital Association are included in the alphabetic and numeric lists of health care systems in sections A and B of this guide. Membership is indicated in the numeric list by a star (★) preceding the name of the system.

Institutional Members / Programs in Health Administration

Type IV

Type IV members of the American Hospital Association include Nonhospital Precute and Postacute Health Care Organizations. These organizations are responsible for delivery or delivery and financing of health care services.
Type IV members also include Associated University Programs in Health Administration and Hospital Schools of Nursing.

Associated University Programs in Health Administration

ALABAMA
Birmingham: UNIVERSITY OF ALABAMA AT BIRMINGHAM, Zip 35294; tel. 205/934–5661; Keith D. Blayney, Dean

ARIZONA
Tempe: SCHOOL OF HEALTH ADMINISTRATION AND POLICY, COLLEGE OF BUSINESS, ARIZONA STATE UNIVERSITY, College & Lemon Streets, Zip 85287; tel. 602/965–7778; Frank G. Williams, Director

CALIFORNIA
Los Angeles: UCLA, SCHOOL OF PUBLIC HEALTH, PROGRAM IN HEALTH SERVICES MANAGEMENT, University of California, Zip 90024; Ronald Andersen, Chairman
San Francisco: GOLDEN GATE UNIVERSITY, 536 Mission Street, General Library, Zip 94105; tel. 415/442–0777; Steven Dunlap, Assistant Librarian

DISTRICT OF COLUMBIA
Washington: DEPARTMENT OF HEALTH SERVICES ADMINISTRATION, GEORGE WASHINGTON UNIVERSITY, The George Washington University, Zip 20052; tel. 202/676–6220; Richard F. Southby, Professor and Chairman

GEORGIA
Atlanta: GEORGIA STATE UNIVERSITY, INSTITUTE OF HEALTH ADMINISTRATION, University Plaza, Zip 30303; tel. 404/651–2000; Everett A. Johnson, Director

ILLINOIS
Carbondale: SOUTHERN ILLINOIS UNIVERSITY, COLLEGE OF TECHNICAL CAREERS, College of Technical Careers, Zip 62901; tel. 618/536–6682; Frederic L. Morgan, Chair and Health Care Professor
Chicago: UNIVERSITY OF CHICAGO, GRADUATE PROGRAM IN HEALTH ADMINISTRATION AND POLICY, 969 East 60th Street, Zip 60637; tel. 312/753–4191; Edward Lawlor, Director

Evanston: PROGRAM HOSPITAL AND HEALTH SERVICE MANAGEMENT, KELLOGG GRADUATE SCHOOL OF MANAGEMENT, NORTHWESTERN UNIVERSITY, Leverone Hall, Zip 60208; tel. 708/492–5540; Joel Shalowitz, Professor
University Park: PROGRAM IN HEALTH SERVICE ADMINISTRATION, SCHOOL OF HEALTH PROFESSIONS, GOVERNORS STATE UNIVERSITY, Zip 60466; tel. 708/534–4030; Sang–O Rhee, Chairman

IOWA
Calmar: NORTHEAST IOWA COMMUNITY COLLEGE, Box 400, Zip 52132; tel. 319/562–3263; Melinda Hanson, Chairperson Health and Human Services
Iowa City: GRADUATE PROGRAM IN HOSPITAL AND HEALTH ADMINISTRATION, UNIVERSITY OF IOWA, 2700 Steindler Building, Zip 52242; tel. 319/356–2593; James E. Rohrer, Program Head

MARYLAND
Bethesda: NAVAL SCHOOL OF HEALTH SCIENCES, Naval Medical Command, National Region, Zip 20889–5611; tel. 202/545–6700

MICHIGAN
Ann Arbor: UNIVERSITY OF MICHIGAN, 1420 Washington Heights, Zip 48109; tel. 313/764–1382

MISSOURI
Saint Louis: PROGRAM IN HOSPITAL AND HEALTH CARE ADMINISTRATION, ST. LOUIS UNIVERSITY, 3525 Caroline Street, Zip 63104; tel. 314/577–8000; James Kimmey, Director
WASHINGTON UNIVERSITY, SCHOOL OF MEDICINE, 4547 Clayton Avenue, Zip 63110; tel. 314/362–2477; James O. Hepner, Director Health

NEW YORK
Rochester: ROCHESTER INSTITUTE OF TECHNOLOGY, One Lomb Memorial Drive, Zip 14623; tel. 716/475–6365; Beverly J. Price, Associate Professor

Valhalla: NEW YORK MEDICAL COLLEGE, Zip 10595; tel. 914/347–5044; Reverend Harry C. Barrett, President and Chief Executive Officer

NORTH CAROLINA
Durham: DUKE UNIVERSITY, DEPARTMENT OF HEALTH ADMINISTRATION, Box 3018, Zip 27710; tel. 919/660–7847

OHIO
Columbus: GRADUATE PROGRAM IN HEALTH SERVICES MANAGEMENT AND POLICY, OHIO STATE UNIVERSITY, 1583 Perry St, Room 246 Samp, Zip 43210; tel. 614/292–9708; Stephen F. Loebs, Chairman and Associate Professor

PENNSYLVANIA
Philadelphia: TEMPLE UNIVERSITY, DEPARTMENT OF HEALTH ADMINISTRATION, SCHOOL OF BUSINESS ADMINISTRATION, Department of Health Administration, Zip 19122; tel. 215/787–8082; William Aaronson, President and Chairman
University Park: PENNSYLVANIA STATE UNIVERSITY, 115 Henderson Building, Zip 16802; tel. 814/863–2859; Frederick R. Eisele, Department Head

TEXAS
Fort Sam Houston: ARMY–BAYLOR UNIVERSITY PROGRAM IN HEALTH CARE ADMINISTRATION, Academy of Health Sciences–USA, Zip 78234; tel. 512/221–5009
San Antonio: OUR LADY OF THE LAKE UNIVERSITY – GRADUATE PROGRAM IN HEALTH CARE MANAGEMENT, 411 S.W. 24th Street, Zip 78207–4666; tel. 512/434–6711; William J. Lambert Jr., Coordinator
TRINITY UNIVERSITY, 715 Stadium Drive, Zip 78212–7200; tel. 210/736–8107; Mary E. Stefl, Chairman
Sheppard Air Force Base: U.S. AIR FORCE SCHOOL OF HEALTH CARE SCIENCES, Building 1900 MSTL/114 Academy Library, Zip 76311; tel. 817/851–2511

PUERTO RICO
San Juan: SCHOOL OF PUBLIC HEALTH, P.O. Box 5067, Zip 00936; tel. 809/767–9626; Orlando Nieves, Dean

Institutional Members / Schools of Nursing

Hospital Schools of Nursing

ARKANSAS

Little Rock: BAPTIST MEDICAL SYSTEM School of Nursing
Pine Bluff: JEFFERSON REGIONAL MEDICAL CENTER School of Nursing

CALIFORNIA

Los Angeles: LOS ANGELES COUNTY–UNIVERSITY OF SOUTHERN CALIFORNIA MEDICAL CENTER School of Nursing

CONNECTICUT

Bridgeport: ST. VINCENT'S COLLEGE OF NURSING
Hartford: SAINT FRANCIS HOSPITAL AND MEDICAL CENTER School of Nursing
Middletown: MIDDLESEX MEMORIAL HOSPITAL ONA M. WILCOX School of Nursing
Waterbury: ST. MARY'S HOSPITAL School of Nursing

DELAWARE

Lewes: BEEBE MEDICAL CENTER School of Nursing

FLORIDA

Miami: JAMES M. JACKSON MEMORIAL HOSPITAL School of Nursing

GEORGIA

Atlanta: GEORGIA BAPTIST MEDICAL CENTER School of Nursing

ILLINOIS

Canton: GRAHAM HOSPITAL School of Nursing
Chicago: RAVENSWOOD HOSPITAL MEDICAL CENTER School of Nursing
Danville: LAKEVIEW MEDICAL CENTER School of Nursing
Evanston: ST. FRANCIS HOSPITAL School of Nursing
Moline: UNITED MEDICAL CENTER School of Nursing
Peoria: METHODIST HOSPITAL OF CENTRAL ILLINOIS School of Nursing

INDIANA

Lafayette: ST. ELIZABETH HOSPITAL MEDICAL CENTER School of Nursing

IOWA

Council Bluffs: JENNIE EDMUNDSON MEMORIAL HOSPITAL School of Nursing
Des Moines: IOWA METHODIST HOSPITAL School of Nursing
  MERCY HOSPITAL MEDICAL CENTER School of Nursing
Sioux City: ST. LUKE'S REGIONAL MEDICAL CENTER School of Nursing

LOUISIANA

Baton Rouge: BATON ROUGE GENERAL MEDICAL CENTER School of Nursing
  OUR LADY OF LAKE REGIONAL MEDICAL CENTER School of Nursing

MAINE

Lewiston: CENTRAL MAINE MEDICAL CENTER School of Nursing

MARYLAND

Baltimore: UNION MEMORIAL HOSPITAL School of Nursing
Easton: MEMORIAL HOSPITAL AT EASTON MARYLAND School of Nursing

MASSACHUSETTS

Boston: NEW ENGLAND BAPTIST HOSPITAL School of Nursing
Brockton: BROCKTON HOSPITAL School of Nursing
Medford: LAWRENCE MEMORIAL HOSPITAL OF MEDFORD School of Nursing
Springfield: BAYSTATE MEDICAL CENTER School of Nursing

MICHIGAN

Detroit: HENRY FORD HOSPITAL School of Nursing
Kalamazoo: BRONSON METHODIST HOSPITAL School of Nursing

MISSOURI

Cape Girardeau: SOUTHEAST MISSOURI HOSPITAL School of Nursing
Saint Louis: BARNES HOSPITAL School of Nursing
  DEACONESS COLLEGE OF NURSING School of Nursing
  JEWISH HOSPITAL OF ST. LOUIS School of Nursing
  LUTHERAN MEDICAL CENTER School of Nursing
Springfield: LESTER E. COX MEDICAL CENTERS School of Nursing
  ST. JOHN'S School of Nursing
Town & Country: MISSOURI BAPTIST MEDICAL CENTER School of Nursing

NEBRASKA

Lincoln: BRYAN MEMORIAL HOSPITAL School of Nursing
Omaha: BISHOP CLARKSON COLLEGE

NEW JERSEY

Camden: OUR LADY OF LOURDES MEDICAL CENTER School of Nursing
Elizabeth: ELIZABETH GENERAL MEDICAL CENTER School of Nursing
Englewood: ENGLEWOOD HOSPITAL AND MEDICAL CENTER School of Nursing
Jersey City: CHRIST HOSPITAL School of Nursing
Montclair: MOUNTAINSIDE HOSPITAL School of Nursing
Neptune: ANN MAY School of Nursing
Orange: HOSPITAL CENTER AT ORANGE WINIFRED B. BALDWIN School of Nursing
Plainfield: MUHLENBERG REGIONAL MEDICAL CENTER School of Nursing
Teaneck: HOLY NAME HOSPITAL School of Nursing
Trenton: HELENE FULD MEDICAL CENTER School of Nursing
  MERCER MEDICAL CENTER School of Nursing
  ST. FRANCIS MEDICAL CENTER School of Nursing

NEW YORK

Buffalo: SISTERS OF CHARITY HOSPITAL School of Nursing
Elmira: ARNOT–OGDEN MEMORIAL HOSPITAL School of Nursing
Jamaica: CATHOLIC MEDICAL CENTER OF BROOKLYN & QUEENS School of Nursing
New York: ST. VINCENT'S HOSPITAL AND MEDICAL CENTER OF NEW YORK School of Nursing
Staten Island: ST. VINCENT'S MEDICAL CENTER School of Nursing
Utica: ST. ELIZABETH HOSPITAL School of Nursing
Yonkers: ST. JOHN'S RIVERSIDE HOSPITAL COCHRAN School of Nursing

NORTH CAROLINA

Charlotte: MERCY HOSPITAL School of Nursing
  PRESBYTERIAN HOSPITAL School of Nursing
Concord: CABARRUS MEMORIAL HOSPITAL School of Nursing
Durham: WATTS School of Nursing

NORTH DAKOTA

Bismarck: MEDCENTER ONE School of Nursing
Minot: TRINITY MEDICAL CENTER School of Nursing

OHIO

Akron: AKRON CITY HOSPITAL IDABELLE FIRESTONE School of Nursing
  SUMMA ST. THOMAS School of Nursing
Canton: AULTMAN HOSPITAL School of Nursing
Cincinnati: CHRIST HOSPITAL School of Nursing
  GOOD SAMARITAN HOSPITAL School of Nursing
Cleveland: FAIRVIEW GENERAL HOSPITAL School of Nursing
  METROHEALTH MEDICAL CENTER School of Nursing
Sandusky: PROVIDENCE HOSPITAL School of Nursing
Springfield: COMMUNITY HOSPITAL OF SPRINGFIELD AND CLARK COUNTY School of Nursing
Toledo: MERCY HOSPITAL School of Nursing
  ST. VINCENT MEDICAL CENTER School of Nursing

PENNSYLVANIA

Abington: ABINGTON MEMORIAL HOSPITAL School of Nursing
Altoona: ALTOONA HOSPITAL School of Nursing
Caln Township: BRANDYWINE HOSPITAL School of Nursing
Johnstown: CONEMAUGH VALLEY MEMORIAL HOSPITAL School of Nursing
New Castle: JAMESON MEMORIAL HOSPITAL School of Nursing
  ST. FRANCIS HOSPITAL OF NEW CASTLE School of Nursing
Philadelphia: EPISCOPAL HOSPITAL School of Nursing
  FRANKFORD HOSPITAL School of Nursing
  GERMANTOWN HOSPITAL AND MEDICAL CENTER School of Nursing
  METHODIST HOSPITAL School of Nursing
Pittsburgh: MERCY HOSPITAL OF PITTSBURGH School of Nursing
  SHADYSIDE HOSPITAL School of Nursing
  ST. FRANCIS MEDICAL CENTER School of Nursing
  ST. MARGARET MEMORIAL HOSPITAL LOUISE SUYDAM MCCLINTIC School of Nursing
  WESTERN PENNSYLVANIA HOSPITAL School of Nursing
Pottsville: POTTSVILLE HOSPITAL AND WARNE CLINIC School of Nursing
Reading: READING HOSPITAL AND MEDICAL CENTER School of Nursing
Scranton: COMMUNITY MEDICAL CENTER School of Nursing
Sewickley: SEWICKLEY VALLEY HOSPITAL School of Nursing
Sharon: SHARON REGIONAL HEALTH SYSTEM School of Nursing
Washington: WASHINGTON HOSPITAL School of Nursing
West Chester: CHESTER COUNTY HOSPITAL School of Nursing

RHODE ISLAND

North Providence: ST. JOSEPH HOSPITAL School of Nursing

TENNESSEE

Knoxville: FORT SANDERS REGIONAL MEDICAL CENTER School of Nursing
Memphis: BAPTIST MEMORIAL HOSPITAL School of Nursing
  METHODIST HOSPITALS OF MEMPHIS–CENTRAL School of Nursing
  ST. JOSEPH HOSPITAL School of Nursing

TEXAS

Lubbock: METHODIST HOSPITAL School of Nursing
San Antonio: BAPTIST MEDICAL CENTER School of Nursing

© 1995 AHA Guide

Institutional Members / Schools of Nursing—Preacute and Postacute Care Facilities

VIRGINIA
Danville: MEMORIAL HOSPITAL OF DANVILLE School of Nursing
Lynchburg: LYNCHBURG GENERAL–MARSHALL LODGE HOSPITAL School of Nursing
Newport News: RIVERSIDE REGIONAL MEDICAL CENTER School of Nursing
Norfolk: DEPAUL MEDICAL CENTER School of Nursing
SENTARA NORFOLK GENERAL HOSPITAL School of Nursing
Petersburg: SOUTHSIDE REGIONAL MEDICAL CENTER School of Nursing
Richmond: RICHMOND MEMORIAL HOSPITAL School of Nursing
Suffolk: OBICI HOSPITAL School of Nursing

WEST VIRGINIA
Huntington: ST. MARY'S HOSPITAL School of Nursing

WISCONSIN
Green Bay: BELLIN MEMORIAL HOSPITAL COLLEGE OF NURSING

Nonhospital Preacute and Postacute Care Facilities

ALABAMA
Birmingham: HEALTH PARTNERS OF ALABAMA, INC, 600 Beacon Parkway West, Zip 35209; tel. 205/942–5787; Robert R. Vogel, President and Chief Executive Officer

ALASKA
Anchorage: DEPARTMENT OF VETERANS AFFAIRS REGIONAL OFFICE AND OUTPATIENT CLINIC, 2925 Debarr Road, Zip 99508–2989; tel. 907/257–6930; John J. Conway, Director

ARIZONA
Phoenix: CAMELBACK FAMILY MEDICINE, 5040 North 15th Avenue, Zip 85015; tel. 602/238–3314
JESSE OWENS MEMORIAL MEDICAL CENTER, 325 East Baseline Road, Zip 85040; tel. 602/238–3314
WEST MCDOWELL FAMILY MEDICAL CENTER, 5030 West McDowell Road, Zip 85035; tel. 602/2383314; Peter J. Martin, Chief Executive Officer
San Carlos: U.S. PUBLIC HEALTH SERVICE INDIAN HOSPITAL, P.O. Box 208, Zip 85550; tel. 602/475–2381; Nella Ben, Administrator

ARKANSAS
Little Rock: CENTRAL ARKANSAS RADIATION THERAPY INSTITUTE, P.O. Box 5210, Zip 72215; tel. 501/664–8573; Janice E. Burford, Director

CALIFORNIA
Long Beach: NAVAL MEDICAL CLINIC, Reeves Avenue, Building 831, Zip 90822–5073; tel. 310/521–4201; Captain J. M. Lamdin, Commanding Officer
Los Angeles: AESTHETICA SURGICAL CENTER, 5757 Wilshire Boulevard, Zip 90036; tel. 213/935–2357; Laurence A. Reich, Chairman
VETERANS AFFAIRS OUTPATIENT CLINIC, 351 East Temple St, Room A–102, Zip 90012–3328; tel. 213/253–5000
Port Hueneme: NAVAL MEDICAL CLINIC, Zip 93043; tel. 805/982–4501
San Francisco: VETERANS AFFAIRS OUTPATIENT CLINIC, 4150 Clement Street, Zip 94121

FLORIDA
Key West: NAVAL REGIONAL MEDICAL CLINIC, Roosevelt Boulevard, Zip 33040; tel. 305/296–2461; W. A. Nacrelli, Commanding Officer
Miami: VITAS HEALTHCARE CORPORATION, 100 South Biscayne Boulevard, Zip 33131; tel. 305/374–4143; J. R. Williams, Executive Director
Riverview: TAMPA BAY ACADEMY, 12012 Boyette Road, Zip 33569; tel. 813/677–6700; Edward C. Hoefle, Administrator

HAWAII
Pearl Harbor: NAVAL REGIONAL MEDICAL CLINIC, Box 121, Building 1750, Zip 96860; tel. 808/471–3025

ILLINOIS
Des Plaines: GOLF SURGICAL CENTER, 8901 Golf Road, Zip 60616; tel. 708/299–2273; Mary Lou Emmons, Administrator

KANSAS
Wichita: U.S. AIR FORCE HOSPITAL, McConnell AFB, Zip 67221–5300; tel. 316/652–5000; Major Theodore B. McFarland, Administrator

LOUISIANA
New Orleans: NAVAL MEDICAL CLINIC, Zip 70142; tel. 504/361–2400

MARYLAND
Annapolis: NAVAL MEDICAL CLINIC, Zip 21402; tel. 410/267–2501
Baltimore: TOTAL HEALTH CARE, INC., 1501 Division Street, Zip 21217; tel. 410/383–8300; Claude D. Hill, Chief Executive Officer

MASSACHUSETTS
Falmouth: GOSNOLD ON CAPE COD, 200 Ter Heun Drive, Box CC, Zip 02540; tel. 508/540–6550; Raymond Tamasi, Chief Executive Officer
Fort Devens: CUTLER ARMY COMMUNITY HOSPITAL, US Army Medical Department Activity, Zip 01433–6401; tel. 508/796–6745; Dewey R. Miller, Deputy Commander

MICHIGAN
Kincheloe: SAULT STE. MARIE TRIBAL HEALTH CLINIC, 312 Water Tower Drive, Zip 49788; tel. 906/495–5651; Russell Vizina, Director Health and Social Services
Port Huron: TRI–HOSPITAL E.M.S., 1001 Karney Street, Zip 48060; tel. 313/985–7115; Ken Cummings, Chief Executive Officer
WILLOW ENTERPRISES, INC., 1001 Kearney Street, Zip 48060; tel. 313/989–3737; James B. Bridge, Chief Executive Officer
Traverse City: MUNSON COMMUNITY HEALTH SERVICES, 550 Munson Avenue, Zip 49684; tel. 616/922–8400

MISSOURI
Independence: SURGI–CARE CENTER OF INDEPENDENCE, 2311 Redwood Avenue, Zip 64057; tel. 816/373–7995; Mike Chappelow, President and Chief Executive Officer
Saint Louis: IRENE WALTER JOHNSON INSTITUTE OF REHABILITATION, P.O. Box 8062, Zip 63110; tel. 314/362–6979; Denise McCartney, Administrative Director

MONTANA
Malmstrom Air Force Base: U.S. AIR FORCE CLINIC, Zip 59402–5300; tel. 406/731–3863

NEVADA
Las Vegas: VETERANS AFFAIRS–OUTPATIENT CLINIC, 1703 West Charleston Boulevard, Zip 89102; tel. 702/389–3700; Ramon J. Reevey, Director
Schurz: U.S. PUBLIC HEALTH SERVICE INDIAN CLINIC, P.O. Box Drawer A, Zip 89427; tel. 702/773–2345; Elmer Brewster, Director

NEW HAMPSHIRE
Portsmouth: NAVAL MEDICAL CLINIC, Building H–1, Zip 03801; tel. 207/439–1000; Captain F. M. Richardson, Commanding Officer

NEW JERSEY
Orange: ST. MARY'S AMBULATORY CARE HOSPITAL, 135 South Center Street, Zip 07050; tel. 201/266–3000; Bertha L. Peters–Stokes, Administrator
Trenton: WALSON AIR FORCE COMMUNITY HOSPITAL, 5250 New Jersey Avenue, Zip 08640–5027; tel. 609/562–2852; Major Frederick L. Woods, Administrator

NEW YORK
Lake Placid: CAMELOT, 50 Riverside Drive, Zip 12946; tel. 518/523–3605; Reverend Carlos J. Caguiat, Vice President
New York: STATE UNIVERSITY OF NEW YORK, UNIVERSITY OPTOMETRIC CENTER, 100 East 24th Street, Zip 10010; tel. 212/780–4930; Richard C. Weber, Executive Director

NORTH CAROLINA
Winston Salem: QUALCHOICE OF NORTH CAROLINA, INC., 2000 West First St, Ste 210, Zip 27104; tel. 910/716–0900; Douglas G. Cueny, President

OHIO
Columbus: VETERANS AFFAIRS OUTPATIENT CLINIC, 2090 Kenny Road, Zip 43221; tel. 614/469–5663; Troy E. Page, Director
Parma: KAISER PERMANENTE, 12301 Snow Road, Zip 44130–1099; tel. 216/362–2000

OKLAHOMA
Enid: U.S. AIR FORCE CLINIC, Vance Air Force Base, Building 810, Zip 73705–5000; tel. 405/249–7494; LTC Andrew F. Love, USAF, MSC, Commander Medical Group

PENNSYLVANIA
Philadelphia: NAVAL MEDICAL CLINIC, Zip 19145–5199; tel. 215/897–8232; Captain Donald F. Eversmann, Commanding Officer
Pittsburgh: HEALTH ASSISTANCE PROGRAM FOR PERSONNEL IN INDUSTRY, 4221 Penn Avenue, Zip 15224; tel. 412/622–4994; Eugene Ginchereau, Director

Institutional Members / Preacute and Postacute Care Facilities—Provisional

PENNSYLVANIA
Pittsburgh: HEALTHAMERICA PENNSYLVANIA, INC., Five Gateway Center, Zip 15222; tel. 412/553–7305; Michael Blackwood, President and Chief Executive Officer
York: YORK HEALTH CARE SERVICES, 25 Monument Road, Ste 195, Zip 17403; tel. 717/851–2121; Bruce M. Bartels, President
YORK HEALTH PLAN, 140 Pine Grove Commons, Zip 17403; tel. 717/741–9511; Charles H. Chodroff, Executive Director
YORK HEALTH SYSTEM MEDICAL GROUP, 25 Monument Road, Ste 190, Zip 17403; tel. 717/741–8125; William R. Richards, Executive Director

RHODE ISLAND
Newport: NAVAL HOSPITAL, Zip 02841–1002; tel. 401/841–3915; Captain C. Henderson III, Commanding Officer

SOUTH DAKOTA
Wagner: U.S. PUBLIC HEALTH SERVICE INDIAN HOSPITAL, Box 490, Zip 57380–4090; tel. 605/384–3621

TEXAS
Bedford: RESIDENTIAL TREATMENT CENTER AT BREDFORD, 2904 Bedford Road, Zip 76021; tel. 817/540–5222; Linda Gunn–Jones, Administrator
El Paso: VETERANS AFFAIRS OUTPATIENT CLINIC, 5919 Brook Hollow Drive, Zip 79925; tel. 915/541–7876; Bruce W. Glover, Director
San Antonio: U.S. AIR FORCE CLINIC BROOKS, Building 615, Zip 78235–5300; tel. 512/536–2087; Michael J. Poulsen, Administrator

UTAH
Salt Lake City: FHP HEALTH CARE–UTAH REGION, 35 West Broadway, Zip 84101; tel. 801/355–1236; Michael A. Graham, Associate Regional Vice President

VIRGINIA
Marshall: MARSHALL MANOR–INTERNATIONAL HEALTH SERVICES, P.O. Box 749, Zip 22115; tel. 703/222–3900; Charles V. Rice, President and Chief Executive Officer
Quantico: NAVAL REGIONAL MEDICAL CLINIC, Zip 22134; tel. 703/640–2236; Commander R. A. Payton, Commanding Officer

WASHINGTON
Seattle: NAVAL REGIONAL MEDICAL CLINIC, 7500 Sand Point Way, Zip 98105; tel. 206/527–3827; Robert A. Jeffs, Commanding Officer

WEST VIRGINIA
Clarksburg: SUMMIT CENTER FOR HUMAN DEVELOPMENT, INC., 6 Hospital Plaza, Zip 26301; tel. 304/623–5666; Les Delpizzo, Executive Director

WISCONSIN
Green Bay: UNITY HOSPICE, P.O. Box 22395, Zip 54305–2395; tel. 414/433–7470; Donald Seibel, Executive Director

Provisional

The listing includes organizations that, as of June 1, 1995, were in the planning or construction stage and that, on completion, will be eligible for institutional membership of type I or II. Some hospitals are granted provisional membership for reasons related to other Association requirements. Hospitals classified as provisional members for reasons other than being under construction are indicated by a bullet (•).

California
Victorville: DESERT VALLEY HOSPITAL, 16850 Bear Valley Road, Zip 92392; tel. 619/241–8000; John Rossfeld, Administrator

Florida
Palm Beach Gardens: VETERANS AFFAIRS MEDICAL CENTER, P.O. Box 33207, Zip 33420–3207; tel. 407/844–8115; Richard D. Isaac, Administrator

Texas
Austin: AUSTIN DIAGNOSTIC MEDICAL CENTER, 12221 MoPac Expressway North, Zip 78758; tel. 512/901–1000; Richard E. Salerno, Chief Executive Officer

Associate Members

Ambulatory Centers and Home Care Agencies

PHILIPPINES
  DEPARTMENT OF VETERANS AFFAIRS, OUTPATIENT CLINIC, Manila, Zip 96440; tel. 632/521-7116

FLORIDA
  NEMOURS CHILDREN'S CLINIC, 807 Nira Street, Jacksonville, Zip 32207; tel. 904/390-3600; Barry P. Sales, Administrator

ILLINOIS
  NATIONAL ASSOCIATION OF HOSPITAL AFFILIATED CHILDREN CARE PROGRAMS, 9375 Church Street, Des Plaines, Zip 60016; tel. 708/824-5180; Josie Disterhoft, President

MICHIGAN
  ST. JOHN AMBULATORY CARE CORPORATION, 22151 Moross Road, Detroit, Zip 48236; tel. 313/343-3325

NEW YORK
  INTERNATIONAL CENTER FOR THE DISABLED, 340 East 24th Street, New York, Zip 10010; tel. 212/679-0100
  VISITING NURSING ASSOCIATION GROUP, INC., 2929 Walden Avenue, Depew, Zip 14043-2602; tel. 716/685-2650; Alexine L. Janiszewski, President
  WESTFALL SURGERY CENTER, 919 Westfall Road, Rochester, Zip 14618; tel. 716/256-1330; Gary J. Scott, Administrative Director

PENNSYLVANIA
  CRAIG HOUSE-TECHNOMA, 751 North Negley Avenue, Pittsburgh, Zip 15206; tel. 412/361-2801; Richard L. Kerchnner, Administrator
  NORTHEAST COMMUNITY CENTER FOR MENTAL HEALTH AND MENTAL RETARDATION, Roosevelt Boulevard & Adams Avenue, Philadelphia, Zip 19124; tel. 215/743-1600; Howard J. Kaufman, Executive Director

TENNESSEE
  SMYRNA HOSPITAL, Box 819, Smyrna, Zip 37167; tel. 615/453-8771; Lawrence L. Pieretti, Chief Executive Officer

TEXAS
  CANCER THERAPY AND RESEARCH FOUNDATION OF SOUTH TEXAS, 4450 Medical Drive, San Antonio, Zip 78229; tel. 512/690-1111; Diane Roberts, Associate Director

WISCONSIN
  CURATIVE REHABILITATION CENTER, 1000 North 92nd Street, Wauwatosa, Zip 53226; tel. 414/259-1414; Robert H. Coons Jr., President

Blue Cross Plans

ALBERTA
  ALBERTA BLUE CROSS PLAN, 10025 108th Street, Edmonton, tel. 403/429-5221; V. G. Ward, President

ONTARIO
  ONTARIO BLUE CROSS, 150 Ferrand Drive, Don Mills, tel. 416/429-2670; H. Dunbar Russel, President

ARIZONA
  BLUE CROSS AND BLUE SHIELD OF ARIZONA, Box 13466, Phoenix, Zip 85002-3466; tel. 602/864-4400; Robert Bulla, President and Chief Executive Officer

DISTRICT OF COLUMBIA
  BLUE CROSS AND BLUE SHIELD OF WASHINGTON, 550 12th Street S.W., Washington, Zip 20065; tel. 202/479-6368; Kirk McLean

FLORIDA
  BLUE CROSS AND BLUE SHIELD OF FLORIDA, INC., P.O. Box 60729, Jacksonville, Zip 32236-0729; tel. 904/791-6111; William E. Flaherty, President

ILLINOIS
  BLUE CROSS-BLUE SHIELD, 233 North Michigan Avenue, Chicago, Zip 60601; tel. 312/661-2500; Raymond D. McCaskey, President

IOWA
  IASD HEALTH SERVICES CORPORATION, 636 Grand Avenue, Des Moines, Zip 50309; tel. 515/244-8961; Robert D. Ray, President and Chief Executive Officer

KANSAS
  BLUE CROSS AND BLUE SHIELD OF KANSAS, Box 239, Topeka, Zip 66629; tel. 913/234-9592; John W. Knack, Executive Vice President

MARYLAND
  BLUE CROSS-BLUE SHIELD OF MARYLAND, 11500 Cronridge Drive, Owings Mills, Zip 21117; tel. 301/494-4800; Thomas J. Durel, Vice President New Products and Systems

MISSOURI
  BLUE CROSS AND BLUE SHIELD OF MISSOURI, 1831 Chestnut Street, Saint Louis, Zip 63103-2275; tel. 314/241-1800; R. R. Heimburger, President and Chief Executive Officer

NEW YORK
  BLUE CROSS AND BLUE SHIELD OF CENTRAL NEW YORK, Box 4809, Syracuse, Zip 13221-4809; tel. 315/424-3801; Albert F. Antonini, President & Chief Executive Officer
  BLUE CROSS AND BLUE SHIELD OF THE ROCHESTER AREA, 150 East Main Street, Rochester, Zip 14647; tel. 716/454-1700; Glenda Lusk, Supervisor

OHIO
  BLUE CROSS AND BLUE SHIELD OF OHIO, P.O. Box 94624, Cleveland, Zip 44101; tel. 216/687-7000; John Burry Jr., Chairman and Chief Executive Officer
  COMMUNITY MUTUAL INSURANCE COMPANY, 1351 William Howard Taft Road, Cincinnati, Zip 45206; tel. 513/872-8100

OKLAHOMA
  BLUE CROSS AND BLUE SHIELD OF OKLAHOMA, Box 3283, Tulsa, Zip 74102; tel. 918/583-0861; Ralph Rhoades, President

PENNSYLVANIA
  BLUE CROSS OF NORTHEASTERN PENNSYLVANIA, 70 North Main Street, Wilkes-Barre, Zip 18711; tel. 717/824-5741; Art Menichillo, Senior Director
  BLUE CROSS OF WESTERN PENNSYLVANIA, 120 Fifth Avenue Place, Pittsburgh, Zip 15222; tel. 412/255-7000
  CAPITAL BLUE CROSS, 2500 Elmerton Avenue, Harrisburg, Zip 17110; tel. 717/541-7000; James M. Mead, President
  INDEPENDENCE BLUE CROSS, 1901 Market Street, Philadelphia, Zip 19103; tel. 215/241-3300; Vail P. Garvin, Senior Vice President Corporate Affairs

TENNESSEE
  BLUE CROSS AND BLUE SHIELD OF MEMPHIS, P.O. Box 98, Memphis, Zip 38101; tel. 901/529-3111; Arthur P. Waymire, President and Chief Executive Officer
  BLUE CROSS-BLUE SHIELD OF TENNESSEE, 801 Pine Street, Chattanooga, Zip 37402; tel. 615/755-5600; Thomas Kinser, President

TEXAS
  BLUE CROSS AND BLUE SHIELD OF TEXAS, INC., Box 655730, Dallas, Zip 75265-5730; tel. 214/669-6900; Rogers Coleman, President

Institutional Members / Blue Cross Plans—HMO's—Health System—Inpatient Care—Shared Services

VIRGINIA
TRIGON MUTUAL INSURANCE COMPANY, P.O. Box 27401, Richmond, Zip 23279; tel. 804/354-7000; Richardson Grinnan, Senior Vice President Healthcare Management

WASHINGTON
KING COUNTY MEDICAL BLUE SHIELD, 1800 Ninth Avenue, Seattle, Zip 98111; tel. 206/464-3635; Stephanie I. Hunter, Vice President, Provider Affairs

Health Maintenance Organizations/Health Care Corporations

HAWAII
KAISER FOUNDATION HEALTH PLAN, INC., 711 Kapiolani Boulevard, Honolulu, Zip 96813; tel. 808/529-5296; Cora M. Tellez, Vice President

NEW YORK
PREFERRED CARE, 259 Monroe Avenue, Rochester, Zip 14607; tel. 716/325-3920; Dawn Richardson, Drug Related Group Analyst

Health System Agencies

MICHIGAN
ALLIANCE FOR HEALTH, 72 Monroe Center N.W., Ste 200, Grand Rapids, Zip 49503; tel. 616/459-1323; Phillip E. Van Heest, President

GREATER DETROIT HEALTH HOSPITAL COUNCIL, INC., 645 Griswold Street, Ste 4100, Detroit, Zip 48226-4209; tel. 313/963-4990; James B. Kenney, President and Chief Executive Officer

Other Inpatient Care Institutions

ONTARIO

HILLCREST HOSPITAL, 47 Austin Terrace, Toronto, Zip MR5 1Y8; tel. 416/537-3421; Frank Martin Markel, President and Chief Executive Officer

Shared Services Organizations

ILLINOIS
PREMIER HEALTH ALLIANCE, INC., 3 Westbrook Corporate Center, 9th Fl, Westchester, Zip 60154-5735; tel. 708/409-4100; Alan Weinstein, President

INDIANA
HOLY CROSS SHARED SERVICES, INC., Saint Mary's-Bertrand Hall, Notre Dame, Zip 46556; tel. 219/284-4615; David L. Burk, Chief Executive Officer

IOWA
MIDWEST HEALTHCARE GROUP, 1221 Center Street, Suite 13, Des Moines, Zip 50309; tel. 515/283-2708; Donald W. Cordes, Executive Director

KENTUCKY
WESTERN KENTUCKY HOSPITAL SERVICES, P.O. Box 1127, Madisonville, Zip 42431; Richard V. Harris, Executive Vice President

MARYLAND
DAUGHTERS OF CHARITY HEALTH SYSTEM EAST, 1302 Concourse Drive, Ste 300, Linthicum, Zip 21090-1014; tel. 301/850-9000; James E. Small, President and Chief Executive Officer

MASSACHUSETTS
MASCO SERVICES, INC., 375 Longwood Avenue, Boston, Zip 02215; tel. 617/632-2310; Alan R. Shoolman, President

PENNSYLVANIA
HOSPITAL CENTRAL SERVICES, INC., 2171 28th Street S.W., Allentown, Zip 18103; tel. 215/791-2222; J. Michael Lee, President

RHODE ISLAND
VECTOR HEALTHSYSTEMS, INC., Box 9427, Providence, Zip 02940; tel. 401/453-8300; Gerald G. McClure, President

TEXAS
TEXAS HOSPITAL ASSOCIATION, Box 15587, Austin, Zip 78761-5587; tel. 512/453-7204; Terry Townsend, President and Chief Executive Officer

Associate Members / Other

Other Associate Members

United States

U.S. government hospitals in areas outside the United States that are members of the American Hospital Association are not shown here, but are included in the list of such hospitals in section A of this guide, where membership is indicated by a star (★) preceeding the name of the individual hospital.

Architecture

3D INTERNATIONAL, INC., 9990 Lee Highway, Suite 400, Fairfax, Virginia Zip 22030–1720; tel. 703/218–8100; David A. Clark, Senior Vice President

AGUIRRE ASSOCIATES, INC., 12700 Park Central Dr, 1508, Dallas, Texas Zip 75251; tel. 214/788–1508; Neil D. Alcorn, Project Manager Healthcare

BURT HILL KOSAR RITTELMANN ASSOCIATES, 400 Morgan Center, Butler, Pennsylvania Zip 16001–5977; tel. 412/285–4761; John E. Brock, Principal

CODINA DEVELOPMENT CORPORATION, 2 Alhambra Plaza, PH2, Coral Gables, Florida Zip 33134; tel. 305/520–2380; Robert E. Bales Sr., Vice President

COOPER MEDICAL BUILDINGS, INC., 7100 N Classen Boulevard, Ste 500, Oklahoma City, Oklahoma Zip 73116; tel. 405/842–6653; Steven Cooper, President

CRSS CONSTRUCTORS, INC., 2500 Michelson Drive, Ste 100, Irvine, California Zip 92715; tel. 714/476–2900; Tisha Luderman, Manager Project Development and Healthcare

EASON, EARL AND ASSOCIATES, INC., One Insignia Financial Plaza, 501, Greenville, South Carolina Zip 29681; tel. 803/233–0003; Richard R. Earl, Principal

ENGBERG ANDERSON, 611 North Broadway, Suite 517, Milwaukee, Wisconsin Zip 53202; tel. 414/276–6600; Scott Smith, Architect

FLUOR DANIEL, INC., 3333 Michelson Drive, C3E, Irvine, California Zip 92730; tel. 714/975–2706

FRANKFURT SHORT BRUZA, 5701 North Shartel, Suite 210, Oklahoma City, Oklahoma Zip 73118; tel. 405/840–2931; Heath J. Barclay, Vice President

HENNINGSON, DURHAM AND RICHARDSON, 8404 Indian Hills Drive, Omaha, Nebraska Zip 68114; tel. 402/391–0123; Lynn E. Bonge, Executive Vice President

INTERNATIONAL TEST AND BALANCE, INC., 3801 West Lake Avenue, Glenview, Illinois Zip 60025; tel. 708/657–1077; Waleed Tarazi, Vice–President

IPS, 10 East Sixth Avenue, Conshohocken, Pennsylvania Zip 19428; tel. 610/828–4090; Andy Signore, President

JCM GROUP, 10866 Wilshire Boulevard, Ste 600, Los Angeles, California Zip 90024; tel. 310/474–6868; Wayne C. Twedell, President

LEGAT MEDICAL ARCHITECTS, 24 North Chapel, Waukegan, Illinois Zip 60085; tel. 708/605–0234; Casimir Frankiewicz, President

MARSHALL CRAFT ASSOCIATES, INC., 6112 York Road, Baltimore, Maryland Zip 21212; tel. 301/532–3131; Richard S. Abbott, Secretary

MATTHEI AND COLIN ASSOCIATES, 332 S Michigan Ave, Ste 614, Chicago, Illinois Zip 60604; tel. 312/939–4002; Ron Kobolt, Vice President

PERINI CORPORATION, 73 Mount Wayte Avenue, Framingham, Massachusetts Zip 01701; tel. 508/628–2214; John R. Rizzo, Vice President Corporate Development

PERKINS & WILL, One Park Avenue, New York, New York Zip 10016; tel. 212/251–7000; Richard Sonder, Partner

QUANTRELL MULLINS AND ASSOCIATES, INC., 999 Peachtree St N.E., Ste 1690, Atlanta, Georgia Zip 30309; tel. 404/874–6048; Libby Laguta, Director Healthcare

SKIDMORE, OWINGS & MERRILL, 220 East 42nd Street, New York, New York Zip 10017; tel. 212/309–9500; Edward A. Carroll, Associate Partner

SVERDRUP FACILITIES CORPORATION, 801 North 11th Street, Saint Louis, Missouri Zip 63101–1015; tel. 314/997–0300; Nicholas J. Varrone, Vice President

THE RITCHIE ORGANIZATION, 80 Bridge Street, Newton, Massachusetts Zip 02158; tel. 617/969–9400; Wendell R. Morgan Jr., President

THE SCHEIN GROUP, 23 East Street, Cambridge, Massachusetts Zip 02141; tel. 617/225–0214; Philip R. Gaudreau, Principal

WILLIAM A. BERRY & SON, INC., 100 Conifer Hill Drive, Danvers, Massachusetts Zip 01923; tel. 508/774–1057; Ronda Paradis, Program Development Manager

Bank

TORONTO DOMINION BANK, 31 West 52nd Street, New York, New York Zip 10019–6101; tel. 212/468–0600; Robert Maloney III, Managing Director Healthcare Finance

Certified Public Accountant

DELOITTE & TOUCHE, 2200 Ross Avenue, Ste 1600, Dallas, Texas Zip 75201; tel. 214/777–7655; Karen Earwood, Senior Manager

HERBERTH AND NETTLETON, 4447 Stoneridge Drive, Pleasanton, California Zip 94588–8325; tel. 510/417–0900; Leonard Herberth, Principal

MITCHELL, TITUS AND COMPANY, 1 Battery Park Plaza, 27th Fl, New York, New York Zip 10004; tel. 212/709–4500; Kenneth Jackson, Partner

WATKINS, WATKINS AND KEENAN, 850 Ridge Lake Boulevard, Ste 101, Memphis, Tennessee Zip 38120–0413; tel. 901/761–2720; Wayne Addison, Managing Partner

Communication Systems Org

A. T. & T. CONSUMER COMMUNICATIONS SERVICES, 20 Independence Boulevard, Rm 3A38, Warren, New Jersey Zip 07059; tel. 908/580–8883; Joe Cornicelli, Staff Manager

A. T. & T., 211 Mount Airy Road, Rm 2C142, Basking Ridge, New Jersey Zip 07920; tel. 908/953–6427; Julie Bilinkas, Healthcare Marketing Manager

AMERITECH SERVICES, INC., 2000 W Ameritech Ctr Dr, 4B47D, Hoffman Estates, Illinois Zip 60196; tel. 708/248–4437; Janice M. Bellman, Industry Manager

COMMONWEALTH COMMUNICATIONS, 256 North Sherman Street, Wilkes Barre, Pennsylvania Zip 18702; tel. 717/820–5000; Barbara Miller, Sales Manager

ERICSSON BUSINESS COMMUNICATIONS, 5757 Plaza Drive, Cypress, California Zip 90630–5029; tel. 714/236–6500

GREENHOUSE COMMUNICATIONS, 303 West Erie, Chicago, Illinois Zip 60610; tel. 312/335–0010; Sandra M. House, President

GTE HEALTH SYSTEMS, 175 Southwest Temple, Salt Lake City, Utah Zip 84101; tel. 801/539–4699; Greg Taylor, Vice President and General Manager

NEC AMERICA, INC., Eight Old Sod Farm Road, Melville, New York Zip 11747; tel. 516/753–7480; Peter Harris, Marketing Director

NORTHERN TELECOM, 4001 E Chapel Hill–Nelson Hwy, Research Triangle Pk, North Carolina Zip 27709; tel. 919/922–7748; Jay Shuler, Marketing Advisor

SOUTHWESTERN BELL TELEPHONE COMPANY, One Bell Center, Room 8–U–1, Saint Louis, Missouri Zip 63101–3099; tel. 314/235–2446

SPRINT, 3100 Cumberland Circle, Atlanta, Georgia Zip 30339; tel. 404/859–6762; Diane D. Brown, National Marketing Manager Healthcare

U.S. SPRINT, 3100 Cumberland Circle, Atlanta, Georgia Zip 30339; tel. 404/859–5056

UNGERMANN–BASS, 3990 Freedom Circle, Santa Clara, California Zip 95052; tel. 408/562–5525; Bruce W. Brown, Executive Vice President

UNITED TELECOMMUNICATIONS, INC., 2330 Shawnee Mission Parkway, Westwood, Kansas Zip 66205; tel. 913/676–6473; Rod Corn, Healthcare Market Manager

Construction Firm

ELLERBE BECKET, 800 La Salle Avenue, Minneapolis, Minnesota Zip 55402–2014; tel. 612/853–2537; James E. Jenkins, Senior Vice President and Director Medical Division

H. J. DEGENKOLB ASSOCIATES, ENGINEERS., 350 Sansome Street, Suite 900, San Francisco, California Zip 94104; tel. 415/392–6952; Maryann T. Phipps, Principal

HBE CORPORATION, P.O. Box 27339, Saint Louis, Missouri Zip 63141; tel. 314/567–9000; John Wodoslawsky, Executive Vice President Sales

LEO A. DALY COMPANY, 8600 Indian Hills Drive, Omaha, Nebraska Zip 68114; tel. 402/391–8111; James M. Ingram, Sr Vice–President

MEDIPLEX MEDICAL BUILDING CORPORATION, 14755 Preston Road, Suite 600, Dallas, Texas Zip 75240–7873; tel. 214/991–6622; Alan J. Guerin, Senior Development Director

PBS BUILDING SYSTEMS, 3031 East La Jolla Street, Anaheim, California Zip 92806–1303; tel. 714/998–4777; James W. Gasper, Senior Vice President

Consulting Firm

A.P.M., INCORPORATED, 1675 Broadway, 18th Floor, New York, New York Zip 10019; tel. 212/903–9300; Karen Flaherty, Coordinator Marketing

AIG CONSULTANTS, INC., 72 Wall Street, 9th Floor, New York, New York Zip 10270; tel. 212/770–3745; Charles G. Benda Ph.D., A.R.M.,, Vice President & National Director Health Care Services

ALTILA REHABILITATION, INC., 3172 N Rainbow Boulevard, Ste 55, Las Vegas, Nevada Zip 89108; tel. 702/266–9205; Jeffrey B. Klein, President and Principal

AMERICAN BIOMEDICAL GROUP, INC., 6220 N Classen Boulevard, Ste 200, Oklahoma City, Oklahoma Zip 73118; tel. 405/848–0081; James K. Burgess, President

ANTHONY J. J. ROURKE, INC., 550 Mamaroneck Avenue, Harrison, New York Zip 10528; tel. 914/698–9100; Anthony J J. Rourke Jr., President

APPLIED MANAGEMENT SYSTEMS, INC., 5 New England Executive Park, Burlington, Massachusetts Zip 01803; tel. 617/272–8001; Alan J. Goldberg, President

ARAMARK HEALTHCARE NUTRITION SERVICES, 1101 Market Street, Philadelphia, Pennsylvania Zip 19107; tel. 215/238–3000; Constance B. Girard–DiCarlo, President

ARTHUR ANDERSEN & COMPANY, 33 West Monroe Street, Chicago, Illinois Zip 60603; tel. 312/580–0033

ARTHUR D. LITTLE, INC., 35–302A Acorn Park, Cambridge, Massachusetts Zip 02140; tel. 617/864–5770; Douglass J. Seaver, National Director Health Care Delivery Practice

AXIS RECEIVABLES SOLUTIONS, INC, 999 East Touhy Ave, Suite 225, Des Plaines, Illinois Zip 60018; tel. 708/635–3300; Brad Gustin, Executive Vice President

B.E. SMITH ASSOCIATES, INC., 10100 Santa Fe Drive, Ste 204, Overland Park, Kansas Zip 66212; tel. 913/341–9116; J. Doug Smith, President

BOOZ–ALLEN & HAMILTON, INC., 8251 Greensboro Drive, Mc Lean, Virginia Zip 22102; tel. 703/917–2594; Debbie Canty, Business Operations Manager

BOSTON CONSULTING GROUP, 135 East 57th Street, New York, New York Zip 10022; tel. 212/446–2800; Abby Klieman, Practice Area Coordinator

CAMPBELL WILSON, 9400 Central Expwy, Suite 613, Dallas, Texas Zip 75231; tel. 214/373–7077; Danna J. Wilson, Principal

CAREMARK, INC., 2211 Sanders Road, Northbrook, Illinois Zip 60062; tel. 708/559–3518

CENTRAL HEALTH SERVICES, INC., 6600 Powers Ferry Rd, Ste 300, Atlanta, Georgia Zip 30339; tel. 404/956–6500; Kay Wetherbee, Director Management Services

CEPHALON, INC., 145 Brandywine Parkway, West Chester, Pennsylvania Zip 19382–4245; tel. 610/344–0200; Beverly L. Cantor, Supervisor Information Services

CHANCELLOR GROUP, INCORPORATED, 3601 Minnesota Drive, Ste 430, Bloomington, Minnesota Zip 55435; tel. 612/835–5123; David Allen, Partner

CHI LABORATORY SYSTEMS, INC, 3135 South State St, Ste 300, Ann Arbor, Michigan Zip 48108; tel. 313/662–6363; John W. Craft, Principal

CHI SYSTEMS, INC., 130 South First Street, Ann Arbor, Michigan Zip 48104; tel. 313/761–3912; Karl G. Bartscht, Chief Executive Officer

COASTAL PHYSICIAN CONTRACT SERVICES GROUP, INC., 3708 Mayfair Street, Suite 103, Durham, North Carolina Zip 27707; tel. 919/382–7551; G. Scott Dillon, Executive Vice President

Associate Members / Other

COFFEY COMMUNICATIONS, INC., 1505 Business One Circle, Walla Walla, Washington Zip 99362; tel. 509/525-0101; Alan H. Coffey, Chief Executive Officer

D.J. SULLIVAN & ASSOCIATES, INC., 2155 Jackson Avenue, Ann Arbor, Michigan Zip 48103-3917; tel. 313/662-7500

DELOITTE & TOUCHE, 180 North Stetson Avenue, Chicago, Illinois Zip 60601; tel. 312/946-3215; Michael A. Engelhart, National Director Health Care Services

DELOITTE AND TOUCHE, 1560 Broadway, Suite 1800, Denver, Colorado Zip 80202; tel. 303/837-3000; Tim Davis, Senior Manager

DIAMONDS AND PEARLS CORPORATE CONSULTANTS, P.O. Box 821, Greensboro, Georgia Zip 30642-0821; tel. 706/453-1169; James E. Tullos Jr., Owner and Senior Systems Consultant

E. M. S. A. LIMITED PARTNERSHIP, 1200 S Pine Island Rd, Ste 600, Fort Lauderdale, Florida Zip 33324; tel. 305/475-1300; Marta Prado, Vice President

EJJ OLSON & ASSOCIATES, 2266 North Prospect Avenue, Milwaukee, Wisconsin Zip 53202; tel. 414/271-3553; Edward Olson, President

ENVIRONMENTAL COMPLIANCE TESTING, INC., 565 Rounseville Road, Box 7, Rochester, Massachusetts Zip 02770; tel. 508/763-5919; Ann Fournier, President

ERNST & YOUNG, 2000 National City Center, Cleveland, Ohio Zip 44114; tel. 216/861-5000; Richard L. Marrapese, Partner

ERNST AND YOUNG, 2001 Market Street, Ste 4000, Philadelphia, Pennsylvania Zip 19103-7096; tel. 215/448-5000; Thomas K. Shaffert, Partner

FHC MANAGEMENT SERVICES, 11876 Sunrise Valley Dr, 200, Reston, Virginia Zip 22091; tel. 703/715-9626; David F. Cawley, President and Chief Executive Officer

FIRST CONSULTING GROUP, 100 East Wadlow Road, Long Beach, California Zip 90807; tel. 213/595-5291; Patricia Robinson, Director Training and Education

FMC CORPORATION – AMHS DIVISION, 400 Highpoint Drive, Chalfont, Pennsylvania Zip 18914; tel. 215/822-4448; B. W. Baum, Manager Engineering

FUTURES GROUP, 80 Glastonbury Boulevard, Glastonbury, Connecticut Zip 06033-4409; tel. 203/633-3501; Maria C. Robotham, Manager Healthcare and Aging Studies

GLS ASSOCIATES, INC., 1500 Chestnut Street, Ste 1004, Philadelphia, Pennsylvania Zip 19102; tel. 215/564-3600

GOBBELL HAYS PARTNERS, INC., 217 Fifth Avenue North, Nashville, Tennessee Zip 37219; tel. 615/254-8500; Nicholas R. Ganick, Vice President

HAMILTON-KSA, 1355 Peachtree St N.E., Ste 900, Atlanta, Georgia Zip 30309-0900; tel. 404/892-0321; W. Barry Moore, National Director

HBO & COMPANY, 301 Perimeter Center North, Atlanta, Georgia Zip 30346; tel. 404/393-6000; Arthur J. Keegan, Vice-President Marketing

HCX, INC., P.O. Box 3088, Naperville, Illinois Zip 60566-7088; tel. 708/420-6800; Barbara Beck Dickson, Vice President and General Counsel

HEALTH DIMENSIONS ALTERNATIVE CARE SYSTEMS, 7100 Northland Circle, Ste 205, Minneapolis, Minnesota Zip 55428; Betty Ice, Director Client Relations

HEALTHCARE FINANCIAL ENTERPRISES, INC, 2717 West Cypress Creek Road, Fort Lauderdale, Florida Zip 33309; tel. 305/970-9600; Peter A. Carvalho, President

HEALTHCARE LINEN AND LAUNDRY, INC., 303 South Broadway, Room 229, Tarrytown, New York Zip 10591; tel. 914/332-4900

HEIDRICK AND STRUGGLES, INCORPORATED, 125 South Wacker Drive, Chicago, Illinois Zip 60606; tel. 312/372-8811; Richard P. Gustafson, Partner

HELLMUTH, OBATA AND KASSABAUM, INC., 1655 26th Street, Suite 200, Santa Monica, California Zip 90404; tel. 310/453-0100; Michael Fejes, Senior Vice President

HERMAN SMITH ASSOCIATES, 203 North LaSalle Street, Chicago, Illinois Zip 60601; tel. 312/701-5893; Jeffrey J. Frommelt, Partner

HEWITT ASSOCIATES, 100 Half Day Road, Lincolnshire, Illinois Zip 60069; tel. 708/295-5000; Wilma Tuthill, Libarian

HOSPICORE, INC., 4378 Wolff Street, Denver, Colorado Zip 80212; tel. 303/458-5337; Mary Neal Lycett, President

HRADVANTAGE, 305 Granada Boulevard, Ste 2, Lake Villa, Illinois Zip 60046; tel. 708/356-1717; Scott Hamilton, Managing Director

INFUSION MANAGEMENT SERVICES, 105 North Detroit, Buchanan, Michigan Zip 49107; tel. 616/695-6640; Thomas R. Hoetger, Director Reimbursement and Controller

JAMES RUSSELL, INC., P.O. Box 427, Bloomington, Illinois Zip 61702-0427; tel. 309/663-9467; Billy D. Adkisson, Pres

JANNOTTA, BRAY AND ASSOCIATES, 30 Oak Hollow, Suite 100, Southfield, Michigan Zip 48034-7467; tel. 313/827-4510; Joan Hanpeter, Managing Director

JAROS, BAUM AND BOLLES, 345 Park Avenue, New York, New York Zip 10154; Richard T. Baum, Consultant

JOHN NUVEEN AND COMPANY, INCORPORATED, 333 West Wacker Drive, Chicago, Illinois Zip 60606; tel. 312/917-7700; Terence M. Mieling, Vice President and National Health Care Director

JURAN INSTITUTE, 11 River Road, Wilton, Connecticut Zip 06896; tel. 203/834-1700; Sally Georgen Archer, Account Executive

KASET INTERNATIONAL, 8875 Hidden River Parkway, 400, Tampa, Florida Zip 33637; tel. 813/977-8875; Beth Z. Potter, Marketing Manager

LAMMERS & GERSHON ASSOCIATES, INC., 1801 Alexander Bell Dr, 600, Reston, Virginia Zip 22091; tel. 703/476-8400; Howard J. Gershon, Executive Vice-President

LOGISTICS MANAGEMENT CORPORATION, 306-1/2 Riverview Avenue, Annapolis, Maryland Zip 21403; tel. 800/562-0051; Robert D. Nolker, Executive Vice President

M. S. CAPITAL RESOURCES, INC., 4225 Executive Square, Ste 250, La Jolla, California Zip 92037; tel. 619/535-9494; Mark Steinberg, President

MARITZ PERFORMANCE IMPROVEMENT COMPANY, 1400 South Highway Drive, Fenton, Missouri Zip 63099; tel. 314/827-2473; Barbara Sutton, Process Manager

MARSHALL ERDMAN & ASSOCIATES, INC., 5117 University Avenue, Madison, Wisconsin Zip 53705; tel. 608/238-0211; William D. Wakefield, Director Marketing

MCFAUL & LYONS, INC., 306 Horizon Center, Trenton, New Jersey Zip 08691; tel. 609/588-4900; William McFaul, President

MEDICAL INTERCEPT SYSTEMS, 500 Turtle Cove, Suite 150, Rockwall, Texas Zip 75087; tel. 214/771-6643; Joe Davis, President

MEDQUIST, INC., State Highway 73 North, Marlton, New Jersey Zip 08053-3422; tel. 609/596-8877; James R. Emshoff, President and Chief Executive Officer

METRICOR, INC., 620 West Main Street, Ste 200, Louisville, Kentucky Zip 40202-2922; tel. 502/561-8400; Craig M. Johnson, Vice President Finance

MMI COMPANIES, INC., 540 Lake Cook Road, Deerfield, Illinois Zip 60015-5290; tel. 708/940-7550; Anna Marie Hajek, Senior Vice President

MRA STAFFING SYSTEMS, INC., 7771 W Oakland Park Boulevard, 100, Fort Lauderdale, Florida Zip 33351; tel. 305/748-3300; Greg Mikkelsen, Vice Pres Mktg

OLDFIELD DAVIS, INC., 211 N Record St, Ste 500 Lb11, Dallas, Texas Zip 75202; tel. 214/745-4545; Rachel M. Davis, President

PEDIATRIX MEDICAL GROUP, 1455 North Park Drive, Fort Lauderdale, Florida Zip 33326; tel. 305/384-0175; Karen Allison, Director Business Development

PRESS, GANEY ASSOCIATES, INC., 1657 Commerce Drive, South Bend, Indiana Zip 46628; tel. 219/232-3387; Mary Patricia Malone MS, J.D.,, Vice President Corporate Development

RURAL HEALTH CONSULTANTS, 2500 West Sixth, Suite H, Lawrence, Kansas Zip 66049; tel. 913/832-8778; Tina Shoemaker, Senior Consultant

SHELDON I. DORENFEST AND ASSOCIATES, LTD., 515 North State St, Suite 1801, Chicago, Illinois Zip 60610; tel. 312/464-3000; Mitchell Work, Senior Vice President Marketing and Sales

SHERLOCK, SMITH AND ADAMS, INC., 3047 Carter Hill Road, Montgomery, Alabama Zip 36111; tel. 205/263-6481; Roland H. Vaughan, President

SIMIONE & SIMIONE, P.O. Box 5248, New Haven, Connecticut Zip 06518; tel. 203/281-0540; William J. Simione Jr., President

SOUTHWEST CONSULTING ASSOCIATES, 4701 West Park Boulevard, Ste 204, Plano, Texas Zip 75093; tel. 214/964-5050; David P. Pfeil, President

SRA CORPORATION, 2000 15th Street North, Arlington, Virginia Zip 22201; tel. 703/824-4442; Mary H. Lambert R.N.,, Deputy Director Health Program

ST. ANTHONY PUBLISHING, INC., 11410 Isaac Newton Sq, Ste 200, Reston, Virginia Zip 22090; tel. 703/904-3900; Michael A. Grambo

TERRA SOL CONSULTANTS, 2020 Paseo Cresta, Vista, California Zip 92084; tel. 619/941-5621; Martin S. Kleckner III, President

THE CIT GROUP, INDUSTRIAL FINANCING, 650 Cit Drive, Livingston, New Jersey Zip 07039; tel. 201/740-5594; Anthony Pacchiano, Vice President

THE COKER GROUP, 3150 Holcomb Bridge Rd, 200, Norcross, Georgia Zip 30071-1312; tel. 404/242-0118; Jackson C. Coker, President

TIBER GROUP, INC., 200 South Wacker Dr, Ste 2620, Chicago, Illinois Zip 60606; tel. 312/902-9990

TOFT WOLFF FARROW, INC., 282 Second Street, San Francisco, California Zip 94105; tel. 415/247-8700; Lawrence S. Wolff, President

TOWERS PERRIN, 100 Summit Lake Drive, Valhalla, New York Zip 10595; tel. 212/309-3400; Julia Blanchard, Information Specialist

VICTOR KRAMER COMPANY, INC., 405 Murray Hill Parkway, Ste 1040, East Rutherford, New Jersey Zip 07073; tel. 201/935-0414; Thomas Mara, President

WEST HUDSON AND COMPANY, INC., 5230 Pacific Concourse Dr, 400, Los Angeles, California Zip 90045; tel. 310/297-4200; Adrianne Court, Operations Manager

WHITMAN GARVEY, INC., 1191 Second Avenue, Suite 1800, Seattle, Washington Zip 98101-2939; tel. 206/628-3763; James T. Whitman, President

WYATT COMPANY RESOURCE & INFORMATION CENTER, 601 13th Street N.W., Ste 1000, Washington, District of Columbia Zip 20005; tel. 202/887-4600; Herbert A. Miller Jr., Library

YAFFE AND COMPANY, INC., 2119 Caves Road, Owings Mills, Maryland Zip 21117; tel. 301/332-1166; Rian M. Yaffe, President

Educational Services

AMERICAN ASSOCIATION FOR MEDICAL TRANSCRIPTION, P.O. Box 576187, Modesto, California Zip 95357-6187; tel. 209/551-0883; Claudia J. Tessier, Executive Director

AMERICAN OVERSEAS BOOK COMPANY, INCORPORATED, 550 Walnut Street, Norwood, New Jersey Zip 07648; tel. 201/767-7600; Hale R. Gaffney, President

CALIFORNIA COLLEGE FOR HEALTH SCIENCES, 222 West 24th Street, National City, California Zip 91950; tel. 619/477-4800; Dale K. Bean, Program Director

GRANADA HOSPITAL GROUP, INC., 21 B Street, Burlington, Massachusetts Zip 01803; tel. 617/270-0074

WESTCOTT COMMUNICATIONS, INC., 1303 Marsh Lane, Carrollton, Texas Zip 75006; tel. 214/716-5100; William H. Fueller Ph.D.,, Vice President and General Manager

Facilities Management

ALLIANCE HOME CARE MANAGEMENT, INCORPORATED, 309 Lennon Lane, Suite 200, Walnut Creek, California Zip 94598; tel. 510/937-8680; Gregory M. Capson, President

AMERICAN UTILITIES, P.O. Box 1214, Orem, Utah Zip 84059-1214; Ellen Burkett, President

DYNAMIC HEALTH, INC., 777 S Harbor Island Boulevard, 890, Tampa, Florida Zip 33602; tel. 813/228-8844; John J. Silver Jr., President and Chief Executive Officer

FORMATIONS IN HEALTH CARE, INC., 155 North Wacker Dr, Ste 725, Chicago, Illinois Zip 60606; tel. 312/849-4200; Pamella Leiter, President

GUARDIAN FOUNDATION, 5725 E Paradise Drive, Ste 550, Corte Madera, California Zip 94925-1219; tel. 412/945-2228; Mary L. Lubily, Director Hospital Services

JOHNSON CONTROLS, INC., 3354 Perimeter Hill Dr, 105, Nashville, Tennessee Zip 37211; tel. 615/333-9304; Larry G. Cox, Business Development Manager

MEDICAL PLANNING ASSOCIATES, 1601 Rambla Pacifico, Malibu, California Zip 90265; tel. 310/456-2084; Daniel Logan, President

PRISON HEALTH SERVICES, INC., 3565 Piedmont Rd, Bldg 2-410, Atlanta, Georgia Zip 30305; tel. 404/816-7471; Gloria Blake, Manager Marketing Services

Associate Members / Other

SCRIBCOR, INC., 400 North Michigan Avenue, Chicago, Illinois Zip 60611; tel. 312/923-8000; Stephen T. Kardel, Chief Operating Officer

SERVICEMASTER MANAGEMENT SERVICES, One Servicemaster Way, Downers Grove, Illinois Zip 60515; tel. 708/964-1300; C. William Pollard, President

SPECTRUM EMERGENCY CARE, INC., 999 Executive Parkway, Saint Louis, Missouri Zip 63141-6395; tel. 314/878-2280; Tony Bevilacqua, Vice President

Information Systems

3M HEALTH INFORMATION SYSTEMS, P.O. Box 57900, Murray, Utah Zip 84157; tel. 801/265-4400; Scott Slivka, Marketing Manager

3NET SYSTEMS, INC., 629 J Street, Sacramento, California Zip 95814-2418; tel. 916/498-3900; Susan Wall, Coordinator Marketing

ALLTELL INFORMATION SERVICES, INC., 200 Ashford Center North, Atlanta, Georgia Zip 30338; tel. 404/847-5000; Katie G. Mazzuckelli, Director Planning and Research

ARKIVE INFORMATION SYSTEM, INC., 4725 Reedley Terrace, San Diego, California Zip 92130; tel. 619/481-7313; Philip W. Faris Jr., Chief Executive Officer

CCSI, 8612 Watershed Court, Gaithersburg, Maryland Zip 20877-3751; tel. 301/948-3579; Brigadier General Carlos B. Arostegui, President

CERNER CORPORATION, 2800 Rockcreek Parkway, Kansas City, Missouri Zip 64117; tel. 816/221-1024; C. S. Runnion III, Executive Vice President

CHC, INC., 5 Greenway Plaza, Ste 1900, Houston, Texas Zip 77046; tel. 713/850-2114

DATIS CORPORATION, 1875 South Grant St, Ste 400, San Mateo, California Zip 94402; tel. 415/571-0931; Mark Collins, President

EMTEK HEALTH CARE SYSTEMS, INC., 1501 W Fountainhead Parkway, 190, Tempe, Arizona Zip 85282; tel. 602/431-9343

FIRST COAST SYSTEMS, 6430 Southpoint Parkway, Ste 250, Jacksonville, Florida Zip 32216-0978; tel. 904/296-4200; Charles,R. Gibbs, President

FIRST DATA CORPORATION, HEALTH SYSTEMS GROUP, P.O. Box 1037, Charlotte, North Carolina Zip 28201-1037; tel. 704/549-7000; Darryl G. Bowles, Senior Vice President

H.C.I.A., P.O. Box 303, Ann Arbor, Michigan Zip 48106-0303; tel. 313/930-7830; Jean Chenoweth, Vice President Business Development

HEALTH DATA SCIENCES CORPORATION, 268 West Hospitality Lane, San Bernardino, California Zip 92408; tel. 714/888-3282; Lynn E. Fordham, Manager Marketing and Communications

HEWLETT-PACKARD, 3000 Minuteman Road, Andover, Massachusetts Zip 01810-1085; tel. 508/687-1501; Peter Gladkin, General Manager Healthcare Information Systems

I. B. M. CORPORATION, 122 Morningside Circle, Parkersburg, West Virginia Zip 26101; tel. 304/428-3268; Jeff Lantz, Health Industry Specialist

I.B.M. CORPORATION, 2345 Grand Avenue, Kansas City, Missouri Zip 64108; tel. 816/556-6696; Donna K. Long, Manager

I.B.M. CORPORATION, P.O. Box 2150, Atlanta, Georgia Zip 30301-2150; tel. 404/238-4671; Wendy Rubel, Communications Senior Program Administrator

IBAX HEALTHCARE SYSTEMS, 587 East Sanlando Springs Dr, Longwood, Florida Zip 32750; tel. 407/831-8444; Walter Suika, Director Business Partner Relations

IDX SYSTEMS CORPORATION, P.O. Box 1070, Burlington, Vermont Zip 05402-1070; tel. 802/862-1022; Richard Tarrant, President

IHS REGULATORY PRODUCTS, INC., 15 Inverness Way East, Englewood, Colorado Zip 80112; tel. 303/267-1497; Douglas T. Stuart, National Sales Manager

IMS AMERICA, LTD., 660 West Germantown Pike, Plymouth Meeting, Pennsylvania Zip 19462; tel. 215/834-5000; Kevin Kelly, National Field Manager

J.D. EDWARDS AND COMPANY, 8055 East Tufts Ave, 12th Fl, Denver, Colorado Zip 80237; tel. 303/488-4000; T. Gayle Sheppard, Director Public Services

KPMG PEAT MARWICK, 303 East Wacker Drive, Chicago, Illinois Zip 60601; tel. 312/938-1000; Robert E. Schimmel, Partner

KURZWEIL APPLIED INTELLIGENCE, INCORPORATED, 411 Waverley Oaks Road, Waltham, Massachusetts Zip 02154; tel. 617/893-5151; Beverly Jill Albiani, Marketing Specialist

LAMBERT COMMUNICATIONS, P.O. Box 305, Brookfield, Connecticut Zip 06804; tel. 203/740-9404; Rebecca Lambert, Chairman and Chief Executive Officer

MANAGEMENT SYSTEMS ASSOCIATES, INC., 5580 Centerview Drive, Raleigh, North Carolina Zip 27606; tel. 919/851-6177; Thomas Campbell Jr., Product Planner

MEDICUS SYSTEMS CORPORATION, One Rotary Center, Suite 400, Evanston, Illinois Zip 60201; tel. 708/570-7500

MEDIMATCH, P.O. Box 270, Sonoma, California Zip 95476; tel. 707/939-9930; Pat Powers, Principal

MICROMEDEX, INC., 6200 S Syracuse Way, Ste 300, Englewood, Colorado Zip 80111-4740; tel. 303/486-6400; A. C. Howerton, Vice President Sales and Marketing

MOTOROLA, INC., 1301 Algonquin Road, Schaumburg, Illinois Zip 60196; tel. 708/576-2412; Ann Jenkins

NEON HEALTHCARE SOFTWARE AND SYSTEMS, 7400 East Orchard Rd, Ste 230, Englewood, Colorado Zip 80111; tel. 303/649-3933; Rick Adam, President

OACIS HEALTHCARE SYSTEMS, 7960 Donegan Drive, Ste 240, Manassas, Virginia Zip 22110; tel. 703/330-8830; Jim Wilson, Director Sales and Marketing

OPTIMARK CORPORATION, 9 Dekay Road, Warwick, New York Zip 10990; tel. 914/986-4554; Jennifer Brodheim, Director Marketing

PHAMIS, INC., 401 Second Ave South, Ste 200, Seattle, Washington Zip 98104-2862; tel. 206/622-9558; Douglas W. Brown, Executive Vice President

PROFESSIONAL HEALTHCARE SYSTEMS, INC., 12960 Coral Tree Place, Los Angeles, California Zip 90066; tel. 310/578-7000; Bradley K. Overby, Senior Vice President

PROFESSIONAL ON-LINE COMPUTERS, INCORPORATED, 4835 Towne Centre Rd, Ste 201, Saginaw, Michigan Zip 48604; tel. 517/790-0970; Trisha Hegler, Marketing Representative

RESOURCE INFORMATION MANAGEMENT SYSTEMS, P.O. Box 3094, Naperville, Illinois Zip 60566-2599; tel. 708/369-5300; Ellen J. Lockwald, Manager Marketing Developmen

REUTERS HEALTH INFORMATION SERVICES, 825 Eighth Avenue, Ste 3100, New York, New York Zip 10019; tel. 212/474-6000; Kathy Bogomolov, Manager Sales Information

SCIENCE APPLICATIONS INTERNATIONAL CORPORATION, 5107 Leesburg Pike, Suite 2200, Falls Church, Virginia Zip 22041; tel. 703/824-5800; David Cox, Group Senior Vice President

SMART CLIPBOARD CORPORATION, 9666 Olive Boulevard, Ste 370, Saint Louis, Missouri Zip 63132; tel. 314/993-0665; Charles N. Mead M.D.,, President

SOCIETE WATKINS LIMITED, P.O. Box 908, Roswell, Georgia Zip 30077; tel. 404/998-0900; Thomas H. Watkins, Managing Principal

SUNQUEST INFORMATION SYSTEMS, INC., 4801 East Broadway, Tucson, Arizona Zip 85711; tel. 602/570-2000; Dennis Morley, Vice President Marketing

SUPERIOR CONSULTANT COMPANY, INC., 31731 Northwestern Hwy, 250W, Farmington Hills, Michigan Zip 48334; tel. 313/855-0960; Richard D. Helppie, President

TANDEM COMPUTERS, INC., 1302 Concourse Drive, Ste 200, Linthicum Heights, Maryland Zip 21090-2916; tel. 410/859-8800; Gloria Parker, Manager Healthcare Solutions

TEKLOGIX, 1102 Peters Road, Troy, Ohio Zip 45373; tel. 513/335-8277; Leib Lurie, Director Marketing

TEUBNER AND ASSOCIATES, 623 South Main Street, Stillwater, Oklahoma Zip 74076; tel. 405/624-2254; Bob Chamberlain, Sales Manager

THE COMPUCARE COMPANY, 12110 Sunset Hills Road, Reston, Virginia Zip 22090; tel. 703/709-2300; Ronald V. Aprahamian, Chairman

TRANSQUICK, INC., 4848 Riverdale Road, Atlanta, Georgia Zip 30337; tel. 404/991-2220; Michael F. Clark, Executive Director

VECTOR RESEARCH, INC., P.O. Box 1506, Ann Arbor, Michigan Zip 48106; tel. 313/973-9210; Kevin J. Dombkowski, Program Scientist

XEROX CORPORATION, 7900 Westpark Drive, Ste 400, Mc Lean, Virginia Zip 22101; tel. 703/442-6704; Jack Bowie, Healthcare Marketing Manager

Insurance Broker

ACORDIA HEALTH INDUSTRY BENEFITS, INC., 6802 Hillsdale Court, Indianapolis, Indiana Zip 46250-2001; tel. 317/488-6000

AETNA LIFE INSURANCE AND ANNUITY COMPANY, 151 Farmington Avenue–RW13, Hartford, Connecticut Zip 06156; tel. 203/273-3291; Robert H. Barley, Assistant Vice President

AFLAC, 1932 Wynnton Road, Columbus, Georgia Zip 31999; tel. 706/660-7034; R. Duke Miller, Vice President

AMERICAN HOME ASSURANCE COMPANY, 70 Pine Street, 7th Floor, New York, New York Zip 10270; tel. 212/770-7060

CLAIMS ADMINISTRATION CORPORATION, 7361 Calhoun Place, Rockville, Maryland Zip 20855; tel. 301/738-1216; Andrea Andrus, Vice President Operations

COPELAND COMPANIES, Two Tower Center Boulevard, East Brunswick, New Jersey Zip 08816-1100; tel. 201/214-2000; Paul J. Cheng, Vice President

HEALTHCARE UNDERWRITERS MUTUAL INSURANCE COMPANY, 8 British American Boulevard, Latham, New York Zip 12110; tel. 518/786-2700

HELMSTAR FUNDING, 206 South Fourth Street, Philadelphia, Pennsylvania Zip 19106; tel. 215/629-5600; Richard Harris, President

JOHN ALDEN LIFE INSURANCE COMPANY, 5200 Blue Lagoon Dr, Ste 470, Miami, Florida Zip 33126; tel. 305/263-8166; James S. Wells, Director Product Development

KEMPER NATIONAL INSURANCE COMPANIES, One Kemper Drive, D-7, Long Grove, Illinois Zip 60049-0001; tel. 708/540-2059; Richard C. Lunt, Manager Property Valuation and Appraisal

KEMPER NATIONAL SERVICES, 1601 S.W. 80th Terrace, Plantation, Florida Zip 33324; tel. 305/452-4000; David K. Patterson, President

LOCKTON COMPANIES, 7400 State Line Road, Prairie Village, Kansas Zip 66208; tel. 913/676-9546; Becky Sullivan, Vice President Unit Manager

MUTUAL OF OMAHA INSURANCE COMPANY, Mutual of Omaha Plaza, Omaha, Nebraska Zip 68175-1008; tel. 402/342-7600; Bill Norris, Vice President

NATIONWIDE MUTUAL INSURANCE COMPANY, One Nationwide Plaza, Columbus, Ohio Zip 43215; tel. 614/249-6153; Victoria Blackford, Corporate Librarian

PHICO INSURANCE COMPANY, P.O. Box 85, Mechanicsburg, Pennsylvania Zip 17055-0085; tel. 717/766-1122; Maynard R. Stufft, President

PRINCIPAL FINANCIAL GROUP, 711 High Street, Des Moines, Iowa Zip 50392-4600; tel. 515/247-5222; Chris Finken, Manual Specialist

PROVIDENT LIFE & ACCIDENT INSURANCE COMPANY, One Fountain Square, Chattanooga, Tennessee Zip 37402; tel. 615/755-3967; Pat G. Veltman, Vice-President Group Field Claims

PRUDENTIAL INSURANCE COMPANY, P.O. Box 1567, Houston, Texas Zip 77251-1567; tel. 713/276-4950; Peggy Goldman, Claims Manager

ROLLINS HUDIG HALL HEALTHCARE RISK, INC., 201 Alhambra Circle, Suite 800, Coral Gables, Florida Zip 33134; tel. 305/441-8770

SULLIVAN, KELLY AND ASSOCIATES, INC., 135 North Los Robles, Pasadena, California Zip 91101; tel. 818/564-1600; Stephanie A. Cafiero, Senior Vice President

VALIC, 2929 Allen Parkway (A7-26), Houston, Texas Zip 77019; tel. 713/831-5311; Carol Melville, Associate Director Healthcare Marketing

WASHINGTON CASUALTY COMPANY–WASHINGTON HOSPITAL INSURANCE FUND, 14100 S.E. 36th Street, Bellevue, Washington Zip 98006-1568; tel. 206/455-2282; Donald G. Steffes, President

Investment Broker

ALEX BROWN AND SONS, INC., 101 Federal Street, 15th Floor, Boston, Massachusetts Zip 02110; tel. 617/727-8100; Jonathan Osgood, Managing Director

GARDNER, CARTON AND DOUGLAS, 1301 K Street N.W., Suite 900E, Washington, District of Columbia Zip 20005; tel. 202/408-8122; Scott Johnson J.D.,, Attorney

GEORGE K. BAUM & COMPANY, 745 Craig Road, Suite 220, Saint Louis, Missouri Zip 63141; tel. 314/872-8884; Arlan Dohrmann, Manager Healthcare

Associate Members / Other

NORWEST FINANCIAL LEASING, INC, 3221 McKelvey Road, Suite 107, Bridgeton, Missouri Zip 63044; tel. 314/298–1735; Linda Rafanello, Vice President Marketing

STEPHENS, INC., 111 Center Street, Little Rock, Arkansas Zip 72201; tel. 501/377–8125; Nancy Weaver, Research Analyst

Manufacturer / Supplier

3M, 3M Center, Building 275–4E–01, Saint Paul, Minnesota Zip 55144–1000; tel. 612/733–8183; Donald R. Brewer, Director Medical Surgical-Markets

ABBOTT LABORATORIES, One Abbott Park Road, Abbott Park, Illinois Zip 60064; tel. 708/937–2692; Michelle Sellers, Coordinator Marketing Relations

ALM SURGICAL EQUIPMENT, INC., 1820 North Lemon Street, Anaheim, California Zip 92801–1009; tel. 714/578–1234; George E. Crispin, President

AMERICAN SEATING COMPANY, 401 American Seating Center, Grand Rapids, Michigan Zip 49504; tel. 616/732–6597; Paul Warren, Manager Healthcare Markets

AMGEN, 1840 Dehavilland Dr, Dept 631, Thousand Oaks, California Zip 91320–1789; tel. 805/499–5725; Chris Ludlow, Data Manager

ASTRA USA, INC., 50 Otis Street, Westboro, Massachusetts Zip 01581; tel. 508/366–1100; Julia Urwin, Librarian

AVCOR HEALTH CARE PRODUCTS, INC., P.O. Box 40500, Fort Worth, Texas Zip 76140; tel. 817/551–0595; Jerry L. Wilson, Operation Manager

BAXTER HEALTHCARE CORPORATION, 26 Wiggins Avenue, Bedford, Massachusetts Zip 01730; tel. 617/275–1100; Stewart Randle, New England Regional President

BAXTER HEALTHCARE CORPORATION, One Baxter Parkway Df3–3W, Deerfield, Illinois Zip 60015; tel. 708/940–6511; Deborah A. Heidecke, Vice President Corporate Marketing

BECKMAN INSTRUMENTS, INC., 200 South Kraemer Boulevard, Brea, California Zip 92621; tel. 714/993–5821; David E. Todd, Manager Market Research

BERLEX LABORATORIES, 300 Fairfield Road, Wayne, New Jersey Zip 07470–7358; tel. 201/695–4100; Larry W. Tobias, Vice President Operations

BFI MEDICAL WASTE SYSTEMS, 757 North Eldridge, Houston, Texas Zip 77077; tel. 713/870–7013; Steven Fields, Vice President

BIC CORPORATION, 500 Bic Drive, Milford, Connecticut Zip 06460; tel. 203/783–2105; Gregory D. Young, Assistant Product Manager

BIOCRAFT LABORATORIES, INC., 18–01 River Road, Fair Lawn, New Jersey Zip 07410; tel. 201/796–3434; Jerry Moskowitz, Vice President Sales

BOEHRINGER INGELHEIM PHARMACEUTICALS, INC., P.O. Box 368, Ridgefield, Connecticut Zip 06877; tel. 203/798–9988; Nancy A. Cunniff

BOSTON SCIENTIFIC CORPORATION, 480 Pleasant Street, Watertown, Massachusetts Zip 02172; tel. 617/972–4406; John Abele, Co-Chairman

CANNON MILLS COMPANY, 1271 Avenue of the Americas, New York, New York Zip 10020; tel. 212/957–2590; J. G. Coles, Vice President

CARL ZEISS, INC., One Zeiss Drive, Thornwood, New York Zip 10594; tel. 914/747–1800; Cathy Lewis, Manager

CIBA-GEIGY CORPORATION, 556 Morris Avenue, D3114, Summit, New Jersey Zip 07901; tel. 908/277–7363; William J. Hix, Head Headquarters Sales

CINE–CATH IMAGING, INC., 17601 Fitch, Irvine, California Zip 92714; Donald R. Burkhead, Director Marketing

COLGATE PALMOLIVE COMPANY SPECIAL MARKETS, P.O. Box 1928, Morristown, New Jersey Zip 07962–1926; tel. 800/75287153; Brian Fisher, Manager

CRITIKON, INC., P.O. Box 31800, Tampa, Florida Zip 33631–3800; tel. 813/887–2000

DEPUY, P.O. Box 988, Warsaw, Indiana Zip 46581–0988; tel. 219/267–8143; Jan Deaton, Manager Marketing Resources

DEVON INDUSTRIES, INC., 9530 Desoto Avenue, Chatsworth, California Zip 91311; tel. 818/709–6880; Kathleen Baffone, Market Research Analyst

DIAGNOSTIC HEALTH SERVICES, 2777 Stemmons Frwy, Ste 1525, Dallas, Texas Zip 75207; tel. 214/634–0403; James Kirker, Vice President

DIGITAL EQUIPMENT CORPORATION, 4 Results Way, MRO4–2/C15, Marlboro, Massachusetts Zip 01752; tel. 508/467–2319; Ava Schutzman, Manager Marketing

DUPONT MERCK PHARMACEUTICAL COMPANY, P.O. Box 80723, Wilmington, Delaware Zip 19880–0723; tel. 302/992–5040; Celesteen Scott, Section Manager

EASTMAN KODAK COMPANY, 343 State Street, Rochester, New York Zip 14650–0868; tel. 716/724–6888

ELI LILLY AND COMPANY, Lilly Corporate Cntr, 1837, Indianapolis, Indiana Zip 46285; tel. 317/276–2000; Mark Nagy, Manager

FISONS PHARMACEUTICALS, P.O. Box 1766, Rochester, New York Zip 14603; tel. 716/274–3994; Judy V. Cometa, Senior Manager

GENERAL ELECTRIC MEDICAL SYSTEMS, P.O. Box 414, W–428, Milwaukee, Wisconsin Zip 53201–0414; tel. 414/548–2369; Tim Butler, Manager Marketing

GRAPHIC CONTROLS CORPORATION, 189 Van Rensselaer Street, Buffalo, New York Zip 14210; tel. 716/849–6418; June Brenan, Market Analyst

HAEMONETICS CORPORATION, 400 Wood Road, Braintree, Massachusetts Zip 02184; tel. 617/848–7100; David M. Sheehan, Director Marketing

HEALTH CARE MICROSYSTEMS, INC., 11911 U.S. Highway One, Ste 201, North Palm Beach, Florida Zip 33408; tel. 407/775–7698; Vicki Miller, Vice President Marketing

HILL-ROM, 1069 State Route 46 East, Batesville, Indiana Zip 47006; tel. 812/934–8285; Fay Bohlke, Marketing

HOLLISTER INCORPORATED, 2000 Hollister Drive, Libertyville, Illinois Zip 60048; tel. 708/680–1000; Elizabeth Cunningham, Librarian

HONEYWELL, INC, P.O. Box 524, Mn27–7246, Minneapolis, Minnesota Zip 55440; tel. 612/951–3718; Mark Shunk, Director Healthcare Business Unit

I-STAT CORPORATION, 303 College Road East, Princeton, New Jersey Zip 08540; tel. 800/827–7828; Maria E. Grant, Production Manager

IMMUNEX CORPORATION, 51 University Street, Seattle, Washington Zip 98101; tel. 206/587–0430; Michael L. Kleinberg, Director Professional Services

INTERMEDICS, INC., 4000 Technology Drive, Angleton, Texas Zip 77515; tel. 409/848–4000; Richard R. Ames, Vice President Sales

JOHNSON AND JOHNSON, P.O. Box 4000, New Brunswick, New Jersey Zip 08903; tel. 201/524–9293

LIFELINE SHELTER SYSTEMS, 250 Lowery Court, Groveport, Ohio Zip 43125; tel. 614/836–1948; K. Lee Guse, Executive Vice President

MANAGEMENT SCIENCE ASSOCIATES, INC., 4801 Cliff Avenue, Independence, Missouri Zip 64055; tel. 816/795–1947; James C. Velghe, President

MARKCARE MEDICAL SYSTEMS, 87 Route 17 North, Maywood, New Jersey Zip 07607; tel. 201/368–8118; Michael Rosenberg, Vice President Sales and Marketing

MEDTRONIC, INC., 7000 Central Avenue N.E., Minneapolis, Minnesota Zip 55440; tel. 612/574–3499; Steve Rasmussen, Manager Information Resources

MERCK U.S. HUMAN HEALTH, Wp35–150, West Point, Pennsylvania Zip 19486; tel. 215/652–5000; Phyllis Rausch, President

MICROTEK MEDICAL, INC., 512 Lehmberg Road, Columbus, Mississippi Zip 39702; tel. 601/327–1863; Kathy W. Zachry, Vice President Marketing and Sales

MILCARE, INC., A. HERMAN MILLER COMPANY, 8500 Byron Road, Zeeland, Michigan Zip 49464; tel. 616/654–8000; David Reid, Vice President Marketing and Human Resources

MILLIKEN AND COMPANY, 201 Lubben Industrial Dr West, La Grange, Georgia Zip 30240; tel. 706/880–5500; Charles R. Ball, Vice President

NEMSCHOFF CHAIRS, INC., P.O. Box 129, Sheboygan, Wisconsin Zip 53082–0129; tel. 414/457–7726; David Goodlund, Vice President Commercial Sales

NEOSTAR MEDICAL TECHNOLOGIES, INC., 201 North Center Drive, North Brunswick, New Jersey Zip 08902; tel. 908/821–2600; David A. Souerwine, Vice President

NICHOLS INSTITUTE, 33608 Ortega Highway, San Juan Capistrano, California Zip 92690; tel. 714/728–4000; Judy Kildow, Associate Director Market Development

OHMEDA, P.O. Box 7550, Madison, Wisconsin Zip 53707–7550; tel. 608/221–1551; Paul J. Gibler, Marketing Communications Manager

OTSUKA AMERICA PHARMACEUTICAL, INC., 2440 Research Boulevard, Ste 500, Rockville, Maryland Zip 20850; tel. 301/990–0030; Rio Iwanaga, Vice President Sales

PACESETTER, INC., P.O. Box 9221, Sylmar, California Zip 91392–9221; tel. 818/362–6822; Lori Hallmark

PFIZER PHARMACEUTICALS, 235 East 42nd Street, New York, New York Zip 10017; tel. 212/573–7877; Daniel J. Coakley, Director Affairs

PROCTER & GAMBLE PATIENT CARE, One Procter & Gamble Plaza, Cincinnati, Ohio Zip 45202; tel. 513/983–6248; James L. Knepler, Manager Professional Relations

PSICOR, INC., 16818 Via Del Campo Court, San Diego, California Zip 92127; tel. 619/485–5599; Michael W. Dunaway, Chief Executive Officer

ROCHE LABORATORIES, 340 Kingsland Street, Nutley, New Jersey Zip 07110; tel. 201/235–4353; Roy Thrush, Market Segment Manager

SANDOZ PHARMACEUTICALS CORPORATION, 59 Route 10, East Hanover, New Jersey Zip 07936–1080; tel. 201/503–8701; Gary Eastwood, Director Institutional Alliances

SHERWOOD MEDICAL COMPANY, 1915 Olive Street, Saint Louis, Missouri Zip 63103–1642; tel. 314/241–5700; Robert C. Egan, Executive Vice President Domestic Marketing

SIEMENS MEDICAL SYSTEMS, INC., 186 Wood Avenue South, Iselin, New Jersey Zip 08830; tel. 908/321–3427; James Mazalewski, Manager Market and Sales Analysis

SIGMA-TAU PHARMACEUTICALS, INC., 800 S Frederick Ave, Ste 300, Gaithersburg, Maryland Zip 20877; tel. 301/948–1041; C. Kenneth Mehrling, Director Sales and Marketing

SMITH & NEPHEW INC. CORPORATE MARKETING, 1875 Harsh Avenue S.E., Massillon, Ohio Zip 44646; tel. 216/833–2811; Judy Becker, Director Marketing and International Sales

STRYKER CORPORATION, 4100 East Milham, Kalamazoo, Michigan Zip 49001; tel. 616/329–2100; Jan L. Rabbers, Marketing Communications Manager

SYNERGEN, INC., 1885 33rd Street, Boulder, Colorado Zip 80301; tel. 303/541–1440; Dennis Houghton, Associate Director Managed Care

TEXAS INSTRUMENTS, INC., P.O. Box 655474, Dallas, Texas Zip 75265; tel. 214/995–6702; Dixie Garr, Manager New Business Assessment

TIMEMED LABELING SYSTEMS, INC., 144 Tower Drive, Burr Ridge, Illinois Zip 60521; tel. 708/986–1800; Nancy Finigan, Director Marketing

TREMCO, INC., 10701 Shaker Boulevard, Cleveland, Ohio Zip 44104; tel. 216/292–5000; Dick McOwen, National Sales Manager

UARCO NATIONAL HEALTH CARE, 10 S Riverside Plaza, Ste 747, Chicago, Illinois Zip 60606–3709; tel. 312/466–1010

W. W. GRAINGER, INC., 333 Knightsbridge Parkway, Lincolnshire, Illinois Zip 60069; tel. 708/913–8333; Kolleen K. Schulze, Associate Marketing Manager

WYETH-AYERST LABS DIVISION, 555 East Lancaster Avenue, Saint Davids, Pennsylvania Zip 19087; tel. 215/971–4541

ZELLERBACH, 12770 East 39th Avenue, Denver, Colorado Zip 80239; tel. 303/373–3524; Patty Frye, Marketing Manager

ZENECA PHARMACEUTICALS GROUP, P.O. Box 15437, Wilmington, Delaware Zip 19850–5437; tel. 302/886–3167; Richard D. Mann, Strategy Manager Government and Distribution

ZENITH CONTROLS, INC., 830 West 40th Street, Chicago, Illinois Zip 60609; tel. 312/247–6400; Thomas Ferry, Director Quality

Other

ABTOX, INC., 104 Terrace Drive, Mundelein, Illinois Zip 60060; tel. 708/949–0552; Robert Riley, President

ADVANCE REHABILITATION RESOURCES, INC., 7733 Forsyth Boulevard, Ste 1700, Clayton, Missouri Zip 63105–1817; David Cross, President

ADVANCED LASER SERVICES CORPORATION, 819 Phillipi Road, Columbus, Ohio Zip 43228; Christopher Zelich, President

ADVISORY BOARD COMPANY, 600 New Hampshire Avenue N.W., Washington, District of Columbia Zip 20037–2403; tel. 202/672–5600; David Bradley, President

AFFILIATED HEALTHCARE, INC., 11200 Westheimer, Suite 700, Houston, Texas Zip 77042; tel. 713/782–4555; Scott A. Hendry, Vice President

ALADDIN SYNERGETICS, INC., P.O. Box 100888, Nashville, Tennessee Zip 37224; tel. 615/748–3000

ALDEN MANAGEMENT SERVICES, 4200 Peterson, Chicago, Illinois Zip 60646; tel. 312/286–3883; Karen L. Scales, Vice President Operations

Associate Members / Other

AMERICAN ASSOCIATION OF NURSE ANESTHETISTS, 222 South Prospect Avenue, Park Ridge, Illinois Zip 60068-5790; tel. 708/692-7050; John F. Garde, Executive Director

AMERICAN BOARD OF MEDICAL SPECIALTIES, 1007 Church Street, Ste 404, Evanston, Illinois Zip 60201-5913; tel. 708/491-9091; J. Lee Dockery M.D.,, Executive Vice President

AMERICAN HEALTH PROPERTIES, INC., 6400 S Fiddlers Green Cr, 1800, Englewood, Colorado Zip 80111-4961; tel. 303/796-9793; Greg Schonert, Vice-President

AMERICAN HEALTHCARE SYSTEMS, 12730 High Bluff Dr, Ste 300, San Diego, California Zip 92130-2099; tel. 619/481-2727; Robert O'Leary, Chairman and Chief Executive Officer

AMERICAN MEDICAL RECOVERY, INC., 2537 South Gessner Rd, Ste 114, Houston, Texas Zip 77063-2026; tel. 713/260-7270; Don Kelly, President

AMERICAN SOCIETY OF HOSPITAL PHARMACISTS, 7272 Wisconsin Avenue, Bethesda, Maryland Zip 20814; tel. 301/657-3000; Joseph A. Oddis, Executive Vice President

ANNASHAE CORPORATION, 230 Alpha Park, Cleveland, Ohio Zip 44143-2202; tel. 216/449-2662; Barbara L. Rieker-Miller, Coordinator Marketing

ANTHEM HEALTH COMPANIES, 4040 Vincennes Circle, Indianapolis, Indiana Zip 46268-3027; tel. 317/298-6600; Jeannine Lewer, Communications Specialist

ARMED FORCES INSTITUTE OF PATHOLOGY, Washington, District of Columbia Zip 20306; tel. 202/576-2900

ARMED FORCES MEDICAL LIBRARY, 4301 Leesburg Pike, Room 670, Falls Church, Virginia Zip 22041-3258; tel. 703/756-8028; D. Zehnpfennig, Administrative Librarian

ASSOCIATION OF OPERATING ROOM NURSES, 2170 South Parker Rd, Ste 300, Denver, Colorado Zip 80231-5711; tel. 303/755-6304; Sara Katsh, Librarian

ASSOCIATION OF UNIVERSITY PROGRAMS IN HEALTH ADMINISTRATION, 1911 N Fort Myer Dr, Ste 503, Arlington, Virginia Zip 22209; tel. 703/524-0511; Henry Fernandez, President

B R + A CONSULTING ENGINEERS, INC., 333 West Wacker Drive, Ste 420, Chicago, Illinois Zip 60606; tel. 312/781-6900; Jeffery Wolfe, Branch Manager

BEECH STREET, 2 Ada, Suite 200, Irvine, California Zip 92718; tel. 714/727-1359; Doreen Corwin, Vice President Network Development

BELL ENVIRONMENTAL SERVICES, INC., 229 New Road, Parsippany, New Jersey Zip 07054; tel. 201/575-7800; Philip M. Waldorf, President

BLATTNER AND BRUNNER, INC., One Oxford Centre, 6th Floor, Pittsburgh, Pennsylvania Zip 15219; tel. 412/263-2979; Scott J. Morgan, Manager Health Care Services Group

BLUE CROSS AND BLUE SHIELD ASSOCIATION, 676 North St Clair, Chicago, Illinois Zip 60611; tel. 312/440-6000; Patrick G. Hays, President

BLUE SHIELD OF CALIFORNIA, 6701 Center Drive West, 800, Los Angeles, California Zip 90045; tel. 310/568-5460; Andrew Allocco, Senior Vice President Provider Relations

BMI, 320 West 57th Street, New York, New York Zip 10019; tel. 212/830-2514; Michael Bath, Manager Industry Relations

BREITNER, CLARK AND HALL, INC., 304 Victory Road, Quincy, Massachusetts Zip 02171; tel. 617/328-0011; Owen Breitner, Partner

BROCKTON MULTI SERVICE CENTER, 165 Quincy Street, Brockton, Massachusetts Zip 02402; tel. 508/580-0800; John P. Sullivan Ph.D.,, Area Director

BUSINESS AND LEGAL REPORTS, 39 Acedemy Street, Madison, Connecticut Zip 06443; tel. 203/245-7448; Peggy Vece, Booklet Editor

CARDINAL DISTRIBUTION, INC., 655 Metro Place South, Ste 925, Dublin, Ohio Zip 43017; tel. 614/761-8700; Gregory A. Serrao, President

CARTER HEALTHCARE FACILITIES, 1275 Peachtree Street N.E., Atlanta, Georgia Zip 30367-1801; tel. 404/888-3148; Charles G. Houston III, Vice President

CBE ENVIRONMENTAL, INC., 2065 Liddell Drive N.E., Atlanta, Georgia Zip 30324-4148; tel. 404/872-3005; Ronald E. Barmore, President

CITATION COMPUTER SYSTEMS, 424 S Woods Mill Rd, Ste 200, Chesterfield, Missouri Zip 63017; tel. 314/579-7900; Kenneth R. Brown, Chairman and Chief Executive Officer

CLINICA RICARDO PALMA, P.O. Box 52-6350, Miami, Florida Zip 33152-6350; Edwardo Salas M.D.,, Executive President

COMMONWEALTH OF VIRGINIA, DEPARTMENT OF MENTAL HEALTH AND MENTAL RETARDATION, Box 1797, Richmond, Virginia Zip 23214; tel. 804/770-3915; King E. Davis Ph.D.,, Commissioner

COMMUNITY BLOOD CENTER, 349 South Main Street, Dayton, Ohio Zip 45402; tel. 513/461-3450; Michael J. Barlow, Administrator

COMMUNITY CARE NETWORK, 5251 Viewridge Court, San Diego, California Zip 92123; tel. 619/278-2273; Jean Timmons, Technical Manager

COMPASS PSYCH-ASSOCIATES, INC., 2010 Corporate Ridge, Ste 700, McLean, Virginia Zip 22102; tel. 703/749-0543; Donald B. Morgan, President

CONNECTICUT HOSPITAL ASSOCIATION, Box 90, Wallingford, Connecticut Zip 06492; tel. 203/265-7611; Dennis P. May, President

COON AND ASSOCIATES, INC., P.O. Box 70, Phoenicia, New York Zip 12464; tel. 914/688-5776; Michael W. Coon, Chief Executive Officer

COOPERS AND LYBRAND L.L.P., 2400 Eleven Penn Center, Philadelphia, Pennsylvania Zip 19103; Glenn Shively, Chairman Healthcare Industry

COPELCO LEASING CORPORATION, 1700 Suckle Plaza, Pennsauken, New Jersey Zip 08110-1495; tel. 609/665-2178; Kevin Ward, Division Manager

CORNERSTONE HEALTH MANAGEMENT, 5080 Spectrum Dr, Ste 920 West, Dallas, Texas Zip 75248; tel. 214/960-0808; Dennis Johnston, President

COUNTRY VILLA SERVICE CORPORATION, 11266 Washington Place, Culver City, California Zip 90230; Stuart Mary Lander, Vice President Hospital Services

CROSS COUNTRY HEALTHCARE PERSONNEL, 1515 South Federal Hwy, 210, Boca Raton, Florida Zip 33432; tel. 407/394-0088; Joe Boshart, President

CROWN OF TEXAS SURGICAL HOSPITAL, 3501 Soncy Road, Suite 118, Amarillo, Texas Zip 79121; tel. 806/359-7999; John C. Coulter, Administrator

DATA GENERAL CORPORATION, 3400 Computer Dr, Mail Stop 9S, Westboro, Massachusetts Zip 01580; tel. 617/898-4196; Debbie Cream, Healthcare Industry Manager

DEPARTMENT OF AIR FORCE MEDICAL SERVICE, Hq Usaf/Sg, Bolling Air Force Base, District of Columbia Zip 20332-6188; tel. 202/545-6700

DEPARTMENT OF THE ARMY, OFFICE OF THE SURGEON GENERAL, Washington, District of Columbia Zip 20310; tel. 202/545-6700

DEPARTMENT OF THE NAVY, BUREAU OF MEDICINE AND SURGERY, Navy Department, Washington, District of Columbia Zip 20372; tel. 202/545-6700

DEPARTMENT OF VETERANS AFFAIRS, 810 Vermont Avenue N.W., Washington, District of Columbia Zip 20420; tel. 202/393-4120

DHHS, PUBLIC HEALTH SERVICE, DIVISION OF INDIAN HEALTH, HEALTH CARE ADMINISTRATION BRANCH, 5600 Fisher Lane, Room 6A-25, Rockville, Maryland Zip 20857; tel. 301/443-1085; Susanne Caviness M.D.,, Chief Patient Registration and Quality Management

DIAMOND CRYSTAL SPECIALTY FOODS, INC., 10 Burlington Avenue, Wilmington, Massachusetts Zip 01887-3997; tel. 617/944-3977; Denise C. Kelly R.D.,, Marketing Manager

DISCOVER CARD SERVICES, 2500 Lake Cook Road, 2-South, Riverwoods, Illinois Zip 60015; tel. 708/405-3429; Sherril Cavaletto, Vice President Medical Services Industry

DIVERSIFIED INVESTMENT ADVISORS, 4 Manhattanville Road, Purchase, New York Zip 10577; tel. 914/697-8552; Cherith Harrison, Director Marketing

DOCTORS CLINIC, P.O. Box 617, Alton, Illinois Zip 62002; tel. 618/474-7850; T. Bruce Vest M.D.,, Administrator

DU PONT CORIAN, P.O. Box 80702, Room 1243, Wilmington, Delaware Zip 19880-0702; tel. 302/999-5447; Todd Sutton, Manager

DUKE ENDOWMENT, 100 N Tryon Street, Suite 3500, Charlotte, North Carolina Zip 28202-4000; tel. 704/376-0291; Jere W. Witherspoon, Executive Director

DUN & BRADSTREET, 899 Eaton Avenue, Bethlehem, Pennsylvania Zip 18025; tel. 610/882-6502; Pat Scardaccione, Manager Analytical Services

DUN AND BRADSTREET, 899 Eaton Avenue, Bethlehem, Pennsylvania Zip 18025-0001; tel. 215/882-7689; Kathleen Attinello, Divisional Manager

ECOLAB INC., Ecolab Center, Saint Paul, Minnesota Zip 55102; tel. 612/293-2233; D. W. Kallgren, Manager Support Functions

EMERGENCY PRACTICE ASSOCIATES, P.O. Box 1260, Waterloo, Iowa Zip 50706; tel. 319/236-3858; Perry J. Miller, Director Development

ENTERPRISE SYSTEMS, INC., 1400 South Wolf Road, Ste 500, Wheeling, Illinois Zip 60090; tel. 708/537-4800; Thomas Pirelli, Chief Executive Officer

ERGODYNE, 1410 Energy Park Drive, Ste 1, Saint Paul, Minnesota Zip 55108; tel. 612/642-9889; Michelle Lee, Marketing Manager

EXECUTIVE RISK MANAGEMENT ASSOCIATES, 82 Hopmeadow Street, Simsbury, Connecticut Zip 06070; tel. 203/244-8900; David Lapin, Manager, Non-Profit Union

FITCH INVESTORS SERVICE, One State Plaza, New York, New York Zip 10004; tel. 212/908-0674; Daniel Decelles, Analyst

FITNESS FORUM, 6800 East Genesee Street, Fayetteville, New York Zip 13066; tel. 315/446-3141; James A. Smith, President

GAS MONITORING, INC., P.O. Box 1285, Cary, North Carolina Zip 27512-1285; tel. 919/469-9326; Keith T. Ferrari, Director Medical Piping

GATX LOGISTICS, INC., 1301 Gulf Life Drive, Jacksonville, Florida Zip 32207; tel. 904/396-2517; Katherine Canipelli, Marketing Director

GENESYS SOFTWARE SYSTEMS, INC., 5 Branch Street, Methuen, Massachusetts Zip 01844; Jayna Smith, Manager

GERIATRIC HEALTH VENTURES, INC., 3626 North Hall St, Ste 826, Dallas, Texas Zip 75219-5133; tel. 214/522-2544; Wilkes L. Kothmann, President

GILBERT TWEED ASSOCIATES, INC., 3411 Silverside Road, Wilmington, Delaware Zip 19810; tel. 302/479-5144; Patricia A. Hoffmeir, Vice President

GLAXO, INC., 5 Moore Drive, Research Triangle Pk, North Carolina Zip 27709; tel. 919/248-7797; Candy Hodge, Senior Manager

GRANCARE, INC., 1051 East Ogden Avenue, Milwaukee, Wisconsin Zip 53202; tel. 414/273-1212; La Vrene Norton, Vice President Executive Development

GROUP HEALTH INC., 330 West 42nd Street, New York, New York Zip 10036; tel. 212/760-6488; Michael F. Shepherd, Director Credentialing and Review

HAL W. SANDERS AND ASSOCIATES, INC, P.O. Box 4009, Eastman, Georgia Zip 31023; Hal W. Sanders, President

HARRIS ADVERTISING, 617 East Huron, Ann Arbor, Michigan Zip 48104; tel. 313/662-3442; Janice Shukle, President

HAWAII STATE DEPARTMENT OF HEALTH, Box 3378, Honolulu, Hawaii Zip 96801; tel. 808/961-4255; Bertrand Kobayashi, Deputy Director

HEALTH CARE PROPERTY INVESTORS, INC., 10990 Wilshire Boulevard, Ste 1200, Los Angeles, California Zip 90024; tel. 213/473-1990; Kenneth B. Roath, President and Chief Executive Officer

HEALTH FOUNDATION OF SOUTH FLORIDA, 1400 N.W. 12th Avenue, Miami, Florida Zip 33136; tel. 305/325-5405; Anthony C. Defurio, Managing Director

HEALTH MANAGEMENT SYSTEMS, INC., 401 Park Avenue South, New York, New York Zip 10016; tel. 212/685-4545

HEALTH NET, 21600 Oxnard Street, 18th Fl, Woodland Hills, California Zip 91367; tel. 818/719-6876

HEALTH PARTNERS OF PHILADELPHIA, 4700 Wissahickon Ave, Ste 118, Philadelphia, Pennsylvania Zip 19144-4283; tel. 215/849-9606; Barbara Plager, President and Chief Executive Officer

HEALTHCARE ASSOCIATION OF SOUTHERN CALIFORNIA, 201 North Figueroa St, 4th Fl, Los Angeles, California Zip 90012; tel. 213/250-5600; Stephen W. Gamble, President

HEALTHCARE COMPARE, 750 Riverpoint Drive, West Sacramento, California Zip 95605; tel. 916/374-4838; Fawn Holeman, Procurement Specialist

HEALTHCARE REALTY TRUST, INC., 3310 West End Avenue, Nashville, Tennessee Zip 37203; tel. 615/269-8175; David R. Emery, Chairman

HEALTHCARE STRATEGIES, INC., 2055 Redondo Place, Salt Lake City, Utah Zip 84108-3123; tel. 801/596-7501; David C. Pittam, Executive Consultant

HORIZON MENTAL HEALTH SERVICES, 4560 Beltline Road, Suite 400, Dallas, Texas Zip 75244; tel. 214/991-0112; Gary A. Kagan, Executive Vice President

Associate Members / Other

IMPAC HEALTH CARE, DIVISION OF INTERGRATED CONTROL SYSTEMS, INC., 231 Beach Street, Litchfield, Connecticut Zip 06759; tel. 203/567–0135; Rose Marie McCafferty, Vice President Health Care

INMAN ASSOCIATES, INC., 1808 West End Avenue, Ste 1400, Nashville, Tennessee Zip 37203; tel. 615/321–5591; William M. Inman, President

INSTITUTE OF PHYSICAL MEDICINE AND REHABILITATION, 6501 North Sheridan Road, Peoria, Illinois Zip 61614; tel. 309/692–8110; James W. Roodhouse, Administrator

INTERMEDICS ORTHOPEDICS, INC., 9900 Spectrum Drive, Austin, Texas Zip 78717; tel. 512/432–9400; Cindy Zhang, Research Analyst

INTERNATIONAL ASSOCIATION FOR HEALTHCARE SECURITY AND SAFETY, P.O. Box 637, Lombard, Illinois Zip 60148; tel. 708/953–0990; Nancy Felesena, Executive Assistant

J. STEPHENS MAYHUGH AND ASSOCIATES, INC., P.O. Box 900, New Roads, Louisiana Zip 70760; tel. 800/426–2349; Janet Stephens Mayhugh C.R.N.A.,, Chief Executive Officer

JANZEN, JOHNSTON AND ROCKWELL, EMERGENCY MEDICINE MANAGEMENT SERVICES, INC., 4551 Glencoe Avenue, Ste 260, Marina Del Rey, California Zip 90292; tel. 310/301–2030; Richard W. Sanders, Vice President Marketing

JOMAR INTERNATIONAL, 31831 Sherman Drive, Madison Heights, Michigan Zip 48071; tel. 313/585–5260; Edward T. Rourke, President

KANSAS HEALTH FOUNDATION, 309 East Douglas, Wichita, Kansas Zip 67202; tel. 316/262–7676; Don Stewart, Vice President and Senior Advisor

KIMBERLY CLARK CORPORATION PROFESSIONAL HEALTH CARE, 1400 Holcomb Bridge RD, Roswell, Georgia Zip 30076; tel. 404/587–8991; Joanne B. Bauer, Director

KNOWLEDGE DATA SYSTEMS, INC., 80 E Sir Francis Drake Boulevard, 2, Larkspur, California Zip 94939; tel. 415/461–5374; C. Lydon Neumann, President

KNOWLEDGE ENTERPRISES, 86 N Main Street, Ste 201, Chagrin Falls, Ohio Zip 44022–3011; tel. 216/543–7077; Shirley Engelhardt, President

KUHN AND WITTENBORN ADVERTISING, 2405 Grand Avenue, Suite 600, Kansas City, Missouri Zip 64108; tel. 816/471–7888; Julie Seifer, Account Supervisor

LANDIS AND GYR POWERS, INC., 1000 Deerfield Parkway, Buffalo Grove, Illinois Zip 60089; tel. 708/215–1000; Timothy M. O'Connor, Manager Healthcare Marketing

LIBERTY HEALTHCARE CORPORATION, 401 City Avenue, Ste 820, Bala Cynwyd, Pennsylvania Zip 19004; tel. 610/668–8800; Danielle Thompson, Administrative Assistant

LINC GROUP, INC., 303 East Wacker Drive, 1000, Chicago, Illinois Zip 60601; tel. 312/946–5500; Martin E. Zimmerman, President

LIVING HOPE INSTITUTE, 600 South McKinley, Ste 400, Little Rock, Arkansas Zip 72205; tel. 501/663–7878; D. Kimbro Stephens, Vice President

LOGIN BROTHERS BOOK COMPANY, INC., 1436 West Randolph Street, Chicago, Illinois Zip 60607; tel. 312/733–6424; Geoff Gustafson, Manager Operations

MARION MERRELL DOW INCORPORATED, P.O. Box 8480, Kansas City, Missouri Zip 64114–0480; tel. 816/966–4000

MARQUETTE ELECTRONICS, INC., 8200 West Tower Avenue, Milwaukee, Wisconsin Zip 53223; tel. 414/355–5000; Don Holt, Vice President National Sales

MASSACHUSETTS HALF–WAY HOUSES, INC., P.O. Box 34 – Back Bay Annex, Boston, Massachusetts Zip 02117; tel. 617/482–2580; J. Bryan Riley

MATRIX MEDICAL SERVICES, INC., 5735 Pineland, Suite 215, Dallas, Texas Zip 75231; tel. 214/361–6455

MAXUM HEALTH CORPORATION, 14850 Quorum Drive, Suite 400, Dallas, Texas Zip 75240–7012; tel. 214/716–6234; Kate Evans, Director Marketing

MCDERMOTT, WILL AND EMERY, 227 West Monroe St, Ste 3100, Chicago, Illinois Zip 60606; tel. 312/984–7765; Louis J. Corotsos, Partner

MCDONALD'S CORPORATION, Cob 2 North, Kroc Dr, Dept 090, Oak Brook, Illinois Zip 60521; tel. 708/575–3000; Elizabeth Blanco, Senior Manager Specials

MCGAW, INC., 2525 McGaw Avenue, Irvine, California Zip 92713–9791; tel. 714/660–2369; Bobby Y. Kutteh, Vice President Sales

MEDFORCE, A DIVISION OF MJP, INC., 3501 N Causeway, 6th Floor, Metairie, Louisiana Zip 70002; tel. 504/833–4796; Patrick E. Haggerty, Pres

MEDICAL EMERGENCY SERVICES ASSOCIATES, 4215 Kirchoff Road, Rolling Meadows, Illinois Zip 60008; tel. 708/925–8300; Michael Muhlenfeld, Vice President Administrative Services

MEDICAL MANAGEMENT DEVELOPMENT ASSOCIATES, INC., 10929 Technology Place, Ste A, San Diego, California Zip 92127; tel. 818/446–0979; Mary Ann Martin, Chief Operating Officer

MEDICAL PROTECTIVE COMPANY, 5814 Reed Road, Fort Wayne, Indiana Zip 46815; tel. 219/486–0424; Kathleen M. Roman, Director Risk Management

MEDICLEAN TECHNOLOGY, INC., 108 Roddy Avenue, South Attleboro, Massachusetts Zip 02703–7976; tel. 508/399–6400; Michael Kelly, President

MEDICODE, INC., 5225 Wiley Post Way, Ste 500, Salt Lake City, Utah Zip 84116–2889; tel. 801/536–1000; Eileen Shanon, President

MENTAL HEALTH MANAGEMENT, INC., 7601 Lewinsville Rd, Ste 200, McLean, Virginia Zip 22102; tel. 703/749–4600; Michael S. Pinkert, President and Chief Executive Officer

METPATH, One Malcolm Avenue, Teterboro, New Jersey Zip 07608; tel. 201/393–5166; Michael R. Napolitano, Director Hospital Partnership

METRIPLEX, INC., 25 First Street, Cambridge, Massachusetts Zip 02141; tel. 617/566–4358; Marc Stutman, Vice President

METRO MEDICAL GROUP, 1800 Tuxedo, Detroit, Michigan Zip 48206; tel. 313/252–1038

MIDMARK CORPORATION, 60 Vista Drive, Versailles, Ohio Zip 45380; tel. 513/526–3662; Robert Lammers, Trade Show Manager

MIRICH MEDICAL CORPORATION, 9001 Broadway, Merrillville, Indiana Zip 46410; tel. 219/769–3570; Eleanor Kay–Mirich R.N., B.S., MS,, Chief Executive Officer

MODERN HEALTHCARE, 740 North Rush Street, Chicago, Illinois Zip 60611; tel. 312/368–6644; Charles S. Lauer, Corporate Vice President

MODERN MANAGEMENT, INC., 101 Waukegan Road, Ste 90000, Lake Bluff, Illinois Zip 60044–1665; tel. 708/945–7400; Gus Martinucci, Director Information Services

MONARCH MARKING, P.O. Box 608, Dayton, Ohio Zip 45401; tel. 513/865–2161; Doug Fergusson, Marketing Manager

MUDGE ROSE GUTHRIE ALEXANDER & FERDON, 180 Maiden Lane, New York, New York Zip 10038; tel. 212/510–7000; Joseph J. Carroll Esq.,, Partner

NALC HEALTH BENEFIT PLAN, 20547 Waverly Court, Ashburn, Virginia Zip 22093–0001; tel. 703/729–4677; Harry D. Boteler, Administrator

NATIONAL ASSOCIATION OF HEALTH UNIT COORDINATORS, INC., 1821 University Ave, 162 S, Saint Paul, Minnesota Zip 55104–2869; tel. 612/641–8095; Florence Frye, President and Chief Execcutive Officer

NATIONAL ASSOCIATION OF HEALTHCARE ACCESS MANAGEMENT, 1200 19th Street N.W., Suite 300, Washington, District of Columbia Zip 20036; tel. 202/857–1125; Carol A. Lively, Executive Director

NATIONAL HEALTHCARE LINEN SERVICES, 1420 Peachtree Street N.E., Atlanta, Georgia Zip 30309; tel. 404/853–6142; William Gallagher, Business Manager

NATIONAL HEALTHCORP, L.P., P.O. Box 1398, Murfreesboro, Tennessee Zip 37130; tel. 615/890–2020; Laura E. McCoy, Manager Census Development

NORTH DAKOTA STATE DEPARTMENT OF HEALTH, DIVISION OF HEALTH FACILITIES, 600 East Boulevard Avenue, Bismarck, North Dakota Zip 58505–0200; tel. 701/224–2352; Fred Gladden, Chief

NURSE ON CALL, 3080 Northwoods Circle, 110, Norcross, Georgia Zip 30071; tel. 404/453–9170; Marty Branch, Director Sales

NURSING MANAGEMENT SERVICES, INC., 3423 Piedmont Road, Suite 500, Atlanta, Georgia Zip 30305; tel. 404/816–8678

OFFICE OF CIVILIAN HEALTH & MEDICAL PROGRAMS OF THE UNIFORMED SERVICES, Ochampus Library, Aurora, Colorado Zip 80045; tel. 303/361–3901; Paul T. McDavid

OLSTEN KIMBERLY QUALITY CARE, 175 Broadhollow Road, Melville, New York Zip 11747–4902; tel. 516/844–7800; Susan Sender, Director Clinical Practice

OMNIFLIGHT HELICOPTERS, INC., 4650 Airport Parkway, Dallas, Texas Zip 75248; tel. 214/233–6464; Lura Donnelly, Manager Healthcare Resource

ORGANON, INC., 375 Mount Pleasant Avenue, West Orange, New Jersey Zip 07052; tel. 201/325–4610; Jeanne Lampasona, Senior Market Research Analyst

OWEN HEALTHCARE, INC., 9800 Centre Parkway, Ste 1100, Houston, Texas Zip 77036; tel. 713/777–8173; Wendy Gold, Communications Coordinator

PDI COMMUNICATION SYSTEMS DIVISION, 40 Greenwood Lane, Springboro, Ohio Zip 45066; tel. 513/743–6010; Donald R. Rettich, Executive Vice President

PHYSICIAN INTERNATIONAL, 4 Vermont Street, Buffalo, New York Zip 14213; tel. 716/884–3700; Charles R. Cimasi, Chairman

PONDER AND COMPANY, P.O. Box 579, Herrin, Illinois Zip 62948–0579; tel. 618/942–7321; John Timmermann, Controller

POTOMAC POINT HEALTH CENTER, P.O. Box 39, Stafford, Virginia Zip 22555; tel. 703/659–4000; C. C. Adams Ph.D.,, President & Director

PREFERRED MEDICAL SERVICES, INC., P.O. Box 1474, Blue Bell, Pennsylvania Zip 19422–0439; tel. 215/641–9530; Dean M. Becker, President

PRIVATE HEALTHCARE SYSTEMS, INC., 15 Ledge Hill Road, Southborough, Massachusetts Zip 01772; tel. 617/895–7500; Dan Malloy, Director Research

QUANTUM SOLUTIONS, 1250 Capital of Texas Hwy S, Austin, Texas Zip 78746; tel. 512/329–8880; Kevin Rioux, Associate

QUARLES AND BRADY, 411 East Wisconsin Avenue, Milwaukee, Wisconsin Zip 53202; tel. 414/277–5000; Alyce C. Katayama, Partner

RATH AND STRONG, INC., 3820 Del Amo Boulevard, Ste 208, Torrance, California Zip 90503–2148; Dean Michelson, Senior Consultant

REHABCARE CORPORATION, 7733 Forsyth Boulevard, Suite 1700, Saint Louis, Missouri Zip 63105–1817; tel. 314/863–7422; James M. Usdan, President and Chief Executive Officer

REHABWORKS, 521 South Greenwood Avenues, Clearwater, Florida Zip 34616; tel. 813/442–6450; Jack Egan, President

RENFREW CENTER, 475 Spring Lane, Philadelphia, Pennsylvania Zip 19128; tel. 215/482–5353; Samuel Menaged, President

RENFREW CENTER, 7700 Renfrew Lane, Coconut Creek, Florida Zip 33073; tel. 305/698–9222; Barbara Peterson, Administrator

RESOURCE PRODUCTIVITY INSTITUTE, 158 Mt Vernon Drive, Boston, Pennsylvania Zip 15135; tel. 412/751–0807; James R. Surman, President

RURAL/METRO CORPORATION, 8401 East Indian School Road, Scottsdale, Arizona Zip 85251; tel. 602/994–3886; Michel A. Sucher M.D.,, Vice President, Medical Affairs

S. L. WABER, INC., 520 Fellowship Road, Ste 306, Mount Laurel, New Jersey Zip 08054; tel. 609/866–8888; Arthur H. Blumenthal, President

S.E.I. CORPORATION–HEALTHCARE PRACTICE, 680 East Swedesford Road, Wayne, Pennsylvania Zip 19087; tel. 215/254–1747; Dave Hendrix, Senior Marketing Manager

SAINT JOSEPH'S CARE GROUP, INC., P.O. Box 1935, South Bend, Indiana Zip 46634; tel. 219/237–7111; Dennis W. Heck, Chief Executive Officer

SHAND MORAHAN AND COMPANY, INC., 1007 Church Street, Evanston, Illinois Zip 60202; tel. 708/866–0713; Frances E. O'Connell R.N.,, Associate Product Manager

SHARED MEDICAL SYSTEMS, 51 Valley Stream Parkway, Malvern, Pennsylvania Zip 19355; tel. 215/296–6300; Susan B. West, Manager Communications

SHERIDAN HEALTHCORPORATION, 4651 Sheridan Street, Ste 400, Hollywood, Florida Zip 33021; tel. 305/987–3077; Charles Fotsch, Executive Vice President

SIGNAL MEDICAL SERVICES, INCORPORATED, 74 Batterson Park Road, Farmington, Connecticut Zip 06032; tel. 203/674–9991; Barry E. O'Brien, President

STEPHENS, LYNN, KLEIN AND MCNICHOLAS, P.A., 9130 S Dadeland Boulevard, Miami, Florida Zip 33156; tel. 305/670–3700; Oscar J. Cabanas, Partner

STEVENS AND LEE, P.O. Box 679, Reading, Pennsylvania Zip 19603; tel. 215/478–2203; David A. Vind

SUPPORT SYSTEMS INTERNATIONAL, 4349 Corporate Road, Charleston, South Carolina Zip 29405; tel. 803/740–8088; Roger E. Harris, Manager Market Research

SYNDICATED OFFICE SYSTEMS, 3 Imperial Promenade, Ste 1100, Santa Ana, California Zip 92707; tel. 714/438–6500; Arnold M. Robin, President

Associate Members / Other

TELERADIOLOGY SERVICES, INC., 950 Winter Street, Ste 3400, Waltham, Massachusetts Zip 02154; tel. 617/890-0060; Richard Wingard, Vice President

TEXAS MEDICAL CENTER, 406 Jesse Jones Library Bldg, Houston, Texas Zip 77030; tel. 713/791-8805; Richard E. Wainerdi, President

THE AON ALLIANCE, 101 Westpark Drive, Ste 160, Brentwood, Tennessee Zip 37027; tel. 615/371-5449; Corbette S. Doyle C.P.C.U., A.R.M.,, President and Chief Executive Officer

THE CANNON CORPORATION, 2170 Whitehaven Road, Grand Island, New York Zip 14072; tel. 716/773-6800; Christopher B. Miovski, Principal

THE MEADOWS, P.O. Box 97, Wickenburg, Arizona Zip 85358; tel. 602/684-3926; Patrick Mellody, Executive Director

TISSUE BANKS INTERNATIONAL, 815 Park Avenue, Baltimore, Maryland Zip 21201; tel. 301/752-3800; Richard L. Fuller, Chief Executive Officer

U.S. ARMY MEDICAL COMMAND, Fort Sam Houston, Texas Zip 78234; tel. 210/221-1211

U.S. AIR FORCE SCHOOL OF AEROSPACE MEDICINE, Usafsam-Cce, Brooks Air Force Base, Texas Zip 78235-5301; tel. 512/536-3342

U.S. NURSING CORPORATION, 3888 East Mexico Ave, Ste 129, Denver, Colorado Zip 80210; tel. 303/692-8550; Thomas D. Frey R.N.,, Director Nursing

U.S. ARMY AND AIR FORCE JOINT MEDICAL LIBRARY, 5109 Leesburg Pike, Ste 670, Falls Church, Virginia Zip 22041; tel. 703/756-8032; Timothy Gasper, Library Technician

UNITED HOSPITAL FUND OF NEW YORK, 350 Fifth Avenue, 23rd Floor, New York, New York Zip 10118; tel. 212/494-0700; James R. Tallon Jr., President

UNIVERSITY HOSPITAL CONSORTIUM, INC., 2001 Spring Road, Suite 700, Oak Brook, Illinois Zip 60521; tel. 708/954-1700; Robert J. Baker, President & Chief Executive Officer

V.D.I. TECHNOLOGIES, INC., 540 Lafayette Road, Hampton, New Hampshire Zip 03842; tel. 603/926-3100; Michael Lachapelle, Manager

VANTAGE HEALTH GROUP, 265 Conneaut Lake Road, Meadville, Pennsylvania Zip 16335; tel. 814/337-0000; David C. Petno, Vice President Business Development

VETERANS AFFAIRS - WESTERN REGION, 301 Howard Street, Suite 700, San Francisco, California Zip 94105

VETERANS AFFAIRS CENTRAL REGION OFFICE, P.O. Box 134002, Ann Arbor, Michigan Zip 48113-4002

VETERANS AFFAIRS EASTERN REGION OFFICE, 9600 North Point Road, Fort Howard, Maryland Zip 21052

VETERANS AFFAIRS MEDICAL REGIONAL OFFICE, P.O. Box 50188, Honolulu, Hawaii Zip 96850; tel. 808/541-1582

VETERANS AFFAIRS SOUTHERN REGION, 1461 Lakeover Road, Jackson, Mississippi Zip 39213; tel. 601/364-7920

VHA, INC., P.O. Box 140909, Irving, Texas Zip 75014-0909; tel. 214/830-0000; C. Thomas Smith, President and Chief Executive Officer

VILLAGE SOUTH, INC., 3180 Biscayne Boulevard, Miami, Florida Zip 33137; tel. 305/573-4357; Matthew Gissen, President

VISITING NURSES ASSOCIATION, 1710 Union Boulevard, Allentown, Pennsylvania Zip 18103; tel. 610/434-6134; Patricia Frenbuto, President

WICKWIRE GAVIN, P.C., 8100 Boone Boulevard, Ste 700, Vienna, Virginia Zip 22182-2642; tel. 703/790-8750; Michael C. Loulakis, Senior Manager

WOOD COMPANY, 6081 Hamilton Boulevard, Allentown, Pennsylvania Zip 18106; tel. 215/366-5295; Mitchell G. Possinger, Vice President Food and Nutrition Services

YAMANOUCHI USA, INC., 10 Bank Street, Ste 790, White Plains, New York Zip 10606; tel. 914/686-0556; Koki Ohashi, Marketing Manager

YANKEE ALLIANCE, 300 Brickstone Square, 5th Fl, Andover, Massachusetts Zip 01810-1429; tel. 508/475-2000; R. Paul O'Neill, President

ZIEGLER SECURITIES, One South Wacker Dr, Ste 3080, Chicago, Illinois Zip 60606; tel. 708/328-3637; Don A. Carlson Jr., President

Other Ambulatory Care

WESTERN NEW YORK AMBULATORY SERVICES, 550 Orchard Park Road, Buffalo, New York Zip 14224; tel. 716/675-7473; Ronald J. Esposito, Administrator

Other Health Care Educ Program

GEORGIA CENTER FOR CONTINUING EDUCATION, University of Georgia, Ste 298, Athens, Georgia Zip 30602; tel. 404/542-7553; Bonnie H. Lawson Ph.D.,, Head Human Relations Section

Preferred Provider Org

USA HEALTHNET, INC, 7301 N 16th Street, Ste 201, Phoenix, Arizona Zip 85020; tel. 602/371-3880; Beatrice E. Hughes, Executive Vice-President

Psychiatric Services Facility

CARON FOUNDATION, Box A, Wernersville, Pennsylvania Zip 19565-0501; tel. 215/678-2332; Leo C. McLaughlin, President and Chief Executive Officer

Recruitment Services

AMERICAN MEDSEARCH, INC., 555 West Madison, Suite 371, Chicago, Illinois Zip 60661; tel. 312/559-7878; Suk Graham, President

AMERICAN NURSE RECRUITERS CORPORATION, Medial Arts Building, Ste 307, Charleston, West Virginia Zip 25301; tel. 304/342-0144; David J. Lewis, President

DIVERSIFIED SEARCH INCORPORATED, 2005 Market Street, 33rd Floor, Philadelphia, Pennsylvania Zip 19103; tel. 215/732-6666; Judith M. Von Seldeneck, President

DURHAM MEDICAL SEARCH, INCORPORATED, P.O. Box 478, Depew, New York Zip 14043; tel. 716/618-7402; Rosemary Blando, Vice President Administration

JACKSON AND COKER, 115 Perimeter Ctr Pl, Ste 380, Atlanta, Georgia Zip 30346; tel. 404/393-1210; Robert J. Minton, Executive Vice President

School of Nursing

NORTHEASTERN HOSPITAL OF PHILADELPHIA SCHOOL OF NURSING, 2301 East Allegheny Avenue, Philadelphia, Pennsylvania Zip 19134; tel. 215/291-3000; Shirley L. Hickman Ph.D.,, Director School of Nursing

State Agency for Health

HOSPITAL DATA SYSTEMS-WASHINGTON STATE DEPARTMENT OF HEALTH, P.O. Box 47811, Olympia, Washington Zip 98504-7811; tel. 206/705-6000; Hank Brown, Acting Office Director

Waste Management

BIOMEDICAL WASTE SYSTEMS, INC., 200 High Street, Boston, Massachusetts Zip 02110; tel. 617/556-4033; Robert A. Pirragua, Director Operations

GTH ROLAND NORTH AMERICA, 8582 Katy Freeway, Suite 200, Houston, Texas Zip 77024; tel. 713/973-1467

WASTE MANAGEMENT OF NORTH AMERICA, 3003 Butterfield Road, Oakbrook, Illinois Zip 60521; tel. 708/572-8800; Bill Plunkett, Vice President

Information Systems

INFOMEDIKA, INC., 40 Mayaguez Street, Hato Rey, Puerto Rico Zip 00918; tel. 809/751-2080; Luis M Ramirez Ronda, President

Australia

Consulting Firm

KOLBACK ENVIRONMENTAL SERVICES AND CLINICAL WASTE, 2 Wiblen Street, Silverwater Nsw, Zip 2128; Paul F. Howlett, Chief Executive

Other

AUSTRALIAN HOSPITAL ASSOCIATION, 42 Thesiger Court, Deakin,

AUSTRALIAN INSTITUTE OF HEALTH AND WELFER, GPO Box 570, Canberra,; Judith Abercromby, Librarian

AUSTRALIAN PRIVATE HOSPITALS ASSOCIATION LTD, 25 Napier Close, Suite 1, Deakin,; M. M. Herring M.D.,, Executive Director

CEDAR COURT PRIVATE PHYSICAL REHABILITATION HOSPITAL, 370 Burke Road, Glen Iris, Victoria, Zip 3146; tel. 613/809-2444; Rodney G. Nissen, General Manager

THE VICTORIAN HOSPITALS' ASSOCIATION LIMITED, P.O. Box 365, South Melbourne, Zip 3205; tel. 613/266-3691; Allan D. Hughes, Executive Director

Provincial Hospital Assn

HEALTH SERVICES ASSOCIATION OF NEW SOUTH WALES, 1/3 Wharf Road, Leichhardt, Sydney, Zip 2040; Rod Young, Executive Director

Bahrain

Other

INTERNATIONAL HOSPITAL OF BAHRAIN, P.O. Box 1084, Manama,; F. S. Zeerah, President

Bermuda

Other

KING EDWARD VII MEMORIAL HOSPITAL, P.O. Box HM1023, Hamilton,; L. Keitha Walker, Health Sciences Librarian

Brazil

Consulting Firm

ADMINISTRACAO PLANEJAMENTO E PARTICIPACAO EM HOSPITAIS, Ave Angelica 2029, Sao Paulo SP, Zip 01227-200; Francisco Balestrin, Director Operations

CARE-HOSPITAL CONSULTANTS, R Cardoso De Almeida 60, S-61, Sao Paulo, Zip 05013-000; Edson G. Santos M.B.A.,, Director and Partner

MEDICAL ENTERPRISE PARTICIPACOES E ADMINISTRACAO, Rua da Assembleia, 10-GR 2920, Rio De Janeiro, Zip 20119-900; Ciro De Freitas Eloy, President

Other

CLINICA SAO VICENTE, Rua Joao Borges 204 - Gavea, Dogue,; Luiz Roberto Londres, President

SOC BEN SAO CAMILO-GHSUL, R Prof Ivocorsevil, 273, Porto Algre-RS, Zip 90 460-051; Nairio A Augusto P. Santos, Director

SOCIEDADE HOSPITAL SAMARITANO, Rua Conselheiro Brotero, 1486, Sao Paulo,; tel. 000/825-1122; Edson M. Dos Santos, General Superintendent

Canada

Architecture

CULHAM, PEDERSEN & VALENTINE, ARCHITECTS & ENGINEERS, 500 404 Sixth Avenue S.W., Calgery, Alberta Zip T2P 059; tel. 403/262-5511; Peter Traverso, Partner

WAISMAN DEWAR GROUT CARTER, INC., 300-1505 West Second Avenue, Vancouver, British Columbia Zip V6H 3Y4; tel. 604/737-7000; Ian Carter, Principal

Manufacturer / Supplier

IBEX TECHNOLOGIES, 5485 Pare, Montreal, Quebec Zip H4P 1P7; tel. 514/344-4004; Celine Houser, Product Director

Other

ALBERTA HEALTH-LIBRARY SERVICES BRANCH, P.O. Box 2222, Edmonton, Alberta Zip T5J 2P4; tel. 403/427-8720

ALBERTA HEALTHCARE ASSOCIATION, 10009-108th Street, Edmonton, Alberta Zip T5J 3C5; tel. 403/498-8400; Larry W. Odegard, President

CANADIAN COORDINATING OFFICE FOR HEALTH TECHNOLOGY ASSESSMENT, 110-Green Valley Crescent, Ottawa, Ontario Zip K2C 3V4; tel. 613/226-2553; Annie Hill, Librarian

COMCARE CANADA, LTD., 744 East Broadway, Vancouver V5L 2X9, British Columbia; tel. 604/873-6451; Patricia Turner, Administrator

COMCARE SOCIETE DU QUEBEC, INC., 4619 Rue St-Denis, Montreal, Quebec Zip H2J 2L4; tel. 514/932-1481; Kristine Audette, Corporate Supervisor

COMCARE, LTD, 18 Spadina Road, Toronto, Ontario Zip M5R 2S7; tel. 416/929-3364; Doris A. Nickerson, Executive Vice-President

Associate Members / Other

CONSPEC CONTROLS LIMITED, 44 Martin Ross Avenue, Downsview, Ontario Zip M3J 2KB; tel. 416/661–0500; Steve Hodges, General Manager

DARCOR CASTERS, INC, 7 Staffordshire Place, Toronto, Ontario Zip MlJ 3L3; tel. 416/255–8563; Cyril J. Muhic, Regional Sales Manager

DESJARDINS LIFE INSURANCE, 200 Avenue Des Commandeurs, Levis, Quebec Zip G6V 6R2; tel. 800/465–6390; Lucie Auger, Director

ELECTROLINE EQUIPMENT, 8265 St Michel, Montreal, Quebec Zip H12 3E4; tel. 514/374–6335; Beth Leve, Manager

FEDERATION DES MEDECINS OMNIPRATICIENS DU QUEBEC, 1440 Ouest Ste Catherine, 1100, Montreal, Quebec Zip H3G 1R8; tel. 514/878–1911; Ghislaine Lincourt, Librarian

FIRST GROUP. INC, 1611 Cremazie East Boulevard, Montreal, Quebec Zip H2M 2P2; tel. 514/383–1611; Lise Boivin, Adm Asst

MEDIREX SYSTEMS, 499 Queen Street East, Toronto M5A 1V1, Ontario; tel. 416/363–9313; Mark D. Caskenette, Consultant

MITEL CORPORATION, P.O. Box 13089, Kanata, Ontario Zip K2K 1X3; tel. 613/592–2122; Michael F. Branchaud, Health Care Manager

PEOPLE AND PROCESS SOLUTIONS, INC., 1120 Finch Ave West, Ste 604, North York, Ontario Zip MEJ 3H7; tel. 416/661–1946; Eileen P. Page, President

SASKATCHEWAN ASSOCIATION OF HEALTH ORGANIZATIONS, 1445 Park Street, Regina, Saskatchewan Zip S4N 4C5; tel. 306/525–2741; John Carter, Education Services Director

SASKATCHEWAN HOSPITAL SERVICES PLAN, 3475 Albert Street, Regina S4S 6X6, Saskatchewan; tel. 306/565–2345

ST. JOSEPH'S HEALTH CARE SYSTEM, P.O. Box 155, Station A, Hamilton, Ontario Zip L8N 3A2; tel. 905/528–0138; Brian Guest, Executive Director

THERMAL ENERGY INTERNATIONAL, 14N Chatsworth Avenue, Ste 4D, Larchmont, Ontario Zip 10538; tel. 613/723–6776; Nick Maiorino, Vice President Sales

TOTAL CARE TECHNOLOGIES, INC., 200–1909 Bredin Road, Kewwna, British Columbia Zip VIY 759; tel. 604/763–0034; Al Hildebrandt, President

UNIVERSITY OF MANITOBA ELIZABETH DAFOE LIBRARY, University of Manitoba, Winnipeg, Manitoba Zip R3T 2N2; tel. 204/474–9881; Bob Lincoln, Head Acquisitions

State Health Planning/Development Agency

GREATER VANCOUVER REGIONAL HOSPITAL DISTRICT, 4330 Kingsway Street, Burnaby V5H 4G8, British Columbia; tel. 604/731–1155; Greg Stump, Administrator

Cayman Islands

Other

CAYMAN ISLANDS GENERAL HOSPITAL, P.O. Box 915, Grand Cayman Islands,; tel. 809/949–8604; Mervyn Conolly, Administrator

INDIAN HOSPITAL CORPORATION LIMITED, Appollo Hosps Complex, Hyderabad, Andhra, Zip 500 034; E. Kumar, General Manager Projects

Chile

Other

CLINICA SANTA MARIA, Avenida Santa Maria 0410, Santiago,; Pedro Navarrete, Chief Executive Officer

School of Medicine

PONTIFICIA UNIVERSIDAD CATOLICA DE CHILE FACULTAD DE MEDICINA, Lira 44, Santiago,; Jamie Bellolio Rodriguez, Administrator

Columbia

Other

FUNDACION SANTA FE DE BOGOTA, Calle 116 9–02, Santa Fe De Bogota,; Ana Catalina Vesquez Quintero, Manager

FUNDACION SANTA FE DE BOGOTA, Apartado Aereo, Bogota,; Roberto Esguerra M.D.,, Director

France

Other

THE AMERICAN HOSPITAL OF PARIS, 63 Boulevard Victor Hugo, Neuilly–S/Sein 92202,; Patrice Triaureau, General Director

Greece

Other

DIAGNOSTIC AND THERAPEUTIC CENTRE OF ATHENS HYGEIA, S A, 4 Erythrou Stavrou & Kifissiap, Athens, Zip 15233; C. Kitsionas, Executive Director

India

Other

MANGALAM HOSPITALS PVT. LTD., Baker Junction, Kottayam 68606,; Saji Varghese M.D.,, President

Israel

Other

HADASSAH MEDICAL ORGANIZATION, Box 12000, Jerusalem, Zip 01120; Samuel Penchas M.D.,, Director General

Japan

Other

NAVAL REGIONAL MEDICAL CENTER, FPO, Zip 96362

ST. LUKE'S INTERNATIONAL HOSPITAL, 10–1 Akashi–Cho, Chuo–Ku, Tokyo,; Shigeaki Hinohara M.D.,, President

Kuwait

Consulting Firm

INTERNATIONAL HEALTH SERVICES, K.S.C.C., P.O. Box 29729 Safat Code 13158, Kuwait City,; Richard Beadleston, Chief Operating Officer

Lebanon

Other

AMERICAN UNIVERSITY OF BEIRUT MEDICAL CENTER, 850 Third Avenue, 18th Floor, New York, Zip 10022; Faysal B. Najjar M.D.,, Director

Malaysia

Other

GLENEAGLES MEDICAL CENTRE, 1 Jalan Pangkor, Penang 10050,; Ronald Koh, Administrator

JOHOR SPECIALIST HOSPITAL, 39–B, Jalan Abdul Samad, 80100 Johor Bahru,; tel. 07/227–8118; Puan Siti Sa'diah Sa–Diah Bakir, Director & Administrator

Mexico

Other

HOSPITAL MEXICO–AMERICANO, Calle Colomos 2110, Guadalajara,; Jorge Angel Rodriquez, Administrator

SHRINERS HOSPITAL FOR CRIPPLED CHILDREN, Suchil 152, Col El Rosario, Mexico City,; Carmen G. Solorzano, Administrator

UNIVERSIDAD LA SALLE, Francia 5, Col Florida, Zip 01030; Maximiliano Villanueva, Associate

Other Inpatient Care

HOSPITAL ERNESTO CONTRERAS R., 2505 Congress St, Ste 120, San Diego, Zip 92110; tel. 619/297–6191; J. Ernesto Contreras Jr. M.D.,, Medical Director

Pakistan

Facilities Management

SHAUKAT KHANUM MEMORIAL CANCER HOSPITAL AND RESEARCH CENTER, 29 Shah Jamal, Lahore 54600,; David Wood, Director

Panama

Other

CLINICA SAN FERNANDO, Panama Exp A100 P.O. Box 527948, Miami, Zip 33152–7948; Ernesto Arosemena M.D.,, Medical Director

Peru

Other

ASOCIACION BENEFICA ANGLO AMERICANA, Ave Alfredo Salazar 3 Era, Lima 27,; Gonzalo Garrido–Lecca, Director

SOUTHERN PERU COPPER CORPORATION, 180 Maiden Lane, 22nd Floor, New York, Zip 10038; tel. 515/476–1148; Rod G. Guzman, General Director of Hospitals

Philippines

Facilities Management

WATEROUS MEDICAL CORPORATION, 166 Pilar Street, San Juan, Manila,; Eleanor M. Santiago M.D., M.P.H.,, Vice Chairperson

Other

ST. LUKE'S MEDICAL CENTER, 279 E Rodriguez Sr Boulevard, Quezon City,; Jose F G. Ledesma, Chief Executive Officer

Qatar

Other

HAMAD GENERAL HOSPITAL, Box 3050, Doha,

Saudi Arabia

Facilities Management

DR. SULAIMAN MEDICAL CENTER, P.O. Box 58586, Riyadh, Zip 11515; Sulaiman Al–Alawait, Director General

Associate Members / Other

Saudi Arabia

Facilities Management
SAUDI CATERING AND CONTRACTING, P.O. Box 308, Riyadh 11411,; Samir S. Layous, Regional Regional Manager

Other
ABDUL RAHMAN AL MISHARI GENERAL HOSPITAL, Olaya, Riyadh 11564,; Abdul Rahman Al Mishari M.D.,, President
AL-HAWRAA CLINICS, Civil Defense Street, Hofuf,; Talal Bu Khamsin, President
AL-SALAMA HOSPITAL, P.O. Box 40030, Jeddah,; Atef S. Salloum M.D.,, Director Development and Planning
GREEN CRESCENT HEALTH SERVICES, P.O. Box 3096, Riyadh, Zip 11471; Wail Buraik M.D.,, President
KING FAHAD HOSPITAL AT AL BAHA, P.O. Box 204, Al Baha,; Mustafa Abdirahman Ahmed, Buyer
MUHAMMAD S BASHARAHIL HOSPITAL, P.O. Box 10505, Makkah,; Sameer M. Basharahil, Vice-President
PRINCE FAHD BIN SULTAN HOSPITAL, P.O. Box 254, Tabuk,; Rajai M. Dajani, Director
SAUDI ARAMCO MEDICAL SERVICES, 9009 West Loop South, Houston, Zip 77096; Daniel Blucker, Medical Library Supervisor
SAUDI TRADING AND SERVICES INTERNATIONAL COMPANY, P.O. Box 90401, Riyadh, Zip 11613; Eli A. Chedid, Division Manager

Singapore

Other
BIOMEDICAL ENGINEERING DEPARTMENT, Outram Road, Singapore 0316,; tel. 065/321-4608; R. Chandrasekhar, Manager

Taiwan

Other
CHANG GUNG MEMORIAL HOSPITAL, 199 Tun Hwa North Road, Taipei,; Yi-Chou Chuang, Director Administration Center
MACKAY MEMORIAL HOSPITAL, 92-Sec-2 North Chung San Road, Taipei,; Rick C C. Huang, Vice Superintendent
NATIONAL TAIWAN UNIVERSITY HOSPITAL, 1 Chang-Te Street, Taipei,; Tung-Yuan Tai M.D.,, Director
VETERANS GENERAL HOSPITAL, 201 Shihpai Rd, Sec Ii, Peitou, Taipei,

Trinidad & Tobago

Other
ERIC WILLIAMS MEDICAL SCIENCES COMPLEX AUTHORITY, Uriah Butler Highway, Trinidad,; tel. 809/645-2940; Trevor J. Romano, Chief Executive Officer

Turkey

Other
BAYMER A. S. CHILDREN'S AND WOMEN'S HOSPITAL, Fisekhane Cad, 18, Bakirkoy-Istanbul,; A. Oktay Cini M.D.,, President

United Arab Emirates

Other
AMERICAN HOSPITAL-DUBAI, P.O. Box 59, Dubai,; Saeed M. Almulla, Chief Executive Officer

Venezuela

Other
ASOCIACION CIVIL COROMOTO, HOSPITAL COROMOTO, P.O. Box 422, Maracaibo-Zulia,; Luis A. Parejo M.D.,, Medical Directro
COLIMODIO, S.A., P.O. Box 52-1308, Miami, Zip 33152; Fernando Colimodio, Pres

B Health Care Systems

- **B2** Introduction
- 3 Integrated Health Delivery Networks
- 8 Statistics for Multihospital Health Care Systems and Their Hospitals
- 9 Health Care Systems and Their Hospitals
- 84 Headquarters of Health Care Systems, Alphabetically
- 85 Headquarters of Health Care Systems, By System Code
- 92 Headquarters of Health Care Systems, Geographically
- 100 Alliances

Introduction

This section includes listings for Integrated Health Delivery Networks, Health Care Systems and Alliances.

Integrated Health Delivery Networks

New in this edition of the *AHA Guide* is a listing of integrated health delivery networks. An integrated health delivery network (network) is defined as a group of hospitals, physicians, other providers, insurers and/or community agencies that work together to coordinate and deliver a broad spectrum of services to their community. Organizations listed represent the lead or hub of the network activity. Networks are listed by state, then alphabetically by name.

The network identification process has purposely been designed to capture networks of varying organization type. Sources include but are not limited to the following: *AHA Annual Survey*, national, state and metropolitan associations, national news and periodical searches, and the networks and their health care providers themselves. Therefore, networks are included regardless of whether a hospital or health care system is the network lead. When an individual hospital does appear in the listing, it is indicative of the role the hospital plays as the network lead. In addition, the network listing is **not** mutually exclusive of the hospital, health care system or alliance listings within this publication.

Networks are very fluid in their composition as goals evolve and partners change. Therefore, some of the networks included in this listing may have dissolved, reformed, or simply been renamed as this section was being produced for publication. It is our hope that you will use the integrated health delivery network update/correction form provided to keep us informed of any changes that have occurred. Simply tear out the perforated form, complete and return to the address listed at the bottom.

The network identification process is an on-going and responsive initiative. As more information is collected and validated, it will be made available in other venues, in addition to the *AHA Guide*. In the future, we hope to provide information on the specific partners included within each network. For more information concerning the network identification process, please contact the AHA at 312/422-3511.

Health Care Systems

To reflect the diversity that exists among health care organizations, the AHA uses the term health care system to identify both multihospital and diversified single hospital systems.

Multihospital Systems

A multihospital health care system is two or more hospitals owned, leased, sponsored, or contract managed by a central organization.

The AHA's data reflects the known universe of multihospital health care systems, despite membership status.

Single Hospital Systems

Single, freestanding member hospitals may be categorized as health care systems by bringing into Type IV-A membership three or more, and at least 25 percent, of their owned or leased non-hospital preacute and postacute health care organizations. (For purposes of definition, health care delivery is the availability of professional health care staff during all hours of the organization's operations). Type IV-A organizations provide, or provide and finance, diagnostic, therapeutic, and/or consultative patient or client services that normally precede or follow acute, inpatient, hospitalization; or that serve to prevent or substitute for such hospitalization. These services are provided in either a freestanding facility not eligible for licensure as a hospital under state statue or through one that is a subsidiary of a hospital. The AHA's data on single-hospital health care systems reflects membership information and not the universe of all such hospitals that may be eligible for classification as a single hospital system.

The first part of this section is an alphabetical list of multihospital systems. Each system listed contains two or more hospitals, which are listed under the system by state. Data for this section were compiled from the 1994 *Annual Survey* and the membership information base as published in section A of the *AHA Guide*.

One of the following codes appears after the name of each system listed to indicate the type of organizational control reported by that system:

- **CC** Catholic (Roman) church-related system, not-for-profit
- **CO** Other church-related system, not-for-profit
- **NP** Other not-for-profit system, including nonfederal, governmental systems
- **IO** Investor-owned, for profit system
- **FG** Federal Government

One of the following codes appears after the name of each hospital to indicate how that hospital is related to the system:

- **O** Owned
- **L** Leased
- **S** Sponsored
- **CM** Contract-managed

The second part of this section lists health care systems in three ways: by system code, alphabetically, and geographically by state and city. Every effort has been made to be as inclusive and accurate as possible. However, as in all efforts of this type, there may be omissions. For further information, write to the section for Health Care Systems, American Hospital Association, One North Franklin, Chicago, IL 60606-3401.

Alliances

An alliance is a formal organization, usually owned by shareholders/members, that works on behalf of its individual members inthe provision of services and products and in the promotion of activities and ventures. The organization functions under a set of bylaws or other written rules to which each member agrees to abide.

Alliances are listed alphabetically by name. Its members are listed alphabetically by state, city, and then by member name.

Integrated Health Delivery Network Update/Correction Form

Please complete and return this form with updates, corrections or additional information on any of the integrated health delivery networks listed.

Name _____

Title _____

Organization _____

Mailing Address _____

City_____ State_____ Zip _____

Telephone (_____) - _____

Signature _____

To report an update/correction please follow these steps.

- Make a photocopy of the page containing the listing
- Highlight the information that needs to be updated
- Staple the highlighted photocopy to this form
- Provide the correct or additional information below (PLEASE TYPE OR PRINT NEATLY)

Page #	Printed Information	Correct/Additional Information
_____	_____	_____
	_____	_____
	_____	_____
_____	_____	_____
	_____	_____
	_____	_____

Return this form by October 31, 1995 to:

Dale Matthews
Health Statistics Group
American Hospital Association
One North Franklin
29th Floor
Chicago, IL 60606-3401

Listing of Network Type Arrangements

ALABAMA
Alabama Health Services, P.O. Box 12407, Birmingham, 35202-2407

Provider of Rural Health Network, P.O. Box 11126, Montgomery, 36111

ALASKA
Ketchikan General Hospital, 3100 Tongass Avenue, Ketchikan, 99901

Norton Sound Regional Hospital, P.O. Box 966, Nome, 99762

ARIZONA
Arizona Voluntary Hospital Federation, 1430 West Broadway, Suite A110, Tempe, 85282

Carondelet Integrated Delivery System, 1601 West Saint Mary's Road, Tucson, 85745

Health Partners of Southern Arizona, 5301 East Grant, Tucson, 85712

Lutheran Healthcare Network, 500 West 10th Place, Mesa, 85201

Maricopa Health System, 2601 East Roosevelt Street, Phoenix, 85008

Samaritan Health Services, 1441 North 12th Street, Phoenix, 85006

Saint Luke's Health System, 1800 East Van Buren Street, Phoenix, 85006

ARKANSAS
Arkansas Network, 5106 McClanahan, Suite E, North Little Rock, 72116

Baptist Health, 9601 Interstate 630, Exit 7, Little Rock, 72205

First Source of Arkansas, P.O. Box 2181, Little Rock, 72203-2181

CALIFORNIA
Adventist Health System–Loma Linda, 11161 Anderson Street, Loma Linda, 93250

Adventist Health System–West, 2100 Douglas Boulevard, Roseville, 95661-3898

Catholic HealthCare West, 1700 Montgomery Street, San Francisco, 94111

CCN, Inc., 8911 Balboa Avenue, San Diego, 92123

Cedars Sinai Medical Center, 8700 Beverly Boulevard–Rm2802, Los Angeles, 90048

East Bay Medical Network, 2000 Powell Street, 9th Floor, Emeryville, 94608

Essential HealthCare Network, 525 North Garfield Park, Montery Park, 91754

Fremont–Rideout Health Group, 970 Plumas Street, Yuba City, 95991

Friendly Hills HealthCare Network, 931 South Beach, LaHabra, 90631

HCP/Mulliken Medical Centers, 26000 Altamont Road, Los Altos Hills, 94022-4398

Health First Network, 4020 5th Avenue, 3rd Floor, San Diego, 92103

InterMountain Healthcare Network, 228 McDowell Street, Alturas, 96101

Kaiser Foundation Health Plan of Northern California, 1950 Franklin Street, Oakland, 94612

Little Company of Mary Health Services, 4101 Torrance Boulevard, Torrance, 90503

Los Angeles Integrated Delivery Network, 501 South Buena Vista Street, Burbank, 91505

NorthBay Healthcare Services, 1200 B Gale Wilson Boulevard, Fairfield, 94533

Saint Joseph Health System, 440 South Batavia Street, Orange, 92668-3995

ScrippsHealth, 4275 Campus Point Court, San Diego, 92121

Sharp Healthcare, 3131 Berger Avenue, Suite 100, San Diego, 92123

Southern California Healthcare, 1300 East Green Street, Pasadena, 91106

Sutter Health, 2800 L Street, Sacramento, 95816

Tenet Healthcare Corporation, 2700 Colorado Avenue, Santa Monica, 90404

UniHealth, 4100 West Alameda, Burbank, 91505

COLORADO
Community Health Providers Organization, 2021 North 12th Street, Grand Junction, 81501

Health & Medical Network of Colorado, 555 East Pikes Peak, Suite 108, Colorado Springs, 80903

Health One, 8200 East Belleview Avenue, Suite 202, Englewood, 80111

High Plains Rural Health Network, 218 East Kiowa Avenue, Fort Morgan, 80701

Penrose–Saint Francis Healthcare, P.O. Box 7021, Colorado Springs, 80917

Primera Health Care, 600 Grant Street, Suite 700, Denver, 80203-3525

Quorum Health Network of Colorado, 4450 Arapahoe Avenue, Suite 200, Boulder, 80303

The Children's Hospital, 1056 East 19th Avenue, Denver, 80218

CONNECTICUT
Connecticut Health System, 55 Farmington Boulevard, Hartford, 06105

Saint Francis Network, 114 Woodland Street, Hartford, 06105

Saint Mary's Hospital, 56 Franklin Street, Waterbury, 06706

DELAWARE
Delaware Network Health Plan, 801 Middlefield Road, Seaford, 19973

Medical Center of Delaware Foundation, P.O. Box 1668, Wilmington, 19899

FLORIDA
Adventist Health Care–Sunbelt Health Care, 2400 Bedford Road, Orlando, 32803

Allegany Health System, 6200 Courtney Campbell Causeway, Tampa, 33607-1458

Baptist Health Care, Inc., 1000 West Moreno, Pensacola, 32501

Baptist/Saint Vincent's Health System, 800 Prudential Drive, Jacksonville, 32207-8244

Bay Care Health Network, 17757 U.S. Highway 19, Tampa Bay, 34524

Columbia/HCA Central Florida Division, 2111 Glenwood Drive, Suite 100, Winter Park, 32792-3309

Columbia/HCA North Florida Division, 3627 University Boulevard South, Suite 810, Jacksonville, 32216

Columbia/HCA NorthEast Florida Division, 3627 University Boulevard South, Suite 810, Jacksonville, 32216

Columbia/HCA South Florida Division, 7975 NorthWest 154th Street, Suite 400A, Miami Lakes, 33106

Columbia/HCA SouthWest Florida Division, Barnett Center, 2000 Main Street, Suite 600, Fort Myers, 33901

Columbia/HCA Tampa Bay Division, 6200 Courtney Campbell Causeway, Suite 100, Tampa, 33607

Community Care Network of Indian River, 1000 36th Street, Vero Beach, 32960

Community Health Network of South Florida, 4725 North Federal Highway, Fort Lauderdale, 33308

Dimensions Heatlh/Baptist Health System, 8900 North Kendall Drive, Miami, 33176

Florida Health Choice, 800 Meadows Road, Boca Raton, 33486

Florida Hospital Health Network, 601 East Rollins Street, Orlando, 32803

Genesis Health, Inc., 3627 University Boulevard South, Jacksonville, 32216

Heartland Rural Health Network, 2010 East Georgia Street, Bartow, 33830

Med Connect, 4901 NorthWest 17th Way, Suite 304, Fort Lauderdale, 33309

Methodist Health Systems, 580 West Eighth Street, Jacksonville, 32209

Orlando Regional Healthcare, 1414 Kuhl Avenue, Orlando, 32806

The Health Advantage Network, 2111 Glenwood Drive, Winter Park, 32792

GEORGIA
Candler Health System, 5353 Reynolds Street, Savannah, 31412

Chattahoochie Health Network, P.O. Box 3274, Gainesville, 30505

Columbus Regional HealthCare Network, 2000 10th Avenue, Suite 200, Columbus, 31901

Community Healthcare Network, 707 Center Street, Suite 400, Columbus, 31902-0790

Emory University System of Healthcare Affiliate Network, 1365 Clifton Road Northeast, Atlanta, 30322

Georgia First Network, 101 West Ponce De Leon, Suite 320, Decatur, 30030

Grady Health System, 80 Butler Street, Atlanta, 30335

Medical Resource Network, 900 Circle, 75 Parkway, Suite 1450, Atlanta, 30339

National Cardiovascular Network, 6 Concourse Parkway, Suite 2950, Atlanta, 30328

Northwest Georgia Healthcare Partnership, P.O. Box 308, Dalton, 30722

Saint Joseph's Hospital of Atlanta, 5665 Peachtree Dunwoody Road, Atlanta, 30342

SouthCare Medical Alliance, 400 North Creek, Suite 300, Atlanta, 30327

University Hospital, 1350 Walton Way, Augusta, 30911

HAWAII
Pacific Health Care, 1946 Young Street, Honolulu, 96826

Queens Health Systems, 1301 Punchbowl Street, Honolulu, 96813

IDAHO
North Idaho Rural Health Consortium, 700 Ironwood Drive, Suite 310, Coeur d'Alene, 83814

ILLINOIS
Advocate Health Care, 2025 Windsor Drive, Oak Brook, 60521-0222

Alexian Brothers Health Systems, 600 Alexian Way, Elk Grove Village, 60007

Columbus Cabrini Medical System, 2520 North Lakeview Avenue, Chicago, 60614

Family Health Network, 205 North Michigan Avenue, Chicago, 60611

Listing of Network Type Arrangements

Freeport Regional Health Alliance, 1045 West Stephenson Street, Freeport, 61032

MEDACOM Tri-State, 1315 West 22nd Street Suite 405, Oakbrook, 60521

Mercer County Community Care Network, 409 NorthWest Ninth Avenue, Aledo, 61231

Northwestern Health Care Network, 980 North Michigan Avenue, Suite 1500, Chicago, 60611

Rush System for Health, 1725 West Congress Parkway, Chicago, 60612

Servantcor, 335 East Fifth Avenue, Clifton, 60927

Southern Illini Healthcare Network, P.O. Box 1588, Mount Vernon, 62864

SwedishAmerican Health System, 1400 Charles Street, Rockford, 61104

Synergon Health System, 520 South Maple Avenue, Oak Park, 60160

The Carle Foundation, 611 West Park Street, Urbana, 61801

University of Chicago Hospitals & Health Network, 5841 South Maryland Avenue, Chicago, 60637

INDIANA

HealthQuest, One Caylor–Nickel Square, Bluffton, 46714

Holy Cross Health System, 3606 East Jefferson Boulevard, South Bend, 46615–3097

Memorial Health System, Inc., 707 North Michigan Street, Suite 100, South Bend, 46601

Methodist Hospital of Indiana, P.O. Box 1367, Indianapolis, 46202

Midwest Health Net, Inc., 6407 Constitution Drive, Fort Wayne, 46804

Sagamore Health Network, Inc., 11555 North Meridian, Suite 400, Carmel, 46032

Saint Vincent Community Health Network, 2001 West 86th Street, Indianapolis, 40970

Suburban Health Organization, 1 American Square, Indianapolis, 46282

IOWA

Genesis Medical Center, 1227 East Rushmore Street, Davenport, 52803

Mercy Network, 400 University Avenue, Des Moines, 50309

Health Network of Iowa, 1200 Pleasant Street, Des Moines, 50304

North Iowa Mercy Health Network, 84 Beaumont Drive, Mason City, 50401

Saint Lukes/Iowa Health System, P.O. Box 3026, Cedar Rapids, 52406–3026

KANSAS

Great Plains Health Alliance, P.O. Box 366, Phillipsburg, 67661

Hays Medical Center, 2220 Canterbury Road, Hays, 67601

JayHawk Health Alliance, 215 West 151st Street, Olathe, 66061

SouthEast Kansas Network, 1400 West 4th Street, Coffeyville, 67337

Sunflower Health Network, 400 South Santa Fe Avenue, Salina, 67401

KENTUCKY

Alliant Health System, 1200 East Gray Street, Louisville, 40202

Baptist Healthcare System, 4007 Kresge Way, Louisville, 40207

Blue Grass Family Health Plan, 651 Perimeter Park, Suite 2B, Lexington, 40517

Caritas Health Services, 1850 Bluegrass Avenue, Louisville, 40215–1199

Centercare, 800 Park Street, BowlingGreen, 42101

Community Health Delivery System, Inc., 2020 Newburg Road, Louisville, 40205

Saint Elizabeth Medical Center, 1 Medical Village Drive, Covington, 41017

LOUISIANA

Healthcare Advantage, Inc., 4427 Robertson, New Orleans, 70115

Lakeview Regional Health Network, 95 East Fairway Drive, Covington, 70433

Louisiana Health Care Authority, 8550 United Plaza Boulevard, Baton Rouge, 70809

Ochsner/Sisters of Charity Health Network, One Galleria Boulevard, Suite 1224, New Orleans, 70001

Peoples Health Network, 111 Veterans Memorial Boulevard, Metaire, 70005

MAINE

Blue Hill Memorial Hospital, Water Street, Blue Hill, 04614

Healthnet, 268 Stillwater Avenue, Bangor, 04401

Synernet, Inc., 222 Saint John Street, Suite 329, Portland, 04102

MARYLAND

Dimensions HealthCare System, 9200 Basil Court, Landover, 20785

Helix Health System, 2330 West Joppa Road, Suite 301, Lutherville, 21093

Johns Hopkins Health System, 600 North Wolfe Street, Baltimore, 21287

Maryland Health Network, 10440 Little Patuxent, Columbia, 21044

University Medical Network, 14 University of Maryland Avenue, Baltimore, 21201

MASSACHUSETTS

Baystate Health System, 759 Chestnut Street, Springfield, 01199

Beth Israel HealthCare, 330 Brookline Avenue, Boston, 02215

Children's Hospital, 300 Longwood Avenue, Boston, 02115

Continuum of Care Network, 57 Union Street, Marlborough, 01752

Fallon Healthcare System, Chestnut Place, 10 Chestnut Street, Worcester, 01608

Lahey Network, 41 Mall Road, Burlington, 01805

New England Health Partnership, 34 Washington Street, Suite 320, Waltham, 02181–1903

Partners HealthCare System, 32 Fruit Street, Boston, 02114

Pathway Health Network, 1 Deaconess Road, Boston, 02215

MICHIGAN

Battle Creek Health System, 300 North Avenue, Battle Creek, 49016

Butterworth Health System, 100 Michigan Street, S.E., Grand Rapids, 49503

Detroit–Macomb Hospital Corporation, 11800 East Twelve Mile Road, Warren, 48093

Detroit Medical Center, 4201 Saint Antoine Boulevard, Detroit, 48201

Genesys Health System, 302 Kensington Avenue, Flint, 48503–2000

Great Lakes Health Network, P.O. Box 5153, Southfield, 48086

Henry Ford Health System, 600 Fisher Boulevard, Detroit, 48202

Hospital Network, Inc., One Healthcare Plaza, Kalamazoo, 49007

Lakeland Regional Health System, 1234 Napier Avenue, Saint Joseph, 49085

Mercy Health Services, 34605 Twelve Mile Road, Farmington Hill, 48331–3221

Munson Health Care System, 1105 Sixth Street, Traverse City, 49684

Muskegon Mercy Community Health Care System, 1500 East Sherman Boulevard, Muskegon, 49443

William Beaumont Hospital Corporation, 3601 West Thirteen Mile Road, Royal Oak, 48073

MINNESOTA

Affiliated Community Health Network, Inc., 101 Wilmar Avenue, S.W., Willmar, 56201

Allina Health System, 5601 Smetana Drive, Minnetonka, 55430

Criterion HealthCare Network, 100 Washington Square, Suite 748, Minneapolis, 55401

Dakota Clinic, P.O. Box 65460, Saint Paul, 55164

Fairview Health System, 2450 Riverside Avenue, Minneapolis, 53454

Healtheast, 1450 Energy Park Drive, Saint Paul, 55108

HealthPartners, 8100 34th Avenue South, Minneapolis, 55440

I–35 Corridor Health Network, 760 West Fourth Street, Rush City, 55069

Itasca Partnership for Quality Healthcare, 501 Pokegama Avenue, Grand Rapids, 55744

Mayo Foundation, 200 SouthWest First Street, Rochester, 55905

Minnesota Rural Health Cooperative, P.O. Box 104, Willmar, 56201

Northern Lakes Health Consortium, 600 East Superior Street, Suite 404, Duluth, 55802

Northstar Health Consortium, 715 Delmore Drive, Roseau, 56751

Quality Health Alliance, 501 Holly Lane, Mankato, 56001

Quality Health Network, 910 Main Street, Suite 202, Redwing, 55066

Southwest Minnesota Health Alliance, 305 East Luverne Street, Luverne, 56156

MISSISSIPPI

North Mississippi Health Services, 830 South Gloster Street, Tupelo, 38801

MISSOURI

BJC Health System, 4444 Forest Park Avenue, Suite 500, Saint Louis, 63108–2259

Health Midwest, 2304 East Meyer Boulevard, A–20, Kansas City, 64132

Mid–America Health First, Inc., 1000 Carondelet Drive, Kansas City, 64114

Northwest Missouri Healthcare Agenda, 705 North College Avenue, Albany, 64402

Saint Louis Health Care Network, 477 North Lindbergh Boulevard, Saint Louis, 63141

Unity Health Network, 425 South Woods Mill Road, Suite 150, Chesterfield, 63017

MONTANA

Montana Health Network, Inc., 11 South 7th Street, Suite 160, Miles City, 59301

Northern Rockies Healthcare Network, P.O. Box 4587, Missoula, 59806

NEBRASKA

Community Health Vision, 10250 Regency Circle, Suite 350, Omaha, 68144

Rural Healthcare Network, 821 Morehead Street, Chadron, 69337

Rural Health Partners, P.O. Box 980, Lexington, 68850

NEW HAMPSHIRE

Partners In Caring, 243 Elm Street, Claremont, 03743

Tri–County Community Care Network, Aiken Avenue, Franklin, 03102

HealthLink, 80 Highland Street, Laconia, 03246

Saint Joseph Health Care, 172 Kinsley Street, Nashua, 03061

Listing of Network Type Arrangements

NEW JERSEY
AtlantiCare Health System, P.O. Box 1460, Pleasantville, 08232
Cape Advantage Health Alliance, Two Stone Habor Boulevard, Cape May, 08210
Clara Maass Health System, One Franklin Avenue, Belleville, 07109
Community/Kimball Health Care System, 99 Highway 37 West, Toms River, 08755
First Option Health Plan, 2 Bridge Street, Red Bank, 07701
General Hospital Center Health Network, 350 Boulevard, Passaic, 07055
Healthcare Network of New Jersey, 253 Withspoon Street, Princeton, 08540–3213
Qualcare, Inc., 242 Old Brunswick Road, Piscataway, 08854
Seton Health Network, Inc., 703 Main Street, Paterson, 07503
SSM Health Care Ministry Corporation, 22 Bloomfield Avenue, Denville, 07834

NEW MEXICO
Lovelace, 5400 Gibson Boulevard, S.E., Albuquerque, 87108
Medical Network of New Mexico, 700 Lomas Boulevard, N.E., Suite 200, Albuquerque, 87102
Presbyterian HealthCare Services, Inc., P.O. Box 26666–6666, Albuquerque, 87125–6666
University of New Mexico Health Science Center, 2211 Lomas Boulevard, N.E., Albuquerque, 87106

NEVADA
Saint Mary's Health Network, 235 West Sixth Street, Reno, 89520

NEW YORK
Adirondack Rural Health Network, 100 Park Street, Glens Falls, 12801
Allegany Rural Health Network, 191 North Main Street, Wellsville, 14895
Bassett Healthcare, 1 Atwell Road, Cooperstown, 13326
Beth Israel Health Care System, 16th Street & 1st Avenue, New York, 10003
Buffalo General Health System, 100 High Street, Buffalo, 14203
Catholic Health Care Network, 75 Vanderbilt Avenue, Staten Island, 10304
Chemung County Rural Health Network, 600 Roe Avenue, Elmira, 14905
Chenango County Rural Health Network, 179 North Broad Street, Norwich, 13815
Columbia–Presbyterian Med Center Health Alliance, Columbia–Presbyterian Med Center, New York, 10032
Community Memorial Hospital, 150 South Broad Street, Hamilton, 13346
Cortland Area Rural Health Network, 134 Homer Avenue, Cortland, 13045
Eastern Adirondack Health Care Network, P.O. Box 466, Westport, 12993
Episcopal Health Services, Inc., 333 Earle Ovington Boulevard, Uniondale, 11787
First Choice Network, Inc ., 165 EAB Plaza, West Tower 6, Uniondale, 11556–1165
Four Lakes Rural Health Network, 196 North Street, Geneva, 14456
Franciscan Health System,Tri–State Region, 160 East Main Street, Port Jervis, 12771
Greater Rochester Health System, 1040 University Avenue, Rochester, 14607
Greene County Rural Health Network, 71 Prospect Avenue, Catskill, 12534
Health First, 555 West 57th Street, Suite 1520, New York, 10019
Lake Ontario Rural Health Network, 200 Ohio Street, Medina, 14103
MercyCare Corporation, 315 South Manning Boulevard, Albany, 12208
MoHawk Valley Network, Inc., P.O. Box 5068, Utica, 13502–5068
Mount Sinai Health System, P.O. Box 1068, New York, 10029
New York Hospital Care Network, 525 East 68th Street, New York, 10021
North Shore Regional Health Systems, 300 Community Drive, Manhasset, 11030
Northern NY Rural Health Care Alliance, 200 Woolworth Building, Watertown, 13601
Oswego County Rural Health Network, 110 West Sixth Ave, Oswego, 13126
Park Ridge Health System, 1555 Long Pond Road, Rochester, 14626
Preferred Health Network, Inc., 45 Avenue & Parsons Boulevard, Flushing, 11355
Premier Preferred Care, 441 Lexington Avenue, New York, 10017
Queens Regional Health Network, 79–01 Broadway, Elmhurst, 11373
Seton Health Care System, 1300 Massachusetts Avenue, Troy, 12180
Shared Health Network, 125 Wolf Road, Suite 404, Albany, 12205
Sisters of Charity Health Care System, 75 Vanderbilt Avenue, Staten Island, 10304
Sullivan County Rural Health Network, Bushville Road, Harris, 12742
The Brooklyn Health Network, 121 DeKalb Avenue, Brooklyn, 11201
The Excelcare System, Inc., 33 Palmer Avenue, Bronxville, 10708
UHS Healthcare System–Binghamton, P.O. Box 540, Johnson City, 13790
Westchester Health Services Network, 116 Radio Circle Drive, Mount Kisco, 10549

NORTH CAROLINA
Alliance For Community Health, 10 Sunnybrook Road, Raleigh, 27620
Bladen County Hospital, Clarkton Road, Elizabethtown, 28337
Carolinas Hospital Network, P.O. Box 32861, Charlotte, 28232
Central Carolina Rural Hospital Alliance, P.O. Box 938, Albemarle, 28002
Duke Health Network, 3100 Tower Building, Suite 600, Durham, 27707
Eastern Carolina Health Network, P.O. Box 6028, Greenville, 27835
North Carolina Baptist Hospitals, Inc., Medical Center Boulevard, Winston–Salem, 27157
UNC Health Network, 101 Manning Drive, Chapel Hill, 27514
Western North Carolina Health Network, 509 Biltmore Avenue, Asheville, 28801

NORTH DAKOTA
MeritCare Health System, 720 Fourth Street North, Fargo, 58122

OHIO
Cleveland Health Network, 9500 Euclid Avenue, H18, Cleveland, 44195
Community Care Network in Akron, P.O. Box 2090, Akron, 44309–2090
Community Hospitals of Ohio, 1320 West Main Street, Newark, 43055–3699
Comprehensive Healthcare of Ohio, Inc., 630 East River Street, Elyria, 44035
County Based Healthcare Network, 2420 Lake Avenue, Ashtabula, 44004
First Interhealth Network, 3454 Oak Alley Court, Suite 510, Toledo, 43606
Health Care Alliance, 6001 East Broad Street, Columbus, 43213
Healthcare Alliance of Greater Cincinnati, 2139 Auburn Avenue, Cincinnati, 45219
HealthCare Consortium of Ohio, 410 West Tenth Avenue, Columbus, 43210
Health Cleveland, 18101 Lorain Avenue, Cleveland, 44111
Lake Erie Health Alliance, 2142 North Cove Boulevard, Toledo, 43606
Lake Hospital System, 10 East Washington, Painesville, 44077
Merida Health System, 6700 Beta Drive, Suite 200, Mayfield Village, 44143
Northeast Ohio Health Network, 400 Wabash Avenue, Akron, 44307
Promedica Network, 2142 North Cove Boulevard, Toledo, 43606
Saint Lukes Medical Center, 11311 Shaker Boulevard, Cleveland, 44104
Summa Health System, 525 East Market Street, Akron, 44309
TriHealth, 619 Oak Street, Cincinnati, 45206
The MetroHealth System, 2500 MetroHealth Drive, Cleveland, 44109–1998
The Mount Sinai Health Care System, One Mount Sinai Drive, Cleveland, 44106
United Health Partners, 2213 Cherry Street, Toledo, 43608
University Hospitals of Cleveland, 11000 Euclid Avenue, Cleveland, 44106
West Central Ohio Regional Health Alliance, 730 West Market Street, Lima, 4580–4670

OKLAHOMA
Eastern Oklahoma Health Network, P.O. Box 14147, Tulsa, 74114
First Health West, 4411 West Gore Boulevard, Lawton, 73505
Oklahoma Health System, 3300 NorthWest Expressway, Oklahoma City, 73112
Mercy Health System, 4300 West Memorial Road, Oklahoma City, 73120
Presbyterian Hospital Network, 700 NorthEast 13th Street, Oklahoma City, 73104
University Hospitals, P.O. Box 26307, Oklahoma City, 73104

OREGON
Central Oregon Hosp Network (CONET), 2500 NorthEast Neff Road, Bend, 97701
Coordinated HealthCare Network, 3030 SouthWest Moody, Suite 230, Portland, 97201–4897
Health Future, Inc., 825 East Main Street, Suite D, Medford, 97504
Inter Community Health Network, 3600 North Samaritan Drive, Corvallis, 97339
Legacy Health System, 1919 NorthWest Lovejoy Street, Portland, 97209
Oregon Health System in Collaboration, 4000 Kruse Way Place, Lake Oswego, 97035
Peace Health, 770 East 11th Avenue, Eugene, 97440–1479
Providence Health System, 1235 NorthEast 47th Avenue, Portland, 97213

PENNSYLVANIA
Albert Einstein Health Care Network, 1200 West Tabor Road, Philadelphia, 19141
Alpha Health Network, Foster Plaza, Pittsburgh, 15220
Community Benefits Strategy, P.O. Box 447, DuBois, 15801
Community Health Net, 1202 State Street, Erie, 16501
Crozer–Keystone Health System, 1400 North Providence Road, Media, 19063

Listing of Network Type Arrangements

First Health Alliance, 10 Duff Road, Suite 211, Pittsburgh, 15235

Fox Chase Network, 7701 Burholme Avenue, Philadelphia, 19111

Geisinger Health Care System, 100 North Academy Avenue, Danville, 17822–3311

Great Lakes Health Network, 201 State Street, Erie, 16550

Laurel Health System, 15 Meade Street, Wellsboro, 16901–1813

Main Line Health, 259 Radnor–Chestnut Road, Radnor, 19087

Partnership for Community Health–Lehigh Valley, P.O. Box 689, Allentown, 18105

Prime Care, 2601 North 3rd Street, Harrisburg, 17110

Providence Health System, 1100 Grampian Boulevard, Williamsport, 17701

QualMed Plans for Health of Pennnsylvania, 500 North Gulph Road, Suite 200, King of Prussia, 19406

Sacred Heart Healthcare Systems, Fourth & Chew Streets, Allentown, 18102

Saint Francis Health System, 4410 Penn Avenue, Pittsburgh, 15224

Saint Margaret Health System, 815 Freeport Road, Pittsburgh, 15215

Saint Vincent Health System, 311 West 24th Street, Suite 304, Erie, 16544

Temple Univeristy Health Network, Broad & Ontario Streets, Philadelphia, 19140

Health Share, 111 South 11th Street, Philadelphia, 19107

University of Pennsylvania Health System, 3400 Spruce Street, Philadelphia, 19104

University of Pittsburgh Medical Center, 3811 O'Hara Street, Pittsburgh, 15213

Vantage Health Care Network, Inc., 265 Conneaut Lake Road, Meadville, 16335

RHODE ISLAND

Saint Joseph Hospital, 200 High Service Avenue, Providence, 02904

Lifespan, 167 Point Street, Providence, 02903

SOUTH CAROLINA

Carolina HealthChoice Network, 4408 Forest Drive, Suite 200, Columbia, 29206

Healthfirst of the Greenville Hospital System, 701 Grove Road, Greenville, 29605

Palmetto Community Health Network, 900 C Main Street, Conway, 29526

Premier Health System, Inc., Taylor at Marion Streets, Columbia, 29220

Richland Community Health Partners, 3 Medical Park, Suite 100, Columbia, 29203

Saint Francis Health System, One St. Francis Drive, Greeneville, 29601

SOUTH DAKOTA

Black Hills Healthcare Network, 430 Oriole Drive, Suite 1A, Spearfish, 57783

Missouri Valley Healthcare Network, 1017 West 5th Street, Yankton, 57078

TENNESSEE

Bristol Healthcare Network, Inc., P.O. Box 989, Bristol, 37621

Columbia Healthcare Network, 310 25th Avenue North, Suite 109, Nashville, 37203

Chattanooga Healthcare Network, 401 Chestnut Street, Suite 222, Chattanooga, 37402

Methodist Health Systems, Inc., 1211 Union Avenue, Memphis, 38104

Mountain States Healthcare Network, 400 North State of Franklin Road, Johnson City, 37604

Nashville Healthcare Partnership, 161 Fourth Avenue North, Nashville, 37219

Premier Health Network, 313 Princeton Road, Suite 7, Johnson City, 37601

Saint Thomas Hospital, 4220 Harding Road, Nashville, 37205

Middle Tennessee Healthcare, Inc., 2000 Church Street, Nashville, 37236

TEXAS

Bay Area Healthcare Group, LTD, 5650 South Staples, Suite 108, Corpus Christi, 78411

Baylor Health Care Network, 2625 Elm Street, Suite 204, Dallas, 75226

Brazo's Valley Health Network, 3115 Pine Avenue, Waco, 76708

Care Alliance of the Southwest, 14901 Quorum Drive, Suite 200, Dallas, 75240

Central Texas Rural Health Network, 503 East 4th Street, Harrietsville, 77964–2824

Good Shepard Health Network, 700 East Marshall Avenue, Longview, 75601

Gulf Coast Provider Network, 2900 North Loop West, Suite 1230, Houston, 77092

Gulf Health Network, 701 University Boulevard, Suite 229, Galveston, 77550

Harris Methodist Network, 611 Ryan Park Plaza, Arlington, 76011

HealthCare Partners of East Texas, Inc., P.O. Box 6340, Tyler, 75711

Lubbock Methodist Hospital System, 3615 19th Street, Lubbock, 79410

Memorial/Sisters of Charity Health Network, 7737 SouthWest Freeway, Suite 200, Houston, 77074

Methodist Health Care System, 7700 Floyd Curl Drive, San Antonio, 78229

Metroplex Health Network, 2201 South Cleer Creek Road, Kileen, 75642

North Texas Health Network, 5601 MacArthur, Suite 300, Irving, 75038

North Texas Healthcare Network, 3333 Lee Parkway, Suite 900, Dallas, 75919

Permian Basin Rural Health Network, P.O. Box 1648, Fort Stockton, 79735

Presbyterian Healthcare System, 8200 Walnut Hill Lane, Dallas, 75231

Primary Care Network of Texas, 62443 IH 10 West, Suite 1001, San Antonio, 78201

Regional Healthcare Alliance, 800 East Dawson Street, Tyler, 75701

SouthEast Texas Hospital System, 233 West 10th Street, Dallas, 75208

SouthEast Texas Integrated Community Health Network, 2600 North Loop, Houston, 77092

SouthWest Texas Rural Health Alliance, 143 East Garza, New Braunfels, 78130

Saint David's Health Network, P.O. Box 49192, Austin, 78765

Saint Paul Medical Center Affiliate Network, 5909 Harry Hines Boulevard, Dallas, 75235

Texoma Health Network, 1600 11th Street, Wichita Falls, 76301

The Heart Network of Texas, 101 East Park Boulevard, Plano, 75074

UTAH

Intermountain HealthCare/Amerinet, 36 South State Street, 22nd Floor, Salt Lake City, 84111

VERMONT

Fletcher Allen Health Care, 111 Colchester Avenue, Burlington, 05401

VIRGINIA

Carilion Health System, 1212 Third Street, S.W., Roanoke, 24016

Central Virginia Health Network, 8100 Three Chopt Street, Suite 209, Richmond, 23229

DePaul Medical Center Group, 150 Kingsley Lane, Norfolk, 23505

Inova Health System, 8001 Braddock Road, Springfield, 22151

Preferred Care of Richmond, 9100 Arboretum Parkway, Richmond, 23236

Sentara Health System, 6015 Poplar Hall Drive, Suite 306, Norfolk, 23502

Valley Health System, P.O. Box 3340, Winchester, 22604

Virginia Health Network, 7400 Beaufont Springs Drive, Richmond, 23225

WASHINGTON

Columbian Basin Health Network, P.O. Box 185, Mead, 99021

Dominican Network, 5633 North Lidgerwood, Spokane, 99207

Group Health Cooperative of Pugent Sound, 521 Wall Street, Seattle, 98121

Health Washington, 700 Fifth Avenue, Suite 4500, Seattle, 98104–5044

PeaceHealth, 15325 SouthEast 30th Place, Suite 300, Bellevue, 98007

Multicare Health System, 315 South K Street, Tacoma, 98405

Providence Services, 9 East Ninth Street, Spokane, 99202

WEST VIRGINIA

Camcare, P.O. Box 1547, Charleston, 25326

Eastern West Virginia Health Services Network, P.O. Box 1019, Petersburg, 26847

Integrated Provider Network, 7000 Hampton Center, Suite F, Morgantown, 26505

Mid–Ohio Valley Rural Health Network, P.O. Box 718, Parkersburg, 26102

Morgan City Primary Care Network, 1124 Fairfax Street, Berkeley Spring, 25411

North Central West Virginia Rural Health Network, P.O. Box 1680, Clarksburg, 26302

Southern Virginia Rural Health Network, 500 Cherry Street, Bluefield, 24701

Tri–State Community Care Network, 601 Colliers Way, Weirton, 26062

Webster Memorial/United Hospital Center, 324 Miller Mountain Drive, Webster Springs, 26288

WISCONSIN

Affinity Health System, Inc., 631 Hazel Street, Oshkosh, 54902–5677

All Saints Healthcare System, 3801 Spring Street, Racine, 53405

Aurora Health Care, P.O. Box 343910, Milwaukee, 53234–3910

Columbia Health System, Inc., 2025 East Newport Avenue, Milwaukee, 53211

Community Health Care, Inc., 425 Pine Ridge Boulevard, Wausau, 54401

Community Health Network, Inc., 225 Memorial Drive, Berlin, 54923

Covenant Healthcare Systems, Inc., 1126 South 70th Street, Suite S306, Milwaukee, 53214–0970

Felician Health Care–Milwaukee Region, 3237 South 16th Street, Milwaukee, 53215

Franciscan Health System, Inc., 615 South Tenth Street, LaCrosse, 54601

Health Care Network of Wisconsin, 250 Bishops Way, Suite 300, Brookfield, 53005

Horizon Healthcare, Inc., 2300 North Mayfair Road, Suite 550, Milwaukee, 53226

Lutheran Health System, 1910 South Avenue, LaCrosse, 54601

Luther/Midelfort/Mayo Health System, 733 West Clairmont, Eau Claire, 54701

Marshfield Clinic's Regional System, 1000 North Oak Avenue, Marshfield, 54449

Prairie du Chien Partnership, 705 East Taylor Street, Prairie du Chie, 53821

Southern Wisconsin Health Care System, 1000 Mineral Point Avenue, Janesville, 53545–5003

University of Wisconsin Hospital & Clinics, 600 Highland Avenue, Madison, 53792

Waukesha Hospital System, Inc., 725 American Avenue, Waukesha, 53188

WYOMING

Jackson Hole Community Health Network, P.O. Box 428, Jackson, 83001

Wyoming Integrated Network, 1233 East 2nd Street, Casper, 82601

Statistics for Multihospital Health Care Systems and their Hospitals

The following tables describing multihospital health care systems refer to information in section B of the 1995 *AHA Guide*.

Table 1 shows the number of multihospital health care systems by type of control. Table 2 provides a breakdown of the number of systems that own, lease, sponsor or contract manage hospitals within each control category. Table 3 gives the number of hospitals and beds in each control category as well as total hospitals and beds. Finally, Table 4 shows the percentage of hospitals and beds in each control category.

For more information on multihospital health care systems, please write to the Section for Health Care Systems, One North Franklin, Chicago, Illinois 60606–3401 or call 312/422–3000.

Table 1. Multihospital Health Care Systems, by Type of Organizational Control

Type of Control	Code	Number of Systems
Catholic (Roman) church–related	CC	62
Other church–related	CO	13
Subtotal, church–related		75
Other not–for–profit	NP	162
Subtotal, not–for–profit		237
Investor owned	IO	37
Federal Government	FG	5
Total		279

Table 2. Multihospital Health Care Systems, by Type of Ownership and Control

Type of Ownership	Catholic Church–Related (CC)	Other Church–Related (CO)	Total Church–Related (CC + CO)	Other Not–for–Profit (NP)	Total Not-for-Profit (CC, CO, + NP)	Investor–Owned (IO)	Federal Government	All Systems
Systems that only own, lease or sponsor	51	8	59	132	191	26	5	222
Systems that only contract–manage	0	0	0	2	2	1	0	3
Systems that manage, own, lease, or sponsor	11	5	16	28	44	10	0	54
Total	62	13	75	162	237	37	5	279

Table 3. Hospitals and Beds in Multihospital Health Care Systems, by Type of Ownership and Control

Type of Ownership	Catholic Church–Related (CC)		Other Church–Related (CO)		Total Church–Related (CC + CO)		Other Not–for–Profit (NP)		Total Not-for-Profit (CC, CO, + NP)		Investor–Owned (IO)		Federal Government		All Systems	
	H	B	H	B	H	B	H	B	H	B	H	B	H	B	H	B
Owned, leased or sponsored	430	106,985	88	17,710	518	124,695	714	178,026	1,232	302,721	771	105,582	311	84,780	2,314	493,083
Contract–managed	57	5,717	9	857	66	6,574	111	8,361	177	14,935	317	30,346	0	0	494	45,281
Total	487	112,702	97	18,567	584	131,269	825	186,387	1,409	317,656	1,088	135,928	311	84,780	2,808	538,364

H = hospitals; B = beds.

Table 4. Hospitals and Beds in Multihospital Health Care Systems, by Type of Ownership and Control, as a Percentage of All Systems

Type of Ownership	Catholic Church–Related (CC)		Other Church–Related (CO)		Total Church–Related (CC + CO)		Other Not–for–Profit (NP)		Total Not-for-Profit (CC, CO, + NP)		Investor–Owned (IO)		Federal Government		All Systems	
	H	B	H	B	H	B	H	B	H	B	H	B	H	B	H	B
Owned, leased or sponsored	18.6	21.7	3.8	3.6	22.4	25.3	30.9	36.1	53.2	61.4	33.3	21.4	13.4	17.2	100.0	100.0
Contract–managed	11.5	12.6	1.8	1.9	13.4	14.5	22.5	18.5	35.8	33.0	64.2	67.0	0.0	0.0	100.0	100.0
Total	17.3	20.9	3.5	3.4	20.8	24.4	29.4	34.6	50.2	59.0	38.7	25.2	11.1	15.7	100.0	100.0

H = hospitals; B = beds.
*Please note that figures may not always equal the provided subtotal or total percentages due to rounding.

Health Care Systems and Their Hospitals

2175: ADVENTIST HEALTH SYSTEM–LOMA LINDA (NP)
11161 Anderson Street, Loma Linda, CA Zip 92350; tel. 909/824-4459; David B. Hinshaw Sr. M.D., President

CALIFORNIA: LOMA LINDA UNIVERSITY BEHAVIORAL MEDICINE CENTER (O, 89 beds) 1710 Barton Road, Redlands, CA Zip 92373; tel. 714/793-9333; Edward H. Weiss, Administrator

LOMA LINDA UNIVERSITY COMMUNITY MEDICAL CENTER (O, 850 beds) 11234 Anderson Street, Loma Linda, CA Zip 92354-2870, Mailing Address: P.O. Box 2000, Zip 92354-0200; tel. 909/824-0800; J. David Moorhead M.D., President and Chief Executive Officer

Owned, leased, sponsored:	2 hospitals	939 beds
Contract–managed:	0 hospitals	0 beds
Totals:	2 hospitals	939 beds

★4165: ADVENTIST HEALTH SYSTEM–SUNBELT HEALTH CARE CORPORATION (CO)
111 North Orlando Avenue, Winter Park, FL Zip 32789-3675; tel. 407/897-1919; Mardian J. Blair, President

FLORIDA: EAST PASCO MEDICAL CENTER (O, 96 beds) 7050 Gall Boulevard, Zephyrhills, FL Zip 33541-1399; tel. 813/788-0411; Bob A. Dodd, President

FLORIDA HOSPITAL KISSIMMEE (O, 120 beds) 200 Hilda Street, Kissimmee, FL Zip 34741-2301; tel. 407/933-6600; Eugene K. Wedel, Administrator

FLORIDA HOSPITAL MEDICAL CENTER (O, 1394 beds) 601 East Rollins Street, Orlando, FL Zip 32803-1489; tel. 407/896-6611; Thomas L. Werner, President

FLORIDA HOSPITAL–WALKER (O, 151 beds) 2501 U.S. Highway 27 North, Avon Park, FL Zip 33825-1200, Mailing Address: P.O. Box 1200, Zip 33825-1200; tel. 813/453-7511; Samuel Leonor, President

FLORIDA HOSPITAL–WATERMAN (O, 182 beds) 201 North Eustis, Eustis, FL Zip 32726, Mailing Address: P.O. Box B, Zip 32727-0377; tel. 904/589-3333; Royce C. Thompson, President

GEORGIA: GORDON HOSPITAL (O, 50 beds) 1035 Red Bud Road, Calhoun, GA Zip 30701, Mailing Address: P.O. Box 12938, Zip 30703-7013; tel. 706/629-2895; Dennis Kiley, President

SMYRNA HOSPITAL (O, 100 beds) 3949 South Cobb Drive, Smyrna, GA Zip 30080; tel. 404/434-0710

KENTUCKY: MEMORIAL HOSPITAL (O, 63 beds) 401 Memorial Drive, Manchester, KY Zip 40962-9156; tel. 606/598-5104; T. Henry Scoggins FACHE, President

NORTH CAROLINA: PARK RIDGE HOSPITAL (O, 87 beds) Naples Road, Fletcher, NC Zip 28732, Mailing Address: P.O. Box 1569, Zip 28732-1569; tel. 704/684-8501; Robert W. Burchard, President

TENNESSEE: JELLICO COMMUNITY HOSPITAL (L, 54 beds) Jellico, TN, Mailing Address: Route 1, Box 197, Zip 37762; tel. 615/784-7252; Kenneth R. Mattison, President

TAKOMA ADVENTIST HOSPITAL (O, 116 beds) 401 Takoma Avenue, Greeneville, TN Zip 37743; tel. 615/639-3151; Paul Michael Norman, President

TENNESSEE CHRISTIAN MEDICAL CENTER (O, 289 beds) 500 Hospital Drive, Madison, TN Zip 37115; tel. 615/865-2373; Milton R. Siepman, President and Chief Executive Officer

TEXAS: CENTRAL TEXAS MEDICAL CENTER (CM, 109 beds) 1301 Wonder World Drive, San Marcos, TX Zip 78666, Mailing Address: Box 1169, Zip 78667; tel. 512/353-8979; Joel W. Hass, President and Chief Executive Officer

HUGULEY MEMORIAL MEDICAL CENTER (O, 213 beds) 11801 South Freeway, Fort Worth, TX Zip 76115, Mailing Address: Box 6337, Zip 76115-0337; tel. 817/293-9110; A. David Jimenez, President and Chief Executive Officer

METROPLEX HOSPITAL (CM, 198 beds) 2201 South Clear Creek Road, Killeen, TX Zip 76542-9305; tel. 817/526-7523; Ernie W. Sadau, President and Chief Executive Officer

WILLOW CREEK HOSPITAL (O, 92 beds) 7000 Highway 287 South, Arlington, TX Zip 76017-2805; tel. 817/561-1600; Donald K. Sykes, Jr., Chief Executive Officer

Owned, leased, sponsored:	14 hospitals	3007 beds
Contract–managed:	2 hospitals	307 beds
Totals:	16 hospitals	3314 beds

0235: ADVENTIST HEALTH SYSTEM/WEST (CO)
2100 Douglas Boulevard, Roseville, CA Zip 95661-3898, Mailing Address: P.O. Box 619002, Zip 95661-9002; tel. 916/781-2000; Frank F. Dupper, President

CALIFORNIA: ANACAPA HOSPITAL (O, 24 beds) 307 East Clara Street, Port Hueneme, CA Zip 93041; tel. 805/488-3661; Dennis N. Fliegelman, Administrator

FEATHER RIVER HOSPITAL (O, 121 beds) 5974 Pentz Road, Paradise, CA Zip 95969-5593; tel. 916/877-9361; George Pifer, President

FRANK R. HOWARD MEMORIAL HOSPITAL (L, 28 beds) Madrone and Manzanita Streets, Willits, CA Zip 95490, Mailing Address: Box 1430, Zip 95490; tel. 707/459-6801; Robert J. Walker, President

GLENDALE ADVENTIST MEDICAL CENTER (O, 463 beds) 1509 Wilson Terrace, Glendale, CA Zip 91206-4007; tel. 818/409-8000; Robert G. Carmen, President

HANFORD COMMUNITY MEDICAL CENTER (O, 54 beds) 450 Greenfield Avenue, Hanford, CA Zip 93230-0240, Mailing Address: Box 240, Zip 93232-0240; tel. 209/582-9000; Stan B. Berry FACHE, Chief Executive Officer

PARADISE VALLEY HOSPITAL (O, 130 beds) 2400 East Fourth Street, National City, CA Zip 91950; tel. 619/470-4321; Fred M. Harder, President

SAN JOAQUIN COMMUNITY HOSPITAL (O, 178 beds) 2615 Eye Street, Bakersfield, CA Zip 93301, Mailing Address: Box 2615, Zip 93303-2615; tel. 805/395-3000; Fred Manchur, President

SIMI VALLEY HOSPITAL AND HEALTH CARE SERVICES (O, 209 beds) 2975 North Sycamore Drive, Simi Valley, CA Zip 93065-1277; tel. 805/527-2462; Alan J. Rice, President and Chief Executive Officer

SONORA COMMUNITY HOSPITAL (O, 112 beds) 1 South Forest Road, Sonora, CA Zip 95370; tel. 209/532-3161; Lary Davis, President

ST. HELENA HOSPITAL (O, 168 beds) 650 Sanitarium Road, Deer Park, CA Zip 94576, Mailing Address: P.O. Box 250, Zip 94576; tel. 707/963-3611; Lenard Heffner M.D., President and Chief Executive Officer

UKIAH VALLEY MEDICAL CENTER (O, 116 beds) 275 Hospital Drive, Ukiah, CA Zip 95482; tel. 707/462-3111; ValGene Devitt, President and Chief Executive Officer

WHITE MEMORIAL MEDICAL CENTER (O, 354 beds) 1720 Brooklyn Avenue, Los Angeles, CA Zip 90033-2481; tel. 213/268-5000

HAWAII: CASTLE MEDICAL CENTER (O, 160 beds) 640 Ulukahiki Street, Kailua, HI Zip 96734-4498; tel. 808/263-5500; Kenneth A. Finch, President and Administrator

OREGON: PIONEER MEMORIAL HOSPITAL (CM, 32 beds) 564 East Pioneer Drive, Heppner, OR Zip 97836, Mailing Address: P.O. Box 9, Zip 97836; tel. 503/676-9133; Kevin R. Erich, Administrator

PIONEER MEMORIAL HOSPITAL (CM, 25 beds) 1201 North Elm Street, Prineville, OR Zip 97754; tel. 503/447-6254; Roger W. Strobel, President and Chief Executive Officer

PORTLAND ADVENTIST MEDICAL CENTER (O, 270 beds) 10123 Southeast Market, Portland, OR Zip 97216-9966; tel. 503/257-2500; Larry D. Dodds, President

TILLAMOOK COUNTY GENERAL HOSPITAL (L, 20 beds) 1000 Third Street, Tillamook, OR Zip 97141-3430; tel. 503/842-4444; Wendell Hesseltine, President

UTAH: MONUMENT VALLEY HOSPITAL (CM, 20 beds) 4 Rock Door Canyon, Monument Valley, UT Zip 84536, Mailing Address: P.O. Box 360004, Zip 84536; tel. 801/727-3241; Raymond T. Carney, Chief Executive Officer

WASHINGTON: WALLA WALLA GENERAL HOSPITAL (O, 72 beds) 1025 South Second Avenue, Walla Walla, WA Zip 99362, Mailing Address: Box 1398, Zip 99362; tel. 509/525-0480; Rodney T. Applegate, President

Owned, leased, sponsored:	16 hospitals	2479 beds
Contract–managed:	3 hospitals	77 beds
Totals:	19 hospitals	2556 beds

For explanation of codes following names, see page B2.
★Indicates Type III membership in the American Hospital Association.

Systems / Advocate Health Care

★0064: **ADVOCATE HEALTH CARE** (NP)
2025 Windsor Drive, Oakbrook, IL Zip 60521-0222;
tel. 708/990-5002; Richard R. Risk, President and Co-Chief
Executive Officer
ILLINOIS: BETHANY HOSPITAL (O, 138 beds) 3435 West Van Buren, Chicago, IL Zip 60624; tel. 312/265-7700; Johnny C. Brown, President
CHRIST HOSPITAL AND MEDICAL CENTER (O, 827 beds) 4440 West 95th Street, Oak Lawn, IL Zip 60453-2699; tel. 708/425-8000; Carol Schneider, Chief Executive
GOOD SAMARITAN HOSPITAL (O, 307 beds) 3815 Highland Avenue, Downers Grove, IL Zip 60515; tel. 708/275-5900; David M. McConkey, President
GOOD SHEPHERD HOSPITAL (O, 154 beds) 450 West Highway 22, Barrington, IL Zip 60010-1999; tel. 708/381-9600; Russell E. Feurer, Chief Executive
LUTHERAN GENERAL HOSPITAL (O, 800 beds) 1775 Dempster Street, Park Ridge, IL Zip 60068-1174; tel. 708/696-8446; Kenneth J. Rojek, Chief Executive
RAVENSWOOD HOSPITAL MEDICAL CENTER (O, 321 beds) 4550 North Winchester Avenue, Chicago, IL Zip 60640-5205; tel. 312/878-4300; John E. Blair, President
SOUTH SUBURBAN HOSPITAL (O, 240 beds) 17800 South Kedzie Avenue, Hazel Crest, IL Zip 60429; tel. 708/799-8000; Robert Rutkowski, President and Chief Executive Officer
TRINITY HOSPITAL (O, 228 beds) 2320 East 93rd Street, Chicago, IL Zip 60617; tel. 312/978-2000; John N. Schwartz, Chief Executive Officer

Owned, leased, sponsored:	8 hospitals	3015 beds
Contract-managed:	0 hospitals	0 beds
Totals:	8 hospitals	3015 beds

0225: **ALAMEDA COUNTY HEALTH CARE SERVICES AGENCY** (NP)
499 Fifth Street, Oakland, CA Zip 94607; tel. 510/268-2722; David J. Kears, Director
CALIFORNIA: FAIRMONT HOSPITAL (O, 193 beds) 15400 Foothill Boulevard, San Leandro, CA Zip 94578-1091; tel. 510/667-7800; Mike Smart, Administrator
HIGHLAND GENERAL HOSPITAL (O, 247 beds) 1411 East 31st Street, Oakland, CA Zip 94602; tel. 510/437-4397; Ophelia Long R.N., Administrator

Owned, leased, sponsored:	2 hospitals	440 beds
Contract-managed:	0 hospitals	0 beds
Totals:	2 hospitals	440 beds

1685: **ALBERT EINSTEIN HEALTHCARE NETWORK** (NP)
5501 Old York Road, Philadelphia, PA Zip 19141-3098; tel. 215/456-7890; Martin Goldsmith, President
PENNSYLVANIA: ALBERT EINSTEIN MEDICAL CENTER (O, 767 beds) 5501 Old York Road, Philadelphia, PA Zip 19141-3098; tel. 215/456-7890; Martin Goldsmith, President
BELMONT CENTER FOR COMPREHENSIVE TREATMENT (O, 146 beds) 4200 Monument Road, Philadelphia, PA Zip 19131-1689; tel. 215/877-2000; Jack H. Dembow, General Director

Owned, leased, sponsored:	2 hospitals	913 beds
Contract-managed:	0 hospitals	0 beds
Totals:	2 hospitals	913 beds

0065: **ALEXIAN BROTHERS HEALTH SYSTEM, INC.** (CC)
600 Alexian Way, Elk Grove Village, IL Zip 60007-3395; tel. 708/640-7550; Brother Felix Bettendorf, President
CALIFORNIA: ALEXIAN BROTHERS HOSPITAL (O, 188 beds) 225 North Jackson Avenue, San Jose, CA Zip 95116-1691; tel. 408/259-5000; Steven R. Barron, Chief Executive Officer
ILLINOIS: ALEXIAN BROTHERS MEDICAL CENTER (O, 378 beds) 800 Biesterfield Road, Elk Grove Village, IL Zip 60007-3397; tel. 708/437-5500; Brother Philip Kennedy, President and Chief Executive Officer
MISSOURI: ALEXIAN BROTHERS HOSPITAL (O, 182 beds) 3933 South Broadway, Saint Louis, MO Zip 63118-9984; tel. 314/865-3333; Deno E. Fabbre, President and Chief Executive Officer

Owned, leased, sponsored:	3 hospitals	748 beds
Contract-managed:	0 hospitals	0 beds
Totals:	3 hospitals	748 beds

★1385: **ALLEGANY HEALTH SYSTEM** (CC)
6200 Courtney Campbell Cswy, Tampa, FL Zip 33607-1458; tel. 813/281-9098; Sister Marie Celeste Sullivan, President and Chief Executive Officer
FLORIDA: ST. ANTHONY'S HOSPITAL (S, 279 beds) 1200 Seventh Avenue North, Saint Petersburg, FL Zip 33705, Mailing Address: P.O. Box 12588, Zip 33733; tel. 813/825-1100; Revonda L. Shumaker R.N., President
ST. JOSEPH'S HOSPITALS (S, 883 beds) 3001 W Martin Luther King Boulevard, Tampa, FL Zip 33607-6387, Mailing Address: P.O. Box 4227, Zip 33677-4227; tel. 813/870-4000; Charles Francis Scott, President
ST. MARY'S HOSPITAL (S, 430 beds) 901 45th Street, West Palm Beach, FL Zip 33407-2495, Mailing Address: P.O. Box 24620, Zip 33416-4620; tel. 407/844-6300; Michael French, President and Chief Executive
NEW JERSEY: OUR LADY OF LOURDES MEDICAL CENTER (S, 327 beds) 1600 Haddon Avenue, Camden, NJ Zip 08103; tel. 609/757-3500; Alexander J. Hatala, Chief Executive Officer

Owned, leased, sponsored:	4 hospitals	1919 beds
Contract-managed:	0 hospitals	0 beds
Totals:	4 hospitals	1919 beds

2305: **ALLEGHENY HEALTH, EDUCATION AND RESEARCH FOUNDATION** (NP)
120 Fifth Avenue, Pittsburgh, PA Zip 15222; tel. 412/359-6000; Sherif S. Abdelhak, President
OHIO: EAST OHIO REGIONAL HOSPITAL (CM, 201 beds) 90 North Fourth Street, Martins Ferry, OH Zip 43935; tel. 614/633-1100; Brian K. Felici, Vice President and Administrator
PENNSYLVANIA: ALLEGHENY GENERAL HOSPITAL (O, 843 beds) 320 East North Avenue, Pittsburgh, PA Zip 15212-4772; tel. 412/359-3131; Anthony M. Sanzo, President and Chief Executive Officer
ALLEGHENY NEUROPSYCHIATRIC INSTITUTE (O, 60 beds) 7777 Steubenville Pike, Oakdale, PA Zip 15071; tel. 412/747-2015; Trevor R P Price M.D., President
BUCKS COUNTY HOSPITAL (O, 166 beds) 225 Newtown Road, Warminster, PA Zip 18974; tel. 215/441-6600; Margaret M. McGoldrick, Executive Director and Chief Executive Officer
HAHNEMANN UNIVERSITY HOSPITAL (O, 618 beds) Broad and Vine Streets, Philadelphia, PA Zip 19102-1192; tel. 215/762-1650; Shelley Gebar, Executive Director and Chief Executive Officer
MEDICAL COLLEGE HOSPITALS – ELKINS PARK CAMPUS (O, 217 beds) 60 East Township Line Road, Elkins Park, PA Zip 19117; tel. 215/663-6000; Margaret M. McGoldrick, Executive Director and Chief Executive Officer
MEDICAL COLLEGE HOSPITALS, MAIN CLINICAL CAMPUS (O, 374 beds) 3300 Henry Avenue, Philadelphia, PA Zip 19129; tel. 215/842-6000; Margaret M. McGoldrick, Executive Director and Chief Executive Officer
ST. CHRISTOPHER'S HOSPITAL FOR CHILDREN (O, 175 beds) Erie Avenue At Front Street, Philadelphia, PA Zip 19134-1095; tel. 215/427-5000; Calvin Bland, President and Chief Executive Officer
WEST VIRGINIA: OHIO VALLEY MEDICAL CENTER (CM, 417 beds) 2000 Eoff Street, Wheeling, WV Zip 26003; tel. 304/234-0123; Thomas P. Galinski, President and Chief Executive Officer

Owned, leased, sponsored:	7 hospitals	2453 beds
Contract-managed:	2 hospitals	618 beds
Totals:	9 hospitals	3071 beds

★2285: **ALLIANT HEALTH SYSTEM** (NP)
234 East Gray Street, Ste 225, Louisville, KY Zip 40202, Mailing Address: P.O. Box 35070, Zip 40232-5070; tel. 502/629-2000; Stephen A. Williams, President
ILLINOIS: FAIRFIELD MEMORIAL HOSPITAL (CM, 185 beds) 303 N.W. 11th Street, Fairfield, IL Zip 62837; tel. 618/842-2611; Albert Ban, Jr., Chief Executive Officer

For explanation of codes following names, see page B2.
★Indicates Type III membership in the American Hospital Association.

Systems / Amerihealth, Inc.

MASSAC MEMORIAL HOSPITAL (CM, 31 beds) 28 Chick Street, Metropolis, IL Zip 62960–2481, Mailing Address: P.O. Box 850, Zip 62960–0850; tel. 618/524–2176; Jim Marshall, Interim Chief Executive Officer

PARIS COMMUNITY HOSPITAL (CM, 49 beds) 721 East Court Street, Paris, IL Zip 61944–2420; tel. 217/465–4141; John M. Dillon, Chief Executive Officer

WABASH GENERAL HOSPITAL DISTRICT (CM, 56 beds) 1418 College Drive, Mount Carmel, IL Zip 62863; tel. 618/262–8621; J. Jay Purvis, Interim Chief Executive Officer

WEST FRANKFORT UNITED MINE WORKERS OF AMERICA UNION HOSPITAL (CM, 34 beds) 507 West St. Louis Street, West Frankfort, IL Zip 62896–1999; tel. 618/932–2155; John D. Groves, Chief Executive Officer

INDIANA: BLACKFORD COUNTY HOSPITAL (CM, 36 beds) 503 East Van Cleve Street, Hartford City, IN Zip 47348; tel. 317/348–0300; Mark A. Edwards, Chief Executive Officer

CLAY COUNTY HOSPITAL (CM, 53 beds) 1206 East National Avenue, Brazil, IN Zip 47834–2797; tel. 812/448–2675; Jay P. Jolly, Chief Executive Officer

COMMUNITY HOSPITAL (CM, 35 beds) 412 North Monroe Street, Williamsport, IN Zip 47993–0215; tel. 317/762–2496; Jane Craigin, Chief Executive Officer

DECATUR COUNTY MEMORIAL HOSPITAL (CM, 71 beds) 720 North Lincoln Street, Greensburg, IN Zip 47240–1398; tel. 812/663–4331; Dalton L. Smart, Chief Executive Director

GIBSON GENERAL HOSPITAL (CM, 109 beds) 1808 Sherman Drive, Princeton, IN Zip 47670–1000; tel. 812/385–3401; Michael J. Budnick, Administrator and Chief Executive Officer

HARRISON COUNTY HOSPITAL (CM, 50 beds) 245 Atwood Street, Corydon, IN Zip 47112–0245; tel. 812/738–4251; Steven L. Taylor, Chief Executive Officer

JAY COUNTY HOSPITAL (CM, 55 beds) 500 West Votaw Street, Portland, IN Zip 47371–1322; tel. 219/726–7131; Thomas J. Valerius, Chief Executive Officer

JENNINGS COMMUNITY HOSPITAL (CM, 48 beds) 301 Henry Street, North Vernon, IN Zip 47265; tel. 812/346–6200; Todd L. Stallings, Chief Executive Officer

PERRY COUNTY MEMORIAL HOSPITAL (CM, 38 beds) 1 Hospital Road, Tell City, IN Zip 47586–0362; tel. 812/547–7011; Bradford W. Dykes, Administrator

RANDOLPH COUNTY HOSPITAL (CM, 27 beds) 325 South Oak Street, Winchester, IN Zip 47394, Mailing Address: P.O. Box 407, Zip 47394; tel. 317/584–9001; James M. Full, Chief Executive Officer

RUSH MEMORIAL HOSPITAL (CM, 52 beds) 1300 North Main Street, Rushville, IN Zip 46173–1198; tel. 317/932–4111; H. William Hartley, Chief Executive Officer

KENTUCKY: ALLIANT HOSPITALS (O, 714 beds) 200 East Chestnut Street, Louisville, KY Zip 40202, Mailing Address: Box 35070, Zip 40232–5070; tel. 502/629–8000; Shirley B. Powers, Senior Executive Officer

BRECKINRIDGE MEMORIAL HOSPITAL (CM, 45 beds) 1011 Old Highway 60, Hardinsburg, KY Zip 40143–9732; tel. 502/756–2124; George Walz CHE, Chief Executive Officer

CALDWELL COUNTY HOSPITAL (CM, 20 beds) 101 Hospital Drive, Princeton, KY Zip 42445–0410, Mailing Address: Box 410, Zip 42445–0410; tel. 502/365–0300; John Svoboda, Administrator

CARROLL COUNTY MEMORIAL HOSPITAL (CM, 39 beds) 309 11th Street, Carrollton, KY Zip 41008; tel. 502/732–4321; Roger Williams, Chief Executive Officer

CAVERNA MEMORIAL HOSPITAL (CM, 28 beds) 1501 South Dixie Street, Horse Cave, KY Zip 42749, Mailing Address: P.O. Box 120, Zip 42749–0120; tel. 502/786–2191; James J. Kerins, Sr., Administrator

JAMES B. HAGGIN MEMORIAL HOSPITAL (CM, 59 beds) 464 Linden Avenue, Harrodsburg, KY Zip 40330–1862; tel. 606/734–5441; Earl James Motzer Ph.D., FACHE, Chief Executive Officer

JANE TODD CRAWFORD MEMORIAL HOSPITAL (CM, 64 beds) 202–206 Milby Street, Greensburg, KY Zip 42743, Mailing Address: P.O. Box 220, Zip 42743; tel. 502/932–4211; Larry Craig, Chief Executive Officer

TRIGG COUNTY HOSPITAL (CM, 40 beds) Highway 68 East, Cadiz, KY Zip 42211, Mailing Address: Box 312, Zip 42211; tel. 502/522–3215; David M. Goodcase, Chief Executive Officer

TWIN LAKES REGIONAL MEDICAL CENTER (CM, 75 beds) 910 Wallace Avenue, Leitchfield, KY Zip 42754; tel. 502/259–9400; Stephen L. Meredith, Chief Executive Officer

Owned, leased, sponsored:	1 hospitals	714 beds
Contract–managed:	24 hospitals	1299 beds
Totals:	25 hospitals	2013 beds

★**0041: ALLINA HEALTH SYSTEM** (NP)
5601 Smetana Drive, Minneapolis, MN Zip 55440, Mailing Address: P.O. Box 9310, Zip 55440–9310; tel. 612/992–2000; Gordon M. Sprenger, Executive Officer

MINNESOTA: ABBOTT NORTHWESTERN HOSPITAL (O, 607 beds) 800 East 28th Street, Minneapolis, MN Zip 55407–3799; tel. 612/863–4000; Robert K. Spinner, President

BUFFALO HOSPITAL (O, 43 beds) 303 Catlin Street, Buffalo, MN Zip 55313–0609, Mailing Address: P.O. Box 609, Zip 55313–0609; tel. 612/682–7180; Mary Ellen Wells, President

CAMBRIDGE MEDICAL CENTER (O, 86 beds) 725 South Dellwood Street, Cambridge, MN Zip 55008–1920; tel. 612/689–1500; Lowell L. Becker M.D., President

GRANITE FALLS MUNICIPAL HOSPITAL AND MANOR (CM, 94 beds) 345 Tenth Avenue, Granite Falls, MN Zip 56241–1499; tel. 612/564–3111; George Gerlach, Administrator

HUTCHINSON COMMUNITY HOSPITAL (CM, 187 beds) 1095 Highway 15 South, Hutchinson, MN Zip 55350–3500; tel. 612/234–5000; Philip G. Graves, President

LONG PRAIRIE MEMORIAL HOSPITAL AND HOME (O, 138 beds) 20 Ninth Street S.E., Long Prairie, MN Zip 56347–1225; tel. 612/732–2141; Kevin J. Smith, President

MILLE LACS HEALTH SYSTEM (CM, 108 beds) 200 North Elm Street, Onamia, MN Zip 56359–0800; tel. 612/532–3154; Frederick W. Haack, Chief Executive Officer

NORTHFIELD HOSPITAL (CM, 69 beds) 801 West First Street, Northfield, MN Zip 55057–1697; tel. 507/645–6661; Kendall C. Bank, Chief Executive Officer

OWATONNA HOSPITAL (O, 65 beds) 903 South Oak Avenue, Owatonna, MN Zip 55060–3296; tel. 507/451–3850; Richard G. Slieter, President

PHILLIPS EYE INSTITUTE (O, 10 beds) 2215 Park Avenue, Minneapolis, MN Zip 55404; tel. 612/336–6000; Shari E. Levy, President

SIOUX VALLEY HOSPITAL (O, 85 beds) 1324 Fifth Street North, New Ulm, MN Zip 56073, Mailing Address: Box 577, Zip 56073; tel. 507/354–2111; Robert Stevens, President

ST. FRANCIS REGIONAL MEDICAL CENTER (O, 63 beds) 325 West Fifth Avenue, Shakopee, MN Zip 55379–1200; tel. 612/445–2322; Donald J. Leivermann, President and Chief Executive Officer

STEVENS COMMUNITY MEDICAL CENTER (CM, 37 beds) 400 East First Street, Morris, MN Zip 56267, Mailing Address: P.O. Box 660, Zip 56267; tel. 612/589–1313; John Rau, President and Chief Executive Officer

UNITED HOSPITAL (O, 366 beds) 333 North Smith Street, Saint Paul, MN Zip 55102–2389; tel. 612/220–8000; David B. M. Jones, President

UNITY HOSPITAL (O, 462 beds) 550 Osborne Road N.E., Fridley, MN Zip 55432–2791; tel. 612/421–2222; William T. MacNally, President

SOUTH DAKOTA: PRAIRIE LAKES HOSPITAL AND CARE CENTER (CM, 119 beds) 400 Tenth Avenue N.W., Watertown, SD Zip 57201, Mailing Address: P.O. Box 1210, Zip 57201–1210; tel. 605/882–7000; Edmond L. Weiland, Administrator

WISCONSIN: RIVER FALLS AREA HOSPITAL (O, 36 beds) 1629 East Division Street, River Falls, WI Zip 54022; tel. 715/425–6155; Sharon Whelan, President

Owned, leased, sponsored:	11 hospitals	1961 beds
Contract–managed:	6 hospitals	614 beds
Totals:	17 hospitals	2575 beds

0985: AMERIHEALTH, INC. (IO)
100 Galeria Parkway, Ste 605, Atlanta, GA Zip 30339; tel. 404/953–9600; William G. White, President

ALABAMA: AUTAUGA MEDICAL CENTER (O, 50 beds) 124 South Memorial Drive, Prattville, AL Zip 36067; tel. 334/365–0651; William C. Bentley, Administrator

GEORGIA: CHARLTON MEMORIAL HOSPITAL (CM, 50 beds) 1203 Third Street, Folkston, GA Zip 31537, Mailing Address: Box 188, Zip 31537; tel. 912/496–2531; James L. Leis, Jr., Administrator and Chief Executive Officer

For explanation of codes following names, see page B2.
★Indicates Type III membership in the American Hospital Association.

Systems / Amerihealth, Inc.

PENNSYLVANIA: MONSOUR MEDICAL CENTER (CM, 151 beds) 70 Lincoln Way East, Jeannette, PA Zip 15644; tel. 412/527-1511; Jerry Joseph, Chief Executive Officer

VIRGINIA: METROPOLITAN HOSPITAL (O, 180 beds) 701 West Grace Street, Richmond, VA Zip 23220; tel. 804/775-4100

Owned, leased, sponsored:	2 hospitals	230 beds
Contract-managed:	2 hospitals	201 beds
Totals:	4 hospitals	431 beds

★**0135:** **ANCILLA SYSTEMS INC.** (CC)
1000 South Lake Park Avenue, Hobart, IN Zip 46342; tel. 219/947-8500; William D. Harkins, President

ILLINOIS: ST. ELIZABETH'S HOSPITAL (O, 240 beds) 1431 North Claremont Avenue, Chicago, IL Zip 60622; tel. 312/633-5930; Joann Birdzell, President

ST. MARY'S HOSPITAL (O, 135 beds) 129 North Eighth Street, East Saint Louis, IL Zip 62201-2999; tel. 618/274-1900; Richard J. Mark, President and Chief Executive Officer

INDIANA: COMMUNITY HOSPITAL OF BREMEN (CM, 28 beds) 411 South Whitlock Street, Bremen, IN Zip 46506-1699; tel. 219/546-2211; Scott R. Graybill, Administrator and Chief Executive Officer

MICHIANA COMMUNITY HOSPITAL (O, 90 beds) 2515 East Jefferson Boulevard, South Bend, IN Zip 46615-2691; tel. 219/288-8311; Stephen Crain, President

ST. CATHERINE HOSPITAL (O, 158 beds) 4321 Fir Street, East Chicago, IN Zip 46312; tel. 219/392-7000; Joseph M. Mark, President and Chief Executive Officer

ST. JOSEPH HOSPITAL (O, 117 beds) 215 West Fourth Street, Mishawaka, IN Zip 46544; tel. 219/259-2431; Douglas L. Elwell, President and Chief Executive Officer

ST. JOSEPH MEDICAL CENTER OF FORT WAYNE (O, 262 beds) 700 Broadway, Fort Wayne, IN Zip 46802; tel. 219/425-3000; John T. Farrell, Sr., President and Chief Executive Officer

ST. MARY MEDICAL CENTER (O, 179 beds) 1500 South Lake Park Avenue, Hobart, IN Zip 46342; tel. 219/947-6000; Joseph M. Mark, President and Chief Executive Officer

Owned, leased, sponsored:	7 hospitals	1181 beds
Contract-managed:	1 hospitals	28 beds
Totals:	8 hospitals	1209 beds

0145: **APPALACHIAN REGIONAL HEALTHCARE** (NP)
1220 Harrodsburg Road, Lexington, KY Zip 40533, Mailing Address: Box 8086, Zip 40533-8086; tel. 606/281-2440; Forrest Calico M.D., President

KENTUCKY: ARH REGIONAL MEDICAL CENTER (O, 284 beds) 100 Medical Center Drive, Hazard, KY Zip 41701-1000; tel. 606/439-6610; David R. Lyon, Administrator

HARLAN ARH HOSPITAL (O, 125 beds) 81 Ball Park Road, Harlan, KY Zip 40831-1792; tel. 606/573-8100; Vernon L. Rucks, Administrator

MCDOWELL ARH HOSPITAL (O, 60 beds) Route 122, McDowell, KY Zip 41647, Mailing Address: Box 247, Zip 41647; tel. 606/377-3400; Jerry Haynes, Administrator

MIDDLESBORO APPALACHIAN REGIONAL HOSPITAL (O, 96 beds) 3600 West Cumberland Avenue, Middlesboro, KY Zip 40965, Mailing Address: Box 340, Zip 40965-0340; tel. 606/242-1101; Paul V. Miles, Administrator

MORGAN COUNTY APPALACHIAN REGIONAL HOSPITAL (L, 55 beds) Wells Hill Road, West Liberty, KY Zip 41472, Mailing Address: Box 579, Zip 41472-0579; tel. 606/743-3186; Dennis R. Chaney, Administrator

WHITESBURG APPALACHIAN REGIONAL HOSPITAL (O, 71 beds) 550 Jenkins Road, Whitesburg, KY Zip 41858; tel. 606/633-3500; Nick Lewis, Administrator

WILLIAMSON ARH HOSPITAL (O, 173 beds) 260 Hospital Drive, South Williamson, KY Zip 41503; tel. 606/237-1700; John A. Grah, Administrator

VIRGINIA: WISE ARH HOSPITAL (O, 67 beds) Wise, VA, Mailing Address: P.O. Box 3267, Zip 24293-3267; tel. 703/328-2511; Dan Fitzpatrick, Administrator

WEST VIRGINIA: BECKLEY APPALACHIAN REGIONAL HOSPITAL (O, 173 beds) 306 Stanaford Road, Beckley, WV Zip 25801; tel. 304/255-3000; Wilbur D. Crosley, Administrator

MAN ARH HOSPITAL (O, 42 beds) 700 East McDonald Avenue, Man, WV Zip 25635-1011; tel. 304/583-8421; Adrian Farmer, Administrator

SUMMERS COUNTY APPALACHIAN REGIONAL HOSPITAL (L, 95 beds) Terrace Street, Hinton, WV Zip 25951, Mailing Address: Drawer 940, Zip 25951-0940; tel. 304/466-1000; Scot Mitchell, Administrator

Owned, leased, sponsored:	11 hospitals	1241 beds
Contract-managed:	0 hospitals	0 beds
Totals:	11 hospitals	1241 beds

★**0205:** **ASC HEALTH SYSTEM** (CC)
6 Eagle Center, Suite 4, O'Fallon, IL Zip 62269-0406, Mailing Address: P.O. Box 670, Zip 62269-0670; tel. 618/632-1284; Gregory F. Yank, President and Chief Executive Officer

ILLINOIS: ST. CLEMENT HOSPITAL (O, 105 beds) 1 St Clement Boulevard, Red Bud, IL Zip 62278-1194; tel. 618/282-3831; Michael Thomas McManus, President

ST. VINCENT MEMORIAL HOSPITAL (O, 152 beds) 201 East Pleasant Street, Taylorville, IL Zip 62568-1597; tel. 217/824-3331; Dan Colby, President and Chief Executive Officer

Owned, leased, sponsored:	2 hospitals	257 beds
Contract-managed:	0 hospitals	0 beds
Totals:	2 hospitals	257 beds

★**2215:** **AURORA HEALTH CARE, INC.** (NP)
3000 West Montana, Milwaukee, WI Zip 53215-3268, Mailing Address: P.O. Box 343910, Zip 53234-3910; tel. 414/647-3000; G. Edwin Howe, President

WISCONSIN: SHEBOYGAN MEMORIAL MEDICAL CENTER (O, 138 beds) 2629 North Seventh Street, Sheboygan, WI Zip 53083-4998; tel. 414/451-5000; Patrick J. Trotter, President

SINAI SAMARITAN MEDICAL CENTER (O, 209 beds) 945 North 12th Street, Milwaukee, WI Zip 53233, Mailing Address: P.O. Box 342, Zip 53201-0342; tel. 414/345-3400; William I. Jenkins, President and Chief Executive Officer

ST. LUKE'S MEDICAL CENTER (O, 368 beds) 2900 West Oklahoma Avenue, Milwaukee, WI Zip 53215, Mailing Address: P.O. Box 2901, Zip 53201; tel. 414/649-6000; Mark R. Ambrosius, President

VALLEY VIEW MEDICAL CENTER (O, 98 beds) 901 Reed Street, Plymouth, WI Zip 53073-2409; tel. 414/893-1771; Patrick J. Trotter, President

Owned, leased, sponsored:	4 hospitals	813 beds
Contract-managed:	0 hospitals	0 beds
Totals:	4 hospitals	813 beds

★**7895:** **AVMED-SANTA FE** (NP)
8930 Northwest 39th Avenue, Gainesville, FL Zip 32606, Mailing Address: P.O. Box 749, Zip 32602-0749; tel. 904/372-8400; Edward C. Peddie, President

FLORIDA: ALACHUA GENERAL HOSPITAL (O, 350 beds) 801 Southwest Second Avenue, Gainesville, FL Zip 32601; tel. 904/372-4321; Les C. Rankin, Chief Executive Officer

BRADFORD HOSPITAL (O, 23 beds) 922 East Call Street, Starke, FL Zip 32091, Mailing Address: P.O. Box 1210, Zip 32091-1210; tel. 904/964-6000; Jeannie Baker, Chief Operating Officer

LAKE SHORE HOSPITAL (L, 60 beds) 560 East Franklin Street, Lake City, FL Zip 32055, Mailing Address: Box 1989, Zip 32056-1989; tel. 904/755-3200; Linda A. McKnew R.N., Chief Operating Officer

SUWANNEE HOSPITAL (O, 16 beds) 1100 Southwest 11th Avenue, Live Oak, FL Zip 32060, Mailing Address: P.O. Drawer X, Zip 32060; tel. 904/362-1413; Rhonda Sherrod, Administrator

UPREACH REHABILITATION HOSPITAL (O, 40 beds) 8900 Northwest 39th Avenue, Gainesville, FL Zip 32606-5625; tel. 904/338-0091; Barry G. Wagner, Chief Executive Officer

Owned, leased, sponsored:	5 hospitals	489 beds
Contract-managed:	0 hospitals	0 beds
Totals:	5 hospitals	489 beds

For explanation of codes following names, see page B2.
★Indicates Type III membership in the American Hospital Association.

Systems / Baptist Medical System

0185: BAPTIST HEALTH CARE CORPORATION (NP)
1717 North E Street, Ste 320, Pensacola, FL Zip 32501–6335;
tel. 904/469–2337; James F. Vickery, President

ALABAMA: MIZELL MEMORIAL HOSPITAL (O, 57 beds) 702 Main Street, Opp, AL Zip 36467–1626, Mailing Address: P.O. Box 429, Zip 36467–0429; tel. 205/493–3541; Allen Foster, Interim Administrator

FLORIDA: BAPTIST HOSPITAL (O, 546 beds) 1000 West Moreno, Pensacola, FL Zip 32501–2393, Mailing Address: P.O. Box 17500, Zip 32522–7500; tel. 904/434–4011; Alfred G. Stubblefield, Senior Vice President and Administrator
GULF BREEZE HOSPITAL (O, 43 beds) 1110 Gulf Breeze Parkway, Gulf Breeze, FL Zip 32561–1110, Mailing Address: P.O. Box 159, Zip 32562–0159; tel. 904/934–2000; Richard C. Fulford, Administrator
JAY HOSPITAL (L, 36 beds) 221 South Alabama Street, Jay, FL Zip 32565; tel. 904/675–4532; William Allen Foster, Administrator

Owned, leased, sponsored:	4 hospitals	682 beds
Contract–managed:	0 hospitals	0 beds
Totals:	4 hospitals	682 beds

★4155: BAPTIST HEALTH CARE SYSTEM OF SOUTH CAROLINA (CO)
Taylor At Marion Street, Columbia, SC Zip 29220;
tel. 803/771–5010; Charles D. Beaman Jr., President and Chief Executive Officer

SOUTH CAROLINA: BAPTIST MEDICAL CENTER EASLEY (O, 90 beds) 200 Fleetwood Drive, Easley, SC Zip 29640, Mailing Address: P.O. Box 2129, Zip 29641–2129; tel. 803/855–7603; Roddey E. Gettys III, Executive Vice President
BAPTIST MEDICAL CENTER–COLUMBIA (O, 411 beds) Taylor At Marion Street, Columbia, SC Zip 29220; tel. 803/771–5010; Charles D. Beaman, Jr., President and Chief Executive Officer

Owned, leased, sponsored:	2 hospitals	501 beds
Contract–managed:	0 hospitals	0 beds
Totals:	2 hospitals	501 beds

★0345: BAPTIST HEALTH SYSTEM (CO)
3500 Blue Lake Drive, Ste 100, Birmingham, AL Zip 35243, Mailing Address: P.O. Box 830605, Zip 35283–0605; tel. 205/715–5319; Dennis A. Hall, President

ALABAMA: BIRMINGHAM BAPTIST MEDICAL CENTER–MONTCLAIR CAMPUS (O, 596 beds) 800 Montclair Road, Birmingham, AL Zip 35213; tel. 205/592–1000; Dana S. Hensley, President
BIRMINGHAM BAPTIST MEDICAL CENTER–PRINCETON (O, 356 beds) 701 Princeton Avenue S.W., Birmingham, AL Zip 35211–1305; tel. 205/783–3000; Dana S. Hensley, President and Chief Executive Officer
CHEROKEE BAPTIST MEDICAL CENTER (O, 45 beds) 400 Northwood Drive, Centre, AL Zip 35960–1023; tel. 205/927–5531; Barry S. Cochran, President
CITIZENS BAPTIST MEDICAL CENTER (O, 97 beds) 604 Stone Avenue, Talladega, AL Zip 35160, Mailing Address: P.O. Box 978, Zip 35160; tel. 205/362–8111; Jack B. Hethcox, President
COOSA VALLEY BAPTIST MEDICAL CENTER (O, 178 beds) 315 West Hickory Street, Sylacauga, AL Zip 35150–2996; tel. 205/249–5000; Steven M. Johnson, Administrator
CULLMAN REGIONAL MEDICAL CENTER (O, 99 beds) 1912 Alabama Highway 157, Cullman, AL Zip 35055, Mailing Address: P.O. Box 1108, Zip 35056–1108; tel. 205/737–2000; Jesse O. Weatherly, President
DEKALB BAPTIST MEDICAL CENTER (O, 103 beds) 200 Medical Center Drive, Fort Payne, AL Zip 35967, Mailing Address: P.O. Box 778, Zip 35967–0778; tel. 205/845–3150; Barry S. Cochran, President
LAWRENCE BAPTIST MEDICAL CENTER (L, 30 beds) 202 Hospital Street, Moulton, AL Zip 35650–0039, Mailing Address: P.O. Box 39, Zip 35650–0039; tel. 205/974–2200; Ronald L. Sparkman, Administrator
MARION BAPTIST MEDICAL CENTER (L, 126 beds) 1315 Military Street South, Hamilton, AL Zip 35570; tel. 205/921–7861
SHELBY MEDICAL CENTER (CM, 228 beds) 1000 First Street North, Alabaster, AL Zip 35007–0488, Mailing Address: Box 488, Zip 35007–0488; tel. 205/620–8100; Charles C. Colvert, President
WALKER BAPTIST MEDICAL CENTER (O, 267 beds) 3400 Highway 78 East, Jasper, AL Zip 35501, Mailing Address: Box 3547, Zip 35502–3547; tel. 205/387–4000; Jeff Brewer, President

Owned, leased, sponsored:	10 hospitals	1897 beds
Contract–managed:	1 hospitals	228 beds
Totals:	11 hospitals	2125 beds

2155: BAPTIST HEALTH SYSTEM OF TENNESSEE (NP)
137 Blount Avenue S.E., Knoxville, TN Zip 37920, Mailing Address: Box 1788, Zip 37901; tel. 615/632–5099; Dale Collins, President & Chief Executive Officer

TENNESSEE: BAPTIST HOSPITAL OF COCKE COUNTY (O, 109 beds) 435 Second Street, Newport, TN Zip 37821; tel. 615/625–2200; Wayne Buckner, Administrator
BAPTIST HOSPITAL OF EAST TENNESSEE (O, 345 beds) 137 Blount Avenue S.E., Knoxville, TN Zip 37920, Mailing Address: Box 1788, Zip 37901–1788; tel. 615/632–5011; Michael Williams, President and Chief Operating Officer
BAPTIST HOSPITAL OF ROANE COUNTY (L, 66 beds) 241 South Chamberlain Avenue, Rockwood, TN Zip 37854, Mailing Address: P.O. Box 388, Zip 37854; tel. 615/354–1121; William E. Torrence, Jr., Chief Executive Officer

Owned, leased, sponsored:	3 hospitals	520 beds
Contract–managed:	0 hospitals	0 beds
Totals:	3 hospitals	520 beds

★0315: BAPTIST HEALTHCARE SYSTEM (CO)
4007 Kresge Way, Louisville, KY Zip 40207–4677;
tel. 502/896–5000; Tommy J. Smith, President and Chief Executive Officer

KENTUCKY: BAPTIST HOSPITAL EAST (O, 407 beds) 4000 Kresge Way, Louisville, KY Zip 40207–4676; tel. 502/897–8100; Susan Stout Tamme, President
BAPTIST REGIONAL MEDICAL CENTER (O, 263 beds) 1 Trillium Way, Corbin, KY Zip 40701–8420; tel. 606/528–1212; John S. Henson, President
CENTRAL BAPTIST HOSPITAL (O, 324 beds) 1740 Nicholasville Road, Lexington, KY Zip 40503; tel. 606/275–6100; William G. Sisson, President
TRI COUNTY BAPTIST HOSPITAL (O, 120 beds) 1025 New Moody Lane, La Grange, KY Zip 40031–0559, Mailing Address: P.O. Box 559, Zip 40031–0559; tel. 502/222–5388; David L. Gray, Administrator
WESTERN BAPTIST HOSPITAL (O, 309 beds) 2501 Kentucky Avenue, Paducah, KY Zip 42003; tel. 502/575–2100; Larry O. Barton, President

Owned, leased, sponsored:	5 hospitals	1423 beds
Contract–managed:	0 hospitals	0 beds
Totals:	5 hospitals	1423 beds

★8810: BAPTIST HOSPITALS AND HEALTH SYSTEMS, INC. (NP)
2224 West Northern Ave, Ste D–300, Phoenix, AZ Zip 85021; tel. 602/864–1184; Gerald L. Wissink, President and Chief Executive Officer

ARIZONA: ARROWHEAD COMMUNITY HOSPITAL AND MEDICAL CENTER (O, 80 beds) 18701 North 67th Avenue, Glendale, AZ Zip 85308–5722; tel. 602/561–1000; Richard S. Alley, Administrator
BULLHEAD COMMUNITY HOSPITAL (O, 62 beds) 2735 Silver Creek Road, Bullhead City, AZ Zip 86442; tel. 602/763–2273; Ronald W. Tenbarge, Executive Vice President and Chief Executive Officer
PHOENIX BAPTIST HOSPITAL AND MEDICAL CENTER (O, 222 beds) 6025 North 20th Avenue, Phoenix, AZ Zip 85015; tel. 602/249–0212; Michael Purvis, Chief Executive Officer

FLORIDA: MANATEE MEMORIAL HOSPITAL (O, 512 beds) 206 Second Street East, Bradenton, FL Zip 34208; tel. 813/746–5111; Karl R. Tague, President and Chief Executive Officer

Owned, leased, sponsored:	4 hospitals	876 beds
Contract–managed:	0 hospitals	0 beds
Totals:	4 hospitals	876 beds

★0355: BAPTIST MEDICAL SYSTEM (NP)
9601 Interstate 630, Exit 7, Little Rock, AR Zip 72205–7299;
tel. 501/227–2000; Russell D. Harrington Jr., President

For explanation of codes following names, see page B2.
★Indicates Type III membership in the American Hospital Association.

Systems / Baptist Medical System

ARKANSAS: BAPTIST MEDICAL CENTER (O, 641 beds) 9601 Interstate 630, Exit 7, Little Rock, AR Zip 72205-7299; tel. 501/227-2000; Steven B. Lampkin, Senior Vice President and Administrator

BAPTIST MEDICAL CENTER ARKADELPHIA (L, 57 beds) 3050 Twin Rivers Drive, Arkadelphia, AR Zip 71923; tel. 501/245-1100; Dan Gathright, Senior Vice President and Administrator

BAPTIST MEMORIAL MEDICAL CENTER (L, 200 beds) One Pershing Circle, North Little Rock, AR Zip 72114-1899; tel. 501/771-3000; Harrison M. Dean, Senior Vice President & Administrator

BAPTIST REHABILITATION INSTITUTE OF ARKANSAS (O, 120 beds) 9601 Interstate 630, Exit 7, Little Rock, AR Zip 72205-7249; tel. 501/223-7000; Doug Weeks, Vice President and Administrator

Owned, leased, sponsored:	4 hospitals	1018 beds
Contract-managed:	0 hospitals	0 beds
Totals:	4 hospitals	1018 beds

★1625: BAPTIST MEMORIAL HEALTH CARE SYSTEM, INC. (NP)
899 Madison Avenue, Memphis, TN Zip 38146; tel. 901/227-2727; Stephen Curtis Reynolds, President and Chief Executive Officer

ARKANSAS: BAPTIST MEMORIAL HOSPITAL-BLYTHEVILLE (L, 198 beds) 1520 North Division Street, Blytheville, AR Zip 72315, Mailing Address: P.O. Box 108, Zip 72316-0108; tel. 501/762-3300; Randy King, Administrator

BAPTIST MEMORIAL HOSPITAL-EASTERN OZARKS (O, 40 beds) 122 South Allegheny Drive, Cherokee Village, AR Zip 72542; tel. 501/257-4101; Jerry L. Lee, Administrator

BAPTIST MEMORIAL HOSPITAL-FORREST CITY (L, 76 beds) 1601 Newcastle Road, Forrest City, AR Zip 72335, Mailing Address: P.O. Box 667, Zip 72335; tel. 501/633-2020; George S. Fray, Administrator

BAPTIST MEMORIAL HOSPITAL-OSCEOLA (L, 72 beds) 611 West Lee Avenue, Osceola, AR Zip 72370, Mailing Address: Box 607, Zip 72370-0607; tel. 501/563-7000; Al Sypniewski, Administrator

MISSISSIPPI: BAPTIST MEMORIAL HOSPITAL-BOONEVILLE (L, 78 beds) 100 Hospital Street, Booneville, MS Zip 38829; tel. 601/728-5331; William A. Tuttle, Administrator

BAPTIST MEMORIAL HOSPITAL-DESOTO (O, 130 beds) 7601 Southcrest Parkway, Southaven, MS Zip 38671; tel. 601/349-4000; Melvin E. Walker, Administrator

BAPTIST MEMORIAL HOSPITAL-GOLDEN TRIANGLE (L, 328 beds) 2520 Fifth Street North, Columbus, MS Zip 39703-2095, Mailing Address: P.O. Box 1307, Zip 39701-1307; tel. 601/243-1000; J. Stuart Mitchell III, Administrator

BAPTIST MEMORIAL HOSPITAL-NORTH MISSISSIPPI (L, 150 beds) 2301 South Lamar Boulevard, Oxford, MS Zip 38655, Mailing Address: Box 946, Zip 38655; tel. 601/232-8100; Stephen L. Mansfield, Administrator

BAPTIST MEMORIAL HOSPITAL-UNION COUNTY (L, 153 beds) Highway 30 West, New Albany, MS Zip 38652-3197; tel. 601/538-7631; John Tompkins, Administrator

TIPPAH COUNTY HOSPITAL (CM, 106 beds) 1005 City Avenue North, Ripley, MS Zip 38663-0499; tel. 601/837-9221; Jerry Green, Administrator

TENNESSEE: BAPTIST MEMORIAL HOSPITAL (O, 1261 beds) 899 Madison Avenue, Memphis, TN Zip 38146; tel. 901/227-2727; Stephen Curtis Reynolds, President and Chief Executive Officer

BAPTIST MEMORIAL HOSPITAL-HUNTINGDON (O, 70 beds) 631 R B Wilson Drive, Huntingdon, TN Zip 38344; tel. 901/986-4461; Jamie Townsend, Administrator

BAPTIST MEMORIAL HOSPITAL-LAUDERDALE (O, 70 beds) 326 Asbury Road, Ripley, TN Zip 38063-9701; tel. 901/635-1331; W. Tate Moorer, Administrator

BAPTIST MEMORIAL HOSPITAL-TIPTON (O, 100 beds) 1995 Highway 51 South, Covington, TN Zip 38019; tel. 901/476-2621; William T. Moorer, Administrator

BAPTIST MEMORIAL HOSPITAL-UNION CITY (O, 95 beds) 1201 Bishop Street, Union City, TN Zip 38261, Mailing Address: Box 310, Zip 38281-0310; tel. 901/884-8601; Mike Perryman, Administrator

Owned, leased, sponsored:	14 hospitals	2821 beds
Contract-managed:	1 hospitals	106 beds
Totals:	15 hospitals	2927 beds

0265: BAPTIST MEMORIAL HOSPITAL SYSTEM (CO)
660 North Main St, Ste 300, San Antonio, TX Zip 78205-1222; tel. 210/222-8431; Callie W. Smith, President and Chief Executive Officer

TEXAS: BAPTIST MEDICAL CENTER (O, 483 beds) 111 Dallas Street, San Antonio, TX Zip 78205-1230; tel. 210/222-8431; William L. Chessher, Administrator

NORTHEAST BAPTIST HOSPITAL (O, 208 beds) 8811 Village Drive, San Antonio, TX Zip 78217; tel. 210/653-2330; Morris R. Harris, Jr., Administrator

SOUTHEAST BAPTIST HOSPITAL (O, 153 beds) 4214 East Southcross, San Antonio, TX Zip 78222; tel. 210/337-6900; Harry E. Smith, Administrator

ST. LUKE'S BAPTIST HOSPITAL (O, 225 beds) 7930 Floyd Curl Drive, San Antonio, TX Zip 78229-0100, Mailing Address: Box 29100, Zip 78229-0100; tel. 210/692-8703; Peggy W. Brown, Administrator

Owned, leased, sponsored:	4 hospitals	1069 beds
Contract-managed:	0 hospitals	0 beds
Totals:	4 hospitals	1069 beds

★0095: BAYLOR HEALTH CARE SYSTEM (CO)
3500 Gaston Avenue, Dallas, TX Zip 75226; tel. 214/820-0111; Boone Powell Jr., President

TEXAS: BAYLOR CENTER FOR RESTORATIVE CARE (O, 74 beds) 3504 Swiss Avenue, Dallas, TX Zip 75204; tel. 214/823-1684; Gerry Brueckner R.N., Administrator

BAYLOR INSTITUTE FOR REHABILITATION (O, 75 beds) 3505 Gaston Avenue, Dallas, TX Zip 75246-2018; tel. 214/826-7030; Judith C. Waterston, Administrator

BAYLOR MEDICAL CENTER – ELLIS COUNTY (O, 73 beds) 1405 West Jefferson Street, Waxahachie, TX Zip 75165; tel. 214/923-7000; J. Michael Lee, Executive Director

BAYLOR MEDICAL CENTER AT GARLAND (O, 159 beds) 2300 Marie Curie Boulevard, Garland, TX Zip 75042-5706; tel. 214/487-5000; Gary D. Brock, Executive Director

BAYLOR MEDICAL CENTER AT GRAPEVINE (O, 58 beds) 1650 West College Street, Grapevine, TX Zip 76051-1650; tel. 817/329-2500; Mark C. Hood, Director

BAYLOR RICHARDSON MEDICAL CENTER (CM, 163 beds) 401 West Campbell Road, Richardson, TX Zip 75080; tel. 214/498-4000; Ronald L. Boring, President and Chief Executive Officer

BAYLOR UNIVERSITY MEDICAL CENTER (O, 922 beds) 3500 Gaston Avenue, Dallas, TX Zip 75246-2088; tel. 214/820-0111; Boone Powell, Jr., President

Owned, leased, sponsored:	6 hospitals	1361 beds
Contract-managed:	1 hospitals	163 beds
Totals:	7 hospitals	1524 beds

★1095: BAYSTATE HEALTH SYSTEMS, INC. (NP)
759 Chestnut Street, Springfield, MA Zip 01199-0001; tel. 413/784-0000; Michael J. Daly, President

MASSACHUSETTS: BAYSTATE MEDICAL CENTER (O, 669 beds) 759 Chestnut Street, Springfield, MA Zip 01199-0001; tel. 413/784-0000; Mark R. Tolosky, Chief Executive Officer

FRANKLIN MEDICAL CENTER (O, 115 beds) 164 High Street, Greenfield, MA Zip 01301; tel. 413/773-0211; Harlan J. Smith, President

MARY LANE HOSPITAL (O, 40 beds) 85 South Street, Ware, MA Zip 01082; tel. 413/967-6211; Christine Shirtcliff, Executive Vice President

Owned, leased, sponsored:	3 hospitals	824 beds
Contract-managed:	0 hospitals	0 beds
Totals:	3 hospitals	824 beds

0515: BENEDICTINE HEALTH SYSTEM (CC)
503 East Third Street, Duluth, MN Zip 55805-1964; tel. 218/720-2370; Sister Kathleen Hofer, Chair Person and Chief Executive Officer

IDAHO: ST. MARY'S HOSPITAL (O, 28 beds) Lewiston and North Streets, Cottonwood, ID Zip 83522, Mailing Address: P.O. Box 137, Zip 83522-0137; tel. 208/962-3251; Casey Uhling, Administrator

---

For explanation of codes following names, see page B2.
★Indicates Type III membership in the American Hospital Association.

Systems / Bon Secours Health System, Inc.

MINNESOTA: ST. JOSEPH'S MEDICAL CENTER (O, 162 beds) 523 North Third Street, Brainerd, MN Zip 56401–3098; tel. 218/829–2861; Thomas K. Prusak, President

ST. MARY'S MEDICAL CENTER (O, 283 beds) 407 East Third Street, Duluth, MN Zip 55805–1984; tel. 218/726–4000; Sister Kathleen Hofer, President

ST. MARY'S REGIONAL HEALTH CENTER (O, 165 beds) 1027 Washington Avenue, Detroit Lakes, MN Zip 56501–3598; tel. 218/847–5611; John H. Solheim, Chief Executive Officer

Owned, leased, sponsored:	4 hospitals	638 beds
Contract–managed:	0 hospitals	0 beds
Totals:	4 hospitals	638 beds

0535: BENEDICTINE SISTERS (CC)
St Benedicts Convent, Saint Joseph, MN Zip 56374–0277; tel. 612/363–7100; Sister Ephrem Hollermann, Prioress

MINNESOTA: QUEEN OF PEACE HOSPITAL (S, 28 beds) 301 Second Street N.E., New Prague, MN Zip 56071–1799; tel. 612/758–4431; Sister Jean Juenemann, Chief Executive Officer

ST. CLOUD HOSPITAL (S, 335 beds) 1406 Sixth Avenue North, Saint Cloud, MN Zip 56303–0016; tel. 612/251–2700; John R. Frobenius, President and Chief Executive Officer

Owned, leased, sponsored:	2 hospitals	363 beds
Contract–managed:	0 hospitals	0 beds
Totals:	2 hospitals	363 beds

0545: BENEDICTINE SISTERS OF THE ANNUNCIATION (CC)
7520 University Drive, Bismarck, ND Zip 58504–9653; tel. 701/255–1520; Sister Susan Lardy, Prioress

NORTH DAKOTA: GARRISON MEMORIAL HOSPITAL (O, 49 beds) 407 Third Avenue S.E., Garrison, ND Zip 58540–0039; tel. 701/463–2275; Richard Spilovoy, Administrator

ST. ALEXIUS MEDICAL CENTER (O, 291 beds) 900 East Broadway, Bismarck, ND Zip 58501, Mailing Address: P.O. Box 5510, Zip 58506–5510; tel. 701/224–7000; Richard A. Tschider FACHE, Administrator and Chief Executive Officer

Owned, leased, sponsored:	2 hospitals	340 beds
Contract–managed:	0 hospitals	0 beds
Totals:	2 hospitals	340 beds

★**2435: BERKSHIRE HEALTH SYSTEMS, INC.** (NP)
725 North Street, Pittsfield, MA Zip 01201; tel. 413/447–2743; David E. Phelps, President and Chief Executive Officer

MASSACHUSETTS: BERKSHIRE MEDICAL CENTER (O, 330 beds) 725 North Street, Pittsfield, MA Zip 01201; tel. 413/447–2000; Kevin E. Nolan, President

FAIRVIEW HOSPITAL (O, 40 beds) 29 Lewis Avenue, Great Barrington, MA Zip 01230–1713; tel. 413/528–0790; Claire L. Bowen, President

Owned, leased, sponsored:	2 hospitals	370 beds
Contract–managed:	0 hospitals	0 beds
Totals:	2 hospitals	370 beds

★**0415: BETHESDA HOSPITAL, INC.** (NP)
619 Oak Street, Cincinnati, OH Zip 45206–1690; tel. 513/569–6141; L. Thomas Wilburn Jr., Chairman

OHIO: BETHESDA NORTH HOSPITAL (O, 244 beds) 10500 Montgomery Road, Cincinnati, OH Zip 45242; tel. 513/745–1111; William F. Groneman, Executive Vice President and System Leader

BETHESDA OAK HOSPITAL (O, 310 beds) 619 Oak Street, Cincinnati, OH Zip 45206–1690; tel. 513/569–6111; William F. Groneman, Executive Vice President and System Leader

Owned, leased, sponsored:	2 hospitals	554 beds
Contract–managed:	0 hospitals	0 beds
Totals:	2 hospitals	554 beds

★**0051: BJC HEALTH SYSTEM** (NP)
4444 Forest Park Avenue, Saint Louis, MO Zip 63108–2259; tel. 314/286–2030; Frederick L. Brown, President & Chief Executive Officer

ILLINOIS: ALTON MEMORIAL HOSPITAL (O, 232 beds) One Memorial Drive, Alton, IL Zip 62002–6722; tel. 618/463–7311; Ronald B. McMullen, President

CLAY COUNTY HOSPITAL (CM, 40 beds) 700 North Mill Street, Flora, IL Zip 62839, Mailing Address: P.O. Box 280, Zip 62839; tel. 618/662–2131; John E. Monnahan, Administrator

FAYETTE COUNTY HOSPITAL (L, 133 beds) Seventh and Taylor Streets, Vandalia, IL Zip 62471–1296; tel. 618/283–1231; Jerome J. Bozek, Administrator

MISSOURI: BARNES HOSPITAL (O, 1088 beds) One Barnes Hospital Plaza, Saint Louis, MO Zip 63110–1094; tel. 314/362–5000; John J. Finan, President and Senior Executive Officer

BARNES ST. PETERS HOSPITAL (O, 103 beds) 10 Hospital Drive, Saint Peters, MO Zip 63376–1659; tel. 314/447–6600; John Gloss, President and Chief Executive Officer

BARNES WEST COUNTY HOSPITAL (O, 87 beds) 12634 Olive Street Road, Saint Louis, MO Zip 63141–6354; tel. 314/434–0600; Gregory T. Wozniak, Administrator

BOONE HOSPITAL CENTER (L, 303 beds) 1600 East Broadway, Columbia, MO Zip 65201; tel. 314/875–4545; Michael Shirk, President

CHRISTIAN HOSPITAL NORTHEAST–NORTHWEST (O, 575 beds) 11133 Dunn Road, Saint Louis, MO Zip 63136–6192; tel. 314/653–5729; W. R. Van Bokkelen, President and Senior Executive Officer

HEDRICK MEDICAL CENTER (L, 64 beds) 100 Central Avenue, Chillicothe, MO Zip 64601–1599; tel. 816/646–1480; Richard L. Conklin, President and Senior Executive Officer

JEWISH HOSPITAL OF ST. LOUIS (O, 358 beds) 216 S Kingshighway Boulevard, Saint Louis, MO Zip 63110; tel. 314/454–7000; Wayne M. Lerner Dr.P.H., President

MISSOURI BAPTIST HOSPITAL OF SULLIVAN (O, 58 beds) 751 Sappington Bridge Road, Sullivan, MO Zip 63080, Mailing Address: P.O. Box 190, Zip 63080; tel. 314/468–4186; Davis D. Skinner, Administrator

MISSOURI BAPTIST MEDICAL CENTER (O, 331 beds) 3015 North Ballas Road, Town and Country, MO Zip 63131–2374; tel. 314/432–1212; Fred R. Mills, President

PARKLAND HEALTH CENTER (O, 87 beds) 1101 West Liberty Street, Farmington, MO Zip 63640–1997; tel. 314/756–6451; William D. Blair, President and Senior Executive Officer

ST. LOUIS CHILDREN'S HOSPITAL (O, 235 beds) One Children's Place, Saint Louis, MO Zip 63110–1077; tel. 314/454–6000; Alan W. Brass, President

Owned, leased, sponsored:	13 hospitals	3654 beds
Contract–managed:	1 hospitals	40 beds
Totals:	14 hospitals	3694 beds

• ★**0053: BLUE WATER HEALTH SERVICES CORPORATION** (NP)
1001 Kearney, Port Huron, MI Zip 48060; tel. 810/989–3717; Donald C. Fletcher, President and Chief Executive Officer

MICHIGAN: PORT HURON HOSPITAL (O, 184 beds) 1001 Kearney Street, Port Huron, MI Zip 48061–5011; tel. 313/987–5000; Donald C. Fletcher, President

Owned, leased, sponsored:	1 hospitals	184 beds
Contract–managed:	0 hospitals	0 beds
Totals:	1 hospitals	184 beds

★**5085: BON SECOURS HEALTH SYSTEM, INC.** (CC)
1505 Marriottsville Road, Marriottsville, MD Zip 21104–1399; tel. 410/442–5511; John L. Fitzgerald, President & Chief Executive Officer

FLORIDA: BON SECOURS–ST. JOSEPH HOSPITAL (O, 216 beds) 2500 Harbor Boulevard, Port Charlotte, FL Zip 33952–5396; tel. 813/625–4122; Kevin T. Potter, Chief Executive Officer

MARYLAND: BON SECOURS HOSPITAL (O, 150 beds) 2000 West Baltimore Street, Baltimore, MD Zip 21223–1597; tel. 410/362–3000; Jane R. Durney, Chief Executive Officer

---

For explanation of codes following names, see page B2.
★Indicates Type III membership in the American Hospital Association.
•Single hospital health care system

Systems / Bon Secours Health System, Inc.

MICHIGAN: BON SECOURS HOSPITAL (O, 256 beds) 468 Cadieux Road, Grosse Pointe, MI Zip 48230; tel. 313/343-1000; Henry Devries, Jr., Chief Executive Officer

SOUTH CAROLINA: BON SECOURS–ST. FRANCIS XAVIER HOSPITAL (O, 214 beds) 135 Rutledge Avenue, Charleston, SC Zip 29401-1399; tel. 803/577-1000; Creighton E. Likes, Jr., Chief Executive Officer

VIRGINIA: BON SECOURS–MARYVIEW MEDICAL CENTER (O, 403 beds) 3636 High Street, Portsmouth, VA Zip 23707-3236; tel. 804/398-2200; Gary J. Herbek, Chief Executive Officer

BON SECOURS–STUART CIRCLE (O, 153 beds) 413 Stuart Circle, Richmond, VA Zip 23220; tel. 804/358-7051; Ann Honeycutt, Administrator

ST. MARY'S HOSPITAL (O, 391 beds) 5801 Bremo Road, Richmond, VA Zip 23226-1900; tel. 804/285-2011; Christopher M. Carney, Chief Executive Officer

Owned, leased, sponsored:	7 hospitals	1783 beds
Contract–managed:	0 hospitals	0 beds
Totals:	7 hospitals	1783 beds

2455: BRADFORD PARKSIDE (IO)

2101 Magnolia Ave S, Ste 518, Birmingham, AL Zip 35205; tel. 205/251-7753; Jerry W. Crowder, President and Chief Executive Officer

ALABAMA: BRADFORD PARKSIDE AT BIRMINGHAM (O, 90 beds) 1221 Alton Drive, Birmingham, AL Zip 35210; tel. 205/833-4000; W. Clay Simmons, Executive Director

BRADFORD PARKSIDE AT MADISON (O, 84 beds) 1600 Browns Ferry Road, Madison, AL Zip 35758, Mailing Address: P.O. Box 176, Zip 35758-0176; tel. 205/461-7272; Bob Hinds, Executive Director

BRADFORD–PARKSIDE ADOLESCENT AT OAK MOUNTAIN (O, 84 beds) 2280 Highway 35, Pelham, AL Zip 35124; tel. 205/664-3460; Joseph Roche, Acting Executive Director

Owned, leased, sponsored:	3 hospitals	258 beds
Contract–managed:	0 hospitals	0 beds
Totals:	3 hospitals	258 beds

★0585: BRIM, INC. (IO)

305 Northeast 102nd Avenue, Portland, OR Zip 97220-4199; tel. 503/256-2070; Armand E. Brim, Chairman & Chief Executive Officer

ARIZONA: COBRE VALLEY COMMUNITY HOSPIAL (CM, 42 beds) One Hospital Drive, Claypool, AZ Zip 85532, Mailing Address: P.O. Box 3261, Zip 85532-3261; tel. 602/425-3261; John L. Hoopes, Chief Executive Officer and Administrator

NAVAPACHE REGIONAL MEDICAL CENTER (CM, 44 beds) 2200 Show Low Lake Road, Show Low, AZ Zip 85901; tel. 602/537-4375; Leigh Cox, Chief Executive Officer

NORTHERN COCHISE COMMUNITY HOSPITAL (CM, 48 beds) 901 West Rex Allen Drive, Willcox, AZ Zip 85643, Mailing Address: P.O. Drawer D, Zip 85643; tel. 520/384-3541; Chris Cronberg, Interim Chief Executive Officer

CALIFORNIA: BEAR VALLEY COMMUNITY HOSPITAL (CM, 30 beds) 41870 Garstin Road, Big Bear Lake, CA Zip 92315, Mailing Address: P.O. Box 1649, Zip 92315-1649; tel. 909/866-6501; Robert M. Baden, Chief Executive Officer

EASTERN PLUMAS DISTRICT HOSPITAL (CM, 24 beds) 500 First Avenue, Portola, CA Zip 96122; tel. 916/832-4277; Charles Gunther, Chief Executive Officer

GENERAL HOSPITAL (O, 83 beds) 2200 Harrison Avenue, Eureka, CA Zip 95501; tel. 707/445-5111; Gary A. McCormack, Chief Executive Officer

OJAI VALLEY COMMUNITY HOSPITAL (O, 116 beds) 1306 Maricopa Highway, Ojai, CA Zip 93023-3180; tel. 805/646-1401; James Van Duzer, Chief Executive Officer

PALO VERDE HOSPITAL (O, 55 beds) 250 North First Street, Blythe, CA Zip 92225, Mailing Address: P.O. Drawer Z, Zip 92226; tel. 619/922-4115; Vern Reed, Chief Executive Officer

PIONEERS MEMORIAL HOSPITAL (CM, 80 beds) 207 West Legion Road, Brawley, CA Zip 92227-9699; tel. 619/351-3333; William W. Daniel, Administrator and Chief Executive Officer

SAN BENITO HOSPITAL DISTRICT (CM, 86 beds) 911 Sunset Drive, Hollister, CA Zip 95023-5695; tel. 408/637-5711; Louis D. Kraml, Administrator

COLORADO: COLORADO PLAINS MEDICAL CENTER (O, 40 beds) 1000 Lincoln Street, Fort Morgan, CO Zip 80701; tel. 303/867-3391; Keith Mesmer, Administrator and Chief Executive Officer

FLORIDA: EVERGLADES REGIONAL MEDICAL CENTER (CM, 63 beds) 200 South Barfield Highway, Pahokee, FL Zip 33476-1897; tel. 407/924-5200; Donald A. Anderson, President and Chief Executive Officer

IDAHO: CLEARWATER VALLEY HOSPITAL (CM, 26 beds) 301 Cedar, Orofino, ID Zip 83544-9029; tel. 208/476-4555; Warner H. Bartleson, Administrator

ILLINOIS: HAMMOND–HENRY HOSPITAL (CM, 105 beds) 210 West Elk Street, Geneseo, IL Zip 61254-1099; tel. 309/944-6431; William Price, Interim Administrator

HILLSBORO AREA HOSPITAL (CM, 100 beds) 1200 East Tremont Street, Hillsboro, IL Zip 62049; tel. 217/532-6111; Rex H. Brown, President

INDIANA: WIRTH OSTEOPATHIC HOSPITAL (CM, 11 beds) Highway 64 West, Oakland City, IN Zip 47660-9379, Mailing Address: Rural Route 3, Box 14A, Zip 47660-9379; tel. 812/749-6111; James A. Schindler, Administrator

IOWA: GUTTENBERG MUNICIPAL HOSPITAL (CM, 29 beds) Second and Main Street, Guttenberg, IA Zip 52052-0550, Mailing Address: Box 550, Zip 52052-0550; tel. 319/252-1121; Timothy J. Wick, Chief Executive Officer

LOUISIANA: JACKSON PARISH HOSPITAL (CM, 59 beds) 600 Beech Springs Road, Jonesboro, LA Zip 71251, Mailing Address: Box 685, Zip 71251; tel. 318/259-4435; Judy Andrews, Acting Administrator

LADY OF THE SEA GENERAL HOSPITAL (CM, 55 beds) 200 West 134th Place, Cut Off, LA Zip 70345; tel. 504/632-6401; Lane Cheramie, Chief Executive Officer

MICHIGAN: CHIPPEWA COUNTY WAR MEMORIAL HOSPITAL (CM, 137 beds) 500 Osborn Boulevard, Sault Sainte Marie, MI Zip 49783-4467; tel. 906/635-4460; Jerry Popowski, Chief Executive Officer

MINNESOTA: SWIFT COUNTY–BENSON HOSPITAL (CM, 31 beds) 1815 Wisconsin Avenue, Benson, MN Zip 56215-1653; tel. 612/843-4232; John Stindt, Chief Executive Officer

MISSOURI: SULLIVAN COUNTY MEMORIAL HOSPITAL (CM, 47 beds) 630 West Third Street, Milan, MO Zip 63556; tel. 816/265-4212; Nancy Bauman, Chief Executive Officer

MONTANA: BARRETT MEMORIAL HOSPITAL (CM, 31 beds) 1260 South Atlantic Street, Dillon, MT Zip 59725; tel. 406/683-2324; Jim D. Le Brun, Chief Executive Officer

BIG HORN COUNTY MEMORIAL HOSPITAL (CM, 53 beds) 17 North Miles Street, Hardin, MT Zip 59034, Mailing Address: P.O. Box 430, Zip 59034; tel. 406/665-2310; Raymond T. Hino, Chief Executive Officer

CLARK FORK VALLEY HOSPITAL (CM, 44 beds) Plains, MT, Mailing Address: P.O. Box 768, Zip 59859-0768; tel. 406/826-3601; Tom Mitchell, Chief Executive Officer

COMMUNITY MEDICAL CENTER (CM, 123 beds) 2827 Fort Missoula Road, Missoula, MT Zip 59801-7493; tel. 406/728-4100; Grant M. Winn, President

MINERAL COMMUNITY HOSPITAL (CM, 30 beds) Roosevelt and Brooklyn, Superior, MT Zip 59872, Mailing Address: Box 66, Zip 59872-0066; tel. 406/822-4841; Madelyn Faller, Executive Director

POWELL COUNTY MEMORIAL HOSPITAL (CM, 35 beds) 1101 Texas Avenue, Deer Lodge, MT Zip 59722-1828; tel. 406/846-2212; Tony Pfaff, Chief Executive Officer

ROSEBUD HEALTH CARE CENTER (CM, 75 beds) 383 North 17th Avenue, Forsyth, MT Zip 59327-0268; tel. 406/356-2161; John M. Chioutsis, Chief Executive Officer

ROUNDUP MEMORIAL HOSPITAL (CM, 54 beds) 1202 Third Street West, Roundup, MT Zip 59072, Mailing Address: P.O. Box 627, Zip 59072-0627; tel. 406/323-2302; Donna Beane, Administrator

ST. JOHN'S LUTHERAN HOSPITAL (CM, 26 beds) 350 Louisiana Avenue, Libby, MT Zip 59923; tel. 406/293-7761; Richard L. Palagi, Chief Executive Officer

NEW MEXICO: NORTHEASTERN REGIONAL HOSPITAL (CM, 62 beds) 1235 Eighth Street, Las Vegas, NM Zip 87701, Mailing Address: P.O. Box 238, Zip 87701-0238; tel. 505/425-6751; Richard L. Mendoza, Chief Executive Officer

NEW YORK: ADIRONDACK MEDICAL CENTER (CM, 100 beds) Lake Colby Drive, Saranac Lake, NY Zip 12983, Mailing Address: P.O. Box 471, Zip 12983; tel. 518/891-4141; Chandler M. Ralph, President and Chief Executive Officer

LEWIS COUNTY GENERAL HOSPITAL (CM, 214 beds) 7785 North State Street, Lowville, NY Zip 13367-1297; tel. 315/376-5200; G. William Udovich, Chief Executive Officer and Administrator

---

For explanation of codes following names, see page B2.
★Indicates Type III membership in the American Hospital Association.

THE HOSPITAL (CM, 87 beds) Pearl Street, Sidney, NY Zip 13838; tel. 607/563-3512; Thomas J. Graham, Chief Executive Officer

NORTH CAROLINA: BERTIE COUNTY MEMORIAL HOSPITAL (CM, 49 beds) 401 Sterlingworth Street, Windsor, NC Zip 27983-1726, Mailing Address: P.O. Box 40, Zip 27983-1726; tel. 919/794-3141; Anthony F. Mullen, Administrator

OKLAHOMA: MISSION HILL MEMORIAL HOSPITAL (CM, 78 beds) 1900 Gordon Cooper Drive, Shawnee, OK Zip 74801; tel. 405/273-2240; Thomas G. Honaker III, Administrator

OREGON: BLUE MOUNTAIN HOSPITAL (CM, 68 beds) 170 Ford Road, John Day, OR Zip 97845; tel. 503/575-1311; David G. Triebes, Administrator

COTTAGE GROVE HOSPITAL (CM, 71 beds) 1340 Birch Avenue, Cottage Grove, OR Zip 97424; tel. 503/942-0511; William N. Wilber, Chief Executive Officer

MOUNTAIN VIEW HOSPITAL DISTRICT (CM, 102 beds) 470 Northeast A Street, Madras, OR Zip 97741; tel. 503/475-3882; Ronald W. Barnes, Executive Director

TEXAS: GOLDEN PLAINS COMMUNITY HOSPITAL (CM, 55 beds) 200 South McGee Street, Borger, TX Zip 79007; tel. 806/273-1100; Larry J. Lehner, Chief Executive Officer

PARKVIEW REGIONAL HOSPITAL (CM, 36 beds) 312 East Glendale Street, Mexia, TX Zip 76667-3699; tel. 817/562-5332; Karl R. Stinson, Administrator

WASHINGTON: COULEE COMMUNITY HOSPITAL (CM, 48 beds) 411 Fortuyn Road, Grand Coulee, WA Zip 99133-0840, Mailing Address: P.O. Box H, Zip 99133; tel. 509/633-1753; Michael C. Wiltermood, Chief Executive Officer

PULLMAN MEMORIAL HOSPITAL (CM, 36 beds) N.E. 1125 Washington Avenue, Pullman, WA Zip 99163-4742; tel. 509/332-2541; Scott K. Adams, Administrator

SUNNYSIDE COMMUNITY HOSPITAL (CM, 38 beds) 10th and Tacoma Avenue, Sunnyside, WA Zip 98944, Mailing Address: P.O. Box 719, Zip 98944-0719; tel. 509/837-1500; Jon D. Smiley, Chief Executive Officer

WISCONSIN: COMMUNITY MEMORIAL HOSPITAL AND NURSING HOME (CM, 136 beds) 819 Ash Street, Spooner, WI Zip 54801; tel. 715/635-2111; Michael Schafer, Administrator

DIVINE SAVIOR HOSPITAL AND NURSING HOME (CM, 160 beds) 1015 West Pleasant Street, Portage, WI Zip 53901-9987, Mailing Address: P.O. Box 387, Zip 53901; tel. 608/742-4131; Delmar Medill, Chief Executive Officer

LANCASTER MEMORIAL HOSPITAL (CM, 31 beds) 507 South Monroe Street, Lancaster, WI Zip 53813; tel. 608/723-2143; Gregory E. Patten, Administrator

MEMORIAL HOSPITAL OF IOWA COUNTY (CM, 82 beds) 825 South Iowa Street, Dodgeville, WI Zip 53533-1999; tel. 608/935-2711; Ray Marmorstone, Administrator

RIPON MEDICAL CENTER (CM, 29 beds) 933 Newbury Street, Ripon, WI Zip 54971, Mailing Address: P.O. Box 390, Zip 54971-0390; tel. 414/748-3101; Jon W. Baker, Administrator and Chief Executive Officer

SHAWANO MEDICAL CENTER (CM, 53 beds) 309 North Bartlette Street, Shawano, WI Zip 54166-2199; tel. 715/526-2111; John J. Kestly, Administrator

SOUTHWEST HEALTH CENTER (CM, 100 beds) 1100 Fifth Avenue, Platteville, WI Zip 53818; tel. 608/348-2331; Anne K. Klawiter, Chief Executive Officer

ST. JOSEPH'S MEMORIAL HOSPITAL AND NURSING HOME (CM, 85 beds) 400 Water Avenue, Hillsboro, WI Zip 54634-0527, Mailing Address: P.O. Box 527, Zip 54634-0527; tel. 608/489-2211; Jacqueline Pavelski, Chief Executive Officer

SUPERIOR MEMORIAL HOSPITAL (CM, 42 beds) 3500 Tower Avenue, Superior, WI Zip 54880-5395; tel. 715/392-8281; Paul E. Gurgel, Chief Executive Officer

WYOMING: POWELL HOSPITAL (CM, 138 beds) 777 Avenue H, Powell, WY Zip 82435; tel. 307/754-2267; Greg Roraff, Chief Executive Officer

Owned, leased, sponsored:	4 hospitals	294 beds
Contract-managed:	51 hospitals	3388 beds
Totals:	55 hospitals	3682 beds

★**0595: BRONSON HEALTHCARE GROUP, INC.** (NP)
One Healthcare Plaza, Kalamazoo, MI Zip 49007-5345; tel. 616/341-6000; Patric E. Ludwig, President

MICHIGAN: BRONSON METHODIST HOSPITAL (O, 312 beds) 252 East Lovell Street, Kalamazoo, MI Zip 49007-5345; tel. 616/341-6000; Patric E. Ludwig, President

BRONSON VICKSBURG HOSPITAL (O, 41 beds) 13326 North Boulevard, Vicksburg, MI Zip 49097-1099; tel. 616/649-2321

Owned, leased, sponsored:	2 hospitals	353 beds
Contract-managed:	0 hospitals	0 beds
Totals:	2 hospitals	353 beds

★**0955: CAMCARE, INC.** (NP)
501 Morris Street, Charleston, WV Zip 25301, Mailing Address: Box 1547, Zip 25326; tel. 304/348-5432; Phillip H. Goodwin, President

WEST VIRGINIA: BRAXTON COUNTY MEMORIAL HOSPITAL (CM, 30 beds) 100 Hoylman Drive, Gassaway, WV Zip 26624-9308; tel. 304/364-5156; Tony E. Atkins, Administrator

CHARLESTON AREA MEDICAL CENTER (O, 776 beds) 501 Morris Street, Charleston, WV Zip 25301, Mailing Address: Box 1547, Zip 25326; tel. 304/348-5432; Phillip H. Goodwin, President and Chief Executive Officer

Owned, leased, sponsored:	1 hospitals	776 beds
Contract-managed:	1 hospitals	30 beds
Totals:	2 hospitals	806 beds

★**2135: CAPITAL HEALTH SYSTEM** (NP)
17 South Market Square, Harrisburg, PA Zip 17101, Mailing Address: P.O. Box 8700, Zip 17105-8700; tel. 717/782-3366; John S. Cramer FACHE, President and Chief Executive Officer

PENNSYLVANIA: HARRISBURG HOSPITAL (O, 398 beds) 111 South Front Street, Harrisburg, PA Zip 17101-2099; tel. 717/782-3131; Susan Edwards, Senior Vice President and Chief Operating Officer

SEIDLE MEMORIAL HOSPITAL (O, 52 beds) 120 South Filbert Street, Mechanicsburg, PA Zip 17055-6591; tel. 717/795-6760; Susan Edwards, Senior Vice President and Chief Operating Officer

Owned, leased, sponsored:	2 hospitals	450 beds
Contract-managed:	0 hospitals	0 beds
Totals:	2 hospitals	450 beds

★**0070: CARILION HEALTH SYSTEM** (NP)
1212 Third Street S.W., Roanoke, VA Zip 24016, Mailing Address: P.O. Box 13727, Zip 24036-3727; tel. 703/981-7347; Thomas L. Robertson, President and Chief Executive Officer

VIRGINIA: BEDFORD COUNTY MEMORIAL HOSPITAL (O, 166 beds) Oakwood Street, Bedford, VA Zip 24523-0688, Mailing Address: P.O. Box 688, Zip 24523-0688; tel. 703/586-2441; John H. Fretz, Administrator

COMMUNITY HOSPITAL OF ROANOKE VALLEY (O, 232 beds) 101 Elm Avenue S.E., Roanoke, VA Zip 24013, Mailing Address: P.O. Box 12946, Zip 24029; tel. 703/985-8000; Dorman Fawley, President and Chief Executive Officer

FRANKLIN MEMORIAL HOSPITAL (O, 37 beds) 124 Floyd Avenue S.W., Rocky Mount, VA Zip 24151-1389; tel. 703/483-5277; Rayburn A. Thompson, Jr., Administrator

GILES MEMORIAL HOSPITAL (O, 53 beds) 1 Taylor Avenue, Pearisburg, VA Zip 24134, Mailing Address: P.O. Box K, Zip 24134; tel. 703/921-6000; Morris D. Reece, Administrator

GILL MEMORIAL EYE, EAR, NOSE AND THROAT HOSPITAL (O, 12 beds) 711 South Jefferson Street, Roanoke, VA Zip 24016-5103, Mailing Address: P.O. Box 1560, Zip 24007-1560; tel. 703/343-3368; Donald J. Love, Administrator

LONESOME PINE HOSPITAL (CM, 60 beds) 1990 Holton Avenue East, Big Stone Gap, VA Zip 24219-0230, Mailing Address: Drawer I, Zip 24219; tel. 703/523-8609; John L. Thorsten, Administrator

RADFORD COMMUNITY HOSPITAL (O, 155 beds) 700 Randolph Street, Radford, VA Zip 24141-2430; tel. 703/731-2000; Lester L. Lamb, President

ROANOKE MEMORIAL HOSPITALS (O, 454 beds) Belleview at Jefferson Street, Roanoke, VA Zip 24014, Mailing Address: P.O. Box 13367, Zip 24033-3367; tel. 703/981-7000; Houston L. Bell, Jr., President and Chief Executive Officer

---

For explanation of codes following names, see page B2.
★Indicates Type III membership in the American Hospital Association.

Systems / Carilion Health System

SOUTHSIDE COMMUNITY HOSPITAL (CM, 136 beds) 800 Oak Street, Farmville, VA Zip 23901-1199; tel. 804/392-8811; Robert E. Huch, President

ST. ALBANS PSYCHIATRIC HOSPITAL (O, 122 beds) Route 11, Lee Highway, Radford, VA Zip 24141, Mailing Address: Box 3608, Zip 24143; tel. 703/639-2481; Janet K. McKinney, Administrator

STONEWALL JACKSON HOSPITAL (CM, 130 beds) 102 Spotswood Drive, Lexington, VA Zip 24450-2492; tel. 703/463-9141; William Mahone, Administrator

TAZEWELL COMMUNITY HOSPITAL (CM, 56 beds) 141 Ben Bolt Avenue, Tazewell, VA Zip 24651; tel. 703/988-2506; John H. Greer, Administrator

WYTHE COUNTY COMMUNITY HOSPITAL (CM, 90 beds) 600 West Ridge Road, Wytheville, VA Zip 24382; tel. 703/228-0200; Howard Newman Ainsley, Chief Executive Officer

Owned, leased, sponsored:	8 hospitals	1231 beds
Contract-managed:	5 hospitals	472 beds
Totals:	13 hospitals	1703 beds

★1125: **CARITAS CHRISTI HEALTH CARE SYSTEM** (NP)
125 Technology Drive, Suite 5, Waltham, MA Zip 02154-8930; tel. 617/893-8544; Michael F. Collins M.D., President

MASSACHUSETTS: GOOD SAMARITAN MEDICAL CENTER (S, 473 beds) 909 Sumner Street, Stoughton, MA Zip 02072; tel. 617/344-5100; Frank J. Larkin, Chief Executive Officer

HOLY FAMILY HOSPITAL AND MEDICAL CENTER (S, 261 beds) 70 East Street, Methuen, MA Zip 01844-4597; tel. 508/687-0151; William L. Lane, President

SAINT ANNE'S HOSPITAL (S, 175 beds) 795 Middle Street, Fall River, MA Zip 02721-1798; tel. 508/674-5741; Joseph W. Wilczek, Acting President

ST. ELIZABETH'S MEDICAL CENTER OF BOSTON (S, 415 beds) 736 Cambridge Street, Boston, MA Zip 02135; tel. 617/789-3000; Michael F. Collins M.D., President

ST. JOHN OF GOD HOSPITAL (S, 50 beds) Boston, MA, Mailing Address: 296 Allston Street, Brighton, Zip 02146; tel. 617/277-5750; William K. Brinkert, President

Owned, leased, sponsored:	5 hospitals	1374 beds
Contract-managed:	0 hospitals	0 beds
Totals:	5 hospitals	1374 beds

2575: **CARLE FOUNDATION** (NP)
611 West Park Street, Urbana, IL Zip 61801-2595; tel. 217/383-3311; Michael H. Fritz, President

ILLINOIS: CARLE FOUNDATION HOSPITAL (O, 540 beds) 611 West Park Street, Urbana, IL Zip 61801-2595; tel. 217/383-3311; Michael H. Fritz, President

THE PAVILION (O, 38 beds) 809 West Church Street, Champaign, IL Zip 61820; tel. 217/373-1700; Nina Wanchic Eisner, Chief Executive Officer

Owned, leased, sponsored:	2 hospitals	578 beds
Contract-managed:	0 hospitals	0 beds
Totals:	2 hospitals	578 beds

★5945: **CARONDELET HEALTH SYSTEM** (CC)
13801 Riverport Drive, Ste 300, Saint Louis, MO Zip 63043-4810; tel. 314/770-0333; Gary Christiansen, President

ARIZONA: CARONDELET ST. JOSEPH'S HOSPITAL (O, 223 beds) 350 North Wilmot Road, Tucson, AZ Zip 85711; tel. 520/296-3211; Thomas C. Gagen, Chief Operating Officer

CARONDELET ST. MARY'S HOSPITAL (O, 332 beds) 1601 West St Mary's Road, Tucson, AZ Zip 85745-2682; tel. 602/622-5833; Sister St Joan Willert, President and Chief Executive Officer

CARONDELET HOLY CROSS HOSPITAL (O, 80 beds) 1171 Target Range Road, Nogales, AZ Zip 85621; tel. 520/287-2771; C. Ray Honaker, Administrator

CALIFORNIA: DANIEL FREEMAN MARINA HOSPITAL (O, 179 beds) 4650 Lincoln Boulevard, Marina Del Rey, CA Zip 90292-6360; tel. 310/823-8911; Joseph W. Dunn Ph.D., Administrator

DANIEL FREEMAN MEMORIAL HOSPITAL (O, 181 beds) 333 North Prairie Avenue, Inglewood, CA Zip 90301-4514; tel. 310/674-7050; Peter F. Bastone, Chief Executive Officer

SANTA MARTA HOSPITAL (O, 110 beds) 319 North Humphreys Avenue, Los Angeles, CA Zip 90022; tel. 213/266-6500; Wilfred G. Mallari, President and Chief Executive Officer

GEORGIA: ST. JOSEPH HOSPITAL (O, 148 beds) 2260 Wrightsboro Road, Augusta, GA Zip 30904-4726; tel. 706/481-7000; J. William Paugh, President and Chief Executive Officer

WALTON REHABILITATION HOSPITAL (P, 58 beds) 1355 Independence Drive, Augusta, GA Zip 30901-1037; tel. 706/823-8505; Dennis B. Skelley, President and Chief Executive Officer

IDAHO: ST. JOSEPH REGIONAL MEDICAL CENTER (O, 141 beds) 415 Sixth Street, Lewiston, ID Zip 83501-0816; tel. 208/743-2511; Howard A. Hayes, President and Chief Executive Officer

MISSOURI: SAINT JOSEPH HEALTH CENTER (O, 254 beds) 1000 Carondelet Drive, Kansas City, MO Zip 64114-4673; tel. 816/942-4400; Richard M. Abell, President

ST. MARY'S HOSPITAL OF BLUE SPRINGS (O, 110 beds) 201 West R D Mize Road, Blue Springs, MO Zip 64014; tel. 816/228-5900; N. Gary Wages, President

NEW YORK: ST. MARY'S HOSPITAL (O, 143 beds) 427 Guy Park Avenue, Amsterdam, NY Zip 12010-1095; tel. 518/842-1900; Peter E. Capobianco, President and Chief Executive Officer

WASHINGTON: OUR LADY OF LOURDES HEALTH CENTER (O, 132 beds) 520 North Fourth Avenue, Pasco, WA Zip 99301, Mailing Address: P.O. Box 2568, Zip 99302; tel. 509/547-7704; Thomas Corley, Administrator

Owned, leased, sponsored:	12 hospitals	2033 beds
Contract-managed:	0 hospitals	0 beds
Totals:	12 hospitals	2033 beds

★6545: **CATHEDRAL HEALTHCARE SYSTEM, INC.** (CC)
219 Chestnut Street, Newark, NJ Zip 07105-1558; tel. 201/690-3600; Frank L. Fumai, President and Chief Executive Officer

NEW JERSEY: SAINT JAMES HOSPITAL OF NEWARK (O, 189 beds) 155 Jefferson Street, Newark, NJ Zip 07105; tel. 201/589-1300; Dominick R. Calgi, Administrator

SAINT MICHAEL'S MEDICAL CENTER (O, 419 beds) 268 Dr Martin Luther King Jr Boulevard, Newark, NJ Zip 07102-2094; tel. 201/877-5000; Dominick R. Calgi, Administrator

Owned, leased, sponsored:	2 hospitals	608 beds
Contract-managed:	0 hospitals	0 beds
Totals:	2 hospitals	608 beds

★5175: **CATHOLIC HEALTH CORPORATION** (CC)
920 South 107th Avenue, Omaha, NE Zip 68114-4719; tel. 402/393-7661; A. Diane Moeller, Chief Executive Officer

CALIFORNIA: MERCY HOSPITAL AND HEALTH SERVICES (CM, 101 beds) 2740 M Street, Merced, CA Zip 95340-2880; tel. 209/384-6444; Kelly C. Morgan, President and Chief Executive Officer

COLORADO: MERCY MEDICAL CENTER (CM, 105 beds) 375 East Park Avenue, Durango, CO Zip 81301; tel. 303/247-4311; G. Dale Jessup, President and Chief Executive Officer

IDAHO: MERCY MEDICAL CENTER (CM, 152 beds) 1512 12th Avenue Road, Nampa, ID Zip 83686-6008; tel. 208/467-1171; Robert A. Fale, President and Chief Executive Officer

IOWA: MERCY HOSPITAL (CM, 22 beds) Rosary Drive, Corning, IA Zip 50841, Mailing Address: Box 368, Zip 50841; tel. 515/322-3121; James C. Ruppert, President

MERCY HOSPITAL (CM, 210 beds) 800 Mercy Drive, Council Bluffs, IA Zip 51503, Mailing Address: Box 1C, Zip 51502; tel. 712/328-5000; Richard A. Hachten II, President

MERCY HOSPITAL MEDICAL CENTER (CM, 638 beds) 400 University Avenue, Des Moines, IA Zip 50314; tel. 515/247-4278; Thomas A. Reitinger, President and Chief Executive Officer

ST. JOSEPH'S MERCY HOSPITAL (CM, 58 beds) 1 St Joseph's Drive, Centerville, IA Zip 52544; tel. 515/437-4111; William C. Assell, President and Chief Executive Officer

---

For explanation of codes following names, see page B2.
★Indicates Type III membership in the American Hospital Association.

KANSAS: CENTRAL KANSAS MEDICAL CENTER (CM, 121 beds) 3515 Broadway Street, Great Bend, KS Zip 67530; tel. 316/792-2511; Gary L. Barnett, President and Chief Executive Officer

ST. CATHERINE HOSPITAL (CM, 99 beds) 410 East Walnut, Garden City, KS Zip 67846-5672; tel. 316/272-2222; Steven D. Wilkinson, President and Chief Executive Officer

MINNESOTA: ALBANY AREA HOSPITAL AND MEDICAL CENTER (S, 17 beds) 300 Third Avenue, Albany, MN Zip 56307; tel. 612/845-2121; Fred Struzyk, Chief Operating Officer

LAKEWOOD HEALTH CENTER (S, 73 beds) 600 South Main Avenue, Baudette, MN Zip 56623, Mailing Address: Route 1, Box 2120, Zip 56623; tel. 218/634-2120; David A. Nelson, President and Chief Executive Officer

ST. FRANCIS MEDICAL CENTER (S, 171 beds) 415 Oak Street, Breckenridge, MN Zip 56520; tel. 218/643-3000; Mark C. McNelly, President and Chief Executive Officer

ST. GABRIEL'S HOSPITAL (S, 205 beds) 815 Second Street S.E., Little Falls, MN Zip 56345-3596; tel. 612/632-5441; Larry A. Schulz, President and Chief Executive Officer

ST. JOSEPH'S HOSPITAL (S, 42 beds) 600 Pleasant Avenue, Park Rapids, MN Zip 56470; tel. 218/732-3311; David R. Hove, President

MISSOURI: ST. JOHN'S REGIONAL MEDICAL CENTER (CM, 331 beds) 2727 McClelland Boulevard, Joplin, MO Zip 64804; tel. 417/781-2727; Robert G. Brueckner, President and Chief Executive Officer

NEBRASKA: BERGAN MERCY MEDICAL CENTER (CM, 607 beds) 7500 Mercy Road, Omaha, NE Zip 68124; tel. 402/398-6060; Richard A. Hachten II, President

NORTH DAKOTA: CARRINGTON HEALTH CENTER (CM, 70 beds) 800 North Fourth Street, Carrington, ND Zip 58421; tel. 701/652-3141; Michael A. Baumgartner, President

MERCY HOSPITAL (CM, 55 beds) 1031 Seventh Street, Devils Lake, ND Zip 58301-2798; tel. 701/662-2131; Marlene Krein, President and Chief Executive Officer

MERCY HOSPITAL (CM, 50 beds) 570 Chautauqua Boulevard, Valley City, ND Zip 58072-3199; tel. 701/845-0440; Greg Hanson, President

MERCY MEDICAL CENTER (CM, 113 beds) 1301 15th Avenue West, Williston, ND Zip 58801-3896; tel. 701/774-7400; Duane D. Jerde, President and Chief Executive Officer

ST. ANSGAR'S HOSPITAL (CM, 20 beds) 115 Vivian Street, Park River, ND Zip 58270-9998; tel. 701/284-7500; Michael D. Mahrer, President

ST. JOSEPH'S HOSPITAL AND HEALTH CENTER (S, 85 beds) 30 Seventh Street West, Dickinson, ND Zip 58601; tel. 701/225-7200; John S. Studsrud, President

OREGON: HOLY ROSARY MEDICAL CENTER (CM, 74 beds) 351 Southwest Ninth Street, Ontario, OR Zip 97914-2693; tel. 503/889-5331; Bruce Jensen, President and Chief Executive Officer

MERCY MEDICAL CENTER (CM, 96 beds) 2700 Stewart Parkway, Roseburg, OR Zip 97470; tel. 503/673-0611; Jacquetta Taylor, President and Chief Executive Officer

SOUTH DAKOTA: GETTYSBURG MEDICAL CENTER (CM, 12 beds) 606 East Garfield, Gettysburg, SD Zip 57442; tel. 605/765-2488; Brian J. McDermott, Administrator

SACRED HEART HEALTH SERVICES (CM, 257 beds) 501 Summit, Yankton, SD Zip 57078-3899; tel. 605/665-9371; Dennis A. Sokol, President and Chief Executive Officer

ST. BENEDICT HEALTH CENTER (CM, 105 beds) Glynn Drive, Parkston, SD Zip 57366, Mailing Address: P.O. Box B, 57366; tel. 605/928-3311; Gale Walker, Administrator

ST. MARY'S HOSPITAL (CM, 191 beds) 800 East Dakota Avenue, Pierre, SD Zip 57501-3313; tel. 605/224-3100; James D. M. Russell, Chief Executive Officer

WISCONSIN: GOOD SAMARITAN HEALTH CENTER OF MERRILL (S, 63 beds) 601 Center Avenue South, Merrill, WI Zip 54452; tel. 715/536-5511; Michael Hammer, President and Chief Executive Officer

ST. CATHERINE'S HOSPITAL (CM, 170 beds) 3556 Seventh Avenue, Kenosha, WI Zip 53140-2595; tel. 414/656-3011; Bruce Rampage, President and Chief Executive Officer

TRINITY MEMORIAL HOSPITAL (S, 178 beds) 5900 South Lake Drive, Cudahy, WI Zip 53110-8903; tel. 414/769-9000; Terrance E. Wilson, Interim Chief Operating Officer

Owned, leased, sponsored:	8 hospitals	834 beds
Contract-managed:	23 hospitals	3657 beds
Totals:	31 hospitals	4491 beds

★**5205:** **CATHOLIC HEALTHCARE WEST** (CC)
1700 Montgomery Street, Suite 300, San Francisco, CA Zip 94111-9603; tel. 415/397-9000; Richard J. Kramer, President and Chief Executive Officer

ARIZONA: ST. JOSEPH'S HOSPITAL AND MEDICAL CENTER (S, 493 beds) 350 West Thomas Road, Phoenix, AZ Zip 85013, Mailing Address: Box 2071, Zip 85001-2071; tel. 602/285-3000; Mary G. Yarbrough, Chief Executive Officer

CALIFORNIA: DOMINICAN SANTA CRUZ HOSPITAL (S, 284 beds) 1555 Soquel Drive, Santa Cruz, CA Zip 95065-1794; tel. 408/462-7700; Sister Julie Hyer, President and Chief Executive Officer

MERCY GENERAL HOSPITAL (S, 404 beds) 4001 J Street, Sacramento, CA Zip 95819; tel. 916/453-4950; Thomas A. Petersen, Vice President and Chief Operating Officer

MERCY HEALTHCARE SACRAMENTO (S, 354 beds) 6501 Coyle Avenue, Carmichael, CA Zip 95608, Mailing Address: P.O. Box 479, Zip 95608; tel. 916/537-5000; Sister Bridget McCarthy, President

MERCY HOSPITAL (S, 261 beds) 2215 Truxtun Avenue, Bakersfield, CA Zip 93301, Mailing Address: Box 119, Zip 93302; tel. 805/632-5000; Bernard J. Herman, President

MERCY HOSPITAL AND MEDICAL CENTER (S, 417 beds) 4077 Fifth Avenue, San Diego, CA Zip 92103-2180; tel. 619/294-8111; Ralph George M.D., President and Chief Executive Officer

MERCY HOSPITAL OF FOLSOM (S, 89 beds) 1650 Creekside Drive, Folsom, CA Zip 95630-3405; tel. 916/983-7400; Donald C. Hudson, Vice President and Chief Operating Officer

MERCY MEDICAL CENTER (S, 220 beds) 2175 Rosaline Avenue, Redding, CA Zip 96001, Mailing Address: Box 496009, Zip 96049-6009; tel. 916/225-6000; George A. Govier, President

MERCY MEDICAL CENTER MOUNT SHASTA (S, 80 beds) 914 Pine Street, Mount Shasta, CA Zip 96067, Mailing Address: P.O. Box 239, Zip 96067-0239; tel. 916/926-6111; James R. Hoss, President

METHODIST HOSPITAL (S, 309 beds) 7500 Hospital Drive, Sacramento, CA Zip 95823-5477; tel. 916/423-3000; Stanley C. Oppegard, Vice President and Chief Operating Officer

SAINT FRANCIS MEMORIAL HOSPITAL (S, 221 beds) 900 Hyde Street, San Francisco, CA Zip 94109, Mailing Address: Box 7726, Zip 94120-7726; tel. 415/353-6000; John G. Williams, President

ST. JOHN'S PLEASANT VALLEY HOSPITAL (S, 158 beds) 2309 Antonio Avenue, Camarillo, CA Zip 93010-1459; tel. 805/389-5800; Charles Padilla, Vice President and Administrator

ST. MARY'S MEDICAL CENTER (S, 309 beds) 450 Stanyan Street, San Francisco, CA Zip 94117-1079; tel. 415/668-1000; Mary Ann Thode, President and Chief Executive Officer

ST. JOHN'S REGIONAL MEDICAL CENTER (S, 240 beds) 1600 North Rose Avenue, Oxnard, CA Zip 93030; tel. 805/988-2500; Daniel R. Herlinger, President and Chief Executive Officer

NEVADA: ST. ROSE DOMINICAN HOSPITAL (S, 117 beds) 102 Lake Mead Drive, Henderson, NV Zip 89015; tel. 702/564-2622; Rod A. Davis, President and Chief Executive Officer

Owned, leased, sponsored:	15 hospitals	3956 beds
Contract-managed:	0 hospitals	0 beds
Totals:	15 hospitals	3956 beds

★**2265:** **CENTRA HEALTH, INC.** (NP)
1920 Atherholt Road, Lynchburg, VA Zip 24501-1104; tel. 804/947-4700; George W. Dawson, President and Chief Executive Officer

VIRGINIA: LYNCHBURG GENERAL HOSPITAL (O, 320 beds) 1901 Tate Springs Road, Lynchburg, VA Zip 24501-1167; tel. 804/947-3000; L. Darrell Powers, President

VIRGINIA BAPTIST HOSPITAL (O, 344 beds) 3300 Rivermont Avenue, Lynchburg, VA Zip 24503-9989; tel. 804/947-4000; Thomas C. Jividen, President

Owned, leased, sponsored:	2 hospitals	664 beds
Contract-managed:	0 hospitals	0 beds
Totals:	2 hospitals	664 beds

0665: **CENTURY HEALTHCARE CORPORATION** (IO)
5555 East 71st Street, Suite 9220, Tulsa, OK Zip 74136-6540; tel. 918/491-0775; Jerry D. Dillon, President & Chief Executive Officer

---

For explanation of codes following names, see page B2.
★Indicates Type III membership in the American Hospital Association.

Systems / Century Healthcare Corporation

ARIZONA: WESTBRIDGE TREATMENT CENTER (O, 83 beds) 1830 East Roosevelt, Phoenix, AZ Zip 85006; tel. 602/254–0884; Jeffrey M. Kaplan, Chief Executive Officer

WESTBRIDGE TREATMENT CENTER – NORTH CAMPUS (O, 45 beds) 720 East Montebello, Phoenix, AZ 85014–2599; tel. 602/277–KIDS; Jeffrey M. Kaplan, Chief Executive Officer

OKLAHOMA: HIGH POINTE (O, 68 beds) 6501 Northeast 50th Street, Oklahoma City, OK Zip 73141–9613; tel. 405/424–3383; Charlene Arnett, Chief Executive Officer

Owned, leased, sponsored:	3 hospitals	196 beds
Contract–managed:	0 hospitals	0 beds
Totals:	3 hospitals	196 beds

0705: CHARLOTTE–MECKLENBURG HOSPITAL AUTHORITY (NP)

1000 Blythe Boulevard, Charlotte, NC Zip 28203, Mailing Address: Box 32861, Zip 28232–2861; tel. 704/355–2000; Harry A. Nurkin Ph.D., President

NORTH CAROLINA: CAROLINAS MEDICAL CENTER (O, 843 beds) 1000 Blythe Boulevard, Charlotte, NC Zip 28203, Mailing Address: P.O. Box 32861, Zip 28232–2861; tel. 704/355–2000; Harry A. Nurkin Ph.D., President

CHARLOTTE INSTITUTE OF REHABILITATION (O, 114 beds) 1100 Blythe Boulevard, Charlotte, NC Zip 28203; tel. 704/355–4300; Hollis Hamilton, Administrator

UNIVERSITY HOSPITAL (O, 107 beds) 8800 North Tryon Street, Charlotte, NC Zip 28262, Mailing Address: P.O. Box 560727, Zip 28256; tel. 704/548–6000; W. Spencer Lilly, Administrator

Owned, leased, sponsored:	3 hospitals	1064 beds
Contract–managed:	0 hospitals	0 beds
Totals:	3 hospitals	1064 beds

0695: CHARTER MEDICAL CORPORATION (IO)

3414 Peachtree Road N.E., Ste 1400, Atlanta, GA Zip 30326; tel. 404/841–9200; E. Mac Crawford, President and Chief Operating Officer

ALABAMA: CHARTER HOSPITAL OF MOBILE (O, 84 beds) 5800 Southland Drive, Mobile, AL Zip 36693, Mailing Address: P.O. Box 991800, Zip 36691; tel. 205/661–3001; Keith Cox, Chief Executive Officer

CHARTER WOODS BEHAVIORAL HEALTH SYSTEM (O, 75 beds) 700 Cottonwood Road, Dothan, AL Zip 36301, Mailing Address: P.O. Box 6138, Zip 36302; tel. 334/794–4357; Charles Whitson, Chief Executive Officer

ALASKA: CHARTER NORTH HOSPITAL (O, 80 beds) 2530 Debarr Road, Anchorage, AK Zip 99508; tel. 907/258–7575; Kathleen Cronen, Administrator

ARIZONA: CHARTER BEHAVIORAL HEALTH SYSTEM (O, 80 beds) 2190 North Grace Boulevard, Chandler, AZ Zip 85224; tel. 602/899–8989; Kim Hall, Administrator

CHARTER BEHAVIORAL HEALTH SYSTEM (O, 90 beds) 6015 West Peoria Avenue, Glendale, AZ Zip 85302; tel. 602/878–7878; Kimbrough Hall, Chief Executive Officer

CHARTER BEHAVIORAL HEALTH SYSTEM–TUCSON (O, 54 beds) 7220 E. Rosewood Street, Tucson, AZ Zip 85710; tel. 520/745–5100; Mary Jean Geroulo, Chief Executive Officer

ARKANSAS: CHARTER HOSPITAL OF LITTLE ROCK (O, 60 beds) 1601 Murphy Drive, Maumelle, AR Zip 72113; tel. 501/851–8700; Joseph Fischer, Administrator

CHARTER VISTA HOSPITAL (O, 65 beds) 4253 Crossover Road, Fayetteville, AR Zip 72702; tel. 501/521–5731; Lucinda DeBruce, Administrator

CALIFORNIA: CANYON SPRINGS HOSPITAL (O, 80 beds) 69–696 Ramon Road, Cathedral City, CA Zip 92234; tel. 619/321–2000; Michael A. Dougherty Ph.D., Chief Executive Officer

CHARTER BEHAVIORAL HEALTH SYSTEM OF SOUTHERN CALIFORNIA–CHARTER OAK (O, 95 beds) 1161 East Covina Boulevard, Covina, CA Zip 91724–1161; tel. 818/966–1632; Todd A. Smith, Chief Executive Officer

CHARTER BEHAVIORAL HEALTH SYSTEM OF SOUTHERN CALIFORNIA–LONG BEACH (O, 50 beds) 6060 Paramount Boulevard, Long Beach, CA Zip 90805; tel. 310/220–1000

CHARTER BEHAVIORAL HEALTH SYSTEM OF SOUTHERN CALIFORNIA–LOS ALTOS (O, 46 beds) 3340 Los Coyotes Diagonal, Long Beach, CA Zip 90808–3999; tel. 310/421–9311; Larry Steudle, Chief Executive Officer

CHARTER BEHAVIORAL HEALTH SYSTEM OF SOUTHERN CALIFORNIA–THOUSAND OAKS (O, 35 beds) 150 Via Merida, Thousand Oaks, CA Zip 91361; tel. 805/495–3292; Michelle Egerer, Chief Executive Officer

CHARTER BEHAVIORAL HEALTH SYSTEM OF THE INLAND EMPIRE (O, 158 beds) 2055 Kellogg Avenue, Corona, CA Zip 91719; tel. 909/735–2910; Diana C. Hanyak, Chief Executive Officer

CHARTER HOSPITAL OF MISSION VIEJO (O, 80 beds) 23228 Madero, Mission Viejo, CA Zip 92691; tel. 714/830–4800; Jeffrey A. Thrash, Administrator

COLORADO: CHARTER BEHAVIORAL HEALTH SYSTEM AT CENTENNIAL PEAKS (O, 72 beds) 2255 South 88th Street, Louisville, CO Zip 80027; tel. 303/673–9990; Sharon Worsham, Administrator

CONNECTICUT: ELMCREST PSYCHIATRIC INSTITUTE (O, 105 beds) 25 Marlborough Street, Portland, CT Zip 06480; tel. 203/342–0480; Ralph Sperry, Chief Executive Officer

FLORIDA: CHARTER BEHAVIORAL HEALTH SYSTEM AT MEDFIELD (O, 64 beds) 12891 Seminole Boulevard, Largo, FL Zip 34648–2300; tel. 813/587–6000; Laura M. Schuck, Chief Executive Officer

CHARTER GLADE BEHAVIORAL HEALTH SYSTEM (O, 104 beds) 3550 Colonial Boulevard, Fort Myers, FL Zip 33912, Mailing Address: P.O. Box 06120, Zip 33906; tel. 813/939–0403; Martin Schappell, Administrator

CHARTER HOSPITAL OF JACKSONVILLE (O, 64 beds) 3947 Salisbury Road, Jacksonville, FL Zip 32216; tel. 904/296–2447; Douglas Joiner, Chief Executive Officer

CHARTER HOSPITAL OF MIAMI (O, 88 beds) 11100 Northwest 27th Street, Miami, FL Zip 33172; tel. 305/591–3230; Amanda Hopkins–Alexiadis, Chief Executive Officer

CHARTER HOSPITAL OF PASCO (O, 72 beds) 21808 State Road 54, Lutz, FL Zip 33549; tel. 813/948–2441; Miriam K. Williams, Administrator

CHARTER HOSPITAL OF TAMPA BAY (O, 146 beds) 4004 North Riverside Drive, Tampa, FL Zip 33603; tel. 813/238–8671; Terry Fields, Administrator

CHARTER HOSPITAL ORLANDO SOUTH (O, 60 beds) 206 Park Place Drive, Kissimmee, FL Zip 34741; tel. 407/846–0444; Michael L. Harrington, Group Chief Executive Officer

CHARTER SPRINGS HOSPITAL (O, 92 beds) 3130 Southwest 27th Avenue, Ocala, FL Zip 34474, Mailing Address: P.O. Box 3338, Zip 34478; tel. 904/237–7293; James Duff, Administrator

GEORGIA: CHARTER BY–THE–SEA HOSPITAL (O, 101 beds) 2927 Demere Road, Saint Simons Island, GA Zip 31522–1620; tel. 912/638–1999; Olivia A. Erbele, Chief Executive Officer

CHARTER LAKE HOSPITAL (O, 118 beds) 3500 Riverside Drive, Macon, GA Zip 31210; tel. 912/474–6200; Blair R. Johanson, Administrator

CHARTER PEACHFORD HOSPITAL (O, 294 beds) 2151 Peachford Road, Atlanta, GA Zip 30338; tel. 404/455–3200; James F. Button, Administrator

CHARTER SAVANNAH BEHAVIORAL HEALTH SYSTEM (O, 112 beds) 1150 Cornell Avenue, Savannah, GA Zip 31406, Mailing Address: P.O. Box 13817, Zip 31416; tel. 912/354–3911; Ron Fincher, Chief Executive Officer

CHARTER WINDS HOSPITAL (O, 80 beds) 240 Mitchell Bridge Road, Athens, GA Zip 30606, Mailing Address: P.O. Box 6297, Zip 30604; tel. 706/546–7277; Mark Snow, Chief Executive Officer

PSYCHIATRIC INSTITUTE OF ATLANTA (O, 40 beds) 811 Juniper Street N.E., Atlanta, GA Zip 30308; tel. 404/881–5800; Dennis Workman M.D., Medical Director

ILLINOIS: CHARTER BARCLAY HOSPITAL (O, 123 beds) 4700 North Clarendon Avenue, Chicago, IL Zip 60640; tel. 312/728–7100; John F. Buckley, Administrator

INDIANA: CHARTER BEACON (O, 97 beds) 1720 Beacon Street, Fort Wayne, IN Zip 46805; tel. 219/423–3651; Wendy Swisher, Chief Executive Officer

CHARTER BEHAVIORAL HEALTH SYSTEM OF MICHIGAN CITY (O, 89 beds) 3714 South Franklin Street, Michigan City, IN Zip 46360; tel. 219/872–0531; Michael J. Brown, Administrator

CHARTER BEHAVIORAL HEALTH SYSTEM OF NORTHWEST INDIANA (O, 60 beds) 101 W 61st Avenue & State Road 51, Hobart, IN Zip 46342; tel. 219/947–4464; Barry W. Woodward, Chief Executive Officer

CHARTER BEHAVIORAL HEALTH SYSTEMS (O, 64 beds) 3700 Rome Drive, Lafayette, IN Zip 47905, Mailing Address: P.O. Box 5969, Zip 47903; tel. 317/448–6999; Stewart Graham, Administrator

---

For explanation of codes following names, see page B2.
★Indicates Type III membership in the American Hospital Association.

Systems / Columbia/HCA Healthcare Corporation

CHARTER INDIANAPOLIS BEHAVIORAL HEALTH SYSTEM (O, 60 beds) 5602 Caito Drive, Indianapolis, IN Zip 46226; tel. 317/545-2111; Daniel J. Body, Chief Executive Officer

KENTUCKY: CHARTER BEHAVIORAL HEALTH SYSTEM OF PADUCAH (O, 51 beds) 435 Berger Road, Paducah, KY Zip 42001, Mailing Address: P.O. Box 7609, Zip 42002-7609; tel. 502/444-0444; Pat Harrod, Chief Executive Officer

CHARTER HOSPITAL OF LOUISVILLE (O, 66 beds) 1405 Browns Lane, Louisville, KY Zip 40207; tel. 502/896-0495; Todd B. Graybill, Administrator

CHARTER RIDGE HOSPITAL (O, 110 beds) 3050 Rio Dosa Drive, Lexington, KY Zip 40509-9990; tel. 606/269-2325; Scott W. Kardenetz, Chief Executive Officer

LOUISIANA: CHARTER BEHAVIORAL HEALTH SYSTEM AT ACADIAN OAKS HOSPITAL (O, 39 beds) 310 Youngsville Highway, Lafayette, LA Zip 70508; tel. 318/837-8787; Joseph A. Dunston, Interim Chief Executive Officer

CHARTER FOREST BEHAVIORAL HEALTH SYSTEM (O, 65 beds) 9320 Linwood Avenue, Shreveport, LA Zip 71106, Mailing Address: P.O. Box 18130, Zip 71138-1130; tel. 318/688-3930; Randy J. Watson, Administrator

CHARTER HOSPITAL OF LAKE CHARLES (O, 60 beds) 4250 Fifth Avenue South, Lake Charles, LA Zip 70605-3812; tel. 318/474-6133; Peter Lomonte, Chief Executive Officer

MARYLAND: CHARTER BEHAVIORAL HEALTH SYSTEM (O, 48 beds) 522 Thomas Run Road, Bel Air, MD Zip 21014-7607; tel. 410/879-1919

CHARTER BEHAVIORAL HEALTH SYSTEM OF POTOMAC RIDGE (O, 88 beds) 14901 Broschart Road, Rockville, MD Zip 20850; tel. 301/251-4500; Jonathan A. Garber, Administrator and Chief Executive Officer

MISSISSIPPI: CHARTER HOSPITAL OF JACKSON (O, 111 beds) 3531 Lakeland Drive, Jackson, MS Zip 39208, Mailing Address: Box 4297, Zip 39296; tel. 601/939-9030; Jim R. Johnson, Administrator

NEVADA: CHARTER BEHAVIORAL HEALTH SYSTEM OF NEVADA (O, 84 beds) 7000 W Spring Mountain Road, Las Vegas, NV Zip 89117; tel. 702/876-4357; Gerald A. Greene, Chief Executive Officer

NEW HAMPSHIRE: CHARTER BROOKSIDE BEHAVIORAL HEALTH SYSTEM OF NEW ENGLAND (O, 100 beds) 29 Northwest Boulevard, Nashua, NH Zip 03063; tel. 603/886-5000; Joel Rosenhaus, Administrator

NEW JERSEY: CHARTER BEHAVIORAL HEALTH SYSTEM OF NEW JERSEY–SUMMIT (O, 80 beds) 19 Prospect Street, Summit, NJ Zip 07902-0100; tel. 908/522-7000

NEW MEXICO: CHARTER HOSPITAL OF ALBUQUERQUE (O, 80 beds) 5901 Zuni Road S.E., Albuquerque, NM Zip 87108; tel. 505/265-8800; Joel A. Hart FACHE, Chief Executive Officer

NORTH CAROLINA: CHARTER ASHEVILLE (O, 100 beds) 60 Caledonia Road, Asheville, NC Zip 28803, Mailing Address: P.O. Box 5534, Zip 28813; tel. 704/253-3681; Jay Cutspec, Chief Executive Officer

CHARTER GREENSBORO BEHAVIORAL HEALTH SYSTEM (O, 68 beds) 700 Walter Reed Drive, Greensboro, NC Zip 27403-1129, Mailing Address: P.O. Box 10399, Zip 27404-0399; tel. 910/852-4821; Joe Crabtree, Chief Executive Officer

CHARTER HOSPITAL OF WINSTON–SALEM (O, 99 beds) 3637 Old Vineyard Road, Winston–Salem, NC Zip 27104; tel. 910/768-7710; Marina Cecchini, Chief Executive Officer

CHARTER PINES HOSPITAL (O, 60 beds) 3621 Randolph Road, Charlotte, NC Zip 28211, Mailing Address: P.O. Box 221709, Zip 28222-1709; tel. 704/365-5368; Edward Payton, Chief Executive Officer

OHIO: CHARTER HOSPITAL OF TOLEDO (O, 38 beds) 1725 Timber Line Road, Maumee, OH Zip 43537-4015; tel. 419/891-9333; Michael Cornelison, Chief Executive Officer

PENNSYLVANIA: CHARTER BEHAVIORAL HEALTH SYSTEM AT COVE FORGE (O, 100 beds) Route 1, Box 79, Williamsburg, PA Zip 16693, Mailing Address: P.O. Box B, Zip 16693; tel. 814/832-2121; Jonathan Wolf, Chief Executive Officer

CHARTER FAIRMOUNT INSTITUTE (O, 146 beds) 561 Fairthorne Avenue, Philadelphia, PA Zip 19128-2499; tel. 215/487-4000; Paul B. Henry, Administrator

SOUTH CAROLINA: CHARTER HOSPITAL OF CHARLESTON (O, 102 beds) 2777 Speissegger Drive, Charleston, SC Zip 29405-8299; tel. 803/747-5830; James E. Ledbetter Ph.D., Administrator

CHARTER HOSPITAL OF GREENVILLE (O, 60 beds) 2700 East Phillips Road, Greer, SC Zip 29650; tel. 803/879-3402; Louis R. Joseph III, Administrator

CHARTER RIVERS HOSPITAL (O, 80 beds) 2900 Sunset Boulevard, West Columbia, SC Zip 29169, Mailing Address: P.O. Box 4116, Zip 29171-4116; tel. 803/796-9911; Janet N. Chubb, Chief Executive Officer

SOUTH DAKOTA: CHARTER SIOUX FALLS BEHAVIORAL HEALTH SYSTEM (O, 60 beds) 2812 South Louise Avenue, Sioux Falls, SD Zip 57106; tel. 605/361-8111; John N. Olson, Administrator

TENNESSEE: CHARTER LAKESIDE HOSPITAL (O, 174 beds) 2911 Brunswick Road, Memphis, TN Zip 38133, Mailing Address: P.O. Box 341308, Zip 38134; tel. 901/377-4700; Sherry C. Thornton, Chief Executive Officer

TEXAS: CHARTER BEHAVIORAL HEALTH SYSTEM (O, 80 beds) 6201 Overton Ridge Boulevard, Fort Worth, TX Zip 76132-3699; tel. 817/292-6844; Liam J. Mulvaney, Chief Executive Officer

CHARTER BEHAVIORAL HEALTH SYSTEM (O, 72 beds) 801 North Quaker, Lubbock, TX Zip 79416, Mailing Address: P.O. Box 10560, Zip 79408; tel. 806/744-5505; Liam J. Mulvaney, Chief Executive Officer and Administrator

CHARTER BEHAVIORAL HEALTH SYSTEM (O, 72 beds) 1421 East Jackson Avenue, McAllen, TX Zip 78501, Mailing Address: P.O. Box 5239, Zip 78502; tel. 512/631-5421; Leslie B. Hedfelt, Chief Executive Officer

CHARTER BEHAVIORAL HEALTH SYSTEM (O, 96 beds) 8550 Huebner Road, San Antonio, TX Zip 78240, Mailing Address: P.O. Box 380157, Zip 78280; tel. 210/699-8585; Michael Lee, Administrator

CHARTER BEHAVIORAL HEALTH SYSTEM (O, 80 beds) 2001 Ladbrook Drive, Kingwood, TX Zip 77339-3004; tel. 713/358-4501; Mark Micheletti, Chief Executive Officer

CHARTER BEHAVIORAL HEALTH SYSTEM OF AUSTIN (O, 70 beds) 8402 Cross Park Drive, Austin, TX Zip 78754, Mailing Address: P.O. Box 140585, Zip 78714-0585; tel. 512/837-1800; Trish Mitchell, Network Chief Executive Officer

CHARTER BEHAVIORAL HEALTH SYSTEM OF CLEAR LAKE (O, 84 beds) 709 Medical Center Boulevard, Webster, TX Zip 77598; tel. 713/332-9550; Chris Duello, Administrator and Chief Executive Officer

CHARTER BEHAVIORAL HEALTH SYSTEM–CORPUS CHRISTI (O, 80 beds) 3126 Rodd Field Road, Corpus Christi, TX Zip 78414; tel. 512/993-8893; Steve Kamber, Administrator

CHARTER GRAPEVINE BEHAVIORAL HEALTH SYSTEM (O, 80 beds) 2300 William D Tate Avenue, Grapevine, TX Zip 76051-9964; tel. 817/481-1900; Richard C. Gibson, Chief Executive Officer

VIRGINIA: CHARTER BEHAVIORAL HEALTH SYSTEM AT SPRINGWOOD (O, 77 beds) Leesburg, VA, Mailing Address: Route 4, Box 50, Zip 22075; tel. 703/777-0800; Sybil Potts, Chief Executive Officer

CHARTER BEHAVIORAL HEALTH SYSTEM OF CHARLOTTESVILLE (O, 75 beds) 2101 Arlington Boulevard, Charlottesville, VA Zip 22903-1593; tel. 804/977-1120; David W. Pedrick, Chief Executive Officer

CHARTER WESTBROOK BEHAVIORAL HEALTH SYSTEM (O, 210 beds) 1500 Westbrook Avenue, Richmond, VA Zip 23227; tel. 804/266-9671; Edward Owen, Jr., Chief Executive Officer

PSYCHIATRIC INSTITUTE OF RICHMOND (O, 84 beds) 12800 West Creek Parkway, Richmond, VA Zip 23238; tel. 804/784-2200; Mark S. Roth, Chief Executive Officer

TIDEWATER PSYCHIATRIC INSTITUTE (O, 65 beds) 1701 Will-O-Wisp Drive, Virginia Beach, VA Zip 23454; tel. 804/481-1211; Richard Warden, Chief Executive Officer

TIDEWATER PSYCHIATRIC INSTITUTE–NORFOLK (O, 61 beds) 860 Kempsville Road, Norfolk, VA Zip 23502-3980; tel. 804/461-4565; Richard Warden, Chief Executive Officer

WISCONSIN: CHARTER HOSPITAL OF MILWAUKEE (O, 80 beds) 11101 West Lincoln Avenue, Milwaukee, WI Zip 53227; tel. 414/327-3000; Gary M. Gilberti, Chief Executive Officer

Owned, leased, sponsored:	78 hospitals	6672 beds
Contract-managed:	0 hospitals	0 beds
Totals:	78 hospitals	6672 beds

★**0048:** **COLUMBIA/HCA HEALTHCARE CORPORATION** (IO) One Park Plaza, Nashville, TN Zip 37203; tel. 615/320-2000; Richard Scott, President and Chief Executive Officer

ALABAMA: ANDALUSIA HOSPITAL (O, 101 beds) South Three Notch Street, Andalusia, AL Zip 36420-0760, Mailing Address: Box 760, Zip 36420; tel. 205/222-8466; Joel O. Montgomery, Interim Chief Executive Officer

CRESTWOOD HOSPITAL (O, 120 beds) One Hospital Drive, Huntsville, AL Zip 35801-3403; tel. 205/882-3100; Thomas M. Weiss, Chief Executive Officer

EAST MONTGOMERY MEDICAL CENTER (O, 150 beds) 400 Taylor Road, Montgomery, AL Zip 36117, Mailing Address: P.O. Box 241267, Zip 36124-1267; tel. 334/277-8330; John W. Melton, Chief Executive Officer

---

For explanation of codes following names, see page B2.
★Indicates Type III membership in the American Hospital Association.

Systems / Columbia/HCA Healthcare Corporation

FLORENCE HOSPITAL (O, 155 beds) 2111 Cloyd Boulevard, Florence, AL Zip 35630, Mailing Address: Box 2010, Zip 35631; tel. 205/766–5091; Glen M. Jones, Chief Executive Officer

FOUR RIVERS MEDICAL CENTER (O, 214 beds) 1015 Medical Center Parkway, Selma, AL Zip 36701; tel. 334/872–8461; J. Glenn Brown, Jr., Chief Executive Officer

MEDICAL CENTER SHOALS (O, 128 beds) 201 Avalon Avenue, Muscle Shoals, AL Zip 35661, Mailing Address: P.O. Box 3359, Zip 35662; tel. 205/386–1600; Connie Hawthorne, Chief Executive Officer

MONTGOMERY REGIONAL MEDICAL CENTER (O, 250 beds) 301 South Ripley Street, Montgomery, AL Zip 36104–4495; tel. 205/269–8000; Larry Montgomery, Interim Chief Executive Officer

NORTHWEST MEDICAL CENTER (O, 100 beds) Highway 43 By-Pass, Russellville, AL Zip 35653, Mailing Address: P.O. Box 1089, Zip 35653; tel. 205/332–1611; Christine R. Stewart, Chief Executive Officer

ALASKA: ALASKA REGIONAL HOSPITAL (O, 238 beds) 2801 Debarr Road, Anchorage, AK Zip 99508, Mailing Address: P.O. Box 143889, Zip 99514–3189; tel. 907/276–1131; Sharon A. Anderson, Chief Executive Officer

ARIZONA: EL DORADO HOSPITAL AND MEDICAL CENTER (O, 166 beds) 1400 North Wilmot, Tucson, AZ Zip 85712, Mailing Address: Box 13070, Zip 85732; tel. 520/886–6361; Rhonda Dean, Chief Executive Officer

HEALTHWEST REGIONAL MEDICAL CENTER (O, 302 beds) 1947 East Thomas Road, Phoenix, AZ Zip 85016; tel. 602/241–7600; John D. Hicks, Chief Executive Officer

NORTHWEST HOSPITAL (O, 144 beds) 6200 North La Cholla Boulevard, Tucson, AZ Zip 85741; tel. 602/742–9000; Mark T. Brenzel, Chief Executive Officer

PARADISE VALLEY HOSPITAL (O, 140 beds) 3929 East Bell Road, Phoenix, AZ Zip 85032; tel. 602/867–1881; Gary Grover, Chief Executive Officer

ARKANSAS: COLUMBIA DOCTORS HOSPITAL (O, 189 beds) 6101 West Capitol, Little Rock, AR Zip 72205–5331; tel. 501/661–4000; W. Perry Kinder, President and Chief Executive Officer

DE QUEEN REGIONAL MEDICAL CENTER (O, 75 beds) Collins Raye Drive, De Queen, AR Zip 71832–2198; tel. 501/584–4111; Steve Nichols, Chief Executive Officer

MEDICAL PARK HOSPITAL (O, 91 beds) 2001 South Main Street, Hope, AR Zip 71801; tel. 501/777–2323; Allen Golson, Executive Director

CALIFORNIA: CHINO VALLEY MEDICAL CENTER (O, 126 beds) 5451 Walnut Avenue, Chino, CA Zip 91710; tel. 909/464–8600; Kenneth Westbrook, Chief Executive Officer

HEALDSBURG GENERAL HOSPITAL (O, 49 beds) 1375 University Street, Healdsburg, CA Zip 95448; tel. 707/431–6500; Brad Mitchell, Executive Director

HUNTINGTON BEACH HOSPITAL AND MEDICAL CENTER (O, 135 beds) 17772 Beach Boulevard, Huntington Beach, CA Zip 92647–9932; tel. 714/842–1473; Carol B. Freeman, Chief Executive Officer

LAS ENCINAS HOSPITAL (O, 147 beds) 2900 East Del Mar Boulevard, Pasadena, CA Zip 91107–4375; tel. 818/795–9901; Roland Metivier, Chief Executive Officer

LOS ROBLES REGIONAL MEDICAL CENTER (O, 187 beds) 215 West Janss Road, Thousand Oaks, CA Zip 91360–1899; tel. 805/497–2727; Ronald P. Phelps, Chief Executive Officer

MISSION BAY MEMORIAL HOSPITAL (O, 128 beds) 3030 Bunker Hill Street, San Diego, CA Zip 92109–5780; tel. 619/274–7721; Britt Berrett, Chief Executive Officer

PALM DRIVE HOSPITAL (O, 48 beds) 501 Petaluma Avenue, Sebastopol, CA Zip 95472; tel. 707/823–8511; Brian E. Dunn, Chief Executive Officer

SAN LEANDRO HOSPITAL (O, 136 beds) 13855 East 14th Street, San Leandro, CA Zip 94578–0398; tel. 510/667–4510; Steve Monaghan, President and Chief Executive Officer

WEST ANAHEIM MEDICAL CENTER (O, 243 beds) 3033 West Orange Avenue, Anaheim, CA Zip 92804–3184; tel. 714/827–3000; David Culberson, Chief Executive Officer

WEST HILLS REGIONAL MEDICAL CENTER (O, 236 beds) 7300 Medical Center Drive, West Hills, CA Zip 91307, Mailing Address: P.O. Box 7937, Zip 91309–7937; tel. 818/712–4110; Dan Brothman, Chief Executive Officer

WESTSIDE HOSPITAL (O, 66 beds) 910 South Fairfax Avenue, Los Angeles, CA Zip 90036; tel. 213/938–3431; Jerry Gillman, President and Chief Executive Officer

COLORADO: AURORA REGIONAL MEDICAL CENTER (O, 180 beds) 1501 South Potomac, Aurora, CO Zip 80012; tel. 303/695–2600; William K. Atkinson, Chief Executive Officer

COLUMBINE PSYCHIATRIC CENTER (O, 70 beds) 8565 South Poplar Way, Littleton, CO Zip 80126; tel. 303/470–9500; Jonathan Bartlett, Chief Financial Officer and Interim Chief Executive Officer

NORTH SUBURBAN MEDICAL CENTER (O, 160 beds) 9191 Grant Street, Thornton, CO Zip 80229; tel. 303/451–7800; Jay S. Weinstein, Chief Executive Officer

ROSE MEDICAL CENTER (O, 285 beds) 4567 East Ninth Avenue, Denver, CO Zip 80220; tel. 303/320–2121; Philip A. Kalin, Executive Vice President

DELAWARE: ROCKFORD CENTER (O, 74 beds) 100 Rockford Drive, Newark, DE Zip 19713; tel. 302/996–5480; Walter J. Yokobosky, Jr., Chief Executive Officer

FLORIDA: AVENTURA HOSPITAL AND MEDICAL CENTER (O, 458 beds) 20900 Biscayne Boulevard, Miami, FL Zip 33180–1407; tel. 305/932–0250; Davide M. Carbone, Chief Executive Officer

BRANDON HOSPITAL (O, 250 beds) 119 Oakfield Drive, Brandon, FL Zip 33511–5799; tel. 813/681–5551; H. Rex Etheredge, Chief Executive Officer

CEDARS MEDICAL CENTER (O, 885 beds) 1400 Northwest 12th Avenue, Miami, FL Zip 33136–1003; tel. 305/325–5511; Ralph A. Aleman, Chief Executive Officer

CENTRAL FLORIDA REGIONAL HOSPITAL (O, 226 beds) 1401 West Seminole Boulevard, Sanford, FL Zip 32771–6764; tel. 407/321–4500; Doug Sills, President and Chief Executive Officer

CLEARWATER COMMUNITY HOSPITAL (O, 133 beds) 1521 East Druid Road, Clearwater, FL Zip 34616–6193; tel. 813/447–4571; Richard H. Katzeff, Executive Director

COLUMBIA HOSPITAL (O, 250 beds) 2201 45th Street, West Palm Beach, FL Zip 33407–2069; tel. 407/842–6141; Michael M. Fencel, Chief Executive Officer

COLUMBIA PARK MEDICAL CENTER (O, 267 beds) 818 South Main Lane, Orlando, FL Zip 32801–9964; tel. 407/649–6111; Roy C. Vinson, Chief Executive Officer

COLUMBIA REGIONAL MEDICAL CENTER AT BAYONET POINT (O, 256 beds) 14000 Fivay Road, Hudson, FL Zip 34667–7199; tel. 813/863–2411; J. Daniel Miller, President and Chief Executive Officer

DADE CITY HOSPITAL (O, 120 beds) 1550 Fort King Road, Dade City, FL Zip 33525–5294; tel. 904/521–1100; Robert Meade, Chief Executive Officer

DAYTONA MEDICAL CENTER (O, 214 beds) 400 North Clyde Morris Boulevard, Daytona Beach, FL Zip 32114, Mailing Address: Box 9000, Zip 32120; tel. 904/239–5000

DEERING HOSPITAL (O, 233 beds) 9333 Southwest 152nd Street, Miami, FL Zip 33157; tel. 305/251–2500; Anthony Degina, Chief Executive Officer

DOCTORS HOSPITAL OF SARASOTA (O, 168 beds) 5731 Bee Ridge Road, Sarasota, FL Zip 34233; tel. 813/342–1100; William C. Lievense, Chief Executive Officer

EAST POINTE HOSPITAL (O, 75 beds) 1500 Lee Boulevard, Lehigh Acres, FL Zip 33936; tel. 813/369–2101; Valerie A. Jackson, Chief Executive Officer

EDWARD WHITE HOSPITAL (O, 167 beds) 2323 Ninth Avenue North, Saint Petersburg, FL Zip 33713, Mailing Address: P.O. Box 12018, Zip 33733–2018; tel. 813/323–1111; Lindell W. Orr, Chief Executive Officer

ENGLEWOOD COMMUNITY HOSPITAL (O, 100 beds) 700 Medical Boulevard, Englewood, FL Zip 34223; tel. 813/475–6571; Terry L. Moore, Chief Executive Officer

FAWCETT MEMORIAL HOSPITAL (O, 249 beds) 21298 Olean Boulevard, Port Charlotte, FL Zip 33952–6765; tel. 813/629–1181; Ward Boston, Chief Executive Officer

FORT WALTON BEACH MEDICAL CENTER (O, 247 beds) 1000 Mar-Walt Drive, Fort Walton Beach, FL Zip 32547–6708; tel. 904/862–1111; David A. McClellan, Chief Executive Officer

GRANT CENTER OF DEERING HOSPITAL (O, 140 beds) 20601 Southwest 157th Avenue, Miami, FL Zip 33187, Mailing Address: Box 1159, Zip 33187–1159; tel. 305/251–0710; Anthony Degina, Chief Executive Officer

GULF COAST HOSPITAL (O, 120 beds) 13681 Doctors Way, Fort Myers, FL Zip 33912; tel. 813/768–5000; Denny W. Powell, Chief Executive Officer

GULF COAST HOSPITAL (O, 176 beds) 449 West 23rd Street, Panama City, FL Zip 32405, Mailing Address: P.O. Box 15309, Zip 32406–5309; tel. 904/769–8341; Donald E. Butts, Chief Executive Officer

HAMILTON MEMORIAL HOSPITAL (O, 42 beds) 506 Northwest Fourth Street, Jasper, FL Zip 32052–1300, Mailing Address: Box 1300, Zip 32052–1300; tel. 904/792–2101; Amelia Tuten R.N., Administrator

For explanation of codes following names, see page B2.
★Indicates Type III membership in the American Hospital Association.

Systems / Columbia/HCA Healthcare Corporation

KENDALL REGIONAL MEDICAL CENTER (O, 230 beds) 11750 Bird Road, Miami, FL Zip 33175–3530; tel. 305/223–3000; Victor Maya, Chief Executive Officer

L. W. BLAKE HOSPITAL (O, 292 beds) 2020 59th Street West, Bradenton, FL Zip 34209, Mailing Address: P.O. Box 25004, Zip 34206–5004; tel. 813/792–6611; Lindell W. Orr, Chief Executive Officer

LAKE CITY MEDICAL CENTER (O, 75 beds) 1701 West Duval Street, Lake City, FL Zip 32055; tel. 904/752–2922; David P. Steitz, Chief Executive Officer

LARGO MEDICAL CENTER (O, 256 beds) 201 14th Street S.W., Largo, FL Zip 34640, Mailing Address: P.O. Box 2905, Zip 34649–2905; tel. 813/586–1411; Jon C. Trezona, Administrator

LAWNWOOD REGIONAL MEDICAL CENTER (O, 320 beds) 1700 South 23rd Street, Fort Pierce, FL Zip 34950–0188; tel. 407/461–4000; Jon C. Trezona, Chief Executive Officer

MARION COMMUNITY HOSPITAL (O, 230 beds) 1431 Southwest First Avenue, Ocala, FL Zip 34474, Mailing Address: Box 2200, Zip 34478–2200; tel. 904/732–2700; Terry Upton, Chief Executive Officer

MEDICAL CENTER OF PORT ST. LUCIE (O, 150 beds) 1800 Southeast Tiffany Avenue, Port Saint Lucie, FL Zip 34952–7580; tel. 407/335–4000; Michael P. Joyce, Chief Executive Officer

MEMORIAL HOSPITAL JACKSONVILLE (O, 311 beds) 3625 University Boulevard S, Jacksonville, FL Zip 32216, Mailing Address: Box 16325, Zip 32216; tel. 904/399–6111; Winston Rushing, President

MEMORIAL HOSPITAL PEMBROKE (O, 301 beds) 2301 University Drive, Pembroke Pines, FL Zip 33024; tel. 305/962–9650; J. E. Piriz, Administrator

MIAMI HEART INSTITUTE (O, 531 beds) 4701 Meridian Avenue, Miami, FL Zip 33140–2910; tel. 305/672–1111; Stephen Bernstein, Chief Executive Officer

NEW PORT RICHEY HOSPITAL (O, 414 beds) 5637 Marine Parkway, New Port Richey, FL Zip 34652, Mailing Address: Box 996, Zip 34656–0996; tel. 813/848–1733; Andrew Oravec, Jr., Administrator

NORTH FLORIDA REGIONAL MEDICAL CENTER (O, 267 beds) 6500 Newberry Road, Gainesville, FL Zip 32605–4392, Mailing Address: P.O. Box 147006, Zip 32614–7006; tel. 904/333–4000; Patrick J. Gray, Chief Executive Officer

NORTH OKALOOSA MEDICAL CENTER (O, 110 beds) 151 Redstone Avenue S.E., Crestview, FL Zip 32539–7304; tel. 904/689–8100; Rodney R. Smith, Chief Executive Officer

NORTHSIDE HOSPITAL (O, 301 beds) 6000 49th Street North, Saint Petersburg, FL Zip 33709; tel. 813/521–4411; Bradley K. Grover, Sr., Chief Executive Officer

NORTHWEST MEDICAL CENTER (O, 150 beds) 2801 North State Road 7, Margate, FL Zip 33063, Mailing Address: P.O. Box 639002, Zip 33063–9002; tel. 305/978–4000; Kenneth H. Feiler, Chief Executive Officer

OAK HILL HOSPITAL (O, 150 beds) 11375 Cortez Boulevard, Spring Hill, FL Zip 34613, Mailing Address: P.O. Box 5300, Zip 34606; tel. 904/596–6632; Robert K. Peterson, Administrator

ORANGE PARK MEDICAL CENTER (O, 224 beds) 2001 Kingsley Avenue, Orange Park, FL Zip 32073–5156; tel. 904/276–8500; Robert M. Krieger, Chief Executive Officer

OSCEOLA REGIONAL HOSPITAL (O, 169 beds) 700 West Oak Street, Kissimmee, FL Zip 34741, Mailing Address: P.O. Box 422589, Zip 34742–2589; tel. 407/846–2266; Mark Aanonson, Chief Executive Officer

PALM BEACH REGIONAL HOSPITAL (O, 200 beds) 2829 Tenth Avenue North, Lake Worth, FL Zip 33461; tel. 407/967–7800; Wayne Campbell, Chief Executive Officer

PALMS WEST HOSPITAL (O, 117 beds) 13001 Southern Boulevard, Loxahatchee, FL Zip 33470–1150; tel. 305/798–3300; Paul M. Pugh, Chief Executive Officer

PLANTATION GENERAL HOSPITAL (O, 264 beds) 401 Northwest 42nd Avenue, Plantation, FL Zip 33317–2882; tel. 305/587–5010

POMPANO BEACH MEDICAL CENTER (O, 273 beds) 600 Southwest Third Street, Pompano Beach, FL Zip 33060–6979; tel. 305/782–2000; Heather J. Rohan, Chief Executive Officer

PUTNAM COMMUNITY HOSPITAL (O, 161 beds) Highway 20 West, Palatka, FL Zip 32177, Mailing Address: P.O. Box 778, Zip 32178–0778; tel. 904/328–5711; Rick Palombo, Chief Executive Officer

RAULERSON HOSPITAL (O, 101 beds) 1796 Highway 441 North, Okeechobee, FL Zip 34972, Mailing Address: Box 1307, Zip 34973–1307; tel. 813/763–2151; Frank Irby, Chief Executive Officer

SANTA ROSA MEDICAL CENTER (O, 129 beds) 1450 Berryhill Road, Milton, FL Zip 32570, Mailing Address: P.O. Box 648, Zip 32572; tel. 904/626–7762; Barbara H. Thames, Chief Executive Officer

SOUTH BAY HOSPITAL (O, 112 beds) 4016 State Road 674, Sun City Center, FL Zip 33573–5298; tel. 813/634–3301; Tracy A. Chelf, Chief Executive Officer

SOUTH SEMINOLE HOSPITAL (O, 206 beds) 555 West State Road 434, Longwood, FL Zip 32750; tel. 407/767–1200; Steve Grimm, Executive Director and Chief Executive Officer

SOUTHWEST FLORIDA REGIONAL MEDICAL CENTER (O, 400 beds) 2727 Winkler Avenue, Fort Myers, FL Zip 33901–9396; tel. 813/939–1147; Nick Carbone, Chief Executive Officer

ST. PETERSBURG GENERAL HOSPITAL (O, 219 beds) 6500 38th Avenue North, Saint Petersburg, FL Zip 33710; tel. 813/384–1414; Thomas L. Herron, Chief Executive Officer

TALLAHASSEE COMMUNITY HOSPITAL (O, 180 beds) 2626 Capital Medical Boulevard, Tallahassee, FL Zip 32308; tel. 904/656–5000; Gary L. Brewer, Chief Executive Officer

TWIN CITIES HOSPITAL (O, 75 beds) 2190 Highway 85 North, Niceville, FL Zip 32578; tel. 904/678–4131; David Whalen, Chief Executive Officer

UNIVERSITY HOSPITAL (O, 211 beds) 7201 North University Drive, Tamarac, FL Zip 33321; tel. 305/721–2200; Robert L. Newman, Chief Executive Officer

WEST FLORIDA REGIONAL MEDICAL CENTER (O, 547 beds) 8383 North Davis Highway, Pensacola, FL Zip 32514, Mailing Address: P.O. Box 18900, Zip 32523–8900; tel. 904/494–4000; John Kausch, Chief Executive Officer

WESTSIDE REGIONAL MEDICAL CENTER (O, 204 beds) 8201 West Broward Boulevard, Plantation, FL Zip 33324–9937; tel. 305/473–6600; David E. Bussone, Chief Executive Officer

WINTER PARK MEMORIAL HOSPITAL (O, 339 beds) 200 North Lakemont Avenue, Winter Park, FL Zip 32792–3273; tel. 407/646–7000; Pete Lawson, Chief Executive Officer

GEORGIA: AUGUSTA REGIONAL MEDICAL CENTER (O, 252 beds) 3651 Wheeler Road, Augusta, GA Zip 30909–1499; tel. 706/863–3232; Jesse G. Smith, Chief Executive Officer

BARROW MEDICAL CENTER (O, 60 beds) 316 North Broad Street, Winder, GA Zip 30680, Mailing Address: Box 768, Zip 30680; tel. 404/867–3400; Jeffrey T. Whitehorn, Chief Executive Officer

CARTERSVILLE MEDICAL CENTER (O, 80 beds) 960 Joe Frank Harris Parkway, Cartersville, GA Zip 30120, Mailing Address: Box 1008, Zip 30120; tel. 404/382–1530; Keith Sandlin, Chief Executive Officer

COLISEUM MEDICAL CENTERS (O, 188 beds) 350 Hospital Drive, Macon, GA Zip 31213; tel. 912/745–9461; Michael S. Boggs, Chief Executive Officer

COLISEUM PSYCHIATRIC HOSPITAL (O, 92 beds) 340 Hospital Drive, Macon, GA Zip 31201–8002; tel. 912/741–1355; James G. Helgeson, Chief Executive Officer

DOCTORS HOSPITAL (O, 248 beds) 616 19th Street, Columbus, GA Zip 31901–1528, Mailing Address: P.O. Box 2188, Zip 31902–2188; tel. 706/571–4262; Kent Vaughn, Chief Executive Officer

DUNWOODY MEDICAL CENTER (O, 168 beds) 4575 North Shallowford Road, Atlanta, GA Zip 30338; tel. 404/454–2000; Thomas D. Gilbert, President and Chief Executive Officer

EASTSIDE MEDICAL CENTER (O, 114 beds) 1700 Medical Way, Snellville, GA Zip 30278, Mailing Address: P.O. Box 587, Zip 30278; tel. 404/736–2498; Michael K. Kerner, Chief Executive Officer

FAIRVIEW PARK HOSPITAL (O, 190 beds) 200 Industrial Boulevard, Dublin, GA Zip 31021, Mailing Address: Box 1408, Zip 31040; tel. 912/275–2000; Steve C. Hoelscher, Chief Executive Officer

HUGHSTON SPORTS MEDICINE HOSPITAL (O, 100 beds) 100 Frist Court, Columbus, GA Zip 31908–7188, Mailing Address: P.O. Box 7188, Zip 31908–7188; tel. 706/576–2100; Charles Keaton, Chief Executive Officer

LANIER PARK REGIONAL HOSPITAL (O, 124 beds) 675 White Sulphur Road, Gainesville, GA Zip 30505, Mailing Address: P.O. Box 1354, Zip 30503; tel. 404/503–3000; Jerry Fulks, Chief Executive Officer

METROPOLITAN HOSPITAL (O, 64 beds) 3223 Howell Mill Road N.W., Atlanta, GA Zip 30327; tel. 404/351–0500; R. Stan Lentz, Chief Executive Officer

MURRAY MEDICAL CENTER (O, 42 beds) 707 Old Ellijay Road, Chatsworth, GA Zip 30705, Mailing Address: P.O. Box 1406, Zip 30705; tel. 706/695–4564; Richard Cook, Administrator

NORTHLAKE REGIONAL MEDICAL CENTER (O, 120 beds) 1455 Montreal Road, Atlanta, GA Zip 30084, Mailing Address: P.O. Box 450000, Zip 31145; tel. 404/270–3000; Michael K. Kerner, Chief Executive Officer

For explanation of codes following names, see page B2.
★Indicates Type III membership in the American Hospital Association.

Systems / Columbia/HCA Healthcare Corporation

PALMYRA MEDICAL CENTERS (O, 145 beds) 2000 Palmyra Road, Albany, GA Zip 31701, Mailing Address: Box 1908, Zip 31702–1908; tel. 912/434–2000; Douglas M. Parker, Chief Executive Officer

PARKWAY MEDICAL CENTER (O, 233 beds) 1000 Thornton Road, Lithia Springs, GA Zip 30057, Mailing Address: P.O. Box 570, Zip 30057; tel. 404/732–7777; Deborah S. Guthrie, Chief Operating Officer

PEACHTREE REGIONAL HOSPITAL (O, 144 beds) 60 Hospital Road, Newnan, GA Zip 30263, Mailing Address: Box 2228, Zip 30264; tel. 404/253–1912; Linda Jubinsky, Chief Executive Officer

REDMOND REGIONAL MEDICAL CENTER (O, 201 beds) 501 Redmond Road, Rome, GA Zip 30165–7001, Mailing Address: Box 107001, Zip 30164–7001; tel. 706/291–0291; James R. Thomas, Chief Executive Officer

WEST PACES MEDICAL CENTER (O, 294 beds) 3200 Howell Mill Road N.W., Atlanta, GA Zip 30327–4101; tel. 404/351–0351; Stuart Voelpel, President and Chief Executive Officer

IDAHO: EASTERN IDAHO REGIONAL MEDICAL CENTER (O, 286 beds) 3100 Channing Way, Idaho Falls, ID Zip 83404, Mailing Address: P.O. Box 2077, Zip 83403–2077; tel. 208/529–6111; Ronald G. Butler, Chief Executive Officer

WEST VALLEY MEDICAL CENTER (O, 118 beds) 1717 Arlington, Caldwell, ID Zip 83605–4864; tel. 208/459–4641; Mark Adams, Chief Executive Officer

ILLINOIS: CHICAGO LAKESHORE HOSPITAL (O, 102 beds) 4840 North Marine Drive, Chicago, IL Zip 60640; tel. 312/878–9700; Marcia S. Shapiro, Chief Executive Officer

GRANT HOSPITAL (O, 232 beds) 550 West Webster Avenue, Chicago, IL Zip 60614–9980; tel. 312/883–2000; Timothy J. Crowley, Chief Executive Officer

HOFFMAN ESTATES MEDICAL CENTER (O, 193 beds) 1555 North Barrington Road, Hoffman Estates, IL Zip 60194; tel. 708/843–2000; Edward Goldberg, Chief Executive Officer

MICHAEL REESE HOSPITAL AND MEDICAL CENTER (O, 565 beds) 2929 South Ellis Avenue, Chicago, IL Zip 60616; tel. 312/791–2000; Nancy S. Carlstedt, Chief Executive Officer

RIVEREDGE HOSPITAL (O, 164 beds) 8311 West Roosevelt Road, Forest Park, IL Zip 60130–2500; tel. 708/771–7000; Joyce W. Washington, President and Chief Executive Officer

WOODLAND HOSPITAL (O, 100 beds) 1650 Moon Lake Boulevard, Hoffman Estates, IL Zip 60194–5000; tel. 708/882–1600; Patrick Waugh, Chief Executive Officer

INDIANA: TERRE HAUTE REGIONAL HOSPITAL (O, 236 beds) 3901 South Seventh Street, Terre Haute, IN Zip 47802–4299; tel. 812/232–0021; Jerry Dooley, Chief Executive Officer

WOMEN'S HOSPITAL–INDIANAPOLIS (O, 132 beds) 8111 Township Line Road, Indianapolis, IN Zip 46260–8043; tel. 317/875–5994; Steven B. Reed, President and Chief Executive Officer

KANSAS: OVERLAND PARK REGIONAL MEDICAL CENTER (O, 250 beds) 10500 Quivira Road, Overland Park, KS Zip 66215–2373, Mailing Address: P.O. Box 15959, Zip 66215; tel. 913/541–5000; Kevin J. Hicks, Chief Executive Officer

WESLEY MEDICAL CENTER (O, 460 beds) 550 North Hillside Avenue, Wichita, KS Zip 67214–4976; tel. 316/688–2468; James R. Kelly, Jr., Chief Executive Officer

WESTERN PLAINS REGIONAL HOSPITAL (O, 84 beds) 3001 Avenue A, Dodge City, KS Zip 67801, Mailing Address: Box 1478, Zip 67801; tel. 316/225–8401; Greg J. Simmons, Interim President and Chief Executive Officer

KENTUCKY: AUDUBON REGIONAL MEDICAL CENTER (O, 480 beds) One Audubon Plaza Drive, Louisville, KY Zip 40217–1397, Mailing Address: Box 17550, Zip 40217–0550; tel. 502/636–7111; Ronald J. Vigus, President and Chief Executive Officer

BLUEGRASS REGIONAL MEDICAL CENTER (O, 146 beds) 299 King's Daughters Drive, Frankfort, KY Zip 40601–4186; tel. 502/875–5240; Ronald T. Tyrer, Chief Executive Officer

BOURBON GENERAL HOSPITAL (O, 58 beds) 9 Linville Drive, Paris, KY Zip 40361; tel. 606/987–3600; John R. Grant, Chief Executive Officer

GREENVIEW HOSPITAL (O, 211 beds) 1801 Ashley Circle, Bowling Green, KY Zip 42104, Mailing Address: Box 90024, Zip 42102–9024; tel. 502/793–1000; Mary T. Brasseaux, Chief Executive Officer

LAKE CUMBERLAND REGIONAL HOSPITAL (O, 227 beds) 305 Langdon Street, Somerset, KY Zip 42501, Mailing Address: Box 620, Zip 42502–2750; tel. 606/679–7441; Derek W. Cimala, Chief Executive Officer

LOGAN MEMORIAL HOSPITAL (O, 100 beds) 1625 South Nashville Road, Russellville, KY Zip 42276–0010, Mailing Address: P.O. Box 10, Zip 42276; tel. 502/726–4011; Jeffrey Manley, Chief Executive Officer

MEADOWVIEW REGIONAL HOSPITAL (O, 111 beds) 989 Medical Park Drive, Maysville, KY Zip 41056; tel. 606/759–5311; Michael L. Graue, Chief Executive Officer

PINELAKE MEDICAL CENTER (O, 106 beds) 1099 Medical Center Circle, Mayfield, KY Zip 42066, Mailing Address: P.O. Box 1099, Zip 42066; tel. 502/251–4100; Harry Alvis, Chief Executive Officer

SCOTT GENERAL HOSPITAL (O, 61 beds) 1140 Lexington Road, Georgetown, KY Zip 40324; tel. 502/868–1100; Kenneth R. Unger, Chief Executive Officer

SOUTHWEST HOSPITAL (O, 150 beds) 9820 Third Street Road, Louisville, KY Zip 40272–9984; tel. 502/933–8100; Jack Wheatley, Chief Executive Officer

SPRING VIEW MEDICAL CENTER (O, 113 beds) 320 Loretto Road, Lebanon, KY Zip 40033–0320; tel. 502/692–3161; Russell Goldberg, Chief Executive Officer

SUBURBAN MEDICAL CENTER (O, 380 beds) 4001 Dutchmans Lane, Louisville, KY Zip 40207; tel. 502/893–1000; Patricia A. Davis, Chief Executive Officer

UNIVERSITY OF LOUISVILLE HOSPITAL (L, 315 beds) 530 South Jackson Street, Louisville, KY Zip 40202–3611; tel. 502/562–3000; Ronald A. Hytoff, Chief Executive Officer

LOUISIANA: AVOYELLES HOSPITAL (O, 55 beds) 4231 Highway 1192, Marksville, LA Zip 71351, Mailing Address: Box 255, Zip 71351; tel. 318/253–8611; David Mitchel, Chief Executive Officer

CYPRESS HOSPITAL (O, 116 beds) 302 Dulles Drive, Lafayette, LA Zip 70506; tel. 318/233–9024; James B. Juneau, Chief Executive Officer

DAUTERIVE HOSPITAL (O, 113 beds) 600 North Lewis Street, New Iberia, LA Zip 70560, Mailing Address: P.O. Box 11210, Zip 70562–1210; tel. 318/365–7311; Kyle J. Viator, Chief Executive Officer

DEPAUL HOSPITAL (O, 102 beds) 1040 Calhoun Street, New Orleans, LA Zip 70118; tel. 504/899–8282; David Hoidal, Chief Executive Officer

DOCTORS' HOSPITAL OF OPELOUSAS (O, 105 beds) 5101 Highway 167 South, Opelousas, LA Zip 70570; tel. 318/948–2100; Gregory L. Gibson, Administrator

HIGHLAND HOSPITAL (O, 120 beds) 1453 East Bert Kouns Industrial Loop, Shreveport, LA Zip 71105–6050; tel. 318/798–4300; Ronald J. Elder, Chief Executive Officer

LAKE AREA MEDICAL CENTER (O, 80 beds) 4200 Nelson Road, Lake Charles, LA Zip 70605; tel. 318/474–6370; James E. Richardson FACHE, Chief Executive Officer

LAKELAND MEDICAL CENTER (O, 150 beds) 6000 Bullard Avenue, New Orleans, LA Zip 70128; tel. 504/241–6335; M. P. Gandy, Jr., Chief Executive Officer

LAKESIDE HOSPITAL (O, 122 beds) 4700 I-10 Service Road, Metairie, LA Zip 70001–1269; tel. 504/885–3333; Hugh D. Wilson, Chief Executive Officer

LAKEVIEW REGIONAL MEDICAL CENTER (O, 163 beds) 95 East Fairway Drive, Covington, LA Zip 70433, Mailing Address: P.O. Box 99, Mandeville, Zip 70470; tel. 504/876–3800; James E. Rogers, Chief Executive Officer

MEDICAL CENTER OF BATON ROUGE (O, 175 beds) 17000 Medical Center Drive, Baton Rouge, LA Zip 70816–3224; tel. 504/755–4800; William L. Anderson, Chief Executive Officer

MEDICAL CENTER OF SOUTHWEST LOUISIANA (O, 105 beds) 2810 Ambassador Caffery Parkway, Lafayette, LA Zip 70506; tel. 318/981–2949; Gerald A. Fornoff, Chief Executive Officer

NORTH MONROE HOSPITAL (O, 130 beds) 3421 Medical Park Drive, Monroe, LA Zip 71203; tel. 318/388–1946; George E. Miller, Chief Executive Officer

OAKDALE COMMUNITY HOSPITAL (O, 60 beds) 130 North Hospital Drive, Oakdale, LA Zip 71463, Mailing Address: Box 629, Zip 71463; tel. 318/335–3700; Robert Bauer, Chief Executive Officer

RAPIDES REGIONAL MEDICAL CENTER (O, 359 beds) Box 30101, 211 Fourth Street, Alexandria, LA Zip 71301–8421; tel. 318/473–3000; James T. Montgomery, President

RIVERVIEW MEDICAL CENTER (O, 104 beds) 1125 West Louisiana Highway 30, Gonzales, LA Zip 70737; tel. 504/647–5000; Glenn L. Craig, Chief Executive Officer

SPRINGHILL MEDICAL CENTER (O, 86 beds) 2001 Doctors Drive, Springhill, LA Zip 71075, Mailing Address: Box 917, Zip 71075–0917; tel. 318/539–9161; James B. Warren, Chief Executive Officer

---

For explanation of codes following names, see page B2.
★Indicates Type III membership in the American Hospital Association.

Systems / Columbia/HCA Healthcare Corporation

TULANE UNIVERSITY HOSPITAL AND CLINICS (O, 259 beds) 1415 Tulane Avenue, New Orleans, LA Zip 70112–2632; tel. 504/588–5263; Stephen A. Pickett, Administrator and Chief Operating Officer

VILLE PLATTE MEDICAL CENTER (O, 116 beds) 800 East Main Street, Ville Platte, LA Zip 70586, Mailing Address: Box 349, Zip 70586; tel. 318/363–5684

WINN PARISH MEDICAL CENTER (O, 103 beds) 301 West Boundary Street, Winnfield, LA Zip 71483, Mailing Address: Box 152, Zip 71483; tel. 318/628–2721; Bobby Jordan, Chief Executive Officer

WOMEN'S AND CHILDREN'S HOSPITAL (O, 93 beds) 4600 Ambassador Caffery Parkway, Lafayette, LA Zip 70508, Mailing Address: P.O. Box 81607, Zip 70598–1607; tel. 318/981–9100; Mimi Roberson, Chief Executive Officer

MISSISSIPPI: GARDEN PARK COMMUNITY HOSPITAL (O, 120 beds) 1520 Broad Avenue, Gulfport, MS Zip 39501, Mailing Address: P.O. Box 1240, Zip 39502; tel. 601/864–4210; William E. Peaks, Executive Director

VICKSBURG MEDICAL CENTER (O, 154 beds) 1111 Frontage Road, Vicksburg, MS Zip 39181–5298; tel. 601/636–2611; G. Thomas Usher, Administrator

MISSOURI: INDEPENDENCE REGIONAL HEALTH CENTER (O, 335 beds) 1509 West Truman Road, Independence, MO Zip 64050; tel. 816/836–8100; Paul F. Herzog, Chief Executive Officer

RESEARCH PSYCHIATRIC CENTER (O, 100 beds) 2323 East 63rd Street, Kansas City, MO Zip 64130; tel. 816/444–8161; Steven R. Newton, Administrator and Chief Executive Officer

SPRINGFIELD COMMUNITY HOSPITAL (O, 114 beds) 3535 South National Avenue, Springfield, MO Zip 65807; tel. 417/882–4700; Fred Woody, Chief Executive Officer

NEVADA: SUNRISE HOSPITAL AND MEDICAL CENTER (O, 688 beds) 3186 Maryland Parkway, Las Vegas, NV Zip 89109–2306, Mailing Address: P.O. Box 98530, Zip 89193–8530; tel. 702/731–8000; A. Allan Stipe, President and Chief Executive Officer

NEW HAMPSHIRE: PARKLAND MEDICAL CENTER (O, 86 beds) One Parkland Drive, Derry, NH Zip 03038; tel. 603/432–1500; Steven R. Gordon, Chief Executive Officer

PORTSMOUTH REGIONAL HOSPITAL (O, 181 beds) 333 Borthwick Avenue, Portsmouth, NH Zip 03802–7004; tel. 603/436–5110; William J. Schuler, Chief Executive Officer

NEW MEXICO: GUADALUPE MEDICAL CENTER (O, 115 beds) 2430 West Pierce Street, Carlsbad, NM Zip 88220–3597; tel. 505/887–4100; Thomas H. Steel, Chief Executive Officer

HEIGHTS PSYCHIATRIC HOSPITAL (O, 92 beds) 103 Hospital Loop N.E., Albuquerque, NM Zip 87109; tel. 505/883–8777; Andrea Brightwell, Chief Executive Officer

LEA REGIONAL HOSPITAL (O, 250 beds) Lovington Highway 18, Hobbs, NM Zip 88240, Mailing Address: P.O. Box 3000, Zip 88240; tel. 505/392–6581; R. Gordon Taylor, Chief Executive Officer

NORTH CAROLINA: BRUNSWICK HOSPITAL (O, 60 beds) 1 Medical Center Drive, Supply, NC Zip 28462, Mailing Address: P.O. Box 139, Zip 28462; tel. 910/754–8121; C. Mark Gregson, Chief Executive Officer

DAVIS COMMUNITY HOSPITAL (O, 149 beds) Old Mocksville Road, Statesville, NC Zip 28677, Mailing Address: P.O. Box 1800, Zip 28677; tel. 704/873–0281; Stephen J. Aragon, Chief Executive Officer

HERITAGE HOSPITAL (O, 127 beds) 111 Hospital Drive, Tarboro, NC Zip 27886; tel. 919/641–7700; James Raynor, Chief Executive Officer

HIGHSMITH–RAINEY MEMORIAL HOSPITAL (O, 150 beds) 150 Robeson Street, Fayetteville, NC Zip 28301–5570; tel. 910/609–1000; William A. Adams, Chief Executive Officer

HOLLY HILL MENTAL HEALTH SERVICES (O, 70 beds) 3019 Falstaff Road, Raleigh, NC Zip 27610; tel. 919/250–7000; Grayce M. Crockett, Chief Executive Officer

PRESBYTERIAN–ORTHOPEDIC HOSPITAL (O, 166 beds) 1901 Randolph Road, Charlotte, NC Zip 28207; tel. 704/375–6792; Tom Pemberton, President

RALEIGH COMMUNITY HOSPITAL (O, 162 beds) 3400 Wake Forest Road, Raleigh, NC Zip 27609–7373, Mailing Address: P.O. Box 28280, Zip 27611; tel. 919/954–3000; G. Michael Girone, Chief Executive Officer

OKLAHOMA: CLAREMORE REGIONAL HOSPITAL (O, 74 beds) 1202 North Muskogee Place, Claremore, OK Zip 74017; tel. 918/341–2556; Ken Seidel, Executive Director

DOCTORS' HOSPITAL (O, 148 beds) 2323 South Harvard Avenue, Tulsa, OK Zip 74114–3370; tel. 918/744–4000; Anthony R. Young, President and Chief Executive Officer

EDMOND REGIONAL MEDICAL CENTER (O, 79 beds) 1 South Bryant Street, Edmond, OK Zip 73034–4798; tel. 405/359–5530; Stanley D. Tatum, Chief Executive Officer

PRESBYTERIAN HOSPITAL (O, 354 beds) 700 Northeast 13th Street, Oklahoma City, OK Zip 73104–5070; tel. 405/271–5100; David L. Dunlap, Chief Executive Officer

SOUTHWESTERN MEDICAL CENTER (O, 110 beds) 5602 Southwest Lee Boulevard, Lawton, OK Zip 73505–9635, Mailing Address: P.O. Box 7290, Zip 73506–7290; tel. 405/531–4700; Ben White, Executive Director

ST. MARY'S MEDICAL CENTER (O, 177 beds) 305 South Fifth Street, Enid, OK Zip 73701–5899, Mailing Address: Box 232, Zip 73702–0232; tel. 405/233–6100; Jim O'Loughlin, Chief Executive Officer

WAGONER COMMUNITY HOSPITAL (O, 100 beds) 1200 West Cherokee, Wagoner, OK Zip 74467–4681, Mailing Address: Box 407, Zip 74477–0407; tel. 918/485–5514; John W. Crawford, Chief Executive Officer

OREGON: DOUGLAS COMMUNITY HOSPITAL (O, 118 beds) 738 West Harvard Boulevard, Roseburg, OR Zip 97470–2996; tel. 503/673–6641; Christopher L. Boyd, Chief Executive Officer

MCMINNVILLE COMMUNITY HOSPITAL (O, 67 beds) 603 South Baker Street, McMinnville, OR Zip 97128–6498; tel. 503/472–6131

SOUTH CAROLINA: AIKEN REGIONAL MEDICAL CENTERS (O, 233 beds) 202 University Parkway, Aiken, SC Zip 29801–2757, Mailing Address: P.O. Box 1117, Zip 29802–1117; tel. 803/641–5000; Richard H. Satcher, Interim Chief Executive Officer

CHESTERFIELD GENERAL HOSPITAL (O, 66 beds) Highway 9, Cheraw, SC Zip 29520, Mailing Address: Box 151, Zip 29520–0151; tel. 803/537–7881; Steve Dean, Chief Executive Officer

COLLETON REGIONAL HOSPITAL (O, 116 beds) 501 Robertson Boulevard, Walterboro, SC Zip 29488; tel. 803/549–6371; Michael H. Greene, Chief Executive Officer

GRAND STRAND REGIONAL MEDICAL CENTER (O, 151 beds) 809 82nd Parkway, Myrtle Beach, SC Zip 29572–1413; tel. 803/449–4411; Doug White, Chief Executive Officer

MARLBORO PARK HOSPITAL (O, 101 beds) 1138 Cheraw Highway, Bennettsville, SC Zip 29512–0738, Mailing Address: Box 738, Zip 29512–0738; tel. 803/479–2881; James W. White, Chief Executive Officer

SUMMERVILLE MEDICAL CENTER (O, 80 beds) 295 Midland Parkway, Summerville, SC Zip 29485; tel. 803/875–3993; James G. Thaw, President and Chief Executive Officer

TRIDENT REGIONAL MEDICAL CENTER (O, 282 beds) 9330 Medical Plaza Drive, Charleston, SC Zip 29406–9195; tel. 803/797–7000; Frank B. Murphy, President and Chief Executive Officer

TENNESSEE: ATHENS COMMUNITY HOSPITAL (O, 97 beds) 1114 West Madison Avenue, Athens, TN Zip 37303, Mailing Address: Box 250, Zip 37371–0250; tel. 615/745–1411; Brenda M. Waltz, Administrator

CENTENNIAL MEDICAL CENTER (O, 680 beds) 2300 Patterson Street, Nashville, TN Zip 37203; tel. 615/342–1000; William Paul Rutledge, President and Chief Executive Officer

CROCKETT HOSPITAL (O, 83 beds) U.S. Highway 43 South, Lawrenceburg, TN Zip 38464–0847, Mailing Address: Box 847, Zip 38464–0847; tel. 615/762–6571; John A. Marshall, Chief Executive Officer

EAST RIDGE HOSPITAL (O, 128 beds) 941 Spring Creek Road, East Ridge, TN Zip 37412, Mailing Address: P.O. Box 91229, Zip 37412–6229; tel. 615/894–7870; William M. Donohoo FACHE, Chief Executive Officer

HENDERSONVILLE HOSPITAL (O, 63 beds) 355 New Shackle Island Road, Hendersonville, TN Zip 37075–2393; tel. 615/264–4000; Lawrence H. Kloess III, Chief Executive Officer

INDIAN PATH MEDICAL CENTER (O, 140 beds) 2000 Brookside Drive, Kingsport, TN Zip 37660–4604; tel. 615/392–7000; Robert Benson, Chief Executive Officer

INDIAN PATH PAVILION (O, 61 beds) 2300 Pavilion Drive, Kingsport, TN Zip 37660–4672; tel. 615/378–7500; Robert Benson, Chief Executive Officer

JOHNSON CITY SPECIALTY HOSPITAL (O, 49 beds) 203 East Watauga Avenue, Johnson City, TN Zip 37601; tel. 615/926–1111; Lori Caudell Fatherree, Chief Executive Officer

LIVINGSTON REGIONAL HOSPITAL (O, 111 beds) 315 Oak Street, Livingston, TN Zip 38570, Mailing Address: P.O. Box 550, Zip 38570; tel. 615/823–5611; Timothy W. McGill, Chief Executive Officer

NASHVILLE MEMORIAL HOSPITAL (O, 250 beds) 612 West Due West Avenue, Madison, TN Zip 37115–4474; tel. 615/865–3511; Thomas R. Pentz, Chief Executive Officer

---

For explanation of codes following names, see page B2.
★Indicates Type III membership in the American Hospital Association.

Systems / Columbia/HCA Healthcare Corporation

NORTH SIDE HOSPITAL (O, 127 beds) 401 Princeton Road, Johnson City, TN Zip 37601, Mailing Address: P.O. Box 4900, Zip 37602; tel. 615/854–5900; John B. Crysel, Chief Executive Officer

PARKRIDGE MEDICAL CENTER (O, 271 beds) 2333 McCallie Avenue, Chattanooga, TN Zip 37404–3285; tel. 615/698–6061; Kelly E. McBryde, Chief Executive Officer

PSYCHIATRIC HOSPITAL AT VANDERBILT (O, 80 beds) 1601 23rd Avenue South, Nashville, TN Zip 37212; tel. 615/320–7770; Robert England, Administrator and Chief Executive Officer

REGIONAL HOSPITAL OF JACKSON (O, 139 beds) 367 Hospital Boulevard, Jackson, TN Zip 38305–4518, Mailing Address: P.O. Box 3310, Zip 38303–0310; tel. 901/661–2000; Donald H. Wilkerson, Chief Executive Officer

RIVER PARK HOSPITAL (O, 90 beds) 1560 Sparta Road, McMinnville, TN Zip 37110; tel. 615/473–8411; William Russell Spray, Chief Executive Officer

SMITH COUNTY MEMORIAL HOSPITAL (O, 63 beds) 158 Hospital Drive, Carthage, TN Zip 37030–1096; tel. 615/735–1560; Jerry H. Futrell, Chief Executive Officer

SOUTH PITTSBURG MUNICIPAL HOSPITAL (O, 47 beds) 210 West 12th Street, South Pittsburg, TN Zip 37380, Mailing Address: P.O. Box 349, Zip 37380–0349; tel. 615/837–6781; Greg Griffith, Chief Executive Officer

SOUTHERN HILLS MEDICAL CENTER (O, 146 beds) 391 Wallace Road, Nashville, TN Zip 37211; tel. 615/781–4100; Lawrence L. Pieretti, Chief Executive Officer

SOUTHERN TENNESSEE MEDICAL CENTER (O, 216 beds) 185 Hospital Road, Winchester, TN Zip 37398; tel. 615/967–8200; Michael W. Garfield, Administrator

STONES RIVER HOSPITAL (O, 55 beds) Doolittle Road, Woodbury, TN Zip 37190, Mailing Address: P.O. Box 458, Zip 37190–0458; tel. 615/563–4001; Ron Walker, Chief Executive Officer

SUMMIT MEDICAL CENTER (O, 204 beds) 5655 Frist Boulevard, Hermitage, TN Zip 37076; tel. 615/316–3000; Bryan Dearing, Chief Executive Officer

SYCAMORE SHOALS HOSPITAL (O, 112 beds) 1501 West Elk Avenue, Elizabethton, TN Zip 37643–1368; tel. 615/542–1300; Larry R. Jeter, Chief Executive Officer

TRINITY HOSPITAL (O, 35 beds) 353 Main Street, Erin, TN Zip 37061, Mailing Address: P.O. Box 489, Zip 37061–0489; tel. 615/289–4211; Jack S. Buck, Chief Executive Officer

VALLEY PSYCHIATRIC HOSPITAL (O, 118 beds) 2200 Morris Hill Road, Chattanooga, TN Zip 37421; tel. 615/894–4220; Mary Palmer, Chief Executive Officer

VOLUNTEER GENERAL HOSPITAL (O, 65 beds) 161 Mount Pelia Road, Martin, TN Zip 38237, Mailing Address: Box 967, Zip 38237; tel. 901/587–4261; Donald E. Annis, Chief Executive Officer

TEXAS: ALICE PHYSICIANS AND SURGEONS HOSPITAL (O, 118 beds) 300 East Third Street, Alice, TX Zip 78332–4794; tel. 512/664–4376; Earl S. Whiteley CHE, Chief Executive Officer

ALVIN COMMUNITY HOSPITAL (O, 41 beds) 301 Medic Lane, Alvin, TX Zip 77511; tel. 713/331–6141; Betsy Postlethwait, Executive Director

ARLINGTON MEDICAL CENTER (O, 223 beds) 3301 Matlock Road, Arlington, TX Zip 76015; tel. 817/465–3241; Michael S. Spurlock, Chief Executive Officer

BAY AREA MEDICAL CENTER (O, 149 beds) 7101 South Padre Island Drive, Corpus Christi, TX Zip 78412; tel. 512/985–1200; Stephen M. Erixon, Chief Executive Officer

BAYSHORE MEDICAL CENTER (O, 352 beds) 4000 Spencer Highway, Pasadena, TX Zip 77504–1294; tel. 713/944–6666; Karen Poole, Chief Executive Officer

BAYVIEW HOSPITAL (O, 68 beds) 6629 Wooldridge Road, Corpus Christi, TX Zip 78414; tel. 512/993–9700; Janie L. Harwood, Chief Executive Officer

BEAUMONT REGIONAL MEDICAL CENTER (O, 362 beds) 3080 College, Beaumont, TX Zip 77701, Mailing Address: P.O. Box 5817, Zip 77726–5817; tel. 409/833–1411; Michael S. Miller, Chief Executive Officer

BELLAIRE HOSPITAL (O, 191 beds) 5314 Dashwood Street, Houston, TX Zip 77081–4689; tel. 713/669–4000; Thomas M. Keefe, Chief Executive Officer

BRAZOS VALLEY MEDICAL CENTER (O, 100 beds) 1604 Rock Prairie Road, College Station, TX Zip 77845, Mailing Address: P.O. Box 10000, Zip 77842–3500; tel. 409/764–5100; Steve Koran, Interim Chief Executive Officer

BROWNWOOD REGIONAL MEDICAL CENTER (O, 164 beds) 1501 Burnet Drive, Brownwood, TX Zip 76801, Mailing Address: Box 760, Zip 76804; tel. 915/646–8541; Art Layne, Administrator and Chief Executive Officer

CLEAR LAKE REGIONAL MEDICAL CENTER (O, 431 beds) 500 Medical Center Boulevard, Webster, TX Zip 77598; tel. 713/332–2511; Donald A. Shaffett, Chief Executive Officer

COASTAL BEND HOSPITAL (O, 68 beds) 1711 West Wheeler Street, Aransas Pass, TX Zip 78336; tel. 512/758–8585; Shirley Gallagher, Chief Executive Officer

COLUMBIA BEHAVIORAL CENTER (O, 117 beds) 1155 Idaho Street, El Paso, TX Zip 79902–1699; tel. 915/544–4000; David M. Polunas, Administrator

COLUMBIA MEDICAL CENTER–EAST (O, 266 beds) 10301 Gateway West, El Paso, TX Zip 79925–7798, Mailing Address: P.O. Box 937003, Zip 79937–1690; tel. 915/595–9000; Douglas A. Matney, Chief Executive Officer

COLUMBIA MEDICAL CENTER–WEST (O, 212 beds) 1801 North Oregon Street, El Paso, TX Zip 79902; tel. 915/521–1200; Ray Fusco, Chief Executive Officer

COLUMBIA REHABILITATION HOSPITAL (O, 40 beds) 300 Waymore, El Paso, TX Zip 77902; tel. 915/577–2600; William G. Collins, Chief Executive Officer

CORONADO HOSPITAL (O, 96 beds) One Medical Plaza, Pampa, TX Zip 79065; tel. 806/665–3721; H. Douglas Garner, Chief Executive Officer

DENTON COMMUNITY HOSPITAL (O, 110 beds) 207 North Bonnie Brae, Denton, TX Zip 76201; tel. 817/898–7000; Scott Koenig, Chief Executive Officer

DENTON REGIONAL MEDICAL CENTER (O, 297 beds) 4405 North Interstate 35, Denton, TX Zip 76207; tel. 817/566–4000; Bob J. Haley, Executive Director

DETAR HOSPITAL (O, 224 beds) 506 East San Antonio Street, Victoria, TX Zip 77901–6060, Mailing Address: Box 2089, Zip 77902–2089; tel. 512/575–7441; William R. Blanchard, Chief Executive Officer

DOCTORS HOSPITAL (O, 84 beds) 3205 West Davis, Conroe, TX Zip 77304, Mailing Address: Box 1349, Zip 77305; tel. 409/756–0631; Duane K. Rossmann, Chief Executive Officer

DOCTORS HOSPITAL OF LAREDO (O, 90 beds) 500 East Mann Road, Laredo, TX Zip 78041; tel. 210/723–1131; David Hodgson, Chief Executive Officer

DOCTORS REGIONAL MEDICAL CENTER (O, 270 beds) 3315 South Alameda, Corpus Christi, TX Zip 78411, Mailing Address: P.O. Box 3828, Zip 78463–3828; tel. 512/857–1501; Steven Woerner, Chief Executive Officer

EL CAMPO MEMORIAL HOSPITAL (O, 60 beds) 303 Sandy Corner Road, El Campo, TX Zip 77437; tel. 409/543–6251; Corinne L. Maib, Interim Administrator

FORT BEND HOSPITAL (O, 64 beds) 3803 FM 1092 At Highway 6, Missouri City, TX Zip 77459; tel. 713/499–4800; Wilson J. Weber, Executive Director

GILMER MEDICAL CENTER (O, 40 beds) 712 North Wood Street, Gilmer, TX Zip 75644; tel. 903/843–5611; Al Chapa, Administrator

GULF COAST MEDICAL CENTER (O, 161 beds) 1400 Highway 59, Wharton, TX Zip 77488–3004, Mailing Address: P.O. Box 3004, Zip 77488–3004; tel. 409/532–2500; Craig B. Watson, Chief Executive Officer

KATY MEDICAL CENTER (O, 73 beds) 5602 Medical Center Drive, Katy, TX Zip 77494; tel. 713/392–1111; Brian S. Barbe, Executive Director

LEWISVILLE MEDICAL CENTER HOSPITAL (O, 105 beds) 500 West Main, Lewisville, TX Zip 75057–3699; tel. 214/420–1000; Raymond M. Dunning, Jr., Chief Executive Officer

LONGVIEW REGIONAL HOSPITAL (O, 95 beds) 2901 North Fourth Street, Longview, TX Zip 75601–1903, Mailing Address: P.O. Box 15000, Zip 75607–5000; tel. 903/758–1818; Velinda Stevens, Administrator and Chief Executive Officer

MAINLAND CENTER HOSPITAL (O, 277 beds) 6801 E F Lowry Expressway, Texas City, TX Zip 77591; tel. 409/938–5000; Sally E. Jeffcoat, Chief Executive Officer

MEDICAL ARTS HOSPITAL (O, 32 beds) 6161 Harry Hines Boulevard, Dallas, TX Zip 75235; tel. 214/688–1111; Thomas Permetti, Chief Executive Officer

MEDICAL ARTS HOSPITAL (O, 76 beds) 2501 College Drive, Texarkana, TX Zip 75501–2703, Mailing Address: P.O. Box 6045, Zip 75505–6045; tel. 903/798–5100; Jerry Kincade, Chief Executive Officer

MEDICAL CENTER HOSPITAL (O, 178 beds) 504 Medical Center Boulevard, Conroe, TX Zip 77304, Mailing Address: Box 1538, Zip 77305–1538; tel. 409/539–1111; Duane K. Rossmann, Chief Executive Officer

MEDICAL CENTER HOSPITAL (O, 165 beds) 8081 Greenbriar, Houston, TX Zip 77054–1900; tel. 713/790–8100; Edward W. Myers, Chief Executive Officer

For explanation of codes following names, see page B2.
★Indicates Type III membership in the American Hospital Association.

Systems / Columbia/HCA Healthcare Corporation

MEDICAL CENTER OF PLANO (O, 233 beds) 3901 West 15th Street, Plano, TX Zip 75075–7799; tel. 214/596–6800; Allyn Harris, President and Chief Executive Officer

MEDICAL CITY DALLAS HOSPITAL (O, 491 beds) 7777 Forest Lane, Dallas, TX Zip 75230–2598; tel. 214/661–7000; C. W. Smith, Chief Operating Officer

MEDICAL PLAZA HOSPITAL (O, 162 beds) 1111 Gallagher Road, Sherman, TX Zip 75090; tel. 903/870–7000; J. F. Adams, Chief Executive Officer

METROPOLITAN HOSPITAL (O, 263 beds) 1310 McCullough Avenue, San Antonio, TX Zip 78212–2617; tel. 210/208–2900; John Hanshaw, Chief Executive Officer

MIDWAY PARK MEDICAL CENTER (O, 87 beds) 2600 West Pleasant Run Road, Lancaster, TX Zip 75146–1199, Mailing Address: 2600 West Pleasant Run Road, Zip 75146–1199; tel. 214/223–9600; Douglas P. DeGraaf, Chief Executive Officer

NAVARRO REGIONAL HOSPITAL (O, 148 beds) 3201 West Highway 22, Corsicana, TX Zip 75110; tel. 903/872–4861; Harvey L. Fishero, Administrator

NORTH HILLS HOSPITAL (O, 151 beds) 4401 Booth Calloway Road, North Richland Hills, TX Zip 76180–7399; tel. 817/284–1431; Randy Moresi, Chief Executive Officer

NORTH TEXAS MEDICAL CENTER (O, 172 beds) 1800 North Graves Street, McKinney, TX Zip 75069; tel. 214/548–3000; Don S. Ciulla, Chief Executive Officer

NORTHEAST COMMUNITY HOSPITAL (O, 122 beds) 1301 Airport Freeway, Bedford, TX Zip 76021–5698; tel. 817/868–5600; Ernie Meier, Chief Executive Officer

PARKWAY HOSPITAL (O, 197 beds) 233 West Parker Road, Houston, TX Zip 77076; tel. 713/697–2831; Mel Bishop, Chief Executive Officer

PLAZA MEDICAL CENTER–EAST (O, 228 beds) 1401 South Main Street, Fort Worth, TX Zip 76104–4945; tel. 817/347–4700; Wayne S. Heatherly, President and Chief Executive Officer

PLAZA MEDICAL CENTER–WEST (O, 599 beds) 900 Eighth Avenue, Fort Worth, TX Zip 76104–3986; tel. 817/336–2100; Wayne S. Heatherly, Chief Executive Officer

REHABILITATION HOSPITAL OF SOUTH TEXAS (O, 80 beds) 6226 Saratoga Boulevard, Corpus Christi, TX Zip 78414–3499; tel. 512/991–9690; Jonny F. Hipp, Chief Executive Officer

RIO GRANDE REGIONAL HOSPITAL (O, 198 beds) 101 East Ridge Road, McAllen, TX Zip 78503; tel. 210/632–6000; Randall M. Everts, Chief Executive Officer

RIVERSIDE COMMUNITY HOSPITAL (O, 81 beds) 13725 Farm Road 624, Corpus Christi, TX Zip 78410; tel. 512/767–4300; Winston Borland, Chief Executive Officer

ROSEWOOD MEDICAL CENTER (O, 184 beds) 9200 Westheimer Road, Houston, TX Zip 77063; tel. 713/780–7900; Pat Currie, Chief Executive Officer

ROUND ROCK HOSPITAL (O, 75 beds) 2400 Round Rock Avenue, Round Rock, TX Zip 78681; tel. 512/255–6066; Larry M. Graham, Administrator

SAN ANTONIO REGIONAL HOSPITAL (O, 297 beds) 8026 Floyd Curl Drive, San Antonio, TX Zip 78229–3915; tel. 210/692–8110; Earl H. Denning, Chief Executive Officer

SILSBEE DOCTORS HOSPITAL (O, 57 beds) Highway 418, Silsbee, TX Zip 77656, Mailing Address: Box 1208, Zip 77656; tel. 409/385–5531; David Cottey, Chief Executive Officer

SOUTH AUSTIN MEDICAL CENTER (O, 150 beds) 901 West Ben White Boulevard, Austin, TX Zip 78704–6903; tel. 512/447–2211; Richard W. Klusmann, Chief Executive Officer

SOUTHWEST TEXAS METHODIST HOSPITAL (O, 553 beds) 7700 Floyd Curl Drive, San Antonio, TX Zip 78229–3993; tel. 210/692–4000; James C. Scoggin, Jr., Chief Executive Officer

SPRING BRANCH MEDICAL CENTER (O, 331 beds) 8850 Long Point Road, Houston, TX Zip 77055; tel. 713/467–6555; Stephen L. Royal, President and Chief Executive Officer

SUN BELT REGIONAL MEDICAL CENTER (O, 136 beds) 13111 East Freeway, Houston, TX Zip 77015; tel. 713/455–6911; John Smithhisler, Chief Executive Officer

TERRELL COMMUNITY HOSPITAL (O, 101 beds) 1551 Highway 34 South, Terrell, TX Zip 75160–4833; tel. 214/563–7611; I. Douglas Streckert, Chief Executive Officer

TEXAS ORTHOPEDIC HOSPITAL (O, 46 beds) 7401 South Main Street, Houston, TX Zip 77030; tel. 713/799–8600; Kathy Sunderland, Administrative Assistant

VALLEY REGIONAL MEDICAL CENTER (O, 167 beds) 1 Ted Hunt Boulevard, Brownsville, TX Zip 78521, Mailing Address: Box 3710, Zip 78521; tel. 210/831–9611; David Butler, Interim Chief Executive Officer

VILLAGE OAKS MEDICAL CENTER (O, 100 beds) 12412 Judson Road, San Antonio, TX Zip 78233, Mailing Address: P.O. Box 659510, Zip 78265–9510; tel. 210/650–4949; John R. Nickens III, Chief Executive Officer

WEST HOUSTON MEDICAL CENTER (O, 169 beds) 12141 Richmond Avenue, Houston, TX Zip 77082–2499; tel. 713/558–3444; Janie R. Kauffman, Chief Executive Officer

WESTBURY HOSPITAL (O, 100 beds) 5556 Gasmer Road, Houston, TX Zip 77035–4598; tel. 713/729–1111; Larry C. Andrews, Chief Executive Officer

WOMAN'S HOSPITAL OF TEXAS (O, 138 beds) 7600 Fannin Street, Houston, TX Zip 77054–1900; tel. 713/790–1234; Linda B. Russell, Chief Executive Officer

WOMEN'S AND CHILDREN'S HOSPITAL (O, 150 beds) 8109 Fredericksburg Road, San Antonio, TX Zip 78229–3383; tel. 210/692–5000; Angeline M. Marano, Chief Executive Officer

WOODLAND HEIGHTS MEDICAL CENTER (O, 116 beds) 500 Gaslight Boulevard, Lufkin, TX Zip 75901, Mailing Address: Box 150610, Zip 75915–0610; tel. 409/634–8311; Don H. McBride, Chief Executive Officer

UTAH: ALLEN MEMORIAL HOSPITAL (O, 38 beds) 719 West 400 North Street, Moab, UT Zip 84532, Mailing Address: Box 998, Zip 84532; tel. 801/259–7191; Charles A. Davis, Administrator

ASHLEY VALLEY MEDICAL CENTER (O, 29 beds) 151 West 200 North, Vernal, UT Zip 84078; tel. 801/789–3342; Ronald J. Perry, Chief Executive Officer

BRIGHAM CITY COMMUNITY HOSPITAL (O, 53 beds) 950 South 500 West, Brigham City, UT Zip 84302; tel. 801/734–9471; Robert H. Parker, Jr., Chief Executive Officer

CASTLEVIEW HOSPITAL (O, 84 beds) 300 North Hospital Drive, Price, UT Zip 84501; tel. 801/637–4800; R. Alan Larson, Administrator and Chief Executive Officer

DAVIS HOSPITAL AND MEDICAL CENTER (O, 120 beds) 1600 West Antelope Drive, Layton, UT Zip 84041–1142; tel. 801/825–9561; Floyd D. Morgan, Chief Executive Officer

JORDAN VALLEY HOSPITAL (O, 50 beds) 3580 West 9000 South, West Jordan, UT Zip 84088–8811; tel. 801/561–8888; Keith Alexander, Chief Executive Officer

LAKEVIEW HOSPITAL (O, 128 beds) 630 East Medical Drive, Bountiful, UT Zip 84010–4996; tel. 801/299–2500; Kay Matsumura, Chief Executive Officer

MOUNTAIN VIEW HOSPITAL (O, 121 beds) 1000 East Highway 6, Payson, UT Zip 84651–1690; tel. 801/465–7101; Don Larsen, Chief Executive Officer

OGDEN REGIONAL MEDICAL CENTER (O, 151 beds) 5475 South 500 East, Ogden, UT Zip 84405–6978; tel. 801/479–2111; Les Beard, Chief Executive Officer

PIONEER VALLEY HOSPITAL (O, 127 beds) 3460 South Pioneer Parkway, West Valley City, UT Zip 84120; tel. 801/964–3100; Steven B. Bateman, Chief Executive Officer

SALT LAKE REGIONAL MEDICAL CENTER (O, 200 beds) 1050 East South Temple, Salt Lake City, UT Zip 84102–1599; tel. 801/350–4111; David L. Jones, Chief Executive Officer

ST. MARK'S HOSPITAL (O, 223 beds) 1200 East 3900 South, Salt Lake City, UT Zip 84124; tel. 801/268–7000; Larry Hancock, Chief Executive Officer

VIRGINIA: CHIPPENHAM MEDICAL CENTER (O, 447 beds) 7101 Jahnke Road, Richmond, VA Zip 23225; tel. 804/320–3911; Marilyn B. Tavenner, Chief Executive Officer

CLINCH VALLEY MEDICAL CENTER (O, 200 beds) 2949 West Front Street, Richlands, VA Zip 24641; tel. 703/596–6000; James W. Thweatt, Chief Executive Officer

DOMINION HOSPITAL (O, 100 beds) 2960 Sleepy Hollow Road, Falls Church, VA Zip 22044–2001; tel. 703/536–2000; Barbara D. S. Hekimian, Chief Executive Officer

HENRICO DOCTOR'S HOSPITAL (O, 340 beds) 1602 Skipwith Road, Richmond, VA Zip 23229; tel. 804/289–4500; Mark W. Clayton, Chief Executive Officer

JOHNSTON–WILLIS HOSPITAL (O, 292 beds) 1401 Johnston–Willis Drive, Richmond, VA Zip 23235; tel. 804/330–2000; Marilyn B. Tavenner, Chief Executive Officer

For explanation of codes following names, see page B2.
★Indicates Type III membership in the American Hospital Association.

© 1995 AHA Guide   Integrated Health Delivery Networks, Health Care Systems and Alliances   B27

Systems / Columbia/HCA Healthcare Corporation

LEWIS–GALE HOSPITAL (O, 376 beds) 1900 Electric Road, Salem, VA Zip 24153; tel. 703/776–4000; Karl N. Miller, Chief Executive Officer

LEWIS–GALE PSYCHIATRIC CENTER (O, 144 beds) 1902 Braeburn Drive, Salem, VA Zip 24153–7391; tel. 703/772–2800; James Sholes, Chief Executive Officer

MONTGOMERY REGIONAL HOSPITAL (O, 146 beds) 3700 South Main Street, Blacksburg, VA Zip 24060, Mailing Address: P.O. Box 90004, Zip 24062–9004; tel. 703/953–5101; Gene B. Wright, Chief Executive Officer

NORTHERN VIRGINIA DOCTORS' HOSPITAL (O, 211 beds) 601 South Carlin Springs Road, Arlington, VA Zip 22204–1096; tel. 703/671–1200

PENINSULA PSYCHIATRIC HOSPITAL (O, 125 beds) 2244 Executive Drive, Hampton, VA Zip 23666; tel. 804/827–1001; Jack B. Wheatley, Jr., Chief Executive Officer

POPLAR SPRINGS HOSPITAL (O, 100 beds) 350 Poplar Drive, Petersburg, VA Zip 23805–4657; tel. 804/733–6874; Anthony J. Vadella, Chief Executive Officer

PULASKI COMMUNITY HOSPITAL (O, 74 beds) 2400 Lee Highway, Pulaski, VA Zip 24301, Mailing Address: P.O. Box 759, Zip 24301–0759; tel. 703/980–6822; Christopher W. Dux, Administrator and Chief Executive Officer

RESTON HOSPITAL CENTER (O, 127 beds) 1850 Town Center Parkway, Reston, VA Zip 22090; tel. 703/689–9023; Thomas D. Miller, President and Chief Executive Officer

RETREAT HOSPITAL (O, 227 beds) 2621 Grove Avenue, Richmond, VA Zip 23220–4308; tel. 804/254–5100; W. Trent Crable, President and Chief Executive Officer

WASHINGTON: CAPITAL MEDICAL CENTER (O, 110 beds) 3900 Capital Mall Drive S.W., Olympia, WA Zip 98502–8654, Mailing Address: P.O. Box 19002, Zip 98507–0013; tel. 360/754–5858; Kelly H. Adams, Chief Executive Officer

WEST VIRGINIA: GREENBRIER VALLEY MEDICAL CENTER (O, 122 beds) 202 Maplewood Avenue, Ronceverte, WV Zip 24970–0497, Mailing Address: P.O. Box 497, Zip 24970–0497; tel. 304/647–4411; James B. Wood, Chief Executive Officer

PUTNAM GENERAL HOSPITAL (O, 55 beds) 1400 Hospital Drive, Hurricane, WV Zip 25526–9210, Mailing Address: P.O. Box 900, Zip 25526–0900; tel. 304/757–1700; Stephens M. Mundy, Chief Executive Officer

RALEIGH GENERAL HOSPITAL (O, 293 beds) 1710 Harper Road, Beckley, WV Zip 25801–3397; tel. 304/256–4100; Kenneth M. Holt, Chief Executive Officer

RIVER PARK HOSPITAL (O, 165 beds) 1230 Sixth Avenue, Huntington, WV Zip 25701, Mailing Address: Box 1875, Zip 25719; tel. 304/526–9111; Ronald E. Yates, Chief Executive Officer

SAINT FRANCIS HOSPITAL (O, 145 beds) 333 Laidley Street, Charleston, WV Zip 25301, Mailing Address: Box 471, Zip 25322; tel. 304/347–6500; David R. Sirk, President and Chief Executive Officer

ST. LUKE'S HOSPITAL (O, 79 beds) 1333 Southview Drive, Bluefield, WV Zip 24701, Mailing Address: P.O. Box 1190, Zip 24701; tel. 304/327–2900; Barry A. Papania, Chief Executive Officer

WYOMING: RIVERTON MEMORIAL HOSPITAL (O, 70 beds) 2100 West Sunset Drive, Riverton, WY Zip 82501; tel. 307/856–4161; Kenneth H. Armstrong, Chief Executive Officer

Owned, leased, sponsored:	314 hospitals	54341 beds
Contract–managed:	0 hospitals	0 beds
Totals:	314 hospitals	54341 beds

8805: COLUMBUS–CABRINI MEDICAL CENTER (CC)
2520 North Lakeview Avenue, Chicago, IL Zip 60614; tel. 312/883–8366; Lee Domanico, Chief Executive Officer

ILLINOIS: COLUMBUS HOSPITAL (O, 290 beds) 2520 North Lakeview Avenue, Chicago, IL Zip 60614; tel. 312/883–7300; Lee Domanico, Chief Executive Officer

SAINT ANTHONY HOSPITAL (O, 159 beds) 2875 West 19th Street, Chicago, IL Zip 60623; tel. 312/521–1710; F. Scott Winslow, Regional Chief Operating Officer

SAINT CABRINI HOSPITAL (O, 190 beds) 811 South Lytle Street, Chicago, IL Zip 60607; tel. 312/883–4300; F. Scott Winslow, Chief Operating Officer

Owned, leased, sponsored:	3 hospitals	639 beds
Contract–managed:	0 hospitals	0 beds
Totals:	3 hospitals	639 beds

0215: COMMUNITY CARE SYSTEMS, INC. (IO)
203 Grove Street, Wellesley, MA Zip 02181; tel. 617/239–0871; Frederick J. Thacher, Chairman

MAINE: JACKSON BROOK INSTITUTE (O, 106 beds) 175 Running Hill Road, South Portland, ME Zip 04106; tel. 207/761–2200; Vincent Furey, President

MASSACHUSETTS: CHARLES RIVER HOSPITAL (O, 62 beds) 203 Grove Street, Wellesley, MA Zip 02181; tel. 617/235–8400; E. Lorraine Baugh, President and Chief Executive Officer

Owned, leased, sponsored:	2 hospitals	168 beds
Contract–managed:	0 hospitals	0 beds
Totals:	2 hospitals	168 beds

0875: COMMUNITY HEALTH SYSTEMS, INC. (IO)
3707 FM 1960 West, Suite 500, Houston, TX Zip 77068; tel. 713/537–5230; E. Thomas Chaney, President

CALIFORNIA: BARSTOW COMMUNITY HOSPITAL (L, 48 beds) 555 South Seventh Avenue, Barstow, CA Zip 92311; tel. 619/256–1761; John V. Villanueva, Executive Director

FLORIDA: UNIVERSITY GENERAL HOSPITAL (O, 140 beds) 10200 Seminole Boulevard, Seminole, FL Zip 34642–0005, Mailing Address: P.O. Box 4005, Zip 34642–0005; tel. 813/397–5511; Emil Miller, Chief Executive Officer

WOMEN'S HOSPITAL AND MEDICAL CENTER (O, 99 beds) 9675 Seminole Boulevard, Seminole, FL Zip 34642–2526, Mailing Address: P.O. Box 4001, Zip 34642; tel. 813/393–4646; Emil Miller, Chief Executive Officer

GEORGIA: FANNIN REGIONAL HOSPITAL (O, 51 beds) Highway 5 North, Blue Ridge, GA Zip 30513, Mailing Address: Box 1549, Zip 30513; tel. 706/632–3711; Marvin Stern, Administrator

KENTUCKY: PARKWAY REGIONAL HOSPITAL (O, 80 beds) 2000 Holiday Lane, Fulton, KY Zip 42041; tel. 502/472–2522; Mary Jo Lewis, Administrator

THREE RIVERS MEDICAL CENTER (O, 90 beds) Highway 644, Louisa, KY Zip 41230, Mailing Address: Box 769, Zip 41230; tel. 606/638–9451; Kiser Greg, Executive Director

MISSISSIPPI: PARKWOOD HOSPITAL (O, 66 beds) 8135 Goodman Road, Olive Branch, MS Zip 38654–2199; tel. 601/895–4900; Thomas I. Hayes, Jr., Administrator

MISSOURI: MOBERLY REGIONAL MEDICAL CENTER (O, 101 beds) 1515 Union Avenue, Moberly, MO Zip 65270–9449, Mailing Address: P.O. Box 3000, Zip 65270–3000; tel. 816/263–8400; Jack P. Nyiri, Executive Director

NORTH CAROLINA: COMMUNITY HOSPITAL OF ROCKY MOUNT (O, 50 beds) 1031 Noell Lane, Rocky Mount, NC Zip 27804; tel. 919/937–5100; Roger L. Hall, Administrator

OKLAHOMA: ENID REGIONAL HOSPITAL (L, 109 beds) 401 South Third, Enid, OK Zip 73701, Mailing Address: Box 3467, Zip 73702; tel. 405/234–3371; John E. Walker, Administrator

TENNESSEE: HILLSIDE HOSPITAL (O, 95 beds) 1265 East College Street, Pulaski, TN Zip 38478; tel. 615/363–7531; Rex Macklin, Chief Executive Officer and Administrator

LAKEWAY REGIONAL HOSPITAL (O, 135 beds) 726 McFarland Street, Morristown, TN Zip 37814–3990; tel. 615/586–2302; Stephen L. Taylor, Executive Director

SCOTT COUNTY HOSPITAL (L, 77 beds) U.S. Highway 27, Oneida, TN Zip 37841–4939, Mailing Address: Box 4939, Zip 37841–4939; tel. 615/569–8521; Doug Dailey, Administrator

TEXAS: HIGHLAND MEDICAL CENTER (O, 76 beds) 2412 50th Street, Lubbock, TX Zip 79412; tel. 806/795–8251; David Conejo, Administrator

VIRGINIA: RUSSELL COUNTY MEDICAL CENTER (O, 78 beds) Carroll and Tate Streets, Lebanon, VA Zip 24266; tel. 703/889–1224; Jerry E. Lowery M.S.H.A., Executive Director

Owned, leased, sponsored:	15 hospitals	1295 beds
Contract–managed:	0 hospitals	0 beds
Totals:	15 hospitals	1295 beds

1085: COMMUNITY HOSPITALS OF CENTRAL CALIFORNIA (NP)
Fresno and R Streets, Fresno, CA Zip 93715, Mailing Address: P.O. Box 1232, Zip 93715; tel. 209/442–6000; Bruce M. Perry, Chief Executive Officer

CALIFORNIA: CLOVIS COMMUNITY HOSPITAL (O, 143 beds) 2755 Herndon Avenue, Clovis, CA Zip 93611; tel. 209/323–4060; Paul F. Dyer, Administrator

---

For explanation of codes following names, see page B2.
★Indicates Type III membership in the American Hospital Association.

Systems / Connecticut State Department of Mental Health

FRESNO COMMUNITY HOSPITAL AND MEDICAL CENTER (O, 359 beds) Fresno and R Streets, Fresno, CA Zip 93721, Mailing Address: Box 1232, Zip 93715; tel. 209/442–6000; Bruce M. Perry, Chief Executive Officer

SIERRA COMMUNITY HOSPITAL (O, 77 beds) 2025 East Dakota Avenue, Fresno, CA Zip 93726–4896; tel. 209/221–5600; Bruce M. Perry, Chief Executive Officer

Owned, leased, sponsored:	3 hospitals	579 beds
Contract–managed:	0 hospitals	0 beds
Totals:	3 hospitals	579 beds

0785: COMMUNITY PSYCHIATRIC CENTERS (IO)
6600 West Charleston Boulevard, 1800, Las Vegas, NV Zip 89102; tel. 702/259–3600

ARKANSAS: CPC PINNACLE POINTE HOSPITAL (O, 102 beds) 11501 Financial Center Parkway, Little Rock, AR Zip 72211–3715; tel. 501/223–3322; Pat Perry, Chief Executive Officer

CALIFORNIA: CPC ALHAMBRA HOSPITAL (O, 98 beds) 4619 North Rosemead Boulevard, Rosemead, CA Zip 91770–1498, Mailing Address: P.O. Box 369, Zip 91770; tel. 818/286–1191; Peggy Minnick, Administrator

CPC BELMONT HILLS HOSPITAL (O, 53 beds) 1301 Ralston Avenue, Belmont, CA Zip 94002; tel. 415/593–2143; Bill Bay, Administrator

CPC FREMONT HOSPITAL (O, 78 beds) 39001 Sundale Drive, Fremont, CA Zip 94538; tel. 510/796–1100; Alan M. Gitlin, Chief Executive Officer

CPC HERITAGE OAKS HOSPITAL (O, 76 beds) 4250 Auburn Boulevard, Sacramento, CA Zip 95841; tel. 916/489–3336; Ingrid L. Whipple, Chief Executive Officer

CPC RANCHO LINDO HOSPITAL (O, 74 beds) 7625 East Avenue, Fontana, CA Zip 92336; tel. 714/899–3233; Bruce Waldo, Chief Executive Officer

CPC SAN LUIS REY HOSPITAL (O, 123 beds) 335 Saxony Road, Encinitas, CA Zip 92024–2723; tel. 619/753–1245; William T. Sparrow, Administrator

CPC SANTA ANA HOSPITAL (O, 100 beds) 2212 East Fourth Street, Santa Ana, CA Zip 92705–3873; tel. 714/543–8481; Gilbert Carmona, Regional Chief Executive Officer

CPC SIERRA VISTA HOSPITAL (O, 72 beds) 8001 Bruceville Road, Sacramento, CA Zip 95823; tel. 916/423–2000; Kenneth A. Meibert, Chief Executive Officer

CPC VISTA DEL MAR HOSPITAL (O, 87 beds) 801 Seneca Street, Ventura, CA Zip 93001; tel. 805/653–6434; Jerry Conway, Chief Executive Officer

CPC WALNUT CREEK HOSPITAL (O, 108 beds) 175 La Casa Via, Walnut Creek, CA Zip 94598; tel. 510/933–7990; Lee L. Haber, Chief Executive Officer

LAGUNA HILLS HOSPITAL AND MENTAL HEALTH CENTER (O, 78 beds) 24552 Pacific Park Drive, Laguna Beach, CA Zip 92656; tel. 714/831–1800; Gilbert Carmona, Regional Chief Executive Officer

FLORIDA: CPC FORT LAUDERDALE HOSPITAL (O, 100 beds) 1601 East Las Olas Boulevard, Fort Lauderdale, FL Zip 33301–2393; tel. 305/463–4321; Eric Trafals, Chief Executive Officer

CPC PALM BAY HOSPITAL (O, 60 beds) 4400 Dixie Highway N.E., Palm Bay, FL Zip 32905–4396; tel. 407/729–0500; Harold G. Marohn, Administrator

CPC ST. JOHNS RIVER HOSPITAL (O, 99 beds) 6300 Beach Boulevard, Jacksonville, FL Zip 32216; tel. 904/724–9202; Doug Gifford, Administrator

GEORGIA: CPC PARKWOOD HOSPITAL (O, 145 beds) 1999 Cliff Valley Way N.E., Atlanta, GA Zip 30329–2448; tel. 404/633–8431; J. Shawn O'Connor, Administrator and Chief Executive Officer

IDAHO: CPC INTERMOUNTAIN HOSPITAL OF BOISE (O, 75 beds) 303 North Allumbaugh Street, Boise, ID Zip 83704–9266; tel. 208/377–8400; Vernon G. Garrett, Administrator

ILLINOIS: CPC OLD ORCHARD HOSPITAL (O, 133 beds) 9700 North Kenton Avenue, Skokie, IL Zip 60076–1218; tel. 708/679–0760; Sheila Mishler, Chief Executive Officer

CPC STREAMWOOD HOSPITAL (O, 100 beds) 1400 East Irving Park Road, Streamwood, IL Zip 60107; tel. 708/837–9000; Suzanne Barry, Administrator

INDIANA: CPC VALLE VISTA HOSPITAL (O, 96 beds) 898 East Main Street, Greenwood, IN Zip 46143; tel. 317/887–1348

KANSAS: CPC COLLEGE MEADOWS HOSPITAL (O, 120 beds) 14425 College Boulevard, Lenexa, KS Zip 66215; tel. 913/469–1100; Stephen Chesney, Chief Executive Officer

LOUISIANA: CPC BRENTWOOD HOSPITAL (O, 88 beds) 1800 Irving Place, Shreveport, LA Zip 71101–4698; tel. 318/424–6761; Michael Amador, Chief Executive Officer

CPC COLISEUM MEDICAL CENTER (O, 109 beds) 3601 Coliseum Street, New Orleans, LA Zip 70115; tel. 504/897–9700; Darlene Salvant, Chief Executive Officer

CPC EAST LAKE HOSPITAL (O, 72 beds) 5650 Read Boulevard, New Orleans, LA Zip 70127–3145; tel. 504/241–0888; Darlene Salvant, Chief Executive Officer

CPC MEADOW WOOD HOSPITAL (O, 85 beds) 9032 Perkins Road, Baton Rouge, LA Zip 70810; tel. 504/766–8553; Charles J. Hooker III, Chief Executive Officer

MISSISSIPPI: CPC SAND HILL HOSPITAL (O, 60 beds) 11150 Highway 49 North, Gulfport, MS Zip 39503–4110; tel. 601/831–1700; Michael A. Zieman, Chief Executive Officer

MISSOURI: CPC SPIRIT OF ST. LOUIS HOSPITAL (O, 104 beds) 5931 Highway 94 South, Saint Charles, MO Zip 63304–5601; tel. 314/441–7300

NORTH CAROLINA: CPC CEDAR SPRING HOSPITAL (O, 70 beds) 9600 Pineville–Matthews Road, Pineville, NC Zip 28134–7548; tel. 704/541–6676; David G. Blackburn, Chief Executive Officer

TEXAS: CPC CAPITAL HOSPITAL (O, 86 beds) 12151 Hunters Chase Drive, Austin, TX Zip 78729; tel. 512/250–8667; Kevin E. Blackwell, Chief Executive Officer

CPC MILLWOOD HOSPITAL (O, 98 beds) 1011 North Cooper Street, Arlington, TX Zip 76011; tel. 817/261–3121; Wayne Hallford, Chief Executive Officer

UTAH: CPC OLYMPUS VIEW HOSPITAL (O, 102 beds) 1430 East 4500 South, Salt Lake City, UT Zip 84117–4208; tel. 801/272–8000; Susan Kosta, Administrator

WASHINGTON: CPC FAIRFAX HOSPITAL (O, 133 beds) 10200 Northeast 132nd Street, Kirkland, WA Zip 98034; tel. 206/821–2000; Robert C. Hails, Chief Executive Officer

WISCONSIN: CPC GREENBRIAR BEHAVIORAL HEALTH CENTER (O, 44 beds) 5015 South 110th Street, Milwaukee, WI Zip 53228–3134; tel. 414/425–8000; Jeff Bergren, Chief Executive Officer and Administrator

PUERTO RICO: CPC HOSPITAL SAN JUAN CAPESTRANO (O, 88 beds) Rio Piedras, PR, Mailing Address: Rural Route 2, Box 11, Zip 00928; tel. 809/760–0222; Laura Vargas, Administrator

Owned, leased, sponsored:	34 hospitals	3116 beds
Contract–managed:	0 hospitals	0 beds
Totals:	34 hospitals	3116 beds

5695: CONGREGATION OF ST. AGNES (CC)
475 Gillett Street, Fond Du Lac, WI Zip 54935–4598; tel. 414/923–0804; Rosann Geiser, Corporate Director

WISCONSIN: ST. AGNES HOSPITAL (S, 161 beds) 430 East Division Street, Fond Du Lac, WI Zip 54936–0385; tel. 414/929–2300; James J. Sexton, President and Chief Executive Officer

THE MONROE CLINIC (S, 139 beds) 515 22nd Avenue, Monroe, WI Zip 53566–1598; tel. 608/324–1000; James D. Beyers, President

WAUPUN MEMORIAL HOSPITAL (S, 49 beds) 620 West Brown Street, Waupun, WI Zip 53963–1799; tel. 414/324–5581; James J. Sexton, President and Chief Executive Officer

Owned, leased, sponsored:	3 hospitals	349 beds
Contract–managed:	0 hospitals	0 beds
Totals:	3 hospitals	349 beds

0014: CONNECTICUT STATE DEPARTMENT OF MENTAL HEALTH (NP)
90 Washington Street, Hartford, CT Zip 06106; tel. 203/566–3650; Albert J. Solnit M.D., Commissioner

CONNECTICUT: CEDARCREST REGIONAL HOSPITAL (O, 73 beds) 525 Russell Road, Newington, CT Zip 06111–1595; tel. 203/666–4613; David E. K. Hunter Ph.D., Superintendent

CONNECTICUT MENTAL HEALTH CENTER (O, 54 beds) 34 Park Street, New Haven, CT Zip 06519, Mailing Address: Box 1842, Zip 06508–1842; tel. 203/789–7290; Ezra Griffith M.D., Director

CONNECTICUT VALLEY HOSPITAL (O, 318 beds) Eastern Drive, Middletown, CT Zip 06457–7023, Mailing Address: P.O. Box 351, Zip 06457–7024; tel. 203/344–2666; Judith Normandin, Chief Executive Officer

FAIRFIELD HILLS HOSPITAL (O, 212 beds) Mile Hill Road, Newtown, CT Zip 06470–5525, Mailing Address: Box 5525, Zip 06470–5525; tel. 203/426–2531; Andrew J. Phillips Ed.D., Superintendent

For explanation of codes following names, see page B2.
★Indicates Type III membership in the American Hospital Association.

Systems / Connecticut State Department of Mental Health

GREATER BRIDGEPORT COMMUNITY MENTAL HEALTH CENTER (O, 22 beds) 1635 Central Avenue, Bridgeport, CT Zip 06610-0902, Mailing Address: Box 5117, Zip 06610; tel. 203/579-6646; James M. Lehane III, Director
NORWICH HOSPITAL (O, 314 beds) Route 12, Norwich, CT Zip 06360, Mailing Address: Box 508, Zip 06360-0508; tel. 203/823-5200; Garrell S. Mullaney, Superintendent
WHITING FORENSIC INSTITUTE (O, 100 beds) O'Brien Drive, Middletown, CT Zip 06457, Mailing Address: Box 70, Zip 06457-3942; tel. 203/344-2541; Michael A. Norko M.D., Director

Owned, leased, sponsored:	7 hospitals	1093 beds
Contract-managed:	0 hospitals	0 beds
Totals:	7 hospitals	1093 beds

1715: CONTINENTAL MEDICAL SYSTEMS, INC. (IO)
600 Wilson Lane, Mechanicsburg, PA Zip 17055-0715, Mailing Address: P.O. Box 715, Zip 17055-0715; tel. 717/790-8300; R. A. Ortenzio, Chairman and Chief Executive Officer

ARKANSAS: CENTRAL ARKANSAS REHABILITATION HOSPITAL (O, 60 beds) 2201 Wildwood Avenue, Sherwood, AR Zip 72116, Mailing Address: P.O. Box 6930, North Little Rock, Zip 72116-6930; tel. 501/834-1800; Douglas W. Parker, Chief Executive Officer
NORTHWEST ARKANSAS REHABILITATION HOSPITAL (O, 60 beds) 153 Monte Painter Drive, Fayetteville, AR Zip 72703; tel. 501/444-2200; Dennis R. Shelby, Administrator
CALIFORNIA: KENTFIELD REHABILITATION HOSPITAL (O, 60 beds) 1125 Sir Francis Drake Boulevard, Kentfield, CA Zip 94904, Mailing Address: P.O. Box 338, Zip 94914-0338; tel. 415/456-9680; William O. Mitchell, Jr., Administrator
KANSAS: WESLEY REHABILITATION HOSPITAL (O, 65 beds) 8338 West 13th Street North, Wichita, KS Zip 67212-2900; tel. 316/729-9999; G. Curt Meyer, Chief Executive Officer
MASSACHUSETTS: BRAINTREE HOSPITAL REHABILITATION NETWORK (O, 166 beds) 250 Pond Street, Braintree, MA Zip 02185; tel. 617/848-5353; Ernest J. Broadbent, President and Chief Executive Officer
TENNESSEE: REHABILITATION HOSPITAL-MIDSOUTH (CM, 50 beds) 2100 Exeter Road, Germantown, TN Zip 38138; tel. 901/757-1350; B. Richard Moseley, Chief Executive Officer
TEXAS: SOUTHEAST TEXAS REHABILITATION HOSPITAL (O, 60 beds) 3340 Plaza 10 Boulevard, Beaumont, TX Zip 77707; tel. 409/835-0835; David J. Holly, Chief Executive Officer

Owned, leased, sponsored:	6 hospitals	471 beds
Contract-managed:	1 hospitals	50 beds
Totals:	7 hospitals	521 beds

0016: COOK COUNTY BUREAU OF HEALTH SERVICES (NP)
1835 West Harrison Street, Chicago, IL Zip 60612; tel. 312/633-3070; Ruth M. Rothstein, Chief

ILLINOIS: COOK COUNTY HOSPITAL (O, 842 beds) 1835 West Harrison Street, Chicago, IL Zip 60612; tel. 312/633-6000; Ruth M. Rothstein, Director
OAK FOREST HOSPITAL OF COOK COUNTY (O, 838 beds) 15900 South Cicero Avenue, Oak Forest, IL Zip 60452; tel. 708/687-7200; Patricia Rush M.D., Director
PROVIDENT HOSPITAL OF COOK COUNTY (O, 96 beds) 500 East 51st Street, Chicago, IL Zip 60615; tel. 312/572-1200; Shirley Bomar-Cole, Acting Chief Operating Officer

Owned, leased, sponsored:	3 hospitals	1776 beds
Contract-managed:	0 hospitals	0 beds
Totals:	3 hospitals	1776 beds

★5885: COVENANT HEALTH SYSTEMS, INC. (CC)
10 Pelham Road, Lexington, MA Zip 02173-5799; tel. 617/862-1634; David R. Lincoln, President

MAINE: ST. MARY'S REGIONAL MEDICAL CENTER (O, 233 beds) 45 Golder Street, Lewiston, ME Zip 04240, Mailing Address: P.O. Box 291, Zip 04243-0291; tel. 207/777-8100; James E. Cassidy, President and Chief Executive Officer
MASSACHUSETTS: YOUVILLE HOSPITAL AND REHABILITATION CENTER (O, 305 beds) 1575 Cambridge Street, Cambridge, MA Zip 02138-4398; tel. 617/876-4344; T. Richard Quigley, President and Chief Executive Officer

---

NEW HAMPSHIRE: ST. JOSEPH HOSPITAL AND TRAUMA CENTER (O, 208 beds) 172 Kinsley Street, Nashua, NH Zip 03061, Mailing Address: Caller Service 2013, Zip 03061; tel. 603/882-3000; Peter B. Davis, President and Chief Executive Officer
OHIO: ST. VINCENT MEDICAL CENTER (O, 472 beds) 2213 Cherry Street, Toledo, OH Zip 43608-2691; tel. 419/321-3232; Darryl R. Lippman, President

Owned, leased, sponsored:	4 hospitals	1218 beds
Contract-managed:	0 hospitals	0 beds
Totals:	4 hospitals	1218 beds

★0008: CROZER-KEYSTONE HEALTH SYSTEM (NP)
1400 North Providence Road, Ste 4010, Media, PA Zip 19063-2049; tel. 610/447-2000; John C. McMeekin, President and Chief Executive Officer

PENNSYLVANIA: CROZER-CHESTER MEDICAL CENTER (O, 478 beds) One Medical Center Boulevard, Upland, PA Zip 19013-3995; tel. 215/447-2000; Gerald Miller, President
DELAWARE COUNTY MEMORIAL HOSPITAL (O, 285 beds) 501 North Lansdowne Avenue, Drexel Hill, PA Zip 19026-1186; tel. 610/284-8100; Dante Caruso, Jr., President and Chief Executive Officer
SPRINGFIELD HOSPITAL (O, 32 beds) 190 West Sproul Road, Springfield, PA Zip 19064-2097; tel. 215/328-8700; Stephen A. Robbins, Executive Director

Owned, leased, sponsored:	3 hospitals	795 beds
Contract-managed:	0 hospitals	0 beds
Totals:	3 hospitals	795 beds

★5435: CSJ HEALTH SYSTEM OF WICHITA (CC)
3720 East Bayley, Wichita, KS Zip 67218-3087; tel. 316/689-4000; LeRoy E. Rheault, President and Chief Executive Officer

CALIFORNIA: ST. ROSE HOSPITAL (O, 175 beds) 27200 Calaroga Avenue, Hayward, CA Zip 94545-4383; tel. 510/264-4000; Michael P. Mahoney, President and Chief Executive Officer
KANSAS: MOUNT CARMEL MEDICAL CENTER (O, 169 beds) Centennial and Rouse Streets, Pittsburg, KS Zip 66762-6686; tel. 316/231-6100; Dan Lingor, President
SAINT MARY HOSPITAL (O, 106 beds) 1823 College Avenue, Manhattan, KS Zip 66502, Mailing Address: Box 1047, Zip 66502-0041; tel. 913/776-3322; J. H. Seitz, President and Chief Executive Officer
ST. JOHN'S REGIONAL HEALTH CENTER (O, 120 beds) 139 North Penn Street, Salina, KS Zip 67401-3057, Mailing Address: P.O. Box 5201, Zip 67402-5201; tel. 913/827-5591; John R. Broberg, Interim President and Chief Executive Officer
ST. JOSEPH HOSPITAL (O, 57 beds) 1100 Highland Drive, Concordia, KS Zip 66901-3997; tel. 913/243-8500; Daniel R. Bartz, Acting Administrator
ST. JOSEPH MEDICAL CENTER (O, 480 beds) 3600 East Harry Street, Wichita, KS Zip 67218-3713; tel. 316/685-1111; LeRoy E. Rheault, President and Chief Executive Officer
OKLAHOMA: ST. JOSEPH REGIONAL MEDICAL CENTER OF NORTHERN OKLAHOMA (O, 75 beds) 14th Street & Hartford Avenue, Ponca City, OK Zip 74601-2035, Mailing Address: Box 1270, Zip 74602-1270; tel. 405/765-3321; Garry L. England, President and Chief Executive Officer

Owned, leased, sponsored:	7 hospitals	1182 beds
Contract-managed:	0 hospitals	0 beds
Totals:	7 hospitals	1182 beds

0075: CUMBERLAND HEALTH SYSTEMS, INC. (IO)
2100 West End Avenue, Ste 900, Nashville, TN Zip 37203; tel. 615/327-2200; Samuel W. Owen, President and Chief Executive Officer

MASSACHUSETTS: HERITAGE HOSPITAL (O, 93 beds) 26 Central Street, Somerville, MA Zip 02143; tel. 617/625-8900; Jay Mitchell, Administrator
TENNESSEE: LEWIS COMMUNITY HOSPITAL (CM, 52 beds) 617 West Main, Hohenwald, TN Zip 38462, Mailing Address: P.O. Box 879, Zip 38462; tel. 615/796-4901; Stephen Chapman, Chief Executive Officer

---

For explanation of codes following names, see page B2.
★Indicates Type III membership in the American Hospital Association.

OAKWOOD MEDICAL CENTER (O, 23 beds) 5310 Ball Camp, Knoxville, TN Zip 37921; tel. 615/584–9191; Steve Petty, Administrator

PERRY MEMORIAL HOSPITAL (CM, 53 beds) Highway 13 South, Linden, TN Zip 37096, Mailing Address: Route 10, Box 8, Zip 37096; tel. 615/589–2121; Judy G. Eads R.N., Administrator

VIRGINIA: DICKENSON COUNTY MEDICAL CENTER (CM, 50 beds) Hospital Drive, Clintwood, VA Zip 24228, Mailing Address: Box 1390, Zip 24228–1390; tel. 703/926–0300; John F. Davis FACHE, Interim Administrator

Owned, leased, sponsored:	2 hospitals	116 beds
Contract–managed:	3 hospitals	155 beds
Totals:	5 hospitals	271 beds

★**1855: DAUGHTERS OF CHARITY NATIONAL HEALTH SYSTEM** (CC)
4600 Edmundson Road, Saint Louis, MO Zip 63134, Mailing Address: P.O. Box 45998, Zip 63145–5998; tel. 314/253–6700; F. Dale Whitten, Interim President

ALABAMA: PROVIDENCE HOSPITAL (S, 349 beds) 6801 Airport Boulevard, Mobile, AL Zip 36608, Mailing Address: P.O. Box 850429, Zip 36685; tel. 334/633–1000; John R. Roeder, President and Chief Executive Officer

ST. VINCENT'S HOSPITAL (S, 338 beds) 810 St. Vincent's Drive, Birmingham, AL Zip 35205, Mailing Address: P.O. Box 12407, Zip 35202–2407; tel. 205/939–7000; Vincent Caponi, President

CALIFORNIA: O'CONNOR HOSPITAL (S, 138 beds) 2105 Forest Avenue, San Jose, CA Zip 95128–1471; tel. 408/947–2500; William C. Finlayson, President and Chief Executive Officer

SAINT LOUISE HOSPITAL (S, 32 beds) 18500 Saint Louise Drive, Morgan Hill, CA Zip 95037; tel. 408/779–1500; William C. Finlayson, President and Chief Executive Officer

SETON MEDICAL CENTER (S, 275 beds) 1900 Sullivan Avenue, Daly City, CA Zip 94015–2229; tel. 415/992–4000; Deborah E. Stebbins FACHE, Acting President and Chief Executive Officer

SETON MEDICAL CENTER COASTSIDE (S, 123 beds) 600 Marine Boulevard, Moss Beach, CA Zip 94038; tel. 415/728–5521; Deborah E. Stebbins FACHE, Acting President and Chief Executive Officer

ST. FRANCIS MEDICAL CENTER (S, 356 beds) 3630 East Imperial Highway, Lynwood, CA Zip 90262; tel. 310/603–6000; Sister Elizabeth Joseph Keaveney, President and Chief Executive Officer

ST. VINCENT MEDICAL CENTER (S, 313 beds) 2131 West Third Street, Los Angeles, CA Zip 90057–0992, Mailing Address: P.O. Box 57992, Zip 90057; tel. 213/484–7111; Vincent F. Guinan, President

CONNECTICUT: ST. VINCENT'S MEDICAL CENTER (S, 289 beds) 2800 Main Street, Bridgeport, CT Zip 06606–4201; tel. 203/576–6000; William J. Riordan, President and Chief Executive Officer

DISTRICT OF COLUMBIA: PROVIDENCE HOSPITAL (S, 333 beds) 1150 Varnum Street N.E., Washington, DC Zip 20017–2180; tel. 202/269–7000; Sister Carol Keehan, President

FLORIDA: RIVERSIDE HOSPITAL (S, 108 beds) 2033 Riverside Avenue, Jacksonville, FL Zip 32204; tel. 904/387–7000; Charles S. Kinney, Executive Vice President

SACRED HEART HOSPITAL OF PENSACOLA (S, 391 beds) 5151 North Ninth Avenue, Pensacola, FL Zip 32504, Mailing Address: P.O. Box 2700, Zip 32513–2700; tel. 904/474–7000; Sister Irene Kraus, President and Chief Executive Officer

ST. VINCENT'S MEDICAL CENTER (S, 528 beds) 1800 Barrs Street, Jacksonville, FL Zip 32204, Mailing Address: P.O. Box 2982, Zip 32203–2982; tel. 904/387–7300; Everett M. Devaney, President

ILLINOIS: ST. JOSEPH HEALTH CENTERS AND HOSPITAL (S, 493 beds) 2900 North Lake Shore Drive, Chicago, IL Zip 60657–6274; tel. 312/665–3000; Sister Theresa Peck, President and Chief Executive Officer

INDIANA: SAINT JOSEPH HOSPITAL AND HEALTH CENTER (S, 160 beds) 1907 West Sycamore Street, Kokomo, IN Zip 46901–9010; tel. 317/452–5611; Sister M. Martin McEntee, President and Chief Executive Officer

ST. MARY'S MEDICAL CENTER OF EVANSVILLE (S, 575 beds) 3700 Washington Avenue, Evansville, IN Zip 47750; tel. 812/479–4000; Richard C. Breon, President and Chief Executive Officer

ST. VINCENT HOSPITAL AND HEALTH CARE CENTER (S, 836 beds) 2001 West 86th Street, Indianapolis, IN Zip 46260, Mailing Address: Box 40970, Zip 46240–0970; tel. 317/338–2345; Douglas D. French, President and Chief Executive Officer

WARRICK HOSPITAL (S, 36 beds) 1116 Millis Avenue, Boonville, IN Zip 47601–0629, Mailing Address: Box 629, Zip 47601–0629; tel. 812/897–4800; John D. O'Neil, Chief Operating Officer

MARYLAND: SACRED HEART HOSPITAL (S, 240 beds) 900 Seton Drive, Cumberland, MD Zip 21502; tel. 301/759–4200; Edward M. Dinan, President

ST. AGNES HOSPITAL OF THE CITY OF BALTIMORE (S, 424 beds) 900 Caton Avenue, Baltimore, MD Zip 21229–5299; tel. 410/368–6000; Robert E. Pezzoli, President and Chief Executive Officer

MASSACHUSETTS: CARNEY HOSPITAL (S, 221 beds) 2100 Dorchester Avenue, Boston, MA Zip 02124–5666; tel. 617/296–4000; Matthias D. Maguire, President

MICHIGAN: PROVIDENCE HOSPITAL AND MEDICAL CENTERS (S, 459 beds) 16001 West Nine Mile Road, Southfield, MI Zip 48075–4854, Mailing Address: Box 2043, Zip 48037–2043; tel. 810/424–3000; Michael A. Slubowski, Chief Executive Officer

ST. MARY'S MEDICAL CENTER (S, 268 beds) 830 South Jefferson Avenue, Saginaw, MI Zip 48601–2594; tel. 517/776–8000; Frederic L. Fraizer, President and Chief Executive Officer

MISSOURI: DEPAUL HEALTH CENTER (S, 466 beds) 12303 DePaul Drive, Saint Louis, MO Zip 63044–2588; tel. 314/344–6000; Robert J. Henkel, President and Chief Executive Officer

NEW YORK: OUR LADY OF LOURDES MEMORIAL HOSPITAL (S, 202 beds) 169 Riverside Drive, Binghamton, NY Zip 13905–4198; tel. 607/798–5111; Michael G. Guley, President and Chief Executive Officer

SETON HEALTH SYSTEM (S, 444 beds) 1300 Massachusetts Avenue, Troy, NY Zip 12180; tel. 518/272–5000; Edward G. Murphy M.D., President and Chief Executive Officer

SISTERS OF CHARITY HOSPITAL OF BUFFALO (S, 493 beds) 2157 Main Street, Buffalo, NY Zip 14214–2692; tel. 716/862–2000; John J. Maher, President and Chief Executive Officer

ST. MARY'S HOSPITAL (S, 227 beds) 89 Genesee Street, Rochester, NY Zip 14611–3285; tel. 716/464–3000; Patrick Madden, President

PENNSYLVANIA: GOOD SAMARITAN REGIONAL MEDICAL CENTER (S, 221 beds) 700 East Norwegian Street, Pottsville, PA Zip 17901–2798; tel. 717/621–4000; Gino J. Pazzaglini, President and Chief Executive Officer

TENNESSEE: ST. THOMAS HOSPITAL (S, 571 beds) 4220 Harding Road, Nashville, TN Zip 37205, Mailing Address: Box 380, Zip 37202; tel. 615/222–2111; John F. Tighe, President and Chief Executive Officer

TEXAS: PROVIDENCE HEALTH CENTER (S, 415 beds) 6901 Medical Parkway, Waco, TX Zip 76712, Mailing Address: P.O. Box 2589, Zip 76702–2589; tel. 817/751–4000; Kent A. Keahey, President

SETON MEDICAL CENTER (S, 532 beds) 1201 West 38th Street, Austin, TX Zip 78705–1056; tel. 512/323–1000; Charles J. Barnett, President

ST. PAUL MEDICAL CENTER (S, 383 beds) 5909 Harry Hines Boulevard, Dallas, TX Zip 75235; tel. 214/879–1000; Anthony L. Bunker, President

VIRGINIA: DEPAUL MEDICAL CENTER (S, 260 beds) 150 Kingsley Lane, Norfolk, VA Zip 23505; tel. 804/889–5000; Kevin P. Conlin, President and Chief Executive Officer

WISCONSIN: ST. MARY'S HILL HOSPITAL (S, 20 beds) 2350 North Lake Drive, Milwaukee, WI Zip 53211–4581; tel. 414/291–1650; Sister Renee Rose, President and Chief Executive Officer

ST. MARY'S HOSPITAL (S, 331 beds) 2323 North Lake Drive, Milwaukee, WI Zip 53211–9682, Mailing Address: Box 503, Zip 53201–0503; tel. 414/291–1000; Sister Renee Rose, President and Chief Executive Officer

ST. MARY'S HOSPITAL OZAUKEE (S, 82 beds) 13111 North Port Washington Road, Mequon, WI Zip 53097–2416; tel. 414/243–7300; Sister Renee Rose, President and Chief Executive Officer

Owned, leased, sponsored:	37 hospitals	11932 beds
Contract–managed:	0 hospitals	0 beds
Totals:	37 hospitals	11932 beds

★**1825: DCH HEALTHCARE AUTHORITY** (NP)
809 University Boulevard East, Tuscaloosa, AL Zip 35401; tel. 205/759–7111; J. H. Ford Jr., Chief Executive Officer

ALABAMA: DCH REGIONAL MEDICAL CENTER (O, 523 beds) 809 University Boulevard East, Tuscaloosa, AL Zip 35401–9961; tel. 205/759–7111; J. H. Ford, Jr., Chief Executive Officer

DCH REHABILITATION PAVILION (O, 65 beds) 1101 Sixth Avenue East, Tuscaloosa, AL Zip 35401–3297; tel. 205/759–7375; Ann Loggins, Vice President Rehabilitation Services

For explanation of codes following names, see page B2.
★Indicates Type III membership in the American Hospital Association.

Systems / DCH Healthcare Authority

FAYETTE COUNTY HOSPITAL AND NURSING HOME (L, 166 beds) 1653 Temple Avenue North, Fayette, AL Zip 35555, Mailing Address: P.O. Drawer 878, Zip 35555; tel. 205/932–5966; Harold Reed, Administrator

NORTHPORT HOSPITAL–DCH (O, 133 beds) 2700 Hospital Drive, Northport, AL Zip 35476; tel. 205/333–4500; Wendell Briggs, Administrator

Owned, leased, sponsored:	4 hospitals	887 beds
Contract–managed:	0 hospitals	0 beds
Totals:	4 hospitals	887 beds

6995: DEPARTMENT OF HEALTH AND HOSPITALS (NP)
818 Harrison Avenue, Boston, MA Zip 02118; tel. 617/534–5365; Lawrence Dwyer, Commissioner

MASSACHUSETTS: BOSTON CITY HOSPITAL (O, 282 beds) 818 Harrison Avenue, Boston, MA Zip 02118; tel. 617/534–5000; Lawrence Dwyer, Commissioner

BOSTON SPECIALTY AND REHABILITATION HOSPITAL (O, 87 beds) 249 River Street, Boston, MA Zip 02126; tel. 617/534–2000; Dorothy L. Turner–Small R.N., Administrator

Owned, leased, sponsored:	2 hospitals	369 beds
Contract–managed:	0 hospitals	0 beds
Totals:	2 hospitals	369 beds

9655: DEPARTMENT OF NAVY (FG)
Washington, DC Zip 20066

CALIFORNIA: NAVAL HOSPITAL (O, 29 beds) 930 Franklin Avenue, Lemoore, CA Zip 93246–5000; tel. 209/998–4201; Lieutenant Commander Sharon R. Thomas MSC, Administrator

NAVAL HOSPITAL (O, 260 beds) Oakland, CA Zip 94627; tel. 510/633–5019; Captain R. E. McKee MSC, USN, Director Administration

NAVAL HOSPITAL (O, 127 beds) Camp Pendleton, CA, Mailing Address: Box 555191, Zip 92055–5191; tel. 619/725–1288; Captain James Staiger, Commanding Officer

NAVAL HOSPITAL (O, 29 beds) Twentynine Palms, CA, Mailing Address: Box 788250, MCAGCC, Zip 92278–8250; tel. 619/830–2188; Captain C. S. Chitwood MSC, USN, Commanding Officer

NAVAL MEDICAL CENTER (O, 422 beds) San Diego, CA Zip 92134–5000; tel. 619/532–6400; Rear Admiral R. A. Nelson MC, USN, Commander

CONNECTICUT: NAVAL HOSPITAL (O, 25 beds) Groton, CT Zip 06349–5600; tel. 203/449–3261; Lieutenant, Junior Grade T. L. Sauvigne' MSC, U.S.N.R., Administrator

FLORIDA: NAVAL HOSPITAL (O, 117 beds) 2080 Child Street, Jacksonville, FL Zip 32214–5000; tel. 904/777–7300; Captain D. Vertrees Hollingsworth MSC, USN, Commanding Officer

NAVAL HOSPITAL (O, 143 beds) Orlando, FL Zip 32813–8221; tel. 407/643–2477

NAVAL HOSPITAL (O, 104 beds) 6000 West Highway 98, Pensacola, FL Zip 32512–0003; tel. 904/452–6611; Commander H. M. Chinnery, Director, Administration

ILLINOIS: NAVAL HOSPITAL (O, 136 beds) Great Lakes, IL Zip 60088–5230; tel. 708/688–4560

MARYLAND: NATIONAL NAVAL MEDICAL CENTER (O, 362 beds) Bethesda, MD Zip 20889–5600; tel. 301/295–5800; Rear Admiral David M. Lichtman MC, USN, Commander

NAVAL HOSPITAL (O, 20 beds) Patuxent River, MD Zip 20670–5370; tel. 301/826–1418

NORTH CAROLINA: NAVAL HOSPITAL (O, 176 beds) Camp Lejeune, NC Zip 28547–0100; tel. 910/451–4300; Captain Michael L. Cowan MC, USN, Commanding Officer

NAVAL HOSPITAL (O, 43 beds) Cherry Point, NC Zip 28533–5008; tel. 919/466–3620; Captain V. Peters MSC, USN, Commanding Officer

SOUTH CAROLINA: NAVAL HOSPITAL (O, 49 beds) 1 Pinckney Boulevard, Beaufort, SC Zip 29902–6148; tel. 803/525–5301; Captain Mark V. Brown MC, USN, Commanding Officer

NAVAL HOSPITAL (O, 160 beds) Charleston, SC Zip 29405; tel. 803/743–7000; Captain H. B. Etienne MC, Commanding Officer

TENNESSEE: NAVAL HOSPITAL (O, 36 beds) Millington, TN Zip 38054–5201; tel. 901/873–5804; Captain Michael Kilpatrick MSC, USN, Commanding Officer

TEXAS: NAVAL HOSPITAL (O, 25 beds) Corpus Christi, TX Zip 78419–5200; tel. 512/939–2685; Captain F. G. Barina, Jr., Commanding Officer

VIRGINIA: NAVAL MEDICAL CENTER (O, 387 beds) 620 John Paul Jones Circle, Portsmouth, VA Zip 23708–5100; tel. 804/398–5008; Rear Admiral William J. McDaniel MC, USN, Commander

WASHINGTON: NAVAL HOSPITAL (O, 106 beds) Boone Road, Bremerton, WA Zip 98312–1898; tel. 206/479–9344; Captain Richard A. Mayo MSC, Commanding Officer

NAVAL HOSPITAL (O, 27 beds) 3475 North Saratoga Street, Oak Harbor, WA Zip 98278–8800; tel. 360/257–9500

GUAM: U.S. NAVAL HOSPITAL (O, 55 beds) Agana, GU, Mailing Address: Box 7607, FPO, AP Zip 96538–1600; tel. 671/344–9340; J. M. Ricciardi, Commanding Officer

PUERTO RICO: U.S. NAVAL HOSPITAL (O, 35 beds) Roosevelt Roads, PR, Mailing Address: Box 3007, FPO, AA Zip 34051–8100; tel. 809/865–6171; M. G. Ashamalla, Commanding Officer

Owned, leased, sponsored:	23 hospitals	2873 beds
Contract–managed:	0 hospitals	0 beds
Totals:	23 hospitals	2873 beds

9495: DEPARTMENT OF THE AIR FORCE (FG)
Washington, DC Zip 20333; tel. 202/767–5066

ALABAMA: MAXWELL HOSPITAL (O, 40 beds) 330 Kirkpatrick Avenue East, Montgomery, AL Zip 36112–6219; tel. 205/953–7801; James J. Gallman, Administrator

ALASKA: U.S. AIR FORCE REGIONAL HOSPITAL (O, 75 beds) 24800 Hospital Drive, Elmendorf Air Force Base, AK Zip 99506–3700; tel. 907/552–4033; Colonel Larry J. Sutterer MSC, Administrator

ARIZONA: U.S. AIR FORCE HOSPITAL (O, 30 beds) 4175 South Alamo Avenue, Davis–Monthan Air Force Base, AZ Zip 85707–4405; tel. 520/750–2930; Colonel Richard C. Storey, Jr. USAF, MSC, Commander

U.S. AIR FORCE HOSPITAL LUKE (O, 40 beds) Luke AFB, Glendale, AZ Zip 85309–1525; tel. 602/856–7501; Colonel Robert P. Edwards, Administrator

ARKANSAS: U.S. AIR FORCE HOSPITAL LITTLE ROCK (O, 20 beds) Little Rock AFB, Jacksonville, AR Zip 72099–5057; tel. 501/988–7411; Colonel Norman L. Sims MSC, USAF, Commander

CALIFORNIA: DAVID GRANT MEDICAL CENTER (O, 195 beds) 101 Bodin Circle, Travis Air Force Base, CA Zip 94535–1800; tel. 707/423–7300; Colonel P. E. Jacobson, Jr. USAF, MSC, Administrator

U.S. AIR FORCE HOSPITAL (O, 32 beds) 338 South Dakota, Vandenberg Air Force Base, CA Zip 93437–6307; tel. 805/734–8232; Colonel Claude H. Chan MSC, Commander

U.S. AIR FORCE HOSPITAL (O, 9 beds) 15301 Warren Shingle Road, Beale Air Force Base, CA Zip 95903–1907; tel. 916/634–4838; Major Ty J. Obenoskey MSC, USAF, Administrator

U.S. AIR FORCE HOSPITAL (O, 28 beds) Edwards Air Force Base, CA, Mailing Address: Building 5500, Zip 93524–1730; tel. 805/277–2010; Colonel Paul H. Lilly, Jr. USAF, MC, Commander

U.S. AIR FORCE REGIONAL HOSPITAL (O, 70 beds) 1500 Hospital Way, Ste 1019, March Air Force Base, CA Zip 92518–2032; tel. 909/655–4461; Lieutenant Colonel George W. Sherman MSC, USAF, Administrator

COLORADO: U.S. AIR FORCE ACADEMY HOSPITAL (O, 82 beds) 4102 Pinion Drive, USAF Academy, CO Zip 80840–4000; tel. 719/472–5101; Colonel Charles K. Maffet MC, Commander

DELAWARE: U.S. AIR FORCE HOSPITAL DOVER (O, 31 beds) 307 Dover Street, Dover Air Force Base, DE Zip 19902–7307; tel. 302/677–2525; Lieutenant Colonel Larry W. Thornhill MSC, Administrator

FLORIDA: U.S. AIR FORCE HOSPITAL (O, 15 beds) 1381 South Patrick Drive, Patrick Air Force Base, FL Zip 32925–3606; tel. 407/494–8102; Colonel William Trent MSC, Commanding Officer

U.S. AIR FORCE HOSPITAL (O, 25 beds) Tyndall AFB, Panama City, FL Zip 32403–5300; tel. 904/283–7515; Colonel Forrest Giles MSC, USAF, Commander

U.S. AIR FORCE HOSPITAL (O, 50 beds) 8415 Bayshore Boulevard, MacDill Air Force Base, FL Zip 33621–1607; tel. 813/828–3258; Colonel Roger H. Bower USAF, MC, Commander

U.S. AIR FORCE REGIONAL HOSPITAL (O, 105 beds) 307 Boatner Road, Suite 114, Eglin Air Force Base, FL Zip 32542–1282; tel. 904/882–7221; Colonel Joseph E. Melchiorre, Jr. MSC, Administrator

GEORGIA: U.S. AIR FORCE HOSPITAL MOODY (O, 30 beds) 3278 Mitchell Boulevard, Moody Air Force Base, GA Zip 31699–1500; tel. 912/333–3772; Colonel P. R. Martin MC, USAF, Commander

---

For explanation of codes following names, see page B2.
★Indicates Type III membership in the American Hospital Association.

U.S. AIR FORCE HOSPITAL ROBINS (O, 32 beds) Robins Air Force Base, GA Zip 31098–2227; tel. 912/926–9381; Lieutenant Colonel Don C. Brown MSC, USAF, Administrator

IDAHO: U.S. AIR FORCE HOSPITAL MOUNTAIN HOME (O, 20 beds) Mountain Home Air Force Base, ID Zip 83648–5300; tel. 208/828–7600; Lieutenant Colonel Roy U. Tweedle, Administrator

ILLINOIS: SCOTT MEDICAL CENTER (O, 85 beds) Scott Air Force Base, IL Zip 62225–5252; tel. 618/256–7012; Colonel Talbot N. Vivian MSC, USAF, Administrator

LOUISIANA: U.S. AIR FORCE HOSPITAL (O, 25 beds) Barksdale AFB, Shreveport, LA Zip 71110–5300; tel. 318/456–6004; Lieutenant Colonel Allen Middleton MSC, USAF, Administrator

MARYLAND: MALCOLM GROW MEDICAL CENTER (O, 185 beds) 1050 West Perimeter, Ste A1–9, Andrews Air Force Base, MD Zip 20748, Mailing Address: Andrews AFB, Washington, DC Zip 20331–6600; tel. 301/981–3002; Colonel Ray J. Chappelle MSC, USAF, Administrator

MISSISSIPPI: U.S. AIR FORCE HOSPITAL (O, 7 beds) 201 Independence, Ste 101, Columbus, MS Zip 39701–5300; tel. 601/434–2297; Lieutenant Colonel Karen A. Bradway USAF, MSC, Administrator

U.S. AIR FORCE MEDICAL CENTER KEESLER (O, 270 beds) 301 Fisher Street, Suite 101, Keesler Air Force Base, MS Zip 39534–2519; tel. 601/377–6510; Brigadier General Pedro N. Rivera MC, USAF, Commander

MISSOURI: U.S. AIR FORCE HOSPITAL WHITEMAN (O, 22 beds) Whiteman Air Force Base, MO Zip 65305–5001; tel. 816/687–2109; Major Thomas E. Fewell, Administrator

NEBRASKA: EHRLING BERGQUIST HOSPITAL (O, 50 beds) 2501 Capehart Road, Offutt Air Force Base, NE Zip 68113–2160; tel. 402/294–7312; Colonel Gary J. Seitz MSC, USAF, Administrator

NEVADA: NELLIS FEDERAL HOSPITAL (O, 35 beds) Nellis AFB, Las Vegas, NV Zip 89191–7007; tel. 702/653–2000; Lieutenant Colonel D. Creager Brown MSC, USAF, Administrator

NEW MEXICO: U.S. AIR FORCE HOSPITAL (O, 8 beds) 280 First Street, Holloman Air Force Base, NM Zip 88330–8273; tel. 505/475–5587; Colonel Willy I. Huyghe MSC, Commander

U.S. AIR FORCE HOSPITAL–KIRTLAND (O, 35 beds) Kirtland Air Force Base, NM Zip 87117–5559; tel. 505/846–3547; Colonel George Seignious MSC, USAF, Commander

U.S. AIR FORCE HOSPITAL (O, 29 beds) Cannon Air Force Base, NM Zip 88103–5300; tel. 505/784–4582; Lieutenant Colonel James E. Tart USAF, MSC, Administrator

NEW YORK: U.S. AIR FORCE HOSPITAL (O, 5 beds) Plattsburgh AFB, Plattsburgh, NY Zip 12903; tel. 518/565–7414; Steven C. Mirick, Administrator

U.S. AIR FORCE HOSPITAL (O, 30 beds) Griffiss AFB, Rome, NY Zip 13441; tel. 315/330–7711; Thomas A. Rupp, Administrator

NORTH CAROLINA: U.S. AIR FORCE HOSPITAL SEYMOUR JOHNSON (O, 15 beds) 1050 Curtiss Avenue, Seymour Johnson Air Force Base, NC Zip 27531–5300; tel. 919/736–5201; Colonel David G. Young USAF, MC, Commander

NORTH DAKOTA: U.S. AIR FORCE HOSPITAL (O, 15 beds) Grand Forks SAC, Grand Forks Air Force Base, ND Zip 58205–6332; tel. 701/747–5391; Major Norman J. Latini MSC, USAF, Administrator

U.S. AIR FORCE REGIONAL HOSPITAL (O, 47 beds) 10 Missle Avenue, Minot, ND Zip 58705–5024; tel. 701/723–5103; Lieutenant Colonel David Houglum MC, Chief of Medical Staff

OHIO: U.S. AIR FORCE MEDICAL CENTER WRIGHT–PATTERSON (O, 165 beds) 4881 Sugar Maple Drive, Wright-Patterson Air Force Base, OH Zip 45433–5529; tel. 513/257–9133; Colonel Timothy J. Elders, Administrator

OKLAHOMA: U.S. AIR FORCE HOSPITAL TINKER (O, 25 beds) 5700 Arnold Street, Tinker Air Force Base, OK Zip 73145; tel. 405/734–8211; Colonel David D. Bissell USAF, MC, Commander

U.S. AIR FORCE HOSPITAL ALTUS (O, 28 beds) Altus AFB, Altus, OK Zip 73523–5005; tel. 405/481–5205; Colonel Jack A. Gupton MSC, USAF, Commander

SOUTH CAROLINA: U.S. AIR FORCE HOSPITAL SHAW (O, 25 beds) 431 Meadowlark Street, Shaw Air Force Base, SC Zip 29152–5300; tel. 803/668–2639; Lieutenant Colonel William R. Renwick MSC, USAF, Administrator

SOUTH DAKOTA: U.S. AIR FORCE HOSPITAL (O, 38 beds) Ellsworth Air Force Base, SD Zip 57706; tel. 605/385–3201; Colonel Ted J. W. Rodgers, Administrator

TEXAS: U.S. AIR FORCE HOSPITAL (O, 15 beds) Dyess AFB, Abilene, TX Zip 79607–1367; tel. 915/696–5427; Colonel Robert Blum MSC, Administrator

U.S. AIR FORCE HOSPITAL (O, 7 beds) 590 Mitchell Boulevard, Laughlin Air Force Base, TX Zip 78843–5200; tel. 210/298–6311; Major Roy J. Ruff MSC, Administrator

U.S. AIR FORCE HOSPITAL (O, 10 beds) 250 13th Street, Reese Air Force Base, TX Zip 79489–5008; tel. 806/885–3542; Major Randy Borg MSC, USAF, Administrator

U.S. AIR FORCE REGIONAL HOSPITAL–SHEPPARD (O, 115 beds) 149 Hart Street, Suite 1, Sheppard Air Force Base, TX Zip 76311–3478; tel. 817/676–2010; Lieutenant Colonel James J. Hooper III MC, USAF, Director Base Medical Services

WILFORD HALL U.S. AIR FORCE MEDICAL CENTER (O, 747 beds) Lackland Air Force Base, TX Zip 78236–5300; tel. 210/670–7100; James T. Vande Hey, Administrator

UTAH: U.S. AIR FORCE HOSPITAL (O, 25 beds) 7321 11th Street, Hill Air Force Base, UT Zip 84056–5012; tel. 801/777–5457; Colonel George P. Taylor, Jr., Commander

VIRGINIA: U.S. AIR FORCE HOSPITAL (O, 52 beds) Langley AFB, Hampton, VA Zip 23665–5300; tel. 804/764–6825; Colonel Neil G. Patterson MSC, Administrator

WASHINGTON: U.S. AIR FORCE HOSPITAL (O, 35 beds) 701 Hospital Loop, Fairchild Air Force Base, WA Zip 99011–8701; tel. 509/247–5216; Colonel Gary L. Mueller M.D., MSC, Commander

WYOMING: U.S. AIR FORCE HOSPITAL (O, 15 beds) Francis E Warren AFB, Cheyenne, WY Zip 82005–3913; tel. 307/775–2045; Major Gary S. Forthman MSC, Administrator

Owned, leased, sponsored:	49 hospitals	3094 beds
Contract–managed:	0 hospitals	0 beds
Totals:	49 hospitals	3094 beds

9395: DEPARTMENT OF THE ARMY (FG)
Washington, DC Zip 20314; tel. 703/756–8210

ALABAMA: FOX ARMY COMMUNITY HOSPITAL (O, 41 beds) Redstone Arsenal, AL Zip 35809–7000; tel. 205/876–4147; Lieutenant Colonel Cary J. Payne, Deputy Commander Administration

LYSTER U.S. ARMY COMMUNITY HOSPITAL (O, 58 beds) U.S. Army Aeromedical Center, Fort Rucker, AL Zip 36362–5333; tel. 334/255–7360; Colonel Glenn W. Mitchell M.D., Commander

NOBLE ARMY COMMUNITY HOSPITAL (O, 48 beds) Fort McClellan, AL Zip 36205–5083; tel. 205/848–2232; Lieutenant Colonel Ed Wacy, Deputy Commander Administration

ALASKA: BASSETT ARMY COMMUNITY HOSPITAL (O, 43 beds) Fort Wainwright, Fairbanks, AK Zip 99703–7300; tel. 907/353–5108; Colonel Charles C. Franz, Deputy Commander Administration

ARIZONA: RAYMOND W. BLISS ARMY COMMUNITY HOSPITAL (O, 30 beds) Fort Huachuca, AZ Zip 85613–7040; tel. 602/533–2026; Lieutenant Colonel Al Santos, Deputy Commander, Administration

CALIFORNIA: WEED ARMY COMMUNITY HOSPITAL (O, 27 beds) Fort Irwin, CA Zip 92310–5065; tel. 619/380–3108; Colonel Alan Mease, Commander

COLORADO: EVANS U.S. ARMY COMMUNITY HOSPITAL (O, 139 beds) Fort Carson, CO Zip 80913–5101; tel. 719/526–7200; Colonel Homer J. Wright MC, Commander

FITZSIMONS ARMY MEDICAL CENTER (O, 237 beds) Aurora, CO Zip 80045–5000; tel. 303/361–8313; Colonel Van R. Booth, Chief of Staff

DISTRICT OF COLUMBIA: WALTER REED ARMY MEDICAL CENTER (O, 738 beds) Washington, DC Zip 20307–5001; tel. 202/782–1104; Major General Ronald R. Blanck MS, Commander

GEORGIA: DWIGHT DAVID EISENHOWER ARMY MEDICAL CENTER (O, 396 beds) Fort Gordon, GA Zip 30905–5650; tel. 706/787–8192; Colonel John E. Vigna, Chief of Staff

MARTIN ARMY COMMUNITY HOSPITAL (O, 152 beds) Fort Benning, GA Zip 31905–6100; tel. 706/544–2041; Colonel Ira F. Walton III MSC, USA, Deputy Commander for Administration

WINN ARMY COMMUNITY HOSPITAL (O, 100 beds) Fort Stewart, GA Zip 31314–5300; tel. 912/767–6001

HAWAII: TRIPLER ARMY MEDICAL CENTER (O, 358 beds) Honolulu, HI Zip 96859–5000; tel. 808/433–5716; Brigadier General James E. Hastings, Commanding General

INDIANA: HAWLEY U.S. ARMY COMMUNITY HOSPITAL (O, 20 beds) Fort Benjamin Harrison, Indianapolis, IN Zip 46216–7000; tel. 317/549–5153; Charles H. Lewis, Deputy Commander Administration

For explanation of codes following names, see page B2.
★Indicates Type III membership in the American Hospital Association.

Systems / Department of the Army

KANSAS: IRWIN ARMY COMMUNITY HOSPITAL (O, 97 beds) Building 600, Fort Riley, KS Zip 66442; tel. 913/239-7101; Colonel James W. Kirkpatrick, Commanding Officer

MUNSON ARMY COMMUNITY HOSPITAL (O, 20 beds) Pope and Biddle Avenue, Fort Leavenworth, KS Zip 66027-5400; tel. 913/684-6420; Colonel Arthur Hadley MSC, USA, Executive Officer

KENTUCKY: COLONEL FLORENCE A. BLANCHFIELD ARMY COMMUNITY HOSPITAL (O, 155 beds) Fort Campbell, KY Zip 42223-5349; tel. 502/798-8040

IRELAND ARMY COMMUNITY HOSPITAL (O, 97 beds) 851 Ireland Loop, Fort Knox, KY Zip 40121-5520; tel. 502/624-9020; Colonel Edward Burkhalter, Commander

LOUISIANA: BAYNE-JONES ARMY COMMUNITY HOSPITAL (O, 52 beds) Fort Polk, LA Zip 71459-6000; tel. 318/531-3928; Colonel Joseph Gonzales, Deputy Commander and Administrator

MARYLAND: KIMBROUGH ARMY COMMUNITY HOSPITAL (O, 47 beds) Fort George G Meade, MD Zip 20755; tel. 301/677-4171; Colonel Robert R. McMeekin, Commanding Officer

MISSOURI: GENERAL LEONARD WOOD ARMY COMMUNITY HOSPITAL (O, 88 beds) Fort Leonard Wood, MO Zip 65473; tel. 314/596-0414; Colonel Dennis Dohanos, Administrator

NEW JERSEY: PATTERSON ARMY COMMUNITY HOSPITAL (O, 35 beds) Fort Monmouth, NJ Zip 07703-5607; tel. 908/532-1266; Colonel Royal C. Hudson, Jr., Commander

NEW YORK: KELLER ARMY COMMUNITY HOSPITAL (O, 65 beds) U.S. Military Academy, West Point, NY Zip 10996-1197; tel. 914/938-3305; Livio F. Pardi MC, Commander

NORTH CAROLINA: WOMACK ARMY MEDICAL CENTER (O, 264 beds) Fort Bragg, NC Zip 28307-5000; tel. 919/432-4802; Colonel Harold L. Timboe, Commander

OKLAHOMA: REYNOLDS ARMY COMMUNITY HOSPITAL (O, 116 beds) 4700 Hartell Boulevard, Fort Sill, OK Zip 73503-6300; tel. 405/458-2000; Colonel Joseph Andronaco, Administrator

SOUTH CAROLINA: MONCRIEF ARMY COMMUNITY HOSPITAL (O, 90 beds) Fort Jackson, SC, Mailing Address: P.O. Box 500, Zip 29207-5720; tel. 803/751-2648; Colonel Robert T. Hawkins MSC, Deputy Commander Administration

TEXAS: BROOKE ARMY MEDICAL CENTER (O, 464 beds) Fort Sam Houston, San Antonio, TX Zip 78234-6213; tel. 210/916-8225; Colonel Herbert K. Reamey III, Chief of Staff

DARNALL ARMY COMMUNITY HOSPITAL (O, 220 beds) Fort Hood, TX Zip 76544-5063; tel. 817/288-8000; Colonel William F. Hughes MC, USA, Commander

WILLIAM BEAUMONT ARMY MEDICAL CENTER (O, 320 beds) El Paso, TX Zip 79920-5001; tel. 915/569-2121; Colonel Thomas J. Scully, MC Commander

VIRGINIA: DEWITT ARMY COMMUNITY HOSPITAL (O, 68 beds) Fort Belvoir, VA Zip 22060-5901; tel. 703/805-0510; Colonel Warren A. Todd, Jr. MSC, Commander

KENNER ARMY COMMUNITY HOSPITAL (O, 48 beds) Fort Lee, VA Zip 23801-5260; tel. 804/734-9256; Colonel Charles M. Ellis, Jr. MSC, Commanding Officer

MCDONALD ARMY COMMUNITY HOSPITAL (O, 37 beds) Fort Eustis, Newport News, VA Zip 23604-5548; tel. 804/878-7501; Colonel John W. Kolmer MSC, Commander

WASHINGTON: MADIGAN ARMY MEDICAL CENTER (O, 334 beds) Tacoma, WA Zip 98431-5000; tel. 206/968-1110; Major General James B. Peake M.D., MSC, USA, Commanding General

MARSHALL ISLANDS: USAKA HOSPITAL (O, 14 beds) Kwajalein Island, MH, Mailing Address: Box 1702, APO, AP Zip 96555-5000; tel. 805/238-7994; Mike Mathews, Administrator

Owned, leased, sponsored:	34 hospitals	5018 beds
Contract-managed:	0 hospitals	0 beds
Totals:	34 hospitals	5018 beds

9295: DEPARTMENT OF VETERANS AFFAIRS (FG) 810 Vermont Avenue N.W., Washington, DC Zip 20420; tel. 202/273-5786; Kenneth W. Kizer M.D., M.P.H., Under Secretary for Health

ALABAMA: VETERANS AFFAIRS MEDICAL CENTER (O, 257 beds) 700 South 19th Street, Birmingham, AL Zip 35233-1996; tel. 205/933-8101; William A. Mountcastle, Director

VETERANS AFFAIRS MEDICAL CENTER (O, 162 beds) 215 Perry Hill Road, Montgomery, AL Zip 36109-3798; tel. 334/272-4670; John R. Rowan, Director

VETERANS AFFAIRS MEDICAL CENTER (O, 649 beds) 3701 Loop Road, Tuscaloosa, AL Zip 35404-9983; tel. 205/554-2000; Robert P. Blair, Director

VETERANS AFFAIRS MEDICAL CENTER (O, 769 beds) 2400 Hospital Road, Tuskegee, AL Zip 36083-5001; tel. 334/727-0550; Jim Clay, Director

ARIZONA: CARL T. HAYDEN VETERANS AFFAIRS MEDICAL CENTER (O, 530 beds) 650 East Indian School Road, Phoenix, AZ Zip 85012-1894; tel. 602/277-5551; John R. Fears, Director

VETERANS AFFAIRS MEDICAL CENTER (O, 286 beds) 3601 South 6th Avenue, Tucson, AZ Zip 85723; tel. 520/792-1450; Jonathan H. Gardner, Director

VETERANS AFFAIRS MEDICAL CENTER (O, 369 beds) 500 Highway 89 North, Prescott, AZ Zip 86313; tel. 520/445-4860; Patricia A. McKlem, Director

ARKANSAS: VETERANS AFFAIRS MEDICAL CENTER (O, 152 beds) 1100 North College Avenue, Fayetteville, AR Zip 72703-6995; tel. 501/443-4301; Richard F. Robinson, Director

VETERANS AFFAIRS MEDICAL CENTER (O, 958 beds) 4300 West Seventh Street, Little Rock, AR Zip 72205-5484; tel. 501/661-1202; Robert D. Shimp, Associate Director

CALIFORNIA: JERRY L. PETTIS MEMORIAL VETERANS HOSPITAL (O, 393 beds) 11201 Benton Street, Loma Linda, CA Zip 92357; tel. 909/825-7084; Dean R. Stordahl, Director

VETERANS AFFAIRS MEDICAL CENTER (O, 219 beds) 2615 East Clinton Avenue, Fresno, CA Zip 93703; tel. 209/225-6100; James C. DeNiro, Director

VETERANS AFFAIRS MEDICAL CENTER (O, 165 beds) 4951 Arroyo Road, Livermore, CA Zip 94550; tel. 510/447-2560; Clarence H. Nixon, Director

VETERANS AFFAIRS MEDICAL CENTER (O, 1131 beds) 5901 East Seventh Street, Long Beach, CA Zip 90822-5201; tel. 310/494-5400; Jerry B. Boyd, Director

VETERANS AFFAIRS MEDICAL CENTER (O, 1062 beds) 3801 Miranda Avenue, Palo Alto, CA Zip 94304-1207; tel. 415/493-5000; James A. Goff FACHE, Director

VETERANS AFFAIRS MEDICAL CENTER (O, 336 beds) 3350 LaJolla Village Drive, San Diego, CA Zip 92161; tel. 619/552-8585; Leonard C. Rogers, Director

VETERANS AFFAIRS MEDICAL CENTER (O, 372 beds) 4150 Clement Street, San Francisco, CA Zip 94121-1598; tel. 415/750-2041; Lawrence C. Stewart, Director

VETERANS AFFAIRS MEDICAL CENTER-WEST LOS ANGELES (O, 1588 beds) 11301 Wilshire Boulevard, Los Angeles, CA Zip 90073-0275; tel. 310/824-3132; Kenneth Clark, Director

COLORADO: VETERANS AFFAIRS MEDICAL CENTER (O, 336 beds) 1055 Clermont Street, Denver, CO Zip 80220-3877; tel. 303/393-2800; Thomas A. Trujillo, Director

VETERANS AFFAIRS MEDICAL CENTER (O, 289 beds) Fort Lyon, CO Zip 81038; tel. 719/456-1260; W. David Smith, Director

VETERANS AFFAIRS MEDICAL CENTER (O, 126 beds) 2121 North Avenue, Grand Junction, CO Zip 81501-6499; tel. 970/242-0731; Robert R. Rhyne D.D.S., Director

CONNECTICUT: VETERANS AFFAIRS MEDICAL CENTER (O, 101 beds) 555 Willard Avenue, Newington, CT Zip 06111-2600; tel. 203/666-6951; Vincent Ng, Director

VETERANS AFFAIRS MEDICAL CENTER (O, 550 beds) 950 Campbell Avenue, West Haven, CT Zip 06516-2700; tel. 203/932-5711; Vincent Ng, Director

DELAWARE: VETERANS AFFAIRS MEDICAL CENTER (O, 210 beds) 1601 Kirkwood Highway, Wilmington, DE Zip 19805-4989; tel. 302/633-5201; Dexter D. Dix, Director

DISTRICT OF COLUMBIA: VETERANS AFFAIRS MEDICAL CENTER (O, 699 beds) 50 Irving Street N.W., Washington, DC Zip 20422; tel. 202/745-8000; Sanford M. Garfunkel, Director

FLORIDA: JAMES A. HALEY VETERANS HOSPITAL (O, 778 beds) 13000 Bruce B Downs Boulevard, Tampa, FL Zip 33612-4798; tel. 813/972-2000; Richard A. Silver, Director

VETERANS AFFAIRS MEDICAL CENTER (O, 1021 beds) 10000 Bay Pines Boulevard, Bay Pines, FL Zip 33504; tel. 813/398-6661; Thomas H. Weaver, Director

VETERANS AFFAIRS MEDICAL CENTER (O, 870 beds) 1201 Northwest 16th Street, Miami, FL Zip 33125-1624; tel. 305/324-4455; Thomas C. Doherty, Medical Director

---

For explanation of codes following names, see page B2.
★Indicates Type III membership in the American Hospital Association.

Systems / Department of Veterans Affairs

VETERANS AFFAIRS MEDICAL CENTER (O, 469 beds) 1601 Southwest Archer Road, Gainesville, FL Zip 32608–1197; tel. 904/376–1611; Malcom Randall, Director

VETERANS AFFAIRS MEDICAL CENTER (O, 387 beds) 801 South Marion Street, Lake City, FL Zip 32025–5898; tel. 904/755–3016; Alline L. Norman, Director

GEORGIA: VETERANS AFFAIRS MEDICAL CENTER (O, 486 beds) 1670 Clairmont Road, Decatur, GA Zip 30033–4098; tel. 404/728–7600; Larry R. Deal, Medical Director

VETERANS AFFAIRS MEDICAL CENTER (O, 732 beds) 1 Freedom Way, Augusta, GA Zip 30904–6285; tel. 706/733–0188; Thomas L. Ayres, Director

VETERANS AFFAIRS MEDICAL CENTER (O, 722 beds) 1826 Veterans Boulevard, Dublin, GA Zip 31021; tel. 912/272–1210; William O. Edgar, Director

IDAHO: VETERANS AFFAIRS MEDICAL CENTER (O, 181 beds) 500 West Fort Street, Boise, ID Zip 83702–4598; tel. 208/336–5100; Wayne C. Tippets, Director

ILLINOIS: VETERANS AFFAIRS EDWARD HINES, JR. HOSPITAL (O, 1022 beds) Fifth Avenue & Roosevelt Road, Hines, IL Zip 60141–5000, Mailing Address: P.O. Box 5000, Zip 60141–5000; tel. 708/343–7200; Joan E. Cummings M.D., Director

VETERANS AFFAIRS LAKESIDE MEDICAL CENTER (O, 252 beds) 333 East Huron Street, Chicago, IL Zip 60611–3004; tel. 312/640–2100; Joseph L. Moore, Director

VETERANS AFFAIRS MEDICAL CENTER (O, 776 beds) 1900 East Main Street, Danville, IL Zip 61832; tel. 217/442–8000; James S. Jones, Director

VETERANS AFFAIRS MEDICAL CENTER (O, 947 beds) 3001 Green Bay Road, North Chicago, IL Zip 60064; tel. 708/578–3700; Alfred S. Pate, Director

VETERANS AFFAIRS MEDICAL CENTER (O, 163 beds) 2401 West Main Street, Marion, IL Zip 62959–1194; tel. 618/997–5311; Linda K. Kurz, Director

VETERANS AFFAIRS WEST SIDE MEDICAL CENTER (O, 337 beds) 820 South Damen Avenue, Chicago, IL Zip 60612, Mailing Address: Box 8195, Zip 60680; tel. 312/666–6500; John J. DeNardo, Director

INDIANA: RICHARD L. ROUDEBUSH VETERANS AFFAIRS MEDICAL CENTER (O, 354 beds) 1481 West Tenth Street, Indianapolis, IN Zip 46202; tel. 317/635–7401

VETERANS AFFAIRS MEDICAL CENTER (O, 151 beds) 2121 Lake Avenue, Fort Wayne, IN Zip 46805–5347; tel. 219/426–5431; Jonathan D. Hawk, Director

VETERANS AFFAIRS MEDICAL CENTER (O, 580 beds) East 38th Street, Marion, IN Zip 46953–4589; tel. 317/674–3321; Jon E. Crisman, Director

IOWA: VETERANS AFFAIRS MEDICAL CENTER (O, 129 beds) 3600 30th Street, Des Moines, IA Zip 50310–5774; tel. 515/255–2173; Ellen DeGeorge-Smith, Director

VETERANS AFFAIRS MEDICAL CENTER (O, 198 beds) Highway 6 West, Iowa City, IA Zip 52246–2208; tel. 319/338–0581; Gary L. Wilkinson, Director

VETERANS AFFAIRS MEDICAL CENTER (O, 637 beds) 1515 West Pleasant, Knoxville, IA Zip 50138–3399; tel. 515/842–3101; Donald D. Ziska, Director

KANSAS: COLMERY-O'NEIL VETERANS AFFAIRS MEDICAL CENTER (O, 622 beds) 2200 Gage Boulevard, Topeka, KS Zip 66622; tel. 913/272–3111

DWIGHT D. EISENHOWER VETERANS AFFAIRS MEDICAL CENTER (O, 318 beds) 4101 South Fourth St Trafficway, Leavenworth, KS Zip 66048–5055; tel. 913/682–2000; Carole Bishop Smith, Director

VETERANS AFFAIRS MEDICAL AND REGIONAL OFFICE CENTER (O, 156 beds) 5500 East Kellogg, Wichita, KS Zip 67218; tel. 316/685–2221; Jerry Mayhall Ph.D., Director

KENTUCKY: VETERANS AFFAIRS MEDICAL CENTER–LEXINGTON (O, 620 beds) 2250 Leestown Pike, Lexington, KY Zip 40511–1093; tel. 606/233–4511; Helen K. Cornish, Director

VETERANS AFFAIRS MEDICAL CENTER–LOUISVILLE (O, 246 beds) 800 Zorn Avenue, Louisville, KY Zip 40206–1499; tel. 502/895–3401; Larry J. Sander, Director

LOUISIANA: OVERTON BROOKS VETERANS AFFAIRS MEDICAL CENTER (O, 259 beds) 510 East Stoner Avenue, Shreveport, LA Zip 71101–4295; tel. 318/221–8411; Michael E. Hamilton, Director

VETERANS AFFAIRS MEDICAL CENTER (O, 468 beds) Shreveport Highway, Alexandria, LA Zip 71301; tel. 318/473–0010; Billy M. Valentine, Director

VETERANS AFFAIRS MEDICAL CENTER (O, 255 beds) 1601 Perdido Street, New Orleans, LA Zip 70146; tel. 504/568–0811; John D. Church, Jr., Director

MAINE: VETERANS AFFAIRS MEDICAL CENTER (O, 315 beds) Togus, ME Zip 04330; tel. 207/623–8411; John H. Sims, Jr., Director

MARYLAND: VETERANS AFFAIRS MEDICAL CENTER (O, 236 beds) 10 North Greene Street, Baltimore, MD Zip 21201–1524; tel. 410/605–7001; Michael B. Phaup, Director

VETERANS AFFAIRS MEDICAL CENTER (O, 221 beds) 9600 North Point Road, Fort Howard, MD Zip 21052–9989; tel. 410/477–1800; Charles Clark, Director

VETERANS AFFAIRS MEDICAL CENTER (O, 634 beds) Circle Drive, Perry Point, MD Zip 21902; tel. 410/642–2411; Allan S. Goss, Director

MASSACHUSETTS: BROCKTON–WEST ROXBURY VETERANS AFFAIRS MEDICAL CENTER (O, 765 beds) 940 Belmont Street, Brockton, MA Zip 02401; tel. 508/583–4500; Michael E. Lawson, Director

EDITH NOURSE ROGERS MEMORIAL VETERANS HOSPITAL (O, 725 beds) 200 Springs Road, Bedford, MA Zip 01730; tel. 617/275–7500; William A. Conte, Director

VETERANS AFFAIRS MEDICAL CENTER (O, 448 beds) Boston, MA, Mailing Address: 150 South Huntington Avenue, Jamaica Plain Station, Zip 02130–4820; tel. 617/232–9500; Smith Jenkins, Jr., Director

VETERANS AFFAIRS MEDICAL CENTER (O, 379 beds) Route 9, Northampton, MA Zip 01060–1288; tel. 413/584–4040; Gary J. Rossio, Chief Executive Officer

MICHIGAN: VETERANS AFFAIRS MEDICAL CENTER (O, 311 beds) 2215 Fuller Road, Ann Arbor, MI Zip 48105; tel. 313/769–7100; Edward L. Gamache, Director

VETERANS AFFAIRS MEDICAL CENTER (O, 806 beds) 5500 Armstrong Road, Battle Creek, MI Zip 49016; tel. 616/966–5600

VETERANS AFFAIRS MEDICAL CENTER (O, 464 beds) Southfield and Outer Drive, Allen Park, MI Zip 48101; tel. 313/562–6000; Carlos B. Lott, Jr., Acting Director

VETERANS AFFAIRS MEDICAL CENTER (O, 160 beds) H Street, Iron Mountain, MI Zip 49801; tel. 906/774–3300; Glen W. Grippen, Director

VETERANS AFFAIRS MEDICAL CENTER (O, 215 beds) 1500 Weiss Street, Saginaw, MI Zip 48602; tel. 517/793–2340; Robert H. Sabin, Medical Center Director

MINNESOTA: VETERANS AFFAIRS MEDICAL CENTER (O, 604 beds) One Veterans Drive, Minneapolis, MN Zip 55417–2399; tel. 612/725–2000; Charles A. Milbrandt, Director

VETERANS AFFAIRS MEDICAL CENTER (O, 566 beds) 4801 Eighth Street North, Saint Cloud, MN Zip 56303–2099; tel. 612/252–1670; Thomas A. Holthaus, Director

MISSISSIPPI: VETERANS AFFAIRS MEDICAL CENTER (O, 510 beds) 400 Veterans Avenue, Biloxi, MS Zip 39531–2410; tel. 601/388–5541

VETERANS AFFAIRS MEDICAL CENTER (O, 492 beds) 1500 East Woodrow Wilson Drive, Jackson, MS Zip 39216–5199; tel. 601/364–1201; Richard P. Miller, Director

MISSOURI: HARRY S. TRUMAN MEMORIAL VETERANS HOSPITAL (O, 291 beds) 800 Hospital Drive, Columbia, MO Zip 65201–5297; tel. 314/443–2511; John T. Carson, Director

JOHN J. PERSHING VETERANS AFFAIRS MEDICAL CENTER (O, 174 beds) 1500 North Westwood Boulevard, Poplar Bluff, MO Zip 63901; tel. 314/686–4151

VETERANS AFFAIRS MEDICAL CENTER (O, 629 beds) Saint Louis, MO Zip 63125; tel. 314/894–6661; Donald L. Ziegenhorn, Director

VETERANS AFFAIRS MEDICAL CENTER (O, 273 beds) 4801 Linwood Boulevard, Kansas City, MO Zip 64128–2295; tel. 816/922–2048; Hugh F. Doran, Director

MONTANA: VETERANS AFFAIRS HOSPITAL (O, 113 beds) Fort Harrison, MT Zip 59636; tel. 406/442–6410; Joe Underkofler, Director

VETERANS AFFAIRS MEDICAL CENTER (O, 41 beds) 210 South Winchester Avenue, Miles City, MT Zip 59301–4798; tel. 406/232–3060; Richard J. Stanley, Director

NEBRASKA: VETERANS AFFAIRS MEDICAL CENTER (O, 154 beds) 2201 North Broadwell Avenue, Grand Island, NE Zip 68803–2196; tel. 308/382–3660

VETERANS AFFAIRS MEDICAL CENTER (O, 113 beds) 600 South 70th Street, Lincoln, NE Zip 68510–2493; tel. 402/489–3802

VETERANS AFFAIRS MEDICAL CENTER (O, 226 beds) 4101 Woolworth Avenue, Omaha, NE Zip 68105–1873; tel. 402/449–0600; John J. Phillips, Director

For explanation of codes following names, see page B2.
★Indicates Type III membership in the American Hospital Association.

Systems / Department of Veterans Affairs

NEVADA: IOANNIS A. LOUGARIS VETERANS AFFAIRS MEDICAL CENTER (O, 167 beds) 1000 Locust Street, Reno, NV Zip 89520–0100; tel. 702/786–7200; Gary R. Whitfield, Director

NEW HAMPSHIRE: VETERANS AFFAIRS MEDICAL CENTER (O, 228 beds) 718 Smyth Road, Manchester, NH Zip 03104–4098; tel. 603/624–4366; Eugene L. Ochocki, Director

NEW JERSEY: VETERANS AFFAIRS MEDICAL CENTER (O, 602 beds) 385 Tremont Avenue, East Orange, NJ Zip 07018–1095; tel. 201/676–1000; Kenneth H. Mizrach, Director

VETERANS AFFAIRS MEDICAL CENTER (O, 937 beds) 151 Knollcroft Road, Lyons, NJ Zip 07939–9998; tel. 908/647–0180; A. Paul Kidd FACHE, Director

NEW MEXICO: VETERANS AFFAIRS MEDICAL CENTER (O, 468 beds) 2100 Ridgecrest Drive S.E., Albuquerque, NM Zip 87108; tel. 505/265–1711; Bruce A. Gordon, Acting Director

NEW YORK: FRANKLIN DELANO ROOSEVELT VETERANS AFFAIRS HOSPITAL (O, 698 beds) Route 9A, Montrose, NY Zip 10548, Mailing Address: P.O. Box 100, Zip 10548; tel. 914/737–4400; Lee J. Kauper, Director

VETERANS AFFAIRS MEDICAL CENTER (O, 406 beds) 113 Holland Avenue, Albany, NY Zip 12208–3473; tel. 518/462–3311; Frederick L. Malphurs, Director

VETERANS AFFAIRS MEDICAL CENTER (O, 158 beds) 222 Richmond Avenue, Batavia, NY Zip 14020; tel. 716/343–7500; Paul J. McCool, Director

VETERANS AFFAIRS MEDICAL CENTER (O, 850 beds) 76 Veterans Avenue, Bath, NY Zip 14810–0842; tel. 607/776–2111; Mel A. Gores FACHE, Director

VETERANS AFFAIRS MEDICAL CENTER (O, 886 beds) 800 Poly Place, Brooklyn, NY Zip 11209; tel. 718/630–3500; James J. Farsetta FACHE, Director

VETERANS AFFAIRS MEDICAL CENTER (O, 472 beds) 3495 Bailey Avenue, Buffalo, NY Zip 14215–1129; tel. 716/834–9200; Richard S. Droske, Director

VETERANS AFFAIRS MEDICAL CENTER (O, 661 beds) 400 Fort Hill Avenue, Canandaigua, NY Zip 14424–1197; tel. 716/396–3601; Stuart C. Collyer, Director

VETERANS AFFAIRS MEDICAL CENTER (O, 235 beds) Castle Point, NY Zip 12511–9999; tel. 914/831–2000; Ronald F. Lipp, Director

VETERANS AFFAIRS MEDICAL CENTER (O, 620 beds) 130 West Kingsbridge Road, Bronx, NY Zip 10468–7511; tel. 718/584–9000; Maryann Musumeci, Director

VETERANS AFFAIRS MEDICAL CENTER (O, 492 beds) 423 East 23rd Street, New York, NY Zip 10010–0070; tel. 212/686–7500; John J. Donnellan, Jr., Director

VETERANS AFFAIRS MEDICAL CENTER (O, 698 beds) 79 Middleville Road, Northport, NY Zip 11768–2293; tel. 516/261–4400; E. M. Travers M.D., Medical Center Director

VETERANS AFFAIRS MEDICAL CENTER (O, 255 beds) 800 Irving Avenue, Syracuse, NY Zip 13210; tel. 315/476–7461; Philip P. Thomas, Associate Director

NORTH CAROLINA: VETERANS AFFAIRS MEDICAL CENTER (O, 376 beds) 508 Fulton Street, Durham, NC Zip 27705; tel. 919/286–0411; Barbara A. Small, Director

VETERANS AFFAIRS MEDICAL CENTER (O, 220 beds) 2300 Ramsey Street, Fayetteville, NC Zip 28301–3899; tel. 919/822–7059; Jerome Calhoun, Director

VETERANS AFFAIRS MEDICAL CENTER (O, 358 beds) 1100 Tunnel Road, Asheville, NC Zip 28805–2087; tel. 704/298–7911; James A. Christian, Director

VETERANS AFFAIRS MEDICAL CENTER (O, 695 beds) 1601 Brenner Avenue, Salisbury, NC Zip 28144; tel. 704/638–9000; R. Eugene Konik, Director

NORTH DAKOTA: VETERANS AFFAIRS MEDICAL AND REGIONAL OFFICE CENTER (O, 163 beds) 2101 Elm Street, Fargo, ND Zip 58102–2498; tel. 701/232–3241; Douglas M. Kenyon, Director

OHIO: VETERANS AFFAIRS MEDICAL CENTER (O, 914 beds) 10701 East Boulevard, Cleveland, OH Zip 44106; tel. 216/791–3800; Krista Ludenia Ph.D., Director

VETERANS AFFAIRS MEDICAL CENTER (O, 587 beds) 17273 State Route 104, Chillicothe, OH Zip 45601–0999; tel. 614/773–1141; Michael W. Walton, Director

VETERANS AFFAIRS MEDICAL CENTER (O, 352 beds) 3200 Vine Street, Cincinnati, OH Zip 45220–2288; tel. 513/861–3100; Gary N. Nugent, Medical Director

VETERANS AFFAIRS MEDICAL CENTER (O, 991 beds) 4100 West Third Street, Dayton, OH Zip 45428–1002; tel. 513/268–6511; Ed Thorsland, Jr., Director

OKLAHOMA: VETERANS AFFAIRS MEDICAL CENTER (O, 140 beds) Honor Heights Drive, Muskogee, OK Zip 74401–1399; tel. 918/683–3261

VETERANS AFFAIRS MEDICAL CENTER (O, 297 beds) 921 N.E. 13th Street, Oklahoma City, OK Zip 73104–5028; tel. 405/270–0501; Steven J. Gentling, Director

OREGON: VETERANS AFFAIRS MEDICAL CENTER (O, 622 beds) 3710 S.W. U.S. Veterans Hospital Road, Portland, OR Zip 97201; tel. 503/220–8262; Barry L. Bell, Director

VETERANS AFFAIRS MEDICAL CENTER (O, 272 beds) 913 N.W. Garden Valley Boulevard, Roseburg, OR Zip 97470–6513; tel. 503/440–1000; Alan S. Perry, Medical Center Director

PENNSYLVANIA: JAMES E. VAN ZANDT VETERANS AFFAIRS MEDICAL CENTER (O, 135 beds) 2907 Pleasant Valley Boulevard, Altoona, PA Zip 16602–4377; tel. 814/943–8164; Gerald L. Williams, Director

VETERANS AFFAIRS MEDICAL CENTER (O, 333 beds) 325 New Castle Road, Butler, PA Zip 16001–2480; tel. 412/287–4781; P. Stajduhar M.D., Director

VETERANS AFFAIRS MEDICAL CENTER (O, 792 beds) Black Horse Hill Road, Coatesville, PA Zip 19320–9985; tel. 610/380–4303; Gary W. Devansky, Director

VETERANS AFFAIRS MEDICAL CENTER (O, 159 beds) 135 East 38th Street, Erie, PA Zip 16504–1596; tel. 814/868–6210; Stephen M. Lucas, Director

VETERANS AFFAIRS MEDICAL CENTER (O, 646 beds) 1700 South Lincoln Avenue, Lebanon, PA Zip 17042–7597; tel. 717/272–6621; Leonard Washington, Jr., Director

VETERANS AFFAIRS MEDICAL CENTER (O, 656 beds) University & Woodland Avenues, Philadelphia, PA Zip 19104–4594; tel. 215/823–5800; Earl F. Falast, Director

VETERANS AFFAIRS MEDICAL CENTER (O, 574 beds) 7180 Highland Drive, Pittsburgh, PA Zip 15206–1297; tel. 412/365–4900; Laura Miller, Director

VETERANS AFFAIRS MEDICAL CENTER (O, 698 beds) University Drive C, Pittsburgh, PA Zip 15240–1001; tel. 412/692–3200; Thomas A. Cappello, Director

VETERANS AFFAIRS MEDICAL CENTER (O, 517 beds) 1111 East End Boulevard, Wilkes-Barre, PA Zip 18711–0026; tel. 717/824–3521; Reedes Hurt, Director

RHODE ISLAND: VETERANS AFFAIRS MEDICAL CENTER (O, 136 beds) 830 Chalkstone Avenue, Providence, RI Zip 02908–4799; tel. 401/457–3042; Edward H. Seiler, Director

SOUTH CAROLINA: VETERANS AFFAIRS MEDICAL CENTER (O, 265 beds) 109 Bee Street, Charleston, SC Zip 29401–5799; tel. 803/577–5011; Dean S. Billik, Director

WILLIAM JENNINGS BRYAN DORN VETERANS HOSPITAL (O, 370 beds) 6439 Garners Ferry Road, Columbia, SC Zip 29201; tel. 803/776–4000; Robert M. Athey, Director

SOUTH DAKOTA: ROYAL C. JOHNSON VETERANS MEMORIAL HOSPITAL (O, 217 beds) 2501 West 22nd Street, Sioux Falls, SD Zip 57105, Mailing Address: P.O. Box 5046, Zip 57117–5046; tel. 605/336–3230; R. Vincent Crawford, Director

VETERANS AFFAIRS MEDICAL CENTER (O, 260 beds) 113 Comanche Road, Fort Meade, SD Zip 57741–1099; tel. 605/347–2511; Peter P. Henry, Director

VETERANS AFFAIRS MEDICAL CENTER (O, 148 beds) 500 North Fifth, Hot Springs, SD Zip 57747; tel. 605/745–2052; Daniel L. Marsh, Director

TENNESSEE: ALVIN C. YORK VETERANS AFFAIRS MEDICAL CENTER (O, 676 beds) 3400 Lebanon Road, Murfreesboro, TN Zip 37129; tel. 615/893–1360; Brian Heckert, Director

VETERANS AFFAIRS MEDICAL CENTER (O, 684 beds) 1030 Jefferson Avenue, Memphis, TN Zip 38104–2193; tel. 901/523–8990; K. L. Mulholland, Jr., Director

VETERANS AFFAIRS MEDICAL CENTER (O, 994 beds) Mountain Home, TN Zip 37684; tel. 615/926–1171; Carl J. Gerber M.D., Ph.D., Director

VETERANS AFFAIRS MEDICAL CENTER (O, 334 beds) 1310 24th Avenue South, Nashville, TN Zip 37212–2637; tel. 615/327–4751; Larry E. Deters, Director

TEXAS: AUDIE L. MURPHY MEMORIAL VETERANS HOSPITAL (O, 732 beds) 7400 Merton Minter Boulevard, San Antonio, TX Zip 78284–5799; tel. 210/617–5140; Jose R. Coronado FACHE, Director

OLIN E. TEAGUE VETERANS' CENTER (O, 914 beds) 1901 South First Street, Temple, TX Zip 76504; tel. 817/778–4811

For explanation of codes following names, see page B2.
★Indicates Type III membership in the American Hospital Association.

Systems / Devereux Foundation

SAM RAYBURN MEMORIAL VETERANS CENTER (O, 391 beds) 1201 East Ninth Street, Bonham, TX Zip 75418; tel. 903/583-2111; Charles C. Freeman, Director
VETERANS AFFAIRS MEDICAL CENTER (O, 246 beds) 6010 Amarillo Boulevard West, Amarillo, TX Zip 79106; tel. 806/355-9703; Y. C. Parris, Director
VETERANS AFFAIRS MEDICAL CENTER (O, 249 beds) 300 Veterans Boulevard, Big Spring, TX Zip 79720-5500; tel. 915/263-7361; Cary D. Brown, Director
VETERANS AFFAIRS MEDICAL CENTER (O, 644 beds) 4500 South Lancaster Road, Dallas, TX Zip 75216-7167; tel. 214/376-5451; Alan G. Harper, Director
VETERANS AFFAIRS MEDICAL CENTER (O, 899 beds) 2002 Holcombe Boulevard, Houston, TX Zip 77030-4298; tel. 713/791-1414; Robert F. Stott, Director
VETERANS AFFAIRS MEDICAL CENTER (O, 345 beds) 3600 Memorial Boulevard, Kerrville, TX Zip 78028; tel. 210/896-2020; Arnold E. Mouish, Director
VETERANS AFFAIRS MEDICAL CENTER (O, 134 beds) 1016 Ward Street, Marlin, TX Zip 76661-2162; tel. 817/883-3511; Melvin E. Baker, Director
VETERANS AFFAIRS MEDICAL CENTER (O, 804 beds) 4800 Memorial Drive, Waco, TX Zip 76711-1397; tel. 817/752-6581; Wallace M. Hopkins FACHE, Director
UTAH: VETERANS AFFAIRS MEDICAL CENTER (O, 294 beds) 500 Foothill Drive, Salt Lake City, UT Zip 84148; tel. 801/582-1565; William L. Hodson, Administrator
VERMONT: VETERANS AFFAIRS MEDICAL CENTER (O, 150 beds) North Hartland Road, White River Junction, VT Zip 05009-0001; tel. 802/295-9363; Gary M. De Gasta, Director
VIRGINIA: HUNTER HOLMES MCGUIRE VETERANS AFFAIRS MEDICAL CENTER (O, 640 beds) 1201 Broad Rock Boulevard, Richmond, VA Zip 23249; tel. 804/230-0001; James W. Dudley, Director
VETERANS AFFAIRS MEDICAL CENTER (O, 590 beds) 100 Emancipation Drive, Hampton, VA Zip 23667-0001; tel. 804/722-9961; William G. Wright, Director
VETERANS AFFAIRS MEDICAL CENTER (O, 500 beds) 1970 Roanoke Boulevard, Salem, VA Zip 24153; tel. 703/982-2463; John M. Presley Ph.D., Director
WASHINGTON: VETERANS AFFAIRS MEDICAL CENTER (O, 339 beds) Tacoma, WA Zip 98493; tel. 206/582-8440; Frank Taylor, Director
VETERANS AFFAIRS MEDICAL CENTER (O, 408 beds) 1660 South Columbian Way, Seattle, WA Zip 98108-1597; tel. 206/762-1010; Timothy B. Williams, Director
VETERANS AFFAIRS MEDICAL CENTER (O, 192 beds) North 4815 Assembly Street, Spokane, WA Zip 99205-6197; tel. 509/328-4521; Joseph M. Manley, Director
VETERANS AFFAIRS MEDICAL CENTER (O, 132 beds) 77 Wainwright Drive, Walla Walla, WA Zip 99362-3975; tel. 509/525-5200; George Marnell, Director
WEST VIRGINIA: LOUIS A. JOHNSON VETERANS AFFAIRS MEDICAL CENTER (O, 160 beds) Clarksburg, WV Zip 26301-4199; tel. 304/623-3461; Michael W. Neusch FACHE, Director
VETERANS AFFAIRS MEDICAL CENTER (O, 186 beds) 200 Veterans Avenue, Beckley, WV Zip 25801-6499; tel. 304/255-2121; G. P. Husson, Director
VETERANS AFFAIRS MEDICAL CENTER (O, 159 beds) 1540 Spring Valley Drive, Huntington, WV Zip 25704; tel. 304/429-6741; Philip S. Elkins, Director
VETERANS AFFAIRS MEDICAL CENTER (O, 771 beds) Charles Town Road, Martinsburg, WV Zip 25401-0205; tel. 304/263-0811; Richard Pell, Jr., Director
WISCONSIN: CLEMENT J. ZABLOCKI VETERANS AFFAIRS MEDICAL CENTER (O, 566 beds) 5000 West National Avenue, Milwaukee, WI Zip 53295-1000; tel. 414/384-2000; R. E. Struble, Director
VETERANS AFFAIRS MEDICAL CENTER (O, 601 beds) 500 East Veterans Street, Tomah, WI Zip 54660-9225; tel. 608/372-3971; Stan Johnson, Director
WILLIAM S. MIDDLETON MEMORIAL VETERANS HOSPITAL (O, 200 beds) 2500 Overlook Terrace, Madison, WI Zip 53705-2286; tel. 608/256-1901; Nathan L. Geraths, Director
WYOMING: VETERANS AFFAIRS CENTER (O, 125 beds) 2360 East Pershing Boulevard, Cheyenne, WY Zip 82001-5392; tel. 307/778-7550; Frank Drake, Director

VETERANS AFFAIRS MEDICAL CENTER (O, 292 beds) Sheridan, WY Zip 82801; tel. 307/672-3473; J. A. Brinkers, Director
PUERTO RICO: VETERANS AFFAIRS MEDICAL CENTER (O, 728 beds) One Veterans Plaza, San Juan, PR Zip 00927-5800; tel. 809/766-5665; Edward Valenzuela, Director

Owned, leased, sponsored:	157 hospitals	71515 beds
Contract-managed:	0 hospitals	0 beds
Totals:	157 hospitals	71515 beds

★**2145: DETROIT MEDICAL CENTER** (NP)
4201 St. Antoine Boulevard, Detroit, MI Zip 48201-2194; tel. 313/745-5192; David J. Campbell, President and Chief Executive Officer
MICHIGAN: CHILDREN'S HOSPITAL OF MICHIGAN (O, 257 beds) 3901 Beaubien, Detroit, MI Zip 48201-9985; tel. 313/745-0073; Thomas M. Rozek, President
DETROIT RECEIVING HOSPITAL AND UNIVERSITY HEALTH CENTER (O, 310 beds) 4201 St. Antoine Boulevard, Detroit, MI Zip 48201-2194; tel. 313/745-3605; Edward S. Thomas, President
GRACE HOSPITAL (O, 476 beds) 6071 West Outer Drive, Detroit, MI Zip 48235; tel. 313/966-3300; Mark A. Eustis, President
HARPER HOSPITAL (O, 549 beds) 3990 John R, Detroit, MI Zip 48201-9027; tel. 313/745-8040; Paul L. Broughton, President
HURON VALLEY HOSPITAL (O, 137 beds) 1601 East Commerce Road, Commerce Township, MI Zip 48382; tel. 810/360-3300; Elliot Joseph, President
HUTZEL HOSPITAL (O, 296 beds) 4707 St. Antoine Boulevard, Detroit, MI Zip 48201-0154; tel. 313/745-7174; Frank P. Iacobell, President
REHABILITATION INSTITUTE OF MICHIGAN (O, 128 beds) 261 Mack Boulevard, Detroit, MI Zip 48201; tel. 313/745-1203; Bruce M. Gans M.D., President

Owned, leased, sponsored:	7 hospitals	2153 beds
Contract-managed:	0 hospitals	0 beds
Totals:	7 hospitals	2153 beds

★**0042: DETROIT-MACOMB HOSPITAL CORPORATION** (NP)
12000 East Twelve Mile Road, Warren, MI Zip 48093; tel. 313/573-5910; Jack Ryan M.D., President and Chief Executive Officer
MICHIGAN: DETROIT RIVERVIEW HOSPITAL (O, 230 beds) 7733 East Jefferson Avenue, Detroit, MI Zip 48214; tel. 313/499-3000; Richard T. Young, Administrator
MACOMB HOSPITAL CENTER (O, 288 beds) 11800 East Twelve Mile Road, Warren, MI Zip 48093; tel. 810/573-5000; George P. Caralis, Administrator

Owned, leased, sponsored:	2 hospitals	518 beds
Contract-managed:	0 hospitals	0 beds
Totals:	2 hospitals	518 beds

0845: DEVEREUX FOUNDATION (NP)
19 South Waterloo Road, Devon, PA Zip 19333, Mailing Address: Box 400, Zip 19333; tel. 610/964-3000; Ronald P. Burd, President and Chief Exeuctive Officer
FLORIDA: DEVEREUX HOSPITAL AND CHILDREN'S CENTER OF FLORIDA (O, 100 beds) 8000 Devereux Drive, Melbourne, FL Zip 32940-7907; tel. 407/242-9100; James E. Colvin, Administrator
GEORGIA: DEVEREUX CENTER-GEORGIA (O, 115 beds) 1291 Stanley Road, Kennesaw, GA Zip 30144-4359; tel. 404/427-0147; Ralph L. Comerford, Director
PENNSYLVANIA: DEVEREUX MAPLETON PSYCHIATRIC INSTITUTE-MAPLETON CENTER (O, 24 beds) 655 Sugartown Road, Malvern, PA Zip 19355-0297, Mailing Address: Box 297, Zip 19355-0297; tel. 610/296-6923; Kenneth Tenley, Director
TEXAS: DEVEREUX TEXAS TREATMENT NETWORK (O, 84 beds) 1150 Devereux Drive, League City, TX Zip 77573; tel. 713/335-1000; Gail Atkinson, Executive Director
DEVEREUX-VICTORIA (O, 88 beds) 120 David Wade Drive, Victoria, TX Zip 77902-2666; tel. 512/575-8271; L. Gail Atkinson, Executive Director

Owned, leased, sponsored:	5 hospitals	411 beds
Contract-managed:	0 hospitals	0 beds
Totals:	5 hospitals	411 beds

For explanation of codes following names, see page B2.
★Indicates Type III membership in the American Hospital Association.

Systems / Dimensions Health Corporation

★0029: **DIMENSIONS HEALTH CORPORATION** (NP)
9200 Basil Court, Landover, MD Zip 20785; tel. 301/925-7000
MARYLAND: LAUREL REGIONAL HOSPITAL (O, 185 beds) 7300 Van Dusen Road, Laurel, MD Zip 20707-9266; tel. 301/725-4300; Patrick F. Mutch, President

PRINCE GEORGE'S HOSPITAL CENTER (O, 394 beds) 3001 Hospital Drive, Cheverly, MD Zip 20785; tel. 301/618-2000; Allan Earl Atzrott, President

Owned, leased, sponsored:	2 hospitals	579 beds
Contract-managed:	0 hospitals	0 beds
Totals:	2 hospitals	579 beds

0010: **DIVISION OF MENTAL HEALTH SERVICES, DEPARTMENT OF HUMAN SERVICES, STATE OF NEW JERSEY** (NP)
Capital Center, CN 727, Trenton, NJ Zip 08625-0727; Alan G. Kaufman, Director
NEW JERSEY: ANCORA PSYCHIATRIC HOSPITAL (O, 626 beds) 202 Spring Garden Road, Hammonton, NJ Zip 08037-9699; tel. 609/561-1700; William J. Camarota, Chief Executive Officer

GREYSTONE PARK PSYCHIATRIC HOSPITAL (O, 607 beds) Central Avenue, Greystone Park, NJ Zip 07950, Mailing Address: P.O. Box A, Zip 07950; tel. 201/538-1800; George A. Waters, Jr. FACHE, Chief Executive Officer

MARLBORO PSYCHIATRIC HOSPITAL (O, 869 beds) 546 County Road 520, Marlboro, NJ Zip 07746-1099; tel. 908/946-8100; Michael Ross Ph.D., Chief Executive Officer

SENATOR GARRET T. W. HAGEDORN GERO PSYCHIATRIC HOSPITAL (O, 181 beds) 200 Sanitorium Road, Glen Gardner, NJ Zip 08826-9752; tel. 908/537-2141; Edna Volpe-Way, Chief Executive Officer

TRENTON PSYCHIATRIC HOSPITAL (O, 379 beds) Sullivan Way, Station A, Trenton, NJ Zip 08625, Mailing Address: P.O. Box 7500, West Trenton, Zip 08628; tel. 609/633-1500; Joseph Jupin, Jr., Chief Executive Officer

Owned, leased, sponsored:	5 hospitals	2662 beds
Contract-managed:	0 hospitals	0 beds
Totals:	5 hospitals	2662 beds

1045: **DOCTORS HOSPITAL** (NP)
1087 Dennison Avenue, Columbus, OH Zip 43201; tel. 614/297-4000; Richard A. Vincent, President
OHIO: DOCTORS HOSPITAL (O, 407 beds) 1087 Dennison Avenue, Columbus, OH Zip 43201; tel. 614/297-4000; Richard A. Vincent, President

DOCTORS HOSPITAL OF NELSONVILLE (O, 77 beds) 1950 Mount Saint Mary Drive, Nelsonville, OH Zip 45764; tel. 614/753-1931; Mark R. Seckinger, Administrator

Owned, leased, sponsored:	2 hospitals	484 beds
Contract-managed:	0 hospitals	0 beds
Totals:	2 hospitals	484 beds

1195: **DOMINICAN SISTERS CONGREGATION OF THE MOST HOLY NAME** (CC)
1520 Grand Avenue, San Rafael, CA Zip 94901-2236; tel. 415/453-8303; Sister Kristin Wombacher, Prioress General
CALIFORNIA: ST. JOSEPH'S MEDICAL CENTER (O, 319 beds) 1800 North California Street, Stockton, CA Zip 95204-6088, Mailing Address: P.O. Box 213008, Zip 95213-9008; tel. 209/943-2000; Edward G. Schroeder, President

NEVADA: ST. MARY'S REGIONAL MEDICAL CENTER (O, 341 beds) 235 West Sixth Street, Reno, NV Zip 89520; tel. 702/323-2041; Jeff K. Bills, President

Owned, leased, sponsored:	2 hospitals	660 beds
Contract-managed:	0 hospitals	0 beds
Totals:	2 hospitals	660 beds

1295: **DOMINICAN SISTERS OF SPRINGFIELD** (CC)
1237 West Monroe Street, Springfield, IL Zip 62704-1680; tel. 217/787-0481; Sister Rose Miriam Schulte, Prioress General

ARKANSAS: ST. MARY-ROGERS MEMORIAL HOSPITAL (S, 92 beds) 1200 West Walnut Street, Rogers, AR Zip 72756-3599; tel. 501/636-0200; Sister Sharon Therese Zayac, President
MISSISSIPPI: ST. DOMINIC-JACKSON MEMORIAL HOSPITAL (S, 571 beds) 969 Lakeland Drive, Jackson, MS Zip 39216-4699; tel. 601/982-0121; Claude W. Harbarger, President

Owned, leased, sponsored:	2 hospitals	663 beds
Contract-managed:	0 hospitals	0 beds
Totals:	2 hospitals	663 beds

1895: **EAST TEXAS MEDICAL CENTER REGIONAL HEALTHCARE SYSTEM** (NP)
1000 South Beckham Street, Tyler, TX Zip 75701-1996, Mailing Address: P.O. Drawer 6400, Zip 75711-6400; tel. 903/597-0351; Elmer G. Ellis, President and Chief Executive Officer
TEXAS: EAST TEXAS MEDICAL CENTER ATHENS (L, 108 beds) 2000 South Palestine, Athens, TX Zip 75751; tel. 903/675-2216; Patrick L. Wallace, Administrator

EAST TEXAS MEDICAL CENTER PITTSBURG (L, 42 beds) 414 Quitman Street, Pittsburg, TX Zip 75686-1032; tel. 903/856-6663; Charles N. Butts, Administrator

EAST TEXAS MEDICAL CENTER RUSK (L, 25 beds) Copeland and Bonner Streets, Rusk, TX Zip 75785, Mailing Address: P.O. Box 317, Zip 75785; tel. 903/683-2273; Donna S. Gunter B.S.N., R.N., C.P.H.Q., Administrator

EAST TEXAS MEDICAL CENTER-MOUNT VERNON (L, 30 beds) Highway 37 South, Mount Vernon, TX Zip 75457, Mailing Address: Box 477, Zip 75457-0477; tel. 903/537-4552; Perry Henderson, Administrator

Owned, leased, sponsored:	4 hospitals	205 beds
Contract-managed:	0 hospitals	0 beds
Totals:	4 hospitals	205 beds

★0555: **EASTERN MAINE HEALTHCARE** (NP)
489 State Street, Bangor, ME Zip 04401; tel. 207/973-7051; Norman A. Ledwin, President
MAINE: ACADIA HOSPITAL (O, 72 beds) 286 Stillwater Avenue, Bangor, ME Zip 04401, Mailing Address: P.O. Box 422, Zip 04402-0422; tel. 207/973-6100; Dennis P. King, President

EASTERN MAINE MEDICAL CENTER (O, 347 beds) 489 State Street, Bangor, ME Zip 04401; tel. 207/945-7000; Norman A. Ledwin, President and Chief Executive Officer

Owned, leased, sponsored:	2 hospitals	419 beds
Contract-managed:	0 hospitals	0 beds
Totals:	2 hospitals	419 beds

★3595: **EASTERN MERCY HEALTH SYSTEM** (CC)
3 Radnor Corporate Center, Suite 220, Radnor, PA Zip 19087; tel. 610/971-9770; Daniel F. Russell, President
ALABAMA: MERCY MEDICAL (S, 157 beds) 101 Villa Drive, Daphne, AL Zip 36526, Mailing Address: P.O. Box 1090, Zip 36526; tel. 334/626-2694; Sister Mary Eileen Wilhelm, President and Chief Executive Officer
FLORIDA: HOLY CROSS HOSPITAL (S, 437 beds) 4725 North Federal Highway, Fort Lauderdale, FL Zip 33308, Mailing Address: Box 23460, Zip 33307; tel. 305/771-8000; Ray Budrys, President and Chief Executive Officer
GEORGIA: SAINT JOSEPH'S HOSPITAL OF ATLANTA (S, 346 beds) 5665 Peachtree Dunwoody Road N.E., Atlanta, GA Zip 30342-1764; tel. 404/851-7001; Kathryn J. McDonagh, President
MAINE: MERCY HOSPITAL (S, 158 beds) 144 State Street, Portland, ME Zip 04101-3795; tel. 207/879-3000; Howard R. Buckley, President
NEW YORK: KENMORE MERCY HOSPITAL (S, 219 beds) 2950 Elmwood Avenue, Kenmore, NY Zip 14217-1390; tel. 716/879-6100; Sister Mary Joel Schimscheiner, Chief Executive Officer

MERCY HOSPITAL (S, 423 beds) 565 Abbott Road, Buffalo, NY Zip 14220; tel. 716/828-2001; Sister Kathi Sweeney, Chief Executive Officer

ST. JAMES MERCY HOSPITAL (S, 220 beds) 411 Canisteo Street, Hornell, NY Zip 14843-2197; tel. 607/324-8000; Paul E. Shephard, President and Chief Executive Officer

For explanation of codes following names, see page B2.
★*Indicates Type III membership in the American Hospital Association.*

Systems / First Hospital Corporation

ST. JEROME HOSPITAL (S, 96 beds) 16 Bank Street, Batavia, NY Zip 14020–2260; tel. 716/343–3131; Charles W. Smith, Jr., Chief Executive Officer

ST. PETER'S HOSPITAL (S, 437 beds) 315 South Manning Boulevard, Albany, NY Zip 12208–1789; tel. 518/454–1550; Steven P. Boyle, President and Chief Executive Officer

PENNSYLVANIA: MERCY HAVERFORD HOSPITAL (S, 107 beds) 2000 Old West Chester Pike, Havertown, PA Zip 19083; tel. 610/645–3600; Andrew E. Harris, Chief Executive Director

MERCY HEALTH CORPORATION OF SOUTHEASTERN PENNSYLVANIA (S, 530 beds) One Bala Plaza, Suite 402, Bala Cynwyd, PA Zip 19004; tel. 215/237–4000; Plato A. Marinakos, President and Chief Executive Officer

MERCY HOSPITAL OF PITTSBURGH (S, 465 beds) 1400 Locust Street, Pittsburgh, PA Zip 15219–5166; tel. 412/232–8111; Sister Joanne Marie, President and Chief Executive Officer

MERCY PROVIDENCE HOSPITAL (S, 130 beds) 1004 Arch Street, Pittsburgh, PA Zip 15212; tel. 412/323–5600; Norman F. Mitry, Chief Operating Officer

MERCY PSYCHIATRIC INSTITUTE (S, 88 beds) 3339 McClure Avenue, Pittsburgh, PA Zip 15212–2197; tel. 412/766–8300; Robert W. Kocent, President

Owned, leased, sponsored:	14 hospitals	3813 beds
Contract–managed:	0 hospitals	0 beds
Totals:	14 hospitals	3813 beds

0945: EMPIRE HEALTH CENTERS GROUP (NP)
West 800 Fifth Avenue, Spokane, WA Zip 99204, Mailing Address: P.O. Box 248, Zip 99210–0248; tel. 509/458–7965; Thomas M. White, President

WASHINGTON: DEACONESS MEDICAL CENTER–SPOKANE (O, 326 beds) 800 West Fifth Avenue, Spokane, WA Zip 99204, Mailing Address: P.O. Box 248, Zip 99210–0248; tel. 509/458–5800; Thomas J. Zellers, Chief Operating Officer

ST. LUKES REHABILITATION INSTITUTE (O, 87 beds) 711 South Cowley Street, Spokane, WA Zip 99202, Mailing Address: P.O. Box 288, Zip 99210–0288; tel. 509/838–4771; Debra D. Hanks, Administrator

VALLEY HOSPITAL AND MEDICAL CENTER (O, 117 beds) 12606 East Mission Avenue, Spokane, WA Zip 99216–9969; tel. 509/924–6650; Michael T. Liepman, Chief Operating Officer

Owned, leased, sponsored:	3 hospitals	530 beds
Contract–managed:	0 hospitals	0 beds
Totals:	3 hospitals	530 beds

★0735: EPISCOPAL HEALTH SERVICES INC. (CO)
333 Earle Ovington Boulevard, Uniondale, NY Zip 11553–3645; tel. 516/228–6100; Jack N. Farrington Ph.D., Executive Vice President

NEW YORK: ST. JOHN'S EPISCOPAL HOSPITAL–SMITHTOWN (O, 366 beds) 50 Route 25–A, Smithtown, NY Zip 11787–1398; tel. 516/862–3000; Laura Righter, Administrator

ST. JOHN'S EPISCOPAL HOSPITAL–SOUTH SHORE (O, 314 beds) 327 Beach 19th Street, Far Rockaway, NY Zip 11691–4424; tel. 718/868–7000; Paul J. Connor III, Administrator

Owned, leased, sponsored:	2 hospitals	680 beds
Contract–managed:	0 hospitals	0 beds
Totals:	2 hospitals	680 beds

1255: ESCAMBIA COUNTY HEALTH CARE AUTHORITY (NP)
1301 Belleville Avenue, Brewton, AL Zip 36426; tel. 334/368–2500; Phillip L. Parker, Administrator

ALABAMA: ATMORE COMMUNITY HOSPITAL (O, 51 beds) 401 Medical Park Drive, Atmore, AL Zip 36502; tel. 205/368–2500; Lavon Henley, Administrator

D. W. MCMILLAN MEMORIAL HOSPITAL (O, 83 beds) 1301 Belleville Avenue, Brewton, AL Zip 36426, Mailing Address: Box 908, Zip 36427; tel. 334/867–8061; Phillip L. Parker, Administrator

Owned, leased, sponsored:	2 hospitals	134 beds
Contract–managed:	0 hospitals	0 beds
Totals:	2 hospitals	134 beds

2515: FAIRVIEW HEALTH SYSTEM (NP)
18101 Lorain Avenue, Cleveland, OH Zip 44111–5656; tel. 216/476–4040; Thomas M. LaMotte, President and Chief Executive Officer

OHIO: FAIRVIEW GENERAL HOSPITAL (O, 453 beds) 18101 Lorain Avenue, Cleveland, OH Zip 44111–5656; tel. 216/476–4040; Thomas M. LaMotte, President and Chief Executive Officer

LUTHERAN MEDICAL CENTER (O, 174 beds) 2609 Franklin Boulevard, Cleveland, OH Zip 44113–2992; tel. 216/696–4300; Thomas M. LaMotte, President and Chief Executive Officer

Owned, leased, sponsored:	2 hospitals	627 beds
Contract–managed:	0 hospitals	0 beds
Totals:	2 hospitals	627 beds

★1325: FAIRVIEW HOSPITAL AND HEALTHCARE SERVICES (NP)
2450 Riverside Avenue, Minneapolis, MN Zip 55454–1400; tel. 612/672–6735; Richard A. Norling, President and Chief Executive Officer

MINNESOTA: FAIRVIEW NORTHLAND REGIONAL HOSPITAL (O, 41 beds) 911 Northland Drive, Princeton, MN Zip 55371; tel. 612/389–1313; Glenn G. Erickson, Vice President and Administrator

FAIRVIEW RIDGES HOSPITAL (O, 123 beds) 201 East Nicollet Boulevard, Burnsville, MN Zip 55337–5799; tel. 612/892–2000; Donald C. Berglund, Senior Vice President and Administrator

FAIRVIEW RIVERSIDE MEDICAL CENTER (O, 808 beds) 2450 Riverside Avenue, Minneapolis, MN Zip 55454–9978; tel. 612/672–6300; Pamela L. Tibbetts, Senior Vice President and Administrator

FAIRVIEW SOUTHDALE HOSPITAL (O, 390 beds) 6401 France Avenue South, Minneapolis, MN Zip 55435–2199; tel. 612/924–5000; Mark M. Enger, Senior Vice President and Administrator

Owned, leased, sponsored:	4 hospitals	1362 beds
Contract–managed:	0 hospitals	0 beds
Totals:	4 hospitals	1362 beds

1275: FIRST HEALTH, INC. (IO)
107 Public Square, Batesville, MS Zip 38606; tel. 601/563–7676

KENTUCKY: JENKINS COMMUNITY HOSPITAL A SUBSIDIARY OF FIRST HEALTH, INC. (O, 60 beds) Main Street, Jenkins, KY Zip 41537, Mailing Address: P.O. Box 472, Zip 41537; tel. 606/832–2171; Jason Staggs, Administrator

MISSISSIPPI: BRUCE HOSPITAL (O, 47 beds) Highway 9 South, Bruce, MS Zip 38915, Mailing Address: Box 429, Zip 38915–0429; tel. 601/983–5100; Robert M. Perry, Administrator

Owned, leased, sponsored:	2 hospitals	107 beds
Contract–managed:	0 hospitals	0 beds
Totals:	2 hospitals	107 beds

2635: FIRST HOSPITAL CORPORATION (IO)
240 Corporate Boulevard, Norfolk, VA Zip 23502; tel. 804/459–5100; Ronald Dozoretz M.D., Chairman

CALIFORNIA: FIRST HOSPITAL VALLEJO (O, 61 beds) 525 Oregon Street, Vallejo, CA Zip 94590; tel. 707/648–2200; Bill F. Dye, Chief Executive Officer and Administrator

FLORIDA: ST. AUGUSTINE PSYCHIATRIC CENTER (O, 50 beds) 200 River Haven Way, Saint Augustine, FL Zip 32086; tel. 904/824–9800; Greg Steele, Administrator

PENNSYLVANIA: CLARION PSYCHIATRIC CENTER (O, 52 beds) 2 Hospital Drive, R D 3, Clarion, PA Zip 16214; tel. 814/226–9545; Michael R. Keefer, Administrator and Chief Executive Officer

FIRST HOSPITAL WYOMING VALLEY (O, 96 beds) 149 Dana Street, Wilkes–Barre, PA Zip 18702; tel. 717/829–7900; John Kasenchak, Administrator

For explanation of codes following names, see page B2.
★Indicates Type III membership in the American Hospital Association.

Integrated Health Delivery Networks, Health Care Systems and Alliances

Systems / First Hospital Corporation

HORSHAM CLINIC (O, 138 beds) 722 East Butler Pike, Ambler, PA Zip 19002; tel. 215/643–7800; David A. Baron D.O., Medical Director

MEADOWS PSYCHIATRIC CENTER (O, 101 beds) Centre Hall, PA, Mailing Address: Rural Delivery 1, Box 259, Zip 16828; tel. 814/364–2161; Joseph Barszczewski, Chief Executive Officer

SOUTHWOOD PSYCHIATRIC HOSPITAL (O, 50 beds) 2575 Boyce Plaza Road, Pittsburgh, PA Zip 15241–3925; tel. 412/257–2290; Alan A. Axelson M.D., Chief Executive Officer

VIRGINIA: NORFOLK PSYCHIATRIC CENTER (O, 62 beds) 100 Kingsley Lane, Norfolk, VA Zip 23505; tel. 804/489–1072; Cheryl Watson, Administrator

PUERTO RICO: FIRST HOSPITAL PANAMERICANO (O, 165 beds) State Road 787 KM 1 5, Cidra, PR Zip 00739, Mailing Address: P.O. Box 1398, Zip 00739; tel. 809/739–5555; Marina Diaz, Administrator

Owned, leased, sponsored:	9 hospitals	775 beds
Contract–managed:	0 hospitals	0 beds
Totals:	9 hospitals	775 beds

★1355: FORBES HEALTH SYSTEM (NP)

500 Finley Street, Pittsburgh, PA Zip 15206; tel. 412/665–3320; Barry H. Roth, President

PENNSYLVANIA: FORBES METROPOLITAN HOSPITAL (O, 152 beds) 225 Penn Avenue, Pittsburgh, PA Zip 15221–2173; tel. 412/247–2424; Dana W. Ramish, Senior Vice President Operations

FORBES REGIONAL HOSPITAL (O, 353 beds) 2570 Haymaker Road, Monroeville, PA Zip 15146–3592; tel. 412/858–2000; Dana W. Ramish, Senior Vice President Operations

Owned, leased, sponsored:	2 hospitals	505 beds
Contract–managed:	0 hospitals	0 beds
Totals:	2 hospitals	505 beds

★5325: FRANCISCAN HEALTH SYSTEM (CC)

One MacIntyre Drive, Chester, PA Zip 19014–1196; tel. 610/358–4223; Ronald R. Aldrich, President and Chief Executive Officer

DELAWARE: ST. FRANCIS HOSPITAL (O, 283 beds) Seventh and Clayton Streets, Wilmington, DE Zip 19805–0500, Mailing Address: P.O. Box 2500, Zip 19805–0500; tel. 302/575–8301; Paul C. King, Jr., President

MARYLAND: ST. JOSEPH MEDICAL CENTER (O, 460 beds) 7620 York Road, Towson, MD Zip 21204; tel. 410/337–1000; John S. Prout, President and Chief Executive Officer

NEW JERSEY: ST. FRANCIS MEDICAL CENTER (O, 344 beds) 601 Hamilton Avenue, Trenton, NJ Zip 08629–1986; tel. 609/599–5000; Patrick F. Roche, President

OREGON: ST. ELIZABETH HEALTH SERVICES (O, 154 beds) 3325 Pocahontas Road, Baker City, OR Zip 97814; tel. 503/523–6461; Rod Barton, President and Chief Operating Officer

ST. ANTHONY HOSPITAL (O, 49 beds) 1601 S.E. Court Avenue, Pendleton, OR Zip 97801–3297; tel. 503/276–5121; Jeffrey S. Drop, President

PENNSYLVANIA: NAZARETH HOSPITAL (O, 214 beds) 2601 Holme Avenue, Philadelphia, PA Zip 19152–2096; tel. 215/335–6000; Sister M. Therese, President

ST. AGNES MEDICAL CENTER (O, 210 beds) 1900 South Broad Street, Philadelphia, PA Zip 19145; tel. 215/339–4100; Daniel J. Sinnott, President and Chief Operating Officer

ST. JOSEPH HOSPITAL (O, 246 beds) 250 College Avenue, Lancaster, PA Zip 17604; tel. 717/291–8211; John Kerr Tolmie, Interim President and Chief Executive Officer

ST. JOSEPH MEDICAL CENTER (O, 257 beds) Twelfth & Walnut Streets, Reading, PA Zip 19603–0316, Mailing Address: P.O. Box 316, Zip 19603–0316; tel. 610/378–2000; David A. Ferrell, President and Chief Executive Officer

ST. MARY MEDICAL CENTER (O, 287 beds) Langhorne–Newtown Road, Langhorne, PA Zip 19047–1295; tel. 215/750–2000; Sister Clare Carty, President

WASHINGTON: ST. CLARE HOSPITAL (O, 60 beds) 11315 Bridgeport Way S.W., Tacoma, WA Zip 98499–0998, Mailing Address: P.O. Box 99998, Zip 98499–0998; tel. 206/588–1711; Craig L. Hendrickson, President

ST. FRANCIS HOSPITAL (O, 67 beds) 34515 Ninth Avenue South, Federal Way, WA Zip 98003–9710; tel. 206/838–9700; Craig L. Hendrickson, Chief Operating Officer

ST. JOSEPH MEDICAL CENTER (O, 271 beds) 1717 South J Street, Tacoma, WA Zip 98405, Mailing Address: P.O. Box 2197, Zip 98401–2197; tel. 206/627–4101; Philip G. Dionne, President and Chief Operating Officer

Owned, leased, sponsored:	13 hospitals	2902 beds
Contract–managed:	0 hospitals	0 beds
Totals:	13 hospitals	2902 beds

★9650: FRANCISCAN HEALTH SYSTEM, INC. (CC)

615 South Tenth Street, La Crosse, WI Zip 54601–4786; tel. 608/791–9710; Brian C. Campion M.D., Chief Executive Officer

WISCONSIN: ST. FRANCIS MEDICAL CENTER (O, 226 beds) 700 West Avenue South, La Crosse, WI Zip 54601–4783; tel. 608/785–0940; Ronald R. Paczkowski, Chief Executive Officer

ST. JOSEPH'S HOSPITAL (O, 101 beds) 464 South St. Joseph Avenue, Arcadia, WI Zip 54612–1401; tel. 608/323–3341; Eugene E. Molitor, Chief Administrative Officer

ST. MARY'S HOSPITAL (O, 60 beds) West Main and K Streets, Sparta, WI Zip 54656, Mailing Address: P.O. Box 529, Zip 54656; tel. 608/269–2132; Bill Sexton, Chief Executive Officer and Administrator

Owned, leased, sponsored:	3 hospitals	387 beds
Contract–managed:	0 hospitals	0 beds
Totals:	3 hospitals	387 beds

★1475: FRANCISCAN MISSIONARIES OF OUR LADY HEALTH SYSTEM, INC. (CC)

4200 Essen Lane, Baton Rouge, LA Zip 70809; tel. 504/923–2701; Sister Brendan Mary Ronayne, President

LOUISIANA: OUR LADY OF LAKE REGIONAL MEDICAL CENTER (O, 676 beds) 5000 Hennessy Boulevard, Baton Rouge, LA Zip 70808–4350; tel. 504/765–6565; Robert C. Davidge, President and Chief Executive Officer

OUR LADY OF LOURDES REGIONAL MEDICAL CENTER (O, 317 beds) 611 St. Landry Street, Lafayette, LA Zip 70506–4697, Mailing Address: Box 4027, Zip 70502–4027; tel. 318/289–2000; Dudley Romero, President and Chief Executive Officer

ST. FRANCIS MEDICAL CENTER (O, 425 beds) 309 Jackson Street, Monroe, LA Zip 71201, Mailing Address: Box 1901, Zip 71210–1901; tel. 318/327–4000; H. Gerald Smith, President and Chief Executive Officer

Owned, leased, sponsored:	3 hospitals	1418 beds
Contract–managed:	0 hospitals	0 beds
Totals:	3 hospitals	1418 beds

★5375: FRANCISCAN SERVICES CORPORATION (CC)

6832 Convent Boulevard, Sylvania, OH Zip 43560–2897; tel. 419/882–8373; John W. O'Connell, President

MICHIGAN: HOLY CROSS HOSPITAL (S, 214 beds) 4777 East Outer Drive, Detroit, MI Zip 48234–0401; tel. 313/369–9100; James E. Koerper, President and Chief Executive Officer

OHIO: PROVIDENCE HOSPITAL (S, 261 beds) 1912 Hayes Avenue, Sandusky, OH Zip 44870–4788; tel. 419/621–7000; Sister Nancy Linenkugel FACHE, President and Chief Executive Officer

ST. JOHN MEDICAL CENTER (S, 161 beds) St. John Heights, Steubenville, OH Zip 43952–2393; tel. 614/264–8000; Angelo G. Calbone, President and Chief Executive Officer

TEXAS: ST. JOSEPH REGIONAL HEALTH CENTER (S, 172 beds) 2801 Franciscan Drive, Bryan, TX Zip 77802; tel. 409/776–3777; Sister Gretchen Kunz, President

TRINITY COMMUNITY MEDICAL CENTER OF BRENHAM (S, 60 beds) 700 Medical Parkway, Brenham, TX Zip 77833; tel. 409/836–6173; John L. Simms, President

Owned, leased, sponsored:	5 hospitals	868 beds
Contract–managed:	0 hospitals	0 beds
Totals:	5 hospitals	868 beds

★1415: FRANCISCAN SISTERS HEALTH CARE CORPORATION (CC)

9223 West Francis Road, Frankfort, IL Zip 60423–8334; tel. 815/469–4888; Gerald P. Pearson, President

For explanation of codes following names, see page B2.
★Indicates Type III membership in the American Hospital Association.

ILLINOIS: SAINT JOSEPH HOSPITAL (O, 97 beds) 77 North Airlite Street, Elgin, IL Zip 60123–4912; tel. 708/695–3200; Larry Narum, President
SAINT JOSEPH MEDICAL CENTER (O, 500 beds) 333 North Madison Street, Joliet, IL Zip 60435–6595; tel. 815/725–7133; David W. Benfer, President and Chief Executive Officer
SAINT THERESE MEDICAL CENTER (O, 254 beds) 2615 Washington Street, Waukegan, IL Zip 60085–4988; tel. 708/249–3900; Timothy P. Selz, President
UNITED SAMARITANS MEDICAL CENTER (O, 332 beds) Danville, IL; Dennis J. Doran, President

Owned, leased, sponsored:	4 hospitals	1183 beds
Contract–managed:	0 hospitals	0 beds
Totals:	4 hospitals	1183 beds

★1455: **FRANCISCAN SISTERS OF CHRISTIAN CHARITY HEALTHCARE MINISTRY, INC** (CC)
2409 South Alverno Road, Manitowoc, WI Zip 54220–9320; tel. 414/684–7071; Sister Laura J. Wolf, President

NEBRASKA: ST. FRANCIS MEMORIAL HOSPITAL (O, 32 beds) 430 North Monitor Street, West Point, NE Zip 68788–1595; tel. 402/372–2404; Sister Helena Young, President
OHIO: GOOD SAMARITAN MEDICAL AND REHABILITATION CENTER (O, 281 beds) 800 Forest Avenue, Zanesville, OH Zip 43701; tel. 614/454–5000; Thomas A. Barone, President
WISCONSIN: HOLY FAMILY MEMORIAL MEDICAL CENTER (O, 216 beds) 2300 Western Avenue, Manitowoc, WI Zip 54220, Mailing Address: P.O. Box 1450, Zip 54221–1450; tel. 414/684–2011; Daniel B. McGinty, President and Chief Operating Officer

Owned, leased, sponsored:	3 hospitals	529 beds
Contract–managed:	0 hospitals	0 beds
Totals:	3 hospitals	529 beds

★1485: **FRANCISCAN SISTERS OF THE POOR HEALTH SYSTEM, INC.** (CC)
186 Joralemon Street, New York, NY Zip 11201–4326; tel. 718/625–6530; Sister Joanne Schuster, President

KENTUCKY: OUR LADY OF BELLEFONTE HOSPITAL (S, 189 beds) St. Christopher Drive, Ashland, KY Zip 41105–0789, Mailing Address: P.O. Box 789, Zip 41105–0789; tel. 606/833–3333; Robert J. Maher, President
NEW JERSEY: ST. FRANCIS HOSPITAL (S, 243 beds) 25 McWilliams Place, Jersey City, NJ Zip 07302–1698; tel. 201/418–1000; Ulrich J. Rosa, President and Chief Executive Officer
ST. MARY HOSPITAL (S, 328 beds) 308 Willow Avenue, Hoboken, NJ Zip 07030–3889; tel. 201/418–1000; Ulrich J. Rosa, President and Chief Executive Officer
NEW YORK: ST. ANTHONY COMMUNITY HOSPITAL (S, 73 beds) 15–19 Maple Avenue, Warwick, NY Zip 10990; tel. 914/986–2276; F. Dennis Harrington, President
OHIO: PROVIDENCE HOSPITAL (S, 238 beds) 2446 Kipling Avenue, Cincinnati, OH Zip 45239–6695; tel. 513/853–5000; R. Christopher West, President and Chief Executive Officer
ST. ELIZABETH MEDICAL CENTER (S, 379 beds) 601 Edwin C. Moses Boulevard, Dayton, OH Zip 45408–1498; tel. 513/229–6000; James M. Strieby, President and Chief Executive Officer
ST. FRANCIS–ST. GEORGE HOSPITAL (S, 229 beds) 3131 Queen City Avenue, Cincinnati, OH Zip 45238–2396; tel. 513/389–5000; R. Christopher West, President
SOUTH CAROLINA: ST. FRANCIS HEALTH SYSTEM (S, 237 beds) One St. Francis Drive, Greenville, SC Zip 29601–3207; tel. 803/255–1000; Richard C. Neugent, President

Owned, leased, sponsored:	8 hospitals	1916 beds
Contract–managed:	0 hospitals	0 beds
Totals:	8 hospitals	1916 beds

2115: **FREMONT–RIDEOUT HEALTH GROUP** (NP)
989 Plumas Street, Yuba City, CA Zip 95991; tel. 916/751–4010; Thomas P. Hayes, Chief Executive Officer

CALIFORNIA: FREMONT MEDICAL CENTER (O, 132 beds) 970 Plumas Street, Yuba City, CA Zip 95991; tel. 916/751–4000; Thomas P. Hayes, Chief Executive Officer
RIDEOUT MEMORIAL HOSPITAL (O, 128 beds) 726 Fourth Street, Marysville, CA Zip 95901–2128, Mailing Address: Box 2128, Zip 95901–2128; tel. 916/749–4300; Thomas P. Hayes, Chief Executive Officer

Owned, leased, sponsored:	2 hospitals	260 beds
Contract–managed:	0 hospitals	0 beds
Totals:	2 hospitals	260 beds

★5570: **GEISINGER HEALTH CARE SYSTEM** (NP)
100 North Academy Avenue, Danville, PA Zip 17822–3311; tel. 717/271–6211; Frank J. Trembulak, Chief Operating Officer

PENNSYLVANIA: GEISINGER MEDICAL CENTER (O, 577 beds) 100 North Academy Avenue, Danville, PA Zip 17822–2201; tel. 717/271–6168; Stuart Heydt, Chief Executive Officer
GEISINGER WYOMING VALLEY MEDICAL CENTER (O, 195 beds) 1000 East Mountain Drive, Wilkes-Barre, PA Zip 18711–0025; tel. 717/826–7300; Conrad W. Schintz, Senior Vice President Operations

Owned, leased, sponsored:	2 hospitals	772 beds
Contract–managed:	0 hospitals	0 beds
Totals:	2 hospitals	772 beds

★0775: **GENERAL HEALTH SYSTEM** (NP)
3849 North Boulevard, Suite 200, Baton Rouge, LA Zip 70806; tel. 504/387–7806; Thomas H. Sawyer, President and Chief Executive Officer

LOUISIANA: BATON ROUGE GENERAL HEALTH CENTER (O, 72 beds) 8585 Picardy Avenue, Baton Rouge, LA Zip 70809, Mailing Address: P.O. Box 84330, Zip 70884–4330; tel. 504/763–4000; Linda Kay Matessino R.N., President and Chief Executive Officer
BATON ROUGE GENERAL MEDICAL CENTER (O, 389 beds) 3600 Florida Street, Baton Rouge, LA Zip 70806, Mailing Address: P.O. Box 2511, Zip 70821–2511; tel. 504/387–7000; James L. Brexler, President and Chief Executive Officer
VERMILION HOSPITAL (O, 54 beds) 2520 North University, Lafayette, LA Zip 70507, Mailing Address: P.O. Box 91526, Zip 70509–1526; tel. 318/234–5614; John Patout, Administrator

Owned, leased, sponsored:	3 hospitals	515 beds
Contract–managed:	0 hospitals	0 beds
Totals:	3 hospitals	515 beds

0645: **GLENBEIGH, INC.** (IO)
4700 Congress Avenue, West Palm Beach, FL Zip 33407–3229; tel. 407/863–4747; G. Norman McCann, President

OHIO: GLENBEIGH HOSPITAL OF CLEVELAND (O, 50 beds) 18120 Puritas Avenue, Cleveland, OH Zip 44135; tel. 216/476–0222; John Sajan R.N., Executive Director
GLENBEIGH HOSPITAL OF ROCK CREEK (O, 80 beds) Route 45, Rock Creek, OH Zip 44084, Mailing Address: Route 45, P.O. Box 298, Zip 44084; tel. 216/563–3400; Patricia Weston-Hall, Executive Director

Owned, leased, sponsored:	2 hospitals	130 beds
Contract–managed:	0 hospitals	0 beds
Totals:	2 hospitals	130 beds

★0965: **GOOD SAMARITAN HEALTH SYSTEM** (NP)
532 Race Street, San Jose, CA Zip 95126–3432; tel. 408/280–5660; Michael B. Guthrie M.D., President and Chief Executive Officer

CALIFORNIA: GOOD SAMARITAN HOSPITAL OF SANTA CLARA VALLEY (O, 348 beds) 2425 Samaritan Drive, San Jose, CA Zip 95124; tel. 408/559–2011; Joan White, Vice President and Administrator
GOOD SAMARITAN HOSPITAL–MISSION OAKS (O, 551 beds) 15891 Los Gatos–Almaden Road, Los Gatos, CA Zip 95032; tel. 408/356–4111; Michael B. Guthrie M.D., President and Chief Executive Officer
SAN JOSE MEDICAL CENTER (O, 327 beds) 675 East Santa Clara Street, San Jose, CA Zip 95112; tel. 408/998–3212

For explanation of codes following names, see page B2.
★Indicates Type III membership in the American Hospital Association.

Systems / Good Samaritan Health System

SOUTH VALLEY HOSPITAL (O, 93 beds) 9400 No Name Uno, Gilroy, CA Zip 95020-2368; tel. 408/848-2000; James M. Davis, Vice President and Administrator

Owned, leased, sponsored:	4 hospitals	1319 beds
Contract–managed:	0 hospitals	0 beds
Totals:	4 hospitals	1319 beds

0006: GRADUATE HEALTH SYSTEM (NP)
2129 Chestnut Street, Philadelphia, PA Zip 19103; tel. 215/448-1500; Harold Cramer, Chairman and Chief Executive Officer

NEW JERSEY: RANCOCAS HOSPITAL (O, 246 beds) 218-A Sunset Road, Willingboro, NJ Zip 08046-1162; tel. 609/835-2900; Garry L. Scheib, President

ZURBRUGG MEMORIAL HOSPITAL (O, 54 beds) Hospital Plaza, Riverside, NJ Zip 08075; tel. 609/461-6700; Garry L. Scheib, President

PENNSYLVANIA: COMMUNITY GENERAL HOSPITAL (O, 161 beds) 145 North Sixth Street, Reading, PA Zip 19601, Mailing Address: P.O. Box 1728, Zip 19603-1728; tel. 610/376-2100; S. Michael Francis, President and Chief Executive Officer

GRADUATE HEALTH SYSTEM–CITY AVENUE HOSPITAL (O, 190 beds) 4150 City Avenue, Philadelphia, PA Zip 19131-1696; tel. 215/871-1000; Melvyn E. Smith, Executive Director and Chief Executive Officer

GRADUATE HEALTH SYSTEM–PARKVIEW HOSPITAL (O, 181 beds) 1331 East Wyoming Avenue, Philadelphia, PA Zip 19124; tel. 215/537-7400; Bernadette M. Mangan, President

GRADUATE HOSPITAL (O, 306 beds) One Graduate Plaza, Philadelphia, PA Zip 19146-1497; tel. 215/893-2000; Samuel H. Steinberg, President

MT. SINAI HOSPITAL (O, 160 beds) 1429 South Fifth Street, Philadelphia, PA Zip 19147-5999; tel. 215/339-3456; Michele M. Volpe, President

Owned, leased, sponsored:	7 hospitals	1298 beds
Contract–managed:	0 hospitals	0 beds
Totals:	7 hospitals	1298 beds

★1535: GREAT PLAINS HEALTH ALLIANCE, INC. (NP)
625 Third, Phillipsburg, KS Zip 67661, Mailing Address: Box 366, Zip 67661-0366; tel. 913/543-2111; Roger S. John, President and Chief Executive Officer

KANSAS: ASHLAND DISTRICT HOSPITAL (CM, 52 beds) 709 Oak Street, Ashland, KS Zip 67831, Mailing Address: P.O. Box 188, Zip 67831; tel. 316/635-2241; Leanne Pike, Administrator

CHEYENNE COUNTY HOSPITAL (L, 23 beds) 210 West First Street, Saint Francis, KS Zip 67756, Mailing Address: P.O. Box 547, Zip 67756-0547; tel. 913/332-2104; Leslie Lacy, Administrator

ELLINWOOD DISTRICT HOSPITAL (L, 24 beds) 605 North Main Street, Ellinwood, KS Zip 67526; tel. 316/564-2548; Marge Ney R.N., Administrator

FREDONIA REGIONAL HOSPITAL (CM, 42 beds) 1527 Madison Street, Fredonia, KS Zip 66736, Mailing Address: Box 579, Zip 66736; tel. 316/378-2121; Terry Deschaine, Administrator

GREELEY COUNTY HOSPITAL (L, 50 beds) 506 Third Street, Tribune, KS Zip 67879, Mailing Address: Box 338, Zip 67879; tel. 316/376-4221; Thomas A. Keeffer, Administrator

GREENWOOD COUNTY HOSPITAL (L, 46 beds) 100 West 16th Street, Eureka, KS Zip 67045; tel. 316/583-7451; Jerry Aldridge, Administrator

GRISELL MEMORIAL HOSPITAL DISTRICT ONE (CM, 46 beds) 210 South Vermont, Ransom, KS Zip 67572-0268, Mailing Address: P.O. Box 268, Zip 67572-0268; tel. 913/731-2231; Kristine Ochs R.N., Administrator

LANE COUNTY HOSPITAL (CM, 31 beds) 243 South Second, Dighton, KS Zip 67839, Mailing Address: Box 969, Zip 67839; tel. 316/397-5321; Donna McGowan R.N., Administrator

LINCOLN COUNTY HOSPITAL (CM, 34 beds) 624 North Second Street, Lincoln, KS Zip 67455, Mailing Address: P.O. Box 406, Zip 67455; tel. 913/524-4403; Jolene Yager R.N., Administrator

MEDICINE LODGE MEMORIAL HOSPITAL (CM, 42 beds) 710 North Walnut Street, Medicine Lodge, KS Zip 67104, Mailing Address: P.O. Drawer C, Zip 67104; tel. 316/886-3771; Kevin A. White, Administrator

MINNEOLA DISTRICT HOSPITAL (CM, 15 beds) 212 Main Street, Minneola, KS Zip 67865; tel. 316/885-4264; Blaine K. Miller, Administrator

MITCHELL COUNTY COMMUNITY HOSPITAL (L, 89 beds) 400 West Eighth, Beloit, KS Zip 67420, Mailing Address: P.O. Box 399, Zip 67420; tel. 913/738-2266; Jeffrey S. Tarrant, Administrator

OSBORNE COUNTY MEMORIAL HOSPITAL (CM, 29 beds) 424 West New Hampshire Street, Osborne, KS Zip 67473-0070, Mailing Address: P.O. Box 70, Zip 67473-0070; tel. 913/346-2121; Patricia Bernard R.N., Administrator

OTTAWA COUNTY HOSPITAL (L, 53 beds) 215 East Eighth, Minneapolis, KS Zip 67467, Mailing Address: Box 209, Zip 67467; tel. 913/392-2122; Joy Reed R.N., Administrator

PHILLIPS COUNTY HOSPITAL (L, 62 beds) 1150 State Street, Phillipsburg, KS Zip 67661, Mailing Address: Box 607, Zip 67661; tel. 913/543-5226; James L. Giedd, Administrator

REPUBLIC COUNTY HOSPITAL (L, 86 beds) 2420 G Street, Belleville, KS Zip 66935; tel. 913/527-2255; Charles A. Westin FACHE, Administrator

SABETHA COMMUNITY HOSPITAL (L, 27 beds) 14th And Oregon Streets, Sabetha, KS Zip 66534, Mailing Address: P.O. Box 229, Zip 66534; tel. 913/284-2121; Rita K. Buurman, Administrator

SATANTA DISTRICT HOSPITAL (CM, 42 beds) Cheyenne and Apache, Satanta, KS Zip 67870, Mailing Address: P.O. Box 159, Zip 67870-0159; tel. 316/649-2761; T. G. Lee, Administrator

SMITH COUNTY MEMORIAL HOSPITAL (L, 54 beds) 614 South Main Street, Smith Center, KS Zip 66967-0349, Mailing Address: P.O. Box 349, Zip 66967-0349; tel. 913/282-6845; John Terrill, Administrator

TREGO COUNTY–LEMKE MEMORIAL HOSPITAL (CM, 73 beds) 320 13th Street, Wakeeney, KS Zip 67672-2099; tel. 913/743-2182; James Wahlmeier, Administrator

NEBRASKA: COMMUNITY HOSPITAL (CM, 49 beds) 2307 Barada Street, Falls City, NE Zip 68355-1599; tel. 402/245-2428; Victor Lee, Chief Executive Officer and Administrator

HARLAN COUNTY HOSPITAL (CM, 25 beds) 717 North Brown, Alma, NE Zip 68920, Mailing Address: P.O. Box 836, Zip 68920; tel. 308/928-2151; Allen Van Driel, Administrator

Owned, leased, sponsored:	10 hospitals	514 beds
Contract–managed:	12 hospitals	480 beds
Totals:	22 hospitals	994 beds

0046: GREATER ROCHESTER HEALTH SYSTEM, INC. (NP)
1040 University Avenue, Rochester, NY Zip 14607; tel. 716/266-0720; Arthur E. Liebert, President

NEW YORK: GENESEE HOSPITAL (O, 385 beds) 224 Alexander Street, Rochester, NY Zip 14607-4055; tel. 716/263-6000; Joseph J. DeSilva FACHE, President and Chief Executive Officer

NEWARK–WAYNE COMMUNITY HOSPITAL (O, 280 beds) Driving Park Avenue, Newark, NY Zip 14513, Mailing Address: P.O. Box 111, Zip 14513-0111; tel. 315/332-2022; L. J. Danehy, President

ROCHESTER GENERAL HOSPITAL (O, 526 beds) 1425 Portland Avenue, Rochester, NY Zip 14621-3099; tel. 716/338-4000; Steven I. Goldstein, President and Chief Executive Officer

Owned, leased, sponsored:	3 hospitals	1191 beds
Contract–managed:	0 hospitals	0 beds
Totals:	3 hospitals	1191 beds

1155: GREENLEAF HEALTH SYSTEMS, INC. (IO)
One Northgate Park, Chattanooga, TN Zip 37415; tel. 615/870-5110; Dan B. Page, President

ARKANSAS: GREENLEAF CENTER (O, 48 beds) 2712 East Johnson, Jonesboro, AR Zip 72401; tel. 501/932-2800; John S. Hart, Administrator

GEORGIA: GREENLEAF CENTER (O, 90 beds) 500 Greenleaf Circle, Fort Oglethorpe, GA Zip 30742; tel. 706/861-4357; Richard A. Waxler, Administrator

GREENLEAF CENTER (O, 70 beds) 2209 Pineview Drive, Valdosta, GA Zip 31602; tel. 912/247-4357; Michael Lane, Administrator and Chief Executive Officer

Owned, leased, sponsored:	3 hospitals	208 beds
Contract–managed:	0 hospitals	0 beds
Totals:	3 hospitals	208 beds

For explanation of codes following names, see page B2.
★Indicates Type III membership in the American Hospital Association.

★1555: GREENVILLE HOSPITAL SYSTEM (NP)
701 Grove Road, Greenville, SC Zip 29605–4211; tel. 803/455–7000; Frank D. Pinckney, President

SOUTH CAROLINA: ALLEN BENNETT HOSPITAL (O, 158 beds) Greer, SC, Mailing Address: Box 1149, Zip 29652–1149; tel. 803/848–8130; Michael W. Massey, Administrator

GREENVILLE GENERAL HOSPITAL (O, 14 beds) 100 Mallard Street, Greenville, SC Zip 29601–4211, Mailing Address: 701 Grove Road, Zip 29605–4295; tel. 803/455–8609; William W. Heizer, Administrator

GREENVILLE MEMORIAL HOSPITAL (O, 843 beds) 701 Grove Road, Greenville, SC Zip 29605–4295; tel. 803/455–7000; J. Bland Burkhardt, Jr., Senior Vice President and Administrator

HILLCREST HOSPITAL (O, 46 beds) 729 Southeast Main Street, Simpsonville, SC Zip 29681, Mailing Address: Box 279, Zip 29681–0279; tel. 803/967–6100; James Dover, Administrator

MARSHALL I. PICKENS HOSPITAL (O, 106 beds) 701 Grove Road, Greenville, SC Zip 29605–4295; tel. 803/455–7836; Ryan D. Beaty, Administrator

NORTH GREENVILLE HOSPITAL (O, 53 beds) 807 North Main Street, Travelers Rest, SC Zip 29690–0628; tel. 803/834–5131; Ryan D. Beaty, Administrator

ROGER C. PEACE REHABILITATION HOSPITAL (O, 50 beds) 701 Grove Road, Greenville, SC Zip 29605–4295; tel. 803/455–7000

Owned, leased, sponsored:	7 hospitals	1270 beds
Contract–managed:	0 hospitals	0 beds
Totals:	7 hospitals	1270 beds

★9995: GROUP HEALTH COOPERATIVE OF PUGET SOUND (NP)
521 Wall Street, Seattle, WA Zip 98121–1536; tel. 206/326–3000; Phil Nudelman Ph.D., President and Chief Executive Officer

WASHINGTON: GROUP HEALTH COOPERATIVE CENTRAL HOSPITAL (O, 222 beds) 201 16th Avenue East, Seattle, WA Zip 98112–5298; tel. 206/326–3000; Sue Hennessy, Regional Vice President

THE EASTSIDE HOSPITAL (O, 142 beds) 2700 152nd Avenue N.E., Redmond, WA Zip 98052–5560; tel. 206/883–5151; Janice Jones, East Region Vice President

Owned, leased, sponsored:	2 hospitals	364 beds
Contract–managed:	0 hospitals	0 beds
Totals:	2 hospitals	364 beds

★0675: GUTHRIE HEALTHCARE SYSTEM (NP)
Guthrie Square, Sayre, PA Zip 18840; tel. 717/882–4312; Ralph H. Meyer, President

PENNSYLVANIA: ROBERT PACKER HOSPITAL (O, 366 beds) Guthrie Square, Sayre, PA Zip 18840; tel. 717/888–6666; Russell M. Knight, President

TROY COMMUNITY HOSPITAL (O, 35 beds) 100 John Street, Troy, PA Zip 16947; tel. 717/297–2121; Mark A. Webster, President

Owned, leased, sponsored:	2 hospitals	401 beds
Contract–managed:	0 hospitals	0 beds
Totals:	2 hospitals	401 beds

5895: HALLMARK HEALTHCARE CORPORATION (IO)
300 Galleria Parkway, Suite 650, Atlanta, GA Zip 30339–5949, Mailing Address: P.O. Box 723049, Zip 30339–0049; tel. 404/933–5500; James T. McAfee Jr., Chairman and Chief Executive Officer

ALABAMA: HARTSELLE MEDICAL CENTER (O, 119 beds) 201 Pine Street N.W., Hartselle, AL Zip 35640, Mailing Address: P.O. Box 969, Zip 35640; tel. 205/773–6511; David E. Loving, Managing Director

L. V. STABLER MEMORIAL HOSPITAL (O, 67 beds) Highway 10 West, Greenville, AL Zip 36037–0915, Mailing Address: Box 1000, Zip 36037–0915; tel. 334/382–2671; Steve Southerland, Executive Director

PARKWAY MEDICAL CENTER HOSPITAL (O, 94 beds) 1874 Beltline Road S.W., Decatur, AL Zip 35601, Mailing Address: P.O. Box 2211, Zip 35609; tel. 205/350–2211; Philip J. Mazzuca, Managing Director

WOODLAND COMMUNITY HOSPITAL (O, 100 beds) 1910 Cherokee Avenue S.W., Cullman, AL Zip 35055; tel. 205/739–3500; Lowell Benton, Executive Director

ARKANSAS: HARRIS HOSPITAL (O, 88 beds) 1205 McLain Street, Newport, AR Zip 72112; tel. 501/523–8911; Ronald T. Seal, Executive Director

RANDOLPH COUNTY MEDICAL CENTER (L, 50 beds) 2801 Medical Center Drive, Pocahontas, AR Zip 72455; tel. 501/892–4511; Michael J. McBride, Executive Director

FLORIDA: DOCTORS MEMORIAL HOSPITAL (L, 34 beds) 401 East Byrd Avenue, Bonifay, FL Zip 32425, Mailing Address: Box 188, Zip 32425; tel. 904/547–1120; Robert E. Winkler, Aministrator

GEORGIA: BERRIEN COUNTY HOSPITAL (O, 167 beds) 1221 East McPherson Street, Nashville, GA Zip 31639, Mailing Address: P.O. Box 665, Zip 31639; tel. 912/686–7471; James P. Seward, Jr., Executive Director

ILLINOIS: CROSSROADS COMMUNITY HOSPITAL (O, 49 beds) 8 Doctors Park, Mount Vernon, IL Zip 62864; tel. 618/244–5500; Chris Wearmouth, Managing Director

LOUISIANA: BYRD REGIONAL HOSPITAL (O, 59 beds) 1020 Fertitta Boulevard, Leesville, LA Zip 71446; tel. 318/239–9041; Robert J. Trautman, Executive Director

RIVERNORTH HOSPITAL CENTER (O, 53 beds) 5505 Shreveport Highway, Pineville, LA Zip 71360; tel. 318/640–0222; Daniel W. Johnson, Chief Executive Officer

SABINE MEDICAL CENTER (O, 68 beds) 240 Highland Drive, Many, LA Zip 71449–3718; tel. 318/256–5691; Frances F. Hopkins, Administrator

TENNESSEE: CLEVELAND COMMUNITY HOSPITAL (O, 70 beds) 2800 Westside Drive N.W., Cleveland, TN Zip 37312; tel. 615/339–4100; Stanley G. Hilliard, Administrator

WHITE COUNTY COMMUNITY HOSPITAL (O, 60 beds) 401 Sewell Road, Sparta, TN Zip 38583; tel. 615/738–9211; Raymond W. Acker, Administrator

TEXAS: HILL REGIONAL HOSPITAL (O, 92 beds) 101 Circle Drive, Hillsboro, TX Zip 76645; tel. 817/582–8425; Jan McClure, Chief Executive Officer

SCENIC MOUNTAIN MEDICAL CENTER (O, 153 beds) 1601 West 11th Place, Big Spring, TX Zip 79720; tel. 915/263–1211; Kenneth W. Randall, Administrator

Owned, leased, sponsored:	16 hospitals	1323 beds
Contract–managed:	0 hospitals	0 beds
Totals:	16 hospitals	1323 beds

★2345: HARRIS METHODIST HEALTH SYSTEM (CO)
6000 Western Place, Suite 200, Fort Worth, TX Zip 76107; tel. 817/570–8900; Ronald L. Smith, President

TEXAS: HARRIS CONTINUED CARE HOSPITAL (O, 10 beds) 1301 Pennsylvania Ave, 4th Floor, Fort Worth, TX Zip 76104, Mailing Address: P.O. Box 3471, Zip 76113; tel. 817/878–5500; Karen Van Wagner Ph.D., Administrator

HARRIS METHODIST FORT WORTH (O, 581 beds) 1301 Pennsylvania Avenue, Fort Worth, TX Zip 76104–2895; tel. 817/882–2000; Barclay E. Berdan, Administrator

HARRIS METHODIST SOUTHWEST (O, 58 beds) 6100 Harris Parkway, Fort Worth, TX Zip 76132; tel. 817/346–5050; Kim Callanan, Senior Vice President and Administrator

HARRIS METHODIST–ERATH COUNTY (O, 72 beds) 411 North Belknap Street, Stephenville, TX Zip 76401–1399, Mailing Address: Box 1399, Zip 76401; tel. 817/965–1500; Michael D. Murphy, Administrator

HARRIS METHODIST–HEB (O, 177 beds) 1600 Hospital Parkway, Bedford, TX Zip 76022–6913, Mailing Address: P.O. Box 669, Zip 76095; tel. 817/685–4000

HARRIS METHODIST–NORTHWEST (O, 38 beds) 108 Denver Trail, Azle, TX Zip 76020; tel. 817/444–8600; Larry Thompson, Vice President and Administrator

WALLS REGIONAL HOSPITAL (O, 102 beds) 201 Walls Drive, Cleburne, TX Zip 76031; tel. 817/641–2551; Brent D. Magers, Administrator

Owned, leased, sponsored:	7 hospitals	1038 beds
Contract–managed:	0 hospitals	0 beds
Totals:	7 hospitals	1038 beds

1775: HEALTH MANAGEMENT ASSOCIATES (IO)
5811 Pelican Bay Boulevard, Suite 500, Naples, FL Zip 33963–2710; tel. 813/598–3175; William J. Schoen, President

---

For explanation of codes following names, see page B2.
★Indicates Type III membership in the American Hospital Association.

Systems / Health Management Associates

ALABAMA: RIVERVIEW REGIONAL MEDICAL CENTER (O, 281 beds) 600 South Third Street, Gadsden, AL Zip 35901, Mailing Address: P.O. Box 268, Zip 35999-0268; tel. 205/543-5200; Jon P. Vollmer, Executive Director
STRINGFELLOW MEMORIAL HOSPITAL (CM, 45 beds) 301 East 18th Street, Anniston, AL Zip 36201; tel. 205/235-8900; Michael E. Cassidy, Administrator and Chief Executive Officer

ARKANSAS: CRAWFORD MEMORIAL HOSPITAL (O, 103 beds) East Main & South 20th Streets, Van Buren, AR Zip 72956, Mailing Address: Box 409, Zip 72956; tel. 501/474-3401; J. Phillip Young, Administrator

FLORIDA: FISHERMEN'S HOSPITAL (L, 58 beds) 3301 Overseas Highway, Marathon, FL Zip 33050-0068; tel. 305/743-5533; Kevin Van Hoose, Administrator
HIGHLANDS REGIONAL MEDICAL CENTER (L, 126 beds) 3600 South Highlands Avenue, Sebring, FL Zip 33870-5495, Mailing Address: Drawer 2066, Zip 33871-2066; tel. 813/385-6101; C. Scott Campbell, Executive Director
PALMVIEW HOSPITAL (O, 66 beds) 2510 North Florida Avenue, Lakeland, FL Zip 33805; tel. 813/682-6105; Michael Terry, Administrator and Chief Executive Officer
SEBASTIAN RIVER MEDICAL CENTER (O, 133 beds) 13695 North U.S. Hwy 1, Sebastian, FL Zip 32958, Mailing Address: Box 780838, Zip 32978; tel. 407/589-3186; David McCormack, Executive Director

KENTUCKY: PAUL B. HALL REGIONAL MEDICAL CENTER (O, 72 beds) 625 James S Trimble Boulevard, Paintsville, KY Zip 41240, Mailing Address: P.O. Box 1487, Zip 41240; tel. 606/789-3511; Deborah T. Meadows, Administrator

MISSISSIPPI: BILOXI REGIONAL MEDICAL CENTER (O, 153 beds) 150 Reynoir Street, Biloxi, MS Zip 39530, Mailing Address: Box 128, Zip 39533; tel. 601/432-1571; James D. Baker, Executive Director
NATCHEZ COMMUNITY HOSPITAL (O, 101 beds) 129 Jefferson Davis Boulevard, Natchez, MS Zip 39120, Mailing Address: Box 1203, Zip 39121; tel. 601/445-6200; Raymond Bane, Executive Director

NORTH CAROLINA: FRANKLIN REGIONAL MEDICAL CENTER (O, 85 beds) 100 Hospital Drive, Louisburg, NC Zip 27549, Mailing Address: Box 609, Zip 27549; tel. 919/496-5131; Mike H. McNair, Administrator
HAMLET HOSPITAL (L, 64 beds) Rice and Vance Streets, Hamlet, NC Zip 28345, Mailing Address: Box 1109, Zip 28345; tel. 910/582-3611; Page Vaughan, Administrator
LAKE NORMAN REGIONAL MEDICAL CENTER (O, 100 beds) 610 East Center Avenue, Mooresville, NC Zip 28115, Mailing Address: Box 360, Zip 28115; tel. 704/663-1113; David L. Miller, Executive Director

OKLAHOMA: MEDICAL CENTER OF SOUTHEASTERN OKLAHOMA (O, 103 beds) 1800 University, Durant, OK Zip 74701, Mailing Address: P.O. Box 1207, Zip 74702; tel. 405/924-3080; Gary D. Newsome, Chief Executive Director

SOUTH CAROLINA: UPSTATE CAROLINA MEDICAL CENTER (O, 125 beds) 1530 North Limestone Street, Gaffney, SC Zip 29340; tel. 803/487-4271; Steve Midkiff, Executive Director

TEXAS: NORTHEAST MEDICAL CENTER (O, 65 beds) 504 Lipscomb Boulevard, Bonham, TX Zip 75418-4096, Mailing Address: P.O. Drawer C, Zip 75418; tel. 903/583-8585

WEST VIRGINIA: WILLIAMSON MEMORIAL HOSPITAL (O, 76 beds) 859 Alderson Street, Williamson, WV Zip 25661, Mailing Address: P.O. Box 1980, Zip 25661; tel. 304/235-2500; Roger C. LeDoux, Administrator

Owned, leased, sponsored:	16 hospitals	1711 beds
Contract-managed:	1 hospitals	45 beds
Totals:	17 hospitals	1756 beds

★8815: HEALTH MIDWEST (NP)
2304 East Meyer Boulevard, Suite A-20, Kansas City, MO Zip 64132-4104; tel. 816/276-9181; Richard W. Brown, President and Chief Executive Officer

KANSAS: ALLEN COUNTY HOSPITAL (L, 49 beds) 101 South First Street, Iola, KS Zip 66749, Mailing Address: P.O. Box 540, Zip 66749-0540; tel. 316/365-3131; Franklin K. Wilson, Administrator

MISSOURI: BAPTIST MEDICAL CENTER (O, 315 beds) 6601 Rockhill Road, Kansas City, MO Zip 64131-1197; tel. 816/276-7000; Dan H. Anderson, President and Chief Executive Officer
CASS MEDICAL CENTER (CM, 42 beds) 1800 East Mechanic Street, Harrisonville, MO Zip 64701; tel. 816/884-3291; David G. Couser, Administrator
LAFAYETTE REGIONAL HEALTH CENTER (L, 37 beds) 1500 State Street, Lexington, MO Zip 64067-1199; tel. 816/259-2203; Michael S. McCoy, Administrator
LEE'S SUMMIT HOSPITAL (O, 77 beds) 530 North Murray Road, Lees Summit, MO Zip 64081-1497; tel. 816/251-7000; John L. Jacobson, President and Chief Executive Officer
MEDICAL CENTER OF INDEPENDENCE (O, 133 beds) 17203 East 23rd Street, Independence, MO Zip 64057; tel. 816/478-5000; Mike Chappelow, President and Chief Executive Officer
MENORAH MEDICAL CENTER (O, 259 beds) 4949 Rockhill Road, Kansas City, MO Zip 64110-2298; tel. 816/276-8000; Roy A. Powell, President
REHABILITATION INSTITUTE (O, 20 beds) 3011 Baltimore, Kansas City, MO Zip 64108-3465; tel. 816/756-2250; John H. Parker, President
RESEARCH BELTON HOSPITAL (O, 40 beds) 17065 South 71 Highway, Belton, MO Zip 64012-0487; tel. 816/348-1200; Daniel F. Sheehan, Administrator
RESEARCH MEDICAL CENTER (O, 480 beds) 2316 East Meyer Boulevard, Kansas City, MO Zip 64132-1199; tel. 816/276-4000; Dan H. Anderson, President and Chief Executive Officer
TRINITY LUTHERAN HOSPITAL (O, 358 beds) 3030 Baltimore Avenue, Kansas City, MO Zip 64108-3404; tel. 816/751-4600; Ronald A. Ommen, President

Owned, leased, sponsored:	10 hospitals	1768 beds
Contract-managed:	1 hospitals	42 beds
Totals:	11 hospitals	1810 beds

0395: HEALTHCARE INTERNATIONAL, INC. (IO)
912 South Capital of Texas Highway, Austin, TX Zip 78765-5210, Mailing Address: P.O. Box 4008, Zip 78765-4008; tel. 512/329-8821; Kevin Sheehan, President and Chief Executive Officer

COLORADO: CEDAR SPRINGS PSYCHIATRIC HOSPITAL (O, 100 beds) 2135 Southgate Road, Colorado Springs, CO Zip 80906, Mailing Address: Box 640, Zip 80901; tel. 719/633-4114

TEXAS: CYPRESS CREEK HOSPITAL (O, 78 beds) 17750 Cali Drive, Houston, TX Zip 77090-2700; tel. 713/586-7600; Dan R. Riley, Administrator
GREEN OAKS HOSPITAL (O, 106 beds) 7808 Clodus Fields Drive, Dallas, TX Zip 75251; tel. 214/991-9504; Thomas M. Collins, Administrator
HEALTHCARE REHABILITATION CENTER (O, 149 beds) 1106 West Dittmar, Austin, TX Zip 78745-9990, Mailing Address: P.O. Box 43148, Zip 78745-9990; tel. 512/444-4835; Cindy McLendon, Administrator
OAKS TREATMENT CENTER (O, 98 beds) 1407 West Stassney Lane, Austin, TX Zip 78745; tel. 512/444-9561; Richard R. Hardin, Executive Director
SAN MARCOS TREATMENT CENTER (O, 152 beds) San Marcos, TX, Mailing Address: P.O. Box 768, Zip 78667-0768; tel. 512/396-8500; Armin Steege, Administrator
WEST OAKS HOSPITAL (O, 150 beds) 6500 Hornwood, Houston, TX Zip 77074, Mailing Address: Box 741389, Zip 77274; tel. 713/995-0909; Margo Bonner, Administrator

VIRGINIA: CUMBERLAND HOSPITAL FOR CHILDREN AND ADOLESCENTS (O, 71 beds) 9407 Cumberland Road, New Kent, VA Zip 23124; tel. 804/966-2242; Leslie Wyatt, Administrator

Owned, leased, sponsored:	8 hospitals	904 beds
Contract-managed:	0 hospitals	0 beds
Totals:	8 hospitals	904 beds

1585: HEALTHCARE MANAGEMENT GROUP, INC. (IO)
776 Baconsfield Drive, Suite 209, Macon, GA Zip 31211-0101; tel. 912/743-5606; Earl Bonds Jr., Chief Executive Officer

GEORGIA: MORGAN MEMORIAL HOSPITAL (L, 26 beds) Canterbury Park, Madison, GA Zip 30650, Mailing Address: Box 860, Zip 30650; tel. 706/342-1667; Shirley C. Harridge, Administrator
SYLVAN GROVE HOSPITAL (L, 28 beds) 1050 McDonough Road, Jackson, GA Zip 30233; tel. 404/775-7861; Jack S. Frayer, Administrator

Owned, leased, sponsored:	2 hospitals	54 beds
Contract-managed:	0 hospitals	0 beds
Totals:	2 hospitals	54 beds

2795: HEALTHCORP OF TENNESSEE, INC. (IO)
735 Broad Street, Chattanooga, TN Zip 37402; tel. 615/267-8406; T. Farrell Hayes, President

---

For explanation of codes following names, see page B2.
★Indicates Type III membership in the American Hospital Association.

Systems / Healthsouth Corporation

ALABAMA: LAKESHORE COMMUNITY HOSPITAL (CM, 27 beds) 201 Mariarden Road, Dadeville, AL Zip 36853, Mailing Address: P.O. Box 248, Zip 36853; tel. 205/825–7821; Mavis B. Halko, Administrator

LAKEVIEW COMMUNITY HOSPITAL (CM, 74 beds) 820 West Washington Street, Eufaula, AL Zip 36027; tel. 205/687–5761; Carl D. Brown, Associate Administrator

VAUGHAN CHILTON MEDICAL CENTER (L, 25 beds) 1010 Lay Dam Road, Clanton, AL Zip 35045; tel. 205/755–2500; Jeffrey Potts, Administrator

ARKANSAS: DALLAS COUNTY HOSPITAL (O, 83 beds) 201 Clifton Street, Fordyce, AR Zip 71742; tel. 501/352–3155; Greg R. McNeil, Administrator

TENNESSEE: NORTH PARK HOSPITAL (CM, 83 beds) 2051 Hamill Road, Chattanooga, TN Zip 37343–4096; tel. 615/870–1300; Roger W. Glass, Administrator

Owned, leased, sponsored:	2 hospitals	108 beds
Contract-managed:	3 hospitals	184 beds
Totals:	5 hospitals	292 beds

★**2185: HEALTHEAST** (NP)
559 Capitol Boulevard, 6–South, Saint Paul, MN Zip 55103–0000; tel. 612/232–2300; Tim Hanson, President and Chief Executive Officer

MINNESOTA: HEALTHEAST BETHESDA LUTHERAN HOSPITAL AND REHABILITATION CENTER (O, 135 beds) 559 Capitol Boulevard, Saint Paul, MN Zip 55103; tel. 612/232–2133; Bonnie Watkins, Administrator

HEALTHEAST MIDWAY HOSPITAL (O, 201 beds) 1700 University Avenue, Saint Paul, MN Zip 55104–2791; tel. 612/232–5000; Douglas P. Cropper, Vice President and Administrator

HEALTHEAST ST. JOHN'S HOSPITAL (O, 179 beds) 1575 Beam Avenue, Maplewood, MN Zip 55109; tel. 612/232–7000; William Knutson, Administrator

HEALTHEAST ST. JOSEPH'S HOSPITAL (O, 297 beds) 69 West Exchange Street, Saint Paul, MN Zip 55102; tel. 612/232–3000; Milton Hertel, Administrator

Owned, leased, sponsored:	4 hospitals	812 beds
Contract–managed:	0 hospitals	0 beds
Totals:	4 hospitals	812 beds

★**0935: HEALTHONE HEALTHCARE SYSTEM** (NP)
501 East Hampden Avenue, Englewood, CO Zip 80110, Mailing Address: P.O. Box 2901, Zip 80150–0101; tel. 303/788–6484; Nick Hilger, President and Chief Executive Officer

COLORADO: AURORA PRESBYTERIAN HOSPITAL (O, 138 beds) 700 Potomac Street, Aurora, CO Zip 80011–6792; tel. 303/363–7200; H. Phil Herre, Administrator

HEALTHONE–BEHAVIORAL HEALTH SERVICES, BETHESDA CAMPUS (O, 82 beds) 4400 East Iliff Avenue, Denver, CO Zip 80222; tel. 303/758–1514; William Kent Ph.D., Vice President Behavioral Health

PRESBYTERIAN–ST. LUKE'S MEDICAL CENTER (O, 558 beds) 1719 East 19th Avenue, Denver, CO Zip 80218; tel. 303/839–6000; H. Phil Herre, Chief Operating Officer

ROCKY MOUNTAIN REHABILITATION INSTITUTE (O, 76 beds) 900 Potomac Street, Aurora, CO Zip 80011–6716; tel. 303/367–1166; Russell W. York, President and Chief Executive Officer

SWEDISH MEDICAL CENTER (O, 310 beds) 501 East Hampden Avenue, Englewood, CO Zip 80110–0101, Mailing Address: P.O. Box 2901, Zip 80150–0101; tel. 303/788–5000; Margaret D. Sabin, Vice President and Administrator

Owned, leased, sponsored:	5 hospitals	1164 beds
Contract–managed:	0 hospitals	0 beds
Totals:	5 hospitals	1164 beds

0023: HEALTHSOUTH CORPORATION (IO)
Two Perimeter Park South, Birmingham, AL Zip 35243; tel. 205/967–7116; Anthony J. Tanner, Executive Vice President

ALABAMA: HEALTHSOUTH MEDICAL CENTER (O, 177 beds) 1201 11th Avenue South, Birmingham, AL Zip 35205; tel. 205/930–7000; Frank R. Gannon, Administrator

HEALTHSOUTH REHABILITATION HOSPITAL OF MONTGOMERY (O, 80 beds) 4465 Narrow Lane Road, Montgomery, AL Zip 36116; tel. 334/284–7700; Arnold F. McRae, Administrator and Chief Executive Officer

ARKANSAS: HEALTHSOUTH REHABILITATION HOSPITAL OF FORT SMITH (O, 80 beds) 1401 South J Street, Fort Smith, AR Zip 72901; tel. 501/785–3300; Stan Johnson, Administrator and Chief Executive Officer

FLORIDA: HEALTHSOUTH DOCTORS' HOSPITAL (O, 157 beds) 5000 University Drive, Coral Gables, FL Zip 33146–2094; tel. 305/666–2111; E. Tim Cook, Chief Executive Officer

HEALTHSOUTH LARKIN HOSPITAL (O, 112 beds) 7031 Southwest 62nd Avenue, South Miami, FL Zip 33143; tel. 305/284–7700; Mel D. Deutsch, Administrator

HEALTHSOUTH REHABILITATION HOSPITAL (O, 40 beds) 901 North Clearwater–Largo Rd, Largo, FL Zip 34640–1955; tel. 813/586–2999; Vincent O. Nico, Administrator

HEALTHSOUTH REHABILITATION HOSPITAL OF TALLAHASSEE (O, 70 beds) 1675 Riggins Road, Tallahassee, FL Zip 32308–5315; tel. 904/656–4800; Mike Marshall, Chief Executive Officer

HEALTHSOUTH REHABILITATION INSTITUTE OF SARASOTA (O, 60 beds) 3251 Proctor Road, Sarasota, FL Zip 34231–8538; tel. 813/921–8600; Jeff Garber, Administrator and Chief Executive Officer

HEALTHSOUTH SEA PINES REHABILITATION HOSPITAL (O, 80 beds) 101 East Florida Avenue, Melbourne, FL Zip 32901–9966; tel. 407/984–4600; Robert M. Smart, Administrator and Chief Executive Officer

HEALTHSOUTH SUNRISE REHABILITATION HOSPITAL (O, 108 beds) 4399 Nob Hill Road, Fort Lauderdale, FL Zip 33351–5899; tel. 305/749–0300; Barbara D. Hayes, Administrator

HEALTHSOUTH TREASURE COAST REHABILITATION HOSPITAL (O, 70 beds) 1600 37th Street, Vero Beach, FL Zip 32960–6549; tel. 407/778–2100; Mark J. Tarr, Administrator and Chief Executive Officer

NEW HAMPSHIRE: HEALTHSOUTH REHABILITATION HOSPITAL (O, 53 beds) 254 Pleasant Street, Concord, NH Zip 03301; tel. 603/226–9800

NEW JERSEY: HEALTHSOUTH REHABILITATION HOSPITAL OF NEW JERSEY (O, 119 beds) 14 Hospital Drive, Toms River, NJ Zip 08755; tel. 908/244–3100; David Coluzzi, Administrator and Chief Executive Officer

NEW MEXICO: HEALTHSOUTH REHABILITATION HOSPITAL (O, 60 beds) 7000 Jefferson N.E., Albuquerque, NM Zip 87109; tel. 505/344–9478; Darby Brockette, Administrator

OKLAHOMA: HEALTHSOUTH REHABILITATION HOSPITAL (O, 46 beds) 700 Northwest Seventh Street, Oklahoma City, OK Zip 73102–1295; tel. 405/236–3131; Ronald J. Castagnl FACHE, Administrator and Chief Executive Officer

PENNSYLVANIA: HEALTHSOUTH GREAT LAKES REHABILITATION HOSPITAL (O, 108 beds) 143 East Second Street, Erie, PA Zip 16507; tel. 814/878–1200; William R. Fox, Chief Executive Officer

HEALTHSOUTH GREATER PITTSBURGH REHAB HOSPITAL (O, 89 beds) 2380 McGinley Road, Monroeville, PA Zip 15146; tel. 412/856–2400; Faith A. Deigan, Administrator

HEALTHSOUTH LAKE ERIE INSTITUTE OF REHABILITATION (O, 99 beds) 137 West Second Street, Erie, PA Zip 16507–1403; tel. 814/453–5602; William R. Fox, Chief Executive Officer

HEALTHSOUTH NITTANY VALLEY REHABILITATION HOSPITAL (O, 88 beds) 550 West College Avenue, Pleasant Gap, PA Zip 16823–8808; tel. 814/359–3421; Mary Jane Hawkins, Administrator and Chief Executive Officer

HEALTHSOUTH REHABILITATION HOSPITAL OF ALTOONA (O, 66 beds) 2005 Valley View Boulevard, Altoona, PA Zip 16602; tel. 814/944–3535; Felix Mariani, Administrator

HEALTHSOUTH REHABILITATION HOSPITAL OF YORK (O, 88 beds) 1850 Normandie Drive, York, PA Zip 17404–1534; tel. 717/767–6941; Patricia McMurry, Administrator

HEALTHSOUTH REHABILITATION OF MECHANICSBURG (O, 103 beds) 175 Lancaster Boulevard, Mechanicsburg, PA Zip 17055–2016, Mailing Address: P.O. Box 2016, Zip 17055–2016; tel. 717/691–3700; Glen R. Davis, Administrator and Chief Executive Officer

SOUTH CAROLINA: HEALTHSOUTH REHABILITATION HOSPITAL (O, 89 beds) 2935 Colonial Drive, Columbia, SC Zip 29203; tel. 803/254–7777; Mark J. Stepanik, Administrator

TEXAS: HEALTHSOUTH DALLAS REHABILITATION INSTITUTE (O, 126 beds) 9713 Harry Hines Boulevard, Dallas, TX Zip 75220–5441; tel. 214/358–6000; Phillip L. Coppage, Administrator

HEALTHSOUTH MEDICAL CENTER (O, 96 beds) 2124 Research Row, Dallas, TX Zip 75235; tel. 214/904–6100

For explanation of codes following names, see page B2.
★Indicates Type III membership in the American Hospital Association.

Systems / Healthsouth Corporation

HEALTHSOUTH REHABILITATION HOSPITAL (O, 60 beds) 1212 West Lancaster, Fort Worth, TX Zip 76102; tel. 817/870–2336; Laura J. Lycan, Administrator

HEALTHSOUTH REHABILITATION HOSPITAL (O, 69 beds) 19002 McKay Drive, Humble, TX Zip 77338; tel. 713/446–6148; Jessica A. Nantz, Chief Executive Officer

HEALTHSOUTH REHABILITATION HOSPITAL OF AUSTIN (O, 80 beds) 1215 Red River Street, Austin, TX Zip 78701, Mailing Address: P.O. Box 13366, Zip 78711–3366; tel. 512/474–5700; Mike Munnerlyn, Chief Executive Officer

HEALTHSOUTH REHABILITATION HOSPITAL OF TEXARKANA (O, 60 beds) 515 West 12th Street, Texarkana, TX Zip 75501; tel. 903/793–0088; Hank Ross, Chief Executive Officer

HEALTHSOUTH REHABILITATION INSTITUTE OF SAN ANTONIO (O, 108 beds) 9119 Cinnamon Hill, San Antonio, TX Zip 78240; tel. 210/691–0737; Diane B. Lampe R.N., Administrator and Chief Executive Officer

UTAH: HEALTHSOUTH REHABILITATION HOSPITAL OF UTAH (O, 73 beds) 8074 South 1300 East, Sandy, UT Zip 84094; tel. 801/561–3400; Robert Cash, Administrator and Chief Executive Officer

VIRGINIA: HEALTHSOUTH MEDICAL CENTER (O, 127 beds) 7700 East Parham Road, Richmond, VA Zip 23294–1999; tel. 804/747–5600; Charles A. Stark CHE, Administrator and Chief Executive Officer

Owned, leased, sponsored:	32 hospitals	2841 beds
Contract–managed:	0 hospitals	0 beds
Totals:	32 hospitals	2841 beds

1985: HEALTHSYSTEM MINNESOTA (NP)
6500 Excelsior Boulevard, Saint Louis Park, MN Zip 55426–4702; tel. 612/932–6300; Robert L. Galloway, President and Administrative Officer

MINNESOTA: GLENCOE AREA HEALTH CENTER (CM, 149 beds) 705 East 18th Street, Glencoe, MN Zip 55336–1499; tel. 612/864–3121; Jon D. Braband, Chief Executive Officer

METHODIST HOSPITAL (O, 355 beds) 6500 Excelsior Boulevard, Saint Louis Park, MN Zip 55426–4702, Mailing Address: Box 650, Minneapolis, Zip 55440–9946; tel. 612/932–5000; Terry S. Finzen, Senior Vice President and Chief Operating Officer

Owned, leased, sponsored:	1 hospitals	355 beds
Contract–managed:	1 hospitals	149 beds
Totals:	2 hospitals	504 beds

★**2485: HEARTLAND HEALTH SYSTEM** (NP)
5325 Faraon, Saint Joseph, MO Zip 64506; tel. 816/271–6000; Lowell C. Kruse, President

MISSOURI: HEARTLAND HOSPITAL EAST (O, 205 beds) 5325 Faraon Street, Saint Joseph, MO Zip 64506; tel. 816/271–6000; Lowell C. Kruse, President

HEARTLAND HOSPITAL WEST (O, 341 beds) 801 Faraon Street, Saint Joseph, MO Zip 64501; tel. 816/271–7111; Lowell C. Kruse, President

Owned, leased, sponsored:	2 hospitals	546 beds
Contract–managed:	0 hospitals	0 beds
Totals:	2 hospitals	546 beds

★**2355: HELIX HEALTH SYSTEM** (NP)
2330 West Joppa Road, Ste 301, Lutherville, MD Zip 21093; tel. 410/296–6050; James A. Oakey, President

MARYLAND: CHURCH HOSPITAL CORPORATION (O, 247 beds) 100 North Broadway, Baltimore, MD Zip 21231–1593; tel. 410/522–8000; James R. Bobb, President

FRANKLIN SQUARE HOSPITAL CENTER (O, 405 beds) 9000 Franklin Square Drive, Baltimore, MD Zip 21237; tel. 410/682–7000; Charles D. Mross, President

GOOD SAMARITAN HOSPITAL OF MARYLAND (O, 273 beds) 5601 Loch Raven Boulevard, Baltimore, MD Zip 21239–2995; tel. 410/532–8000; Lawrence M. Beck, President

UNION MEMORIAL HOSPITAL (O, 376 beds) 201 East University Parkway, Baltimore, MD Zip 21218–2391; tel. 410/554–2000; Edward J. Kelly III, President and Chief Executive Officer

Owned, leased, sponsored:	4 hospitals	1301 beds
Contract–managed:	0 hospitals	0 beds
Totals:	4 hospitals	1301 beds

★**9505: HENRY FORD HEALTH SYSTEM** (NP)
One Ford Place, Detroit, MI Zip 48202; tel. 313/876–8700; Gail L. Warden, President and Chief Executive Officer

MICHIGAN: HENRY FORD COTTAGE HOSPITAL (O, 175 beds) 159 Kercheval Avenue, Grosse Pointe Farms, MI Zip 48236–3692; tel. 313/884–8600; Gregory J. Vasse, President and Chief Executive Officer

HENRY FORD HOSPITAL (O, 903 beds) 2799 West Grand Boulevard, Detroit, MI Zip 48202–2689; tel. 313/876–2600; Stephen H. Velick, Group Vice President, Henry Ford Health System and Chief Operating Officer

KINGSWOOD HOSPITAL (O, 64 beds) 10300 West Eight Mile Road, Ferndale, MI Zip 48220; tel. 810/398–3200; Kathleen Emrich Ed.D., R.N., Assistant Vice President

WYANDOTTE HOSPITAL AND MEDICAL CENTER (O, 355 beds) 2333 Biddle Avenue, Wyandotte, MI Zip 48192; tel. 313/284–2400; William R. Alvin, President

Owned, leased, sponsored:	4 hospitals	1497 beds
Contract–managed:	0 hospitals	0 beds
Totals:	4 hospitals	1497 beds

★**5585: HOLY CROSS HEALTH SYSTEM CORPORATION** (CC)
3606 East Jefferson Boulevard, South Bend, IN Zip 46615–3097; tel. 219/233–8558; Sister Patricia Vandenberg, President and Chief Executive Officer

CALIFORNIA: HOLY CROSS MEDICAL CENTER (O, 257 beds) 15031 Rinaldi Street, Mission Hills, CA Zip 91345–1285; tel. 818/365–8051; Carl W. Fitch, Sr., President and Chief Executive Officer

ST. AGNES MEDICAL CENTER (O, 326 beds) 1303 East Herndon Avenue, Fresno, CA Zip 93720–3397; tel. 209/449–3000; Sister Ruth Marie Nickerson, President

IDAHO: ELMORE MEDICAL CENTER (CM, 75 beds) 895 North Sixth East Street, Mountain Home, ID Zip 83647, Mailing Address: P.O. Box 1270, Zip 83647–0348; tel. 208/587–8401; Jan G. Cox, Administrator

MCCALL MEMORIAL HOSPITAL (CM, 17 beds) 1000 State Street, McCall, ID Zip 83638, Mailing Address: P.O. Box 906, Zip 83638; tel. 208/634–2221; Karen J. Kellie, President

SAINT ALPHONSUS REGIONAL MEDICAL CENTER (O, 248 beds) 1055 North Curtis Road, Boise, ID Zip 83706–1370; tel. 208/378–2121; Chris J. Anton, President

ST. BENEDICTS FAMILY MEDICAL CENTER (CM, 80 beds) 709 North Lincoln Avenue, Jerome, ID Zip 83338, Mailing Address: Box 586, Zip 83338–0586; tel. 208/324–4301; David Farnes, Administrator

VALLEY COUNTY HOSPITAL (CM, 10 beds) 402 Old State Highway, Cascade, ID Zip 83611, Mailing Address: P.O. Box 151, Zip 83611; tel. 208/382–4242; Richard Holm, Administrator

INDIANA: SAINT JOHN'S HEALTH SYSTEM (O, 371 beds) 2015 Jackson Street, Anderson, IN Zip 46016–4339; tel. 317/649–2511; James H. Stephens, President and Chief Executive Officer

ST. JOSEPH'S HOSPITAL OF MARSHALL COUNTY (O, 58 beds) 1915 Lake Avenue, Plymouth, IN Zip 46563–9905, Mailing Address: P.O. Box 670, Zip 46563–9905; tel. 219/936–3181; Brian E. Dietz, President

ST. JOSEPH'S MEDICAL CENTER (O, 297 beds) 801 East LaSalle, South Bend, IN Zip 46617, Mailing Address: Box 1935, Zip 46634; tel. 219/237–7111; Dennis W. Heck, Chief Executive Officer

MARYLAND: HOLY CROSS HOSPITAL OF SILVER SPRING (O, 366 beds) 1500 Forest Glen Road, Silver Spring, MD Zip 20910; tel. 301/905–0100; James P. Hamill, President

OHIO: MOUNT CARMEL HEALTH (O, 749 beds) 793 West State Street, Columbus, OH Zip 43222–9988; tel. 614/225–5000; Dale St Arnold, President and Chief Executive Officer

Owned, leased, sponsored:	8 hospitals	2672 beds
Contract–managed:	4 hospitals	182 beds
Totals:	12 hospitals	2854 beds

For explanation of codes following names, see page B2.
★Indicates Type III membership in the American Hospital Association.

Systems / Incarnate Word Health Services

1035: HORIZON HEALTH SYSTEM (NP)
26100 American Drive, Southfield, MI Zip 48086, Mailing Address: P.O. Box 5153, Zip 48086-5153; tel. 810/746-4460; Thomas W. Caulfield, President
MICHIGAN: BI-COUNTY COMMUNITY HOSPITAL (O, 185 beds) 13355 East Ten Mile Road, Warren, MI Zip 48089-2065; tel. 810/759-7300; Gary W. Popiel, Chief Executive Officer
RIVERSIDE OSTEOPATHIC HOSPITAL (O, 185 beds) 150 Truax Street, Trenton, MI Zip 48183-2151; tel. 313/676-4200; Dennis A. Christen, Vice President and Administrator

Owned, leased, sponsored:	2 hospitals	370 beds
Contract-managed:	0 hospitals	0 beds
Totals:	2 hospitals	370 beds

★0027: HORIZON HEALTHCARE, INC. (NP)
2300 North Mayfair Road, Suite 550, Milwaukee, WI Zip 53226-1508; tel. 414/257-3888; Kurt W. Metzner, President and Chief Executive Officer
WISCONSIN: COLUMBIA HOSPITAL (O, 339 beds) 2025 East Newport Avenue, Milwaukee, WI Zip 53211-2990; tel. 414/961-3300; John F. Schuler, President
COMMUNITY MEMORIAL HOSPITAL (O, 153 beds) W180 N8085 Town Hall Road, Menomonee Falls, WI Zip 53051, Mailing Address: P.O. Box 408, Zip 53052-0408; tel. 414/251-1000; Robert Eugene Drisner, President and Chief Executive Officer
FROEDTERT MEMORIAL LUTHERAN HOSPITAL (O, 241 beds) 9200 West Wisconsin Avenue, Milwaukee, WI Zip 53226-3596; tel. 414/259-3000; William D. Petasnick, President
KENOSHA HOSPITAL AND MEDICAL CENTER (O, 128 beds) 6308 Eighth Avenue, Kenosha, WI Zip 53143; tel. 414/656-2011; Richard O. Schmidt, Jr., President and Chief Executive Officer

Owned, leased, sponsored:	4 hospitals	861 beds
Contract-managed:	0 hospitals	0 beds
Totals:	4 hospitals	861 beds

0455: HOSPITAL GROUP OF AMERICA (IO)
1265 Drummers Lane, Suite 107, Wayne, PA Zip 19087; tel. 610/687-5151; Mark R. Russell, President and Chief Executive Officer
DELAWARE: MEADOW WOOD HOSPITAL (O, 50 beds) 575 South Dupont Highway, New Castle, DE Zip 19720; tel. 302/328-3330; Arris S. Veronie, Administrator and Chief Executive Officer
ILLINOIS: HARTGROVE HOSPITAL (O, 109 beds) 520 North Ridgeway Avenue, Chicago, IL Zip 60624; tel. 312/722-3113; Karen E. Johnson, Administrator
NEW JERSEY: HAMPTON HOSPITAL (O, 100 beds) Rancocas Road, Westampton Township, NJ Zip 08073, Mailing Address: P.O. Box 7000, Zip 08073; tel. 609/267-7000; Michael Terwilliger, Acting Chief Executive Officer
PENNSYLVANIA: MALVERN INSTITUTE (CM, 36 beds) 940 King Road, Malvern, PA Zip 19355-2058; tel. 610/647-0330; Valerie Craig, Administrator and Chief Executive Officer
NORTHWESTERN INSTITUTE (CM, 146 beds) 450 Bethlehem Pike, Fort Washington, PA Zip 19034-0209; tel. 215/641-5300; Richard Jensen, Administrator
TEXAS: PINELANDS HOSPITAL (CM, 38 beds) 4632 Northeast Stallings Drive, Nacogdoches, TX Zip 75961, Mailing Address: P.O. Box 1004, Zip 79563-1004; tel. 409/560-5900; Jerry Wilson, Administrator

Owned, leased, sponsored:	3 hospitals	259 beds
Contract-managed:	3 hospitals	220 beds
Totals:	6 hospitals	479 beds

★5355: HOSPITAL SISTERS HEALTH SYSTEM (CC)
Sangamon Avenue Road, Springfield, IL Zip 62794, Mailing Address: Box 19431, Zip 62794-9431; tel. 217/522-6969; Sister Jomary Trstensky, President
ILLINOIS: ST. ANTHONY'S MEMORIAL HOSPITAL (O, 146 beds) 503 North Maple Street, Effingham, IL Zip 62401-2099; tel. 217/342-2121; Anthony D. Pfitzer, Executive Vice President and Chief Executive Officer

ST. ELIZABETH'S HOSPITAL (O, 379 beds) 211 South Third Street, Belleville, IL Zip 62222-0694; tel. 618/234-2120; Gerald M. Harman, Chief Executive Officer and Executive Vice President
ST. FRANCIS HOSPITAL (O, 101 beds) 1215 East Union Avenue, Litchfield, IL Zip 62056-1215, Mailing Address: P.O. Box 1215, Zip 62056-1215; tel. 217/324-2191; Michael Sipkoski, Executive Vice President
ST. JOHN'S HOSPITAL (O, 633 beds) 800 East Carpenter Street, Springfield, IL Zip 62769; tel. 217/544-6464; Allison C. Laabs, Executive Vice President
ST. JOSEPH'S HOSPITAL (O, 85 beds) 9515 Holy Cross Lane, Breese, IL Zip 62230-0099, Mailing Address: P.O. Box 99, Zip 62230-0099; tel. 618/526-4511; Jacolyn M. Schlautman, Executive Vice President and Administrator
ST. JOSEPH'S HOSPITAL (O, 76 beds) 1515 Main Street, Highland, IL Zip 62249-1656; tel. 618/654-7421; Anthony G. Mastrangelo, Executive Vice President and Chief Executive Officer
ST. MARY'S HOSPITAL (O, 290 beds) 1800 East Lake Shore Drive, Decatur, IL Zip 62521-3883; tel. 217/464-2966; Rex D. Conger, Acting Administrator
ST. MARY'S HOSPITAL (O, 170 beds) 111 East Spring Street, Streator, IL Zip 61364; tel. 815/673-2311; Jimmie D. Lansford, Executive Vice President
WISCONSIN: SACRED HEART HOSPITAL (O, 301 beds) 900 West Clairemont Avenue, Eau Claire, WI Zip 54701-5105; tel. 715/839-4121; Matthew W. Hubler, Executive Vice President
ST. JOSEPH'S HOSPITAL (O, 127 beds) 2661 County Road I, Chippewa Falls, WI Zip 54729-1498; tel. 715/723-1811; David B. Fish, Executive Vice President
ST. MARY'S HOSPITAL MEDICAL CENTER (O, 120 beds) 1726 Shawano Avenue, Green Bay, WI Zip 54303-3282; tel. 414/498-4200; James G. Coller, Executive Vice President and Administrator
ST. NICHOLAS HOSPITAL (O, 112 beds) 1601 North Taylor Drive, Sheboygan, WI Zip 53081-2496; tel. 414/459-8300; Thomas W. Laux, Executive Vice President and Administrator
ST. VINCENT HOSPITAL (O, 349 beds) 835 South Van Buren Street, Green Bay, WI Zip 54301, Mailing Address: P.O. Box 13508, Zip 54307-3508; tel. 414/433-0111; Joseph J. Neidenbach, Administrator and Executive Vice President

Owned, leased, sponsored:	13 hospitals	2889 beds
Contract-managed:	0 hospitals	0 beds
Totals:	13 hospitals	2889 beds

★5645: HUMILITY OF MARY HEALTH CARE CORPORATION (CC)
1919 Reid Avenue, Lorain, OH Zip 44052, Mailing Address: P.O. Box 841, Zip 44052-0841; tel. 216/245-3569; Sister Frances Flanigan, President and Chief Executive Officer
OHIO: LORAIN COMMUNITY/ST. JOSEPH REGIONAL HEALTH CENTER (S, 484 beds) 3700 Kolbe Road, Lorain, OH Zip 44053-1697; tel. 216/960-3000; Paul C. Balcom, President and Chief Executive Officer
ST. ELIZABETH HOSPITAL MEDICAL CENTER (S, 430 beds) 1044 Belmont Avenue, Youngstown, OH Zip 44501-1790, Mailing Address: Box 1790, Zip 44501-1790; tel. 216/746-7211; Andrew W. Allen, President and Chief Executive Officer
ST. JOSEPH RIVERSIDE HOSPITAL (S, 203 beds) 1400 Tod Avenue N.W., Warren, OH Zip 44485; tel. 216/841-4000; Sister Mildred Ely, President and Chief Executive Officer

Owned, leased, sponsored:	3 hospitals	1117 beds
Contract-managed:	0 hospitals	0 beds
Totals:	3 hospitals	1117 beds

★5565: INCARNATE WORD HEALTH SERVICES (CC)
9311 San Pedro, Suite 1250, San Antonio, TX Zip 78216-4469; tel. 210/524-4100; Joseph Blasko Jr., President and Chief Executive Officer
MISSOURI: INCARNATE WORD HOSPITAL (O, 296 beds) 3545 Lafayette Avenue, Saint Louis, MO Zip 63104-9984; tel. 314/865-6500; Linda M. Allin, President and Chief Executive Officer
TEXAS: SANTA ROSA HEALTH CARE CORPORATION (O, 702 beds) 519 West Houston Street, San Antonio, TX Zip 78207-3108, Mailing Address: Box 7330, Station A, Zip 78207-3108; tel. 210/704-2011; Robert J. Nolan, President and Chief Executive Officer

For explanation of codes following names, see page B2.
★Indicates Type III membership in the American Hospital Association.

Integrated Health Delivery Networks, Health Care Systems and Alliances

Systems / Incarnate Word Health Services

SPOHN HEALTH SYSTEM (O, 428 beds) 600 Elizabeth Street, Corpus Christi, TX Zip 78404–2235; tel. 512/881–3000; Sister Kathleen Coughlin, President

SPOHN KLEBERG MEMORIAL HOSPITAL (O, 100 beds) 1300 General Cavazos Boulevard, Kingsville, TX Zip 78363, Mailing Address: P.O. Box 1197, Zip 78363–1197; tel. 512/595–1661; Andrew M. Harris, Administrator

ST. ANTHONY'S HOSPITAL (O, 290 beds) 200 Northwest Seventh, Amarillo, TX Zip 79107–9872, Mailing Address: Box 950, Zip 79176–0950; tel. 806/376–4411; John D. Koobs, President and Chief Executive Officer

ST. JOSEPH'S HOSPITAL AND HEALTH CENTER (O, 177 beds) 820 Clarksville Street, Paris, TX Zip 75460–9070, Mailing Address: P.O. Box 9070, Zip 75461–9070; tel. 903/785–4521; Monty E. McLaurin, President

Owned, leased, sponsored:	6 hospitals	1993 beds
Contract–managed:	0 hospitals	0 beds
Totals:	6 hospitals	1993 beds

2025: INFIRMARY HEALTH SYSTEM, INC. (NP)
3 Mobile Infirmary Circle, Mobile, AL Zip 36607; tel. 334/431–5500; E. Chandler Bramlett Jr., President

ALABAMA: GROVE HILL MEMORIAL HOSPITAL (CM, 32 beds) Jackson Highway, Grove Hill, AL Zip 36451, Mailing Address: P.O. Box 935, Zip 36451; tel. 205/275–3191; Darrell M. Butler, Administrator

MOBILE INFIRMARY MEDICAL CENTER (O, 633 beds) 5 Mobile Infirmary Circle, Mobile, AL Zip 36607, Mailing Address: P.O. Box 2144, Zip 36652–2144; tel. 334/431–2408; E. Chandler Bramlett, Jr., President and Chief Executive Officer

WASHINGTON COUNTY INFIRMARY AND NURSING HOME (CM, 103 beds) St Stephens Avenue, Chatom, AL Zip 36518, Mailing Address: Box 597, Zip 36518–0597; tel. 334/847–2223; Howard C. Holcomb, Administrator

Owned, leased, sponsored:	1 hospitals	633 beds
Contract–managed:	2 hospitals	135 beds
Totals:	3 hospitals	768 beds

★1305: INOVA HEALTH SYSTEM (NP)
8001 Braddock Road, Springfield, VA Zip 22151; tel. 703/321–4213; J. Knox Singleton, President

VIRGINIA: FAIR OAKS HOSPITAL (O, 136 beds) 3600 Joseph Siewick Drive, Fairfax, VA Zip 22033; tel. 703/391–3600; Steven E. Brown, Administrator

FAIRFAX HOSPITAL (O, 656 beds) 3300 Gallows Road, Falls Church, VA Zip 22046–3300; tel. 703/698–3372; Jolene Tornabeni, Administrator

MOUNT VERNON HOSPITAL (O, 229 beds) 2501 Parker's Lane, Alexandria, VA Zip 22306–3209; tel. 703/664–7000; Joanne Carrocino, Administrator

Owned, leased, sponsored:	3 hospitals	1021 beds
Contract–managed:	0 hospitals	0 beds
Totals:	3 hospitals	1021 beds

★1815: INTERMOUNTAIN HEALTH CARE, INC. (NP)
36 South State Street, 22nd Floor, Salt Lake City, UT Zip 84111; tel. 801/533–8282; Scott S. Parker, President

IDAHO: CASSIA REGIONAL MEDICAL CENTER (L, 83 beds) 1501 Hiland Avenue, Burley, ID Zip 83318, Mailing Address: Box 489, Zip 83318; tel. 208/678–4444; Richard Packer, Administrator

POCATELLO REGIONAL MEDICAL CENTER (O, 110 beds) 777 Hospital Way, Pocatello, ID Zip 83201; tel. 208/234–0777; Earl L. Christison, Administrator

UTAH: ALTA VIEW HOSPITAL (O, 70 beds) 9660 South 1300 East, Sandy, UT Zip 84094; tel. 801/576–2600; Wes Thompson, Administrator

AMERICAN FORK HOSPITAL (O, 67 beds) 1100 East 170 North, American Fork, UT Zip 84003–9787; tel. 801/763–3300; Craig M. Smedley, Administrator

BEAR RIVER VALLEY HOSPITAL (O, 20 beds) 440 West 600 North, Tremonton, UT Zip 84337; tel. 801/257–7441; Robert F. Jex, Administrator

COTTONWOOD HOSPITAL MEDICAL CENTER (O, 163 beds) 5770 South 300 East, Murray, UT Zip 84107; tel. 801/262–3461; Douglas R. Fonnesbeck, Administrator

DELTA COMMUNITY MEDICAL CENTER (O, 20 beds) 126 South White Sage Avenue, Delta, UT Zip 84624; tel. 801/864–5591; James E. Beckstrand, Administrator

DIXIE REGIONAL MEDICAL CENTER (O, 137 beds) 544 South 400 East, Saint George, UT Zip 84770; tel. 801/634–4000; L. Steven Wilson, Administrator

FILLMORE COMMUNITY MEDICAL CENTER (O, 20 beds) 674 South Highway 99, Fillmore, UT Zip 84631; tel. 801/743–5591; James E. Beckstrand, Administrator

GARFIELD MEMORIAL HOSPITAL AND CLINICS (O, 20 beds) 200 North Fourth East, Panguitch, UT Zip 84759, Mailing Address: P.O. Box 389, Zip 84759–0389; tel. 801/676–8811; Wayne R. Ross, Administrator

LDS HOSPITAL (O, 440 beds) Eighth Avenue and C Street, Salt Lake City, UT Zip 84143; tel. 801/321–1100; Richard M. Cagen, Administrator

LOGAN REGIONAL HOSPITAL (O, 133 beds) 1400 North 500 East, Logan, UT Zip 84321–2499; tel. 801/752–2050; Richard Smith, Administrator

MCKAY–DEE HOSPITAL CENTER (O, 340 beds) 3939 Harrison Boulevard, Ogden, UT Zip 84409–2386, Mailing Address: Box 9370, Zip 84409–0370; tel. 801/627–2800; Thomas Hanrahan, Administrator and Chief Executive Officer

OREM COMMUNITY HOSPITAL (O, 20 beds) 331 North 400 West, Orem, UT Zip 84057; tel. 801/224–4080; Mark F. Dalley, Administrator and Chief Operating Officer

PRIMARY CHILDREN'S MEDICAL CENTER (O, 208 beds) 100 North Medical Drive, Salt Lake City, UT Zip 84113–1100; tel. 801/588–2000; Joseph R. Horton, Chief Executive Officer and Administrator

SANPETE VALLEY HOSPITAL (O, 20 beds) 1100 South Medical Drive, Mount Pleasant, UT Zip 84647; tel. 801/462–2441; George Winn, Administrator

SEVIER VALLEY HOSPITAL (O, 42 beds) 1100 North Main Street, Richfield, UT Zip 84701; tel. 801/896–8271; Gary E. Beck, Administrator

UTAH VALLEY REGIONAL MEDICAL CENTER (O, 343 beds) 1034 North 500 West, Provo, UT Zip 84605–0390; tel. 801/373–7850; Larry R. Dursteler, Administrator and Chief Operating Officer

VALLEY VIEW MEDICAL CENTER (O, 36 beds) 595 South 75 East, Cedar City, UT Zip 84720; tel. 801/586–6587; Margaret Holm, Administrator

WASATCH CANYONS HOSPITAL (O, 44 beds) 5770 South 1500 West, Salt Lake City, UT Zip 84123; tel. 801/262–6199; Jill Green, Administrator

WASATCH COUNTY HOSPITAL (L, 40 beds) 55 South Fifth East, Heber City, UT Zip 84032–1848; tel. 801/654–2500; Randall K. Probst, Administrator

WYOMING: IHC EVANSTON REGIONAL HOSPITAL (O, 42 beds) 190 Arrowhead Drive, Evanston, WY Zip 82930; tel. 307/789–3636; Robert W. Allen, Administrator

STAR VALLEY HOSPITAL (CM, 15 beds) 110 Hospital Lane, Afton, WY Zip 83110, Mailing Address: P.O. Box 579, Zip 83110; tel. 307/886–3841; Carolyne Jo Allen, Chief Executive Officer

Owned, leased, sponsored:	22 hospitals	2418 beds
Contract–managed:	1 hospitals	15 beds
Totals:	23 hospitals	2433 beds

★0061: IOWA HEALTH SYSTEM (NP)
1200 Pleasant Street, Des Moines, IA Zip 50309–1453; Samuel T. Wallace, President

IOWA: ANAMOSA COMMUNITY HOSPITAL (L, 24 beds) 104 Broadway Place, Anamosa, IA Zip 52205; tel. 319/462–6131; Julie May, Administrator

CLARKE COUNTY HOSPITAL (CM, 48 beds) 800 South Fillmore Street, Osceola, IA Zip 50213–0427, Mailing Address: P.O. Box 427, Zip 50213–0427; tel. 515/342–2184; Kris Baumgart, Administrator

COMMUNITY MEMORIAL HOSPITAL (CM, 33 beds) 1316 South Main Street, Clarion, IA Zip 50525–0429; tel. 515/532–2811; Richard W. Rhiner, Interim Administrator

DALLAS COUNTY HOSPITAL (CM, 30 beds) 610 10th Street, Perry, IA Zip 50220, Mailing Address: P.O. Box 608, Zip 50220; tel. 515/465–3547; Vernette Riley, Administrator

IOWA LUTHERAN HOSPITAL (O, 275 beds) 700 East University Avenue, Des Moines, IA Zip 50316–2392; tel. 515/263–5612; James H. Skogsbergh, President

IOWA METHODIST MEDICAL CENTER (O, 573 beds) 1200 Pleasant Street, Des Moines, IA Zip 50309–9976; tel. 515/241–6212; James H. Skogsbergh, President

LORING HOSPITAL (CM, 54 beds) Highland Avenue, Sac City, IA Zip 50583–0217; tel. 712/662–7105; Greg Miner, Administrator

For explanation of codes following names, see page B2.
★Indicates Type III membership in the American Hospital Association.

Systems / Kaiser Foundation Hospitals

MAHASKA COUNTY HOSPITAL (CM, 53 beds) 1229 C Avenue East, Oskaloosa, IA Zip 52577; tel. 515/673-3431; David E. Rutter, Administrator

ST. LUKE'S HOSPITAL (O, 428 beds) 1026 A Avenue N.E., Cedar Rapids, IA Zip 52402-3026, Mailing Address: P.O. Box 3026, Zip 52406-3026; tel. 319/369-7211; Samuel T. Wallace, President

VIRGINIA GAY HOSPITAL (CM, 87 beds) 502 North Ninth Avenue, Vinton, IA Zip 52349; tel. 319/472-2348; Michael J. Riege, Administrator

Owned, leased, sponsored:	4 hospitals	1300 beds
Contract-managed:	6 hospitals	305 beds
Totals:	10 hospitals	1605 beds

2415: JEWISH HEALTH SYSTEMS, INC. (NP)
3200 Burnet Avenue, Cincinnati, OH Zip 45229-3099; tel. 513/569-2434; Warren C. Falberg, President

OHIO: JEWISH HOSPITAL KENWOOD (O, 60 beds) 8000 Kenwood Road, Cincinnati, OH Zip 45236-2891; tel. 513/745-2200; M. Aurora Lambert, Executive Vice President

JEWISH HOSPITAL OF CINCINNATI (O, 489 beds) 3200 Burnet Avenue, Cincinnati, OH Zip 45229-3099; tel. 513/569-2000; Warren C. Falberg, President and Chief Executive Officer

Owned, leased, sponsored:	2 hospitals	549 beds
Contract-managed:	0 hospitals	0 beds
Totals:	2 hospitals	549 beds

★0052: JEWISH HOSPITAL HEALTHCARE SERVICES (NP)
217 East Chestnut Street, Louisville, KY Zip 40202; tel. 502/587-4011; Henry C. Wagner, President

INDIANA: CLARK MEMORIAL HOSPITAL (CM, 280 beds) 1220 Missouri Avenue, Jeffersonville, IN Zip 47130-3743, Mailing Address: Box 69, Zip 47131-0069; tel. 812/282-6631; Merle E. Stepp, President

SCOTT MEMORIAL HOSPITAL (CM, 40 beds) 1415 North Gardner Street, Scottsburg, IN Zip 47170-0456, Mailing Address: Box 456, Zip 47170-0456; tel. 812/752-8500; Clifford D. Nay, Administrator

WASHINGTON COUNTY MEMORIAL HOSPITAL (CM, 70 beds) 911 North Shelby Street, Salem, IN Zip 47167; tel. 812/883-5881; Rodney M. Coats, Executive Director

KENTUCKY: FRAZIER REHABILITATION CENTER (O, 95 beds) 220 Abraham Flexner Way, Louisville, KY Zip 40202-1887; tel. 502/582-7400; Joanne Berryman, President

HUMANA HOSPITAL-LEXINGTON (CM, 174 beds) 150 North Eagle Creek Drive, Lexington, KY Zip 40509-1807, Mailing Address: P.O. Box 23260, Zip 40523-3260; tel. 606/268-4800; Jeffrey Helton, Executive Director

JEWISH HOSPITAL (O, 408 beds) 217 East Chestnut Street, Louisville, KY Zip 40202-1886; tel. 502/587-4011; Douglas E. Shaw, President

JEWISH HOSPITAL-SHELBYVILLE (O, 72 beds) 727 Hospital Drive, Shelbyville, KY Zip 40065; tel. 502/647-4301; Timothy L. Jarm, President and Chief Executive Officer

PATTIE A. CLAY HOSPITAL (CM, 105 beds) EKU By-Pass, Richmond, KY Zip 40475, Mailing Address: P.O. Box 1600, Zip 40476-2603; tel. 606/623-3131; Richard M. Thomas, Administrator

Owned, leased, sponsored:	3 hospitals	575 beds
Contract-managed:	5 hospitals	669 beds
Totals:	8 hospitals	1244 beds

★8855: JFK HEALTH SYSTEMS, INC. (NP)
80 James Street, 2nd Floor, Edison, NJ Zip 08820-3998; tel. 908/632-1500; John P. McGee, President and Chief Executive Officer

NEW JERSEY: JFK JOHNSON REHABILITATION INSTITUTE (O, 90 beds) 65 James Street, Edison, NJ Zip 08818-3059; tel. 908/321-7050; Scott Gebhard, Administrator

JFK MEDICAL CENTER (O, 417 beds) 65 James Street, Edison, NJ Zip 08818-3059; tel. 908/321-7000; John P. McGee, President and Chief Executive Officer

Owned, leased, sponsored:	2 hospitals	507 beds
Contract-managed:	0 hospitals	0 beds
Totals:	2 hospitals	507 beds

★1015: JOHNS HOPKINS HEALTH SYSTEM (NP)
600 North Wolfe Street, Baltimore, MD Zip 21287-1160; tel. 410/955-0428; James A. Block M.D., President

MARYLAND: JOHNS HOPKINS BAYVIEW MEDICAL CENTER (O, 667 beds) 4940 Eastern Avenue, Baltimore, MD Zip 21224; tel. 410/550-0100; Ronald R. Peterson, President

JOHNS HOPKINS HOSPITAL (O, 954 beds) 600 North Wolfe Street, Baltimore, MD Zip 21287; tel. 410/955-5000; James A. Block M.D., President and Chief Executive Officer

Owned, leased, sponsored:	2 hospitals	1621 beds
Contract-managed:	0 hospitals	0 beds
Totals:	2 hospitals	1621 beds

★2105: KAISER FOUNDATION HOSPITALS (NP)
One Kaiser Plaza, Oakland, CA Zip 94612-3600; tel. 510/271-5990; David M. Lawrence M.D., Chairman and Chief Executive Officer

CALIFORNIA: KAISER FOUNDATION HOSPITAL (O, 149 beds) 2425 Geary Boulevard, San Francisco, CA Zip 94115; tel. 415/202-2000; Frank D. Alvarez, Administrator

KAISER FOUNDATION HOSPITAL (O, 110 beds) 401 Bicentennial Way, Santa Rosa, CA Zip 95403; tel. 707/571-4000; Pete Delgado, Vice President and Area Manager

KAISER FOUNDATION HOSPITAL (O, 496 beds) 4867 Sunset Boulevard, Los Angeles, CA Zip 90027; tel. 213/667-4011; Joseph William Hummel, Administrator

KAISER FOUNDATION HOSPITAL (O, 41 beds) 7300 North Fresno Street, Fresno, CA Zip 93720; tel. 209/448-4000; Edward S. Glavis, Vice President and Area Administrator

KAISER FOUNDATION HOSPITAL (O, 158 beds) 441 North Lakeview Avenue, Anaheim, CA Zip 92807; tel. 714/978-4100; Gerald A. McCall, Administrator

KAISER FOUNDATION HOSPITAL (O, 210 beds) 9400 East Rosecrans Avenue, Bellflower, CA Zip 90706-2246; tel. 310/461-3000; Timothy A. Reed, Administrator

KAISER FOUNDATION HOSPITAL (O, 233 beds) 9961 Sierra Avenue, Fontana, CA Zip 92335-6794; tel. 909/427-5000; Patricia Siegel, Administrator

KAISER FOUNDATION HOSPITAL (O, 223 beds) 25825 South Vermont Avenue, Harbor City, CA Zip 90710; tel. 310/517-2770; Mary Ann Barnes, Administrator

KAISER FOUNDATION HOSPITAL (O, 224 beds) 27400 Hesperian Boulevard, Hayward, CA Zip 94545-4297; tel. 510/784-4313

KAISER FOUNDATION HOSPITAL (O, 326 beds) 4647 Zion Avenue, San Diego, CA Zip 92120; tel. 619/528-5000; Kenneth F. Colling, Administrator

KAISER FOUNDATION HOSPITAL (O, 134 beds) 200 Muir Road, Martinez, CA Zip 94553-4696; tel. 510/372-1000; Joyce M. Berger, Administrator

KAISER FOUNDATION HOSPITAL (O, 220 beds) 280 West MacArthur Boulevard, Oakland, CA Zip 94611; tel. 510/596-1000; Donald Oxley, Vice President and Area Manager

KAISER FOUNDATION HOSPITAL (O, 147 beds) 1150 Veterans Boulevard, Redwood City, CA Zip 94063-2087; tel. 415/299-2000; Carol Kiecker, Administrator

KAISER FOUNDATION HOSPITAL (O, 43 beds) 1330 Cutting Boulevard, Richmond, CA Zip 94804-2555; tel. 510/596-6000; Donald Oxley, Administrator

KAISER FOUNDATION HOSPITAL (O, 304 beds) 2025 Morse Avenue, Sacramento, CA Zip 95825-2115; tel. 916/973-5000; Sarah Krevans, Area Manager

KAISER FOUNDATION HOSPITAL (O, 221 beds) 6600 Bruceville Road, Sacramento, CA Zip 95823; tel. 916/688-2430; Sarah Krevans, Area Manager

KAISER FOUNDATION HOSPITAL (O, 119 beds) 99 Montecillo Road, San Rafael, CA Zip 94903-3397; tel. 415/499-2227; Pete Delgado, Vice President and Area Manager

For explanation of codes following names, see page B2.
★Indicates Type III membership in the American Hospital Association.

Systems / Kaiser Foundation Hospitals

KAISER FOUNDATION HOSPITAL (O, 287 beds) 900 Kiely Boulevard, Santa Clara, CA Zip 95051–5386; tel. 408/236–6400; Carol Kiecker, Vice President and Area Manager

KAISER FOUNDATION HOSPITAL (O, 127 beds) 1200 El Camino Real, South San Francisco, CA Zip 94080–3299; tel. 415/742–2547; Frank D. Alvarez, Administrator

KAISER FOUNDATION HOSPITAL (O, 269 beds) 13652 Cantara Street, Panorama City, CA Zip 91402; tel. 818/375–2000; Dev Mahadevan, Administrator

KAISER FOUNDATION HOSPITAL (O, 134 beds) 1425 South Main Street, Walnut Creek, CA Zip 94596; tel. 510/295–4000

KAISER FOUNDATION HOSPITAL (O, 134 beds) 5601 DeSoto Avenue, Woodland Hills, CA Zip 91365–4084; tel. 818/719–2000; James L. Breeden, Administrator

KAISER FOUNDATION HOSPITAL AND REHABILITATION CENTER (O, 231 beds) 975 Sereno Drive, Vallejo, CA Zip 94589; tel. 707/648–6230; Joyce M. Berger, Area Manager

KAISER FOUNDATION HOSPITAL–RIVERSIDE (O, 215 beds) 10800 Magnolia Avenue, Riverside, CA Zip 92505–3000; tel. 909/353–4600; Robert S. Lund, Administrator

KAISER FOUNDATION HOSPITAL–WEST LOS ANGELES (O, 191 beds) 6041 Cadillac Avenue, Los Angeles, CA 90034; tel. 213/857–2201; Ivette Estrada, Administrator

SANTA TERESA COMMUNITY HOSPITAL (O, 208 beds) 250 Hospital Parkway, San Jose, CA Zip 95119; tel. 408/972–7000; Nancy Madsen R.N., Patient Care Services Leader

HAWAII: KAISER FOUNDATION HOSPITAL (O, 194 beds) 3288 Moanalua Road, Honolulu, HI Zip 96819; tel. 808/834–5333; Bruce Behnke, Administrator

OREGON: BESS KAISER MEDICAL CENTER (O, 216 beds) 5055 North Greeley Avenue, Portland, OR Zip 97217–3591; tel. 503/285–9321; Alide Chase, Administrator

KAISER FOUNDATION HOSPITAL (O, 177 beds) 10200 Southeast Sunnyside Road, Clackamas, OR Zip 97015–9303; tel. 503/652–2880; Alide Chase, Administrator

Owned, leased, sponsored:	29 hospitals	5741 beds
Contract–managed:	0 hospitals	0 beds
Totals:	29 hospitals	5741 beds

★0056: LAKELAND REGIONAL HEALTH SYSTEM, INC. (NP)
1234 Napier Avenue, Saint Joseph, MI Zip 49085–2158; tel. 616/983–8300; Joseph A. Wasserman, President and Chief Executive Officer

MICHIGAN: BERRIEN GENERAL HOSPITAL (O, 248 beds) 6418 Dean's Hill Road, Berrien Center, MI Zip 49102–9704; tel. 616/471–5610; Linda Wegener, Vice President Operations and Patient Services

MERCY–MEMORIAL MEDICAL CENTER (O, 254 beds) 1234 Napier Avenue, Saint Joseph, MI Zip 49085; tel. 616/983–8300; Joseph A. Wasserman, President and Chief Executive Officer

PAWATING HOSPITAL (O, 106 beds) 31 North St Joseph Avenue, Niles, MI Zip 49120–2287; tel. 616/683–5510; Gerald W. Dechert, Senior Vice President and Chief Operating Officer

Owned, leased, sponsored:	3 hospitals	608 beds
Contract–managed:	0 hospitals	0 beds
Totals:	3 hospitals	608 beds

★2755: LEGACY HEALTH SYSTEM (NP)
1919 N.W. Lovejoy Street, Portland, OR Zip 97209–1503; tel. 503/225–8600; John G. King, President and Chief Executive Officer

OREGON: LEGACY EMANUEL HOSPITAL AND HEALTH CENTER (O, 346 beds) 2801 North Gantenbein Avenue, Portland, OR Zip 97227–1674; tel. 503/280–3200; James E. May, President

LEGACY GOOD SAMARITAN HOSPITAL AND HEALTH CENTER (O, 393 beds) 1015 Northwest 22nd Avenue, Portland, OR Zip 97210; tel. 503/229–7711; James E. May, President

LEGACY MERIDIAN PARK HOSPITAL (O, 108 beds) 19300 Southwest 65th Avenue, Tualatin, OR Zip 97062–9741; tel. 503/692–1212; Jane C. Cummins, President and Chief Executive Officer

LEGACY MOUNT HOOD MEDICAL CENTER (O, 97 beds) 24800 Southeast Stark, Gresham, OR Zip 97030–3399; tel. 503/667–1122; Barbara A. Zappas, President

Owned, leased, sponsored:	4 hospitals	944 beds
Contract–managed:	0 hospitals	0 beds
Totals:	4 hospitals	944 beds

★0060: LIFESPAN CORPORATION (NP)
167 Point Street, Providence, RI Zip 02903; tel. 401/444–6699; William Kreykes, President and Chief Executive Officer

RHODE ISLAND: MIRIAM HOSPITAL (O, 247 beds) 164 Summit Avenue, Providence, RI Zip 02906–2895; tel. 401/331–8500; Steven D. Baron, President and Chief Executive Officer

RHODE ISLAND HOSPITAL (O, 655 beds) 593 Eddy Street, Providence, RI Zip 02903; tel. 401/444–4000; Steven D. Baron, President and Chief Executive Officer

Owned, leased, sponsored:	2 hospitals	902 beds
Contract–managed:	0 hospitals	0 beds
Totals:	2 hospitals	902 beds

2295: LITTLE COMPANY OF MARY SISTERS HEALTHCARE SYSTEM (CC)
9350 South California Avenue, Evergreen Park, IL Zip 60642; tel. 708/422–6200; Sister Nancy Boyle, Provincialate Superior

CALIFORNIA: LITTLE COMPANY OF MARY HEALTH SERVICES (O, 345 beds) 4101 Torrance Boulevard, Torrance, CA Zip 90503–4698; tel. 310/540–7676; Mark Costa, President

ILLINOIS: LITTLE COMPANY OF MARY HOSPITAL AND HEALTH CARE CENTERS (O, 367 beds) 2800 West 95th Street, Evergreen Park, IL Zip 60642–2795; tel. 708/422–6200; Sister Kathleen McIntyre, President

INDIANA: MEMORIAL HOSPITAL AND HEALTH CARE CENTER (O, 122 beds) 800 West Ninth Street, Jasper, IN Zip 47546–2516; tel. 812/482–2345; Sister M. Adrian Davis Ph.D., President and Chief Executive Officer

Owned, leased, sponsored:	3 hospitals	834 beds
Contract–managed:	0 hospitals	0 beds
Totals:	3 hospitals	834 beds

5755: LOS ANGELES COUNTY–DEPARTMENT OF HEALTH SERVICES (NP)
313 North Figueroa Street, Room 936, Los Angeles, CA Zip 90012; tel. 213/240–8101; Robert C. Gates, Director Health

CALIFORNIA: LAC–UNIVERSITY OF SOUTHERN CALIFORNIA MEDICAL CENTER (O, 1236 beds) 1200 North State Street, Los Angeles, CA Zip 90033–1084; tel. 213/226–2622

LAC–HARBOR–UNIVERSITY OF CALIFORNIA AT LOS ANGELES MEDICAL CENTER (O, 493 beds) 1000 West Carson Street, Torrance, CA Zip 90509; tel. 310/222–2101; Tecla A. Mickoseff, Administrator

LAC–HIGH DESERT HOSPITAL (O, 114 beds) 44900 North 60th Street West, Lancaster, CA Zip 93536; tel. 805/945–8461; A. Roy Fleischman, Administrator

LAC–KING–DREW MEDICAL CENTER (O, 444 beds) 12021 South Wilmington Avenue, Los Angeles, CA Zip 90059; tel. 310/668–5201; Jaron Gammons, Administrator

LAC–RANCHO LOS AMIGOS MEDICAL CENTER (O, 369 beds) 7601 East Imperial Highway, Downey, CA Zip 90242; tel. 310/940–7022; Consuelo C. Diaz, Chief Executive Officer

OLIVE VIEW MEDICAL CENTER (O, 253 beds) 14445 Olive View Drive, Sylmar, CA Zip 91342–1495; tel. 818/364–1555; Melinda Anderson, Acting Administrator

Owned, leased, sponsored:	6 hospitals	2909 beds
Contract–managed:	0 hospitals	0 beds
Totals:	6 hospitals	2909 beds

0715: LOUISIANA HEALTH CARE AUTHORITY (NP)
8550 United Plaza Boulevard, 4th Floor, Baton Rouge, LA Zip 70809; tel. 504/922–0488; William Cherry M.D., Chief Executive Officer

LOUISIANA: E. A. CONWAY MEDICAL CENTER (O, 210 beds) 4864 Jackson Street, Monroe, LA Zip 71201, Mailing Address: P.O. Box 1881, Zip 71210–1881; tel. 318/388–7000; Roy D. Bostick, Director

---

For explanation of codes following names, see page B2.
★Indicates Type III membership in the American Hospital Association.

EARL K. LONG MEDICAL CENTER (O, 204 beds) 5825 Airline Highway, Baton Rouge, LA Zip 70805; tel. 504/358–1000; Steven L. Smith, Administrator

HUEY P. LONG MEDICAL CENTER (O, 123 beds) 352 Hospital Boulevard, Pineville, LA Zip 71360, Mailing Address: Box 5352, Zip 71361–5352; tel. 318/448–0811; James E. Morgan, Director

LALLIE KEMP MEDICAL CENTER (O, 60 beds) 900 Highway 51 South, Independence, LA Zip 70443; tel. 504/878–9421; William C. Bankston, Administrator

LEONARD J. CHABERT MEDICAL CENTER (O, 151 beds) 1978 Industrial Boulevard, Houma, LA Zip 70363; tel. 504/873–2200; William B. Mohon, Chief Executive Officer

MEDICAL CENTER OF LOUISIANA–EAST (O, 611 beds) 1532 Tulane Avenue, New Orleans, LA Zip 70140; tel. 504/568–3201; Jonathan Roberts, Chief Executive Officer

MEDICAL CENTER OF LOUISIANA–UNIVERSITY HOSPITAL CAMPUS (L, 272 beds) 2021 Perdido Street, New Orleans, LA Zip 70112–1396, Mailing Address: Box 61262, Zip 70161–1262; tel. 504/588–3000; Robert L. Marier M.D., Chief Administrative Officer

UNIVERSITY MEDICAL CENTER (O, 166 beds) 2390 West Congress Street, Lafayette, LA Zip 70506, Mailing Address: P.O. Box 4016–C, Zip 70502–4016; tel. 318/261–6004; Larry T. Dorsey, Administrator

WALTER OLIN MOSS REGIONAL MEDICAL CENTER (O, 66 beds) 1000 Walters Street, Lake Charles, LA Zip 70605; tel. 318/475–8100; Philip H. Rome, Administrator

WASHINGTON–ST. TAMMANY REGIONAL MEDICAL CENTER (O, 55 beds) 400 Memphis Street, Bogalusa, LA Zip 70427–0040, Mailing Address: Box 40, Zip 70429–0040; tel. 504/735–1322; Larry King, Acting Administrator

Owned, leased, sponsored:	10 hospitals	1918 beds
Contract–managed:	0 hospitals	0 beds
Totals:	10 hospitals	1918 beds

0047: LOUISIANA STATE HOSPITALS (NP)
210 State Street, New Orleans, LA Zip 70118; M. E. Teague, Chief Executive Officer

LOUISIANA: CENTRAL LOUISIANA STATE HOSPITAL (O, 280 beds) 242 West Shamrock Avenue, Pineville, LA Zip 71360–6439, Mailing Address: P.O. Box 5031, Zip 71361–5031; tel. 318/484–6200; Gary S. Grand, Chief Executive Officer

EAST LOUISIANA STATE HOSPITAL (O, 452 beds) Jackson, LA, Mailing Address: P.O. Box 498, Zip 70748; tel. 504/634–2651; Fred E. Calcote, Jr., Chief Executive Officer

GREENWELL SPRINGS HOSPITAL (O, 79 beds) 23260 Greenwell Springs Road, Greenwell Springs, LA Zip 70739, Mailing Address: P.O. Box 549, Zip 70739–0549; tel. 504/261–2730; Wilbur A. Smith, Chief Executive Officer

NEW ORLEANS ADOLESCENT HOSPITAL (O, 104 beds) 210 State Street, New Orleans, LA Zip 70118; tel. 504/897–3400

SOUTHEAST LOUISIANA HOSPITAL (O, 357 beds) Mandeville, LA, Mailing Address: P.O. Box 3850, Zip 70470–3850; tel. 504/626–8161; Joseph C. Vinturella B.C.S.W., Chief Executive Officer

Owned, leased, sponsored:	5 hospitals	1272 beds
Contract–managed:	0 hospitals	0 beds
Totals:	5 hospitals	1272 beds

★0036: LUBBOCK METHODIST HOSPITAL SYSTEM (NP)
3615 19th Street, Lubbock, TX Zip 79410–1201; tel. 806/792–1011; William D. Poteet III FACHE, President and Chief Executive Officer

TEXAS: FISHER COUNTY HOSPITAL DISTRICT (CM, 30 beds) Roby Highway, Rotan, TX Zip 79546, Mailing Address: Drawer F, Zip 79546; tel. 915/735–2256; Ella Raye Helms, Administrator

GARZA MEMORIAL HOSPITAL (CM, 13 beds) 608 West Sixth Street, Post, TX Zip 79356–3699; tel. 806/495–2828; Maritta Reed, Administrator

HEREFORD REGIONAL MEDICAL CENTER (CM, 40 beds) 801 East Third Street, Hereford, TX Zip 79045, Mailing Address: Box 1858, Zip 79045; tel. 806/364–2141; James M. Robinson, Sr., Administrator

LAMB HEALTHCARE CENTER (CM, 41 beds) 1500 South Sunset, Littlefield, TX Zip 79339; tel. 806/385–6411; Randall A. Young, Administrator

METHODIST CHILDREN'S HOSPITAL (O, 50 beds) 3610 21st Street, Lubbock, TX Zip 79410; tel. 806/784–5040; William D. Poteet III FACHE, President and Chief Executive Officer

METHODIST HOSPITAL (O, 635 beds) 3615 19th Street, Lubbock, TX Zip 79410–1201, Mailing Address: Box 1201, Zip 79408–1201; tel. 806/792–1011; William D. Poteet III FACHE, President and Chief Executive Officer

METHODIST HOSPITAL PLAINVIEW (CM, 90 beds) 2601 Dimmitt Road, Plainview, TX Zip 79072–1833; tel. 806/296–5531; Donald W. Shouse, Administrator

METHODIST HOSPITAL–LEVELLAND (L, 44 beds) 1900 South College Avenue, Levelland, TX Zip 79336; tel. 806/894–4963; Jerry Osburn, Administrator

MITCHELL COUNTY HOSPITAL (CM, 33 beds) 1543 Chestnut Street, Colorado City, TX Zip 79512–3998; tel. 915/728–3431; Wendell Alford, Administrator

MULESHOE AREA MEDICAL CENTER (CM, 31 beds) 708 South First Street, Muleshoe, TX Zip 79347; tel. 806/272–4524; Richard Murphy, Administrator

PERMIAN GENERAL HOSPITAL (CM, 76 beds) N.E. By–Pass, Andrews, TX Zip 79714, Mailing Address: Box 2108, Zip 79714; tel. 915/523–2200; Terry R. Andris CHE, Chief Executive Officer

Owned, leased, sponsored:	3 hospitals	729 beds
Contract–managed:	8 hospitals	354 beds
Totals:	11 hospitals	1083 beds

★2235: LUTHERAN HEALTH SYSTEMS (NP)
4310 17th Avenue S.W., Fargo, ND Zip 58103, Mailing Address: P.O. Box 6200, Zip 58106–6200; tel. 701/277–7500; Steven R. Orr, President

ALASKA: CENTRAL PENINSULA GENERAL HOSPITAL (CM, 62 beds) 250 Hospital Place, Soldotna, AK Zip 99669; tel. 907/262–4404; Randy Wirick, Administrator

FAIRBANKS MEMORIAL HOSPITAL (L, 206 beds) 1650 Cowles Street, Fairbanks, AK Zip 99701; tel. 907/452–8181; James Gingerich, Administrator

KODIAK ISLAND HOSPITAL AND CARE CENTER (CM, 44 beds) 1915 East Rezanof Drive, Kodiak, AK Zip 99615; tel. 907/486–3281; Edmon W. Myers, Administrator

VALDEZ COMMUNITY HOSPITAL (CM, 15 beds) 911 Meals Avenue, Valdez, AK Zip 99686–0550, Mailing Address: Box 550, Zip 99686–0550; tel. 907/835–2249; Daniel R. Mohler, Administrator

ARIZONA: MESA LUTHERAN HOSPITAL (O, 278 beds) 525 West Brown Road, Mesa, AZ Zip 85201–3299; tel. 602/834–1211; Robert A. Rundio, Executive Director

VALLEY LUTHERAN HOSPITAL (O, 172 beds) 6644 Baywood Avenue, Mesa, AZ Zip 85206; tel. 602/981–4100; Robert A. Rundio, Executive Director

COLORADO: EAST MORGAN COUNTY HOSPITAL (L, 29 beds) 2400 West Edison, Brush, CO Zip 80723; tel. 303/842–5151; Anne Platt, Administrator

MCKEE MEDICAL CENTER (O, 106 beds) 2000 Boise Avenue, Loveland, CO Zip 80538–4281; tel. 303/635–4000; Charles F. Harms, Administrator

NORTH COLORADO MEDICAL CENTER (L, 326 beds) 1801 16th Street, Greeley, CO Zip 80631–5199; tel. 970/352–4121; Karl Benjamin Gills, Administrator

STERLING REGIONAL MEDCENTER (O, 36 beds) 615 Fairhurst, Sterling, CO Zip 80751–0500, Mailing Address: Box 3500, Zip 80751; tel. 303/522–0122; James O. Pernau, Administrator

IOWA: CENTRAL COMMUNITY HOSPITAL (CM, 29 beds) Elkader, IA, Mailing Address: Rural Route 1, Box 269A, Zip 52043–9799; tel. 319/245–2250; Lisa Manson, Co–Administrator

KANSAS: DECATUR COUNTY HOSPITAL (L, 74 beds) 810 West Columbia, Oberlin, KS Zip 67749, Mailing Address: P.O. Box 268, Zip 67749; tel. 913/475–2208; R. Kim Hardman, Administrator

ST. LUKE HOSPITAL (L, 54 beds) 1014 East Melvin, Marion, KS Zip 66861; tel. 316/382–2179; Craig Hanson, Administrator

MINNESOTA: ORTONVILLE AREA HEALTH SERVICES (CM, 105 beds) 750 Eastvold Avenue, Ortonville, MN Zip 56278; tel. 612/839–2502; Donald Wee, Administrator

NEBRASKA: OGALLALA COMMUNITY HOSPITAL (L, 41 beds) 300 East Tenth Street, Ogallala, NE Zip 69153; tel. 308/284–4011; Linda Morris, Administrator

For explanation of codes following names, see page B2.
★Indicates Type III membership in the American Hospital Association.

Systems / Lutheran Health Systems

NEVADA: CHURCHILL COMMUNITY HOSPITAL (L, 40 beds) 155 North Taylor Street, Fallon, NV Zip 89406–2797; tel. 702/423–3151; Jeffrey Feike, Administrator and Chief Executive Officer

PERSHING GENERAL HOSPITAL (CM, 34 beds) 855 Sixth Street, Lovelock, NV Zip 89419, Mailing Address: P.O. Box 661, Zip 89419; tel. 702/273–2621; John Schaper, Administrator

NEW MEXICO: LOS ALAMOS MEDICAL CENTER (O, 53 beds) 3917 West Road, Los Alamos, NM Zip 87544; tel. 505/662–4201; Paul J. Wilson, Administrator

UNION COUNTY GENERAL HOSPITAL (L, 28 beds) 301 Harding Street, Clayton, NM Zip 88415, Mailing Address: P.O. Box 489, Zip 88415–0489; tel. 505/374–2585; Carrell R. Blakely, Administrator

NORTH DAKOTA: COMMUNITY MEMORIAL HOSPITAL (O, 70 beds) 905 Main, Lisbon, ND Zip 58054–0353; tel. 701/683–5241; Deb J. Krmpotic R.N., Administrator

PEMBINA COUNTY MEMORIAL HOSPITAL AND WEDGEWOOD MANOR (L, 89 beds) 205 East Third Avenue, Cavalier, ND Zip 58220, Mailing Address: Box M, Zip 58220; tel. 701/265–8461; Glen Gray, Chief Executive Officer

OREGON: CENTRAL OREGON DISTRICT HOSPITAL (CM, 47 beds) 1253 North Canal Boulevard, Redmond, OR Zip 97756–1395; tel. 503/548–8131; James A. Diegel, Administrator

SOUTH DAKOTA: BELLE FOURCHE HEALTH CARE CENTER (O, 128 beds) 2200 13th Avenue, Belle Fourche, SD Zip 57717; tel. 605/892–3331; Stephen G. Carlson, Administrator

GREGORY COMMUNITY HOSPITAL (O, 90 beds) 400 Park Street, Gregory, SD Zip 57533–0400, Mailing Address: Box 408, Zip 57533–0408; tel. 605/835–8394; Carol A. Varland, Administrator

LOOKOUT MEMORIAL HOSPITAL (O, 34 beds) 1440 North Main Street, Spearfish, SD Zip 57783–1504; tel. 605/642–2617; Stephen G. Carlson, Administrator

SOUTHERN HILLS GENERAL HOSPITAL (O, 74 beds) 209 North 16th Street, Hot Springs, SD Zip 57747–1375; tel. 605/745–3159; Linda Iverson, Administrator

STURGIS COMMUNITY HEALTH CARE CENTER (O, 114 beds) 949 Harmon Street, Sturgis, SD Zip 57785–0279, Mailing Address: P.O. Box 279, Zip 57785–0279; tel. 605/347–2536; Roger R. Heidt, Administrator

UTAH: SAN JUAN HOSPITAL (CM, 33 beds) 364 West First North, Monticello, UT Zip 84535, Mailing Address: Box 308, Zip 84535–0308; tel. 801/587–2116; Dana K. Barnett, Executive Director

WYOMING: COMMUNITY HOSPITAL (O, 36 beds) 2000 Campbell Drive, Torrington, WY Zip 82240; tel. 307/532–4181; Charles Myers, Administrator

PLATTE COUNTY MEMORIAL HOSPITAL (L, 86 beds) 201 14th Street, Wheatland, WY Zip 82201, Mailing Address: P.O. Box 848, Zip 82201; tel. 307/322–3636; Jon Frantsvog, Administrator

WASHAKIE MEMORIAL HOSPITAL (L, 30 beds) 400 South 15th Street, Worland, WY Zip 82401, Mailing Address: Box 700, Zip 82401; tel. 307/347–3221; John Johnson, Administrator

Owned, leased, sponsored:	23 hospitals	2194 beds
Contract–managed:	8 hospitals	369 beds
Totals:	31 hospitals	2563 beds

★7775: MAIN LINE HEALTH (NP)

259 Radnor–Chester Road, Suite 290, Radnor, PA Zip 19087–5260; tel. 610/293–8200; Douglas S. Peters, President and Chief Executive Officer

PENNSYLVANIA: BRYN MAWR HOSPITAL (O, 281 beds) 130 South Bryn Mawr Avenue, Bryn Mawr, PA Zip 19010–3160; tel. 610/526–3000; Kenneth Hanover, President and Chief Executive Officer

BRYN MAWR REHABILITATION HOSPITAL (O, 131 beds) 414 Paoli Pike, Malvern, PA Zip 19355–3300, Mailing Address: P.O. Box 3007, Zip 19355–3007; tel. 610/251–5400; Barry S. Rabner, President and Chief Executive Officer

LANKENAU HOSPITAL (O, 350 beds) 100 Lancaster Avenue, Wynnewood, PA Zip 19096; tel. 610/645–2000; Kenneth Hanover, President and Chief Executive Officer

PAOLI MEMORIAL HOSPITAL (O, 146 beds) 255 West Lancaster Avenue, Paoli, PA Zip 19301–1792; tel. 610/648–1201; Leland White, President

Owned, leased, sponsored:	4 hospitals	908 beds
Contract–managed:	0 hospitals	0 beds
Totals:	4 hospitals	908 beds

1975: MARSHALL COUNTY HEALTH CARE AUTHORITY (NP)

8000 Alabama Highway 69, Guntersville, AL Zip 35976; tel. 205/753–8000; L. C. Couch, Board Chairman

ALABAMA: BOAZ–ALBERTVILLE MEDICAL CENTER (O, 102 beds) U.S. Highway 431 North, Boaz, AL Zip 35957–0999, Mailing Address: Drawer Z, Zip 35957–0999; tel. 205/593–8310; Marlin Hanson, Administrator

GUNTERSVILLE–ARAB MEDICAL CENTER (O, 90 beds) 8000 Alabama Highway 69, Guntersville, AL Zip 35976; tel. 205/753–8000; Gary R. Gore, Administrator

Owned, leased, sponsored:	2 hospitals	192 beds
Contract–managed:	0 hospitals	0 beds
Totals:	2 hospitals	192 beds

0013: MASSACHUSETTS DEPARTMENT OF MENTAL HEALTH (NP)

25 Staniford Street, Boston, MA Zip 02114; tel. 617/727–5500; Eileen Elias, Commissioner

MASSACHUSETTS: LEMUEL SHATTUCK HOSPITAL (O, 230 beds) 170 Morton St, Jamaica Plain, Boston, MA Zip 02130–3787; tel. 617/522–8110; Robert Wakefield, Jr., Executive Director

MASSACHUSETTS HOSPITAL SCHOOL (O, 143 beds) 3 Randolph Street, Canton, MA Zip 02021–2397; tel. 617/828–2440; John H. Britt, Chief Executive Officer

MASSACHUSETTS MENTAL HEALTH CENTER (O, 27 beds) 74 Fenwood Road, Boston, MA Zip 02115; tel. 617/734–1300; Catherine Howard, Chief Executive Officer

MEDFIELD STATE HOSPITAL (O, 212 beds) 45 Hospital Road, Medfield, MA Zip 02052; tel. 508/359–7312; Barbara A. Leadholm, Area Director

SOLDIERS' HOME IN HOLYOKE (O, 336 beds) 110 Cherry Street, Holyoke, MA Zip 01040; tel. 413/532–9475; Rudy Chmura, Superintendent

TEWKSBURY HOSPITAL (O, 720 beds) East Street, Tewksbury, MA Zip 01876–1998; tel. 508/851–7321; Raymond D. Sanzone, Executive Director

WESTBOROUGH STATE HOSPITAL (O, 267 beds) Westborough, MA, Mailing Address: P.O. Box 288, Zip 01581; tel. 508/366–4401; Steven Scheibel, Chief Operating Officer

Owned, leased, sponsored:	7 hospitals	1935 beds
Contract–managed:	0 hospitals	0 beds
Totals:	7 hospitals	1935 beds

★1785: MASSACHUSETTS GENERAL HOSPITAL CORPORATION (NP)

32 Fruit Street, Boston, MA Zip 02114–2696; tel. 617/726–2100; Samuel O. Thier M.D., President

MASSACHUSETTS: MASSACHUSETTS GENERAL HOSPITAL (O, 899 beds) 32 Fruit Street, Boston, MA Zip 02114; tel. 617/726–2000; Richard Crater, Chief Executive Officer

MCLEAN HOSPITAL (O, 205 beds) 115 Mill Street, Belmont, MA Zip 02178–9106; tel. 617/855–2000; Steven M. Mirin M.D., Chief Executive Officer and Psychiatrist in Chief

SPAULDING REHABILITATION HOSPITAL (O, 284 beds) 125 Nashua Street, Boston, MA Zip 02114; tel. 617/720–6400; Manuel J. Lipson M.D., Chief Executive Officer

Owned, leased, sponsored:	3 hospitals	1388 beds
Contract–managed:	0 hospitals	0 beds
Totals:	3 hospitals	1388 beds

★1875: MAYO FOUNDATION (NP)

200 Southwest First Street, Rochester, MN Zip 55905; tel. 507/284–2511; Robert R. Waller M.D., President and Chief Executive Officer

FLORIDA: ST. LUKE'S HOSPITAL (O, 226 beds) 4201 Belfort Road, Jacksonville, FL Zip 32216; tel. 904/296–3700; J. Larry Read, President

MINNESOTA: ROCHESTER METHODIST HOSPITAL (O, 350 beds) 201 West Center Street, Rochester, MN Zip 55902–3084; tel. 507/266–7890; Stephen C. Waldhoff, Administrator

SAINT MARYS HOSPITAL OF ROCHESTER (O, 903 beds) 1216 Second Street S.W., Rochester, MN Zip 55902–1970; tel. 507/255–5123; Gerald T. Mahoney, Administrator

---

For explanation of codes following names, see page B2.
★Indicates Type III membership in the American Hospital Association.

Systems / Mercy Health Services

WISCONSIN: LUTHER HOSPITAL (O, 207 beds) 1221 Whipple Street, Eau Claire, WI Zip 54702–4105; tel. 715/839–3311; William Rupp M.D., President and Chief Executive Officer

Owned, leased, sponsored:	4 hospitals	1686 beds
Contract–managed:	0 hospitals	0 beds
Totals:	4 hospitals	1686 beds

1335: MEASE HEALTH CARE (NP)
135 Annwood Road, Palm Harbor, FL Zip 34648; tel. 813/733–1111; Philip K. Beauchamp FACHE, President and Chief Executive Officer

FLORIDA: MEASE COUNTRYSIDE HOSPITAL (O, 100 beds) 3231 McMullen–Booth Road, Safety Harbor, FL Zip 34695–1098, Mailing Address: P.O. 1098, Zip 34695–1098; tel. 813/725–6222; James A. Pfeiffer, Chief Administrative Officer

MEASE HOSPITAL DUNEDIN (O, 258 beds) 601 Main Street, Dunedin, FL Zip 34698, Mailing Address: P.O. Box 760, Zip 34697–0760; tel. 813/733–1111; Philip K. Beauchamp FACHE, President and Chief Executive Officer

Owned, leased, sponsored:	2 hospitals	358 beds
Contract–managed:	0 hospitals	0 beds
Totals:	2 hospitals	358 beds

★6615: MEDLANTIC HEALTHCARE GROUP (NP)
100 Irving Street N.W., Washington, DC Zip 20010–2975; tel. 202/877–6006; John P. McDaniel, Chief Executive Officer

DISTRICT OF COLUMBIA: NATIONAL REHABILITATION HOSPITAL (O, 160 beds) 102 Irving Street N.W., Washington, DC Zip 20010–2949; tel. 202/877–1000; Edward A. Eckenhoff, President and Chief Executive Officer

WASHINGTON HOSPITAL CENTER (O, 874 beds) 110 Irving Street N.W., Washington, DC Zip 20010–2975; tel. 202/877–7000; Kenneth A. Samet, President

Owned, leased, sponsored:	2 hospitals	1034 beds
Contract–managed:	0 hospitals	0 beds
Totals:	2 hospitals	1034 beds

2335: MEMORIAL HEALTH SERVICES (IO)
706 North Parrish Avenue, Adel, GA Zip 31620, Mailing Address: Box 677, Zip 31620; tel. 912/896–2251; James E. Cunningham, Chief Executive Officer

GEORGIA: BLECKLEY MEMORIAL HOSPITAL (CM, 45 beds) 408 Peacock Street, Cochran, GA Zip 31014–1559, Mailing Address: Box 536, Zip 31014–0536; tel. 912/934–6211; Henry T. Gibbs, Administrator

BURKE COUNTY HOSPITAL (CM, 40 beds) 351 Liberty Street, Waynesboro, GA Zip 30830; tel. 706/554–4435; Gloria Cochran, Administrator

IRWIN COUNTY HOSPITAL (CM, 64 beds) 710 North Irwin Avenue, Ocilla, GA Zip 31774; tel. 912/468–7411; H. Richard Murphy, Administrator

MEMORIAL HOSPITAL OF ADEL (CM, 161 beds) 706 North Parrish Avenue, Adel, GA Zip 31620–0677, Mailing Address: Box 677, Zip 31620–0677; tel. 912/896–2251; James E. Cunningham, Administrator

SMITH HOSPITAL (CM, 71 beds) 117 East Main Street, Hahira, GA Zip 31632; tel. 912/794–2502; Amanda M. Hall, Administrator

TELFAIR COUNTY HOSPITAL (CM, 52 beds) U.S. 341 South, McRae, GA Zip 31055, Mailing Address: P.O. Box 150, Zip 31055; tel. 912/868–5621; Gail B. Norris, Administrator

WORTH COUNTY HOSPITAL (CM, 50 beds) 807 South Isabella Street, Sylvester, GA Zip 31791–0545, Mailing Address: Box 545, Zip 31791–0545; tel. 912/776–6961; Loron H. Coxwell, Administrator

Owned, leased, sponsored:	0 hospitals	0 beds
Contract–managed:	7 hospitals	483 beds
Totals:	7 hospitals	483 beds

★2615: MEMORIAL HEALTH SYSTEMS (NP)
875 Sterthaus Avenue, Ormond Beach, FL Zip 32174–5197; tel. 904/676–6114; Richard A. Lind, President and Chief Executive Officer

FLORIDA: MEMORIAL HOSPITAL–FLAGLER (O, 81 beds) Moody Boulevard, Bunnell, FL Zip 32110, Mailing Address: HCR1, Box 2, Zip 32110; tel. 904/437–2211; Clark P. Christianson, Senior Vice President and Administrator

MEMORIAL HOSPITAL–ORMOND BEACH (O, 205 beds) 875 Sterthaus Avenue, Ormond Beach, FL Zip 32174–5197; tel. 904/676–6000; Clark P. Christianson, Senior Vice President and Administrator

MEMORIAL HOSPITAL–WEST VOLUSIA (L, 138 beds) 701 West Plymouth Avenue, De Land, FL Zip 32720, Mailing Address: Box 509, Zip 32721–0509; tel. 904/734–3320; Mark B. Van Fleet, Chief Executive Officer

Owned, leased, sponsored:	3 hospitals	424 beds
Contract–managed:	0 hospitals	0 beds
Totals:	3 hospitals	424 beds

★2645: MEMORIAL HEALTHCARE SYSTEM (NP)
7737 Southwest Freeway, Ste 200, Houston, TX Zip 77074–1800; tel. 713/776–6992; Dan S. Wilford, President

TEXAS: ANGLETON–DANBURY GENERAL HOSPITAL (CM, 64 beds) 132 Hospital Drive, Angleton, TX Zip 77515; tel. 409/849–7721; David A. Bleakney, Administrator

MEMORIAL HOSPITAL – MEMORIAL CITY (L, 340 beds) 920 Frostwood Drive, Houston, TX Zip 77024–9173; tel. 713/932–3055; Gerel T. Humphrey, Vice President and Chief Executive Officer

MEMORIAL HOSPITAL SYSTEM (O, 1480 beds) 7600 Beechnut, Houston, TX Zip 77074–1850; tel. 713/776–5111; Dan S. Wilford, President and Chief Executive Officer

MEMORIAL HOSPITAL–THE WOODLANDS (O, 68 beds) 9250 Pinecroft, The Woodlands, TX Zip 77380; tel. 713/364–2300; Steve Sanders, Vice President and Chief Executive Officer

MEMORIAL SPRING SHADOWS GLEN (O, 104 beds) 2801 Gessner, Houston, TX Zip 77080–2599; tel. 713/462–4000; G Jerry Mueck, Vice President and Chief Executive Officer

VAL VERDE MEMORIAL HOSPITAL (CM, 78 beds) 801 Bedell Avenue, Del Rio, TX Zip 78840, Mailing Address: P.O. Box 1527, Zip 78840; tel. 210/775–8566; Scott D. Evans FACHE, Administrator

Owned, leased, sponsored:	4 hospitals	1992 beds
Contract–managed:	2 hospitals	142 beds
Totals:	6 hospitals	2134 beds

★5165: MERCY HEALTH SERVICES (CC)
34605 Twelve Mile Road, Farmington Hills, MI Zip 48331–3221; tel. 810/489–6000; Judith Pelham, President and Chief Executive Officer

ILLINOIS: MORRISON COMMUNITY HOSPITAL (CM, 114 beds) 303 North Jackson Street, Morrison, IL Zip 61270–3042; tel. 815/772–4003; Mark F. Fedyk, Chief Executive Officer

IOWA: BAUM HARMON MEMORIAL HOSPITAL (CM, 19 beds) 255 North Welch Avenue, Primghar, IA Zip 51245; tel. 712/757–3905; Dan Ellis, Administrator

BELMOND COMMUNITY HOSPITAL (CM, 22 beds) 403 First Street S.E., Belmond, IA Zip 50421–0326, Mailing Address: P.O. Box 326, Zip 50421; tel. 515/444–3223; Douglas E. Morse, Interim Administrator

ELDORA REGIONAL MEDICAL CENTER (CM, 18 beds) 2413 Edgington Avenue, Eldora, IA Zip 50627–1541; tel. 515/858–5416; Jeffrey C. Brittain, Administrator

FRANKLIN GENERAL HOSPITAL (CM, 92 beds) 1720 Central Avenue East, Hampton, IA Zip 50441–0417, Mailing Address: P.O. Box 417, Zip 50441–0417; tel. 515/456–4721; Scott Curtis, Interim Chief Executive Officer

HANCOCK COUNTY MEMORIAL HOSPITAL (CM, 30 beds) 531 Second Street N.W., Britt, IA Zip 50423, Mailing Address: Box 68, Zip 50423–0068; tel. 515/843–3801; Lawrence N. Crail, Administrator

HAWARDEN COMMUNITY HOSPITAL (CM, 19 beds) 1111 11th Street, Hawarden, IA Zip 51023; tel. 712/552–1121; Omar L. Voran, Administrator

HOWARD COUNTY HOSPITAL (CM, 42 beds) 235 Eighth Avenue West, Cresco, IA Zip 52136–1098; tel. 319/547–2101; Elizabeth Doty, Administrator

KOSSUTH COUNTY HOSPITAL (CM, 29 beds) 1515 South Phillips Street, Algona, IA Zip 50511; tel. 515/295–2451; James G. Fitzpatrick, Administrator

For explanation of codes following names, see page B2.
★Indicates Type III membership in the American Hospital Association.

Integrated Health Delivery Networks, Health Care Systems and Alliances

Systems / Mercy Health Services

MARIAN HEALTH CENTER (O, 328 beds) 801 Fifth Street, Sioux City, IA Zip 51101, Mailing Address: Box 3168, Zip 51102; tel. 712/279-2010; Douglas V. Johnson, President

MERCY HEALTH CENTER (O, 363 beds) 250 Mercy Drive, Dubuque, IA Zip 52001-7360; tel. 319/589-8000; Sister Helen Huewe, President

MITCHELL COUNTY REGIONAL HEALTH CENTER (CM, 40 beds) 616 North Eighth Street, Osage, IA Zip 50461-1498; tel. 515/732-3781; Richard C. Hamilton, Chief Executive Officer

NORTH IOWA MERCY HEALTH CENTER (O, 285 beds) 84 Beaumont Drive, Mason City, IA Zip 50401-2999; tel. 515/424-7211; David H. Vellinga, President and Chief Executive Officer

SAINT JOSEPH COMMUNITY HOSPITAL (O, 55 beds) 308 North Maple Avenue, New Hampton, IA Zip 50659; tel. 515/394-4121; Thomas Thompson, President

SAMARITAN HEALTH SYSTEM (O, 194 beds) 1410 North Fourth Street, Clinton, IA Zip 52732, Mailing Address: P.O. Box 2960, Zip 52733-2960; tel. 319/244-5555; Thomas J. Hesselmann, President

MICHIGAN: BATTLE CREEK HEALTH SYSTEM (O, 358 beds) 300 North Avenue, Battle Creek, MI Zip 49016-3396; tel. 616/966-8000; Stephen L. Abbott, President and Chief Executive Officer

CATHERINE MCAULEY HEALTH SYSTEM (O, 530 beds) 5305 East Huron River Drive, Ann Arbor, MI Zip 48106, Mailing Address: Box 992, Zip 48106-0992; tel. 313/712-3456; Garry C. Faja, President and Chief Executive Officer

DECKERVILLE COMMUNITY HOSPITAL (CM, 17 beds) 3559 Pine Street, Deckerville, MI Zip 48427-0126; tel. 810/376-2835; David M. Simmons, Administrator

MCPHERSON HOSPITAL (O, 85 beds) 620 Byron Road, Howell, MI Zip 48843-1093; tel. 517/545-6000; Robert B. Carbeck M.D., President and Chief Executive Officer

MERCY HOSPITAL (O, 133 beds) 400 Hobart Street, Cadillac, MI Zip 49601-9596; tel. 616/779-7200; Dennis J. Renander, President and Chief Executive Officer

MERCY HOSPITAL (O, 268 beds) 5555 Conner Avenue, Detroit, MI Zip 48213-3499; tel. 313/579-4000; Brenita Crawford, President and Chief Executive Officer

MERCY HOSPITAL (O, 130 beds) 1100 Michigan Avenue, Grayling, MI Zip 49738-1398; tel. 517/348-5461; Dennis J. Renander, President and Chief Executive Officer

MERCY HOSPITAL (O, 119 beds) 2601 Electric Avenue, Port Huron, MI Zip 48061-6518; tel. 313/985-1510; Mary R. Trimmer, President and Chief Executive Officer

MUSKEGON MERCY COMMUNITY HEALTHCARE SYSTEM (O, 217 beds) 1500 East Sherman Boulevard, Muskegon, MI Zip 49443, Mailing Address: P.O. Box 358, Zip 49443-0358; tel. 616/739-9341; Sandra Bennett Bruce, President and Chief Executive Officer

SAINT MARY'S HEALTH SERVICES (O, 250 beds) 200 Jefferson Avenue S.E., Grand Rapids, MI Zip 49503; tel. 616/774-6399; Nancy Conlee Hart, President and Chief Executive Officer

SALINE COMMUNITY HOSPITAL (O, 54 beds) 400 West Russell Street, Saline, MI Zip 48176-1101; tel. 313/429-1500; James F. Harns, Chief Operating Officer

ST. JOSEPH MERCY COMMUNITY HEALTHCARE SYSTEM (O, 421 beds) 900 Woodward Avenue, Pontiac, MI Zip 48341-2985; tel. 313/858-3000; John P. Cullen, President and Chief Executive Officer

ST. JOSEPH'S MERCY HOSPITALS AND HEALTH SERVICES (O, 855 beds) 15855 19 Mile Road, Clinton Township, MI Zip 48038; tel. 810/263-2707; Robert L. Beyer, President and Chief Executive Officer

ST. LAWRENCE HOSPITAL AND HEALTHCARE SERVICES (O, 389 beds) 1210 West Saginaw Street, Lansing, MI Zip 48915-1999; tel. 517/372-3610; Arthur Knueppel, President

NEBRASKA: PENDER COMMUNITY HOSPITAL (CM, 24 beds) 603 Earl Street, Pender, NE Zip 68047-0100, Mailing Address: Box 100, Zip 68047-0100; tel. 402/385-3083; Ryan Baldwin, Administrator

NEW YORK: MERCY COMMUNITY HOSPITAL (CM, 180 beds) 160 East Main Street, Port Jervis, NY Zip 12771-0268, Mailing Address: P.O. Box 1014, Zip 12771; tel. 914/856-5351; Thomas J. Moakler, President and Chief Executive Officer

Owned, leased, sponsored:	18 hospitals	5034 beds
Contract-managed:	13 hospitals	646 beds
Totals:	31 hospitals	5680 beds

★**5155:** **MERCY HEALTH SYSTEM** (CC)
2335 Grandview Ave, 4th Floor, Cincinnati, OH Zip 45206-2280; tel. 513/221-2736; Michael D. Connelly, President and Chief Executive Officer

KENTUCKY: LOURDES HOSPITAL (S, 370 beds) 1530 Lone Oak Road, Paducah, KY Zip 42001, Mailing Address: P.O. Box 7100, Zip 42002-7100; tel. 502/444-2444; Gerald J. Lagesse, President and Chief Executive Officer

MARCUM AND WALLACE MEMORIAL HOSPITAL (S, 26 beds) 201 Richmond Avenue, Irvine, KY Zip 40336; tel. 606/723-2115; Christopher M. Goddard, Administrator

MERCY HOSPITAL (S, 149 beds) 1006 Ford Avenue, Owensboro, KY Zip 42301, Mailing Address: P.O. Box 2839, Zip 42302; tel. 502/686-6100; Douglas Borders, President and Chief Executive Officer

OHIO: CLERMONT MERCY HOSPITAL (S, 151 beds) 3000 Hospital Drive, Batavia, OH Zip 45103-1998; tel. 513/732-8200; Karen S. Ehrat Ph.D., President and Chief Executive Officer

MERCY HOSPITAL (S, 260 beds) 100 River Front Plaza, Hamilton, OH Zip 45012, Mailing Address: P.O. Box 418, Zip 45012-0418; tel. 513/870-7080; Thomas S. Urban, President and Chief Executive Officer

MERCY HOSPITAL (S, 70 beds) 485 West Market Street, Tiffin, OH Zip 44883, Mailing Address: Box 727, Zip 44883-0727; tel. 419/447-3130; Mark David Shugarman, President

MERCY HOSPITAL (S, 170 beds) 2200 Jefferson Avenue, Toledo, OH Zip 43624-9988; tel. 419/259-1500; Randall D. Kordash, President and Chief Executive Officer

MERCY HOSPITAL ANDERSON (S, 186 beds) 7500 State Road, Cincinnati, OH Zip 45255-2492; tel. 513/624-4500; Karen S. Ehrat Ph.D., President and Chief Executive Officer

MERCY HOSPITAL-WILLARD (S, 30 beds) 110 East Howard Street, Willard, OH Zip 44890-1699; tel. 419/933-2931; James O. Detwiler, President

MERCY MEDICAL CENTER (S, 218 beds) 1343 North Fountain Boulevard, Springfield, OH Zip 45501-1380; tel. 513/390-5000; David C. Hunter, Administrator

MERCY MEMORIAL HOSPITAL (S, 43 beds) 904 Scioto Street, Urbana, OH Zip 43078-2200; tel. 513/653-5231; David C. Hunter, Administrator

ST. CHARLES HOSPITAL (S, 234 beds) 2600 Navarre Avenue, Oregon, OH Zip 43616-3297; tel. 419/698-7200; Randall D. Kordash, President

ST. RITA'S MEDICAL CENTER (S, 360 beds) 730 West Market Street, Lima, OH Zip 45801-4667; tel. 419/227-3361; James P. Reber, President

PENNSYLVANIA: MERCY HOSPITAL OF NANTICOKE (S, 18 beds) 128 West Washington Street, Nanticoke, PA Zip 18634; tel. 717/735-5000; Robert D. Williams, Administrator

MERCY HOSPITAL OF SCRANTON (S, 293 beds) 746 Jefferson Avenue, Scranton, PA Zip 18501-0994; tel. 717/348-7100; John L. Nespoli, President and Chief Executive Officer

MERCY HOSPITAL OF WILKES-BARRE (S, 226 beds) 25 Church Street, Wilkes-Barre, PA Zip 18765, Mailing Address: Box 658, Zip 18765; tel. 717/826-3100; Robert P. Goodwin, President and Chief Executive Officer

TENNESSEE: ST. MARY'S HEALTH SYSTEM (S, 377 beds) 900 East Oak Hill Avenue, Knoxville, TN Zip 37917-4556; tel. 615/545-8000; Richard C. Williams, President and Chief Executive Officer

Owned, leased, sponsored:	17 hospitals	3181 beds
Contract-managed:	0 hospitals	0 beds
Totals:	17 hospitals	3181 beds

★**5215:** **MERCY-CHICAGO REGION HEALTHCARE SYSTEM** (CC)
55 Shuman Boulevard, Ste 150, Naperville, IL Zip 60563-8469; tel. 708/355-6310; Sister Catherine C. Gallagher, President

ILLINOIS: MERCY CENTER FOR HEALTH CARE SERVICES (S, 262 beds) 1325 North Highland Avenue, Aurora, IL Zip 60506; tel. 708/801-2601; Sister Dorothy Burns, President

MERCY HOSPITAL AND MEDICAL CENTER (S, 487 beds) Stevenson Expressway at King Drive, Chicago, IL Zip 60616-2477; tel. 312/567-2100; Winkle Lee, Chief Executive Officer

IOWA: MERCY HOSPITAL (S, 240 beds) 500 East Market Street, Iowa City, IA Zip 52245; tel. 319/339-0300

For explanation of codes following names, see page B2.
★Indicates Type III membership in the American Hospital Association.

Systems / Metropolitan Nashville General Hospital

Owned, leased, sponsored:	3 hospitals	989 beds
Contract–managed:	0 hospitals	0 beds
Totals:	3 hospitals	989 beds

★**8835: MERIDIA HEALTH SYSTEM** (NP)
6700 Beta Drive, Suite 200, Mayfield Village, OH Zip 44143; tel. 216/446–8000; Richard J. McCann, President

OHIO: MERIDIA EUCLID HOSPITAL (O, 224 beds) 18901 Lake Shore Boulevard, Euclid, OH Zip 44119–1090; tel. 216/531–9000; Fred L. Jackson, President

MERIDIA HILLCREST HOSPITAL (O, 263 beds) 6780 Mayfield Road, Mayfield Heights, OH Zip 44124–2294; tel. 216/449–4500; Charles B. Miner, President

MERIDIA HURON HOSPITAL (O, 289 beds) 13951 Terrace Road, Cleveland, OH Zip 44112; tel. 216/761–3300; Charles B. Miner, President and Chief Operating Officer

MERIDIA SOUTH POINTE (O, 152 beds) 4110 Warrensville Center Road, Warrensville Heights, OH Zip 44122–7099; tel. 216/283–2900; Thomas J. Strauss, President and Chief Operating Officer

MERIDIA SOUTH POINTE HOSPITAL (O, 291 beds) 4180 Warrensville Center Road, Warrensville Heights, OH Zip 44122–7098; tel. 216/491–6000; Thomas J. Strauss, President and Chief Operating Officer

Owned, leased, sponsored:	5 hospitals	1219 beds
Contract–managed:	0 hospitals	0 beds
Totals:	5 hospitals	1219 beds

8875: METHODIST HEALTH SERVICES CORPORATION (NP)
221 N.E. Glen Oak Avenue, Peoria, IL Zip 61636; tel. 309/672–4826; Robert E. Wierman, President

ILLINOIS: COMMUNITY MEMORIAL HOSPITAL (CM, 69 beds) 1000 West Harlem Avenue, Monmouth, IL Zip 61462–1099; tel. 309/734–3141; Mary K. Robbins, Co–Administrator

METHODIST MEDICAL CENTER OF ILLINOIS (O, 346 beds) 221 Northeast Glen Oak Avenue, Peoria, IL Zip 61636; tel. 309/672–5522; James K. Knoble, President

Owned, leased, sponsored:	1 hospitals	346 beds
Contract–managed:	1 hospitals	69 beds
Totals:	2 hospitals	415 beds

2715: METHODIST HEALTH SYSTEM (CO)
580 West Eighth Street, Jacksonville, FL Zip 32209–6553; tel. 904/798–8000; Marcus E. Drewa, President

FLORIDA: METHODIST MEDICAL CENTER (O, 269 beds) 580 West Eighth Street, Jacksonville, FL Zip 32209–6553; tel. 904/798–8000; Marcus E. Drewa, President

METHODIST PATHWAY CENTER (O, 25 beds) 580 West Eighth Street, Jacksonville, FL Zip 32209–6553; tel. 904/798–8250; Marcus E. Drewa, President

Owned, leased, sponsored:	2 hospitals	294 beds
Contract–managed:	0 hospitals	0 beds
Totals:	2 hospitals	294 beds

★**9345: METHODIST HEALTH SYSTEMS, INC.** (CO)
1211 Union Avenue, Suite 700, Memphis, TN Zip 38104; tel. 901/726–2300; Maurice W. Elliott, President

ARKANSAS: METHODIST HOSPITAL OF JONESBORO (O, 104 beds) 3024 Stadium Boulevard, Jonesboro, AR Zip 72401; tel. 501/972–7000; Philip H. Walkley, Jr., Administrator

MISSISSIPPI: METHODIST HOSPITAL OF MIDDLE MISSISSIPPI (O, 84 beds) 1 Bowling Green Street, Lexington, MS Zip 39095, Mailing Address: Box 641, Zip 39095; tel. 601/834–1321; Joe Dan Edwards, Administrator

METHODIST MEDICAL CENTER (L, 277 beds) 1850 Chadwick Drive, Jackson, MS Zip 39204–3479, Mailing Address: P.O. Box 59001, Zip 39204–9001; tel. 601/376–1000; Thomas L. Harper, President and Chief Executive Officer

TENNESSEE: METHODIST HOSPITAL OF DYERSBURG (O, 125 beds) 400 Tickle Street, Dyersburg, TN Zip 38024–3182; tel. 901/285–2410; Richard McCormick, Administrator

METHODIST HOSPITAL OF FAYETTE (O, 38 beds) 214 Lakeview Road, Somerville, TN Zip 38068–0001, Mailing Address: Box 909, Zip 38068–0001; tel. 901/465–3594; Stan Caummisar, Administrator

METHODIST HOSPITAL OF LEXINGTON (O, 35 beds) 200 West Church Street, Lexington, TN Zip 38351, Mailing Address: Box 160, Zip 38351; tel. 901/968–3646; Gene Ragghianti, Administrator

METHODIST HOSPITAL OF MCKENZIE (O, 27 beds) 161 Hospital Drive, McKenzie, TN Zip 38201; tel. 901/352–4170; Randal E. Carson, Administrator

METHODIST HOSPITALS OF MEMPHIS (O, 1051 beds) 1265 Union Avenue, Memphis, TN Zip 38104–3499; tel. 901/726–7000; Gary S. Shorb, President

METHODIST–HAYWOOD PARK HOSPITAL (O, 44 beds) 2545 North Washington Avenue, Brownsville, TN Zip 38012; tel. 901/772–4110; H. Lee Kirk, Jr., Administrator

Owned, leased, sponsored:	9 hospitals	1785 beds
Contract–managed:	0 hospitals	0 beds
Totals:	9 hospitals	1785 beds

★**7235: METHODIST HOSPITAL SYSTEM** (CO)
6565 Fannin Street, Houston, TX Zip 77030; tel. 713/790–2221; Larry L. Mathis FACHE, President & Chief Executive Officer

TEXAS: DIAGNOSTIC CENTER HOSPITAL (O, 145 beds) 6447 Main Street, Houston, TX Zip 77030; tel. 713/790–0790; William A. Gregory, Chief Executive Officer

SAN JACINTO METHODIST HOSPITAL (O, 266 beds) 4401 Garth Road, Baytown, TX Zip 77521; tel. 713/420–8600; Rod Seidel, President and Chief Executive Officer

THE METHODIST HOSPITAL (O, 845 beds) 6565 Fannin, Houston, TX Zip 77030; tel. 713/790–3311; Larry L. Mathis FACHE, President and Chief Executive Officer

Owned, leased, sponsored:	3 hospitals	1256 beds
Contract–managed:	0 hospitals	0 beds
Totals:	3 hospitals	1256 beds

★**2735: METHODIST HOSPITALS OF DALLAS** (NP)
1441 North Beckley, Dallas, TX Zip 75203, Mailing Address: P.O. Box 655999, Zip 75265–5999; tel. 214/947–8181; David H. Hitt, President and Chief Executive Officer

TEXAS: CHARLTON METHODIST HOSPITAL (O, 105 beds) 3500 West Wheatland Road, Dallas, TX Zip 75237–3460, Mailing Address: Box 225357, Zip 75222–5357; tel. 214/296–2511; Kim N. Hollon, Executive Director and Senior Vice President

METHODIST MEDICAL CENTER (O, 362 beds) 1441 North Beckley Avenue, Dallas, TX Zip 75203, Mailing Address: Box 655999, Zip 75265–5999; tel. 214/947–8181; John W. Carver FACHE, Executive Director

Owned, leased, sponsored:	2 hospitals	467 beds
Contract–managed:	0 hospitals	0 beds
Totals:	2 hospitals	467 beds

• ★**8285: METROHEALTH SYSTEM** (NP)
2500 Metrohealth Drive, Cleveland, OH Zip 44109; tel. 216/459–8050; Terry R. White, President and Chief Executive Officer

OHIO: METROHEALTH MEDICAL CENTER (O, 1000 beds) 2500 Metrohealth Drive, Cleveland, OH Zip 44109–1998; tel. 216/398–6000; Terry R. White, President and Chief Executive Officer

Owned, leased, sponsored:	1 hospitals	1000 beds
Contract–managed:	0 hospitals	0 beds
Totals:	1 hospitals	1000 beds

0022: METROPOLITAN NASHVILLE GENERAL HOSPITAL (NP)
215 Second Avenue North, Nashville, TN Zip 37201; tel. 615/862–4000; Tom Deweese, Administrator

TENNESSEE: METROPOLITAN NASHVILLE GENERAL HOSPITAL (O, 105 beds) 72 Hermitage Avenue, Nashville, TN Zip 37210–2110; tel. 615/862–4490; John M. Stone, Director

For explanation of codes following names, see page B2.
★Indicates Type III membership in the American Hospital Association.
•Single hospital health care system

Systems / Metropolitan...

NASHVILLE METROPOLITAN BORDEAUX ...(... beds)
1414 County Hospital Road, Nashville, TN Zip 37218-3001;
tel. 615/862-7000; Wayne Hayes, Administrator

Owned, leased, sponsored:	2 hospitals	660 beds
Contract-managed:	0 hospitals	0 beds
Totals:	2 hospitals	660 beds

- **1515: MICHIGAN CAPITAL HEALTHCARE** (NP)
  401 West Greenlawn, Lansing, MI Zip 48910-2819;
  tel. 517/334-2967; Dennis M. Litos, President and Chief Executive Officer

MICHIGAN: EATON RAPIDS COMMUNITY HOSPITAL (CM, 21 beds) 1500 South Main Street, Eaton Rapids, MI Zip 48827-0130, Mailing Address: P.O. Box 130, Zip 48827-0130; tel. 517/663-2671; Jeffrey S. Allison, Chief Executive Officer

Owned, leased, sponsored:	0 hospitals	0 beds
Contract-managed:	1 hospitals	21 beds
Totals:	1 hospitals	21 beds

2055: MICHIGAN HEALTH CARE CORPORATION (NP)
7430 Second Avenue, Ste 610, Detroit, MI Zip 48202;
tel. 313/874-9110; Charles E. Housley FACHE, President and Chief Executive Officer

MICHIGAN: AURORA HOSPITAL FOR CHILDREN (O, 80 beds) 3737 Lawton, Detroit, MI Zip 48208; tel. 313/361-7600

MARGARET W. MONTGOMERY HOSPITAL (O, 60 beds) 28303 Joy Road, Detroit, MI Zip 48185; tel. 313/458-9208; Barbara J. Clark, Vice President and Chief Operating Officer

MICHIGAN HOSPITAL AND MEDICAL CENTER (O, 416 beds) 2700 Martin Luther King Jr. Boulevard, Detroit, MI Zip 48208, Mailing Address: 2700 Martin Luther King Jr Boulevard, Zip 48208; tel. 313/361-8112; Patricia Kennedy-Scott, Vice President and Chief Operating Officer

Owned, leased, sponsored:	3 hospitals	556 beds
Contract-managed:	0 hospitals	0 beds
Totals:	3 hospitals	556 beds

★**0001: MIDMICHIGAN REGIONAL HEALTH SYSTEM** (NP)
4005 Orchard Drive, Midland, MI Zip 48670; tel. 517/839-3399;
Terence F. Moore, President

MICHIGAN: MIDMICHIGAN REGIONAL MEDICAL CENTER (O, 221 beds) 4005 Orchard Drive, Midland, MI Zip 48670; tel. 517/839-3000; David A. Reece, President

MIDMICHIGAN REGIONAL MEDICAL CENTER-CLARE (O, 64 beds) 104 West Sixth Street, Clare, MI Zip 48617-1409; tel. 517/386-9951; Lawrence F. Barco, President

MIDMICHIGAN REGIONAL MEDICAL CENTER-GLADWIN (O, 42 beds) 455 South Quarter Street, Gladwin, MI Zip 48624; tel. 517/426-9286; Mark E. Bush, Vice President and Controller

Owned, leased, sponsored:	3 hospitals	327 beds
Contract-managed:	0 hospitals	0 beds
Totals:	3 hospitals	327 beds

3775: MILWAUKEE COUNTY BOARD OF SUPERVISORS (NP)
901 North Ninth Street, Milwaukee, WI Zip 53233;
tel. 414/278-4244; F. Thomas Ament, County Executive

WISCONSIN: JOHN L. DOYNE HOSPITAL (O, 339 beds) 8700 West Wisconsin Avenue, Milwaukee, WI Zip 53226; tel. 414/257-7996; Thomas Brophy, Director

MILWAUKEE COUNTY MENTAL HEALTH COMPLEX (O, 726 beds) 9455 Watertown Plank Road, Milwaukee, WI Zip 53226-3559; tel. 414/257-6995; M. Kathleen Eilers, Administrator

Owned, leased, sponsored:	2 hospitals	1065 beds
Contract-managed:	0 hospitals	0 beds
Totals:	2 hospitals	1065 beds

2855: MISSIONARY BENEDICTINE SISTERS AMERICAN PROVINCE (CC)
300 North 18th Street, Norfolk, NE Zip 68701;
tel. 402/371-3438; Sister M. Agnes Falber, Prioress

NEBRASKA: OUR LADY OF LOURDES HOSPITAL (O, 76 beds) 1500 Koenigstein Avenue, Norfolk, NE Zip 68701-3698; tel. 402/371-3402; Randall Richards, President and Chief Executive Officer

PROVIDENCE MEDICAL CENTER (O, 34 beds) 1200 Providence Road, Wayne, NE Zip 68787; tel. 402/375-3800; Marcile Thomas, Administrator

Owned, leased, sponsored:	2 hospitals	110 beds
Contract-managed:	0 hospitals	0 beds
Totals:	2 hospitals	110 beds

0017: MISSISSIPPI STATE DEPARTMENT OF MENTAL HEALTH (NP)
1101 Robert E. Lee Building, Jackson, MS Zip 39201-1101;
tel. 601/359-1288; Roger McMurtry, Chief Mental Health Bureau

MISSISSIPPI: EAST MISSISSIPPI STATE HOSPITAL (O, 657 beds) 4555 Highland Park Drive, Meridian, MS Zip 39307, Mailing Address: Box 4128, West Station, Zip 39304-4128; tel. 601/482-6186; Ramiro J. Martinez M.D., Director

MISSISSIPPI STATE HOSPITAL (O, 1293 beds) Whitfield, MS, Mailing Address: P.O. Box 157-A, Zip 39193-0157; tel. 601/351-8000; James G. Chastain, Director

Owned, leased, sponsored:	2 hospitals	1950 beds
Contract-managed:	0 hospitals	0 beds
Totals:	2 hospitals	1950 beds

6555: MULTICARE HEALTH SYSTEM (NP)
315 Martin Luther King Jr Way, Tacoma, WA Zip 98405, Mailing Address: P.O. Box 5299, Zip 98405-0299; tel. 206/552-1000; William B. Connoley, President

WASHINGTON: ALLENMORE HOSPITAL (O, 82 beds) South 19th And Union Streets, Tacoma, WA Zip 98405, Mailing Address: P.O. Box 11414, Zip 98411-0414; tel. 206/572-2323; Charles Hoffman, Administrator

MARY BRIDGE CHILDREN'S HOSPITAL AND HEALTH CENTER (O, 72 beds) 317 Martin Luther King Jr Way, Tacoma, WA Zip 98405, Mailing Address: Box 5299, Zip 98405-0299; tel. 206/552-1400; William B. Connoley, President and Chief Executive Officer

TACOMA GENERAL HOSPITAL (O, 306 beds) 315 South K Street, Tacoma, WA Zip 98405, Mailing Address: P.O. Box 5299, Zip 98405-0299; tel. 206/552-1000; William B. Connoley, President and Chief Executive Officer

Owned, leased, sponsored:	3 hospitals	460 beds
Contract-managed:	0 hospitals	0 beds
Totals:	3 hospitals	460 beds

★**1465: MUNSON HEALTHCARE** (NP)
1105 Sixth Street, Traverse City, MI Zip 49684-2386;
tel. 616/935-5000; John M. Rockwood Jr., President

MICHIGAN: KALKASKA MEMORIAL HEALTH CENTER (CM, 81 beds) 419 Coral Street, Kalkaska, MI Zip 49646, Mailing Address: P.O. Box 249, Zip 49646-0249; tel. 616/258-9142; James D. Austin, Administrator

LEELANAU MEMORIAL HOSPITAL (CM, 95 beds) 215 South High Street, Northport, MI Zip 49670, Mailing Address: P.O. Box 217, Zip 49670; tel. 616/386-5101; James Packard, Administrator

PAUL OLIVER MEMORIAL HOSPITAL (O, 48 beds) 224 Park Avenue, Frankfort, MI Zip 49635; tel. 616/352-9621; James D. Austin, Administrator

Owned, leased, sponsored:	1 hospitals	48 beds
Contract-managed:	2 hospitals	176 beds
Totals:	3 hospitals	224 beds

3175: NEPONSET VALLEY HEALTH SYSTEM (NP)
800 Washington Street, Norwood, MA Zip 02062-3487;
tel. 617/769-4000; Yolanda Landrau R.N., Ed.D., President and Chief Executive Officer

---

For explanation of codes following names, see page B2.
★Indicates Type III membership in the American Hospital Association.
•Single hospital health care system

Systems / North Broward Hospital District

MASSACHUSETTS: NORWOOD HOSPITAL (O, 201 beds) 800 Washington Street, Norwood, MA Zip 02062; tel. 617/769-4000; Yolanda Landrau R.N., Ed.D., President
SOUTHWOOD COMMUNITY HOSPITAL (O, 182 beds) 111 Dedham Street, Norfolk, MA Zip 02056; tel. 508/668-0385

Owned, leased, sponsored:	2 hospitals	383 beds
Contract-managed:	0 hospitals	0 beds
Totals:	2 hospitals	383 beds

3075: NEW YORK CITY HEALTH AND HOSPITALS CORPORATION (NP)
125 Worth Street, Room 514, New York, NY Zip 10013; tel. 212/788-3321; Bruce Siegel M.D., M.P.H., President

NEW YORK: BELLEVUE HOSPITAL CENTER (O, 1150 beds) First Avenue and 27th Street, New York, NY Zip 10016; tel. 212/562-4141; Howard C. Cohen, Acting Executive Director
BRONX MUNICIPAL HOSPITAL CENTER (O, 725 beds) Pelham Parkway S & Eastchester Road, Bronx, NY Zip 10461; tel. 718/918-6000; Lorraine C. Tregde, Executive Director
COLER MEMORIAL HOSPITAL (O, 1025 beds) Franklin D. Roosevelt Island, New York, NY Zip 10044; tel. 212/848-6000; Mark J. Kator, Executive Director
CONEY ISLAND HOSPITAL (O, 462 beds) 2601 Ocean Parkway, Brooklyn, NY Zip 11235-7795; tel. 718/615-4000; Howard C. Cohen, Executive Director
ELMHURST HOSPITAL CENTER (O, 574 beds) 79-01 Broadway, Elmhurst, NY Zip 11373; tel. 718/334-4000; Pete Velez, Executive Director
GOLDWATER MEMORIAL HOSPITAL (O, 952 beds) Franklin D. Roosevelt Island, New York, NY Zip 10044; tel. 212/318-8000; Samuel Lehrfeld, Executive Director
HARLEM HOSPITAL CENTER (O, 688 beds) 506 Lenox Avenue, New York, NY Zip 10037-1894; tel. 212/939-1340; Bruce Goldman, Executive Director
KINGS COUNTY HOSPITAL CENTER (O, 1150 beds) 451 Clarkson Avenue, Brooklyn, NY Zip 11203-2097; tel. 718/245-3131; Jean G. Leon R.N., M.P.A., Interim Executive Director
LINCOLN MEDICAL AND MENTAL HEALTH CENTER (O, 554 beds) 234 East 149th Street, Bronx, NY Zip 10451-9998; tel. 718/579-5700; Roberto Rodriguez, Executive Director
METROPOLITAN HOSPITAL CENTER (O, 607 beds) 1901 First Avenue, New York, NY Zip 10029; tel. 212/230-6262; Lorraine C. Tregde, Acting Executive Director
NORTH CENTRAL BRONX HOSPITAL (O, 403 beds) 3424 Kossuth Avenue, Bronx, NY Zip 10467; tel. 718/519-3500; Lorraine C. Tregde, Acting Executive Director
QUEENS HOSPITAL CENTER (O, 483 beds) 82-68 164 Street, Jamaica, NY Zip 11432; tel. 718/883-3000; Arnoline W. Jones, Executive Director
WOODHULL MEDICAL AND MENTAL HEALTH CENTER (O, 558 beds) 760 Broadway, Brooklyn, NY Zip 11206; tel. 718/963-8101; Norma Noriega, Executive Director

Owned, leased, sponsored:	13 hospitals	9331 beds
Contract-managed:	0 hospitals	0 beds
Totals:	13 hospitals	9331 beds

0009: NEW YORK STATE DEPARTMENT OF MENTAL HEALTH (NP)
44 Holland Avenue, Albany, NY Zip 12229; tel. 518/447-9611; Jesse Nixon Jr. Ph.D., Director

NEW YORK: BINGHAMTON PSYCHIATRIC CENTER (O, 250 beds) 425 Robinson Street, Binghamton, NY Zip 13901; tel. 607/773-4022; David J. Woodlock, Acting Executive Director
BRONX CHILDREN'S PSYCHIATRIC CENTER (O, 75 beds) 1000 Waters Place, Bronx, NY Zip 10461-2799; tel. 718/892-0808; E. Richard Feinberg M.D., Executive Director
BRONX PSYCHIATRIC CENTER (O, 658 beds) 1500 Waters Place, Bronx, NY Zip 10461; tel. 718/931-0600; Marlene Lopez, Executive Director
BUFFALO PSYCHIATRIC CENTER (O, 436 beds) 400 Forest Avenue, Buffalo, NY Zip 14213-1298; tel. 716/885-2261; George Molnar M.D., Executive Director
CAPITAL DISTRICT PSYCHIATRIC CENTER (O, 225 beds) 75 New Scotland Avenue, Albany, NY Zip 12208; tel. 518/447-9611; Jesse Nixon, Jr. Ph.D., Director
CENTRAL ISLIP PSYCHIATRIC CENTER (O, 375 beds) Carleton Avenue, Central Islip, NY Zip 11722-4598; tel. 516/234-6262; James E. Ramseur, Exeuctive Director
CREEDMOOR PSYCHIATRIC CENTER (O, 955 beds) Jamaica, NY, Mailing Address: 80-45 Winchester Boulevard, Queens Village, Zip 11427; tel. 718/264-3300; Charlotte Seltzer, Chief Executive Officer
ELMIRA PSYCHIATRIC CENTER (O, 122 beds) 100 Washington Street, Elmira, NY Zip 14902-1527; tel. 607/737-4739; Bert W. Pyle, Jr., Director
HUDSON RIVER PSYCHIATRIC CENTER (O, 1258 beds) Branch B, Poughkeepsie, NY Zip 12601-1197; tel. 914/452-8000; Wendy P. Acrish M.P.S., Executive Director
KINGS PARK PSYCHIATRIC CENTER (O, 990 beds) Kings Park, NY, Mailing Address: Box 9000, Zip 11754-9000; tel. 516/544-2957; Alan M. Weinstock MS, M.P.A., Chief Executive Officer
KINGSBORO PSYCHIATRIC CENTER (O, 526 beds) 681 Clarkson Avenue, Brooklyn, NY Zip 11203; tel. 718/221-7395; Colga B. Hylton MS, Acting Executive Director
MANHATTAN PSYCHIATRIC CENTER–WARD'S ISLAND (O, 875 beds) 600 East 125th Street, New York, NY Zip 10035-9998; tel. 212/369-0500; Michael H. Ford M.D., Executive Director
MIDDLETOWN PSYCHIATRIC CENTER (O, 423 beds) 141 Monhagen Avenue, Middletown, NY Zip 10940-6198, Mailing Address: Box 1453, Zip 10940; tel. 914/342-5511; James Bopp, Executive Director
MOHAWK VALLEY PSYCHIATRIC CENTER (O, 614 beds) 1400 Noyes At York, Utica, NY Zip 13502-3803; tel. 315/797-6800; Sarah F. Rudes, Executive Director
NEW YORK STATE PSYCHIATRIC INSTITUTE (O, 70 beds) 722 West 168th Street, New York, NY Zip 10032; tel. 212/960-2200; John M. Oldham M.D., Director
PILGRIM PSYCHIATRIC CENTER (O, 1478 beds) Crooked Hill Road, West Brentwood, NY Zip 11717, Mailing Address: Box A, Zip 11717; tel. 516/434-7500; Peggy O'Neill R.N., Executive Director
QUEENS CHILDREN'S PSYCHIATRIC CENTER (O, 70 beds) 74-03 Commonwealth Boulevard, Bellerose, NY Zip 11426; tel. 718/264-4506; Gloria Faretra M.D., Executive Director
RICHARD H. HUTCHINGS PSYCHIATRIC CENTER (O, 184 beds) 620 Madison Street, Syracuse, NY Zip 13210-2319; tel. 315/473-4980; Bryan F. Rudes, Executive Director
ROCHESTER PSYCHIATRIC CENTER (O, 345 beds) 1111 Elmwood Avenue, Rochester, NY Zip 14620-3005; tel. 716/473-3230; Martin H. Vonholden, Executive Director
ROCKLAND CHILDREN'S PSYCHIATRIC CENTER (O, 69 beds) Convent Road, Orangeburg, NY Zip 10962; tel. 914/359-7400; James McDermott, Administrator
ROCKLAND PSYCHIATRIC CENTER (O, 902 beds) 140 Old Orangeburg Road, Orangeburg, NY Zip 10962-0071; tel. 914/359-1000; Stephen N. Lawrence Ph.D., M.P.A., Chief Executive Officer
SAGAMORE CHILDREN'S PSYCHIATRIC CENTER (O, 69 beds) 197 Half Hollow Road, Dix Hills, NY Zip 11746; tel. 516/673-7700; Robert Schweitzer Ed.D., Executive Director
SOUTH BEACH PSYCHIATRIC CENTER (O, 342 beds) 777 Seaview Avenue, Staten Island, NY Zip 10305; tel. 718/667-2300; Lucy Sarkis M.D., Executive Director
ST. LAWRENCE PSYCHIATRIC CENTER (O, 418 beds) Ogdensburg, NY, Mailing Address: Station A, Zip 13669; tel. 315/393-3000; John R. Scott, Acting Director
WESTERN NEW YORK CHILDREN'S PSYCHIATRIC CENTER (O, 46 beds) 1010 East and West Road, West Seneca, NY Zip 14224; tel. 716/674-9730; Allen R. Morganstein M.D., Clinical Director

Owned, leased, sponsored:	25 hospitals	11775 beds
Contract-managed:	0 hospitals	0 beds
Totals:	25 hospitals	11775 beds

★3115: NORTH BROWARD HOSPITAL DISTRICT (NP)
303 Southeast 17th Street, Fort Lauderdale, FL Zip 33316-2510; tel. 305/355-5100; G. Wil Trower, President and Chief Executive Officer

FLORIDA: BROWARD GENERAL MEDICAL CENTER (O, 577 beds) 1600 South Andrews Avenue, Fort Lauderdale, FL Zip 33316-2510; tel. 305/355-5610; Ruth A. Eldridge R.N., Interim Vice President, Hospital Administration

For explanation of codes following names, see page B2.
★Indicates Type III membership in the American Hospital Association.

Systems / North Broward Hospital District

CORAL SPRINGS MEDICAL CENTER (O, 167 beds) 3000 Coral Hills Drive, Coral Springs, FL Zip 33065; tel. 305/344-3000; Jason H. Moore, Administrator

IMPERIAL POINT MEDICAL CENTER (O, 154 beds) 6401 North Federal Highway, Fort Lauderdale, FL Zip 33308-1495; tel. 305/776-8500; A. Gary Muller, Administrator

NORTH BROWARD MEDICAL CENTER (O, 316 beds) 201 Sample Road, Pompano Beach, FL Zip 33064-3502; tel. 305/941-8300; James R. Chromik, Administrator

Owned, leased, sponsored:	4 hospitals	1214 beds
Contract-managed:	0 hospitals	0 beds
Totals:	4 hospitals	1214 beds

0032: NORTH MISSISSIPPI HEALTH SERVICES, INC. (NP)
830 South Gloster Street, Tupelo, MS Zip 38801; tel. 601/841-3136; Jeffrey B. Barber Ph.D., Dr.P.H., President and Chief Executive Officer

MISSISSIPPI: CLAY COUNTY MEDICAL CENTER (O, 60 beds) 835 Medical Center Drive, West Point, MS Zip 39773; tel. 601/495-2300; David M. Reid, Administrator

IUKA HOSPITAL & NURSING FACILITY (O, 88 beds) 1410 West Quitman, Iuka, MS Zip 38852, Mailing Address: P.O. Box 860, Zip 38852; tel. 601/423-6051; Glendon Spigner, Administrator

NORTH MISSISSIPPI MEDICAL CENTER (O, 610 beds) 830 South Gloster Street, Tupelo, MS Zip 38801-4934; tel. 601/841-3000; Jeffrey B. Barber Ph.D., Dr.P.H., President and Chief Executive Officer

PONTOTOC HOSPITAL AND EXTENDED CARE FACILITY (L, 61 beds) 176 South Main Street, Pontotoc, MS Zip 38863, Mailing Address: P.O. Box C, Zip 38863; tel. 601/489-5510; Fred B. Hood, Administrator

WEBSTER HEALTH SERVICES (L, 76 beds) 500 Highway 9 South, Eupora, MS Zip 39744; tel. 601/258-6221; Harold L. Whitaker, Sr., Administrator

Owned, leased, sponsored:	5 hospitals	895 beds
Contract-managed:	0 hospitals	0 beds
Totals:	5 hospitals	895 beds

★0062: NORTH SHORE HEALTH SYSTEM (NP)
300 Community Drive, Manhasset, NY 11030; tel. 516/562-4060; John S. T. Gallagher, President

NEW YORK: HUNTINGTON HOSPITAL (CM, 314 beds) 270 Park Avenue, Huntington, NY Zip 11743-2799; tel. 516/351-2000; J. Ronald Gaudreault, President and Chief Executive Officer

NORTH SHORE UNIVERSITY HOSPITAL (O, 958 beds) 300 Community Drive, Manhasset, NY Zip 11030; tel. 516/562-0100; John S T. Gallagher, President

NORTH SHORE UNIVERSITY HOSPITAL AT GLEN COVE (O, 265 beds) St Andrews Lane, Glen Cove, NY Zip 11542; tel. 516/676-5000; John S. T. Gallagher, President

NORTH SHORE UNIVERSITY HOSPITAL AT PLAINVIEW (O, 279 beds) 888 Old Country Road, Plainview, NY Zip 11803-4978; tel. 516/681-8900; Glenn S. Hirsch, Administrator

Owned, leased, sponsored:	3 hospitals	1502 beds
Contract-managed:	1 hospitals	314 beds
Totals:	4 hospitals	1816 beds

★2075: NORTHBAY HEALTHCARE SYSTEM (NP)
1200 B Gale Wilson Boulevard, Fairfield, CA Zip 94533-3587; tel. 707/429-3600; Gary J. Passama, President

CALIFORNIA: NORTHBAY MEDICAL CENTER (O, 89 beds) 1200 B Gale Wilson Boulevard, Fairfield, CA Zip 94533-3587; tel. 707/429-3600; Deborah Sugiyama, Administrator

VACAVALLEY HOSPITAL (O, 35 beds) 1000 Nut Tree Road, Vacaville, CA Zip 95687; tel. 707/446-5716; Deborah Sugiyama, Administrator

Owned, leased, sponsored:	2 hospitals	124 beds
Contract-managed:	0 hospitals	0 beds
Totals:	2 hospitals	124 beds

★1165: OAKWOOD HEALTHCARE SYSTEM (NP)
18101 Oakwood Boulevard, Dearborn, MI Zip 48124, Mailing Address: P.O. Box 2500, Zip 48123-2500; tel. 313/593-7000; Gerald D. Fitzgerald, President

MICHIGAN: OAKWOOD HOSPITAL AND MEDICAL CENTER – DEARBORN (O, 615 beds) 18101 Oakwood Boulevard, Dearborn, MI Zip 48124, Mailing Address: P.O. Box 2500, Zip 48123-2500; tel. 313/593-7000; Gerald D. Fitzgerald, President

OAKWOOD HOSPITAL ANNAPOLIS CENTER (O, 381 beds) 33155 Annapolis Road, Wayne, MI Zip 48184; tel. 313/467-4000; Carla O'Malley, Senior Vice President, Acute Care Services

OAKWOOD HOSPITAL BEYER CENTER–YPSILANTI (O, 78 beds) 135 South Prospect Street, Ypsilanti, MI Zip 48198-5693; tel. 313/484-2200; Mary A. Finn, Vice President and Administrator

OAKWOOD HOSPITAL DOWNRIVER CENTER – LINCOLN PARK (O, 49 beds) 25750 West Outer Drive, Lincoln Park, MI Zip 48146-1574; tel. 313/382-6000; Mindy L. Richards, Administrator

OAKWOOD HOSPITAL SEAWAY CENTER (O, 97 beds) 5450 Fort Street, Trenton, MI Zip 48183; tel. 313/671-3800; Edward E. Freysinger, Vice President and Administrator

OAKWOOD HOSPITAL–HERITAGE CENTER (O, 245 beds) 10000 Telegraph Road, Taylor, MI Zip 48180-3349; tel. 313/295-5232; Thomas E. Johnson, Vice President, Administrator

Owned, leased, sponsored:	6 hospitals	1465 beds
Contract-managed:	0 hospitals	0 beds
Totals:	6 hospitals	1465 beds

★0305: OKLAHOMA HEALTH SYSTEM (NP)
3300 Northwest Expressway, Oklahoma City, OK Zip 73112; tel. 405/949-6068; Stanley F. Hupfeld, President and Chief Executive Officer

OKLAHOMA: BAPTIST MEDICAL CENTER OF OKLAHOMA (O, 529 beds) 3300 Northwest Expressway, Oklahoma City, OK Zip 73112-4481; tel. 405/949-3011; Stanley F. Hupfeld, President

BAPTIST REGIONAL HEALTH CENTER (O, 124 beds) 200 Second Street S.W., Miami, OK Zip 74354, Mailing Address: Box 1207, Zip 74355-1207; tel. 918/542-6611; Randy DuBois, Administrator

BASS MEMORIAL BAPTIST HOSPITAL (O, 119 beds) 600 South Monroe, Enid, OK Zip 73701, Mailing Address: Box 3168, Zip 73702; tel. 405/233-2300; W. Eugene Baxter Dr.P.H., Administrator

BLACKWELL REGIONAL HOSPITAL (L, 34 beds) 710 South 13th Street, Blackwell, OK Zip 74631; tel. 405/363-2311; Greg Martin, Administrator

BRISTOW MEMORIAL HOSPITAL (L, 32 beds) Seventh and Spruce Streets, Bristow, OK Zip 74010, Mailing Address: Box 780, Zip 74010; tel. 918/367-2215; William L. Legate, Administrator

CHOCTAW MEMORIAL HOSPITAL (CM, 52 beds) 1405 East Kirk Road, Hugo, OK Zip 74743; tel. 405/326-6414; Michael R. Morel, Administrator

DRUMRIGHT MEMORIAL HOSPITAL (L, 43 beds) 501 South Lou Allard Drive, Drumright, OK Zip 74030-4899; tel. 918/352-2525; Jerry Jones, Administrator

GROVE GENERAL HOSPITAL (O, 62 beds) 1310 South Main Street, Grove, OK Zip 74344-1310, Mailing Address: Box 1348, Zip 74344-1348; tel. 918/786-2243; Randy DuBois, Administrator

LOGAN HOSPITAL AND MEDICAL CENTER (CM, 50 beds) Hwy 33 West at Academy Road, Guthrie, OK Zip 73044, Mailing Address: P.O. Box 1017, Zip 73044; tel. 405/282-6700

MARSHALL MEMORIAL HOSPITAL (CM, 25 beds) 1 Hospital Drive, Madill, OK Zip 73446, Mailing Address: P.O. Box 827, Zip 73446; tel. 405/795-3384; Norma Howard, Administrator

MAYES COUNTY MEDICAL CENTER (L, 43 beds) 129 North Kentucky, Pryor, OK Zip 74361, Mailing Address: Box 278, Zip 74362-0278; tel. 918/825-1600; Charles Jordan, Administrator

MEMORIAL HOSPITAL OF TEXAS COUNTY (CM, 27 beds) 520 Medical Drive, Guymon, OK Zip 73942-4438; tel. 405/338-6515; Lu Ann Weldon, Administrator

PAWNEE MUNICIPAL HOSPITAL (L, 40 beds) 1212 Fourth Street, Pawnee, OK Zip 74058, Mailing Address: Box 467, Zip 74058; tel. 918/762-2577; Dan A. Clements, Administrator

SOUTHWEST MEDICAL CENTER OF OKLAHOMA (CM, 298 beds) 4401 South Western, Oklahoma City, OK Zip 73109-3413; tel. 405/636-7000; Bob Phillips, President and Chief Executive Officer

---

For explanation of codes following names, see page B2.
★Indicates Type III membership in the American Hospital Association.

Systems / Ornda Healthcorp

STROUD MUNICIPAL HOSPITAL (L, 30 beds) Highway 66 West, Stroud, OK Zip 74079, Mailing Address: P.O. Box 530, Zip 74079; tel. 918/968–3571; Jerrell J. Horton, Chief Executive Officer

WATONGA MUNICIPAL HOSPITAL (CM, 25 beds) 500 North Nash Boulevard, Watonga, OK Zip 73772–0370, Mailing Address: Box 370, Zip 73772–0370; tel. 405/623–7211; Frank D. Loveless, Administrator

Owned, leased, sponsored:	10 hospitals	1056 beds
Contract–managed:	6 hospitals	477 beds
Totals:	16 hospitals	1533 beds

0018: OKLAHOMA STATE DEPARTMENT OF MENTAL HEALTH AND SUBSTANCE ABUSE SERVICES (NP)
1000 Northeast Tenth, Oklahoma City, OK Zip 73152, Mailing Address: P.O. Box 53277, Zip 73152; tel. 405/271–6868; Thomas Peace Ph.D., Commissioner

OKLAHOMA: GRIFFIN MEMORIAL HOSPITAL (O, 215 beds) 900 East Main Street, Norman, OK Zip 73070–0101, Mailing Address: Box 151, Zip 73070; tel. 405/321–4880; Stand LaBoon, Superintendent

WESTERN STATE PSYCHIATRIC CENTER (O, 178 beds) Fort Supply, OK, Mailing Address: P.O. Box 1, Zip 73841–0001; tel. 405/766–2311; Steve Norwood, Director

Owned, leased, sponsored:	2 hospitals	393 beds
Contract–managed:	0 hospitals	0 beds
Totals:	2 hospitals	393 beds

★3355: ORLANDO REGIONAL HEALTHCARE SYSTEM (NP)
1414 Kuhl Avenue, Orlando, FL Zip 32806–2093; tel. 407/841–5111; J. Gary Strack, President and Chief Executive Officer

FLORIDA: ORLANDO REGIONAL MEDICAL CENTER (O, 790 beds) 1414 Kuhl Avenue, Orlando, FL Zip 32806–2093; tel. 407/841–5111; J. Gary Strack, President and Chief Executive Officer

ST. CLOUD HOSPITAL, A DIVISION OF ORLANDO REGIONAL HEALTHCARE SYSTEM (O, 68 beds) 2906 17th Street, Saint Cloud, FL Zip 34769–6099; tel. 407/892–2135; Jim Norris, Executive Director

Owned, leased, sponsored:	2 hospitals	858 beds
Contract–managed:	0 hospitals	0 beds
Totals:	2 hospitals	858 beds

6525: ORNDA HEALTHCORP (IO)
3401 West End Avenue, Suite 700, Nashville, TN Zip 37203; tel. 615/383–8599; Elizabeth A. Berryman, Assistant Vice President and General Counsel

ARIZONA: COMMUNITY HOSPITAL MEDICAL CENTER (O, 59 beds) 6501 North 19th Avenue, Phoenix, AZ Zip 85015; tel. 602/249–3434; Michael Miglis, Chief Executive Officer

MESA GENERAL HOSPITAL MEDICAL CENTER (O, 138 beds) 515 North Mesa Drive, Mesa, AZ Zip 85201; tel. 602/969–9111; Jeffrey A. Ashin, Chief Executive Officer

ST. LUKE'S BEHAVIORAL HEALTH CENTER (O, 86 beds) 1800 East Van Buren, Phoenix, AZ Zip 85006–3742; tel. 602/251–8484; Edward H. Lamb, Chief Executive Officer

ST. LUKE'S MEDICAL CENTER (O, 296 beds) 1800 East Van Buren Street, Phoenix, AZ Zip 85006–3742; tel. 602/251–8100; Mary Starmann–Harrison FACHE, President

TEMPE ST. LUKE'S HOSPITAL (O, 102 beds) 1500 South Mill Avenue, Tempe, AZ Zip 85281–6699; tel. 602/968–9411; Brian S. Bentley, President

TUCSON GENERAL HOSPITAL (O, 94 beds) 3838 North Campbell Avenue, Tucson, AZ Zip 85719–1497, Mailing Address: P.O. Box 40360, Zip 85717–0360; tel. 520/318–6302; William C. Behnke, Jr., Chief Executive Officer

CALIFORNIA: BROTMAN MEDICAL CENTER (O, 240 beds) 3828 Delmas Terrace, Culver City, CA Zip 90231–2459, Mailing Address: Box 2459, Zip 90231–2459; tel. 310/836–7000; Daniel P. McLean, Chief Executive Officer

CHAPMAN GENERAL HOSPITAL (O, 104 beds) 2601 East Chapman Avenue, Orange, CA Zip 92669; tel. 714/633–0011; Howard H. Levine, Executive Director

COASTAL COMMUNITIES HOSPITAL (O, 165 beds) 2701 South Bristol Street, Santa Ana, CA Zip 92704–9911, Mailing Address: P.O. Box 5240, Zip 92704–0240; tel. 714/754–5454

COMMUNITY AND MISSION HOSPITALS OF HUNTINGTON (O, 226 beds) 2623 East Slauson Avenue, Huntington Park, CA Zip 90255; tel. 213/583–1931; Jeffrey K. Stadnik, Administrator

DOCTORS HOSPITAL OF SANTA ANA (O, 54 beds) 1901 North College Avenue, Santa Ana, CA Zip 92706; tel. 714/547–2565; R. Michael Hartman, Chief Executive Officer

FOUNTAIN VALLEY REGIONAL HOSPITAL AND MEDICAL CENTER (O, 359 beds) 17100 Euclid, Fountain Valley, CA Zip 92708; tel. 714/966–7200; Richard Butler, Administrator

FRENCH HOSPITAL MEDICAL CENTER (O, 124 beds) 1911 Johnson Avenue, San Luis Obispo, CA Zip 93401; tel. 805/543–5353

GREATER EL MONTE COMMUNITY HOSPITAL (O, 115 beds) 1701 South Santa Anita Avenue, South El Monte, CA Zip 91733–9918; tel. 818/579–7777; Sandra M. Chester, Chief Executive Officer

HARBOR VIEW MEDICAL CENTER (O, 130 beds) 120 Elm Street, San Diego, CA Zip 92101; tel. 619/235–3102; Roger W. Kielman, Administrator

MIDWAY HOSPITAL MEDICAL CENTER (O, 225 beds) 5925 San Vicente Boulevard, Los Angeles, CA Zip 90019, Mailing Address: Box 35909, Zip 90035; tel. 213/938–3161; John V. Fenton, Chief Executive Officer

MONTEREY PARK HOSPITAL (O, 95 beds) 900 South Atlantic Boulevard, Monterey Park, CA Zip 91754; tel. 818/570–9000; Dan F. Ausman, Chief Executive Officer

SANTA ANA HOSPITAL MEDICAL CENTER (O, 99 beds) 1901 North Fairview Street, Santa Ana, CA Zip 92706; tel. 714/554–1653; R. Michael Hartman, Chief Executive Officer

ST. LUKE MEDICAL CENTER (O, 120 beds) 2632 East Washington Boulevard, Pasadena, CA Zip 91107–1494, Mailing Address: Bin 7021, Zip 91109; tel. 818/797–1141; Robert S. Freymuller, Chief Executive Officer

SUBURBAN MEDICAL CENTER (O, 140 beds) 16453 South Colorado Avenue, Paramount, CA Zip 90723; tel. 310/531–3110; Marc A. Furstman, Chief Executive Officer

VALLEY COMMUNITY HOSPITAL (O, 70 beds) 505 East Plaza Drive, Santa Maria, CA Zip 93454–9943; tel. 805/925–0935; William C. Rasmussen, Chief Executive Officer

WHITTIER HOSPITAL MEDICAL CENTER (O, 159 beds) 15151 Janine Drive, Whittier, CA Zip 90605; tel. 310/945–3561; Michael H. Sussman, Chief Executive Officer

WOODRUFF COMMUNITY HOSPITAL (O, 96 beds) 3800 Woodruff Avenue, Long Beach, CA Zip 90808; tel. 310/421–8241; Robert Glass, Administrator

FLORIDA: CORAL GABLES HOSPITAL (O, 205 beds) 3100 Douglas Road, Coral Gables, FL Zip 33134–6990; tel. 305/445–8461; Nick Bianco, Chief Executive Officer

FLORIDA MEDICAL CENTER HOSPITAL (O, 459 beds) 5000 West Oakland Park Boulevard, Fort Lauderdale, FL Zip 33313–1585; tel. 305/735–6000; Denny De Narvaez, Chief Executive Officer

GOLDEN GLADES REGIONAL MEDICAL CENTER (O, 128 beds) 17300 Northwest Seventh Avenue, Miami, FL Zip 33169; tel. 305/652–4200; Martha Garcia, Acting Chief Executive Officer

NORTH BAY MEDICAL CENTER (O, 122 beds) 6600 Madison Street, New Port Richey, FL Zip 34652; tel. 813/842–8468; Michael G. Layfield, Administrator

PARKWAY REGIONAL MEDICAL CENTER (O, 299 beds) 160 Northwest 170th Street, North Miami Beach, FL Zip 33169; tel. 305/654–5050; David S. Catlin, Chief Executive Officer

INDIANA: WINONA MEMORIAL HOSPITAL (O, 170 beds) 3232 North Meridian Street, Indianapolis, IN Zip 46208–4693; tel. 317/924–3392; Keith R. King, Chief Executive Officer

IOWA: DAVENPORT MEDICAL CENTER (O, 150 beds) 1111 West Kimberly Road, Davenport, IA Zip 52806; tel. 319/391–2020; Richard A. Seidler, Chief Executive Officer

LOUISIANA: MINDEN MEDICAL CENTER (O, 108 beds) 1 Medical Plaza, Minden, LA Zip 71055; tel. 318/377–2321; George E. French III, Administrator

MISSISSIPPI: GULF COAST MEDICAL CENTER (O, 189 beds) 180–A Debuys Road, Biloxi, MS Zip 39531–4405, Mailing Address: Box 4518, Zip 39531–4518; tel. 601/388–6711; C. L. Smith, Chief Executive Officer

GULF OAKS HOSPITAL (O, 45 beds) 180–C Debuys Road, Biloxi, MS Zip 39531; tel. 601/388–0600; Hugh S. Simcoe III, Administrator

For explanation of codes following names, see page B2.
★Indicates Type III membership in the American Hospital Association.

Systems / Ornda Healthcorp

MISSOURI: TWIN RIVERS REGIONAL MEDICAL CENTER (O, 116 beds) 1301 First Street, Kennett, MO Zip 63857; tel. 314/888–4522; Cliff Yeager, Chief Executive Officer

NEVADA: LAKE MEAD HOSPITAL MEDICAL CENTER (O, 140 beds) 1409 East Lake Mead Boulevard, North Las Vegas, NV Zip 89030; tel. 702/649–7711; Ernest Libman, Administrator and Chief Executive Officer

OREGON: EASTMORELAND HOSPITAL (O, 77 beds) 2900 Southeast Steele Street, Portland, OR Zip 97202; tel. 503/234–0411; Ken Giles, Administrator

WOODLAND PARK HOSPITAL (O, 123 beds) 10300 Northeast Hancock, Portland, OR Zip 97220; tel. 503/257–5500; William E. Price, Chief Executive Officer

TEXAS: GARLAND COMMUNITY HOSPITAL (O, 113 beds) 2696 West Walnut Street, Garland, TX Zip 75042; tel. 214/276–7116; Gary L. Stokes, Administrator and Chief Executive Officer

LAKE POINTE MEDICAL CENTER (L, 92 beds) 6800 Scenic Drive, Rowlett, TX Zip 75088–1550, Mailing Address: P.O. Box 1550, Zip 75030–1500; tel. 214/412–2273; Kenneth R. Teel, Administrator

SHARPSTOWN GENERAL HOSPITAL (O, 53 beds) 6700 Bellaire At Tarnef, Houston, TX Zip 77074–4999, Mailing Address: P.O. Box 740389, Zip 77274–0389; tel. 713/774–7611; J. O. Lewis, Administrator

SOUTH PARK HOSPITAL (O, 61 beds) 6610 Quaker Avenue, Lubbock, TX Zip 79413–5938; tel. 806/791–8000; Steve Rowley, Chief Executive Officer

SOUTHWEST GENERAL HOSPITAL (O, 199 beds) 7400 Barlite Boulevard, San Antonio, TX Zip 78224–1399; tel. 210/921–2000; Mark L. Bernard, Chief Executive Officer

TRINITY VALLEY MEDICAL CENTER (O, 126 beds) 2900 South Loop 256, Palestine, TX Zip 75801; tel. 903/731–1000; Larry C. Bozeman, Chief Executive Officer

WASHINGTON: PUGET SOUND HOSPITAL (O, 146 beds) 215 South 36th Street, Tacoma, WA Zip 98408, Mailing Address: P.O. Box 11412, Zip 98411–0412; tel. 206/474–0561; Bruce Brandler, Administrator

WEST VIRGINIA: PLATEAU MEDICAL CENTER (O, 80 beds) 430 Main Street, Oak Hill, WV Zip 25901; tel. 304/469–8600; Albert H. Michaels, Administrator

WYOMING: LANDER VALLEY MEDICAL CENTER (O, 102 beds) 1320 Bishop Randall Drive, Lander, WY Zip 82520; tel. 307/332–4420; Andrew Gramlich, Chief Executive Officer

Owned, leased, sponsored:	46 hospitals	6599 beds
Contract–managed:	0 hospitals	0 beds
Totals:	46 hospitals	6599 beds

★**5335: OSF HEALTHCARE SYSTEM** (CC)
800 Northeast Glen Oak Avenue, Peoria, IL Zip 61603–3200; tel. 309/655–2850; Sister Frances Marie Masching, President

ILLINOIS: SAINT ANTHONY MEDICAL CENTER (O, 210 beds) 5666 East State Street, Rockford, IL Zip 61108–2472; tel. 815/226–2000; Jerry A. Nash, Administrator

SAINT FRANCIS MEDICAL CENTER (O, 560 beds) 530 Northeast Glen Oak Avenue, Peoria, IL Zip 61637; tel. 309/655–2000; Sister M. Canisia, Administrator

SAINT JAMES HOSPITAL (O, 84 beds) 610 East Water Street, Pontiac, IL Zip 61764; tel. 815/842–2828; David Ochs, Administrator

SAINT JOSEPH HOSPITAL (O, 48 beds) 1005 Julien Street, Belvidere, IL Zip 61008–9932; tel. 815/544–3411; Kevin D. Schoplein, Administrator

ST. JOSEPH MEDICAL CENTER (O, 164 beds) 2200 East Washington Street, Bloomington, IL Zip 61701–4364, Mailing Address: Box 1287, Zip 61702–1287; tel. 309/662–3311; Kenneth J. Natzke, Administrator

ST. MARY MEDICAL CENTER (O, 156 beds) 3333 North Seminary Street, Galesburg, IL Zip 61401–1299; tel. 309/344–3161; Richard S. Kowalski, Chief Executive Officer

MICHIGAN: ST. FRANCIS HOSPITAL (O, 66 beds) 3401 Ludington Street, Escanaba, MI Zip 49829; tel. 906/786–3311; Roger M. Burgess, Administrator

Owned, leased, sponsored:	7 hospitals	1288 beds
Contract–managed:	0 hospitals	0 beds
Totals:	7 hospitals	1288 beds

0435: PACIFIC HEALTH CORPORATION (IO)
249 East Ocean Boulevard, Long Beach, CA Zip 90802; tel. 310/435–1300; Jens Mueller, Chairman

CALIFORNIA: ANAHEIM GENERAL HOSPITAL (O, 99 beds) 3350 West Ball Road, Anaheim, CA Zip 92804–9998; tel. 714/827–6700; Peter A. Szekrenyi Ph.D., Executive Director

BELLFLOWER MEDICAL CENTER (O, 145 beds) 9542 East Artesia Boulevard, Bellflower, CA Zip 90706; tel. 310/925–8355; Stanley Otake, Administrator and Chief Executive Officer

BUENA PARK MEDICAL CENTER (O, 58 beds) 5742 Beach Boulevard, Buena Park, CA Zip 90621; tel. 714/521–4770

HAWTHORNE HOSPITAL (O, 73 beds) 13300 South Hawthorne Boulevard, Hawthorne, CA Zip 90250; tel. 310/679–3321; Marvin Herschberg, Administrator

LOS ANGELES METROPOLITAN MEDICAL CENTER (O, 100 beds) 2231 South Western Avenue, Los Angeles, CA Zip 90018–1399; tel. 213/737–7372; Marvin Herschberg, Chief Executive Officer

Owned, leased, sponsored:	5 hospitals	475 beds
Contract–managed:	0 hospitals	0 beds
Totals:	5 hospitals	475 beds

★**7555: PALOMAR POMERADO HEALTH SYSTEM** (NP)
15255 Innovation Drive, Suite 204, San Diego, CA Zip 92128–3410; tel. 619/675–5100; Andrew W. Deems, President and Chief Executive Officer

CALIFORNIA: PALOMAR MEDICAL CENTER (O, 395 beds) 555 East Valley Parkway, Escondido, CA Zip 92025–3084; tel. 619/739–3000; Victoria M. Penland, Administrator and Chief Operating Officer

POMERADO HOSPITAL (O, 279 beds) 15615 Pomerado Road, Poway, CA Zip 92064; tel. 619/485–4600; Mark R. Middlebrook, Administrator and Chief Operating Officer

Owned, leased, sponsored:	2 hospitals	674 beds
Contract–managed:	0 hospitals	0 beds
Totals:	2 hospitals	674 beds

5765: PARACELSUS HEALTHCARE CORPORATION (IO)
155 North Lake Ave, Suite 1100, Pasadena, CA Zip 91101; tel. 818/792–8600; R. J. Messenger, President and Chief Executive Officer

CALIFORNIA: BELLWOOD GENERAL HOSPITAL (O, 85 beds) 10250 East Artesia Boulevard, Bellflower, CA Zip 90706; tel. 310/866–9028; Roger W. Wessels, Chief Executive Officer and Administrator

CHICO COMMUNITY HOSPITAL (O, 129 beds) 560 Cohasset Road, Chico, CA Zip 95926; tel. 916/896–5000; Fredrick W. Hodges, Chief Executive Officer

DESERT PALMS COMMUNITY HOSPITAL (O, 123 beds) 1212 East Avenue South, Palmdale, CA Zip 93550; tel. 805/273–2211; Elizabeth Scarcelli, Interim Administrator

HOLLYWOOD COMMUNITY HOSPITAL OF HOLLYWOOD (O, 99 beds) 6245 De Longpre Avenue, Hollywood, CA Zip 90028; tel. 213/462–2271; Maxine Cooper, Chief Executive Officer

HOLLYWOOD COMMUNITY HOSPITAL OF VAN NUYS (O, 61 beds) 14433 Emelita Street, Van Nuys, CA Zip 91401, Mailing Address: P.O. Box 2698, Zip 91401; tel. 818/787–1511; Elizabeth Scarcelli, Administrator

LANCASTER COMMUNITY HOSPITAL (O, 132 beds) 43830 North Tenth Street West, Lancaster, CA Zip 93534; tel. 805/948–4781; Steve Schmidt, Chief Executive Officer

LOS ANGELES COMMUNITY HOSPITAL (O, 136 beds) 4081 East Olympic Boulevard, Los Angeles, CA Zip 90023; tel. 213/267–0477; Sandra J. Anaya R.N., Administrator

LOS ANGELES COMMUNITY HOSPITAL OF NORWALK (O, 50 beds) 13222 Bloomfield Avenue, Norwalk, CA Zip 90650; tel. 310/863–4763; Sandra J. Anaya R.N., Administrator

MONROVIA COMMUNITY HOSPITAL (O, 49 beds) 323 South Heliotrope Avenue, Monrovia, CA Zip 91016, Mailing Address: Box 707, Zip 91017–0707; tel. 818/359–8341; Steve Courtier, Administrator

ORANGE COUNTY COMMUNITY HOSPITAL OF BUENA PARK (O, 159 beds) 6850 Lincoln Avenue, Buena Park, CA Zip 90620–5703; tel. 714/827–1161; Joseph Sharp, Acting Administrator

FLORIDA: PENINSULA MEDICAL CENTER (O, 119 beds) 264 South Atlantic Avenue, Ormond Beach, FL Zip 32176–8192; tel. 904/672–4161; Peter A. Marmerstein, Chief Executive Officer

For explanation of codes following names, see page B2.
★*Indicates Type III membership in the American Hospital Association.*

Systems / Presbyterian Healthcare System

GEORGIA: FLINT RIVER COMMUNITY HOSPITAL (O, 50 beds) 509 Sumter Street, Montezuma, GA 31063-0770, Mailing Address: P.O. Box 770, Zip 31063-0770; tel. 912/472-3100; Michael Clark, Administrator

KANSAS: HALSTEAD HOSPITAL (L, 137 beds) 328 Poplar Street, Halstead, KS Zip 67056-2099; tel. 316/835-2651; Jeffrey A. Feeney, President and Chief Executive Officer

LOUISIANA: ELMWOOD MEDICAL CENTER (L, 108 beds) 1221 South Clearview Parkway, Jefferson, LA Zip 70121; tel. 504/734-1900; Deborah C. Keel, Acting Administrator

MISSISSIPPI: SENATOBIA COMMUNITY HOSPITAL (O, 52 beds) 401 Getwell Drive, Senatobia, MS Zip 38668, Mailing Address: P.O. Box 648, Zip 38668; tel. 601/562-3100; James D. Tesar, Administrator

TENNESSEE: BLEDSOE COUNTY GENERAL HOSPITAL (O, 32 beds) Pikeville, TN, Mailing Address: P.O. Box 428, Zip 37367-0428; tel. 615/447-2112; Gary Burton, Administrator

CLAY COUNTY HOSPITAL (O, 36 beds) McArthur Street, Celina, TN Zip 38551, Mailing Address: Box 427, Zip 38551; tel. 615/243-3581; Donald E. Downey, Administrator

FENTRESS COUNTY GENERAL HOSPITAL (O, 73 beds) Highway 52-W, Jamestown, TN Zip 38556, Mailing Address: P.O. Box 1500, Zip 38556; tel. 615/879-8171; Curtis B. Courtney, Administrator

TEXAS: MEDICAL CENTER OF MESQUITE (O, 152 beds) 1011 North Galloway Avenue, Mesquite, TX Zip 75149; tel. 214/320-7000; Terry J. Fontenot, Administrator

Owned, leased, sponsored:	19 hospitals	1782 beds
Contract-managed:	0 hospitals	0 beds
Totals:	19 hospitals	1782 beds

0335: PARK HEALTHCARE COMPANY (IO)
4015 Travis Drive, Nashville, TN Zip 37211; tel. 615/833-1077; Jerry E. Gilliland, President

KENTUCKY: LINCOLN TRAIL HOSPITAL (O, 67 beds) 3909 South Wilson Road, Radcliff, KY Zip 40160-9714, Mailing Address: P.O. Box 369, Zip 40159-0369; tel. 502/351-9444; Melvin E. Modderman, Administrator

TEXAS: MEMORIAL HOSPITAL (O, 42 beds) 602 Hurst Street, Center, TX Zip 75935, Mailing Address: Box 1749, Zip 75935; tel. 409/598-2781; Anton P. Zurbrugg CHE, Administrator and Chief Executive Officer

Owned, leased, sponsored:	2 hospitals	109 beds
Contract-managed:	0 hospitals	0 beds
Totals:	2 hospitals	109 beds

★5415: PEACEHEALTH (CC)
15325 Southeast 30th Place, Suite 300, Bellevue, WA Zip 98007; tel. 206/747-1711; Sister Monica Heeran, President

ALASKA: KETCHIKAN GENERAL HOSPITAL (L, 60 beds) 3100 Tongass Avenue, Ketchikan, AK Zip 99901-5746; tel. 907/225-5171; Edward F. Mahn, Chief Executive Officer

OREGON: PEACE HARBOR HOSPITAL (O, 21 beds) 400 Ninth Street, Florence, OR Zip 97439, Mailing Address: Box 580, Zip 97439; tel. 503/997-8412; James Barnhart, Administrator

SACRED HEART MEDICAL CENTER (O, 396 beds) 1255 Hilyard Street, Eugene, OR Zip 97401, Mailing Address: Box 10905, Zip 97440; tel. 503/686-7300; Andrew R. McCulloch, Administrator

WASHINGTON: ST. JOHN'S MEDICAL CENTER (O, 200 beds) 1614 East Kessler Boulevard, Longview, WA Zip 98632, Mailing Address: P.O. Box 3002, Zip 98632-0302; tel. 206/423-1530; Mark E. McGourty, Regional Chief Executive Officer

ST. JOSEPH HOSPITAL (O, 195 beds) 2901 Squalicum Parkway, Bellingham, WA Zip 98225-1898; tel. 206/734-5400; John Hayward, Administrator

Owned, leased, sponsored:	5 hospitals	872 beds
Contract-managed:	0 hospitals	0 beds
Totals:	5 hospitals	872 beds

• ★0034: PMH HEALTH RESOURCES, INC. (NP)
1201 South Seventh Avenue, Phoenix, AZ Zip 85007-3913, Mailing Address: P.O. Box 21207, Zip 85036-1207; tel. 602/238-3321; Reginald M. Ballantyne III, President

ARIZONA: PMH HEALTH SERVICES NETWORK (O, 183 beds) 1201 South Seventh Avenue, Phoenix, AZ Zip 85007-3995; tel. 602/258-5111; Jeffrey Norman, Chief Executive Officer

Owned, leased, sponsored:	1 hospitals	183 beds
Contract-managed:	0 hospitals	0 beds
Totals:	1 hospitals	183 beds

★3505: PRESBYTERIAN HEALTHCARE SERVICES (CO)
5901 Harper Drive N.E., Albuquerque, NM Zip 87109, Mailing Address: P.O. Box 26666, Zip 87125-6666; tel. 505/260-6300; James Hinton, President and Chief Executive Officer

COLORADO: DELTA COUNTY MEMORIAL HOSPITAL (CM, 44 beds) 100 Stafford Lane, Delta, CO Zip 81416-5003, Mailing Address: P.O. Box 10100, Zip 81416-5003; tel. 303/874-7681; Kevin McMullan, Administrator

NEW MEXICO: ARTESIA GENERAL HOSPITAL (CM, 38 beds) 702 North 13th Street, Artesia, NM Zip 88210; tel. 505/748-3333; William D. Haddock FACHE, Administrator

DR. DAN C. TRIGG MEMORIAL HOSPITAL (L, 29 beds) 301 East Miel De Luna Avenue, Tucumcari, NM Zip 88401, Mailing Address: P.O. Box 608, Zip 88401; tel. 505/461-0141; Dan Noteware, Administrator

ESPANOLA HOSPITAL (O, 61 beds) 1010 Spruce Street, Espanola, NM Zip 87532; tel. 505/753-7111; Marcella A. Romero, Administrator

LINCOLN COUNTY MEDICAL CENTER (L, 38 beds) 211 Sudderth Drive, Ruidoso, NM Zip 88345, Mailing Address: P.O. Drawer 3C/D, Hollywood Station, Zip 88345; tel. 505/257-7381; Valerie Miller, Administrator

PLAINS REGIONAL MEDICAL CENTER – CLOVIS (O, 106 beds) 2100 North Thomas Street, Clovis, NM Zip 88101, Mailing Address: P.O. Box 1688, Zip 88101-1688; tel. 505/769-2141; Grant H. Nelson, Administrator

PLAINS REGIONAL MEDICAL CENTER–PORTALES (O, 103 beds) 1700 South Avenue O, Portales, NM Zip 88130, Mailing Address: P.O. Drawer 60, Zip 88130; tel. 505/356-4411; Grant H. Nelson, Administrator

PRESBYTERIAN HOSPITAL (O, 433 beds) 1100 Central Avenue S.E., Albuquerque, NM Zip 87102, Mailing Address: P.O. Box 26666, Zip 87125-6666; tel. 505/841-1234; James Hinton, Vice President Operations

PRESBYTERIAN KASEMAN HOSPITAL (O, 120 beds) 8300 Constitution Avenue N.E., Albuquerque, NM Zip 87110; tel. 505/291-2000; Jim Purdy, Administrative Director

SOCORRO GENERAL HOSPITAL (O, 30 beds) 1202 Highway 60 West, Socorro, NM Zip 87801, Mailing Address: P.O. Box 1009, Zip 87801-1009; tel. 505/835-1140; Jeff Dye, Administrator

Owned, leased, sponsored:	8 hospitals	920 beds
Contract-managed:	2 hospitals	82 beds
Totals:	10 hospitals	1002 beds

★1130: PRESBYTERIAN HEALTHCARE SYSTEM (NP)
8220 Walnut Hill Lane, Suite 700, Dallas, TX Zip 75231; tel. 214/345-8500; Douglas D. Hawthorne, President and Chief Executive Officer

TEXAS: PRESBYTERIAN HOSPITAL OF DALLAS (O, 558 beds) 8200 Walnut Hill Lane, Dallas, TX Zip 75231-4402; tel. 214/345-6789; Mark H. Merrill, Executive Director

PRESBYTERIAN HOSPITAL OF KAUFMAN (O, 72 beds) Highway 243 West At Highway 175, Kaufman, TX Zip 75142-9998, Mailing Address: Box 310, Zip 75142; tel. 214/932-7200; Argus D. Forrest, Executive Vice President and Executive Director

PRESBYTERIAN HOSPITAL OF PLANO (O, 87 beds) 6200 West Parker Road, Plano, TX Zip 75093-7914; tel. 214/608-8000; Philip M. Wentworth FACHE, President and Chief Executive Officer

PRESBYTERIAN HOSPITAL OF WINNSBORO (O, 50 beds) 719 West Coke Road, Winnsboro, TX Zip 75494-3098, Mailing Address: P.O. Box 628, Zip 75494-0628; tel. 903/342-5227; Jerry Hopper, Vice President and Executive Director

Owned, leased, sponsored:	4 hospitals	767 beds
Contract-managed:	0 hospitals	0 beds
Totals:	4 hospitals	767 beds

For explanation of codes following names, see page B2.
★Indicates Type III membership in the American Hospital Association.
•Single hospital health care system

Integrated Health Delivery Networks, Health Care Systems and Alliances

Systems / Presentation Health System

★**5255: PRESENTATION HEALTH SYSTEM** (CC)
1301 South Ninth Ave, Suite 102, Sioux Falls, SD Zip 57105–1043; tel. 605/331–4999; John T. Porter, President

MINNESOTA: A.L. VADHEIM MEMORIAL HOSPITAL (CM, 63 beds) 240 Willow Street, Tyler, MN Zip 56178–0280; tel. 507/247–5521; James Rotert, Administrator

MONTANA: HOLY ROSARY HOSPITAL (O, 146 beds) 2101 Clark Street, Miles City, MT Zip 59301–2796; tel. 406/232–2540; H. Ray Gibbons, President and Chief Executive Officer

SOUTH DAKOTA: DEUEL COUNTY MEMORIAL HOSPITAL (CM, 20 beds) 701 Third Avenue South, Clear Lake, SD Zip 57226–1037, Mailing Address: P.O. Box 1037, Zip 57226–1037; tel. 605/874–2141

FLANDREAU MUNICIPAL HOSPITAL (CM, 20 beds) 214 North Prairie Avenue, Flandreau, SD Zip 57028–1243; tel. 605/997–2433; Kent Olson, Administrator

HAND COUNTY MEMORIAL HOSPITAL (CM, 30 beds) 300 West Fifth Street, Miller, SD Zip 57362; tel. 605/853–2421; Clarence A. Lee, Administrator

MARSHALL COUNTY MEMORIAL HOSPITAL (CM, 38 beds) 413 Ninth Street, Britton, SD Zip 57430–0230, Mailing Address: Box 230, Zip 57430–0230; tel. 605/448–2253; Jeff R. Dorn, Administrator

MCKENNAN HOSPITAL (O, 429 beds) 800 East 21st Street, Sioux Falls, SD Zip 57105, Mailing Address: P.O. Box 5045, Zip 57117–5045; tel. 605/339–8000; Fredrick Slunecka, President and Chief Executive Officer

QUEEN OF PEACE HOSPITAL (O, 99 beds) 525 North Foster, Mitchell, SD Zip 57301–2999; tel. 605/995–2000; Ronald L. Jacobson, President and Chief Executive Officer

ST. LUKE'S MIDLAND REGIONAL MEDICAL CENTER (O, 225 beds) 305 South State Street, Aberdeen, SD Zip 57402–4450; tel. 605/622–5000; Dale J. Stein, President and Chief Executive Officer

Owned, leased, sponsored:	4 hospitals	899 beds
Contract–managed:	5 hospitals	171 beds
Totals:	9 hospitals	1070 beds

★**0995: PROMINA NORTHWEST HEALTH SYSTEM** (NP)
1791 Mulkey Road, Suite 102, Austell, GA Zip 30001–1124; tel. 404/732–5501; Thomas E. Hill, President and Chief Executive Officer

GEORGIA: COBB HOSPITAL AND MEDICAL CENTER (O, 303 beds) 3950 Austell Road, Austell, GA Zip 30001–1121; tel. 404/732–4000; Paul F. Johnson, President

KENNESTONE HOSPITAL (O, 505 beds) 677 Church Street, Marietta, GA Zip 30060; tel. 404/793–5000; Edward J. Bonn, President

PROMINA DOUGLAS HOSPITAL (O, 98 beds) 8954 Hospital Drive, Douglasville, GA Zip 30134–2282; tel. 404/949–1500; T. Mark Haney, President and Chief Executive Officer

PROMINA PAULDING MEMORIAL MEDICAL CENTER (O, 175 beds) 600 West Memorial Drive, Dallas, GA Zip 30132–1335; tel. 404/445–4411; James Roy Orr, Jr., Administrator

PROMINA R. T. JONES HOSPITAL (O, 84 beds) 201 Hospital Road, Canton, GA Zip 30114, Mailing Address: P.O. Box 906, Zip 30114; tel. 404/720–5100; Duane Thompson, Chief Executive Officer

PROMINA WINDY HILL HOSPITAL (O, 100 beds) 2540 Windy Hill Road, Marietta, GA Zip 30067; tel. 404/644–1000; John H. Richards, Administrator

Owned, leased, sponsored:	6 hospitals	1265 beds
Contract–managed:	0 hospitals	0 beds
Totals:	6 hospitals	1265 beds

★**5265: PROVIDENCE SERVICES** (CC)
9 East Ninth Avenue, Spokane, WA Zip 99202; tel. 509/455–4884; Richard J. Umbdenstock, President and Chief Executive Officer

MONTANA: COLUMBUS HOSPITAL (S, 145 beds) 500 15th Avenue South, Great Falls, MT Zip 59403, Mailing Address: Box 5013, Zip 59403–5013; tel. 406/727–3333; Daniel W. Boatman, Executive Vice President and Chief Operating Officer

ST. JOSEPH HOSPITAL (S, 22 beds) Skyline Drive & 14th Avenue, Polson, MT Zip 59860, Mailing Address: Box 1010, Zip 59860–1010; tel. 406/883–5377; John W. Glueckert, President

ST. PATRICK HOSPITAL (S, 213 beds) 500 West Broadway, Missoula, MT Zip 59802–4096, Mailing Address: Box 4587, Zip 59806–4587; tel. 406/543–7271; Lawrence L. White, Jr., President

WASHINGTON: HOLY FAMILY HOSPITAL (S, 190 beds) North 5633 Lidgerwood Avenue, Spokane, WA Zip 99220; tel. 509/482–0111; Ronald J. Schurra, Chief Executive Officer

MOUNT CARMEL HOSPITAL (S, 33 beds) 982 East Columbia Street, Colville, WA Zip 99114–0351, Mailing Address: Box 351, Zip 99114–0351; tel. 509/684–2561; Gloria Cooper, Chief Executive Officer

SACRED HEART MEDICAL CENTER (S, 623 beds) West 101 Eighth Avenue, Spokane, WA Zip 99220, Mailing Address: P.O. Box 2555, Zip 99220–2555; tel. 509/455–3040; Gerald P. Leahy, President

ST. JOSEPH'S HOSPITAL (S, 65 beds) 500 East Webster Street, Chewelah, WA Zip 99109, Mailing Address: P.O. Box 197, Zip 99109; tel. 509/935–8211; Gary V. Peck, Chief Executive Officer

ST. MARY MEDICAL CENTER (S, 120 beds) 401 West Poplar Street, Walla Walla, WA Zip 99362, Mailing Address: Box 1477, Zip 99362–0312; tel. 509/525–3320; John A. Isely, President

Owned, leased, sponsored:	8 hospitals	1411 beds
Contract–managed:	0 hospitals	0 beds
Totals:	8 hospitals	1411 beds

0011: PUERTO RICO DEPARTMENT OF HEALTH (NP)
Building A – Medical Center, San Juan, PR Zip 00936, Mailing Address: Call Box 70184, Zip 00936; tel. 809/274–7676; Carmen Feliciano De Melecio M.D., Secretary of Health

PUERTO RICO: AGUADILLA GENERAL HOSPITAL (O, 104 beds) Carr Aguadilla San Juan, Aguadilla, PR Zip 00605, Mailing Address: P.O. Box 3968, Zip 00605; tel. 809/891–3000; Luis Acevedo, Executive Director

ARECIBO REGIONAL HOSPITAL (O, 183 beds) San Luis Avenue, Arecibo, PR Zip 00612, Mailing Address: Call Box 1500, Zip 00612; tel. 809/878–7272; Jose L. Mirauda M.D., Executive Director

DR. JOSE RAMOS LEBRON HOSPITAL (O, 180 beds) General Valero Ave, #194, Fajardo, PR Zip 00738, Mailing Address: P.O. Box 1283, Zip 00738–1283; tel. 809/863–0505; Domingo Velez M.H.S.A., Executive Administrator

HOSPITAL UNIVERSITARIO DR. RAMON RUIZ ARNAU (O, 340 beds) Avenue Laurel, Santa Juanita, Bayamon, PR Zip 00956; tel. 809/787–5151; Ivan Millon, Executive Director

PONCE REGIONAL HOSPITAL (O, 407 beds) Barrio Machuelo, Ponce, PR Zip 00731; tel. 809/844–2080; Jose Toro Font M.D., Medical Director

STATE PSYCHIATRIC HOSPITAL (O, 425 beds) San Juan, PR, Mailing Address: Call Box 2100, Caparra Heights Station, Zip 00922–2100; tel. 809/766–4646; Judy Fernandez M.D., Medical Director

UNIVERSITY HOSPITAL (O, 297 beds) Puerto Rico Medical Center, Rio Piedras Station, San Juan, PR Zip 00935; tel. 809/754–3654; Gorye Sanchez M.D., Director

Owned, leased, sponsored:	7 hospitals	1936 beds
Contract–managed:	0 hospitals	0 beds
Totals:	7 hospitals	1936 beds

★**0040: QUEEN'S HEALTH SYSTEMS** (NP)
201 Merchant Street, Suite 2450, Honolulu, HI Zip 96813–2929; tel. 808/532–6102; Richard L. Griffith, Chief Executive Officer

HAWAII: MOLOKAI GENERAL HOSPITAL (O, 30 beds) Kaunakakai, HI, Mailing Address: P.O. Box 408, Zip 96748–0408; tel. 808/553–5331; W. C. McElhannon, President and Chief Executive Officer

QUEEN'S MEDICAL CENTER (O, 541 beds) 1301 Punchbowl Street, Honolulu, HI Zip 96813; tel. 808/538–9011; Arthur A. Ushijima, President and Chief Executive Officer

Owned, leased, sponsored:	2 hospitals	571 beds
Contract–managed:	0 hospitals	0 beds
Totals:	2 hospitals	571 beds

★**0002: QUORUM HEALTH GROUP/QUORUM HEALTH RESOURCES** (IO)
155 Franklin Road, Suite 401, Brentwood, TN Zip 37027; tel. 615/371–7979; James E. Dalton Jr., President and Chief Executive Officer

For explanation of codes following names, see page B2.
★Indicates Type III membership in the American Hospital Association.

Systems / Quorum Health Group/Quorum Health Resources

ALABAMA: GADSDEN REGIONAL MEDICAL CENTER (O, 287 beds) 1007 Goodyear Avenue, Gadsden, AL Zip 35999; tel. 205/494–4648; Michael R. Blackburn, Chief Executive Officer

JACKSONVILLE HOSPITAL (CM, 56 beds) 1701 Pelham Road South, Jacksonville, AL Zip 36265, Mailing Address: P.O. Box 999, Zip 36265; tel. 205/435–4970; Richard L. McConahy, Administrator

MEDICAL CENTER ENTERPRISE (O, 113 beds) 400 North Edwards Street, Enterprise, AL Zip 36330–9981; tel. 334/347–0584; John L. Robertson, Chief Executive Officer

WIREGRASS HOSPITAL (CM, 151 beds) 1200 West Maple Avenue, Geneva, AL Zip 36340; tel. 334/684–3655; H. Randolph Smith, Administrator

ALASKA: BARTLETT MEMORIAL HOSPITAL (CM, 64 beds) 3260 Hospital Drive, Juneau, AK Zip 99801; tel. 907/586–8438; Robert F. Valliant, Administrator

ARIZONA: PHOENIX GENERAL HOSPITAL AND MEDICAL CENTER (CM, 97 beds) 19829 North 27th Avenue, Phoenix, AZ Zip 85027–4002; tel. 602/879–6100; Robert Duncan, Chief Executive Officer

ARKANSAS: BATES MEDICAL CENTER (CM, 40 beds) 602 North Walton Boulevard, Bentonville, AR Zip 72712; tel. 501/273–2481; Thomas P. O'Neal, President

CHICOT MEMORIAL HOSPITAL (CM, 54 beds) Highway 65 and 82, Lake Village, AR Zip 71653–0000, Mailing Address: Box 512, Zip 71653–0441; tel. 501/265–5351; Robert R. Reddish, Administrator

DELTA MEMORIAL HOSPITAL (CM, 35 beds) 300 East Pickens Street, Dumas, AR Zip 71639, Mailing Address: Box 128, Zip 71639–0126; tel. 501/382–4303; Rodney McPherson, Administrator

DREW MEMORIAL HOSPITAL (CM, 50 beds) 778 Scogin Drive, Monticello, AR Zip 71655–5728; tel. 501/367–2411; Jerry W. Bradshaw, Chief Executive Officer

HELENA REGIONAL MEDICAL CENTER (CM, 100 beds) 1801 Martin Luther King, Helena, AR Zip 72342, Mailing Address: Box 788, Zip 72342–0788; tel. 501/338–5800; Steve Reeder, Chief Executive Officer

HOWARD MEMORIAL HOSPITAL (CM, 50 beds) 800 West Leslie Street, Nashville, AR Zip 71852–0381, Mailing Address: Box 381, Zip 71852 0381; tel. 501/845–4400; Lynn Crowell, Chief Executive Officer

MEMORIAL HOSPITAL (CM, 73 beds) 205 East Jefferson Street, Siloam Springs, AR Zip 72761; tel. 501/524–4141; Donald E. Patterson, Administrator

REBSAMEN REGIONAL MEDICAL CENTER (CM, 113 beds) 1400 West Braden Street, Jacksonville, AR Zip 72076, Mailing Address: Box 159, Zip 72078–0159; tel. 501/985–7000; Thomas R. Siemers, Administrator

SALINE MEMORIAL HOSPITAL (CM, 141 beds) 1 Medical Park Drive, Benton, AR Zip 72015; tel. 501/776–6000; Terry G. Whittington, Chief Executive Officer

COLORADO: CLAGETT MEMORIAL HOSPITAL (CM, 75 beds) 701 East Fifth Street, Rifle, CO Zip 81650–2970, Mailing Address: P.O. Box 912, Zip 81650–0912; tel. 303/625–1510; Edwin A. Gast, Administrator

HEART OF THE ROCKIES REGIONAL MEDICAL CENTER (CM, 35 beds) 448 East First Street, Salida, CO Zip 81201–0429, Mailing Address: P.O. Box 429, Zip 81201–0429; tel. 719/539–6661; Howard D. Turner, Administrator and Chief Executive Officer

MEMORIAL HOSPITAL (CM, 27 beds) 785 Russell Street, Craig, CO Zip 81625–9906; tel. 303/824–9411; M. Randell Phelps, Administrator

MONTEZUMA COUNTY HOSPITAL DISTRICT (CM, 123 beds) 1311 North Mildred Road, Cortez, CO Zip 81321; tel. 303/565–6666; Stephen R. Selzer, Administrator

MONTROSE MEMORIAL HOSPITAL (CM, 68 beds) 800 South Third Street, Montrose, CO Zip 81401–4291; tel. 303/249–2211; Tyler Erickson, Administrator

MOUNT SAN RAFAEL HOSPITAL (CM, 31 beds) 410 Benedicta Avenue, Trinidad, CO Zip 81082–2093; tel. 719/846–9213; James P. D'Agostino, Chief Executive Officer

PARKVIEW EPISCOPAL MEDICAL CENTER (CM, 249 beds) 400 West 16th Street, Pueblo, CO Zip 81003; tel. 719/584–4000; C. W. Smith, President and Chief Operating Officer

PIONEERS HOSPITAL OF RIO BLANCO COUNTY (CM, 42 beds) 345 Cleveland Street, Meeker, CO Zip 81641–0000; tel. 303/878–5047; Jim Murphy, Administrator

PROWERS MEDICAL CENTER (CM, 40 beds) 401 Kendall Drive, Lamar, CO Zip 81052–3993; tel. 719/336–4343; Earl J. Steinhoff, Chief Executive Officer

VALLEY VIEW HOSPITAL (CM, 59 beds) 1906 Blake Avenue, Glenwood Springs, CO Zip 81601, Mailing Address: Box 1970, Zip 81602; tel. 303/945–6535; Norman L. McBride, Chief Executive Officer

FLORIDA: BARTOW MEMORIAL HOSPITAL (CM, 56 beds) 1239 East Main Street, Bartow, FL Zip 33830–5005, Mailing Address: Box 1050, Zip 33830–1050; tel. 813/533–8111; David M. Klein, Administrator

BASCOM PALMER EYE INSTITUTE–ANNE BATES LEACH EYE HOSPITAL (CM, 34 beds) 900 Northwest 17th Street, Miami, FL Zip 33136–1199, Mailing Address: Box 016880, Zip 33101–6880; tel. 305/326–6000; David Bixler, Administrator

BERT FISH MEDICAL CENTER (CM, 82 beds) 401 Palmetto, New Smyrna Beach, FL Zip 32168; tel. 904/427–3401; James R. Foster, Administrator

BROOKSVILLE REGIONAL HOSPITAL (CM, 91 beds) 55 Ponce De Leon Boulevard, Brooksville, FL Zip 34601–0037, Mailing Address: Box 37, Zip 34605–0037; tel. 904/796–5111; Hal W. Leftwich FACHE, Administrator

DESOTO MEMORIAL HOSPITAL (CM, 82 beds) 900 North Robert Avenue, Arcadia, FL Zip 33821–2180, Mailing Address: P.O. Box 2180, Zip 33821–2180; tel. 813/494–3535; Gary M. Moore, Administrator

GLADES GENERAL HOSPITAL (CM, 73 beds) 1201 South Main Street, Belle Glade, FL Zip 33430–8002, Mailing Address: Box 8002, Zip 33430–8002; tel. 407/996–6571; Neil Whipkey, Administrator

HENDRY GENERAL HOSPITAL (CM, 48 beds) 500 West Sugarland Highway, Clewiston, FL Zip 33440; tel. 813/983–9121; J. Rudy Reinhardt, Administrator

HIALEAH HOSPITAL (CM, 411 beds) 651 East 25th Street, Hialeah, FL Zip 33013–3878; tel. 305/693–6100; Clifford J. Bauer, Chief Executive Officer

JACKSON HOSPITAL (CM, 107 beds) 4250 Hospital Drive, Marianna, FL Zip 32446, Mailing Address: P.O. Box 1608, Zip 32447–1608; tel. 904/526–2200; Chuck Ellis, Administrator

JUPITER MEDICAL CENTER (CM, 276 beds) 1210 South Old Dixie Highway, Jupiter, FL Zip 33458; tel. 407/747–2234; Donald A. Mayer, Chief Executive Officer

LEESBURG REGIONAL MEDICAL CENTER (CM, 414 beds) 600 East Dixie Avenue, Leesburg, FL Zip 34748; tel. 904/323–5000; James R. Giffin, President and Chief Executive Officer

SOUTH LAKE MEMORIAL HOSPITAL (CM, 68 beds) 847 Eighth Street, Clermont, FL Zip 34711; tel. 904/394–4071; P. Shannon Elswick, Administrator and Chief Executive Officer

SPRING HILL REGIONAL HOSPITAL (CM, 75 beds) 10461 Quality Drive, Spring Hill, FL Zip 34609; tel. 904/688–3053; Michael J. Stenger, Administrator and Chief Executive Officer

UNIVERSITY OF MIAMI HOSPITAL AND CLINICS (CM, 40 beds) 1475 Northwest 12th Avenue, Miami, FL Zip 33136–1002; tel. 305/548–4382; David L. Stansberry, Administrator

GEORGIA: CAMDEN MEDICAL CENTER (CM, 40 beds) 2000 Dan Proctor Drive, Saint Marys, GA Zip 31558–0805, Mailing Address: Box 805, Zip 31558–0805; tel. 912/576–4200

ELBERT MEMORIAL HOSPITAL (CM, 53 beds) 4 Medical Drive, Elberton, GA Zip 30635–1897; tel. 706/283–3151; Tim Merritt, Administrator

EMANUEL COUNTY HOSPITAL (CM, 119 beds) 117 Kite Road, Swainsboro, GA Zip 30401, Mailing Address: P.O. Box 879, Zip 30401; tel. 912/237–9911; James Jarrett, Administrator

HABERSHAM COUNTY MEDICAL CENTER (CM, 137 beds) Highway 441, Demorest, GA Zip 30535, Mailing Address: Box 37, Zip 30535; tel. 706/754–2161; C. Richard Dwozan, President

HANCOCK MEMORIAL HOSPITAL (CM, 30 beds) 453 Boland Street, Sparta, GA Zip 31087, Mailing Address: P.O. Box 490, Zip 31087; tel. 706/444–7006; Daniel D. Holtz FACHE, Administrator and Chief Executive Officer

MCDUFFIE COUNTY HOSPITAL (CM, 47 beds) 521 Hill Street S.W., Thomson, GA Zip 30824; tel. 706/595–1411; Douglas C. Keir, Chief Executive Officer

OCONEE REGIONAL MEDICAL CENTER (CM, 145 beds) 821 North Cobb Street, Milledgeville, GA Zip 31061, Mailing Address: Box 690, Zip 31061; tel. 912/454–3500; Brian L. Riddle, Chief Executive Officer

RIDGECREST HOSPITAL (CM, 45 beds) 393 Ridgecrest Circle, Clayton, GA Zip 30525; tel. 706/782–4297; Gerald E. Knepp, Chief Executive Officer

SOUTHEAST GEORGIA REGIONAL MEDICAL CENTER (CM, 337 beds) 3100 Kemble Avenue, Brunswick, GA Zip 31520, Mailing Address: Box 1518, Zip 31521; tel. 912/264–7000; Ted R. Whitten, Acting Chief Executive Officer

TANNER MEDICAL CENTER (CM, 183 beds) 705 Dixie Street, Carrollton, GA Zip 30117–3818; tel. 404/836–9666; Loy M. Howard, Chief Executive Officer

For explanation of codes following names, see page B2.
★Indicates Type III membership in the American Hospital Association.

Systems / Quorum Health Group/Quorum Health Resources

TANNER MEDICAL CENTER–VILLA RICA (CM, 53 beds) 601 Dallas Road, Villa Rica, GA Zip 30180, Mailing Address: Box 638, Zip 30180; tel. 404/459-7100; J. M. McCollum, Administrator

UPSON REGIONAL MEDICAL CENTER (CM, 119 beds) 801 West Gordon Street, Thomaston, GA Zip 30286-2831, Mailing Address: Box 1059, Zip 30286; tel. 706/647-8111; Samuel S. Gregory, Administrator

WALTON MEDICAL CENTER (CM, 115 beds) 330 Alcova Street, Monroe, GA Zip 30655, Mailing Address: Box 1346, Zip 30655; tel. 404/267-8461; Edgar L. Belcher, Administrator

WAYNE MEMORIAL HOSPITAL (CM, 138 beds) 865 South First Street, Jesup, GA Zip 31545, Mailing Address: Box 408, Zip 31545; tel. 912/427-6811; Charles R. Morgan, Administrator

WOODRIDGE HOSPITAL (CM, 42 beds) 394 Ridgecrest Circle, Clayton, GA Zip 30525; tel. 706/782-3100; Gerald E. Knepp, Chief Executive Officer

IDAHO: BINGHAM MEMORIAL HOSPITAL (CM, 120 beds) 98 Poplar Street, Blackfoot, ID Zip 83221-1799; tel. 208/785-4100; Robert M. Peterson, Administrator

GRITMAN MEDICAL CENTER (CM, 45 beds) 700 South Washington Street, Moscow, ID Zip 83843; tel. 208/882-4511; Robert A. Colvin, President and Chief Executive Officer

MAGIC VALLEY REGIONAL MEDICAL CENTER (CM, 147 beds) 650 Addison Avenue West, Twin Falls, ID Zip 83301, Mailing Address: Box 409, Zip 83303-0409; tel. 208/737-2000; John Bingham, Administrator

ILLINOIS: COMMUNITY MEMORIAL HOSPITAL (CM, 57 beds) 400 Caldwell Street, Staunton, IL Zip 62088-1499; tel. 618/635-2200; Patrick B. Heise, Chief Executive Officer

CRAWFORD MEMORIAL HOSPITAL (CM, 107 beds) 1000 North Allen Street, Robinson, IL Zip 62454, Mailing Address: P.O. Box 151, Zip 62454; tel. 618/544-3131; Roger D. Feldt, Chief Executive Officer

GIBSON COMMUNITY HOSPITAL (CM, 82 beds) 1120 North Melvin Street, Gibson City, IL Zip 60936, Mailing Address: P.O. Box 429, Zip 60936-0429; tel. 217/784-4251; Terry Thompson, Administrator

HARRISBURG MEDICAL CENTER (CM, 78 beds) 17 Country Club Court, Harrisburg, IL Zip 62946-0017, Mailing Address: P.O. Box 428, Zip 62946-0428; tel. 618/253-7671; John T. Graves, Chief Executive Officer

ILLINI COMMUNITY HOSPITAL (CM, 48 beds) 640 West Washington Street, Pittsfield, IL Zip 62363; tel. 217/285-2113; Kathleen E. Millgard, President and Chief Executive Officer

KEWANEE HOSPITAL (CM, 55 beds) 719 Elliott Street, Kewanee, IL Zip 61443-2711, Mailing Address: P.O. Box 747, Zip 61443-0747; tel. 309/853-3361; Charles Duffy, President

MEMORIAL HOSPITAL (CM, 67 beds) South Adams Street, Carthage, IL Zip 62321, Mailing Address: P.O. Box 160, Zip 62321; tel. 217/357-3131; Joseph Murrell, Chief Executive Officer

PANA COMMUNITY HOSPITAL (CM, 44 beds) South Locust Street, Pana, IL Zip 62557-0169; tel. 217/562-2131; David Faulkner, Administrator and Chief Executive Officer

SANDWICH COMMUNITY HOSPITAL (CM, 50 beds) 11 East Pleasant Avenue, Sandwich, IL Zip 60548-0901; tel. 815/786-8484; Loren D. Slade, Administrator

WHITE COUNTY HOSPITAL (CM, 130 beds) 400 Plum Street, Carmi, IL Zip 62821-1799; tel. 618/382-4171; Craig A. Jesiolowski, Chief Executive Officer

INDIANA: DAVIESS COUNTY HOSPITAL (CM, 85 beds) 1314 Grand Avenue, Washington, IN Zip 47501-2198, Mailing Address: P.O. Box 760, Zip 47501-0760; tel. 812/254-2760; Marc Chircop, Chief Executive Officer

MARY SHERMAN HOSPITAL (CM, 53 beds) 320 North Section Street, Sullivan, IN Zip 47882, Mailing Address: P.O. Box 10, Zip 47882-0010; tel. 812/268-4311; Thomas J. Hudgins, Administrator

STARKE MEMORIAL HOSPITAL (CM, 35 beds) 102 East Culver Road, Knox, IN Zip 46534-2299; tel. 219/772-6231; Leonard W. Daugherty, Executive Director

IOWA: BOONE COUNTY HOSPITAL (CM, 57 beds) 1015 Union Street, Boone, IA Zip 50036-4898; tel. 515/432-3140; Joseph S. Smith, Chief Executive Officer

DES MOINES GENERAL HOSPITAL (CM, 113 beds) 603 East 12th Street, Des Moines, IA Zip 50309-5515; tel. 515/263-4200; Roy W. Wright, Chief Executive Officer

FORT MADISON COMMUNITY HOSPITAL (CM, 50 beds) 5445 Avenue O, Fort Madison, IA Zip 52627-0174, Mailing Address: P.O. Box 174, Zip 52627-0174; tel. 319/372-6530; C. James Platt, Administrator

KNOXVILLE AREA COMMUNITY HOSPITAL (CM, 59 beds) 1002 South Lincoln Street, Knoxville, IA Zip 50138-3121; tel. 515/842-2151; Terry R. Lambert, Administrator

WASHINGTON COUNTY HOSPITAL (CM, 83 beds) 400 East Polk Street, Washington, IA Zip 52353, Mailing Address: P.O. Box 909, Zip 52353; tel. 319/653-5481; E. Patrick Smith III, Administrator

KANSAS: COFFEYVILLE REGIONAL MEDICAL CENTER (CM, 123 beds) 1400 West Fourth, Coffeyville, KS Zip 67337-3306; tel. 316/251-1200; Jerry Marquette, Jr., Administrator

KINGMAN COMMUNITY HOSPITAL (CM, 49 beds) 750 Avenue D West, Kingman, KS Zip 67068; tel. 316/532-3147; Sam J. Allen, Chief Executive Officer

NEOSHO MEMORIAL REGIONAL MEDICAL CENTER (CM, 60 beds) 629 South Plummer, Chanute, KS Zip 66720; tel. 316/431-4000; Murray L. Brown, Administrator

NEWMAN MEMORIAL HOSPITAL (CM, 152 beds) 1201 West 12th Avenue, Emporia, KS Zip 66801-2597; tel. 316/343-6800; David Christiansen, Chief Executive Officer

KENTUCKY: CRITTENDEN COUNTY HOSPITAL (CM, 100 beds) Highway 60 South, Marion, KY Zip 42064-0386, Mailing Address: Box 386, Zip 42064; tel. 502/965-5281; Rick Napper, Chief Executive Officer

CUMBERLAND COUNTY HOSPITAL (CM, 31 beds) Highway 90 West, Burkesville, KY Zip 42717-0280, Mailing Address: P.O. Box 280, Zip 42717-0280; tel. 502/864-2511; Mark Thompson, Chief Executive Officer

FLEMING COUNTY HOSPITAL (CM, 52 beds) 920 Elizaville Avenue, Flemingsburg, KY Zip 41041, Mailing Address: Box 388, Zip 41041-0388; tel. 606/849-2351; Bobby B. Emmons, Administrator

FRANKLIN–SIMPSON MEMORIAL HOSPITAL (CM, 36 beds) Brookhaven Road, Franklin, KY Zip 42135-2929, Mailing Address: P.O. Box 2929, Zip 42135-2929; tel. 502/586-3253; William P. Macri, Administrator

HARDIN MEMORIAL HOSPITAL (CM, 276 beds) 913 North Dixie Highway, Elizabethtown, KY Zip 42701-2599; tel. 502/737-1212; Gary Colberg, Administrator

MARSHALL COUNTY HOSPITAL (CM, 80 beds) 503 George McClain Drive, Benton, KY Zip 42025, Mailing Address: P.O. Box 630, Zip 42025; tel. 502/527-4800; David Fuqua, Administrator

MONROE COUNTY MEDICAL CENTER (CM, 49 beds) 529 Capp Harlan Road, Tompkinsville, KY Zip 42167; tel. 502/487-9231; John B. Millstead, Chief Executive Officer

MUHLENBERG COMMUNITY HOSPITAL (CM, 135 beds) 440 Hopkinsville Street, Greenville, KY Zip 42345, Mailing Address: P.O. Box 387, Zip 42345; tel. 502/338-8000; Charles D. Lovell, Jr., Chief Executive Officer

OHIO COUNTY HOSPITAL (CM, 54 beds) 1211 Main Street, Hartford, KY Zip 42347; tel. 502/298-7411; Blaine Pieper, Administrator

LOUISIANA: FRANKLIN FOUNDATION HOSPITAL (CM, 43 beds) 1501 Hospital Avenue, Franklin, LA Zip 70538, Mailing Address: Box 577, Zip 70538-0577; tel. 318/828-0760; A. Dale Morgan, Administrator

LAKEWOOD HOSPITAL (CM, 99 beds) 1125 Marguerite Street, Morgan City, LA Zip 70380, Mailing Address: Drawer 2308, Zip 70381; tel. 504/384-2200; Joyce Grove Hein, Chief Executive Officer

LANE MEMORIAL HOSPITAL (CM, 136 beds) 6300 Main Street, Zachary, LA Zip 70791-9990; tel. 504/658-4000; Charlie L. Massey, Administrator

NORTH OAKS MEDICAL CENTER (CM, 240 beds) 15790 Medical Center Drive, Hammond, LA Zip 70403, Mailing Address: Box 2668, Zip 70404; tel. 504/345-2700; James E. Cathey, Jr., Chief Executive Officer

OPELOUSAS GENERAL HOSPITAL (CM, 131 beds) 520 Prudhomme Lane, Opelousas, LA Zip 70570, Mailing Address: Box 1208, Zip 70571-1208; tel. 318/948-3011; Patrick Brian Carrier, Administrator

RIVERSIDE MEDICAL CENTER (CM, 48 beds) Enon Highway, Franklinton, LA Zip 70438, Mailing Address: Box 528, Zip 70438; tel. 504/839-4431; Craig R. Cudworth, Administrator

THIBODAUX HOSPITAL AND HEALTH CENTERS (CM, 100 beds) 602 North Acadia Road, Thibodaux, LA Zip 70301, Mailing Address: Box 1118, Zip 70302-1118; tel. 504/447-5500; Greg K. Stock, Chief Executive Officer

MAINE: CALAIS REGIONAL HOSPITAL (CM, 49 beds) 50 Franklin Street, Calais, ME Zip 04619-1398; tel. 207/454-7521; Ray H. Davis, Jr., Chief Executive Officer

CARY MEDICAL CENTER (CM, 74 beds) 37 Van Buren Road, Caribou, ME Zip 04736-2599; tel. 207/498-3111; John J. McCormack, Executive Director

For explanation of codes following names, see page B2.
★Indicates Type III membership in the American Hospital Association.

Systems / Quorum Health Group/Quorum Health Resources

DOWN EAST COMMUNITY HOSPITAL (CM, 38 beds) Upper Court Street, Machias, ME 04654, Mailing Address: Rural Route 1, Box 11, Zip 04654; tel. 207/255-3356; George Avery, Administrator

HOULTON REGIONAL HOSPITAL (CM, 77 beds) 20 Hartford Street, Houlton, ME Zip 04730-9998; tel. 207/532-9471; Bradley C. Bean, Administrator

MAINE COAST MEMORIAL HOSPITAL (CM, 55 beds) 50 Union Street, Ellsworth, ME Zip 04605-1599; tel. 207/667-5311; David L. Hample, President

MAYO REGIONAL HOSPITAL (CM, 48 beds) 75 West Main Street, Dover-Foxcroft, ME Zip 04426; tel. 207/564-8401; William J. Thompson, Interim Chief Executive Officer

MILLINOCKET REGIONAL HOSPITAL (CM, 29 beds) 200 Somerset Street, Millinocket, ME Zip 04462; tel. 207/723-5161; Craig A. Kantos, Chief Executive Officer

PENOBSCOT VALLEY HOSPITAL (CM, 42 beds) Transalpine Road, Lincoln, ME Zip 04457-0368, Mailing Address: P.O. Box 368, Zip 04457-0368; tel. 207/794-3321; Ronald D. Victory, Administrator

ST. ANDREWS HOSPITAL (CM, 52 beds) 3 St. Andrews Lane, Boothbay Harbor, ME Zip 04538, Mailing Address: P.O. Box 417, Zip 04538-0417; tel. 207/633-2121; Donald A. Keller, Chief Executive Officer

WATERVILLE OSTEOPATHIC HOSPITAL (CM, 42 beds) Kennedy Memorial Drive, Waterville, ME Zip 04901; tel. 207/873-0731; Wilfred J. Addison, Administrator

MARYLAND: ATLANTIC GENERAL HOSPITAL (CM, 62 beds) 9733 Healthway Drive, Berlin, MD Zip 21811; tel. 410/641-1100; William B. Donatelli, President

MASSACHUSETTS: HALE HOSPITAL (CM, 153 beds) 140 Lincoln Avenue, Haverhill, MA Zip 01830; tel. 508/374-2000; John J. Buckley, Chief Executive Officer and Administrator

HUBBARD REGIONAL HOSPITAL (CM, 37 beds) 340 Thompson Road, Webster, MA Zip 01570-0608; tel. 508/943-2600; Gerald J. Barbini, Administrator and Chief Executive Officer

JORDAN HOSPITAL (CM, 145 beds) 275 Sandwich Street, Plymouth, MA Zip 02360-2196; tel. 508/746-2001; Elliot L. Schwartz, Acting President and Chief Executive Officer

MASSACHUSETTS RESPIRATORY HOSPITAL (CM, 98 beds) 2001 Washington Street, Braintree, MA Zip 02184; tel. 617/848-2600; Edward F. Kittredge, Chief Executive Officer

QUINCY HOSPITAL (CM, 286 beds) 114 Whitwell Street, Quincy, MA Zip 02169-1899; tel. 617/773-6100; Ralph Dipisa, Chief Executive Officer

MICHIGAN: COMMUNITY HEALTH CENTER OF BRANCH COUNTY (CM, 96 beds) 274 East Chicago Street, Coldwater, MI Zip 49036-2088; tel. 517/279-5400; Earl Tamar, Chief Executive Officer

COMMUNITY HOSPITAL (CM, 54 beds) Medical Park Drive, Watervliet, MI Zip 49098-0158, Mailing Address: Box 158, Zip 49098; tel. 616/463-3111; Douglas L. Rahn, Administrator

LAKE VIEW COMMUNITY HOSPITAL (CM, 174 beds) 408 Hazen Street, Paw Paw, MI Zip 49079, Mailing Address: Box 209, Zip 49079-0209; tel. 616/657-3141; Sue E. Johnson, President and Chief Executive Officer

MARLETTE COMMUNITY HOSPITAL (CM, 71 beds) 2770 Main Street, Marlette, MI Zip 48453-0307, Mailing Address: P.O. Box 307, Zip 48453-0307; tel. 517/635-7491; David S. McEwen, Administrator

MECOSTA COUNTY GENERAL HOSPITAL (CM, 74 beds) 405 Winter Avenue, Big Rapids, MI Zip 49307-2099; tel. 616/796-8691; Thomas E. Daugherty, Chief Executive Officer

STURGIS HOSPITAL (CM, 53 beds) 916 Myrtle, Sturgis, MI Zip 49091-2001; tel. 616/659-4400; David James, Chief Executive Officer

THREE RIVERS AREA HOSPITAL (CM, 60 beds) 1111 West Broadway, Three Rivers, MI Zip 49093-9362; tel. 616/278-1145; Brad Solberg, President and Chief Executive Officer

MINNESOTA: FALLS MEMORIAL HOSPITAL (CM, 42 beds) 1400 Highway 11-71, International Falls, MN Zip 56649-2189; tel. 218/283-4481; James F. Hanko, Administrator and Chief Executive Officer

ITASCA MEDICAL CENTER (CM, 112 beds) 126 First Avenue S.E., Grand Rapids, MN Zip 55744-3698; tel. 218/326-3401; Darwin Root, Administrator

VIRGINIA REGIONAL MEDICAL CENTER (CM, 199 beds) 901 Ninth Street North, Virginia, MN Zip 55792-2398; tel. 218/741-3340; Gerald R. Lundberg, Administrator

MISSISSIPPI: BOLIVAR COUNTY HOSPITAL (CM, 143 beds) Highway 8 East, Cleveland, MS Zip 38732, Mailing Address: P.O. Box 1380, Zip 38732; tel. 601/846-0061; Robert L. Hawley, Jr., Chief Executive Officer

DELTA REGIONAL MEDICAL CENTER (CM, 150 beds) 1400 East Union Street, Greenville, MS Zip 38703-3246, Mailing Address: Box 5247, Zip 38704-5247; tel. 601/378-3783; E. Berton Whitaker, Administrator and Chief Executive Officer

FIELD MEMORIAL COMMUNITY HOSPITAL (CM, 66 beds) 270 West Main Street, Centreville, MS Zip 39631, Mailing Address: Box 639, Zip 39631-0639; tel. 601/645-5221; Brock A. Slabach, Administrator

H.C. WATKINS MEMORIAL HOSPITAL (CM, 42 beds) 605 South Archusa Avenue, Quitman, MS Zip 39355-2398; tel. 601/776-6925; Thomas G. Bartlett, President and Chief Executive Officer

HANCOCK MEDICAL CENTER (CM, 66 beds) 149 Drinkwater Boulevard, Bay Saint Louis, MS Zip 39520, Mailing Address: P.O. Box 2790, Zip 39521; tel. 601/467-9081; Donald G. Henderson, Administrator

KING'S DAUGHTERS HOSPITAL (CM, 95 beds) Highway 51 North, Brookhaven, MS Zip 39601, Mailing Address: P.O. Box 948, Zip 39601; tel. 601/833-6011; Wallace Cooper, Chief Executive Officer

MAGNOLIA REGIONAL HEALTH CENTER (CM, 150 beds) 611 Alcorn Drive, Corinth, MS Zip 38834; tel. 601/286-6961; Rohn J. Butterfield, Chief Executive Officer

NATCHEZ REGIONAL MEDICAL CENTER (CM, 137 beds) Seargent S Prentiss Drive, Natchez, MS Zip 39120, Mailing Address: Box 1488, Zip 39121-1488; tel. 601/443-2100; Jonathan F. Godfrey FACHE, Chief Executive Officer

PARKVIEW REGIONAL MEDICAL CENTER (O, 189 beds) 100 McAuley Drive, Vicksburg, MS Zip 39180-2897, Mailing Address: P.O. Box 590, Zip 39181-0590; tel. 601/631-2131; Lewis T. Peeples, Administrator and Chief Executive Officer

UNIVERSITY HOSPITALS AND CLINICS, UNIVERSITY OF MISSISSIPPI MEDICAL CENTER (CM, 485 beds) 2500 North State Street, Jackson, MS Zip 39216-4505; tel. 601/984-1000; Frederick Woodrell, Director

MISSOURI: BREECH MEDICAL CENTER (CM, 42 beds) 325 Harwood Avenue, Lebanon, MO Zip 65536, Mailing Address: P.O. Box N, Zip 65536; tel. 417/532-2136; Gary W. Pulsipher, Chief Executive Officer

NEVADA REGIONAL MEDICAL CENTER (CM, 97 beds) 800 South Ash Street, Nevada, MO Zip 64772; tel. 417/667-3355; Michael L. Mullins, President

PHELPS COUNTY REGIONAL MEDICAL CENTER (CM, 245 beds) 1000 West Tenth Street, Rolla, MO Zip 65401; tel. 314/364-3100; Dan Smigelski, Chief Executive Officer

MONTANA: CENTRAL MONTANA MEDICAL CENTER (CM, 126 beds) 408 Wendell Avenue, Lewistown, MT Zip 59457, Mailing Address: Box 580, Zip 59457; tel. 406/538-6201; Kyle Hopstad, Administrator and Chief Executive Officer

COMMUNITY HOSPITAL OF ANACONDA (CM, 102 beds) 401 West Pennsylvania Avenue, Anaconda, MT Zip 59711; tel. 406/563-5261; James J. Cliborne, Jr., Interim Administrator

NORTH VALLEY HOSPITAL (CM, 100 beds) 6575 Highway 93 South, Whitefish, MT Zip 59937-2990; tel. 406/863-2501; Kenneth E S Platou, Chief Executive Officer

NEBRASKA: CRETE MUNICIPAL HOSPITAL (CM, 57 beds) 1540 Grove Streets, Crete, NE Zip 68333, Mailing Address: P.O. Box 220, Zip 68333; tel. 402/826-2154; Tony Staynings, Chief Executive Officer

GREAT PLAINS REGIONAL MEDICAL CENTER (CM, 113 beds) 601 West Leota Street, North Platte, NE Zip 69101, Mailing Address: Box 1167, Zip 69103; tel. 308/534-9310; Lucinda A. Bradley, President

MIDLANDS COMMUNITY HOSPITAL (O, 160 beds) 11111 South 84th Street, Papillion, NE Zip 68046; tel. 402/593-3000; Don M. Chase, Administrator

PHELPS MEMORIAL HEALTH CENTER (CM, 55 beds) 1220 Miller Street, Holdrege, NE Zip 68949, Mailing Address: P.O. Box 828, Zip 68949-0828; tel. 308/995-2211; Jerome Jr Seigfried, Chief Executive Officer

NEW HAMPSHIRE: LITTLETON REGIONAL HOSPITAL (CM, 54 beds) 107 Cottage Street, Littleton, NH Zip 03561; tel. 603/444-7731; Robert S. Pearson, Administrator

MONADNOCK COMMUNITY HOSPITAL (CM, 62 beds) 452 Old Street Road, Peterborough, NH Zip 03458; tel. 603/924-7191; Frank A. Niro, Chief Executive Officer

NEW MEXICO: CIBOLA GENERAL HOSPITAL (CM, 43 beds) 1212 Bonita Avenue, Grants, NM Zip 87020; tel. 505/287-4446; Polly Pine, Administrator

GERALD CHAMPION MEMORIAL HOSPITAL (CM, 74 beds) 1209 Ninth Street, Alamogordo, NM Zip 88310-0597, Mailing Address: P.O. Box 597, Zip 88311-0597; tel. 505/439-2100; Carl W. Mantey, Chief Executive Officer

GILA REGIONAL MEDICAL CENTER (CM, 68 beds) 1313 East 32nd Street, Silver City, NM Zip 88061; tel. 505/538-4000; Steve Jacobson, Administrator

For explanation of codes following names, see page B2.
★Indicates Type III membership in the American Hospital Association.

Systems / Quorum Health Group/Quorum Health Resources

HOLY CROSS HOSPITAL (CM, 29 beds) 630 Paseo De Pueblo Sur, Taos, NM Zip 87571, Mailing Address: P.O. Box Dd, Zip 87571; tel. 505/751–2234; Rita Campbell, Administrator

NEW YORK: ELLIS HOSPITAL (CM, 434 beds) 1101 Nott Street, Schenectady, NY Zip 12308–2487; tel. 518/382–4124; G. B. Serrill, President and Chief Executive Officer

NORTH CAROLINA: ALEXANDER COMMUNITY HOSPITAL (CM, 36 beds) 326 Third Street S.W., Taylorsville, NC Zip 28681–3096; tel. 704/632–4282; Robert D. Jones, Administrator

ALLEGHANY MEMORIAL HOSPITAL (CM, 46 beds) 617 Doctor's Street, Sparta, NC Zip 28675–0009, Mailing Address: P.O. Box 9, Zip 28675–0009; tel. 910/372–5511; James Yarborough, Chief Executive Officer

ANGEL COMMUNITY HOSPITAL (CM, 59 beds) Riverview & White Oak Streets, Franklin, NC Zip 28734, Mailing Address: P.O. Box 1209, Zip 28734–1209; tel. 704/524–8411; Michael E. Zuliani, Administrator

ASHE MEMORIAL HOSPITAL (CM, 115 beds) 200 Hospital Avenue, Jefferson, NC Zip 28640–0008, Mailing Address: P.O. Box 8, Zip 28640–0008; tel. 910/246–7101; R. D. Williams, Administrator

CHATHAM HOSPITAL (CM, 42 beds) West Third Street & Ivy Avenue, Siler City, NC Zip 27344–2343, Mailing Address: P.O. Box 649, Zip 27344; tel. 919/663–2113; Ted G. Chapin, Chief Executive Officer

COLUMBUS COUNTY HOSPITAL (CM, 136 beds) 500 Jefferson Street, Whiteville, NC Zip 28472–9987; tel. 910/642–8011; William S. Clark, Chief Executive Officer

GRANVILLE MEDICAL CENTER (CM, 146 beds) 1010 College Street, Oxford, NC Zip 27565–2507, Mailing Address: Box 947, Zip 27565–0947; tel. 919/690–3000; Andrew Mannich, Administrator

HUGH CHATHAM MEMORIAL HOSPITAL (CM, 160 beds) Parkwood Drive, Elkin, NC Zip 28621–0560, Mailing Address: P.O. Box 560, Zip 28621–0560; tel. 910/835–3722; Richard D. Osmus, Chief Executive Officer

JOHNSTON MEMORIAL HOSPITAL (CM, 127 beds) 509 North Bright Leaf Boulevard, Smithfield, NC Zip 27577–1376, Mailing Address: P.O. Box 1376, Zip 27577–1376; tel. 919/934–8171; Leland E. Farnell, President

MOREHEAD MEMORIAL HOSPITAL (CM, 213 beds) 117 East King's Highway, Eden, NC Zip 27288–5299; tel. 910/623–9711; Robert Enders, President

NORTHERN HOSPITAL OF SURRY COUNTY (CM, 129 beds) 830 Rockford Street, Mount Airy, NC Zip 27030, Mailing Address: Box 1101, Zip 27030–1101; tel. 910/719–7000; Charles K. Van Sluyter, President and Chief Executive Officer

PERSON COUNTY MEMORIAL HOSPITAL (CM, 85 beds) 615 Ridge Road, Roxboro, NC Zip 27573–4630; tel. 910/599–2121; H. James Graham, Administrator

RUTHERFORD HOSPITAL (CM, 260 beds) 308 South Ridgecrest Avenue, Rutherfordton, NC Zip 28139–3097; tel. 704/286–5000; Larry H. Chewning III, President

WASHINGTON COUNTY HOSPITAL (CM, 49 beds) 1 Medical Plaza, Plymouth, NC Zip 27962; tel. 919/793–4135; Jack Floyd, Interim Administrator

OHIO: AMHERST HOSPITAL (CM, 71 beds) 254 Cleveland Avenue, Amherst, OH Zip 44001–1699; tel. 216/988–2831; Bradley P. Smith, President and Chief Executive Officer

DEFIANCE HOSPITAL (CM, 96 beds) 1206 East Second Street, Defiance, OH Zip 43512–2495; tel. 419/783–6955; Richard C. Sommer, Administrator

FAYETTE COUNTY MEMORIAL HOSPITAL (CM, 35 beds) 1430 Columbus Avenue, Washington Court House, OH Zip 43160–1791; tel. 614/333–2705; Francis G. Albarano, Administrator

GREENFIELD AREA MEDICAL CENTER (CM, 36 beds) 545 South Street, Greenfield, OH Zip 45123–0545; tel. 513/981–2116; Mark E. Marchetti, Chief Executive Officer

KNOX COMMUNITY HOSPITAL (CM, 117 beds) 1330 Coshocton Road, Mount Vernon, OH Zip 43050; tel. 614/393–9000; Robert G. Polahar, Chief Executive Officer

MEMORIAL HOSPITAL (CM, 132 beds) 715 South Taft Avenue, Fremont, OH Zip 43420–3296; tel. 419/332–7321; John A. Gorman, Chief Executive Officer

MEMORIAL HOSPITAL OF GENEVA (CM, 46 beds) 870 West Main Street, Geneva, OH Zip 44041; tel. 216/466–1141; Gerard D. Klein, Chief Executive Officer

PAULDING COUNTY HOSPITAL (CM, 51 beds) 11558 S R 111, Paulding, OH Zip 45879–9605; tel. 419/399–4080; Joseph M. Dorko, Chief Executive Officer

SELBY GENERAL HOSPITAL (CM, 75 beds) 1106 Colgate Drive, Marietta, OH Zip 45750–1323; tel. 614/373–0582; William M. Greene, Chief Executive Officer

WARREN GENERAL HOSPITAL (CM, 139 beds) 667 Eastland Avenue S.E., Warren, OH Zip 44484–0128; tel. 216/373–9000; Kevin R. Andrews, Chief Executive Officer

WOOSTER COMMUNITY HOSPITAL (CM, 90 beds) 1761 Beall Avenue, Wooster, OH Zip 44691; tel. 216/263–8100; William E. Sheron, Chief Executive Officer

OKLAHOMA: ATOKA MEMORIAL HOSPITAL (CM, 37 beds) 1501 South Virginia, Atoka, OK Zip 74525; tel. 405/889–3333; J. R. Caton, Administrator

CUSHING REGIONAL HOSPITAL (CM, 75 beds) 1027 East Cherry, Cushing, OK Zip 74023, Mailing Address: Box 1409, Zip 74023–1409; tel. 918/225–2915; Ron Cackler, Chief Executive Officer

HENRYETTA MEDICAL CENTER (CM, 52 beds) Dewey Bartlett & Main Streets, Henryetta, OK Zip 74437, Mailing Address: P.O. Box 1269, Zip 74437–1269; tel. 918/652–4463; James P. Bailey, Administrator and Chief Executive Officer

HOLDENVILLE GENERAL HOSPITAL (CM, 27 beds) 100 Crestview Drive, Holdenville, OK Zip 74848–9700; tel. 405/379–6631; Charles M. Smith, Administrator

KINGFISHER REGIONAL HOSPITAL (CM, 24 beds) 500 South Ninth Street, Kingfisher, OK Zip 73750, Mailing Address: Box 59, Zip 73750–0059; tel. 405/375–3342; Steven G. Daniel, Administrator

PERRY MEMORIAL HOSPITAL (CM, 28 beds) 501 14th Street, Perry, OK Zip 73077–5099; tel. 405/336–3541; Judith K. Feuquay, Chief Executive Officer

PURCELL MUNICIPAL HOSPITAL (CM, 36 beds) 1500 North Green Avenue, Purcell, OK Zip 73080, Mailing Address: P.O. Box 511, Zip 73080–0511; tel. 405/527–6524; Joe Duerr, Administrator

SEMINOLE MUNICIPAL HOSPITAL (CM, 39 beds) 606 West Evans Street, Seminole, OK Zip 74868, Mailing Address: P.O. Box 2130, Zip 74818–2130; tel. 405/382–0600; Bruce A. Bennett, President and Chief Executive Officer

SHARE MEDICAL CENTER (CM, 120 beds) 800 Share Drive, Alva, OK Zip 73717, Mailing Address: P.O. Box 727, Zip 73717–0727; tel. 405/327–2800; Michael McCoy, Chief Executive Officer

TAHLEQUAH CITY HOSPITAL (CM, 65 beds) 1400 East Downing Street, Tahlequah, OK Zip 74464, Mailing Address: Box 1008, Zip 74465–1008; tel. 918/456–0641; L. Gene Matthews, Chief Executive Officer

WILLOW VIEW MENTAL HEALTH SYSTEM (CM, 74 beds) 2601 Spencer Road, Spencer, OK Zip 73084–3699, Mailing Address: P.O. Box 11137, Oklahoma City, Zip 73136–0137; tel. 405/427–2441; Gary L. Watson, Chief Executive Officer

WOODWARD HOSPITAL AND HEALTH CENTER (CM, 68 beds) 900 17th Street, Woodward, OK Zip 73801; tel. 405/256–5511; Warren K. Spellman, Administrator

PENNSYLVANIA: ALIQUIPPA HOSPITAL (CM, 183 beds) 2500 Hospital Drive, Aliquippa, PA Zip 15001–2191; tel. 412/857–1212; Charles Lonchar, President and Chief Executive Officer

BERWICK HOSPITAL CENTER (CM, 409 beds) 701 East 16th Street, Berwick, PA Zip 18603–2397; tel. 717/759–5000; Thomas R. Sphatt, President and Chief Executive Officer

BROWNSVILLE GENERAL HOSPITAL (CM, 115 beds) 125 Simpson Road, Brownsville, PA Zip 15417; tel. 412/785–7200; Alvin W. Allison, Jr., Interim Chief Executive Officer

CANONSBURG GENERAL HOSPITAL (CM, 120 beds) 100 Medical Boulevard, Canonsburg, PA Zip 15317; tel. 412/745–6100; Robert R. Tracht, President and Chief Executive Officer

CARLISLE HOSPITAL (CM, 183 beds) 246 Parker Street, Carlisle, PA Zip 17013–0310; tel. 717/249–1212; Michael J. Halstead, Interim President and Chief Executive Officer

CLARION HOSPITAL (CM, 88 beds) One Hospital Drive, Clarion, PA Zip 16214; tel. 814/226–9500; John J. Shepard, President and Chief Executive Officer

GREENE COUNTY MEMORIAL HOSPITAL (CM, 78 beds) Seventh Street & Bonar Avenue, Waynesburg, PA Zip 15370; tel. 412/627–3101; Raoul Walsh, Chief Executive Officer

J.C. BLAIR MEMORIAL HOSPITAL (CM, 104 beds) Warm Springs Avenue, Huntingdon, PA Zip 16652; tel. 814/643–2290; Stephen Schoaps, Chief Executive Officer

JERSEY SHORE HOSPITAL (CM, 55 beds) 1020 Thompson Street, Jersey Shore, PA Zip 17740–0689; tel. 717/398–0100; Louis A. Ditzel, Jr., President and Chief Executive Officer

---

For explanation of codes following names, see page B2.
★Indicates Type III membership in the American Hospital Association.

Systems / Quorum Health Group/Quorum Health Resources

LOCK HAVEN HOSPITAL (CM, 250 beds) 24 Cree Drive, Lock Haven, PA Zip 17745; tel. 717/893–5000; Gary R. Rhoads, President and Chief Executive Officer

MEMORIAL HOSPITAL (CM, 104 beds) One Hospital Drive, Towanda, PA Zip 18848–9767; tel. 717/265–2191; Gary A. Baker, President

METRO HEALTH CENTER (CM, 101 beds) 252 West 11th Street, Erie, PA Zip 16501; tel. 814/870–3400; J. B. Frith, Chief Executive Officer

MINERS HOSPITAL NORTHERN CAMBRIA (CM, 40 beds) 2205 Crawford Avenue, Spangler, PA Zip 15775, Mailing Address: P.O. Box 490, Zip 15775; tel. 814/948–7171; Roger P. Winn, Administrator

OHIO VALLEY GENERAL HOSPITAL (CM, 135 beds) 25 Heckel Road, McKees Rocks, PA Zip 15136–1694; tel. 412/777–6161; William Provenzano, President

POTTSVILLE HOSPITAL AND WARNE CLINIC (CM, 195 beds) 420 South Jackson Street, Pottsville, PA Zip 17901–3692; tel. 717/621–5000; Donald R. Gintzig, President and Chief Executive Officer

TYRONE HOSPITAL (CM, 59 beds) One Hospital Drive, Tyrone, PA Zip 16686–1898; tel. 814/684–1255; Philip J. Stoner, Chief Executive Officer

SOUTH CAROLINA: BEAUFORT MEMORIAL HOSPITAL (CM, 141 beds) 121 South Ribaut Road, Beaufort, SC Zip 29902, Mailing Address: P.O. Box 1068, Zip 29901–1068; tel. 803/522–5200; Charles W. Elliott, Jr., Chief Executive Officer

BYERLY HOSPITAL (CM, 100 beds) 413 East Carolina Avenue, Hartsville, SC Zip 29550–4309; tel. 803/339–2100

GEORGETOWN MEMORIAL HOSPITAL (CM, 141 beds) 606 Black River Road, Georgetown, SC Zip 29440, Mailing Address: Drawer 1718, Zip 29442–1718; tel. 803/527–7000; Paul D. Gatens, Sr., Administrator

LAURENS COUNTY HEALTHCARE SYSTEM (CM, 203 beds) Highway 76 West, Clinton, SC Zip 29325, Mailing Address: P.O. Box 976, Zip 29325–0976; tel. 803/833–9100; Randall M. Olson, Chief Executive Officer

MARY BLACK MEMORIAL HOSPITAL (CM, 201 beds) 1700 Skylyn Drive, Spartanburg, SC Zip 29307, Mailing Address: Box 3217, Zip 29304–3217; tel. 803/573–3000; Gerald W. Landis, President

NEWBERRY COUNTY MEMORIAL HOSPITAL (CM, 64 beds) 2669 Kinard Street, Newberry, SC Zip 29108–0497, Mailing Address: P.O. Box 497, Zip 29108–0497; tel. 803/276–7570; Lynn W. Beasley, President and Chief Executive Officer

REGIONAL MEDICAL CENTER OF ORANGEBURG AND CALHOUN COUNTIES (CM, 295 beds) 3000 St. Matthews Road, Orangeburg, SC Zip 29115–1498; tel. 803/533–2200; Thomas C. Dandridge, President

TUOMEY REGIONAL MEDICAL CENTER (CM, 230 beds) 129 North Washington Street, Sumter, SC Zip 29150–4983; tel. 803/778–9000; Jay Cox, President and Chief Executive Officer

WALLACE THOMSON HOSPITAL (CM, 107 beds) 322 West South Street, Union, SC Zip 29379–0789, Mailing Address: Box 789, Zip 29379; tel. 803/429–2600; Mark H. Petermann, Chief Executive Officer

SOUTH DAKOTA: HURON REGIONAL MEDICAL CENTER (CM, 91 beds) 172 Fourth Street S.E., Huron, SD Zip 57350–2590; tel. 605/353–6200; John L. Single, Chief Executive Officer

MID DAKOTA HOSPITAL (CM, 54 beds) 300 South Byron Boulevard, Chamberlain, SD Zip 57325; tel. 605/734–5511; Mick Penticoff, Administrator

TENNESSEE: BOLIVAR COMMUNITY HOSPITAL (CM, 47 beds) 650 Nuckolls Road, Bolivar, TN Zip 38008; tel. 901/658–3100; George L. Austin, Chief Executive Officer

BRISTOL REGIONAL MEDICAL CENTER (CM, 336 beds) 1 Medical Park Boulevard, Bristol, TN Zip 37620; tel. 615/844–4200; Eddie A. George, President

CITY OF MILAN HOSPITAL (CM, 61 beds) 4039 South Highland, Milan, TN Zip 38358; tel. 901/686–1591; Mark D. Le Neave, Chief Executive Officer

COFFEE MEDICAL CENTER (CM, 106 beds) 1001 McArthur Drive, Manchester, TN Zip 37355, Mailing Address: P.O. Box 1079, Zip 37355; tel. 615/728–3586; Keith Heuser, Administrator

LINCOLN REGIONAL HOSPITAL (CM, 63 beds) 700 West Maple Street, Fayetteville, TN Zip 37334; tel. 615/438–1111; George Repa, Chief Executive Officer

MACON COUNTY GENERAL HOSPITAL (CM, 43 beds) 204 Medical Drive, Lafayette, TN Zip 37083, Mailing Address: P.O. Box 378, Zip 37083; tel. 615/666–2147; Dennis Wolford, Administrator

RHEA MEDICAL CENTER (CM, 125 beds) 7900 Rhea County Highway, Dayton, TN Zip 37321; tel. 615/775–1121; Kennedy L. Croom, Jr., Administrator and Chief Executive Officer

TEXAS: ABILENE REGIONAL MEDICAL CENTER (O, 145 beds) 6250 Highway 83–84 at Antilley Road, Abilene, TX Zip 79606; tel. 915/695–9900; David M. Collins, President and Chief Executive Officer

BRAZOSPORT MEMORIAL HOSPITAL (CM, 134 beds) 100 Medical Drive, Lake Jackson, TX Zip 77566–9983; tel. 409/297–4411; Wesley W. Oswald, Chief Executive Officer

DALLAS–FORT WORTH MEDICAL CENTER (CM, 124 beds) 2709 Hospital Boulevard, Grand Prairie, TX Zip 75051–1083; tel. 214/641–5000; Timothy Baylor, Chief Executive Officer

DOCTORS HOSPITAL (CM, 84 beds) 5500 39th Street, Groves, TX Zip 77619–9805; tel. 409/962–5733; John Isbell, Chief Executive Officer

FORT DUNCAN MEDICAL CENTER (CM, 57 beds) 350 South Adams Street, Eagle Pass, TX Zip 78852; tel. 210/757–7501; Don Spaulding, Administrator and Chief Executive Officer

HENDERSON MEMORIAL HOSPITAL (CM, 96 beds) 300 Wilson Street, Henderson, TX Zip 75652; tel. 903/657–7541; George T. Roberts, Jr., Chief Executive Officer

HOOD GENERAL HOSPITAL (CM, 56 beds) 1310 Paluxy Road, Granbury, TX Zip 76048; tel. 817/573–2683; Michael A. Kozar, Administrator

HOUSTON COUNTY HOSPITAL (CM, 50 beds) 1100 Loop 304 East, Crockett, TX Zip 75835–1810; tel. 409/544–2002; Kathleen S. Wegener, Administrator and Chief Executive Officer

HUNTSVILLE MEMORIAL HOSPITAL (CM, 119 beds) 3000 I-45, Huntsville, TX Zip 77340, Mailing Address: P.O. Box 4001, Zip 77342–4001; tel. 409/291–3411; Ralph E. Beaty, Administrator

MISSION HOSPITAL (CM, 110 beds) 900 South Bryan Road, Mission, TX Zip 78572; tel. 210/580–9000; Thomas B. Symonds, Administrator

REEVES COUNTY HOSPITAL (CM, 46 beds) 2323 Texas Street, Pecos, TX Zip 79772; tel. 915/447–3551; Bruce K. Brichell, Administrator

TITUS REGIONAL MEDICAL CENTER (CM, 165 beds) 2001 North Jefferson, Mount Pleasant, TX Zip 75455; tel. 903/577–6000; Wayne L. Ogburn FACHE, Chief Executive Officer and Administrator

UTAH: TOOELE VALLEY REGIONAL MEDICAL CENTER (CM, 107 beds) 211 South 100 East, Tooele, UT Zip 84074–2794; tel. 801/882–1697; Matthew Chambers, Chief Executive Officer

VERMONT: NORTHEASTERN VERMONT REGIONAL HOSPITAL (CM, 72 beds) Hospital Drive, Saint Johnsbury, VT Zip 05819–9962; tel. 802/748–8141; Paul R. Bengtson, Chief Executive Officer

NORTHWESTERN MEDICAL CENTER (CM, 70 beds) Fairfield Street, Saint Albans, VT Zip 05478–1004, Mailing Address: Box 1370, Zip 05478; tel. 802/524–5911; Peter A. Hofstetter, Chief Executive Officer

VIRGINIA: ALLEGHANY REGIONAL HOSPITAL (CM, 190 beds) One ARH Lane, Low Moor, VA Zip 24457, Mailing Address: P.O. Box 7, Zip 24457–0007; tel. 703/862–6200; William B. James, Administrator

GREENSVILLE MEMORIAL HOSPITAL (CM, 182 beds) 214 Weaver Avenue, Emporia, VA Zip 23847–1288; tel. 804/348–2000; Charles Mitchener, Jr., Chief Executive Officer

HALIFAX REGIONAL HOSPITAL (CM, 192 beds) 2204 Wilborn Avenue, South Boston, VA Zip 24592; tel. 804/575–3100; Chris A. Lumsden, Administrator

MEMORIAL HOSPITAL OF MARTINSVILLE AND HENRY COUNTY (CM, 182 beds) 310 Hospital Drive, Martinsville, VA Zip 24112–1981, Mailing Address: Box 4788, Zip 24115–4788; tel. 703/666–7200; Joseph Roach, Executive Director

RICHMOND EYE AND EAR HOSPITAL (CM, 33 beds) 1001 East Marshall Street, Richmond, VA Zip 23219; tel. 804/775–4500; Karen A. Fiducia, Chief Executive Officer

SOUTHSIDE REGIONAL MEDICAL CENTER (CM, 296 beds) 801 South Adams Street, Petersburg, VA Zip 23803–5133; tel. 804/862–5000; David S. Dunham, President

WASHINGTON: KADLEC MEDICAL CENTER (CM, 135 beds) 888 Swift Boulevard, Richland, WA Zip 99352–9974; tel. 509/946–4611; Marcel Loh, Chief Executive Officer

WEST VIRGINIA: CITY HOSPITAL (CM, 182 beds) Dry Run Road, Martinsburg, WV Zip 25401, Mailing Address: P.O. Box 1418, Zip 25401–1418; tel. 304/264–1000; Peter L. Mulford, Administrator

FAIRMONT GENERAL HOSPITAL (CM, 238 beds) 1325 Locust Avenue, Fairmont, WV Zip 26554–0000; tel. 304/367–7100; Richard W. Graham FACHE, President

WISCONSIN: APPLE RIVER HOSPITAL (CM, 13 beds) 230 Deronda Street, Amery, WI Zip 54001–1412; tel. 715/268–7151; Michael Karuschak, Jr., Administrator

For explanation of codes following names, see page B2.
★Indicates Type III membership in the American Hospital Association.

Systems / Quorum Health Group/Quorum Health Resources

BAY AREA MEDICAL CENTER (CM, 115 beds) 3100 Shore Drive, Marinette, WI Zip 54143–4297; tel. 715/735–6621; Rick Ament, Chief Executive Officer

OCONTO MEMORIAL HOSPITAL (CM, 25 beds) 405 First Street, Oconto, WI Zip 54153; tel. 414/834–8800; Steve Dewoody, Chief Executive Officer

RIVERSIDE MEDICAL CENTER (CM, 40 beds) 800 Riverside Drive, Waupaca, WI Zip 54981–1999; tel. 715/258–1000; Jan V. Carrell, Administrator

WYOMING: CAMPBELL COUNTY MEMORIAL HOSPITAL (CM, 119 beds) 501 South Burma Avenue, Gillette, WY Zip 82716, Mailing Address: Box 3011, Zip 82717; tel. 307/682–8811; Jack F. Houghton, Chief Executive Officer

WEST PARK HOSPITAL (CM, 202 beds) 707 Sheridan Avenue, Cody, WY Zip 82414; tel. 307/527–7501; Gary Bishop, Administrator

Owned, leased, sponsored:	5 hospitals	894 beds
Contract–managed:	244 hospitals	25246 beds
Totals:	249 hospitals	26140 beds

0405: RAMSAY HEALTH CARE, INC. (IO)
639 Loyola Avenue, Suite 1400, New Orleans, LA Zip 70113; tel. 504/585–2505; Gregory H. Browne, President and Chief Executive Officer

ALABAMA: HILL CREST BEHAVIORAL HEALTH SERVICES (O, 130 beds) 6869 Fifth Avenue South, Birmingham, AL Zip 35212; tel. 205/833–9000; Guy A. Barg, Chief Executive Officer

ARIZONA: DESERT VISTA HOSPITAL (O, 98 beds) 570 West Brown Road, Mesa, AZ Zip 85201; tel. 602/962–3900; Allen S. Nohre, Chief Executive Officer

LOUISIANA: BAYOU OAKS HOSPITAL (O, 88 beds) 934 East Main Street, Houma, LA Zip 70360, Mailing Address: P.O. Box 4374, Zip 70361–4374; tel. 504/876–2020; George H. Perry Ph.D., Chief Executive Officer

GREENBRIER HOSPITAL (O, 61 beds) 201 Greenbrier Boulevard, Covington, LA Zip 70433; tel. 504/893–2970; Craig B. Koele, Chief Executive Officer

MICHIGAN: HAVENWYCK HOSPITAL (O, 120 beds) 1525 University Drive, Auburn Hills, MI Zip 48326–2675; tel. 810/373–9200; Robert A. Kercorian, Chief Executive Officer

MISSOURI: HEARTLAND HOSPITAL (O, 60 beds) 1500 West Ashland, Nevada, MO Zip 64772; tel. 417/667–2666; Eugene Hastings, Administrator

NORTH CAROLINA: BRYNN MARR HOSPITAL (O, 76 beds) 192 Village Drive, Jacksonville, NC Zip 28546; tel. 919/577–1400; Dale Armstrong, Administrator

OKLAHOMA: MEADOWLAKE HOSPITAL (O, 50 beds) 2216 South Van Buren, Enid, OK Zip 73703, Mailing Address: P.O. Box 5409, Zip 73702; tel. 405/234–2220; Dave Lamerton, Chief Executive Officer

SOUTH CAROLINA: COASTAL CAROLINA HOSPITAL (O, 80 beds) 152 Waccamaw Medical Park Drive, Conway, SC Zip 29526; tel. 803/347–7156; Shawn J. O'Connor, Administrator and Chief Executive Officer

TEXAS: HAVEN HOSPITAL (O, 46 beds) 800 Kirnwood Drive, De Soto, TX Zip 75115–2092; tel. 214/709–3700; Dan Aranda, Chief Executive Officer

MISSION VISTA HOSPITAL (O, 48 beds) 14747 Jones Maltsberger, San Antonio, TX Zip 78247–3713; tel. 210/490–0000; Dan Aranda, Chief Executive Officer

UTAH: BENCHMARK REGIONAL HOSPITAL (O, 68 beds) 592 West 1350 South, Woods Cross, UT Zip 84087–1665; tel. 801/299–5300; Richard O. Hurt, Jr., Chief Executive Officer

WEST VIRGINIA: CHESTNUT RIDGE HOSPITAL (O, 62 beds) 930 Chestnut Ridge Road, Morgantown, WV Zip 26505; tel. 304/293–4000; Lawrence J. Drake, Chief Executive Officer

Owned, leased, sponsored:	13 hospitals	987 beds
Contract–managed:	0 hospitals	0 beds
Totals:	13 hospitals	987 beds

4810: RIVERSIDE HEALTH SYSTEM (NP)
606 Denbigh Boulevard, Suite 601, Newport News, VA Zip 23602; tel. 804/875–7500; Nelson L. St. Clair, President

VIRGINIA: LAKE TAYLOR HOSPITAL (CM, 332 beds) 1309 Kempsville Road, Norfolk, VA Zip 23502–2286; tel. 804/461–5001; David B. Tate, Jr., President and Chief Executive Officer

RIVERSIDE REGIONAL MEDICAL CENTER (O, 576 beds) 500 J Clyde Morris Boulevard, Newport News, VA Zip 23601–1976; tel. 804/594–2000; Gerald R. Brink, President and Chief Executive Officer

RIVERSIDE TAPPAHANNOCK HOSPITAL (O, 100 beds) Tappahannock, VA, Mailing Address: Route 2, Box 612, Zip 22560; tel. 804/443–3311; Glenn D. Waters, Administrator

RIVERSIDE WALTER REED HOSPITAL (O, 71 beds) Gloucester, VA, Mailing Address: Route 17, Box 1130, Zip 23061–1130; tel. 804/693–8800; Grady W. Philips III, Administrator

Owned, leased, sponsored:	3 hospitals	747 beds
Contract–managed:	1 hospitals	332 beds
Totals:	4 hospitals	1079 beds

★**3855: RUSH–PRESBYTERIAN–ST. LUKE'S MEDICAL CENTER** (NP)
1653 West Congress Parkway, Chicago, IL Zip 60612–3864; tel. 312/942–5000; Leo M. Henikoff M.D., President

ILLINOIS: COPLEY MEMORIAL HOSPITAL (O, 152 beds) 502 South Lincoln Avenue, Aurora, IL Zip 60505–4690; tel. 708/844–1030; D. Chet McKee, President

RUSH NORTH SHORE MEDICAL CENTER (O, 245 beds) 9600 Gross Point Road, Skokie, IL Zip 60076–1257; tel. 708/677–9600; John S. Frigo, President

RUSH–PRESBYTERIAN–ST. LUKE'S MEDICAL CENTER (O, 829 beds) 1653 West Congress Parkway, Chicago, IL Zip 60612–3833; tel. 312/942–5000; Leo M. Henikoff M.D., President and Chief Executive Officer

Owned, leased, sponsored:	3 hospitals	1226 beds
Contract–managed:	0 hospitals	0 beds
Totals:	3 hospitals	1226 beds

★**2535: SAMARITAN HEALTH SYSTEM** (NP)
1441 North 12th Street, Phoenix, AZ Zip 85006–2666; tel. 602/495–4000; James C. Crews, President and Chief Executive Officer

ARIZONA: DESERT SAMARITAN MEDICAL CENTER (O, 324 beds) 1400 South Dobson Road, Mesa, AZ Zip 85202–9879; tel. 602/835–3000; Steven L. Seiler, Senior Vice President and Chief Executive Officer

GOOD SAMARITAN REGIONAL MEDICAL CENTER (O, 576 beds) 1111 East McDowell Road, Phoenix, AZ Zip 85006, Mailing Address: Box 2989, Zip 85062; tel. 602/239–2000; Steven L. Seiler, Senior Vice President and Chief Executive Officer

HAVASU SAMARITAN REGIONAL HOSPITAL (O, 118 beds) 101 Civic Center Lane, Lake Havasu City, AZ Zip 86403; tel. 602/855–8185; Dennis G. Zielinski, Vice President and Chief Executive Officer

MARYVALE SAMARITAN MEDICAL CENTER (O, 213 beds) 5102 West Campbell Avenue, Phoenix, AZ Zip 85031; tel. 602/848–5101; Robert H. Curry, Sr., Senior Vice President and Chief Executive Officer

PAGE HOSPITAL (CM, 25 beds) North Navajo Drive and Vista Avenue, Page, AZ Zip 86040, Mailing Address: P.O. Box 1447, Zip 86040; tel. 602/645–2424; Kevin P. Poorten, Chief Executive Officer

SAMARITAN BEHAVIORAL HEALTH CENTER – DESERT SAMARITAN CAMPUS (O, 26 beds) 2225 West Southern Avenue, Mesa, AZ Zip 85202; tel. 602/464–4000; Steven L. Seiler, Senior Vice President and Chief Executive Officer

SAMARITAN BEHAVIORAL HEALTH CENTER – SCOTTSDALE (O, 60 beds) 7575 East Earll Drive, Scottsdale, AZ Zip 85251–6998; tel. 602/941–7500; Robert F. Meyer M.D., Vice President, Chief Executive Officer and Medical Director

SAMARITAN–WENDY PAINE O'BRIEN TREATMENT CENTER (O, 23 beds) 5055 North 34th Street, Phoenix, AZ Zip 85018; tel. 602/955–6200; Mike Todd, Chief Executive Officer

THUNDERBIRD SAMARITAN MEDICAL CENTER (O, 290 beds) 5555 West Thunderbird Road, Glendale, AZ Zip 85306; tel. 602/588–5555; Robert H. Curry, Sr., Senior Vice President and Chief Executive Officer

CALIFORNIA: SAMARITAN MEDICAL CENTER SAN CLEMENTE (O, 86 beds) 654 Camino De Los Mares, San Clemente, CA Zip 92673; tel. 714/496–1122; Tony Struthers, Chief Executive Officer

Owned, leased, sponsored:	9 hospitals	1716 beds
Contract–managed:	1 hospitals	25 beds
Totals:	10 hospitals	1741 beds

For explanation of codes following names, see page B2.
★Indicates Type III membership in the American Hospital Association.

Systems / Shriners Hospitals for Crippled Children

0575: SCHICK LABORATORIES, INC. (IO)
15760 Ventura Boulevard, Suite 1201, Los Angeles, CA Zip 91436; tel. 818/382-3682; Patrick J. Frawley Jr., Chairman

CALIFORNIA: ALAMAR HOSPITAL (O, 30 beds) 45 East Alamar, Santa Barbara, CA Zip 93105-3495; tel. 805/687-2411; Pamela J. Pratt, Administrator and Chief Executive Officer

WASHINGTON: SCHICK SHADEL HOSPITAL (O, 63 beds) 12101 Ambaum Boulevard S.W., Seattle, WA Zip 98146-2699, Mailing Address: Box 48149, Zip 98148-0149; tel. 206/244-8100; Mary Ellen Stewart, Administrator

Owned, leased, sponsored:	2 hospitals	93 beds
Contract-managed:	0 hospitals	0 beds
Totals:	2 hospitals	93 beds

0037: SCOTTSDALE MEMORIAL HEALTH SYSTEMS, INC. (NP)
3621 Wells Fargo Avenue, Scottsdale, AZ Zip 85251; tel. 602/481-4324; Max Poll, President and Chief Executive Officer

ARIZONA: SCOTTSDALE MEMORIAL HOSPITAL (O, 318 beds) 7400 East Osborn Road, Scottsdale, AZ Zip 85251; tel. 602/481-4000; David R. Carpenter, Senior Vice President and Administrator

SCOTTSDALE MEMORIAL HOSPITAL-NORTH (O, 242 beds) 10450 North 92nd Street, Scottsdale, AZ Zip 85258-4514, Mailing Address: P.O. Box 4500, Zip 85261-9930; tel. 602/860-3000; Thomas J. Sadvary, Senior Vice President and Administrator

Owned, leased, sponsored:	2 hospitals	560 beds
Contract-managed:	0 hospitals	0 beds
Totals:	2 hospitals	560 beds

★1505: SCRIPPS HOSPITALS (NP)
4275 Campus Point Court, San Diego, CA Zip 92121, Mailing Address: P.O. Box 28, La Jolla, Zip 92038; tel. 619/678-7470; Martin B. Buser, President and Chief Executive Officer

CALIFORNIA: GREEN HOSPITAL OF SCRIPPS CLINIC (O, 165 beds) 10666 North Torrey Pines Road, La Jolla, CA Zip 92037-1093; tel. 619/455-9100; Glenn W. Chong, Senior Vice President and Director

SCRIPPS HOSPITAL-EAST COUNTY (O, 158 beds) 1688 East Main Street, El Cajon, CA Zip 92021; tel. 619/440-1122; Robin B. Brown, Vice President and Administrator

SCRIPPS MEMORIAL HOSPITAL – LA JOLLA (O, 433 beds) 9888 Genesee Avenue, La Jolla, CA Zip 92037-1276, Mailing Address: Box 28, Zip 92038-0028; tel. 619/457-4123

SCRIPPS MEMORIAL HOSPITAL-CHULA VISTA (O, 159 beds) 435 H Street, Chula Vista, CA Zip 91912-1537, Mailing Address: Box 1537, Zip 91910-1537; tel. 619/691-7000; Thomas A. Gammiere, Vice President, Administration

SCRIPPS MEMORIAL HOSPITAL-ENCINITAS (O, 145 beds) 354 Santa Fe Drive, Encinitas, CA Zip 92023, Mailing Address: P.O. Box 817, Zip 92023; tel. 619/753-6501; Steven J. Goe, Vice President and Administrator

Owned, leased, sponsored:	5 hospitals	1060 beds
Contract-managed:	0 hospitals	0 beds
Totals:	5 hospitals	1060 beds

★2565: SENTARA HEALTH SYSTEM (NP)
6015 Poplar Hall Drive, Norfolk, VA Zip 23502; tel. 804/455-7000; David L. Bernd, President and Chief Executive Officer

VIRGINIA: SENTARA BAYSIDE HOSPITAL (O, 170 beds) 800 Independence Boulevard, Virginia Beach, VA Zip 23455-6076; tel. 804/363-6100; Edward L. Berdick, President

SENTARA HAMPTON GENERAL HOSPITAL (O, 255 beds) 3120 Victoria Boulevard, Hampton, VA Zip 23661, Mailing Address: Drawer 640, Zip 23669; tel. 804/727-7000; Richard A. Hanson, President

SENTARA LEIGH HOSPITAL (O, 220 beds) 830 Kempsville Road, Norfolk, VA Zip 23502; tel. 804/466-6000; Roger M. Eitelman, Administrator

SENTARA NORFOLK GENERAL HOSPITAL (O, 613 beds) 600 Gresham Drive, Norfolk, VA Zip 23507-1999; tel. 804/668-3000; Howard P. Kern, Administrator and Executive Vice President

Owned, leased, sponsored:	4 hospitals	1258 beds
Contract-managed:	0 hospitals	0 beds
Totals:	4 hospitals	1258 beds

★4025: SERVANTCOR (CC)
175 South Wall Street, Kankakee, IL Zip 60901-3470; tel. 815/937-2034; Joseph S. Feth, President

ILLINOIS: CENTRAL COMMUNITY HOSPITAL (CM, 33 beds) 335 East Fifth Avenue, Clifton, IL Zip 60927, Mailing Address: Box 68, Zip 60927; tel. 815/694-2392; John F. Kuhn, Chief Executive Officer

COVENANT MEDICAL CENTER (O, 268 beds) 1400 West Park Street, Urbana, IL Zip 61801; tel. 217/337-2000; Joseph W. Beard, President

ST. MARY'S HOSPITAL OF KANKAKEE (O, 214 beds) 500 West Court Street, Kankakee, IL Zip 60901; tel. 815/937-2400; Allan C. Sonduck, President and Chief Executive Officer

Owned, leased, sponsored:	2 hospitals	482 beds
Contract-managed:	1 hospitals	33 beds
Totals:	3 hospitals	515 beds

★2065: SHARP HEALTHCARE (NP)
3131 Berger Avenue, Suite 100, San Diego, CA Zip 92123; tel. 619/541-4000; Peter K. Ellsworth, President

CALIFORNIA: GROSSMONT HOSPITAL (O, 377 beds) 5555 Grossmont Center Drive, La Mesa, CA Zip 91942, Mailing Address: Box 158, Zip 91944-0158; tel. 619/465-0711; Thomas F. Spindler, Interim Chief Executive Officer

SHARP CABRILLO HOSPITAL (O, 227 beds) 3475 Kenyon Street, San Diego, CA Zip 92110-5067; tel. 619/221-3400; James M. Schibanoff M.D., Chief Executive Officer

SHARP CHULA VISTA MEDICAL CENTER (O, 306 beds) 751 Medical Center Court, Chula Vista, CA Zip 91911, Mailing Address: Box 1297, Zip 91912; tel. 619/482-5800; Thomas F. Spindler, Chief Executive Officer

SHARP HEALTHCARE MURRIETA (O, 91 beds) 25500 Medical Center Drive, Murrieta, CA Zip 92562-5966; tel. 909/696-6000; Robert M. Edwards, Senior Vice President and Administrator

SHARP MEMORIAL HOSPITAL (O, 488 beds) 7901 Frost Street, San Diego, CA Zip 92123-2788; tel. 619/541-3400; James M. Schibanoff M.D., Chief Executive Officer

Owned, leased, sponsored:	5 hospitals	1489 beds
Contract-managed:	0 hospitals	0 beds
Totals:	5 hospitals	1489 beds

★4125: SHRINERS HOSPITALS FOR CRIPPLED CHILDREN (NP)
2900 Rocky Point Drive, Tampa, FL Zip 33607-1435, Mailing Address: Box 31356, Zip 33631-3356; tel. 813/281-0300; Jack D. Hoard, Executive Administrator

CALIFORNIA: SHRINERS HOSPITALS FOR CRIPPLED CHILDREN, LOS ANGELES UNIT (O, 50 beds) 3160 Geneva Street, Los Angeles, CA Zip 90020-1199; tel. 213/388-3151; Paul D. Hargis, Administrator

SHRINERS HOSPITALS FOR CRIPPLED CHILDREN, SAN FRANCISCO UNIT (O, 48 beds) 1701 19th Avenue, San Francisco, CA Zip 94122-4599; tel. 415/759-4000; Margaret Bryan-Williams, Administrator

FLORIDA: SHRINERS HOSPITALS FOR CRIPPLED CHILDREN, TAMPA UNIT (O, 60 beds) 12502 North Pine Drive, Tampa, FL Zip 33612-9499; tel. 813/972-2250; John Holtz, Administrator

HAWAII: SHRINERS HOSPITALS FOR CRIPPLED CHILDREN, HONOLULU UNIT (O, 40 beds) 1310 Punahou Street, Honolulu, HI Zip 96826; tel. 808/941-4466; James B. Brasel, Administrator

ILLINOIS: SHRINERS HOSPITALS FOR CRIPPLED CHILDREN, CHICAGO UNIT (O, 60 beds) 2211 North Oak Park Avenue, Chicago, IL Zip 60635-3392; tel. 312/622-5400; A. James Spang, Administrator

KENTUCKY: SHRINERS HOSPITALS FOR CRIPPLED CHILDREN, LEXINGTON UNIT (O, 50 beds) 1900 Richmond Road, Lexington, KY Zip 40502; tel. 606/266-2101; Tony Lewgood, Administrator

LOUISIANA: SHRINERS HOSPITALS FOR CRIPPLED CHILDREN, SHREVEPORT UNIT (O, 45 beds) 3100 Samford Avenue, Shreveport, LA Zip 71103; tel. 318/222-5704; Thomas R. Schneider, Administrator

MASSACHUSETTS: SHRINERS HOSPITAL FOR CRIPPLED CHILDREN, BURNS INSTITUTE BOSTON UNIT (O, 30 beds) 51 Blossom Street, Boston, MA Zip 02114-2699; tel. 617/722-3000; Robert F. Bories, Administrator

---

For explanation of codes following names, see page B2.
★Indicates Type III membership in the American Hospital Association.

Systems / Shriners Hospitals for Crippled Children

SHRINERS HOSPITALS FOR CRIPPLED CHILDREN, SPRINGFIELD UNIT (O, 40 beds) 516 Carew Street, Springfield, MA Zip 01104–2396; tel. 413/787–2000; Mark L. Niederpruem, Administrator

MINNESOTA: SHRINERS HOSPITALS FOR CRIPPLED CHILDREN, TWIN CITIES UNIT (O, 40 beds) 2025 East River Road, Minneapolis, MN Zip 55414–3696; tel. 612/335–5300; Laurence E. Johnson, Administrator

MISSOURI: SHRINERS HOSPITALS FOR CRIPPLED CHILDREN, ST. LOUIS UNIT (O, 80 beds) 2001 South Lindbergh Boulevard, Saint Louis, MO Zip 63131–3597; tel. 314/432–3600; Patricia E. Carey FACHE, Administrator

OHIO: SHRINERS HOSPITALS FOR CRIPPLED CHILDREN, CINCINNATI BURNS INSTITUTE (O, 30 beds) 3229 Burnet Avenue, Cincinnati, OH Zip 45229–3095; tel. 513/872–6000; Ronald R. Hitzler, Administrator

OREGON: SHRINERS HOSPITALS FOR CRIPPLED CHILDREN, PORTLAND UNIT (O, 40 beds) 3101 Southwest Sam Jackson Park Road, Portland, OR Zip 97201; tel. 503/241–5090; Patricia J. Sadowski, Administrator

PENNSYLVANIA: SHRINERS HOSPITALS FOR CRIPPLED CHILDREN, ERIE UNIT (O, 30 beds) 1645 West 8th Street, Erie, PA Zip 16505; tel. 814/875–8700; Richard W. Brzuz, Administrator

SHRINERS HOSPITALS FOR CRIPPLED CHILDREN, PHILADELPHIA UNIT (O, 80 beds) 8400 Roosevelt Boulevard, Philadelphia, PA Zip 19152–1299; tel. 215/332–4500; Sharon J. Rajnic, Administrator

SOUTH CAROLINA: SHRINERS HOSPITALS FOR CRIPPLED CHILDREN, GREENVILLE UNIT (O, 60 beds) 950 West Faris Road, Greenville, SC Zip 29605–4277; tel. 803/271–3444; Gary F. Fraley, Administrator

TEXAS: SHRINERS HOSPITALS FOR CRIPPLED CHILDREN, GALVESTON BURNS INSTITUTE (O, 30 beds) 815 Market Street, Galveston, TX Zip 77550–2725; tel. 409/770–6600; John A. Swartwout, Administrator

SHRINERS HOSPITALS FOR CRIPPLED CHILDREN, HOUSTON UNIT (O, 40 beds) 1402 North MacGregor Drive, Houston, TX Zip 77030–1695; tel. 713/797–1616; Steven B. Reiter, Administrator

UTAH: SHRINERS HOSPITALS FOR CRIPPLED CHILDREN, INTERMOUNTAIN UNIT (O, 40 beds) Fairfax Road & Virginia Street, Salt Lake City, UT Zip 84103–4399; tel. 801/532–5307; Douglas P. Schweikhart, Administrator

WASHINGTON: SHRINERS HOSPITALS FOR CRIPPLED CHILDREN–SPOKANE UNIT (O, 30 beds) 911 West Fifth Avenue, Spokane, WA Zip 99204–2901, Mailing Address: P.O. Box 2472, Zip 99210–2472; tel. 509/455–7844; Charles R. Young, Administrator

Owned, leased, sponsored:	20 hospitals	923 beds
Contract–managed:	0 hospitals	0 beds
Totals:	20 hospitals	923 beds

0067: SINGING RIVER HOSPITAL SYSTEM (NP)
2809 Denny Avenue, Pascagoula, MS Zip 39581; tel. 601/938–5062; Robert L. Lingle, Executive Director

MISSISSIPPI: OCEAN SPRINGS HOSPITAL (O, 124 beds) 3109 Bienville Boulevard, Ocean Springs, MS Zip 39564; tel. 601/872–1111; Dwight Rimes, Administrator

SINGING RIVER HOSPITAL (O, 322 beds) 2809 Denny Avenue, Pascagoula, MS Zip 39581; tel. 601/938–5000; James S. Kaigler FACHE, Administrator

Owned, leased, sponsored:	2 hospitals	446 beds
Contract–managed:	0 hospitals	0 beds
Totals:	2 hospitals	446 beds

5995: SISTERS OF CHARITY CENTER (CC)
Mount St Vincent on Hudson, New York, NY Zip 10471–1093; tel. 718/549–9200; Sister Carol Barnes, President

NEW YORK: ST. JOSEPH'S MEDICAL CENTER (S, 394 beds) 127 South Broadway, Yonkers, NY Zip 10701–4080; tel. 914/378–7000; Sister Mary Linehan, President

ST. VINCENT'S HOSPITAL AND MEDICAL CENTER OF NEW YORK (S, 978 beds) 153 West 11th Street, New York, NY Zip 10011–8397; tel. 212/604–7000; Karl P. Adler M.D., President and Chief Executive Officer

Owned, leased, sponsored:	2 hospitals	1372 beds
Contract–managed:	0 hospitals	0 beds
Totals:	2 hospitals	1372 beds

★**6095: SISTERS OF CHARITY HEALTH CARE SYSTEM CORPORATION** (CC)
75 Vanderbilt Avenue, New York, NY Zip 10304–3850; tel. 718/390–5080; John J. DePierro, President and Chief Executive Officer

NEW YORK: BAYLEY SETON HOSPITAL (S, 191 beds) 75 Vanderbilt Avenue, Staten Island, NY Zip 10304–3850; tel. 718/390–6000; John N. Kastanis FACHE, Executive Vice President

ST. VINCENT'S MEDICAL CENTER OF RICHMOND (S, 440 beds) 355 Bard Avenue, Staten Island, NY Zip 10310–1699; tel. 718/876–1234; Dominick M. Stanzione, Executive Vice President

Owned, leased, sponsored:	2 hospitals	631 beds
Contract–managed:	0 hospitals	0 beds
Totals:	2 hospitals	631 beds

★**5115: SISTERS OF CHARITY HEALTH CARE SYSTEMS, INC.** (CC)
345 Neeb Road, Cincinnati, OH Zip 45233–5102; tel. 513/347–1000; Sister Celestia Koebel, President

COLORADO: PENROSE–ST. FRANCIS HEALTHCARE SYSTEM (S, 522 beds) 2215 North Cascade Avenue, Colorado Springs, CO Zip 80907, Mailing Address: P.O. Box 7021, Zip 80933–7021; tel. 719/776–5000; Leonard A. Farr, President and Chief Executive Officer

PROVENANT ST. ANTHONY HOSPITAL CENTRAL (S, 364 beds) 4231 West 16th Avenue, Denver, CO Zip 80204–4098; tel. 303/629–3511; Michael H. Erne, Chief Executive Officer and Executive Vice President

PROVENANT ST. ANTHONY HOSPITAL NORTH (S, 130 beds) 2551 West 84th Avenue, Westminster, CO Zip 80030; tel. 303/426–2151; Michael H. Erne, Chief Executive Officer and Executive Vice President

ST. MARY–CORWIN REGIONAL MEDICAL CENTER (S, 307 beds) 1008 Minnequa Avenue, Pueblo, CO Zip 81004–3798; tel. 719/560–4000; William G. Turman M.D., President and Chief Executive Officer

ST. THOMAS MORE HOSPITAL AND PROGRESSIVE CARE CENTER (O, 218 beds) 1338 Phay Avenue, Canon City, CO Zip 81212–2221; tel. 719/269–2021; William A. Burns, Chief Executive Officer

KENTUCKY: OUR LADY OF THE WAY HOSPITAL (S, 35 beds) Route 1428, Main Street, Martin, KY Zip 41649–0910; tel. 606/285–5181; Lowell Jones, Chief Executive Officer

NEBRASKA: GOOD SAMARITAN HEALTH SYSTEMS (S, 267 beds) 10 East 31st Street, Kearney, NE Zip 68847–2926, Mailing Address: P.O. Box 1990, Zip 68848–1990; tel. 308/236–8511; William Wilson Hendrickson, President

SAINT FRANCIS MEDICAL CENTER (S, 165 beds) 2620 West Faidley Avenue, Grand Island, NE Zip 68803–, Mailing Address: Box 9804, Zip 68802–9804; tel. 308/384–4600; Michael R. Gloor, President and Chief Executive Officer

ST. ELIZABETH COMMUNITY HEALTH CENTER (S, 177 beds) 555 South 70th Street, Lincoln, NE Zip 68510–2494; tel. 402/489–7181; Robert J. Lanik, President

ST. MARY'S HOSPITAL (S, 28 beds) 1314 Third Avenue, Nebraska City, NE Zip 68410; tel. 402/873–3321; Richard W. Waller, Interim Administrator

NEW MEXICO: ST. JOSEPH MEDICAL CENTER (S, 275 beds) 601 Martin Luther King Drive N.E., Albuquerque, NM Zip 87102, Mailing Address: P.O. Box 25555, Zip 87125; tel. 505/244–8000; Ray H. Barton III, President and Chief Executive Officer

ST. JOSEPH NORTHEAST HEIGHTS HOSPITAL (S, 112 beds) 4701 Montgomery N.E., Albuquerque, NM Zip 87109, Mailing Address: P.O. Box 25555, Zip 87125–0555; tel. 505/888–7800; C. Vincent Townsend, Jr., Vice President

ST. JOSEPH REHABILITATION HOSPITAL AND OUTPATIENT CENTER (S, 63 beds) 505 Elm Street N.E., Albuquerque, NM Zip 87102, Mailing Address: P.O. Box 25555, Zip 87125–2500; tel. 505/244–4700; Mary Lou Coors, Administrator

ST. JOSEPH WEST MESA HOSPITAL (S, 128 beds) 10501 Golf Course Road N.W., Albuquerque, NM Zip 87114, Mailing Address: P.O. Box 25555, Zip 87125–0555; tel. 505/893–2003; C. Vincent Townsend, Jr., Vice President

OHIO: GOOD SAMARITAN HOSPITAL (S, 479 beds) 375 Dixmyth Avenue, Cincinnati, OH Zip 45220–2489; tel. 513/872–1400; Sister Myra James Bradley, Chairman of the Executive Board and Chief Executive Officer

GOOD SAMARITAN HOSPITAL AND HEALTH CENTER (S, 560 beds) 2222 Philadelphia Drive, Dayton, OH Zip 45406–1891; tel. 513/278–2612; K. Douglas Deck, President and Chief Executive Officer

---

For explanation of codes following names, see page B2.
★Indicates Type III membership in the American Hospital Association.

Systems / Sisters of Mary of the Presentation Health Corporation

Owned, leased, sponsored:	16 hospitals	3830 beds
Contract–managed:	0 hospitals	0 beds
Totals:	16 hospitals	3830 beds

★**5095: SISTERS OF CHARITY OF LEAVENWORTH HEALTH SERVICES CORPORATION** (CC)
4200 South Fourth Street, Leavenworth, KS Zip 66048–5054; tel. 913/682–1338; Sister Marie Damian Glatt, President

CALIFORNIA: SAINT JOHN'S HOSPITAL AND HEALTH CENTER (O, 353 beds) 1328 22nd Street, Santa Monica, CA Zip 90404; tel. 310/829–5511; Sister Marie Madeleine Shonka, President

COLORADO: SAINT JOSEPH HOSPITAL (O, 437 beds) 1835 Franklin Street, Denver, CO Zip 80218; tel. 303/837–7111; Sister Marianna Bauder, President and Chief Executive Officer

ST. MARY'S HOSPITAL AND MEDICAL CENTER (O, 200 beds) 2635 North 7th Street, Grand Junction, CO Zip 81501–1628, Mailing Address: P.O. Box 3433, Zip 81502; tel. 303/244–2273; Sister Lynn Casey, President

KANSAS: PROVIDENCE MEDICAL CENTER (O, 209 beds) 8929 Parallel Parkway, Kansas City, KS Zip 66112–0430; tel. 913/596–4000; Sister Ann Marita Loosen, President and Chief Executive Officer

SAINT JOHN HOSPITAL (O, 30 beds) 3500 South Fourth Street, Leavenworth, KS Zip 66048–5092; tel. 913/682–3721; Frank Creeden, Chief Operating Officer

ST. FRANCIS HOSPITAL AND MEDICAL CENTER (O, 320 beds) 1700 West Seventh Street, Topeka, KS Zip 66606–1690; tel. 913/295–8000; Sister Loretto Marie Colwell, President

MONTANA: SAINT VINCENT HOSPITAL AND HEALTH CENTER (O, 285 beds) 1233 North 30th Street, Billings, MT Zip 59101, Mailing Address: P.O. Box 35200, Zip 59107–5200; tel. 406/657–7000; James T. Paquette, President and Chief Executive Officer

ST. JAMES COMMUNITY HOSPITAL (O, 103 beds) 400 South Clark Street, Butte, MT Zip 59701, Mailing Address: P.O. Box 3300, Zip 59702; tel. 406/782–8361; Thomas R. Hochwalt, Chief Executive Officer

Owned, leased, sponsored:	8 hospitals	1937 beds
Contract–managed:	0 hospitals	0 beds
Totals:	8 hospitals	1937 beds

★**3045: SISTERS OF CHARITY OF NAZARETH HEALTH SYSTEM** (CC)
135 West Drive, Nazareth, KY Zip 40048, Mailing Address: P.O. Box 171, Zip 40048–0171; tel. 502/349–6250; Mark W. Dundon, President and Chief Executive Officer

ARKANSAS: ST. VINCENT INFIRMARY MEDICAL CENTER (O, 566 beds) Two St. Vincent Circle, Little Rock, AR Zip 72205–5499; tel. 501/660–3000; Thomas L. Feurig, President and Chief Executive Officer

KENTUCKY: CARITAS PEACE CENTER (O, 156 beds) 2020 Newburg Road, Louisville, KY Zip 40232; tel. 502/451–3330; Peter J. Bernard, President and Chief Executive Officer

FLAGET MEMORIAL HOSPITAL (O, 52 beds) 201 Cathedral Manor, Bardstown, KY Zip 40004–1299; tel. 502/348–3923; Suzanne Reasbeck, Acting President and Chief Executive Officer

MARYMOUNT HOSPITAL (O, 95 beds) 310 East Ninth Street, London, KY Zip 40741–1299; tel. 606/878–6520; Lowell Jones, President

SAINTS MARY AND ELIZABETH HOSPITAL (O, 177 beds) 1850 Bluegrass Avenue, Louisville, KY Zip 40215–1199; tel. 502/361–6000; Peter J. Bernard, President and Chief Executive Officer

ST. JOSEPH HOSPITAL (O, 325 beds) One St. Joseph Drive, Lexington, KY Zip 40504; tel. 606/278–3436; William D. Fuchs, President

TENNESSEE: MEMORIAL HOSPITAL (O, 296 beds) 2525 De Sales Avenue, Chattanooga, TN Zip 37404–3322; tel. 615/495–2525; L. Clark Taylor, Jr., President and Chief Executive Officer

Owned, leased, sponsored:	7 hospitals	1667 beds
Contract–managed:	0 hospitals	0 beds
Totals:	7 hospitals	1667 beds

5125: SISTERS OF CHARITY OF ST. AUGUSTINE HEALTH SYSTEM (CC)
2351 East 22nd Street, Cleveland, OH Zip 44115; tel. 216/696–5560; Peter G. Reibold, President

OHIO: ST. JOHN WEST SHORE HOSPITAL (S, 183 beds) 29000 Center Ridge Road, Westlake, OH Zip 44145–5294; tel. 216/835–8000; Fred M. Degrandis, President

ST. VINCENT CHARITY HOSPITAL (S, 266 beds) 2351 East 22nd Street, Cleveland, OH Zip 44115; tel. 216/861–6200; Samuel H. Turner, President

TIMKEN MERCY MEDICAL CENTER (S, 416 beds) 1320 Timken Mercy Drive N.W., Canton, OH Zip 44708–2641; tel. 216/489–1000; Jack W. Topoleski, President and Chief Executive Officer

SOUTH CAROLINA: PROVIDENCE HOSPITAL (S, 211 beds) 2435 Forest Drive, Columbia, SC Zip 29204–2098; tel. 803/256–5313; M. John Heydel, President and Chief Executive Officer

Owned, leased, sponsored:	4 hospitals	1076 beds
Contract–managed:	0 hospitals	0 beds
Totals:	4 hospitals	1076 beds

★**0605: SISTERS OF CHARITY OF THE INCARNATE WORD HEALTHCARE SYSTEM** (CC)
2600 North Loop West, Houston, TX Zip 77092; tel. 713/681–8877; Stanley T. Urban, President and Chief Executive Officer

CALIFORNIA: ST. BERNARDINE MEDICAL CENTER (O, 447 beds) 2101 North Waterman Avenue, San Bernardino, CA Zip 92404; tel. 909/883–8711; Gregory A. Adams, Administrator and Chief Executive Officer

ST. MARY MEDICAL CENTER (O, 484 beds) 1050 Linden Avenue, Long Beach, CA Zip 90801, Mailing Address: P.O. Box 887, Zip 90801; tel. 310/491–9000; David Tillman M.D., President

LOUISIANA: SCHUMPERT MEDICAL CENTER (O, 486 beds) One St. Mary Place, Shreveport, LA Zip 71101, Mailing Address: P.O. Box 21976, Zip 71120–1076; tel. 318/227–4500; Arthur A. Gonzalez Dr.P.H., Chief Executive Officer

ST. FRANCES CABRINI HOSPITAL (O, 264 beds) 3330 Masonic Drive, Alexandria, LA Zip 71301; tel. 318/487–1122; L. Rene' Goux, Chief Executive Officer

ST. PATRICK HOSPITAL OF LAKE CHARLES (O, 298 beds) 524 South Ryan Street, Lake Charles, LA Zip 70601, Mailing Address: P.O. Box 3401, Zip 70602–3401; tel. 318/436–2511; J. William Hankins, Administrator and Chief Executive Officer

TEXAS: ST. ELIZABETH HOSPITAL (O, 483 beds) 2830 Calder Avenue, Beaumont, TX Zip 77702, Mailing Address: P.O. Box 5405, Zip 77726–5405; tel. 409/892–7171; Sister M. Fatima McCarthy, Administrator

ST. JOHN HOSPITAL (O, 133 beds) 2050 Space Park Drive, Nassau Bay, TX Zip 77058; tel. 713/333–5503

ST. JOSEPH HOSPITAL (O, 611 beds) 1919 Labranch Street, Houston, TX Zip 77002; tel. 713/757–1000; Raymond J. Khoury, Administrator

ST. MARY HOSPITAL (O, 226 beds) 3600 Gates Boulevard, Port Arthur, TX Zip 77642–3601, Mailing Address: P.O. Box 3696, Zip 77643–3696; tel. 409/985–7431; John K. Barto, Jr., Administrator

ST. MARY'S HOSPITAL (O, 235 beds) 404 St. Mary's Boulevard, Galveston, TX Zip 77550; tel. 409/763–5301; James E. Gardner, Jr., Administrator

ST. MICHAEL HEALTH CARE CENTER (O, 239 beds) 2600 St. Michael Drive, Texarkana, TX Zip 75503; tel. 903/614–1000; Stephen F. Wright, Interim Administrator and Chief Executive Officer

ST. MICHAEL REHABILITATION HOSPITAL (O, 80 beds) 2400 St Michael Drive, Texarkana, TX Zip 75503; tel. 903/614–4000; Freeman P. Lockhart, Administrator

Owned, leased, sponsored:	12 hospitals	3986 beds
Contract–managed:	0 hospitals	0 beds
Totals:	12 hospitals	3986 beds

5805: SISTERS OF MARY OF THE PRESENTATION HEALTH CORPORATION (CC)
1102 Page Drive S.W., Fargo, ND Zip 58106–0007, Mailing Address: P.O. Box 10007, Zip 58106–0007; tel. 701/237–9290; Aaron Alton, President

ILLINOIS: ST. MARGARET'S HOSPITAL (O, 127 beds) 600 East First Street, Spring Valley, IL Zip 61362–2034; tel. 815/664–5311; Tim Muntz, President

IOWA: VAN BUREN COUNTY HOSPITAL (CM, 40 beds) Highway 1 North, Keosauqua, IA Zip 52565, Mailing Address: Box 70, Zip 52565; tel. 319/293–3171; Lisa Wagner Schnedler, Administrator

For explanation of codes following names, see page B2.
★Indicates Type III membership in the American Hospital Association.

Systems / Sisters of Mary of the Presentation Health Corporation

NORTH DAKOTA: PRESENTATION MEDICAL CENTER (O, 102 beds) 213 Second Avenue N.E., Rolla, ND Zip 58367, Mailing Address: P.O. Box 759, Zip 58367-0759; tel. 701/477-3161; Kimber Wraalstad, Chief Executive Officer

ST. ALOISIUS MEDICAL CENTER (O, 165 beds) 325 East Brewster Street, Harvey, ND Zip 58341-1605; tel. 701/324-4651; Ronald J. Volk, President

ST. ANDREW'S HEALTH CENTER (O, 67 beds) 316 Ohmer Street, Bottineau, ND Zip 58318-1018; tel. 701/228-2255; Keith Korman, President

Owned, leased, sponsored:	4 hospitals	461 beds
Contract-managed:	1 hospitals	40 beds
Totals:	5 hospitals	501 beds

5985: SISTERS OF MERCY (CC)
431 East Wilkinson Boulevard, Belmont, NC Zip 28012; tel. 704/829-5103; Sister Pauline Clifford, Regional President

NORTH CAROLINA: MERCY HOSPITAL (O, 276 beds) 2001 Vail Avenue, Charlotte, NC Zip 28207; tel. 704/379-5000; C. Curtis Copenhaver, President

ST. JOSEPH'S HOSPITAL (O, 292 beds) 428 Biltmore Avenue, Asheville, NC Zip 28801-4502; tel. 704/255-3100; J. Lewis Daniels, President and Chief Executive Officer

Owned, leased, sponsored:	2 hospitals	568 beds
Contract-managed:	0 hospitals	0 beds
Totals:	2 hospitals	568 beds

★**5185: SISTERS OF MERCY HEALTH SYSTEM–ST. LOUIS** (CC)
2039 North Geyer Road, Saint Louis, MO Zip 63131-3399; tel. 314/965-6100; Sister Mary Roch Rocklage, Chief Executive Officer

ARKANSAS: HARBOR VIEW MERCY HOSPITAL (O, 80 beds) 10301 Mayo Road, Fort Smith, AR Zip 72903, Mailing Address: P.O. Box 17000, Zip 72917-7000; tel. 501/484-5550; Ron Summerhill, Administrator

MERCY HOSPITAL OF SCOTT COUNTY (O, 129 beds) Highways 71 and 80, Waldron, AR Zip 72958-9984, Mailing Address: Box 2230, Zip 72958-2230; tel. 501/637-4135; Sister Mary Alvera Simon, Administrator

MERCY HOSPITAL-TURNER MEMORIAL (O, 39 beds) 801 West River, Ozark, AR Zip 72949; tel. 501/667-4138; Sister Mary Werner Keith, Administrator

NORTH LOGAN MERCY HOSPITAL (O, 16 beds) 500 East Academy, Paris, AR Zip 72855-4099; tel. 501/963-6101; Jim L. Maddox, Chief Administrative Officer

ST. EDWARD MERCY MEDICAL CENTER (O, 260 beds) 7301 Rogers Avenue, Fort Smith, AR Zip 72903, Mailing Address: P.O. Box 17000, Zip 72917-7000; tel. 501/484-6000; Sister Judith Marie Keith, President and Chief Executive Officer

ST. JOSEPH'S REGIONAL HEALTH CENTER (O, 276 beds) 300 Werner Street, Hot Springs, AR Zip 71913; tel. 501/622-1000; Randall J. Fale, President and Chief Executive Officer

KANSAS: MERCY HOSPITALS OF KANSAS (O, 105 beds) 821 Burke Street, Fort Scott, KS Zip 66701; tel. 316/223-2200; Susan Barrett, President and Chief Executive Officer

MERCY HOSPITALS OF KANSAS (O, 58 beds) 800 West Myrtle Street, Independence, KS Zip 67301, Mailing Address: Box 388, Zip 67301-0388; tel. 316/331-2200; Susan Barrett, President and Chief Executive Officer

MISSOURI: ST. JOHN'S MERCY MEDICAL CENTER (O, 867 beds) 615 South New Ballas Road, Saint Louis, MO Zip 63141-8277; tel. 314/239-8000; Charles Thoele, Chief Executive Officer

ST. JOHN'S REGIONAL HEALTH CENTER (O, 866 beds) 1235 East Cherokee Street, Springfield, MO Zip 65804-2263; tel. 417/885-2000; Allen L. Shockley, President and Chief Executive Officer

OKLAHOMA: MERCY HEALTH CENTER (O, 385 beds) 4300 West Memorial Road, Oklahoma City, OK Zip 73120-8362; tel. 405/755-1515; Bruce Forrest Buchanan FACHE, President and Chief Executive Officer

TEXAS: MERCY REGIONAL MEDICAL CENTER (O, 309 beds) 1515 Logan Avenue, Laredo, TX Zip 78040, Mailing Address: Drawer 2068, Zip 78044-2068; tel. 210/718-6230; Michael L. Morgan, President and Chief Executive Officer

Owned, leased, sponsored:	12 hospitals	3390 beds
Contract-managed:	0 hospitals	0 beds
Totals:	12 hospitals	3390 beds

6015: SISTERS OF MERCY OF THE AMERICAS–REGIONAL COMMUNITY OF BALTIMORE (CC)
1300 Northern Parkway, Baltimore, MD Zip 21239, Mailing Address: P.O. Box 11448, Zip 21239; tel. 410/435-4400; Sister Margaret Beatty, President

GEORGIA: ST. JOSEPH'S HOSPITAL (O, 305 beds) 11705 Mercy Boulevard, Savannah, GA Zip 31419-1791; tel. 912/927-5404; Paul H. Hinchey, President and Chief Executive Officer

MARYLAND: MERCY MEDICAL CENTER (O, 245 beds) 301 St. Paul Place, Baltimore, MD Zip 21202-2165; tel. 410/332-9000; Sister Helen Amos, President and Chief Executive Officer

Owned, leased, sponsored:	2 hospitals	550 beds
Contract-managed:	0 hospitals	0 beds
Totals:	2 hospitals	550 beds

★**5285: SISTERS OF PROVIDENCE HEALTH SYSTEM** (CC)
146 Chestnut Street, Springfield, MA Zip 01103; tel. 413/737-3981; Sister Kathleen Popko, President and Chief Executive Officer

MASSACHUSETTS: MERCY HOSPITAL (O, 276 beds) 271 Carew Street, Springfield, MA Zip 01104, Mailing Address: P.O. Box 9012, Zip 01102-9012; tel. 413/748-9000; Vincent J. McCorkle, President and Chief Executive Officer

PROVIDENCE HOSPITAL (O, 202 beds) 1233 Main Street, Holyoke, MA Zip 01040-5381; tel. 413/536-5111; Vincent J. McCorkle, President and Chief Executive Officer

Owned, leased, sponsored:	2 hospitals	478 beds
Contract-managed:	0 hospitals	0 beds
Totals:	2 hospitals	478 beds

★**5275: SISTERS OF PROVIDENCE HEALTH SYSTEM** (CC)
520 Pike Street, Seattle, WA Zip 98101, Mailing Address: P.O. Box 11038, Zip 98111-9038; tel. 206/464-3355; Sister Dona Taylor, President and Chief Executive Officer

ALASKA: PROVIDENCE ALASKA MEDICAL CENTER (O, 341 beds) 3200 Providence Drive, Anchorage, AK Zip 99508, Mailing Address: P.O. Box 196604, Zip 99519-6604; tel. 907/562-2211; Douglas A. Bruce, Chief Executive

CALIFORNIA: SAINT JOSEPH MEDICAL CENTER (O, 423 beds) 501 South Buena Vista Street, Burbank, CA Zip 91505-4866; tel. 818/843-5111; Michael J. Madden, Administrator and Chief Executive Officer

OREGON: PROVIDENCE MEDFORD MEDICAL CENTER (O, 118 beds) 1111 Crater Lake Avenue, Medford, OR Zip 97504-6241; tel. 503/773-6611; Andrea Y. Coleman, Chief Executive, Southern Oregon Service Area and Administrator

PROVIDENCE MILWAUKIE HOSPITAL (O, 56 beds) 10150 Southeast 32nd Avenue, Milwaukie, OR Zip 97222-6593; tel. 503/652-8300; Sister Betsy Mickel, Chief Operating Officer

PROVIDENCE NEWBERG HOSPITAL (O, 35 beds) 501 Villa Road, Newberg, OR Zip 97132; tel. 503/537-1555; Mark W. Meinert CHE, Chief Executive, Yamhill Service Area

PROVIDENCE PORTLAND MEDICAL CENTER (O, 449 beds) 4805 Northeast Glisan Street, Portland, OR Zip 97213-2967; tel. 503/230-1111; Marvin O'Quinn, Chief Operating Officer

PROVIDENCE SEASIDE HOSPITAL (L, 29 beds) 725 South Wahanna Road, Seaside, OR Zip 97138, Mailing Address: Box 740, Zip 97138-0740; tel. 503/738-8463; Ronald Swanson, Administrator

PROVIDENCE ST. VINCENT MEDICAL CENTER (O, 275 beds) 9205 Southwest Barnes Road, Portland, OR Zip 97225-6661; tel. 503/297-4411; Donald Elsom, Chief Operating Officer

WASHINGTON: MARK REED HOSPITAL (CM, 8 beds) 322 South Birch Street, McCleary, WA Zip 98557, Mailing Address: P.O. Box 1300, Zip 98557-1300; tel. 360/495-3244; Jean E. Roberts, Administrator

---

For explanation of codes following names, see page B2.
★Indicates Type III membership in the American Hospital Association.

Systems / Sisters of the Sorrowful Mother United States Health System

MORTON GENERAL HOSPITAL (CM, 46 beds) 521 Adams Street, Morton, WA Zip 98356, Mailing Address: Drawer C, Zip 98356; tel. 360/496-5112

PROVIDENCE CENTRALIA HOSPITAL (O, 149 beds) 1820 Cooks Hill Road, Centralia, WA Zip 98531; tel. 360/736-2803; Sister Maureen Comer, Administrator

PROVIDENCE GENERAL MEDICAL CENTER (O, 327 beds) Pacific and Nassau Streets, Everett, WA Zip 98201, Mailing Address: P.O. Box 1067, Zip 98206-1067; tel. 206/258-7267; John P. Rinset, President and Chief Executive Officer

PROVIDENCE SEATTLE MEDICAL CENTER (O, 334 beds) 500 17th Avenue, Seattle, WA Zip 98122, Mailing Address: P.O. Box 34008, Zip 98124-1008; tel. 206/320-2000; Nancy A. Giunto, Administrator

PROVIDENCE ST. PETER HOSPITAL (O, 327 beds) 413 Lilly Road N.E., Olympia, WA Zip 98506-5166; tel. 206/491-9480; C. Scott Bond, Administrator

PROVIDENCE TOPPENISH HOSPITAL (O, 48 beds) 504 West Fourth Avenue, Toppenish, WA Zip 98948, Mailing Address: P.O. Box 672, Zip 98948-0672; tel. 509/865-3105; Roy W. Holmes, Administrator

PROVIDENCE YAKIMA MEDICAL CENTER (O, 184 beds) 110 South Ninth Avenue, Yakima, WA Zip 98902-3397; tel. 509/575-5000; Barbara A. Hood, Acting Administrator

Owned, leased, sponsored:	14 hospitals	3095 beds
Contract-managed:	2 hospitals	54 beds
Totals:	16 hospitals	3149 beds

★**5345: SISTERS OF ST. FRANCIS HEALTH SERVICES, INC.** (CC)
1515 Dragoon Trail, Mishawaka, IN Zip 46546-1290, Mailing Address: P.O. Box 1290, Zip 46546-1290; tel. 219/256-3935; Sister Jane Marie Klein, President

ILLINOIS: ST. FRANCIS HOSPITAL (O, 555 beds) 355 Ridge Avenue, Evanston, IL Zip 60202-3399; tel. 708/316-4000; James C. Gizzi, President and Chief Executive Officer

ST. JAMES HOSPITAL AND HEALTH CENTERS (O, 348 beds) 1423 Chicago Road, Chicago Heights, IL Zip 60411-9934; tel. 708/756-1000; Peter J. Murphy, President and Chief Executive Officer

INDIANA: SAINT ANTHONY HOSPITAL AND HEALTH CENTERS (O, 141 beds) 301 West Homer Street, Michigan City, IN Zip 46360-4358; tel. 219/879-8511; Edel Dunne-O'Toole, President and Chief Executive Officer

SAINT MARGARET MERCY HEALTHCARE CENTERS (O, 592 beds) 5454 Hohman Avenue, Hammond, IN Zip 46320; tel. 219/933-2074; Gene Diamond, President and Chief Executive Officer

ST. ELIZABETH HOSPITAL MEDICAL CENTER (O, 212 beds) 1501 Hartford Street, Lafayette, IN Zip 47904-2126, Mailing Address: Box 7501, Zip 47903-7501; tel. 317/423-6011; Douglas W. Eberle, President and Chief Executive Officer

ST. FRANCIS HOSPITAL AND HEALTH CENTERS (O, 428 beds) 1600 Albany Street, Beech Grove, IN Zip 46107-1593; tel. 317/787-3311; Kevin D. Leahy, President and Chief Executive Officer

TENNESSEE: ST. JOSEPH HOSPITAL AND HEALTH CENTERS (O, 372 beds) 220 Overton Avenue, Memphis, TN Zip 38105-2789; tel. 901/577-2700; Joan M. Carlson, President and Chief Executive Officer

Owned, leased, sponsored:	7 hospitals	2648 beds
Contract-managed:	0 hospitals	0 beds
Totals:	7 hospitals	2648 beds

★**5555: SISTERS OF ST. JOSEPH HEALTH SYSTEM** (CC)
455 East Eisenhower Parkway, Suite 300, Ann Arbor, MI Zip 48108-3304; tel. 313/741-1160; John S. Lore, President and Chief Executive Officer

MICHIGAN: BORGESS MEDICAL CENTER (O, 351 beds) 1521 Gull Road, Kalamazoo, MI Zip 49001-1640; tel. 616/383-7000; R. Timothy Stack FACHE, President

GENESYS REGIONAL MEDICAL CENTER-FLINT OSTEOPATHIC CAMPUS (O, 263 beds) 3921 Beecher Road, Flint, MI Zip 48532-3699; tel. 810/762-4000; Young S. Suh, President

GENESYS REGIONAL MEDICAL CENTER-GENESEE MEMORIAL CAMPUS (O, 40 beds) 702 South Ballenger Highway, Flint, MI Zip 48532-3899; tel. 810/766-8800; Young S. Suh, President and Chief Executive Officer

GENESYS REGIONAL MEDICAL CENTER-ST. JOSEPH CAMPUS (O, 337 beds) 302 Kensington Avenue, Flint, MI Zip 48503-2000; tel. 810/762-8000; Young S. Suh, President

GENESYS REGIONAL MEDICAL CENTER-WHEELOCK MEMORIAL CAMPUS (O, 31 beds) 7280 State Road, Goodrich, MI Zip 48438; tel. 810/636-2221; Joseph W. Kyle, Vice President

LEE MEMORIAL HOSPITAL (O, 57 beds) 420 West High Street, Dowagiac, MI Zip 49047-1907; tel. 616/782-8681; Merrill A. Frank, Chief Executive Officer

RIVER DISTRICT HOSPITAL (O, 68 beds) 4100 South River Road, East China, MI Zip 48054; tel. 810/329-7111; John E. Knox, President and Chief Executive Officer

ST. JOHN HOSPITAL AND MEDICAL CENTER (O, 589 beds) 22101 Moross Road, Detroit, MI Zip 48236-2172; tel. 313/343-4000; Timothy J. Grajewski, President and Chief Executive Officer

ST. JOHN HOSPITAL-MACOMB CENTER (O, 65 beds) 26755 Ballard Road, Harrison Township, MI Zip 48045-2458; tel. 810/465-5501; David Sessions, Administrator

TAWAS ST. JOSEPH HOSPITAL (O, 69 beds) 200 Hemlock, Tawas City, MI Zip 48763, Mailing Address: P.O. Box 659, Zip 48764-0659; tel. 517/362-3411; Paul R. Schmidt, President and Chief Executive Officer

Owned, leased, sponsored:	10 hospitals	1870 beds
Contract-managed:	0 hospitals	0 beds
Totals:	10 hospitals	1870 beds

5955: SISTERS OF THE 3RD FRANCISCAN ORDER (CC)
2500 Grant Boulevard, Syracuse, NY Zip 13208-1713; tel. 315/425-0115; Sister Grace Anne Dillenschneider, General Superior

HAWAII: ST. FRANCIS MEDICAL CENTER (O, 217 beds) 2230 Liliha Street, Honolulu, HI Zip 96817-9979, Mailing Address: P.O. Box 30100, Zip 96820-0100; tel. 808/547-6011; Sister Beatrice Tom, President and Chief Executive Officer

NEW YORK: ST. ELIZABETH HOSPITAL (O, 217 beds) 2209 Genesee Street, Utica, NY Zip 13501-5999; tel. 315/798-8100; Sister Rose Vincent, President and Chief Executive Officer

ST. JOSEPH'S HOSPITAL HEALTH CENTER (O, 431 beds) 301 Prospect Avenue, Syracuse, NY Zip 13203; tel. 315/448-5111; William J. Watt, President

Owned, leased, sponsored:	3 hospitals	865 beds
Contract-managed:	0 hospitals	0 beds
Totals:	3 hospitals	865 beds

5575: SISTERS OF THE HOLY FAMILY OF NAZARETH-SACRED HEART PROVINCE (CC)
353 North River Road, Des Plaines, IL Zip 60016-1291; tel. 708/298-6760; Sister M. Lucille Madura, Provincial Superior

ILLINOIS: HOLY FAMILY MEDICAL CENTER (O, 183 beds) 100 North River Road, Des Plaines, IL Zip 60016; tel. 708/297-1800; Sister Patricia Ann Koschalke, President and Chief Executive Officer

SAINT MARY OF NAZARETH HOSPITAL CENTER (O, 305 beds) 2233 West Division Street, Chicago, IL Zip 60622-3086; tel. 312/770-2000; Sister Stella Louise, President and Chief Executive Officer

Owned, leased, sponsored:	2 hospitals	488 beds
Contract-managed:	0 hospitals	0 beds
Totals:	2 hospitals	488 beds

★**5305: SISTERS OF THE SORROWFUL MOTHER UNITED STATES HEALTH SYSTEM** (CC)
P.O. Box 4753, Tulsa, OK Zip 74159-0753; tel. 918/742-9988; Sister M. Therese Gottschalk, President

IOWA: HOLY FAMILY HOSPITAL (O, 58 beds) 826 North Eighth Street, Estherville, IA Zip 51334-1598; tel. 712/362-2631; Thomas Nordwick, President and Chief Executive Officer

KANSAS: ST. FRANCIS REGIONAL MEDICAL CENTER (O, 681 beds) 929 North St. Francis Street, Wichita, KS Zip 67214-3882; tel. 316/268-5000; Sister M. Sylvia Egan, President and Chief Executive Officer

---

For explanation of codes following names, see page B2.
★Indicates Type III membership in the American Hospital Association.

Systems / Sisters of the Sorrowful Mother United States Health System

MINNESOTA: ST. ELIZABETH HOSPITAL (O, 198 beds) 1200 Fifth Grand Boulevard W, Wabasha, MN Zip 55981; tel. 612/565-4531; Thomas Crowley, President

NEW JERSEY: NORTHWEST COVENANT MEDICAL CENTER (O, 504 beds) 25 Pocono Road, Denville, NJ Zip 07834-2995; tel. 201/625-6000; Joseph A. Trunfio Ph.D., President and Chief Executive Officer

OKLAHOMA: ST. JOHN MEDICAL CENTER (O, 597 beds) 1923 South Utica Avenue, Tulsa, OK Zip 74104-5445; tel. 918/744-2345; Sister M. Therese Gottschalk, President

WISCONSIN: MERCY MEDICAL CENTER (O, 236 beds) 631 Hazel Street, Oshkosh, WI Zip 54902, Mailing Address: Box 1100, Zip 54902-1100; tel. 414/236-2000; Otto L. Cox, President

SACRED HEART-ST. MARY'S HOSPITALS (O, 62 beds) 1044 Kabel Avenue, Rhinelander, WI Zip 54501-3998, Mailing Address: P.O. Box 20, Zip 54501; tel. 715/369-6600; Kevin J. O'Donnell, President and Chief Executive Officer

SAINT JOSEPH'S HOSPITAL (O, 524 beds) 611 St. Joseph Avenue, Marshfield, WI Zip 54449-1898; tel. 715/387-1713; Michael A. Schmidt, President and Chief Executive Officer

SAINT MICHAEL'S HOSPITAL (O, 115 beds) 900 Illinois Avenue, Stevens Point, WI Zip 54481; tel. 715/346-5000; Jeffrey L. Martin, President and Chief Executive Officer

Owned, leased, sponsored:	9 hospitals	2975 beds
Contract-managed:	0 hospitals	0 beds
Totals:	9 hospitals	2975 beds

★4175: **SOUTHERN ILLINOIS HOSPITAL SERVICES** (NP)
608 East College Street, Carbondale, IL Zip 62901, Mailing Address: P.O. Box 3988, Zip 62902-3988; tel. 618/457-5200; John J. Buckley Jr., President

ILLINOIS: HERRIN HOSPITAL (O, 78 beds) 201 South 14th Street, Herrin, IL Zip 62948; tel. 618/942-2171; Virgil Hannig, Administrator

MEMORIAL HOSPITAL OF CARBONDALE (O, 137 beds) 405 West Jackson Street, Carbondale, IL Zip 62902, Mailing Address: P.O. Box 10000, Zip 62902-9000; tel. 618/549-0721; George Maroney, Administrator

ST. JOSEPH MEMORIAL HOSPITAL (O, 59 beds) 800 North Second Street, Murphysboro, IL Zip 62966, Mailing Address: P.O. Box 580, Zip 62966-0580; tel. 618/684-3156; Virgil Hannig, President

Owned, leased, sponsored:	3 hospitals	274 beds
Contract-managed:	0 hospitals	0 beds
Totals:	3 hospitals	274 beds

★4195: **SPARTANBURG HOSPITAL SYSTEM** (NP)
101 East Wood Street, Spartanburg, SC Zip 29303-3016; tel. 803/560-6000; Joseph Michael Oddis, President

SOUTH CAROLINA: B.J. WORKMAN MEMORIAL HOSPITAL (O, 32 beds) 751 East Georgia Street, Woodruff, SC Zip 29388, Mailing Address: P.O. Box 699, Zip 29388-0699; tel. 803/476-8122; G. Curtis Walker R.N., Administrator

SPARTANBURG REGIONAL MEDICAL CENTER (O, 448 beds) 101 East Wood Street, Spartanburg, SC Zip 29303-3016; tel. 803/560-6000; Joseph Michael Oddis, President

Owned, leased, sponsored:	2 hospitals	480 beds
Contract-managed:	0 hospitals	0 beds
Totals:	2 hospitals	480 beds

★5455: **SSM HEALTH CARE SYSTEM** (CC)
477 North Lindbergh Boulevard, Saint Louis, MO Zip 63141-7813; tel. 314/994-7800; Sister Mary Jean Ryan, President and Chief Executive Officer

GEORGIA: ST. FRANCIS HOSPITAL (CM, 201 beds) Manchester Expressway & Woodruff Road, Columbus, GA Zip 31904-6878, Mailing Address: Box 7000, Zip 31908-7000; tel. 706/596-4000; Michael E. Garrigan, President

ILLINOIS: GOOD SAMARITAN REGIONAL HEALTH CENTER (O, 141 beds) 605 North 12th Street, Mount Vernon, IL Zip 62864; tel. 618/242-4600; Leo F. Childers, Jr. FACHE, President

ST. FRANCIS HOSPITAL AND HEALTH CENTER (O, 306 beds) 12935 South Gregory Street, Blue Island, IL Zip 60406-2470; tel. 708/597-2000; Jay E. Kreuzer, President

WASHINGTON COUNTY HOSPITAL (CM, 56 beds) 705 South Grand Street, Nashville, IL Zip 62263-1532; tel. 618/327-8236; Michael P. Ellermann, Administrator and Chief Executive Officer

MISSOURI: ARCADIA VALLEY HOSPITAL (O, 50 beds) Highway 21, Pilot Knob, MO Zip 63663, Mailing Address: P.O. Box 548, Zip 63663-0548; tel. 314/546-3924; H. Clark Duncan, Administrator

CARDINAL GLENNON CHILDREN'S HOSPITAL (L, 190 beds) 1465 South Grand Boulevard, Saint Louis, MO Zip 63104-1095; tel. 314/577-5600; Douglas A. Ries, President

PIKE COUNTY MEMORIAL HOSPITAL (CM, 25 beds) 2305 West Georgia Street, Louisiana, MO Zip 63353-0020; tel. 314/754-5531; Thomas E. Lefebvre, President

SSM REHABILITATION INSTITUTE (O, 100 beds) 555 North New Ballas Road, Suite 150, Saint Louis, MO Zip 63141-6827; tel. 314/994-0157; Carla S. Baum, President

ST. FRANCIS HOSPITAL (O, 55 beds) 2016 South Main Street, Maryville, MO Zip 64468-2693; tel. 816/562-2600; Ray Brazier, President

ST. JOSEPH HEALTH CENTER (O, 362 beds) 300 First Capitol Drive, Saint Charles, MO Zip 63301-2835; tel. 314/947-5000; Kevin F. Kast, President

ST. JOSEPH HOSPITAL (O, 240 beds) 525 Couch Avenue, Saint Louis, MO Zip 63122-5594; tel. 314/966-1500; Michael E. Zilm, President

ST. JOSEPH HOSPITAL WEST (O, 100 beds) 100 Medical Plaza, Lake Saint Louis, MO Zip 63367-1395; tel. 314/625-5200; Kevin F. Kast, President

ST. MARY'S HEALTH CENTER (O, 515 beds) 6420 Clayton Road, Saint Louis, MO Zip 63117-1811; tel. 314/768-8000; Ronald J. Levy, President

ST. MARYS HEALTH CENTER (O, 263 beds) 100 St Marys Medical Plaza, Jefferson City, MO Zip 65101; tel. 314/761-7151; John S. Dubis, President

OKLAHOMA: ST. ANTHONY HOSPITAL (O, 247 beds) 1000 North Lee Street, Oklahoma City, OK Zip 73102, Mailing Address: Box 205, Zip 73101-0205; tel. 405/272-7000; Steven L. Hunter, President

SOUTH CAROLINA: SAINT EUGENE COMMUNITY HOSPITAL (O, 85 beds) 301 East Jackson Street, Dillon, SC Zip 29536-2509; tel. 803/774-4111; Ronald W. Webb, President

WISCONSIN: ST. CLARE HOSPITAL AND HEALTH SERVICES (O, 78 beds) 707 14th Street, Baraboo, WI Zip 53913-1597; tel. 608/356-5561; Thomas R. Warwick, President

ST. MARYS HOSPITAL MEDICAL CENTER (O, 340 beds) 707 South Mills Street, Madison, WI Zip 53715-0450; tel. 608/251-6100; Gerald W. Lefert, President

Owned, leased, sponsored:	15 hospitals	3072 beds
Contract-managed:	3 hospitals	282 beds
Totals:	18 hospitals	3354 beds

★0003: **ST. DAVID'S HEALTH CARE SYSTEM** (NP)
919 East 32nd Street, Austin, TX Zip 78705, Mailing Address: P.O. Box 4039, Zip 78765; tel. 512/476-7111; Jack L. Campbell, President

TEXAS: ST. DAVID'S HEALTH CARE SYSTEM (O, 296 beds) 919 East 32nd Street, Austin, TX Zip 78705, Mailing Address: Box 4039, Zip 78765-4039; tel. 512/476-7111; Jack L. Campbell, President

ST. DAVID'S PAVILION (O, 38 beds) 1025 East 32nd Street, Austin, TX Zip 78765; tel. 512/867-5800; Deborah L. Ryle, Administrator

ST. DAVID'S REHABILITATION CENTER (O, 103 beds) 1005 East 32nd Street, Austin, TX Zip 78705, Mailing Address: P.O. Box 4270, Zip 78765-4270; tel. 512/867-5100; Deborah L. Ryle, Administrator

Owned, leased, sponsored:	3 hospitals	437 beds
Contract-managed:	0 hospitals	0 beds
Totals:	3 hospitals	437 beds

★2255: **ST. FRANCIS HEALTH SYSTEM** (NP)
4401 Penn Avenue, Pittsburgh, PA Zip 15224-1334; tel. 412/622-4212; Sister M. Rosita Wellinger, President

PENNSYLVANIA: ST. FRANCIS CENTRAL HOSPITAL (O, 143 beds) 1200 Centre Avenue, Pittsburgh, PA Zip 15219-3594; tel. 412/562-3000; Kenneth F. Sample, Chief Executive Officer

For explanation of codes following names, see page B2.
★Indicates Type III membership in the American Hospital Association.

ST. FRANCIS HOSPITAL OF NEW CASTLE (O, 193 beds) 1000 South Mercer Street, New Castle, PA Zip 16101–4673; tel. 412/658–3511; Sister Donna Zwigart, Chief Executive Officer

ST. FRANCIS MEDICAL CENTER (O, 965 beds) 400 45th Street, Pittsburgh, PA Zip 15201–1198; tel. 412/622–4343; Sister Florence Brandt, Chief Executive Officer

Owned, leased, sponsored:	3 hospitals	1301 beds
Contract–managed:	0 hospitals	0 beds
Totals:	3 hospitals	1301 beds

★5425: **ST. JOSEPH HEALTH SYSTEM** (CC)
440 South Batavia Street, Orange, CA Zip 92668–3995, Mailing Address: P.O. Box 14132, Zip 92613–1532; tel. 714/997–7690; Richard Statuto, Chief Executive Officer

CALIFORNIA: MISSION HOSPITAL REGIONAL MEDICAL CENTER (O, 202 beds) 27700 Medical Center Road, Mission Viejo, CA Zip 92691; tel. 714/364–1400; Reynold R. Welch, President

QUEEN OF THE VALLEY HOSPITAL (O, 176 beds) 1000 Trancas Street, Napa, CA Zip 94558, Mailing Address: Box 2340, Zip 94558; tel. 707/252–4411; Joseph A. Stewart, President and Chief Executive Officer

REDWOOD MEMORIAL HOSPITAL (O, 35 beds) 3300 Renner Drive, Fortuna, CA Zip 95540; tel. 707/725–3361; Paul J. Chodkowski, President and Chief Executive Officer

SANTA ROSA MEMORIAL HOSPITAL (O, 225 beds) 1165 Montgomery Drive, Santa Rosa, CA Zip 95405, Mailing Address: Box 522, Zip 95402; tel. 707/546–3210; James P. Houser, Regional President

ST. JOSEPH HOSPITAL (O, 65 beds) 2700 Dolbeer Street, Eureka, CA Zip 95501; tel. 707/445–8121; Paul J. Chodkowski, President and Chief Executive Officer

ST. JOSEPH HOSPITAL (O, 411 beds) 1100 West Stewart Drive, Orange, CA Zip 92668, Mailing Address: P.O. Box 5600, Zip 92613–5600; tel. 714/633–9111; Larry K. Ainsworth, Chief Executive Officer

ST. JUDE MEDICAL CENTER (O, 317 beds) 101 East Valencia Mesa Drive, Fullerton, CA Zip 92635; tel. 714/992–3000; Patty Maysent, President and Chief Executive Officer

ST. MARY DESERT VALLEY HOSPITAL (O, 109 beds) 18300 Highway 18, Apple Valley, CA Zip 92307–0725, Mailing Address: Box 7025, Zip 92307–0725; tel. 619/242–2311; Thomas G. Neff, President

TEXAS: CROSBYTON CLINIC HOSPITAL (CM, 35 beds) 710 West Main Street, Crosbyton, TX Zip 79322; tel. 806/675–2382; Michael Johnson, Administrator and Chief Executive Officer

D. M. COGDELL MEMORIAL HOSPITAL (CM, 72 beds) 1700 Cogdell Boulevard, Snyder, TX Zip 79549–6198; tel. 915/573–6374; Jeff Reecer, Chief Executive Officer

ST. MARY OF THE PLAINS HOSPITAL (O, 410 beds) 4000 24th Street, Lubbock, TX Zip 79410; tel. 806/796–6000; Charley O. Trimble, President and Chief Executive Officer

Owned, leased, sponsored:	9 hospitals	1950 beds
Contract–managed:	2 hospitals	107 beds
Totals:	11 hospitals	2057 beds

5845: **ST. LUKE'S HEALTH SYSTEM, INC.** (NP)
2720 Stone Park Boulevard, Sioux City, IA Zip 51104–2000; tel. 712/279–3500; David O. Biorn FACHE, President and Chief Executive Officer

IOWA: FLOYD VALLEY HOSPITAL (CM, 44 beds) Highway 3 East, Le Mars, IA Zip 51031, Mailing Address: P.O. Box 10, Zip 51031; tel. 712/546–7871; G. Frank Labonte, Chief Executive Officer

ORANGE CITY MUNICIPAL HOSPITAL (CM, 63 beds) 400 Central Avenue N.W., Orange City, IA Zip 51041–1398; tel. 712/737–4984; Martin W. Guthmiller, Administrator

ST. LUKE'S REGIONAL MEDICAL CENTER (O, 242 beds) 2720 Stone Park Boulevard, Sioux City, IA Zip 51104–2000; tel. 712/279–3500; David O. Biorn FACHE, President and Chief Executive Officer

Owned, leased, sponsored:	1 hospitals	242 beds
Contract–managed:	2 hospitals	107 beds
Totals:	3 hospitals	349 beds

3555: **STATE OF HAWAII, DEPARTMENT OF HEALTH** (NP)
1250 Punchbowl Street, Honolulu, HI Zip 96813; tel. 808/586–4416; Fred D. Horwitz, Deputy Director

HAWAII: HILO MEDICAL CENTER (O, 274 beds) 1190 Waianuenue Avenue, Hilo, HI Zip 96720–2095; tel. 808/969–4111; John H. Westerman, Administrator

HONOKAA HOSPITAL (O, 30 beds) Honokaa, HI, Mailing Address: P.O. Box 237, Zip 96727–0237; tel. 808/775–7211; Ivan S. Yamamoto, Administrator

KAU HOSPITAL (O, 15 beds) Pahala, HI, Mailing Address: P.O. Box 40, Zip 96777; tel. 808/928–8331; Dawn S. Pung, Administrator

KAUAI VETERANS MEMORIAL HOSPITAL (O, 49 beds) Waimea Canyon Road, Waimea, HI Zip 96796, Mailing Address: Box 337, Zip 96796–0337; tel. 808/338–9431; Orianna A. Skomoroch, Administrator

KOHALA HOSPITAL (O, 26 beds) Kohala, HI, Mailing Address: P.O. Box 10, Kapaau, Zip 96755–0010; tel. 808/889–6211; Manuel Anduha, Administrator

KONA COMMUNITY HOSPITAL (O, 71 beds) Kealakekua, HI, Mailing Address: P.O. Box 69, Zip 96750–0069; tel. 808/322–4429; David W. Patton, President

KULA HOSPITAL (O, 105 beds) 204 Kula Highway, Kula, HI Zip 96790–9499; tel. 808/878–1221; Shirley K. Takahashi R.N., Administrator

LANAI COMMUNITY HOSPITAL (O, 14 beds) 628 Seventh Street, Lanai City, HI Zip 96763–0797, Mailing Address: P.O. Box 797, Zip 96763–0797; tel. 808/565–6411; Herbert K. Yim, Administrator

LEAHI HOSPITAL (O, 192 beds) 3675 Kilauea Avenue, Honolulu, HI Zip 96816; tel. 808/733–8000; Fred D. Horwitz, Administrator

MAUI MEMORIAL HOSPITAL (O, 145 beds) 221 Mahalani Street, Wailuku, HI Zip 96793–2581; tel. 808/244–9056; Marian Hanlon M.D., Acting Administrator

SAMUEL MAHELONA MEMORIAL HOSPITAL (O, 82 beds) 4800 Kawaihau Road, Kapaa, HI Zip 96746–1998; tel. 808/822–4961; Neva M. Olson, Administrator

Owned, leased, sponsored:	11 hospitals	1003 beds
Contract–managed:	0 hospitals	0 beds
Totals:	11 hospitals	1003 beds

0044: **STERLING HEALTHCARE CORPORATION** (IO)
1500 114th Avenue S.E., Suite 100, Bellevue, WA Zip 98004; tel. 206/453–5445; David Jacobsen, President

ALASKA: NORTH STAR HOSPITAL AND COUNSELING CENTER (O, 34 beds) 1650 South Bragaw, Anchorage, AK Zip 99508–3467; tel. 907/277–1522; Bob Marshall, Administrator

IDAHO: PINE CREST HOSPITAL AND COUNSELING CENTER (O, 48 beds) 2301 North Ironwood Place, Coeur D'Alene, ID Zip 83814; tel. 208/666–1441; Ron Mays, Administrator

INDIANA: KOALA HOSPITAL AND COUNSELING CENTER (O, 80 beds) 1800 North Oak Road, Plymouth, IN Zip 46563; tel. 219/936–3784; Wayne T. Miller, Administrator

KOALA HOSPITAL AND COUNSELING CENTER (O, 60 beds) 2223 Poshard Drive, Columbus, IN Zip 47203; tel. 812/376–1711; Thomas N. Theroult, Administrator

OKLAHOMA: OAK CREST HOSPITAL (O, 50 beds) 1601 Gordon Cooper Drive, Shawnee, OK Zip 74801; tel. 405/275–9610; Rodger Hopkins, Administrator

WILLOW CREST HOSPITAL (O, 50 beds) 130 A Street S.W., Miami, OK Zip 74354; tel. 918/542–1836; Kenneth O'Rourke, Administrator and Chief Executive Officer

Owned, leased, sponsored:	6 hospitals	322 beds
Contract–managed:	0 hospitals	0 beds
Totals:	6 hospitals	322 beds

0805: **STORMONT–VAIL HEALTH SERVICES CORPORATION** (NP)
1500 Southwest Tenth Street, Topeka, KS Zip 66604–1353; tel. 913/354–6112; Howard M. Chase, President

KANSAS: DECHAIRO HOSPITAL (O, 13 beds) First and North Streets, Westmoreland, KS Zip 66549; tel. 913/457–3311; Donn Demaree, Administrator

For explanation of codes following names, see page B2.
★Indicates Type III membership in the American Hospital Association.

Systems / Stormont–Vail Health Services Corporation

HIAWATHA COMMUNITY HOSPITAL (CM, 29 beds) 300 Utah Street, Hiawatha, KS Zip 66434; tel. 913/742–2131; J. Michael Frost, Administrator

MEMORIAL HOSPITAL (CM, 81 beds) 1105 Sunset Avenue, Manhattan, KS Zip 66502, Mailing Address: Box 1208, Zip 66502; tel. 913/776–3300; E. Michael Nunamaker, Chief Executive Officer

STORMONT–VAIL REGIONAL MEDICAL CENTER (O, 313 beds) 1500 Southwest Tenth Street, Topeka, KS Zip 66604–1353; tel. 913/354–6000; Howard M. Chase, President and Chief Executive Officer

WAMEGO CITY HOSPITAL (CM, 18 beds) 711 Genn Drive, Wamego, KS Zip 66547; tel. 913/456–2295; Lisa J. Freeborn, Administrator

Owned, leased, sponsored:	2 hospitals	326 beds
Contract–managed:	3 hospitals	128 beds
Totals:	5 hospitals	454 beds

0905: SUMMIT MEDICAL MANAGEMENT, INC. (IO)
5 Concourse Parkway, Suite 800, Atlanta, GA Zip 30328–6111; tel. 404/392–1454; Ken Couch, Chief Executive Officer

ILLINOIS: LORETTO HOSPITAL (CM, 222 beds) 645 South Central Avenue, Chicago, IL Zip 60644–5088; tel. 312/626–4300; Dallas Keith Larson, President and Chief Executive Officer

INDIANA: NORTHWEST FAMILY HOSPITAL (O, 140 beds) 501 Family Plaza, Gary, IN Zip 46402; tel. 219/882–9411; Willie C. White III, President and Chief Executive Officer

LOUISIANA: SUMMIT INSTITUTE FOR PULMONARY MEDICINE AND REHABILITATION (O, 54 beds) 4900 Medical Drive, Bossier City, LA Zip 71112, Mailing Address: P.O. Box 8450, Zip 71112–8450; tel. 318/747–9500; Danny Edwards, Administrator

Owned, leased, sponsored:	2 hospitals	194 beds
Contract–managed:	1 hospitals	222 beds
Totals:	3 hospitals	416 beds

★0030: SUN HEALTH CORPORATION (NP)
13180 North 103rd Drive, Sun City, AZ Zip 85351, Mailing Address: P.O. Box 1278, Zip 85372–1278; tel. 602/876–5352; Leland W. Peterson, President and Chief Executive Officer

ARIZONA: DEL E. WEBB MEMORIAL HOSPITAL (O, 241 beds) 14502 West Meeker Boulevard, Sun City West, AZ Zip 85375, Mailing Address: P.O. Box 5169, Zip 85375; tel. 602/214–4000; Thomas C. Dickson, Chief Operating Officer and Executive Vice President

WALTER O. BOSWELL MEMORIAL HOSPITAL (O, 317 beds) 10401 W. Thunderbird Boulevard, Sun City, AZ Zip 85351, Mailing Address: Box 1690, Zip 85372; tel. 602/977–7211; George Perez, Executive Vice President and Chief Executive Officer

Owned, leased, sponsored:	2 hospitals	558 beds
Contract–managed:	0 hospitals	0 beds
Totals:	2 hospitals	558 beds

★0066: SUSQUEHANNA HEALTH SYSTEM (NP)
1001 Grampian Boulevard, Williamsport, PA Zip 17701–1946; tel. 717/320–7000; Donald R. Creamer, President and Chief Executive Officer

PENNSYLVANIA: DIVINE PROVIDENCE HOSPITAL (O, 194 beds) 1100 Grampian Boulevard, Williamsport, PA Zip 17701–1995; tel. 717/326–8181; Kirby O. Smith, President

MUNCY VALLEY HOSPITAL (O, 120 beds) 215 East Water Street, Muncy, PA Zip 17756–8700; tel. 717/546–8282; Diane M. Burfeindt, Assistant Administrator

WILLIAMSPORT HOSPITAL AND MEDICAL CENTER (O, 252 beds) 777 Rural Avenue, Williamsport, PA Zip 17701–3198; tel. 717/321–1000; Steven P. Johnson, Senior Vice President and Chief Operating Officer

Owned, leased, sponsored:	3 hospitals	566 beds
Contract–managed:	0 hospitals	0 beds
Totals:	3 hospitals	566 beds

8795: SUTTER HEALTH (NP)
2800 L Street, Sacramento, CA Zip 95816, Mailing Address: P.O. Box 160727, Zip 95816; tel. 916/733–8800; Van R. Johnson, President and Chief Executive Officer

CALIFORNIA: AUBURN FAITH COMMUNITY HOSPITAL (O, 106 beds) 11815 Education Street, Auburn, CA Zip 95604, Mailing Address: Box 8992, Zip 95604–8992; tel. 916/888–4518; Joel E. Grey, Administrator

DELTA MEMORIAL HOSPITAL (O, 111 beds) 3901 Lone Tree Way, Antioch, CA Zip 94509; tel. 510/779–7200; Linda Horn, Administrator

NOVATO COMMUNITY HOSPITAL (O, 52 beds) 1625 Hill Road, Novato, CA Zip 94947, Mailing Address: P.O. Box 1108, Zip 94948; tel. 415/897–3111; Lowell W. Smith, Administrator

PLUMAS DISTRICT HOSPITAL (O, 32 beds) 1065 Bucks Lake Road, Quincy, CA Zip 95971–9599; tel. 916/283–2121; R. Michael Barry, Administrator

ROSEVILLE HOSPITAL (O, 201 beds) 333 Sunrise Avenue, Roseville, CA Zip 95661–3477; tel. 916/781–1000; W. Jefferson Comer, Administrator

SUTTER AMADOR HOSPITAL (O, 85 beds) 810 Court Street, Jackson, CA Zip 95642–2379; tel. 209/223–7500; Scott Stenberg, Administrator

SUTTER CENTER FOR PSYCHIATRY (O, 69 beds) 7700 Folsom Boulevard, Sacramento, CA Zip 95826–2608; tel. 916/386–3000; Diane Gail Stewart, Administrator

SUTTER COAST HOSPITAL (L, 47 beds) 800 East Washington Boulevard, Crescent City, CA Zip 95531; tel. 707/464–8511; John E. Menaugh, Administrator

SUTTER DAVIS HOSPITAL (O, 48 beds) 2000 Sutter Place, Davis, CA Zip 95616, Mailing Address: P.O. Box 1617, Zip 95617; tel. 916/756–6440; Lawrence A. Maas, Administrator

SUTTER GENERAL HOSPITAL (O, 438 beds) 2801 L Street, Sacramento, CA Zip 95816; tel. 916/454–2222; Patrick E. Fry, Administrator

SUTTER LAKESIDE HOSPITAL (O, 50 beds) 5176 Hill Road East, Lakeport, CA Zip 95453–6112; tel. 707/262–5001; Paul J. Hensler, Administrator

SUTTER MEMORIAL HOSPITAL (O, 346 beds) 5151 F Street, Sacramento, CA Zip 95819–3295; tel. 916/454–3333; Patrick E. Fry, Chief Operating Officer

SUTTER SOLANO MEDICAL CENTER (O, 108 beds) 300 Hospital Drive, Vallejo, CA Zip 94589–2517, Mailing Address: P.O. Box 3189, Zip 94589; tel. 707/554–4444; Patrick R. Brady, Administrator

TRACY COMMUNITY MEMORIAL HOSPITAL (O, 79 beds) 1420 North Tracy Boulevard, Tracy, CA Zip 95376–3497; tel. 209/835–1500; Terry G. Mack, Vice President and Administrator

Owned, leased, sponsored:	14 hospitals	1772 beds
Contract–managed:	0 hospitals	0 beds
Totals:	14 hospitals	1772 beds

★0039: TARRANT COUNTY HOSPITAL DISTRICT (NP)
1500 South Main Street, Fort Worth, TX Zip 76104; tel. 817/927–1230; Marion Timothy Philpot, President and Chief Executive Officer

TEXAS: TARRANT COUNTY HOSPITAL DISTRICT (O, 360 beds) 1500 South Main Street, Fort Worth, TX Zip 76104–4941; tel. 817/921–3431; Marion Timothy Philpot, President and Chief Executive Officer

TRINITY SPRINGS PAVILION–EAST (O, 39 beds) 1500 South Main Street, Fort Worth, TX Zip 76104–4917; tel. 817/927–3636; Robert Bourassa, Executive Director

Owned, leased, sponsored:	2 hospitals	399 beds
Contract–managed:	0 hospitals	0 beds
Totals:	2 hospitals	399 beds

0063: TENET HEALTHCARE CORPORATION (IO)
2700 Colorado Avenue, Santa Monica, CA Zip 90404, Mailing Address: P.O. Box 4070, Zip 90404; tel. 310/998–8000; Jeffrey Barbakow, Chairman and Chief Executive Officer

ALABAMA: BROOKWOOD MEDICAL CENTER (O, 515 beds) 2010 Brookwood Medical Center Drive, Birmingham, AL Zip 35209; tel. 205/877–1000; Gregory H. Burfitt, Chief Executive Officer

ARKANSAS: CENTRAL ARKANSAS HOSPITAL (O, 149 beds) 1200 South Main, Searcy, AR Zip 72143; tel. 501/278–3131; David C. Laffoon, Executive Director

---

For explanation of codes following names, see page B2.
★Indicates Type III membership in the American Hospital Association.

Systems / Tenet Healthcare Corporation

NATIONAL PARK MEDICAL CENTER (O, 166 beds) 1910 Malvern Avenue, Hot Springs, AR Zip 71901; tel. 501/321-1000; Jerry D. Mabry, Executive Director

ST. MARY'S REGIONAL MEDICAL CENTER (O, 155 beds) 1808 West Main Street, Russellville, AR Zip 72801; tel. 501/968-2841; William L. Bradley, Executive Director

CALIFORNIA: ALVARADO HOSPITAL MEDICAL CENTER (O, 231 beds) 6655 Alvarado Road, San Diego, CA Zip 92120-5298; tel. 619/229-3100; Barry G. Weinbaum, Executive Director

CENTURY CITY HOSPITAL (L, 135 beds) 2070 Century Park East, Los Angeles, CA Zip 90067; tel. 310/553-6211; Kenneth Berg, Chief Executive Officer

COMMUNITY HOSPITAL AND REHABILITATION CENTER OF LOS GATOS-SARATOGA (L, 209 beds) 815 Pollard Road, Los Gatos, CA Zip 95030; tel. 408/378-6131; Truman L. Gates, Chief Executive Officer

DOCTORS HOSPITAL OF MANTECA (O, 73 beds) 1205 East North Street, Manteca, CA Zip 95336, Mailing Address: Box 191, Zip 95336; tel. 209/823-3111; Richard H. Robinson, Administrator

DOCTORS HOSPITAL OF PINOLE (L, 137 beds) 2151 Appian Way, Pinole, CA Zip 94564; tel. 510/724-5000; Gary Sloan, Chief Executive Officer

DOCTORS MEDICAL CENTER (O, 364 beds) 1441 Florida Avenue, Modesto, CA Zip 95350-4418, Mailing Address: P.O. Box 4138, Zip 95352-4138; tel. 209/578-1211; Chris DiCicco, Chief Executive Officer

ENCINO-TARZANA REGIONAL MEDICAL CENTER (O, 391 beds) 18321 Clark Street, Tarzana, CA Zip 91356; tel. 818/881-0800; William H. Comte, Chief Executive Officer

GARDEN GROVE HOSPITAL AND MEDICAL CENTER (O, 167 beds) 12601 Garden Grove Boulevard, Garden Grove, CA Zip 92643-1959; tel. 714/741-2700; Timothy Smith, Executive Director

GARFIELD MEDICAL CENTER (O, 223 beds) 525 North Garfield Avenue, Monterey Park, CA Zip 91754; tel. 818/573-2222; Arnold R. Schaffer, Chief Executive Officer

IRVINE MEDICAL CENTER (O, 176 beds) 16200 Sand Canyon Avenue, Irvine, CA Zip 92718-3701; tel. 714/753-2000; Robert C. Shaw, Executive Director

LAKEWOOD REGIONAL MEDICAL CENTER (O, 175 beds) 3700 East South Street, Lakewood, CA Zip 90712; tel. 310/531-2550; Gustavo A. Valdespino, Chief Executive Officer

LOS ALAMITOS MEDICAL CENTER (O, 173 beds) 3751 Katella Avenue, Los Alamitos, CA Zip 90720; tel. 310/598-1311; Gustavo A. Valdespino, Executive Director

MEDICAL CENTER OF NORTH HOLLYWOOD (O, 163 beds) 12629 Riverside Drive, North Hollywood, CA Zip 91607-3495; tel. 818/980-9200; Dale Surowitz, Chief Executive Officer

PLACENTIA-LINDA COMMUNITY HOSPITAL (O, 114 beds) 1301 Rose Drive, Placentia, CA Zip 92670; tel. 714/993-2000; Michael A. Kelly, Chief Executive Officer

SAN DIMAS COMMUNITY HOSPITAL (O, 99 beds) 1350 West Covina Boulevard, San Dimas, CA Zip 91773-0308; tel. 909/599-6811; Larry Peterson, Chief Executive Officer

SOUTH BAY MEDICAL CENTER (O, 201 beds) 514 North Prospect Avenue, Redondo Beach, CA Zip 90277; tel. 310/376-9474; Jerald R. Happel, Administrator

TENET SIERRA VISTA REGIONAL MEDICAL CENTER (O, 178 beds) 1010 Murray Street, San Luis Obispo, CA Zip 93405, Mailing Address: Box 1367, Zip 93406-1367; tel. 805/546-7600; Philip R. Wolfe, Executive Director

TWIN CITIES COMMUNITY HOSPITAL (O, 84 beds) 1100 Las Tablas Road, Templeton, CA Zip 93465; tel. 805/434-3500; Harold E. Chilton, Chief Executive Officer

FLORIDA: DELRAY COMMUNITY HOSPITAL (O, 211 beds) 5352 Linton Boulevard, Delray Beach, FL Zip 33484; tel. 407/498-4440

HOLLYWOOD MEDICAL CENTER (O, 334 beds) 3600 Washington Street, Hollywood, FL Zip 33021; tel. 305/966-4500; Holly L. Lerner, Chief Executive Officer

MEMORIAL HOSPITAL OF TAMPA (O, 174 beds) 2901 Swann Avenue, Tampa, FL Zip 33609-4057; tel. 813/873-6400; Keith Henthorne, President

NORTH RIDGE MEDICAL CENTER (O, 280 beds) 5757 North Dixie Highway, Fort Lauderdale, FL Zip 33334; tel. 305/776-6000; Don S. Steigman, Executive Director

PALM BEACH GARDENS MEDICAL CENTER (O, 189 beds) 3360 Burns Road, Palm Beach Gardens, FL Zip 33410-4304; tel. 407/622-1411; Thomas G. Hennessy, Chief Executive Officer

PALMETTO GENERAL HOSPITAL (O, 360 beds) 2001 West 68th Street, Hialeah, FL Zip 33016; tel. 305/823-5000

PALMS OF PASADENA HOSPITAL (O, 276 beds) 1501 Pasadena Avenue South, Saint Petersburg, FL Zip 33707; tel. 813/381-1000; Daniel J. Bonk, Interim Chief Executive Officer

SEVEN RIVERS COMMUNITY HOSPITAL (O, 128 beds) 6201 North Suncoast Boulevard, Crystal River, FL Zip 34428; tel. 904/795-6560; Frank T. Beirne, Chief Executive Officer

TOWN AND COUNTRY HOSPITAL (O, 148 beds) 6001 Webb Road, Tampa, FL Zip 33615-3291; tel. 813/885-6666; Keith Henthorne, Executive Director

WEST BOCA MEDICAL CENTER (O, 185 beds) 21644 State Road 7, Boca Raton, FL Zip 33428-1899; tel. 407/488-8000; Richard S. Freeman, Chief Executive Officer

GEORGIA: NORTH FULTON REGIONAL HOSPITAL (O, 168 beds) 3000 Hospital Boulevard, Roswell, GA Zip 30076-9930; tel. 404/751-2500; Frederick R. Bailey, Chief Executive Officer

SPALDING REGIONAL HOSPITAL (O, 162 beds) South Eighth Street, Griffin, GA Zip 30223, Mailing Address: P.O. Drawer V, Zip 30224-1168; tel. 404/228-2721; Phil Shaw, Executive Director

INDIANA: CULVER UNION HOSPITAL (O, 101 beds) 1710 Lafayette Road, Crawfordsville, IN Zip 47933; tel. 317/362-2800; Michael Collins, Executive Director

LOUISIANA: DOCTORS HOSPITAL OF JEFFERSON (L, 114 beds) 4320 Houma Boulevard, Metairie, LA Zip 70006-2973; tel. 504/456-5800; Michael D. Snow, Chief Executive Officer

JO ELLEN SMITH MEDICAL CENTER (O, 186 beds) 4444 General Meyer Avenue, New Orleans, LA Zip 70131; tel. 504/363-7011; Stan Morton, Administrator and Chief Executive Officer

KENNER REGIONAL MEDICAL CENTER (O, 124 beds) 180 West Esplanade Avenue, Kenner, LA Zip 70065; tel. 504/468-8600; Steven J. Greene, Administrator

MEADOWCREST HOSPITAL (O, 161 beds) 2500 Belle Chase Highway, Gretna, LA Zip 70056; tel. 504/392-3131; Jaime A. Wesolowski, Chief Executive Officer

NORTHSHORE REGIONAL MEDICAL CENTER (L, 147 beds) 100 Medical Center Drive, Slidell, LA Zip 70461-8572; tel. 504/649-7070; Nicholas J. Marzocco, Executive Director

ST. CHARLES GENERAL HOSPITAL (O, 173 beds) 3700 St. Charles Avenue, New Orleans, LA Zip 70115; tel. 504/899-7441; Lynn C. Orfgen, Chief Executive Officer

MISSOURI: COLUMBIA REGIONAL HOSPITAL (O, 274 beds) 404 Keene Street, Columbia, MO Zip 65201; tel. 314/875-9000; Richard A. Royer, Chief Executive Officer

KIRKSVILLE OSTEOPATHIC MEDICAL CENTER (L, 238 beds) 800 West Jefferson Street, Kirksville, MO Zip 63501-1497; tel. 816/626-2121; Herbert F. Dorsett, Chief Executive Officer

LUCY LEE HOSPITAL (O, 189 beds) 2620 North Westwood Boulevard, Poplar Bluff, MO Zip 63901-2341; tel. 314/785-7721; David L. Archer, Chief Executive Officer

LUTHERAN MEDICAL CENTER (O, 294 beds) 2639 Miami Street, Saint Louis, MO Zip 63118-3999; tel. 314/772-1456; William T. Moore, Chief Executive Officer

NEBRASKA: SAINT JOSEPH HOSPITAL (O, 299 beds) 601 North 30th Street, Omaha, NE Zip 68131-2197; tel. 402/449-5021; Matthew A. Kurs, President and Chief Executive Officer

NORTH CAROLINA: CENTRAL CAROLINA HOSPITAL (O, 137 beds) 1135 Carthage Street, Sanford, NC Zip 27330; tel. 919/774-2100; James E. Lathren, Executive Director

FRYE REGIONAL MEDICAL CENTER (O, 314 beds) 420 North Center Street, Hickory, NC Zip 28601; tel. 704/322-6070; Dennis Phillips, Chief Executive Officer

SOUTH CAROLINA: EAST COOPER COMMUNITY HOSPITAL (O, 100 beds) 1200 Johnnie Dodds Boulevard, Mount Pleasant, SC Zip 29464; tel. 803/881-0100; John Holland, Executive Director

HILTON HEAD HOSPITAL (O, 68 beds) Hilton Head Island, SC, Mailing Address: P.O. Box 21117, Zip 29925-1117; tel. 803/681-6122; Dennis Ray Bruns, President and Chief Executive Officer

PIEDMONT MEDICAL CENTER (O, 276 beds) 222 Herlong Avenue, Rock Hill, SC Zip 29732; tel. 803/329-1234; Paul A. Walker, President

TENNESSEE: HARTON REGIONAL MEDICAL CENTER (O, 137 beds) 1801 North Jackson Street, Tullahoma, TN Zip 37388, Mailing Address: P.O. Box 460, Zip 37388; tel. 615/393-3000; Brian T. Flynn, Administrator and Chief Executive Officer

For explanation of codes following names, see page B2.
★Indicates Type III membership in the American Hospital Association.

Systems / Tenet Healthcare Corporation

ST. FRANCIS HOSPITAL (O, 609 beds) 5959 Park Avenue, Memphis, TN Zip 38119-5198, Mailing Address: P.O. Box 171808, Zip 38187-1808; tel. 901/765-1000; Jake Henry, Jr., President

UNIVERSITY MEDICAL CENTER (O, 260 beds) 1411 Baddour Parkway, Lebanon, TN Zip 37087; tel. 615/444-8262; Larry W. Keller, Chief Executive Officer

TEXAS: BROWNSVILLE MEDICAL CENTER (O, 168 beds) 1040 West Jefferson Street, Brownsville, TX Zip 78520-5829, Mailing Address: Box 3590, Zip 78523-3590; tel. 210/544-1400; Robert Collette, Executive Director

DOCTORS HOSPITAL OF DALLAS (O, 231 beds) 9440 Poppy Drive, Dallas, TX Zip 75218; tel. 214/324-6100; C. E. Ward, Administrator

MID-JEFFERSON HOSPITAL (O, 138 beds) Highway 365 and 27th Street, Nederland, TX Zip 77627, Mailing Address: P.O. Box 1917, Zip 77627-1917; tel. 409/727-2321; Luis G. Silva, Chief Executive Officer

NACOGDOCHES MEDICAL CENTER (O, 142 beds) 4920 Northeast Stallings, Nacogdoches, TX Zip 75961, Mailing Address: Box 631604, Zip 75963-1604; tel. 409/569-9481; Bryant H. Krenek, Jr., Director

ODESSA REGIONAL HOSPITAL (O, 100 beds) 520 East Sixth Street, Odessa, TX Zip 79761, Mailing Address: Box 4859, Zip 79760; tel. 915/334-8200; Lex A. Guinn, Chief Executive Officer

PARK PLACE MEDICAL CENTER (O, 233 beds) 3050 39th Street, Port Arthur, TX Zip 77642, Mailing Address: Box 1648, Zip 77641; tel. 409/983-4951; Luis G. Silva, Chief Executive Officer

RHD MEMORIAL MEDICAL CENTER (O, 136 beds) Seven Medical Parkway, Dallas, TX Zip 75234, Mailing Address: P.O. Box 819094, Zip 75381-9094; tel. 214/247-1000; James R. Shafer, Executive Director

SIERRA MEDICAL CENTER (O, 365 beds) 1625 Medical Center Drive, El Paso, TX Zip 79902-5044; tel. 915/747-4000; L. Marcus Fry, Jr., Chief Executive Officer

TENET PARK PLAZA HOSPITAL (O, 382 beds) 1313 Hermann Drive, Houston, TX Zip 77004; tel. 713/527-5000; Judith Novak, President and Chief Executive Officer

TRINITY MEDICAL CENTER (L, 125 beds) 4343 North Josey Lane, Carrollton, TX Zip 75010; tel. 214/492-1010; Thomas E. Casaday, Chief Executive Officer

TWELVE OAKS HOSPITAL (O, 336 beds) 4200 Portsmouth Street, Houston, TX Zip 77027; tel. 713/623-2500; Walter J. Ornsteen, Executive Director

Owned, leased, sponsored:	65 hospitals	13450 beds
Contract-managed:	0 hospitals	0 beds
Totals:	65 hospitals	13450 beds

0020: TEXAS DEPARTMENT OF HEALTH (NP)
1100 West 49th Street, Austin, TX Zip 78756; tel. 512/458-7111; David R. Smith M.D., Commissioner

TEXAS: SOUTH TEXAS HOSPITAL (O, 85 beds) 1301 Rangerville Road, Harlingen, TX 78552-7609, Mailing Address: P.O. Box 592, Zip 78551-0592; tel. 210/423-3420; James N. Elkins FACHE, Director

TEXAS CENTER FOR INFECTIOUS DESEASE (O, 129 beds) 2303 Southeast Military Drive, San Antonio, TX Zip 78223-2334, Mailing Address: Box 23340, Zip 78223-2334; tel. 210/534-8857; Hugh N. Keel, Chief Administrative Officer

Owned, leased, sponsored:	2 hospitals	214 beds
Contract-managed:	0 hospitals	0 beds
Totals:	2 hospitals	214 beds

★2205: TIDEWATER HEALTH CARE, INC. (NP)
1080 First Colonial Road, Virginia Beach, VA Zip 23454-3001; tel. 804/496-6200; Douglas L. Johnson Ph.D., President and Chief Executive Officer

VIRGINIA: PORTSMOUTH GENERAL HOSPITAL (O, 184 beds) 850 Crawford Parkway, Portsmouth, VA Zip 23704-2386; tel. 804/398-4000; Carl F. Medley, Jr., Administrator

VIRGINIA BEACH GENERAL HOSPITAL (O, 274 beds) 1060 First Colonial Road, Virginia Beach, VA Zip 23454-9000; tel. 804/481-8000; Robert L. Graves, Administrator

Owned, leased, sponsored:	2 hospitals	458 beds
Contract-managed:	0 hospitals	0 beds
Totals:	2 hospitals	458 beds

★9255: TRUMAN MEDICAL CENTER (NP)
2301 Holmes Street, Kansas City, MO Zip 64108-2677; tel. 816/556-3153; James J. Mongan M.D., Director

MISSOURI: TRUMAN MEDICAL CENTER-EAST (CM, 300 beds) 7900 Lee's Summit Road, Kansas City, MO Zip 64139-1241; tel. 816/373-4415; Ross P. Marine, Administrator and Chief Executive Officer

TRUMAN MEDICAL CENTER-WEST (CM, 225 beds) 2301 Holmes Street, Kansas City, MO Zip 64108; tel. 816/556-3000; Rosa L. Miller R.N., Administrator

Owned, leased, sponsored:	0 hospitals	0 beds
Contract-managed:	2 hospitals	525 beds
Totals:	2 hospitals	525 beds

★9095: U.S. HEALTH CORPORATION (NP)
3555 Olentangy River Rd, 4000, Columbus, OH Zip 43214; tel. 614/566-5424; Erie Chapman, President and Chief Executive Officer

OHIO: BUCYRUS COMMUNITY HOSPITAL (CM, 55 beds) 629 North Sandusky Avenue, Bucyrus, OH Zip 44820-0627, Mailing Address: Box 627, Zip 44820-0627; tel. 419/562-4677; V. Richard Stelzer, Administrator and Chief Executive Officer

GALION COMMUNITY HOSPITAL (CM, 120 beds) Portland Way South, Galion, OH Zip 44833; tel. 419/468-4841; Mark E. Marley, Chief Executive Officer

GRANT MEDICAL CENTER (O, 439 beds) 111 South Grant Avenue, Columbus, OH Zip 43215-1898; tel. 614/461-3232; David Paul Blom, President and Chief Executive Officer

HARDIN MEMORIAL HOSPITAL (O, 51 beds) 921 East Franklin Street, Kenton, OH Zip 43326-2099, Mailing Address: P.O. Box 710, Zip 43326-0710; tel. 419/673-0761; Don J. Sabol, Administrator

MARION GENERAL HOSPITAL (O, 151 beds) McKinley Park Drive, Marion, OH Zip 43302-6397; tel. 614/383-8400; Frank V. Swinehart, President and Chief Executive Officer

MORROW COUNTY HOSPITAL (CM, 56 beds) 651 West Marion Road, Mount Gilead, OH Zip 43338; tel. 419/946-5015; Alan C. Pauley, Administrator

RIVERSIDE METHODIST HOSPITALS (O, 884 beds) 3535 Olentangy River Road, Columbus, OH Zip 43214; tel. 614/566-5000; Nancy M. Schlichting, President and Chief Executive Officer

SOUTHERN OHIO MEDICAL CENTER (O, 281 beds) 1805 27th Street, Portsmouth, OH Zip 45662-2654; tel. 614/354-5000; Randal M. Arnett, President and Chief Executive Officer

Owned, leased, sponsored:	5 hospitals	1806 beds
Contract-managed:	3 hospitals	231 beds
Totals:	8 hospitals	2037 beds

9195: U.S. PUBLIC HEALTH SERVICE INDIAN HEALTH SERVICE (FG)
2275 Research Boulevard, Rockville, MD Zip 20850

ALASKA: KANAKANAK HOSPITAL (O, 16 beds) Dillingham, AK, Mailing Address: P.O. Box 130, Zip 99576; tel. 907/842-5201; Darrel C. Richardson, Administrator

MANIILAQ HEALTH CENTER (O, 25 beds) Kotzebue, AK Zip 99752-0043; tel. 907/442-3321; Jan Harris, Administrator

NORTON SOUND REGIONAL HOSPITAL (O, 34 beds) Bering Street, Nome, AK Zip 99762, Mailing Address: Box 966, Zip 99762; tel. 907/443-3311; Gail Atchnson, Administrator

SEARHC MOUNTAIN EDGECUMBE HOSPITAL (O, 72 beds) 222 Tongass Drive, Sitka, AK Zip 99835-9416; tel. 907/966-2411; Arthur C. Willman, Vice President Operations

U.S. PUBLIC HEALTH SERVICE ALASKA NATIVE HOSPITAL (O, 15 beds) Barrow, AK Zip 99723; tel. 907/852-4611

U.S. PUBLIC HEALTH SERVICE ALASKA NATIVE MEDICAL CENTER (O, 146 beds) 255 Gambell Street, Anchorage, AK Zip 99501, Mailing Address: P.O. Box 107741, Zip 99510; tel. 907/279-6661; Frank H. Williams, Executive Officer

YUKON-KUSKOKWIM DELTA REGIONAL HOSPITAL (O, 50 beds) P.O. Box 528, Bethel, AK Zip 99559-3000; tel. 907/543-2220; Edwin L. Hansen, Administrator

ARIZONA: CHINLE COMPREHENSIVE HEALTH CARE FACILITY (O, 60 beds) Highway 191, Chinle, AZ Zip 86503, Mailing Address: P.O. Drawer PH, Zip 86503; tel. 602/674-5281; Ronald Tso, Chief Executive Officer

---

For explanation of codes following names, see page B2.
★Indicates Type III membership in the American Hospital Association.

Systems / Unihealth

HUHUKAM MEMORIAL HOSPITAL (O, 20 beds) Seed Farm Road, Sacaton, AZ Zip 85247–0038, Mailing Address: P.O. Box 38, Zip 85247; tel. 602/562–3321; Viola Johnson, Service Unit Director

TUBA CITY INDIAN MEDICAL CENTER (O, 85 beds) Main Street, Tuba City, AZ Zip 86045–6211, Mailing Address: P.O. Box 600, Zip 86045–6211; tel. 602/283–7201; Rosalyn Curtis, Chief Executive Officer

U.S. PUBLIC HEALTH SERVICE FORT DEFIANCE INDIAN HEALTH SERVICE HOSPITAL (O, 49 beds) Fort Defiance, AZ, Mailing Address: P.O. Box 649, Zip 86504; tel. 602/729–3223; Franklin Freeland Ph.D., Ed.D., Chief Executive Officer

U.S. PUBLIC HEALTH SERVICE INDIAN HOSPITAL (O, 20 beds) Parker, AZ, Mailing Address: Route 1, Box 12, Zip 85344; tel. 602/669–2137

U.S. PUBLIC HEALTH SERVICE INDIAN HOSPITAL (O, 36 beds) Sells, AZ, Mailing Address: P.O. Box 548, Zip 85634; tel. 602/383–7251; Darrell Rumley, Director

U.S. PUBLIC HEALTH SERVICE INDIAN HOSPITAL (O, 45 beds) State Route 73, Box 860, Whiteriver, AZ Zip 85941–0860; tel. 520/338–4911; Carla Alchesay-Nachu, Service Unit Director

U.S. PUBLIC HEALTH SERVICE PHOENIX INDIAN MEDICAL CENTER (O, 147 beds) 4212 North 16th Street, Phoenix, AZ Zip 85016–5389; tel. 602/263–1200; Anna Albert, Chief Executive Officer

U.S. PUBLIC HEALTH SERVICES INDIAN HOSPITAL (O, 26 beds) Keams Canyon, AZ, Mailing Address: P.O. Box 98, Zip 86034; tel. 602/738–2211; Taylor Satala, Service Unit Director

CALIFORNIA: U.S. PUBLIC HEALTH SERVICE INDIAN HOSPITAL (O, 17 beds) Winterhaven, CA, Mailing Address: P.O. Box 1368, Yuma, AZ Zip 85366–8368; tel. 619/572–0217; Kenneth W. Hernasy M.P.H., Service Unit Director

MARYLAND: CLINICAL CENTER, NATIONAL INSTITUTES OF HEALTH (O, 385 beds) 9000 Rockville Pike, Bethesda, MD Zip 20892–1504; tel. 301/496–4114; John I. Gallin M.D., Director

MINNESOTA: U.S. PUBLIC HEALTH SERVICE INDIAN HOSPITAL (O, 13 beds) 7th Street & Grant Utley Avenue N.W., Cass Lake, MN Zip 56633; tel. 218/335–2293; Luella Brown, Service Unit Director

U.S. PUBLIC HEALTH SERVICE INDIAN HOSPITAL (O, 23 beds) Redlake, MN Zip 56671; tel. 218/679–3912; Essimae Stevens, Service Unit Director

MISSISSIPPI: CHOCTAW HEALTH CENTER (O, 35 beds) Hospital Street, Philadelphia, MS Zip 39350, Mailing Address: Route 7, Box R–50, Zip 39350; tel. 601/656–2211; Jim Wallace, Executive Director

MONTANA: U.S. PUBLIC HEALTH SERVICE INDIAN HOSPITAL (O, 25 beds) Browning, MT, Mailing Address: P.O. Box 7, Zip 59417–0760; tel. 406/338–6100; Mary Ellen Lafromboise, Unit Director

U.S. PUBLIC HEALTH SERVICE INDIAN HOSPITAL (O, 34 beds) Crow Agency, MT, Mailing Address: Box 9, Zip 59022; tel. 406/638–2626; Tennyson Doney, Service Unit Director

U.S. PUBLIC HEALTH SERVICE INDIAN HOSPITAL (O, 12 beds) Rural Route 1, Box 67, Harlem, MT Zip 59526; tel. 406/353–2651; Charles D. Plumage, Director

NEBRASKA: U.S. PUBLIC HEALTH SERVICE INDIAN HOSPITAL (O, 30 beds) Winnebago, NE Zip 68071; tel. 402/878–2231; Wehnona St. Cyr, Service Unit Director

NEVADA: U.S. PUBLIC HEALTH SERVICE OWYHEE COMMUNITY HEALTH FACILITY (O, 15 beds) Owyhee, NV, Mailing Address: P.O. Box 130, Zip 89832–0130; tel. 702/757–2415; Kay C. Jewett, Acting Service Unit Director

NEW MEXICO: ACOMA–CANONCITO–LAGUNA HOSPITAL (O, 25 beds) San Fidel, NM, Mailing Address: P.O. Box 130, Zip 87049; tel. 505/552–6634; Richard L. Zephier Ph.D., Service Unit Director

GALLUP INDIAN MEDICAL CENTER (O, 107 beds) 516 East Nizhoni Boulevard, Gallup, NM Zip 87301–1334, Mailing Address: Box 1337, Zip 87301–1344; tel. 505/722–1000; Timothy G. Fleming M.D., Chief Executive Officer

PHS SANTA FE INDIAN HOSPITAL (O, 39 beds) 1700 Cerrillos Road, Santa Fe, NM Zip 87505; tel. 505/988–9821; Lawrence A. Jordan, Director

PUBLIC HEALTH SERVICE INDIAN HOSPITAL (O, 28 beds) 801 Vassar Drive N.E., Albuquerque, NM Zip 87106–2799; tel. 505/256–4000; Raymond L. Rodgers, Administrator

SHIPROCK INDIAN HOSPITAL (O, 50 beds) Shiprock, NM, Mailing Address: Box 160, Zip 87420; tel. 505/368–4971; Dee Hutchison, Chief Executive Officer

U.S. PUBLIC HEALTH SERVICE INDIAN HOSPITAL (O, 37 beds) Zuni, NM, Mailing Address: P.O. Box 467, Zip 87327; tel. 505/782–4431; Jean Othole, Service Unit Director

U.S. PUBLIC HEALTH SERVICE INDIAN HOSPITAL (O, 13 beds) Mescalero, NM, Mailing Address: Box 210, Zip 88340–0210; tel. 505/671–4441; Joe Wahnee, Jr., Service Unit Director

U.S. PUBLIC HEALTH SERVICE INDIAN HOSPITAL (O, 32 beds) Crownpoint, NM, Mailing Address: Box 358, Zip 87313–0358; tel. 505/786–5291; Anita Muneta, Chief Executive Officer

NORTH CAROLINA: U.S. PUBLIC HEALTH SERVICE INDIAN HOSPITAL (O, 30 beds) Hospital Road, Cherokee, NC Zip 28719; tel. 704/497–9163; G. E. Graning M.D., Administrator

NORTH DAKOTA: U.S. PUBLIC HEALTH SERVICE INDIAN HOSPITAL (O, 42 beds) Belcourt, ND, Mailing Address: P.O. Box 130, Zip 58316–0130; tel. 701/477–6111; Clarence Frederick, Director

U.S. PUBLIC HEALTH SERVICE INDIAN HOSPITAL (O, 16 beds) Fort Yates, ND, Mailing Address: P.O. Box J, Zip 58538; tel. 701/854–3831; Terry Pourier, Service Unit Director

OKLAHOMA: CARL ALBERT INDIAN HEALTH FACILITY (O, 53 beds) 1001 North Country Club Road, Ada, OK Zip 74820–2847; tel. 405/436–3980; Catherine E. Hanley FACHE, Director, Chickasaw Nation Health System

CHOCTAW NATION INDIAN HOSPITAL (O, 52 beds) Route 2, Box 1725, Talihina, OK Zip 74571; tel. 918/567–2211; Bat Shunatona, Administrator

U.S. PUBLIC HEALTH SERVICE COMPREHENSIVE INDIAN HEALTH FACILITY (O, 50 beds) 101 South Moore Avenue, Claremore, OK Zip 74017–5091; tel. 918/341–8430; John Daugherty, Jr., Service Unit Director

U.S. PUBLIC HEALTH SERVICE INDIAN HOSPITAL (O, 11 beds) Clinton, OK, Mailing Address: P.O. Box 279, Zip 73601; tel. 405/323–2884; Thedis V. Mitchell, Director

U.S. PUBLIC HEALTH SERVICE INDIAN HOSPITAL (O, 42 beds) 1515 Lawrie Tatum Road, Lawton, OK Zip 73507; tel. 405/353–0350; George F. Howell, Chief Executive Officer

WILLIAM W. HASTINGS INDIAN HOSPITAL (O, 60 beds) 100 South Bliss Avenue, Tahlequah, OK Zip 74464–3399; tel. 918/458–3100; John A. Boren, Acting Administrator

SOUTH DAKOTA: INDIAN HEALTH SERVICE–SIOUX SAN HOSPITAL (O, 32 beds) 3200 Canyon Lake Drive, Rapid City, SD Zip 57702; tel. 605/355–2280; James Cournoyer, Director

U.S. PUBLIC HEALTH SERVICE INDIAN HOSPITAL (O, 27 beds) Eagle Butte, SD, Mailing Address: P.O. Box 1012, Zip 57625–1012; tel. 605/964–7030; Terry Pourier, Administrator

U.S. PUBLIC HEALTH SERVICE INDIAN HOSPITAL (O, 46 beds) Pine Ridge, SD 57770–1201; tel. 605/867–5131; George E. Howell, Unit Director

U.S. PUBLIC HEALTH SERVICE INDIAN HOSPITAL (O, 35 beds) Rosebud, SD Zip 57570; tel. 605/747–2231; Gayla J. Twiss, Service Unit Director

U.S. PUBLIC HEALTH SERVICE INDIAN HOSPITAL (O, 18 beds) Chestnut Street, Sisseton, SD Zip 57262, Mailing Address: P.O. Box 189, Zip 57262; tel. 605/698–7606; Richard Huff, Administrator

Owned, leased, sponsored:	48 hospitals	2280 beds
Contract–managed:	0 hospitals	0 beds
Totals:	48 hospitals	2280 beds

★**2315: UNIHEALTH** (NP)
3400 Riverside Drive, Burbank, CA Zip 91505; tel. 818/238–6000; Terry Hartshorn, President and Chief Executive Officer

CALIFORNIA: CALIFORNIA HOSPITAL MEDICAL CENTER (O, 279 beds) 1401 South Grand Avenue, Los Angeles, CA Zip 90015; tel. 213/748–2411; James T. Yoshioka, President and Chief Executive Officer

GLENDALE MEMORIAL HOSPITAL AND HEALTH CENTER (O, 273 beds) 1420 South Central Avenue, Glendale, CA Zip 91204; tel. 818/502–1900; Roger E. Seaver, President and Chief Executive Officer

LA PALMA INTERCOMMUNITY HOSPITAL (O, 139 beds) 7901 Walker Street, La Palma, CA Zip 90623–5850, Mailing Address: P.O. Box 5850, Buena Park, Zip 90622; tel. 714/670–7400; Stephen Dixon, President and Chief Executive Officer

LINDSAY HOSPITAL MEDICAL CENTER (O, 106 beds) 740 North Sequoia Avenue, Lindsay, CA Zip 93247, Mailing Address: Box 40, Zip 93247; tel. 209/562–4955; Frank F. Jordan, President and Chief Executive Officer

LONG BEACH COMMUNITY HOSPITAL AND MEDICAL CENTER (O, 302 beds) 1720 Termino Avenue, Long Beach, CA Zip 90804; tel. 310/498–1000; Janet Parodi, President and Chief Executive Officer

MARTIN LUTHER HOSPITAL– ANEHEIM (O, 200 beds) 1830 West Romneya Drive, Anaheim, CA Zip 92801–1854, Mailing Address: Box 3304, Zip 92803–3304; tel. 714/491–5200; John R. Cochran III, President and Chief Executive Officer

For explanation of codes following names, see page B2.
★Indicates Type III membership in the American Hospital Association.

Systems / Unihealth

NORTHRIDGE HOSPITAL MEDICAL CENTER (O, 385 beds) 18300 Roscoe Boulevard, Northridge, CA Zip 91328; tel. 818/885–8500; Jeffery E. Flocken, President and Chief Executive Officer

SAN GABRIEL VALLEY MEDICAL CENTER (O, 266 beds) 218 South Santa Anita Street, San Gabriel, CA Zip 91776, Mailing Address: P.O. Box 1507, Zip 91778–1507; tel. 818/289–5454; Makoto Nakayama, President

SANTA MONICA HOSPITAL MEDICAL CENTER (O, 178 beds) 1250 16th Street, Santa Monica, CA Zip 90404–1200; tel. 310/319–4000; William D. Parente, President and Chief Executive Officer

VALLEY HOSPITAL MEDICAL CENTER (O, 163 beds) 14500 Sherman Circle, Van Nuys, CA Zip 91405; tel. 818/997–0101; Richard D. Lyons, President and Chief Executive Officer

Owned, leased, sponsored:	10 hospitals	2291 beds
Contract–managed:	0 hospitals	0 beds
Totals:	10 hospitals	2291 beds

★2445: UNITED HEALTH GROUP (NP)

Five Innovation Court, Appleton, WI Zip 54914, Mailing Address: P.O. Box 8025, Zip 54913–8025; tel. 414/730–0330; James Edward Raney, President and Chief Executive Officer

WISCONSIN: APPLETON MEDICAL CENTER (O, 161 beds) 1818 North Meade Street, Appleton, WI Zip 54911; tel. 414/731–4101; Walter L. Edwards, President

THEDA CLARK REGIONAL MEDICAL CENTER (O, 223 beds) 130 Second Street, Neenah, WI Zip 54956, Mailing Address: P.O. Box 2021, Zip 54957–2021; tel. 414/729–3100; Paul E. Macek, President

Owned, leased, sponsored:	2 hospitals	384 beds
Contract–managed:	0 hospitals	0 beds
Totals:	2 hospitals	384 beds

1765: UNITED HOSPITAL CORPORATION (IO)

6189 East Shelby Drive, Memphis, TN Zip 38115; tel. 901/794–8440; James C. Henson, President

ALABAMA: FLORALA MEMORIAL HOSPITAL (O, 23 beds) 515 East Fifth, Florala, AL Zip 36442–0206, Mailing Address: Box 206, Zip 36442–0206; tel. 205/858–3287; James N. York, Administrator

ARKANSAS: VAN BUREN COUNTY MEMORIAL HOSPITAL (CM, 152 beds) Highway 65 South, Clinton, AR Zip 72031, Mailing Address: Box 206, Zip 72031; tel. 501/745–2401; Alan Finley, Administrator

Owned, leased, sponsored:	1 hospitals	23 beds
Contract–managed:	1 hospitals	152 beds
Totals:	2 hospitals	175 beds

9605: UNITED MEDICAL CORPORATION (IO)

603 Main Street, Windermere, FL Zip 34786, Mailing Address: P.O. Box 1100, Zip 34786–1100; tel. 407/876–2200; Donald R. Dizney, Chairman

KENTUCKY: TEN BROECK HOSPITAL (O, 94 beds) 8521 Old LaGrange Road, Louisville, KY Zip 40242; tel. 502/426–6380; Don S. McLendon, Executive Director

LOUISIANA: UNITED MEDICAL CENTER NEW ORLEANS (O, 136 beds) 3419 St. Claude Avenue, New Orleans, LA Zip 70117; tel. 504/948–8200; Romona Baudy, Executive Director

PUERTO RICO: HOSPITAL PAVIA (O, 165 beds) 1462 Asia Street, San Juan, PR Zip 00909, Mailing Address: Box 11137, Santurce Station, Zip 00910; tel. 809/727–6060; Alfredo E. Volckers, Executive Director

SAN JORGE CHILDREN'S HOSPITAL (O, 85 beds) 258 San Jorge Avenue, San Juan, PR Zip 00912; tel. 809/727–1000; Domingo Cruz Vivaldi, Administrator

Owned, leased, sponsored:	4 hospitals	480 beds
Contract–managed:	0 hospitals	0 beds
Totals:	4 hospitals	480 beds

2085: UNITED WESTERN MEDICAL CENTERS (NP)

1001 North Tustin Avenue, Santa Ana, CA Zip 92705–3502; tel. 714/953–3610; David E. Morgan, Chief Executive Officer

CALIFORNIA: WESTERN MEDICAL CENTER HOSPITAL ANAHEIM (O, 171 beds) 1025 South Anaheim Boulevard, Anaheim, CA Zip 92805; tel. 714/533–6220; Daniel L. Frank, Chief Executive Officer

WESTERN MEDICAL CENTER–SANTA ANA (O, 288 beds) 1001 North Tustin Avenue, Santa Ana, CA Zip 92705–3502; tel. 714/835–3555; Daniel L. Frank, Chief Executive Officer

Owned, leased, sponsored:	2 hospitals	459 beds
Contract–managed:	0 hospitals	0 beds
Totals:	2 hospitals	459 beds

9555: UNIVERSAL HEALTH SERVICES, INC. (IO)

367 South Gulph Road, King of Prussia, PA Zip 19406; tel. 610/768–3300; Alan B. Miller, President and Chief Executive Officer

ARKANSAS: BRIDGEWAY (O, 70 beds) 21 Bridgeway Road, North Little Rock, AR Zip 72113; tel. 501/771–1500; Barry Pipkin, Director

CALIFORNIA: DEL AMO HOSPITAL (O, 166 beds) 23700 Camino Del Sol, Torrance, CA Zip 90505; tel. 310/530–1151; Michael Hunn, Administrator and Chief Executive Officer

INLAND VALLEY REGIONAL MEDICAL CENTER (O, 80 beds) 36485 Inland Valley Drive, Wildomar, CA Zip 92595; tel. 909/677–1111; B. Ann Kuss, Chief Executive Officer and Managing Director

WESTLAKE MEDICAL CENTER (O, 60 beds) 4415 South Lakeview Canyon Road, Westlake Village, CA Zip 91361; tel. 818/706–8000; K. D. Justyn, Managing Director

FLORIDA: UNIVERSAL MEDICAL CENTER (O, 80 beds) 6701 West Sunrise Boulevard, Plantation, FL Zip 33313; tel. 305/581–7800; Gregory E. Boyer, Administrator

WELLINGTON REGIONAL MEDICAL CENTER (O, 87 beds) 10101 Forest Hill Boulevard, West Palm Beach, FL Zip 33414; tel. 407/798–8500; Michael Marquez, Chief Executive Officer

GEORGIA: TURNING POINT HOSPITAL (O, 59 beds) 319 By-Pass, Moultrie, GA Zip 31776, Mailing Address: P.O. Box 1177, Zip 31768; tel. 912/985–4815; Larry J. Burge, Managing Director

LOUISIANA: CHALMETTE MEDICAL CENTERS (O, 196 beds) 9001 Patricia Street, Chalmette, LA Zip 70043; tel. 504/277–8011; James M. Reilly, Acting Managing Director

DOCTORS' HOSPITAL OF SHREVEPORT (L, 142 beds) 1130 Louisiana Avenue, Shreveport, LA Zip 71165, Mailing Address: Box 1526, Zip 71101; tel. 318/227–1211; Charles E. Boyd, Administrator

RIVER OAKS HOSPITAL (O, 94 beds) 1525 River Oaks Road West, New Orleans, LA Zip 70123; tel. 504/734–1740; Daryl Sue White R.N., Managing Director

RIVER PARISHES HOSPITAL (O, 120 beds) 500 Rue De Sante, Laplace, LA Zip 70068; tel. 504/652–7000; John Lloyd Hummer, Chief Executive Officer and Managing Director

MASSACHUSETTS: ARBOUR HOSPITAL (O, 118 beds) 49 Robinwood Avenue, Boston, MA Zip 02130, Mailing Address: P.O. Box 9, Zip 02130; tel. 617/522–4400; Roy A. Ettlinger, Managing Director

H.R.I. HOSPITAL (O, 68 beds) 227 Babcock Street, Brookline, MA Zip 02146; tel. 617/731–3200; Roy A. Ettlinger, Managing Director

MICHIGAN: FOREST VIEW HOSPITAL (O, 62 beds) 1055 Medical Park Drive S.E., Grand Rapids, MI Zip 49546; tel. 616/942–9610; Gerard Cyranowski, Managing Director

MISSOURI: TWO RIVERS PSYCHIATRIC HOSPITAL (O, 80 beds) 5121 Raytown Road, Kansas City, MO Zip 64133–2141; tel. 816/356–5688; Craig Nuckles, Administrator

NEVADA: NORTHERN NEVADA MEDICAL CENTER (O, 138 beds) 2375 East Prater Way, Sparks, NV Zip 89434–9645; tel. 702/331–7000; Michael Callahan, Chief Executive Officer

VALLEY HOSPITAL MEDICAL CENTER (O, 390 beds) 620 Shadow Lane, Las Vegas, NV Zip 89106; tel. 702/388–4000; Claus Eggers, Managing Director

PENNSYLVANIA: KEYSTONE CENTER (O, 76 beds) 2001 Providence Avenue, Chester, PA Zip 19013–5504; tel. 610/876–9000; Daniel A. Kidd, Chief Executive Officer and Managing Director

TEXAS: DALLAS FAMILY HOSPITAL (O, 104 beds) 2929 South Hampton Road, Dallas, TX Zip 75224; tel. 214/330–4611; Gary A. Saff, Administrator

EDINBURG HOSPITAL (O, 112 beds) 333 West Freddy Gonzalez Drive, Edinburg, TX Zip 78539–6199; tel. 210/383–6211; Leon J. Belila, Administrator

---

For explanation of codes following names, see page B2.
★Indicates Type III membership in the American Hospital Association.

GLEN OAKS HOSPITAL (O, 54 beds) 301 East Division, Greenville, TX Zip 75401; tel. 903/454-6000; Jerry W. Echols, Administrator

MCALLEN MEDICAL CENTER (L, 408 beds) 301 West Expressway 83, McAllen, TX Zip 78503; tel. 210/632-4000; John L. Mims, Executive Director

MERIDELL ACHIEVEMENT CENTER (L, 78 beds) Austin, TX, Mailing Address: Box 203638, Zip 78720-3638; tel. 512/259-5107; Mark Snow, Managing Director

RIVER CREST HOSPITAL (O, 80 beds) 1636 Hunters Glen Road, San Angelo, TX Zip 76901-5016; tel. 915/949-5722

VICTORIA REGIONAL MEDICAL CENTER (O, 105 beds) 101 Medical Drive, Victoria, TX Zip 77904; tel. 512/573-6100; J. Michael Mastej, Chief Executive Officer and Managing Director

WASHINGTON: AUBURN GENERAL HOSPITAL (O, 100 beds) 20 Second Street N.E., Auburn, WA Zip 98002-0000; tel. 206/833-7711; Michael M. Gherardini, Managing Director

Owned, leased, sponsored:	26 hospitals	3127 beds
Contract-managed:	0 hospitals	0 beds
Totals:	26 hospitals	3127 beds

★**9105: UNIVERSITY OF ALABAMA HOSPITALS** (NP)
619 South 19th Street, Birmingham, AL Zip 35233; tel. 205/975-7545; Kevin E. Lofton, Executive Director

ALABAMA: ST. CLAIR REGIONAL HOSPITAL (CM, 72 beds) 2805 Hospital Drive, Pell City, AL Zip 35125; tel. 205/338-3301; Martin Nowak, Administrator

UNIVERSITY OF ALABAMA HOSPITAL (O, 783 beds) 619 South 19th Street, Birmingham, AL Zip 35233-6505; tel. 205/975-7545; Kevin E. Lofton, Executive Director and Chief Executive Officer

Owned, leased, sponsored:	1 hospitals	783 beds
Contract-managed:	1 hospitals	72 beds
Totals:	2 hospitals	855 beds

6405: UNIVERSITY OF CALIFORNIA-SYSTEMWIDE ADMINISTRATION (NP)
300 Lakeside Drive, 18th Floor, Oakland, CA Zip 94612-3550; tel. 510/987-9701; Cornelius L. Hopper M.D., Vice President Health Affairs

CALIFORNIA: MOUNT ZION MEDICAL CENTER OF UNIVERSITY OF CALIFORNIA-SAN FRANCISCO (O, 290 beds) 1600 Divisadero Street, San Francisco, CA Zip 94115, Mailing Address: Box 7921, Zip 94120; tel. 415/567-6600; Martin H. Diamond, Director

UNIVERSITY OF CALIFORNIA LOS ANGELES MEDICAL CENTER (L, 610 beds) 10833 Le Conte Avenue, Los Angeles, CA Zip 90024-1730; tel. 310/825-5041; Raymond G. Schultze M.D., Director

UNIVERSITY OF CALIFORNIA LOS ANGELES NEUROPSYCHIATRIC HOSPITAL (O, 117 beds) 760 Westwood Plaza, Los Angeles, CA Zip 90024-1759; tel. 310/825-9548; Don A. Rockwell M.D., Director

UNIVERSITY OF CALIFORNIA SAN DIEGO MEDICAL CENTER (O, 412 beds) 200 West Arbor Drive, San Diego, CA Zip 92103-8970; tel. 619/543-6222; Michael R. Stringer, Director

UNIVERSITY OF CALIFORNIA SAN FRANCISCO MEDICAL CENTER (O, 706 beds) 500 Parnassus, San Francisco, CA Zip 94143-0296; tel. 415/476-1000; William B. Kerr, Director

UNIVERSITY OF CALIFORNIA, DAVIS MEDICAL CENTER (O, 474 beds) 2315 Stockton Boulevard, Sacramento, CA Zip 95817-2282; tel. 916/734-3096; Frank J. Loge, Director

UNIVERSITY OF CALIFORNIA, IRVINE MEDICAL CENTER (O, 383 beds) 101 The City Drive, Orange, CA Zip 92668-3298; tel. 714/456-5678; Mary A. Piccione, Executive Director

Owned, leased, sponsored:	7 hospitals	2992 beds
Contract-managed:	0 hospitals	0 beds
Totals:	7 hospitals	2992 beds

0021: UNIVERSITY OF NEW MEXICO (NP)
915 Camino De Salud, Albuquerque, NM Zip 87131; tel. 505/277-5849; Jane E. Henney M.D., Vice President Health Sciences

NEW MEXICO: CARRIE TINGLEY HOSPITAL (O, 18 beds) 1127 University Boulevard N.E., Albuquerque, NM Zip 87102-1715; tel. 505/272-5200; James C. Drennan M.S.H.A., M.D., Medical Director and Chief Executive Officer

UNIVERSITY HOSPITAL (O, 318 beds) 2211 Lomas Boulevard N.E., Albuquerque, NM Zip 87106; tel. 505/843-2121; William H. Johnson, Jr., Chief Executive Officer

UNIVERSITY OF NEW MEXICO CHILDREN'S PSYCHIATRIC HOSPITAL (O, 53 beds) 1001 Yale Boulevard N.E., Albuquerque, NM Zip 87131; tel. 505/843-2945; Christina B. Gunn, Chief Executive Officer

UNIVERSITY OF NEW MEXICO MENTAL HEALTH CENTER (O, 60 beds) 2600 Marble N.E., Albuquerque, NM Zip 87131-2600; tel. 505/843-2870; Christina B. Gunn, Chief Executive Officer

Owned, leased, sponsored:	4 hospitals	449 beds
Contract-managed:	0 hospitals	0 beds
Totals:	4 hospitals	449 beds

0057: UNIVERSITY OF SOUTH ALABAMA HOSPITALS (NP)
2451 Fillingim Street, Mobile, AL Zip 36617-2293; tel. 205/471-7110; Don Ikner, Assistant Administrator Finance

ALABAMA: UNIVERSITY OF SOUTH ALABAMA DOCTORS HOSPITAL (O, 124 beds) 1700 Center Street, Mobile, AL Zip 36604-3391; tel. 205/415-1000; Thomas J. Gibson, Administrator

UNIVERSITY OF SOUTH ALABAMA KNOLLWOOD PARK HOSPITAL (O, 201 beds) 5600 Girby Road, Mobile, AL Zip 36693-3398; tel. 205/660-5120; Stanley K. Hammack, Administrator

UNIVERSITY OF SOUTH ALABAMA MEDICAL CENTER (O, 316 beds) 2451 Fillingim Street, Mobile, AL Zip 36617; tel. 205/471-7000; Stephen H. Simmons, Senior Administrator

Owned, leased, sponsored:	3 hospitals	641 beds
Contract-managed:	0 hospitals	0 beds
Totals:	3 hospitals	641 beds

0033: UNIVERSITY OF TEXAS HOSPITALS (NP)
601 Colorado Avenue, Austin, TX Zip 78701; tel. 512/471-4224

TEXAS: UNIVERSITY OF TEXAS HEALTH CENTER AT TYLER (O, 146 beds) Gladewater Highway, Tyler, TX Zip 75708, Mailing Address: Box 2003, Zip 75710-2003; tel. 903/877-7750; George A. Hurst M.D., Director

UNIVERSITY OF TEXAS M. D. ANDERSON CANCER CENTER (O, 467 beds) 1515 Holcombe Boulevard, Houston, TX Zip 77030-4096; tel. 713/792-6170; Donna K. Sollenberger, Vice President

UNIVERSITY OF TEXAS MEDICAL BRANCH HOSPITALS (O, 860 beds) 301 University Boulevard, Galveston, TX Zip 77555-0138; tel. 409/772-1011; James F. Arens M.D., Vice President Clinical Affairs and Chief Executive Officer

Owned, leased, sponsored:	3 hospitals	1473 beds
Contract-managed:	0 hospitals	0 beds
Totals:	3 hospitals	1473 beds

★**0038: UPPER CHESAPEAKE HEALTH SYSTEM** (NP)
1916 Belair Road, Fallston, MD Zip 21047; tel. 410/893-0322; Lyle Ernest Sheldon, President and Chief Executive Officer

MARYLAND: FALLSTON GENERAL HOSPITAL (O, 148 beds) 200 Milton Avenue, Fallston, MD Zip 21047-2777; tel. 410/877-3700

HARFORD MEMORIAL HOSPITAL (O, 175 beds) 501 South Union Avenue, Havre De Grace, MD Zip 21078-3493; tel. 410/939-2400; Linda S. Widra R.N., Ph.D., Senior Vice President and Chief Operating Officer

Owned, leased, sponsored:	2 hospitals	323 beds
Contract-managed:	0 hospitals	0 beds
Totals:	2 hospitals	323 beds

★**1965: UPPER VALLEY MEDICAL CENTERS** (NP)
3130 North Dixie Highway, Troy, OH Zip 45373; tel. 513/332-7500; David J. Meckstroth, President

OHIO: DETTMER HOSPITAL (O, 105 beds) 3130 North Dixie Highway, Troy, OH Zip 45373-1039; tel. 513/332-7500; Michael J. Maiberger, Vice President and Chief Operating Officer

---

For explanation of codes following names, see page B2.
★Indicates Type III membership in the American Hospital Association.

Systems / Upper Valley Medical Centers

PIQUA MEMORIAL MEDICAL CENTER (O, 149 beds) 624 Park Avenue, Piqua, OH Zip 45356-2098; tel. 513/778-6500; Michael J. Maiberger, Administrator

STOUDER MEMORIAL HOSPITAL (O, 138 beds) 920 Summit Avenue, Troy, OH Zip 45373; tel. 513/332-8500; Michael J. Maiberger, Vice President and Chief Operating Officer

Owned, leased, sponsored:	3 hospitals	392 beds
Contract-managed:	0 hospitals	0 beds
Totals:	3 hospitals	392 beds

0043: VALLEY HEALTH SYSTEM (NP)

1117 East Devonshire Avenue, Hemet, CA Zip 92543; tel. 909/652-2811; Geoffrey Lang, Chief Executive Officer

CALIFORNIA: HEMET VALLEY MEDICAL CENTER (O, 295 beds) 1117 East Devonshire Avenue, Hemet, CA Zip 92543; tel. 909/652-2811; Edward C. Burke, Administrator

MENIFEE VALLEY MEDICAL CENTER (O, 84 beds) 28400 McCall Boulevard, Sun City, CA Zip 92585-9537; tel. 909/679-8888; Susan Ballard, Administrator

MORENO VALLEY COMMUNITY HOSPITAL (O, 66 beds) 27300 Iris Avenue, Moreno Valley, CA Zip 92555; tel. 909/243-0811; Thomas McClintock, Administrator

Owned, leased, sponsored:	3 hospitals	445 beds
Contract-managed:	0 hospitals	0 beds
Totals:	3 hospitals	445 beds

0026: VENCOR, INCORPORATED (IO)

400 West Market Street, Suite 3300, Louisville, KY Zip 40202-3360; tel. 502/569-7300; W. Bruce Lunsford, Board Chairman

ARIZONA: VENCOR HOSPITAL – PHOENIX (O, 104 beds) 40 East Indianola, Phoenix, AZ Zip 85012; tel. 602/280-7000; John L. Harrington, Jr. FACHE, Administrator

CALIFORNIA: VENCOR HOSPITAL-SACRAMENTO (O, 32 beds) 223 Fargo Way, Folsom, CA Zip 95630; tel. 916/351-9151; Kenneth H. Smith, Administrator

VENCOR HOSPITAL-SAN DIEGO (O, 133 beds) 1940 El Cajon Boulevard, San Diego, CA Zip 92104; tel. 619/543-4500

VENCOR HOSPITAL-SAN LEANDRO (O, 62 beds) 2800 Benedict Drive, San Leandro, CA Zip 94577; tel. 510/357-8300; Jan E. Nielsen, Administrator

FLORIDA: VENCOR HOSPITAL – TAMPA (O, 73 beds) 4555 South Manhattan Avenue, Tampa, FL Zip 33611; tel. 813/839-6341; Frank J. Battafarano, Administrator

VENCOR HOSPITAL-CORAL GABLES (O, 53 beds) 5190 Southwest Eighth Street, Coral Gables, FL Zip 33134; tel. 305/445-1364; Theodore Welding, Chief Executive Officer

VENCOR HOSPITAL-FORT LAUDERDALE (O, 64 beds) 1516 East Las Olas Boulevard, Fort Lauderdale, FL Zip 33301-2399; tel. 305/764-8900; Lewis A. Ransdell, Administrator

GEORGIA: VENCOR HOSPITAL-ATLANTA (O, 66 beds) 705 Juniper Street N.E., Atlanta, GA Zip 30365; tel. 404/873-2871; Skip Wright, Administrator

ILLINOIS: VENCOR HOSPITAL-CHICAGO NORTH (O, 94 beds) 2544 West Montrose Avenue, Chicago, IL Zip 60618; tel. 312/267-2200; Jack Nathan Shapiro, Administrator

VENCOR HOSPITAL-SYCAMORE (O, 50 beds) 225 Edward Street, Sycamore, IL Zip 60178; tel. 815/895-2144; Donald Van Voorhis, Administrator

INDIANA: VENCOR HOSPITAL-LAGRANGE (O, 62 beds) 0300N 00EW Townline Road, LaGrange, IN Zip 46761; tel. 219/463-2143; Joseph A. Stuber, Administrator

MICHIGAN: VENCOR HOSPITAL-DETROIT (O, 218 beds) 26400 West Outer Drive, Lincoln Park, MI Zip 48146; tel. 313/594-6000; Joseph R. Gordon, Administrator

MISSOURI: VENCOR HOSPITAL-KANSAS CITY (O, 167 beds) 8701 Troost Avenue, Kansas City, MO Zip 64131; tel. 816/995-2000; Suzanne R. Wilsey R.N., Administrator

TENNESSEE: VENCOR HOSPITAL-CHATTANOOGA (O, 49 beds) 709 Walnut Street, Chattanooga, TN Zip 37402; tel. 615/266-7721; Doug Sundlof, Administrator

TEXAS: VENCOR HOSPITAL – DALLAS (O, 55 beds) 1600 Abrams Road, Dallas, TX Zip 75214-4499; tel. 214/818-2401

VENCOR HOSPITAL-FORT WORTH SOUTH (O, 94 beds) 1802 Highway 157 North, Mansfield, TX Zip 76063-9555; tel. 817/473-6101; James L. Ashbaugh, Administrator

VENCOR HOSPITAL-HOUSTON (O, 94 beds) 6441 Main Street, Houston, TX Zip 77030; tel. 713/790-0500; Darrell L. Pile, Administrator

Owned, leased, sponsored:	17 hospitals	1470 beds
Contract-managed:	0 hospitals	0 beds
Totals:	17 hospitals	1470 beds

0012: VIRGINIA DEPARTMENT OF MENTAL HEALTH (NP)

109 Governor Street, Richmond, VA Zip 23219, Mailing Address: P.O. Box 1797, Zip 23214; tel. 804/786-3915; King E. Davis Ph.D., Commissioner

VIRGINIA: CENTRAL VIRGINIA TRAINING CENTER (O, 1093 beds) 210 East Colony Road, Madison Heights, VA Zip 24572, Mailing Address: P.O. Box 1098, Lynchburg, VA Zip 24505; tel. 804/947-6326; S. J. Butkus Ph.D., Director

DE JARNETTE CENTER (O, 60 beds) 1290 Richmond Road, Staunton, VA Zip 24401-1091, Mailing Address: Box 2309, Zip 24402-2309; tel. 703/332-8800; Andrea C. Newsome FACHE, Director

EASTERN STATE HOSPITAL (O, 727 beds) Williamsburg, VA, Mailing Address: P.O. Box 8791, Zip 23187-8791; tel. 804/253-5161; John M. Favret, Director

NORTHERN VIRGINIA MENTAL HEALTH INSTITUTE (O, 114 beds) 3302 Gallows Road, Falls Church, VA Zip 22042-3398; tel. 703/207-7111; David A. Rosenquist M.H.A., Acting Facility Director

PIEDMONT GERIATRIC HOSPITAL (O, 210 beds) Highway 460/360, Burkeville, VA Zip 23922-9999; tel. 804/767-4401; Willard R. Pierce, Jr., Director

SOUTHERN VIRGINIA MENTAL HEALTH INSTITUTE (O, 96 beds) 382 Taylor Drive, Danville, VA Zip 24541-4023; tel. 804/799-6220; Constance N. Fletcher Ph.D., Director

SOUTHWESTERN VIRGINIA MENTAL HEALTH INSTITUTE (O, 266 beds) 502 East Main Street, Marion, VA Zip 24354; tel. 703/783-1200; Gerald E. Deans, Director

WESTERN STATE HOSPITAL (O, 460 beds) 1301 Richmond Avenue, Staunton, VA Zip 24401, Mailing Address: Box 2500, Zip 24402-2500; tel. 703/332-8000; L. F. Harding, Director

Owned, leased, sponsored:	8 hospitals	3026 beds
Contract-managed:	0 hospitals	0 beds
Totals:	8 hospitals	3026 beds

8895: VISTA HILL FOUNDATION (NP)

2355 Northside Drive, 3rd Floor, San Diego, CA Zip 92108; tel. 619/563-1770; Ronald E. Fickle, President

CALIFORNIA: MESA VISTA HOSPITAL (O, 150 beds) 7850 Vista Hill Avenue, San Diego, CA Zip 92123-2790; tel. 619/694-8300; Donald K. Allen, Administrator and Chief Executive Officer

VISTA HILL HOSPITAL (O, 77 beds) 730 Medical Center Court, Chula Vista, CA Zip 91911-6618; tel. 619/421-6900; Shawn Miyake, Administrator

Owned, leased, sponsored:	2 hospitals	227 beds
Contract-managed:	0 hospitals	0 beds
Totals:	2 hospitals	227 beds

★6725: WEST JERSEY HEALTH SYSTEM (NP)

1000 Atlantic Avenue, Camden, NJ Zip 08104; tel. 609/342-4604; Barry D. Brown, President and Chief Executive Officer

NEW JERSEY: WEST JERSEY HOSPITAL-BERLIN (O, 95 beds) 100 Townsend Avenue, Berlin, NJ Zip 08009; tel. 609/768-6006; Martin B. Idler, Executive Director

WEST JERSEY HOSPITAL-CAMDEN (O, 222 beds) 1000 Atlantic Avenue, Camden, NJ Zip 08104-1595; tel. 609/342-4000; Joan T. Meyers R.N., Executive Director

WEST JERSEY HOSPITAL-MARLTON (O, 202 beds) Route 73 and Brick Road, Marlton, NJ Zip 08053; tel. 609/596-3500; Kevin M. Manley, Executive Director

---

For explanation of codes following names, see page B2.
★Indicates Type III membership in the American Hospital Association.

Systems / York Health System

WEST JERSEY HOSPITAL–VOORHEES (O, 262 beds) 101 Carnie Boulevard, Voorhees, NJ Zip 08043–1597; tel. 609/772–5000; James R. Shedno, Executive Director

Owned, leased, sponsored:	4 hospitals	781 beds
Contract–managed:	0 hospitals	0 beds
Totals:	4 hospitals	781 beds

★0004: **WEST TENNESSEE HEALTHCARE, INC.** (NP)
708 West Forest Avenue, Jackson, TN Zip 38301; tel. 901/425–5000; James T. Moss, President
TENNESSEE: HUMBOLDT GENERAL HOSPITAL (O, 42 beds) 3525 Chere Carol Road, Humboldt, TN Zip 38343–3699; tel. 901/784–0301; Billy Alred, Administrator
JACKSON–MADISON COUNTY GENERAL HOSPITAL (O, 636 beds) 708 West Forest Avenue, Jackson, TN Zip 38301–3855; tel. 901/425–5000; James T. Moss, President
VALLEY REGIONAL HOSPITAL (CM, 45 beds) Hospital Street, Camden, TN Zip 38320, Mailing Address: P.O. Box 468, Zip 38320–1696; tel. 901/584–6135; Alfred P. Taylor, Administrator and Chief Executive Officer
WEST TENNESSEE BEHAVIORAL CENTER (O, 25 beds) 238 Summar Drive, Jackson, TN Zip 38301; tel. 901/935–8200

Owned, leased, sponsored:	3 hospitals	703 beds
Contract–managed:	1 hospitals	45 beds
Totals:	4 hospitals	748 beds

★6745: **WHEATON FRANCISCAN SERVICES, INC.** (CC)
26W171 Roosevelt Road, Wheaton, IL Zip 60189–0667, Mailing Address: P.O. Box 667, Zip 60189–0667; tel. 708/462–9271; Wilfred F. Loebig Jr., President and Chief Executive Officer
ILLINOIS: MARIANJOY REHABILITATION HOSPITAL AND CLINICS (O, 107 beds) 26 West 171 Roosevelt Road, Wheaton, IL Zip 60187, Mailing Address: P.O. Box 795, Zip 60189–0795; tel. 708/462–4000; Bruce A. Schurman, President
OAK PARK HOSPITAL (O, 186 beds) 520 South Maple Avenue, Oak Park, IL Zip 60304–1097; tel. 708/383–9300; Leonard J. Muller, President
IOWA: COVENANT MEDICAL CENTER (O, 346 beds) 3421 West Ninth Street, Waterloo, IA Zip 50702–5499; tel. 319/236–4111; Raymond F. Burfeind, President
MERCY HOSPITAL OF FRANCISCAN SISTERS (O, 64 beds) 201 Eighth Avenue S.E., Oelwein, IA Zip 50662; tel. 319/283–2314; Judith Blake, President and Chief Executive Officer
WISCONSIN: ELMBROOK MEMORIAL HOSPITAL (O, 136 beds) 19333 West North Avenue, Brookfield, WI Zip 53045–4198; tel. 414/785–2000; Kimry A. Johnsrud, President
KAUKAUNA COMMUNITY HOSPITAL (O, 40 beds) 308 East 14th Street, Kaukauna, WI Zip 54130; tel. 414/766–4211; Gregory S. Holub, President and Chief Executive Officer
SAINT MARY'S MEDICAL CENTER (O, 226 beds) 3801 Spring Street, Racine, WI Zip 53405; tel. 414/636–4011; Edward P. Demeulenaere, President and Chief Executive Officer
ST. ELIZABETH HOSPITAL (O, 218 beds) 1506 South Oneida Street, Appleton, WI Zip 54915–1397; tel. 414/738–2000; Otto L. Cox, President
ST. FRANCIS HOSPITAL (CM, 279 beds) 3237 South 16th Street, Milwaukee, WI Zip 53215–4592; tel. 414/647–5000; Gregory A. Banaszynski, President
ST. JOSEPH'S HOSPITAL (O, 495 beds) 5000 West Chambers Street, Milwaukee, WI Zip 53210–9988; tel. 414/447–2000; Jon L. Wachs, President and Chief Operating Officer
ST. LUKE'S MEMORIAL HOSPITAL (CM, 238 beds) 1320 Wisconsin Avenue, Racine, WI Zip 53403–1987; tel. 414/636–2011; Ray Di Iulio, President and Chief Executive Officer
ST. MICHAEL HOSPITAL (O, 168 beds) 2400 West Villard Avenue, Milwaukee, WI Zip 53209; tel. 414/527–8000; Stephen R. Young, President and Chief Executive Officer

Owned, leased, sponsored:	10 hospitals	1986 beds
Contract–managed:	2 hospitals	517 beds
Totals:	12 hospitals	2503 beds

★9575: **WILLIAM BEAUMONT HOSPITAL CORPORATION** (NP)
3601 West Thirteen Mile Road, Royal Oak, MI Zip 48073–6769; tel. 810/551–5000; Kenneth E. Myers, President
MICHIGAN: WILLIAM BEAUMONT HOSPITAL (O, 894 beds) 3601 West Thirteen Mile Road, Royal Oak, MI Zip 48073–6769; tel. 810/551–5000; Kenneth J. Matzick, Vice President and Director
WILLIAM BEAUMONT HOSPITAL–TROY (O, 189 beds) 44201 Dequindre Road, Troy, MI Zip 48098–1198; tel. 810/828–5100; John D. Labriola, Vice President and Director

Owned, leased, sponsored:	2 hospitals	1083 beds
Contract–managed:	0 hospitals	0 beds
Totals:	2 hospitals	1083 beds

• ★0068: **YORK HEALTH SYSTEM** (NP)
1001 South George Street, York, PA Zip 17405; tel. 717/851–2121; Bruce M. Bartels, President
PENNSYLVANIA: YORK HOSPITAL (O, 428 beds) 1001 South George Street, York, PA Zip 17405–3676; tel. 717/851–2345; Bruce M. Bartels, President

Owned, leased, sponsored:	1 hospitals	428 beds
Contract–managed:	0 hospitals	0 beds
Totals:	1 hospitals	428 beds

For explanation of codes following names, see page B2.
★Indicates Type III membership in the American Hospital Association.
• Single hospital health care system

Headquarters of Health Care Systems

Alphabetically

2175 ADVENTIST HEALTH SYSTEM–LOMA LINDA, p. B9
4165 ADVENTIST HEALTH SYSTEM–SUNBELT HEALTH CARE CORPORATION, p. B9
0235 ADVENTIST HEALTH SYSTEM/WEST, p. B9
0064 ADVOCATE HEALTH CARE, p. B10
0225 ALAMEDA COUNTY HEALTH CARE SERVICES AGENCY, p. B10
1685 ALBERT EINSTEIN HEALTHCARE NETWORK, p. B10
0065 ALEXIAN BROTHERS HEALTH SYSTEM, INC., p. B10
1385 ALLEGANY HEALTH SYSTEM, p. B10
2305 ALLEGHENY HEALTH, EDUCATION AND RESEARCH FOUNDATION, p. B10
2285 ALLIANT HEALTH SYSTEM, p. B10
0041 ALLINA HEALTH SYSTEM, p. B11
0985 AMERIHEALTH, INC., p. B11
0135 ANCILLA SYSTEMS INC., p. B12
0145 APPALACHIAN REGIONAL HEALTHCARE, p. B12
0205 ASC HEALTH SYSTEM, p. B12
2215 AURORA HEALTH CARE, INC., p. B12
7895 AVMED–SANTA FE, p. B12
0185 BAPTIST HEALTH CARE CORPORATION, p. B13
4155 BAPTIST HEALTH CARE SYSTEM OF SOUTH CAROLINA, p. B13
0345 BAPTIST HEALTH SYSTEM, p. B13
2155 BAPTIST HEALTH SYSTEM OF TENNESSEE, p. B13
0315 BAPTIST HEALTHCARE SYSTEM, p. B13
8810 BAPTIST HOSPITALS AND HEALTH SYSTEMS, INC., p. B13
0355 BAPTIST MEDICAL SYSTEM, p. B13
1625 BAPTIST MEMORIAL HEALTH CARE SYSTEM, INC., p. B14
0265 BAPTIST MEMORIAL HOSPITAL SYSTEM, p. B14
0095 BAYLOR HEALTH CARE SYSTEM, p. B14
1095 BAYSTATE HEALTH SYSTEMS, INC., p. B14
0515 BENEDICTINE HEALTH SYSTEM, p. B14
0535 BENEDICTINE SISTERS, p. B15
0545 BENEDICTINE SISTERS OF THE ANNUNCIATION, p. B15
2435 BERKSHIRE HEALTH SYSTEMS, INC., p. B15
0415 BETHESDA HOSPITAL, INC., p. B15
0051 BJC HEALTH SYSTEM, p. B15
0053 BLUE WATER HEALTH SERVICES CORPORATION, p. B15
5085 BON SECOURS HEALTH SYSTEM, INC., p. B15
2455 BRADFORD PARKSIDE, p. B16
0585 BRIM, INC., p. B16
0595 BRONSON HEALTHCARE GROUP, INC., p. B17
0955 CAMCARE, INC., p. B17
2135 CAPITAL HEALTH SYSTEM, p. B17
0070 CARILION HEALTH SYSTEM, p. B17
1125 CARITAS CHRISTI HEALTH CARE SYSTEM, p. B18
2575 CARLE FOUNDATION, p. B18
5945 CARONDELET HEALTH SYSTEM, p. B18
6545 CATHEDRAL HEALTHCARE SYSTEM, INC., p. B18
5175 CATHOLIC HEALTH CORPORATION, p. B18
5205 CATHOLIC HEALTHCARE WEST, p. B19
2265 CENTRA HEALTH, INC., p. B19
0665 CENTURY HEALTHCARE CORPORATION, p. B19
0705 CHARLOTTE–MECKLENBURG HOSPITAL AUTHORITY, p. B20
0695 CHARTER MEDICAL CORPORATION, p. B20
0048 COLUMBIA/HCA HEALTHCARE CORPORATION, p. B21
8805 COLUMBUS–CABRINI MEDICAL CENTER, p. B28
0215 COMMUNITY CARE SYSTEMS, INC., p. B28
0875 COMMUNITY HEALTH SYSTEMS, INC., p. B28
1085 COMMUNITY HOSPITALS OF CENTRAL CALIFORNIA, p. B28

0785 COMMUNITY PSYCHIATRIC CENTERS, p. B29
5695 CONGREGATION OF ST. AGNES, p. B29
0014 CONNECTICUT STATE DEPARTMENT OF MENTAL HEALTH, p. B29
1715 CONTINENTAL MEDICAL SYSTEMS, INC., p. B30
0016 COOK COUNTY BUREAU OF HEALTH SERVICES, p. B30
5885 COVENANT HEALTH SYSTEMS, INC., p. B30
0008 CROZER–KEYSTONE HEALTH SYSTEM, p. B30
5435 CSJ HEALTH SYSTEM OF WICHITA, p. B30
0075 CUMBERLAND HEALTH SYSTEMS, INC., p. B30
1855 DAUGHTERS OF CHARITY NATIONAL HEALTH SYSTEM, p. B31
1825 DCH HEALTHCARE AUTHORITY, p. B31
6995 DEPARTMENT OF HEALTH AND HOSPITALS, p. B32
9655 DEPARTMENT OF NAVY, p. B32
9495 DEPARTMENT OF THE AIR FORCE, p. B32
9395 DEPARTMENT OF THE ARMY, p. B33
9295 DEPARTMENT OF VETERANS AFFAIRS, p. B34
2145 DETROIT MEDICAL CENTER, p. B37
0042 DETROIT–MACOMB HOSPITAL CORPORATION, p. B37
0845 DEVEREUX FOUNDATION, p. B37
0029 DIMENSIONS HEALTH CORPORATION, p. B38
0010 DIVISION OF MENTAL HEALTH SERVICES, DEPARTMENT OF HUMAN SERVICES, STATE OF NEW JERSEY, p. B38
1045 DOCTORS HOSPITAL, p. B38
1195 DOMINICAN SISTERS CONGREGATION OF THE MOST HOLY NAME, p. B38
1295 DOMINICAN SISTERS OF SPRINGFIELD, p. B38
1895 EAST TEXAS MEDICAL CENTER REGIONAL HEALTHCARE SYSTEM, p. B38
0555 EASTERN MAINE HEALTHCARE, p. B38
3595 EASTERN MERCY HEALTH SYSTEM, p. B38
0945 EMPIRE HEALTH CENTERS GROUP, p. B39
0735 EPISCOPAL HEALTH SERVICES INC., p. B39
1255 ESCAMBIA COUNTY HEALTH CARE AUTHORITY, p. B39
2515 FAIRVIEW HEALTH SYSTEM, p. B39
1325 FAIRVIEW HOSPITAL AND HEALTHCARE SERVICES, p. B39
1275 FIRST HEALTH, INC., p. B39
2635 FIRST HOSPITAL CORPORATION, p. B39
1355 FORBES HEALTH SYSTEM, p. B40
5325 FRANCISCAN HEALTH SYSTEM, p. B40
9650 FRANCISCAN HEALTH SYSTEM, INC., p. B40
1475 FRANCISCAN MISSIONARIES OF OUR LADY HEALTH SYSTEM, INC., p. B40
5375 FRANCISCAN SERVICES CORPORATION, p. B40
1415 FRANCISCAN SISTERS HEALTH CARE CORPORATION, p. B40
1455 FRANCISCAN SISTERS OF CHRISTIAN CHARITY HEALTHCARE MINISTRY, INC, p. B41
1485 FRANCISCAN SISTERS OF THE POOR HEALTH SYSTEM, INC., p. B41
2115 FREMONT–RIDEOUT HEALTH GROUP, p. B41
5570 GEISINGER HEALTH CARE SYSTEM, p. B41
0775 GENERAL HEALTH SYSTEM, p. B41
0645 GLENBEIGH, INC., p. B41
0965 GOOD SAMARITAN HEALTH SYSTEM, p. B41
0006 GRADUATE HEALTH SYSTEM, p. B42
1535 GREAT PLAINS HEALTH ALLIANCE, INC., p. B42
0046 GREATER ROCHESTER HEALTH SYSTEM, INC., p. B42
1155 GREENLEAF HEALTH SYSTEMS, INC., p. B42
1555 GREENVILLE HOSPITAL SYSTEM, p. B43
9995 GROUP HEALTH COOPERATIVE OF PUGET SOUND, p. B43
0675 GUTHRIE HEALTHCARE SYSTEM, p. B43
5895 HALLMARK HEALTHCARE CORPORATION, p. B43
2345 HARRIS METHODIST HEALTH SYSTEM, p. B43

1775 HEALTH MANAGEMENT ASSOCIATES, p. B43
8815 HEALTH MIDWEST, p. B44
0395 HEALTHCARE INTERNATIONAL, INC., p. B44
1585 HEALTHCARE MANAGEMENT GROUP, INC., p. B44
2795 HEALTHCORP OF TENNESSEE, INC., p. B44
2185 HEALTHEAST, p. B45
0935 HEALTHONE HEALTHCARE SYSTEM, p. B45
0023 HEALTHSOUTH CORPORATION, p. B45
1985 HEALTHSYSTEM MINNESOTA, p. B46
2485 HEARTLAND HEALTH SYSTEM, p. B46
2355 HELIX HEALTH SYSTEM, p. B46
9505 HENRY FORD HEALTH SYSTEM, p. B46
5585 HOLY CROSS HEALTH SYSTEM CORPORATION, p. B46
1035 HORIZON HEALTH SYSTEM, p. B47
0027 HORIZON HEALTHCARE, INC., p. B47
0455 HOSPITAL GROUP OF AMERICA, p. B47
5355 HOSPITAL SISTERS HEALTH SYSTEM, p. B47
5645 HUMILITY OF MARY HEALTH CARE CORPORATION, p. B47
5565 INCARNATE WORD HEALTH SERVICES, p. B47
2025 INFIRMARY HEALTH SYSTEM, INC., p. B48
1305 INOVA HEALTH SYSTEM, p. B48
1815 INTERMOUNTAIN HEALTH CARE, INC., p. B48
0061 IOWA HEALTH SYSTEM, p. B48
2415 JEWISH HEALTH SYSTEMS, INC., p. B49
0052 JEWISH HOSPITAL HEALTHCARE SERVICES, p. B49
8855 JFK HEALTH SYSTEMS, INC., p. B49
1015 JOHNS HOPKINS HEALTH SYSTEM, p. B49
2105 KAISER FOUNDATION HOSPITALS, p. B49
0056 LAKELAND REGIONAL HEALTH SYSTEM, INC., p. B50
2755 LEGACY HEALTH SYSTEM, p. B50
0060 LIFESPAN CORPORATION, p. B50
2295 LITTLE COMPANY OF MARY SISTERS HEALTHCARE SYSTEM, p. B50
5755 LOS ANGELES COUNTY–DEPARTMENT OF HEALTH SERVICES, p. B50
0715 LOUISIANA HEALTH CARE AUTHORITY, p. B50
0047 LOUISIANA STATE HOSPITALS, p. B51
0036 LUBBOCK METHODIST HOSPITAL SYSTEM, p. B51
2235 LUTHERAN HEALTH SYSTEMS, p. B51
7775 MAIN LINE HEALTH, p. B52
1975 MARSHALL COUNTY HEALTH CARE AUTHORITY, p. B52
0013 MASSACHUSETTS DEPARTMENT OF MENTAL HEALTH, p. B52
1785 MASSACHUSETTS GENERAL HOSPITAL CORPORATION, p. B52
1875 MAYO FOUNDATION, p. B52
1335 MEASE HEALTH CARE, p. B53
6615 MEDLANTIC HEALTHCARE GROUP, p. B53
2335 MEMORIAL HEALTH SERVICES, p. B53
2615 MEMORIAL HEALTH SYSTEMS, p. B53
2645 MEMORIAL HEALTHCARE SYSTEM, p. B53
5165 MERCY HEALTH SERVICES, p. B53
5155 MERCY HEALTH SYSTEM, p. B54
5215 MERCY–CHICAGO REGION HEALTHCARE SYSTEM, p. B54
8835 MERIDIA HEALTH SYSTEM, p. B55
8875 METHODIST HEALTH SERVICES CORPORATION, p. B55
2715 METHODIST HEALTH SYSTEM, p. B55
9345 METHODIST HEALTH SYSTEMS, INC., p. B55
7235 METHODIST HOSPITAL SYSTEM, p. B55
2735 METHODIST HOSPITALS OF DALLAS, p. B55
8285 METROHEALTH SYSTEM, p. B55
0022 METROPOLITAN NASHVILLE GENERAL HOSPITAL, p. B55
1515 MICHIGAN CAPITAL HEALTHCARE, p. B56

Headquarters of Health Care Systems / Alphabetically—By System Code

2055 MICHIGAN HEALTH CARE CORPORATION, p. B56
0001 MIDMICHIGAN REGIONAL HEALTH SYSTEM, p. B56
3775 MILWAUKEE COUNTY BOARD OF SUPERVISORS, p. B56
2855 MISSIONARY BENEDICTINE SISTERS AMERICAN PROVINCE, p. B56
0017 MISSISSIPPI STATE DEPARTMENT OF MENTAL HEALTH, p. B56
6555 MULTICARE HEALTH SYSTEM, p. B56
1465 MUNSON HEALTHCARE, p. B56
3175 NEPONSET VALLEY HEALTH SYSTEM, p. B56
3075 NEW YORK CITY HEALTH AND HOSPITALS CORPORATION, p. B57
0009 NEW YORK STATE DEPARTMENT OF MENTAL HEALTH, p. B57
3115 NORTH BROWARD HOSPITAL DISTRICT, p. B57
0032 NORTH MISSISSIPPI HEALTH SERVICES, INC., p. B58
0062 NORTH SHORE HEALTH SYSTEM, p. B58
2075 NORTHBAY HEALTHCARE SYSTEM, p. B58
1165 OAKWOOD HEALTHCARE SYSTEM, p. B58
0305 OKLAHOMA HEALTH SYSTEM, p. B58
0018 OKLAHOMA STATE DEPARTMENT OF MENTAL HEALTH AND SUBSTANCE ABUSE SERVICES, p. B59
3355 ORLANDO REGIONAL HEALTHCARE SYSTEM, p. B59
6525 ORNDA HEALTHCORP, p. B59
5335 OSF HEALTHCARE SYSTEM, p. B60
0435 PACIFIC HEALTH CORPORATION, p. B60
7555 PALOMAR POMERADO HEALTH SYSTEM, p. B60
5765 PARACELSUS HEALTHCARE CORPORATION, p. B60
0335 PARK HEALTHCARE COMPANY, p. B61
5415 PEACEHEALTH, p. B61
0034 PMH HEALTH RESOURCES, INC., p. B61
3505 PRESBYTERIAN HEALTHCARE SERVICES, p. B61
1130 PRESBYTERIAN HEALTHCARE SYSTEM, p. B61
5255 PRESENTATION HEALTH SYSTEM, p. B62
0995 PROMINA NORTHWEST HEALTH SYSTEM, p. B62
5265 PROVIDENCE SERVICES, p. B62
0011 PUERTO RICO DEPARTMENT OF HEALTH, p. B62
0040 QUEEN'S HEALTH SYSTEMS, p. B62
0002 QUORUM HEALTH GROUP/QUORUM HEALTH RESOURCES, p. B62
0405 RAMSAY HEALTH CARE, INC., p. B68
4810 RIVERSIDE HEALTH SYSTEM, p. B68
3855 RUSH–PRESBYTERIAN–ST. LUKE'S MEDICAL CENTER, p. B68

2535 SAMARITAN HEALTH SYSTEM, p. B68
0575 SCHICK LABORATORIES, INC., p. B69
0037 SCOTTSDALE MEMORIAL HEALTH SYSTEMS, INC., p. B69
1505 SCRIPPS HOSPITALS, p. B69
2565 SENTARA HEALTH SYSTEM, p. B69
4025 SERVANTCOR, p. B69
2065 SHARP HEALTHCARE, p. B69
4125 SHRINERS HOSPITALS FOR CRIPPLED CHILDREN, p. B69
0067 SINGING RIVER HOSPITAL SYSTEM, p. B70
5995 SISTERS OF CHARITY CENTER, p. B70
6095 SISTERS OF CHARITY HEALTH CARE SYSTEM CORPORATION, p. B70
5115 SISTERS OF CHARITY HEALTH CARE SYSTEMS, INC., p. B70
5095 SISTERS OF CHARITY OF LEAVENWORTH HEALTH SERVICES CORPORATION, p. B71
3045 SISTERS OF CHARITY OF NAZARETH HEALTH SYSTEM, p. B71
5125 SISTERS OF CHARITY OF ST. AUGUSTINE HEALTH SYSTEM, p. B71
0605 SISTERS OF CHARITY OF THE INCARNATE WORD HEALTHCARE SYSTEM, p. B71
5805 SISTERS OF MARY OF THE PRESENTATION HEALTH CORPORATION, p. B71
5985 SISTERS OF MERCY, p. B72
5185 SISTERS OF MERCY HEALTH SYSTEM–ST. LOUIS, p. B72
6015 SISTERS OF MERCY OF THE AMERICAS–REGIONAL COMMUNITY OF BALTIMORE, p. B72
5285 SISTERS OF PROVIDENCE HEALTH SYSTEM, p. B72
5275 SISTERS OF PROVIDENCE HEALTH SYSTEM, p. B72
5345 SISTERS OF ST. FRANCIS HEALTH SERVICES, INC., p. B73
5555 SISTERS OF ST. JOSEPH HEALTH SYSTEM, p. B73
5955 SISTERS OF THE 3RD FRANCISCAN ORDER, p. B73
5575 SISTERS OF THE HOLY FAMILY OF NAZARETH–SACRED HEART PROVINCE, p. B73
5305 SISTERS OF THE SORROWFUL MOTHER UNITED STATES HEALTH SYSTEM, p. B73
4175 SOUTHERN ILLINOIS HOSPITAL SERVICES, p. B74
4195 SPARTANBURG HOSPITAL SYSTEM, p. B74

5455 SSM HEALTH CARE SYSTEM, p. B74
0003 ST. DAVID'S HEALTH CARE SYSTEM, p. B74
2255 ST. FRANCIS HEALTH SYSTEM, p. B74
5425 ST. JOSEPH HEALTH SYSTEM, p. B75
5845 ST. LUKE'S HEALTH SYSTEM, INC., p. B75
3555 STATE OF HAWAII, DEPARTMENT OF HEALTH, p. B75
0044 STERLING HEALTHCARE CORPORATION, p. B75
0805 STORMONT–VAIL HEALTH SERVICES CORPORATION, p. B75
0905 SUMMIT MEDICAL MANAGEMENT, INC., p. B76
0030 SUN HEALTH CORPORATION, p. B76
0066 SUSQUEHANNA HEALTH SYSTEM, p. B76
8795 SUTTER HEALTH, p. B76
0039 TARRANT COUNTY HOSPITAL DISTRICT, p. B76
0063 TENET HEALTHCARE CORPORATION, p. B76
0020 TEXAS DEPARTMENT OF HEALTH, p. B78
2205 TIDEWATER HEALTH CARE, INC., p. B78
9255 TRUMAN MEDICAL CENTER, p. B78
9095 U.S. HEALTH CORPORATION, p. B78
9195 U.S. PUBLIC HEALTH SERVICE INDIAN HEALTH SERVICE, p. B78
2315 UNIHEALTH, p. B79
2445 UNITED HEALTH GROUP, p. B80
1765 UNITED HOSPITAL CORPORATION, p. B80
9605 UNITED MEDICAL CORPORATION, p. B80
2085 UNITED WESTERN MEDICAL CENTERS, p. B80
9555 UNIVERSAL HEALTH SERVICES, INC., p. B80
9105 UNIVERSITY OF ALABAMA HOSPITALS, p. B81
6405 UNIVERSITY OF CALIFORNIA–SYSTEMWIDE ADMINISTRATION, p. B81
0021 UNIVERSITY OF NEW MEXICO, p. B81
0057 UNIVERSITY OF SOUTH ALABAMA HOSPITALS, p. B81
0033 UNIVERSITY OF TEXAS HOSPITALS, p. B81
0038 UPPER CHESAPEAKE HEALTH SYSTEM, p. B81
1965 UPPER VALLEY MEDICAL CENTERS, p. B81
0043 VALLEY HEALTH SYSTEM, p. B82
0026 VENCOR, INCORPORATED, p. B82
0012 VIRGINIA DEPARTMENT OF MENTAL HEALTH, p. B82
8895 VISTA HILL FOUNDATION, p. B82
6725 WEST JERSEY HEALTH SYSTEM, p. B82
0004 WEST TENNESSEE HEALTHCARE, INC., p. B83
6745 WHEATON FRANCISCAN SERVICES, INC., p. B83
9575 WILLIAM BEAUMONT HOSPITAL CORPORATION, p. B83
0068 YORK HEALTH SYSTEM, p. B83

By System Code

0001 ★ MIDMICHIGAN REGIONAL HEALTH SYSTEM 4005 Orchard Drive, Midland, MI Zip 48670; tel. 517/839-3399; Terence F. Moore, President, p. B56

0002 ★ QUORUM HEALTH GROUP/QUORUM HEALTH RESOURCES 155 Franklin Road, Suite 401, Brentwood, TN Zip 37027; tel. 615/371-7979; James E. Dalton Jr., President and Chief Executive Officer, p. B62

0003 ★ ST. DAVID'S HEALTH CARE SYSTEM 919 East 32nd Street, Austin, TX Zip 78705, Mailing Address: P.O. Box 4039, Zip 78765; tel. 512/476-7111; Jack L. Campbell, President, p. B74

0004 ★ WEST TENNESSEE HEALTHCARE, INC. 708 West Forest Avenue, Jackson, TN Zip 38301; tel. 901/425-5000; James T. Moss, President, p. B83

0006 GRADUATE HEALTH SYSTEM 2129 Chestnut Street, Philadelphia, PA Zip 19103; tel. 215/448-1500; Harold Cramer, Chairman and Chief Executive Officer, p. B42

0008 ★ CROZER–KEYSTONE HEALTH SYSTEM 1400 North Providence Road, Ste 4010, Media, PA Zip 19063-2049; tel. 610/447-2000; John C. McMeekin, President and Chief Executive Officer, p. B30

0009 NEW YORK STATE DEPARTMENT OF MENTAL HEALTH 44 Holland Avenue, Albany, NY Zip 12229; tel. 518/447-9611; Jesse Nixon Jr. Ph.D., Director, p. B57

0010 DIVISION OF MENTAL HEALTH SERVICES, DEPARTMENT OF HUMAN SERVICES, STATE OF NEW JERSEY Capital Center, CN 727, Trenton, NJ Zip 08625-0727; Alan G. Kaufman, Director, p. B38

0011 PUERTO RICO DEPARTMENT OF HEALTH Building A – Medical Center, San Juan, PR Zip 00936, Mailing Address: Call Box 70184, Zip 00936; tel. 809/274-7676; Carmen Feliciano De Melecio M.D., Secretary of Health, p. B62

0012 VIRGINIA DEPARTMENT OF MENTAL HEALTH 109 Governor Street, Richmond, VA Zip 23219, Mailing Address: P.O. Box 1797, Zip 23214; tel. 804/786-3915; King E. Davis Ph.D., Commissioner, p. B82

0013 MASSACHUSETTS DEPARTMENT OF MENTAL HEALTH 25 Staniford Street, Boston, MA Zip 02114; tel. 617/727-5500; Eileen Elias, Commissioner, p. B52

0014 CONNECTICUT STATE DEPARTMENT OF MENTAL HEALTH 90 Washington Street, Hartford, CT Zip 06106; tel. 203/566-3650; Albert J. Solnit M.D., Commissioner, p. B29

Headquarters of Health Care Systems / By System Code

0016 COOK COUNTY BUREAU OF HEALTH SERVICES 1835 West Harrison Street, Chicago, IL Zip 60612; tel. 312/633-3070; Ruth M. Rothstein, Chief, p. B30

0017 MISSISSIPPI STATE DEPARTMENT OF MENTAL HEALTH 1101 Robert E. Lee Building, Jackson, MS Zip 39201-1101; tel. 601/359-1288; Roger McMurtry, Chief Mental Health Bureau, p. B56

0018 OKLAHOMA STATE DEPARTMENT OF MENTAL HEALTH AND SUBSTANCE ABUSE SERVICES 1000 Northeast Tenth, Oklahoma City, OK Zip 73152, Mailing Address: P.O. Box 53277, Zip 73152; tel. 405/271-6868; Thomas Peace Ph.D., Commissioner, p. B59

0020 TEXAS DEPARTMENT OF HEALTH 1100 West 49th Street, Austin, TX Zip 78756; tel. 512/458-7111; David R. Smith M.D., Commissioner, p. B78

0021 UNIVERSITY OF NEW MEXICO 915 Camino De Salud, Albuquerque, NM Zip 87131; tel. 505/277-5849; Jane E. Henney M.D., Vice President Health Sciences, p. B81

0022 METROPOLITAN NASHVILLE GENERAL HOSPITAL 215 Second Avenue North, Nashville, TN Zip 37201; tel. 615/862-4000; Tom Deweese, Administrator, p. B55

0023 HEALTHSOUTH CORPORATION Two Perimeter Park South, Birmingham, AL Zip 35243; tel. 205/967-7116; Anthony J. Tanner, Executive Vice President, p. B45

0026 VENCOR, INCORPORATED 400 West Market Street, Suite 3300, Louisville, KY Zip 40202-3360; tel. 502/569-7300; W. Bruce Lunsford, Board Chairman, p. B82

0027 ★ HORIZON HEALTHCARE, INC. 2300 North Mayfair Road, Suite 550, Milwaukee, WI Zip 53226-1508; tel. 414/257-3888; Kurt W. Metzner, President and Chief Executive Officer, p. B47

0029 ★ DIMENSIONS HEALTH CORPORATION 9200 Basil Court, Landover, MD Zip 20785; tel. 301/925-7000, p. B38

0030 ★ SUN HEALTH CORPORATION 13180 North 103rd Drive, Sun City, AZ Zip 85351, Mailing Address: P.O. Box 1278, Zip 85372-1278; tel. 602/876-5352; Leland W. Peterson, President and Chief Executive Officer, p. B76

0032 NORTH MISSISSIPPI HEALTH SERVICES, INC. 830 South Gloster Street, Tupelo, MS Zip 38801; tel. 601/841-3136; Jeffrey B. Barber Ph.D., Dr.P.H., President and Chief Executive Officer, p. B58

0033 UNIVERSITY OF TEXAS HOSPITALS 601 Colorado Avenue, Austin, TX Zip 78701; tel. 512/471-4224, p. B81

0034 ★ PMH HEALTH RESOURCES, INC. 1201 South Seventh Avenue, Phoenix, AZ Zip 85007-3913, Mailing Address: P.O. Box 21207, Zip 85036-1207; tel. 602/238-3321; Reginald M. Ballantyne, President, p. B61

0036 ★ LUBBOCK METHODIST HOSPITAL SYSTEM 3615 19th Street, Lubbock, TX Zip 79410-1201; tel. 806/792-1011; William D. Poteet III FACHE, President and Chief Executive Officer, p. B51

0037 SCOTTSDALE MEMORIAL HEALTH SYSTEMS, INC. 3621 Wells Fargo Avenue, Scottsdale, AZ Zip 85251; tel. 602/481-4324; Max Poll, President and Chief Executive Officer, p. B69

0038 ★ UPPER CHESAPEAKE HEALTH SYSTEM 1916 Belair Road, Fallston, MD Zip 21047; tel. 410/893-0322; Lyle Ernest Sheldon, President and Chief Executive Officer, p. B81

0039 ★ TARRANT COUNTY HOSPITAL DISTRICT 1500 South Main Street, Fort Worth, TX Zip 76104; tel. 817/927-1230; Marion Timothy Philpot, President and Chief Executive Officer, p. B76

0040 ★ QUEEN'S HEALTH SYSTEMS 201 Merchant Street, Suite 2450, Honolulu, HI Zip 96813-2929; tel. 808/532-6102; Richard L. Griffith, Chief Executive Officer, p. B62

0041 ★ ALLINA HEALTH SYSTEM 5601 Smetana Drive, Minneapolis, MN Zip 55440, Mailing Address: P.O. Box 9310, Zip 55440-9310; tel. 612/992-2000; Gordon M. Sprenger, Executive Officer, p. B11

0042 ★ DETROIT-MACOMB HOSPITAL CORPORATION 12000 East Twelve Mile Road, Warren, MI Zip 48093; tel. 313/573-5910; Jack Ryan M.D., President and Chief Executive Officer, p. B37

0043 VALLEY HEALTH SYSTEM 1117 East Devonshire Avenue, Hemet, CA Zip 92543; tel. 909/652-2811; Geoffrey Lang, Chief Executive Officer, p. B82

0044 STERLING HEALTHCARE CORPORATION 1500 114th Avenue S.E., Suite 100, Bellevue, WA Zip 98004; tel. 206/453-5445; David Jacobsen, President, p. B75

0046 GREATER ROCHESTER HEALTH SYSTEM, INC. 1040 University Avenue, Rochester, NY Zip 14607; tel. 716/266-0720; Arthur E. Liebert, President, p. B42

0047 LOUISIANA STATE HOSPITALS 210 State Street, New Orleans, LA Zip 70118; M. E. Teague, Chief Executive Officer, p. B51

0048 ★ COLUMBIA/HCA HEALTHCARE CORPORATION One Park Plaza, Nashville, TN Zip 37203; tel. 615/320-2000; Richard Scott, President and Chief Executive Officer, p. B21

0051 ★ BJC HEALTH SYSTEM 4444 Forest Park Avenue, Saint Louis, MO Zip 63108-2259; tel. 314/286-2030; Frederick L. Brown, President & Chief Executive Officer, p. B15

0052 ★ JEWISH HOSPITAL HEALTHCARE SERVICES 217 East Chestnut Street, Louisville, KY Zip 40202; tel. 502/587-4011; Henry C. Wagner, President, p. B49

0053 ★ BLUE WATER HEALTH SERVICES CORPORATION 1001 Kearney, Port Huron, MI Zip 48060; tel. 810/989-3717; Donald C. Fletcher, President and Chief Executive Officer, p. B15

0056 ★ LAKELAND REGIONAL HEALTH SYSTEM, INC. 1234 Napier Avenue, Saint Joseph, MI Zip 49085-2158; tel. 616/983-8300; Joseph A. Wasserman, President and Chief Executive Officer, p. B50

0057 UNIVERSITY OF SOUTH ALABAMA HOSPITALS 2451 Fillingim Street, Mobile, AL Zip 36617-2293; tel. 205/471-7110; Don Ikner, Assistant Administrator Finance, p. B81

0060 ★ LIFESPAN CORPORATION 167 Point Street, Providence, RI Zip 02903; tel. 401/444-6699; William Kreykes, President and Chief Executive Officer, p. B50

0061 ★ IOWA HEALTH SYSTEM 1200 Pleasant Street, Des Moines, IA Zip 50309-1453; Samuel T. Wallace, President, p. B48

0062 ★ NORTH SHORE HEALTH SYSTEM 300 Community Drive, Manhasset, NY Zip 11030; tel. 516/562-4060; John S. T. Gallagher, President, p. B58

0063 ★ TENET HEALTHCARE CORPORATION 2700 Colorado Avenue, Santa Monica, CA Zip 90404, Mailing Address: P.O. Box 4070, Zip 90404; tel. 310/998-8000; Jeffrey Barbakow, Chairman and Chief Executive Officer, p. B76

0064 ★ ADVOCATE HEALTH CARE 2025 Windsor Drive, Oakbrook, IL Zip 60521-0222; tel. 708/990-5002; Richard R. Risk, President and Co-Chief Executive Officer, p. B10

0065 ALEXIAN BROTHERS HEALTH SYSTEM, INC. 600 Alexian Way, Elk Grove Village, IL Zip 60007-3395; tel. 708/640-7550; Brother Felix Bettendorf, President, p. B10

0066 ★ SUSQUEHANNA HEALTH SYSTEM 1001 Grampian Boulevard, Williamsport, PA Zip 17701-1946; tel. 717/320-7000; Donald R. Creamer, President and Chief Executive Officer, p. B76

0067 SINGING RIVER HOSPITAL SYSTEM 2809 Denny Avenue, Pascagoula, MS Zip 39581; tel. 601/938-5062; Robert L. Lingle, Executive Director, p. B70

0068 ★ YORK HEALTH SYSTEM 1001 South George Street, York, PA Zip 17405; tel. 717/851-2121; Bruce M. Bartels, President, p. B83

0070 ★ CARILION HEALTH SYSTEM 1212 Third Street S.W., Roanoke, VA Zip 24016, Mailing Address: P.O. Box 13727, Zip 24036-3727; tel. 703/981-7347; Thomas L. Robertson, President and Chief Executive Officer, p. B17

0075 CUMBERLAND HEALTH SYSTEMS, INC. 2100 West End Avenue, Ste 900, Nashville, TN Zip 37203; tel. 615/327-2200; Samuel W. Owen, President and Chief Executive Officer, p. B30

Headquarters of Health Care Systems / By System Code

0095 ★ BAYLOR HEALTH CARE SYSTEM 3500 Gaston Avenue, Dallas, TX Zip 75226; tel. 214/820–0111; Boone Powell Jr., President, p. B14

0135 ★ ANCILLA SYSTEMS INC. 1000 South Lake Park Avenue, Hobart, IN Zip 46342; tel. 219/947–8500; William D. Harkins, President, p. B12

0145 APPALACHIAN REGIONAL HEALTHCARE 1220 Harrodsburg Road, Lexington, KY Zip 40533, Mailing Address: Box 8086, Zip 40533–8086; tel. 606/281–2440; Forrest Calico M.D., President, p. B12

0185 BAPTIST HEALTH CARE CORPORATION 1717 North E Street, Ste 320, Pensacola, FL Zip 32501–6335; tel. 904/469–2337; James F. Vickery, President, p. B13

0205 ★ ASC HEALTH SYSTEM 6 Eagle Center, Suite 4, O'Fallon, IL Zip 62269–0406, Mailing Address: P.O. Box 670, Zip 62269–0670; tel. 618/632–1284; Gregory F. Yank, President and Chief Executive Officer, p. B12

0215 COMMUNITY CARE SYSTEMS, INC. 203 Grove Street, Wellesley, MA Zip 02181; tel. 617/239–0871; Frederick J. Thacher, Chairman, p. B28

0225 ALAMEDA COUNTY HEALTH CARE SERVICES AGENCY 499 Fifth Street, Oakland, CA Zip 94607; tel. 510/268–2722; David J. Kears, Director, p. B10

0235 ADVENTIST HEALTH SYSTEM/WEST 2100 Douglas Boulevard, Roseville, CA Zip 95661–3898, Mailing Address: P.O. Box 619002, Zip 95661–9002; tel. 916/781–2000; Frank F. Dupper, President, p. B9

0265 BAPTIST MEMORIAL HOSPITAL SYSTEM 660 North Main St, Ste 300, San Antonio, TX Zip 78205–1222; tel. 210/222–8431; Callie W. Smith, President and Chief Executive Officer, p. B14

0305 ★ OKLAHOMA HEALTH SYSTEM 3300 Northwest Expressway, Oklahoma City, OK Zip 73112; tel. 405/949–6068; Stanley F. Hupfeld, President and Chief Executive Officer, p. B58

0315 ★ BAPTIST HEALTHCARE SYSTEM 4007 Kresge Way, Louisville, KY Zip 40207–4677; tel. 502/896–5000; Tommy J. Smith, President and Chief Executive Officer, p. B13

0335 PARK HEALTHCARE COMPANY 4015 Travis Drive, Nashville, TN Zip 37211; tel. 615/833–1077; Jerry E. Gilliland, President, p. B61

0345 ★ BAPTIST HEALTH SYSTEM 3500 Blue Lake Drive, Ste 100, Birmingham, AL Zip 35243, Mailing Address: P.O. Box 830605, Zip 35283–0605; tel. 205/715–5319; Dennis A. Hall, President, p. B13

0355 ★ BAPTIST MEDICAL SYSTEM 9601 Interstate 630, Exit 7, Little Rock, AR Zip 72205–7299; tel. 501/227–2000; Russell D. Harrington Jr., President, p. B13

0395 HEALTHCARE INTERNATIONAL, INC. 912 South Capital of Texas Highway, Austin, TX Zip 78765–5210, Mailing Address: P.O. Box 4008, Zip 78765–4008; tel. 512/329–8821; Kevin Sheehan, President and Chief Executive Officer, p. B44

0405 RAMSAY HEALTH CARE, INC. 639 Loyola Avenue, Suite 1400, New Orleans, LA Zip 70113; tel. 504/585–2505; Gregory H. Browne, President and Chief Executive Officer, p. B68

0415 ★ BETHESDA HOSPITAL, INC. 619 Oak Street, Cincinnati, OH Zip 45206–1690; tel. 513/569–6141; L. Thomas Wilburn Jr., Chairman, p. B15

0435 PACIFIC HEALTH CORPORATION 249 East Ocean Boulevard, Long Beach, CA Zip 90802; tel. 310/435–1300; Jens Mueller, Chairman, p. B60

0455 HOSPITAL GROUP OF AMERICA 1265 Drummers Lane, Suite 107, Wayne, PA Zip 19087; tel. 610/687–5151; Mark R. Russell, President and Chief Executive Officer, p. B47

0515 BENEDICTINE HEALTH SYSTEM 503 East Third Street, Duluth, MN Zip 55805–1964; tel. 218/720–2370; Sister Kathleen Hofer, Chair Person and Chief Executive Officer, p. B14

0535 BENEDICTINE SISTERS St Benedicts Convent, Saint Joseph, MN Zip 56374–0277; tel. 612/363–7100; Sister Ephrem Hollermann, Prioress, p. B15

0545 BENEDICTINE SISTERS OF THE ANNUNCIATION 7520 University Drive, Bismarck, ND Zip 58504–9653; tel. 701/255–1520; Sister Susan Lardy, Prioress, p. B15

0555 ★ EASTERN MAINE HEALTHCARE 489 State Street, Bangor, ME Zip 04401; tel. 207/973–7051; Norman A. Ledwin, President, p. B38

0575 SCHICK LABORATORIES, INC. 15760 Ventura Boulevard, Suite 1201, Los Angeles, CA Zip 91436; tel. 818/382–3682; Patrick J. Frawley Jr., Chairman, p. B69

0585 ★ BRIM, INC. 305 Northeast 102nd Avenue, Portland, OR Zip 97220–4199; tel. 503/256–2070; Armand E. Brim, Chairman & Chief Executive Officer, p. B16

0595 ★ BRONSON HEALTHCARE GROUP, INC. One Healthcare Plaza, Kalamazoo, MI Zip 49007–5345; tel. 616/341–6000; Patric E. Ludwig, President, p. B17

0605 ★ SISTERS OF CHARITY OF THE INCARNATE WORD HEALTHCARE SYSTEM 2600 North Loop West, Houston, TX Zip 77092; tel. 713/681–8877; Stanley T. Urban, President and Chief Executive Officer, p. B71

0645 GLENBEIGH, INC. 4700 Congress Avenue, West Palm Beach, FL Zip 33407–3229; tel. 407/863–4747; G. Norman McCann, President, p. B41

0665 CENTURY HEALTHCARE CORPORATION 5555 East 71st Street, Suite 9220, Tulsa, OK Zip 74136–6540; tel. 918/491–0775; Jerry D. Dillon, President & Chief Executive Officer, p. B19

0675 ★ GUTHRIE HEALTHCARE SYSTEM Guthrie Square, Sayre, PA Zip 18840; tel. 717/882–4312; Ralph H. Meyer, President, p. B43

0695 CHARTER MEDICAL CORPORATION 3414 Peachtree Road N.E., Ste 1400, Atlanta, GA Zip 30326; tel. 404/841–9200; E. Mac Crawford, President and Chief Operating Officer, p. B20

0705 CHARLOTTE–MECKLENBURG HOSPITAL AUTHORITY 1000 Blythe Boulevard, Charlotte, NC Zip 28203, Mailing Address: Box 32861, Zip 28232–2861; tel. 704/355–2000; Harry A. Nurkin Ph.D., President, p. B20

0715 LOUISIANA HEALTH CARE AUTHORITY 8550 United Plaza Boulevard, 4th Floor, Baton Rouge, LA Zip 70809; tel. 504/922–0488; William Cherry M.D., Chief Executive Officer, p. B50

0735 ★ EPISCOPAL HEALTH SERVICES INC. 333 Earle Ovington Boulevard, Uniondale, NY Zip 11553–3645; tel. 516/228–6100; Jack N. Farrington Ph.D., Executive Vice President, p. B39

0775 ★ GENERAL HEALTH SYSTEM 3849 North Boulevard, Suite 200, Baton Rouge, LA Zip 70806; tel. 504/387–7806; Thomas H. Sawyer, President and Chief Executive Officer, p. B41

0785 COMMUNITY PSYCHIATRIC CENTERS 6600 West Charleston Boulevard, 1800, Las Vegas, NV Zip 89102; tel. 702/259–3600, p. B29

0805 STORMONT–VAIL HEALTH SERVICES CORPORATION 1500 Southwest Tenth Street, Topeka, KS Zip 66604–1353; tel. 913/354–6112; Howard M. Chase, President, p. B75

0845 DEVEREUX FOUNDATION 19 South Waterloo Road, Devon, PA Zip 19333, Mailing Address: Box 400, Zip 19333; tel. 610/964–3000; Ronald P. Burd, President and Chief Exeuctive Officer, p. B37

0875 COMMUNITY HEALTH SYSTEMS, INC. 3707 FM 1960 West, Suite 500, Houston, TX Zip 77068; tel. 713/537–5230; E. Thomas Chaney, President, p. B28

0905 SUMMIT MEDICAL MANAGEMENT, INC. 5 Concourse Parkway, Suite 800, Atlanta, GA Zip 30328–6111; tel. 404/392–1454; Ken Couch, Chief Executive Officer, p. B76

0935 ★ HEALTHONE HEALTHCARE SYSTEM 501 East Hampden Avenue, Englewood, CO Zip 80110, Mailing Address: P.O. Box 2901, Zip 80150–0101; tel. 303/788–6484; Nick Hilger, President and Chief Executive Officer, p. B45

Section B Index

© 1995 AHA Guide

Health Care Systems **B87**

Headquarters of Health Care Systems / By System Code

0945 EMPIRE HEALTH CENTERS GROUP West 800 Fifth Avenue, Spokane, WA Zip 99204, Mailing Address: P.O. Box 248, Zip 99210-0248; tel. 509/458-7965; Thomas M. White, President, p. B39

0955 ★ CAMCARE, INC. 501 Morris Street, Charleston, WV Zip 25301, Mailing Address: Box 1547, Zip 25326; tel. 304/348-5432; Phillip H. Goodwin, President, p. B17

0965 ★ GOOD SAMARITAN HEALTH SYSTEM 532 Race Street, San Jose, CA Zip 95126-3432; tel. 408/280-5660; Michael B. Guthrie M.D., President and Chief Executive Officer, p. B41

0985 ★ AMERIHEALTH, INC. 100 Galeria Parkway, Ste 605, Atlanta, GA Zip 30339; tel. 404/953-9600; William G. White, President, p. B11

0995 ★ PROMINA NORTHWEST HEALTH SYSTEM 1791 Mulkey Road, Suite 102, Austell, GA Zip 30001-1124; tel. 404/732-5501; Thomas E. Hill, President and Chief Executive Officer, p. B62

1015 ★ JOHNS HOPKINS HEALTH SYSTEM 600 North Wolfe Street, Baltimore, MD Zip 21287-1160; tel. 410/955-0428; James A. Block M.D., President, p. B49

1035 HORIZON HEALTH SYSTEM 26100 American Drive, Southfield, MI Zip 48086, Mailing Address: P.O. Box 5153, Zip 48086-5153; tel. 810/746-4460; Thomas W. Caulfield, President, p. B47

1045 DOCTORS HOSPITAL 1087 Dennison Avenue, Columbus, OH Zip 43201; tel. 614/297-4000; Richard A. Vincent, President, p. B38

1085 COMMUNITY HOSPITALS OF CENTRAL CALIFORNIA Fresno and R Streets, Fresno, CA Zip 93715, Mailing Address: P.O. Box 1232, Zip 93715; tel. 209/442-6000; Bruce M. Perry, Chief Executive Officer, p. B28

1095 ★ BAYSTATE HEALTH SYSTEMS, INC. 759 Chestnut Street, Springfield, MA Zip 01199-0001; tel. 413/784-0000; Michael J. Daly, President, p. B14

1125 ★ CARITAS CHRISTI HEALTH CARE SYSTEM 125 Technology Drive, Suite 5, Waltham, MA Zip 02154-8930; tel. 617/893-8544; Michael F. Collins M.D., President, p. B18

1130 ★ PRESBYTERIAN HEALTHCARE SYSTEM 8220 Walnut Hill Lane, Suite 700, Dallas, TX Zip 75231; tel. 214/345-8500; Douglas D. Hawthorne, President and Chief Executive Officer, p. B61

1155 GREENLEAF HEALTH SYSTEMS, INC. One Northgate Park, Chattanooga, TN Zip 37415; tel. 615/870-5110; Dan B. Page, President, p. B42

1165 ★ OAKWOOD HEALTHCARE SYSTEM 18101 Oakwood Boulevard, Dearborn, MI Zip 48124, Mailing Address: P.O. Box 2500, Zip 48123-2500; tel. 313/593-7000; Gerald D. Fitzgerald, President, p. B58

1195 DOMINICAN SISTERS CONGREGATION OF THE MOST HOLY NAME 1520 Grand Avenue, San Rafael, CA Zip 94901-2236; tel. 415/453-8303; Sister Kristin Wombacher, Prioress General, p. B38

1255 ESCAMBIA COUNTY HEALTH CARE AUTHORITY 1301 Belleville Avenue, Brewton, AL Zip 36426; tel. 334/368-2500; Phillip L. Parker, Administrator, p. B39

1275 FIRST HEALTH, INC. 107 Public Square, Batesville, MS Zip 38606; tel. 601/563-7676, p. B39

1295 DOMINICAN SISTERS OF SPRINGFIELD 1237 West Monroe Street, Springfield, IL Zip 62704-1680; tel. 217/787-0481; Sister Rose Miriam Schulte, Prioress General, p. B38

1305 ★ INOVA HEALTH SYSTEM 8001 Braddock Road, Springfield, VA Zip 22151; tel. 703/321-4213; J. Knox Singleton, President, p. B48

1325 ★ FAIRVIEW HOSPITAL AND HEALTHCARE SERVICES 2450 Riverside Avenue, Minneapolis, MN Zip 55454-1400; tel. 612/672-6735; Richard A. Norling, President and Chief Executive Officer, p. B39

1335 MEASE HEALTH CARE 135 Annwood Road, Palm Harbor, FL Zip 34648; tel. 813/733-1111; Philip K. Beauchamp FACHE, President and Chief Executive Officer, p. B53

1355 ★ FORBES HEALTH SYSTEM 500 Finley Street, Pittsburgh, PA Zip 15206; tel. 412/665-3320; Barry H. Roth, President, p. B40

1385 ★ ALLEGANY HEALTH SYSTEM 6200 Courtney Campbell Cswy, Tampa, FL Zip 33607-1458; tel. 813/281-9098; Sister Marie Celeste Sullivan, President and Chief Executive Officer, p. B10

1415 ★ FRANCISCAN SISTERS HEALTH CARE CORPORATION 9223 West Francis Road, Frankfort, IL Zip 60423-8334; tel. 815/469-4888; Gerald P. Pearson, President, p. B40

1455 ★ FRANCISCAN SISTERS OF CHRISTIAN CHARITY HEALTHCARE MINISTRY, INC 2409 South Alverno Road, Manitowoc, WI Zip 54220-9320; tel. 414/684-7071; Sister Laura J. Wolf, President, p. B41

1465 ★ MUNSON HEALTHCARE 1105 Sixth Street, Traverse City, MI Zip 49684-2386; tel. 616/935-5000; John M. Rockwood Jr., President, p. B56

1475 ★ FRANCISCAN MISSIONARIES OF OUR LADY HEALTH SYSTEM, INC. 4200 Essen Lane, Baton Rouge, LA Zip 70809; tel. 504/923-2701; Sister Brendan Mary Ronayne, President, p. B40

1485 ★ FRANCISCAN SISTERS OF THE POOR HEALTH SYSTEM, INC. 186 Joralemon Street, New York, NY Zip 11201-4326; tel. 718/625-6530; Sister Joanne Schuster, President, p. B41

1505 ★ SCRIPPS HOSPITALS 4275 Campus Point Court, San Diego, CA Zip 92121, Mailing Address: P.O. Box 28, La Jolla, Zip 92038; tel. 619/678-7470; Martin B. Buser, President and Chief Executive Officer, p. B69

1515 MICHIGAN CAPITAL HEALTHCARE 401 West Greenlawn, Lansing, MI Zip 48910-2819; tel. 517/334-2967; Dennis M. Litos, President and Chief Executive Officer, p. B56

1535 ★ GREAT PLAINS HEALTH ALLIANCE, INC. 625 Third, Phillipsburg, KS Zip 67661, Mailing Address: Box 366, Zip 67661-0366; tel. 913/543-2111; Roger S. John, President and Chief Executive Officer, p. B42

1555 ★ GREENVILLE HOSPITAL SYSTEM 701 Grove Road, Greenville, SC Zip 29605-4211; tel. 803/455-7000; Frank D. Pinckney, President, p. B43

1585 HEALTHCARE MANAGEMENT GROUP, INC. 776 Baconsfield Drive, Suite 209, Macon, GA Zip 31211-0101; tel. 912/743-5606; Earl Bonds Jr., Chief Executive Officer, p. B44

1625 ★ BAPTIST MEMORIAL HEALTH CARE SYSTEM, INC. 899 Madison Avenue, Memphis, TN Zip 38146; tel. 901/227-2727; Stephen Curtis Reynolds, President and Chief Executive Officer, p. B14

1685 ALBERT EINSTEIN HEALTHCARE NETWORK 5501 Old York Road, Philadelphia, PA Zip 19141-3098; tel. 215/456-7890; Martin Goldsmith, President, p. B10

1715 CONTINENTAL MEDICAL SYSTEMS, INC. 600 Wilson Lane, Mechanicsburg, PA Zip 17055-0715, Mailing Address: P.O. Box 715, Zip 17055-0715; tel. 717/790-8300; R. A. Ortenzio, Chairman and Chief Executive Officer, p. B30

1765 UNITED HOSPITAL CORPORATION 6189 East Shelby Drive, Memphis, TN Zip 38115; tel. 901/794-8440; James C. Henson, President, p. B80

1775 HEALTH MANAGEMENT ASSOCIATES 5811 Pelican Bay Boulevard, Suite 500, Naples, FL Zip 33963-2710; tel. 813/598-3175; William J. Schoen, President, p. B43

1785 ★ MASSACHUSETTS GENERAL HOSPITAL CORPORATION 32 Fruit Street, Boston, MA Zip 02114-2696; tel. 617/726-2100; Samuel O. Thier M.D., President, p. B52

1815 ★ INTERMOUNTAIN HEALTH CARE, INC. 36 South State Street, 22nd Floor, Salt Lake City, UT Zip 84111; tel. 801/533-8282; Scott S. Parker, President, p. B48

1825 ★ DCH HEALTHCARE AUTHORITY 809 University Boulevard East, Tuscaloosa, AL Zip 35401; tel. 205/759-7111; J. H. Ford Jr., Chief Executive Officer, p. B31

1855 ★ DAUGHTERS OF CHARITY NATIONAL HEALTH SYSTEM 4600 Edmundson Road, Saint Louis, MO Zip 63134, Mailing Address: P.O. Box 45998, Zip 63145-5998; tel. 314/253-6700; F. Dale Whitten, Interim President, p. B31

Headquarters of Health Care Systems / By System Code

1875 ★ MAYO FOUNDATION 200 Southwest First Street, Rochester, MN Zip 55905; tel. 507/284–2511; Robert R. Waller M.D., President and Chief Executive Officer, p. B52

1895 EAST TEXAS MEDICAL CENTER REGIONAL HEALTHCARE SYSTEM 1000 South Beckham Street, Tyler, TX Zip 75701–1996, Mailing Address: P.O. Drawer 6400, Zip 75711–6400; tel. 903/597–0351; Elmer G. Ellis, President and Chief Executive Officer, p. B38

1965 ★ UPPER VALLEY MEDICAL CENTERS 3130 North Dixie Highway, Troy, OH Zip 45373; tel. 513/332–7500; David J. Meckstroth, President, p. B81

1975 MARSHALL COUNTY HEALTH CARE AUTHORITY 8000 Alabama Highway 69, Guntersville, AL Zip 35976; tel. 205/753–8000; L. C. Couch, Board Chairman, p. B52

1985 HEALTHSYSTEM MINNESOTA 6500 Excelsior Boulevard, Saint Louis Park, MN Zip 55426–4702; tel. 612/932–6300; Robert L. Galloway, President and Administrative Officer, p. B46

2025 INFIRMARY HEALTH SYSTEM, INC. 3 Mobile Infirmary Circle, Mobile, AL Zip 36607; tel. 334/431–5500; E. Chandler Bramlett Jr., President, p. B48

2055 MICHIGAN HEALTH CARE CORPORATION 7430 Second Avenue, Ste 610, Detroit, MI Zip 48202; tel. 313/874–9110; Charles E. Housley FACHE, President and Chief Executive Officer, p. B56

2065 ★ SHARP HEALTHCARE 3131 Berger Avenue, Suite 100, San Diego, CA Zip 92123; tel. 619/541–4000; Peter K. Ellsworth, President, p. B69

2075 ★ NORTHBAY HEALTHCARE SYSTEM 1200 B Gale Wilson Boulevard, Fairfield, CA Zip 94533–3587; tel. 707/429–3600; Gary J. Passama, President, p. B58

2085 UNITED WESTERN MEDICAL CENTERS 1001 North Tustin Avenue, Santa Ana, CA Zip 92705–3502; tel. 714/953–3610; David E. Morgan, Chief Executive Officer, p. B80

2105 ★ KAISER FOUNDATION HOSPITALS One Kaiser Plaza, Oakland, CA Zip 94612–3600; tel. 510/271–5990; David M. Lawrence M.D., Chairman and Chief Executive Officer, p. B49

2115 FREMONT–RIDEOUT HEALTH GROUP 989 Plumas Street, Yuba City, CA Zip 95991; tel. 916/751–4010; Thomas P. Hayes, Chief Executive Officer, p. B41

2135 ★ CAPITAL HEALTH SYSTEM 17 South Market Square, Harrisburg, PA Zip 17101, Mailing Address: P.O. Box 8700, Zip 17105–8700; tel. 717/782–3366; John S. Cramer FACHE, President and Chief Executive Officer, p. B17

2145 ★ DETROIT MEDICAL CENTER 4201 St. Antoine Boulevard, Detroit, MI Zip 48201–2194; tel. 313/745–5192; David J. Campbell, President and Chief Executive Officer, p. B37

2155 BAPTIST HEALTH SYSTEM OF TENNESSEE 137 Blount Avenue S.E., Knoxville, TN Zip 37920, Mailing Address: Box 1788, Zip 37901; tel. 615/632–5099; Dale Collins, President & Chief Executive Officer, p. B13

2175 ADVENTIST HEALTH SYSTEM–LOMA LINDA 11161 Anderson Street, Loma Linda, CA Zip 92350; tel. 909/824–4459; David B. Hinshaw Sr. M.D., President, p. B9

2185 ★ HEALTHEAST 559 Capitol Boulevard, 6–South, Saint Paul, MN Zip 55103–0000; tel. 612/232–2300; Tim Hanson, President and Chief Executive Officer, p. B45

2205 ★ TIDEWATER HEALTH CARE, INC. 1080 First Colonial Road, Virginia Beach, VA Zip 23454–3001; tel. 804/496–6200; Douglas L. Johnson Ph.D., President and Chief Executive Officer, p. B78

2215 ★ AURORA HEALTH CARE, INC. 3000 West Montana, Milwaukee, WI Zip 53215–3268, Mailing Address: P.O. Box 343910, Zip 53234–3910; tel. 414/647–3000; G. Edwin Howe, President, p. B12

2235 ★ LUTHERAN HEALTH SYSTEMS 4310 17th Avenue S.W., Fargo, ND Zip 58103, Mailing Address: P.O. Box 6200, Zip 58106–6200; tel. 701/277–7500; Steven R. Orr, President, p. B51

2255 ★ ST. FRANCIS HEALTH SYSTEM 4401 Penn Avenue, Pittsburgh, PA Zip 15224–1334; tel. 412/622–4212; Sister M. Rosita Wellinger, President, p. B74

2265 ★ CENTRA HEALTH, INC. 1920 Atherholt Road, Lynchburg, VA Zip 24501–1104; tel. 804/947–4700; George W. Dawson, President and Chief Executive Officer, p. B19

2285 ★ ALLIANT HEALTH SYSTEM 234 East Gray Street, Ste 225, Louisville, KY Zip 40202, Mailing Address: P.O. Box 35070, Zip 40232–5070; tel. 502/629–2000; Stephen A. Williams, President, p. B10

2295 LITTLE COMPANY OF MARY SISTERS HEALTHCARE SYSTEM 9350 South California Avenue, Evergreen Park, IL Zip 60642; tel. 708/422–6200; Sister Nancy Boyle, Provincialate Superior, p. B50

2305 ALLEGHENY HEALTH, EDUCATION AND RESEARCH FOUNDATION 120 Fifth Avenue, Pittsburgh, PA Zip 15222; tel. 412/359–6000; Sherif S. Abdelhak, President, p. B10

2315 ★ UNIHEALTH 3400 Riverside Drive, Burbank, CA Zip 91505; tel. 818/238–6000; Terry Hartshorn, President and Chief Executive Officer, p. B79

2335 MEMORIAL HEALTH SERVICES 706 North Parrish Avenue, Adel, GA Zip 31620, Mailing Address: Box 677, Zip 31620; tel. 912/896–2251; James E. Cunningham, Chief Executive Officer, p. B53

2345 ★ HARRIS METHODIST HEALTH SYSTEM 6000 Western Place, Suite 200, Fort Worth, TX Zip 76107; tel. 817/570–8900; Ronald L. Smith, President, p. B43

2355 ★ HELIX HEALTH SYSTEM 2330 West Joppa Road, Ste 301, Lutherville, MD Zip 21093; tel. 410/296–6050; James A. Oakey, President, p. B46

2415 JEWISH HEALTH SYSTEMS, INC. 3200 Burnet Avenue, Cincinnati, OH Zip 45229–3099; tel. 513/569–2434; Warren C. Falberg, President, p. B49

2435 ★ BERKSHIRE HEALTH SYSTEMS, INC. 725 North Street, Pittsfield, MA Zip 01201; tel. 413/447–2743; David E. Phelps, President and Chief Executive Officer, p. B15

2445 ★ UNITED HEALTH GROUP Five Innovation Court, Appleton, WI Zip 54914, Mailing Address: P.O. Box 8025, Zip 54913–8025; tel. 414/730–0330; James Edward Raney, President and Chief Executive Officer, p. B80

2455 BRADFORD PARKSIDE 2101 Magnolia Ave S, Ste 518, Birmingham, AL Zip 35205; tel. 205/251–7753; Jerry W. Crowder, President and Chief Executive Officer, p. B16

2485 ★ HEARTLAND HEALTH SYSTEM 5325 Faraon, Saint Joseph, MO Zip 64506; tel. 816/271–6000; Lowell C. Kruse, President, p. B46

2515 FAIRVIEW HEALTH SYSTEM 18101 Lorain Avenue, Cleveland, OH Zip 44111–5656; tel. 216/476–4040; Thomas M. LaMotte, President and Chief Executive Officer, p. B39

2535 ★ SAMARITAN HEALTH SYSTEM 1441 North 12th Street, Phoenix, AZ Zip 85006–2666; tel. 602/495–4000; James C. Crews, President and Chief Executive Officer, p. B68

2565 ★ SENTARA HEALTH SYSTEM 6015 Poplar Hall Drive, Norfolk, VA Zip 23502; tel. 804/455–7000; David L. Bernd, President and Chief Executive Officer, p. B69

2575 CARLE FOUNDATION 611 West Park Street, Urbana, IL Zip 61801–2595; tel. 217/383–3311; Michael H. Fritz, President, p. B18

2615 ★ MEMORIAL HEALTH SYSTEMS 875 Sterthaus Avenue, Ormond Beach, FL Zip 32174–5197; tel. 904/676–6114; Richard A. Lind, President and Chief Executive Officer, p. B53

2635 FIRST HOSPITAL CORPORATION 240 Corporate Boulevard, Norfolk, VA Zip 23502; tel. 804/459–5100; Ronald Dozoretz M.D., Chairman, p. B39

2645 ★ MEMORIAL HEALTHCARE SYSTEM 7737 Southwest Freeway, Ste 200, Houston, TX Zip 77074–1800; tel. 713/776–6992; Dan S. Wilford, President, p. B53

Headquarters of Health Care Systems / By System Code

2715 METHODIST HEALTH SYSTEM 580 West Eighth Street, Jacksonville, FL Zip 32209–6553; tel. 904/798–8000; Marcus E. Drewa, President, p. B55

2735 ★ METHODIST HOSPITALS OF DALLAS 1441 North Beckley, Dallas, TX Zip 75203, Mailing Address: P.O. Box 655999, Zip 75265–5999; tel. 214/947–8181; David H. Hitt, President and Chief Executive Officer, p. B55

2755 ★ LEGACY HEALTH SYSTEM 1919 N.W. Lovejoy Street, Portland, OR Zip 97209–1503; tel. 503/225–8600; John G. King, President and Chief Executive Officer, p. B50

2795 HEALTHCORP OF TENNESSEE, INC. 735 Broad Street, Chattanooga, TN Zip 37402; tel. 615/267–8406; T. Farrell Hayes, President, p. B44

2855 MISSIONARY BENEDICTINE SISTERS AMERICAN PROVINCE 300 North 18th Street, Norfolk, NE Zip 68701; tel. 402/371–3438; Sister M. Agnes Falber, Prioress, p. B56

3045 ★ SISTERS OF CHARITY OF NAZARETH HEALTH SYSTEM 135 West Drive, Nazareth, KY Zip 40048, Mailing Address: P.O. Box 171, Zip 40048–0171; tel. 502/349–6250; Mark W. Dundon, President and Chief Executive Officer, p. B71

3075 NEW YORK CITY HEALTH AND HOSPITALS CORPORATION 125 Worth Street, Room 514, New York, NY Zip 10013; tel. 212/788–3321; Bruce Siegel M.D., M.P.H., President, p. B57

3115 ★ NORTH BROWARD HOSPITAL DISTRICT 303 Southeast 17th Street, Fort Lauderdale, FL Zip 33316–2510; tel. 305/355–5100; G. Wil Trower, President and Chief Executive Officer, p. B57

3175 NEPONSET VALLEY HEALTH SYSTEM 800 Washington Street, Norwood, MA Zip 02062–3487; tel. 617/769–4000; Yolanda Landrau R.N., Ed.D., President and Chief Executive Officer, p. B56

3355 ★ ORLANDO REGIONAL HEALTHCARE SYSTEM 1414 Kuhl Avenue, Orlando, FL Zip 32806–2093; tel. 407/841–5111; J. Gary Strack, President and Chief Executive Officer, p. B59

3505 ★ PRESBYTERIAN HEALTHCARE SERVICES 5901 Harper Drive N.E., Albuquerque, NM Zip 87109, Mailing Address: P.O. Box 26666, Zip 87125–6666; tel. 505/260–6300; James Hinton, President and Chief Executive Officer, p. B61

3555 STATE OF HAWAII, DEPARTMENT OF HEALTH 1250 Punchbowl Street, Honolulu, HI Zip 96813; tel. 808/586–4416; Fred D. Horwitz, Deputy Director, p. B75

3595 ★ EASTERN MERCY HEALTH SYSTEM 3 Radnor Corporate Center, Suite 220, Radnor, PA Zip 19087; tel. 610/971–9770; Daniel F. Russell, President, p. B38

3775 MILWAUKEE COUNTY BOARD OF SUPERVISORS 901 North Ninth Street, Milwaukee, WI Zip 53233; tel. 414/278–4244; F. Thomas Ament, County Executive, p. B56

3855 ★ RUSH–PRESBYTERIAN–ST. LUKE'S MEDICAL CENTER 1653 West Congress Parkway, Chicago, IL Zip 60612–3864; tel. 312/942–5000; Leo M. Henikoff M.D., President, p. B68

4025 ★ SERVANTCOR 175 South Wall Street, Kankakee, IL Zip 60901–3470; tel. 815/937–2034; Joseph S. Feth, President, p. B69

4125 ★ SHRINERS HOSPITALS FOR CRIPPLED CHILDREN 2900 Rocky Point Drive, Tampa, FL Zip 33607–1435, Mailing Address: Box 31356, Zip 33631–3356; tel. 813/281–0300; Jack D. Hoard, Executive Administrator, p. B69

4155 ★ BAPTIST HEALTH CARE SYSTEM OF SOUTH CAROLINA Taylor At Marion Street, Columbia, SC Zip 29220; tel. 803/771–5010; Charles D. Beaman Jr., President and Chief Executive Officer, p. B13

4165 ★ ADVENTIST HEALTH SYSTEM–SUNBELT HEALTH CARE CORPORATION 111 North Orlando Avenue, Winter Park, FL Zip 32789–3675; tel. 407/897–1919; Mardian J. Blair, President, p. B9

4175 ★ SOUTHERN ILLINOIS HOSPITAL SERVICES 608 East College Street, Carbondale, IL Zip 62901, Mailing Address: P.O. Box 3988, Zip 62902–3988; tel. 618/457–5200; John J. Buckley Jr., President, p. B74

4195 ★ SPARTANBURG HOSPITAL SYSTEM 101 East Wood Street, Spartanburg, SC Zip 29303–3016; tel. 803/560–6000; Joseph Michael Oddis, President, p. B74

4810 RIVERSIDE HEALTH SYSTEM 606 Denbigh Boulevard, Suite 601, Newport News, VA Zip 23602; tel. 804/875–7500; Nelson L. St. Clair, President, p. B68

5085 ★ BON SECOURS HEALTH SYSTEM, INC. 1505 Marriottsville Road, Marriottsville, MD Zip 21104–1399; tel. 410/442–5511; John L. Fitzgerald, President & Chief Executive Officer, p. B15

5095 ★ SISTERS OF CHARITY OF LEAVENWORTH HEALTH SERVICES CORPORATION 4200 South Fourth Street, Leavenworth, KS Zip 66048–5054; tel. 913/682–1338; Sister Marie Damian Glatt, President, p. B71

5115 ★ SISTERS OF CHARITY HEALTH CARE SYSTEMS, INC. 345 Neeb Road, Cincinnati, OH Zip 45233–5102; tel. 513/347–1000; Sister Celestia Koebel, President, p. B70

5125 SISTERS OF CHARITY OF ST. AUGUSTINE HEALTH SYSTEM 2351 East 22nd Street, Cleveland, OH Zip 44115; tel. 216/696–5560; Peter G. Reibold, President, p. B71

5155 ★ MERCY HEALTH SYSTEM 2335 Grandview Ave, 4th Floor, Cincinnati, OH Zip 45206–2280; tel. 513/221–2736; Michael D. Connelly, President and Chief Executive Officer, p. B54

5165 ★ MERCY HEALTH SERVICES 34605 Twelve Mile Road, Farmington Hills, MI Zip 48331–3221; tel. 810/489–6000; Judith Pelham, President and Chief Executive Officer, p. B53

5175 ★ CATHOLIC HEALTH CORPORATION 920 South 107th Avenue, Omaha, NE Zip 68114–4719; tel. 402/393–7661; A. Diane Moeller, Chief Executive Officer, p. B18

5185 ★ SISTERS OF MERCY HEALTH SYSTEM–ST. LOUIS 2039 North Geyer Road, Saint Louis, MO Zip 63131–3399; tel. 314/965–6100; Sister Mary Roch Rocklage, Chief Executive Officer, p. B72

5205 ★ CATHOLIC HEALTHCARE WEST 1700 Montgomery Street, Suite 300, San Francisco, CA Zip 94111–9603; tel. 415/397–9000; Richard J. Kramer, President and Chief Executive Officer, p. B19

5215 ★ MERCY–CHICAGO REGION HEALTHCARE SYSTEM 55 Shuman Boulevard, Ste 150, Naperville, IL Zip 60563–8469; tel. 708/355–6310; Sister Catherine C. Gallagher, President, p. B54

5255 ★ PRESENTATION HEALTH SYSTEM 1301 South Ninth Ave, Suite 102, Sioux Falls, SD Zip 57105–1043; tel. 605/331–4999; John T. Porter, President, p. B62

5265 ★ PROVIDENCE SERVICES 9 East Ninth Avenue, Spokane, WA Zip 99202; tel. 509/455–4884; Richard J. Umbdenstock, President and Chief Executive Officer, p. B62

5275 ★ SISTERS OF PROVIDENCE HEALTH SYSTEM 520 Pike Street, Seattle, WA Zip 98101, Mailing Address: P.O. Box 11038, Zip 98111–9038; tel. 206/464–3355; Sister Dona Taylor, President and Chief Executive Officer, p. B72

5285 ★ SISTERS OF PROVIDENCE HEALTH SYSTEM 146 Chestnut Street, Springfield, MA Zip 01103; tel. 413/737–3981; Sister Kathleen Popko, President and Chief Executive Officer, p. B72

5305 ★ SISTERS OF THE SORROWFUL MOTHER UNITED STATES HEALTH SYSTEM P.O. Box 4753, Tulsa, OK Zip 74159–0753; tel. 918/742–9988; Sister M. Therese Gottschalk, President, p. B73

5325 ★ FRANCISCAN HEALTH SYSTEM One MacIntyre Drive, Chester, PA Zip 19014–1196; tel. 610/358–4223; Ronald R. Aldrich, President and Chief Executive Officer, p. B40

5335 ★ OSF HEALTHCARE SYSTEM 800 Northeast Glen Oak Avenue, Peoria, IL Zip 61603–3200; tel. 309/655–2850; Sister Frances Marie Masching, President, p. B60

Headquarters of Health Care Systems / By System Code

5345 ★ SISTERS OF ST. FRANCIS HEALTH SERVICES, INC. 1515 Dragoon Trail, Mishawaka, IN Zip 46546–1290, Mailing Address: P.O. Box 1290, Zip 46546–1290; tel. 219/256–3935; Sister Jane Marie Klein, President, p. B73

5355 ★ HOSPITAL SISTERS HEALTH SYSTEM Sangamon Avenue Road, Springfield, IL Zip 62794, Mailing Address: Box 19431, Zip 62794–9431; tel. 217/522–6969; Sister Jomary Trstensky, President, p. B47

5375 ★ FRANCISCAN SERVICES CORPORATION 6832 Convent Boulevard, Sylvania, OH Zip 43560–2897; tel. 419/882–8373; John W. O'Connell, President, p. B40

5415 ★ PEACEHEALTH 15325 Southeast 30th Place, Suite 300, Bellevue, WA Zip 98007; tel. 206/747–1711; Sister Monica Heeran, President, p. B61

5425 ★ ST. JOSEPH HEALTH SYSTEM 440 South Batavia Street, Orange, CA Zip 92668–3995, Mailing Address: P.O. Box 14132, Zip 92613–1532; tel. 714/997–7690; Richard Statuto, Chief Executive Officer, p. B75

5435 ★ CSJ HEALTH SYSTEM OF WICHITA 3720 East Bayley, Wichita, KS Zip 67218–3087; tel. 316/689–4000; LeRoy E. Rheault, President and Chief Executive Officer, p. B30

5455 ★ SSM HEALTH CARE SYSTEM 477 North Lindbergh Boulevard, Saint Louis, MO Zip 63141–7813; tel. 314/994–7800; Sister Mary Jean Ryan, President and Chief Executive Officer, p. B74

5555 ★ SISTERS OF ST. JOSEPH HEALTH SYSTEM 455 East Eisenhower Parkway, Suite 300, Ann Arbor, MI Zip 48108–3304; tel. 313/741–1160; John S. Lore, President and Chief Executive Officer, p. B73

5565 ★ INCARNATE WORD HEALTH SERVICES 9311 San Pedro, Suite 1250, San Antonio, TX Zip 78216–4469; tel. 210/524–4100; Joseph Blasko Jr., President and Chief Executive Officer, p. B47

5570 ★ GEISINGER HEALTH CARE SYSTEM 100 North Academy Avenue, Danville, PA Zip 17822–3311; tel. 717/271–6211; Frank J. Trembulak, Chief Operating Officer, p. B41

5575 SISTERS OF THE HOLY FAMILY OF NAZARETH–SACRED HEART PROVINCE 353 North River Road, Des Plaines, IL Zip 60016–1291; tel. 708/298–6760; Sister M. Lucille Madura, Provincial Superior, p. B73

5585 ★ HOLY CROSS HEALTH SYSTEM CORPORATION 3606 East Jefferson Boulevard, South Bend, IN Zip 46615–3097; tel. 219/233–8558; Sister Patricia Vandenberg, President and Chief Executive Officer, p. B46

5645 ★ HUMILITY OF MARY HEALTH CARE CORPORATION 1919 Reid Avenue, Lorain, OH Zip 44052, Mailing Address: P.O. Box 841, Zip 44052–0841; tel. 216/245–3569; Sister Frances Flanigan, President and Chief Executive Officer, p. B47

5695 CONGREGATION OF ST. AGNES 475 Gillett Street, Fond Du Lac, WI Zip 54935–4598; tel. 414/923–0804; Rosann Geiser, Corporate Director, p. B29

5755 LOS ANGELES COUNTY–DEPARTMENT OF HEALTH SERVICES 313 North Figueroa Street, Room 936, Los Angeles, CA Zip 90012; tel. 213/240–8101; Robert C. Gates, Director Health, p. B50

5765 PARACELSUS HEALTHCARE CORPORATION 155 North Lake Ave, Suite 1100, Pasadena, CA Zip 91101; tel. 818/792–8600; R. J. Messenger, President and Chief Executive Officer, p. B60

5805 SISTERS OF MARY OF THE PRESENTATION HEALTH CORPORATION 1102 Page Drive S.W., Fargo, ND Zip 58106–0007, Mailing Address: P.O. Box 10007, Zip 58106–0007; tel. 701/237–9290; Aaron Alton, President, p. B71

5845 ST. LUKE'S HEALTH SYSTEM, INC. 2720 Stone Park Boulevard, Sioux City, IA Zip 51104–2000; tel. 712/279–3500; David O. Biorn FACHE, President and Chief Executive Officer, p. B75

5885 ★ COVENANT HEALTH SYSTEMS, INC. 10 Pelham Road, Lexington, MA Zip 02173–5799; tel. 617/862–1634; David R. Lincoln, President, p. B30

5895 HALLMARK HEALTHCARE CORPORATION 300 Galleria Parkway, Suite 650, Atlanta, GA Zip 30339–5949, Mailing Address: P.O. Box 723049, Zip 30339–0049; tel. 404/933–5500; James T. McAfee Jr., Chairman and Chief Executive Officer, p. B43

5945 ★ CARONDELET HEALTH SYSTEM 13801 Riverport Drive, Ste 300, Saint Louis, MO Zip 63043–4810; tel. 314/770–0333; Gary Christiansen, President, p. B18

5955 SISTERS OF THE 3RD FRANCISCAN ORDER 2500 Grant Boulevard, Syracuse, NY Zip 13208–1713; tel. 315/425–0115; Sister Grace Anne Dillenschneider, General Superior, p. B73

5985 SISTERS OF MERCY 431 East Wilkinson Boulevard, Belmont, NC Zip 28012; tel. 704/829–5103; Sister Pauline Clifford, Regional President, p. B72

5995 SISTERS OF CHARITY CENTER Mount St Vincent on Hudson, New York, NY Zip 10471–1093; tel. 718/549–9200; Sister Carol Barnes, President, p. B70

6015 SISTERS OF MERCY OF THE AMERICAS–REGIONAL COMMUNITY OF BALTIMORE 1300 Northern Parkway, Baltimore, MD Zip 21239, Mailing Address: P.O. Box 11448, Zip 21239; tel. 410/435–4400; Sister Margaret Beatty, President, p. B72

6095 ★ SISTERS OF CHARITY HEALTH CARE SYSTEM CORPORATION 75 Vanderbilt Avenue, New York, NY Zip 10304–3850; tel. 718/390–5080; John J. DePierro, President and Chief Executive Officer, p. B70

6405 UNIVERSITY OF CALIFORNIA–SYSTEMWIDE ADMINISTRATION 300 Lakeside Drive, 18th Floor, Oakland, CA Zip 94612–3550; tel. 510/987–9701; Cornelius L. Hopper M.D., Vice President Health Affairs, p. B81

6525 ORNDA HEALTHCORP 3401 West End Avenue, Suite 700, Nashville, TN Zip 37203; tel. 615/383–8599; Elizabeth A. Berryman, Assistant Vice President and General Counsel, p. B59

6545 ★ CATHEDRAL HEALTHCARE SYSTEM, INC. 219 Chestnut Street, Newark, NJ Zip 07105–1558; tel. 201/690–3600; Frank L. Fumai, President and Chief Executive Officer, p. B18

6555 MULTICARE HEALTH SYSTEM 315 Martin Luther King Jr Way, Tacoma, WA Zip 98405, Mailing Address: P.O. Box 5299, Zip 98405–0299; tel. 206/552–1000; William B. Connoley, President, p. B56

6615 ★ MEDLANTIC HEALTHCARE GROUP 100 Irving Street N.W., Washington, DC Zip 20010–2975; tel. 202/877–6006; John P. McDaniel, Chief Executive Officer, p. B53

6725 ★ WEST JERSEY HEALTH SYSTEM 1000 Atlantic Avenue, Camden, NJ Zip 08104; tel. 609/342–4604; Barry D. Brown, President and Chief Executive Officer, p. B82

6745 ★ WHEATON FRANCISCAN SERVICES, INC. 26W171 Roosevelt Road, Wheaton, IL Zip 60189–0667, Mailing Address: P.O. Box 667, Zip 60189–0667; tel. 708/462–9271; Wilfred F. Loebig Jr., President and Chief Executive Officer, p. B83

6995 DEPARTMENT OF HEALTH AND HOSPITALS 818 Harrison Avenue, Boston, MA Zip 02118; tel. 617/534–5365; Lawrence Dwyer, Commissioner, p. B32

7235 ★ METHODIST HOSPITAL SYSTEM 6565 Fannin Street, Houston, TX Zip 77030; tel. 713/790–2221; Larry L. Mathis FACHE, President & Chief Executive Officer, p. B55

7555 ★ PALOMAR POMERADO HEALTH SYSTEM 15255 Innovation Drive, Suite 204, San Diego, CA Zip 92128–3410; tel. 619/675–5100; Andrew W. Deems, President and Chief Executive Officer, p. B60

7775 ★ MAIN LINE HEALTH 259 Radnor–Chester Road, Suite 290, Radnor, PA Zip 19087–5260; tel. 610/293–8200; Douglas S. Peters, President and Chief Executive Officer, p. B52

7895 ★ AVMED–SANTA FE 8930 Northwest 39th Avenue, Gainesville, FL Zip 32606, Mailing Address: P.O. Box 749, Zip 32602–0749; tel. 904/372–8400; Edward C. Peddie, President, p. B12

8285 ★ METROHEALTH SYSTEM 2500 Metrohealth Drive, Cleveland, OH Zip 44109; tel. 216/459–8050; Terry R. White, President and Chief Executive Officer, p. B55

Section B Index

© 1995 AHA Guide

Health Care Systems B91

Headquarters of Health Care Systems / By System Code—Geographically by City and State

8795 SUTTER HEALTH 2800 L Street, Sacramento, CA Zip 95816, Mailing Address: P.O. Box 160727, Zip 95816; tel. 916/733–8800; Van R. Johnson, President and Chief Executive Officer, p. B76

8805 COLUMBUS–CABRINI MEDICAL CENTER 2520 North Lakeview Avenue, Chicago, IL Zip 60614; tel. 312/883–8366; Lee Domanico, Chief Executive Officer, p. B28

8810 ★ BAPTIST HOSPITALS AND HEALTH SYSTEMS, INC. 2224 West Northern Ave, Ste D–300, Phoenix, AZ Zip 85021; tel. 602/864–1184; Gerald L. Wissink, President and Chief Executive Officer, p. B13

8815 ★ HEALTH MIDWEST 2304 East Meyer Boulevard, Suite A–20, Kansas City, MO Zip 64132–4104; tel. 816/276–9181; Richard W. Brown, President and Chief Executive Officer, p. B44

8835 ★ MERIDIA HEALTH SYSTEM 6700 Beta Drive, Suite 200, Mayfield Village, OH Zip 44143; tel. 216/446–8000; Richard J. McCann, President, p. B55

8855 ★ JFK HEALTH SYSTEMS, INC. 80 James Street, 2nd Floor, Edison, NJ Zip 08820–3998; tel. 908/632–1500; John P. McGee, President and Chief Executive Officer, p. B49

8875 METHODIST HEALTH SERVICES CORPORATION 221 N.E. Glen Oak Avenue, Peoria, IL Zip 61636; tel. 309/672–4826; Robert E. Wierman, President, p. B55

8895 VISTA HILL FOUNDATION 2355 Northside Drive, 3rd Floor, San Diego, CA Zip 92108; tel. 619/563–1770; Ronald E. Fickle, President, p. B82

9095 ★ U.S. HEALTH CORPORATION 3555 Olentangy River Rd, 4000, Columbus, OH Zip 43214; tel. 614/566–5424; Erie Chapman, President and Chief Executive Officer, p. B78

9105 ★ UNIVERSITY OF ALABAMA HOSPITALS 619 South 19th Street, Birmingham, AL Zip 35233; tel. 205/975–7545; Kevin E. Lofton, Executive Director, p. B81

9195 U.S. PUBLIC HEALTH SERVICE INDIAN HEALTH SERVICE 2275 Research Boulevard, Rockville, MD Zip 20850, p. B78

9255 ★ TRUMAN MEDICAL CENTER 2301 Holmes Street, Kansas City, MO Zip 64108–2677; tel. 816/556–3153; James J. Mongan M.D., Director, p. B78

9295 DEPARTMENT OF VETERANS AFFAIRS 810 Vermont Avenue N.W., Washington, DC Zip 20420; tel. 202/273–5786; Kenneth W. Kizer M.D., M.P.H., Under Secretary for Health, p. B34

9345 ★ METHODIST HEALTH SYSTEMS, INC. 1211 Union Avenue, Suite 700, Memphis, TN Zip 38104; tel. 901/726–2300; Maurice W. Elliott, President, p. B55

9395 DEPARTMENT OF THE ARMY Washington, DC Zip 20314; tel. 703/756–8210, p. B33

9495 DEPARTMENT OF THE AIR FORCE Washington, DC Zip 20333; tel. 202/767–5066, p. B32

9505 ★ HENRY FORD HEALTH SYSTEM One Ford Place, Detroit, MI Zip 48202; tel. 313/876–8700; Gail L. Warden, President and Chief Executive Officer, p. B46

9555 UNIVERSAL HEALTH SERVICES, INC. 367 South Gulph Road, King of Prussia, PA Zip 19406; tel. 610/768–3300; Alan B. Miller, President and Chief Executive Officer, p. B80

9575 ★ WILLIAM BEAUMONT HOSPITAL CORPORATION 3601 West Thirteen Mile Road, Royal Oak, MI Zip 48073–6769; tel. 810/551–5000; Kenneth E. Myers, President, p. B83

9605 UNITED MEDICAL CORPORATION 603 Main Street, Windermere, FL Zip 34786, Mailing Address: P.O. Box 1100, Zip 34786–1100; tel. 407/876–2200; Donald R. Dizney, Chairman, p. B80

9650 ★ FRANCISCAN HEALTH SYSTEM, INC. 615 South Tenth Street, La Crosse, WI Zip 54601–4786; tel. 608/791–9710; Brian C. Campion M.D., Chief Executive Officer, p. B40

9655 DEPARTMENT OF NAVY Washington, DC Zip 20066, p. B32

9995 ★ GROUP HEALTH COOPERATIVE OF PUGET SOUND 521 Wall Street, Seattle, WA Zip 98121–1536; tel. 206/326–3000; Phil Nudelman Ph.D., President and Chief Executive Officer, p. B43

Geographically

United States

ALABAMA

Birmingham: 0345 ★ BAPTIST HEALTH SYSTEM 3500 Blue Lake Drive, Ste 100, Zip 35243, Mailing Address: P.O. Box 830605, Zip 35283–0605; tel. 205/715–5319; Dennis A. Hall, President, p. B13

2455 BRADFORD PARKSIDE 2101 Magnolia Ave S, Ste 518, Zip 35205; tel. 205/251–7753; Jerry W. Crowder, President and Chief Executive Officer, p. B16

0023 HEALTHSOUTH CORPORATION Two Perimeter Park South, Zip 35243; tel. 205/967–7116; Anthony J. Tanner, Executive Vice President, p. B45

9105 ★ UNIVERSITY OF ALABAMA HOSPITALS 619 South 19th Street, Zip 35233; tel. 205/975–7545; Kevin E. Lofton, Executive Director, p. B81

Brewton: 1255 ESCAMBIA COUNTY HEALTH CARE AUTHORITY 1301 Belleville Avenue, Zip 36426; tel. 334/368–2500; Phillip L. Parker, Administrator, p. B39

Guntersville: 1975 MARSHALL COUNTY HEALTH CARE AUTHORITY 8000 Alabama Highway 69, Zip 35976; tel. 205/753–8000; L. C. Couch, Board Chairman, p. B52

Mobile: 2025 INFIRMARY HEALTH SYSTEM, INC. 3 Mobile Infirmary Circle, Zip 36607; tel. 334/431–5500; E. Chandler Bramlett Jr., President, p. B48

0057 UNIVERSITY OF SOUTH ALABAMA HOSPITALS 2451 Fillingim Street, Zip 36617–2293; tel. 205/471–7110; Don Ikner, Assistant Administrator Finance, p. B81

Tuscaloosa: 1825 ★ DCH HEALTHCARE AUTHORITY 809 University Boulevard East, Zip 35401; tel. 205/759–7111; J. H. Ford Jr., Chief Executive Officer, p. B31

ARIZONA

Phoenix: 8810 ★ BAPTIST HOSPITALS AND HEALTH SYSTEMS, INC. 2224 West Northern Ave, Ste D–300, Zip 85021; tel. 602/864–1184; Gerald L. Wissink, President and Chief Executive Officer, p. B13

0034 ★ PMH HEALTH RESOURCES, INC. 1201 South Seventh Avenue, Zip 85007–3913, Mailing Address: P.O. Box 21207, Zip 85036–1207; tel. 602/238–3321; Reginald M. Ballantyne III, President, p. B61

2535 ★ SAMARITAN HEALTH SYSTEM 1441 North 12th Street, Zip 85006–2666; tel. 602/495–4000; James C. Crews, President and Chief Executive Officer, p. B68

Scottsdale: 0037 SCOTTSDALE MEMORIAL HEALTH SYSTEMS, INC. 3621 Wells Fargo Avenue, Zip 85251; tel. 602/481–4324; Max Poll, President and Chief Executive Officer, p. B69

Sun City: 0030 ★ SUN HEALTH CORPORATION 13180 North 103rd Drive, Zip 85351, Mailing Address: P.O. Box 1278, Zip 85372–1278; tel. 602/876–5352; Leland W. Peterson, President and Chief Executive Officer, p. B76

Headquarters of Health Care Systems / Geographically by City and State

ARKANSAS

Little Rock: 0355 ★ BAPTIST MEDICAL SYSTEM 9601 Interstate 630, Exit 7, Zip 72205-7299; tel. 501/227-2000; Russell D. Harrington Jr., President, p. B13

CALIFORNIA

Burbank: 2315 ★ UNIHEALTH 3400 Riverside Drive, Zip 91505; tel. 818/238-6000; Terry Hartshorn, President and Chief Executive Officer, p. B79

Fairfield: 2075 ★ NORTHBAY HEALTHCARE SYSTEM 1200 B Gale Wilson Boulevard, Zip 94533-3587; tel. 707/429-3600; Gary J. Passama, President, p. B58

Fresno: 1085 COMMUNITY HOSPITALS OF CENTRAL CALIFORNIA Fresno and R Streets, Zip 93715, Mailing Address: P.O. Box 1232, Zip 93715; tel. 209/442-6000; Bruce M. Perry, Chief Executive Officer, p. B28

Hemet: 0043 VALLEY HEALTH SYSTEM 1117 East Devonshire Avenue, Zip 92543; tel. 909/652-2811; Geoffrey Lang, Chief Executive Officer, p. B82

Loma Linda: 2175 ADVENTIST HEALTH SYSTEM–LOMA LINDA 11161 Anderson Street, Zip 92350; tel. 909/824-4459; David B. Hinshaw Sr. M.D., President, p. B9

Long Beach: 0435 PACIFIC HEALTH CORPORATION 249 East Ocean Boulevard, Zip 90802; tel. 310/435-1300; Jens Mueller, Chairman, p. B60

Los Angeles: 5755 LOS ANGELES COUNTY–DEPARTMENT OF HEALTH SERVICES 313 North Figueroa Street, Room 936, Zip 90012; tel. 213/240-8101; Robert C. Gates, Director Health, p. B50
0575 SCHICK LABORATORIES, INC. 15760 Ventura Boulevard, Suite 1201, Zip 91436; tel. 818/382-3682; Patrick J. Frawley Jr., Chairman, p. B69

Oakland: 0225 ALAMEDA COUNTY HEALTH CARE SERVICES AGENCY 499 Fifth Street, Zip 94607; tel. 510/268-2722; David J. Kears, Director, p. B10
2105 ★ KAISER FOUNDATION HOSPITALS One Kaiser Plaza, Zip 94612-3600; tel. 510/271-5990; David M. Lawrence M.D., Chairman and Chief Executive Officer, p. B49
6405 UNIVERSITY OF CALIFORNIA–SYSTEMWIDE ADMINISTRATION 300 Lakeside Drive, 18th Floor, Zip 94612-3550; tel. 510/987-9701; Cornelius L. Hopper M.D., Vice President Health Affairs, p. B81

Orange: 5425 ★ ST. JOSEPH HEALTH SYSTEM 440 South Batavia Street, Zip 92668-3995, Mailing Address: P.O. Box 14132, Zip 92613-1532; tel. 714/997-7690; Richard Statuto, Chief Executive Officer, p. B75

Pasadena: 5765 PARACELSUS HEALTHCARE CORPORATION 155 North Lake Ave, Suite 1100, Zip 91101; tel. 818/792-8600; R. J. Messenger, President and Chief Executive Officer, p. B60

Roseville: 0235 ADVENTIST HEALTH SYSTEM/WEST 2100 Douglas Boulevard, Zip 95661-3898, Mailing Address: P.O. Box 619002, Zip 95661-9002; tel. 916/781-2000; Frank F. Dupper, President, p. B9

Sacramento: 8795 SUTTER HEALTH 2800 L Street, Zip 95816, Mailing Address: P.O. Box 160727, Zip 95816; tel. 916/733-8800; Van R. Johnson, President and Chief Executive Officer, p. B76

San Diego: 7555 ★ PALOMAR POMERADO HEALTH SYSTEM 15255 Innovation Drive, Suite 204, Zip 92128-3410; tel. 619/675-5100; Andrew W. Deems, President and Chief Executive Officer, p. B60
1505 ★ SCRIPPS HOSPITALS 4275 Campus Point Court, Zip 92121, Mailing Address: P.O. Box 28, La Jolla, Zip 92038; tel. 619/678-7470; Martin B. Buser, President and Chief Executive Officer, p. B69
2065 ★ SHARP HEALTHCARE 3131 Berger Avenue, Suite 100, Zip 92123; tel. 619/541-4000; Peter K. Ellsworth, President, p. B69
8895 VISTA HILL FOUNDATION 2355 Northside Drive, 3rd Floor, Zip 92108; tel. 619/563-1770; Ronald E. Fickle, President, p. B82

San Francisco: 5205 ★ CATHOLIC HEALTHCARE WEST 1700 Montgomery Street, Suite 300, Zip 94111-9603; tel. 415/397-9000; Richard J. Kramer, President and Chief Executive Officer, p. B19

San Jose: 0965 ★ GOOD SAMARITAN HEALTH SYSTEM 532 Race Street, Zip 95126-3432; tel. 408/280-5660; Michael B. Guthrie M.D., President and Chief Executive Officer, p. B41

San Rafael: 1195 DOMINICAN SISTERS CONGREGATION OF THE MOST HOLY NAME 1520 Grand Avenue, Zip 94901-2236; tel. 415/453-8303; Sister Kristin Wombacher, Prioress General, p. B38

Santa Ana: 2085 UNITED WESTERN MEDICAL CENTERS 1001 North Tustin Avenue, Zip 92705-3502; tel. 714/953-3610; David E. Morgan, Chief Executive Officer, p. B80

Santa Monica: 0063 TENET HEALTHCARE CORPORATION 2700 Colorado Avenue, Zip 90404, Mailing Address: P.O. Box 4070, Zip 90404; tel. 310/998-8000; Jeffrey Barbakow, Chairman and Chief Executive Officer, p. B76

Yuba City: 2115 FREMONT–RIDEOUT HEALTH GROUP 989 Plumas Street, Zip 95991; tel. 916/751-4010; Thomas P. Hayes, Chief Executive Officer, p. B41

COLORADO

Englewood: 0935 ★ HEALTHONE HEALTHCARE SYSTEM 501 East Hampden Avenue, Zip 80110, Mailing Address: P.O. Box 2901, Zip 80150-0101; tel. 303/788-6484; Nick Hilger, President and Chief Executive Officer, p. B45

CONNECTICUT

Hartford: 0014 CONNECTICUT STATE DEPARTMENT OF MENTAL HEALTH 90 Washington Street, Zip 06106; tel. 203/566-3650; Albert J. Solnit M.D., Commissioner, p. B29

DISTRICT OF COLUMBIA

Washington: 9655 DEPARTMENT OF NAVY Zip 20066, p. B32
9495 DEPARTMENT OF THE AIR FORCE Zip 20333; tel. 202/767-5066, p. B32
9395 DEPARTMENT OF THE ARMY Zip 20314; tel. 703/756-8210, p. B33
9295 DEPARTMENT OF VETERANS AFFAIRS 810 Vermont Avenue N.W., Zip 20420; tel. 202/273-5786; Kenneth W. Kizer M.D., M.P.H., Under Secretary for Health, p. B34
6615 ★ MEDLANTIC HEALTHCARE GROUP 100 Irving Street N.W., Zip 20010-2975; tel. 202/877-6006; John P. McDaniel, Chief Executive Officer, p. B53

FLORIDA

Fort Lauderdale: 3115 ★ NORTH BROWARD HOSPITAL DISTRICT 303 Southeast 17th Street, Zip 33316-2510; tel. 305/355-5100; G. Wil Trower, President and Chief Executive Officer, p. B57

Gainesville: 7895 ★ AVMED–SANTA FE 8930 Northwest 39th Avenue, Zip 32606, Mailing Address: P.O. Box 749, Zip 32602-0749; tel. 904/372-8400; Edward C. Peddie, President, p. B12

Jacksonville: 2715 METHODIST HEALTH SYSTEM 580 West Eighth Street, Zip 32209-6553; tel. 904/798-8000; Marcus E. Drewa, President, p. B55

Naples: 1775 HEALTH MANAGEMENT ASSOCIATES 5811 Pelican Bay Boulevard, Suite 500, Zip 33963-2710; tel. 813/598-3175; William J. Schoen, President, p. B43

Orlando: 3355 ★ ORLANDO REGIONAL HEALTHCARE SYSTEM 1414 Kuhl Avenue, Zip 32806-2093; tel. 407/841-5111; J. Gary Strack, President and Chief Executive Officer, p. B59

Ormond Beach: 2615 ★ MEMORIAL HEALTH SYSTEMS 875 Sterthaus Avenue, Zip 32174-5197; tel. 904/676-6114; Richard A. Lind, President and Chief Executive Officer, p. B53

Headquarters of Health Care Systems / Geographically by City and State

Palm Harbor: 1335 MEASE HEALTH CARE 135 Annwood Road, Zip 34648; tel. 813/733-1111; Philip K. Beauchamp FACHE, President and Chief Executive Officer, p. B53

Pensacola: 0185 BAPTIST HEALTH CARE CORPORATION 1717 North E Street, Ste 320, Zip 32501-6335; tel. 904/469-2337; James F. Vickery, President, p. B13

Tampa: 1385 ★ ALLEGANY HEALTH SYSTEM 6200 Courtney Campbell Cswy, Zip 33607-1458; tel. 813/281-9098; Sister Marie Celeste Sullivan, President and Chief Executive Officer, p. B10

4125 ★ SHRINERS HOSPITALS FOR CRIPPLED CHILDREN 2900 Rocky Point Drive, Zip 33607-1435, Mailing Address: Box 31356, Zip 33631-3356; tel. 813/281-0300; Jack D. Hoard, Executive Administrator, p. B69

West Palm Beach: 0645 GLENBEIGH, INC. 4700 Congress Avenue, Zip 33407-3229; tel. 407/863-4747; G. Norman McCann, President, p. B41

Windermere: 9605 UNITED MEDICAL CORPORATION 603 Main Street, Zip 34786, Mailing Address: P.O. Box 1100, Zip 34786-1100; tel. 407/876-2200; Donald R. Dizney, Chairman, p. B80

Winter Park: 4165 ★ ADVENTIST HEALTH SYSTEM-SUNBELT HEALTH CARE CORPORATION 111 North Orlando Avenue, Zip 32789-3675; tel. 407/897-1919; Mardian J. Blair, President, p. B9

GEORGIA

Adel: 2335 MEMORIAL HEALTH SERVICES 706 North Parrish Avenue, Zip 31620, Mailing Address: Box 677, Zip 31620; tel. 912/896-2251; James E. Cunningham, Chief Executive Officer, p. B53

Atlanta: 0985 AMERIHEALTH, INC. 100 Galeria Parkway, Ste 605, Zip 30339; tel. 404/953-9600; William G. White, President, p. B11

0695 CHARTER MEDICAL CORPORATION 3414 Peachtree Road N.E., Ste 1400, Zip 30326; tel. 404/841-9200; E. Mac Crawford, President and Chief Operating Officer, p. B20

5895 HALLMARK HEALTHCARE CORPORATION 300 Galleria Parkway, Suite 650, Zip 30339-5949, Mailing Address: P.O. Box 723049, Zip 30339-0049; tel. 404/933-5500; James T. McAfee Jr., Chairman and Chief Executive Officer, p. B43

0905 SUMMIT MEDICAL MANAGEMENT, INC. 5 Concourse Parkway, Suite 800, Zip 30328-6111; tel. 404/392-1454; Ken Couch, Chief Executive Officer, p. B76

Austell: 0995 ★ PROMINA NORTHWEST HEALTH SYSTEM 1791 Mulkey Road, Suite 102, Zip 30001-1124; tel. 404/732-5501; Thomas E. Hill, President and Chief Executive Officer, p. B62

Macon: 1585 HEALTHCARE MANAGEMENT GROUP, INC. 776 Baconsfield Drive, Suite 209, Zip 31211-0101; tel. 912/743-5606; Earl Bonds Jr., Chief Executive Officer, p. B44

HAWAII

Honolulu: 0040 ★ QUEEN'S HEALTH SYSTEMS 201 Merchant Street, Suite 2450, Zip 96813-2929; tel. 808/532-6102; Richard L. Griffith, Chief Executive Officer, p. B62

3555 STATE OF HAWAII, DEPARTMENT OF HEALTH 1250 Punchbowl Street, Zip 96813; tel. 808/586-4416; Fred D. Horwitz, Deputy Director, p. B75

ILLINOIS

Carbondale: 4175 ★ SOUTHERN ILLINOIS HOSPITAL SERVICES 608 East College Street, Zip 62901, Mailing Address: P.O. Box 3988, Zip 62902-3988; tel. 618/457-5200; John J. Buckley Jr., President, p. B74

Chicago: 8805 COLUMBUS-CABRINI MEDICAL CENTER 2520 North Lakeview Avenue, Zip 60614; tel. 312/883-8366; Lee Domanico, Chief Executive Officer, p. B28

0016 COOK COUNTY BUREAU OF HEALTH SERVICES 1835 West Harrison Street, Zip 60612; tel. 312/633-3070; Ruth M. Rothstein, Chief, p. B30

3855 ★ RUSH-PRESBYTERIAN-ST. LUKE'S MEDICAL CENTER 1653 West Congress Parkway, Zip 60612-3864; tel. 312/942-5000; Leo M. Henikoff M.D., President, p. B68

Des Plaines: 5575 SISTERS OF THE HOLY FAMILY OF NAZARETH-SACRED HEART PROVINCE 353 North River Road, Zip 60016-1291; tel. 708/298-6760; Sister M. Lucille Madura, Provincial Superior, p. B73

Elk Grove Village: 0065 ALEXIAN BROTHERS HEALTH SYSTEM, INC. 600 Alexian Way, Zip 60007-3395; tel. 708/640-7550; Brother Felix Bettendorf, President, p. B10

Evergreen Park: 2295 LITTLE COMPANY OF MARY SISTERS HEALTHCARE SYSTEM 9350 South California Avenue, Zip 60642; tel. 708/422-6200; Sister Nancy Boyle, Provincialate Superior, p. B50

Frankfort: 1415 ★ FRANCISCAN SISTERS HEALTH CARE CORPORATION 9223 West Francis Road, Zip 60423-8334; tel. 815/469-4888; Gerald P. Pearson, President, p. B40

Kankakee: 4025 ★ SERVANTCOR 175 South Wall Street, Zip 60901-3470; tel. 815/937-2034; Joseph S. Feth, President, p. B69

Naperville: 5215 ★ MERCY-CHICAGO REGION HEALTHCARE SYSTEM 55 Shuman Boulevard, Ste 150, Zip 60563-8469; tel. 708/355-6310; Sister Catherine C. Gallagher, President, p. B54

O'Fallon: 0205 ★ ASC HEALTH SYSTEM 6 Eagle Center, Suite 4, Zip 62269-0406, Mailing Address: P.O. Box 670, Zip 62269-0670; tel. 618/632-1284; Gregory F. Yank, President and Chief Executive Officer, p. B12

Oakbrook: 0064 ★ ADVOCATE HEALTH CARE 2025 Windsor Drive, Zip 60521-0222; tel. 708/990-5002; Richard R. Risk, President and Co-Chief Executive Officer, p. B10

Peoria: 8875 METHODIST HEALTH SERVICES CORPORATION 221 N.E. Glen Oak Avenue, Zip 61636; tel. 309/672-4826; Robert E. Wierman, President, p. B55

5335 ★ OSF HEALTHCARE SYSTEM 800 Northeast Glen Oak Avenue, Zip 61603-3200; tel. 309/655-2850; Sister Frances Marie Masching, President, p. B60

Springfield: 1295 DOMINICAN SISTERS OF SPRINGFIELD 1237 West Monroe Street, Zip 62704-1680; tel. 217/787-0481; Sister Rose Miriam Schulte, Prioress General, p. B38

5355 ★ HOSPITAL SISTERS HEALTH SYSTEM Sangamon Avenue Road, Zip 62794, Mailing Address: Box 19431, Zip 62794-9431; tel. 217/522-6969; Sister Jomary Trstensky, President, p. B47

Urbana: 2575 CARLE FOUNDATION 611 West Park Street, Zip 61801-2595; tel. 217/383-3311; Michael H. Fritz, President, p. B18

Wheaton: 6745 ★ WHEATON FRANCISCAN SERVICES, INC. 26W171 Roosevelt Road, Zip 60189-0667, Mailing Address: P.O. Box 667, Zip 60189-0667; tel. 708/462-9271; Wilfred F. Loebig Jr., President and Chief Executive Officer, p. B83

INDIANA

Hobart: 0135 ★ ANCILLA SYSTEMS INC. 1000 South Lake Park Avenue, Zip 46342; tel. 219/947-8500; William D. Harkins, President, p. B12

Mishawaka: 5345 ★ SISTERS OF ST. FRANCIS HEALTH SERVICES, INC. 1515 Dragoon Trail, Zip 46546-1290, Mailing Address: P.O. Box 1290, Zip 46546-1290; tel. 219/256-3935; Sister Jane Marie Klein, President, p. B73

South Bend: 5585 ★ HOLY CROSS HEALTH SYSTEM CORPORATION 3606 East Jefferson Boulevard, Zip 46615-3097; tel. 219/233-8558; Sister Patricia Vandenberg, President and Chief Executive Officer, p. B46

IOWA

Des Moines: 0061 ★ IOWA HEALTH SYSTEM 1200 Pleasant Street, Zip 50309-1453; Samuel T. Wallace, President, p. B48

Sioux City: 5845 ST. LUKE'S HEALTH SYSTEM, INC. 2720 Stone Park Boulevard, Zip 51104-2000; tel. 712/279-3500; David O. Biorn FACHE, President and Chief Executive Officer, p. B75

KANSAS

Leavenworth: 5095 ★ SISTERS OF CHARITY OF LEAVENWORTH HEALTH SERVICES CORPORATION 4200 South Fourth Street, Zip 66048-5054; tel. 913/682-1338; Sister Marie Damian Glatt, President, p. B71

Phillipsburg: 1535 ★ GREAT PLAINS HEALTH ALLIANCE, INC. 625 Third, Zip 67661, Mailing Address: Box 366, Zip 67661-0366; tel. 913/543-2111; Roger S. John, President and Chief Executive Officer, p. B42

Topeka: 0805 STORMONT-VAIL HEALTH SERVICES CORPORATION 1500 Southwest Tenth Street, Zip 66604-1353; tel. 913/354-6112; Howard M. Chase, President, p. B75

Wichita: 5435 ★ CSJ HEALTH SYSTEM OF WICHITA 3720 East Bayley, Zip 67218-3087; tel. 316/689-4000; LeRoy E. Rheault, President and Chief Executive Officer, p. B30

KENTUCKY

Lexington: 0145 APPALACHIAN REGIONAL HEALTHCARE 1220 Harrodsburg Road, Zip 40533, Mailing Address: Box 8086, Zip 40533-8086; tel. 606/281-2440; Forrest Calico M.D., President, p. B12

Louisville: 2285 ★ ALLIANT HEALTH SYSTEM 234 East Gray Street, Ste 225, Zip 40202, Mailing Address: P.O. Box 35070, Zip 40232-5070; tel. 502/629-2000; Stephen A. Williams, President, p. B10

0315 ★ BAPTIST HEALTHCARE SYSTEM 4007 Kresge Way, Zip 40207-4677; tel. 502/896-5000; Tommy J. Smith, President and Chief Executive Officer, p. B13

0052 ★ JEWISH HOSPITAL HEALTHCARE SERVICES 217 East Chestnut Street, Zip 40202; tel. 502/587-4011; Henry C. Wagner, President, p. B49

0026 VENCOR, INCORPORATED 400 West Market Street, Suite 3300, Zip 40202-3360; tel. 502/569-7300; W. Bruce Lunsford, Board Chairman, p. B82

Nazareth: 3045 ★ SISTERS OF CHARITY OF NAZARETH HEALTH SYSTEM 135 West Drive, Zip 40048, Mailing Address: P.O. Box 171, Zip 40048-0171; tel. 502/349-6250; Mark W. Dundon, President and Chief Executive Officer, p. B71

LOUISIANA

Baton Rouge: 1475 ★ FRANCISCAN MISSIONARIES OF OUR LADY HEALTH SYSTEM, INC. 4200 Essen Lane, Zip 70809; tel. 504/923-2701; Sister Brendan Mary Ronayne, President, p. B40

0775 ★ GENERAL HEALTH SYSTEM 3849 North Boulevard, Suite 200, Zip 70806; tel. 504/387-7806; Thomas H. Sawyer, President and Chief Executive Officer, p. B41

0715 LOUISIANA HEALTH CARE AUTHORITY 8550 United Plaza Boulevard, 4th Floor, Zip 70809; tel. 504/922-0488; William Cherry M.D., Chief Executive Officer, p. B50

New Orleans: 0047 LOUISIANA STATE HOSPITALS 210 State Street, Zip 70118; M. E. Teague, Chief Executive Officer, p. B51

0405 RAMSAY HEALTH CARE, INC. 639 Loyola Avenue, Suite 1400, Zip 70113; tel. 504/585-2505; Gregory H. Browne, President and Chief Executive Officer, p. B68

MAINE

Bangor: 0555 ★ EASTERN MAINE HEALTHCARE 489 State Street, Zip 04401; tel. 207/973-7051; Norman A. Ledwin, President, p. B38

MARYLAND

Baltimore: 1015 ★ JOHNS HOPKINS HEALTH SYSTEM 600 North Wolfe Street, Zip 21287-1160; tel. 410/955-0428; James A. Block M.D., President, p. B49

6015 SISTERS OF MERCY OF THE AMERICAS–REGIONAL COMMUNITY OF BALTIMORE 1300 Northern Parkway, Zip 21239, Mailing Address: P.O. Box 11448, Zip 21239; tel. 410/435-4400; Sister Margaret Beatty, President, p. B72

Fallston: 0038 ★ UPPER CHESAPEAKE HEALTH SYSTEM 1916 Belair Road, Zip 21047; tel. 410/893-0322; Lyle Ernest Sheldon, President and Chief Executive Officer, p. B81

Landover: 0029 ★ DIMENSIONS HEALTH CORPORATION 9200 Basil Court, Zip 20785; tel. 301/925-7000, p. B38

Lutherville: 2355 ★ HELIX HEALTH SYSTEM 2330 West Joppa Road, Ste 301, Zip 21093; tel. 410/296-6050; James A. Oakey, President, p. B46

Marriottsville: 5085 ★ BON SECOURS HEALTH SYSTEM, INC. 1505 Marriottsville Road, Zip 21104-1399; tel. 410/442-5511; John L. Fitzgerald, President & Chief Executive Officer, p. B15

Rockville: 9195 U.S. PUBLIC HEALTH SERVICE INDIAN HEALTH SERVICE 2275 Research Boulevard, Zip 20850, p. B78

MASSACHUSETTS

Boston: 6995 DEPARTMENT OF HEALTH AND HOSPITALS 818 Harrison Avenue, Zip 02118; tel. 617/534-5365; Lawrence Dwyer, Commissioner, p. B32

0013 MASSACHUSETTS DEPARTMENT OF MENTAL HEALTH 25 Staniford Street, Zip 02114; tel. 617/727-5500; Eileen Elias, Commissioner, p. B52

1785 ★ MASSACHUSETTS GENERAL HOSPITAL CORPORATION 32 Fruit Street, Zip 02114-2696; tel. 617/726-2100; Samuel O. Thier M.D., President, p. B52

Lexington: 5885 ★ COVENANT HEALTH SYSTEMS, INC. 10 Pelham Road, Zip 02173-5799; tel. 617/862-1634; David R. Lincoln, President, p. B30

Norwood: 3175 NEPONSET VALLEY HEALTH SYSTEM 800 Washington Street, Zip 02062-3487; tel. 617/769-4000; Yolanda Landrau R.N., Ed.D., President and Chief Executive Officer, p. B56

Pittsfield: 2435 ★ BERKSHIRE HEALTH SYSTEMS, INC. 725 North Street, Zip 01201; tel. 413/447-2743; David E. Phelps, President and Chief Executive Officer, p. B15

Springfield: 1095 ★ BAYSTATE HEALTH SYSTEMS, INC. 759 Chestnut Street, Zip 01199-0001; tel. 413/784-0000; Michael J. Daly, President, p. B14

5285 ★ SISTERS OF PROVIDENCE HEALTH SYSTEM 146 Chestnut Street, Zip 01103; tel. 413/737-3981; Sister Kathleen Popko, President and Chief Executive Officer, p. B72

Waltham: 1125 ★ CARITAS CHRISTI HEALTH CARE SYSTEM 125 Technology Drive, Suite 5, Zip 02154-8930; tel. 617/893-8544; Michael F. Collins M.D., President, p. B18

Wellesley: 0215 COMMUNITY CARE SYSTEMS, INC. 203 Grove Street, Zip 02181; tel. 617/239-0871; Frederick J. Thacher, Chairman, p. B28

MICHIGAN

Ann Arbor: 5555 ★ SISTERS OF ST. JOSEPH HEALTH SYSTEM 455 East Eisenhower Parkway, Suite 300, Zip 48108-3304; tel. 313/741-1160; John S. Lore, President and Chief Executive Officer, p. B73

Dearborn: 1165 ★ OAKWOOD HEALTHCARE SYSTEM 18101 Oakwood Boulevard, Zip 48124, Mailing Address: P.O. Box 2500, Zip 48123-2500; tel. 313/593-7000; Gerald D. Fitzgerald, President, p. B58

Detroit: 2145 ★ DETROIT MEDICAL CENTER 4201 St. Antoine Boulevard, Zip 48201-2194; tel. 313/745-5192; David J. Campbell, President and Chief Executive Officer, p. B37

9505 ★ HENRY FORD HEALTH SYSTEM One Ford Place, Zip 48202; tel. 313/876-8700; Gail L. Warden, President and Chief Executive Officer, p. B46

2055 MICHIGAN HEALTH CARE CORPORATION 7430 Second Avenue, Ste 610, Zip 48202; tel. 313/874-9110; Charles E. Housley FACHE, President and Chief Executive Officer, p. B56

Farmington Hills: 5165 ★ MERCY HEALTH SERVICES 34605 Twelve Mile Road, Zip 48331-3221; tel. 810/489-6000; Judith Pelham, President and Chief Executive Officer, p. B53

Headquarters of Health Care Systems / Geographically by City and State

Kalamazoo: 0595 ★ BRONSON HEALTHCARE GROUP, INC. One Healthcare Plaza, Zip 49007–5345; tel. 616/341–6000; Patric E. Ludwig, President, p. B17

Lansing: 1515 MICHIGAN CAPITAL HEALTHCARE 401 West Greenlawn, Zip 48910–2819; tel. 517/334–2967; Dennis M. Litos, President and Chief Executive Officer, p. B56

Midland: 0001 ★ MIDMICHIGAN REGIONAL HEALTH SYSTEM 4005 Orchard Drive, Zip 48670; tel. 517/839–3399; Terence F. Moore, President, p. B56

Port Huron: 0053 ★ BLUE WATER HEALTH SERVICES CORPORATION 1001 Kearney, Zip 48060; tel. 810/989–3717; Donald C. Fletcher, President and Chief Executive Officer, p. B15

Royal Oak: 9575 ★ WILLIAM BEAUMONT HOSPITAL CORPORATION 3601 West Thirteen Mile Road, Zip 48073–6769; tel. 810/551–5000; Kenneth E. Myers, President, p. B83

Saint Joseph: 0056 ★ LAKELAND REGIONAL HEALTH SYSTEM, INC. 1234 Napier Avenue, Zip 49085–2158; tel. 616/983–8300; Joseph A. Wasserman, President and Chief Executive Officer, p. B50

Southfield: 1035 HORIZON HEALTH SYSTEM 26100 American Drive, Zip 48086, Mailing Address: P.O. Box 5153, Zip 48086–5153; tel. 810/746–4460; Thomas W. Caulfield, President, p. B47

Traverse City: 1465 ★ MUNSON HEALTHCARE 1105 Sixth Street, Zip 49684–2386; tel. 616/935–5000; John R. Rockwood Jr., President, p. B56

Warren: 0042 ★ DETROIT–MACOMB HOSPITAL CORPORATION 12000 East Twelve Mile Road, Zip 48093; tel. 313/573–5910; Jack Ryan M.D., President and Chief Executive Officer, p. B37

MINNESOTA

Duluth: 0515 BENEDICTINE HEALTH SYSTEM 503 East Third Street, Zip 55805–1964; tel. 218/720–2370; Sister Kathleen Hofer, Chair Person and Chief Executive Officer, p. B14

Minneapolis: 0041 ★ ALLINA HEALTH SYSTEM 5601 Smetana Drive, Zip 55440, Mailing Address: P.O. Box 9310, Zip 55440–9310; tel. 612/992–2000; Gordon M. Sprenger, Executive Officer, p. B11

1325 ★ FAIRVIEW HOSPITAL AND HEALTHCARE SERVICES 2450 Riverside Avenue, Zip 55454–1400; tel. 612/672–6735; Richard A. Norling, President and Chief Executive Officer, p. B39

Rochester: 1875 ★ MAYO FOUNDATION 200 Southwest First Street, Zip 55905; tel. 507/284–2511; Robert R. Waller M.D., President and Chief Executive Officer, p. B52

Saint Joseph: 0535 BENEDICTINE SISTERS St Benedicts Convent, Zip 56374–0277; tel. 612/363–7100; Sister Ephrem Hollermann, Prioress, p. B15

Saint Louis Park: 1985 HEALTHSYSTEM MINNESOTA 6500 Excelsior Boulevard, Zip 55426–4702; tel. 612/932–6300; Robert L. Galloway, President and Administrative Officer, p. B46

Saint Paul: 2185 ★ HEALTHEAST 559 Capitol Boulevard, 6–South, Zip 55103–0000; tel. 612/232–2300; Tim Hanson, President and Chief Executive Officer, p. B45

MISSISSIPPI

Batesville: 1275 FIRST HEALTH, INC. 107 Public Square, Zip 38606; tel. 601/563–7676, p. B39

Jackson: 0017 MISSISSIPPI STATE DEPARTMENT OF MENTAL HEALTH 1101 Robert E. Lee Building, Zip 39201–1101; tel. 601/359–1288; Roger McMurtry, Chief Mental Health Bureau, p. B56

Pascagoula: 0067 SINGING RIVER HOSPITAL SYSTEM 2809 Denny Avenue, Zip 39581; tel. 601/938–5062; Robert L. Lingle, Executive Director, p. B70

Tupelo: 0032 NORTH MISSISSIPPI HEALTH SERVICES, INC. 830 South Gloster Street, Zip 38801; tel. 601/841–3136; Jeffrey B. Barber Ph.D., Dr.P.H., President and Chief Executive Officer, p. B58

MISSOURI

Kansas City: 8815 ★ HEALTH MIDWEST 2304 East Meyer Boulevard, Suite A–20, Zip 64132–4104; tel. 816/276–9181; Richard W. Brown, President and Chief Executive Officer, p. B44

9255 ★ TRUMAN MEDICAL CENTER 2301 Holmes Street, Zip 64108–2677; tel. 816/556–3153; James J. Mongan M.D., Director, p. B78

Saint Joseph: 2485 ★ HEARTLAND HEALTH SYSTEM 5325 Faraon, Zip 64506; tel. 816/271–6000; Lowell C. Kruse, President, p. B46

Saint Louis: 0051 ★ BJC HEALTH SYSTEM 4444 Forest Park Avenue, Zip 63108–2259; tel. 314/286–2030; Frederick L. Brown, President & Chief Executive Officer, p. B15

5945 ★ CARONDELET HEALTH SYSTEM 13801 Riverport Drive, Ste 300, Zip 63043–4810; tel. 314/770–0333; Gary Christiansen, President, p. B18

1855 ★ DAUGHTERS OF CHARITY NATIONAL HEALTH SYSTEM 4600 Edmundson Road, Zip 63134, Mailing Address: P.O. Box 45998, Zip 63145–5998; tel. 314/253–6700; F. Dale Whitten, Interim President, p. B31

5185 ★ SISTERS OF MERCY HEALTH SYSTEM–ST. LOUIS 2039 North Geyer Road, Zip 63131–3399; tel. 314/965–6100; Sister Mary Roch Rocklage, Chief Executive Officer, p. B72

5455 ★ SSM HEALTH CARE SYSTEM 477 North Lindbergh Boulevard, Zip 63141–7813; tel. 314/994–7800; Sister Mary Jean Ryan, President and Chief Executive Officer, p. B74

NEBRASKA

Norfolk: 2855 MISSIONARY BENEDICTINE SISTERS AMERICAN PROVINCE 300 North 18th Street, Zip 68701; tel. 402/371–3438; Sister M. Agnes Falber, Prioress, p. B56

Omaha: 5175 ★ CATHOLIC HEALTH CORPORATION 920 South 107th Avenue, Zip 68114–4719; tel. 402/393–7661; A. Diane Moeller, Chief Executive Officer, p. B18

NEVADA

Las Vegas: 0785 COMMUNITY PSYCHIATRIC CENTERS 6600 West Charleston Boulevard, 1800, Zip 89102; tel. 702/259–3600, p. B29

NEW JERSEY

Camden: 6725 ★ WEST JERSEY HEALTH SYSTEM 1000 Atlantic Avenue, Zip 08104; tel. 609/342–4604; Barry D. Brown, President and Chief Executive Officer, p. B82

Edison: 8855 ★ JFK HEALTH SYSTEMS, INC. 80 James Street, 2nd Floor, Zip 08820–3998; tel. 908/632–1500; John P. McGee, President and Chief Executive Officer, p. B49

Newark: 6545 ★ CATHEDRAL HEALTHCARE SYSTEM, INC. 219 Chestnut Street, Zip 07105–1558; tel. 201/690–3600; Frank L. Fumai, President and Chief Executive Officer, p. B18

Trenton: 0010 DIVISION OF MENTAL HEALTH SERVICES, DEPARTMENT OF HUMAN SERVICES, STATE OF NEW JERSEY Capital Center, CN 727, Zip 08625–0727; Alan G. Kaufman, Director, p. B38

NEW MEXICO

Albuquerque: 3505 ★ PRESBYTERIAN HEALTHCARE SERVICES 5901 Harper Drive N.E., Zip 87109, Mailing Address: P.O. Box 26666, Zip 87125–6666; tel. 505/260–6300; James Hinton, President and Chief Executive Officer, p. B61

0021 UNIVERSITY OF NEW MEXICO 915 Camino De Salud, Zip 87131; tel. 505/277–5849; Jane E. Henney M.D., Vice President Health Sciences, p. B81

NEW YORK

Albany: 0009 NEW YORK STATE DEPARTMENT OF MENTAL HEALTH 44 Holland Avenue, Zip 12229; tel. 518/447–9611; Jesse Nixon Jr. Ph.D., Director, p. B57

Headquarters of Health Care Systems / Geographically by City and State

Manhasset: 0062 ★ NORTH SHORE HEALTH SYSTEM 300 Community Drive, Zip 11030; tel. 516/562-4060; John S. T. Gallagher, President, p. B58

New York: 1485 ★ FRANCISCAN SISTERS OF THE POOR HEALTH SYSTEM, INC. 186 Joralemon Street, Zip 11201-4326; tel. 718/625-6530; Sister Joanne Schuster, President, p. B41

3075 NEW YORK CITY HEALTH AND HOSPITALS CORPORATION 125 Worth Street, Room 514, Zip 10013; tel. 212/788-3321; Bruce Siegel M.D., M.P.H., President, p. B57

5995 SISTERS OF CHARITY CENTER Mount St Vincent on Hudson, Zip 10471-1093; tel. 718/549-9200; Sister Carol Barnes, President, p. B70

6095 ★ SISTERS OF CHARITY HEALTH CARE SYSTEM CORPORATION 75 Vanderbilt Avenue, Zip 10304-3850; tel. 718/390-5080; John J. DePierro, President and Chief Executive Officer, p. B70

Rochester: 0046 GREATER ROCHESTER HEALTH SYSTEM, INC. 1040 University Avenue, Zip 14607; tel. 716/266-0720; Arthur E. Liebert, President, p. B42

Syracuse: 5955 SISTERS OF THE 3RD FRANCISCAN ORDER 2500 Grant Boulevard, Zip 13208-1713; tel. 315/425-0115; Sister Grace Anne Dillenschneider, General Superior, p. B73

Uniondale: 0735 ★ EPISCOPAL HEALTH SERVICES INC. 333 Earle Ovington Boulevard, Zip 11553-3645; tel. 516/228-6100; Jack N. Farrington Ph.D., Executive Vice President, p. B39

NORTH CAROLINA

Belmont: 5985 SISTERS OF MERCY 431 East Wilkinson Boulevard, Zip 28012; tel. 704/829-5103; Sister Pauline Clifford, Regional President, p. B72

Charlotte: 0705 CHARLOTTE-MECKLENBURG HOSPITAL AUTHORITY 1000 Blythe Boulevard, Zip 28203, Mailing Address: Box 32861, Zip 28232-2861; tel. 704/355-2000; Harry A. Nurkin Ph.D., President, p. B20

NORTH DAKOTA

Bismarck: 0545 BENEDICTINE SISTERS OF THE ANNUNCIATION 7520 University Drive, Zip 58504-9653; tel. 701/255-1520; Sister Susan Lardy, Prioress, p. B15

Fargo: 2235 ★ LUTHERAN HEALTH SYSTEMS 4310 17th Avenue S.W., Zip 58103, Mailing Address: P.O. Box 6200, Zip 58106-6200; tel. 701/277-7500; Steven R. Orr, President, p. B51

5805 SISTERS OF MARY OF THE PRESENTATION HEALTH CORPORATION 1102 Page Drive S.W., Zip 58106-0007, Mailing Address: P.O. Box 10007, Zip 58106-0007; tel. 701/237-9290; Aaron Alton, President, p. B71

OHIO

Cincinnati: 0415 ★ BETHESDA HOSPITAL, INC. 619 Oak Street, Zip 45206-1690; tel. 513/569-6141; L. Thomas Wilburn Jr., Chairman, p. B15

2415 JEWISH HEALTH SYSTEMS, INC. 3200 Burnet Avenue, Zip 45229-3099; tel. 513/569-2434; Warren C. Falberg, President, p. B49

5155 ★ MERCY HEALTH SYSTEM 2335 Grandview Ave, 4th Floor, Zip 45206-2280; tel. 513/221-2736; Michael D. Connelly, President and Chief Executive Officer, p. B54

5115 ★ SISTERS OF CHARITY HEALTH CARE SYSTEMS, INC. 345 Neeb Road, Zip 45233-5102; tel. 513/347-1000; Sister Celestia Koebel, President, p. B70

Cleveland: 2515 FAIRVIEW HEALTH SYSTEM 18101 Lorain Avenue, Zip 44111-5656; tel. 216/476-4040; Thomas M. LaMotte, President and Chief Executive Officer, p. B39

8285 ★ METROHEALTH SYSTEM 2500 Metrohealth Drive, Zip 44109; tel. 216/459-8050; Terry R. White, President and Chief Executive Officer, p. B55

5125 SISTERS OF CHARITY OF ST. AUGUSTINE HEALTH SYSTEM 2351 East 22nd Street, Zip 44115; tel. 216/696-5560; Peter G. Reibold, President, p. B71

Columbus: 1045 DOCTORS HOSPITAL 1087 Dennison Avenue, Zip 43201; tel. 614/297-4000; Richard A. Vincent, President, p. B38

9095 ★ U.S. HEALTH CORPORATION 3555 Olentangy River Rd, 4000, Zip 43214; tel. 614/566-5424; Erie Chapman, President and Chief Executive Officer, p. B78

Lorain: 5645 ★ HUMILITY OF MARY HEALTH CARE CORPORATION 1919 Reid Avenue, Zip 44052, Mailing Address: P.O. Box 841, Zip 44052-0841; tel. 216/245-3569; Sister Frances Flanigan, President and Chief Executive Officer, p. B47

Mayfield Village: 8835 ★ MERIDIA HEALTH SYSTEM 6700 Beta Drive, Suite 200, Zip 44143; tel. 216/446-8000; Richard J. McCann, President, p. B55

Sylvania: 5375 ★ FRANCISCAN SERVICES CORPORATION 6832 Convent Boulevard, Zip 43560-2897; tel. 419/882-8373; John W. O'Connell, President, p. B40

Troy: 1965 ★ UPPER VALLEY MEDICAL CENTERS 3130 North Dixie Highway, Zip 45373; tel. 513/332-7500; David J. Meckstroth, President, p. B81

OKLAHOMA

Oklahoma City: 0305 ★ OKLAHOMA HEALTH SYSTEM 3300 Northwest Expressway, Zip 73112; tel. 405/949-6068; Stanley F. Hupfeld, President and Chief Executive Officer, p. B58

0018 OKLAHOMA STATE DEPARTMENT OF MENTAL HEALTH AND SUBSTANCE ABUSE SERVICES 1000 Northeast Tenth, Zip 73152, Mailing Address: P.O. Box 53277, Zip 73152; tel. 405/271-6868; Thomas Peace Ph.D., Commissioner, p. B59

Tulsa: 0665 CENTURY HEALTHCARE CORPORATION 5555 East 71st Street, Suite 9220, Zip 74136-6540; tel. 918/491-0775; Jerry D. Dillon, President & Chief Executive Officer, p. B19

5305 ★ SISTERS OF THE SORROWFUL MOTHER UNITED STATES HEALTH SYSTEM P.O. Box 4753, Zip 74159-0753; tel. 918/742-9988; Sister M. Therese Gottschalk, President, p. B73

OREGON

Portland: 0585 ★ BRIM, INC. 305 Northeast 102nd Avenue, Zip 97220-4199; tel. 503/256-2070; Armand E. Brim, Chairman & Chief Executive Officer, p. B16

2755 ★ LEGACY HEALTH SYSTEM 1919 N.W. Lovejoy Street, Zip 97209-1503; tel. 503/225-8600; John G. King, President and Chief Executive Officer, p. B50

PENNSYLVANIA

Chester: 5325 ★ FRANCISCAN HEALTH SYSTEM One MacIntyre Drive, Zip 19014-1196; tel. 610/358-4223; Ronald R. Aldrich, President and Chief Executive Officer, p. B40

Danville: 5570 ★ GEISINGER HEALTH CARE SYSTEM 100 North Academy Avenue, Zip 17822-3311; tel. 717/271-6211; Frank J. Trembulak, Chief Operating Officer, p. B41

Devon: 0845 DEVEREUX FOUNDATION 19 South Waterloo Road, Zip 19333, Mailing Address: Box 400, Zip 19333; tel. 610/964-3000; Ronald P. Burd, President and Chief Exeuctive Officer, p. B37

Harrisburg: 2135 ★ CAPITAL HEALTH SYSTEM 17 South Market Square, Zip 17101, Mailing Address: P.O. Box 8700, Zip 17105-8700; tel. 717/782-3366; John S. Cramer FACHE, President and Chief Executive Officer, p. B17

King of Prussia: 9555 UNIVERSAL HEALTH SERVICES, INC. 367 South Gulph Road, Zip 19406; tel. 610/768-3300; Alan B. Miller, President and Chief Executive Officer, p. B80

Mechanicsburg: 1715 CONTINENTAL MEDICAL SYSTEMS, INC. 600 Wilson Lane, Zip 17055-0715, Mailing Address: P.O. Box 715, Zip 17055-0715; tel. 717/790-8300; R. A. Ortenzio, Chairman and Chief Executive Officer, p. B30

Headquarters of Health Care Systems / Geographically by City and State

Media: 0008 ★ CROZER–KEYSTONE HEALTH SYSTEM 1400 North Providence Road, Ste 4010, Zip 19063–2049; tel. 610/447–2000; John C. McMeekin, President and Chief Executive Officer, p. B30

Philadelphia: 1685 ALBERT EINSTEIN HEALTHCARE NETWORK 5501 Old York Road, Zip 19141–3098; tel. 215/456–7890; Martin Goldsmith, President, p. B10

0006 GRADUATE HEALTH SYSTEM 2129 Chestnut Street, Zip 19103; tel. 215/448–1500; Harold Cramer, Chairman and Chief Executive Officer, p. B42

Pittsburgh: 2305 ALLEGHENY HEALTH, EDUCATION AND RESEARCH FOUNDATION 120 Fifth Avenue, Zip 15222; tel. 412/359–6000; Sherif S. Abdelhak, President, p. B10

1355 ★ FORBES HEALTH SYSTEM 500 Finley Street, Zip 15206; tel. 412/665–3320; Barry H. Roth, President, p. B40

2255 ★ ST. FRANCIS HEALTH SYSTEM 4401 Penn Avenue, Zip 15224–1334; tel. 412/622–4212; Sister M. Rosita Wellinger, President, p. B74

Radnor: 3595 ★ EASTERN MERCY HEALTH SYSTEM 3 Radnor Corporate Center, Suite 220, Zip 19087; tel. 610/971–9770; Daniel F. Russell, President, p. B38

7775 ★ MAIN LINE HEALTH 259 Radnor–Chester Road, Suite 290, Zip 19087–5260; tel. 610/293–8200; Douglas S. Peters, President and Chief Executive Officer, p. B52

Sayre: 0675 ★ GUTHRIE HEALTHCARE SYSTEM Guthrie Square, Zip 18840; tel. 717/882–4312; Ralph H. Meyer, President, p. B43

Wayne: 0455 HOSPITAL GROUP OF AMERICA 1265 Drummers Lane, Suite 107, Zip 19087; tel. 610/687–5151; Mark R. Russell, President and Chief Executive Officer, p. B47

Williamsport: 0066 ★ SUSQUEHANNA HEALTH SYSTEM 1001 Grampian Boulevard, Zip 17701–1946; tel. 717/320–7000; Donald R. Creamer, President and Chief Executive Officer, p. B76

York: 0068 ★ YORK HEALTH SYSTEM 1001 South George Street, Zip 17405; tel. 717/851–2121; Bruce M. Bartels, President, p. B83

PUERTO RICO

San Juan: 0011 PUERTO RICO DEPARTMENT OF HEALTH Building A – Medical Center, Zip 00936, Mailing Address: Call Box 70184, Zip 00936; tel. 809/274–7676; Carmen Feliciano De Melecio M.D., Secretary of Health, p. B62

RHODE ISLAND

Providence: 0060 ★ LIFESPAN CORPORATION 167 Point Street, Zip 02903; tel. 401/444–6699; William Kreykes, President and Chief Executive Officer, p. B50

SOUTH CAROLINA

Columbia: 4155 ★ BAPTIST HEALTH CARE SYSTEM OF SOUTH CAROLINA Taylor At Marion Street, Zip 29220; tel. 803/771–5010; Charles D. Beaman Jr., President and Chief Executive Officer, p. B13

Greenville: 1555 ★ GREENVILLE HOSPITAL SYSTEM 701 Grove Road, Zip 29605–4211; tel. 803/455–7000; Frank D. Pinckney, President, p. B43

Spartanburg: 4195 ★ SPARTANBURG HOSPITAL SYSTEM 101 East Wood Street, Zip 29303–3016; tel. 803/560–6000; Joseph Michael Oddis, President, p. B74

SOUTH DAKOTA

Sioux Falls: 5255 ★ PRESENTATION HEALTH SYSTEM 1301 South Ninth Ave, Suite 102, Zip 57105–1043; tel. 605/331–4999; John T. Porter, President, p. B62

TENNESSEE

Brentwood: 0002 ★ QUORUM HEALTH GROUP/QUORUM HEALTH RESOURCES 155 Franklin Road, Suite 401, Zip 37027; tel. 615/371–7979; James E. Dalton Jr., President and Chief Executive Officer, p. B62

Chattanooga: 1155 GREENLEAF HEALTH SYSTEMS, INC. One Northgate Park, Zip 37415; tel. 615/870–5110; Dan B. Page, President, p. B42

2795 HEALTHCORP OF TENNESSEE, INC. 735 Broad Street, Zip 37402; tel. 615/267–8406; T. Farrell Hayes, President, p. B44

Jackson: 0004 ★ WEST TENNESSEE HEALTHCARE, INC. 708 West Forest Avenue, Zip 38301; tel. 901/425–5000; James T. Moss, President, p. B83

Knoxville: 2155 BAPTIST HEALTH SYSTEM OF TENNESSEE 137 Blount Avenue S.E., Zip 37920, Mailing Address: Box 1788, Zip 37901; tel. 615/632–5099; Dale Collins, President & Chief Executive Officer, p. B13

Memphis: 1625 ★ BAPTIST MEMORIAL HEALTH CARE SYSTEM, INC. 899 Madison Avenue, Zip 38146; tel. 901/227–2727; Stephen Curtis Reynolds, President and Chief Executive Officer, p. B14

9345 ★ METHODIST HEALTH SYSTEMS, INC. 1211 Union Avenue, Suite 700, Zip 38104; tel. 901/726–2300; Maurice W. Elliott, President, p. B55

1765 UNITED HOSPITAL CORPORATION 6189 East Shelby Drive, Zip 38115; tel. 901/794–8440; James C. Henson, President, p. B80

Nashville: 0048 ★ COLUMBIA/HCA HEALTHCARE CORPORATION One Park Plaza, Zip 37203; tel. 615/320–2000; Richard Scott, President and Chief Executive Officer, p. B21

0075 CUMBERLAND HEALTH SYSTEMS, INC. 2100 West End Avenue, Ste 900, Zip 37203; tel. 615/327–2200; Samuel W. Owen, President and Chief Executive Officer, p. B30

0022 METROPOLITAN NASHVILLE GENERAL HOSPITAL 215 Second Avenue North, Zip 37201; tel. 615/862–4000; Tom Deweese, Administrator, p. B55

6525 ORNDA HEALTHCORP 3401 West End Avenue, Suite 700, Zip 37203; tel. 615/383–8599; Elizabeth A. Berryman, Assistant Vice President and General Counsel, p. B59

0335 PARK HEALTHCARE COMPANY 4015 Travis Drive, Zip 37211; tel. 615/833–1077; Jerry E. Gilliland, President, p. B61

TEXAS

Austin: 0395 HEALTHCARE INTERNATIONAL, INC. 912 South Capital of Texas Highway, Zip 78765–5210, Mailing Address: P.O. Box 4008, Zip 78765–4008; tel. 512/329–8821; Kevin Sheehan, President and Chief Executive Officer, p. B44

0003 ★ ST. DAVID'S HEALTH CARE SYSTEM 919 East 32nd Street, Zip 78705, Mailing Address: P.O. Box 4039, Zip 78765; tel. 512/476–7111; Jack L. Campbell, President, p. B74

0020 TEXAS DEPARTMENT OF HEALTH 1100 West 49th Street, Zip 78756; tel. 512/458–7111; David R. Smith M.D., Commissioner, p. B78

0033 UNIVERSITY OF TEXAS HOSPITALS 601 Colorado Avenue, Zip 78701; tel. 512/471–4224, p. B81

Dallas: 0095 ★ BAYLOR HEALTH CARE SYSTEM 3500 Gaston Avenue, Zip 75226; tel. 214/820–0111; Boone Powell Jr., President, p. B14

2735 ★ METHODIST HOSPITALS OF DALLAS 1441 North Beckley, Zip 75203, Mailing Address: P.O. Box 655999, Zip 75265–5999; tel. 214/947–8181; David H. Hitt, President and Chief Executive Officer, p. B55

1130 ★ PRESBYTERIAN HEALTHCARE SYSTEM 8220 Walnut Hill Lane, Suite 700, Zip 75231; tel. 214/345–8500; Douglas D. Hawthorne, President and Chief Executive Officer, p. B61

Fort Worth: 2345 ★ HARRIS METHODIST HEALTH SYSTEM 6000 Western Place, Suite 200, Zip 76107; tel. 817/570–8900; Ronald L. Smith, President, p. B43

Headquarters of Health Care Systems / Geographically by City and State

0039 ★ TARRANT COUNTY HOSPITAL DISTRICT 1500 South Main Street, Zip 76104; tel. 817/927–1230; Marion Timothy Philpot, President and Chief Executive Officer, p. B76

Houston: 0875 COMMUNITY HEALTH SYSTEMS, INC. 3707 FM 1960 West, Suite 500, Zip 77068; tel. 713/537–5230; E. Thomas Chaney, President, p. B28

2645 ★ MEMORIAL HEALTHCARE SYSTEM 7737 Southwest Freeway, Ste 200, Zip 77074–1800; tel. 713/776–6992; Dan S. Wilford, President, p. B53

7235 ★ METHODIST HOSPITAL SYSTEM 6565 Fannin Street, Zip 77030; tel. 713/790–2221; Larry L. Mathis FACHE, President & Chief Executive Officer, p. B55

0605 ★ SISTERS OF CHARITY OF THE INCARNATE WORD HEALTHCARE SYSTEM 2600 North Loop West, Zip 77092; tel. 713/681–8877; Stanley T. Urban, President and Chief Executive Officer, p. B71

Lubbock: 0036 ★ LUBBOCK METHODIST HOSPITAL SYSTEM 3615 19th Street, Zip 79410–1201; tel. 806/792–1011; William D. Poteet III FACHE, President and Chief Executive Officer, p. B51

San Antonio: 0265 BAPTIST MEMORIAL HOSPITAL SYSTEM 660 North Main St, Ste 300, Zip 78205–1222; tel. 210/222–8431; Callie W. Smith, President and Chief Executive Officer, p. B14

5565 ★ INCARNATE WORD HEALTH SERVICES 9311 San Pedro, Suite 1250, Zip 78216–4469; tel. 210/524–4100; Joseph Blasko Jr., President and Chief Executive Officer, p. B47

Tyler: 1895 EAST TEXAS MEDICAL CENTER REGIONAL HEALTHCARE SYSTEM 1000 South Beckham Street, Zip 75701–1996, Mailing Address: P.O. Drawer 6400, Zip 75711–6400; tel. 903/597–0351; Elmer G. Ellis, President and Chief Executive Officer, p. B38

UTAH

Salt Lake City: 1815 ★ INTERMOUNTAIN HEALTH CARE, INC. 36 South State Street, 22nd Floor, Zip 84111; tel. 801/533–8282; Scott S. Parker, President, p. B48

VIRGINIA

Lynchburg: 2265 ★ CENTRA HEALTH, INC. 1920 Atherholt Road, Zip 24501–1104; tel. 804/947–4700; George W. Dawson, President and Chief Executive Officer, p. B19

Newport News: 4810 RIVERSIDE HEALTH SYSTEM 606 Denbigh Boulevard, Suite 601, Zip 23602; tel. 804/875–7500; Nelson L. St. Clair, President, p. B68

Norfolk: 2635 FIRST HOSPITAL CORPORATION 240 Corporate Boulevard, Zip 23502; tel. 804/459–5100; Ronald Dozoretz M.D., Chairman, p. B39

2565 ★ SENTARA HEALTH SYSTEM 6015 Poplar Hall Drive, Zip 23502; tel. 804/455–7000; David L. Bernd, President and Chief Executive Officer, p. B69

Richmond: 0012 VIRGINIA DEPARTMENT OF MENTAL HEALTH 109 Governor Street, Zip 23219, Mailing Address: P.O. Box 1797, Zip 23214; tel. 804/786–3915; King E. Davis Ph.D., Commissioner, p. B82

Roanoke: 0070 ★ CARILION HEALTH SYSTEM 1212 Third Street S.W., Zip 24016, Mailing Address: P.O. Box 13727, Zip 24036–3727; tel. 703/981–7347; Thomas L. Robertson, President and Chief Executive Officer, p. B17

Springfield: 1305 ★ INOVA HEALTH SYSTEM 8001 Braddock Road, Zip 22151; tel. 703/321–4213; J. Knox Singleton, President, p. B48

Virginia Beach: 2205 ★ TIDEWATER HEALTH CARE, INC. 1080 First Colonial Road, Zip 23454–3001; tel. 804/496–6200; Douglas L. Johnson Ph.D., President and Chief Executive Officer, p. B78

WASHINGTON

Bellevue: 5415 ★ PEACEHEALTH 15325 Southeast 30th Place, Suite 300, Zip 98007; tel. 206/747–1711; Sister Monica Heeran, President, p. B61

0044 STERLING HEALTHCARE CORPORATION 1500 114th Avenue S.E., Suite 100, Zip 98004; tel. 206/453–5445; David Jacobsen, President, p. B75

Seattle: 9995 ★ GROUP HEALTH COOPERATIVE OF PUGET SOUND 521 Wall Street, Zip 98121–1536; tel. 206/326–3000; Phil Nudelman Ph.D., President and Chief Executive Officer, p. B43

5275 ★ SISTERS OF PROVIDENCE HEALTH SYSTEM 520 Pike Street, Zip 98101, Mailing Address: P.O. Box 11038, Zip 98111–9038; tel. 206/464–3355; Sister Dona Taylor, President and Chief Executive Officer, p. B72

Spokane: 0945 EMPIRE HEALTH CENTERS GROUP West 800 Fifth Avenue, Zip 99204, Mailing Address: P.O. Box 248, Zip 99210–0248; tel. 509/458–7965; Thomas M. White, President, p. B39

5265 ★ PROVIDENCE SERVICES 9 East Ninth Avenue, Zip 99202; tel. 509/455–4884; Richard J. Umbdenstock, President and Chief Executive Officer, p. B62

Tacoma: 6555 MULTICARE HEALTH SYSTEM 315 Martin Luther King Jr Way, Zip 98405, Mailing Address: P.O. Box 5299, Zip 98405–0299; tel. 206/552–1000; William B. Connoley, President, p. B56

WEST VIRGINIA

Charleston: 0955 ★ CAMCARE, INC. 501 Morris Street, Zip 25301, Mailing Address: Box 1547, Zip 25326; tel. 304/348–5432; Phillip H. Goodwin, President, p. B17

WISCONSIN

Appleton: 2445 ★ UNITED HEALTH GROUP Five Innovation Court, Zip 54914, Mailing Address: P.O. Box 8025, Zip 54913–8025; tel. 414/730–0330; James Edward Raney, President and Chief Executive Officer, p. B80

Fond Du Lac: 5695 CONGREGATION OF ST. AGNES 475 Gillett Street, Zip 54935–4598; tel. 414/923–0804; Rosann Geiser, Corporate Director, p. B29

La Crosse: 9650 ★ FRANCISCAN HEALTH SYSTEM, INC. 615 South Tenth Street, Zip 54601–4786; tel. 608/791–9710; Brian C. Campion M.D., Chief Executive Officer, p. B40

Manitowoc: 1455 ★ FRANCISCAN SISTERS OF CHRISTIAN CHARITY HEALTHCARE MINISTRY, INC 2409 South Alverno Road, Zip 54220–9320; tel. 414/684–7071; Sister Laura J. Wolf, President, p. B41

Milwaukee: 2215 ★ AURORA HEALTH CARE, INC. 3000 West Montana, Zip 53215–3268, Mailing Address: P.O. Box 343910, Zip 53234–3910; tel. 414/647–3000; G. Edwin Howe, President, p. B12

0027 ★ HORIZON HEALTHCARE, INC. 2300 North Mayfair Road, Suite 550, Zip 53226–1508; tel. 414/257–3888; Kurt W. Metzner, President and Chief Executive Officer, p. B47

3775 MILWAUKEE COUNTY BOARD OF SUPERVISORS 901 North Ninth Street, Zip 53233; tel. 414/278–4244; F. Thomas Ament, County Executive, p. B56

Alliances

ACADEMIC MEDICAL CENTER CONSORTIUM

30 Corporate Woods, Suite 300, Rochester, NY 14623 716/282-7830; Fax 716/292-7820 David M. Witter Jr., President and Chief Executive Officer

FLORIDA
Affiliate
Jacksonville
   Mayo Foundation/St. Luke's Hospital

CALIFORNIA
General Member
Los Angeles
   University of California at Los Angeles Medical Center

IOWA
General Member
Iowa City
   University of Iowa Hospitals & Clinics

LOUISIANA
General Member
New Orleans
   Alton Ochsner Medical Institutions (including the Ochsner Foundation Hospital)

MASSACHUSETTS
General Member
Boston
   Brigham and Women's Hospital
   Massachusetts General Hospital
   New England Medical Center
Member
Springfield
   Baystate Health Systems–including Baystate Medical Center, Franklin Medical Center, and Mary Lane Hospital

MINNESOTA
General Member
Rochester
   Mayo Foundation–including St. Mary's Hospital of Rochester and Rochester Methodist Hospital

NEW YORK
General Members
Rochester
   University of Rochester Medical Center (including Strong Memorial Hospital)
New York
   Mt. Sinai Medical Center
Affiliate
Rochester
   Rochester General Hospital

NEW HAMPSHIRE
General Member
Lebanon
   Dartmouth–Hitchcock Medical Center–including Mary Hitchcock Memorial Hospital

NORTH CAROLINA
General Member
Durham
   Duke University Medical Center

PENNSYLVANIA
General Member
Philadelphia
   University of Pennsylvania Health System

HOSPITALS	BEDS
15	11,374

AMERICAN HEALTH CARE SYSTEMS

12730 High Bluff Drive, Suite 300, San Diego, CA 92130-2099, 619/481-2727; Robert W. O'Leary, Chairman & CEO

CALIFORNIA
Burbank
   UniHealth
Oakland
   Summit Medical Center
Roseville
   Adventist Health System/West

FLORIDA
Gainesville
   AvMed–SantaFe Health Care

ILLINOIS
Oak Brook
   Advocate Health Care
Peoria
   Methodist Health Services Corp.

IOWA
Des Moines
   Iowa Health System

KENTUCKY
Louisville
   Alliant Health System

MARYLAND
Lutherville
   Helix Health System
Marriottsville
   Bon Secours Health System, Inc.

MASSACHUSETTS
Andover
   Yankee Alliance
Springfield
   Baystate Health Systems, Inc.

MICHIGAN
Detroit
   The Detroit Medical Center
   Henry Ford Health System
Farmington Hills
   Mercy Health Services

MINNESOTA
Minneapolis
   Fairview Hospital and Healthcare Services

MISSOURI
Kansas City
   Health Midwest
St. Louis
   SSM Health Care System

NEBRASKA
Omaha
   Immanuel Healthcare Systems, Inc.

NEW MEXICO
Albuquerque
   Presbyterian Healthcare Services

NEW YORK
Rochester
   Seagate Alliance

NORTH DAKOTA
Fargo
   Lutheran Health Systems

OHIO
Cincinnati
   Bethesda Hospital, Inc.
Cleveland
   The Cleveland Clinic Foundation
Mayfield Village
   Meridia Health System

OREGON
Portland
   Legacy Health System

PENNSYLVANIA
Pittsburgh
   Forbes Health System
Radnor
   Main Line Health

SOUTH CAROLINA
Greenville
   Greenville Hospital System

SOUTH DAKOTA
Rapid City
   Rapid City Regional Hospital, Inc.

TENNESSEE
Knoxville
   The Baptist Health System of East Tennessee
Memphis
   Methodist Health Systems Inc.

TEXAS
Abilene
   Hendrick Medical Center
Dallas
   Presbyterian Healthcare System
Fort Worth
   Harris Methodist Health System
Houston
   The Methodist Hospital System

VIRGINIA
Springfield
   Inova Health System

WASHINGTON
Bellevue
   PeaceHealth
Seattle
   Group Health Cooperative of Puget Sound

WISCONSIN
Milwaukee
   Aurora Health Care

HOSPITALS and HEALTH CARE FACILITIES	BEDS
40 owner systems (397 facilities)	70,744
Affiliated– 528 facilities with 68,535 beds	

ASSOCIATION OF INDEPENDENT HOSPITALS

8300 Troost Avenue, Kansas City, MO 64131; 816/276-7580; Jeff Tindle, President, Chief Executive Officer

ILLINOIS
Nashville
   Washington County Hospital
Woodstock
   Memorial Hospital

KANSAS
Columbus
   Maude Norton Memorial City Hospital
Garnett
   Anderson County Hospital
Girard
   Crawford County Hospital District One
Holton
   Holton Community Hospital
Horton
   Horton Community Hospital, Inc.
Iola
   Allen County Hospital
Junction City
   Geary Community Hospital
Kansas City
   Providence Medical Center
   University of Kansas Medical Center
Lawrence
   Lawrence Memorial Hospital

Alliances

Leavenworth
  Saint John Hospital
Olathe
  Olathe Medical Center
Onaga
  Community Hospital Onaga
Ottawa
  Ranson Memorial Hospital
Paola
  Miami County Medical Center Seneca
  Nemaha Valley Community Hospital
Topeka
  Menninger Clinic
  St. Francis Hospital and Medical Center
Winchester
  Jefferson County Memorial Hospital

MISSOURI
Belton
  Research Belton Hospital
Bethany
  Harrison County Community
Boonville
  Cooper County Memorial Hospital
Brookfield
  Pershing Memorial Hospital
Carrollton
  Carroll County Memorial Hospital
Clinton
  Golden Valley Memorial Hospital
Columbia
  University Hospital and Clinics
Farmington
  Mineral Area Regional Medical
Hannibal
  Hannibal Regional Hospital
Harrisonville
  Cass Medical Center
Hermann
  Hermann Area District Hospital
Independence
  Medical Center of Independence
Jefferson City
  St. Mary's Health Center
Joplin
  St. John's Regional Medical Center
Kansas City
  Baptist Medical Center
  Menorah Medical Center
  Research Medical Center
  Trinity Lutheran Hospital
Kirkwood
  St. Joseph Hospital
Lake Saint Louis
  St. Joseph Hospital West
Lee's Summit
  Lee's Summit Hospital
Lexington
  Lafayette Regional Health Center
Louisiana
  Pike County Memorial Hospital
Macon
  Samaritan Memorial Hospital
Mexico
  Audrain Medical Center
Moberly
  Moberly Regional Medical Center
Nevada
  Nevada Regional Medical Center
North Kansas City
  North Kansas City Hospital
Pilot Knob
  Arcadia Valley Hospital
Raytown
  Park Lane Medical Center
Richmond
  Ray County Memorial Hospital
St. Charles
  St. Joseph Health Center
St. Louis
  Cardinal Glennon Children's Hospital
  DePaul Health Center
  Saint Louis University Hospital
  SSM Rehabilitation Institute
  St. Mary's Health Center

Trenton
  Wright Memorial Hospital
Troy
  Lincoln County Memorial Hospital
Warrensburg
  Western Missouri Medical Center

HOSPITALS	BEDS
61	9,118

CHILD HEALTH CORPORATION OF AMERICA
6803 West 64 Street, Suite 208, Shawnee Mission, KS 66202; 913/262-1436; Don C. Black, President and Chief Executive Officer

ALABAMA
Birmingham
  Children's Hospital of Alabama
ARKANSAS
Little Rock
  Arkansas Children's Hospital
Boston
  Children's Hospital
CALIFORNIA
Fresno
  Valley Children's Hospital
Los Angeles
  Children's Hospital Los Angeles
Oakland
  Children's Hospital Medical Center of Northern California
Orange
  Children's Hospital of Orange County
Palo Alto
  Lucile Salter Packard Children's Hospital at Stanford
San Diego
  Children's Hospital and Health Center
COLORADO
Denver
  The Children's Hospital
DISTRICT OF COLUMBIA
  Children's National Medical Center
FLORIDA
Miami
  Miami Children's Hospital
St. Petersburg
  All Children's Hospital
GEORGIA
Atlanta
  Egleston Children's Hospital at Emory University
ILLINOIS
Chicago
  The Children's Memorial Hospital
LOUISIANA
New Orleans
  Children's Hospital
MASSACHUSETTS
Boston
  Children's Hospital
MISSOURI
Kansas City
  The Children's Mercy Hospital
St. Louis
  St. Louis Children's Hospital
NEW YORK
Buffalo
  Children's Hospital of Buffalo
OHIO
Akron
  Children's Hospital Medical Center of Akron
Cincinnati
  Children's Hospital Medical Center
Columbus
  Children's Hospital

Dayton
  The Children's Medical Center
PENNSYLVANIA
Philadelphia
  The Children's Hospital of Philadelphia
Pittsburgh
  Children's Hospital of Pittsburgh
TENNESSEE
Memphis
  Le Bonheur Children's Medical Center
TEXAS
Corpus Christi
  Driscoll Children's Hospital
Dallas
  Children's Medical Center of Dallas
Ft. Worth
  Cook-Ft. Worth Children's Medical Center
Houston
  Texas Children's Hospital
VIRGINIA
Norfolk
  Children's Hospital of The King's Daughters
WASHINGTON
Seattle
  Children's Hospital and Medical Center
WISCONSIN
Milwaukee
  Children's Hospital of Wisconsin

HOSPITALS	BEDS
33	6,548

CONSOLIDATED CATHOLIC HEALTH CARE
1301 W. 22nd Street, Suite 202. Oak Brook, IL 60521; 708/990-2242 (FAX 708/990-2249; Roger Butler, Executive Director

FLORIDA
Tampa
  Allegany Health System
ILLINOIS
Frankfort
  Franciscan Sisters Health Care Corporation
INDIANA
Mishawaka
  Sisters of St. Francis Health Services, Inc.
South Bend
  Holy Cross Health System
KANSAS
Leavenworth
  Sisters of Charity of Leavenworth Health Services Corporation
MASSACHUSETTS
Springfield
  Sisters of Providence Health System
MICHIGAN
Ann Arbor
  Sisters of St. Joseph Health System
Farmington Hills
  Mercy Health Services
NEW YORK
Brooklyn Heights
  Franciscan Sisters of the Poor Health System, Inc.
OHIO
Cincinnati
  Mercy Health System
  Sisters of Charity Health Care Systems Inc.
Lorain
  Humility of Mary Health Care Corporation
Sylvania
  Franciscan Services Corporation

HOSPITALS	BEDS
150	33,000

© 1995 AHA Guide Integrated Health Delivery Networks, Health Care Systems and Alliances B101

Alliances

HOSPITAL NETWORK, INC.
One Healthcare Plaza, Kalamazoo, MI 49007; 616/341-8888; Fax (616/341-6898 Richard Fluke, President, Chief Executive Officer

MICHIGAN
Allegan
   Allegan General Hospital
Hastings
   Pennock Hospital
Kalamazoo
   Bronson Healthcare Group, Inc.
   Bronson Methodist Hospital
Marshall
   Oaklawn Hospital
Sturgis
   Sturgis Hospital
Vicksburg
   Bronson Vicksburg Hospital

HOSPITALS	BEDS
6	839

INTERHEALTH
2550 University Avenue W., Suite 233-N, St. Paul, MN 55114; 612/646-5574; Benjamin Aune, President, Chief Executive Officer

ALABAMA
Birmingham
   Baptist Health System

FLORIDA
Miami
   Baptist Health System of South Florida, Inc.

ILLINOIS
Bloomington
   BroMenn Healthcare
Chicago
   Covenant Benevolent Institutions
Oak Brook
   Advocate Health Care
Park Ridge
   Lutheran General Medical Group, S.C.
Rock Island
   Trinity Regional Health System

IOWA
Sioux City
   St. Luke's Health System, Inc.

KENTUCKY
Louisville
   Baptist Healthcare System

MINNESOTA
St. Paul
   Lutheran Social Service of MN

MISSISSIPPI
Jackson
   Mississippi Baptist Medical Center

MISSOURI
St. Louis
   Deaconess Health System

OHIO
Columbus
   U.S. Health Corporation
Cleveland
   Health Cleveland

HOSPITALS	BEDS
14 members	12,860
34 hospitals	

PREMIER HEALTH ALLIANCE, INC.
Three Westbrook Corporate Center, Ninth Floor, Westchester, IL 60154-5735; 708/409-4100; Alan Weinstein, President

CALIFORNIA
Affiliate Members
Apple Valley
   St. Mary Desert Valley Hospital
Corona
   Corona Regional Medical Center
Mission Viejo
   Mission Hospital Regional Medical Center
Orange
   St. Joseph Hospital
San Diego
   Palomar-Pomerado Health System
Owners
Rancho Mirage
   Eisenhower Medical Center
San Diego
   Sharp HealthCare

CONNECTICUT
Owners
Hartford
   Saint Francis Hospital and Medical Center
Affiliate Member
   Mount Sinai Hospital

DELAWARE
Owner
Wilmington
   Medical Center of Delaware

DISTRICT OF COLUMBIA
Owner
   The George Washington University Medical Center

FLORIDA
Owners
Miami Beach
   Mount Sinai Medical Center
Affiliate Members
Titusville
   Parrish Medical Center

GEORGIA
Owners
Atlanta
   Georgia Baptist Medical Center
Affiliate Member
Atlanta
   Southwest Hospital and Medical Center
Owner
Savannah
   Memorial Medical Center, Inc.

HAWAII
Owner
Honolulu
   Kuakini Medical Center

ILLINOIS
Owners
Chicago
   Illinois Masonic Medical Center
   Mount Sinai Hospital Medical Center
Affiliate Member
LaGrange
   LaGrange Memorial Health System, Inc.
Owner
Winfield
   Central DuPage Health System
Affiliate Members
Melrose Park
   Gottlieb Memorial Hospital
Oak Park
   West Suburban Hospital Medical Center

INDIANA
Affiliate Member
Evansville
   Welborn Memorial Baptist Hospital
Owner
Ft. Wayne
   The Lutheran Hospital of Indiana, Inc.
Gary
   The Methodist Hospitals, Inc.
Affiliate Members
Jeffersonville
   Clark Memorial Hospital
Salem
   Washington County Memorial Hospital
Scottsburg
   Scott Memorial Hospital

KENTUCKY
Owner
Louisville
   Jewish Hospital HealthCare Services
Affiliate Members
Richmond
   Pattie A. Clay Hospital

LOUISIANA
Owners
New Orleans
   Touro Infirmary
Shreveport
   Schumpert Medical Center

MAINE
Affiliate Member
Lewiston
   St. Mary's Regional Medical Center

MARYLAND
Owner
Baltimore
   Sinai Hospital of Baltimore
Affiliate Members
   The New Children's Hospital
   Maryland Kidney Stone Center
   Mt. Washington Pediatric Hospital

MASSACHUSETTS
Owners
Boston
   Beth Israel Hospital
Worcester
   The Medical Center of Central Massachusetts, Inc.
Affiliate Members
Brockton
   Brockton Hospital, Inc.
Cambridge
   Central New England Health Alliance/Leominster Hospital
   Youville Hospital & Rehabilitation Center
Affiliate Member
Gardner
   Heywood Hospital
Affiliate
Palmer
   Wing Memorial Hospital and Medical Center

MICHIGAN
Owners
Detroit
   Sinai Hospital
Owner
Flint
   McLaren Health Care Corporation
Kalamazoo
   Borgess Medical Center
Lansing
   Sparrow Hospital
Affiliate Member
St. Johns
   Clinton Memorial Hospital

MISSISSIPPI
Affiliate
Greenville
   King's Daughters' Hospital
Owner
Jackson
   Mississippi Baptist Medical Center
Affiliate Members
Brandon
   Rankin Medical Center
Louisville
   Winston County Community Hospital & Nursing Home

Alliances

Affiliate
Magee
  Magee General Hospital
Yazoo City
  King's Daughters' Hospital

MONTANA
Affiliates
Great Falls
  Columbus Hospital
Missoula
  St. Patrick Hospital
Polson
  St. Joseph Hospital

NEBRASKA
Owner
Omaha
  Clarkson Hospital

NEW HAMPSHIRE
Affiliate Member
Nashua
  St. Joseph Hospital

NEW JERSEY
Owners
Englewood
  Englewood Hospital and Medical Center
Long Branch
  Monmouth Medical Center
Newark
  Newark Beth Israel Medical Center
Affiliate Members
East Orange
  East Orange General Hospital
Edison
  JFK Health Systems, Inc.
Freehold
  CentraState Health System
Holmdel
  Bayshore Community Hospital
Irvington
  Irvington General Hospital
Manahawkin
  Southern Ocean County Hospital
Salem
  The Memorial Hospital of Salem County, Inc.
Montclair
  The Mountainside Hospital
Passaic
  Beth Israel Hospital
Paterson
  Barnert Hospital

NEW YORK
Owners
Brooklyn
  St. Mary's Hospital of Brooklyn Division
Buffalo
  Millard Fillmore Health System
Affiliate
Elmhurst
  St. John's Queens Hospital Division
Flushing
  St. Joseph's Hospital Division
Jamaica
  Catholic Medical Center of Brooklyn and Queens, Inc.
  Mary Immaculate Hospital Division
New York City
  Beth Israel Medical Center
  The Long Island College Hospital
  Long Island Jewish Medical Center – (In New York Hyde Park, NY)
  Maimonides Medical Center
  Montefiore Medical Center
  The Mount Sinai Medical Center
Rochester
  Strong Memorial Hospital of the University of Rochester
Staten Island
  Staten Island University Hospital

Affiliate Members
Owner
Uniondale
  Episcopal Health Services
Manhattan
  Jewish Home and Hospital for Aged
Mineola
  Winthrop–University Hospital
Newfane
  Inter-Community Memorial Hospital
Nyack
  Nyack Hospital
Port Jefferson
  St. Charles Hospital and Rehabilitation Center
Poughkeepsie
Affiliate
  St. Francis Hospital
Owner
  Vassar Brothers Hospital
Affiliates
Rhinebeck
  Northern Dutchess Hospital

OHIO
Owners
Akron
  Summa Health System
Affiliate
Bellevue
  The Bellevue Hospital
Bowling Green
  Wood County Hospital
Owners
Cincinnati
  Jewish Hospitals, Inc.
Cleveland
  Mt. Sinai Health Care System
Fostoria
  Fostoria Community Hospital
Affiliate
Greensprings
  St. Francis Health Care Centre
Owner
Toledo
  Covenant Health Systems/St. Vincent Medical Center
Affiliate
Sandusky
  Providence Hospital
Affiliate Member
Sylvania
  Flower Hospital
Tiffin
  Mercy Hospital
Affiliate
Wauseon
  Fulton County Health Center
Willard
  Mercy Hospital

PENNSYLVANIA
Owners
Bethlehem
  St. Luke's Hospital
Harrisburg
  Polyclinic Medical Center
Meadville
  Vantage Health Group
Philadelphia
  Albert Einstein Healthcare Network
Pittsburgh
  The Western Pennsylvania Hospital
Affiliate Members
Allentown
  Allentown Osteopathic Medical Center
Danville
  Geisinger Medical Center
Easton
  Easton Hospital
Hazleton
  Hazleton–Saint Joseph Medical Center

Quakertown
  Quakertown Community Hospital

RHODE ISLAND
Owner
Providence
  The Miriam Hospital

TEXAS
Affiliate
Clifton
  Goodall–Witcher Hospital
Gatesville
  Coryell Memorial Hospital
Hamilton
  Hamilton General Hospital
Owners
Houston
  St. Luke's Episcopal Hospital
  The University of Texas M. D. Anderson Cancer Center
Affiliates
Llano
  Llano Memorial Hospital
Marlin
  Falls Community Hospital and Clinic
Mexia
  Parkview Regional Hospital
Taylor
  Johns Community Hospital
West
  West Community Hospital
Owner
Temple
  Scott and White Memorial Hospital

VERMONT
Affiliate Member
Colchester
  Fanny Allen Hospital

WASHINGTON
Owners
Seattle
  Northwest Hospital
Spokane
  Providence Services/Sacred Heart Medical Center
Affiliate Members
Chewelah
  St. Joseph's Hospital
Colfax
  Whitman Hospital and Medical Center
Colville
  Mount Carmel Hospital
Richland
  Kadlec Medical Center
Spokane
  Holy Family Hospital
Walla Walla
  St. Mary Medical Center

HOSPITALS	BEDS
135	49,418

(54 Owners and 81 Affiliates)

THE SUNHEALTH ALLIANCE

SunHealth Alliance, Inc., 4501 Charlotte Park Drive (28217), P.O. Box 668800, Charlotte, NC 28266–8800; 704/529–3300; Ben W. Latimer, President

ALABAMA
Shareholders
Dothan
  Southeast Alabama Medical Center
Opelika
  East Alabama Health Care Authority (East Alabama Medical Center)
Affiliates
  George H. Lanier Memorial Hospital and Nursing Home

Alliances

ARKANSAS
Shareholders
Batesville
  White River Medical Center, Inc.
Little Rock
  Arkansas Children's Hospital
Pine Bluff
  Jefferson Regional Medical Center
Springdale
  Northwest Health System, Inc. (Northwest Medical Center)
Affiliates
Morrilton
  Conway County Hospital
Sherwood
  Central Arkansas Rehabilitation Hospital
Affiliates
Berryville
  Carroll General Hospital
Harrison
  North Arkansas Medical Center

DELAWARE
Shareholder
Dover
  Kent General Hospital, Inc.
Lewes
  Beebe Medical Center, Inc.

DISTRICT OF COLUMBIA
Shareholders
  Columbia Hospital for Women Medical Center, Inc.
  Sibley Memorial Hospital

FLORIDA
Shareholders
Atlantis
  JFK Medical Center, Inc.
Bradenton
  Manatee Hospitals and Health Systems, Inc. (Manatee Memorial Hospital)
Cape Coral
  The Cape Coral Medical Center, Inc.
Clearwater
  Morton F. Plant Hospital Association, Inc.
Fort Lauderdale
  Foundation Healthcorp, Inc. (North Broward Hospital District)
Gainesville
  Shands Teaching Hospital and Clinics, Inc.
Jacksonville
  Southern Baptist Hospital of Florida, Inc. (d/b/a Baptist Medical Center)
Miami
  Baptist Health Systems of South Florida
Naples
  Community Health Care, Inc. (Naples Community Hospital, Inc.)
Orlando
  Adventist Health System/Sunbelt Health Care Corporation
Ormond Beach
  Memorial Health Systems, Inc.
Pensacola
  Sacred Heart Hospital of Pensacola
Plant City
  South Florida Baptist Hospital
Rockledge
  Wuestoff Health Systems, Inc.
Sarasota
  Community Health Corporation (Sarasota Memorial Hospital)
Tampa
  Franciscan Sisters of Allegany Health System, Inc.
Tarpon Springs
  Tarpon Springs Hospital Foundation, Inc. (d/b/a Helen Ellis Memorial Hospital)
Vero Beach
  Indian River Memorial Hospital, Inc.
Winter Haven
  Mid–Florida Medical Services, Inc. (Winter Haven Hospital, Inc.)

Affiliates
Largo
  Sun Coast Hospital, Inc.

GEORGIA
Shareholders
Athens
  St. Mary's Health Care System, Inc.
Atlanta
  Crawford Long Hospital
  Egleston Children's Hospital at Emory University
  Emory University Hospital
Augusta
  St. Joseph Center for Life, Inc.
  University Health Services, Inc. (University Hospital)
Columbus
  St. Francis Hospital
Fort Oglethorpe
  Hutcheson Medical Center
LaGrange
  West Georgia Medical Center, Inc.
Riverdale
  Georgia Medcorp, Inc. (d/b/a Southern Regional Medical Center)
Savannah
  St. Joseph's Hospital, Inc.
Tifton
  Tift General Hospital

KENTUCKY
Shareholders
Bowling Green
  Commonwealth Health Corporation (The Medical Center at Bowling Green)
Glasgow
  T. J. Samson Community Hospital, Inc.
Henderson
  Community United Methodist Hospital, Inc.
Louisville
  Baptist Healthcare System
Murray
  Murray–Calloway County Hospital
Nazareth
  Sisters of Charity of Nazareth Health Corporation
Pikeville
  The Methodist Hospital of Kentucky, Inc. (Pikeville United Methodist Hospital of Kentucky)
Affiliates
Berea
  Berea Hospital, Inc.
Lancaster
  Garrard County Memorial Hospital
Mt. Sterling
  Mary Chiles Hospital, Inc.
Mt. Vernon
  Rockcastle Hospital/Respiratory Care Center, Inc.
Stanford
  Fort Logan Hospital Foundation, Inc.
Versailles
  Woodford Hospital

LOUISIANA
Shareholders
Baton Rouge
  General Health, Inc.
Bossier City
  Bossier County Medical Center
Houma
  Terrebonne General Medical Center
Lafayette
  Lafayette General Medical Center
Marrero
  West Jefferson Medical Center
New Orleans
  Mercy and Baptist Medical Center
West Monroe
  Glenwood Regional Medical Center
Affiliates
Bastrop
  Morehouse General Hospital
Columbia
  Citizens Medical Center
Delhi
  Richland Parish Hospital

Galliano
  Lady of the Sea General Hospital
Rayville
  Richardson Medical Center
Ruston
  Lincoln General Hospital
Raceland
  St. Anne General Hospital
Winnsboro
  Franklin Medical Center

MARYLAND
Shareholders
Annapolis
  Anne Arundel Health System, Inc.
Baltimore
  Church Hospital Corporation
  Harbor Health System Corporation
  Helix Health System (Franklin Square Hospital and Union Memorial Health Services, Inc.)
Bethesda
  Suburban Hospital, Inc.
Columbia
  Howard County General Hospital, Inc.
Cumberland
  The Memorial Hospital and Medical Center of Cumberland, Inc.
Elkton
  Union Hospital of Cecil County
Frederick
  Frederick Memorial Hospital, Inc.
Hagerstown
  Washington County Hospital Association
Lanham
  Doctors' Hospital, Inc.
Olney
  Montgomery General Hospital
Randallstown
  Northwest Hospital and Health System, Inc.
Salisbury
  Peninsula Regional Medical Center
Westminster
  Carroll County General Hospital, Inc.
Affiliate
Cambridge
  Dorchester General Hospital, Inc.

MISSISSIPPI
Shareholders
Clarksdale
  Northwest Mississippi Regional Medical Center
Grenada
  Grenada Lake Medical Center
Hattiesburg
  Wesley Health System, Inc.
Laurel
  South Central Regional Medical Center
Meridian
  Rush Health Systems, Inc.
Affiliates
Amory
  Gilmore Memorial Hospital

NORTH CAROLINA
Shareholders
Albemarle
  Stanly Memorial Hospital, Inc.
Asheboro
  Randolph Hospital
Asheville
  Memorial Mission Hospital, Inc.
Boone
  Watauga Medical Center, Inc.
Burlington
  Alamance Health Services, Inc.
Charlotte
  Presbyterian Health Services Corporation
Clyde
  Haywood County Hospital
Concord
  Cabarrus Memorial Hospital Development Association
Durham
  Durham County Hospital Corporation

Alliances

Fayetteville
  Cumberland County Health System, Inc. (d/b/a Cape Fear Valley Medical Center)
Gastonia
  Gaston Healthcare Inc.
Goldsboro
  Wayne Memorial Hospital, Inc.
Greensboro
  The Moses H. Cone Memorial Hospital
Hendersonville
  Margaret R. Pardee Memorial Hospital
Hickory
  Catawba Memorial Hospital
High Point
  High Point Regional Hospital
Kinston
  Lenoir Health Services, Inc.
Lenoir
  Caldwell Memorial Hospital, Inc.
Lumberton
  Southeastern Regional Medical Center
Morganton
  Grace Hospital, Inc.
New Bern
  Craven Regional Medical Authority
Pinehurst
  Moore Regional Hospital, Inc.
Raleigh
  Rex Hospital, Inc.
Roanoke Rapids
  Halifax Memorial Hospital
Salisbury
  Rowan Memorial Hospital, Inc.
Shelby
  Cleveland Memorial Hospital, Inc.
Statesville
  Iredell Memorial Hospital, Incorporated
Sylva
  Harris Regional Hospital
Wilmington
  New Hanover Regional Medical Center
Wilson
  Wilson Memorial Hospital
Winston–Salem
  North Carolina Baptist Hospitals, Inc.
Affiliates
Asheville
  Thoms Rehabilitation Hospital
Banner Elk
  Charles A. Cannon Jr. Memorial Hospital, Inc.
Blowing Rock
  Blowing Rock Hospital
Burgaw
  Pender Memorial Hospital
Clinton
  Sampson County Memorial Hospital, Inc.
Crossnore
  Sloop Memorial Hospital, Inc.
Edenton
  Chowan Hospital
Elizabethtown
  Bladen County Hospital
Henderson
  Maria Parham Hospital
Jacksonville
  Onslow Memorial Hospital
Kenansville
  Duplin General Hospital, Inc.
Lexington
  Lexington Memorial Hospital, Inc.
Lincolnton
  Lincoln County Hospital
Marion
  The McDowell Hospital
Mount Airy
  Northern Hospital of Surry County
Marion
  The McDowell Hospital
Murphy
  Murphy Medical Center
North Wilkesboro
  Wilkes Regional Medical Center
Rockingham
  Richmond Memorial Hospital, Inc.
Troy
  Montgomery Memorial Hospital, Inc.
Wadesboro
  Anson County Hospital and Skilled Nursing Facilities
Williamston
  Martin General Hospital
Winston–Salem
  Baptist Retirement Homes of North Carolina, Inc.

SOUTH CAROLINA
Shareholders
Anderson
  Anderson Area Medical Center
Columbia
  Richland Regional Medical Center Foundation
Conway
  Conway Hospital, Inc.
Florence
  McLeod Regional Medical Center
Greenwood
  Self Memorial Hospital
Spartanburg
  Spartanburg Regional Medical Center
West Columbia
  Lexington Medical Center
Affiliates
Camden
  Kershaw County Memorial Hospital
Columbus, N.C.
  St. Luke's Hospital, Inc.
Edgefield
  Edgefield County Hospital
Lake City
  Lake City Community Hospital
Lancaster
  Springs Memorial Hospital, Inc.

TENNESSEE
Shareholders
Chattanooga
  Erlanger Medical Center
Cleveland
  Bradley Memorial Hospital
Gallatin
  Sumner Regional Medical Center
Johnson City
  Johnson City Medical Center Hospital, Inc.
Kingsport
  Holston Valley Health Care, Inc.
Maryville
  Blount Memorial Hospital, Inc.
Nashville
  Vanderbilt University Hospital and the Vanderbilt Clinic
Affiliate
Erwin
  Unicoi County Memorial Hospital, Inc.
Hixon
  North Park Hospital
Johnson City
  Watauga Mental Health Services, Inc.

TEXAS
Shareholders
Bryan
  St. Joseph Hospital and Health Center
Dallas
  Methodist Hospitals of Dallas
Denison
  Texoma Medical Center, Inc.
El Paso
  El Paso County Hospital District (d/b/a Thomason General Hospital)
Galveston
  The University of Texas Medical Branch at Galveston
Lubbock
  University Medical Center Foundation
Lufkin
  Memorial Medical Center of East Texas
Nacogdoches
  Nacogdoches County Hospital District
Paris
  McCuistion Regional Medical Center
Weslaco
  Knapp Medical Center
Affiliate
Caldwell
  Burleson Memorial Hospital
Madisonville
  Madison County Hospital

VIRGINIA
Shareholders
Abingdon
  Johnston Memorial Hospital, Inc.
Chesapeake
  Chesapeake Hospital Authority
Danville
  Danville Regional Medical Center
Galax
  Twin County Community Hospital, Inc.
Hopewell
  Hopewell Hospital Authority (John Randolph Hospital)
Marion
  Smyth County Community Hospital, Inc.
Newport News
  Riverside Health System
Norfolk
  DePaul Hospital
Richmond
  Health Corporation of Virginia (Richmond Memorial Hospital)
  The Retreat Hospital
Roanoke
  Carilion Health System
South Hill
  Community Memorial Healthcenter
Suffolk
  Louise Obici Memorial Hospital
Virginia Beach
  Tidewater Health Care, Inc.
Winchester
  Valley Health System (Winchester Medical Center, Inc.)
Affiliates
Culpeper
  Culpeper Memorial Hospital, Inc.
Luray
  Page Memorial Hospital, Inc.
Nassawdox
  Northampton–Accomack Memorial Hospital
Petersburg
  Grant Memorial Hospital
Romney
  Hampshire Memorial Hospital, Inc.
Stuart
  R.J. Reynolds–Patrick County Memorial
Woodstock
  Shenandoah County Memorial Hospital

WEST VIRGINIA
Shareholders
Bluefield
  Bluefield Community Hospital, Inc.
Clarksburg
  United Hospital Center, Inc.
Elkins
  Davis Memorial Hospital
Morgantown
  Monongalia Health System, Inc. (Monongalia General Hospital)
Parkersburg
  Camden–Clark Memorial Hospital
Point Pleasant
  Pleasant Valley Hospital, Inc.
South Charleston
  Herbert J. Thomas Memorial Hospital Association
Weirton
  Weirton Medical Center, Inc.
Affiliate
Buckhannon
  St. Joseph's Hospital of Buckhannon, Inc.
Huntington
  St. Mary's Hospital
Keyser
  Potomac Valley Hospital of West Virginia, Inc.

Alliances

Kingwood
  Preston Memorial Hospital Corporation
New Martinsville
  Wetzel County Hospital
Ranson
  Jefferson Memorial Hospital
Summersville
  Summersville Memorial Hospital
Weston
  Stonewall Jackson Memorial Hospital

HOSPITALS	BEDS
306	74,000

SYNERNET, Inc.
222 St. John Street, Portland, ME 04102; 207/775-6081; Paul I. Davis III, President

MAINE
Bangor
  St. Joseph Hospital
Bar Harbor
  Mount Desert Island Hospital
Biddeford
  Southern Maine Medical Center
Bridgton
  Northern Cumberland Memorial Hospital
Brunswick
  Mid Coast Hospital
Damariscotta
  Miles Health Care
Farmington
  Franklin Memorial Hospital
Fort Kent
  Northern Maine Medical Center
Lewiston
  St. Mary's General Hospital
Norway
  Stephens Memorial Hospital
Pittsfield
  Sebasticook Valley Hospital
Portland
  Brighton Medical Center
  Mercy Hospital
Rockland
  Penobscot Bay Medical Center
Rumford
  Rumford Community Hospital
Sanford
  H. D. Goodall Hospital
Skowhegan
  Redington-Fairview General Hospital
Waterville
  Waterville Osteopathic Hospital
Westbrook
  Westbrook Community Hospital
York
  York Hospital

HOSPITALS	BEDS
20	2,558
	(includes four nursing facilities)

UNIVERSITY HEALTH SYSTEM OF NEW JERSEY
Plaza 11, 317 George Street, New Brunswick, NJ 08901; 908/235-7000 (FAX 908/235-7010); Thomas E. Terrill, Ph.D., FACHE, Executive Vice President

NEW JERSEY
Atlantic City
  Atlantic City Medical Center
Camden
  Cooper Hospital/University Medical Center
Cherry Hill
  Kennedy Memorial Hospitals-University Medical Center
Hackensack
  Hackensack Medical Center
Neptune
  Jersey Shore Medical Center
Newark
  University of Medicine & Dentistry of New Jersey UMDNJ-University Hospital
New Brunswick
  Robert Wood Johnson University Hospital
Stratford
  Kennedy Memorial Hospitals-University Medical Center
Trenton
  Helene Fuld Medical Center
Washington Twp. (Camden County)
  Kennedy Memorial Hospitals University Medical Center
West Orange
  Kessler Institute for Rehabilitation

HOSPITALS	BEDS
9	4000

UNIVERSITY HOSPITAL CONSORTIUM, INC.
2001 Spring Road, Suite 700, Oak Brook, IL 60521-1890; 708/954-1700; Robert J. Baker, President

ALABAMA
Birmingham
  University of Alabama Hospital
ARIZONA
Tucson
  University Medical Center Corporation
ARKANSAS
Little Rock
  The University Hospital of Arkansas
CALIFORNIA
Los Angeles
  University of California, Los Angeles Medical Center
Orange
  University of California, Irvine Medical Center
Sacramento
  University of California, Davis Medical Center
San Diego
  University of California, San Diego Medical Center
San Francisco
  The Medical Center at UC San Francisco
Stanford
  Stanford University Hospital
COLORADO
Denver
  University of Colorado Hospital
CONNECTICUT
Farmington
  John Dempsey Hospital, The University of Connecticut Health Center
New Haven
  Yale-New Haven Hospital
DISTRICT OF COLUMBIA
  Georgetown University Hospital
  Howard University Hospital
FLORIDA
Gainesville
  Shands Hospital at the University of Florida
GEORGIA
Atlanta
  Emory University System of Health Care
Augusta
  Medical College of Georgia Hospital and Clinics
ILLINOIS
Chicago
  University of Chicago Hospitals
  University of Illinois Hospital and Clinics
Maywood
  Loyola University Medical Center
INDIANA
Indianapolis
  Indiana University Medical Center
IOWA
Iowa City
  The University of Iowa Hospitals and Clinics

KANSAS
Kansas City
  The University of Kansas Hospital
KENTUCKY
Lexington
  University of Kentucky Hospital
LOUISIANA
New Orleans
  Tulane University Hospital and Clinic
Shreveport
  Louisiana State University Medical Center
MARYLAND
Baltimore
  University of Maryland Medical System
MASSACHUSETTS
Worcester
  University of Massachusetts Medical Center
MICHIGAN
Ann Arbor
  University of Michigan Hospitals
MINNESOTA
Minneapolis
  University of Minnesota Hospital and Clinic
MISSOURI
Columbia
  University of Missouri Hospitals and Clinics
St. Louis
  St. Louis University Hospital
NEBRASKA
Omaha
  University of Nebraska Medical Center
NEW JERSEY
Newark
  University of Medicine and Dentistry of New Jersey, University Hospital
New Brunswick
  Robert Wood Johnson University Hospital, UMDNJ
NEW YORK
Albany
  Albany Medical Center
Brooklyn
  SUNY Health Science Center at Brooklyn
New York City
  New York University Medical Center
  The Presbyterian Hospital, Columbia-Presbyterian Medical Center
Stony Brook
  SUNY University Hospital at Stony Brook
Syracuse
  SUNY Health Science Center at Syracuse
NORTH CAROLINA
Chapel Hill
  University of North Carolina Hospitals
Greenville
  University Medical Center of Eastern Carolina-Pitt County
Winston-Salem
  Bowman Gray/Baptist Hospital Medical Center
OHIO
Cincinnati
  University of Cincinnati Hospital
Cleveland
  University Hospitals of Cleveland, Case Western Reserve University
Columbus
  The Ohio State University Hospitals
Toledo
  Medical College of Ohio Hospital
OKLAHOMA
Oklahoma City
  The University Hospitals
OREGON
Portland
  Oregon Health Sciences University Hospital & Clinics

PENNSYLVANIA
Hershey
  Penn State's Milton S. Hershey Medical Center
Philadelphia
  Hahnemann University Hospital
  Hospital of the University of Pennsylvania
  Thomas Jefferson University Hospital
Pittsburgh
  University of Pittsburgh Medical Center

SOUTH CAROLINA
Charleston
  Medical University of South Carolina

TENNESSEE
Nashville
  Vanderbilt University Hospital and Clinic

TEXAS
Dallas
  Zale Lipshy University Hospital, University of Texas Southwestern Medical Center
Galveston
  University of Texas Medical Branch
Houston
  Hermann Hospital at the University of Texas Health Science Center

UTAH
Salt Lake City
  University of Utah Health Sciences Center

VIRGINIA
Charlotteville
  University of Virginia Medical Center
Richmond
  Medical College of Virginia Hospitals, Virginia Commonwealth University

WASHINGTON
Seattle
  University of Washington Academic Medical Center

WEST VIRGINIA
Morgantown
  West Virginia University Hospitals

WISCONSIN
Madison
  Froedtert Memorial Lutheran Hospital, Inc.
  University of Wisconsin Hospital and Clinics

SWITZERLAND
Zurich
  University Hospital of Zurich

HOSPITALS	BEDS
68	39,850

VANTAGE HEALTH GROUP
265 Conneaut Lake Road, Meadville, Pennsylvania 16335; (814) 337–0000; Gerald P. Alonge, Executive Director

PENNSYLVANIA
Erie
  Millcreek Community Hospital
  Saint Vincent Health System
Farrell
  Horizon Hospital System–Shenango Division
Franklin
  Northwest Medical Center–Franklin Campus
Greenville
  Horizon Hospital System–Greenville Division
Grove City
  United Community Hospital
Kane
  The Community Hospital
Meadville
  Meadville Medical Center
Oil City
  Northwest Medical Center–Oil City Campus
Titusville
  Titusville Area Hospital
Union City
  Union City Memorial Hospital
Warren
  Warren General Hospital

Hospitals	Beds
11	1,700

VOLUNTARY HOSPITALS, INC.
220 East Colinas Boulevard, Irving, TX 75039; P.O. Box 140909, Irving TX 75014; 215/830–0000; C. Thomas Smith, President, Chief Executive Officer

ALABAMA
Shareholders
Birmingham
  Baptist Health System, Inc.
Mobile
  Infirmary Health System, Inc.
Montgomery
  Baptist Health Services Corp.
Partners
  Cullman Medical Center
  DCH Healthcare Authority
  Decatur General Hospital
  Eliza Coffee Memorial Hospital
  Jackson County Health Care Authority
  Marshall County Health Care Authority
  Regional Health Services, Inc.
  The Health Care Authority of the City of Huntsville
  Vaughn Regional Medical Center

ARIZONA
Shareholders
Tucson
  Health Partners of Southern Arizona

ARKANSAS
Shareholders
Fort Smith
  Sparks Regional Medical Center
Little Rock
  Baptist Medical System
Partner
  St. Bernard's Regional Medical Center

CALIFORNIA
Shareholders
Emeryville
  Alta Bates Health System
Fresno
  Community Hospitals of Central California
La Jolla
  Scripps Memorial Hospitals
Long Beach
  Memorial Health Services
Los Angeles
  Cedars–Sinai Medical Center
Newport Beach
  Hoag Memorial Hospital Presbyterian
Sacramento
  Sutter Health
San Francisco
  California Pacific Medical Center
San Jose
  Good Samaritan Health System, Inc.
Van Nuys
  Valley Presbyterian Hospital
Partners
  Anaheim Memorial Hospital
  Antelope Valley Hospital Med. Center.
  Bakersfield Memorial Hospital
  Citrus Valley Health Partners
  Emanuel Medical Center, Inc.
  John Muir Medical Center
  Memorial Hospitals Association
  Palomar Pomerado Health System
  Pomona Valley Hospital Medical Center
  Presbyterian Intercommunity Hospital
  Riverside Community Hospital
  Santa Barbara Cottage Hospital
  Santa Clarita Health Care Association, Inc.
  Southern California Healthcare System, Ltd.
  St. Joseph's Regional Health System
  Torrance Memorial Medical Center

COLORADO
Shareholders
Englewood
  HealthOne
Wheat Ridge
  Lutheran Medical Center
Partners
  Arkansas Valley Regional Medical Center
  Aspen Valley Hospital
  Boulder Community Hospital
  Community Hospital
  Longmont United Hospital Association
  Memorial Hospital of Colorado Springs
  Poudre Valley Hospital
  Routt Memorial Hospital, Inc.
  San Luis Valley Regional Medical Center, Inc.
  Vail Valley Medical Center

CONNECTICUT
Shareholders
Hartford
  Hartford Hospital
New Haven
  Yale–New Haven Health Services Corporation
Partners
  Bridgeport Hospital
  Day Kimball Hospital
  Greater Waterbury Health Network, Inc.
  Manchester Memorial Hospital
  Middlesex Hospital
  New Britain General Hospital
  The Charlotte Hungerford Hospital
  The Danbury Hospital
  The Greenwich Hospital Association
  The Stamford Hospital
  Veterans Memorial Medical Center

DELAWARE
Partner
Milford
  Milford Memorial Hospital, Inc.

DISTRICT OF COLUMBIA
Shareholder
  Medlantic Healthcare Group

FLORIDA
Shareholders
Daytona Beach
  Halifax Health Care Systems, Inc.
Gainesville
  SantaFe HealthCare, Inc.
Lakeland
  Lakeland Regional Medical Center
Melbourne
  Holmes Regional Medical Center, Inc.
Orlando
  Orlando Regional Healthcare System
Pensacola
  Baptist Health Care Corporation
Tallahassee
  Tallahassee Memorial Regional Medical Center
Partners
  Bay Medical Center
  Bayfront Medical Center, Inc.
  Bethesda Memorial Hospital, Inc.
  Boca Raton Community Hospital, Inc.
  Citrus Memorial Hospital
  Coastal Health Corporation
  Good Samaritan Medical Center
  Lee Memorial Hospital
  Mease Health Care
  Methodist Hospital, Inc.
  Munroe Regional Medical Center
  South Miami Health System, Inc.
  St. Luke's Hospital
  University Community Hospital, Inc.
  Venice Hospital

GEORGIA
Shareholder
Atlanta
  Piedmont Hospital
Partners
  Athens Regional Medical Center
  Candler Health Services, Inc.
  Cobb Health Services, Inc.
  Columbus Regional Healthcare System, Inc.
  DeKalb Medical Center

Alliances

Floyd Medical Center
Gwinnett Hospital System
Hamilton Medical Center, Inc.
John D. Archbold Memorial Hospital
Kennestone Regional Health Care System, Inc.
Medical Center of Central Georgia
Northeast Georgia Health Services, Inc.
Northside Hospital
Phoebe Putney Memorial Hospital
South Fulton Medical Center
South Georgia Medical Center

HAWAII
Shareholder
Honolulu
  The Queen's Medical Center

IDAHO
Shareholder
Boise
  St. Luke's Regional Medical Center, Ltd.
Partners
  Bannock Regional Medical Center
  Kootenai Medical Center

ILLINOIS
Shareholders
Chicago
  Northwestern Memorial Corporation
  Rush–Presbyterian–St. Luke's Medical Center
Decatur
  DMH Health Systems
Evanston
  Evanston Hospital Corporation
Harvey
  Ingalls Health System
Park Ridge
  Advocate Health Care
Springfield
  Memorial Medical Center System
Partners
  Anderson Hospital
  Blessing Corporate Services, Inc.
  Bromenn HealthCare
  Elmhurst Memorial Hospital
  Freeport Memorial Hospital
  Highland Park Hospital
  Katherine Shaw Bethea Hospital
  Kishwaukee Community Hospital
  Lake Forest Hospital
  Little Company of Mary Hospital and Health Care Center
  MacNeal Hospital
  McDonough District Hospital
  Memorial Hospital
  Passavant Area Hospital
  Riverside Medical Center
  Rockford Memorial Hospital
  Sarah Bush Lincoln Health Center
  Sherman Hospital
  Silver Cross Hospital Corp.
  Southern Illinois Hospital Services
  Trinity Medical Center

INDIANA
Shareholders
Evansville
  Deaconess Development Corp.
Indianapolis
  Community Hospitals of Indiana, Inc.
Muncie
  Ball Memorial Hospital
South Bend
  Memorial Health System, Inc.
Partners
  Bloomington Hospital
  Columbus Regional Hospital
  Community Hospital of Anderson–Madison County, Inc.
  Elkhart General Hospital
  Floyd Memorial Hospital
  Good Samaritan Hospital
  Hendricks County Hospital
  Indiana University Hospitals
  LaPorte Hospital, Inc.

Marion General Hospital
North Central Health Services, Inc.
Parkview Memorial Hospital
Porter Memorial Hospital
Reid Memorial Hospital
Riverview Hospital
The King's Daughters' Hospital
Union Hospital

IOWA
Shareholders
Cedar Rapids
  St. Luke's Methodist Hospital
Partners
  Burlington Medical Center
  Cass County Memorial Hospital
  Covenant Medical Center, Inc.
  Delaware County Memorial Hospital
  Floyd County Memorial Hospital
  Genesis Medical Center
  Grinnell General Hospital
  Henry County Health Center
  Jackson County Public Hospital
  Jefferson County Hospital
  Jennie Edmundson Memorial Hospital
  Keokuk Area Hospital
  Lucas County Health Center
  Mercy Hospital
  Montgomery County Memorial Hospital
  Ottumwa Regional Health Center
  Sartori Memorial Hospital
  Skiff Medical Center
  St. Luke's Regional Medical Center
  The Finley Hospital
  Trinity Regional Hospital of Ft. Dodge

KANSAS
Shareholder
Topeka
  Stormont–Vail Regional Medical Center
Partners
  Asbury–Salina Regional Medical Center
  Atchison Hospital
  Bethany Medical Center, Inc.
  Citizens Medical Center
  Great Plains Health Alliance
  Hays Medical Center
  Hutchinson Hospital Corporation
  Pratt Regional Medical Center
  Shawnee Mission Medical Center
  Southwest Medical Center
  St. Francis Ministry Corporation

KENTUCKY
Partners
  Owensboro–Daviess County Hospital
  Regional Medical Center of Hopkins County
  St. Luke Hospital, Inc.

LOUISIANA
Shareholders
Baton Rouge
  Our Lady of the Lake Regional Medical Center
New Orleans
  Alton Oschner Medical Foundation
Shreveport
  Willis–Knighton Medical Center
Partners
  American Legion Hospital
  Beauregard Memorial Hospital
  Lake Charles Memorial Hospital
  Lincoln General Hospital
  Our Lady of Lourdes Regional Medical Center
  Pendleton Memorial Methodist Hospital
  St. Francis Medical Center, Inc.
  Woman's Hospital

MAINE
Shareholder
Portland
  Maine Medical Center
Partners
  Central Maine Medical Center
  Kennebec Health System
  Mid-Maine Medical Center

Southern Maine Medical Center

MARYLAND
Partners
  The Memorial Hospital at Easton Maryland, Inc.
  Upper Chesapeake Health System, Inc.

MASSACHUSETTS
Shareholders
Boston
  New England Medical Center Hospitals, Inc.
  The General Hospital Corporation
Partners
  Addison Gilbert Hospital
  Beverly Hospital
  Cape Cod Hospital
  Emerson Hospital
  Harrington Memorial Hospital
  Health Alliance
  Lawrence General Hospital
  Lawrence Memorial Hospital of Medford
  Lowell General Hospital
  Massachusetts Eye and Ear Infirmary
  Melrose–Wakefield Hospital Association
  Mount Auburn Hospital
  Newell Health Care System, Inc.
  South Shore Health and Educational Corp.
  St. Luke's Hospital of New Bedford, Inc.
  St. Vincent Healthcare System, Inc.

MICHIGAN
Shareholders
Grand Rapids
  Butterworth Hospital
Royal Oak
  William Beaumont Hospital
Partners
  Bay Medical Center
  Blue Water Health Services Corporation
  Bronson Healthcare Group, Inc.
  Genesys Health System
  Healthshare Group, Inc.
  Holland Community Hospital
  Lakeland Regional Health System
  Lenawee Health Systems
  Mercy Memorial Hospital Foundation
  Michigan Capital Healthcare
  Oakwood Health Services Corporation
  Saginaw General Hospital
  St. John Hospital & Medical Center

MINNESOTA
Shareholders
Minneapolis
  Allina Health System
St. Paul
  HealthEast Inc.
Partners
  Immanuel–St. Joseph's Hospital
  Lake Region Hospital & Nursing Home
  North Country Hospital
  Rice Memorial Hospital
  Ridgeview Medical Center
  Saint Cloud Hospital
  St. Luke's Hospital of Duluth

MISSISSIPPI
Shareholder
Tupelo
  North Mississippi Health Services, Inc.
Partners
  Forrest General Hospital
  Greenwood Leflore Hospital
  Jeff Anderson Regional Medical Center
  Memorial Hospital at Gulfport
  Singing River Hospital System
  Southwest Mississippi Regional Medical Center
  St. Dominic–Jackson Memorial Hospital

MISSOURI
Shareholders
Kansas City
  St. Luke's Hospital of Kansas City
Springfield
  Cox Health Systems

Alliances

St. Louis
  BJC Health System
Partners
  Cameron Community Hospital
  Citizens Memorial Hospital
  Freeman Hospital
  Liberty Hospital
  McCune–Brooks Hospital
  Ozarks Medical Center
  Skaggs Community Health Center
  Southeast Missouri Hospital
  St. Francis Medical Center

MONTANA
Partners
  Deaconess Medical Center of Billings, Inc.
  Montana Deaconess Medical Center
  St. Peter's Community Hospital

NEBRASKA
Shareholder
Omaha
  Nebraska Methodist Health System, Inc.
Partners
  Beatrice Community Hospital and Health Center
  Bryan Memorial Hospital
  Childrens Memorial Hospital
  Columbus Community Hospital
  Lutheran Community Hospital
  Mary Lanning Memorial Hospital
  Memorial Hospital & Home
  Regional West Medical Center

NEW HAMPSHIRE
Shareholder
Lebanon
  Hitchcock Alliance
Partners
  Concord Hospital
  Frisbie Memorial Hospital
  Southern New Hampshire Regional Medical Center
  The Cheshire Medical Center
  Wentworth–Douglass Hospital

NEW JERSEY
Shareholders
Belleville
  Clara Maass Health System, Inc.
Mount Holly
  Memorial Hospital of Burlington County
Toms River
  Community/Kimball Health Care System
Partners
  Chilton Memorial Hospital
  Christ Hospital
  Elizabeth General Medical Center
  Hackettstown Community Hospital
  Hunterdon Medical Center
  Mercer Medical Center
  Morristown Memorial Hospital
  Muhlenberg Regional Medical Center
  Newton Memorial Hospital
  Our Lady of Lourdes Medical Center
  Overlook Hospital
  Rahway Hospital
  Riverview Medical Center
  Shore Memorial Hospital
  Underwood–Memorial Hospital
  Warren Hospital

NEW MEXICO
Partners
  Eastern New Mexico Medical Center
  Memorial Medical Center
  San Juan Regional Medical Center

NEW YORK
Shareholders
Binghamton
  United Health Services, Inc.
New York
  The Presbyterian Hospital in the City of New York
  The Society of the New York Hospital

Partners
  Bassett Healthcare
  Brooklyn Hospital Center
  CVPH Medical Center
  Crouse Irving Companies, Inc.
  DeGraff Memorial Hospital
  Geneva General Hospital
  Highland Hospital of Rochester
  Lenox Hill Hospital
  Mercy Medical Center
  Mohawk Valley Network
  New Rochelle Hospital Medical Center
  New York University Medical Center
  Northern Westchester Hospital Center
  Park Ridge Health System, Inc.
  Samaritan Hospital
  Southampton Hospital
  St. John's Riverside Hospital
  St. Luke's–Roosevelt Hospital Center
  The House of the Good Samaritan
  Tompkins Community Hospital
  White Plains Hospital Center
  Woman's Christian Association Hospital

NORTH CAROLINA
Shareholders
Charlotte
  Charlotte Mecklenburg Hospital Authority
Winston–Salem
  Carolina Medicorp, Inc.
Partners
  Community General Hospital of Thomasville, Inc.
  Nash General Hospital, Inc.
  Wake County Hospital System, Inc.
  Wesley Long Community Hospital, Inc.

NORTH DAKOTA
Shareholders
Fargo
  MeritCare Health Systems
Partners
  Jamestown Hospital
  Medcenter One Health Systems
  Trinity Medical Center
  The United Hospital

OHIO
Shareholders
Akron
  Akron General Medical Center
Cincinnati
  The Christ Hospital
Columbus
  U. S. Health Corporation
Dayton
  MedAmerica Health Systems Corporation
Toledo
  The Toledo Hospital
Partners
  Ashtabula County Medical Center
  Community Hospital of Springfield & Clark County
  Elyria Memorial Hospital
  Ft. Hamilton–Hughes Memorial Hospital Center
  Greene Memorial Hospital
  Guernsey Memorial Hospital
  Lake Hospital System, Inc.
  Lima Memorial Hospital
  Mansfield General Hospital
  Marymount Hospital
  Memorial Hospital
  Middletown Regional Hospital
  Ohio Valley Hospital
  St. Luke's Hospital
  Trumbull Memorial Hospital
  Union Hospital
  Upper Valley Medical Center
  Western Reserve Care System

OKLAHOMA
Shareholders
Oklahoma City
  Oklahoma Health System
Tulsa
  Hillcrest Medical Center

Partners
  Baptist Healthcare of Oklahoma, Inc.
  Deaconess Hospital
  Duncan Regional Hospital, Inc.
  Eastern Oklahoma Medical Center
  Jackson County Memorial Hospital
  Jane Phillips Episcopal Hospital, Inc.
  McAlester Regional Hospital
  Memorial Hospital of Southern Oklahoma
  Midwest City Regional Hospital
  Muskogee Regional Medical Center
  Norman Regional Hospital
  SMC Health Services Corporation
  Stillwater Medical Center
  Valley View Regional Hospital

PENNSYLVANIA
Shareholders
Allentown
  Lehigh Valley Hospital
Erie
  Hamot Health Systems, Inc.
Media
  Crozer–Keystone Health System
Philadelphia
  Pennsylvania Hospital
Pittsburgh
  Allegheny Health, Education & Research Foundation
Sayre
  Guthrie Healthcare System
Partners
  Allegheny Valley Hospital
  Butler Area Health Resources Development Corp.
  Capital Health System Services
  Chestnut Hill Hospital Healthcare
  Community Medical Center
  Conemaugh Valley Memorial Hospital
  Episcopal Hospital
  Frankford Hospital
  Grand View Hospital, Inc.
  Jeanes Health System
  Lancaster General Hospital Foundation
  Latrobe Area Hospital
  Lower Bucks Hospital
  Montgomery Hospital
  Pottstown Memorial Medical Center
  Sewickley Valley Hospital
  Shadyside Hospital
  St. Clair Memorial Hospital
  St. Margaret Memorial Hospital
  Susquehanna Health System
  The Altoona Hospital
  The Chester County Hospital Foundation, Inc.
  The Reading Hospital and Medical Center
  The Washington Hospital
  Uniontown Health Resources, Inc.
  York Health System

RHODE ISLAND
Shareholder
Providence
  Rhode Island Hospital

SOUTH CAROLINA
Shareholder
Columbia
  South Carolina Baptist Hospitals, Inc.
Partner
  Roper Hospital

SOUTH DAKOTA
Shareholder
Sioux Falls
  Sioux Valley Hospital

TENNESSEE
Shareholders
Jacksonville
  West Tennessee Healthcare, Inc.
Knoxville
  Fort Sanders Alliance
Memphis
  Baptist Memorial Hospital
Nashville
  Baptist Hospital, Inc.

Alliances

TEXAS
Shareholders
Dallas
  Baylor Health Care System
Fort Worth
  All Saints Episcopal Hospital
Houston
  Memorial Hospital System
Lubbock
  Lubbock Methodist Hospital System, Inc.
Partners
  Arlington Memorial Hospital
  Baptist Hospital of Southeast Texas, Inc.
  Baptist Memorial Hospital System
  Baylor/Richardson Medical Center
  High Plains Baptist Hospital
  Hillcrest Baptist Medical Center
  Irving Healthcare System
  King's Daughters' Hospital
  Marshall Memorial Hospital
  Memorial Hospital and Medical Center
  Mother Frances Hospital
  Providence Memorial Hospital
  Shannon Medical Center
  St. David's Hospital
  Valley Baptist Medical Center
  Wadley Regional Medical Center
  Wichita General Hospital
  Wilson N. Jones Memorial Hospital

VERMONT
Shareholder
Burlington
  Medical Center Hospital of Vermont
Partners
  Central Vermont Medical Center, Inc.
  Rutland Regional Medical Center

VIRGINIA
Shareholder
Norfolk
  Sentara Health System, Inc.
Partners
  Centra Health, Inc.
  Children's Health System, Inc.
  MWH MediCorp
  Martha Jefferson Hospital
  Rockingham Memorial Hospital
  Southampton Memorial Hospital
  The Alexandria Hospital
  The Arlington Hospital
  The Fauquier Hospital, Inc.

WASHINGTON
Shareholder
Tacoma
  Multicare Medical Center

WEST VIRGINIA
Shareholder
Charleston
  CAMCARE, Inc.

Partners
  Cabell Huntington Hospital
  Princeton Community Hospital
  Reynolds Memorial Hospital
  St. Joseph's Hospital
  West Virginia University Hospitals, Inc.
  Wheeling Hospital

WISCONSIN
Shareholders
La Crosse
  Lutheran Health System
Madison
  Meriter Hospital, Inc.
Partners
  Beaver Dam Community Hospitals, Inc.
  Columbia Hospital
  Community Memorial Hospital of Menomonee Falls, Inc.
  Froedtert Memorial Lutheran Hospital
  Horizon Healthcare, Inc.
  Kenosha Hospital and Medical Center
  Lakeview Medical Center
  Luther Hospital
  St. Joseph's Community Hospital
  Watertown Memorial Hospital
  Waukesha Hospital System, Inc.

WYOMING
Partners
  Ivinson Memorial Hospital
  Memorial Hospital of Sheridan County
  United Medical Center
  Wyoming Medical Center

HOSPITALS	BEDS
744	249,156

116 Other health care providers

YANKEE ALLIANCE
200 Brickstone Square, Andover, MA 01810–1429; 508/470–2000; R. Paul O'Neill, President

CONNECTICUT
Affiliate
Hartford
  Mount Sinai Hospital
Affiliate
  Saint Francis Hospital & Medical Center
New Haven
Member
  Hospital of St. Raphael
Affiliate
Southington
Affiliate
  Bradley Hospital

MAINE
Bangor
  Eastern Maine Healthcare

Affiliate
  Acadia Hospital
Belfast
Affiliate
  Waldo County General Hospital
Blue Hill
Affiliate
  Blue Hill Memorial Hospital
Pittsfield
Affiliate
  Sebasticook Valley Hospital

MASSACHUSETTS
Ayer
  Deaconess–Nashoba Hospital
Boston
  New England Baptist Hospital
  New England Deaconess Hospital
Fall River
  Charlton Memorial Hospital
Framingham/Natick
  MetroWest Medical Center (Framingham Campus/Natick Campus)
Great Barrington
Affiliate
  Fairview Hospital
Lowell
  Saints Memorial Medical Center (Saint John's Campus/Saint Joseph's Campus)
Natick
  Metrowest Health, Inc.
Needham
Affiliate
  Glover Memorial Hospital
Newton
Affiliate
  New England Organ Bank
Pittsfield
  Berkshire Health Systems
Winchester
  Winchester Healthcare Management, Inc.

NEW HAMPSHIRE
Affiliate
Manchester
  Catholic Medical Center
Affiliate
  Elliot Hospital

NEW YORK
Albany
  Albany Memorial Hospital
Cambridge
Affiliate
  Mary McClellan Hospital
Glens Falls
  Glens Falls Hospital

HOSPITALS	BEDS
11	4,800

C

Health Organizations, Agencies, and Providers

C2 Description of Lists
3 National Organizations
13 Healthfinder
25 International Organizations
27 U.S. Government Agencies

State and Local Organizations and Agencies
28 *Blue Cross–Blue Shield Plans*
30 *Health Systems Agencies*
31 *Hospital Associations*
34 *Hospital Licensure Agencies*
36 *Medical and Nursing Licensure Agencies*
39 *Peer Review Organizations*
41 *State Health Planning and Development Agencies*
43 *State and Provincial Government Agencies*

Health Care Providers
60 *Health Maintenance Organizations*
73 *State Government Agencies for Health Maintenance Organizations*
75 *Freestanding Ambulatory Surgery Centers*
100 *State Government Agencies for Freestanding Ambulatory Surgery Centers*
102 *Freestanding Hospices*
121 *State Government Agencies for Freestanding Hospices*
123 *Accredited Freestanding Long–Term Care Facilities†*
129 *Accredited Freestanding Psychiatric Facilities†*
141 *Accredited Freestanding Substance Abuse Programs†*

†List supplied by the Joint Commission on Accreditation of Healthcare Organizations

For more information on membership contact:
Manager, Department of Membership
American Hospital Association
One North Franklin
Chicago, Illinois 60606–3401

Description of Lists

This section was compiled to provide a directory of information useful to the health care field.

National and International Organizations

The national and international lists include many types of voluntary organizations concerned with matters of interest to the health care field. The organizational information includes address, telephone number, FAX number, and the contact person. For organizations that maintain permanent offices, office addresses and telephone numbers are given. For organizations not maintaining offices, the addresses and telephone numbers given are those of their corresponding secretaries. The information was obtained directly from the organizations.

National Organizations are listed alphabetically by their full names. International Organizations are grouped alphabetically by country.

Also included is the Healthfinder listings. The Healthfinder is composed of two listing types: toll-free numbers for health information and federal health information centers and clearinghouses. Organizations are listed alphabetically by topic area.

We present this list simply as a convenient directory. Inclusion or omission of any organization's name indicates neither approval nor disapproval by the American Hospital Association.

United States Government Agencies

National agencies concerned with health-related matters are listed by the major department of government under which the different functions fall.

State and Local Organizations and Agencies

The lists of organizations in states, associated areas, and provinces include Blue Cross-Blue Shield plans, health systems agencies, hospital associations and councils, hospital licensure agencies, medical and nursing licensure agencies, peer review organizations, state health planning and development agencies, and statewide health coordinating councils.

There are many active local organizations that do not fall within these categories. Contact the hospital association of the state or province for information about such additional groups. The hospital association and councils listed have offices with full-time executives.

The selected state and provincial government agencies include those within state departments of health and welfare, and other agencies, such as comprehensive health planning, crippled children's services, maternal and child health, mental health, and vocational rehabilitation.

Health Care Providers

Lists of JCAHO Accredited Freestanding Long-Term Care Facilities, Health Maintenance Organizations, Freestanding Ambulatory Surgery Centers, Freestanding Hospices, JCAHO Accredited Freestanding Substance Abuse Programs, and JCAHO Accredited Freestanding Psychiatric Facilities are provided in this section. The lists were developed from information supplied by the providers themselves.

As with the lists of National and International Organizations, these lists are provided simply as a convenient directory. Inclusion or omission of any organization's name indicates neither approval nor disapproval by the American Hospital Association.

National Organizations

A

ADARA: Professionals Networking for Excellence in Service Delivery, with Individuals Who are Deaf or Hard of Hearing, P.O. Box 251554, Little Rock, AR 72225; tel. 501/868–8850; FAX. 501/868–8812; Steve Larew, President

Academy for Implants and Transplants, P.O. Box 223, Springfield, VA 22150; tel. 703/451–0001; Anthony J. Viscido, D.D.S., Secretary–Treasurer

Academy of Dentistry for Persons with Disabilities, 211 East Chicago Avenue, Suite 948, Chicago, IL 60611; tel. 312/440–2660; FAX. 312/440–2824; John S. Rutkauskas, M.S., D.D.S., Executive Director

Academy of General Dentistry, 211 East Chicago Avenue, Suite 1200, Chicago, IL 60611–2670; tel. 312/440–4300; FAX. 312/440–0559; Harold E. Donnell, Jr., Executive Director

Academy of Oral Dynamics, 5950 Elmer Derr Road, Frederick, MD 21701; tel. 301/473–9719; Joseph P. Skellchock, D.D.S., Secretary

Accreditation Association for Ambulatory Health Care, 9933 Lawler Avenue, Skokie, IL 60077–3708; tel. 708/676–9610; Christopher A. Damon, Executive Director

Aerospace Medical Association, 320 South Henry Street, Alexandria, VA 22314–3579; tel. 703/739–2240; FAX. 703/739–9652; Russell B. Rayman, M.D., Executive Director

Alexander Graham Bell Association for the Deaf, Inc., 3417 Volta Place, N.W., Washington, DC 20007; tel. 202/337–5220; Donna McCord Dickman, Ph.D., Executive Director

Allergy Testing Laboratory, 133 East 58th Street, New York, NY 10022; tel. 212/355–1005; FAX. 212/355–1019; Joseph D'more, M.D.

Alliance for Healthcare Strategy and Marketing, 11 S. LaSalle, Suite 2300, Chicago, IL 60603; tel. 312/704–9700; FAX. 312/704–9709; Carla Windhorst, Executive Director

Alzheimer's Association, (Alzheimer's Disease and Related Disorders Association, Inc.), 919 North Michigan Avenue, Suite 1000, Chicago, IL 60611; tel. 800/272–3900; FAX. 312/335–1110; Edward F. Truschke, President and Chief Executive Officer

Ambulatory Pediatric Association, 6728 Old McLean Village, McLean, VA 22101; tel. 703/556–9222; FAX. 703/556–8729; Marge Degnon, Executive Secretary

American Academy for Cerebral Palsy and Developmental Medicine, 6300 N. River Road, Suite 727, Rosemont, IL 60018–4226; tel. 708/698–1635; FAX. 708/823–0536; Arlene Napolilli, Executive Director

American Academy of Allergy and Immunology, 611 East Wells Street, Milwaukee, WI 53202; tel. 414/272–6071; FAX. 414/276–3349; Donald L. McNeil, Executive Director

American Academy of Child and Adolescent Psychiatry, 3615 Wisconsin Avenue, N.W., Washington, DC 20016; tel. 202/966–7300; FAX. 202/966–2891; Virginia Q. Anthony, Executive Director

American Academy of Dental Electrosurgery, Planetarium Station, P.O. Box 374, New York, NY 10024; tel. 212/595–1925; Maurice J. Oringer, D.D.S., Executive Secretary

American Academy of Dental Practice Administration, 1063 Whippoorwill Lane, Palatine, IL 60067; tel. 708/934–4404; Kathleen Uebel, Executive Director

American Academy of Dermatology, P.O. Box 4014, Schaumburg, IL 60168–4014; tel. 708/330–0230; FAX. 708/330–0050; Bradford W. Claxton, Executive Director

American Academy of Environmental Medicine, 4510 W. 89th Street, Prairie Village, KS 66207; tel. 913/642–6062; FAX. 913/341–3625; Matt Tidwell, Executive Director

American Academy of Facial Plastic and Reconstructive Surgery, Inc., 1110 Vermont Avenue, N.W., Suite 220, Washington, DC 20005; tel. 202/842–4500; FAX. 202/371–1514; Stephen C. Duffy, Executive Vice President

American Academy of Family Physicians, 8880 Ward Parkway, Kansas City, MO 64114; tel. 816/333–9700; FAX. 816/822–0580; Robert Graham, M.D., Executive Vice President

American Academy of Hospital Attorneys (AHA), One North Franklin, Chicago, IL 60606–3491; tel. 312/422–3701; FAX. 312/422–4575; Marietta Gadden, Director

American Academy of Implant Dentistry, 6900 Grove Road, Thorofare, NJ 08086; tel. 609/848–7027; FAX. 609/853–5991; Christine Malin, Executive Secretary

American Academy of Insurance Medicine, 2211 Congress Street, Portland, ME 04122; tel. 207/770–6454; FAX. 207/770–6772; Paul R. Bell, M.D., Secretary

American Academy of Medical Administrators, 30555 Southfield Road, Suite 150, Southfield, MI 48076–7747; tel. 810/540–4310; FAX. 810/645–0590; Thomas R. O'Donovan, Ph.D., President

American Academy of Neurology, 2221 University Avenue, S.E., Suite 335, Minneapolis, MN 55414; tel. 612/623–8115; FAX. 612/623–3504; Jan W. Kolehmainen, Executive Director

American Academy of Ophthalmology, 655 Beach Street, P.O. Box 7424, San Francisco, CA 94120; tel. 415/561–8500; FAX. 415/561–8533; H. Dunbar Hoskins, Jr., M.D., Executive Vice President

American Academy of Optometry, 5530 Wisconsin Avenue, N.W., Suite 1149, Washington, DC 20815; tel. 301/652–0905; FAX. 301/656–0989; David Lewis, Executive Director

American Academy of Oral Medicine, 631 South 29th Street, Arlington, VA 22202; tel. 703/684–6649; FAX. 703/684–2008; Ronald S. Brown, D.D.S., M.S., Secretary

American Academy of Orthodontics for the General Practitioner, 3953 North 76th Street, Milwaukee, WI 53222; tel. 414/464–7870; Maxine Hirmer, Administrative Assistant

American Academy of Orthopaedic Surgeons, 6300 North River Road, Rosemont, IL 60018–4262; tel. 708/823–7186; FAX. 708/823–8125; Thomas C. Nelson, Executive Director

American Academy of Otolaryngic Allergy, 8455 Colesville Road, Suite 745, Silver Spring, MD 20910; tel. 301/588–1800; FAX. 301/588–2454; Donald J. Clark, Executive Director

American Academy of Otolaryngology–Head and Neck Surgery, Inc., One Prince Street, Alexandria, VA 22314; tel. 703/836–4444; FAX. 703/683–5100; Jerome C. Goldstein, M.D., Senior Executive Vice President

American Academy of Pain Management, 3600 Sisk Road, Suite 2D, Modesto, CA 95356; tel. 209/545–0754; FAX. 209/545–2920; Richard S. Weiner, Ph.D., Executive Director

American Academy of Pediatric Dentistry, 211 East Chicago Avenue, Suite 700, Chicago, IL 60611; tel. 312/337–2169; Dr. John A. Bogert, Executive Director

American Academy of Pediatrics, 141 N.W. Point Boulevard, P.O. Box 927, Elk Grove Village, IL 60009–0927; tel. 708/228–5005; FAX. 708/228–5097; Joe M. Sanders, Jr., M.D., Executive Director

American Academy of Physical Medicine and Rehabilitation, One IBM Plaza, Suite 2500, Chicago, IL 60611–3604; tel. 312/464–9700; FAX. 312/464–0227; Ronald A. Henrichs, CAE, Executive Director

American Academy of Physician Assistants, 950 North Washington Street, Alexandria, VA 22314; tel. 703/836–2272; FAX. 703/684–1924; Stephen C. Crane, Ph.D., M.P.H., Executive Vice President

American Academy of Physiologic Dentistry, 567 South Washington Street, Naperville, IL 60540; tel. 708/355–2625; Dr. William Kopperud, Secretary

American Academy of Psychoanalysis, 47 East 19th Street, 6th Floor, New York, NY 10003; tel. 212/475–7980; FAX. 212/475–8101; Vivian Mendelsohn, Executive Director

American Academy of Restorative Dentistry, 1235 Lake Plaza Drive, Suite 251, Colorado Springs, CO 80906; tel. 719/576–8840; Donald H. Downs, D.D.S., Secretary–Treasurer

American Aging Association, 2129 Providence Avenue, Chester, PA 19013–5506; tel. 610/874–7550; FAX. 610/876–7715; Arthur K. Balin, M.D., Ph.D., Executive Director

American Alliance for Health, Physical Education, Recreation, and Dance, 1900 Association Drive, Reston, VA 22091; tel. 703/476–3400; FAX. 703/476–9527; A. Gilson Brown, Executive Vice President

American Ambulance Association, 3814 Auburn Boulevard, Suite 70, Sacramento, CA 95821; tel. 916/483–3827; FAX. 916/482–5473; David A. Nevins, Executive Vice President

American Art Therapy Association, 505 East Hawley Street, Mundelein, IL 60060; tel. 708/949–6064; Edward J. Stygar, Jr., Executive Director

American Assembly for Men in Nursing, P.O. Box 31753, Independence, OH 44131; tel. 216/524–3504; David O. Sprouse, President

American Association for Accreditation of Laboratory Animal Care (AAALAC), 11300 Rockville Pike, Suite 1211, Rockville, MD 20852–3035; tel. 301/231–5353; FAX. 301/231–8282; Dr. Albert E. New, Executive Director

American Association for Adult and Continuing Education, 1200 19th Street, N.W., Suite 300, Washington, DC 20036; tel. 202/429–5131; FAX. 202/223–4579; Dr. Drew Allbritten, Executive Director

American Association for Clinical Chemistry, Inc., 2101 L Street, N.W., Suite 202, Washington, DC 20037; tel. 202/857–0717; FAX. 202/887–5093; Richard Flaherty, Executive Vice President

American Association for Dental Research, 1619 Duke Street, Alexandria, VA 22314–3406; tel. 202/898–1050; FAX. 202/789–1033; John J. Clarkson, BDS, Ph.D., Executive Director

American Association for Laboratory Animal Science, 70 Timber Creek Drive, Cordova, TN 38018; tel. 901/754–8620; FAX. 901/753–0046; Michael R. Sondag, Executive Director

American Association for Rehabilitation Therapy, P.O. Box 93, North Little Rock, AR 72115; tel. 601/863–1972; Woody Cavalier, President

American Association for Respiratory Care, 11030 Ables Lane, Dallas, TX 75229; tel. 214/243–2272; FAX. 214/484–2720; Sam P. Giordano, Executive Director

American Association for the Advancement of Science, 1333 H Street, N.W., Washington, DC 20005; tel. 202/326–6400; William D. Carey, Executive Officer

American Association for the Study of Headache, 875 Kings Highway, Suite 200, Woodbury, NJ 08096; tel. 609/845–0322; FAX. 609/384–5811; Robert K. Talley, Executive Director

American Association for the Surgery of Trauma, c/o Anthony A. Meyer, M.D., Secretary Treasurer, AAST/Department of Surgery, UNC, CB #7210, 167 Burnett Womack, Chapel Hill, NC 27599–7210; tel. 919/966–7842; FAX. 919/966–7841; Anthony A. Meyer, M.D.

American Association of Anatomists, Department of Anatomy, Tulane Medical School, 1430 Tulane Avenue, New Orleans, LA 70112; FAX. 504/584–1687; Robert Yates, Secretary–Treasurer

American Association of Bioanalysts, 818 Olive Street, Suite 918, St. Louis, MO 63101–1598; tel. 314/241–1445; FAX. 314/241–1449; Mark S. Birenbaum, Ph.D., Administrator

Organizations / National Organizations

American Association of Blood Banks, 1117 North 19th Street, Suite 600, Arlington, VA 22209; tel. 703/528-8200; FAX. 703/527-8036; Joel M. Solomon, Executive Director

American Association of Certified Orthoptists, Herman Eye Center/UTHSC, 6411 Fannin, 17th Floor-Jones, Houston, TX 77030-1697; tel. 713/797-1777; FAX. 713/799-4325; Patricia Jenkins, President

American Association of Colleges of Nursing, One Dupont Circle, Suite 530, Washington, DC 20036; tel. 202/463-6930; FAX. 202/785-8320; Geraldine Bednash, Ph.D., RN, FAAN, Executive Director

American Association of Colleges of Pharmacy, 1426 Prince Street, Alexandria, VA 22314-2841; tel. 703/739-2330; FAX. 703/836-8982; Carl E. Trinca, Ph.D., Executive Director

American Association of Colleges of Podiatric Medicine, 1350 Piccard Drive, Suite 322, Rockville, MD 20850-4307; tel. 301/990-7400; FAX. 301/990-2807; Anthony J. McNevin, CAE, President

American Association of Critical-Care Nurses, 101 Columbia, Aliso Viejo, CA 92656-1491; tel. 714/362-2000; FAX. 714/362-2020; Sarah J. Sanford, RN, M.A., CNAA, FAAN, Chief Executive Officer

American Association of Dental Consultants, Inc., P.O. Box 3345, Lawrence, KS 66046; tel. 913/749-2727; FAX. 913/749-1140; Alan M. Helerstein, D.D.S., Secretary-Treasurer

American Association of Dental Schools, 1625 Massachusetts Avenue, N.W., Washington, DC 20036; tel. 202/667-9433; FAX. 202/667-0642; Preston A. Littleton, Jr., D.D.S., Ph.D., Executive Director

American Association of Endodontists, 211 East Chicago Avenue, Suite 1100, Chicago, IL 60611; tel. 312/266-7255; FAX. 312/266-9867; Irma S. Kudo, Executive Director

American Association of Fund-Raising Counsel, Inc., 25 West 43rd Street, New York, NY 10036; tel. 212/354-5799; FAX. 212/768-1795; Ann Kaplan, Research Director

American Association of Healthcare Consultants, 11208 Waples Mill Road, Suite 109, Fairfax, VA 22030; tel. 703/691-2242; FAX. 703/691-2247; Vaughan A. Smith, President

American Association of Homes and Services for the Aging, 901 E Street, N.W., Suite 500, Washington, DC 20004-2037; tel. 202/783-2242; FAX. 202/783-2255; Sheldon L. Goldberg, President

American Association of Hospital Dentists, Inc., 211 East Chicago Avenue, Suite 948, Chicago, IL 60611; tel. 312/440-2661; FAX. 312/440-2824; John S. Rutkauskas, M.S., D.D.S., Executive Director

American Association of Kidney Patients, 100 South Ashley Drive, Suite 280, Tampa, FL 33602; tel. 800/749-2257; FAX. 813/223-7099; Kris Robinson, Executive Director

American Association of Medical Assistants, 20 North Wacker Drive, Suite 1575, Chicago, IL 60606; tel. 312/899-1500; Edward J. Collins, CAE, Executive Director

American Association of Neuroscience Nurses, 224 North DesPlaines, Suite 601, Chicago, IL 60661; tel. 312/993-0043; FAX. 312/993-0362; John F. Settich, Executive Director

American Association of Nurse Anesthetists, 222 South Prospect Avenue, Park Ridge, IL 60068-4001; tel. 708/692-7050, ext. 302; FAX. 708/692-6968; John F. Garde, CRNA, M.S., FAAN, Executive Director

American Association of Nutritional Consultants, 880 Canarios Court, Suite 210, Chula Vista, CA 91910; tel. 619/482-8533; FAX. 619/482-0938; Dr. Kurt W. Donsbach, Administrator

American Association of Occupational Health Nurses, Inc., 50 Lenox Pointe, Atlanta, GA 30324; tel. 404/262-1162; FAX. 404/262-1165; Ann R. Cox, CAE, Executive Director

American Association of Oral and Maxillofacial Surgeons, 9700 West Bryn Mawr Avenue, Rosemont, IL 60018-5701; tel. 708/678-6200; FAX. 708/678-6286; Jeff Flood, Executive Director

American Association of Orthodontists, 401 North Lindbergh Boulevard, St. Louis, MO 63141-7816; tel. 314/993-1700; FAX. 314/997-1745; Ronald S. Moen, Executive Director

American Association of Pastoral Counselors, 9504A Lee Highway, Fairfax, VA 22031-2303; tel. 703/385-6967; FAX. 703/352-7725; C. Roy Woodruff, Ph.D., Executive Director

American Association of Physicists in Medicine, One Physics Ellipse, College Park, MD 20740; tel. 301/209-3350; FAX. 301/209-0862; Salvatore Trofi, Jr., Executive Director

American Association of Plastic Surgeons, 2317 Seminole Road, Atlantic Beach, FL 32233; tel. 904/359-3759; FAX. 904/359-3789; Francis A. Harris, Executive Secretary

American Association of Poison Control Centers, Arizona Poison Information Center, Arizona Health Sciences Center, Suite 3204-K, 1501 North Campbell, Tucson, AZ 85724; tel. 602/626-7899; FAX. 602/626-2720; Theodore Tong, Ph.D., Secretary

American Association of Preferred Provider Organizations, 1101 Connecticut Avenue, N.W., Suite 700, Washington, DC 20036; tel. 202/429-5133; FAX. 202/429-5108; Gordon Wheeler, President, Chief Operating Officer

American Association of Psychiatric Technicians, A.A.P.T., 2030 East Broadway, Suite 218, P.O. Box 13912, Tucson, AZ 85732; tel. 520/623-0522; FAX. 520/748-0458; George Blake, Ph.D., Director, President

American Association of Psychiatric Technicians, A.A.R.T, P.O. Box 13912, Tucson, AZ 85732; tel. 602/321-2075; FAX. 602/622-5029; George Blake, Ph.D., Director, President

American Association of Public Health Dentistry, A.A.P.H.D. National Office, 10619 Jousting Lane, Richmond, VA 23235-3838; tel. 804/272-8344; FAX. 804/272-0802; Rhys Jones, D.D.S, M.S., President

American Association of Public Health Physicians, Texas Department of Criminal Justice, P.O. Box 99, Huntsville, TX 77342-0099; tel. 409/294-2214; FAX. 409/294-2911; Charles R. Webb, Jr., M.D.

American Association on Mental Retardation, 444 N. Capitol Street, N.W., Suite 846, Washington, DC 20001-1512; tel. 202/387-1968; FAX. 202/387-2193; M. Doreen Croser, Executive Director

American Baptist Homes and Hospitals Association, P.O. Box 851, Valley Forge, PA 19482-0851; tel. 215/768-2382; FAX. 215/768-2470; Milton E. Owens, Jr., Executive Director

American Board of Allergy and Immunology, A Conjoint Board of the American Board of Internal Medicine and the American Board of Pediatrics, University City Science Center, 3624 Market Street, Philadelphia, PA 19104; tel. 215/349-9466; FAX. 215/222-8669; John W. Yunginger, M.D., Executive Secretary

American Board of Anesthesiology, 100 Constitution Plaza, Suite 1668, Hartford, CT 06103; tel. 203/522-9857; FAX. 203/522-6626; D. David Glass, M.D., Secretary-Treasurer

American Board of Cardiovascular Perfusion, 207 North 25th Avenue, Hattiesburg, MS 39401; tel. 601/582-3309; Beth A. Richmond, Ph.D., Mark G. Richmond, Ed.D., Co-Executive Directors

American Board of Colon and Rectal Surgery, 20600 Eureka Road, Suite 713, Taylor, MI 48180; tel. 313/282-9400; FAX. 313/282-9402; Herand Abcarian, M.D., Executive Director

American Board of Dermatology, Inc., Henry Ford Hospital, One Ford Place, Detroit, MI 48202-3450; tel. 313/874-1088; FAX. 313/872-3221; Harry J. Hurley, M.D., Executive Director

American Board of Emergency Medicine, 3000 Coolidge Road, East Lansing, MI 48823; tel. 517/332-4800; FAX. 517/332-2234; Benson S. Munger, Ph.D., Executive Director

American Board of Family Practice, Inc., 2228 Young Drive, Lexington, KY 40505; tel. 606/269-5626; FAX. 606/266-9699; Paul R. Young, M.D., Executive Director

American Board of Internal Medicine, 3624 Market Street, Philadelphia, PA 19104; tel. 215/243-1500; FAX. 215/382-4702; Harry R. Kimball, M.D., President

American Board of Medical Management, 4890 West Kennedy Boulevard, Suite 200, Tampa, FL 33609-2575; tel. 813/287-2815; FAX. 813/287-8993; Roger S. Schenke, Executive Vice President

American Board of Medical Specialties, 1007 Church Street, Suite 404, Evanston, IL 60201-5913; tel. 708/491-9091; FAX. 708/328-3596; J. Lee Dockery, M.D., Executive Vice President

American Board of Neurological Surgery, 6550 Fannin Street, Suite 2139, Houston, TX 77030; tel. 713/790-6015; Howard M. Eisenberg, M.D., Secretary-Treasurer

American Board of Nuclear Medicine, 900 Veteran Avenue, Los Angeles, CA 90024; tel. 310/825-6787; FAX. 310/825-9433; Joseph F. Ross, M.D., President

American Board of Obstetrics and Gynecology, Inc., 936 North 34th Street, Suite 200, Seattle, WA 98103; tel. 206/547-4884; Norman F. Gant, M.D., Executive Director

American Board of Ophthalmology, 111 Presidential Boulevard, Suite 241, Bala Cynwyd, PA 19004; tel. 610/664-1175; William H. Spencer, M.D., Executive Director

American Board of Oral and Maxillofacial Surgery, 625 North Michigan Avenue, Suite 1820, Chicago, IL 60611; tel. 312/642-0070; FAX. 312/642-8584; Cheryl E. Mounts, Executive Secretary

American Board of Orthopaedic Surgery, Inc., 400 Silver Cedar Court, Chapel Hill, NC 27514; tel. 919/929-7103; FAX. 919/942-8988; G. Paul De Rosa, M.D., Executive Director

American Board of Otolaryngology, 5615 Kirby Drive, Suite 936, Houston, TX 77005-2452; tel. 713/528-6200; FAX. 713/528-1171; Robert W. Cantrell, M.D., Executive Vice President

American Board of Pathology, Lincoln Center, 4830 West Kennedy Boulevard, P.O. Box 25915, Tampa, FL 33622-5915; tel. 813/286-2444; FAX. 813/289-5279; William H. Hartmann, M.D., Executive Vice President

American Board of Pediatric Dentistry, 1193 Woodgate Drive, Carmel, IN 46033-9232; tel. 317/573-0877; FAX. 317/846-7235; James R. Roche, D.D.S., Executive Secretary-Treasurer

American Board of Pediatrics, Inc., 111 Silver Cedar Court, Chapel Hill, NC 27514; tel. 919/929-0461; FAX. 919/929-9255; James A. Stockman III, M.D., President

American Board of Physical Medicine and Rehabilitation, Norwest Center, Suite 674, 21 First Street, S.W., Rochester, MN 55902; tel. 507/282-1776; FAX. 507/282-9242; Joachim L. Opitz, M.D., Executive Director

American Board of Podiatric Orthopedics and Primary Podiatric Medicine, 401 N. Michigan Avenue, Suite 2400, P.O. Box 39, Chicago, IL 60611-4267; tel. 312/321-5139; FAX. 312/881-1815; Jeffrey P. Knezovich, Executive Director

American Board of Podiatric Surgery, 1601 Dolores Street, San Francisco, CA 94110-4906; tel. 415/826-3200; FAX. 415/826-4640; John L. Bennett, Executive Director

American Board of Preventive Medicine, Inc., 9950 West Lawrence Avenue, Suite 106, Schiller Park, IL 60176; tel. 708/671-1750; FAX. 708/671-1751; Alice R. Ring, M.D., M.P.H., Executive Director

American Board of Prosthodontics, P.O. Box 8437, Atlanta, GA 31106; tel. 404/876-2625; FAX. 404/872-8804; William D. Culpepper, D.D.S., M.S.D., Executive Director

American Board of Psychiatry and Neurology, Inc., 500 Lake Cook Road, Suite 335, Deerfield, IL 60015; tel. 708/945-7900; FAX. 708/945-1146; Stephen C. Scheiber, M.D., Executive Vice President

American Board of Quality Assurance and Utilization Review Physicians, 4890 West Kennedy Boulevard, Suite 260, Tampa, FL 33609; tel. 813/286-4411; FAX. 813/286-4387; Joseph L. Murphy, M.D., President

Organizations / National Organizations

American Board of Radiology, Inc., 5255 East Williams Circle, Suite 6800, Tucson, AZ 85711; tel. 520/790-2900; FAX. 520/790-3200; M. Paul Capp, M.D., Executive Director

American Board of Science in Nuclear Medicine, Society of Nuclear Medicine, 136 Madison Avenue, New York, NY 10016-6760; tel. 212/889-0717, ext. 250; FAX. 212/545-0221; Christine Santos, Associate Coordinator

American Board of Surgery, Inc., 1617 John F. Kennedy Boulevard, Suite 860, Philadelphia, PA 19103; tel. 215/568-4000; FAX. 215/563-5718; Wallace P. Ritchie, Jr., M.D., Executive Director

American Board of Thoracic Surgery, One Rotary Center, Suite 803, Evanston, IL 60201; tel. 708/475-1520; FAX. 708/475-6240; Richard J. Cleveland, M.D., Secretary-Treasurer

American Board of Urology, 31700 Telegraph Road, Suite 150, Bingham Farms, MI 48025; tel. 810/646-9720; FAX. 810/644-0039; Alan D. Perlmutter, M.D., Executive Secretary

American Broncho-Esophagological Association, St. Louis Children's Hospital, Department of Otolaryngology, Room 3S35, One Children's Place, St. Louis, MO 63110; tel. 314/454-2138; FAX. 314/454-2174; Rodney P. Lusk, M.D., Secretary

American Burn Association, 525 East 68th Street, Room L-706, New York, NY 10021; tel. 800/548-2876; Cleon Goodwin, M.D., Secretary

American Cancer Society, 1599 Clifton Road, N.E., Atlanta, GA 30329; tel. 404/320-3333; Gerald P. Murphy, M.D., Senior Vice President, Medical Affairs

American Center for the Alexander Technique, Inc., 129 West 67th Street, New York, NY 10023; tel. 212/799-0468; Kathryn Miranda, Executive Director

American Chiropractic Association, 1701 Clarendon Boulevard, Arlington, VA 22209; tel. 703/276-8800; FAX. 703/243-2593; Ray Morgan, Executive Vice President

American Cleft Palate-Craniofacial Association, 1218 Grandview Avenue, Pittsburgh, PA 15211; tel. 412/481-1376; FAX. 412/481-0847; Nancy C. Smythe, Executive Director

American College Health Association, P.O. Box 28937, Baltimore, MD 21240-8937; tel. 410/859-1500; FAX. 410/859-1510; Charles H. Hartman, Ed.D, CAE, Executive Director

American College of Addiction Treatment Administrators, 5700 Old Orchard Road, First Floor, Skokie, IL 60077-1057; tel. 708/966-0181; FAX. 708/966-9418; David Stumph, CAE, Executive Vice President

American College of Allergy, Asthma and Immunology, 85 West Algonquin Road, Suite 550, Arlington Heights, IL 60005; tel. 708/427-1200; FAX. 708/427-1294; James R. Slawny, Executive Director

American College of Apothecaries, 205 Daingerfield Road, Alexandria, VA 22314; tel. 703/684-8603; FAX. 703/683-3619; D. C. Huffman, Jr., Ph.D., Executive Vice President

American College of Cardiology, 9111 Old Georgetown Road, Bethesda, MD 20814; tel. 301/897-2622; FAX. 301/897-9745; Penny S. Mills, Associate Executive Vice President

American College of Cardiovascular Administrators, 30555 Southfield Road, Suite 150, Southfield, MI 48076-7747; tel. 810/540-4598; FAX. 810/645-0590; James Reinhardt, FAAMA, FACCA

American College of Chest Physicians, 3300 Dundee Road, Northbrook, IL 60062-2348; tel. 708/498-1400; FAX. 708/498-5460; Alvin Lever, Executive Director

American College of Dentists, 839 Quince Orchard Boulevard, Suite J, Gaithersburg, MD 20878-1603; tel. 301/977-3223; FAX. 301/977-3330; Sherry Keramidas, Ph.D., CAE

American College of Emergency Physicians, P.O. Box 619911, Dallas, TX 75261-9911; tel. 214/550-0911; FAX. 214/580-2816; Colin C. Rorrie, Jr., Ph.D., Executive Director

American College of Foot and Ankle Orthopedics and Medicine (ACFAOM), 4603 Highway 95 South, P.O. Box 39, Cocolalla, ID 83813-0039; tel. 208/683-3900; FAX. 208/683-3700; Judith A. Baerg, Executive Director

American College of Foot and Ankle Surgeons, 515 Busse Highway, Park Ridge, IL 60068; tel. 708/292-2237; FAX. 708/292-2022; Teri Gargano Barabash, Manager, Communications

American College of Health Care Administrators, 325 South Patrick Street, Alexandria, VA 22314; tel. 703/549-5822; FAX. 703/739-7901; Richard L. Thorpe, CAE, Executive Vice President

American College of Healthcare Executives, One North Franklin, Suite 1700, Chicago, IL 60606-3491; tel. 312/424-2800; FAX. 312/424-0023; Thomas C. Dolan, Ph.D., FACHE, CAE, President/Chief Executive Officer

American College of Healthcare Inforamtion Administrator, 30555 Southfield Road, Suite 150, Southfield, MI 48076-7747; tel. 810/540-4310; FAX. 810/645-0590; Shyam Heda, President

American College of Legal Medicine, 5700 Old Orchard Road, First Floor, Skokie, IL 60077-1024; tel. 800/433-9137; FAX. 708/966-9418; Jay A. Gold, M.D., J.D., M.P.H., FUM, Executive Director

American College of MOHS Micrographic Surgery and Cutaneous Oncology, 930 North Meacham, Schaumburg, IL 60173-4965; tel. 708/330-0230, ext. 371; FAX. 708/330-0050; Michael Thompson, Staff Coordinator

American College of Managed Care Administrators, 30555 Southfield Road, Suite 150, Southfield, MI 48076-7747; tel. 810/540-4310; FAX. 810/645-0590; Eugene Migilaccio, Dr.P.H., President

American College of Medical Staff Development, 3150 Holcomb Bridge Road, Suite 205, Norcross, GA 30071; tel. 800/897-9494; FAX. 404/417-2176; Karen Kelley-Black, Executive Director

American College of Medicine, 4711 West Gulf Road, Suited 408, Skokie, IL 60076; tel. 708/568-1500; Randall T. Bellows, M.D., Director

American College of Nurse-Midwives, 818 Connecticut Avenue, N.W., Suite 900, Washington, DC 20006; tel. 202/728-9860; FAX. 202/728-9897; Ronald E. Nitzsche, Chief Operating Officer

American College of Obstetricians and Gynecologists, 409 12th Street, S.W., Washington, DC 20024-2188; tel. 202/638-5577; FAX. 202/484-5107; Ralph W. Hale, M.D., Executive Director

American College of Occupational and Environmental Medicine, (Includes ACOEM Research and Education Fund, and Occupational Physicians Scholarship Fund OPSF), 55 West Seegers, Arlington Heights, IL 60005; tel. 708/228-6850, ext. 11; FAX. 708/228-1856; Donald L. Hoops, Ph.D., Executive Vice President

American College of Oncology Administrators, 30555 Southfield Road, Suite 150, Southfield, MI 48076-7747; tel. 810/540-4310; FAX. 810/645-0590; Arthur T. Porter, M.D., President

American College of Osteopathic Pediatricians, 5301 Wisconsin Avenue, NW, Suite 630, Washington, DC 20015; tel. 202/362-3229; FAX. 202/537-1362; David Kushner, Executive Director

American College of Physician Executives, 4890 West Kennedy Boulevard, Suite 200, Tampa, FL 33609-2575; tel. 813/287-2000; FAX. 813/287-8993; Roger S. Schenke, Executive Vice President

American College of Physicians, Independence Mall West, Sixth Street at Race, Philadelphia, PA 19106; tel. 215/351-2400; FAX. 215/351-2799; Joseph E. Johnson III, M.D. Executive Vice President

American College of Preventive Medicine, 1015 15th Street, N.W., Suite 403, Washington, DC 20005; tel. 202/789-0003; FAX. 202/289-8274; Hazel K. Keimowitz, M.A., Executive Director

American College of Radiology, 1891 Preston White Drive, Reston, VA 22091; tel. 703/648-8900; FAX. 703/648-9176; John J. Curry, Executive Director

American College of Rheumatology, 60 Executive Park, S., Suite 150, Atlanta, GA 30329; tel. 404/633-3777; FAX. 404/633-1870; Lynn Bonfiglio, Director, Membership

American College of Sports Medicine, P.O. Box 1440, Indianapolis, IN 46206-1440; tel. 317/637-9200; FAX. 317/634-7817, ext. 100; James R. Whitehead, Executive Vice President

American College of Surgeons, 55 East Erie Street, Chicago, IL 60611; tel. 312/664-4050, ext. 201; FAX. 312/440-7014; Paul A. Ebert, M.D., Director

American Congress of Rehabilitation Medicine, 5700 Old Orchard Road, First Floor, Skokie, IL 60077-1057; tel. 708/966-0095; FAX. 708/966-9418; Richard Muir, Executive Director

American Council on Pharmaceutical Education, Inc., 311 West Superior Street, Suite 512, Chicago, IL 60610; tel. 312/664-3575; FAX. 312/664-4652; Daniel A. Nona, Ph.D., Executive Director

American Dental Assistants Association, 203 North LaSalle, Suite 1320, Chicago, IL 60601; tel. 312/541-1550, ext. 204; FAX. 312/541-1496; Lawrence H. Sepin, Executive Director

American Dental Association, 211 East Chicago Avenue, Chicago, IL 60611; tel. 312/440-2700; FAX. 312/440-7488; John S. Zapp, D.D.S., Executive Director

American Dental Society of Anesthesiology, Inc., 211 East Chicago Avenue, Suite 810, Chicago, IL 60611; tel. 312/664-8270; FAX. 312/642-9713; Christopher LoFrisco, D.M.D., Executive Director

American Diabetes Association, Inc., 1660 Duke Street, Alexandria, VA 22314; tel. 703/549-1500; FAX. 703/836-7439; John H. Graham IV, Chief Executive Officer

American Dietetic Association, 216 West Jackson Boulevard, Suite 800, Chicago, IL 60606-6995; tel. 312/899-0040, ext. 4889; FAX. 312/899-1758; Beverly Bajus, Chief Operating Officer

American Electroencephalographic Society, One Regency Drive, P.O. Box 30, Bloomfield, CT 06002; tel. 203/243-3977; FAX. 203/286-0787; Jacquelyn T. Coleman, Executive Director

American Epilepsy Society, 638 Prospect Avenue, Hartford, CT 06105-4298; tel. 203/232-4825; FAX. 203/232-0819; Suzanne C. Berry, Executive Director

American Federation for Clinical Research, 6900 Grove Road, Thorofare, NJ 08086; tel. 609/848-7072, ext. 212; FAX. 609/384-6504; Jean M. Haddock, Executive Director

American Foundation for Aging Research, North Carolina State University, Biochemistry Department, P.O. Box 7622, Raleigh, NC 27695-7622; tel. 919/515-5679; FAX. 919/515-2047; Paul F. Agris, President

American Foundation for Aids Research, 5900 Wilshire Boulevard, 2nd Floor, E., Los Angeles, CA 90036; tel. 213/857-5900; Mathilde Krim, Ph.D., Founding Co-Chair

American Foundation for the Blind, Inc., 11 Penn Plaza, Suite 300, New York, NY 10001; tel. 212/502-7600; Liz Greco, Vice President, Communications

American Fracture Association, 2416 East Washington Street, Suite D, Bloomington, IL 61704-4472; tel. 309/663-6272; Barbara Dehority, Executive Director

American Geriatrics Society, 770 Lexington Avenue, Suite 300, New York, NY 10021; tel. 212/308-1414; FAX. 212/832-8646; Linda Hiddemen Barondess, Executive Vice President

American Group Practice Association, Inc., 1422 Duke Street, Alexandria, VA 22314-3430; tel. 703/838-0033; FAX. 703/548-1890; Donald W. Fisher, Ph.D., Exec. Vice President and Chief Executive Officer

Organizations / National Organizations

American Group Psychotherapy Association, Inc., 25 East 21st Street, 6th Floor, New York, NY 10010; tel. 212/477-2677; FAX. 212/979-6627; Marsha S. Block, CAE, Chief Executive Officer

American Guild of Patient Account Management, 1101 Connecticut Avenue, N.W., Suite 700, Washington, DC 20036; tel. 202/857-1179; FAX. 202/223-4579; Dennis E. Smeage, Executive Director

American Gynecological and Obstetrical Society, Department of OB–GYN, University of Virginia, Charlottesville, VA 22908; tel. 804/924-9937; FAX. 804/982-1840; Paul Underwood, M.D., Secretary

American Health Care Association, 1201 L Street, N.W., Washington, DC 20005; tel. 202/842-4444; FAX. 202/842-3860; Paul R. Willging, Ph.D., Executive Vice President

American Health Foundation, One Dana Road, Valhalla, NY 10595; tel. 914/789-7191; Dr. Gordon C. Hard, Director of Administration

American Health Information Management Association, 919 North Michigan Avenue, Suite 1400, Chicago, IL 60611; tel. 312/787-2672, ext. 210; FAX. 312/787-9793; Pamela K. Wear, M.B.A., R.R.A., Executive Director

American Health Planning Association, 1110 Vermont Avenue, N.W., Suite LL-4, Washington, DC 20005; tel. 202/861-1200; James O'Donnell, Executive Director

American Healthcare Radiology Administrators, P.O. Box 334, Sudbury, MA 01776; tel. 508/443-7591; FAX. 508/443-8046; Teresa Cryan, Office Administrator

American Heart Association, Inc., Office of Scientific Affairs, 7320 Greenville Avenue, Dallas, TX 75231; tel. 214/706-1446; Mary Jane Jesse, M.D., Senior Vice President

American Hospital Association, One North Franklin, Chicago, IL 60606-3491; tel. 312/422-3000; Office of the President: 325 Seventh Street, N.W., Washington, DC 20004; tel. 202/638-1100; FAX. 202/626-2345; Richard J. Davidson, President

American Hospital Association, Washington Office, 325 Seventh Street, N.W., Suite 700, Washington, DC 20004; tel. 202/638-1100; FAX. 202/626-2345; Richard Pollack, Executive Vice President, Federal Relations

American Institute of Architects, Committee on Architecture for Health, 1735 New York Avenue, N.W., Washington, DC 20006; tel. 202/626-7366; FAX. 206/626-7518; Todd S. Phillips, Ph.D., Director

American Juvenile Arthritis Organization, a Council of the Arthritis Foundation, 1314 Spring Street, N.W., Atlanta, GA 30309; tel. 404/872-7100, ext. 6271; FAX. 404/872-0457; Patricia Harrington, CAE, Vice President

American Kinesiotherapy Association, Inc., P.O. Box 611, Wright Brothers Station, Dayton, OH 45409-0611; tel. 800/326-0268; FAX. 513/293-0958; Edmund C. Reiling, Executive Director

American Laryngological Association, 300 Longwood Avenue, Fegan 9, Boston, MA 02115; tel. 617/735-6417; FAX. 617/735-8041

American Laryngological, Rhinological, and Otological Society, Inc., (The Triological Society), 10 South Broadway, Suite 1401, St. Louis, MO 63102-1741; tel. 314/621-6580; FAX. 314/621-6688; Daniel Henroid, Sr., Executive Director

American Library Association, 50 East Huron Street, Chicago, IL 60611; tel. 312/280-3205; FAX. 312/944-3897; Elizabeth Martinez, Executive Director

American Lung Association, 1740 Broadway, New York, NY 10019-4374; tel. 212/315-8700; FAX. 212/265-5642; John R. Garrison, Managing Director

American Lung Association of Ohio, Dayton Office, 7560 McEwen Road, Dayton, OH 45459; tel. 513/291-0451; FAX. 513/291-0453; Roberta M. Taylor, Director

American Managed Care and Review Association (A.M.C.R.A.), 1200 19th Street, N.W., Suite 200, Washington, DC 20036; tel. 202/728-0506; FAX. 202/728-0609; Charles W. Stellar, President

American Medical Association, 515 North State Street, Chicago, IL 60610; tel. 312/464-5000; FAX. 312/464-4184; James S. Todd, M.D., Executive Vice President

American Medical Association Alliance, 515 North State Street, Chicago, IL 60610; tel. 312/464-4470; FAX. 312/464-5839; Hazel J. Lewis, Executive Director

American Medical Student Association/Foundation, 1902 Association Drive, Reston, VA 22091; tel. 703/620-6600; FAX. 703/620-5873; Paul R. Wright, Executive Director

American Medical Technologists, 710 Higgins Road, Park Ridge, IL 60068; tel. 708/823-5169; FAX. 708/823-0458; Gerard P. Boe, Ph.D., Executive Director

American Medical Women's Association, Inc., 800 North Fairfax Street, Suite 400, Alexandria, VA 22314; tel. 703/838-0500; FAX. 703/549-3864; Eileen McGrath, J.D., CAE, Executive Director

American Medical Writers Association, 9650 Rockville Pike, Bethesda, MD 20814; tel. 301/493-0003; FAX. 301/493-6384; Lillian Sablack, Executive Director

American National Standards Institute, 11 West 42nd Street, New York, NY 10036; tel. 212/642-4900; FAX. 212/398-0023; Manuel Peralta, President

American Nephrology Nurses' Association, East Holly Avenue, P.O. Box 56, Pitman, NJ 08071; tel. 609/256-2320; FAX. 609/589-7463; Ron P. Brady, Executive Director

American Neurological Association, 2221 University Avenue, S.E., Suite 350, Minneapolis, MN 55414; tel. 612/623-2401; FAX. 612/623-3504; Carol Hamel, Association Manager

American Nurses' Association, 600 Maryland Avenue, S.W., Suite 100 W, Washington, DC 20024-2571; tel. 202/651-7012; FAX. 202/651-7006; Geri Marullo, MS, RN, Executive Director

American Occupational Therapy Association, Inc., 4720 Montgomery Lane, P.O. Box 31220, Bethesda, MD 20824-1220; tel. 301/652-2682, ext. 2101; FAX. 301/652-7711; Jeanette Bair, M.B.A., O.T.R., F.A.O.T.A.

American Ophthalmological Society, Duke University Eye Center, Box 3802, Durham, NC 27710-3802; tel. 919/684-5365; FAX. 919/684-2230; W. Banks Anderson, Jr., M.D., Secretary–Treasurer

American Optometric Association, 243 North Lindbergh Boulevard, St. Louis, MO 63141; tel. 314/991-4100; FAX. 314/991-4101; Earle L. Hunter, O.D. Executive Director

American Organization of Nurse Executives (AONE), One North Franklin, 34th Floor, Chicago, IL 60606; tel. 312/422-2800; FAX. 312/422-4503; Marjorie Beyers, RN, Ph.D., FAAN

American Orthopsychiatric Association, Inc., 330 Seventh Avenue, 18th Floor, New York, NY 10001; tel. 212/564-5930; FAX. 212/564-6180; Ernest Herman, Executive Director

American Orthoptic Council, 3914 Nakoma Road, Madison, WI 53711; tel. 608/233-5383; FAX. 608/263-7694; Leslie France, Administrator

American Osteopathic Academy of Addictionology, Inc., 5301 Wisconsin Avenue, NW, Suite 630, Washington, DC 20015; tel. 202/966-7732; FAX. 202/537-1362; David Kushner, Executive Director

American Osteopathic Association, 142 East Ontario Street, Chicago, IL 60611; tel. 312/280-5800; FAX. 312/280-3860; Robert E. Draba, Ph.D., Executive Director

American Osteopathic Healthcare Association, 5301 Wisconsin Avenue, N.W., Suite 630, Washington, DC 20015; tel. 202/686-1700; FAX. 202/686-7615; David Kushner, President and Chief Executive Officer

American Otological Society, Inc., Loyola University Medical Center, 2160 South First Avenue, Building 105, Number 1870, Maywood, IL 60153; tel. 708/216-8526; FAX. 708/696-0769; Gregory J. Matz, M.D., Secretary–Treasurer

American Parkinson Disease Association, 60 Bay Street, Suite 401, Staten Island, NY 10301; tel. 800/223-2732; FAX. 718/981-4399; G. Maestrome, D.V.M., Scientific and Medical Affairs Director

American Pediatric Society, Inc., 141 N.W. Point Boulevard, P.O. Box 675, Elk Grove Village, IL 60009-0675; tel. 708/427-0205; FAX. 708/427-1305; Norman J. Siegel, M.D., Secretary–Treasurer

American Pharmaceutical Association, 2215 Constitution Avenue, N.W., Washington, DC 20037; tel. 202/628-4410; FAX. 202/783-2351; John A. Gans, Pharm.D., Executive Vice President

American Physical Therapy Association, 1111 North Fairfax Street, Alexandria, VA 22314; tel. 703/706-3252; FAX. 703/706-8519; Francis J. Mallon, Esq., Chief Executive Officer

American Physiological Society, 9650 Rockville Pike, Bethesda, MD 20814-3991; tel. 301/530-7118; FAX. 301/571-8305; Martin Frank, Ph.D., Executive Director

American Podiatric Medical Association, 9312 Old Georgetown Road, Bethesda, MD 20814-1698; tel. 301/571-9200; FAX. 301/530-2752; Frank J. Malouff, Executive Director

American Psychiatric Association, 1400 K Street, N.W., Washington, DC 20005; tel. 202/682-6000; FAX. 202/682-6114; Melvin Sabshin, M.D., Medical Director

American Psychoanalytic Association, 309 East 49th Street, New York, NY 10017; tel. 212/752-0450; Doris L. Eder, Administrative Director

American Psychological Association, 750 First Street, N.E., Washington, DC 20002-4242; tel. 202/336-5500; FAX. 202/336-6069; Raymond D. Fowler, Ph.D., Chief Executive Officer

American Psychosomatic Society, 6728 Old McLean Village Drive, McLean, VA 22101; tel. 703/556-9222; George K. Degnon, Executive Director

American Public Health Association, 1015 15th Street, N.W., Washington, DC 20005; tel. 202/789-5600; FAX. 202/789-5681; Fernando M. Trevino, Ph.D., M.P.H., Executive Director

American Public Welfare Association, 810 First Street, N.E., Suite 500, Washington, DC 20002; tel. 202/682-0100; FAX. 202/289-6555; Sidney Johnson III, Executive Director

American Red Cross, National Headquarters, 8111 Gatehouse Road, Falls Church, VA 22042; tel. 703/206-7764; FAX. 703/206-7765; Susan M. Livingstone, Vice President, Health and Safety Services

American Registry of Clinical Radiography Technologists, 710 Higgins Road, Park Ridge, IL 60068; tel. 708/318-9050; Joe Johns, President

American Registry of Medical Assistants, 69 Southwick Road, Suite A, Westfield, MA 01085-4729; tel. 413/562-7336; Annette H. Heyman, R.M.A., Director

American Registry of Radiologic Technologists, 1255 Northland Drive, St. Paul, MN 55120; tel. 612/687-0048; Jerry B. Reid, Ph.D., Executive Director

American Rhinologic Society, Long Island College Hospital, Department of Otolaryngology, Brooklyn, NY 11201; tel. 718/780-1281; FAX. 718/780-1488; Frank E. Lucente, M.D., Secretary

American Roentgen Ray Society, 1891 Preston White Drive, Reston, VA 22091; tel. 703/648-8992; FAX. 703/264-8863; Paul R. Fullagar, Executive Director

American School Health Association, Box 708, Kent, OH 44240; tel. 216/678-1601; FAX. 216/678-4526; Diane D. Allensworth, Ph.D., RN, Executive Director

American Society for Adolescent Psychiatry, 5530 Wisconsin Avenue, N.W., Suite 1149, Washington, DC 20815; tel. 301/652-0646; FAX. 301/656-0989; David Lewis, Executive Director

Organizations / National Organizations

American Society for Biochemistry and Molecular Biology, Inc., 9650 Rockville Pike, Bethesda, MD 20814–3996; tel. 301/530–7145; FAX. 301/571–1824; Charles C. Hancock, Executive Officer

American Society for Clinical Laboratory Science, 7910 Woodmont Avenue, Suite 1301, Bethesda, MD 20814; tel. 301/657–2768; Lynn Podell Robinson, Executive Director

American Society for Clinical Pharmacology and Therapeutics, 1718 Gallagher Road, Norristown, PA 19401–2800; tel. 610/825–3838; FAX. 610/834–8652; Elaine Galasso, Executive Director

American Society for Cytotechnology, 920 Paverstone Drive, Suite D, Raleigh, NC 27615; tel. 919/848–9911; FAX. 919/848–9853; Margaret Bundy, Secretary–Treasurer

American Society for Head and Neck Surgery, John Hopkins Hospital, Carnegie Building, 600 North Wolfe Street, Suite 466, Baltimore, MD 21205; tel. 410/955–7400; Charles Cummings, M.D., Secretary

American Society for Health Care Marketing and Public Relations (AHA), One North Franklin, 31st Floor, Chicago, IL 60606; tel. 312/422–3737; FAX. 312/422–4579; Lauren A. Barnett, Executive Director

American Society for Healthcare Central Service Personnel (AHA), One North Franklin, 30th Floor, Chicago, IL 60606; tel. 312/422–3570; FAX. 312/422–4571; Lorna Dizon, Administrative Assistant

American Society for Healthcare Education and Training (AHA), One North Franklin, Chicago, IL 60606; tel. 312/422–3720; FAX. 312/422–4579; Linda H. Brooks, Executive Director

American Society for Healthcare Engineering (AHA), One North Franklin, Chicago, IL 60606; tel. 312/422–3850; FAX. 312/422–4572; V. James McLarney, Acting Executive Director

American Society for Healthcare Food Service Administrators (AHA), One North Franklin, Chicago, IL 60606; tel. 312/422–3870; FAX. 312/422–4581; Kathleen Pontius, Executive Director

American Society for Healthcare Human Resources Administration (AHA), One North Franklin, 31st Floor, Chicago, IL 60606; tel. 312/422–3720; FAX. 312/422–4579; Linda H. Brooks, Executive Director

American Society for Healthcare Risk Management (AHA), One North Franklin, Chicago, IL 60606; tel. 312/422–3980; FAX. 312/422–4580; Trudy Goldman, Executive Director

American Society for Hospital Materials Management (AHA), One North Franklin, Chicago, IL 60606–3491; tel. 312/422–3840; FAX. 312/422–4573; Shelly Johnson, Director

American Society for Investigative Pathology, 9650 Rockville Pike, Bethesda, MD 20814–3993; tel. 301/530–7130; Frances A. Pitlick, Ph.D., Executive Officer

American Society for Laser Medicine and Surgery, Inc., 2404 Stewart Square, Wausau, WI 54401; tel. 715/845–9283; FAX. 715/848–2493; Richard O. Gregory, M.D.

American Society for Microbiology, 1325 Massachusetts Avenue, N.W., Washington, DC 20005; tel. 202/924–9265; FAX. 202/942–9333; Michael I. Goldberg, Ph.D., Executive Director

American Society for Pharmacology and Experimental Therapeutics, Inc., 9650 Rockville Pike, Bethesda, MD 20814–3995; tel. 301/530–7060; Kay A. Croker, Executive Officer

American Society for Psychoprophylaxis in Obstetrics, Inc. (ASPO/LAMAZE), 1200 19th Street, N.W., Suite 300, Washington, DC 20036; tel. 202/857–1128; FAX. 202/223–4579; Linda L. Harmon, Executive Director

American Society for Public Administration, 1120 G Street, N.W., Suite 700, Washington, DC 20005; tel. 202/393–7878; FAX. 202/638–4952; John P. Thomas, Executive Director

American Society for Reproductive Medicine, (formerly The American Fertility Society), 1209 Montgomery Highway, Birmingham, AL 35216–2809; tel. 205/978–5000; FAX. 205/978–5005; Robert D. Visscher, M.D., Executive Director

American Society for Therapeutic Radiology and Oncology, 1891 Preston White Drive, Reston, VA 22091; tel. 800/962–7876; FAX. 703/476–8167; Gregg Robinson, Chief Operating Officer

American Society for Training and Development, 1640 King Street, P.O. Box 1443, Alexandria, VA 22313–2043; tel. 703/683–8150; FAX. 703/548–2383; Anthony P. Carnevale, Chief Economist

American Society for the Advancement of Anesthesia in Dentistry, 6 East Union Avenue, P.O. Box 551, Bound Brook, NJ 08805; tel. 201/469–9050; David Crystal, D.D.S., Executive Secretary

American Society of Anesthesiologists, 520 North Northwest Highway, Park Ridge, IL 60068; tel. 708/825–5586; FAX. 708/825–1692; Glenn W. Johnson, Executive Director

American Society of Cardiovascular Professionals, 120 Falcon Drive, Suite 3, Fredericksburg, VA 22408; tel. 703/891–0079; FAX. 703/898–2393; Peggy McElgunn, Executive Director

American Society of Clinical Oncology, 435 North Michigan Avenue, Suite 1717, Chicago, IL 60611–4067; tel. 312/644–0828; FAX. 312/644–8557; Robert E. Becker, J.D., CAE, Executive Director

American Society of Clinical Pathologists., (Includes Board of Registry), 2100 West Harrison Street, Chicago, IL 60612–3798; tel. 312/738–1336; FAX. 312/738–9798; Robert C. Rock, M.D., Senior Vice President

American Society of Colon and Rectal Surgeons, 85 West Algonquin Road, Suite 550, Arlington Heights, IL 60005; tel. 708/290–9184; FAX. 708/290–9203; Ira J. Kodner, M.D., Secretary

American Society of Consultant Pharmacists, 1321 Duke Street, Alexandria, VA 22314–3563; tel. 703/739–1300; FAX. 703/739–1321; R. Timothy Webster, Executive Director

American Society of Contemporary Medicine and Surgery, 233 East Erie Street, Suite 710, Chicago, IL 60611; tel. 312/951–1400; FAX. 312/951–1410; Randall T. Bellows, M.D., Director

American Society of Contemporary Ophthalmology, 4711 West Golf Road, Suite 408, Skokie, IL 60076; tel. 708/568–1500; Randall T. Bellows, M.D., Director

American Society of Cytopathology, 400 West 9th Street, Suite 201, Wilmington, DE 19801; tel. 302/429–8802; FAX. 302/429–8807; Petrina M. Smith, RN, M.B.A., Executive Secretary

American Society of Dentistry for Children, John Hancock Center, 875 North Michigan Avenue, Suite 4040, Chicago, IL 60611; tel. 312/943–1244; FAX. 312/943–5341; Dr. Norman H. Olsen, Executive Director

American Society of Directors of Volunteer Services (AHA), One North Franklin, Chicago, IL 60606; tel. 312/422–3938; FAX. 312/422–4575; Nancy A. Brown, Executive Director

American Society of Electroneurodiagnostic Technologists, Inc., 204 West 7th Street, Carroll, IA 51401; tel. 712/792–2978; FAX. 712/792–6962; M. Fran Pedelty, Executive Director

American Society of Extra–Corporeal Technology, Inc., 11480 Sunset Hills Road, Suite 210E, Reston, VA 22090; tel. 703/435–8556; FAX. 703/435–0056; George M. Cate, Executive Director

American Society of Hospital Pharmacists, 7272 Wisconsin Avenue, Bethesda, MD 20814; tel. 301/657–3000; FAX. 301/652–8278; Joseph A. Oddis, Executive Vice President

American Society of Internal Medicine, 2011 Pennsylvania Avenue, N.W., Suite 800, Washington, DC 20006–1808; tel. 202/835–2746; FAX. 202/835–0443; Alan R. Nelson, M.D., Executive Vice President

American Society of Law, Medicine and Ethics, 765 Commonwealth Avenue, 16th Floor, Boston, MA 02215; tel. 617/262–4990; FAX. 617/437–7596; Benjamin Moulton, J.D., M.P.H., Executive Director

American Society of Lipo–Suction Surgery, 159 East Live Oak, Suite 204, Arcadia, CA 91006–5249; tel. 818/447–1579; FAX. 818/447–7880; Thomas H. Alt, M.D., President

American Society of Maxillofacial Surgeons, 444 East Algonquin Road, Arlington Heights, IL 60005; tel. 708/228–3327; FAX. 708/228–6509; Mary S. Feeley, Executive Director

American Society of Neuroimaging, 2221 University Avenue, S.E., Suite 340, Minneapolis, MN 55414; tel. 612/623–2404; FAX. 612/623–3504; Carol Hamel, Society Manager

American Society of Plastic and Reconstructive Surgeons, 444 East Algonquin Road, Arlington Heights, IL 60005; tel. 708/228–9900; FAX. 708/228–9131; Dave Fellers, CAE, Executive Director

American Society of Radiologic Technologists, 15000 Central Avenue, S.E., Albuquerque, NM 87123–3917; tel. 505/298–4500; FAX. 505/298–5063; Ward M. Keller, Chief Executive Officer

American Speech–Language–Hearing Association, Consumer Division, 10801 Rockville Pike, Rockville, MD 20852; tel. 800/638–8255; FAX. 301/571–0457; Frederick T. Spahr, Ph.D., Executive Director

American Surgical Association, 13 Elm Street, Manchester, MA 01944; tel. 508/526–8330; FAX. 508/526–4018; John L. Cameron, M.D., Secretary

American Thoracic Society, 1740 Broadway, New York, NY 10019–4374; tel. 212/315–8700, ext. 778; FAX. 212/315–6498; Marilyn Hansen, Executive Director

American Thyroid Association, Inc., Montefiore Medical Center, 111 East 210th Street, Room 311, Bronx, NY 10467; tel. 718/882–6047; FAX. 718/882–6085; Martin I. Surks, M.D., F.A.C.P., Secretary

American Trauma Society, 8903 Presidential Parkway, Suite 512, Upper Marlboro, MD 20772–2656; tel. 800/556–7890; FAX. 301/420–0617; Harry Teter, Executive Director

American Urological Association, Inc., 1120 North Charles Street, Baltimore, MD 21201; tel. 410/727–1100; FAX. 410/625–2390; G. James Gallagher, Executive Director

Arthritis Foundation, 1314 Spring Street, N.W., Atlanta, GA 30309; tel. 404/872–7100, ext. 6200; FAX. 404/872–0457; Don L. Riggin, President and Chief Executive Officer

Association for Applied Psychophysiology and Biofeedback, 10200 West 44th Avenue, Suite 304, Wheat Ridge, CO 80033; tel. 303/422–8436; FAX. 303/422–8894; Francine Butler, Ph.D.

Association for Clinical Pastoral Education, Inc., 1549 Clairmont Road, Suite 103, Decatur, GA 30033; tel. 404/320–1472; FAX. 404/320–0849; Duane Parker, Executive Director

Association for Healthcare Philanthropy, 313 Park Avenue, Suite 400, Falls Church, VA 22046; tel. 703/532–6243; FAX. 703/532–7170; Dr. William C. McGinly, CAE, President

Association for Hospital Medical Education, 1200 19th Street, N.W., Suite 300, Washington, DC 20036–2401; tel. 202/857–1196; FAX. 202/223–4579; Michael S. Hamm, Executive Director

Association for Professionals in Infection Control and Epidemiology, Inc., 1016 16th Street, Washington, DC 20036; tel. 202/296–2742; FAX. 202/296–5645; Robert B. Willis, Executive Director

Association for Quality HealthCare, Inc., P.O. Box 670, Columbus, GA 31902; tel. 404/571–2122; FAX. 404/571–2650; L. B. Skip Teaster, Executive Director

Association for Voluntary Surgical Contraception, Inc., 122 East 42nd Street, New York, NY 10168; tel. 212/351–2561; Janel Halpern, Public Information Manager

Organizations / National Organizations

Association for Volunteer Administration, P.O. Box 4584, Boulder, CO 80306; tel. 303/541-0238; FAX. 303/541-0277; Martha N. Martin, Member Services Manager

Association for the Advancement of Automotive Medicine, 2350 East Devon Avenue, Suite 205, Des Plaines, IL 60018; tel. 708/390-8927; Elaine Petrucelli, Executive Director

Association for the Advancement of Medical Instrumentation, 3330 Washington Boulevard, Suite 400, Arlington, VA 22201-4598; tel. 703/525-4890; Michael J. Miller, J.D., President

Association for the Care of Children's Health (ACCH), 7910 Woodmont Avenue, Suite 300, Bethesda, MD 20814; tel. 301/654-6549; FAX. 301/986-4553; William Sciarillo, Sc.D., Executive Director

Association of American Medical Colleges, 2450 N Street, N.W., Washington, DC 20037-1125; tel. 202/828-0400; FAX. 202/828-1125; Jordan J. Cohen, M.D., President

Association of American Physicians, Krannert Institute of Cardiology, Indiana University School of Medicine, 1111 West 10th Street, Indianapolis, IN 46202-4800; tel. 317/630-7712; FAX. 317/274-9697; David R. Hathaway, M.D., Secretary

Association of American Physicians and Surgeons, Inc., 1601 North Tucson Boulevard, Suite 9, Tucson, AZ 85716; tel. 602/327-4885; FAX. 602/326-3529; Jane M. Orient, M.D., Executive Director

Association of Birth Defect Children, 827 Irma Avenue, Orlando, FL 32803; tel. 407/245-7035; FAX. 407/245-7035; Betty Mekdeci, Executive Director

Association of Community Cancer Centers, 11600 Nebel Street, Suite 201, Rockville, MD 20852; tel. 301/984-9496; FAX. 301/770-1949; Lee E. Mortenson, DPA, Executive Director

Association of Mental Health Administrators, 60 Revere Drive, Suite 500, Northbrook, IL 60062; tel. 708/480-9626; FAX. 708/480-9282; Maria R. Helm, Executive Director

Association of Mental Health Clergy, Inc., 12320 River Oaks Point, Knoxville, TN 37922; tel. 615/544-9704; FAX. 615/544-8888; George E. Doebler, Executive Director

Association of Military Surgeons of the U.S., 9320 Old Georgetown Road, Bethesda, MD 20814; tel. 301/897-8800; FAX. 301/530-5446; Lt. General Max B. Bralliar, USAF MC Ret., Executive Director

Association of Operating Room Nurses, Inc., 2170 South Parker Road, Suite 300, Denver, CO 80231-5711; tel. 303/755-6300; FAX. 303/750-2927; Lola M. Fehr, RN, M.S., CAE, Executive Director

Association of Osteopathic Directors and Medical Educators, 5301 Wisconsin Avenue, NW, Suite 630, Washington, DC 20015; tel. 202/537-1021; FAX. 202/537-1362; David Kushner, Executive Director

Association of Schools of Allied Health Professions, 1730 M Street, N.W., Suite 500, Washington, DC 20036; tel. 202/293-4848; FAX. 202/293-4852; Carolyn M. Freeland, Ph.D., Executive Director

Association of Schools of Public Health, Inc., 1015 Fifteenth Street, N.W., Suite 404, Washington, DC 20005; tel. 202/842-4668; FAX. 202/289-8274; Michael K. Gemmell, CAE, Executive Director

Association of Specialized and Cooperative Library Agencies, 50 East Huron Street, Chicago, IL 60611; tel. 312/280-4399; FAX. 312/944-8085; Cathleen Bourdon, ASCLA, Executive Director

Association of State and Territorial Health Officials, (Includes Association of Health Facility Licensure and Certification Directors.), 6728 Old McLean Village Drive, McLean, VA 22101; tel. 703/556-9222; George K. Degnon, Executive Vice President

Association of Surgical Technologists, Inc., 7108-C South Alton Way, Englewood, CO 80112-2106; tel. 303/694-9130; FAX. 303/694-9169; William J. Teutsch, Executive Director

Association of University Anesthesiologists, 2033 Sixth Avenue, Suite 804, Seattle, WA 98121-2586; tel. 206/441-6020; FAX. 206/441-8262; Shirley Bishop

Association of University Programs in Health Administration, 1911 North Fort Myer Drive, Suite 503, Arlington, VA 22209; tel. 703/524-5500; FAX. 703/525-4791; Henry A. Fernandez, J.D., President/Chief Executive Director

Asthma Foundation of Southern Arizona, P.O. Box 30069, Tucson, AZ 85751-0069; tel. 602/323-6046; FAX. 602/324-1137; Lynn Krust, Executive Director

Asthma and Allergy Foundation of America, 1125 Fifteenth Street, N.W., Suite 502, Washington, DC 20005; tel. 202/466-7643; FAX. 202/466-8940; Mary E. Worstell, M.P.H., Executive Director

B

BCS Financial Corporation, 676 North St. Clair, Chicago, IL 60611; tel. 312/951-7700; FAX. 312/951-7876; Edward J. Baran, President

Biological Photographic Association, Inc., 1819 Peachtree Road, N.E., Suite 620, Atlanta, GA 30309; tel. 404/351-6300; FAX. 404/351-3348; William Just, Executive Director

Biological Stain Commission, Inc., University of Rochester Medical Center, Rochester, NY 14642-0001; tel. 716/275-6335; FAX. 716/273-1042; David P. Penney, Ph.D., Treasurer

Blinded Veterans Association, 477 H Street, N.W., Washington, DC 20001; tel. 800/669-7079; FAX. 202/371-8258; Ronald L. Miller, Ph.D., Executive Director

Blue Cross and Blue Shield Association, 676 North St. Clair Street, Chicago, IL 60611; tel. 312/440-6000; FAX. 312/440-6609; Harry P. Cain, Acting President, Chief Executive Officer

C

Catholic Health Association of the United States, 4455 Woodson Road, St. Louis, MO 63134-3797; tel. 314/427-2500; FAX. 314/427-0029; John E. Curley, Jr., President, Chief Executive Officer

Center for Health Administration Studies, University of Chicago, 969 East 60th Street, Chicago, IL 60637; tel. 312/702-7104; FAX. 312/702-7222; Edward F. Lawlor, Ph.D., Director

Central Neuropsychiatric Association, 720 West 34th Street, Austin, TX 78705; tel. 512/454-7741; FAX. 512/451-7245; Robert L. Zapalac, M.D., Secretary-Treasurer

Central Society for Clinical Research, Inc., 1228 West Nelson Street, Chicago, IL 60657; tel. 312/871-1618; Morton F. Arnsdorf, M.D., Secretary-Treasurer

Central Surgical Association, Northwestern University School of Medicine, Department of Surgery, 250 E. Superior Street, Suite 201, Chicago, IL 60611-2950; tel. 312/908-8060; FAX. 312/908-7404; David L. Nahrwold, M.D., Secretary

Children's Rights Council (CRC), a/k/a National Council for Children's Rights, 220 Eye Street, N.E., Suite 230, Washington, DC 20002; tel. 202/547-6227; FAX. 202/546-4272; David L. Levy, Esq., President

Christian Record Services, Inc., 4444 South 52nd Street, Lincoln, NE 68516; tel. 402/488-0981; FAX. 402/488-7582; Rikki Stenbakken, Assistant to the President

College of American Pathologists, 325 Waukegan Road, Northfield, IL 60093-2750; tel. 708/446-8800; FAX. 708/446-8807; Lee VanBremen, Ph.D., Executive Vice President

College of Osteopathic Healthcare Executives, 5301 Wisconsin Avenue, NW, Suite 630, Washington, DC 20015; tel. 202/686-1700; FAX. 202/686-7615; David Kushner, President

Commission on Accreditation of Rehabilitation Facilities, 101 North Wilmot Road, Suite 500, Tucson, AZ 85711; tel. 520/748-1212; FAX. 520/571-1601; Donald E. Galvin, Ph.D., President, Chief Executive Officer

Commission on Professional and Hospital Activities, P.O. Box 304, Ann Arbor, MI 48106-0304; tel. 313/995-9800; FAX. 313/995-9845; William F. Jessee, M.D., Chairman

Commission on Recognition of Postsecondary Accreditation, Inc., One Dupont Circle, N.W., Suite 305, Washington, DC 20036; tel. 202/452-1433; FAX. 202/331-9571; Dorothy Fenwick, Ph.D., Executive Director

Committee of Interns and Residents, 386 Park Avenue, S., New York, NY 10016; tel. 212/725-5500; FAX. 212/779-2413; John Ronches, Executive Director

Cooley's Anemia Foundation, Inc., 129-09 26th Avenue, Suite 203, Flushing, NY 11354; tel. 800/522-7222; FAX. 718/321-3340; Gina Cioffi, Esq. National Executive Director

Corporate Angel Network, Inc., CAN (Arranges Free Air Transportation for Cancer Patients), Westchester County Airport, Building One, White Plains, NY 10604; tel. 914/328-1313; FAX. 914/328-3938

Council of Community Blood Centers, 725 15th Street, N.W., Suite 700, Washington, DC 20005-2109; tel. 202/393-5725; FAX. 202/393-1282; James L. MacPherson, Executive Director

Council of Jewish Federations, Inc., 730 Broadway, New York, NY 10003; tel. 212/475-5000; FAX. 212/529-5842; Martin S. Kraar, Executive Vice President

Council of Medical Specialty Societies, 51 Sherwood Terrace, Suite Y, Lake Bluff, IL 60044; tel. 708/295-3456; FAX. 708/295-3759; Rebecca R. Gschwend, M.A., M.B.A., Executive Vice President

Council of State Administrators of Vocational Rehabilitation, P.O. Box 3776, Washington, DC 20007; tel. 202/638-4634; Jack G. Duncan, General Counsel, Rehabilitation Policy

Council on Education for Public Health, 1015 Fifteenth Street, N.W., Washington, DC 20005; tel. 202/789-1050; Patricia P. Evans, Executive Director

Council on Social Work Education, 1600 Duke Street, Alexandria, VA 22314; tel. 703/683-8080; FAX. 703/683-8099; Donald W. Beless, Ph.D., Executive Director

Crohn's and Colitis Foundation of America, Inc, 386 Park Avenue South, 17th Floor, New York, NY 10016-8804; tel. 800/343-3637; FAX. 212/779-4098; Barbara T. Boyle, National Executive Director

Cystic Fibrosis Foundation, 6931 Arlington Road, Bethesda, MD 20814; tel. 301/951-4422; FAX. 301/951-6378; Robert J. Beall, Ph.D., President/Chief Executive Officer

D

Damien Dutton Society for Leprosy Aid, Inc., 616 Bedford Avenue, Bellmore, NY 11710; tel. 516/221-5829; Howard E. Crouch, President

Delta Dental Plans Association, 211 East Chicago Avenue, Suite 800, Chicago, IL 60611; tel. 312/337-4707; FAX. 312/337-7991; James Bonk, President

Organizations / National Organizations

Dermatology Foundation, 1560 Sherman Avenue, Evanston, IL 60201-4802; tel. 708/328-2256; FAX. 708/328-0509; Sandra Rahn Goldman, Executive Director

Dietary Managers Association, One Pierce Place, Suite 1220W, Itasca, IL 60143; tel. 708/775-9200; FAX. 708/775-9250; William St. John, Executive Director

Dysautonomia Foundation, Inc., 20 East 46th Street, Suite 302, New York, NY 10017; tel. 212/949-6644; FAX. 212/682-7625; Lenore F. Roseman, Executive Director

E

ECRI, 5200 Butler Pike, Plymouth Meeting, PA 19462; tel. 610/825-6000, ext. 140; FAX. 610/834-1275; Joel J. Nobel, M.D., President

Eastern Orthopaedic Association, Inc., Pier 5 North, Suite 5D, 7 North Columbus Boulevard, Philadelphia, PA 19106-1486; tel. 215/351-4110; FAX. 215/351-1825; Elizabeth F. Capella, Executive Director

Educational Commission for Foreign Medical Graduates, 3624 Market Street, Philadelphia, PA 19104-2685; tel. 215/386-5900; FAX. 215/387-9963; Marjorie P. Wilson, M.D., President, Chief Executive Officer

Ehlers-Danlos National Foundation, P.O. Box 13157, Richmond, VA 23225; tel. 804/320-8192; FAX. 804/320-8192; Susan L. Stephenson, Vice President, Patient Advocate

Emergency Nurses Association, 216 Higgins Road, Park Ridge, IL 60068-5736; tel. 708/698-9400; FAX. 708/698-9406; H. Stephen Lieber, CAE, Executive Director

Environmental Management Association, 4350 Dipaolo Center, Suite C, Glenview, IL 60025; tel. 708/699-6362; FAX. 708/699-6369; Carl Wangman, President

Epilepsy Foundation of America, 4351 Garden City Drive, Landover, MD 20785; tel. 301/459-3700; FAX. 301/577-2684; William M. McLin, Executive Vice President

Episcopal Guild for the Blind, 561 Pacific Street, Brooklyn, NY 11217; tel. 718/625-4886; Rev. Harry J. Sutcliffe

F

Family Service America, Inc., 11700 West Lake Park Drive, Milwaukee, WI 53224; tel. 414/359-1040; FAX. 414/359-1074; Geneva B. Johnson, President, Chief Executive Officer

Federation of American Health Systems, 1111 19th Street, N.W., Suite 402, Washington, DC 20036; tel. 202/833-3090; FAX. 202/833-0063; Anne-Louise Oliphant, Assistant Vice President, Communications

Federation of State Medical Boards of the United States, Inc., 6000 Western Place, Suite 707, Fort Worth, TX 76107-4695; tel. 817/735-8445; FAX. 817/738-6629; James R. Winn, M.D., Executive Vice President

Financial Accounting Standards Board, 401 Merritt 7, P.O. Box 5116, Norwalk, CT 06856-5116; tel. 203/847-0700; FAX. 203/849-9714; Timothy S. Lucas, Director, Research, Technical Activities

Forum for Health Care Planning, 1101 Connecticut Avenue, N.W., Suite 700, Washington, DC 20036; tel. 202/857-1162; Cornelia Hinz, Executive Director

Foundation for Chiropractic Education and Research, 1701 Clarendon Boulevard, Arlington, VA 22209; tel. 703/276-7445; FAX. 703/276-8178; Stephen R. Seaten, CAE, Executive Director

Foundation for Osteopathic Health Services, 5301 Wisconsin Avenue, NW, Suite 630, Washington, DC 20015; tel. 202/686-1700; FAX. 202/686-7615; David Kushner, President

G

Gerontological Society of America, 1275 K Street, N.W., Suite 350, Washington, DC 20005-4006; tel. 202/842-1275; FAX. 202/842-1150; Carol A. Schultz, Executive Director

Great Plains Health Alliance, Inc., 625 Third Street, Box 366, Phillipsburg, KS 67661; tel. 913/543-2111; FAX. 913/543-5098; Roger S. John, President, Chief Executive Officer

Greater Flint Area Hospital Assembly, 702 South Ballenger Highway, Flint, MI 48532-3803; tel. 810/766-8898; FAX. 810/766-6422; Marlene Soderstrom, Executive Director

Group Health Association of America, Inc., 1129 20th Street, N.W., Suite 600, Washington, DC 20036; tel. 202/778-3200; FAX. 202/331-7487; Karen Ignagni, President, Chief Executive Officer

Guide Dog Users, Inc., 57 Grandview Avenue, Watertown, MA 02172; tel. 617/926-9198; Kim Charlson, Editor

H

HEAR Center, 301 East Del Mar Boulevard, Pasadena, CA 91101; tel. 818/796-2016; FAX. 818/796-2320; Josephine Wilson, Executive Director

Health Industry Distributors Association, 225 Reinekers Lane, Suite 650, Alexandria, VA 22314-2875; tel. 703/549-4432; FAX. 703/549-6495; Tom Deckert, Chairman

Health Industry Manufacturers Association, 1200 G Street, N.W., Suite 400, Washington, DC 20005; tel. 202/783-8700; FAX. 202/783-8750; Alan H. Magazine, President

Health Insurance Association of America, 1025 Connecticut Avenue, N.W., Suite 1200, Washington, DC 20036-3998; tel. 202/223-7780; FAX. 202/223-7897; Gloria Tibby, Administrative Assistant

Health and Education Resources, Inc., 4733 Bethesda Avenue, Suite 700, Bethesda, MD 20814; tel. 301/656-3178; FAX. 301/656-3179; Dallas Johnson, President

Healthcare Financial Management Association, Two Westbrook Corporate Center, Suite 700, Westchester, IL 60154; tel. 708/531-9600; FAX. 708/531-0032; Richard L. Clarke, F.H.F.M.A., President

Healthcare Information and Management Systems Society, 230 East Ohio Street, Suite 600, Chicago, IL 60611-3201; tel. 312/664-4467; FAX. 312/664-6143; John A. Page, Executive Director

Hispanic American Geriatrics Society, 1 Cutts Road, Durham, NH 03824-3102; tel. 603/868-5757; Eugene E. Tillock, Ed.D., President

Histochemical Society, Inc., 204 Woods Hole Road, P.O. Box 294, Woods Hole, MA 02543; tel. 508/457-7680; FAX. 508/548-9053

Hospital Research and Educational Trust, One North Franklin, Chicago, IL 60606; tel. 312/422-2624; FAX. 312/422-4568; Deborah Bohr, Vice President

Huntington's Disease Society of America, Inc., 140 West 22nd Street, 6th floor, New York, NY 10011-2420; tel. 212/242-1968; FAX. 212/243-2443; Stephen Bajardi, Executive Director

I

Institute for the Achievement of Human Potential, 8801 Stenton Avenue, Philadelphia, PA 19118; tel. 215/233-2050; FAX. 215/233-3940; Roselise H. Wilkinson, M.D., Medical Director

InterHealth, 2550 University Avenue West, St. Paul, MN 55114; tel. 612/646-5574; FAX. 612/646-2559; Benjamin Aune, President, Chief Executive Officer

International Association of Ocular Surgeons, 233 East Erie Street, Suite 710, Chicago, IL 60611; tel. 312/951-1400; FAX. 312/951-1410; Randall T. Bellows, M.D., Director

International Childbirth Education Association, Inc., P.O. Box 20048, Minneapolis, MN 55420-0048; tel. 612/854-8660; FAX. 612/854-8772; Doris Olson, Office Manager

International College of Surgeons/United States Section, 1516 North Lake Shore Drive, Chicago, IL 60610-1694; tel. 312/787-6274; FAX. 312/787-9289; Melissa Feinleib, Meeting and Convention Manager

International Council for Health, Physical Education, Recreation, Sport and Dance, 1900 Association Drive, Reston, VA 22091; tel. 703/476-3486; FAX. 703/476-9527; Dr. Dong Ja Yang, Secretary General

International Council on Social Welfare/U. S. Committee, 750 First Street, N.E., Washington, DC 20002; tel. 202/336-8274; FAX. 202/336-8311; Toshio Tatara, Chair

International Society for Clinical Laboratory Technology, 818 Olive Street, Suite 918, St. Louis, MO 63101; tel. 314/241-1445; FAX. 314/241-1449; Mark S. Birenbaum, Ph.D., Administrator

Intravenous Nurses Society, Inc., Two Brighton Street, Belmont, MA 02178; tel. 617/489-5205; FAX. 617/489-0656; Mary Larkin, Chief Executive Officer

J

John Milton Society for the Blind, 475 Riverside Drive, Suite 455, New York, NY 10115; tel. 212/870-3335; FAX. 212/870-3229; Richard R. Preston, Executive Director

Joint Commission on Accreditation of Healthcare Organizations, One Renaissance Boulevard, Oakbrook Terrace, IL 60181; tel. 708/916-5600; FAX. 708/916-5644; Dennis S. O'Leary, M.D., President

Juvenile Diabetes Foundation International, 432 Park Avenue, S., New York, NY 10016; tel. 212/889-7575; Gloria Pennington, Executive Director

L

Leukemia Society of America, Inc., 733 Third Avenue, New York, NY 10017; tel. 212/573-8484; FAX. 212/972-5776; Peter N. Cakridas, President, Chief Executive Officer

Lutheran Health Systems/Lutheran Hospitals and Homes Society of America, Western Health Network, Inc., Box 6200, 4310 17th Avenue, S.W., Fargo, ND 58106-6200; tel. 701/277-7629; FAX. 701/277-7636; Steven R. Orr, President, Chief Executive Officer

Organizations / National Organizations

M

March of Dimes Birth Defects Foundation, 1275 Mamaroneck Avenue, White Plains, NY 10605; tel. 914/428-7100; FAX. 914/428-8203; Jennifer L. Howse, Ph.D., President

Maternity Center Association, 48 East 92nd Street, New York, NY 10128; tel. 212/369-7300; FAX. 212/369-8747; Ruth Watson Lubic, C.N.M., Ed.D., General Director

Medic Alert Foundation International, 2323 Colorado Avenue, Turlock, CA 95381-1009; tel. 209/668-3333; FAX. 209/668-8752; Donald G. Nichols, Senior Vice President

Medical Group Management Association, 104 Inverness Terrace East, Englewood, CO 80112-5306; tel. 303/799-1111; FAX. 303/643-4427; Frederick J. Wenzel, Executive Director, Chief Executive Officer

Medical Library Association, Six North Michigan Avenue, Suite 300, Chicago, IL 60602; tel. 312/419-9094; FAX. 312/419-8950; Carla J. Funk, Executive Director

Medical Staff Recruitment Certification Program, 3150 Holcomb Road, Suite 205, Norcross, GA 30071; tel. 800/258-4081; FAX. 404/417-2176; Susan Woodbury, Vice President

Mended Hearts, Inc., 7272 Greenville Avenue, Dallas, TX 75231; tel. 214/706-1442; Darla Bonham, Executive Director

Minnesota Healthcare Conference, 2221 University Avenue, S.E., Suite 425, Minneapolis, MN 55414; tel. 612/331-5571; FAX. 612/331-1001; Peggy Westby, Manager

Muscular Dystrophy Association, 3300 East Sunrise Drive, Tucson, AZ 85718; tel. 602/529-2000; FAX. 602/529-5300; Robert Ross, Senior Vice President and Executive Director

N

NSF International, 3475 Plymouth Road, P.O. Box 130140, Ann Arbor, MI 48113-0140; tel. 313/769-8010, ext. 201; FAX. 313/769-0109; Nina I. McClelland, Ph.D., President, Chief Executive Officer

National Academy of Sciences, National Research Council/Commission on Life Sciences, 2101 Constitution Avenue, N.W., NAS 343, Washington, DC 20418; tel. 202/334-2500; FAX. 202/334-1639; Paul Gilman, Ph.D., Executive Director

National Accreditation Council for Agencies Serving the Blind and Visually Handicapped, 15 East 40th Street, Suite 1004, New York, NY 10016; tel. 212/683-5068; FAX. 212/683-4475; Ruth Westman, Executive Director

National Accrediting Agency for Clinical Laboratory Sciences, 8410 West Bryn Mawr, Suite 670, Chicago, IL 60631; tel. 312/714-8880; FAX. 312/714-8886; Olive M. Kimball, Executive Director

National Alliance for the Mentally Ill, 2101 Wilson Boulevard, Suite 302, Arlington, VA 22201; tel. 703/524-7600; FAX. 703/524-9094; Laurie Flynn, Executive Director

National Association Medical Staff Services, P.O. Box 23350, Knoxville, TN 37933-1350; tel. 615/531-3571; FAX. 615/531-9939; Margaret F. Nicholson, Executive Director

National Association for Home Care, 519 C Street, N.E., Stanton Park, Washington, DC 20002; tel. 202/547-7424; FAX. 202/547-3540; Val J. Halamandaris, President

National Association for Medical Equipment Services, 625 Slaters Lane, Suite 200, Alexandria, VA 22314-1171; tel. 703/836-6263; FAX. 703/836-6730; Steve Haracznak, Vice President, Professional Relations

National Association for Music Therapy, Inc., 8455 Colesville Road, Suite 930, Silver Spring, MD 20910; tel. 301/589-3300; FAX. 301/589-5175; Andrea Farbman, Ed.D., Executive Director

National Association for Practical Nurse Education and Service, Inc. (NAPNES), 1400 Spring Street, Suite 310, Silver Spring, MD 20910; tel. 301/588-2491; FAX. 301/588-2839; John H. Word, LPN, Executive Director

National Association of Boards of Pharmacy, 700 Busse Highway, Park Ridge, IL 60068; tel. 708/698-6227; FAX. 708/698-0124; Carmen A. Catizone, R.Ph., M.S.

National Association of Children's Hospitals and Related Institutions, Inc., 401 Wythe Street, Alexandria, VA 22314; tel. 703/684-1355; FAX. 703/684-1589; Lawrence A. McAndrews, President, Chief Executive Officer

National Association of Dental Assistants, 900 South Washington, Suite G13, Falls Church, VA 22046; tel. 703/237-8616; S. Young, Director

National Association of Dental Laboratories, (Includes National Board for Certification in Dental Laboratory Technology), 555 East Braddock Road, Alexandria, VA 22314-2106; tel. 703/683-5263; FAX. 703/549-4788; Robert W. Stanley, Executive Director

National Association of Health Services Executives, 8630 Fenton Street, Suite 328, Silver Spring, MD 20910; tel. 202/628-3953; FAX. 301/588-0011; Ozzie Jenkins, CMP, Association Director

National Association of Hospital Hospitality Houses, Inc., 4013 West Jackson Street, Muncie, IN 47304; tel. 800/542-9730; FAX. 317/287-0321; Josephine Lee, Chairperson

National Association of Institutional Laundry Managers, 781 Twin Oaks Avenue, Chula Vista, CA 92010; tel. 619/420-1396; FAX. 619/420-1396; Robert J. Conard, Executive Secretary

National Association of Psychiatric Health Systems, 1319 F Street, N.W., Suite 1000, Washington, DC 20004; tel. 202/393-6700; FAX. 202/783-6041; Robert L. Trachtenberg, Executive Director

National Association of Rehabilitation Facilities, 5530 Wisconsin Avenue, Suite 955, Washington, DC 20015; tel. 703/648-9300; James Allen Cox, Jr., Executive Director

National Association of Social Workers, Inc., 750 First Street, N.E., Suite 700, Washington, DC 20002; tel. 202/408-8600, ext. 233; FAX. 202/336-8311; James P. Brennan, LISW, ACSW, Senior Staff Associate, Health, Mental Health

National Association of State Mental Health Program Directors, 66 Canal Center Plaza, Suite 302, Alexandria, VA 22314; tel. 703/739-9333; FAX. 703/548-9517; Robert W. Glover, Ph.D., Executive Director

National Board for Respiratory Care, 8310 Nieman Road, Lenexa, KS 66214; tel. 913/599-4200; FAX. 913/541-0156; Steven K. Bryant, Executive Director

National Board of Medical Examiners, 3750 Market Street, Philadelphia, PA 19104; tel. 215/590-9500; FAX. 215/590-9755; L. Thompson Bowles, M.D., Ph.D., President

National Children's Eye Care Foundation, P.O. Box 795069, Dallas, TX 75379-5069; tel. 214/407-0404; FAX. 214/407-0616; Suzanne C. Beauchamp, Executive Director

National Commission on Certification of Physician Assistants, 2845 Henderson Mill Road, N.E., Atlanta, GA 30341; tel. 404/493-9100; FAX. 404/493-7316; David L. Glazer, Executive Vice President, Managing Director

National Council on Alcoholism and Drug Dependence, Inc., 12 West 21st Street, New York, NY 10010; tel. 212/206-6770, ext. 222; FAX. 212/645-1690

National Council on Radiation Protection and Measurements, 7910 Woodmont Avenue, Suite 800, Bethesda, MD 20814; tel. 301/657-2652; FAX. 301/907-8768; W. Roger Ney, J.D., Executive Director

National Council on the Aging, Inc., 409 Third Street, S.W., Suite 200, Washington, DC 20024; tel. 202/479-1200; FAX. 202/479-0735; James Firman, President

National Dental Association, 5506 Connecticut Avenue, N.W., Suite 24–25, Washington, DC 20015; tel. 202/244-7555; FAX. 202/244-5992; Robert S. Johns, Executive Director

National Depressive and Manic-Depressive Association, 730 North Franklin Street, Suite 501, Chicago, IL 60610; tel. 312/642-0049; FAX. 312/642-7243; Susan Dime-Meenan, Executive Director

National Easter Seal Society, 70 East Lake Street, Chicago, IL 60601; tel. 312/726-6200; FAX. 312/726-1494; James E. Williams, Jr., President

National Environmental Health Association, 720 South Colorado Boulevard, South Tower, Suite 970, Denver, CO 80222; tel. 303/756-9090; FAX. 303/691-9490; Nelson Fabian, Executive Director

National Executive Housekeepers Association, Inc., 1001 Eastwind Drive, Suite 301, Westerville, OH 43081-3361; tel. 614/895-7166; FAX. 614/895-1248; Beth Risinger, Chief Executive Officer, Executive Director

National Federation of Catholic Physicians' Guilds, 850 Elm Grove Road, Elm Grove, WI 53122; tel. 414/784-3435; FAX. 414/782-8788; Robert H. Herzog, Executive Director

National Federation of Licensed Practical Nurses, 1418 Aversboro Road, Garner, NC 27529; tel. 919/779-0046; FAX. 919/779-5642; Charlene Barbour, Executive Director

National Fire Protection Association, P.O. Box 9101, One Batterymarch Park, Quincy, MA 02269-9101; tel. 617/770-3000; FAX. 617/770-0700; Burton R. Klein, Health Care Fire Protection Engineer

National Gaucher Foundation, 19241 Montgomery Village Avenue, Suite E 21, Gaithersburg, MD 20879; tel. 301/990-3800; FAX. 301/990-4898; Karen Cohen, Executive Director

National Headache Foundation, 5252 North Western Avenue, Chicago, IL 60625; tel. 800/843-2256; FAX. 312/907-6278; Suzanne Simons, Director, Administration and Development

National Health Council, Inc., 1730 M Street, N.W., Suite 500, Washington, DC 20036; tel. 202/785-3910; FAX. 202/785-5923; Joseph C. Isaacs, President

National Health Lawyers Association, 1120 Connecticut Avenue, N.W., Suite 950, Washington, DC 20036; tel. 202/833-1100; FAX. 202/833-1105; Marilou M. King, Esq., Executive Vice President, Chief Executive Officer

National Hemophilia Foundation, 110 Greene Street, Manhattan, NY 10012; tel. 212/219-8180; Allan Brownstein, Executive Director

National Institute for Jewish Hospice, Central Telephone Network, 8723 Alden Drive, Suite 652, Los Angeles, CA 90048; tel. 213/467-7423; Levana Lev, Executive Director

National Kidney Foundation, 30 East 33rd Street, New York, NY 10016; tel. 800/622-9010; FAX. 212/689-9261; John Davis, Executive Director

National League for Nursing, 350 Hudson Street, New York, NY 10014; tel. 212/989-9393; FAX. 212/989-9256; Patricia Moccia, Ph.D., RN, FAAN, Chief Executive Officer

National Medical Association, 1012 10th Street, N.W., Washington, DC 20001; tel. 202/347-1895; FAX. 202/842-3293; Rosemary A. Davis, Executive Vice President, Administrative Affairs

National Mental Health Association, Inc., 1021 Prince Street, Alexandria, VA 22314-2971; tel. 703/684-7722; FAX. 703/684-5968; Michael M. Faenza, President, Chief Executive Officer

National Multiple Sclerosis Society, 733 Third Avenue, New York, NY 10017; tel. 212/986-3240; FAX. 212/986-7981; Dwayne Howell, Executive Vice President

National Nutrition Consortium, Inc., 24 Third Street, N.E., Suite 200, Washington, DC 20002; tel. 202/547-4819; Betty B. Blouin, Executive Director

National Osteopathic Women Physicians Association, 5301 Wisconsin Avenue, NW, Suite 630, Washington, DC 20015; tel. 202/686-1700; FAX. 202/537-1362; David Kushner, Executive Director

Organizations / National Organizations

National Parkinson Foundation, Inc., 1501 N.W. Ninth Avenue, Miami, FL 33136–1494; tel. 305/547–6666; FAX. 305/548–4403; Brian Morton, Controller

National Perinatal Association, 3500 East Fletcher Avenue, Suite 209, Tampa, FL 33613–4709; tel. 813/971–1008; FAX. 813/971–9306; Julie Leachman, Executive Director

National Pharmaceutical Association, 1288 Route 73, 456, Mt. Laurel, NJ 08540; tel. 609/722–0902; FAX. 609/866–1050; Jordan D. Johnson, Jr., Executive Vice President

National Recreation and Park Association, (Includes National Therapeutic Recreation Society), 2775 South Quincy Street, Suite 300, Arlington, VA 22206; tel. 703/820–4940; FAX. 703/671–6772; R. Dean Tice, Executive Director

National Registry in Clinical Chemistry, 1155 16th Street, N.W., Washington, DC 20036; tel. 202/745–1698; FAX. 202/872–4615; Gilbert E. Smith, Ph.D, Executive Director

National Registry of Emergency Medical Technicians, 6610 Busch Boulevard, P.O. Box 29233, Columbus, OH 43229; tel. 614/888–4484; William E. Brown, Jr., Executive Director

National Rehabilitation Association, (Includes Nine National Associations and Sixty Affiliate Chapters), 633 South Washington Street, Alexandria, VA 22314; tel. 703/836–0850; FAX. 703/836–0848; Ann Tourigny, Ph.D., CAE, Executive Director

National Renal Administrators Association, 1527 Wisconsin Avenue, N.W., Washington, DC 20007; tel. 202/342–2733; Gloria Smith Justice, Executive Director

National Resident Matching Program, 2450 N Street, N.W., Suite 201, Washington, DC 20037–1141; tel. 202/828–0676; FAX. 202/828–1121; Richard R. Randlett, Deputy Executive Director

National Rural Health Association, 1320 19th Street, N.W., Suite 350, Washington, DC 20036; tel. 202/232–6200; FAX. 202/232–1133; Millicent Gorham, Government Affairs Director

National Safety Council, 1121 Spring Lake Drive, Itasca, IL 60143–3201; tel. 708/285–1121; FAX. 708/285–0797

National Society for Medical Research, 1029 Vermont Avenue, N.W., Suite 700, Washington, DC 20005; tel. 202/347–9565

National Society for Patient Representation (AHA) and Consumer Affairs, One North Franklin, Chicago, IL 60606; tel. 312/422–3999; FAX. 312/422–4580; Alexandra B. Gekas, Director

National Spinal Cord Injury Association, 545 Concord Avenue, Suite 29, Cambridge, MA 02138; tel. 617/441–8500; FAX. 617/441–3449; Janna Jacobs, Executive Director

National Student Nurses' Association, Inc., 555 West 57th Street, Suite 1327, New York, NY 10019; tel. 212/581–2211; FAX. 212/581–2368; Robert V. Piemonte, Ed.D, RN, CAE, FAAN, Executive Director

National Tay–Sachs and Allied Diseases Association, 2001 Beacon Street, Brookline, MA 02146; tel. 617/277–4463; FAX. 617/277–0134; Debi Gutter, Executive Director

Neurosurgical Society of America, UCLA Division of Neurosurgery, 10833 Le Conte Avenue, Los Angeles, CA 90024; tel. 310/825–5111; FAX. 310/825–7245; Donald P. Becker, M.D., President

Neurotics Anonymous, 11140 Bainbridge Drive, Little Rock, AR 72212; tel. 501/221–2809; FAX. 501/221–2809; Grover Boydston, Chairman

New England Gerontological Association, 1 Cutts Road, Durham, NH 03824–3102; tel. 603/868–5757; Eugene F. Tillock, Ed.D., Executive Director

New England Healthcare Assembly, Inc., 125 Technology Drive, Durham, NH 03824–4724; tel. 603/862–1903; FAX. 603/862–0583; James S. Dolph, President

O

Osteogenesis Imperfecta Foundation, Inc., 5005 West Laurel Street, Suite 210, Tampa, FL 33607–3836; tel. 813/282–1161; FAX. 813/287–8214; Vonnie Coleman, Executive Director

Otosclerosis Study Group, 6465 Yale, Tulsa, OK 74136; Roger E. Wehrs, M.D., Secretary–Treasurer

P

Pan American Health Organization, 525 23rd Street, N.W., Washington, DC 20037; tel. 202/861–3200; Jose M. Paganini, Director HSS

Pathology Practice Association, 1225 8th Street, Suite 590, Sacramento, CA 95814; tel. 916/446–2651; J. Michael Allen, Executive Secretary

Physician Executive Management Center, 4014 Gunn Highway, Suite 160, Tampa, FL 33624–4787; tel. 813/963–1800; FAX. 813/264–2207; David R. Kirschman, President

Pilot Dogs, Inc., 625 West Town Street, Columbus, OH 43215; tel. 614/221–6367; FAX. 614/221–1577; J. Jay Gray, Executive Director

Prevent Blindness America, 500 East Remington Road, Schaumburg, IL 60173–4557; tel. 708/843–2020; FAX. 708/843–8458; Richard T. Hellner, Executive Director

Public Relations Society of America, 33 Irving Place, New York, NY 10003–2376; tel. 212/995–2230; FAX. 212/995–0757; Ray Gaulke, Chief Operating Officer

Puerto Rico Hospital Association, Villa Nevarez Professional Center, Suite 101, Rio Piedras, PR 00927; tel. 809/764–0290; FAX. 809/753–9748; Juan Rivera, Chief Executive Officer

R

RTS Bereavement Services, 1910 South Avenue, La Crosse, WI 54601; tel. 800/362–9567, ext. 4747; FAX. 608/791–5137; Fran Rybarik, Director

Radiological Society of North America, Inc., 2021 Spring Road, Suite 600, Oak Brook, IL 60521; tel. 708/571–2670; FAX. 708/571–7837; Delmar J. Stauffer, Executive Director

Recording for the Blind, Inc., 20 Roszel Road, Princeton, NJ 08540; tel. 609/452–0606; FAX. 609/520–7990; Ritchie L. Geisel, President, Chief Executive Officer

Renal Physicians Association, 2011 Pennsylvania Avenue, N.W., Suite 800, Washington, DC 20006–1808; tel. 202/835–0436; FAX. 202/835–0443; Carol Cooper Chadsey, Executive Director

Robert Wood Johnson Foundation, P.O. Box 2316, Route One and College Road East, Princeton, NJ 08543–2316; tel. 609/452–8701; FAX. 609/987–8845; Edward Robbins, Proposal Manager

Rochester Regional Hospital Association, 3445 Winton Place, Rochester, NY 14623; tel. 716/273–8180; FAX. 716/273–8189; Seth M. Gordon, President

S

Seeing Eye, Inc., Box 375, Morristown, NJ 07963–0375; tel. 201/539–4425; FAX. 201/539–0922; Dennis J. Murphy, President, David Loux, Director, Admissions

Shriners Hospitals for Crippled Children, P.O. Box 31356, Tampa, FL 33631–3356; tel. 813/281–0300, ext. 8163; FAX. 813/281–8113; Jack D. Hoard, Executive Administrator

Sickle Cell Disease Foundation of Greater New York, 127 West 127th Street, Suite 421, New York, NY 10027; tel. 212/865–1500; Dick Campbell, Executive Director

Society for Academic Emergency Medicine, 901 North Washington Avenue, Lansing, MI 48906; tel. 517/485–5484; FAX. 517/485–0801; Mary Ann Schropp, Executive Director

Society for Adolescent Medicine, Inc., 19401 East 40 Highway, Suite 120, Independence, MO 64055; tel. 816/795–8336; Edie Moore, Administrative Director

Society for Healthcare Planning and Marketing (AHA), 840 North Lake Shore Drive, Chicago, IL 60611–2431; tel. 312/280–6086; FAX. 312/280–6252; Peter M. Columbus, Associate Director

Society for Social Work Administrators in Health Care, One North Franklin, Chicago, IL 60606–3401; tel. 312/422–3771; FAX. 312/422–4580; Richard Koepke, Executive Director

Society of Critical Care Medicine, 8101 East Kaiser Boulevard, Anaheim, CA 92808–2214; tel. 714/282–6000; FAX. 714/282–6050; Norma J. Shoemaker, M.N., Executive Director

Society of Neurological Surgeons, New England Medical Center, Department of Neurosurgery, 750 Washington Street, P.O. Box 178, Boston, MA 02111; tel. 617/636–5858; William Shucart, M.D., Secretary

Society of Nuclear Medicine, 1850 Samuel Morse Drive, Reston, VA 22090; tel. 703/708–9000; FAX. 703/708–9015; Torry Mark Sansone, Executive Director

Society of University Otolaryngologists–Head and Neck Surgeons, Joint Center for Otolaryngology, Harvard Medical School, 333 Longwood Avenue, Boston, MA 02115; tel. 617/732–7003; FAX. 617/217–1372; Marvin Fried, M.D., Secretary–Treasurer

Southeastern Healthcare Association, 1345 Carmichael Way, P.O. Box 11126, Montgomery, AL 36111–0126; tel. 800/246–8762; FAX. 205/260–0023; Tommy R. McDougal, FACHE, President

Southeastern Surgical Congress, 1776 Peachtree Road, N.W., Suite 410N, Atlanta, GA 30309; tel. 404/607–8958; FAX. 404/607–8972; R. Phillip Burns, M.D., Secretary–Director

T

Technologist Section, Society of Nuclear Medicine, 1850 Samuel Morse Drive, Reston, VA 22090; tel. 703/708–9000, ext. 241; FAX. 703/708–9015; Virginia M. Pappas, Administrator

The American Association of Immunologists, 9650 Rockville Pike, Bethesda, MD 20814; tel. 301/530–7178; FAX. 301/571–1816; Raymond A. Palmer, Executive Director

The American Board of Plastic Surgery, Inc., Seven Penn Center, Suite 400, 1635 Market Street, Philadelphia, PA 19103–2204; tel. 215/587–9322; Kathleen H. Lemly, Gwen A. Hanuscin, Administrative Assistants

Organizations / National Organizations

The American Board of Professional Disability Consultants, 1350 Beverly Road, Suite 115–327, McLean, VA 22101; tel. 703/790–8644; Taras J. Cerkevitch, Ph.D., Director, Operations

The American Lupus Society, 260 Maple Court, Suite 123, Ventura, CA 93003; tel. 805/339–0443; Charlean Wakefield, Administrator

The American Orthopaedic Association, 6300 North River Road, Suite 300, Rosemont, IL 60018–4263; tel. 708/318–7330; FAX. 708/318–7339; Hildegard A. Weiler, Executive Director

The Arc, Formerly Association for Retarded Citizens, 500 East Border Street, Suite 300, Arlington, TX 76011; tel. 817/640–0204; FAX. 817/633–6459; Al Abeson, Ed.D., Executive Director

The Association for Research in Vision and Ophthalmology, 9650 Rockville Pike, Suite 1500, Bethesda, MD 20814–3998; tel. 301/571–1844; FAX. 301/571–8311; Ann M. Diven, Conference Manager

The Association of Medical Illustrators, 1819 Peachtree Street, N.E., Suite 712, Atlanta, GA 30309; tel. 404/350–7900; FAX. 404/351–3348; William H. Just, Executive Director

The Association of Women's Health, Obstetric, and Neonatal Nurses, 700 14th Street, N.W., Suite 600, Washington, DC 20005–2019; tel. 202/662–1600, ext. 1608; FAX. 202/737–0575; Gail G. Kincaid, Executive Director

The Duke Endowment, 100 North Tryon Street, Suite 3500, Charlotte, NC 28202; tel. 704/376–0291; FAX. 704/376–9336; Jere W. Witherspoon, Executive Director

The Endocrine Society, 4350 East West Highway, Suite 500, Bethesda, MD 20814–4410; tel. 301/941–0200; FAX. 301/941–0259; Sean Tipton, Director, Public Affairs

The Foundation Fighting Blindness, 1401 Mount Royal Avenue, Fourth floor, Baltimore, MD 21217–4245; tel. 800/683–5555; FAX. 410/225–3936; Robert M. Gray, Executive Director

The Foundation for Ichthyosis & Related Skin Types, Inc., (F.I.R.S.T.), P.O. Box 20921, Raleigh, NC 27619–0921; tel. 919/782–5728; FAX. 919/781–0679; Nicholas Gattuccio, Executive Director

The Healthcare Forum, 425 Market Street, 16th Floor, San Francisco, CA 94105; tel. 415/356–4300; FAX. 415/356–9300; Kathryn E. Johnson, President, Chief Executive Officer

The Institute for Rehabilitation and Research, Administration, 1333 Moursund, Houston, TX 77030; tel. 713/799–5000; FAX. 713/799–7095; Louisa Adelung, Executive Vice President

The National Association of Children's Hospitals and Related Institutions, Inc., 401 Wythe Street, Alexandria, VA 22314; tel. 703/684–1355; FAX. 703/684–1589; Robert H. Sweeney, President

The Orton Dyslexia Society, Chester Building, Suite 382, 8600 LaSalle Road, Baltimore, MD 21286; tel. 410/296–0232; FAX. 410/321–5069; Dr. Steve Laubacher, Executive Director

The Points of Light Foundation, 1737 H Street, N.W., Washington, DC 20006; tel. 202/223–9186, ext. 146; FAX. 202/223–9256; Catherine Q. Soffin, Manager, Information Services

The Salvation Army National Corporation, 615 Slaters Lane, P.O. Box 269, Alexandria, VA 22313; tel. 703/684–5500; FAX. 703/684–3478; Commissioner James Osborne, National Commander

The Southwestern Surgical Congress, 401 North Michigan Avenue, Chicago, IL 60611–4267; tel. 312/527–6667; FAX. 312/321–6869; James A. Edney, M.D., Secretary–Treasurer

U

United Cerebral Palsy Associations, Inc., 1660 L Street, N.W., 7th Floor, Washington, DC 20005; tel. 800/872–5827; John D. Kemp, Executive Director

United Methodist Association of Health and Welfare Ministries, 601 West Riverview Avenue, Dayton, OH 45406–5543; tel. 513/227–9494; FAX. 513/227–9493; Dean W. Pulliam, President, Chief Executive Officer

United Ostomy Association, Inc., 36 Executive Park, Suite 120, Irvine, CA 92714; tel. 800/826–0826; FAX. 714/660–9262; Darlene A. Smith, Executive Director

United Parkinson Foundation, 220 South State Street, Suite 1806–08, Chicago, IL 60604; tel. 312/922–9734; Judy Rosner, Executive Director

United States Pharmacopeial Convention, Inc., 12601 Twinbrook Parkway, Rockville, MD 20852; tel. 301/881–0666; FAX. 301/816–8299; Jerome A. Halperin, Executive Director

United Way of America, 701 North Fairfax Street, Alexandria, VA 22314–2045; tel. 703/836–7100; FAX. 703/683–7840; William Aramony, President

W

W. K. Kellogg Foundation, One Michigan Avenue East, Battle Creek, MI 49017–4058; tel. 616/968–1611; FAX. 616/968–0413; Robert A. DeVries, Program Director

Western Orthopaedic Association, 2975 Treat Boulevard, Building D–4, Concord, CA 94518; tel. 510/671–2164; FAX. 510/671–2012; H. Jacqueline Martin, Executive Director

Western Surgical Association, Mayo Clinic, 200 First Street, S.W., Rochester, MN 55905; Jon A. VanHeerden, M.D., Secretary

Healthfinder

The Healthfinder is composed of two listing types: toll-free numbers for health information and federal health information centers and clearinghouses. Toll-free numbers are denoted with the letter T and federal numbers are denoted with the letter F. Toll-free numbers are listed first, followed by the federal numbers.

This file was released in March 1995. This document is revised annually.

This Federal document is in the public domain, but is distributed subject to two conditions: 1) Any person or organization posting and/or distributing this document in electronic or paper form MUST respect the integrity of the document and post or distribute it ONLY in its entirety, including this paragraph, and without any change whatsoever; and 2) Any person or organization either posting or distributing this document MUST agree to post and/or distribute future editions of the document in the same manner as this edition to ensure that the most current information is made available to those parties who received the earlier version.

TOLL-FREE NUMBERS FOR HEALTH INFORMATION

This Healthfinder lists selected toll-free numbers and describes organizations that provide health-related information. The numbers do not diagnose or recommend treatment for any disease. Some offer recorded information; others provide personalized counseling, referrals, and/or written materials. Unless otherwise stated, numbers can be reached within the continental United States Monday through Friday, and hours of operation are eastern time. Numbers that operate 24 hours a day can be reached 7 days a week unless otherwise noted.

This Healthfinder is one in a series of publications, on a variety of topics, prepared by the National Health Information Center (NHIC). NHIC is a service of the Office of Disease Prevention and Health Promotion, Public Health Service, U.S. Department of Health and Human Services. The information contained on the following pages in no way should be construed as an endorsement, real or implied, by the U.S. Department of Health and Human Services.

ADOPTION

Bethany Christian Services (T-1)
(800)238-4269
Services for women considering adoption as an option. Free counseling. Housing is available. 8 a.m.-1 a.m., every day. (See also F-24)

National Adoption Center (T-2)
(800)TO-ADOPT
(215)735-9988
Expands adoption opportunities throughout the United States, particularly for children with special needs. Links all State adoption agencies through a telecommunication network. Addresses adoption and child welfare issues. 9 a.m.-5 p.m.

AGING

National Institute on Aging Information Center (T-3)
(800)222-2225
(800)222-4225 (TTY)
(301)589-3014 (Fax)
Provides information and publications on health topics of interest to older adults, to the public, and to doctors, nurses, social activities directors, and health educators. 8:30 a.m.-5 p.m. (See also T-16, T-17, T-18, T-81, F-1)

AIDS/HIV

See SEXUALLY TRANSMITTED DISEASES

AIDS Clinical Trials Information Service (T-4)
(800)874-2572
(800)243-7012 (TDD)
Sponsored by the Centers for Disease Control and Prevention, the Food and Drug Administration, the National Institute of Allergy and Infectious Diseases, and the National Library of Medicine. Provides current information on federally and privately sponsored clinical trials for AIDS patients and others with HIV infection and on the drugs used in those trials. All calls are confidential. Spanish-speaking operators available. 9 a.m.-7 p.m.

CDC National AIDS Clearinghouse (T-5)
(800)458-5231
(800)243-7012 (TDD)
(301)738-6616 (Fax)
Sponsored by the Centers for Disease Control and Prevention. Collects, classifies, and distributes up-to-date information and educational materials; provides expert assistance to HIV and AIDS prevention professionals. Makes referrals nationally to AIDS organizations for publications and HIV/AIDS-related services. Provides information and publications in English and Spanish. 9 a.m.-7 p.m. (See also F-3)

CDC National AIDS Hotline (T-6)
(800)342-2437
(800)344-7432 (Spanish)
(800)243-7889 (TDD)
Sponsored by the Centers for Disease Control and Prevention. Provides information to the public on the prevention and spread of HIV/AIDS. The first toll-free number provides 24-hour service; the second number provides service in Spanish 8 a.m.-2 a.m., everyday except holidays. The third toll-free number is available 10 a.m.-10 p.m., Monday-Friday.

National Indian AIDS Hotline (T-7)
(800)283-2437
Sponsored by the National Native American AIDS Prevention Center. Provides printed materials and information about AIDS and AIDS prevention in the Indian community. 8:30 a.m.-12 p.m. and 1 p.m.-5 p.m. (Pacific). Leave recorded message after hours.

Project Inform HIV/AIDS Treatment Hotline (T-8)
(800)822-7422
(415)558-9051
Provides treatment information and referral for HIV-infected individuals. Information on clinical trials. No diagnosis. 10 a.m.-4 p.m., Monday-Saturday (Pacific).

ALCOHOL ABUSE

See also DRUG ABUSE

ADCARE Hospital Helpline (T-9)
(800)ALCOHOL
Provides information and referral for alcohol and other drug concerns. Operates 24 hours.

Al-Anon Family Group Headquarters (T-10)
(800)356-9996
Al-Anon and Alateen provide help for families and friends of alcoholics. The headquarters provides literature and refers people who need assistance to local meetings. 9 a.m.-4:30 p.m.

Alcohol and Drug Helpline (T-11)
(800)821-4357
(801)272-4357
Sponsored by Pioneer Health Care. Provides referrals to local facilities where adolescents and adults can seek help. Operates 24 hours.

American Council on Alcoholism (T-12)
(800)527-5344
Offers treatment referrals, counseling, and advice for recovering alcoholics and provides information on alcohol-related topics. 9 a.m.-5 p.m.

CSAP's National Clearinghouse for Alcohol and Drug Information (T-13)
(800)729-6686
(800)487-4889 (TTY/TDD)
(301)230-2867 (TTY/TDD)
(301)468-2600
Sponsored by the Center for Substance Abuse Prevention, Substance Abuse and Mental Health Services Administration. Provides Federal publications, especially those oriented to prevention and education, to the public. Also provides literature searches. 8 a.m.-7 p.m. (See also F-4)

CSAT's National Drug Information Treatment and Referral Hotline (T-14)
(800)662-HELP (English)
(800)66-AYUDA (Spanish)
(800)228-0427 (TDD)
Sponsored by the Center for Substance Abuse Treatment, Substance Abuse and Mental Health Services Administration. Provides information on alcohol/drug abuse and on HIV/AIDS as it relates to substance abuse. Offers referrals to alcohol/drug treatment programs and to self-help groups. The hotline is a confidential service available to all 50 States and U.S. Territories. 9 a.m.-3 a.m., Monday-Friday; 12 p.m.-3 a.m., Saturday-Sunday.

National Council on Alcoholism and Drug Dependence, Inc. (T-15)
(800)622-2255
(212)206-6770
(212)645-1690 (Fax)
Refers to local affiliates for counseling and provides written information on alcoholism and drug dependence. The toll-free number operates 24 hours; the other number is staffed 9 a.m.-5 p.m.

ALLERGY/ASTHMA

See LUNG DISEASE/ASTHMA/ALLERGY

ALZHEIMER'S DISEASE

See also AGING

Alzheimer's Association (T-16)
(800)272-3900
Refers to local chapters and support groups. Offers information on publications available from the association. 9 a.m.-5 p.m. (Central).

Alzheimer's Disease Education and Referral Center (T-17)
(800)438-4380
(301)495-3334
Sponsored by the National Institute on Aging. Provides information and publications on Alzheimer's disease. 8:30 a.m.-5 p.m.

Organizations / Healthfinder

ARTHRITIS

Arthritis Foundation Information Line (T-18)
(800)283-7800
Provides information about arthritis and referrals to local chapters. 24 hours. (See also F-7)

AUDIOVISUALS

See LIBRARY SERVICES

BONE MARROW

See CANCER

CANCER

American Cancer Society Response Line (T-19)
(800)227-2345
(301)929-8243
Provides publications and information about cancer and coping with cancer. Refers callers to local chapters for support ser ices. 8:30 a.m.–5 p.m. (See also F-10)

Cancer Information Service (T-20)
(800)4-CANCER
(800)422-6237
Sponsored by the National Cancer Institute. Answers cancer-related questions from the public, cancer patients and families, and health professionals. Spanish-speaking operators available. 9 a.m.–7 p.m.

National Marrow Donor Program (T-21)
(800)MARROW-2
Sponsored by the National Heart, Lung, and Blood Institute and the Department of the Navy. Provides multilingual information on donating marrow and the transplant process. Also provides information on donor centers in the caller's area. Professional staff answer questions from 8 a.m.–6 p.m. (Central); recorded message at all other times. (See also T-117)

Y-Me National Organization for Breast Cancer Information Support Program (T-22)
(800)221-2141
(312)986-8228
Provides breast cancer patients with presurgery counseling, treatment information, peer support, self-help counseling, and patient literature. Also provides information to any and all women concerned about breast health and breast cancer. Y-ME has a matching caller program for men whose partners have been diagnosed with breast cancer. 9 a.m.–5 p.m. (Central). Local number operates 24 hours.

CEREBRAL PALSY

See RARE DISORDERS

CHEMICAL PRODUCTS/PESTICIDES

See also HOUSING

Chemtrec Non-Emergency Services Hotline (T-23)
(800)262-8200
Provides nonemergency referrals to companies that manufacture chemicals and to Federal and State agencies for health and safety information and information regarding chemical regulations. 9 a.m.–6 p.m.

National Pesticide Telecommunications Network (T-24)
(800)858-7378
Sponsored by the U.S. Environmental Protection Agency and Texas Tech University. Responds to nonemergency questions about the effects of pesticides, toxicology and symptoms, environmental effects, disposal and cleanup, and safe use of pesticides. Also responds to emergency questions from homeowners, medical professionals, and veterinarians. TDD capability. 8 a.m.–6 p.m. (Central). (See also F-23)

CHILD ABUSE/MISSING CHILDREN

Boys Town National Hotline (T-25)
(800)448-3000
(800)448-1833 (TDD)
Provides short-term intervention and counseling and refers callers to local community resources. Counsels on parent-child conflicts, family issues, suicide, pregnancy, runaway youth, physical and sexual abuse, and other issues that impact children and families. Spanish-speaking operators are available. TDD capability. Operates 24 hours.

Child Find of America, Inc. (T-26)
(800)426-5678 (I AM LOST)
Searches for missing children under age 18 who are victims of parental abduction, stranger abduction, or who have run away. Provides safety prevention information. Operates 24 hours.

(800)292 9688 (A WAY OUT)
Provides unique crisis mediation program for parents contemplating abduction of their children, or who have already abducted their children and want to use Child Find Volunteer Family Mediators to resolve their custody dispute. Operates 24 hours.

CHILDHELP/IOF Foresters National Child Abuse Hotline (T-27)
(800)4-A-CHILD
(800)2-A-CHILD (TDD)
Provides multilingual crisis intervention and professional counseling on child abuse. Gives referrals to local social service groups offering counseling on child abuse. Provides literature on child abuse in English and Spanish. Operates 24 hours.

Covenant House Nineline (T-28)
(800)999-9999
(800)999-9915 (TDD)
Crisis line for youth, teens, and families. Locally based referrals throughout the United States. Help for youth and parents regarding drugs, abuse, homelessness, runaway children, and message relays. Operates 24 hours.

National Child Safety Council Childwatch (T-29)
(800)222-1464
Answers questions and distributes literature on safety, including drug abuse, household dangers, and electricity. Provides safety information to local police departments. Sponsor of the missing kids milk carton program. Operates 24 hours.

National Clearinghouse on Child Abuse and Neglect Information (T-30)
(800)394-3366
(703)385-7565
(703)385-3206 (Fax)
Serves as a national resource for the acquisition and dissemination of child abuse and neglect materials and distributes a free publications catalog upon request. Maintains bibliographic databases of documents, audiovisuals, and national organizations. Services include searches of databases and annotated bibliographies on frequently requested topics. CD-ROM containing Clearinghouse databases is available free to qualified institutions. Spanish-speaking operators available. 8:30 a.m.–5 p.m. (See also F-11, F-12)

National Hotline for Missing Children (T-31)
(800)843-5678
(703)235-3900
(703)235-4067 (Fax)
Sponsored by the National Center for Missing and Exploited Children. Operates a hotline for reporting missing children and sightings of missing children. Offers assistance to law enforcement agents. 7:30 a.m.–11 p.m.

National Resource Center on Child Abuse and Neglect (T-32)
(800)227-5242
Sponsored by the American Humane Association. Provides general information and statistics about child abuse. 8:30 a.m.–4:30 p.m.

National Runaway Switchboard (T-33)
(800)621-4000
(800)621-0394 (TDD)
(312)929-5150 (Fax)
Provides crisis intervention and travel assistance to runaways. Gives referrals to shelters nationwide. Also relays messages to, or sets up conference calls with, parents at the request of the child. Has access to AT&T-Language Line. Operates 24 hours.

National Youth Crisis Hotline (T-34)
(800)448-4663
Provides counseling and referrals to local drug treatment centers, shelters, and counseling services. Responds to youth dealing with pregnancy, molestation, suicide, and child abuse. Operates 24 hours.

Runaway Hotline (T-35)
(800)231-6946
Provides information and referral for shelter, counseling, medical and legal services, and transportation back home. Operates a personal, confidential message relay service between runaways and their families. Operates 24 hours.

CHILD DEVELOPMENT

Human Growth Foundation (T-36)
(800)451-6434
(703)883-1773
Provides parent education and mutual support, funds research, and promotes public awareness of the physical and emotional problems of short-statured people. Offers brochures on child growth abnormalities. 8:30 a.m.–5 p.m.

CHILD EDUCATION

National Association for the Education of Young Children (T-37)
(800)424-2460
(202)232-8777
(202)328-1846 (Fax)
The National Association for the Education of Young Children is neither a help-line nor hotline. The association publishes books, posters, and brochures for teachers and parents of young children, birth through age 8. Sponsors conferences and public awareness activities concerning quality programs for the education of young children. 9 a.m.–5 p.m.

CLEFT PALATE

See RARE DISORDERS

CYSTIC FIBROSIS

See RARE DISORDERS

DIABETES/DIGESTIVE DISEASES

American Diabetes Association (T-38)
(800)232-3472, (800)DIABETES
(703)549-1500
(703)549-6995 (Fax, Customer Service)
(703)519-5674 (Fax, Order Fulfillment)
Offers patient assistance in many areas, including general information about diabetes, nutrition, exercise, treatment, and referrals to diabetes medical professionals. For people with diabetes facing discrimination, the association offers referrals from a nationwide attorney s network and information on how to influence public leaders. The association also conducts a variety of patient activities, including educational seminars and workshops, culturally diverse programs, support groups, and youth programs. Spanish-speaking operators available. 8:30 a.m.–5 p.m. (See also F-16)

Crohn's and Colitis Foundation of America, Inc. (T-39)
(800)932-2423
(800)343-3637 (Warehouse)
Provides educational materials on Crohn's disease and ulcerative colitis. Refers to local support groups and physicians. 9 a.m.–5 p.m. Recording after hours. Warehouse is open 8 a.m.–5 p.m.

Organizations / Healthfinder

Juvenile Diabetes Foundation International Hotline (T–40)
(800)223–1138
(212)889–7575
Answers questions and provides brochures on diabetes. Refers to local chapters, physicians, and clinics. Chapters located worldwide. 9 a.m.–5 p.m.

DISABLING CONDITIONS

See also HEARING AND SPEECH

Handicapped Media, Inc. (T–41)
(800)321–8708 (Voice/TDD)
Provides information, referral on services, and advocacy. Operates 8 a.m.–5 p.m. (Mountain).

Heath Resource Center (T–42)
(800)544–3284
(202)939–9320
Operates the national clearinghouse on postsecondary education for individuals with disabilities and on learning disabilities. 9 a.m.–5 p.m.

Job Accommodation Network (T–43)
(800)ADA–Work (Voice/TDD)
(800)526–7234 (Voice/TDD)
(800)526–2262 (in Canada)
(800)DIAL–JAN (Electronic Bulletin Board)
(304)293–5407 (Fax)
Sponsored by the President's Commission on the Employment of People with Disabilities. Offers ideas for accommodating disabled persons in the workplace and information on the availability of accommodation aids and procedures. Services available in English, Spanish, and French. 8 a.m.–8 p.m., Monday–Thursday; 8 a.m.–5 p.m., Friday.

Medical Rehabilitation Education Foundation (T–44)
(800)GET–REHAB
Provides medical rehabilitation information and a referral service for help in locating rehabilitation facilities throughout the country. 8 a.m.–6 p.m.

National Center for Youth with Disabilities Adolescent Health Program (T–45)
University of Minnesota
(800)333–6293
(612)626–2825
(612)626–2134 (Fax)
(612)624–3939 (TDD)
NCYD is an information, policy, and resource center focusing on adolescents with chronic illnesses and disabilities and the issues surrounding their transition to adult life. Offers a number of publications, including a newsletter, Connections, and a series of annotated bibliographies, CYDLINE Reviews. Maintains the National Resource Library, a database containing abstracts of current research literature, information about model programs, training/educational materials, and a list of consultants. 8 a.m.–4:30 p.m. (Central). (See also F–18, F–19)

National Clearinghouse on Family Support and Children's Mental Health (T–46)
(800)628–1696
(503)725–4040
(503)725–4165 (Fax)
(503)725–4180 (TDD)
Sponsored by the National Institute on Disability and Rehabilitation Research, U.S. Department of Education, and the Center for Mental Health Services, U.S. Department of Health and Human Services. Provides publications on parent/family support groups, financing, early intervention, various mental disorders, and other topics concerning children's mental health. Also offers a computerized databank and a state-by-state resource file. Recording is operated 24 hours.

National Easter Seal Society (T–47)
(800)221–6827
(312)726–6200
(312)726–1494 (Fax)
(312)726–4258 (TDD)
Through its 160 affiliates nationwide, provides rehabilitative and other support services to assist children and adults with disabilities to achieve their maximum independence. 8:30 a.m.–5 p.m. (Central).

National Information Center for Children and Youth with Disabilities (T–48)
(800)695–0285 (Voice/TT)
(202)884–8200 (Voice/TT)
(202)884–8441 (Fax)
nichcy@capcon.net (Internet)
Sponsored by the U.S. Department of Education. Information and referral service dedicated to disabled children. 8:30 a.m.–5 p.m. or leave recorded message after hours.

National Information Clearinghouse for Infants with Disabilities and Life–Threatening Conditions (T–49)
(800)922–9234, ext. 201
Sponsored by the National Clearinghouse on Child Abuse and Neglect Information, Administration on Children and Families, U.S. Department of Health and Human Services. Makes referrals to support groups and sources of financial, medical, and educational assistance for families having infants with disabilities (birth to age 3). Spanish–speaking operators available. 9 a.m.–5 p.m.

National Information System for Vietnam Veterans and their Families (T–50)
(800)922–9234, ext. 401 (Voice/TDD)
Provides information and referrals for Vietnam veterans having children with disabilities or special health care needs. Produces and disseminates fact sheets on health conditions common to Vietnam veterans' children and on advocacy topics. 9 a.m.–5 p.m.

National Rehabilitation Information Center (NARIC) (T–51)
(800)346–2742 (Voice/TDD)
(301)588–9284 (Voice/TDD)
(301)587–1967 (Fax)
Sponsored by the National Institute on Disability and Rehabilitation Research. Collects and disseminates the results of federally funded research projects. The collection includes commercially published books, journal articles, and audiovisuals. Spanish–speaking operators available. 8 a.m.–6 p.m. (See also T–49)

DOWN SYNDROME

See RARE DISORDERS

DRINKING WATER SAFETY

Safe Drinking Water Hotline (T–52)
(800)426–4791
Sponsored by the U.S. Environmental Protection Agency. Provides general and technical information on the Federal drinking water program and referrals to other organizations when appropriate. Does not provide site–specific information on local water quality, bottled water, or home water treatment units. 9 a.m.–5:30 p.m., weekdays, except Federal holidays.

DRUG ABUSE

See also ALCOHOL ABUSE

CSAP Drug–Free Workplace Helpline (T–53)
(800)843–4971
Sponsored by the Center for Substance Abuse Prevention, Substance Abuse and Mental Health Services Administration. Offers information, publications, and referrals to corporations, businesses, industry, and national organizations on assessing drug abuse within an organization and developing and implementing drug abuse policy and programs. 9 a.m.–7 p.m.

Housing and Urban Development Drug Information and Strategy Clearinghouse (T–54)
(800)578–3472
Promotes strategies for eradicating drugs and drug trafficking from public housing. Provides housing officials, residents, and community leaders a source for information and assistance on drug abuse prevention and trafficking control techniques. Maintains a database system consisting of national and community program descriptions, publications, research, and news articles. Provides resource lists. 8 a.m.–5 p.m. (See also F–21)

"Just Say No" International (T–55)
(800)258–2766
(510)451–6666
Thirteen thousand clubs. Founded in 1985. Provides materials, technical assistance, and training to help children and teenagers lead healthy, productive, drug–free lives. The New Youth Power program builds on young people's resiliency, drawing on and encouraging the skills and attributes that allow young people to cope with challenges and adversity. Youth Power empowers youth to discover and hone their assets to succeed in all areas of their lives. 7 a.m.–5 p.m. (Pacific).

National Cocaine Hotline (T–56)
(800)262–2463
Sponsored by the Phoenix House Foundation. Answers questions on cocaine, alcohol, and other drugs from users, their friends, and families. Provides referrals to drug rehabilitation centers. Operates 24 hours.

Target Resource Center (T–57)
(800)366–6667
(816)464–5400
Sponsored by the National Federation of State High School Associations. Provides education and prevention materials on tobacco, alcohol, and other drugs, including steroids and other performance–enhancing drugs, and on other healthy life–style issues surrounding high school athletics and activities. 8 a.m.–4:30 p.m. (Central).

DYSLEXIA

See LEARNING DISORDERS

ENDOMETRIOSIS

See WOMEN

ENVIRONMENT

Indoor Air Quality Information Clearinghouse (T–58)
(800)438–4318
Provides information on indoor air quality, including the health effects of passive smoke, formaldehyde, and various indoor air pollutants. 9 a.m.–5 p.m. (See also F–23, F–35)

EPILEPSY

See RARE DISORDERS

ETHICS

Joseph and Rose Kennedy Institute of Ethics National Reference Center for Bioethics Literature Georgetown University (T–59)
(800)633–3849
(202)687–3885
(202)687–6770 (Fax)
Provides reference assistance and conducts free searches on bioethical topics. 9 a.m.–5 p.m., Monday, Wednesday, Thursday, Friday; 9 a.m.–9 p.m., Tuesday; 10 a.m.–3 p.m., Saturday, except summers and holidays.

FIRE PREVENTION

National Fire Protection Association (T–60)
(800)344–3555 (Customer Service)
(617)770–3000
(617)984–7880 (TDD)
Develops fire protection codes and standards and provides technical information on fire prevention, firefighting procedures, and the fire loss experience. 8:30 a.m.–5 p.m.

FITNESS

Aerobics and Fitness Foundation of America (T–61)
(800)446–2322 (for Professionals)
(800)YOUR–BODY (for Consumers)
Answers questions regarding safe and effective exercise programs and practices. Written health and fitness guidelines also available (shipping and handling charges may apply). 7:30 a.m.–5:30 p.m. (Pacific).

YMCA of the USA (T–62)
(800)872–9622
Provides information about YMCA services and locations of Ys in, residential areas. 8 a.m.–5 p.m. (Central).

Organizations / Healthfinder

FOOD SAFETY

Food Labeling Hotline Meat and Poultry Hotline (T–63)
(800)535–4555
Sponsored by the U.S. Department of Agriculture. Provides information on safe handling, preparation, and storage of meat, poultry, and eggs. Also provides tips on buying a turkey, holiday food safety, and understanding labels on meat and poultry. 10 a.m.–4 p.m. (See also F–26)

Seafood Hotline (T–64)
(800)FDA–4010
(202)205–4314
Sponsored by the Food and Drug Administration. Provides information on seafood buying, handling, and storage for home consumption and labeling. Also provides seafood publications and prerecorded seafood safety messages. Items and information not related to seafood are available also. To receive publications on food labeling and nutrition, callers can press "1" if using a touch tone telephone and then "2" for a list of available publications. 12 p.m. 4 p.m.

GENERAL HEALTH

Agency for Health Care Policy and Research Clearinghouse (T–65)
(800)358–9295
(301)495–3453
Distributes lay and scientific publications produced by the agency, including clinical practice guidelines on a variety of topics, reports from the National Medical Expenditure Survey, and health care technology assessment reports. 9 a.m.–5 p.m. (See also F–28)

MedicAlert Foundation (T–66)
(800)432–5378
(800)344–3226
(209)669–2495 (Fax)
Provides emergency service for people who cannot speak for themselves by means of a unique member number on a MedicAlert bracelet or necklace. Operates 24 hours.

National Health Information Center (T–67)
(800)336–4797
(301)565–4167
(301)984–4256 (Fax)
Sponsored by the Office of Disease Prevention and Health Promotion, U.S. Department of Health and Human Services. Provides a central source of information and referral for health questions from health educators, health professionals, and the public. Spanish-speaking operators available. 9 a.m.–5 p.m. (See also F–29)

GRIEF

Grief Recovery Helpline (T–68)
(800)445–4808
Provides educational services on recovering from loss. 9 a.m.–5 p.m. (Pacific).

HEADACHE/HEAD INJURY

National Headache Foundation (T–69)
(800)843–2256
Disseminates free information on headache causes and treatments, funds research, and sponsors public and professional education programs nationwide. Offers audio and videotapes, brochures, and other helpful materials for purchase. Organized a nationwide network of local support groups. 9 a.m.–5 p.m. (Central).

National Head Injury Foundation Family Helpline (T–70)
(800)444–6443
(202)296–6443
(202)296–8850 (Fax)
Dedicated to improving the quality of life of people with head injuries and promoting prevention of head injury. Provides information and resources for people with head injury, their families, and the professionals who provide rehabilitative care. Offers educational materials on the impact of brain injury, location of rehabilitative facilities, and availability of community services. 9 a.m.–5 p.m.

HEARING AND SPEECH

American Speech–Language–Hearing Association (T–71)
(800)638–8255
(301)897–5700
Offers information on speech, language, and hearing disabilities. Also provides referrals to speech language pathologists and audiologists certified by the American Speech–Language–Hearing Association. 9:30 a.m.–4:30 p.m.

Deafness Research Foundation (T–72)
(800)535–3323
(212)684–6556 (Voice/TDD)
(212)779–2125 (Fax)
Funds research into causes, treatment, and prevention of hearing loss and other ear disorders. Also offers resource and referral information on ear-related problems. 9 a.m.–5 p.m.

Dial A Hearing Screening Test (T–73)
(800)222–3277
(215)543–2802 (Fax)
Sponsored by Occupational Hearing Services. Answers questions on hearing problems and makes referrals to local numbers for a 2-minute telephone hearing screening test, as well as for ear, nose, and throat specialists. Also makes referrals to organizations that have information on ear-related problems, including broken hearing aids. 9 a.m.–5 p.m.

The Ear Foundation at Baptist Hospital (T–74)
(800)545–4327
(615)329–7849
(615)329–7935 (Fax)
Committed to integration of hearing and balance impaired people into the mainstream of society through public awareness and medical education. Includes the Meniere's Network and Young EAR's Program. Provides brochure about Meniere's disease and other literature, including newsletters. 8:30 a.m.–4:30 p.m. (Central) or leave recorded message after hours.

Hear Now (T–75)
(800)648–4327 (Voice/TDD)
(303)695–7797 (Voice/TDD)
(303)695–7789 (Fax)
Provides hearing aids and cochlear implants for deaf and hard of hearing individuals with limited financial resources. Collects used hearing aids. Applications for assistance available. 8 a.m.–4 p.m. (Mountain).

Hearing HelpLine (T–76)
(800)EAR–WELL
(703)642–0580
(703)750–9302 (Fax)
Sponsored by the Better Hearing Institute. Implements national public information programs on hearing loss and available medical, surgical, hearing aid, and rehabilitation assistance for millions with uncorrected hearing problems. Provides information on hearing loss and hearing help. 9 a.m.–5 p.m.

John Tracy Clinic (T–77)
(800)522–4582
(213)749–1651 (Fax)
Provides free diagnostic, habilitative, and educational services to preschool deaf children and their families through onsite services and to the preschool deaf and deaf-blind children through worldwide correspondence courses in Spanish and English. 8 a.m.–4 p.m. (Pacific). Leave recorded message after hours.

International Hearing Society (T–78)
(800)521–5247
(810)478–4520 (Fax)
Provides general information on hearing aids and a listing of local hearing aid specialists. 9 a.m.–5 p.m.

National Institute on Deafness and Other Communication Disorders Information Clearinghouse (T–79)
(800)241–1044
(800)241–1055 (TT)
Collects and disseminates information on hearing, balance, smell, taste, voice, speech, and language for health professionals, patients, people in industry, and the public. Maintains a database of references to brochures, books, articles, fact sheets, organizations, and educational materials, which is a subfile on the Combined Health Information Database (CHID). Develops publications. 8:30 a.m.–5 p.m.

Tripod Grapevine (T–80)
(800)352–8888 (Voice/TDD)
(800)287–4763 (Voice/TDD)
Offers information on deafness, including raising and educating a deaf child. Refers callers to parents, professionals, and other resources in their own communities nationwide. 8 a.m.–5 p.m. (Pacific) or leave recorded message after hours.

HEART DISEASE

American Heart Association (T–81)
(800)242–8721
Provides English and Spanish publications and information about heart and blood vessel diseases, exercise, nutrition, and smoking cessation. Additional information is available for minority and senior citizen audiences. Callers are routed to local AHA offices for additional local information. 9 a.m.–5 p.m.

HISTIOCYTOSIS

See RARE DISORDERS

HOMELESSNESS

National Resource Center on Homelessness and Mental Illness (T–82)
(800)444–7415
Sponsored by the Center for Mental Health Services, Substance Abuse and Mental Health Services Administration. Provides technical assistance and information about services and housing for the homeless and mentally ill population. 8 a.m.–5 p.m. (See also F–33, F–41)

HOSPITAL/HOSPICE CARE

Children's Hospice International (T–83)
(800)242–4453
(703)684–0330
Within a community, provides support system and information for health care professionals, families, and the network of organizations that offer hospice care to terminally ill children. Distributes educational materials. 9 a.m.–5 p.m.

Hill–Burton Hospital Free Care (T–84)
(800)638–0742
(800)492–0359
Sponsored by the Bureau of Health Resources Development, Health Resources and Services Administration. Provides information on hospitals and other health facilities participating in the Hill-Burton Hospital Free Care Program. 9:30 a.m.–5:30 p.m. or leave recorded message after hours.

Hospice Education Institute Hospice Link (T–85)
(800)331–1620
Offers information and advice about hospice and palliative care, makes referrals to local hospice and palliative care programs nationwide, and offers information and advice on grief support programs. Maintains a current database of hospices and palliative care units, publishes books and pamphlets, offers continuing education. No medical advice or psychological counseling offered, but sympathetic listening is available to patients and families coping with advanced illness and loss. 9 a.m.–4 p.m.

Shriners Hospital Referral Line (T–86)
(800)237–5055
Gives information on free hospital care available to children under 18 who need orthopedic care or burn treatment. Sends application forms to requesters who meet eligibility requirements for treatment provided by 22 Shriners Hospitals in the United States, Mexico, and Canada. 8 a.m.–5 p.m.

Organizations / Healthfinder

HOUSING

See also CHEMICAL PRODUCTS/PESTICIDES, LEAD

Housing and Urban Development User (T-87)
(800)245-2691
Disseminates publications for U.S. Department of Housing and Urban Development's Office of Policy Development and Research. Offers database searches on housing research. Provides reports on housing safety, housing for elderly and handicapped persons, and lead-based paint. 8:30 a.m.–5:15 p.m. (See also F-34)

HUNTINGTON'S DISEASE

See RARE DISORDERS

IMPOTENCE

Impotence Information Center (T-88)
(800)843-4315
(800)543-9632
Provides free information to prospective patients regarding the causes of and treatments for impotence. 8:30 a.m.–5 p.m. (Central) or leave recorded message after hours.

INCOME TAX

Internal Revenue Service for TDD Users (T-89)
(800)829-4059 (TDD)
(800)829-1040 (Voice tax information)
(800)829-3676 (Forms, publications)
Answers questions on Federal income tax, including medical deductions for the cost of telecommunication devices for the deaf, hearing aids, trained hearing-ear dogs, and questions about sending deaf children to special schools. Accepts orders for Tax Information for Handicapped and Disabled Individuals and other publications. Times for the first number are: Jan. 1 Apr. 2: 8 a.m.–6:30 p.m., Apr. 3 15: 9 a.m.–7:30 p.m., Apr. 16 Oct. 29: 9 a.m.–5:30 p.m., Oct. 30 Dec 31: 8 a.m.–4:30 p.m.; the second number is staffed during regular business hours; and the third number is staffed 8 a.m.–5 p.m. on weekdays, and 9 a.m.–3 p.m. on Saturdays.

INSURANCE/MEDICARE/MEDICAID

DHHS Inspector General's Hotline (T-90)
(800)368-5779
Handles complaints regarding fraud, employee misconduct, and waste and abuse of U.S. Department of Health and Human Services' funds, including medicare, medicaid, and Social Security. 10 a.m.–4 p.m.

Medicare Telephone Hotline (T-91)
(800)638-6833
Sponsored by the Health Care Financing Administration. Gives information on medicare/medigap insurance and policies, answers general questions on medicare problems, and sends free medicare publications. 8 a.m.–8 p.m.

National Insurance Consumer Helpline (T-92)
(800)942-4242
(202)223-7896 (Fax)
Provides general information and answers questions regarding life, health, and home and automobile insurance. Free consumer publications available. Spanish-speaking operators available. 8 a.m.–8 p.m.

JUSTICE

National Criminal Justice Reference Service (NCJRS) (T-93)
(800)851-3420
(301)738-8895 (Electronic Bulletin Board)
Provides criminal justice research findings and documents from bureaus within the Office of Justice Programs, U.S. Department of Justice. The NCJRS library collection contains more than 130,000 documents and is accessible online. Clearinghouse resources and activities also can be accessed via the NCJRS electronic bulletin board. 8:30 a.m.–7 p.m.

KIDNEY DISEASE

See UROLOGICAL DISORDERS

LEAD

See also HOUSING

National Lead Information Hotline (T-94)
(800)LEAD-FYI (Hotline)
(800)424-LEAD (Clearinghouse)
(800)526-5456 (TDD)
Hotline supplies a basic information packet to the public in English or Spanish on lead poisoning and prevention through a 24-hour automated response system. Clearinghouse provides technical information and answers in English or Spanish to specific lead-related questions for private citizens and professionals. 8:30 a.m.–5 p.m. (See also F-34)

LEARNING DISORDERS

See also DISABLING CONDITIONS

The Orton Dyslexia Society (T-95)
(800)222-3123
(410)296-0232
Clearinghouse that provides information on testing; tutoring; and computers used to aid people with dyslexia and related disorders and general information. 8:30 a.m.–4:30 p.m.

LIBRARY SERVICES

See also DISABLING CONDITIONS

Modern Talking Picture Service, Inc. Captioned Films/Videos (T-96)
(800)237-6213 (Voice/TDD)
(813)545-8782 (Fax)
Provides free loan of captioned films and videos for deaf and hearing impaired people. 8:30 a.m.–5 p.m.

National Audiovisual Center (T-97)
(800)788-6282
Provides information on a variety of Government-produced materials, including slides, videotapes, 16mm films, books, and cassettes. 8 a.m.–5 p.m. (See also F-8)

National Library of Medicine (T-98)
(800)272-4787
(301)496-6308
Information service for the National Library of Medicine, National Institutes of Health. Reference services available. Memorial Day Labor Day, 8:30 a.m.–5 p.m., Monday–Friday; 8:30 a.m.–12:30 p.m., Saturday; Labor Day–Memorial Day, 8:30 a.m.–5 p.m., Monday and Friday; 8:30 a.m.–9 p.m., Tuesday–Thursday; and 8:30 a.m.–12:30 p.m., Saturday.

National Library Service for the Blind and Physically Handicapped (T-99)
(800)424-8567
(202)707-5100
(202)707-0744 (TDD)
A total of over 140 network libraries that work in cooperation with the Library of Congress to provide free library service to anyone who is unable to read standard print because of visual or physical impairment. Provides both audio and braille formats through a network of regional libraries. 8 a.m.–4:30 p.m.

Recording for the Blind (T-100)
(800)221-4792
Serves people who cannot read standard print because of a visual, learning, or physical disability. Service includes free lending library of academic textbooks on audio cassette and sale of books on computer diskette and specially adapted tape players and recorders. One-time registration fee of $37.50. 9 a.m.–9 p.m. Leave recorded message after hours.

LIVER DISEASES

American Liver Foundation (T-101)
(800)223-0179
(201)256-2550
Provides information, including fact sheets, and makes physician and support group referrals. Liver disease information brochures and information sheets available upon request. 8:30 a.m.–4:30 p.m.

LUNG DISEASE/ASTHMA/ALLERGY

Asthma and Allergy Foundation of America (T-102)
(800) 7-ASTHMA (727-8462)
Provides general information, publications and videotapes. Operates 24 hours.

Asthma Information Line (T-103)
(800)822-2762
Sponsored by the American Academy of Allergy and Immunology.
Provides written materials on asthma and allergies and offers a printed listing of physician referrals. Operates 24 hours.

Lung Line (T-104)
National Jewish Center for Immunology and Respiratory Medicine
(800)222-5864
(303)355-5864
(800)552-LUNG (LUNG FACTS)
Answers questions about asthma, emphysema, chronic bronchitis, allergies, juvenile rheumatoid arthritis, smoking, and other respiratory and immune system disorders. Questions answered by registered nurses. 8 a.m.–5 p.m. (Mountain). LUNG FACTS, a companion to LUNG LINE, is a 24-hour, 7-days-a-week automated information service. Using a touch-tone telephone, callers can choose among a selection of recorded topics on lung disease and immunological disorders.

MATERNAL AND INFANT-HEALTH

La Leche League International (T-105)
(800)LA-LECHE
(708)519-7730
(708)519-0035 (Fax)
Provides breastfeeding information and mother-to-mother support for women who wish to breastfeed. Distributes and sells a wide variety of materials on breastfeeding and parenting. Also organizes training for health professionals and provides a reliable source for current breastfeeding research information through the Breastfeeding Reference Library and Database. Catalogue free of charge upon request. 9 a.m.–5 p.m. (Central).

MEDICARE/MEDICAID

See INSURANCE/MEDICARE/MEDICAID

MENTAL HEALTH

See also CHILD ABUSE/MISSING CHILDREN

Depression Awareness, Recognition, and Treatment (D/ART) (T-106)
(800)421-4211
Sponsored by the National Institute of Mental Health. Provides free information and literature on depressive disorders, symptoms, treatments, and sources of help. Publications available in Spanish, Asian languages, and Russian.

National Clearinghouse on Family Support and Children's Mental Health (T-107)
(800)628-1696
(503)725-4165 (TDD)
(503)725-4180 (Fax)
Sponsored by the National Institute on Disability and Rehabilitation Research, U.S. Department of Education, and the Center for Mental Health Services, U.S. Department of Health and Human Services. Provides publications on parent/family support groups, financing, early intervention, various mental disorders, and other topics concerning children's mental health. Also offers a computerized data bank and a state-by-state resource file. Recording operates 24 hours a day. (See also F-12, F-41)

Organizations / Healthfinder

National Foundation for Depressive Illness (T-108)
(800)248-4344
A 24-hour recorded message describes symptoms of depression and manic depression and gives an address for more information and physician and support group referrals by state.

National Mental Health Association (T-109)
(800)969-6642
(703)684-5968 (Fax)
Provides brochures on clinical depression and the warning signs of illness and pamphlets regarding women and stress. Offers additional assistance and a referral service to mental health organizations. Makes referrals to mental health groups. Educational brochures available. 9 a.m.–5 p.m.

National Resource Center on Homelessness and Mental Illness (T-110)
(800)444-7415
Abuse and Mental Health Services Administration. Provides technical assistance and information about services and housing for the homeless and mentally ill population. 8 a.m.–5 p.m.

Panic Disorder Information Line (T-111)
(800)64-PANIC
Sponsored by the National Institute of Mental Health. Provides educational materials on panic disorder symptoms, diagnosis, referral, and treatment to health care and mental health professionals and the public. Also disseminates lists of additional resource materials and organizations that can help callers locate a treatment professional. Spanish-speaking operators available. Operates 24 hours a day.

MINORITY HEALTH

Office of Minority Health Resource Center (T-112)
(800)444-6472
Responds to consumer and professional inquiries on minority health–related topics by distributing materials, providing referrals, and identifying sources of technical assistance. Spanish- and Asian-speaking operators available. 9 a.m.–5 p.m. (See also F-42)

NUTRITION

American Dietetic Association's Consumer Nutrition Hotline (T-113)
(800)366-1655
Provides consumers with direct and immediate access to reliable nutrition information. Free publications about a wide range of nutrition topics available. Callers may listen to recorded nutrition messages in English or Spanish, 8 a.m.–8 p.m. (Central). Registered dietitians (RDs) answer food and nutrition questions and provide referrals to RDs in the caller's area 9 a.m.–4 p.m. (Central). TDD available. (See also F-27)

American Institute for Cancer Research (T-114)
(800)843-8114
Provides free educational publications about diet, nutrition, and cancer prevention, as well as a Nutrition Hotline staffed by registered dietitians. 9 a.m.–5 p.m.

National Dairy Council (T-115)
(800)426-8271
(708)803-2077 (Fax)
Develops and provides educational materials on nutrition. 8:30 a.m.–4:30 p.m. (Central).

ORGAN DONATION

See also VISION and UROLOGICAL DISORDERS

The Living Bank (T-116)
(800)528-2971
National registry and referral service for people wanting to donate their tissues and vital organs for transplantation. Informs the public about organ donation and transplantation. Operates 24 hours.

National Marrow Donor Program (T-117)
(800)MARROW-2
Sponsored by the National Heart, Lung, and Blood Institute and the Department of the Navy. Offers information on becoming a bone marrow donor. 8 a.m.–6 p.m. (Central).

United Network for Organ Sharing (T-118)
(800)243-6667
(804)330-8507 (Fax)
Offers information and referrals for organ donation and transplantation. Answers requests for organ donor cards. Operates 24 hours.

PARALYSIS AND SPINAL CORD INJURY

See also DISABLING CONDITIONS AND STROKE

American Paralysis Association (T-119)
(800)225-0292
(201)912-9433 (Fax)
Raises money to fund research to find a cure for paralysis caused by spinal injuries and other central nervous system disorders. Provides information about spinal cord research. 9 a.m.–5 p.m.

National Rehabilitation Information Center (T-120)
(800)346-2742 (Voice/TDD)
(301)588-9284 (Voice/TDD)
(301)587-1967 (Fax)
Provides research referrals and information on rehabilitation issues and concerns. Spanish-speaking operators available. 8 a.m.–6 p.m.

National Spinal Cord Injury Association (T-121)
(800)962-9629 (Members/individuals with spinal cord injuries; no vendors)
(617)441-8500 (Nonmembers, public, professionals)
Provides peer counseling to those with spinal cord injuries through local chapters and organizations. Provides information and referral service. 9 a.m.–5 p.m.

National Spinal Cord Injury Hotline (T-122)
(800)526-3456
Sponsored by the Paralyzed Veterans of America. Offers information on spinal cord injuries and peer support to those with spinal cord injuries and their families. Answering service will page for emergency. 9 a.m.–5 p.m.

PARKINSON'S DISEASE

American Parkinson's Disease Association (T-123)
(800)223-2732
(718)981-4399 (Fax)
Operates 51 information and referral centers throughout the United States. Raises funds for Parkinson's disease research and education. Provides information and referrals to patients and families. Multilingual educational literature available. 9 a.m.–5 p.m. Leave recorded message after hours.

National Parkinson Foundation, Inc. (T-124)
(800)327-4545
(800)433-7022
(305)548-4403 (Fax)
A worldwide research, clinical, and therapeutic organization. Also provides physician references, support group systems, and educational materials in both English and Spanish. Professional staff answer questions about the disease from 9 a.m.–5 p.m. Monday–Friday; recorded messages at all other times.

Parkinson's Educational Program (T-125)
(800)344-7872 (Leave recorded message)
(714)250-2975 (Voice)
(714)250-8530 (Fax)
Provides materials, such as newsletters, glossary of definitions, videotape, and publications catalog. Offers patient-support group information and physician referrals. Operates 24 hours.

PESTICIDES

See CHEMICAL PRODUCTS/PESTICIDES

PHYSICIANS

American Board of Medical Specialties (T-126)
(800)776-2378
Verifies board certification of physicians. 9 a.m.–6 p.m.

PRACTITIONER REPORTING

USP Practitioners Reporting Network (T-127)
(800)4-USP-PRN (487-7776)
(800)23-ERROR (Medication error)
Offers a service for health professionals to report problems with drugs, medical devices, radiopharmaceuticals, animal drugs, and actual or potential medication errors. Recording operates 24 hours a day; staff available 9 a.m.–4:30 p.m., Monday–Friday. Medication error telephone number records information 24 hours a day.

PREGNANCY/MISCARRIAGE

American Academy of Husband-Coached Childbirth (T-128)
(800)4A-BIRTH
Provides free listing of teachers of the Bradley Method, including package of information and referral for local classes in natural childbirth. Books and videotapes may be ordered also. Operates 24 hours.

ASPO/Lamaze (American Society for Psychoprophylaxis in Obstetrics) (T-129)
(800)368-4404
(202)857-1128
(202)223-4579 (Fax)
Operates a toll-free telephone service to provide consumers with information about prepared childbirth and how to locate a local ASPO-Certified Childbirth Educator. 9 a.m.–5 p.m.

International Childbirth Education Association (T-130)
(800)624-4934 (Book Center orders)
(612)854-8660 (General information)
Provides referrals to local chapters and support groups, membership information, certification, and mail-order service. 7 a.m.–4:30 p.m. (Central).

Liberty Godparent Home (T-131)
(800)542-4453
Provides a residential program for adolescent single mothers. Provides counseling referrals to local and national organizations and distributes brochures on request. Operates 24 hours.

RADON

Radon Hotline (T-132)
(800)SOS-RADON
(800)526-5456 (TDD)
Operated by the National Safety Council. Provides packet of information, including brochure on reducing radon risks. Provides a 24-hour recording. (See also F-23, F-34)

RARE DISORDERS*

*A rare disorder is defined as a disorder that affects less than 1 percent of the population at any given time.

American Leprosy Missions (Hansen's Disease) (T-133)
(800)543 3131
(803)271 7040
(803)271 7062 (Fax)
Answers questions and distributes materials. Also assists in raising funds for people with this disease. 8 a.m.–5 p.m.

The American Lupus Society (T-134)
(800)331-1802
Provides a 24-hour recording for callers to leave their names and addresses to receive information on services provided.

American SIDS Institute (T-135)
(800)232-7437
(800)847-7437
Answers inquiries about Sudden Infant Death Syndrome from families and physicians, distributes literature, and makes referrals to other organizations. Operates 24 hours. (See F-53)

Amyotrophic Lateral Sclerosis Association (ALS, Lou Gehrig's Disease) (T-136)
(800)782-4747
(818)340-2060 (Fax)
Provides names of support groups and locations of clinics and distributes literature. 8 a.m.–5 p.m. (Pacific). Leave recorded message after hours.

Batten Disease Support (T-137)
(800)448-4570
Provides telephone counseling, newsletter, support groups, literature, and referrals to other organizations. Operates 24 hours.

Cleft Palate Foundation (T-138)
(800)242-5338 (CLEFTLINE)
(412)481-1376
(412)481-0847 (Fax)
Provides information and referral to individuals and families affected by cleft lip, cleft palate, or other craniofacial birth defects. Referrals are made to local cleft palate/craniofacial teams for treatment and to parent/patient support groups. Free information on various aspects of clefting is available; some available in Spanish. CLEFTLINE operates 24 hours. Spanish-speaking operators available 8:30 a.m.–4:30 p.m., Monday–Friday.

Cooley's Anemia Foundation (T-139)
(800)522-7222
(718)321-CURE
(718)321-3340 (Fax)
Provides information on patient care, research, fundraising, patient-support groups, and research grants. Makes referrals to local chapters and screening centers. 9 a.m.–5 p.m.

Cornelia de Lange Syndrome Foundation (T-140)
(800)223-8355
(203)693-0159
(203)693-6819 (Fax)
Provides a variety of materials for families, friends, and professionals about this syndrome. 9 a.m.–5 p.m. Leave recorded message after hours.

Cystic Fibrosis Foundation (T-141)
(800)344-4823
(301)951-6378 (Fax)
Responds to patient and family questions, offers literature, and provides referrals to local clinics. 8:30 a.m.–5:30 p.m.

Epilepsy Foundation of America (T-142)
(800)332-1000
(301)459-3700
(301)577-2684 or 4941 (Fax)
Provides information on epilepsy and makes referrals to local chapters. Spanish-speaking operators available. 9 a.m.–5 p.m.

Histiocytosis Association (T-143)
(800)548-2758
(609)589-6614 (Fax)
Provides patient and family support, quarterly newsletter, information, brochures, directory, and list of regional meetings, and promotes research. Operates 8:30 a.m.–4 p.m., Monday–Friday. Leave recorded message after hours.

Huntington's Disease Society of America (T-144)
(800)345-4372 (Patients and family members)
(212)242-1968
(212)243-2443 (Fax)
Provides information and referrals to physicians, support groups, chapters, and long-term care facilities. Answers questions on testing. 9 a.m.–5 p.m.

Lupus Foundation of America (T-145)
(800)558-0121
(301)670-9292
Answers basic questions about the disease and provides health professionals, patients and their families with information and literature. Refers to local affiliates. 9 a.m.–5 p.m. Recording 24 hours a day.

Meniere's Network (T-146)
(800)545-4327
See T-74.

Myasthenia Gravis Foundation (T-147)
(800)541-5454
(312)258-0461 (Fax)
Provides information regarding services for myasthenia patients. Promotes public awareness. Funds research. 8:45 a.m.–4:45 p.m. (Central).

National Down Syndrome Congress (T-148)
(800)232-6372
(404)633-2 817 (Fax)
Responds to questions concerning all aspects of Down syndrome. Refers to local organizations. 9 a.m.–5 p.m. Recording after hours.

National Down Syndrome Society Hotline (T-149)
(800)221-4602
(212)460-9330
Provides information about Down syndrome, a genetic disorder that affects 250,000 people in the United States, through its printed and video materials, information referral services, 24-hour toll-free hotline, and research. 9 a.m.–5 p.m.

National Information Center for Orphan Drugs and Rare Diseases (T-150)
(800)300-7469
Disseminates information to patients, health professionals, and the public. 9 a.m.–4 p.m.

National Lymphedema Network (T-151)
(800)541-3259
Provides information on the prevention and management of primary and secondary lymphedema to the public and professionals. Offers referrals to health care professionals and treatment centers, local support groups, and exercise programs. Provides quarterly newsletter, resource guide, and information on support groups, conferences, and professional training courses. 9 a.m.–5 p.m. (Pacific). Leave recorded message after hours.

National Multiple Sclerosis Society (T-152)
(800)FIGHT-MS
(212)986-7981 (Fax)
Offers a 24-hour telephone message line. Staff members available to answer questions 11 a.m.–5 p.m., Monday Thursday.

National Neurofibromatosis Foundation (T-153)
(800)323-7938
(212)460-8980
(212)529-6094 (Fax)
Responds to inquiries from health professionals, patients, and families. Makes referrals to physicians on clinical advisory board. 9 a.m.–5 p.m.

National Organization for Rare Disorders (T-154)
(800)999-6673
(203)746-6518
(203)746-6481 (Fax)
(203)746-6927 (TDD)
Provides information on 5,000 rare disorders and their symptoms, standard and investigative therapies, statistics, voluntary agencies for rare disorders, and networking programs. Offers referrals to organizations for specific disorders. 9 a.m.–5 p.m. Leave recorded message after hours.

National Reye's Syndrome Foundation (T-155)
(800)233-7393
(419)636-2679
Provides awareness materials to the public and medical community, raises funds for research, and offers guidance and counseling to victims. 8 a.m.–5 p.m. Leave recorded message after hours.

National Tuberous Sclerosis Association (T-156)
(800)225-6872
(301)459-9888
(301)459-0394 (Fax)
ntsa@capcon.net (Internet)
Answers questions about the disease and makes parent-to-parent contact referrals. Literature is provided to families and professionals. 8:30 a.m.–5 p.m.

Sarcoidosis Family Aid and Research Foundation (T-157)
(800)223-6429 (Leave recorded message)
(201)923-8818 (Voice)
Information mailed to callers. Staff available for counseling. 1 p.m.–5 p.m., Tuesday–Friday.

Sickle Cell Disease Association of America, Inc. (T-158)
(800)421-8453
Offers educational materials, referrals for client services, research support, and public awareness. 8:30 a.m.–5 p.m. (Pacific). Recording after hours and weekends.

SIDS Alliance (T-159)
(800)221-7437
(410)964-8000
(410)964-8009 (Fax)
Provides medical information on Sudden Infant Death Syndrome and referrals, as well as support groups. 9 a.m.–5 p.m. or leave a recorded message after hours on the emergency line. (See also F-53)

Spina Bifida Information and Referral (T-160)
(800)621-3141
(202)944-3285
(202)944-3295 (Fax)
Sponsored by the Spina Bifida Association of America. Provides information to consumers and health professionals and referrals to local chapters. 9 a.m.–5 p.m.

Spondylitis Association of America (formerly the Ankylosing Association of America) (T-161)
(800)777-8189
(818)981-1616
Provides information on ankylosing spondylitis, psoriatic arthritis, and Reiter's syndrome. 9 a.m.–5 p.m. (Pacific). Leave recorded message after hours.

Sturge-Weber Foundation (T-162)
(800)627-5482
Provides list of publications, long-distance support groups, and referrals for families, friends, and professionals. 10 a.m.–3 p.m., Monday–Thursday.

Tourette Syndrome Association, Inc. (T-163)
(800)237-0717
(718)224-2999
(718)279-9596 (Fax)
Provides a 24-hour recording for callers to request information and leave name and address. To speak with a staff member, call the local number between 9 a.m.–5 p.m.

United Cerebral Palsy Association (T-164)
(800)872-5827
(202)842-1266
(202)842-3519 (Fax)
Provides literature about cerebral palsy. Responds to inquiries from people with cerebral palsy, their families, and the public. Makes referrals to local affiliates. 8:30 a.m.–5:30 p.m.

United Scleroderma Foundation (T-165)
(800)722-HOPE
(408)728-2202
(408)728-3328 (Fax)
Provides list of publications, chapters throughout the United States, and general information. 8 a.m.–5 p.m. (Pacific).

REHABILITATION

See DISABLING CONDITIONS, PARALYSIS AND SPINAL CORD INJURY

RETINITIS PIGMENTOSA

See VISION

RURAL

Rural Information Center Health Service (T-166)
(800)633-7701
(301)504-5547
(301)504-6856 (TTY/TDD)
(301)504-5181 (Fax)
Provides information and referrals to the public and to professionals on rural health issues. Performs brief, complimentary literature searches. 8 a.m.–4:30 p.m. (See also F-51)

Organizations / Healthfinder

SAFETY

See CHEMICAL PRODUCTS/PESTICIDES; CHILD ABUSE/MISSING CHILDREN

National Highway Traffic Safety Administration Auto Safety Hotline (T-167)
(800)424-9393
(202)366-0123
Provides information and referral on the effectiveness of occupant protection, such as safety belt use, child safety seats, and automobile recalls. Gives referrals to other Government agencies for consumer questions on warranties, service, automobile safety regulations, and reporting safety problems. 8 a.m.–4 p.m. (See also F-32)

National Institute for Occupational Safety and Health Technical Information Branch (T-168)
(800)356-4674
Provides information on chemical and physical hazards in the workplace, training courses, publications, and the health hazard evaluation program. 9 a.m.–4 p.m. (See also F-36, F-44, F-49)

Office of Navigation Safety and Waterway Services U.S. Coast Guard Boating Safety Hotline (T-169)
(800)368-5647
(202)267-0780
Provides information on boating safety, including a kit for consumers, recalls on boating products, and makes referrals to their organizations. 8 a.m.–4 p.m.

U.S. Consumer Product Safety Commission Hotline (T-170)
(800)638-2772
(800)638-8270 (TDD)
info@cpsc.gov (Internet)
Provides 24-hour messages on consumer product safety, including product hazards and product recalls. Covers only products used n and around the home, excluding automobiles, child safety eats, health care products, warranties, foods, drugs, cosmetics, oats, and firearms. (See also F-36, F-49)

SEXUAL EDUCATION

Planned Parenthood Federation of America, Inc. (T-171)
(800)230-PLAN (To schedule appointment at the closest clinic)
(800)669-0156 (For health information)
Provides family planning, reproductive, and sexual health care and information. Callers will reach the nearest Planned Parenthood center for clinical appointments or education staff. (See also F-24)

SEXUALLY TRANSMITTED DISEASES

See AIDS/HIV

Centers for Disease Control and Prevention National STD Hotline (T-172)
(800)227-8922
Information regarding all sexually transmitted diseases. Referral to community clinics offering free or low-cost examination and treatment. 8 a.m.–11 p.m.

SPINAL CORD INJURY

See PARALYSIS AND SPINAL CORD INJURY

STROKE

See PARALYSIS AND SPINAL CORD INJURY

American Heart Association Stroke Connection (T-173)
(800)553-6321
(214)696-5211 (Fax)
Maintains a listing of more than 900 groups across the Nation for referral to stroke survivors, their families, care givers, and interested professionals. Publishes Stroke Connection magazine, a forum for stroke survivors and their families to share information about coping with stroke. Provides information and referral and carries stroke-related books, videotapes, and literature available for purchase. 8:30 a.m.–5 p.m. (Central).

National Stroke Association (T-174)
(800)STROKES
(303)771-1700
(303)771-1887 (TDD)
Provides both written and referral information to individuals, including stroke survivors, families, and health care providers on prevention, treatment, and rehabilitation. 8 a.m.–4:30 p.m., Monday–Thursday; 8 a.m.–4 p.m., Friday (Mountain).

STUTTERING

National Center for Stuttering (T-175)
(800)221-2483
Provides treatment for older children (above age 7) and adults, training for professionals, and information for parents with children below age 7. 9 a.m.–6 p.m.

Stuttering Foundation of America (T-176)
(800)992-9392
Provides materials and makes referrals to speech-language pathologists. 9 a.m.–5 p.m.

SUDDEN INFANT-DEATH SYNDROME

See RARE DISORDERS

SURGERY/FACIAL PLASTIC SURGERY

American Society for Dermatologic Surgery, Inc. (T-177)
(800)441-2737
Provides information about various dermatologic surgical procedures, as well as referrals to dermatologic surgeons in local areas. 8:30 a.m.–5 p.m. (Central).

American Society of Plastic and Reconstructive Surgeons, Inc. (T-178)
(800)635-0635
Provides referrals to board-certified plastic surgeons nationwide and in Canada. 8:30 a.m.–4:30 p.m. (Central). Leave recorded message after hours.

Facial Plastic Surgery Information Service (T-179)
(800)332-3223
(202)842-4500
Provides physician referral list and brochures. 24 hours.

TRAUMA

American Trauma Society (ATS) (T-180)
(800)556-7890
(301)420-4189
(301)420-0617 (Fax)
Offers information to health professionals and the public; answers questions about trauma and medical emergencies. 9 a.m.–5 p.m.

UROLOGICAL DISORDERS

American Association of Kidney Patients (T-181)
(800)749-2257
(813)223-0001 (Fax)
Helps renal patients and their families to deal with the physical and emotional impact of kidney disease. Supplies information on renal conditions. 9 a.m.–5 p.m.

American Foundation for Urologic Disease (T-182)
(800)242-2383
(410)528-0550 (Fax)
Provides educational materials about urologic diseases and dysfunctions to the public and health care professionals. Referrals and support group information furnished upon request. 8:30 a.m.–9 p.m. (See also F-37)

American Kidney Fund (T-183)
(800)638 8299
Offers financial assistance to kidney patients who are unable to pay treatment-related costs. Also provides information on organ donations and kidney-related diseases. 8 a.m.–5 p.m.

National Kidney Foundation (T-184)
(800)622-9010
(212)689-9261 (Fax)
Provides information and referrals to the public and health professionals regarding kidney disorders. 9 a.m.–5 p.m.

The Simon Foundation for Continence (T-185)
(800)237-4666 (Patient information)
(708)864-3913
Provides information on continence and ordering a quarterly newsletter and other publications. Also has a community-based education program/self-help group and informational videotape. Toll-free number operates 24 hours; second number is staffed 8 a.m.–5 p.m. (Central).

VENEREAL DISEASES

See SEXUALLY TRANSMITTED DISEASES

VISION

See LIBRARY SERVICES

American Council of the Blind (T-186)
(800)424-8666
(202)467-5081
(202)467-5085 (Fax)
(202)331-1058 (Electronic Bulletin Board)
Offers information on blindness and referrals to rehabilitation organizations, research centers, and chapters. Publishes resource lists. 3 p.m. 5:30 p.m. Leave recorded message after hours.

Blind Children's Center (T-187)
(800)222-3566
(800)222-3567
Nonprofit early intervention program and educational preschool. Family support services. Information and referral line. Educational booklets for parents, educators, and specialists. 7 a.m.–5 p.m. (Pacific).

Guide Dog Foundation for the Blind, Inc. (T-188)
(800)548-4337
(516)265-2121
(516)361-5192 (Fax)
(516)366-4462 (Electronic Bulletin Board)
School for blind individuals requiring guide dogs. Operates 24 hours.

The Lighthouse National Center for Vision and Aging (T-189)
(800)334-5497
(212)808-0077
(212)821-9713 (TDD)
(212)821-9705 (Fax)
Provides educational materials and information on vision and child development and age-related vision loss to professionals and consumers. Some materials in Spanish. 9 a.m.–5 p.m. Leave recorded message after hours.

Louisiana Center for the Blind (T-190)
(800)234-4166
(318)251-2891
(318)251-0109 (Fax)
Private, residential training program for legally blind adults and children. 8 a.m.–5 p.m. (Central).

National Association for Parents of the Visually Impaired (T-191)
(800)562-6265
(617)972-7444 (Fax)
Provides support and information to parents of visually impaired, blind, deaf-blind, and blind multi-handicapped children. 9 a.m.–5 p.m. (Central).

National Eye Care Project Helpline (T-192)
(800)222-EYES (3937)
Provides medical and surgical eye care to disadvantaged elderly people who can no longer access the ophthalmologists they have visited in the past. 8 a.m.–4 p.m. (Pacific).

National Eye Research Foundation (T-193)
(800)621-2258
(708)564-4652
(708)564-0807 (Fax)
Recording provides patient and membership information. Publishes the Green Directory, an international listing of member optometrists for patient referrals. 8:30 a.m.–5 p.m. Leave recorded message after hours.

The National Eye Research Foundation's Memorial Eye Clinic (T-194)
(800)621-2258
Provides low-vision care, orthokeratology, and problem contact lens care. 9 a.m.–5 p.m.,

Monday, Tuesday, Wednesday; 9 a.m.–2 p.m., Friday; closed Thursday. Leave recorded message after hours.

National Federation of the Blind: Job Opportunities for the Blind (JOB) (T–195)
(800)638–7518
Offers support and factual information to blind individuals seeking jobs, employers, parents, and teachers. Also provides a free sample package and job magazine on cassette. 8 a.m.–5 p.m.

Prevent Blindness Center for Sight (T–196)
(800)331–2020
Sponsored by Prevent Blindness America. Provides information on a broad range of eye health and safety topics. 8 a.m.–5 p.m. (Central).

RP Foundation Fighting Blindness (T–197)
(800)683–5555
(800)683–5551 (TDD)
(410)225–3936 (Fax)
Funds medical research and provides information on retinitis pigmentosa and other inherited retinal degenerations. Scope of information includes current research, genetics, retina donor program, and practical resources available throughout the United States. 8:30 a.m.–5 p.m.

VIOLENCE

Family Violence Prevention Fund (T–198)
(800)313–1310
Provides information and resources on how to diagnose, treat, and prevent domestic violence.

WOMEN

Endometriosis Association (T–199)
(800)992–3636
Provides a 24-hour recording for callers to request information and leave name and address.

PMS Access (T–200)
(800)222–4767
(608)833–7412 (Fax)
Sponsored by Madison Pharmacy Associates, Inc. Provides information, literature, and counseling on premenstrual syndrome (PMS). Gives referrals to physicians and clinics in the caller's area. 9 a.m.–5 p.m. (Central).

Women's Sports Foundation (T–201)
(800)227–3988
Provides information on funding opportunities and educational materials for girls and women in sports and fitness. 9 a.m.–5 p.m.

FEDERAL HEALTH INFORMATION CENTERS AND CLEARINGHOUSES

The Federal Government operates many clearinghouses and information centers that focus on specific topics. Their services include distributing publications, providing referrals, and answering inquiries. Many offer toll–free numbers. Unless otherwise stated, numbers can be reached within the continental United States Monday through Friday, during normal business hours, and hours of operation are eastern time. The clearinghouses are listed below by keyword.

National Institute on AGING Information Center (F–1)
P.O. Box 8057
Gaithersburg, MD 20898–8057
(800)222–2225 (Voice/TTY)
(800)222–4225 (TTD)
(301)589–3014 (Fax)
Provides information and publications on health topics of interest to older adults, to the public, and to doctors, nurses, social activities directors, and health educators. (See also T–3, T–16, T–17, T–18, T–81).

U.S. Department of AGRICULTURE Extension Service (F–2)
See the listing in the Government section of your telephone book for your local extension office. Provides information on health, nutrition, fitness, and family well–being.

CDC National AIDS Clearinghouse (F–3)
P.O. Box 6003
Rockville, MD 20849–6003
(800)458–5231 (Clearinghouse; Business Responds to AIDS Resource Service)
(800)342–AIDS (English)
(800)344–SIDA (Spanish)
(800)243–7012 (TTY/TDD)
(800)TRIALS A (AIDS Clinical Trials Information Service)
(301)738–6616 (Fax)
(301)217–0023 (International)
A service of the Centers for Disease Control and Prevention. Offers reference and referral assistance; distributes HIV/AIDS educational materials; and maintains databases on AIDS service organizations and HIV/AIDS materials. Operates the AIDS Clinical Trials Information Service (ACTIS) to provide up–to–date information on federally and privately sponsored HIV/AIDS clinical trials. Operates the CDC Business Responds to AIDS Resource Service (BRTA). BRTA is a centralized information service and referral service that links the business and labor communities with resources for developing HIV/AIDS in workplace programs. BRTA reference specialists refer callers to relevant local, State, and national programs and services, and identify HIV/AIDS educational materials for workplace programs and services. Callers may order CDC–approved HIV/AIDS educational materials brochures, posters, and videotapes directly from the Clearinghouse. Some materials available in Spanish. Some materials available free of charge. 9 a.m.–7 p.m. (See also T–5)

CSAP's National Clearinghouse for ALCOHOL and DRUG Information (F–4)
P.O. Box 2345
Rockville, MD 20847–2345
(800)729–6686
(301)468–2600
(800)487–4889 (TTY/TDD)
(301)230–2867 (TTY/TDD)
(301)468–6433 (Fax)
Sponsored by the Center for Substance Abuse Prevention, Substance Abuse and Mental Health Services Administration. Gathers and disseminates information on alcohol and other drug–related subjects, including tobacco. Distributes publications. Services include subject searches and provision of statistics and other information. Operates the Regional Alcohol and Drug Awareness Resource (RADAR) Network, a nationwide linkage of alcohol and other drug information centers. Maintains a library open to the public. 8 a.m.–7 p.m. (See also T–13, T–53, F–51)

National Institute of ALLERGY and INFECTIOUS DISEASES (F–5)
Office of Communications
Building 31, Room 7A50
9000 Rockville Pike
Bethesda, MD 20892
(301)496–5717
Distributes publications to the public and to doctors, nurses, and researchers.

ALZHEIMER's DISEASE Education and Referral Center (F–6)
P.O. Box 8250
Silver Spring, MD 20907–8250
(800)438–4380
(301)495–3334 (Fax)
Sponsored by the National Institute on Aging. Provides information and publications on Alzheimer's disease to health and service professionals, patients and their families, care givers, and the public. (See also T–3, T–16, T–17)

National ARTHRITIS and Musculoskeletal and Skin Diseases Information Clearinghouse (F–7)
P.O. Box AMS
9000 Rockville Pike
Bethesda, MD 20892
(301)495–4484
(301)587–4352 (Fax)
Identifies educational materials about arthritis and musculoskeletal and skin diseases and serves as an information exchange for individuals and organizations involved in public, professional, and patient education. Conducts subject searches and makes resource referrals. (See also T–3, T–18)

National AUDIOVISUAL Center (F–8)
National Technical Information Service
U.S. Department of Commerce
Springfield, VA 22161
(703)487–4780
(703)321–8547 (Fax)
Sells more than 8,000 federally produced audiovisual programs. Provides catalogs and referrals to free–loan sources at no cost. Several catalogs cover health–related topics, including alcohol and other drug abuse, dentistry, emergency medical services, industrial safety, medicine, nursing, and occupational health. (See also T–97)

National Library Service for the BLIND and Physically Handicapped (F–9)
Library of Congress
1291 Taylor Street, NW.
Washington, DC 20542
(800)424–8567
(202)707–5100
(202)707–0744 (TDD)
(202)707–0712 (Fax)
A network of 56 regional and 87 local libraries that work in cooperation with the Library of Congress to provide free library service to anyone who is unable to read standard print due to visual or physical disabilities. Delivers recorded and Braille books and magazines to eligible readers. Specially designed phonographs and cassette players also are loaned. A list of participating local and regional libraries is available.

CANCER Information Service (F–10)
Office of Cancer Communications
National Cancer Institute
Building 31, Room 10A16
9000 Rockville Pike
Bethesda, MD 20892
(800)4–CANCER
(301)496–5583
(301)402–2594 (Fax)
Provides information about cancer and cancer–related resources to patients, the public, and health professionals. Inquiries are handled by trained information specialists. Spanish–speaking staff members are available. Distributes free publications from the National Cancer Institute. Operates 9 a.m.–7 p.m. (See also T–19, T–20, T–21, T–22)

National Clearinghouse on CHILD ABUSE and Neglect Information (F–11)
P.O. Box 1182
Washington, DC 20013–1182
(800)FYI 3366
(703)385–7565
(703)385–3206 (Fax)
Serves as a national resource for the acquisition and dissemination on child abuse and neglect materials and distributes a free publications catalog upon request. Maintains bibliographic databases of documents, audiovisuals, and national organizations. Services include searches of databases and annotated bibliographies on frequently requested topics. Spanish–speaking staff is available. (See also T–30)

National Clearinghouse on Family Support and CHILDREN's MENTAL HEALTH (F–12)
Portland State University
P.O. Box 751
Portland, OR 97207–0751
(800)628–1696
(503)725–4040
(503)725–4165 (TTD)
(503)725–4180 (Fax)
Sponsored by the National Institute on Disability and Rehabilitation Research, U.S. Department of Education, and the Center for Mental Health Services, U.S. Department of Health and Human Services. Provides publications on parent/family support groups, financing, early intervention, various mental disorders, and other topics concerning children's mental health. Also offers a computerized databank and a state–by–state resource file. Recording operates 24 hours a day. (See also T–107, F–41)

Organizations / Healthfinder

COMBINED HEALTH INFORMATION DATABASE (CHID) (F–13)
(800)955–0906 (BRS Online, to subscribe to CHID)
Available only on BRS Online. The Combined Health Information Database (CHID) is a computerized, bibliographic database developed and managed by health–related agencies of the Federal Government. CHID contains more than 93,350 abstracted items and references to many diverse health education resources. The database is available to the public and can be accessed by many university, medical, and public libraries. The database is updated quarterly, and coverage dates back to 1973.

CONSUMER INFORMATION Center (F–14)
General Services Administration
P.O. Box 100
Pueblo, CO 81009
(719)948–4000
Distributes Federal agency publications. Publishes quarterly catalog of available materials.

National Institute on DEAFNESS and Other Communication Disorders Information Clearinghouse (F–15)
1 Communication Avenue
Bethesda, MD 20892–3456 (800)241–1044 (Voice)
(800)241–1055 (TT)
(301)907–8830 (Fax)
Collects and disseminates information on hearing, balance, smell, taste, voice, speech, and language for health professionals, patients, people in industry, and the public. Maintains a database of references to brochures, books, articles, fact sheets, organizations, and educational materials, which is a subfile on CHID. Develops publications, including directories, fact sheets, brochures, information packets, and newsletters.

National DIABETES Information Clearinghouse (F–16)
1 Information Way
Bethesda, MD 20892–3560
(301)654–3327
(301)907–8906 (Fax)
Sponsored by the National Institute of Diabetes and Digestive and Kidney Diseases. Collects and disseminates information about patient and professional education materials related to diabetes and its complications. Distributes its own publications and other diabetes–related materials. Maintains a registry of meetings pertaining to diabetes and an automated database of patient and professional materials. (See also T–38, T–40)

National DIGESTIVE DISEASES Information Clearinghouse (F–17)
2 Information Way
Bethesda, MD 20892–3570
(301)654–3810
(301)907–8906 (Fax)
Sponsored by the National Institute of Diabetes and Digestive and Kidney Diseases. Provides a central information resource on the prevention and management of digestive diseases. Develops, identifies, and distributes educational materials and responds to requests for information. Maintains an automated database of patient and professional education materials about digestive diseases. (See also T–39)

National Information Center for Children and Youth with DISABILITIES (F–18)
P.O. Box 1492
Washington, DC 20013–1492
(800)695–0285 (Voice/TT)
(202)884–8200 (Voice/TT)
(202)884–8441 (Fax)
nichcy@capcon.net (Internet)
Sponsored by the U.S. Department of Education. Assists individuals by providing information on disabilities and disability–related issues, with a special focus on children and youth with disabilities (birth to age 22). Services include responses to questions, referrals, and technical assistance to parents, educators, care givers, and advocates. Develops and distributes fact sheets on disability and general information on parent support groups and public advocacy. All information and services are provided free of charge. (See also T–46, T–48, T–49)

Clearinghouse on DISABILITY INFORMATION (F–19)
Office of Special Education and Rehabilitative Services
U.S. Department of Education
330 C Street, SW.
Switzer Building, Room 3132
Washington, DC 20202–2524
(202)205–8241
(202)205–9252 (Fax)
Responds to inquiries on a wide range of topics, especially in the areas of Federal funding, legislation, programs benefiting people with disabling conditions, and the Americans With Disabilities Act. Provides referrals. (See also T–46)

Centers for Disease Control and Prevention (F–20)
National Center for Chronic DISEASE PREVENTION and Health Promotion (NCCDPHP)
Technical Information Service Branch
4770 Buford Highway, MS K13
Atlanta, GA 30341–3724
(404)488–5080
Provides information and referrals to the public and to professionals. Gathers information on chronic disease prevention and health promotion. Develops bibliographic databases focusing on health promotion program information: the Health Promotion and Education Database, the Cancer Prevention and Control Database, and the Comprehensive School Health Database with an AIDS school health component. Produces bibliographies on topics of interest in chronic disease prevention and health promotion. The NCCDPHP Information Center collections include approximately 400 periodical subscriptions, 4,000 books, and 400 reference books. Visitors may use the collection by appointment.

Housing and Urban Development DRUG INFORMATION and Strategy Clearinghouse (F–21)
P.O. Box 6424
Rockville, MD 20850
(800)955–2232
Sponsored by the U.S. Department of Housing and Urban Development. Promotes strategies for eradicating drugs and drug trafficking from public housing. Provides housing officials, residents, and community leaders a source for information and assistance on drug abuse prevention and trafficking control techniques. Maintains an automated database system consisting of national and community program descriptions, publications, research, and news articles. Provides resource lists. (See also T–54)

ERIC Clearinghouse on Teaching and Teacher EDUCATION (F–22)
One Dupont Circle, NW.
Suite 610
Washington, DC 20036–1186
(202)293–2450
(202)457–8095 (Fax)
Sponsored by the U.S. Department of Education. Acquires, evaluates, abstracts, and indexes literature on the preparation and development of education personnel and on selected aspects of health and physical education, recreation, and dance. Publishes monographs, trends and issues papers, ERIC Digests and ERIC Recent Resources (annotated bibliographies from the ERIC database). Performs computer searches of the ERIC database and sponsors workshops on searching the ERIC database.

U.S. ENVIRONMENTAL PROTECTION Agency (F–23)
Public Information Center
401 M Street, SW.
Washington, DC 20460
(202)260–2080
(202)260–6257 (Fax)
Offers general information about the Agency and nontechnical publications on various environmental topics, such as air quality, pesticides, radon, indoor air, drinking water, water quality, and Superfund. Refers inquiries for technical information to the appropriate regional or program office. The public may visit the PIC Visitor Center 9 a.m. 4:30 p.m., Monday–Friday, except Federal holidays. (See also T–24, T–58, T–132, F–35)

FAMILY LIFE Information Exchange (F–24)
P.O. Box 37299
Washington, DC 20013–7299
(301)585–6636
(301)588–3408 (Fax)
Sponsored by the Office of Population Affairs. Provides information and distributes publications to health professionals and the public in the areas of family planning, adolescent pregnancy, and adoption. Makes referrals to other information on centers in related subject areas. (See also T–1, T–2, T–171)

FEDERAL INFORMATION Center Program (F–25)
General Services Administration
18th and F–Streets, NW.
Washington, DC 20405
(202)501–0308
(800)347–1997 (East Coast)
(800)726–4995 (West Coast)
Provides information about the Federal Government's agencies, programs, and services. Current Government reference materials and service directories are used to respond to inquiries. A list of the Federal Information Center's toll–free 800 telephone numbers and addresses is available free from the Consumer Information Center (see F–14).

FOOD AND DRUG Administration (F–26)
Office of Consumer Affairs
5600 Fishers Lane, HFE 50
Rockville, MD 20857
(301)443–3170
(301)443–9767 (Fax)
Responds to consumer requests for information and publications on foods, drugs, cosmetics, medical devices, radiation–emitting products, and veterinary products. (See also T–63, T–64)

FOOD AND NUTRITION Information Center (F–27)
U.S. Department of Agriculture
National Agricultural Library
10301 Baltimore Boulevard
Room 304
Beltsville, MD 20705–2351
(301)504–5719
(301)504–6409 (Fax)
fnic@nalusda.gov (Internet)
Provides information on human nutrition, food service management, and food technology. Acquires and lends books and audiovisual materials. Offers database searching and access through electronic mail. (See also T–113, T–114)

Agency for HEALTH CARE POLICY and Research Clearinghouse (F–28)
P.O. Box 8547
Silver Spring, MD 20907–8547
(800)358–9295
(301)495–3453
Distributes publications produced by the agency, including clinical practice guidelines on a variety of topics, reports from the National Medical Expenditure Survey, and health care technology assessment reports. (See also T–65)

National HEALTH INFORMATION Center (F–29)
P.O. Box 1133
Washington, DC 20013–1133
(800)336–4797
(301)565–4167
(301)984–4256 (Fax)
Helps the public and health professionals locate health information through identification of health information resources, an information and referral system, and publications. Uses a database containing descriptions of health–related organizations to refer inquirers to the most appropriate resources. Does not diagnose medical conditions or give medical advice. Prepares and distributes publications and directories on health promotion and disease prevention topics. (See also T–67)

National Center for HEALTH STATISTICS (F–30)
Data Dissemination Branch
6525 Belcrest Road, Room 1064
Hyattsville, MD 20782
(301)436–8500
The Data Dissemination Branch of the National Center for Health Statistics answers requests for catalogs of publications and electronic data

products; single copies of publications, such as Advance Data reports; ordering information for publications and electronic products sold through the Government Printing Office and National Technical Information Service; adding addresses to the mailing list for new publications; and specific statistical data collected by the National Center for Health Statistics.

National HEART, LUNG, AND BLOOD Institute Information Center (NHLBI) (F–31)
P.O. Box 30105
Bethesda, MD 20824–0105
(301)251–1222
(301)251–1223 (Fax)
NHLBI serves as a source of information and materials on risk factors for cardiovascular disease. Services include dissemination of public education materials, programmatic and scientific information for health professionals, and materials on worksite health, as well as responses to information requests. Materials on cardiovascular health are available to consumers and professionals. (See also F–44)

National HIGHWAY TRAFFIC SAFETY Administration (F–32)
U.S. Department of Transportation
400 Seventh Street, SW.
Washington, DC 20590
(800)424–9393
(202)366–0123
(202)366–5962 (Fax)
Provides information and referral on the effectiveness of occupant protection, such as safety belt use, child safety seats, and automobile recalls. Gives referrals to other Government agencies for con–consumer questions on warranties, service, automobile safety regulations, and re-porting safety problems. Works with private organizations to promote safety programs. Provides technical and financial assistance to state and local governments and awards grants for highway safety. (See also T–170)

The National Resource Center on HOMELESSNESS and Mental Illness (F–33)
262 Delaware Avenue
Delmar, NY 12054
(800)444–7415
(518)439–7415
(518)439–7612 (Fax)
Collects, synthesizes, and disseminates information on the services, supports, and housing needs of homeless people with serious mental illnesses. Maintains extensive database of published and unpublished materials, prepares customized database searches, holds workshops and national conferences, provides technical assistance. (See also T–82, F–41)

HOUSING AND URBAN DEVELOPMENT–(HUD) User (F–34)
P.O. Box 6091
Rockville, MD 20850
(800)245–2691
(301)251–5154
(800)877–8339 (TDD)
Disseminates publications for U.S. Department of Housing and Urban Development's Office of Policy Development and Research. Offers database searches on housing research. Provides reports on housing safety, housing for elderly and disabled persons, and lead–based paint. (See also T–87, T–94, T–132)

INDOOR AIR Quality Information Clearinghouse (F–35)
P.O. Box 37133
Washington, DC 20013–7133
(800)438–4318
(202)484–1307
(202)484–1510 (Fax)
Provides information, referrals, publications, and database searches on indoor air quality. Information is provided about pollutants and sources, health effects, control methods, commercial building operations and maintenance, standards and guidelines, and Federal and state legislation. (See also T–58, F–23)

National INJURY Information Clearinghouse (F–36)
c/o U.S. Consumer Product Safety Commission
Washington, DC 20207–0001
(301)504–0424
(301)504–0124 (Fax)
Sponsored by the U.S. Consumer Product Safety Commission (CPSC). Collects, investigates, analyzes, and disseminates information on the causes and prevention of death, injury, and illness associated with consumer products. Compiles data obtained from accident reports, consumer complaints, death certificates, news clips, and the National Electronic Injury Surveillance System operated by the CPSC. Publications include statistical analyses of data and hazard and accident patterns. (See also T–168, F–48)

National KIDNEY AND UROLOGIC Diseases Information Clearinghouse (F–37)
3 Information Way
Bethesda, MD 20892–3580
(301)654–4415
(301)907–8906 (Fax)
Provides education and information on kidney and urologic diseases to professionals and the public. Makes referrals to other appropriate organizations. Maintains the kidney and urologic diseases subfile of the Combined Health Information Database (CHID). Provides publications and audiovisual materials on kidney and urologic diseases. (See also T–181, T–182, T–183, T–184, T–185)

National LEAD Information Center (F–38)
1019 19th Street, NW.
Suite 401
Washington, DC 20036
(800)424–LEAD (Clearinghouse)
(800)LEAD FYI (Hotline)
(800)526–5456 (TDD)
(202)659–1192 (Fax)
Sponsored by the National Safety Council. Responds to inquiries regarding lead and lead poisoning. Provides information on lead poisoning and children, lead–based paint, a list of local and state contacts who can help, and other lead–related questions. (See also T–87, T–94)

National Center for Education in MATERNAL AND CHILD HEALTH (F–39)
2000 15th Street, North
Suite 701
Arlington, VA 22201–2617
(703)524–7802
(703)524–9335 (Fax)
Sponsored by the Maternal and Child Health Bureau, Health Resources and Services Administration. Provides information to health professionals and the public, develops educational and reference materials, and provides technical assistance in program development. Subjects covered are women's health including pregnancy and childbirth; infant, child, and adolescent health; nutrition; children with special health needs; injury and violence prevention; health and safety in day care; and maternal and child health programs and services. Types of materials include professional literature, curricula, patient education materials, audiovisuals, and information about organizations and programs. Appointment preferred for on–site visits. (See also T–105)

National MATERNAL AND CHILD HEALTH Clearinghouse (F–40)
8201 Greensboro Drive
Suite 600
McLean, VA 22102
(703)821–8955, ext. 254 or 265
(703)821–2098 (Fax)
Sponsored by the Maternal and Child Health Bureau, Health Resources and Services Administration. Centralized source of materials and information in the areas of human genetics and maternal and child health. Distributes publications and provides referrals. (See also T–105)

National Institute of MENTAL HEALTH (F–41)
Information Resources and Inquiries Branch
5600 Fishers Lane, Room 7C 02
Rockville, MD 20857
(301)443–4513
(301)443–8431 (TDD)
(301)443–0008 (Fax)
(301)443–5158 (MENTAL HEALTH FAX4U Fax Information System)
(800)64–PANIC (PANIC DISORDER Information)
(800)421–4211 (D/ART–Information)

Responds to information requests from the public, clinicians, and the scientific community, with a variety of printed materials on such subjects as children's mental disorders, schizophrenia, depression, bipolar disorder, seasonal affective disorder, anxiety and panic disorders, obsessive–compulsive disorder, eating disorders, learning disabilities, and Alzheimer's disease. Information and publications on the Depression/Awareness, Recognition, and Treatment Program (D/ART) and on the Panic Disorder Education Program, NIMH–sponsored educational programs on depressive and panic disorders, their symptoms and treatment, are distributed. Single copies of publications are free of charge. A list of NIMH publications, including several in Spanish, is available upon request. (See also T–106)

Office of MINORITY HEALTH Resource Center (F–42)
P.O. Box 37337
Washington, DC 20013–7337
(800)444–6472
(301)565–5112 (Fax)
Responds to information requests from health professionals and consumers on minority health issues and locates sources of technical assistance. Provides referrals to relevant organizations and distributes materials. Spanish– and Asian–speaking operators are available. (See also T–112)

Office of NAVIGATION SAFETY and Waterway Services (F–43)
U.S. Coast Guard Consumer Affairs and Analysis Branch
2100 Second Street, SW.
Washington, DC 20593–0001
(800)368–5647 (Boating Safety Hotline)
(202)267–0780
(202)267–4285 (Fax)
Provides safety information to recreational boaters; assists the public in finding boating education classes; answers technical questions; and distributes literature on boating safety, Federal laws, and the prevention of recreational boating casualties.

Clearinghouse for OCCUPATIONAL SAFETY AND HEALTH INFORMATION (F–44)
4676 Columbia Parkway
Cincinnati, OH 45226
(800)35–NIOSH
(513)533–8326
(513)533–8573 (Fax)
Provides technical information support for National Institute for Occupational Health and Safety (NIOSH) research programs and disseminates information to others on request. Services include reference and referral, interlibrary loans, and information about NIOSH studies. Distributes a subject–indexed catalog of NIOSH materials with information about availability. Publications list issued periodically. Maintains automated data-base covering the field of occupational safety and health and a library open to the public. (See also T–168)

National Oral Health Information Clearinghouse (F–45)
1 NOHIC Way
Bethesda, MD 20892–3500
(301)402–7364
nidr@aerie.com (Internet)
Sponsored by the National Institute of Dental Research, NOHIC provides information to dentists about treatment and to patients and their families about appropriate oral health care. Maintains a computerized catalog of publications and other materials.

President's Council on PHYSICAL FITNESS and Sports (F–46)
701 Pennsylvania Avenue, NW.
Suite 250
Washington, DC 20004
(202)272–3430
(202)504–2064 (Fax)
Conducts a public service advertising program, prepares educational materials, and works to promote the development of physical fitness leadership, facilities, and programs. Helps schools, clubs, recreation agencies, employers, and Federal

Organizations / Healthfinder

agencies design and implement programs. Offers a variety of testing, recognition, and incentive programs for individuals, institutions, and organizations. Materials on exercise and physical fitness for all ages are available.

POLICY Information Center (F–47)
Office of the Assistant Secretary for Planning and Evaluation
U.S. Department of Health and Human Services
Hubert H. Humphrey Building
Room 438F
200 Independence Avenue, SW.
Washington, DC 20201
(202)690–6445
(202)690–6518 (Fax)
A centralized repository of evaluations, short-term evaluative research reports and program inspections/audits relevant to the Department's operations, programs, and policies. It also includes relevant reports from the General Accounting Office (GAO), Congressional Budget Office (CBO), Office of Technology Assessment (OTA), and the Institute of Medicine and the National Research Council's Committee on National Statistics, both part of the National Academy of Sciences, Departments of Agriculture, Labor, and Education, as well as from the private sector. Final reports and executive summaries are available for review at the facility, or final reports may be purchased from the National Technical Information Service (NTIS). In addition, the PIC online data-base of evaluation abstracts are accessible on Internet through HHS HomePage, http://www.os.dhhs.gov or gopher.os.dhhs.gov. The database includes over 6,000 project descriptions of both in-process and completed studies. PIC Highlights, a quarterly publication, features recently completed studies.

National Clearinghouse for PRIMARY CARE Information (F–48)
8201 Greensboro Drive
Suite 600
McLean, VA 22102
(703)821–8955, ext. 245
(703)821–2098 (Fax)
Sponsored by the Bureau of Primary Health Care (BPHC), Health Resources and Services Administration. Provides information services to support the planning, development, and delivery of ambulatory health care to urban and rural areas that have shortages of medical personnel and services. A primary role of the clearinghouse is to identify, obtain, and disseminate information to community and migrant health centers. Distributes publications focusing on ambulatory care, financial management, primary health care, and health services administration of special interest to professionals working in primary care centers funded by BPHC. Materials are available on health education, governing boards, financial management, administrative management, and clinical care. Bilingual medical phrase books, a directory of federally funded health centers, and an annotated bibliography are available also.

U.S. Consumer PRODUCT SAFETY Commission Hotline (F–49)
Washington, DC 20207
(800)638–2772
(800)638–8270 (TT)
(301)504–0580
(301)504–0399 (Fax)
Maintains the National Injury Information Clearinghouse, conducts investigations of alleged unsafe/defective products, and establishes product safety standards. Assists consumers in evaluating the comparative safety of products and conducts educational programs to increase consumer awareness. Operates the National Electronic Inquiry Surveillance System, which monitors a statistical sample of hospital emergency rooms for injuries associated with consumer products. Maintains free hotline to provide information about recalls and to receive reports on unsafe products and product-related injuries. Publications describe hazards associated with electrical products and children's toys. Spanish-speaking operator available through the toll-free number. (See also T–168, T–170, F–36)

National REHABILITATION Information Center (F–50)
8455 Colesville Road
Suite 935
Silver Spring, MD 20910
(800)346–2742 (Voice/TT)
(301)588–9284 (Voice/TT)
(301)587–1967 (Fax)
The National Rehabilitation Information Center (NARIC) is a library and information center on disability and rehabilitation. Funded by the National Institute on Disability and Rehabilitation Research, NARIC collects and disseminates the results of federally funded research projects. The collection, which also includes commercially published books, journal articles, and audiovisuals, grows at a rate of about 300 documents per month. (See also T–51)

RURAL Information Center Health Service (RICHS) (F–51)
National Agricultural Library
10301 Baltimore Boulevard
Room 304
Beltsville, MD 20705
(800)633–7701
(301)504–5547
(301)504–6856 (TDD)
(301)504–5181 (Fax)
Sponsored by the U.S. Department of Agriculture. Disseminates information on a variety of rural health issues including health professions, health care financing, special populations and the delivery of health care services. Provides information, referrals, publications, brief complimentary literature searches and access to an electronic bulletin board to professionals and the public. RICHS is funded by the Federal Office of Rural Health Policy, DHHS and is part of the USDA Rural Information Center, which provides information on rural issues such as economic development, local government viability and community well-being. (See also T–166)

Centers for Disease Control and Prevention (F–52)
Office on SMOKING and Health
4770 Buford Highway, NE.
Mail Stop K 50
Atlanta, GA 30341–3724
(800)CDC 1311
(404)488–5705
(404)488–5939 (Fax)
Leads and coordinates strategic efforts aimed at the prevention and cessation of tobacco use and the protection of non-smokers by: expanding the science base of tobacco control; building capacity to conduct tobacco control programs; communicating information to constituents and the public; and facilitating concerted action with and among partners. Develops and distributes the Surgeon General's Report on Smoking and Health. Coordinates a national public information and education program on tobacco use and health. A publication list is available upon request by calling (404)488–5705. Maintains a Technical Information Center with a Smoking and Health database comprised of over 60,000 records. The database is available both online and on CD-ROM. Call (404)488–5708 for additional electronic information. (See also F–4, F–10, F–23)

National SUDDEN INFANT–DEATH SYNDROME Resource Center (F–53)
8201 Greensboro Drive
Suite 600
McLean, VA 22102
(703)821–8955
(703)821–2098 (Fax)
Sponsored by the Maternal and Child Health Bureau, Health Resources and Services Administration. Provides information and educational materials on sudden infant death syndrome (SIDS), apnea, and other related issues. Responds to information requests from professionals and from the public. Maintains a library of standard reference materials on topics related to SIDS. Maintains and updates mailing lists of State programs, groups, and individuals concerned with SIDS. Also develops fact sheets, catalogs, and bibliographies on areas of special interest to the community. Conducts customized searches of database on SIDS, and SIDS-related materials. (See also T–135, T–159)

The YOUTH DEVELOPMENT Information Center (F–54)
National Agricultural Library
U.S. Department of Agriculture
10301 Baltimore Boulevard
Room 304
Beltsville, MD 20705
(301)504–6400
(301)504–6409 (Fax)
jkane@nalusda.gov (Internet)
Provides information services to professionals who plan, develop, implement, and evaluate programs designed to meet the changing needs of America's youth. Acquires print and audiovisual resources and develops resource lists and bibliographies. Collaborates with the National Extension Service in CYFERNET (Child, Youth and Family Education and Research Network) to use fully computer and communications technology in organizational collaborations and information management, so that a greater variety and amount of information will be made available to a larger proportion of the child, youth, and family serving community.

International Organizations

ARGENTINA

Argentinan Association of Dermatology, Asociacion Argentina De Dermatologia, Mexico 1720, 1100 Buenos Aires, Argentina; tel. 381–2737; FAX. 381–2737; Dr. Pedro H. Magnin, Chairman

BELGIUM

European Association of Poison, Centres and Clinical Toxicologists (EAPCCT), 1, rue Joseph Stallaert, 15, B–1060 Brussels, Belgium; tel. 2 3459474; FAX. 2 3475860; Dr. Allister Vale, President

International Federation of Oto–Rhino–Laryngological Societies, 1FOS–MISA–NKO Oosterweldlaan 24, 2610 WKRIJK, Belgium; tel. 3 4433611; Ms. Gadeyne, Administrator, Publication Manager

Verbond der Verzorgingsinstellingen V.Z.W., 1, Guimardstraat, Brussels 1040, Belgium; tel. 2 5118008; FAX. 2 5135269; Mrs. C. Boonen, M.D., General Director

BRAZIL

Fraternidade Crista De Doentes E Deficientes, Cap. Correa Pacheco 134, Americana, SP, 13470, Brazil; tel. 0 194 619754; Celso Zoppi

CANADA

Association des Medecins de Langue Francaise du Canada, 8355 St. Laurent Boulevard, Montreal, PQ H2P 2Z6, Canada; tel. 514/388–2228; FAX. 514/388–5335; Andre de Seve, Administrative Director

Canadian Anaesthetists' Society, One Eglinton Avenue East, Suite 208, Toronto, ON M4P 3A1, Canada; tel. 416/480–0602; FAX. 416/480–0320; Ann Andrews, Executive Director

Canadian Association of Medical Radiation Technologists, 280 Metcalfe Street, Suite 410, Ottawa, ON K2P 1R7, Canada; tel. 613/234–0012; FAX. 613/234–1097; Earl P. Rooney, Executive Director

Canadian Association of Pathologists, Office of the Secretariat, 190 Railway Street, P.O. Box 1570, Kingston, ON KZL 5C8, Canada; tel. 613–531–8889; FAX. 613–531–0626; Dr. Joan Sweet, Secretary-Treasurer

Canadian Association of Social Workers, 383 Parkdale Avenue, Suite 402, Ottawa, ON K1Y 4R4, Canada; tel. 613/729–6668; FAX. 613/725–3720; Eugenia Repetur Moreno, Executive Director

Canadian Cancer Society, 10 Alcorn Avenue, Suite 200, Toronto, ON M4V 3B1, Canada; tel. 416/961–7223; FAX. 416/961–4189; Dorothy Lamont, Chief Executive Officer

Canadian Cardiovascular Society, 360 Victoria Avenue, Suite 401, Westmount, PQ H3Z 2N4, Canada; tel. 514/482–3407; Dolores Lourenco, Executive Secretary

Canadian College of Health Record Administrators, Canadian Health Record Association, 250 Ferrand Drive, Suite 909, Don Mills, ON M3C 3G8, Canada; tel. 416/429–5835; FAX. 416/429–2967; Deborah Del Duca, Executive Director

Canadian Council of the Blind, 396 Cooper Street, Suite 405, Ottawa, ON K2P 2H7, Canada; tel. 613/567–0311; FAX. 613/567–2728; Mary Lee Moran, Executive Director

Canadian Council on Social Development, 441 Maclaren, Fourth Floor, Ottawa, ON K2P 2H3, Canada; tel. 613/236–8977; FAX. 613/236–2750; Nancy Perkins, Communications Coordinator

Canadian Dental Association, 1815 Alta Vista Drive, Ottawa, ON K1G 3Y6, Canada; tel. 613/523–1770; FAX. 613/523–7736; Jardine Neilson, Executive Director

Canadian Hospital Association/Association des hopitaux du Canada, 17 York Street, Suite 100, Ottawa, ON K1N 9J6, Canada; tel. 613/241–8005; FAX. 613/241–5055; Carol Clemenhagen, President

Canadian Medical Engineering Consultants, 594 Bush Street, Belfountain, ON L0N 1B0, Canada; tel. 519/927–3286; FAX. 519/927–9440; A. M. Dolan, President

Canadian Mental Health Association, 2160 Yonge Street, Toronto, ON M4S 2Z3, Canada; tel. 416/484–7750; FAX. 416/484–4617; Edward J. Pennington, General Director

Canadian National Institute for the Blind, 1931 Bayview Avenue, Toronto, ON M4G 4C8, Canada; tel. 416/480–7588; FAX. 416/480–7677; Euclid J. Herie, President, Chief Executive Officer

Canadian Nurses Association, 50 Driveway, Ottawa, ON K2P 1E2, Canada; tel. 613/237–2133; FAX. 613/237–3520; Judith Oulton, Executive Director

Canadian Orthopaedic Association, 1440 Ste. Catherine Street, W., Suite 421, Montreal, PQ H3G 1R8, Canada; tel. 514/874–9003; FAX. 514/874–0464; Robert F. Martin, M.D., Secretary

Canadian Pharmaceutical Association, 1785 Alta Vista Drive, Ottawa, ON K1G 3Y6, Canada; tel. 613/523–7877; FAX. 613/523–0445; Leroy C. Fevang, Executive Director

Canadian Physiotherapy Association, 890 Yonge Street, 9th Floor, Toronto, ON M4W 3P4, Canada; tel. 416/924–5312; FAX. 416/924–7335; Brenda Myers, Executive Director

Canadian Psychiatric Association, 237 Argyle Street, Suite 200, Ottawa, ON K2P 1B8, Canada; tel. 613/234–2815; FAX. 613/234–9857; Alex Saunders, Chief Executive Officer

Canadian Public Health Association, 1565 Carling Avenue, Suite 400, Ottawa, ON K1Z 8R1, Canada; tel. 613/725–3769; FAX. 613/725–9826; Gerald H. Dafoe, M.H.A., Executive Director

Canadian Rehabilitation Council for the Disabled, 45 Sheppard Avenue, E., Suite 801, Toronto, ON M2N 5W9, Canada; tel. 416/250–7490; FAX. 416/229–1371; Henry Botchford, National Executive Director

Canadian Society of Hospital Pharmacists, 1145 Hunt Club Road, Suite 350, Ottawa, ON K1V 0Y3, Canada; tel. 613/736–9733; FAX. 613/736–5660; Bill Leslie, Executive Director

Canadian Society of Laboratory Technologists, Box 2830, LCD 1, Hamilton, ON L8N 3N8, Canada; tel. 905/528–8642; FAX. 905/528–4968; E. Valerie Booth, Executive Director

Catholic Health Association of Canada, 1247 Kilborn Place, Ottawa, ON K1H 6K9, Canada; tel. 613/731–7148; FAX. 613/731–7797; Maryse Blollin, Director, Programs and Communications

College des medecins du Quebec, 2170, boul. Rene–Levesque Quest, Montreal, PQ H3H 2T8, Canada; tel. 514/933–4441; FAX. 514/993–3112; Joelle Lescop, MD, Secretary General

College of Family Physicians of Canada, 2630 Skymark Avenue, Mississauga, ON L4W 5A4, Canada; tel. 905/629–0900; FAX. 905/629–0893; Dr. Claude A. Renaud, Director, Professional Affairs

College of Physicians and Surgeons of New Brunswick, 400 Main Street, Suite 1078, Saint John, NB E2K 4N5, Canada; tel. 506/658–0959; FAX. 506/658–0859; Victor D. McLaughlin, M.D., FRCSC, Registrar

National Cancer Institute of Canada, 10 Alcorn Avenue, Suite 200, Toronto, ON M4V 3B1, Canada; tel. 416/961–7223; FAX. 416/961–4189; J. David Beatty, M.D., Executive Director

The Canadian Dietetic Association, 480 University Avenue, Suite 601, Toronto, ON M5G 1V2, Canada; tel. 416/596–0857, ext. 314; FAX. 416/596–0603; Marsha Sharp, Chief Executive Officer

The Canadian Hearing Society, 271 Spadina Road, Toronto, ON M5R 2V3, Canada; tel. 416/964–9595; FAX. 416/964–2066; Gordon Ryall, Executive Director

The Canadian Medical Association, Box 8650, Ottawa, ON K1G 0G8, Canada; tel. 613/731–9331; FAX. 613/731–7314; Leo-Paul Landry, M.D., Secretary General

The Canadian Red Cross Society, National Office, 1800 Alta Vista Drive, Ottawa, ON K1G 4J5, Canada; tel. 613/739–3000; FAX. 613/731–1411; M. T. Aye, M.B., Ph.D., FRCPC, National Director, Blood Services

The Royal College of Physicians and Surgeons of Canada, 774 Echo Drive, Ottawa, ON K1S 5N8, Canada; tel. 613/730–8177; FAX. 613/730–8830; Mrs. Pierrette Leonard, APR, Head Communications Section

World Federation of Hemophilia, 4616 St. Catherine Street, W., Montreal, PQ H3Z 1S3, Canada; tel. 514/933–7944; FAX. 514/933–8916; The Rev. Prebendary Alan J. Tanner

DENMARK

Amstraadsforeningen I Danmark, Landemaerket 10, P.O. Box 1144, DK–1010 Copenhagen K, Denmark; tel. 45 33 91 21 61; FAX. 45 33 11 21 15; Ida Sofie Jensen, Assistant Director

Danish Dental Association, Amaliegade 17, Postboks 143, DK–1004, Copenhagen, Denmark; tel. 45 33157711; FAX. 45 33151637; Karsten Thuen, Executive

National Committee for Danish Hospitals, Amtsraadsforeningen i Danmark, Landemaerket 10, P.O. Box 1144, DK–1010 Copenhagen K., Denmark; tel. 45 33 91 21 61; FAX. 45 33 11 21 15; Torben Stentoft, Assistant Director

ENGLAND

British Medical Association, B.M.A. House Tavistock Square, London, WCH1 9JP, England; tel. 0171/387–4499; FAX. 0171/383–6400; Dr. E. M. Armstrong, B.Sc., FRCP(Glas), FRCGP, Secretary

Institute of Health Services Management (United Kingdom and International), 39 Chalton Street, London, NW1 1JD, England; tel. 071/388–2626; FAX. 071/388–2386; Ray Rowden, SRN, RMN, MHSM

International Hospital Federation, Four Abbots Place, London, NW6 4NP, England; tel. 071–372 7181; FAX. 071/328 7433; Dr. Errol N. Pickering, Director General

King Edward's Hospital Fund for London, Two Palace Court, London, W2 4H5, England; tel. 071/727–0581; FAX. 071/727–7603; R. J. Maxwell, Chief Executive Officer, Secretary

Nuffield Provincial Hospitals Trust, 59 New Cavendish Street, London W1M 7RD, England; tel. 071/485–6632; FAX. 071/485–8215; Dr. Michael Ashley–Miller, Secretary

FRANCE

World Medical Association, 28 avenue des Alpes–01210 Ferney–Voltaire, France, P.O. Box 63, 01212 Ferney–Voltaire, France; tel. 50 407575; FAX. 50 405937; Dr. Ian Field, Secretary General

GERMANY

Deutsche Krankenhausgesellschaft, (German Hospital Federation), Tersteegenstrasse 9, D40474, Dusseldorf, Germany; tel. 211 454730; FAX. 211 4547361; Dr. Klaus Proessdorf, Director General

International Academy of Cytology, Universitaets–Frauenklinik, Hugstetterstrausse 55, D–79106 Freiburg i. Br., Germany; tel. 761 2703012; FAX. 761 2703112; Manuel Hilgarth, M.D., F.I.A.C.

HUNGARY

Magyar Korhazszovetseg, Furedi utca 9/c. VIII.34., 1144 Hungary, Budapest, Hungary; tel. (36–1) 163-52–73; FAX. (36–1) 163–52–73; Dr. I. Mikola, President

Organizations / International Organizations

KOREA

Korean Hospital Association, (Mapo Hyun Dai Building), 35-1 Mapo-dong, Mapo-gu, Seoul 121-050, Korea; tel. 2 7187521; FAX. 2 7187522; Ho Uk Ha, Ph.D., Vice President

MEXICO

Federacion Latinoamericana de Hospitales, Apartado Postal 107-076, C.P. 06741, Mexico D.F., Mexico; tel. 5 482650; Dr. Guillermo Fajardo, Representative

NETHERLANDS

Federation of Health Care Organizations in the Netherlands, Postbus 9696, NL-3506 GR Utrecht, Netherlands; tel. 30 739911; FAX. 30 739438

International Society of General Practice, Societas Internationalis Medicinae Generalis (SIMG), Helvoirtseweg 183 A, NL-5263 EC Vught, Netherlands; tel. +31 73 564242; FAX. +31 73 570156

NEW ZEALAND

Health Boards New Zealand Incorporated, P.O. Box 714, Wellington One, FA, New Zealand; tel. 4 736181; FAX. 4 711227; John M. Rennie, Executive Director

PERU

Peruvian Hospital Association, Av. Dos De Mayo 8502 Of. 203, San Isidro, Lima 27, Peru; tel. 14 419546; Arturo Vasi Paez, President

PHILIPPINES

Philippine Hospital Association, 14 Kamias Rd., Quezon City-1102 Metro Ma, Philippines; tel. 2 9227674/75; Thelma Navarrete-Clemente, M.D., M.H.A., President

SOUTH AFRICA

Provincial Administration, Health Services Branch, P.O. Box 517, Bloemfontein 9300, South Africa, South Africa; tel. 051/4055818; FAX. 051/304958; Dr. J. H. Kotze

SWITZERLAND

Vereinigung Schweizerischer Krankenhaeuser, (VESKA—Swiss Hospital Association.), Box 4202, Rain 32, CH-5001, Aarau, Switzerland; tel. 64 24 12 22; FAX. 64 22 33 35; Mr. N. Undritz, Secretary General

World Health Organization, 20 Avenue Appia, CH-1211 Geneva 27, Switzerland; tel. 22 791 21 11; FAX. 22 791 07 46; Hiroshi Nakajima, M.D., Ph.D., Director-General

UNITED STATES

American College of Gastroenterology, 4900B South 31st Street, Arlington, VA 22206, United States; tel. 703/820-7400; FAX. 703/931-4520; Thomas F. Fise, Executive Director

American Society for Testing and Materials, 1916 Race Street, Philadelphia, PA 19103, United States; tel. 215/299-5520; FAX. 215/299-2630; Kenneth C. Pearson, Vice President

International Academy of Podiatric Medicine (IAPM), 4603 Highway 95 South, P.O. Box 39, Cocolalla, ID 83813-0039, United States; tel. 208/683-3900; FAX. 208/683-3700; Judith A. Baerg, Executive Director

International Association for Dental Research, 1111 14th Street, N.W., Suite 1000, Washington, DC 20005, United States; tel. 202/898-1050; FAX. 202/789-1033; John J. Clarkson, BDS, Ph.D., Executive Director

Rehabilitation International, 25 East 21st Street, New York, NY 10010, United States; tel. 212/420-1500; FAX. 212/505-0871; John Stott, President

Sigma Theta Tau International Honor Society of Nursing, 550 West North Street, Indianapolis, IN 46202, United States; tel. 317/634-8171; FAX. 317/634-8188; Nancy A. Dickenson-Hazard, Executive Officer

World Federation of Public Health Associations, c/o APHA, 1015 15th Street, N.W., Washington, DC 20005, United States; tel. 202/789-5696; FAX. 202/789-5681; Diane Kuntz, M.P.H., Executive Secretary

VENEZUELA

Latin American Association for the Study of the Liver (LAASL), P.O. Box 51890, Sabana Grande, Caracas, 1050-A, Venezuela; tel. 58-2-9799380; FAX. 58-2-9799380; Dr. Miguel A. Garassini, President

U.S. GOVERNMENT AGENCIES

Specific addresses have been omitted because of the many changes presently occurring, and scheduled for the future among federal agencies. The telephone numbers given are general public information numbers, unless specifically identified with the officials listed.
The following information is based on data available as of March 1995.
For more information about U.S. government agencies, consult the U.S. Government Manual, *available from the Office of the* Federal Register, *National Archives and Records Service, Washington, DC 20408. A telephone directory of the U.S. Department of Health and Human Services is available from the Superintendent of Documents, Government Printing Office, Washington, DC 20402. Additional assistance may be obtained by contacting the American Hospital Association's Washington office, 325 Seventh Street, N.W., Washington, DC 20004.*

Executive Office of the President
tel. 202/456-1414
Counsel to the President: Abner Mikva; 202/456-2632
Chief of Staff: Leon Panetta; 202/456-6797
Assistant to the President for Economic Policy: Robert Rubin; 202/456-2174
Assistant to the President for Domestic Policy: Carol Rasco; 202/456-2216
Assistant to the President and Director of Public Liaison: Alexis M. Herman; 202/456-2930
COUNCIL OF ECONOMIC ADVISORS
Chairman: Laura D'Andra Tyson; 202/395-5042
OFFICE OF MANAGEMENT AND BUDGET
Director: Alice Rivlin; 202/395-4840

Department of Agriculture
tel. 202/720-8732
Secretary: Dan Glickman; 202/720-3631

Department of Commerce
tel. 202/482-2000
Secretary: Ronald H. Brown; 202/482-2112
BUREAU OF ECONOMIC ANALYSIS
Director: Carol S. Carson; 202/606-9606
ECONOMIC DEVELOPMENT ADMINISTRATION
Acting Assistant Secretary: Wilbur F. Hawkins; 202/482-5067
NATIONAL BUREAU OF STANDARDS
Director: Arati Prabhakar; 301/975-2300

Department of Defense
tel. 202/545-6700
Secretary: William J. Perry; 703/695-5261
Assistant Secretary of Defense (Health Affairs): Dr. Stephen Joseph; 703/697-2111
CIVILIAN HEALTH AND MEDICAL PROGRAMS OF THE UNIFORMED SERVICES (CHAMPUS) (Denver, CO)
Director: Capt. Paul T. McDavid; 303/361-8606
UNIFORMED SERVICES UNIVERSITY OF THE HEALTH SCIENCES
President: James A. Zimble; 301/295-3013
DEPARTMENT OF THE AIR FORCE
Surgeon General: Lt. Gen. Edgar R. Anderson, Jr.; 202/767-4343
DEPARTMENT OF THE ARMY
Surgeon General: Lt. Gen. Alcide M. LaNoue; 703/756-0000
DEPARTMENT OF THE NAVY
Surgeon General of the Navy: V.ADM. Donald F. Hagen; 202/653-1144

Department of Education
tel. 202/708-5366
Secretary: Richard W. Riley; 202/401-3000

Department of Health and Human Services
tel. 202/619-0257
Secretary: Donna E. Shalala; 202/690-7000
General Counsel: Harriet Rabb; 202/690-7741
MANAGEMENT AND BUDGET
Assistant Secretary: Kenneth Apfel; 202/690-6396
HEALTH
Assistant Secretary: Dr. Philip Lee; 202/690-7694
ADMINISTRATION FOR CHILDREN AND FAMILIES
Assistant Secretary: Mary Jo Bane; 202/401-2337
LEGISLATION
Assistant Secretary: Jerry D. Klepner; 202/690-7627
PLANNING AND EVALUATION
Assistant Secretary: David T. Ellwood; 202/690-7858
PUBLIC AFFAIRS
Assistant Secretary: Avis La Velle; 202/690-7850
PUBLIC HEALTH SERVICE
Acting Surgeon General: Audrey F. Manely, M.D., M.P.H.; 202/690-6467
Alcohol, Drug Abuse, and Mental Health Administration, Rockville, MD
Administrator: Nelba Chavez, Ph.D.; 301/443-4795
Center for Disease Control, Atlanta 30333
Deputy Director: Dr. Claire V. Broome; 404/639-3291
Food and Drug Administration, Rockville, MD 20857
Commissioner: David Kessler, M.D.; 301/443-2410
Health Resources and Services Administration, Hyattsville, MD 20782
Administrator: Ciro Sumaya, Ph.D.; 301/443-2216
National Institutes of Health, Bethesda, MD 20014
Director: Harold Varmus, M.D.; 301/496-2433
HEALTH CARE FINANCING ADMINISTRATION
Administrator: Bruce C. Vladeck; 202/690-6726
SOCIAL SECURITY ADMINISTRATION: Baltimore, MD 21235
Commissioner: Dr. Shirley S. Chater; 410/965-7700
Regional Commissioners telephone: 1-800/772-1213
(1) Boston
Robert C. Green
(2) New York
Peter P. DiSturco
(3) Philadelphia
Larry G. Massanari
(4) Atlanta
Gordon M. Sherman
(5) Chicago
Paul D. Barnes
(6) Dallas
Noel D. Wall
(7) Kansas City
Peggy Foertschbeck
(8) Denver
Guadalupe Salinas
(9) San Francisco
Linda S. McMahon
(10) Seattle
Donald N. Mings

Department of Housing and Urban Development
tel. 202/708-1112
Secretary: Henry Cisneros; 202/708-0417

Department of Justice
tel. 202/514-2000
Attorney General: Janet Reno; 202/514-2001
DRUG ENFORCEMENT ADMINISTRATION
Administrator: Thomas A. Constantine; 202/307-8000

Department of Labor
tel. 202/219-5000
Secretary: Robert Reich (Honorable); 202/219-8271
BUREAU OF LABOR STATISTICS
Commissioner: Katharine G. Abraham; 202/606-7800
EMPLOYMENT AND TRAINING ADMINISTRATION
Assistant Secretary: Doug Ross; 202/219-6050
OCCUPATIONAL SAFETY AND HEALTH ADMINISTRATION
Assistant Secretary: Joseph A. Dear; 202/219-7162

Department of State
tel. 202/647-4000
Secretary: Warren Christopher: 202/647-6575
AGENCY FOR INTERNATIONAL DEVELOPMENT
Administrator: J. Brian Atwood; 202/647-9620

Independent Agencies
U.S. COMMISSION ON CIVIL RIGHTS
Chairperson: Mary F. Berry; 202/376-7572
CONSUMER PRODUCT SAFETY COMMISSION
Chairperson: Ann Brown; 301/504-0500
ENVIRONMENTAL PROTECTION AGENCY
Administrator: Carol M. Browner; 202/260-4700
EQUAL EMPLOYMENT OPPORTUNITY COMMISSION
Chairman: Gilbert Casellas; 202/663-4001
FEDERAL EMERGENCY MANAGEMENT AGENCY
Director: James Lee Witt; 202/646-3923

Government-Related Groups
Federally aided corporations and quasi-official agencies, such as American Red Cross, National Academy of Sciences and World Health Organization, are listed with International, National, and Regional Organizations beginning on page C3.

State and Local Organizations and Agencies

Blue Cross–Blue Shield Plans

The following list of Blue Cross and Blue Shield Plans is based on the Winter 1995 edition of the Directory Blue Cross and Blue Shield Plans, obtained from Blue Cross and Blue Shield Association, 676 North St. Clair, Chicago, IL 60611; tel. 312/440–6000. When addressing mail to a plan, use the post office box number.

United States

ALABAMA: Blue Cross and Blue Shield of Alabama, 450 Riverchase Parkway, E., P.O. Box 995, Birmingham, AL 35298; tel. 205/988–2200; FAX. 205/988–2949; E. Gene Thrasher, President, Chief Executive Officer

ALASKA: Blue Cross of Washington and Alaska, Blue Cross and Blue Shield of Alaska, 7001 220th Street, S.W., Mountlake Terrace, WA 98045–2124, P.O. Box 327, Seattle, WA 98111–0327; tel. 206/670–5900; FAX. 206/670–4900; Betty Woods, President, Chief Executive Officer

ARIZONA: Blue Cross and Blue Shield of Arizona, Inc., 2444 West Las Palmaritas Drive, Zip 85021, P.O. Box 13466, Phoenix, AZ 85002–3466; tel. 602/864–4400; FAX. 602/864–4242; Robert B. Bulla, President, Chief Executive Officer

ARKANSAS: Arkansas Blue Cross and Blue Shield, a Mutual Insurance Company, 601 Gaines Street, Zip 72201, P.O. Box 2181, Little Rock, AR 72203; tel. 501/378–2010; FAX. 501/378–2037; Robert L. Shoptaw, President, Chief Executive Officer

CALIFORNIA: Blue Cross of California, 21555 Oxnard Street, Woodland Hills, CA 91367, P.O. Box 70000, Van Nuys, CA 91470; tel. 818/703–2345; FAX. 818/703–2848; Leonard D. Schaeffer, Chairman, Chief Executive Officer

Blue Shield of California, California Physicians' Service Corporation, Two North Point, Zip 94133, P.O. Box 7168, San Francisco, CA 94120; tel. 209/634–9121; FAX. 415/445–5056; Thomas C. Paton, Chairman

COLORADO: Blue Cross and Blue Shield of Colorado, Rocky Mountain Hospital and Medical Service, 700 Broadway, Denver, CO 80273–0002; tel. 303/831–2131; FAX. 303/830–0887; C. David Kikumoto, President, Chief Executive Officer

CONNECTICUT: Blue Cross and Blue Shield of Connecticut, Inc., 370 Bassett Road, P.O. Box 504, North Haven, CT 06473; tel. 203/239–4911; FAX. 203/239–7742; John F. Croweak, Chairman, Chief Executive Officer

DELAWARE: Blue Cross and Blue Shield of Delaware, Blue Cross and Blue Shield of Delaware, Inc., One Brandywine Gateway, P.O. Box 1991, Wilmington, DE 19899; tel. 302/429–0260; FAX. 302/421–2089; Robert C. Cole, Jr., President, Chief Executive Officer

DISTRICT OF COLUMBIA: Blue Cross and Blue Shield of the National Capital Area, 550 12th Street, S.W., Washington, DC 20065; tel. 202/479–8000; FAX. 202/479–3520; Larry C. Glasscock, President, Chief Executive Officer

FLORIDA: Blue Cross and Blue Shield of Florida, Inc., 532 Riverside Avenue, Zip 32202, P.O. Box 1798, Jacksonville, FL 32231–0014; tel. 904/354–3331; FAX. 904/791–8738; William E. Flaherty, President

GEORGIA: Blue Cross and Blue Shield of Georgia, Inc., Capital City Plaza, 3350 Peachtree Road, N.E., Zip 30326, P.O. Box 4445, Atlanta, GA 30302–4445; tel. 404/842–8000; FAX. 404/842–8010; Richard D. Shirk, President, Chief Executive Officer

HAWAII: Hawaii Medical Service Association, P.O. Box 860, Honolulu, HI 96808; tel. 808/948–5110; FAX. 808/948–6555; Robert P. Hiam, President

IDAHO: Blue Cross of Idaho Health Service, Inc., 1501 Federal Way, Zip 83705, P.O. Box 7408, Boise, ID 83707; tel. 208/345–4550; FAX. 208/331–7311; David L. Barnett, President, Chief Executive Officer

Blue Shield of Idaho, Medical Service Bureau of Idaho, Inc., 1602 21st Avenue, P.O. Box 1106, Lewiston, ID 83501; tel. 208/746–2671; FAX. 208/743–7091; Rich D. Nelson, President, Chief Executive Officer

ILLINOIS: Blue Cross and Blue Shield of Illinois, Health Care Service Corporation, a Mutual Legal Reserve Company, 233 North Michigan Avenue, Zip 60601, P.O. Box 1364, Chicago, IL 60690; tel. 312/938–7500; FAX. 312/819–1220; Raymond F. McCaskey, President, Chief Executive Officer

INDIANA: Blue Cross and Blue Shield of Indiana, Associated Insurance Companies, Inc., Blue Cross and Blue Shield of Kentucky, 120 Monument Circle, Indianapolis, IN 46204; tel. 317/488–6489; FAX. 317/488–6477; L. Ben Lytle, President, Chief Executive Officer, Chairman

IOWA: Blue Cross and Blue Shield of Iowa, IASD Health Services Corp., Blue Cross of South Dakota, 636 Grand Avenue, Des Moines, IA 50309; tel. 515/245–4545; FAX. 515/245–5090; Robert D. Ray, President, Chief Executive Officer

KANSAS: Blue Cross and Blue Shield of Kansas, Inc., 1133 Topeka Boulevard, Zip 66629–0001, P.O. Box 239, Topeka, KS 66601–0239; tel. 800/432–3990; FAX. 913/291–8465; Thomas L. Miller, President, Chief Executive Officer

KENTUCKY: Blue Cross and Blue Shield of Kentucky, Associated Insurance Companies, Inc., 9901 Linn Station Road, Louisville, KY 40223; tel. 502/423–2011; FAX. 502/423–6632; James T. Murphy, President, Chief Executive Officer

LOUISIANA: Blue Cross and Blue Shield of Louisiana, Louisiana Health Service and Indemnity Company, 5525 Reitz Avenue, Zip 70809–3802, P.O. Box 98029, Baton Rouge, LA 70898–9029; tel. 504/295–2511; FAX. 504/295–2506; P. J. Mills, President, Chief Executive Officer

MAINE: Blue Cross and Blue Shield of Maine, Associated Hospital Service of Maine, Two Gannett Drive, South Portland, ME 04106–6911; tel. 207/822–7000; FAX. 207/822–7350; Andrew W. Greene, President, Chief Executive Officer

MARYLAND: Blue Cross and Blue Shield of Maryland, Inc., 10455 Mill Run Circle, P.O. Box 1010, Owings Mills, MD 21117; tel. 800/524–4555; FAX. 410/998–5576; William L. Jews, President, Chief Executive Officer

MASSACHUSETTS: Blue Cross and Blue Shield of Massachusetts, Inc., 100 Summer Street, Boston, MA 02110; tel. 617/956–4000; FAX. 617/832–3355; William C. Van Faasen, President, Chief Executive Officer

MICHIGAN: Blue Cross and Blue Shield of Michigan, 600 Lafayette East, Detroit, MI 48226–2998; tel. 313/225–8000; FAX. 313/225–6239; Richard E. Whitmer, President, Chief Executive Officer

MINNESOTA: Blue Cross and Blue Shield of Minnesota, 3535 Blue Cross Road, Zip 55122, P.O. Box 64560, St. Paul, MN 55164; tel. 612/456–5210; FAX. 612/456–1657; Andrew P. Czajkowski, President, Chief Executive Officer

MISSISSIPPI: Blue Cross and Blue Shield of Mississippi, Inc., 3545 Lakeland Drive, E., Zip 39208, P.O. Box 1043, Jackson, MS 39215–1043; tel. 601/932–3800; FAX. 601/939–7035; Richard J. Hale, Executive Vice President, Chief Executive Officer

MISSOURI: Blue Cross and Blue Shield of Kansas City, 2301 Main, Zip 64108, P.O. Box 419169, Kansas City, MO 64141–6169; tel. 816/395–2222; FAX. 816/395–2035; Richard P. Krecker, President, Chief Executive Officer

Blue Cross and Blue Shield of Missouri, Alliance Blue Cross Blue Shield, RightChoice Managed Care, Inc., 1831 Chestnut Street, St. Louis, MO 63103–2275; tel. 314/923–4444; FAX. 314/923–5002; Roy R. Heimburger, President, Chief Executive Officer

MONTANA: Blue Cross and Blue Shield of Montana, Inc., 404 Fuller Avenue, Zip 59601, P.O. Box 4309, Helena, MT 59604; tel. 406/447–8600; FAX. 406/442–6946; Alan F. Cain, President, Chief Executive Officer

NEBRASKA: Blue Cross and Blue Shield of Nebraska, 7261 Mercy Road, P.O. Box 3248 Main P.O. Station, Omaha, NE 68180–0001; tel. 402/390–1800; FAX. 402/392–2141; Richard L. Guffey, Chairman of the Board, Chief Executive Officer

NEVADA: Blue Cross and Blue Shield of Nevada, 5250 South Virginia Street, Zip 89502, P.O. Box 10330, Reno, NV 89520–0330; tel. 702/829–4040; FAX. 702/829–4101; C. David Kikumoto, President, Chief Executive Officer

NEW HAMPSHIRE: Blue Cross and Blue Shield of New Hampshire, New Hampshire–Vermont Health Service, 3000 Goffs Falls Road, Manchester, NH 03111–0001; tel. 800/225–2666; FAX. 603/695–7304; Joseph L. Marcille, CLU, President, Chief Executive Officer

NEW JERSEY: Blue Cross and Blue Shield of New Jersey, Inc., Three Penn Plaza East, P.O. Box 420, Newark, NJ 07105–2200; tel. 201/466–4000; William J. Marino, President, Chief Executive Officer

NEW MEXICO: Blue Cross and Blue Shield of New Mexico, New Mexico Blue Cross and Blue Shield, Inc., 12800 Indian School Road, N.E., Zip 87112, P.O. Box 27630, Albuquerque, NM 87125–7630; tel. 505/292–2600; FAX. 505/291–3541; C. David Kikumoto, President, Chief Executive Officer

NEW YORK: Blue Cross and Blue Shield of Central New York, Inc., 344 South Warren Street, Zip 13202, P.O. Box 4809, Syracuse, NY 13221–4809; tel. 315/448–3902; FAX. 315/448–6763; Albert F. Antonini, President, Chief Executive Officer

Blue Cross and Blue Shield of Utica–Watertown, Inc., 12 Rhoads Drive, Utica Business Park, Utica, NY 13502–6398; tel. 315/798–4238; FAX. 315/797–4298; Sondra L. Rafferty, President

Blue Cross and Blue Shield of Western New York, Inc., 1901 Main Street, Zip 14208, P.O. Box 80, Buffalo, NY 14240–0080; tel. 716/884–2911; FAX. 716/887–8981; Richard A. Villari, CLU, CHC, President

Blue Cross of the Rochester Area, Inc., a Finger Lakes Company, Blue Shield of the Rochester Area, Inc., a Finger Lakes Company, 150 East Main Street, Rochester, NY 14647; tel. 716/325–3630; FAX. 716/238–4400; Howard J. Berman, President, Chief Executive Officer

Organizations / Blue Cross–Blue Shield Plans

Empire Blue Cross and Blue Shield, 622 Third Avenue, Zip 10017-6758, P.O. Box 345, New York, NY 10163-0345; tel. 212/261-5962; FAX. 212/983-7615; Michael A. Stocker, M.D., President, Chief Executive Offic

NORTH CAROLINA: Blue Cross and Blue Shield of North Carolina, 5901 Chapel Hill Road, Zip 27707-0718, P.O. Box 2291, Durham, NC 27702; tel. 919/489-7431; FAX. 919/490-0171; Kenneth C. Otis II, President

NORTH DAKOTA: Blue Cross Blue Shield of North Dakota, 4510 13th Avenue, S.W., Fargo, ND 58121-0001; tel. 800/342-4718; FAX. 701/282-1866; Michael B. Unhjem, President, Chief Executive Officer

OHIO: Blue Cross and Blue Shield of Ohio, Blue Cross and Blue Shield Mutual of Ohio, 2060 East Ninth Street, Cleveland, OH 44115-1355; tel. 216/687-7000; FAX. 216/687-6044; John Burry, Jr., Chairman of the Board, Chief Executive Officer

The Community Mutual Insurance Company, 1351 William Howard Taft Road, Cincinnati, OH 45206; tel. 513/977-8811; FAX. 513/977-8812; Dwane R. Houser, Chairman of the Board, Chief Executive Officer

OKLAHOMA: Blue Cross and Blue Shield of Oklahoma, (Group Health Service of Oklahoma, Inc.), 1215 South Boulder Avenue, Zip 74119-2800, P.O. Box 3283, Tulsa, OK 74102-3283; tel. 918/560-3500; FAX. 918/560-2095; Ralph S. Rhoades, Chief Executive Officer

OREGON: Blue Cross and Blue Shield of Oregon, 100 S.W. Market Street, Zip 97201, P.O. Box 1271, Portland, OR 97207; tel. 800/452-7390; FAX. 503/225-5232; Richard L. Woolworth, President, Chief Executive Officer

PENNSYLVANIA: Blue Cross of Northeastern Pennsylvania, Hospital Service Association of Northeastern Pennsylvania, 70 North Main Street, Wilkes Barre, PA 18711; tel. 717/829-8500; FAX. 717/829-0188; Thomas J. Ward, President, Chief Executive Officer

Blue Cross of Western Pennsylvania, Veritus, Inc., 120 Fifth Avenue, Pittsburgh, PA 15222-3099; tel. 412/255-7000; FAX. 412/255-8240; William Lowry, President

Capital Blue Cross, 2500 Elmerton Avenue, Harrisburg, PA 17177-1032; tel. 717/255-0820; FAX. 717/541-6072; James M. Mead, President, Chief Executive Officer

Independence Blue Cross, 1901 Market Street, Philadelphia, PA 19103; tel. 800/358-0050; FAX. 215/241-3824; G. Fred DiBona, Jr., Esq., President, Chief Executive Officer

Pennsylvania Blue Shield, Medical Service Association of Pennsylvania, 1800 Center Street, Zip 17011, P.O.Box 890089, Camp Hill, PA 17089-0089; tel. 800/637-3493; FAX. 717/763-3544; Samuel D. Ross, Jr., President, Chief Executive Officer

RHODE ISLAND: Blue Cross and Blue Shield of Rhode Island, 444 Westminster Street, Providence, RI 02903-3279; tel. 401/831-7300; FAX. 401/351-2050; Douglas J. McIntosh, President

SOUTH CAROLINA: Blue Cross and Blue Shield of South Carolina, I-20 East at Alpine Road, Columbia, SC 29219; tel. 803/788-3860; FAX. 803/736-3420; M. Edward Sellers, President, Chief Executive Officer

SOUTH DAKOTA: Blue Cross of South Dakota, IASD Health Services Corp., Regional Service Center, Hamilton Boulevard and I-29, P.O. Box 1677, Sioux City, IA 51102; tel. 712/279-8400; FAX. 712/279-8450; Bob O'Connell Vice President, General Manager, Regional Service Center

South Dakota Blue Shield, South Dakota Medical Service, Inc., 1601 West Madison Street, Sioux Falls, SD 57104; tel. 605/336-1976; FAX. 605/336-5613; Ben R. Johnson, President

TENNESSEE: Blue Cross and Blue Shield of Memphis, Memphis Hospital Service and Surgical Association, Inc., 85 North Danny Thomas Boulevard, Zip 38103, P.O. Box 98, Memphis, TN 38101; tel. 901/544-2111; FAX. 901/544-2440; Gene Holcomb, President, Chief Executive Officer

Blue Cross and Blue Shield of Tennessee, 801 Pine Street, Chattanooga, TN 37402; tel. 615/755-5600; FAX. 615/755-2178; Thomas Kinser, Chief Executive Officer

TEXAS: Blue Cross and Blue Shield of Texas, Inc., 901 South Central Expressway, Richardson, TX 75080, P.O. Box 655730, Dallas, TX 75265-5730; tel. 214/766-6900; FAX. 214/766-6060; Rogers K. Coleman, M.D., President, Chief Executive Officer

UTAH: Blue Cross and Blue Shield of Utah, 2455 Parley's Way, P.O. Box 30270, Salt Lake City, UT 84130-0270; tel. 801/481-6198; FAX. 801/481-6994; Jed H. Pitcher, Chairman of the Board, President, Chief Executive Officer

VERMONT: Blue Cross and Blue Shield of Vermont, One East Road, Berlin, VT 05602, P.O. Box 186, Montpelier, VT 05601; tel. 802/223-6131; FAX. 802/229-0511; Preston Jordan, President, Chief Executive Officer

VIRGINIA: Trigon Blue Cross Blue Shield, Blue Cross and Blue Shield of Virginia, 2015 Staples Mill Road, Zip 23230, P.O. Box 27401, Richmond, VA 23279; tel. 804/354-7173; FAX. 804/354-7044; Norwood H. Davis, Jr., Chairman of the Board, Chief Executive Officer

WASHINGTON: Blue Cross of Washington and Alaska, Blue Shield in North Central Washington, 7001 220th Street, S.W., Mountlake Terrace, WA 98043-2124, P.O. Box 327, Seattle, WA 98111-0327; tel. 206/670-5900; FAX. 206/670-4900; Betty Woods, President, Chief Executive Officer

King County Medical Blue Shield, 1800 Ninth Avenue, Zip 98101-1322, P.O. Box 21267, Seattle, WA 98111-3267; tel. 206/464-3600; FAX. 206/389-6778; Dale M. Francis, President, Chief Executive Officer

Medical Service Corporation of Eastern Washington, 3900 East Sprague Avenue, Zip 99202, P.O. Box 3048, Spokane, WA 99220-3048; tel. 509/536-4500; FAX. 509/536-4770; Fred A. Jacot, President, Chief Executive Officer

Pierce County Medical Bureau, Inc., 1501 Market Street, Zip 98402, P.O. Box 2354, Tacoma, WA 98401-2354; tel. 206/597-6557; FAX. 206/597-7475; Donald P. Sacco, President

Washington Physicians Service Association, 1800 Ninth Avenue, Zip 98101, P.O. Box 2010, Seattle, WA 98111; tel. 206/389-7520; FAX. 206/389-7521; William Van Hollebeke, Executive Director

WEST VIRGINIA: Mountain State Blue Cross and Blue Shield, Inc., 700 Market Square, Zip 26101, P.O. Box 1948, Parkersburg, WV 26102; tel. 304/424-7701; FAX. 304/424-7730; Kent W. Clapp, Chief Executive Officer

WISCONSIN: Blue Cross and Blue Shield United of Wisconsin, 401 West Michigan Street, Zip 53203, P.O. Box 2025, Milwaukee, WI 53201; tel. 414/224-6100; FAX. 414/226-5488; Thomas R. Hefty, Chairman, Chief Executive Officer

WYOMING: Blue Cross and Blue Shield of Wyoming, 4000 House Avenue, P.O. Box 2266, Cheyenne, WY 82003-2266; tel. 307/634-1393; FAX. 307/778-8582; C. E. Chapman, President

U.S. Associated Areas

JAMAICA: Blue Cross of Jamaica, 85 Hope Road, Kingston 6, JA, West Indies; tel. 809/927-9821, ext. 224; FAX. 809/927-9817; Henry Lowe, Ph.D., C.D., J.P., President, Chief Executive Officer

PUERTO RICO: La Cruz Azul de Puerto Rico, Blue Cross of Puerto Rico, Carretera Estatal 1, K.M. 17.3–Rio Piedras, PR 00927, P.O. Box 366068, San Juan, PR 00936-6068; tel. 809/272-9898; FAX. 809/272-7817; Jose Julian Alvarez, Executive President

Triple-S, Inc., Avenida F.D. Roosevelt 1441, Caparra, PR 00920, P.O. Box 363628, San Juan, PR 00936-3628; tel. 809/749-4114; FAX. 809/749-4191; Miguel A. Vazquez-Deynes, President

Canada

ALBERTA: Alberta Blue Cross Plan, 10009–108th Street, Edmonton, AB T5J 3C5, CANADA; tel. 403/428-1100; FAX. 403/498-8532; V. George Ward, President, Chief Executive Officer

BRITISH COLUMBIA: Medical Services Association, 2025 West Broadway, P.O. Box 9300, Vancouver, BC V6B 5M1, CANADA; tel. 604/737-5700; FAX. 604/737-5781; John D. Seney, President, Chief Executive Officer

MANITOBA: Manitoba Blue Cross, United Health Services Corporation, 100A Polo Park Centre, 1485 Portage Avenue, Zip R3G 0W4, P.O. Box 1046, Winnipeg, MB R3C 2X7, CANADA; tel. 204/775-0151; FAX. 204/774-1761; Kerry V. Bittner, President

NEW BRUNSWICK: Blue Cross of Atlantic Canada, 644 Main Street, Zip E1C 1E2, P.O. Box 220, Moncton, NB E1C 8L3, CANADA; tel. 506/853-1811; FAX. 506/853-4651; Leon R. Furlong, President, Chief Executive Officer

NEWFOUNDLAND: Blue Cross of Atlantic Canada, 644 Main Street, Zip E1C 1E2, P.O. Box 220, Moncton, NB E1C 8L3; tel. 506/853-1811; FAX. 506/853-4651; Leon R. Furlong, President, Chief Executive Officer

NOVA SCOTIA: Blue Cross of Atlantic Canada, 644 Main Street, Zip E1C 1E2, P.O. Box 220, Moncton, NB E1C 8L3; tel. 506/853-1811; FAX. 506/853-4651; Leon R. Furlong, President, Chief Executive Officer

ONTARIO: Liberty Health, 150 Ferrand Drive, Toronto, ON M3C 1H6, CANADA; tel. 416/429-2670; FAX. 416/429-7255; Brian G. Johnston, President, Chief Executive Officer

PRINCE EDWARD ISLAND: Blue Cross of Atlantic Canada, 644 Main Street, Zip E1C 1E2, P.O. Box 220, Moncton, NB E1C 8L3; tel. 506/853-1811; FAX. 506/853-4651; Leon R. Furlong, President, Chief Executive Officer

QUEBEC: Quebec Blue Cross Quebec Hospital Service Association, 550 Sherbrooke Street, W., Montreal, PQ H3A 1B9, CANADA; tel. 514/286-8472; FAX. 514/286-8475; Claude Ferron, CA, President

SASKATCHEWAN: Group Medical Services, 1992 Hamilton Street, Regina, SK S4P 2C6, CANADA; tel. 306/352-7638; FAX. 306/525-3825; Harold N. Hoffman, President

Saskatchewan Blue Cross, (MSI) Medical Services Incorporated, 516 Second Avenue, N., Zip S7K 2C5, P.O. Box 4030, Saskatoon, SK S7K 3T2, CANADA; tel. 306/244-2662; FAX. 306/652-5751; Terry R. Brash, President, Chief Executive Officer

Health Systems Agencies

The following is a list of federally funded Health Systems Agencies. The information was obtained from the National Directory of Health Planning Policy and Regulatory Agencies, published by the Missouri Department of Health, Certificate of Need Program. States not listed do not have HSAs. For information about other local agencies and organizations that fulfill similar functions, contact the state or metropolitan hospital associations; see also the list of State Health Planning and Development Agencies in section C.

United States

FLORIDA: Big Bend Health Council, Inc. (District Two), 2629 West 10th Street, Panama City, FL 32401; tel. 904/872-4128; FAX. 904/872-4131; David W. Carter, Executive Director

Broward Regional Health Planning Council (District 10), 915 Middle River Drive, Suite 521, Fort Lauderdale, FL 33304; tel. 305/561-9681; FAX. 305/561-9685; John H. Werner, Executive Director

Health Council of South Florida, Inc. (District 11), 5757 Blue Lagoon Drive, Suite 170, Miami, FL 33126; tel. 305/263-9020; Sonya Albury, Executive Director

Health Council of West Central Florida (District Six), 9721 Executive Center Drive, N., Suite 114, St. Petersburg, FL 33702-2438; tel. 813/576-7772; Donald D. Lamb, Director

Health Planning Council of Northeast Florida, Inc., 2236 St. Johns Avenue, Jacksonville, FL 32204; tel. 904/381-6035; FAX. 904/381-6067; Fred J. Huerkamp, Executive Director

Health Planning Council of Southwest Florida, Inc., 12811 Kenwood Lane, Suite 105, Fort Myers, FL 33907; tel. 813/278-7160; FAX. 813/278-7231; Mary W. Schulthess, Planner, Coordinator

Local Health Council of East Central Florida (District Seven), 1155 South Semoran Boulevard, Suite 1137, Winter Park, FL 32792; tel. 407/671-2005; FAX. 407/671-5474; Steve Windham, Executive Director

North Central Florida Health Planning Council, 11 West University Avenue, Suite Seven, Gainesville, FL 32601; tel. 904/955-2264; FAX. 904/955-3109; Carol J. Gormley, Executive Director

Northwest Florida Health Council, Inc. (District One), 2629 West 10th Street, Panama City, FL 32401; tel. 904/872-4128; FAX. 904/872-4131; David W. Carter, Executive Director

Suncoast Health Council, Inc., 9721 Executive Center Drive, N., Suite 114, St. Petersburg, FL 33702-2451; tel. 813/576-7772; FAX. 813/570-3033; Donald D. Lamb, Executive Director

Treasure Coast Health Council (District Nine and 15), 8895 North Military Trail, Suite 300E, Palm Beach Gardens, FL 33410-6263; tel. 407/624-1100; FAX. 407/624-1137; Herbert Hooven, Executive Director

MARYLAND: Chesapeake Health Planning System, Inc., P.O. Box 773, Cambridge, MD 21613; tel. 410/221-0907; FAX. 410/228-1321; Jake Frego, Executive Director

Western Maryland Health Planning Agency, 153 Baltimore Street, Cumberland, MD 21502; tel. 301/724-1616; FAX. 301/724-2860; Glenda J. McCreary, Acting Executive Director

NEW JERSEY: Essex and Union Advisory Board for Health Planning, Inc., 14 South Orange Avenue, South Orange, NJ 07079; tel. 201/761-6969; FAX. 201/761-7401; Sharon Pastel, Executive Director

Fairleigh Dickinson University, Region Two Health Planning Advisory Board, Inc., 1000 River Road, Teaneck, NJ 07666; tel. 201/692-7180; FAX. 201/692-7189; Thomas Pavlak, Ph.D., Executive Director

Health Visions, Inc., 6981 North Park Drive, East Building, Suite 307, Pennsauken, NJ 08109; tel. 609/662-2050; FAX. 609/662-2261; Robert Culleton, Ph.D., Director

Jersey Coast Health Planning Council, Inc., 515 Route 70, Suite 208, Brick, NJ 08723; tel. 908/262-9047; FAX. 908/262-9049; Eleanor Jaeger, Executive Director

Mid-State Health Advisory Corporation, Rutgers University, Livingston Campus, Building 4161, New Brunswick, NJ 08903; tel. 908/445-5143; FAX. 908/445-5144; Bernadette West, Director

Region One Health Planning Advisory Board, Five Emery Avenue, Randolph, NJ 07869-1368; tel. 201/361-3390; FAX. 201/361-3864; Robert Schermer, Executive Director

NEW YORK: Central New York Health Systems Agency, 101 Intrepid Lane, Syracuse, NY 13205; tel. 315/492-8557; FAX. 315/492-8563; Timothy J. Bobo, Executive Director

Finger Lakes Health Systems Agency, 1150 University Avenue, Rochester, NY 14607; tel. 716/461-3520; FAX. 716/461-0997; Rene H. Reixach, Executive Director

Health Systems Agency of New York City, 450 Seventh Avenue, 13th Floor, New York, NY 10001; tel. 212/244-8100; FAX. 212/244-8120; Robert D. Gumbs, Executive Director

Health Systems Agency of Northeastern New York, Pine West Plaza, One United Way, Washington Avenue Extension, Albany, NY 12205-5558; tel. 518/452-3300; FAX. 518/452-5943; Bruce R. Stanley, Executive Director

Health Systems Agency of Western New York, 2070 Sheridan Drive, Buffalo, NY 14223; tel. 716/876-7131; FAX. 716/876-4968; Brian G. McBride, Ph.D., Executive Director

Hudson Valley Health Systems Agency, P.O. Box 696, Tuxedo, NY 10987; tel. 914/351-5146; Regina M. Kelly, Executive Director

NY Penn Health Systems Agency, 84 Court Street, Suite 300, Binghamton, NY 13901; tel. 607/772-0336; FAX. 607/772-0158; Denise Murray, Executive Director

Nassau-Suffolk Health Systems Agency, 1537 Old Country Road, Plainview, NY 11803; tel. 516/293-5740; FAX. 516/293-6288; Renee Pekmezaris, Ph.D., Executive Director

OHIO: Health Coalition of Central Ohio, 261 East Livingston Avenue, Columbus, OH 43215; tel. 614/221-1381; FAX. 614/221-7016; Franklin Hirsch, President, Chief Executive Officer

Health Planning and Resource Development Association of Central Ohio River Valley, 35 East Seventh Street, Suite 311, Cincinnati, OH 45202; tel. 513/621-2434; FAX. 513/621-4307; James F. Sandmann, President

Health Systems Agency, 415 Bulkley Building, 1501 Euclid Avenue, Cleveland, OH 44115; tel. 216/771-6814; FAX. 216/771-2939; Nancy J. Roth, Executive Director

Lake to River Health Care Coalition, 106 Robbins Avenue, Niles, OH 44446; tel. 216/652-8111; FAX. 216/652-0003; Thomas J. Flynn, Executive Director

Miami Valley Health Improvement Council, 7039 Taylorsville Road, Huber Heights, OH 45424-3103; tel. 513/236-5358; FAX. 513/236-5358; Robert P. Thimmes, President, Chief Executive Officer

Northwest Ohio Health Planning, Inc., 635 North Erie Street, Toledo, OH 43624; tel. 419/255-1190; FAX. 419/255-2900; David G. Pollick, Executive Director

VIRGINIA: Central Virginia Health Planning Agency, Inc., P.O. Box 24287, Richmond, VA 23224; tel. 804/233-6206; FAX. 804/233-8834; Karen L. Cameron, Executive Director

Eastern Virginia Health Systems Agency, Inc., 18 Koger Executive Center, Suite 232, Norfolk, VA 23502; tel. 804/461-4834; FAX. 804/461-3255; Paul M. Boynton, Executive Director

Health Systems Agency of Northern Virginia, 7245 Arlington Boulevard, Suite 300, Falls Church, VA 22042; tel. 703/573-3100, ext. 1500; FAX. 703/573-1276; Dean Montgomery, Executive Director

Northwestern Virginia Health Systems Agency, c/o Blue Ridge Hospital, Charlottesville, VA 22901; tel. 804/977-6010; FAX. 804/977-0748; Margaret P. King, Executive Director

Southwestern Virginia Health Systems Agency, 3100-A Peters Creek Road, N.W., Roanoke, VA 24019; tel. 703/362-9528; FAX. 703/362-9676; Richard S. Roark, Executive Director

Hospital Associations

United States

The following list of state and metropolitan hospital associations is derived from the American Hospital Association's 1995 Directory of Hospital Associations.

ALABAMA: Alabama Hospital Association, 500 North East Boulevard, Zip 36117, P.O. Box 210759, Montgomery, AL 36121-0759; tel. 334/272-8781; FAX. 334/270-9527; J. Michael Horsley, President, Chief Executive Officer

ALASKA: Alaska State Hospital and Nursing Home Association, 319 Seward Street, Suite 11, Juneau, AK 99801; tel. 907/586-1790; FAX. 907/463-3573; Harlan R. Knudson, President, Chief Executive Officer

ARIZONA: Arizona Hospital and Healthcare Association, 1501 West Fountainhead Parkway, Suite 650, Tempe, AZ 85282; tel. 602/968-1083; FAX. 602/967-2029; John R. Rivers, President, Chief Executive Officer

ARKANSAS: Arkansas Hospital Association, 419 Natural Resources Drive, Little Rock, AR 72205-1539; tel. 501/224-7878; FAX. 501/224-0519; James R. Teeter, President, Chief Executive Officer

CALIFORNIA: California Association of Hospitals and Health Systems (CAHHS), 1201 K Street, Suite 800, Sacramento, CA 95814, P.O. Box 1100, Sacramento, CA 95812-1100; tel. 916/443-7401; FAX. 916/552-7596; C. Duane Dauner, President

Healthcare Association of Southern California, 201 North Figueroa Street, Fourth Floor, Los Angeles, CA 90012; tel. 213/250-5600; FAX. 213/250-4863; James D. Barber, President

Hospital Council of Northern and Central California, 7901 Stoneridge Drive, Suite 500, Pleasanton, CA 93710; tel. 510/460-5444; FAX. 510/460-5457; J. Michael Gallagher, President

Hospital Council of San Diego and Imperial Counties, 2333 Camino Del Rio, S., Suite 200, San Diego, CA 92108-3607; tel. 619/298-0777; FAX. 619/298-1054; William Moseley, President, Chief Executive Officer

COLORADO: Colorado Hospital Association, 2140 South Holly Street, Denver, CO 80222-5607; tel. 303/758-1630; FAX. 303/758-0047; Larry Wall, President

CONNECTICUT: Connecticut Hospital Association, Incorporated, 110 Barnes Road, P.O. Box 90, Wallingford, CT 06492-0090; tel. 203/265-7611; FAX. 203/284-9318; Dennis P. May, President

DELAWARE: Association of Delaware Hospitals, 1280 South Governors Avenue, Dover, DE 19904-4802; tel. 302/674-2853; FAX. 302/734-2731; Joseph M. Letnaunchyn, President

DISTRICT OF COLUMBIA: District of Columbia Hospital Association, 1250 Eye Street, N.W., Suite 700, Washington, DC 20005-3930; tel. 202/682-1581; FAX. 202/371-8151; Howard T. Jessamy, President

FLORIDA: Florida Hospital Association, 307 Park Lake Circle, Zip 32803, P.O. Box 531107, Orlando, FL 32853-1107; tel. 407/841-6230; FAX. 407/422-5948; Charles F. Pierce, Jr., President

South Florida Hospital Association, Inc., 8181 Miami Lakes Drive, W., Suite 200, Miami Lakes, FL 33016-5817; tel. 305/825-4007; FAX. 305/825-8697; Linda S. Quick, President

The Tampa Bay Hospital Association, Inc., 9455 Koger Boulevard, Suite 118, St. Petersburg, FL 33702; tel. 813/579-0252; FAX. 813/579-9494; Willard E. Wisler, FACHE, President

GEORGIA: Georgia Hospital Association, 1675 Terrell Mill Road, Marietta, GA 30067; tel. 404/955-0324; FAX. 404/955-5801; Joseph A. Parker, President

HAWAII: Healthcare Association of Hawaii, 932 Ward Avenue, Suite 430, Honolulu, HI 96814-2126; tel. 808/521-8961; FAX. 808/599-2879; Richard E. Meiers, President, Chief Executive Officer

IDAHO: Idaho Hospital Association, 802 West Bannock Street, Suite 500, P.O. Box 1278, Boise, ID 83701; tel. 208/338-5100; FAX. 208/338-7800; Steven A. Millard, President

ILLINOIS: Illinois Hospital and HealthSystems Association, Center for Health Affairs, 1151 East Warrenville Road, P.O. Box 3015, Naperville, IL 60566-7015; tel. 708/505-7777; FAX. 708/505-9457; Kenneth C. Robbins, President

Metropolitan Chicago Healthcare Council, 222 South Riverside Plaza, 17th Floor, Chicago, IL 60606; tel. 312/906-6000; FAX. 312/993-0779; Earl C. Bird, President

INDIANA: Indiana Hospital Association, One American Square, P.O. Box 82063, Indianapolis, IN 46282; tel. 317/633-4870; FAX. 317/633-4875; Kenneth G. Stella, President

IOWA: Hospital Association of Greater Des Moines, 100 East Grand Avenue, Suite 100, Des Moines, IA 50309; tel. 515/243-8077; FAX. 515/283-9366; Arthur J. Spies, Executive Director

The Iowa Hospital Association, Inc., 100 East Grand Avenue, Suite 100, Des Moines, IA 50309; tel. 515/288-1955; FAX. 515/283-9366; Stephen F. Brenton, President

KANSAS: Kansas Hospital Association, 1263 Topeka Avenue, P.O. Box 2308, Topeka, KS 66601-2308; tel. 913/233-7436; FAX. 913/233-6955; Donald A. Wilson, President

KENTUCKY: Kentucky Hospital Association, 1302 Clear Spring Trace, P.O. Box 24163, Louisville, KY 40224; tel. 502/426-6220; FAX. 502/426-6226; William S. Conn, Jr., President

LOUISIANA: Louisiana Hospital Association, 9521 Brookline Avenue, P.O. Box 80720, Baton Rouge, LA 70898-0720; tel. 504/928-0026; FAX. 504/923-1004; Robert D. Merkel, President

Metropolitan Hospital Council of New Orleans, 2450 Severn Avenue, Suite 210, Metairie, LA 70001; tel. 504/837-1171; FAX. 504/837-1174; John J. Finn, Ph.D., President

MAINE: Maine Hospital Association, 150 Capitol Street, Augusta, ME 04330; tel. 207/622-4794; FAX. 207/622-3073; Bruce J. Rueben, President

MARYLAND: Healthcare Council of the National Capital Area, 8201 Corporate Drive, Suite 410, Landover, MD 20785-2229; tel. 301/731-4700; FAX. 301/731-8286; Anthony J. Monaco, President

The Maryland Hospital Association, Inc., 1301 York Road, Suite 800, Lutherville, MD 21093-6087; tel. 410/321-6200; FAX. 410/321-6268; Calvin M. Pierson, President

MASSACHUSETTS: Massachusetts Hospital Association, Five New England Executive Park, Burlington, MA 01803; tel. 617/272-8000; FAX. 617/272-0466; Stephen J. Hegarty, President

MICHIGAN: Greater Flint Area Hospital Assembly, 702 South Ballenger Highway, Flint, MI 48532-3803; tel. 810/766-8898; FAX. 810/766-6422; Marlene Soderstrom, Executive Director

Hospital Council of East Central Michigan, 141 Harrow Lane, Suite 11, Saginaw, MI 48603; tel. 517/792-1725; FAX. 517/792-3099; Randolph K. Flechsig, President

Hospital Council/Center for Health Affairs, 3075 Charlevoix Drive, S.E., Grand Rapids, MI 49546; tel. 616/940-3337; FAX. 616/940-0723; Edward A. Rode, President

Michigan Health & Hospital Association, 6215 West St. Joseph Highway, Lansing, MI 48917; tel. 517/323-3443; FAX. 517/323-0946; Spencer Johnson, President

North Central Council of the Michigan Health and Hospital Association, 200 South Court Street, Gaylord, MI 49735; tel. 517/732-7002; FAX. 517/732-3059; Mary E. Fox, Executive Director

South Central Michigan Hospital Council, 6215 West St. Joseph Highway, Lansing, MI 48917; tel. 517/323-3443; FAX. 517/323-0946; Marlene Soderstrom, President

Southeast Michigan Hospital Council, 24725 West Twelve Mile Road, Suite 104A, Southfield, MI 48034; tel. 810/358-2950; FAX. 810/358-1098; Donald P. Potter, President

Southwestern Michigan Hospital Council, 6215 West St. Joseph Highway, Lansing, MI 48917; tel. 517/323-3443; FAX. 517/323-0946; Clark Ballard, President

MINNESOTA: Metropolitan Healthcare Council, 2550 University Avenue, W., Suite 221-N, St. Paul, MN 55114; tel. 612/641-1121; FAX. 612/659-1477; Allan N. Johnson, Ph.D., President

Minnesota Hospital Association, University Office Plaza, Suite 425, 2221 University Avenue, S.E., Minneapolis, MN 55414-3085; tel. 612/331-5571; FAX. 612/331-1001; Stephen Rogness, President

MISSISSIPPI: Mississippi Hospital Association, 6425 Lakeover Road, Zip 39213, P.O. Box 16444, Jackson, MS 39236-6444; tel. 601/982-3251; FAX. 601/982-2992; Sam W. Cameron, President, Chief Executive Officer

MISSOURI: Kansas City Area Hospital Association, 10401 Holmes Road, Suite 280, Kansas City, MO 64131-3368; tel. 816/941-3800; FAX. 816/941-0818; Cheryl L. Jernigan, President

Missouri Hospital Association, 4712 Country Club Drive, Zip 65109-4544, P.O. Box 60, Jefferson City, MO 65102-0060; tel. 314/893-3700; FAX. 314/893-2809; Charles L. Bowman, President

MONTANA: Montana Hospital Association, 1720 Ninth Avenue, Zip 59601, P.O. Box 5119, Helena, MT 59604; tel. 406/442-1911; FAX. 406/443-3894; James F. Ahrens, President

NEBRASKA: Nebraska Association of Hospitals and Health Systems, 1640 L Street, Suite D, Lincoln, NE 68508-2509; tel. 402/476-0141; FAX. 402/475-4091; Harlan M. Heald, Ph.D., President

NEVADA: Nevada Association of Hospitals and Health Systems, 4600 Kietzke Lane, Suite A-108, Reno, NV 89502; tel. 702/827-0184; FAX. 702/827-0190; James Lamb, Interim Chief Executive Officer

NEW HAMPSHIRE: New England Healthcare Assembly, Inc., 125 Technology Drive, Durham, NH 03824-4724; tel. 603/862-1903; FAX. 603/862-0583; James S. Dolph, President

New Hampshire Hospital Association, 125 Airport Road, Concord, NH 03301-7300; tel. 603/225-0900; FAX. 603/225-4346; Michael J. Hill, President

Organizations / Hospital Associations

NEW JERSEY: Hospital Alliance of New Jersey, Inc., 150 West State Street, Trenton, NJ 08608; tel. 609/989-8200; FAX. 609/989-7768; Mary K. Brennan, Executive Director

Middle Atlantic Health Congress, Center for Health Affairs, 760 Alexander Road, CN-1, Princeton, NJ 08543-0001; tel. 609/924-0049; FAX. 609/275-4114; Lisa Heher, Convention Manager

New Jersey Hospital Association, 760 Alexander Road, CN-1, Princeton, NJ 08543-0001; tel. 609/275-4000; FAX. 609/452-8097; Gary S. Carter, President, Chief Executive Officer

NEW MEXICO: New Mexico Hospitals and Health Systems Association, 2121 Osuna Road, N.E., Albuquerque, NM 87113; tel. 505/343-0010; FAX. 505/343-0012; Maureen L. Boshier, President

NEW YORK: Central New York Hospital Association, Inc., 5740 Commons Park, P.O. Box 160, East Syracuse, NY 13057; tel. 315/445-1851; FAX. 315/445-2293; Richard E. Benoit, President

Greater New York Hospital Association, Subsidiaries and Affiliates, 555 West 57th Street, 15th Floor, New York, NY 10019; tel. 212/246-7100; FAX. 212/262-6350; Kenneth E. Raske, President

Healthcare Association of New York State, 74 North Pearl Street, Albany, NY 12207; tel. 518/431-7600; FAX. 518/431-7915; Daniel Sisto, President

Nassau-Suffolk Hospital Council, Inc., 888 Veterans Highway, Suite 310, Hauppauge, NY 11788; tel. 516/435-3000; FAX. 516/435-2343; Peter M. Sullivan, Executive Vice President, Chief Executive Officer

Northeastern New York Hospital Council, 74 North Pearl Street, Albany, NY 12207; tel. 518/431-7900; FAX. 518/431-7975; Gary J. Fitzgerald, President

Northern Metropolitan Hospital Association, 400 Stony Brook Court, Newburgh, NY 12550; tel. 914/562-7520; FAX. 914/562-0187; Arthur E. Weintraub, President

Rochester Regional Hospital Association, 3445 Winton Place, Rochester, NY 14623; tel. 716/273-8180; FAX. 716/273-8189; Diane Ashley, Interim President

Western New York Healthcare Association, 1876 Niagara Falls Boulevard, Tonawanda, NY 14150-6439; tel. 716/695-0843; FAX. 716/695-0073; William D. Pike, President

NORTH CAROLINA: North Carolina Hospital Association, P.O. Box 80428, Raleigh, NC 27623-0428; tel. 919/677-2400; FAX. 919/677-4200; C. Edward McCauley, President

NORTH DAKOTA: North Dakota Hospital Association, 1120 College Drive, P.O. Box 7340, Bismarck, ND 58507-7340; tel. 701/224-9732; FAX. 701/224-9529; Arnold R. Thomas, President

OHIO: Akron Regional Hospital Association, 326 Locust Street, Suite 14, Akron, OH 44302-1801; tel. 216/379-8989; FAX. 216/379-8189; Robin Louis, Executive Director

Greater Cincinnati Hospital Council, 2100 Sherman Avenue, Suite 100, Cincinnati, OH 45212-2736; tel. 513/531-0200; FAX. 513/531-0278; Lynn R. Olman, President

Greater Cleveland Hospital Association, 1226 Huron Road, Playhouse Square, Cleveland, OH 44115; tel. 216/696-6900; FAX. 216/696-1875; C. Wayne Rice, Ph.D., President, Chief Executive Officer

Greater Dayton Area Hospital Association, Society Bank Building, 32 North Main Street, Suite 1441, Dayton, OH 45402; tel. 513/228-1000; FAX. 513/228-1035; Joseph M. Krella, President

Hospital Association of Central Ohio, 155 East Broad Street, 14th Floor, Columbus, OH 43215-3600; tel. 614/222-6500; FAX. 614/222-6504; John T. Snyder, President

Hospital Council of Northwest Ohio, 5515 Southwyck Boulevard, Suite 203, Toledo, OH 43614; tel. 419/865-1274; FAX. 419/867-4425; W. Scott Fry, President, Chief Executive Officer

Ohio Hospital Association, 155 East Broad Street, Columbus, OH 43215; tel. 614/221-7614; FAX. 614/221-4771; James R. Castle, President

OKLAHOMA: Greater Oklahoma City Hospital Council, 4000 Lincoln Boulevard, Oklahoma City, OK 73105; tel. 405/427-9537; FAX. 405/424-4507; Sheryl Ray, Executive Director

Oklahoma Hospital Association, 4000 Lincoln Boulevard, Oklahoma City, OK 73105; tel. 405/427-9537; FAX. 405/424-4507; John C. Coffey, President

Tulsa Hospital Council, 4120 East 51st Street, Suite A, Tulsa, OK 74135; tel. 918/742-1284; FAX. 918/747-4563; James D. Stansbarger, President

OREGON: Oregon Association of Hospitals and Health Systems, 4000 Kruse Way Place, Building 2, Suite 100, Lake Oswego, OR 97035-2543; tel. 503/636-2204; FAX. 503/636-8310; Kenneth M. Rutledge, President

PENNSYLVANIA: Hospital Association of Pennsylvania, Northeast Regional Council, One Montage Mountain Road, Suite A, Moosic, PA 18507-1776; tel. 717/344-1196; FAX. 717/344-8553; John D. Francis, Regional Director

Hospital Council of Western Pennsylvania, 500 Commonwealth Drive, Warrendale, PA 15086; tel. 412/776-6400; FAX. 412/776-6969; Jack C. Robinette, President

The Delaware Valley Hospital Council, Inc., 1315 Walnut Street, Suite 200, Philadelphia, PA 19107; tel. 215/735-9695; FAX. 215/790-1267; Andrew B. Wigglesworth, President

The Hospital Association of Pennsylvania, 4750 Lindle Road, P.O. Box 8600, Harrisburg, PA 17105-8600; tel. 717/564-9200; FAX. 717/561-5333; Carolyn F. Scanlon, President

RHODE ISLAND: Hospital Association of Rhode Island, Weld Building, 2nd Floor, 880 Butler Drive, Suite One, Providence, RI 02906; tel. 401/453-8400; FAX. 401/453-8411; Gerald G. McClure, President

SOUTH CAROLINA: South Carolina Hospital Association, 101 Medical Circle, P.O. Box 6009, West Columbia, SC 29171-6009; tel. 803/796-3080; FAX. 803/796-2938; William L. Yates, President

SOUTH DAKOTA: South Dakota Hospital Association, 3708 Brooks Place, Suite 1, Sioux Falls, SD 57106; tel. 605/361-2281; FAX. 605/361-5175; Frank M. Drew, President

TENNESSEE: Tennessee Hospital Association, 500 Interstate Boulevard, S., Nashville, TN 37210-4634; tel. 615/256-8240; FAX. 615/242-4803; Craig A. Becker, President

TEXAS: Dallas-Fort Worth Hospital Council, 250 Decker Court, Irving, TX 75062; tel. 214/719-4900; FAX. 214/719-4009; John C. Gavras, President

Greater Houston Hospital Council, 3333 Eastside, Suite 130, Zip 77098, P.O. Box 66962, Houston, TX 77266-6962; tel. 713/526-9031; FAX. 713/526-1351; Eugene P. Beck, President

Greater San Antonio Hospital Council, 530 McCullough, Suite 900, San Antonio, TX 78215-2104; tel. 210/246-2500; FAX. 210/246-2515; William Dean Rasco, President, Chief Executive Officer

Texas Hospital Association, 6225 U.S. Highway 290, E., P.O. Box 15587, Austin, TX 78761-5587; tel. 512/465-1000; FAX. 512/465-1090; Terry Townsend, CAE, FACHE, President, Chief Executive Officer

UTAH: Utah Association of Healthcare Providers, 127 South 500 East, Suite 625, Salt Lake City, UT 84102; tel. 801/364-1515; FAX. 801/532-4806; Richard B. Kinnersley, President

VERMONT: Vermont Hospital Association, 148 Main Street, Montpelier, VT 05602; tel. 802/223-3461; FAX. 802/223-0364; Norman E. Wright, President

VIRGINIA: Virginia Hospital Association, 4200 Innslake Drive, Glen Allen, VA 23060, P.O. Box 31394, Richmond, VA 23294; tel. 804/747-8600; FAX. 804/965-0475; Laurens Sartoris, President

WASHINGTON: Washington State Hospital Association, 300 Elliott Avenue, W., Suite 300, Seattle, WA 98119-4118; tel. 206/281-7211; FAX. 206/283-6122; Leo F. Greenawalt, President, Chief Executive Officer

WEST VIRGINIA: West Virginia Hospital Association, 600 D Street, Second Level, South Charleston, WV 25303-3112; tel. 304/744-9842; FAX. 304/744-9889; Steven J. Summer, President

WISCONSIN: Hospital Council of Greater Milwaukee Area, 2300 North Mayfair Road, Milwaukee, WI 53226; tel. 414/258-9610; FAX. 414/258-2103; Marvin F. Neely, Jr., President

Wisconsin Hospital Association, 5721 Odana Road, Madison, WI 53719-1289; tel. 608/274-1820; FAX. 608/274-8554; Robert C. Taylor, President, Chief Executive Officer

WYOMING: Wyoming Hospital Association, 2005 Warren Avenue, Zip 82001, P.O. Box 5539, Cheyenne, WY 82003; tel. 307/632-9344; FAX. 307/632-9347; Robert C. Kidd II, President

U.S. Associated Areas

PUERTO RICO: Puerto Rico Hospital Association, Officina 101-103, Villa Nevarez Professional Center, Centro Commercial Villa Nevarez, San Juan, PR 00927; tel. 809/764-0290; FAX. 809/753-9748; Eduardo Sotomayor, President

Canada

ALBERTA: Alberta Healthcare Association, 10009 108th Street, Edmonton, AB T5J 3C5; tel. 403/498-8400; FAX. 403/498-8465; Michael Higgins, Executive Director

BRITISH COLUMBIA: British Columbia Health Association, 600-1333 West Broadway, Vancouver, BC V6H 4C7; tel. 604/734-2423; FAX. 604/734-7202; Mary Collins, President

MANITOBA: Manitoba Health Organizations, 600-360 Broadway, Winnipeg, MB R3C 4G6; tel. 204/942-6591; FAX. 204/956-1373; R. G. Birt, President

NEW BRUNSWICK: New Brunswick Healthcare Association, 861 Woodstock Road, Fredericton, NB E3B 4X4; tel. 506/451-0750; FAX. 506/451-0760; Michel J. Poirier, Executive Director

NEWFOUNDLAND: Newfoundland Hospital and Nursing Home Association, P.O. Box 8234, Post Station A, St. John's, NF A1B 3N4; tel. 709/364-7701; FAX. 709/364-6460; Robin J. Burnell, Executive Director

NORTHWEST TERRITORY: Northwest Territories Health Care Association, P.O. Box 1709, Yellowknife, NT X1A 2P3; tel. 403/873-9253; FAX. 403/873-9254; Wendy MacDonald, Executive Director

NOVA SCOTIA: Nova Scotia Association of Health Organizations, Bedford Professional Centre, Two Dartmouth Road, Bedford, NS B4A 2K7; tel. 902/832-8500; FAX. 902/832-8505; Sharon C. Oliver, J.D., President, Chief Executive Officer

Organizations / Hospital Associations

ONTARIO: Ontario Hospital Association, 150 Ferrand Drive, Don Mills, ON M3C 1H6; tel. 416/429-2661, ext. 2285; FAX. 416/429-6748; Dennis R. Timbrell, President

PRINCE EDWARD ISLAND: Health Association of Prince Edward Island, 10 Pownel Street, P.O. Box 490, Charlottetown, PE C1A 3V6; tel. 902/368-3901; FAX. 902/368-3231; Carol Gabanna, Executive Director

QUEBEC: The Quebec Hospital Association, 505 boulevard de Maisonneuve, W., Suite 400, Montreal, PQ H3A 3C2; tel. 514/842-4861; FAX. 514/282-4271; Jacques A. Nadeau, Executive Vice President

SASKATCHEWAN: Saskatchewan Association of Health Organizations, 1445 Park Street, Regina, SK S4N 4C5; tel. 306/347-5500; FAX. 306/525-1960; Arliss Wright, President, Chief Executive Officer

Hospital Licensure Agencies

Information for the following list of state hospital licensure agencies was obtained directly from the agencies.

United States

ALABAMA: Division of Licensure and Certification, Alabama Department of Public Health, 434 Monroe Street, Montgomery, AL 36130-1701; tel. 334/240-3503; FAX. 334/240-3147; L. O'Neal Green, Director

ALASKA: Health Facilities Licensing and Certification, 4730 Business Park Boulevard, Building H, Suite 18, Anchorage, AK 99503-7137; tel. 907/561-8081; FAX. 907/561-3011; Karen Martz, Administrator

ARIZONA: Arizona Department of Health Services, Office of Health Care Licensure, Medical Facilities Section, 1647 East Morten Avenue, Suite 110, Phoenix, AZ 85020; tel. 602/255-1144; FAX. 602/255-1109; Virginia Blair, Program Manager

ARKANSAS: Division of Health Facility Services, Arkansas Department of Health–Area 2300, Slot Nine, 4815 West Markham Street, Little Rock, AR 72205-3867; tel. 501/661-2201; FAX. 501/661-2468; Valetta M. Buck, Director

CALIFORNIA: Licensing and Certification, Department of Health Services, 1800 3rd Street, Suite 210, Zip 95814, P.O. Box 942732, Sacramento, CA 94234-7320; tel. 916/445-2070; Margaret DeBow, Deputy Director

COLORADO: Health Facilities Division, Colorado Department of Public Health and Environment, 4300 Cherry Creek Drive, S., Denver, CO 80222-1530; tel. 303/692-2800; FAX. 303/782-4883; Susan E. Rehak, Deputy Director

CONNECTICUT: Department of Public Health and Addiction Service, Connecticut State Department of Health Services, 150 Washington Street, Hartford, CT 06106; tel. 203/566-1073; FAX. 203/566-1097; Elizabeth M. Burns, RN, M.S., Director

DELAWARE: Office of Health Facilities Licensing and Certification, Department of Health and Social Services, Three Mill Road, Suite 308, Wilmington, DE 19806; tel. 302/577-6666; FAX. 302/577-6672; Ellen T. Reap, Director

DISTRICT OF COLUMBIA: Service Facility Regulation Administration, 614 H Street, N.W., Suite 1007, Washington, DC 20001; tel. 202/727-7190; FAX. 202/727-7780; James R. Murphy, Administrator

FLORIDA: Division of Health Quality Assurance, Agency for Health Care Administration, 2727 Mahan Drive, Tallahassee, FL 32308; tel. 904/487-2717; FAX. 904/487-6240; Gloria Crawford-Henderson, Director

GEORGIA: Health Care Section, Office of Regulatory Services, Department of Human Resources, Two Peachtree Street, N.W., Suite 19.204, Atlanta, GA 30303-3167; tel. 404/657-5550; FAX. 404/657-8934; Susie M. Woods, Director

HAWAII: Hawaii Department of Health, Hospital and Medical Facilities Branch, P.O. Box 3378, Honolulu, HI 96801; tel. 808/586-4080; FAX. 808/586-4747; Helen K. Yoshimi, B.S.N., M.P.H., Chief, HMFB

IDAHO: Bureau of Facility Standards, Department of Health and Welfare, P.O. Box 83720, Boise, ID 83720-0036; tel. 208/334-6626; FAX. 208/334-0657; Loyal Perry, Supervisor, Non–Long Term Care

ILLINOIS: Division of Health Care Facilities and Programs, Illinois Department of Public Health, 525 West Jefferson Street, Springfield, IL 62671; tel. 217/782-7412; FAX. 217/782-0382; Joseph L. Voss, Adminstrator, Central Office Operations Section

INDIANA: Division of Acute Care, Indiana State Department of Health, 1330 West Michigan Street, P.O. Box 1964, Indianapolis, IN 46206-1964; tel. 317/383-6472; FAX. 317/383-6750; John A. Braeckel, Director

IOWA: Division of Health Facilities, Iowa State Department of Inspections and Appeals, Lucas State Office Building, Des Moines, IA 50319; tel. 515/281-4115; FAX. 515/242-5022; Pearl Johnson, Administrator

KANSAS: Kansas Department of Health and Environment, Bureau of Adult and Child Care Facilities, 900 S.W. Jackson, Suite 1001, Topeka, KS 66620-0001; tel. 913/296-1240; George Dugger, Medical Facilities Certification Administrator

KENTUCKY: Division of Licensing and Regulation, Cabinet for Human Resources, Cabinet for Human Resources Building, 275 East Main Street, 4th Floor, E., Frankfort, KY 40621; tel. 502/564-2800; FAX. 502/564-6546; Timothy L. Veno, Director

LOUISIANA: Health Standards Section, Louisiana Department of Health and Hospitals, P.O. Box 3767, Baton Rouge, LA 70821; tel. 504/342-5782; FAX. 504/342-5292; Lily W. McAlister, RN, Manager

MAINE: Division of Licensing and Certification, Department of Human Services, State House, Station 11, Augusta, ME 04333; tel. 207/624-5443; FAX. 207/624-5378; Louis Dorogi, Director

MARYLAND: Department of Health and Mental Hygiene, Office of Licensing and Certification Programs, 4201 Patterson Avenue, Baltimore, MD 21215; tel. 410/764-4980; FAX. 410/764-5969; William Dorrill, Deputy Director

MASSACHUSETTS: Division of Health Care Quality, Massachusetts Department of Public Health, 10 West Street, Fifth Floor, Boston, MA 02111; tel. 617/727-5860; FAX. 617/727-1414; Virginia C. Sullivan, Director

MICHIGAN: Bureau of Health Systems, Michigan Department of Public Health, 3423 North Logan Street, P.O. Box 30195, Lansing, MI 48909; tel. 517/335-8505; FAX. 517/335-8510; Walter S. Wheeler III, Chief

MINNESOTA: Facility and Provider Compliance Division, Minnesota Department of Health, 393 North Dunlap Street, P.O. Box 64900, St. Paul, MN 55164-0900; tel. 612/643-2100; FAX. 612/643-2593; Linda G. Sutherland, Director

MISSISSIPPI: Division of Health Facilities Licensure and Certification, Mississippi State Department of Health, 421 West Pascagoula Street, Jackson, MS 39203; tel. 601/354-7300; FAX. 601/354-7230; Vanessa Breckenridge, Director

MISSOURI: Bureau of Hospital Licensing and Certification, Missouri Department of Health, P.O. Box 570, Jefferson City, MO 65102; tel. 314/751-6302; FAX. 314/526-3621; Darrell Hendrickson, Administrator

MONTANA: Health Facilities Division, Montana Department of Health and Environmental Sciences, Cogswell Building, Helena, MT 59620; tel. 406/444-2037; FAX. 406/444-1742; Denzel Davis, Administrator

NEBRASKA: Bureau of Health Facilities Standards, State Department of Health, 301 Centennial Mall, S., P.O. Box 95007, Lincoln, NE 68509-5007; tel. 402/471-2946; FAX. 402/471-0555; Frederick M. Wright, Director

NEVADA: Bureau of Licensure and Certification, Nevada Health Division, 505 East King Street, Suite 202, Carson City, NV 89710; tel. 702/687-4475; FAX. 702/687-5751; Sharon M. Ezell, Chief

NEW HAMPSHIRE: Bureau of Health Facilities Administration, Division of Public Health Services, Health and Human Services Building, Six Hazen Drive, Concord, NH 03301; tel. 603/271-4592; FAX. 602/271-3745; Eleanor B. Robinson, Bureau Chief

NEW JERSEY: Licensing, Certification, and Standards, New Jersey State Department of Health, CN-367, Trenton, NJ 08625; tel. 609/588-7726; FAX. 609/588-7823; Robert J. Fogg, Esq., Director

NEW MEXICO: Department of Health, Licensing and Certification Bureau, 525 Camino de los Marquez, Suite 2, Santa Fe, NM 87501; tel. 505/827-4200; FAX. 505/827-4222; Sue K. Morris, Bureau Chief

NEW YORK: Bureau of Hospital Services, Office of Health Systems Management, Empire State Plaza, Albany, NY 12237; tel. 518/474-5013; FAX. 518/474-2031; Frederick J. Heigel, Director

NORTH CAROLINA: Division of Facility Services, Department of Human Resources, 701 Barbour Drive, P.O. Box 29530, Raleigh, NC 27626-0530; tel. 919/733-1610; FAX. 919/733-3207; Jesse Goodman, Chief, Licensure Section

NORTH DAKOTA: Health Resources Section, State Department of Health, 600 East Boulevard Avenue, Bismarck, ND 58505-0200; tel. 701/328-2352; FAX. 701/328-4727; Fred Gladden, Chief

OHIO: Office of Health Systems Planning, Primary Care and Rural Health, Department of Health, P.O. Box 118, Columbus, OH 43266-0118; tel. 614/466-3325; FAX. 614/644-8661; Louis Pomerantz, Chief, Health Systems Planning, Primary Care, Rural Health

OKLAHOMA: State Department of Health, 1000 N.E. 10th, Oklahoma City, OK 73117; tel. 405/271-4200; FAX. 405/271-3431; Jerry R. Nida, M.D., Commissioner, Health

OREGON: Health Care Licensure and Certification, Oregon Health Division, P.O. Box 14450, Portland, OR 97214-0450; tel. 503/731-4013; FAX. 503/731-4080; Kathleen Smail, Manager

PENNSYLVANIA: Division of Acute and Ambulatory Care Facilities, Bureau of Quality Assurance, Health and Welfare Building, Suite 532, Harrisburg, PA 17120; tel. 717/783-8980; FAX. 717/772-2163; William White, Director

RHODE ISLAND: Rhode Island Department of Health, Three Capitol Hill, Providence, RI 02908-5097; tel. 401/277-2231; FAX. 401/277-6548; Barbara A. DeBuono, M.D., M.P.H., Director

SOUTH CAROLINA: Department of Health and Environmental Control, Division of Health Licensing, 2600 Bull Street, Columbia, SC 29201; tel. 803/737-7202; FAX. 803/737-7212; Alan Samuels, Director

Organizations / Hospital Licensure Agencies

SOUTH DAKOTA: Office of Health Care Facilities Licensure and Certification, State Department of Health, Anderson Building, 445 East Capitol, Pierre, SD 57501; tel. 605/773-3364; FAX. 605/773-5904; Joan Bachman, Program Director

TENNESSEE: Tennessee Department of Health, Division of Health Care Facilities, 283 Plus Park Boulevard, Nashville, TN 37247-0530; tel. 615/367-6316; Leslie A. Brown, Director

TEXAS: Health Facility Certification Division, Texas Department of Health, 1100 West 49th Street, Austin, TX 78756-3199; tel. 512/834-6650; Nance Stearman, Division Director

UTAH: Utah State Department of Health, Bureau of Health Facility Licensure, P.O. Box 16990, Salt Lake City, UT 84116-0990; tel. 801/538-6152; FAX. 801/538-6325; Debra Wynkoop-Green, Director

VERMONT: Medical Care Regulation Division, Vermont Department of Health, 60 Main Street, P.O. Box 70, Burlington, VT 05402; tel. 802/863-7272; Robert Aiken, Director

VIRGINIA: Office of Health Facilities Regulation, Virginia Department of Health, 3600 Centre, Suite 216, 3600 West Broad Street, Richmond, VA 23230; tel. 804/367-2102; FAX. 804/367-2149; Nancy R. Hofheimer, Director

WASHINGTON: Acute Care and Construction Review Services, Washington Department of Health, Target Plaza, Suite 500, 2725 Harrison Avenue, N.W., P.O. Box 7852, Olympia, WA 98504-7852; tel. 206/705-6622; FAX. 206/705-6654; Byron Plan, Manager

WEST VIRGINIA: Office of Health Facility Licensure and Certification, West Virginia Division of Health, State Capitol Complex, Building Three, Suite 550, Charleston, WV 25305; tel. 304/558-0050; FAX. 304/558-2515; Nancy Tyler, Director

WISCONSIN: Bureau of Quality Compliance, Division of Health, One West Wilson Street, P.O. Box 309, Madison, WI 53701; tel. 608/267-7185; FAX. 608/267-0352; Judy Fryback, Director, Bureau of Quality Compliance

WYOMING: Department of Health, Health Facilities Licensing, Metropolitan Bank Building, Eighth Floor, Cheyenne, WY 82002; tel. 307/777-7123; FAX. 307/777-5970; Charlie Simineo, Program Manager

Medical and Nursing Licensure Agencies

Information for the following list of state medical licensure agencies was obtained from the Federation of State Medical Board and nursing licensure agencies was obtained from the National League for Nursing.

United States

ALABAMA
  Alabama Board of Nursing, RSA Plaza, Suite 250, 770 Washington Avenue, Montgomery, AL 36130-3900; tel. 334/242-4060; FAX. 334/242-4360; Judi Crume, Executive Officer
  Alabama State Board of Medical Examiners, 848 Washington Avenue, Zip 36104, P.O. Box 946, Montgomery, AL 36101-0946; tel. 334/242-4116; FAX. 334/242-4155; Larry D. Dixon, Executive Director

ALASKA
  Alaska Board of Nursing, 3601 C Street, Suite 722, Anchorage, AK 99503; tel. 907/561-2878; FAX. 907/562-5781; Gail M. McGuill, RN, M.S., Executive Secretary
  Alaska State Medical Board, Division of Occupational Licensing, 3601 C Street, Suite 722, Anchorage, AK 99503; tel. 907/561-2878; FAX. 907/562-5781; Leslie G. Haywood, Executive Secretary

ARIZONA
  Arizona Board of Medical Examiners, 1651 East Morton, Suite 210, Phoenix, AZ 85020; tel. 602/255-3751; FAX. 602/255-1848; Mark R. Speicher, Executive Director
  Arizona Board of Osteopathic Examiners in Medicine and Surgery, 141 East Palm Lane, Suite 205, Phoenix, AZ 85004; tel. 602/255-1747; FAX. 602/255-1756; Robert J. Miller, Ph.D., Executive Director
  Arizona State Board of Nursing, 2001 West Camelback Road, Suite 350, Phoenix, AZ 85015; tel. 602/255-5092; FAX. 602/255-5130; Fran Roberts, RN, M.S., Executive Director

ARKANSAS
  Arkansas State Board of Nursing, University Tower Building, Suite 800, 1123 South University Avenue, Little Rock, AR 72204; tel. 501/686-2700; Linda C. Murphey, RN, M.N., Executive Director
  Arkansas State Medical Board, 2100 Riverfront Drive, Suite 200, Little Rock, AR 72202; tel. 501/296-1802; FAX. 501/296-1805; Peggy P. Cryer, Executive Director

CALIFORNIA
  California Board of Registered Nursing, 400 R Street, Suite 4030, Zip 95814, P.O. Box 944210, Sacramento, CA 94244-2100; tel. 916/322-3350; Ruth Ann Terry, RN, M.P.H., Executive Officer
  Medical Board of California, 1426 Howe Avenue, Suite 54, Sacramento, CA 95825; tel. 916/263-2344; FAX. 916/263-2487; Douglas Laue, Deputy Director
  Osteopathic Medical Board of California, 444 North Third Street, Suite A-200, Sacramento, CA 95814; tel. 916/322-4306; FAX. 916/327-6119; Linda J. Bergmann, Executive Director

COLORADO
  Colorado State Board of Medical Examiners, 1560 Broadway, Suite 1300, Denver, CO 80202-5140; tel. 303/894-7690; FAX. 303/894-7692; Susan Miller, Program Administrator
  Colorado State Board of Nursing, 1560 Broadway, Suite 670, Denver, CO 80202; tel. 303/894-2430; Karen Brumley, Program Administrator

CONNECTICUT
  Connecticut Board of Examiners for Nursing, Department of Public Health and Addiction Services, 150 Washington Street, Hartford, CT 06106; tel. 203/566-1041; FAX. 203/566-1464; Marie Hilliard, Ph.D., RN, Executive Officer
  Connecticut Division of Medical Quality Assurance, 150 Washington Street, Hartford, CT 06106; tel. 203/566-7398; FAX. 203/566-2774; Stanley K. Peck, J.D., Director

DELAWARE
  Delaware Board of Medical Practice, Cannon Building, 861 Silver Lake Boulevard, Suite 203, P.O. Box 1401, Dover, DE 19903; tel. 302/739-4522; FAX. 302/739-2711; Wayne Martz, M.D., Executive Director
  Delaware Board of Nursing, Cannon Building, 861 Silver Lake Boulevard, Suite 203, P.O. Box 1401, Dover, DE 19903; tel. 302/739-4522, ext. 216; FAX. 302/739-2711; Iva J. Boardman, RN, M.S.N., Executive Director

DISTRICT OF COLUMBIA
  District of Columbia Board of Medicine, 605 G Street, N.W., Suite 202, Lower Level, Washington, DC 20001; tel. 202/727-7454; FAX. 202/727-4087; James R. Granger, Jr., Acting Executive Director
  District of Columbia Board of Nursing, 614 H Street, N.W., Washington, DC 20001; tel. 202/727-7461; FAX. 202/727-8030; Barbara Hatcher, Chairperson

FLORIDA
  Florida Board of Medicine, 1940 North Monroe Street, Northwood Centre, Suite 60, Tallahassee, FL 32399-0750; tel. 904/488-0595; FAX. 904/922-3040; Marm M. Harris, Executive Director
  Florida Board of Osteopathic Medicine, 1940 North Monroe Street, Northwood Centre, Suite 60, Tallahassee, FL 32399-0757; tel. 904/922-6725; FAX. 904/921-6184; Melissa Coggins, Staff Assistant
  Florida State Board of Nursing, 111 Coast Line Drive, E., Suite 516, Jacksonville, FL 32202; tel. 904/359-6331; FAX. 904/359-6323; Judie K. Ritter, RN, Executive Director

GEORGIA
  Georgia Board of Nursing, 166 Pryor Street, S.W., Atlanta, GA 30303; tel. 404/656-3943; FAX. 404/651-9532; Carolyn Hutcherson, Executive Director
  Georgia Composite State Board of Medical Examiners, 166 Pryor Street, S.W., Atlanta, GA 30303; tel. 404/656-3913; FAX. 404/651-9532; Andrew Watry, Executive Director

HAWAII
  Hawaii Board of Medical Examiners, Department of Commerce and Consumer Affairs, 1010 Richards Street, Zip 96813, P.O. Box 3469, Honolulu, HI 96801; tel. 808/586-2708; June Kamioka, Executive Secretary
  Hawaii Board of Nursing, P.O. Box 3469, Honolulu, HI 96801; tel. 808/586-2695; FAX. 808/586-2689; Kathy Yokouchi, Executive Officer

IDAHO
  Idaho State Board of Medicine, State House Mail, 280 North Eighth, Suite 202, P.O. Box 83720, Boise, ID 83720-0058; tel. 208/334-2822; FAX. 203/334-2801; Donald L. Deleski, Executive Director
  Idaho State Board of Nursing, 280 North Eighth Street, Suite 210, P.O. Box 83720, Boise, ID 83720-0061; tel. 208/334-3110; FAX. 208/334-3262; Leola Daniels, Executive Director

ILLINOIS
  Illinois Department of Professional Regulation, 320 West Washington Street, Springfield, IL 62786; tel. 217/782-0458; FAX. 217/782-7645; Tony Sanders, Deputy Director's Staff
  Illinois Department of Professional Regulation, James R. Thompson, 100 West Randolph Street, Suite 9-300, Chicago, IL 60601; tel. 312/814-4500; FAX. 312/814-1837; Nikki Zollar, Director

INDIANA
  Indiana Health Professions Bureau, Medical Licensing Board of Indiana, 402 West Washington, Room 041, Indianapolis, IN 46204; tel. 317/233-4401; FAX. 317/233-4236; Laura Langford, Executive Director
  Indiana State Board of Nursing, Health Professions Bureau, 402 West Washington, Suite 041, Indianapolis, IN 46282; tel. 317/233-4405; FAX. 317/233-4236; Barbara Powers, Board Administrator

IOWA
  Iowa Board of Nursing, State Capitol Complex, 1223 East Court Avenue, Des Moines, IA 50319; tel. 515/281-3255; Lorinda K. Inman, RN, M.S.N., Executive Director
  Iowa State Board of Medical Examiners, State Capitol Complex, Executive Hills West, 1209 East Court Avenue, Des Moines, IA 50319-0180; tel. 515/281-5171; FAX. 515/242-5908; Ann M. Martino, Ph.D., Executive Director

KANSAS
  Kansas State Board of Healing Arts, 235 S.W. Topeka Boulevard, Topeka, KS 66603-3068; tel. 913/296-7413; FAX. 913/296-0852; Lawrence T. Buening, Jr., J.D., Executive Director
  Kansas State Board of Nursing, Landon State Office Building, 900 S.W. Jackson, Suite 551-S, Topeka, KS 66612-1230; tel. 913/296-4929; FAX. 913/296-3929; Patsy Johnson, RN, M.N., Executive Administrator

KENTUCKY
  Kentucky Board of Medical Licensure, The Hurstbourne Office Park, 310 Whittington Parkway, Suite 1B, Louisville, KY 40222; tel. 502/429-8046; FAX. 502/429-9923; C. William Schmidt, Executive Director
  Kentucky Board of Nursing, 312 Whittington Parkway, Suite 300, Louisville, KY 40222; tel. 502/329-7000; FAX. 502/329-7011; Sharon M. Weisenbeck, M.S., RN, Executive Director

LOUISIANA
  Louisiana State Board of Medical Examiners, P.O. Box 30250, New Orleans, LA 70190-0250; tel. 504/524-6763; FAX. 504/568-8893; Mrs. Delmar Rorison, Executive Director
  Louisiana State Board of Nursing, 912 Pere Marquette Building, New Orleans, LA 70112; tel. 504/568-5464; FAX. 504/568-5467; Barbara L. Morvant, RN, M.N., Executive Director

MAINE
  Maine Board of Licensure in Medicine, Two Bangor Street, State House Station, #137, Augusta, ME 04333; tel. 207/287-3601; Randal C. Manning, Executive Director
  Maine Board of Osteopathic Licensure, State House Station, # 142, Two Bangor Street, Augusta, ME 04333; tel. 207/287-2480; FAX. 207/287-2480; Susan E. Stout, Executive Secretary
  Maine State Board of Nursing, 35 Anthony Avenue, State House Station, #158, Augusta, ME 04333; tel. 207/624-5275; FAX. 207/624-5290; Jean C. Caron, RN, Executive Director

MARYLAND
  Maryland Board of Physician Quality Assurance, 4201 Patterson Avenue, Third Floor, Zip 21215-0095, P.O. Box 2571, Baltimore, MD 21215-0095; tel. 800/492-6836; FAX. 410/764-2478; J. Michael Compton, Executive Director

Organizations / Medical and Nursing Licensure Agencies

Maryland State Board of Nursing, 4140 Patterson Avenue, Baltimore, MD 21215; tel. 410/764-5124; FAX. 410/358-3530; Donna M. Dorsey, RN, M.S., Executive Director

MASSACHUSETTS
Massachusetts Board of Registration in Medicine, 10 West Street, Third Floor, Boston, MA 02111; tel. 617/727-3086; FAX. 617/451-9568; Alexander F. Fleming, J.D., Executive Director

Massachusetts Board of Registration in Nursing, 100 Cambridge Street, Suite 1517, Boston, MA 02202; tel. 617/727-9961; FAX. 617/727-2197; Theresa M. Bonanno, M.S.N., RN, Executive Secretary

MICHIGAN
Michigan Board of Medicine, 611 West Ottawa Street, 4th Floor, Box 30192, Lansing, MI 48909; tel. 517/373-9102; FAX. 517/373-2179; Carol S. Johnson, Licensing Administrator

Michigan Board of Nursing, Department of Commerce, 611 West Ottawa Street, P.O. Box 30018, Lansing, MI 48909; tel. 517/373-1600; Doris Foley, Licensing Administrator

Michigan Board of Osteopathic Medicine and Surgery, 611 West Ottawa Street, 4th Floor, P.O. Box 30018, Lansing, MI 48909; tel. 517/373-9102; FAX. 517/373-2179; Carol S. Johnson, Licensing Administrator

MINNESOTA
Minnesota Board of Medical Practice, 2700 University Avenue, W., Suite 106, St. Paul, MN 55114-1080; tel. 612/642-0538; FAX. 612/642-0393; H. Leonard Boche, Executive Director

Minnesota Board of Nursing, 2700 University Avenue, W., Suite 108, St. Paul, MN 55114; tel. 612/642-0567; FAX. 612/642-0574; Joyce M. Schowalter, Executive Director

MISSISSIPPI
Mississippi Board of Nursing, 239 North Lamar Street, Suite 401, Jackson, MS 39201-1397; tel. 601/359-6170; FAX. 601/359-6185; Marcia M. Rachel, Ph.D., RN, Executive Director

Mississippi State Board of Medical Licensure, 2688-D Insurance Center Drive, Jackson, MS 39216; tel. 601/354-6645; FAX. 601/987-4159; P. Doyle Bradshaw, Executive Officer

MISSOURI
Missouri State Board of Nursing, 3605 Missouri Boulevard, P.O. Box 656, Jefferson City, MO 65102; tel. 314/751-0681; FAX. 314/751-0075

Missouri State Board of Registration for the Healing Arts, 3605 Missouri Boulevard, Zip 65109, P.O. Box 4, Jefferson City, MO 65102; tel. 314/751-0098; FAX. 314/751-3166; Alden Henrickson, Executive Director

MONTANA
Montana Board of Medical Examiners, 111 North Jackson, P.O. Box 200513, Helena, MT 59620-0513; tel. 406/444-4284; FAX. 406/444-1667; Patricia I. England, J.D., Executive Director, Board Attorney

Montana State Board of Nursing, 111 North Jackson, P.O. Box 200513, Arcade Building, Helena, MT 59620-0513; tel. 406/444-2071; FAX. 406/444-7759; Dianne Wickham, RN, M.N., Executive Director

NEBRASKA
Nebraska State Board of Examiners in Medicine and Surgery, 301 Centennial Mall, S., P.O. Box 95007, Lincoln, NE 68509-5007; tel. 402/471-2115; FAX. 402/471-0383; Katherine A. Brown, Associate Director

NEVADA
Nevada State Board of Medical Examiners, 1105 Terminal Way, Suite 301, Zip 89502, P.O. Box 7238, Reno, NV 89510; tel. 702/688-2559; FAX. 702/688-2321; Patricia R. Perry, Executive Director

Nevada State Board of Nursing, 4335 South Industrial Road, Suite 430, Las Vegas, NV 89103; tel. 702/739-1575; FAX. 702/739-0298; Lonna Burress, Executive Director

Nevada State Board of Osteopathic Medicine, 2950 East Flamingo Road, Suite E-3, Las Vegas, NV 89121; tel. 702/732-9670; Larry J. Tarno, D.O., Executive Director

NEW HAMPSHIRE
New Hampshire Board of Registration in Medicine, 2 Industrial Park Drive, Concord, NH 03301; tel. 603/271-1203; Karen LaCroix, Administrator

New Hampshire State Board of Nursing, Division of Public Health Services, 6 Hazen Drive, Concord, NH 03301; tel. 603/271-2323; Doris G. Nuttelman, RN, Ed.D., Executive Director

NEW JERSEY
New Jersey Board of Nursing, 124 Halsey Street, Zip 07102, P.O. Box 45010, Newark, NJ 07101; tel. 201/504-6430; FAX. 201/648-3481; Sister Teresa L. Harris, Executive Director

New Jersey State Board of Medical Examiners, 140 East Front Street, 2nd Floor, Trenton, NJ 08608; tel. 609/826-7100; FAX. 609/984-3930; Kevin B. Earle, Executive Director

NEW MEXICO
New Mexico Board of Osteopathic Medical Examiners, 725 St. Michaels Drive, Zip 87501, P.O. Box 25101, Santa Fe, NM 87504; tel. 505/827-7171; FAX. 505/827-7095; Michelle McGinnis, Executive Director

New Mexico State Board of Medical Examiners, 491 Old Santa Fe Trail, Lamy Building, 2nd Floor, P.O. Box 20001, Santa Fe, NM 87501; tel. 505/827-7317; FAX. 505/827-7377; Dorothy Lane Welby, Executive Secretary

State of New Mexico, Board of Nursing, 4206 Louisiana NE, Suite A, Albuquerque, NM 87109; tel. 505/841-8340; Nancy L. Twigg, Executive Director

NEW YORK
New York Board for Professional Medical Conduct, State Department of Health, Corning Tower Building, Suite 438, Empire State Plaza, Albany, NY 12237-0061; tel. 518/474-8357; FAX. 518/473-8905; Kathleen Tanner, Director

New York State Board for Nursing, State Education Department, The Cultural Center, Suite 3023, Albany, NY 12230; tel. 518/474-3845; FAX. 518/473-0578; Milene A. Megel, RN, Ph.D., Executive Secretary

New York State Division of Professional Licensing Services, Cultural Education Center, Suite 3021, Empire State Plaza, Albany, NY 12230; tel. 518/474-3817; Robert G. Bentley, Director, Professional Licensing

NORTH CAROLINA
North Carolina Board of Medical Examiners, 1203 Front Street, Zip 27609, P.O. Box 26808, Raleigh, NC 27611-6808; tel. 919/828-1212; FAX. 919/828-1295; Bryant D. Paris, Jr., Executive Secretary

North Carolina Board of Nursing, P.O. Box 2129, Raleigh, NC 27602-2129; tel. 919/782-3211; FAX. 919/781-9461; Carol A. Osman, RN, Ed.D., Executive Director

NORTH DAKOTA
North Dakota Board of Nursing, 919 South 7th Street, Suite 504, Bismarck, ND 58504-5881; tel. 701/328-2974; FAX. 701/328-4614; Karen Macdonald, RN, Executive Director

North Dakota State Board of Medical Examiners, City Center Plaza, Suite 12, 418 East Broadway Avenue, Bismarck, ND 58501; tel. 701/223-9485; FAX. 701/223-9756; Rolf P. Sletten, Executive Secretary-Treasurer

OHIO
Ohio Board of Nursing, 77 South High Street, 17th Floor, Columbus, OH 43266-0316; tel. 614/466-3947; Rosa Lee Weinert, RN, Executive Director

Ohio State Medical Board, 77 South High Street, 17th Floor, Columbus, OH 43266-0315; tel. 614/466-3934; Ray Q. Bumgarner, Executive Director

OKLAHOMA
Oklahoma Board of Nursing, 2915 North Classen Boulevard, Suite 524, Oklahoma City, OK 73106; tel. 405/525-2076; FAX. 405/521-6089; Sulinda Moffett, M.S.N., RN, Executive Director

Oklahoma Board of Osteopathic Examiners, 4848 North Lincoln Boulevard, Suite 100, Oklahoma City, OK 73105-3321; tel. 405/528-8625; FAX. 405/528-6102; Gary R. Clark, Executive Director

Oklahoma State Board of Medical Licensure and Supervision, 5104 North Francis, Suite C, Zip 73118, P.O. Box 18256, Oklahoma City, OK 73154-0256; tel. 405/848-2189; FAX. 405/848-8240; Carole A. Smith, Executive Director

OREGON
Oregon Board of Medical Examiners, 620 Crown Plaza, 1500 S.W. First Avenue, Portland, OR 97201-5826; tel. 503/229-5770; FAX. 503/229-6543; Kathleen Haley, J.D., Executive Director

Oregon State Board of Nursing, 800 N.E. Oregon Street, Suite 465, Portland, OR 97232-2162; tel. 503/731-4745; FAX. 503/731-4755; Joan C. Bouchard, Executive Director

PENNSYLVANIA
Pennsylvania State Board of Medicine, 116 Pine Street, Zip 17101, P.O. Box 2649, Harrisburg, PA 17105-2649; tel. 717/783-1400; FAX. 717/787-7769; Cindy L. Warner, Administrative Assistant

Pennsylvania State Board of Nursing, Department of State, P.O. Box 2649, Harrisburg, PA 17105-2649; tel. 717/783-7142; FAX. 717/787-7769; Miriam H. Limo, Executive Secretary

Pennsylvania State Board of Osteopathic Medicine, P.O. Box 2649, Harrisburg, PA 17105-2649; tel. 717/783-4858; Gina Bittner, Administrative Assistant

RHODE ISLAND
Board of Nursing Education and Nurse Registration, Three Capitol Hill, Room 104, Providence, RI 02908-5097; tel. 401/277-2827; FAX. 401/277-1272; Patricia Molloy, RN, M.S.N., Director

Rhode Island Board of Medical Licensure and Discipline, Rhode Island Department of Health, Cannon Building, Room 205, Three Capitol Hill, Providence, RI 02908-5097; tel. 401/277-3855; FAX. 401/277-2158; Milton W. Hamolsky, M.D., Chief Administrative Officer

SOUTH CAROLINA
Department of Labor, Licensing and Regulation, State Board of Nursing for South Carolina, 220 Executive Center Drive, Suite 220, Columbia, SC 29210; tel. 803/731-1648; FAX. 803/731-1647; Renatta S. Loquist, RN, Executive Director

South Carolina Department of Labor, Licensing and Regulation, Board of Medical Examiners, 101 Executive Center Drive, Saluda Building, Suite 120, Zip 29210, P.O. Box 212269, Columbia, SC 29221-2269; tel. 803/731-1650; FAX. 803/731-1660; Henry D. Foster, Jr., J.D., Executive Director

SOUTH DAKOTA
South Dakota Board of Nursing, 3307 South Lincoln, Sioux Falls, SD 57105; tel. 605/335-4973; FAX. 605/335-2977; Diana Vander Woude, Executive Secretary

South Dakota State Board of Medical and Osteopathic Examiners, 1323 South Minnesota Avenue, Sioux Falls, SD 57105; tel. 605/336-1965; FAX. 605/336-0270; Robert D. Johnson, Executive Secretary

TENNESSEE
Tennessee Board of Nursing, 283 Plus Park Boulevard, Nashville, TN 37217; tel. 615/367-6232; FAX. 615/367-6397; Elizabeth J. Lund, RN, Executive Director

Tennessee State Board of Medical Examiners, 283 Plus Park Boulevard, Nashville, TN 37247-1010; tel. 615/367-6231; FAX. 615/367-6210; Jerry Kosten, Administrator

Organizations / Medical and Nursing Licensure Agencies

Tennessee State Board of Osteopathic Examiners, 283 Plus Park Boulevard, Nashville, TN 37247-1010; tel. 615/367-6281; FAX. 615/367-6210; Judy Hartman, Administrator

TEXAS
Texas Board of Nurse Examiners, 9101 Burnet Road, Suite 104, Austin, TX 78758; tel. 512/835-4880; Louise Waddill, RN, Ph.D., Executive Director

Texas State Board of Medical Examiners, 1812 Centre Creek, Suite 300, Zip 78754, P.O. Box 149134, Austin, TX 78714-9134; tel. 512/834-7728; FAX. 512/834-4597; Bruce A. Levy, M.D., J.D., Executive Director

UTAH
Utah Physicians Licensing Board, Division of Occupational and Professional Licensing, Heber M. Wells Building, 4th Floor, 160 East 300 South, Zip 84145, P.O. Box 45805, Salt Lake City, UT 84145-0805; tel. 801/530-6628; FAX. 801/530-6511; David E. Robinson, Director

Utah State Board of Nursing, 160 East 300 South, P.O. Box 45805, Salt Lake City, UT 84145-0805; tel. 801/530-6628; FAX. 801/530-6511; Laura Poe, Executive Administrator

VERMONT
Vermont Board of Medical Practice, 109 State Street, Montpelier, VT 05609-1106; tel. 802/828-2673; FAX. 802/828-2496; Barbara Newman, J.D., Executive Director

Vermont Board of Nursing Licensure and Regulation Division, 109 State Street, Montpelier, VT 05609-1106; tel. 802/828-3180; FAX. 802/828-2496; Claire LeFrancois, M.P.H., RN, Executive Director

VIRGINIA
Virginia Board of Medicine, 6606 West Broad Street, Fourth Floor, Richmond, VA 23230-1717; tel. 804/662-9925; FAX. 804/662-9943; Warren W. Koontz, Jr., M.D., Executive Director

Virginia Board of Nursing, 6606 West Broad Street, Fourth Floor, Richmond, VA 23230; tel. 804/662-9909; FAX. 804/662-9943; Corinne F. Dorsey, RN, Executive Director

WASHINGTON
State of Washington Board of Osteopathic Medicine and Surgery, Department of Health, 1300 S.E. Quince Street, P.O. Box 47868, Olympia, WA 98504-7868; tel. 206/586-8438; FAX. 206/753-0657; Robert Nicoloff, Executive Director

Washington Medical Quality Assurance Commission, 1300 S.E. Quince Street, P.O Box 47866, Olympia, WA 98504-7866; tel. 206/753-2844; FAX. 206/664-8686; Keith O. Shafer, Executive Director

Washington State Nursing Care Quality Assurance Commission, Department of Health, 1300 S.E. Quince Street, P.O. Box 47864, Olympia, WA 98504-7864; tel. 206/753-2686; FAX. 206/586-5935; Patricia O. Brown, RN, M.S.N., Executive Director

WEST VIRGINIA
West Virginia Board of Examiners for Registered Professional Nurses, 101 Dee Drive, Charleston, WV 25311-1620; tel. 304/558-3596; FAX. 304/558-3666; Janet H. Fairchild, M.S., RN, Executive Secretary

West Virginia Board of Medicine, 101 Dee Drive, Charleston, WV 25311; tel. 304/558-2921; FAX. 304/558-2084; Ronald D. Walton, Executive Director

West Virginia Board of Osteopathy, 334 Penco Road, Weirton, WV 26062; tel. 304/723-4638; Cheryl D. Schreiber, Executive Secretary

WISCONSIN
Bureau of Health Service Professions, 1400 East Washington Avenue, Suite 174, P.O. Box 8935, Madison, WI 53708-8935; tel. 608/266-0257; FAX. 608/267-0644; Cathy Pond, Administrative Assistant

Wisconsin Medical Examining Board, 1400 East Washington Avenue, Zip 53702, P.O. Box 8935, Madison, WI 53708; tel. 608/266-2811; FAX. 608/267-0644; Patrick D. Braatz, Bureau Director

WYOMING
Wyoming Board of Medicine, Barrett Building, Suite 208, 2301 Central Avenue, Cheyenne, WY 82002; tel. 307/777-6463; FAX. 307/777-6478; Carole Shotwell, Executive Secretary

Wyoming State Board of Nursing, Barrett Building, Second Floor, 2301 Central Avenue, Cheyenne, WY 82002; tel. 307/777-7601; FAX. 307/777-6005; Toma A. Nisbet, RN, M.S., Executive Director

U.S. Associated Areas

AMERICAN SAMOA-GUAM
American Samoa Health Services Regulatory Board, LBJ Tropical Medical Center, Pago Pago, AS 96799; tel. 684/633-1222, ext. 206; FAX. 684/633-1869; Marie F. Mao, RN, M.S., Executive Secretary

GUAM
Guam Board of Nurse Examiners, Department of Public Health and Social Services, P.O. Box 2816, Agana, GU 96910; tel. 671/734-7296; FAX. 671/734-2066; Teofila P. Cruz, RN, M.S., Administrator

Health Professional Licensing Office, Department of Public Health and Social Services, Route 10, Mangilao, Zip 96923, P.O. Box 2816, Agana, GU 96910; tel. 671/734-7304; FAX. 671/734-2066; Teofila P. Cruz, Administrator

PUERTO RICO
Council on Higher Education of Puerto Rico, UPR Station, P.O. Box 23305, San Juan, PR 00931-3305; tel. 809/758-3356; Madeline Quilichini Paz, Director, Office of Licensing and Accreditation

Puerto Rico Board of Medical Examiners, Kennedy Avenue, ILA Building, Hogar del Obrero Portuario, Piso 8, Puerto Nuevo, Zip 00920, Call Box 13969, San Juan, PR 00908; tel. 809/793-1333; FAX. 809/782-8733; Pablo Valentin Torres, J.D., Executive Director

VIRGIN ISLANDS
Virgin Islands Board of Medical Examiners, Virgin Islands Department of Health, 48 Sugar Estate, St. Thomas, VI 00802; tel. 809/774-0117; FAX. 809/777-4001; Jane Aubain, Office Manager

Virgin Islands Board of Nursing Licensure, P.O. Box 4247, St. Thomas, VI 00803; tel. 809/776-7397; FAX. 809/777-4003; Winifred L. Garfield, CRNA, Executive Secretary

Canada

ALBERTA
College of Physicians and Surgeons of Alberta, 9901 108th Street, Edmonton, AB T5K 1G9; tel. 403/423-4764; L. H. le Riche, M.B., CH.B., Registrar

MANITOBA
College of Physicians and Surgeons of Manitoba, 494 St. James Street, Winnipeg, MB R3G 3J4; tel. 204/774-4344; FAX. 204/774-0750; Kenneth R. Brown, M.D., Registrar

NEW BRUNSWICK
College of Physicians and Surgeons of New Brunswick, 10 Prince Edward Street, Saint John, NB E2L 4M5

NOVA SCOTIA
Provincial Medical Board of Nova Scotia, Office of the Registrar, 5248 Morris Street, Halifax, NS B3J 1B4; tel. 902/422-5823; FAX. 902/422-5035; Dr. Cameron Little, Registrar, Secretary

PRINCE EDWARD ISLAND
College of Physicians and Surgeons of Prince Edward Island, 199 Grafton Street, Charlottetown, PE C1A 1L2; tel. 902/566-3861; FAX. 902/566-3861; H. E. Ross, M.D., Registrar

QUEBEC
Corporation Professionnelle des Medecins du Quebec, College des medecins du Quebec, 1440 Ste. Catherine Street, W., Suite 914, Zip H3G 1S5, 2170, boul. Rene-Levesque Quest, Montreal, PQ H3H 2T8; tel. 514/933-4441; FAX. 514/933-3112; Joelle Lescop, M.D., Secretary General

SASKATCHEWAN
College of Physicians and Surgeons of Saskatchewan, 211 Fourth Avenue, S., Saskatoon, SK S7K 1N1; tel. 306/244-7355; FAX. 306/244-0090; D. A. Kendel, M.D., Registrar

Peer Review Organizations

The following list of PROs was obtained from the Office of Medical Review, Division of Program Operation, HCFA. For more information, contact the office at 410/966-7201.

United States

ALABAMA: Alabama Quality Assurance Foundation, Inc., One Perimeter Park, S., Suite 200 North, Birmingham, AL 35243-2327; tel. 205/970-1600; FAX. 205/970-1616; H. Terrell Lindsey, President, Chief Executive Officer

ALASKA: PRO-WEST, 10700 Meridian Avenue, N., Suite 100, Seattle, WA 98133-9075; tel. 206/364-9700; FAX. 206/368-2419; John W. Daise, Chief Executive Officer

ARIZONA: Health Services Advisory Group, Inc., 301 East Bethany Home Road, Suite B-157, Phoenix, AZ 85012; tel. 602/264-6382; FAX. 602/241-0757; Lawrence J. Shapiro, M.D., President, Chief Executive Officer

ARKANSAS: Arkansas Foundation for Medical Care, Inc., 809 Garrision Avenue, P.O. Box 2424, Fort Smith, AR 72902; tel. 501/785-2471; FAX. 501/785-3460; Russell G. Brasher, Ph.D., Chief Executive Officer

CALIFORNIA: California Medical Review, Inc., 60 Spear Street, Suite 500, San Francisco, CA 94105; tel. 415/882-5800; FAX. 415/882-5995; Jo Ellen H. Ross, Chief Executive Officer

COLORADO: Colorado Foundation for Medical Care, 2821 South Parker Road, Suite 605, Aurora, CO 80014-2713; tel. 303/695-3300; FAX. 303/695-3350; Arja P. Adair, Jr., Executive Director

CONNECTICUT: Connecticut Peer Review Organization, Inc., 100 Roscommon Drive, Suite 200, Middletown, CT 06457; tel. 203/632-2008; FAX. 203/632-5865; Neil Dreyer, M.D., President

DELAWARE: West Virginia Medical Institute, Inc., 3001 Chesterfield Place, Charleston, WV 25304; tel. 304/346-9864, ext. 269; FAX. 304/346-9863; Harry S. Weeks, Jr., M.D., President

DISTRICT OF COLUMBIA: Delmarva Foundation for Medical Care, Inc., 9240 Centreville Road, Easton, MD 21601; tel. 410/822-0697; FAX. 410/822-1997; Jean E. Edwards, Vice President, External Relations

FLORIDA: Florida Medical Quality Assurance, Inc., 1211 North Westshore Boulevard, Suite 700, Tampa, FL 33607; tel. 813/281-9024; FAX. 813/281-2195; Jennifer Barnett, President, Chief Executive Officer

GEORGIA: Georgia Medical Care Foundation, 57 Executive Park, S., Suite 200, Atlanta, GA 30329; tel. 404/982-0411; FAX. 404/982-7591; Tom W. Williams, Chief Executive Officer

HAWAII: Hawaii Medical Service Association, 818 Keeaumoku Street, P.O. Box 860, Honolulu, HI 96808-0860; tel. 808/944-3586; FAX. 808/943-8811; Sandra J. Wells, Assistant Vice President

IDAHO: PRO-WEST, 10700 Meridian Avenue, N., Suite 100, Seattle, WA 98133-9075; tel. 206/364-9700; FAX. 208/343-4705; John W. Daise, Chief Executive Officer

ILLINOIS: Crescent Counties Foundation for Medical Care, 1001 Warrenville Road, Suite 500, Lisle, IL 60532; tel. 708/769-9600; FAX. 708/769-5595; Gary Button, M.D., President

INDIANA: Indiana Medical Review Organization, 2901 Ohio Boulevard, P.O. Box 3713, Terre Haute, IN 47803; tel. 812/234-1499; FAX. 812/232-6167; Philip L. Morphew, Chief Executive Officer

IOWA: Iowa Foundation for Medical Care, 6000 Westown Parkway, Suite 350 E, West Des Moines, IA 50266-7771; tel. 515/223-2900; FAX. 515/222-2407; Fred A. Ferree, Executive Vice President

KANSAS: The Kansas Foundation for Medical Care, Inc., 2947 S.W. Wanamaker Drive, Topeka, KS 66614; tel. 913/273-2552, ext. 363; FAX. 913/273-5130; Larry W. Pitman, Chief Executive Officer

KENTUCKY: Kentucky Medical Review Organization, 10503 Timberwood Circle, Suite 200, P.O. Box 23540, Louisville, KY 40223; tel. 502/339-7442; FAX. 502/339-8641; Philip L. Morphew, Executive Director

LOUISIANA: Louisiana Health Care Review, Inc., 8591 United Plaza Boulevard, Suite 270, Baton Rouge, LA 70809; tel. 504/926-6353; FAX. 504/923-0957; Leo Stanley, Chief Executive Officer

MAINE: Health Care Review, Inc. (Maine), Moshassuck Square, 528 North Main Street, Suite 4, Providence, RI 02904; tel. 401/331-6661; FAX. 401/331-4438; Edward J. Lynch, President

MARYLAND: Delmarva Foundation for Medical Care, Inc., 9240 Centreville Road, Easton, MD 21601; tel. 410/822-0697; FAX. 410/822-1997; Linda E. Clark, RN, Executive Vice President

MASSACHUSETTS: Massachusetts Peer Review Organization, Inc., 235 Wyman Street, Waltham, MA 02154-1231; tel. 617/890-0011; FAX. 617/487-0083; Brenda E. Richardson, M.D., President

MICHIGAN: Michigan Peer Review Organization, 40600 Ann Arbor Road, Suite 200, Plymouth, MI 48170-4495; tel. 313/459-0900; Gary Horvat, Chief Executive Officer

MINNESOTA: Foundation for Health Care Evaluation, 2901 Metro Drive, Suite 400, Bloomington, MN 55425; tel. 612/854-3306; FAX. 612/853-8503; David M. Ziegenhagen, Chief Executive Officer

MISSISSIPPI: Mississippi Foundation for Medical Care, Inc., 735 Riverside Drive, P.O. Box 4665, Jackson, MS 39296-4665; tel. 601/948-8894; FAX. 601/948-8917; W. Lamar Weems, M.D., President

MISSOURI: Missouri Patient Care Review Foundation, 505 Hobbs Road, Suite 100, Jefferson City, MO 65109; tel. 314/893-7900; FAX. 314/893-5827; Dan Jaco, Chief Executive Officer

MONTANA: Montana-Wyoming Foundation for Medical Care, 400 North Park Avenue, 2nd Floor, Helena, MT 59601; tel. 406/443-4020; FAX. 406/443-4585; Robert Henderson, M.D., President

NEBRASKA: Iowa Foundation for Medical Care/The Sunderbruch Corporation/Nebraska, CTU Building, 1221 N Street, Suite 800, Lincoln, NE 68508; tel. 402/474-7471; FAX. 402/474-7410; Fred Ferree, Executive Vice President

NEVADA: Nevada Peer Review, 675 East 2100 South, Suite 270, Salt Lake City, UT 84106-1864; tel. 702/385-9933; FAX. 702/385-4586; Gary D. Lower, M.D., President

NEW HAMPSHIRE: New Hampshire Foundation for Medical Care, 15 Old Rollinsford Road, Suite 302, Dover, NH 03820-2830; tel. 603/749-1641; FAX. 603/749-1195; Robert A. Aurilio, Chief Executive Officer

NEW JERSEY: The Peer Review Organization of New Jersey, Inc., Central Division, Brier Hill Court, Building J, East Brunswick, NJ 08816; tel. 908/238-5570; FAX. 908/238-7766; Martin P. Margolies, Chief Executive Officer

NEW MEXICO: New Mexico Medical Review Association, 707 Broadway, N.E., Suite 200, P.O. Box 27449, Albuquerque, NM 87125-7449; tel. 505/842-6236; FAX. 505/764-9093; Ernest D. Cuaron, Chief Executive Officer

NEW YORK: IPRO, 1979 Marcus Avenue, First Floor, Lake Success, NY 11042-1002; tel. 516/326-7767, ext. 540; FAX. 516/328-2310; Theodore O. Will, Executive Vice President

NORTH CAROLINA: Medical Review of North Carolina, Inc., 5625 Dillard Drive, Suite 203, Cary, NC 27511-9227; tel. 919/851-2955; FAX. 919/851-8457; Charles Riddick, Executive Director

NORTH DAKOTA: North Dakota Health Care Review Inc., 800 31st Avenue S.W., Minot, ND 58701; tel. 701/852-4231; FAX. 701/838-6009; David Remillard, Chief Executive Officer

OHIO: Peer Review Systems, Inc., 757 Brooksedge Plaza Drive, P.O. Box 6174, Westerville, OH 43086-6174; tel. 614/895-9900; FAX. 614/895-6784; Gregory J. Dykes, Chief Executive Officer

OKLAHOMA: Oklahoma Foundation for Peer Review, Inc., The Paragon Building, 5801 Broadway Extension, Suite 400, Oklahoma City, OK 73118-7489; tel. 405/840-2891; FAX. 405/840-1343; Jim L. Williams, Chief Executive Officer

OREGON: Oregon Medical Professional Review Organization, 1220 S.W. Morrison, Suite 200, Portland, OR 97205; tel. 503/279-0100; FAX. 503/279-0190; Robert S. Kinoshita, President

PENNSYLVANIA: Keystone Peer Review Organization, Inc., 777 East Park Drive, P.O. Box 8310, Harrisburg, PA 17105-8310; tel. 717/564-8288; FAX. 717/564-4188; John DiNardi III, Executive Director

RHODE ISLAND: Health Care Review, Inc., Henry C. Hall Building, 345 Blackstone Boulevard, Providence, RI 02906; tel. 401/331-6661; FAX. 401/331-4438; Edward J. Lynch, President

SOUTH CAROLINA: Medical Review of North Carolina (PRO for South Carolina), 5625 Dillard Drive, Suite 203, Cary, NC 27511-9227; tel. 919/851-2955; FAX. 919/851-8457; Charles Riddick, Executive Director

SOUTH DAKOTA: South Dakota Foundation for Medical Care, 1323 South Minnesota Avenue, Sioux Falls, SD 57105; tel. 605/336-3505; FAX. 605/336-0270; Robert D. Johnson, Chief Executive Director

TENNESSEE: Mid-South Foundation for Medical Care, Inc., 6401 Poplar Avenue, Suite 400, Memphis, TN 38119; tel. 901/682-0381; FAX. 901/761-3786; Logan Malone, Chief Executive Officer

TEXAS: Texas Medical Foundation, Barton Oaks Plaza Two, Suite 200, 901 Mopac Expressway, S., Austin, TX 78746-5799; tel. 512/329-6610; FAX. 512/327-7159; Phil Dunne, Executive Director

Organizations / Peer Review Organizations

UTAH: HealthInsight, 675 East 2100 South, Suite 270, Salt Lake City, UT 84106-1864; tel. 801/487-2290; FAX. 801/487-2296; Nina M. Egbert, Executive Assistant

VERMONT: New Hampshire Foundation for Medical Care, 15 Old Rollinsford Road, Suite 302, Dover, NH 03820-2830; tel. 603/749-1641; FAX. 603/749-1195; Robert A. Aurilio, Chief Executive Officer

VIRGINIA: Medical Society of Virginia Review Organization, 1604 Santa Rosa Road, Suite 200, Zip 23229-5008, P.O. Box K-70, Richmond, VA 23288-0070; tel. 804/289-5320; FAX. 804/289-5324; Terrence E. Dwyer, Executive Director

WASHINGTON: PRO-WEST, 10700 Meridian Avenue, N., Suite 100, Seattle, WA 98133-9075; tel. 206/364-9700; FAX. 206/368-2419; John W. Daise, Chief Executive Officer

WEST VIRGINIA: West Virginia Medical Institute, Inc., 3001 Chesterfield Place, Charleston, WV 25304; tel. 304/346-9864, ext. 269; FAX. 304/346-9863; Harry S. Weeks, Jr., M.D., President

WISCONSIN: Wisconsin Peer Review Organization, 2909 Landmark Place, Madison, WI 53713; tel. 608/274-1940; FAX. 608/274-5008; Greg E. Simmons, Chief Executive Officer

WYOMING: Montana-Wyoming Foundation for Medical Care, 400 North Park Avenue, 2nd Floor, Helena, MT 59601; tel. 406/443-4020; FAX. 406/443-4585; Robert Henderson, M.D., President

U.S. Associated Areas

AMERICAN SAMOA-GUAM: Hawaii Medical Service Association (PRO for Hawaii American Samoa/Guam), P.O. Box 860, Honolulu, HI 96808-0860; tel. 808/944-3586; FAX. 808/943-8811; Sandra J. Wells, Assistant Vice President

PUERTO RICO: Puerto Rico Foundation for Medical Care, Inc., Quality Improvement Professional Research Organization (QIPRO), Mercantile Plaza Building, Suite 605, Hato Rey, PR 00918; tel. 809/753-6705; FAX. 809/753-6885; Sylvia Fuertes, M.D., President

VIRGIN ISLANDS: Virgin Islands Medical Institute, Inc., 1AD Estate Diamond Ruby, P.O. Box 1566, Christiansted, St. Croix, U.S., VI 00821-1566; tel. 809/778-6470; FAX. 809/778-6801; Denyce E. Singleton, Chief Executive Officer

State Health Planning and Development Agencies

United States

The following is a list of state health planning and development agencies. The information was obtained from the Missouri Department of Health, Certificate of Need Program. For information about other state agencies and organizations that fulfill many of the same functions, contact the state or metropolitan hospital associations.

ALABAMA: State Health Planning Agency, State of Alabama, 312 Montgomery Street, Seventh Floor, Montgomery, AL 36104; tel. 334/242–4103; FAX. 334/242–4113; Gary L. Jordan, Director, Office of Health Planning

ALASKA: Facilities and Planning Section, Department of Health and Social Services, P.O. Box 110650, Juneau, AK 99811–0650; tel. 907/465–3015; FAX. 907/465–2499; Larry J. Streuber, Section Chief

ARIZONA: Office of Health Planning, Evaluation and Statistics, 1740 West Adams, Suite 312, Phoenix, AZ 85007; tel. 602/542–1216; FAX. 602/542–1244; Phil Lopes, Chief

CALIFORNIA: Office of Statewide Health Planning and Development, 1600 Ninth Street, Suite 440, Sacramento, CA 95814; tel. 916/654–2032; FAX. 916/654–3138; Paul Cerles, Chief, Professions Development and Assistance Section

COLORADO: Department of Health, Office of Health, 4300 Cherry Creek Drive, S., Denver, CO 80222–1530; tel. 303/692–2858; Susan Rehak, Planner

CONNECTICUT: Connecticut Department of Public Health and Addiction Services, Health Research and Data Analysis Unit, 150 Washington Street, Hartford, CT 06106; tel. 203/566–1120; FAX. 203/566–8801; Donald Iodice, Health Program Associate

DELAWARE: Bureau of Health Planning and Resources Management, Department of Health and Social Services, P.O. Box 637, Dover, DE 19903; tel. 302/739–4776; FAX. 302/739–3008; Robert I. Welch, Director

DISTRICT OF COLUMBIA: Plan Development and Data Coordination, 613 G Street, N.W., Suite 311, Washington, DC 20001; tel. 202/727–0744; Gail Smith, Interim Chief

FLORIDA: Agency for Health Care Administration, Office of Health Policy, 2727 Mahan Drive, Tallahassee, FL 32308–5403; tel. 904/488–8394; FAX. 904/922–2897; H. Robert Sharpe, Chief

GEORGIA: State Health Planning Agency, Planning and Implementation Division, Four Executive Park Drive, N.E., Suite 2100, Atlanta, GA 30329; tel. 404/679–4829; FAX. 404/679–4914; Karen Butler–Decker, Director, Division of Planning and Implementation

HAWAII: State Health Planning and Development Agency, 335 Merchant Street, Suite 214–E, Honolulu, HI 96813; tel. 808/587–0788; FAX. 808/587–0783; Patricia Hunter, Chief Planning Branch

IDAHO: Center for Vital Statistics and Health Policy, Division of Health, Idaho Department of Health and Welfare, 450 West State Street, First Floor, P.O. Box 83720, Boise, ID 83720–0036; tel. 208/334–5976; FAX. 208/334–0685; Jane Smith, Chief

ILLINOIS: Illinois Department of Public Health, Division of Health Policy, 525 West Jefferson, Springfield, IL 62761; tel. 217/782–6235; Angela Oldfield, Chief

INDIANA: Indiana State Board of Health, Office of Policy and Research, 1330 West Michigan Street, Indianapolis, IN 46206–1964; tel. 317/683–6521; FAX. 317/633–0776; Keith Main, Ed.D.

IOWA: Department of Public Health, Division of Substance Abuse and Health Promotion, Lucas State Office Building, Des Moines, IA 50319; tel. 515/281–5914; FAX. 515/281–4958; Ronald Eckoff

KENTUCKY: Interim Office of Health Planning and Certification, Cabinet for Human Resources, 275 East Main Street, Health Services Building, Frankfort, KY 40621; tel. 502/564–3386; FAX. 502/564–6533; Don Coffey, Manager, Health Planning Branch

MAINE: Division of Health Planning, Office of Health Planning, and Development, Department of Human Services, State House Station 11, 35 Anthony Avenue, Augusta, ME 04333–0011; tel. 207/624–5424; FAX. 207/624–5431; Stephen LaForge, Director

MARYLAND: Maryland Health Resources Planning Commission, 4201 Patterson Avenue, P.O. Box 2679, Baltimore, MD 21215–2299; tel. 410/764–3255; FAX. 410/764–5996; James Stanton, Executive Director

MICHIGAN: Office of Policy, Planning and Evaluation, Division of Policy and Planning, 3423 North Martin Luther King Jr. Boulevard, Lansing, MI 48909; tel. 517/335–9372; FAX. 517/335–8560; Jan Ruff, Chief

MINNESOTA: Division of Community Health Services, Health Systems Development Bureau, Metro Square Building, 121 East Seventh Place, Suite 460, Minneapolis, MN 55164–0075; tel. 612/296–9720; FAX. 612/296–9362; Ryan Church, Director

MISSISSIPPI: Mississippi State Department of Health, Health Planning and Resource Development Division, 2423 North State Street, P.O. Box 1700, Jackson, MS 39215–1700; tel. 601/960–7874; FAX. 601/354–6123; Jill E. Knight, Senior Health Planner

MISSOURI: Missouri Department of Health, Office of Planning, 1738 East Elm Street, P.O. Box 570, Jefferson City, MO 65102; tel. 314/751–6005; FAX. 314/751–6041; Linda Hillemann, Chief

MONTANA: Health Services Division, Department of Health and Environmental Sciences, Cogswell Building, P.O. Box 200901, Helena, MT 59620–0901; tel. 406/444–4349; FAX. 406/444–2606; Gary T. Rose, Health Planner

NEBRASKA: Division of Health Policy/Planning, Nebraska Department of Health, P.O. Box 95007, Lincoln, NE 68509; tel. 402/471–2337; FAX. 402/471–0180; John Sahs, Director

NEVADA: State Health Division, Bureau of Health Planning, 505 East King Street, Suite 203, Carson City, NV 89710; tel. 702/687–4720; FAX. 702/687–3859; Emil DeJan, Chief

NEW HAMPSHIRE: Office of Health Services Planning and Review, Six Hazen Drive, Concord, NH 03301–6527; tel. 603/271–4606; FAX. 603/271–3745; Edmond Duchesne, Administrator, Planning Coordination

NEW JERSEY: Health Care Planning Services, New Jersey Department of Health, CN 360, John Fitch Plaza, Trenton, NJ 08625–0360; tel. 609/292–5960; FAX. 609/292–3780; John Gontarski, Director

NEW MEXICO: New Mexico Health Policy Commission, 435 St. Michael's Drive, Suite A–202, Santa Fe, NM 87505; tel. 505/827–7500; FAX. 505/827–4481; Katherine Ganz, M.D., Director

NEW YORK: New York State Department of Health, Division of Planning, Policy and Resource Development, Corning Tower, Suite 1619, Empire State Plaza, Albany, NY 12237; tel. 518/473–7541; FAX. 518/473–6195; Ronald L. Rouse, Acting Director

NORTH CAROLINA: State Medical Facilities Planning Section, 701 Barbour Drive, 27603, P.O. Box 29530, Raleigh, NC 27626–0530; tel. 919/733–4130; FAX. 919/715–4413; Curtis Jackson, Chief

NORTH DAKOTA: Division of Health Resource Analysis, State Capitol, Judicial Wing, 600 East Boulevard Avenue, Bismarck, ND 58505–0200; tel. 701/328–2894; FAX. 701/328–4727; Fred Larson, Project Review Administrator

OHIO: Ohio Department of Health, Health Systems Planning, Primary Care and Rural Health, 246 North High Street, P.O. Box 118, Columbus, OH 43266–0118; tel. 614/466–3325; FAX. 614/644–8661; Louis Pomerantz, Chief, Health Systems Planning, Primary Care, Rural Health

OKLAHOMA: Oklahoma State Department of Health, Health Promotion and Policy Analysis, 1000 N.E. 10th Street, Oklahoma City, OK 73117–1299; tel. 405/271–1110; Jerry Prilliman, Director Planning

PENNSYLVANIA: Division of Planning and Technical Assistance, Pennsylvania Department of Health, Health and Welfare Building, Suite 1027, P.O. Box 90, Harrisburg, PA 17108; tel. 717/783–1410; FAX. 717/783–3794; William Dethlefs, Director

RHODE ISLAND: Health Policy and Planning, Rhode Island Department of Health, Cannon Building, Three Capitol Hill, Suite 401, Providence, RI 02908; tel. 401/277–2231; FAX. 401/277–6548; William J. Waters, Jr., Ph.D., Deputy Director

SOUTH CAROLINA: DHEC, Division of Planning and Certificate of Need, 2600 Bull Street, Columbia, SC 29201; tel. 803/737–7200; FAX. 803/737–7212; Albert Whiteside, Director

SOUTH DAKOTA: Health Policy and External Affairs, South Dakota Department of Health, 445 East Capitol Avenue, Pierre, SD 57501–3185; tel. 605/773–3361; FAX. 605/773–5683; Terrance L. Dosch, Assistant Secretary

TENNESSEE: Office of Health Policy, Tennessee Tower, 312 Eighth Avenue, N., Ninth Floor, Nashville, TN 37247–0150; tel. 615/741–9395; FAX. 615/741–2491; Gary Miles, Health Planner

TEXAS: Bureau of State Health Data and Policy Analysis, Texas Department of Health, 1100 West 49th Street, Austin, TX 78756; tel. 512/458–7261; FAX. 512/458–7344; Trish O'Day, Planning Director

UTAH: Office of Strategic Planning and Evaluation, Utah Department of Health, 288 North 1460 West, P.O. Box 16700, Salt Lake City, UT 84116–0700; tel. 801/538–6352; FAX. 801/538–6694; Laverne Snow, Director

VERMONT: Vermont Health Care Authority, 89 Main Street, Drawer 20, Montpelier, VT 05620–3601; tel. 802/828–2900; FAX. 802/828–2949; Stan Lane, Policy Analyst

Organizations / State Health Planning and Development Agencies

VIRGINIA: Virginia Department of Health, Office of Resources Development, 1500 East Main Street, Suite 105, P.O. Box 2448, Richmond, VA 23219; tel. 804/786-7463; FAX. 804/786-6776; Paul E. Parker, Director

WASHINGTON: Washington State Board of Health, 1102 S. E. Quince, P.O. Box 47990, Olympia, WA 98504-7990; tel. 360/586-0399; FAX. 206/586-6033; Sylvia I. Beck, Executive Director

WEST VIRGINIA: West Virginia Office of Health Reform, 1018 Kanawha Boulevard, E., Suite 901, Charleston, WV 25301-2827; tel. 304/558-0530; FAX. 304/558-0532; Renate E. Pore, Ph.D., Director

WYOMING: Department of Health, 133 Hathaway Building, Suite 117, Cheyenne, WY 82002; tel. 307/777-7656; FAX. 307/777-7439; Earl DeGroot, HP 2000 Coordinator

State and Provincial Government Agencies

The following list includes state departments of health and welfare, and their subagencies as well as such independent agencies as those for crippled children's services, maternal and child health, mental health, and vocational rehabilitation. The information was obtained directly from the agencies.

United States

ALABAMA
The Honorable Jim Folsom, Governor, 334/242-7100

Health
- **Department of Public Health,** 434 Monroe Street, Montgomery, AL 36130-3017; tel. 334/613-5200; FAX. 334/240-3387; Donald E. Williamson, M.D., State Health Officer

Family
- **Alabama Department of Public Health, Bureau of Family Health Services,** 434 Monroe Street, Montgomery, AL 36130-3017; tel. 334/242-5661; FAX. 334/269-4865; Thomas M. Miller, M.D., M.P.H., Director

Licensing
- **Alabama Department of Public Health, Division of Licensure and Certification,** 434 Monroe Street, Montgomery, AL 36130-1701; tel. 334/240-3503; FAX. 334/240-3147; L. O'Neal Green, Director

Welfare
- **Department of Human Resources,** Gordon Persons Building, 50 Ripley Street, Montgomery, AL 36130; tel. 334/242-1160; FAX. 334/242-0198; Andrew P. Hornsby, Jr., Commissioner

Medical Services
- **Alabama Medicaid Agency,** 501 Dexter Avenue, P.O. Box 5264, Montgomery, AL 36103-5624; tel. 334/242-5600; FAX. 334/242-5097; David G. Toney, Commissioner

Insurance
- **Department of Insurance,** 135 South Union Street, Montgomery, AL 36130; tel. 334/269-3550; FAX. 334/269-3213; James H. Dill, Commissioner

Other

Education
- **State Department of Education,** Gordon Persons Building, Suite 5114, P.O. Box 302101, Montgomery, AL 36130-2101; tel. 334/242-9700; FAX. 334/242-9708; Wayne Teague, Superintendent

Mental Health
- **State Department of Mental Health and Mental Retardation,** 200 Interstate Park Drive, P.O. Box 3710, Montgomery, AL 36109-0710; tel. 334/271-9207; FAX. 334/270-4629; Richard E. Hanan, Commissioner

Nursing
- **Alabama Board of Nursing,** RSA Plaza, 770 Washington Avenue, Suite 250, Montgomery, AL 36130; tel. 334/242-4060; FAX. 334/242-4360; Judi Crume, RN, M.S.N., Executive Officer

Rehabilitation
- **Department of Rehabilitation Services,** 2129 East South Boulevard, Montgomery, AL 36111; tel. 334/281-8780; FAX. 334/281-1973; Lamona Lucas, Commissioner

ALASKA
The Honorable Tony Knowles, Governor, 907/465-3500

Health
- **Department of Health and Social Services,** 350 Main Street, Room 229, P.O. Box 110601, Juneau, AK 99811-0601; tel. 907/465-3030; FAX. 907/465-3068; Jay A. Livey, Acting Commissioner

Assistance
- **State of Alaska, Division of Public Assistance,** P.O. 110640, Juneau, AK 99811-0640; tel. 907/465-3347; FAX. 907/463-5154; Jan Hansen, Director

Family
- **Division of Family and Youth Services,** P.O. Box 110630, Juneau, AK 99811; tel. 907/465-3191; FAX. 907/465-3397; Michael L. Price, Director

Finance
- **Division of Administrative Services, Department of Health and Social Services,** P.O. Box 110650, Juneau, AK 99811-0650; tel. 907/465-3082; FAX. 907/465-2499; Janet E. Clarke, Director

Licensing
- **Health Facilities Licensing and Certification,** 4730 Business Park Boulevard, Suite 18, Building H, Anchorage, AK 99503-7137; tel. 907/561-8081; FAX. 907/561-3011; Karen Martz, Administrator

Medical Assistance
- **Division of Medical Assistance,** P.O. Box 110660, Juneau, AK 99811-0660; tel. 907/465-3355; FAX. 907/465-2204; Kimberly Busch, Director

Mental Health
- **Division of Mental Health and Developmental Disabilities,** P.O. Box 110620, Juneau, AK 99811-0620; tel. 907/465-3370; FAX. 907/465-2668

Substance Abuse
- **Division of Alcoholism and Drug Abuse,** P.O. Box 110607, Juneau, AK 99811-0607; tel. 907/465-2071; FAX. 907/465-2185; Loren A. Jones, Director

Other
- **State of Alaska, Department of Health and Social Services,** 350 Main Street, Room 229, P.O. Box 110601, Juneau, AK 99811-0601; tel. 907/465-3030; FAX. 907/465-3068; Jay A. Livey, Deputy Commissioner

Other

Education
- **Department of Education,** 801 West 10th Street, Suite 200, Juneau, AK 99801-1894; tel. 907/465-2800; FAX. 907/465-4156; Jerry Covey, Commissioner

Licensing
- **Department of Commerce and Economic Development, Division of Occupational Licensing, State Medical Board,** 3601 C Street, Suite 722, Anchorage, AK 99503; tel. 907/561-2878; FAX. 907/562-5781; Leslie G. Haywood, Executive Secretary

Nursing
- **Alaska Board of Nursing,** 3601 C Street, Suite 722, Anchorage, AK 99503; tel. 907/561-2878; FAX. 907/562-5781; Dorothy P. Fulton, RN, M.A., Executive Secretary

Rehabilitation
- **Division of Vocational Rehabilitation,** 801 West 10th Street, Suite 200, Juneau, AK 99801-1894; tel. 907/465-2814; FAX. 907/465-2856; Keith J. Anderson, Director

ARIZONA
The Honorable Fife Symington, Governor, 602/542-4331

Health
- **Arizona Department of Health Services,** 1740 West Adams Street, Suite 407, Phoenix, AZ 85007; tel. 602/542-1025; FAX. 602/542-1062; Jack Dillenberg, D.D.S., M.P.H., Director

Children
- **Children's Rehabilitative Services,** Administrative Offices, 1740 West Adams Street, Suite 300, Phoenix, AZ 85007; tel. 602/542-1860; FAX. 602/542-2589; Lynda Miller, Chief

Environment
- **Arizona Department of Environmental Quality,** 3033 North Central Avenue, Phoenix, AZ 85012; tel. 602/207-2300; FAX. 602/207-2218, ext. 2200; Edward Z. Fox

Family
- **Community and Family Health Services,** 1740 West Adams Street, Suite 307, Phoenix, AZ 85007; tel. 602/542-1223; FAX. 602/542-1265; Jane Pearson, RN, Assistant Director

Health
- **Behavioral Health Services, Arizona Department of Health Services,** 2122 East Highland, Suite 100, Phoenix, AZ 85016; tel. 602/381-8999; FAX. 602/553-9140; Charles P. Carbone, Associate Director

Licensing
- **Arizona Department of Health Services, Division of Health and Child Care Review Services, Office of Health Care Licensure,** 1647 East Morten, Phoenix, AZ 85020; tel. 602/255-1177; FAX. 602/255-1109; Lynda Rahi, Associate Director

Prevention
- **Arizona Department of Health Services, Disease Prevention Services,** 3815 North Black Canyon Highway, Phoenix, AZ 85015; tel. 602/230-5808; FAX. 602/230-5959; Norman J. Petersen, Assistant Director

- **Department of Economic Security,** Site Code 010A, P.O. Box 6123, Phoenix, AZ 85005; tel. 602/542-5678; FAX. 602/542-5339; Linda J. Blessing, Director

Rehabilitation
- **Rehabilitation Services Administration (930A),** 1789 West Jefferson, 2nd Floor Northwest, Phoenix, AZ 85007; tel. 602/542-3332; FAX. 602/542-3778; Roger J. Hodges, Administrator

Insurance
- **Department of Insurance,** 3030 North Third Street, Suite 1100, Phoenix, AZ 85012; tel. 602/255-5400; FAX. 602/255-5316

Other

Medical Examiners
- **Arizona Board of Medical Examiners,** 1651 East Morten, Suite 210, Phoenix, AZ 85020; tel. 602/255-3751; Mark R. Speicher, Executive Director

Nursing
- **Arizona State Board of Nursing,** 1651 East Morten, Suite 150, Phoenix, AZ 85020; tel. 602/255-5092; FAX. 602/255-5130; Fran Roberts, RN, Ph.D., Executive Director

ARKANSAS
The Honorable Jim Guy Tucker, Governor, 501/682-2345

Health
- **Department of Health,** 4815 West Markham Street, Slot 39, Little Rock, AR 72205-3867; tel. 501/661-2111; FAX. 501/661-2601; Sandra B. Nichols, M.D., Director

Administration
- **Bureau of Administrative Support,** State Health Building, Little Rock, AR 72205-3867; tel. 501/661-2252; Tom Butler, Director

Community
- **Bureau of Community Health Services, Arkansas Department of Health,** 4815 West Markham Street, Slot 2, Little Rock, AR 72205-3867; tel. 501/661-2167; FAX. 501/661-2601; Jim Mills, Director

Facilities
- **Division of Health Facility Services,** 4815 West Markham Street, Slot 9, Little Rock, AR 72205-3867; tel. 501/661-2201; FAX. 501/661-2165; Valetta M. Buck, Director

Organizations / State and Provincial Government Agencies

Health
Bureau of Public Health Programs, Arkansas Department of Health, 4815 West Markham Street, Slot 41, Little Rock, AR 72205; tel. 501/661–2243; FAX. 501/661–2055; Martha Hiett, Director

Planning
Planning and Policy Development, Arkansas Department of Health, 4815 W. Markham, Slot 55, Little Rock, AR 72205; tel. 501/661–2238; FAX. 501/661–2414; Nancy Kirsch, Deputy Director

Resources
Bureau of Health Resources, 4815 West Markham Street, Slot 21, Little Rock, AR 72205-3867; tel. 501/661–2268; FAX. 501/661–2544; Robert L. Robinette, B.S., M.S.E.H., Director

Welfare
Arkansas Department of Human Services, P.O. Box 1437, Little Rock, AR 72203-1437; tel. 501/682–8650; FAX. 501/682–6836; Tom Dalton, Director

Aging
Division of Aging and Adult Services, P.O. Box 1437, Little Rock, AR 72203-1437; tel. 501/682–2441; FAX. 501/682–8155; Herb Sanderson, Director

Children
Children's Medical Service, Donaghey Plaza South, Seventh and Main Streets, P.O. Box 1437, Slot 526, Little Rock, AR 72203; tel. 501/682–2277; FAX. 501/682–8247; G. A. Buchanan, M.D., Medical Director

Long Term Care
Office of Long–Term Care, Lafayette Building, Sixth and Louisiana Streets, P.O. Box 8059, Slot 400, Little Rock, AR 72203–8059; tel. 501/682–8487; FAX. 501/682–6955; Shirley Gamble, Director

Medical Services
Division of Economic and Medical Services, Donaghey Building, Suite 1100, Seventh and Main Streets, P.O. Box 1437, Little Rock, AR 72203; tel. 501/682–8292; FAX. 501/682–8013; Ray Hanley, Director

Mental Health
Division of Mental Health Services, Arkansas State Hospital, 4313 West Markham, Little Rock, AR 72205-4096; tel. 501/686–9000; FAX. 501/686–9182; Pamela Marshall, Director

Rehabilitation
Arkansas Rehabilitation Services, 1616 Brookwood, P.O. Box 3781, Little Rock, AR 72203; tel. 501/296–1616; FAX. 501/296–1675; Bobby C. Simpson, Commissioner

Substance Abuse
Bureau of Alcohol & Drug Abuse Prevention, Freeway Medical Center, Suite 907, 5800 West 10th Street, Little Rock, AR 72204; tel. 501/280–4500; FAX. 501/280–4519; Joe M. Hill, Director

Insurance
Arkansas Insurance Department, 1123 South University Avenue, Suite 400, Little Rock, AR 72204; tel. 501/686–2900; FAX. 501/686–2913; Lee Douglass, Commissioner

Other
Nursing
Arkansas State Board of Nursing, University Tower Building, Suite 800, 1123 South University, Little Rock, AR 72204; tel. 501/686–2700; Linda C. Murphey, RN, M.N., Executive Director

CALIFORNIA
The Honorable Pete Wilson, Governor, 916/445–2841
Health
Department of Health Services, 714 P Street, Suite 1253, Sacramento, CA 95814; tel. 916/657–1425; FAX. 916/657–1156; S. Kimberly Belshe, Director

Welfare
Health and Welfare Agency, Office of the Secretary, 1600 Ninth Street, Suite 460, Sacramento, CA 95814; tel. 916/654–3454; FAX. 916/654–3343

Community
Community Resources Development Section, California Department of Rehabilitation, 830 K Street Mall, Sacramento, CA 95814; tel. 916/323–0390; FAX. 916/322–0503; Sig Brivkalns, Chief

Developmental Disabilities
Department of Developmental Services, 1600 Ninth Street, Suite 240, Sacramento, CA 95814; tel. 916/654–1897; FAX. 916/654–2167; Dennis G. Amundson, Director

Mental Health
Department of Mental Health, 1600 Ninth Street, Room 151, Sacramento, CA 95814; tel. 916/654–2309; FAX. 916/654–3198; Stephen W. Mayberg, Ph.D., Director

Rehabilitation
Department of Rehabilitation, 830 K Street Mall, Sacramento, CA 95814; tel. 916/445–8638

Social Services
Department of Social Services, 744 P Street, MS 17–11, Sacramento, CA 95814; tel. 916/657–2598; FAX. 916/654–6012; Eloise Anderson, Director

Substance Abuse
Department of Alcohol and Drug Programs, 111 Capitol Mall, Suite 450, Sacramento, CA 95814; tel. 916/445–1943; FAX. 916/323–5873; Chauncey L. Veatch III, Director

Other
Nurse Examiners
Board of Vocational Nurse and Psychiatric Technician Examiners, 2535 Capitol Oaks Drive, Suite 205, Sacramento, CA 95833; tel. 916/263–7845; FAX. 916/263–7859; Teresa Bello–Jones, J.D., M.S.N., RN, Executive Officer

Nursing
Board of Registered Nursing, 400 R Street, Suite 4030, P.O. Box 944210, Sacramento, CA 94244-2100; tel. 916/322–3350; Ruth Ann Terry, M.P.H., R.N., Executive Officer

Quality Assurance
Medical Board of California, 1426 Howe Avenue, Suite 54, Sacramento, CA 95825-3236; tel. 916/263–2389; FAX. 916/263–2387; Dixon Arnett, Executive Director

Other
Department of Corporations, Health Care Service Plan Division, 3700 Wilshire Boulevard, 2nd Floor, Los Angeles, CA 90010; tel. 213/376-2776

COLORADO
The Honorable Roy Romer, Governor, 303/866–2471
Health
Colorado Department of Public Health and Environment, 4300 Cherry Creek Drive S., Denver, CO 80222-1530; tel. 303/692–2000; FAX. 303/782–0095; Patricia A. Nolan, M.D., M.P.H., Executive Director

Facilities
Colorado Department of Public Health and Environment, Health Facilities Division, 4300 Cherry Creek Drive S., Denver, CO 80222-1530; tel. 303/692–2800; FAX. 303/782–4883; Susan E. Rehak, Deputy Director

Family
Family and Community Health Services Division, Colorado Department of Public Health and Environment, 4300 Cherry Creek Drive South, Denver, CO 80222-1530; tel. 303/692–2310; FAX. 303/753–9249; Daniel J. Gossert, ACSW, M.P.H., Director

Substance Abuse
Alcohol and Drug Abuse Division, Colorado Department of Health, 4300 Cherry Creek Drive South, Denver, CO 80222; tel. 303/692–2932; FAX. 303/782–4883; Robert Aukerman, Director

Welfare
State Department of Health Care Policy and Financing, 1575 Sherman Street, Denver, CO 80203; tel. 303/866–6092; FAX. 303/866–4214; Richard Allen, Acting Manager, Health Plans and Medical Services

Aging
Division of Aging and Adult Services, Colorado Department of Human Services, 110 16th Street, 2nd Floor, Denver, CO 80202; tel. 303/620–4127; FAX. 303/620–4189; Rita A. Barreras, Director

Rehabilitation
State Department of Health Care Policy and Financing, 1575 Sherman Street, 10th Floor, Denver, CO 80203–1714; tel. 303/866–2993; FAX. 303/866–4411; Alan R. Weil, Executive Director

Other
Finance
Colorado Division of Insurance, Corporate Affairs Section, 1560 Broadway, Suite 850, Denver, CO 80202; tel. 303/894–7499, ext. 322; Frank Dino, Chief Actuary

Insurance
Division of Insurance, 1560 Broadway, Suite 850, Denver, CO 80202; tel. 303/894–7499, ext. 311; FAX. 303/894–7455; Jack Ehnes, Commissioner

Medical Examiners
Colorado Board of Medical Examiners, 1560 Broadway, Suite 1300, Denver, CO 80202–5140; tel. 303/894–7690; Susan Miller, Program Administrator

Mental Health
Division of Mental Health, 3520 West Oxford Avenue, Denver, CO 80236; tel. 303/762–4088; FAX. 303/762–4373; Thomas J. Barrett, Ph.D., Acting Director

Regulatory
Department of Regulatory Agencies, 1560 Broadway, Suite 1550, Denver, CO 80202; tel. 303/894–7855; Steven V. Berson, Executive Director

Other
Department of Institutions, 3550 West Oxford Avenue, Denver, CO 80236; tel. 303/762–4404; FAX. 303/762–4686; Barbara McDonnell, Executive Director

CONNECTICUT
The Honorable John G. Rowland, Governor, 203/566–4840
Health
Department of Health Services, 150 Washington Street, Hartford, CT 06106; tel. 203/566–2038; Frederick G. Adams, D.D.S., M.P.H., Commissioner

Health
Connecticut Department of Public Health and Addiction Services, Bureau of Health Promotion, 150 Washington Street, Hartford, CT 06106; tel. 203/566–5475; FAX. 203/566–1400; Peter Galbraith, D.M.D., Bureau Chief

Quality
Division of Medical Quality Assurance, Department of Public Health and Addiction Services, 150 Washington Street, Hartford, CT 06106; tel. 203/566–7398; FAX. 203/566–8401; Stanley K. Peck, Esq., Director

Regulation
Department of Public Health and Addiction Services, Bureau of Health System Regulation, 150 Washington Street, Hartford, CT 06106; tel. 203/566–1174; FAX. 203/566–1097; Stephen A. Harriman, Bureau Chief

Other
Department of Public Health and Addiction Services, Division of Hospital and Medical Care, 150 Washington Street, Hartford, CT 06106; tel. 203/566–1073; FAX. 203/566–1097; Elizabeth M. Burns, RN, M.S., Director

Welfare
Department of Social Services, 25 Sigourney Street, Hartford, CT 06106; tel. 203/424–5008; Patricia Giardi, Commissioner

Insurance
Department of Insurance, P.O. Box 816, Hartford, CT 06142–0816; tel. 203/297–3800; FAX. 203/566–7410; Allan B. Roby, Jr., Director, Life and Health Division

Other
Aging
Elderly Services, Division of the Department of Social Services, 25 Sigourney Street, Hartford, CT 06106–5033; tel. 203/424–5274; FAX. 203/424–4966; Tom Corrigan, Director

Organizations / State and Provincial Government Agencies

Education
Department of Education, 165 Capitol Avenue, Hartford, CT 06145; tel. 203/566-5061; FAX. 203/566-8964

Mental Health
State Department of Mental Health, 90 Washington Street, Hartford, CT 06106; tel. 203/566-3650; FAX. 203/566-6195; Albert J. Solnit, M.D., Commissioner

Nurse Examiners
Connecticut Board of Examiners for Nursing, Department of Public Health and Addiction Services, 150 Washington Street, Hartford, CT 06106; tel. 203/566-1041; FAX. 203/566-1464; Marie Hilliard, Ph.D., RN, Executive Officer

Rehabilitation
Department of Social Services, Bureau of Rehabilitation Services, Division of Organizational Support, 10 Griffin Road, N., Windsor, CT 06095; tel. 203/298-2032; FAX. 203/298-9590; John J. Galiette, Chief

DELAWARE
The Honorable Tom Carper, Governor, 302/739-4101
Health
Department of Health and Social Services, 1901 North DuPont Highway, New Castle, DE 19720; tel. 302/577-4500; FAX. 302/577-4510; Office of the Secretary

Aging
Division of Services for Aging and Adults with Physical Disabilities, 1901 North DuPont Highway, New Castle, DE 19720; tel. 302/577-4791, ext. 21; FAX. 302/577-4793; Eleanor Cain, Director

Children
Division of Public Health, Community Health Care Access Section, Jesse S. Cooper Building, Federal Street, P.O. Box 637, Dover, DE 19903; tel. 302/739-4785; FAX. 302/739-6617; Gregg Sylvester, M.D., M.P.H., Chief, Community Health Care Access Section
Maternal and Child Health, Division of Public Health, P.O. Box 637, Dover, DE 19903; tel. 302/739-4735; FAX. 302/739-6617; Sathyavathi Lingaraju, M.D., Director

Health
Bureau of Personal Health Service, Jesse Cooper Building, P.O. Box 637, Dover, DE 19901; tel. 302/739-4768; FAX. 302/739-6617; John A. J. Forest, M.D., Chief
Division of Public Health, P.O. Box 637, Dover, DE 19903; tel. 302/739-4701; FAX. 302/739-6659; Charles Konigsberg, Jr., M.D., M.P.H., Director, Division of Public Health

Laboratories
Delaware Public Health Laboratory, 30 Sunnyside Road, P.O. Box 1047, Smyrna, DE 19977-1047; tel. 302/653-2870; FAX. 302/653-2877; Mahadeo P. Verma, Ph.D., M.P.H., C.L.D., Director

Licensing
Office of Health Facilities Licensing and Certification, Department of Health and Social Services, 3000 Newport Gap Pike, Wilmington, DE 19808; tel. 302/995-6674; FAX. 302/995-8332; Ellen Reap, Director

Medical Assistance
Division of Social Services, P.O. Box 906, New Castle, DE 19720; tel. 302/577-4400; FAX. 302/577-4405; Elaine Archangelo, Director

Medical Services
Emergency Medical Services, Jesse Cooper Building, P.O. Box 637, Dover, DE 19903; tel. 302/739-6637; FAX. 302/739-3008; Ruth Oates-Graham, Director

Other
Medicine
Board of Medical Practice of Delaware, Cannon Building, Suite 203, 861 Silver Lake Boulevard, P.O. Box 1401, Dover, DE 19903; tel. 302/739-4522; FAX. 302/739-2711; Rosemarie S. Vanderhoogt, Office Manager

Nursing
Delaware Board of Nursing, Cannon Building, Suite 203, P.O. Box 1401, Dover, DE 19903; tel. 302/739-4522, ext. 216; FAX. 302/739-2711; Iva J. Boardman, RN, M.S.N., Executive Director

Rehabilitation
Department of Labor, Division of Vocational Rehabilitation, 321 East 11th Street, Wilmington, DE 19801; tel. 302/577-2850; Michelle P. Pointer, Director

Substance Abuse
Delaware State Hospital, Division of Alcoholism, Drug Abuse and Mental Health, 1901 North DuPont Highway, New Castle, DE 19720; tel. 302/577-4000; FAX. 302/577-4359; Charles H. Debnam, Interim Director

DISTRICT OF COLUMBIA
Government Switchboard, 202/727-1000
Health
Department of Human Services, 801 East Building, P.O. Box 54047, Washington, DC 20032; tel. 202/279-6002; FAX. 202/279-6014; Vincent C. Gray, Director

Children
Bureau of Maternal and Child Health Services, Commission of Public Health, DC, 1660 L Street, N.W., Suite 904, Washington, DC 20036; tel. 202/673-6665; FAX. 202/727-2386; Harry C. Lynch, M.D., Administrator

Health
D.C. Commission of Public Health, 1660 L Street, N.W., Washington, DC 20036; tel. 202/673-6700; Reed V. Tuckson, M.D., Commissioner

Long Term Care
Long-Term Care Administration, 1660 L Street, N.W., 10th Floor, Washington, DC 20036; tel. 202/673-3597; A. Sue Brown, Administrator

Prevention
Preventive Health Services Administration, 1875 Connecticut Avenue, N.W., Suite 818, Washington, DC 20009; tel. 202/673-6756; Martin E. Levy, M.P.H., Administrator

Rehabilitation
Rehabilitation Services Administration, 605 G Street, N.W., Washington, DC 20001; tel. 202/727-3211; FAX. 202/727-1707

Substance Abuse
Alcohol and Drug Abuse Services Administration, 1300 1st Street, N.E., Washington, DC 20002; tel. 202/727-1762, ext. 223; FAX. 202/535-2028

Welfare
Social Services
Commission on Social Services, 609 H Street, N.E., 5th Floor, Washington, DC 20002; tel. 202/727-5930; FAX. 202/727-1687; Clarice Dibble Walker, Commissioner of Social Services

Department of Consumer and Regulatory Affairs, 614 H Street, N.W., Suite 1120, Washington, DC 20001; tel. 202/727-7120; FAX. 202/727-7842; Hampton Cross, Director

Facility
Department of Consumer and Regulatory Affairs, Service Facility Regulation Administration, 614 H Street, N.W., Suite 1007, Washington, DC 20001; tel. 202/727-7190; FAX. 202/727-7780; James R. Murphy, Administrator

Licensing
Occupational and Professional Licensing Administration, Department of Consumer and Regulatory Affairs, 614 H Street, N.W., Suite 903, Washington, DC 20001; tel. 202/727-7480; FAX. 202/727-7662; Winnie R. Huston, Administrator

Mental Health
Commission on Mental Health Services, St. Elizabeths Campus, 2700 Martin Luther King Jr. Avenue, S.E., A Building, Suite 105, Washington, DC 20032; tel. 202/373-7166; FAX. 202/373-6484; Guido R. Zanni, Ph.D., Commissioner

FLORIDA
The Honorable Lawton Chiles, Governor, 904/488-2272
Health
State Health Office, Department of Health & Rehabilitative Services, 1323 Winewood Boulevard, Tallahassee, FL 32399-0700; tel. 904/487-2705; FAX. 904/487-3729; Charles S. Mahan, M.D., State Health Officer

Welfare
Department of Health and Rehabilitative Services, 1317 Winewood Boulevard, Tallahassee, FL 32399-0700; tel. 904/488-7721; FAX. 904/922-2993; Robert B. Williams, Secretary

Aging
Adult Services, 1317 Winewood Boulevard, Building 2, Suite 323-A, Tallahassee, FL 32399-0700; tel. 904/488-8922; Ms. Conchy T. Bretos, Assistant Secretary

Children
Children's Medical Services, 1317 Winewood Boulevard, Tallahassee, FL 32399-0700; tel. 904/487-2690; FAX. 904/488-3813; J. Michael Cupoli, M.D., Assistant Secretary, CMS

Facilities
Certificate of Need Office, Agency for Health Care Administration, 2727 Mahan Drive, Tallahassee, FL 32308; tel. 904/488-8673; FAX. 904/922-6964; Elizabeth Dudek, Chief

Licensing
Division of Health Quality Assurance, 2727 Mahan Drive, Tallahassee, FL 32308; tel. 904/487-2527; FAX. 904/487-6240; Gloria Crawford Henderson, Director

Mental Health
Department of Health and Rehabilitative Services, Alcohol, Drug Abuse and Mental Health Program Office, 1317 Winewood Boulevard, Tallahassee, FL 32399-0700; tel. 904/488-8304; FAX. 904/487-2239; Robert J. Constantine, Ph.D., Assistant Secretary

Insurance
Department of Insurance, Bureau of Specialty Insurers, 200 East Gaines Street, Tallahassee, FL 32399; tel. 904/488-6766; FAX. 904/488-0313; Al Willis, Chief

Other
Medicine
Florida Board of Medicine, 1940 North Monroe Street, Tallahassee, FL 32399-0750; tel. 904/488-0595; Marm M. Harris, Executive Director

Nursing
Board of Nursing, 111 Coast Line Drive, E., Suite 516, Jacksonville, FL 32202; tel. 904/359-6331; FAX. 904/359-6323; Judie K. Ritter, RN, Executive Director

Rehabilitation
Division of Vocational Rehabilitation, 2002 Old St. Augustine Road, Building A, Tallahassee, FL 32399-0696; tel. 904/488-6210; FAX. 904/488-8062; Tamara Allen Bibb, Director

Other
Department of Labor and Employment Security, 2012 Capital Circle, S.E., 303 Hartman Building, Tallahassee, FL 32399-2152; tel. 904/922-7021; FAX. 904/488-8930; Shirley O. Gooding, Secretary

GEORGIA
The Honorable Zell Miller, Governor, 404/656-1776
Health
Department of Human Resources, 47 Trinity Avenue, S.W., Suite 522H, Atlanta, GA 30334; tel. 404/656-5680; FAX. 404/651-8669; Tommy C. Olmstead, Commissioner

Health
Division of Public Health, 2 Peachtree Street, S.W., Suite 7-300, Atlanta, GA 30303; tel. 404/657-2700; FAX. 404/657-2715; Patrick Meehan, M.D., Director

Organizations / State and Provincial Government Agencies

Laboratories
Diagnostic Services Unit, Health Care Section, Office of Regulatory Services, 2 Peachtree Street, N.W., 19th Floor, Room 320, Atlanta, GA 30303-3167; tel. 404/657-5449; FAX. 404/657-8934; Betty J. Logan, Regional Director, Diagnostic Services Unit

Licensing
Child Care Licensing Section, 2 Peachtree Street, N.W., 20th Floor, Atlanta, GA 30303; tel. 404/657-5562; FAX. 404/657-8936; Jo Cato, Director

Department of Human Resources, Office of Regulatory Services, Health Care Section, 2 Peachtree Street, N.W., Suite 19.204, Atlanta, GA 30303-3167; tel. 404/657-5550; FAX. 404/657-8934; Susie M. Woods, Director

Mental Health
Division of Mental Health, Mental Retardation and Substance Abuse, 2 Peachtree Street, Fourth Floor, Atlanta, GA 30303; tel. 404/657-2252; FAX. 404/657-2256; Carl E. Roland, Jr., Director

Radiology
Diagnostic Services Unit, 878 Peachtree Street, N.E., Suite 719, Atlanta, GA 30309-3997; tel. 404/894-4747; FAX. 404/894-2185; Betty Logan, Director

Regulation
Office of Regulatory Services, Georgia Department of Human Resources, 2 Peachtree Street, N.W., 21st Floor, Suite 325, Atlanta, GA 30303-3167; tel. 404/657-5700; FAX. 404/657-5708; Martin J. Rotter, Director

Rehabilitation
Division of Rehabilitation Services, 2 Peachtree Street, N.W., Suite 23.319, Atlanta, GA 30303-3166; tel. 404/657-3000; FAX. 404/657-3079; Yvonne Johnson, Director

Other
Personal Care Home Program, 2 Peachtree Street, 21st Floor, Atlanta, GA 30303-3167; tel. 404/657-4076; Victoria L. Flynn, Director

Insurance
Georgia Department of Insurance, 2 Martin Luther King, Jr. Drive, 7th Floor, West Tower, Floyd Building, Atlanta, GA 30334; tel. 404/656-2056; FAX. 404/657-7743; John W. Oxendiner, Commissioner, Insurance

Other
Medical Examiners
Composite State Board of Medical Examiners, 166 Pryor Street, S.W., Atlanta, GA 30303; tel. 404/656-3913; FAX. 404/656-9723; Andrew Watry, Executive Director

Nursing
Georgia Board of Nursing, 166 Pryor Street, S.W., Atlanta, GA 30303; tel. 404/656-3943; FAX. 404/651-9532; Carolyn Hutcherson, Executive Director

Planning
State Health Planning Agency, 4 Executive Park Drive, N.E., Suite 2100, Atlanta, GA 30329; tel. 404/679-4821; FAX. 404/679-4914; Dotty W. Roach, Executive Director

HAWAII
The Honorable Ben Cayetano, Governor, 808/586-0034
Health
Hawaii Department of Health, P.O. Box 3378, Honolulu, HI 96801; tel. 808/586-4410; FAX. 808/586-4444; Lawrence Miike, Director

Chronic Disease
Communicable Disease Division, P.O. Box 3378, Honolulu, HI 96801; tel. 808/586-4580; FAX. 808/586-4595

Dental
Dental Health Division, 1700 Lanakila Avenue, Suite 203, Honolulu, HI 96817-2199; tel. 808/832-5700; FAX. 808/832-5722; Mark H.K. Greer, D.M.D., M.P.H., Chief

Environment
Environmental Health, P.O. Box 3378, Honolulu, HI 96801; Shinji Soneda, Chief

Family
Family Health Services Division, Hawaii State Department of Health, 3652 Kilauea Avenue, Honolulu, HI 96816; tel. 808/733-9017; FAX. 808/733-8369; Nancy L. Kuntz, M.D, Chief, Family Health Services Division

Licensing
Department of Health/Hospital and Medical Facilities, Licensing and Certification, P.O. Box 3378, Honolulu, HI 96801; tel. 808/586-4080; FAX. 808/586-4747; Helen K. Yoshimi, B.S.N., M.P.H., Chief, H.M.F.B.

Medical Services
Health Quality Assurance Division, P.O. Box 3378, Honolulu, HI 96801; tel. 808/586-4531; FAX. 800/586-4745; Elisabeth Anderson, M.D., M.P.H., Chief

Mental Health
Adult Mental Health Division, P.O. Box 3378, Honolulu, HI 96801-9984; tel. 808/586-4686; FAX. 808/586-4745; Sherry Harrison, RN, M.A., Chief

Planning
State Health Planning and Development Agency, 335 Merchant Street, Suite 214 E, Honolulu, HI 96813; tel. 808/587-0788; FAX. 808/587-0783; Patrick J. Boland, Administrator

Substance Abuse
Alcohol and Drug Abuse Division, 1270 Queen Emma Street, Suite 305, Honolulu, HI 96813; tel. 808/586-3961; FAX. 808/586-4016; Elaine Wilson, Chief

Welfare
Medical Services
Department of Human Services, Med-Quest Division, 820 Mililani Street, Suite 606, Box 339, Honolulu, HI 96813; tel. 808/586-5391; FAX. 808/586-5389; Winifred N. Odo, Administrator

Rehabilitation
Vocational Rehabilitation, 1000 Bishop Street, Suite 605, Honolulu, HI 96813; tel. 808/586-5355; FAX. 808/586-5377; Neil Shim, Administrator

Other
Disability
Department of Labor and Industrial Relations, Disability Compensation Division, P.O. Box 3769, Honolulu, HI 96812; tel. 808/586-9151; FAX. 808/586-9219; Gary S. Hamada, Administrator

Medical Examiners
Department of Commerce and Consumer Affairs, Board of Medical Examiners, P.O. Box 3469, Honolulu, HI 96801; tel. 808/586-2708; June Kamioka, Executive Secretary

IDAHO
The Honorable Phillip E. Batt, Governor, 208/334-2100
Health
Children
Bureau of Maternal and Child Health, P.O. Box 83720, Boise, ID 83720; tel. 208/334-5967; FAX. 208/334-6581; Susan Ault, Acting Chief

Health
Department of Health and Welfare, Division of Health, 450 West State, 4th Floor, P.O. Box 83720, Boise, ID 83720-0036; tel. 208/334-5945; FAX. 208/334-6581; Richard H. Schultz, Administrator

Laboratories
Bureau of Laboratories, 2220 Old Penitentiary Road, Boise, ID 83712; tel. 208/334-2235; FAX. 208/334-2382; Richard F. Hudson, Ph.D., Chief

Licensing
Bureau of Facility Standards, Department of Health and Welfare, 450 West State, 2nd Floor, Boise, ID 83720-5450; tel. 208/334-6626; FAX. 208/334-0657; Loyal Perry, Supervisor-Non LTC

Medical Services
Bureau of Emergency Medical Services, P.O. Box 83720, Boise, ID 83720-0036; tel. 208/334-4000; FAX. 208/334-4015; Dia Gainor, Bureau Chief

Prevention
Bureau of Communicable Disease Prevention, Division of Health, P.O. Box 83720, Boise, ID 83720-0036; tel. 208/334-5930; FAX. 208/334-6581; Roger A. Perotto, Chief

Statistics
Center for Vital Statistics and Health Policy, 450 West State, 1st Floor, P.O. Box 83720, Boise, ID 83720-0036; tel. 208/334-5976; FAX. 208/334-0685; Jane S. Smith, State Registrar, Chief

Substance Abuse
Division of Family and Community Services, Bureau of Substance Abuse, 450 West State, Boise, ID 83720; tel. 208/334-5700; FAX. 208/334-6699; Tina Klamt, Bureau of Substance Abuse, Chief

Insurance
Department of Insurance, Division of Examinations, 700 West State Street, P.O. Box 83720, Boise, ID 83720-0043; tel. 208/334-4250; FAX. 208/334-4398; James M. Alcorn, Acting Director

Other
Medicine
Idaho State Board of Medicine, 280 North 8th Street, Suite 202, P.O. Box 83720, Boise, ID 83720-0058; tel. 208/334-2822; FAX. 208/334-2801; Darleene Thorsted, Executive Director

Nursing
Idaho State Board of Nursing, 280 North 8th Street Suite 210, Boise, ID 83720; tel. 208/334-3110; FAX. 208/334-3262; Leola Daniels, RN, M.S., Executive Director

Rehabilitation
Vocational Rehabilitation, 650 West State, P.O. Box 83720, Len B. Jordan Building, Suite 150, Boise, ID 83720-0096; tel. 208/334-3390; FAX. 208/334-5315; George J. Pelletier, Jr., Administrator

ILLINOIS
The Honorable Jim Edgar, Governor, 217/782-6830
Health
Illinois Department of Public Health, 535 West Jefferson Street, Springfield, IL 62761; tel. 217/782-4977; FAX. 217/782-3987; John R. Lumpkin, M.D. Director

Administration
Office of Finance and Administration, 535 West Jefferson Street, Springfield, IL 62761; tel. 217/785-2033; FAX. 217/782-3987; Gary Robinson, Deputy Director

Facilities
Illinois Department of Public Health, Division of Health Care Facilities and Programs, 525 West Jefferson Street, 4th Floor, Springfield, IL 62761; tel. 217/782-7412; FAX. 217/782-0382; Catherine M. Stokes, Chief

Health
Illinois Department of Public Health, Office of Health Protection, 525 West Jefferson Street, Springfield, IL 62761; tel. 217/782-3984; FAX. 217/524-0802; Dave King, Deputy Director

Laboratories
Illinois Department of Public Health Laboratories, 825 North Rutledge Street, P.O. Box 19435, Springfield, IL 62794-9435; tel. 217/782-6562; FAX. 217/524-7924; David Carpenter, Ph.D., State Laboratory Director

Medical Services
Illinois Department of Public Health, 535 West Jefferson Street, Springfield, IL 62761; tel. 217/785-0245; FAX. 217/524-2491; James R. Nelson, Deputy Director, Community Health

Policy
Office of Epidemiology and Health Systems Development, 525 West Jefferson Street, Springfield, IL 62761; tel. 217/785-2040; FAX. 217/785-4308; Laura B. Landrum, Deputy Director

Regulation
Illinois Department of Public Health, Office of Health Care Regulation, 525 West Jefferson Street, Springfield, IL 62761; tel. 217/782-2913; FAX. 217/524-6292; William A. Bell, Deputy Director

Organizations / State and Provincial Government Agencies

Welfare
Department of Public Aid, 100 South Grand Avenue, E., Springfield, IL 62762; tel. 217/782-1200; FAX. 217/524-7979; Robert W. Wright, Director

Insurance
Department of Insurance, 320 West Washington Street, 4th Floor, Springfield, IL 62767; tel. 217/782-4515; FAX. 217/782-5020; James W. Schacht, Acting Director

Other
Children
Division of Specialized Care for Children, University of Illinois at Chicago, (Illinois' Title V Program for Children with Special Health Care Needs), 2815 West Washington, Suite 300, Springfield, IL 62794-9481; tel. 217/793-2350; FAX. 217/793-0773; Robert F. Biehl, M.D., Director

Mental Health
Illinois Department of Mental Health and Developmental Disabilities, 401 William G. Stratton Building, Springfield, IL 62765; tel. 217/782-7179; FAX. 217/524-0835; Jess McDonald, Director

Regulatory
Department of Professional Regulation, 100 West Randolph, Suite 9-300, Chicago, IL 60601; tel. 312/814-4934; FAX. 312/814-1837; Nikki M. Zollar, Director

Rehabilitation
Department of Rehabilitation Services, 623 East Adams Street, P.O. Box 19429, Springfield, IL 62794-9429; tel. 217/782-2722; FAX. 217/524-2471; Sharon Banks, Field Operations Manager, Home Service Program

INDIANA
The Honorable Evan Bayh, Governor, 317/232-4567
Health
Indiana State Department of Health, 1330 West Michigan Street, P.O. Box 1964, Indianapolis, IN 46206-1964; tel. 317/383-6400; FAX. 317/383-6779; John C. Bailey, M.D., State Health Commissioner

Children
Maternal and Child Health Services, Indiana State Department of Health, 1330 West Michigan Street, P.O. Box 1964, Indianapolis, IN 46206-1964; tel. 317/383-6478; FAX. 317/383-6757; Judith A. Ganser, M.D., M.P.H., Director

Facilities
Division of Long Term Care, 1330 West Michigan Street, Box 1964, Indianapolis, IN 46206-1964; tel. 317/633-8442; FAX. 317/633-0750; Suzanne Hornstein, Director

Other
Indiana State Department of Health, Division of Acute Care, 1330 West Michigan Street, P.O. Box 1964, Indianapolis, IN 46206-1964; tel. 317/383-6472; FAX. 317/383-6750; John A. Braeckel, Director

Welfare
Office of Medicaid Policy and Planning, Indiana Family and Social Services Administration, Indiana Government Center-South, 402 West Washington, Room W 382, Indianapolis, IN 46204-2739; tel. 317/233-4455; FAX. 317/232-7382; James M. Verdier, Assistant Secretary

Children
Children's Special Health Care Services, 1330 West Michigan Street, P.O. Box 1964, Indianapolis, IN 46206-1964; tel. 317/383-6273; FAX. 317/383-6757; Joni Albright, Director

Insurance
Department of Insurance, 311 West Washington Street, Suite 300, Indianapolis, IN 46204; tel. 317/232-2385; FAX. 317/232-5251; David B. Reddick, Chief Deputy

Other
Human Services
Indiana Department of Human Services, 150 West Market, P.O. Box 7083, Indianapolis, IN 46207-7083; tel. 317/232-7000; FAX. 317/232-1240; Jeff Richardson, Commissioner

Licensing
Medical Licensing Board of Indiana, Health Professions Bureau, 402 West Washington, Suite 041, Indianapolis, IN 46204; tel. 317/232-2960; FAX. 317/233-4236; Lisa A. Perius, Board Director

Mental Health
Indiana Family and Social Services Administration, Division of Mental Health, Indiana Government Center-South West, 353, 402 West Washington Street, Indianapolis, IN 46204; tel. 317/232-7800; FAX. 317/233-3472; Patrick Sullivan, Ph.D., Director

Nursing
Indiana State Board of Nursing, Health Professions Bureau, 402 West Washington Street, Room 041, Indianapolis, IN 46204; tel. 317/232-1105; FAX. 317/233-4236; Barbara Powers, Director

IOWA
The Honorable Terry E. Branstad, Governor, 515/281-5211
Health
Department of Public Health, Lucas State Office Building, 1st, 3rd and 4th Floors, Des Moines, IA 50319-0075; tel. 515/281-5605; FAX. 515/281-4958; Christopher G. Atchison, Director

Planning
Center for Health Policy, Iowa Department of Public Health, Lucas State Office Building, 4th Floor, Des Moines, IA 50319; tel. 515/281-4346; FAX. 515/281-4958; Gerd Clabaugh, Director

Prevention
Division of Health Protection, Lucas State Office Building, 1st Floor, Des Moines, IA 50319; tel. 515/281-7785; FAX. 515/242-6284; John R. Kelly, Director

Substance Abuse
Division of Substance Abuse and Health Promotion, Iowa Department of Public Health, Lucas State Office Building, 3rd Floor, Des Moines, IA 50319-0075; tel. 515/281-3641; FAX. 515/281-4535; Janet Zwick, Director
Governor's Alliance on Substance Abuse, Lucas State Office Building, Des Moines, IA 50319; tel. 515/281-4518; FAX. 515/242-6390; Martha Crist, Administrator

Welfare
Department of Human Services, Hoover State Office Building, Des Moines, IA 50319; tel. 515/281-5452; FAX. 515/281-4597; Charles M. Palmer, Director

Mental Health
Division of Mental Health/Developmental Disabilities, Hoover State Office Building, Des Moines, IA 50319-0114; tel. 515/281-5874; FAX. 515/281-4597; Division Administrator

Insurance
Division of Insurance, Lucas State Office Building, Des Moines, IA 50319; tel. 515/281-5705; FAX. 515/281-3059; Therese M. Vaughan, Commissioner

Other
Aging
Iowa Department of Elder Affairs, 236 Jewett Building, 914 Grand Avenue, Des Moines, IA 50309-2801; tel. 515/281-5187; FAX. 515/281-4036; Betty L. Grandquist, Executive Director

Children
Child Health Specialty Clinics, 247 Hospital School, University of Iowa, Iowa City, IA 52242-1011; tel. 319/356-1469; FAX. 319/356-3715; Richard Nelson, M.D., Director

Facility
Department of Inspection and Appeals, Division of Health Facilities, Lucas State Office Building, Des Moines, IA 50319; tel. 515/281-4115; FAX. 515/242-5022; Pearl Johnson, Administrator

Medical Examiners
Iowa State Board of Medical Examiners, State Capital Complex, Executive Hills West, Des Moines, IA 50319; tel. 515/281-5171; FAX. 515/242-5908; Ann M. Martino, Ph.D., Executive Director

Nursing
Iowa Board of Nursing, State Capital Complex, 1223 East Court Avenue, Des Moines, IA 50319; tel. 515/281-3255; Lorinda K. Inman, RN, M.S.N., Executive Director

Rehabilitation
Department of Education, Division of Vocational Rehabilitation Services, 510 East 12th Street, Des Moines, IA 50319; tel. 515/281-4311; Marge Knudsen, Administrator

KANSAS
The Honorable Bill Graves, Governor, 913/296-3232
Health
Kansas Department of Health and Environment, Landon State Office Building, 900 SW Jackson, Topeka, KS 66612-1290; tel. 913/296-0461; FAX. 912/296-1231; Robert C. Harder, Secretary, Kansas Health and Environment

Children
Hospital and Medical Programs, Kansas Department of Health and Environment, Bureau of Adult and Child Care Facilities, 900 S.W. Jackson, Suite 1001, Topeka, KS 66612-1290; tel. 913/296-3362; FAX. 913/296-1266; William C. Rein, J.D., Director, Hospital and Medical Programs

Welfare
State Department of Social and Rehabilitation Services, Docking State Office Building, Suite 628-S, Topeka, KS 66612; tel. 913/296-6750; FAX. 913/296-4813; Robert L. Epps, Commissioner

Medical Services
Income Support and Medical Services, Docking State Office Building, Topeka, KS 66612; tel. 913/296-6750; FAX. 913/296-4813; Robert L. Epps, Commissioner

Mental Health
Mental Health and Retardation Services, Docking State Office Building, 5th Floor-N, Topeka, KS 66612; tel. 913/296-3773; FAX. 913/296-6142; George D. Vega, Commissioner

Rehabilitation
Rehabilitation Services, Biddle Building, 300 S.W. Oakley, 1st Floor, Topeka, KS 66606; tel. 913/296-3911; FAX. 913/296-0511; Glen Yancey, Commissioner

Insurance
Kansas Insurance Department, 420 S.W. 9th, Topeka, KS 66612; tel. 913/296-3071; FAX. 913/296-2283; Kathleen Sebelius, Commissioner of Insurance

Health
Kansas Insurance Department, Accident and Health Division, 420 S.W. 9th, Topeka, KS 66612; tel. 913/296-7850; FAX. 913/296-2283; Richard G. Huncker, Supervisor

Other
Nursing
Kansas State Board of Nursing, Landon State Office Building, 900 S.W. Jackson, Suite 551-S, Topeka, KS 66612-1230; tel. 913/296-4929; FAX. 913/296-3929; Patsy Johnson, RN, M.N., Executive Administrator

Other
Kansas State Board of Healing Arts, 235 South Topeka Boulevard, Topeka, KS 66603-3068; tel. 913/296-7413; FAX. 913/296-0852; Lawrence T. Buening, Jr., Executive Director

KENTUCKY
The Honorable Brereton C. Jones, Governor, 502/564-2611
Health
Department for Health Services, Cabinet for Human Resources, 275 East Main Street, Frankfort, KY 40621; tel. 502/564-3970; FAX. 502/564-6533; Rice C. Leach, M.D., MSHSA, Commissioner

Licensing
Division of Licensing and Regulation, Cabinet for Human Resources, C.H.R. Building, 4th Floor, E., 275 East Main Street, Frankfort, KY 40621; tel. 502/564-2800; FAX. 502/565-6546; Timothy L. Veno, Director

Organizations / State and Provincial Government Agencies

Policy
Health Data Branch, 275 East Main Street, Frankfort, KY 40621; tel. 502/564–2757; FAX. 502/564–6533; George Robertson, Manager
Interim Office of Health Planning and Certification, 275 East Main Street, Frankfort, KY 40621; tel. 502/564–6620; FAX. 502/564–8975; Greg Lawther, Acting Executive Director

Welfare
Department for Social Insurance, 275 East Main Street, Frankfort, KY 40621; tel. 502/564–3703; FAX. 502/564–6907; John L. Clayton, Commissioner

Insurance
Department of Insurance, Life and Health Division, 215 West Main Street, P.O. Box 517, Frankfort, KY 40602; tel. 502/564–6088; FAX. 502/564–6090; Paula Isaacs, Program Manager, Health Care

Other

Children
Commission for Children with Special Health Care Needs, 982 Eastern Parkway, Louisville, KY 40217; tel. 502/595–4459; FAX. 502/595–4673; Denzle L. Hill, Executive Director

Medical Services
Department for Medicaid Services, 275 East Main Street, Frankfort, KY 40621; tel. 502/564–4321; FAX. 502/564–3232; Tom Graham, Deputy Commissioner

Mental Health
Department For Mental Health/Mental Retardation Services, 275 East Main Street, Frankfort, KY 40621; tel. 502/564–4527; FAX. 502/564–3844; Elizabeth Rehm Wachtel, Ph.D., Commissioner

Nursing
Kentucky Board of Nursing, 312 Whittington Parkway, Suite 300, Louisville, KY 40222–5172; tel. 502/329–7000, ext. 226; FAX. 502/329–7011; Sharon M. Weisenbeck, M.S., RN, Executive Director

Rehabilitation
Department of Vocational Rehabilitation, Capital Plaza Tower, 9th Floor, 500 Mero Street, Frankfort, KY 40601; tel. 502/564–4440; FAX. 502/564–6745; Carroll Burchett, Commissioner

Other
Commission for Health Economics Control, 275 East Main Street, Frankfort, KY 40621; tel. 502/564–6620; W. R. Hourigan, Ph.D., Chairman

LOUISIANA
The Honorable Edwin W. Edwards, Governor, 504/342–7015

Health
Louisiana Department of Health and Hospitals, P.O. Box 629 Bin #2, Baton Rouge, LA 70821; tel. 504/342–9509; FAX. 504/342–9508; Rose V. Forrest, Secretary

Family
Office of Family Support, P.O. Box 94065, Baton Rouge, LA 70804–4065; tel. 504/342–3950; Howard L. Prejean, Assistant Secretary

Finance
Office of The Secretary, P.O. Box 629 Bin #2, Baton Rouge, LA 70821; tel. 504/342–9500; FAX. 504/342–9508; Rose V. Forrest, Secretary

Health
Louisiana Healthcare Authority, Medical Center of Louisiana at New Orleans, 1532 Tulane Avenue, New Orleans, LA 70140; tel. 504/568–3201; FAX. 504/568–2028; Elliott C. Roberts, Sr., Chief Executive Officer

Licensing
Department of Health and Hospitals, Bureau of Health Services Financing, Health Standards Section, Box 3767, Baton Rouge, LA 70821; tel. 504/342–0138; FAX. 504/342–5292; Lily W. McAlister, RN, Manager, Health Standards Section

Mental Health
Office of Alcohol and Drug Abuse, P.O. Box 2790, Bin #18, Baton Rouge, LA 70821–2790; tel. 504/342–6717; FAX. 504/342–3931; Joseph Williams, Jr., Assistant Secretary

Substance Abuse
Office for Prevention and Recovery from Alcohol and Drug Abuse, P.O. Box 53129, Baton Rouge, LA 70892; tel. 504/922–0730; Vern Ridgeway, Assistant Secretary

Other
Office of Community Services, P.O. Box 3318, Baton Rouge, LA 70821; tel. 504/342–2297; FAX. 504/342–2268; Brenda L. Kelley, Assistant Secretary
Office of Hospitals, 455 North Boulevard, Baton Rouge, LA 70806; tel. 504/922–1325; A. Jack Edwards, Assistant Secretary

Insurance
Department of Insurance, P.O. Box 94214, Baton Rouge, LA 70804; tel. 504/342–5900; FAX. 504/342–8622; James H. Brown, Commissioner

Other

Medical Examiners
Louisiana State Board of Medical Examiners, 630 Camp Street, Zip 70130, P.O. Box 30250, New Orleans, LA 70190–0250; tel. 504/524–6763; FAX. 504/568–8893; Paula M. Mensen, Administrative Manager II

Nurse Examiners
Louisiana State Board of Practical Nurse Examiners, 3421 North Causeway Boulevard, Suite 203, Metairie, LA 70002; tel. 504/838–5791; FAX. 504/838–5279; Terry L. De Marcay, RN, Executive Director

Nursing
Louisiana State Board of Nursing, 150 Baronne Street, 912 Pere Marquette Building, New Orleans, LA 70112; tel. 504/568–5464; Barbara L. Movant, RN, M.N.

MAINE
The Honorable Bill Angus, Jr., Governor, 207/287–3531

Health
Maine Department of Human Services, State House, Station 11, Augusta, ME 04333; tel. 207/287–2736; FAX. 207/287–3005; Jane Sheehan, Commissioner

Aging
Bureau of Elder and Adult Services, State House, Station 11, Augusta, ME 04333; tel. 207/624–5335; FAX. 207/624–5361; Christine Gianopoulos, Director

Children
Division of Maternal and Child Health, 151 Capitol Street, State House, Station 11, Augusta, ME 04333; tel. 207/287–3311; FAX. 207/287–5355; Zsolt Koppanyi, M.D., M.P.H.

Health
Bureau of Health, Department of Human Services, State House, Station 11, Augusta, ME 04333; tel. 207/287–3201; FAX. 207/287–4631; Lani Graham, M.D., MPH, Director

Licensing
Division of Licensing and Certification, Department of Human Services, 35 Anthony Avenue, Station #11, Augusta, ME 04333; tel. 207/624–5443; FAX. 207/624–5378; Louis Dorogi, Director

Medical Services
Department of Human Services, Bureau of Medical Services, State House, Station 11, Augusta, ME 04333; tel. 207/287–2674; FAX. 207/287–2675; Elaine E. Fuller, Director

Insurance
Bureau of Insurance, Department of Professional and Financial Regulation, State House, Station 34, Augusta, ME 04333; tel. 207/582–8707; FAX. 207/582–8716

Financial
Department of Professional and Financial Regulation, State House, Station 35, Augusta, ME 04333; tel. 207/582–8700; FAX. 207/582–5415; Jane E. Titcomb, Commissioner

Other

Medicine
Board of Registration in Medicine, 2 Bangor Street, State House, Station 137, Augusta, ME 04333; tel. 207/287–3601; Randal C. Manning, Executive Director

Mental Health
Division of Mental Health, State House, Station 165, Augusta, ME 04333; tel. 207/287–4230; FAX. 207/287–7286; Linda Breslin, Director

Mental Retardation
Department of Mental Health and Mental Retardation, 411 State Office Building, Station Number 40, Augusta, ME 04333; tel. 207/287–4223; FAX. 207/287–4268; Sue W. Davenport, Commissioner

Nursing
Maine State Board of Nursing, 35 Anthony Avenue, State House Station 158, Augusta, ME 04333; tel. 207/624–5275; FAX. 207/624–5290; Jean C. Caron, RN, Executive Director

Rehabilitation
Office of Rehabilitation Services, 35 Anthony Avenue, Augusta, ME 04333–0150; tel. 207/624–5300; FAX. 207/624–5302; Dr. Pamela A. Tetley, Director

Other
Division for the Blind and Visually Impaired, State House, Station 150, Augusta, ME 04333–0150; tel. 207/624–5323; FAX. 207/624–5302; Harold Lewis, Director
Division of Deafness, 35 Anthony Avenue, Augusta, ME 04333–0011; tel. 207/624–5318; FAX. 207/624–5361; Norman Perrin, Director

MARYLAND
The Honorable William Donald Schaefer, Governor, 410/974–3901

Health
Department of Health and Mental Hygiene, 201 West Preston Street, Baltimore, MD 21201; tel. 410/225–6500; FAX. 410/225–6489; Nelson J. Sabatini, Secretary

Developmental Disabilities
Developmental Disabilities Administration, 201 West Preston Street., Baltimore, MD 21201; tel. 410/225–5600; FAX. 410/225–5850; Lois M. Meszaros, Ph.D., Director

Environment
Maryland Department of the Environment, Office of Environmental Health Coordination, 2500 Broening Highway, Baltimore, MD 21224; tel. 410/631–3851; FAX. 410/631–4112; Tom Allen, Director

Family
Local and Family Health Administration, 201 West Preston Street, Baltimore, MD 21201; tel. 410/225–5300; FAX. 410/333–7106; Dr. C. Devadason, Director

Health
Local and Family Health Administration, 201 West Preston Street, Baltimore, MD 21201; tel. 410/225–5300; FAX. 410/333–7106; Dr. C. Devadason, Director

Laboratories
Laboratories Administration, 201 West Preston Street, Baltimore, MD 21201; tel. 410/225–6100; FAX. 410/333–5403; J. Mehsen Joseph, Ph.D., Director

Licensing
Licensing and Certification Programs, 4201 West Patterson Avenue, Baltimore, MD 21215; tel. 410/764–2750; FAX. 410/764–5969; Carol Benner, Director

Mental Health
Mental Hygiene Administration, 201 West Preston Street, Baltimore, MD 21201; tel. 410/225–6611; FAX. 410/333–5402; Dr. Stuart B. Silver, Director

Planning
Office of Planning and Capital Financing, 201 West Preston Street, Baltimore, MD 21201; tel. 410/225–6816; FAX. 410/225–6489; Elizabeth G. Barnard, Director

Policy
Department of Health and Mental Hygiene, 201 West Preston Street, Room 500, Baltimore, MD 21201; tel. 410/225–6500; FAX. 410/225–6489; Nelson J. Sabatini, Secretary

Organizations / State and Provincial Government Agencies

Rehabilitation
Office of Chronic and Rehabilitation Services, 201 West Preston Street, Baltimore, MD 21201; tel. 410/225–5736; Patricia Smith, M.D., M.P.H., Director

Substance Abuse
Alcohol and Drug Abuse Administration, 201 West Preston Street, Baltimore, MD 21201; tel. 410/225–6925; FAX. 410/333–7206; Rick Sampson, Director

Welfare
Social Services Administration, 311 West Saratoga Street, 5th Floor, Baltimore, MD 21201; tel. 410/767–7216; FAX. 410/333–0099; Diane Gordy, Executive Director

Insurance
Maryland Insurance Administration, 501 St. Paul Place, Baltimore, MD 21202; tel. 410/333–2521; FAX. 410/333–6650; Dwight K. Bartlett, III, Insurance Commissioner

Other
Education
Department of Education, 200 West Baltimore Street, Baltimore, MD 21201–1595; tel. 410/767–0100; FAX. 410/333–6033; Nancy S. Grasmick, State Superintendent of Schools

Medical Examiners
Board of Physician Quality Assurance, 4201 Patterson Avenue, Baltimore, MD 21215; tel. 800/492–6836; FAX. 410/764–2478; J. Michael Compton, Executive Director

Nursing
Maryland State Board of Nursing, 4140 Patterson Avenue, Baltimore, MD 21215; tel. 410/764–5124; FAX. 410/368–3530; Donna M. Dorsey, RN, M.S., Executive Director

Rehabilitation
Division of Rehabilitation Services, 2301 Argonne Drive, Baltimore, MD 21218; tel. 410/554–3000; FAX. 410/554–3299; Robert A. Burns, Assistant State Superintendent

MASSACHUSETTS
The Honorable William F. Weld, Governor, 617/727–9173

Health
Massachusetts Department of Public Health, 150 Tremont Street, 10th Floor, Boston, MA 02111; tel. 617/727–2700; FAX. 617/727–2559; David H. Mulligan, Commissioner

Environment
Division of Environmental Health, 150 Tremont Street, Boston, MA 02111; tel. 617/727–70999; Gerald Parker, Assistant Commissioner

Medical Services
Office of Emergency Medical Services, 150 Tremont Street, Boston, MA 02111; tel. 617/727–8338; FAX. 617/727–3172; Louise Goyette, Director

Quality
Division of Health Care Quality, 10 West Street, 5th Floor, Boston, MA 02111; tel. 617/727–5860, ext. 335; FAX. 617/727–1414; Virginia C. Sullivan, Director

Statistics
Bureau of Health Statistics, Research and Evaluation, Massachusetts Department of Public Health, 150 Tremont Street, 8th Floor, Boston, MA 02111–1197; tel. 617/727–6452; FAX. 617/727–6584; Daniel J. Friedman, Ph.D., Assistant Commissioner

Systems
Bureau of Health Quality Management, Massachusetts Department of Public Health, 150 Tremont Street, Boston, MA 02111; tel. 617/727–7023; FAX. 617/727–6496; Nancy Ridley, Assistant Commissioner

Welfare
Department of Public Welfare, 600 Washington Street, Boston, MA 02111; tel. 617/348–8500; FAX. 617/348–8575; Joseph Gallant, Commissioner

Insurance
Division of Insurance, 470 Atlantic Avenue, Sixth Floor, Boston, MA 02210–2223; tel. 617/727–7189; FAX. 617/727–7189, ext. 299; Linda Ruthardt, Commissioner

Other
Blind
Commission for the Blind, 110 Tremont Street, Boston, MA 02108; tel. 617/727–5550; Charles Crawford, Commissioner

Medicine
Board of Registration in Medicine, Commonwealth of Massachusetts, Ten West Street, Boston, MA 02111; tel. 617/727–3086; FAX. 617/451–9568; Alexander F. Fleming, Executive Director

Mental Health
Massachusetts Department of Mental Health, Central Office, 25 Staniford Street, Boston, MA 02114; tel. 617/727–5600, ext. 447; FAX. 617/727–4530, ext. 426; Eileen Elias, Commissioner

Nursing
Board of Registration in Nursing, 100 Cambridge Street, Suite 1519, Boston, MA 02202; tel. 617/727–9961; FAX. 617/727–2197; Theresa M. Bonanno, M.S.N., RN, Executive Director

Rehabilitation
Massachusetts Rehabilitation Commission, Fort Point Place, 27–43 Wormwood Street, Boston, MA 02210–1606; tel. 617/727–2172; FAX. 617/727–1354; Elmer C. Bartels, Commissioner

Substance Abuse
Bureau of Substance Abuse Services, 150 Tremont Street, 6th Floor, Boston, MA 02111; tel. 617/727–1960; FAX. 617/727–9288; Dennis McCarty, Director

MICHIGAN
The Honorable John Engler, Governor, 517/373–3400

Health
Michigan Department of Public Health, 3423 North Logan Street, Martin Luther King Jr. Boulevard, P.O. Box 30195, Lansing, MI 48909; tel. 517/335–8024; FAX. 517/335–9476; Vernice Davis Anthony, M.P.H., Director

Community
Michigan Department of Public Health, Office of Policy, Planning and Evaluation, 3423 North Martin Luther King, Jr. Boulevard, P.O. Box 30195, Lansing, MI 48906; tel. 517/335–9371; FAX. 517/335–8560; Denise Holmes, Chief

Environment
Division of Environmental Health, Medical Waste Regulatory Program, 3423 North Logan Street, Lansing, MI 48909; tel. 517/335–8637; FAX. 517/335–9033; Lawrence Chadzynski, R.S., M.P.H., Environmental Quality Specialist

Facilities
Bureau of Health Systems, 3423 Martin Luther King, Jr. Boulevard, Lansing, MI 48909; tel. 517/335–8505; FAX. 517/335–8510; Walter S. Wheeler III, Chief

Health
Center for Health Promotion and Chronic Disease Prevention, 3423 Martin Luther King, Jr. Boulevard, P.O. Box 30195, Lansing, MI 48909; tel. 517/335–8368; FAX. 517/335–8395; Jean Chabut, Chief

Laboratories
Michigan Department of Public Health, Laboratory Improvement Section, Division of Health Facility Licensing & Certification, Bureau of Health Systems, 3500 North Martin Luther King, Jr., Boulevard, P.O. Box 30035, Lansing, MI 48909; tel. 517/321–6816; FAX. 517/321–3430; Gladys M. Thomas, Ph.D., Chief

Licensing
Division of Licensing and Certification, 3500 North Logan Street, Lansing, MI 48909; tel. 517/335–8505; Nancy Graham, Supervisor

Medical Services
Division of Managed Care, Michigan Department of Public Health, P.O. Box 30195, Lansing, MI 48909; tel. 517/335–8566; FAX. 517/335–8582; Nancy A. Koert, Chief

Substance Abuse
Center for Substance Abuse Services, Michigan Department of Public Health, 3423 North Martin Luther King, Jr. Boulevard, P.O. Box 30195, Lansing, MI 48909; tel. 517/335–8808; FAX. 517/335–8837; Karen Schrock, Chief

Welfare
Michigan Department of Social Services, 235 South Cesar Chavez Avenue, P.O. Box 30037, Lansing, MI 48909; tel. 517/373–2035; FAX. 517/373–8471; Gerald H. Miller, Director

Medical Services
Medical Services Administration, 400 South Pine, P.O. Box 30037, Lansing, MI 48909; tel. 517/335–5000; FAX. 517/335–5007; Vernon K. Smith, Ph.D., Director

Insurance
Department of Commerce Michigan Insurance Bureau, P.O. Box 30220, Lansing, MI 48909; tel. 517/373–9273; FAX. 517/335–4978; David J. Dykhouse, Commissioner of Insurance

Other
Aging
Office of Services to the Aging, P.O. Box 30026, Lansing, MI 48909; tel. 517/373–8230; FAX. 517/373–4092; Diane K. Braunstein, Director

Education
Department of Education, Box 30008, Lansing, MI 48909; tel. 517/373–2589; FAX. 517/373–1233; Patricia Nichols, Supervisor, Comprehensive Programs

Licensing
Bureau of Occupational and Professional Regulation, P.O. Box 30018, Lansing, MI 48909; tel. 517/373–1870; FAX. 517/335–6696; Kathleen M. Wilbur, Director

Medical Services
Office of Health Services, Bureau of Occupational and Professional Regulation, Michigan Department of Commerce, Box 30018, Lansing, MI 48909; tel. 517/373–8068; FAX. 517/373–2179; Thomas C. Lindsay II, Director

Medicine
Michigan Board of Medicine, 611 West Ottawa Street, Box 30018, Lansing, MI 48909; tel. 517/373–6873; FAX. 517/373–2179; Robert Ulieru, Director, Licensing

Mental Health
Michigan Department of Mental Health, Lewis Cass Building, 320 South Walnut, Lansing, MI 48913; tel. 517/373–3500; FAX. 517/335–3090; James K. Haveman, Jr., Director

Nursing
Michigan Board of Nursing, 611 West Ottawa Street, Box 30018, Lansing, MI 48909; tel. 517/373–1600; FAX. 517/373–2179; Doris Foley, Licensing Administrator

Rehabilitation
Bureau of Rehabilitation and Disability Determination, Box 30010, Lansing, MI 48909; tel. 517/373–3390; Ivan L. Cotman, Associate Superintendent

Other
Office of Health and Human Services, Michigan Department of Management and Budget, Lewis Cass Building, Box 30026, Lansing, MI 48909; tel. 517/373–1076; FAX. 517/373–3624; Paul Reinhart, Director

MINNESOTA
The Honorable Arne H. Carlson, Governor, 612/296–3391

Health
Department of Health, 717 Delaware Street S.E., P.O. Box 9441, Minneapolis, MN 55440–9441; tel. 612/623–5712; FAX. 612/623–5794; Mary Jo O'Brien, Commissioner

Administration
Minnesota Department of Health, Division of Finance and Administration, 717 S.E. Delaware Street, P.O. Box 9441, Minneapolis, MN 55440; tel. 612/623–5465; Thomas Maloy, Director

Organizations / State and Provincial Government Agencies

Children
Minnesota Department of Health, Division of Family Health, 717 S.E. Delaware Street, P.O. Box 9441, Minneapolis, MN 55440; tel. 612/623-5167; FAX. 612/623-5442; Donna Petersen, Sc.D., Director

Community
Minnesota Department of Health, Division of Community Health Services, Metro Square Building, Suite 460, P.O. Box 64975, St. Paul, MN 55164-0975; tel. 612/296-9720; FAX. 612/296-9362; Ryan Church, Director

Environment
Division of Environmental Health, 925 S.E. Delaware Street, P.O. Box 59040, Minneapolis, MN 55459-0040; tel. 612/627-5100; FAX. 612/627-5479; Patricia A. Bloomgren, Director

Laboratories
Public Health Laboratory Division, 717 S.E. Delaware Street, P.O. Box 9441, Minneapolis, MN 55440; tel. 612/623-5331; FAX. 612/623-5514; Pauline Bouchard, J.D., Director

Prevention
Minnesota Department of Health, Division of Disease Prevention and Control, 717 S.E. Delaware Street, P.O. Box 9441, Minneapolis, MN 55440-9441; tel. 612/623-5363; FAX. 612/623-5743; Michael Moen, Director

Resources
Facility and Provider Compliance Division, Minnesota Department of Health, 393 North Dunlap Street, P.O. Box 64900, St. Paul, MN 55164-0900; tel. 612/643-2100; FAX. 612/643-2593; Linda G. Sutherland, Director

Systems
Minnesota Department of Health, Health Care Delivery Systems, 121 East 7th Place, P.O. Box 64975, St. Paul, MN 55164-0975; tel. 612/282-5627; FAX. 612/282-5628; Nanette M. Schroeder, Director

Other
Survey and Compliance Section, 393 North Dunlap Street, P.O. Box 64900, St. Paul, MN 55164-0900; tel. 612/643-2130; FAX. 612/643-3534; Carol Hirschfeld, Supervisor Record and Information Unit

Welfare
Department of Human Services, 444 Lafayette Road, St. Paul, MN 55155-3815; tel. 612/296-6117; FAX. 612/296-6244; Maria R. Gomez, Commissioner

Other
Medical Examiners
Minnesota Board of Medical Practice, 2700 University Avenue, W., Suite 106, St. Paul, MN 55114-1080; tel. 612/642-0538; FAX. 612/642-0393; H. Leonard Boche, Executive Director

Nursing
Minnesota Board of Nursing, 2700 University Avenue, W., Suite 108, St. Paul, MN 55114; tel. 612/642-0567; FAX. 612/642-0574; Joyce M. Schowalter, Executive Director

Rehabilitation
Division of Rehabilitation Services, 390 North Robert Street, 5th Floor, St. Paul, MN 55101; tel. 612/296-1822; FAX. 612/297-5159; David A. Schwartzkopf, Asssistant Commissioner

Other
Department of Commerce, 133 East 7th Street, St. Paul, MN 55101; tel. 612/296-4026; FAX. 612/296-4328; James E. Ulland

MISSISSIPPI
The Honorable Kirk Fordice, Governor, 601/359-3100
Health
Department of Health, Felix J. Underwood State Board of Health Building, P.O. Box 1700, Jackson, MS 32915-1700; tel. 601/960-7634; FAX. 601/960-7931; F.E. Thompson, M.D., M.P.H., State Health Officer

Children
Children's Medical Program, 421 Stadium Circle, P.O. Box 1700, Jackson, MS 39215-1700; tel. 601/987-3965; FAX. 601/987-5560; Sam Valentine, Director

Environment
Bureau of Environmental Health, Felix J. Underwood State Board of Health Building, P.O. Box 1700, Jackson, MS 32915; tel. 601/960-7518; Joe Brown, Director

Health
Bureau of Health Services, Felix J. Underwood State Board of Health Building Annex, P.O. Box 1700, Jackson, MS 32915; tel. 601/960-7472; FAX. 601/960-7480; Michael J. Gandy, Ed.D., Bureau Director, Deputy

Licensing
Division of Health Facility Licensure and Certification, P.O. Box 1700, Jackson, MS 39215; tel. 601/987-3775; FAX. 601/987-4888; Mendal G. Kemp, Director

Medical Services
Mississippi State Department of Health, Felix J. Underwood State Board of Health Building, P.O. Box 1700, Jackson, MS 32915-1700; tel. 601/960-7873; Betty Jane Phillips, Dr.P.H. Deputy State Health Officer

Planning
Health Planning and Resources Development Division, Mississippi State Department of Health, Felix J. Underwood State Board of Health Building, 2423 North State Street, P.O. Box 1700, Jackson, MS 39215-1700; tel. 601/960-7874; FAX. 601/960-7748; Harold B. Armstrong, Chief

Statistics
Public Health Statistics, Felix J. Underwood State Board of Health Building, Box 1700, Jackson, MS 39215-1700; tel. 601/960-7960; FAX. 601/960-7948; Nita C. Gunter, Director

Other
State Epidemiologist, Underwood Annex, P.O Box 1700, Jackson, MS 39215-1700; tel. 601/960-7725; FAX. 601/960-7909; Mary Currier, M.D., M.P.H.

Welfare
Mississippi Department of Human Services, 750 North State Street, Box 352, Jackson, MS 39202; tel. 601/359-4480; FAX. 601/359-4477; Gregg Phillips, Executive Director

Other
Mental Health
Department of Mental Health, 1101 Robert E. Lee Building, Jackson, MS 39201; tel. 601/359-1288; FAX. 601/359-6295; Randy Hendrix, Ph.D., Director

Nursing
Mississippi Board of Nursing, 239 North Lamar Street, Suite 401, Jackson, MS 39201-1397; tel. 601/359-6170; FAX. 601/359-6185; Marcia M. Rachel, Ph.D., RN, M.S.N., Executive Director

Rehabilitation
State Department of Rehabilitation Services, P.O. Box 22806, Jackson, MS 39225-2806; tel. 601/853-5100; FAX. 601/853-5205; Nell C. Carney, L.H.D., Executive Director

MISSOURI
The Honorable Mel Carnahan, Governor, 314/751-3222
Health
Department of Health, Box 570, Jefferson City, MO 65102; tel. 314/751-6001; FAX. 314/751-6010; Coleen Kivlahan, M.D., M.S.P.H., Director

Licensing
Bureau of Hospital Licensing and Certification, Missouri Department of Health, Box 570, Jefferson City, MO 65102; tel. 314/751-6302; FAX. 314/526-3621; Darrell Hendrickson, Administrator

Resources
Division of Health Resources, Box 570, Jefferson City, MO 65102; tel. 314/751-6272; FAX. 314/526-4102; Garland H. Land, Director

Insurance
Department of Insurance, P.O. Box 690, Jefferson City, MO 65102; tel. 314/751-4126; FAX. 314/751-1165; Jay Angoff, Director

Health
Life and Health Section, Missouri Department of Insurance, P.O. Box 690, Jefferson City, MO 65102; tel. 314/751-4363; James W. Casey, Supervisor

Other
Children
Division of Maternal, Child and Family Health, 1730 East Elm, Box 570, Jefferson City, MO 65102; tel. 314/751-6174; FAX. 314/526-5348; Darlinda Smith-Van Buren, B.S.N., M.P.H.

Education
Department of Elementary and Secondary Education, 205 Jefferson, P.O. Box 480, Jefferson City, MO 65102; tel. 314/751-4446; FAX. 314/751-1179; Dr. Robert E. Bartman, Commissioner of Education

Mental Health
Department of Mental Health, 1706 East Elm Street, P.O. Box 687, Jefferson City, MO 65102; tel. 314/751-4122; FAX. 314/751-8224; Roy C. Wilson, M.D., Director

Rehabilitation
Vocational Rehabilitation, 2401 East McCarty, Jefferson City, MO 65101; tel. 314/751-3251; FAX. 314/751-1441; Don L. Gann, Assistant Commissioner

Other
Bureau of Special Health Care Needs, 1730 East Elm, P.O. Box 570, Jefferson City, MO 65102; tel. 314/751-6246; FAX. 314/751-6447; L. L. Hancock, Bureau Chief
Missouri State Board of Registration for the Healing Arts, 3605 Missouri Boulevard, Zip 65109, P.O. Box 4, Jefferson City, MO 65102; tel. 314/751-0098; FAX. 314/751-3166; Alden Henrickson, Executive Director

MONTANA
The Honorable Marc Racicot, Governor, 406/444-3111
Health
State Department of Health and Environmental Sciences, W. F. Cogswell Building, Helena, MT 59620-0901; tel. 406/444-2544; FAX. 406/444-1804; Robert J. Robinson, Director

Family
Family/Maternal and Child Health Services Bureau, W. F. Cogswell Building, Helena, MT 59620; tel. 406/444-4740; FAX. 406/444-2606; Maxine B. Ferguson, RN, M.N., Chief

Licensing
Health Facilities Division, Department of Health and Environmental Sciences, Bureau of Certification, W. F. Cogswell Building, Helena, MT 59620; tel. 406/444-2037; FAX. 406/444-1742; Linda Sandman, Chief

Medical Services
Health Services Division, Montana Department of Health and Environmental Sciences, W. F. Cogswell Building, Helena, MT 59620; tel. 406/444-4472; FAX. 406/444-2606; J. Dale Taliaferro, Administrator

Welfare
Department of Social and Rehabilitation Services, 111 Sanders Street, Box 4210, Helena, MT 59604; tel. 406/444-5622; FAX. 406/444-1970; Peter S. Blouke, Director

Aging
Office on Aging, Department of Family Services, P.O. Box 8005, Helena, MT 59620; tel. 406/444-5900; FAX. 406/444-7743; Robert E. Bartholomew, Program Manager

Community
Department of Family Services, P.O. Box 8005, Helena, MT 59604-8005; tel. 406/444-5902; FAX. 406/444-5956; Hank Hudson, Director

Rehabilitation
Rehabilitative/Visual Services Divisions, P.O. Box 4210, Helena, MT 59604; tel. 406/444-2590; FAX. 406/444-3632; Joel A. Mathews, Administrator

Organizations / State and Provincial Government Agencies

Other
Nursing
Department of Commerce, Montana State Board of Nursing, Arcade Building – Lower Level, 111 North Jackson, Helena, MT 59620-0407; tel. 406/444-4279; FAX. 406/444-1667; Dianne Wickham, RN, M.N., Executive Director

NEBRASKA
The Honorable E. Benjamin Nelson, Governor, 402/471-2244
Health
State Department of Health, 301 Centennial Mall South, Lincoln, NE 68509; tel. 402/471-2133; FAX. 402/471-0383; Mark B. Horton, M.D., M.S.P.H., Director of Health
Children
Division of Maternal and Child Health, Nebraska Department of Health, 301 Centennial Mall South, P.O. Box 95007, Lincoln, NE 68509-9007; tel. 402/471-2907; FAX. 402/471-0383; David P. Schor, M.D., F.A.A.P., Director
Facilities
Nebraska Department of Health, Section of Hospital and Medical Facilities, P.O. Box 95007, Lincoln, NE 68509-5007; tel. 402/471-2105; FAX. 402/471-0555; Charlene Gondring, Director
Health
Nutrition Division, Nebraska Department of Health, 301 Centennial Mall, S., P.O. Box 95007, Lincoln, NE 68509; tel. 402/471-2781; Sue Medinger, Director
Licensing
Department of Health, Bureau of Health Facilities Standards, 301 Centennial Mall, S., P.O. Box 95007, Lincoln, NE 68509-5007; tel. 402/471-2946; FAX. 402/471-0555; Frederick M. Wright, Director
Policy
Division of Health Policy and Planning, 301 Centennial Mall, S., P.O. Box 95007, Lincoln, NE 68509; tel. 402/471-2337; David Palm, Ph.D., Director
Radiology
Nebraska Department of Health, Division of Radiological Health, 301 Centennial Mall, S., P.O. Box 95007, Lincoln, NE 68509; tel. 402/471-2168; FAX. 402/471-0169; Harold Borchert, Director
Welfare
Nebraska Department of Social Services, 301 Centennial Mall, S., P.O. Box 95026, Lincoln, NE 68509-5026; tel. 402/471-3121; FAX. 401/471-9449; Mary Dean Harvey, Director
Children
Nebraska Department of Social Services, Special Services for Children and Adults, 301 Centennial Mall, S., P.O. Box 95026, Lincoln, NE 68509; tel. 402/471-9345; FAX. 402/471-9455; Mary Jo Iwan, Administrator
Medical Services
Nebraska Department of Social Services, Medical Services Division, 301 Centennial Mall, S., P.O. Box 95026, Lincoln, NE 68509; tel. 402/471-9147; FAX. 402/471-9092; Robert Seiffert, Administrator
Insurance
Department of Insurance, 941 O Street, Suite 400, Lincoln, NE 68508; tel. 402/471-2201; FAX. 402/471-4610; Robert G. Lange, Acting Director
Other
Rehabilitation
Department of Education, Vocational Rehabilitation, 301 Centennial Mall, S., P.O. Box 94987, Lincoln, NE 68509; tel. 402/471-3652; Frank Lloyd, Director
Other
Bureau of Examining Boards, 301 Centennial Mall, S., Box 95007, Lincoln, NE 68509; tel. 402/471-2115; FAX. 402/471-0383; Helen L. Meeks, Director

NEVADA
The Honorable Bob Miller, Governor, 702/687-5670
Health
Department of Human Resources, Kinkead Building, 505 East King, Suite 600, Carson City, NV 89710; tel. 702/687-4400; FAX. 702/687-4733; Jerry Griepentrog-Carlin, Director

Children
Children With Special Health Care Needs Program, Kinkead Building, 505 East King, Suite 205, Carson City, NV 89710; tel. 702/687-4885; FAX. 702/687-3859; Gloria Deyhle, MCH Nurse Consultant
Community
Bureau of Community Health Services, 3656 Research Way, Carson City, NV 89706; tel. 702/687-6944; FAX. 702/687-7693; Sandra Fairburn, Bureau Chief
Health
Division of Health, Capitol Complex, 505 East King, Suite 201, Carson City, NV 89710; tel. 702/687-3786; FAX. 702/687-3859; Yvonne Sylva, Administrator
Laboratories
Nevada State Health Laboratory, 1660 North Virginia Street, Reno, NV 89503; tel. 702/688-1335; FAX. 702/688-1460; Arthur F. DiSalvo, M.D., Director
Medical Services
Medicaid, 2527 North Carson Street, Carson City, NV 89710; tel. 702/687-4775; FAX. 702/687-5080; April Townley, Deputy Administrator
Mental Health
Mental Hygiene and Mental Retardation Division, Kinkead Building, Suite 603, 505 East King Street, Carson City, NV 89710; tel. 702/687-5943; FAX. 702/687-4773; Jerry Zadny, Ph.D., Administrator
Regulation
Bureau of Licensure and Certification, Nevada Health Division, 1550 College Parkway, Capitol Complex, Suite 158, Carson City, NV 89710; tel. 702/687-4475; FAX. 702/687-5751; Sharon M. Ezell, Chief
Rehabilitation
Rehabilitation Division, Kinkead Building, 505 East King, Suite 502, Carson City, NV 89710; tel. 702/687-4440; FAX. 702/687-5980; Stephen A. Shaw, Administrator
Resources
Bureau of Health Planning, 406 East Second Street, Carson City, NV 89710; tel. 702/687-4720; FAX. 702/687-6732; Emil DeJan, Chief
Other
Welfare Division, 2527 North Carson Street, Carson City, NV 89710; tel. 702/687-4770; FAX. 702/687-5080; Myla C. Florence, Administrator
Insurance
Department of Business and Industry, Director's Office, 2500 West Washington Boulevard, Suite 100, Las Vegas, NV 89106; tel. 702/486-5330; FAX. 702/486-5018; Rose McKinney-James, Director
Insurance
Division of Insurance, Capitol Complex, 1665 Hot Springs Road, Suite 152, Carson City, NV 89710; tel. 702/687-4270; FAX. 702/687-3937; Alice Molasky, Commissioner
Other
Medical Examiners
Nevada State Board of Medical Examiners, P.O. Box 7238, Reno, NV 89510; tel. 702/688-2559; FAX. 702/688-2321; Patricia R. Perry, Executive Director
Nursing
Nevada State Board of Nursing, 4335 South Industrial Road, Suite 430, Las Vegas, NV 89103; tel. 702/739-1575; FAX. 702/739-0298; Lonna Burress, M.S., RN, Executive Director

NEW HAMPSHIRE
The Honorable Stephen Merrill, Governor, 603/271-2121
Health
Department of Health and Human Services, 6 Hazen Drive, Concord, NH 03301; tel. 603/271-4334; FAX. 603/271-4232; Kathleen G. Sgambati, Acting Commissioner

Community
Division of Public Health Services, Office of Family and Community Health, Health and Welfare Building, 6 Hazen Drive, Concord, NH 03301; tel. 603/271-4726; FAX. 603/271-3745; Roger Taillefer, Assistant Director
Facilities
Division of Public Health Services, Bureau of Health Facilities Administration, 6 Hazen Drive, Concord, NH 03301; tel. 603/271-4592; FAX. 603/271-3745; Eleanor Robinson, Chief
Health
Department of Health and Human Services, Division of Public Health Services, 6 Hazen Drive, Concord, NH 03301-6527; tel. 603/271-4501; FAX. 603/271-3745; Charles E. Danielson, M.D., M.P.H., Director
Mental Health
Division of Mental Health and Developmental Services, State Office Park, S., 105 Pleasant Street, Concord, NH 03301; tel. 603/271-5007; FAX. 603/271-5058; Donald L. Shumway, Director
Prevention
New Hampshire Division of Public Health Services, Office of Disease Prevention and Control, 6 Hazen Drive, Concord, NH 03301; tel. 603/271-4671; FAX. 603/225-2325; Richard DiPentima, Assistant Director
Welfare
Division of Human Services, 6 Hazen Drive, Concord, NH 03301-6521; tel. 603/271-4321; FAX. 603/271-4727; Richard A. Chevrefils, Director
Health
Department of Health and Human Services, Division of Public Health Services, 6 Hazen Drive, Concord, NH 03301-6527; tel. 603/271-4501; FAX. 603/271-3745
Insurance
Department of Insurance, 169 Manchester Street, Concord, NH 03301; tel. 603/271-2661; FAX. 603/271-1406; Sylvio L. Dupuis, O.D., Commissioner
Other
Examination Division, 169 Manchester Street, Concord, NH 03301; tel. 603/271-2241; FAX. 603/271-1406; Thomas S. Burke, Director
Other
Education
State Department of Education, 101 Pleasant Street, State Office Park, S., Concord, NH 03301; tel. 603/271-3494; FAX. 603/271-1953; Charles H. Marston, Commissioner
Environment
Department of Environmental Services, 6 Hazen Drive, Concord, NH 03301; tel. 603/271-3503; FAX. 603/271-2867; Robert W. Varney, Commissioner
Medicine
New Hampshire Board of Registration in Medicine, Board of Registration in Medicine, 2 Industrial Park Drive, Concord, NH 03301; tel. 603/271-1203; FAX. 603/271-6702; Karen LaCroix, Administrator
Nursing
Division of Public Health Services, New Hampshire Board of Nursing, 6 Hazen Drive, Concord, NH 03301-6527; tel. 603/271-3823; Doris G. Nuttelman, RN, Ed.D., Executive Director
Rehabilitation
Vocational Rehabilitation Division, 78 Regional Drive, Concord, NH 03301; tel. 603/271-3471; Bruce A. Archambault, Director

NEW JERSEY
The Honorable Christine T. Whitman, Governor, 609/292-6000
Health
New Jersey Department of Health, Office of the Commissioner, CN-360, Trenton, NJ 08625-0360; tel. 609/292-7837; FAX. 609/984-5474; Len Fishman, State Commissioner of Health

Organizations / State and Provincial Government Agencies

Children
Maternal and Child Health Planning and Regional Services, 50 East State Street, CN 364, Trenton, NJ 08625; tel. 609/292-5656; FAX. 609/292-3580; Roberta B. McDonough, RN, M.A., Director

Facilities
Health Facilities Construction Service, CN-367, 300 Whitehead Road, Trenton, NJ 08625; tel. 609/588-7731; FAX. 609/588-7823; Kenneth A. Hess, Director
Office of the Commissioner, CN-360, Trenton, NJ 08625; tel. 609/292-7874; FAX. 609/984-5474; Paul R. Langevin, Jr., Senior Assistant Commissioner

Family
Division of Family Health Services, 50 East State Street, CN-364, Trenton, NJ 08625; tel. 609/292-4043; FAX. 609/292-3580; Jean R. Marshall, M.S.N., RN., FAAN, Assistant Commissioner

Licensing
Division of Health Facilities Evaluation and Licensing, Licensing, Certification, and Standards, CN-367, Trenton, NJ 08625; tel. 609/588-7726; FAX. 609/588-7823; Robert J. Fogg, Esq., Director

Planning
Division of Health Planning, Financing and Information Services, CN-360, Trenton, NJ 08625; tel. 609/292-8772; FAX. 609/292-3780; Pamela S. Dickson, Assistant Commissioner

Systems
Office of Managed Care, New Jersey State Department of Health, CN-367, Trenton, NJ 08625; tel. 609/588-2510; FAX. 609/588-7823; Edwin V. Kelleher, Chief

Welfare
Division of Family Development, CN-716, Hamilton Township, NJ 08625; tel. 609/588-2000; FAX. 609/588-3369; Karen D. Highsmith, Acting Director

Other
Medical Examiners
State Board of Medical Examiners, 140 E. Front Street, 2nd Floor, Trenton, NJ 08608; tel. 609/826-7100; Charles Janousek, Executive Director

Nursing
New Jersey Board of Nursing, P.O. Box 45010, Newark, NJ 07101; tel. 201/504-6430; FAX. 201/648-3481; Sister Teresa L. Harris, Executive Director

Other
Department of Law and Public Safety, 25 Market Street, Trenton, NJ 08625; tel. 609/292-4925; W. Cary Edwards, Attorney General
Division of Consumer Affairs, 124 Halsey Street, P.O. Box 45027, Newark, NJ 07101; tel. 201/504-6534; FAX. 201/648-3538; Emma N. Byrne, Director

NEW MEXICO
The Honorable Gary E. Johnson, Governor, 505/827-3000
Health
Department of Health, 1190 St. Francis Drive, Santa Fe, NM 87502; tel. 505/827-2613; FAX. 505/827-2530; Michael J. Burkhart, Secretary

Health
Public Health Division, Department of Health, 1190 St. Francis Drive, P.O. Box 26110, Santa Fe, NM 87502-6110; tel. 505/827-2389; FAX. 505/827-2329; Pat Cleaveland, Director

Other
Federal Program Certification Section, 525 Camino de los Marquez, Suite 2, Santa Fe, NM 87501; tel. 505/827-4200; FAX. 505/827-4222; Sue K. Morris, Bureau Chief

Welfare
Human Services Department, P.O. Box 2348, Santa Fe, NM 87504-2348; tel. 505/827-7750; FAX. 505/827-6286; Dick Heim, Secretary

Social Services
Social Services Division, P.O. Box 2348, Santa Fe, NM 87504-2348; tel. 505/827-4439; Jack Callaghan, Ph.D., Director

Other
Income Support Division, P.O. Box 2348, Santa Fe, NM 87504-2348; tel. 505/827-7252

Insurance
New Mexico Department of Insurance, P.O. Drawer 1269, Santa Fe, NM 87504-1269; tel. 505/827-4500; FAX. 505/827-4734; Helen Hordes, Director, Life and Health Division

Other
State Corporation Commission, P.O. Drawer 1269, Santa Fe, NM 87504; tel. 505/827-4529; Eric P. Serna, Chairman

Other
Education
State Department of Education, Education Building, 300 Don Gaspar, Santa Fe, NM 87501-2786; tel. 505/827-6516; FAX. 505/827-6696; Alan D. Morgan, State Superintendent of Public Instruction

Medical Examiners
New Mexico Board of Medical Examiners, 491 Old Santa Fe Trail, Lamy Building, Second Floor, Santa Fe, NM 87501; tel. 505/827-5022; FAX. 505/827-7377; Dorothy L. Welby, Executive Secretary

Nursing
State of New Mexico, Board of Nursing, 4206 Louisiana NE, Suite A, Albuquerque, NM 87109; tel. 505/841-8340; Nancy Twigg, Executive Director

Rehabilitation
Division of Vocational Rehabilitation, 435 St. Michaels Drive, Building D, Santa Fe, NM 87505; tel. 505/827-3511; FAX. 505/827-3746; Terry Brigance, Director

NEW YORK
The Honorable George E. Pataki, Governor, 518/474-7516
Health
State Department of Health, Tower Building, Empire State Plaza, Albany, NY 12237; tel. 518/474-7354; FAX. 518/473-7071; Mark R. Chassin, M.D., Commissioner

Health
Bureau of Home Health Care Services, New York State Department of Health, Tower Building, Room 1970, Empire State Plaza, Albany, NY 12237; tel. 518/474-2006; FAX. 518/474-2031; Dr. Nancy Barhydt, Director
New York State Department of Health, Office of Public Health, Tower Building, Empire State Plaza, Room 1482, Albany, NY 12237; tel. 518/474-6462; FAX. 518/473-3824; Diana Jones Ritter, Executive Deputy Director

Laboratories
Wadsworth Center for Laboratories and Research, Clinical Lab Evaluation, P.O. Box 509, Empire State Plaza, Albany, NY 12201-0509; tel. 518/474-7592; Dr. Herbert W. Dickerman, M.D., Ph.D., Director

Systems
New York State Department of Health, Office of Health Systems Management, Bureau of Alternative Delivery Systems, 1911 Corning Tower Building, Empire State Plaza, Albany, NY 12237; tel. 518/474-5515; FAX. 518/474-2031; Gary Riviello, Director
Office of Health Systems Management, Tower Building, Empire State Plaza, Room 1441, Albany, NY 12237-0701; tel. 518/474-7028; Raymond Sweeney, Director

Other
Bureau of Project Management, New York State Department of Health, Tower Building, Empire State Plaza, Albany, NY 12237; tel. 518/473-7915; FAX. 518/474-3209; Robert J. Stackrow, Director

Welfare
New York State Department of Social Services, 40 North Pearl Street, Albany, NY 12243; tel. 518/474-9003; FAX. 518/474-9004; Cesar A. Perales, Commissioner

Other
Education
New York State Education Department, Main Education Building, Room 111, 89 Washington Avenue, Albany, NY 12234; tel. 518/474-5844; FAX. 518/473-4909

Medicine
New York State Board for Medicine, Cultural Education Center, Albany, NY 12230; tel. 518/474-3841; FAX. 518/473-6995; Thomas J. Monahan, Executive Secretary

Mental Health
New York State Office of Mental Health, 44 Holland Avenue, Albany, NY 12229; tel. 518/474-4403; FAX. 518/474-2149; Richard C. Surles, Ph.D. Commissioner

Mental Retardation
Office of Mental Retardation and Developmental Disabilities, 44 Holland Avenue, Albany, NY 12229; tel. 518/473-1997; FAX. 518/473-1271; Thomas A. Maul, Commissioner

Nursing
State Board for Nursing, New York State Education Department, Cultural Education Center, Room 3023, Albany, NY 12230; tel. 518/474-3843; FAX. 518/473-0578; Milene A. Megel, Ph.D., RN, Executive Secretary

Rehabilitation
New York State Education Department, Vocational and Educational Services for Individuals with Disabilities, One Commerce Plaza, Suite 1606, Albany, NY 12234; tel. 518/474-2714; Lawrence C. Gloeckler, Deputy Commissioner

Substance Abuse
New York State Office of Alcoholism and Substance Abuse Services, 1450 Western Avenue, Albany, NY 12203; tel. 518/457-2061; FAX. 518/457-5474; Marguerite T. Saunders, Commissioner

NORTH CAROLINA
The Honorable James B. Hunt, Governor, 919/733-4240
Health
Department of Human Resources, 101 Blair Drive, Raleigh, NC 27603; tel. 919/733-4534; FAX. 919/715-4645; C. Robin Britt, Sr., Secretary

Facilities
Department of Human Resources, Division of Facility Services, 701 Barbour Drive, Raleigh, NC 27603; tel. 919/733-2342; FAX. 919/733-2757; John M. Syria, Director

Health
Department of Environment, Health and Natural Resources, P.O. Box 27687, Raleigh, NC 27611-7687; tel. 919/715-4126; FAX. 919/715-3060; Ronald H. Levine, M.D., M.P.H., State Health Director

Mental Health
Division of Mental Health, Developmental Disabilities, and Substance Abuse Services, 325 North Salisbury Street, Raleigh, NC 27603; tel. 919/733-7011; FAX. 919/733-9455; Michael S. Pedneau, Director

Rehabilitation
Division of Vocational Rehabilitation Services, 805 Ruggles Drive, P.O. Box 26053, Raleigh, NC 27611; tel. 919/733-3364; Bob H. Philbeck, Director

Welfare
Medical Assistance
Division of Medical Assistance, 1985 Umstead Drive, P.O. Box 29529, Raleigh, NC 27626-0529; tel. 919/733-2060; FAX. 919/733-6608; Barbara D. Matula, Director

Insurance
Department of Insurance, P.O. Box 26387, Raleigh, NC 27611; tel. 919/733-7343; FAX. 919/733-6495; James E. Long, Commissioner

Other
Medical Examiners
North Carolina Board of Medical Examiners, 1313 Navaho Drive, Raleigh, NC 27609; tel. 919/876-3885; Bryant D. Paris, Jr., Executive Secretary

Nursing
North Carolina Board of Nursing, P.O. Box 2129, Raleigh, NC 27602; tel. 919/782-3211; FAX. 919/781-9461; Carol A. Osman, RN, Ed.D., Executive Director

NORTH DAKOTA
The Honorable Edward T. Schafer, Governor, 701/328-2200

Health
State Department of Health and Consolidated Laboratories, 2nd Floor Judicial Wing, State Capitol, 600 East Boulevard Avenue, Bismarck, ND 58505-0200; tel. 701/328-2372; FAX. 701/328-4727

Children
Division of Maternal and Child Health, North Dakota State Department of Health and Consolidated Laboratories, State Capitol, 600 East Boulevard Avenue, Bismarck, ND 58505-0200; tel. 701/328-2493; FAX. 701/328-4727; David Cunningham, Director, Division of Maternal and Child Health

Facilities
Division of Health Facilities, North Dakota Department of Health, 600 East Boulevard Avenue, Bismarck, ND 58505-0200; tel. 701/328-2352; FAX. 701/328-4727; Fred Gladden, Director

Resources
Health Resources Section, North Dakota Department of Health, 600 East Boulevard Avenue, Bismarck, ND 58505-0200; tel. 701/328-2352; FAX. 701/328-4727; Fred Gladden, Chief

Welfare
Children
Children's Special Health Services (Formerly Crippled Children's Services), Department of Human Services, State Capitol, 600 East Boulevard Avenue, Bismarck, ND 58505-0269; tel. 701/328-2436; FAX. 701/328-2359; Robert W. Nelson, Director

Developmental Disabilities
Developmental Disabilities Division, Department of Human Services, State Capitol, 600 East Boulevard Avenue, Bismarck, ND 58505-0270; tel. 701/328-2768; FAX. 701/328-2359; Sandra Noble, Director

Medical Services
Medical Services Division, North Dakota Department of Human Services, 600 East Boulevard Avenue, Bismarck, ND 58505-0216; tel. 701/328-2321; FAX. 701/328-2359; David J. Zentner, Director

Mental Retardation
Mental Health Services, Department of Human Services, Judicial Wing, Third Floor, 600 East Boulevard Avenue, Bismarck, ND 58505-0271; tel. 701/224-2766; FAX. 701/224-2359; Samih Ismir, Director

Rehabilitation
Office of Vocational Rehabilitation, Department of Human Services, 400 East Broadway Avenue, Suite 303, Bismarck, ND 58501-4038; tel. 701/328-3999; FAX. 701/328-3976; Gene Hysjulien, Director

Substance Abuse
Division of Alcoholism and Drug Abuse, 1839 East Capitol Avenue, Professional Building, Bismarck, ND 58501-2152; tel. 701/328-2769; FAX. 701/328-3008; John J. Allen, Director

Other
Office of Economic Assistance, North Dakota Department of Human Services, 600 East Boulevard Avenue, Bismarck, ND 58505-0250; tel. 701/328-2310; FAX. 701/328-2359; Wayne Anderson, Deputy Director
Program and Policy, State Capitol, 600 East Boulevard Avenue, Bismarck, ND 58505-0265; tel. 701/224-4217; FAX. 701/224-2359; Lori Wightman, Deputy Director

Insurance
Department of Insurance, State Capitol, 600 East Boulevard Avenue, Bismarck, ND 58505-0320; tel. 701/328-2440; FAX. 701/328-4880; Glenn Pomeroy, Commissioner

Other
Medical Examiners
North Dakota State Board of Medical Examiners, City Center Plaza, 418 East Broadway Avenue, Suite 12, Bismarck, ND 58501; tel. 701/223-9485; FAX. 701/223-9756; Rolf P. Sletten, Executive Secretary, Treasurer

Nurse Examiners
North Dakota Board of Nursing, 919 South 7th Street, Suite 504, Bismarck, ND 58504-5881; tel. 701/224-2974; FAX. 701/224-4614; Karen Macdonald, RN, Executive Director

Other
Facility Management Division, Office of Management and Budget, 600 East Boulevard, State Capital, Bismarck, ND 58505; tel. 701/224-2471; Rodney Backman, Director

OHIO
The Honorable George V. Voinovich, Governor, 614/466-3555

Health
Ohio Department of Health, 246 North High Street, Columbus, OH 43266-0588; tel. 614/466-2253; FAX. 614/644-0085; Peter Somani, M.D., Ph.D., Director

Children
Division of Maternal and Child Health, 246 North High Street, P.O. Box 118, Columbus, OH 43266-0118; tel. 614/466-3263; FAX. 614/644-8526; Kathryn K. Peppe, RN, M.S., Acting Chief

Licensing
Division of Health Facilities Regulation, Ohio Department of Health, 246 North High Street, Columbus, OH 43266-0588; tel. 614/466-8739; FAX. 614/644-0208; Rebecca S. Maust, Chief

Nursing
Ohio Department of Health, Bureau of Nursing, 246 North High Street, Columbus, OH 43266-0118; tel. 614/466-2205; FAX. 614/728-3616; Joya Neff, RN, M.P.H., Chief

Resources
Ohio Department of Health, Office of Health Systems Planning, Primary Care and Rural Health, 246 North High Street, Columbus, OH 43266-0118; tel. 614/466-3325; FAX. 614/644-8661; Louis Pomerantz, Chief, Health Systems Planning, Primary Care, Rural Health

Substance Abuse
Ohio Department of Alcohol and Drug Addiction Services, Two Nationwide Plaza, 280 North High Street, 12th Floor, Columbus, OH 43215-2537; tel. 614/466-3445; FAX. 614/752-8645; Luceille Fleming, Director

Welfare
Ohio Department of Human Services, 30 East Broad Street, 32nd Floor, Columbus, OH 43266-0423; tel. 614/466-6282; FAX. 614/466-1504; Arnold R. Tompkins, Director

Medical Assistance
Bureau of Medical Assistance, 30 East Broad Street, 31st Floor, Columbus, OH 43266-0423; tel. 614/466-2365; John J. Nichols, Acting Chief

Medical Services
Ohio Department of Human Services, Office of Medicaid, 30 East Broad Street, 31st Floor, Columbus, OH 43266-0423; tel. 614/644-0140; FAX. 614/752-3986; Kathryn Glynn, Deputy Director

Insurance
Department of Insurance, 2100 Stella Court, Columbus, OH 43215-1067; tel. 614/644-2658; FAX. 614/644-3743; Harold T. Duryee, Director

Other
Managed Care Division, 2100 Stella Court, Columbus, OH 43215-1067; tel. 614/644-2661; FAX. 614/644-3741; Teresa Reedus, Senior Contract Analyst

Other
Disability
Bureau of Disability Determination, 1944 Morse Road, Columbus, OH 43229; tel. 614/438-1500; Leonard F. Herman, Director

Medicine
State Medical Board of Ohio, 77 South High Street, 17th floor, Columbus, OH 43266-0315; tel. 614/466-3934; Ray Q. Bumgarner, Executive Director

Mental Health
Department of Mental Health, 30 East Broad Street, 8th Floor, Columbus, OH 43266-0414; tel. 614/466-2596; FAX. 614/752-9453; Michael F. Hogan, Ph.D. Director

Mental Retardation
Department of Mental Retardation and Developmental Disabilities, 30 East Broad Street, Suite 1280, Columbus, OH 43266-0415; tel. 614/466-5214; FAX. 614/644-5013; Jerome C. Manuel, Director

Nursing
Ohio Board of Nursing, 77 South High Street, 17th Floor, Columbus, OH 43266-0316; tel. 614/466-3947; Rosa Lee Weinert, RN, Executive Director

Rehabilitation
Ohio Rehabilitation Services Commission, Bureau of Vocational Rehabilitation, 400 East Campus View Boulevard (SW3), Columbus, OH 43235-4604; tel. 614/438-1250; FAX. 614/438-1257; June K. Gutterman, Ed.D., Director
Rehabilitation Services Commission, 400 East Campus View Boulevard, Columbus, OH 43235-4604; tel. 614/438-1210; FAX. 614/438-1257; Robert L. Rabe, Administrator

Other
Ohio Rehabilitatioin Services Commission,, Bureau of Services for the Visually Impaired, 400 East Campus View Boulevard, Columbus, OH 43235-4604; tel. 614/438-1255; FAX. 614/438-1257; William A. Casto II, Director

OKLAHOMA
The Honorable Frank Keating, Governor, 405/521-2342

Oklahoma State Board of Medical Licensure and Supervision, P.O. Box 18256, Oklahoma City, OK 73154-0256; tel. 405/848-6841; FAX. 405/848-8240; Carole A. Smith, Executive Director
State Department of Health, 1000 N.E. 10th, Oklahoma City, OK 73117-1299; tel. 405/271-4200; FAX. 405/271-3431; Jerry R. Nida, M.D., Commissioner of Health

Children
Child Health and Guidance Service, 1000 N.E. 10th Street, Oklahoma City, OK 73117-1299; tel. 405/271-4477; FAX. 405/271-1011; Edd D. Rhoades, M.D., M.P.H., Chief
Maternal and Infant Health Service, 1000 N.E. 10th Street, Oklahoma City, OK 73117-1299; tel. 405/271-4476; FAX. 405/271-6199; Tisha Dowe Webb, M.D., M.P.H., Medical Director

Dental
State Department of Health, Dental Services, 1000 N.E. 10th Street, Oklahoma City, OK 73117-1299; tel. 405/271-5502; FAX. 405/271-6199; Michael L. Morgan, D.D.S., Chief

Facilities
Special Health Services, 1000 N.E. 10th, Oklahoma City, OK 73152; tel. 405/271-6576; FAX. 405/271-3442; Gary Glover, Chief, Medical Facilities

Health
State Department of Health, Special Health Services, 1000 N.E. 10th, OKlahoma City, OK 73117-1299; tel. 405/271-4200; FAX. 405/271-3442; Brent E. VanMeter, Deputy Commissioner

Laboratories
Public Health Laboratory Services, 1000 N.E. 10th, Oklahoma City, OK 73117-1299; tel. 405/271-5070; FAX. 405/271-4850; Garry McKee, Ph.D., Chief

Organizations / State and Provincial Government Agencies

Nursing
State Department of Health, Nursing Service, 1000 N.E. 10th, Oklahoma City, OK 73117-1299; tel. 405/271-5183; FAX. 405/271-5493; Toni Frioux, R.N.C., M.S.

Welfare
Oklahoma Health Care Authority, 4545 N. Lincoln, Suite 124, Oklahoma City, OK 73105; tel. 405/530-3439; FAX. 405/521-6684; Garth L. Splinter, M.D., M.B.A., Chief Executive Officer

Aging
Aging Services Division, 312 N.E. 28th, Oklahoma City, OK 73105; tel. 405/521-2327; FAX. 405/521-2086; Roy R. Keen, Division Administrator

Children
Oklahoma Health Care Authority, Special Health Care Needs Unit, 4545 North Lincoln Boulevard, Suite 124, Oklahoma City, OK 73105; tel. 405/530-3373; FAX. 405/528-4786; Jim Igo, State Medicaid Director

Medical Services
Department of Human Services, Medical Services Division, P.O. Box 25352, Oklahoma City, OK 73125; tel. 405/557-2539; FAX. 405/528-4786; Jim Igo, Acting Division Administrator

Rehabilitation
Don H. O'Donoghue Rehabilitation Institute, P.O. Box 26307, Oklahoma City, OK 73126; tel. 405/271-6955; FAX. 405/271-3746; John Mohr, M.D., Chief of Staff

Rehabilitation Services, P.O. Box 36659, Oklahoma City, OK 73136; tel. 405/522-2840; FAX. 405/427-3027; Jerry Dunlap, Director

Other
Mental Health
Department of Mental Health and Substance Abuse Services, P.O. Box 53277, Oklahoma City, OK 73152; tel. 405/522-3877; FAX. 405/522-3650; Sharron D. Boehler, Commissioner

Nursing
Oklahoma Board of Nursing, 2915 North Classen Boulevard, Suite 524, Oklahoma City, OK 73106; tel. 405/525-2076; FAX. 405/521-6089; Sulinda Moffett, RN, Executive Director

OREGON
The Honorable John A. Kitzhaber, Governor, 503/378-3111

Health
Oregon Health Division, 800 Oregon Street, Suite 21, Portland, OR 97232; tel. 503/731-4000; FAX. 503/731-4078; Jono Hildner, Acting Administrator

Facilities
Oregon Health Division, Health Care Licensure and Certification, P.O. Box 14450, Portland, OR 97214-0450; tel. 503/731-4013; FAX. 503/731-4080; Kathleen Smail, Manager

Laboratories
Center for Public Health Laboratories, P.O. Box 275, Portland, OR 97207-0275; tel. 503/229-5882; FAX. 503/229-5682; Michael R. Skeel, Ph.D., M.P.H.

Welfare
Family
Adult and Family Services Division, 500 Summer Street, N.E., Salem, OR 97310-1013; tel. 503/945-5601; Stephen D. Minnich, Administrator

Insurance
Department of Consumer and Business Services, 21 Labor and Industries Building, Salem, OR 97310; tel. 503/378-4120; FAX. 503/378-6444; Kerry Barnett

Other
Children
Child Development and Rehabilitation Center, Oregon Health Sciences University, Box 574, Portland, OR 97207; tel. 503/494-8362; FAX. 503/494-6868; Clifford J. Sells, M.D., Director

Mental Health
Mental Health and Developmental Disability Services Division, 2575 Bittern Street, N.E., Salem, OR 97310; tel. 503/945-9449; FAX. 503/378-3796; Barry S. Kast, M.S.W., Administrator

Nursing
Oregon State Board of Nursing, 800 N.E. Oregon Street #25, Suite 465, Portland, OR 97232; tel. 503/731-4745; FAX. 503/731-4755; Joan C. Bouchard, RN, Executive Director

Rehabilitation
Vocational Rehabilitation Division, Human Resources Building, 500 Summer Street N.E., Salem, OR 97310-1018; tel. 503/945-5880; FAX. 503/378-3318; Mr. Joil A. Southwell, Administrator

Substance Abuse
Office of Alcohol and Drug Abuse Programs, 500 Summer Street, N.E., Salem, OR 97310-1016; tel. 503/945-5763; FAX. 503/378-8467; Jeffrey N. Kushner, Director

PENNSYLVANIA
The Honorable Robert P. Casey, Governor, 717/787-2500

Health
Pennsylvania Department of Health, Health and Welfare Building, Suite 802, Harrisburg, PA 17120; tel. 717/787-6436; FAX. 717/787-0191; Allan S. Noonan, M.D., M.P.H., Secretary

Administration
Pennsylvania Department of Health, Health and Welfare Building, Suite 806, Harrisburg, PA 17120; tel. 717/783-8770; FAX. 717/772-6959; Terrence L. Spaar, Executive Deputy Secretary, Administration, Management

Community
Office for Community Health Systems Development, 815 Health and Welfare Building, Harrisburg, PA 17120; tel. 717/787-4366; Joseph B. May, Deputy Secretary

Health
Division of Primary Care and Home Health, 132 Kline Plaza, Suite A, Harrisburg, PA 17104; tel. 717/783-1379; FAX. 717/787-3188; Robert Bastian, Director

Pennsylvania Department of Health, Public Health Programs, 801 Health and Welfare Building, Harrisburg, PA 17120; tel. 717/783-8804; FAX. 717/783-3794; Jeannie D. Peterson, M.P.A., Deputy Secretary

Laboratories
Department of Health, Bureau of Laboratories, P.O. Box 500, Exton, PA 19341-0500; tel. 610/363-8500; FAX. 610/436-3346; Dr. Bruce Kleger, Director

Planning
Pennsylvania Department of Health, Planning and Quality Assurance, Health and Welfare Building, Room 805, P.O. Box 90, Harrisburg, PA 17108; tel. 717/783-1078; FAX. 717/783-3794; Carol Cochran, Deputy Secretary

Quality
Bureau of Quality Assurance, Health and Welfare Building, Room 907, Harrisburg, PA 17120; tel. 717/787-8015; FAX. 717/787-1491; Andrew Major, Director

Substance Abuse
Drug and Alcohol Programs, Health and Welfare Building, Lionville, PA 19353; tel. 717/787-9857; Luceille Fleming, Deputy Secretary

Other
Division of Acute and Ambulatory Care Facilities, Health and Welfare Building, Room 532, Harrisburg, PA 17120; tel. 717/783-8980; William White, Director

Welfare
Pennsylvania Department of Public Welfare, Health and Welfare Building, Harrisburg, PA 17120; tel. 717/787-2600; Karen F. Snider, Secretary

Family
Office of Children, Youth, and Families, Department of Public Welfare, P.O. Box 2675, Harrisburg, PA 17105-2675; tel. 717/787-4756; FAX. 717/787-0414; George B. Taylor, Deputy Secretary

Medical Assistance
Office of Medical Assistance, Health and Welfare Building, Harrisburg, PA 17120; tel. 717/787-1870; FAX. 717/787-4639; Sherry Knowlton, Deputy Secretary

Mental Health
Mental Health, Health and Welfare Building, Room 502, P.O. Box 2675, Harrisburg, PA 17120; tel. 717/787-6443; FAX. 717/787-5394; Ford S. Thompson, Jr., Deputy Secretary, Mental Health

Other
Office of Income Maintenance, Health and Welfare Building, Room 432, Harrisburg, PA 17120, P.O. Box 2675, Harrisburg, PA 17105; tel. 717/783-3063; FAX. 717/787-6765; Christine M. Bowser, Acting Deputy Secretary

Insurance
Department of Insurance, 1326 Strawberry Square, Harrisburg, PA 17120; tel. 717/783-0442; FAX. 717/783-1059; Cynthia M. Maleski, Insurance Commissioner

Business Regulation
Pennsylvania Insurance Department, Office of Company Regulation, 1311 Strawberry Square, Harrisburg, PA 17120; tel. 717/787-2735; FAX. 717/783-7059; Gregory Martino, Deputy Insurance Commissioner

Other
Laboratories
Division of Laboratory Improvement, Bureau of Laboratories, P.O. Box 500, Exton, PA 19341-0500; tel. 610/363-8500; FAX. 610/436-3346; Joseph W. Gasiewski, Director

Medicine
State Board of Medicine, P.O. Box 2649, Harrisburg, PA 17105-2649; tel. 717/783-1400; FAX. 717/787-7769; Cindy L. Warner, Administrative Assistant

Nursing
State Board of Nursing, Department of State, P.O. Box 2649, Harrisburg, PA 17105-2649; tel. 717/783-7142; FAX. 717/787-7769; Miriam H. Limo, Executive Secretary

Rehabilitation
Office of Vocational Rehabilitation, Labor and Industry Building, Room 1300, Seventh and Forster Streets, Harrisburg, PA 17120; tel. 717/787-5244; FAX. 717/783-5221; Gil Selders, Executive Director

RHODE ISLAND
The Honorable Lincoln Almond, Governor, 401/277-2080

Health
Department of Health, 3 Capitol Hill, Providence, RI 02908-5097; tel. 401/277-2231; FAX. 401/277-6548; Barbara A. DeBuono, M.D., M.P.H., Director, Health

Facilities
Rhode Island Department of Health, Division of Facilities Regulation, 3 Capitol Hill, Providence, RI 02908-5097; tel. 401/277-2566; FAX. 401/277-3999; Wayne I. Farrington, Chief

Family
Rhode Island Department of Health, Division of Family Health, 3 Capitol Hill, Room 302, Providence, RI 02908-5097; tel. 401/277-1185, ext. 142; FAX. 401/277-1442; William H. Hollinshead, M.D., M.P.H., Medical Director

Mental Health
Rhode Island Department of Mental Health, Retardation and Hospitals, Aime J. Forand Building, 600 New London Avenue, Cranston, RI 02920; tel. 401/464-3201; FAX. 401/464-3204; A. Kathryn Power, Director

Policy
Rhode Island Department of Health, 3 Capitol Hill, Providence, RI 02908-5097; tel. 401/277-2231; FAX. 401/277-6548; William J. Waters, Jr., Ph.D., Deputy Director

Regulation
Division of Professional Regulation, 3 Capitol Hill, Suite 104, Providence, RI 02908-5097; tel. 401/277-2827; FAX. 401/277-1272; Russell J. Spaight, Administrator

Organizations / State and Provincial Government Agencies

Systems
Rhode Island Department of Health, Office of Health Systems Development, 3 Capitol Hill, Providence, RI 02908-5097; tel. 401/277-2788; FAX. 401/273-4350; John X. Donahue, Chief

Insurance
Division of Insurance, 233 Richmond Street, Suite 233, Providence, RI 02903-4233; tel. 401/277-2223; FAX. 401/751-4887; Charles P. Kwolek, Jr, CPA, Associate Director, Superintendent of Insurance

Business Regulation
Department of Business Regulation, 233 Richmond Street, Suite 237, Providence, RI 02903-4237; tel. 401/277-2246; FAX. 401/277-6098; Barry G. Hittner, Director

Other

Human Services
Department of Human Services, 600 New London Avenue, Cranston, RI 02920; tel. 401/464-3575; FAX. 401/464-1876; Robert J. Palumbo, Associate Director, Division of Medical Services

Rehabilitation
Office of Rehabilitation Services, 40 Fountain Street, Providence, RI 02903; tel. 401/421-7005; FAX. 401/421-9259; Raymond A. Carroll, Acting Administrator

Other
Division of Medical Services, 600 New London Avenue, Cranston, RI 02920; tel. 401/464-3575; FAX. 401/464-1876; Robert J. Palumbo, Associate Director

SOUTH CAROLINA
The Honorable Carroll A. Campbell, Jr., Governor, 803/734-9818

Health
Department of Health and Environmental Control, 2600 Bull Street, Columbia, SC 29201; tel. 803/734-4880; FAX. 803/734-4620; Douglas E. Bryant, Commissioner

Children
Bureau of Maternal and Child Health, South Carolina Department of Health and Environmental Control, Robert Mills Complex, P.O. Box 101106, Columbia, SC 29211; tel. 803/737-4190; FAX. 803/734-4442; Marie Meglen, M.S., C.N.M., Bureau Director

Environment
Bureau of Environmental Health, 2600 Bull Street, Columbia, SC 29201; tel. 803/935-7945; FAX. 803/935-7825; Jack H. Vaughan, Jr., Chief

Laboratories
Bureau of Laboratories, P.O. Box 2202, Columbia, SC 29202; tel. 803/935-7045; FAX. 803/935-7357; Sarah J. Robinson, Acting Chief

Licensing
Department of Health and Environmental Control, Division of Health Licensing, 2600 Bull Street, Columbia, SC 29201; tel. 803/737-7202; FAX. 803/737-7212; Alan Samuels, Director

Long Term Care
South Carolina Department of Health and Environmental Control, Bureau of Home Health Services and Long Term Care, 2600 Bull Street, Columbia, SC 29201; tel. 803/737-3955; FAX. 803/734-3352; Michael Byrd, Chief

Prevention
Bureau of Preventive Health Services, South Carolina Department of Health and Environmental Control, 2600 Bull Street, Columbia, SC 29201; tel. 803/737-4040; FAX. 803/737-4036; Dee C. Breeden, M.D., M.P.H., Bureau Chief

Substance Abuse
Bureau of Drug Control, South Carolina Department of Health and Environmental Control, 2600 Bull Street, Columbia, SC 29201; tel. 803/935-7817; FAX. 803/935-7820; Wilbur L. Harling, Jr., Director

Welfare
South Carolina Department of Social Services, P.O. Box 1520, Columbia, SC 29202; tel. 803/734-5760; FAX. 803/734-5597; Dr. J. Samuel Grisold, Acting Commissioner

Other

Aging
South Carolina Governor's Office, Division on Aging, 202 Arbor Lake Drive, Suite 301, Columbia, SC 29223; tel. 803/737-7500; FAX. 803/737-7501; Ruth Q. Seigler, Director

Blind
South Carolina Commission for the Blind, 1430 Confederate Avenue, Columbia, SC 29201; tel. 803/734-7522; FAX. 803/734-7885; Donald Gist, Commissioner

Medical Examiners
State Board of Medical Examiners of South Carolina, 101 Executive Center Drive, Suite 120, Columbia, SC 29210-8412; tel. 803/731-1650; FAX. 803/731-1660; Henry D. Foster, Jr., Executive Director

Mental Health
State Department of Mental Health, 2414 Bull Street, P.O. Box 485, Columbia, SC 29202; tel. 803/734-7780; FAX. 803/734-7879; Joseph J. Bevilacqua, Ph.D., State Director

Mental Retardation
South Carolina Department of Disabilities and Special Needs, 3440 Harden Street Extension, P.O. Box 4706, Columbia, SC 29240; tel. 803/737-6444; FAX. 803/737-6323; Philip S. Massey, Ph.D, State Director

Nursing
Department of Labor, Licensing and Regulation, State Board of Nursing for South Carolina, 220 Executive Center Drive, Suite 220, Columbia, SC 29210; tel. 803/731-1648; FAX. 803/731-1647; Renatta S. Loquist, RN, Executive Director

Rehabilitation
Vocational Rehabilitation Department, 1410 Boston Avenue, P.O. Box 15, West Columbia, SC 29171-0015; tel. 803/822-4300; P. Charles LaRosa, Jr., Commissioner

Services
State Health and Human Services Finance Commission, 1801 Main Street, P.O. Box 8206, Columbia, SC 29202-8206; tel. 803/253-6100; FAX. 803/253-4137; Eugene A. Laurent, Ph.D., Executive Director

Substance Abuse
South Carolina Department of Alcohol and Drug Abuse Services, 3700 Forest Drive, Suite 300, Columbia, SC 29204; tel. 803/734-9520; FAX. 803/734-9663; William J. McCord, Director

SOUTH DAKOTA
The Honorable William J. Janklow, Governor, 605/773-3212

Health
Department of Health, 445 East Capitol, Pierre, SD 57501-3185; tel. 605/773-3361; FAX. 605/773-5683; Barbara A. Smith, Secretary, Health

Health
Regulation and Quality Assurance, Anderson Building, 445 East Capitol, Pierre, SD 57501; tel. 605/773-3364; FAX. 605/773-5904; Kevin Forsch, Director

Licensing
Office of Health Care Facilities Licensure and Certification, State Department of Health, Anderson Building, 445 East Capitol, Pierre, SD 57501; tel. 605/773-3364; FAX. 605/773-5904; Joan Bachman, Director

Medical Services
Division of Health and Medical Services, 445 East Capitol, Pierre, SD 57501-3185; tel. 605/773-3737; FAX. 605/773-5509; Sandra Van Gerpen, M.D., M.P.H.

Policy
Office of Administrative Services, South Dakota Department of Health, 445 East Capitol Avenue, Pierre, SD 57501-3185; tel. 605/773-3693; FAX. 605/773-5683; Brian Williams, Director

Substance Abuse
Division of Alcohol and Drug Abuse, 3800 East Highway 34, Hillsview Plaza, c/o 500 East Capital, Pierre, SD 57501; tel. 605/773-3123; FAX. 605/773-5483; Gilbert Sudbeck, Director

Welfare

Developmental Disabilities
Division of Developmental Disabilities, Hillsview Plaza, E. Highway 34, c/o 500 East Capitol, Pierre, SD 57501-5070; tel. 605/773-3438; FAX. 605/773-5483; Deborah K. Bowman, Director

Medical Services
Office of Medical Services, 700 Governor's Drive, Pierre, SD 57501-2291; tel. 605/773-3495; FAX. 605/773-4855; David Christensen, Program Administrator

Social Services
Department of Social Services, 700 Governor's Drive, Pierre, SD 57501-2291; tel. 605/773-3165; FAX. 605/773-4855; James W. Ellenbecker, Secretary

Other

Medical Examiners
State Board of Medical and Osteopathic Examiners, 1323 South Minnesota Avenue, Sioux Falls, SD 57105; tel. 605/336-1965; FAX. 605/336-0270; Robert D. Johnson, Executive Secretary

Rehabilitation
Department of Human Services, East Highway 34, Hillsview Plaza, c/o 500 East Capital, Pierre, SD 57501; tel. 605/773-5990; FAX. 605/773-5483; William Podhradsky, Secretary

TENNESSEE
The Honorable Ned Ray McWherter, Governor, 615/741-2001

Health
Department of Health, 312 Eighth Avenue, N., 9th Floor, Tennessee Tower, Nashville, TN 37247-0101; tel. 615/741-3111; FAX. 615/741-2491; Fredia Wadley, Commissioner

Administration
Bureau of Administrative Services, Tennessee Department of Health, Tennessee Tower, 9th Floor, 312 Eighth Avenue, N., Nashville, TN 37247-0301; tel. 615/741-3824; FAX. 615/741-2491; Robert G. Maxwell, Director

Environment
Bureau of Environment, L & C TOWER-21st Floor, 401 Church Street, Nashville, TN 37243-1530; tel. 615/532-0220; FAX. 615/532-0120; Wayne K. Scharber, Assistant Commissioner

Facilities
Department of Health, Bureau of Manpower and Facilities, 283 Plus Park Boulevard, Nashville, TN 37247-0501; tel. 615/367-6204; FAX. 615/367-6397; Richard Long, Assistant Commissioner

Division of Health Care Facilities, 283 Plus Park Boulevard, Nashville, TN 37247-0530; tel. 615/367-6316; FAX. 615/367-6397; Leslie A. Brown, Director

Health
Tennessee Department of Health, Commissioner's Office, Tennessee Tower, 9th Floor, 312 Eighth Avenue, N., Nashville, TN 37247-0101; tel. 615/741-3111; FAX. 615/741-2491

Laboratories
Medical Laboratory Board, 283 Plus Park Boulevard, Nashville, TN 37219-5407; tel. 615/367-6281; FAX. 615/367-6397; Leslie Brown, Director

Licensing
Board for Licensing Health Care Facilities, 283 Plus Park Boulevard, Nashville, TN 37247-0530; tel. 615/367-6316; FAX. 615/367-6397; Carol A. Mace, Director

Medical Services
Medicaid, 729 Church Street, Nashville, TN 37247-6501; tel. 615/741-0213; FAX. 615/741-0882; Manuel Martins, Assistant Commissioner

Welfare
Tennessee Department of Human Services, 400 Deaderick Street, Nashville, TN 37248; tel. 615/741-3241; FAX. 615/741-4165; Robert A. Grunow, Commissioner

Organizations / State and Provincial Government Agencies

Family
Family Assistance, 400 Deaderick Street, Nashville, TN 37248–0070; tel. 615/741–5463; FAX. 615/741–4165; Michael O'Hara, Assistant Commissioner

Rehabilitation
Division of Rehabilitation Services, Citizens Plaza State Office Building, 15th Floor, 400 Deaderick Street, Nashville, TN 37248–0060; tel. 615/741–2019; FAX. 615/741–4165; Patsy Mathews, Assistant Commissioner

Tennessee Rehabilitation Center, 460 9th Avenue, Smyrna, TN 37167; tel. 615/741–4921; FAX. 615/355–1373; Joseph J. DiDomenico, Superintendent

Social Services
Social Services, 400 Deaderick Street, Nashville, TN 37248–0090; tel. 615/741–5924; FAX. 615/741–4165; Betty Gayle Lankford, Assistant Commissioner

Other

Aging
Tennessee Commission on Aging, 500 Deaderick Street, 9th Floor, Nashville, TN 37243–0860; tel. 615/741–2056; FAX. 615/741–3309; Emily Wiseman, Director

Medical Examiners
Tennessee Board of Medical Examiners, 283 Plus Park Boulevard, Nashville, TN 37247–1010; tel. 615/367–6231; Jerry Kosten, Administrator

Mental Health
Tennessee Department of Mental Health and Mental Retardation, 710 James Robertson Parkway, Nashville, TN 37243–0675; tel. 615/532–6500; FAX. 615/532–6514; Evelyn C. Robertson, Jr., Commissioner

Nursing
Tennessee Board of Nursing, 283 Plus Park Boulevard, Nashville, TN 37217; tel. 615/367–6232; FAX. 615/367–6397; Elizabeth J. Lund, RN, Executive Director

Substance Abuse
Bureau of Alcohol and Drug Abuse Services, Tennessee Tower, 12th Floor, 312 8th Avenue, N., Nashville, TN 37247–4401; tel. 615/741–1921; FAX. 615/532–2286; Robbie M. Jackman, Assistant Commissioner

TEXAS
The Honorable Ann W. Richards, Governor, 512/463–2000

Health
Department of Health, 1100 West 49th Street, Austin, TX 78756; tel. 512/458–7111, ext. 7375; FAX. 512/458–7477; David R. Smith, M.D., Commissioner

Children
Bureau of Women and Children, (Texas Department of Health), 1100 West 49th Street, Austin, TX 78756; tel. 512/458–7700; FAX. 512/458–7350; Patti Patterson, M.D., Chief

Texas Department of Health, Centers for Minority Health Initiatives and Cultural Competency, 1100 West 49th Street, Suite M543, Austin, TX 78756; tel. 512/458–7555, ext. 3005; FAX. 512/458–7713; John E. Evans, Executive Director

Data Analysis
Bureau of State Health Data and Policy Analysis, 1100 West 49th Street, Austin, TX 78756; tel. 512/458–7261; FAX. 512/458–7344

Licensing
Bureau of Licensing and Certification, Texas Department of Health, 1100 West 49th Street, Austin, TX 78756–3199; tel. 512/834–6645; FAX. 512/834–6653; Maurice B. Shaw, Chief

Health Facility Licensure and Certification Division, 8407 Wall Street, Austin, TX 78754, 1100 West 49th Street, Austin, TX 78756; tel. 512/834–6650; FAX. 512/834–6653; Nance Stearman, RN, M.S.N., Director

Welfare
Texas Department of Health, 1100 West 49th Street, Austin, TX 78756–3167; tel. 512/338–6501; FAX. 512/338–6945; Randy P. Washington, Associate Commissioner, Health Care Financing

Insurance
Texas Department of Insurance, P.O. Box 149104, Mail Code 106–1A, Austin, TX 78714–9104; tel. 512/322–3401; FAX. 512/322–3552; Rhonda C. Myron, Deputy Insurance Commissioner, Life/Health Group

Other

Mental Health
Texas Department of Mental Health and Mental Retardation, 909 West 45th Street, P.O. Box 12668, Capitol Station, Austin, TX 78711; tel. 512/454–3761; FAX. 512/206–4836; Tex Killion, Deputy Medical Director for Administration

Nurse Examiners
Board of Nurse Examiners for the State of Texas, P.O. Box 140466, Austin, TX 78714; tel. 512/835–4880; Louise Waddill, RN, Ph.D., Executive Director

Texas Board of Vocational Nurse Examiners, 9101 Burnet Road, Suite 105, Austin, TX 78758; tel. 512/835–2071; FAX. 512/835–1367; Marjorie Bronk, Executive Director

UTAH
The Honorable Mike Leavitt, Governor, 801/538–1500

Health
Utah Department of Health, 288 North 1460 West, Salt Lake City, UT 84116; tel. 801/538–6111; FAX. 801/538–6694; Rod Betit, Interim Executive Director

Community
Utah Department of Health, Division of Community Health Services, P.O. Box 16660, Salt Lake City, UT 84116–0660; tel. 801/538–6129; FAX. 801/538–6036; Doug Vilnius, Director

Environment
Department of Environmental Quality, 288 North, 1460 West, Salt Lake City, UT 84116; tel. 801/538–6121; FAX. 801/538–6016; Kenneth Alkema, Executive Director

Family
Family Health Services Division, P.O. Box 144100, Salt Lake City, UT 84114–4100; tel. 801/538–6901; FAX. 801/538–6510; Scott D. Williams, M.D., M.P.H., Director

Finance
Division of Health Care Financing (Utah Medicaid), P.O. Box 16580, Salt Lake City, UT 84116–0580; tel. 801/538–6406; FAX. 801/538–6478; Joan M. Gallegos, Director

Health
Utah Department of Health, Bureau of Primary Care and Rural Health Systems, P.O. Box 16990, Salt Lake City, UT 84116–0900; tel. 801/538–6113; FAX. 801/538–6387; Robert W. Sherwood, Jr., Bureau Director

Laboratories
Utah Department of Health, Division of Laboratory Services, 46 North Medical Drive, Salt Lake City, UT 84113; tel. 801/584–8400; FAX. 801/584–8486; Charles D. Brokopp, Dr.P.H., Director

Licensing
Utah Department of Health, Bureau of Health Facility Licensure, P.O. Box 16990, Salt Lake City, UT 84116–0990; tel. 801/538–6152; FAX. 801/538–6325; Debra Wynkoop-Green, Director

Medical Examiner
Office of The Medical Examiners, State of Utah, 48 North Medical Drive, Salt Lake City, UT 84113; tel. 801/584–8410; FAX. 801/584–8435; Todd C. Grey, M.D., Director

Insurance
Insurance Department, State Office Building, Suite 3110, Salt Lake City, UT 84114; tel. 801/538–3800; FAX. 801/538–3829; Robert E. Wilcox, Commissioner

Other

Aging
Division of Aging and Adult Services, 120 North 200 West, Room 401, Salt Lake City, UT 84103; tel. 801/538–3910; FAX. 801/538–4395; James G. Quast, Director

Children
Youth Corrections, P.O. Box 45500, Salt Lake City, UT 84145–0500; tel. 801/538–4330; FAX. 801/538–4334; Gary K. Dalton, Director

Education
State Office of Education, 250 East 500 South, Salt Lake City, UT 84111; tel. 801/538–7500; FAX. 801/538–7521; Scott W. Bean, Superintendent

Family
Family Services, P.O. Box 45500, Salt Lake City, UT 84145–0500; tel. 801/538–4100; FAX. 801/538–4016; Lynn A. Samsel, Director

Licensing
Division of Occupational and Professional Licensing, Heber M. Wells Building, 160 East 300 South, P.O. Box 45805, Salt Lake City, UT 84145–0805; tel. 801/530–6628; FAX. 801/530–6511; David E. Robinson, Director

Mental Health
Mental Health, P.O. Box 45500, Salt Lake City, UT 84145–0500; tel. 801/538–4270; Paul Thorpe, Director

Rehabilitation
Utah State Office of Rehabilitation, 250 East 500 South, Salt Lake City, UT 84111; tel. 801/538–7530; FAX. 801/538–7522; Blaine Petersen, Ed.D., Executive Director

Services
Department of Human Services, 120 North 200 West, P.O. Box 45500, Salt Lake City, UT 84145–0500; tel. 801/538–4001; FAX. 801/538–4016; Norman G. Angus, Executive Director

Division of Services for People With Disabilities, 120 North 200 West, Suite 201, P.O. Box 45500, Salt Lake City, UT 84103; tel. 801/538–4190; FAX. 801/538–4279; Ric Zaharia, Ph.D., Director

Substance Abuse
Division of Substance Abuse, 120 North 200 West, P.O. Box 45500, Salt Lake City, UT 84145; tel. 801/538–3939; FAX. 801/538–4334; F. Leon PoVey, Director

VERMONT
The Honorable Howard Dean, Governor, 802/828–3333

Health
Vermont Department of Health, 108 Cherry Street, P.O. Box 70, Burlington, VT 05402; tel. 802/863–7280; FAX. 802/863–7425; Jan K. Carney, M.D., M.P.H., Commissioner

Environment
Environmental Health Division, 108 Cherry Street, P.O. Box 70, Burlington, VT 05402; tel. 802/863–7220; FAX. 802/863–7425; Robert O'Grady, Director

Laboratories
Vermont Department of Health Laboratory, 195 Colchester Avenue, P.O. Box 1125, Burlington, VT 05402–1125; tel. 802/863–7335; FAX. 802/863–7632; Burton W. Wilcke, Jr., Ph.D., Laboratory Director

Licensing
Licensing and Protection, Ladd Hall, 103 South Main Street, Waterbury, VT 05671–2306; tel. 802/241–2345; FAX. 802/241–2358; Patrick Flood, Director

Medical Services
Vermont Department of Health, Division of Local Health, P.O. Box 70, Burlington, VT 05402; tel. 802/863–7347; FAX. 802/863–7425; Patricia Berry, Director

Regulation
Vermont Department of Aging and Disabilities, Division of Licensing and Protection, Ladd Hall, 103 South Main Street, Waterbury, VT 05671–2306; tel. 802/241–2345; FAX. 802/241–2358; Robert Aiken, Director

Statistics
Vermont Department of Health, Division of Public Health Analysis and Policy, 108 Cherry Street, P.O. Box 70, Burlington, VT 05402; tel. 802/863–7300; FAX. 802/865–7701; Stefan Rosenstreich, Director

Organizations / State and Provincial Government Agencies

Other
Vermont Department of Health Epidemiology and Disease Prevention, 108 Cherry Street, P.O. Box 70, Burlington, VT 05402; tel. 802/863-7240; FAX. 802/865-7701; Bob O'Grady, Acting Division Director

Welfare
Agency of Human Services, 103 South Main Street, Waterbury, VT 05676; tel. 802/241-2220; FAX. 802/244-8103; Cornelius Hogan, Secretary
Department of Social Welfare, 103 South Main Street, Waterbury, VT 05676; tel. 802/241-2853; FAX. 802/241-2830; M. Jane Kitchel, Commissioner

Medical Services
Medicaid Division, D.S.W., 103 South Main Street, Waterbury, VT 05671-1201; tel. 802/241-2880; FAX. 802/241-2974; Kent Stoneman, Director

Mental Health
Department of Mental Health and Mental Retardation, Weeks Building, 103 South Main Street, Waterbury, VT 05671-1601; tel. 802/241-2610; FAX. 802/241-3052; William A. Dalton, Commissioner

Rehabilitation
Department of Social and Rehabilitation Services, 103 South Main Street, Waterbury, VT 05671-2401; tel. 802/241-2100; FAX. 802/241-2980; William M. Young, Commissioner
Vocational Rehabilitation Division, 103 South Main Street, Osgood Building, Waterbury, VT 05671-2303; tel. 802/241-2186; FAX. 802/241-3359; Diane P. Dalmasse, Director

Substance Abuse
Office of Alcohol and Drug Abuse Programs, 103 South Main Street, Waterbury, VT 05671-1701; tel. 802/241-2170; FAX. 802/241-3095; Thomas E. Perras, Director

Insurance
Department of Banking, Insurance and Securities, 89 Main Street, Drawer 20, Montpelier, VT 05620-3101; tel. 802/828-3301; FAX. 802/828-3306; Elizabeth R. Costle, Commissioner

Other
Nursing
Vermont State Board of Nursing, 109 State Street, Montpelier, VT 05609-1106; tel. 802/828-2396; FAX. 802/828-2853; Anita Ristau, RN, M.S., Executive Director

VIRGINIA
The Honorable George F. Allen, Governor, 804/786-2211

Health
State Department of Health, Main Street Station, P.O. Box 2448, Richmond, VA 23218; tel. 804/786-3561; FAX. 804/786-4616; Robert B. Strouhe, M.D. M.P.H., Commissioner

Children
Division of Children's Specialty Services, Virginia Department of Health, P.O. Box 2448, Room 135, Richmond, VA 23218; tel. 804/786-3691; FAX. 804/225-3307; Nancy R. Bullock, RN, M.P.H., Acting Director
Division of Women's and Infants' Health, 1500 East Main Street, Suite 136, P.O. Box 2448, Richmond, VA 23218-2448; tel. 804/786-5916; FAX. 804/371-6032; Barbara E. Parker, RN, M.P.H., Acting Director

Licensing
Office of Health Facilities Regulation, Virginia Department of Health, 3600 Centre, Suite 216, 3600 West Broad Street, Richmond, VA 23230; tel. 804/367-2102; FAX. 804/367-2149; Nancy R. Hofheimer, Director

Welfare
Virginia Department of Social Services, 730 East Broad Street, Richmond, VA 23219-1949; tel. 804/692-1900; FAX. 804/692-1849; Carol A. Brunty, Commissioner

Insurance
State Corporation Commission–Bureau of Insurance, P.O. Box 1157, Richmond, VA 23209; tel. 804/371-9869; FAX. 804/371-9511; Alfred W. Gross, Deputy Insurance Commissioner

Business Regulation
State Corporation Commission Bureau of Insurance, Company Licensing and Regulatory Compliance Section, P.O. Box 1157, Richmond, VA 23209; tel. 904/371-9636; FAX. 904/371-9396; Andy Delbridge, Supervisor

Insurance
Bureau of Insurance, Virginia State Corporation Commission, P.O. Box 1157, Richmond, VA 23209; tel. 804/371-9691; FAX. 804/371-9944; Life and Health Consumer Services Section

Other
Aging
Department for the Aging, 700 East Franklin Street, 10th Floor, 700 Centre, Richmond, VA 23219-2327; tel. 804/225-2271; FAX. 804/371-8381; Thelma Bland, Commissioner

Medical Assistance
Department of Medical Assistance Services, 600 East Broad Street, Suite 1300, Richmond, VA 23219; tel. 804/786-8099; FAX. 804/371-4981; Robert C. Metcalf, Director

Medicine
Virginia State Board of Medicine, 6606 West Board Street, 4th Floor, Richmond, VA 23230-1717; tel. 804/662-9925; FAX. 804/662-9943; Warren W. Koonzt, Jr., M.D., Executive Director

Mental Health
Department of Mental Health, Mental Retardation and Substance Abuse Services, P.O. Box 1797, Richmond, VA 23214; tel. 804/786-3921; FAX. 804/371-6638; Timothy A. Kelly, Ph.D., Commissioner

Rehabilitation
Department of Rehabilitative Services, 4901 Fitzhugh Avenue, Box 11045, Richmond, VA 23230; tel. 804/367-0318; FAX. 804/367-9256; Susan Urofsky, Commissioner

WASHINGTON
The Honorable Mike Lowry, Governor, 206/753-6780

Health
State Department of Social and Health Services, P.O. Box 45500, Olympia, WA 98504; tel. 206/753-1777; FAX. 206/586-7498; Jane Beyer, Assistant Secretary, Medical Assistance, Administration

Facilities
Office of Field Services, Department of Health, Target Plaza, 2725 Harrison Avenue, N.W., Suite 500, P.O. Box 47852, Olympia, WA 98504-7852; tel. 206/705-6622; FAX. 206/705-6654; Fern Bettridge, Program Manager

Health
Department of Health, Facilities and Services Licensing, P.O. Box 47852, Olympia, WA 98504-7852; tel. 206/705-6652; FAX. 206/705-6654; Kathy Stout, Director
Department of Health, Office of Emergency Medical Services and Trauma Systems, P.O. Box 47853, Olympia, WA 98504-7853; tel. 206/705-6700; FAX. 206/705-6706; Janet Griffith, Director

Medical Assistance
Medical Assistance Administration, P.O. Box 45080, Olympia, WA 98504-5080; tel. 206/753-1777; FAX. 206/586-5874; Jane Beyer, Assistant Secretary

Policy
Medical Assistance Administration, P.O. Box 45500, Olympia, WA 98504-5500; tel. 206/753-5839; FAX. 206/664-2186; Eric Houghton, M.D., Acting Medical Director

Rehabilitation
Division of Vocational Rehabilitation, P.O. Box 45340, Olympia, WA 98504-5340; tel. 206/438-8000; FAX. 206/438-8007; Jeanne Munro, Director

Substance Abuse
Division of Alcohol and Substance Abuse, P.O. Box 45330, Mail Stop 5330, Olympia, WA 98504-5330; tel. 206/438-8200; FAX. 206/438-8078; Ken Stark, Director

Other
Washington State Department of Health, P.O. Box 47812, Mail Stop 7812, Olympia, WA 98504-7812; tel. 206/705-6060; FAX. 206/705-6043; Dan Rubin, Director, Special Projects Office

Insurance
Office of the Insurance Commissioner, Insurance Building, P.O. Box 40255, Olympia, WA 98504-0255; tel. 206/586-3535; Deborah Senn, Commissioner

Other
Licensing
Health Systems Quality Assurance, Department of Health, 1112 Quince, Mail Stop 7850, Olympia, WA 98504-7850; tel. 360/753-2241; FAX. 360/664-0398; Sherman Cox, Assistant Secretary

Nursing
Washington State Nursing Care Quality Assurance Commission, 1300 Southeast Quince Street, P.O. Box 47864, Olympia, WA 98504-7864; tel. 206/753-2686; FAX. 206/586-5935; Patricia O. Brown, RN, M.S.N., Executive Director

WEST VIRGINIA
The Honorable Gaston Caperton, Governor, 304/558-2000

Health
Bureau of Public Health, Building 3, Room 518, State Capitol Complex, Charleston, WV 25305; tel. 304/558-2971; FAX. 304/558-1035; William T. Wallace, Jr., M.D., M.P.H., Commissioner
Department of Health and Human Resources, Bureau of Public Health, Capitol Complex, Building 3, Room 518, Charleston, WV 25305; tel. 304/558-9116; FAX. 304/558-1035; Nancy J. Tolliver, Deputy Commissioner

Community
Office of Community and Rural Health Services, Bureau for Public Health, 1411 Virginia Street, E., Charleston, WV 25301-3013; tel. 304/558-0580; FAX. 304/558-1437

Environment
Office of Environmental Health Services, Morrison Building, 815 Quarrier Street, Suite 418, Charleston, WV 25301-2616; tel. 304/558-2981; FAX. 304/558-0691; Joseph P. Schock, M.P.H., P.E., Director

Licensing
Office of Health Facility Licensure and Certification, West Virginia Division of Health, Capitol Complex, 1900 Kanawha Boulevard, E., Building 3, Suite 550, Charleston, WV 25305; tel. 304/558-0050; FAX. 304/558-2515; Lynda Kramer, Director

Medical Examiner
Office of Chief Medical Examiner, State of West Virginia, 701 Jefferson Road, South Charleston, WV 25309; tel. 304/558-3920; FAX. 304/558-7886; Irvin Sopher, M.D., Chief Medical Examiner

Substance Abuse
Division on Alcoholism and Drug Abuse, Capitol Complex, Building 6, Room B-738, Charleston, WV 25305; tel. 304/558-2276; FAX. 304/558-1008; Jack C. Clohan, Jr., Director

Other
West Virginia Department of Health and Human Resources, Division of Primary Care and Recruitment, 1411 Virginia Street, E., Charleston, WV 25301; tel. 304/558-4007; FAX. 304/558-1437; Charles W. Dawkins, Director

Welfare
Department of Health and Human Resources, Capitol Complex, Building 3, Room 206, Charleston, WV 25305; tel. 304/558-0684; FAX. 304/558-1130; Gretchen O. Lewis, Secretary

Children
Handicapped Children's Services, 1116 Quarrier Street, Charleston, WV 25301; tel. 304/558-3071; FAX. 304/558-2866; Patricia Kent, Administrative Director

Organizations / State and Provincial Government Agencies

Other
Division of Medical Care, Department of Human Services, 1900 Washington Street, E., Charleston, WV 25305; tel. 304/348-8990; Helen Condry, Director

Insurance
Insurance Commissioners Office, 2019 Washington Street, E., P.O. Box 50540, Charleston, WV 25305-0540; tel. 304/558-3354; FAX. 304/558-0412; Hanley C. Clark, Commissioner

Financial
Insurance Commissioner's Office, 2019 Washington Street, E., Charleston, WV 25305-0540; tel. 304/558-2100; FAX. 304/558-0412; John Collins, Director, Chief Examiner

Other

Education
West Virginia Department of Education, Division of Technical and Adult Education, State Capitol, 1900 Kanawha Boulevard, E., Charleston, WV 25305; tel. 304/558-2346; FAX. 304/558-0048; Adam Sponaugle, Assistant State Superintendent

Medicine
West Virginia Board of Medicine, 101 Dee Drive, Charleston, WV 25311; tel. 304/558-2921; FAX. 304/558-2084; Ronald D. Walton, Executive Director

Nurse Examiners
West Virginia Board of Examiners for Registered Professional Nurses, 101 Dee Drive, Charleston, WV 25311-1620; tel. 304/558-3596; FAX. 304/558-3666; Janet H. Fairchild, M.S., RN, Executive Secretary

West Virginia State Board of Examiners for Licensed Practical Nurses, 101 Dee Drive, Charleston, WV 25311-1688; tel. 304/558-3572; Nancy R. Wilson, RN, Executive Secretary

Rehabilitation
Division of Rehabilitation Services, P.O. Box 50890, State Capitol Complex, Charleston, WV 25305-0890; tel. 304/766-4601; FAX. 304/766-4671; William C. Dearien, Director

WISCONSIN
The Honorable Tommy G. Thompson, Governor, 608/266-1212

Health
Department of Health and Social Services, P.O. Box 7850, Madison, WI 53707; tel. 608/266-9622; FAX. 608/266-7882; Richard W. Lorang, Acting Secretary

Environment
Bureau of Public Health, P.O. Box 309, Madison, WI 53701; tel. 608/266-1704; FAX. 608/267-4853

Finance
Bureau of Health Care Financing (Wisconsin Medicaid), One West Wilson Street, Suite 250, P.O. Box 309, Madison, WI 53701-0309; tel. 608/266-2522; FAX. 608/266-1096; Kevin B. Piper, Director

Health
Bureau of Health Services, P.O. Box 7925, Madison, WI 53707-7925; tel. 608/267-1720; FAX. 608/267-1751; Sharon Zunker, Director
Division of Health, 1 West Wilson Street, Room 218, P.O. Box 309, Madison, WI 53701-0309; tel. 608/266-1511; FAX. 608/267-2832; Ann J. Haney, Administrator

Policy
Office of Management and Policy, Division of Health, P.O. Box 309, Madison, WI 53701; tel. 608/266-7384; FAX. 608/266-2832

Prevention
Bureau of Public Health, 1414 East Washington Avenue, Room 167,, Madison, WI 53703; tel. 608/266-1251; FAX. 608/264-6078; Kenneth Baldwin, Director

Quality
Bureau of Quality Compliance, Division of Health, P.O. Box 309, Madison, WI 53701; tel. 608/267-7185; FAX. 608/267-0352; Judy Fryback, Director, Bureau of Quality Compliance

Rehabilitation
Division of Vocational Rehabilitation, 1 West Wilson Street, Room 850, Box 7852, Madison, WI 53707-7852; tel. 608/266-1281; FAX. 608/267-3657; Judy Norman-Nunnery, Administrator

Statistics
Center for Health Statistics, P.O. Box 309, Madison, WI 53701; tel. 608/266-1334; FAX. 608/267-0352; R. D. Nashold, Ph.D., Director

Insurance
Office of the Commissioner of Insurance, P.O. Box 7873, Madison, WI 53707-7873; tel. 608/266-3585; FAX. 608/266-9835

Other

Children
Division for Learning Support: Equity and Advocacy, 125 South Webster Street, P.O. Box 7841, Madison, WI 53707-7841; tel. 608/266-8960; FAX. 608/267-1052; Nancy F. Holloway, Director, Divisionwide Policy and Human Resources

Medical Examiners
Wisconsin Medical Examining Board, 1400 East Washington Avenue, P.O. Box 8935, Madison, WI 53708; tel. 608/266-2811; FAX. 608/267-0644; Patrick D. Braatz, Bureau Director

Professions
Bureau of Health Service Professions, 1400 East Washington Avenue, Suite 174, P.O. Box 8935, Madison, WI 53708-8935; tel. 608/266-0257; FAX. 608/267-0644; Cathy Pond, Administrative Assistant

Regulatory
State of Wisconsin, Department of Regulation and Licensing, 1400 East Washington Avenue, Suite 173, P.O. Box 8935, Madison, WI 53708-8935; tel. 608/266-8609; FAX. 608/267-0644; Marlene A. Cummings, Secretary

Other
State Department of Public Instruction, 125 South Webster Street, P.O. Box 7841, Madison, WI 53707; tel. 608/266-1771; FAX. 608/267-1052; John T. Benson, State Superintendent

WYOMING
The Honorable Jim Geringer, Governor, 307/777-7434

Health
Department of Health, 117 Hathaway Building, Cheyenne, WY 82002; tel. 307/777-7656; FAX. 307/777-7439

Children
Childrens Health Service, Department of Health, Hathaway Building, 4th Floor, Cheyenne, WY 82002; tel. 307/777-7941; FAX. 307/777-5402; Cathy Parish, Program Manager
Division of Public Health, Hathaway Building, 2300 Capitol Avenue, Cheyenne, WY 82002; tel. 307/777-6186; FAX. 307/777-5402; Bill Letson, M.D., Administrator

Facilities
Health Facilities Licensing, Department of Health, Metropolitan Bank Building, 8th Floor, Cheyenne, WY 82002; tel. 307/777-7123; FAX. 307/777-5970; Charlie Simineo, Program Manager

Medical Assistance
Division of Health Care Financing, 6101 Yellowstone, Cheyenne, WY 82002; tel. 307/777-7531; FAX. 307/777-6964; Kenneth C. Kamis, Administrator

Medical Services
Department of Health, 117 Hathaway Building, Cheyenne, WY 82002; tel. 307/777-7656; FAX. 307/777-7439

Prevention
Preventive Medicine, Hathaway Building, 2300 Capitol Avenue, Cheyenne, WY 82002; tel. 307/777-6004; FAX. 307/777-5402

Welfare
Department of Family Services, Hathaway Building, Third Floor, Cheyenne, WY 82002-0490; tel. 307/777-7561; FAX. 307/777-7747; George Lovato, Director

Other

Aging
Wyoming Division on Aging, Hathaway Building, Suite 139, Cheyenne, WY 82002-0480; tel. 307/777-7986; FAX. 307/777-5340; Morris L. Gardner, Administrator

Community
Division of Behavioral Health, 447 Hathaway Building, Cheyenne, WY 82002-0480; tel. 307/777-7094; FAX. 307/777-5580

Medical Examiners
Wyoming Board of Medicine, Barrett Building, 2nd Floor, Cheyenne, WY 82002; tel. 307/777-6463; FAX. 307/777-6478; Carole Shotwell, Executive Secretary

Nursing
Wyoming State Board of Nursing, Barrett Building, 2301 Central Avenue, 2nd Floor, Cheyenne, WY 82002; tel. 307/777-7601; FAX. 307/777-6005; Toma A. Nisbet, RN, M.S., Executive Director

Rehabilitation
Division of Vocational Rehabilitation, Herschler Building, Room 1128, Cheyenne, WY 82002; tel. 307/777-7385; FAX. 307/777-5939; Gary W. Child, Administrator

U.S. Associated Areas

GUAM
The Honorable Carl C. T. Gutierrez, Governor, 011 671/472-8931

Health
Department of Public Health and Social Services, Box 2816, Agana, GU 96910; tel. 671/734-7102; FAX. 671/734-5910; Leticia V. Espaldon, M.D., Director

Planning
Health Planning and Development Agency, 212 West Aspinall Avenue, Administration Building, Suite 155, Agana, GU 96910; tel. 671/472-6831; Aida Z. Fernandez, Acting Administrator

Welfare
Division of Public Welfare, Box 2816, Agana, GU 96910; tel. 671/734-7262; FAX. 671/734-5910; Jesse Catahay, Chief Human Services Administrator

Other

Rehabilitation
Department of Vocational Rehabilitation, Government of Guam, 122 Harmon Plaza, Suite B201, Harmon Industrial Park, GU 96911; tel. 671/646-9468; FAX. 671/649-7672; Albert San Agustin, Acting Director

PUERTO RICO
The Honorable Pedro J. Rossello, Governor, 809/721-7000

Health
Puerto Rico Department of Health, Building A-Medical Center, Call Box 70184, San Juan, PR 00936; tel. 809/766-1616; FAX. 809/766-2240; Enrique Vazquez Quintana, M.D., Secretary, Health

Administration
Administration, Building A-Medical Center, Call Box 70184, San Juan, PR 00936; tel. 809/765-0585; FAX. 809/250-6547, ext. 2006; Icelia Medina Medina, Assistant Secretary for Administration

Dental
Dental Health, Building A-Medical Center, Call Box 70184, San Juan, PR 00936; tel. 809/751-4750; FAX. 809/765-5675; Wanda Urbiztondo, D.M.D., Oral Health Coordinator

Environment
Environmental Health, Department of Health, Building A-Medical Center, Call Box 70184, San Juan, PR 00936; tel. 809/765-7580; FAX. 809/758-6285; Hernan Horta, Assistant Secretary

Organizations / State and Provincial Government Agencies

Health
U.S. Public Health, Building A–Medical Center, Call Box 70184, San Juan, PR 00936; Anibal Marin, M.D., Director

Mental Health
Mental Health and Antiaddiction Services Administration, P.O. Box 1414, San Juan, PR 00928–1414; tel. 809/764–3670; FAX. 809/765–5895; Nestor J. Galarza, M.D., Administrator

Prevention
Department of Health, Secretaryship for Preventive Medicine and Family Health, Building E–Medical Center, Call Box 70184, San Juan, PR 00936; tel. 809/765–0482; FAX. 809/765–5675; Dr. Raul G. Castellanos Bran, Director, Division of Family Health

Other
Legal Services, Building A–Medical Center, Call Box 70184, San Juan, PR 00936; tel. 809/766–1616; FAX. 809/766–2240; Ricardo L. Torres–Munoz, Esquire Director

Welfare
Department of Social Services, Call Box 11398–Fernandez Juncos Street, Santurce, PR 00910; tel. 809/727–4624; FAX. 809/723–1223; Carmen L. Rodriguez de Rivera, Secretary

Other
Rehabilitation
Vocational Rehabilitation Program, Department of Social Services, Apartado 191118, San Juan, PR 00919–1118; tel. 809/725–1792; FAX. 809/721–6286; Sr. Francisco Vallejo, Assistant Secretary

VIRGIN ISLANDS
The Honorable Roy L. Schneider, Governor, 809/774–0001

Health
Virgin Islands Department of Health, St. Thomas Hospital, Charlotte Amalie, St. Thomas, VI 00802; tel. 809/774–0117; FAX. 809/777–4001; Olaf Hendricks, M.D., Acting Commissioner

Children
Division of Maternal and Child Health Services, Virgin Islands Department of Health, Nisky Center Suite 21Q, St. Thomas, VI 00801; tel. 809/776–3580; FAX. 809/774–8633; Dr. Mavis Matthew, Director

Environment
Division of Environmental Health, Old Hospital Complex, Charlotte Amalie, St. Thomas, VI 00802; tel. 809/774–9000, ext. 4644; FAX. 809/776–7899; Lorna W. Smith, Director

Medical Services
Division of Hospitals and Medical Services, St. Thomas Hospital, Sugar Estate, St. Thomas, VI 00802; tel. 809/774–0117; FAX. 809/776–0610; Evelyn McLaughlin, Acting Chief Executive Officer

Mental Health
Division of Mental Health, Alcoholism, and Drug Dependency Services, Oswald Harris Court, Street C, St. Thomas, VI 00801; tel. 809/774–4888; FAX. 809/774–4701

Prevention
Prevention, Health, Promotion and Protection, Department of Health, Charles Harwood Hospital, 3500 Richmond Christiansted, St. Croix, VI 00820–4300; tel. 809/773–1311; FAX. 809/772–5895; Olaf G. Hendricks, M.D., Assistant Commissioner

Other
Division of Financial Services, Knud Hansen Complex, St. Thomas, VI 00802; tel. 809/774–3171; FAX. 809/777–5120; Alphonse J. Stalliard, Deputy Commissioner

Welfare
Virgin Islands Department of Human Services, Barbel Plaza, S., St. Thomas, VI 00802; tel. 809/774–1166; FAX. 809/774–3466; Juel T. R. Molloy, Commissioner

Other
Rehabilitation
Disabilities and Rehabilitation Services, Department of Human Services, Knud Hansen Complex–Building A, 1303 Hospital Ground, St. Thomas, VI 00802; tel. 809/774–0930; FAX. 809/774–3466; Sedonie Halbert, Administrator

Canada

ALBERTA
Health
Department of Family and Social Services, 109 Street and 97 Avenue, 104 Legislature Building, Edmonton, AB T5K 2B6; tel. 403/427–2606; FAX. 403/427–0954; The Honorable Mike Cardinal

BRITISH COLUMBIA
Health
Ministry of Health, Parliament Building, Room 310, Victoria, BC V8V 1X4; tel. 604/387–5394; FAX. 604/387–3696; The Honorable Paul Ramsey

MANITOBA
Health
Department of Health, 302 Legislative Building, Winnipeg, MB R3C 0V8; tel. 204/945–3731; FAX. 204/945–0441; The Honorable James C. McCrae, Minister

Other
Community
Department of Manitoba Family Services, 450 Broadway, Room 357, Legislative Building, Winnipeg, MB R3C 0V8; tel. 204/945–4173; FAX. 204/945–5149; The Honorable Bonnie Mitchelson, Minister

NEW BRUNSWICK
Health
Department of Health and Community Services, Box 5100, Fredericton, NB E3B 5G8; tel. 506/453–3454; FAX. 506/453–5243; The Honorable Russell H. T. King, M.D.

NEWFOUNDLAND
Health
Department of Health, Confederation Building, P.O. Box 8700, St. John's, NF A1B 4J6; tel. 709/729–3124; FAX. 709/729–0121; The Honorable Lloyd Matthews, Minister, Health

NOVA SCOTIA
Health
Department of Health, P.O. Box 488, Halifax, NS B3J 2R8; tel. 902/424–4310; FAX. 902/424–0559; The Honorable Ronald D. Stewart, M.D.

PRINCE EDWARD ISLAND
Health
Department of Health and Social Services, Sullivan Building, 2nd Floor, P.O. Box 2000, Charlottetown, PE C1A 7N8; tel. 902/368–4930; FAX. 902/368–4969; The Honorable Walter A. McEwen, Q.C./Minister

QUEBEC
Health
Ministry of Health and Social Services, Ministere de la Sante et des Services Sociaux, 1075 Chemin Ste–Foy, 15e Etage, Quebec, PQ G1S 2M1; tel. 418/643–3160; FAX. 418/644–4534; Jean Rochon, Minister

SASKATCHEWAN
Health
Department of Health, Legislative Building, Room 334, Regina, SK S4S 0B3; tel. 306/787–1895; FAX. 306/787–8677; The Honorable Louise Simard, Minister

Health Care Providers

Health Maintenance Organizations

The following is a list of Health Maintenance Organizations developed with the assistance of state government agencies and the individual facilities listed. The list is current as of January 1, 1995.

We present this list simply as a convenient directory. Inclusion or omission of any organization indicates neither approval nor disapproval by the American Hospital Association.

United States

ALABAMA

Complete Health of Alabama, Inc., 2160 Highland Avenue, Birmingham, AL 35205; tel. 205/933-7661

Complete Health, Inc., 2160 Highland Avenue, Birmingham, AL 35205; tel. 205/933-7661; FAX. 205/933-0083; William W. Featheringill, President, Chief Executive Officer

Health Advantage Plans, Inc., 701 Lloyd Noland Parkway, Fairfield, AL 35064; tel. 205/786-0211; FAX. 205/783-6917; Mike Caputo, Executive Director

Health Maintenance Group of Birmingham, 495 Wynn Drive, Huntsville, AL 35805; tel. 205/729-9100; FAX. 205/726-9117; Adina Bishop, Director

Health Options, Inc., 532 Riverside Avenue, Jacksonville, FL 32203; tel. 904/791-6086; Harvey Matoren, President

Health Partners of Alabama, Inc., 600 Beacon Parkway, W., Suite 500, Birmingham, AL 35209; tel. 205/942-5787; FAX. 205/945-9450; Carole Zimbrolt, Vice President, Chief Operating Officer

Health Services of Alabama, 2117 Second Avenue, N., Birmingham, AL 35203; tel. 205/328-4100

Humana Health Plan of Alabama, Inc., 303 Williams Avenue, S.W., Suite 121, Huntsville, AL 35801; tel. 205/532-2000; FAX. 205/532-2025; Rene Moret, Executive Director

Mobile Health Plan, d/b/a Prime Health, 124 South University Boulevard, Mobile, AL 36608; tel. 334/342-0022; FAX. 334/342-1176

Mobile Health Plan of Alabama, Inc., 124 South University Boulevard, Mobile, AL 36608; tel. 334/342-0022; Walter L. Hovell, Chairman

Principal Health Care of Florida, Inc., 1200 Gulf Life Drive, Suite 100, Jacksonville, FL 32207-1802; tel. 904/390-0935, ext. 200; FAX. 904/390-0950; James F. H. Henry, Regional Director

Southeast Health Plans of Alabama, Inc., 104 Inverness Parkway West, Suite 280, Birmingham, AL 35242; tel. 205/991-6000; George Salem, President, Chief Executive Officer

ARIZONA

Aetna Health Plan of Arizona, Inc., 7878 North 16th Street, Suite 210, Phoenix, AZ 85020; tel. 602/395-8800; FAX. 602/395-8813; James W. Jones, Acting Vice President, Market Manager

CIGNA HealthCare of Arizona, Inc., 11001 North Black Canyon Highway, Suite 400, Phoenix, AZ 85029; tel. 602/371-2500; FAX. 602/371-2625; Clyde Wright, M.D., President, General Manager

FHP Inc., 410 North 44th Street, P.O. Box 52078, Phoenix, AZ 85072-2078; tel. 602/244-8200; FAX. 602/681-7680; Clifford Klima, President, Arizona Region

First Health of Arizona, Inc., 10448 West Coggins Drive, Sun City, AZ 85351; tel. 602/933-1344; FAX. 602/977-8808; Donald J. Hinnen, Plan Director

HMO Arizona, 2444 West Las Palmaritas, P.O. Box 13466, Phoenix, AZ 85002-3466; tel. 602/864-4252; FAX. 602/864-4035; Julie Pressley, Executive Director

Humana Health Plan, Inc., Anchor Centre III, 2231 East Camelback Road, Suite 208, Phoenix, AZ 85016; tel. 602/381-4300; FAX. 602/381-4381; Elizabeth Kelly, Associate Executive Director

Intergroup Prepaid Health Plan of Arizona, Inc., 1010 North Finance Center Drive, Suite 100, Tucson, AZ 85710; tel. 602/290-7400; FAX. 602/290-7585; Edward J. Munno, Jr., President, Chief Operating Officer

MetLife Healthcare Network of Arizona, Inc., MetraHealth, 3020 East Camelback, Suite 100, Phoenix, AZ 85016; tel. 602/553-1300; FAX. 602/553-1331; Kathleen Garast, President, Chief Executive Officer

Partners Health Plan of Arizona, Inc., 5210 East Williams Circle, Suite 300, Tucson, AZ 85711; tel. 602/748-8020; FAX. 602/748-4289; Paul A. Zucarelli, President, Chief Executive Officer

The Samaritan Health Plan, Inc., 5300 North Central Avenue, Phoenix, AZ 85012; tel. 602/230-1555; FAX. 602/266-9580; Phyllis Biedess, President, Chief Executive Officer

ARKANSAS

American Dental Providers, Inc., 103 West Capitol, Suite 617, Little Rock, AR 72201-0000; tel. 501/376-0544; FAX. 501/375-5021; Dale Beeber, Vice President

American Health Care Providers, Inc., 4801 Southwick Drive, Suite 500, Matteson, IL 60443-2254; tel. 708/503-5000; FAX. 708/503-5001; Asif Sayeed, President

Complete Health of Arkansas, Inc., 415 North McKinley Street, Plaza West Building, Suite 820, Little Rock, AR 72205; tel. 501/664-7700; FAX. 501/664-7768; V. Rob Herndon III

DentiCare of Arkansas, Inc., Regional Administration Office, 7112 South Mingo, Suite 108, Tulsa, OK 74133; tel. 918/254-9055; FAX. 918/254-9076; Robert E. Acklin, President

HMO Arkansas, 601 Gaines, Little Rock, AR 72201-0000; tel. 501/378-2201; FAX. 501/378-3732; David Bridges, Executive Director

HMO Partners, Inc., d/b/a HEALTH ADVANTAGE, 26 Corporate Hill Drive, Little Rock, AR 72205; tel. 501/221-1800; FAX. 501/221-7103; Marlon J. Doucet, M.D., Medical Director

Prudential Health Care Plan Inc., 24 Greenway Plaza, Suite 500, P.O. Box 2884, Houston, TX 77252-2884

CALIFORNIA

Access Dental Plan, Inc., 555 University Avenue, Suite 182, Sacramento, CA 95825; tel. 916/922-5000, ext. 310; FAX. 916/646-9000; Reza Abbaszaden, D.D.S., Chief Executive Officer

Advanced Dental Systems, Inc., 3162 Newberry Drive, San Jose, CA 95118; tel. 800/448-1942; FAX. 408/448-5418; Dr. Roy Ingram, President

Aetna Dental Care of California, Inc., 201 North Civic Drive, Suite 300, Walnut Creek, CA 94596; tel. 510/977-7865; FAX. 510/746-6560; Bryan J. Geremia, Chief Executive Officer

Aetna Health Plans of California, 7676 Hazard Center Drive, San Diego, CA 92108; tel. 619/497-0046; FAX. 619/497-4251; Dean M. Hosmer, Market Vice President

Aetna Health Plans of California, 201 North Civic Drive, Suite 300, Walnut Creek, CA 94596; tel. 909/386-3145; FAX. 909/386-3330; Michael Dobbs, Market Vice President

Alternative Dental Care of California, Inc., 21700 Oxnard Street, Suite 500, Woodland Hills, CA 91367; tel. 818/710-9400, ext. 451; FAX. 510/416-7390; William E. Gregor, Chief Finance Officer

American Chiropractic Network Health Plan, Inc., 8989 Rio San Diego Drive, Suite 250, San Diego, CA 92108; tel. 619/297-8100; FAX. 619/297-8189; George DeVries, President

American Healthguard Corporation, Centaguard Dental Plan, 21031 Ventura Boulevard, Suite 506, Woodland Hills, CA 91364-1836; tel. 818/884-7645; David Kutner, M.D., President

American Psychmanagement of California, Inc., 4640 Admiralty Way, Suite 600, Marina Del Rey, CA 90292; tel. 310/822-4811, ext. 6001; FAX. 310/574-6130; Charlton C. Tooke III, Chief Operating Officer

Ameritas Managed Dental Plan, Inc., 151 Kalmus Drive, Suite B-250, Costa Mesa, CA 92626; tel. 714/437-5966; FAX. 714/437-5967; Skip Gray, President

Baycare Health Plan, 101 Skyport Drive, Suite B, San Jose, CA 95110; tel. 408/441-9340; Tracy K. Herta, D.D.S., President

Blue Cross of California/Wellpoint Health Network Inc./, CaliforniaCare Health Plans, 21555 Oxnard Street, Woodland Hills, CA 91367; tel. 818/703-2497; Brian J. Donnelly, Senior Vice President

CIGNA Dental Health of California, Inc., 5990 Sepulveda Boulevard, Suite 500, Van Nuys, CA 91411; tel. 818/756-2900; FAX. 818/756-2997; Claire Marie Burchill, President, Chief Executive Officer

CMG Behavioral Health of California, Inc., 865 South Figueroa Street, Suite 1450, Los Angeles, CA 90017; tel. 213/312-9400; FAX. 213/312-9413; Michael L. Jospe, Ph.D., Executive Director

California Benefits Dental Plan, 4911 Warner Avenue, Suite 208, Huntington Beach, CA 92649; tel. 714/840-2852; FAX. 714/840-3213; Robert F. Gosin, D.D.S., President

California Dental Health Plan, 14471 Chambers Road, 92680, P.O. Box 899, Tustin, CA 92681-0899; tel. 714/731-4751; FAX. 714/731-2049; James R. Lindsey, President

California Physicians' Service, Blue Shield of California, Two NorthPoint, San Francisco, CA 94133; tel. 415/445-5195; FAX. 415/445-3596; Patricia Ernsberger, Corporate Regulatory Counsel

California Psychological Health Plan, 5750 Wilshire Boulevard, Suite 490, Los Angeles, CA 90036; tel. 213/965-4870; David L. Auchterlonie, Chief Executive Officer, Administrator

Californiacare Health Plans, 21555 Oxnard Street, Suite 8A, Woodland Hills, CA 91367; tel. 818/703-2872; FAX. 818/703-4332; Andrew Allocco, Sneior Vice President, Provider, Association Relations

CareAmerican Southern California, Inc., 6300 Canoga Avenue, Woodland Hills, CA 91367; tel. 818/228-2229; FAX. 818/228-5117; Arthur Southam, M.D., Chief Executive Officer

Chinese Community Health Plan, 170 Columbus Avenue, Suite 210, San Francisco, CA 94133; tel. 415/397-3190; FAX. 415/677-2488; Thomas M. Harlan, Chief Executive Officer

City of San Jose, 801 North First Street, Suite 207, San Jose, CA 95110; tel. 408/277-5137; Jay Castellano, Senior Administrative Officer

Community Dental Services, Smilecare, 18101 Von Karman Avenue, Irvine, CA 92715; tel. 714/756-1111; M. E. Hardin, President, Chief Executive Officer

Community Health Group, 740 Bay Boulevard, Chula Vista, CA 91910; tel. 619/422-0422; FAX. 619/422-5930; Gabriel Arce, Chief Executive Officer

Providers / Health Maintenance Organizations

ConsumerHealth, Inc., d/b/a Newport Dental Plan, 1401 Dove Street, Suite 290, Newport Beach, CA 92660; tel. 714/752–8522, ext. 220; FAX. 714/833–9172; Stephen R. Casey, President

Continental Dental Plan, 300 Corporate Pointe, Suite 385, Culver City, CA 90230; tel. 310/216–1154; James M. Hubbard, President

Contra Costa Health Plan, 595 Center Avenue, Suite 100, Martinez, CA 94553; tel. 510/313–6000; FAX. 510/313–6002; Milton Camhi, Executive Director

County of Los Angeles, Department of Health Services, d/b/a Community Health Plan, 313 North Figueroa Street, Los Angeles, CA 90012; tel. 213/974–8136; Westley Sholes, Deputy Director, Administrative Services

Dedicated Dental Systems, Inc., 3990 Ming Avenue, Bakersfield, CA 93309; tel. 805/397–5513; FAX. 805/397–2888; Robert J. Newman, Administrator

Dental Benefit Providers of California, Inc., d/b/a Dental Choice of California, Inc., 1999 Harrison Street, Suite 2750, Oakland, CA 94612; tel. 510/832–2611; FAX. 510/832–2405; Paul Brown, Chief Operating Officer

Dental Health Services, 3833 Atlantic Avenue, Long Beach, CA 90807–3505; tel. 310/595–6000; FAX. 310/424–0150; Godfrey Pernell, President

Denticare of California, Inc., 28202 Cabot Road, Suite 600, Zip 92677, P.O. Box 30019, Laguna Niguel, CA 92607–0019; tel. 714/365–8010, ext. 229; FAX. 714/347–7612; Steven D. Bonham, Chief Operating Officer

Dr. Leventhal's Vision Care Centers of America, 3680 Rosecrans Street, Zip 92110, P.O. Box 87808, San Diego, CA 92138; tel. 619/223–5656; FAX. 619/223–2318; Debra Brant, Chief Operating Officer

Eyecare Service Plan, Inc., 9090 Burton Way, Beverly Hills, CA 90211; tel. 310/271–0145; Matthew Rips, Vice President

Eyexam 2000 of California, Inc., 951 Mariner's Island Boulevard, Suite 310, San Mateo, CA 94404; tel. 415/349–4417; FAX. 415/572–9313; Evyn L. Shomer, Corporate Counsel

FHP, Inc., 18000 Studebaker Road, Suite 750, Cerritos, CA 90701; tel. 213/809–5399; FAX. 714/968–7159; Stuart Byer, Associate Vice President, Consumer, Government Affairs

Foundation Health, a California Health Plan, 3400 Data Drive, Rancho Cordova, CA 95670; tel. 916/631–5299; FAX. 916/631–5294; Marshall Bentley, Vice President, Counsel

Foundation Health Psychcare Services, Inc., 125 East Sir Francis Drake Boulevard, Suite 300, Larkspur, CA 94939–1860; tel. 510/655–0535; Cathy Clement, Administrator

Fountain Valley Vision Services, AVP Vision Plans, 155 DuBois Street, 95060, P.O. Box 8425, Santa Cruz, CA 95061–8425; tel. 408/425–0989; FAX. 408/425–3805; D. K. Kim

Freedom Plan, Inc., 201 North Salsipuedes, Suite 206, Santa Barbara, CA 93103–3256; tel. 805/564–0072; FAX. 805/564–4167; Leeba R. Lessin, Chief Executive Officer

Golden West Health Plan, Inc., Ventura Dental Health Plan, 888 West Ventura Boulevard, Suite 7, Camarillo, CA 93010; tel. 805/987–8941; Karl H. Lehmann, Executive Director

Greater California Dental Plan, Smilesaver, Signature Dental Plan, 22144 Clarendon Street, First Floor, P.O. Box 4281, Woodland Hills, CA 91365–4281; tel. 818/348–1500; Mark Johnson, President

HMO California, 4675 MacArthur Court, Suite 1400, Newport Beach, CA 92660; tel. 800/795–8755; FAX. 714/756–5550; Mitchell J. Goodstein, Chief Executive Officer

Health Benefits, Inc., H.B.I. Prepaid Dental Plans, 4557 Quail Lakes Drive, Stockton, CA 95207; tel. 800/331–0903; FAX. 209/478–2918; Sherri E. Crowl, Vice President

Health Net, 21600 Oxnard Street, Woodland Hills, CA 91367, P.O. Box 9103, Van Nuys, CA 91409–9103; tel. 818/593–7203; FAX. 818/719–7126; Sam Ho, M.D., Senior Vice President, Health Care Services

Health Plan of the Redwoods, 3033 Cleveland Avenue, Santa Rosa, CA 95403; tel. 707/544–2273; FAX. 707/544–0312; John W. Baxter, Executive Director

Health and Human Resource Center, 7798 Starling Drive, San Diego, CA 92123; tel. 619/571–1698; Stephen H. Heidel, M.D., President, Chief Executive Officer

Healthdent of California, Inc., 2848 Arden Way, Suite 100, Sacramento, CA 95825; tel. 916/486–0749; FAX. 916/486–3642; Edward L. Cruchley, D.D.S., President

Holman Professional Counseling Centers, 21050 Van Owen Street, Canoga Park, CA 91303; tel. 818/704–1444, ext. 235; FAX. 818/704–9339; Ron Holman, Ph.D., President

Human Affairs International of California, 300 North Continental Boulevard, Suite 200, El Segundo, CA 90245; tel. 310/414–0066; FAX. 310/414–9282; Jonathan Wormhoudt, Ph.D., Chief Executive Officer

Ideal Dental Health Plan, 1720 South San Gabriel Boulevard, Suite 102, San Gabriel, CA 91776; tel. 818/288–2203; Richard Sun, D.D.S., President

Inter Valley Health Plan, 300 South Park Avenue, Suite 300, Pomona, CA 91766; tel. 909/623–6333; FAX. 909/622–2907; James E. Taylor, President

Jaslie, Inc., 3415 South Sepulveda Boulevard, Suite 112, Los Angeles, CA 90034; tel. 310/915–7266; Mark Fisher, President

Kaiser Foundation Added Choice Health Plan, 2770 Ordway Building, One Kaiser Plaza, Oakland, CA 94612; tel. 510/271–2680; FAX. 510/271–5917; H. Paul Brandes, Assistant Secretary, Senior Counsel

Kaiser Foundation Health Plan, Inc., 2770 Ordway Building, One Kaiser Plaza, Oakland, CA 94612; tel. 510/271–2680; FAX. 510/271–5917; H. Paul Brandes, Assistant Secretary, Senior Counsel

Laurel Dental Plan, Inc., 5451 Laurel Canyon Boulevard, Suite 209, North Hollywood, CA 91607; tel. 818/980–0929; FAX. 818/980–4668; Dr. Victor Sands, President

LifeLink, Inc., 23046 Avenida de la Carlota, Suite 700, Laguna Hills, CA 92653; tel. 714/859–7971; Ron Stock, Director, Sales, Marketing

Lifeguard, Inc., 1851 McCarthy Boulevard, Milpitas, CA 95035; tel. 408/943–9400; FAX. 408/383–4259; Mark G. Hyde, President, Chief Executive Director

MAXICARE, 1149 South Broadway Street, Los Angeles, CA 90015; tel. 213/765–2000, ext. 2101; FAX. 213/765–2694; Peter J. Ratican, Chairman, President, Chief Executive Officer

MCC Behavioral Care of California, Inc., 801 North Brand Boulevard, Suite 1150, Glendale, CA 91203; tel. 818/551–2200; Bernhild E. Quintero, Vice President

Managed Dental Care of California, 6312 Variel Avenue, Suite 220, Woodland Hills, CA 91367; tel. 818/587–9420; FAX. 818/347–7302; Michael Gould, President, Chief Executive Officer

Managed Health Network, Inc., 5100 West Goldleaf Circle, Suite 300, Los Angeles, CA 90056; tel. 213/299–0999; FAX. 213/298–2765; Alethea Caldwell, President

Medco Behavioral Care of California, Inc., 400 Oyster Point Boulevard, Suite 306, South San Francisco, CA 94080; tel. 415/742–0980; FAX. 415/742–0988; Douglas Studebaker, President

MetLife Healthcare Network of California, Inc., 4500 East Pacific Coast Highway, Suite 120, Long Beach, CA 90804–6441; tel. 310/597–9932; FAX. 310/498–5137; Bud Volberding, President, Chief Executive Officer

Molina Medical Centers, One Golden Shore, Long Beach, CA 90802; tel. 310/435–3666; John Molina, J.D., Vice President

National Dental Health, The Dental Advantage, 3111 Camino Del Rio North, Suite 1000, San Diego, CA 92108; tel. 800/288–9992; FAX. 619/283–9437; Keith C. Macumber, Senior Vice President, Western Regional Manager

National Health Plans, 1005 West Orangeburg Avenue, Suite B, Modesto, CA 95350–4163; tel. 209/527–3350; FAX. 209/527–6773; Clive Riddle, Senior Vice President, Chief Executive Officer

National Resource Consultants, Inc., 2835 Camino Del Rio, S., Suite 300, San Diego, CA 92108; tel. 619/291–0330; Jordan Goldrich, Vice President, Operations

Omni Health Care, 1776 West March Lane, Suite 240, Stockton, CA 95207–6425; tel. 209/474–6664; FAX. 209/955–7533; Robert E. Edmonson, President, Chief Executive Officer

Oral Health Services, Inc., Mida Dental Plan, 21700 Oxnard Street, Suite 500, Woodland Hills, CA 91367; tel. 818/710–9400, ext. 451; FAX. 818/710–9400; William E. Gregor, Chief Financial Officer

PMI Dental Health Plan, (an affiliate of Delta Dental Plan of California), 12898 Towne Center Drive, Cerritos, CA 90703; tel. 310/403–4040; FAX. 310/924–8039; Jeff Album, Public Relations Associate

PacifiCare of California, Secure Horizons, 5701 Katella Avenue, Zip 90630–5019, P.O. Box 6006, Cypress, CA 90630–6006; tel. 714/952–1121; FAX. 714/236–7887; Jeff Folick, President

Pacific Union Dental, Inc., 2200 Powell Street, Suite 805, Emeryville, CA 94608; tel. 510/547–8227; FAX. 510/547–7305; Carl Legreca, Vice President, Marketing

Pearle Vision Care, Inc., 12625 High Bluff Drive, Suite 108, San Diego, CA 92130; tel. 800/843–6706; FAX. 619/793–4090; Nan Johnson, President

Preferred Health Care of California, Inc., PHC–Cal, 5 Park Plaza, Suite 500, Irvine, CA 92714; tel. 203/761–7239; Lisa M. Lopez, Secretary

Preferred Health Plan, Inc., Personal Dental Services, 4034 Park Boulevard, San Diego, CA 92103; tel. 619/297–6670; FAX. 619/297–0317; Philip G. Menna, D.D.S., President

Preventive Dental Systems, Inc., 2000 L Street, Sacramento, CA 95814; tel. 916/448–2994; FAX. 916/448–2997; Carolyn Brodt, Executive Director

Priority Health Services, Central Valley Health Plan, Inc., P.O. Box 25790, Fresno, CA 93729–5790; tel. 209/435–8366; FAX. 209/435–7693; John M. Cronin, President, Chief Executive Officer

Private Medical–Care, Inc., PMI, 12898 Towne Center Drive, Cerritos, CA 90701; tel. 213/493–6661; FAX. 310/924–8311; Robert B. Elliott, President

Prudential Health Care Plan of California, Inc., 5800 Canoga Avenue, Woodland Hills, CA 91367; tel. 818/712–5001; FAX. 818/992–2474; Kathleen Swenson, President

Psychology Systems, Inc., The Psych/Care Plan, 615 South Main Street, Milpitas, CA 95035; tel. 408/263–8046; FAX. 408/942–0264; John C. Brady II, Ph.D., President

Ross–Loos Health Plan of California, Inc., d/b/a CIGNA HealthCare of California, 505 North Brand Boulevard, P.O. Box 2125, Glendale, CA 91203; tel. 818/500–6726; FAX. 818/500–6831; Leslie A. Margolin, Chief Counsel

Safeguard Health Plans, 505 North Euclid Street, P.O. Box 3210, Anaheim, CA 92803–3210; tel. 714/778–1005; FAX. 714/778–4517; Ronald I. Brendzel, Senior Vice President

Santa Clara Valley Medical Center, Valley Health Plan, 750 South Bascom Avenue, San Jose, CA 95128; tel. 408/885–5704; FAX. 408/885–4050; Roger Wells, Executive Director

Scan Health Plan, 521 East Fourth Street, Long Beach, CA 90802–2502; tel. 310/435–0380; FAX. 310/491–0020; Sam L. Ervin, President, Chief Executive Officer

Sharp Health Plan, 9325 Sky Park Court, Suite 300, San Diego, CA 92123; tel. 619/637–6536; FAX. 619/637–6504; Jayne Chaffin, Vice President, Administration and Product Development

TakeCare Health Plan, Inc., 2300 Clayton Road, Suite 1000, Concord, CA 94520; tel. 510/246–1300; FAX. 510/246–1490; R. Judd Jessup, President

Providers / Health Maintenance Organizations

Takecare of California, Inc., 3875 Hopyard Road, Pleasanton, CA 94588; tel. 510/847–7284; FAX. 510/847–6075; Terry P. Bayer, President, General Manager

U. S. Behavioral Health Plan, California, 2000 Powell, Suite 1180, Emeryville, CA 94608; tel. 510/601–2200; FAX. 510/547–2336; Ann McClanathan, Vice President, Client Services and Sales

Universal Care, 1600 East Hill Street, Signal Hill, CA 90806; tel. 310/424–6200, ext. 4003; FAX. 310/427–4634; Howard E. Davis, President, Chief Executive Officer

Vision Plan of America, 8111 Beverly Boulevard, Suite 306, Los Angeles, CA 90048; tel. 213/658–6113; FAX. 213/658–8611; Dr. Stuart Needleman

Vision Service Plan, 3333 Quality Drive, Rancho Cordova, CA 95670; tel. 800/852–7600; Al Schubert, Vice President, Managed Care

Visioncare of California, 3512 Breakwater Court, Hayward, CA 94545; tel. 415/732–8900; Dr. Garold Edwards, President

Vista Hill Foundation, Vista Health Plans, 2355 Northside Drive, Suite 300, San Diego, CA 92108; tel. 619/521–4440; Keith Dixon, President, Chief Executive Officer, Vista Health Plans

Viva Health Plan, 17 Cupania Circle, Monterey Park, CA 91754; tel. 213/724–8770; Mitchell Zevin, President

Watts Health Foundation, Inc., United Health Plan, 10300 Compton Avenue, Los Angeles, CA 90002; tel. 213/564–4331; Clyde W. Oden, M.P.H., O.D., President, Chief Executive Officer

Wellpoint Dental Plan, 21555 Oxnard Street, Woodland Hills, CA 91367; tel. 818/703–2412; Thomas C. Geiser, Senior Vice President, General Counsel

Wellpoint Pharmacy Plan, 21555 Oxnard Street, Woodland Hills, CA 91367; tel. 818/703–2412; Thomas C. Geiser, Senior Vice President, General Counsel

Western Dental Services, Inc., Western Dental Plan, 300 Plaza Alicante, Suite 800, Garden Grove, CA 92640; tel. 714/938–1600; FAX. 714/938–1611; Frank F. Pellkofer, President

COLORADO

CIGNA HealthCare of Colorado, Inc., 3900 East Mexico Avenue, Suite 1100, Denver, CO 80210–3946; tel. 303/782–1500; FAX. 303/782–1577; Dennis Mouras, General Manager

Colorado Dental Service, Inc., d/b/a Delta Dental, 2675 South Abilene Street, Aurora, CO 80014; tel. 303/671–0200

Colorado Vision Service, Inc., 7878 Wadsworth Boulevard, Suite 300, Arvada, CO 80003; tel. 303/420–2052

Comprecare Health Care Services, Inc., 12100 East Iliff Avenue, P.O. Box 441170, Aurora, CO 80014; tel. 303/695–6685; FAX. 303/751–4432; Eric D. Sipf, President, Chief Executive Officer

Exclusive Healthcare of Colorado, Inc., Stanford Place Three, Suite 202, 4582 South Ulster Street Parkway, Denver, CO 80237; tel. 303/694–6919; FAX. 303/694–3204; Donald L. Shovein, Executive Director

FHP of Colorado, Inc., 6312 South Fiddlers Green Circle, Suite 230 E, Englewood, CO 80111; tel. 303/689–9646

FHP of Colorado, Inc., 12100 East Iliff Avenue, Aurora, CO 80014; tel. 303/695–6685

HMO Colorado, Inc., 700 Broadway, Suite 612, Denver, CO 80203; tel. 303/831–2131

HMO Health Plans, Inc., d/b/a San Luis Valley HMO, Inc., 95 West First Avenue, Monte Vista, CO 81144; tel. 719/852–4055; FAX. 719/852–3481; Douglas Johnson, Executive Director, Chief Executive Officer

HSI Health Plans, Inc., 200 South College Avenue, Fort Collins, CO 80524; tel. 303/482–8403; FAX. 303/482–8911; Leslie Mussetter, Vice President, Healthcare Services

Health Network of Colorado Springs, Inc., 555 East Pikes Peaks Avenue, Suite 108, Colorado Springs, CO 80903; tel. 719/475–5025; FAX. 719/475–5004; Ron Burnside, Chief Executive Officer

Humana Health Plan, Inc., P.O. Box 740036, Louisville, KY 40201; tel. 502/580–1000; FAX. 502/580–2099; Wayne T. Smith, President

Kaiser Foundation Health Plan of Colorado, 2045 Franklin, Denver, CO 80205; tel. 303/344–7200; FAX. 303/344–7290; James A. Vohs, President

MetLife HealthCare Network of Colorado, Inc., 1512 Larimer Street, Denver, CO 80202; tel. 303/629–5331; FAX. 303/899–4190; Nancy W. Ashbach, M.D., M.B.A., President, Chief Executive Officer

Prudential Health Care Plan, Inc., d/b/a Prucare of Colorado, Inc., 4643 South Ulster Street, Suite 1000, Denver, CO 80237; tel. 303/796–6161

Qual–Med Plans for Health of Colorado, Inc., P.O. Box 1986, Pueblo, CO 81002–1986; tel. 719/542–0500; FAX. 719/542–4921; Malik Hasan, M.D., Chairman, President

Rocky Mountain, P.O. Box 60129, Grand Junction, CO 81506; tel. 303/244–7760; FAX. 303/244–7880; Michael J. Weber, Executive Director

Rocky Mountain Healthcare Options, Inc., 2775 Crossroads Boulevard, Grand Junction, CO 81506; tel. 303/245–0060

Rocky Mountain Hospital and Medical Service, 700 Broadway, Denver, CO 80203; tel. 303/831–2670

Southern Colorado Health Plan, Inc., (a subsidiary of Foundation Health Corporation), 41 Montebello, Suite H, Pueblo, CO 81001; tel. 719/545–6272; FAX. 719/545–6282; Byron Cairns, President

CONNECTICUT

Aetna Health Plans of Southern New England, 80 Lamberton Road, Conveyor LB2B, Windsor, CT 06095; tel. 203/298–4000; Craig W. Gage, M.D., Vice President, Health Services Management

CIGNA HealthCare of Connecticut, Inc., 900 Cottage Grove Road, A–118, Hartford, CT 06152–1118; tel. 800/345–9458; FAX. 203/769–2399; Ellen C. Harrison, General Manager

Community Health Care Plan, 221 Whitney Avenue, New Haven, CT 06511; tel. 203/773–8359; FAX. 203/787–5917; Carl Maleri, President, Chief Executive Officer

ConnectiCare, Inc., 30 Batterson Park Road, Farmington, CT 06032–3006; tel. 203/674–5700; FAX. 203/674–5728; Marcel Gamache, President, Chief Executive Officer

Constitution HealthCare, Inc., 370 Bassett Road, P.O. Box 720, North Haven, CT 06473–0720; tel. 800/227–3246; FAX. 203/234–8573

Enterprise Health Plans, Inc., 370 Bassett Road, North Haven, CT 06473

Kaiser Foundation Health Plan, 76 Batterson Park Road, P.O. Box 4011, Farmington, CT 06034–4011; tel. 203/678–6178; FAX. 203/678–6160; Pat Parkerton, Area Operations Manager

M.D. Health Plan, 6 Devine Street, North Haven, CT 06473; tel. 203/776–5789; FAX. 203/288–6667; Douglas A. Hayward, President

Oxford Health Plans, 800 Connecticut Avenue, Norwalk, CT 06854; tel. 800/444–6222; Melissa McCormick, Marketing Associate

Physicians Health Services, Inc., 120 Hawley Lane, Trumbull, CT 06611–5343; tel. 203/381–6400; FAX. 203/381–6683; Amy Rich, Vice President, Research

Prudential Health Care of Connecticut, Inc., 101 Merritt Seven, Norwalk, CT 06851; tel. 203/849–1800; FAX. 203/849–8387; Lewis E. Devendorf, Executive Director

Suburban Health Plan, Inc., 680 Bridgeport Avenue, Shelton, CT 06484; tel. 203/926–8882; FAX. 203/925–1202; Teresa Guidone, Vice President, Sales and Marketing

U.S. Healthcare, Inc., 55 Lane Road, Fairfield, NJ 07004; tel. 201/244–3911; Leonard Abramson, President

DELAWARE

AETNA Health Plans, 3541 Winchester Road, Allentown, PA 18195; tel. 800/624–4478; FAX. 610/391–9309

CIGNA HealthCare of Pennsylvania, New Jersey and Delaware, One Beaver Valley Road, Suite CHP, Wilmington, DE 19803; tel. 302/477–3000, ext. 3725; FAX. 302/477–3707; Norman Scott, M.D., Medical Director

Delaware Network Health Plan, 121 South Front Street, Seaford, DE 19973; tel. 302/629–8005; FAX. 302/629–8927; Donald Pinner, Vice President, Managed Care Services

Delaware Valley HMO, Concord Industrial Park, 925 Baltimore Pike, P.O. Box 1111, Concordville, PA 19931; tel. 215/358–5650; FAX. 215/358–5238; Alfred F. Meyer, President

Delmarva Health Plan, Inc., 106 Marlboro Road, Easton, MD 21601; tel. 410/822–7223; Richard Moore, Chief Executive Officer

Healthcare Delaware, Inc., P.O. Box 7498, Wilmington, DE 19803; tel. 302/652–8038, ext. 4799; FAX. 215/358–5238; James J. Thomas III, Senior Vice President

Optimum Choice Inc./MDIPA, Inc./Alliance PPO, Inc., Four Taft Court, Rockville, MD 20850; tel. 301/762–8205, ext. 3994; Gloria Stem, Human Resource, Senior Director

Principal Health Care of Delaware, Inc., One Corporate Commons, 100 West Commons Boulevard, Suite 300, New Castle, DE 19720; tel. 302/322–4700; FAX. 302/322–9007; Max Kenyon, Executive Director

The Health Care Centers, Inc., The Health Care Center at Christiana, 200 Hygeia Drive, P.O. Box 6008, Newark, DE 19714; tel. 302/421–2466; FAX. 302/421–2577; R. Walter Powell, M.D., Medical Director

Total Health, Inc., One Brandywine Gateway, P.O. Box 8792, Wilmington, DE 19899; tel. 302/421–3034; FAX. 302/421–2577; Robert C. Cole, Jr., President

U.S. Healthcare, Inc., 980 Jolly Road, P.O. Box 1109, Blue Bell, PA 19422; tel. 215/628–4800; Leonard Abramson, President

DISTRICT OF COLUMBIA

CIGNA HealthCare Mid–Atlantic, Inc., 9700 Patuxent Woods Drive, Columbia, MD 21046; tel. 410/720–5800; Linda Hacker

George Washington University Health Plan, Inc., 4550 Montgomery Avenue, Suite 800, Bethesda, MD 20814; tel. 301/941–2000, ext. 2100; FAX. 301/941–2005; Dr. John E. Ott, Executive Director, Chief Executive Officer

HealthPlus, Inc., 7601 Ora Glen Drive, Suite 200, Greenbelt, MD 20770–3641; tel. 301/441–1600, ext. 3308; FAX. 301/489–5284; Jeff D. Emerson, Chief Executive Officer

Humana Group Health Association, Inc., 4301 Connecticut Avenue, N.W., Washington, DC 20008; tel. 202/364–2000; FAX. 202/364–7418; Robert Pfotenhauer, President, Chief Executive Officer

Kaiser Foundation Health Plan of the Mid–Atlantic States, 2101 East Jefferson Street, Rockville, MD 20849; tel. 301/468–6000, ext. 3018; FAX. 301/816–7482; Alan J. Silverstone, President

Maryland–IPA, Inc., MAMSI, Four Taft Court, Rockville, MD 20850; tel. 301/294–5100; FAX. 301/309–1709; Richard K. Slater, President

Physicians Health Plan, Inc./Physicians Care, d/b/a Health Keepers, 2111 Wilson Boulevard, Suite 11510, Arlington, VA 22201; tel. 703/525–0602; Wyndahm Kidd

United Mine Workers of America, 4455 Connecticut Avenue, N.W., Washington, DC 20008; tel. 202/895–3960; Robert Condra

FLORIDA

Aetna Health Plans of Florida, Inc., 4890 West Kennedy, Suite 545, Tampa, FL 33630–3123; tel. 813/287–7820; FAX. 813/282–0893; James R. Gilmour, Administrator

Anthem Health Plan of Florida, Inc., 10199 Southside Boulevard, Suite 301, Jacksonville, FL 32256; tel. 904/363–7601; FAX. 904/363–7627; Ann F. Dehgan, Senior Vice President, Chief Operating Officer

Providers / Health Maintenance Organizations

AvMed Health Plan, P.O. Box 749, Gainesville, FL 32606–0749; tel. 904/372–8400; FAX. 904/372–5155; Edward C. Peddie, President, Chief Executive Officer

C.A.C. Ramsay, Inc., 75 Valencia Avenue, Coral Gables, FL 33134; tel. 305/441–1140; Luis E. Lamela, President, Chief Executive Officer

CAC–Ramsay Health Plans, Inc., 75 Valencia Avenue, Coral Gables, FL 33134; tel. 305/441–1140

CIGNA Health Care of Florida, Inc., 5404 Cypress Center Drive, Suite 200, P.O. Box 24203, Tampa, FL 33623; tel. 813/281–1000; FAX. 813/282–0356; Edward M. Dillabough, Vice President, Healthplan Manager

Capital Group Health Services of Florida, Inc., 2140 Centerville Place, P.O. Box 13267, Tallahassee, FL 32317; tel. 904/386–3161; FAX. 904/385–3193; John Hogan, Administrator

CareFlorida, Inc., 7950 N.W. 53rd Street, Suite 300, Miami, FL 33166; tel. 305/591–3311, ext. 1997; FAX. 305/470–1996; Warren Stowell, President

Century Medical Health Plan, Inc., 6101 Blue Lagoon Drive, Suite 300, Miami, FL 33126; tel. 305/267–6633; FAX. 305/264–2771; Peter Kilissanly, President, Chief Executive Officer

Complete Health of Florida, Inc., 5201 West Kennedy Boulevard, Suite 712, Tampa, FL 33609; tel. 813/286–8429; FAX. 813/289–2707; Brad Green, Vice President, General Manager

Dimension Physician–Hospital Organization, Inc., 6303 Blue Lagoon Drive, Suite 225, Miami, FL 33126; tel. 305/266–2166; FAX. 305/266–9903; Robert W. Carmack, President, Chief Executive Officer

Family Health Plan, Inc., 7975 Miami Lakes Drive, Suite 300, Miami Lakes, FL 33016; tel. 305/364–8100; FAX. 305/364–8136; Catherine P. Hill, Executive Vice President

Florida Health Care Plan, Inc., 1340 Ridgewood Avenue, Holly Hill, FL 32117; tel. 904/676–7193; FAX. 904/676–7196; Edward F. Simpson, Jr., President, Chief Executive Officer

Florida lst Health Plan, Inc., 1201 First Street, S., P.O. Box 9126, Winter Haven, FL 33883–9126; tel. 813/293–0785, ext. 5125; FAX. 813/297–9095; Jack Bradley, President

Foundation Health, A Florida Health Plan, Inc., 901 Lake Destiny Drive, Suite 265, Maitland, FL 32751; tel. 407/660–2589; FAX. 407/660–2750; Gary Lewison, Executive Director

HIP Health Plan of Florida, Inc., 200 South Park Road, Hollywood, FL 333021; tel. 305/962–3008, ext. 4100; FAX. 305/985–4379; Steven M. Cohen, President, Chief Executive Officer

Health Options, Inc., 532 Riverside Avenue, P.O. Box 2210, Jacksonville, FL 32202–2210; tel. 904/791–6105; FAX. 904/791–8082; William E. Flaherty, President

Healthplan Southeast, Inc., 3520 Thomasville Road, Suite 200, Tallahassee, FL 32308; tel. 904/668–3000; FAX. 904/668–3133; Bonnie C. Bailey, Chief Operating Officer

Humana Health Plan of Florida, Inc., 3400 Lakeside Drive, Miramar, FL 33027; tel. 305/626–5616; FAX. 305/626–5297; Joe Berding, Administrator

Humana Medical Plan, Inc., 3400 Lakeside Drive, Miramar, FL 33027; tel. 305/626–5619; FAX. 305/626–5297; Joe Berding, Vice President, South Florida Market Operations

Max A Med Health Plans, Inc., 1515 N.W. 167th Street, Suite 104, Miami, FL 33169; tel. 305/626–0135; FAX. 305/626–0887; Carolina G. Sierra, M.D., President

Metlife Healthcare Network of Florida, Inc., 2600 Lake Lucien Drive, Suite 300, Maitland, FL 32751; tel. 407/660–0444; FAX. 407/875–5518; Donna M. Blexrud, Network Director

PCA Health Plans of Florida, Inc., 6101 Blue Lagoon Drive, Suite 300, Miami, FL 33126; tel. 305/267–6633; FAX. 305/264–2771; Neil A. Natkow, D.O., President

PacifiCare of Florida, Inc., One Alhambra Plaza, Suite 1000, Coral Gables, FL 33134; tel. 800/887–6888; FAX. 305/447–6625; David Spivack, Vice President, Planning and Development

Physicians Healthcare Plans, Inc., One Harbour Place, 777 South Harbor Island Boulevard, Tampa, FL 33602; tel. 813/229–5300; FAX. 813/229–5301; Miguel B. Fernandez, Administrator

Preferred Medical Plan, Inc., 2500 S.W. 75th Avenue, Miami, FL 33155; tel. 305/669–1501; FAX. 305/669–3957; Sylvia Urlich, President

Principal Health Care of Florida, Inc., 1200 Riverplace Boulevard, Jacksonville, FL 32207; tel. 904/390–0935, ext. 200; FAX. 904/390–0948; James F. H. Henry, Regional Director

Prudential Health Care Plan, Inc., d/b/a PruCare, 2301 Lucien Way, Suite 230, Maitland, FL 32751–7086; tel. 404/933–6700; FAX. 404/933–6885; David A. George, Administrator

Suncare HMO, Inc., 9424 Baymeadows Road, Suite 200, Jacksonville, FL 32256; tel. 904/733–8159; FAX. 904/372–5155; Douglas G. Cueny, Chief Executive Officer

GEORGIA

AETNA Health Plans of Georgia, Inc., 300 Interstate North Parkway, Suite 630, Atlanta, GA 30346; tel. 404/396–2111; FAX. 404/814–4218; Theresa L. Kline, Executive Director

CIGNA Healthcare of Georgia, Inc., 1349 West Peachtree Street, NE, Suite 1300, Atlanta, GA 30309; tel. 404/881–9779; FAX. 404/898–4832; Terri L. Branning, Healthplan Manager

Complete Health of Georgia, Inc., 1455 Lincoln Parkway, Suite 730, Atlanta, GA 30346; tel. 404/698–8600

HMO Georgia, Inc., 3350 Peachtree Road, N.E., Atlanta, GA 30326; tel. 404/842–8422; FAX. 404/842–8451; John Harris, President

Healthsource Savannah, Inc., 7130 Hodgson Memorial Drive, Suite 4000, Savannah, GA 31406; tel. 912/351–2140; FAX. 912/351–2416; Charles A. Holley, Chief Operating Officer

Kaiser Foundation Health Plan of Georgia, Inc., Nine Piedmont Center, 3565 Piedmont Road, N.E., Atlanta, GA 30305; tel. 404/233–0555; Ron Hostettler, Health Plan Manager

Master Health Plan, Inc., 1456 Walton Way, Suite B, Augusta, GA 30904; tel. 404/722–6337; FAX. 404/722–6571; John B. O'Neal, Executive Director

Metlife Healthcare Network of Georgia, Inc., Perimeter Center, E., Suite 650, Atlanta, GA 30346–2092; tel. 404/396–2111; FAX. 404/953–4365; Alvin John Hollkamp, Administrator

PCA Health Plans of Georgia, Inc., 1349 West Peachtree Street, Suite 1000, Atlanta, GA 30309; tel. 404/815–7160; FAX. 404/815–7228; T.E. Garner, Jr. President

Prudential Health Care Plan of Georgia, Inc., PRUCARE, 2859 Paces Ferry Road, Suite 770, Atlanta, GA 30339; tel. 404/801–7700; FAX. 404/801–7885; David Andrew George, Vice President

United Healthcare of Georgia, Inc., 3390 Peachtree Road, N.E., Suite 600, Atlanta, GA 30326; tel. 404/364–8800; FAX. 404/364–8818; A. Kelly Atkinson, Executive Director

HAWAII

Health Plan Hawaii (HMSA), 818 Keeaumoku Street, P.O. Box 860, Honolulu, HI 96814; tel. 808/948–5481; FAX. 808/948–5063; Cliff Cisco, Vice President

Island Care (HMO), Queen's Hawaii Care (HMO), Two Waterfront Plaza, Suite 200, 500 Ala Moana Boulevard, Honolulu, HI 96813; tel. 808/532–6982; FAX. 808/532–3396; Nate Nygaard, Director, Network Management

Kaiser Foundation Health Plan, Inc., 711 Kapiolani Boulevard, Honolulu, HI 96813; tel. 808/834–5333; FAX. 808/529–5495; Cora M. Tellez, Vice President, Regional Manager

Pacific Health Care, 1946 Young Street, Suite 450, Honolulu, HI 96826; tel. 808/973–3000; FAX. 808/949–3259; John Kim, M.D., President, Medical Director

Straub Plan, 888 South King Street, Honolulu, HI 96813; tel. 808/522–4540; FAX. 808/522–4544; Karen Lennox, Executive Director

IDAHO

Group Health Northwest, 5615 West Sunset Highway, Spokane, WA 99204; tel. 509/838–9100; FAX. 509/838–3823; Henry S. Berman, M.D., President, Chief Executive Officer

Healthplus, P.O. Box 2113, Seattle, WA 98111–2113; tel. 206/670–4700; FAX. 206/670–4505; Gary Meade, President, Chief Executive Officer

Healthsense, P.O. Box 1106, Lewiston, ID 83501; tel. 208/746–6621; FAX. 208/746–1030

Idaho Preferred Healthcare, P.O. Box 8262, Boise, ID 83707; tel. 208/345–4550; FAX. 208/336–6311

Peak Health Plan of Idaho, Inc., c/o Takecare, Inc., P.O. Box 7803, Fort Wayne, IN 46801

Qual–Med Washington Health Plan, Inc., West 201 North River Drive, Suite 300, Spokane, WA 99201–2262; tel. 509/326–8820, ext. 229; FAX. 509/325–1655; Eileen Walter, Provider Relations

ILLINOIS

Aetna Health Plans of Illinois, 100 North Riverside Plaza, 20th Floor, Chicago, IL 60606; tel. 312/441–3000, ext. 3231; FAX. 312/441–3000, ext. 3215; Kevin F. Hickey, President

American Health Care Providers, Inc., 4801 Southwick Drive, Suite 500, Matteson, IL 60443; tel. 708/503–5000; Joe Garrett, Chief Operating Officer

BCI HMO, Inc., 233 North Michigan Avenue, Zip 60601–5655, P.O. Box A3694, Chicago, IL 60690; tel. 312/938–7491; Eileen Holderbaum, Director

CIGNA HealthCare of Illinois, Inc., 1700 East Higgins Road, Suite 600, Des Plaines, IL 60018; tel. 708/699–5600; FAX. 708/699–5675; Bert B. Wagener, General Manager

Chicago HMO, 540 North LaSalle Street, Chicago, IL 60610; tel. 312/751–4460; FAX. 312/751–7685; Judith Brown, Vice President, Chief Operating Officer

Cigna HealthCare of St. Louis, Inc., 8182 Maryland Avenue, Suite 900, St. Louis, MO 63105; tel. 314/726–7860; FAX. 314/726–7819; Eric Schultz, Executive Director

CliniCare, Inc., 7124 Windsor Lake Parkway, Rockford, IL 61111; tel. 815/654–3600; FAX. 815/654–5186; John W. Zilavy, President, Chief Executive Officer

Compass Health Care Plans, 310 South Michigan Avenue, Chicago, IL 60604; tel. 312/294–0200; FAX. 312/294–5826; Aldo Giacchino, Chief Executive Officer

Dreyer Health Plans, 1877 West Downer Place, Aurora, IL 60506; tel. 708/859–1100, ext. 5501; FAX. 708/906–5100; Richard A. Lutz, President

GenCare Health Systems, Inc., d/b/a Sanus Health Plan, Inc., 969 Executive Parkway, Suite 100, P.O. Box 27379, St. Louis, MO 63141–6301; tel. 314/434–6114; FAX. 314/434–8461; Tom Zorumski, President, Chief Executive Officer

Group Health Plan, 940 Westport Plaza, Suite 300, St. Louis, MO 63146; tel. 314/453–1700; FAX. 314/453–1958; Jerry R. Hansen, President, Chief Executive Officer

HMO Illinois a product of Health Care Services Corporation, 233 North Michigan Avenue, Chicago, IL 60601–5655; tel. 312/938–6359; Don Pebworth, J.D., Director

HMO Missouri (Blue Choice), 1831 Chestnut Street, P.O. Box 66828, St. Louis, MO 63166–6828; tel. 314/923–6198; FAX. 314/923–8958; Peter E. Clay, President, Chief Executive Officer

Health Alliance Medical Plans, Inc., d/b/a Health Alliance HMO, 102 East Main, Suite 200, P.O. Box 6003, Urbana, IL 61801; tel. 217/337–8010; FAX. 217/337–8093; C. Carleton King, Chief Executive Officer

Health Direct Insurance, Inc., 1011 East Touhy Avenue, Suite 500, Des Plaines, IL 60018–2808; tel. 708/391–9500; Charles R. Stark, Chief Executive Officer

Providers / Health Maintenance Organizations

Heritage National Healthplan, Inc., 1515 Fifth Avenue, Suite 600, Moline, IL 61265-1368; tel. 309/765-1200; G. Michael Hammes, President

Humana Health Chicago, Inc., 2545 South Dr. Martin Luther King Drive, Chicago, IL 60616; tel. 312/808-3810; Barry Averill, Vice President, Illinois

Humana Health Plan, Inc. (Formerly Michael Reese Health Plan), 2545 South King Drive, Chicago, IL 60616; tel. 312/808-3810; FAX. 312/808-9245; Barry Averill, Vice President, Illinois

Illinois Masonic Community Health Plan, 836 West Wellington, Chicago, IL 60657; tel. 312/975-1600; Bruce C. Campbell, President

John Deere Family Healthplan, Inc., 1515 Fifth Avenue, Suite 600, Moline, IL 61265-1368; tel. 309/765-1287; James K. Thomson, Operations

Maxicare Health Plans of the Midwest, Inc., 111 East Wacker Drive, Suite 1500, Chicago, IL 60601; tel. 312/616-4700; FAX. 312/616-4998; William P. Donahue, Vice President, General Manager

Medical Associates Health Plan, Inc., 700 Locust Street, Suite 230, Dubuque, IA 52001-6800; tel. 319/556-8070; FAX. 319/556-5134; Lawrence E. Cremer, Executive Director

Medical Center Health Plan, d/b/a Partners HMO, One City Place Drive, Suite 670, St. Louis, MO 63141; Dalbert E. Snoberger, Chief Executive Officer

Metlife Healthcare Network of Illinois, Inc., 1900 East Golf Road, Suite 501, Schaumburg, IL 60173; tel. 708/619-2222; FAX. 708/619-3160; Claudia Bjerre, President, Chief Executive Officer

Metlife Healthcare Network, Inc., 14500 South Outer Forty Road, Suite 333, Chesterfield, MO 63017; tel. 314/542-1400; FAX. 314/576-8365; Barbara C. Buenemann, President

New York Life/Sanus Health Plan, Inc., 1111 West 22nd Street, Suite 810, Oak Brook, IL 60521; tel. 708/368-1800; Joseph T. Lynaugh, President

Personal Care Insurance of Illinois, Inc., 510 Devonshire Drive, Suite G, Champaign, IL 61820; tel. 217/351-1226; FAX. 217/373-5410; Alan L. Mytty, President

Principal Health Care of Illinois, Inc., One Lincoln Center, Suite 1040, Oakbrook Terrace, IL 60181-4267; tel. 708/916-6622; FAX. 708/916-9595; Lee Green, Executive Director

Prudential Health Care Plan, Inc., Prucare, 10845 Olive Street Road, St. Louis, MO 63141; tel. 314/567-1100; Richard Rivers, Vice President

Prudential Healthcare Plan of Illinois (PruCare), Columbia Centre II, 9450 West Bryn Mawr, Rosemont, IL 60018; tel. 708/671-8770; FAX. 708/671-6958; Scott P. Serota, Vice President, Chief Executive Officer

Rush Prudential HMO, Inc., 233 South Wacker Drive, Suite 3900, Chicago, IL 60606; tel. 312/234-7000; Scott Serota, President, Chief Executive Officer

SHARE Health Plan of Illinois, Inc., One South Wacker Drive, P.O. Box 909714, Chicago, IL 60690-9714; tel. 312/424-4813; FAX. 312/424-4914; John G. Ruther, President

Take Care Great Lakes, 747 East 22nd Street, Suite 100, Lombard, IL 60148; tel. 708/916-4270; FAX. 708/916-0852; Tony Van Roekel, Vice President

Travelers Health Network of Illinois, Inc., 184 Shuman Boulvard, Suite 500, Naperville, IL 60563; tel. 800/253-0497; FAX. 708/357-1807; Timothy F. Dickman, Executive Director

Union Health Service, 1634 West Polk, Chicago, IL 60612; tel. 312/829-4224; FAX. 312/829-8241; Helen M. Hrynkiw, Executive Director

University of Illinois Health Plan, 2023 West Ogden Avenue, Suite 205, M/C 692, Chicago, IL 60612-3741; tel. 312/996-3553; FAX. 312/413-7872; Diane S. Eng, Interim Director

INDIANA

Alternative Dental Care of Indiana, Inc., One Penmark, Suite 200, 11595 Meridian Street, Carmel, IN 46032; tel. 800/237-7727; David P. McSweeney, President

Alternative Health Delivery Systems, Inc., 9901 Linn Station Road, Louisville, KY 40223; tel. 502/425-8324; FAX. 502/339-5471; Kathleen M. Wiljanen, President, Chief Executive Officer

American Health Care Providers, Inc., 4801 Southwick Drive, Matteson, IL 60443; tel. 708/503-5000; Asif Sayeed, President

Anthem Health Plan of Indiana, Inc., 333 North Alabama, Indianapolis, IN 46204; tel. 317/262-4501; John D. Cuny, President, Chief Executive Officer

Arnett HMO, Inc., 3768 Rome Drive, Lafayette, IN 47905; tel. 317/448-8200; FAX. 317/448-8660; James T. Poulos, M.D., President

BCI HMO, Inc. (Formerly HMO Illinois, Inc.), 233 North Michigan Avenue, Chicago, IL 60601; tel. 312/938-6347; FAX. 312/819-1220; Simeon Martin Hickman, President

CIGNA Healthplan of Illinois, Inc., 1700 Higgins, Suite 600, Des Plaines, IL 60018; tel. 708/699-5600; FAX. 708/699-5675; John W. Rohfritch, Senior Vice President

CompDent Corporation, 1930 Bishop Lane, 16th Floor, Louisville, KY 40218; tel. 800/456-5500, ext. 201; FAX. 502/456-2772; Allan Brockway Morris, President, Chief Executive Officer

First Commonwealth, Inc., 444 North Wells, Suite 600, Chicago, IL 60610; tel. 312/644-1800; Mark R. Lundberg, Vice President, Sales

Great Lakes Health Plan, Inc., 747 East 22nd Street, Suite 100, Lombard, IL 60148; tel. 708/916-8400

HMO Kentucky, Inc., 9901 Linn Station Road, Louisville, KY 40223; tel. 502/423-2282; FAX. 502/423-6979; G. Douglas Sutherland, President

HPLAN, Inc., 101 East Main Street, Louisville, KY 40202; tel. 505/580-5061

Health Maintenance of Indiana, Inc., 333 North Alabama, Indianapolis, IN 46204; tel. 317/262-4501; FAX. 317/262-4603; John D. Cuny, President, Chief Executive Officer

Health Resources, Inc., 420 N.W. Fifth Street, Suite 1-C, Evansville, IN 47708; tel. 812/424-I444; FAX. 812/428-6725; Edward L. Fritz, D.D.S., President

Healthsource Indiana Managed Care Plan, Inc., 225 South East Street, Suite 100, P.O. Box 6115, Indianapolis, IN 46206-6115; tel. 800/933-3466; FAX. 317/687-8500; David H. Smith, President

Humana Gold Plus Plan, 101 East Main Street, 12th Floor, Louisville, KY 40204; tel. 800/245-4446

Humana HealthChicago, Inc., 950 Warrenville Road, Lisle, IN 60532; tel. 708/964-6200; FAX. 708/964-8904; Norman J. Beles, President

Humana Inc., 500 West Main Street, Louisville, KY 40202; tel. 502/580-1860; FAX. 502/580-3127; Greg Donaldson, Director, Corporate Communications

Indiana Vision Services, Inc., 494 South Emerson Avenue, Suite G, Greenwood, IN 46142; tel. 317/888-6005

M Plan, Inc., 8802 North Meridian Street, Suite 100, Indianapolis, IN 46260; tel. 317/571-5300; FAX. 317/571-5306; Alex Slabosky, President

MIDA Dental Plans, Inc., 2000 Town Center, Suite 2200, Southfield, MI 48075; tel. 810/353-6410; Walter Knysz, Jr., D.D.S., President

Maxicare Health Plans of the Midwest, Maxicare Illinois, 111 East Wacker Dr., Suite 1500, Chicago, IL 60601; tel. 312/616-4700

Maxicare Indiana, Inc., 9480 Priority Way, West Drive, Indianapolis, IN 46240-3899; tel. 317/844-5775; FAX. 317/574-0713; Vicki F. Perry, Vice President, General Manager

MetLife Healthcare Network of Illinois, Inc., 1900 East Golf Road, Suite 501, Schaumburg, IL 60173; tel. 708/619-2222

Metlife Health Care Network of Kentucky, Inc., Northmark Business Center III, 4501 Erskin, Suite 100, Cincinnati, OH 45242-4713; tel. 513/745-9700; Charles Stark, President

Midwest Foundation Independent Physicians Assoc., Choicecare, 655 Eden Park Drive, Suite 400, Cincinnati, OH 45202; tel. 513/784-5200

National Foot Care Program, Inc., Pinewood Plaza, 22255 Greenfield, Suite 550, Southfield, MI 48075; tel. 313/559-2579

Partners National Health Plans of Indiana, Inc., One Michiana Square, 100 East Wayne, Suite 502, South Bend, IN 46601; tel. 219/233-4899; FAX. 219/234-7484; James J. Ewing, Vice President, Chief Financial Officer

Physicians Health Network, Inc., One Riverfront Place, Suite 400, P.O. Box 3357, Evansville, IN 47732; tel. 812/465-6000; FAX. 812/465-6014; Russell W. Sherlock, Chairman, President, Chief Executive Officer

Physicians Health Plan of Northern Indiana, Inc., 7222 Engle Road, Suite 120, Fort Wayne, IN 46804; tel. 219/432-6690; FAX. 219/432-0493; John P. Smith, M.D., President

Physicians Health Plan of Northern Indiana, Inc., 8101 West Jefferson Boulevard, Fort Wayne, IN 46804-4163; tel. 800/982-6257; FAX. 219/432-0493

Principal Health Care of Indiana, Inc., 415 East Cook Road, Fort Wayne, IN 46825; tel. 219/455-2081

Prudential Health Care Plan, Inc., PruCare, 24 Greenway Plaza, Suite 500, Houston, TX 77046; tel. 201/716-8174

Riverside Dental Care of Indiana, Inc., 1100 Dennison Avenue, Columbus, OH 43201; tel. 614/297-4870; Richard A. Mitchell, President

Rush Prudential HMO, Inc., 33 East Congress Parkway, Suite 600, Chicago, IL 60605; tel. 312/347-3430

Southeastern Indiana Health Organization, Inc. (SIHO), 432 Washington Street, P.O. Box I787, Columbus, IN 47202-1787; tel. 812/378-7000; Roy H. Flaherty, President, Chief Executive Officer

TDC/The Dental Concern, Ltd., 222 North LaSalle Street, Suite 2140, Chicago, IL 60601; tel. 312/201-1260; FAX. 312/201-0743; Fred L. Horowitz, D.M.D., President

The Dental Advantage, Inc., 3111 Camino Del Rio, N., Suite 1000, San Diego, CA 92108; tel. 619/283-8611; Robert Nettinga, President

Universal Health Services, Inc., 403 West 14th Street, Chicago Heights, IL 60411-2498; tel. 708/755-2462; Ralph R. Crescenzo, President

Welborn Clinic/Welborn HMO, Welborn Health Options, 421 Chestnut Street, Evansville, IN 47713; tel. 812/425-3939; John C. Huus, M.D., Chairman of the Board

Welborn HMO, 19 N.W. Fourth Street, Suite 600, Evansville, IN 47708; tel. 812/426-9319

IOWA

Care Choices HMO, 600 Fourth Street, Terra Centre, Suite 401, Sioux City, IA 51101; tel. 712/252-2344; FAX. 712/233-3684; Karen Pederson, Executive Director

Exclusive Healthcare, Mutual of Omaha Plaza, Omaha, NE 68175; tel. 402/978-2700; FAX. 402/978-2999; Dick L. Easley, President

Heritage National Healthplan, 11 Corporate East, 1910 East Kimberley Road, Davenport, IA 52807; tel. 319/344-4400; FAX. 319/344-4486; G. Michael Hammes, President

John Deere Family Health Plan, 1515 Fifth Avenue, Suite 200, Moline, IL 61265-1368; tel. 309/765-1600; Richard Van Bell, President

Medical Associates Health Plan, One Cycare Plaza, Suite 230, Dubuque, IA 5200l; tel. 319/556-8070; FAX. 319/556-5134; Lawrence Cremer, Executive Director

Principal Health Care of Iowa, Inc., 4600 Westown Parkway, Suite 301, West Des Moines, IA 50266-1099; tel. 515/225-1234; FAX. 515/223-0097; Louis Garcia, Executive Director

Principal Health Care of Nebraska, Inc., 10810 Farnam Drive, Suite 425, Omaha, NE 68154; tel. 402/333-1720; FAX. 402/333-1116; Louis B. Garcia, Executive Director

Share Health Plan of Nebraska, 302 South 36th Street, Suite 300, Omaha, NE 68131; tel. 402/345-9900; FAX. 402/345-7904; John M. Braasch, President, Chief Executive Officer

Providers / Health Maintenance Organizations

KANSAS

BMA Selectcare, Inc., One Penn Valley Park, Zip 64108, P.O. Box 419458, Kansas City, MO 64141; tel. 816/753-8000, ext. 5309; FAX. 816/751-5571; John R. Barton, President

Blue-Care, Inc., 2301 Main, Zip 64108-2428, P.O. Box 413163, Kansas City, MO 64141-6163; tel. 816/395-2222; Richard P. Krecker, President

CIGNA Healthcare of Kansas/Missouri, Inc., 101 South Webb Road, Suite 200, Wichita, KS 67207; tel. 316/687-5606; FAX. 316/681-4329; D. Douglas Stratton, Vice President, Executive Director

Exclusive Healthcare, Inc., 7300 College Boulevard, Suite 208, Overland Park, KS 66210; tel. 913/451-1777; FAX. 913/451-7742; Robert Vaupell, Executive Director

HMO Kansas, Inc., 1133 Topeka Boulevard, P.O. Box 110, Topeka, KS 66601-0110; tel. 913/291-8600; Thomas Miller, President

Healthcare America Plans, Inc., 331 East Douglas, Wichita, KS 67202; tel. 316/262-7400; FAX. 316/262-1395; Garland L. Bugg, President

Humana Health Plan, Inc., 10450 Holmes, Suite 330, Kansas City, MO 64131-1471; tel. 816/941-8900; FAX. 816/941-8630; David Fields, Executive Director

Humana Kansas City, Inc., 10450 Holmes, Suite 330, Kansas City, MO 64134-1471; tel. 816/941-8900; David Fields, Executive Director

Kaiser Foundation Health Plan of Kansas City, Inc., 10561 Barkley, Suite 200, Overland Park, KS 66212-1886; tel. 913/967-4600; FAX. 913/642-0209; Kathryn Paul, President, Regional Manager

Metlife Healthcare Network Of Kansas City, Inc., 9200 Indian Creek Parkway, Suite 185, Overland Park, KS 66210; tel. 913/451-5656; FAX. 913/451-0492; Barbara C. Buenemann, President

Preferred Plus of Kansas, Inc., 345 Riverview, Suite 103, P.O. Box 49288, Wichita, KS 67203; tel. 316/268-0390; Marlon Dauner, President

Principal Health Care of Kansas City, Inc., 1001 East 101st Terrace, Suite 230, Kansas City, MO 64131; tel. 816/941-3030; FAX. 816/941-8516; Kenneth J. Linde, President

Prudential Health Care Plan, Inc., 4600 Madison Avenue, Suite 300, Kansas City, MO 64112; tel. 816/756-5588; FAX. 816/756-5667; David W. Dingley, Executive Director

Total Health Care, 2301 Main Street, 64108-2428, P.O. Box 413613, Kansas City, MO 64141-6163; tel. 816/395-2222; Richard P. Krecker, President

TriSource HealthCare, Inc., d/b/a Blue Advantage, 2301 Main Street, P.O. Box 419130, Kansas City, MO 64141-6130; tel. 816/395-3636; FAX. 816/395-3811; Larry K. Chastain, President, Chief Executive Officer

KENTUCKY

Alternative Health Delivery Systems, 11003 Bluegrass Parkway, Suite 600, Louisville, KY 40299; tel. 502/261-2102; Cheryl Kutchinski, Vice President, Operations

Blue Cross/Blue Shield of Kentucky, Inc., 9901 Linn Station Road, Louisville, KY 40223; tel. 502/423-2011; Stephen T. Bow, Administrator

ChoiceCare, 655 Eden Park Drive, Cincinnati, OH 45202; tel. 513/784-5200; FAX. 513/784-5300; Daniel Gregorie, M.D., President, Chief Executive Officer

HMO Kentucky, 10100 Linn Station Road, Louisville, KY 40223; tel. 502/329-5537; FAX. 502/423-2094; Brenda Luckett, Executive Director

HPLAN, 101 East Main Street, Louisville, KY 40222; tel. 502/580-5005; FAX. 502/580-4516; James Nadler, M.D., Medical Director

Healthwise of Kentucky, Ltd., 489 East Main Street, Suite 200, Lexington, KY 40507; tel. 606/259-1771; FAX. 606/255-9134; Harold Bischoff, Executive Director

Humana Health Plan, 101 East Main Street, Louisville, KY 40202; tel. 502/580-5005; FAX. 502/580-5044; Vicky Hatfield, Executive Director

Humana Medical Plan of Kentucky, 101 East Main Street, Louisville, KY 40202; tel. 502/580-5005; Vicky Hatfield, Administrator

Lexington Health Advantage, 701 Bob-O-Link Drive, Suite 120, Lexington, KY 40504-3760; tel. 606/276-0306; FAX. 606/278-2839; Nileen Verbeten, Chief Operating Officer

MetLife HealthCare Network of Kentucky, 4501 Erskine Road, Suite 150, Cincinnati, OH 45242; tel. 502/339-8481; Charles Stark, Administrator

Prucare, 312 Elm Street, Suite 1400, Cincinnati, OH 45202; tel. 513/784-7795; FAX. 513/784-7007; Kim Bellard, Executive Director

Southeastern United Medigroup, Inc., 9901 Linn Station Road, Louisville, KY 40223; tel. 502/423-2277; FAX. 502/423-2729; Robert McIntire, President, Chief Executive Officer

TakeCare Healthplan, 11260 Chester Road, Suite 800, Cincinnati, OH 45246; tel. 513/772-7325; FAX. 513/772-1466; Robert Sheedy, Administrator

LOUISIANA

Advantage Health Plan, Inc., 4427 South Robertson Street, New Orleans, LA 70115; tel. 504/899-8686

Aetna Health Plans of Louisiana, Inc., 3900 North Causeway Boulevard, Suite 410, Metairie, LA 70002-7283; tel. 504/830-5600; FAX. 504/837-6571; Michael L. Rogers, President

CIGNA HealthCare of Louisiana, Inc., 4354 South Sherwood Forest Boulevard, Suite D240, Baton Rouge, LA 70816; tel. 504/295-2800; FAX. 504/295-2888; John D. Davis, Executive Director

CIGNA HealthCare of North Louisiana, Inc., 4354 South Sherwood Forest Boulevard, Suite D240, Baton Rouge, LA 70816; tel. 504/295-2800; FAX. 504/295-2888; John D. Davis, Executive Director

Community Health Network of Louisiana, 2431 South Acadian Thruway, Suite 350, P.O. Box 80159, Baton Rouge, LA 70898-0159; tel. 504/923-0550; FAX. 504/928-7026; G. Larry Mitchum, President, Chief Executive Officer

Foundation Health, Louisiana Health Plan, Inc., 3400 Data Drive, Rancho Cordova, CA 95670; tel. 916/631-5000

Gulf South Health Plans, Inc., 5615 Corporate Boulevard, Suite Three, P.O. Box 80339, Baton Rouge, LA 70898-0339; tel. 504/927-7212; FAX. 504/922-9241; Jack W. Walker, President, Chief Executive Officer

Gulf South Preferred Health Plan, 5615 Corporate Boulevard, Suite Three, Baton Rouge, LA 70808; tel. 504/927-7212; FAX. 504/929-6560; Pattie Jackson, RN, C.P.H.Q., Vice President, Medical Management

HMO of Louisiana, Inc., P.O. Box 98029, Baton Rouge, LA 70898-8024; tel. 504/922-1801

Humana Health Plan of Louisiana, Inc., Galleria One, Suite 1713, Metairie, LA 70001; tel. 504/835-5474; FAX. 504/835-6224; David P. Giles, Executive Director

Louisiana Health Service and Indemnity Company, 5525 Reitz Avenue, Zip 70809, P.O. Box 98029, Baton Rouge, LA 70898

Maxicare Louisiana, Inc., 3850 North Causeway Boulevard, Suite 990, Metairie, LA 70002; tel. 504/836-2022; FAX. 504/835-0493; Alan M. Preston, Vice President, General Manager

Ochsner/Sisters of Charity Health Plan, Inc. (HMO), One Galleria Boulevard, Suite 1224, Metairie, LA 70001; tel. 504/836-6600; FAX. 504/836-6566; Richard Todd, President, Chief Executive Officer

Principal Health Care of Louisiana, 3421 North Causeway Boulevard, Suite 600, Metairie, LA 70002; tel. 504/834-0840; FAX. 504/834-2694; Jan Stallmeyer, Executive Director

Travelers Health Network of Louisiana, Galleria One, Suite 2100, One Galleria Boulevard, Metairie, LA 70001; tel. 504/836-5555; FAX. 504/836-5506; Elizabeth M. Mitchell, RN, Vice President, Executive Director

MAINE

HMO Maine, Two Gannett Drive, South Portland, ME 04106; tel. 800/527-7706; FAX. 207/822-7375; Stephen Dunn, Executive Director

Harvard Community Health Plan, Inc., 10 Brookline Place West, Brookline, MA 02146; tel. 617/421-6400

Health Plans, Inc., 202 US Route One, Falmouth, ME 04105; tel. 207/774-5801

Healthsource Maine, Inc., 174 South Freeport Road, P.O. Box 447, Freeport, ME 04032-0447; tel. 207/865-6161, ext. 5201; FAX. 207/865-1812; Richard White, Chief Executive Officer

Healthsource New Hampshire, Donovan Street Extension, P.O. Box 2041, Concord, NH 03302; tel. 603/225-5077; FAX. 603/225-7621; Susan Berry, Director, Marketing

Lincoln National Health Plan, Inc., 75 John Roberts Road, Suite One C, South Portland, ME 04106; tel. 800/544-5007

MARYLAND

Aetna Health Plans of the Mid-Atlantic, Inc., 7799 Leesburg Pike, Suite 1100-South, Falls Church, VA 22043; tel. 703/903-7100; Mary Ann Eull, Director, Health Services Management Operation

CFS, Care First-Free State Potomac, Equitable Bank Center's Tower-II, 100 South Charles Street, Baltimore, MD 21201; tel. 410/528-7025; FAX. 410/528-7013; David Wolf, President

CIGNA Healthplan of the MidAtlantic, Inc., 9700 Patuxent Woods Drive, Columbia, MD 21046; tel. 410/720-5800; FAX. 410/720-5860

Capital Care, Inc., 550 12th Street, S.W., Washington, DC 20065; tel. 202/479-3678; FAX. 202/479-3660; M. Bruce Edwards, President

Chesapeake Health Plan, Inc., Executive Office, 814 Light Street, Baltimore, MD 21230; tel. 410/539-8622; FAX. 410/752-0271; Leon Kaplan, President, Chief Executive Officer

Columbia Medical Plan, Inc., Two Knoll North Drive, Columbia, MD 21045; tel. 410/997-8500; FAX. 410/964-4563; Marilyn M. Levinson, Director, Patient Services

Delmarva Health Care Plan, 106 Marlboro Road, P.O. Box 2410, Easton, MD 21601; tel. 410/822-7223; FAX. 410/822-8152; Richard Moore, President

George Washington University Health Plan, Inc., 4550 Montgomery Avenue, Suite 800, Bethesda, MD 20814; tel. 301/941-2000; FAX. 301/941-2005; Lawrence E. Berman, Director, Government Relations and Legal Affairs

HealthPlus, Inc., 7601 Ora Glen Drive, Suite 200, Greenbelt, MD 20770; tel. 301/982-0098, ext. 3308; FAX. 301/489-5284; Jeff D. Emerson, Chief Executive Officer

Humana Group Health Association, Inc., 4301 Connecticut Avenue, N.W., Washington, DC 20008; tel. 202/364-2000; FAX. 202/364-7418; Robert P. Pfotenhauer, President, Chief Executive Officer

Kaiser Foundation Health Plan of the Mid-Atlantic States, Inc., 2101 East Jefferson Street, Rockville, MD 20852; tel. 301/816-2424; FAX. 301/816-7478; Alan J. Silverston, President

MD Individual Practice Association, MDIPA/Optimum, Four Taft Court, Rockville, MD 20850; tel. 301/762-8205; FAX. 301/762-2479; Steve B. Griffin, President

PHN-HMO, Inc., 5700 Executive Drive, Suite 104, Baltimore, MD 21228-1798; tel. 410/747-9060; FAX. 410/788-7543; L. David Taylor, President, Chief Executive Officer

Physicians Health Plan, Inc., 2111 Wilson Boulevard, Suite 1150, Arlington, VA 22201; tel. 703/525-0602; FAX. 703/243-3066; Suellen Rainey, Executive Director

Principal Health Care of Delaware, Inc., One Corporate Commons, 100 West Commons Boulevard, Suite 300, New Castle, DE 19720; tel. 302/322-4700

Principal Health Care of the Mid-Atlantic, Inc., 1801 Rockville Pike, Suite 110, Rockville, MD 20852; tel. 301/881-4903; FAX. 301/881-9808; Fran Soistman, Executive Director

Prudential Health Care Plan of the Mid-Atlantic, Seton Court, 2800 North Charles Street, Baltimore, MD 21218; tel. 410/554-7000; FAX. 410/554-7070

© 1995 AHA Guide — Health Organizations, Agencies and Providers

Providers / Health Maintenance Organizations

Total Health Care, Inc., 2305 North Charles Street, Baltimore, MD 21218; tel. 410/383-8300; FAX. 410/554-9012; Jesse L. Thomas, Jr., President

U.S. Healthcare, 980 Jolly Road, Blue Bell, PA 19422; tel. 215/628-4800; FAX. 215/283-6858

MASSACHUSETTS

Bay State Health Care, 101 Main Street, Cambridge, MA 02142; tel. 617/868-7000; FAX. 617/499-6620; Donald B. Smallwood, Executive Director

CIGNA HealthCare of Connecticut, Inc., 900 Cottage Grove Road, A118, Hartford, CT 06152-1118; tel. 203/769-9800; FAX. 203/769-2399; Ellen C. Harrison, General Manager

Central Massachusetts Health Care, Mechanics Tower, 100 Front Street, Suite 300, Worcester, MA 01608; tel. 508/798-8667; FAX. 508/798-3069; Benjamin R. Schenck, President

Community Health Plan, 163 Conz Street, Northampton, MA 01060; tel. 413/584-0600; Frederick H. Hooven, Regional Administrator

Fallon Community Health Plan, Chestnut Place, 10 Chestnut Street, Worcester, MA 01608; tel. 508/799-2100; FAX. 508/831-0921; Christy W. Bell, Executive Director

HMO Blue, 100 Summer Street, Boston, MA 02110; tel. 617/832-7797; FAX. 617/832-7973; Maureen Coneys, Executive Director

HMO Rhode Island, 30 Chestnut Street, Providence, RI 02903; tel. 401/274-6674; FAX. 401/453-2533; Michael Gerhardt, President

Harvard Community Health Plan, 10 Brookline Place West, Brookline, MA 02146; tel. 617/731-8240; FAX. 617/730-4695; Manuel M. Ferris, President, Chief Executive Officer

Harvard Community Health Plan of New England, One Hoppin Street, Providence, RI 02903-4199; tel. 401/331-3000; Stephen Schoen Baum, M.D., Medical Director

Health New England, One Monarch Place, Springfield, MA 01144; tel. 413/787-4000; FAX. 413/731-7498; Richard Belloff, President

Healthsource New Hampshire, 54 Regional Drive, P.O. Box 2041, Concord, NH 03302-2041; tel. 603/225-5077; FAX. 603/225-2610; Donna K. Lencki, Chief Executive Director

Kaiser Foundation Health Plan, 170 University Drive, P.O. Box 862, Amherst, MA 01002; tel. 413/256-0151, ext. 5162; FAX. 413/549-1601; Linda Todaro, Massachusetts Area Administrator

Matthew Thornton Health Plan, 410 Amherst Street, Nashua, NH 03063; tel. 603/595-4441, ext. 609; FAX. 603/880-9410; Everett Page, Chief Operating Officer

MetLife HealthCare Network of Massachusetts, 99 High Street, 21st Floor, Boston, MA 02110-2310; tel. 800/444-7855; FAX. 617/574-3972; Daniel Bigelow, Vice President

Neighborhood Health Plan, 253 Summer Street, Boston, MA 02210; tel. 617/772-5500; FAX. 617/772-5513; Jay Harrington, Chief Executive Officer

Pilgrim Health Care, 10 Accord Executive Drive, P.O. Box 9102, Norwell, MA 02061; tel. 617/871-3950; FAX. 617/982-9668; Allan Greenberg, Chief Executive Officer

PruCare of Massachusetts, 10 New England Business Center, Suite 200, P.O. Box 1827, Andover, MA 01810; tel. 508/681-4723; FAX. 508/609-4198; Ernest R. Bourassa, Director

Tufts Associated Health Plan, 333 Wyman Street, P.O. Box 9112, Waltham, MA 02254-9112; tel. 617/466-9400; FAX. 617/466-9430; Harris A. Berman, M.D., President, Chief Executive Officer

U.S. Healthcare, Inc., Three Burlington Woods Drive, Burlington, MA 01803; tel. 617/273-5600; Richard Cornell, Medical Director

United Health Plans of NE, Inc., Metro Center, 475 Kilvert Street, Suite 310, Warwick, RI 02886

MICHIGAN

Blue Care Network of East Michigan, 4200 Fashion Square Boulevard, Saginaw, MI 48603; tel. 517/791-3200; FAX. 517/791-3237; Arnold C. Dufort, President, Chief Executive Officer

Blue Care Network of East Michigan, G-3245 Beecher Road, Flint, MI 48532; tel. 800/527-1906; FAX. 810/733-0422; Arnold C. Dufort, Executive Director

Blue Care Network of Southeast Michigan, 25925 Telegraph, P.O. Box 5043, Southfield, MI 48086-5043; tel. 313/354-7450; FAX. 313/799-6970; David H. Smith, President, Chief Executive Officer

Blue Care Network–Great Lakes, 1769 South Garfield Avenue, Suite B, Traverse City, MI 49684; tel. 616/941-6000, ext. 6030; FAX. 616/941-6012; Sharon Carlin, Regional Director

Blue Care Network–Great Lakes, 3624 South Westnedge, Kalamazoo, MI 49008; tel. 616/388-9500; FAX. 616/388-5156; Marcia Lallaman, Regional Manager

Blue Care Network–Great Lakes, 611 Cascade West Parkway, S.E., Grand Rapids, MI 49546; tel. 616/957-5057; FAX. 616/956-5866; Sharon Carlin, President, Chief Executive Officer

Blue Care Network–Great Lakes, 3375 Merriam Avenue, Muskegon Heights, MI 49444-3173; tel. 616/739-6600; FAX. 616/739-6670; Barbara Carlson, Regional Manager

Blue Care Network–Great Lakes, 67 West Michigan Mall, Suite 400, Battle Creek, MI 49017; tel. 616/965-2442; Ruth Clark, Regional Manager

Blue Care Network–Health Central, 1403 South Creyts Road, Lansing, MI 48917; tel. 517/322-9000; FAX. 517/322-8015; Arnold C. DuFort, President, Chief Executive Officer

Care Choices HMO, Mercy Health Plans, 34605 Twelve Mile Road, Farmington Hills, MI 48331; tel. 313/489-6203; FAX. 810/489-6278; Robert J. Flanagan, Ph.D., President, Chief Executive Officer

Care Choices–Eastern Michigan, 2000 Hogback Road, Suite 15, Ann Arbor, MI 48105; tel. 313/971-7667; FAX. 313/971-7455; Robert J. Brown, Regional Director, Eastern Michigan

Care Choices–Grand Rapids, 1500 East Beltline S.E., Suite 300, Grand Rapids, MI 49506; tel. 616/285-3801; FAX. 616/285-3810; Janie Begeman, Site Manager

Care Choices–Lansing, 2111 University Park, Suite 100, Okemos, MI 48864; tel. 517/349-2111; FAX. 517/349-6449; Jeffrey Ash, Executive Director

Care Choices–Muskegon, 950 West Norton Avenue, Suite 500, Muskegon, MI 49441; tel. 616/737-0307; FAX. 616/733-6352; Molly McCarthy, Site Manager

Community Health Plan, Inc., 2401 20th Street, Detroit, MI 48216; tel. 313/496-0610; FAX. 313/496-0525; Robin Barclay, President, Chief Executive Officer

Family Health Plan, 1001 Madison Street, Toledo, OH 43624; tel. 419/241-6501; Rose Myers, Manager, Marketing Services

Grand Valley Health Plan, 829 Forest Hill Avenue, S.E., Grand Rapids, MI 49546; tel. 616/949-2410; FAX. 616/949-4978; Roland Palmer, President

Health Alliance Plan, 2850 West Grand Boulevard, Detroit, MI 48202; tel. 313/874-8310; FAX. 313/874-8301; Roman Kulich, Chief Operating Officer

HealthPlus of Michigan, 2050 South Linden Road, P.O. Box 1700, Flint, MI 48501-1700; tel. 313/230-2000; FAX. 313/230-2208; Paul F. Fuhs, Ph.D., President, Chief Executive Officer

HealthPlus of Michigan–Saginaw, 4800 Fashion Square Boulevard, Suite 250, Saginaw, MI 48604; tel. 517/799-6451

M-Care, 3601 Plymouth Road, Ann Arbor, MI 48105; tel. 313/747-8700; FAX. 313/747-7152; Peter W. Roberts, President

Mercy Health Plans–Livingston County, 7990 West Grand River, Brighton, MI 48116; tel. 810/229-6866; Richard Nowakowski, Site Director

NorthMed HMO, 109 East Front Street, Suite 204, Traverse City, MI 49684; tel. 616/935-0500; FAX. 616/935-0505; Walter J. Hooper III, President

OmniCare, 1155 Brewery Park, Suite 250, Detroit, MI 48207-2602; tel. 313/259-4000, ext. 4570; FAX. 313/393-7944; Ronald R. Dobbins, President, Chief Executive Officer

PHP–Kalamazoo, 150 East Crosstown Parkway, Suite 205, Kalamazoo, MI 49008; tel. 616/349-6692; FAX. 616/349-1476; Michael Koehler, Acting Regional Director

Physicians Health Plan, P.O. Box 30377, Lansing, MI 48909-7877; tel. 517/349-2101; FAX. 517/347-9460; James Savage, President

Physicians Health Plan–Jackson, 209 East Washington Avenue, Suite 315 E, Jackson, MI 49201; tel. 517/782-7154; FAX. 517/782-4512; Janice Dubey Messeroff, Chief Executive Officer

Physicians Health Plan–Muskegon, Terrace Plaza, 250 Morris Avenue, Suite 550, Muskegon, MI 49440-1143; tel. 616/728-3900; FAX. 616/728-5189; Ronald Franzese, Chief Executive Officer

Priority Health, 1231 East Beltline, Suite 300, Grand Rapids, MI 49505; tel. 616/942-0954; FAX. 616/942-0145; Vic Turvey, President, Chief Executive Officer

SelectCare HMO, Inc., 2401 West Big Beaver Road, Suite 700, Troy, MI 48084; tel. 810/637-5300, ext. 5571; FAX. 810/637-6710; Mark T. Bertolini, President, Chief Executive Officer

The Wellness Plan, Comprehensive Health Services, Inc., 6500 John C. Lodge, Detroit, MI 48202; tel. 313/875-6960; FAX. 313/875-7416; Sharon P. Matthews, Regional Administrator

The Wellness Plan, 1060 West Norton Avenue, Suite Four B, Muskegon, MI 49442; tel. 616/780-4722; FAX. 616/780-3557; Evangeline Zimmerman, Health Systems Manager

Total Health Care, Inc., 1600 Fisher Building, Detroit, MI 48202; tel. 313/871-7800; FAX. 313/871-0196; Kenneth G. Rimmer, Executive Director

MINNESOTA

Blue Plus, P.O. Box 64179, St. Paul, MN 55164; tel. 612/456-8438; FAX. 612/683-2905; Mary Banks, M.D., President, Chief Executive Officer

Central Minnesota Group Health Plan, 1245 15th Street, N., St. Cloud, MN 56303; tel. 612/259-2410; FAX. 612/259-7345; John Hoefs, Executive Director, Chief Executive Officer

First Plan HMO, 1010 Fourth Street, Two Harbors, MN 55616; tel. 218/834-7210; John Bjorum, Executive Director

Group Health, Inc., 8100–34th Avenue South, P.O. Box 1309, Minneapolis, MN 55440-1309; tel. 612/883-7000; George Halvorson, President, Chief Executive Officer

HealthPartners, 2829 University Avenue, S.E., Minneapolis, MN 55414; tel. 612/623-8400; FAX. 612/623-8560; George C. Halvorson, President, Chief Executive Officer

Mayo Health Plan, 21 First Street S.W., Suite 401, Rochester, MN 55902; tel. 507/284-8274; FAX. 507/284-0528; Kathleen Kelly, Administrator

MedCenters Health Plan, 8100–34th Avenue S, P.O. Box 1309, Minneapolis, MN 55440-1309; tel. 612/883-5382; FAX. 612/883-5120; Mary Brainerd, Executive Director, Chief Operating Officer

Medica, 5601 Smetana Drive, P.O. Box 1587, Minneapolis, MN 55440; tel. 612/992-3839; FAX. 612/992-3998; K. James Ehlen, M.D., Chairman, Chief Executive Officer

Metropolitan Health Plan, 822 South Third Street, Suite 140, Minneapolis, MN 55415; tel. 612/347-2340; FAX. 612/347-6142; John Bluford, Executive Director

NWNL Health Network, Inc., 1295 Bandana Boulevard N., Suite 220, St. Paul, MN 55108; tel. 612/647-0558; FAX. 612/659-2309; Fred Sattler, President, Chief Executive Officer

Northern Plains Health Plan, 1001 South Columbia Road, Grand Forks, ND 58201; tel. 800/675-2467; Tim Sayler, Executive Director

UCARE Minnesota, 2550 University Avenue, W., Suite 201 S, St. Paul, MN 55114; tel. 612/627-4301; FAX. 612/627-4143; E. W. Ciriacy, M.D., Acting Chief Executive Officer

Providers / Health Maintenance Organizations

MISSISSIPPI

Cigna Healthcare of Tennessee, Inc., 6555 Quince Road, Suite 215, Memphis, TN 38119; tel. 901/755-7411

Complete Health of Mississippi, Inc., 713 South Pear Orchard Road, Suite 205, Ridgeland, MS 39157; tel. 601/956-8030; FAX. 601/957-1306; Charles C. Pitts, Vice President, General Manager

Progressive Health Management, 1421 East Peace Street, Canton, MS 39046

MISSOURI

Alliance for Community Health, Inc., 3556 Caroline Street, Suite 207, St. Louis, MO 63104; tel. 314/577-8105

BMA Selectcare, Inc., One Penn Valley Park, P.O. Box 419458, Kansas City, MO 64141; tel. 816/751-5336; FAX. 816/751-5571; Sara L. Adams, Vice President

CIGNA HealthCare of Kansas/Missouri, Inc., 7400 West 110th Street, Suite 600, Overland Park, KS 66210; tel. 913/339-4700; Cynthia Finter, Executive Director

CIGNA Healthplan of St. Louis, Inc., 8182 Maryland Avenue, Suite 900, St. Louis, MO 63105-3721; tel. 314/726-7860; FAX. 314/726-7819

Exclusive Healthcare, Inc., Mutual of Omaha Plaza, Omaha, NE 68175; tel. 402/978-2869; FAX. 402/978-2999; Kurt Irlbeck, Administrative Services Coordinator

Gencare Health Systems, Inc., d/b/a Sanus Health Plan, Inc., P.O.Box 27379, St. Louis, MO 63141-6301; tel. 800/627-0687, ext. 3307; FAX. 314/469-9854; Thomas Zorumski, Chief Executive Officer

Good Health HMO, Inc., d/b/a Blue-care, Inc., One Pershing Square, 2301 Main Street, Kansas City, MO 64108; tel. 816/395-3636; FAX. 816/395-3811; Larry K. Chastain, President, Chief Operating Officer

Group Health Plan, Inc., 940 West Port Plaza, Suite 300, St. Louis, MO 63146; tel. 314/453-1700; FAX. 314/453-1956; Mark H. Tabak, President, Chief Executive Officer

HMO Missouri, Inc., d/b/a BlueChoice, 4444 Forest Park, St. Louis, MO 63108-2292; tel. 314/658-4444; FAX. 314/289-6239; Seymour Kaplan, President, Chief Executive Officer

HealthLink HMO, Inc., d/b/a HealthLink HMO, 777 Craig Road, Suite 110, Creve Coeur, MO 63141; tel. 314/569-7200; FAX. 314/569-3268; Dennis McCart, Executive Director

HealthNet, Inc., 2300 Main, Suite 700, Kansas City, MO 64108; tel. 816/221-8400; Andrew Dahl, Sc.D., Chief Executive Officer

Healthmark Health Plan, Inc., 10955 Lowell Avenue, Suite 800, Overland Park, KS 66210; tel. 913/345-2240

Humana Health Plan, Inc., 101 East Main Street, 11th Floor, 40202, P.O. Box 1438, Louisville, KY 40201-1438; tel. 502/580-1000; FAX. 502/580-5043

Humana Kansas City, Inc., 10450 Holmes Road, Kansas City, MO 64131-3471; tel. 816/941-8900; FAX. 816/941-3910; David W. Fields, Executive Director

Kaiser Foundation Health Plan of Kansas City, Inc., 10561 Barkley, Suite 200, Overland Park, KS 66212-1886; tel. 913/967-4600; Robert Biblo, Regional Manager

Medical Center Health Plan, d/b/a Partners HMO, One City Place Drive, Suite 670, St. Louis, MO 63141; tel. 314/567-6660; FAX. 314/567-3627; Del Snoberger, Executive Director

MetLife HealthCare Network, Inc., 14500 South Outer 40 Road, Suite 333, Chesterfield, MO 63017; tel. 314/542-1400; FAX. 314/576-8365; Barbara C. Buenemann, President

Metlife Healthcare Network of Kansas City, Inc., Nine Corporate Woods, Suite 185, Overland Park, KS 66210; tel. 312/882-4470; Charles Stark, Chief Executive Officer

Physicians Health Plan of Greater St. Louis, Inc., 77 West Port Plaza, Suite 500, St. Louis, MO 63146; tel. 314/275-7000; FAX. 314/542-1155; Michael F. Neidorff, President, Chief Executive Officer

Physicians Health Plan of Midwest, Inc., 77 Westport Plaza, Suite 500, St. Louis, MO 63146; tel. 314/275-7000; FAX. 314/542-1155

Principal Health Care of Kansas City, Inc., 1001 East 101st Terrace, Suite 300, P.O. Box 410976, Kansas City, MO 64131; tel. 816/941-3030; FAX. 816/941-8516; Jan Stallmeyer, Executive Director

Prudential Health Care Plan, Inc., 12312 Olive Boulevard, Suite 500, St. Louis, MO 63141; tel. 314/567-1100; Lesley Ralson, Chief Executive Officer

Total Health Care, 2301 Main Street, P.O. Box 413163, Kansas City, MO 64141-3163; tel. 816/395-3636; FAX. 816/395-3811; Larry Chastain, President, Chief Executive Officer

TriSource HealthCare, Inc., d/b/a Blue Advantage HMO, P.O. Box 419130, Kansas City, MO 64141-6130; tel. 816/395-3616; FAX. 816/395-3811; David R. Gentile, Vice President, Chief Operating Officer, HMO Programs

Truman Medical Center, Inc., 2301 Holmes Street, Kansas City, MO 64108; tel. 816/556-3094; James J. Mongan, M.D., Executive Director

MONTANA

HMO Montana, 404 Fuller Avenue, Helena, MT 59604; tel. 406/444-8250; Keith Wolcott, Director

NEBRASKA

Exclusive Healthcare, Inc., Mutual of Omaha Plaza, Omaha, NE 68175; tel. 402/978-2700; Dick L. Easley, President

HMO Nebraska, Inc., 2421 South 73rd Street, Omaha, NE 68124; tel. 402/392-2800; FAX. 402/392-2761; Maxine E. Crossley, Executive Vice President, Chief Operating Officer

HealthAmerica of Lincoln, 220 South 17th Street, Lincoln, NE 68508; FAX. 402/475-6003

Principal Health Care of Nebraska, Inc., 10810 Farnum Drive, Suite 425, Omaha, NE 68154; tel. 402/333-1720; FAX. 402/333-1116; Ronald Chaffin, Executive Director

Share Health Plan, 302 South 36th Street, Suite 300, Omaha, NE 68131; tel. 402/345-9900; FAX. 402/345-7904; John Braasch, Chief Executive Officer

NEVADA

Exclusive Healthcare, Inc., Mutual of Omaha Plaza, Omaha, NE 68175

FHP, Inc., 2300 West Sahara, Suite 700, Box 14, Las Vegas, NV 89102; tel. 702/222-4641; FAX. 702/222-4705; R. Lyle Luman, President, Nevada Region

HMO Colorado, Inc., d/b/a HMO Nevada, 6900 Westcliff Drive, Suite 600, Las Vegas, NV 89128; tel. 702/228-2583; Norman P. Becker, CLU, Regional Vice President

Health Plan of Nevada, Inc., P.O. Box 15645, Las Vegas, NV 89114-5645; tel. 702/242-7148; FAX. 702/242-6559; Larry Howard, President

Holaman Mental Health Care Service Plan, Inc., 21050 Van Owen Street, Canoga Park, CA 91303; B. Billstein

Hospital Health Plan, Inc., 400 South Wells Avenue, Reno, NV 89502; tel. 702/329-0101, ext. 258; FAX. 702/329-3723; Ed Holme, Executive Director

Humana Health Plan, Inc., 3107 South Maryland Parkway, Las Vegas, NV 89109; tel. 702/737-7211; FAX. 702/791-5826; Craig A. Drablos, Executive Director

Mutual of Omaha Dental Plans of Nevada, Inc., 3720 Howard Hughes Parkway, Suite 140, Las Vegas, NV 89109

Nevada Health Visions, Inc., 1050 East Flamingo Road, Suite E-120, Las Vegas, NV 89119; tel. 702/693-5250; FAX. 702/693-5399; Jeff Allen, Director, Provider Relations

St. Mary's HealthFirst, 5290 Neil Road, Reno, NV 89502; tel. 702/829-6000; FAX. 702/829-6010; David Briere, Chief Operating Officer

NEW HAMPSHIRE

Harvard Community Health Plan of New England, Inc., 10 Brookline Place, W., Brookline, MA 02146; tel. 617/731-8250

Healthsource New Hampshire, Inc., Donovan Street Extension, P.O. Box 2041, Concord, NH 03302-2041; tel. 603/225-5077; FAX. 603/225-7621; Sally Crawford, Chief Executive Officer

Matthew Thornton Health Plan, 410 Amherst Street, Nashua, NH 03063; tel. 603/595-4441, ext. 609; FAX. 603/883-9410; Everett Page, Chief Operating Officer

U.S. Healthcare New Hampshire, Inc., U.S. Healthcare Massachusetts, Inc., Three Burlington Woods Drive, Burlington, MA 01803; tel. 617/273-5600; FAX. 617/238-8999; James J. Broderick, General Manager

NEW JERSEY

Aetna Health Plans, 3541 Winchester Road, Allentown, PA 18195; tel. 800/624-4478; FAX. 610/391-9309

CIGNA Health Plan of Southern New Jersey, CIGNA HealthCare of PA, NJ & DE, One Beaver Valley Road, Suite CHP, Wilmington, DE 19803; tel. 302/477-3700; FAX. 302/477-3707; Norman Scott, M.D.

CIGNA of Northern New Jersey, Inc., Three Stewart Court, Denville, NJ 07834-1028; tel. 201/262-7700; FAX. 201/262-9135; Diane Foy-Noa, Vice President, General Manager

First Option Health Plan, The Galleria, Two Bridge Avenue, Building Six, Second Floor, Red Bank, NJ 07701; tel. 908/842-5000; John L. Adessa, President, Chief Executive Officer

Garden State Health Plan, CN-712, Trenton, NJ 08625-0712; tel. 800/525-0047; FAX. 609/588-4643; Beverly Blacher, EIDG, Chief Executive Officer

Greater Atlantic Health Services, 3550 Market Street, Philadelphia, PA 19106; tel. 215/823-8600; FAX. 215/823-8617; Emily A. Zuzelo, Vice President

HIP Health Plan of New Jersey, One HIP Plaza, North Brunswick, NJ 08902; tel. 908/937-7861; FAX. 908/937-7870; Victoria A. Wicks, President, Chief Executive Officer

HMO Blue, 416 Bellevue Avenue, Trenton, NJ 08618; tel. 609/396-4600; FAX. 609/599-1095; Sharon J. Hayman, Chief Operating Officer

HMO Blue, 341 Roseville Avenue, Newark, NJ 07107; tel. 201/481-0004; David Dintenfass, Executive Director

HMO Blue, 111 Howard Boulevard, Suite 105, Mt. Arlington, NJ 07856; tel. 201/398-6700; Lawrence Tyson, Executive Director

HMO Blue, Four Greentree Center, Marlton, NJ 08053; tel. 609/983-8808; Carol Thomas, Executive Director

HMO Blue, Three Penn Plaza East, Newark, NJ 07105-2000; tel. 201/466-8120; FAX. 201/456-6745; Dan Drasalin, M.D., President

HMO New Jersey, U.S. HealthCare, 55 Lane Road, Fairfield, NJ 07004; tel. 201/575-5600; Andrew Schuyler, M.D., Medical Director

Keystone Health Plan of New Jersey, 925 Baltimore Pike, P.O. Box 1111, Concordville, PA 19331; tel. 215/358-5650, ext. 4799; FAX. 215/558-2289; James J. Thomas III, Senior Vice President

Liberty Health Plan, 50 Baldwin Avenue, Jersey City, NJ 07304; tel. 201/915-2203; Stephen Schneider, Executive Director

Metlife Health Care Network, 485 B. Route One, Suite 120, Iselin, NJ 08830; tel. 908/602-6500; FAX. 908/602-6519; William Van Gieson, Director

Oxford Health Plans, 320 Post Road, Darien, CT 06820; tel. 212/656-1442; Stephen Wiggins, Chief Executive Officer

PruCare of New Jersey, (Northern Division), 200 Wood Avenue, S., Iselin, NJ 08830; tel. 908/632-6188; FAX. 908/632-6128; Paul Conlin, Vice President, Group Operations

Quakerbridge Center, Three Quakerbridge Plaza, Mercerville, NJ 08619; tel. 609/586-6700; Sharon J. Hayman, Chief Operating Officer

Sanus Health Plans of Greater New York and New Jersey, 75-20 Astoria Boulevard, Jackson Heights, NY 11370; tel. 718/899-5200, ext. 7376; FAX. 718/458-2912; Ramon J. Rodriguez, Executive Director

Providers / Health Maintenance Organizations

Travelers Health Plan Network of New York, Inc., Northern New Jersey Division, 701 Westchester Avenue, Suite 310 E, White Plains, NY 10604-3001; tel. 914/761-9102; Mr. McNair, Executive Director

University Health Plans, Inc., 60 Park Place, 15th Floor, Newark, NJ 07102; tel. 201/623-8700; FAX. 201/623-3635; Steven Marcus, Chief Executive Officer

NEW MEXICO

F.H.P. of New Mexico, Inc., 4700 Montgomery Boulevard, N.E., Albuquerque, NM 87109; tel. 505/881-7900; FAX. 505/883-0102; Christobel Shedd, Associate Vice President

HMO New Mexico, 12800 Indian School Road, N.E., zip 87112, P.O. Box 11968, Albuquerque, NM 87192; tel. 505/291-6902; FAX. 505/291-3586; Blair Christensen, President, HMO New Mexico

Health Plus of New Mexico, Inc., 7500 Jefferson, N.E., Building Two, Albuquerque, NM 87109; tel. 505/823-0700; FAX. 505/823-0718; Robert L. Simmons, President

Lovelace, Inc., P.O. Box 27107, Albuquerque, NM 87125-7107; tel. 505/262-7363; Derick Pasternak, M.D., President

Qual-Med, Inc.-New Mexico Health Plan, 6100 Uptown Boulevard, N.E., Suite 400, Albuquerque, NM 87110; tel. 505/889-8800; FAX. 505/889-8819; Michael J. Mayer, President

NEW YORK

Aetna Health Plans of New York, Inc., 2700 Westchester Avenue, Purchase, NY 10577; tel. 914/251-0600; FAX. 914/251-0260; Kathryn L. Pizzano, Executive Director

Blue Cross and Blue Shield of Western New York, Inc., Community Blue, 1901 Main Street, P.O. Box 159, Buffalo, NY 14240-0159; tel. 716/887-8790; FAX. 716/887-7911; Mary Lee Campbell-Wisley, Vice President

Blue Cross and Blue Shield of the Rochester Area, Blue Choice, 150 East Main Street, Rochester, NY 14647; tel. 716/454-1700; FAX. 716/238-4400; Peter Wood, Vice President

BlueCARE Plus, The Utica Business Park, 12 Rhoads Drive, Utica, NY 13502; tel. 315/798-4358; FAX. 315/797-4298; Thomas Flannery, M.D.

CIGNA Health Care of New York, Inc., 1010 Northern Boulevard, Suite 324, Great Neck, NY 11021; tel. 516/466-1000; FAX. 516/466-1125; Tom Garvey, Executive Director

Capital Area Community Health Plans, Inc., 1201 Troy-Schenectady Road, Latham, NY 12110; tel. 518/783-1864, ext. 4216; FAX. 518/783-0234; John Baackes, President, Chief Executive Officer

Capital District Physicians' Health Plan, One Columbia Circle, Albany, NY 12203; tel. 518/452-1941; FAX. 518/452-0003; Diane E. Bergman, Executive Director

ChoiceCare Long Island, Corporate Center, 395 North Service Road, Melville, NY 11747-3127; tel. 516/694-4000; FAX. 516/694-5780; David S. Reynolds, Ph.D., President

ChubbHealth, Inc., 380 Madison Avenue, 20th Floor, New York, NY 10017; tel. 212/880-5400; FAX. 212/880-5454; Stephen A. Rogers, President, Chief Executive Officer

Elderplan, Inc., 6323 Seventh Avenue, Brooklyn, NY 11220; tel. 718/921-7990; FAX. 718/921-7962; Eli S. Feldman, Executive Vice President, Chief Executive Officer

Empire Blue Cross and Blue Shield Healthnet/Blue Choice, Three Park Avenue, New York, NY 10016; tel. 212/251-2623; FAX. 212/779-7876; Victor Botnick, Vice President, Managed Care

HIP Health Insurance Plan of Greater New York, Seven West 34th Street, New York, NY l000l; tel. 212/630-5110; FAX. 212/630-5078; Anthony Watson, President

HMO-CNY, Inc., 344 South Warren Street, P.O. Box 4809, Syracuse, NY 13221; tel. 315/448-4931; FAX. 315/448-6802; George W. Manton, President, Chief Executive Officer

Health Care Plan, Inc., 900 Guaranty Building, Buffalo, NY 14202; tel. 716/847-1480; FAX. 716/847-1817; Arthur R. Goshin, M.D., Plan President, Chief Executive Officer

Health Services Medical Corporation of Central New York, Inc., a/k/a Prepaid Health Plan (PHP) in Syracuse, NY, PHP/SDMN in Utica, NY, 8278 Willett Parkway, Baldwinsville, NY 13027; tel. 315/638-2133; FAX. 315/638-0985; Frederick F. Yanni, Jr., President, Chief Executive Officer

Independent Health Association, Inc., 511 Farber Lakes Drive, Buffalo, NY 14221; tel. 716/631-3001; FAX. 716/635-3838; Frank Colantuono, President

Kaiser Foundation Health Plan of New York, 210 Westchester Avenue, White Plains, NY l0604; tel. 914/682-6401; FAX. 914/682-6403; Maura Carley, New York Area Operations Manager

Managed Health, Inc., EAB Plaza, Uniondale, NY 11556-0162; tel. 516/683-1010; FAX. 516/683-1034; James Molbihill, M.D., President

Metlife Healthcare Network of New York, Inc., 2929 Express Drive, N., Hauppauge, NY ll788-5390; tel. 516/348-4200; FAX. 516/348-4299

Metropolitan Health Plan, 500 Fifth Avenue, 27th Floor, New York, NY 10110; tel. 212/626-8300; FAX. 212/626-8378; Jerome Gibbs, Ph.D., Acting Executive Director

Mohawk Valley Physicians' Health Plan, Inc., MVP Health Plan, 111 Liberty Street, Schenectady, NY 12305; tel. 518/370-4793; FAX. 518/370-0852; David W. Oliker, President, Chief Executive Officer

Oxford Health Plans of New York, 521 Fifth Avenue, 15th Floor, New York, NY 10175; tel. 212/599-2266; FAX. 212/599-3552; Stephen F. Wiggins, Chief Executive Officer

Patients' Choice, Inc., P.O. Box 1498, Syracuse, NY 132011498; tel. 315/449-1100; FAX. 315/449-2200; Ron Harms, Chief Executive Officer

Physicians Health Services of New York, Inc., Crosswest Office Center, 399 Knollwood Road, Suite 212, White Plains, NY 10603; tel. 914/682-8006; FAX. 914/682-5692; Philip J. Passantino, President

PruCare of New York, Federal Plaza II, 140 Fell Court, Hauppauge, NY 11788; tel. 516/232-1943; FAX. 516/232-2181; Ray Allen, Vice President

Rochester Area HMO, Inc., a/k/a Preferred Care, 259 Monroe Avenue, Suite A, Rochester, NY 14607; tel. 716/327-2210; FAX. 716/325-3122; John Urban, President

Sanus Health Plan of Greater New York, Inc., 75-20 Astoria Boulevard, Jackson Heights, NY 11370; tel. 718/899-5200; Harry Blair, Executive Director

Travelers Health Network of New York, Inc., Metropolitan Division, 701 Westchester Avenue, Suite 310 E, White Plains, NY 10604-3001; tel. 914/761-9102; Gerald L. McNair, Executive Director

U.S. Healthcare, Inc., Nassau Omni West, 333 Earle Ovington Boulevard, Suite 502, Uniondale, NY 11553; tel. 516/794-6565; Michael A. Stocker, M.D., President

WellCare of New York, Inc., 130 Meadow Avenue, Newburgh, NY 12550; tel. 914/566-0700; FAX. 914/566-9046; Robert Goff, Chief Executive Officer

NORTH CAROLINA

Aetna Health Plans of the Carolinas, Inc., 1010 Charlotte Plaza, Charlotte, NC 28244; tel. 704/353-7176; FAX. 704/353-7180; Patrick Dowd, President

American Dental Plan of North Carolina, Inc., 130 Edinburgh South, Suite 107, Cary, NC 27511; tel. 919/380-9267; FAX. 919/380-1729; Mark Fischman

Blue Cross Blue Shield of North Carolina, P.O. Box 2291, Durham, NC 27702; tel. 919/489-7431, ext. 9194; FAX. 191/338-; Earl Ridout, Senior Director

CIGNA Dental Health of North Carolina, Inc., 300 N.W. 82nd Court, Suite 700, P.O. Box 189060, Plantation, FL 33318-9060; tel. 305/423-5800; FAX. 305/423-5488; David O. Cannady, President

CIGNA Health Plan of North Carolina, Inc., 7400 Carmel Executive Park, Charlotte, NC 28235; tel. 800/235-5707; FAX. 704/544-4375; Debbie Walters, Manager

Coastal Health Plan of North Carolina, Inc., 2828 Croasdaile Drive, P.O. Box 15309, Durham, NC 27704; Richard W. Kaplan, President

Health Maintenance Organization of North Carolina, Inc., P.O. Box 2291, Durham, NC 27702; tel. 919/489-7431; FAX. 919/419-1338; Earl Ridout, Senior Director

Healthsource North Carolina, Inc., 4000 Aerial Center Parkway, Morrisville, NC 27560; tel. 919/460-1610, ext. 7700; FAX. 919/460-9522; Robert J. Greczyn, Jr., President, Chief Executive Officer

Kaiser Foundation Health Plan of North Carolina, 3120 Highwoods Boulevard, Suite 300, Raleigh, NC 27604-1038; tel. 919/878-9870; FAX. 919/878-5835; Alvin W. Washington, Vice President, Regional Manager

Maxicare North Carolina, Inc., 5550 77 Center Drive, Suite 380, Charlotte, NC 28217-0700; tel. 704/525-0880, ext. 6451; FAX. 704/529-0382; Richard T. Hedlund, Vice President, General Manager

PARTNERS National Health Plans of North Carolina, Inc., P.O. Box 24907, Winston-Salem, NC 27114-4907; tel. 919/760-4822; FAX. 919/760-3198; John W. Jones, President

PHP, Inc., Northwestern Plaza, 2307 West Cone Boulevard, Greensboro, NC 27408; tel. 910/282-0900; FAX. 910/545-5099; Frank R. Mascia, President, Chief Executive Officer

Personal Care Plan of North Carolina, Inc., Blue Cross and Blue Shield of North Carolina Personal Care Plan, P.O. Box 30004, Durham, NC 27702; tel. 919/490-4003; FAX. 919/419-1338; Don W. Bradley, M.D., Executive Director

Provident Health Care Plans, Inc. of North Carolina, 6101 Carnegie Boulevard, Suite 400, Charlotte, NC 28209; tel. 704/556-5400; FAX. 704/344-4660; Dennis E. Edmonds, Vice President

Prudential Health Care Plan, Inc., 2701 Coltsgate Road, Suite 100, Charlotte, NC 28211; tel. 704/367-3044; FAX. 704/365-9959; David Patterson, Executive Director

Qualchoice of North Carolina, Inc., 2000 West First Street, Suite 201, Winston-Salem, NC 27104; tel. 919/716-0900; FAX. 910/716-0920; Douglas Cueny, President

NORTH DAKOTA

Blue Cross Blue Shield of North Dakota, 4510 13th Avenue, S., Fargo, ND 58121; tel. 701/282-1100; Michael B. Unhjem, President

Employers Health Insurance Company, (Life Co. Licensed for HMO), 1100 Employers Boulevard, Green Bay, WI 54344; tel. 414/337-8127; FAX. 414/337-8187; Jonathan M. Fuchs, FACHE, Vice President, Managed Care

Heart of America HMO, 802 South Main, Rugby, ND 58368; tel. 701/776-5848; FAX. 701/776-5235; Mary Ann Jaeger, Office Manager

Medica Choice, 5601 Smetana Drive, Minneapolis, MN 55440-7001; tel. 612/936-1200; FAX. 612/936-6858; Peter Fish, Manager, Public Relations

Northern Plains Health Plan, 1000 South Columbia Road, Grand Forks, ND 58201; tel. 701/780-1600; Raymond Kuntz

OHIO

Aetna Health Plans of Ohio, Inc., 3690 Orange Place, Suite 200, Cleveland, OH 44122-4438; tel. 216/464-2722; FAX. 216/464-2723; David K. Ellwanger, Executive Director

Aultcare HMO, 2600 Sixth Street, S.W., Canton, OH 44710; tel. 216/438-6360; Rick L. Haines, Vice President, Managed Care

CIGNA HealthCare of Ohio, Inc., 3700 Corporate Drive, Suite 200, Columbus, OH 43231; tel. 614/823-7500; FAX. 614/823-7519; James D. Massie, Executive Director

ChoiceCare, 655 Eden Park Drive, Suite 400, Cincinnati, OH 45202; tel. 513/784-5200; FAX. 513/784-5300; Daniel A. Gregorie, M.D., Chief Executive Officer

Providers / Health Maintenance Organizations

Cigna Health Care of Ohio, 5005 Rockside Road, Suite 700, Cleveland, OH 44131-9720; tel. 216/642-2920; FAX. 216/642-2990

Day-Med Health Maintenance Plan, 9797 Springboro Pike, Miamisburg, OH 45342; tel. 513/847-5646, ext. 120; FAX. 513/847-5620; Jeanette Prear, President, Chief Executive Officer

Dayton Area Health Plan, One Dayton Centre, One South Main Street, Suite 440, Dayton, OH 45402-9794; tel. 513/224-3300; FAX. 513/224-8587; Pamela B. Morris, President, Chief Executive Officer

Emerald HMO, Inc., Diamond Building, 1100 Superior Avenue, 16th Floor, Cleveland, OH 44114-2591; tel. 216/241-4133; FAX. 216/241-4158; Randolph C. Hoffman, Chief Operations Officer

Family Health Plan, Inc., 1001 Madison Avenue, Toledo, OH 43264-1916; tel. 419/241-6501; FAX. 419/241-5441; David Bick, Vice President, Sales and Marketing

HMO Health Ohio, 2060 East Ninth Street, Cleveland, OH 44115-1353; tel. 216/687-6092; FAX. 216/687-7787; Gerry P. Long, Director, Health Care Services Administrative Support

Health Guard, d/b/a Advantage Health Plan, 3000 Guernsey Street, Bellaire, OH 43906-1598; tel. 614/676-4623; FAX. 614/676-3319; Elizabeth Stolkowski, Acting Chief Operating Officer

Health Maintenance Plan, 4665 Cornell Road, Suite 351, Cincinnati, OH 45241; tel. 513/247-6688; FAX. 513/247-6789; Bradford A. Buxton, Executive Director

Health Power HMO, Inc., 560 East Town Street, Columbus, OH 43215-0346; tel. 614/461-9900; FAX. 614/461-0960; Thomas Beaty, Jr., President

Health Power HMO, Inc., Newmark Center, Suite 200, 3131 Newmark Drive, Miamisburg, OH 45342-5400; tel. 614/461-9900; FAX. 513/438-9024; Thomas E. Beaty, President

HealthFirst, 372 East Center Street, Marion, OH 43302-3831; tel. 614/387-6355; FAX. 614/387-0665; N. Robert Jones, President, Chief Executive Officer

HomeTown Hospital Health Plan, 876 Amherst Road, N.E., Massillon, OH 44646-8508; tel. 216/837-6880; FAX. 216/837-6869; William C. Epling, Vice President, Chief Operating Officer

Humana Health Plan of Ohio, Inc., 8044 Montgomery Road, Suite 460, Cincinnati, OH 45236; tel. 513/792-0511; FAX. 513/792-0520; Bill Wakefield, Executive Director

InHealth, Inc., 200 East Campus View Boulevard, Worthington, OH 43235; tel. 614/888-2223; Jeralyn Green, President

Kaiser Permanente, North Point Tower, 1001 Lakeside Avenue, Suite 1200, Cleveland, OH 44114-1153; tel. 216/621-5600, ext. 5138; FAX. 216/623-8776; Robert Baker, Director, Government Relations and Corporate Communications

Licking Memorial Hospital Health Plan, 1320 West Main Street, Suite HP, Newark, OH 43055-3699; tel. 614/366-0533; FAX. 614/366-0256; Kitty Martin, Director

Medical Value Plan, 405 Madison Avenue, P.O. Box 2147, Toledo, OH 43603-2147; tel. 419/244-2900; FAX. 419/244-0532; Hal A. White, M.D. Medical Director

Metlife Healthcare Network of Ohio, Inc., 4501 Erskine Road, Suite 150, Cincinnati, OH 45242-4713; tel. 216/464-8446; FAX. 513/745-9878; Marilyn McMichael, Chief Operating Officer

Paramount Health Care, 1715 Indian Wood Circle, Suite 200, P.O. Box 928, Toledo, OH 43697-0928; tel. 419/891-2500; FAX. 419/891-2530; John C. Randolph, President

Personal Physician Care, Inc., Sterling Building, 1255 Euclid Avenue, Suite 500, Cleveland, OH 44115-1807; tel. 216/687-0015; FAX. 216/687-9484; Wilton A. Savage, Executive Director

Physicians Health Plan Benefit Systems, P.H.P./Medplan-P.H.P./Clinicare, 3650 Olentangy River Road, P.O. Box 1138, Columbus, OH 43216-1138; tel. 614/442-6139; FAX. 614/442-3902; Mark Ridenour, Manager, Contracting, Compliance, Provider

Principal Health Care of Ohio, Inc., 8101 North High Street, Suite 380, Columbus, OH 43235; tel. 614/841-1240; FAX. 614/841-1245; Vernon A. Perry, Jr., Executive Director

Prudential Health Care Plan, Inc., PruCare of Central Ohio, 485 Metro Place S., Suite 450, Dublin, OH 43017; tel. 614/761-0002; FAX. 614/761-1757; Budd Fisher, Director, Group Operations

Prudential Health Care System, Inc., PruCare of Northern Ohio, Halle Building, Suite 750, 1228 Euclid Avenue, Cleveland, OH 44115-3858; tel. 216/241-5623; FAX. 216/241-7561; Linda Somers, Director, Health Care Management

Qualchoice HMO, 6000 Parkland Boulevard, Cleveland, OH 44124; tel. 216/460-4040; FAX. 216/460-4004; Michael L. Cotton, Senior Vice President, Government Programs

SummaCare, Inc., 400 West Market Street, P.O. Box 3620, Akron, OH 44309-3620; tel. 216/996-8410; FAX. 216/996-8415; Martin P. Hauser, President

Super Blue HMO, 2060 East Ninth Street, Cleveland, OH 44115

Takecare Health Plan of Ohio, Inc., Spectrum Office Tower, 11260 Chester Road, Suite 800, Cincinnati, OH 45246-9928; tel. 513/772-9191; FAX. 513/772-1466; John Davren, M.D., Plan Director

The Health Plan of the Upper Ohio Valley, Inc., 52160 National Road, E., St. Clairsville, OH 43950-9365; tel. 614/695-3585; FAX. 614/695-5297; Philip D. Wright, President

Total Health Care Plan, Inc., 12800 Shaker Boulevard, Cleveland, OH 44120; tel. 216/991-3000; FAX. 216/991-3010; James G. Turner, President, Chief Executive Officer

Western Ohio Health Care Plan, 6601 Centerville Business Parkway, P.O. Box 591208, Dayton, OH 45459-8028; tel. 513/439-8903; Jon D. Rahman, Chairman

OKLAHOMA

CIGNA HealthCare of Oklahoma, Inc., Cigna Center, 5100 North Brookline, Ninth Floor, Oklahoma City, OK 73112; tel. 405/943-7711; FAX. 405/946-9568; Lawrence Filosa, General Manager

Community Care HMO, Inc., 4720 South Harvard, Suite 202, Tulsa, OK 74135; tel. 918/749-1171; FAX. 918/749-7970; David J. Pynn, President

GHS Health Maintenance Organization, Inc., d/b/a BlueLincs HMO, Tulsa Service Area, 1400 South Boston, Tulsa, OK 74119-3630; tel. 918/560-2195; FAX. 918/560-2095; Ronald F. King, Executive Vice President

MULTIMED Health Plan, Inc., d/b/a Pacificare, 525 Central Park Drive, Suite 350, Oklahoma City, OK 73105; tel. 405/525-9200; FAX. 405/521-8349; I. David Kibbe, President

PacifiCare of Oklahoma, 7666 East 61st Street, Tulsa, OK 74133-1112; tel. 918/459-1100; FAX. 918/459-1451; Chris Whitty, Vice President, General Manager

Prudential Health Care Plan, Inc., d/b/a Prucare of Oklahoma City, 4005 N.W. Expressway, Suite 300, Oklahoma City, OK 73116; tel. 405/858-1780; Gary Hawkins, Executive Director

Prudential Health Care Plan, Inc., d/b/a Prucare of Tulsa, 7912 East 31st Court, Suite 300, Tulsa, OK 74145; tel. 918/624-4600; FAX. 918/627-9759; John Kennedy, Executive Director

OREGON

HMO Oregon, Inc., P.O. Box 12625, Salem, OR 97309; tel. 503/364-4868; FAX. 503/588-4350; Roger B. Lyman, President, Chief Executive Officer

Health Maintenance of Oregon, Inc., P.O. Box 139, Portland, OR 97207-0139; tel. 503/274-0755; FAX. 501/223-5993; Richard Woolworth, President, Chief Executive Officer

Health Masters of Oregon, Inc., 201 High Street, S.E., Salem, OR 97301; tel. 503/779-9468; FAX. 503/779-3238; Jud Holtey, Chief Operating Officer, Southern Regional Office, BCBSO

HealthGuard Services, Inc., d/b/a SelectCare, P.O. Box 10106, Eugene, OR 97440; tel. 503/485-1850; FAX. 503/686-2572; David Slade, President

Kaiser Foundation Health Plan of the Northwest, 500 N.E. Multnomah Street, Suite 100, Portland, OR 97232-2099; tel. 503/813-2800; Michael H. Katcher, President

Liberty Health Plan, Inc., 825 N.E. Multnomah Street, Suite 1600, Portland, OR 97232; tel. 503/234-5345; FAX. 503/234-5381; Kristen A. Fassenfelt, Vice President

PACC, P.O. Box 286, Clackamas, OR 97015-0286; tel. 503/659-4212; FAX. 503/794-3409; Martin A. Preizler, President, Chief Executive Officer

Pacificare of Oregon, Five Centerpointe Drive, Suite 600, Lake Oswego, OR 97035-8650; tel. 503/620-9324; FAX. 503/624-5162; Mary O. McWilliams, President

Providence Health Plans, l235 N.E. 47th Avenue, Suite 220, Portland, OR 97213; tel. 503/249-2981; FAX. 503/280-7655; Jack Friedman, Executive Director

Qual-Med Oregon Health Plan, Inc., 4800 S.W. Macadam, Suite 400, Portland, OR 97201; tel. 503/222-5217; FAX. 503/796-6366; Tom Jovick, Ph.D, Executive Director

PENNSYLVANIA

Aetna Health Plan of Western Pennsylvania, Inc., 5700 Corporate Drive, Suite 300, P.O. Box 101769, Pittsburgh, PA 15237; tel. 412/369-4650; FAX. 412/364-2393; C. Timothy Brown, Market Vice President

Aetna Health Plans of Central and Eastern Pennsylvania, Inc., 150 Monument Road, Suite 106, Bala Cynwyd, PA 19004; tel. 215/668-1440; Gene R. Heath, Chief Executive Officer

Alliance Health Network, 1700 Peach Street, Suite 244, Erie, PA 16501; tel. 814/878-1700; FAX. 814/452-4358; Rose A. Sleptzoff, Administrative Assistant

Central Medical Health Plan, d/b/a Advantage Health, 121 Seventh Avenue, Suite 500, Pittsburgh, PA 15222-3408; tel. 412/391-9300, ext. 509; FAX. 412/391-0377; Elizabeth Stolkowski, Executive Vice President, Chief Operating Officer

Cigna Health Plan of Pennsylvania, Inc., One Beaver Valley Road, Suite CHP, Wilmington, DE 19803

Geisinger Health Plan, Geisinger Office Building, 100 North Academy Avenue, Danville, PA 17822-3020; tel. 717/271-8760; FAX. 717/271-5268; Howard G. Hughes, M.D., Senior Vice President Health Plans

Greater Atlantic Health Service, Inc., 3550 Market Street, Philadelphia, PA 19104; tel. 215/823-8600; Ernest Monfiletto, President, Chief Executive Officer

HMO of Northeastern Pennsylvania, 70 North Main Street, Wilkes-Barre, PA 18711; tel. 717/829-6044; FAX. 717/829-6910; Denise S. Cesare, Vice President, Chief Operating Officer

HMO of Pennsylvania, 980 Jolly Road, P.O. Box 1109, Blue Bell, PA 19422; tel. 215/628-4800; Leonard Abramson, President

HealthAmerica of Central Pennsylvania, Inc., 2601 Market Place Street, Second Floor, Harrisburg, PA 17110-9339; tel. 717/540-4260; FAX. 717/540-6316; F. G. Chip Merkel, President

HealthAmerica of Pittsburgh, Five Gateway Center, Pittsburgh, PA 15222; tel. 412/553-7300; FAX. 412/553-7384; Mike Blackwood, Chief Executive Officer

HealthGuard of Lancaster, Inc., 280 Granite Run Drive, Suite 105, Lancaster, PA 17601-6810; tel. 717/560-9049; FAX. 717/581-4580; James R. Godfrey, President

Keystone Health Plan Central, Inc., 300 Corporate Center Drive, P.O. Box 898812, Camp Hill, PA 17089-8812; tel. 717/763-3458; FAX. 717/975-6895; Joseph M. Pfister, President, Chief Executive Officer

Keystone Health Plan East, Inc., 1901 Market Street, Philadelphia, PA l9101-7516; tel. 215/241-2001; John Daddis, Executive Vice President, Chief Operating Officer

Providers / Health Maintenance Organizations

Keystone Health Plan West, Inc., Foster Plaza Six, Fifth and Sixth Floor, 681 Andersen Drive, Pittsburgh, PA 15220-2771; tel. 412/937-4300; FAX. 412/937-0111; Kenneth R. Melani, M.D., President

Oaktree Health Plan of Pennsylvania, Inc., Scott Plaza 2, Suite 640, Philadelphia, PA 19113; tel. 610/595-8631; FAX. 610/521-8635; Felicia T. Neczypor, President, Chief Executive Officer

Prudential Health Care Plan, Inc., PruCare of Philadelphia, 220 Gibralter Road, Suite 200, P.O. Box 901, Horsham, PA 19044-0901; tel. 215/672-1944; FAX. 215/442-2946; Kenneth W. Janda, Executive Director

U.S. HealthCare Systems, Inc., Two Marquis Plaza, Suite 300, 5313 Campbells Run Road, Pittsburgh, PA 15205; tel. 412/788-0500; Leonard Abramson, President

RHODE ISLAND

HMO Rhode Island, 30 Chestnut Street, Providence, RI 02903; tel. 401/274-6644; FAX. 401/453-2533; Michael Gerhardt, President

Harvard Community Health Plan of New England, One Hoppin Street, Providence, RI 02903; tel. 401/331-3000; Stephen Schoenbaum, M.D., Medical Director

Pilgrim Health Care, 10 Accord Executive Drive, P.O. Box 200, Norwell, MA 02061; tel. 617/871-3950; FAX. 617/982-9668; Allan Greenberg, Executive Vice President

United Health Plans of New England, Inc., 475 Kilvert Street, Suite 310, Warwick, RI 02886-1392; tel. 401/737-6900; FAX. 401/737-6957; Max Powell, Chief Executive Officer

SOUTH CAROLINA

Companion HealthCare Corporation, I-20 at Alpine Road, Columbia, SC 29219-2401; tel. 803/786-8466; FAX. 803/699-2374; Harvey L. Galloway, Executive Vice President, Chief Operating Officer

Healthsource South Carolina, Inc., 215 East Bay Street, Suite 401, Charleston, SC 29401; tel. 803/723-5520; FAX. 803/723-7715; Michael V. Clark, President, Chief Executive Officer

Maxicare Southeast Health Plans, Inc., d/b/a Maxicare South Carolina, 535 Pleasantburg Drive, Suite 210, Greenville, SC 29607; tel. 803/233-7437; Richard T. Hedlund, Vice President, General Manager

Physicians Health Plan of South Carolina, Inc., 110 Centerview Drive, Suite 301, Columbia, SC 29210-8438; tel. 803/750-7400, ext. 4; FAX. 803/750-7486; William E. Martin, Chief Executive Officer

Preferred Health Systems, Inc., I-20 at Alpine Road, Columbus, SC 29219; tel. 803/788-0222

Provident Health Care Plan, Inc. of South Carolina, 201 Brookfield Parkway, Suite 100, Greenville, SC 29607; tel. 803/987-3100

SOUTH DAKOTA

Dakota Care, 1323 South Minnesota Avenue, Sioux Falls, SD 57105; tel. 605/334-4000; FAX. 605/336-0270; Robert D. Johnson, Chief Executive Officer

TENNESSEE

Aetna Health Plans of Tennessee, 1801 West End Avenue, Suite 500, Nashville, TN 37203; tel. 615/322-1600; FAX. 615/322-1217; David R. Field, President

CIGNA HealthCare of Tennessee, Inc., Palmer Plaza, Suite 800, 1801 West End Avenue, Nashville, TN 37203; tel. 615/340-3059; FAX. 615/340-3590; Sherri A. Silvas, Administrative Assistant

Complete Health of Tennessee, Inc., 2160 Highland Avenue, Birmingham, AL 35205

HealthWise of Tennessee, Inc., 404 BNA Drive, Suite 204, Nashville, TN 37217; tel. 615/366-5800; FAX. 615/367-5008; Len Cantrell, Chief Executive Officer

Healthsource Tennessee, Inc., Two Centre Square, Suite 300, 625 South Gay Street, Knoxville, TN 37902-1656; tel. 615/546-2529; FAX. 615/522-5422; Catherine N. Ferry, Chief Executive Officer

Heritage National Healthplan of Tennessee, Inc., 1515 Fifth Avenue, Suite 600, Moline, IL 61265; tel. 615/584-1127; FAX. 615/584-1141; Cynthia A. Winker

Memphis Managed Care Corporation, P.O. Box 49, Memphis, TN 38101; tel. 901/725-7100, ext. 3009; FAX. 901/725-5208

Phoenix Healthcare of Tennessee, Inc., 3401 West End Avenue, Suite 470, Nashville, TN 37203; tel. 615/298-3666, ext. 260; FAX. 615/297-2036; Samuel H. Howard, Chairman

Provident Health Care Plan, Inc. of Tennessee, Two Northgate Park, Chattanooga, TN 37415

Southern Health Plan, Inc., 600 Jefferson, Memphis, TN 38105; tel. 901/544-2202; FAX. 901/544-2250; Tim J. Hogan, Executive Director

Tennessee Health Care Network, Inc., P.O. Box 1407, Chattanooga, TN 37402; tel. 615/755-5744; FAX. 615/755-5630; Wayne E. Willison, President

Tennessee Primary Care Network, Inc., 205 Reidhurst Avenue, Suite N-104, Nashville, TN 37203; tel. 615/329-2016; FAX. 615/329-5835; Anthony J. Cebrun, J.D., M.P.H., President, Chief Executive Officer

TotalCare, Inc., 44 Vantage Way, Suite 300, Nashville, TN 37228

University of Tennessee Health Plan, Inc., 1111 Northshore Drive, Suite N-400, Knoxville, TN 37919; tel. 615/450-9000; FAX. 615/450-9099; Steven W. Roads, General Council, Chief Operating Officer

Vanderbilt Health Plans, Inc., Baker Building, Suite 1100, 110 21st Avenue South, Nashville, TN 37203; tel. 615/343-2670; FAX. 615/343-2823; Randal B. Farr, Executive Vice President

TEXAS

Aetna Dental Care of Texas, Inc., 2350 Lakeside Boulevard, Suite 740, Richardson, TX 75082; tel. 214/470-7990; Carol Eakin, Chief Operating Officer

Aetna Health Plans of Texas, Inc., 2900 North Loop West, Suite 200, Houston, TX 77092; tel. 713/683-7500; FAX. 713/683-5819; Joseph T. Blanford III, Vice President, Health Services Management

Alpha Dental Programs, Inc., d/b/a Delta Care, 5525 MacArthur, Suite 810, Irving, TX 75038; tel. 214/580-1616; FAX. 214/580-1333; Vicki A. Harden, Operations Manager

Alternative Dental Care of Texas, Inc., 1300 Waterway Tower, 433 East Las Colinas Boulevard, Irving, TX 75039; tel. 800/237-7727; David P. McSweeney, M.D., President

Anthem Health Plan of Texas, Inc., 5055 Keller Springs Road, Dallas, TX 75243; tel. 214/732-2000; FAX. 214/250-0834; Francis Browning, Executive Vice President

Anthem Health Plans of Texas, Inc., 2727 Allen Parkway, Suite W-265, Houston, TX 77019; tel. 713/630-6400; FAX. 713/522-5389; Kathy Morgan, Operations Manager

Anthem Health Plans of Texas, Inc., 5414 Fredericksburg Road, Suite 100, San Antonio, TX 78229; tel. 210/530-3220; FAX. 210/530-3232; Peggy Duvall, Chief Operating Officer

CIGNA Dental Health of Texas, Inc., d/b/a CIGNA Dental Health, 600 East Las Colinas Boulevard, Suite 1000, Irving, TX 75039; tel. 800/367-1037; Brent Martin, D.D.S., M.B.A., Chief Executive Officer, Regional Vice President

CIGNA HealthCare of North Texas, Inc., 600 East Las Colinas Boulevard, Suite 1100, Irving, TX 75039; tel. 214/401-5200; FAX. 214/401-5209; Lawrence H. Levy, M.D., Executive Director, Vice President

CIGNA HealthCare of Texas, Inc., Houston Division, 1360 Post Oak Boulevard, Suite 1100, Houston, TX 77056; tel. 713/552-7600; FAX. 713/552-7041; Dennis E. Edmonds, Executive Director

Coastal Bend Health Plan, Inc., 2502 Morgan, Corpus Christi, TX 78405; tel. 800/622-3881; FAX. 512/887-8115; Diana Tchida, Executive Director

Denticare, Inc., 14141 Southwest Freeway, Suite 1300, Sugarland, TX 77478-9990; tel. 713/242-1099; FAX. 713/242-1007; Henry New, President

Exclusive Healthcare, Inc., 12790 Merit Drive, Suite 714, Dallas, TX 75251; Robert Robidou, Plan Manager

FHP of Texas, Inc., 12 Greenway Plaza, Suite 500, Houston, TX 77046-1201; tel. 800/455-4156; FAX. 713/621-9647; Patrick Stewart, President

First American Dental Benefits, Inc., 14800 Landmark Boulevard, Suite 700, Dallas, TX 75240; tel. 214/661-5848; Jim Davenport, President, Acting Chief Executive Officer

Foundation Health, a Texas Health Plan, Inc., 110 Wild Basin Road, Suite 230, Austin, TX 78746; tel. 512/314-8421; Penny Zagroba, Operations Manager

Harris Health Plan, Inc., 1300 Summit Avenue, Suite 300, Fort Worth, TX 76102; tel. 817/878-5800; FAX. 817/878-3959; Robert Watkins, Executive Director

Humana Health Plan of Texas, Inc., d/b/a Humana Health Plan of San Antonio, 8431 Fredericksburg Road, Suite 360, San Antonio, TX 78229; tel. 210/617-1000; FAX. 210/617-1045; Michael A. Seltzer, Executive Director

Humana Health Plan of Texas, Inc., d/b/a Humana Health Plan of Dallas, 8431 Fredericksburg Road, San Antonio, TX 78229; tel. 512/617-1000; Brenda Luckett, Executive Director

Humana Health Plan of Texas, Inc., d/b/a Humana Health Plan of Corpus Christi, 5350 South Staples, Suite 301, Corpus Christi, TX 78411; tel. 512/994-2000; Richard Willis, Executive Director

Humana Health Plan of Texas, Inc., d/b/a Humana Health Plan of Houston, 1980 Post Oak Boulevard, Suite 1900, Houston, TX 77056; tel. 713/622-6639; FAX. 713/622-6649; Robert Horrar, Associate Executive Director

Kaiser Foundation Health Plan of Texas, 12720 Hillcrest Road, Suite 600, Dallas, TX 75230; tel. 214/458-5000; FAX. 214/233-5281; Sharon Flaherty, President

MetLife Healthcare Network of Texas, Inc., 1320 Greenway Drive, Suite 400, Irving, TX 75038; tel. 214/751-7777; FAX. 214/550-6395; Gregorio Cortez III, Chief Operating Officer

Metlife Healthcare Network of Texas, Inc., Houston Division, Five Post Oak Park, Suite 550, Houston, TX 77027-3416; tel. 713/961-4300; FAX. 713/961-4431; Donald M. Ledden, President

PCA Health Plans of Texas, Inc., 8303 MoPac, Suite 450, Austin, TX 78759; tel. 512/338-6100; FAX. 512/338-6137; Donald Gessler, M.D., President, Chief Executive Officer

PCA Health Plans of Texas, Inc., Dallas/Fort Worth Region, 14800 Landmark Boulevard, Suite 500, Dallas, TX 75240; tel. 214/448-1100; John Pinkney, Executive Director

PCA Health Plans of Texas, Inc., San Antonio Region, 85 N.W. Loop 410, Fifth Floor, San Antonio, TX 78216; tel. 210/979-4000; FAX. 210/979-4100; Tom Jackson, Executive Director

PCA Health Plans of Texas, Inc., Houston Region, 13100 Northwest Freeway, Suite 400, Houston, TX 77040; tel. 713/329-5000; FAX. 713/329-5010; Beverly Sepulveda, Executive Director

Pacificare of Texas, Inc., 8200 I.H. 10 West, Suite 1000, San Antonio, TX 78230-3878; tel. 210/524-9800; FAX. 210/979-6311; Jeannie Hinman, J.D., Legal Services

Pacificare of Texas, Inc., Dallas Region, 2911 Turtle Creek Boulevard, Suite 300, Dallas, TX 75219; tel. 214/520-8333; Linda Gordon, General Manager

Pacificare of Texas, Inc., Houston Region, 1800 West Loop South, Suite 350, Houston, TX 77027-3210; tel. 800/947-8646; Stephen Zeger, Vice President, General Manager

Parliament Dental Plans, Inc., 2909 Hillcroft, Suite 515, Houston, TX 77057; tel. 713/784-6262; FAX. 713/784-0488; Paul H. Michael, President

Prudential Dental Maintenance Organization, Inc., 24 Greenway Plaza, Suite 1900, Houston, TX 77046; tel. 713/993-3687; Anne Bossi, President

Providers / Health Maintenance Organizations

Prudential Health Care Plan, Inc., PruCare of Austin, P.O. Box 26725, Austin, TX 78752–1562; tel. 512/323–0440; FAX. 512/323–5908; Ron Yarbrough, Executive Director

Prudential Health Care Plan, Inc., PruCare of San Antonio, 40 N.E. Loop 410, Suite 600, San Antonio, TX 78216; tel. 512/366–1921; FAX. 512/366–1209; Robert L. Smith, Jr., Executive Director

Prudential Health Care Plan, Inc., d/b/a PruCare of North Texas, 4100 Alpha Road, Suite 400, Dallas, TX 75244–4327; tel. 214/991–0014; FAX. 214/448–3892; Victor Lazzaro, Jr., Vice President, Health Care Management

Prudential Health Care Plan, Inc., Prucare of El Paso, 300 East Main, Suite 924, El Paso, TX 79901; tel. 915/532–0700; Russell Kent Hill, Executive Director

Prudential Health Care Plan, Inc. of Houston, Stop 300–D, One Prudential Circle, Sugarland, TX 77478; tel. 713/276–3850; FAX. 713/276–8254; Raymond Flachbart, Executive Director

Rio Grande HMO, Inc., HMO Blue, Central Texas, 3445 Executive Center Drive, Suite 150, Austin, TX 78731; tel. 512/345–0089; FAX. 512/345–0889; Larry J. Bowermon, President, Chief Executive Officer

Rio Grande HMO, Inc., 4150 Pinnacle, Suite 203, El Paso, TX 79902; tel. 800/831–0576; Anne McDow, Vice President, Operations

Rio Grande HMO, Inc., HMO Blue DFW Metroplex, 901 South Central Expressway, Richardson, TX 75080; tel. 214/766–1610; Pat Hemingway, Vice President, Operations

Rio Grande HMO, Inc., HMO Blue Southeast Texas, 4888 Loop Central Drive, Suite 970, Houston, TX 77081–2214; tel. 713/664–9048; J. Darren Rodgers, Vice President, Operations

SOUTHWEST Health Plan, Inc., 2350 Lakeside Boulevard, Suite 500, Richardson, TX 75082; tel. 214/470–7878; FAX. 214/970–2881; John W. Coyle, President

Safeguard Health Plans, Inc., 6688 North Central Expressway, Suite 970, Dallas, TX 75206; tel. 214/265–7041; FAX. 214/265–7702; David Branstetter, Executive Director

Sanus Dental Plan of Texas, Inc., 4500 Fuller Drive, Irving, TX 75038; tel. 214/650–5500; FAX. 214/650–5707; Steve Yerxa, Chief Executive Officer, Executive Director

Sanus Dental Plan of Texas, Inc., Houston Division, 3800 Buffalo Speedway, Suite 200, Houston, TX 77098; tel. 713/993–9520; FAX. 713/963–9417; Don Triano, Executive Director

Sanus Health Plan, Inc., 3800 Buffalo Speedway, Suite 200, Houston, TX 77098; tel. 713/624–5000; FAX. 713/963–9417; Thomas S. Lucksinger, President, Chief Executive Officer

Sanus Texas Health Plan, Inc., 8600 Freeport Parkway, Suite 3040, Irving, TX 75063; tel. 214/929–0376; Max Brown, Jr., Executive Director

Scott & White Health Plan, 2401 South 31st Street, Temple, TX 76508; tel. 817/742–3030; Deny Radefeld, Executive Director

Southwest Health Alliances, Inc., d/b/a Firstcare, 3310 Danvers, Amarillo, TX 79109; tel. 806/358–5151; Gary Gerard, Chief Executive Officer

Travelers Health Network of Texas, Inc., Aboretum Plaza Building Two, Suite 600, 9442 Capital of Texas Highway N., Austin, TX 78759; tel. 800/424–6480; FAX. 512/338–6812; Laura Kabay, Executive Director

Travelers Health Network of Texas, Inc., Dallas/Fort Worth Division, 2270 Lakeside Boulevard, Suite 600, Richardson, TX 75082; tel. 214/437–3074; FAX. 214/470–5855; Dave Barker, Executive Director

Travelers Health Network of Texas, Inc., Houston Division, 10800 Richmond Avenue, Suite 500, Houston, TX 77042; tel. 713/268–7800; FAX. 713/268–7820; Denise Palmer, Executive Director

United Dental Care of Texas, Inc., 14755 Preston Road, Suite 300, Dallas, TX 75240; tel. 214/458–7474; James B. Kingston, President

United Healthcare Dental, Inc., 1445 North Loop West, Suite 1000, Houston, TX 77008; tel. 713/861–3231; Arlene Sheldon, Executive Director

UTAH

Associated Health Plans, Inc., 2525 East Broadway Suite 100, Tucson, AZ 85716; tel. 602/325–0691; FAX. 602/325–5212; Timothy J. Moncher, Chief Executive Officer

CIGNA Health Plan of Utah, Inc., 5295 South 320 West, Suite 280, Salt Lake City, UT 84107; tel. 801/265–2777, ext. 7501; FAX. 801/261–5349; Robert Immitt, Vice President

Educators Health Care, 852 East Arrowhead Lane, Murray, UT 84107–5298; tel. 801/262–7476; FAX. 801/269–9734; Donald W. Ulmer, President

Employees Choice Health Option, 35 West Broadway, Salt Lake City, UT 84101; tel. 801/355–1234; Westcott W. Price III, President

FHP of Utah, Inc., 35 West Broadway, Salt Lake City, UT 84101; tel. 801/355–1234; FAX. 801/351–9005; Westcott W. Price III, President

HealthWise, 2455 Parley's Way, P.O. Box 30270, Salt Lake City, UT 84130–0270; tel. 801/481–6184; FAX. 801/481–6994; Jed H. Pitcher, Chairman

IHC Care, Inc., 36 South State Street, Salt Lake City, UT 84111; tel. 801/538–5000; FAX. 801/538–5003; William H. Nelson, President

IHC Group, Inc., 36 South State Street, Salt Lake City, UT 84111; tel. 801/538–5000; William H. Nelson, President

IHC Health Plans, Inc., 36 South State Street, Salt Lake City, UT 84111; tel. 801/538–5000; William H. Nelson, President

Intergroup Healthcare Corporation of Utah, 127 South 500 East, Suite 410, Salt Lake City, UT 84102; tel. 801/532–7665; FAX. 801/297–4585; Elden Mitchell, President

Opticare of Utah, 159 1/2 South Main Street, Salt Lake City, UT 84111; tel. 801/363–0950; Stephen H. Schubach, President

Safeguard Health Plans, Inc., P.O. Box 3210, Anaheim, CA 92803–3210; tel. 714/778–1005; Steven J. Baileys, D.D.S., President

United HealthCare of Utah, 7910 South 3500 East, Salt Lake City, UT 84121; tel. 801/942–6200; FAX. 801/944–0940; Colin Gardner, Chief Executive Officer

Utah Community Health Plan, 36 South State Street, Suite 1020, Salt Lake City, UT 84111–1418; tel. 801/442–3780; FAX. 801/442–3791; William K. Willson, Executive Director

VERMONT

Capital Area Community Health Plan, Inc., 120l Troy–Schenectady Road, Latham, NY l2110; tel. 518/783–1864; FAX. 518/783–0234; John Baackes, President, Chief Executive Officer

Harvard Community Health Plan, 60 Walnut Street, Wellesley, MA 02181; tel. 800/338–4247

MVP Health Plan, 111 Liberty Street, P.O. Box 2207, Schenectady, NY 12301–2207; tel. 518/370–4793; David W. Chlikes, President MVP Health Plan

Matthew Thornton Health Plan, 410 Amherst Street, Nashua, NH 03063; tel. 603/595–4441, ext. 609; FAX. 603/886–3392; Everett Page, Chief Operating Officer

VIRGINIA

Aetna Health Plans of the Mid–Atlantic, Inc., 7799 Leesburg Pike, Suite 1100 South, Falls Church, VA 22043; tel. 703/903–7100; FAX. 703/903–0316; Russell R. Dickhart, President, Executive Director

CIGNA HealthCare of Virginia, Inc., 4050 Innslake Drive, Glen Allen, VA 23060; tel. 804/273–1100; John E. Sharp, Vice President, Executive Director

CIGNA Healthplan Mid–Atlantic, Inc., 9700 Patuxent Woods Drive, Columbia, MD 21046; tel. 301/720–5800; Timothy P. Fitzgerald, President

CapitalCare, Inc., Tysons International Plaza, 1921 Gallows Road, Suite 900, Vienna, VA 22182; tel. 703/761–5400; FAX. 703/761–5576; David L. Ward, President, Chief Executive Officer

HMO Virginia, Inc., Health Keepers, 2220 Edward Holland Drive, Richmond, VA 23230; tel. 804/354–3844; FAX. 804/354–3936; Sam Weidman, Vice President Finance

Health First, Inc., 621 Lynnhaven Parkway, Suite 450, Virginia Beach, VA 23452–7330; tel. 804/431–5298; Russell F. Mohawk, Executive Director

HealthKeepers, Inc., 2220 Edward Holland Drive, P.O. Box 26623, Richmond, VA 23230; tel. 804/354–3844; FAX. 804/354–3936; Sam Weidman, Vice President, Finance

HealthPlus, Inc., 7601 Ora Glen Drive, Suite 200, Greenbelt, MD 20770; tel. 301/982–0098, ext. 3308; FAX. 301/489–5284; Jeff D. Emerson, Chief Executive Officer

Humana Group Health Plan, Inc., 4301 Connecticut Avenue, N.W., Washington, DC 20008; tel. 202/364–2000; Ted W. LaBedz

Kaiser Foundation Health Plan of the Mid–Atlantic States, Inc., 2101 East Jefferson Street, Rockville, MD 20852; tel. 301/816–2424; FAX. 301/816–7478; Alan J. Silverstone, President

MD–Individual Practice Association, Inc., Four Taft Court, Rockville, MD 20850; tel. 301/294–5100; FAX. 301/309–1709; Susan Goff, President

Optima Health Plan, 4417 Corporation Lane, Virginia Beach, VA 23462; tel. 804/552–7400; FAX. 804/552–7396; Theodore Morgan Wille, Jr., President

Optimum Choice, Inc., Four Taft Court, Rockville, MD 20850; tel. 301/738–7920; FAX. 301/309–3782; George T. Jochum, President, Chief Executive Officer

Peninsula Health Care, Inc., 606 Denbigh Boulevard, Suite 500, Newport News, VA 23602; tel. 804/875–5760; FAX. 804/875–5785; John F. McIntyre, President

Physicians Health Plan, Inc., Health Keepers, 2220 Edward Holland Drive, Richmond, VA 23230; tel. 804/354–3844; FAX. 804/354–3936; Sam Weidman, Vice President, Finance

Principal Health Care of the Mid–Atlantic, Inc., 1801 Rockville Pike, Suite 110, Rockville, MD 20852; tel. 301/881–1033; Kenneth J. Linde, President

Priority Health Plan, Inc., 621 Lynnhaven Parkway, Suite 450, Virginia Beach, VA 23452–7330; tel. 804/463–4600; Russell F. Mohawk, Executive Director

Prudential Health Care Plan, Inc., d/b/a PruCare and Prudential Health Care Plan of the Mid–Atlantic, 1000 Boulders Parkway, Richmond, VA 23225; tel. 804/323–0900; William Patrick Link, President

Sentara Health Plans, Inc., d/b/a Sentara Health Plan, 4417 Corporation Lane, Virginia Beach, VA 23462; tel. 804/552–7100; FAX. 804/552–7396; John E. McNamara III, President

Southern Health Services, 9881 Mayland Drive, P.O. Box 85603, Richmond, VA 23285–5603; tel. 804/747–3700; FAX. 804/747–8723; James L. Gore, President

The George Washington University Health Plan, Inc., 1901 Pennsylvania Avenue, N.W., Suite 600, Washington, DC 20006; tel. 202/416–0410; FAX. 202/296–7348; Roger E. Meyer, M.D., President

WASHINGTON

CIGNA Healthplan of Washington, Inc., 2940 Columbia Center, 701 Fifth Avenue, Seattle, WA 98104; tel. 206/625–8800; Nina Auger, Vice President, General Manager

Good Health Plan of Washington, Century Square, 1501 Fourth Avenue, Suite 500, Seattle, WA 98101; tel. 206/622–6111; FAX. 206/292–4370; Gerald Coe, President

Group Health Cooperative of Puget Sound, Administration and Conference Center, 521 Wall Street, Seattle, WA 98121–1535; tel. 206/448–6460; FAX. 206/448–5844; Phil Nudelman, Ph.D., President, Chief Executive Officer

Group Health Northwest, 5615 West Sunset Highway, Spokane, WA 99204; tel. 509/838–9100; FAX. 509/838–3823; Henry S. Berman, M.D., President, Chief Executive Officer

Providers / Health Maintenance Organizations

HMO Washington, 1800 Ninth Avenue, P.O. Box 2088, Seattle, WA 98111–2088; tel. 206/340–6600; FAX. 206/389–6719; Mark S. Hawkins, President, Chief Executive Officer

Health Maintenance of Oregon, Inc., 100 S.W. Market Street, P.O. Box 1271, Portland, OR 97207–1271; tel. 503/226–8715; FAX. 503/223–5993; Roger B. Lyman, President, Chief Executive Officer

HealthGuard Services, Inc., d/b/a SelectCare, 600 Country Club Road, P.O. Box 10106, Eugene, OR 97401–2240; tel. 503/686–2501; FAX. 503/686–2504; David Slade, President, Chief Executive Officer

HealthPlus, P.O. Box 2113, Seattle, WA 98111–2113; tel. 206/670–4700; FAX. 206/670–4766; Gary L. Meade, President, Chief Executive Officer

Humana Health Plan of Washington, Inc., P.O. Box 1438, Louisville, KY 40201–1438; tel. 502/580–1854; Heidi Margulis, Licensure Manager

Kaiser Foundation Health Plan of the Northwest, 2701 N.W. Vaughn, Suite 300, Portland, OR 97210–5398; tel. 503/280–2000; FAX. 503/721–6838; Denise L. Honzel, Vice President

PACC, d/b/a PACC Health Plans of Washington, 12901 S.E. 97th Avenue, P.O. Box 286, Clackamas, OR 97015–0286; tel. 503/659–4212; FAX. 503/794–3409; Martin A. Preizler, President, Chief Executive Officer

PacifiCare of Washington, Inc., 7525 S.E. 24th Street, Suite 200, Mercer Island, WA 98040; tel. 206/236–2500; FAX. 206/232–3099; Mary O. McWilliams, President

Pacific Health Plans, 401 Second Avenue South, Suite 300, Seattle, WA 98104; tel. 206/326–4645; FAX. 206/624–5790; Michael P. Fleck, President

QualMed Washington Health Plan, Inc, d/b/a Qual–Med Health Plan, 2331 130th Avenue, N.E., Suite 200, Zip 98005, P.O. Box 3387, Bellevue, WA 98009–3387; tel. 206/869–3500; FAX. 206/869–3568; C.F. du Laney, Executive Director

Sisters of Providence, Good Health Plan of Oregon, Inc., 1235 N.E. 47th Avenue, Suite 220, Portland, OR 97213; tel. 503/249–2981; FAX. 503/280–7655; Mary O. McWilliams, Chief Executive Officer

Virginia Mason Health Plan, Inc., Metropolitan Park West, 1100 Olive Way, Suite 1580, Seattle, WA 98101–1828; tel. 206/223–8844; FAX. 206/223–7506; John Clarke, Director, Operations

WEST VIRGINIA

Anthem Health Plan of West Virginia, Inc., d/b/a Prime One, One Players Club, P.O. Box 1551, Charleston, WV 25326–1551; tel. 304/340–0253; Robert Harris

Charleston Area Health Plan, Inc., d/b/a Carelink, Kanawha Valley Building, 300 Capitol Street, P.O. Box 1711, Charleston, WV 25326–1711; tel. 304/348–2901; FAX. 304/348–2948; Alan L. Mytty

Health Guard, Inc., d/b/a Advantage Health Plan, Inc., 300 Guernsey Street, Bellaire, OH 43906; tel. 614/676–4623; Dan Splain

Optimum Choice, Four Taft Court, Rockville, MD 20850; tel. 703/207–6570; Susan Hrubes

The Health Plan of the Upper Ohio Valley, 52160 National Road, E., St. Clairsville, OH 43950; tel. 614/695–3585; Phillip D. Wright, Contact Person

WISCONSIN

Compcare Health Services Insurance Corp., 401 West Michigan Street, P.O. Box 2947, Milwaukee, WI 53201–2025; tel. 414/226–6171; FAX. 414/226–6229; Jeffrey J. Nohl, President, Chief Operating Officer

Dean Health Plan, Inc., P.O. Box 56099, Madison, WI 53705–9399; tel. 608/836–1400; FAX. 608/836–9620; John A. Turcott, President

Family Health Plan Cooperative, 11524 West Theo Trecker Way, Milwaukee, WI 53214–7260; tel. 414/256–0006; FAX. 414/256–5681; Conrad Sobczak, Executive Director

Greater La Crosse Health Plans, Inc., 1285 Rudy Street, Onalaska, WI 54650; tel. 608/782–2638; FAX. 608/781–8862; Steven M. Kunes, Plan Administrator

Group Health Cooperative of Eau Claire, P.O. Box 3217, Eau Claire, WI 54702–3217; tel. 715/836–8552; FAX. 715/836–7683; Joanne P. Rafferty, General Manager

Group Health Cooperative of South Central Wisconsin, One South Park Street, Madison, WI 53715; tel. 608/251–4156; FAX. 608/257–3842; John Parr, Executive Director

HMO Midwest, P.O. Box 64179, 3535 Blue Cross Road, St. Paul, MN 55164; tel. 612/456–8429; FAX. 612/456–1004; Deborah Glass, Chief Operating Officer

HMO of Wisconsin Insurance Corp., 840 Carolina Street, Sauk City, WI 53583; tel. 800/362–3308; FAX. 608/643–2564; Devon W. Barrix, President

Managed Health Services Corp., 10607 West Oklahoma Avenue, Milwaukee, WI 53227; tel. 414/321–9001; FAX. 414/321–9724; Thomas M. Gazzana, President, Chief Executive Officer

Maxicare Health Insurance Company, 790 North Milwaukee Street, Milwaukee, WI 53202; tel. 414/271–6371; John F. Southworth, Administrator

Medical Associates Clinic Health Plan of Wisconsin, One Dubuque Plaza, Suite 230, Dubuque, IA 52001; tel. 319/556–8070; FAX. 319/556–5134; Ross A. Madden, Chairman of the Board, Director

MercyCare Health Plan, Inc., One Parker Place, Suite 750, Janesville, WI 53545; tel. 608/752–3431; FAX. 608/752–3751

MetLife Healthcare Network of Wisconsin, Inc., 1900 East Golf Road, Suite 501, Schaumburg, IL 60173–5463; tel. 708/619–2222; Claudia Bjerre, Network Director

Network Health Plan of Wisconsin, Inc., 1165 Appleton Road, P.O. Box 120, Menasha, WI 54952–0120; tel. 414/727–0100; FAX. 414/727–5634; Michael D. Wolff, Chief Executive Officer

North Central Health Protection Plan, 2000 Westwood Drive, Zip 54401, P.O. Box 969, Wausau, WI 54402–0969; tel. 715/847–8866; Larry A. Baker, Administrator

Physicians Plus Insurance Corporation, 340 West Washington Avenue, P.O. Box 2078, Madison, WI 53703; tel. 608/282–8900; FAX. 608/282–8365; Michael Mohoney, Acting President, Chief Executive Officer

PrimeCare Health Plan, Inc., 1233 North Mayfair Road, Suite 301, Wauwatosa, WI 53226; tel. 414/453–9070; FAX. 414/471–8626; James Schultz, Administrator

Security Health Plan of Wisconsin, Inc., 1000 North Oak Avenue, Marshfield, WI 54449; tel. 715/387–5534; FAX. 715/387–5240; Richard A. Leer, President

United Health of Wisconsin Insurance Company, Inc., P.O. Box 507, Appleton, WI 54912–0507; tel. 414/735–6440; FAX. 414/731–7232; Jay Fulkerson, Chief Executive Officer

Valley Health Plan, 2270 Highland Mall, P.O. Box 3128, Eau Claire, WI 54701–3128; tel. 715/832–3235; FAX. 715/836–1298; Kathyrn R. Teeters, Director

Wisconsin Health Organization Insurance Corp., 111 West Pleasant Street, P.O.Box 12359, Milwaukee, WI 53212–0359; tel. 414/223–3300; FAX. 414/223–7777; William L. Carr, Executive Director

WYOMING

IHC Care, Inc., 36 South State Street, Salt Lake City, UT 84111; tel. 801/538–5000; FAX. 801/538–5003; William H. Nelson, President

U.S. Associated Areas

GUAM

F.H.P., Inc., P.O. Box 6578, Tamunig, GU 96911; tel. 671/646–5824; FAX. 671/646–6923; Edward English, Associate Regional Vice President

Guam Memorial Health Plan, 142 West Seaton Boulevard, Agana, GU 96910; tel. 671/472–4647; FAX. 671/477–1784; James W. Gillan, Chief Operating Officer

PUERTO RICO

Cooperativa de Servicios de Salud Castaner, Apartado 1025, Castaner, PR 00631; tel. 809/829–5770; FAX. 809/829–5740; Miguel A. Gonzalez, Administrator

Damas Health Plan, Inc., Hospital Damas–Ponce By Pass, Ponce, PR 00731; tel. 809/840–8722; FAX. 809/840–8772

Golden Cross HMO Health Plan Corporation, Antes HMO Medical System Corporation, Apartado 1727, Estacion Viejo San Juan, San Juan, PR 00902; tel. 809/721–0427; FAX. 809/724–7249; Maria J. Gonzalez

Group Sales and Service of Puerto Rico, Inc., Carr. Estatal #165, Esq., Calle 1, Rexco Office Park, Guaynabo, PR 00968; tel. 809/782–7005; FAX. 809/782–5269; Luis A. Salgado Munoz, Executive Vice President

Health Plus, Inc., Metro Office Park–Texaco Plaza, Suite 200-Calle 1 Numero 2, Guaynabo, PR 00968–1705; tel. 809/782–7900; FAX. 809/793–1450; Jose A. Cuevas, President, Chief Executive Officer

Medical Card System, Inc., Royal Bank Center, Avenida Ponce de Leon 255, Suite 1600, Hato Rey, PR 00917; tel. 809/758–2500; FAX. 809/250–0380; Felipe Benedit, President

Mennonite General Hospital, Inc., Calle Jose C. Vazquez, Apartado 1379, Aibonito, PR 00705; tel. 809/735–8001; FAX. 809/735–8073; Domingo Torres Zayas, Chief Executive Officer

Plan Comprensivo de Salud, Inc., Avenida Ponce de Leon 328, Avenida de Diego 301–Pda. 22, Santurce, PR 00909; tel. 809/723–6061; FAX. 809/723–6014; J. A. Soler, President

Plan De Salud De La Federacion De Maestros, De Puerto Rico, Inc., Call Box 71336, San Juan, PR 00936; tel. 809/758–5610

Plan Medico Doctor Gubern, Inc., Calle General Valero Numero 267, Apartado 846, Fajardo, PR 00738; tel. 809/863–0924; FAX. 809/863–1071; Montserrat G. de Garcia, Chief Executive Officer

Plan Medico U.T.I. de Puerto Rico, Inc., Calle Maximo Aloman 1167, Unb. San Agustin, Rio Piedras, PR 00924; tel. 809/758–1500; FAX. 809/758–3210; David Munoz, President

Plan Medico, Servicios de Salud Bella Vista, Inc., Bella Vista Gardens Numero 43, Mayaguez, PR 00680; tel. 809/833–8070; FAX. 809/831–6315; Jose E. Sanabria, President

Plan de Salud Hospital Metropolitano, Inc., Apartado 11981–Caparra Heights, San Juan, PR 00922; tel. 809/783–2600; FAX. 809/782–0280; Jorge Meneses, Treasurer

Plan de Salud Hospital de la Concepcion, Inc., Calle Luna, Numero 41, Apartado 39, San German, PR 00683; tel. 809/892–1830; Ivonne Montaluo, Executive Director

Ryder Health Plan, Inc., Call Box 859, Humacao, PR 00792; tel. 809/852–0768, ext. 4686; FAX. 809/852–0428; Juan L. De Le Rosa, Director

Servi Medical, Inc., Avenida Munoz Rivera 402, Parada 31, Hato Rey, PR 00917; tel. 809/758–5555; FAX. 809/250–1425; Lexie Gomez

State Government Agencies for HMO's

Information for the following list was obtained directly from the agencies.

United States

ALABAMA: Department of Insurance, Department of Public Health, 135 South Union Street, Montgomery, AL 36130; tel. 334/269-3550; FAX. 334/240-3194; James D. Dill, Commissioner of Insurance

ARIZONA: Department of Insurance, 2910 North 44th Street, Suite 210, Phoenix, AZ 85018; tel. 602/912-8451, ext. 4305; FAX. 602/255-5316; Sandra Lewis, Executive Assistant

ARKANSAS: Arkansas Insurance Department, 1123 South University Avenue, Suite 400, University Tower Building, Little Rock, AR 72204-1699; tel. 501/686-2900; FAX. 501/686-2913; Lee Douglass, Insurance Commissioner

CALIFORNIA: Department of Corporations, Health Care Service Plan Division, 3700 Wilshire Boulevard, Los Angeles, CA 90010; tel. 213/736-2776; Richard M. Murakami, Assistant Commissioner

COLORADO: Department of Regulatory Agencies, Colorado Division of Insurance, 1560 Broadway, Suite 850, Denver, CO 80202; tel. 303/894-7499; FAX. 303/894-7455, ext. 322; Frank Dino, Chief, Corporate Affairs

CONNECTICUT: Department of Insurance, P.O. Box 816, Hartford, CT 06142-0816; tel. 203/297-3800; FAX. 203/566-7410; Allan B. Roby, Jr., Director, Life and Health Division

DELAWARE: Department of Health and Social Services, Office of Health Facilities Licensure and Certification, 3000 Newport Gap Pike, Wilmington, DE 19808; tel. 302/995-6674; FAX. 302/995-8332; Ellen T. Reap, Director

DISTRICT OF COLUMBIA: Department of Health and Human Services, Health Care Financing Administration, Washington, DC 20201; tel. 202/245-0758

FLORIDA: Florida Department of Insurance, Bureau of Life and Health Insurer Solvency and Market Conduct, 200 East Gaines, Larson Building, Tallahassee, FL 32399-0327; tel. 904/922-3153, ext. 2460; FAX. 904/488-7061; Larry Daniels, HMO Administrator

GEORGIA: Department of Insurance, 716 West Tower, Floyd Building, 2 Martin Luther King Jr. Drive, Atlanta, GA 30334; tel. 404/656-5826; FAX. 404/657-7743; Tim Ryles, Commissioner

HAWAII: State of Hawaii Department of Labor and Industrial Relations, Disability Compensation Division, P.O. Box 3769, Honolulu, HI 96812; tel. 808/586-9151; Gary S. Hamada, Administrator

IDAHO: Department of Insurance, 700 West State Street, Third Floor, Boise, ID 83720; tel. 208/334-4250; FAX. 208/334-4398; Cynthia Sikorski, Chief Examiner

ILLINOIS: Department of Insurance, 320 West Washington Street, 4th Floor, Springfield, IL 62767; tel. 217/782-6369; FAX. 217/782-5020; David E. Grant, Health Care Coordinator

INDIANA: Department of Insurance, 311 West Washington Street, Suite 300, Indianapolis, IN 46204; tel. 317/232-2408; FAX. 317/232-5251; Shelly Hitch, Supervising Life and Health Auditor, HMO Coordinator

IOWA: Iowa Department of Commerce, Division of Insurance, Lucas State Office Building, Des Moines, IA 50319; tel. 515/281-5705; FAX. 515/281-3059; Therese M. Vaughan, Commissioner

KANSAS: Kansas Insurance Department, 420 S.W. Ninth Street, Topeka, KS 66612; tel. 913/296-3071; FAX. 913/296-2283; Kathleen Sebelius, Commissioner

KENTUCKY: Department of Insurance, Life and Health Division, 229 West Main Street, P.O. Box 517, Frankfort, KY 40602; tel. 502/564-6088; Matthew Johnson, Director

LOUISIANA: Department of Insurance, P.O. Box 94214, Baton Rouge, LA 70804; tel. 504/342-5900; FAX. 504/342-7401; James H. Brown, Commissioner

MAINE: Department of Professional and Financial Regulation, Bureau of Insurance, State House, Station 34, Augusta, ME 04333; tel. 207/582-8707; FAX. 207/582-8716; Nancy Johnson, Deputy Superintendent

MARYLAND: Department of Health and Mental Hygiene, Insurance Division, 201 West Preston Street, Baltimore, MD 21201-2399; tel. 410/225-5430; Edward J. Muhl, Commissioner

MASSACHUSETTS: Division of Insurance, 470 Atlantic Avenue, Boston, MA 02210; tel. 617/521-7794; FAX. 617/521-7770; Linda Ruthardt, Commissioner

MICHIGAN: Department of Public Health, Bureau of Health Systems, Division of Managed Care, 3423 North Logan/Martin Luther King Boulevard, P.O. Box 30195, Lansing, MI 48909; tel. 517/335-8551; FAX. 517/335-8582; Janet Olszewski, Chief, Managed Care Division

MINNESOTA: Department of Health, Health Systems Development Division, 121 East Seventh Place, Suite 450, P.O. Box 64975, St. Paul, MN 55164-0975; tel. 612/282-5627; Nanette M. Schroeder, Director

MISSISSIPPI: State Department of Health, 2423 North State Street, 39216, P.O. Box 1700, Jackson, MS 39215-1700; tel. 601/354-7300; FAX. 601/354-7230; F. E. Thompson, Jr., M.D., M.P.H., State Health Officer

MISSOURI: Department of Insurance, Division of Company Regulation Life and Health Section, P.O. Box 690, Jefferson City, MO 65102; tel. 314/751-4363; FAX. 314/751-1165; James W. Casey, Supervisor

MONTANA: Department of Health and Environmental Sciences, Cogswell Building, Helena, MT 59620; tel. 406/444-3121; FAX. 406/444-2606; Charles Aagenes, Assistant Administrator, Health Services Division

NEBRASKA: Department of Insurance, 941 O Street, Suite 400, Lincoln, NE 68508; tel. 402/471-2201; FAX. 402/471-4610; Robert G. Lange, Acting Director

NEVADA: Nevada Division of Insurance, Capitol Complex, 1665 Hot Springs Road, Suite 152, Carson City, NV 89710; tel. 702/687-4270; FAX. 702/687-3937

NEW HAMPSHIRE: Department of Health and Human Services, Office of Medical Services, Hazen Drive, Concord, NH 03301-6521; tel. 603/271-4365; Diane Kemp, Program Specialist

NEW JERSEY: Department of Health, Division of Health Facilities, Evaluation, Licensing and Resource Development, Alternative Health Systems, CN-367, Trenton, NJ 08625; tel. 609/588-2510; FAX. 609/588-7823; Edwin V. Kelleher, Chief

NEW MEXICO: State Corporation Commission, Department of Insurance, P.O. Drawer 1269, Santa Fe, NM 87504; tel. 505/827-4601; FAX. 505/827-4734; Helen S. Hordes, Insurance Specialist

NEW YORK: Department of Health, Office of Health Systems Management, Empire State Plaza, Corning Tower Building, Albany, NY 12237; tel. 518/474-5515

NORTH CAROLINA: Department of Insurance, Financial Evaluation Division, P.O. Box 26387, Raleigh, NC 27611; tel. 919/733-5633; L. W. Cannady, Alternative Healthcare Administrator

NORTH DAKOTA: North Dakota Department of Insurance, State Capitol, 600 East Boulevard, Bismarck, ND 58505-0320; tel. 701/328-2440; FAX. 701/328-4880; Glenn Pomeroy, Commissioner

OHIO: Department of Insurance, Managed Care Division, 2100 Stella Court, Columbus, OH 43215-1067; tel. 614/644-2661; FAX. 614/644-3741; Kip May, Assistant Director

OREGON: Department of Consumer and Business Services, Insurance Division, 440 Labor and Industries Building, Salem, OR 97310; tel. 503/378-4271, ext. 640; FAX. 503/378-4351; Mary Alice Bjork, Administrator

PENNSYLVANIA: Department of Insurance, Company Division System, 1311 Strawberry Square, Harrisburg, PA 17120; tel. 717/787-7701; Edward A. Thomas, Supervisor, HMO-PPO Division

RHODE ISLAND: Department of Business Regulation, Division of Insurance, 233 Richmond Street, Suite 233, Providence, RI 02903-4233; tel. 401/277-2223; FAX. 401/751-4887; Alfonso E. Mastrostefano, Associate Director, Superintendent, Insurance

SOUTH CAROLINA: Financial Condition Division, South Carolina Department of Insurance, 1612 Marion Street, Columbia, SC 29201; tel. 803/737-6200; Cecil W. Thomas, Division Director

SOUTH DAKOTA: Health Policy and External Affairs, South Dakota Department of Health, 445 East Capitol Avenue, Pierre, SD 57501-3185; tel. 605/773-3361; FAX. 605/773-5683; Terrance L. Dosch, Division Director

TENNESSEE: Department of Health, Bureau of Manpower and Facilities, 283 Plus Park Boulevard, Nashville, TN 37247-0501; tel. 615/367-6204; FAX. 615/367-6397; Richard Long, Assistant Commissioner

TEXAS: Texas Department of Insurance, Mail Code 106-3A, P.O. Box 149104, Austin, TX 78714-9104; tel. 512/322-4266; FAX. 512/322-3552; Leah Rummel, Director, HMO/URA

UTAH: Utah Insurance Department, 3110 State Office Building, Salt Lake City, UT 84114; tel. 801/538-3800; FAX. 801/538-3829; Robert E. Wilcox, Commissioner

VERMONT: Department of Banking, Insurance and Securities, 89 Main Street, Drawer 20, Montpelier, VT 05620-3101; tel. 802/828-3301; FAX. 802/828-3306; Elizabeth R. Costle, Commissioner

Providers / State Government Agencies for HMO's

VIRGINIA: State Corporation Commission, Bureau of Insurance, P.O. Box 1157, Richmond, VA 23209; tel. 804/371-9636; FAX. 804/371-9511; Susan Smith, Senior Financial Examiner

WASHINGTON: Office of the Insurance Commissioner, Insurance Building, P.O. Box 40255, Olympia, WA 98504-0255; tel. 206/664-8002; FAX. 206/586-3535; Paula M. Strain, Manager, Health Care Contract

WEST VIRGINIA: Insurance Commissioner's Office, Financial Conditions Division, 2019 Washington Street, E., Charleston, WV 25305; tel. 304/348-2100; FAX. 304/348-0412; John Collins, Director, Chief Examiner

WISCONSIN: Office of the Commissioner of Insurance, P.O. Box 7873, Madison, WI 53707-7873; tel. 608/266-3585; FAX. 608/266-9935; Josephine W. Musser, Commissioner

WYOMING: Department of Insurance, Herschler Building, Third Floor East, 122 West 25th Street, Cheyenne, WY 82002; tel. 307/777-6888; FAX. 307/777-5895; Mark A. Pring, Insurance Standards Consultant

U.S. Associated Areas

GUAM: Department of Public Health and Social Services, Government of Guam, P.O. Box 2816, Agana, GU 96910; tel. 671/734-7102; FAX. 671/734-5910; Leticia V. Espaldon, M.D., Director

PUERTO RICO: Aurea Lopez, Chief Examiners Division, Office of the Commissioner of Insurance, P.O. Box 8330, Fernandez Juncos Station, Santurce, PR 00910-8330; tel. 809/722-8686, ext. 2212; FAX. 809/722-4400; Aurea Lopez, Chief, Examiners Division

Freestanding Ambulatory Surgery Centers

The following list of freestanding ambulatory surgery centers was developed with the assistance of state government agencies and the individual facilities listed. It is current as of January 1, 1995.

The AHA Guide contains two types of ambulatory surgery center listings; those that are hospital based and those that are freestanding. Hospital based ambulatory surgery centers are listed in section A of the AHA Guide and are identified by Facility Code F44. Please refer to that section for information on the over 5,000 hospital based ambulatory surgery centers.

Those freestanding ambulatory surgery centers accredited by the Joint Commission on Accreditation of Healthcare Organizations (JCAHO) are identified by a hollow square (□). These surgery centers have been found to be in substantial compliance with the Joint Commission standards for ambulatory health care facilities, as found in the Ambulatory Health Care Standards Manual.

We present this list simply as a convenient directory. Inclusion or omission of any organization's name indicates neither approval nor disapproval by the American Hospital Association.

United States

ALABAMA

Birmingham Outpatient Surgery Center, Ltd., 2720 University Boulevard, Birmingham, AL 35233; tel. 205/933–0050; FAX. 205/933–8212; Jackie Harrison, RN, Administrator

Cullman Outpatient Services, Inc., 909 Graham Street, S.W., Cullman, AL 35055; tel. 205/739–9090; FAX. 205/739–3079; Marcus F. Thublin, Jr., Administrator

Dauphin West Surgery Center, 3701 Dauphin Street, Mobile, AL 36608; tel. 334/341–3405; James L. Spires, Executive Director

Decatur Ambulatory Surgery Center, 2828 Highway 31, S., Decatur, AL 35603; tel. 205/340–1212; FAX. 205/340–0252; Andrew Hetrick, Administrator

Dothan Surgery Center, 1450 Ross Clark Circle, S.E., Dothan, AL 36301; tel. 334/793–3442; FAX. 334/793–3318; Donna Bernstrom, Facility Administrator

□ **Eye Surgery Center,** 2802 Ross Clark Circle, S.W., Dothan, AL 36301; tel. 334/793–3411; FAX. 334/793–7161; Marnix E. Heersink, M.D., Administrator

Florence Surgery Center, 103 Helton Court, Florence, AL 35630; tel. 205/760–0672; FAX. 205/766–4547; Levonne Rhodes, CPA, Administrator

Gadsden Surgery Center, 418 South Fifth Street, Gadsden, AL 35901; tel. 205/543–1253; FAX. 205/543–1260; Lisa LeQuire, RN, B.S.N., Administrator

Huntsville Endoscopy Center, Inc., 119 Longwood Drive, Huntsville, AL 35801; tel. 205/533–6488; FAX. 205/533–6495; Michael W. Brown, M.D.

Medplex Outpatient Medical Centers, Inc., 4511 Southlake Parkway, Birmingham, AL 32544; tel. 205/985–4398; FAX. 205/985–4486; Dawn Ousley, RN, Administrator

Mobile Surgery Center, 1721 Springhill Avenue, Mobile, AL 36604; tel. 334/438–3614; Julie Saucier, RN, B.S.N., Facility Administrator

Montgomery Surgical Center, Ltd., 855 East South Boulevard, Montgomery, AL 36116; tel. 334/284–9600; FAX. 334/284–4233; Victoria S. Kearley, Administrator

□ **Outpatient Services East, Inc.,** 52 Medical Park Drive, E., Suite 401, Birmingham, AL 35235; tel. 205/838–3888, ext. 211; FAX. 205/838–3875; James E. Stidham, Chief Executive Officer, President

Surgicare of Mobile, Ltd., 2882 Dauphin Street, Mobile, AL 36606; tel. 334/473–2020; FAX. 334/478–6737; Sandy Bunch, Administrator

The Kirklin Clinic Ambulatory Surgical Center, 2000 Sixth Avenue, S., Birmingham, AL 35233; tel. 205/801–8000; Steven C. Schultz, Executive Vice President

The Surgery Center of Huntsville, 721 Madison Street, Huntsville, AL 35801; tel. 205/533–4888; FAX. 205/532–9510; Bobbye H. Riggs, Chief Executive Officer

Tuscaloosa Endoscopy Center, 100 Rice Mine Road, N.E., Suite E, Tuscaloosa, AL 35406; tel. 205/345–0010; FAX. 205/752–1175; A. B. Reddy, M.D., Medical Director

Tuscaloosa Surgical Center, 1400 McFarland Boulevard, N., Tuscaloosa, AL 35406; tel. 205/345–5500; J. Russell Peake, Administrator

ALASKA

Alaska Surgery Center, 4001 Laurel Street, Anchorage, AK 99508; tel. 907/563–3327, ext. 226; FAX. 907/562–7042; Louise M. Bjornstad, Executive Director

Alaska Women's Health Services, Inc., 4115 Lake Otis Drive, Anchorage, AK 99508; tel. 907/563–7228; FAX. 907/563–6278; Lisa Weston, Administrator

Geneva Woods Surgical Center, 3730 Rhone Circle, Suite 100, Anchorage, AK 99508; tel. 907/562–4764; J. David Williams, M.D.

ARIZONA

A.I.M.S. Outpatient Surgery, 3636 Stockton Hill Road, Kingman, AZ 86401; tel. 602/757–3636; Bill Margita

Academy Eye Surgery Center, 310 North Wilmot Road, Suite 106, Tucson, AZ 85711; tel. 602/885–6783; FAX. 602/885–5366; Joseph L. McCready, M.D., Administrator

Adobe Plastic Surgery, 2635 North Wyatt Drive, Tucson, AZ 85712; tel. 602/322–5295; Lucricia Banks

Aesthetic Reconstructive Associates, P.C., 4222 East Camelback, Suite H–150, Phoenix, AZ 85018; tel. 602/952–8100; FAX. 602/952–9519; Martin L. Johnson, M.D.

All–Med Surgical Center, 1107 East Bell Road, Suite 13, Phoenix, AZ 85022; tel. 602/789–9015; FAX. 602/789–8499; Alan Nickamin

Ambulatory Surgicenter, Inc., 1940 East Southern Avenue, Tempe, AZ 85282; tel. 602/820–7101; FAX. 602/820–9291; Sarann Hughes, RN, M.B.A., Administrator

Arizona Diagnostic and Surgical Center, 545 North Mesa Drive, Mesa, AZ 85201; tel. 602/461–4407; FAX. 602/461–4401; Lynnette King, RN, Administrator

Arizona Foot Institute, P.C., 1901 West Glendale Avenue, Phoenix, AZ 85021; tel. 602/246–0816; FAX. 602/433–2257; Barry Kaplan

Arizona Medical Clinic, 13640 North Plaza Del Rio Boulevard, Peoria, AZ 85381; tel. 602/876–3800; Larry D. Schwartz

Arizona Surgical Arts, Inc., 1245 North Wilmot Road, Tucson, AZ 85712; tel. 602/296–7550; Susan Bell, RN, Administrator

Barnet Dulaney Eye Center, 13760 North 93rd Avenue, Peoria, AZ 85381; tel. 602/977–4291; Ronald W. Barnet, M.D.

Barnet Dulaney Eye Center–Phoenix, 3333 East Camelback Road, Suite 122, Phoenix, AZ 85018; tel. 602/955–1000; FAX. 602/957–9202; Ronald W. Barnet, M.D.

Barnet Eye Center–Mesa, 6335 East Main Street, Mesa, AZ 85205; tel. 602/981–1000; FAX. 602/981–0467; Carolyn Miller, Administrator

Boswell Eye Institute, 10541 West Thunderbird Boulevard, Sun City, AZ 85351; tel. 602/933–3402; FAX. 602/972–5014; Jan Zellmann, Administrator

CIGNA Healthplan of Arizona, Outpatient Surgery, 755 East McDowell Road, Phoenix, AZ 85006; tel. 602/371–2500; Clifton Worsham, M.D., Administrator

Carriker Eye Center, 6425 North 16th Street, Phoenix, AZ 85106; tel. 602/274–1703; Richard G. Carriker, M.D.

Casa Blanca Clinic Ltd., 4001 East Baseline Road, Gilbert, AZ 85234, P.O. Box 11000, Mesa, AZ 85214–1000; tel. 602/926–6200; FAX. 602/926–6222; Stanley W. Decker, Administrator

Cataract Surgery Clinic, 215 South Power Road, Suite 112, Mesa, AZ 85208; tel. 602/981–1345; Robert P. Gervais, M.D., Administrator

Cochise Eye and Laser, PC, 2445 East Wilcox Drive, Sierra Vista, AZ 85635; tel. 602/458–8131; FAX. 602/458–0422; Julie A. Passwaters, Administrator

Desert Mountain Surgicenter, Ltd., 7776 Pointe Parkway West, Suite 135, Phoenix, AZ 85044; tel. 602/431–8500; FAX. 602/431–1677; David M. Creech, M.D.

Dooley Outpatient Surgery Center, 151 Riviera Drive, Lake Havasu City, AZ 86403; tel. 602/855–9477; FAX. 602/855–2983; William J. Dooley, Jr., M.D., Medical Director

East Valley Surgical Associates, Ltd., 6424 East Broadway Road, Suite 102, Mesa, AZ 85206; tel. 602/833–2216; Manuel J. Chee

Fifty–Ninth Avenue Surgical Facility, Ltd., 8608 North 59th Avenue, Glendale, AZ 85302; tel. 602/934–0272; FAX. 602/930–1891; Mark Gorman, Administrator

Fishkind and Bakewell Eye Care and Surgery Center, 5599 North Oracle Road, Tucson, AZ 85704; tel. 602/293–6740; Sally A. Sylvester, Administrator

Flagstaff Outpatient Surgery Center, 77 West Forest Avenue, Suite 306, Flagstaff, AZ 86001; tel. 520/773–2597; FAX. 520/773–2327; Jackie Mosier, RN

Footcare Surgi Center, 10249 West Thunderbird Suite 100, Sun City, AZ 85351; tel. 602/979–4466; Gary N. Friedlander, D.P.M.

Footcare Surgi Center of Northern Arizona, 10 West Columbus Avenue, Flagstaff, AZ 86001; tel. 602/774–4191; Dr. Edward L. Wiebe

Gary Hall Eye Surgery Institute, 2501 North 32nd Street, Phoenix, AZ 85008; tel. 602/957–6799; FAX. 602/957–0172; Gary W. Hall, M.D., Medical Director

Health Organizations, Agencies and Providers

Providers / Freestanding Ambulatory Surgery Centers

Glendale Surgicenter, 5757 West Thunderbird Road, Suite E–150, Glendale, AZ 85306; tel. 602/843–1900; FAX. 602/843–5607; Douglas G. Merrill, M.D., Medical Director

Grimm Eye Clinic and Cataract Institute, P.C., 1502 North Tucson Boulevard, Tucson, AZ 85716; tel. 602/326–4321; Stephen F. Grimm, M.D.; Eleanor M. Grimm, M.D.

Havasu Arthritis and Sports Medicine Institute, 1840 Mesquite Avenue, Suite G, Lake Havasu, AZ 86403; tel. 602/453–2663; Marc H. Zimmerman, M.D., Administrator

Havasu Foot and Ankle Surgi–Center, 90 Riviera Drive, Lake Havasu, AZ 86403; tel. 602/855–7800; FAX. 602/855–5392; Robert Novack, D.P.M., Director

Lear Surgery Clinic–Scottsdale, 7351 East Osborn Road, Suite 104, Scottsdale, AZ 85251–6452; tel. 602/990–9400; FAX. 602/990–2664; David E. Marine, Executive Director

Lear Surgery Clinic–Sun City, 10615 West Thunderbird, Suite A–100, Sun City, AZ 85351; tel. 602/974–9375; FAX. 602/977–2598; David E. Marine, Executive Director

M. Kent Moore, M.D. Ambulatory Surgical Centre, 605 West 10th Street, Mesa, AZ 85201; tel. 602/834–3868; M. Kent Moore

Mayo Clinic Scottsdale Ambulatory Surgery Center, 13400 East Shea Boulevard, Scottsdale, AZ 85259; tel. 602/301–8188; FAX. 602/301–8367; Duane H. Anderson, Administrator

Medivision of Tucson, Inc., 5632 East Fifth Street, Tucson, AZ 85711; tel. 602/790–8888; FAX. 602/790–1427; Clara Dupnik

Metro Ambulatory Surgery, Inc., a/k/a Metro Recovery Care Center, 3131 West Peoria Avenue, Phoenix, AZ 85029; tel. 602/375–1083; FAX. 602/789–6833; Virginia F. Palazzetti, RN, Chief Executive Officer

Mohave Surgery Center, Inc., 1919 Florence Avenue, Kingman, AZ 86401; tel. 602/753–5454; FAX. 602/753–4283; Frank Brown, Administrator

Moon Valley Surgery Center, Inc., 14045 North Seventh Street, Suite Two, Phoenix, AZ 85022; tel. 602/942–3966; Andrew E. Lowy

National Surgery Centers, Las Palmas Medical Plaza, 16620 North 40th Street, Building F–1, Phoenix, AZ 85032; tel. 602/867–7106; Virgina French, Administrator

Nogales Medical Clinic Outpatient Surgery, 480 North Morley Avenue, Nogales, AZ 85621; tel. 602/287–2726; FAX. 602/287–5959; Imogene A. Bell, Administrator

Osborn Ambulatory Surgical Center, 3330 North Second Street, Suite 300, Phoenix, AZ 85012; tel. 602/265–0113; FAX. 602/277–8580; Donna Klamm, RN, Administrator

Outpatient Surgical Care, Ltd., 1530 West Glendale, Suite 105, Phoenix, AZ 85021; tel. 602/995–3395; FAX. 602/995–1853; James Kennedy, Administrator

Outpatient Surgical Center, 456 North Mesa Drive, Mesa, AZ 85201; tel. 602/464–8000; FAX. 602/969–7107; Maddie Dauernheim, Administrator

Outpatient Surgical and Recovery Care Center, 3624 Wells Fargo Avenue, Scottsdale, AZ 85251; tel. 602/481–4958; Barbara Hazel, Administrator

Phoenix Center for Outpatient Surgery, 1950 West Heatherbrae Drive, Suite Seven, Phoenix, AZ 85015; tel. 602/230–0437; Eric Reimts, Administrator

Porter, Michael, D.P.M., 3620 East Campbell, Suite B, Phoenix, AZ 85018; tel. 602/954–6224; Michael Porter

Prescott Outpatient Surgery Center, Inc., 815 Ainsworth Drive, Prescott, AZ 86301; tel. 602/778–9770; Gail Reidhead, Administrative Director

Prescott Urocenter, Ltd., 811 Ainsworth, Suite 101, Prescott, AZ 86301; tel. 602/771–5282; Gregory Oldani

Romania Eyecare, P.C., 2820 North Glassford Hill Road, Suite 106, Prescott Valley, AZ 86314; tel. 602/775–5606; FAX. 602/772–4999; Linda Talerico, Administrator

Safford Surgi–Care, 825 20th Avenue, Safford, AZ 85546; tel. 602/428–6930; FAX. 602/428–7272; James Holder, O.D.

Santa Cruz Ambulatory Surgical Center, 699 West Ajo Way, Tucson, AZ 85713; tel. 602/746–1711; Richard Edward Quint, Administrator

Scottsdale Eye Surgery Center, P.C., 3320 North Miller Road, Scottsdale, AZ 85251; tel. 602/949–1208; Karen Borowiak, Administrator

Scottsdale Outpatient Surgery Center, P.C., 3501 North Scottsdale Road, Suite 230, Scottsdale, AZ 85251; tel. 602/946–5665; James McDowell

Southwestern Eye Center–Casa Grande, 1515 East Florence Boulevard, Casa Grande, AZ 85222; tel. 602/426–9224; FAX. 602/396–6362; Karen Buck, Administrator

Southwestern Eye Center–Yuma, 2179 West 24th Street, Yuma, AZ 85364; tel. 602/726–4120; FAX. 602/341–0315; Dr. Lothaire Bluth, Administrator

Southwestern Eye Surgicenter–Dobson Ranch, 2150 South Dobson Road, Mesa, AZ 85202; tel. 602/839–2862; FAX. 602/839–2862; Pat Bray, RN, CRNA, Director, Surgical and Medical Services

Southwestern Eye Surgicenter–Flagstaff, 1355 North Beaver, Flagstaff, AZ 86001; tel. 602/773–1184; Robbie Hughes, RN, Director, Surgical Services

Sun City Endoscopy Center, Inc., 13203 North 103rd Avenue, Suite C 3, Sun City, AZ 85351; tel. 602/972–2116; John E. Phelps, M.D., Medical Director

Sun City Surgical Center, 13260 North 94th Drive, Suite 300, Peoria, AZ 85381; tel. 602/277–0619; FAX. 602/933–5787; H. William Reese, D.P.M., Director

Surgi–Care, 5115 North Central Avenue, Suite B, Phoenix, AZ 85012; tel. 602/264–1818; FAX. 602/264–2172; Ellison F. Herro, M.D., Administrator

Surgi–Tech Centers, 3271 North Civic Center Plaza, Suite Three, Scottsdale, AZ 85251; tel. 602/994–5978; FAX. 602/990–9397; Richard Jacoby, D.P.M., President

SurgiCenter, 1040 East McDowell Road, Phoenix, AZ 85006; tel. 602/258–1521; FAX. 602/340–0889; Sharon Shafer, RN, Administrator

Surgical Eye Center of Arizona, Inc., 555 West Catalina Drive, Suite 100, Phoenix, AZ 85013; tel. 602/277–7997; FAX. 602/277–0772; Donald R. Miles, M.D., Administrator

Sutter Tucson Surgery Center, 310 North Wilmot Road, Suite 309, Tucson, AZ 85711; tel. 602/296–7080; FAX. 602/886–6518; Aaron Chatterson, Administrative Director

Swagel Wootton Eye Center, 220 South 63rd Street, Mesa, AZ 85206; tel. 602/641–3937; FAX. 602/924–5096; S. Joyce Graham

T.A.S.I. Surgery Center, 5585 North Oracle Road, Suite B, Tucson, AZ 85704; tel. 602/293–4730; John A. Pierce, M.D., Medical Director

Tempe Surgical Center, Inc., 2000 East Southern Avenue, Suite 101, Tempe, AZ 85282; tel. 602/838–9313; Richard F. Pavese, M.D.

The Cataract Institute, Ltd.–Sun City, 9425 West Bell Road, Sun City, AZ 85351; tel. 602/974–1000; FAX. 602/933–5462; David D. Dulaney, Executive Director

The Cataract Institute–Mesa, 6335 East Main Street, Mesa, AZ 85205; tel. 602/981–1000; David D. Dulaney, M.D., Medical Director

Thomas–Davis SurgiCenter, P.C., 750 North Alvernon Way, Tucson, AZ 85711; tel. 602/322–8440; FAX. 602/322–2653; Vicki Gagnier, RN, Manager

Valley Outpatient Surgery Center, 160 West University Drive, Mesa, AZ 85201; tel. 602/835–7373; FAX. 602/969–7981; Craig R. Cassidy, D.O., President

Warner Medical Park Outpatient Surgery, Inc., 604 West Warner Road, Building A, Chandler, AZ 85224; tel. 602/899–2571; FAX. 602/899–4263; Robert Thunberg, Managing Director

White Mountain Ambulatory Surgery Center, 2650 East Show Low Lake Road, Suite Two, Show Low, AZ 85901; tel. 602/537–4240; William J. Waldo

Yuma Outpatient Surgery Center, L.P., 2475 Avenue A, Suite B, Yuma, AZ 85364; tel. 602/726–6910; FAX. 602/726–7423; Cairne–Lee Larson, Facility Manager

ARKANSAS

Ambulatory Surgical Center, Inc., d/b/a Fort Smith Surgi–Center, 7306A Rogers Avenue, Fort Smith, AR 72903; tel. 501/452–7333; A. Joy Hyden

Arkansas Ear, Nose and Throat Clinic, P.A., Ambulatory Surgery Center, Medical Towers I, Suite 900, 9601 Lile Drive, Little Rock, AR 72205; tel. 501/227–8501; Donna Pool, RN, Administrator

Arkansas Endoscopy Center, P.A., 9501 Lile Drive, Suite 100, Little Rock, AR 72205; tel. 501/224–9100; FAX. 501/224–0420; Ronald D. Hardin, M.D.

Arkansas Surgery Center, 10 Hospital Circle, Batesville, AR 72501; tel. 501/793–4040; Fredric J. Sloan, M.D., Administrator

BEC Surgery Center, One Mercy Lane, Suite 201, P.O. Box 6409, Hot Springs, AR 71902; tel. 501/623–0755; Terry D. Brown

Central Arkansas Surgery Center, Inc., d/b/a Physicians Surgery Center, 1024 North University Avenue, Little Rock, AR 72207; tel. 501/663–0158; FAX. 501/663–4652; Caroline Williams, Administrator

Dempsey–McKee, Inc., d/b/a McKee Outpatient Surgery Center, 601 East Matthews, Jonesboro, AR 72401; tel. 501/935–6396; FAX. 501/935–4063; Terry V. DePriest, Administrator

Doctors Surgery Center, 303 West Polk Street, Suite B, West Memphis, AR 72301; tel. 501/732–2100; Doris Davis, Administrator

Gastroenterology and Surgery Center Of Arkansas, P.A., 8908 Kanis Road, Little Rock, AR 72205; tel. 501/227–7688; FAX. 501/225–2930; Alonzo D. Williams, M.D., Medical Director

Head and Neck Surgery Clinic, P.A., 8500 West Markham Street, Suite 316, Little Rock, AR 72205–2456; tel. 501/224–1044; FAX. 501/224–0447; Ellery C. Gay, M.D., Administrator

Holt–Krock Clinic, 1500 Dodson Avenue, Fort Smith, AR 72901; tel. 501/788–4000; Harold H. Mings, M.D., Chief Executive Officer

Hot Springs Outpatient Surgery, P.A., 100 Ridgeway Boulevard, Suite Seven, Hot Springs, AR 71901; tel. 501/624–4464; FAX. 501/624–4602; Edwin L. Harper, M.D., Administrator

Little Rock Diagnostic Clinic ASC, 10001 Lile Drive, Little Rock, AR 72205; tel. 501/227–8000, ext. 845; Roger J. St. Onge, Administrator

Little Rock Surgery Center, 8820 Knoedl Court, Little Rock, AR 72205; tel. 501/224–6767; FAX. 501/224–8203; Pamela J. Hooper, Administrator

Lowery Medical/Surgical Eye Center, P.A., 105 Central Avenue, Searcy, AR 72143; tel. 501/268–7154; FAX. 501/268–9071; Benjamin R. Lowery, M.D., Administrator

North Hills Gastroenterology Endoscopy Center, Inc., 3344 North Futrall Drive, Fayetteville, AR 72703; tel. 501/582–7280; William C. Martin, M.D.

Northeast Arkansas Surgery Center, Inc., 505 East Matthews, Jonesboro, AR 72401; tel. 501/972–1723; FAX. 501/972–5941; Carol D. Crawford, Administrator

Ozark Eye Center, 360 Highway Five North, Mountain Home, AR 72653; tel. 501/425–2277; Rick Galkoski, Administrator

Physicians Day Surgery Center, 3805 West 28th, Pine Bluff, AR 71603; tel. 501/536–4100; FAX. 501/536–3100; Joan Fletcher, Administrator

South Arkansas Outpatient Surgi–Center, 4800 South Hazel, Suite B, Pine Bluff, AR 71603; tel. 501/536–0798; FAX. 501/536–0865; Jim Stewart, Administrator

South Arkansas Surgery Center, 4310 South Mulberry, Pine Bluff, AR 71603; tel. 501/535–5719; Gayle B. Shelton, CMA Administrator

Providers / Freestanding Ambulatory Surgery Centers

Springdale Ambulatory Surgery Center, P.A., 800 Searcy Street, Springdale, AR 72764; tel. 501/756–2720; Cathy Battle, Administrator

The Center for Day Surgery, 4200 Jenny Lind, Suite A, Fort Smith, AR 72901; tel. 501/648–9496; Deena Lee, RN, Administrator

☐ **The Ear and Nose–Throat Clinic, P.A. Outpatient Surgery Center,** 1200 Medical Towers Building, 9601 Lile Drive, Little Rock, AR 72205; tel. 501/227–5050; Joseph R. Phillips, RN, Administrator

The Gastro–Intestinal Center, 405 North University, Little Rock, AR 72205; tel. 501/663–1074; James G. Dunlap, Administrator

CALIFORNIA

A New You Plastic Surgery Center, 250 East Yale Loop, Suite A, Irvine, CA 92714; tel. 714/857–5002; Martin Elliott, M.D., Administrator

Aesthetic Facial Surgery Center of Menlo Park, 2200 Sand Hill Road, Suite 130, Menlo Park, CA 94025; tel. 415/854–6444; Harry Mittleman

Aestheticare Outpatient Surgery Center, 30260 Rancho Viejo Road, San Juan Capistrano, CA 92675; tel. 714/661–1700; FAX. 714/661–4913; Ronald E. Moser, M.D.

Ambulatory Surgery Center of Santa Cruz Medical Clinic, 2025 Soquel Avenue, Santa Cruz, CA 95062; tel. 408/423–4111; FAX. 408/423–4515; Wayne V. Boss, President, Chief Executive Officer

Ambulatory Surgical Center of Chico, 1950 East 20th Street, Suite 102, Chico, CA 95928; tel. 916/343–1674; Robert G. Basinger, D.P.M.

Ambulatory Surgical Center of Southern California, 880 South Atlantic Boulevard, Monterey Park, CA 91754; tel. 213/483–9080; Marco Sprintis, M.D.

Ambulatory Surgical Center of the Zeiter Eye, 117 North San Joaquin Street, Stockton, CA 95202; tel. 209/466–5566; Donna M. Tschirky

Ambulatory Surgical Center, Inc., 14400 Bear Valley Road, Victorville, CA 92392; tel. 916/951–5162; FAX. 818/368–2290; Garey L. Weber, D.P.M., Administrator

Ambulatory Surgical Centers, Inc., 18952 Mac Arthur Boulevard, Suite 102, Irvine, CA 92715; tel. 714/833–3406; FAX. 818/368–2290; Garey L. Weber, D.P.M., Administrator

Anacapa Ambulatory Surgical Center, 2460 Ponderosa Drive, Suite A–116, Camarillo, CA 93010; tel. 805/484–4226; Carol Beckton, Manager

Anaheim Surgical Center, 1324 South Euclid Street, Anaheim, CA 92802; tel. 714/533–9880; FAX. 714/533–1802; Robert W. Brown, Administrator

Antelope Valley Surgery Center, 44301 North Lorimer Avenue, Lancaster, CA 93534; tel. 805/940–1112; FAX. 805/940–6856; Silvia Penna

Apple Valley Surgery Center, 18122 Outer Highway 18, Apple Valley, CA 92307; tel. 619/946–1170; FAX. 619/946–2646; Virginia L. Budington, Administrator

Arcadia Outpatient Surgery, Inc., 614 West Duarte Road, Arcadia, CA 91007; tel. 818/445–4714; Sandy Lazare, Administrator

Arlington Podiatry Surgery Center, 7310 Magnolia Avenue, Riverside, CA 92504; tel. 909/354–8787; FAX. 909/354–0350; James A. De Silva, Administrator

Arrowhead Surgical Center, Inc., 29099 Hospital Road, Suite 110, P.O. Box 1130, Lake Arrowhead, CA 92352; tel. 909/336–3778; FAX. 909/336–3202; Basil N. Spitros, M.D.

Aspen Outpatient Center, 2750 North Sycamore Drive, Simi Valley, CA 93065; tel. 805/583–5923; FAX. 805/583–0652; Jay Evans, Administrator

Atherton Plastic Surgery Center, 3351 El Camino Real, Suite 201, Atherton, CA 94027; tel. 415/363–0300; FAX. 415/363–0302; David Apfelberg

Auburn Outpatient Surgery and Diagnostic Center, 3123 Professional Drive, Suite 100, Auburn, CA 95603; tel. 916/888–8899; FAX. 916/888–1464; Charles Smith, Administrator

Bakersfield Surgery Center, 2120 19th Street, Bakersfield, CA 93301; tel. 805/323–2020; FAX. 805/323–6552; Betty J. Thomas, Administrator

Barr Eye Surgery Center,, an EquiVision, Inc, affiliate, 1805 North California Street, Stockton, CA 95204; tel. 209/948–3241; FAX. 209/948–9321; Richard G. Barr, M.D.

Beverly Surgical Center, 105 West Beverly Boulevard, Montebello, CA 90640–4375; tel. 213/728–5400; FAX. 213/887–0058; James G. Ovieda, Administrator

Blackhawk Surgery Center, Inc., 4165 Blackhawk, Danville, CA 94506; tel. 510/736–7881; Juris Bunkis, Administrator

Bonaventure Surgery Center, 221 North Jackson Avenue, San Jose, CA 95116; tel. 408/729–2848; FAX. 408/729–2884; Virginia Field

Brockton Surgical Center, 5905 Brockton Avenue, Suite B, Riverside, CA 92506; tel. 909/686–5373; Michael N. Durrant, D.P.M.

Bruce A. Kaplan, M.D., 39000 Bob Hope Drive, Wright Building, Suite 209, Rancho Mirage, CA 92270; tel. 619/346–5603; FAX. 619/346–5604; Jessie Schumaker

Camden Surgery Center of Beverly Hills, 414 North. Camden Drive, Suite 800, Beverly Hills, CA 90210; tel. 310/859–3991; FAX. 310/275–5079; Yasmin Sibulo

Capistrano Surgicenter, Inc., 30280 Rancho Viejo Road, San Juan Capistrano, CA 92675; tel. 714/248–5757; FAX. 714/248–9339; Jacqueline P. Klein, President

Cataract Surgery Center, 433 North Prairie Avenue, Inglewood, CA 90301; tel. 213/671–7172; Leroy W. Vaughn, M.D., Administrator

Center for Ambulatory Medicine and Surgery, 111 East Noble Avenue, Visalia, CA 93277; tel. 209/739–8383; FAX. 209/739–7929; James J. Shea, M.D., Administrator

Center for Endoscopy, 3921 Waring Road, Suite B, Oceanside, CA 92056; tel. 619/940–6300; FAX. 619/724–2909; Barbara Bockover, RN

Center for Sight, Northern California, 900 Butte Street, Redding, CA 96001; tel. 916/241–4044; FAX. 916/241–1408; Jan McEwen, Administrator

☐ **Center for Surgery of Encinitas,** 477 North El Camino Real, Suite C–100, Encinitas, CA 92024; tel. 619/942–8800; FAX. 619/942–0106; Joseph Grover, RN, Administrator

Central Coast Surgery Center, 1941 Johnson Avenue, Suite 103, San Luis Obispo, CA 93401; tel. 805/546–9999; FAX. 804/546–8904; Terri Nefores, RN, Administrator

Channel Islands Surgicenter, 2300 Wankel Way, Oxnard, CA 93030; tel. 805/485–1908; FAX. 805/485–5767; Mary K. Fish, Administrator

Children's Surgery Center, 744 Fifty–Second Street, Oakland, CA 94609; tel. 510/428–3133; Tony Paap

Community Surgery Centre, 17190 Bernado Center Drive, Suite 100, San Diego, CA 92128; tel. 619/675–3270; FAX. 619/675–3260; Regina S. Boore, B.S.N., M.S.

Corona Del Mar Plastic Surgery, 1101 Bayside Drive, Suite 100, Corona Del Mar, CA 92625; tel. 714/644–5000; W. Graham Wood, M.D.

Corona Outpatient Surgicenter, Surgery Center of Corona, 1124 South Main Street, Suite 102, Corona, CA 91720; tel. 909/737–9091; FAX. 909/737–9093; Teri Lynn Ransbury, Administrator

Cypress Outpatient Surgical Center, Inc., 1665 Dominican Way, Suite 120, Santa Cruz, CA 95065; tel. 408/476–6943; FAX. 408/475–0733; William L. Adams, M.D., President, Medical Director

Cypress Surgery Center, 842 South Akers Road, Visalia, CA 93277; tel. 209/740–4094; FAX. 209/740–4100; Jack Waller

Danville Ambulatory Surgery Center, 905 San Ramon Valley Boulevard, Suite 110B, Danville, CA 94526; tel. 510/831–1317; FAX. 510/831–3609; Kay Ellis, RN, Clinical Coordinator

De La Vina Surgicenter Medical Group, 2323 De La Vina, Suite 103, Santa Barbara, CA 93105; tel. 805/682–5065; FAX. 805/682–5921; Susan Robuck, Administrator

Doctors Surgery Center of Whittier, 8135 South Painter Avenue, Suite 103, Whittier, CA 90602; tel. 310/945–8961; FAX. 310/698–3578; Veronica Coughenour, RN

Doctors Surgical Center, Inc., 9461 Grindlay Street, Suite 102, Cypress, CA 90630; tel. 714/995–3001; R. Wayne Ives, Administrator

E. N. T. Facial Surgery Center, 1351 East Spruce, Fresno, CA 93720; tel. 209/432–3724; FAX. 209/432–8759; JoAnn Loforti, RN, Division of Nursing

East Bay Medical Surgical Center, 20998 Redwood Road, Castro Valley, CA 94546; tel. 510/538–2828; FAX. 510/538–2508; Yoshitsugu Teramoto, M.D., Administrator

El Camino Surgery Center, 2480 Grant Road, Mountain View, CA 94040–4300; tel. 415/961–1200; FAX. 415/960–7041; Nancy Webb

Endoscopy Center of Southern California, 2336 Santa Monica Boulevard, Suite 204, Santa Monica, CA 90404; tel. 310/453–4477; FAX. 310/453–4811; Parviz D. Afshani

Escondido Surgery Center, 343 East Second Avenue, Escondido, CA 92025; tel. 619/480–6606; FAX. 619/480–6671; Marvin W. Levenson, M.D., Managing Medical Director

Estudillo Ambulatory Surgery Center, 345 Estudillo Avenue, P.O. Box 1090, San Leandro, CA 94577–0126; tel. 510/483–5114; FAX. 510/483–0396; Sheila L. Cook, Chief Executive Officer

Eye Center of Northern California Surgicenter, 6500 Fairmount Avenue, Suite Two, El Cerrito, CA 94530; tel. 510/525–2600; FAX. 510/524–1887; William Ellis

Eye Life Institute, 6283 Clark Road, Suite Seven, Paradise, CA 95969; tel. 916/877–2020; Almary Hivale, RN

Eye Surgery Center of Southern California, Inc./Med. Group, 2023 W. Vista Way, Suite E, Vista, CA 92083; tel. 619/941–8152; FAX. 619/726–4822; Regg V. Antle, M.D., Medical Director

FHP Outpatient Surgery Center, 19066 Magnolia Avenue, Huntington Beach, CA 92646; tel. 714/968–0068; FAX. 714/968–4967; Raelynn Price, Administrator

Feather River Surgery Center, 370 Del Norte Avenue, Yuba City, CA 95991; tel. 916/751–4800; FAX. 916/751–4884; Valerie Macpherson, Preoperative Coordinator

Foothill Ambulatory Surgery Center, 1030 East Foothill Boulevard, Suite 101B, Upland, CA 91786; tel. 909/981–5859; FAX. 909/981–8293; Montra M. Kanok, M.D.

Forest Surgery Center, 2110 Forest Avenue, San Jose, CA 95128; tel. 408/297–3432; FAX. 408/298–3338; Bonnie J. Weinert, RN, Administrator

Fort Sutter Surgery Center, 2801 K Street, Suite 525, Sacramento, CA 95816; tel. 916/733–5017; FAX. 916/733–8738; Bill Davis, Administrator

Fountain Valley Outpatient Surgical Center, 11160 Warner Avenue, Suite 421, Fountain Valley, CA 92708; tel. 714/751–5621; Eugene Elliott, M.D.

Four Thirty–Six North Bedford Surgicenter, Inc., 436 North Bedford, Suite 101, Beverly Hills, CA 90210; tel. 310/278–0188; FAX. 310/278–1791; Robert Kotler, M.D.

Fritch Eye Care Center, 2525 Eye Street, Suite A and B, Bakersfield, CA 93301; tel. 805/327–8511; FAX. 805/327–9809; Charles D. Fritch, M.D.

Frost Street Outpatient Surgical Center, Inc., 8008 Frost Street, Suite 200, San Diego, CA 92123; tel. 619/576–8320; Jacqueline McWilliams

GastroDiagnostics, A Medical Group, 1140 West La Veta, Suite 550, Orange, CA 92668; tel. 714/835–5100; FAX. 714/835–5567; Stephanie Quinn, Administrator

Glendale Eye Medical Group, Inc., 607 North Central, Suite 103, Glendale, CA 91203; tel. 818/956–1010; FAX. 818/543–6083; James M. McCaffery, M.D.

Glenwood Surgical Center, L.P., 8945 Magnolia Avenue, Suite 200, Riverside, CA 92503; tel. 909/688–7270; Calvin Nash

Golden Empire Surgical Center, 1519 Graces Highway, Suite 103, Delano, CA 93215; tel. 805/721–7900; Lucy Lara

Providers / Freestanding Ambulatory Surgery Centers

Golden State Eye Center, 1001 Tower Way, Suite 150 B, Bakersfield, CA 93309; tel. 805/324–6406; FAX. 805/327–4381; Ronald Morton, M.D., F.A.C.S.

Golden Triangle Surgicenter, 25405 Hancock Avenue, Suite 103, Murrieta, CA 92562; tel. 714/698–4670; FAX. 714/698–4675; Marc Jones

Golden West Pain Therapy Center, 25405 Hancock Avenue, Suite 110, Murrieta, CA 92562–5964; tel. 909/698–4710; FAX. 909/698–4715; Marlene Wilson, Office Manager

Greater Long Beach Endoscopy Center, 2880 Atlantic Avenue, Suite 180, Long Beach, CA 90806; tel. 310/426–2606; FAX. 310/426–5866; Diane Pandora–Lass, RN, Director, Nursing

Greater Sacramento Surgery Center, 2288 Auburn Boulevard, Suite 201, Sacramento, CA 95821; tel. 916/929–7229; FAX. 916/929–2590; Susan Brunone, MHS, Administrator

Grossmont Surgery Center, 8881 Fletcher Parkway, Suite 100, La Mesa, CA 92041; tel. 619/698–0930; Jacqueline McWilliams, Administrator

Hemet Cataract Surgery Clinic, 162 North Santa Fe, Hemet, CA 92343; tel. 714/929–3200; Stephen K. Schaller, M.D., Administrator

Hemet Endoscopy Center, 2390 East Florida Avenue, Suite 101, Hemet, CA 92544; tel. 909/652–2252; FAX. 909/925–9252; Milan S. Chakrabarty, M.D.

Hemet Healthcare Surgicenter, 301 North San Jacinto Avenue, Hemet, CA 92543; tel. 909/765–1717; Kali Chaudhuri, M.D.

Henry Tahl, M.D., 790 East Latham, Hemet, CA 92343; tel. 714/658–3224

Hesperia Podiatry Surgery Center, 14661 Main Street, Hesperia, CA 92345; tel. 619/244–0222; William S. Beal

Hi–Desert Surgery Center, 18002 Outer Highway 18, Apple Valley, CA 92307; tel. 619/242–5505; FAX. 619/242–3502; Venkat R. Vangala, M.D.

High Desert Endoscopy, 18523 Corwin Road, Suite H2, Apple Valley, CA 92307; tel. 619/242–3000; FAX. 619/262–1802; Raman S. Poola, M.D., Administrator

Holy Cross Surgery Center, 11550 Indian Hills Road, Suite 160, Mission Hills, CA 91345; tel. 818/898–1061; FAX. 818/898–3866; Laura Moore, Administrator

Huntington Outpatient Surgery Center, 797 South Fair Oaks Avenue, Pasadena, CA 91105; tel. 818/397–3173; FAX. 818/397–8003; Sandra Bidlack, Administrator

Imperial Valley Surgery Center, 608 G Street, Brawley, CA 92227; tel. 619/344–IIOl; FAX. 619/344–4985; Vida C. Baron, M.D., Administrator

Inland Endoscopy Center, 10408 Industrial Circle, Redlands, CA 92374; tel. 909/796–0363; FAX. 909/796–0762; Khushal Stanisai

Inland Eye Surgicenter, 361 North San Jacinto, Hemet, CA 92543; tel. 909/652–4343; R. Michael Duffin, M.D., Medical Director

Inland Midwife Services–The Birth Center, 251 Cajon Street, Suite B, Redlands, CA 92373; tel. 909/335–6241; Leonette Clayson

Inland Surgery Center, 1620 Laurel Avenue, Redlands, CA 92373; tel. 909/793–4701; FAX. 909/792–6397; Janet Greenfield

Irvine Plastic Surgery Center, 16300 San Canyon Avenue, Suite 1011, Irvine, CA 92717; tel. 714/727–3999; Donald I. Altman, M.D.

Kaiser Ambulatory Surgical Center, 2025 Morse Avenue, Sacramento, CA 95825; tel. 916/973–7675

Kaiser Ambulatory Surgical Center, 10725 International Drive, Rancho Cordova, CA 95670; tel. 916/973–7675; FAX. 916/631–2013; Angela Hardiman, RN, M.S., Manager

Kaiser Permanente Ambulatory Surgery Center, 7300 North Fresno Street, Fresno, CA 93720; tel. 209/448–4500, ext. 4040; FAX. 209/448–4142; Edward Glavis, Vice President, Area Manager

Kaiser Permanente Medical Facility–Stockton, 7373 West Lane, Stockton, CA 95210; tel. 209/476–3300; Jose R. Rivera, Administrator

Klaus Kuehn, M.D., Inc.–Eye Center, 1920 North Waterman Avenue, San Bernardino, CA 92404; tel. 714/882–3728; FAX. 714/882–3019; Klaus Kuehn, M.D., Director

L.A. Surgery Center, 12660 Riverside Drive, Suite 300, North Hollywood, CA 91607; tel. 818/985–1100; FAX. 818/985–1915; Dale Bowman, RN, Administrator

La Jolla Cosmetic Surgery Centre, 484 Prospect Street, La Jolla, CA 92037; tel. 619/456–0484; Melvin I. Dinner

La Jolla Gastroenterology Medical Group, Inc., Endoscopy Center, 9850 Genesee Avenue, Suite 980, La Jolla, CA 92037; tel. 619/453–5200; FAX. 619/453–5753; Otto T. Nebel, M.D., Medical Director

La Veta Surgical Center, 725 West La Veta, Suite 270, Orange, CA 92668; tel. 714/744–0900; Jamie Torrez, Manager

Laser and Skin Surgery Center of La Jolla, 9850 Genesee Avenue, Suite 480, La Jolla, CA 92037; tel. 619/558–2424; Nancy Fritzenkotter

Lassen Surgery Center, 103 Fair Drive, P.O. Box 1150, Susanville, CA 96130; tel. 916/257–7773; FAX. 916/257–2939; Deborah L. Sutton, Medical Staff Secretary

Lodi Outpatient Surgical Center, 521 South Ham Lane, Suite F, Lodi, CA 95242; tel. 209/333–0905; FAX. 209/333–0219; Marklin E. Brown, Administrator

Loma Linda Foot Clinic, Ambulatory Surgical Center, 11332 Mount View Avenue, Suite A, Loma Linda, CA 92354; tel. 714/796–3707; FAX. 909/796–3709; Sheldon Collis, D.P.M., Administrator

Los Gatos Surgical Center, 15195 National Avenue, Los Gatos, CA 95032; tel. 408/356–0454; Alan E. Bickel, M.D., Medical Director

Los Robles Surgicenter, 2190 Lynn Road, Suite 100, Thousand Oaks, CA 91360; tel. 805/497–3737; FAX. 805/373–8878; Le Anne Schai, Administrative Director

Lynn Eye Surgery Center, 2230 Lynn Road, Thousand Oaks, CA 91360; tel. 805/495–0458

M/S Surgery Center, 3510 Martin Luther King Boulevard, Lynwood, CA 90262; tel. 310/635–7550; FAX. 310/603–8749; John H. Shammas, M.D., Medical Director

Madera Ambulatory Endoscopy Center, 1015 West Yosemite Avenue, Suite 101, Madera, CA 93637; tel. 209/673–4000; FAX. 209/673–1430; Naeem M. Akhtar, M.D.

Magnolia Outpatient Surgery Center, 14571 Magnolia Street, Suite 107, Westminster, CA 92683; tel. 714/898–6448; Arthur Lu, M.D., Administrator

Magnolia Plastic Surgery Center, 10694 Magnolia Avenue, Riverside, CA 92503; tel. 909/688–8660; Alexander Carli

Martel Eye Surgical Center, 11216 Trinity River, Suite G, Rancho Cordova, CA 95670; tel. 916/635–6161; FAX. 916/635–5145; Joseph Martel, M.D.

McHenry Surgery Center, 1524 McHenry Street, Suite 240, Modesto, CA 95350; tel. 209/576–2900; FAX. 209/575–5815; Syd Fuentes, RN, Director

Medical Arts Ambulatory Surgery Center, 205 South West Street, Suite B, Visalia, CA 93291; tel. 209/625–9601; FAX. 209/625–3124; Thomas F. Mitts, M.D., Administrator

Medical Plaza Orthopedic Surgery Center, 1301 20th Street, Suite 140, Santa Monica, CA 90404; tel. 310/315–0333; FAX. 310/315–0341; Kevin M. Ehrhart, M.D., Medical Director

Merced Ambulatory Endoscopy Center, 750 W. Olive Avenue, Suite 107A, Merced, CA 95348; tel. 209/384–3116; Madhu K. Kris, M.D.

Mercy Surgical and Diagnostic Center, 3303 North M Street, Merced, CA 95348; tel. 209/384–3533; FAX. 209/384–3929; Lynda Pitts, Administrator

Mirage Center Outpatient Surgery, 39–935 Vista Del Sol, P.O. Box 6000, Rancho Mirage, CA 92270; tel. 619/779–9989; James Merson, M.D.

Mission Ambulatory Surgicenter, Ltd., 26730 Crown Valley Parkway, First Floor, Mission Viejo, CA 92691; tel. 714/364–6880; FAX. 714/364–5372; Thomas H. Catlett, Administrator

Mission Valley Surgery Centre, 39263 Mission Boulevard, Fremont, CA 94539; tel. 510/796–4500; FAX. 510/796–4573; Sarb S. Hundal, M.D.

Mission Viejo Surgi Center, 26732 Crown Valley Parkway, Suite 331, Mission Viejo, CA 92691; tel. 714/364–1007; Suuan Christiansen

Monterey Bay Endoscopy Center, 833 Cass Street, Suite B, Monterey, CA 93940; tel. 408/375–3598; FAX. 408/375–1478; James Farrow, Administrator

Moreno Valley Ambulatory Surgery Center, 24384 Sunnymead Boulevard, Moreno Valley, CA 92388; tel. 714/247–8080; FAX. 714/247–9381; Ahmad Javaheri, M.D., Administrator

Mt. Diablo Surgery Center, d/b/a Diablo Valley Surgery, 2222 East Street, Suite 200, Concord, CA 94520; tel. 510/671–2222; FAX. 510/671–2672; Virginia Goodrich, Administrator

Napa Surgery Center, 3444 Valle Verde Drive, Napa, CA 94558; tel. 707/252–9660; Eric Grigsby, M.D., Medical Director

Newport Beach Orange Coast Endoscopy Center, 1525 Superior Avenue, Suite 114, Newport Beach, CA 92663; tel. 714/646–6999; Donald Abrahm

Newport Beach Surgery Center, 361 Hospital Road, Suite 124, Newport Beach, CA 92663; tel. 714/631–0988, ext. 3002; FAX. 714/631–2036; Brad DeGeorge, Administrator

North Anaheim Surgicenter, 1154 North Euclid, Anaheim, CA 92801; tel. 714/635–6272; FAX. 714/635–0943; Donna Burkhalter

North Coast Surgery Center, 3903 Waring Road, Oceanside, CA 92056; tel. 619/940–0997; FAX. 619/940–0407; Donna Danley, Administrator

North County Outpatient Surgery Center, 1101 Las Tablas Road, P.O. Box 147, Templeton, CA 93465; tel. 805/434–1333; FAX. 805/434–3171; Carol Alexander, RN, Director of Nursing

Northern California Kidney Stone Center, 15195 National Avenue, Suite 204, Los Gatos, CA 95032; tel. 408/358–2111; FAX. 408/356–2359; John Kersten Kraft, Medical Director

Northridge Surgery Center, 8327 Reseda Boulevard, Northridge, CA 91324; tel. 818/993–3131; FAX. 818/993–3347; Cindy B. Gerstl, Executive Director

Optima Ophthalmic Medical Associates, Inc., 1237 B Street, Hayward, CA 94541–2977; tel. 510/886–3937; Nora J. McQuinn

Orange County Litho Center, Inc., 12555 Garden Grove Boulevard, Suite 200, Garden Grove, CA 92643; tel. 714/530–6000; Guy A. Biagiotti, M.D.

Orange County Nasal and Sinus Surgery Center, 3420 Bristol Street, Suite 751, Costa Mesa, CA 92626; tel. 714/432–1438; Robert Beltran, M.D.

Orange Surgical Services, 302 West La Veta Avenue, Suite 100, Orange, CA 92666; tel. 714/771–3432; Elizabeth E. Grant, RN, M.S.

Out–Patient Surgery Center, 17752 Beach Boulevard, Huntington Beach, CA 92647; tel. 714/842–1426; FAX. 714/847–1503; Madelyn Tinkler, Administrator

Outpatient Care Surgery Center North, 5225 Kearney Villa Way, San Diego, CA 92123; tel. 619/278–1661; Ronald L. Gertsch, M.D.

Outpatient Care Surgery Center South, 5205 Kearny Villa Way, Suite 110, San Diego, CA 92123; tel. 619/278–1611; FAX. 619/278–5853; Ronald Gertsch, M.D.

Outpatient Eye Surgery Center of the Desert, 39700 Bob Hope Drive, Suite 111, Rancho Mirage, CA 92270; tel. 619/340–3937; FAX. 619/340–1940; Dorothy Milauskas, Administrator

Outpatient Surgical Center, 999 North Tustin Avenue, Suite 105, Santa Ana, CA 92705; tel. 714/547–5376; FAX. 714/835–4735; C. H. Baick, M.D.

PFC Surgicenter, 3445 Pacific Court Highway, Suite 110, Torrance, CA 90505; tel. 213/539–9100; Rifaat Salem, M.D., Ph.D.

Pacific Eye Institute, 555 North 13th Avenue, Upland, CA 91786; tel. 909/982–8846; FAX. 909/994–3967; Robert Fabricant, M.D., FACS, Medical Director

Providers / Freestanding Ambulatory Surgery Centers

Pacific Hills Surgery Center, Inc., 24022 Calle De La Plata, Suite 180, Laguna Hills, CA 92653; tel. 714/951–9470; FAX. 714/951–9478; Norman D. Peterson, M.D., Medical Director

Pacific Surgicenter, Inc., 1301 20th Street, Suite 470, Santa Monica, CA 90404; tel. 310/315–0222; FAX. 310/828–8852; Jocelyne Rosenthal, RN, Administrator

Palm Desert Ambulatory Surgery Center, 73–345 Highway 111, Palm Desert, CA 92260; tel. 619/346–4780; FAX. 619/340–4650; S. C. Shah, M.D., Administrator

Petaluma Surgicenter, 1400 Professional Drive, Suite 102, Petaluma, CA 94954; tel. 707/763–9325; FAX. 707/769–0751; Ronald M. La Vigna, D.P.M.

Physician Care L. P., 603 South Valencia Avenue, Brea, CA 92621; tel. 714/996–7600; FAX. 714/524–5648; Cyndi Chick, Administrative Assistant

Physician's Surgery Center, 901 Campus Drive, Suite 102, Daly City, CA 94015; tel. 415/991–2000; FAX. 415/755–8638; Phillip G. Grassia, Executive Director

Physicians Plaza Surgical Center, 6000 Physicians Boulevard, Bakersfield, CA 93301; tel. 805/322–4744, ext. 26; FAX. 805/322–2938; Michael G. Clark, Administrator

Plastic Surgery Center, 1515 El Camino Real, Palo Alto, CA 94304; tel. 415/322–2723; FAX. 415/322–3260; Donald R. Laub, M.D.

Plaza Surgical Center, Inc., 168 North Brent Street, Suite 403B, Ventura, CA 93003; tel. 805/643–5438; FAX. 805/643–1625; Dale P. Armstrong, M.D.

Podiatric Surgery Center, 255 North Gilbert, Suite B, Hemet, CA 92543; tel. 909/925–2186; FAX. 909/925–4947; Robert Drake, D.P.M., Administrator

Point Loma Surgical Center, 3434 Midway Drive, Suite 1006, San Diego, CA 92110; tel. 619/223–0910; Monica Pfiitzner, Administrator

Premier Surgery of Palm Desert, 73–180 El Paseo, Palm Desert, CA 92660; tel. 619/776–7580; Phillip R. Roy

Premiere Surgery Center, Inc., 700 West El Norte Parkway, Escondido, CA 92026; tel. 619/738–7830; FAX. 619/738–7841; Esther Massengill, Administrator

Providence Ambulatory Surgical Center, 1310 West Stewart Drive, Suite 310, Orange, CA 92680; tel. 714/771–6363; Carol R. Stevenson, Manager

Rabkin Eye Institute, 275 West Hospitality, Suite 106, San Bernardino, CA 92408; tel. 714/885–0180; Sally Rabkin, M.D., Administrator

Rainin Eye Center, 1455 Montego Drive, Suite 102, Walnut Creek, CA 94598; tel. 510/932–1050; Edgar A. Rainin, M.D., Medical Director

Redlands Dental Surgery Center, 1180 Nevada Street, Suite 100, Redlands, CA 92373; tel. 909/335–0474; Russell O. Seheult, D.D.S.

Richburg Valley Eye Institute Ambulatory Surgical Center, 1680 East Herndon Avenue, Fresno, CA 93710–1234; tel. 209/432–4200; FAX. 209/432–0147; Donald J. McCrumb, Administrator

Riverside Community Surgi–Center, 3980 14th Street, Riverside, CA 92501; tel. 909/787–0580; FAX. 909/787–8201; Jan Maddox, M.D., Medical Director

Riverside Eye, Ear, Nose and Throat Institute Surgery Center, 4500 Brockton Avenue, Suite 105, Riverside, CA 92501; tel. 714/788–2788; FAX. 909/788–4374; B. G. Smith, M.D., Medical Director

Riverside Medical Clinic Surgery Center, 7160 Brockton Avenue, Riverside, CA 92506; tel. 714/782–3801; FAX. 909/782–3861

Riverside Podiatry Group Ambulatory Surgery Center, 6896 Magnolia Avenue, Riverside, CA 92506; tel. 714/684–9102; Robert E. Parker

Robert M. Sinskey, M.D., Inc., 2232 Santa Monica Boulevard, Santa Monica, CA 90411; tel. 310/453–8911; FAX. 310/453–2519; Cindy Miller, Administrator

Ross Valley Medical Group, 1350 South Eliseo Drive, Greenbrae, CA 94904; tel. 415/461–1350; Edward J. Boland, Administrator

Sacramento Eye Surgicenter, 3150 J Street, Sacramento, CA 95816; tel. 916/446–2020; Keith A. Baldwin

Sacramento Midtown Endoscopy Center, 3941 J Street, Suite 460, Sacramento, CA 95819; tel. 916/453–4913; FAX. 916/453–4587; Tommy Poirer

Saddleback Eye Center, 23161 Moulton Parkway, Laguna Hills, CA 92653; tel. 714/951–4641; FAX. 714/951–4601; Tracy Takatsuka

Saddleback Valley Outpatient Surgery, 24302 Paseo De Valencia, Laguna Hills, CA 92653; tel. 714/472–0244; FAX. 714/472–0380; Mary Parker, Administrator

Saint John's Ambulatory Surgery Center–Beverly Hills, 9675 Brighton Way, Beverly Hills, CA 90210; tel. 213/281–4950; FAX. 213/273–6639; Paul E. Banta, M.D., Medical Director

Salinas Surgery Center, 955–A Blanco Circle, Salinas, CA 93901; tel. 408/753–5800; FAX. 408/753–5808; Andrew W. Miller, Executive Director

Samaritan Breast Center, 2520 Samaritan Drive, San Jose, CA 95124; tel. 408/358–2778; Jamal Modir, M.D.

Samaritan Pain Management Center, 2520 Samaritan Drive, San Jose, CA 95124; tel. 408/356–2731; FAX. 408/356–6366; Robert W. Presley, M.D., Medical Director

San Buenaventura Surgery Center, A Partnership, 3525 Loma Vista Road, Ventura, CA 93003; tel. 805/641–6434; FAX. 805/641–6437; M. P. Bacon, Medical Director

San Diego Endoscopy Center, A Partnership, 4033 Third Avenue, Suite 106, San Diego, CA 92103; tel. 619/291–6064; John D. Goodman, M.D.

San Diego Outpatient Surgical Center, 770 Washington Street, Suite 101, San Diego, CA 92103; tel. 619/299–9530; FAX. 619/296–5316; Lisa A. Harrington, Executive Director

San Francisco Surgi Center, 1635 Divisidero Street, Suite 200, San Francisco, CA 94115; tel. 415/346–1218; FAX. 415/346–1819; Elizabeth Mollner, Administrator

San Gabriel Valley Surgical Center, 1250 South Sunset Avenue, West Covina, CA 91790; tel. 818/960–6623; FAX. 818/962–4341; Susan Raub, Administrator

Sani Eye Surgery Center, 1315 Las Tablas Road, Templeton, CA 93465; tel. 805/434–2533; FAX. 805/434–3037

Sansum Medical Clinic, Inc., 317 West Pueblo, Santa Barbara, CA 93105; tel. 805/682–2621; Lowell G. McLellan, M.D.

Santa Cruz Surgery Center, 3003 Paul Sweet Road, Santa Cruz, CA 95065; tel. 408/462–5512; FAX. 408/462–2451; Donald S. Harner, M.D.

Santa Rosa Podiatry Group Surgical Center, 528 B Street, Santa Rosa, CA 95401; tel. 707/575–5026; Dr. Michael Prado

Sebastopol Ambulatory Surgery Center, 6880 Palm Avenue, Sebastopol, CA 95472; tel. 707/823–7628; Edward J. Boland, Administrator

Sereno Surgery Center, 14601 South Bascom Avenue, Suite 100, Los Gatos, CA 95032–2043; tel. 408/358–2727; FAX. 408/358–2950; Cathleen McCallister, Administrator

Shepard Eye Center Medical Group, 1414 East Main Street, Santa Maria, CA 93454–4806; tel. 805/925–2637; FAX. 809/928–2067; Dennis D. Shepard, M.D.

Sierra Plastic Surgery Center, 6153 North Thesta, Fresno, CA 93710; tel. 209/432–5156; FAX. 209/432–2247; Terry A. Gillian, M.D., Medical Director

Sierra Surgi–Center, 1601 Ygnacio Valley Road, Walnut Creek, CA 94598; tel. 510/947–5276; Martha H. Plante, Administrator

Simi Health Center, 1350 Los Angeles Avenue, Simi Valley, CA 93065; tel. 805/522–3782; FAX. 805/522–1283; Lorna Holland, Administrator

Solano Surgery Center, 991 Nut Tree Road, Vacaville, CA 95687; tel. 707/447–5400; FAX. 707/447–2356; Ronald D. Fike, Jr.

Sonora Eye Surgery Center, 940 Sylva Lane, Suite G, Sonora, CA 95370; tel. 209/532–8191; FAX. 209/532–1687; Pamela Donaldson

South Bay Ambulatory Surgical Center, 251 Landis Street, Chula Vista, CA 91910; tel. 619/585–1020; FAX. 619/585–0247; Arthur E. Casey, Administrator

South Coast Eye Institute, A Medical Clinic, 3420 Bristol Street, Suite 701, Costa Mesa, CA 92626; tel. 714/957–0272; FAX. 714/641–2020; Gary E. Feldman, M.D., Administrator

Southland Endoscopy Center, 949 East Calhoun Place, Suite B, Hemet, CA 92543; tel. 909/929–1177; Sreenivasa R. Nakka, M.D.

Southwest Surgical Clinic, Inc., 4201 Torrance Boulevard, Torrance, CA 90503; tel. 310/540–7803; FAX. 310/316–3903; Otto Munchow, M.D., Director

Spencer Eye Surgery and Laser Center, 2486 Ponderosa Drive, N., Camarillo, CA 93010; tel. 805/987–2942

Stanislaus Surgery Center, 1421 Oakdale Road, Modesto, CA 95355; tel. 209/572–2700; Michael Lipomi, Administrator

Stevenson Surgery Center, 2675 Stevenson Boulevard, Fremont, CA 94538; tel. 510/793–4987; FAX. 510/745–0136; Margaret Holmes, Director, Nursing

Stockton Eye Surgery Center, 36 West Yokuts Avenue, Stockton, CA 95207; tel. 209/473–2940; FAX. 209/474–1181

Surgecenter of Palo Alto, 400 Forest Avenue, Palo Alto, CA 94301; tel. 415/324–1832; FAX. 415/324–2282; Rose Parkes, Chief Executive Officer

Surgery Center of Northern California, 950 Butte Street, Redding, CA 96001; tel. 916/241–4044; FAX. 916/241–1408; Jan McEwen, Administrator

Surgery Center of San Bernardino, 2150 North Sierra Way, San Bernardino, CA 92405; tel. 909/881–2595; FAX. 909/881–1146; Sharon Segui, RN, Administrator

Surgery Center of San Luis Obispo, 1304–C Ella Street, San Luis Obispo, CA 93401; tel. 805/544–7874; FAX. 805/544–6057; Linda M. Harris, RN, M.S.N., Administrator

Surgery Center of Santa Monica, 2121 Wilshire Boulevard, Santa Monica, CA 90403; tel. 310/260–5577; Carolyn G. Catton

Surgery Centers of the Desert, 1180 North Palm Canyon, Palm Springs, CA 92262; tel. 619/320–7600; FAX. 619/320–1694; Rosemary Coombs, Executive Director

Surgery Centers of the Desert, 39700 Bob Hope Drive, Suite 301, Rancho Mirage, CA 92270; tel. 619/346–7696; Rosemary Coombs, Executive Director

Surgi–Med Center, 1332 West Herndon Avenue, Suite 102, Fresno, CA 93711–0431; tel. 209/439–3100; Danette Sailer

Surgical Eye Care Center, 655 Laguna Drive, Carlsbad, CA 92008; tel. 619/729–7101; James A. Davies, M.D.

Surgicenter of South Bay, 23500 Madison Street, Torrance, CA 90505; tel. 213/539–5120; Debra Saxton

Sutter Alhambra Surgery Center, 1201 Alhambra Boulevard, Sacramento, CA 95816; tel. 916/733–8222; FAX. 916/733–8224; Bill Davis, Administrator

Sutter Street Surgery Center, 450 Sutter Street, San Francisco, CA 94108; tel. 415/981–1666; FAX. 415/616–6829; Susan Abell, Acting Administrator

Sutter Surgery Center, 75 Scripps Drive, Sacramento, CA 95825; tel. 916/929–9431; FAX. 916/929–0132; Charlene Nakayama, Administrator

Sutter Surgery Center–J Street, 3810 J Street, Sacramento, CA 95816; tel. 916/929–9431; FAX. 916/929–0132; Charlene Nakayama, Administrator

Templeton Surgicenter, 1105 Las Tablas Road, Suite E, Templeton, CA 93465; tel. 805/434–2822; D. Larry Stanton, M.D.

The Centre for Plastic Surgery, 401 East Highland Avenue, Suite 352, San Bernardino, CA 92404; tel. 909/883–8686; FAX. 909/881–6537; Dennis K. Anderson, Administrator

The Darr Eye Clinic Surgical Medical Group, Inc., 44139 Monterey Avenue, Suite A, Palm Desert, CA 92260; tel. 619/773–3099; FAX. 619/341–6863; William Lou Lozano, Administrator

Providers / Freestanding Ambulatory Surgery Centers

The Endoscopy Center, 870 Shasta Street, Suite 100, Yuba City, CA 95991; tel. 916/671-3636; FAX. 916/671-4099; Floyd V. Burton, M.D.

The Endoscopy Center of the South Bay, 23560 Madison Street, Suite 109, Torrance, CA 90505; tel. 310/325-6331; FAX. 310/325-6335; Norman M. Panitch, M.D.

The Eye Surgery Center (Colton), 1900 East Washington, Colton, CA 92324; tel. 909/825-3524; FAX. 909/824-0356

The Eye Surgery Center of Northern California, 5959 Greenback Lane, Citrus Heights, CA 95621; tel. 916/723-7400; Shari Sloan, Administrator

The Eye Surgery Center of Riverside, Inc., 8990 Garfield, Suite One, Riverside, CA 92503; tel. 909/785-5421; FAX. 909/785-0130

The Montebello Surgery Center, 229 East Beverly Boulevard, Montebello, CA 90640; tel. 213/728-7998; Clifton M. Baker, Administrator

The Palos Verdes Plastic Surgery Medical Center, 3400 West Lomita Boulevard, Suite 307, Torrance, CA 90505; tel. 310/539-5888; FAX. 310/517-9916; Valerie McZeal, Office Manager

The Plastic Surgery Center Medical Group, Inc., 95 Scripps Drive, Sacramento, CA 95825; tel. 916/929-1833; FAX. 916/929-6730; Mark L. Ross

The Specialists Surgery Center, 2450 Martin Road, Fairfield, CA 94533; tel. 707/422-2325; FAX. 707/429-6088; Ronald D. Fike, Jr.

The Surgery Center, 1111 Sonoma Avenue, Santa Rosa, CA 95405; tel. 707/578-4100; Ken Alban, Administrator

The Surgery Center, 6840 Sepulveda Boulevard, Van Nuys, CA 91405; tel. 818/785-6840; FAX. 818/785-3931; Gail Morales, RN, Nurse Manager

The Surgery Center, 3875 Telegraph Avenue, Oakland, CA 94609; tel. 510/547-2244; Peggy S. Wellman

The Valley Endoscopy Center, 18425 Burbank Boulevard, Suite 525, Tarzana, CA 91356; tel. 818/708-6050; FAX. 818/708-6009; John Trocino, RN, Clinical Director

Tri-Valley Surgery Center, 4487 Stoneridge Drive, Pleasanton, CA 94588; tel. 510/484-3100; FAX. 510/484-3113; Karen Stevens, RN, CNOR, Administrator

Twin Cities Surgicenter, Inc., 812 Fourth Street, Suite A, Marysville, CA 95901; tel. 916/741-3937; FAX. 916/743-0427; Bonnie Archuleta

☐ **UTC Surgicenter,** 8929 University Center Lane, Suite 103, San Diego, CA 92122; tel. 619/554-0220; FAX. 619/554-0458; Dawn Ainsworth, RN, Administrator

Upland Outpatient Surgical Center, Inc., 1330 San Bernardino Road, Upland, CA 91786; tel. 909/981-8755; FAX. 909/981-9462; Roger E. Murken, M.D., President

Valencia/Holy Cross Outpatient Surgical Center, 24355 Lyons Avenue, Suite 120, Santa Clarita, CA 91321; tel. 805/255-6644; FAX. 805/255-6717; Nina Turner, Acting Administrative Director

Valley Surgical Center, 5555 West Las Positas Boulevard, Pleasanton, CA 94566; tel. 510/734-3300; FAX. 510/734-3358; Beth Combs, RN, Director, Nursing

Ventura Out-patient Surgery, Inc., 3555 Loma Vista Road, Suite 204, Ventura, CA 93003; tel. 805/653-5460; FAX. 805/653-1470; Brian P. Brantner, M.D.

Victorville Ambulatory Surgery Center, 15030 Seventh Street, Victorville, CA 92392; tel. 619/241-2273; FAX. 619/245-6798; John D. Amar, M.D., Medical Director

Vision Care Surgery Center, 1045 S Street, Fresno, CA 93721; tel. 209/486-2000; Ken Lasbury, Executive Director

Walnut Creek Ambulatory Surgery Center, Ltd., 2021 Ygnacio Valley Road, Walnut Creek, CA 94598; tel. 510/933-0290; FAX. 510/933-7034; Lori Fried, Administrator

Wardlow Surgery Center, 200 West Wardlow Road, Long Beach, CA 90806; tel. 310/424-3574; FAX. 310/490-0329; Marisol Magana, Administrator

Washington Outpatient Surgery Center, 2299 Mowry Avenue, First Floor, Fremont, CA 94538; tel. 510/791-5374; FAX. 510/790-8916; Gerald G. Pousho, M.D.

West Valley Surgery Center, 3803 South Bascom Avenue, Suite 106, Campbell, CA 95008; tel. 408/559-4886; FAX. 408/559-4908; Virginia M. Crane, RN, Administrator

Westlake Eye Surgery Center, 2900 Townsgate Road, Suite 201, Westlake Village, CA 91361; tel. 805/496-6789; FAX. 805/494-8392; Don Hirschman, M.H.A., Administrator

Woodland Surgery Center, 1321 Cottonwood Street, Woodland, CA 95695; tel. 916/662-9112; FAX. 916/668-5783; LaRue Shaw

Woodward Park Surgicenter, 7055 North Fresno Street, Suite 100, Fresno, CA 93710; tel. 209/442-9977; FAX. 209/449-9350; Lori Ruffner, RN

COLORADO

Ambulatory Surgery, Ltd., 320 East Fontanero, Colorado Springs, CO 80907; tel. 719/634-8878; John McKiernan, Administrator

Aurora Outpatient Surgery, 2900 South Peoria Street, Suite D, Aurora, CO 80014; tel. 303/752-2496; FAX. 303/752-2577; L. F. Peede, Jr., M.D., Administrator

Aurora Surgery Center, Ltd., 13701 Mississippi Avenue, Suite 200, Aurora, CO 80012; tel. 303/363-8646; FAX. 303/363-8689; Beverly Kirchner, RN, Administrator

Boulder Medical Center, P.C., 2750 Broadway, Boulder, CO 80304; tel. 303/440-3000; Bradford B. McKane

Centennial Healthcare Plaza, a Division of Healthone, 14200 East Arapahoe Road, Englewood, CO 80112; tel. 303/699-3000; FAX. 303/699-3182; Ginger McNally, Administrator

Center for Reproductive Surgery, 799 East Hampden Avenue, Suite 300, Englewood, CO 80110; tel. 303/788-8309; FAX. 303/788-8310; Dr. William Schoolcraft, Administrator

Centrum Surgical Center, 8200 East Belleview, Suite 300, Englewood, CO 80111; tel. 303/999-9999; Connie Holtz, Administrator

Cherry Creek Eye Surgery Center, (Rose Medical Center), 4999 East Kentucky Avenue, Denver, CO 80222; tel. 303/692-0903; Jeffrey Dorsey, Administrator

Colorado Outpatient Eye Surgical Center, 2480 South Downing, Suite G-20, Denver, CO 80210; tel. 303/777-3852; FAX. 300/778-0738; Thomas P. Larkin

Colorado Springs Eye Surgery Center, 2920 North Cascade Avenue, Colorado Springs, CO 80907; tel. 719/636-5054; Paul Angotti, Administrator

Colorado Springs Medical Center Ambulatory Surgery Unit, 209 South Nevada Avenue, Colorado Springs, CO 80903; tel. 719/475-7700; FAX. 719/475-1241; Gary Trunnell, Executive Vice President

Colorado Springs Surgery Center, Ltd., 1615 Medical Center Point, Colorado Springs, CO 80907; tel. 719/635-7740; FAX. 719/635-7750; B. J. Schott, Administrator

DTC Eye Surgery Center, 8400 East Prentice Avenue, Suite 1200, Englewood, CO 80111; tel. 303/793-3000; Jon Dishler, M.D., President

Denver Eye Surgery Center, Inc., 13772 Denver West Parkway, Building 55, Golden, CO 80401; tel. 303/279-6600; Larry W. Kreider, M.D., Administrator

Denver West Surgery Center, 13952 Denver West Parkway, Building 53, Suite 100, Golden, CO 80401; tel. 303/271-1112; FAX. 303/271-1117; Annette Kancilia, Facility Manager

ENT Surgicenter, Inc., 1032 Luke, Fort Collins, CO 80524; tel. 303/484-8686; FAX. 303/484-1064; Debbie Brown, Manager

Eye Surgery Center of Colorado, 8403 Bryant Street, Westminster, CO 80030; tel. 303/426-4810; FAX. 303/426-8708; William G. Self, Jr., M.D., Administrator

Kaiser Permanente Ambulatory Surgery Center, 2045 Franklin Street, Denver, CO 80205; tel. 303/764-4444; Rosemarie Polemi, Director

Lakewood Surgical Center, 2201 Wadsworth Boulevard, Lakewood, CO 80215; tel. 303/234-0445; FAX. 303/232-7182; Kenneth R. Richardson, Medical Director

Littleton Day Surgery Center, 8381 South Park Lane, Littleton, CO 80120; tel. 303/795-2244; FAX. 303/730-6163; Tony Piccone, M.D., Medical Director

North Denver Surgical Center, Ltd., 10001 North Washington, Thornton, CO 80229; tel. 303/252-0083; FAX. 303/252-9095; Charlotte Santoro, Administrator

Orthopaedic Center of the Rockies Ambulatory Surgery Center, 2500 East Prospect, Fort Collins, CO 80525; tel. 303/493-0112; FAX. 303/493-0521; Scott M. Thomas, Executive Director

Provenant Medical Center at Summit Surgical Services, Highway Nine at School Road, Frisco, CO 80443; tel. 303/668-1458; Carol Turrin, Administrator

Pueblo Ambulatory Surgery Center, 25 Montebello Road, Pueblo, CO 81001; tel. 719/544-1600; FAX. 719/544-2599; Marlene Keithley

Rocky Mountain Surgery Center, LTD., 2405 Broadway, Boulder, CO 80304-4108; tel. 303/449-2020; FAX. 303/440-6893; James R. Schubert, Executive Director

Southern Colorado Center for Endoscopy and Surgery, 2002 Lake Avenue, Pueblo, CO 81004; tel. 719/560-7111; Glenn Scott, Executive Director

Spring Creek Surgery Center, Spring Creek Medical Park, 2001 South Shields Street, Building H, Suite 100, Fort Collins, CO 80526; tel. 303/221-9363; FAX. 303/221-9636; Sharyn Salmen, Facility Administrator, Director of Nursing

Sterling Eye Surgical Center, 1410 South Seventh Avenue, Sterling, CO 80751; tel. 303/522-1833; FAX. 303/522-1832; Inez C. Plank, General Manager

Surgery Center of Fort Collins, 1100 East Prospect Road, P.O. Box 548, Fort Collins, CO 80525; tel. 303/493-7200; FAX. 303/493-2380; Alice Fischer, Administrator

Surgicenter of the San Luis Valley, 2115 Stuart, Alamosa, CO 81101; tel. 719/589-8010; Gwen Heller, Administrator

Western Rockies Surgery Center, Inc., 1000 Wellington Avenue, Grand Junction, CO 81501; tel. 303/243-9000; FAX. 303/245-4936; Marilyn M. Smith, RN, Surgery Center Administrator

CONNECTICUT

Bridgeport Surgical Center, 4920 Main Street, Bridgeport, CT 06606; tel. 203/374-1515; FAX. 203/374-4702; Anthony German, Administrative Director

☐ **Connecticut Surgical Center,** 81 Gillett Street, Hartford, CT 06105; tel. 203/247-5555; FAX. 203/249-5860; Margaret Rubino, President

Danbury Surgical Center, 73 Sandpit Road, Suite 101, Danbury, CT 06810; tel. 203/743-2400; Bernard A. Kershner, President

Hartford Surgical Center, 100 Retreat Avenue, Hartford, CT 06106; tel. 203/549-7970; FAX. 203/247-4121; Christine M. Quallen, Administrative Director

Johnson Surgery Center, 148 Hazard Avenue, P.O. Box 909, Enfield, CT 06083; tel. 203/749-8365; FAX. 203/749-8833; Anthony T. Valente, Vice President, Chief Operating Officer

Middlesex Surgical Center, 530 Saybrook Road, Middletown, CT 06457; tel. 203/343-0400; FAX. 203/343-0396; Louise DeChesser, RN, CNOR,M.S.

Naugatuck Valley Surgical Center, Ltd., 160 Robbins Street, Waterbury, CT 06708; tel. 203/755-6663; FAX. 203/756-9645; Bernard A. Kershner, President

Stamford Surgical Center, 1290 Summer Street, Stamford, CT 06905; tel. 203/961-1345; FAX. 213/324-1470; Charles Tienken, Administrative Director

Woman's Surgical Center, 40 Temple Street, New Haven, CT 06510; tel. 203/624-3080; Bruce I. Fisher, Administrator

Providers / Freestanding Ambulatory Surgery Centers

Yale–New Haven Ambulatory Services Corporation, d/b/a Temple Surgical Center, 60 Temple Street, New Haven, CT 06510; tel. 203/624–6008; Alvin D. Greenberg, M.D., Administrator

DELAWARE

Central Delaware Surgery Center, 100 Scull Terrace, Dover, DE 19901; tel. 302/735–8290; Paul Fransisco, Administrator

Limestone Medical Center, 1941 Limestone Road, Wilmington, DE 19808; tel. 302/836–8350; FAX. 302/992–9248; Joseph M. Rule, Ph.D., Director

DISTRICT OF COLUMBIA

Capitol Women's Center, 1339 22nd Street, N.W., Washington, DC 20037; tel. 202/338–2772; Kelly Turner–Minor, Administrator

Endoscopy Center, 2021 K Street, N.W., Suite T–115, Washington, DC 20006; tel. 202/775–8692; FAX. 202/296–9122; Ms. P. J. Krchma, Administrator

Hillcrest Northwest, 7603 Georgia Avenue, N.W., Washington, DC 20012; tel. 202/829–5620; FAX. 202/882–8387; Alice Harper, Administrator

Hillcrest Women's Surgi–Center, 3233 Pennsylvania Avenue, S.E., Washington, DC 20020; tel. 202/584–6500; Ms. Caridad V. Wright, Administrator

Medlantic Center for Ambulatory Surgery, Inc., 1145 19th Street, N.W., Suite 850, Washington, DC 20036; tel. 202/223–9040; FAX. 202/223–9047; Marcia F. Gundy, President

Metropolitan Ambulatory Surgery Center, 6323 Georgia Avenue, N.W., Washington, DC 20011; tel. 202/291–0036; Gwen S. Robinson–Terry, Chief Operating Officer

New Summit Medical Center II, Inc., 1630 Euclid Street, N.W., Suite 130, Washington, DC 20037; tel. 202/337–7200; Johnette Anderson, RNC, Administrator

Planned Parenthood of Metropolitan Washington, D.C., Schumacher Center, 1108 16th Street, N.W., Washington, DC 20036; tel. 202/483–3999; FAX. 202/783–1007; Claudia Allers, Center Manager

Washington Surgi–Clinic, 1018 22nd Street, N.W., Washington, DC 20037; tel. 202/659–9403; FAX. 202/467–0056; Maria Barrera, Administrator

Women's Health Care, 3543 16th Street, N.W., Washington, DC 20010; tel. 202/462–5455; Ellen Neblett, Administrator

FLORIDA

Aker–Kasten Cataract and Laser Institute, 1445 N.W. Boca Raton Boulevard, Boca Raton, FL 33432; tel. 407/338–7722, ext. 238; FAX. 407/338–7785; Kim Harrington, Administrator

Alpha Ambulatory Surgery, Inc., 2160 Capital Circle, N.E., Tallahassee, FL 32308; tel. 904/385–0033; FAX. 904/422–0201; Gloria Jeter, Office Manager

Ambulatory Ankle and Foot Center of Florida, 1509 South Orange Avenue, 32806, P.O. Box 36951, Orlando, FL 32853–6951; tel. 407/895–2432; Craig C. Maguire, D.P.M.

Ambulatory Surgery Center, 4500 East Fletcher Avenue, Tampa, FL 33613; tel. 813/977–8550; FAX. 813/977–7941; Marcy Barrie, Administrator

Ambulatory Surgery Center of Brevard, 719 East New Haven Avenue, Melbourne, FL 32901; tel. 407/984–4411; FAX. 407/728–3001; Dwight J. Miller, General Manager

Ambulatory Surgery Center of Naples, 1351 Pine Street, Naples, FL 33942; tel. 813/793–0664; FAX. 813/793–4318; L. Christian Mogelvang, M.D., Medical Director

☐ Ambulatory Surgery Center/Bradenton, 5817 21st Avenue, W., Bradenton, FL 34209; tel. 813/794–0379; J. Leikensohn, M.D. Medical Director

Ambulatory Surgical Care, 1045 North Courtenay Parkway, Merritt Island, FL 32953; tel. 407/452–4448; FAX. 407/452–5404; Bill Bernhardt, Administrative Director

Ambulatory Surgical Center of Central Florida, Inc., 801 North Stone Street, Deland, FL 32720; tel. 904/734–4431; FAX. 904/738–1045; Albert C. Neumann, M.D., Medical Director

Ambulatory Surgical Center of Lake County, Inc., 803 East Dixie Avenue, Leesburg, FL 32748; tel. 904/787–6656; FAX. 904/787–9008; Patricia R. Hux, RN, Business Manager

Ambulatory Surgical Centre, 8700 North Kendall Drive, Suite 100, Miami, FL 33176; tel. 305/595–9511; FAX. 305/271–0383; Gail Tauriello, Administrator

Ayers Surgery Center, 720 S.W. Second Avenue, Suite 101, Gainesville, FL 32601; tel. 904/338–7100; FAX. 904/338–7102; Barbara Hyder, RN, Nurse Manager

Bay Eye and Surgical Center, 1600 Jenks Avenue, Panama City, FL 32405; tel. 904/769–5248; FAX. 904/763–6665; O. Lee Mullis, M.D., Administrator

☐ Belleair Surgi–Center, 1130 Ponce de Leon Boulevard, Clearwater, FL 34616; tel. 813/581–4800; FAX. 813/585–0319; Lee Youngblood, Administrator

Boca Raton Outpatient Surgery and Laser Center, 501 Glades Road, Boca Raton, FL 33432; tel. 407/362–4400; FAX. 407/362–4440; Thomas Harrington, Administrator

☐ Brandon Surgi–Center, 711 South Parsons, Brandon, FL 33511; tel. 813/654–7771; Charlene Harrell, RN, Administrator

☐ Cape Surgery Center, 1941 Waldemere Street, Sarasota, FL 34239–3555; tel. 813/953–1900; FAX. 813/952–2356; Lynda L. Herndon, RN, M.B.A., Director

Central Florida Eye Institute, 3133 S.W. 32nd Avenue, Ocala, FL 34474; tel. 904/237–8400; Thomas L. Croley, M.D.

Central Florida Outpatient Surgery Center, 11140 West Colonial Drive, Suite Three, Ocoee, FL 34761; tel. 407/656–2700; FAX. 407/877–9432; Antonio Caos, M.D., Medical Director

Clearwater Endoscopy Center, 401 Corbett Street, Suite 220, Clearwater, FL 34616; tel. 813/443–0100; Donna M. Carron, RN, Clinical Director

Collier Surgical Center, 800 Goodlette Road, N., Suite 120, Naples, FL 33940; tel. 813/262–5757; FAX. 813/262–6073; Donna Rae Malone, Administrator

Coral View Ambulatory Surgery, 8390 West Flager, Suite 216, Miami, FL 33144; tel. 305/226–5574; Victor Suarez, M.D., President

Cordova Ambulatory Surgical Center, 545 Brent Lane, Pensacola, FL 32503; tel. 904/477–5437; Cynthia Blake, Assistant Administrator

Cortez Foot Surgery Center, PA, 1800 Cortez Road, W., Suite B, Bradenton, FL 34207; tel. 813/758–4608; FAX. 813/753–6062; Margaret Provencher, Administrator

Countryside Surgi–Center, 3291 North McMullen Booth Road, Clearwater, FL 34621; tel. 813/725–5800; FAX. 813/797–4002

Day Surgery, Inc., 1715 S.E. Tiffany Avenue, Port St. Lucie, FL 34952; tel. 407/335–7005

Dermatologic and Cosmetic Surgery Center, 2668 Swamp Cabbage Court, Fort Myers, FL 33901; tel. 813/275–7546; FAX. 813/275–5074; Charles Eby, M.D.

Diagnostic Clinic Center for Outpatient Surgery, 1401 West Bay Drive, Largo, FL 34640; tel. 813/581–8767; FAX. 813/584–1938; Robert R. Dippong, Administrator, Chief Executive Officer

Endoscopy Center of Ocala, Inc., 1160 S.E. 18th Place, Ocala, FL 34471; tel. 904/732–2662; Carol Hiatt, RN, Administrator

Eye Care and Surgery Center of Ft. Lauderdale, 2540 N.E. Ninth Street, Ft. Lauderdale, FL 33304; tel. 305/561–3533; FAX. 305/565–9706; Michael Goldstone, Technical Administrator

Eye Surgery Facility, Inc., 2808 West Martin Luther King Boulevard, Tampa, FL 33607; tel. 813/876–1331; FAX. 813/872–0647; Phyllis S. Chisholm, RN, M.A., Executive Director

Eye Surgery and Laser Center, 4120 Del Prado Boulevard, Cape Coral, FL 33904; tel. 813/542–2020; FAX. 813/542–0704; Louise Bennett, RN, Administrator

Eye Surgery and Laser Center of Mid-Florida, Inc., 409 Avenue K, S.E., Winter Haven, FL 33880; tel. 813/294–3504, ext. 303; FAX. 813/294–8305; Sue Koha, ASC Supervisor

Eye Surgicenter, 2521 N.W. 41st Street, Gainesville, FL 32606; tel. 904/377–7733; William A. Newsome, M.D.

Florida Eye Care, Inc. of Lakeland, 814 Griffin Road, Lakeland, FL 33805; tel. 813/686–1010

Florida Eye Clinic Ambulatory Surgical Center, 160 Boston Avenue, Altamonte Springs, FL 32701; tel. 407/834–7776; FAX. 407/831–8607; Genevieve Parm, Chief Executive Officer

Florida Eye Institute Surgicenter, Inc., 2750 Indian River Boulevard, Vero Beach, FL 32960; tel. 407/569–9500; FAX. 407/569–9507; Mary Lynne Schlitt, Administrator

Florida Surgery Center, 180 Boston Avenue, Altamonte Springs, FL 32701; tel. 407/830–0573; FAX. 407/830–4373; Paige L. Adams, Administrator

Florida Surgical Center, Shands at University of Florida, 2001 S.W. 13th Street, Gainesville, FL 32608; tel. 904/375–7373; FAX. 904/375–1599; Deborah Lombardi, Executive Director

Forest Oaks Ambulatory Surgical Center, Inc., 7320 Forest Oaks Boulevard, Spring Hill, FL 34606; tel. 904/683–5666; Thomas D. Stelnicki, D.P.M.

Foundation for Advanced Eye Care, 3737 Pine Island Road, Sunrise, FL 33351; tel. 305/572–5888; FAX. 305/572–5994; Andrea B. Lettman, Administrator

Gaskins Eye Care and Surgery Center, 2335 Ninth Street, N., Suite 304, Naples, FL 33940; tel. 813/263–7750; FAX. 813/263–1754; Cindy Gaskins, RN, M.S.N., R.M.

Gulf Coast Endoscopy Center, Inc., 665 Del Prado Boulevard, Cape Coral, FL 33990; tel. 813/772–3800; FAX. 813/772–5073; Mrs. Lee Caruso, Administrator

Gulf Coast Gastroenterology and Surgical Center, 1936 Jenks Avenue, Panama City, FL 32405; tel. 904/763–6700; FAX. 904/763–5779; Riyad Albibi, M.D., Director

Gulf Coast Surgery Center, 411 Second Street, E., Bradenton, FL 34208; tel. 813/746–1121; FAX. 813/746–7816; Carlene Bailey, RN, Administrator

Hialeah Ambulatory Care Center, 445 East 25th Street, Hialeah, FL 33176; tel. 305/691–4450; FAX. 305/693–0823; Jose Kone, Administrative Director

Indian River Surgery Center, 1200 37th Street, Vero Beach, FL 32960; tel. 407/770–5600; FAX. 407/770–1793; Thomas S. Lally, Administrator

Institute for Plastic and Reconstructive Surgery, 820 Arthur Godfrey Road, Third Floor, Miami Beach, FL 33140; tel. 305/673–6164; FAX. 305/534–9759; Lawrence B. Robbins, M.D.

Jacksonville Surgery Center, 4253 Salisbury Road, Jacksonville, FL 32216; tel. 904/281–0021; FAX. 904/281–0988; Katherine Anderson, RN, B.S.N., Center Director

Johnson Eye Institute Surgery Center, Inc., 5923 Seventh Street, Zephyrhills, FL 33539; tel. 813/788–7656; FAX. 813/788–6011; Linda Ward, Administrator

Kissimmee Surgery Center, 2275 North Central Avenue, Kissimmee, FL 34741; tel. 407/870–0573; FAX. 407/870–1859; Lou Warmijak, Administrator

Lazenby Cataract and Eye Care Center, 1109 U.S. Highway 19, Suite B, Holiday, FL 34691; tel. 813/934–5705; Laverne Peyton, Administrator

Leesburg Regional Day Surgery Center, 601 East Dixie Avenue, Plaza 501, Leesburg, FL 34748; tel. 904/365–0700; FAX. 904/365–0758; Kim Anderson, RN, CAPA, Clinical Coordinator

Lowrey Eye Clinic, 1840 North Highlands Avenue, Clearwater, FL 34615; tel. 813/442–4147; FAX. 813/446–9297; Miquel E. Mulet, Jr., M.D.

Manatee Endoscopy Center, Inc., 6010 Pointe West Boulevard, Bradenton, FL 34209; tel. 813/792–4239

Martin Memorial SurgiCenter, P.O. Box 9010, Stuart, FL 34995; tel. 407/223–5920; FAX. 407/288–1821

Mayo Clinic Jacksonville Ambulatory Surgery Center for G.I., 4500 San Pablo Road, Jacksonville, FL 32224; tel. 904/223–2000; Judy Pearce, ASC for GI Coordinator

Providers / Freestanding Ambulatory Surgery Centers

Mease Countryside Ambulatory Care Center, 1880 Mease Drive, Safety Harbor, FL 34695; tel. 813/726-2873; FAX. 813/791-4317; William G. Harger, Administrator

Medical Development Corporation of Pasco County, 7315 Hudson Avenue, Hudson, FL 34667; tel. 813/868-9563, ext. 251; FAX. 813/869-6918; Dawn M. Ernst, Director, Nursing

Medivision of Northern Palm Beach County, 2889 10th Avenue, N., Suite 304, Lake Worth, FL 33461; tel. 407/969-0139; FAX. 407/642-1167; Denise Brower, Administrator

Medivision of Orange County, 116 West Sturtevant Street, Orlando, FL 32806; tel. 407/423-4090; Eric Kriss, Chief Executive Officer

Memorial Same Day Surgery Center, 4470 Sheridan Street, Hollywood, FL 33021; tel. 305/962-3210; FAX. 305/962-3466; Ross S. Ackerman, Executive Director, Administrator

Miami Eye Center, 619 N.W. 12th Avenue, Miami, FL 33136; tel. 305/326-0260; FAX. 305/326-1907; Edward C. Gelber, M.D.

Mid Florida Surgery Center, 17564 West Highway 441, Mt. Dora, FL 32757; tel. 904/735-4100; FAX. 904/735-2444; Patsy Lentz, RN, Administrative Director

Montgomery Eye Center, 700 Neapolitan Way, Naples, FL 33940; tel. 813/261-8383; FAX. 813/261-8443; Mary Lee Montgomery, Administrator

☐ **Naples Day Surgery,** 790 Fourth Avenue, N., Naples, FL 33940; tel. 813/263-3863; FAX. 813/263-7429; Sara May McCallum, Executive Director

Naples Day Surgery North, 11161 Health Park Boulevard, Naples, FL 33963; tel. 813/598-3111; FAX. 813/598-1707; Sara May McCallum, Executive Director

☐ **New Port Richey Surgi-Center,** 5415 Gulf Drive, New Port Richey, FL 34652; tel. 813/848-0446; FAX. 813/842-3166; Sandra McFarland, RN, Administrator

New Smyrna Beach Ambulatory Care Center, Inc., 612 Palmetto Street, New Smyrna Beach, FL 32168; tel. 904/423-5500

North County Surgicenter, 4000 Burns Road, Palm Beach, FL 33410; tel. 407/626-6446; Steve Sergi, Business Manager

North Florida Eye Clinic Surgicenter, 590 Dundas Drive, Jacksonville, FL 32218; tel. 904/751-3600; FAX. 904/757-8922; Mary Miller, RN, Director Surgical Services

North Florida Surgical Pavilion, 6705 N.W. 10th Place, Gainesville, FL 32605; tel. 904/333-4555; FAX. 904/333-4569; Becky Hite, Administrative Director

North Miami Beach Surgical Center, 120 N.E. 167th Street, North Miami Beach, FL 33162; tel. 305/940-5100; FAX. 305/956-3961; Deborah M. O'Connor, Executive Officer

Oak Hill Ambulatory Surgery and Endoscopy Center, 11377 Cortez Boulevard, Spring Hill, FL 34613; tel. 904/597-3060; FAX. 904/597-3077

Oakwater Outpatient Surgery Center, 3885 Oakwater Circle, Suite B, Orlando, FL 32806; tel. 407/438-9533; FAX. 407/438-9542; Mary Pohlman, Office Manager

Obi Plastic Surgery Clinic, Inc., 3599 University Boulevard, S., Suite 604, Jacksonville, FL 32216; tel. 904/399-0905; FAX. 904/346-0757; Faye T. Evans, Administrator

Orange Park Surgery Center, 2050 Professional Center Drive, Orange Park, FL 32073; tel. 904/272-2550; FAX. 904/272-7911; Charles J. Jacobson, Executive Director

☐ **Orlando Center for Outpatient Surgery,** 1405 South Orange Avenue, Suite 400, Orlando, FL 32806; tel. 407/426-8331; FAX. 407/425-9582

Ormond Eye Surgi Center, 26 North Beach Street, Suite A, Ormond Beach, FL 32174; tel. 904/673-3341; FAX. 904/672-1854; Karen S. LaMotte, RN, Assistant Administrator

Outpatient Surgical Services, Ltd., 301 N.W. 82nd Avenue, Plantation, FL 33324; tel. 305/424-1766; FAX. 305/424-1966; John J. Singletary, Administrator

Pal-Med Same Day Surgery, 6950 West 20th Avenue, Hialeah, FL 33016; tel. 305/821-0079, ext. 321; FAX. 305/558-7494; Roseann Burdman, Director

Palm Bay Surgery Center, 5191 Babcock Street, Palm Bay, FL 32905; tel. 407/676-4700; FAX. 407/952-4481

Palm Beach Endoscopy Center, 2015 North Flagler Drive, West Palm Beach, FL 33407; tel. 407/659-6543

Palm Beach Eye Clinic, 130 Butler Street, West Palm Beach, FL 33407; tel. 407/832-6113; FAX. 407/833-3003; Andre J. Golino, M.D.

Palm Beach Lakes Surgery Center, 2047 Palm Beach Lakes Boulevard, West Palm Beach, FL 33409; tel. 407/683-0004; FAX. 407/683-0332; Mrs. Patti Marotta, Administrator

Palms Wellington Surgical Center, 460 State Road Seven, West Palm Beach, FL 33411; tel. 407/791-9500; FAX. 407/795-7574; Mary A. Perry, RN, Administrator

Parikh Volusia Ambulatory Surgery Center, 598 Sterthaus Avenue, Ormond Beach, FL 32174; tel. 904/673-2262; FAX. 904/677-3808; Robin Hess, Administrator

Parkside Surgery Center, 2731 Park Street, Jacksonville, FL 32205; tel. 904/389-1077; FAX. 904/389-9959; Jim Rardin, Administrator

☐ **Physicians Surgery Center, Ltd.,** 4035 Evans Avenue, Fort Myers, FL 33901; tel. 813/939-3456; Caryl A. Serbin, RN, Administrator

Pinebrook Surgery Center, 14540 Cortez Boulevard, Brooksville, FL 34613; tel. 904/596-1130, ext. 7260; FAX. 904/596-1063

Premier Medical Group, P.A., Florida Eye Microsurgical Institute, 1717 Woolbright Road, Boynton Beach, FL 33426; tel. 407/737-5500; FAX. 407/737-7055; Aida Zin, Office Manager

Presidential Surgicenter, Inc., 1501 Presidential Way, Suite Nine, West Palm Beach, FL 33401; tel. 407/689-7255; FAX. 407/683-7342; Steve S. Spector, M.D.

Rand Surgical Pavillion Corp., Five West Sample Road, Pompano Beach, FL 33064; tel. 305/782-1700; FAX. 305/782-7490; Deborah Rand, Administrator

Riverside Park Surgicenter, 2001 College Street, Jacksonville, FL 32204; tel. 904/355-9800; Janice Carter, RN, Director, Nursing

☐ **Same–Day Surgicenter of Orlando, Ltd.,** 88 West Kaley Street, Orlando, FL 32806; tel. 407/423-0573; Barbara Starr, Administrator

☐ **Sarasota Surgery Center,** 983 South Beneva Road, Sarasota, FL 34232; tel. 813/365-5355; FAX. 813/953-7080; Margo Kallio, Administrator

Seven Springs Surgery Center, Inc., 2024 Seven Springs Boulevard, New Port Richey, FL 34655; tel. 813/376-7000; Barbara Perich, Administrator

Single Day Surgery, 6629 Beach Boulevard, Jacksonville, FL 32216; tel. 904/721-3096

South Miami Ambulatory Care Center, 6250 Sunset Drive, South Miami, FL 33143; tel. 305/662-5353

Southeastern Eyecare Surgicenter, 4131 University Boulevard, S., Building Three, Jacksonville, FL 32216; tel. 904/737-6888; FAX. 904/448-2020; Robert F. Hook, M.D.

Southwest Florida Endoscopy Center, 5050 Mason Corbin Court, Ft. Myers, FL 33907; tel. 813/275-6678; FAX. 813/275-8404

Southwest Florida Institute of Ambulatory Surgery, 3700 Central Avenue, Suite Two, Ft. Myers, FL 33901; tel. 813/275-0665; Rick L. Hale, Executive Director

Space Coast Surgical Center, Inc., 270 North Sykes Creek Parkway, Merritt Island, FL 32953; tel. 407/459-0015

St. Augustine Endoscopy Center, 212 South Park Circle, E., St. Augustine, FL 32086; tel. 904/824-6108; Michael D. Schiff, M.D., President

St. Joseph's Same Day Surgery Center, 3003 West Martin Luther King Boulevard, Tampa, FL 33607; tel. 813/870-4711; FAX. 813/870-4907; Paula McGuiness, Executive Director

St. Lucy's Outpatient Surgery Center, 21275 Olean Boulevard, Port Charlotte, FL 33952; tel. 813/625-1325; FAX. 813/625-6482; Anthony Limoncelli, M.D., P.A.

St. Luke's Surgical Center, 43309 U.S. Highway 19, N., P.O. Box 5000, Tarpon Springs, FL 34688-5000; tel. 813/938-2020; FAX. 813/938-5606; Glenn S. Wolfson, M.D., Medical Director

St. Petersburg Medical Clinic P.A., Ambulatory Surgery Center, 1099 Fifth Avenue, N., St. Petersburg, FL 33705-1419; tel. 813/821-1221, ext. 8740; FAX. 813/892-8754; Iverson Pace, RN, Facility Manager, Director, Nursing

St. Petersburg Surgery Center, 539 Pasadena Avenue, S., St. Petersburg, FL 33707; tel. 813/345-8337; FAX. 813/347-4675; Donna Gelardi-Slosburg, RN, B.S.N., Administrator

Stuart Outpatient Surgery, Center, 2096 S.E. Ocean Boulevard, Stuart, FL 34996; tel. 407/287-8777; FAX. 407/287-1996; Jill Logan, Administrative Director

Suburban Medical Ambulatory Surgical Center, 17615 S.W. 97th Avenue, Miami, FL 33157; tel. 305/255-3950; FAX. 305/233-2503; Jules G. Minkes, D.O., Administrator

Suncoast Eye Center, Eye Surgery Institute, 14003 Lakeshore Boulevard, Hudson, FL 34667; tel. 813/868-9442; FAX. 813/862-6210; Lawrence A. Seigel, M.D., P.A., Medical Director

Suncoast Outpatient Surgery Center, 4519 U.S. Highway 19, New Port Richey, FL 34652; tel. 813/849-8922; FAX. 813/841-7553; Bethany Carvallo, Administrator

Suncoast Surgery Center of Hernando, Inc., 5060 Commercial Way, Spring Hill, FL 34606; tel. 904/596-3696; FAX. 904/596-2707; Bethany Carvallo, Administrator

Surgery Center of Jupiter, Inc., 102 Coastal Way, Jupiter, FL 33477; tel. 407/747-1111; FAX. 407/747-4151; Jane MacDonald, Administrator

Surgical Center of Central Florida, 3601 South Highlands Avenue, Sebring, FL 33870; tel. 813/382-7500; FAX. 813/385-7332; Sharon Keiber, RN, Administrator

Surgical Park Center, Ltd., 9100 S.W. 87th Avenue, Miami, FL 33176; tel. 305/271-9100; Anthony Degina, Administrator

Surgicare Center, 4101 Evans Avenue, Ft. Myers, FL 33901; tel. 813/939-3456; FAX. 813/939-1164; Robin Fox, Administrative Coordinator

Surgicenter of the Palm Beaches, 2808 Australian Avenue, West Palm Beach, FL 33407; tel. 407/848-5700; Laurence Kustin, Executive Director

Tallahassee Cataract Surgery Center, 3411 Capital Medical Boulevard, P.O. Box 13675, Tallahassee, FL 32317; tel. 904/878-3834; FAX. 904/656-1692; James R. Copeland, M.D., Medical Director

Tallahassee Endoscopy Center, 2400 Miccosukee Road, Tallahassee, FL 32308; tel. 904/877-2105; FAX. 904/942-1761; Noel Withers, Administrator

☐ **Tallahassee Outpatient Surgery Center, Inc.,** 3334 Capital Medical Boulevard, Suite 500, Tallahassee, FL 32308; tel. 904/877-4688; FAX. 904/877-0368; Martin Shipman, Administrator

☐ **Tallahassee Single Day Surgery,** 1661 Phillips Road, Tallahassee, FL 32308; tel. 904/878-5165; FAX. 904/942-9711; Susan Kizirian, Executive Director

Tampa Bay Surgery Center, Inc., 11811 North Dale Mabry, Tampa, FL 33618; tel. 813/961-8500; FAX. 813/968-6818; Jay L. Rosen, M.D., Executive Director

Tampa Eye Surgery Center, 4302 North Gomez, Tampa, FL 33607; tel. 813/870-6330; FAX. 813/871-3956; Margie Brill, Administrator

Tampa Outpatient Surgical Facility, 5013 North Armenia Avenue, Tampa, FL 33603; tel. 813/875-0562; FAX. 813/875-1983; Dianne Pugh, Facility Administrator

The Aesthetic Plastic Surgery Center, 135 San Marco Drive, Venice, FL 34285; tel. 813/484-6836; FAX. 813/484-9690; Claudell Crowe, Administrative Director

Providers / Freestanding Ambulatory Surgery Centers

The Endoscopy Center of Naples, 150 Tamiami Trail, N., Suite One, Naples, FL 33940; tel. 813/262-6665; Marjorie Rogers, Office Manager

The Eye Associates Surgery Center, 6002 Pointe West Boulevard, Bradenton, FL 34209; tel. 813/792-2020; FAX. 813/792-2832; Linda Colson, RN, Director

The Gastrointestinal Center of Hialeah, 135 West 49th Street, Hialeah, FL 33012; tel. 305/825-0500; FAX. 305/826-6910; Darlene Boytell, B.S.N,, RN

The Miami Vision Center, 2441 S.W. 37th Avenue, Miami, FL 33145; tel. 305/442-0066

The Treasure Coast Cosmetic Surgery Center, 1901 Port St. Lucie Boulevard, Port St. Lucie, FL 34952; tel. 407/335-3954; Donato A. Viggiano, M.D.

Urological Ambulatory Surgery Center, Inc., 1812 North Mills Avenue, Orlando, FL 32803; tel. 407/897-5499; FAX. 407/894-8746; Susan A. Wuerz, Administrator

Urology Center of Florida, Inc., 3201 S.W. 34th Street, Ocala, FL 34474; tel. 904/237-8100; FAX. 904/237-5684; Christopher S. Hill, Administrator

Urology Health Center, 5652 Meadow Lane, New Port Richey, FL 34652; tel. 813/842-9561; FAX. 813/848-7270; Greg Toney, Administrator

Venice Same Day Surgery, 950 Cooper Street, Venice, FL 34285; tel. 813/485-4868; FAX. 813/484-4084; Randy Malaska, Administrator

Venice Surgery Center, 600 Nokomis Avenue, S., Suite 102, Venice, FL 34285; tel. 813/484-9773; FAX. 813/488-4578; Mary Rogers, Acting Administrator

Venture Ambulatory Surgery Center, 16853 N.E. Second Avenue, Suite 400, North Miami Beach, FL 33162; tel. 305/652-2999; FAX. 305/652-8156; Mary A. Perry, RN, Administrator

Vero Eye Center, 70 Royal Palm Boulevard, Vero Beach, FL 32960; tel. 407/569-6600

☐ **Winter Park Ambulatory Surgical Center,** 1000 South Orlando Avenue, Winter Park, FL 32789; tel. 407/629-1500; FAX. 407/629-1741; James Branon, Administrator

GEORGIA

Albany Ambulatory Surgery Center, 531 Seventh Avenue, Albany, GA 31701; tel. 912/883-3535; J. Kenneth Durham, Medical Director

Ambulatory Foot and Leg Surgical Center, 1652 Mulkey Road, Austell, GA 30001; tel. 912/941-3633; Alan Shaw, D.P.M., Chief Executive Officer

Ambulatory Laser and Surgery Center, 425 Forest Parkway, Suite 103, Forest Park, GA 30050; tel. 404/363-1087; Dr. Paul A. Colon, Administrator

Ambulatory Surgical Facility of Brunswick, Eight Tower Medical Park, 3215 Shrine Road, Brunswick, GA 31520; tel. 912/264-4882; Jimmy L. Dixon, Administrator

Athens Plastic Surgery Clinic, 2325 Prince Avenue, Athens, GA 30606; tel. 706/546-0280; FAX. 404/548-0258; James C. Moore, M.D., Administrator

Atlanta Aesthetic Surgery Center, Inc., 4200 Northside Parkway, Building 8, Atlanta, GA 30327; tel. 404/233-3833; Debbie Clotfelter, Administrator

Atlanta Arthoscopic Surgical Center, 600 West Peachtree Street, Suite 620, Atlanta, GA 30308; tel. 404/874-4878

Atlanta Eye Surgery Center, P.C., 3200 Downwood Circle, Suite 200, Atlanta, GA 30327; tel. 404/355-8721; Robert J. Allen, Administrator

Atlanta Outpatient Peachtree Dunwoody Center, 5505 Peachtree-Dunwoody Road, Suite 150, Atlanta, GA 30342; tel. 404/847-0893; FAX. 404/843-8664; Janie Ellison, Administrator

Atlanta Outpatient Surgery Center, 993 Johnson Ferry Road, Suite 300, Atlanta, GA 30342; tel. 404/252-3074; FAX. 404/843-2089; Marjane Ellison, Administrator

Atlanta Plastic Surgery Clinic, P.C., 975 Johnson Ferry Road, Suite 500, Atlanta, GA 30342; tel. 404/256-1311; Walter G. Elliott, Administrator

Atlanta Surgi-Center, Inc., 1113 Spring Street, Atlanta, GA 30309; tel. 404/892-8608; FAX. 404/892-8143; Elizabeth Petzelt, Administrator

Atlanta Women's Medical Center, Inc., 3316 Piedmont Road, N.E., Suite 220, Atlanta, GA 30305; tel. 404/262-3920; Ann Garzia, Administrator

Augusta Surgical Center, 915 Russell Street, Augusta, GA 30904; tel. 404/738-4925; FAX. 706/738-7224; Beryl Barrett, RN, Administrator

Center for Plastic Surgery, Inc., 365 East Paces Ferry Road, Atlanta, GA 30305; tel. 404/814-0868; Dr. Vincent Zubowicz, Medical Director

Center for Reconstructive Surgery, 5335 Old National Highway, College Park, GA 30349; tel. 404/768-3668; Gregory Alvarez, D.P.M.

Clayton Outpatient Surgical Center, P.C., 6911 Tara Boulevard, Jonesboro, GA 30236; tel. 404/477-9535; Jane Rimmer, Administrator

Cobb Foot and Leg Surgery Center, 792 Church Street, Suite Two, Marietta, GA 30060; tel. 404/422-9864; FAX. 404/984-0303; Anthony Gatti, Administrator

Coliseum Same Day Surgery, 310 Hospital Drive, P.O. Box 6154, Macon, GA 31208; tel. 912/742-1403; FAX. 912/742-1671; Michael Boggs, Chief Executive Officer, Executive Director

Columbia County Medical Plaza - Surgery, 635 Washington West, Evans, GA 30809; tel. 706/868-1050; Jack Clark, Vice President

Columbus Women's Health Organization, Inc., 3850 Rosemont Drive, Columbus, GA 31901; tel. 404/323-8363; Amelia Morelane, Administrator

DeKalb Gastroenterology Associates, 2675 North Decatur Road, Decatur, GA 30033; tel. 404/299-1679; FAX. 404/501-7558; Peter Leff, M.D.

Decatur Urological Clinic-Ambulatory Surgery Center, Inc., 428 Winn Court, Decatur, GA 30030; tel. 404/292-3727; FAX. 404/294-9674; Diane Moore, RN, M.B.A., Administrator

Dennis Surgery Center, Inc., 3193 Howell Mill Road, Suite 215, Atlanta, GA 30327; tel. 404/355-1312; Kim A. Wolfe, Administrator

Dunwoody Outpatient Surgicenter, Inc., 4553 North Shallowford Road, Suite 60-C, Atlanta, GA 30338; tel. 404/457-6303; Theresa Scott, Administrator

Endoscopy Center of Southeast Georgia, Inc., 200 Maple Drive, Vidalia, GA 30474; tel. 912/537-9851; Dixie Calhoun, RN, Administrator

Feminist Women's Health Center, 580 14th Street, N.W., Atlanta, GA 30318; tel. 404/874-7551; FAX. 404/875-7644; Nancy Boothe, Executive Director

Friedrich Surgical Center, 2916 Glynn Avenue, Brunswick, GA 31530

☐ **G.I. Endoscopy Center,** 6555 Professional Place, Suite B, Riverdale, GA 30274; tel. 404/996-8830; FAX. 404/991-1596; Aruna Jaya Prakash, Administrator

Georgia Lithotripsy Center, 120 Trinity Place, Athens, GA 30607; tel. 404/543-2718; David C. Allen, M.D., Administrator

Gwinnet Endoscopy Center, 696 Pike Street, Suite 150, Lawrenceville, GA 30245; tel. 404/822-5560; Kerry H. King, M.D., President

Gwinnett Center for Outpatient Surgery, L.P., 2131 Fountain Drive, Snellville, GA 30278; tel. 404/979-8200; FAX. 404/979-1327; Laura Perez, RN, Administrator

☐ **Hollis Eye Surgery Center, Inc.,** 7351 Old Moon Road, Columbus, GA 31909; tel. 706/323-8127; Kenneth Hopkins, Administrator

Marietta Surgical Center, Ambulatory Surgery Division, Columbia Healthcare Corporation, 796 Church Street, Marietta, GA 30060; tel. 404/422-1579; FAX. 404/422-1057; Charlotte Bellantoni, Administrator

Medical Eye Associates, Inc., 1429 Oglethorpe Street, Macon, GA 31201; tel. 912/743-7061; FAX. 912/743-6296; Emmy Smallwood, Office Manager

Newton Rockdale Ambulatory Surgery Center, 4167 Hospital Drive, Covington, GA 30209; tel. 404/786-1234; Lori Goff, Administrator

North Atlanta Endoscopy Center, L.P., 5555 Peachtree-Dunwoody Road, Suite G-70, Atlanta, GA 30342; tel. 404/843-0500; Laura Dixon, Clinical Supervisor

North Atlanta Head and Neck Surgery Center, 980 Johnson Ferry Road, Northside Doctors Building, Suite 110, Atlanta, GA 30342; tel. 404/256-5428; Ramon S. Franco, M.D.

North Georgia Outpatient Surgery Center, 795 Red Bud Road, Calhoun, GA 30701; tel. 706/629-1852; Herbert E. Kosmahl, President

North Metro Day Surgery, 220 Hospital Road, Canton, GA 30114; tel. 404/479-2202; Robert E. Cole, Chief Executive Officer

North Oak Ambulatory Surgical Center, 2718 North Oak Street, Valdosta, GA 31602; tel. 912/242-3668; FAX. 912/242-9905; William Kevin Pearson

Northeast Georgia Plastic Surgery Center, 1296 Sims Street, Gainesville, GA 30501; tel. 404/534-1856; FAX. 404/531-0355; Sam Richwine, Medical Director

Northlake Ambulatory Surgical Center, 2193 Northlake Parkway, Building 12, Suite 114, Tucker, GA 30084-4193; tel. 404/938-4860; Winfield Butlin, Administrator

Northlake Endoscopy Center, 1459 Montreal Road, Suite 204, Tucker, GA 30084; tel. 404/939-4721; Gayle Carter, Administrator

Northlake-Tucker Ambulatory Surgery Center, 1491 Montreal, Tucker, GA 30084; tel. 404/934-1984; FAX. 404/493-4900; Doris Boye-Mintz

Northside Foot and Ankle Outpatient Surgical Center, 3415 Holcomb Bridge Road, Norcross, GA 30091; tel. 404/449-1122; FAX. 404/242-8709; Steven T. Arminio, Administrator

Northside Women's Clinic, Inc., 3543 Chamblee-Dunwoody Road, Atlanta, GA 30341; tel. 404/455-4210; FAX. 404/451-9529; James W. Gay, M.D., Administrator

Perimeter Center for Outpatient Surgery, 1140 Hammond Drive, Building F, Suite 6100, Atlanta, GA 30328; tel. 404/551-9944; Teressa Sowel, Administrator

☐ **Perimeter Center for Outpatient Surgery, L.P.,** 1140 Hammond Drive, Building F, Suite 6100, Atlanta, GA 30328; tel. 404/551-9944; Doris Boye-Mintz

Piedmont Surgery Center, 4660 Riverside Park Boulevard, Macon, GA 31210; tel. 912/471-6300; Stephen N. Barnes, M.D.

Planned Parenthood of East Central Georgia, 1289 Broad Street, Augusta, GA 30911; tel. 404/724-5557; FAX. 706/724-5293; Dale Brown, Administrator

Podiatric Surgi Center, 215 Clairmont Avenue, Decatur, GA 30030; tel. 404/373-2529; Jerald N. Kramer, President

Resurgens Surgical Center, 5671 Peachtree Dunwoody Road, Suite 800, Atlanta, GA 30342; tel. 404/847-9999; Kay F. Elliott, RN

Roderique Centre for Hand and Upper Extremity Surgery, 730 Peachtree Street, Suite 105, Atlanta, GA 30308; tel. 404/872-4263

Savannah Medical Clinic, 120 East 34th Street, Savannah, GA 31401; tel. 912/236-1603; Leonard Berger, Administrator

Savannah Outpatient Foot Surgery Center, 310 Eisenhower Drive, Suite Seven, Savannah, GA 31406; tel. 912/355-6503; Dr. Kalman Baruch, President

Savannah Plastic Surgicenter, 4750 Waters Avenue, Suite 505, Savannah, GA 31404; tel. 912/351-5050; Dr. E. D. Deloach

Southeastern Fertility Institute, 5505 Peachtree Dunwood Road, Suite 400, Atlanta, GA 30342; tel. 404/257-1900; Randy L. Haviland, Administrator

Southlake Orthopedic Center, 6635 Lake Drive, Morrow, GA 30260

☐ **Surgery Center of Rome,** 16 John Maddox Drive, Rome, GA 30161; tel. 404/234-0315; Jan Routledge, Director

Providers / Freestanding Ambulatory Surgery Centers

The Cosmetic and Plastic Surgicenter of South Atlanta, 6524 Professional Place, Riverdale, GA 30274; tel. 404/991–1733; FAX. 404/997–7204; Nabil Elsahy, M.D.

☐ **The Emory Clinic Ambulatory Surgery Center,** 1327 Clifton Road, N.E., Atlanta, GA 30322; tel. 404/321–0111; J. Lee Tribble, Administrator

The Foot Surgery Center, 2520 Windy Hill Road, Suite 105, Marietta, GA 30067; tel. 404/952–0868; L. Susan Rothstein, Administrator

The Rome Endoscopy Center, Inc., 11 John Maddox Drive, Rome, GA 30165; tel. 706/295–3992; FAX. 706/295–3979; Stephen M. Patton, Administrator

Tifton Medical Clinic Outpatient Services, 712 East 18 Street, Tifton, GA 31794; tel. 912/382–3814; Sheila M. Ridley

HAWAII

Aloha Eye Clinic and Surgical Center Ltd., 239 Wakea Avenue, Kahului, HI 96732; tel. 808/877–3984; FAX. 808/871–6498; Russell T. Stodd, M.D., Administrator

Ambulatory Surgical Center, Kauai, Kauai Medical Group, 4366 Kukui Grove Street, Lihue, HI 96766; Thatcher Magoun, Administrator

Cataract and Retina Center of Hawaii, 1712 Liliha Street, Suite 400, Honolulu, HI 96817; Worldster Lee, M.D., Administrator

Faulkner Institute for Eye Care and Surgery, 1100 Ward Avenue, Suite 1001, Honolulu, HI 96814; tel. 808/521–2305; FAX. 808/599–4818; Gerald D. Faulkner, M.D., President

Hawaiian Eye Center, 606 Kilani Avenue, Wahiawa, HI 96786; tel. 808/621–8448; FAX. 808/621–2082; John M. Corboy, M.D., Administrator

Kaiser Honolulu Clinic, 1010 Pensacola Street, Honolulu, HI 96814; tel. 808/593–2950; Jonathan Gans, Administrator

Surgicare of Hawaii, Inc., 226 North Kuakini Street, Suite 200, Honolulu, HI 96817; tel. 808/528–2511; FAX. 808/526–0651; Eileen M. Peyton, Facility Manager

The Honolulu Medical Group, Inc., 550 South Beretania Street, Honolulu, HI 96813; tel. 808/537–2211; FAX. 808/531–4179; Kimberly Rocha, Administrator

IDAHO

Boise Center for Foot Surgery, 1400 West Bannock, Boise, ID 83702; tel. 208/345–1871; FAX. 208/368–9707; Marshall D. Ogden, D.P.M., Medical Director

Boise Gastroenterology Associates, P.A., Idaho Endoscopy Center, 5680 West Gage, Boise, ID 83706; tel. 208/378–2894; R. Brent Archibald, M.D., President

Coeur d'Alene Surgery Center, 2121 Ironwood Center Drive, Coeur d'Alene, ID 83814; tel. 208/765–9059; FAX. 208/664–9998; Peter C. Jones, M.D., President

Idaho Ambucare Center, Inc., 211 West Iowa, Nampa, ID 83651; tel. 208/467–4222; FAX. 208/466–0328; Gary Botimer, Administrator

Idaho Eye Surgicenter, 2025 East 17th Street, Idaho Falls, ID 83404; tel. 208/524–2025; FAX. 208/529–1924; Kenneth W. Turley, M.D., Medical Director

Idaho Falls Surgical Center, 1945 East 17th Street, Idaho Falls, ID 83404; tel. 208/529–1945; James A. Haney, M.D., Medical Director

Idaho Foot Surgery Center, 782 South Woodruff, Idaho Falls, ID 83401; tel. 208/529–8393; FAX. 208/529–8078; Bruce G. Tolman, D.P.M., Facility Director

Jefferson Day Surgery Center, 220 West Jefferson, Boise, ID 83702; tel. 208/343–3802; William Stano, President

Lake City Surgery Center, 2201 Ironwood Place, Suite B, Coeur d'Alene, ID 83814; tel. 208/667–9362; FAX. 208/765–1310; Rachel Muthersbaugh, Director

North Idaho Cataract and Laser Center, Inc., 1814 Lincoln Way, Coeur d'Alene, ID 83814; tel. 208/667–2531; Marilyn Miller, Administrator

North Idaho Day Surgery and Laser Center, Inc., 2205 North Ironwood Drive, Coeur d'Alene, ID 83814; tel. 208/664–0543; FAX. 208/765–2867; Michael P. Christensen, M.D., President

Surgicare Center of Idaho, L.C., 360 East Mallard Drive, Suite 125, Boise, ID 83706; tel. 208/336–8700; W. Andrew Lyle, M.D., Medical Director

The Surgery Center, 115 Falls Avenue, W., P.O. Box 1864, Twin Falls, ID 83303–1864; tel. 208/733–1662; FAX. 208/734–3632; Larry Maxwell, M.D., Administrator

ILLINOIS

25 East Same Day Surgery, 25 East Washington, Chicago, IL 60602; tel. 312/726–3329; FAX. 312/726–3823; Tom Mallon, Administrator

A.C.T. Medical Center, 5714 West Division Street, Chicago, IL 60651; tel. 312/921–4300; Anthony Centrachio

Access Health Center, Ltd., 1700 75th Street, Downers Grove, IL 60516; tel. 708/964–0000; FAX. 708/964–0047; Anne V. Baginski, Administrative Director

Albany Medical Surgical Center, 5086 North Elston, Chicago, IL 60630; tel. 312/725–0200; FAX. 312/725–6152; Diana Lammon, Administrator

☐ **AmSurg,** 330 North Madison Street, Joliet, IL 60435; tel. 815/744–3000; FAX. 815/744–7916; Anne M. Cole, Administrator

American Women's Medical Center, 2744 North Western, Chicago, IL 60647; tel. 312/772–7726; Jan Barton, M.D., Administrator

Bel-Clair Ambulatory Surgical Treatment, 325 West Lincoln, Belleville, IL 62220; tel. 618/235–2299; David Horace

Bio Enterprises, Ltd., 520 North Michigan Avenue, Suite 1100, Chicago, IL 60611; tel. 312/266–1235; Laura Palomino

CMP Surgicenter, 3412 West Fullerton Avenue, Chicago, IL 60647; tel. 312/235–8000; FAX. 312/235–7018; Carlos G. Baldoceda, M.D., Medical Director

Carbondale Clinic Ambulatory Surgical Treatment Center, 2601 West Main Street, Carbondale, IL 62901; tel. 618/549–5361, ext. 218; FAX. 618/549–5128; William R. Hamilton, M.D., Chief Executive Officer, Medical Director

Center for Reconstructive Surgery, 6309 West 95th Street, Oak Lawn, IL 60453; tel. 708/499–3355; FAX. 708/423–2305; James D. Schlenker, M.D., Administrator

Chang's Medical Arts Building, 2809 North Center Street, Collinsville, IL 62234; tel. 618/288–1882; FAX. 618/288–3575; Donna Evans, RN

Children's New Specialty Pediatric Center, 2301 Enterprise Drive, Westchester, IL 60154; tel. 708/947–4000; Kathleen Majetich, Administrator

Community Health and Emergency Services, R.R. 1, Box 11, P.O. Box 233, Cairo, IL 62914; tel. 618/734–4400, ext. 303; FAX. 618/734–2884; Frederick L. Bernstein, Executvie Director

☐ **Concord Medical Center,** 17 West Grand, Chicago, IL 60610; tel. 312/467–6555; FAX. 312/467–9683; Faramarz Farahati, Managing Director

Concord West Medical Center, Ltd., 530 North Cass Avenue, Westmont, IL 60559; tel. 708/963–2500; Faramarz Farahati, Managing Director

Day SurgiCenters, Inc., 18 South Michigan Avenue, Suite 700, Chicago, IL 60603; tel. 312/726–2000; FAX. 312/726–3921; Paul Sussman, President, Chief Executive Officer

Day Surgicenters, Inc., One South 224 Summit Avenue, Suite 201, Oakbrook Terrace, IL 60181; tel. 708/916–7008, Andrew Andrikos, Administrator

☐ **Dimensions Medical Center, Ltd.,** 1455 East Golf Road, Suite 108, Des Plaines, IL 60016; tel. 708/390–9300; FAX. 708/390–0035; Alan Snider, Executive Director

Doctor's Clinic, 4325 Alby, P.O. Box 3195, Alton, IL 62002; tel. 618/474–8000, ext. 8052; FAX. 618/474–8054; Dr. Bruce T. Vest, Jr., M.D., Director, Surgery

Doctors Surgicenter, Ltd., 1045 Martin Luther King Jr. Drive, Centralia, IL 62801; tel. 618/532–3110; Charles K. Fischer, M.D., Medical Director

Dreyer Ambulatory Surgery Center, 1221 North Highland Avenue, Aurora, IL 60506; tel. 708/264–8400; James Shear

Eastland Medical Plaza SurgiCenter, 1505 Eastland Drive, Bloomington, IL 61701; tel. 309/662–2500, ext. 1284; FAX. 309/662–7143; Anna Lee Fenger, B.S.N., M.A., Administrator

Eyecare Physicians of America, 3101 North Harlem Avenue, Chicago, IL 60634; tel. 312/282–6840; Sandra Ankebrant, Executive Director

Eyes of Illinois Surgery Center, SC, 12 Maryville Professional Center, Maryville, IL 62062; tel. 618/288–7483; Melinda Smith, RN, Administrator

Foot and Ankle Surgical Center, 1455 Golf Road, Suite 134, Des Plaines, IL 60016; tel. 708/390–7666; Michelle Gormish, Administrator

Golf Surgical Center, 8901 Golf Road, Des Plaines, IL 60016; tel. 708/299–2273; FAX. 708/299–2297; Mary Lou Emmons, Administrator

☐ **Hauser-Ross Surgicenter, Inc.,** 2240 Gateway Drive, Sycamore, IL 60115; tel. 815/756–8571; FAX. 815/756–1226; Barbara Lauger, Administrator

Hawthorn Place Surgical Center, 1900 Hollister Drive, Libertyville, IL 60048; tel. 708/367–8100; FAX. 708/367–8335; Maury Kulwin, Administrator

Hinsdale Surgical Center, Inc., 40 South Clay Street, Hinsdale, IL 60521; tel. 708/325–5035; FAX. 708/325–5134; Judith L. McCammon, M.S., RN, Administrator

Hope Clinic for Women, Ltd., 1602 21st Street, Granite City, IL 62040; tel. 618/451–5722; Sally Burgess-Griffin, Director

Horizons Ambulatory Surgery Center, 630 Locust Street, Carthage, IL 62321; tel. 217/357–2173; James E. Coeur, M.D., Administrator

Hugar Surgery Center, 1614 North Harlem Avenue, Elmwood Park, IL 60635; tel. 708/452–6102; FAX. 708/452–1614; Frank A. Salvino, FACHA, Administrator

Illinois Eye Surgeons Cataract Surgery, 3990 North Illinois Street, Belleville, IL 62221; tel. 618/277–1130; Cathy Vieluf, Administrator

☐ **Ingalls Same Day Surgery,** 6701 West 159th Street, Tinley Park, IL 60477; tel. 708/429–0222; FAX. 708/429–0293; Joseph J. Maschek, Administrator

Kirk Eye Center, S.C., 7427 Lake Street, River Forest, IL 60305; tel. 708/771–3334; FAX. 708/771–0841; Steven T. Schwartz, Administrator

Lakeshore Physicians and Surgery Center, 7200 North Western Avenue, Chicago, IL 60645; tel. 312/743–6700; FAX. 312/761–9226; Phyllis J. Allen, Administrator

☐ **Magna Surgical Center,** 9831 South Western Avenue, Chicago, IL 60643; tel. 312/445–9696; FAX. 312/445–9590; Nader Bozorgi, M.D., Medical Director

McLean County Surgicenter, Ltd., 2502-B East Empire, Bloomington, IL 61704; tel. 309/662–6120; FAX. 309/663–8972; Tracy J. Silver, RN, Administrator

Metro Surgical Center, 201 North Wells Street, Chicago, IL 60606; tel. 312/263–5300; FAX. 312/263–7873; Nasiruddin Rana, M.D., Administrator

Michael Reese North-One Day Surgery, 60 East Delaware, 15th Floor, Chicago, IL 60611; tel. 312/440–5100; FAX. 312/440–5114; Cheryl Dancey, Vice President

Midwest Ambulatory Surgicenter, 7340 West College Drive, Palos Heights, IL 60463; tel. 708/361–3233; FAX. 708/361–4876; Thomas A. Evans, Administrator

☐ **Midwest Center for Day Surgery,** 3811 Highland Avenue, Downers Grove, IL 60515; tel. 708/852–9300; FAX. 708/852–7773; Ronald P. Ladniak, Administrator

Midwest Eye Center, 1700 East West Road, Calumet City, IL 60409; tel. 708/891–3330; FAX. 708/891–0904; Jill Stevenson, Administrator

C84 Health Organizations, Agencies and Providers

Providers / Freestanding Ambulatory Surgery Centers

Naperville Surgical Centre, 1263 Rickert Drive, Naperville, IL 60540; tel. 708/305-3300; FAX. 708/305-3301; Ronald P. Ladniak

Natioinal Health Care Services of Peoria, Inc., 7501 N. University Road, Suite 200, Peoria, IL 61614; tel. 309/691-9073; Margaret A. Vanduyn

North Shore Outpatient Surgicenter, L.P., 815 Howard Street, Evanston, IL 60202; tel. 708/869-8500; FAX. 708/869-0028; Edward Atkins, M.D., Medical Director

Northern Illinois Surgery Center, 1620 Sauk Road, Dixon, IL 61021; tel. 815/288-7722; Gail Hanson, Director, Nursing

Northern Illinois Women's Center, Ltd., 1400 Broadway Street, Suite 201, Rockford, IL 61104; tel. 815/963-4101; FAX. 815/963-6122; Richard Ragsdale

Northshore Eye Surgicenter, Ltd., 3034 West Peterson Avenue, Chicago, IL 60659; tel. 312/973-7432; FAX. 312/973-1119; Hilde Schoonmaker, Director of Nursing

Northwest Community Day Surgery Center, 675 West Kirchoff Road, Arlington Heights, IL 60005; tel. 708/506-4361; FAX. 708/577-4001; Karen Zillgitt, RN, Administrative Director

Northwest Surgicare, Inc., 1100 West Central Road, Arlington Heights, IL 60005; tel. 708/259-3080; FAX. 708/259-3190; Barbara Cerwin, RN, Administrator

Notre Dame Hills Surgical Center, 28 North 64th Street, Belleville, IL 62223; tel. 618/398-5705; FAX. 618/398-5764; Kathleen Claunch, RN, Administrator

Oak Brook Surgical Center, Inc., 2425 West 22nd Street, Oak Brook, IL 60521; tel. 708/990-2212, ext. 2022; FAX. 708/990-3130; Dr. K. Jafari, President, Medical Director

One Day Surgery Center, 4211 North Cicero Avenue, Chicago, IL 60641; tel. 312/794-1000, ext. 228; FAX. 312/794-9738; Andrew P. Cameron, Administrator

Orthopedic Institute of Illinois Ambulatory Surgery Center, 303 North Kumpf Boulevard, Peoria, IL 61605; tel. 309/676-5559; FAX. 309/676-5045; Donna Adair, Administrator

Paulina Surgi-Center, Inc., 7616 North Paulina, Chicago, IL 60626; tel. 312/761-0500; Sheldon Schecter, Administrator

Peoria Ambulatory Surgery Center, 4909 North Glen Park Place, Peoria, IL 61514; tel. 309/691-9069

Peoria Day Surgery Center, 7309 North Knoxville, Peoria, IL 61614; tel. 309/692-9210; FAX. 309/692-9055; Wanda Spacht, RN, CNOR, Nursing Administrator

Physicians' Surgical Center, Ltd., 311 West Lincoln, Suite 300, Belleville, IL 62220; tel. 618/233-7077; Cindy Chapman, RN, Administrator

Poplar Creek Surgical Center, 1800 McDonough Road, Hoffman Estates, IL 60192; tel. 708/742-7272; JoAnn Uteg, Administrative Director

Quad City Ambulatory Surgery Center, 520 Valley View Drive, Moline, IL 61265; tel. 309/762-1952; FAX. 309/762-3642

Quad City Endoscopy, 2525 24th Street, Rock Island, IL 61201; tel. 309/788-5624; FAX. 309/788-5668; Najwa Bayrakdar, Administrator

Regional Surgicenter, Ltd., 545 Valley View Drive, Moline, IL 61265; tel. 309/762-5560; FAX. 309/762-7351; Donna Lyons, Administrator

River North Surgery Center, One East Erie, Suite 115, Chicago, IL 60611; tel. 312/649-3939; FAX. 312/649-3943; Patricia Wamsley, Administrator

Rockford Endoscopy Center, 401 Roxbury Road, Rockford, IL 61107; tel. 815/397-7340

South Shore Surgicenter, Inc., 8300 South Brandon Avenue, Chicago, IL 60617; tel. 312/721-6000; FAX. 312/721-9861; Lucy Morales, RN, Administrator

Southeast Suburban Ambulatory Surgery Center, Ltd., 15643 Lincoln Avenue, Harvey, IL 60426; tel. 708/339-7000; FAX. 708/339-7026; James Kuyper, RN, Administrator

Southwestern Illinois Outpatient Surgical Center, 12 Ginger Creek Professional Park, Edwardsville, IL 62025; tel. 618/656-8200; FAX. 618/656-8204; Deborah Ashley-Petroff, RN, B.S.N., SNA, Administrator

Spiritus Dei Eye Surgery Center, 7600 West College Drive, Palos Heights, IL 60463; tel. 708/361-0010; Peggy A. Toth, Administrator

Springfield Clinic Ambulatory Surgical Treatment Center, Inc., 1025 South Seventh Street, Springfield, IL 62794-9248; tel. 217/528-7541; Michael Maynard

Suburban Otolaryngology SurgiCenter, 3340 South Oak Park Avenue, Berwyn, IL 60402; tel. 708/749-3070; FAX. 708/749-3410; Edward A. Razim, M.D., Administrator

Surgicare Center, Inc., 333 Dixie Highway, Chicago Heights, IL 60411; tel. 708/754-4890; Franz J. Herpok, Administrator

Surgicare, Inc., 10547 South Ewing Avenue, Chicago, IL 60617; tel. 312/375-0791; William Wood, Medical Director

The Center for Surgery, 475 East Diehl Road, Naperville, IL 60563-1253; tel. 708/505-7733; FAX. 708/505-0656; Eric Myers

The Surgery Center of Southern Illinois, New Route 13 West, Marion, IL 62959; tel. 618/993-2113; FAX. 618/993-2041; Linda Bickers, RN, Administrator

Valley Ambulatory Surgery Center, 2210 Dean Street, St. Charles, IL 60175; tel. 708/584-9800; FAX. 708/584-9805; Mark Mayo, Facility Director

Watertower Surgicenter Corp., 845 North Michigan Avenue, Suite 994-W, Chicago, IL 60611; tel. 312/944-2929; FAX. 312/944-7769; John M. Sevcik, President, Chief Executive Officer

Women's Aid Clinic, 4751 West Touhy Avenue, Lincolnwood, IL 60646; tel. 708/676-2428; Iris Schneider

INDIANA

☐ **Akin Medical Center,** 2019 State Street, New Albany, IN 47150-4963; tel. 812/945-3557; FAX. 812/949-3469; Alice M. Bryant, RN, Administrator

American Eye Institute Surgical Division, 520 West First Street, New Albany, IN 47150-3603; tel. 812/949-3442; FAX. 812/949-3447; John M. Schmitt, Executive Director

Bloomington Surgery Center, 1011 West Second Street, Bloomington, IN 47403-2216; tel. 812/334-1213, ext. 250; FAX. 812/333-5039; Teresa Mathis, RN, Administrator

Brodersen-Williams Eye Institute, 6836 Hohman Avenue, Hammond, IN 46324; tel. 219/931-7509; James D. Brodersen, M.D., Administrator

Calumet Surgery Center, 7847 Calumet Avenue, Munster, IN 46321-1296; tel. 219/836-5102; FAX. 219/836-2249; Gloria J. Portney, RN, Chief Administrative Officer

Columbus Surgery Center, 940 North Marr Road, Columbus, IN 47201; tel. 812/372-1370; Patricia A. Tackett-Barnard, Administrator

Digestive Health Center, 1120 AAA Way, Suite A, Carmel, IN 46032-3210; tel. 317/848-5494; FAX. 317/575-0392; Melissa Berry, Administrative Assistant

Evansville Surgery Center Associates, 1212 Lincoln Avenue, Evansville, IN 47714-1076; tel. 812/428-0810; FAX. 812/421-6070; LaDonna Joergens, B.S.N., Facility Manager

Eye Specialist Surgery Center, 1901 North Meridian Street, Indianapolis, IN 46202-1303; tel. 317/925-2200; Dan Bradford, Administrator

Fort Wayne Ophthalmic Surgical Center, 321 East Wayne Street, Ft. Wayne, IN 46802-2713; tel. 219/422-5976; FAX. 219/424-4511; J. Rex Parent, M.D., Chief Executive Officer

Gastrointestinal Endoscopy Center, 801 St. Mary's Drive, Suite 110, West, Evansville, IN 47714; tel. 812/477-6103; FAX. 812/477-4897; Christine Wittman, Practice Administrator

Grossnickle Eye Surgery Center, Inc., 2251 DuBois Drive, Warsaw, IN 46580-3292; tel. 219/269-3777; FAX. 219/269-9828; Shirley Rhodes, RN, Administrative Director

IMA Endoscopy Surgicenter, P.C., 8895 Broadway, Merrillville, IN 46410; tel. 219/738-2081; FAX. 219/736-4658; Sandra K. Shaw, Administrator

Indiana Eye Clinic, 30 North Emerson Avenue, Greenwood, IN 46143-9760; tel. 317/881-3937; FAX. 317/887-4008; Mr. B. H. Draffen, Executive Director

Indiana Surgery Center, 8040 Clearvista Parkway, Indianapolis, IN 46256-1695; tel. 317/841-2000; Amy Glover, Administrator

Indianapolis Breast Center and Consulting Services, 1950 West 86th Street, Indianapolis, IN 46260-2064; tel. 317/871-6874; FAX. 317/872-9856; Pat Harper, M.D., Executive Director

Indianapolis Surgery Center, 2007 North Capitol Avenue, Indianapolis, IN 46202-1254; tel. 317/926-4359; FAX. 317/927-3880; Judy Rodocker, RN, M.A., Facility Administrator

Lafayette Ambulatory Surgery Center, 3733 Rome Drive, Box 6477, Lafayette, IN 47903-6477; tel. 317/449-5272; FAX. 317/477-8723; Dale T. Krynak, Executive Director

Laser Surgery Center, 8514 Broadway, Merrillville, IN 46410; tel. 219/756-5010; Eldi E. Deschamps, M.D., Executive Director

MHC Surgical Center Associates, Inc., d/b/a Broadwest Surgical Center, 315 West 89th Avenue, Merrillville, IN 46410-2904; tel. 219/757-5275; FAX. 219/980-7804; Lisa M. Goranovich, Administrator

MediVision, Inc., 1305 Wall Street, Suite 101, Jeffersonville, IN 47130-3898; tel. 812/288-9674; FAX. 812/283-6955; Marsha Parker, Administrator

Meridian Plastic Surgery Center, 170 West 106th Street, Indianapolis, IN 46290-1004; tel. 317/575-0110; FAX. 317/846-5719; Sally Gentner, Director

Muncie Ambulatory Surgicenter, LLC, 200 North Tillotson Avenue, Muncie, IN 47304-3988; tel. 317/286-8888; FAX. 317/747-7962; L. Marshall Roch, M.D., Administrator

Nasser Smith and Pinkerton Cardiac Cath Lab, 8333 Naab Road, Indianapolis, IN 46260; tel. 317/338-6094; FAX. 317/338-6066; Rodger P. Pinto, Ph.D., Administrator

North Indianapolis Surgery Center, 8651 North Township Line Road, Indianapolis, IN 46260-1578; tel. 317/876-2090; FAX. 317/876-2097; Judy Rodocker, RN, M.A., Facility Administrator

Northside Cardiac Cath Lab, 8333 Naab Road, Suite 180, Indianapolis, IN 46260; tel. 317/338-9001; FAX. 317/338-9045; Mary Ellen Boyd, Administrator

Outpatient Surgery Center of Indiana, Inc., 711 Gardner Drive, Marion, IN 46952; tel. 317/664-2000; FAX. 317/668-6797; Valerie Walls, RN, Administrator

Physiciancare Outpatient Surgery Center, Inc., 7460 North Shadeland, Indianapolis, IN 46250; tel. 317/577-7450; FAX. 317/577-7462; Rick S. Mohler, Administrator

Premier Ambulatory Surgery of Fort Wayne, 1333 Maycrest Drive, Fort Wayne, IN 46805-5478; tel. 219/423-3339; FAX. 219/423-6344; Mary Schafer, Administrator

Sagamore Surgical Services, Inc., 2320 Concord Road, Suite B, Lafayette, IN 47905; tel. 317/474-7838; FAX. 317/474-7853; Carol Blanar, Administrator

South Bend Clinic Surgicenter, 211 North Eddy Street, P.O. Box 4061, South Bend, IN 46634-4061; tel. 219/237-9366; FAX. 219/237-9329; Teresa Roberts, Executive Officer

Southern Indiana Infusion Therapy Clinic, 1120 Spring Street, Jeffersonville, IN 47130; tel. 502/429-5500; FAX. 502/429-5141; Kevin R. Burk, Administrator

Southern Indiana Surgery Center, 2800 Rex Grossman Boulevard, Bloomington, IN 47403; tel. 812/333-8969; FAX. 812/335-2309; Miriam Malone, RN, B.S.N., Executive Director

Surgery Center Plus, 7430 North Shadeland Avenue, Suite 100, Indianapolis, IN 46250-2025; tel. 317/841-8005; FAX. 317/577-7538; James Hansen, Administrator

Providers / Freestanding Ambulatory Surgery Centers

Surgery One, Inc., 5052 North Clinton, Fort Wayne, IN 46825–5822; tel. 219/482–5194; William H. Couch, Jr., M.D., Executive Officer

Surgical Care Center, Inc., 8103 Clearvista Parkway, Indianapolis, IN 46256–4600; tel. 317/842–5173; FAX. 317/576–9644; Larry Gardner, Executive Director

Surgical Center of New Albany, 2201 Green Valley Road, New Albany, IN 47150–4648; tel. 812/949–1223; Tamara E. Hay, RN, Administrator

The Center for Specialty Surgery of Ft. Wayne, Inc., 2730 East State Boulevard, Fort Wayne, IN 46805–4731; tel. 219/483–2540; FAX. 219/483–3097, ext. 2; Andrea Kelley, RN, Director of Nursing

The Indiana Hand Surgery Center, 8501 Harcourt Road, P.O. Box 80434, Indianapolis, IN 46280–0434; tel. 317/875–9105; FAX. 317/875–8638; Mark S. Fritz, Chief Executive Officer

Valparaiso Physican and Surgery Center, 1700 Pointe Drive, Valparaiso, IN 46383; tel. 219/757–6496; FAX. 219/531–5060; Ray Ingham, Administrator

Wabash Valley Surgery Center, 422 Poplar, Terre Haute, IN 47807–4214; tel. 812/232–0564; FAX. 812/234–3565; James P. McNeely, Executive Director

Zollman Surgery Center, Inc., 7439 Woodland Drive, Indianapolis, IN 46268; tel. 317/328–1100; FAX. 317/328–6948; Susan Matouk, RN, B.S.N., Clinical Administrator

IOWA

Iowa Eye Institute, 1721 West 18th Street, Spencer, IA 51301; tel. 712/262–8878; FAX. 712/262–8807; Dennis D. Gordy, M.D., Administrator

Jones Eye Clinic, 4405 Hamilton Boulevard, Sioux City, IA 51104; tel. 712/239–3937; Charles E. Jones, M.D., Medical Director

Land–Barowsky Eye Center, 931 13th Avenue, N., P.O. Box 608, Clinton, IA 52733–0608; tel. 319/242–3937; FAX. 319/242–3845; Patricia McEachron, Administrator

Surgery Center of Des Moines, 1301 Penn Avenue, Suite 100, Des Moines, IA 50312; tel. 515/266–3140; FAX. 515/266–3073; Kathleen Supplee, RN, Administrator

Surgery Center of Des Moines, 974 73rd Street, Suite Nine, Des Moines, IA 50312; tel. 515/224–1984; FAX. 515/224–6827; Jackie Schram

Tower Surgical Center, 3200 Grand Avenue, Des Moines, IA 50312; tel. 515/271–1735; FAX. 515/271–1726; L. Duane Murray, Administrator

Uro Surgery Center, 3319 Spring Street, Suite 202–A, Davenport, IA 52807; tel. 319/359–1641; FAX. 319/359–9492; Paul Rohlf, M.D., Administrator

KANSAS

Cataract Surgery Center, 6100 East Central Street, Suite Five, Wichita, KS 67208–4237; tel. 316/684–8013; Linda S. Buettner, Vice President

College Park Family Care Center, 11725 West 112th Street, Overland Park, KS 66210–2761; tel. 913/469–5579; Thomas Miller, M.D., Administrator

Comprehensive Health for Women, 4401 West 109th Street, Overland Park, KS 66211–1303; tel. 913/345–1400; Sheila Kostas, Director, Human Resources

Cotton–O'Neil Clinic Endoscopy Center, 823 S.W. Mulvane Street, Suite 375, Topeka, KS 66606–1666; tel. 913/354–9591, ext. 741; FAX. 913/354–0547; Irene Hasenbank, R.N., Administrator

Dodge City Surgicenter, 100 Ross Boulevard, Dodge City, KS 67801–2131; tel. 316/225–2200; Denise Mayhew, Administrator

Emporia Ambulatory Surgery Center, 2528 West 15th Avenue, Emporia, KS 66801–6102; tel. 316/343–2233; J. E. Bosiljevac, M.D., Administrator

Endoscopic Services, P.A., 1431 South Bluffview Street, Suite 215, Wichita, KS 67218–3000; tel. 316/687–0234; FAX. 316/687–0360; Jace Hyder, M.D.

Endoscopy Center of Topeka, L.P., 2200 S.W. Sixth Avenue, Suite 103, Topeka, KS 66606–1707; tel. 913/354–1254; FAX. 913/354–1255; Ashraf M. Sufi, M.D., Medical Director

EyeSurg of Kansas City, 5520 College Boulevard, Overland Park, KS 66211–1600; tel. 913/491–3757; FAX. 913/469–6686; Phillip Hoopes, M.D., Medical Administrator

Great Plains Clinic, 201 East 7th, Hays, KS 67601; tel. 913/628–8251; William Norris, Administrator

Kansas Ambulatory Surgery Center, 7015 East Central Street, Wichita, KS 67206–1940; tel. 316/684–9300; FAX. 316/652–7618; Robert G. Clark, M.D., Medical Director

Laser Center, 1518A East Iron Avenue, Salina, KS 67401–3236; tel. 913/825–6016; Brian E. Conner, M.D., Administrator

Microsurgery, Inc., 920 S.W. Washburn Avenue, Topeka, KS 66606–1527; tel. 913/233–3939; Adrienne V. Prokop, Administrator

Newman–Young Clinic-A.S.C., 710 West Eighth Street, Fort Scott, KS 66701–2404; tel. 316/223–3100; FAX. 316/223–5390; Thomas W. Smith, Administrator

Newton Surgery Centre, 215 South Pine Street, Newton, KS 67114–3761; tel. 316/283–4400; Sherry White, Administrator

Ochsner Eye Medical/Surgical Center, 1100 North Topeka Street, Wichita, KS 67214–2810; tel. 316/263–6273; FAX. 316/263–5568; Bruce B. Ochsner, Medical Director

South Pointe Surgery Center, 151 West 151st Street, Suite 200, Olathe, KS 66061–5351; tel. 913/782–3631; FAX. 913/782–2606; Shelley Eisenbeisz, RN, Administrator

Surgery Center of Kansas, Inc., 1507 West 21st Street, Wichita, KS 67203–2449; tel. 316/838–8388; FAX. 316/838–2999; Thomas Potts, Associate Director, Chief Operating Officer

☐ **Surgicare of Wichita, Inc.,** 810 North Lorraine, Wichita, KS 67214–4841; tel. 316/685–2207; FAX. 316/685–2861; Carolyn J. Exley, Administrator

Surgicenter of Johnson County, 8800 Ballentine Street, Overland Park, KS 66214–1985; tel. 913/894–4050; FAX. 913/894–0384; Nancy E. Sturgeon, Administrator

The Center for Same Day Surgery, 818 North Emporia Street, Suite 108, Wichita, KS 67214–3725; tel. 316/262–7263; Shelly LeGate, RN, B.S., Administrator

The Headache and Pain Center, 11111 Nall Avenue, Suite 222, Leawood, KS 66211–1625; tel. 913/491–3999; FAX. 913/491–6453; Steven D. Waldman, Administrator

The Wichita Clinic DaySurgery, 3311 East Murdock Street, Wichita, KS 67208–3054; tel. 316/689–9349; James A. Greer, Jr., Administrator

Topeka Single Day Surgery, 823 S.W. Mulvane Street, Suite 101, Topeka, KS 66606–1679; tel. 913/354–8737; FAX. 913/354–1440; Linda Daniel, Executive Director

KENTUCKY

Ambulatory Surgery Center, 2831 Lone Oak Road, Paducah, KY 42003; tel. 502/554–8373; FAX. 502/554–8987; Laxmaiah Manchikanti, M.D.

Bio–Medical Appl of East Louisville, 5620 Bardstown Road, Louisville, KY 40291; tel. 502/239–8221; Deborah A. Downs

Center For Surgical Care, 7575 U.S. 42, Florence, KY 41042; tel. 606/283–6048; Thomas Mayer, M.D., Medical Director

Dupont Surgery Center, 4004 Dupont Circle, Louisville, KY 40207; tel. 502/896–6428; FAX. 502/895–6787; Vicki Lococo, Nurse Manager

E.M.W. Women's Surgical Center, 138 West Market Street, Louisville, KY 40202; tel. 502/589–2124; FAX. 502/589–1588; Dona F. Wells, Administrator

East Bernstadt Outpatient Surgery Center, Highway 25, P.O. Box 248, East Bernstadt, KY 40729; tel. 606/843–7704; Lowell Jones, Administrator

Iroquois Surgical Center, 4414 Churchman Avenue, Louisville, KY 40215; tel. 502/366–9525; FAX. 502/366–9520; Norman Stiefler, Administrative Director

Lexington Clinic, 1221 South Broadway, Lexington, KY 40504; tel. 606/255–6841; FAX. 606/253–0561; Brian A. McAlpin, Executive Director

Lexington Surgery Center, 1725 Harrodsburg Road, Lexington, KY 40504; tel. 606/276–2525; FAX. 606/277–6497; Bemedji Asher, Administrator

Louisville Surgery Center, 614 East Chestnut Street, Louisville, KY 40202; tel. 502/589–9488; FAX. 502/589–9928; Jane E. Burbank, Administrator

McPeak Center For Eye Care, 1507 Bravo Boulevard, Glasgow, KY 42141; tel. 502/651–2181; FAX. 502/651–2183; Nancy McPeak, Administrator

Medical Heights Surgery Center, 2374 Nicholasville Road, Lexington, KY 40503; tel. 606/278–1460; Ben Crawford, M.D., Administrator

Outpatient Care Center at Jewish Hospital, 225 Abraham Flexner Way, Louisville, KY 40202; tel. 502/587–4709; FAX. 502/587–4323; Kim Tharp, Administrator

Owensboro Ambulatory Surgical Facility, 1100 Walnut Street, Owensboro, KY 42301; tel. 502/683–2751; FAX. 502/926–1618; Lisa D. Revlett, Administrator

Pikeville United Methodist Hospital of Kentucky, Inc., 911 South By-Pass Road, Pikeville, KY 41501; tel. 606/437–3500; Martha O'Regan Chill, Administrator, Chief Executive Officer

Surgecenter of Louisville, 4005 DuPont Circle, Louisville, KY 40207; tel. 502/897–7401; Sheila S. Stinnett, Administrator

Surgical Center of Elizabethtown, 708 Westport Road, Elizabethtown, KY 42701; tel. 502/737–5200; FAX. 502/765–5362; Suzanne Broadwater, Administrator

The Eye Surgery Center of Paducah, 100 Medical Center Drive, P.O. Box 8269, Paducah, KY 42002–8269; tel. 502/442–1024; FAX. 502/442–1001; Kelly Harris, RN, Administrator

The Pain Treatment Center, 280 Stone Road, Lexington, KY 40503; tel. 606/278–1316; Ballard Wright

Tri–State Digestive Disorder Center Ambulatory Surgery Center, 196 Barnwood Drive, Edgewood, KY 41017; tel. 606/341–3575; Stephen W. Hiltz, M.D.

Walk In and Out Surgery Center, Inc., 353 Bogle Street, Suite 101, Somerset, KY 42501; tel. 606/679–9322; Sally Mullins, Administrator

LOUISIANA

Acadiana Endoscopy Center, 113 St. Louis Street, Lafayette, LA 70506; tel. 318/269–1126; FAX. 318/269–0553; Stephen M. Person, M.D., Administrator

Baton Rouge Ambulatory Surgicare Services, 5328 Didesse Drive, Baton Rouge, LA 70808; tel. 504/766–1718; FAX. 504/767–3034; Laura B. Cronin, Administrator

Broussard Surgery Institute, 1250 Pecanland Road, Suite E–1, Monroe, LA 71203; tel. 318/387–2015; Gerald Broussard, M.D., Administrator

Browne–McHardy Outpatient Surgery Center, 4315 Houma Boulevard, Metairie, LA 70006–2981; tel. 504/887–5500; FAX. 504/889–5297; Robert L. Goldstein, Chief Administrative Officer

Central Louisiana Ambulatory Surgical Center, 720 Madison Street, P.O. Box 8646, Alexandria, LA 71301; tel. 318/443–3511; Louise Barker, RN, Administrator

Colonnade Surgery, 555 South Ryan Street, Lake Charles, LA 70601; tel. 318/439–6226; FAX. 312/436–6223; Pam Ragusa, Administrator

Eye Care and Surgery Center, 10423 Old Hammond Highway, Baton Rouge, LA 70816; tel. 504/923–0960; Carl N. Doggette, Administrator

Foot Surgery Center of Shreveport, 9308 Mansfield Road, Suite 300, Shreveport, LA 71118; tel. 318/686–9622; Arnold M. Castellano, Administrator

Providers / Freestanding Ambulatory Surgery Centers

Gamble Ambulatory Surgery Center, 2601 Line Avenue, Suite B, Shreveport, LA 71104; tel. 318/424–3291; Michael Drews, D.P.M., Administrator

Green Clinic Surgery Center, 1200 South Farmerville Street, Ruston, LA 71270; tel. 318/255–3690; FAX. 318/251–6116; Glenn Scott, Executive Director

Hedgewood Surgical Center, 2427 St. Charles Avenue, New Orleans, LA 70130; tel. 504/895–7642; FAX. 504/895–0728; Calvin M. Johnson, Jr., M.D.

Houma Outpatient Surgery Center, Ltd., 3800 Houma Boulevard, Suite 250, Metairie, LA 70006; tel. 504/456–1515; Jay Weil III, President, Chief Executive Officer

Houma Surgi Center, Inc., 1020 School Street, Houma, LA 70360; tel. 504/868–4320; FAX. 504/868–3617; Robert M. Alexander, M.D., Administrator

☐ **Institute for Cardiovascular Studies,** 4413 Wichers Drive, Marrero, LA 70072; tel. 504/347–5914; Patrick N. Stewart, Administrator

LSU Eye Surgery Center, 2020 Gravier Street, Suite B, New Orleans, LA 70112; tel. 504/568–6700; W. L. Blackwell, Chief Executive Officer

LaHaye Center for Advanced Care, 201 Rue Iberville, Lafayette, LA 70508; tel. 318/235–2149; Darryl Wagley

LaHaye Eye and Ambulatory Surgical Center, 100 Harry Guilbeau Road, Opelousas, LA 70570; tel. 318/942–2024; FAX. 318/948–8869; Dana Cockran, Administrator

Lakeview Surgery and Diagnostic Center, Inc., 800 Heavens Drive, Mandeville, LA 70471; tel. 504/845–7100; Glenda P. Escudero, Administrator

Laser and Surgery Center, 4100 Parliment Drive, Alexandria, LA 71303; tel. 318/448–4488, ext. 318; FAX. 318/448–9731; M. L. Revelett, Administrator

Louisiana Endoscopy Center, Inc., 8150 Jefferson Highway, Baton Rouge, LA 70809; tel. 504/927–0970; FAX. 504/927–0988; Lorrie Rogerson, Administrator

Louisville Plaza Surgery Center, 3101 Kilpatrick Boulevard, P.O. Box 4335, Monroe, LA 71201; tel. 318/322–5916; FAX. 318/322–5916; Frank Wilderman, D.P.M., Administrator

MGA GI Diagnostic and Therapeutic Center, 1111 Medical Center Boulevard, Suite 310, Marrero, LA 70072; tel. 504/349–6401; Thomas D. McCaffery, Jr., President

MGA GI Diagnostic and Therapeutic Center, 2633 Napolean Avenue, Suite 707, New Orleans, LA 70115; tel. 504/349–6401; Thomas D. McCaffery, Jr., Administrator

Magnolia Surgical Facility, 3939 Houma Boulevard, Suite 216, Metairie, LA 70006; tel. 504/455–7771; FAX. 504/885–5063; Hamid Massiha, M.D., Administrator

Marrero SurgiCenter, Inc., 4511 Westbank Expressway, Suite B, Marrero, LA 70072; tel. 504/340–1993; John Schiro, M.D., Administrator

Ochsner Clinic–Plastic Surgery Department, 1514 Jefferson Highway, Fifth Floor, New Orleans, LA 70121; tel. 504/838–3950; Amy Freeman, Administrator

Outpatient Eye Surgery Center, 4324 Veterans Boulevard, Metairie, LA 70006; tel. 504/455–4046; FAX. 504/889–0399; Cheryl Crouse, Administrator

Outpatient Surgery Center for Sight, 550 Connell's Park Lane, Baton Rouge, LA 70809; tel. 504/924–2020; Alan DeCorte, Administrator

P and S Surgery Center, 312 Grammont Street, P.O. Box 3187, Monroe, LA 71201–3187; tel. 318/388–4040; FAX. 318/388–4099; Hank Atherton, Administrator

Prytania Surgery, Inc., 3525 Prytania Street, New Orleans, LA 70115; tel. 504/897–1515; Jay Weil III, Administrator

Saints Streets ASC Endoscopy Center, Inc., 201 St. Patrick Street, Suite 202, Lafayette, LA 70506; tel. 318/232–6697; FAX. 318/233–8065; Stephen G. Abshire, M.D., Administrator

Shreveport Endoscopy Center, A.M.C., 3217 Mabel Street, P.O. Box 37045, Shreveport, LA 71133–7045; tel. 318/631–0072; FAX. 318/631–9688; Linda Sibley, Administrator

Shreveport Surgery Center, 745 Olive Street, Suite 100, Shreveport, LA 71104; tel. 318/227–1163; FAX. 318/227–0413; Mary Jones, Administrator

St. Charles Avenue Surgical Facility, Inc., 3600 St. Charles Avenue, New Orleans, LA 70115; tel. 504/897–2237; George W. Hoffman, Administrator

Surgery Center, Inc., 1101 South College Road, Suite 100, Lafayette, LA 70503; tel. 318/233–8603; FAX. 318/234–0341; Russell J. Arceneaux, Administrator

☐ **Surgi–Center of Baton Rouge,** 5222 Brittany Drive, Baton Rouge, LA 70809; tel. 504/767–5636; FAX. 504/769–9107; Celeste M. Wiggins, Administrator

Surgicare of Lake Charles, 214 South Ryan Street, Lake Charles, LA 70601; tel. 318/436–6941; Debbie Boudreaux, Clinical Administrator

Surgiunit, Inc., 4204 Teuton Street, Metairie, LA 70006; tel. 504/888–3836; Gustavo A. Colon, M.D., Administrator

The Endoscopy Center of Monroe, 316 South Sixth Street, Monroe, LA 71201; tel. 318/325–2649; FAX. 318/325–0717; David R. Raines, M.D., Administrator

The Endoscopy Clinic of Lake Charles Medical and Surgical, 501 South Ryan, Lake Charles, LA 70601; tel. 318/478–2210; Robert Oates, Administrator

The Greater New Orleans Surgery Center, 3434 Houma Boulevard, Metairie, LA 70006; tel. 504/888–7100; David R. Vela, M.D., Administrator

☐ **The Iberia Endoscopy Center, Inc.,** 1100 Andre Street, Suite 12, New Iberia, LA 70560; tel. 318/364–9680; Alice M. Broussard, Administrator

The Outpatient Surgery Center of Baton Rouge, 505 East Airport Drive, Baton Rouge, LA 70806; tel. 504/925–2031; FAX. 504/924–2809; Lorraine Caraway, Administrator

The Plastic Surgery Center, Inc., 4224 Houma Boulevard, Suite 430, Metairie, LA 70006; tel. 504/456–5150; FAX. 504/456–5055; James B. Johnson, M.D., Administrator

The Surgery Suite, 103 Medical Center Drive, Slidell, LA 70461; tel. 504/646–4466; Allison F. Maestri, RN, Administrator

Urology Specialty and Surgery Center, 234 South Ryan Street, Lake Charles, LA 70601; tel. 318/433–5282; FAX. 318/433–1159; Charles Enright, Administrator

Willis-Knighton, d/b/a Northwest Louisiana Surgical Center, 2401 Greenwood Road, Shreveport, LA 71103; tel. 318/632–8222; FAX. 318/632–8230; Sharon C. Elias, Department Head

Young Eye Surgery Center, Inc., 204 North Magdalen Square, Abbeville, LA 70510; tel. 318/893–4452; FAX. 318/893–7870; Virginia Y. Herbert, Administrator

MAINE

Acadia Medical Arts Ambulatory Surgical Suite, 404 State Street, Bangor, ME 04401; tel. 207/990–0928; Jordan J. Shubert, M.D., President

Aroostook County Regional Opthalmology Center, 148 Academy Street, Presque Isle, ME 04769–0151; tel. 207/764–0376; FAX. 207/764–7612; Craig W. Young, M.D., Director

Eye Care and Surgery Center of Maine, P.A., 53 Sewall Street, Portland, ME 04102; tel. 207/773–6336; FAX. 207/773–7034; William S. Holt, M.D., President

Maine Cataract and Eye Center, 386 Bridgton Road, Route 302, Westbrook, ME 04092; tel. 207/797–9214; FAX. 207/797–8236; Elliot Schweid, D.O., Director

Maine Eye Center, P.A., 15 Lowell Street, Portland, ME 04102; tel. 207/774–8277; FAX. 207/871–1415; Frank Read, M.D., Director

Orthopaedic Surgery Center, 33 Sewall Street, Portland, ME 04102; tel. 207/828–2130; FAX. 207/828–2190; Linda M. Ruterbories, Medical Director

Portland Endoscopy Center, 131 Chadwick Street, Portland, ME 04102–3266; tel. 207/773–7964; Newell Augur, M.D., President

Western Avenue Day Surgery Center, a/k/a Plastic and Hand Surgical Associates, P.A., 244 Western Avenue, South Portland, ME 04106; tel. 207/775–3446; FAX. 207/879–1646; Jean J. Labelle, M.D., President

MARYLAND

Albert Shoumer, D.P.M., Dundalk Professional Center, 40 South Dundalk Avenue, Dundalk, MD 21222; tel. 410/282–6434

Albert Shoumer, D.P.M., 1645 Liberty Road, Eldersburg, MD 21784; tel. 310/795–2889

Amber Meadows Ambulatory Care Center, Inc., 198 Thomas Johnson Drive, Suite Three, Frederick, MD 21702; tel. 301/695–9669; FAX. 301/695–0346

Amber Ridge Operating Room Center, 1475 Taney Avenue, Suite 101, Frederick, MD 21702; tel. 301/694–5656; FAX. 301/846–4117; Lorin F. Busselberg, M.D., Director

Ambulatory Plastic Surgery–Robert Conrad, M.D., 9715 Medical Center Drive, Rockville, MD 20850; tel. 301/948–5670; FAX. 301/948–5598; Linda Quesenberry, Assistant Office Manager

American Podiatric Surgery, 10236 River Road, Potomac, MD 20854; tel. 301/983–9873; Amy Meehan, Administrator

Annapolis Plastic Surgery Center, 1300 Ritchie Highway, Arnold, MD 21012; tel. 410/544–0707; FAX. 410/544–0724; Jack Frost, M.D., President

Anne Arundel Gastroenterology Endoscopy Center, 703 Giddings Avenue, Annapolis, MD 21401; tel. 410/280–2242; Nancy L. Reynolds, Office Manager

Armiger, William G., M.D., P.A., d/b/a Chesapeake Plastic Surgery Associates, 1421 South Caton Avenue, Suite 203, Baltimore, MD 21227; tel. 410/646–3226; FAX. 410/644–2134; Sharon H. Oakley, Administrator

Arundel Ambulatory Center for Endoscopy, 621 Ridgley Avenue, Suite 101, Annapolis, MD 21401; tel. 410/224–3636

Ashok K. Narang, M.D., P.A., Two North Avenue, Suite 102, Belair, MD 21014; tel. 410/877–7595

Baltimore County Out–Patient Plastic Surgery Center, 1205 York Road, Suite 36, Lutherville, MD 21093; tel. 410/828–9570; FAX. 410/583–9120; Bernard McGibbon, M.D.

Baltimore Podiatry Group, 5205 East Drive, Suite I, Arbutus, MD 21227; tel. 410/247–5333; FAX. 410/242–5449; Neil Scheffler, D.P.M., President

Baltimore Washington Eye Center, 200 Hospital Drive, Suite 600, Glen Burnie, MD 21061; tel. 410/761–1267; FAX. 410/761–4386; Phillip L. Harrington, Administrator

Beitler, Samuel D., D.P.M. Ambulatory Surgery Center, 795 Aquahart Road, Suite 125, Glen Burnie, MD 21061; tel. 410/768–0702; Samuel D. Beitler, D.P.M.

☐ **Benson Surgery Center, Inc.,** 3421 Benson Avenue, Baltimore, MD 21227; tel. 410/644–3311; FAX. 410/247–9446; Ann Rogowski, Assistant Administrator

Bowie Health Center, 15001 Health Center Drive, Bowie, MD 20716; tel. 301/262–5511; FAX. 301/464–3572

Carroll Medicine, d/b/a Steven Shaffer, M.D., 211 Hanover Pike, Hampstead, MD 21074; tel. 410/239–7073

Central Maryland Surgery, 1500 Joh Avenue, Baltimore, MD 21227; tel. 410/536–0012; FAX. 410/536–0016

Cheasapeake Ambulatory Surgery Center, 8028 Governor Ritchie Highway, Suite 100, Pasadena, MD 21122; tel. 410/768–5800; FAX. 410/768–5806; Dr. Ira J. Gottlieb

Clinical Associates, 515 Fairmont Avenue, Suite 500, Towson, MD 21286; tel. 410/494–1335

Cockeysville Ambulatory Surgical Center, 10400 Ridgland Road, Suite Three, Cockeysville, MD 21030; tel. 410/666–3338; FAX. 410/666–3877

Providers / Freestanding Ambulatory Surgery Centers

Dr. Michael K. Schwartz, D.D.S., P.A., 25 Crossroads Drive, Owings Mills, MD 21117; tel. 410/363-7780; FAX. 410/581-9724

Dr. Michael K. Schwartz, D.D.S., P.A., 723 South Charles Street, Baltimore, MD 21230; tel. 410/727-4886

Dr. W. Alan Hopson, P.A., 560 Riverside Drive, Suite A-101, Salisbury, MD 21801; tel. 410/749-0121; FAX. 410/749-6807; Pat Timmons, Office Manager

Drs. Smith and Schwartz, D.D.S., P.A., 10 Warren Road, Suite 330, Cockeysville, MD 21030; tel. 410/666-5225; FAX. 410/666-7220; Mary Thompson, Office Manager

Dubroff Eye Center, 8905 Fairview Road, Silver Spring, MD 20910; tel. 301/588-8300

Dundalk Ambulatory Surgery Center, 1123 Merritt Boulevard, Baltimore, MD 21222; tel. 410/282-6666

Ear, Nose and Throat, P.A., 201 B-1212 York Road, Lutherville, MD 21093; tel. 410/821-6130

Endocenter of Baltimore, 7211 Park Heights Avenue, Baltimore, MD 21208; tel. 410/764-6107; FAX. 410/358-4167

Facial Plastic Surgicenter, Ltd., 21 Crossroads Drive, Owings Mills, MD 21117; tel. 410/356-1100; N. Edward Nachlas, Secretary

Family Foot Health Specialists, P.C., 339 East Antietam Street, Hagerstown, MD 21740; tel. 301/797-7272

Foot Care Associates Ambulatory Care Center at Hamilton Foot Care, 5508 Harford Road, Baltimore, MD 21214; tel. 410/426-5508

Foot Care Associates Ambulatory Care Center at Joppa Foot Care, 2316 East Joppa Road, Baltimore, MD 21234; tel. 410/882-5100

Foot Surgery, Inc., 8023 Ritchie Highway, Pasadena, MD 21122; tel. 301/761-3338; Coordinator

Foot and Ankle Associates, 2415 Musgrove Road, Suite 103, Silver Spring, MD 20904; tel. 301/384-6500

Four Corners Ambulatory Surgical Center, 10101 Lorain Avenue, Silver Spring, MD 20901; tel. 301/681-8400

Frederick Surgical Center, 915 Toll House Avenue, Suite 103, Frederick, MD 21701; tel. 301/694-3400; FAX. 301/694-3620; Barbara Smith, Administrator

Gaurdino and Glubo, P.A., 4660 Wilkens Avenue, Baltimore, MD 21229; tel. 410/242-7066; FAX. 410/242-4126; Eileen Giardina, RN

Johns Hopkins Plastic Surgery Associates, JHOC 8, 601 North Caroline Street, Baltimore, MD 21287; tel. 410/955-6897; FAX. 410/614-1296

Kaiser–Permanente–Kensington, 10810 Connecticut Avenue, Kensington, MD 20895; tel. 301/929-7100; FAX. 301/929-7599

Kalash, MD, Suhayl, M.D., Ambulatory Surgery Center, 3455 Wilkens Avenue, Suite 203, Baltimore, MD 21229; tel. 410/646-0330

Kenneth Margolis, M.D., P.A., Ambulatory Endoscopy Center, 9101 Franklin Square Drive, Suite 213, Baltimore, MD 21237; tel. 410/687-0202; FAX. 410/687-0202

Klatsky Plastic Surgery Facility, 122 Slade Avenue, Pikesville, MD 21208; tel. 410/484-0400; FAX. 410/484-2993; Stanley A. Klatsky, M.D., Director

Laser Surgery Center, 484A Ritchie Highway, Severna Park, MD 21146; tel. 410/544-4600

Maclean, Kishel, Applestein, M.D., 3450 Fort Meade Road, Laurel, MD 20724; tel. 301/725-8880

Maple Springs Podiatric Surgery Center, 10810 Darnstown Road, Suite 101, Gaithersburg, MD 20878; tel. 301/762-3338; FAX. 301/762-1585

Maryland Digestive Disease Center, 7350 Van Ducen Road, Suite 230, Laurel, MD 20707; tel. 301/498-5500

Maryland Ear, Nose and Throat, P.A., 2112 Bel Air Road, Fallston, MD 21047; tel. 410/879-7049

Maryland Outpatient Foot Surgery Center, Dennis M. Weber D.P.M., 4701 Randolph Road, Suite 115, Rockville, MD 20852; tel. 301/770-5741; FAX. 301/468-1093; Dennis M. Weber, D.P.M., Director

McCone, Jonathan, Jr., M.D., 6196 Oxon Hill Road, Suite 640, Oxon Hill, MD 20745; tel. 301/567-2400

Metropolitan Ambulatory Urologic Institute Inc., 7753 Belle Point Drive, Greenbelt, MD 20770; tel. 301/474-5583; FAX. 301/513-5087; Eleanor Adams, Director

Mid Shore Surgical Eye Center, 8420 Ocean Gateway, Suite One, Easton, MD 21601; tel. 410/822-0424; FAX. 410/822-2283; Adrienne Welch, RN

Montgomery Endoscopy Center, Drs. Doman, Goldberg & Golding P.A., 12012 Veirs Mill Road, Wheaton, MD 20906; tel. 301/942-3550; FAX. 301/933-3621; Howard Goldberg, M.D., A.S.C Director

☐ **Montgomery Surgical Center,** 46 West Gude Drive, Rockville, MD 20850; tel. 301/424-6901; FAX. 301/294-7847; Jeannie M. Lohmeyer, RN, CNOR, Administrative Director

Neil J. Napora, D.P.M., 7809 Wise Avenue, Baltimore, MD 21222; tel. 410/285-0310; FAX. 410/288-1569; Neil J. Napora, D.P.M.

North Arundel Plastic Surgery Specialists, 203 Hospital Drive, Suite 308, Glen Burnie, MD 21061; tel. 410/841-5355; FAX. 410/841-6589; Ajia S. Layman, Administrator

Parris–Castro Eye Association, Six North Boulton Street, Bel Air, MD 21014; tel. 410/836-7010; Michael Grasham, Administrator

Peninsula Obstetrics and Gynecology, 314 West Carroll Street, Salisbury, MD 21801; tel. 410/546-3125

Peninsula Surgery Center, P.A., 145 East Carroll Street, Salisbury, MD 21801; tel. 410/548-1108; FAX. 410/548-2607; Joseph G. Walters, PA–C Administrative Director

Plastic Surgery Specialists, 2448 Holly Avenue, Suite 400, Annapolis, MD 21401; tel. 410/841-5355; FAX. 410/841-6589; Ajia S. Layman, Administrator

Plastic and Aesthetic, Surgical Center of Maryland, Orchard Square, 1212 York Road, Suite B101, Lutherville, MD 21093; tel. 410/337-2551; FAX. 410/321-1550; Oscar M. Ramirez, M.D., Medical Director

Podiatry Associates of Hagerstown, 12821 Oak Hill Avenue, Hagerstown, MD 21742; tel. 301/739-1575; FAX. 301/739-1578; Crystal Shockey, Office Manager

Podiatry Associates, P.A., 9712 Bel Air Road, Baltimore, MD 21236; tel. 410/574-6060; FAX. 410/256-2727; Anthony Costa, Treasurer

Podiatry Associates, P.A., One North Main Street, Bel Air, MD 21014; tel. 410/879-1212; FAX. 410/838-0213

Podiatry Associates, P.A., 10840 Little Patuxent Parkway, Columbia, MD 21045; tel. 410/730-0970; FAX. 410/730-0161; Dr. Cappello, Podiatrist

Podiatry Associates, P.A., 6569 North Charles Street, Suite 702, Towson, MD 21204; tel. 410/828-5420; Nancy L. Patterson, Billing Manager

Podiatry Associates, P.A., 9101 Franklin Square Drive, Baltimore, MD 21237; tel. 410/574-3900; FAX. 410/574-3902; Vincent J. Martorana, D.P.M.

☐ **Prince George's Ambulatory Care Center/Endoscopy Suites, Inc.,** 6001 Landover Road, Cheverly, MD 20785; tel. 301/773-1111

Prince George's Ambulatory Foot Surgical Centre, Inc., 8700 Central Avenue, Suite 106, Landover, MD 20785; tel. 301/808-9298; FAX. 301/499-1266; Gloria H. Nelson, Administrator

Prince George's Center for Plastic Surgery, 6196 Oxon Hill Road, Suite 650, Oxon Hill, MD 20745; tel. 301/839-7497; FAX. 301/839-8726

Professional Village Surgical Center, 356 Mill Street, Hagerstown, MD 21740; tel. 301/791-1800

Queen Anne Plastic, L.L.C., 2110 Red Apple Plaza, Chester, MD 2161; tel. 410/643-7207; FAX. 410/643-6945

Queen Anne Podiatry, L.L.C., 2108 Red Apple Plaza, Chester, MD 21619; tel. 410/643-7207; FAX. 410/643-6945

Rafiq Patel, M.D., Ambulatory Surgery Center, 1952 Pulaski Highway, Edgewood, MD 21040; tel. 410/679-5800

River Reach Outpatient Surgery Center, 790 Governor Ritchie Highway, Suite E-35, Severna Park, MD 21146; tel. 410/544-2487

Robinwood Surgery, 11110 Medical Campus Road, Hagerstown, MD 21742; tel. 301/714-4300; FAX. 301/714-4324; Niki Showe, Office Supervisor

Roger J. Oldham, M.D., Ambulatory Surgery Center, 1025 Fernwood Road, Suite 412, Bethesda, MD 20817; tel. 301/530-6100

Rotunda Ambulatory Surgery Center, 711 West 40th Street, Suite 410, Baltimore, MD 21211; tel. 410/889-4885

Santiago L. Padilla, M.D., d/b/a Fertility Center of Maryland, 110 West Road, Suite 102, Towson, MD 21204; tel. 410/296-6400; FAX. 410/296-6405; Vicki Maruschak, Charge Nurse

Silver Spring Ambulatory Surgical Center, Inc., 1104 Spring Street, Suite T110, Silver Spring, MD 20910; tel. 301/589-7664; FAX. 301/589-3410

Smith and Harne, M.D., P.A., 2005 Rock Spring Road, Suite One, Forest Hill, MD 21050; tel. 410/879-4879; FAX. 410/893-4763; Louise Pollard, Office Manager

St. Agnes Surgery Center of Ellicott City, 2850 North Ridge Road, Ellicott City, MD 21043; tel. 410/461-1600; FAX. 410/750-7615

SurgiCenter of Baltimore, Formerly Health Specialists, P.A., 23 Crossroads Drive, Suite 100, Owings Mills, MD 21117; tel. 410/356-0300; FAX. 410/356-0309; Donna M. Kincaid, Administrator

Surgical Center of Greater Annapolis, Inc., 83 Church Road, Arnold, MD 21012; tel. 410/757-5018; FAX. 410/757-0632; LoRain Potter, RN, Administrator

The Ambulatory Urosurgical Center, 401 East Jefferson Street, Suite 105, Rockville, MD 20850; tel. 301/309-8219; FAX. 301/309-9370; Tricia Flanagan, RN, Director, Nursing

The Endoscopy Center, 7402 York Road, Suite 101, Towson, MD 21204; tel. 410/494-0156; FAX. 410/828-1706; Carole Custer, General Manager

Total Foot Care Surgery Center, Inc., 7525 Greenway Center Drive, Suite 112, Greenbelt, MD 20770; tel. 301/345-4087; FAX. 301/345-0482; Dale Scoville, Office Manager

Towson Ambulatory Surgical Center, 912 A Tower Avenue, Towson, MD 21204; tel. 410/583-8637

Tri County Endoscopy, Shanti Medical Center, P.O. Box 664, Leonardstown, MD 20650; tel. 301/475-5579; Dr. A. Shah

Tri County Endoscopy, Charlotte Hall, Route Five, Charlotte Hall, MD 20622; tel. 301/884-7322; Dr. Shah

Tri County Endoscopy, Calvert Medical Office Building, Suite 303, 110 Hospital Road, Prince Frederick, MD 20678; tel. 410/535-4333; Dr. A. Shah

Urology Center at Charles North, 1104 Kenilworth Avenue, Suite 300, Towson, MD 21204; tel. 410/823-1565

Vahos Aesthetic Surgery Institute, 1001 Pine Heights Avenue, Suite 100, Baltimore, MD 21229; tel. 410/644-4877; FAX. 410/525-1346

Waldorf Endoscopy Center, 11340 Pembrooke Square, Suite 202, Waldorf, MD 20603; tel. 301/645-7220; Joan Barker, Office Manager

Washington Surgi Center, 6228 Oxon Hill Road, Oxon Hill, MD 20745; tel. 301/839-0770; FAX. 301/839-1350

Western Maryland Eye Center, 1003 West Seventh Street, Suite 401, Frederick, MD 21701

MASSACHUSETTS

Andover Surgical Day Care Clinic, Inc., 38 Haverhill Street, Andover, MA 01810; tel. 508/475-2880

Boston Center for Ambulatory Surgery, Inc., 170 Commonwealth Avenue, Boston, MA 02116; tel. 617/267-0701; FAX. 617/236-8704

Boston Eye Surgery & Laser Center, P.C., 50 Staniford Street, Boston, MA 02114; tel. 617/723-2015; FAX. 617/723-7787; Maureen Whitney, Business Manager

Providers / Freestanding Ambulatory Surgery Centers

Eye Institute of the Merrimack Valley, 280 Haverhill Street, Lawrence, MA 01840; tel. 508/685–5366
Greater New Bedford Surgicare, Inc., 540 Hawthorne Street, North Dartmouth, MA 02747; tel. 508/997–1271; FAX. 508/992–7701; George A. Picord, Administrator
Maple Surgery Center, 298 Carew Street, Springfield, MA 01104; tel. 413/739–9668; FAX. 413/781–3652; Angela S. Kramer, RN, M.S., Facility Administrator
McGowan Eye Care Center, 297 Union Street, Framingham, MA 01701; tel. 508/872–4590; Bernard L. McGowan, M.D.
New England Eye Surgery Center, 696 Main Street, Weymouth, MA 02190; tel. 617/331–3820; FAX. 617/331–1076; Kenneth Camerota
New England Surgicare, One Brookline Place, Suite 201, Brookline, MA 02146; tel. 617/730–9650; Gratia S. Chase, RN, Administrator
☐ **Same Day SurgiClinic,** 272 Stanley Street, Fall River, MA 02720; tel. 508/672–2290; FAX. 508/679–3766; John Harries, M.D., Chief Executive Officer
Suburban Surgicare, 23 Warren Avenue, Woburn, MA 01801; tel. 617/938–6700; Karen J. Byrne, Administrator
The Eye Center, Florence Street, Route 128, Danvers, MA 01923; tel. 508/774–2040; FAX. 508/750–4463
Worcester Surgical Center, Inc., 300 Grove Street, Worcester, MA 01650; tel. 508/754–0700; FAX. 508/831–9989; Shauna P. Baker, Administrative Director

ICHIGAN

Balian Eye Center, 432 West University Drive, Rochester, MI 48307; tel. 313/651–6122; John V. Balian, M.D.
Birth Control Center, Inc., 2783 Fourteen Mile Road, Sterling Height, MI 48310; tel. 810/939–4000
Blodgett Memorial Medical Center, 1000 East Paris S.E., Suite 100, Grand Rapids, MI 49506
Bronson Outpatient Surgery–Crosstown Center, 150 East Crosstown Parkway, Suite One, Kalamazoo, MI 49007
Castleman Eye Center, 14050 Dix–Toledo Road, Southgate, MI 48195; tel. 313/283–0500; FAX. 313/283–2720
Community Surgical Center, 30671 Stephenson Highway, Madison Heights, MI 48071; tel. 810/588–8000; FAX. 810/588–9140; C. F. Pinkerman, Administrator
East Michigan Eye Surgery Center, 701 South Ballenger, Flint, MI 48532; tel. 810/238–3603; FAX. 810/767–5194; Judith A. Kirby, RN, Administrative Director
Feminine Health Care Clinic of Flint, 2032 South Saginaw Street, Flint, MI 48503; tel. 800/323–6205; FAX. 313/232–8071; Dawn LoRec, Director
Health Alliance Plan/Metro Medical Group, 1800 Tuxedo, Detroit, MI 48206; tel. 313/252–1381; FAX. 313/252–1522; Wallace E. Brown, Jr., Associate Vice President, Ambulatory Services
Hemmorrhoid Clinics of America, 22000 Greenfield Road, Oak Park, MI 48237; tel. 810/967–4140; FAX. 810/967–0745; Max Ali, M.D. President
Heritage Clinic for Women, 320 East Fulton, Grand Rapids, MI 49503; tel. 616/456–5727; Elaine Bower, Administrator
Holland Eye Clinic, 999 South Washington, Holland, MI 49423; tel. 616/396–2316
Horizon Surgery Center, 19900 Haggerty Road, Livonia, MI 48152; tel. 313/462–1888; FAX. 313/462–1944; Pamela A. Cittan, Administrator
Hutzel Health Center, 4050 East 12 Mile Road, Warren, MI 48237; tel. 810/573–3140
John Michael Garrett, P.C., 1301 Carpenter Avenue, Iron Mountain, MI 49801; tel. 906/774–1404; FAX. 906/774–8132; Sharon Nickels, Administrator
Lee Eye Center, Inc., 750 Stewart Road, Monroe, MI 48161; tel. 313/241–1106
M.D. Surgicenter, 375 Barclay Circle, Rochester Hills, MI 48307; tel. 810/852–3636; FAX. 810/852–3631; Robert Swartz, Administrator

Metropolitan Eye Center, 21711 Greater Mack, St. Clair Shores, MI 48080; tel. 313/774–6820; FAX. 313/777–2214; Richard C. Mertz, Jr., M.D., Director
Michigan Center for Outpatient Ocular Surgery, 33080 Utica Road, P.O. Box 26010, Fraser, MI 48026; tel. 810/296–7250; FAX. 810/296–0276; Norbert P. Czajkowski, M.D., Professional Corporation
Midwest Health Center, 5050 Schaefer Avenue, Dearborn, MI 48126; tel. 313/581–2600, ext. 286; FAX. 313/581–6013; Mark B. Saffer, M.D., President, Chief Executive Officer
Oakwood Health Center – Dearborn, 10151 Michigan Avenue, Dearborn, MI 48126; tel. 313/436–2430; FAX. 313/436–2411; Dan West, Director
Park Eye and Surgicenter, 5014 Villa Linde Parkway, Flint, MI 48532
Planned Parenthood League, Inc., 25932 Dequindre, Warren, MI 48091; tel. 810/758–2100; FAX. 810/758–2104; Pam Johnson, Administrator
Planned Parenthood of Mid–Michigan, 3100 Professional Drive, 48104, P.O. Box 3673, Ann Arbor, MI 48106–3673; tel. 313/973–0710, ext. 131; FAX. 313/973–0595; Cindy Bourland, Clinic Manager
Planned Parenthood of South Central Michigan, 4201 West Michigan Avenue, Kalamazoo, MI 49006–5833; tel. 616/372–1205; FAX. 616/372–1279; Louise D. Safron, Executive Director
Port Huron Eye Surgery Center, 1131 Erie Street, Port Huron, MI 48060; tel. 313/984–2681; Paul DeGrow, Administrator
Reconstructive Surgery Center, 125 West Walnut, Kalamazoo, MI 49007; tel. 616/343–1381; Frank J. Newman, M.D., Medical Director
Sinai Surgery Center, 28500 Orchard Lake Road, Farmington Hills, MI 48334; tel. 313/851–9215; FAX. 313/851–2077; Michael K. Rosenberg, M.D., Medical Director
St. Mary's Ambulatory Surgery Center, 4599 Towne Centre, Sagniaw, MI 48604
Summit Medical Center, 15800 West McNichols, Detroit, MI 48235; tel. 313/272–8450
Surgical Care Center of Michigan, 750 East Beltline, N.E., Grand Rapids, MI 49506; tel. 616/940–3600; FAX. 616/954–0216; Kris Kilgore, RN, B.S.N, Administrative Director
Troy Obstetrics and Gynecology, P.C., 1565 West Big Beaver Road, Building F, Troy, MI 48084; tel. 810/643–7775; FAX. 810/643–0999; Reza S. Mohajer, M.D., Administrator
Waterford Ambulatory Surgi–Center, 1305 North Oakland Boulevard, Waterford, MI 48327; tel. 810/666–5519; FAX. 810/666–5550; Sandra K. Parrott, General Manager

MINNESOTA

Centennial Lakes Same Day Surgery Center, 7373 France Avenue, S., Suite 400, Edina, MN 55435; tel. 612/920–9100; FAX. 612/920–0925; Kathleen L. Whatley, Administrator
Children's Health Care – West, 6050 Clearwater Drive, Minnetonka, MN 55343; tel. 612/930–8600; FAX. 612/930–8650; Jane Price, Director
Dakota Clinic, Ltd, 125 East Frazee Street, Detroit Lakes, MN 56501; tel. 218/847–3181; FAX. 218/847–2795; Linda L. Walz, Division Manager
First Eye Care Center, Inc., 9117 Lyndale Avenue, S., Bloomington, MN 55420; tel. 612/884–7568; FAX. 612/884–2656; Barbara McGovern, Administrator
☐ **Gastrointestinal Diagnostic Center,** 2545 Chicago Avenue, S., Suite 601, Minneapolis, MN 55404; tel. 612/871–1722; FAX. 612/871–4566; Karen Laing, Administrator
Healtheast Maplewood Surgery Center, 1655 Beam Avenue, Maplewood, MN 55109; tel. 612/232–2780; FAX. 612/232–7786; Sandra Todd, Administrator
Midwest Surgicenter, d/b/a Midwest Eye and Ear Institute, 393 North Dunlap Street, Suite 900, St. Paul, MN 55104; tel. 612/642–9199; FAX. 612/641–0704; H. Joseph Drannen, Administrator

Ridgedale Surgery Center, 2000 South Plymouth Road, Minnetonka, MN 55343; tel. 612/541–1045; Robin R. Goihl, Administrator
St. Cloud Surgical Center, 1526 Northway Drive, St. Cloud, MN 56303; tel. 612/251–8385; FAX. 612/251–1267; Jeanette I. Stack, Administrator
St. Paul Endoscopy Center, 17 West Exchange Street, Suite 215, St. Paul, MN 55102; tel. 612/224–9677; Glenda Tims, RN, Clinical Manager
Surgicare of Minneapolis, 6525 Barrie Road, Edina, MN 55435; tel. 612/920–9100; FAX. 612/920–0925; Kathleen L. Whatley, Administrator
WestHealth, Inc., 2855 Campus Drive, Plymouth, MN 55441; tel. 612/577–7000, ext. 7120; FAX. 612/577–7130; Paula Witke, Administrator
Willmar Surgery Center, 1320 South First Street, P.O. Box 773, Willmar, MN 56201; tel. 612/235–6506; Janelle Hanson, Manager

MISSISSIPPI

Ambu–Care Outpatient Surgery Center, 6204 North State Street, Jackson, MS 39213; tel. 601/956–3251; FAX. 601/957–8456; Frank McCune, M.D., Administrator
Biloxi Outpatient Surgery and Endoscopy Center, 111 Lameuse Street, Suite 104, Biloxi, MS 39530; tel. 601/374–2130; FAX. 601/374–0938; Shirley Gunter, Director, Nursing
Gulf South Outpatient Center, 1206 31st Avenue, P.O. Box 1778, Gulfport, MS 39501; tel. 601/864–0008; FAX. 601/863–1747; Jason V. Smith, M.D., President
Gulfport Outpatient Surgical Center, 1240 Broad Avenue, Gulfport, MS 39501; tel. 601/868–1120; William Peaks, Administrator
Lowery A. Woodall Outpatient Surgery Facility, 105 South 28th Avenue, Hattiesburg, MS 39401; tel. 601/288–1072; FAX. 601/288–8911; Lowery A. Woodall, Administrator
Mississippi Surgical Center, Inc., 1421 North State Street, Jackson, MS 39202; tel. 601/353–8000; Virginia Brown, Administrator
North Mississippi Surgery Center, 500 West Eason Boulevard, Tupelo, MS 38801; tel. 601/841–4700; FAX. 601/841–3101; Beth Taylor, RN, Director
Southern Eye Center of Excellence, 1420 South 28th Avenue, Hattiesburg, MS 39402; tel. 601/264–3937; Lynn McMahan, M.D., Medical Director
Southwest Ambulatory Surgery Center, 215 Marion Avenue, McComb, MS 39648; tel. 601/249–1477; FAX. 601/249–1700; Norman M. Price, Administrator
Surgicare of Jackson, 766 Lakeland Drive, Jackson, MS 39216; tel. 601/362–8700; FAX. 601/362–6439; Sheila Grillis, RN, Administrator

MISSOURI

Arnold Eye Surgery Center, Inc., 1265 East Primrose, Springfield, MO 65804; tel. 417/886–3937; FAX. 417/886–1285; Stephen C. Sheppard, Administrator
Associated Plastic Surgeons Ambulatory Surgical Center, 6420 Prospect, Suite 115, Kansas City, MO 64132; tel. 816/333–5524; Joni Reist, RN
BarnesCare, 401 Pine Street, St. Louis, MO 63102; tel. 314/621–4300; FAX. 314/241–2663; Elizabeth Lenke, Administrator
Cataract Surgery Center of St. Louis, Inc., 900 North Highway 67 (Lindbergh), Florissant, MO 63031; tel. 314/838–0321; FAX. 314/838–4682; Antoinette E. Varner, RN, Administrator
Cataract Surgery Center of Young Eye Clinic, Inc., 3201 Ashland Avenue, St. Joseph, MO 64506; tel. 816/279–0079; Judy Watowa, RN, B.S.N., Administrator
Cataract and Glaucoma Outpatient Surgicenter, 7220 Watson Road, St. Louis, MO 63119; tel. 314/352–5515; Stanley C. Becker, M.D.
Cave Springs Surgery Center, 4203 South Cloverleaf Drive, St. Peters, MO 63376; tel. 314/928–0087; FAX. 314/928–1242; Mary Scharf, Administrator

Providers / Freestanding Ambulatory Surgery Centers

Center for Eye Surgery, 6650 Troost, Suite 301, Kansas City, MO 64131; tel. 816/276–7757; Richard B. Klein, Administrator

Creekwood Surgery Center, 211 N.E. 54th Street, Suite 100, Kansas City, MO 64118; tel. 816/455–4214; FAX. 816/455–4216; Carol Ohmes, Administrator

Creve Coeur Surgery Center, 633 Emerson, Creve Coeur, MO 63141; tel. 314/872–7100; Judy Henderson, Nursing Administrator

Doctors' Park Surgery, Inc., 30 Doctors' Park, Cape Girardeau, MO 63701; tel. 314/334–9606; FAX. 314/334–9608; Ronald G. Wittmer, President

Eye Care Surgery Center, Inc., 4801 Cliff Avenue, Suite 100, Independence, MO 64055; tel. 816/478–4400; FAX. 816/478–4413; Patricia Thomas, RN, Director, Nursing

G.I. Diagnostics, Inc., 4321 Washington, Suite 5700, Kansas City, MO 64111; tel. 816/561–2000; FAX. 816/931–7559; Craig B. Reeves, Administrator

Hunkeler Eye Surgery Center, Inc., 4321 Washington, Suite 6000, Kansas City, MO 64111; tel. 816/753–6511; FAX. 816/931–9498; Debby Milliken, LPN

Kansas City Surgicenter, Ltd., 1800 East Meyer Boulevard, Kansas City, MO 64132; tel. 816/523–0100; FAX. 816/523–6241; Barbara Klein, RN

Laser Surgery Center North, 1028 South Kirkwood Road, St. Louis, MO 63122; tel. 314/261–2020; FAX. 314/821–4080; Tim Welsh, Administrator

Laser Surgery Center West, 1028 South Kirkwood, St. Louis, MO 63122; tel. 314/984–0080; FAX. 314/821–4080; Francis E. O'Donnell, Jr., M.D., President

Midwest Eye Institute, 5139 Mattis Road, St. Louis, MO 63128; tel. 314/849–8400; Anwar Shah, M.D.

Missouri Surgery Center, Inc., 300 South Mount Auburn Road, Suite 200, Cape Girardeau, MO 63701; tel. 314/339–7575; FAX. 314/339–7887; Steve Telford, Administrator

Outpatient Surgery Center, 450 North New Ballas Road, Suite 103, St. Louis, MO 63141; tel. 314/991–0776; FAX. 314/991–3076; Karen Barrow, Administrator

Regional Surgery Center, P.C., 1531 West 32nd Street, Suite 107, Joplin, MO 64804; tel. 417/781–9595; FAX. 417/781–9814; Cynthia Shofner, Administrator

Surgery Center of Springfield, L.P., 1350 East Woodhurst Drive, Springfield, MO 65804; tel. 417/887–5243; FAX. 417/887–6507; Celine Snyder, RN, Administrator

☐ **Surgi-Care Center of Independence,** 2311 Redwood Avenue, Independence, MO 64057; tel. 816/373–9312; FAX. 816/373–8580; Dolores Sabia, Administrator

The Ambulatory Head and Neck Surgical Center, 1965 South Fremont, Suite 1940, Springfield, MO 65804; tel. 417/887–5750; FAX. 417/887–6612; Charles R. Taylor, Administrator

The Tobin Eye Institute, 3902 Sherman, St. Joseph, MO 64506; tel. 816/279–1363; FAX. 816/233–8936; Linda S. Wildhagen, Administrator

Tri County Outpatient Surgery Center, Inc., 1111 East Sixth Street, Washington, MO 63090; tel. 314/239-1766; FAX. 314/239–2964; Beverly Connor, RN, Administrator

West County Surgery Center, 1130 Town and Country Commons, Chesterfield, MO 63017; tel. 314/394–0698; FAX. 314/394–7493; Sherry Mohr, Administrator

MONTANA

Billings Cataract and Laser Surgicenter, 1221 North 26th Street, Billings, MT 59101; tel. 406/252–5681

Eye Microsurgery Center, Inc., 1232 North 30th Street, Billings, MT 59101; tel. 406/256–9006; Nancy Oliphant, Office Manager

Flathead Outpatient Surgical Center, 66 Claremont Street, Kalispell, MT 59901; tel. 406/752–8484; FAX. 406/756–8008; Victoria L. Johnson, RN, Facility Manager

Great Falls Eye Surgery Center, Inc., 1717 Fourth Street, South, Great Falls, MT 59405; tel. 406/727–9920; FAX. 406/727–9904

Highland View Outpatient Surgical Center, Inc., 840 South Montana, Butte, MT 59701; tel. 406/782–2391; Richard O. York, Business Administrator

Northern Rockies Surgicenter, Inc., 1020 North 27th Street, Suite 100, Billings, MT 59101; tel. 406/248–7186; FAX. 406/248–6889; Sharon McLeod, RN, OR Supervisor

Same Day Surgery Center, Inc., 300 North Willson, Bozeman, MT 59715; tel. 406/586–1956; Kenneth Younger, M.D., Medical Director

The Eye Surgicenter, 1600 Poly Drive, Billings, MT 59102; tel. 406/252–6608; FAX. 406/252–6600; Sara Coleman, Supervisor

NEBRASKA

Aesthetic Surgical Images, P.C., 8900 West Dodge Road, Omaha, NE 68114; tel. 402/390–0100; FAX. 402/390–2711; Carl H. Dahl, M.D.

Anis Eye Institute, P.C., d/b/a The Nebraska Eye Surgical Center, 1500 South 48th Street, Suite 610, Lincoln, NE 68506; tel. 402/483–4448; Dr. Aziz Y. Anis

Bergan Mercy Surgical Center, 11704 West Center Road, Omaha, NE 68124; tel. 402/333–3111; Richard A. Hachten, III

Clarkson Hospital Outpatient Surgery, 4353 Dodge Street, Omaha, NE 68131; tel. 402/442–2000; D. Max Francis

Clarkson West Medical Center–Outpatient Surgery, 14505 West Center Road, Omaha, NE 68144; tel. 402/334–1243; Cindy Alloway, Director

Omaha Surgical Center, 8051 West Center Road, Omaha, NE 68124; tel. 402/391–3333; James Quinn, M.D., Administrator

The Urology Center, P.C., 111 South 90th Street, Omaha, NE 68114; tel. 402/397–9800; Laura Forehead

NEVADA

Aesthetic Associates Day Surgery Center, 1580 East Desert Inn Road, Las Vegas, NV 89109; tel. 702/735–6755; FAX. 702/733–8221; Charles A. Vinnik, M.D., Administrator

☐ **Carson Ambulatory Surgery Center, Inc.,** 1299 Mountain Street, Carson City, NV 89703; tel. 702/883–1700; FAX. 702/883–8905; Joan P. Lapham, RN, Administrator

Center for Outpatient Surgery, 343 Elm Street, Suite 100, Reno, NV 89503; tel. 702/789–6500; FAX. 702/789–6535; Christine Kreger, Executive Director

Desert Surgery Center, 1569 East Flamingo Road, Suite B, Las Vegas, NV 89119; tel. 792/735–5177; FAX. 702/735–3140; Dale Kirby, Administrator

Digestive Disease Center, 2136 East Desert Inn Road, Suite B, Las Vegas, NV 89109; tel. 702/734–0075; Osama Haikal, M.D., Administrator

Eye Surgery Center of Nevada, 3839 North Carson Street, Carson City, NV 89706; tel. 702/882–3950; FAX. 708/882–1726; Michael J. Fischer, M.D., Administrator

Foot Surgery Center of Northern Nevada, 1300 East Plumb Lane, Suite A, Reno, NV 89502; tel. 702/829–8066; FAX. 702/829–8069; Dr. Frank M. Davis, Jr., Administrator

Ford Center for Foot Surgery, 2321 Pyramid Way, Sparks, NV 89431; tel. 702/331–1919; FAX. 702/331–2008; Dr. L. Bruce Ford, Administrator

Gastrointestinal Diagnostic Clinic, 3196 South Maryland Parkway, Suite 207, Las Vegas, NV 89109; tel. 702/369–3400; Luis Tupal, Administrator

Institute for Pain Surgery, 630 South Rancho Drive, Suite A, Las Vegas, NV 89106; tel. 702/870–1111; Pat Nicholson, Administrator

Las Vegas Surgicare, Ltd., 870 South Rancho Drive, Las Vegas, NV 89106; tel. 702/870–2090; FAX. 702/870–5468; Stephanie Finkelstein, Administrator

NMC–Red Rock Surgical Center, 5701 West Charleston Boulevard, Suite 102, Las Vegas, NV 89102; tel. 702/870–3443; FAX. 702/258–8238; Diane McNamee, Administrator

Nellis/Craig Ambulatory G. I. Surgery Center, 4333 Las Vegas Boulevard, N., Las Vegas, NV 89115; tel. 702/643–0500; Nathan Ozobia, M.D., Administrator

Nevada Institute of Ambulatory Surgery, 2316 West Charleston, Suite 120, Las Vegas, NV 89102; tel. 702/878–5668; FAX. 702/878–0265; Lois M. Webb, RN, Administrator

Nevada Surgery Center, 4187 Pecos Road, Las Vegas, NV 89121; tel. 702/458–3179; Lyndell Kewley, Administrator

Northern Nevada Plastic Surgery Associates, 932 Ryland Street, Reno, NV 89502; tel. 702/322–3446; FAX. 702/322–4529; Karen Holcher, Office Manager

Rancho Surgical Plaza, 888 South Rancho Drive, Las Vegas, NV 89106; tel. 702/877–8660; Steve Evans, M.D., Medical Director

Reno Endoscopy Center, Inc., 753 Ryland Street, Reno, NV 89502; tel. 702/329–1009; FAX. 702/329–4297; Timothy P. Wiever, Administrator

Reno Medical Plaza, 2005 Silverada Boulevard, Suite 100, Reno, NV 89512; tel. 702/359–0212; FAX. 702/359–0645; Sandra Walker–Wright, Administrator

Sahara–Lindell Surgery Center, 2575 Lindell Road, Las Vegas, NV 89102; tel. 702/362–3937; FAX. 702/362–7935; Elizabeth Sayers, Administrator

Shepherd Eye Surgicenter, 3575 Pecos McLeod, Las Vegas, NV 89121; tel. 702/731–2088; FAX. 702/734–7836; John R. Shepherd, M.D., Medical Director

Sierra Center for Foot Surgery, 1801 North Carson, Suite B, Carson City, NV 89701; tel. 702/885–1790; FAX. 702/882–6844; Beverlee J. Gillette, RN, B.S.N. CNOR, OCN, Administrator

Valley View Surgery Center, 1330 Valley View Boulevard, Las Vegas, NV 89102; tel. 702/870–7101; FAX. 702/870–7118; Dale A. Kirby

NEW HAMPSHIRE

Bedford Ambulatory Surgical Center, 11 Washington Place, Bedford, NH 03110; tel. 603/622–3670; FAX. 603/626–9750; Linda Dwyer, RN, B.S.N., Director

Dunning Street Ambulatory Care Center, Seven Dunning Street, Claremont, NH 03743; tel. 603/543–3501; Jyl Bradley, Administrator

Elliot One Day Surgery Center, Formerly Northeast One Day Surgery Center, 445 Cypress Street, Manchester, NH 03103; tel. 603/627–4889; FAX. 603/626–4300; Donna Quinn, RN, B.S.N., M.B.A., Director

Nashua Eye Surgery Center, Inc., Five Coliseum Avenue, Nashua, NH 03063; tel. 603/882–9800; FAX. 603/882–0556; Paul O'Leary, Administrator

New Hampshire Eye Surgicenter, 19 Riverway Place, Building One, Bedford, NH 03110; tel. 603/627–9540; Paul Pender, M.D.

Northeast Pain Consultation and Management PC, 255 State Route 16, Somersworth, NH 03878; tel. 603/692–3166; FAX. 603/692–3168; Michael J. O'Connell, M.D., Director

Nutfield Surgicenter, Inc., 44 Birch Street, Suite 304, Derry, NH 03038; tel. 603/432–8104; Dr. Keith D. Jorgensen, Director

Salem Surgery Center, 32 Stiles Road, Salem, NH 03079; tel. 603/898–3610; FAX. 603/890–6673; Rita Fairbanks, O.R., Administrator

Seacoast Outpatient Surgical Center, 200 Route 108, Suite II, Somersworth, NH 03878; tel. 603/749–4327; FAX. 603/749–5296; Cynthia S. Rawski, RN, Nursing Director

The Clinic Surgery Center, 253 Pleasant Street, Concord, NH 03301; tel. 603/226–2200; Kevin Appleton, Administrator

NEW JERSEY

Garden State Surgi-Center, 550 Newark Avenue, Jersey City, NJ 07306; tel. 201/795–0646; FAX. 201/795–0744; James B. Berg, President

☐ **Mediplex Surgery Center,** 98 James Street, Suite 108, Edison, NJ 08820–3998; tel. 908/632–1600; FAX. 908/632–1678; Ruth Mosher, Administrator

Providers / Freestanding Ambulatory Surgery Centers

Middlesex Same Day Surgical Center, 561 Cranbury Road, East Brunswick, NJ 08816; tel. 908/390–4300; FAX. 908/390–4405; Charles Indelicato, Administrator

Newark Mini–Surgi Site, Inc., 145 Roseville Avenue, Newark, NJ 07107; tel. 201/485–3300; FAX. 201/485–2404; Monica Chomsky

North Jersey Women's Medical Center, Inc., 6000 Kennedy Boulevard, West New York, NJ 07093; tel. 201/869–9293; Saul Luchs, M.D.

Pilgrim Medical Group, 393 Bloomfield Avenue, Montclair, NJ 07042; tel. 201/746–1500; Herbert Wiskind, M.D.

Planned Parenthood of Greater Northern New Jersey, 196 Speedwell Avenue, Morristown, NJ 07960; tel. 201/539–9580, ext. 136; FAX. 201/539–3828; Carole M. Harper, M.A., RN, Senior Associate Executive Director

Planned Parenthood of Monmouth County, Inc., 69 East Newman Springs Road, Shrewsbury, NJ 07702; tel. 908/842–9300; FAX. 908/842–9338; Phyllis Kinsler

Princeton Ambulatory Surgery Center, Inc., 281 Witherspoon Street, Third Floor, Princeton, NJ 08542; tel. 609/497–4380; FAX. 609/497–4986; Dennis Doody, President

Roseland Surgery Center, 556 Eagle Rock Avenue, Roseland, NJ 07068; tel. 201/226–1717; FAX. 201/403–9034; Joseph Brandspiegel, Executive Director

St. Barnabas Outpatient Centers, Same Day Surgery Center, 101 Old Short Hills Road, West Orange, NJ 07052; tel. 201/325–6565; FAX. 201/325–6551; Sheila Bloom, Administrative Director

Summit Surgical Center, 110 Carnie Boulevard, Voorhees, NJ 08043; tel. 609/770–5813; Maureen Miller, Executive Director

Surgicare of Central Jersey, Inc., 40 Stirling Road, Watchung, NJ 07060; tel. 908/769–8000; FAX. 908/668–3139; Jacqueline Jerko, Executive Director

United Hospital Community Health Center, 194 Clinton Avenue, Newark, NJ 07108; tel. 201/242–2300; Delores Henderson

NEW MEXICO

Alamogordo Eye Clinic and Surgical Center, 1124 Tenth Street, Alamogordo, NM 88310; tel. 505/434–1200; FAX. 505/437–3947; Donald J. Ham, Administrator

Cibola Medical Foundation, 2111 College Drive, Gallup, NM 87305; tel. 505/722–4483; FAX. 502/722–5214; Claudia Klesert, Administrator

Eastern New Mexico Eye Clinic, 1820 West 21st Street, Clovis, NM 88101; tel. 505/762–2207; Dik S. Cheung, M.D.

Lazaro Eye Surgical Center, 1131 Mall Drive, Las Cruces, NM 88011; tel. 505/522–7676; Corine B. Lazaro, M.D., Administrator

St. Joseph Eye Surgery Center Partnership, P.O. Box 25555, Albuquerque, NM 87125; tel. 505/244–8454; FAX. 505/244–8397; Julie Nunley, Director

Surgery Center of Albuquerque, 1720 Wyoming Boulevard, N.E., Albuquerque, NM 87112; tel. 505/292–9200; FAX. 505/292–1398; Amy Miller, Administrator

The Endoscopy Center of Santa Fe, 1650 Hospital Drive, Suite 900, Santa Fe, NM 87505; tel. 505/988–3373; FAX. 505/984–1858; Jim Howlett, Administrator

Valley Eye Surgery Center, 110 North Coronado Avenue, Espanola, NM 87532; tel. 505/753–7391; Dr. Gary Puro

NEW YORK

Ambulatory Surgery Center of Brooklyn, 313 43rd Street, Brooklyn, NY 11232; tel. 718/369–1900; FAX. 718/965–4157

Ambulatory Surgery Center of Greater New York, Inc., 1101 Pelham Parkway, N., Bronx, NY 10469; tel. 718/515–3500; FAX. 718/655–1795, ext. 3204; Joanne McLaughlin, Administrator

Brook Plaza Ambulatory Surgical Center, 1901 Utica Avenue, Brooklyn, NY 11234; tel. 718/968–8700; Sharron Resnick, Office Manager

Buffalo Ambulatory Services, Inc., 3095 Harlem Road, Cheektowaga, NY 14225; tel. 716/896–7234

Day–Op Center of Long Island, Inc., 110 Willis Avenue, Mineola, NY 11501; tel. 516/294–0030; FAX. 516/294–0228; Robin Fishman, Executive Director

Fifth Avenue Surgery Center, 1049 Fifth Avenue, New York, NY 10028; tel. 212/772–6667; Francois Simon, Vice President

Harrison Center Outpatient Surgery, Inc., 550 Harrison Street, Suite 230, Syracuse, NY 13202; tel. 315/472–4424; FAX. 315/475–8056; Margaret M. Alteri, Administrator, Chief Executive Officer

Hurley Avenue Surgical Center, Inc., 40 Hurley Avenue, Kingston, NY 12401; tel. 914/338–4777; FAX. 914/339–7339; Maher Sarrag, Administrator

Kings Highway Surgi–Center, 3121 Kings Highway, Brooklyn, NY 11234; tel. 718/258–9200; Rhetta Felton, Executive Director

Kochman Eye Surgical Facility, 1301–1311 Avenue J, Brooklyn, NY 11230; tel. 718/645–0600; FAX. 718/692–4456; Rosalind A. Kochman, Administrator

Lattimore Community Surgicenter, 125 Lattimore Road, Rochester, NY 14620; tel. 716/473–9000; FAX. 716/473–9018; Deborah G. Spratt, RN, M.P.A., CNOR, CNAA, Clinical Director

☐ **Long Island Surgi–Center,** 1895 Walt Whitman Road, Melville, NY 11747; tel. 516/293–9700; FAX. 516/293–1018; Howard Leemon, D.D.S.

Millard Fillmore Ambulatory Surgery Center, 215 Klein Road, Williamsville, NY 14221; tel. 716/689–2300; FAX. 716/689–2385; Gary Schultz, Fiscal Officer

Nassau Center for Ambulatory Surgery, Inc., 400 Endo Boulevard, Garden City, NY 11530; tel. 516/832–8504; FAX. 516/832–8379; Miriam DeJesus, RN, Operating Room Supervisor

New York Institute for Same Day Surgery, Inc., 99 Dutch Hill Plaza, Orangeburg, NY 10994; tel. 914/359–9000; FAX. 914/359–0729; Richard Sherman, Director of Finance and Business Development

North Shore Surgi Center, Inc., 989 Jericho Turnpike, Smithtown, NY 11787; tel. 516/864–7100; FAX. 516/864–7129; Gerald Mazzola, Administrator

Our Lady of Victory Primary Care and Surgery Center, 6300 Powers Road, Orchard Park, NY 14127; tel. 716/667–3200; FAX. 716/667–3120; Dana M. Mata, Administrative Director

Queens Surgi–Center, 83–40 Woodhaven Boulevard, Glendale, NY 11385; tel. 718/849–8700; FAX. 718/849–6523; Stanley H. Kornhauser, Ph.D., Administrator

Queens Surgical Community Center, 46–04 31st Avenue, Long Island City, NY 11103; tel. 718/721–9100

Same Day Surgery of Latham, Inc., Seven Century Hill Drive, Latham, NY 12110; tel. 518/785–5741

Westfall Surgery Center, 919 Westfall Road, Rochester, NY 14618; tel. 716/256–1330; FAX. 716/256–3823; Gary J. Scott, Administrative Director

NORTH CAROLINA

☐ **Asheboro Endoscopy Center,** 700 Sunset Avenue, P.O. Box 4830, Asheboro, NC 27203; tel. 910/626–4328; Trudy Hogan, RN, Clinical Director

Asheville Hand Ambulatory Surgery Center, 34 Granby Street, P.O. Box 1980, Asheville, NC 28802; tel. 704/258–0847; FAX. 704/258–0374; E. Brown Crosby, M.D., Executive Officer

Blue Ridge Day Surgery Center, 2308 Wesvill Court, Raleigh, NC 27607; tel. 919/781–4311; FAX. 919/781–0625; Susan S. Swift, Facility Manager

Chapel Hill Surgical Center, 109 Conner Drive, Suite 1201, Chapel Hill, NC 27514; tel. 919/968–0611; FAX. 919/967–8637; Gary S. Berger, M.D., President

Charlotte Surgery and Laser Center, 2825 Randolph Road, Charlotte, NC 28211; tel. 704/377–1647; FAX. 704/358–8267; Margaret Slattery, Manager

Christenbury Ambulatory Surgical Center, 449 North Wendover Road Park Place, Charlotte, NC 28211; tel. 704/332–9365; Terry Coman

Durham Ambulatory Surgical Center, 120 Carver Street, P.O. Box 15727, Durham, NC 27704; tel. 919/477–9677; FAX. 919/479–6755; Joseph T. Jordan, Director

Eye Surgery and Laser Clinic, 500 Lake Concord Road, N.E., Concord, NC 28025; tel. 704/782–1127; FAX. 704/782–1207; J. W. Wheatley, Co-Chief Administrator

Fayetteville Ambulatory Surgery Center, 1781 Metromedical Drive, Fayetteville, NC 28304; tel. 910/323–1647; FAX. 910/323–4142; John T. Henley, Jr., M.D., Director

FemCare, 62 Orange Street, Asheville, NC 28801; tel. 704/255–8400; Philip J. Kittner, M.D., Executive Director

Gaston Ambulatory Surgery, 2511 Court Drive, Gastonia, NC 28054; tel. 704/834–2086; FAX. 704/834–2085; Elizabeth Kohli, Director

Goldsboro Endoscopy Center, 2705 Medical Office Place, Goldsboro, NC 27534; tel. 919/580–9111; FAX. 919/580–0988; Venkata C. Motaparthy, Chief Executive Officer

Greensboro Center for Digestive Diseases, 520 North Elam Avenue, P.O. Box 10829, Greensboro, NC 27403; tel. 910/547–1741; FAX. 910/547–1711; Robert Rosso, Administrator

Greensboro Specialty Surgical Center, 522 North Elam Avenue, Greensboro, NC 27403; tel. 910/294–1833; FAX. 910/292–9423; L. L. Patseavouras, M.D., President

☐ **Hawthorne Surgical Center,** 1999 South Hawthorne Road, Winston–Salem, NC 27103; tel. 919/760–3880; FAX. 919/659–1071; Teresa L. Carter, Facility Director

High Point Endoscopy Center, Inc., 624 Quaker Lane, Suite C–106, High Point, NC 27262; tel. 910/885–1400; Lester E. Hurrelbrink

High Point Surgery Center, 600 Lindsay Street, P.O. Box 2476, High Point, NC 27261; tel. 910/884–6068; FAX. 910/888–6111; Joan Gayle, Administrator

Iredell Head, Neck and Ear Ambulatory Surgery Center, 707 Bryant Street, Statesville, NC 28677; tel. 704/873–5224; FAX. 704/873–5984; Rob Wilson, Administrator

Iredell Surgical Center, 1720 Davie Avenue, Statesville, NC 28677; tel. 704/871–0081; Jeannie Naylor, Administrator

Lexington Ambulatory Surgery, Inc., Seven Medical Park Drive, Lexington, NC 27292; tel. 704/243–2431; FAX. 704/243–2359; Lloyd D. Lohr, President

MediVision Inc., 2200 East Seventh Street, Charlotte, NC 28204; tel. 704/334–4317; Cathy G. Houck, Administrator

MediVision of Hickory, Outpatient Surgery Center, 27 Thirteenth Avenue, N.E., Hickory, NC 28601; tel. 704/328–1493; FAX. 704/322–6097; Marie Hudson, Nurse Manager

MediVision, Inc., 3312 Battleground Avenue, Greensboro, NC 27410; tel. 919/282–8330; Jeanne Justice, Administrator

MediVision, Inc., 2170 Midland Road, Southern Pines, NC 28387; tel. 910/295–1221; FAX. 910/295–0512; Dottie Laton, Administrator

New Bern Outpatient Surgery Center, 801 College Court, P.O. Box 12446, New Bern, NC 28561; tel. 919/633–2000; FAX. 919/633–0096; Danny Jackson, Administrator

Piedmont Gastroenterology Center, Inc., 1901 South Hawthorne Road, Suite 308, Winston–Salem, NC 27103; tel. 910/760–4340; FAX. 919/765–2869; Charles H. Hauser, Administrator

Plastic Surgery Center of North Carolina, Inc., 2901 Maplewood Avenue, Winston–Salem, NC 27103; tel. 910/768–6210; FAX. 910/768–6236; Ronald C. Stewart, M.D., Chief of Staff

Quandrangle Endoscopy Center, 620 South Memorial Drive, Greenville, NC 27834; tel. 919/757–3636; Mark Dellasega

RMS Surgery Center, 5200 North Croatan Highway, Kitty Hawk, NC 27949; tel. 919/261–9009; FAX. 919/261–4329; Jane Plough, RN, Clinical Manager

Providers / Freestanding Ambulatory Surgery Centers

☐ **Raleigh Endoscopy Center,** 3320 Wake Forest Road, Raleigh, NC 27609; tel. 919/878-1151; Robert N. Harper, Jr., Medical Director

Raleigh Plastic Surgery Center, Inc., 1112 Dresser Court, Raleigh, NC 27609; tel. 919/872-2616; FAX. 919/872-2771; Arlene Roessler, Administrator

Raleigh Women's Health Organization, Inc., 3613 Haworth Drive, Raleigh, NC 27609; tel. 919/783-0444; FAX. 919/781-8432; Susan Hill, Vice President

SameDay Surgery Center at Presbyterian, 1800 East Fourth Street, P.O. Box 34425, Charlotte, NC 28234; tel. 704/384-4200; Anne McKelvey, Vice President, Nursing

Southern Eye Associates, P.A., Ophthalmic Surgery Center, 2801 Blue Ridge Road, Suite 200, Raleigh, NC 27607; tel. 919/571-0081; Gloria Johnson, Executive Director

Surgery Center of Morganton Eye Physicians, P.A., 335 East Parker Road, Morganton, NC 28655; tel. 704/433-6225; L. A. Raynor, M.D., Medical Director

SurgiCenter of Wilson, 209 Richards Street, Wilson, NC 27893; tel. 919/237-5649; FAX. 919/237-4977; Phyllis Renfrow, President

Surgical Center of Greensboro, Inc., 1211 Virginia Street, P.O. Box 29347, Greensboro, NC 27429; tel. 919/272-0012; FAX. 919/272-4063; Donald E. Linder, M.D., Medical Director

☐ **Surgicenter Services of Pitt, Inc.,** 102 Bethesda Drive, Greenville, NC 27834; tel. 919/816-7700; FAX. 919/816-7733; Anna Letchworth, RN, B.S.N., Administrator

The Endoscopy Center, 191 Biltmore Avenue, Asheville, NC 28801; tel. 704/254-0881; Michael Grier, M.D.

The Eye Surgery Center of Shelby, 507 North Morgan Street, Shelby, NC 28150; tel. 704/482-0696; FAX. 704/482-7707; Frank Hannah, M.D., Medical Director

The Surgery Center, 166 Memorial Court, Jacksonville, NC 28546; tel. 910/353-9565; FAX. 919/353-5497; Takey Crist, M.D., President

Wilmington Health Associates, P.A., 1202 Medical Center Drive, Wilmington, NC 28401; tel. 910/341-3433; Diane A. Atkinson, Administrator

Wilmington SurgCare, Inc., 1801 South 17th Street, Wilmington, NC 28401; tel. 910/763-4555; Catherine Peterman, President, Chief Executive Officer

Wilson OB-GYN, 2500 Horton Boulevard, Zip 27893, P.O. Box 7639, Wilson, NC 27895; tel. 919/206-1000; FAX. 919/206-1000; Kay Long,, RN

Woman Care and Carolina Birth Center, 712 North Elm Street, High Point, NC 27262; tel. 910/889-3646; Robert C. Crawford, M.D., Chief Executive Officer

NORTH DAKOTA

Ambulatory Surgical Center of Fargo, 321 Eighth Avenue, N., P.O. Box 6016, Fargo, ND 58102; tel. 701/234-6400; FAX. 701/234-5854; Ron Beare, Administrator

Centennial Medical Center, 1500 24th Avenue, S.W., Minot, ND 58702; tel. 701/852-0777; John C. Tescher, Controller

Dakota Day Surgery, 1717 South University Drive, P.O. Box 6014, Fargo, ND 58103; tel. 701/280-4700; Lynn R. Wold, Business Manager

Day Surgery - Wahpeton, 275 South 11th Street, Wahpeton, ND 58075; tel. 701/642-2000; FAX. 701/671-4153; Keith Robberstad, Administrator

Great Plains Clinic Surgery Center, 33 Ninth Street, W., Dickinson, ND 58601; tel. 701/225-6017; Joel Frey, Administrator

Western Dakota Medical Group, P.C., 1102 Main, Williston, ND 58801; tel. 701/572-7711; Jeff Neuberger, Administrator

OHIO

Amend Center for Eye Surgery, 5939 Colerain Avenue, Cincinnati, OH 45239; tel. 513/923-3900; FAX. 513/923-3012

Aultman Center for One Day Surgery, 4715 Whipple Avenue, N.W., Canton, OH 44718; tel. 216/492-3050; James Davis, Administrator

Austintown Ambulatory Surgical Center, 45 North Canfield-Niles Road, Youngstown, OH 44515; tel. 216/792-2722; FAX. 216/793-4883; Ralph J. Reese, Jr., Executive Director

Bloomberg Eye Center, 1651 West Main Street, Newark, OH 43055; tel. 614/344-2151; FAX. 614/522-6766; John M. Faulk, Executive Director

Carnegie Surgery Center, 10681 Carnegie Avenue, Cleveland, OH 44106; tel. 216/231-3300; FAX. 216/231-1441; K. L. Rosacco, RN, CNOR, Nurse Administrator

Cincinnati Eye Institute and Outpatient Eye Surgery Center, 10494 Montgomery Road, Cincinnati, OH 45242; tel. 513/984-5133; FAX. 513/984-4240; Doris Holton, Administrator

Cincinnati Foot Clinic, Inc., 9600 Colerain Avenue, Suite 400, Cincinnati, OH 45239; tel. 513/385-6946; Robert Hayman, M.D., President

Consultants in Gastroenterology, Inc., 29001 Cedar Road, Suite 110, Lyndhurst, OH 44124; tel. 216/461-2550; FAX. 216/461-5319; Gloria Bradshaw, Office Manager

☐ **Crystal Clinic Surgery Center,** 3975 Embassy Parkway, Akron, OH 44313; tel. 216/668-4085; Katherine L. McNeal, RN, Administrator

Dayton Ear, Nose and Throat Surgeons, Inc., 7076 Corporate Way, Centerville, OH 45459; tel. 513/434-0555; FAX. 513/434-7413; K. Jean Christian, Administrator

Digestivecare Endoscopy Unit, 75 Sylvania Drive, Dayton, OH 45440; tel. 513/325-5065; FAX. 513/325-5060; Patty Mannix, Endoscopy Coordinator

Eye Care Center of Cincinnati, 5300 Cornell Road, Cincinnati, OH 45242; tel. 513/489-6161; FAX. 513/489-6442; Amy D. Riegler, Coordinator

Eye Institute of Northwestern Ohio, Inc., 5555 Airport Highway, Suite 110, Toledo, OH 43615; tel. 419/865-3866; FAX. 419/865-3451; Carol R. Kollarits, M.D., President

Eye Surgery Center of Wooster, 3519 Friendsville Road, Wooster, OH 44691; tel. 216/345-6371; FAX. 216/345-8029; Michelle Morrison, Director

Franciscan Center for Sight, 2841 Boudinot Avenue, Cincinnati, OH 45238; tel. 513/389-5900; FAX. 513/389-5911; Kris Hoffman, RN, Nurse Manager

GI and Liver Disease Endoscopy Center, 4200 Indian Ripple Road, Beaver Creek, OH 45440; tel. 513/427-1680

Gastroenterology Associates of Cleveland, 6801 Mayfield Road, Suite 142, Mayfield Heights, OH 44124; tel. 216/461-8800; James Andrassy, Administrator

Gastroenterology Specialists, Inc., 2732 Fulton Drive, N.W., Canton, OH 44718; tel. 216/455-5011; Melissa Smith, RN, C.G.C.

Gastroenterology, Inc. Endoscopy Center, 777 West State Street, Suite 402, Columbus, OH 43222; tel. 614/221-4960; FAX. 614/221-4108; Joyce McLaughlan, RN

Halpin-Poweleit Eye Surgery Center, 8044 Montgomery Road, Suite 155, Cincinnati, OH 45236; tel. 513/791-3937; FAX. 513/791-1473

Innova Surgery Center East, d/b/a Eastside Surgical Center, 3755 Orange Place, Beachwood, OH 44122; tel. 216/464-7300; FAX. 216/467-3050; Nancy Halkerston, RN, Director Clinical Services

Kaiser Foundation Health Plan of Ohio, 12301 Snow Road, Parma, OH 44130; tel. 216/362-2000

Kunesh Eye Surgery Center, 2601 Far Hills Avenue, Dayton, OH 45419-1665; tel. 513/298-1093; FAX. 513/298-6344; Lucy Helmers, Administrator

Levin Eye Institute, 119 West Kemper Road, Cincinnati, OH 45246; tel. 513/671-6112

Mercy Ambulatory Surgery Center, 2990 Mack Road, Fairfield, OH 45014; tel. 513/874-6440; FAX. 513/874-6005

Mid-Ohio Outpatient Surgery Center, 245 Taylor Station Road, Columbus, OH 43213; tel. 614/861-0448; FAX. 614/861-7717; Dr. Grace L. Kim

North Coast Endoscopy, Inc., 9500 Mentor Avenue, Suite 380, Mentor, OH 44060; tel. 216/942-0004; FAX. 216/352-9407; Ahmad Ascha, M.D.

Northwest Ohio Urologic, P.O. Box 351837, Toledo, OH 43635-6254; tel. 419/535-1837; FAX. 419/535-6254; Carl V. Dreyer, M.D., President

Ohio Eye Associates Surgery Center, 466 South Trimble Road, Mansfield, OH 44906; tel. 419/756-8000; FAX. 419/756-7100; John L. Marquardt, M.D.

Parkside Women's Center, Inc., 1011 Boardman-Canfield Road, Boardman, OH 44512; tel. 216/758-0975; FAX. 216/758-8453

☐ **Parkway Urology Center, Inc.,** 3500 Executive Parkway, Toledo, OH 43606; tel. 419/531-8349; FAX. 419/531-8798; Gregor K. Emmert, Sr., M.D., Chief Executive Officer

Plastic Surgery Center, 3030 Streetsboro Road, Richfield, OH 44286; tel. 216/659-6868

Ram Bandi M.D. A.S.C., 1037 North Main Street, Akron, OH 44310; tel. 216/923-0094; FAX. 216/923-0094; Susan Barron

Restorative Vision Center, 4452 Eastgate Boulevard, Suite 305, Cincinnati, OH 45245; tel. 513/752-5700; FAX. 513/752-5716; Holly Schwab, RN, Surgery Manager

☐ **Sandusky Surgeons, Inc.,** 1221 Hayes Avenue, Sandusky, OH 44870; tel. 419/625-1374; Donald Lenhart, M.D., President

Sidney Foot and Ankle Surgical Center, 1000 Michigan, Sidney, OH 45365; tel. 513/492-1211

South Dayton Urological Associates, Inc., 10 Southmoor Circle, N.W., Kettering, OH 45429; tel. 513/294-1489; FAX. 513/294-7999; Donald Bailey, Practice Administrator

Stoneridge Endoscopy Center, 3900 Stoneridge Lane, Dublin, OH 43017; tel. 614/889-5001, ext. 1236; FAX. 614/889-5913; Cheryl Miller, Clinic Manager

☐ **Surgery Center,** 19250 East Bagley Road, Middleburg Heights, OH 44130; tel. 216/826-3240; FAX. 216/826-3250

Surgiplex, 950 Clague Road, Westlake, OH 44145; tel. 216/333-1020; FAX. 216/333-3278

The Surgical Center of East Liverpool, 16480 St. Clair Avenue, P.O. Box 62, East Liverpool, OH 43920; tel. 216/386-9000; JoAnn Bradfield, Chief Executive Officer

The Zeeba Clinic, A Meridia Outpatient and Laser Surgery Center, 29017 Cedar Road, Lyndhurst, OH 44124; tel. 216/461-7774; FAX. 216/461-5401; Esther Zeitz, Administrative Director

Toledo Clinic, Inc., 4235 Secor Road, Toledo, OH 43623; tel. 419/473-3561; FAX. 419/472-0838; David J. Sobczak, Chief Financial Officer

Toledo Community Lithotripter Center, 3158 West Central Avenue, Toledo, OH 43606; tel. 419/531-3538

Toledo Plastic Surgeons Center, 2865 North Reynolds Road, Toledo, OH 43615; tel. 419/534-3330; FAX. 419/534-5716; Charles E. Jaeger, General Manager, Chief Executive Officer

Tri-State Endoscopy Center, 2925 Vernon Place, Suite 101, Cincinnati, OH 45219; tel. 513/751-6125; FAX. 513/751-4532; Patti Murphy, RN, Director

Western Reserve Medical Center, 1930 State Route 59, Kent, OH 44240; tel. 216/677-3620

Wilson Eye Clinic Surgicenter, Inc., 300 West National Road, Vandalia, OH 45377; tel. 513/890-8992; FAX. 513/890-0763

☐ **Wright Surgery Center,** 1611 South Green Road, Suite 124, South Euclid, OH 44121; tel. 216/291-0056; Barbara McCann, Director of Marketing, Communication

OKLAHOMA

Ambulatory Surgery Associates, 6160 South Yale Avenue, Tulsa, OK 74136; tel. 918/495-2625; FAX. 918/495-2601; Jaquelyn S. Moore, RN, Director

Central Oklahoma Ambulatory Surgical Center, Inc., 3301 N.W. 63rd Street, Oklahoma City, OK 73116; tel. 405/842-9732; FAX. 405/842-9771; Paul Silverstein, M.D., Administrator

Digestive Disease Specialists, Inc., 3366 N.W. Expressway, Suite 400, P.O. Box 99521, Oklahoma City, OK 73199; tel. 405/948–7834; Larry A. Bookman, M.D.
Eastern Oklahoma Surgery Center, L. L. C., 5020 East 68th Street, Tulsa, OK 74136; tel. 918/492–1539, ext. 138; FAX. 918/494–4683; Bobbie Huff, RN, Director
Grisham Eye Surgery Center, P.O. Box 1437, Bartlesville, OK 74005; tel. 918/333–1990, ext. 119; Dennis McKinley
Heritage Eye Surgicenter of Oklahoma, 6922 South Western, Suite 104, Oklahoma City, OK 73139; tel. 405/636–1508; Edward D. Glinski, D.O., Administrator
Lawton Physician's Surgery Center, 3617 West Gore Boulevard, Suite D, Lawton, OK 73505; tel. 405/357–1900; FAX. 405/357–1775; Roxanne H. Gibson, Executive Director
Medical Plaza Endoscopy Unit, 1125 N. Porter, Suite 304, Norman, OK 73071; tel. 405/360–2799; FAX. 405/447–0321; Philip C. Bird, M.D.
Oklahoma Ambulatory Surgery Center, 6908–B East Reno, Midwest City, OK 73110; tel. 405/737–6900; FAX. 405/732–0885; Richard E. Donner, M.D., Administrator
Oklahoma City Clinic, 701 N.W. 10th Street, Oklahoma City, OK 73104; tel. 405/271–2700; A. Wayne Coventon, FACMPE, Executive Director
Oklahoma Surgicare, 13313 North Meridian, Suite B, Oklahoma City, OK 73120; tel. 405/755–6240; FAX. 405/752–1819; Lindie Slater, Administrator
Orthopedic Associates Ambulatory Surgery Center, Inc., 3301 N.W. 50th Street, P.O. Box 57027, Oklahoma City, OK 73157–7027; tel. 405/947–5610; Thomas H. Flesher, Administrator
Outpatient Surgical Center of Ponca City, 400 Fairview, Ponca City, OK 74601; tel. 405/762–0695; FAX. 405/762–0770; Peggy Maples, RN, Executive Director
Physicians Surgical Center, 805 East Robinson, Norman, OK 73071–6610; tel. 405/364–9789; FAX. 405/366–8081; Ruth Beller, RN, Director
Southern Oklahoma Surgical Center, Inc., 2412 North Commerce, Ardmore, OK 73401; tel. 405/226–5000; Ann Willis, RN, Administrator
Southern Plains Ambulatory Surgery Center, 2222 Iowa Avenue, P.O. Box 1069, Chickasha, OK 73023; tel. 405/224–8111; FAX. 405/222–5359; Daniel N. Vaughan, Executive Director
☐ **Southwest Orthopedic Ambulatory Surgery Center, Inc.,** 8125 South Walker Avenue, Oklahoma City, OK 73139; tel. 405/631–1014; Anthony L. Cruse, D.O., President
Surgery Center of Edmond, 1700 South State Street, Edmon, OK 73013; tel. 405/330–1003; FAX. 405/330–1087; Timothy A. Gee, Administrator
Surgery Center of Midwest City, 8121 National Avenue, Suite 108, Midwest City, OK 73110; tel. 405/732–7905; FAX. 405/732–3561; Jackie Reed, Administrator
Surgery Center of Oklahoma, 815 N.W 12th Street, Oklahoma City, OK 73106; tel. 405/235–4525; Joy Babich, Administrator
Surgicare of Tulsa, 4415 South Harvard Avenue, Suite 100, Tulsa, OK 74135; tel. 918/742–2502; FAX. 918/745–9750; Dirk Foxworthy, Administrator
Three Rivers Surgery Center, 3800 West Okmulgee, Muskogee, OK 74401; tel. 918/682–9899; Doug Blessen, Chief Executive Officer
Tower Day Surgery, 1044 S.W. 44th Street, Suite 100, Oklahoma City, OK 73109; tel. 405/636–1701; FAX. 405/636–4314; Marie Smith, RN, Director
Triad Eye Medical Clinic and Cataract Institute, 6140 South Memorial, Tulsa, OK 74133; tel. 918/252–2020; FAX. 918/252–7466; Marc L. Abel, D.O., Administrator
Wilson Surgery Center, 5404 West Lee Boulevard, Lawton, OK 73505; tel. 405/357–2020; Gary Wilson, M.D., Administrator
Young Eye Institute, 4214 S.W. Lee Boulevard, Lawton, OK 73505; tel. 405/353–5860; Stephen W. Gilkeson, Executive Administrator

OREGON

Aesthetic Breast Care Center, 10201 S.E. Main, Suite 20, Portland, OR 97216; tel. 503/253–3458; FAX. 503/253–0856; Mary K. Barnhart, M.D., Administrator
Cascade Gastroenterology, 24900 S.E. Stark, Suite 205, Gresham, OR 97030; tel. 503/661–2000; FAX. 503/661–2001; Jeffrey S. Albaugh, M.D., Administrator
Center for Cosmetic and Plastic Surgery, 1353 East McAndrews Road, Medford, OR 97504; tel. 503/770–6776; Robert M. Jensen, M.D., Administrator
Eye Surgery Center, 2925 Siskiyou Boulevard, Medford, OR 97504; tel. 503/779–2020; Loren R. Barrus, M.D., Administrator
Futures Outpatient Surgical Center, Inc., 1849 N.W. Kearney, Suite 302, Portland, OR 97209; tel. 503/224–0723; FAX. 503/224–0722; Bryce E. Potter, M.D.
GI Endoscopy Center, 2560 N.W. Medical Park Drive, Roseburg, OR 97470; tel. 503/673–2046; Ruth E. Harpole, RN, Administrator
Lawrence W. O'Dell, d/b/a Northwest Eye Center, 9975 S.W. Nimbus Avenue, Beaverton, OR 97005; tel. 503/646–7644; Jim Heath, Administrator
Lovejoy Surgicenter, Inc., 933 N.W. 25th Avenue, Portland, OR 97210; tel. 503/221–1870; FAX. 503/221–1488; Allene M. Klass, Administrator
Medford Clinic, P.C., 555 Black Oak Drive, Medford, OR 97504; tel. 503/734–3434; Carol Flinn, Acting Executive Officer
North Bend Medical Center, Inc., 1900 Woodland Drive, Coos Bay, OR 97420; tel. 503/267–5151, ext. 298; FAX. 503/269–0797; Frederick L. Saunders, Jr., Executive Director
Northbank Surgical Center, 700 Bellevue Street, S., Suite 300, Salem, OR 97301; tel. 503/364–3704; Peggy Seidler, Administrator
Northwest Eye Center, 1700 Valley River Drive, Eugene, OR 97401; tel. 503/343–3900; FAX. 503/343–3913; Jim Health, Administrator
Oregon Cataract and Laser Institute, 2700 S.E. 14th Avenue, Albany, OR 97321; tel. 503/928–1666; Darrell Genstler, M.D., Administrator
Oregon Eye Surgery Center, Inc., 1550 Oak Street, Eugene, OR 97401; tel. 503/683–8771; William E. Spangler, M.D., Medical Director
Roseburg Surgicenter, 631 West Stanton, Roseburg, OR 97470; tel. 503/440–6311; FAX. 503/440–6394; Marlin Larsen, Ph.D., Executive Officer
The Gastroenterology Endoscopy Center, 6464 S.W. Borland Road, Suite D–4, Tualatin, OR 97062; tel. 503/692–4537; Robert Wollmuth, M.D., Administrator
The Portland Clinic Surgical Center, 800 S.W. 13th Avenue, Portland, OR 97205; tel. 503/221–0161; FAX. 503/274–1697; J. Michael Schwab, Administrator
Tigard Surgery Center, 13240 S.W. Pacific Highway, Suite 200, Tigard, OR 97223; tel. 503/639–6571; FAX. 503/624–6037; Ivan L. Bakos, M.D., Administrator
Willamette Valley Eye SurgiCenter, 2001 Commercial Street, S.E., Salem, OR 97302; tel. 503/363–1500; FAX. 503/588–2028; Gordon Miller, M.D., Administrator

PENNSYLVANIA

☐ **Abington Surgical Center,** 2701 Blair Mill Road, Suite 35, Willow Grove, PA 19090; tel. 215/443–8505; FAX. 215/443–0565; Deborah S. Kitz, Ph.D., Executive Director
Aesthetic and Reconstructive Surgery, 816 Belvedere Street, Carlisle, PA 17013
Aestique Ambulatory Surgical Center, One Aesthetic Way, Greensburg, PA 15601; tel. 412/832–7555; FAX. 412/832–7568; Theordore A. Lazzaro, M.D., Medical Director
Apple Hill Surgical Center, 25 Monument Road, Suite 270, York, PA 17403; tel. 717/741–8250; FAX. 717/741–8254; Gwendolyn J. Grothouse, RN, Administrative Director
Cottman Eye Surgery Center, 1815 Cottman Avenue, Philadelphia, PA 19111; tel. 215/722–2505; FAX. 215/742–6386; Lawrence S. Schaffzin, M.D., Medical Director
Dermatologic SurgiCenter, 1200 Locust Street, Philadelphia, PA 19107; tel. 215/546–3666; FAX. 215/546–6688; Anthony V. Benedetto, D.O., FACP, Medical Director
Dermatologic SurgiCenter, 2221 Garrett Road, Drexel Hill, PA 19026; tel. 610/623–5885; FAX. 610/623–7276; Anthony V. Beneetto, D.O. Medical Director
Digestive Disease Institute, 897 Poplar Church Road, Camp Hill, PA 17011; tel. 717/763–1239; FAX. 717/763–0768; Iris Garman, Administrator
Eye Clinic Ambulatory Surgical Center, Inc., 601 Wyoming Avenue, Kingston, PA 18704; tel. 717/288–7405; Mark Kelly, Administrator
Eye Surgery Center, 558 East Lancaster Avenue, Radnor, PA 19087; tel. 215/688–9333; FAX. 215/688–4227; Linda Kremer, Administrator
Fairgrounds Surgical Center, 400 North 17th Street, Suite 300, Allentown, PA 18104; tel. 610/821–2020; FAX. 610/821–2016; Barbara Ann Harmer, Administrative Director
Grandview Surgery & Laser Center, 205 Grandview Avenue, Camp Hill, PA 17011; tel. 717/731–5444; FAX. 717/731–0415; Cheryl L. Graybill, RN, Administrative Director
Hanover Surgicenter, Inc., 3130 Grandview Road, Building B, Hanover, PA 17331; tel. 717/633–1600; FAX. 717/633–6556; Melvin L. Brooks, Jr., CRNA, Director
☐ **Jefferson Surgery Center,** Coal Valley Road, P.O. Box 18420, Pittsburgh, PA 15236; tel. 412/469–6060; Sheran Sullivan, Manager
John A. Zitelli, M.D., P.C., Ambulatory Surgery Facility, 5200 Centre Avenue, Suite 303, Pittsburgh, PA 15232; tel. 412/681–9400; FAX. 412/681–5240; John A. Zitelli, M.D.
☐ **Lancaster Surgery Center,** 217 Harrisburg Avenue, Lancaster, PA 17603; tel. 717/295–2500; FAX. 717/295–4898; Debra K. Sanders, RN, Administrative Director
Lebanon Outpatient Surgical Center, L.P., 830 Tuck Street, Lebanon, PA 17042; tel. 717/228–1620; FAX. 717/228–1642; Anita Gingrich, Manager
Lowry SurgiCenter, 1115 Lowry Avenue, Jeannette, PA 15644; tel. 412/527–2885; K. Diddle, M.D., Medical Director
Mt. Lebanon Surgical Center, Professional Office Building, 1050 Bower Hill Road, Suite 102, Pittsburgh, PA 15243; tel. 412/563–6808; FAX. 412/563–6857; Patricia Strosnider, Director, Nursing
N.E.I. Ambulatory Surgery, Inc., 204 Mifflin Avenue, Scranton, PA 18503; tel. 717/342–3145, ext. 2400; FAX. 717/342–3136
North Shore Surgi–Center, Two Allegheny Center, Suite 530, Pittsburgh, PA 15212–5493; tel. 412/231–0200; FAX. 412/231–0613; Jack Demos, M.D., FACS
Ophtalmology Surgical Center, Inc., 92 Tuscarora Street, Harrisburg, PA 17104; tel. 717/233–2020; FAX. 717/232–3294; Marcia A. Lammando, B.S.N, RN, Director
Paoli Surgery Center, One Industrial Boulevard, Paoli, PA 19301; tel. 610/408–0822
Pennsylvania College of Podiatric Medicine, Foot and Ankle Institute, 8th and Race Streets, Philadelphia, PA 19107; tel. 215/629–0300; James E. Bates, D.P.M., President
Pennsylvania Eye Surgery Center, 4100 Linglestown Road, Harrisburg, PA 17112; tel. 717/657–2020; Jacklyn R. Linehart, RN, Director, Surgical Services
Pennsylvania Eye Surgery Institute, Two Bala Plaza, Pl 33, Bala Cynwd, PA 19004; tel. 215/668–2935; FAX. 215/668–1509; Herbert J. Nevyas, M.D., Medical Director
☐ **Plastic Surgery Center, Inc.,** 1130 Highway 315, Wilkes-Barre, PA 18702; tel. 717/821–2820; FAX. 717/825–7962; David N. Culp, Chief Executive Officer
Pocono Ambulatory Surgery Center, One Veterans Place, Stroudsburg, PA 18360; tel. 717/421–4978; Mary P. Hayden RN, B.S., A.S.C. Coordinator

Providers / Freestanding Ambulatory Surgery Centers

Ridgeway Esper Medical Center Ambulatory Surgical Center, 5050 West Ridge Road, Erie, PA 16506-1298; tel. 814/833-8800; FAX. 814/833-2079; Deborah Hartmann, RN, Director, Nursing

☐ **Saint Vincent Surgery Center,** 312 West 25th Street, Erie, PA 16502; tel. 814/452-7000; FAX. 814/452-7136; James J. Tarasovitch, Executive Director

Sewickley Surgical Center at Edgeworth Commons, 301 Ohio River Boulevard, Edgeworth, Suite 100, Sewickley, PA 15143; tel. 412/741-5866; FAX. 412/741-5884; Carol Figas, RN, CNOR, Supervisor

Shadyside Surgi-Center, Inc., 5727 Centre Avenue, Pittsburgh, PA 15206; tel. 412/363-6626; FAX. 412/363-7008; Ralph J. Falvo, RN, Director

☐ **Southwestern Ambulatory Surgery Center,** 500 Lewis Run Road, Pittsburgh, PA 15236; tel. 412/469-6964; FAX. 412/469-6948; Philip P. Ripepi, M.D., President

Southwestern Pennsylvania Eye Surgery Center, 750 East Beau Street, Washington, PA 15301; tel. 412/228-7477; FAX. 412/228-8117; Karen A. Dynice, Clinical Director

Specialists Health Care Clinic of Monroeville, 125 Daugherty Drive, Monroeville, PA 15146

St. Francis Surgery Center-North, One St. Francis Way, Cranberry Township, PA 16066; tel. 412/772-5360; Mark R. LaRosa, Director Surgery Center-North

☐ **Surgical Center of York,** 1750 Fifth Avenue, P.O. Box 290, York, PA 17405; tel. 717/843-7613; Thomas R. Harlow, Director, Management Services

Surgical Eye Institute of Western Pennsylvania, 618 Monongahela Avenue, Glassport, PA 15045; tel. 412/664-7874; FAX. 412/673-5720; Shirley A. Smith, RN

The Medical Skin Care and Surgery Center, 6415 Bustleton Avenue, Philadelphia, PA 19149

The Scranton Surgery Center, 425 Adams Street, Scranton, PA 18510; tel. 717/348-1114; FAX. 717/347-4351; Nancy A. Nealon, RN, B.S.N., Administrative Director

The Surgery Center of Chester County, Oaklands Corporate Center, 460 Creamery Way, Exton, PA 19341-2500; tel. 610/594-8900; FAX. 215/594-8907; Stephen P. Barainyak, Executive Director

The SurgiCenter at Ligonier, 221 West Main Street, Ligonier, PA 15658; tel. 412/238-9573; FAX. 412/238-4709; Kim Kenney-Ciarimboli, Director, Operations

West Shore Endoscopy Center, 423 North 21st Street, Camp Hill, PA 17011; tel. 717/975-2430; Marilee Ball, RN, Director

Westmoreland Surgery Center, 200 Beggemer Road, Mt. Pleasant, PA 15666; tel. 412/547-5432; FAX. 412/547-2435; Janet Mahn, Administrative Director

York Road Ambulatory Surgical Center, 399 North York Road, Warminster, PA 18974; tel. 215/672-3222; FAX. 215/672-6634; Linda Rothenberger, Regional Director

RHODE ISLAND

Bayside Endoscopy Center, 120 Dudley Street, Suite 103, Providence, RI 02905; tel. 401/274-1810; FAX. 401/273-9689; Nicholas Califano, M.D., Administrator

Blackstone Valley Surgicare, Inc., 333 School Street, Pawtucket, RI 02860; tel. 401/728-3800; FAX. 401/723-2440; Ann Dugan, Administrator

Koch Eye Surgi Center, Inc., 566 Tollgate Road, Warwick, RI 02886; tel. 401/738-4800; FAX. 401/738-8153; Paul S. Koch, M.D., Administrator

Planned Parenthood of Rhode Island, 111 Point Street, Providence, RI 02903; tel. 401/421-9620; FAX. 401/621-6250; Barbara Baldwin, Executive Director

Wayland Square Surgicare, 17 Seekonk Street, Providence, RI 02906; tel. 401/453-3311; Ann Dugan, Administrator

Women's Medical Center, 1725 Broad Street, Cranston, RI 02905; tel. 401/272-1440; FAX. 401/461-1390; Mary Elizabeth Nicolace, Administrator

SOUTH CAROLINA

Bay Microsurgical Unit, Inc., 400 Marina Drive, P.O. Drawer L, Georgetown, SC 29442; tel. 803/546-8421; FAX. 803/546-1173; Rebecca Lammonds, Administrator, Director, Nursing

Bearwood Plastic & Reconstructive Surgery Center, 3031 Highway 81, N., Anderson, SC 29621; tel. 803/226-7371; Patricia P. Smith, Administrator

Carolina Eye Ambulatory Surgery Center, 210 University Parkway, Suite 1500 B, Aiken, SC 29801; tel. 803/649-3953; FAX. 803/641-3801; Stephen K. VanDerVliet, M.D.

Carolina Surgical Center, 198 South Herlong Avenue, P.O. Box 4491, Rock Hill, SC 29732; tel. 803/327-4664; FAX. 803/327-7456; Don Rivers, Jr., Administrator

Charleston Plastic Surgery Center, 159 Rutledge Avenue, Charleston, SC 29403; tel. 803/722-1985; FAX. 803/722-4840; Pamela L. Fisher, Office Manager

Charleston Surgery Center, 2690 Lake Park Drive, North Charleston, SC 29418; tel. 803/764-0992; FAX. 803/764-3187; Donna Padgette, RN, M.S.N., Facility Manager

Columbia Ambulatory Plastic Surgery Center, Inc., 338 Harbison Boulevard, Columbia, SC 29212; tel. 803/732-6655; FAX. 803/732-6644; Vickie H. Ott, Administrator

Columbia Eye Surgery Center, Inc., 1920 Pickens Street, P.O. Box 1754, Columbia, SC 29202; tel. 803/254-7732; FAX. 803/771-7639; Kenneth W. Gibbons, Administrator

Columbia Gastrointestinal Endoscopy Center, 2739 Laurel Street, Suite One-B, Columbia, SC 29240; tel. 803/254-9588; FAX. 803/252-0052; Frederick F. DuRant, III, Administrator

Eastern Carolina Regional Ambulatory Surgical Center, 900 Medical Circle, Myrtle Beach, SC 29572; tel. 803/449-6414; FAX. 803/497-0357; Tony Rovinsky, Administrator

Greenville Endoscopy Center, Inc., 317 St. Francis Drive, Suite 150, Greenville, SC 29601; tel. 803/232-7338; Rebecca K. Swoyer, Administrator

Greenville Surgery Center, Five Memorial Medical Court, Greenville, SC 29605; tel. 803/295-3067; Vicki Puckett, Executive Director

Palmetto Eye Associates and Surgery Center, 9297 Medical Plaza Drive, Charleston, SC 29418; tel. 803/572-2888; FAX. 803/572-2765; Margaret A. Thompson, Administrative Director

Pee Dee Ambulatory Surgery Center, 604 East Cheves Street, Box F-17, Florence, SC 29506; tel. 803/669-3822; Joseph J. McEvoy, Administrator

Roper West Ashley Surgery Center, 18 Farmfield Avenue, Charleston, SC 29407; tel. 803/763-3763; FAX. 803/763-3881; Maria I. Sample, Administrator

Same Day Surgery East, 10 Enterprise Boulevard, Suite 104, Greenville, SC 29615; tel. 803/458-7141; FAX. 803/676-9116; Linda Zavasnik, Clinical Nurse Manager

Spartanburg Urology Surgicenter, Inc., 391 Serpentine Drive, Suite 330, Spartanburg, SC 29303; tel. 803/585-2002; Charles Davis

Surgery Center on Forest, 2631 Forest Drive, Columbia, SC 29204; tel. 803/253-7570; Norenne B. Harris

The Eye Surgery Center of Greenville Hospital System, Nine Doctors Drive, Crosscreek Medical Park, Greenville, SC 29605; tel. 803/455-8400; Joe Pollard, Administrator

The Greenwood Endoscopy Center, 103 Liner Drive, Greenwood, SC 29646; tel. 803/227-3838; FAX. 803/227-6116; A. A. Ramage, M.D., Administrator

The MicroSurgery Center, Inc., 1655 East Greenville Street, P.O. Box 1886, Anderson, SC 29622-1886; tel. 803/225-1933; FAX. 803/225-9035; Ann Geier, Administrator

Trident Surgery Center, 9313 Medical Plaza Drive, Suite 102, Charleston, SC 29406; tel. 803/797-8992; FAX. 803/797-4094; Scott R. Jones

SOUTH DAKOTA

Aberdeen Surgical Center, 1200 South Main, Box 1150, Aberdeen, SD 57401-1150; tel. 605/225-2466; Scott H. Berry, M.D., Administrator

Black Hills Regional Eye Surgery Center, 2800 Third Street, Rapid City, SD 57701-7394; tel. 605/341-4100; FAX. 605/341-0278; Richard B. Hanafin, Executive Director

Jones Eye Clinic, 3801 South Elmwood, Sioux Falls, SD 57105-6565; tel. 605/336-3142; Charles E. Jones, M.D.

Medical Associates Surgi Center, 772 East Dakota, Pierre, SD 57501-3399; tel. 605/224-5901; Dennis C. Decker, Administrator

Sioux Falls Surgical Center, 910 East 20th Street, Sioux Falls, SD 57105-1012; tel. 605/334-6730; Donald A. Schellpfeffer, M.D., Ph.D., Medical Director

SurgiClinic, 1010 Ninth Street, Rapid City, SD 57701-3599; tel. 605/348-7607; FAX. 605/342-1359; Ray G. Burnett, M.D., Medical Director

Yankton Medical Clinic P.C., 1104 West Eighth Street, Yankton, SD 57078-3306; tel. 605/665-7841; FAX. 605/665-0546; Don P. Lake, Administrator

TENNESSEE

Appalachian Ambulatory Surgical Center, Medical Arts Building, 106 Rogosin Drive, Elizabethton, TN 37643; tel. 615/543-5888

Arrowsmith Eye Surgery Center, Parkview Tower, Suite 900, 210 25th Avenue, N., Nashville, TN 37203; tel. 615/327-2244; FAX. 615/321-3175; Barbara K. Arrowsmith, Administrator

Atrium Memorial Surgical Center, 1949 Gunbarrel Road, Suite 290, Chattanooga, TN 37421; tel. 615/495-3550; FAX. 615/495-3580; Susan Deakins, Administrator

Bristol Surgery Center, 350 Blountville Highway, Suite 108, Bristol, TN 37620; tel. 615/844-6120; FAX. 615/844-6126; David Paul Gross, Administrator

Cataract Surgery Center, 5406 Knight Arnold Road, Memphis, TN 38115; tel. 901/360-8081

☐ **Centennial Surgery Center,** 340 23rd Avenue, N., Nashville, TN 37203; tel. 615/327-1123; FAX. 615/327-0261; Cynthia S. Duvall, RN, B.S., Administrator

☐ **Chattanooga Surgery Center,** 400 North Holtzclaw Avenue, Chattanooga, TN 37404; tel. 615/698-6871; Becky Myers, Facility Manager

Clarksville Encoscopy Center, 132 Hillcrest, Clarksville, TN 37043; tel. 615/552-0180; FAX. 615/572-0915

Cleveland Surgery Center, L.P., 137 25th Street, N.E., Cleveland, TN 37311; tel. 615/472-7874

Columbia Endoscopy Center, Inc., 1510 1/2 Hatcher Lane, Columbia, TN 38401; tel. 615/381-7818

Columbia Outpatient Surgery, Inc., 1405 Hatcher Lane, Columbia, TN 38401; tel. 615/381-3700; Deborah Woodard, Administrator

Digestive Disease Endoscopy Center, 2021 Church Street, Suite 303, Nashville, TN 37203; tel. 615/340-4625; FAX. 615/340-4628

East Memphis Surgery Center, 80 Humphreys Center Drive, Memphis, TN 38120; tel. 901/747-3233

Endoscopy Center of Kingsport, 2204 Pavilion Drive, Kingsport, TN 37660; tel. 615/392-6100; FAX. 615/392-6159; Barbara Light, Office Manager

Endoscopy Center of Northeast Tennessee, 310 State of Franklin Road, Suite 202, Johnson City, TN 37604; tel. 615/929-7111

Fort Sanders West Outpatient Surgery Center, Ltd., 210 Fort Sanders West Boulevard, Knoxville, TN 37922; tel. 615/531-5222; FAX. 615/531-5043; Leslie Irwin, Administrator

Franklin Surgery Center at MedCore, 2105 Edward Curd Lane, Franklin, TN 37064; tel. 615/794-7320

G. Baker Hubbard Ambulatory Surgery Center, 616 West Forest Avenue, Jackson, TN 38301; tel. 901/422-0330

Providers / Freestanding Ambulatory Surgery Centers

G. I. Diagnostic and Therapeutic Center, 1068 Cresthaven Road, Suite 300, Memphis, TN 38119; tel. 901/682-6700; FAX. 901/683-3046; Randolph M. McCloy, M.D., Medical Director

Germantown Ambulatory Surgical Center, Inc., 7499 Old Poplar Pike, Germantown, TN 38138; tel. 901/755-6465; FAX. 901/757-5543

Heritage Surgery Center of Clarksville, 121 Hillcrest Drive, Clarksville, TN 37043; tel. 615/552-9992

Kingsport Bronchoscopy Center, Inc., 135 West Ravine Road, Suite Eight–A, Kingsport, TN 37660; tel. 615/247-5197; FAX. 615/247-5254; Shirley Hawkins, Administrator

Kingsport Endoscopy Corporation, 135 West Ravine Road, Suite Seven–A, Kingsport, TN 37660; tel. 615/246-9752; Bettye E. Reed, Administrator

Knoxville Surgery Center, 9300 Park West Boulevard, Knoxville, TN 37923; tel. 615/691-2725; FAX. 615/691-3090; Ranae Thompson, RN, Facility Administrator

LeBonheur East Surgery Center, L.P., 786 Estate Place, Memphis, TN 38120; tel. 901/681-4100; FAX. 901/681-4140; Diane Swain, Director

Lebanon Surgery Center, Inc., 1414 Baddour Parkway, P.O. Box 549, Lebanon, TN 37088; tel. 615/444-8944; Sheena Sloan, Administrator

Memphis Eye and Cataract Ambulatory Surgery Center, 6485 Poplar Avenue, Memphis, TN 38119; tel. 901/767-3937

Memphis Gastroenterology Group, 80 Humphrey's Blvd., Suite 220, Memphis, TN 38120; tel. 901/747-3630; FAX. 901/747-4039; Sylvia Hawkins, RN, Nurse Manager

Memphis Surgery Center, 1044 Cresthaven Road, Memphis, TN 38119; tel. 901/682-1516; FAX. 901/682-1545; Barbara Hopper, RN, B.S., CNOR, Facility Manager

Mid-State Endoscopy Center, 2010 Church Street, Suite 320, Nashville, TN 37203; tel. 615/329-2141; FAX. 615/321-0522; Robert W. Herring, Jr. M.D., Medical Director

Nashville Endoscopy Center, 300 20th N., Eighth Floor, Nashville, TN 37203; tel. 615/284-1335; FAX. 615/284-1316

Nashville Gastrointestinal Endoscopy Center, 4230 Harding Road, Suite 309, Nashville, TN 37205; tel. 615/383-0165; Ron E. Pruitt, M.D.

Nashville Surgery Center, 1717 Patterson Street, Nashville, TN 37203; tel. 615/329-1888; FAX. 615/329-0179; Patricia Middleton, Facility Manager

Ophthalmic Ambulatory Surgery Center, P.C., 2001 Hayes Street, Nashville, TN 37203; tel. 615/327-2001; FAX. 615/327-2069; Alec Dryden, Administrator

Oral Facial Surgery Center, 322 22nd Avenue, N., Nashville, TN 37203; tel. 615/321-6160

PRISM Aesthetic Surgery Center, 80 Humphreys Center, Suite 310, Memphis, TN 38120; tel. 901/747-0446; FAX. 901/747-4406; Linda M. Economides, Director, PRISM ASC

Physicians Pavilion, 360 Wallace Road, Nashville, TN 37222; tel. 615/781-9020; FAX. 615/781-9144; Sandra Holshouser, Administrator

Ridge Lake Ambulatory Surgery Center, 825 Ridge Lake Boulevard, Memphis, TN 38119; tel. 901/685-0777

☐ **Rivergate Surgery Center,** 647 Myatt Drive, Madison, TN 37115; tel. 615/868-8942; Brenda Cruse, Director

Southern Endoscopy Center, 397 Wallace Road, Suite 407, Nashville, TN 37211; tel. 615/832-5530; FAX. 615/832-5713; Robert W. Herring, Jr., M.D., Medical Director

St. Thomas Medical Group Endoscopy Center, 4230 Harding Road, Suite 400, Nashville, TN 37205; tel. 615/297-2700

Surgical Services, P.C., 604 South Main Street, Sweetwater, TN 37874; tel. 615/337-4508

Surgicenter Of Murfreesboro Medical Clinic, P.A., 1004 North Highland Avenue, Murfreesboro, TN 37130; tel. 615/893-4480, ext. 351; FAX. 615/895-6212

Tennessee Endoscopy Center, 1706 East Lamar Alexander Parkway, Maryville, TN 37811; tel. 615/983-0073; FAX. 615/984-1731; Craig Jarvis, M.D., Administrator

The Cookville Surgery Center, 100 West Fourth Street, Suite 100, Cookville, TN 38501; tel. 615/528-6115; FAX. 615/526-2962; Diana Welch, RN, Administrator

The Endoscopy Center, 801 Weisgarber Road, Suite 100, 37909, P.O. Box 59002, Knoxville, TN 37950-9002; tel. 615/588-5121; Gayle Mahan, Office Manager

The Gastrointestinal Endoscopy Center, 250 25th Avenue N., Suite 301, Nashville, TN 37203; tel. 615/327-2111; FAX. 615/327-9292; Dawn Lynn Gray, RN, B.S., Endoscopy Administrator

The Pain Clinic and Rehabilitation Center, 55 Humphreys Center Drive, Suite 200, Memphis, TN 38120; tel. 901/747-0040; FAX. 901/747-3424; Lori Parris, RN, Administrator

The Surgery Center, 2761 Sullins Street, Knoxville, TN 37919; tel. 615/522-2949; FAX. 615/637-3259; Carolyn Liles–Gillespie, RN, Executive Director

Tullahoma Outpatient Surgery Center, 1918 North Jackson, Tullahoma, TN 37388; tel. 615/455-2006

Urology Surgery Center, Inc., 2011 Church Street, Sixth Floor, Nashville, TN 37203; tel. 615/329-7700; Robert B. Barnett, M.D., Medical Director

Van Dyke Ambulatory Surgery Center, 400 Hospital Drive, Paris, TN 38242; tel. 901/642-5003; FAX. 901/642-8756; John T. VanDyck III, M.D., Owner

Wesberry Eye, Dental Institute and Surgery Center, Inc., 2900 South Perkins Road, Memphis, TN 38118; tel. 901/362-3100; J.M. Wesberry, Sr., M.D., Chairman, Chief Executive Officer

West Tennessee Surgery Center, 637 Skyline Drive, Jackson, TN 38301; tel. 901/424-1211; Judy Haskins, RN, Administrator

TEXAS

AHCA–Mainland Outpatient Surgery Center, 3810 Hughes Court, Dickinson, TX 77539; tel. 713/337-7001; FAX. 713/337-7091; Terry R. Williams, Administrator

Abilene Cataract and Refractive Surgery Center, 2120 Antilley Road, Abilene, TX 79606; tel. 915/695-2020; FAX. 915/695-2326; Robert W. Cameron, M.D., Administrator

Amarillo Cataract and Eye Surgery Center, Inc., 7310 Fleming Avenue, Amarillo, TX 79106; tel. 806/354-8891; FAX. 806/354-2591; Carol T. Carpenter, Administrator

Ambulatory Endoscopy Center of Dallas, Ltd., 6390 LBJ Freeway, Suite 200, Dallas, TX 75240; tel. 214/934-3691; Andrew Schueck, Administrator

Ambulatory Urological Surgery Center, Inc., 1149 Ambler, Abilene, TX 79601; tel. 915/676-3557; FAX. 915/673-2143; Angela X. Young, RN, Manager

American Surgery Centers of South Texas, LTD, 7810 Louis Pasteur, Suite 101, San Antonio, TX 78229; tel. 210/692-0218; Robert Poirier, Administrator

Arlington Day Surgery, 918 North Davis Street, Arlington, TX 76012; tel. 817/860-9933; FAX. 817/860-2314; James Pilano, M.D., Administrator

Bailey Square Surgical Center, Ltd., 1111 West 34th Street, Austin, TX 78705; tel. 512/454-6753; FAX. 512/454-4314; Katherine S. Wilson, RN, M.H.A.

Barbara Jean Bartlett Memorial Surgery Center, 4200 Andrews Highway, Midland, TX 79707; tel. 915/520-5777; Sylvan Bartlett, M.D., Administrator

Bay Area Surgery, 7101 South Padre Island Drive, Corpus Christi, TX 78412; tel. 512/985-3500; FAX. 512/985-3754; Gene Hybner, Administrator

Bay Area Surgicare Center, Inc., 200 Medical Center Boulevard, Suite 106, Webster, TX 77598; tel. 713/332-2433; FAX. 713/332-0619; Mary P. Colombo, Administrator

Baylor SurgiCare, 3920 Worth Street, Dallas, TX 75246; tel. 214/820-2581; Patty Crabb, Administrative Director

Beaumont Surgical Center, 3050 Liberty, Beaumont, TX 77702; tel. 409/895-0100; Susan Almquist, Administrator

Brazos Valley Surgical Center, 2800 East 29th Street, Zip 77802, P.O. Box 2700, Bryan, TX 77805; tel. 409/776-4300; FAX. 409/774-7149; Pat Cornelison, Executive Director

Brazosport Eye Institute, 103 Parking Way, P.O. Box 369, Lake Jackson, TX 77566; tel. 409/297-2961; FAX. 409/297-2395; Frank J. Grady, M.D., Ph.D., FACS, Director

Brownsville Surgicare, 1024 Los Ebanos Boulevard, Brownsville, TX 78520; tel. 210/548-0101; FAX. 210/541-3752; Robert H. Carey, Administrator

Central Texas Day Surgery Center, L.P., 1817 S.W. Dodgen, Loop, Temple, TX 76502; tel. 817/773-7785; FAX. 817/773-9333; Stephen Earnhardt

Coastal Bend Ambulatory Surgical Center, 900 Morgan, Corpus Christi, TX 78404; tel. 512/888-4288; Barbara VandenBout

Conroe Surgery Center, 233 Interstate 45 N., P.O. Box 3091, Conroe, TX 77304; tel. 409/760-3443; FAX. 409/760-1322; Cindy Grundler, RN, Facility Manager

Crystal Outpatient Surgery Center, Inc., 215 Oak Drive, S., Suite J, Lake Jackson, TX 77566; tel. 409/299-6118; FAX. 409/299-1007; R. Scott Yarish, M.D., Administrator

Cy-Fair Surgery Center, 11250 Fallbrook Drive, Houston, TX 77065; tel. 713/955-7194; Cheryl Smith, Administrator

Dallas Day Surgery Center, Inc., 411 North Washington, Suite 5400, Dallas, TX 75246; tel. 214/821-8613; Henry S. Byrd, President

Dallas Eye Surgicenter, Inc., 720 South Cedar Ridge Road, Duncanville, TX 75137; tel. 214/296-6634; William Hamilton, Administrator

Dallas Opthalmology Center, Inc., 2811 Lemmon Avenue, Suite 102, Dallas, TX 75204; tel. 214/520-7444; James A. Bentley, Jr., M.D.

Dallas Surgi Center, 8230 Walnut Hill Lane, Suite 808, Dallas, TX 75231; tel. 214/696-8828; FAX. 214/696-1444

DeHaven Surgical Center, Inc., 1424 East Front Street, Tyler, TX 75702; tel. 903/595-4168; FAX. 903/595-6821; Barbara Shamburger, RN, Administrator

Diagnostic Clinic of San Antonio Ambulatory Surgical Center, 4647 Medical Drive, P.O. Box 29249, San Antonio, TX 78224-3100; tel. 210/615-1300; FAX. 512/692-3397; Dan Cogdill, Administrator

Doctors Surgery Center, Inc., 5300 North Street, Nacogdoches, TX 75961; tel. 409/569-8278; Robert P. Lehman, M.D., Director

Eagle Pass Surgicenter, 345 South Adams Street, Suite Eight, P.O. Box 2546, 78852-2546, Eagle Pass, TX 78852; tel. 210/773-5338; Cynthia G. Villa, Business Office Manager

East El Paso Surgery Center, 7835 Corral Drive, El Paso, TX 79915; tel. 915/595-3353; FAX. 915/595-6796; Ruth Robertson, Administrator

East Texas Eye Associates Surgery Center, 1306 Frank Avenue, Lufkin, TX 75901; tel. 409/634-8381; Jo Ann O'Neill, C.O.T., Administrator

El Paso Institute of Eye Surgery, Inc., 1717 North Brown Street, Building Three, El Paso, TX 79902; tel. 915/544-0526; FAX. 915/544-2877; Esthern A. Calderon, Administrator

Elm Place Ambulatory Surgical Center, 2217 South Danville Drive, Abilene, TX 79605; tel. 915/695-0600; FAX. 915/695-3908; Susan King, RN, Director

Eye Surgery Center, 2001 Ed Carey Drive, Suite Three, Harlingen, TX 78550; tel. 210/423-2100; Michael Laney, C.O.M.T., Administrator

Facial Plastic and Cosmetic Surgical Center, 6300 Humana Plaza, Suite 475, Abilene, TX 79606; tel. 915/695-3630; FAX. 915/695-3633; Howard A. Tobin, M.D., FACS, Medical Director

Forest Park Surgery Pavilion, 5920 Forest Park Road, Suite 700, Dallas, TX 75235; tel. 214/350-2400; FAX. 214/352-3853; David Yoder, Administrator

Garland Surgery Center L.P., 777 Walter Reed Boulevard, Suite 105, Garland, TX 75042; tel. 214/494-2400; FAX. 214/494-3873; Dan Nicholson, President

© 1995 AHA Guide — Health Organizations, Agencies and Providers — C95

Providers / Freestanding Ambulatory Surgery Centers

Gastroenterology Consultants Outpatient Surgical Center, 8214 Wurzbach, San Antonio, TX 78229; tel. 210/614-1234; FAX. 210/614-7749; Wanda Batch, B.S.N., RN, C.G.R.N., Clinical Nurse Director

Gonzaba Surgical Center, 720 Pleasanton Road, San Antonio, TX 78214; tel. 210/921-3826; FAX. 512/921-3825; William Gonzaba, M.D., Chief Executive Officer

Gramercy Outpatient Surgery Center, LTD, 2727 Gramercy, Houston, TX 77025; tel. 713/660-6900; FAX. 713/660-0704; Elaine Hand, RN, CNOR, Clinical Director

Greenpark Surgery Center, 7515 South Main Street, Suite 800, Houston, TX 77030; tel. 713/796-9666; FAX. 713/796-9660; Joan M. Culberson, RN, Administrator

Greenville Surgery Center, 7150 Greenville Avenue, Suite 200, Dallas, TX 75231; tel. 214/891-0466; FAX. 214/739-4702; Carla J. Holden, Administrator

Heart of Texas Outpatient Cataract Center, 100 South Park Drive, Brownwood, TX 76801; tel. 915/643-3561; FAX. 915/646-0670; Larry Smith, CRNA, Administrator

Heritage Surgery Center, 1501 Redbud, McKinney, TX 75069; tel. 214/548-0771; FAX. 214/562-2300; Rudolf Churner, M.D., Administrator

Houston Eye Clinic Partnership, 1200 Binz, Suite 1000, Houston, TX 77004; tel. 713/526-1600; FAX. 713/529-5254; Dan Chambers, Executive Director

Howerton Eye and Laser Surgical Center, 2610 I.H. 35 South, Austin, TX 78704-5703; tel. 512/443-9715; FAX. 512/443-9845; Ernest E. Howerton, M.D., Administrator

Institute of Eye Surgery, Houston, Inc., 6699 Chimney Rock, Second Floor, Houston, TX 77081; tel. 713/665-1406; Michael B. Files, Administrator

☐ **Key Eye Surgery Center,** 2801 Lemmon Avenue, W., Dallas, TX 75204; tel. 214/754-0000; FAX. 214/754-0079; Charles B. Key, M.D.

Knolle Ocular Surgery Center, 4126 S.W. Freeway, Suite 108, Houston, TX 77027; tel. 713/621-3920; FAX. 713/621-7217; Guy E. Knolle, Jr., M.D., Administrator

Lipsky Sight Center, 1060 Hercules, Houston, TX 77058; tel. 713/488-7213; Ed Bercier, Administrator

Lufkin Endoscopy Center, 317 Gaslight Boulevard, Lufkin, TX 75901; tel. 409/634-3713; FAX. 409/634-8136; Bhagvan R. Malladi, M.D., Administrator

Maddox Outpatient Eye Surgery Center, 1755 Curie Drive, El Paso, TX 79902; tel. 915/544-9597; FAX. 915/533-3460; Robert M. Maddox, M.D., Administrator

Mann Cataract Surgery Center, 18850 South Memorial Boulevard, Humble, TX 77338; tel. 713/446-9164; Elpidio Fahel, Administrator

Medical City Dallas Ambulatory Surgery Center, 7777 Forest Lane, Suite C-150, Dallas, TX 75230; tel. 214/661-7000; FAX. 214/788-6181; Pam J. Burgess, Vice President, Chief Operating Officer

Medical Mall Surgery Center, Inc., 1665 Antilley Road, Suite 170, Abilene, TX 79606; tel. 915/692-6694; FAX. 915/691-1568; Cindy Edgington, RN

☐ **Memorial Health Center,** 1211 Highway Six, Suite One, Sugarland, TX 77478; tel. 713/242-7220; Deborah Ganelin, Administrator

Methodist Malone and Hogan – Texas Surgery, 1501 West 11th Place, Suite A, Big Spring, TX 79720-4199; tel. 915/267-1623; FAX. 915/267-1137; Penny Phillips, Administrator

Metroplex Ambulatory Surgical Center, 2717 Osler Drive, Suite 102, Grand Prairie, TX 75051; tel. 214/647-6272; FAX. 214/660-1822; Glenda Daniels, RN, Director

Mid-Town Surgical Center, Inc., 2105 Jackson Street, Suite 200, Houston, TX 77003; tel. 713/659-3050; FAX. 713/659-3037; Glory Gee, Administrator

North Carrier Surgicenter, 517 North Carrier Parkway, Suite A, Grand Prairie, TX 75050-5494; tel. 214/264-0533; FAX. 214/262-5974; Abraham F. Syrquin, M.D., Medical Director

North Dallas Surgicare, Inc., 375 North Municipal Drive, Suite 214, Richardson, TX 75080; tel. 214/918-9400; FAX. 214/918-9749; Dawnette Anderson, Administrator

North Texas Surgi-Center, 917 Midwestern Parkway, E., Wichita Falls, TX 76302; tel. 817/767-7273; Barbara Dawson, Administrator

One Day Surgery Center, Inc., 1001 Haskell Street, Fort Worth, TX 76107; tel. 817/735-3555; FAX. 817/737-6084; Deborah G. Adams, RN, B.S.N.

Outpatient Surgical Center, 2507 Medical Row, Suite 101, Grand Prairie, TX 75051; tel. 214/647-8520; Jack Gray, Administrator

Outpatient Surgisite, 401-A East Pinecrest Drive, Marshall, TX 75670; tel. 903/938-3110; Carol C. Hall

Park Central Surgical Center, 12200 Park Central Drive, Third Floor, Dallas, TX 75251; tel. 214/661-0505; G. Lynn Warren, Administrator

☐ **Physicians Daysurgery Center,** 3930 Crutcher Street, Dallas, TX 75246; tel. 214/827-0760; FAX. 214/827-0944; Vickie Roberts, RN, Administrator

Plaza Day Surgery, 909 Ninth Avenue, Fort Worth, TX 76104-3986; tel. 817/336-6060; Steven L. Smith, Administrator

Port Arthur Day Surgery Center, 3449 Gates Boulevard, Port Arthur, TX 77642; tel. 409/983-6144; Betty Murchison, Administrative Director

Premier Ambulatory Surgery of Austin, 4207 James Casey, Suite 203, Austin, TX 78745; tel. 512/440-7894; FAX. 512/440-1932; Danica Frost, Executive Director

Premier Ambulatory Surgery of Duncanville, 1018 East Wheatland Road, Duncanville, TX 75116; tel. 214/296-6912; Robert C. Williams, Vice President

Regional Eye Surgery Center, 107 West 30th Street, Pampa, TX 79065; tel. 806/665-0051; FAX. 806/665-0640; George R. Walters, M.D., President

Rio Grande Surgery Center, 1809 South Cynthia, McAllen, TX 78503; tel. 512/618-4402; FAX. 210/618-4174; Janet R. West, Director

San Antonio Eye Surgicenter, 800 McCullough, San Antonio, TX 78215; tel. 210/226-6169; FAX. 210/226-6383; Carol Harris, Administrator

San Antonio Surgery Center, Inc., 5290 Medical Drive, San Antonio, TX 78229; tel. 210/614-0187; FAX. 210/692-7757; Ann Finney, RN, Facility Administrator

Santa Rose Diagnostic and Surgical Center, 315 North San Saba, San Antonio, TX 78207; tel. 210/704-4000; FAX. 210/704-4014; Julie Meador, Clinical Manager

Santa Rose Northwest Ambulatory Center, 2833 Babcock Road, San Antonio, TX 78229; tel. 210/705-5101; Kathleen A. Rubano, Department Head

South Plains Endoscopy Center, 3610 24th Street, Lubbock, TX 79410; tel. 806/797-1015; Bill R. Davis, Administrator

South Texas Eye Surgicenter, Inc., 4406 North Laurent, Victoria, TX 77901; tel. 800/352-5928; Robert T. McMahon, M.D., Chief Executive Officer

South Texas Outpatient Surgical Center, Inc., 4025 East Southcross Boulevard, Building Three, Suite 15, San Antonio, TX 78222; tel. 210/333-0633; FAX. 210/333-0671; Michael P. Lewis, Administrator

Southwest Houston Surgical Center, 8111 Southwest Freeway, Houston, TX 77074; tel. 713/988-7600; FAX. 713/988-4070; Patsy Elsaifi, Administrator

St. Mary Surgicenter, Ltd., 2301 Quaker Avenue, Lubbock, TX 79410; tel. 806/793-8801; David S. Weil, Executive Director

SurgEyeCare, Inc., 5421 La Sierra Drive, Dallas, TX 75231; tel. 214/361-1443; FAX. 214/691-3299; Sandra J. Yankee, Administrator

Surgery Center Southwest, 8230 Walnut Hill Lane, Suite 102, Dallas, TX 75231; tel. 214/345-4090; FAX. 214/345-4055; Odelia Peters, Administrator

Surgery Center of Fort Worth, 2001 West Rosedale, Fort Worth, TX 76104; tel. 817/877-4777; Debra Delain, RN, Administrator

☐ **Surgery Center of Texas,** 155 East Loop 338, Suite 500, Odessa, TX 79762; tel. 915/367-3906; FAX. 915/367-3895; Ann Wilson, Clinical Director

Surgi-Care Center of Midland, Inc., 3001 West Illinois, Suite Five-A, Midland, TX 79701; tel. 915/697-1067; Geneva Ridgeway, RN, B.S.N., Director

SurgiSystems, Inc., 427 West 20th Street, Houston, TX 77008; tel. 713/868-3641; FAX. 713/865-5460; Jo McBeth, RN

Surgical Center of El Paso, 1815 North Stanton, El Paso, TX 79902; tel. 915/533-8412; FAX. 915/542-0367; Thomas Reynolds, Managing Director

Surgical Center of Southeast Texas, 3127 College Street, Beaumont, TX 77701; tel. 409/835-2607; Jim Hoeks, Administrator

Surgical and Diagnostic Center, Inc., 729 Bedford Euless Road West 100, Hurst, TX 76053; tel. 817/282-6905; FAX. 817/285-8114; Edward William Smith, D.O., Medical Director

Surgicare Outpatient Center of Victoria, 1903 East Sabine, Victoria, TX 77901; tel. 512/576-4105; M. Margaret Coleman, Administrator

Surgicare of Central San Antonio, 1008 Brooklyn Avenue, San Antonio, TX 78215-1600; tel. 210/225-0496; Carl J. Collazo, Administrator

☐ **Surgicare of Travis Centre, Inc.,** 6655 Travis, Suite 200, Houston, TX 77030; tel. 713/526-5100; Carol Simons, Administrator

Surgicare, Ltd., 3534 Vista, Pasadena, TX 77504; tel. 713/947-0330; Evelyn Grimes, Administrator

Surgicenter of San Antonio, L.P., 7902 Ewing Halsell Drive, San Antonio, TX 78229; tel. 210/614-7372; FAX. 210/614-7362; Russell Furth, Executive Director

Tarrant Outpatient Center, Inc., 1717 Precinct Line Road, Suite 101, Hurst, TX 76054; tel. 817/498-0525; FAX. 817/656-1490; Tracy Anderson, Business Manager

Texas Ambulatory Surgical Center, Inc., 2505 North Shepherd, Houston, TX 77008; tel. 713/880-3940; FAX. 713/880-1923; Kwang S. Park, Administrator

Texas Institute of Surgery, 12700 North Featherwood Drive, Suite 100, Houston, TX 77034; tel. 713/481-9303; FAX. 713/481-4263; Glenn Rodriguez, Administrator

The Birth Center of Southeast Texas, Inc., 2400 Highway 96 S., Lumberton, TX 77656; tel. 409/755-0252; Dennis D. Riston, M.D., Administrator

The Cataract Center of East Texas, Inc., 802 Turtle Creek Drive, Tyler, TX 75701; tel. 903/595-4333; FAX. 903/535-9845, ext. 1988; Judy Lanier, Administrator

The Center for Sight, Two Medical Center Boulevard, Lufkin, TX 75904; tel. 409/634-8434; FAX. 409/639-2581; Donn E. Sapp, Administrator

The Eye Surgery Center of the Rio Grande Valley, 1402 East Sixth Street, Weslaco, TX 78596; tel. 210/968-6155; FAX. 210/968-8291; Linda Kelley, Administrator

The Ocular Surgery Center, Inc., 1100 North Main Avenue, San Antonio, TX 78212; tel. 210/222-2154; FAX. 512/222-0706; Gloria Panagua, Administrator

The Surgery Center of the Woodlands, 1441 Woodstead Court, Suite 100, The Woodlands, TX 77380; tel. 713/363-0058; Teresa Danna, Administrator

Thorstenson Eye Clinic Surgery Center, 3302 N.E. Stallings Drive, Nacogdoches, TX 75963-2020; tel. 409/564-2411; FAX. 409/564-1280; Lyle S. Thorstenson, M.D., FACS, Administrator

University Surgery Center, Inc., 311 University Drive, Fort Worth, TX 76107; tel. 817/877-1002; FAX. 817/877-1006; Lori Schooler, Administrator

Urological Surgery Center of Fort Worth, 418 South Henderson, Fort Worth, TX 76104; tel. 817/338-4637; Charles Bamberger, M.D.

Valley Eye Surgery Center, 1515 North Ed Carey Drive, Harlingen, TX 78550; tel. 512/423-2772; Michael D. Laney, Administrator

Valley View Surgery Center, 5744 LBJ Freeway, Suite 200, Dallas, TX 75240; tel. 214/490-4333; Ronald W. Disney, Chief Executive Officer

Providers / Freestanding Ambulatory Surgery Centers

Vista Healthcare, Inc., 4301 Vista, Pasadena, TX 77504; tel. 713/947-0891; FAX. 713/947-1377; Chiu M. Chan, Administrator

Waco Medical Surgical Center, 2911 Herring, Waco, TX 76708; tel. 817/755-4430; FAX. 817/755-4590; William R. Bowen, Administrator

West Houston Surgicare, 970 Campbell Road, Houston, TX 77024-2804; tel. 713/461-3547; FAX. 713/461-2017; Shirley Schoener, RN, Administrator

WestPark Surgery Center, 130 South Central Expressway, McKinney, TX 75070; tel. 214/542-9382; FAX. 214/548-5303; Debbie Taylor

Westside Surgery Center, Ltd., 16100 Cairnway, Houston, TX 77084; tel. 713/550-5556; FAX. 713/550-7888; Harold F. Taylor, President, Chief Executive Officer

Wilson Surgicenter, 4315 28th Street, Lubbock, TX 79410; tel. 806/792-2104; Bill W. Wilson, M.D., Chief Executive

Woodhill Surgery Center, 8315 Walnut Hill Lane, Suite 120, Dallas, TX 75231; tel. 214/363-4093; FAX. 214/750-1512; Thomas Simonton, M.D.

UTAH

Institute of Facial Surgery, 5929 Fashion Boulevard, Murray, UT 84107; tel. 801/261-3637; FAX. 801/261-4096; Pam J. Groves, O.R. Supervisor

Intermountain Surgical Center, 359 Eighth Avenue, Salt Lake City, UT 84103; tel. 801/321-3200; FAX. 801/321-3035; Joan W. Lelis, Administrative Director

McKay-Dee Surgical Center, 3903 Harrison Boulevard, Suite 100, Ogden, UT 84403; tel. 801/625-2809; FAX. 801/629-5938; Suzanne Richins, Administrator

Provo Surgical Center, 585 North 500 West, Provo, UT 84601; tel. 801/375-0983; Brent K. Ashby, Administrator

Salt Lake Endoscopy Center, 24 South 1100 East, Salt Lake City, UT 84102; tel. 801/355-2987; FAX. 801/531-9704; Clifford G. Harmon, M.D., Administrator

☐ **Salt Lake Surgical Center,** 617 East 3900 South, Salt Lake City, UT 84107; tel. 801/261-3141; FAX. 801/268-2599; Jay T. Lighthall, Administrator

St. George Surgical Center, 676 South Bluff Street, St. George, UT 84770; tel. 801/673-8080; FAX. 801/673-0096; Michael L. Staheli, Administrator

☐ **St. Mark's Outpatient Surgery Center,** 1250 East 3900 South, Suite 100, Salt Lake City, UT 84124; tel. 801/262-0358; FAX. 801/262-0901; Marjorie Kimes, Administrator

The SurgiCare Center of Utah, 755 East 3900 South, Salt Lake City, UT 84107; tel. 801/266-2283, ext. 712; FAX. 801/268-6151; Lori Brewer, R.N.

Western Surgery Center, Inc., 850 East 1200 North, Logan, UT 84341; tel. 801/797-3670; FAX. 801/797-3848; Steven V. Hodson, Administrator

VIRGINIA

Ambulatory Surgery Center, 844 Kempsville Road, Norfolk, VA 23502; tel. 804/466-6900; FAX. 804/461-6796; Roger M. Eitelman, Administrator

Cataract and Refractive Surgery Center, 2010 Bremo Road, Suite 128, Richmond, VA 23226; tel. 804/285-0680; Jeffrey A. Staples, Administrator

CountrySide Ambulatory Surgery Center, 4 Pidgeon Hill Drive, Sterling, VA 20165; tel. 703/444-6060; FAX. 703/444-2278; Deborah F. Fox, RN, Director

Fairfax Surgery Center, 10730 Main Street, Fairfax, VA 22030; tel. 703/691-0670; Sharon B. Johnson, RN, Administrator

Fredericksburg Ambulatory Surgery Center, Inc., 2216 Princess Anne Street, Fredericksburg, VA 22401; tel. 703/899-3403; FAX. 703/899-6893; Felix Fraraccio, Administrator

Kaiser Permanente Falls Church Medical Center Ambulatory Surgery Center, 201 North Washington Street, Falls Church, VA 22046; tel. 703/237-4020; Debbie Bland, Director, Surgical Services

Lakeview Medical Center, Inc., 2000 Meade Parkway, Suffolk, VA 23424; tel. 804/539-0251; FAX. 804/934-2620; Michael B. Stout, Administrator

Lewis-Gale Clinic, Inc., Same Day Surgery, 1802 Braeburn Drive, Salem, VA 24153; tel. 703/772-3671; FAX. 703/989-0879; Darrell D. Whitt, President

Piedmont Day Surgery Center, Inc., 1040 Main Street, Danville, VA 24541; tel. 804/792-1433, ext. 64; FAX. 804/797-2807; Ruth McGregor, Administrator

Retreat Regional Medical Center, 7016 Lee Park Road, Mechanicsville, VA 23111; tel. 804/730-9000; FAX. 804/730-1460; Patricia E. Walker, Director, Outpatient Services

Riverside Surgery Center-Warwick, 12420 Warwick Boulevard, Building ThreeSuite C, Newport News, VA 23606; tel. 804/594-2796; FAX. 804/594-3911; M. Caroline Martin, Executive Vice President

Sentara Care Plex, 3000 Coliseum Drive, Hampton, VA 23666; tel. 804/827-2000; FAX. 804/827-6748; Richard A. Hanson, President

Surgi Center of Central Virginia, Inc., 223 Willow Street, Fredericksburg, VA 22405; tel. 703/371-5349; FAX. 703/373-1745; Gwyneth A. Chubb, Facility Administrator

Surgi-Center of Winchester, Inc., 1860 Amherst Street, Winchester, VA 22601; tel. 703/722-8934; FAX. 703/722-8936; H. Emerson Poling, M.D., Administrator

Tuckahoe Surgery Center, Inc., 8919 Three Chopt Road, Richmond, VA 23229; tel. 804/285-4763; FAX. 804/288-2850; Charles A. Stark, CHE, Administrator

Urosurgical Center of Richmond, 5224 Monument Avenue, Richmond, VA 23226; tel. 804/288-4137; FAX. 804/288-3529; Terry W. Coffey, Administrator

Urosurgical Center of Richmond-North, 6120 Meadowbridge Road, Mechanicsville, VA 23111; tel. 804/730-5023; FAX. 804/746-4015; Terry W. Coffey, Administrator

Urosurgical Center of Richmond-South, 7001 Jahnke Road, Richmond, VA 23225; tel. 804/287-1027; FAX. 804/272-1178; Terry W. Coffey, Administrator

☐ **Virginia Ambulatory Surgery Center,** 337-15th Street, S.W., Charlottesville, VA 22903; tel. 804/295-4800; FAX. 804/977-0544; Gerry Dobrasz, Administrator

Virginia Beach Ambulatory Surgery Center, 1700 Will-o-Wisp Drive, Virginia Beach, VA 23454; tel. 804/496-6400; FAX. 804/496-3137; Brian Murray, M.D., Administrator/Director

Virginia Eye Institute/Eye Surgeons of Richmond, Inc., 400 Westhampton Station, Richmond, VA 23226; tel. 804/282-3931; FAX. 804/287-4256; Kenneth J. Newell, Administrator

Virginia Heart Institute, LTD., 205 North Hamilton Street, Richmond, VA 23221; tel. 804/359-9265; Charles L. Baird, Jr., M.D., Director

WASHINGTON

Aesteem Outpatient Surgery Center, 1200 North Northgate Way, Seattle, WA 98133-8916; tel. 206/522-0200; Peter R. N. Chatard, Jr., M.D., Medical Director

Bel-Red Ambulatory Surgical Facility, 1370 116th Avenue, N.E., Suite 209, Bellevue, WA 98004; tel. 206/455-7225; FAX. 206/455-0045

Bellingham Surgery Center, 2980 Squalicum Parkway, Bellingham, WA 98225; tel. 206/671-6933; Richard Brumenschenkel, Managing Agent

Boyd Davis Eye Center, 1051 116th Avenue, N.E., Bellevue, WA 98004; tel. 206/454-2018; Herschell H. Boyd, M.D.

CIM Center, 5335 Cordata Parkway, Bellingham, WA 98226; tel. 360/676-1712; Ken Herwerden, Clinic Administrator

Cascade Ambulatory Surgery Center, 407 N.E. 87th Street, Vancouver, WA 98664; tel. 360/253-9201

Cascade Regional Eye Surgery Center, 16404 Smokey Point Boulevard, Suite 111, Arlington, WA 98223; tel. 206/653-4000; FAX. 206/658-1266; Cathie Berglund, RN, Director

Central Washington Cataract Surgery, 1450 North 16th Avenue, Building J, Yakima, WA 98902; tel. 509/457-5000; FAX. 509/457-6498; Paul Almeida, CRNA

Covington Day Surgery Center, 17700 S.E. 272nd Street, Kent, WA 98042; tel. 206/639-8302

Dietrich Von Feldmann, M.D., Inc., 16259 Sylvester S.W., Suite 401, Seattle, WA 98166; tel. 206/242-7947; FAX. 206/244-4147; Dietrich Von Feldmann, M.D.

Eastside Podiatry Ambulatory Surgery Center, 15617 Bel-Red Road, Bellevue, WA 98008; tel. 206/881-5592; G. Curda, D.P.M.

Everett Surgical Center, Inc., 3025 Rucker Avenue, Everett, WA 98201; tel. 206/339-2464; FAX. 206/252-4700; Rita Sweeney, RNFA, CNOR, Administrator

Evergreen Surgical Center, 12034 N.E. 130th Lane, Kirkland, WA 98034; tel. 206/821-3131; Ronald E. Abrams, M.D.

☐ **Good Samaritan Surgery Center,** 1322 Third Street S.E., Suite 100, Puyallup, WA 98372; tel. 206/840-2200; FAX. 206/840-2352; Roger D. Robinett, M.D.

Green River Surgical Center, 126 Auburn Avenue, Suite 200, Auburn, WA 98002; tel. 206/735-0500

Group Health Tacoma Specialty Center, Ambulatory Surgery Unit, 209 Martin Luther King, Jr. Way, Tacoma, WA 98405; tel. 206/596-3590; FAX. 206/596-3603; Linda Bradley, Manager, ASU

Inland Empire Endoscopy Center, South 820 McClellan, Suite 314, Spokane, WA 99204; tel. 509/747-0143; J. D. Fitterer, M.D.

Inland Eye Center, South 842 Cowley, Spokane, WA 99202; tel. 509/624-5300; FAX. 509/747-1348; Michael H. Cunningham, M.D., President

Lomas Surgery Center, 17800 Talbot Road, S., Renton, WA 98055; tel. 206/255-0986; FAX. 206/271-5703; Inese A. Lomas, Administrator

Mark A. Kuzel, D.P.M., PS, 21229 84th Avenue W., Edmonds, WA 98026; tel. 206/775-1505

McIntyre Eye Surgical Center, 1920 116th Avenue, N.E., Bellevue, WA 98004; tel. 206/454-3937; FAX. 206/646-5914; David McIntyre, M.D., FACS

☐ **Mid-Columbia Surgical Suite, Inc.,** 471 Williams Boulevard, Suite Four, Richland, WA 99352; tel. 509/943-1134; Robert C. Luckey, M.D., Medical Director

Minor and James Medical, 515 Minor Avenue, Suite 200, Seattle, WA 98104; tel. 206/386-9500

Monroe Foot Care Associates Ambulatory Surgery Center, 14692 179th Avenue, S.E., Suite 300, Monroe, WA 98272; tel. 206/794-1266; Dr. Brunsman, Medical Director

NW Aesthetic Surgery Center, 550 16th Avenue, Suite 404, Seattle, WA 98122; tel. 206/328-2250

North Cascade ENT and Facial Plastic Surgery, 111 South 13th Street, Mount Vernon, WA 98273; tel. 206/336-2178

North Kitsap Ambulatory Surgical Center, 20696 Bond Road, N.E., Poulsbo, WA 98370; tel. 206/779-6527; FAX. 206/779-3093; Thomas D. Case, M.D.

North Kitsap Gastrointestinal Endoscopy Center, 20700 Bond Road, N.E., Suite 101, Poulsbo, WA 98370; tel. 206/697-1116; FAX. 206/697-9277; Thomas Steffens, D.O., Medical Director

Northwest Eye Surgery Center, 10330 Meridian Avenue N., Suite 370, Seattle, WA 98125; tel. 206/528-6000, ext. 114; FAX. 206/528-0014; Linda M. Duncan, Administrator

Northwest Eye Surgery, P.C., N1120 Pines Road, Spokane, WA 99206; tel. 509/927-0700

Northwest Gastroenterology, d/b/a Northwest Endoscopy, 2930 Squalicum, Suite 202, Bellingham, WA 98225

Northwest Nasal Sinus Center, 10330 Meridan Avenue, N., Suite 240, Seattle, WA 98133; tel. 206/525-2525; FAX. 206/525-0346

Providers / Freestanding Ambulatory Surgery Centers

Northwest Surgery Center, Inc., West 123 Francis, Spokane, WA 99205; tel. 509/483–9363; Douglas P. Romney

Olympic Ambulatory Surgery Center, Inc., 2601 Cherry Avenue, Suite 115, Bremerton, WA 98310; tel. 206/479–5990; Audrey E. Harris, RN

Olympic Plastic Surgery Suite, 2600 Cherry Avenue, Suite 201, Bremerton, WA 98310; tel. 206/479-4370

Pacific Cataract and Laser Institute, 2517 N.E. Kresky, Chehalis, WA 98532; tel. 206/748–8632; Wayne Carlson, Administrator

Pacific Cataract and Laser Institute, 10500 N.E. Eighth Street, Suite 1650, Bellevue, WA 98004–4332; tel. 206/462–7664; FAX. 206/462–6429; Maynard Pohl, O.D., Clinical Director

Pacific Cataract and Laser Institute, 8200 West Grandridge, Kennewick, WA 99336

Pacific Medical Center, 1200 12th Avenue, S., Seventh Floor, Seattle, WA 98144; tel. 206/326–4000, ext. 2469; Carolyn Bodeen, RN, Clinic Director

Pacific NW Facial Plastic Ambulatory Surgery Center, 600 Broadway, Suite 280, Seattle, WA 98122; tel. 206/386–3550; FAX. 206/386–3553

Parkway Surgical Center, 2940 Squalicum Parkway, Suite 204, Bellingham, WA 98225; tel. 206/676–8350; FAX: 206/676–8351; Orville Vandergriend, M.D., Administrator

Physicians Eye Surgical Center, 3930 Hoyt Avenue, Everett, WA 98201; tel. 206/259–2020; Carol Schoenfelder, Administrator

Plastic Surgicenter of Olympia, 400 Lilly Road, N.E., Building Four, Olympia, WA 98506; tel. 360/456–4400; FAX. 360/491–7619; Wayne L. Dickason, M.D.

Plastic and Reconstructive Surgeons, 17930 Talbot Road, S., Renton, WA 98055; tel. 206/228–3187; Mack D. Richey, M.D.

Plastic and Reconstructive Surgery, 105 27th Avenue, S.E., Puyallup, WA 98374; tel. 206/848–8110; FAX. 206/845–3561; Karen Smith, RN

Professional Surgical Specialists, 1609 South Meridian, Puyallup, WA 98371; tel. 206/841–1331

Rockwood Clinic, d/b/a Gastrointestinal Endoscopy Unit, East 400 5th Avenue, Spokane, WA 99202; tel. 509/838–2531; FAX. 509/459–1527; Stephen Burgert, M.D., Administrator

Rockwood Clinic, PS, East 400 Fifth Avenue, Spokane, WA 99202; tel. 509/838–2531; FAX. 509/455–5315; William R. Poppy, Chief Executive Officer, Administrator

SW Washington Ambulatory Surgery Center, Inc., 416 N.E. 87th Avenue, Vancouver, WA 98664; tel. 206/696–4000; FAX. 206/696–4287

Seattle Eye Plastic Surgery Center, 1229 Madison Street, Suite 1190, Seattle, WA 98104; tel. 206/621–0800; FAX. 206/621–7023; R. Toby Sutcliffe, M.D.

Seattle Hand Surgery Group, P.C., 600 Broadway, Suite 440, Seattle, WA 98122; tel. 206/292–6252; FAX. 206/292–7893; Suzann H. Demianew, Administrator

Seattle Head and Neck Office Surgery, 515 Minor Avenue, Suite 130, Seattle, WA 98104; tel. 206/682–6103; Adrienne C. Peach, RN, Director

Seattle Microsurgical Eyecare Center, 5300 17th Avenue, N.W., Seattle, WA 98107; tel. 206/783–3929; Jack C. Bunn, M.D., Medical Director

Seattle Plastic Surgery Center, 600 Broadway, Suite 320, Seattle, WA 98122; tel. 206/324–1120; FAX. 206/720–0800; Nancy Spencer, Manager

Seattle Surgery Center, Columbus Pavilion, 900 Terry Avenue, Fourth Floor, Seattle, WA 98104–1240; tel. 206/382–1021; FAX. 206/382–1026; Linda Williams, Administrator

Sequim Same Day Surgery, 777 North Fifth Avenue, Sequim, WA 98382; tel. 360/681–0358; Tammy Paolini, Surgical Technician

South Hill Ambulatory Surgical Center, South 3028 Grand Boulevard, Spokane, WA 99203; tel. 509/747–0279

Southwest Washington Ambulatory Surgery Center, Inc., 102 West Fourth Plain Boulevard, Vancouver, WA 98666; tel. 206/696–4400

Spokane Digestive Disease Center, 105 West Eighth Avenue, Suite 6010, Spokane, WA 99204–2318; tel. 509/838–5950; FAX. 509/838–5961; Margie Troske–Johnson, RN, B.S.N., Director

Spokane Eye Surgery Center, West 208 Fifth Street, Spokane, WA 99204; tel. 509/456–8150; FAX. 509/455–9887; Donald Ellingsen, M.D.

Spokane Foot and Ankle Surgery Center, 9405 East Sprague Avenue, Spokane, WA 99206; tel. 509/922–3199

Spokane Surgery Center, North 1120 Pines Road, Spokane, WA 99206; tel. 509/924–3235; Steward P. Brim, D.P.M.

St. Mark's Micro Surgical Center, Inc., 502 South M Street, Tacoma, WA 98405; tel. 206/627–8266; Douglas MacLeod, M.D., Administrator

Tacoma Ambulatory Surgery Center, 1112 Sixth Avenue, Suite 100, Tacoma, WA 98405; tel. 206/272–3916, ext. 324; FAX. 206/627–1713; Joan Hoover, Administrator

The Plastic SurgiCentre, Inc., 535 South Pine Street, Spokane, WA 99202; tel. 509/623–2160; Pamala Silvers, RN, Manager

The Polyclinic, Inc., 1145 Broadway, Seattle, WA 98122; tel. 206/329–1760

Trenton J. Spolar, 505 N.E. 87th Avenue, Suite 203, Vancouver, WA 98664; tel. 206/254–8596

VM Clinic Plastic and Reconstructive Surgery, 1100 Ninth Avenue, Suite 1100, Seattle, WA 98111; tel. 206/223–6837

Valley Outpatient Surgery Center, North 1414 Houk Road, Suite 204, Spokane, WA 99216; tel. 509/922–0362; FAX. 509/927–8316; Dr. Douglas Norquist, President

Valley Surgi Centre, Five South 14th Avenue, Yakima, WA 98902; tel. 509/248–6813; FAX. 509/457–9691

Virginia Mason Clinic South, 33501 First Way South, Federal Way, WA 98003; tel. 206/874–1635

Virginia Mason GI Endoscopy/Gastric Lab, 1100 Ninth Avenue, Seattle, WA 98111; tel. 206/583–6440

Virginia Mason–Issaquah, 100 N.E. Gilman Boulevard, Issaquah, WA 98027; tel. 206/557–8000

Washington Orthopaedic Center, Inc., PS, 1900 Cooks Hill Road, Centralia, WA 98531; tel. 206/736–2889, ext. 400; Kathleen Alves, Director

Wenatchee Surgical Center, 600 Orondo Avenue, Wenatchee, WA 98807; tel. 509/662–8956; Shirley DeWitz, RN, Manager

Wenatchee Valley Clinic, 820 North Chelan, Wenatchee, WA 98801; tel. 509/663–8711; FAX. 509/664–4860; Dr. Steven Kerr, Chief Day Surgery, Director Quality Management

Westlake Surgical Center, 509 Olive Way, Third Floor, Seattle, WA 98101; tel. 206/623–4755; Alex R. Jordan, M.B.A., Administrator

Whidbey SurgiCare, 5373 500th Avenue, W., Suite B, Oak Harbor, WA 98277–2334; tel. 360/679–3117; FAX. 360/679–3118

Whitehorse Surgical Center, 875 Wesley Street, Suite 60, Arlington, WA 98223; tel. 360/435–6969

WEST VIRGINIA

Anwar Eye Center, 1500 Lafayette Avenue, Moundsville, WV 26041; tel. 304/845–0908; M. F. Anwar, M.D.

Cabell Huntington Surgery Center, 1201 Hal Greer Boulevard, Huntington, WV 25701; tel. 304/523–1885; FAX. 304/523–8942; Ann Allen, Facility Director

Cook Eye Center, 1300 Third Avenue, Huntington, WV 25701; tel. 304/522–1802; FAX. 304/529–6752; David W. Cook, M.D., President

Jerry N. Black, M.D., Surgical Suite, 10 Amalia Drive, Buckhannon, WV 26201; tel. 304/472–2100; Jerry N. Black, M.D., Medical Director

Kanawha Valley Surgi–Center, 4803 MacCorkle Avenue, S.E., Charleston, WV 25304; tel. 304/925–6390; Gorli Harish, M.D., Medical Director

Lee's Surgi–Center, 415 Morris Street, Suite 200, Charleston, WV 25301; tel. 304/342–1113; FAX. 304/346–2271; Hans Lee, M.D., President

SurgiCare, 3200 MacCorkle Avenue, S.E., Charleston, WV 25304; tel. 304/348–9556; C. E. Arthur, III, President

West Virginia Surgery Center, Inc., 425 Greenway Avenue, South Charleston, WV 25309; tel. 304/768–7310; FAX. 304/768–8211; Nancy Jo Vinson, Administrator

WISCONSIN

Bay Lake Outpatient Surgery Center, 1843 Michigan Street, P.O. Box 678, Sturgeon Bay, WI 54235; tel. 414/746–1070; FAX. 414/746–1072; Michael Herlache, Administrator

Baycare Surgery and Endoscopy Center, 1843 Michigan Street, Box 678, Sturgeon Bay, WI 54235; tel. 414/746–1070; Michael Herlache

Center for Digestive Health, 2901 West Kinnickinnic River Parkway, Suite 560, Milwaukee, WI 53215; tel. 414/649–3522; Robert Chang, Administrator

Davis Duehr Day Surgery, 1025 Regent Street, Madison, WI 53715; tel. 608/282–2050; Rodney Sturm, M.D., President

Dean St. Mary's Surgery Center, 800 South Brooks Street, Madison, WI 53715; tel. 608/259–3510; FAX. 608/255–1272; Patricia Klitzman, Director

Eau Claire Surgery Center, 950 West Clairemont Avenue, Eau Claire, WI 54701; tel. 715/839–9339; FAX. 715/839–9033; Jane Louden, RN, Facility Manager

Green Bay Surgical Center, Ltd., 704 South Webster Avenue, Green Bay, WI 54301; tel. 414/432–7433; FAX. 414/432–6313; Herbert F. Sandmire, Administrator

Kenosha Surgery Center, Inc., 3505 30th Avenue, Kenosha, WI 53144; tel. 414/654–8877; FAX. 414/654–8819; Anthony T. Safranski, FACMPE, Executive Director

LaSalle Surgery Center, 1550 Midway Place, Menasha, WI 54952; tel. 414/727–8200; FAX. 414/727–8703; Eileen Leinweber

Marshfield Clinic Ambulatory Surgery Center, 1000 North Oak Avenue, Marshfield, WI 54449; tel. 715/387–5315; FAX. 715/387–5240; Robert J. DeVita, Executive Director

Menomonee Falls Ambulatory Surgery Center, W180 N8045 Town Hall Road, Menomonee Falls, WI 53051; tel. 414/250–0950; FAX. 414/250–0955; Robert W. Scheller Jr, CPA, Business Manager

Meriter Ambulatory Surgery Center, 20 South Park Street, Madison, WI 53715; tel. 608/267–6479; FAX. 608/267–6370; Robert L. Coats, President

North Shore Surgical Center, 7007 North Range Line Road, Milwaukee, WI 53209; tel. 414/352–3341; FAX. 414/352–3218; Robert Lonergan, Executive Director

Northlake Surgery Center, 2110 Medical Drive, Box 636, Menomonee, WI 54751; tel. 715/235–8884; Joe Mack

Northwest Surgery Center, 2300 North Mayfair Road, Wauwatosa, WI 53226; tel. 414/257–3322; Nancy Jones, Administrator

Oshkosh Surgery Center, 1925 Surgery Center Drive, Oshkosh, WI 54901; tel. 414/233–1233; FAX. 414/233–2101; Jean Cox, Administrator

Riverview Surgery Center, 616 North Washington Street, Janesville, WI 53545; tel. 608/758–7300; FAX. 608/758–1050; Cheryl A. Wilson, Director

Surgery Center of Wisconsin, 10401 West Lincoln Avenue, Suite 210, West Allis, WI 53227; tel. 414/321–7850; Penny Leinbeck, Administrator

Surgi-Center of Racine, 5802 Washington Avenue, Racine, WI 53406; tel. 414/886–9100; Randy Procknow, Administrator

Surgicenter of Greater Milwaukee, 3223 South 103rd Street, Milwaukee, WI 53227; tel. 414/328–5800; Raymond E. Grundman, General Manager

Wausau Surgery Center, 2809 Westhill Drive, Wausau, WI 54401; tel. 715/842–4490; Kathy Eisenschink, RN, Facility Manager

Providers / Freestanding Ambulatory Surgery Centers

Wauwatosa Surgery Center, 10900 West Potter Road, Wauwatosa, WI 53226; tel. 414/774–9227; FAX. 414/774–0957; Kathleen Owens, RN, M.S.N., Facility Manager

WYOMING

Casper Surgical Center, 245 South Fenway Street, Casper, WY 82601; tel. 307/577–2950; FAX. 307/577–2954; Nancy Pingel, RN, Team Leader

Wyoming Endoscopy Center, 1200 East 20th Street, Cheyenne, WY 82001; tel. 307/635–5439; John W. Beckman

Wyoming Outpatient Services, 5050 Powderhouse Road, Cheyenne, WY 82009; tel. 307/634–1311; FAX. 307/638–6820; Peter Perakos, Director

Yellowstone Surgery Center, Ltd., 5201 Yellowstone Road, Cheyenne, WY 82009; tel. 307/635–7070; FAX. 307/632–9920; Colleen Bridenstine, RN, Director

State Government Agencies for Freestanding Ambulatory Surgery Centers

Information for the following list was obtained directly from the agencies.

United States

ALABAMA
Alabama Department of Public Health, Division of Licensure and Certification, 434 Monroe Street, Montgomery, AL 36130-1701; tel. 334/240-3503; FAX. 334/240-3147; L. O'Neal Green, Director

ALASKA
Health Facilities Licensing and Certification, 4730 Business Park Boulevard, Suite 18, Anchorage, AK 99503-7137; tel. 907/561-8081; FAX. 907/561-3011; Karen Martz, Administrator

ARIZONA
Arizona Department of Health Services, Health and Child Care Review Services, 1647 East Morten, Phoenix, AZ 85020; tel. 602/255-1221; FAX. 602/255-1109; Virginia Blair, Acting Assistant Director

ARKANSAS
Department of Health, Division of Health Facility Services, 4815 West Markham Street, Little Rock, AR 72205-3867; tel. 501/661-2201; FAX. 501/661-2165; Valetta Buck, Director

CALIFORNIA
Department of Health Services, Licensing and Certification Division, 1800 Third Street, Suite 210, P.O. Box 942732, Sacramento, CA 94234-7320; tel. 916/445-2070; FAX. 916/445-6979; Michael Rodrian, Branch Manager

COLORADO
Department of Health, Division of Health Facilities, 4210 East 11th Avenue, Denver, CO 80220; tel. 303/331-6600; FAX. 303/331-6559; Diane Carter, Deputy, Director

CONNECTICUT
Department of Health and Addiction Services, Hospital and Medical Care Division, 150 Washington Street, Hartford, CT 06106; tel. 203/566-1073; FAX. 203/566-1097; Elizabeth M. Burns, RN, M.S., Director

DELAWARE
Department of Health and Social Services, Licensing and Certification, Office of Health Facilities, 3000 Newport Gap Pike, Wilmington, DE 19808; tel. 302/995-6674; FAX. 302/995-8332; Ellen T. Reap, Director

DISTRICT OF COLUMBIA
Department of Consumer and Regulatory Affairs, Service Facility Regulation Administration, 614 H Street, N.W., Suite 1003, Washington, DC 20001; tel. 202/727-7190; FAX. 202/727-7780; James R. Murphy, Administrator

FLORIDA
Division of Health Quality Assurance, Agency for Health Care Administration, Fort Knox Executive Office Center, 2727 Mahan Drive, Suite 214, Tallahassee, FL 32308-5407; tel. 904/487-2527; FAX. 904/487-6240; Gloria Crawford-Henderson, Director

GEORGIA
Health Care Section, Office of Regulatory Services, Department of Human Resources, Two Peachtree Street, N.W., Suite 19.204, Atlanta, GA 30303-3167; tel. 404/657-5550; FAX. 404/657-8934; Susie M. Woods, Director

HAWAII
Hawaii Department of Health, Health Quality Assurance Division, Hospital and Medical Facilities Branch, P.O. Box 3378, Honolulu, HI 96801; tel. 808/586-4080; FAX. 808/586-4747; Helen K. Yoshimi, B.S.N., M.P.H., Chief, HMFB

IDAHO
Bureau of Facility Standards, Department of Health and Welfare, P.O. Box 83720, Boise, ID 83720-0036; tel. 208/334-6626; FAX. 208/334-0657; Loyal Perry, Supervisor-Non Long Term Care

ILLINOIS
Department of Public Health, Division of Health Care Facilities and Programs, 525 West Jefferson Street, Springfield, IL 62761; tel. 217/782-7412; FAX. 217/782-0382; Catherine M. Stokes, Acting Chief

INDIANA
Indiana State Department of Health, Division of Acute Care, 1330 West Michigan Street, P.O. Box 1964, Indianapolis, IN 46206-1964; tel. 317/383-6472; FAX. 317/383-6750; John A. Braeckel, Director

IOWA
Department of Inspection and Appeals, Division of Health Facilities, Lucas State Office Building, Des Moines, IA 50319; tel. 515/281-4115; FAX. 515/242-5022; Pearl Johnson, Administrator

KANSAS
Kansas Department of Health and Environment, Bureau of Adult and Child Care, 900 S.W. Jackson, Suite 1001, Topeka, KS 66612-1290; tel. 913/296-3362; FAX. 913/296-1266; George A. Dugger, Medical Facilities Certification Administrator

KENTUCKY
Cabinet for Human Resources, Division of Licensing and Regulation, C.H.R. Building, 275 East Main Street, 4th Floor East, Frankfort, KY 40621; tel. 502/564-2800; FAX. 502/564-6546; Timothy L. Veno, Director

LOUISIANA
Department of Health and Hospitals, Bureau of Health Services Financing-Health Standards Section, P.O. Box 3767, Baton Rouge, LA 70821; tel. 504/342-0138; FAX. 504/342-5292; Lily W. McAlister, RN, Manager

MAINE
Division of Licensing and Certification, Department of Human Services, 35 Anthony Avenue, Station 11, Augusta, ME 04333; tel. 207/624-5443; FAX. 207/624-5378; Louis Dorogi, Director

MARYLAND
Department of Health and Mental Hygiene, Office of Licensing and Certification, 4201 Patterson Avenue, Baltimore, MD 21215; tel. 410/764-4980; FAX. 410/764-5969

MASSACHUSETTS
Department of Public Health, Division of Health Care Quality, 80 Boylston Street, Suite 1100, Boston, MA 02116; tel. 617/727-5860; Irene McManus, Director

MICHIGAN
Department of Public Health, Division of Licensing and Certification, 3500 North Logan, Lansing, MI 48909; tel. 517/335-8505; Nancy Graham, Superior

MINNESOTA
Department of Health, Facility and Provider Compliance Division, Licensing and Certification Section, 393 North Dunlap Street, P.O. Box 64900, St. Paul, MN 55164-0900; tel. 612/643-2130; FAX. 612/643-3534; Carol Hirschfeld, Supervisor, Records and Information Unit

MISSISSIPPI
Department of Health, Division of Health Facilities Licensure and Certification, P.O. Box 1700, Jackson, MS 39215; tel. 601/987-3775; FAX. 601/987-4888; Mendal G. Kemp, Director

MISSOURI
Missouri Department of Health, Bureau of Hospital Licensing and Certification, P.O. Box 570, Jefferson City, MO 65102; tel. 314/751-6302; FAX. 314/526-3621; Darrell Hendrickson, Administrator

MONTANA
Health Facilities Division, Department of Health and Environmental Sciences, Cogswell Building, Helena, MT 59620; tel. 406/444-2037; FAX. 406/444-1742; Denzel C. Davis, Division Administrator

NEBRASKA
Department of Health, Bureau of Health Facilities Standards, 301 Centennial Mall, S., P.O. Box 95007, Lincoln, NE 68509-5007; tel. 402/471-4961; FAX. 402/471-0555; Frederick M. Wright, Director

NEVADA
Bureau of Licensure & Certification, Nevada Health Divison, 505 East King Street, Suite 202, Carson City, NV 89710; tel. 702/687-4475; FAX. 702/687-5751; Sharon M. Ezell, Chief

NEW HAMPSHIRE
Division of Public Health Services, Bureau of Health Facilities Administration, Six Hazen Drive, Concord, NH 03301; tel. 603/271-4592; FAX. 603/271-3745; Eleanor Robinson, Chief

NEW JERSEY
Division of Health Facilities Evaluation, Licensing, Certification, and Standards, CN-367, Trenton, NJ 08625; tel. 609/588-7725; FAX. 609/588-7823; Robert J. Fogg, Esq., Director

NEW MEXICO
Department of Health and Environment, Health Facility Licensing and Certification Bureau, 525 Camino de los Marquez, Suite Two, Santa Fe, NM 87501; tel. 505/727-4200; FAX. 505/827-4222; Sue K. Morris, Chief, Licensing and Certification Bureau

NEW YORK
Department of Health, Office of Health Systems Management, Empire State Plaza, Corning Tower Building, Albany, NY 12237; tel. 518/474-5515

NORTH CAROLINA
Department of Human Resources, Division of Facility Services, 701 Barbour Drive, P.O. Box 29530, Raleigh, NC 27626-0530; tel. 919/733-1610; FAX. 919/733-3207; Jesse Goodman, Chief, Licensure Section

NORTH DAKOTA
North Dakota Department of Health, Health Resources Section, 600 East Boulevard Avenue, Bismarck, ND 58505-0200; tel. 701/328-2352; FAX. 701/328-4727; Fred Gladden, Chief

Providers / State Government Agencies for Freestanding Ambulatory Surgery Centers

OHIO
Division of Health Facilities Regulation, Ohio Department of Health, 246 North High Street, Columbus, OH 43266-0588; tel. 614/466-7857; FAX. 614/644-0208; Rebecca Maust, Chief

OKLAHOMA
Department of Health, Special Health Services, 1000 N.E. 10th Street, P.O. Box 53551, Oklahoma City, OK 73152; tel. 405/271-6576; FAX. 405/271-3442; Gary Glover, Chief, Medical Facilities

OREGON
Health Care Licensure and Certification, Oregon Health Division, 800 N.E. Oregon Street, Suite 640, # 21, Portland, OR 97232; tel. 503/731-4013; FAX. 503/731-4080; Kathleen Smail, Manager

PENNSYLVANIA
Bureau of Quality Assurance, Division of Acute and Ambulatory Care Facilities, Health and Welfare Building, Suite 532, Harrisburg, PA 17120; tel. 717/783-8980; FAX. 717/772-2163; William White, Director

RHODE ISLAND
Rhode Island Department of Health, Division of Facilities Regulation, 3 Capitol Hill, Providence, RI 02908-5097; tel. 401/277-2566; FAX. 401/277-3999; Wayne I. Farrington, Chief

SOUTH CAROLINA
Department of Health and Environmental Control, Division of Health Licensing, 2600 Bull Street, Columbia, SC 29201; tel. 803/737-7202; FAX. 803/737-7212; Alan Samuels, Director

SOUTH DAKOTA
Department of Health, Licensure and Certification Program, 445 East Capitol, Pierre, SD 57501; tel. 605/773-3364; Joann Bachman, Program Director

TENNESSEE
Department of Health, Division of Health Care Facilities, 283 Plus Park Boulevard, Nashville, TN 37247-0530; tel. 615/367-6316; FAX. 615/367-6397; Leslie A. Brown, Director

TEXAS
Department of Health, Health Facility Licensure and Certification Division, 8407 Wall Street, Zip 78754, 1100 West 49th Street, Austin, TX 78756; tel. 512/834-6650; FAX. 512/834-6653; Nance Stearman, RN, M.S.N., Director

UTAH
Utah Department of Health, Bureau of Health Facility Licensure, P.O. Box 16990, Salt Lake City, UT 84116-0990; tel. 801/538-6152; FAX. 801/538-6325; Debra Wynkoop-Green, Director

VIRGINIA
Virginia Department of Health, Office of Health Facilities Regulation, 3600 Centre, Suite 216, 3600 West Broad Street, Richmond, VA 23230; tel. 804/367-2102; FAX. 804/367-2149; Nancy R. Hofheimer, Director

WASHINGTON
Office of Field Services, Washington Department of Health, Target Plaza, Suite 500, 2725 Harrison Avenue N.W., P.O. Box 47852, Olympia, WA 98504-7852; tel. 206/705-6622; FAX. 206/705-6654; Fern Bettridge, Program Manager

WEST VIRGINIA
Office of Health Facility Licensure and Certification, West Virginia Division of Health, 1900 Kanawha Boulevard, E., Charleston, WV 25305; tel. 304/558-0050; FAX. 304/588-2515; Dianne Anderson, Program Manager

WISCONSIN
Department of Health and Social Services, Division of Health, P.O. Box 309, Madison, WI 53701; tel. 608/267-7185; FAX. 608/267-0352; Judy Fryback, Director, Bureau of Quality Compliance

WYOMING
Wyoming Department of Health, Health Facilities Licensing, Metropolitan Bank Building, Eighth Floor, Cheyenne, WY 82001; tel. 307/777-7123; FAX. 307/777-5970; Charlie Simineo, Program Manager

U.S. Associated Areas

PUERTO RICO
Department of Health, P. O. Box 70184, San Juan, PR 00936; tel. 809/766-1616; FAX. 809/766-2240; Carmen Feliciano de Melecio, M.D., Secretary of Health

Freestanding Hospices

The following list of freestanding hospices was developed with the assistance of state government agencies and the individual facilities listed. The list is current as of January 1, 1995. For a complete list of hospital based hospice programs please refer to Section A. In Section A, hospice programs are identified by Facility Code F33.

We present this list simply as a convenient directory. Inclusion or omission of any organization's name indicates neither approval nor disapproval by the American Hospital Association.

United States

ALABAMA

Baptist Hospice, 2055 Normandie Drive, Suite 214, Montgomery, AL 36111–2732; tel. 334/286–3321; FAX. 334/286–3306; Margaret Wells, Clinical Manager

Birmingham Area Hospice, 1400 Sixth Avenue, S., P.O. Box 2648, Birmingham, AL 35233; tel. 205/930–1330; FAX. 205/930–1390; Flora Y. Blackledge, Director

Chattahoochee Hospice, Inc., 604 Cusseta Road, Valley, AL 36854; tel. 334/756–8043; FAX. 334/756–8059; Judy Guin, RN, Administrator

Community Hospice, Medical Arts Tower, Suite 510, Jasper, AL 35501; tel. 205/387–4514; FAX. 205/387–4519; Patrick Willingham

Health Services East, Inc., Hospice Care, 7916 Second Avenue, S., Birmingham, AL 35206; tel. 205/838–5730; FAX. 205/838–5757; Jeff Johnson, Director, Home Care Services

Hospice Care, Division of St. Clair Care, A Hospice, Inc., 17 Lake Plaza, P.O. Box 544, Pell City, AL 35125; tel. 205/884–1111; FAX. 205/884–1114; Phyllis A. Brown, Director

Hospice of Cullman County, Inc., 402 Fourth Avenue, N.E., P.O. Box 435, Cullman, AL 35055; tel. 205/739–5185; Jackie H. Cook

Hospice of East Alabama, Inc., 825 Keith Avenue, Anniston, AL 36207; tel. 205/236–5334; FAX. 205/231–4558; Jeannie Stanko, RN, M.S.N., Executive Director

Hospice of Huntsville, Inc., 806 Governors Drive, Suite 202, Huntsville, AL 35801; tel. 205/536–1889; FAX. 205/536–9541; Jim Higgins, Executive Director

Hospice of Limestone County, 307 North Beaty Street, P.O. Box 626, Athens, AL 35611; tel. 205/232–5017; Patricia P. Jackson, Administrator

Hospice of Marshall County, 501 Blount Avenue, Guntersville, AL 35976; tel. 205/582–2111; FAX. 205/582–5072; Rhonda Floyd, RN, B.S.N., OCN, Patient Care Coordinator

Hospice of Montgomery, 1111 Holloway Park, Montgomery, AL 36117; tel. 334/279–6677; FAX. 334/277–2223; Jan Niel, Executive Director

Hospice of Northeast Alabama, 112 College Street, P.O. Box 981, Scottsboro, AL 35768; tel. 205/574–4622; FAX. 205/259–3772; Virginia Stone, Executive Director

Hospice of Northwest Alabama, Forty East First Avenue, Winfield, AL 35594; tel. 205/487–8140; FAX. 205/487–8740; Linda Martin Sewell, Executive Director

Hospice of West Alabama, 1800 McFarland Boulevard, N., Suite 310, Tuscaloosa, AL 35406; tel. 205/345–0067; Julie Sittason, Executive Director

Hospice of the Shoals, Inc., 1106 Bradshaw Drive, P.O. Box 307, Florence, AL 35630–0000; tel. 205/767–6699; FAX. 205/767–6695; Bill Crowson, Administrator

Hospice of the Valley, Inc., 216 Johnston Street, N.E., P.O. Box 2745, Decatur, AL 35602; tel. 205/350–5585; FAX. 205/350–5567; Carolyn Dobson, Executive Director

Huntsville Hospice Cares, Inc., 509 Madison Street, Huntsville, AL 35801–0000; tel. 205/534–1095; FAX. 205/534–1096; Florence M. Helman

Mercy Medical Hospice–Escambia, 1665 Wilkerson Street, P.O. Box 638, Flomaton, AL 36441; tel. 334/296–5496; FAX. 334/296–3594; Scotti Dixon, Director

Mercy Medical Hospice–Mobile, 3712 Dauphin Street, Mobile, AL 36608–5917; tel. 334/344–7126; FAX. 334/304–3012; Paul A. Shorrosh, M.S.W., M.B.A., Facility Director

Providence Hospice of Bay Area Home Health, 6051 Airport Boulevard, Building B, Suite Two, Mobile, AL 36608; tel. 334/344–2234; Roberta Norris

Saad's Hospice Services, Inc., 3725 Airport Boulevard, Suite 180, Mobile, AL 36608; tel. 334/343–9600; FAX. 334/380–3328; Barbara S. Fulgham

St. Vincent's Hospice, 2112 11th Avenue, S., Suite 335, Birmingham, AL 35205; tel. 205/252–9727; Sue Cacioppo

Tombigbee Hospice, Inc., 112 Marshall Street, P.O. Box 219, Livingston, AL 35470; tel. 205/652–2451; FAX. 205/652–5212; Bobby T. Williams, Ph.D., M.B.A., Chief Executive Officer

Warrior Area Hospice, Inc., 718 1/2 Boligee Street, Eutaw, AL 35462; tel. 205/372–0888; Patricia H. Rankin, RN, Director

Wiregrass Hospice, Inc., 1211 West Main Street, Dothan, AL 36301; tel. 334/792–1100; Ray L. Shrout, Administrator

ALASKA

Hospice of Mat–Su, 950 East Bogard Road, Suite 133, Wasilla, AK 99654; tel. 907/352–2845; FAX. 907/352–2844; James Walsh

ARIZONA

Carondelet Hospice Services, 1802 West St. Mary's Road, Tucson, AZ 85745; tel. 602/623–5982; FAX. 602/740–6042; Pete Briguglio, Director

Cigna Companies Hospice, 7600 North 15th Street, Suite 185, Phoenix, AZ 85020; tel. 602/942–4462; FAX. 602/678–3106; Hilda Keogh, Director

Community Hospice, 4330 North Campbell Avenue, Suite 256, Tucson, AZ 85718; tel. 602/544–2273; Bonnie Lindstrom

Community Hospice, 340 East Palm Lane, Suite 150, Phoenix, AZ 85004; tel. 602/252–2273; FAX. 602/254–6166; Kristy Thompson, Administrator

Dignita Home Hospice, 202 East Earll Drive, Suite 478, Phoenix, AZ 85012; tel. 602/279–0677; FAX. 602/279–1085; Gary Polsky

East Valley Samaritan Hospice, 1450 South Dobson Road, Suite B–322, Mesa, AZ 85202; tel. 602/835–0711; Sandra Rose Hancin

Hospice Family Care Inc., 3443 East Fort Lowell Road, Tucson, AZ 85716; tel. 602/325–2339; Nancy Smith, Acting Administrator

Hospice Family Care Inpatient Unit, 5037 East Broadway Road, Mesa, AZ 85206; tel. 602/807–2655; Donna Jazz

Hospice Family Care Inpatient Unit–Sonora, 1920 West Rudasill, Tucson, AZ 85704; tel. 602/797–3442; Nancy Smith

Hospice Family Care, Inc., 7330 North 16th Street, Suite A100, Phoenix, AZ 85020; tel. 602/331–9200; FAX. 602/331–9222; Mike Reimann, Administrator

Hospice Family Care, Inc.–Green Valley, 210 West Continental Road, Suite 134, Green Valley, AZ 85614; tel. 602/648–6166; FAX. 602/648–6165; Suzanne Kroll or Patricia Irons

Hospice of Havasu, Inc., 1685 Mesquite Avenue, Suite F, Lake Havasu City, AZ 86403; tel. 602/453–2111; FAX. 605/453–3003; Shirley Stephan, Administrator

Hospice of Yuma, 1824 South Eighth Avenue, Yuma, AZ 85364; tel. 602/343–2222; FAX. 602/343–0688; Phyllis K. Swanson, Executive Director

Hospice of the Valley, 2601 East Thomas Road, Suite 100, Phoenix, AZ 85016; tel. 602/956–9040; FAX. 602/956–6377; Susan Goldwater, Administrator

In Home Health, 4600 South Hill, Suite 170, Tempe, AZ 85282; tel. 602/839–5686; FAX. 602/839–3872; Tracy May

Jacob C. Fruchthendler Jewish Community Hospice, 5100 East Grant Road, P.O. Box 13090, Tucson, AZ 85732–3090; tel. 602/881–5300; FAX. 602/322–3620; Bonnie Ransom, Administrator

LHS Home and Community Care–Hospice, 325 East Elliot Road, Suite 27, Chandler, AZ 85225; tel. 602/497–5535; Jennifer P. Huppenthal

Mt. Graham Community Hospital–Hospice Services, 1879 Peppertree Drive, Suite A–28, Safford, AZ 85546; tel. 602/348–4045; FAX. 602/428–3868; Theresa M. Kiser, Administrator

Northland Hospice, 702 North Beaver, P.O. Box 997, Flagstaff, AZ 86001; tel. 520/779–1227; FAX. 520/779–5884; Marilyn J. Pate, Executive Director

RTA Hospice, 134 East Highway 260, Payson, AZ 85541; tel. 602/472–6340, ext. 12; FAX. 602/472–6464; Vicki Dietz, RN, B.S.N., Administrator

RTA Hospice, 1275 East Florence Boulevard, Suite 10, Casa Grande, AZ 85222; tel. 602/421–7143; FAX. 602/421–7315; Susan Hapak, Administrator

Special Care Hospice, 1514 C Gold Rush Road, Suite 236, Bullhead City, AZ 86442; tel. 602/758–3800; FAX. 602/758–4403; Jayne Knox, Director

St. Joseph's Mercy Hospice, 2700 North Central, Suite 600, Phoenix, AZ 85004; tel. 602/406–5709; FAX. 602/406–5719; Carolyn Stephenson, Director

Sun Health Hospice, 13101 North 103rd Avenue, Sun City, AZ 85351; tel. 602/974–7810; FAX. 602/974–7894; Nathalie Rennell, Administrator

ARKANSAS

Area Agency on Aging Hospice of Western Arkansas, Inc., 115 North 10th Street, Suite H119, P.O. Box 1724, Fort Smith, AR 72902; tel. 501/783–4500; FAX. 501/783–0029; Mary Keith, RNC, Vice President

Area Agency on Aging of Western Arkansas, Inc., Mena Hospice, 600 Seventh Street, Mena, AR 71953; tel. 501/394–5458; FAX. 501/394–7675; Mary Keith, RNC, Vice President

Arkansas Department of Health Hospice, 5800 West 10th, Suite 30, Little Rock, AR 72204; tel. 501/661–2951; FAX. 501/661–2725; Gayla Lanum, Hospice Director

Baptist Memorial Regional Home Health Care, d/b/a Arkansas Home Health and Hospice, P.O. Box 90, Forrest City, AR 72335; tel. 501/633–6184; Gary Hughes, Administrator

Baptist Memorial Regional Home Health Care, Inc., d/b/a Arkansas Home Health and Hospice–West Memphis, 310 Mid–Continent Building, Suite 400, P.O. Box 2013, West Memphis, AR 72303; tel. 501/735–0363; FAX. 501/735–7156; Gary Hughes, Administrator

Central Arkansas Area Agency on Aging, d/b/a Hospice of Central Arkansas, 706 West Fourth Street, P.O. Box 5988, North Little Rock, AR 72119; tel. 501/372–5300, ext. 223; FAX. 501/688–7443; Ann Patterson, Director

Providers / Freestanding Hospices

Heart of the Lake Hospice, Inc., P.O. Box 314, Greers Ferry, AR 72067; tel. 501/723–4655; Irene Krueger, Administrator

Hospice Care of Carroll Regional Medical Center, 214 Center Street, P.O. Box 387, Berryville, AR 72616; tel. 501/423–5259; FAX. 501/423–5268; Rudy Darling, Administrator

Hospice of Cherokee Village, Inc., 13 Minentonka, P.O. Box 986, Cherokee Village, AR 72525; tel. 501/257–3108; Sally Lindemood, Administrator

Visiting Nurses Agency of Western Arkansas, Inc., 207 College Avenue, Clarksville, AR 72830; tel. 501/754–8280; Lois Phillips, RNC, Regional Nursing Supervisor

CALIFORNIA

AIDS Healthcare Foundation, 6255 Sunset Boulevard, Los Angeles, CA 90028; tel. 213/462–2273; FAX. 213/962–8513; Tay Aston, Cesar Mier, Admissions Officers

Assisted Home Hospice, 468 Pennsfeld Place, Suite 100, Thousand Oaks, CA 91360; tel. 805/371–9988; FAX. 805/371–9987; Susan K. Rice, RN, Executive Director

Carl Bean Aids Care Center, 2146 West Adams Boulevard, Los Angeles, CA 90018; tel. 213/766–2326; FAX. 213/730–8244; Leslie Burke, RN, M.P.H., J.D., Executive Director

Catered Living, Inc., Home Health and Hospice, 1060 Eight Avenue, Suite 405, San Diego, CA 92101; tel. 619/234–4323; FAX. 619/234–4380; Laura Baker, President, Chief Operating Officer

Children's Homecare–Hospice, 9550 Chesapeake Drive, Suite 201, San Diego, CA 92123; tel. 619/495–4941; James Rodisch, Director

Community Home Care Services/Hospice, 1925 East Dakota, Suite 208, Fresno, CA 93726; tel. 209/221–5615; FAX. 209/221–5798; John Thomas, Service Integrator

Community Hospice of the Bay Area, d/b/a Hospice by the Bay, 1540 Market Street, Suite 350, San Francisco, CA 94102–6035; tel. 415/626–5900; FAX. 415/626–7800; Constance L. Borden, Executive Director

Community Hospice, Inc., 601 McHenry Avenue, Suite C, Modesto, CA 95350; tel. 209/577–0615; FAX. 209/577–0738; W. Kay Wray, Executive Director

Community Hospice–San Diego, 8880 Rio San Diego Drive, Suite 950, San Diego, CA 92108; tel. 619/280–2273; Catherine Estherheld, RN

Companion Hospice, 12072 Trask Avenue, Suite 100, Garden Grove, CA 92643; tel. 714/741–0953; FAX. 714/534–0998; Michael Uranga, Administrator

Coordinated Hospice, 13800 Arizona Street, Suite 202, Westminster, CA 92683; tel. 714/898–7106; Susan Willet, RN, Director

Elizabeth Hospice, 1845 East Valley Parkway, Escondido, CA 92027; tel. 619/737–2050; FAX. 619/737–2088; Pamela Winch–Matayoshi, Executive Director

Helping Hands–Hospice, 1310 South Imperial Avenue, El Centro, CA 92243; tel. 619/352–7100; FAX. 619/352–7448; Linda Marrs, Administrator

Home Health/Hospice of San Luis Obispo, 285 South Street, Suite J, P.O. Box 1489, San Luis Obispo, CA 93406; tel. 805/781–4141; FAX. 805/781–1236; Michelle S. Groff, Administrator

Home Hospice, 888 Prospect Street, Suite 201, LaJolla, CA 92037; tel. 619/456–9703; Robert Cohn, Administrator

Home Hospice of Sonoma County, 1110 North Dutton Avenue, Santa Rosa, CA 95401–4606; tel. 707/542–5045; FAX. 707/542–6731; True Ryndes, President, Chief Executive Officer

Horizon Hospice, 12709 Poway Road, Suite E2, Poway, CA 92064; tel. 619/748–3030; Thomas Dusmu–Johnson

Hospice Care of California, 377 East Chapman Avenue, Suite 280, Placentia, CA 92670; tel. 714/577–9656; FAX. 714/577–9679; Ann Hablitzl, Director of Operations

Hospice Services of Lake County, 14642 Clakeshore Drive, P.O. Box 1430, Clearlake, CA 95422; tel. 707/994–8820; FAX. 707/994–1356; Michael Brooks, Executive Director

Hospice Services of Santa Barbara, a Division of the Santa Barbara Visiting Nurse Association, 222 East Canon Perdido, Santa Barbara, CA 93101; tel. 805/963–6794; Patricia Abler, Hospice Director

Hospice of Contra Costa, 3480 Buskirk Avenue, Suite 225, Pleasant Hill, CA 94523; tel. 510/295–1930; FAX. 510/934–1707; Cindy Siljestrom, Executive Director

Hospice of East County, 3835 Railroad Avenue, Pittsburg, CA 94565; tel. 510/439–4115; FAX. 510/439–4602; Peggy Nichols, Executive Director

Hospice of Grossmont Hospital, 8881 Flether Parkway, Suite 310, La Mesa, CA 91942; tel. 619/463–9911; Deirdre Holst, Vice President Home Care

Hospice of Humboldt, Inc., 2010 Myrtle Avenue, Eureka, CA 95501; tel. 707/445–8443; FAX. 707/445–2209; Jacqueline Berry, Executive Director

Hospice of Marin, 150 Nellen Avenue, Corte Madera, CA 94925; tel. 415/927–2273; FAX. 415/927–2284; Mary Tavema, President

Hospice of Napa Valley, Three Woodland Lane, Deer Park, CA 94576; tel. 707/963–3691; FAX. 707/963–6295; Marla Kae Stahlnecker, Administrator

Hospice of San Joaquin, 2609 East Hammer Lane, Stockton, CA 95210; tel. 209/957–3888; FAX. 209/957–3986; Barbara Tognoli, Administrator

Hospice of the Canyon, 5045 Parkway Calabasas, Calabasas, CA 91302; tel. 818/591–1459; FAX. 815/591–1486; David Bernstein, D.D.S., Executive Director

Hospice of the Central Coast, 100 Barnet Segal Lane, Monterey, CA 93940; tel. 408/648–7744; Patricia Cincone

Hospice of the East San Gabriel Valley, d/b/a Home Care Advantage, 820 North Phillips Avenue, West Covina, CA 91791; tel. 818/915–6200; FAX. 818/859–2272

Hospice of the North Coast, 4002 Vista Way, Oceanside, CA 92056; tel. 619/724–8411; John P. Lauri, Chief Executive Officer

Hospital Home Health Care–Hospice, 2601 Airport Drive, Suite 110, Torrance, CA 90505; tel. 310/530–3800; FAX. 310/534–1754; Kaye Daniels, President

Kaiser Foundation Hospital Hospice Program, 12500 Hoxie Avenue, Room 650, Norwalk, CA 90650; tel. 213/925–7511; Tim Reed, Administrator

Kaiser Foundation Hospital Panorama City–Hospice, 9140 Van Nuys Boulevard, Panorama City, CA 91402; tel. 818/908–2400

Kern Hospice, 4300 Stine Road, Suite 720, Bakersfield, CA 93313; tel. 805/327–1012; David Christen, Administrator

Lifecare Solutions, Inc.–Hospice, 9823 Pacific Heights Boulevard, Suite N, San Diego, CA 92121; tel. 619/546–3834; David Golman, Administrator

Livingston Memorial VNA and Hospice, 1996 Eastman Avenue, Suite 101, Ventura, CA 93003; tel. 805/642–0239; FAX. 805/642–2320; A. Lee Hickman, President, Chief Executive Officer

Madeleine Healthcare Services, 2277 Fair Oaks Boulevard, Suite 350, Sacramento, CA 95825–5533; tel. 916/565–8181; FAX. 916/565–1417; Cynthia Clayton, Administrator

Marian Hospital Homecare and Hospice, 1300 East Cypress, Suite G, Santa Maria, CA 93454; tel. 805/922–9609; FAX. 805/349–9229; Marie Whitford, Vice President, Alternate Care Services

Mercy Hospice, 9940 Business Park Drive, Suite 165, Sacramento, CA 95827; tel. 916/854–3900; FAX. 916/854–3948; Janice Campbell, Hospice Manager

Metropolitan Hospice, 4904 Crenshaw Boulevard, Los Angeles, CA 90043; tel. 213/293–6163; FAX. 213/296–3913; Kathleen I. Jones, RN, B.S., Director

Midpeninsula Hospice, 201 San Antonio Circle, Suite 135, Mountain View, CA 94040; tel. 415/949–3029; FAX. 415/949–4317; John D. Hart, Executive Director

Olsten Kimberly Quality Care–Hospice, 1850 West Main Street, Suite C, El Centro, CA 92243; tel. 619/353–3773; FAX. 619/353–5128; Ruth Dixon, Administrator

Orangegrove Hospice, 12332 Garden Grove Boulevard, Garden Grove, CA 92643; tel. 714/534–1041; FAX. 714/534–7921; Maria Aguilar, Director, Hospice Services

San Diego Hospice Corporation, 9797 Aero Drive, Suite B, San Diego, CA 92123; tel. 619/560–0302; FAX. 619/688–1599; Donna Spaulding

San Pedro Peninsula Home Care/Hospice, 1386 B West Seventh Street, San Pedro, CA 90732; tel. 310/548–4106; FAX. 310/514–5328; Susan Nowinski, M.S.N., Executive Director

Spectrum Health and Hospice Services, 2421 Mendacino Avenue, Suite 150, Santa Rosa, CA 95403; tel. 707/528–4663, ext. 318; FAX. 707/528–2301; Kimberly Allpress, Administrative Assistant

St. Ambros Hospice Care, 15022 Pacific Street, Suite #A, Midway City, CA 92655; tel. 714/379–6738; Mike Peiton, Director, Operations

St. Joseph Medical Center Home Hospice, 2101 West Alameda Avenue, Burbank, CA 91506; tel. 213/555–5555

The Miller Project, 970 North Van Ness, Fresno, CA 93728; tel. 209/264–0061

The Visiting Nurse Service Hospice, 212 Carman Lane, P.O. Box 1029, Santa Maria, CA 93456; tel. 800/870–3108; FAX. 805/925–1387; John W. Puryear, Executive Director

University of California, Davis Medical Center–Hospice, 1771 Stockton Boulevard, Sacramento, CA 95826; tel. 916/734–2458; Mary E. Kennedy, Home Care Services Manager

Valley of the Moon Hospice, 370 West Napa Street, Sonoma, CA 95476–0600; tel. 707/938–4545; FAX. 707/935–7590; Christine Gruhn, RN, Team Coordinator

Verdugo Hills VNA Hospice in the Home, 1101 East Broadway, Suite 201, Glendale, CA 91205–1386; tel. 818/956–1860; FAX. 818/956–1881; Marie Reynolds, RN, Executive Director

Visiting Nurse Association Home Health Care, Inc., Hospice at Home, 2025 Gateway Place, Suite 270, San Jose, CA 95110; tel. 408/452–1224; Ellen Allen, Vice President

Visiting Nurse Association Los Angeles, Inc., 2461 208th Street, Torrance, CA 90501; tel. 310/782–8886; FAX. 310/782–9172; Judy Regotti, PHN

Visiting Nurse Association and Hospice of Northern California, 1900 Powell Street, Suite 300, Emeryville, CA 94608; tel. 510/450–8596; FAX. 510/450–8532; Pat Sussman, Director

Visiting Nurse Association and Hospice of Pomona/San Bernardino, Inc., 170 West San Jose, Suite 200, P.O. Box 908, Claremont, CA 91711; tel. 714/624–3574; FAX. 714/624–8904; Karen H. Green, President

Visiting Nurse Association of Long Beach–Hospice, 3295 Pacific Avenue, Long Beach, CA 90807; tel. 310/426–8856; FAX. 310/988–9474; Susanne B. Fairman

Yvette Luque Hospice, 520 South Lafayette Park Place, Suite 540, Los Angeles, CA 90057; tel. 213/386–7200; FAX. 213/386–4227; Sharon Grigsby, President

COLORADO

Arkansas Valley Hospice, 118 West Fourth Street, Box 1067, LaJunta, CO 81050; tel. 719/384–8827; FAX. 719/384–2045; Erma J. Isaac, Executive Director

Boulder County Hospice, 2825 Marine Street, Boulder, CO 80303; tel. 303/449–7740; FAX. 303/449–6961; Constance Holden, Director

Bristlecone Hospice, Highway Nine and School Road, P.O. Box 1327, Frisco, CO 80443; tel. 303/668–5604; FAX. 303/668–3189; Linda Jones, Administrator

Caring Unlimited Hospice Services, 1012 Cherry Street, P.O. Box 88, La Veta, CO 81055; tel. 719/742–3028; FAX. 719/742–3048; Karen Clouse, Patient Care Coordinator

© 1995 AHA Guide — Health Organizations, Agencies and Providers — C103

Providers / Freestanding Hospices

Caring Unlimited Hospice Services, Inc., 328 North Bonaventure, Trinidad, CO 81082; tel. 719/846-6224; FAX. 719/846-0799; Karen Clouse, Director

Community Hospice, Inc., 1401 17th Street, Suite 700, Denver, CO 80202; tel. 303/293-2273; FAX. 303/293-2262; Edward Lowe, Administrator

Community Hospice/Roaring Fork Valley, P.O. Box 5016, Aspen, CO 81612; tel. 303/925-4885; FAX. 303/963-4566; Marie Browne, Executive Director

Estes Park Hospice, 555 Prospect, P.O. Box 2740, Estes Park, CO 80517-2740; tel. 303/586-2273; FAX. 303/586-3895; Andrew Wills

Grand Valley Hospice, Inc., d/b/a Hospice of the Grand Valley, 2784 Crossroads Boulevard, Grand Junction, CO 81506; tel. 303/241-2212; Christy Whitney, Executive Director

Hospice Del Valle, Inc., 231 State Avenue, P.O. Box 1554, Alamosa, CO 81101; tel. 719/589-9019; Greta L. Roberts, Executive Director

Hospice at the Mount, 7550 Assisi Heights, Colorado Springs, CO 80919; tel. 719/633-3400; FAX. 719/633-1150; Martha Barton, RN, Executive Director

Hospice of Larimer County, 5205 South College Avenue, Fort Collins, CO 80525; tel. 303/226-6533; FAX. 303/226-6999; Brian Hoag, Executive Director

Hospice of Mercy Medical Center, 3801 North Main Avenue, Durango, CO 81301; tel. 303/259-4121; Dale Jessup, Administrator

Hospice of Metro Denver, Inc., 3955 East Exposition Avenue, Suite 500, Denver, CO 80209; tel. 303/778-1010; FAX. 303/722-4524; Jacob S. Blass, President, Chief Executive Officer

Hospice of Montezuma, Inc., 44 North Ash, Cortez, CO 81321; tel. 303/565-4400; FAX. 303/565-9543; Brenda Dunn, RN, Administrator

Hospice of Northern Colorado, 1403 10th Avenue, Greeley, CO 80631; tel. 303/352-8487; FAX. 303/352-6685; Jane M. Schnell, RN, Executive Director

Hospice of Peace, 1620 Meade Street, Denver, CO 80204; tel. 303/575-8393; FAX. 303/575-8390; Ann Luke, Supervisor

Hospice of St. John, 1320 Everett Court, Lakewood, CO 80215; tel. 303/232-7900; FAX. 303/232-3614; Bernard C. Heese, Administrator

Hospice of Steamboat, 135 Sixth Street, P.O. Box 775816, Steamboat Springs, CO 80477; tel. 303/879-9218; Janet Fritz, Executive Director

Hospice of the Comforter, 3715 Parkmoor Village Drive, Suite 108, Colorado Springs, CO 80917; tel. 719/573-4166; Ronald Coffin, Ph.D., M.B.A., Executive Director

Lamar Area Hospice Association, Inc., 1001 South Main, P.O. Box 843, Lamar, CO 81052; tel. 719/336-2100; Linda Earl, Executive Director

Mount Evans Hospice, 3721 Evergreen Parkway, P.O. Box 2770, Evergreen, CO 80439; tel. 303/674-6400; Louisa B. Walthers, Executive Director

Pikes Peak Hospice, Inc., 3630 Sinton Road, Suite 302, Colorado Springs, CO 80907; tel. 719/633-3400; FAX. 719/633-1150; Martha Barton, RN, Executive Director

Porter Hospice, 2465 South Downing Street, Suite 202, Denver, CO 80210; tel. 303/871-0835; FAX. 303/778-5859; Terri Walter, Director

Prospect Home Care Hospice, Inc., 321 West Henrietta Avenue, Suite E, P.O. Box 6278, Woodland Park, CO 80866; tel. 719/687-0549; FAX. 719/687-8558; Joleen Bailey, Executive Director

Sangre de Cristo Hospice, 704 Elmhurst Place, Pueblo, CO 81004; tel. 719/542-0032; FAX. 719/542-1486; Joni Fair, President, Chief Executive Officer

Visiting Nurse Association Hospice at Home, 3801 East Florida, Suite 800, Denver, CO 80210; tel. 303/757-6363, ext. 413; FAX. 303/782-2573; Judith Sutherland, President

CONNECTICUT

The Connecticut Hospice, Inc., 61 Burban Drive, Branford, CT 06405; tel. 203/481-6231; FAX. 203/483-9539; Rosemary J. Hurzeler, President, Chief Executive Officer

DELAWARE

Delaware Hospice Northern Division, 100 Clayton Building, 3515 Silverside Road, Wilmington, DE 19810; tel. 302/478-5707; FAX. 302/479-2586; Susan D. Lloyd, RN, M.S.N., Executive Director

Delaware Hospice, Inc.–Georgetown, 600 Dupont Highway, Suite 107, Georgetown Professional Park, Georgetown, DE 19947; tel. 302/856-7717; Susan D. Lloyd, RN, M.S.N., Executive Director

Delaware Hospice–Central Division, Lotus Plaza, 911 South Dupont Highway, Dover, DE 19901; tel. 302/678-4444; FAX. 302/678-4451; Susan D. Lloyd, RN, M.S.N., Executive Director

Hospice of the Tri State Area, Oxford Building, Suite 201-A, University Plaza, Newark, DE 19700; tel. 302/454-7002; FAX. 302/454-7003; Sharon Garrick, RN, B.S.N., Administrator

DISTRICT OF COLUMBIA

Children's Hospice Service, 216 Michigan Avenue, N.E., Washington, DC 20017; tel. 202/884-4663; FAX. 202/884-6897; Janice Miller-Thiel, Clinical Services Director

Hospice Care of District of Columbia, 1325 Massachusetts Avenue, N.W., Suite 606, Washington, DC 20005-4171; tel. 202/347-1700; FAX. 202/347-4285; Darla Schueth, Acting Director

Hospice of Washington, 3720 Upton Street, N.W., Washington, DC 20016; tel. 202/966-3720; FAX. 202/895-0177; Molly Sherwood, Acting Interim Administrator

FLORIDA

Bay Medical Center Hospice, 608 N. Cove Boulevard, Panama City, FL 32401; tel. 904/747-5400, ext. 21; FAX. 904/747-5415

Big Bend Hospice, Inc., 1982 Capital Circle, N.E., Tallahassee, FL 32308-4422; tel. 904/878-5310; FAX. 904/385-5850; Elaine C. Bartelt, M.S., Executive Director

Brevard Hospice, 14 Suntree Place, Melbourne, FL 32940; tel. 407/253-2222; FAX. 407/253-2238; Marilyn H. Cromer, M.S.W., LCSW, Executive Director

Catholic Hospice, Inc., 14100 Palmetto Frontage Road, Suite 370, Miami Lakes, FL 33016; tel. 305/822-2380; FAX. 305/824-0665; Janet L. Jones, President, Chief Executive Officer

Good Shepherd Hospice of Mid-Florida, Inc., 245 South Commerce, Sebring, FL 33870; tel. 813/471-3700; FAX. 813/471-9452; Jane Turner, RN, Patient Care Coordinator

Good Shepherd Hospice of Mid-Florida/Winter Haven, Inc., 105 Arneson Avenue, Auburndale, FL 33823; tel. 813/297-1880; FAX. 813/965-5601; Nancy J. Meyer, Administrator

Hernando-Pasco Hospice, Inc., 12107 Majestic Boulevard, Hudson, FL 34667; tel. 813/863-7971; FAX. 813/868-9261; Rodney Taylor, Executive Director

Holmes Regional Hospice, Inc., 1900 Dairy Road, West Melbourne, FL 32904; tel. 407/952-0494; FAX. 407/952-0382; Roberta Van Dusen, Director

Hope Hospice of Lee County, Inc., 9470 Health Park Circle, Ft. Myers, FL 33908; tel. 813/482-4673; FAX. 813/482-2488; Samira K. Beckwith, President, Chief Executive Officer

Hospice By The Sea, Inc., 1531 West Palmetto Park Road, Boca Raton, FL 33486; tel. 407/395-5031; FAX. 407/393-7137; Trudi Webb, Executive Director

Hospice Care of Broward County, Inc., 309 S.E. 18th Street, Ft. Lauderdale, FL 33316; tel. 305/467-7423; FAX. 305/524-6067; Susan G. Telli, Chief Executive Officer

Hospice Care of South Florida, 7270 N.W. 12th Street, Penthouse 6, Miami, FL 33126; tel. 305/591-1606; FAX. 305/591-1618; Rose Marie R. Marty, Executive Director

Hospice of Central Florida, Inc., 2500 Maitland Center Parkway, Suite 300, Maitland, FL 32751; tel. 407/875-0028; FAX. 407/875-2074; Brenda K. Horne, President, Chief Executive Officer

Hospice of Citrus County, Inc., 3350 West Audubon Park Path, Lecanto, FL 34461-8450; tel. 904/527-2020; FAX. 904/527-0386; William J. Murphy, Interim Executive Director

Hospice of Gold Coast H.H.S., 911 East Atlantic Boulevard, Suite 200, Pompano Beach, FL 33060; tel. 305/785-2990; FAX. 305/785-2993; Mary Fay Verville, Vice President, Administrator

Hospice of Hillsborough, Inc., 3010 West Azeele Street, Tampa, FL 33609-3139; tel. 813/877-2200; FAX. 813/872-7037; Anne E. Thal, Executive Director

Hospice of Lake and Sumter, Inc., 12300 Lane Park Road, Taveres, FL 32778-9660; tel. 904/343-1341; FAX. 904/343-6115; Kenneth O. Drees, Chief Executive Officer

Hospice of Marion County, Inc., 317 N.E. 36th Avenue, P.O. Box 4860, Ocala, FL 34478-4860; tel. 904/694-7158; FAX. 904/694-6524; Alice J. Privett, Executive Director

Hospice of Martin, Inc., 2030 S.E. Ocean Boulevard, Stuart, FL 34996; tel. 407/287-7860; FAX. 407/287-7928; Mary C. Knox, Executive Director

Hospice of Naples, Inc., 1095 Whippoorwill Lane, Naples, FL 33940; tel. 813/261-4404; FAX. 813/262-2429; Diane S. Cox, Executive Director

Hospice of Northeast Florida, Inc., 841 Prudential Drive, 1 Prudential Plaza, Jacksonville, FL 32207-8331; tel. 904/398-4724; FAX. 904/398-3027; Susan Ponder-Stansel, President, Chief Executive Officer

Hospice of Northwest Florida, Inc., 2001 North Palafox Street, Pensacola, FL 32501; tel. 904/433-2155; FAX. 904/438-5861; Dale O. Knee, Chief Executive Officer

Hospice of Okeechobee, Inc., 411 S.E. Fourth Street, P.O. Box 1548, Okeechobee, FL 34973; tel. 813/467-2321; FAX. 813/467-8330; Donna L. Watson, Executive Director

Hospice of Palm Beach County, Inc., 5300 East Avenue, West Palm Beach, FL 33407; tel. 407/848-5200; FAX. 407/863-2955; Deborah S. Dailey, President, Chief Executive Officer

Hospice of Pasco, Inc., 6224-6230 Lafayette Street, New Port Richey, FL 34652-2626; tel. 813/845-5707; Michael Wilson, Executive Director

Hospice of Southwest Florida, Inc., 6055 Rand Boulevard, Sarasota, FL 34238; tel. 813/923-5822; FAX. 813/921-7431; Bonnie Harvey, President, Chief Executive Officer

Hospice of St. Francis, Nine South Palm Avenue, P.O. Box 5563, Titusville, FL 32796; tel. 407/269-4240; FAX. 407/269-5428; Cheryl M. Parker, Executive Director

Hospice of Treasure Coast, Inc., 600 Atlantic Avenue, P.O. Box 1748, Ft. Pierce, FL 34954-1748; tel. 407/465-0504; FAX. 407/465-6309; Carol W. Pendeleton, President, Chief Executive Officer

Hospice of Volusia and Flagler, 3800 Woodbriar Trail, Port Orange, FL; tel. 904/322-4701; Rebecca McDonald, Administrator

Hospice of the Comforter, 595 Montgomery Road, Altamonte Springs, FL 32714; tel. 407/682-0808; FAX. 407/682-5787; Robert G. Wilson, President, Director

Hospice of the Florida Keys, 1319 William Street, Key West, FL 33040; tel. 305/294-8812; FAX. 305/292-9466; Liz Kern, Chief Executive Officer

Hospice of the Florida Suncoast, Inc., 300 East Bay Drive, Largo, FL 34640; tel. 813/586-4432; FAX. 813/581-5846; Mary Labyak, M.S.S.W., L.C.S.W., President

The Hospice of North Central Florida, 3615 S.W. 13th Street, Gainesville, FL 32608; tel. 904/378-2121; FAX. 904/378-4111; Patrice Moore, Administrator

Visiting Nurse Association Hospice of Indian River County, 1111 36th Street, Vero Beach, FL 32960; tel. 407/567-5551; FAX. 407/569-1444; Sharon L. Kennedy, President, Chief Executive Officer

Vitas Healthcare Corporation of Florida, 3323 West Commercial Boulevard, Suite 200, Ft. Lauderdale, FL 33309; tel. 305/486-4085; FAX. 305/777-5328; Deirdre Lawe, Regional Vice President

Providers / Freestanding Hospices

Vitas Healthcare Corporation of Florida, 4770 Biscayane Boulevard, Suite 500, Miami, FL 33137; tel. 305/576-9333; FAX. 305/571-9471; Barbara Gray, Director of Operations

GEORGIA

Central Hospice Care, 1150 Hammond Drive, Suite B-2100, Atlanta, GA 30328; tel. 404/391-9531; FAX. 404/391-9732; Brenda Clarkson, Administrator

Columbus Hospice, Inc., Physician's Building, Suite 104, 1315 Delauney Avenue, Columbus, GA 31901; tel. 706/327-5153; FAX. 706/660-0162; Mike Smajd, Executive Director

Elysium House, 6490 West Fayetteville Road, Riverdale, GA 30274; tel. 404/997-0889; FAX. 404/997-8559; Kimberly K. Partain, Administrator

Georgia Mountains Hospice, Inc., 1426 Church Street, P.O. Box 881, Jasper, GA 30143; tel. 706/692-3125; FAX. 706/692-4300; Lynn Corliss, Executive Director

Hamilton Medical Center–Hospice, P.O. Box 1168, 1103 Memorial Drive, Dalton, GA 30720-1168; tel. 404/226-2848; Johnnie Bradley, Vice President

Hand In Hand Hospice, 2150 Limestone Parkway, Gainesville, GA 30501; tel. 404/536-0497; FAX. 404/536-0157; Teresa J. Warren, Director

Haven House at Midtown, Inc., 250 14th Street, Atlanta, GA 30309; tel. 404/874-8313; FAX. 404/875-4363; Clyde W. Johnson, Jr., President, Chief Executive Officer

Helping Hands Community Hospice, Inc., 622 16th Avenue, E., P.O. Box 398, Cordele, GA 31015; tel. 912/273-2957; FAX. 912/276-1491; Jackie Perlis, Chairman

Hospice Atlanta, 100 Edgewood Avenue, N.E., Atlanta, GA 30303-9748; tel. 404/577-6989; FAX. 404/527-0697; Kathy Ziegler, Administrator

Hospice Care of Carroll County, Inc., 710 Dixie Street, Carrollton, GA 30117; tel. 404/214-2355; Ann Rossomondo, Administrator

Hospice Satilla of Memorial Hospital, Inc., 1906 Tebeau Street, Waycross, GA 31501; tel. 912/287-2664; Betty Gant, Director

Hospice Savannah, Inc., 1352 Eisenhower Drive, Zip 31406, P.O. Box 13190, Savannah, GA 31416; tel. 912/355-2289; FAX. 912/355-2376; Judith B. Brunger, Executive Director

Hospice of Americus and Sumter County, 121 Brannan Street, P.O. Box 1434, Americus, GA 31709; tel. 912/928-4000; Chris Chrismon, Executive Director

Hospice of Central Georgia, 3312 Northside Drive, Building D, Suite 100, Macon, GA 31201; tel. 912/477-0335; FAX. 912/477-0690; Gary Thomas, Director

Hospice of Georgia, Inc., P.O. Box 190, High Shoals, GA 30645; tel. 404/769-7730; Magda D. Bennett, President

Hospice of Houston Co., Inc., 2066 Watson Boulevard, P.O. Box 1023, Warner Robins, GA 31099; tel. 912/922-1777; FAX. 912/922-9433; Jackie Connors, Administrator

Hospice of Laurens County, 1205 Bellevue Avenue, P.O. Box 1344, Dublin, GA 31040; tel. 912/272-8333; Kaye Bracewell, Executive Director

Hospice of Northeast Georgia, Highway 76 West, Parks and Recreation Building, Clayton, GA 30526; tel. 404/782-7505; Hazel Stone, Executive Director

Hospice of South Georgia, 201 Pendleton Drive, Suite 207, Valdosta, GA 31603-1727; tel. 912/333-1661; Frances Rowell, Director

Hospice of Southeast Georgia, Inc., P.O. Box 1077, Kingsland, GA 31548; tel. 912/673-7000; Susan Ponder-Stansel, President, Chief Executive Officer

Hospice of Southwest Georgia, 808 Gordon Avenue, Thomasville, GA 31798; tel. 912/227-5520; FAX. 912/227-5526; Patricia Whetsell, Director

Hospice of the Golden Isles, Inc., 2311 Heron Street, Brunswick, GA 31520; tel. 912/265-4735; Cheryl Johns, RN, Executive Director

Hospice of the Upstate, Inc., 506 Summit Avenue, Anderson, SC 29621; tel. 803/261-1594; FAX. 803/261-1523; Nancy Boyle, Executive Director

Metro Hospice, Inc., 2045 Peachtree Road, N.E., Suite 110, Atlanta, GA 30309; tel. 404/355-3134; FAX. 404/352-5193; Shari Silvers, Administrator

Northside Hospice, 5825 Glenridge Drive, Building Four, Atlanta, GA 30328-5544; tel. 404/851-6300; JoAnn Doyle, Patient Care Coordinator

Olsten Kimberly Quality Care Hospice, 3355 Northeast Expressway, Suite 150, Atlanta, GA 30341; tel. 404/936-5100; FAX. 404/936-5110; Joan Richters, RN, M.N.

Peachtree Hospice, 3125 Presidential Drive, Box 48839, Suite 220, Altanta, GA 30340; tel. 404/451-1903; FAX. 404/451-0021; Edwin R. Morgan, Jr., Administrator

Shepherd's Gate Hospice, Inc., 2149 Pace Street, Covington, GA 30209; tel. 404/784-9200; FAX. 404/784-9200; John J. McBride, Executive Director

Southwest Christian Hospice, 7225 Lester Road, East Point, GA 30344; tel. 404/969-8354; Ira P. Sanderson, Executive Director

United Hospice, Inc., 3945 Lawrenceville Highway, Lilburn, GA 30247; tel. 800/544-4788; Scott Shull, Vice President

HAWAII

Hospice Hawaii, 445 Seaside Avenue, Suite 604, Honolulu, HI 96815; tel. 808/924-9255; FAX. 808/922-9161; Stephen A. Kula, President, Chief Executive Officer

Hospice Maui, 400 Mahalani Street, Wailuku, HI 96793; tel. 808/244-5555; Dr. Gregory LaGoy, Executive Director

Hospice of Hilo, 1266 Waianuenue Avenue, Hilo, HI 96720; tel. 808/969-1733; FAX. 808/969-4863; Brenda Nichols, Executive Director

Hospice of Kona, 74-5620A Palani Road, Suite 105, Kailua-Kona, HI 96740; tel. 808/334-0334; FAX. 808/334-0365; Ester Ramos, Executive Director

North Hawaii Hospice, Inc., P.O. Box 1236, Kamuela, HI 96743; tel. 808/885-7547; FAX. 808/885-6902; Nancy Bouvet, Executive Director

St. Francis Hospice, 24 Puiwa Road, Honolulu, HI 96817; tel. 808/595-7566; FAX. 808/595-6996; Sister Francine Gries, Executive Director

IDAHO

Family Hospice, 608 Fifth Avenue, Lewiston, ID 83501; tel. 208/799-5275; FAX. 208/799-5343; Rebecca Witt, RN, Director

Good Samaritan Hospice, 840 East Elva, Idaho Falls, ID 83401; tel. 208/523-4795; FAX. 208/522-9175; James W. Barta, Administrator

Hospice of Idaho, Idaho Home Health, 1910 Channing Way, Idaho Falls, ID 83404; tel. 800/491-2224; FAX. 800/464-2877; Frank Dalley, President

Hospice of North Idaho, West 280 Prairie Avenue, Coeur d'Alene, ID 83814; tel. 208/772-7994; John Nugent, Administrator

Hospice of the Palouse, P.O. Box 9461, Moscow, ID 83843; tel. 208/882-1228; FAX. 208/883-2239; Irma Laskowski, Administrator

Life's Doors Hospice, Inc., 1111 South Orchard, Suite 209A, P.O. Box 5754, Boise, ID 83705; tel. 208/344-6500; FAX. 208/344-6590; Mary L. Langenfeld, Chief Executive Officer

MSTI–Hospice of Boise, 151 East Bannock, Boise, ID 83712; tel. 208/386-2721; FAX. 208/384-4675; Diane Records, Director

Magic Valley Staffing Service, Inc., 200 Second Avenue, N., Twin Falls, ID 83301; tel. 208/734-0600; FAX. 208/733-5980; Gary L. Thietten, RN, President

Mercy Hospice, 111 Third Street, S., Nampa, ID 83651; tel. 208/465-5235; Robert A. Fale, Chief Executive Officer

Southeastern District Hospice, 465 Memorial Drive, Pocatello, ID 83201; tel. 208/239-5210; FAX. 208/234-7169; Judy Moyer, Administrator

XL Hospice, Inc., 1401 N. Whitley Drive, Suite 16, Fruitland, ID 83619; tel. 208/452-5911; FAX. 208/452-4090; Leon C. Felder, President

ILLINOIS

Community Hospices of America Northwest Illinois, 256 South Soangetaha Road, Suite 103, Galesburg, IL 61401-5586; tel. 309/342-3007; FAX. 309/342-6973; Susan Myer, Program Director

Cork Willow Tree Healthcare, 9730 South Western Avenue, Suite 426, Evergreen, IL 60642; tel. 708/422-8575; Dorothy L. Sims

DeKalb County Hospice, 615 North First Street, Suite 204, DeKalb, IL 60115; tel. 815/756-3000; Karen Hagen, RN, M.S., Executive Director

EHS Hospice/Meridian Team, 8704 South Constance Avenue, Third Floor, Chicago, IL 60617; tel. 312/768-2500; FAX. 312/768-5782

Family Hospice of Belleville Area, 11B Park Place, Professional Center, Swansea, IL 62221; tel. 618/277-1800; Diane Smith, Administrator

Fox Valley Hospice, 200 Whitfield Drive, P.O. Box 707, Geneva, IL 60134; tel. 708/232-2233; FAX. 708/232-0023; Vivian J. Nimmo, Executive Director

Grundy Community Hospice, 1802 North Division Street, Suite 307, Morris, IL 60450; tel. 815/942-8525; Joan Sereno

Horizon Hospice, Inc., 833 West Chicago Avenue, Chicago, IL 60622; tel. 312/733-2233; FAX. 312/871-7642; Kathryn A. Meshenberg, President, Chief Executive Officer

Hospice Alliance, Inc., 3747 Grand Avenue, Gurnee, IL 60031; tel. 708/263-1180; Ken Dowdell

Hospice Suburban South, 2609 Flossmoor Road, Flossmoor, IL 60422; tel. 708/957-7177; Susie Zavodngik, Executive Director

Hospice of Kankakee Valley, Inc., 1015 North Fifth Avenue, P.O. Box 202, Kankakee, IL 60901; tel. 815/939-4141; FAX. 815/939-1501; Dorothea MacDonald–Lagesse, Executive Director

Hospice of Lincolnland, Inc., 75 Professional Plaza, Mattoon, IL 61938; tel. 217/234-4044; FAX. 217/345-3231; Rebecca Wisdom, Executive Director

Hospice of Northeastern Illinois, Inc., 410 South Hager Avenue, Barrington, IL 60010; tel. 708/381-5599; FAX. 708/381-5713; Jane Bilyeu, Executive Director

Hospice of Northwest Illinois, Inc., 155 West Front Street, P.O. Box 185, Stockton, IL 61085-0185; tel. 815/947-3260; FAX. 815/947-3257; Les Graham

Hospice of Southern Illinois, Inc., 305 South Illinois Street, Belleville, IL 62220; tel. 618/235-1703; FAX. 618/235-2828; Merle L. Aukamp, President, Chief Executive Officer

Hospice of the Calumet Area, Inc., 3224 Ridge Road, Suite 202 and 204, Lansing, IL 60438; tel. 708/895-8332; FAX. 219/922-1947; Walter M. Knish, Executive Director

Hospice of the North Shore, A Division of Palliative Center of the North Shore, 2821 Central Street, Evanston, IL 60201; tel. 708/467-7423; FAX. 708/866-6023; Dorothy L. Pitner, RN, B.S.N., MM, President

Joliet Area Community Hospice, Inc., 335 West Jefferson Street, Joliet, IL 60435; tel. 815/740-4104; FAX. 815/740-4107; Duane A. Krieger, Executive Director

Lourdes Hospice, 600 Market Street, Metropolis, IL 62960; tel. 618/524-3647; FAX. 618/524-3920; Donna Stewart, Director

Northern Illinois Hospice Association, 4215 Newburg Road, Rockford, IL 61108; tel. 815/398-0500; FAX. 815/964-0255; Judith A. Engblom, Executive Director

Ogle County Hospice Association, 421 Pines Road, P.O. Box 462, Oregon, IL 61061; tel. 815/732-2499; Lorrie Bearrows, RN, Executive Director

Samaritan Care, Inc., 1955 Bernice Road, Suite One N, Lansing, IL 60438; tel. 708/418-0100; Linda Mendoza

Sauk Valley Hospice, 321 West First Street, P.O. Box 82, Dixon, IL 61021; tel. 815/288-3673; Cheryl Price, Administrator

St. Thomas Hospice, Inc., Seven Salt Creek Lane, Suite 101, Hinsdale, IL 60521; tel. 708/850-3990; FAX. 708/850-3553; Bruce G. Harlow, Executive Director

Providers / Freestanding Hospices

Tip of Illinois Hospice Program, 103 North Market, Marion, IL 62959; tel. 618/993–6100; Jodell Wheeler, Chief Executive Officer

Unity Hospice, 8142 North Lawndale, Skokie, IL 60076; tel. 708/982–2300; FAX. 312/752–6194; Michael Klein, President

Whiteside County Hospice Association, 212 – Fourth Avenue, P.O. Box 918, Rock Falls, IL 61071; tel. 815/626–9242; FAX. 815/626–7438; Mary Bohlken

Woodhaven Hospice and Special Support Services, 800 Hoagland Boulevard, Jacksonville, IL 62650; tel. 217/245–0838; Bette Jackson, Administrator

INDIANA

Allen Hospice, 1315 Directors Row, Suite 206, Fort Wayne, IN 46808; tel. 219/484–7622; FAX. 219/484–5662; Tim Boon, Administrator

Bartholomew County Area Hospice, Inc., 2400 East 17th Street, Columbus, IN 47201–5351; tel. 812/376–5813; FAX. 812/376–5929; Sandra Carmichael, Executive Director

Hospice of Indianapolis, 2601 Fortune Circle East Drive, Suite 105B, Indianapolis, IN 46241; tel. 317/484–9400; FAX. 317/484–9500; Dianna Pandak, Administrator

Hospice of Southern Indiana, 624 East Market Street, P.O. Box 17, New Albany, IN 47150–4621; tel. 812/945–4596; FAX. 812/945–4733; Pat Payne, Executive Director

Hospice of St. Joseph County, Inc., JMS Building, 108 North Main Street, Suite 111–113, South Bend, IN 46601–1625; tel. 219/237–0340; FAX. 219/237–0349; Thomas Burzynski, Executive Director

Hospice of Wabash Valley, 686 Wabash Avenue, Terre Haute, IN 47807; tel. 812/234–2515; FAX. 812/232–2047; Jacquelyn Fox, Vice President, Chief Operating Officer

Hospice of the Calumet Area, Inc., 600 Superior Avenue, Munster, IN 46321–4032; tel. 219/922–2732; FAX. 219/922–1947; Walter M. Knish, Executive Director

Methodist Home Health and Hospice Service, 2039 North Capitol Avenue, Indianapolis, IN 46202; tel. 317/927–3800, ext. 239; FAX. 317/927–3815; Tena Barker, Administrator

Samaritan Care, Inc., 1101 East Coolspring Avenue, Michigan City, IN 46360; tel. 219/879–3411

St. Francis Hospice, 438 South Emerson, Greenwood, IN 46143; tel. 317/865–2095; Pamela Franklin, Administrator

VNA Home Care Services – Hospice, 1719 State Street, Suite One, LaPorte, IN 46350; tel. 219/325–8153; FAX. 219/325–8616; Trudie Hahn, RN, Hospice Coordinator

VNA Home Care Services Hospice, Inc., 1719 State Street, Suite I, LaPorte, IN 46350–3172; tel. 219/325–8153; FAX. 219/325–8616; Mary Craymer, Administrator

VNA Hospice, 600 S.E. Sixth Street, Evansville, IN 47713; tel. 812/425–3561; FAX. 812/428–5771; Intake and Referral Department

VNA Hospice Home Care, 501 Marquette Street, Valparaiso, IN 46383–2058; tel. 219/462–5195; FAX. 219/462–6020; Laura Harting, Administrator

VNA Hospice of Southeastern Indiana, 1806 East 10th Street, Jeffersonville, IN 47130; tel. 812/288–2700; Nora Newman, Hospice Director

Visiting Nurse Association of Northwest Indiana, Inc., 201 West 89th Avenue, Merrillville, IN 46410; tel. 219/769–3644; FAX. 219/756–7372; Susan Rehrer, Executive Director

Visiting Nurse Home Health Service, Inc., 2323 Shoshone Court, Lafayette, IN 47905; tel. 317/448–6171; FAX. 317/474–7292; Marguerite Boerger, Executive Director

Visiting Nurse Service Hospice of Central Indiana, 4701 North Keystone Avenue, Indianapolis, IN 46205; tel. 317/722–8200; Harriett H. Olson, President, Chief Executive Officer

Visiting Nurse Service and Hospice, Inc., 3015 South Wayne Avenue, Fort Wayne, IN 46807; tel. 219/456–9888, ext. 232; FAX. 219/458–3089; Karen Gardner, President

Vitas Healthcare Corporation, 5240 Fountain Drive, Suite E, Crown Point, IN 46307; tel. 219/736–8921; FAX. 219/736–0972; Jay Koeper, General Manager

IOWA

Bremer–Butler Hospice, 406 West Bremer Avenue, Suites C and D, Waverly, IA 50677; tel. 319/352–1274; FAX. 319/352–9001; Rod Meyer, Director

Cedar Valley Hospice, 2101 Kimball Avenue, Suite 401, Waterloo, IA 50702; tel. 319/292–1450; FAX. 319/292–1256; Cheryl A. Hoerner, Executive Director

Community Hospice of Iowa, 508 East Broadway, Council Bluffs, IA 51503; tel. 712/325–1751; FAX. 712/325–1895; Barbara Coppa, Administrator

Green Valley Hospice, 1700 West Townline Road, Creston, IA 50801; tel. 515/782–7091; FAX. 515/782–2191; Marlys Scherlin, Administrator

Hamilton County PHNS – Hospice Division, 821 Seneca Street, Webster City, IA 50595; tel. 515/832–9555; FAX. 515/832–9554; Jacqueline Butler, Administrator

Homeward Hospice, 1111 Duff, Ames, IA 50010; tel. 515/239–6730; FAX. 515/239–6891

Hospice of Central Iowa, 3619 1/2 Douglas Avenue, Des Moines, IA 50310; tel. 515/274–3400; FAX. 515/271–1302; Kathleen A. Colburn, Executive Director

Hospice of Compassion, 406 Court, P.O. Box 1034, Williamsburg, IA 52361–1034; tel. 319/668–2262; Carole Moore, Executive Director

Hospice of Dubuque County, 3448 Hillcrest Road, Dubuque, IA 52002; tel. 319/582–1220; FAX. 319/582–8089; Barbara Zoeller, Director

Hospice of Jasper County, 204 North Fourth Avenue, E., Newton, IA 50208; tel. 515/792–5086; Ronald R. Ross, Administrator

Hospice of Lee County, Lee County Health Department–Community Nursing, 2218 Avenue H, Fort Madison, IA 52627; tel. 319/372–5225; FAX. 319/372–4374; M. Therese O'Brian, Administrator

Hospice of Mahaska County, 1229 C Avenue, E., Oskaloosa, IA 52577; tel. 515/673–3431; David E. Rutter, Administrator

Hospice of North Iowa, 232 Second Street, S.E., Mason City, IA 50401; tel. 515/423–3508; FAX. 515/423–5250; Ann MacGregor, Administrator

Hospice of Siouxland, 500 11th Street, Sioux City, IA 51101; tel. 712/233–1298; FAX. 712/233–1123; Linda Todd, Hospice Director

Hospice of VNA, 242 North Bluff Boulevard, Clinton, IA 52732; tel. 319/242–7165; Denise Schrader, Executive Director

Hospice of Wapello County, 312 East Alta Vista Avenue, Ottumwa, IA 52501; tel. 515/682–0684; Mary Moreland, Administrator

Iowa City Hospice, Inc., 613 Bloomington Street, Iowa City, IA 52245; tel. 319/351–5665; FAX. 319/351–5729; William P. Havekost, Interim Executive Director

Iowa River Hospice, Inc., 206 West Linn Street, Marshalltown, IA 50158; tel. 515/753–7704; FAX. 515/753–0379; Brent D. Blackwell, Executive Director

Northwest Iowa Home Health Care and Hospice, 160 South Hayes Avenue, Primghar, IA 51245; tel. 800/745–8506; FAX. 712/757–0060; Joanne Heerde, Administrator

KANSAS

Central Homecare & Hospice, 427 S.E. Second, P.O. Box 645, Newton, KS 67114; tel. 316/283–8220; FAX. 316/283–8576; Robert E. Carlton, Executive Director

Community Hospice, 100 West Eighth, Onaga, KS 66521; tel. 913/889–7200; FAX. 913/889–4808; Mary Abitz, Director

Friends of Hospice, 416 1/2 Pennsylvania, Holton, KS 66436; tel. 913/364–4828; Cathleen Reed, Director

Home Health and Hospice of Dickinson County, 1015 North Brady, 511 N.E. 10th Street (Mailing Address), Abilene, KS 67410; tel. 913/263–2100, ext. 405; FAX. 913/263–4105; Pam Jackson, Director

Homecare and Hospice, Inc., 323 Poyntz Avenue, Suite A, Manhattan, KS 66502; tel. 913/537–0688; FAX. 913/537–1309; Sandy Rogers, Hospice Director

Hospice Care in Douglas County, 336 Missouri, Lower Level, Lawrence, KS 66044; tel. 913/749–5006; FAX. 913/843–0757; L. Kay Metzger, Director

Hospice Care of VNA, 413 Division Street, Kansas City, KS 66103; tel. 913/262–6068, ext. 37; FAX. 913/262–2237; Darlene Carraher, Executive Director

Hospice Care, Inc., 402 West Eighth Street, Coffeyville, KS 67337; tel. 316/251–1640; FAX. 316/251–2774; Karan Nugent, Administrator

Hospice Inc., 313 South Market, P.O. Box 3267, Wichita, KS 67201–3267; tel. 316/265–9441; FAX. 316/265–6066; John G. Carney, President

Hospice Services, Inc., P.O. Box 116, Phillipsburg, KS 67661; tel. 913/543–2900; FAX. 913/543–5688; Sandy Kuhlman

Hospice of Ellsworth County, A Service of Hays Medical Center, 401 East First, Apartment B, Ellsworth, KS 67439; tel. 800/248–0073; FAX. 913/623–5902; Jill Lawson, RN, B.S.N., Hospice Care Coordinator

Hospice of Jefferson County, 1212 Walnut, Highway 59, P.O. Box 324, Oskaloosa, KS 66066–0275; tel. 913/863–2447; FAX. 913/863–2652; Marilyn Zieg, RN, Hospice Coordinator

Hospice of Leavenworth, 920 Sixth Avenue, Leavenworth, KS 66048; tel. 913/684–1305; FAX. 913/684–1182; Toni Rich, Director

Hospice of North Central Kansas, P.O. Box 272, Concordia, KS 66901; tel. 913/243–8138; FAX. 913/243–2841; Jim Haritatos, President

Hospice of Oswego, 800 Barker Drive, Oswego, KS 67356; tel. 316/795–4400; FAX. 316/795–4802; Tom Heflin, Supervisor

Hospice of Ottawa County, 307 North Concord, Suite 200, Minneapolis, KS 67467; tel. 913/392–2822; FAX. 913/392–3659; June Clark, Director

Hospice of Reno County, Inc., Three Compound Drive, Hutchinson, KS 67502; tel. 316/665–2473; FAX. 316/669–5959; Carolyn Carter, RN, M.N., Executive Director

Hospice of Salina, Inc., 333 South Santa Fe, P.O. Box 2238, Salina, KS 67402–2238; tel. 913/825–1717; FAX. 913/825–4949; Kim Fair, Administrator

Hospice of the Flint Hills, 527 Commercial, Suite 501, P.O. Box 102, Emporia, KS 66801; tel. 316/342–6640; FAX. 316/342–9424; Sandra Grendahl–Jefferis, Director

Hospice of the Heartland, Inc., 400 West Eighth, Suite 207, P.O. Box 21, Beloit, KS 67420; tel. 913/738–9227; FAX. 913/738–9227; Martha McCabe, Executive Director

Hospice of the Prairie, Inc., 2012 A First Avenue, P.O. Box 1294, Dodge City, KS 67801–2623; tel. 316/227–7209; FAX. 316/227–7429; Jeannie Reinert–Schuette, Executive Director

Kansas City Hospice, 1625 West 92nd Street, Kansas City, MO 64114; tel. 816/363–2600; FAX. 816/523–0068; Elaine McIntosh, Executive Director

Lincoln County Hospice, Inc., 218 West School, P.O. Box 32, Lincoln, KS 67455; tel. 913/524–4027; Shirley Ronan, Director

Midland Hospice Care, Inc., 200 Southwest Frazier Circle, Topeka, KS 66606–2800; tel. 913/232–2044; FAX. 913/232–5567; Karren Weichert, Executive Director

Mobile Agency of Southwest Hospice, 617 North Main, Garden City, KS 67846; tel. 316/275–4077; FAX. 316/275–0147; Jacque Sue, Administrator

Smith County Hospice, 220 North Brandon, Smith Center, KS 66967; tel. 913/282–3506; FAX. 913/282–6331; Debra Evangelidis, Hospice Coordinator

South Wind Hospice, 413 South Main, P.O. Box 862, Pratt, KS 67124; tel. 316/672–7553; FAX. 316/672–7554; Diane L. Johnson, B.S.W., Director

Providers / Freestanding Hospices

Southwest Homecare and Hospice, 103 East 11th Street, Liberal, KS 67901; tel. 316/629-2456; FAX. 316/629-2486; Ida Rodkey, Administrator

KENTUCKY
Barren River Home Care, 1133 Adams Street, P.O. Box 1157, Bowling Green, KY 42101; tel. 502/781-2490; FAX. 502/796-8946, ext. 301; Connie Jones, Administrator
Community Hospice, 1538 Carter Avenue, Ashland, KY 41101; tel. 606/329-1890; FAX. 606/329-0018; Susan Hunt, Administrator
Cumberland Valley District Health Department Hospice, 102 South Court Street, Manchester, KY 40962; tel. 606/287-8437; Dottie Dunsil, RN, Nursing Supervisor
Green River Hospice, 210 West Second Street, P.O. Box 449, Calhoun, KY 42327; tel. 502/273-3486; Tim Dempsey
Heritage Hospice, 337 West Broadway, P.O. Box 1213, Danville, KY 40422; tel. 606/236-2425; FAX. 606/236-6152; Andy Baker, Executive Director
Hospice Association, Inc., 2225 Frederica Street, P.O. Box 1403, Owensboro, KY 42301; tel. 502/926-7565; FAX. 502/926-1223; Dr. Linda Domerese, Executive Director
Hospice East, 24 West Lexington Avenue, P.O. Box 115, Winchester, KY 40392; tel. 606/744-9866; FAX. 606/744-1971; Carol Richardson, Director
Hospice of Big Sandy, 236 College Street, Paintsville, KY 41240-1747; tel. 606/789-3841; FAX. 667/789-1527; Claire Arsenault, Executive Director
Hospice of Central Kentucky, 105 Diecks Drive, P.O. Box 2149, Elizabethtown, KY 42701-2444; tel. 502/737-6300; FAX. 502/737-4053; Stephen Connor, Ph.D., Executive Director
Hospice of Hope, One West McDonald Parkway, Maysville, KY 41056; tel. 606/564-4848; FAX. 606/564-7615; Norman McRae, Chief Executive Officer
Hospice of Lake Cumberland, P.O. Box 651, Somerset, KY 42502; tel. 606/679-4389; FAX. 606/678-0191; Connie K. McCracken, Executive Director
Hospice of Louisville, 3532 Ephraim McDowell Drive, Louisville, KY 40205-3224; tel. 502/456-6200; FAX. 502/456-6655; Randall DuFour, Executive Director
Hospice of Nelson County, 118 East Broadway, Bardstown, KY 40004; tel. 502/348-3660; FAX. 502/349-1292; Sharon Bade, Administrator
Hospice of Ohio County, 1211 Main Street, Hartford, KY 42347; tel. 502/298-5451; FAX. 502/298-3758; Holly Reneer, RN, Director
Hospice of Pike County, 546 South Mayo Trail, Harris Building, Pikeville, KY 41501; tel. 606/432-2112; FAX. 606/437-1000; Sharon Bailey, Administrator
Hospice of Southern Kentucky, Inc., 1027 Broadway, Bowling Green, KY 42104; tel. 502/782-3402; FAX. 502/782-3496; Connie Jones, Associate Director
Hospice of the Bluegrass, 2312 Alexandria Drive, Lexington, KY 40504; tel. 606/276-5344; FAX. 606/223-0490; Gretchen M. Brown, President, Chief Executive Officer
Hospice of the Kentucky River, Inc., 210 St. George Street, Richmond, KY 40475-2376; tel. 606/624-8820; FAX. 606/624-9230; Gail McGillis, MSN, Chief Executive Officer
Jessamine County Hospice, 109 Shannon Parkway, P.O. Box 873, Nicholasville, KY 40356; tel. 606/887-2696; FAX. 606/885-1474; Susan G. Swinford, M.S.W., Executive Director
Lourdes Hospice, 2855 Jackson, Paducah, KY 42001; tel. 502/444-2262; FAX. 502/444-2380; Donna Stewart, Administrator
Mountain Community Hospice, Old Hospital Road, P.O. Box 1234, Hazard, KY 41702; tel. 606/439-2111; E. Pearl Anderson, RN, Administrator
Mountain Heritage Hospice, Inc., Office Building 2, Village Center, P.O. Box 189, Harlan, KY 40831-0189; tel. 606/573-6144; FAX. 606/573-7964; Bernice Reynolds, Administrator

Pennyroyal Hospice, Inc., 1821 East Ninth Street, Suite A, Hopkinsville, KY 42240; tel. 502/885-6428; Hanna Sabel, Executive Director
St. Anthony's Hospice, Inc., 739 South Main Street, P.O. Box 351, Henderson, KY 42420; tel. 502/826-2326; FAX. 502/831-2169; Rebecca S. Curry, Administrator
Tri County Hospice, 530 North Laurel Road, P.O. Box 395, London, KY 40741; tel. 606/864-2208; FAX. 606/878-8525; Clara Benge, Administrator

LOUISIANA
Avoyelles Hospice, Inc., P.O. Box 506, Marksville, LA 71351; tel. 318/253-8844; FAX. 318/253-0806; Cleon Guillot, Administrator
Best Hospice and Palliative Care, 10001 Lake Forest Boulevard, Suite 1000, New Orleans, LA 70127; tel. 504/245-1138; Carolyn H. Best, Administrator
Community Hospice of Bossier Medical Center, 2285 Benton Road, Suite 201D, Bossier, LA 71111; tel. 318/741-6032; FAX. 318/747-0142; Linda McMillan, Director
Friendship Hospice of New Orleans, Inc., 1406 Esplanade Avenue, New Orleans, LA 70116; tel. 504/522-3183; Valarie Davis, Administrator
Hospice Home Care of Lake Charles Memorial Hospital, 3050 Aster Street, Lake Charles, LA 70601; tel. 318/494-6444; FAX. 318/494-6451; Carol A. Markisch, B.S.N., M.B.A., Administrator
Hospice of Acadiana, Inc., 125 South Buchanan, P.O. Box 3467, Lafayette, LA 70501; tel. 318/232-1234; FAX. 318/232-1297; Nelson Waguespack, Jr., Executive Director
Hospice of Jefferson, 2200 Veterans Highway, Suite 209, Kenner, LA 70062; tel. 504/464-7357; Anne Hedberg, Administrator
Hospice of Louisiana, 2915 Missouri Avenue, Shreveport, LA 71109; tel. 318/632-4697; FAX. 318/632-2382; Peggy Gavin, Hospice Administrative Representative
Hospice of North Louisiana, 511 South Trenton, Ruston, LA 71270; tel. 318/251-2559; Joan Gordon, Director
Hospice of South Louisiana, 210 Mystic Boulevard, Houma, LA 70360; tel. 504/851-4273; FAX. 504/872-6543; Dottie Landry, RN, Administration
Hospice of St. Luke, 235 North Second Street, Eunice, LA 70535; tel. 800/673-5724; Willadean McWhorter, Administrator
North Oaks Hospice, 15790 Medical Center Drive, P.O. Box 2668, Hammond, LA 70404; tel. 504/543-6412; James E. Cathey, Administrator
North Shore Regional Medical Center Hospice, 104 Smart Place, Slidell, LA 70458; tel. 504/641-7373; FAX. 504/641-4772; Aubrey Price, Director
Olsten Kimberly Quality Care Hospice, 2404 Edenborn Avenue, Metairie, LA 70001; tel. 504/835-9127; FAX. 504/838-0488; Nancy Bottoms, RN, Administrator
Peoples Hospice, 1743 Stumpf Boulevard, Gretna, LA 70056; tel. 504/364-1494; FAX. 504/362-1056; Maggie Faucheux, RN, Administrator
Schumpert Medical Center Hospice, One Saint Mary Place, Shreveport, LA 71101; tel. 318/227-4605; FAX. 318/227-6839; Janet Laney, RN
The Hospice Foundation of Greater Baton Rouge, 8322 One Calais Avenue, Suite A, Baton Rouge, LA 70809-3412; tel. 504/767-4673; FAX. 504/769-8113; Kathryn Grigsby, Executive Director
The Hospice of Greater New Orleans, 3616 South I-10 Service Road, Suite 109, Metairie, LA 70001; tel. 504/838-8944; FAX. 504/838-9034; Jo-Ann Mueller, Chief Executive Officer
University Hospital, 2021 Perdido Street, New Orleans, LA 70112; tel. 504/588-3130; FAX. 504/588-3870; Robert O. Nugent, Administrator

MAINE
CHS Hospice, 98 Chestnut Street, P.O. Box 8250, Portland, ME 04104; tel. 207/775-7231; FAX. 207/775-5521; Robert P. Liversidge, Jr., President, Chief Executive Officer

Community Health And Nursing Services, d/b/a Hospice Care, 50 Baribeau Drive, Brunswick, ME 04011; tel. 207/729-6782; FAX. 207/725-5640; Jeanne St. Amand, RN, Executive Director
Health Reach Home Care and Hospice, Eighth Highwood Street, P.O. Box 1568, Waterville, ME 04903-1568; tel. 207/873-1127; FAX. 207/873-2059; Rebecca K. Colwell, Vice President, Home Care
Hospice of Aroostook, Route 89 Access Highway, P.O. Box 688, Caribou, ME 04736; tel. 207/498-2578; FAX. 207/493-3111; Philip A. Cyr, Executive Director
Hospice of Eastern Maine, 412 State Street, Bangor, ME 04401; tel. 800/350-8269; Christel Lingenfelter, Executive Director
Hospice of St. Joseph, 12 Stillwater Avenue, P.O. Box 934, Bangor, ME 04402; tel. 207/947-0177; Elaine Gerard, Director
Kno-Wal-Lin Coastal Family Hospice, One Park Drive, Rockland, ME 04841; tel. 207/594-9561; FAX. 207/594-2527; Kathleen Deupree, RN, Patient Care Coordinator
Miles Home Health Hospice Division, R.R. 2, P.O. Box 4500, Damariscotta, ME 04543-8903; tel. 207/563-1709; Judith C. Tarr, Chief Executive Officer
Visiting Nurse Association and Hospice, 50 Foden Road, South Portland, ME 04106; tel. 207/780-8624; FAX. 207/756-8676; Delthia Vilasuso, Executive Director
Visiting Nurse Service of Southern Maine, 15 Industrial Park Road, Saco, ME 04072; tel. 207/284-4566; FAX. 207/282-4148; Maryanna Arsenault, Executive Director

MARYLAND
Bon Secours Home Health/Hospice, 1138 Hollins Street, Baltimore, MD 21223; tel. 410/837-8500; FAX. 410/837-4239
Calvert Hospice, 310 Main Street, Prince Frederick, MD 20678; tel. 410/535-0892; Carolyn S. Lewis, Executive Director
Caroline County Home Health/Hospice, 601 North Sixth Street, (P.O. Box 10 mailing address), Denton, MD 21629; tel. 410/479-3500; FAX. 410/479-3425; L. Carol Smith, Administrator
Carroll Hospice, 95 Carroll Street, Westminster, MD 21157; tel. 410/857-1838; Julie Flaherty, Executive Director
Coastal Hospice, Inc., 2604 Old Ocean City Road, P.O. Box 1733, Salisbury, MD 21802-1733; tel. 410/742-6044; FAX. 410/548-5669; Marion F. Keenan, President
Dorchester County Home Health Hospice, 751 Woods Road, Cambridge, MD 21613; tel. 410/228-5860; FAX. 410/228-4475; Mary B. Clifton, RN, Director
Harford Hospice, Inc., 56 East Bel Air Avenue, Aberdeen, MD 21001-3759; tel. 410/272-2266; FAX. 410/272-8413; Barry E. Yingling, President, Chief Executive Officer
Hospice Caring, Inc., Volunteer Hospice, P.O. Box 2220, Gaithersburg, MD 20879; tel. 301/869-4673; Carol Sheehan, Executive Director
Hospice Services of Howard County, 5537 Twin Knoll Road, Suite 433, Columbia, MD 21045; tel. 410/730-5072; FAX. 410/730-5284; Elaine Patico
Hospice of Charles County, 616 East Charles Street, Suite 101, P.O. Box 1703, LaPlata, MD 20646; tel. 301/934-1268; FAX. 301/934-2237; Wendell Chappell, FACHE, Executive Director
Hospice of Frederick County, 1730 North Market Street, P.O. Box 1799, Frederick, MD 21702; tel. 301/694-6444; FAX. 301/694-9012; Laurel A. Cucchi, Executive Director
Hospice of Prince George's County, 96 Harry Truman Drive, Largo, MD 20772; tel. 301/499-0550; FAX. 301/350-7844; Lois Kimber, Director, Nursing Services
Hospice of St. Mary's, Inc., 100 Courthouse Drive, Leonardtown, MD 20650; tel. 301/475-2023; FAX. 301/475-3497; Dana McGarity, Executive Director
Hospice of Washington County, 101 East Baltimore, Hagerstown, MD 21740; tel. 301/791-6360; FAX. 301/791-6579; Shelby J. Higgins, M.H.S.A., Executive Director

Providers / Freestanding Hospices

Hospice of the Chesapeake, Inc., 8424 Veterans Highway, Millersville, MD 21108; tel. 410/987-2003; FAX. 410/987-3961; Erwin E. Abrams, President

Jewish Community Hospice, 6123 Montrose Road, Rockville, MD 20852; tel. 301/816-2674; FAX. 301/990-0257; Laura Freiden, Director, Home Care Services

Joseph Richey Hospice, 828 North Eutaw Street, Baltimore, MD 21201; tel. 410/523-2150; FAX. 410/523-1146; Ruth E. Eger, Executive Director

Kent Home Health/Hospice, 125 Lynchburg Street, P.O. Box 359, Chestertown, MD 21620; tel. 410/778-1050; FAX. 410/778-7399; Karen Russum, RN, Director

Montgomery Hospice Society, 1450 Research Boulevard, Suite 310, Rockville, MD 20850; tel. 301/279-2566; Nancy Taylor, Executive Director

Northern Chesapeake Hospice, Inc., 239 South Bridge Street, Elkton, MD 21921; tel. 410/392-4742; FAX. 410/392-6448; Cathy Stouffer Kimble, Executive Director

Queen Anne's Hospice Volunteers, Inc., 206 North Commerce Street, P.O. Box 179, Centerville, MD 21617; tel. 410/758-3043; FAX. 410/758-2838; Joni Sadler, Nursing Supervisor

Saint Joseph Hospital Home Care/Hospice, 7620 York Road, Towson, MD 21204; tel. 410/337-1549

Stella Maris Hospice, Dulaney Valley Road, Towson, MD 21204; tel. 410/252-4500; FAX. 410/560-9675; Sister Karen McNally, R.S.M., Associate Administrator

Talbot County Home Health Hospice, 100 South Hanson Street, Easton, MD 21601; tel. 410/822-3855

The Union Memorial Hospital Home Health Care Program, 201 East University Parkway, Baltimore, MD 21218; tel. 410/554-2950; Romaine L. Eyler, Administrator

Tri–Home Health Care and Services, 2000 Rock Springs Road, P.O. Box 240, Forest Hills, MD 21050; tel. 301/893-0544; Susan Parks, RN, Hospice Coordinator

VNA Hospice of Maryland L.L.C., Inc., 6000 Metro Drive, Baltimore, MD 21215; tel. 410/358-7300; FAX. 410/358-7326; Janet Melancon, RN, Hospice Director

MASSACHUSETTS

Cranberry Area Hospice, Inc., 161 Summer Street, Kingston, MA 02364-1224; tel. 617/585-1881; FAX. 617/585-1898

Diversified Home Services Hospice, 316 Nichols Road, Fitchburg, MA 01420; tel. 508/342-6013; FAX. 508/343-5629; Noreen Basque, Administrator

Good Samaritan Hospice, Inc., 310 Allston Street, Brighton, MA 02146; tel. 617/566-6242; FAX. 617/566-3055; Helen Marino Connolly, Executive Director

Hampshire County Hospice, Inc., Seven Denniston Place, P.O. Box 1087, Northampton, MA 01061; tel. 413/586-8288; FAX. 413/584-9615; Joan Keochakian, Executive Director

Hospice Care in The Berkshires, Inc., 235 East Street, Pittsfield, MA 01201; tel. 413/443-2994; FAX. 413/433-7814; Margaret M. Anthony, Executive Director

Hospice Care, Inc., 21 Maple Street, Arlington, MA 02174; tel. 617/648-3172; FAX. 617/641-1526; Sheila Scott, Executive Director

Hospice Community Services V.N.A., Inc., 1100 High Street, Dedham, MA 02026; tel. 617/329-8603; Kathleen S. Wright, President

Hospice Life Care, P.O. Box 10428, Holyoke, MA 01041; tel. 413/533-3923; FAX. 413/536-4513; Patricia Cavanaugh, Director

Hospice VNA of Central and Outer Cape Cod, 434 Route 134, South Dennis, MA 02660; tel. 508/760-5650; FAX. 508/394-8329; Janice C. Emrich, President, Chief Executive Officer

Hospice West, Inc., 254 South Street, Waltham, MA 02154-2707; tel. 617/894-1100; FAX. 617/736-0908; Patricia A. Field, Executive Director

Hospice of Boston, Inc., Long Island Hospice, Administration Building, 2nd Floor, Boston Harbor, Boston, MA 02169; tel. 617/328-8039; FAX. 617/774-1755; Ruth Capernaros, Executive Director

Hospice of Cambridge, Inc., 186 Alewife Brook Parkway, Suite 206, Cambridge, MA 02138; tel. 617/547-0025; FAX. 617/547-2329; Arlene Lowney, Director

Hospice of Cape Cod, Inc., 923 Route 6A, Yarmouthport, MA 02675; tel. 508/362-1103; FAX. 508/362-6885; Marilyn Hannus, RN, Director

Hospice of Community Visiting Nurse Agency, 141 Park Street, Attleboro, MA 02703; tel. 800/220-0110; FAX. 508/226-8939; Kathleen M. Trier, Executive Director

Hospice of Northern Berkshire, Inc., 329 Eagle Street, North Adams, MA 01247; tel. 413/664-6526; FAX. 413/664-0010; Marcia G. Doran, Executive Director

Hospice of the Good Shepherd, 2042 Beacon Street, Waban, MA 02168; tel. 617/969-6130; FAX. 617/928-1450; Ellen Rudikoff, Ph.D., Executive Director

Hospice of the North Shore, Inc., 10 Elm Street, Danvers, MA 01923; tel. 508/774-7566; FAX. 508/774-4389; Diane Stringer, Executive Director

Lighthouse Hospice Association, Inc., 166 Main Street, P.O. Box 448, Wareham, MA 02571-0448; tel. 508/295-8544; FAX. 508/295-0930; Phyllis G. Pheeney, Executive Director

Merrimack Valley Hospice, Inc., One Union Street, Andover, MA 01810; tel. 508/470-1615; FAX. 508/475-1128; Raymond Brockill, Director

Metrowest Hospice of the VNA of South Middlesex, Inc., 475 Franklin Street, Framingham, MA 01701; tel. 508/383-7000; FAX. 508/626-8053; Connie Walsh, Manager

Old Colony Hospice, Inc., 14 Page Terrace, Stoughton, MA 02072; tel. 617/341-4145; FAX. 617/297-7345; Analee Wuhkule, Executive Director

Quaboag Valley Hospice–V.N.A. Home Care Program, 103 Fairview Street, Palmer, MA 01069-1105; tel. 413/283-9715; FAX. 413/283-8084; Jane B. Wordsworth, Director

South Shore Visiting Nurse and Health Services, Inc., d/b/a Hospice of the South Shore, 100 Bay State Drive, P.O. Box 334, Braintree, MA 02184; tel. 617/849-1710; FAX. 617/843-6465; Susan A. Distasio, Director

Trinity Hospice of Greater Boston, Inc., 111 Cypress Street, Brookline, MA 02146; tel. 617/232-0111; FAX. 617/232-2482; Nancy Euchner, Executive Director

V.N.A. of Central Massachusetts, Inc., 120 Thomas Street, Worcester, MA 01608; tel. 508/756-7176; FAX. 508/751-6878; Gloria Powaza, President

V.N.A. of Greater Gardner Hospice, 95 Mechanic Street, Gardner, MA 01440; tel. 508/632-1230, ext. 60; FAX. 508/632-4513; Donna J. Menger, Administrator

VNA Hospice of Greater Milford, 391 South Main Street, P.O. Box 122, Hopedale, MA 01747; tel. 508/634-8382; FAX. 508/634-8738; Renee Merolli, RN, Supervisor

Visiting Nurse Association of Greater Lowell Hospice, 336 Central Street, P.O. Box 1965, Lowell, MA 01853-1965; tel. 508/459-9343; FAX. 508/459-0981; Shirley M. Cyronis, Executive Director

Visiting Nurse Hospice of Pioneer Valley, Inc., 50 Maple Street, P.O. Box 9058, Springfield, MA 01102-9058; tel. 413/781-2317; FAX. 413/781-3342; Maureen Skipper, President

Wayside Hospice, Parmenter Health Services, 266 Cochituate Road, Wayland, MA 01778; tel. 508/358-3000; FAX. 508/358-3005; Edith L. Murray, Director

Wayside Hospice, Parmenter Health Center, Inc., 266 Cochituate Road, Wayland, MA 01778; tel. 508/653-1111; FAX. 508/650-9276; Edith L. Murray

MICHIGAN

Allen Hospice, 814 Adams, Suite 109, Bay City, MI 48708; tel. 517/892-0355; Corinne Douglas, RN, Director

Angela Hospice Home Care, Inc., 14100 Newburgh Road, Livonia, MI 48154-5010; tel. 313/464-7810; FAX. 313/464-6930; Clare McAuliffe, Admissions

Arbor Hospice, 7445 Allen Road, Suite 230, Allen Park, MI 48101; tel. 313/383-8800; FAX. 313/383-0115; Sue Andres, Director, Clinical Services

Arbor Hospice, Home Care, and Care–ousel, 3810 Packard Road, Suite 200, Ann Arbor, MI 48108; tel. 313/677-0500; FAX. 313/677-2014; Mary Lindquist, President

Barry Community Hospice–Good Samaritan, 301 South Michigan, Hastings, MI 49058; tel. 616/948-8452; FAX. 616/948-9545; Deb Winkler, Division Manager

Blue Water Hospices, Inc., 1422 Lyon Street, Port Huron, MI 48060; tel. 313/982-8809; FAX. 313/984-1612; Brenda K. Clark, Vice President, Operations

Branch–Hillsdale–St. Joseph, 1123 West Broadway, Suite Six, Three Rivers, MI 49093; tel. 616/273-2161; FAX. 616/273-2452; Helen Jakstas, RN, M.P.H., Director

Branch–Hillsdale–St. Joseph DHD, 155 West Fayette Street, Hillsdale, MI 49242

Branch–Hillsdale–St. Joseph District, Health Department Hospice, 809 Marshall Road, Coldwater, MI 49036; tel. 517/279-5961; FAX. 517/278-2923; Helen Jakstas, RN, B.S.N., M.P.H., Director

Cass Branch Hospice Program, 201 M–62 North, Cassopolis, MI 49031

Community Hospice Services, 32932 Warren Road, Suite 100, Westland, MI 48185; tel. 313/522-4244; FAX. 313/522-2099; Maureen Beutrico, Executive Director

Cottage Hospice, 159 Kercheval, Grosse Pointe Farms, MI 48236; tel. 313/884-8600; FAX. 313/885-7023; Sondra L. Seely, Director

Cottage Hospice–HFH (The), 2921 W. Grand Boulevard, New Pavilion Center, Suite 412, Detroit, MI 48202

Cranbrook Hospice Care, 281 Enterprise Court, Suite 300, Bloomfield, MI 48302-0313; tel. 313/334-6700; FAX. 313/334-7064; Beth Johnson, RN, Director

District Health Department, #3, 220 West Garfield Street, Charleviox, MI 49720; tel. 616/547-6092; FAX. 616/547-1164; Nancy Bottomley, RN, M.S., Director, Adult Health

Genesys Home Health and Hospice, Inc., 100 South Dort Highway, Flint, MI 48503; tel. 810/762-3875; FAX. 810/762-0027; LaVerne McCombs, Administrator

Good Samaritan Hospice Care, Inc., 80 North 20th Street, P.O. Box 30195, Battle Creek, MI 49016; tel. 616/965-1391; FAX. 616/965-2833; Jo Cunningham, Executive Director

Grand Traverse Area Hospice, 1105 Sixth Street, Traverse City, MI 49684; tel. 616/935-6395; Kay Benisek, Manager

Helping Hands/Hospice of Ionia County, 1108 West Lincoln Avenue, Ionia, MI 48846; tel. 616/527-5550; FAX. 616/527-5683; Becky Mason

Henry Ford Hospice–West Bloomfield, 6777 West Maple Road, West Bloomfield, MI 48322; tel. 810/661-6454; FAX. 810/661-6453; Laura Zeile, RN, B.S.N., Manager

Home Health Services, 150 Mill Wood Road, P.O. Box 325, Caro, MI 48723

Home Hospice, 315 Ives, Big Rapids, MI 49307; tel. 616/796-7371; FAX. 616/796-4841; Kathy Shefferly, RN, Director

Hope Hospice, 127 Phillips Place, Royal Oak, MI 48067; tel. 810/543-7500; FAX. 810/543-3599

Hospice at Home, Inc., 2626 West John Beers Road, P.O. Box 297, Stevensville, MI 49127; tel. 616/429-7100; FAX. 616/428-3499; Stephen S. Towns, Director

Hospice for Communities, G–3499 South Linden Road, Flint, MI 48507; tel. 313/733-7250; FAX. 313/733-8424; Donna Lloyd, Administrator

Providers / Freestanding Hospices

Hospice of Bay Area, 820 South Lincoln, Bay City, MI 48708; tel. 517/893-7471; FAX. 517/894-2704; Chris Chesny, Administrator

Hospice of Central Michigan, Inc., 210 North Court Street, Suite C, Mt. Pleasant, MI 48858; tel. 517/773-6137; FAX. 517/773-1072; Brian L. Hansen, Executive Director

Hospice of Chippewa County/Chippewa County Health Department, 125 Arlington Street, Sault Ste. Marie, MI 49783; tel. 906/632-2202; FAX. 906/635-1701; Judy Jones, Supportive Services Director

Hospice of Clinton Memorial and Sparrow, 805 South Oakland Street, St. Johns, MI 48879; tel. 517/224-5650; FAX. 517/224-1501, ext. 330; Michelle Wiseman, Director

Hospice of Greater Kalamazoo, Inc., 301 West Cedar Street, Kalamazoo, MI 49007-5106; tel. 616/345-0273; FAX. 616/345-8522; Jean Maile, Executive Director

Hospice of Helping Hands, Inc., 801 East Houghton Avenue, West Branch, MI 48661; tel. 517/345-4700; Ernie Spencer, Interim Director

Hospice of Holland, Inc., 270 Hoover Boulevard, Holland, MI 49423; tel. 616/396-2972; FAX. 616/396-2808; Judith A. Zylman, RN, Executive Director

Hospice of Jackson, 915 Airport Road, Jackson, MI 49202; tel. 517/783-2648; FAX. 517/783-2674; Michael L. Freytag, MA, LPC, Executive Director

Hospice of Lake County, 735 Third Street, P.O. Box 699, Baldwin, MI 49304; tel. 616/745-6161; FAX. 616/745-7676; Margaret Horner, RN, Program Director

Hospice of Lansing, Inc., 6035 Executive Drive, Suite 103, Lansing, MI 48911; tel. 517/882-4500; FAX. 517/882-3010; Barbara A. Kowalski, M.P.A., Executive Director

Hospice of Lenawee, 415 Mill Road, Adrian, MI 49221; tel. 517/263-2323; FAX. 517/263-1279; Mary Fowler, RN, Patient Care Coordinator

Hospice of Little Traverse Bay, 416 Connable, P.O. Box 2117, Petoskey, MI 49770; tel. 616/347-9700; FAX. 616/348-4552; Steve D. Averill, Executive Director

Hospice of MI Cancer Foundation, 18831 Twelve Mile Road, Lathrup Village, MI 48076

Hospice of Mason County, Inc., 10 Atkinson Drive, Suite Three, Ludington, MI 49431; tel. 616/845-0321; Glenna Lou Nelson, RN, B.S.N., Interim Executive Director

Hospice of Monroe/Hospice of Washtenaw, 502 West Elm Street, Monroe, MI 48161; tel. 313/457-3220; FAX. 313/457-5060; Paul Doerfler, B.S.N., Manager

Hospice of Muskegon County, 1095 Third Street, Suite 209, Muskegon, MI 49441; tel. 616/728-3442; FAX. 616/722-0708; Mary Anne Gorman, Executive Director

Hospice of Newaygo County, A division of Hospice of Michigan, Inc., 212 Sullivan, Fremont, MI 49412; tel. 616/924-6123; Marie Malone, RN, B.S.N., Hospice Director

Hospice of North Ottawa Community, Inc., 1515 South Despelder, Grand Haven, MI 49417; tel. 616/846-2015; FAX. 616/846-7227; Carolyn K. Howes, Executive Director

Hospice of Northeastern Michigan, Inc., 112 West Chisholm, Alpena, MI 49707; tel. 517/354-5258; Jeraldyne Habermehl, Executive Director

Hospice of Southeastern Michigan, Crossroads Building, 16250 Northland Drive, Suite 212, Southfield, MI 48075-5200; tel. 810/559-9209; FAX. 810/559-6489; Carolyn Fitzpatrick-Cassin, President, Chief Executive Officer

Hospice of Southeastern Michigan – North Oakland, 1695 South Woodward Avenue, Suite 208, Bloomfield Hill, MI 48302; tel. 810/253-2580; Rita Ann Mahon, RN, Director

Hospice of Southeastern Michigan–St. Clair Shores, 22811 Greater Mack Avenue, St. Clair Shore, MI 48080; tel. 810/445-6855

Hospice of Van Buren County/Greater Kalamazoo, 404 North Hazen Street, Suite L3, Paw Paw, MI 49079; tel. 616/657-7769; FAX. 616/657-7225; Genevieve Dykehouse, Division Manager

Hospice of Washtenaw, 806 Airport Boulevard, Ann Arbor, MI 48108; tel. 313/741-5777; FAX. 313/741-5757; Stephanie Gilbert, Admissions Coordinator

Hospice of Western Michigan, Inc., 750 Fuller, N.E., Suite Five, P.O. Box 2427, Grand Rapids, MI 49501-2427; tel. 616/454-1426; FAX. 616/454-9413; Thomas J. Nobel, Executive Director

Hospice of Wexford–Missaukee, A Program of Hospice of Michigan, 828 Oak Street, Cadillac, MI 49601; tel. 616/779-9570; FAX. 616/779-0717; Pat Spragg, RN, Director

Hospice of the Straits/Vital Care, 748 South Main Street, Cheboygan, MI 49721; tel. 616/627-4774; FAX. 616/627-4416; Kimberly L. Sangster, Executive Director

Hospice–Partners in Caring, Division of VNA of Saginaw, 500 South Hamilton, Saginaw, MI 48602; tel. 517/799-6020; FAX. 517/799-6062; S. J. Schultz, B.S.N., M.S., President, Chief Executive Officer

Individualized Hospice, 3003 Washtenaw Avenue, Suite Two, Ann Arbor, MI 48104; tel. 313/971-0444; FAX. 313/971-1980; Patricia Love, Clinical Director

Keweenaw Home Nursing and Hospice, 414 Hecla Street, Laurium, MI 49913; tel. 906/337-5700; FAX. 906/337-9929; Diane Tibery, RN, Director

LMAS DHD Hospice/St. Ignace, 749 Hombach Street, St. Ignace, MI 49781

Lake Superior Hospice Association, 102 West Washington, Suite 225, Marquette, MI 49855; tel. 906/226-2646; FAX. 906/226-2044; Jill Baker, Executive Director

MI Home Health Care/Terminal Care, 955 E. Commerce Drive, Traverse City, MI 49684; tel. 616/943-8451; FAX. 616/943-4515

McLaren Hospice Service, 237 Davis Lake Road, Lapeer, MI 48446; tel. 810/667-0042; Terry Morgan, Executive Director

Michigan Home Health Care, Terminal Care and Bereavement Hospice Program, 5097 South Straits Highway, Indian River, MI 49749; tel. 616/238-8971; FAX. 616/238-9949; Carol Best, M.S., RN, Director, Indian River Subunit

Mid Michigan VNA Hospice/Clare, 1438 North McEwan, Clare, MI 48617; tel. 800/852-9350; FAX. 517/631-7718; Miriam Markowitz, Director

MidMichigan Visiting Nurses Association–Hospice/Midland, 3007 North Saginaw Road, Midland, MI 48640; tel. 517/631-7510; FAX. 517/631-7718; Miriam Markowitz, Hospice Director

North Woods Home Nursing and Hospice, P.O. Box 307, Manistique, MI 49854; tel. 906/341-6963; FAX. 906/341-2490; Susan Bjorne, Administrator

R. P. Hicks Memorial Hospice, Inc., LMAS District Health Department, P.O. Box 398, Co. Road 378, Newberry, MI 49868; tel. 906/293-5107; Kathleen Nyeste, Clinical Coordinator

Samaritan Care, Inc., 24445 Northwestern Highway, Suite 209, Southfield, MI 48075; tel. 810/355-9900

South Haven Area Hospice, 05055 Blue Star Highway, P.O. Box 990, South Haven, MI 49090-0990; tel. 616/637-3825; FAX. 616/637-6777; Barbara Reicherts, Executive Director

St. Joseph Huron Home Health and Hospice, P.O. Box 208, 716 German Street, Suite B, Tawas City, MI 48763; tel. 517/362-4611; FAX. 517/362-8771; Ann Balfour, Administrator

St. Joseph's Hospice/Cottage Hospice, 17001 19 Mile Road, Clinton Township, MI 48038; tel. 810/263-2840; FAX. 810/263-2895; Patti Ciechanovski, RN, Manager

Upper Peninsula Home Nursing/Hospice, 1414 Fair, Suite 44, Marquette, MI 49855; tel. 906/225-4545; FAX. 906/225-4544; Cynthia A. Nyquist, RN, B.S.N., Administrator, Chief Executive Officer

VNA of Southwestern Michigan – Hospice Program, 57418 County Road #681, Suite D, Hartford, MI 49054-9634; tel. 616/621-3154; FAX. 616/621-4956

VNA of Southwestern Michigan Hospice Program, 348 North Burdick, Kalamazoo, MI 49007; tel. 616/343-1396; FAX. 616/382-8686; Lou Hildebrandt, CRN, Hospice Director

Visiting Nurse Hospice, 4801 Willoughby, Suite Seven, Holt, MI 48842; tel. 517/694-8300; FAX. 517/694-4968; Jeanne Zabihaylo, Admissions Coordinator

Visiting Nurse Service of Western Michigan Hospice Program, 1401 Cedar, N.E., Grand Rapids, MI 49503; tel. 616/774-2702; FAX. 616/774-7017; Laurie Sefton, RN, M.S.N., Hospice Program Director

West Oakland Hospice/Living Community, 801 East Commerce, Milford, MI 48042

Wings of Hope Hospice, Inc., 189 South 10th Street, Plainwell, MI 49080; tel. 616/685-1645; FAX. 616/685-2105; Marie Tucker, Executive Director

MINNESOTA

Aitkin County Hospice Program, 208 Second Avenue Northwest, Aitkin, MN 56431; tel. 218/927-6895

Coram Healthcare Hospice, 1301 Corporate Center Drive, Suite 170, Eagan, MN 55121; tel. 612/452-4115; FAX. 612/452-7370; Pam Schmitt, RN, Oncology/Hospice Manager

Douglas County Public Health NS, 305 Eighth Avenue West, Alexandria, MN 56308; tel. 612/763-6018; FAX. 612/763-4127; Mark Lundin, Administrator

Fosston Hospice, 220 East First Street, Fosston, MN 56542; tel. 218/435-1500; Carole Larson, Director

HealthSpan Home Care and Hospice, 3030 Centre Point Drive, Suite 100, Roseville, MN 55113; tel. 612/628-4200; FAX. 612/635-9074; Nancy Rehkamp, President

Homecaring Hospice, 11685 Lake Boulevard North, Chisago City, MN 55013; tel. 612/257-8402; Scott Wordelman, Administrator

Hospice Partners, Inc., 201 North Concord Exchange, Suite 250, South St. Paul, MN 55075-1150; tel. 612/457-5161; FAX. 612/457-5168; Roberta S. Cline, Chief Executive Officer, President

Hospice of Morrison County, 200 East Broadway, Little Falls, MN 56345; tel. 612/632-6664; FAX. 612/632-0392; Elaine Westerdahl-Delaney

Hospice of Murray County, 2042 Juniper Avenue, Slayton, MN 56172; tel. 507/836-8114

Hospice of The Twin Cities Inc., 7100 Northland Circle, Suite 205, Minneapolis, MN 55428; tel. 612/531-2424; FAX. 612/531-2422; Lisa Abicht-Swensen, Administrator

Hospice of the Lakes, 8100 34th Avenue, S., P.O. Box 1309, Minneapolis, MN 55440-1309; tel. 612/883-6872; FAX. 612/883-6883; Barry Baines, M.D., Medical Director

In Home Health Hospice Program, 2250 County Road C, Roseville, MN 55113; tel. 612/633-6522; FAX. 612/633-5733; Kris Teigen, RN

Itasca Hospice Project Inc., 123 Fourth Street Northeast, P.O. Box 74, Grand Rapids, MN 55744; tel. 218/327-2851, ext. 372; FAX. 218/327-2848, ext. 348

Kittson County Hospice, Inc., P.O. Box 581, Hallock, MN 56728; tel. 218/843-3612

Koochiching Hospice, Inc., P.O. Box 1105, International Falls, MN 56649; tel. 218/283-6458

Lakeland Hospice, Inc., 117 East Vasa, P.O. Box 824, Fergus Falls, MN 56538; tel. 218/736-7885; FAX. 218/736-2231

Lakeview Hospice, 927 West Churchill Street, Stillwater, MN 55082; tel. 612/430-4521; FAX. 612/430-4734; Geri Wagner, Director

Litchfield Area Hospice, 218 North Holcombe, Litchfield, MN 55355; tel. 612/693-7233; FAX. 612/693-7418

Martin County Hospice, Inc., 610 Summit Drive, Fairmont, MN 56031; tel. 507/235-6606; FAX. 507/235-8363

Mayo Hospice Program, 200 First Street, S.W., Rochester, MN 55905; tel. 507/284-4002; FAX. 507/284-0161; Margaret Gillard, RN, Program Coodinator

Midwest Community Hospice, 5527 Penn Avenue South, Minneapolis, MN 55419; tel. 612/926-2243; FAX. 612/926-2716; Marlene Gerber, Executive Director

Providers / Freestanding Hospices

Nobles Community Hospice, 1018 Sixth Avenue, P.O. Box 997, Worthington, MN 56187; tel. 507/372–2941; Melvin J. Platt, Administrator

North Memorial Medical Center Hospice, 3500 France Avenue North, Suite 101, Robbinsdale, MN 55422; tel. 612/520–5770; FAX. 612/520–3920; Elizabeth A. Woll, Manager

Pine To Prairie Hospice, Inc., P.O. Box 83, Karlstad, MN 56732; tel. 800/494–6081; FAX. 218/436–4665

Pope County Hospice, 10 Fourth Avenue, S.E., Glenwood, MN 56334; tel. 612/634–4521; FAX. 612/634–4521; Douglas J. Reker, Chief Executive Officer, Administrator

Prairie Home Hospice, Inc., 300 South Bruce, Marshall, MN 56258; tel. 507/537–9247; Lynn Yueill, Administrative Director

Red Wing Hospice, 434 West Fourth Street, Suite 200, Red Wing, MN 55066; tel. 612/385–3410; FAX. 612/385–3414; Beth Krehbiel, Director

Rum River Area Hospice, P.O. Box 225, Princeton, MN 55371; tel. 612/389–5080; Brenda Hoffman, CHES, Director

Shamrock Seasons Hospice, 1242 Whitewater Avenue, St. Charles, MN 55972; tel. 507/932–3949; FAX. 507/932–5125; Doris Oehlke, Director

The Lutheran Home – Home Health Agency, 425 North Badger Street, Caledonia, MN 55921; tel. 507/724–3351; FAX. 507/724–5142

Waseca Area Hospice, Inc., 107 Fifth Avenue NW, P.O. Box 94, Waseca, MN 56093; tel. 507/835–8737; FAX. 507/837–4280; Linda Grant, Director

MISSISSIPPI

Bienville Clinic, PA, 221 South Street, Morton, MS 39117; tel. 601/732–7202; Michael Reddix, M.D., Patricia M. McLain, F.N.P.

Comfort Care Hospice, 1220 Jefferson Street, P.O. Box 607, Laurel, MS 39440; tel. 601/426–4416; G. Douglas Higginbotham, Executive Director

Delta Area Hospice Care, Ltd., 522 Arnold Avenue, P.O. Box 5915, Greenville, MS 38704–5915; tel. 601/335–7040; FAX. 601/335–7048; Gloria Blakely, Administrator

Hospice Care Foundation, Inc., P.O. Box 2056, Vicksburg, MS 39181; tel. 800/380–3070; FAX. 601/634–6688; Rachel Y. Goodman, RN, Coordinator

Hospice of Central Mississippi, Inc., 2600 Insurance Center Drive, Suite B–124, Jackson, MS 39216–4911; tel. 601/366–9881; FAX. 601/981–0150; John Fletcher, Executive Director

Hospice of Central Mississippi, Inc., 224 South First, Brookhaven, MS 39601; tel. 601/835–1020; FAX. 601/835–1063; Jean Berch, Branch Director

Hospice of Light, 4341 Gautier & Vancleave Road, Gautier, MS 39553; tel. 601/497–2400; FAX. 601/497–5287

Hospice–North Mississippi Medical Center, 600 West Main, Tupelo, MS 38801; tel. 601/841–3612; Laura Kelley, Administrator

Laird Hospice Care, Route Nine, Box One–B, Philadelphia, MS 39350; tel. 601/656–4238; Georgia Buchanan, President

Laird Hospice Care, 1101 22nd Street, Meridan, MS 39301; tel. 601/485–6709; LaRue Miles, RN, Administrator, Dr. Leon Park, Director

Physician's Hospice, Inc., 862 Goodman Road East, P.O. Box 744, Southaven, MS 38671; tel. 601/349–6711; FAX. 601/349–8826; Roy Myrick, General Manager

Rush Hospital Hospice, Highway 15, Route Nine, Box 28, Philadelphia, MS 39350; tel. 601/656–8388; Ken Boyette, Patient Care Coordinator/Supervisor

Sta–Home Hospice, 105 North Van Buren, Carthage, MS 39051; tel. 800/898–1159; Gail Rawson, Administrator

Sta–Home Hospice, 205 Walthall, P.O. Box 777, Greenwood, MS 38930; tel. 800/898–1064; Gail Rawson, Administrator

Superior Home Health and Hospice, 611 Alcorn Drive, Corinth, MS 38834; tel. 601/287–8001; Gary J. Blan, FACHE, President

Whispering Pines Hospice, 1480 Raymond Road, Jackson, MS 39204; tel. 601/373–2472; Jean Jones, Administrator

MISSOURI

American Heartland Hospice, 7555 South Lindbergh, St. Louis, MO 63125; tel. 314/894–8189; Susan O'Kane, Administrator

Bates County Hospice, 501 North Orange, Butler, MO 64730; tel. 816/679–6108; George Taylor, Administrator

Beacon of Hope Hospice, Inc., 4191 Crescent Drive, St. Louis, MO 63129; tel. 314/842–7544; FAX. 314/842–7229; Kenneth G. Barber, Executive Director

Christian Hospital Northeast–Northwest Hospice, 12444 Lusher Road, St. Louis, MO 63138; tel. 314/355–2729; Ruth N. Sedano, RN, B.S.N., Administrator

Comfort Care Hospice, 1015 West Fourth Street, Cameron, MO 64429; tel. 816/632–5124; FAX. 816/632–6121; Pam Walker, RN, Administrator

Community Hospice of America–Tri Lakes, 1756 Bee Creek Road, Suite G, Branson, MO 65616; tel. 417/335–2004; Janet Gard, Administrator

Community Hospices of America–South Central, 101 East 2nd Street, Mountain Grove, MO 65711; tel. 417/926–4146; FAX. 417/926–6123; Don Whitworth, Administrator

Comprehealth, Inc., Hospice Services Division, 2001 South Hanley Road, Suite 450, St. Louis, MO 63144; tel. 314/781–2800; FAX. 314/781–4844

Hands of Hope Hospice, 416 North Seventh, St. Joseph, MO 64501; tel. 816/271–7190; Debbie Parker, Vice President

Hartline Hospice, Inc., 3322 South Campbell, Suite T, Springfield, MO 65807; tel. 417/886–9600; FAX. 417/886–0082; Robert Stauff, Executive Director

Heart of America Hospice, L.C., 9229 Ward Parkway, Suite 350, Kansas City, MO 64114; tel. 816/333–1980; FAX. 816/333–2421; Jacquelin Tuohig, Executive Director

Hospice Care of Mid–America, 3435 Broadway, Suite 104, Kansas City, MO 64111–2415; tel. 816/931–4276; FAX. 816/931–9147; Sharil L. Baxter, Administrator

Hospice Care of Visiting Nurse Association (VNA), 600 West 39th Street, Kansas City, MO 64111; tel. 816/561–1221; FAX. 816/531–8231; Richard Roberson, Administrator

Hospice of Care, 1333 Highway 63, Houston, MO 65483; tel. 417/967–3311; Beverly Derrickson, Administrator

Hospice of Southwest Missouri, Inc., 3653 South Avenue, Springfield, MO 65807; tel. 417/882–0453; FAX. 417/882–1245; Richard Williams, Administrator

Hospice of Visiting Nurse Association, 531 B South Union, Springfield, MO 65802; tel. 417/866–6670; FAX. 417/866–3310; Suzanne Dollar, Chief Executive Officer

Kansas City Hospice, 1625 W. 92nd Street, Kansas City, MO 64114; tel. 816/363–2600; FAX. 816/523–0068; Elaine McIntosh, President

Kathy–Jim Roberts Hospice, 117 East Broadway, Sedalia, MO 65301; tel. 816/827–3122; Tamara Wilson, RN, B.S.N., Administrator

Kendallwood Hospice, 7000 N.W. Prairie View Road, Suite 200, Kansas City, MO 64151; tel. 816/746–5900; FAX. 816/587–5888; Charlotte Bruyn, Administrator

Meramec Hospice, 200 North Main, Rolla, MO 65401; tel. 314/364–2425; FAX. 314/364–1575; Shirley Rutz, Administrator

Missouri River Hospice, 1440 Aaron Court, Jefferson City, MO 65101; tel. 314/635–5643; FAX. 314/635–6552; Marge Borst, Administrator

Pike County Home Health Agency and Hospice, 19 North Main Cross, Bowling Green, MO 63334; tel. 314/324–2111; FAX. 314/324–5517; LuAnn Meyer, RN, Administrator

Providence Hospice Group, Inc., 510 North Main, Sikeston, MO 63801; tel. 314/472–4041; FAX. 314/472–4043; Matthew Brauss, Administrator

Randolph County Health Department, Home Care and Hospice, 425 East Logan, P.O. Box 488, Moberly, MO 65270; tel. 816/263–6643; FAX. 816/263–0333; Ross W. McKinstry, Administrator

Regional Hospice of Central Missouri, 1000 West Nifong, Suite 210, Columbia, MO 65203–5680; tel. 314/499–6070; FAX. 314/499–6038; Ellen Lynch, Director

Riverways Hospice of Ozarks Medical Center, 114 East Main, West Plains, MO 65775; tel. 417/256–3133; Mary Dyck, Administrator

Southeast Hospice, 760 South Kingshighway, Suite C, Cape Girardeau, MO 63701; tel. 314/335–6208; FAX. 314/335–5864; Judy Aslin, Director

Twin Lakes Hospice, Inc., 304 Main, P.O. Box 211, Warsaw, MO 65355; tel. 816/438–9700; FAX. 816/438–6404; Sandra Lindsay, Administrator

VNA of Southeast Missouri Hospice, 100 East Harrison, Kennett, MO 63857; tel. 314/888–5892; Teresa McCulloch, Administrator

Visiting Nurse Association Hospice Care, 1260 Andes Boulevard, St. Louis, MO 63132; tel. 314/993–6800; Susan Pettit, Administrator

MONTANA

Anaconda Pintler Hospice of Community Hospital of Anaconda, 112 Oak Street, P.O. Box 596, Anaconda, MT 59711; tel. 406/563–5422; Alice Cortright, Director

Big Sky Hospice, 1041 North 29th Street, Zip 59101, P.O. Box 1049, Billings, MT 59103–1049; tel. 406/248–7442; FAX. 406/248–2572; Bernice Bjertness, RN, M.N., Executive Director

Dillon Hospice, 1260 South Atlantic, Dillon, MT 59725; tel. 406/683–2324; Debbie Hawkins, RN, Program Director

Flathead Hospice, 1280 Burns Way, Suite Three, Kalispell, MT 59901; tel. 406/752–8667; FAX. 406/257–0355; Judy Graham, RN, Administrative Manager

Hearts and Hands Hospice, P.O. Box 1337, Big Timber, MT 59011; tel. 406/932–5918

Helping Hands Hospice, P.O. Box 81, Roundup, MT 59072; tel. 406/323–1342

Highlands Hospice, 2121 Amherst–505 Centennial Avenue, Butte, MT 59701; tel. 406/723–5780; FAX. 406/723–9595; Virginia Mick, Director

Hospice of Powell County, 310 Milwaukee Avenue, P.O. Box 808, Deer Lodge, MT 59722; tel. 406/846–3975; Nora E. Meier, Office Manager

Kootenai Volunteer Hospice, P.O. Box 781, Libby, MT 59923; tel. 406/293–3923; Theresa Schneider, Director

Partners in Home Care Home Health & Hospice, Inc.–Hospice, 500 North Higgins, Suite 201, Missoula, MT 59801; tel. 406/728–8848; Teresa Smith, RN, Patient Care Coordinator

Peace Hospice of Montana, 125 Northwest Bypass H, Great Falls, MT 59404; tel. 406/727–6161; FAX. 406/727–9758; Mary Gray, RNCS, Director

Pondera Hospice, 300 North Virginia, Suite 305, Conrad, MT 59425; tel. 406/278–5566; FAX. 406/278–5569

Stillwater Convalescent Center Hospice, 350 West Pike Avenue, P.O. Box 898, Columbus, MT 59019; tel. 406/322–5342; FAX. 406/322–5737; Sharon Marten, Chairperson

NEBRASKA

Visiting Nurse Association of the Midlands, 10840 Harney Street, Omaha, NE 68154; tel. 402/334–1820; FAX. 402/342–4587; Marlene Tully, Acting Administrator

NEVADA

Family Home Hospice, 1701 West Charleston, Suite 150, Zip 89102, P.O. Box 15645, Las Vegas, NV 89114–5645; tel. 702/383–0887; FAX. 702/383–1173; Jerilyn D. Hudgens, Administrator

Home Care Connection, 1000 Ryland, Suite 410, Reno, NV 89502; tel. 702/785–4711; Linda Rosewarne, Administrator

Nathan Adelson Hospice, 4141 South Swenson Street, Las Vegas, NV 89119; tel. 702/733–0320; FAX. 702/796–3195; Betsy Peirson-Gornet, Chief Executive Officer

Providers / Freestanding Hospices

PRN Home Hospice, 3022 West Post Road, Las Vegas, NV 89118; tel. 702/361-6801; Marti Norris, Administrator

NEW HAMPSHIRE

Community Health and Hospice, Inc., 780 North Main Street, P.O. Box 578, Lanconia, NH 03247-0578; tel. 603/524-8444; FAX. 603/524-8217; Alida Millham, Executive Director

Concord Regional VNA–Hospice, 250 Pleasant Street, Concord, NH 03301; tel. 603/224-4093; FAX. 603/224-4093; Joanne Fadale Wagner, ACSW, Director

Elliot Home Care & Hospice, 25 South Maple Street, Manchester, NH 03103; tel. 603/628-4430; FAX. 603/622-4800; Diane LaBossiere, M.S.W.

Home Health and Hospice Care, 22 Prospect Street, Nashua, NH 03060; tel. 603/882-2941; FAX. 603/883-1515; Margaret Gilmour, Chief Executive Officer

Hospice Alliance, VNA at HCS, Inc., 69L Island Street, P.O. Box 564, Keene, NH 03431; tel. 603/352-2253; FAX. 603/358-3904; Lois Hopkins, Hospice Program Coordinator

Hospice of the Monadnock Region, 64 Main Street, Keene, NH 03431; tel. 603/357-1314; FAX. 603/357-6004; Molly M. Kelly, Director

Hospice of the Upper Valley, Inc., Hospice VNH, 20 South Main Street, White River, VT 05001; tel. 603/448-5182; FAX. 603/448-1599; Marie Kirn, Executive Director, Chief Executive Officer

Lake Sunapee Home Care and Hospice, 290 County Road, P.O. Box 2209, New London, NH 03257; tel. 603/526-4077; FAX. 603/526-4272; Andrea F. Steel, B.S.N., RN, Vice President

Merrimack Valley Hospice, Inc., One Union Street, Andover, MA 01810; tel. 508/623-3100; FAX. 508/470-4690; Raymond Brockhill, Administrator

Portsmouth Regional Visitng Nurses Association and Hospice, 127 Parrott Avenue, Portsmouth, NH 03801; tel. 603/436-0815; FAX. 603/431-5457; Joan P. Nickell, President

Rockingham VNA and Hospice, 11 Wall Street, Derry, NH 03038; tel. 603/432-7776; FAX. 603/432-0068; Barbara Leake, Director

Seacoast Hospice, 10 Hampton Road, Exeter, NH 03833; tel. 603/778-7391; FAX. 603/778-1434; Walter Phinney, Executive Director

Squamscott Visiting Nurse and Hospice Care, 89 Old Rochester Road, Dover, NH 03820; tel. 603/742-7921; Barbara Brock, Director

Strafford Hospice Care, Inc., Southeast Bank Building, Front Street, Rollinsford, NH 03869; tel. 603/749-4300; Susan E. Cole, Director

Tri-Area VNA Hospice, 301 High Street, Somersworth, NH 03878; tel. 603/692-2112; FAX. 603/692-9940

VNA Home Health and Hospice Services, Inc., 1850 Elm Street, Manchester, NH 03104; tel. 603/622-3781; FAX. 603/622-3781; Mary McKillop, Director, Home Health Services

NEW JERSEY

Atlantic City Medical Center Hospice, 1406 Doughty Road, Pleasantville, NJ 08232; tel. 609/272-2424; FAX. 609/272-2414; Diana Ciurczak, Director

Barbara E. Cheung Memorial Hospice at Roosevelt Hospital, P.O. Box 151, CN4003 and Parsonage Road, Metuchen, NJ 08840-0151; tel. 908/321-9334; FAX. 908/321-9044; Enory Coughlin, RN, Supervisor

Center for Hope Hospice, Inc., 176 Hussa Street, Linden, NJ 07036; tel. 908/486-0700; FAX. 201/241-9628; Margaret J. Coloney, President

Cumberland County Hospice, Inc., 2848 South Delsea Drive, Vineland, NJ 08360; tel. 609/794-1515; FAX. 609/691-7660; Yvonne Crouch, Executive Director

Greater Monmouth VNA Hospice, 111 Union Avenue, Long Branch, NJ 07740

Hackensack Medical Center Hospice, 385 Prospect Avenue, Hackensack, NJ 07601; tel. 201/342-7766; FAX. 201/996-5993

Holy Redeemer Hospice, 1801 Route Nine North, P.O. Box 280A, Swainton, NJ 08210; tel. 609/465-2082; FAX. 609/465-6185; Arleen Moffitt, ACSW

Home Care Resources Hospice, 615 Hope Road, Building 3, First Floor, Eatontown, NJ 07724; tel. 908/935-1797; FAX. 908/935-0949

Hospice at Bergen Community Health Care, 400 Old Hook Road, Westwood, NJ 07675-3131; tel. 201/358-2900; FAX. 201/358-0836; Patricia Hutzelman, RN, Hospice Coordinator

Hospice of Morris County, 282 West Hanover Avenue, Morristown, NJ 07960; tel. 201/539-6l2l; FAX. 201/539-3975; Ann Liebers, Executive Director

Hospice of the VNA of the Delaware Valley, P.O. Box 441, 325 Jersey Street, Trenton, NJ 08611; tel. 609/695-3461; FAX. 609/771-8010

Hospice, Inc., Three High Street, Glen Ridge, NJ 07028-2306; tel. 201/429-0300; FAX. 201/429-9274; Lorraine M. Sciara, President

Hunterdon Hospice, Inc., 2100 Wescott Drive, Flemington, NJ 08822; tel. 901/788-3050; FAX. 901/788-6370; Catherine M. Keevey, President

Karen Ann Quinlan Center of Hope Hospice, 136 Woodside Avenue, Newton, NJ 07860; tel. 201/383-0115; FAX. 201/383-6889; Jackie Petrazzelli, Executive Director

Overlook Hospital Hospice, 33 Bleeker Street, Millburn, NJ 07041; tel. 201/379-8440; FAX. 201/379-8412

Passaic Valley Hospice, VHS of New Jersey, Inc., 783 Riverview Drive, P.O. Box 1007, Totowa, NJ 07511-1007; tel. 201/256-4636, ext. 257; FAX. 201/256-6757; Carol Lee O'Shea, Associate Director

Samaritan Hospice, 214 West Second Street, Moorestown, NJ 08057; tel. 800/229-8183; FAX. 609/778-0237; Clark D. Dingman, President, Chief Executive Officer

Somerset Valley Visiting Nurse Association Hospice, 586 East Main Street, Bridgewater, NJ 08807; tel. 201/725-9355; Maureen Bassinger, RN, MPA, Hospice Director

Trinity Hospice, 150 Ninth Street, Runnemede, NJ 08078; tel. 609/939-9000, ext. 157; FAX. 609/939-9010; Patricia Bevlock, Administrator

VNA of Central Jersey Hospice Program, 1100 Wayside Road, Tinton Falls, NJ 07712; tel. 908/493-2220; FAX. 908/493-4256; Barbara Buczny, Director

Valley Hospice, a Division of Valley Home, Inc., 505 Goffle Road, Ridgewood, NJ 07450; tel. 201/447-8822; FAX. 201/447-0105; Joan E. Schaper, Director

Visiting Nurse Association Somerset Hills Hospice, 12 Olcott Avenue, Bernardsville, NJ 07924; tel. 908/766-0180; FAX. 908/766-2268; Barbara Fox, Hospice Coordinator

Visiting Nurse and Health Services Hospice, 354 Union Avenue, P.O. Box 170, Elizabeth, NJ 07208; tel. 908/352-5694; FAX. 908/352-9216; Shirley Altman, Hospice Administrator

Vitas Health Care Corporation of Penn, Two Executive Campus, Route 70 & Cuthbert Road, Cherry Hill, NJ 08002; tel. 609/661-5600; FAX. 609/661-5650; Emily Fedullo, Director, Operations

West Essex Hospice, 799 Bloomfield Avenue, Verona, NJ 07044; tel. 201/857-7300; FAX. 201/857-3433; Janice Breen, President, Chief Executive Officer

NEW MEXICO

Caring Unlimited Hospice Services, 200 South Third, Raton, NM 87740; tel. 505/445-5113; Jo Ellen Ferguson, Administrator

Carlsbad Hospice, Inc., 1003 West Riverside Drive, P.O. Drawer PP, Carlsbad, NM 88220; tel. 505/885-8257; Nancy Flanagan, Administrator

Chaves County Home Health Services Hospice, 107 South Union Avenue, P.O. Box 237, Roswell, NM 88201; tel. 505/623-8000; John H. Taylor, L.N.H.A., Executive Director

Esperanza Home Health Care Hospice, Inc., Highway 518 Buena Vista, P.O. Box 270, Mora, NM 87732; tel. 505/387-2215; Josephine P. Garcia

Guadalupe Hospice, 110 South Halagueno, Carlsbad, NM 88220; tel. 505/887-7690; Brenda K. Jones, Administrator

Hospice Services, Inc., 90l East Bender, P.O. Box 249, Hobbs, NM 88241; tel. 800/658-6844; FAX. 505/393-3985; Brenda Chambers

Hospice of Artesia, 702 North 13th, Artesia, NM 88210; tel. 505/748-3333, ext. 306; Joyce Munoz

Lovelace Health Systems Inc. Hospice, 4308 Carlisle, Suite 101, Albuquerque, NM 87107; tel. 505/262-7745; Helen Karns, Administrator

Mesilla Valley Hospice, Inc., 125 Wyatt Drive, Las Cruces, NM 88005; tel. 505/523-4700; FAX. 505/527-2204; Margaret L. Connealy, M.S.W., Executive Director

Northwest New Mexico Hospice, 608 Reilly Avenue, P.O. Box 3336, Farmington, NM 87499; tel. 505/327-0301; FAX. 505/325-2477; Lizette Vannest, Program Coordinator

Professional Home Health Care, Inc., 1345 Pacheco Street, Santa Fe, NM 87505; tel. 505/982-8581; Debbie Conway

Roswell Hospice Home Care, 600 North Richardson, Roswell, NM 88201; tel. 505/623-5887; FAX. 505/624-8566; John Taylor, Executive Director

The Hospice Center, 1422 Paseo De Peralta, Santa Fe, NM 87501; tel. 505/988-2211; FAX. 505/986-1833; Ann Gerber, Executive Director

Victory Home Health Hospice, 1112 Fourth Street, Las Vegas, NM 87701; tel. 505/454-0499; Maria Luisa Padilla, Administrator

Visiting Nurse Service Hospice, 811 St. Michaels Drive, Santa Fe, NM 87505; tel. 505/984-2571; Janet Rose, Chief Executive Officer

NEW YORK

Brookhaven Memorial Hospital Medical Center Hospice, Four Phyllis Drive, Patchogue, NY 11772; tel. 516/758-3620; FAX. 516/758-3619

Capital District Hospice, Inc., a/k/a Hospice of Schenectady, Hospice of Saratoga, Hospice of Amsterdam, 1411 Union Street, Schenectady, NY 12308; tel. 518/377-8846; FAX. 518/377-8868; Philip G. Di Sorbo, Executive Director

Caring Community Hospice of Cortland, 4281 North Homer Avenue, Cortland, NY 13045; tel. 607/753-9105; Mary Beach, Administrator, Patient Care Coordinator

Catskill Area Hospice, Inc., 542 Main Street, Oneonta, NY 13820; tel. 607/432-6773; FAX. 607/432-7741; Lesley Deleski, Executive Director

Comstock Hospice Care Network, 1225 West State Street, Olean, NY 14760; tel. 716/372-2106; FAX. 716/372-4635; Kathleen Mack, Hospice Director

East End Hospice, Inc., 1111 Riverhead Road, P.O. Box 1048, Westhampton Beach, NY 11978; tel. 516/288-8400; FAX. 512/288-8492; Priscilla Ruffin, Executive Director

Good Samaritan Hospice, 175 Beach Drive, West Islip, NY 11795; tel. 516/321-7602; FAX. 516/321-7624; Kathleen Coffey, Administrator

Herkimer County Hospice, 267 North Main Street, Herkimer, NY 13350; tel. 315/867-1317; FAX. 315/867-1371; Sue Campagna, Administrator

High Peaks Hospice, Inc., P.O. Box 131, Old Lake Colby Drive, Saranac Lake, NY 12983; tel. 518/891-0606; FAX. 518/891-0657; Frances Filshie, Executive Director

Hospicare of Tompkins County, 301 Harris B Dates Drive, Ithaca, NY 14850; tel. 607/272-0212; FAX. 607/272-0237; Brenton C. Phillis, Executive Director

Hospice Buffalo, Inc., 4226 Ridge Lea Road, Amherst, NY 14226; tel. 716/838-4438; FAX. 716/837-1682; J. Donald Schumacher, Psy.D., President, Chief Executive Officer

Hospice Care of Long Island, Inc., 900 Ellison Avenue, Westbury, NY 11590; tel. 516/832-7100; FAX. 516/832-7160; Maureen Hinkleman, Chief Executive Officer

Providers / Freestanding Hospices

Hospice Care, Inc., 4277 Middlesettlement Road, New Hartford, NY 13413; tel. 315/735-6484; FAX. 315/735-8545; Sandra S. Huegel, Executive Director

Hospice Chautauqua County, Inc., Nine Park Street, P.O. Box 503, Sinclairville, NY 14782-0503; tel. 716/962-2010; FAX. 716/962-2020; Susan Schwartz, M.P.A., Executive Director

Hospice Family Care, 550 East Main Street, Batavia, NY 14020; tel. 716/343-7596; FAX. 716/343-7629; Deborah Schafer, Operating Director

Hospice VNSW/WPHC, Inc., d/b/a Hospice of Westchester, 360 Mamaroneck Avenue, White Plains, NY 10605; tel. 914/682-1484; FAX. 914/682-9425; Emily R. Giannattasio, Administrator

Hospice of Central New York, 1118 B Court Street, P.O. Box 69, Syracuse, NY 13208; tel. 315/476-5552; FAX. 315/476-5559; Peter Moberg-Sarver, Executive Director

Hospice of Chenango County, Inc., 156 North Broad Street, Norwich, NY 13815; tel. 607/334-3556; FAX. 607/336-1824; Laurie Vogel, Executive Director

Hospice of Dutchess County, 70 South Hamilton Street, Poughkeepsie, NY 12601; tel. 914/485-2273; Wayne Herron, Chief Executive Officer

Hospice of Jefferson County, Inc., 425 Washington Street, Watertown, NY 13601; tel. 315/788-7323; FAX. 315/785-9932; Frances Calabrese, Executive Director

Hospice of Northern Westchester and Putnam, VNA of Hudson Valley, 43 Kensico Drive, Mount Kisco, NY 10549; tel. 914/666-7616; FAX. 914/666-0378; Cornelia Schimert, Director

Hospice of Orange in Hudson Valley, Inc., 70 Dubois Street, Newburgh, NY 12550; tel. 914/561-6111; FAX. 914/561-2179; Daniel Grady, Executive Director

Hospice of Rochester and Hospice of Wayne and Seneca Counties, 49 Stone Street, Rochester, NY 14604; tel. 716/325-1880, ext. 1155; FAX. 716/325-7678; Sue Greer, RN, B.S.N., Vice President, Hospice Services

Hospice of South Shore, 14 Shore Lane, Bay Shore, NY 11706; tel. 516/666-4804; FAX. 516/666-4823; Lucille McCue, Executive Director

Hospice of St. Lawrence Valley, Inc., 6439 State Highway 56, P.O. Box 469, Potsdam, NY 13676; tel. 315/265-3105; FAX. 315/265-0323; Jonathan I. Lawrence, Executive Director

Hospice of the Finger Lakes, 25 William Street, Auburn, NY 13021; tel. 315/255-2733; FAX. 315/252-9080; Theresa A. Kenny, Executive Director

Hospice of the North Country, Inc., 386 Rugar Street, Plattsburgh, NY 12901; tel. 518/561-8465; FAX. 518/561-3182; Helena Madison, Executive Director

Jacob Perlow Hospice, Inc., 10 Nathan Perlman Place, New York, NY 10003; tel. 212/420-2844; FAX. 212/420-2420; Paul Brenner, Executive Director

Jansen Memorial Hospice/Home Nursing Association of Westchester, 69 Main Street, Tuckahoe, NY 10707; tel. 914/961-2818, ext. 307; FAX. 914/961-8654; Lucille D. Winton, Director

Livingston County Hospice, Two Livingston County Campus, Mount Morris, NY 14510; tel. 716/243-7290; FAX. 716/243-7287

Mercy Hospice, St. Pius X Service Center, 1220 Front Street, Uniondale, NY 11553; tel. 516/485-3060; FAX. 516/485-1007; Sister Dolores Castellano, Executive Director

Mountain Valley Hospice, 34 West Fulton Street, Gloversville, NY 12078; tel. 518/725-4545; FAX. 518/725-8066; Nancy Dowd, Executive Director

Niagara Hospice, Inc., 460 Wheatfield Street, Suite 201, North Tonawanda, NY 14120; tel. 716/695-7448; FAX. 716/695-7514; Carol E. Gettings, M.S., Executive Director

Oswego County Hospice, H. Douglas Barclay Court House, Pulaski, NY 13142; tel. 315/298-2233; FAX. 315/298-2718; Rupert J. Collins, Administrator

Pax Christi Hospice, 355 Bard Avenue, Staten Island, NY 10310; tel. 718/876-1022

Southern Tier Hospice, Inc., 244 West Water Street, Elmira, NY 14901; tel. 607/734-1570; FAX. 607/734-1902; Mary Ann Starbuck, Executive Director

St. Charles Hospice, 222 Belle Terre Road, Port Jefferson, NY 11777; tel. 516/474-4040; FAX. 516/474-4058; Marianne Gillan, Executive Director

The Brooklyn Hospice, 6323 Seventh Avenue, Brooklyn, NY 11220; tel. 718/921-7900; FAX. 718/921-0752; Abby Gordon, Administrator

Tioga County Hospice, 231 Main Street, Owego, NY 13827; tel. 607/687-0682; Janette Swindell, Administrator

United Hospice of Rockland, 18 Thiells-Mount Ivy Road, Pomona, NY 10970; tel. 914/354-5100; FAX. 914/354-2128; Amy Stern, Executive Director

V.N.S. Hospice of Suffolk, 505 Main Street, Northport, NY 11768; tel. 516/261-7200; FAX. 516/261-7364; Virginia Stein, RN, B.S.N., CRNI, Nurse Coordinator

VNSNY Hospice Care, 350 Fifth Avenue, New York, NY 10118; tel. 212/560-5952; FAX. 212/560-5836; Eileen Hanley, RN, M.B.A., Administrator

Visiting Nurse Hospice, 2180 Empire Boulevard, Webster, NY 14580; tel. 716/787-8315; FAX. 716/787-9726

NORTH CAROLINA

Albemarle Home Care, 103 Charles Street, P.O. Box 189, Elizabeth City, NC 27907; tel. 919/426-5488; Paula Vanhorn, Administrator

Albemarle Home Care, County Office Building, P.O. Box 189, Elizabeth City, NC 27907; tel. 919/482-7001; Angie Layden, Administrator

Albemarle Home Care, Highway 168, P.O. Box 189, Elizabeth City, NC 27907; tel. 919/232-2026; Victoria Rentrop, Administrator

Albemarle Home Care, South 343, Courthouse Complex, P.O. Box 189, Elizabeth City, NC 27907; tel. 919/338-4460; Kay Cherry, Administrator

Albemarle Home Care, 400 South Road Street, P.O. Box 189, Elizabeth City, NC 27907; tel. 919/338-4066; Wendy Bizzell

Caldwell County Hospice, Inc., 902 Kirkwood Street, N.W., Lenoir, NC 28645; tel. 704/754-0101; Cathy S. Simmons, Executive Director

Cashiers Home Health, Highway 107 South, 59 Hospital Road, Sylva, NC 28779; tel. 704/586-7410

Comprehensive Home Health Care, 3104 Randall Parkway, Wilmington, NC 28403; tel. 910/251-8111; Carolyn Mise, RN, Director, Operations

Comprehensive Home Health Care, 3840 Henderson Drive, Jacksonville, NC 28456; tel. 910/346-4800; Angela Brooks, Administrator

Comprehensive Home Health Care, 902 Jefferson Street, P.O. Box 366, Whiteville, NC 28472; tel. 910/642-5808; Kim Smith, Administrator

Comprehensive Home Health Care, 1120 Ocean Highway W, P.O. Box 200, Supply, NC 28462; tel. 910/754-8133, ext. 212; FAX. 910/754-2096; Crystal Floyd, RN, Director

Comprehensive Home Health Care and Comprehensive Hospice, Inc., 101 South Craig Street, P.O. Drawer 2540, Elizabethtown, NC 28337; tel. 910/862-8538; Sherry Hester, Administrator

Comprehensive Home Health Care/Comprehensive Hospice, 1800 Skibo Road, Suite 228, Fayetteville, NC 28303; tel. 910/864-8411; Jody Yaeger, Patient Care Coordinator

Craven County Home Health–Hospice Agency, 2818 Neuse Boulevard, P.O. Drawer 12610, New Bern, NC 28561; tel. 919/636-4930; FAX. 919/636-5301

Dare Hospice, (Dare Hospice, Inc.), P.O. Box 2511, Kill Devil Hills, NC 27948; tel. 919/441-6242; Mary A. Burrus, Administrator

Davie County Health Department, and Home Health, Hospice of Davie County, 210 Hospital Street, P.O. Box 665, Mocksville, NC 27028; tel. 704/634-8770; FAX. 704/634-0335; Janet Blair, RN, B.S.H.E., Nursing Supervisor

Duplin Home Care and Hospice Inc., Duplin Street, Kenansville, Box 887, Kenansville, NC 28349; tel. 919/296-0819; Janet B. Jones, RN, Director, Home Care Services

Duplin Homecare Hospice Inc., 101 East Main St., Wallace, NC 28466; tel. 919/285-1100; Tina Davis, Nursing Supervisor

Edgecombe County Home Care and Hospice, 2909 Main Street, Tarboro, NC 27886; tel. 919/641-7558; FAX. 919/641-7004; Jessie Worthington, Coordinator

Good Shepherd Home Health and Hospice Agency, 203 Hiawassee Street, P.O. Box 465, Hayesville, NC 28904; tel. 704/837-3430; Thomas J. Taaffe, Administrator

Health Horizons Home Health, 202 North Cedar Street, Suite B, Lumberton, NC 28358; tel. 910/671-5614; Alice Singletary, Administrator

Home Health Agency of Chapel Hill, Inc., 1101 Weaver Dairy Road, P.O. Box 4126, Chapel Hill, NC 27514; tel. 919/929-7149; Charles Milch, Administrator

Home Health Services of Cumberland County, Inc., 711 Executive Place, Suite 207, Fayetteville, NC 28305; tel. 910/483-3489; Elizabeth Hudspeth, Administrator

Home Health and Hospice Care, Inc., 1004 Jenkins Avenue, P.O. Box 190, Maysville, NC 28555; tel. 919/743-2800; Janet Haddow-Green, Administrator

Home Health and Hospice Care, Inc., 1023 Beaman Street, P.O. Box 852, Clinton, NC 28328; tel. 800/695-4442; FAX. 910/592-7392; Richard Stone, Administrator

Home Health and Hospice Care, Inc., 2419 East Ash Street, P.O. Box 11418, Goldsboro, NC 27532; tel. 800/879-4442; FAX. 919/731-4985; Tim Baker, Administrator

Home Health and Hospice Care, Inc., 702 B. W. H. Smith Boulevard, P.O. Box 795, Greenville, NC 27835; tel. 919/758-8212; Debbie Wampler, Administrator

Home Health and Hospice Care, Inc., 2305 Wellington Drive, Suite G, P.O. Box 3673, Wilson, NC 27895; tel. 919/291-4400; Debbie Wampler, Administrator

Home Health and Hospice Care, Inc., 15 Noble Street, P.O. Box 1524, Smithfield, NC 27577; tel. 919/934-0664; Michelle Fox, Administrator

Home Health and Hospice Care, Inc., 2419 East Ash Street, Suites Four and Five, P.O. Box 11418, Goldsboro, NC 27532; tel. 919/658-5036; FAX. 919/731-4985; Beverly Withrow, President

Home Health and Hospice Care, Inc., 2402 Wayne Memorial Drive, P.O. Box 88, Goldsboro, NC 27533-0088; tel. 919/735-1387; FAX. 919/735-8460; Beverly Withrow, President

Home Health and Hospice of Halifax, 1229 Weldon Road, Roanoke Rapids, NC 27870; tel. 919/308-0700; Sheila Alford, RN, Home Care Director

Homehealth and Hospice Care, Inc., 744 Airport Road, P.O. Box 1396, Kinston, NC 28503; tel. 919/527-9561; Ann Harrison, Clinical Director

Hometown Hospice, Inc., 1704 South Tarboro Street, P.O. Box 2303, Wilson, NC 27894; tel. 919/237-4333; FAX. 919/237-1125; Pattie Lotts, Administrator

Hospice Home, 918 Chapel Hill Road, Burlington, NC 27217; tel. 910/513-4460; FAX. 910/513-4471; Judy Bowman, Manager

Hospice at Charlotte, Inc., 1420 East Seventh Street, Charlotte, NC 28204; tel. 704/375-0100; FAX. 704/375-8623; Janet Fortner, President

Hospice at Greensboro, Inc., 2500 Summit Avenue, Greensboro, NC 27405; tel. 910/621-2500; FAX. 910/621-4516; Pamela Barrett, Executive Director

Hospice of Alamance-Caswell, 317 North Graham Hopedale Road, Burlington, NC 27217; tel. 919/570-5200; FAX. 919/570-3767; Peter Barcus, Executive Director

Hospice of Alexander County, Inc., 412 Third Street, S.W., Taylorsville, NC 28681; tel. 704/632-5026; FAX. 704/632-3707; Donna W. AuBuchon, Executive Director

Hospice of Alleghany, P.O. Box 1278, Sparta, NC 28675; tel. 910/373-8018; Wanda Branch, Administrator

Providers / Freestanding Hospices

Hospice of Ashe, Highway 88-16, P.O. Box 421, Jefferson City, NC 28640; tel. 704/265-3926; Wanda Branch, Administrator

Hospice of Avery County, Inc., P.O. Box 221, Newland, NC 28657; tel. 704/898-8581; FAX. 704/898-8582; Sharon Cole, RN, Patient Care Coordinator

Hospice of Burke County, Inc., P.O. Box 1579, Morganton, NC 28680; tel. 704/879-1601; FAX. 704/879-3500; A. Malanie Price, Executive Director

Hospice of Cabarrus County, Inc., 1060 Diploma Place, S.W., P.O. Box 1235, Concord, NC 28026-1235; tel. 704/788-9434; FAX. 704/788-6013; Shirley McDowell, Executive Director

Hospice of Carteret County, Inc., Eighth and Evans St. Webb, P.O. Box 3598, Morehead City, NC 28557; tel. 919/247-2808; Emily Nobles, Administrator

Hospice of Catawba Valley, Inc., 263 Third Avenue, N.W., Hickory, NC 28601; tel. 704/328-4200; FAX. 704/328-3031; Peter R. Prunkl, Executive Director

Hospice of Chatham County, Inc., 211 East Street, P.O. Box 1077, Pittsboro, NC 27312; tel. 919/542-5545; FAX. 919/542-6232; Susan H. Balfour, RN, Executive Director

Hospice of Cleveland County, Inc., 201 West Marion Street, Suite 306, Shelby, NC 28150; tel. 704/487-4677; FAX. 704/481-8050; Myra McGinnis Hamrick, Executive Director

Hospice of Davidson County, Inc., 524 South State Street, P.O. Box 1941, Lexington, NC 27293-1941; tel. 704/246-6185; FAX. 704/246-4574; Gary Drake, Executive Director

Hospice of Gaston County, Inc., 717 North New Hope Road Gastonia, Gastonia, NC 28054; tel. 704/861-8405; Eleanor Beasley, Executive Director

Hospice of Harnett County, Inc., 111A North Ellis Avenue, Dunn, NC, 28334, P.O. Box 373, Erwin, NC 28339; tel. 910/892-1213; FAX. 910/892-1229; Grace E. Tart, Administrator

Hospice of Henderson County, Inc., 802 Old Spartanburg Highway, P.O. Box 2395, Hendersonville, NC 28739; tel. 704/692-6178; FAX. 704/692-2365; Barbara W. Stewart, Executive Director

Hospice of Iredell County, Inc., 2347 Simonton Road, P.O. Box 822, Statesville, NC 28687; tel. 704/873-4719; FAX. 704/872-1810; Judy Snowden, Executive Director

Hospice of Lee County, Inc., P.O. Box 1181, Sanford, NC 27331-1181; tel. 919/774-4169; FAX. 919/774-6348; Janet MacLaren Scovil, Executive Director

Hospice of Lincoln County, Inc., 107 North Cedar Street, P.O. Box 1526, Lincolnton, NC 28093-1526; tel. 704/732-6146; FAX. 704/732-9808; Leona C. Ormand, Executive Director

Hospice of Macon County, Inc., 30 Roller Mill Road, P.O. Box 1594, Franklin, NC 28734; tel. 704/369-6641; Suzanne A. Owens, Executive Director

Hospice of McDowell County, Inc., East Court Street (County Administrative Building), P.O. Box 1072, Marion, NC 28752; tel. 704/652-1318

Hospice of Mitchell County, Inc., 188 C Highway 226 South, Bakersville, NC 28705; tel. 704/688-4090; FAX. 704/688-3566; Gloria Schulman, Executive Director

Hospice of Pamlico County, Inc., Main Street, Highway 55, P.O. Box 827, Bayboro, NC 28515; tel. 919/745-5171; Diane McDaniel, Executive Director

Hospice of Polk County, Inc., 423 Trade Street, Suite B, P.O. Box Y, Tryon, NC 28782; tel. 704/859-2270; FAX. 704/859-2731; Jean H. Eckert, Executive Director

Hospice of Randolph County, Inc., d/b/a Center of Living Healthcare, 416 Vision Drive, Zip 27203, P.O. Box 9, Asheboro, NC 27204-0009; tel. 910/672-9300, ext. 263; FAX. 910/672-0868; Billie Vuncannon, Chief Executive Officer, President

Hospice of Rockingham County, Inc., 2150 NC 65, P.O. Box 281, Wentworth, NC 27375; tel. 910/427-9022; FAX. 919/427-9030; Fran Hughes, Director

Hospice of Rowan County, Inc., 1410 North Main Street, P.O. Box 1603, Salisbury, NC 28144-1603; tel. 704/637-7645; FAX. 704/637-9901; Patricia A. Ashworth, Executive Director

Hospice of Rutherford County, Inc., 11 North Powell Street, P.O. Box 336, Forest City, NC 28043; tel. 704/245-0095; FAX. 704/248-1035; Rita Burch, Executive Director

Hospice of Scotland County, 600 South Main Street, Suite F, P.O. Box 1033, Laurinburg, NC 28353; tel. 910/276-7176; FAX. 910/276-1941; Linda McQueen, RN, Executive Director

Hospice of Stanly County, Inc., 620 North First Street, Albermarle, NC 28001-3405; tel. 704/983-4216; FAX. 704/983-6662; Elvin T. Henry, Executive Director

Hospice of Surry County, Inc., 1326 North Main Street, Mt. Airy, NC 27030; tel. 910/789-2922; FAX. 910/789-0856; Laney Johnson, Director

Hospice of Surry County, Inc., 827 North Bridge Street, Elkin, NC 28621; tel. 910/526-2650; FAX. 910/526-2383

Hospice of Tar Heel, 1003 South Clark Street, P.O. Box 1645, Greenville, NC 27835; tel. 919/758-4622; FAX. 919/758-7006; Judy Chaplinski, Patient Care Manager

Hospice of Union County, Inc., 700 West Roosevelt Boulevard, Monroe, NC 28110; tel. 704/292-2100; FAX. 704/292-2193; Lana R. McGuirt, Executive Director

Hospice of Wake County, Inc., 4513 Creedmoor Road, Suite 400, Raleigh, NC 27612; tel. 919/782-3959; FAX. 919/782-3598; Karolyn H. Kaye, Executive Director

Hospice of Watauga, 136 Furman Road, Route Five, Box 199, Boone, NC 28607; tel. 704/265-3926; Wanda Branch, Administrator

Hospice of Winston-Salem/Forsyth Co., Inc., 1100 South Stratford Road, Building C, Winston-Salem, NC 27103-3212; tel. 910/768-3972; FAX. 910/659-0461; Jo Ann Davis, Director, Operations

Hospice of Yancey County, 314 West Main Street, P.O. Box 471, Burnsville, NC 28714; tel. 704/682-9675; FAX. 704/682-4713; Donna Messenger, Executive Director

Hospice of the Piedmont, Inc., 213 North Lindsay, Suite 110, High Point, NC 27262; tel. 919/889-8446; Judy Frazier, RN, Patient Care Coordinator

Johnston Memorial Home Care and Hospice, 509 North Bright Leaf Boulevard, P.O. Box 1376, Smithfield, NC 27577; tel. 919/989-1560; Ann L. Jessup, Administrator

Lower Cape Fear Hospice, Inc., 810 Princess Street, Wilmington, NC 28401; tel. 910/762-0200; FAX. 910/762-9146; Eloise Thomas, Executive Director

Lower Cape Fear Hospice, Inc., 121 West Main Street, P.O. Box 636, Whiteville, NC 28472; tel. 919/642-9051; Barbara Godwin, RN, BSN, Patient Care Coordinator

Lower Cape Fear Hospice, Inc., 2507-B North Marine Boulevard, Jacksonville, NC 28546; tel. 919/347-6266; FAX. 910/347-9279; Lori Griffin, Patient Care Coordinator

Lower Cape Fear Hospice, Inc., 112 Pine Street, P.O. Box 1926, Shallotte, NC 28459; tel. 910/754-5356; Jeff Hickey, Director, Operations

Madison Home Care and Hospice, P.O. Box 909, 170 Carl Eller Road, Mars Hill, NC 28754; tel. 704/689-3491; FAX. 704/689-3496; John H. Estes, Executive Director

Medvisit, Inc., 1924 Ruin Creek Road, Suite 207, Henderson, NC 27536; tel. 919/492-6046; Sue Lightell, Administrator

Medvisit, Inc., Highway 39 North, Route Three, Box 48, Louisburg, NC 27549; tel. 919/496-1900; Sherry Watson, Administrator

Mountain Area Hospice, Inc., 75 Livingston Street, P.O. Box 16, Asheville, NC 28802; tel. 704/255-0231; FAX. 704/255-2880; Kit Cosgrove, Associate Director

Northern Hospital Home Care and Hospice, 933 Old Rockford Street, P.O. Box 1605, Mount Airy, NC 27030; tel. 910/719-7434; Mary Alice Culler, Administrator

Person County Home Health and Hospice, 325 South Morgan Street, Roxboro, NC 27573; tel. 910/597-2542; FAX. 910/597-4804; Joyce Franke, Administrator

Richmond County Hospice, Inc., 230 South Lawrence Street, P.O. Box 2136, Rockingham, NC 28379; tel. 910/997-4464; Lydia P. Talbert, RN, Patient Care Coordinator

Roanoke Home Care, 210 West Liberty Street, Williamston, NC 27892; tel. 919/792-5899; Barbara Owens, Administrator

Roanoke Home Care-Hospice, 408 Bridge Street, P.O. Box 238, Columbia, NC 27925; tel. 919/796-2681; Rena Grimsley, Administrator

Roanoke Home Care-Hospice, Route Two, Box 78R, Highway 45 North, Plymouth, NC 27962; tel. 919/793-3023; Phyllis McCombs, Administrator

Roanoke-Chowan Hospice, Inc., 521 Myers Street, P.O. Box 272, Ahoskie, NC 27910; tel. 919/332-3392; FAX. 919/332-5705; Brenda Hoggard, Director

Sandhills Hospice, Inc., Inverness Park, Five Aviemore Drive, P.O. Box 1956, Pinehurst, NC 28374; tel. 910/295-2220; FAX. 910/295-3720; Carole White, RN, Executive Director

St. Joseph Hospital Home Health Agency, 117 Worthan Street, P.O. Box 974, Wadesboro, NC 28170; tel. 704/694-5992; Kathy Appenzeller, Director, Daily Operations

St. Joseph Hospital Home Health Agency, Highway 24/27 South, Montgomery Square, Route Two, Box MS4, Troy, NC 27371; tel. 910/572-4962; Cynthia Furr, RN, Coordinator

St. Joseph Hospital Home Health Agency, 336 South Main Street, P.O. Box 879, Raeford, NC 28376; tel. 910/875-8198; Ronda Pickler, Administrator

Swain County Home Health Agency, 100 Teptal Terrance, P.O. Box 546, Bryson City, NC 28713; tel. 704/488-3198; R.D. Childers, Jr., Administrator

Swain County Home Health Agency, Serving Graham and Swain Counties, P.O. Box 546, Bryson City, NC 28713; tel. 704/488-3198; FAX. 704/488-8672; Betty DeHart, RN

Triangle Hospice, Inc., 1804 West Southern Parkway, Suite 112, Durham, NC 27707; tel. 919/490-8480; FAX. 919/493-0242; Carol Minton, M.S.W., M.P.H., Executive Director

Yadkin County Home Health/Hospice Agency, 217 Willow Street, P.O. Box 457, Yadkinville, NC 27055; tel. 910/679-4207; FAX. 910/679-6005

Your Hometown Hospice, 301 South Church Street, Suite 254, Rocky Mount, NC 27804; tel. 919/442-2531; Pattie Lotts, Administrator

Your Hometown Hospice, 101 A. West Freen Street, P.O. Box 2303, Wilson, NC 27894; tel. 919/747-4110; Pattie Lotts, Administrator

NORTH DAKOTA

Hospice of the Red River Valley, 702 28th Avenue, N., Fargo, ND 58102; tel. 701/237-4629; FAX. 701/280-9069; Dick Markstrom, Executive Director

Hospice of the Red River Valley, 702 28th Avenue North, Fargo, ND 58102; tel. 701/237-4629; FAX. 701/280-9069; Ann Malmberg, RN, Director, Patient Services

Trinity Hospice, 300 S.W. First Street, Minot, ND 58701; tel. 701/857-5083; Marilyn Bader, Administrator

OHIO

Allen Hospice, 5700 Southwyck Boulevard, Suite 111, Toledo, OH 43614; tel. 419/867-4655; FAX. 419/865-1601; Jane Wilcox, RN, Executive Director

Aultman Hospice Program, 4510 Dressler Road, N.W., Canton, OH 44718; tel. 216/493-3344; Kathy Cummings, RN, Program Coordinator

Bridge of Hope Hospice Inc., 317 Howell Avenue, Suite B, Cincinnati, OH 45220; tel. 513/221-5800

Providers / Freestanding Hospices

Community Hospice Care, 182 St. Francis Avenue, Rear Suite, Tiffin, OH 44883; tel. 800/834-8100; FAX. 419/447-4657; Rebecca S. Shank, Executive Director

Community Hospitals of Williams County–Hospice Care, 909 Snyder Avenue, Montpelier, OH 43543; tel. 419/485-3154, ext. 2378; FAX. 419/485-3833; Chris Kuehne, RN, Director

Crawford County Hospice, 1810 East Mansfield Street, Bucyrus, OH 44820; tel. 419/562-2001; FAX. 419/562-2803; Bert Maglott, RN, Executive Director

Home Nursing Service and Hospice, 900 Third Street, Second Floor, Marietta, OH 45750; tel. 614/373-8549; FAX. 614/373-3995; Pamela Parr, Director

Hospice Care Bethesda Division Buckeye HH, 2529 Maple Avenue, Zanesville, OH 43701; tel. 614/454-3384; FAX. 614/454-9470

Hospice Care of Williams Co., Inc., 127 West Butler Street, Bryan, OH 43506; tel. 419/636-8034; FAX. 419/636-8221; Kim M. Smith, RN, Executive Director

Hospice Home Care, Inc., 2055 Reading Road, Suite 240, Cincinnati, OH 45202; tel. 513/241-9209; FAX. 513/241-4012; Anthony Chase, President, Chief Executive Officer

Hospice Homecare, 341 South Third Street, Suite 301, Columbus, OH 43215; tel. 614/228-4414; FAX. 614/228-6278; Belinda R. Shaw, RN, Clinical Manager

Hospice Service of Licking County, Inc., 1435 B West Main Street, Newark, OH 43055; tel. 614/344-0311; FAX. 614/344-6577; James H. Moss, Executive Director

Hospice and Health Services of Fairfield County, 1111 East Main Street, Lancaster, OH 43130; tel. 614/654-7077; FAX. 614/654-6321; Donna J. Householder, Executive Director

Hospice at Riverside, 3595 Olentangy River Road, Columbus, OH 43214; tel. 614/261-5377; FAX. 614/566-4391

Hospice of Appalachia, 282 East State Street, P.O. Box 873, Athens, OH 45701; tel. 619/592-3493

Hospice of Care Corporation, 831 South Street, Chardon, OH 44024; tel. 216/338-6628; FAX. 216/286-7662; Elizabeth A. Petersen, RN, Vice President, Operations

Hospice of Cincinnati, Inc., 2710 Reading Road, Cincinnati, OH 45206; tel. 513/569-3100

Hospice of Columbus, 181 South Washington Boulevard, Columbus, OH 43215; tel. 614/645-6471; Jody Harper, Director

Hospice of Coshocton County, Inc., 1501 Walnut Street, P.O. Box 1284, Coshocton, OH 43812; tel. 614/623-4450; FAX. 614/623-4146; Barbara Brooks-Emmons, Director

Hospice of Darke County, Inc., 122 West Martz Street, Greenville, OH 45331; tel. 513/548-2999; FAX. 513/548-7144; Joy Marchal, Executive Director

Hospice of Dayton, Inc., 324 Wilmington Avenue, Dayton, OH 45420; tel. 513/256-4490; Betty Schmoll, President

Hospice of Fayette County, Inc., 216 West Court Street, Rear, P.O. Box 849, Washington Court House, OH 43160-0149; tel. 614/335-0149; FAX. 614/335-3489; Anne Bonzo, Executive Director

Hospice of Guernsey, Inc., 1300 Clark Street, P.O. Box 1537, Cambridge, OH 43725; tel. 614/432-7440; Patricia Howell, RN, Administrator

Hospice of Henry County, 104 East Washington, Suite 302, Napoleon, OH 43545; tel. 419/599-5545

Hospice of Knox County, 302 East High Street, Mount Vernon, OH 43050; tel. 614/397-5188; FAX. 614/397-5189; Anne Storan Mankins, Executive Director

Hospice of Medina County, 797 North Court Street, Medina, OH 44256; tel. 216/722-4771; FAX. 216/722-5266; Patricia M. Stropko-O'Leary, Executive Director

Hospice of Miami County, Inc., P.O. Box 502, Troy, OH 45373; tel. 513/335-5191; FAX. 513/335-8841; Sidney J. Pinkus, Chief Executive Officer

Hospice of Morrow County, P.O. Box 272, 851 West Marion Road, Mount Gilead, OH 43338; tel. 419/946-9822; Frances Turner, RN, Executive Director

Hospice of North Central Ohio, Inc., 1200 East Main Street, Ashland, OH 44805; tel. 419/281-7107; Ruth A. Lindsey, Executive Director

Hospice of Pickaway County, 702 Pickaway Street, Circleville, OH 43113; tel. 614/474-3525

Hospice of Stark County, 1445 Harrison Avenue, N.W., Suite 201, Canton, OH 44708; tel. 216/489-6855; FAX. 216/489-6868; Patricia Filigno, Clinical Specialist

Hospice of The Valley, Inc., 5190 Market Street, Youngstown, OH 44512; tel. 216/788-1992; FAX. 216/788-1998; Paul Easton, Executive Director

Hospice of Tuscarawas County, Inc., 125 East Second Street, Dover, OH 44622; tel. 216/343-7605; FAX. 216/343-3542; Janie Jones, Administrator

Hospice of V.N.A., 1195-C Professional Drive, Van Wert, OH 45891; tel. 419/238-9223; FAX. 419/238-9391; Donna Grimm, Director

Hospice of Visiting Nurse Service, 3358 Ridgewood Road, Akron, OH 44333; tel. 800/335-1455; Kathy Lukity, RN, OCN, Hospice Program Director

Hospice of Wayne County, Ohio, 2330 Cleveland Road, Wooster, OH 44691; tel. 216/264-4899; FAX. 216/264-4874; Mary Ellen Walsh, Executive Director

Hospice of Wyandot County, 320 West Maple Street, Suite C, Upper Sandusky, OH 43351; tel. 419/294-5787

Hospice of the Miami Valley, Inc., 930 Laurel Avenue, Hamilton, OH 45015; tel. 513/863-3433; FAX. 513/867-7444; Rebecca Hight, RN, President, Chief Executive Officer

Hospice of the Western Reserve, 300 East 185, Cleveland, OH 44110; tel. 216/383-2222; FAX. 216/383-3750; David A. Simpson, Executive Director

Hospice, The Caring Way of Defiance County, 197-C Island Park Avenue, Defiance, OH 43512; tel. 419/784-3818; FAX. 419/782-4979; Ruthann Czartoski, Hospice Coordinator

Loving Care Hospice, Inc., 106 West High Street, P.O. Box 445, London, OH 43140; tel. 614/852-7755

M J Nursing Registry, 2534 Victory Parkway, Cincinnati, OH 45206; tel. 513/961-1000; FAX. 513/872-7550; Jan Brown, RN, Assistant Administrator, Home Care

Madison County Home Health Hospice Inc., 212 North Main, London, OH 43140; tel. 614/852-3915; FAX. 614/852-5125

Mercy Hospice, 5350 Cornell Road, Cincinnati, OH 45242; tel. 513/489-6600

NCJW/Montefiore Hospice, One David N. Myers Parkway, Beachwood, OH 44122; tel. 216/360-9080, ext. 297; FAX. 216/360-9697; Jennifer Hooks, Hospice Director

New Life Hospice, Inc., 1212 North Abbe Road, Suite D, Elyria, OH 44035; tel. 216/365-5767; FAX. 216/365-4392; Micki M. Tubbs, President, Chief Executive Officer

Northwest Ohio Hospice Association, 3930 Sunforest Court, Toledo, OH 43623; tel. 419/479-3115; FAX. 419/479-3122; Virginia Clifford, Executive Director

Northwest Ohio Hospice Association, 3930 Sunforest Court, Suite 200, Toledo, OH 43623; tel. 419/479-3115; FAX. 419/479-3122

Southwest Hospice Services, 17951 Jefferson Park Road, Middleburg Heights, OH 44130; tel. 216/243-4082

Stein Hospice Service, Inc., 1200 Sycamore Line, Sandusky, OH 44870; tel. 419/625-5269; FAX. 419/625-5761; Rosalie A. Perry, Executive Director

The Bridge Hospice Care Center, 1815 South Main Street, Findlay, OH 45840; tel. 419/424-1050; Karen Mallett, RN, Ph.D., Executive Director

The Mount Carmel Hospice, 1144 Dublin Road, Columbus, OH 43215; tel. 614/234-0200; FAX. 614/234-0201; Mary Ann Gill, Director

Tricare Hospice, 701 Park Road, Bellefontaine, OH 43311; tel. 800/886-5936; FAX. 513/593-9783; Karen Byler, Director

United Home Care Hospice, 2400 Reading Road, Cincinnati, OH 45202-1468; tel. 513/345-8091; FAX. 513/345-8010

VNA of Cleveland Hospice, 2500 East 22nd Street, Cleveland, OH 44115; tel. 216/931-1450; FAX. 216/694-6355; Roberta Laurie, Executive Director, Hospice

Valley Hospice, Inc., One Ross Park, Steubenville, OH 43952; tel. 614/283-7487; FAX. 614/283-7507; Karen Nichols, RN, B.S.N., Executive Director

Visiting Nurse Service, Inc., Geauga County, 13221 Ravenna Road, Chardon, OH 44024; tel. 216/286-9461

Vitas Health Care Corporation of Ohio, 4700 Smith Road, Suite M, Cincinnati, OH 45212; tel. 513/531-6317; FAX. 513/531-7551; Dennis C. Bottonari, General Manager

Wilson Hospice Care, 915 West Michigan, Sidney, OH 45365; tel. 513/498-2311, ext. 2533; FAX. 513/498-4669; Martha Ernst, Director

OKLAHOMA

Blaine County Hospice, 203 North Weigle, P.O. Box 370, Watonga, OK 73772; tel. 405/623-7414; Pam Miller, RN

Carter Hospice Care, Inc., 1231 Sovereign Row, Suite A-1, Oklahoma City, OK 73108; tel. 405/942-1161; Carrie Mailand, RN

Community Hospice of Moore/Norman, 2424 Springer, Suite 105, Norman, OK 73069; tel. 405/360-4913; Vivian H. Davis

Community Hospice, Inc., 1400 South Broadway, Suite 100, Edmond, OK 73034; tel. 405/359-4884; L. Jim Anthis, Ph.D., Chief Executive Officer

Family Hospice of Greater Oklahoma City, 4900 Richmond Square, Suite 203, Oklahoma City, OK 73118; tel. 405/843-4097; FAX. 405/843-5629; Margaret Back, RN, Executive Director

Family Hospice of Tulsa, 7030 South Yale Avenue, Suite 412, Tulsa, OK 74136; tel. 918/488-9477; FAX. 918/488-9506; Bill Beck, B.A., Executive Director

Four Square Hospice, P.O. Box 544, Madill, OK 73446; tel. 405/795-9917; FAX. 405/795-5861; Sharron Watts

HealthWatch Home Health and Hospice, P.O. Box 374, Hydro, OK 73601; tel. 800/777-2735; FAX. 405/774-2251; Sharon Collins, RN, Hospice Coordinator

Hospice Care of Oklahoma, 5901 North Western, Suite 101, Oklahoma City, OK 73118; tel. 405/848-2324; Jean Calder, RN

Hospice Circle of Love, 605 South Monroe, Enid, OK 73701; tel. 405/234-2273; Cathy Graber, Director

Hospice of Central Oklahoma, 4549 Northwest 36th Street, Oklahoma City, OK 73122; tel. 405/491-0828; Sharon Holland, President

Hospice of Green Country, Inc., 3010 South Harvard, Suite 110, Tulsa, OK 74114-6136; tel. 918/747-2273; FAX. 918/747-2573; Becky Armstrong, Patient Care Coordinator

Hospice of Lawton Area, Inc., 1011 C Avenue, Suite One, Lawton, OK 73502; tel. 405/248-5885; FAX. 405/355-2446; Lee Young, Executive Director

Hospice of McAlester, First National Center, Suite 112, McAlester, OK 74501; tel. 918/423-3911; FAX. 918/426-6335; Vicki Schaff, Executive Director

Hospice of Oklahoma County, Inc., 4334 N.W. Expressway, Suite 106, Oklahoma City, OK 73116-1515; tel. 405/848-8884; FAX. 405/841-4899; Douglas M. Gibson, Executive Director

Hospice of Ponca City, 1904 North Union, Suite 103, Ponca City, OK 74601; tel. 405/762-9102; FAX. 405/762-9111; Melody Lahann, Director

Hospice of Woodard Pioneers, Inc., 1115 18th Street, Woodward, OK 73801; tel. 405/254-3024; Jackie Branson, RN, B.S.N., Executive Director

Providers / Freestanding Hospices

Judith Karman Hospice, Inc., 824 South Main Street, P.O. Box 818, Stillwater, OK 74076; tel. 405/377–8012; Mary Lee Warren, Executive Director

Mission Hospice, Inc., 7301 North Broadway, Suite 225, Oklahoma City, OK 73116; tel. 405/848–3779; FAX. 405/848–8481; Susan Osborne, RN, President

New Hope Hospice of Oklahoma, Inc., 6539 East 31st Street, Suite 14, Tulsa, OK 74145; tel. 918/622–7744; Jay Tipps, Director

Russell–Murray Hospice, Inc., 117 North Bickford, P.O. Box 1423, El Reno, OK 73036; tel. 405/262–3088; Cathie Sales, Administrator

The Hospice, 2023 West Broadway, Muskogee, OK 74401; tel. 918/683–1192; FAX. 918/687–0750; Jamie Bridgewater, Executive Director

Visiting Nurses Agency of Eastern Oklahoma, Inc., #2 Eastern Heights Shopping Center, P.O. Box 1647, Muldrow, OK 74948; tel. 918/427–1010; Mary Keith, RNC, Vice President

OREGON

Benton Hospice Service, Inc., 917 N.W. Grant Street, P.O. Box 100, Corvallis, OR 97333; tel. 503/757–9616; FAX. 503/757–1760; Judy List, Executive Director

Harney County Home Health/Hospice, 420 North Fairview, Burns, OR 97720; tel. 503/573–8360; FAX. 503/573–8389; Angela Ivey, Director

Hospice of Bend, 1303 N.W. Galveston, Bend, OR 97709; tel. 503/383–3910; FAX. 503/388–4221; Robert W. Luck, Executive Director

Hospice of Lebanon Community Hospital, 400 North Main Street, P.O. Box 611, Lebanon, OR 97355; tel. 503/451–7103; Alan Yordy, Chief Executive Officer

Hospice of Providence, 1180 Crater Lake Avenue, P.O. Box 4548, Medford, OR 97504; tel. 503/779–5033; FAX. 503/776–3980; James Beers, Administrator

Hospice of Redmond and Sisters, P.O. Box 1092, Redmond, OR 97756; tel. 503/548–7483; FAX. 503/548–1507; Ellen Garcia, Executive Director

Hospice of the Gorge, Inc., 13th and May Streets, P.O. Box 36, Hood River, OR 97031; tel. 503/387–6449; FAX. 503/387–6462; Ina Holman, Executive Director

Kaiser Permanente, Home Health/Hospice, 2701 N. W. Vaughn Street, Suite 140, Portland, OR 97210; tel. 503/499–5200; FAX. 503/499–5213; Linda Van Buren, RN, Administrator

Legacy VNA Hospice, 2701 N.W. Vaughn, Suite 720, P.O. Box 3426, Portland, OR 97208; tel. 503/220–1000; FAX. 503/225–6398; Linda Downey, Administrator

Lovejoy Hospice, Inc., 132 N.E. B Street, Suite 23, P.O. Box 356, Grants Pass, OR 97526; tel. 503/474–1193; FAX. 503/474–3035; Charlotte Carroll, RN, P.H.N., Executive Director

Lower Columbia Hospice, 2111 Exchange Street, Astoria, OR 97103; tel. 503/338–7540; FAX. 503/338–7590; Brenda Penner, RN, Manager

Lower Umpqua Hospice, 600 Ranch Road, Reedsport, OR 97467; tel. 503/271–2171, ext. 273; Geraldine Simms, RN, Manager

Mid–Willamette Valley Hospice, 1467 13th Street, S.E., Salem, OR 97302; tel. 503/588–3600; FAX. 503/363–3891; Simon B. Paquette, M.S.W., Administrator

Mt. Hood Hospice, 17270 S.E. Bluff Road, P.O. Box 835, Sandy, OR 97055; tel. 503/668–5545; FAX. 503/668–7951; Judith Wesley, Executive Director

Portland Adventist Hospice, 10201 S.E. Main Street, Suite One, Portland, OR 97216; tel. 503/251–6192; Jeanne Rowe, RN, Hospice Coordinator

Providence Hospice, 1235 N.E. 47th, Suite 215, 4805 N.E. Glisan (Mailing Address), Portland, OR 97213; tel. 503/331–4601; Beverly Bruender, Administrator

Providence Hospice at St. Vincent, 9340 S.W. Barnes Road, Suite M, Portland, OR 97225; tel. 503/297–6109; FAX. 503/297–6251; Karen Bell, RN, Regional Manager

South Coast Hospice, 371 West Anderson, Suite 218, Coos Bay, OR 97420; tel. 503/269–2986; FAX. 503/267–0458; Linda J. Furman, Administrator

Washington County Hospice, Inc., 427 S.E. Eighth Avenue, Hillsboro, OR 97123–4519; tel. 503/648–9565; FAX. 503/648–1282; Christine Larch, Administrator

Willamette Falls Hospice, 1678 Beavercreek Road, Suite K, Oregon City, OR 97045; tel. 503/655–0550; FAX. 503/655–7585; Robert Steed, Administrator

PENNSYLVANIA

Above All Home Health Care and Hospice, Inc., 808 South Main Street, Taylor, PA 18517; tel. 717/562–0422; Rosemary Blum, Administrator

Albert Gallatin Hospice Program, 20 Highland Park Drive, Suite 203, Uniontown, PA 15401; tel. 412/438–6660; FAX. 412/438–4468; Chris Constantine, RN, Administrator

Allegheny Hospice, Four Allegheny Center, Sixth Floor, Pittsburgh, PA 15212; tel. 412/330–4200; FAX. 412/330–4112; Earl Ash Evens, Administrator

Berks Visiting Nurse Association, Inc., 1170 Berkshire Boulevard, Wyomissing, PA 19610; tel. 610/378–0481; FAX. 610/378–9762; Lucille D. Gough, RN, M.S.N., M.B.A., President, Chief Executive Officer

Brandywine Hospice, 1219 East Lincoln Highway, Coatesville, PA 19320; tel. 610/384–4200; FAX. 610/384–6871; Dottie Anderson, Coordinator

Centre Hospice, A Program of Centre HomeCare, Inc., 221 West High Street, Bellefonte, PA 16823–1385; tel. 814/355–2273; FAX. 814/353–9292; Maureen Snedden, Coordinator

Chandler Hall Hospice, 99 Barclay Street, Newtown, PA 18940; tel. 215/860–4000; FAX. 215/860–3458; Jane W. Fox, Executive Director

Clarion Forest VNA Hospice, R.D. #3, Box 186, Clarion, PA 16214; tel. 814/226–1140; Jill R. Over, Administrator

Clearfield Hospital Home Health Service Hospice, 220 Merrill Street, P.O. Box 992, Clearfield, PA 16830; tel. 814/768–2012; Amelia Samuelson, Manager

Columbia–Montour Home Hospice, 480 Central Road, Bloomsburg, PA 17815; tel. 717/784–1723; FAX. 717/784–8512; Jane Gittler, Administrator

Community Nurses Professional Health Services/Hospice, 99 Erie Avenue, St. Marys, PA 15857; tel. 814/781–1415; FAX. 814/781–6987; Elizabeth A. Roberts, RN

Community Nursing Hospice, 119 Walnut Street, Walnut Plaza, 4th Floor, Johnstown, PA 15901; tel. 814/535–1817; FAX. 814/536–6101; Donna L. Russian, Administrator

Community Visiting Nurse Services Hospice, 1288 Valley Forge Road, Suite 57, Phoenixville, PA 19460; tel. 215/933–1263; Gerri Kucharik, RN, M.S.A., OCN, Hospice Supervisor

Compassionate Care Hospice, 100 Granite Drive, Suite 200, Media, PA 19063; tel. 610/892–7741; FAX. 610/892–7721; Catherine A. Stevens, Administrator

Crozer Hospice, One Medical Center Boulevard, Chester, PA 19013; tel. 215/447–6141; FAX. 215/447–6027; Patricia T. McCabe, RN, B.S.N., M.P.A., Director

Family Hospice, a/k/a South Hills Family Hospice, Inc., 1910 Cochran Road, Suite 500, Pittsburgh, PA 15220; tel. 412/572–8800; FAX. 412/572–8827; Baylee Gordon, Executive Director

Family Hospice of Indiana County, 119 Professional Center, 1265 Wayne Avenue, Indiana, PA 15701; tel. 412/463–8711; FAX. 412/463–8907; Susan K. Burkholder, RN, Director, Special Care Services

Forbes Hospice–Forbes Health System, 6655 Frankstown Avenue, Pittsburgh, PA 15206; tel. 412/665–3301; FAX. 412/665–3234; Maryanne Fello, RN, Manager

General Care Services, d/b/a Hospice of Warren County, Two Crescent Park, W., Warren, PA 16365; tel. 814/723–2455; FAX. 814/723–1177; Elsa L. Redding, Director

Guthrie Hospice, R.R. 4, P.O. Box 60A, Towanda, PA 18848; tel. 800/327–8039; FAX. 717/265–3570; Jocelyn O'Donnell, Administrator

HealthReach Home Care and Hospice, 409 South Second Street, Harrisburg, PA 17104; tel. 717/231–6363; Janet T. Foreman, RN, M.S., Director

Holy Redeemer, Nazarath and St. Mary Hospice Program, 12265 Townsend Road, Philadelphia, PA 19154; tel. 215/671–9200; FAX. 215/671–1950; Jerold S. Cohen, President

Home Hospice Agency of St. Francis, 131 Columbus Innerbelt, New Castle, PA 16101; tel. 412/652–8847; FAX. 412/656–0876; Sister Carmen Puhl

Home Nursing Agency/VNA Hospice Program, 201 Chestnut Avenue, P.O. Box 352, Altoona, PA 16603–0352; tel. 814/946–5411; FAX. 814/941–2482; Sylvia H. Schraff, RN, Chief Executive Officer

Hospice – The Bridge, Lewistown Hospital, 1126 W. Fourth Street, Lewistown, PA 17044–1909; tel. 717/242–5000; FAX. 717/242–7245; Shirley McNeal, RN, Manager

Hospice Care, Inc., 59 South Washington Street, P.O. Box 168, Waynesburg, PA 15370; tel. 412/627–8118; FAX. 412/627–3898; Catherine R. Shultz, M.S.W., L.S.W., Executive Director

Hospice Community Care, Inc., 385 Wyoming Avenue, Kingston, PA 18704; tel. 717/288–2288; FAX. 717/288–7424; Philip Decker, President

Hospice Program/VNA of Hanover and Spring Grove, 440 N. Madison Street, Hanover, PA 17331; tel. 717/637–1227; Sandra L. Wojtkowiak

Hospice Saint John, 665 Carey Avenue, Wilkes-Barre, PA 18702; tel. 717/823–2114; FAX. 717/823–6438; Thomas Pregent, Administrator

Hospice Services of the VNA of York County, 218 East Market Street, York, PA 17403; tel. 717/846–9900; FAX. 717/846–1933; Marie V. Fraser, President, Chief Executive Officer

Hospice Services, Inc., 154 Hindman Road, Butler, PA 16001; tel. 412/282–6806; FAX. 412/282–7517; Kristy Wright, RN, M.B.A., Vice President

Hospice of Central Pennsylvania, 98 South Enola Drive, P.O. Box 266, Enola, PA 17025; tel. 717/732–1000; FAX. 717/732–5348; Karen M. Paris, Chief Executive Officer

Hospice of Community and Home Health Services, 117 North Hanover Street, Carlisle, PA 17013; tel. 717/245–5600; FAX. 717/249–9346; Elizabeth Hain, RN, Administrator

Hospice of Crawford County, Inc., 747 Terrace Street, Meadville, PA 16335; tel. 814/337–8701; John E. Brown, Chief Executive Officer

Hospice of Lancaster County, 120 West Airport Road, P.O. Box 5179, Lancaster, PA 17606–5179; tel. 717/569–3900; FAX. 717/569–6787; Mary Graner, Executive Director

Hospice of North Penn Visiting Nurse Association, 51 Medical Campus Drive, Lansdale, PA 19446; tel. 215/855–8296; FAX. 215/855–1305; Ruth Anne Fritz, Director

Hospice of the Delaware Valley, 527 Plymouth Road, Suite 417, Plymouth Meeting, PA 19462; tel. 610/941–6700; FAX. 610/941–6440; Marcia M. Cook, Administrator

Hospice of the VNA of Bethlehem and Vicinity, 1510 Valley Center Parkway, Suite 200, Bethlehem, PA 18017; tel. 215/691–1100; FAX. 610/691–2271; Jean Fiore, RN, Administrator

Hospice of the VNA of Greater Philadelphia, One Winding Way, Philadelphia, PA 19131; tel. 215/581–2046; FAX. 215/473–5047; Beverly Paukstis, Administrator

HospiceCare of Pittsburgh, 11 Parkway Center, Suite 275, Pittsburgh, PA 15220; tel. 412/937–8088; Pat Myers, RN, Administrator

Lehigh Valley Hospice, 2166 South 12th Street, Allentown, PA 18103; tel. 610/402–7400; FAX. 610/402–7382; William V. Dunstan, Administrator

Providers / Freestanding Hospices

Lutheran Home Health Care Services/Hospice, 2700 Luther Drive, Chambersburg, PA 17201; tel. 717/264-8178; FAX. 717/264-6347; Diane M. Howell, Executive Director

McKean County VNA Hospice, 20 School Street, P.O. Box 465, Bradford, PA 16701-0465; tel. 814/362-7466; FAX. 814/362-2916; Elizabeth M. Costello, Administrator

Montgomery Hospital Hospice Program, 25 West Fornance Street, Norristown, PA 19401; tel. 610/272-1080; Jane M. Feinman, M.S.N.

Neighborhood Visiting Nurse Association, 795 East Marshall Street, West Chester, PA 19380; tel. 610/696-6511; FAX. 610/429-2470; Mahlon R. Fiscel, Chief Executive Officer

North Penn HH Agency/Hospice Program, 520 Rush Street, P.O. Box Eight, Blossburg, PA 16912; tel. 717/638-2141; Elaine Hickey, Administrator

Northeast Health and Hospice Care, Inc., 38 North Main Street, Pittston, PA 18640; tel. 717/457-2020; FAX. 717/654-0360; Stephan Hannon, Administrator

Olsten Kimberly QualityCare Hospice, 749 Northern Boulevard, Clarks Summit, PA 18411; tel. 800/870-0085; Peggy Durkin, Administrator

Professional Hospice Care, 3605 Vartan Way, Harrisburg, PA 17110; tel. 717/671-3700; FAX. 717/671-3713; Denise K. Harris, M.S.W., Director

Regional Home Health Service/Hospice, 1201 Grampian Boulevard, Suite Three A, Williamsport, PA 17701; tel. 717/323-9891; FAX. 717/323-0716; Carol J. Greene, RN, Executive Director

Ridgway Community Nurse Service, Inc., Hospice, 200 West Main Street, P.O. Box 179, Ridgway, PA 15853; tel. 814/773-5705; FAX. 814/776-6246; Catherine M. Grove, RN, Executive Director

SUN Home Hospice, 61 Duke Street, Northumberland, PA 17857; tel. 717/473-8320; FAX. 717/473-3070; Pat Campbell, Director

Sharon Regional Health System, Hospice Home Care, 490 North Kerrwood Drive, Suite 204, Hermitage, PA 16148; tel. 412/983-3878; Carole D. Welch, RN

St. Gregory's Hospice, Inc., R.D. Four, Box 314, Burgettstown, PA 15021; tel. 412/729-3051; FAX. 412/729-3820; Bernadine J. Eschner, RN, Administrator

Three Rivers Family Hospice, Inc., 3001 Jacks Run Road, White Oak, PA 15131; tel. 412/672-6737; FAX. 412/672-5823; Margaret K. Dennis, Executive Director

Unlimited Home Care, Inc., Hospice, P.O. Box 1070, Uniontown, PA 15401; tel. 412/439-1610; FAX. 412/439-1650; Diane Sanner, Director

Upper Bucks Hospice, 124 South Tenth Street, Quakertown, PA 18951; tel. 215/538-2232; R. Timothy Shimer, Administrator

VNA Community Services Hospice, 354 North Prince Street, P.O. Box 4304, Lancaster, PA 17604-4304; tel. 717/397-8251; FAX. 717/397-8666; Ann Burden, President

VNA Hospice, 334 Jefferson Avenue, Scranton, PA 18501; tel. 717/341-6840; Nancy S. Menapace, RN, M.A., Administrator

VNA Hospice Services of Erie County, 1305 Peach Street, Erie, PA 16501; tel. 814/454-2831; James J. Jaruszewicz, Administrator

VNA of Easton Hospice, 3421 Nightingale Drive, Easton, PA 18042; tel. 215/258-7189; Theresa P. Onorath

VNA of Pottstown and Vicinity Comprehensive Hospice Program, 1610 Medical Drive, First Floor, Pottstown, PA 19464; tel. 610/327-5700; FAX. 610/327-5701; Sandra Levengood, Executive Director

VNA/Hospice of Monroe County, Inc., R.R. Two, P.O. Box 2159A, Stroudsburg, PA 18360; tel. 717/421-5390; FAX. 717/421-7423; Mark Hodgson, Administrator

Visiting Nurse Association of Eastern Montgomery County, Department of Abington Memorial Hospital, 2510 Maryland Road, Suite 250, Willow Grove, PA 19090-0520; tel. 215/881-5800; FAX. 215/881-5850; Marilyn D. Harris, Administrator

Visiting Nurse Association of Northumberland County, 101 South Market Street, Shamokin, PA 17872; tel. 800/732-2486; FAX. 717/648-9590; Joseph L. Scopelliti, Jr., Executive Director

Visiting Nurses Association of the Lehigh Valley, Inc., 1710 Union Boulevard, Allentown, PA 18103; tel. 215/434-6134; Patricia Frenduto, President, Chief Executive Officer

Vitas Health Care Corporation, 805 East Germantown Pike, Suite 805, Norristown, PA 19401; tel. 215/275-2370; Emily B. Fedullo, RN, Director, Development

White Rose Hospice, 2870 Eastern Boulevard, York, PA 17402; tel. 717/840-0782; FAX. 717/849-5630; Susan M. Gordon, RN, Manager

Wissahickon Hospice, 8835 Germantown Avenue, Philadelphia, PA 19118; tel. 215/247-0277; FAX. 215/248-3253; Priscilla D. Kissick, RN, M.N., Executive Director

RHODE ISLAND

Hospice Care of Rhode Island, 169 George Street, Pawtucket, RI 02860-3868; tel. 401/727-7070; FAX. 401/727-7080; David Rehm, Executive Director

Hospice Care of the Visiting Nurse Service of Greater Woonsocket, Marquette Plaza, Woonsocket, RI 02895; tel. 401/769-5670; FAX. 401/762-2966; Elaine D. Bartro, RN, M.P.H., Chief Executive Officer

Hospice of VNS Washington County and Jamestown, 14 Woodruff Avenue, Naragansett, RI 02882-3467; tel. 401/788-2000; FAX. 401/788-2064; Lyle Mook, Director, Hospice Services

Kent County Visiting Nurse Association Hospice, Health Lane, Warwick, RI 02886; tel. 401/737-6050; FAX. 401/738-0247; Claire S. Connor, RN, Executive Director

VNA, Inc., 157 Waterman Avenue, Providence, RI 02906; tel. 401/444-9400; FAX. 401/444-9430; Sandra L. Hooper, RN, M.B.A., CNAA, Director, Adult Services

VNS Hospice of Newport County, 21 Chapel Street, Newport, RI 02840; tel. 800/849-2100; FAX. 401/849-7720; Florence M. Tankevich, RN, M.S., Director

Valley Hospice–VNS of Pawtucket, Central Falls, Lincoln and Cumberland, 172 Armistice Boulevard, Pawtucket, RI 02860; tel. 401/725-3414; FAX. 401/728-4999; Christopher L. Boys, Chief Executive Officer

SOUTH CAROLINA

Hitchcock Rehabilitation Center Home Health and Hospice, 690 Medical Park Drive, Aiken, SC 29801; tel. 803/648-8344, ext. 460; FAX. 803/649-4639; Gayle Jones, Director, Home Health, Hospice

Hospice Volunteers of the Low Country, 20 Palmetto Parkway, Hilton Head Island, SC 29926; tel. 803/681-7814; FAX. 803/681-7821; Carole B. Klein, Administrator

Hospice of Anderson, Inc., 800 North Fant Street, Anderson, SC 29621; tel. 803/261-1594; Nancy Garrett-Boyle, Administrator

Hospice of Charleston, Inc., 3896 Leeds Avenue, North Charleston, SC 29405; tel. 803/529-3100; FAX. 803/529-3111; Carol Younker, Executive Director

Hospice of Chesterfield County, Inc., 140 South Page Street, P.O. Box 293, Chesterfield, SC 29709; tel. 803/623-9155; FAX. 803/623-3833; Monnie W. Bittle, Executive Director

Hospice of Colleton County, Inc., 336 Walter Street, Walterboro, SC 29488; tel. 803/549-7337; FAX. 803/549-1451; Alfred S. Givens, Administrator

Hospice of Georgetown County, Inc., 1018 Huger Drive, P.O. Box 1436, Georgetown, SC 29442; tel. 803/546-3410; FAX. 803/527-6964; Brenda Stroup, RN, Executive Director

Hospice of Laurens County, Inc., 16 Peachtree Street, P.O. Box 178, Clinton, SC 29325; tel. 803/833-6287; FAX. 803/833-0556; Martha Ficklin, RN, Executive Director

Hospice of the Foothills, Inc., 807 Bypass 123, Suite 30, P.O. Box 245, Seneca, SC 29679; tel. 803/882-8940; Tenna W. Sines, Executive Director

Hospice of the Midlands, P.O. Box 7275, Columbia, SC 29202; tel. 803/364-9300; Jeanne Conrad

HospiceCare of the Piedmont, 303 West Alexander Street, Greenwood, SC 29646; tel. 803/227-9393; FAX. 803/227-9377; Nancy B. Corley, Director

Island Hospice, P.O. Box 6765, Hilton Head Island, SC 29938; tel. 803/842-6123; FAX. 803/842-4316; Mary Rose VanDeWeghe, Administrator

Mercy Hospice of Horry County, Columbus Plaza, 131 Wesley Street, P.O. Box 1409, Myrtle Beach, SC 29578; tel. 803/347-2282; FAX. 803/236-4306; Connie Fahey, FSM, Executive Director

Palmetto Hospice, 2711 Middleburg Drive, Suite 316, Columbia, SC 29204; Eve Barth

St. Francis Hospital Home Care – Hospice Services, 414 Pettigru Street, Greenville, SC 29601; tel. 803/233-5300; FAX. 803/233-4873; Paul H. Grier, Administrator

Tri–County Hospice, 29 Leinbach Drive, Building D, Charleston, SC 29407; tel. 803/852-2177; FAX. 803/769-0148; Louise T. Barnes, Chief Executive Officer

United Hospice, Inc., Third Street, Ridgeway, SC 29130; Jean Tilley

York County Hospice, Inc./Home Health, (Serving York and Chester Counties), 325 South Oakland Avenue, Rock Hill, SC 29730; tel. 803/329-4663; FAX. 803/329-5935; Tamra N. West, Director

TENNESSEE

A Plus Hospice, Inc., 116 Wilson Pike Circle, Suite 103, Brentwood, TN 37027; tel. 615/377-6276; FAX. 615/377-6287; Jessie Bynum, Director

Alive Hospice, Inc., 1718 Patterson Road, Nashville, TN 37203; tel. 615/327-1085; FAX. 615/327-1166; Sarah Gorodezky, Executive Director

Blount Memorial Hospital Hospice, 1095 East Lamar Alexander Parkway, Maryville, TN 37801

Bradley Memorial Hospital Hospice, 175 24th Street, Cleveland, TN 37311; tel. 615/559-6092, ext. 6969; FAX. 615/559-6093; Carolyn Marr, RN, CNA, Director

Comprehensive HHC Hospice Services, Inc., 208 A Court Street, Tazewell, TN 37879; tel. 615/626-0388; FAX. 615/626-0300; Jan Hamlin, Administrator, Coordinator

Friendship Hospice of Nashville, Inc., 1326 Eighth Avenue, N., Nashville, TN 37203; tel. 615/327-3950; Andre L. Lee, DPA, Chairman of the Board

Homecare Hospice, 211 Lee Avenue East, P.O. Box 308, McKenzie, TN 38201; tel. 901/352-2240; FAX. 901/352-5203; Renee Guerrero, RN, Hospice Coordinator

Homeward Bound Hospice, 1084 Bradford Hicks Drive, Livingston, TN 38570; tel. 615/823-2050; FAX. 615/823-1338; Denise Elder, RN

Hospice of Chattanooga, Inc., 165 Hamm Road, Chattanooga, TN 37405; tel. 615/267-6828; FAX. 615/756-4765; Viston Taylor III, Executive Director

Hospice of Cumberland County, Inc., 638 Rockwood Highway, P.O. Box 542, Crossville, TN 38557; tel. 615/484-4748; Lorraine Young, Executive Director

Hospice of Murfreesboro, 417 North Highland Avenue, Murfreesboro, TN 37130; tel. 615/896-4663; FAX. 615/896-4976; Sandra Jones, M.A., Director

Hospice of Tennessee, 521 West Main Street, Lebanon, TN 37087; tel. 800/889-4673; FAX. 615/444-2547

Hospice of Tennessee, Inc., 112 Louise Avenue, Nashville, TN 37203; tel. 615/320-9224

Housecall Hospice, 117 Center Park Drive, Suite 200, Knoxville, TN 37918; tel. 615/693-2474; FAX. 615/693-4031; Becki VanGuilder, Provider Relations Coordinator

Providers / Freestanding Hospices

Housecall Hospice, 100 Rogosin Drive, Suite B, Elizabethton, TN 37643; tel. 615/547-0852; FAX. 615/543-6449; Ed Peters, Assistant Regional Administrator

Housecall Hospice, 6025 Lee Highway, Executive Business Park, Chattanooga, TN 37421; tel. 615/892-2561; Caroline McBrayer

Housecall Hospice, 3343 Perimeter Hill Drive, Suite 102, Nashville, TN 37211; tel. 615/333-3995; FAX. 615/333-6997; Ray Acker, Administrator

Housecall Hospice, 630 South Cooper, Memphis, TN 38104; tel. 901/276-4948; FAX. 901/276-5785

Jackson Area Hospice, Madison Square Business Park, 77 Executive Drive, N., I-40 and Ridgecrest Road, Jackson, TN 38305; tel. 901/664-4220; FAX. 901/664-4231; Shirley Rowe, RN, Director

Jem Health Care Inc., 315 10th Avenue, N., Suite 109, Nashville, TN 37207; tel. 615/726-8668; FAX. 615/726-8665; Marilyn McClain, Administrator

Jesse Holman Jones Hospital HHA Hospice, 512 A Hill Street, Springfield, TN 37172; tel. 615/384-6323; FAX. 615/384-5102; Judy Suter, Hospice Coordinator

Lazarus House Hospice, Inc., 260 West Fifth Street, Cookeville, TN 38501; tel: 615/528-5133; J. Steve Mathias, Executive Director

Methodist Hospice and Health Care Services, Inc., d/b/a Methodist Hospice, 930 South White Station Road, Suite 100, Memphis, TN 38117; tel. 901/680-0169; FAX. 901/537-2109; Caby Byrne, Director

Procare Support Services, Inc., 374 North Parkway, Suite 7, Jackson, TN 38305; tel. 800/467-3480; FAX. 901/664-7399; Elaine Kirk, Director

Smoky Mountain Hospice, Inc., 324 West Broadway, Newport, TN 37821

Tennessee Nursing Services of Knoxville, 1530 West Andrew Johnson Highway, Morristown, TN 37816; tel. 615/586-6808

Tennessee Nursing Services of Morristown, Coldwell Bank Building, 415 North Fairmont, Morristown, TN 37816

Tri-County Home Health and Hospice, 115 Vicksburg Avenue, Camden, TN 38320; tel. 901/584-1927; FAX. 901/584-0401

Trinity Hospice, 1049 Cresthaven Road, Memphis, TN 38119; tel. 901/767-6767; FAX. 901/767-4627; Bradford A. Austin, RN, Hospice Director

UTMK Home Care Services Hospice Program, 2200 Sutherland Avenue, 1924 Alcoa Highway 42, Knoxville, TN 37920; tel. 615/544-6200; FAX. 615/544-6240; Carolyn Foster, RN, Director

University Home Health and Hospice, Inc., 135 Kennedy Drive, Martin, TN 38237; tel. 901/587-2996; FAX. 800/627-3228; Joann Newbill, RN, Executive Director

Willowbrook Hospice, Inc., 220 Second Avenue South, Franklin, TN 37064; tel. 800/790-8499; Jim Herrod, Director

TEXAS

AIM Hospice, 703 East Concho, P.O. Box 2300, Rockport, TX 78381-2300; tel. 512/729-0507; FAX. 512/790-0243; Kathleen J. Akin, Administrator

Ann's Haven Hospice, 216 West Mulberry, Denton, TX 76201; tel. 817/566-6550; FAX. 817/383-4000; Rebecca S. Rabinowitz, Chief Executive Officer

Ark-La-Tex Health and Hospice Care, 6500 Summerhill Road, Three Crown Center, Texarkana, TX 75503; tel. 903/792-6430; FAX. 903/792-5537; Doyle Land, Administrator

Burton Hospice Care, Inc., 6640 Eastex Freeway, Suite 140, Beaumont, TX 77708; tel. 409/892-7476; FAX. 409/892-7740; Vergie A. Burton, Administrator

Circle of Life Hospice, 2512 A Grandview, Odesa, TX 79761; tel. 915/367-7771; Jo Cheryl Miller, Administrator

Community Care Services, Inc., 403 East Blackjack, Dublin, TX 76446; tel. 817/445-4675; Bobbie Nichols, Administrator

Community Hospice of Waco, 3215 Pine Avenue, Waco, TX 76708; tel. 817/756-6911; FAX. 817/756-0029; Richard E. Scott, President

Country Nurses, Inc. Hospice, 608 A North Rockwall Street, Terrell, TX 75160; tel. 214/563-2415; FAX. 214/563-4042; Carla Menasco, RN, B.S.N.

Cross Timbers Hospice, 103 East Frey, Stephenville, TX 76401; tel. 817/968-6142; FAX. 817/965-2388; Jan Hoover, RN, Administrator

Crown of Texas Hospice, 1000 South Jefferson, Amarillo, TX 79101; tel. 806/372-7696; FAX. 806/372-2825; Sharla Roselius, B.S.N., RN, President

Crown of Texas Hospice, 100 I-45 North, Suite 100, P.O. Box 103, Conroe, TX 77301; tel. 409/788-7707; FAX. 409/788-7708; Elizabeth Tilley, RN, Patient/Family Care Coordinator

Cypress Basin Hospice, Inc., 414 North Van Buren Street, P.O. Box 544, Mount Pleasant, TX 75455; tel. 903/577-1510; FAX. 903/577-9377; Edd C. Hess, Executive Director

Denson Community Hospice, 1100 Gulf Freeway, N., Suite 122, League City, TX 77573; tel. 713/332-4970; FAX. 713/338-1766; Suzanne Denson, Administrator

Family Hospice of Dallas, 1140 Empire Central, Suite 235, Dallas, TX 75247; tel. 214/631-7273; FAX. 214/630-4032; Jim Grant, RN, B.S.N., Executive Director

Family Hospice of Fort Worth, 4040 Fossil Creek Boulevard, Suite 204, Fort Worth, TX 76137; tel. 817/232-3492; FAX. 817/232-3499; Sally Day, RN, B.S.N., Executive Director

Family Hospice of San Antonio, 6800 Park Ten Boulevard, Suite 110 North, San Antonio, TX 78213-4201; tel. 210/738-8141; FAX. 210/738-3507; Bernadine Dailey, RN, B.S.N., Executive Director

Family Service, Inc., 1424 Hemphill Street, Fort Worth, TX 76104-4790; tel. 817/927-8884, ext. 219; FAX. 817/926-0701; Glen J. Good, President

Harris Hospice, 1418 Rosedale, Fort Worth, TX 76104; tel. 817/877-0307; Serene Smith, Administrator

Heart of Texas Hospice, Inc., 17 N. 25th, Temple, TX 76504; tel. 800/643-5139; FAX. 817/742-2023; Bob Fisher, Administrator

Heart of the Valley Hospice, 320 North Williams Road, San Benito, TX 78586; tel. 800/333-6131; FAX. 210/399-3553; Rebecca Hernandez, RN, Administrator

Home Health Specialists, Inc., 813 South Palestine, Athens, TX 75751; tel. 800/801-8126; FAX. 903/657-9513; Donna Isabell, Administrator

Home Hospice, 505 West Center Street, P.O. Box 2306, Sherman, TX 75091; tel. 903/868-9315; FAX. 903/893-2772; Marty Barr, Executive Director

HospiCenter of Texas, Inc., d/b/a HospiCenter of Houston, 8203 Willow Place South, Suite 530, Houston, TX 77070; tel. 713/469-7990; FAX. 713/894-1294; Melven R. Nehleber, Administrator

Hospice Austin, 3710 Cedar Street, Suite 299, Austin, TX 78705; tel. 512/458-3261; FAX. 512/467-0767; Marjorie D. Mulanax, Executive Director

Hospice Family Care, Inc., 1408 19th Street, Lubbock, TX 79401; tel. 806/765-6111; Marjorie Calvert, Administrator

Hospice Highland Lakes, 2001 South Water Street, Burnet, TX 78611; tel. 512/756-8003; FAX. 512/756-8046; Pam Reagor, RN, Director

Hospice Kerrville, 28710 IH 10 West, Boerne, TX 78006; tel. 210/755-9011; Mark J. Bigott, Administrator

Hospice New Braunfels, 613 North Walnut, New Braunfels, TX 78130; tel. 512/625-7500; Jack Melton, Administrator

Hospice San Antonio, Inc., 8207 Callaghan, Suite 355, San Antonio, TX 78230; tel. 210/377-3882; FAX. 210/349-4896; Frederick W. Hines, Executive Director

Hospice Uvalde Area, (a program of Hospice San Antonio), P.O. Box 5280, Uvalde, TX 78802-5280; tel. 210/278-6691; FAX. 210/278-8925; Rene Hill, Administrative Assistant

Hospice in the Pines, 116 South Raguet, Lufkin, TX 75904; tel. 800/324-8557; FAX. 409/632-1352; Cheryl Lindsey, Intake Coordinator

Hospice of Abilene, Inc., 1682 Hickory, P.O. Box 1922, Abilene, TX 79601; tel. 915/677-8516; FAX. 915/675-5031; Sandi Saringer, Executive Director

Hospice of Brazos Valley, Inc., 2729 A East 29th Street, Bryan, TX 77802; tel. 409/776-0793; FAX. 409/774-0041; John Foster, B.S., M.S., CPM, Executive Director

Hospice of Canyon, Two Hospital Drive, Canyon, TX 79015; tel. 806/655-3062; FAX. 806/655-4784; Michele Webb, Director

Hospice of Cedar Lake, 114 South Gun Barrel Lane, Suite One, Gun Barrel City, TX 75147; tel. 903/887-3772; FAX. 903/887-3700; Karen Gilmore, Director

Hospice of Central Texas, 2007 B Medical Parkway, San Marcos, TX 78666; tel. 512/754-7584; FAX. 512/754-7521; Pat Huber, L.M.S.W., A.C.P, Team Leader

Hospice of East Texas, 3800 Paluxy, Suite 560, Tyler, TX 75703; tel. 903/581-5585; FAX. 903/581-5293; Michael C. Couch, Executive Director

Hospice of El Paso, Inc., 3901 North Mesa, Suite 400, El Paso, TX 79902; tel. 915/532-5699; FAX. 915/532-7822; Charles E. Roark, FACHE

Hospice of Galveston County, Inc., 1708 Amburn Road, Suite C, Texas City, TX 77591; tel. 409/938-0070; FAX. 409/938-1509; Sue Mistretta, Executive Director

Hospice of Hope, 801 East Campbell, Suite 300, Richardson, TX 75081; tel. 214/680-5010; Price Daniel, Administrator

Hospice of Longview, Inc., 802 Medical Circle, Suite C, Longview, TX 75601; tel. 903/753-7870; Stephanie Foster, Executive Director

Hospice of Lubbock, Inc., 4314 South Loop 289, Zip 79413, P.O. Box 53276, Lubbock, TX 79453; tel. 806/795-2751; FAX. 806/795-8464; Lee Battey, RN, M.S.

Hospice of Mercy, 500 West Third Avenue, Suite Two, Corsicana, TX 75110; tel. 800/852-5526; FAX. 903/872-4499; Ann Massey, Administrator

Hospice of Midland, Inc., 911 West Texas, Midland, TX 79701; tel. 915/682-2855; FAX. 915/682-2989; Carol Armstrong, Executive Director

Hospice of North Texas, 1420 Pioneer Road, Mesquite, TX 75149; tel. 214/285-8081; FAX. 214/288-0742; Beckie Ferguson, Administrator

Hospice of North Texas, 700 Elm, Graham, TX 76450; tel. 817/549-9704; Ruby Jeffreys, Administrator

Hospice of San Angelo, Inc., 16A East Beauregard, P.O. Box 471, San Angelo, TX 76902; tel. 915/658-6524; David McBride, Executive Director

Hospice of South Texas, 2001 East Sabine, Suite 102, Victoria, TX 77901; tel. 512/572-4300; FAX. 512/572-4532; Doug Eaves, Executive Director

Hospice of St. Michael Hospital of Texarkana, 1425–A College Drive, Texarkana, TX 75501; tel. 903/793-3303; Tommy McGee, Administrator

Hospice of Texarkana, Inc., 803 Spruce Street, Texarkana, TX 75501; tel. 214/794-4263; FAX. 501/744-1108; Cynthia L. Marsh, Administrator

Hospice of V.N.A., 2905 Sackett, Houston, TX 77098; tel. 713/520-8115; FAX. 713/520-6054; Dr. Maggie Kao, Executive Director

Hospice of Wichita Falls, 4909 Johnson, Wichita Falls, TX 76310; tel. 817/691-0982; FAX. 817/691-1608; Jan Banta, Executive Director

Hospice of the Big Bend, 611 East Avenue E, Alpine, TX 79830-4817; tel. 915/837-7286; FAX. 915/837-1132; Marvie Burton, RN, Patient Care Coordinator, Executive Director

Hospice of the Big Country, Inc., 3113 Oldham Lane, Abilene, TX 79602; tel. 915/677-1191; FAX. 915/677-1808; Danna L. Clouse, Administrator

© 1995 AHA Guide — Health Organizations, Agencies and Providers

Providers / Freestanding Hospices

Hospice of the Panhandle, 120 West Kingsmill, P.O. Box 2782, 79066–2782, Pampa, TX 79065; tel. 806/665–6677; Sherry McCavit, Executive Director

Hospice of the Plains, Inc., 7109 Olton Road, Plainview, TX 79072; tel. 806/293–5127; FAX. 806/293–5902; Roxey Williams, Executive Director

Hospice of the Southwest, Inc., 3800 East 42nd Street, Suite 500, P.O. Box 14710, Odessa, TX 79768–4710; tel. 915/362–1431; FAX. 915/362–1468; Connie Brinker, Executive Director

Houston Hospice, 8811 Gaylord, Suite 100, Houston, TX 77024; tel. 713/468–2441; FAX. 713/468–0879; Margaret Caddy, RN, Executive Director

Huguley Hospice Care, 11801 South Freeway, Ft. Worth, TX 76115; tel. 817/551–2545; FAX. 817/568–3294; Donna Reddell, RN, Director

La Mariposa Hospice, 2001 North Oregon, El Paso, TX 79902; tel. 915/452–6802; Frances Witt, Director

Lakes Area Hospice, 254 Ethel Street, Jasper, TX 75951; tel. 409/384–5995; Jeanette Coffield, Executive Director

Lifeline Home Health Services, Inc., 4301 Saturn Road, Suite 200, Garland, TX 75041; tel. 214/271–2022; Deanna Beauchamp, Administrator

Lone Star Hospice, 1212 Palm Valley Boulevard, Round Rock, TX 78664; tel. 512/218–9890; FAX. 512/218–9288; Janet A. Baker, Administrator

Managed Home Health Care, 4675–A Washington Boulevard, Beaumont, TX 77707; tel. 409/842–2255; FAX. 409/842–2369; J. Clayton Moore, Administrator

McCuistion Hospice, 2875 Lewis Lane, Paris, TX 75460; tel. 903/784–3359; FAX. 903/737–0903; Linda Kennedy, RN, Director

Mediplex Hospice, Inc., Two Village Drive, Suite 500, Abilene, TX 79606; tel. 915/691–5747; William O. Ulmer, Chief Executive Officer

Memorial Hospice, 115 West First Street, Dumas, TX 79029; tel. 806/935–7171; David D. Clark, CHE, Administrator, Chief Executive Officer

Ochiltree Hospital District, d/b/a Hospice of Ochiltree County, 2402 South Main, Perryton, TX 79070–5223; tel. 806/435–2122; FAX. 806/435–2318; Wallace Boyd, Administrator

Santa Rosa Hospice, 5115 Medical Drive, Villa Rosa Hospital, Cottage E, San Antonio, TX 78229; tel. 210/705–5252; FAX. 210/705–5270; Debra Garcia, Director

Spohn Hospice, 1660 South Staples, Corpus Christi, TX 78404; tel. 512/881–3159; FAX. 512/881–3755; Rita Mueller, RN, Director

St. Anthony's Hospice and Life Enrichment Program, 600 North Tyler, Zip 79107, P.O. Box 950, Amarillo, TX 79176–0001; tel. 806/378–6777; FAX. 806/378–5031; Lezlie Roberson, Executive Director

Stephen's Hospice, 353 West Live Oak, Dublin, TX 76446; tel. 817/445–4620; Lavinia Ann Stephen, Administrator

The Hospice at the Texas Medical Center, 1905 Holcombe Boulevard, Houston, TX 77030; tel. 713/467–7423; FAX. 713/799–9227; Randal A. Condit, Director, Operations

The Southeast Texas Hospice, Inc., 912 West Cherry, P.O. Box 2385, Orange, TX 77630; tel. 409/886–0622; FAX. 409/886–0623; Mary McKenna, Administrator

The Visiting Nurse Association of Texas Hospice, 1440 West Mockingbird Lane, Suite 500, Dallas, TX 75247–4929; tel. 214/689–0000; FAX. 214/689–0010; Mary C. Suther, President

Thee Hospice, P.O. Box 6548, Huntsville, TX 77342–6548; tel. 800/999–5935; FAX. 409/291–8582; Marilyn Louther, Administrator

Tomlinson Health Services, Hospice Program, 1300 West Mockingbird, Suite 160, Dallas, TX 75247; tel. 214/630–8847; FAX. 817/573–3160; Reba Tomlinson, Chief Executive Officer

Tyler Hospice, 423 South Beckham Avenue, Tyler, TX 75701; tel. 903/592–9703; FAX. 903/593–0639; Sandra L. Bunch, Administrator

Ultimate Hospice Care, 2300 Highway 365, Suite 510, Nederland, TX 77627; tel. 409/727–2885; Lewanna D. Jones, Administrator

VNA Hospice of Brazoria County, 112 N. Munson, Angleton, TX 77515; tel. 409/848–8441; FAX. 409/848–8572; Jenny Carswell, Administrator

Visiting Nurse Association Hospice, 212 Brown Street, Brownwood, TX 76801; tel. 915/646–6500; FAX. 915/646–6412; Mary Suther, President, Chief Executive Officer

Vitas Healthcare Corporation, 5001 LBJ Freeway, Suite 1050, Dallas, TX 75244; tel. 214/661–2004; FAX. 214/661–3474; David C. Gasmire, General Manager

Vitas Healthcare Corporation, 4828 Loop Central Drive, Suite 890, Houston, TX 77081; tel. 713/663–7777; FAX. 713/663–4990, ext. 4912; Diane Incognito, General Manager

Vitas Healthcare Corporation, 801 West Freeway, Suite 620, Grand Prairie, TX 75051; tel. 214/269–4200; Gene Schulle, Director, Operations

Vitas Healthcare Corporation, 4241 Piedras Drive East, Suite 111, San Antonio, TX 78228; tel. 210/731–4300; FAX. 210/731–4380; Ruth R. Castillo, Administrator

Vitas Healthcare Corporation, 211 East Parkwood, Suite 211, Friendswood, TX 77546; tel. 713/996–4400; Diane A. Incognito

UTAH

CNS Community Hospice, 2970 South Main, Suite 300, Salt Lake City, UT 84115; tel. 801/461–9500; FAX. 801/486–2193; Grant C. Howarth, Administrator

Creekside Hospice Care, 1935 East Vine Street, Suite 350, Salt Lake City, UT 84123; tel. 801/272–8617; FAX. 801/277–3790; Maryann Pales, Administrator

Dixie Regional Home Health Hospice, 354 East 400 North, Suite 304, St. George, UT 84770; tel. 801/634–4567; FAX. 801/634–4564; Kathy Andrus, RN, Administrator

Hospice of Cache Valley, 1400 North 500 East, Logan, UT 84341; tel. 801/750–5477; FAX. 801/750–5361; Neil C. Perkes, RN, M.B.A., Administrator

Hospice of Northern Utah, 2404 Washington Boulevard, Suite 304, Ogden, UT 84401; tel. 801/399–5232; FAX. 801/399–2742; Suzanne Phillips, Administrator

IHC Home Health Agency–Hospice of IHC, 2250 South 1300 West, Suite A, Salt Lake City, UT 84119; tel. 801/977–9900; FAX. 801/977–9956; Shauna Einerson, Administrator

VERMONT

Addison County Hospice, Inc., Charter House, P.O. Box 772, Middlebury, VT 05753; tel. 802/388–4111; Catherine Studley, Executive Director

Bennington Area Home Health Agency, Inc., 324 Main Street, Box 603, Bennington, VT 05201; tel. 802/442–5502; Pat Hurley, Executive Director

Brattleboro Area Hospice, P.O. Box l053, 40 High Street, Brattleboro, VT 05301; tel. 802/257–0775; Amy Martyn, Administrator

Caledonia Home Health Agency–Hospice, Sherman Drive, P.O. Box 383, St. Johnsbury, VT 05819; tel. 802/748–9405; FAX. 802/748–4540; Brenda B. Smith, Director, Home Care, Hospice

Central Vermont Home Health and Hospice, Inc., R.R. Three, Box 6694, Barre, VT 05641; tel. 802/223–1878; Diana Peirce, RN, CRNH, Director

Franklin County Home Health and Hospice, Three Home Health Circle, St. Albans, VT 05478; tel. 802/527–7531; FAX. 802/527–7533; Janet McCarthy, Executive Director

Hospice of Bennington County, Inc., P.O. Box 1231, Bennington, VT 05201; tel. 802/447–0307; Amy Barber–Thomas, Executive Director

Hospice of Champlain Valley, 25 Prim Road, Colchester, VT 05446; tel. 802/860–4410; FAX. 802/860–6149; Barbara Segal, RN, M.S., Program Director

Hospice of the Upper Valley, Inc./Hospice VNH, 20 South Main Street, White River Junction, VT 05001; tel. 603/448–5182; FAX. 603/448–1599; Marie Kirn, Executive Director, Chief Executive Officer

Lamoille Home Health and Hospice, R.R. Three, Box 790, Farr Avenue, Morrisville, VT 05661; tel. 802/888–4651; Linda Taft, Home Care Supervisor

Orleans Essex VNA and Hospice, Inc., Three Lakemont Road, Newport, VT 05855–1550; tel. 802/334–5213, ext. 19; FAX. 802/334–8822, ext. 45; Diana Hamilton, RN, Director

Randolph Area Hospice, Five Maple Street, Randolph, VT 05060; tel. 802/728–5059, ext. 2273; Carol Reid

Rutland Area Hospice, Inc., P.O. Box 924, Rutland, VT 05702; tel. 802/775–3009; Jane Taylor, Director, Hospice Programs, Coordinator, Hospice Volunteers

Rutland Area Visiting Nurse Association, Seven Albert Cree Drive, Rutland, VT 05701; tel. 802/775–0568; FAX. 802/775–2304; Sally Tobin, Associate Director, Community Health Programs

Southern Vermont Home Health Agency, Five Belmont Avenue, Brattleboro, VT 05301; tel. 802/257–4390; FAX. 802/257–8831; Ellen Bristol, RN

Springfield Area Hospice, Inc., 366 River Street, Springfield, VT 05156; tel. 802/886–2525; Marisa Bolognese, Volunteer Coordinator

Visiting Nurse Alliance of Vermont and New Hampshire, 20 South Main Street, Old Court House, White River Junction, VT 05001; tel. 802/295–2604; FAX. 802/295–3163; Betsy Davis

VIRGINIA

Blue Ridge Hospice, Inc., 333 West Cork Street, Winchester, VA 22601; tel. 703/665–5210; FAX. 703/678–0584; Carol A. Horne, Executive Director

Blue Ridge Hospice, Inc., 1870 Amherst Street, Level G, Winchester, VA 22601; tel. 703/667–8464; Carol A. Horne, Executive Director

Cana Hospice, Route One, P.O. Box Nine, Cana, VA 24317; tel. 800/719–7434; Dee Eadie, Manager

Commonwealth Home Nursing and Hospice, Inc., 990 Main Street, Danville, VA 24541; tel. 804/792–4663; Robert S. McFarland, Chief Administrator

Edmarc Hospice for Children, 1131 Crawford Parkway, P.O. Box 7188, Portsmouth, VA 23707; tel. 804/397–0432; FAX. 804/397–5827; Julie S. Sligh, Executive Director

Familycare Home Care and Hospice Services, 610 Laurel Street, P.O. Box 592, Culpeper, VA 22701; tel. 703/829–4140; FAX. 703/825–0307; William A. Gravely, President

Good Samaritan Hospice, Inc., 3528 Electric Road, Suite A, Roanoke, VA 24018; tel. 703/776–0198; FAX. 703/776–0841; Sue Moore, President

Hospice Choice, Inc., 444 Orby Cantrell Highway, South, P.O. Box 359, Big Stone Gap, VA 24219; tel. 703/523–7208; FAX. 703/523–1103; Wesley T. Polly, Administrator

Hospice of Central Virginia, 406 Chatham Square Office Park, 312 Butler Road, Falmouth, VA 22405; tel. 703/899–6433; FAX. 703/899–6328; Susan Tamburro, Administrator

Hospice of Northern Virginia, Inc., 6400 Arlington Boulevard, Suite 1000, Falls Church, VA 22042; tel. 703/534–7070; FAX. 703/538–2163; David J. English, President, Chief Executive Officer

Hospice of Northern Virginia, Inc., 11166 Main Street, Suite 401, Fairfax, VA 22030; tel. 703/525–7070; Karen Price Woods, Acting Administrator

Hospice of Northern Virginia, Inc., 885 Harrison Street, S.E., Leesburg, VA 22075; tel. 703/777–7866; FAX. 703/771–8904; Elisabeth A. Murphy, NP, CRNH, Regional Vice President

Hospice of Roanoke Memorial Hospitals, 127 McClanahan Street, Suite 101, Roanoke, VA 24014; tel. 703/981–7802; Robert E. Lee, Jr., Vice President

Providers / Freestanding Hospices

Hospice of Wythe–Bland, Inc., 275 East Main Street, P.O. Box 381, Wytheville, VA 24382; tel. 703/228–5424; Rita C. Cobbs, Executive Director

Hospice of the Hills, 3300 Rivermont Avenue, Lynchburg, VA 24503; tel. 804/947–3204; Linda H. Vitale, Director

Hospice of the Piedmont, Inc., 1290 Seminole Trail, Charlottesville, VA 22901; tel. 804/975–5500; FAX. 804/975–4040; Victoria Todd, Executive Director

Hospice of the Piedmont, Inc., 1002 East Jefferson Street, Charlottesville, VA 22901; tel. 804/971–3995; Virginia Kelly, Executive Director

Hospice of the Rapidan, Inc., 763 Madison Road, Suite 203, P.O. Box 715, Culpeper, VA 22701; tel. 703/825–4840; Jean Falk Morgan, Executive Director

Hospice of the Rapidan, Inc., 1200 Sunset Lane, Suite 2320, Culpeper, VA 22701; tel. 703/825–4840; FAX. 703/825–7752; Jean Falk Morgan, Executive Director

House Call Hospice, 603–605 King Street, Fourth Floor, Alexandria, VA 22314; tel. 703/548–2197; Ray Evans, President

Housecall Hospice, 2167 Apperson Drive, Salem, VA 24153; tel. 703/776–3207; FAX. 703/776–3215; Nancy Kelderhouse, Regional Administrator

Housecall Hospice, Two Main Street, P.O. Box 850, Jonesville, VA 24263; tel. 703/346–1095; Faye Carson, Administrator

New River Valley Hospice, Inc., 111 West Main Street, Christiansburg, VA 24073; tel. 703/381–5001; FAX. 703/381–5008; Judith B. Brach, Executive Director

Rockbridge Area Hospice, Inc., 129 South Randolph Street, P.O. Box 948, Lexington, VA 24450; tel. 703/463–1848; FAX. 703/463–1848; Susan Hogg, Executive Director

Thomas Hospice of Retreat Hospital, 2922 West Marshal Street, Richmond, VA 23230; tel. 804/254–9700; Florence M. Weierbach, RNC, B.S.N., Director

VNA Community Hospice, 2775 South Quincy Street, Suite 260, Arlington, VA 22206; tel. 703/824–5200; FAX. 703/824–5228; Eileen L. Dohmann, Executive Director

WASHINGTON

Associated Health Services, 737 South Fawcett Street, Tacoma, WA 98402; tel. 206/552–1825, ext. 1819; FAX. 206/552–1838; Pam Knudsen, Associate Administrator

Assured Home Health Agency Hospice, 1817 South Market Boulevard, Chehalis, WA 98532; tel. 360/748–0151; FAX. 360/748–0518; Wilma Wayson, RN, B.S.N., Director

Central Basin Home Health and Hospice, 410 West Third Avenue, Moses Lake, WA 98837; tel. 509/765–1856; FAX. 509/765–3323; Joanne C. Petersen, Executive Director

Community Home Health and Hospice, 1035 11th Avenue, Longview, WA 98632; tel. 360/425–8510; FAX. 360/425–7180

Community Hospice, 5610 Kitsap Way, Suite 301, Bremerton, WA 98312; tel. 206/373–5280; FAX. 206/373–5398

Evergreen Home Health and Hospice, 12910 Totem Lake Boulevard, N.E., Suite 217, Kirkland, WA 98034; tel. 206/899–3300; FAX. 206/899–1033

Group Health Cooperative Hospice Program, 2100 124th, N.E., Suite 110, Bellevue, WA 98005; tel. 206/882–2022; FAX. 206/881–7147; Marcia Harding, Program Administrator

Harbors Home Health and Hospice, 201 Seventh Street, Hoquiam, WA 98550; tel. 360/532–5454; DeLila Thorp

Home Health Plus Hospice, 13810 Southeast Eastgate Way, Suite 100, Bellevue, WA 98005; tel. 206/644–3027; FAX. 206/644–3286; Carrie Malmberg, RN

Home Health and Hospice of Southeastern Washington, South 106 Mill Street, Colfax, WA 99111; tel. 509/334–6016; FAX. 509/397–4650; Terri Maldonado, Chief Executive Officer

Hospice Northwest, 1550 North 115th, Seattle, WA 98133; tel. 206/368–1794

Hospice of Kitsap County, 1007 Scott Avenue, Suite D, Bremerton, WA 98310; tel. 206/479–1749; FAX. 206/479–5800; Don Tarbutton, MHA, Executive Director

Hospice of Snohomish County, 2731 Wetmore Avenue, Suite 520, Everett, WA 98201–3581; tel. 206/261–4800; FAX. 206/258–1097; Mary L. Brueggeman, Executive Director

Hospice of Spokane, West 1325 First Avenue, Suite 200, P.O. Box 2215, Spokane, WA 99210; tel. 509/456–0438; FAX. 509/458–0359

Hospice of Whatcom County, 600 Birchwood Avenue, Bellingham, WA 98225; tel. 206/733–5877; FAX. 360/734–9621

Hospice of the Palouse, 803 South Jefferson, P.O. Box 9461, Moscow, ID 83843–0119; tel. 208/882–1228; FAX. 208/883–2239

Kaiser Permanente Home Health/Hospice, 2701 N.W. Vaughn Street, Suite 140, Portland, OR 97210–5398; tel. 503/499–5200; FAX. 503/499–5213; Linda Van Buren, Administrator

Lower Valley Hospice, P.O. Box 719/10th and Tacoma, Sunnyside, WA 98944; tel. 509/837–1676; FAX. 509/837–8622; Geoff Piper, Executive Director

Okanogan Regional Home Health Care Agency, 217 Second Avenue South, Okanogan, WA 98840; tel. 509/422–6721; Bernice Hartzell, Executive Director

Providence Homecare/Hospice of Seattle, 425 Pontius Avenue, N., Suite 300, Seattle, WA 98109; tel. 206/320–4000; FAX. 206/320–3804; Robert Anderson, Administrator, Home Services

Providence Hospice of Yakima, 110 South Ninth Avenue, Yakima, WA 98902; tel. 509/575–5093; Glenda Abercrombie, RN, Manager

SoundHomeCare, 3706 Griffin Lane, S.E., Olympia, WA 98501; tel. 360/459–8311; FAX. 360/493–4657; Alice G. Armstrong, Chief Executive Officer

Swedish Home Health and Hospice and Infusion, 5701 Sixth Avenue, S., Suite 504, Seattle, WA 98108–2522; tel. 206/386–6602; FAX. 206/386–6613

Tri-Cities Chaplaincy/Hospice, 7525 West Deschutes Place, Suite–Two A, Kennewick, WA 99336; tel. 509/783–7416; FAX. 509/735–7850; Thomas H. Halazon, Executive Director

Walla Walla Community Hospice, P.O. Box 2026, 35 Jade Street, Walla Walla, WA 99362; tel. 509/525–5561; Marlow B. Wootton, Executive Director

WEST VIRGINIA

Albert Gallatin Hospice, 3280 University Avenue, Morgantown, WV 25605; tel. 304/598–0226; Christine Constantine, Administrator

Community Home Care and Hospice, 1209 Warwood Avenue, Wheeling, WV 26003; tel. 304/277–1503; FAX. 304/277–1507; Katherine Holstein, RN, Administrator

Dignity Hospice, P.O. Box 4455, Chapmanville, WV 25508; tel. 304/855–7104; Regina Bias, RN, M.S.N., OCN, Director

GlenWood Park Hospice, c/o GlenWood Park, Inc., Route One, Box 464, Princeton, WV 24740; tel. 304/425–8128; Daniel W. Farley, Ph.D., CNHA, President, Chief Executive Officer

Greenbrier Valley Hospice, Inc., 400 North Lee Street, Lewisburg, WV 24901; tel. 304/645–2700; Tim Bailes, Executive Director

Hospice Care Corporation, 321 Garden Towers, P.O. Box 229, Kingwood, WV 26537; tel. 304/329–1161; FAX. 304/329–3285; Malene J. Davis, RN, Executive Director

Hospice Care of the Virginias, Inc., P.O. Box 328, Bluefield, WV 24701; tel. 304/325–7220; Vicki Webb, Executive Director

Hospice of Huntington, 1101 Sixth Avenue, P.O. Box 464, Huntington, WV 25709; tel. 304/529–4217; FAX. 304/523–6051; Charlene Farrell, Executive Director

Hospice of Marion County, P.O. Box 1112, Fairmont, WV 26555–1112; tel. 304/366–0700, ext. 312; FAX. 304/366–9529; Karen Cummins, Administrator

Hospice of South West Virginia, P.O. Box 1472, Beckley, WV 25802; tel. 304/255–6404; FAX. 304/255–6494; Thomas A. Williams, Executive Director

Hospice of the Panhandle, Inc., 306 West Burke Street, Martinsburg, WV 25401; tel. 304/264–0406; FAX. 304/264–0409; Margaret Cogswell, RN, Executive Director

House Calls Hospice, Inc., 914 Market Street, Suite 301, Parkersburg, WV 26101; tel. 304/422–7225; FAX. 304/422–7902; Penny Bauer, Director

Jackson County Community Hospice, Walnut Street, P.O. Box 754, Ravenswood, WV 26164; tel. 304/273–9520; Uda Wiggins, Program Director

Journey Hospice, 314 South Wells Street, Sisterville, WV 26175; tel. 304/652–2611; Robert L. Kunz, Administrator

Kanawha Hospice Care, Inc., 1143 Dunbar Avenue, Dunbar, WV 25064; tel. 304/768–8523; FAX. 304/768–8627; Linda Y. Stevens, Executive Director

Monongalia County Health Department Hospice, 453 Van Voorhis Road, Morgantown, WV 26505–3408; tel. 304/598–5500; FAX. 304/598–5167; Gabriele Votta, Coordinator

Morgantown Hospice, 1159 Van Voorhis Road, Suite B, P.O. Box 4222, Morgantown, WV 26505; tel. 304/285–2777; Margaret M. Kearney, Executive Director

Mountain Hospice, Inc., P.O. Box 661, Philippi, WV 26416; tel. 304/457–2180, ext. 323; FAX. 304/457–1516; Dorothy Hayhurst, Director

People's Hospice, United Hospital Center, P.O. Box 1680, Clarksburg, WV 26302–1680; tel. 304/623–0524; FAX. 304/623–3399; William R. VanGieson, Director

St. Gregory's Hospice, Inc., 836 Charles Street, Wellsburg, WV 26070; tel. 800/252–7290; FAX. 304/737–0871; Patricia Murphy, RN, M.S.N., Director

St. Joseph's Hospice, 92 West Main Street, Buckannon, WV 26201; tel. 304/472–6846; Sandra Knotts, Director

Unity Hospice, 24 Garton Plaza, Weston, WV 26452; tel. 304/269–6432; Chryl Drummond, Supervisor

Valley Hospice, One Ross Park, Steubenville, OK 43952; tel. 614/264–7161; Karen Nichols, Executive Director

WISCONSIN

All Saints VNA–Hospice/Racine, 4000 Spring Street, P.O. Box 4045, Racine, WI 53404; tel. 414/635–7580; FAX. 414/633–7332; Debra Ostroski, Administrator

Beloit Hospice, Inc., 2958 Prairie Avenue, Beloit, WI 53511; tel. 608/363–7421; Virginia Young–Meyer, Administrator

C. Ross Hospice Home Care, 4041 North Richards Street, Suite 100, Milwaukee, WI 53212; tel. 414/963–7600; Lee D. Critchfield

Community Home Hospice, 3149 Saemann Avenue, Sheboygan, WI 53081; tel. 414/457–5770; FAX. 414/457–5951; M. Kaye Christman, Administrator

Dr. Kate–Lakeland Hospice, P.O. Box 770, Woodruff, WI 54568; tel. 715/356–8805; FAX. 715/358–7299; Karen Jeselun, RN, Administrator

Grancare Hospice, W136 N5283 Campbell Court, Menomonee Falls, WI 53051; tel. 414/252–5303; Phyllis Locicero, Administrator

Grant County Coping/Hospice, 111 South Jefferson Street, Lancaster, WI 53813; tel. 608/723–6416; FAX. 608/723–6501; Linda S. Adrian, Director, Health Officer

Hillside Homecare/Hospice, 709 South University Avenue, Beaver Dam, WI 53916; tel. 414/887–4050, ext. 4182; FAX. 414/887–6815; Jane Belongie

Holy Family Memorial Medical Center–Hospice, 2300 Wollmer, P.O. Box 1450, Manitowoc, WI 54221; tel. 414/684–2417; FAX. 414/684–2489; Karen Deehr, Director

Home Health United Hospice, 520 South Boulevard, P.O. Box 527, Baraboo, WI 53913; tel. 608/356–2288; FAX. 608/356–2290; Thomas H. Brown, President

Providers / Freestanding Hospices

Hope Hospice, Inc., 709 McComb Avenue, P.O. Box 237, Rib Lake, WI 54470; tel. 715/427-3532; FAX. 715/427-3537; Barbara Meyer, Director

Horizon Home Care and Hospice, Inc., 1720 West Florist Avenue, Glendale, WI 53209; tel. 414/351-8300; FAX. 414/351-8338; Cathy D. Ott, Associate Administrator

Hospice Alliance, Inc., 3410 80th Street, Kenosha, WI 53142; tel. 414/942-1630; Ron DeGolier, Executive Director

Hospice Program, 333 Pine Ridge Boulevard, Wausau, WI 54401; tel. 715/847-2702; Linda F. Grilley

Hospice Program of Waupaca County, 811 Harding Street, Waupaca, WI 54981; tel. 715/258-6323; Barbara J. Black

Hospice Team Care, Inc., 2100 East Milwaukee Street, Janesville, WI 53545; tel. 608/755-1871; Judith Balcitis, Administrator

Hospice of Portage County, 2232 Prais, P.O. Box 1017, Stevens Point, WI 54481; tel. 715/346-5355; FAX. 715/345-1304; Judy N. Mason

HospiceCare, Inc., 2802 Coho Street, Suite 100, Madison, WI 53713-4521; tel. 608/276-4660; FAX. 608/276-4672; Susan Phillips, Executive Director

Jefferson Home Health and Hospice, 1203 Eighth Street, P.O. Box 117, Baraboo, WI 53913; tel. 608/356-7570; FAX. 608/356-2629; William J. Hamilton, Jr., Managing Director

LaCrosse Visiting Nurses Hospice, 900 Monitor Street, LaCrosse, WI 54601; tel. 608/796-1666; FAX. 608/787-4655; Sandra J. Holter, Administrator

Lafayette County Hospice, 740 East Street, Darlington, WI 53530; tel. 608/776-4895; Kristi Lueck, RN, Coordinator

Manitowoc County Community Hospice, 1004 Washington Street, Manitowoc, WI 54220; tel. 414/684-7155; FAX. 414/684-1991; Lynn Seidl-Babcock, RN, B.S.N., Administrator

Mayo Hospice Program, 200 First Street, S.W., Rochester, MN 55905; tel. 507/284-4002; Margaret M. Gillard, RN, Program Director

Memorial Hospice, Inc., 320 Detroit Avenue, Iron Mountain, MI 49801; tel. 906/774-5589; Peter Carli, Director

Mercy Medical Center V.N. Hospice, 515 South Washburn, Suite 206, Oshkosh, WI 54904; tel. 414/236-8820; Michael Drees, Administrator

Milwaukee Hospice Home Care and Residence, 4067 North 92nd Street, Wauwatosa, WI 53222; tel. 414/438-8000; FAX. 414/438-8010; James Ewens, Mary New, Co-Directors

Mount Carmel Home Hospice, 5700 West Layton Avenue, Milwaukee, WI 53220; tel. 414/281-7200, ext. 350; FAX. 414/281-1666; Donna Borgealt, Hospice Director

Northwest Wisconsin HomeCare/Hospice, 2321 East Clairemont Parkway, P.O. Box 2060, Eau Claire, WI 54702-2060; tel. 715/831-0100; FAX. 715/831-0108; Faith Garnatz, RN, Director, Hospice Services

Rainbow Hospice Care, LLC, 147 West Rockwell Street, Jefferson, WI 53549; tel. 414/674-6255; FAX. 414/674-5288; Ingrid A. Forgy, Administrator

Red Wing Hospice, 434 West Fourth, Suite 200, Red Wing, MN 55066; tel. 612/385-3410; FAX. 612/385-3414; Peggy Wolner, B.S.N., L.S.W.

Regional Hospice, 2101 Beaser Avenue, Ashland, WI 54806; tel. 715/682-8677; FAX. 715/682-6404; Phil Garrison, Executive Director

Rolland Nelson Memorial Home Hospice, 419 Frederick Street, Waukesha, WI 53186; tel. 414/542-0724; FAX. 414/542-0608; Jacalyn Burdick, Program Manager

Seton Hospice, 2266 North Prospect Avenue, Milwaukee, WI 53202; tel. 414/291-1300; FAX. 414/291-1319; Judith Lindsey, Manager

Unity Hospice, 801 East Walnut, Green Bay, WI 54301; tel. 414/433-7470; FAX. 414/437-1934; Donald W. Seibel

Unity Hospice, 212 South 11th Street, LaCrosse, WI 54601; tel. 608/791-9790; FAX. 608/791-9548; Marilyn Viehl, Administrator

V.N.A. Home Care and Hospice, 201 East Bell Street, Neenah, WI 54956; tel. 414/727-5555; FAX. 414/727-5552; Judith Eberhardy, President, Chief Executive Officer

VNA Community Hospice, 11333 West National Avenue, Milwaukee, WI 53227; tel. 414/327-2295; FAX. 414/328-4499; Mary Runge, Chief Operating Officer

Visiting Nurse Association Comfortcare Hospice, 3306 Superior Avenue, Sheboygan, WI 53081; tel. 414/458-4314; FAX. 414/458-1819; Robert W. Walters, President

Visiting Nurse Association of the Fox Cities, 820 Association Drive, Appleton, WI 54914; tel. 414/733-8562; FAX. 414/733-2845; Susan Kostka, RN, Director

Visiting Nurse Health Care Services, 901 Mineral Point Avenue, Jariesville, WI 53545; tel. 608/754-2201; FAX. 608/754-1147; Anne M. Adams, Administrator

Vitas Healthcare, 450 North Sunny Slope Road, Brookfield, WI 53005; tel. 414/789-6886; Dwayne Ostrom, Administrator

WYOMING

Central Wyoming Hospice Program, 233 South Jackson, Casper, WY 82601; tel. 307/577-4832; FAX. 307/577-4841; Janace Chapman, RN, Director

Hospice of Sweetwater County, 809 Thompson, Rock Springs, WY 82901; tel. 307/362-1990; FAX. 307/352-6769; Pamela L. Jelaca, Executive Director

Hospice of the Tetons, 555 East Broadway, P.O. Box 428, Jackson, WY 83001; Pamela Maples, Director

Northeast Wyoming Hospice, 720 West Seventh Street Annex J, Gillette, WY 82801; tel. 307/682-6570; Kathy L. Austin, Executive Director

State Government Agencies for Freestanding Hospices

Information for the following list was obtained directly from the agencies.

United States

ALABAMA
Alabama Department of Public Health, Division of Licensure and Certification, 434 Monroe Street, Montgomery, AL 36130-1701; tel. 334/240-3503; FAX. 334/240-3147; L. O'Neal Green, Director

ALASKA
Division of Medical Assistance, Health Facilities Licensing and Certification Section, 4041 B Street, Suite 101, Anchorage, AK 99503; tel. 907/561-2171; Karen Martz, Superior

ARIZONA
Arizona Department of Health Services, Divison of Emergency Medical Services, Health Care Facilities, 701 East Jefferson, 3rd Floor, Phoenix, AZ 85034; tel. 602/255-1177; FAX. 602/255-1109; Catherine Rosenthal, Acting Chief

ARKANSAS
Department of Health, Division of Health Facility Services, 4815 West Markham Street, Slot Nine, Little Rock, AR 72205-3867; tel. 501/661-2201; FAX. 501/661-2165; Valetta M. Buck, Director

CALIFORNIA
Department of Health Services, Licensing and Certification Division, 1800 Third Street, Suite 210, Sacramento, CA 95814, P.O. Box 942732, Sacramento, CA 94234-7320; tel. 916/327-4306; Joyce Fukui, Chief, Policy Section

COLORADO
Colorado Department of Public Health and Environment, Health Facilities Division A-2, 4300 Cherry Creek Drive, S., Denver, CO 80222-1530; tel. 303/692-2800; FAX. 303/782-4883; Peggy Waldon, RN, Program Administrator

CONNECTICUT
Department of Public Health and Addiction Services, Hospital and Medical Care Division, 150 Washington Street, Hartford, CT 06106; tel. 203/566-1073; FAX. 203/566-1097; Elizabeth M. Burns, RN, M.S., Director

DELAWARE
Department of Health and Social Services, Office of Health Facilities Licensure and Certification, 3000 Newport Gap Pike, Wilmington, DE 19808; tel. 302/995-6674; FAX. 302/995-8332; Ellen T. Reap, Director

DISTRICT OF COLUMBIA
Department of Consumer and Regulatory Affairs, Service Facility Regulation Administration, 614 H Street, N.W., Suite 1007, Washington, DC 20001; tel. 202/727-7190; FAX. 202/727-7780; James R. Murphy, Administrator

FLORIDA
Agency for HealthCare Administration, Division of Health Quality Assurance, Fort Knox Executive Center, 2727 Mahan Drive, Suite 212, Tallahassee, FL 32308-5407; tel. 904/487-3513; FAX. 904/487-6240; Gloria Henderson, Director

GEORGIA
Health Care Section, Office of Regulatory Services, Two Peachtree Street, N.W., Suite 19-204, Atlanta, GA 30303-3167; tel. 404/657-5550; FAX. 404/657-8934; Susie M. Woods, Director

HAWAII
Department of Health, Licensing and Certification, Health Quality Assurance Division, Hospital and Medical Facilities Branch, P.O. Box 3378, Honolulu, HI 96801; tel. 808/586-4080; FAX. 808/586-4747; Helen K. Yoshimi, B.S.N., M.P.H., HMF Branch, Chief

ILLINOIS
Department of Public Health, Division of Health Facilities Standards, 525 West Jefferson Street, Fourth Floor, Springfield, IL 62761; tel. 217/782-7412; FAX. 217/782-0382; Joseph Voss, Administrator, Central Office Operation Section

INDIANA
Indiana State Department of Health, Division of Acute Care, 1330 West Michigan Street, P.O. Box 1964, Indianapolis, IN 46206-1964; tel. 317/383-6472; FAX. 317/383-6750; John A. Braeckel, Director

IOWA
Department of Inspection and Appeals, Division of Health Facilities, Lucas State Office Building, Des Moines, IA 50319; tel. 515/281-4115; FAX. 515/242-5022; Pearl Johnson, Adiministrator

KANSAS
Department of Health and Environment, Bureau of Adult and Child Care Facilities, 900 S.W. Jackson, Suite 1001, Topeka, KS 66620-0001; tel. 913/296-1240; Greg L. Reser, Director, Hospital and Medical Programs

KENTUCKY
Cabinet for Human Resources, Division of Licensing and Regulation, C.H.R. Building, 275 East Main Street, 4th Floor, East, Frankfort, KY 40621; tel. 502/564-2800; FAX. 502/564-6546; Timothy L. Veno, Director

LOUISIANA
Department of Health and Hospitals, Bureau of Health Services Financing, Health Standards Section Licensing Unit, P.O. Box 3767, Baton Rouge, LA 70821; tel. 504/342-0138; FAX. 504/342-5292; Lily W. McAlister, RN, Manager

MAINE
Division of Licensing and Certification, Department of Human Services, State House, Station 11, Augusta, ME 04333; tel. 207/624-5443; FAX. 207/624-5378; Louis Dorogi, Director

MARYLAND
Department of Health and Mental Hygiene, Office of Licensing and Certification Programs, 4201 Patterson Avenue, Baltimore, MD 21215; tel. 410/764-4980; FAX. 410/764-5969; William Dorrill, Deputy Director

MASSACHUSETTS
Department of Public Health, Division of Health Care Quality, 80 Boylston Street, Suite 1100, Boston, MA 02116; tel. 617/727-5860; Irene McManus, Director

MICHIGAN
Department of Public Health, Division of Licensing and Certification, 3500 North Logan, Lansing, MI 48909; tel. 517/335-8505; Nancy Graham, Superior

MINNESOTA
Department of Health, Facility and Provider Compliance Division, Licensing and Certification Section, 393 North Dunlap Street, P.O. Box 64900, St. Paul, MN 55164-0900; tel. 612/643-2130; FAX. 612/643-3534; Carol Hirschfeld, Supervisor, Records Information Unit

MISSISSIPPI
Department of Health, Division of Health Facilities, Licensure and Certification, P.O. Box 1700, Jackson, MS 39215; tel. 601/987-3775; FAX. 301/987-4888; Mendal G. Kemp, Director

MISSOURI
Department of Health, Bureau of Home Health Licensing and Certification, P.O. Box 570, Jefferson City, MO 65102; tel. 314/751-6336; FAX. 314/526-3621; Lois Kollmeyer, RN, Administrator

MONTANA
Department of Health and Environmental Sciences, Bureau of Licensing, Health Facilities Division, Cogswell Building, P.O. Box 200901, Helena, MT 59620-0901; tel. 406/444-2037; FAX. 406/444-1742; Roy P. Kemp, Chief

NEBRASKA
Department of Health, Bureau of Health Facilities Standards, 301 Centennial Mall, S., P.O. Box 95007, Lincoln, NE 68509-5007; tel. 402/471-2946; FAX. 402/471-0555; Frederick M. Wright, Director

NEVADA
Nevada State Health Division, Bureau of Licensure and Certification, 505 East King Street, Suite 202, Carson City, NV 89710; tel. 702/687-4475; FAX. 702/687-6588; Sharon M. Ezell, Chief

NEW HAMPSHIRE
Division of Public Health Services, Bureau of Health Facilities Administration, Six Hazen Drive, Concord, NH 03301; tel. 603/271-4592; FAX. 603/271-3745; Eleanor B. Robinson, Bureau Chief

NEW JERSEY
Department of Health, Health Facilities Evaluations and Licensing, CN-367, Trenton, NJ 08625-0367; tel. 609/588-7735; FAX. 609/588-7823; Henry T. Kozek, CPM, Assistant Director

NEW MEXICO
Department of Health, Health Facility Licensing and Certification Bureau, 525 Camino de los Marquez, Suite Two, Santa Fe, NM 87501; tel. 505/827-4200; FAX. 505/827-4222; Sue K. Morris, Bureau Chief

NEW YORK
Bureau of Home Health Care Services, Department of Health, Empire State Plaza, Corning Tower, Room 1970, Albany, NY 12237; tel. 518/474-2006; FAX. 518/474-2031; Dr. Nancy Barhydt, Director

NORTH CAROLINA
Department of Human Resources, Division of Facility Services, 701 Barbour Drive, Raleigh, NC 27603; tel. 919/733-1610; FAX. 919/733-3207; Jesse Goodman, Chief, Licensure Section

NORTH DAKOTA
Department of Health, Health Resources Section, 600 East Boulevard Avenue, Bismarck, ND 58505; tel. 701/328-2352; FAX. 701/328-4727; Fred Gladden, Chief

OHIO
Division of Health Facilities Regulation, Ohio Department of Health, 246 North High Street, Columbus, OH 43266-0588; tel. 614/466-7857; FAX. 614/644-0208; Rebecca Maust, Chief

Providers / State Government Agencies for Freestanding Hospices

OKLAHOMA
Department of Health, Special Health Services, 1000 N.E. 10th Street, P.O. Box 53551, Oklahoma City, OK 73152; tel. 405/271-6868; FAX. 405/271-3442; Gary Glover, Director of Hospitals and Related Institutions

OREGON
Health Care Licensing and Certification, Oregon Health Division, 800 S.E. Oregon Street, # 21, Suite 640, Portland, OR 97232; tel. 503/731-4013; FAX. 503/731-4080; Kathleen Smail, Manager

PENNSYLVANIA
Department of Health, Division of Primary Care and Home Health, 132 Kline Plaza, Suite A, Harrisburg, PA 17104; tel. 717/783-1379; FAX. 717/787-3188; Robert Bastian, Director

RHODE ISLAND
Rhode Island Department of Health, Division of Facilities Regulation, 3 Capitol Hill, Providence, RI 02908-5097; tel. 401/277-2566; FAX. 401/277-3999; Wayne I. Farrington, Chief

SOUTH CAROLINA
Department of Health and Environmental Control, Bureau of Certification, 2600 Bull Street, Columbia, SC 29201; tel. 803/737-7205; FAX. 803/737-7292; Florence Tumboken, RN, M.S.N., Program Manager, Medicare Insurance Benefits

SOUTH DAKOTA
Department of Health, Office of Health Care Facilities, 523 East Capitol, Joe Foss Building, Pierre, SD 57501; tel. 605/773-3364; FAX. 605/773-5904; Joan Bachman, Program Director

TENNESSEE
Department of Health, Division of Health Care Facilities, 283 Plus Park Boulevard, Nashville, TN 37247-0530; tel. 615/367-6316; FAX. 615/367-6397; Leslie A. Brown, Director

TEXAS
Department of Health, Health Facility Licensure and Certification Division, 8407 Wall Street, Zip 78754, 1100 West 49th Street, Austin, TX 78756; tel. 512/834-6647; FAX. 512/834-6653; Nance Stearman, RN, M.S.N., Director

UTAH
Utah Department of Health, Bureau of Health Facility Licensure, P.O. Box 16990, Salt Lake City, UT 84116-0990; tel. 801/538-6152; FAX. 801/538-6325; Debra Wynkoop-Green, Director

VERMONT
Hospice Council of Vermont, 52 State Street, Montpelier, VT 05602; tel. 802/229-0579; FAX. 802/229-0579; Virginia L. Fry, Director

VIRGINIA
Virginia Department of Health, Office of Health Facilities Regulation, 3600 Centre, Suite 216, 3600 West Broad Street, Richmond, VA 23230; tel. 804/367-2102; FAX. 804/367-2149; Nancy R. Hofheimer, Director

WASHINGTON
Office of Field Services, Department of Health, Target Plaza, Suite 500, 2725 Harrison Avenue, NW, P.O. Box 47852, Olympia, WA 98504-7852; tel. 206/705-6622; FAX. 206/705-6654; Fern Bettridge, Program Manager

WEST VIRGINIA
Office of Health Facility Licensure and Certification, West Virginia Division of Health, 1900 Kanawha Boulevard, E., Building 3, Suite 550, Charleston, WV 25305; tel. 304/558-0050; FAX. 304/558-2515; Robert P. Brauner, R.Ph., D.P.M., Program Administrator

WISCONSIN
Department of Health and Social Services, Division of Health, P.O. Box 309, Madison, WI 53701; tel. 608/267-7185; FAX. 608/267-0352; Judy Fryback, Director, Bureau of Quality Compliance

WYOMING
Department of Health, Health Facilities Licensing, Metropolitan Bank Building, Eighth Floor, Cheyenne, WY 82002; tel. 307/777-7123; FAX. 307/777-5402; Charlie Simineo, Program Manager

U.S. Associated Areas

PUERTO RICO
Puerto Rico Department of Health, Call Box 70184, San Juan, PR 00936; tel. 809/766-1616; FAX. 809/274-7608; Carmen Feliciano de Melecio, M.D., Secretary of Health

Accredited Freestanding Long-Term Care Facilities

The accredited freestanding long-term care facilities listed have been accredited as of January 1, 1995, by the Joint Commission on Accreditation of Healthcare Organizations by decision of the Accreditation Committee of the Board of Commissioners.

The facilities listed here have been found to be in substantial compliance with the Joint Commission standards for long-term care facilities, as found in the Accreditation Manual for the Long-Term Care Facilities.

Please refer to section A of the AHA Guide for information on hospitals with Long-Term Care services. These hospitals are identified by Facility Code 64. In Section A, those hospitals identified by Approval Code 1 are JCAHO accredited.

We present this list simply as a convenient directory. Inclusion or omission of any organization's name indicates neither approval nor disapproval by the American Hospital Association.

United States

ALABAMA

Canterbury Health Facility, 1720 Knowles Road, Phenix City, AL 36869; tel. 334/291–0485; FAX. 334/297–5816; Joyce Spivey, Administrator

Integrated Health Services at Briarcliff, 850 N.W. Ninth Street, Alabaster, AL 35007; tel. 205/663–3859; FAX. 205/663–9791; Frances Eddings, Administrator

Northside Health Care, 700 Hutchins Avenue, Gadsen, AL 35901; tel. 205/543–7101; FAX. 205/546–3924; Sherry D. Barton, Administrator

ARIZONA

Casa Delmar Nursing and Rehabilitation Center, 3333 North Civic Center Plaza, Scottsdale, AZ 85251; tel. 602/994–1333; FAX. 602/990–3895; Patricia A. Phillips

Catalina Care Center, 2611 North Warren, Tucson, AZ 85719; tel. 602/795–9574; FAX. 602/795–9850; James K. Kinsey, Administrator

Coronado Care Center, 11411 North 19th Avenue, Phoenix, AZ 85029; tel. 602/256–7500; FAX. 602/943–7697; Jacqueline Lanter, Administrator

Desert Samaritan Care Center, 2145 West Southern Avenue, Mesa, AZ 85202; tel. 602/890–4800; FAX. 602/890–4829; Steven D. Bakken, Administrator

East Mesa Care Center, 51 South 48th Street, Mesa, AZ 85206; tel. 602/832–8333; FAX. 602/830–2466; W. H. Syckes, Administrator

Good Samaritan Care Center, 901 East Willetta Street, Phoenix, AZ 85006; tel. 602/223–3000; FAX. 602/223–3197; Michael J. Oliver, Administrator

St. Joseph's Care Center, 531 West Thomas Road, Phoenix, AZ 85013; tel. 602/406–6800; FAX. 602/406–7146; Mary M. Klein, Administrator

CALIFORNIA

Brittany Healthcare Center, Inc., 3900 Garfield Avenue, Carmichael, CA 95608; tel. 916/481–6455; Diane Hoyt, Administrator

Calistoga Care Nursing and Rehab Center, 1715 Washington Street, Calistoga, CA 94515; tel. 707/942–6253; FAX. 707/942–6288; Dottie Dowswell, Director of Nursing

CareWest Huntington Valley Nursing and Rehabilitation, 8382 Newman Avenue, Huntington Valley, CA 92647; tel. 714/842–5551; Tish Gamboni, Director, Nursing

CareWest La Mariposa, 1244 Travis Boulevard, Fairfield, CA 94533; tel. 707/422–7750; FAX. 707/422–8102; Joanne Lewis, Director, Nursing

Carmichael Convalescent Hospital Center, 8336 Fair Oaks Boulevard, Carmichael, CA 95608; tel. 916/944–3100; Kathy Spake, Administrator

Casa Colina Peninsula Rehabilitation Center, 26303 Western Avenue, Lomita, CA 90717; tel. 310/325–3202; FAX. 310/534–2782; Terry Banta Winkowski, Administrator

Casa Palmera Care Center, 14750 El Camino Real, Del Mar, CA 92014; tel. 619/481–4411; FAX. 619/792–7356; Lee Johnson, Administrator

Chapman Harbor Skilled Nursing Facility, 12232 West Chapman Avenue, Garden Grove, CA 92640; tel. 714/971–5517; Genman Kaw, Mds. Coordinator

Clear View Sanitarium and Convalescent Center, 15823 South Western Avenue, Gardena, CA 90247–7378; tel. 310/538–2323; FAX. 310/538–3509; W. Lee Towns, President

Covina Rehabilitation Center, 261 West Badillo, Covina, CA 91723; tel. 813/967–3874; Alan M. Hull, Administrator

Driftwood Health Care Center, 4109 Emerald Street, Torrance, CA 90503; tel. 310/371–4628; Yasmin Murphy, Director, Case Management

English Oaks Convalescent and Rehabilitation Center, 2633 West Rumble Road, Modesto, CA 95350; tel. 209/577–1001, ext. 7601; FAX. 209/577–0366; Michael A. Wray, Administrator

Evergreen Convalescent Hospital and Rehabilitation Center, 2030 Evergreen Avenue, Modesto, CA 95350; tel. 209/577–1055; Daniel J. Cipponeri, Vice President

FHP Westminister, 206 Hospital Circle, Westminister, CA 92683; tel. 714/891–2769; FAX. 714/893–1014; Kim Phan, Administrator

Fairfield Health Care Center, 1255 Travis Boulevard, Fairfield, CA 94533; tel. 707/425–0623; Annette Eugenis, Administrator

Gateway Nursing and Rehabilitation Center, 26660 Patrick Avenue, Hayward, CA 94544; tel. 510/782–1845; Helen Jones, Director, Nursing

Glendora Rehabilitation Center, 435 East Gladstone, Glendora, CA 91740; tel. 818/963–5955; Gerald R. Hardy, Administrator

Grand Terrace Convalescent Hospital, 12000 Mt. Vernon Avenue, Grand Terrace, CA 92324; tel. 909/825–5221; FAX. 909/783–4811; Irma Cooper, RN, M.S., Administrator

Greenery Rehabilitation Center, 385 Esplanade, Pacifica, CA 94044; tel. 415/993–5576; FAX. 415/359–9388; Janet T. Kempis, Ed.D

Heritage Rehabilitation Center, 21414 South Vermont Avenue, Torrance, CA 90502; tel. 310/320–8714; FAX. 310/320–1809; Doug Nelson, Administrator

Heritage of Stockton, A Convalescent and Rehab Center, 9107 North Davis Road, Stockton, CA 95209; tel. 209/478–6488; Edward J. Garrison, Administrator

Hillhaven San Francisco, 1359 Pine Street, San Francisco, CA 94109; tel. 415/673–8405; Paul Tunnell, Administrator

Huntington Beach Convalescent Hospital, 18811 Florida Street, Huntington Beach, CA 92648; tel. 714/847–3515; Carolyn E. Paul, Ph.D., Administrator

Integrated Health Services at Orange Hills, 5017 East Chapman Avenue, Orange, CA 92669; tel. 714/997–7090; Retha Tyler, Controller for Quality

Integrated Health Services of Park Regency, 1770 West La Habra Boulevard, La Habra, CA 90631; tel. 310/691–8810; FAX. 310/697–8478; Marianne J. Schultz, Administrator

Lacey Manor Convalescent Hospital, 1007 West Lacey Boulevard, Hanford, CA 93230; tel. 209/582–2871; Brian Kallio, Administrator

Orinda Rehabilitation and Convalescent Hospital, 11 Altarinda Road, Orinda, CA 94563; tel. 510/254–6500; FAX. 510/254–9063; Charles Speers, Administrator

Park Anaheim Healthcare Center, 3435 West Ball Road, Anaheim, CA 92804; tel. 714/827–5880; Gregory D. Hirst, Administrator

Park Tustin Rehabilitation Healthcare, 2210 East First Street, Santa Ana, CA 92705; tel. 714/547–7091; FAX. 714/547–4516; Rachel Bennett, Administrator

Regency Hills Convalescent Hospital, 2351 Loveridge Road, Pittsburg, CA 94565; tel. 510/432–2200; James K. Osborn, Administrator

San Bruno Skilled Nursing Hospital, 890 El Camino Real, San Bruno, CA 94066; tel. 415/583–7768; FAX. 415/583–9710; Jeremy Grimes, Administrator

Scripps Memorial Ocean View Convalescent Hospital, 900 Santa Fe Drive, Encinitas, CA 92024; tel. 619/753–6423; Pamela I. Turner, Administrator

Scripps Memorial Torrey Pines Convalescent Hospital, 2552 Torrey Pines Road, La Jolla, CA 92037; tel. 619/453–5810; FAX. 619/452–4301; Elena M. Gulla, Administrator

Simi Valley Rehabilitation and Nursing Center Valley, 5270 Los Angeles Avenue, Simi Valley, CA 93063; tel. 805/527–6204; Janiece M. Lackey, Administrator

Skilled Nursing Facility Memorial Hospitals Association, 1905 Memorial Drive, Ceres, CA 95307; tel. 209/526–4500; Betty Lopez, Manager

Springs Road Living Center, 1527 Springs Road, Vallejo, CA 94591; tel. 707/643–2793; Georgia Otterson, Administrator

St. Luke's Subacute Hospital and Nursing Centre, 1652 Mono Avenue, San Leandro, CA 94578; tel. 415/357–5351; FAX. 415/278–7912; Guy R. Seaton, President

Subacute Saratoga Hospital, 18611 Sousa Lane, Saratoga, CA 95070; tel. 408/378–8875; Connie Rolfe, Vice President

Western Medical Center Bartlett, 600 East Washington Avenue, Santa Ana, CA 92701; tel. 714/973–1656, ext. 408; FAX. 714/836–4349; Page Van Hoy, Chief Executive Officer

COLORADO

Boulder Manor, 4685 East Baseline Road, Boulder, CO 80303; tel. 303/494–0535; Elizabeth Lee, Administrator

Colorado State Veterans Nursing Home – Walsenburg, 23500 US Highway 60, Walsenburg, CO 81089; tel. 719/738–5144; Sandra Ledbetter

CONNECTICUT

Ashlar of Newtown, Toddy Hill Road, Newtown, CT 06470; tel. 203/426–5847; FAX. 203/270–0695; Thomas Gutner, Administrator

Providers / Accredited Freestanding Long–Term Care Facilities

Avon Convalescent Home, 652 West Avon Road, Avon, CT 06001; tel. 203/673–2521; FAX. 203/675–1587; Laura L. Nelson, Administrator

Bloomfield Manor, 160 Coventry Street, Bloomfield, CT 06002; tel. 203/243–2995; FAX. 203/243–1902; Ellen Saltarella, Administrator

Branford Hills Health Care Center, 189 Alps Road, Branford, CT 06405; tel. 203/481–6221; FAX. 203/483–1893; Charles F. Shelton, Jr., Administrator

Brook Hollow Health Care Center, 55 Kondracki Lane, Wallingford, CT 06492; tel. 203/265–6771; Regina King, Administrator

Brookview Health Care Facility, 130 Loomis Drive, West Hartford, CT 06017; tel. 203/521–8700; FAX. 203/521–7452; Clifton P. Mix, Administrator

Cedar Lane Rehabilitation and Health Care Center, 128 Cedar Avenue, Waterbury, CT 06705; tel. 203/757–9271; FAX. 203/757–2988; Peter J. Belval, Administrator

Cheshire Convalescent Center, 745 Highland Avenue, Cheshire, CT 06410; tel. 203/272–7285; Lawrence J. Condon, Administrator

Clifton House Rehabilitation Center, 181 Clifton Street, New Haven, CT 06513; tel. 203/467–1666; FAX. 203/469–7213; Peter M. Madden, Administrator

Forestville Health and Rehabilitation Center, 23 Fair Street, Forestville, CT 06010; tel. 203/589–2923; FAX. 203/589–3148; Linda Bradigo, Administrator

Glen Hill Convalescent Center, One Glen Hill Road, Danbury, CT 06811; tel. 203/744–2840; FAX. 203/792–1521; James Malloy, Administrator

Greenery Extended Care Center at Cheshire, 50 Hazel Drive, Cheshire, CT 06410; tel. 203/272–7204; FAX. 203/272–4607; Denis Twigg, Administrator

Greenery Rehabilitation Center at Waterbury, 177 Whitewood Road, Waterbury, CT 06708; tel. 203/757–9491; FAX. 203/575–1714; Charles Chidester, Administrator

Jewish Home for the Elderly of Fairfield County, 175 Jefferson Street, Fairfield, CT 06432; tel. 203/374–9461; Donna Joyce, Vice President

Mariner Health Care of Pendleton Rehabilitation, Inc., 44 Maritime Drive, Mystic, CT 06355; tel. 203/572–1700; Louise Rief, Director of Nursing

Mediplex Rehabilitation and Skilled Nursing Center of Southern Connecticut, 2028 Bridgeport Avenue, Milford, CT 06460; tel. 203/877–0371; FAX. 203/877–6185; Mary Grabell, Executive Director

Mediplex Rehabilitation and Skilled Nursing Center of Central Connecticut, 261 Summit Street, Plantsville, CT 06479; tel. 203/628–0364; Raymond C. DeBlasio, Administrator

Mediplex of Danbury, 107 Osborne Street, Danbury, CT 06810; tel. 203/792–8102; FAX. 203/731–5306; Michael E. Osyczka, Administrator

Mediplex of Darien Rehabilitation Center, 599 Boston Post Road, Darien, CT 06820; tel. 203/655–7727, ext. 202; FAX. 203/655–6718; Samuel S. Hamilton, Chief Executive Officer

Mediplex of Milford, 245 Orange Avenue, Milford, CT 06460; tel. 203/876–5123; Donna C. Stango, Administrator

Mediplex of Newington, 240 Church Street, Newington, CT 06111; tel. 203/667–2256; FAX. 203/667–6367; Linda Odaynik, Administrator

Mediplex of Southbury, South Britain Road, Southbury, CT 06488; tel. 203/264–9600; Ann M. Rogers, Administrator

Mediplex of Westport, One Burr Road, Westport, CT 06880; tel. 203/226–4201; FAX. 203/221–4766; Dorothy H. Feigin, Administrator

Mediplex of Wethersfield, 341 Jordan Lane, Wethersfield, CT 06109; tel. 203/563–0101; J. Kevin Prisco, Administrator

Miller Memorial Community, 360 Broad Street, Meriden, CT 06450; tel. 203/237–8815; FAX. 203/630–3714; Sister Ann Noonan, R.S.M., Administrator, Chief Operating Officer

Montowese Health and Rehabilitation, Inc., 163 Quinnipiac Avenue, North Haven, CT 06473; tel. 203/624–3303; Judith Andrews, Admissions Director

Noble Horizons, 17 Cobble Road, Salisbury, CT 06068; tel. 203/435–9851; FAX. 203/435–0636; Eileen M. Mulligan, Administrator

Sound View Specialized Care Center, One Care Lane, West Haven, CT 06516; tel. 203/934–7955; FAX. 203/934–1038; Mary Ellen Gaudette, Administrator

Southport Manor Convalescent Center, Inc., 930 Mill Hill Terrace, Southport, CT 06490; tel. 203/259–7894; FAX. 203/254–3720; Anne P. Toth, Administrator, President

The Elim Park Baptist Home, Inc., 140 Cook Hill Road, Cheshire, CT 06410; tel. 203/272–3547; David MacNeill, President

The Kent, Ltd, 46 Maple Street, P.O. Box 212, Kent, CT 06757; tel. 203/927–5368; FAX. 203/927–1594; Patricia Brooks, Administrator

Valerie Manor, 1360 Torringford Street, Route 183, Torrington, CT 06790; tel. 203/489–1008; Anne Marie Murray, RN, Administrator

Waterford Health and Rehabilitation Center, 171 Rope Ferry Road, Waterford, CT 06385; tel. 203/443–8357; Lawrence Condon, Administrator

Waveny Care Center, Three Farm Road, New Canaan, CT 06840; tel. 203/966–8725; FAX. 203/966–1641; Jeremy Vickers, Executive Director

Westcott Care Center, 111 Westcott Road, Danielson, CT 06239; tel. 203/774–9540; FAX. 203/774–9703; E. L. Attella, Administrator

Windham Hills Healthcare Center, 595 Valley Street, Willimantic, CT 06226; tel. 203/423–2597; FAX. 203/450–7070; Richard Kase, Administrator

DELAWARE

Methodist Country House, 4830 Kennett Pike, Wilmington, DE 19807; tel. 302/654–5101; FAX. 302/426–8108; William H. James, Jr.

DISTRICT OF COLUMBIA

Benjamin King Health Center, U.S. Soldiers' and Airmen's Home, 3700 North Capitol Street, N.W., Washington, DC 20317–0001; tel. 202/722–3323; FAX. 202/722–3570; Paul D. Gleason, M.D., Associate Director, Health Care Services

Health Care Institute, 1380 Southern Avenue, S.E., Washington, DC 20032; tel. 202/279–5880; FAX. 202/574–0192; Vanessa Mattox, Administrator

FLORIDA

Arbors at Lakeland, 2020 West Lake Parker Drive, Lakeland, FL 33805; tel. 813/682–7580; FAX. 813/683–4944; Doug Eitel, Administrator

Arbors at Orange Park Nursing and Rehabilitation Center, 1215 Kingsley Avenue, Orange Park, FL 32073; tel. 904/269–8922; Caryl W. Hall, Administrator

Arbors of Tallahassee, 1650 Phillips Road, Tallahassee, FL 32308; tel. 904/942–9868; Kathryn Tarun, Administrator

Bay Pointe Nursing Pavillion, 4201 31st Street, South, St. Petersburg,, FL 33712; tel. 813/867–1104; Marianne Essex, Director of Nursing

Boca Raton Rehabilitation Center, 755 Meadows Road, Boca Raton, FL 33486; tel. 407/391–5200; FAX. 407/391–5487; Maraleita K. Jackson, Administrator

Greynolds Park Manor Rehabilitation Center, 17400 West Dixie Highway, North Miami Beach, FL 33160; tel. 305/944–2361; FAX. 305/949–9464; Martin E. Casper, Executive Director

Heartland Health Care Center Miami Lakes, 5725 186th Street, Hialeah, FL 33015; tel. 305/625–9857; Joyce Ploudre, Administrator

Heartland Health Care and Rehabilitaiton Center, 5401 Sawyer Road, Sarasota, FL 34233; tel. 813/925–3427; John K. Graham, Director, Operation Support

Heartland Healthcare Convalescent Center, 3600 Boynton Road, Boynton Beach, FL 33436; tel. 407/736–9992; Martha A. Davis, Mobile Director of Nursing

Hillhaven Rehabilitation Center of Tampa, 4411 North Habana Avenue, Tampa, FL 33614; tel. 813/872–2771; Rebecca Waggers, Administrator

IHS at Green Briar (Integrated Health Services), 9820 North Kendall Drive, Miami, FL 33176; tel. 305/271–6311; FAX. 305/274–5880; Rosemary Wedderspoon, Administrator

Integrated Health Services of St. Petersburg, 811 Jackson Street, St. Petersburg, FL 33705; tel. 813/896–3651; Kathleen Wesolowski, Administrator

Manor Care Nursing and Rehabilitation Center, 3648 University Boulevard, Jacksonville, FL 32216; tel. 904/733–7440; Norman Durmaskin, Administrator

Manor Care of Carrollwood, Reach Rehabilitation, 3030 West Bearss Avenue, Tampa, FL 33618; tel. 813/968–8777; Mary Bryre, Administrator

Mediplex Rehabilitation of Palm Beach, 6414 13th Road, S., West Palm Beach, FL 33415; tel. 407/478–9900; FAX. 407/478–5067; Gerry Labourene, Administrator

Mediplex Rehabilitation–Bradenton, 5627 Ninth Street, E., Bradenton, FL 34203; tel. 813/753–8941; FAX. 813/753–7576; Dale Bergquist, Chief Executive Officer

River Garden Hebrew Home for the Aged, 11401 Old St. Augustine Road, Jacksonville, FL 32258; tel. 904/260–1818; FAX. 904/260–9733; Martin A. Goetz, Administrator

GEORGIA

Family Life Enrichment Centers, Inc., 3450 New High Shoals Road, High Shoals, GA 30645; tel. 706/769–7738; FAX. 706/769–5944; Magda D. Bennett, Administrator

Georgia War Veterans Nursing Home, 1101 Fifteenth Street, Augusta, GA 30910; tel. 706/721–2531; FAX. 706/721–3892; Charles Esposito, Administrator

Integrated Health Services at Briarcliff Haven, Inc., 1000 Briarcliff Road, Atlanta, GA 30306; tel. 404/875–6456; Andrew J. Morris, Administrator

Oak Manor and Pine Manor Nursing Homes, Inc., 2010 Warm Springs Road, P.O. Box 8828, Columbus, GA 31908–8828; tel. 404/324–0387; Caroline L. Nahley, RN, Administrator

HAWAII

Island Nursing Home, 1205 Alexander Street, Honolulu, HI 96826; tel. 808/946–5027; Leland M. Yagi, President, Administrator

ILLINOIS

Admiral (The Old People's Home of the City of Chicago), 909 West Foster Avenue, Chicago, IL 60640; tel. 312/561–2900; FAX. 312/561–2573; Robert R. Porter, Executive Director

Alma Nelson Manor, Inc., 550 South Mulford, Rockford, IL 61108; tel. 815/399–4914; FAX. 815/399–0054; Judy K. Larson, Administrator

Anchorage of Bensenville Home Society, Lifelink Corporation, 111 East Washington Street, Bensenville, IL 60106; tel. 708/766–5800, ext. 206; FAX. 708/860–5130; Jane M. Muller, Administrator

Apostolic Christian Restmor, Inc., 935 East Jefferson, Morton, IL 61550; tel. 309/266–7141; FAX. 309/266–7877; James L. Metzger, Executive Director

Ballard, A Healthcare Residence, 9300 Ballard Road, Des Plaines, IL 60016; tel. 708/294–2300; FAX. 708/299–4012; Joanne Bedrosian, Administrator

Bethany Terrace Nursing Center, 8425 North Waukegan Road, Morton Grove, IL 60053; tel. 708/965–8100; FAX. 708/965–8104; Myra Webster, Administrator

Brentwood North Nursing and Rehabilitation Center, 3705 Deerfield Road, Riverwoods, IL 60015; tel. 708/459–1200; FAX. 708/459–0113; Jerome J. Aniolowski, Vice President

Community Convalescent Center of Naperville, 1136 North Mill Street, Naperville, IL 60563; tel. 708/355–3300; FAX. 708/355–1417; Elizabeth A. Giacobbe, Executive Vice President, Administrator

Providers / Accredited Freestanding Long-Term Care Facilities

DuPage Convalescent Center, 400 North County Farm Road, Wheaton, IL 60187; tel. 708/665-6400; FAX. 708/665-2446; Ronald R. Reinecke, Administrator

Evenglow Lodge, Inc., 215 East Washington Street, Pontiac, IL 61764; tel. 815/844-6131; FAX. 815/842-3558; Tyler B. Schoenherr, Administrator

Fairview Baptist Home, 250 Village Drive, Downers Grove, IL 60516-3099; tel. 708/769-6200; FAX. 708/769-6226; Robert F. Underwood, Acting President

Friendship Manor, 1209 21st Avenue, Rock Island, IL 61201; tel. 309/782-9667; Michael Kearney, Administrator

Galena Park Home, 5533 North Galena Road, Peoria Heights, IL 61614; tel. 309/682-5428; Jane S. Foster, Administrator

Heartland Health Care Center Canton, 2081 North Main Street, Canton, IL 61520; tel. 309/647-6135

Heartland Health Care Center of Homewood, 940 Maple Avenue, Homewood, IL 60430; tel. 708/799-0244; John K. Graham, Director, Operation Support

Integrated Health Services at Brentwood, 5400 West 87th Street, Burbank, IL 60459; tel. 708/423-1200; FAX. 708/423-8405; John Walton, Chief Executive Officer

John C. Proctor Endowment, 2724 West Reservoir Boulevard, Peoria, IL 61615; tel. 309/685-6580; Andrew Cali, Administrator

Lieberman Geriatric Health Centre, 9700 Gross Point Road, Skokie, IL 60076; tel. 708/674-7210; FAX. 708/674-6366; Barbara Wexler, Administrator

Medbridge Medical and Physical Rehabilitation, 715 West Central Road, Arlington Heights, IL 60005; tel. 708/392-2020; FAX. 708/392-3250; Katharine A. Keane, Executive Director

Medbridge Medical and Physical Rehabilitation Center, 9401 South Kostner Avenue, Oak Lawn, IL 60453; tel. 708/423-7882; Cecilia M. Credille, Executive Director

Norridge Nursing Centre, Inc., 7001 West Cullom Avenue, Norridge, IL 60634; tel. 708/457-0700; FAX. 708/457-8852; Jeff S. Berns, Administrator

North Adams Home, Inc., Rural Route 2, Box 100, Mendon, IL 62351; tel. 217/936-2137; John D. Bainum, Administrator

Oakton Pavilion Healthcare Facility, Inc., 1660 Oakton Place, Des Plaines, IL 60018; tel. 708/299-5588; FAX. 708/298-6017; Jay Lewkowitz, ACSW, Administrator

Park Strathmoor Subacute Hospital, 5668 Strathmoor Drive, Rockford, IL 61107; tel. 815/229-5200; FAX. 815/229-1411; Laura Gruetzmacher, Administrator

Parkway Healthcare Center, 219 East Parkway Drive, Wheaton, IL 60187; tel. 708/668-4635; Beth A. LaPointe, Administrator

Piatt County Nursing Home, 1111 North State Street, Monticello, IL 61856; tel. 217/762-2506; FAX. 217/762-9926; Marilyn E. Benedino, Administrator

Pinecrest Manor, 414 South Wesley Avenue, Mount Morris, IL 61054; tel. 815/734-4103; FAX. 815/734-7318; Vernon C. Showalter, Administrator

Plymouth Place, Inc., 315 North LaGrange Road, LaGrange Park, IL 60525; tel. 708/354-0340; FAX. 708/482-6847; Gloria E. Bialek, Executive Director

Regency Nursing Centre, 6631 North Milwaukee Avenue, Niles, IL 60714; tel. 708/647-7444; FAX. 708/647-6403; Barbara A. Hecht, Administrator

Sherman West Court, 1950 Larkin Avenue, Elgin, IL 60123; tel. 708/742-7070; FAX. 708/742-7248; Stephen Erickson, Administrator

Sherwin Manor Nursing Center, 7350 North Sheridan Road, Chicago, IL 60626; tel. 312/274-1000; FAX. 312/274-2353; Abe Osina, President

St. Matthew Lutheran Home, 1601 North Western Avenue, Park Ridge, IL 60068; tel. 708/825-5531; FAX. 708/318-6659; Scott L. Swanson, Executive Director

INDIANA

Americana Healthcare Center of Indianapolis–North, 8350 Naab Road, Indianapolis, IN 46260; tel. 317/872-4051; Robert J. Couch, Administrator

Arbors at Fort Wayne, 2827 Northgate Boulevard, Fort Wayne, IN 46835; tel. 219/485-9691; Tim Daugherty, Administrator

Covington Manor Health Care Center, 1600 East Liberty Street, Covington, IN 47932; tel. 317/793-4818; Peter L. Grogg, Administrator

Holiday Care Center, 1201 West Buena Vista Road, Evansville, IN 47710; tel. 812/429-0700; Don Hester, Administrator

Integrated Health Services of Indianapolis at Cambridge, 8530 Township Line Road, Indianapolis, IN 46260; tel. 317/876-9955; FAX. 317/876-6016; Michael E. Toral, Executive Director

Lifeline Children's Hospital, 1707 West 86th Street, P.O. Box 40407, Indianapolis, IN 46240-0407; tel. 317/872-0555; FAX. 317/471-0058; David Carter, Executive Director

Miller's Merry Manor, 1500 Grant Street, Huntington, IN 46750; tel. 219/356-5713; FAX. 219/356-8671; Jack Schaefer, Administrator

Miller's Merry Manor, 200 26th Street, Logansport, IN 46947; tel. 219/722-4006; FAX. 219/753-8753; Gregory Fassett, Administrator

Miller's Merry Manor, 612 East 11th Street, Rushville, IN 46173; tel. 317/932-4127; FAX. 317/932-3054; Ron A. Green, Administrator

Northest Manor Health Care Center, 6440 West 34th Street, Indianapolis, IN 46224; tel. 371/293-4930; Jennifer A. Knoll, Administrator

Vermillion Convalescent Center, 1705 South Main Street, Clinton, IN 47842; tel. 317/832-3573; FAX. 317/832-3574; David Olson, Administrator

IOWA

Anamosa Care Center, 1209 East 3rd Street, Anamosa, IA 52205; tel. 319/462-4356; FAX. 319/462-5038; Darlene M. Sissel, Administrator

Bettendorf Health Care Center, 2730 Crow Creek Road, Bettendorf, IA 52722; tel. 319/332-7463; Susan Morton, Administrator

Danville Care Center, Birch and Seymour Streets, Danville, IA 52623; tel. 319/392-4259; Michael W. Hocking, Administrator

Edgewood Convalescent Home, 513 Bell Street, Edgewood, IA 52042; tel. 319/928-6461; Eileen Eilers Dudek, Administrator

Elkader Care Center, 116 Reimer Street, Elkader, IA 52043; tel. 319/245-1620; Eileen Eilers Dudek, Administrator

Great River Care Center, Highway 18 South, McGregor, IA 52157; tel. 319/873-3527; Raletta W. Thomas, Administrator

Health Care Manor, 703 South Fourth Avenue, P.O. Box 428, New Hampton, IA 50659; tel. 515/394-4153; Michael W. Rissien, Administrator

Iowa Veterans Home, 1301 Summit Street, Marshalltown, IA 50158-5485; tel. 515/752-1501; FAX. 515/753-4278; Jack J. Dack, Commandant

Lone Tree Health Care Center, 501 East Pioneer Road, Lone Tree, IA 52755; tel. 319/629-4255; FAX. 319/629-5300; Roberta Shirkey, Administrator

Mill Valley Care Center, 1201 Park Avenue, Bellevue, IA 52031-1911; tel. 319/872-5521; Glinda L. Manternach, Administrator

New London Care Center, South Pine Street, New London, IA 52645; tel. 319/367-5753; Michael W. Hocking, Administrator

Riverview Manor, 17990 Spencer Road, P.O. Box 503, Pleasant Valley, IA 52767; tel. 319/332-4600; Kathy Grimes, Administrator

Senior Home, 500 Pinehaven Drive, Monticello, IA 52310; tel. 319/465-5415; Barbara Himes, Administrator

St. Francis Continuation Care and Nursing Home Center, 210 South Fifth Street, P.O. Box 339, Burlington, IA 52601; tel. 319/752-4564; Sister Bernadette Duman, Chief Executive Officer

St. Luke's Living Center East, 1220 5th Avenue, S.E., Cedar Rapids, IA 52403; tel. 319/366-8701; Thomas L. Wagg, Administrator

St. Luke's Living Center West, 1050 Fourth Avenue, S.E., Cedar Rapids, IA 52403; tel. 319/366-8714; Patrick J. Carmody, Administrator

State Center Manor, 702 Third Street, N.W., State Center, IA 50247; tel. 515/483-2812; FAX. 515/483-2675; Kathleen R. Jones, Administrator

Wheatland Manor, Inc., 515 East Lincolnway, Wheatland, IA 52777; tel. 319/374-1295; Cindy Perdue, RN, Administrator

KENTUCKY

Christopher East Health Care Center, 4200 Brown's Lane, Louisville, KY 40220; tel. 502/459-8900; Thomas J. Martin, Senior Administrator

Winchester Health Care Center, 200 White Drive, Winchester, KY 40391; tel. 606/744-1800; Damie U. Castle, Administrator

LOUISIANA

Gillis W. Long Hansen's Disease Center, 5445 Point Clair Road, Carville, LA 70721-9607; tel. 504/642-4740; FAX. 504/642-4728; Robert R. Jacobson, M.D., Ph.D., Director

Greenery Neurologic Rehabilitation Center at Slidell, 1400 Lindberg Drive, Slidell, LA 70458; tel. 504/641-4985, ext. 3003; FAX. 504/646-0728; James L. McEwen, Ph.D., Executive Director

Lafon Nursing Home of the Holy Family, 6900 Chef Menteur Highway, New Orleans, LA 70126; tel. 504/246-1100; FAX. 504/241-6672; Sister Ann Elise Sonnier, Chief Executive Officer

MAINE

Brewer Rehabilitation and Living Center, 74 Parkway, S., Brewer, ME 04412; tel. 207/989-7300; FAX. 207/989-4240; Michael Skirven, Administrator

MARYLAND

Carriage Hill Nursing Center, 9101 Second Avenue, Silver Spring, MD 20910; tel. 301/588-5544; FAX. 301/588-0788; Teri Karr, Administrator

Fox Chase Rehabilitation and Nursing Center, 2015 East West Highway, Silver Spring, MD 20910; tel. 301/587-2400; FAX. 301/587-2404; Mary Clinton, Administrator

Home for Incurables of Baltimore City (Keswick), 700 West 40th Street, Baltimore, MD 21211; tel. 410/235-8860, ext. 201; FAX. 410/235-7425; Garret A. Falcone, Executive Director

Horizon Specialty Care Center at Canton Harbor, 1300 South Ellwood Avenue, Baltimore, MD 21224; tel. 410/342-6644; FAX. 410/327-3949; Donna Yorkston, Administrator

Manor Care Ruxton Center, 7001 North Charles Street, Towson, MD 21204; tel. 410/821-9600; FAX. 410/337-8313; Robert F. Harris, Administrator

MedBridge Medical and Physical Rehabilitation, 6600 Ridge Road, Baltimore, MD 21237; tel. 410/574-4950; Barry E. Gratic, Administrator

MASSACHUSETTS

Briarwood Healthcare Nursing Center, 150 Lincoln Street, Needham, MA 01292; tel. 617/449-4040; Penny Packard, Director, Nursing Service

Colonial Nursing and Rehabilitation Center, 125 Broad Street, Weymouth, MA 02188; tel. 617/337-3121; FAX. 617/337-9831; Brian J. McKenna, Administrator

Elihu White Nursing and Rehabilitation Center, 95 Commercial Street, Braintree, MA 02184; tel. 617/848-3678; FAX. 617/356-8559; Kenneth M. Logan, Jr., Administrator

Greenery Extended Care Center, 59 Acton Street, Worcester, MA 01604; tel. 508/791-3147; FAX. 508/753-6267; Walter Collins, Administrator

Greenery Extended Care Center at Beverly, 40 Heather Street, Beverly, MA 01915; tel. 508/927-6220; FAX. 508/927-1438; James F. Smith, Administrator

Greenery Extended Care Center at Danvers, A Horizon Healthcare Facility, 56 Liberty Street, Danvers, MA 01923; tel. 508/777-2700; FAX. 508/777-2372; M. Jean Heffernan, Administrator

Providers / Accredited Freestanding Long–Term Care Facilities

Greenery Extended Care Center at North Andover, 75 Park Street, North Andover, MA 01845; tel. 617/685–3372; John H. Keeney, Administrator

Greenery Rehabilitation & Skilled Nursing Center at Hyannis, 89 Lewis Bay Road, Hyannis, MA 02601; tel. 508/775–7601; FAX. 508/790–4239; Emmanuel P. Freddura, Executive Director

Greenery Rehabilitation Center, 99 Chestnut Hill Avenue, Brighton, MA 02135; tel. 617/787–3390; FAX. 617/787–9169; James Brusstar, Administrator

Greenery Rehabilitation and Skilled Nursing Center at Middleboro, Isaac Street, Middleboro, MA 02346; tel. 508/947–9295; FAX. 508/947–7974; Brian K. Sullivan, Administrator

Harrington House Nursing and Rehabilitation Center, 160 Main Street, Walpole, MA 02081; tel. 508/660–3080; FAX. 508/660–1634; William J. McGinley, Administrator

Jewish Nursing Home of Western Massachusetts, 770 Converse Street, Longmeadow, MA 01106–1786; tel. 413/567–6211; FAX. 413/567–0175; Howard Braverman, President

Jml Care Center, Inc., 184 Ter Heun Drive, Falmouth, MA 02540–0250; tel. 508/457–4621; FAX. 508/457–1218; Joyce A. Carroll, Vice President, Nursing

John Scott House Nursing and Rehabilitation Center, 233 Middle Street, Braintree, MA 02184; tel. 617/843–1860; FAX. 617/843–8834; Thomas D. Nolan, Administrator

Mariner Health Care at Longwood, 53 Parker Hill Road, Boston, MA 02120; tel. 617/278–3700; Anne C. Scott, Director, Nursing Services

Mariner Health Care of Metheun, 480 Jackson Street, Methuen, MA 01844; tel. 508/686–3906; FAX. 508/687–6007; Elizabeth W. Rozzi, Director, Nursing

Meadow Green Nursing and Rehabilitation Center, 45 Woburn Street, Waltham, MA 02154; tel. 617/899–8600; FAX. 617/899–3124; David L. Bell, Administrator

Mediplex Rehabilitation and Skilled Nursing Center of the North Shore, 70 Granite Street, Lynn, MA 01904; tel. 617/581–2400; FAX. 617/581–3080; John A. Holt, Executive Director

Mediplex Rehabilitation and Skilled Nursing Facility of Northampton, 548 Elm Street, Northampton, MA 01060; tel. 413/586–3150; FAX. 413/584–7720; David L. Johnson, Executive Director

Mediplex Skilled Nursing and Rehab Center of Boston, 910 Saratoga Street, East Boston, MA 02128; tel. 617/569–1157; FAX. 617/567–2236; Gerald L. MacDonald, Executive Director

Mediplex Skilled Nursing and Rehabilitation Center of Holyoke, 260 Easthampton Road, Holyoke, MA 01040; tel. 413/538–9733; FAX. 413/538–9919; Kevin F. Henry, Administrator

Mediplex Skilled Nursing and Rehabilitation Center of Lowell, 19 Varnum Street, Lowell, MA 01850; tel. 508/454–5644; FAX. 508/459–6520; Robert E. Kneeland, Administrator

Mediplex of Beverly, 265 Essex Street, Beverly, MA 01915; tel. 508/927–3260; FAX. 508/922–8347; John E. Gerety, Jr., Executive Director

Mediplex of Brookline, 99 Park Street, Brookline, MA 02146; tel. 617/731–1050; Gerald Labourene, Administrator

Mediplex of East Longmeadow, 135 Benton Drive, East Longmeadow, MA 01028; tel. 413/525–3336; Lisa Ferreri, Administrator

Mediplex of Lexington, 178 Lowell Street, Lexington, MA 02173; tel. 617/862–7400; FAX. 617/862–9255; Robert Belluche, Administrator

Mediplex of Newton, 2101 Washington Street, Newton, MA 02162; tel. 617/969–4660; FAX. 617/964–4622; Matt Weinstock, Executive Director

Milford Meadows Skilled Nursing and Rehabilitation Center, 10 Veteran's Memorial Drive, Milford, MA 01757; tel. 508/473–6414; FAX. 508/473–9974; Ira M. Schoenberger, Executive Director

Peabody Glen Nursing Center, 199 Andover Street, Peabody, MA 01960; tel. 508/531–0772; FAX. 508/532–4134; Clyde Tyler, Administrator

Port Rehabilitation and Skilled Nursing Center, Hale and Low Streets, Newburyport, MA 01950; tel. 508/462–7373; FAX. 508/462–6510; Kathleen Pepe, RNC, Director, Quality Assurance

Randolph Crossings Nursing Center, 49 Thomas Patten Drive, Randolph, MA 02368; tel. 617/961–1160; FAX. 617/963–5744; Emmanuel P. Freddura, Administrator

Sacred Heart Nursing Home, 359 Summer Street, New Bedford, MA 02740–5599; tel. 508/996–6751; FAX. 508/996–6751, ext. 24; Sister Blandine D'Amours, Administrator

Sherrill House, Inc., 135 South Huntington Avenue, Boston, MA 02130; tel. 617/731–2400; FAX. 617/731–8671; Donald M. Powell, Executive Director

Westridge Health Care Center, 121 Northboro Road, Marlborough, MA 01752; tel. 508/485–4040; FAX. 508/460–6595; William P. Fleming, Executive Director

Willowood Health Care Center, 175 Franklin Street, North Adams, MA 01247; tel. 413/664–4041; FAX. 413/664–8447; Sandra L. Stanek, Administrator

Willowood Healthcare Center, Christian Hill Road, P.O. Box 330, Great Barrington, MA 01230; tel. 413/528–4560; FAX. 413/528–5691; Frank Meyers, Administrator

Willowood of Williamstown, 25 Adams Road, Williamstown, MA 01267; tel. 413/458–2111; Darrell A. Carlson, Administrator

Wilmington Woods Nursing Care Center, 750 Woburn Street, Wilmington, MA 01887; tel. 508/988–0888; Steve DeMaranville, Executive Director

MICHIGAN

Bay County Medical Care Facility, 564 West Hampton Road, Essexville, MI 48732; tel. 517/892–3591; FAX. 517/892–6991; William R. Mahoney, Administrator

Clare Nursing Home, Inc., 600 S.E. 4th Street, Clare, MI 48617; tel. 517/386–7723; FAX. 517/386–4100; Wilma Shurlow, Administrator

Crestmont Nursing Care Center, 111 Trealout Drive, Fenton, MI 48430; tel. 810/629–4105; Barbara L. Lawson, Executive Director

Georgian Bloomfield, Inc., 2975 Adams Road, Bloomfield Hills, MI 48013; tel. 313/645–2900; Mary Caldera, Administrator

Greenery Extended Care Center, 34225 Grand River, Farmington, MI 48335; tel. 313/477–7373; Thomas L. Johnsrud, Administrator

Greenery Health Care Center, 4800 Clintonville Road, Clarkston, MI 48346; tel. 313/674–0903; Maureen L. Hewitt, Executive Director

Greenery Health Care Center, 3003 West Grand River, Howell, MI 48843; tel. 517/546–4210; Darlena Richman, Administrator

Integrated Health Services of Michigan at Riverbend, 11941 Belsay Road, Grand Blanc, MI 48439; tel. 313/694–1970; John F. Beaudrie, Executive Director, Chief Executive Officer

Isabella County Medical Care Facility, 1222 North Drive, Mount Pleasant, MI 48858; tel. 517/772–2957; FAX. 517/772–3669; Vickie S. Block, Administrator

Martha T. Berry Memorial Medical Care Facility, 43533 Elizabeth Road, Mount Clemens, MI 48043; tel. 810/469–5623; FAX. 810/469–6352; Raymond D. Pietrzak, Administrator

Mercy Bellbrook, 873 W. Avon Road, Rochester Hills, MI 48307; tel. 810/656–3239, ext. 203; FAX. 810/656–8160; Ann L. Eastman, Administrator

Mercy Pavilion of Battle Creek, 80 North 20th, Battle Creek, MI 49015; tel. 616/964–5400; FAX. 616/964–5559; Michael Richards, Senior Administrator

Oakland County Medical Care Facility, 1200 North Telegraph Road, Pontiac, MI 48341–0469; tel. 810/858–1415; FAX. 810/858–4026; Shirla F. Kugler, Administrator

Shore Haven, A Mercy Living Center, 900 S. Beacon Boulevard, Grand Haven, MI 49417; tel. 616/846–1850; FAX. 616/846–0971; Nancy J. Ritchie, Administrator

University Health Care Center, 28550 Five Mile Road, Livonia, MI 48154; tel. 313/427–8270; FAX. 313/427–2550; John T. Graham, Director

MISSOURI

Harry S. Truman Restorative Center, 5700 Arsenal Street, St. Louis, MO 63139; tel. 314/768–6600, ext. 13; FAX. 314/645–7628; Shirley E. Herr, RN, Chief Executive Officer

Integrated Health Services at Alpine North, 4700 Cliff View Drive, Kansas City, MO 64150; tel. 816/741–5105; Karen Leverich, Administrator

Integrated Health Services at Big Bend Woods, 110 Highland, Valley Park, MO 63088; tel. 314/225–5144; FAX. 314/225–8427; Melissa J. Watkins, Administrator

Integrated Health Services of St. Louis at Gravois, 10954 Kennerly Road, St. Louis, MO 63128; tel. 314/843–4242; FAX. 314/843–5370; Cathy Deffendall, Administrator

Village North Health Center, 11160 Village North Drive, St. Louis, MO 63136; tel. 314/355–8010; Wes Sperr, Administrator

Village North Manor, 6768 North Highway 67, Florissant, MO 63034; tel. 314/741–9101; Judy R. Mincher, Administrator

Village North Woods, 9500 Bellefontaine Road, St. Louis, MO 63137; tel. 314/868–1400; FAX. 314/868–0170; Gladys A. Sullivan, Administrator

NEVADA

Integrated Health Services of Las Vegas, 2170 East Harmon Avenue, Las Vegas, NV 89119; tel. 702/794–0100; FAX. 702/794–0041; Maryanne Smith, Assistant Vice President

NEW HAMPSHIRE

Good Shepherd Nursing Home, Five Plantation Dive, Joffrey, NH 03452; tel. 603/532–8762; Judith A. LeBlanc, Administrator

Greenbriar Terrace Healthcare, 55 Harris Road, Nashua, NH 03062; tel. 603/888–1573; FAX. 603/888–5089; Arthur O'Leary, Administrator

Integrated Health Services at Derry, 8 Peabody Road, Derry, NH 03038; tel. 603/434–1566; Malcolm Perry, Administrator

Integrated Health Services of New Hampshire at Manchester, 191 Hackett Hill Road, Manchester, NH 03102; tel. 603/668–8161; FAX. 603/622–2584; Marcia S. Couitt, Administrator

Mount Carmel Nursing Home, 235 Myrtle Street, Manchester, NH 03104; tel. 603/627–3811; Sister Jacinta Mary Hirner, Administrator

Saint Ann Home, 195 Dover Point Road, Dover, NH 03820; tel. 603/742–2612; Sister Margaret Therese Jackson, Administrator

St. Francis Home, 406 Court Street, Laconia, NH 03246; tel. 603/524–0466; FAX. 603/527–0884; Julieann Fay, Administrator

St. Teresa's Manor, 519 Bridge Street, Manchester, NH 03104; tel. 603/668–2373; Monique Dosogne, Administrator

St. Vincent de Paul Nursing Home, 29 Providence Avenue, Berlin, NH 03570; tel. 603/752–1820; FAX. 603/752–7149; Stephen V. Fulchino, Administrator

NEW JERSEY

Daughters of Miriam Center for the Aged, 155 Hazel Street, Clifton, NJ 07015; tel. 201/772–3700; FAX. 201/772–5044; Steven Schilsky, L.N.H.A., Executive Vice President

Dunroven Health Care Center, 221 County Road, Cresskill, NJ 07656; tel. 201/567–9310; FAX. 201/567–9239; Donald C. DeVries, Executive Director

Integrated Health Services of New Jersey at Somerset Valley, 1621 Route 22, Bound Brook, NJ 08805; tel. 908/469–2000; Carolyn Allen, Executive Director

King James Care and Rehabilitation Center, 1165 Easton Avenue, Somerset, NJ 08873; tel. 908/246–4100; FAX. 908/246–3926; Egon Scheil, Administrator

Providers / Accredited Freestanding Long-Term Care Facilities

Linwood Convalescent Center, New Road and Central Avenue, Linwood, NJ 08221; tel. 609/927-6131; FAX. 609/927-0069; David G. Wolf, Administrator

MedBridge Medical and Physical Rehabilitation, 1180 Route 22 West, Mountainside, NJ 07092; tel. 908/654-0020; FAX. 908/654-8661; Catherine Engler, Executive Director

MedBridge Physical and Rehabilitation Services, 550 Jessup Road, West Deptford, NJ 08066; tel. 609/848-9551; FAX. 609/848-1817; Paul Goldenberg, Administrator

Morris View Nursing Home, 540 West Hanover Avenue, Morris Plains, NJ 07950; tel. 201/285-2820; FAX. 201/285-6062; Joaquin Deniz, Administrator

The Manor, 689 West Main Street, Freehold, NJ 07728; tel. 908/431-5200, ext. 11; FAX. 908/409-2446; Mrs. J. Escovar, Administrator

Valley Health Care Center, 300 Old Hook Road, Westwood, NJ 07675; tel. 201/664-8888; FAX. 201/664-9577; Dorothy E. Franklin, Administrator

Voorhees Pediatric Facility, 1304 Laurel Oak Road, Voorhees, NJ 08043; tel. 609/346-3300; FAX. 609/435-4223; Carl Underland, Administrator

Woodcrest Center, 800 River Road, New Milford, NJ 07646; tel. 201/967-1700; FAX. 201/967-5423; Jack Ellias, Administrator

NEW YORK

Bainbridge Nursing Home, 3518 Bainbridge Avenue, Bronx, NY 10467; tel. 718/655-1991; FAX. 718/655-3903; Isaac Goldbrenner, Administrator

Community Skilled Nursing Facility, 23 Harper Street, Stamford, NY 12167; tel. 607/652-7521; FAX. 607/652-3362; Jeffry Ruso, Administrator

Dumont Masonic Home, 676 Pelham Road, New Rochelle, NY 10805; tel. 914/632-9600; FAX. 914/632-4766; Beth Goldstein, Administrator

East Haven Nursing Home, 2323 Eastchester Road, Bronx, NY 10469; tel. 718/655-2848; FAX. 718/655-2750; Joseph Brachfeld, Administrator

Golden Gate Health Care Center, Inc., 191 Bradley Avenue, Staten Island, NY 10314; tel. 718/698-8800; FAX. 718/698-5536; Alan Chopp, Administrator

Grace Plaza of Great Neck, Inc., 15 St Paul's Place, Great Neck, NY 11021; tel. 516/466-3001; FAX. 516/829-3854; Celia Strow, Administrator

Haven Manor Health Care Center, 1441 Gateway Boulevard, Far Rockaway, NY 11691; tel. 718/471-1500; FAX. 718/868-0030; Aron Cytryn, Administrator

Highgate Manor of Cortland, Inc., 28 Kellogg Road, Cortland, NY 13045; tel. 607/753-9631; FAX. 607/756-2968; Sue Connors, Chief Executive Officer

Highgate Manor of Rensselaer, Inc., 100 New Turnpike Road, Troy, NY 12182; tel. 518/235-1410; Mark Carden, Administrator

Hilltop Manor of Niskayuna, 1805 Providence Avenue, Niskayuna, NY 12309; tel. 518/374-2212; FAX. 518/374-4330; Jill M. Mozzi, Administrator

Margaret Tietz Center for Nursing Care, 164-11 Chapin Parkway, Jamaica, NY 11432; tel. 718/523-6400, ext. 705; FAX. 718/262-8839; Kenneth M. Brown, President

Mosolu Parkway Nursing Home, 3356 Perry Avenue, Bronx, NY 10467; tel. 718/655-3568; FAX. 718/515-5713; Issac Schapiro, Administrator

Palm Gardens Nursing Home, 615 Avenue C, Brooklyn, NY 11218; tel. 718/633-3300; FAX. 718/633-3320; Shoshana Lefkowitz, Administrator

Promenade Nursing Home, 140 Beach 114th Street, Rockaway Park, NY 11694; tel. 718/945-4600; FAX. 718/634-8237; Stanley Spector, Chief Executive Officer

Providence Rest, 3304 Waterbury Avenue, Bronx, NY 10465; tel. 718/931-3000; FAX. 718/863-0185; Sister Joanne Marruso, C.S.J.B., Chief Executive Officer, Administrtator

Rosewood Gardens Convalescent Home, Inc., 284 Troy Road, Rensselaer, NY 12144; tel. 518/286-1621; Beverly Benno, Administrator

Sea View Hospital and Home, 460 Brielle Avenue, Staten Island, NY 10314; tel. 718/317-3221; FAX. 718/351-7898; Jane M. Lyons, Executive Director

St. Mary's Hospital for Children, Inc., 29-01 216th Street, Bayside, NY 11360; tel. 718/281-8800, ext. 8850; FAX. 718/279-2141; Stuart C. Kaplan, Executive Vice President

Victory Lake Nursing Center, 419 North Quaker Lane, Hyde Park, NY 12538; tel. 914/229-9177; FAX. 914/229-9819; Robert C. Farrow, M.P.H., Administrator

Wayne Nursing Home, 3530 Wayne Avenue, Bronx, NY 10467; tel. 212/655-1700, ext. 541; FAX. 212/515-5650; I. Hartman, Assistant Administrator

Wesley Group, Inc., 630 East Avenue, Rochester, NY 14607-2194; tel. 716/442-0863; FAX. 716/244-1773; Jon R. Zemans, President, Chief Executive Officer

NORTH CAROLINA

Emerald Health Care of Taylorsville, Inc., 539 Third Street, S.W., Taylorsville, NC 28681; tel. 704/632-8146; Richard C. Thompson, Administrator

Hillhaven Rehabilitation and Convalescent Center, 2006 South 16th Street, Wilmington, NC 28401; tel. 910/763-6271; FAX. 910/251-9803; Faye M. Kennedy, Administrator

Horizon Rehabilitation Center, 3100 Erwin Road, Durham, NC 27705; tel. 919/383-1546; FAX. 919/382-0156; Maureen O'Neal, Administrator

Integrated Health Services of Raleigh at Crabtree Valley, 3838 Blue Ridge Road, Raleigh, NC 27612; tel. 919/781-4900; Deo Garlock, Executive Director

North Carolina Special Care Center, Ward Boulevard, Wilson, NC 27893; tel. 919/399-2112; Seth P. Hunt, Jr., Director

OHIO

Arbors East Subacute Nursing and Rehabilitation Center, 5500 East Broad Street, Columbus, OH 43213; tel. 614/575-9003; FAX. 614/575-9101; Alexander Bettinger, Administrator

Arbors West, 375 West Main Street, West Jefferson, OH 43162; tel. 614/879-7661; Thomas C. Widney

Arbors at Canton, 2714 13th Street, N.W., Canton, OH 44708; tel. 216/456-2842; Gary L. Van, Administrator

Arbors at Delaware, 2270 Warrensburg Road, Delaware, OH 43015; tel. 614/369-9614; FAX. 614/363-7677; Kelly Darrow, Administrator

Arbors at Marietta, 400 Seventh Street, Marietta, OH 45750; tel. 614/373-3597; Richard W. Porter, Administrator

Arbors at Toledo Subacute and Rehabilitation Center, 2920 Cherry Street, Toledo, OH 43608; tel. 419/242-7458; FAX. 419/242-6514; Robert D. Brooks, Administrator

Aurora Manor Special Care Centre, 101 Bissell Road, Aurora, OH 44022; tel. 216/562-5000; Debra Kover, Administrator

Centerburg Nursing Center, 212 Fairview Avenue, Centerburg, OH 43011; tel. 614/625-5774; FAX. 614/625-7426; Montell Hutchison, Administrator

Columbus Rehabilitation and Subacute Institute, 44 South Souder Avenue, Columbus, OH 43222; tel. 614/228-9500, ext. 231; FAX. 614/228-3989; Ronald J. Castagno, FACHE, Executive Director

Community Multicare Center, 908 Symmes Road, Fairfield, OH 45014; tel. 513/868-6500; FAX. 513/844-8579; Anne Dahling, Chief Executive Officer

Gateway Health Care Center, Three Gateway Drive, Euclid, OH 44119; tel. 216/486-4949; Linda Bliss, Director, Nursing

Heartland of Beavercreek, 1974 North Fairfield Road, Dayton, OH 45432; tel. 515/429-1106; Jim Kyle, Administrator

Heartland of Marysville, 755 South Plum Street, Marysville, OH 43040; tel. 513/644-8836; FAX. 513/644-1811; James M. Reese, Administrator

Heartland of Perrysburg, 10540 Fremont Pike, Perrysburg, OH 443551; tel. 419/874-3578; John K. Graham, Director, New Product

Hennis Care Center, 1720 Cross Street, Dover, OH 44622; tel. 216/364-8849; FAX. 216/343-2411; H. D. Hennis, Administrator

Horizon Village Nursing and Rehabilitation Center, 2473 North Road, Northeast, Warren, OH 44483; tel. 216/372-2251; Albert C. Parton, Administrator

IHS at Waterford Commons Subacute Care and Rehabilitation Center, 955 Garden Lake Parkway, Toledo, OH 43614; tel. 419/382-2200; FAX. 419/381-0188; Martin M. Jan, Administrator, Executive Director

MedBridge Medical and Physical Rehabilitation, 23225 Lorain Road, North Olmsted, OH 44070; tel. 216/779-6900; Susan M. Doherty, Administrator

Middlebury Manor, 974 East Market Street, Akron, OH 44305; tel. 216/762-9066; Daniel H. Blechschmid, MHA, L.N.H.A., Assistant Administrator

Newark Healthcare Centre, 75 McMillen Drive, Newark, OH 43055; tel. 614/344-0357; Joanne Whiteman, Administrator

Northland Terrace Medical Center for Subacute Care and Rehabilitation, 5700 Karl Road, Columbus, OH 43229; tel. 614/846-5420; FAX. 614/846-3247; Sharon L. Reynolds, Administrator

Secrest/Giffin Long Term Care Facility, 3416 South Columbus Avenue, Sandusky, OH 44870; tel. 419/625-2454, ext. 500; FAX. 419/625-3207; Linda Wagner, Nursing Home Administrator

St. Augustine Manor, 7801 Detroit Avenue, Cleveland, OH 44102; tel. 216/634-7400; FAX. 216/634-7483; Patrick Gareau, President, Chief Executive Officer

Walton Manor Health Care Center, 19859 Alexander Road, Walton Hills, OH 44146; tel. 216/439-4433; Susanne M. Rusnak, Administrator

Whitecliff Manor, 12504 Cedar Road, Cleveland Heights, OH 44106; tel. 216/371-3600; FAX. 216/371-3631; Sam Zimerman, Owner

OKLAHOMA

Oklahoma Veterans Center Claremore Division, 3001 West Blue Starr Drive, Claremore, OK 74018; tel. 918/342-5432; Phillip L. Dirskill, Administrator

Oklahoma Veterans Center Clinton Division, South Highway 183, P.O. Box 1209, Clinton, OK 73601; tel. 405/323-5540; FAX. 405/323-3752; Paul L. Brown, Administrator

Oklahoma Veterans Center Norman Division, 12th and East Main Streets, P.O. Box 1668, Norman, OK 73070; tel. 405/360-5600; FAX. 405/364-8432; Billie D. Taylor, Administrator

OREGON

Cascade Terrace Nursing Center, 5601 Southeast 122nd Avenue, Portland, OR 97236; tel. 503/761-3181; FAX. 503/760-6556; Diane Richardson, Administrator

PENNSYLVANIA

Bishop Nursing Home, Inc., 318 South Orange Street, Media, PA 19063; tel. 215/565-3881; Walter M. Strine, Jr., Chief Executive Officer

Chester Care Center, 15th Street and Shaw Terrace, Chester, PA 19013; tel. 215/499-8800; Geraldine Willmott, Administrator

Dowden Nursing and Rehabilitation Center, 3503 Rhoads Avenue, Newtown, PA 19073; tel. 215/359-0300; FAX. 215/359-1187; Katherine D. Ohline, Administrator

Providers / Accredited Freestanding Long-Term Care Facilities

Greenery Rehabilitation and Skilled Nursing Center at Meadowlands, Road 1, Box 146, Route 519 South, Canonsburg, PA 15317; tel. 412/745–8000, ext. 212; FAX. 412/746–8780; Joseph G. Hugar, Executive Director

Hanover Hall Nursing and Rehabilitation Center, 267 Frederick Street, Hanover, PA 17331; tel. 717/637–8937; FAX. 717/633–5700; Christine F. Lorah, NHA, Administrator

Head Injury Recovery Center at Hillcrest, 404 East Harford Street, Milford, PA 18337; tel. 717/296–9261; FAX. 717/296–3607; David Scarisbrick, Program Director

Heatherbank Rehabilitation and Skilled Nursing Center, 745 Chiques Hill Road, Columbia, PA 17512; tel. 717/684–7555; FAX. 717/684–0571; Nan Kennicutt, Director, Admissions

Integrated Health Services of Greater Pittsburgh, 890 Mount Pleasant Road, Greensboro, PA 15601; tel. 412/837–8076; FAX. 412/837–3152; James Anthony Palmer, Administrator

Jefferson Manor Health Centers, Rural Route 5, Brookville, PA 15825; tel. 814/849–8026; FAX. 814/849–3889; Diane Endress, Assistant Director, Nursing

Laurel Nursing and Rehabilitation Center, 125 Holly Road, Hamburg, PA 19526–6902; tel. 610/562–2284; FAX. 610/562–0775; Sue B. Righter, Director, Nursing

Liberty Nursing Center, 17th and Allen Streets, Allentown, PA 18104; tel. 215/432–4351; John K. Graham, Director, Operational Support

Manchester House Nursing & Convalescent Center, 411 Manchester Avenue, Media, PA 19063; tel. 610/565–1800; FAX. 610/891–0471; Donna L. Doyle, RN, NHA, Administrator

Presbyterian Medical Center of Oakmont, 1215 Hulton Road, Oakmont, PA 15139; tel. 412/828–5600; FAX. 412/826–6121; Paul M. Winkler, NHA, Executive Vice President

Presbyterian Medical Center of Washington, 835 South Main Street, Washington, PA 15301; tel. 412/222–4300; FAX. 412/223–5697; Harvey Brown, Jr., Executive Vice President, Chief Executive Officer

Quincy United Methodist Home, Orphanage Road, P.O. Box 217, Quincy, PA 17247; tel. 717/749–3151; Kathleen R. Hoos, RN, NHA, President

Rest Haven-York, 1050 South George Street, York, PA 17403; tel. 717/843–9866; FAX. 717/846–5894; Nancy A. Underwood, Administrator

South Mountain Restoration Center, 10058 South Mountain Road, South Mountain, PA 17261; tel. 717/749–3121, ext. 316; FAX. 717/749–3946; Thomas A. Buckus, Administrator

St. John Lutheran Care Center, 500 Wittenberg Way, Mars, PA 16046; tel. 412/625–1571, ext. 255; FAX. 412/625–1571, ext. 210; John W. Schrader, Executive Director

The Healthcare Campus at Colonial Manor, 970 Colonial Avenue, York, PA 17403; tel. 717/845–2661; FAX. 717/854–0529; George R. Lorah, Administrator

Twinbrook Medical Center, 3805 Field Street, Erie, PA 16511; tel. 814/899–0651; FAX. 814/899–9829; Elizabeth Seibert, Nursing Home Administrator

Woodhaven Care Center, 2400 McGinley Road, Monroeville, PA 15146; tel. 412/856–4770; Stuart Lindeman, Administrator

RHODE ISLAND

Oak Hill Nursing and Rehabilitation Center, 544 Pleasant Street, Pawtucket, RI 02860; tel. 401/725–8888; Richard E. Gamache, Administrator

Saint Elizabeth Home, 109 Melrose Street, Providence, RI 02907–1898; tel. 401/941–0200; FAX. 401/941–5231; Steven J. Horowitz, Administrator

SOUTH CAROLINA

C. M. Tucker, Jr./Dowdy Gardner Nursing Care Center, 2200 Harden Street, Columbia, SC 29203–7199; tel. 803/737–5302; FAX. 803/737–5342; Lee V. Woodbury, M.D., Director, Administrator

Eagle Landing Health Care Center, 1800 Eagle Landing Boulevard, Hanahan, SC 29406; tel. 803/553–656; John K. Graham, Director, New Product

Integrated Health Services of Charleston at Driftwood, 2375 Baker Hospital Boulevard, North Charleston, SC 29405; tel. 803/744–2750; FAX. 803/747–0406; B. C. Davidson, Administrator

TENNESSEE

Allen Morgan Health Center, 177 North Highland, Memphis, TN 38111; tel. 901/325–4003; FAX. 901/327–8847; Rebecca D. DeRousse, Vice President, Administrator

Briarcliff Health Care Center, 100 Elmhurst Drive, Oak Ridge, TN 37803; tel. 615/481–3367; FAX. 615/483–7121; Billy S. Hunt, Administrator

Manor House of Dover, 537 Spring Street, Dover, TN 37058–8039; tel. 615/232–6902; Sheila K. McArdle, Regional Vice President

TEXAS

American Transitional Hospital–Houston West, Sixth Floor Tower, 8850 Long Point Road, Houston, TX 77055; tel. 713/984–2273; FAX. 713/984–9826; Connie Cowan, Chief Executive Officer, Administrator

Hearthstone of Round Rock, 401 Oakwood Boulevard, Round Rock, TX 78681; tel. 512/388–7494; Stacy Adams, Administrator

Heartland Health Care Center, 11406 Rustic Rock Drive, Austin, TX 78750; tel. 512/335–5028; Mary Lou Clem, Administrator

Heartland Health Care Center–Bedford, 2001 Forst Ridge Drive, Bedford, TX 76021; tel. 817/571–6804; FAX. 817/267–4176; Donna J. Snyder, Administrator

Heartland of San Antonio, One Heartland Drive, San Antonio, TX 78247; tel. 210/653–1219; Guy Bowles, Administrator

Integrated Health Services of Amarillo, 5601 Plum Creek Drive, Amarillo, TX 79124; tel. 806/351–1000; Dalton Stewart, Executive Director

Integrated Health Services of Dallas at Treemont, 5550 Harvest Hill Road, Dallas, TX 75230; tel. 214/661–1862; FAX. 214/715–5557; John W. Conway, Administrator

Normandy Terrace Northeast Nursing and Rehabilitation Center, 8607 Village Drive, San Antonio, TX 78217; tel. 210/656–6733; FAX. 210/656–4507; William M. Moore, Administrator

UTAH

South Davis Community Hospital, 401 South 400 East, Bountiful, UT 84010; tel. 801/295–2361; Gordon W. Bennet, Administrator

Sunshine Terrace Foundation, Inc., 225 North 200 West, Logan, UT 84321–3805; tel. 801/752–0411, ext. 216; FAX. 801/752–1318; Sara V. Sinclair, RN, Administrator

VIRGINIA

Berkshire Health Care Center, 705 Clearview Drive, Vinton, VA 24179; tel. 703/982–6691; FAX. 703/982–6518; Richie Alba, Administrator

Camelot Hall of Lynchburg, 5615 Seminole Avenue, Lynchburg, VA 24502; tel. 804/239–2657; FAX. 804/239–4062; Elizabeth E. Kail, Administrator

Chesterfield County Health Center Commission, Lucy Corr Nursing Home, 6800 Lucy Corr Court, Chesterfield, VA 23832; tel. 804/748–1511; FAX. 804/796–6285; Jacob W. Mast, Chief Executive Officer

Goodwin House West, 3440 South Jefferson Street, Falls Church, VA 22041; tel. 703/578–7230; Fran Casey, Director

Health of Virginia, 2420 Pemberton Road, Richmond, VA 23233–3209; tel. 804/747–9200; FAX. 804/747–1574; Walter W. Regirer, President, General Counsel

Hillcrest Manor Nursing Home, Inc., 110 Lauck Drive, Winchester, VA 22603; tel. 703/667–7830; FAX. 703/662–6557; Doris M. Traylor, Administrator

Hillhaven Rehabilitation Nursing Center of Virginia Beach, 1148 First Colonial Road, Virginia Beach, VA 23454–4249; tel. 804/481–3321; Vicki Fisher, Administrator

Hillhaven Rehabilitation and Nursing Center Norfolk, 1005 Hampton Boulevard, Norfolk, VA 23507; tel. 804/623–5602; FAX. 804/623–4646; Vickie Archer, Administrator

James River Convalescent Center, 540 Aberthaw Avenue, Newport News, VA 23601; tel. 804/595–2273; Nancy Pittman, Administrator, Vice President

Manning Convalescent Home, Inc., 175 Hatton Street, Portsmouth, VA 23705; tel. 804/399–1321; FAX. 804/399–4337; T. W. Manning, President

Manor Care Fair Oaks Nursing and Rehabilitation Center, 12475 Lee Jackson Memorial Highway, Fairfax, VA 22033; tel. 703/352–7172, ext. 3203; FAX. 703/218–3200; Mary Jo Sbitani, Administrator

Manor Care Nursing and Rehabilitation Center, 550 South Carlin Springs Road, Arlington, VA 22204; tel. 703/379–7200; FAX. 703/820–1048; Barry Grofie, Administrator

Riverside Regional Convalescent Center, 1000 Old Denbigh Boulevard, Newport News, VA 23602; tel. 804/875–2020; FAX. 804/875–2036; Patricia A. Iannetta, Administrator

WASHINGTON

Blue Mountain Medical and Rehabilitation Center, 1200 S.E. 12th, College Place, WA 99324; tel. 509/529–4080; FAX. 509/529–2173; Gloria Botimer, Chief Executive Officer

Harmony Gardens Care Center, 10010 Des Moines Way, S., Seattle, WA 98168; tel. 206/762–0166; FAX. 206/762–8612; Marilyn Heger, Ph.D., Administrator

Integrated Health Services of Seattle, 820 Northwest 95th Street; Seattle, WA 98117; tel. 206/782–0100, ext. 228; FAX. 206/781–1448; Kathleen Parry, Administrator

Phoenix Rehabilitation Center, 555 16th Avenue, Seattle, WA 98122; tel. 206/324–8200; FAX. 206/324–0780; Skip McDonald, Ph.D., Executive Director

WEST VIRGINIA

GlenWood Park Retirement Village, Route One, Box 464, Princeton, WV 24740–9244; tel. 304/425–8128; Daniel W. Farley, Ph.D., CNHA, President, Chief Executive Officer

WISCONSIN

Franciscan Villa, 3601 South Chicago Avenue, South Milwaukee, WI 53172; tel. 414/764–4100; FAX. 414/764–0706; Roger L. DeMark, Administrator

Middleton Village Nursing and Rehabilitation Center, 6201 Elmwood Avenue, Middleton, WI 53562; tel. 608/831–8300; Mary Ann Drescher, Administrator

Mount Carmel Health and Rehabilitation Center, 5700 West Layton Avenue, Milwaukee, WI 53220; tel. 414/281–7200; Andrea J. Ludington, Executive Director

Northwest Health Care Center, 7800 West Fond Du Lac Avenue, Milwaukee, WI 53218; tel. 414/464–3950; FAX. 414/464–5110; Candy Gremore, Executive Director

Outagamie County Health Center, 3400 West Brewster Street, Appleton, WI 54914; tel. 414/832–5400; FAX. 414/832–5416; David A. Rothmann, Administrator

Villa Clement and Clement Manor Health Center, 3939 South 92nd Street, Greenfield, WI 53228; tel. 414/321–1800; FAX. 414/546–7305; Joan Carlson, President, Chief Executive Officer

Accredited Freestanding Psychiatric Facilities

The accredited freestanding psychiatric facilities listed have been accredited as of January 1, 1995, by the Joint Commission on Accreditation of Healthcare Organizations by decision of the Accreditation Committee of the Board of Commissioners.

The facilities listed here have been found to be in substantial compliance with the Joint Commissions standards for freestanding pyschiatric facilities, as found in the Consolidated Standards Manual.

Please refer to section A of the AHA Guide for information on hospitals with inpatient and/or outpatient services. These hospitals are identified by Facility Codes F52, F53, F54, F55, F56, F57, F58 and F59. In section A, those hospitals identified by Approval Code 1 are JCAHO accredited.

We present this list simply as a convenient directory. Inclusion or omission of any organization's name indicates neither approval nor disapproval by the American Hospital Association.

United States

ALABAMA

Bradford Adolescent at Oak Mountain, 2280 Highway, Pelham, AL 35124; tel. 205/664-3460; Eve S. Laxer, Chief Executive Officer

Bradford at Birmingham for Adults, 1189 Allbritton Road, Warrior, AL 35180; tel. 205/833-4000; FAX. 205/833-3669; Clay Simmons, Chief Executive Officer

Bradford at Huntsville, 1600 Browns Ferry Road, Madison, AL 35758; tel. 205/461-7272; Benjamin Y. Lee, Ph.D., Chief Executive Officer

Charter Academy of Mobile, 251 Cox Street, Mobile, AL 36604; tel. 334/432-4111; FAX. 334/432-4626; Keith Cox, Chief Executive Officer

Cobblestone Psychiatric Center, 400 14th Street, Suite C, Decatur, AL 35601; tel. 205/351-6858; John C. Hayes, Medical Director

Eufaula Adolescent Center, P.O. Box 1179, Eufaula, AL 36072-1179; tel. 334/687-5741; FAX. 334/687-0693; Carol M. Driggers, Quality Improvement

Mobile Mental Health Center, Inc., 2400 Gordon Smith Drive, Mobile, AL 36617; tel. 334/473-4423; FAX. 334/450-2213; T. Edmund Lakeman, Executive Director

New Perspectives, Inc., 1000 Fairfax Park, Tuscaloosa, AL 35406; tel. 205/759-3229; Martha Hinkle, Administrator

Parkside Lodge of Birmingham, 1189 Allbritton Road, Warrior, AL 35180; tel. 205/647-1945; Jerry W. Crowder, Executive Director

Partial Hospital Institute of America, Inc., 501 Bel Air Boulevard, Mobile, AL 36606; tel. 334/473-6700; James S. Harrold, Chief Executive Officer

Pathway, Inc., Route 2, Box 352-A, New Brockton, AL 36351; tel. 334/894-6322; Norman G. Hemp, Executive Director

Physicians' Psychiatric Clinic, P.C., 10 Mobile Street, Mobile, AL 36607; tel. 334/450-1200; FAX. 334/450-1207; Maureen Driscoll, M.S., Director, Clinical Services

Thomasville Mental Health Rehabilitation Center, Bashi Road, Thomasville, AL 36784; tel. 334/636-5421, ext. 230; FAX. 334/636-5421, ext. 285; Kimberly S. Ingram, M.S.N., Facility Director

Three Springs Residential Treatment Center, 101 Madison Street, P.O. Box 370, Courtland, AL 35618; tel. 205/637-2199; Gregory Martin, Chief Executive Officer

ALASKA

Alaska Children's Services, 4600 Abbott Road, Anchorage, AK 99507; tel. 907/346-2101; FAX. 907/346-2748; James E. Maley, Executive Director

ARIZONA

ABCS Little Canyon Center, Inc., P.O. Box 39239, Phoenix, AZ 85069-9239; tel. 602/943-7760; FAX. 602/943-7864; Bob Garrett, CBSW, Admissions Coordinator

Arizona Children's Home Association, 2700 South 8th Avenue, Tucson, AZ 85725-7277; tel. 602/622-7611; FAX. 602/624-7042; Fred J. Chaffee, Executive Director

Chandler Valley Hope, 501 North Washington, Chandler, AZ 85244-1839; tel. 602/899-3335; FAX. 602/899-6697; Julian S. Pickens, Ed.D., Chief Executive Officer

Cottonwood De Tucson, Inc., 4110 West Sweetwater Drive, Tucson, AZ 85745; tel. 602/743-0411; FAX. 602/743-7991; Ronald B. Welch, President, Chief Executive Officer

Devereux/Arizona, 6436 East Sweetwater Avenue, Scottsdale, AZ 85254; tel. 602/998-2920; FAX. 602/443-5589; Stephen A. Vitali, Executive Director

META Services, 621 West Southern Avenue, Mesa, AZ 85210; tel. 602/649-1111; Eugene Johnson, Executive Director

Mingus Mountain Estate Residential Center, Inc., HC #76, Prescott Valley, AZ 86314; tel. 602/249-1311; Dr. Pauline H. Don Carlos, Chief Executive Officer

Parc Place, 5116 East Thomas Road, Phoenix, AZ 85018; tel. 602/840-4774, ext. 311; FAX. 602/840-7567; Mishele K. Boynton, B.S., Director, Admissions and Intake

Prehab of Arizona, Inc., 868 East University, Mesa, AZ 85203; tel. 602/969-4024; Michael T. Hughes, Executive Director

Remuda Ranch Center for Anorexia and Bulimia, Jack Burden Road, Wickenburg, AZ 85358; tel. 602/684-3913; FAX. 602/684-2908; Ward Keller, President

Sierra Tucson, Inc., 16500 North Lago Del Oro Parkway, Tucson, AZ 85737; tel. 602/624-4000; Ken Whitaker, Executive Director

The Meadows, 1655 North Tegner, P.O. Box 97, Highway 89/93, Wickenburg, AZ 85358; tel. 800/621-4062; FAX. 602/684-3261; J. P. Mellody, Executive Director

The New Foundation, 1200 North 77th Street, Scottsdale, AZ 85271; tel. 602/945-3302; David S. Hedgcock, Executive Director

Touchstone Community, Inc., 4202 East Union Hill Drive, Phoenix, AZ 85024; tel. 602/992-2952; FAX. 602/953-9217; Ida Chiappetta, Director, Admissions

Westbridge Treatment Centers, 1830 East Roosevelt, Phoenix, AZ 85006; tel. 602/254-0884; FAX. 602/258-4033; Jeffrey M. Kaplan, Chief Executive Officer

Westcenter, 2105 East Allen Road, Tucson, AZ 85719; tel. 602/795-0952; FAX. 602/318-6442; Allan Harrington, Executive Director

ARKANSAS

Centers for Youth and Families, 6501 West 12th Street, Little Rock, AR 72204; tel. 501/666-8686; FAX. 501/666-4238; Richard T. Hill, President, Chief Executive Officer

Millcreek of Arkansas, Industrial Park Drive, Highway 79 North, Fordyce, AR 71742; tel. 501/352-8203; Wanda Miles-Bell, Executive Director

Ozark Guidance Center, Inc., 219 South Thompson Street, P.O. Box 1340, Springdale, AR 72765; tel. 501/751-7052; FAX. 501/751-4346; David L. Williams, Ph.D., Executive Director

Timer Ridge Ranch Neurorehabilitation Center, Inc., 15000 Highway 298, Benton, AR 72015-5009; tel. 501/594-5211; Roscoe Gordon Burrows, Program Director

Youth Home, Inc., 20400 Colonel Glenn Road, Little Rock, AR 72210-5323; tel. 501/821-5500; FAX. 501/821-5580; Beth Cartwright, ACSW, L.C.S.W. Executive Director

CALIFORNIA

A Touch of Care, 2231 South Carmelina Avenue, Los Angeles, CA 90064; tel. 310/473-6525; FAX. 310/479-1287; Richard B. Cohen, MFCC, Executive Director

Bellwood Health Center, 17800 Woodruff Avenue, Bellflower, CA 90706; tel. 213/925-9913; Jeff Rice, Administrator

Betty Ford Center at Eisenhower, 39000 Bob Hope Drive, Rancho Mirage, CA 92270; tel. 619/773-4100; FAX. 619/773-4141; Michael S. Neatherton, Vice President, Administrator

Broad Horizons of Ramona, Inc., P.O. Box 1920, Ramona, CA 92065; tel. 619/789-7060; FAX. 619/789-4062; Ellen Wright, LCSW, Chief Executive Officer

Care Options In Home Treatment Program, 874 Katella Street, Laguna Beach, CA 92651; tel. 714/740-8040; FAX. 714/497-6737; David F. Ellisor, Chief Executive Officer

Cornerstone Residential Center for Addictions, 13682 Yorba Street, Tustin, CA 92680; tel. 714/730-5399; Lynda Klinger, Business Development

Creative Care, Inc., 18850 Devonshire Street, Northridge, CA 91324; tel. 818/363-5630; Morteza Khaleghi, Ph.D., Clinical Director

Health Care Children's Campus Lions Gate, 15339 Saticoy Street, Van Nuys, CA 91406; tel. 818/778-6400; Kimberly A. Brandi, Admissions Director

Impact Drug and Alcohol Treatment Center, 1680 North Fair Oaks Avenue, Pasadena, CA 91103; tel. 818/798-0884; James M. Stillwell, Executive Director

Ivy Lea Manor-Parkview, 2120 Paseo Del Mar, San Pedro, CA 90732; tel. 310/832-8511; Casey Smart, Administrator

Kings View Mental Health System, 42675 Road 44, Reedley, CA 93654; tel. 209/638-2505; FAX. 209/638-8279; Michael Waters, Chief Executive Officer

Learning Services – Escondido, 2335 Bear Valley Parkway, Escondido, CA 92027; tel. 619/746-3223; Elizabeth Alexander, Program Director

Learning Services–Northern California, 10855 DeBruin Way, Gilroy, CA 95020; tel. 408/848-4379; Lareen Chonzena, M.S., Program Director

Michael's House, The Treatment Center for Men, 430 South Cahuilla Road, Palm Springs, CA 92262; tel. 619/320-5486; FAX. 619/778-6020; Arlene Rosen, President, Chief Executive Officer

Providers / Accredited Freestanding Psychiatric Facilities

Newport Bay Hospital Acute Geriatric Psychiatry, 1501 East 16th Street, Newport Beach, CA 92663; tel. 714/650-9750; FAX. 714/650-9751; James E. Parichurst, Chief Executive Officer

Oak Grove Institute Foundation, 24275 Jefferson Avenue, Murrieta, CA 92562; tel. 909/677-5599; FAX. 909/698-0461; Elizabeth H. Burnett, Ph.D., Clinical Project Director

Reiss Davis Child Study Center, 3200 Motor Avenue, Los Angeles, CA 90034-3710; tel. 310/204-1666, ext. 316; FAX. 310/204-1405; Gerald D. Zaslaw, Chief Executive Officer

Residential Treatment Centers of America, Inc., 1227 East Shepherd Avenue, Fresno, CA 93720; tel. 209/449-2604; Robert F. Norton, Chief Administrative Officer

S. T. E. P. S., 224 East Clara Street, Port Hueneme, CA 93044; tel. 805/488-6424; FAX. 805/488-6717; John J. Megara, M.B.A., Administrator

San Diego Center for Children, 3002 Armstrong Street, San Diego, CA 92111-5798; tel. 619/277-9550, ext. 114; FAX. 619/279-2763; Mark A. Hopper, Ph.D., ACSW, Chief Executive Officer

SeaBridge, Inc., 30371 Morning View Drive, Malibu, CA 90265; tel. 310/457-5802; FAX. 310/457-6093; Martha Zimmerman, Executive Director

Serendipity Diagnostic and Treatment Center, 6441 Matheney Way, Citrus Heights, CA 95621; tel. 916/969-1240; FAX. 916/726-2921; Robert T. Elliott, Ed.D., Executive Director

Spencer Recovery Centers, Inc., 343 West Foothill Boulevard, Monrovia, CA 91016; tel. 818/358-3662; FAX. 818/357-7405; Cindy Salo Garcia, Chief Operating Officer

Starting Point of Orange County, 350 West Bay Street, Costa Mesa, CA 92627; tel. 714/642-3505; FAX. 714/631-8669; Mike Berman, Assistant Administrator

Substance Abuse Foundation of Long Beach, Inc., 3125 East Seventh Street, Long Beach, CA 90804; tel. 310/439-7755; Ronald H. Banner, Executive Director

The Linden Center, 5750 Wilshire Boulevard, Suite 535, Los Angeles, CA 90036; tel. 213/937-3999, ext. 209; FAX. 213/937-6641; David Amitai, Ph.D., Administrator

Twin Town Treatment Centers, 10741 Los Alamitos Boulevard, Los Alamitos, CA 90720; tel. 310/594-8844; FAX. 310/493-1280; Warren L. Devon, Director

Vista Del Mar Child and Family Services, 3200 Motor Avenue, Los Angeles, CA 90034; tel. 310/836-1223, ext. 201; FAX. 310/204-1405; Gerald D. Zaslaw, ACSW, Chief Executive Officer

Vista Pacifica, 7989 Linda Vista Road, San Diego, CA 92111; tel. 619/576-1200; FAX. 619/576-8362; Daniel R. Valentine, Administrator

Vista San Diego Center, 3003 Armstrong Street, San Diego, CA 92111; tel. 619/268-3343, ext. 204; FAX. 619/268-8737; Joanne Downing, Intake Coordinator

COLORADO

Adolescent and Family Institute of Colorado, Inc., 10001 West 32nd Avenue, Wheat Ridge, CO 80033; tel. 303/238-1231; FAX. 303/238-0500; Alex M. Panio, Jr., Ph.D., Chief Executive Officer

Aurora Behavioral Health Hospital, 1290 South Potomac Street, Aurora, CO 80012; tel. 303/745-2273; FAX. 303/369-9556; Lorry Kenney, Administrator

Cheyenne Mesa, 1301 South Eighth Street, Colorado Springs, CO 80906; tel. 719/520-1400; FAX. 719/475-1527; Barbara E. Thomas, Chief Executive Officer

Colorado Boys Ranch, 28071 Highway 109, La Junta, CO 81050; tel. 719/384-5981; FAX. 719/384-8119; David Zimmerman, Vice President

Forest Heights Lodge, 4801 Forest Hill Road, Evergreen, CO 80439; tel. 303/674-6681; FAX. 303/674-6805; Russell H. Colburn, M.S.W., LCSW, Executive Director

Harmony Foundation, Inc., 1600 Fish Hatchery Road, P.O. Box 1989, Estes Park, CO 80517; tel. 303/586-4491; Howard L. Clarke, Jr., Director

Learning Services–Rocky Mountain Region, Brain Injury and Stroke Rehabilitation Programs, 7201 West Hampden Avenue, Lakewood, CO 80227; tel. 303/989-6660; FAX. 303/989-2830; Kenneth R. Hosack, Program Director

Parker Valley Hope, 22422 East Main Street, Parker, CO 80134; tel. 303/841-7857; FAX. 303/841-6526; John J. Arnold, Ph.D., Program Director

Pikes Peak Mental Health Center Systems, Inc., 875 West Moreno Avenue, Colorado Springs, CO 80905; tel. 719/471-8200, ext. 230; FAX. 719/471-0987; Charles J. Vorwaller, Chief Executive Officer

CONNECTICUT

Berkshire Woods Chemical Dependence Treatment Center, Mile Hill Road, Newtown, CT 06470; tel. 203/426-2531, ext. 2749; FAX. 203/426-6285; Sarah T. Kruel, Chief Executive Officer

Blue Hills Hospital, 51 Coventry Street, Hartford, CT 06112; tel. 203/722-2001; FAX. 203/722-2010; Stephen A. Glass, Acting Superintendent

Cornerstone of Eagle Hill, 32 Alberts Hill Road, Sandy Hook, CT 06482; tel. 203/426-8085; FAX. 203/426-2821; Norman J. Sokolow, President

Dutcher Chemical Dependence Treatment Center, Holmes Drive, P.O. Box 469, Middletown, CT 06457; tel. 203/638-5807; Patrick DeChello, Superintendent

Eugene T. Boneski Chemical Dependence Treatment Center, Route 12, Norwich, CT 06360; tel. 203/823-5237; FAX. 203/823-5446; Anita Ellis Howard, Superintendent

Greater Bridgeport Community Mental Health Center, 1635 Central Avenue, Bridgeport, CT 06610; tel. 203/579-6646; FAX. 203/579-6094; James M. Lehane III, Director

Guenster Rehabilitation Center, Inc., 276 Union Avenue, Bridgeport, CT 06610; tel. 203/384-9301; FAX. 203/336-4395; Sue Roselle, President

High Meadows, 825 Hartford Turnpike, Hamden, CT 06517; tel. 203/281-8300; Ms. Chris Deppen-DeMatteo, RN, Quality Assurance Coordinator

Klingberg Family Centers, Inc., 370 Linwood Street, New Britain, CT 06052; tel. 203/224-9113, ext. 363; FAX. 203/826-1739; Rosemarie A. Burton, President

Reid Treatment Center, Inc., 121 West Avon Road, Avon, CT 06001; tel. 203/673-6115; FAX. 203/673-6115; Mary Ann Reid, Executive Director

Riverview Hospital for Children and Youth, 915 River Road, Middletown, CT 06457-9297; tel. 203/343-6790; FAX. 203/343-6789; Carl H. Sundell, Jr., Superintendent

Rushford Center, Inc., 1250 Silver Street, Middletown, CT 06457; tel. 203/346-0300; John D. Habif, Vice President for Program Operations

Stonington Institute, Swantown Hill Road, North Stonington, CT 06359; tel. 203/535-1010; Michael J. Angelides, President

The Blueridge Center, 1095 Blue Hills Avenue, Bloomfield, CT 06002; tel. 203/243-1331, ext. 517; FAX. 203/242-3265; Joseph G. Nolan, Executive Director

The Center, 4920 Main Street, Suite 310, Bridgeport, CT 06606; tel. 203/365-8400; Susan Dalesandro, Clinical Director

The Children's Center, 1400 Whitney Avenue, Hamden, CT 06517; tel. 203/248-2116; FAX. 203/248-2572; Brian F. Lynch, Chief Executive Officer

The Wellspring Foundation, Inc., 21 Arch Bridge Road, P.O. Box 370, Bethlehem, CT 06751-0370; tel. 203/266-7235; FAX. 203/266-5830; Herbert Hall, M.Ed., Chief Executive Officer

Vitam Center, Inc., 57 West Rocks Road, P.O. Box 730, Norwalk, CT 06852; tel. 203/846-2091; FAX. 203/846-3620; Leonard A. Kenowitz, Ph.D., Executive Director

Wheeler Clinic, Inc., 91 Northwest Drive, Plainville, CT 06062; tel. 203/747-6801; FAX. 203/793-3520; Dennis Keenan, Executive Director

DELAWARE

Brandywine Counseling, Inc., 2713 Lancaster Avenue, Wilmington, DE 19805; tel. 302/656-2348; FAX. 302/656-0746; Sara Taylor Allshouse, Executive Director

Delaware Guidance Services for Children and Youth, Inc., 1213 Delaware Avenue, Wilmington, DE 19806; tel. 302/652-3948; FAX. 302/652-8297; Bruce Kelsey, LCSW, BCD, Acting Executive Officer

Lower Kensington Environmental Center, Inc., Recovery Center of Delaware, P.O. Box 546, Delaware City, DE 19706; tel. 302/836-1615; FAX. 302/836-0412; John Moody, Project Director

Sodat–Delaware, Inc., 625 North Orange Street, Wilmington, DE 19801; tel. 302/656-4044; Thomas C. Maloney, Executive Director

DISTRICT OF COLUMBIA

Devereux Children's Center, 3050 R Street, N.W., Washington, DC 20007; tel. 202/282-1200; FAX. 202/282-1219; Janet Heisse, Director of Management Service

FLORIDA

45th Street Mental Health Center, Inc., 1041 45th Street, West Palm Beach, FL 33407; tel. 407/844-9741; FAX. 407/844-2353; Terry H. Allen, Executive Director

Alternatives in Treatment, Inc., 7601 North Federal Highway, Suite 260B, Boca Raton, FL 33487; tel. 407/998-0866; FAX. 407/241-5042; Jacob Frydman, Executive Director

American Day Treatment Centers of Boca Raton, 2101 Corporate Boulevard, Suite 102, Boca Raton, FL 33431; tel. 407/241-7741; FAX. 407/241-7743; Victor Lugo, Executive Director

Apalachee Center for Human Services, Inc., 625 East Tennessee Street, Tallahassee, FL 32308; tel. 904/487-2930; FAX. 904/487-0851; Ronald P. Kirkland, Chief Executive Officer

CBHS at Bay Harbor, 12895 Seminole Boulevard, Largo, FL 34648; tel. 813/587-1000; FAX. 813/584-1835; Steve McCabe, Administrator

Camelot Care Centers, Inc., 9180 Oakhurst Road, Largo, FL 34646; tel. 813/596-9960; Elizabeth Doyle, Admissions Director

Coastal Recovery Centers, Inc., 3830 Bee Ridge Road, Sarasota, FL 34233; tel. 813/927-8900; FAX. 813/925-3836; James R. Sleeper, President Chief Executive Officer

Crossroads – The Recovery Center, 2121 Lisenby Avenue, Panama City, FL 32406; tel. 904/784-0869; Aubrey White, Chief Executive Officer

Crossroads School, 4650 Southwest 61 Avenue, Fort Lauderdale, FL 33314; tel. 305/584-1100; FAX. 305/584-0150; Aubrey Fein, Administrator

Daniel Memorial Hospital, Inc., 3725 Belfort Road, Jacksonville, FL 32216; tel. 904/737-1677; FAX. 904/448-7700; Daniel H. Cook, LCSW, President

David Lawrence Center, Inc., 6075 Golden Gate Parkway, Naples, FL 33999; tel. 813/455-1031; FAX. 813/455-6561; David Schimmel, Executive Director

Devereux Florida Treatment Network–Campus Programs, 8000 Devereux Drive, Viera, FL 32940-0790; tel. 407/242-9100; Patty Hurst, Director, Quality Management

Disc Village, Inc., Tallahassee/Leon County Human Services Center, 3333 West Pensacola Street, Tallahassee, FL 32304; tel. 904/575-4388; FAX. 904/576-5960; Thomas K. Olk, Executive Director

Providers / Accredited Freestanding Psychiatric Facilities

Eckerd Alternative Treatment Program at E. Hew-Kee, 197 Culbreath Road, Brooksville, FL 34602; tel. 800/554-4357, ext. 456; Dwight Lord, Director, Admissions

Fairwinds, 1569 South Fort Harrison, Clearwater, FL 34616; tel. 813/449-0300; Mazhar Al-Abed, Chief Executive Officer, Administrator

Florida Institute for Neurologic Rehabilitation, Inc., Vandolah Road, Wauchula, FL 33873; tel. 800/697-5390; Anthony J. Chioccarelli, Chief Operating Officer

Florida Mental Health Institute, 13301 North 30th Street, Tampa, FL 33612; tel. 813/974-1990; Jini Hanjnan, Quality Assurance Coordinator

Growing Together, Inc., 1013 Lucerne Avenue, Lake Worth, FL 33460; tel. 407/585-0892; Ivan Goldberg, Chief Executive Officer

Hanley-Hazelden Center at St. Mary's, 5200 East Avenue, West Palm Beach, FL 33407; tel. 407/848-1666; Jerry Singleton, Executive Director

Harbor Oaks Hospital, 1015 Mar Walt Drive, Fort Walton Beach, FL 32547; tel. 904/863-4160; J. Michael Townley, Chief Executive Officer

High Point, 5960 S.W. 106th Avenue, Cooper City, FL 33328; tel. 305/680-2700; Joseph A. Hartl, Chief Financial Officer

InterPhase Recovery Program, Inc., 23120 Sandlefoot Plaza Drive, Boca Raton, FL 33428; tel. 407/487-5400; FAX. 407/852-8872; Janice Wilmoth, M.S., Executive Director

La Amistad Residential Treatment Center, 201 Alpine Drive, Maitland, FL 32751; tel. 407/647-0660; FAX. 407/647-3060; Rosemary Cohen, Chief Executive Officer

Leon F. Stewart-Hal S. Marcham Treatment Center, 120 Michigan Avenue, Daytona Beach, FL 32114; tel. 904/255-0447; FAX. 904/238-0877; Ernest D. Cantley, Executive Director

LifeStream Behavioral Center and Hospital, 515 West Main Street, Leesburg, FL 34749-9100; tel. 904/360-6575; FAX. 904/360-6595; Kurth C. Fatt, Quality Improvement Coordinator

Lifeskills of Boca Raton, Inc., 7301A West Palmetto Park Road, Suite 300B, Boca Raton, FL 33433; tel. 407/392-1199; Carol A. Parks, Administrator

Mainstream Winter Park, 1276 Minnesota Avenue, Winter Park, FL 32789; tel. 407/647-1781; FAX. 407/647-0668; Helen Parker, Executive Director

Manatee Palms Adolescent Specialty Hospital, 1324 37th Avenue, E., Bradenton, FL 34208; tel. 813/746-1388; FAX. 813/746-2690; Ray Heckerman, Administrator/ Chief Executive Officer

Marion Citrus Mental Health Center, Inc., 717 S.W. Martin Luther King, Jr., P.O. Box 1330, Ocala, FL 34478; tel. 904/629-8893; FAX. 904/732-1413; Russell Rasco, Executive Director

Mental Health Care, Inc., 5707 North 22nd Street, Tampa, FL 33610; tel. 813/237-3914; Julian Rice, Executive Director

Mental Health Resource Center, Inc., 11820 Beach Boulevard, Jacksonville, FL 32246; tel. 904/642-9100; FAX. 904/641-6529; David H. Panken, President, Chief Executive Officer

Mental Health Services, Inc. of North Central Florida, 4300 S.W. 13th Street, Gainesville, FL 32608; tel. 904/374-5670; FAX. 904/371-9841; Douglas L. Starr, Ph.D., Chief Executive Officer

Montanari Residential Treatment Center, 291 East 2nd Street, Hialeah, FL 33011-1360; tel. 305/887-7543; FAX. 305/882-1970; Paul Hague, Executive Director

National Recovery Institutes Group, 1000 N.W. 15th Street, Boca Raton, FL 33486; tel. 407/392-8444; FAX. 407/368-0879; Don Russakoff, President, Chief Executive Officer

Northside Mental Health Center, Inc., 12512 Bruce B. Downs Boulevard, Tampa, FL 33612; tel. 813/977-8700; FAX. 813/971-2029; Marsha Lewis Brown, LCSW, Executive Director

Northwest Dade Center, Inc., 4175 West 20th Avenue, Hialeah, FL 33012; tel. 305/825-0300; FAX. 305/824-1006; Mario Jardon, LCSW, Chief Executive Officer

Oak Center, 8889 Corporate Square Court, Jacksonville, FL 32216; tel. 904/725-7073; FAX. 904/727-9777; Diana Sourbrine, Administrator

Pathways to Recovery, Inc., 13132 Barwick Road, Delray Beach, FL 33445; tel. 407/496-7532; Allen Bombart, Executive Director

Peace River Center for Personal Development, Inc., 1745 Highway 17, S., Bartow, FL 33830; tel. 941/534-7020; FAX. 941/534-7028; Roy Gaither, Executive Director

Personal Enrichment through Mental Health Services, Inc., 11254 58th Street, Pinellas Park, FL 34666; tel. 813/784-9444; FAX. 813/545-1537; Debbie Piechocki, Director, Quality Management

Recovery Corner of West Palm Beach, 4440 PGA Boulevard, Suite 203, Palm Beach Gardens, FL 33410; tel. 407/624-1924; FAX. 407/626-1739; Steven M. Petrovich, Executive Director

Renaissance Institute of Palm Beach, Inc., 7300 North Federal Highway, Suite 201, Boca Raton, FL 33487; tel. 407/241-7977; FAX. 407/241-9233; Renee Peacock, Administrator

South County Mental Health Center, Inc., 16158 South Military Trail, Delray Beach, FL 33484; tel. 407/495-0522; FAX. 407/495-7975; Joseph S. Speicher, Executive Director

Spectrum Programs, Inc., 18441 N.W. 2nd Avenue, Suite 218, Miami, FL 33169; tel. 305/653-8288, ext. 19; FAX. 305/653-6787; David Freedman, Vice President, Administrative Services

Tampa Bay Academy, Ltd., 12012 Boyette Road, Riverview, FL 33569; tel. 813/677-6700; FAX. 813/671-3145; Edward C. Hoefle, Administrator

The Beachcomber, 4493 North Ocean Boulevard, Delray Beach, FL 33483; tel. 407/734-1818; FAX. 407/265-1349; James A. Bryan, Director

The Cloisters at Pine Island, 13771 Waterfront Drive, Pineland, FL 33945-1616; tel. 813/283-1019; FAX. 813/283-3079; Edward L. Doherty, MHS, CAC, Executive Director

The Friary of Baptist Health Care, 4400 Hickory Shores Boulevard, Gulf Breeze, FL 32561; tel. 904/932-9375; FAX. 904/932-7144; Darryl Knight, Executive Director

The Inn at Bowling Green Family Recovery Center, 101 North Oak Street, Bowling Green, FL 33834; tel. 800/762-3712; FAX. 813/375-2832; JoAnn Summerlin, Vice President, Administration

The Renfrew Center of Florida, 7700 Renfrew Lane, Coconut Creek, FL 33073; tel. 305/698-9222; FAX. 305/698-9007; Barbara Peterson, Executive Director

The Village South, Inc., 3180 Biscayne Boulevard, Miami, FL 33137; tel. 305/573-3784; FAX. 305/576-1348; Matthew Gissen, Chief Executive Officer

The Willough at Naples, 9001 Tamiami Trail, E., Naples, FL 33962; tel. 813/775-4500; FAX. 813/793-0534; Gary D. Centafanti, Executive Director

Transitions Recovery Program, 2040 N.E. 163rd Street, North Miami Beach, FL 33162; tel. 305/949-9001; Roselyn McGowan, Administrator

Turning Point of Tampa, 6301 Memorial Boulevard, Suite 201, Tampa, FL 33615; tel. 813/882-3003; FAX. 813/885-6974; C. Fred Hill, Chief Executive Officer

Twelve Oaks, 2068 Heathcare Avenue, Navarre, FL 32566; tel. 904/939-1200; FAX. 904/939-1257; James W. Griffis, Administrator

GEORGIA

Anchor Hospital and the Talbott-Marsh Recovery Campus, 5454 Yorktowne Drive, Atlanta, GA 30349; tel. 404/991-6044; FAX. 404/991-3843; Benjamin H. Underwood, FAAMA, President, Chief Executive Officer

Anxiety Disorders Institute of Atlanta Center, One Dunwoody Park, Suite 112, Atlanta, GA 30338; tel. 404/395-6845; Asaf Aleem, Chief Executive Officer

Brightmore Day Hospital, 115 Davis Road, P.O. Box 211849, Martinez, GA 30907-1849; tel. 404/868-1735; FAX. 404/860-6358; R. Adair Blackwood, M.D., Medical Director

Devereux Center In Georgia, 1291 Stanley Road, N.W., Kennesaw, GA 30144; tel. 404/427-0147; FAX. 404/425-1413; Ralph L. Comerford, Executive Director

Inner Harbour Hospitals, Ltd., 4685 Dorsett Shoals Road, Douglasville, GA 30135; tel. 404/942-2391; C. Stevens Izenour III, Chief Executive Officer

Learning Services – Peachtree, 2400 Highway 29 South, Lawrenceville, GA 30245; tel. 404/962-4828; FAX. 404/995-1253; Mark Pavlovich, Director

Murphy-Harpst-Vashti, Inc., 740 Fletcher Street, Cedartown, GA 30125; tel. 404/748-1500; FAX. 404/749-1094; Robert M. Spaulding II, Admissions Coordinator

Perimeter Adolescent Day Treatment Program, Inc., 1140 Hammond Drive, Suite 9150, Atlanta, GA 30328; tel. 404/804-8255; Franci Robertson, Administrator

Safe Recovery Systems, Inc., 2300 Peachtree Road, Suite 2000, Atlanta, GA 30338; tel. 404/455-7233; FAX. 404/458-1481; Henslee Dutton, Chief Executive Officer

Schizophrenia Treatment and Rehabilitation, Inc., 208 Church Street, Decatur, GA 30030; tel. 404/377-9844; FAX. 404/373-5258; Kimberly H. Littrell, RN, M.S., C.S., President, Chief Executive Officer

Turning Point Care Center, Inc., 319 Bypass, Moultrie, GA 31776; tel. 912/985-4815; Michael Cornelison, Chief Executive Officer

Woodridge Hospital, 394 Ridgecrest Circle, Clayton, GA 30525; tel. 404/782-3100; FAX. 404/782-4873; Gerald E. Knepp, Chief Executive Officer

IDAHO

Northview Hospital, 8050 Northview Street, Boise, ID 83704; tel. 208/327-0504; FAX. 208/327-0594; Rick L. Holloway, Administrator

Northwest Children's Home, Inc., P.O. Box 1288, Lewiston, ID 83501-1288; tel. 208/743-9404; FAX. 208/746-4955; A. J. Rusty Cooper, Executive Director

Pine Crest Hospital and Counseling Centers, 2301 North Ironwood Place, Cour d'Alene, ID 83814; tel. 208/765-4800; FAX. 208/664-1805; Ron Mays, Administrator

Walker Center, 1120A Montana Street, Gooding, ID 83330-1858; tel. 208/934-8461; FAX. 208/934-5437; Vayle Mauldin, Program Director

ILLINOIS

Alcholism Treatment Center of Central DuPage Hospital, 27 West 350 High Lake Road, Winfield, IL 60190; tel. 708/653-4000; Paul M. Teodo, Vice President

Allendale Association, Grand Avenue, P.O. Box 1088, Lake Villa, IL 60046; tel. 708/356-2351; FAX. 708/356-0289; Robert Holway, President

American Day Treatment Centers at Highland Park Hospital, 1936 Green Bay Road, Highland Park, IL 60053; tel. 708/480-2625; Monica Megivern, Director of Training

Camelot Care Center, Inc., 1502 North Northwest Highway, Palatine, IL 60067; tel. 708/359-5600; FAX. 708/359-2759; Maria Wywialowski, LCSW, Director, Social Services

Chestnut Health Systems, Inc., 1003 Dr. Martin Luther King Jr. Drive, Bloomington, IL 61701; tel. 309/827-6026; Alan R. Sodetz, Clinical Director

Evergreen Recovery Center, 1055 East State Street, Rockford, IL 61104; tel. 815/965-8600; FAX. 815/965-2348; Philip W. Eaton, President

Gateway Youth Care Foundation, 2200 Lake Victoria Drive, Springfield, IL 62703; tel. 217/529-9266; FAX. 217/529-9151

Gateway Youth Care Foundation, 25480 West Cedarcrest Lane, Lake Villa, IL 60046; tel. 708/356-8292; Michael Darcy, President

Horizons Wellness Center, Inc., 970 South McHenry Avenue, Crystal Lake, IL 60014; tel. 708/854-4357; Linda D. Simko, Clinical Director

Interventions-DuPage Adolescent Center, 11 South 250 Route 53, Hinsdale, IL 60521; tel. 708/325-5050; Anthony Kunkemoeller, Director

Health Organizations, Agencies and Providers

Providers / Accredited Freestanding Psychiatric Facilities

Life Works Chemical Dependency Centers, 404 West Boughton, Suite B, Bolingbrook, IL 60440; tel. 708/759-5750; FAX. 708/759-9446; Loretta L. Berry, Chief Executive Officer

Rosecrance Center, 1505 North Alpine Road, Rockford, IL 61107; tel. 800/383-5351; FAX. 815/398-2641; Lori Berkes-Nelson, Administrator

Sojourn House, Inc., 565 North Turner Avenue, Freeport, IL 61032; tel. 815/232-5121; FAX. 815/233-4591; Brenda J. Bombard, M.S.W., Executive Director

Southeastern Illinois Counseling Centers, Inc., P.O. Drawer M, Olney, IL 62450; tel. 618/395-4306; FAX. 618/395-4507; Gary Robertson, Executive Director

Triangle Center, 120 North 11th Street, Springfield, IL 62703; tel. 217/544-9858; Stephen J. Knox, Executive Director

INDIANA

Comprehensive Mental Health Services, Inc., 240 North Tillotson Avenue, Muncie, IN 47304; tel. 317/288-1928; FAX. 317/741-0310; Suzanne Gresham, Ph.D., Chief Executive Officer

Evansville Psychiatric Children's Center, 3300 East Morgan Avenue, Evansville, IN 47715; tel. 812/477-6436; FAX. 812/474-4248; Thomas C. Andis, Jr., Superintendent

Fairbanks Hospital, Inc., 8102 Clearvista Parkway, Indianapolis, IN 46256-4698; tel. 317/849-8222, ext. 100; FAX. 317/849-1455; Timothy L. Boruff, President

Four-County Counseling Center, 1015 Michigan Avenue, Logansport, IN 46947; tel. 219/722-5151; FAX. 219/722-9523; Umamaheswara Rao Kalapatapu, M.D., Administrator

Grant-Blackford Mental Health, Inc., 505 Wabash Avenue, Marion, IN 46952; tel. 317/662-3971; FAX. 317/662-7480; Paul G. Kuczora, Chief Executive Officer

Hamilton Center, Inc., 620 8th Avenue, Terre Haute, IN 47804; tel. 812/231-8323; FAX. 812/232-8228; Galen Goode, Center Director

Lifespring Mental Health Services, 207 West 13th Street, Jeffersonville, IN 47130; tel. 812/283-4491; John Case, Executive Director

Madison Hospital, 403 East Madison, South Bend, IN 46617; tel. 219/234-0061; FAX. 219/234-0670; John Twardos, Chief Operating Officer

Park Center, Inc., 909 East State Boulevard, Fort Wayne, IN 46805; tel. 219/481-2700; FAX. 219/481-2717; James L. McKee, Ph.D., Chief Executive Officer

Porter-Starke Counseling Centers, 601 Wall Street, Valparaiso, IN 46383; tel. 219/531-3500; FAX. 219/462-3975; Lee E. Grogg, Chief Executive Officer

Quinco Behavioral Health Systems, 1455 N. National Road, Columbus, IN 47201; tel. 812/379-2341; FAX. 812/376-4875; Robert J. Williams, Ph.D., Chief Executive Officer

Southlake Center for Mental Health, 8555 Taft Street, Merrillville, IN 46410; tel. 219/769-4005, ext. 287; FAX. 219/769-2508; Maureen Handley, M.S.W., Director, Quality Improvement

Southwestern Indiana Mental Health Center, Inc., 415 Mulberry Street, Evansville, IN 47713; tel. 812/423-7791; FAX. 812/422-7558; John K. Browning, Executive Director

The Center for Mental Health, Inc., P.O. Box 1258, Anderson, IN 46016; tel. 317/649-8161; FAX. 317/641-8238; C. Richard DeHaven, President

The Children's Campus, 1411 Lincoln Way W., Mishawaka, IN 46544-1690; tel. 219/259-5666, ext. 222; FAX. 219/255-6179; Michael James, Vice President

The Madison Clinic Inc., 303A Alexandria Pike, Anderson, IN 46012; tel. 317/644-1414; FAX. 317/649-6426; Pamela L. Porter, M.A., Executive Director

The Otis R. Bowen Center for Human Services, Inc., 850 North Harrison Street, Warsaw, IN 46581-0497; tel. 219/267-7169; FAX. 219/269-3995; Kurt Carlson, President, Chief Executive Officer

Tri-City Comprehensive Community Mental Health Center, 3903 Indianapolis Boulevard, East Chicago, IN 46312; tel. 219/398-7050; FAX. 219/392-6998; Sandy Appleby, Assistant Director Special Services

Tri-County Center, Inc., 8945 North Meridian Street, Indianapolis, IN 46260; tel. 317/574-0022; FAX. 317/574-1234; Larry L. Burch, ACSW, Executive Director

Wabash Valley Hospital, Inc., 2900 North River Road, West Lafayette, IN 47906; tel. 317/463-2555; R. Craig Lysinger, Administrator

IOWA

Boys and Girls Home And Family Service, Inc., 2601 Douglas Street, Sioux City, IA 51102; tel. 712/277-4031; Robert P. Sheehan, Chief Executive Officer

Children and Families of Iowa, 1111 University, Des Moines, IA 50314; tel. 515/288-1981, ext. 346; FAX. 515/288-1981, ext. 402; Bobbretta M. Brewton, Director, Program Development

Christian Home Association – Children's Square U.S.A., North 6th Street and Avenue E, P.O. Box 8-C, Council Bluffs, IA 51502-3008; tel. 712/322-3700; FAX. 712/325-0913; Carol D. Wood, ACSW, LSW, President, Chief Executive Officer

Four Oaks, Inc. Smith Center, 5400 Kirkwood Boulevard, S.W., Cedar Rapids, IA 52404; tel. 319/364-0259; FAX. 319/364-1162; Anne C. Gruenewald, Director, Family and Children's Services

Gerard Treatment Programs, 980 South Iowa Avenue, Mason City, IA 50401; tel. 515/423-3222; Rita Faxson, Chief Executive Officer

Hillcrest Family Services, 2005 Asbury Road, P.O. Box 1161, Dubuque, IA 52004-1161; tel. 319/583-7357; FAX. 319/583-7026; Gary L. Gansemer, Assistant Executive Director

Lutheran Social Service of Iowa, 1323 Northwestern, Ames, IA 50010; tel. 515/232-7262; FAX. 515/232-7416; Ed Ruppert, LSW, Center Director

Orchard Place, 925 S.W. Porter Avenue, P.O. Box 35425, Des Moines, IA 50315-0304; tel. 515/285-6781, ext. 601; FAX. 515/287-9695; Earl P. Kelly, Chief Executive Officer

Tanager Place, 2309 C Street, S.W., Cedar Rapids, IA 52404; tel. 319/365-9165, ext. 314; FAX. 319/365-6411; Joe Schreder, Program Administrator

KANSAS

Atchison Valley Hope, 1816 North Second Street, Atchison, KS 66002; tel. 913/367-1618; FAX. 913/367-6224; Dennis Gilhousen, Chief Executive Officer

Columbia Health Systems, Inc., 10114 West 105th Street, Overland Park, KS 66212; tel. 913/492-9875; Robert L. Reed, President

Comprehensive Evaluation and Transition Unit, 300 Southwest Oakley, Topeka, KS 66606; tel. 913/296-2196; James Fairchild, Director

Kaw Valley Center, 4300 Brenner Drive, Kansas City, KS 66104; tel. 913/334-0294; B. W. Sims, President, Chief Executive Officer

Norton Valley Hope, 709 West Holme, Norton, KS 67654; tel. 913/877-5101; FAX. 913/877-2322; Dennis R. Gilhousen, President, Chief Executive Officer

S.P.I.R.I.T. Program of United Methodist Youthville, Inc., 900 West Broadway, Newton, KS 67114; tel. 316/283-1950, ext. 305; FAX. 316/283-9540; Karen Baker, Vice President of Programs

The Saint Francis Academy, Inc., 509 East Elm Street, Salina, KS 67401; tel. 913/825-0541; FAX. 913/825-2502; Reverend Phillip J. Rapp, President, Chief Executive Officer

KENTUCKY

Bluegrass Regional Mental Health–Mental Retardation Board, 1351 Newton Pike, Lexington, KY 40511; tel. 606/253-1686; David Hanna, Ph.D., Director, Quality Assurance

Brooklawn, Inc., 2125 Goldsmith Lane, Louisville, KY 40218; tel. 502/451-5177; David A. Graves, President, Chief Executive Officer

Central State Hospital, 10510 LaGrange Road, Louisville, KY 40223; tel. 502/245-4121, ext. 597; FAX. 502/245-4121, ext. 259; Paula Tamme, CSW, Chief Executive Officer

Comprehensive Care Centers of Northern Kentucky, Inc., 503 Farrell Drive, Covington, KY 41011; tel. 606/578-3252; FAX. 606/578-3256; Edward G. Muntel, Ph.D., President

Cumberland River Regional Mental Health and Mental Retardation, Inc., American Greeting Road, P.O. Box 568, Corbin, KY 40702; tel. 606/528-7010; Ralph Lipps, Executive Director

Green River Regional Mental Health and Mental Retardation Board, Inc., 416 West Third Street, P.O. Box 1637, Owensboro, KY 42302; tel. 502/684-0696; FAX. 502/926-6367; Gayle DiCesare, President, Chief Executive Officer

Jefferson Alcohol and Drug Abuse Center, 600 South Preston Street, Louisville, KY 40202; tel. 502/583-3951; FAX. 502/581-9234; Diane E. Hague, Director

Presbyterian Child Welfare Agency, One Buckhorn Lane, Buckhorn, KY 41721; tel. 606/398-7245; Charles Baker, President, Chief Executive Officer

Seven Counties Services, Inc., 137 West Muhammad Ali, Louisville, KY 40202; tel. 502/589-8600; Debra Hino, Quality Improvement Officer

Spectrum Care Academy, 4500 Campbellsville Road, Columbia, KY 42728; tel. 502/384-6444; FAX. 502/384-4883; Beverly K. Harvey, Administrator

The Adanta Group–Behavioral Health Srvices, 259 Parkers Mill Road, Somerset, KY 42501; tel. 606/678-2768; Sandra Renfro, Quality Improvement Coordinator

LOUISIANA

Bowling Green Hospital, 701 Florida Avenue, Mandeville, LA 70448; tel. 504/626-5661; FAX. 504/626-4217; Richard M. Taylor, Executive Director

Hope Haven Center (Residential Treatment), Includes Hope Haven, Madonna Manor, St. Elizabeth's, 1101 Barataria Boulevard, Marrero, LA 70072; tel. 504/347-5581; FAX. 504/340-2075; Robert J. Guasco, Chief Administrative Officer

New Beginnings Residential Program of Opelousas, 1692 Linwood Loop, Opelousas, LA 70570; tel. 318/942-1171; FAX. 318/948-9101; Kim Signorelli, Chief Executive Officer

Vermilion Hospital for Psychiatric and Addictive Medicine, 2520 North University Avenue, Lafayette, LA 70507; tel. 318/234-5614; FAX. 318/235-0696; Johnny Patout, Administrator

Victory House, 12038 Greenwell Springs Point, Zachary, LA 70791; Sheila Howard, Administrative Director

MAINE

Kids Peace National Centers for Kids in Crisis New England, Route 180, P.O. Box 787, Ellsworth, ME 04605; tel. 207/667-0909; FAX. 207/667-6348; John P. Peter, President, Chief Executive Officer

MARYLAND

A. F. Whitsitt Center Rehabilitation Center, P.O. Box 229, Chestertown, MD 21620; tel. 410/778-6404; FAX. 410/778-5431; Terri Dowling, LPN, Admissions Coordinator

Allegany County Health Department Addictions Program, Willowbrook Road, Cumberland, MD 21502; tel. 301/777-5680; Rodger D. Simons, Administrator

American Day Treatment Centers of Chevy Chase, LP, Two Wisconsin Circle, Suite 620, Chevy Chase, MD 20815; tel. 301/656-0151; Heidi Brown, Executive Director

Providers / Accredited Freestanding Psychiatric Facilities

American Day Treatment Centers of Prince Georges County, 7404 Executive Place, Seabrook, MD 20706; tel. 301/805-2900; FAX. 301/805-5510; Randall McKennie

Ashley, Inc., 800 Tydings Lane, Havre DeGrace, MD 21078; tel. 410/273-6600; FAX. 410/272-5617; Leonard Angus Dahl, Executive Director

Baltimore Recovery Center, 16 South Poppleton Street, Baltimore, MD 21201; tel. 410/962-7180; FAX. 410/962-7192; William K. Hathaway, Executive Director

Changing Point, 4100 College Avenue, P.O. Box 396, Ellicott City, MD 21041-0396; tel. 410/465-9500; FAX. 410/465-9500, ext. 320; Beatrice Grant, RN, Program Director

Charter Behavioral Health System of Maryland at Meadows, 730 Maryland, Route 3, Gambrills, MD 21054; tel. 410/923-6022; FAX. 410/923-1433; Wes Fuhrman, Executive Director, Business Development

Charter Behavioral Health Systems at Hidden Brook, 522 Thomas Run Road, P.O. Box 1607, Bel Air, MD 21014; tel. 410/879-1919; FAX. 410/734-6752; Carol Koffinke, Chief Operating Officer

Choptank Center, P.O. Box 1238, Cambridge, MD 21613; tel. 301/221-0288; FAX. 301/228-9588; Jurgen H. Schwermer, Ph.D., President

Crossroads Centers, 2 West Madison Street, Baltimore, MD 21201; tel. 410/752-6505; FAX. 410/385-1237; Barbara Q. McKenna, Executive Director

Edgemeade, 13400 Edgemeade Road, Upper Marlboro, MD 20772; tel. 301/888-1330; FAX. 301/888-2693; James Filipczak, Ph.D., Executive Director

FairBridge Residential Treatment Center, 14907 Broschart Road, Rockville, MD 20850; tel. 301/217-9010; FAX. 301/251-4684; Amanda Hopkins-Alexiadis, Chief Executive Officer

Glass Substance Abuse Programs, Inc., 821 North Eutaw Street, Suite 201, Baltimore, MD 21201; tel. 410/225-9185; FAX. 410/225-7964; Herman Jones, President

Good Shepherd Center, 4100 Maple Avenue, Baltimore, MD 21227-2770; tel. 410/247-2770; FAX. 410/247-3242; Sister Mary Rosaria Baxter, M.S., Administrator

Hope House, Marbury Drive, Building 26, Crownsville, MD 21032; tel. 410/923-6700; FAX. 410/923-6213; William H. Rufenacht, Executive Director

Maryland Treatment Center, Inc., U. S. Route 15, Emmitsburg, MD 21727; tel. 301/447-2361; FAX. 301/447-6504; Mary A. Roby, President

Melwood Farm Treatment Center, 19715 Zion Road, Olney, MD 20832; tel. 800/368-8313; Sue Krantz, Corporate Director of Quality

New Beginnings at Warwick Manor, Warwick Road, Route 1, Box 178, East New Market, MD 21631; tel. 410/943-8108; Charles J. Hooker, Executive Director

New Beginnings at White Oak, 1441 Taylors Island Road, P.O. Box 56, Woolford, MD 21677; tel. 410/228-7000; FAX. 410/228-8609; Charles J. Hooker, Chief Executive Officer

New Life Addiction Counseling Services, Inc., 2528 Mountain Road, Pasadena, MD 21122; tel. 410/255-4475; FAX. 410/255-6277; Thomas S. Porter, Chief Executive Officer

Oakview Treatment Center, 3100 North Ridge Road, Ellicott City, MD 21043; tel. 410/461-9922; David C. Heebner, Administrator

Pathways Services, Inc., 2620 Riva Road, Annapolis, MD 21401; tel. 410/573-5400; FAX. 410/573-5401; Art Sullivan, Director

Psych Systems of Bethesda, 6701 Democracy Boulevard, Bethesda, MD 20817; tel. 301/530-2777; Cindy Lee, Ph.D., J.D., Director, Clinical Services

Regional Institute for Children and Adolescents, 605 South Chapel Gate Lane, Baltimore, MD 21229; tel. 410/368-6500; FAX. 410/368-5885; Clifford A. Palmer, Chief Executive Officer

Regional Institute for Children and Adolescents/Rockville, 15000 Broschart Road, Rockville, MD 20850-3392; tel. 301/251-6800; FAX. 301/309-9004; John L. Gildner, Chief Executive Officer

Regional Institute for Children and Adolescents/Southern Maryland, 9400 Surratts Road, Cheltenham, MD 20623; tel. 301/372-1800; FAX. 301/372-1906; Brenda Harris, Director of Admissions

Saint Luke Institute, Inc., 2420 Brooks Drive, Suitland, MD 20746; tel. 301/967-3700; FAX. 301/967-3953; Canice Connors, OFM, Ph.D., President, Chief Executive Officer

Villa Maria, 2300 Dulaney Valley Road, Timonium, MD 21093; tel. 301/252-4700; John D. Rusinko, M.S.W., Administrator

Walter P. Carter Community Mental Health Center, 630 West Fayette Street, Baltimore, MD 21201; tel. 410/328-2200; FAX. 410/328-0167; P. Whitmore-Kendall, Ph.D., Chief Executive Officer

Woodbourne Center, Inc., 1301 Woodbourne Avenue, Baltimore, MD 21239; tel. 410/433-1000; FAX. 410/433-1459; Patricia Cronin, Executive Vice President

Worcester County Health Department, 6040 Public Landing Road, P.O. Box 249, Snow Hill, MD 21863; tel. 410/632-1100; FAX. 410/632-0906; Deborah Goeller, RN, M.S., Health Officer

MASSACHUSETTS

Adcare Hospital of Worcester, Inc., 107 Lincoln Street, Worcester, MA 01605; tel. 508/799-9000; David W. Hillis, President

Baldpate Hospital, Baldpate Road, Georgetown, MA 01833; tel. 508/352-2131; Subhash C. Mukherjee, Administrator

Brockton Multi Service Center, 165 Quincy Street, Brockton, MA 02402; tel. 508/580-0800; FAX. 508/588-2949; John P. Sullivan, Ph.D., Area Director

Cape Cod Alcoholism Intervention and Rehabilitation Unit, Inc., d/b/a Gosnold on Cape Cod, 200 Ter Heun Drive, Box CC, Falmouth, MA 02541; tel. 508/540-6550; FAX. 508/540-6550; Raymond Tamasi, President, Chief Executive Officer

Cape Cod and the Islands, Community Mental Health Center, 259 North Street, Hyannis, MA 02601; tel. 508/775-1199; Richard Dunnells, Center Director, Superintendent

Centerpoint, Tewksbury Hospital, Southgate, 132 Boylston Street, Tewksbury, MA 01876; tel. 508/858-3776; John Lynch, Program Director

Choate Health Systems, Inc., 23 Warren Avenue, Woburn, MA 01801; tel. 617/279-0200, ext. 304; FAX. 617/279-2804; Margaret A. Moran, Vice President, Marketing & Program Development

Corrigan Mental Health Center, 49 Hillside Street, Fall River, MA 02720; tel. 617/678-2901; FAX. 617/678-2901; Daniel K. Amigone, Superintendent

Dr. Harry C. Solomon Mental Health Center, 391 Varnum Avenue, Lowell, MA 01854; tel. 508/454-8851; FAX. 508/454-7538; Linda D. Sutter, Superintendent, Site Director

Germaine Lawrence Intensive Residential Treatment Program, Cushing Hill Drive, Marlborough, MA 01752; tel. 508/481-0738; David L. Hirshberg, Ed.D., Chief Executive Officer

High Point, 1233 State Road, Route 3A, Plymouth, MA 02360; tel. 508/224-7701; FAX. 508/224-2845; Thomas Salmon, Chief Executive Officer

Meadowridge Behavioral Health Center, Residential Psychiatric Care, 664 Stevens Road, Swansea, MA 02777; tel. 508/676-8740; FAX. 508/678-9059; John Lynch, Program Director

Quincy Mental Health Center, 460 Quincy Avenue, Quincy, MA 02169; tel. 617/770-4000, ext. 253; FAX. 617/770-2953; Christina Browne, Center Director

Spectrum Addiction Services, Inc., 106 East Main Street, Westboro, MA 01581; tel. 508/898-1550; FAX. 508/836-4242; Roy Ross, President

The Grove Adolescent Treatment Center, 320 Riverside Drive, Northampton, MA 01060; tel. 413/586-6210; FAX. 413/586-7852; Victoria Perry, Program Director

The Harbor Schools, Inc., 26 Rolfes Lane, Newbury, MA 01951; tel. 508/462-3151; Arthur C. DiMauro, Executive Director

The Kolburne School, Inc., Southfield Road, New Marlborough, MA 01230; tel. 413/229-8787; FAX. 413/229-7708; Jeane K. Weinstein, M.A., Executive Director

The Three Rivers Treatment Program, 78 Pomeroy Terrace, Northampton, MA 01060; tel. 413/584-1310; FAX. 413/586-1490; Andrew Pollock, Director, Operations

The Whitney Academy, Inc., 85 Doctor Braley Road, P.O. Box 619, East Freetown, MA 02717; tel. 508/763-3737; FAX. 508/763-4200; George E. Harmon, Executive Director

Westlake Academy, 42 Institute Road, P.O. Box 122, North Grafton, MA 01970; tel. 508/839-6281; FAX. 508/839-3084; Don Mosher, Program Director

Wild Acre Inns, 108 Pleasant Street, Arlington, MA 02174-4813; tel. 617/643-0643; Barbara D'Antonio, RN, Director, Development

MICHIGAN

AOS, Inc., 1331 Lake Drive, S.E., Grand Rapids, MI 49506; tel. 616/456-8010; FAX. 616/451-0020; Charles Logie, President

Adult/Youth Developmental Services, P. C., 23133 Orchard Lake Road, Suite 104, Farmington, MI 48336; tel. 810/477-0107; FAX. 810/477-2303; George H. Kates, Ph.D., Executive Director

Alcohol Information and Counseling Center of the Lapeer County Health Department, 1575 Suncrest Drive, Lapeer, MI 48446; tel. 313/667-0391; FAX. 313/667-9399; John D. Niederhauser, M.P.H., Director, Health Officer

Alcohol and Chemical Abuse Consultants, Inc., 2020 Raybrook, S.E., Suite 102, Grand Rapids, MI 49546; tel. 616/957-5850; FAX. 616/957-5853; Joseph Merrell III, Chief Executive Officer

Alger-Marquette Community Mental Health Center, 200 West Spring Street, Marquette, MI 49855; tel. 906/225-7201; FAX. 906/225-7204; William G. Birch, Ed.D., M.S.W., Chief Executive Officer

Ann Arbor Consultation Services, 5331 Plymouth Road, Ann Arbor, MI 48105; tel. 313/996-9111; Steven Sheldon, Director

Auro Medical Center, 2515 Woodward Avenue, Suite 250, Bloomfield Hills, MI 48304; tel. 313/335-1130; FAX. 313/335-4680; Sue Comer, Contact Person

Boniface Human Services, 25050 West Outer Drive, Suite 201, Lincoln Park, MI 48146; tel. 313/928-8940; FAX. 313/928-5152; Ronald G. Berglund, Executive Director

Brighton Hospital, 12851 East Grand River Avenue, Brighton, MI 48116; tel. 810/227-1211, ext. 235; FAX. 810/227-1869; Ivan C. Harner, President, Chief Executive Officer

CFCS-Catholic Charities Diocese of Gaylord, 111 South Michigan Avenue, Gaylord, MI 49735; tel. 517/732-6761; Kathleen Arndt, Administrator

Care Unit of Grand Rapids, 1931 Boston Street, S.E., Grand Rapids, MI 49506; tel. 616/243-3608; FAX. 616/243-5206; Thomas G. Elzinga, Administrator

Catholic Services of Macomb, 235 South Gratiot Avenue, Mount Clemens, MI 48043; tel. 313/468-2616; Linda Stum, Vice President, Client Services

Center for Behavior and Medicine, 2004 Hogback Road, Suite 16, Ann Arbor, MI 48105; tel. 313/677-0809; Gerard M. Schmit, M.D., Chief Executive Officer

Center for Personal Growth, P.C., 817 10th Avenue, Port Huron, MI 48060; tel. 810/984-4550; FAX. 810/984-3737; Fredric B. Roberts, Ed.D., Chief Executive Officer

Center of Behavioral Therapy P.C., 24453 Grand River, Detroit, MI 48219; tel. 313/592-1765; Hollis Evans, Executive Director

Central Therapeutic Services, Inc., 17600 West 8 Mile Road, Southfield, MI 48075; tel. 313/559-4340; K. G. Thimotheose, Ph.D., President, Chief Executive Officer

Children's Home of Detroit, 900 Cook Road, Grosse Pointe Woods, MI 48236; tel. 313/886-0800; FAX. 313/886-9446; Michael R. Horwitz, Executive Director

Providers / Accredited Freestanding Psychiatric Facilities

Chip Counseling Center, Inc., 14695 Park Avenue, Charlevoix, MI 49720; tel. 616/547-6551; Patrick Q. Nestor, Executive Director

Choices Unlimited, Inc., 1012 Professional Drive, Suite 1075, Flint, MI 48532; tel. 313/732-0606; FAX. 313/732-6064; Raymond V. Failer, D.O., Executive Director

Clinton Counseling Center, 2 Crocker Boulevard, Suite 103, Mount Clemens, MI 48043; tel. 313/463-7079; Joanne Smyth, M.A., CSW, Chief Executive Officer

Clinton–Eaton–Ingham Community Mental Health Board, 808–B Southland, Lansing, MI 48910; tel. 517/887-2126; FAX. 517/887-0086; Judith Taylor, Ph.D., Executive Director

Community Care Services, 26184 West Outer Drive, Lincoln Park, MI 48146; tel. 313/389-7525; FAX. 313/389-7515; Mr. Kari Walker, Deputy Director

Community Commission On Drug Abuse, 13325 Farmington Road, Livonia, MI 48150; tel. 313/261-3760; Ruth Barry, Director

Community Human Services, Inc., 332 South Main Street, Romeo, MI 48065; tel. 810/752-9696; Deanna McGraw, Executive Director

Consortium for Human Development, Inc., 1701 Baldwin Avenue, Pontiac, MI 48340; tel. 810/334-0220; FAX. 810/334-0229; Dr. Ronald Fenton, Chief Executive Officer, Director

Cruz Clinic, 17177 North Laurel Park Drive, Suite 131, Livonia, MI 48152; tel. 313/462-3210; FAX. 313/462-1024; Ida Goutman, Administrator, Program Director

Desgranges Psychiatric Center P.C., G-8145 South Saginaw Street, Grand Blanc, MI 48439; tel. 810/694-2730; L. Desgranges, M.D., Chief Executive Officer

Detroit Central City Community Mental Health, Inc., 10 Peterboro, Detroit, MI 48201; tel. 313/831-3160; FAX. 313/831-2604; George D. Gaines, M.S.W., M.P.H., Executive Director

Dimensions of Life, Inc., 3320 West Saginaw Street, Lansing, MI 48917; tel. 517/886-0340; FAX. 517/886-0505; Alfred K. Doering, Director

Dot Caring Centers, Inc., 3190 Hallmark Court, Saginaw, MI 48603; tel. 517/790-3366; Jim Baranski, M.A., LRC, CSW, Corporate Program Director

Downriver Guidance Clinic of Wayne County, 2959 Biddle Avenue, Suite 200, Wyandotte, MI 48192; tel. 313/285-6400; Leroy A. Lott, M.S.W., Executive Director

Downriver Mental Health Clinic, 20600 Eureka Road, Suite 819, Taylor, MI 48180; tel. 313/285-8282; David S. Monhollen, Administrator

Elrose Health Services, Inc., 1475 East Outer Drive, Detroit, MI 48234; tel. 313/892-4244; FAX. 813/892-1457; Ellsworth E. Jackson, M.A., CSW, Program Director

Fairlane Community Mental Health Centre, 23400 Michigan Avenue, Suite P-24, Dearborn, MI 48124; tel. 313/562-6730; FAX. 313/562-8840; Cheryl Anderson-Smith, Deputy Director

Farmington Area Advisory Council, Inc., 23450 Middlebelt Road, Farmington Hills, MI 48336; tel. 810/477-6767; FAX. 810/473-1284; Betty Arnold, Executive Director

Gateway Services, 333 Turwill Lane, Kalamazoo, MI 49006; tel. 616/382-9827; FAX. 616/342-6440; Thomas E. Lucking, Executive Director

Growth Works, Inc., 271 South Main Street, Plymouth, MI 48170; tel. 313/455-4095; Dale F. Yagiela, Executive Director

Harbor Light, 2643 Park Avenue, Detroit, MI 48201; tel. 313/964-0577

Hegira Programs, Inc., 1375 Inkster Road, Inkster, MI 48141; tel. 313/565-7577; FAX. 313/565-6530; Edward L. Forry, Chief Executive Officer

Highland Waterford Center, Inc., 4501 Grange Hall Road, Holly, MI 48442; tel. 810/634-0140; FAX. 810/634-3838; Michael J. Filipek, B.A., Executive Director

Huron Valley Consultation Center, 955 West Eisenhower Circle, Suite B, Ann Arbor, MI 48103; tel. 313/662-6300; Janet Ford, Business Manager

Insight, 1110 Eldon Baker Drive, Flint, MI 48507; tel. 810/744-3600; FAX. 810/744-4703; Stephen N. LeBel, President

Jackson–Hillsdale Community Mental Health Services Board, 1200 North West Avenue, Jackson, MI 49202; tel. 517/789-1200; FAX. 517/789-1276; Christina M. Thompson, Chief Executive Officer

Jensen Counseling Centers P.C., 26105 Orchard Lake Road, Suite 301, Farmington Hills, MI 48334; tel. 313/478-4411; Christine Jensen, Chief Executive Officer

Lake Orion Treatment Center, 1840 West Scripps Road, Lake Orion, MI 48361; tel. 507/288-4693; Erik A. Vagenius, Treatment Center Director

Lakewood Center, 26000 Hoover, Warren, MI 48089-1167; tel. 313/754-2565; Ronald Fenton, Ph.D., Director, Chief Executive Officer

Lapeer County Community Mental Health Center, 1570 Suncrest Drive, Lapeer, MI 48446-1154; tel. 810/667-0500; FAX. 810/664-8728; Richard I. Berman, Ph.D., Executive Director

Livingston Counseling and Assessment Services, 3744 East Grand River Avenue, Howell, MI 48843; tel. 517/546-7070; FAX. 313/227-1869; Ivan C. Harner, President

Macomb Child Guidance Clinic, Inc., 7828 22 Mile Road, Utica, MI 48317; tel. 810/254-3737; Mary Vandia, ACSW, Clinic Director

Macomb Counseling Center, Inc., 221 South Gratiot, Mount Clemens, MI 48043; tel. 810/468-7420; Megan Gallagher, Chief Executive Officer

Mason County Community Mental Health Services, 920 Diana Street, Ludington, MI 49431; tel. 616/845-6294; FAX. 616/845-7095; John Sternberg, Director, Clinical Services

Meridian Professional Psychological Consultants, P.C., 5031 Park Lake Road, East Lansing, MI 48823; tel. 517/332-0811; FAX. 517/332-4452; Thomas S. Gunnings, Ph.D., President, Clinical Director

Metro East Substance Abuse Treatment Corporation, 13929 Harper Avenue, Detroit, MI 48213; tel. 313/371-0055; FAX. 313/371-1409; Leslie B. Carroll, President

Monroe County Community Mental Health Services Board, 1001 South Raisinville Road, Monroe, MI 48161; tel. 313/243-3371; FAX. 313/243-5564; Sheldon M. Rosen, Executive Director

Mount Pleasant Counseling Services, 3480 South Isabella Road, Mount Pleasant, MI 48858; tel. 517/773-9655; FAX. 517/773-1187; Byron J. Doty, Executive Director

NPL, Inc., 18641 West Seven Mile Road, Detroit, MI 48219; tel. 313/532-8015; Ken Wolf, Ph.D., Chief Executive Officer

Nardin Park Outpatient Psychiatric Center, 9605 Grand River, P.O. Box 04506, Detroit, MI 48204; tel. 313/834-5930; FAX. 313/834-4541; Annie B. Scott, Director

National Council on Alcoholism Lansing Regional Area, 3400 South Cedar, Suite 200, Lansing, MI 48910; tel. 517/887-0851; FAX. 517/887-8121; Nancy L. Siegrist, Executive Director

National Council on Alcoholism and Addictions, 202 East Boulevard, Suite 310, Flint, MI 48503; tel. 810/767-0350; FAX. 810/767-4031; James E. Hartz, M.A., Executive Director

National Council on Alcoholism and Drug Dependence, 17330 Northland Park Court, Southfield, MI 48075; tel. 313/443-1676; FAX. 313/443-0988; Benjamin Jones, Program Coordinator

Neighborhood Service Organization, 220 Bagley, Suite 840, Detroit, MI 48226; tel. 313/961-4890; FAX. 313/961-5120; Carita I. Sledge, Executive Director

New Center Community Mental Health Services, 2051 West Grand Boulevard, Detroit, MI 48208; tel. 313/961-3200; FAX. 313/961-3769; Roberta V. Sanders, Executive Director

New Era Alternative Treatment Center, 13700 Woodward Avenue, Suite 200, Highland Park, MI 48203; tel. 313/869-6328, ext. 312; FAX. 313/869-1765; Joseph A. Pitts, Executive Medical Director

New Perspectives Center, Inc., 1321 South Fayette Street, Saginaw, MI 48602; tel. 517/790-0301; Jimmie D. Westbrook, Executive Director

North Point Mental Health Associates, 28595 Orchard Lake Road, Suite 301, Farmington Hills, MI 48334; tel. 810/489-1550; FAX. 810/489-1737; Alan A. Rickfelder, Ph.D., Chief Executive Officer

Northeast Guidance Center, 13340 East Warren, Detroit, MI 48215; tel. 313/824-5641; FAX. 313/824-7779; Cheryl Coleman, Executive Director

Northern Michigan Alcoholism and Addiction Treatment Services, Inc., 116 East Eighth Street, Traverse City, MI 49684; tel. 616/922-4810; FAX. 616/922-2095; David N. Abeel, M.S.W., Executive Director

O. Ganesh, M.D., P.C., 28165 Greenfield, Southfield, MI 48076; tel. 313/569-6642; G. Borovsky, M.A., L.L.P., CSW, Administrator

Oakland Psychological Clinic, P.C., 2000 South Woodward Avenue, Suite 102, Bloomfield Hills, MI 48302; tel. 313/335-6670; Barry H. Tigay, Ph.D., President

Perspectives of Troy, P.C., 2690 Crooks Road, Suite 300, Troy, MI 48084; tel. 810/244-8644; FAX. 810/244-1330; Timothy Coldiron, ACSW, Ph.D., Chief Executive Officer

Program for Alcohol and Substance Treatment, 110 Sanborn, Big Rapids, MI 49307; tel. 616/796-6203; John R. Kelly, Director

Propelled Therapeutic Services, 18820 Woodward Avenue, Detroit, MI 48203; tel. 313/368-2600; FAX. 313/368-2605; Cecelia Wallace, Executive Director/President

Psychological Consultants of Michigan, P.C., 2518 Capital Avenue, S.W., Suite 2, Battle Creek, MI 49015; tel. 616/968-2811; FAX. 616/968-2651; Jeffrey N. Andert, Ph.D., Administrator

Redford Counseling Center, 25945 West Seven Mile Road, Redford, MI 48240; tel. 313/535-6560; FAX. 313/535-5266; Jo Ann Sadler, Director, ACSW, BCD

Regional Mental Health Clinic, P.C., 23100 Cherry Hill Road, Suite 10, Dearborn, MI 48124-4144; tel. 313/277-1300; Gena J. D'Alessandro, Ph.D., Chief Executive Officer

Romulus Help Center, Hegira Programs, Inc, 9340 South Wayne Road, Suite A, Romulus, MI 48174; tel. 313/942-7585; FAX. 313/947-7977; Pat Buchanan, Clinical Services Supervisor

Rose Hill Center, Inc., 5130 Rose Hill Boulevard, Holly, MI 48442; tel. 810/634-5530; FAX. 810/634-7754; Ronald L. Stuursma, President, Executive Director

Rossano Clinic, Inc., 719 Harrison Street, Flint, MI 48502-2161; tel. 810/235-1950; Nicholas A. Rossano, Program Director

Sacred Heart Rehabilitation Center, Inc., 400 Stoddard Road, Memphis, MI 48041; tel. 810/392-2167; Michael Kelly, Director, Treatment Programs

Self Help Addiction Rehabilitation, 1852 West Grand Boulevard, Detroit, MI 48208; tel. 313/894-1445; FAX. 313/894-5542; Anne C. Benion, ACSW, Program Services Manager

Square Lake Corporation, 1750 South Telegraph, Suite 200, Bloomfield Hills, MI 48302; tel. 810/338-0382; FAX. 810/338-3940; M. Diane Vincent, Chief Operating Officer

Substance Abuse Council of St. Joseph County, 222 South Main Street, Three Rivers, MI 49093-1658; tel. 616/279-5187; FAX. 616/273-2083; James Brundirks, MA/LLP, Clinical Director

Suburban West Community Center, 11677 Beech Daly Road, Redford, MI 48239; tel. 313/937-9500; FAX. 313/937-9504; William R. Hart, Clinical Program Director

The Center for Human Resources, 1001 Military Street, Port Huron, MI 48060-0541; tel. 313/985-5168; Thomas P. Pope, Executive Director

The Counseling Center P.C., 1411 South Woodward, Suite 101, Bloomfield Hills, MI 48304; tel. 810/338-2918; FAX. 810/338-1322; Robert L. Bailey, Director

The Salvation Army Substance Abuse Services, 1215 East Fulton, Grand Rapids, MI 49503; tel. 616/451-0432; FAX. 616/459-9640; Robert E. Byrd, M.A., Director

Providers / Accredited Freestanding Psychiatric Facilities

The Vintage Program, 120 Cutler Street, Allegan, MI 49010; tel. 616/673–8735; Paul Mailloux, Acting Executive Director

Tuscola Substance Abuse Services, 1309 Cleaver Road, P.O. Box 365, Caro, MI 48723; tel. 517/673–7575; FAX. 517/673–7579; Susan H. Clara, Program Director

Washtenaw Council on Alcoholism, 2301 Platt Road, Ann Arbor, MI 48104; tel. 313/971–7900; FAX. 313/971–5950; Barry K. Kistner, Executive Director

Wendie D. Lee Center for Life Management, Inc., 11000 West McNichols, Suite 212, Detroit, MI 48221; tel. 313/345–6777; Wendie D. Lee, Director, Chief Executive Officer

MINNESOTA

Anthony Louis Center, 1000 Paul Parkway, Blaine, MN 55434; tel. 612/757–2906; Jon Benson, Chief Executive Officer

Fairview Riverside Woodbury, Extended Care and Halfway House, 1665 Woodbury Drive, Woodbury, MN 55125; tel. 612/436–6623; Richard Peterson, President, Chief Executive Officer

Guest House, 4800 48th Street N.E., P.O. Box 954, Rochester, MN 55903; tel. 507/288–4693; FAX. 507/288–1240; William C. Morgan, Treatment Center Director

Hazelden Foundation, 15245 Pleasant Valley Road, Center City, MN 55012; tel. 612/257–4010; FAX. 612/257–1055; Jerry Spicer, MHA, Chief Executive Officer

Mission Care Detox Center, 3409 East Medicine Lake, Plymouth, MN 55441; tel. 612/559–1402; FAX. 612/559–2559; Judy Retterath, Program Director

Naeve Behavioral Health Services, 414 Park Avenue, Albert Lea, MN 56007; tel. 507/377–6406; Larry W. Pfaff, Chief Executive Officer

New Beginnings at Waverly, 109 North Shore Drive, Waverly, MN 55390; tel. 612/658–4811; FAX. 612/658–4128; Nina T. Johnson, Director, Treatment

Omegon, Inc., 2000 Hopkins Crossroads, Minnetonka, MN 55343; tel. 612/541–4738; Barbara J. Danielsen, Executive Administrator

Pride Institute, 14400 Martin Drive, Eden Prairie, MN 55344; tel. 800/547–7433; Margaret Gordon, RN, Director, Quality Assurance

St. Joseph's Home for Children, 1121 East 46th Street, Minneapolis, MN 55407; tel. 612/827–9366; FAX. 612/827–7954; Lori Squire, Quality Assurance Director

The Gables, 604 Fifth Street, S.W., Rochester, MN 55902–3256; tel. 507/282–2500; Nancy Stofferahn, Chief Executive Officer

Twin Town Treatment Center, 1706 University Avenue, St. Paul, MN 55104; tel. 612/645–3661; FAX. 612/645–0959; Robert Haven, Chief Executive Officer

MISSISSIPPI

Cares Center, Inc., 402 Wesley Avenue, Jackson, MS 39202; tel. 601/352–7784; Charles H. Caperton, Director

Copac, Inc., 3949 Highway 43N, Brandon, MS 39042; tel. 800/446–9727; Jerald Stacy Hughes, Jr., Ph.D., Executive Director

Jackson Recovery Center, 5354 I–55 South Frontage Road, Jackson, MS 39212; tel. 601/372–9788; FAX. 601/372–9505; D. Preston Smith, Jr., President, Chief Executive Officer

Millcreek, 900 First Avenue, N.E., P.O. Box 1160, Magee, MS 39111; tel. 601/849–4221; FAX. 601/849–7183; Karen L. Lister, Ph.D., Administrator

MISSOURI

Boonville Valley Hope, 1415 Ashley Road, Boonville, MO 65233; tel. 816/882–6547; William Leipold, Ph.D., Chief Executive Officer

Boys and Girls Town of Missouri, Route D.D., P.O. Box 189, St. James, MO 65559; tel. 314/265–3251; FAX. 314/265–5370; Richard C. Dunn, ACSW, LCSW, Executive Director

COPE and Twin Town, 777 South New Ballas Road, Suite 230 W, St. Louis, MO 63141; tel. 314/991–1007; FAX. 314/991–9675; Sue McClure, Program Director

Carpenter Recovery Centers, 723 Riverport Drive, Creve Coeur, MO 63141–1706; tel. 314/569–2662; Robert Coerver, Vice President

Centrec–Care, Inc., 12401 Olive Street Road, Suite 103, St Louis, MO 63141; tel. 314/576–9929; Mohammed A. Kabir, M.D., Chief Executive Officer

Child Center of Our Lady, 7900 Natural Bridge Road, St. Louis, MO 63121; tel. 314/383–0200; FAX. 314/383–6334; Milton T. Fujita, M.D., Chief Executive Officer

Comprehensive Mental Health Services, Inc., 10901 Winner Road, P.O. Box 520169, Independence, MO 64052; tel. 816/254–3652; FAX. 816/254–9243; William H. Kyles, M.A., President, Chief Executive Officer

Epworth Children's Home, 110 North Elm, St. Louis, MO 63119; tel. 314/961–5718; FAX. 314/961–3503; Kevin Drollinger, Executive Director

Great Rivers Mental Health Services, 9362 Dielman Industrial Drive, St. Louis, MO 63132; tel. 314/340–6400; Bonnie DiFranco, Director

Industrial Rehabilitation Center, 2701 Rockcreek Parkway, Suite 205, North Kansas City, MO 64117; tel. 816/471–0511; Maurice L. Cummings, Executive Director

Marillac Center, 2826 Main Street, Kansas City, MO 64108; tel. 816/751–4900; FAX. 816/751–4921; R. Michael Bowen, President

Piney Ridge Center, Inc., 1000 Hospital Road, Waynesville, MO 65583; tel. 314/774–5353; FAX. 314/774–2907; Thomas Arnold, President

Provident Counseling, Inc., 2650 Olive Street, St. Louis, MO 63103; tel. 314/371–6500; FAX. 314/371–6510; Kathleen E. Buescher, President, Chief Executive Officer

Research Mental Health Services, 901 N.E. Independence Avenue, Lees Summit, MO 64086; tel. 816/246–8000; FAX. 816/246–8207; Alan Flory, President

St. Louis Mental Health Center, 1508 South Grand, St. Louis, MO 63104; tel. 314/664–6633; David P. Juedemann, Quality Assurance

The Children's Place, 2 East 59th Street, Kansas City, MO 64113; tel. 816/363–1898; FAX. 816/822–7711; Dana Letts, Executive Director

MONTANA

Intermountain Children's Home, 500 South Lamborn, Helena, MT 59601; tel. 406/442–7920; FAX. 406/442–7949; John Wilkinson, Administrator

Rimrock Foundation, 1231 North 29th Street, Billings, MT 59101; tel. 406/248–3175; FAX. 406/248–3821; David W. Cunningham, M.H.A., Chief Executive Officer

Rocky Mountain Treatment Center, 920 Fourth Avenue North, Great Falls, MT 59401; tel. 406/727–8832; FAX. 406/727–8172; Claree Schulte, Administrator

Yellowstone Treatment Centers, 1732 South 72nd Street, W., Billings, MT 59106; tel. 406/655–2100; FAX. 406/656–0021; Trisha Eik, Director, Admissions

NEBRASKA

Epworth Village, Inc., 2119 Division, York, NE 68467; tel. 402/362–3353; FAX. 402/362–3248; Kristi Weber, Admissions Coordinator

Lincoln Lancaster County Child Guidance Center, 215 Centennial Mall South, Lincoln, NE 68508; tel. 402/475–7666; Howard A. Halpern, Executive Director

O'Neill Valley Hope, North Tenth Street, O'Neill, NE 68753; tel. 402/336–3747; FAX. 402/336–3096; Kaye Chohon, Program Director

Uta Halee Girls Village, 10625 Calhoun Road, Omaha, NE 68112; tel. 402/453–0803; FAX. 402/453–1247; Denis McCarville, Executive Director

NEW HAMPSHIRE

Beech Hill Hospital, New Harrisville Road, P.O. Box 254, Dublin, NH 03444; tel. 603/563–8511; FAX. 603/563–8771; Barbara R. Duckett, Chief Executive Officer

Community Council of Nashua, New Hampshire, Inc., 7 Prospect Street, Nashua, NH 03060–3990; tel. 603/889–6147, ext. 1221; FAX. 603/883–1568; Zlatko Kuftinec, M.D., Executive Director, Chief Medical Officer

Lakeview Neuro Rehab Center, 101 Highwatch Road, Effingham Falls, NH 03814; tel. 603/539–7451; Tony Merka, Chief Executive Officer

Seaborne Hospital, Inc., Seaborne Drive, Dover, NH 03820; tel. 603/742–9300; Bud Charest, Administrator

Seacoast Mental Health Center, Inc., 1145 Sagamore Avenue, Portsmouth, NH 03801; tel. 603/431–6703; FAX. 603/433–5078; Susan Turner, Quality Assurance Coordinator

Seminole Point Hospital Corporation, Woodland Road, Sunapee, NH 03782; tel. 603/763–2545; James F. O'Neill, Chief Executive Officer

The Mental Health Center of Greater Manchester, Inc., 401 Cypress Street, Manchester, NH 03103; tel. 603/668–4111; FAX. 603/669–1131; Nicholas Verven, Ph.D., Executive Director

NEW JERSEY

American Day Treatment Center, of West Essex Network, Inc., 799 Bloomfield Avenue, Verona, NJ 07044; tel. 201/857–5200; E. Bonnie Lizzio, Director

Arthur Brisbane Child Treatment Center, Allaire Road, P.O. Box 625, Farmingdale, NJ 07227; tel. 908/938–5061; FAX. 908/938–9202; Vincent Giampeitro, Chief Executive Officer

Cedar Grove Residential Center, 240 Grove Avenue, Cedar Grove, NJ 07009; tel. 201/857–0200; Patrick Lodato, Superintendent

Charter Behavioral Health System, Lakehurst, 440 Beckerville Road, P.O. Box 5, Lakehurst, NJ 08733; tel. 908/657–4800; FAX. 908/657–2719; Allan Boyer, Chief Executive Officer

Discovery, Inc., P.O. Box 177, Marlboro, NJ 07746; tel. 908/946–9444; Henry Crowell, Director, Admissions

Ewing Residential Treatment Center, 1610 Stuyvesant Avenue, Trenton, NJ 08618; tel. 609/530–3350; FAX. 609/530–3467; Julius Campbell, Chief Executive Officer

High Focus Centers, Inc., 41 Grand Avenue, River Edge, NJ 07661; tel. 201/646–0313; FAX. 201/646–0325; David Nyman, Ph.D., Director, Program Development

Holley Child Care and Development Center of Youth Consultation Service, 260 Union Street, Hackensack, NJ 07601; tel. 201/343–8803; FAX. 201/343–8563

Honesty House, 1272 Long Hill Road, Stirling, NJ 07980; tel. 908/647–3211; FAX. 908/647–7864; Charles H. Stucky, N.C.A.D.C., Executive Director

Lighthouse at Mays Landing, Atlantic Avenue, Mays Landing, NJ 08330; tel. 609/625–4900; FAX. 609/625–8058; Henry A. Bennett, Chief Executive Officer

Monmouth Chemical Dependency Treatment Center, Inc., 152 Chelsea Avenue, Long Branch, NJ 07740; tel. 908/222–5190; FAX. 908/222–5577; Timothy Harrington, Chief Executive Officer

New Hope Foundation, Inc., Route 520, Marlboro, NJ 07746; tel. 908/946–3030; FAX. 908/946–3507; George J. Mattie, Chief Executive Officer

Ocean Mental Health Services, Inc., 230 Main Street, Toms River, NJ 08753; tel. 908/349–0838; Charles J. Langan, Chief Executive Officer

Seabrook House, Polk Lane, Seabrook, NJ 08302; tel. 800/582–5968; FAX. 609/451–7669; Matt Wolf, Admissions Coordinator

Sunrise House Foundation, Inc., Sunset Inn Road, Lafayette, NJ 07848; tel. 201/383–6300; FAX. 201/383–8458; Beth Anne Nathans, M.S., Chief Executive Officer

The Harbor, 1405 Clinton Street, Hoboken, NJ 07030; tel. 201/656–4040; John J. Clancy, Chief Executive Officer

U.M.D.N.J–Community Mental Health Center at Piscataway, 671 Hoes Lane, P.O. Box 1392, Piscataway, NJ 08855–1392; tel. 908/235–5900; FAX. 908/235–4594; Gary W. Lamson, Vice President, Chief Executive Officer

Providers / Accredited Freestanding Psychiatric Facilities

Vineland Children's Residential Treatment Center, 2000 Maple Avenue, Vineland, NJ 08360; tel. 609/696-6620; FAX. 609/696-6847; Theodore Allen, Superintendent

Willowgien Academy–New Jersey, Inc., Highway 206, Newton, NJ 07860; tel. 201/579-3700; Leonard F. Dziubla, Chief Executive Officer

Woodbridge Child Diagnostic and Treatment Center, 15 Paddock Street, Avenel, NJ 07001; tel. 908/499-5050; FAX. 908/815-4874; William Falvo, Superintendent

NEW MEXICO

Desert Hills Center for Youth and Families, 5310 Sequoia, N.W., Albuquerque, NM 87120; tel. 505/836-7330; FAX. 505/836-7424; Dan Lopez, Chief Executive Officer

Four Corners Regional Adolescent Treatment Center, P.O. Box 567, Shiprock, NM 87420; tel. 505/368-4712; FAX. 505/368-5457; Hoskie Benally, Chief Executive Officer

NAMASTE, P.O. Box 489, Los Lunas, NM 87031; tel. 505/865-6176; FAX. 505/865-3268; Kevin Alexy, Administrative Director

New Sunrise Regional Treatment Center, Indian Health Service, Department of Health and Human Services, Acoma Indian Reservation, P.O. Box 219, San Fidel, NM 87049-0219; tel. 505/552-6091; FAX. 505/552-6527; Michael B. Smith, Program Director

River's Bend Children's Residential Treatment, 300 East Griggs, Las Cruces, NM 80001; tel. 505/525-2693; FAX. 505/525-2965; Mike Boyce, Chief Executive Officer

Sequoyah Adolescent Treatment Center, 3405 West Pan American Freeway, N.E., Albuquerque, NM 87107; tel. 505/841-4375; FAX. 505/841-4361; W. Henry Gardner, Ph.D., Director

NEW YORK

Baker Hall, Inc., 125 Martin Road, Lackawanna, NY 14218; tel. 716/828-9777; FAX. 716/828-9767; James J. Casion, Director

Bronx Alcoholism Treatment Center, 1500 Waters Place, Bronx, NY 10461; tel. 718/904-0026; FAX. 718/597-9434; Ronald B. Lonesome, M.D., Director

Capital District Psychiatric Center, 75 New Scotland Avenue, Albany, NY 12208; tel. 518/447-9611; Jesse Nixon, Chief Executive Officer

Charles K. Post Alcoholism Treatment Center, Building 1 Pilgrim Psychiatric Center, West Brentwood, NY 11717; tel. 516/434-7209; Phillip A. Dawes, Director

Children's Home RTF, Inc., Squirrel Hill Road, P.O. Box 658, Greene, NY 13778; tel. 607/656-9004; FAX. 607/656-9076; Mary Jo Thorn, Program Director

Conifer Park, Inc., 79 Glenridge Road, Glenville, NY 12302; tel. 518/399-6446; Mr. Gail Harkness, Chief Executive Officer

Conners Residential Treatment Facility, Inc., 824 Delaware Avenue, Buffalo, NY 14209; tel. 716/884-3802; FAX..716/884-8689; James D. Lawson, Director

Cornerstone of Medical Arts Center Hospital, 57 West 57th Street, New York, NY 10019; tel. 212/755-0200; FAX. 212/755-0915; Norman J. Sokolow, President

Cortland Medical, Four Skyline Drive, Hawthorne, NY 10532; tel. 914/347-2990; Jeffery Smith, M.D., Chief Executive Officer

Creedmoor Alcoholism Treatment Center, 80-45 Winchester Boulevard, Queens Village, NY 11427; tel. 718/464-7500; FAX. 718/776-5145; Jose Sarabia, M.D., Medical Director

Crestwood Children's Center, 2075 Scottsville Road, Rochester, NY 14623-2098; tel. 716/436-4442; FAX. 716/436-0169; Denise M. Groesbeck, OTR, M.P.A., Director for Administration

DayBreak Alcoholism Treatment Facility, 435 East Henrietta Road, Rochester, NY 14620; tel. 716/461-4114; Luisa E. Baars, M.A., M.P.A., Division Director

Dick Van Dyke Alcoholism Treatment Center, Building 112, Willard Psychiatric Center, Willard, NY 14588; tel. 607/869-3111, ext. 2306; FAX. 607/869-4711; John R. Cole, CSW, Director

Dutchess County Department of Mental Hygiene, 230 North Road, Poughkeepsie, NY 12601; tel. 914/485-9700; FAX. 914/485-2759; Kenneth M. Glatt, Ph.D., Commissioner

Family Mental Health Clinic, 141 North Central Avenue, Hartsdale, NY 10530-1912; tel. 914/949-6761; FAX. 914/949-3224; Ronald Gaudia, M.S., Executive Director

Freeport Hospital, 267 South Ocean Avenue, Freeport, NY 11520; tel. 516/378-0800; Debbie A. Turkel, Executive Director

Green Chimneys Children's Services, Inc., Putnam Lake Road, Caller Box 719, Brewster, NY 10509; tel. 914/279-2995, ext. 200; FAX. 914/279-2714; Samuel B. Ross, Jr., Ph.D., Chief Executive Officer

Hillside Children's Center, 1183 Monroe Avenue, Rochester, NY 14620; tel. 716/256-7500; FAX. 716/256-7510; Dennis M. Richardson, President, Chief Executive Officer

Hope House, Inc., 44 Tivoli Street, Albany, NY 12207; tel. 518/465-7879; Arelene Murphy, Acting Director

Hopevale, Inc., 3780 Howard Road, Hamburg, NY 14075; tel. 716/648-1964; FAX. 716/648-5266; Stanfort J. Perry, Executive Director

Hutchings Psychiatric Center, 620 Madison Street, Syracuse, NY 13210; tel. 315/473-4980; Thomas Cheney, Director, Quality Assurance

J. L. Norris Alcoholism Treatment Center, 1600 South Avenue, Rochester, NY 14620; tel. 716/461-0410; FAX. 716/461-4545; Thomas E. Nightingale, Director

Jewish Board of Family and Children's Services, Inc., 120 West 57th Street, New York, NY 10019; tel. 212/582-9100, ext. 1750; FAX. 212/956-5676; Alan B. Siskind, Ph.D., Executive Vice President

Kings Park Psychiatric Center, Route 25 A and Kings Park, Kings Park, NY 11754-4900; tel. 516/544-2957; FAX. 516/544-9599; Donna J. McCarthy, Director, Quality Assurance

Kingsboro Alcoholism Treatment Center, 754 Lexington Avenue, Brooklyn, NY 11221; tel. 718/453-6747; FAX. 718/453-7581; Jacqueline Cole, Director

Madonna Heights Services, 151 Burrs Lane, P.O. Box 8020, Dix Hills, NY 11746-9020; tel. 516/643-8800; FAX. 516/491-4440; Robert J. McMahon, Executive Director

Manhattan Alcoholism Treatment Center, 600 East 125th St., Ward's Island, New York, NY 10035; tel. 212/369-0703; K. Santiago-Yazquez, RN, Chief Executive Officer

McPike Alcoholism Treatment Center, 1213 Court Street, Utica, NY 13502; tel. 315/797-6800; FAX. 315/733-0499; John F. Robertson, Ph.D., Director

Middletown Alcoholism Treatment Center, 141 Monahagen Avenue, Middleton, NY 10940; tel. 914/341-2500; FAX. 914/341-2570; Richard C. Ward, Director

National Recovery Institutes, 455 West 50th Street, New York, NY 10019; tel. 212/262-6000; Roger Cohn, Executive Vice President

Parsons Child and Family Center, 60 Academy Road, Albany, NY 12208; tel. 518/426-2600; FAX. 518/426-2792; John W. Carswell, Executive Director

Pilgrim Psychiatric Center, Crooked Hill Road, West Brentwood, NY 11717-7106; tel. 516/434-5033; John P. Iafrate, M.D., Director

Research Institute on Addictions, 1021 Main Street, Buffalo, NY 14203; tel. 716/887-2386; FAX. 716/887-2215; Linda Rotering, Ph.D., CRC Director

Rochester Mental Health Center, Hart Building, 490 East Ridge Road, Rochester, NY 14621; tel. 716/544-5220; FAX. 716/544-6694; Connie Aiello, RN, Vice President

Russell E. Blaisdell Alcoholism Treatment Center, R. P. C. Campus, Orangeburg, NY 10962; tel. 914/359-8500; FAX. 914/359-2016; Louis R. Brandes, M.D., Director

Saint Peter's Addiction Recovery Center (SPARC, Inc.), 2232 Western Avenue, Guiderland, NY 12084; tel. 518/452-6700; Karen A. Giles, Chief Executive Director

Salamanca Hospital District Authority, d/b/a Salamanca Healthcare Complex, 150 Parkway Drive, Salamanca, NY 14779; tel. 716/945-1900; FAX. 716/945-5016; Kenneth Oakley, Administrator

Salvation Army–Wayside Home School For Girls, 1461 Dutch Broadway, Valley Stream, NY 11580; tel. 516/825-1600; FAX. 516/825-1829; Joseph Juliana, Director

Seafield Center, Inc., Seven Seafield Lane, Westhampton Beach, NY 11978; tel. 516/288-1122; John C. Haley, Executive Director

Sleepy Valley Center, Inpatient Alcohol Rehabilitation Center, 117 Sleepy Valley Road, Warwick, NY 10990; tel. 914/986-2545; FAX. 914/986-7882; Joan Pakenham, Chief Executive Officer

South Beach Alcoholism Treatment Center, 777 Seaview Avenue, Building A, 2nd Floor, Staten Island, NY 10305; tel. 718/667-4218; FAX. 718/351-1958; Gerlando A. Verruso, Director

St. Christopher-Ottilie Residential Treatment Facility, 85-70 148th Street, Briarwood, NY 11435; tel. 718/658-4101; Robert J. McMahon, Chief Executive Officer

St. Joseph's Rehabilitation Center, Inc., 99 Glenwood Estates, P.O. Box 470, Saranac Lake, NY 12983-0470; tel. 518/891-3950; FAX. 518/891-3986; Reverend Arthur M. Johnson, Executive Director

St. Joseph's Villa of Rochester, 3300 Dewey Avenue, Rochester, NY 14616-3795; tel. 716/865-1550; FAX. 716/865-5219; M. Judith McKay, ACSW, President, Chief Executive Officer

St. Lawrence Alcoholism Treatment Center, Station A–Hamilton Hall, Ogdensburg, NY 13669; tel. 315/393-1180; FAX. 315/393-6160; Phillip Dranger, Director

St. Mary's Children and Family Services, 525 Convent Road, Syosset, NY 11791-3864; tel. 516/921-0808; FAX. 516/921-0737; Liz Giordano, Executive Director

Stutzman Alcoholism Treatment Center, 360 Forest Avenue, Buffalo, NY 14213; tel. 716/882-4900; FAX. 716/882-4426; Steven Schwartz, Director

The Areba/Casriel Institute, 500 West 57th Street, New York, NY 10019; tel. 212/247-5500; Steven Yohay, Executive Director

The Astor Home for Children, 36 Mill Street, P.O. Box 5005, Rhinebeck, NY 12572-5005; tel. 914/876-4081; FAX. 914/876-2020; Sister Rose Logan, D.C., Executive Director

The August Aichhorn Center for Adolescent Residential Care, Inc., 23 West 106th Street, New York, NY 10025; tel. 212/316-9353; FAX. 212/662-2755; Michael A. Pawel, M.D., Executive Director

The Children's Village, Dobbs Ferry, NY 10522; tel. 914/693-0600, ext. 1383; FAX. 914/693-7708; Nan Dale, Executive Director

The Rhinebeck Lodge for Successful Living, Inpatient Treatment Program, 500 Milan Hollow Road, Rhinebeck, NY 12572; tel. 800/266-4410; Chandra Singh, Ph.D., Executive Director

The Saint Francis Academy, Incorporated, Lake Placid (Camelot, The Knight House, Adirondack Experience), 50 Riverside Drive, Lake Placid, NY 12946; tel. 518/523-3605; FAX. 518/523-1470; Reverend Carlos J. Caguiat, FACHE, Vice President, Executive Director

The Villa Outpatient Center, 290 Madison Avenue, New York, NY 10017; tel. 212/679-4960; Alfonso Tafoya, President

Tully Hill, Route 80, P.O. Box 920, Tully, NY 13159; tel. 315/696-6114; FAX. 315/696-8509; Karl J. Kabza, Chief Executive Officer

Veritas Villa, Inc., R.R. 2, Box 415, Kerhonkson, NY 12446; tel. 914/626-3555; FAX. 914/626-3840; James S. Cusack, President, Owner

Providers / Accredited Freestanding Psychiatric Facilities

NORTH CAROLINA

Alcohol and Drug Abuse Treatment Center, 205 West E Street, Butner, NC 27509; tel. 919/575–7928

Amethyst Charlotte, Inc., 1715 Sharon Road, W., Charlotte, NC 28224; tel. 704/554–8373; Wallace M. Slatinsky, President, Chief Executive Officer

Fellowship Hall, Inc., Highway 29 North, Hicone Road, Greensboro, NC 27415; tel. 919/621–3381; Edmund F. Ward, Executive Director

Forsyth–Stokes Mental Health Center, 725 North Highland Avenue, Winston–Salem, NC 27101; tel. 919/725–7777; Roy H. Haberkern, M.D., Medical Director

Learning Services Carolina Regional Campus, 707 Morehead Avenue, Durham, NC 27707; tel. 919/688–4444; Dr. Randall W. Evans, Program Director

Mary Frances Center, 1212 Recovery Road, Tarboro, NC 27886; tel. 919/641–1111; FAX. 919/641–0297; Richard Herring, Director, Operations

Step One, Inc., 545 North Trade Street, Winston–Salem, NC 27101; tel. 910/725–8389; Selbert M. Wood, President, Chief Executive Officer

The Alcohol and Drug Abuse Treatment Center, 301 Tabernacle Road, Black Mountain, NC 28711; tel. 704/669–3402; FAX. 704/669–3451; Bill Rafter, Director

The Wilmington Treatment Center, 2520 Troy Drive, Wilmington, NC 28401; tel. 919/762–2727; FAX. 919/762–7923; Charles Sharp, Executive Director

Three Springs of North Carolina, P.O. Box 1320, Pittsboro, NC 27312; tel. 919/542–1104; Jonathan Carmel, Administrator

Unity Regional Youth Treatment Center, P.O. Box C–201, Cherokee, NC 28719; tel. 704/497–3958; Mary Anne Farrell, M.D., Director

Walter B. Jones Alcohol and Drug Abuse Treatment Center, 2577 West Fifth Street, Greenville, NC 27834; tel. 919/830–3426; FAX. 919/830–8585; Phillip A. Mooring, Chief Executive Officer

NORTH DAKOTA

Heartview Foundation, 1406 Second Street, N.W., Mandan, ND 58554; tel. 701/663–2321; FAX. 701/663–2598; Allen M. Gillette, Administrator

OHIO

Beech Brook, 3737 Lander Road, Cleveland, OH 44124; tel. 216/831–2255, ext. 309; FAX. 216/831–0436; Mark Groner, Assistant Clinical Director

Bellefaire JCB, 22001 Fairmount Boulevard, Cleveland, OH 44118; tel. 216/932–2800; FAX. 216/932–8520; Margaret M. Culp, ACSW, L.I.S.W., Intake Director

Careunit Hospital of Cincinnati, 3156 Glenmore Avenue, Cincinnati, OH 45211; tel. 513/481–8822; FAX. 513/481–7317; Judith Erwin, Director, Quality Assurance

Center for Chemical Addiction Treatment, 830 Ezzard Charles Drive, Cincinnati, OH 45214; tel. 513/381–6672; Sandra L. Kuel, Executive Director

Central Mental Health, 832 McKinley Avenue, N.W., Canton, OH 44703; tel. 216/455–9407; Richard W. Thompson, Chief Executive Officer

Charles B. Mills Center, Inc., 715 South Plum Street, Marysville, OH 43040; tel. 513/644–9192; FAX. 513/644–3426; Robert C. Mertz, Executive Director

Children's Aid Society, 10427 Detroit Avenue, Cleveland, OH 44102; tel. 216/521–6511; FAX. 216/521–6006; Bob Allenick, Director, Administrative Services

Community Drug Board, Inc., 725 East Market Street, Akron, OH 44305; tel. 216/434–1141; FAX. 216/434–7125; Theodore Paul Ziegler, Chief Executive Officer

Comprehensive Psychiatry Specialists, 955 Windham Court, Suite Two, Boardman, OH 44512; tel. 216/726–9570; FAX. 216/726–9031; Pradeep Mathur, President

Crisis Intervention Center of Stark County, Inc., 2421 13th Street, N.W., Canton, OH 44708; tel. 216/452–9812; FAX. 216/454–4357; Lori S. Lapp, M.B.A., Executive Director

Family Recovery Center, 964 North Market Street, Lisbon, OH 44432; tel. 216/424–1468; FAX. 216/424–9844; Eloise V. Traina, Executive Director

Focus Health, 700 Morse Road, Suite 208, Columbus, OH 43214; tel. 614/885–1944; FAX. 614/885–6665; Jo-Ann Boundy, Operations Manager

Glenbeigh Hospital of Cleveland, 18120 Puritas Avenue, Cleveland, OH 44135; tel. 216/476–0222; FAX. 216/476–2938; Mark Davis, Executive Director

Glenbeigh Hospital of Rock Creek, Route 45, Rock Creek, OH 44084; tel. 216/563–3400; Patricia Weston–Hall, Executive Director

Harbor Behavioral Healthcare, 4334 Secor Road, Toledo, OH 43623–4234; tel. 419/475–4449; FAX. 419/479–3832; Dale E. Shreve, Chief Operating Officer

Health Recovery Services, Inc., 28 North College Street, Athens, OH 45701; tel. 614/594–3511; FAX. 614/593–7258; Kenneth H. Pickering, Executive Director

INTERACT Behavioral Healthcare Services, Inc., Administrative Offices, 1808 East Broad Street, Columbus, OH 43203; tel. 614/251–8242; James M. Shulman, Ph.D., Chief Executive Officer

Interval Brotherhood Home, Alcohol Drug Rehabilitation Center, 3445 South Main Street, Akron, OH 44319; tel. 216/644–4095; FAX. 216/645–2031; Father Samuel R. Ciccolini, Executive Director

Lincoln Center For Prevention and Treatment of Chemical Dependency, 1918 North Main Street, Findlay, OH 45840; tel. 419/423–9242; FAX. 419/423–7854; W. Scott Kibler, Executive Director

Mahoning County Chemical Dependency Programs, Inc., 527 North Meridan Road, Youngstown, OH 44509; tel. 216/797–0070; Martin K. Gaudiose, Chief Executive Officer

McKinley Hall, Inc., 1101 East High Street, Springfield, OH 45505; tel. 513/328–5300; FAX. 513/322–4900; Judith O. Hoy, Chief Executive Officer

Mental Health Center of Western Stark County, Inc., 111 Tremont Avenue, S.W., Massillon, OH 44647; tel. 216/833–4132; FAX. 216/833–6548; Lawrence R. Cook, Executive Director

Mental Health Center, Inc., 111 Glamorgan Avenue, Suite 201, Alliance, OH 44601; tel. 216/821–1995; FAX. 216/821–6080; Carol H. Hales, Chief Executive Officer

Mental Health Services for Clark County, Inc., 1345 Fountain Boulevard, Springfield, OH 45504; tel. 513/399–9500; FAX. 513/399–2701; Suzanne Goodell, Director, Quality Improvement

Miami Valley Labor Management, Health Care Delivery Systems, Inc., 136 Heid Avenue, Dayton, OH 45404; tel. 513/236–1367; Thomas Keen, Director

Neil Kennedy Recovery Clinic, 2151 Rush Boulevard, Youngstown, OH 44507; tel. 216/744–1181; FAX. 216/740–2849; Gerald V. Carter, Executive Director

Neo Psych Consultants, 819 McKay Court, Suite 101, Boardman, OH 44512; tel. 216/726–7785; Charles L. Boris, President

New Directions, Inc., 30800 Chagrin Boulevard, Pepper Pike, OH 44124; tel. 216/591–0324; FAX. 216/591–1243; Sally Newman, Intake Coordinator

Northwest Counseling Services, 1560 Fishinger Road, Columbus, OH 43221; tel. 614/457–7876; FAX. 614/457–7896; Hollie Goldberg, Director, Quality Assurance

Parkside Behavioral Healthcare, Inc., 349 Olde Ridenour Road, Columbus, OH 43230; tel. 614/471–2552; FAX. 614/471–0167; Christine Gerber, President, Chief Executive Officer

Parmadale Family Services, 6753 State Road, Parma, OH 44134; tel. 216/845–7700; FAX. 216/845–5910; Thomas Woll, Executive Director

Portage Path Community Mental Health Center, 340 South Broadway Street, Akron, OH 44308–8159; tel. 216/376–6144; FAX. 216/376–8002; Shelly Obert, Clinical Services Director

Psycare, Inc., 3530 Belmont Avenue, Suite Seven, Youngstown, OH 44505; tel. 216/759–2310; FAX. 216/759–0018; Douglas Darnall, Ph.D., Chief Executive Officer

Psych Systems of Greater Cincinnati, 4243 Hunt Road, Suite 120, Cincinnati, OH 45242; tel. 513/891–9114; R. Sharon Wilson, Director, Nursing

Quest Recovery Services, 1341 Market Avenue, N., Canton, OH 44714; tel. 216/453–8252; FAX. 216/453–6716; Donald C. Davies, Chief Executive Officer

Ravenwood Mental Health Center, 12557 Ravenwood Drive, Chardon, OH 44024; tel. 216/285–3568; David Boyle, Executive Director

Rescue Mental Health Services, 3350 Collingwood Boulevard, Toledo, OH 43610; tel. 419/255–9585; FAX. 419/255–2801; Frank C. Ayers, Executive Director

Serenity Living, Inc., 210 West National Road, P.O. Box 217, Vandalia, OH 45377; tel. 513/898–2788; Joseph J. Trevino, M.D., Chief Executive Officer

Specialty Care Psychiatric Services, 2657 Nives Courtland Road, Warren, OH 44484; tel. 216/652–3533; Donna H. Morse, Chairperson, Quality Assurance

Springview Developmental Center, 3130 East Main Street, Springfield, OH 45505; tel. 513/325–9263; FAX. 513/325–3593; Dominick S. Dennis, Superintendent

The Akron Child Guidance Center, Inc., 312 Locust Street, Akron, OH 44302–1878; tel. 216/762–0591; FAX. 216/762–2242; Charles M. Vehlow, Jr., Executive Director

The Buckeye Ranch, 5665 Hoover Road, Grove City, OH 43123; tel. 614/875–2371; FAX. 614/871–6487; Sally Pedon, L.I.S.W., L.P.C., Director, Admissions

The Campus, 905 South Sunbury Road, Westerville, OH 43081; tel. 614/895–1000, ext. 13; FAX. 614/895–3010; Robert Stevenson, CCDC III, Intake Coordinator

The Lake Area Recovery Center, 2801 C Court, Ashtabula, OH 44004; tel. 216/998–0722; Kathleen Kinney, Executive Director

Two North Park, Inc., 720 Pine Street, S.E., Warren, OH 44483; tel. 216/399–3677; FAX. 216/394–3815; Ken Lloyd, M.S. Ed., L.S.W., CCDC III, Executive Director

Wood County Council on Alcoholism and Drug Abuse, Inc., 320 West Gypsy Lane, Bowling Green, OH 43402; tel. 419/352–2551; Randall J. LaFond, Executive Director

OKLAHOMA

Christopher Youth Center, Inc., 2741 East 7th Street, Tulsa, OK 74104; tel. 918/583–0612; FAX. 918/583–5459; Thomas E. McKee, Ed.D., Director

Drug/Alcohol Residential Treatment Center, 604 South Ninth, Tecumseh, OK 74873; tel. 405/598–2859; Camille Palmer, Acting Program Director

High Pointe, 6501 N.E. 50th Street, Oklahoma City, OK 73141; tel. 405/424–3383; FAX. 405/424–0729; Charlene Arnett, Chief Executive Officer

Jim Taliaferro Community Mental Health Center, 602 S.W. 38th Street, Lawton, OK 73505–6999; tel. 405/248–5780; FAX. 405/248–3610; Ted Debbs, M.S., Executive Director

Mendros Psychiatric Medical Clinic, 2100 North Broadway, Moore, OK 73160; tel. 405/794–7719; Harry G. Mendros, M.D., Chief Executive Officer

Moccasin Bend Ranch, Adolescent Treatment Center, 130 A Street, S.W., Miami, OK 74354; tel. 918/542–1836; FAX. 918/542–8730; Kenneth O'Rourke, Administrator, Chief Executive Officer

Oklahoma Youth Center, 1120 East Main Street, Norman, OK 73071–5300; tel. 405/364–9004; FAX. 405/364–0096, ext. 2802; Paul Bouffard, Director

Providers / Accredited Freestanding Psychiatric Facilities

Parkside, Inc., 1620 East 12th Street, Tulsa, OK 74120; tel. 918/582–2131; FAX. 918/588–8822; Quentin Henley, Chief Executive Officer

Recovery Plus, 817 South Elm Place, Suite 105, Broken Arrow, OK 74012–2537; tel. 918/258–6900; Karen Doney, Executive Director

Valley Hope Alcohol and Drug Treatment Center, 100 South Jones, P.O. Box 472, Cushing, OK 74023; tel. 918/225–1736; FAX. 918/225–7742; Dennis Gilhousen, Chief Executive Officer

OREGON

Children's Farm House, 4455 Northeast Highway 20, Corvallis, OR 97339–9102; tel. 503/757–1852; Kim Scott, Associate Director

Eastern Oregon Adolescent Multi–Treatment Center, 412 S.E. Dorion, Pendleton, OR 97801; tel. 503/276–0057; FAX. 503/276–1704; Ronald Humiston, Executive Director

Edgefield Children's Center, Inc., 2408 S.W. Halsey Street, Troutdale, OR 97060–1097; tel. 503/665–0157; FAX. 503/666–3066; David Fuks, M.S.W., Executive Director

Kerr Youth and Family Center, 722 N.E. 162nd Avenue, Portland, OR 97230; tel. 503/255–4205; James V. Novell, Administrator

Pioneer Trail Adolescent Treatment Center, 4101 N.E. Division Street, Gresham, OR 97030; tel. 503/661–0775; FAX. 503/661–4649; Marcia Hille, ACSW, M.B.A., Administrator

RiverBend Youth Center, 15544 South Clackamas River Drive, Oregon City, OR 97045; tel. 503/656–8005; FAX. 503/656–8929; Marcia L. McClocklin, Executive Director

Serenity Lane, Inc., 616 East 16th Avenue, Eugene, OR 97401; tel. 503/687–1110; Neil H. McNaughton, Executive Director

Southern Oregon Adolescent Study and Treatment Center, Inc., 210 Tacoma Street, Grants Pass, OR 97526; tel. 503/476–3302; FAX. 503/476–2895; Robert Lieberman, Executive Director

Springbook Northwest, 2001 Crestview Drive, Newberg, OR 97132; tel. 503/537–7000; Patti Williamson, Quality Assurance Coordinator

The Christie School, P.O. Box 368, Marylhurst, OR 97036; tel. 503/635–3416; FAX. 503/697–6932; Daniel A. Mahler, M.S.W., LCSW, Executive Director

PENNSYLVANIA

American Day Treatment Center of Bryn Mawr, 950 Haverford Road, Suite D, Bryn Mawr, PA 19010; tel. 610/527–7474; FAX. 610/527–7479; Stacey Solley, Executive Director

Bowling Green Inn–Brandywine, 1375 Newark Road, Kennett Square, PA 19348; tel. 610/268–3588; FAX. 610/268–2334; Jeffrey J. Kegley, Executive Director

Caron Foundation, Galen Hall Road, Box A, Wernersville, PA 19565; tel. 215/678–2332; FAX. 215/678–5704; Joseph K. Lauginiger, Jr., Interim President, Chief Executive Officer

Charter Behavioral Health System at Cove Forge, New Beginnings Road, Williamsburg, PA 16693; tel. 800/873–2131; FAX. 814/832–2882; Jonathan Wolf, Chief Executive Officer

Chit Chat Westfield, 355 Church Street, Westfield, PA 16950; tel. 814/367–5901; FAX. 814/367–5901; Leo C. McLaughlin, Chief Executive Officer

Clear Brook, Inc., 1003 Wyoming Avenue, Forty–Fort, PA 18704; tel. 717/288–6692; Dave Lombard, Chief Executive Officer

College Hill Medical Center, 329 East Brown Street, East Stroudsburg, PA 18301; tel. 717/424–6233; FAX. 717/424–6380; William I. Van Meter, Chief Executive Officer

Devereux Mapleton Psychiatric Institute, 655 Sugartown Road, P.O. Box 297, Malvern, PA 19355–0297; tel. 215/296–6923; FAX. 215/296–6949; Kenneth Tenley, Executive Director

Devereux–Brandywine Center, Devereux Road, P.O. Box 69, Glenmore, PA 19343; tel. 610/942–5964; FAX. 610/942–5979; Fran Laird, Director, Administrative and Quality Management

Eagleville Hospital, 100 Eagleville Road, Eagleville, PA 19403–1800; tel. 610/539–6000, ext. 101; FAX. 610/539–9314; Frederick M. Carey, Chief Executive Officer

Edward L. French Center of The Devereux Foundation, 119 Old Lancaster Road, Devon, PA 19333; tel. 215/964–3214; FAX. 215/971–4603; Joan M. Vermillion, Ph.D., Director, Operations

Friends Recovery Center, 520 North Delaware Avenue, Suite 302, Riverview Place Building, Philadelphia, PA 19123; tel. 215/627–4278; FAX. 215/627–4058; Robyn B. Kulp, M.S., CAC, Director

Friendship House Children's Center, 1615 East Elm Street, Scranton, PA 18505; tel. 717/342–8305; FAX. 717/344–1105; Robert Angeloni, Chief Executive Officer

Gateway Rehabilitation Center, Moffett Run Road, Aliquippa, PA 15001; tel. 412/766–8700, ext. 101; FAX. 412/375–8815; Kenneth S. Ramsey, Ph.D., President

Gaudenzia, Inc.–Common Ground, 2835 North Front Street, Harrisburg, PA 17110; tel. 717/238–5553; Gerald McFarland, Program Director

Greenbriar Treatment Center, 800 Manor Drive, Washington, PA 15301; tel. 412/225–9700; FAX. 412/225–9764; Mary Banaszak, Executive Director

Hoffman Homes for Youth, 815 Orphanage Road, Littlestown, PA 17340; tel. 717/359–7148; FAX. 717/359–9536; Frank Deroba, Director

Lakewood Retreat, Inc., Rural Route Seven, Box 7803, East Stroudsburg, PA 18301; tel. 717/476–4610; FAX. 717/476–4614; Diana C. Reid, Administrator

Livengrin Foundation, Inc., 4833 Hulmeville Road, Bensalem, PA 19020–3099; tel. 215/638–5200; FAX. 215/638–2603; Timothy D. Shanahan, Ph.D., M.A., Assistant Executive Director

Lutheran Youth and Family Services, Beaver Road, P.O. Box 70, Zelienople, PA 16063; tel. 412/452–4453; Charles T. Lockwood, Executive Director

Malvern Institute, 940 King Road, Malvern, PA 19355; tel. 610/647–0330; FAX. 610/647–2572; Valerie Craig, Administrator, Chief Executive Officer

Marworth, Lily Lake Road, Waverly, PA 18471; tel. 717/563–1112; FAX. 717/563–2711; James Dougherty, Senior Vice President

Mirmont Treatment Center, 100 Yearsley Mill Road, Lima, PA 19037; tel. 215/565–9232; FAX. 215/565–7497; Thomas F. Crane, Executive Director

National Hospital for Kids in Crisis, A Division of Kids Peace, 5300 KidsPeace Drive, Orefield, PA 18069–9101; tel. 215/799–8897; FAX. 215/799–8801; Candance Herrman, Hospital Director

New Vitae Partial Hospital, St. Joseph Road and Limeport Park, Limeport, PA 18060; tel. 215/965–9021; David T. Wilson, Executive Director

Penn Foundation, 807 Lawn Avenue, P.O. Box 32, Sellersville, PA 18960; tel. 215/257–6551; FAX. 215/257–9347; Vernon H. Kratz, M.D., President

Philadelphia Center for Young Adult Psychiatry, 111 North 49th Street, Philadelphia, PA 19139; tel. 215/471–2128; FAX. 215/471–2866; Steven H. Weinstein, Chief Executive Officer

Renewal Centers, 2705 Old Bethlehem Pike, Quakertown, PA 18951; tel. 215/536–9070; FAX. 215/536–4788; Theresa E. Walsh, Executive Director

Roxbury, 601 Roxbury Road, P.O. Box L, Shippensburg, PA 17257; tel. 717/532–4217; FAX. 717/532–4003; Claire F. Beckwith, Chief Executive Officer

Serenity Hall, Inc., 414 West Fifth Street, Erie, PA 16507; tel. 814/459–4775; FAX. 814/453–6118; Suzanne C. Mack, Executive Director

The Bridge, 8400 Pine Road, Philadelphia, PA 19111; tel. 215/342–5000; Star Weiss, Program Director

The Ellen O'Brien Gaiser Addiction Center, Inc., 165 Old Plank Road, P.O. Box 2127, Butler, PA 16003; tel. 412/287–8205; FAX. 412/287–6788; Reverand Paul A. Sandusky, Executive Director

The Mercy Center For Chemical Dependency Services, 3350 Fleming Avenue, Pittsburgh, PA 15212; tel. 412/734–7501; Daniel M. Taylor, Executive Director

The Renfrew Center, 475 Spring Lane, Philadelphia, PA 19128; tel. 215/482–5353; FAX. 215/482–7390; Samuel Menaged, Chief Executive Officer

The Residence of Presbyterian, 39th and Market Streets, Philadelphia, PA 19104; tel. 215/662–8880; Elizabeth Dean, Program Administrator

The Terraces, 1170 South State Street, Ephrata, PA 17522; tel. 717/859–4100; FAX. 717/859–2131; Ronald J. Hunsicker, Executive Director

Today, Inc., 1990 North Woodbourne Road, P.O. Box 908, Newtown, PA 18940; tel. 215/968–4713; FAX. 215/968–8742; John E. Howell, Executive Vice President

Twin Lakes Center for Drug and Alcohol Rehabilitation, P.O. Box 909, Somerset, PA 15501–0909; tel. 814/443–3639; Mark T. Pile, ACSW, Chief Executive Officer

UHS Keystone Center, 2001 Providence Road, Chester, PA 19013–5504; tel. 610/876–9000; FAX. 610/876–5441; Daniel A. Kidd, Managing Director

Villa St. John Vianney Hospital, Lincoln Highway at Woodbine Road, P.O. Box 219, Downingtown, PA 19335–0219; tel. 610/269–2600; FAX. 610/873–8028; Louis D. Horvath, Administrator

Westmeade Healthcare, 8765 Stenton Avenue, Wyndmoor, PA 19118; tel. 215/836–9600; FAX. 215/836–9107; Patricia Allen, Executive Director

White Deer Run, Devitt Camp Road, P.O. Box 97, Allenwood, PA 17810–0097; tel. 717/538–2567; FAX. 717/538–5303; Wallace M. Slatinsky, Executive Director

Wordsworth Academy, Pennsylvania Avenue and Camp Hill, Fort Washington, PA 19034; tel. 215/643–5400, ext. 3201; FAX. 215/643–0595; Bernard Cooper, Ph.D., Chief Executive Officer

RHODE ISLAND

Community Counseling Center, 160 Beechwood Avenue, Pawtucket, RI 02860; tel. 401/722–5573; FAX. 401/722–5630; Richard H. Leclerc, President

Good Hope Center, Inc., P.O. Box 470, East Greenwich, RI 02818; tel. 401/826–2750; Alan Willoughby, Ph.D., Chief Executive Officer

Mental Health Services, Inc., 1516 Alwood Avenue, Johnston, RI 02919–9323; tel. 401/273–8756; FAX. 401/454–0148; Stephen DeRosa, Vice President, Management, Technical Operations

SOUTH CAROLINA

Charter Behavioral Health System at Fenwick Hall, 1709 River Road, Johns Island, SC 29457; tel. 803/559–2461; FAX. 803/559–6202; Anne F. Battin, Associate Director

New Hope Treatment Centers, Inc., 225 Midland Parkway, Summerville, SC 29485–8104; tel. 803/851–5010; FAX. 803/851–5020; Katherine W. Grego, President, Chief Operating Officer

York Place–Episcopal Church Home for Children, 234 Kings Mountain Street, York, SC 29745; tel. 803/684–8005; FAX. 803/684–8002; Barry Allison, Treatment Services Director

SOUTH DAKOTA

Black Hills Childrens Home, 24100 South Rockerville Road, Rapid City, SD 57701; tel. 605/343–5422; FAX. 605/343–1411; David P. Loving, Executive Director

Children's Home Society of South Dakota, 801 North Sycamore, P.O. Box 1749, Sioux Falls, SD 57101–1749; tel. 605/334–6004, ext. 46; FAX. 605/335–2776; David P. Loving, Executive Director

Keystone Treatment Center, 1010 East Second Street, Canton, SD 57013; tel. 605/987–2751; Carol A. Regier, RN, CCDC, Executive Director

Providers / Accredited Freestanding Psychiatric Facilities

TENNESSEE

Buffalo Valley, Inc., 501 Park Avenue, S., Hohenwald, TN 38462; tel. 615/796-5427; Jerry T. Risner, Executive Director

Camelot Care Center, Inc., Route 3, Box 267C, 183 Fiddlers Lane, Kingston, TN 37763; tel. 615/376-2296; FAX. 615/376-1850; James E. Spicer, Ph.D., Executive Director

Child and Family Services of Knox County, Inc., 114 Dameron Avenue, Knoxville, TN 37917; tel. 615/524-7483; FAX. 615/524-4790; Charles E. Gentry, ACSW, LCSW, Chief Executive Officer

Cornerstone of Recovery, Inc., 1120 Topside Road, Louisville, TN 37777; tel. 615/970-7747; FAX. 615/681-2266; J. William Hood, President

Council for Alcohol and Drug Abuse Services, Inc., 207 Spears Avenue, Chattanooga, TN 37405; tel. 615/756-7644; FAX. 615/756-7646; James F. Marcotte, Executive Director

Cumberland Hall of Chattanooga, Inc., 7351 Standifer Gap Road, Chattanooga, TN 37421; tel. 615/499-9007; FAX. 615/499-9757; Charles Dickens, Administrator

Cumberland Heights Drug and Alcohol Treatment Center, Route 2, 8283 River Road, Nashville, TN 37209; tel. 615/352-1757; FAX. 615/353-4300; James Moore, Executive Director

Jackson Academy L.L.C., 222 Church Street, Dickson, TN 37055; tel. 615/446-3900; FAX. 615/446-3985; Robert D. Glasner, Psy.D., Chief Executive Officer

Peninsula Village, Jones Bend Road, Louisville, TN 37777; tel. 615/970-1828; Laura J. Thomas, Administrator

Pine Point Center, Inc., 49 Old Hickory Boulevard, Jackson, TN 38305; tel. 901/664-7196; FAX. 901/661-0640; Britt Whitaker, Executive Director

The Harbours at Brentwood, 209 Ward Circle, P.O. Box 1644, Brentwood, TN 37024-1644; tel. 615/373-8700; FAX. 615/373-1899; Melanie Sircy, Controller

The Renewal Center, Methodist Outreach, Inc., 2009 Lamar Avenue, Memphis, TN 38114; tel. 901/276-5401; FAX. 901/272-2551; Louise D. Renfroe, A.R.T., Coordinator, Health Information Services

University of Tennessee Day Treatment Program, 711 Jefferson, Suite 607, Memphis, TN 38105; tel. 901/448-6378; Pamela A. Millsap, Program Director

Youth Villages' Dogwood Village, Memphis Boys Town, Deer Valley Programs, Intercept Families, 2890 Bekemeyer Drive, Arlington, TN 38002; tel. 901/867-8832; Jane Hemphill, Director, Marketing

TEXAS

Austin Child Guidance Center, 810 West 45th Street, Austin, TX 78751; tel. 512/451-2242; FAX. 512/454-9204; Donald J. Zappone, Dr.P.H., Executive Director

Burke Center, 4101 South Medford Drive, Lufkin, TX 75901; tel. 409/639-1141, ext. 215; FAX. 409/634-8601; George Patterson, Director, Operations

Canyon Lakes Residential Treatment Center, 2402 Canyon Lake Drive, Lubbock, TX 79415; tel. 806/762-5782; FAX. 806/762-0838; Ray H. Brown, Ph.D., Administrator

Cedar Crest Residential Treatment Center, 3500 I-35 South, Belton, TX 76513; tel. 800/888-4071; FAX. 817/939-2334; M.J. Caldwell, R.R.A., Director, Information Services

Champions Psychiatric Treatment Center, 14320 Walters Road, Houston, TX 77014; tel. 713/537-5050; FAX. 713/537-2726; April Guillory, RN, Director, Patient Care Services

Child Study Center, 1300 West Lancaster, Fort Worth, TX 76102; tel. 817/336-8611; Larry D. Eason, Ed.D., Administrator

Day Treatment Center of Dallas, 1326 Stemmons Avenue, Dallas, TX 75208; tel. 214/943-1878; FAX. 214/943-9208; Jane M. Baggett, RN, Executive Director

Devereux-Texas Treatment Network, 120 David Wade Drive, Victoria, TX 77902-2666; tel. 512/575-8271; FAX. 512/575-6520; L. Gail Atkinson, Executive Director

Family Opportunity Resources, The F.O.R.G.I.V.E. Program, 1814 45th Street, Suite 106, Galveston, TX 77550; tel. 409/763-1181; Gordon W. McKee, Administrator

Glass Treatment Center, Inc., 18842 Memorial Street, Suite 205, Humble, TX 77338; tel. 713/666-9811; FAX. 713/446-5292; G. Glass, M.D., Medical Director

La Hacienda Treatment Center, FM 1340, Hunt, TX 78024; tel. 512/238-4222; FAX. 512/238-4070; Frank Sadlack, Ph.D., Executive Director

Life Resource, 2750 South Eighth Street, Beaumont, TX 77701; tel. 409/838-6203; FAX. 409/832-3530; N. Charles Harris, Ph.D., Chief Executive Officer

Meridell Achievement Center, Inc., P.O. Box 87, Liberty Hill, TX 78642; tel. 512/515-6650; FAX. 512/515-6710; Debra Lowrance, Managing Director

Minirth-Meier New Life Day Hospital, 2071 North Collins Boulevard, Richardson, TX 75080; tel. 214/437-4697; FAX. 214/690-9309; W. Tom Parker, RNC, Administrative Director

New Dimensions Day Treatment, 18333 Egret Bay Boulevard, Suite 560, Houston, TX 77058; tel. 713/333-2284; FAX. 713/333-2293; Valerie Corbett, Assistant Administrator

New Spirit, 2411 Fountainview, Suite 175, Houston, TX 77057-4803; tel. 713/975-1580; FAX. 717/975-0228; Thomas A. Blocher, M.D., Chief Executive Officer

New View Partial Hospitalization Centre, Inc., 4310 Dowlen Road, Suite 13, Beaumont, TX 77706; tel. 409/892-0009; Darla Tortorice, Nursing Coordinator

Oak Grove Treatment Center, 6436 Mark Drive, Burleson, TX 76028; tel. 817/483-0989; FAX. 817/561-1309; Robert N. Bourassa, Administrator

Rio Grande State Center, 1401 Rangerville Road, Harlingen, TX 78551; tel. 512/425-8900; Sonia H. Hernandez, Director

River Oaks Academy Day Hospital, 8120 Westglen, Houston, TX 77063; tel. 713/783-7200; FAX. 713/783-7286; Sandra E. Phares, Chief Executive Officer

Serenty House of Abilene, Inc., 1546 North Second Street, Abilene, TX 79601; tel. 915/673-6489; FAX. 915/673-1794; Richard L. Spalding, President

St. James Behavioral Health Center, Inc., 1819 St. James Place, Houston, TX 77056; tel. 713/626-7730; FAX. 713/621-1329; Julie Sengstacken, RN, Administrator

Summer Sky Treatment Center, 1100 McCart Street, Stephenville, TX 76401; tel. 817/968-2907; FAX. 817/968-4509; Cathern Brooks, Chief Executive Officer

Sundown Ranch, Inc., Route 4, Box 182, Canton, TX 75103; tel. 903/479-3933; FAX. 903/479-3999; Richard Boardman, Chief Executive Officer

The Country Place Adolescent Residential Treatment Center, 2708 Highway 1378, Wylie, TX 75098; tel. 214/340-1613; FAX. 214/340-1058; Jill Smith, Director, Community Relations

The Patrician Movement, 222 East Mitchell, San Antonio, TX 78210; tel. 512/532-3126; FAX. 512/534-3779; Patrick Clancey, Administrator

Waco Center for Youth, 3501 North 19th Street, Waco, TX 76708; tel. 817/756-2171; FAX. 817/756-2171; Thomas Stidvent, M.D., Clinical Director

Westheimer Psychiatric Day Hospital, 5631 Dolores Street, Houston, TX 77057; tel. 713/780-1229; Bernard Levitt, Chief Executive Officer

UTAH

Brightway at St. George, 115 West 1470 South, St. George, UT 84770; tel. 801/673-0303; FAX. 801/673-8420; Paula O. Bell, Managing Director

Highland Ridge Hospital, 4578 Highland Drive, Salt Lake City, UT 84117; tel. 801/272-9851; FAX. 801/272-9857; Robert Boswell, Executive Vice President, Pioneer Healthcare, Inc.

Provo Canyon School, 4501 North University Avenue, Provo, UT 84604; tel. 801/227-2000; FAX. 801/227-2095; Robert R. Harrison, Chief Executive Officer

Rivendell of Utah, 5899 West Rivendell Drive, West Jordan, UT 84084; tel. 801/561-3377; John T. Young, M.S., Chief Executive Officer

Sorenson's Ranch School, Second East 345 North, Box 440219, Koosharem, UT 84744; tel. 801/638-7318; FAX. 801/638-7582; Burnell D. Sorenson, Owner

The Heritage Center, 5600 North Heritage School Drive, Provo, UT 84604; tel. 801/225-5552; FAX. 801/224-5814; Jerry Spanos, Chief Executive Officer

VIRGINIA

American Day Treatment Center of Virginia, 11200 Waples Mill Road, Suite 100, Fairfax, VA 22030; tel. 703/691-2900; FAX. 703/691-4740; Patricia Petralia, Executive Director

Barry Robinson Center, 443 Kempsville Road, Norfolk, VA 23502; tel. 804/455-6100; FAX. 804/455-6127; Thomas D. Pittman, M.P.H., Executive Director

CATS–Comprehensive Addiction Treatment Services, 3300 Gallows Road, Falls Church, VA 22046; tel. 703/698-1530; Wanda L. Miller, Director, Administration

Colonial Hospital and Recovery Center, 17579 Warwick Boulevard, Newport News, VA 23603-3134; tel. 800/697-0999; Robert Lehmann, Chief Executive Officer

Commonwealth Medical Institute, Koger Executive Center, Building 20, Suite 212, Norfolk, VA 23502; tel. 804/461-1178; FAX. 804/461-8352; Wendy Van Fossen, Business Manager

Diamond Healthcare of Williamsburg Place, 5477 Mooretown Road, Williamsburg, VA 23185; tel. 804/565-0106; FAX. 804/565-0620; Mac McAllister, Administrator

Graydon Manor, 301 Children's Center Road, Leesburg, VA 22075-2598; tel. 703/777-3485; FAX. 703/777-4887; Bernard J. Haberlein, Executive Director, Chairman of the Board

Learning Services-Shenandoah, 9524 Fairview Avenue, Manassas, VA 22110; tel. 703/335-9771; Peter D. Patrick, Program Director

Mount Regis Center, 405 Kimball Avenue, Salem, VA 24153; tel. 703/389-4761; Mark S. Cowell, Administrator

New Beginnings at Serenity Lodge, 2097 South Military Highway, Chesapeake, VA 23320; tel. 804/543-6888; FAX. 804/543-7453; Richard Warden, Chief Executive Officer

New Life Center, Inc., 315 East Cork Street, Winchester, VA 22601; tel. 703/662-8865; S. Terry Rudolph, M.S., Executive Director

Psychiatric Institute of Richmond, Inc., 12800 West Creek Parkway, Richmond, VA 23238; tel. 804/784-2200; Wanda H. Sadler, Assistant Administrator

The Kellar Center, 10396 Democracy Lane, Fairfax, VA 22030-0252; tel. 703/281-8500; Wanda L. Miller, Director, Administration

The Life Center of Galax, 112 Painter Street, Galax, VA 24333; tel. 800/345-6998; FAX. 703/236-8821; Tina R. Bullins, Executive Director

The Pines Residential Treatment Center, 825 Crawford Parkway, Portsmouth, VA 23704; tel. 804/393-0061; FAX. 804/393-1029; Edward C. Irby, Executive Administrative Director

WASHINGTON

Advanced Clinical Services, 34709 Ninth Avenue, South, Federal Way, WA 98003; tel. 206/874-1475; FAX. 206/661-9338; Wayne Watkinson, Executive Director

Careunit Hospital of Kirkland, 10322 N.E. 132nd Street, Kirkland, WA 98034; tel. 206/821-1122; John Thompson, Administrator

Carondelet Psychiatric Care Center, 1175 Carondelet Drive, Richland, WA 99352; tel. 509/943-9104; Barbara Mead, Quality Assurance Coordinator

Providers / Accredited Freestanding Psychiatric Facilities

Martin Center, 2806 Douglas Avenue, Bellingham, WA 98227-5704; tel. 360/733-5804; Michele Hall, M.A., Chief Executive Officer

Pearl Street Center, 815 South Pearl Street, Tacoma, WA 98465; tel. 206/756-5290; FAX. 206/759-7008; Michael Kent Laederich, Ph.D., Director, Children and Family Services

Seattle Children's Home, 2142 Tenth Avenue, W., Seattle, WA 98119; tel. 206/283-3300; FAX. 206/284-7843; R. David Cousineau, Executive Director

Tamarack Center, Inc., 2901 West Fort George Wright Drive, Spokane, WA 99204; tel. 509/326-8100; FAX. 509/326-9358; Chris Dalpra, M.C., Director, Family Services and Development

WEST VIRGINIA

Abraxas Foundation of West Virginia, Inc., Route Two, Box 56-A, Waverly, WV 26184; tel. 304/679-3621, ext. 104; FAX. 304/679-3771; Johanna F. Lampert, Administrator

Olympic Center Preston, Adolescent Alcohol/Drug Treatment, Route Seven West, P.O. Box 158, Kingwood, WV 26537; tel. 304/329-2400; William W. Perkins, Executive Director

Shawnee Hills, Inc., 511 Morris Street, P.O. Box 3698, Charleston, WV 25336-3698; tel. 304/345-4800; FAX. 304/341-0277; John E. Barnette, Ed.D., President, Chief Executive Officer

WISCONSIN

DePaul Hospital, Inc., 4143 South 13th Street, Milwaukee, WI 53221-1170; tel. 414/281-4400; Kathy M. Olewinski, Director

Eau Claire Academy, 550 North Dewey Street, Eau Claire, WI 54702; tel. 715/834-6681; FAX. 715/834-9954; Marcia R. Van Beek, Executive Director

Learning Services Mid-Western Region, 1424 North Highpoint Road, Middleton, WI 53562; tel. 608/836-3339; Chauncey J. Hunker, Program Director

Libertas Treatment Center, 1701 Dousman Street, Green Bay, WI 54303; tel. 414/498-8600; Patrick Ryan, Program Director

St. Rose Residence, Inc., 3801 North 88th Street, Milwaukee, WI 53222; tel. 414/466-9450; FAX. 414/466-0730; Kenneth Czaplewski, President

Accredited Freestanding Substance Abuse Programs

The accredited freestanding substance abuse programs listed have been accredited as of January 1, 1995, by the Joint Commission on Accreditation of Healthcare Organizations by decision of the Accreditation Committee of the Board of Commissioners.

The programs listed here have been found to be in substantial compliance with the Joint Commission standards for substance abuse programs, as found in the Consolidated Standards Manual.

Please refer to section A of the AHA Guide for information on hospitals with inpatient and/or outpatient alcohol and chemical dependency services. These hospitals are identified by Facility Codes F2 and F3. In section A, those hospitals identified by Approval Code 1 are JCAHO accredited.

We present this list simply as a convenient directory. Inclusion or omission of any organization's name indicates neither approval nor disapproval by the American Hospital Association.

United States

ALABAMA

Bradford Adolescent at Oak Mountain, 2280 Highway 35, Pelham, AL 35124; tel. 205/664-3460; FAX. 205/664-8476; Eve S. Laxer, M.S.S.W., Chief Executive Officer

Bradford Parkside Lodge, 1189 Allbritton Road, P.O. Box 129, Warrior, AL 35180; tel. 205/647-1945; FAX. 205/647-3626; Roy M. Ramsey, Executive Director

Bradford at Huntsville, 1600 Browns Ferry Road, Madison, AL 35758; tel. 205/461-7272; FAX. 205/464-9618; Benjamin Y. Lee Ph.D., Chief Executive Officer

Mobile Mental Health Center, Inc., 2400 Gordon Smith Drive, Mobile, AL 36617; tel. 334/473-4423; T. Edmund Lakeman, Executive Director

Partial Hospital Institute of America, Inc., 501 Bel Air Boulevard, Suite 200 A, Mobile, AL 36606; tel. 334/473-6700; FAX. 334/476-0111; James S. Harrold, Chief Executive Officer

ARIZONA

Chandler Valley Hope, 501 North Washington, Chandler, AZ 85244-1839; tel. 602/899-3335; FAX. 602/899-6697; Julian S. Pickens, Ed.D., Chief Executive Officer

Cottonwood de Tucson, 4110 Sweetwater Drive, Tucson, AZ 85745; tel. 602/743-0411, ext. 623; FAX. 602/743-7991; Ron Welch, Chief Executive Officer

Parc Place, 5116 East Thomas Road, Phoenix, AZ 85018; tel. 602/840-4774; FAX. 602/840-7567; Gary Buchik, Program Director

Prehab of Arizona, Inc., 868 East University, Mesa, AZ 85203; tel. 602/969-4024; Michael T. Hughes, Executive Director

Sierra Tucson, Inc., 16500 North Lago Del Oro, Tucson, AZ 85737; tel. 602/624-4000, ext. 2001; FAX. 602/792-2916; Kenneth J. Whitaker, Executive Director

The Meadows Addiction Recovery Corp. West, Inc., 1655 North Tegner, Wickenburg, AZ 85358; tel. 800/621-4062; FAX. 602/684-3261; J. P. Mellody, Executive Director

Westcenter Rehabilitation Facility, Inc., d/b/a Westcenter, 2105 East Allen Road, Tucson, AZ 85719; tel. 602/318-6440; FAX. 602/318-6442; Allan Chip Harrington, Executive Director

ARKANSAS

Ozark Guidance Center, Inc., 219 South Thompson Street, P.O. Box 1340, Springdale, AR 72765; tel. 501/751-7052; FAX. 501/751-4346; David L. Williams, Ph.D., Executive Director

CALIFORNIA

Betty Ford Center at Eisenhower, 39000 Bob Hope Drive, Rancho Mirage, CA 92270; tel. 619/773-4100; FAX. 619/773-4141; Michael S. Neatherton, Vice President, Administrator

Broad Horizons, 1236 H Street, P.O. Box 1920, Ramona, CA 92065; tel. 619/789-7060; Ellen Wright, Administrator

Care Options, 12419 Lewis Street, Suite 103, Garden Grove, CA 92640; tel. 800/700-8040; FAX. 714/740-8053; Patricia A. Ellisor, Chief Operating Officer

Cornerstone Residential Center for Addictions, 13682 Yorba Street, Tustin, CA 92680; tel. 714/730-5399; FAX. 714/730-3505; Michael Stone, M.D., Administrator

Health Care Children's Campus, 15339 Saticoy Street, Van Nuys, CA 91406; tel. 818/778-6400; FAX. 818/778-6434; Kimberly A. Brandi, M.A., MFCC, Clinical Director

Impact Drug and Alcohol Treatment Center, 1680 North Fair Oaks Avenue, Pasadena, CA 91103; tel. 818/798-0884; James M. Stillwell, Executive Director

Michael's House Treatment Center for Men, 430 South Cahuilla Road, Palm Springs, CA 92262; tel. 619/320-5486; FAX. 619/778-6020; Arlene Rosen, President

S.T.E.P.S., 224 East Clara Street, Port Hueneme, CA 93044; tel. 805/488-6424; FAX. 805/488-6717; John J. Megara, Administrator

SeaBridge, Inc., 30371 Morning View Drive, Malibu, CA 90265; tel. 310/457-5802; FAX. 310/457-6093; Martha Zimmerman, Executive Director

Spencer Recovery Centers, Inc., 343 West Foothill Boulevard, Monrovia, CA 91016; tel. 818/358-3662; FAX. 818/357-7405; Chris Spencer, President, Chief Executive Officer

Starting Point of Orange County, 350 West Bay Street, Costa Mesa, CA 92627; tel. 714/642-3505; FAX. 714/631-8669; Richard Vincent, Administrator

Substance Abuse Foundation of Long Beach, Inc., 3125 East Seventh Street, Long Beach, CA 90804; tel. 310/439-7755; Ronald H. Banner, Executive Director

Twin Town Treatment Centers, 2501 Burbank Boulevard, Burbank, CA 91505; tel. 818/840-0806; FAX. 818/840-0845; Stan Galperson, Clinical Coordinator

Vista Pacifica Hospital, 7989 Linda Vista Road, San Diego, CA 92111; tel. 619/576-1200; FAX. 619/576-8362; Daniel R. Valentine, Adminstrator

COLORADO

Adolescent and Family Institute of Colorado, Inc, 10001 West 32nd Avenue, Wheat Ridge, CO 80033; tel. 303/238-1231; FAX. 303/238-0500; Alex M. Panio, Jr., Ph.D., Chief Executive Officer

Aurora Behavioral Health Hospital, 1290 South Potomac, Aurora, CO 80012; tel. 303/745-2273; FAX. 303/369-9556; Lorry Kenney, Administrator

Harmony Foundation, Inc., 1600 Fish Hatchery Road, P.O. Box 1989, Estes Park, CO 80517; tel. 303/586-4491; Howard L. Clarke, Jr., Director

Parker Valley Hope, 22422 East Main Street, Parker, CO 80134; tel. 303/841-7857; FAX. 303/841-6526; John J. Arnold, Ph.D., Program Director

Pikes Peak Mental Health Center Systems, Inc., 875 West Moreno Avenue, Colorado Springs, CO 80905; tel. 719/471-8300; FAX. 719/471-0987; Charles J. Vorwaller, Chief Executive Officer

CONNECTICUT

Berkshire Woods Chemical Dependence Treatment Center, Mile Hill Road, Newtown, CT 06470; tel. 203/426-2531, ext. 2749; FAX. 203/426-6285; Sarah T. Kruel, Chief Executive Officer

Blue Hills Hospital, 51 Coventry Street, Hartford, CT 06112; tel. 203/722-2001; FAX. 203/722-2010; Stephen A. Glass, Acting Superintendent

Cornerstone of Eagle Hill, 28 Alberts Hill Road, Sandy Hook, CT 06482; tel. 203/426-8085; FAX. 203/426-2821; Norman J. Sokolow, Executive Director

Dutcher Chemical Dependence Treatment Center, Holmes Drive, Middletown, CT 06457; tel. 203/638-5800; Patrick DeChello, Superintendent

Eugene T. Boneski Chemical Dependence Treatment Center, Route 12, Norwich, CT 06360; tel. 203/823-5237; FAX. 203/823-5446; Anita Ellis Howard, Superintendent, Chief Executive Officer

Guenster Rehabilitation Center, Inc., 276 Union Avenue, Bridgeport, CT 06607; tel. 203/384-9301; FAX. 203/336-4395; Sue Roselle, President

Reid Treatment Center, Inc., 121 West Avon Road, Avon, CT 06001; tel. 203/673-6115; FAX. 203/675-7433; Mary Ann Reid, Executive Director

Rushford Center, Inc., 1250 Silver Street, Middletown, CT 06457; tel. 203/346-0300; Margaret Crafton, Vice President, Clinical Operations

Stonington Institute, Swantown Hill Road, North Stonington, CT 06359; tel. 203/535-1010; FAX. 203/535-4820; Michael J. Angelides, Chief Executive Officer

The Blueridge Center, 1095 Blue Hills Avenue, Bloomfield, CT 06002; tel. 203/243-1331; FAX. 203/242-3265; Joseph W. Nolan, Executive Director

The Center, 4920 Main Street, Suite 310, Bridgeport, CT 06606; tel. 203/365-8400; Susan Dalesandro, CISW, CAC, Clinical Director

The Children's Center, 1400 Whitney Avenue, Hamden, CT 06517; tel. 203/248-2116; FAX. 203/248-2572; Brian F. Lynch, Executive Director

Vitam Center, Inc., 57 West Rocks Road, P.O. Box 730, Norwalk, CT 06852-0730; tel. 203/846-2091; FAX. 203/846-3620; Leonard A. Kenowitz, Ph.D., Executive Director

Wheeler Clinic, Inc., 91 Northwest Drive, Plainville, CT 06062; tel. 800/793-3588; FAX. 203/793-3520; Dennis Keenan, Executive Director

DELAWARE

Brandywine Counseling, Inc., 2713 Lancaster Avenue, Wilmington, DE 19805; tel. 302/656-2348; FAX. 302/656-0746; Sara Taylor Allshouse, Executive Director

Providers / Accredited Freestanding Substance Abuse Programs

Greenwood, 1000 Old Lancaster Pike, Hockessin, DE 19707; tel. 302/239-3410; Hannah L. Cohen, Chief Executive Officer

Sodat-Delaware, Inc., 625 North Orange Street, Wilmington, DE 19801; tel. 302/656-4044; Thomas C. Maloney, Executive Director

The Recovery Center of Delaware, Inc., Governor Bacon Health Center, Delaware City, DE 19706; tel. 302/836-1615; Terence McSherry, Executive Director

FLORIDA

Alternatives In Treatment, Inc, 7601 North Federal Highway, Suite 260 B, Boca Raton, FL 33487; tel. 407/998-0866; FAX. 407/241-5042; Jacob Frydman, Executive Director

Apalachee Center for Human Services, Inc., 625 East Tennessee Street, Tallahassee, FL 32308; tel. 904/487-2930; Ronald P. Kirkland, Chief Executive Officer

Charter Behavioral Health System at Bay Harbor Treatment Center, 12895 Seminole Boulevard, Largo, FL 34648; tel. 813/587-1000; FAX. 813/584-1835; Steve McCabe, Administrator

Coastal Recovery Centers, Inc., 3830 Bee Ridge Road, Sarasota, FL 34233; tel. 813/927-8900; FAX. 813/925-3836; James R. Sleeper, President, Chief Executive Officer

Crossroads Center, 2121 Lisenby Avenue, Panama City, FL 32406; tel. 800/922-7522; FAX. 904/763-3933; Ernest H. Borders, Chief Executive Officer

DISC Village, Inc., (Tallahassee/Leon County Human Services Center), 3333 West Pensacola Street, Tallahassee, FL 32304; tel. 904/575-4388, ext. 117; FAX. 904/576-5960; Thomas K. Olk, Executive Director

David Lawrence Center, Inc., 6075 Golden Gate Parkway, Naples, FL 33999; tel. 813/455-1031; FAX. 813/455-6561; David Schimmel, Executive Director

Fairwinds Treatment Center, 1569 South Fort Harrison, Clearwater, FL 34616; tel. 800/226-0301; FAX. 813/446-1022; Samuel Teresi, Director, Community Relations

Florida Hospital Center for Psychiatry Partial Hospital Program, 1276 Minnesota Avenue, Winter Park, FL 32789; tel. 407/647-1781; Martin Lazoritz, M.D., Chief Executive Officer

Florida Mental Health Institute, 13301 Bruce B. Downs Boulevard, Tampa, FL 33612-3899; tel. 813/974-4533; FAX. 813/974-4406; Jini Hanjian, Quality Management Facilitator

Growing Together, Inc, 1000 Lucerne Avenue, Lake Worth, FL 33460; tel. 407/585-0892; Ivan Goldberg, Chief Executive Officer

Hanley-Hazelden Center at St. Mary's, 5200 East Avenue, West Palm Beach, FL 33407; tel. 407/848-1666; FAX. 407/848-6333; Jerry Singleton, M.A.

High Point, 5960 Southwest 106th Avenue, Cooper City, FL 33328; tel. 305/680-2700; FAX. 305/680-9941; Alan Sherman, Administrator

Interphase Recovery Program, Inc., 23120 Sandlefoot Square Place Drive, Boca Raton, FL 33428; tel. 407/487-5400; Janice Wilmoth, Executive Director

Leon F. Stewart-Hal S. Marchman Center, 120 Michigan Avenue, Daytona Beach, FL 32114; tel. 904/255-0447, ext. 298; FAX. 904/238-0877; Dr. Ernest D. Cantley, Executive Director

LifeStream Behavioral Center, 515 West Main Street, P.O. Box 491000, Leesburg, FL 34749-1000; tel. 904/360-6575; FAX. 904/360-6595; Tim Camp, Vice President, Clinical Services

Lifeskills of Boca Raton, 7301A West Palmetto Park Road, Boca Raton, FL 33433; tel. 407/392-1199; FAX. 407/392-4341; Carol Parks, Executive Director

Marion-Citrus Mental Health Centers, Inc., 717 S.W. Martin Luther King Jr. Avenue, P.O. Box 1330, Ocala, FL 34478; tel. 904/620-7300; FAX. 904/732-1413; Russell Rasco, Executive Director

Mental Health Resource Center, Inc, 11820 Beach Boulevard, Jacksonville, FL 32246; tel. 904/642-9100; FAX. 904/641-6529; David H. Panken, President, Chief Executive Officer

Mental Health Services, Inc. of North Central Florida, 4300 S.W. 13th Street, Gainesville, FL 32608; tel. 904/374-5600; Douglas L. Starr, Chief Executive Officer

National Recovery Institutes Group, 1000 N.W. 15th Street, Boca Raton, FL 33486; tel. 407/392-8444; Sheldon Russakoff, President, Chief Executive Officer

Northwest Dade Center, Inc., 4175 West 20th Avenue, Hialeah, FL 33012; tel. 305/825-0300; FAX. 305/824-1006; Mario Jardon, LCSW, Chief Executive Officer

Oak Center, 8889 Corporate Square Court, Jacksonville, FL 32216; tel. 904/725-7073; FAX. 904/727-9777; Diana Sourbrine, Administrator

Pathways to Recovery, Inc., 13132 Barwick Road, Delray Beach, FL 33445; tel. 407/496-7532; Allen Bombart, Executive Director

Professional Comprehensive Addiction Services, Inc., 6150 150th Avenue, North, Clearwater, FL 34620; tel. 813/530-1420; FAX. 813/530-3791; Robert A. Maestra, Executive Director

Recovery Corner, 4440 PGA Boulevard, Suite 203, Palm Beach Gardens, FL 33410; tel. 800/435-3668; FAX. 407/626-1739; Steven M. Petrovich, Executive Director

Renaissance Institute of Palm Beach, Inc., 7300 North Federal Highway, Suite 201, Boca Raton, FL 33487; tel. 407/241-7977; FAX. 407/241-9233; Sid Goodman, Executive Director

Rivendell of Fort Walton Beach, 1015 Mar Nalt Drive, Fort Walton Beach, FL 32547; tel. 904/863-4160; Holly Butcher, Chief Executive Officer

South County Mental Health Center, Inc., 16158 South Military Trail, Delray Beach, FL 33484; tel. 407/495-0522; FAX. 407/495-7975; Joseph S. Speicher, Executive Director

Spectrum Programs, Inc., 18441 N.W. Second Avenue, Suite 218, Miami, FL 33169; tel. 305/653-8288, ext. 19; FAX. 305/653-6787; H. Bruce Hayden, President

The Beachcomber, 4493 North Ocean Boulevard, Delray Beach, FL 33483; tel. 407/734-1818; FAX. 407/265-1349; James Bryan, Director

The Cloisters at Pine Island, 13771 Waterfront Drive, Pineland, FL 33945-1616; tel. 813/283-1019; FAX. 813/283-3079; Tom F. Zercher, MHR, Executive Director

The Friary, Inc., 4400 Hickory Shores Boulevard, Gulf Breeze, FL 32561; tel. 800/332-2271; FAX. 904/932-1044; Gayle Piret, M.S., CAP, Chief Executive Officer

The Inn at Bowling Green, 101 North Oak Street, Bowling Green, FL 33834; tel. 813/375-4373; Joann Summerlin, Chief Executive Officer, Administration

The Village South, Inc., 3180 Biscayne Boulevard, Miami, FL 33137; tel. 800/443-3784; FAX. 305/576-1348; Matthew Gissen, Chief Executive Officer

The Willough at Naples, 9001 Tamiami Trail East, Naples, FL 33962; tel. 813/775-4500; FAX. 813/793-0534; Gary D. Centafanti, Executive Director

Transitions Recovery Program, 2040 N.E. 163rd Street, North Miami Beach, FL 33162; tel. 305/949-9001; Roselyn McGowan, Administrator

Turning Point of Tampa, 6301 Memorial Highway, Suite 201, Tampa, FL 33615; tel. 813/882-3003; FAX. 813/885-6974; C. Fred Hill, Chief Executive Officer

Twelve Oaks, 2068 Healthcare Avenue, Navarre, FL 32566; tel. 904/939-1200; FAX. 904/939-1257; James W. Griffis, Administrator

GEORGIA

Anchor Hospital and The Talbott-Marsh Recovery Campus, 5454 Yorktowne Drive, Atlanta, GA 30349; tel. 404/991-6044, ext. 201; FAX. 404/991-6044, ext. 298; Benjamin H. Underwood, FAAMA, President, Chief Executive Officer

Anxiety Disorders Institute of Atlanta Center, One Dunwoody Park, Suite 112, Atlanta, GA 30338; tel. 404/395-6845; Asaf Aleem, Chief Executive Officer

Brightmore Day Hospital, 115 Davis Road, Martinez, GA 30907-7184; tel. 404/868-1735; Ellen Jones, Administrator

Perimeter Adolescent Treatment Program, Inc., 1140 Hammond Drive, Suite 9150, Atlanta, GA 30328; tel. 404/804-8255; Francis Robertson, Administrator

Safe Recovery Systems, Inc., 2300 Peachford Road, Suite 2000, Atlanta, GA 30338; tel. 404/455-7233; FAX. 404/458-1481; Henslee Dutton, Chief Executive Officer

Turning Point Care Center, Inc., 319 Bypass, P.O. Box 1177, Moultrie, GA 31768; tel. 912/985-4815; FAX. 912/890-1614; Sonny McCutcheon, Managing Director

Woodridge Hospital, 394 Ridgecrest Circle, Clayton, GA 30525; tel. 404/782-3100; FAX. 404/782-4873; Lewis A. Ransdell, Executive Director

IDAHO

Northview Hospital, 8050 Northview Street, Boise, ID 83704; tel. 208/327-0504; FAX. 208/327-0594; Rick L. Holloway, Administrator

Walker Center, 1120-A Montana Street, Gooding, ID 83330-1858; tel. 208/934-8461; FAX. 208/934-5437; Vayle Mauldin, Treatment Coordinator

ILLINOIS

Alcoholism Treatment Center of Central DuPage Hospital, 27 West 350 High Lake Road, Winfield, IL 60190; tel. 708/653-4000; FAX. 708/653-0591; Paul M. Teodo, Vice President

Allendale Association's, Edward L. Bradley Counseling Center, Grand Avenue and Offield Road, P.O. Box 1088, Lake Villa, IL 60046; tel. 708/356-2351; FAX. 708/356-0289; Ann Adams, Vice President

Camelot Care Center, Inc., 1502 North Northwest Highway, Palatine, IL 60067; tel. 708/359-5600; Peggy Williams, President, Professional Staff

Chestnut Health Systems, Inc., 1003 Martin Luther King Jr. Drive, Bloomington, IL 61701; tel. 309/827-6026; FAX. 309/827-6496; Alan R. Sodetz, Ph.D., Clinical Director

Evergreen Recovery Center, 1055 East State Street, Rockford, IL 61104-218; tel. 815/965-8600; FAX. 815/965-2348; Judith K. Jobe, Administrator

Gateway Youth Care Foundation, 25480 West Cedarcrest Lane, Lake Villa, IL 60046; tel. 708/356-8292; FAX. 708/356-0414; Janet Mason, Director

Gateway Youth Care Foundation, 2200 Lake Victoria Drive, Springfield, IL 62703-3100; tel. 217/529-9266; FAX. 217/529-9151; Patricia S. Taylor, Director

Interventions-DuPage Adolescent Center, 11 South 250, Route 83, Hinsdale, IL 60521; tel. 708/325-5050; Georgia Ponos, Director

Life Works Chemical Dependency Centers, 404 West Boughton Road, Bolingbrook, IL 60440; tel. 708/759-5750; FAX. 708/759-9446; Loretta L. Berry, Chief Executive Officer

Rosecrance Center, 1505 North Alpine Road, Rockford, IL 61107; tel. 815/399-5351; FAX. 815/398-2641; Philip W. Eaton, President

Sojourn House, Inc., 565 North Turner Avenue, Freeport, IL 61032; tel. 815/232-5121; FAX. 815/233-4591; Brenda J. Bombard, M.S.W., Executive Director

Southeastern Illinois Counseling Centers, Inc., P.O. Drawer M, Olney, IL 62450; tel. 618/395-4306; FAX. 618/395-4507; Glenn Jackson, Clinical Director

Triangle Center, 120 North 11th Street, Springfield, IL 62703; tel. 217/544-9858; FAX. 217/544-0223; Stephen J. Knox, Executive Director

INDIANA

Comprehensive Mental Health Services, Inc., 240 North Tillotson, Muncie, IN 47304; tel. 317/288-1928; FAX. 317/741-0310; Suzanne Gresham, Ph.D., Chief Executive Officer

Providers / Accredited Freestanding Substance Abuse Programs

Fairbanks Hospital, Inc., 8102 Clearvista Parkway, Indianapolis, IN 46256; tel. 317/849-8222; FAX. 317/849-1455; Timothy L. Boruff, President, Administrator

Four County Counseling Center, 1015 Michigan Avenue, Logansport, IN 46947; tel. 219/722-5151; Umamaheswara R. Kalapatapu, Executive Director

Grant-Blackford Mental Health, Inc., d/b/a Cornerstone Professional Treatment Services, 505 Wabash Avenue, Marion, IN 46952; tel. 317/662-3971; FAX. 317/662-7490; Paul G. Kuczora, Chief Executive Officer

Hamilton Center, Inc., 620 Eighth Avenue, Terre Haute, IN 47804; tel. 812/231-8323; FAX. 812/232-8228; Galen Goode, Center Director

Lifespring Mental Health Services, 207 West 13th Street, Jeffersonville, IN 47130; tel. 812/283-4491; John Case, Executive Director

Madison Center and Hospital, Inc., 403 East Madison Street, South Bend, IN 46617; tel. 219/234-0061, ext. 1116; FAX. 219/288-5047; Jack Roberts, Executive Director

Madison Clinic, Inc., 6405 Pendleton Avenue, Anderson, IN 46013; tel. 317/644-1414; Gary L. Porter, Chief Executive Officer

Otis R. Bowen Center For Human Services, Inc., 850 North Harrison Street, Warsaw, IN 46581; tel. 219/267-7169; Cindy Hoover, RN

Park Center, Inc, 909 East State Boulevard, Fort Wayne, IN 46805; tel. 219/481-2700; FAX. 219/481-2717; James L. McKee, Ph.D., Chief Executive Officer

Porter-Starke Services, Inc., 701 Wall Street, Valparaiso, IN 46383; tel. 219/464-8541; FAX. 219/462-3975; Lee E. Grogg, Chief Executive Officer

Quinco Behavioral Health Systems, P.O. Box 628, Columbus, IN 47202; tel. 812/379-2341; Robert J. Williams, Ph.D., Chief Executive Officer

SouthLake Center for Mental Health, 8555 Taft Street, Merrillville, IN 46410; tel. 219/769-4005, ext. 287; FAX. 219/769-2508; Maureen Handley, M.S.W., Director, Quality Improvement

Southwestern Indiana Mental Health Center, Inc, 415 Mulberry Street, Evansville, IN 47713; tel. 812/423-7791; FAX. 812/422-7558; John K. Browning, Executive Director

The Center for Mental Health, Inc., 2020 Brown Street, Anderson, IN 46016; tel. 317/649-8161; FAX. 317/641-8238; Cynthia Goodman, ACSW, Addiction Services Manager

Tri-City Comprehensive Community Mental Health Center, 3903 Indianapolis Boulevard, East Chicago, IN 46312; tel. 219/398-7050; FAX. 219/392-6998; Sandy Appleby, Assistant Director

Tri-County Center, Inc., 8945 North Meridian Street, Indianapolis, IN 46260; tel. 317/574-0022; FAX. 317/574-1234; Larry L. Burch, ACSW, Executive Director

Wabash Valley Hospital, Inc., 2900 North River Road, West Lafayette, IN 47906; tel. 317/463-2555; R. Craig Lysinger, Administrator

IOWA

Children and Families of Iowa, 1111 University, Des Moines, IA 50314; tel. 515/288-1981, ext. 356; FAX. 515/288-1981, ext. 402; Steve Ziebell, Director, Programs

KANSAS

Atchison Valley Hope, 1816 North Second Street, Atchison, KS 66002; tel. 913/367-1618; FAX. 913/367-6224; Dave Ketter, Program Director

Columbia Health Systems, Inc., 10114 West 105th Street, Overland Park, KS 66212; tel. 913/492-9875; FAX. 913/492-0187, ext. 11; Robert L. Reed, President

Norton Valley Hope, 709 West Holme, Norton, KS 67654; tel. 913/877-5101; FAX. 913/877-2322; Dennis Gilhousen, Chief Executive Officer

KENTUCKY

Adanta Group Behavioral Health Services, 259 Parkers Mill Road, Somerset, KY 42501; tel. 606/678-2768; Sandrda Renfro, QI Coordinator

Bluegrass Regional Mental Health-Mental Retardation Board, 1351 Newton Pike, Lexington, KY 40511; tel. 606/253-1686; David Hanna, Director, Quality Assurance

Comprehensive Care Centers of Northern Kentucky, Inc., 722 Scott Boulevard, Covington, KY 41011; tel. 606/431-2225; David Lindemann, M.S.W., Director Substance Abuse Programs

Cumberland River Regional MH/MR Board, Inc. Xiii, American Greeting Road, Corbin, KY 40701; tel. 606/528-7010; FAX. 606/528-5401; Robert Koehler, Substance Abuse Director

Green River Comprehensive Care and Valley Institute of Psychiatry, 416 West Third Street, P.O. Box 1637, Owensboro, KY 42302; tel. 502/684-0696; FAX. 502/926-6367; Gayle DiCesare, President, Chief Executive Officer

Jefferson Alcohol and Drug Abuse Center, 600 South Preston Street, Louisville, KY 40202; tel. 502/583-3951; FAX. 502/581-9234; Diane E. Hague, Director

LOUISIANA

Bowling Green-Hospital of St. Tammany, 701 Florida Avenue, Mandeville, LA 70448; tel. 800/375-5433; FAX. 504/626-4217; Richard M. Taylor, Executive Director

New Beginnings of Opelousas, Inc., 1692 Linwood Loop, Opelousas, LA 70570; tel. 318/942-1171; FAX. 318/948-9101; Kim Signorelli, Administrator

Vermilion Hospital for Psychiatric and Addictive Medicine, 2520 North University Avenue, Lafayette, LA 70507; tel. 318/234-5614; Johnny Patout, Director

Victory House, 12038 Greenwell Springs, Zachary, LA 70791; tel. 504/654-6884; Sheila Howard, Administrative Director

MARYLAND

A. F. Whitsitt Center, 300 Scheeler Road, P.O. Box 229, Chestertown, MD 21620; tel. 410/778-6404; FAX. 410/778-5341; Terri Dowling, Admissions Coordinator

Allegany County Health Department Addictions Program, Willowbrook Road, Cumberland, MD 21502; tel. 301/777-5680; FAX. 301/777-5674; Rodger D. Simons, Administrator

American Day Treatment Centers of Chevy Chase, LP, Two Wisconsin Circle, Suite 620, Chevy Chase, MD 20815; tel. 301/656-0151; FAX. 301/656-3523; Heidi Brown, Executive Director

Ashley, Inc., 800 Tydings Lane, Havre De Grace, MD 21078; tel. 410/273-6600; FAX. 410/272-5617; Leonard Angus Dahl, Executive Director

Baltimore Recovery Center, 16 South Poppleton Street, Baltimore, MD 21201; tel. 410/962-7180; FAX. 410/962-7192; William K. Hathaway, Executive Director

Changing Point, Inc., 4100 College Avenue, P.O. Box 396, Ellicott City, MD 21041-0396; tel. 410/465-9500; FAX. 410/465-9500, ext. 320; Morris L. Scherr, Chief Operating Officer, Executive Vice President

Charter at Hidden Brook, 522 Thomas Run Road, P.O. Box 1607, Bel Air, MD 21014; tel. 410/879-1919; Carol Koffinke, Chief Operating Officer

Crossroads Centers, Two West Madison Street, Baltimore, MD 21201; tel. 410/752-6505; FAX. 410/385-1237; Barbara Q. McKenna, Executive Director

Glass Substance Abuse Program, Inc., 1777 Reisterstown Road, Suite 345, Baltimore, MD 21208; tel. 410/484-2700; FAX. 410/484-1949; Sheldon D. Glass, M.D., President

Hope House, Marbury Drive, Building 26, Crownsville, MD 21032; tel. 410/923-6700; FAX. 410/923-6213; William H. Rufenacht, Executive Director

Maryland Treatment Centers, Inc., U.S. Route 15, Emmitsburg, MD 21727; tel. 301/447-2361; Mary A. Roby, Executive Director

Melwood Farm Treatment Center, 19715 Zion Road, P.O. Box 182, Olney, MD 20832; tel. 800/368-8313; Sue Krantz, Director

New Beginnings at Meadows, 730 Maryland Route 3, P.O. Box 521, Gambrills, MD 21054; tel. 800/333-5353, ext. 603; FAX. 301/923-6539; Ken Broghammer, Chief Operating Officer

New Beginnings at Warwick Manor, 3680 Warwick Road, East New Market, MD 21631; tel. 301/943-8108; FAX. 410/943-3976; Larry V. Foxwell, Chief Executive Officer

New Beginnings at White Oak, 1441 Taylors Island Road, Woolford, MD 21677; tel. 301/228-7000; FAX. 410/228-8609; Larry Foxwell, Chief Executive Officer

New Life Addiction Counseling Services, 2528 Mountain Road, Suite 203, Pasadena, MD 21122; tel. 410/255-4475; FAX. 410/255-6277; Thomas S. Porter, Chief Executive Officer

Oakview Treatment Center, 3100 North Ridge Road, Ellicott City, MD 21043; tel. 301/461-9922; FAX. 301/465-0923; David C. Heebner, Administrator

Pathways Services, Inc., 2620 Riva Road, Annapolis, MD 21401; tel. 410/573-5430; Art Sullivan, Director

Saint Luke Institute, Inc., 2420 Brooks Drive, Suitland, MD 20746; tel. 301/967-3700; FAX. 301/967-3953; Frank L. Valcour, Medical Director

Worcester County Health Department, 6040 Public Landing Road, P.O. Box 249, Snow Hill, MD 21863; tel. 410/632-1100; FAX. 410/632-0906; Deborah Goeller, RN, M.S., Health Officer

MASSACHUSETTS

AdCare Hospital of Worcester, Inc., 107 Lincoln Street, Worcester, MA 01605; tel. 508/799-9000; FAX. 508/753-3733; David W. Hillis, President

Baldpate Hospital, Baldpate Road, Georgetown, MA 01833; tel. 508/352-2131; Subhash C. Mukherjee, Administrator

Cape Cod Alcoholism Intervention & Rehab Unit, Inc., d/b/a Gosnold on Cape Cod, 200 Ter Heun Drive, Box CC, Falmouth, MA 02541; tel. 508/540-6550; FAX. 508/540-6550; Raymond V. Tamasi, President, Chief Executive Officer

Caulfield Center, 23 Warren Avenue, Woburn, MA 01801; tel. 617/933-6700, ext. 328; FAX. 617/933-9119; Gail Hanson-Mayer, RNCS, M.P.H., Chief Operating Officer

High Point, 1233 State Road, Route 3 A, Plymouth, MA 02360; tel. 508/224-7701; FAX. 508/224-2845; Arnold E. Goldie, Chief Executive Officer

Spectrum Addiction Services, Inc., 106 East Main Street, Westboro, MA 01581; tel. 508/898-1550; FAX. 508/836-4242; Roy Ross, President

Wild Acre Inns, 108 Pleasant Street, Arlington, MA 02174-4813; tel. 617/643-0643; John Sciretta, L.I.S.W., Chief Clinical Officer

MICHIGAN

AOS, Inc., Alcohol Outpatient Services, 1331 Lake Drive, S.E., Grand Rapids, MI 49506; tel. 616/456-8010; FAX. 616/451-0020; Charles F. Logie, Jr., President

Adult/Youth Developmental Services, P.C., 23133 Orchard Lake Road, Suite 104, Farmington, MI 48336; tel. 810/477-0107; FAX. 810/477-2303; George H. Kates, Ph.D., Executive Director

Advanced Counseling Services, P.C., 20600 Eureka Road, Suite 819, Taylor, MI 48180; tel. 313/285-8282; David S. Monhollen, Administrator

Alcohol Information and Counseling Center, 1575 Suncrest Drive, Lapeer, MI 48446; tel. 810/667-0243; FAX. 810/667-9399; Stephen L. Cranfield, Director

Alcohol and Chemical Abuse Consultants, Inc., 2020 Raybrook, S.E., Suite 102, Grand Rapids, MI 49546; tel. 616/957-5850; FAX. 616/957-5853; Joseph Merrell III, Chief Executive Officer

Allegan Substance Abuse Agency, 120 Cutler Street, Allegan, MI 49010; tel. 616/673-8735; FAX. 616/673-1572; Paul Mailloux, M.S.W., Executive Director

Providers / Accredited Freestanding Substance Abuse Programs

Ann Arbor Consultation Services, 5331 Plymouth Road, Ann Arbor, MI 48105; tel. 313/996-9111; Steven Sheldon, Director

Auro Medical Center, 2515 Woodard Avenue, Suite 250, Bloomfield Hills, MI 48013; tel. 313/335-1130; Yatinder M. Singhal, M.D., Administrator

Boniface Community Action Corporation, 25050 West Outer Drive, Suite 201, Lincoln Park, MI 48146; tel. 313/928-8940; FAX. 313/928-5152; Margaret Dutka, Interim Executive Director

Brighton Hospital, 12851 East Grand River Avenue, Brighton, MI 48116; tel. 810/227-1211, ext. 235; FAX. 810/227-1869; Ivan C. Harner, President, Chief Executive Officer

Brookfield Clinics, 6245 North Inkster Road, Garden City, MI 48135; tel. 313/421-3374; Elizabeth B. Schrock, Administrator

Care Unit of Grand Rapids, 1931 Boston Street, S.E., Grand Rapids, MI 49506; tel. 616/243-3608; FAX. 616/243-0186; Thomas G. Elzinga, Administrator

Catholic Human Services, Inc., 411 West Main Street, Gaylord, MI 49735; tel. 517/731-2877; FAX. 517/732-8165; Clement C. Veeser, Executive Director

Catholic Services of Macomb, 12434 Twelve Mile Road, Suite 201, Warren, MI 48093; tel. 810/558-7551; Linda Stum, Vice President, Client Services

Center for Behavior and Medicine, 2004 Hogback Road, Suite 16, Ann Arbor, MI 48105; tel. 313/677-0809; Gerard M. Schmit, M.D., Chief Executive Officer

Center for Personal Growth, PC, 817 Tenth Avenue, Port Huron, MI 48060; tel. 810/984-4550; FAX. 810/984-3737; Fredric B. Roberts, Ed.D., Chief Executive Officer

Center of Behavioral Therapy, P.C., 24453 Grand River, Detroit, MI 48219; tel. 313/592-1765; FAX. 313/592-1864; Hollis Evans, Executive Director

Central Therapeutic Services, Inc., 17600 West Eight Mile Road, Suite Seven, Southfield, MI 48075; tel. 810/559-4340; FAX. 810/559-1451; K. G. Thimotheose, Ph.D., President, Chief Executive Officer

Charles Allen Ransom Counseling Center, Inc. (CHIP), 14695 Park Avenue, Charlevoix, MI 49720; tel. 616/547-6551; Patrick Q. Nestor, Executive Officer

Clinton Counseling Center, Two Crocker Boulevard, Suite 103, Mount Clemens, MI 48043; tel. 313/463-7079; FAX. 313/469-5909; Joanne Smyth, M.A., CSW, Chief Executive Officer

Clinton-Eaton-Ingham, Community Mental Health Board, 808 Southland, Suite B, Lansing, MI 48910; tel. 517/887-2126; FAX. 517/887-0086; Judith Taylor, Ph.D., Executive Director

Community Care Services, 8750 Telegraph Road, Suite 420, Taylor, MI 48180; tel. 313/389-7525; FAX. 313/389-7515; Kari Walker, Deputy Director

Community Commission on Drug Abuse, 13325 Farmington Road, Livonia, MI 48150; tel. 313/261-3760, ext. 104; FAX. 313/261-0266; Ruth Barry, Clinical Director

Community Human Services, Inc., 332 South Main Street, Romeo, MI 48065; tel. 810/752-9696; Deanna McGraw, Executive Director

Consortium for Human Development, Inc., 1701 Baldwin Road, Pontiac, MI 48340; tel. 810/334-0220; FAX. 810/334-0229; Dr. Ronald Fenton, Clinic Director

Dearborn Heights Human Service Center, Inc., 25639 Ford Road, Dearborn Heights, MI 48127; tel. 313/277-3293; FAX. 313/277-3656; Marylyn Krzeminski, M.A., Clinical Director

Dimensions of Life, Inc., 3320 West Saginaw Street, Lansing, MI 48917; tel. 517/886-0340; FAX. 517/886-0505; Alfred K. Doering, Director

Dot Caring Centers, Inc., 3190 Hallmark Court, Saginaw, MI 48603; tel. 517/790-3366; FAX. 517/790-9156; William E. Watters, Chief Executive Officer

Downriver Guidance Clinic of Wayne County, 2959 Biddle Avenue, Suite 200, Wyandotte, MI 48192; tel. 313/285-6400; FAX. 313/285-1036; Leroy A. Lott, M.S.W., Executive Director

Elrose Health Services, Inc., 1475 East Outer Drive, Detroit, MI 48234; tel. 313/892-4244; FAX. 313/892-1457; Ellsworth Jackson M.A., CSW, Program Director

Fairlane Community Mental Health Center, 23400 Michigan Avenue, Dearborn, MI 48124; tel. 313/562-5626; Cheryl Anderson-Smith, Deputy Director

Farmington Area Advisory Council, Inc., Youth and Family Services, 23450 Middlebelt Road, Farmington Hills, MI 48336; tel. 810/477-6767; FAX. 810/473-1284; Betty Arnold, Executive Director

Gateway Services, 333 Turwill Lane, Kalamazoo, MI 49006; tel. 616/382-9827; Thomas E. Lucking, Executive Director

Growth Works, Inc., 271 South Main Street, Plymouth, MI 48170; tel. 313/455-4095; Dale F. Yagiela, Executive Director

Guest House, Inc., Lake Orion Treatment Center, 1840 West Scripps Road, Lake Orion, MI 48361; tel. 313/391-3100; Edward Higgins, Director, Education

Harbor Light, 2643 Park Avenue, Detroit, MI 48201; tel. 313/964-0577; FAX. 313/964-2853; Major Geoffrey Allan, Executive Director

Hegira Programs, Inc., Holiday Park Office Plaza, 8623 North Wayne Road, Second Floor, Suite 240, Westland, MI 48185; tel. 313/595-1500; Edward L. Forry, Chief Executive Officer

Highland Waterford Center, Inc, Holly Gardens, 4501 Grange Hall Road, Holly, MI 48442; tel. 810/634-0140; FAX. 810/634-3838; Michael J. Filipek, Executive Director

Huron Valley Consultation Center, 955 West Eisenhower Circle, Suite B, 48103, 2750 Carpenter Road, Suite One, Ann Arbor, MI 48108; tel. 313/662-6300; Carrie Gardner, Administrator

Insight, 1110 Eldon Baker Drive, Flint, MI 48507; tel. 810/744-3600; FAX. 810/744-4703; Stephen N. LeBel, President

Jackson Hillside Community Mental Health Services Board, 1200 North West Avenue, Jackson, MI 49202; tel. 517/789-1208; Christina M. Thompson, Executive Director

Lakewood Substance Abuse Center, 26000 Hoover, Warren, MI 48089; tel. 810/754-2565; FAX. 810/754-2568; Ronald Fenton, Ph.D., Director

Livingston Counseling and Assessment Services, 3744 East Grand River Avenue, Howell, MI 48843; tel. 517/546-7070; FAX. 517/545-0326; Ivan C. Harner, President

Mason County Community Mental Health Services, 920 Diana Street, Ludington, MI 49431; tel. 616/845-6294; FAX. 616/845-7095; Tom Griffer, Coordinator, Counseling and Evaluation Services

Meridian Professional Psychological Consultants, P.C., 5031 Park Lake Road, East Lansing, MI 48823; tel. 517/332-0811; FAX. 517/332-4452; Thomas S. Gunnings, Ph.D., President, Clinical Director

Metro East Substance Abuse Treatment Corporation, Metro East Drug Treatment Corporation, 13929 Harper Avenue, Detroit, MI 48213; tel. 313/371-0055; FAX. 313/371-1409; Leslie B. Carroll, M.S., President

Monroe County Community Mental Health Services Board, 1001 South Raisinville Road, Monroe, MI 48161; tel. 313/243-7340; FAX. 313/243-5564; Pat Heselton

Mount Pleasant Counseling Services, 3480 South Isabella Road, Mount Pleasant, MI 48858; tel. 517/773-9655; Williard E. Last, Executive Director

NPL, Inc., 18641 West Seven Mile Road, Detroit, MI 48219; tel. 313/532-8015; Yvette Woodruff, Chief Executive Officer

Nardin Park Substance Abuse Program, 9605 Grand River, Detroit, MI 48204; tel. 313/834-5930; FAX. 313/834-4541; Annie B. Scott, Director

National Council On Alcholism and Drug Dependencies, 17330 Northland Park Court, Southfield, MI 48075; tel. 313/443-1676; FAX. 313/443-0988; Gilbert A. Kendrick, Director

National Council On Alcoholism Lansing Regional Area, 3400 South Cedar, Suite 200, Lansing, MI 48910; tel. 517/887-0851; FAX. 517/887-8121; Nancy L. Siegrist, Executive Director

National Council On Alcoholism and Addictions, 202 East Boulevard Drive, Suite 310, Flint, MI 48503; tel. 313/767-0350; FAX. 313/767-4031; James E. Hartz, Executive Director

Neighborhood Service Organization, 220 Bagley, Suite 840, Detroit, MI 48226; tel. 313/961-4890; FAX. 313/961-5120; Carita I. Sledge, Executive Director

New Perspectives Center, Inc., 1321 South Fayette Street, Saginaw, MI 48602; tel. 517/790-0301; FAX. 517/790-2333; Jimmie D. Westbrook, Chief Executive Officer

North Point Mental Health Associates, 28595 Orchard Lake Road, Suite 301, Farmington Hills, MI 48334; tel. 810/489-1550; Alan R. Rickfelder, Ph.D., Chief Executive Officer

Northern Michigan Alcoholism and Addiction Treatment Services, Inc., 116 East Eighth Street, Traverse City, MI 49684; tel. 616/922-4810; David N. Abeel, M.S.W., Executive Director

O. Ganesh, M.D., P.C., 28165 Greenfield, Southfield, MI 48076; tel. 810/569-6642; FAX. 810/589-7922; Gerard Borovsky, M.A.

Oakland Psychological Clinic, P.C., 2000 South Woodward Avenue, Suite 102, Bloomfield Hills, MI 48302; tel. 810/335-6670; FAX. 810/334-7581; Barry H. Tigay, Ph.D., President

Perspectives of Troy, P.C., 2690 Crooks Road, Suite 300, Troy, MI 48084; tel. 810/244-8644; FAX. 810/244-1330; Timothy Coldinon, Ph.D., Chief Executive Officer

Program for Alcohol and Substance Treatment, 110 Sanborn, Big Rapids, MI 49307; tel. 616/796-6203; FAX. 616/796-7430; John R. Kelly, Director

Psychological Consultants of Michigan, P.C., 2518 Capital Avenue, S.W., Suite Two, Battle Creek, MI 49015; tel. 616/968-2811; FAX. 616/968-2651; Jeffrey N. Andert, Ph.D. Administrative Director

Redford Counseling Center, 25945 West Seven Mile Road, Redford, MI 48240; tel. 313/535-6560; Jo Ann Sadler, Director

Regional Mental Health Clinic, 23100 Cherry Hill, Suite 10, Dearborn, MI 48124-4144; tel. 313/277-1300; Gena J. D'Alessandro, Ph.D., Chief Executive Officer

Romulus Help Center Division Hegira Programs, Inc., 9340 South Wayne Road, Suite A, Romulus, MI 48174; tel. 313/942-7585; FAX. 313/942-7977; Edward Forry, Chief Executive Officer

Rossano Clinic, Inc., 719 Harrison Street, Flint, MI 48502-2161; tel. 313/235-1950; Nicholas A. Rossano, Program Director

Sacred Heart Rehabilitation Center, Inc., 400 Stoddard Road, P.O. Box 41038, Memphis, MI 48041; tel. 810/392-2167, ext. 231; FAX. 810/392-2057; Michael Kelly, Director, Treatment Programs

Self Help Addiction Rehabilitation, Parent Facility, 1852 West Grand Boulevard, Detroit, MI 48208; tel. 313/894-1445; FAX. 313/894-5542; Anne C. Benion, Program Services Manager

Substance Abuse Council of St. Joseph County, 222 South Main Street, Three Rivers, MI 49093-1658; tel. 616/279-5187; FAX. 616/273-2083; Sally Reames, Administrator

The Center for Human Resources, 1001 Military Street, Port Huron, MI 48060-5418; tel. 313/985-5168; FAX. 313/985-9011; Thomas P. Pope, Chief Executive Officer

The Counseling Center, P.C., 1411 South Woodward, Suite 101, Bloomfield Hills, MI 48302; tel. 313/338-2988; Robert L. Bailey; Kim Kostere, Co-Directors

The Salvation Army Substance Abuse Treatment Services, 1215 East Fulton, Grand Rapids, MI 49503; tel. 616/451-0432; FAX. 616/451-9640; Robert E. Byrd, M.A., Director

Tuscola Substance Abuse Services, 1309 Cleaver Road, P.O. Box 365, Caro, MI 48723; tel. 517/673-7575; FAX. 517/673-7579; Susan H. Clara, Program Director

Providers / Accredited Freestanding Substance Abuse Programs

VBH – Square Lake Corporation, 10 West Square Lake Road, Suite 300, Bloomfield Hills, MI 48302; tel. 313/338–0250; FAX. 313/338–3940; Andrew Blinder, M.A., L.L.P., Site Director

W. D. Lee Center for Life Management, Inc., 11000 West McNichols Road, Suite 212, Detroit, MI 48221; tel. 313/345–6777; Rose Jackson, Quality Assurance Coordinator

Washtenaw Council On Alcoholism, 2301 Platt Road, Ann Arbor, MI 48104; tel. 313/971–7900; FAX. 313/971–5950; Barry K. Kistner, Executive Director

MINNESOTA

Anthony Louis Center, 1000 Paul Parkway, Blaine, MN 55434; tel. 612/757–2906; FAX. 612/757–2059; Jon Benson, Chief Executive Officer

Charter Behavioral Health System of Waverly, 109 North Shore Drive, Waverly, MN 55390; tel. 612/658–4811; FAX. 612/658–4128; Nina T. Johnson, Director, Treatment

Fairview Behavioral Services, Woodbury Primary, Extended Care Treatment and Halfway House, 2450 Riverside Avenue, Minneapolis, MN 55454; tel. 612/672–4283; Beth Zeilinger, Provider Relations Representative

Fountain Lake Treatment Center, 408 Fountain Street, Albert Lea, MN 56007; tel. 507/377–6411; FAX. 507/377–6453; Steve Underdahl, Director, Marketing, Development

Guest House, Inc., 4800 48th Street, N.E., Rochester, MN 55903; tel. 800/634–4155; William C. Morgan, Director

Hazelden Foundation, 15245 Pleasant Valley Road, Center City, MN 55012; tel. 612/257–4010, ext. 4404; FAX. 612/257–1055; Jerry Spicer, MHA, President

Mission Inc. Programs, 3409 East Medicine Lake Boulevard, Plymouth, MN 55441; tel. 612/559–1883; Patricia Murphy, Executive Director

Omegon, Inc., 2000 Hopkins Crossroads, Minnetonka, MN 55343; tel. 612/541–4738; FAX. 612/541–9546; Barbara J. Danielsen, Executive Administrator

Pride Institute, 14400 Martin Drive, Eden Prairie, MN 55344; tel. 800/547–7433; FAX. 612/934–8764; Margaret Gordon, RN, Director, Quality Assurance

The Gables, 604 Fifth Street, S.W., Rochester, MN 55902–3256; tel. 507/282–2500; June Davis, Chief Executive Officer

Twin Town Treatment Center, 1706 University Avenue, St. Paul, MN 55104; tel. 612/645–3661; FAX. 612/645–0959; Robert Haven, Chief Executive Officer

MISSISSIPPI

Copac, Inc., 3949 Highway 43 North, Brandon, MS 39042; tel. 800/446–9727; FAX. 601/829–4278; Jerald Stacy Hughes, Jr., Ph.D., Executive Director

Jackson Recovery Center, 5354 I–55 South Frontage Road, Jackson, MS 39212; tel. 800/237–2122; FAX. 601/372–9505; D. Preston Smith, Jr., Executive Director

MISSOURI

Boonville Valley Hope, 1415 Ashley Road, Boonville, MO 65233; tel. 816/882–6547; FAX. 816/882–2391; Juanita L. Krebsbach, Program Director

Centrec Care, Inc, 12401 Olive Street Road, Suite 103A, St. Louis, MO 63141; tel. 314/576–9929; FAX. 314/576–1253; Mohammed A. Kabir, M.D., Chief Executive Officer

Comprehensive Mental Health Services, Inc., 10901 Winner Road, Independence, MO 64052; tel. 816/254–3652; William H. Kyles, M.A., President, Chief Executive Officer

Cope and Twin Town, 777 South New Ballas Road, St. Louis, MO 63141; tel. 314/991–1007; FAX. 314/991–9675; Sue McClure, Director

Industrial Rehabilitation Center, 2701 Rock Creek Parkway, Suite 205, North Kansas City, MO 64117–7252; tel. 816/471–5013; FAX. 816/471–3808; Maurice L. Cummings, Executive Director

Marillac, 2826 Main Street, Kansas City, MO 64108; tel. 816/751–4900, ext. 62; FAX. 816/751–4921; Sharon A. McGloin, Assistant Clinical Director

Piney Ridge Center, Inc., 1000 Hospital Road, Waynesville, MO 65583; tel. 314/774–5353; FAX. 314/774–2907; Thomas Arnold, President

Provident Counseling, Inc., 2650 Olive Street, St. Louis, MO 63103; tel. 314/371–6500; FAX. 314/371–6510; Kathleen E. Buescher, President, Chief Executive Officer

Research Mental Health Services, 1001 N.E. Independence Avenue, Lee's Summit, MO 64063; tel. 816/246–8000; FAX. 816/246–8207; Melvin D. Fetter, Director, Operations

MONTANA

Rimrock Foundation, 1231 North 29th Street, Billings, MT 59101; tel. 406/248–3175; FAX. 406/248–3821; David W. Cunningham, MHA, Chief Executive Officer

Rocky Mountain Treatment Center, 920 Fourth Avenue, N., Great Falls, MT 59401; tel. 406/727–8832; FAX. 406/727–8172; Claree Schulte, Administrator

NEBRASKA

Lincoln Lancaster County Child Guidance Center, 215 Centennial Mall, S., Lincoln, NE 68508; tel. 402/475–7666; Howard A. Halpern, Executive Director

O'Neill Valley Hope Alcohol and Drug Treatment Center, North 10th Street, P.O. Box 918, O. Neill, NE 68763; tel. 402/336–3747; FAX. 402/336–3096; Kaye Chohon, Program Director

NEW HAMPSHIRE

Beech Hill Hospital, New Harrisville Road, P.O. Box 254, Dublin, NH 03444; tel. 603/563–8511; FAX. 603/563–8771; Barbara R. Duckett, RN, M.S., Chief Executive Officer

Seaborne Hospital, Inc., Seaborne Drive, Dover, NH 03820; tel. 603/742–9300; Bud Charest, Administrator

Seacoast Substance Abuse Associates, a Department/Program of Seacoast Mental Health Center, Inc., Morning Light Bulding Six, 500 Market Street, Suite One–G, Portsmouth, NH 03801; tel. 603/431–8883; Susan Turner, Quality Assurance Coordinator

Seminole Point Hospital Corporation, 1000 Woodland Road, Box 1000, Sunapee, NH 03782; tel. 800/633–4000; FAX. 603/763–4682; James F. O'Neill, Chief Executive Officer

The Mental Health Center of Greater Manchester, 401 Cypress Street, Manchester, NH 03103; tel. 603/668–4111, ext. 187; FAX. 603/669–1131; Jane Gulmette, Quality Management Director

NEW JERSEY

American Day Treatment Center of West Essex Network, Inc., 799 Bloomfield Avenue, Verona, NJ 07044; tel. 201/857–5200; Bonnie Lizzio, Director

Discovery Institute for Addictive Disorders, P.O. Box 177, Marlboro, NJ 07746; tel. 908/946–9444; FAX. 908/946–0758; Robert C. Denes, Chief Executive Officer

High Focus Centers, Inc., 41 Grand Avenue, River Edge, NJ 07661; tel. 201/646–0313; FAX. 201/646–0325; David Nyman, Ph.D., Director, Program Development

Honesty House, 1272 Long Hill Road, Stirling, NJ 07980; tel. 908/647–3211; FAX. 908/647–7684; Charles H. Stucky, N.C.A.D.C., Executive Director

Lighthouse at Mays Landing, 5034 Atlantic Avenue, Mays Landing, NJ 08330; tel. 609/625–4900; C. William Brett, Ph.D., Executive Officer

Monmouth Chemical Dependency Treatment Center, Inc., 152 Chelsea Avenue, Long Branch, NJ 07740; tel. 908/222–5190; FAX. 908/222–5577; Brian J. Rafferty, Executive Director

New Beginnings at Lakehurst, 440 Beckerville Road, P.O. Box Five, Lakehurst, NJ 08733; tel. 908/657–4800; FAX. 908/657–2719; Edmund Bienkowski, Executive Director

New Hope Foundation, Inc., Route 520, P.O. Box 66, Marlboro, NJ 07746; tel. 908/946–3030; FAX. 908/946–3507; George J. Mattie, Chief Executive Officer

Seabrook House, 133 Polk Lane, P.O. Box 5055, Seabrook, NJ 08302; tel. 609/455–7575; FAX. 609/451–7669; Regina Marcacci, Chief Operating Officer

Sunrise House Foundation, Inc., Sunset Inn Road, Lafayette, NJ 07848; tel. 201/383–6300; FAX. 201/383–8458; Beth Anne Nathans, M.S., Chief Executive Officer

The Harbor, 1405 Clinton Street, Hoboken, NJ 07030; tel. 201/656–4040; John J. Clancy, Chief Executive Officer

UMDNJ–Community Mental Health Center at Piscataway, 671 Hoes Lane, P.O. Box 1392, Piscataway, NJ 08855–1392; tel. 201/463–4338; Gary W. Lamson, Vice President, Chief Executive Officer

NEW MEXICO

Four Corners Regional Adolescent Treatment Center, NCC Campus, Dorm Unit Two, P.O. Box 567, Shiprock, NM 87420; tel. 505/368–4712; Hoskie Benally, Chief Executive Officer

New Sunrise Regional Treatment Center, Acoma Indian Reservation, P.O. Box 219, San Fidel, NM 87049–0219; tel. 505/552–6091; FAX. 505/552–6527; Michael B. Smith, Program Director

NEW YORK

Areba Casriel Institute, Inc. (ACI), 500 West 57th Street, New York, NY 10019; tel. 800/724–4444; FAX. 212/765–1879; Steven Yohay, Executive Director

Arms Acres, Inc., 75 Seminary Hill Road, Carmel, NY 10512; tel. 914/225–3400; FAX. 914/225–5660; Eileen Donohue, RN, MSA, Associate Executive Director

Bronx Alcoholism Treatment Center, 1500 Waters Place, Bronx, NY 10461; tel. 718/904–0026; FAX. 718/597–9434; Ronald B. Lonesome, M.D., Director

Charles K. Post Alcoholism Treatment Center, Building One, PPC Campus, West Brentwood, NY 11717; tel. 516/434–7209; Phillip A. Dawes, Director

Conifer Park, Inc., 79 Glenridge Road, Glenville, NY 12302; tel. 518/399–6446; FAX. 518/399–1361, ext. 240; Mr. Gail Harkness, Executive Officer

Cornerstone of Medical Arts Center Hospital, 57 West 57th Street, New York, NY 10019; tel. 212/755–0200, ext. 3100; FAX. 212/755–0915; Norman J. Sokolow, Chief Executive Officer

Cortland Medical, Four Skyline Drive, Hawthorne, NY 10532; tel. 914/347–2990; FAX. 914/347–3074; Jeffery Smith, M.D., Founding Medical Director

Creedmoor Alcoholism Treatment Center, 80–45 Winchester Boulevard, Queens Village, NY 11427; tel. 718/464–7500; FAX. 718/776–5145; Jose Sarabia, M.D., Medical Director

DayBreak Alcoholism Treatment Facility, 435 East Henrietta Road, Rochester, NY 14620; tel. 716/461–4114; FAX. 716/461–3043; Luisa E. Baars, M.A., M.P.A., Division Director

Dick Van Dyke Alcoholism Treatment Center, Building 112, Willard Psychiatric Center, Willard, NY 14588; tel. 607/869–3111, ext. 2306; FAX. 607/869–4711; John R. Cole, C.S.W., Director

Dutchess County Department of Mental Hygiene, 230 North Road, Poughkeepsie, NY 12601; tel. 914/485–9700; FAX. 914/485–2759; Kenneth M. Glatt, Ph.D., Commissioner

Freeport Hospital, 267 South Ocean Avenue, Freeport, NY 11520; tel. 516/378–0800; Debbie Turkel, Chief Executive Officer

Hope House, Inc., 517 Western Avenue, Albany, NY 12203; tel. 518/482–4673; FAX. 518/482–0873; Mary Ann Finn, Executive Director

John L. Norris Alcoholism Treatment Center, 1600 South Avenue, Rochester, NY 14620; tel. 716/461–0410; FAX. 716/461–4545; Thomas E. Nightingale, Director

Kingsboro Alcoholism Treatment Center, 754 Lexington Avenue, Brooklyn, NY 11221; tel. 718/453–3200; FAX. 718/453–4785; Jacqueline Cole, Director

Providers / Accredited Freestanding Substance Abuse Programs

Manhattan Alcoholism Treatment Center and Substance Abuse Services, 600 East 125th Street, New York, NY 10035; tel. 212/369–0500; Vera Ward, Chairperson

McPike Alcoholism Treatment Center, 1213 Court Street, Utica, NY 13502; tel. 315/797–6800, ext. 4801; FAX. 315/738–4437; John F. Robertson, Ph.D., Director

Middletown Alcoholism Treatment Center, 141 Monhagen Avenue, Middletown, NY 10940; tel. 914/341–2500; FAX. 914/341–2570; Richard C. Ward, Director

National Expert Care Consultants, Inc., d/b/a National Recovery Institutes, 455 West 50th Street, New York, NY 10019; tel. 212/262–6000; FAX. 212/262–9378; Roger Cohn, Executive Vice President

Research Institute on Addictions, 1021 Main Street, Buffalo, NY 14203; tel. 716/887–2386; FAX. 716/887–2215; Linda Rotering, Ph.D., Director

Rochester Mental Health Center, 490 Ridge Road, E., Rochester, NY 14621; tel. 716/544–5220; FAX. 716/544–6694; Fred Volpe, President

Russell E. Blaisdell Alcoholism Treatment Center, R.P.C. Campus, Orangeburg, NY 10962; tel. 914/359–8500; FAX. 914/359–2016; Louis R. Brandes, M.D., Director

Saint Peter's Addiction Recovery Center (SPARC, Inc.), 2232 Western Avenue, Guilderland, NY 12084; tel. 518/452–6700; FAX. 518/452–6756; Karen A. Giles, Executive Director

Salamanca Hospital District Authority, d/b/a Salamanca HealthCare Complex, 150 Parkway Drive, Salamanca, NY 14779; tel. 716/945–1900; FAX. 716/945–5016; Kenneth L. Oakley, Ph.D., Administrator

Seafield Center, Inc., Seven Seafield Lane, Westhampton Beach, NY 11978; tel. 516/288–1122; FAX. 516/288–1638; Mark Epley, M.B.A., Assistant Executive Director

Seafield Services, 212 West Main Street, Riverhead, NY 11901; tel. 516/369–7800; Sheryl Stellwagen-Svensson, Executive Director

Sleepy Valley Center, 117 Sleepy Valley Road, Warwick, NY 10990; tel. 914/986–2545; FAX. 914/986–7882; Joan Wegener, Chief Executive Officer

South Beach Alcoholism Treatment Center, 777 Seaview Avenue, Building A, Second Floor, Staten Island, NY 10305; tel. 718/667–4218; FAX. 718/351–1958; Gerlando A. Verruso, Chief Executive Officer

St. Joseph's Rehabilitation Center, Inc., 99 Glenwood Estates, P.O. Box 470, Saranac Lake, NY 12983–0470; tel. 518/891–3950; Rev. Arthur M. Johnson, Executive Director

St. Joseph's Villa of Rochester, 3300 Dewey Avenue, Rochester, NY 14616–3795; tel. 716/865–1550; FAX. 716/865–5219; M. Judith McKay, President, Chief Executive Officer

St. Lawrence Alcoholism Treatment Center, Station A–Hamilton Hall, Ogdensburg, NY 13669; tel. 315/393–1180; FAX. 315/393–6160; Phillip Dranger, Director

Stutzman Alcoholism Treatment Center, 360 Forest Avenue, Buffalo, NY 14213; tel. 716/882–4900; FAX. 716/882–4426; Steven Schwartz, Director

The Rhinebeck Lodge for Successful Living, Inpatient Treatment Program, 500 Milan Hollow Road, Rhinebeck, NY 12572; tel. 914/266–3481; Chandra Singh, Ph.D., Executive Director

Tully Hill Corporation, P.O. Box 920, Tully, NY 13159; tel. 315/696–6114; FAX. 315/696–8509; Karl J. Kabza, Chief Executive Officer

Valley View House, Inc., Swiss Hill Road, P.O. Box 26, Kenoza Lake, NY 12750; tel. 914/482–3400; FAX. 914/482–3516; William J. Coleman, Chief Operations Officer

Veritas Villa, Inc., Route Two, P.O. Box 415, Kerhonkson, NY 12446; tel. 914/626–3555; FAX. 914/626–3840; James Cusack, President

Villa Outpatient Center, 290 Madison Avenue, New York, NY 10017; tel. 212/679–4960; FAX. 212/679–4966; John F. Golden, Executive Director

NORTH CAROLINA

Alcohol and Drug Abuse Treatment Center, 301 Tabernacle Road, Black Mountain, NC 28711; tel. 704/669–3414; FAX. 704/669–3451; William A. Rafter, Director

Alcohol and Drug Abuse Treatment Center, 205 West E Street, Butner, NC 27509; tel. 919/575–7073; FAX. 919/575–7006

Amethyst Charlotte, Inc., 1715 Sharon Road, West, Charlotte, NC 28224; tel. 704/554–8373; FAX. 704/554–8058; William K. Brown, Vice President, Administrator

Fellowship Hall, Inc., 5140 Dunstan Road, P.O. Box 13890, Greensboro, NC 27415; tel. 910/621–3381; FAX. 910/621–7513; Edmund F. Ward, Executive Director

Forsyth-Stokes Mental Health Center, 725 North Highland Avenue, Winston-Salem, NC 27101; tel. 919/725–7777; Roy H. Haberkern, M.D., Area Director

Mary Frances Center, 1212 Recovery Road, Tarboro, NC 27886; tel. 919/641–1111; Richard Herring, Director, Operations

Step One, Inc., 665 West Fourth Street, Winston-Salem, NC 27101; tel. 910/725–8389; FAX. 910/725–6628; Selbert M. Wood, President, Chief Executive Officer

The Wilmington Treatment Center, 2520 Troy Drive, Wilmington, NC 28401; tel. 910/762–2727; FAX. 910/762–7923; Keith G. Lewis, Executive Director

Unity Regional Youth Treatment Center, Highway 441 North, P.O. Box C–201, Cherokee, NC 28719; tel. 704/497–3958; Mary Anne Farrell, M.D., Director

Walter B. Jones Alcohol and Drug Abuse Treatment Center, 2577 West Fifth Street, Greenville, NC 27834; tel. 919/830–3426; Phillip A. Mooring, Director

NORTH DAKOTA

Heartview Foundation, 1406 Second Street, N.W, Mandan, ND 58554; tel. 701/663–2321; FAX. 701/663–2598; Allen Gillette, Executive Director

OHIO

Careunit Hospital of Cincinnati, 3156 Glenmore Avenue, Cincinnati, OH 45211; tel. 513/481–8822; FAX. 513/481–7317; Judith Erwin, Director, Quality, Utilization Management

Center for Comprehensive Alcoholism Treatment, Inc., 830 Ezzard Charles Drive, Cincinnati, OH 45214; tel. 513/381–6672; FAX. 513/381–6086; Sandra L. Kuehn, Associate Executive Director, Chief Operating Officer

Charles B. Mills Center, Inc, 715 South Plum Street, Marysville, OH 43040; tel. 513/644–9192; FAX. 513/644–3426; Robert C. Mertz, Executive Director

Community Drug Board, Inc., 725 East Market Street, Akron, OH 44305; tel. 216/434–4141; FAX. 216/434–7125; Theodore Paul Ziegler, Chief Executive Officer

Crisis Intervention Center of Stark County, Inc., 2421 13th Street, N.W., Canton, OH 44708; tel. 216/452–9812; Lori S. Lapp, Executive Director

Family Recovery Center, 964 North Market Street, Lisbon, OH 44432; tel. 216/424–1468; FAX. 216/424–9844; Eloise V. Traina, Executive Director

Focus Health Care, 700 Morse Road, Suite 208, Columbus, OH 43214; tel. 614/885–1944; FAX. 614/885–6665; Jo-Ann Boundy, Operations Manager

Glenbeigh Hospital of Cleveland, 18120 Puritas Avenue, Cleveland, OH 44135; tel. 216/476–0222; FAX. 216/476–2938; Mark D. Davis, Executive Director

Glenbeigh Hospital of Rock Creek, Route 45, Rock Creek, OH 44084; tel. 216/563–3400; Patricia Weston-Hall, Executive Director

Health Recovery Services, Inc., 28 North College Street, Athens, OH 45701; tel. 614/594–3511; FAX. 614/593–7258; Kenneth H. Pickering, Executive Director

INTERACT Behavioral Healthcare Services, Inc., Administrative Offices, 1808 East Broad Street, Columbus, OH 43203; tel. 614/251–8242; James Shulman, Ph.D., Chief Executive Officer

Interval Brotherhood Home Alcohol-Drug Rehab Center, 3445 South Main Street, Akron, OH 44319; tel. 216/644–4095; Father Samuel R. Ciccolini, Executive Director

Lake Area Recovery Center–Chemical Dependency Treatment, Residential, Outpatient, Adult, and Adolescent, 2801 C Court, Ashtabula, OH 44004; tel. 216/998–0722; FAX. 216/992–2761; Kathleen Kinney, Executive Director

Lincoln Center for Prevention and Treatment of Chemical Dependency, 1918 North Main Street, Findlay, OH 45840; tel. 419/423–9242; FAX. 419/423–7854; W. Scott Kibler, Executive Director

McKinley Hall, Inc., 1101 East High Street, Springfield, OH 45505; tel. 513/328–5300; Judith O. Hoy, Chief Executive Officer

Miami Valley Labor Management Health Care Delivery Systems, Inc., 136 Heid Avenue, Dayton, OH 45404; tel. 513/236–1367; Thomas Keen, Director

Neil Kennedy Recovery Clinic, 2151 Rush Boulevard, Youngstown, OH 44507; tel. 216/744–1181; FAX. 216/740–2849; Gerald V. Carter, Executive Director

New Directions, Inc., 30800 Chagrin Boulevard, PepperPike, OH 44124; tel. 216/591–0324; FAX. 216/591–1243; Michael Matoney, Executive Director

Northwest Counseling Services, 1560 Fishinger Road, Columbus, OH 43221; tel. 614/457–7876; FAX. 614/457–7896; Hollie Goldberg, Director, Quality Assurance

Parkside Behavioral Healthcare, Inc., d/b/a Parkside Recovery Services, 349 Olde Ridenour Road, Columbus, OH 43230; tel. 614/471–2552; FAX. 614/471–0167; Chris Gerber, Ph.D., President, Chief Executive Officer

Parmadale, 6753 State Road, Parma, OH 44134–4459; tel. 216/845–7700; Michael J. Haggerty, Associate Executive Director

PsyCare, Inc., 3530 Belmont Avenue, Suite Seven, Youngstown, OH 44505; tel. 216/759–2310; FAX. 216/759–0018; Douglas Darnall, Ph.D., Chief Executive Officer

Psych Systems of Greater Cincinnati, 4243 Hunt Road, Suite 120, Cincinnati, OH 45242; tel. 513/891–9114; FAX. 513/891–9314; Nora Quinn, Program Coordinator, Addiction Services

Quest Recovery Services, 1341 Market Avenue, N., Canton, OH 44714; tel. 216/453–8252; FAX. 216/453–6716; Joan Arnold, Counseling Services Manager

Ravenwood Mental Health Center, 12557 Ravenwood Drive, Chardon, OH 44024; tel. 216/285–3568; David Boyle, Executive Director

Serenity Living, Inc. and Medical Professional Services, 210 West National Road, P.O. Box 217, Vandalia, OH 45377; tel. 513/898–8979; FAX. 513/898–3258; Justin J. Trevino, M.D., Medical Consultant

Shepherd Hill Hospital, 200 Messimer Drive, P.O. Box 1067, Newark, OH 43058–1067; tel. 614/522–8484; FAX. 614/522–6653; Heather Nicolozakis, Vice President

Specialty Care Psychiatric Services, Inc., 2657 Niles–Courtland Road, Warren, OH 44484; tel. 216/652–3533; William A. Price, M.D., President

The Campus, 905 South Sunbury Road, Westerville, OH 43081; tel. 614/895–1000; FAX. 614/895–3010; Robert J. Stevenson, Ph.B., CCDC, III

Two North Park, Inc., 720 Pine Street, S.E., Warren, OH 44483; tel. 216/399–3677; FAX. 216/394–3815; Robert M. Kaschak, M.Ed., Executive Director

Wood County Council on Alcoholism and Drug Abuse, Inc., 320 West Gypsy Lane, Bowling Green, OH 43402; tel. 419/352–2551; Randall J. LaFond, Executive Director

Providers / Accredited Freestanding Substance Abuse Programs

OKLAHOMA
Cushing Valley Hope, 100 South Jones, Cushing, OK 74023; tel. 918/225-1736; FAX. 918/225-7742; AL Roberts, Program Director

Jim Taliaferro Community Mental Health Center, 602 S.W. 38th Street, Lawton, OK 73505-6999; tel. 405/248-5780; FAX. 405/248-3610; Ted Debbs, Executive Director

Mendros Psychiatric Medical Clinic, 2100 North Broadway, Moore, OK 73160; tel. 405/794-7719; Harry G. Mendros, M.D., Psychiatrist, Chief Executive Officer

Parkside, Inc., 1620 East 12th Street, Tulsa, OK 74120; tel. 918/582-2131; FAX. 918/588-8822; Quentin Henley, Chief Executive Officer

OREGON
Pioneer Trail Adolescent Treatment Center, 4101 N.E. Division Street, Gresham, OR 97030; tel. 503/661-0775; FAX. 503/661-4649; Marcia Hille, Administrator

River Bend Youth Center, Inc., 15544 South Clackamas River Drive, Oregon City, OR 97045; tel. 503/656-8005; FAX. 503/656-8929; Marcia L. McClocklin, Executive Director

Rogue Valley Serenity Lane, 600 South Second Street, Central Point, OR 97502; tel. 800/872-0983; Kristine Kopp, Director

Serenity Lane, Inc., 616 East 16th Avenue, Eugene, OR 97401; tel. 503/687-1110; FAX. 503/687-9041; Neil H. McNaughton, Executive Director

Springbrook Northwest, 2001 Crestview Drive, Newberg, OR 97132; tel. 503/537-7000; Carol Peake, Admissions Coordinator

PENNSYLVANIA
Bowling Green Inn–Brandywine, 1375 Newark Road, Kennett Square, PA 19348; tel. 215/268-3588; FAX. 215/268-2334; Jeffrey J. Kegley, Administrator

Butler A. Center, Inc., 165 Old Plank Road, P.O. Box 2127, Butler, PA 16003; tel. 412/287-8205; FAX. 412/287-6788; Paul A. Sandusky, Executive Director

Caron Foundation, Galen Hall Road, Box A, Wernersville, PA 19565-0501; tel. 610/678-2332; FAX. 610/678-5704; Joseph K. Lauginiger, Jr., Interim President, Chief Executive Officer

Charter Behavioral Health System at Cove Forge, New Beginnings Road, Williamsburg, PA 16693; tel. 800/873-2131; FAX. 814/832-2882; Jonathan Wolf, Chief Executive Officer

Chit Chat Westfield, 355 Church Street, Westfield, PA 16950; tel. 814/367-5901; FAX. 814/367-5666; Peggy Fitzwater, Executive Director

Clear Brook, Inc., 1003 Wyoming Avenue, Forty-Fort, PA 18704; tel. 717/288-6692; Dave Lombard, Chief Executive Officer

College Hill Medical Center, 329 East Brown Street, East Stroudsburg, PA 18301; tel. 717/424-6233; FAX. 717/424-6380; William I. Van Meter, Chief Executive Officer

Eagleville Hospital, 100 Eagleville Road, Eagleville, PA 19403-1800; tel. 610/539-6000, ext. 101; FAX. 610/539-9314; Frederick M. Carey, Chief Executive Officer

Friends Recovery Center at Friends Hospital, 4641 Roosevelt Boulevard, Philadelphia, PA 19124; tel. 215/831-6960; Robyn Kulp, Executive Director

Gateway Rehabilitation Center, Moffett Run Road, Aliquippa, PA 15001; tel. 412/766-8700, ext. 101; FAX. 412/375-8815; Kenneth S. Ramsey Ph.D., President, Chief Executive Officer

Gaudenzia, Inc.–Common Ground, 2835 North Front Street, Harrisburg, PA 17110; tel. 717/238-5553; FAX. 717/232-7362; Jerry McFarland, Program Director

Greenbriar Treatment Center, 800 Manor Drive, Washington, PA 15301; tel. 412/225-9700; FAX. 412/225-9764; Mary Banaszak, Executive Director

Keystone Center, 2001 Providence Road, Chester, PA 19013; tel. 215/876-9000; FAX. 215/876-5441; Daniel A. Kidd, Managing Director

Livengrin Foundation, Inc., 4833 Hulmeville Road, Bensalem, PA 19020-3099; tel. 215/638-5200, ext. 5224; FAX. 215/638-2603; Timothy D. Shanahan, Ph.D., M.A., Assistant Executive Director

Malvern Institute, 940 King Road, Malvern, PA 19355; tel. 610/647-0330; FAX. 610/647-2572; Valerie Craig, Administrator, Chief Executive Officer

Marworth, Lily Lake Road, Waverly, PA 18471; tel. 717/563-1112; FAX. 717/563-1138; James J. Dougherty, President

Mirmont Treatment Center, 100 Yearsley Mill Road, Lima, PA 19037; tel. 215/565-9232; FAX. 215/565-7497; Thomas F. Crane, Executive Director

Penn Foundation, 807 Lawn Avenue, P.O. Box 32, Sellersville, PA 18960; tel. 215/257-6551; FAX. 215/257-9347; Ellen T. Bench, Medical Records Manager

Renewal Centers, 2705 Old Bethlehem Pike, Quakerstown, PA 18951; tel. 215/536-9070; FAX. 215/536-4788; Theresa E. Walsh, Executive Director

Roxbury, 601 Roxbury Road, Shippensburg, PA 17257; tel. 717/532-4217; FAX. 717/532-4003; Claire F. Beckwith, Chief Executive Officer

Serenity Hall, Crossroads Program, 414 West 5th Street, Erie, PA 16507; tel. 814/459-4775; FAX. 814/453-6118; Suzanne C. Mack, Director

The Bridge, 8400 Pine Road, Philadelphia, PA 19111; tel. 215/342-5000; FAX. 215/342-7709; Star Weiss, Chief Executive Officer

The Mercy Center for Chemical Dependency Services, 3334 Fleming Avenue, Pittsburgh, PA 15212; tel. 412/734-7501; Stephanie Murtaugh, Director, Clinical Programs

The Terraces, 1170 South State Street, Ephrata, PA 17522; tel. 717/859-4100; FAX. 717/859-2131; Gerald D. Shulman, M.A., FACATA, Executive Director

Today, Inc., 1990 West Woodbourne Road, P.O. Box 908, Newtown, PA 18940; tel. 215/968-4713; FAX. 215/968-8742; John E. Howell, M.A., CAC, Executive Vice President

Twin Lakes Center for Drug and Alcohol Rehabilitation, P.O. Box 909, Somerset, PA 15501-0909; tel. 814/443-3639; FAX. 814/443-2737; Mark T. Pile, ACSW, Chief Executive Officer

RHODE ISLAND
Community Counseling Center, 160 Beechwood Avenue, Pawtucket, RI 02860; tel. 401/722-7855; FAX. 401/722-5630; Roxanne Arakelian, ACSW, Manager

Good Hope Center, Inc., John Potter Road, East Greenwich, RI 02818; tel. 401/826-2750; Alan Willoughby, Chief Executive Officer

SOUTH CAROLINA
Fenwick Hall Hospital, 1709 River Road, P.O. Box 688, Johns Island, SC 29457; tel. 803/559-2461; FAX. 803/559-6202; John Magill, Executive Director

SOUTH DAKOTA
Keystone Treatment Center, 1010 East Second Street, P.O. Box 159, Canton, SD 57013; tel. 605/987-2751; FAX. 605/987-2365; Carol Regier, Executive Director

TENNESSEE
Cornerstone of Recovery, Inc., 1120 Topside Road, Louisville, TN 37777; tel. 615/970-7747; FAX. 615/681-2266; Dan R. Caldwell, President

Council for Alcohol and Drug Abuse Services, Inc., 207 Spears Avenue, Chattanooga, TN 37405; tel. 615/756-7644; James F. Marcotte, Executive Director

Cumberland Heights Foundation, 8283 River Road, Route Two, Nashville, TN 37209; tel. 615/352-1757; FAX. 615/353-4325; James Moore, Executive Director

Methodist Outreach, Inc., 2009 Lamar Avenue, Memphis, TN 38114; tel. 901/276-5401; FAX. 901/272-2551; Louise Renfroe, Supervisor, Medical Records

The Harbours at Brentwood, 209 Ward Circle, P.O. Box 1644, Brentwood, TN 37027; tel. 615/373-8700; FAX. 615/373-1899; Joe H. McWaters, Executive Director

TEXAS
Burke Center, 4101 South Medford Drive, Lufkin, TX 75901; tel. 409/639-1141; Susan Rushing, Chief Executive Officer

Champions Psychiatric Treatment Center, 14320 Walters Road, Houston, TX 77014; tel. 713/537-5050; FAX. 713/537-2728; Philippa Porter, RN, Associate Administrator

Family Opportunity Resources, The FORGIVE Program, 1814 45th Street, Suite 106, Galveston, TX 77550; tel. 409/763-1181; Gordon W. McKee, Administrator

Glass Treatment Center, 18842 Memorial, Suite 205, Humble, TX 77338; tel. 713/666-9811; FAX. 713/446-5292; George S. Glass, M.D., Medical Director

La Hacienda Treatment Center, FM Road 1340, P.O. Box One, Hunt, TX 78024; tel. 210/238-4222; FAX. 210/238-4070; Frank J. Sadlack, Ph.D., C.A.S., Executive Director

Life Resource, 2750 South Eighth Street, Beaumont, TX 77701; tel. 409/838-6203; FAX. 409/832-3530; N. Charles Harris, Ph.D., Chief Executive Officer

New Dimensions Day Treatment, 18333 Egret Bay Boulevard, Suite 560, Houston, TX 77058; tel. 713/333-2284; FAX. 713/333-2293; Valerie Corbett, Administrative Assistant

New Spirit, 2411 Fountainview Drive, Suite 175, Houston, TX 77057-4803; tel. 713/975-1580; FAX. 713/975-0228; Tom Blocher, M.D., President

New View Partial Hospitalization Centre, Inc., 4310 Dowlen Road, Suite 13, Beaumont, TX 77706; tel. 409/892-0009; Darla Tortorice, Nursing Coordinator

Rio Grande State Center, 1401 Rangerville Road, Harlingen, TX 78551; tel. 512/425-8900; Sonia H. Hernandez, Facility Director

River Oaks Academy Day Hospital, 8120 Westglen, Houston, TX 77063; tel. 713/783-7200; FAX. 713/783-7286; Sandra E. Phares, Chief Executive Officer

Serenity House of Abilene, Inc., 1546 North Second Street, Abilene, TX 79601; tel. 915/673-6489; FAX. 915/673-1794; Richard L. Spalding, President

St. James Center, 1819 St. James Place, Houston, TX 77056; tel. 713/623-6456; FAX. 713/621-1329; Julie Sengstacken, Administrator

Summer Sky Treatment Center, 1100 McCart Street, Stephenville, TX 76401; tel. 800/588-2907; FAX. 817/968-4509; Cathern Brooks, Chief Executive Officer

Sundown Ranch, Inc., Route Four, Box 182, Canton, TX 75103; tel. 903/479-3933; FAX. 903/479-3999; Richard Boardman, Chief Executive Officer

The Country Place Adolescent Residential Treatment Center, 2708 Highway 1378, Wylie, TX 75098; tel. 214/442-6002; FAX. 214/442-4804; William Barabas, Chief Executive Officer

The Patrician Movement, 222 East Mitchell, San Antonio, TX 78210; tel. 512/532-3126; FAX. 512/534-3779; Patrick Clancey, Administrator

UTAH
Brightway at St. George, 115 West 1470 South, St. George, UT 84770; tel. 801/673-0303; FAX. 801/673-8420; Paula O. Bell, Director

Highland Ridge Hospital, 4578 Highland Drive, Salt Lake City, UT 84117; tel. 801/272-9851; FAX. 801/272-9857; Mike Dusoe, Administrator

Sorenson's Ranch School, P.O. Box 440219, Koosharem, UT 84744; tel. 801/638-7318; FAX. 801/638-7582; Burnell D. Sorenson, Owner

VIRGINIA
Colonial Hospital/Colonial Recovery Center, 17579 Warwick Boulevard, Newport News, VA 23603-3134; tel. 800/697-0999; David R. Campbell, Director, Operations Management

Commonwealth Medical Institute, Koger Executive Center, Building 20, Suite 212, Norfolk, VA 23502; tel. 804/461-1178; FAX. 804/461-8352; Wendy Van Fossen, Administrator

Providers / Accredited Freestanding Substance Abuse Programs

Comprehensive Addiction Treatment Services, 3300 Gallows Road, Falls Church, VA 22046; tel. 703/698-1530; FAX. 703/698-1537; Wanda L. Miller, Director, Administration

Mount Regis Center, 405 Kimball Avenue, Salem, VA 24153; tel. 703/389-4761; Mark S. Cowell, Administrator

New Beginnings at Serenity Lodge, 2097 South Military Highway, Chesapeake, VA 23320; tel. 804/543-6888; FAX. 804/543-7453; Katie DeBaun, Executive Administrator

New Life Center, Inc., 315 East Cork Street, Winchester, VA 22601; tel. 703/662-8865; S. Terry Rudolph, M.S., Executive Director

The Kellar Center, 10396 Democracy Lane, Fairfax, VA 22030-0252; tel. 703/281-8500; Wanda L. Miller, Director, Administration

The Life Center of Galax, 112 Painter Street, Galax, VA 24333; tel. 800/345-6998; FAX. 703/236-8821; Tina Bullins, Executive Director

Williamsburg Place, 5477 Mooretown Road, Williamsburg, VA 23185; tel. 800/582-6066; FAX. 804/565-0620; William McAllister, Administrator

WASHINGTON

Advanced Clinical Services, 34709 Ninth Avenue, S., Federal Way, WA 98003; tel. 206/874-1475; Wayne Watkinson, Executive Director

Careunit Hospital of Kirkland, 10322 N.E. 132nd Street, Kirkland, WA 98034; tel. 206/821-1122; FAX. 206/821-1122; John Thompson, Administrator

Mountainview Hospital, 628 South Cowley, Spokane, WA 99202; tel. 509/624-3226; Ron Mays, Administrator

WEST VIRGINIA

Olympic Center–Preston, (Adolescent Treatment Only), Route Seven West Manown, Kingwood, WV 26537; tel. 304/329-2400; FAX. 304/329-2405; William W. Perkins, Executive Director

Shawnee Hills, Inc., P.O. Box 3698, Charleston, WV 25336-3698; tel. 304/345-4800; FAX. 304/341-0277; John E. Barnette, Ed.D., President, Chief Executive Officer

WISCONSIN

DePaul Hospital, Inc., 4143 South 13th Street, Milwaukee, WI 53221-1170; tel. 414/281-4400; Kathy M. Olewinski, Director

Libertas Treatment Center, 1701 Dousman, Green Bay, WI 54303; tel. 414/498-8600; Patrick Ryan, Program Director

Index

Abbreviations Used in AHA Guide, D2
Accredited Freestanding Long–Term Care
    Facilities, C123
Accredited Freestanding Psychiatric Facilities, C129
Accredited Freestanding Substance Abuse
    Programs, C141
Acknowledgements, v
AHA Offices, Officers, and Historical Data, A2
AHA Registered Hospitals, A4
Alliances, B100
    defined, B2
Annual Survey, A8
AOHA Listed Hospitals, A5
Approval Codes, A6
Associate Members, A492
    defined, A492
Blue Cross–Blue Shield Plans, C28
Canadian Hospitals, A487
Classification Codes, A7
Description of Lists, C2
Explanation of Hospital Listings, A6
Facility Codes
    alphabetically, A6
    defines, A8
    numerically, A6
Freestanding Ambulatory Surgery Centers, C75
    state government agencies, C100
Freestanding Hospices, C102
    state government agencies, C121
Headings, A7
    defined, A7
    expense, A7
    facilities, A7
    personnel, A7
    utilization data, A7
Health Care Providers, C60
    defined, C2
Health Care Systems
    alphabetically, B84
    and their hospitals, by state, B9
    by system code, B85
    defined, B2
    geographically, B92
    introduced, B2
Statistics for Multihospital Health Care Systems and
    their Hospitals, B8
Health Maintenance Organizations, C60
    state government agencies, C73
Health System Agencies, A493

Health Systems Agencies, C30
Healthfinder, C13
Hospital Associations, C31
Hospital Licensure Agencies, C34
Hospitals in Areas Associated with the U.S., by
    area, A447
Hospitals in the United States, A13
    alphabetically, A452
    by state, A13
Institutional Members, A487
    defined, A486
Integrated Health Delivery Networks, B3
    defined, B2
International Organizations, C25
    defined, C2
Introduction, vi
Joint Commission on Accreditation of Healthcare
    Organizations
    accredited Freestanding Ambulatory Surgery
        Centers, C75
    accredited Freestanding Long–Term Care
        Facilities, C123
    accredited Freestanding Substance Abuse
        Programs, C141
    accredited Hospitals, A13
Medical and Nursing Licensure Agencies, C36
Membership Categories, A486
National Organizations, C3
Newly Registered defined, A6
Nonhospital Preacute & Postacute Care
    Facilities, A490
Nonreporting defined, A6
Peer Review Organizations, C39
Registration Requirements, A4
Shared Services Organizations, A493
State and Local Organizations and Agencies, C28
    defined, C2
State and Provincial Government Agencies, C43
State Health Planning and Development
    Agencies, C41
Types of Hospitals, A5
    general, A5
    psychiatric, A5
    rehabilitation and chronic disease, A5
    special, A5
U.S. Government Agencies, C27
    defined, C2
U.S. Government Hospitals outside the U.S., by
    area, A451

Abbreviations Used in the AHA Guide

AB, Army Base
ACSW, Academy of Certified Social Workers
AEC, Atomic Energy Commission
AFB, Air Force Base
AHA, American Hospital Association
AK, Alaska
AL, Alabama
AODA, Alcohol and Other Drug Abuse
APO, Army Post Office
AR, Arkansas
A.R.T., Accredited Record Technician
A.S.C., Ambulatory Surgical Center
A.T.C., Alcoholism Treatment Center
Ave., Avenue
AZ, Arizona

B.A., Bachelor of Arts
B.C., British Columbia
Blvd., Boulevard
B.S., Bachelor of Science
B.S.H.S., Bachelor of Science in Health Studies
B.S.N., Bachelor of Science in Nursing
B.S.W., Bachelor of Science and Social Worker

C.A.A.D.A.C., Certified Alcohol and Drug Abuse Counselor
CA, California; Controller of Accounts
CAC, Certified Alcoholism Counselor
CAE, Certified Association Executive
CAP, College of American Pathologists
CAPA, Certified Ambulatory Post Anesthesia
C.A.S., Certificate of Advanced Study
C.D., Commander of the Order of Distinction
CDR, Commander
CDS, Chemical Dependency Specialist
CFACHE, Certified Fellow American College of Healthcare Executives
CCDC, Certified Chemical Dependency Counselor
CFRE, Certified Fund Raising Executive
C.G., Certified Gastroenterology
CHC, Certified Health Consultant
C.L.D., Clinical Laboratory Director
CLU, Certified Life Underwriter, Chartered Life Underwriter
CMA, Certified Medical Assistant
C.M.H.A., Certified Mental Health Administrator
CNHA, Certified Nursing Home Administrator
CNM, Certified Nurse Midwife
CNOR, Certified Operating Room Nurse
C.N.S., Clinical Nurse Specialist
CO, Colorado; Commanding Officer
COA, Certified Ophthalmic Assistant
COMT, Commandant
C.O.M.T., Certified Ophthalmic Medical Technician
Conv., Conventions
C.P.H.Q., Certified Professional in Health Care Quality
Corp., Corporation; Corporate
C.O.T., Certified Ophthalmic Technician
CPA, Certified Public Accountant
CPM, Certified Public Manager
CRNA, Certified Registered Nurse Anesthetist
C.S.J.B, Catholic Saint John the Baptist
CSW, Certified Social Worker
CT, Connecticut
CWO, Chief Warrant Officer

D.B.A., Doctor of Business Administration
DC, District of Columbia

D.D., Doctor of Divinity
D.D.S., Doctor of Dental Surgery
DE, Delaware
Diet, Dietitian; Dietary; Dietetics
D.M.D., Doctor of Dental Medicine
D.MIN., Doctor of Ministry
DPA, Doctorate Public Administration
D.P.M., Doctor of Podiatric Medicine
Dr., Drive
Dr.P.h., Doctor of Public Health
D.Sc., Doctor of Science
D.S.W., Doctor of Social Welfare
D.V.M., Doctor of Veterinary Medicine

E., East
Ed.D., Doctor of Education
Ed.S., Specialist in Education
ENS, Ensign
Esq., Esquire
Expwy., Expressway
ext., extension

FAAN, Fellow of the American Academy of Nursing
FACATA, Fellow of the American College of Addiction Treatment Administrators
FACHE, Fellow of the American College of Healthcare Executives
FACMGA, Fellow of the American College of Medical Group Administrators
FACP, Fellow of the American College of Physicians
FACS, Fellow of the American College of Surgeons
FAX, Facsimile
FL, Florida
FPO, Fleet Post Office
FRCPSC, Fellow of the Royal College of Physicians and Surgeons of Canada
FT, Full-time

GA, Georgia
Govt., Government; Governmental

HHS, Department of Health and Human Services
HI, Hawaii
HM, Helmsman
HMO, Health Maintenance Organization
Hon., Honorable; Honorary
H.S.A., Health System Administrator
Hts., Heights
Hwy., Highway

IA, Iowa
ID, Idaho
IL, Illinois
IN, Indiana
Inc., Incorporated

J.D., Doctor of Law
J.P., Justice of the Peace
Jr., Junior

KS, Kansas
KY, Kentucky

LA, Louisiana
LCDR, Lieutenant Commander
LCSW, Licensed Certified Social Worker
L.H.D., Doctor of Humanities
L.I.S.W., Licensed Independent Social Worker
L.M.H.C., Licensed Master of Health Care
L.M.S.W., Licensed Master of Social Work

L.N.H.A., Licensed Nursing Home Administrator
L.P.C., Licensed Professional Counselor
LPN, Licensed Practical Nurse
L.P.N., Licensed Practical Nurse
Lt., Lieutenant
LTC, Lieutenant Colonel
Ltd., Limited
LL.D., Doctor of Laws
L.L.P., Limited Licensed Practitioner
L.L.T., Limited Licensed Psychologist
L.S.W., Licensed Social Worker
LT.GEN., Lieutenant General
LTJG, Lieutenant (junior grade)

MA, Massachusetts
M.A., Master of Arts
Maj., Major
M.B., Bachelor of Medicine
M.B.A., Masters of Business Administration
M.C., Member of Congress
MC, Medical Corps; Marine Corps
MD, Maryland
M.D., Doctor of Medicine
ME, Maine
M.Ed., Master of Education
MFCC, Marriage/Family/Child Counselor
MHA, Mental Health Association
M.H.S., Masters in Health Science; Masters in Human Service
MI, Michigan
MM, Masters of Management
MN, Minnesota
M.N., Master of Nursing
MO, Missouri
M.P.A., Master of Public Administration; Master Public Affairs
M.P.H., Master of Public Health
M.P.S., Master of Professional Studies; Master of Public Science
M.S., Master of Science
MS, Mississippi
MSC, Medical Service Corps
M.S.D., Doctor of Medical Science
MSHSA, Master of Science Health Service Administration
M.S.N., Master of Science in Nursing
M.S.P.H., Master of Science in Public Health
M.S.S.W., Master of Science in Social Work
M.S.W., Master of Social Work
MT, Montana
Mt., Mount

N., North
NC, North Carolina
N.C.A.D.C., National Certification of Alcohol and Drug Counselors
ND, North Dakota
NE, Nebraska
NH, New Hampshire
NHA, National Hearing Association; Nursing Home Administrator
NJ, New Jersey
NM, New Mexico
NPA, National Perinatal Association
NV, Nevada
NY, New York

OCN, Oncology Certified Nurse
O.D., Doctor of Optometry
O.F.M., Order Franciscan Monks, Order of Friars Minor
OH, Ohio
OK, Oklahoma

OR, Oregon
O.R., Operating Room
O.R.S., Operating Room Supervisor
OSF, Order of St. Francis

PA, Pennsylvania
P.A., Professional Association
P.C., Professional Corporation
Pharm.D., Doctor of Pharmacy
Ph.B., Bachelor of Philosophy
PHS, Public Health Service
Pkwy., Parkway
Pl., Place
PR, Puerto Rico
PS, Professional Services
PSRO, Professional Standards Review Organization

RADM, Rear Admiral
Rd., Road
RD, Rural Delivery
R.F.D., Rural Free Delivery
RI, Rhode Island
R.M., Risk Manager
RN, Registered Nurse
RNC, Republican National Committee; Registered Nurse or Board Certified
R.R.A., Registered Record Administrator
R.S.M., Religious Sisters of Mercy
Rte., Route

S., South
SC, South Carolina
S.C., Surgery Center
SCAC, Senior Certified Addiction Counselor
Sc.D., Doctor of Science
Sci., Science, Scientific
SD, South Dakota
SHCC, Statewide Health Coordinating Council
Sgt., Sergeant
SNA, Surgical Nursing Assistant
SNF, Skilled Nursing Facility
Sq., Square
Sr., Senior, Sister
St., Saint, Street
Sta., Station
Ste., Saint; Suite

Tel., Telephone
Terr., Terrace
TN, Tennessee
Tpke, Turnpike
Twp., Township
TX, Texas

USA, United States Army
USAF, United States Air Force
USMC, United States Marine Corps
USN, United States Navy
USPHS, United States Public Health Service
UT, Utah

VA, Virginia
VADM, Vice Admiral
VI, Virgin Islands
Vlg., Village
VT, Vermont

W., West
WA, Washington
WI, Wisconsin
WV, West Virginia
WY, Wyoming

NOTES

NOTES

NOTES

NOTES

NOTES

NOTES

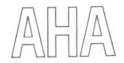

AHA Services, Inc.

Order Form

Ordered by: Please print or type

_____
Name   Title

_____
Organization

_____
Address

_____
City   State   Zip code

_____
Telephone

Please bill my organization

_____
Purchase order no.

_____
For billed order: Bill to attention of

_____
Name of member

Ship to: Complete only if different from ordered by

_____
Name   Title

_____
Organization

_____
Address

_____
City   State   Zip code

Please charge my   ☐ VISA   ☐ MasterCard   ☐ American Express

| | | | | | | | | | | | | | | | | |
Card no.

_____
Cardholder's signature   Expiration date

_____
Purchase order no.   Date of order

_____
For billed order: Bill to attention of

Order Number	Title	Quantity	Institutional Member Price	Associate Member Price	Personal Member Price	Nonmember Price	Extended Price
G02-010095	1995–96 AHA Guide to the Health Care Field		$ 75	$ 75	$195	$195	

Telephone Orders
1-800-AHA-2626

FAX Orders:
312-422-4505

MasterCard, Visa, American Express or institutional/company purchase order number accepted. Telephone orders will usually be shipped within 48 hours.

Orders from individuals must be prepaid or charged to a credit card. Billed orders must be accompanied by a purchase order number.

Mail Orders

Mail all orders to:
AHA Services, Inc.
P.O. Box 92683
Chicago, IL 60675-2683

Foreign Orders

All foreign orders must be pre-paid in U.S. funds only.

For surface mail: add 18% of merchandise price for shipping and handling. Allow 3 to 4 weeks for delivery.

For airmail: add 20% of merchandise price for shipping and handling. Allow 4 weeks for delivery.

Sales tax:
Sales tax must be paid on orders shipped to CA, CO, GA, IL, KS, MA, MO, NY, OH, and TX unless you provide us with a copy of your tax-exempt certificate.

Quantity discounts
Except where otherwise noted in the item description, quantity discounts are:

15%	11 to 50 copies
20%	51 to 100 copies
25%	101 to 1,000 copies

when shipped to one address.

Subtotal

Shipping and Handling

Sales Tax

Total
U.S. Funds Only

Shipping and handling charges apply to all domestic and Canadian orders

$ 1.00 to $19.99 add $ 4.95 $ 75.00 to $ 99.99 add $12.95 $300.00 to $399.99 add $20.95
$20.00 to $34.99 add $ 6.95 $100.00 to $199.99 add $14.95 $400.00 to $499.99 add $27.95
$35.00 to $49.99 add $ 8.95 $200.00 to $299.99 add $17.95 $500.00 and above   add $34.95
$50.00 to $74.99 add $10.95